T3-BOQ-663

PRIMARY PEDIATRIC CARE

PRIMARY PEDIATRIC CARE

SECOND EDITION

Editor-in-Chief

ROBERT A. HOEKELMAN, M.D.

Professor and Chairman, Department of Pediatrics
University of Rochester School of Medicine and Dentistry
Pediatrician-in-Chief, Strong Memorial Hospital
Rochester, New York

Co-Editors

STANFORD B. FRIEDMAN, M.D.

Professor of Pediatrics
Chief, Division of Adolescent Medicine and Behavioral Pediatrics
North Shore University Hospital/Cornell University Medical College
Manhasset, New York

NICHOLAS M. NELSON, M.D.

Professor of Pediatrics
Pennsylvania State University College of Medicine
The Milton S. Hershey Medical Center
Hershey, Pennsylvania

HENRY M. SEIDEL, M.D.

Professor of Pediatrics
The Johns Hopkins University School of Medicine
Attending Pediatrician, The Johns Hopkins Hospital
Baltimore, Maryland

with 258 *Illustrations*

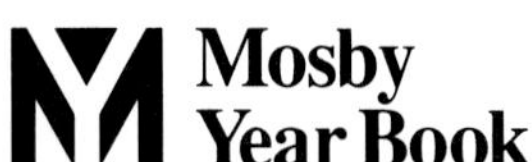

St. Louis Baltimore Boston Chicago London Philadelphia Sydney Toronto

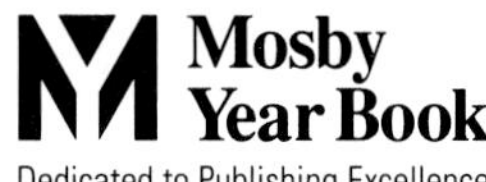

Dedicated to Publishing Excellence

Acquisitions Editor: Stephanie Manning
Developmental Editor: Kathryn H. Falk
Assistant Editor: Ellen Baker Geisel
Project Manager: Karen Edwards
Production Editor: Richard Barber
Production Assistant: Ginny Douglas
Design: Elizabeth Fett
Manuscript Editors: Sylvia Kluth Barnard and Chris O'Neil

SECOND EDITION

Printed in the United States of America

Mosby-Year Book, Inc.
11830 Westline Industrial Drive
St. Louis, MO 63146

Library of Congress Cataloging-in-Publication Data

Primary pediatric care / editor-in-chief, Robert A. Hoekelman ; co
-editors, Stanford B. Friedman, Nicholas M. Nelson, Henry M. Seidel.
—2nd ed.
p. cm.
Includes bibliographical references and index.
ISBN 0-8016-2269-7
1. Pediatrics. I. Hoekelman, Robert A.
[DNLM: 1. Pediatrics. 2. Primary Health Care—in infancy & childhood. WS 100 P9526]
RJ45.P673 1992
618.92—dc20
DNLM/DLC
for Library of Congress 91-21969
CIP

GW/VH 9 8 7 6 5 4 3 2 1

Contributors

Alice D. Ackerman, MD, FAAP, FCCM
Assistant Professor Pediatrics
Head, Division of Pediatric Critical Care Medicine
University of Maryland School of Medicine
Director, Pediatric Critical Care Unit
University of Maryland Medical System
Baltimore, Maryland
(25: Fluid Therapy)

Barbara N. Adams, RN, MS
Associate Professor of Nursing, University of Rochester School of Nursing
Rochester, New York
(107: The Teenage Parent)

Gerald R. Adams, PhD
Professor and Chair, Department of Family Studies
University of Guelph, Guelph, Ontario, Canada
(105: Runaway Youth)

Bayard W. Allmond, Jr., MD
Associate Clinical Professor of Pediatrics
University of California, San Francisco
San Francisco, California
(52: Health Care Management of the Family: The Family as the Focus of Treatment in Pediatrics)

Nick G. Anas, MD
Director, Pediatric Intensive Care Unit
Department of Pediatrics
Children's Hospital of Orange County
University of California, Irvine
Orange, California
(289: Status Asthmaticus)

Thomas F. Anders, MD
Professor and Head, Division of Child & Adolescent Psychiatry
Brown University
Director, Academic Division, Emma Pendleton Bradley Hospital
East Providence, Rhode Island
(86: Nightmares and Other Sleep Disturbances)

Joel M. Andres, MD
Associate Professor and Chief, Pediatric Gastroenterology
Department of Pediatrics, University of Florida College of Medicine
Gainesville, Florida
(147: Jaundice)

Barbara L. Asselin, MD
Director, Hematology/Oncology and Cancer Center
Assistant Professor of Pediatrics
University of Rochester School of Medicine and Dentistry
Rochester, New York
(224: Leukemias)

Lewis A. Barness, MD
Visiting Professor
Department of Pediatrics
University of Wisconsin
Madison, Wisconsin
(82: Failure to Thrive)

Nancy K. Barnett, MD
Director, Pediatric Dermatology
Assistant Professor of Pediatrics and Dermatology
Johns Hopkins University School of Medicine
Baltimore, Maryland
(144: Hyperhidrosis, 159: Pruritus, 160: Rash, 193: Contact Dermatitis, 219: Insect Bites and Infestations)

Ronald G. Barr, MDCM, FRCP(C)
Associate Professor of Pediatrics and Psychiatry
McGill University Faculty of Medicine
Director, Child Development Program
Montreal Children's Hospital
Montreal, Quebec, Canada
(109: Abdominal Pain)

John Baum, MD
Professor of Medicine, Pediatrics, and Rehabilitation Medicine
Strong Memorial Hospital Medical Center
University of Rochester
School of Medicine and Dentistry
Rochester, New York
(148: Joint Pain)

William R. Beardslee, MD
Associate Professor of Psychiatry
Harvard Medical School
Clinical Director
Department of Psychiatry
Children's Hospital
Boston, Massachusetts
(49: Day Care and Preschool Programs, 55: Mental Health of the Young: An Overview)

Avril P. Beckford, MD, FAAP
Instructor in General Pediatrics
Co-Director, Pediatric HIV Disease Services
The Pennsylvania State University Hospital
The Milton S. Hershey Medical Center
Hershey, Pennsylvania
(178: Acquired Immunodeficiency Syndrome (AIDS) and Human Immunodeficiency Virus (HIV) Infection

Mark F. Bellinger, MD
Associate Professor of Surgery
University of Pittsburgh School of Medicine
Chief of Pediatric Urology
Children's Hospital of Pittsburgh
Pittsburgh, Pennsylvania
(226: Meatal Ulceration)

Cheston M. Berlin, Jr., MD
University Professor of Pediatrics and Professor of Pharmacology
Department of Pediatrics
Milton S. Hershey Medical Center
Pennsylvania State University College of Medicine
Hershey, Pennsylvania
(216: Iatrogenic Disease, 274: Drug Overdose)

Wallace F. Berman, MD
Associate Professor of Pediatrics
Department of Pediatrics
Chief, Pediatric Gastroenterology
Medical College of Virginia
Richmond, Virginia
(134: Gastrointestinal Hemorrhage)

William E. Boyle, Jr., MD
Associate Professor of Pediatrics
Department of Maternal and Child Health
Dartmouth Medical School
Hanover, New Hampshire
(6: The Pediatric History)

T. Berry Brazelton, MD
Clinical Professor
Department of Pediatrics
Harvard Medical School
Boston, Massachusetts
(70: Developmental Approach to Behavioral Problems)

David I. Bromberg, MD
Assistant Professor of Pediatrics and Psychiatry
University of Maryland School of Medicine
Baltimore, Maryland
(71: Interviewing Children, 284: Pneumothorax and Pneumomediastinum)

M. Aileen Brown, J.D.
Attorney, Health Services Practice Group of Nixon, Hargrave, Devans, & Doyle
Rochester, New York
(4: Legal Aspects of Pediatric Medicine)

Michael G. Burke, MD
Instructor, Department of Pediatrics
Johns Hopkins University School of Medicine
Director, Inpatient Pediatrics
Francis Scott Key Medical Center
Department of Pediatrics
Baltimore, Maryland
(128: Extremity Pain)

Karen Byrne, MD
Department of Pediatrics
University of Maryland School of Medicine
Baltimore, Maryland
(85: Mental Retardation)

Bill S. Caldwell, MD
Associate Professor, Department of Pediatrics
Department of Psychiatry and Behavioral Sciences
University of Texas Medical Branch
Child Health Center
Galveston, Texas
(59: Overview of School Health)

James R. Campbell, MD
Fellow, Academic General Pediatrics
Strong Memorial Hospital
University of Rochester School of Medicine and Dentistry
Department of Pediatrics
Rochester, New York
(9: The Pediatric Record and Clinical Decision-Making)

Preston W. Campbell, MD
Department of Pediatrics
Vanderbilt University Medical Center
Nashville, Tennessee
(246: Acute Pneumonia)

Virginia Casper, PhD
Graduate Faculty
Department of Teacher Education
Bank Street College of Education
New York, New York
(101: Homosexuality: Challenges of Treating Lesbian and Gay Adolescents)

Robert W. Chamberlin, MD, MPH
Developmental Pediatrician and Consultant in Maternal and Child Health
Exceptional Family Member Program
United States Army
2nd General Hospital
Lanstuhl, Germany
(5: Community-Wide Approaches to Promoting the Health and Development of Families and Children)

Patricia Chute, MA
Director, Cochlear Implant Center
Manhatten Eye, Ear, & Throat Hospital
New York, New York
(136: Hearing Loss)

Edward B. Clark, MD
Professor of Pediatrics
Chief of Pediatric Cardiology
Department of Pediatrics
University of Rochester School of Medicine and Dentistry
Rochester, New York
(114: Cardiac Arrhythmias, 137: Heart Murmurs, 141: High Blood Pressure in Infants, Children, and Adolescents, 192: Congenital Heart Disease)

Harvey J. Cohen, MD, PhD
Professor and Associate Chair, Department of Pediatrics
Associate Director, Cancer Center
Chief, Division of Pediatric Hematology/Oncology
University of Rochester School of Medicine and Dentistry
Rochester, New York
(112: Anemia and Pallor)

Michael W. Cohen, MD
Senior Lecturer
Department of Pediatrics
University of Arizona Medical School
Tucson, Arizona
(81: Enuresis)

Cynthia H. Cole, MD
Assistant Professor of Pediatrics
Department of Pediatrics
Division of Neonatology
The University of Vermont College of Medicine
Burlington, Vermont
(142: Hirsutism, Hypertrichosis, and Precocious Sexual Hair Development, 145: Hypotonia)

Arnold H. Colodny, MD
Clinical Professor of Surgery
Harvard Medical School
Senior Surgeon
Children's Hospital
Boston, Massachusetts
(247: Pyloric Stenosis)

Steven Couch, MD
Assistant Professor of Pediatrics
The Pennsylvania State University
University Hospital Rehabilitation Center
Hershey, Pennsylvania
(188: Cerebral Palsy)

Susan M. Coupey, MD
Associate Professor of Pediatrics
Albert Einstein College of Medicine
Associate Director, Division of Adolescent Medicine
Montefiore Medical Center
Bronx, New York
(100: Drug, Alcohol, and Tobacco Abuse)

David R. Cunningham, PhD
Professor of Surgery (Audiology)
Director, Division of Communicative Disorders
Health Sciences Center
University of Louisville School of Medicine
Louisville, Kentucky
(18: Nine: Screening: Auditory Screening) •

Richard E. Cuskar, JD
(Formerly) Attorney, Health Services Practice Group of Nixon, Hargrave, Devans, & Doyle
Rochester, New York
(4: Legal Aspects of Pediatric Medicine)

Joseph R. Custer, MD
Director, Pediatric Intensive Care Unit
Associate Professor of Pediatrics
C.S. Mott Children's Hospital
University of Michigan Hospital
Ann Arbor, Michigan
(288: Shock, B: Special Procedures)

Philip W. Davidson, PhD
Professor of Pediatrics, and Psychiatry (Psychology)
Director, University Affiliated Program for Developmental Disabilities
University of Rochester School of Medicine and Dentistry
Rochester, New York
(10: Communication with Parents and Patients, D: Common Psychological and Educational Tests)

Jonathan M. Davis, MD
Assistant Professor of Pediatrics
Medical Director, Newborn Intensive Care Unit
Strong Memorial Hospital
University of Rochester School of Medicine and Dentistry
Rochester, New York
(33: The Effects of Drugs and other Substances on the Fetus)

Ross M. Decter, MD
Assistant Professor of Surgery and Pediatrics
Director of Pediatric Urology
The Milton S. Hershey Medical Center
The Pennsylvania State University
Hershey, Pennsylvania
(163: Scrotal Swelling)

David D. DeLawyer, PhD
Private Practice of Clinical Psychology
Tacoma, Washington
(87: Peer Relationship Problems)

Harry C. Dietz, MD
Chief Resident, Department of Pediatrics
The Johns Hopkins Hospital
Baltimore, Maryland
(268: Coma, 270: Dehydration)

Jay N. Dolitsky, MD
Chief Resident, Department of Otolaryngology
Cornell University Medical College
Chief Resident, Department of Otolaryngology
Manhatten Eye, Ear, & Throat Hospital
New York, New York
(203: Foreign Bodies of the Ear, Nose, Airway, and Esophagus)

John H. Dossett, MD
Chief, Division of Infectious Diseases
Co-Director, Pediatric HIV Disease Services
Associate Professor of Pediatrics and Infectious Diseases
M.S. Hershey Medical Center
The Pennsylvania State University College of Medicine
Hershey, Pennsylvania
(17: Immunizations, 161: Recurrent Infections, 178: Acquired Immunodeficiency Syndrome (AIDS) and Human Immunodeficiency Syndrome (HIV) Infection, 194: Contagious Exanthematous Diseases)

David L. Dudgeon, MD
Professor of Surgery and Pediatrics
Children's Medical and Surgical Center
The Johns Hopkins Hospital
Baltimore, Maryland
(206: Gastrointestinal Obstruction)

Reggie E. Duerst, MD
Assistant Professor of Pediatrics
University of Rochester School of Medicine and Dentistry
Rochester, New York
(156: Petechiae and Purpura)

William A. Durbin, Jr. MD
Associate Professor of Pediatrics
University of Massachusetts Medical School
Worcester, Massachusetts
(117: Cough)

Alice G. Dvoskin, PhD
Psychologist, Private Practice
Baltimore, Maryland
(47: Child Custody)

Paul H. Dworkin, MD
Professor and Vice-Chairman
Department of Pediatrics
University of Connecticut School of Medicine
Head, Division of General Pediatrics
University of Connecticut Health Center
Farmington, Connecticut
(67: School Learning Problems and Developmental Differences)

David R. Edlestein, MD
Resident Coordinator, Department of Otolaryngology
Manhatten Eye, Ear, & Throat Hospital
Clinical Assistant Professor
Department of Otorhinolaryngology
Cornell University Medical College
New York, New York
(127: Epistaxis)

Marvin S. Eiger, MD
Director, Breast Feeding Program
Beth Israel Medical Center
New York, New York
(16: Two: The Feeding of Infants and Children)

Allen Eskenazi, MD
Assistant Professor
Department of Pediatrics
University of Maryland
School of Medicine
Baltimore, Maryland
(165: Splenomegaly)

Muki W. Fairchild, MSW, ACSW
Chief Social Worker for the Division of Child and Adolescent Psychiatry
Department of Psychiatry
Clinical Associate
Department of Pediatrics
Duke University Medical Center
Durham, North Carolina
(48: Children of Divorce, 98: Counseling the Parents of Adolescents)

Mary Farren, MS, RN
Clinical Chief, Community Health Nursing
Assistant Professor of Clinical Nursing
University of Rochester
School of Nursing
Strong Memorial Hospital
Rochester, New York
(68: Nursing Roles in School Health)

Marianne E. Felice, MD
Professor, Department of Pediatrics
University of Maryland School of Medicine
Chief, Division of Adolescent Medicine
Department of Pediatrics
University of Maryland Hospital
Baltimore, Maryland
(22: The Ill Child)

Loretta P. Finnegan, MD
Professor of Pediatrics, Psychology, and Human Behavior
Jefferson Medical College
Director, Family Center
Thomas Jefferson University
Philadelphia, Pennsylvania
(229: Neonatal Abstinence Syndrome)

Philip Fireman, MD
Professor of Pediatrics
University of Pittsburgh School of Medicine
Director, Department of Allergy, Immunology, and Rheumatology
Children's Hospital of Pittsburgh
Pittsburgh, Pennsylvania
(183: Asthma)

Martin Fisher, MD
Associate Chief
Division of Adolescent Medicine
North Shore University Hospital
Manhasset, New York
Cornell Medical College
New York, New York
(99: Anorexia Nervosa and Bulimia)

Lois T. Flaherty, MD
Associate Professor
Department of Psychiatry
University of Maryland
Director, Division of Child and Adolescent Psychiatry
Institute of Psychiatry and Human Behavior
Baltimore, Maryland
(167: Strange Behavior)

Thomas P. Foley, Jr. MD
Professor of Pediatrics
University of Pittsburgh School of Medicine
Director, Division of Endocrinology, Metabolism, and Diabetes Mellitus
Children's Hospital of Pittsburgh
Pittsburgh, Pennsylvania
(215: Hypothyroidism)

Gilbert B. Forbes, MD
Professor of Pediatrics
University of Rochester School of Medicine and Dentistry
Rochester, New York
(16: One: Nutrition: Nutritonal Requirements, 16: Three: Nutrition: Obesity)

Rex L. Forehand, PhD
Research Professor
Department of Psychology
University of Georgia
Athens, Georgia
(77: Conduct Disorders)

Donald J. Forrester, DDS
Chairman, Department of Pediatric Dentistry
Children's National Medical Center
Professor, Department of Pediatrics
George Washington University Medical Center
Washington, D.C.
(20: Preventive Aspects of Dental Care)

Sharon L. Foster, PhD
Professor of Psychology
California School of Professional Psychology, San Diego
San Diego, California
(87: Peer Relationship Problems)

Howard R. Foye, Jr., MD
Clinical Associate Professor of Pediatrics
University of Rochester School of Medicine and Dentistry
Attending Physician
Department of Pediatrics
Strong Memorial Hospital
Rochester, New York
(15: Anticipatory Guidance, 76: Colic, 201: Eczema, 252: Seborrheic Dermatitis)

T. Emmett Francoeur, MD, CM, FRCPC
Assistant Professor of Pediatrics
McGill University
Montreal Children's Hospital
Montreal, Quebec, Canada
(116: Constipation)

Carl A. Frankel, MD, FACP
Assistant Professor
Departments of Ophthalmology and Pediatrics
Pennsylvania State University
Director, Pediatric Ophthalmology and Strabismus
Department of Ophthalmology
University Hospital
The Milton S. Hershey Medical Center
Hershey, Pennsylvania
(162: The Red Eye, 166: Strabismus, 234: Ocular Foreign Bodies, 235: Ocular Trauma, 241: Periorbital and Orbital Edema)

William K. Frankenburg, MD
Professor, Department of Pediatrics and Preventive Medicine
University of Colorado School of Medicine
Attending Pediatrician
University Hospital
University of Colorado Health Sciences Center
Denver, Colorado
(18:One: Screening: General Considerations, 18:Thirteen: Screening: Programmatic Considerations in Initiating and Maintaining a Community Screening Program)

Christopher N. Frantz, MD
Professor of Pediatrics
Chief, Division of Hematology/Oncology
Department of Pediatrics
University of Maryland
Baltimore, Maryland
(217: Idiopathic Thrombocytopenia)

Henry S. Friedman, MD
Professor of Pediatrics
Department of Pediatrics
Division of Hematology and Oncology
Duke University School of Medicine
Durham, North Carolina
(168: Stridor)

Stanford B. Friedman, MD
Professor of Pediatrics
Chief, Division of Adolescent Medicine and Behavioral Pediatrics
Department of Pediatrics
North Shore University Hospital/Cornell University Medical College
Manhasset, New York
(22: The Ill Child, 72: Concepts of Psychosomatic Illness, 75: Consultation and Referral for Behavioral and Developmental Problems, 96: Challenges of Health Care Delivery to Adolescents, 97: Conversion Reactions in Adolescents)

John H. Fugate, MD
Associate Director
Neonatal & Pediatric Intensive Care Units
Massachusetts General Hospital
Boston, Massachusetts
(288: Shock)

Donna Futterman, MD
Assistant Professor of Pediatrics
Albert Einstein College of Medicine
Medical Director, Adolescent AIDS Program
Division of Adolescent Medicine
Department of Pediatrics
Montefiore Medical Center
Bronx, New York
(101: Homosexuality: Challenges of Treating Lesbian and Gay Adolescents)

Keith J. Gallaher, MD
Attending Neonatologist
Division of Neonatology
Cape Fear Valley Medical Center
Fayetteville, North Carolina
Clinical Assistant Professor of Pediatrics
University of North Carolina
Chapel Hill, North Carolina
(39: Signs and Symptoms of Neonatal Illness)

Jean M. Garrett, MD
University of Rochester
Department of Pediatrics
Rochester, New York
(D: Common Psychological and Educational Tests)

William F. Gayton, PhD
Professor and Chairman
Department of Psychology
University of Southern Maine
Portland, Maine
(83: Fire-setting)

Harry L. Gewanter, MD, FAAP, FACR
Clinical Assistant Professor of Pediatrics
Medical College of Virginia
Assistant Medical Director
Director of Pediatric Rheumatology
Children's Hospital
Richmond, Virginia
(221: Juvenile Arthritis)

Kathleen L. Gifford, RN
Neonatal Outreach Coordinator
Department of Pediatrics
Milton S. Hershey Medical Center
The Pennsylvania State University
Hershey, Pennsylvania
(36: Four: Neonatal Adaptations: Adjustment Period)

Archie S. Golden, MD
Associate Professor of Pediatrics
Johns Hopkins University School of Medicine
Chief, Department of Pediatrics
Francis Scott Key Medical Center
Baltimore, Maryland
(190: Cleft Lip and Cleft Palate)

Donald A. Goldmann, MD
Associate Professor of Pediatrics
Division of Infectious Diseases
Children's Hospital Medical Center
Harvard Medical School
Boston, Massachusetts
(207: Giardiasis, 245: Pinworm Infestations)

Robert E. Greenberg, MD
Professor and Chairman
Department of Pediatrics
University of New Mexico School of Medicine
Albuquerque, New Mexico
(197: Diabetes Mellitus, 271: Diabetic Ketoacidosis)

Joseph Greensher, MD, FAAP
Professor of Pediatrics
State University of New York School of Medicine
Stony Brook, New York
Medical Director, Associate Chairman
Department of Pediatrics
Winthrop-University Hospital
Mineola, New York
(21: Accident Prevention, A: Pediatric Basic and Advanced Life Support)

Sylvia P. Griffiths, MD
Professor of Clinical Pediatrics
Department of Pediatrics
Columbia University College of Physicians and Surgeons
Attending Pediatrician
Presbyterian Hospital
New York, New York
(249: Rheumatic Fever)

Lindsey K. Grossman, MD
Associate Professor of Pediatrics
Ohio State University College of Medicine
Section Chief, Ambulatory Pediatrics
Children's Hospital
University Hospital Clinics
Columbus, Ohio
(118: Dental Stains, 152: Malocclusion, 212: Herpes Infections)

John H. Gundy, MD
Associate Clinical Professor
Department of Pediatrics
Yale University School of Medicine
New Haven, Connecticut
Attending Physician
Department of Pediatrics
Danbury Hospital
Danbury, Connecticut
(7: The Pediatric Physical Examination)

Caroline Breese Hall, MD
Professor of Pediatrics and Medicine
Infectious Diseases Division
University of Rochester School of Medicine and Dentistry
Rochester, New York
(151: Lymphadenopathy, 186: Bronchiolitis, 269: Croup [Acute Laryngotracheobronchitis], 276: Epiglottitis)

David E. Hall, MD
Private Practice in Pediatrics
Townson, Maryland
Instructor, Department of Pediatrics
Johns Hopkins University School of Medicine
Baltimore, Maryland
(259: Sports Injuries, 278: Head Injuries)

William J. Hall, MD
Professor of Medicine and Pediatrics
University of Rochester School of Medicine and Dentistry
Chief, Department of Medicine
Rochester General Hospital
Rochester, New York
(186: Bronchiolitis, 269: Croup [Acute Laryngotracheobronchitis], 276: Epiglottitis)

J. Alex Haller, Jr., MD
Robert Garrett Professor of Pediatric Surgery
Children's Surgeon-in-Chief
The Johns Hopkins University School of Medicine
Baltimore, Maryland
(240: Pectus Excavatum and Pectus Carinatum, 277: Esophageal Burns)

William E. Hathaway, MD
Professor Emeritus of Pediatrics
University of Colorado School of Medicine
Denver, Colorado
(272: Disseminated Intravascular Coagulation)

Thomas A. Hazanski, MD
Department of Pediatrics
Vanderbilt University Medical Center
Nashville, Tennessee
(176: Wheezing, 246: Acute Pneumonia)

Alice B. Heisler, MD
Assistant Professor of Pediatrics and Child Psychiatry
Walter P. Carter Center
University of Maryland School of Medicine
Baltimore, Maryland
(91: Self-Stimulating Behaviors)

Fred J. Heldrich, MD
Associate Professor of Pediatrics
Johns Hopkins University School of Medicine
Chairman, Department of Pediatrics
St. Agnes Hospital
Baltimore, Maryland
(125: Dysuria, 242: Pertussis (Whooping cough), 250: Rocky Mountain Spotted Fever)

Roberta A. Hibbard, MD
Associate Professor of Pediatrics
Indiana University School of Medicine
James Whitcomb Riley Hospital for Children
Indianapolis, Indiana
(140: Hepatomegaly, 264: Umbilical Anomalies)

Robert A. Hoekelman, MD
Professor and Chairman
Department of Pediatrics
University of Rochester School of Medicine and Dentistry
Pediatrician-in-Chief, Strong Memorial Hospital
Rochester, New York
(Introduction, 3: Child Health Supervision, 6: The Pediatric History, 10: Communication with Parents and Patients, 18:Two: Screening: The Physical Examination as a Screening Test, 133: Foot and Leg Problems, 261: Tonsillectomy and Adenoidectomy)

Neil A. Holtzman, MD
Professor, Department of Pediatrics with Joint appointments in Health Policy and Epidemiology
The Johns Hopkins Medical Institutions
Attending Pediatrician
Johns Hopkins Hospital
Baltimore, Maryland
(18:Three: Screening: Screening for Genetic-Metabolic Disorders)

Barbara J. Howard, MD
University of Massachusetts
Department of Pediatrics
Worcester, Massachusetts
(223: Labial Adhesions)

Sharon Humiston, MD, MPH
Instructor and Fellow
Department of Pediatrics
University of Rochester School of Medicine and Dentistry
Rochester, New York
(275: Envenomations)

Margaret K. Ikeda, MD
Department of Pediatrics
Yale University School of Medicine
New Haven, Connecticut
(228: Meningoencephalitis)

Heidi Inderbitzen-Pisaruk, PhD
Assistant Professor of Psychology
University of Nebraska
Lincoln, Nebraska
(87: Peer Relationship Problems)

Jerri Ann Jenista, MD
Clinical Assistant Professor of Pediatrics and Communicable Diseases
University of Michigan Medical Center Drive
C.S. Mott Children's Hospital
Ann Arbor, Michigan
(202: Enterovirus Infections, 251: Roseola)

Alain Joffe, MD, MPH
Associate Professor of Pediatrics
Director, Adolescent Medicine
Department of Pediatrics
The Johns Hopkins School of Medicine
Baltimore, Maryland
(111: Amenorrhea, 122: Dysmenorrhea, 149: Limp, 171: Vaginal Bleeding, 172: Vaginal Discharge, 255: Sexually Transmitted Diseases)

R. Joseph Jopling, MD
Willow Creek Pediatrics
Salt Lake City, Utah
(19: Physical Fitness in Children)

Linda Juszczak, RN, MS, MPH, PNA
Senior Teaching Associate
Department of Pediatrics
Division of Adolescent Medicine
Clinical Director, Far Rockaway High School Clinic
North Shore University Hospital/Cornell University Medical College
Manhasset, New York
(65: The Chronically Ill and Disabled Child in School)

Helen W. Karl, MD
Assistant Professor of Anesthesia and Pediatrics
The Milton S. Hershey Medical Center
Pennsylvania State University College of Medicine
Hershey, Pennsylvania
(267: Airway Obstruction)

Aubrey J. Katz, MD
Associate Clinical Professor of Pediatrics
Boston University School of Medicine
Boston, Massachusetts
(205: Gastrointestinal Allergy, 208: Gluten-Sensitive Enteropathy [Celiac Sprue])

Karol Kaltenbach, PhD
Assistant Professor of Pediatrics, Psychiatry, and Human Behavior
Jefferson Medical College of Thomas Jefferson University
Philadelphia, Pennsylvania
(229: Neonatal Abstinence Syndrome)

James G. Kavanaugh, Jr., MD
Assistant Professor of Pediatrics
Division of Child and Family Psychiatry
University of Virginia School of Medicine
Charlottesville, Virginia
(88: Phobias)

Alan E. Kazdin, PhD
Professor of Psychology and Child Psychiatry
Department of Psychology
Yale University
New Haven, Connecticut
(79: Depression)

Bradley B. Keller, MD
Assistant Professor of Pediatrics
University of Rochester
School of Medicine & Dentistry
Department of Pediatrics
Rochester, New York
(279: Heart Failure)

John H. Kennell, MD
Professor of Pediatrics
Case Western Reserve University School of Medicine
Chief, Division of Child Development
Department of Pediatrics
Rainbow Babies and Children's Hospital
Cleveland, Ohio
(38: Pediatric Support for Parents)

Thomas J. Kenny, PhD
Professor and Director of Pediatrics and Psychology
The W.P. Carter Center
University of Maryland School of Medicine
Baltimore, Maryland
(85: Mental Retardation)

George R. Kim, MD
Instructor, Department of Pediatrics
Johns Hopkins University School of Medicine
Staff Pediatrician
Francis Scott Key Medical Center
Baltimore, Maryland
(113: Back Pain)

Herb Klar, ACSW
Senior Psychiatric Social Worker
Clinical Associate, Department of Psychiatry
Duke University Medical Center
Duke Day Hospital for Youth
Durham, North Carolina
(51: Family Systems Interventions in Pediatric Practice)

Marshall H. Klaus, MD
Adjunct Professor of Pediatrics
University of California
San Francisco, California
Director, Academic Affairs
Children's Hospital of Oakland
Oakland, California
(38: Pediatric Support for Parents)

Maurice D. Kogut, MD
Professor and Chair
Department of Pediatrics
Wright State University School of Medicine
The Children's Medical Center
Dayton, Ohio
(281: Hypoglycemia)

David N. Korones, MD
Senior Instructor of Pediatrics
Division of Pediatric Hematology/Oncology
University of Rochester
School of Medicine & Dentistry
Rochester, New York
(112: Anemia and Pallor)

Robert K. Kritzler, MD
Physician-in-Chief
Kaiser Permanente Medical Group, Baltimore
Pediatric Endocrinologist
Kaiser Permanente Mid-Atlantic Region
Clinical Assistant Professor of Pediatrics
University of Maryland School of Medicine
Baltimore, Maryland
(164: Sexual Developmental Alterations)

Joanne Kurtzberg, MD
Associate Professor of Pediatrics
Duke University School of Medicine
Durham, North Carolina
(108: Abdominal Distention, 168: Stridor)

Sandra R. Leichtman, PhD
Chief Psychologist and Program Analyst
Mental Hygiene Administration and Office of Licensing and Certification Programs
Department of Health and Mental Hygiene
Baltimore, Maryland
(96: Challenges of Health Care Delivery to Adolescents)

Melvin D. Levine, MD
Professor of Pediatrics
University of North Carolina School of Medicine
Director, Clinical Center for the Study of Development and Learning
University of North Carolina
Chapel Hill, North Carolina
(80: Encopresis)

Susan E. Levitzky, MD, FAAP
Assistant Clinical Professor
Department of Pediatrics
Mount Sinai School of Medicine
Attending Pediatrician
Beth Israel Medical Center
New York, New York
(143: Hoarseness)

Samuel M. Libber, MD
Assistant Professor of Pediatrics
Division of Pediatric Endocrinology
The Johns Hopkins University School of Medicine
Baltimore, Maryland
(157: Polyuria)

Gregory S. Liptak, MD, MPH
Associate Professor of Pediatrics
University of Rochester School of Medicine and Dentistry
Department of Pediatrics
Rochester, New York
(89: Physical Disability and Chronic Illness, 198: Diaper Rash, 257: Spina Bifida)

George A. Little, MD
Professor and Chairman
Department of Maternal and Child Health
Dartmouth Medical School
Hanover, New Hampshire
(31: The Fetus at Risk, 35:Two: Perinatal Medicine: Perinatal Transport)

Louis C. Littlefield, Pharm D
Professor of Pharmacy
College of Pharmacy
The University of Texas
Austin, Texas
Assistant Dean for Pharmacy Education
Graduate School of Biomedical Sciences
The University of Texas Health Science Center at San Antonio
San Antonio, Texas
(23: Management of Fever)

Thomas J. Long, EdD
Associate Professor of Education
The Catholic University of America
Washington, D.C.
(64: Dealing with Common Classroom Behavior Problems)

Donald P. Lookingbill, MD
Chief of Dermatology
Professor of Medicine
Division of Dermatology
Department of Medicine
The Milton S. Hershey Medical Center
The Pennsylvania State University
Hershey, Pennsylvania
(177: Acne, 184: Bacterial Skin Infections, 200: Drug Eruptions, 266: Verrucae [warts])

Paul S. Lubinsky, MD
Assistant Director, Pediatric Intensive Care Unit
Department of Pediatrics
Children's Hospital of Orange County
University of California, Irvine
Orange, California
(289: Status Asthmaticus)

Lois A. Maiman, PhD
Associate Professor, Department of Pediatrics
Associate Professor of Preventive, Family, and Rehabilitation Medicine
University of Rochester School of Medicine and Dentistry
Rochester, New York
(12: Compliance with Pediatric Health Care Recommendations)

M. Jeffrey Maisels, MB, BCh
Clinical Professor of Pediatrics
Wayne State University School of Medicine
University of Michigan Medical School
Chairman, Department of Pediatrics
William Beaumont Hospital
Royal Oak, Michigan
(36:One: Neonatal Adaptations: Peripartum Considerations, 36:Four: Neonatal Adaptations: Adjustment Period, 41: Critical Neonatal Illnesses)

Keith H. Marks, MD, PhD
Professor of Pediatrics
Division of Newborn Medicine
The Milton S. Hershey Medical Center
The Pennsylvania State University College of Medicine
Hershey, Pennsylvania
(41: Critical Neonatal Illnesses)

Harold P. Martin, MD
University of Colorado
Medical School
Department of Psychiatry
Denver, Colorado
(46: Child Abuse and Neglect)

Barry S. Marx, MD
Instructor of Pediatrics
Johns Hopkins University School of Medicine
Associated Program for Primary Care
Baltimore, Maryland
(146: Irritability)

Ake Mattsson, MD
Professor of Psychiatry
East Carolina University School of Medicine
Greenville, North Carolina
(88: Phobias, 104: Mood Disturbance, Mood Disorders, and Suicidal Behavior in Adolescents)

Lynne G. Maxwell, MD
Assistant Professor of Anesthesiology, Critical Care Medicine, and Pediatrics
The Johns Hopkins Medical Institutions
Baltimore, Maryland
(24: The Management of Acute Pain in Children)

Jay H. Mayefsky, MD, MPH
Senior Attending Physician
Division of Ambulatory Pediatrics
Cook County Hospital
Assistant Professor of Pediatrics
University of the Health Sciences/The Chicago Medical School
Chicago, Illinois
(124: Dyspnea)

Elizabeth R. McAnarney, MD
Professor of Pediatrics and Associate Chair of Academic Affairs
University of Rochester School of Medicine and Dentistry
Rochester, New York
(107: The Teenage Parent)

Margaret C. McBride, MD
Associate Professor of Neurology and Pediatrics
University of Rochester School of Medicine and Dentistry
Strong Memorial Hospital
Division of Child Neurology
Rochester, New York
(253: Seizure Disorders, 290: Status Epilepticus)

Hiram L. McDade, PhD
Associate Professor of Speech-Language and Audiology
University of South Carolina
Columbia, South Carolina
(69: Language and Speech Assessment at School Entry)

Diane L. McDonald, MD
Instructor of Pediatrics
Johns Hopkins University School of Medicine
Children's Medical Practice
Francis Scott Key Medical Center
Baltimore, Maryland
(121: Dizziness and Vertigo, 169: Syncope)

Rosemary K. McKevitt, RN, EdD*
San Antonio, Texas
(68: Nursing Roles in School Health)

Robert H. McLean, MD
Associate Professor of Pediatrics
The Johns Hopkins University School of Medicine
Chief, Division of Pediatric Nephrology
Department of Pediatrics
Johns Hopkins Hospital
Baltimore, Maryland
(126: Edema)

*deceased

Charles E. Mercier, MD
Fellow, Neonatology
Department of Pediatrics
University of Rochester School of Medicine and Dentistry
Rochester, New York
(33: The Effects of Drugs and Other Substances on the Fetus)

Ruth Messinger, MSW
Associate, Department of Health Services and Pediatrics
University of Rochester School of Medicine and Dentistry
Chief Social Worker
Department of Pediatrics
Rochester, New York
(10: Communication with Parents and Patients)

Geoffrey Miller, MD, MRCP, FRACP
Associate Professor of Pediatric Neurology
The Milton S. Hershey Medical Center
The Pennsylvania State University
Hershey, Pennsylvania
(188: Cerebral Palsy)

Marvin Elliott Miller, MD
Associate Professor of Pediatrics and Genetics
Department of Pediatrics
University of Rochester School of Medicine and Dentistry
Rochester, New York
(29: Genetic Diseases, 37: Skin Lesions of the Neonate)

Howard C. Mofenson, MD, FAAP, FAACT
Professor of Pediatrics and Emergency Medicine
State University of New York
Stony Brook, New York
Director, Long Island Regional Poison Control Center
Department of Pediatrics
Nassau County Medical Center
East Meadow, New York
(21: Accident Prevention, A: Pediatric Basic and Advanced Life Support)

Dennis Mujsce, MD
Assistant Professor of Pediatrics
The Milton S. Hershey Medical Center
The Pennsylvania State University
Hershey, Pennsylvania
(42: High-Risk Follow-up)

Beverly A. Myers, MD
Assistant Professor of Psychiatry and Pediatrics
Division of Child Psychiatry
Brown University School of Medicine
Providence, Rhode Island
Attending Psychiatrist
Rhode Island Hospital
Pawtucket, Rhode Island
(89: Physical Disability and Chronic Illness)

Philip R. Nader, MD
Professor and Director
Division of General Pediatrics
University of California at San Diego
San Diego, California
(59: Overview of School Health, 60: School Health Program Goals, 62: School Absenteeism, 66: School Refusal [School Avoidance Syndromes])

Nicholas M. Nelson, MD
Professor of Pediatrics
The Pennsylvania State University College of Medicine
The Milton S. Hershey Medical Center
Hershey, Pennsylvania
(8: Structural and Functional Analysis of Body Systems, 35:One: Perinatal Medicine: Overview and Regionalization, 36:One: Neonatal Adaptations: Peripartum Considerations, 36:Two: Physiological Status of the Healthy Infant, 36:Three: Recovery Period, 36:Four: Adjustment Period, 36:Five: Establishment of Equilibrium, 42: High-Risk Follow-up)

Steven L. Nickman, MD
Clinical Assistant Professor of Psychiatry
Harvard Medical School
Assistant in Psychiatry
Child Psychiatry Unit
Massachusetts General Hospital
Boston, Massachusetts
(44: Adoption and Foster Care)

Robert J. Nolan, Jr., MD
Assistant Professor
Assistant Chair for Education and Training
Department of Pediatrics
University of Texas Health Science Center
San Antonio, Texas
(285: Poisoning)

Judith M. Norman, JD
Attorney, Health Services Practice Group of Nixon, Hargrave, Devans, & Doyle
Rochester, New York
(4: Legal Aspects of Pediatric Medicine)

Karen Olness, MD
Professor of Pediatrics
Division of General Academic Pediatrics
Rainbow Babies and Children's Hospital
Professor of Family Medicine
Case Western Reserve University
Cleveland, Ohio
(11: Cultural Issues in Primary Pediatric Care)

J. Ramon Ongkingco, MD
Fellow, Department of Pediatric Nephrology
Children's National Medical Center
Washington, D.C.
(18:Eight: Screening: Use of Urinalysis and the Urine Culture in Screening, 209: Hemolytic-Uremic Syndrome, 233: Obstructive Uropathy and Vesicoureteral Reflex)

Robert B. Page, MD
Professor of Neurosurgery
Milton S. Hershey Medical Center
Pennsylvania State University College of Medicine
Hershey, Pennsylvania
(213: Hydrocephalus)

James Palis, MD
Assistant Professor of Pediatrics
Division of Pediatric Hematology/Oncology
University of Rochester School of Medicine and Dentistry
Rochester, New York
(220: Iron-Deficiency Anemia)

Charles Palmer, MBChB, FCP(SA)
Assistant Professor of Pediatrics
The Milton S. Hershey Medical Center
The Pennsylvania State University College of Medicine
Hershey, Pennsylvania
(40: Common Neonatal Illnesses)

Earl A. Palmer, MD
Professor of Ophthalmology and Pediatrics
The Oregon Health Sciences University
Portland, Oregon
(173: Visual Disturbances)

Guy S. Parcel, PhD
Professor and Director
Center for Health Promotion Research and Development
The University of Texas Health Science Center
Houston, Texas
(59: Overview of School Health, 61: School Health Education)

Simon C. Parisier, MD
Clinical Professor, Department of Otolaryngology
Cornell University Medical College
Chairman, Department of Otolaryngology
Manhattan Eye, Ear, and Throat Hospital
New York, New York
(136: Hearing Loss)

Doris R. Pastore, MD
Clinical Assistant Professor of Pediatrics
Division of Adolescent Medicine
North Shore University Hospital/Cornell University Medical College
Manhasset, New York
The Mt. Sinai Medical Center
New York, New York
(92: Stuttering)

Evan G. Pattishall III, MD
Assistant Professor of Pediatrics
The Milton, S. Hershey Medical Center
The Pennsylvania State University College of Medicine
Hershey, Pennsylvania
(189: Chickenpox)

David S. Pellegrini, PhD
Associate Professor of Psychology
The Catholic University of America
Life Cycle Institute
Washington, D.C.
(73: Prediction of Adult Behavior from Childhood)

Jay A. Perman, MD
Associate Professor of Pediatrics
Division of Pediatric Gastroenterology/Nutrition
The Johns Hopkins University School of Medicine and University of Maryland Medical School
Baltimore, Maryland
(211: Hepatitis)

Sheridan Phillips, PhD
Associate Professor
Department of Psychiatry and Department of Pediatrics
University of Maryland School of Medicine
Baltimore, Maryland
(74: Options for Psychosocial Intervention with Children and Adolescents, 75: Consultation and Referral for Behavioral and Developmental Problems)

Michael E. Pichichero, MD
Clinical Professor of Pediatrics
University of Rochester School of Medicine and Dentistry
Elmwood Pediatric Group
Rochester, New York
(222: Kawasaki Disease, 262: Toxic Shock Syndrome)

Sergio Piomelli, MD
Professor of Pediatrics
Columbia University College of Physicians and Surgeons
New York, New York
(18:Five: Screening: Screening for Anemia, 18:Six: Screening for Lead Poisoning)

S. Michael Plaut, PhD
Associate Professor of Psychiatry
University of Maryland School of Medicine
Baltimore, Maryland
(14: Assessing the Medical Literature)

I. Barry Pless, MD
Professor of Pediatrics, Epidemiology, and Biostatistics
Department of Pediatrics
McGill University School of Medicine
Director, Community Pediatric Research
Montreal Children's Hospital
Montreal, Quebec, Canada
(2: Morbidity and Mortality Among the Young)

Leslie P. Plotnick, MD
Associate Professor of Pediatrics
Johns Hopkins University School of Medicine
Baltimore, Maryland
(157: Polyuria, 164: Sexual Developmental Alterations)

Keith R. Powell, MD
George Washington Goler Professor and Associate Chairman for Clinical Affairs
Department of Pediatrics
Chief, Division of Pediatric Infections Diseases
University of Rochester School of Medicine and Dentistry
Rochester, New York
(28: Antimicrobial Therapy, 227: Meningitis, 283: Meningococcemia)

Gregory E. Prazar, MD
Exeter Pediatric Associates
Exeter, New Hampshire
(84: Lying and Stealing, 93: Temper Tantrums and Breath-Holding Spells, 97: Conversion Reactions in Adolescents)

Richard Owen Proctor, (Brigadier General), MD, MPH, TM
Commanding General
William Beaumont Army Medical Center
El Paso, Texas
(239: Parasitic Infestations)

George A. Rekers, PhD
Professor, Department of Neuropsychiatry & Behavioral Science
University of South Carolina Medical School
Columbia, South Carolina
(78: Cross-Sex Behavior)

Rebecca E. Ribovich, MD
Assistant Professor of Pediatrics
Johns Hopkins University School of Medicine
Baltimore, Maryland
(248: Reye Syndrome)

Julius B. Richmond, MD
John D. MacArthur Professor of Health Policy and Management, Emeritus
Harvard University
Advisor on Child Health Policy
Children's Hospital Medical Center
Boston, Massachusetts
(49: Day Care and PreSchool Programs, 55: Mental Health of the Young)

Sarah M. Roddy, MD
Assistant Professor of Neurology and Pediatrics
University of Rochester School of Medicine and Dentistry
Rochester, New York
(154: Nonconvulsive Periodic Disorders, 253: Seizure Disorders, 290: Status Epilepticus)

Lance E. Rodewald, MD
Assistant Professor of Pediatrics
University of Rochester School of Medicine and Dentistry
Rochester, New York
(12: Compliance with Pediatric Health Care Recommendations)

Alvin Rosenfeld, MD
Director of Psychiatric Services
Jewish Child Care Association of New York
New York, New York
(57: Sexual Abuse of Children)

Beryl J. Rosenstein, MD
Professor of Pediatrics
The Johns Hopkins University School of Medicine
Director, Cystic Fibrosis Center
The Johns Hopkins Hospital
Baltimore, Maryland
(115: Chest Pain, 139: Hemoptysis, 170: Torticollis)

Pedro Rosso, MD
Professor of Pediatrics
Pontifica Universidad Catolica de Chile
Santiago, Chile, South America
(32: Maternal Nutritional Status and Prenatal Growth)

Edward J. Ruley, MD
Professor of Pediatrics
George Washington School of Medicine
Chairman, Department of Nephrology
Children's Hospital National Medical Center
Washington, D.C.
(18:Eight: Screening: Use of Urinalysis and the Urine Culture in Screening, 138: Hematuria, 158: Proteinuria, 181: Anuria/Oliguria, 209: Hemolytic-Uremic Syndrome, 210: Henoch-Schonlein Purpura, 230: Nephritis, 231: Nephrotic Syndrome, 233: Obstructive Uropathy and Vesicoureteral Reflex, 265: Urinary Tract Infections, 280: Hypertensive Emergencies, 287: Acute Renal Failure)

Olle Jane Z. Sahler, MD
Professor of Pediatrics, Psychiatry, Medical Humanities, and Medical Informatics
University of Rochester School of Medicine and Dentistry
Strong Memorial Hospital
Rochester, New York
(43: Theories and Concepts of Development as They Relate to Pediatric Practice, D: Common Psychological and Educational Tests)

Edward J. Saltzman, MD
Clinical Professor of Pediatrics
University of Miami School of Medicine
Hollywood, Florida
(1: The Health Care Delivery System)

John Sargent, MD
Associate Professor of Psychiatry and Pediatrics
Director, Child Psychiatry Training
Philadelphia Child Guidance Clinic
University of Pennsylvania School of Medicine
Philadelphia, Pennsylvania
(50: Family Interactions: Children with Unexplained Physical Symptoms)

Richard M. Sarles, MD
Director, Division of Child and Adolescent Psychiatry
Sheppard and Enoch Pratt Hospital
Clinical Professor of Psychiatry and Pediatrics
University of Maryland School of Medicine
Baltimore, Maryland
(57: Sexual Abuse of Children, 91: Self-Stimulating Behaviors, 153: Nervousness, 286: Rape)

Sharon B. Satterfield, MD
Assistant Professor of Family Practice and Community Health
Attending Physician
Department of Family Practice & Community Health
University of Minnesota Medical School
Minneapolis, Minnesota
(106: Sexual Behavior in Adolescents)

Edward V. Sauris, MD
Clinical Fellow, Department of Otolaryngology
Manhattan Eye, Ear, & Throat Hospital
New York, New York
(127: Epistaxis)

Eric A. Schaff, MD
Associate Professor of Family Medicine and Pediatrics
Department of Family Medicine
University of Rochester School of Medicine and Dentistry
Project Director, Teen Center
Anthony L. Jordan Health Center
Rochester, New York
(30: Contraception, 34: Abortion)

L.R. Scherer III, MD
Assistant Professor of Pediatric Surgery, Pediatrics, and Anesthesia and Critical Care Medicine
The Johns Hopkins University School of Medicine
Baltimore, Maryland
(291: Thermal Injuries)

Therese K. Schmalbach, MD
Research Fellow in Clinical Pharmacology
Laboratory of Clinical Pharmacology
Harvard Medical School
Boston, Massachusetts
(27: Clinical Pharmacology)

Marcie B. Scheider, MD
Assistant Professor of Pediatrics
Department of Pediatrics
Attending Physician in Adolescent Medicine
North Shore University Hospital/Cornell University Medical College
Manhasset, New York
(65: The Chronically Ill and Disabled Child in School)

S. Kenneth Schonberg, MD
Professor of Pediatrics
Albert Einstein College of Medicine
Director, Division of Adolescent Medicine
Montefiore Medical Center
Bronx, New York
(18:Six: Screening: Drug Screening, 100: Drug, Alcohol, and Tobacco Abuse)

Kenneth C. Schuberth, MD
Assistant Professor of Pediatrics
Johns Hopkins University School of Medicine
Baltimore, Maryland
(179: Allergic Rhinitis)

Cindy Schwartz, MD
Assistant Professor of Pediatrics
University of Rochester School of Medicine and Dentistry
Rochester, New York
(187: Cancers in Childhood)

Robert H. Schwartz, MD
Clinical Professor of Pediatrics
University of Rochester School of Medicine and Dentistry
Attending Physician
Director, Clinical Allergy
Department of Pediatrics
Strong Memorial Hospital
Rochester, New York
(195: Cystic Fibrosis)

Kathleen B. Schwartz, MD
Associate Professor of Pediatrics
Department of Pediatrics
Division of Pediatric Gastroenterology and Nutrition
The Johns Hopkins University School of Medicine
University of Maryland Medical School
Baltimore, Maryland
(211: Hepatitis)

Edwards P. Schwentker, MD
Associate Professor of Surgery
The Milton S. Hershey Medical Center
The Pennsylvania State University College of Medicine
Hershey, Pennsylvania
(237: Osteomyelitis, 254: Septic Arthritis)

George B. Segel, MD
Professor of Pediatrics, Medicine, and Genetics
University of Rochester School of Medicine and Dentistry
Director, Division of Pediatric Genetics
Strong Memorial Hospital
Rochester, New York
(151: Lymphadenopathy)

Henry M. Seidel, MD
Professor of Pediatrics
The Johns Hopkins University School of Medicine
Attending Pediatrician
The Johns Hopkins Hospital
Baltimore, Maryland
(13: The Art of Consultation, 53: Health Needs of Parents, 110: Alopecia and Hair Shaft Anomalies, 135: Headache, 153: Nervousness, 214: Hypospadias, Epispadias, and Cryptorchism)

Michael C. Sharp, MD
Associate Professor of Pediatrics
University of North Carolina School of Medicine
Chapel Hill, North Carolina
(119: Developmental Delays)

David M. Siegel, MD, MPH
Assistant Professor of Pediatrics and Medicine
University of Rochester School of Medicine and Dentistry
Co-Director, Pediatric Rheumatology Clinic
Strong Memorial Hospital
Rochester General Hospital
Rochester, New York
(148: Joint Pain, 225: Lyme Disease)

Arnold T. Sigler, MD
Associate Professor of Pediatrics
The Johns Hopkins University School of Medicine
The Johns Hopkins Hospital
Baltimore, Maryland
(130: Fatigue and Weakness)

Edward M. Sills, MD
Associate Professor of Pediatrics
Johns Hopkins University School of Medicine
Director, Pediatrics and Adolescent Collagen-Vascular Service
Department of Pediatrics
Johns Hopkins Hospital
Baltimore, Maryland
(236: Osteochondroses, 258: Spinal Deformities)

Nancy E. Simeonsson, RN, BS, PNP
Pediatric Nurse Practitioner
Department of Medical Research
Frank Porter Graham Child Development Center
University of North Carolina
Chapel Hill, North Carolina
(18:Eleven: Screening: Developmental Assessment)

Rune J. Simeonsson, PhD
Professor of Education
Research Professor of Psychology
Scientist, Frank Porter Graham Child Development Center
University of North Carolina
Chapel Hill, North Carolina
(18:Eleven: Screening: Developmental Assessment, 119: Developmental Delays)

Neil H. Sims, MD*
Little Rock, Arkansas
(190: Cleft Lip and Cleft Palate)

Shirley A. Smoyak, PhD, RN
Professor of Planning
Rutgers—The State University of New Jersey
New Brunswick, New Jersey
(45: Changing American Families)

Linda K. Snelling, MD
Assistant Professor of Pediatrics & Anesthesiology
Yale University School of Medicine
New Haven, Connecticut
(273: Drowning and Near-Drowning)

David M. Snyder, MD
Assistant Clinical Professor of Pediatrics
University of California at San Francisco School of Medicine
San Francisco, California
Director, Developmental and Behavioral Pediatrics
Valley Children's Hospital
Fresno, California
(70: Developmental Approach to Behavioral Problems)

Mary V. Solanto, PhD
Associate Professor of Pediatrics
Albert Einstein College of Medicine
Bronx, New York
Coordinator of Research
Division of Developmental and Behavioral Pediatrics
Schneider Children's Hospital of Long Island
Jewish Medical Center
New Hyde Park, New York
(63: Attention-Deficit Hyperactivity Disorder)

Joyce Sprafkin, PhD
Associate Professor
Department of Psychiatry
State University of New York
Stony Brook, New York
(58: Television and the Family)

Barbara Starfield, MD
Professor and Head, Division of Health Policy
The Johns Hopkins University School of Hygiene and Public Health
Joint Appointment in Pediatrics
The Johns Hopkins University School of Medicine
Baltimore, Maryland
(1: The Health Care Delivery System)

Carole A. Stashwick, MD
Assistant Professor of Maternal & Child Health
Dartmouth Medical School
Director of Pediatric and Adolescent Medicine Clinics
Hitchcock Clinic
Dartmouth-Hitchcock Medical Center
Hanover, New Hampshire
(175: Weight Loss)

*deceased

David M. Steinhorn, MD
Instructor, Pediatric Critical Care
Associate Director, Pediatric Intensive Care Unit
Department of Pediatrics
University of Minnesota
Minneapolis, Minnesota
(134: Gastrointestinal Hemorrhage)

Ellen R. Strahlman, MD, MHS
Medical Officer
Department of Epidemiology Program
National Eye Institute
National Institutes of Health
Bethesda, Maryland
(18:Ten: Screening: Vision Screening)

R. Scott Strahlman, MD
Instructor, Department of Pediatrics
The Johns Hopkins University School of Medicine
Baltimore, Maryland
Pediatrician
The Patuxent Medical Group
Columbia, Maryland
(182: Appendicitis, 204: Fractures and Dislocations in Children)

Ciro V. Sumaya, MD
Professor of Pediatrics and Pathology
The University of Texas Health Science Center
Consultant, Diagnostic District
San Antonio, Texas
(18:Four: Screening: Tuberculin Skin Testing, 218: Infectious Mononucleosis and Epstein-Barr Virus Infections, 263: Tuberculin Skin Test Positivity)

Dennis M. Super, MD, MPH
Assistant Professor of Pediatrics
Case Western Reserve University School of Medicine
Attending Physician
Department of Pediatrics
MetroHealth Medical Center
Cleveland, Ohio
(36:Five: Neonatal Adaptations: Establishment of Equilibrium, 244: Phimosis)

Peter G. Szilagyi, MD, MPH
Assistant Professor of Pediatrics
University of Rochester School of Medicine and Dentistry
Rochester, New York
(180: Animal Bites, 196: Cystic and Solid Masses of the Face and Neck)

Susan M. Thornton, MD
University of Colorado Health Sciences Center
Denver, Colorado
(18:One: Screening: General Considerations)

I. David Todres, MD
Associate Professor of Anesthesia (Pediatrics)
Harvard Medical School
Director, Neonatal and Pediatric Intensive Care Units
Massachusetts General Hospital
Boston, Massachusetts
(288: Shock)

Gail P. Udkow, MD
Staff Pediatrician
The Permanente Medical Group
Oakland, California
(C: Miscellaneous Values)

Martin H. Ulshen, MD
Associate Professor of Pediatrics
Chief, Division of Gastroenterology
University of North Carolina School of Medicine
Chapel Hill, North Carolina
(120: Diarrhea and Steatorrhea, 150: Loss of Appetite, 174: Vomiting)

Élise W. van der Jagt, MD, MPH
Associate Professor of Pediatrics
Director of The Strong Children's Critical Care Center
University of Rochester School of Medicine and Dentistry
Department of Pediatrics
Strong Children's Medical Center
Rochester, New York
(131: Fever, 132: Fever of Unknown Origin)

Robert C. Vannucci, MD
Professor of Pediatrics
Chief, Division of Pediatric Neurology
The Milton S. Hershey Medical Center
The Pennsylvania State University College of Medicine
Hershey, Pennsylvania
(185: Brain Tumors)

Eileen P.G. Vining, MD
Associate Professor of Pediatrics and Neurology
The Johns Hopkins University School of Medicine
Baltimore, Maryland
(199: Down Syndrome)

Robert F. Ward, MD
Assistant Professor of Otolaryngology
Cornell University Medical College
Attending Physician
Department of Otolaryngology
The New York Hospital
Assistant Attending Physician
Manhattan Eye, Ear, and Throat Hospital
New York, New York
(203: Foreign Bodies of the Ear, Nose, Airway, and Esophagus)

Irving B. Weiner, PhD
Professor of Psychiatry and Behavioral Medicine
Director of Psychological Services
University of South Florida
Psychiatry Center
Tampa, Florida
(90: Psychosis, 103: Juvenile Delinquency)

Michael H. Weiss, MD
Clinical Assistant Professor
Department of Otorhinolarynology
Cornell University Medical College
Resident Coordinator of Otolaryngology
Manhattan Eye, Ear, & Throat Hospital
New York, New York
(136: Hearing Loss)

Karen C. Wells, PhD
Associate Professor of Medical Psychology
Director, Family Studies Program and Clinic
Duke University Medical Center
Durham, North Carolina
(77: Conduct Disorders)

Esther H. Wender, MD
Professor of Pediatrics
Albert Einstein College of Medicine
Bronx, New York
Chief, Division of Developmental and Behavioral Pediatrics
Schneider Children's Hospital of Long Island
Jewish Medical Center
New Hyde Park, New York
(63: Attention-Deficit Hyperactivity Disorder, 102: Interviewing Adolescents)

Steven L. Werlin, MD
Associate Professor of Pediatrics
Medical College of Wisconsin
Director of Gastroenterology
Department of Pediatrics
Children's Hospital of Wisconsin
Milwaukee, Wisconsin
(123: Dysphagia)

John S. Werry, MD
Professor of Psychiatry
University of Auckland School of Medicine
Auckland, New Zealand
(94: Tics)

Charles F. Whitten, MD
Distinguished Professor of Pediatrics
Associate Dean for Curricular Affairs
Director, Comprehensive Sickle Cell Center
The Wayne State University School of Medicine
Detroit, Michigan
(18:Twelve: Screening: Sickle Cell Conditions)

Mark D. Widome, MD
Associate Professor of Pediatrics
The Milton S. Hershey Medical Center
The Pennsylvania State University College of Medicine
Hershey, Pennsylvania
(191: The Common Cold, 243: Pharyngitis and Tonsillitis)

Rickey L. Williams, MD
Clinical Lecturer
University of Arizona Health Sciences Center
Tucson, Arizona
(54: Latchkey Children: Children in Self-Care, 238: Otitis Media and Otitis Externa, 256: Sinusitus)

Thomas E. Williams, MD
Associate Professor
The University of Texas Health Science Center at San Antonio
San Antonio, Texas
(26: Blood Products and Their Uses)

Craig M. Wilson, MD
Instructor in Pediatrics
Division of Infectious Diseases
The Children's Hospital
Harvard University
Boston, Massachusetts
(207: Giardiasis, 245: Pinworm Infestations)

Modena Hoover Wilson, MD, MPH
Associate Professor of Pediatrics
The Johns Hopkins School of Medicine
Associate Professor of Health Policy and Management
School of Hygiene and Public Health
Baltimore, Maryland
(155: Odor [Unusual Urine and Body] 232: Obesity)

Kathleen A. Woodin, MD
Assistant Professor of Pediatrics
Divisions of General Pediatrics and Infectious Diseases
University of Rochester School of Medicine and Dentistry
Attending Physician
(C: Miscellaneous Values)

Susan F. Woolsey, RN
Former Assistant Clinical Professor of Behavioral Pediatrics
Director of Maryland SIDS Information and Counseling Program
University of Maryland School of Medicine
Baltimore, Maryland
(260: Sudden Infant Death Syndrome)

Jerome Y. Yager, MD
Assistant Professor of Pediatrics
Department of Pediatric Neurology
The Milton S. Hershey Medical Center
The Pennsylvania State University School of Medicine
Hershey, Pennsylvania
(185: Brain Tumors)

W. Sam Yancy, MD
Clinical Professor of Pediatrics
Associate Clinical Professor of Psychiatry
Duke University Medical Center
Durham, North Carolina
(95: Adolescence, 98: Counseling the Parents of Adolescents)

Myron Yaster, MD
Associate Professor of Anesthesiology/Critical Care Medicine and Pediatrics
Director, Multi-Discipline Pain Service
Children's Center
The Johns Hopkins Hospital
Baltimore, Maryland
(24: The Management of Acute Pain in Children)

Michael W. Yogman, MD
Assistant Professor of Pediatrics
Harvard Medical School
Director, Infant Health and Development Program
Children's Hospital
Boston, Massachusetts
(70: Developmental Approach to Behavioral Problems)

Richard S.K. Young, MD
Associate Professor of Pediatrics and Neurology
Yale University School of Medicine
New Haven, Connecticut
(228: Meningoencephalitis, 273: Drowning and Near-Drowning, 282: Increased Intracranial Pressure)

Bradley H. Zebal, MSW, MBA
Division Administrator
Ambulatory and Ancillary Services
Sheppard Pratt Hospital
Baltimore, Maryland
(48: Children of Divorce)

Foreword

The discipline we know as pediatrics is now just over 100 years of age in the United States. With growth has come development and increasing complexity. Pediatrics has moved from a discipline largely taught with regard to the hospitalized patient to one that is increasingly being learned and studied in the ambulatory setting. The comprehensive textbooks of pediatrics have not kept pace with these changes.

The pathophysiology of the disease, once the focus of all textbooks of pediatrics, now represents a smaller portion of the knowledge base required to practice pediatrics effectively. Familiarity with the determinants of health and disease, from birth through the end of adolescence, is required for the physician providing primary care.

The consummate clinician should be firmly grounded in topics that run the gamut from health care delivery systems, through ethics, to the art of consultation. The effective primary care provider should have a thorough background in the prevention of disease, whether it is through immunization, screening procedures, or dietary counseling, as well as in the recognition of disease and its treatment options. The primary care provider should be as comfortable dealing with problems that confront the normal neonate as with the behavioral problems that often accompany childhood and adolescence.

Textbooks of pediatrics do not adequately address the issues commonly encountered by the primary health care practitioner; nor do they examine the environment in which the problems occur, such as the day-care setting, the school, or the larger community. This textbook does. The authors have accomplished what others have only attempted.

Primary care has a scientific foundation—a foundation as concrete as that encountered when dealing with the pathophysiology of disease. This textbook contains the information that now is an essential part of the fabric of pediatrics. Pediatrics is more robust and vigorous today because of this widened scope.

Frank A. Oski, MD

Chariman and Given Professor of Pediatrics,
Johns Hopkins University School of Medicine,
Baltimore, Maryland

Preface

The practice of pediatrics has become increasingly complicated over the years, as knowledge of the etiology, pathophysiology, and management of physical, emotional, behavioral, and social ills has developed more rapidly and fully.

Although the dimensions of pediatrics have grown, the education of the pediatrician has remained, for the most part, disease-oriented and pathophysiologic in substance. Educators, despite the recommendations made by the Task Force on Pediatric Education in 1978, have demonstrated minimal awareness of the gap between this disease orientation and the actual practice of primary health care, and they have made only token efforts to adjust teaching programs to reflect the actual practice of the majority of pediatricians. In fact, the pathophysiologic priority has been maintained in the belief that, given a sound disease-oriented experience, the primary care provider can acquire the other, softer, "easier" knowledge of health care "on the job." This belief is quite unjustified.

Knowledge of pathophysiology is essential to the understanding of disease and of normalcy; however, it is not sufficient in itself to ensure success in the management of illness. An understanding of illness requires both an understanding of health per se and of the greater complexities of health.

The purpose of this text is to provide much of the pertinent information concerning the *determinants and reflections of health and of disease*. The primary provider of health care to the young should be in command of this information, which constitutes a body of knowledge not now conveniently available to the student and practitioner in one repository. It may seem more subjective than the "harder" pathophysiologic knowledge base and, therefore, less scientific. It is not. Indeed, its variables are infinite and its experiments more difficult to control. Although pathophysiologic knowledge is treated throughout this text, the book focuses on the *determinants* of health and disease; it attempts to be comprehensive only in regard to this body of knowledge. The reader is referred to other sources when information in greater depth in other areas is required. Cited references to scientific publications are used, and contributors have been asked to identify and clarify controversial issues.

The scope of this text, then, is different from that of traditional pediatric texts in that *all* aspects of *health* care are considered. The breadth and depth of the discussion of *illness*, however, are limited to that information which the primary care provider needs to function effectively in his or her role. The rarer diseases and the esoteric points in etiologic, pathophysiologic, and therapeutic considerations of the more common diseases are not included here. The message is that the physical and emotional health of the child can be adequately maintained by the primary care provider (1) through well-child visits, which focus on prevention and early detection of disease and of psychosocial dysfunction, and (2) through competent management of acute and chronic illness with or without the help of other professionals.

In using this text, our readers are asked to keep in mind the following five questions: (1) What does the primary care provider need to know about the condition or disease being described to recognize it? (2) How should the condition be managed? (3) When should consultation be sought or referral to a specialist be made? (4) What can the primary care provider expect the consultant to do for the patient? and (5) What role should the primary care provider play in the management of care after a referral has been made? Certain general considerations to guide one's thinking include prevention, screening, and emergency management, as well as collaborative care, follow-up care, and costs. Family, community, environmental, and political influences on the presentation and outcome of the condition must also be considered.

We hope that this book will provide *all* primary health care practitioners much of the information required to understand and manage the various problems they encounter in caring for the young. It would be extremely difficult, if not impossible, for any one text to provide all the information such practitioners require. We do not pretend to do so but urge the reader (student or practitioner) to seek that information not found herein from the references we have provided or from other comprehensive pediatric textbooks that emphasize different elements of the health care of the young.

This textbook would not have been published without the help and support of many persons. The names and affiliations of the 254 contributing authors are given in the list of contributors.

Our publishers provided us with the essentials editors need: opportunity, direction, proficiency, provocation, criticism, and, above all, reassurance and patience. Stephanie Bircher Manning, Kathryn H. Falk, Richard Barber, and especially Ellen Baker Geisel gave us these and more.

Extensive editorial comment and direction were given by Sydney A. Sutherland. Her assistance in ensuring the seemingly impossible—the smooth and continual communication among authors, editors, and publishers—has been especially appreciated. Secretarial assistance was provided in the revision of manuscripts by Tamara Davies.

We thank all of these good people for their interest, expertise, and understanding.

Robert A. Hoekelman
Stanford B. Friedman
Nicholas M. Nelson
Henry M. Seidel

Contents

Part Eight Specific Clinical Problems

Part Nine Critical Situations

Appendixes

Introduction

Robert A. Hoekelman

There is no doubt that those who are concerned with the delivery of child health care face serious difficulties in finding the resources and mechanisms to ensure that all children in need of preventive, maintenance, and curative services receive them. No matter how the pediatric health care pie is sliced, as it presently exists, all the appetites will not be satisfied. This is true for those who seek these services and even more so for the greater numbers who are in need yet do not recognize that need or do not have the resources to seek the appropriate care.

Any review of health care needs and prospects for meeting them demands an assessment of the services that are required, how these can be organized and delivered effectively and efficiently, who will deliver these services, and how these persons can be prepared to do so.

Traditionally, primary care pediatricians have conducted high-volume practices in solo or small partnership arrangements. They have provided preventive services and health maintenance supervision and have managed acute minor illnesses on an ambulatory basis. Only a small part of their efforts, however, have been spent in the diagnosis and treatment of serious illness in the hospital, for which most of their postgraduate training prepared them. These problems have increasingly been referred to subspecialty pediatricians located in large medical centers, either because primary care pediatricians have not had the time to deal with them or because their knowledge and skills in the management of severe illness have atrophied from disuse.

Most pediatricians learn to do what they do through on-the-job experience rather than through formal training. To many, the content of private practice comes somewhat as a surprise. Some pediatricians are not satisfied with this role and turn to subspecialty training and practice, but most adjust quickly and find primary care practice extremely rewarding.

There are, however, forces coming to bear on the future of primary pediatric practice over which the individual physician has little or no control. These forces are as follows: (1) The incidence of serious disease in childhood is decreasing because of public and individual preventive health measures; therefore the number of these illnesses occurring in a single practice is diminishing. (2) The reproductive behavior of the population is changing. The use of contraceptive devices and the liberalization of abortion laws have decreased the birth rate significantly, particularly in the populations served by most pediatricians. Infant mortality, prematurity, and morbidity have diminished as well, and the regionalization of perinatal care has transferred the management of most high-risk newborn infants from the primary care pediatrician to neonatologists in regional centers. (3) The rapid increase in medical knowledge and technology has produced methods of treatment for many childhood diseases that can only be provided in large institutions by specialists who devote most of their efforts to these problems. The primary care physician, therefore, cannot morally or ethically elect to continue to care for these patients. (4) Other professionals have demonstrated their ability to provide competently much of the care currently undertaken by the practicing pediatrician. Family practitioners, pediatric nurse practitioners, and physicians' assistants are capable of providing those services, working with or independent of the pediatrician. (5) Private practice is moving toward consumer control. Demands are being made on the practitioner to institute new organizational and financial arrangements in the provision of primary care. Issues of cost, availability, acceptability, accountability, and efficacy of care provided must be dealt with by each practitioner.

These forces need not be viewed negatively. Rather, they can be used by pediatric practitioners to improve the health care available to children. Pediatric practice will need to be reorganized to meet the needs of all children, not just those for whom care is sought. Care must also become more continuous and comprehensive and must be coordinated with the health-related needs of children that are met by others. Pediatricians will have to relate to the broader issues that affect the health of children within the family structure, within the community, and within the greater environment.

The list of these issues, long neglected, is extensive and includes specific problems within the areas of education (attaining full intellectual potential), communication (understanding and being understood), socialization (behaving appropriately with others), and normalization (functioning within acceptable limits) for both well and ill children. Efforts to deal with these issues effectively will need to be directed through the community. The prospect for success in effecting improvement in the health of children is probably greater along this avenue than in the provision of individual health care. It is clear that practicing pediatricians cannot accomplish these goals without working collaboratively with other professionals within and outside the practice setting.

This change in the complexion of primary care practice requires changes in our system of undergraduate and graduate medical education. The curriculum must be altered to include educational objectives commensurate with the activities of primary care physicians and to exclude objectives that are no longer pertinent to practice. Early tracking of students who plan to enter primary care versus those who plan on subspecialty practice within academia or outside is needed, and interdisciplinary education with other professionals who will be working collaboratively with physicians in team-oriented care needs to be instituted. In addition, the milieu in which medical education takes place must be supportive of the broader concept of the practice of primary care.

Primary care has finally been defined to the satisfaction of almost everyone, and educational programs to prepare physicians to provide such care to children have emerged in response to reason, demand, and dictum. Questions now arise as to who should provide the bulk of that care and how it can best be organized to ensure that the health care needs of all our children are met. The politics of primary pediatric care begin to occupy more of our thoughts and discussion.

Part One of this book, "Overview of Pediatric Care," presents an analysis of pediatric care in the United States including how it is delivered, the morbidity and mortality that occur, the application of child health supervision designed to promote health and reduce morbidity and mortality, the legal issues that affect the way pediatrics is practiced, and the methods used in delivering pediatric care within the community.

Part Two, "Communication and Evaluation," addresses the diagnostic process, which begins with construction of a data base through the gathering of historical information concerning the patient's illness, the conducting of a complete examination to detect deviations from the normal physical status, and the performing of specific tests to analyze the structure and function of the body systems that may be involved. The process continues with recording of the findings in the medical record and assimilation of the information gathered to reach a provisional or definitive diagnosis, with or without assistance from consulting specialists and the medical literature. It moves to communication of the diagnosis to the patient and parents so that they understand what the problem is, what can be done to solve it, and what their role is in its management.

The management of pediatric patients must be accomplished with the understanding that they are dependent on others to ensure their optimum growth and development, their protection from the acquisition of disease, and their recovery from illness. Those responsible for these assurances are, in turn, dependent on health professionals to guide them in the use of the means by which those assurances can best be realized.

It follows with addressing how practitioners perceive and respond to the cultural issues that affect how medicine is practiced among selected ethnic populations and how compliance with pediatric health care recommendations can be enhanced in general, both at the primary care level and at the level of consultation with subspecialists. It ends with how physicians communicate with each other through the medical literature.

Part Three, "Principles of Patient Care," explores the general principles of prevention and treatment that are applicable to the comprehensive care of the young. It deals with the maintenance of health in well children and with therapies directed to acutely and chronically ill children, stressing aspects of illness care that are unique to the pediatric patient.

Practitioners of medicine in the United States and other highly developed nations often approach health care of children as though it were separate from that of the rest of the family. Yet common sense tells us that attention to the mother, her pregnancy, the fetus, and the birth process is mandatory for optimal care of the child. These are addressed in Part Four of this text, "The Reproductive Process."

Understanding the mother's genetic makeup is essential for the physician who is in the position of giving advice about continuing a pregnancy or undertaking another one. Similarly, an understanding of conception control methods and abortion issues is necessary.

The environment of the developing baby likewise influences the outcome of pregnancy; therefore knowledge of the transfer of noxious substances across the placenta is valuable, as is familiarity with diagnostic methods such as amniocentesis, ultrasound, and fetoscopy.

As the identification of risk during pregnancy becomes better understood, the developing baby can be made safe from adverse intrauterine influences. Nutritional requirements of the fetus are now better understood, one consequence being that most physicians no longer starve the mother to keep her weight down during pregnancy.

Personal adaptation (both emotional and physical) of women to pregnancy has been given new emphasis in an attempt to provide caring, individual prenatal services. The involvement of physicians, nurse practitioners, other health workers, and laypersons in educational programs for pregnant women has led to improved services for women and children.

Development of regional facilities and programs for high-risk perinatal patients has promoted successful pregnancies, just as tertiary care obstetric and newborn services have improved the outcome for newborns and older infants with serious medical problems.

Part Five, "The Newborn," addresses the specifics of the care of the newborn baby from the primary care practitioner's perspective. Even though much of the technology described is applied by neonatologists, the practitioner must be able to recognize those situations in which neonatologists should be consulted and must be able to apply initial therapeutic measures to stabilize the condition of the sick infant until help can be obtained.

Children are the center of a "universe"; they are surrounded in successive rings by the family and the community. In Part Six, "Psychosocial Issues in Child Health Care," we address the theories of psychological development and the influences of the family, the school, and society on the psychological and physical well-being of infants, children, and adolescents.

Although the pediatric patient's demographic characteristics (age, sex, race, socioeconomic status), ethical influences, and geographic and seasonal environments direct practitioner's thoughts to specific diagnoses, the presenting signs and symptoms are more persuasive. They immediately bring to mind many diagnostic possibilities and rule out many others. Differential diagnosis begins with consideration of the potential cause of each sign observed by the examiner and each symptom experienced by the patient. It ends when only one cause remains to explain all of the patient's signs and symptoms—at least this is usually the case.

Sixty-nine signs and symptoms commonly encountered in pediatric practice are discussed in Part Seven, "Presenting Signs and Symptoms." Most are also mentioned in other parts of the book in discussions of specific diseases.

Pediatric practice surveys, among other things, catalog the diagnoses made by pediatricians for patients they care for in their offices. The 89 diagnoses discussed in Part Eight, "Specific Clinical Problems," along with well-child care, constitute the reasons for most office visits made to pediatricians. Almost all the rest of the visits are related to various psychosocial issues discussed in Part Six. These diagnoses also include most of the reasons for hospitalization of pediatric patients beyond the newborn period. The remaining reasons for hospitalization in this age group (except for those due to a small number of rare diseases) are discussed in Part Nine, "Critical Situations."

The primary care pediatric practitioner is seldom called on to intervene in critical situations that threaten the life of an infant, child, or adolescent. However, regardless of the practice location and the availability of subspecialists who assist in such instances, each practitioner should be prepared to make appropriate decisions or to take immediate actions that will lead to positive outcomes in such situations. To this end, the methods for management of emergency life-threatening conditions are presented. Appendix A details the methods required for "Pediatric Basic and Advanced Life Support." Appendix B, "Special Procedures," provides detailed instructions for performing the procedures that may be required in the management of the critical situations described.

Appendix C, "Miscellaneous Values," and Appendix D, "Common Psychological and Educational Tests," provide the balance of the information pediatric practitioners need to aid themselves in the interpretation of data gathered for the assessment and management of their patients.

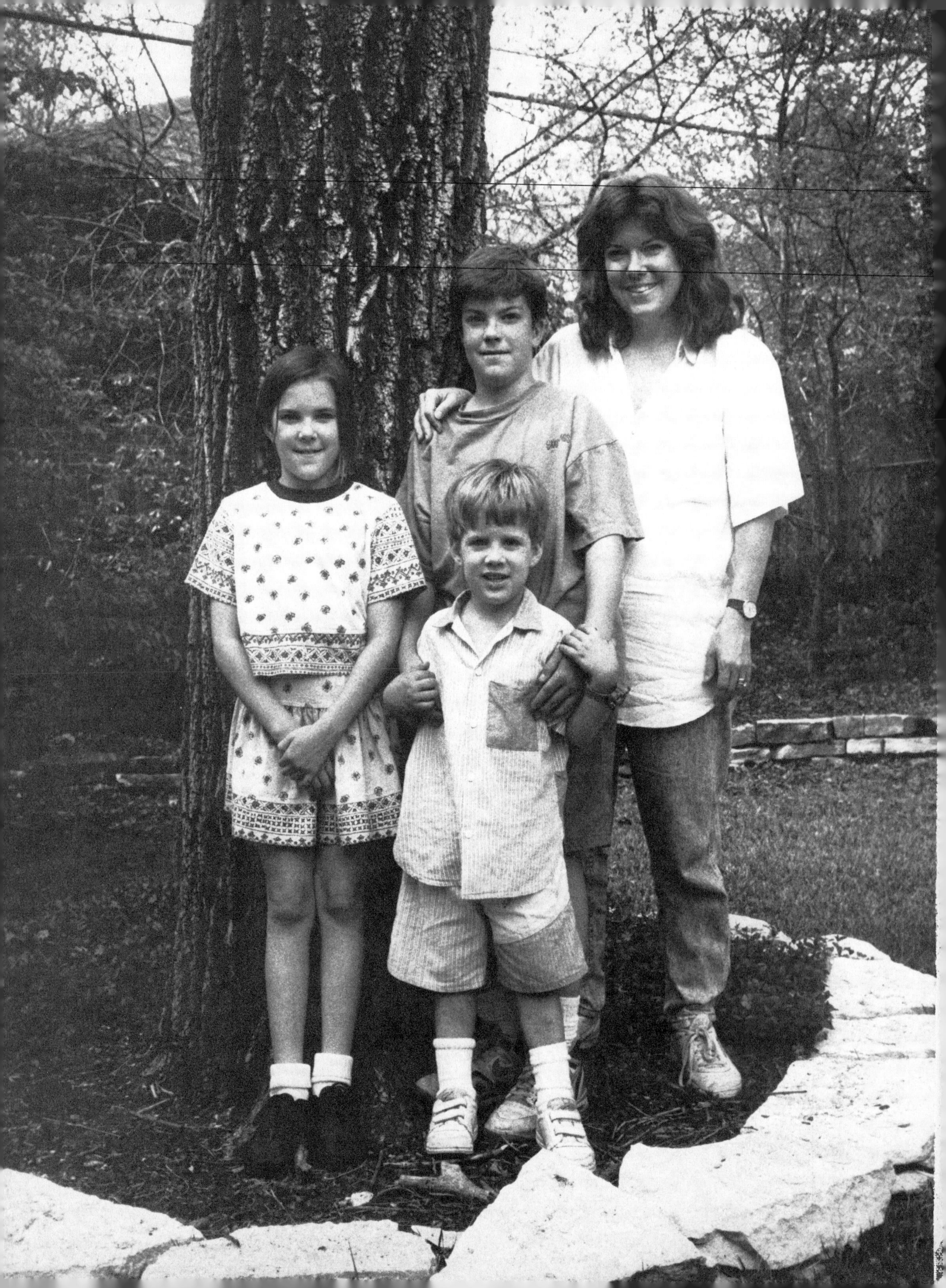

Part One

Overview of Pediatric Care

1

The Health Care Delivery System

Barbara Starfield and Edward Saltzman

PEDIATRICIANS AS PROVIDERS OF HEALTH SERVICES TO CHILDREN

As the specialty devoted solely to the health of children, pediatrics plays an important role in the U.S. health care system. In the past 50 years, the number of pediatricians, the characteristics of pediatricians, and the characteristics of pediatric practice have changed dramatically all in concert with the vast increase in medical knowledge, technical advances, and social change.

Pediatricians constitute a growing share of the physician population—a population of professionals in which growth has far outstripped the general population's total growth. In 1986 there were 43,600 pediatricians (60% male, 40% female) and an additional 1347 subspecialists in pediatric allergy and pediatric cardiology[6] (see Table 1-1).* The number of pediatricians grew by about 140% between 1970 and 1990, in contrast to a 22% growth rate in the population of children under 16 years of age during this period.

While women have always been well represented in pediatrics, their entrance into the specialty has accelerated, relative to the number of women entering medicine overall. Over one third (35%) of all pediatricians are women (an increase from 20% in 1970) with almost 51% of all pediatric residents being women in 1990.[2] About 5% of male medical students choose pediatrics, while 15% of white female students choose pediatrics.

Black physicians comprised 4.9% (312) of the 1990 resident pool, while osteopathic physicians totaled 2.4% (152), and foreign medical graduates 28.8% (1694).[2]

A large proportion of pediatricians are young. In 1987, 34% of all pediatricians and 46% of all female pediatricians were younger than 35 years of age, compared with 25% of all physicians and 41% of all female physicians in this age bracket.

Of the 43,600 pediatricians in 1990, 24,000 were office based; if the annual growth rate of pediatricians in the past 5 years (4%) remains unchanged, it is estimated that there will be 26,800 office-based pediatricians by 1991 (see Table 1-1).[4]

According to data for the year 1982 to 1989, pediatricians practiced 47.4 weeks a year in direct patient care; those pediatricians practicing in a group averaged almost 2 weeks less practice time per year than those who practice alone. Direct patient care includes such activities as interpreting laboratory and roentgenogram studies and consulting with other physicians, but it does not include activities such as medical staff functions, teaching, and research.

Data from 1990 reveal that 91% of pediatricians, 98% of general practitioners, and 97% of family practitioners spent most of their time in patient care, but only 62% of all pediatricians practiced in private offices, compared with 90% of general practitioners and 74% of family practitioners (see Table 1-1).

Despite the increase in numbers of pediatricians, many children in the country receive their regular care from physicians who do not limit their practices to pediatrics; many are seen by general practitioners or family physicians, who provide care to both children and adults. However, the proportion of children who see pediatricians, especially young children, has been increasing. By 1987, approximately 50% of all children, from newborns to teenagers 19 years of age, visited pediatricians (an increase from 38% in 1977). The remainder visited family practitioners, general practitioners, and other physicians. About half of all pediatrician visits are by children under 2 years of age; almost three fourths (72%) of the visits by these children are to pediatricians. Visits by older children are less likely to be to pediatricians: 55% of the visits of 3- to 9-year olds and 24% of the visits by 10- to 19-year-olds are to pediatricians.[4]

It is clear from these data that the pediatric office is the medical home to the majority of children only in the preschool years, and although increases in this respect have been made in the past decade, there is still much potential market share growth for pediatricians in terms of children in older age groups.

It is estimated that if the annual growth rate of the pediatrician population continues to be 4%, the number of newborns whose parents seek pediatric care for them will have declined from 250 per pediatrician in 1986 to 149 by 1991, and the total number of all children will have declined from 3000 in 1976 to 1254 per pediatrician in 1991.[4] If the new alternative health care delivery systems (discussed later in this chapter) rely on other types of practitioners to assume at least part of the care of children, fewer pediatricians per child will be needed to serve the child population in these types of organizations.

A major study by the Graduate Medical Education National

*Editor's note: The American Medical Association, which maintains data on physician numbers and characteristics, places general and subspecialty pediatricians into just three categories—pediatricians, pediatric allergists, and pediatric cardiologists.

Advisory Committee (GMENAC) in 1981 concluded that there would be a surplus of pediatricians by the 1990s. However, the number of pediatricians needed to care for the child population may, in fact, be increasing. Female pediatricians, as a group, work fewer hours than their male counterparts; thus, more pediatricians will be needed in the work force to care for the same number of children. Also the trend toward an increasing assumption of patient care responsibilities by nurse practitioners and child health associates that GMENAC predicted has not materialized. Furthermore, insurers and other third-party payers are likely to increase coverage of well-child care, thus stimulating more such visits. An increasing recognition of a host of health-related behavioral and social problems (such as substance abuse, eating disorders, nonpsychotic mental disorders, suicide attempts, sexually transmitted diseases, and teen sexuality) may also increase the workload of physicians who see children. Other possible changes in the health services system that will affect the need for more pediatricians are universal access to health care for children, a possible national health delivery system for children, Medicaid expansions, and the impact of managed care delivery systems. If society targets children and young adult populations as most in need of an expansion in access to health care and health supervision, the need for pediatricians may increase dramatically.

ORGANIZATION OF PRACTICE

With the exception of pediatric practice in sparsely populated areas of the country with limited hospital and technical support services and few ancillary specialists, pediatricians generally practice similarly throughout the United States.

Pediatrics traditionally has been an office-based specialty; over 85% of patient-care pediatricians (excluding resident physicians) are office-based. Pediatricians practice mostly in individual offices or in small groups in private offices, where they make their own decisions about the focus and scope of their practice, office equipment and arrangements, and method of charging for their services. The vast majority of payment mechanisms involve a fee-for-service arrangement. According to a census by the American Academy of Pediatrics, most pediatricians are self-employed (63%). About one third (34%) receive at least some proportion of their income from salary, and a small percentage (2%) are independent contractors. Of the self-employed, 48% are in solo practice and 52% are in single or multispecialty group practice: 13% in two-physician practices, 9% in three-physician practices, 16% in four- to eight-physician practices, and 13% in practices with more than eight physicians. It is expected that with the explosive growth of managed care (discussed later in this chapter) and the advantage to payers who seek "larger offices" in order to provide more complete medical coverage and greater concentration of patients in fewer offices, the trend toward group practice will increase. The desirable "on-call" schedules, cost savings, and medical camaraderie are also appealing features of group practice. Other modes of organizing services have existed for many decades, but only recently have the alternative health care delivery systems begun to increase in importance and frequency. These systems, which attempt to manage and finance the delivery

Table 1-1 *Number of Physicians in the United States by Specialty and Activity (January 1, 1989)*

		PATIENT CARE				OTHER PROFESSIONAL ACTIVITY			
				HOSPITAL-BASED					
		TOTAL PATIENT CARE	OFFICE-BASED	HOUSE STAFF	FULL-TIME PHYSICIAN STAFF	MEDICAL TEACHING	ADMINISTRATION	RESEARCH	OTHER
Total number of physicians	600,789								
Pediatrics	35,692*	33,205	22,279	7084	2842	671	933	760	123

Modified from Roback G, et al: Physician characteristics and distribution in the U.S., Chicago, 1990, Survey and Data Resources, American Medical Association, p 54.
*Does not include the pediatric subspecialties of allergy, cardiology, or psychiatry.

of health care, comprise the "alphabetizing" of medical care (that is, HMOs, PPOs, IPAs, and the newer form of managed care, EPOs).

Health Maintenance Organizations (HMOs)

In 1932 the Committee on the Costs of Medical Care* recommended that health care be furnished by organized groups of health professionals, preferably in a hospital setting, on a group prepayment basis. The idea was of little interest to the medical profession, which devoted its energies to an alternative mechanism for improving access to care—private insurance, under which physicians were to be reimbursed on a fee-for-service basis for covered services. The prepayment idea grew very slowly, involving only 2% of physicians and less than 5% of the U.S. population by the early 1980s.

Rapidly exploding medical care costs under a fee-for-service insurance system provided impetus, however, for new thinking about prepayment in the 1980s. In 1981 there were 260 HMOs; by 1990 there were 615. By 1990 an estimated 37 million Americans were enrolled in such organizations, with a projection to 52 million enrollees by the early 1990s.

Five characteristics distinguish HMOs: (1) a defined population of enrolled members, (2) payments determined in advance for a specific period of time, (3) a contractual responsibility of the organization to provide or ensure medical services, (4) voluntary enrollment, and (5) medical services provided directly, with the HMO and its physician members assuming at least part of the financial risk of loss in providing services.

Three major types of HMOs exist:

1. Staff-model group practices, in which physicians are salaried members of the organization. These were the earliest prepaid plans, arising from cooperative health care movements in which consumers contributed funds to form nonprofit organizations to provide health care.
2. Group-model group practices (also known as prepaid group practices or PPGPs), in which physicians are organized as separate groups or corporations (usually multispecialty) that contract with HMOs to provide care to their enrollees. The group receives a capitation for each enrollee plus a share of the group's net income, if any; individual physicians may be paid a salary, may share the income equally, or may be paid on the basis of their productivity.
3. Independent practice associations (IPAs), the newest form of HMO, in which practitioners (usually working alone) join and make agreements with organizations to provide services to a defined population. They often continue to practice in their own offices, seeing their own patients as well. The capitation fee is provided to the organization, which then reimburses physicians by a billing mechanism for services rendered according to fixed-fee schedules. A proportion of the fee is usually retained by the IPA to cover any losses at the end of the year; if there is a surplus, it is redistributed to the physicians. IPAs are the dominant model type, accounting for 62% of the HMOs.

*A self-created voluntary committee of government and public health groups.

In the HMO, patient care can be given only by providers (doctors, hospitals, special laboratories, and roentgenogram facilities) who either are employees of the HMO or have contracted with the HMO to provide specific services for a specific dollar payment. Under this system patients cannot choose to receive their care from a physician unless the physician is on the HMO roster. In return for this limitation of freedom, the patients or their employers are guaranteed that their costs for medical care will not exceed a predetermined value. It is the HMO and, through it, the physicians and hospitals who are at risk for excessive expenses.

Although enrollees of HMOs, especially those in prepaid group plans, tend to visit physicians more often, their hospitalization rates are much lower than the rates of those who use other types of services, primarily because their hospitalization rates for common conditions and minor surgery are lower. Drug costs are also lower. The prevalence of health conditions known to be influenced by medical care, such as prematurity, is reduced in populations covered by prepaid group practice plans, and their overall costs of care are lower,[3] presumably because practice in a multispecialty group offers greater ease of consultation and mutual professional support, a strong financial incentive to match facilities to the needs of the population served, economic and professional incentives to match the specialty mix to the needs of the population, and enhanced opportunities for quality control. As noted later in this chapter, studies have found that the organizational arrangement under which physicians work influences the quality of care delivered more than the details of their training or individual characteristics.[5]

Despite its proven ability to hold down costs while ensuring quality, the growth rate of other organizational forms has exceeded the growth rate of HMOs. Given a choice of insurance plans, more people choose a traditional plan over an HMO. Working to the competitive disadvantage of HMOs is their tendency to exclude drug and dental benefits, as well as their restriction on a choice of physician. In the period from 1981 to 1990, the number of HMOs grew from 160 to 615, but another form of organization, PPOs, grew much more (from about 20 to over 500).

Preferred Provider Organizations (PPOs)

A newer type of fee-for-service organization is the preferred provider organization (PPO), an association of physicians or hospitals that contracts with employers or insurers to provide services on a fee-for-service basis. Pediatricians are popular with PPO insurers. The population cared for by pediatricians is generally not costly, and inclusion of young families (with relatively low demands on the health care system) in PPO plans is desirable to insurers. PPOs differ from traditional insured fee-for-service arrangements by contracting to provide services to specific populations and by agreeing to review use and claims experiences to control an overuse of services (visits and procedures). In contrast to health maintenance organizations, PPO physicians incur no financial risk from overuse of services.

One of the mechanisms for containing costs requires a referral by the primary care physician (pediatricians, family practitioners, internists) for specialty care or for laboratory, radiology, and emergency room services. (This is what is known as the "gate-keeper" concept.) Patients have to pay an additional amount if they visit specialists or special facilities without prior authorization from their primary care provider.

Two major factors have stimulated PPO growth: failure of HMOs to stem the rise in health care costs and the limited choice of providers offered. By giving patients a choice of physicians, PPOs place fewer restrictions on patients when they enter the medical care system.

Exclusive Provider Organizations (EPOs)

Combine the restrictive structure of an HMO's provider panel with the flexibility and payment structure of a PPO, and the result is an Exclusive Provider Organization (EPO), the latest addition to the "alphabet soup" of managed care plans.

Insurance companies are luring new enrollees into managed care by using this hybrid that combines the low, out-of-pocket charges of the IPA model HMO with the PPO's option that provides some choice among a panel of providers. EPOs, which restrict members to a select list of providers, are moving opposite the trend among PPOs (which offer choice to customers through open-ended plans and out-of-network provisions). In their purest form, EPOs offer members an all-or-nothing approach to coverage. Unlike PPOs, which require patients to pay part of the cost of care, EPOs usually do not require co-payments, but they also do not pay any bills resulting from the use of unapproved providers, while PPOs still pay for part of out-of-network care. The choice of physicians in an EPO is generally more limited than in a PPO; physicians are selected on the basis of their reputation in the community, cost, and popularity with patients. EPOs also offer companies greater discounts and tighter utilization review than other managed care models. Payment for the exclusive provider is generally by a discounted fee-for-service, as with PPOs and IPAs, rather than by capitation (as in staff or group-model HMOs). Physicians find EPOs' fee-for-service reimbursement attractive.

It is estimated that by the early 1990s, as much as 45% of the population will be enrolled in some form of care (such as HMOs and EPOs) in which the choice of physician will be dictated by the type of insurance.

Tax-Supported Programs

Although governmental agencies have always assumed at least some responsibility for health services of those unable to provide for their own, the need for a more concerted effort became evident as the Depression of the 1930s deepened and access to medical care had not spread to the entire population. Title V of the Social Security Act of 1935 was responsible for the substantial involvement of local health departments in certain aspects of health care delivery.

By 1978 public programs contributed 29% of the total expenditures for the health care of persons under the age of 19 years: 67% of the public expenditures were by the federal government and 33% by state and municipal governments; 55% of the expenditures were in the form of direct payment to physicians through the Medicaid program; and the remainder was divided among services provided through federally supported programs (20%), state and local programs (6%), the Department of Defense (14%), state and local hospitals (2%), and various other programs (3%).[1] Although more recent data are not available for children, the balance of expenditures for the population as a whole has not changed; the federal share has grown slightly, whereas the state and local share has declined.

Health Department Programs. Although local health departments provide a sizable proportion of preventive and case-finding services, particularly in rural and central-city urban areas, the wave of "privatization" in the 1980s resulted in their direct services involvement being reduced markedly. Their efforts are concentrated largely on environmental health and communicable disease control. In many cities, health departments operate a municipal hospital, but even this role has declined. Where such hospitals exist, they are often overwhelmed by the challenges of AIDS (acquired immune deficiency syndrome) and related problems and the difficulty in finding adequate reimbursement for services provided to those lacking insurance.

Some services are provided in schools, particularly in areas where children would not otherwise receive them. These services are often supported by general tax revenues or by direct grants from federal agencies and are administered by local departments of education or health. Preeminent among such services are those related to essential preventive services. For example, all states require some immunization as a prerequisite for school attendance. Many also require a physical examination, which may be required periodically during the years the child is in school.

Community Health Centers. Initiated in the middle of the 1960s as an effort to provide comprehensive health services for underserved populations, these centers have grown into a network of facilities serving several million poor and underserved individuals in 50 states, Puerto Rico, and the District of Columbia. The centers are funded primarily by grants from the federal government through the programs for Community Health Centers, Migrant Health Centers, National Health Services Corps, Maternal and Child Health Block grants to states, and the Urban Indian Health Program, although many centers also try to attract patients with Medicaid or private insurance. However, fewer than one fourth of the country's medically underserved are reached by existing facilities.

Social Security Programs. Two of the Social Security amendments of the middle 1960s have had a significant impact on health care delivery for children. Medicaid, authorized by Title XIX of the Social Security Act, provides a means to pay for medical care through tax dollars for those who cannot afford it. It was intended originally that medical care be provided through existing settings, primarily through independent office practices.

Medicaid is a joint federal-state program, with both federal and state contributions. The federal government requires that a minimum amount of services be provided, although states may limit the duration of the required services. Eligibility for Medicaid is based primarily on low family income. Medicaid accounts for a greater proportion of all expenditures of health services for children than for adults, but the children's share of Medicaid payments has dropped despite an increase in the proportion of children among the eligible.

States vary widely in their eligibility requirements for Medicaid. Nationally, fewer than half of families with incomes below the national poverty level standard are covered. States often do not cover even those children who are eligible for Medicaid; the proportion covered varies from a small minority in some jurisdictions to a substantial majority in others. In response to this situation, Congress has encouraged (and in some cases mandated) incremental additions starting with infants and young children. States must cover children younger than age 6 in families with incomes up to 133% of the poverty level. Effective July 1, 1991, coverage of poor children of ages 6-19 will be required and phased in over the next 10 years.

Title V Amendments. The original Social Security Title V program, enacted in 1935, supported a variety of programs to deliver health services to mothers and children, usually on a state level. The law was amended significantly between 1963 and 1967 to provide funds to support services in low-income and rural areas for maternal and child health clinics, family planning, regionalized infant care, and dental care. In the 1980s, these were replaced by the "new federalism," which provided "block" grants to the states for maternal and child health services, Supplemental Security Income for Disabled Children (for children with chronic health problems), lead-based paint poisoning prevention programs, sudden infant death programs, hemophilia treatment centers, and adolescent pregnancy and genetics services grants. In most Southern, Midwestern, and Western states that have large networks of county and local health departments, services are often provided directly through governmental agencies in schools, local health clinics, well-child clinics, antenatal clinics, health screening services, and immunization services. In other areas, particularly the Northeast, the state maternal and child health agency often contracts with private health centers to provide services.

Hospital-Based Services

In 1988, one in eight physician encounters with persons under 18 years of age took place in a hospital. The number of encounters occurring in these facilities is increasing, particularly by very young children and by the poor. Although numerous studies have been done in individual outpatient departments of teaching hospitals, little is known about the amount, scope, and type of care provided nationwide. Most of the medical services in these facilities are provided by physicians in training who rotate through outpatient departments as part of their postgraduate education. This hospital-based sector of care is particularly prevalent in central city areas near teaching hospitals, through which many children receive most of their health services.

PRACTICE CHARACTERISTICS

Style and Content

A generation ago, the pediatrician was the daily expert: always on call in the office for the family in need, on frequent house calls, or on busy hospital rounds. The practitioner worried about, comforted, and ministered to both well and sick newborns and to premature infants, as well as to sick children out of the hospital and especially in the hospital. Pediatricians had the last word on rheumatic fever, glomerulonephritis, all forms of contagious disease, oncologic diagnosis and treatment, all forms of heart and neurologic disease, and some types of eczema; in short, all "routine" and serious illness was dealt with by pediatricians. The subspecialists were few and were located only in academic centers. Concepts such as "primary," "secondary," and "tertiary" care were unknown, and the hospital-based pediatric intensivist, pediatric neonatologist, or other subspecialist did not yet exist. There was little time for health education because the pediatrician was relied upon to provide definitive care or medical treatment on any subject pertaining to children, and the respected doctor remained constantly busy. With a few exceptions, such an approach to pediatric health care is a thing of the past.

Today, the office-based pediatrician (known as the primary care pediatrician) deals with illnesses that are only potentially serious; the patient is almost always seen in the office, rarely in the hospital, and almost never in the home. The variety of illnesses treated today does not even remotely resemble that in the past. Upper respiratory disease (including ear infections), moderate lower respiratory problems, feeding problems, gastrointestinal upsets, and minor trauma make up 75% to 85% of "see-it-now" illness care. But child health needs are changing. Practice time is needed for wellness care, family dynamics and reassurance, and the new "morbidity," including the following:

- Prenatal counseling.
- Preventing accidents—that is, advice on seat belts, smoke alarms, water safety, home safety, and poison control.
- Discussing the child's education with the family and supporting the fulfillment of educational goals from infancy through adolescence.
- Emphasizing the lifetime importance of reading and proper reading habits from late infancy onward.
- Supporting the new concept of family centers where infants, together with parents, meet and socialize through supervised constructive play.
- Being an expert in abuse-avoidance, whether it be drug abuse, child abuse, or parent abuse.
- Providing advice and support during divorce or other marital problems.
- Advising families on life-style goals, such as the need for family time and for an understanding of work-related time constraints and stresses and how the family copes with them.
- Advising and promoting good health through prudent diet and nutrition, exercise, avoidance of salt, and avoidance of smoking.
- Encouraging community activism: knowledge and use of common resources and involvement with school boards, religious groups, school athletic programs, and community facilities.

More and more time is devoted to the care of adolescents and young adults, with the goal in mind of being able to provide guidance and to anticipate problems as well as being helpful in solving such problems. Pediatricians' time in office practice remains challenging and interesting, although it is channeled differently than in the past.

Because the typical practitioner wants to be (and is becoming) less involved with patients' illnesses that require time-consuming workups or acute-care management either as an outpatient or as an inpatient, care is becoming increasingly limited to the office. Office-based pediatricians are spending less time in the hospital than in the past; during the 1980s, there was a 14% decrease in hospital visits by primary care pediatricians. Referrals to hospital-based pediatricians and neonatologists have become routine. As a result, a new type of pediatrician may be emerging: the hospital-based pediatric generalist, several of whom would be located in the community hospital as well as in the teaching hospital and would provide consultation coverage at all times. This type of pediatrician is known as a consulting or secondary care pediatrician. The office-based pediatrician has assumed a more restricted but important role in the hospital—that is, to provide the family and community linkages necessary for the hospitalized child.

Although little is known about pediatricians' involvement in providing care in community settings, an Academy of Pediatrics survey in 1976 indicated that about one third of the pediatricians in solo or group practice spend less than 1% of their patient-care time in school or community activities; about one fifth of pediatricians spend 1% to 5% of their time in this way. Less than 10% spend more than 5% of their time in schools and community facilities. (The remainder of the pediatricians did not respond and presumably spent no time in these settings.) The extent to which this has changed during the 1980s is unknown.

The newer organizational formats such as HMOs and other managed care settings may facilitate certain changes in the role of pediatricians, since pediatricians have primary care and case management skills that are well matched to the needs of these types of care systems.

Extended Hours and Satellite Offices

Families in which both parents are employed or where there is only one parent now comprise the majority of families in the United States. This has forced groups or solo practices in which physicians share coverage to extend their office hours to provide coverage in the early evening and on weekends, in addition to the traditional on-call coverage at night. This is a radical departure from the office hours traditionally available.

Pediatricians have also embraced the concept of the satellite office as a response to the movement of young families to the suburbs. These offices offer the same complete pediatric office care that the "main" office provides, but they are a response to the consumer demand for accessible professional care with less travel time. These locales are in the new communities that have their own hospital systems, school systems, and community identity. The satellite offices—many times more than one—frequently outgrow the "main" office as communities change in their character or stage of development. Satellite offices enable a pediatric group to prevent the loss of patients to physicians who may locate new practices in the area, because people are familiar with the reputations and method of practice of the older office and its pediatricians. Well-run satellite offices also are inclined to reduce the attractiveness of these new communities to new pediatricians moving into that area. A satellite office does not entail a major financial gamble; rather, because there are many young families and families needing pediatric care in these communities, it affords the main practice the ability to enlarge its professional and ancillary services so that there is less on-call time for the individual physician and possibly more services available in the practice itself. Thus, developing satellite practices has many advantages without risking loss of income.

Professional Liability

Pediatricians are part of a socioeconomic environment of medicine experiencing skyrocketing professional liability claims and, concomitantly, very high professional liability insurance premiums. Some pediatricians are subject to premiums as high as $20,000 to $25,000 annually, which comprises a high percent of gross revenue. In earlier times, litigation almost exclusively involved surgeons and surgical procedures. Today, failure to diagnose illness and anticipate drug reactions is high on the list of causes for suits against pediatricians. Pediatricians who fail to diagnose meningitis or sepsis, who delay in diagnosing congenital dislocation of the hip or congenital hypothyroidism, or who experience problems with managing croup versus epiglottitis, for example, are at a high risk every day for malpractice suits. Because of the variability among states in statutes of limitations for filing malpractice claims on behalf of minors or failure to set limits ("caps") for malpractice awards, pediatricians are at risk not only for high awards but for settlement many years after the alleged malpractice occurrence. Many legal remedies have been proposed to adjust these claims reasonably; so far, except for a few states, these remedies have had little fiscal impact and have provided almost no physical relief.

Pediatricians, in attempting to cope with this litiginous environment, are obtaining additional tests (40%), providing additional procedures (27%), making more referrals (44%), maintaining better records (57%), and spending more time with patients (36%).[7] However, there is no evidence of the effectiveness of these approaches or of annual risk-management educational programs on reducing medical malpractice suits. Such defensive medicine has had its economic effect by increasing expenditures for medical care. Some of these practice changes may constitute improvements in medical care. Others, which are of little or no benefit, may be unnecessary or even harmful. Because of a perceived alteration in physician/patient relationships resulting from the threat of liability, the pleasure of practice is lessening gradually. Hope for a change that is both fair and equitable to the public and the medical profession depends on societal attention to this difficult problem.

Scope of Pediatric Practice

Until recently, the types of services provided by the nation's pediatric practitioners were unknown. Because of the rising

Table 1-2 *Office Visits to Pediatricians: The 10 Most Frequent Patient Problems (United States, 1985)*

RANK	MOST COMMON PATIENT PROBLEMS, COMPLAINTS, OR SYMPTOMS	NUMBER OF VISITS (THOUSANDS)	PERCENTAGE OF VISITS	CUMULATIVE PERCENTAGE
1	Well-baby examination, general medical examination, immunization	19,308	26.15	26.5
2	Ear problems	7006	9.6	36.1
3	Cough	5616	7.7	43.8
4	Fever	5490	7.6	51.4
5	Throat soreness	3567	4.9	56.3
6	Skin rash	2374	3.3	59.6
7	Upper respiratory infection	1788	2.5	62.1
8	Nasal congestion	1815	2.5	64.6
9	Vomiting	1012	1.4	66.0
10	Diarrhea	897	1.2	67.2

From National Center for Health Statistics: National Ambulatory Medical Care Survey, 1985 (special tabulation).

Table 1-3 *Office Visits to Pediatricians: The 10 Most Frequent Diagnoses Rendered by the Physician (United States, 1985)*

RANK (IN 1975)	MOST COMMON PATIENT PROBLEMS, COMPLAINTS, OR SYMPTOMS	NUMBER OF VISITS (THOUSANDS)	PERCENTAGE OF VISITS	CUMULATIVE PERCENTAGE
1	Health supervision medical examination	16,617	22.8	22.8
2	Otitis media	8819	12.1	34.9
3	Acute upper respiratory infection of multiple or unspecified sites	4912	6.8	41.7
4	Acute pharyngitis	2699	3.7	45.4
5	Acute tonsillitis	1888	2.6	48.0
6	Bronchitis, unqualified	1711	2.4	50.4
7	Asthma	1547	2.1	52.5
8	Other nonspecific gastroenteritis and colitis	1448	2.0	54.6
9	Viral infections, unspecified site	1399	1.9	56.4
10	Streptococcal sore throat/scarlet fever	1248	1.7	68.1

From National Center for Health Statistics: National Ambulatory Medical Care Survey, 1985 (special tabulation).

Table 1-4 *Office Visits to Pediatricians: Selected Diagnostic or Therapeutic Services Ordered or Provided (United States, 1985)*

SERVICES	PERCENTAGE
Diagnostic services	
None	65.5
Hematologic survey	10.7
Blood pressure check	9.4
Urinalysis	8.7
Vision test	3.5
Blood chemistry	2.0
Therapeutic services (excluding medication)	
None	80.4
Family or social counseling	13.4
Medical counseling	10.1
Diet counseling	8.7
Office surgery	2.0
Physiotherapy	1.0

From National Center for Health Statistics: National Ambulatory Medical Care Survey, 1985 (special tabulation).

Table 1-5 *Office Visits to Pediatricians: Disposition of Patient and Number of Medications (United States, 1985)*

	PERCENTAGE
Disposition	
No follow-up planned	17.1
Return at specified time	49.4
Return if needed	29.5
Telephone follow-up planned	5.8
Referred to other physician/agency	2.4
Number of medications	
None	33.2
1	44.9
2	17.1
3	3.8
4 or more	1.0

From National Center for Health Statistics: National Ambulatory Medical Care Survey, 1985 (special tabulation).

costs of health care, documentation of services rendered is being required of practitioners more often to determine how the money is being spent and whether increased costs have resulted in improved health. Although sporadic studies of individual practices have appeared since the 1930s, nothing in the way of national practice data existed until the development by the National Center for Health Statistics of the National Ambulatory Medical Care Survey (NAMCS) in the early 1970s. NAMCS is a periodic survey of office-based practices that does not include hospital outpatient departments or tax-supported patient care service programs.

Tables 1-2 to 1-5 provide statistics gathered by the NAMCS in 1985 regarding office-based practices, including the most common complaints, the most frequent diagnoses, and the services provided during office visits. A relatively large proportion of children require a visit to another physician or a repeat visit to the same physician (Table 1-5); this indicates the need to integrate care over several visits, both to consultants and to the original physician. Providing continuity is a major challenge to physicians in primary care.

All children are supposed to have a "medical home" that provides continued and integrated care over time. Even for children who have a "regular source of care," this source of care does not always provide all the required services, nor does it always integrate the services that the child received elsewhere. About one in five children who have a physician whom they identify as their "regular source of care" actually goes to another physician when he or she needs medical care. Moreover, physicians in primary care facilities frequently fail to recognize both the fact of visits elsewhere and what occurred elsewhere, even though this may significantly influence the patient's response to subsequent care.

This fragmented and uncoordinated care constitutes a major challenge to our health care system. If practitioners, health programs, and health institutions continue to function as separate and uncoordinated agencies, and if individuals continue to seek care from as many sources, duplication of services will likely result in ever-increasing costs of care without commensurate gains. In fact, effectiveness is likely to decrease because patients are given conflicting advice and therapies from different practitioners. The extent to which "managed care" systems actually reduce fragmented care is still unknown.

In most other industrialized nations, health services are regionalized: services are organized according to the degree to which they are needed. Services that are required by large proportions of the population or frequently are provided on local or community levels and thus are easily accessible to the population. These are called primary health services.

The experience of prepaid group practices, which by definition provide care for a defined population, is useful in determining how many physicians may be needed to ensure accessibility to primary care services. In general, one child health physician for 2000 children has been satisfactory.

Physicians in primary care (all family physicians and most pediatricians and internists) should assume responsibility for providing a broad spectrum of care (both preventive and curative) over time and for coordinating all the care patients receive, including that from specialists. When primary care physicians require advice with difficult cases, they should refer patients for consultation to secondary health facilities, which are more centralized than the primary care facilities and are usually located in community hospitals. Patients who require care for complicated and unusual illnesses should be referred to tertiary care medical centers, which are even more centralized and carry out training and research functions as well. These tertiary care centers, on referral from primary or secondary health centers, provide services requiring a high degree of technical expertise. Expensive equipment required to support such specialty services should be located only in tertiary centers and not in every health center that desires it and can obtain money to purchase it (as is often the case). To date, however, there is no national priority to develop such a regional system of health services for children.

Reimbursement Issues

An American Academy of Pediatrics survey in 1989 provided information on the sources of income for pediatricians primarily in direct patient care. Two thirds (66%) of these physicians received their income primarily from noncontract fee-for-service practice. Another 3% had their secondary source of income in this category. Eight percent received their primary source of income from contract fee-for-service, with another 13% having their secondary source of income in this category. The remainder came from salary (25% as a primary source, 9% as a secondary source) and from some other source (2% and 6%, respectively). Just over half (52%) reported that they had more than one type of income source. The most common combinations of sources were noncontract fee-for-service and contract fee-for-service (11% of respondents) and noncontract fee-for-service and salary (8%). None of the other combinations were reported by more than 4% of the pediatricians.

Pediatricians typically earn 20% less than the average medical specialist. In suburban and metropolitan areas (in which pediatricians earn 30% more income than in nonmetropolitan areas), self-employed pediatricians earn 36% more than those who are employed by others, and age variations show that pediatricians who are 46 to 55 years earn 42% more than pediatricians younger than 36 years of age.

Because pediatrics is a specialty that requires counseling and listening rather than the performance of procedures, and because reimbursement often favors the performance of procedures, pediatrician income has lagged far behind that of most medical specialties and all surgical specialties.

A new relative value system for reimbursement has been adopted in Congress for use in 1992 to pay physicians for care of the elderly. This system, called the Resource-Based Relative Value Scale (RBRVS), measures work in four dimensions—time, mental effort and judgment, technical skill and physical effort, and psychological stress. Although the RBRVS tends to equalize reimbursement by lowering fees for technical procedures and elevating fees for "cognitive services," there is still much concern about the plan within the medical profession, and the outcome and final form are still under discussion, especially with regard to other age groups, including children. Pediatricians await the outcome with interest, since it is thought that once institutionalized by Medicare, third-party payers will follow, and an entirely new system of compensation for providing health services will evolve.

Impact of Reimbursement on Scope of Services

Services that are not reimbursed are unlikely to be provided in fee-for-service practice. The percentage of the U.S. population covered by some private health insurance increased from 47% in 1950 to 77% in 1982. A smaller percent is covered for ambulatory care, and there are many restrictions on the types of ambulatory care reimbursable by insurance. Moreover, the percentage of persons not covered by any health insurance increased from 12% in 1980 to 16% in 1986; by 1986, 18% of children under age 5 and 16% of all children under age 14 had no insurance coverage for their health care (Table 1-6). During the 1980s, the percentage of children who were not covered by either private insurance or Medicaid rose, while the percentage covered by private insurance fell.

The proportion of the population covered by private insurance varies markedly according to family income. Less than 33% of children in poor families have private health insurance, compared with over 90% of those in higher income families. Some of the cost of care for indigent children is paid directly by the government. This tax-supported contribution to the funding of care for children is composed of two parts: the direct services to mothers and children provided by local, state, and federally supported health care agencies and payment mechanisms (largely Medicaid) channeled through the "private" health care system.

Table 1-6 shows that children are less likely than the population as a whole to have their health care covered by insurance or by Medicaid; preschoolers are much less likely to have private insurance than are other children. Poor children are much less likely than nonpoor children to have any coverage for medical care, whether or not they have disability as a result of medical problems. Children in low-income families are more compromised if they have no insurance coverage than are adults. When family funds are meager, they must be rationed; illness in low-income adults, particularly if they are employed, has greater immediate economic consequences than does illness in children. This explains why children in the "gray" area, in which their families neither qualify for governmental help nor can afford to purchase insurance, are less likely than other children to see a health care practitioner when they are ill.

A minority of insurance plans pay providers for any preventive services. Recent surveys of group indemnity policies written by large and medium-size major insurers show that only 18% provide coverage for annual physical examinations. Small firms are much less likely to provide any health insurance as a benefit. Overall, only a very small proportion (6%) of all private insurance companies pay for well-child care, and these only pay for children up to 1 year of age. Although HMO plans almost always cover such services, a minority of the population is enrolled in HMOs. HMOs limit the ability of physicians to provide one aspect of care that may be important in health promotion—home visits, which are rarely if ever included in the benefit package.

In 1986, Florida, with the help of the American Academy of Pediatrics, became the first state to mandate private health insurance coverage for health supervision. Under the Child Health Incentive Reform Plan (CHIRP), a certain number of visits are covered without a deductible payment by the parents. To the extent that other states follow this trend toward mandating coverage for preventive services, this legislation will enhance the role of the pediatrician in furthering child health. As of the end of 1990, six states had CHIRP legislation, although all had different ages and types of care mandates. Of concern, however, is the growth in industry's attempts to provide employee "self-insurance" health care programs, which are exempted from state laws mandating coverage of certain services. Because the cost of health insurance continues to escalate, small and large businesses are looking for a less costly method of providing health services for their employees. By using self-insurance plans, the employer can save money by eliminating some of the presently mandated-by-law coverages (e.g., coverage of children and other dependents) and create higher deductible cost levels and higher co-payments. Eliminating coverage for dependents in this way could affect children and their pediatricians adversely.

The sustained rise in medical care costs is responsible for much congressional interest in controlling certain aspects of medical practice. However, the debates about whether this control should reside with governmental agencies or be delegated to insurance companies, professional organizations, or hospitals, and the scope of activities to be included under those controls have impeded implementation of any serious federal cost-control proposal.

A major attack on the escalation of medical care costs was instituted by the Department of Health and Human Services through the Social Security Act Amendments of 1983, which mandated the use of diagnosis-related groups (DRGs) as the basis for reimbursing hospitals for care provided to patients. Until then, hospitals were reimbursed on the basis of per diem rates and diagnostic and therapeutic procedures performed. Under the DRG system, care for Medicare recipients (mostly persons over age 65) is reimbursed according to the diagnosis established on admission. All diagnoses have been grouped

Table 1-6 *Health Care Coverage For Persons Under Age 65 (United States, 1986)*

PATIENT'S AGE	PRIVATE INSURANCE	MEDICAID	NOT COVERED
All ages	76	6	15
Children under age 5 years	68	11	18
Children age 5-14 years	73	9	15

From U.S. Government Printing Office: Health, United States, 1988. National Center for Health Statistics. DHHS Pub NO. (PHS) 89-1232. Public Health Services. Washington, D.C., March 1989, p. 171.

into 467 categories, each of which is relatively homogeneous with respect to length of hospital stay and costs. Hospitals receive a specific sum for each DRG regardless of the patient's actual length of stay or the number of procedures performed.

By the end of 1986, at least 10 Medicaid programs and some Blue Shield and commercial insurers also were using DRG-based reimbursement for hospital care. A separate classification of DRGs has been developed for the pediatric age group. By the early 1990s, it is likely that a system of prospective fee-for-service pricing will be used for outpatient as well as inpatient care. It is also likely, as already noted, that physicians will be paid for health services providing counseling and guidance. These changes should facilitate the provision of preventive care, so essential to the practice of pediatrics.

QUALITY OF CARE

The medical profession has always claimed responsibility for regulating entry into its ranks and for assessing the quality of care provided. Although state boards have the legal authority to dispense licenses to practice, this authority in all states is delegated to the profession, which nominates the candidates who are then appointed by the state.

Individuals must merely demonstrate that they graduated from medical school and can achieve a passing grade on a cognitive examination developed by the profession itself, either in the state (state licensing examinations) or nationally (National Board of Medical Examiners or Federation of State Licensing Boards; i.e., "Flex" examinations). Many specialties have their own certifying examinations. Some specialty boards provide a means of periodic recertification in the form of various types of examinations; in some specialties (e.g., family medicine), periodic recertification is required, as it is for pediatricians currently becoming certified in the specialty. There is no requirement, however, that physicians demonstrate competence under the conditions of actual practice, either when they enter the profession or anytime afterward.

Medical School Accreditation

Medical schools are accredited by the Liaison Committee on Medical Education, which is composed of representatives of the American Medical Association and of the Association of American Medical Colleges.

Medical schools qualify for accreditation by demonstrating to the Liaison Committee that they conduct (1) a "sound educational program," including the opportunity to acquire a sound basis of education in medicine and to foster the development of lifelong habits of scholarship and service; (2) scientific research; (3) graduate education through both clinical residency programs and advanced degree programs in the basic medical sciences; and (4) continuing education aimed at maintaining and improving the competence of professionals engaged in caring for patients.

Hospital Accreditation

To be accredited, hospitals must receive approval from the Joint Commission on Accreditation of Health Care Organizations, a council composed of representatives of the American Medical Association, the American Hospital Association, the American College of Surgeons, and the American College of Physicians. Accreditation, both of hospitals and of medical schools, is essential to the financial viability of those institutions. Most "third-party" payers (the government and insurance companies) that reimburse hospitals or contribute to the support of medical schools require them to be accredited as a condition for payment.

Assurance of Quality Care

The passage of federal legislation stimulated the profession to demonstrate its involvement in assuring quality of care. Review of medical activities in hospitals was the first step to be proposed, largely because hospital costs assume a disproportionate share of the health care dollar. Legislation passed in 1972 (the Professional Standards Review Organization [PSRO] Act) required that hospital admission of patients covered by governmental payments be reviewed for justifiability and that hospitals periodically designate individual diagnoses for which all medical records of patients with those diagnoses would be audited to determine adequacy of care. These requirements, although opposed by many physicians, stimulated the profession to specify standards of care for common problems requiring hospitalization. However, continued opposition by the profession, the inability to demonstrate unequivocally that costs were lowered as a result of quality assurance activities, and general governmental policy to greatly reduce governmental regulation led to severe restrictions in the program and eventually to its demise.

A new program, professional review organizations (PROs), was established by the Tax Equity and Fiscal Responsibility Act (TEFRA) of 1982 as a means of reviewing the completeness, adequacy, and quality of care. In contrast to the PSROs, which were nonprofit physician organizations, PROs could be for-profit groups and fiscal intermediaries that won the contracts from the federal government for monitoring health care use. Although these PROs are for the purpose of reviewing diagnostic information, completeness and adequacy of care, and appropriateness of admissions for the elderly (patients covered by Medicare), it is likely that the precedent will spread to other groups of patients covered by governmental and even private insurers.

Studies have shown that the organization within which a physician practices has a greater influence on the quality of practice than the individual characteristics of the physician.[5] Team practice, in which nurses and community health workers share responsibility with the physician for certain aspects of care, is likely to result in both greater recognition of patients' problems and greater likelihood that they will be addressed by the physician. Prepaid group practice in which several physicians share fiscal accountability in their practices is also likely to result in greater consideration of the necessity and justifiability of professional actions.

In a health system in which patients may seek care at any place of their choice, those who fail to obtain relief of their complaints often seek subsequent care elsewhere. Thus physicians may not be in a position to observe the impact of their services. Conversely, there is no mechanism by which patients who are cured can make their physician aware of this. Most physicians are unable to assume responsibility for follow-up care of their patients in the event that the patients do not voluntarily return for care. As the costs of care become an increasing concern of third-party payers (government, insurance companies, employers), duplication of services, as reflected in visits to different providers of care for the same problem, will become evident. As a result, physicians may be encouraged to assume greater responsibility for episodes of illness rather than just for individual visits made by patients; managed care systems will encourage such assumption of responsibility. This is likely to make physicians more aware of deficiencies that may exist in current medical practice.

The historical prerogative by which physicians decide what practices constitute "good quality" also could be altered by a movement toward consumer involvement, control, and ownership of health facilities. Physicians and consumers may differ in the priority they place on the various aspects of health care. The effect of nonprofessional community members assuming responsibility for decision making in the health field is largely unexplored, but increasing interest among some consumers in moving in this direction suggests that this could be an important avenue of control in the future.

It appears likely, however, that certain aspects of practice will remain under the control of physicians. The first is the selection of students for entrance into medical school. Ever since the Flexner Report, the upper social classes have been overrepresented in the profession of medicine compared with their proportion in the general population. The high and continually rising cost of medical education without substantial governmental subsidy of those who cannot afford it is a powerful deterrent to applications from such students.

The second aspect is practice location. In many countries with national health insurance, physicians are not reimbursed for their services if they locate their practices in areas that already have a sufficient number of physicians. In the United States, there are no deterrents to physicians locating wherever they please and wherever they can obtain a license.

The third aspect likely to remain in the professional domain is the disciplining of physicians. In some countries the dissatisfaction and complaints of patients may be addressed to governmental agencies that consider them; these agencies then recommend sanctions (usually financial) against the physician. The medical profession in the United States has been rather impotent in disciplining its members in any meaningful way, because there is no way short of revoking a license (which is hardly ever done) to impose sanctions. To date, both professional and legislative bodies have failed to come to grips with this issue.

The fourth aspect likely to remain in the hands of the profession is control over the technical areas of medical care. As new technology is developed, it is often used without adequate prior assessment of its costs and benefits. Although pressures to reduce the rate of growth in medical care costs (which are largely a result of increased use of technology) will undoubtedly lead to attempts to restrain some of the practices of physicians, actual control over these practices is likely to be assumed by the organizations that employ or pay physicians. The development of policies concerning these controls, however, may be retained by the profession itself.

EFFECTIVENESS OF CARE

Although all practitioners must demonstrate at least a minimal amount of theoretical knowledge as a condition of licensure before they enter practice, the relationship between performance in tests and subsequent quality of practice has never been demonstrated. Even the procedure by which physicians become certified as "specialists" provides dubious assurance of high quality. As noted above, practice organization (group practice, teaching-hospital practice) is more important as a determinant of practice quality than are individual physician characteristics. Board certification, apart from its relationship to longer lengths of postgraduate training, appears to have no relationship to practice quality. Continuing education requirements and periodic recertification procedures imposed by professional organizations are unlikely to improve the situation unless the model of quality of care on which the original educational and certification procedures are based is broadened to encompass assessments of the impact of services on health status.

Improving Health and Well-Being

The significant declines in mortality over the last century can be attributed more to improvements in public health than to specific technologic advances applied to individual patients. The discovery of antibiotics is the only scientific advance applied to individual patients who are ill that has had a major impact in improving length of life; even here, the predominant, albeit not the only, effect seems to have been to reduce deaths in the elderly from acute infectious complications of chronic illness. The marked improvement in life expectancy over the last century has resulted primarily from lowered infant mortality. Infant mortality began to decline long before specific medical interventions were imposed, and the decline resulted from general improvements in sanitation, maternal nutrition, hygiene, and infant feeding.

Perhaps measuring the value of personal health services delivery in terms of a reduction in mortality is too great an expectation. Rather, some say that the measure of the system should be a reduction in the occurrence of disease and its manifestations—morbidity. But even here, it is unclear that physicians make a critical difference. Certainly the introduction of immunization has been responsible for large declines in the incidence of diphtheria, tetanus, pertussis, poliomyelitis, rubeola, and rubella and for the eradication of smallpox. But, once again, it is the public health sector rather than the practice of individual physicians that has been most responsible. Federal funds to support immunizations have been crucial to the effectiveness of these programs; attempts to reduce or eliminate federal support have led to reduced immunization and to disease epidemics among children, particularly the poor.

The impact that health services can be expected to have, even under the best of circumstances, is limited by the role of other forces. At least four factors determine an individual's state of health (Fig. 1-1). Genetic constitution is the basic determinant. People differ in predisposition to specific illnesses and in response to their treatment, largely because of differences in their genotypes.

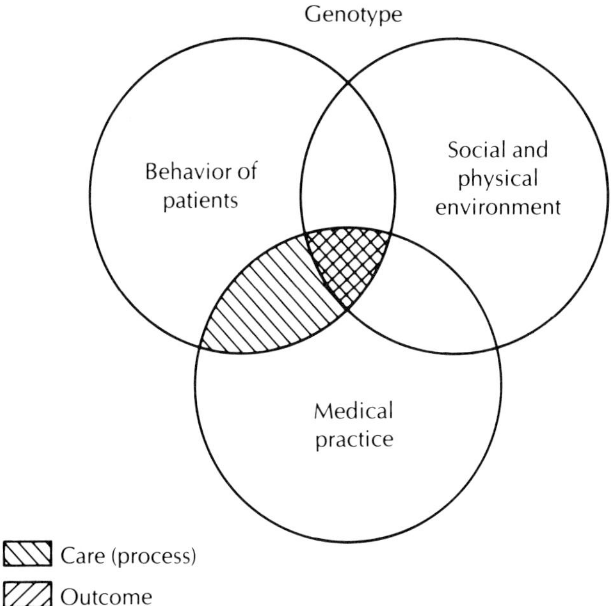

Fig. 1-1 Determinants of health status.

Probably the second most important determinant of an individual's state of health is his or her social and physical environment. Where individuals live, how they work, the food available to them, and the stresses that are imposed upon them by the social system all affect how healthy they are and how well they resist insults to their health. Children are particularly vulnerable to the effects of the physical and social environment because they are even less able to select their surroundings and exposures than are adults.

The third most important ingredient is the role that individuals themselves play. Although young children are less likely to determine their life patterns than are adults (whose smoking, drinking, eating, and driving behaviors are major underlying causes of death), the patterns set for them by their parents influence not only how ill health is dealt with in childhood but also how well they are taught behavior destined to affect their health in later life.

The final and probably least critical determinant of health, except in unusual situations, is the provision of medical services. The following discussion will show why and what might be done to enhance the contribution that these services make to health.

Who Defines What "Good Care" Is?

Consumers and providers of health services differ in the priorities they place on the three main elements of care: access, cost, and quality. Costs of and access to medical care are of prime importance to consumers. In contrast, neither access nor cost is an important component of medical school training, which focuses almost exclusively on how to make a diagnosis, to support this diagnosis with appropriate information from the history, physical examination, and laboratory findings, and to institute treatment appropriate to the diagnosis. The nature of most educational settings (university based, research oriented, generally highly specialized faculty) is responsible for the following important limitations in medical training:

1. The educational process focuses largely on the biochemical and biophysical bases of disease processes. In contrast, relatively little attention is devoted to understanding the social, occupational, and environmental causes of ill health, although these are major determinants of disease.
2. The diagnostic process emphasizes assigning single causes for disease and arriving at a single diagnosis. While appropriate in the past, it is more appropriate today to consider multiple causes of a disease. Moreover, one disease is often complicated and modified by the presence of another disease or a genetic, environmental, or psychosocial factor.
3. Insufficient attention is paid to the concept of human variability. In medical education, little attention is paid to the reasons why some individuals with predispositions to disease stay well while others succumb and why some respond to therapy while others do not.
4. Students' exposures to patients' illnesses are short-term. Education, composed of blocks of time in various specialties, does not prepare students to assume long-term responsibility for patients, as will be required in the subsequent practice of medicine.
5. Students learn about illnesses either through reading about them or by participating in the care of ill patients. In both instances, their knowledge is derived primarily from experiences with patients at university-affiliated hospitals. Patients appearing for care at such institutions are not representative of the population as a whole or even of the patients whom the students will subsequently meet as practitioners.

In the education of physicians, "quality" of care, characterized by the use of optimal techniques in arriving at diagnostic and therapeutic decisions, is virtually the only dictum emphasized. With this limited concept of "quality," it might be expected that at least diagnosis and therapy would be optimum in clinical practice. This, unfortunately, is not the case, as the following situations indicate.

Many well-accepted diagnostic strategies are of unproven usefulness, and some are actually harmful. For example, studies have shown that patterns of laboratory use may bear little or no relation to the needs of the patients. The extent of error, both in clinical observations and in laboratory findings, appears largely unrecognized by physicians.

Many commonly applied therapeutic maneuvers are of unproven usefulness and may be dangerous. For example, several studies demonstrate that surgical rates in the United States are much higher than in other developed countries, in the absence of any demonstrable difference in need for surgery as defined by prevalence of disease or illness. Even within the United States, the number of hospital admissions, the length of stay in the hospital, and the rate of surgical procedures vary markedly from area to area, unrelated to differences in medical need.

Another problem is the misuse of drug therapy. For many physicians, drug manufacturer representatives and advertisements are the primary source of information on new drugs. Several surveys have shown a widespread lack of appreciation

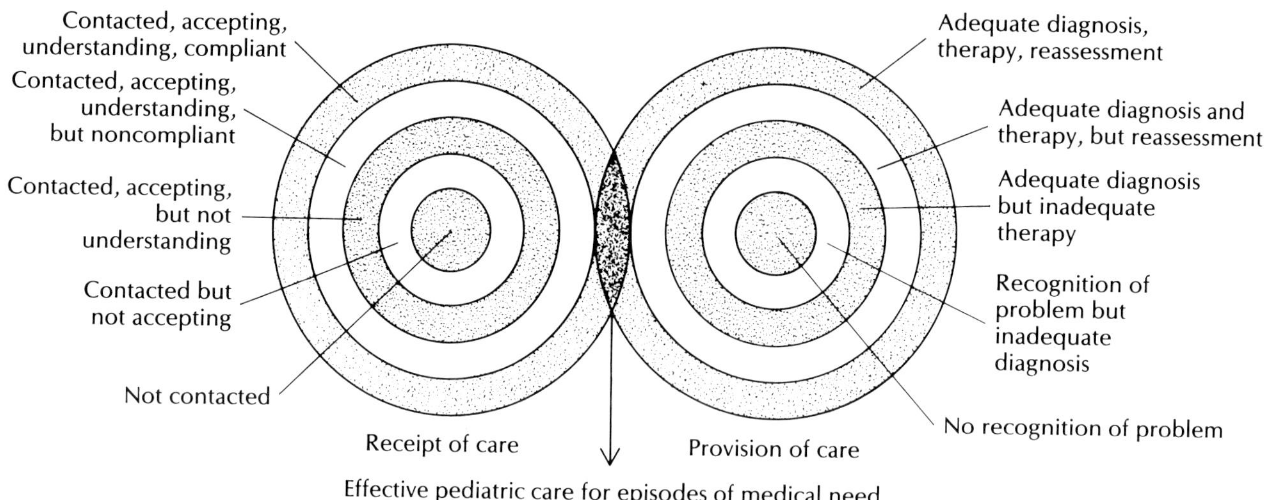

Fig. 1-2 Process of pediatric care.

of the dangers of many drugs and much unwarranted use of drugs.

Even when diagnostic and therapeutic interventions can be shown to be appropriate and efficacious, their application does not necessarily produce the desired outcome. This is because adequate diagnosis and therapy, while necessary for care of high quality, are by themselves insufficient. The treatment of illness and the maintenance of health also require the participation of patients and potential patients and a social and physical environment that is supportive, as Fig. 1-1 shows. The very best quality of care, defined as efficacious diagnosis and treatment, will fail to achieve its effect if those who require it and can benefit from it do not appear for care, if they fail to understand and accept it, or if they are unwilling to comply with the prescribed therapy (Fig. 1-2).

For these reasons, the traditional definition of quality of care should be broadened from its concentration on diagnostic and therapeutic strategies to include two additional facets of medical practice—problem recognition and follow-up with reassessment.

Problem Recognition

The application of diagnostic or therapeutic strategies requires first that problems, or potential problems, be recognized. Evidence indicates that the existence of many types of health problems is often overlooked.

Physicians are consistently poorer at recognizing the existence of significant behavior problems and social factors related to illness than they are at recognizing problems with obvious biophysiologic or anatomic manifestations. But even organic problems may be neglected. Many children and adults too have health conditions that fail to be followed up by their physicians, even when information about them is available. Failure to recognize the problems that patients bring to physicians is a serious shortcoming in the provision of health services, because it has been shown that this failure is associated both with decreased patient satisfaction and with patient failure to follow medical advice. Without recognizing the full range of patients' problems, no diagnostic strategy or therapeutic intervention can be fully effective.

Problem recognition also extends to prevention of disease. One type of prevention, primary prevention, is traditional to pediatricians. It consists of recognizing susceptibility to disease and applying measures to prevent it from occurring. Immunizations are the most obvious example of primary prevention, but prevention goes far beyond this. Sometimes only certain people are at risk of acquiring disease later in life; pediatricians must direct efforts at discovering who these people are, at keeping them under surveillance, and at trying to eliminate the situations that permit the illness to develop. This is known as secondary prevention. As social, occupational, environmental, and behavioral factors become recognized as important antecedents of many chronic illnesses, pediatricians will become more involved in activities directed toward preventing them.

Up to now, secondary prevention has not been a common feature of pediatric practice, and when children at risk have been identified, it generally has been at the initiative of governmental and social agencies. Examples of such efforts include hearing and vision screening in schools, special screening programs for specific disease in special populations (sickle cell anemia, Tay-Sachs disease), and state-mandated neonatal screening for inherited metabolic disorders (such as phenylketonuria). A major challenge for pediatricians is recognizing and dealing with occupational hazards that result in parents, unknowingly exposing their children to toxic materials invisibly carried home from the workplace. Ultimately, pediatricians must assume responsibility for coordinating all of the care of children, including primary prevention and secondary prevention, as well as treatment of manifest illness.

Follow-up and Reassessment

To ensure that diagnostic procedures and instituted therapy are adequate, patients must be monitored to determine if problems are being resolved as expected.

Medical textbooks and teaching rarely include information

that would help the practitioner define appropriate intervals for reassessing particular health problems. Such information would have to come from careful studies of the natural history of patients' problems, with and without intervention, and such studies are rare. Moreover, little is known about the extent to which practitioners do follow up problems that they treat. When the issue has been examined, it has been found that failure to follow up on treated patients results in unresolved health problems. At the very least, it produces a highly inefficient health care system; care is paid for, but no benefit is gained. At the most, it will ultimately lead to societal demands for greater accountability of the profession.

Outcome of Care

This chapter, up to this point, has examined issues relating to the "structure" and "process" of medical care. Manpower, the organization of care, accessibility, and costs reflect the structure, or form, of health services. The process of care has been addressed in the discussion of quality, which involves the recognition of patients' problems, further data gathering to arrive at medical diagnoses, the institution of therapy, and reassessment to ensure optimal response to therapy. As has been shown, patients contribute to the process of care by deciding whether to seek it (utilization), whether to accept it, and to understand it and comply with recommendations. The third means by which care may be evaluated is based on the attainment of goals, or outcomes. Outcomes may be divided into four categories: deaths, illness and injury, disability, and others.

Deaths are uniformly registered and therefore are available and easily tabulated. But after infancy, deaths in childhood are so relatively infrequent that they are an insensitive indicator of the value of medical interventions.

Illness and injury data are obtainable only for those few conditions for which reporting is mandated by law because of their potential public health impact (contagiousness). Some examples of these conditions are rubella, rubeola, and hepatitis; however, these causes of morbidity constitute a small proportion of the health problems of children. National health surveys, including household surveys and surveys of practitioners' offices, are an important source of information about the prevalence of other child health conditions.

The ongoing household survey administered by the National Center for Health Statistics of the U.S. Department of Health and Human Services obtains information about disability from a sample of the population. Disability is ascertained by asking questions regarding limitations of activity as a result of chronic conditions and regarding restrictions on usual daily activity or confinement to bed as a result of acute conditions.

Increasingly, the impact of medical care is being measured; evidence exists that individuals are more or less comfortable, more or less satisfied with their health, more or less able to achieve their physical and intellectual potential, and more or less able to control physical, emotional, and social threats to their health. The pediatric practitioner of the future will be confronted more with these new concepts of disease and health than with the acute illnesses that have preoccupied the child health practitioner of the past.

It seems likely that future physicians will be encouraged, and perhaps even required, to keep certain types of data about the children in their practices. A data set for hospitals to use for each patient admitted and a similar set for ambulatory care have been accepted by the National Committee for Health Statistics and recommended for wide use. These include registration data (patient identification number, name, address, birth date, sex, race, and marital status) and encounter data (facility identification number, provider identification number, patient identification number, source of payment, date of encounter, patient's purpose for visit, physician diagnosis, diagnostic and management procedures, and disposition).

The adoption of this or a similar system for collecting information in a standardized way will facilitate the understanding of health and disease processes and the role medical care plays in influencing them.

A national collaborative research network, under the aegis of the American Academy of Pediatrics, has been developed that as of 1989 involves hundreds of office-based pediatricians in scientifically based inquiry about child health problems and their care. Participation in such networks can provide a stimulating experience for pediatricians and engage them in a lifelong process of continuing education and intellectual renewal. Pediatric practitioners who are involved could contribute in a major way to improving knowledge about the distribution and nature of child health problems and their responsiveness to medical therapy.

REFERENCES

1. Budetti P, Butler J, and McManus P: Federal health program reforms: implications for child health care, Milbank Q 60:155, 1982.
2. Etzel SI, et al: Graduate medical education in the United States, JAMA 262(8):1029, 1989.
3. Luft HS: Health maintenance organizations: dimensions of performance, New York, 1981, John Wiley & Sons Inc.
4. Martinez G and Ryan A: The pediatric market place, Am J Dis Child 143:924, 1989.
5. Palmer RH and Reilly MC: Individual and institutional variables which may serve as indicators of quality of medical care, Med Care 17:693, 1979.
6. Roback G, et al: Physician characteristics and distribution in the U.S., Chicago, 1990, American Medical Association.
7. Robertson WO: Medical malpractice: 1984. Pediatr Rev 6(8):229, 1985.

2

Morbidity and Mortality Among the Young

I. Barry Pless

Understanding the major causes of death, disease, and disability in children and adolescents is central to the efforts of all who serve the young. The goal must be to prevent the preventable with respect to disease and its consequences and to limit the disability resulting from the unpreventable.

The general pattern of morbidity, mortality, and disability over time is the basis for predicting future trends of child health care. The *morbidity* rate is the proportion of children who are affected by any illness or impairment at a given time or over a specified period of time. The *mortality* rate is the proportion of children who die in a given time period; it may be age, sex, or disease specific. *Disability* rates describe the proportion of children who have an illness or impairment judged to be disabling (e.g., resulting in school absence, days in bed, hospitalizations, or limitations in activities).

Such statistics are reasonably similar within small regions but often differ markedly from state to state. They point to two important factors: In part they reveal variations in socioeconomic composition, but they also may indicate differences in the medical care available. Together these factors account for the difference in infant mortality from state to state; for example, the death rate generally is lower in the Northeast than in parts of the Southeast. Likewise, differences between the races persist (Fig. 2-1). In 1960 the infant mortality rate for blacks was 44.3 per 1000 live births, compared with 22.9 per 1000 for whites; in 1985 the respective rates were 18.2 and 9.3 per 1000. Although the difference in the mortality rates for the two groups in the postneonatal period (29 days to 1 year) diminished between 1965 and 1985, the gap between the rates for the neonatal period (birth through 28 days) actually increased.

International data add another perspective to these statistics. For example, the outstanding causes of illness and death vary greatly between the United States and countries in Latin America, where infant mortality ranges from 45 to 80 per 1000 live births. Nonetheless, in 1980 the United States ranked only fifteenth among the 25 countries with the lowest infant death rates, and by 1987 it ranked even lower. In large

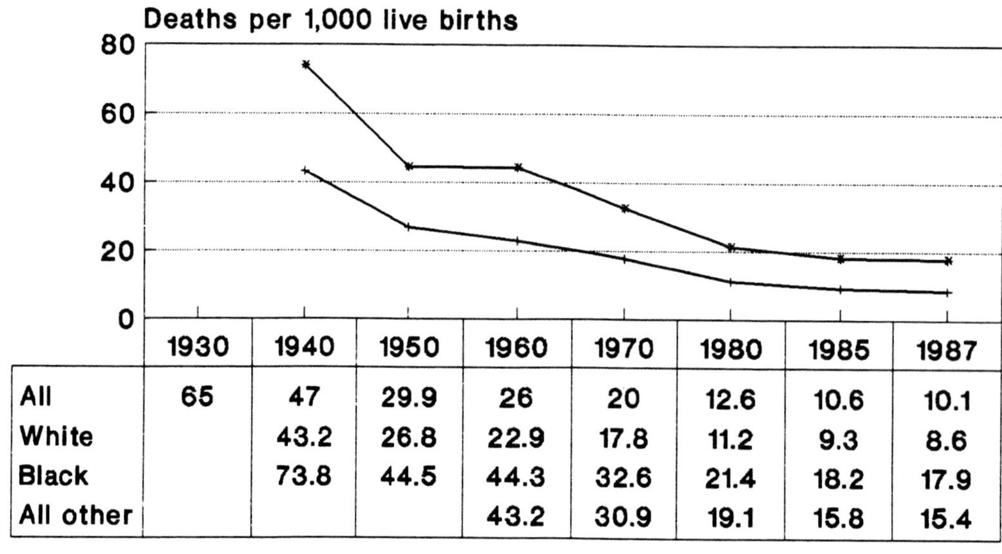

	1930	1940	1950	1960	1970	1980	1985	1987
All	65	47	29.9	26	20	12.6	10.6	10.1
White		43.2	26.8	22.9	17.8	11.2	9.3	8.6
Black		73.8	44.5	44.3	32.6	21.4	18.2	17.9
All other				43.2	30.9	19.1	15.8	15.4

Fig. 2-1 Infant mortality in the United States has declined steadily since 1950 for both whites *(bottom line)* and blacks *(top line)*. The flattening curves beginning in 1980 reflect a slowing of the rate of decline in these dates. Although the differences in postneonatal mortality rates between these two groups diminished between 1965 and 1985, the differences between the neonatal rates increased.
(Data from United States Vital Statistics, Annual Summaries of Vital Statistics.)

measure these differences reflect the major variations in the socioeconomic compositions of the countries, but they are also a function of important differences in health care organization and delivery.

VITAL STATISTICS

An important difference exists between the terms prevalence and incidence. *Prevalence* is the proportion of individuals in a population who have a specific disease at any particular time. *Incidence* is the proportion who develop new cases of a disease over any given period of time. Both rates are expressed only in relation to those individuals who are potentially at risk for a particular disorder. For example, both sexes are not included in the denominator when figures on circumcisions or teenage pregnancies are presented. Most of the rates presented here are prevalence rates, especially in the case of chronic diseases. These are usually expressed as rates per 1000 persons under 18 years of age. Mortality statistics, however, are often presented as rates per 100,000 in view of the much lower frequency of occurrence.

Crude rates, as a rule, give little information about the distribution of events in a particular population or group. They must be compared with a model or standard by statistical methods to allow for differences in age and sex distribution in different populations, countries, or settings.

Still more caution is needed when attempting to apply national statistics to an individual pediatric practice. The composition of a typical pediatric practice of 2500 to 3000 patients can be expected to change by about 10% a year. A physician therefore may expect to provide care for about 60 asthmatic children at any given time; however, even over a 10-year period encompassing perhaps as many as 3000 new faces, the pediatrician will see only one or two cases of any less common disorder.

Birth Rates

Around 1955 a striking decline in the birth rate began in the United States (Fig. 2-2). In 1960 the rate was nearly 24 per 1000 population; by 1970 it had fallen to 18 per 1000. It began to level off in 1974, when it reached 15 per 1000, and by 1987 it had not changed appreciably. The implications of this trend are important in relation to the absolute size of the child population and its size relative to the elderly. Both factors influence the number of people and hospital beds needed to care for children properly.

Two other important factors also should be noted. First, although the fertility rate fell nearly 50% between 1957 and 1987, this has been countered to some degree by the large number of women now of childbearing age as a result of the postwar baby boom. Reasons for the decline in fertility rates are numerous. It is widely believed that the state of the economy plays a large role, alongside the growing desire during this time to limit family size for other reasons. Certainly the widespread availability and popularity of more effective methods of contraception (e.g., the "pill") are also important factors. Second, the growing number of legal abortions must be taken into account. Thus the leveling off of the birth rate may reflect the balancing of these factors, and zero population growth is still an eventuality.

Several studies of the effect of abortion law reform on birth patterns have noted a falling number of low-birth-weight and premature babies. This trend, combined with improved care for such babies in neonatal intensive care nurseries, probably has had a significant impact on both infant mortality and the quality of survival. The net effect may be an appreciable reduction of handicaps that are secondary to birth factors.

Teenage pregnancies, particularly those of girls under 15

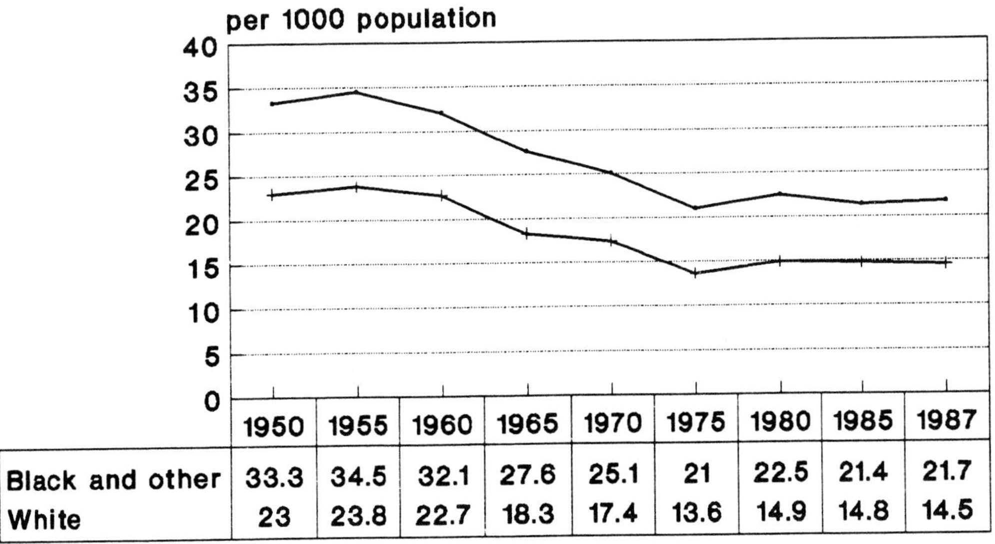

	1950	1955	1960	1965	1970	1975	1980	1985	1987
Black and other	33.3	34.5	32.1	27.6	25.1	21	22.5	21.4	21.7
White	23	23.8	22.7	18.3	17.4	13.6	14.9	14.8	14.5

Fig. 2-2 Birth rates in the United States have declined since 1955 for both whites *(bottom line)* and blacks *(top line)*. Leveling off took place in 1975.

(Data from United States Vital Statistics, Annual Summaries of Vital Statistics.)

Table 2-1 *United States, 1987: Major Causes of Death by Age Birth Through 24 Years of Age*

CAUSE OF DEATH	AGE IN YEARS <1	1-4	5-14	1-14	15-24	0-24	TOTAL NO. OF DEATHS
	(Rates per 100,000 population)						
Accidents and adverse effects (E800-E949)*	25.2 (4)†	20.2 (1)	12.3 (1)	14.7 (1)	48.9 (1)	29.5 (1)	26,688
Certain conditions in the perinatal period (760-779)	479.2 (1)	0.8	0.0	0.0	0.0	20.1 (2)	18,187
Congenital anomalies (740-759)	209.1 (2)	6.4 (2)	1.3 (3)	2.8 (3)	1.3	10.8 (3)	9,750
Homicide (E960-978)	7.2	2.3 (5)	1.2 (4)	1.5 (5)	14.0 (2)	6.9 (4)	6,243
Suicide (E950-959)	. . .	. . .	0.7	0.5	12.9 (3)	5.6 (5)	5,149
Malignant and benign neoplasms (140-208, 210-239)	4.3	4.2 (4)	3.5 (2)	3.7 (2)	5.4 (4)	4.4	4,020
Infectious illnesses (including organ systems) (001-139, 320-322, 466, 480-487, 590)	45.4 (3)	5.2 (3)	1.0 (5)	2.2 (4)	3.2 (5)	4.4	4,024
Cardiovascular diseases (390-398, 402, 404-429)	25.2 (4)	2.2	0.9	1.3	2.8	2.9	2,599
Cerebrovascular diseases (430-438)	3.4	0.4	0.2	0.3	0.6	0.5	481
Chronic obstructive pulmonary diseases and allied conditions (490-496)	1.4	0.3	0.3	0.3	0.5	0.4	387
Renal diseases and renal failure (580-589)	5.8	0.1	0.1	0.1	0.2	0.4	344
Gastrointestinal diseases (531-533, 540-543, 550-553, 560, 571, 574-575)	3.4	0.2	0.0	0.1	0.3	0.3	285
Anemias (280-285)	0.5	0.3	0.2	0.2	0.3	0.3	244
Diabetes mellitus (250)	. . .	0.1	0.1	0.1	0.3	0.2	163
Complications of pregnancy and childbirth (630-676)	. . .	. . .	0.0	0.0	0.2	0.1	76
Nutritional deficiencies (260-269)	0.7	0.1	0.0	0.0	0.0	0.1	41
All other causes	207.7	8.8	3.8	5.5	9.0	15.4	13,930
Total	1,018.5	51.6	25.6	33.3	99.9	102.4	92,611‡
Estimated population (thousands)	3,771	14,483	34,152	48,635	38,061	90,467	
Number of deaths	38,408	7,473	8,743	16,216	38,023	92,647	

*Numbers in parentheses indicate specific illnesses according to the Ninth Revision, International Classification of Diseases, 1975.

†Number in parentheses indicates the rank order for the five leading causes of death in each age group.

‡This total number of deaths figure does not match the actual number (92,647) because of rounding of the death rates for each cause of death. 0.0, < 0.1, 0.0 = < 0.1, . . . = no deaths

(Modified from National Center for Health Statistics: Advance report, final mortality statistics, 1987, Monthly vital statistics report vol 38, no 5, suppl, Hyattsville, Md, Public Health Service.)

years of age, are a major cause of morbidity and mortality for both mother and child. The pregnancy rate in this age group has doubled since 1960. However, the percentage of all live births attributable to women under 20 years of age declined from 17.2% in 1968 to 12.5% in 1987. For those 15 to 17 years of age, this decline was from 5.5% to 4.5%. The general decline in the 15 to 20 age group was initially attributed to the increase in the number of legal abortions, one third of which were performed on women in this age group. With recent proposed changes in legislation prohibiting abortion in some states, this picture may change.

Leading Causes of Death

The prevention of premature death is a priority for all pediatricians. However, in 1987 the causes of death in each stage of childhood differed substantially (as shown in Table 2-1), which should be reflected in the amount of attention devoted to preventing particular causes. This is not always done. For example, accidents comprise the most common cause of death beyond the first year of life, yet the time devoted to their prevention is much less than that given to the care of minor illnesses.

In 1987 the infant mortality rate reached an all-time low of 10.1 per 1000 live births, a drop of 78.5% from the level of 47 per 1000 in 1940 (see Fig. 2-1). This has been the result of improvements in therapy for perinatal disorders (particularly asphyxia and other respiratory conditions), immaturity, and gastrointestinal problems. In spite of this steady record of improvement, almost 50% of all deaths up to 18 years of age still occur during the first year of life.

The causes of death in children over 1 year of age have changed remarkably little over time, although the trend is generally one of consistent improvement. Accidents are followed by neoplasms and congenital anomalies in the age group 1 to 14 years. A particularly disturbing change, however, is the rise in homicides. Between 1968 and 1985 the rates increased from 1.5 to 2.4 per 100,000 for those 1 to 4 years of age, from 0.6 to 1 for those 5 to 9 years of age, and from 0.8 to 1.5 and 6.9 to 8.5 for those 10 to 14 and 15 to 19 years of age, respectively. On average these trends represent a worsening of about 60%.

In the age group 15 to 24 years, the main causes of death are accidents, homicide, suicide, and neoplasms, in that order (see Table 2-1). The first three of these causes account for 75.8% of all deaths in this age group! Hence, across all age groups the most promising opportunities for still further reducing death rates lie with preventing serious injuries and with gaining greater understanding of the social and psychological factors that lead to homicide and suicide. (See Chapter 104.)

Trends in Specific Causes of Death. The rates of infant deaths resulting from pneumonia, bronchitis, and meningitis have changed little in most countries since 1952, and deaths from most congenital abnormalities remain virtually unchanged since 1932. For example, the death rate for congenital heart disease has stabilized at approximately 1.5 per 10,000, probably because improved technology has resulted only in the postponement of death. Mortality beyond the first year of life is chiefly attributed to accidents or violence; these rates showed relatively little improvement over the past several decades—until the mid-1970s, when some positive changes in certain categories (e.g., poisoning) became evident.

Sudden infant death syndrome (SIDS), which has long been of great interest to epidemiologists, now receives far more attention from clinicians. Several studies suggest a fairly consistent incidence of about 2 to 3 in 1000 live births, but little is known about the causes or the prevention of the syndrome. (SIDS is discussed in greater detail in Chapter 260.)

Another area of concern is the number of injuries and deaths resulting from child abuse and neglect, but accurate estimates of this problem are impossible to determine.

Many observers have been troubled by the possibility that efforts to save sick newborns might result in an increasing societal burden to care for more handicapped individuals. However, some reports suggest that there is a decreasing incidence of sequelae among infants who have received good neonatal care.

In Sweden the decrease in the incidence of cerebral palsy, first noted in the early 1960s, appears to have been reversed. Hagberg and colleagues reported in 1989 that the rate for the period between 1967 and 1970, about 1.4 per 1000 live births, has risen sharply since. Between 1979 and 1982 the average crude prevalence was 2.17 per 1000.[5] Although more recent figures are not available, the fears that improved technology might have adverse effects are not without substance and reflect in particular the impact of this technology on ever smaller and younger preterm infants, who are surviving in increased numbers.

An exceptionally illuminating report produced by the National Center for Health Statistics (NCHS) in 1989 describes trends in mortality.[4] As the authors indicate, the findings highlight not only the large decline in death rates during the last half of the twentieth century, but also the large proportion of deaths caused by injuries and violence. They also call attention to the sizable race and sex differences in many causes of death, especially injuries, geographic variations, and cross-national comparisons. This section draws heavily on this report.

Apart from the wealth of information provided, the NCHS report also makes an important semantic contribution. The authors introduce the terms "natural" and "external" causes of death to refer to all noninjury disease categories, rather than "injury" or "accident" (excluding homicide and suicide), respectively.

Deaths in both categories follow a U-shaped pattern by age, so that the lowest rates are found in the middle childhood years, that is, between about 4 and 12. The curve is highest for natural causes among the very young; for external causes it is highest in adolescence.

The trends over time are encouraging. Although most of the dramatic improvements were found in all age groups during the first half of the century, they continued, albeit at a lesser rate, until 1980, except among those 15 to 19 years of age. Since 1970 rates have declined still further, between 37% and 50% in those under 9 years of age and much less (about 25%) among older children and adolescents. But the patterns are quite different between the two major categories;

natural causes have decreased by about 70% in all age groups since the early 1930s, whereas external causes decreased by only about 30%.

Of special interest is the consistent and dramatic shift in relative importance between the two categories. For example, between 1900 and 1950, the proportion of deaths among 5- to 9-year-olds resulting from external causes rose from only 9% to nearly 40%; the same general pattern is seen for the other age groups as well. This reflects both the growing success in combating the natural causes and the absolute increases in deaths from injuries. The data show, too, that the more recent improvements, although widespread, are unequally distributed; the decline in death rates since 1979 has been more rapid among white children than among black children.

The great importance of injuries as a cause of death in the 1980s is underscored by this report, as well as by the data reviewed by Hoekelman and Pless.[7] Although injuries remain the leading cause of death in all age groups over 1 year, the decline since 1975 has been impressive. In the age group 1 to 14 years, the rate has fallen by nearly 30%, whereas among 15- to 24-year-olds the decline has been only about half as great, approximately 18%. By comparison the trends for the natural causes are considerably less impressive. For example, among 5- to 14-year-olds, deaths from infectious illnesses fell by only 20%; much the same is true for deaths from neoplasms over this time period.

Hoekelman and Pless suggest that the trends described are unlikely to be the result of any methodologic artifacts and that in the case of natural or "biologic" causes, much of the credit for the improvement must be given to advances in medical technology such as vaccines, antibiotics, and surgical techniques. In comparison, the external causes reflect societal phenomena, only some of which have been identified: counseling, health education, seat restraint legislation, and reductions in legal speed limits. However, in some age groups death rates have actually increased in some categories since 1975; these categories include cardiovascular and renal diseases, perinatal conditions, homicides, and suicides. In the case of the first two conditions, part of the explanation may be greater diagnostic accuracy and measures that have resulted in prolonging survival so that, in effect, deaths that would have occurred in one age group have been postponed to another. Explanations for the rise in homicides and suicides are, sadly, all too apparent: an increase in societal violence generally, the popularity of firearms, and widespread pessimism among many young people.

Most revealing are the state and international comparisons. Fingerhut and Kleinman[4] noted that the distribution of deaths by states, depending on the broad category of cause of death, is curiously mixed. For example, although states in the South and West generally had high rates among children 1 to 4 years of age for all causes, those in the Northeast (New Hampshire, Connecticut, and New Jersey) were in the lowest quartile; New York was among the lowest for deaths from external causes and highest for deaths from natural causes for this age group. The reverse was seen for Wyoming, Nevada, and Vermont. Conversely, in the 5 to 9 age group only Minnesota and Pennsylvania had consistently low rates for both causes, whereas the rates in the South, as well as in Arizona and Oklahoma, were in the highest quartile for both natural and external causes. The pattern for the 10 to 14 age group is again different. There are no simple explanations for these perplexing variations.

At the international level, the United States in 1985 had the highest injury death rates when compared with those of eight other developed countries; this is true for all age groups, with very few exceptions. The rates for homicide and suicide among teenagers (15 to 19 years of age) are also the highest, except for suicide among male Canadians. In sharp contrast, the differences are much less pronounced for deaths resulting from natural causes, and generally the rankings for the United States are in the midrange for all age groups.

MORBIDITY AND DISABILITY

Clinicians and epidemiologists need to distinguish morbidity from disability. Disability is defined by the National Center for Health Statistics as a "general term used to describe any temporary or long-term reduction of a person's activity as a result of an acute or chronic condition." Children frequently experience an illness (or an episode of morbidity) that is not accompanied by significant disability. Children with colds, for example, may attend school and play actively, and even children with a limb in a plaster cast often participate in vigorous athletics. For practical purposes, days in bed, days off from school, and days of limited activity are the best measures of significant disability.

Ogden Nash defined the family as "a unit composed not only of children, but of men, women, the occasional animal, and the common cold." The cold is the dominant illness of childhood, one that occupies a disproportionate share of the physician's time and skill, in view of its usually self-limiting nature. Upper respiratory and gastrointestinal tract infections together account for more than 60% of all acute childhood illnesses. The average child has one or two colds per year, and one third of all children have at least one episode of some other infection annually. An equal proportion has at least one accident each year, and about 3% require hospitalization. Approximately one child in 10 develops a chronic physical illness by 15 years of age, at least 5% of children have emotional problems, and roughly 3% are handicapped because of low intelligence. A precise figure for the constellation of problems encompassed by the rubric "learning disorder" is impossible to determine; the reported range is 3% to 23%.

Population-Based Morbidity

Earlier surveys (1981) conducted by the National Center for Health Statistics showed that 50% of all acute conditions were caused by respiratory illness, 11% by infections and parasitic diseases, and 15% by injuries; this has changed little in recent years. A study by Hoekelman and colleagues[8] found that although well-child visits still dominate primary care pediatric practice, constituting 28% of all visits, respiratory tract illnesses accounted for only 23% of visits, and other diseases of the ears, nose, mouth, and throat made up a further 24%. Noteworthy at the opposite extreme is the very small proportion of visits characterized as being for emotional or behavioral reasons—1% overall—but this figure rises progressively through the age groups so that among those 15 to 19 years old, the proportion is 3.3%.

Chronic conditions affect children less often than acute conditions, so the rate of occurrence for a chronic condition is usually expressed as the prevalence in 1000 persons under 18 years of age. Various allergic disorders have the highest rate of occurrence (90 to 100 per 1000), followed by other respiratory conditions (50 to 60 per 1000) and orthopedic and paralytic disorders (about 23 per 1000). Disorders of speech, hearing, and vision combined affect between 17 and 28 children per 1000 (the higher figure pertains to boys). Skin diseases affect 15 in 1000, and digestive system disorders affect between 8 and 13 per 1000. Mental and nervous disorders involve 6 or 7 children per 1000. These national figures are consistent with those found at the community level.

Over the past 25 years there has been an impressive decline in the incidence of infectious diseases in the United States because of the development of effective vaccines. The elimination of smallpox and the virtual elimination of both poliomyelitis and the serious sequelae of mumps and measles are excellent examples of the success of vaccine technology. An equally important role in these advances was played by the development of improved, more stringent methods of field-testing procedures essential to ensure the safety and effectiveness of the vaccines. This is one of the major triumphs of public health, and it is one in which the practicing community has played a key role.

The development of effective vaccines, however, illustrates an age-old problem: how to ensure that good technology is implemented fully, promptly, and appropriately. In most parts of the country immunizations are provided by private practitioners, but in some areas public health departments are also involved. As a result, adequate records of these immunizations are difficult to maintain; when this problem is compounded by inadequate financial subsidies, epidemics may follow. Thus on several occasions since the mid-1970s there have been alarming increases in measles, often with serious sequelae. With the help of well-directed government funding, the number of cases fell from 57,000 in 1977 to 3032 in 1981. However, during the subsequent period the case rate rose from 1.4 to 2.6 per 100,000 in 1986 (Williams BC, 1990, unpublished data). It is believed that this reflects the withdrawal of government funding for immunizations. Clearly, success in this area depends heavily on continued federal involvement.

Hospital Morbidity

Another important measure of morbidity is hospitalization. The advantage of this measure is that in many countries statistics based on discharge diagnoses are collected routinely. A report from the National Center for Health Statistics provides such rates for children in the United States compared with the same statistics for Canada.[9] This exercise is of special interest because Canada has a system of comprehensive health insurance that covers all hospital costs. However, in many other respects the populations and systems of care are similar. The report was prompted by the finding that the hospital discharge rate for children in the United States during 1980 was among the lowest of the seven Western countries examined, whereas the rate in Canada was 42% higher (95 per 1000 versus 67 per 1000 population). It was also found that Canada had a longer average length of stay in the hospital (5.3 versus 4.4 days) and that the proportion of sick newborns was considerably higher in the United States.

Large differences were seen for certain diagnostic groups (e.g., tonsillectomy and adenoidectomy, upper respiratory infections), and these in turn varied by age. It is not clear what accounts for these differences, which on the surface appear to suggest that children in the United States are healthier than those in Canada. When the disability rates are compared, however, this explanation seems unlikely, because generally these rates are higher in the United States. In particular, the data do not tell whether the differences represent the greater emphasis placed on ambulatory care in the United States or the existence of financial barriers to hospital care.

Such differences are also noted within the United States. A report by Perrin and colleagues[10] covering a wide range of conditions shows marked variations in hospitalization rates across three urban communities. The rate of admissions in Boston was more than twice the rate in Rochester, New York; the rate for New Haven, Connecticut, fell between the two. Some diagnoses were especially prominent; the relative rate for toxic injuries in Boston was nearly seven times that of Rochester. Although socioeconomic differences may partly explain these variations, it also seems likely that local practices play a significant role.

The NCHS study also used data from comparable National Health Interview Surveys to provide information about other measures of disability. The study found that children in the United States had 28% more disability days and more bed days. There were also important differences in death rates, but these were not consistent across age groups. Although the statistics are not recent, most observers believe the patterns and trends still hold.

Practice-Based Morbidity

Whether pediatricians serve mainly as consultants or as primary care physicians varies greatly from country to country. In Scotland, for example, pediatricians serve almost exclusively as consultants to general practitioners; accordingly, they are involved in fewer than 8% of all child-physician encounters. More than half of their work involves the diagnosis and treatment of serious, complex chronic illnesses, toward which their training is heavily oriented. In contrast, most pediatricians in the United States and Canada provide primary care, and the spectrum of illness they see is quite different from that seen by their Scottish counterparts and from the case mix they encountered during residency training.

Although few data are available, it appears that office practice in most communities in the United States has become increasingly focused on well-child care and the care of children with minor infectious illnesses.[8] One reason may be the growth of pediatric subspecialties and the inclination of the generalist to refer many of the more complex disorders to specialists. Another reason may be the loss of many older children to physicians in internal medicine. Only 15% of pediatric office visits are made by patients over 10 years of age. Starfield and colleagues report that in 1983 pediatricians were involved in only 6% of all medical encounters by those 15 to 19 years of age; even in the 10 to 14 age group, the proportion was only 25.5%.[13] In both age groups general practitioners and other physician specialists saw far more patients than did pediatricians. Nonetheless, most of the common infectious illnesses such as otitis media, throat infections, pneumonia, and diarrhea are managed by pediatricians. Nationally, however, general practitioners provide almost as much preventive and psychosocial care (35.8% and 19.5%, respectively) as do pediatricians (44.2% and 16.5%), and considerably more surgical care.

There are variations from one practice to another, but the general pattern is that the more complex and challenging chronic disorders are rarely seen in everyday practice. On the whole only about one third of the office time in primary care is devoted to the diagnosis and treatment of sick children. In fact, the National Ambulatory Medical Care Survey (NAMCS), conducted periodically by the National Center for Health Statistics, shows that only about 10% of all visits to pediatricians are for serious problems.

Disability

The most important aspect of morbidity is the extent of disability that it produces. Because there is no universally accepted way to assess disability, several indicators are used to describe the extent and manner in which illnesses are manifested. Common to most indicators is an estimate of functional impairment, as reflected in alterations of usual activities.

"Usual activities," of course, depend on age. Moreover, many childhood illnesses such as asthma and epilepsy are episodic. Thus even with a chronic disorder, levels of disability may vary greatly from one day to the next. It is particularly difficult therefore to judge the overall disability of children with chronic disorders. To confuse matters further, parents of handicapped children may fail to distinguish between what is "usual" for their child and what is usual for the child's healthy peers. According to the National Center for Health Statistics, "Persons who have permanently reduced their usual activities because of a chronic condition might not report any restricted activity days during a 2-week period. Therefore, absence of restricted activity days does not imply normal health."

Three commonly used indicators of disability based upon parents' reports of limitations of activities during the preceding 2 weeks are disability days per person per year, bed days per person per year, and percent of persons with limitation of activities. Distinctions depend on whether an illness or injury prevents a child from carrying on the major activity typical of his or her age group (e.g., ordinary play with other children or school attendance); whether it only limits the amount or kind of major activity performed; or whether it restricts only strenuous activities such as athletics. At any given time, over 95% of all children under 17 years of age are not disabled in any way, about 2% have mild or moderate limitations, and 0.2% have severe disabilities. With increasing degrees of limitation there are proportionately more days of restricted activity per child per year and an increasing number of days during which the child stays in bed because of a specific illness or injury. The number of children hospitalized and the length of hospital stay are also proportional to the level of disability, as is the number of physician visits per year.

An average child misses 5.3 days of school per year because of illness or injury. Most such absences (58%) are caused by respiratory disorders. Infective and parasitic diseases account for 20%, injuries for 8.2%, digestive system conditions for 4.5%, and all other acute conditions for 9.5%. Overall, girls miss considerably more school than do boys; however, boys are almost twice as likely to be absent because of injuries.

Use of Health Services. The development of a rational health care system should be based on the results of studies about how health services are used by children.

Patients who have symptoms of equal severity seek medical attention, if at all, at different times. The explanation for this takes into account both what the symptom is and how disruptive it is to the individual and the family. Convenience and finances, as well as a broad range of sociocultural factors, influence this decision. For example, the belief that a perceived symptom is serious or that medical care is appropriate varies considerably among cultural, ethnic, and religious groups. Although little can be done to influence such beliefs, much can be done to affect some of the cost factors involved.

The family is the basis of Andersen's analysis[2] of the use of medical care. He found correlations among the age of the child, the marital status of the mother, maternal education, race, parental occupation, number of children, access to care, and the use of medical services over the course of 1 year. The Andersen study and those of Suchman[14] and Rosenstock[12] found that there are different explanations for short-term (2 weeks or less) and long-term use of health care and for the use of preventive and curative services. The results also suggest that stress may trigger a parent's decision to see a doctor.

Stress resulting from causes other than illness frequently determines the tolerance a parent may have for a child's given symptom. Roghmann and Haggerty[11] distinguish between acute and chronic stress, because each influences the use of medical services to a different degree. For example, poor families live with stress every day, and it has been suggested that they are crisis oriented; that is, only when a symptom becomes extremely severe is the decision made to seek medical advice.

However, many epidemiologists suggest that medical care itself may be less important in determining health than is social class. The pervasiveness of the influence of social class or income on health is evident in countries such as Great Britain. Although Great Britain has had a national health service since 1945, several studies show that social class continues to be correlated significantly with many measures of child health.

Numerous other reports have shown that income-related problems may be ameliorated by reducing barriers to accessibility. In one experiment (by Alpert and his colleagues), low-income families were provided with a model of care similar to that provided in a middle-class group practice.[1] Compared with a control group that received episodic care, the experimental group had fewer hospitalizations, operations, and illness visits, obtained more preventive services and more health supervision visits, and reported greater satisfaction—all at a relatively low cost.

Changes in health care delivery in other countries have yielded similar results. After the introduction of universal health insurance in Canada, for instance, increases were reported in the number of lower-income families seeking early prenatal care, postpartum checkups, and postnatal examinations of infants. Increases in the percentage of individuals consulting physicians for symptoms related to measles, tonsillitis, diarrhea, and vomiting were also noted.

Current Public Health Issues: The New Morbidity

The term *new morbidity* has been used to draw attention to a group of child health problems that assumed growing importance during the 1960s. Although none of the problems were, strictly speaking, "new," they had gained in prominence as many of the causes of the old, traditional morbidity declined. Thus in place of nutritional and vitamin deficiencies, for example, more attention is being paid to school and behavioral problems, accidents, and problems of adolescence, and there is a growing concern for a more comprehensive approach to the care of children with chronic disorders.

The argument for adopting community strategies to deal with these problems is strengthened by the fact that complex, interacting factors characterize much of the new morbidity. No single etiologic factor predominates, nor are these problems amenable to single or simple forms of treatment. Many involve, simultaneously and equally, dysfunction in the child, in the family, and in the community. For example, biologic, psychological, and sociologic forces are at work in most school and behavioral problems. The greatest challenge presented by the new morbidity is the oldest of all—prevention. A group of scientists led by Breslow[3] systematically assessed many preventive measures aimed at children. Much the same sort of exercise was conducted in Canada by a task force responsible for evaluating periodic health examinations (e.g., routine checkups or, in the case of infants, well-baby care). Further assessments of this contentious issue are provided in a 1989 review by Hoekelman[6] and in a report from the Office of Technology Assessment of the U.S. Congress.[15] It is generally agreed that it is not yet possible to prove the value of many procedures listed in the American Academy of Pediatrics' Guidelines for Childhood Health Supervision. Nonetheless, there is some basis for concluding that primary and secondary prevention of conditions such as maladjustment, smoking, dental caries, malnutrition, accidents, communicable diseases, and unwanted pregnancies are warranted but only at specified intervals or ages and in some cases only for well-defined high-risk subgroups. How these procedures can be implemented most effectively, whether certain procedures can be done in private practices, and how the effects are to be evaluated must still be determined. Also to be resolved are questions about how such preventive services are best organized and financed.

Apart from economic issues and those related to organization, one further major obstacle to accomplishing many of the preventive objectives arising from the new morbidity may be the astonishing neglect of one of the most important determinants of a child's health and health care—the family. Practitioners and academicians recognize that the family may either generate the psychological stress that results in dysfunction or provide the child's needed social support. Although much lip service is paid to the need to know more about families, many physicians remain ignorant of many of the most fundamental structural and functional aspects of the families they treat.

REFERENCES

1. Alpert JJ et al: Delivery of health care for children: report of an experiment, Pediatrics 57:917, 1976.
2. Andersen RA: Behavioral model of families' use of health services, Center for Health Administration Studies, Research Series, Chicago, 1968.
3. Breslow L et al: Preventive medicine USA: theory, practice and application of prevention in personal health services, Canton, Mass, 1976, Watson Publishing International.
4. Fingerhut LA and Kleinman JC: Trends and current status in childhood mortality, US Department of Health and Human Services, Public Health Service DHHS Pub No (PHS) 89-1410, Washington, DC, 1989.
5. Hagberg B et al: The changing panorama of cerebral palsy in Sweden. V. The birth year period 1979-82, Acta Paediatr Scand 78:283, 1989.
6. Hoekelman RA: An appraisal of the effectiveness of child health supervision, Curr Opinion Pediatr 1:146, 1989.
7. Hoekelman RA and Pless IB: Decline in mortality among young Americans during the twentieth century: prospects for reaching national mortality-reduction goals for 1990, Pediatrics 82:582, 1988.
8. Hoekelman RA et al: A profile of pediatric practice in the United States, Am J Dis Child 137:1057, 1983.
9. Kozak LJ and McCarthy E: Hospital use by children in the United States and Canada, National Center for Health Statistics, Vital and Health Statistics Series 5, No 1, DHHS Pub No (PHS) 84-1477, Washington, DC, 1984, US Government Printing Office.
10. Perrin JM et al: Variations in rates of hospitalization of children in three urban communities, N Engl J Med 320:1183, 1989.
11. Roghmann KG and Haggerty RJ: Daily stress, illness, and use of health services Pediatr Res 7:520, 1973.
12. Rosenstock IM: Why people use health services. II., Milbank Mem Fund Q 44:94, 1966.
13. Starfield B et al: Who provides health care to children and adolescents in the United States? Pediatrics 74:991, 1984.
14. Suchman EA: Social patterns of illness and medical care, J Health Hum Behav 6:2, 1965.
15. US Congress, Office of Technology Assessment: Healthy children: investing in the future, Pub No OTA-H-345, Washington, DC, 1988, US Government Printing Office.

SUGGESTED READING

Wegman ME: Annual summary of vital statistics, 1987, Pediatrics 82:817, 1988.

3

Child Health Supervision

Robert A. Hoekelman

We credit George Armstrong as the father of ambulatory pediatrics and the champion of health maintenance and disease prevention in the individual child—this at a time in nineteenth century England when most of his colleagues were concerned only with the treatment of illness. In the United States child health supervision had its beginnings in the milk stations and child health conferences of our large cities, where babies were brought to be fed, weighed, examined, and immunized against contagious diseases. It was the conviction of the importance of child health supervision that provided the fundamental impetus for the establishment of the American Academy of Pediatrics (AAP) and that continues to be the principle upon which pediatrics as a special discipline is based. At the American Public Health Association's 1955 conference on health supervision of young children, health was defined as "a state of physical, mental, and social well-being, not merely the absence of disease or infirmity"; the objective of health supervision for children was deemed "to keep the well child well and promote the highest possible level of his complete well-being."[3]

It has not been documented how the frequency and content of well-child visits have evolved. However, in 1967, the AAP established guidelines, based on observed practices and expert opinion, for child health supervision. These were revised in 1974, in 1977, in 1982, in 1985, and most recently in 1988, again based on similar observations and opinions. The guidelines call for 20 health supervision visits during the first 21 years of life (Table 3-1) in addition to a prenatal visit and at least two visits in the hospital following birth. The guidelines are designed for the care of children who are receiving competent parenting, have no manifestations of any important health problems, and are growing and developing satisfactorily. Additional visits may become necessary if circumstances suggest variations from normal.[1]

In the 23 years following the introduction of the initial guidelines, pediatric practitioners and investigators have begun to reexamine the objectives of child health supervision and the methods by which those objectives can be met realistically in terms of needs, costs, and benefits.

OBJECTIVES

The objectives of child health supervision have been categorized in several ways. Basically, there are three:

1. Prevention of disease
    a. Immunization
    b. Health education
2. Early detection and treatment of disease
    a. History
    b. Physical examination
    c. Screening
3. Guidance in psychosocial aspects of child rearing

Disease Prevention

The first objective is accomplished mostly through immunization against specific communicable diseases and through health education initially directed to the parents and later to the child when the age of understanding and reasoning is reached. These educational efforts concern general and dental hygiene, nutrition, and accident prevention. The aim of this approach is the improvement of individual and public health. These elements of disease prevention are discussed in detail in Chapters 16, 17, 20, and 21.

Early Detection and Treatment of Disease

The second objective is based on the presumption that early intervention in identified illnesses will result in increased cure rates and decreased disability.

Through history-taking and physical assessment of how well or poorly an infant or child is growing and developing compared with suggested norms, invaluable criteria are provided for identification of wellness or of underlying disease. In this sense, these activities are screening tests as much as are those specific tests pediatricians use routinely to detect the presence of anemia, urinary tract infections, tuberculosis, phenylketonuria, sickle cell disease, lead intoxication, and other illnesses in asymptomatic, seemingly normal infants and children.

The principles and techniques of history-taking and the physical examination of infants, young children, and adolescents are detailed in Chapters 6 and 7. The use of the physical examination for early detection of disease is discussed in Chapter 18, as are the specific screening tests used and the methods by which motor, intellectual, social, and emotional development are assessed and monitored in well children.

Guidance in Psychosocial Aspects of Child Rearing

The psychosocial aspect of child health supervision is often placed under the rubrics of advice, anticipatory guidance, counseling, and reassuring the parents about their concerns and that they are doing a good job. Well-child visits offer an opportunity to identify potential and real problems in psy-

Table 3-1 *Guidelines for Childhood Health Supervision*

ITEM	INFANCY						EARLY CHILDHOOD					LATE CHILDHOOD					ADOLESCENCE			
Age	By 1 mo	2 mo	4 mo	6 mo	9 mo	12 mo	15 mo	16 mo	24 mo	3 y	4 y	5 y	6 y	8 y	10 y	12 y	14 y	16 y	18 y	20 + y
History																				
Initial/interval	●	●	●	●	●	●	●	●	●	●	●	●	●	●	●	●	●	●	●	●
Measurements																				
Height and weight	●	●	●	●	●	●	●	●	●	●	●	●	●	●	●	●	●	●	●	●
Head circumference	●	●	●	●	●	●						●	●	●	●	●	●	●	●	●
Blood pressure										●	●									
Sensory screening																				
Vision	S	S	S	S	S	S	S	S	S	S	O	O	O	O	S	O	O	S	O	O
Hearing	S	S	S	S	S	S	S	S	S	S	O	O	S	S	S	O	S	S	O	S
Development/behavior assessment	●	●	●	●	●	●	●	●	●	●	●	●	●	●	●	●	●	●	●	●
Physical examination	●	●	●	●	●	●	●	●	●	●	●	●	●	●	●	●	●	●	●	●
Procedures																				
Hereditary/metabolic screening	●																			
Immunization		●	●	●			●	●				●					●			
Tuberculin test	←					● →	←		●		→	←		●		→	←		●	→
Hematocrit or hemoglobin	←				●	→	←		●		→	←		●		→	←		●	→
Urinalysis	←			●		→	←		●		→	←		●		→	←		●	→
Anticipatory guidance	●	●	●	●	●	●	●	●	●	●	●	●	●	●	●	●	●	●	●	●
Initial dental referral										●										

Key: Closed circle indicates to be performed; S, subjective, by history; O, objective, by a standard testing method; arrow, once within that period.
Recommended by the American Academy of Pediatrics' Committee on Practice and Ambulatory Medicine, September 1987; adapted with permission.
From Hoekelman RA: An appraisal of the effectiveness of child health supervision, Current Opinion in Pediatrics 1:146, 1989.

chosocial adjustment, to prevent potential disorders, to treat actual disorders early in their courses, and to make referrals for children and their families with gross interpersonal relationship problems that are beyond the therapeutic scope of the primary care practitioner. Anticipatory guidance in these areas is discussed in Chapter 15.

Continuity of Care

Some feel that there is a fourth objective of well-child care—continuity of care. This actually can be considered more an outcome of well-child care than an objective, since it speaks to the establishment of a meaningful relationship between the pediatrician and the parents and child. It implies that regular visits produce familiarity, trust, and respect and that these enable the physician to be more effective in the management of all aspects of health and illness care.

That continuity of care makes a difference in these respects, however, has not been proven, and although it seems a logical assumption, a physician who demonstrates interest in and concern for the child and family can establish a meaningful relationship instantly without that prior experience of continuity. Conversely, meaningful relationships can dissolve just as quickly if interest and concern are not sustained, regardless of past performance.

EVALUATION OF THE EFFECTIVENESS OF CHILD HEALTH SUPERVISION

The basis of the effectiveness of child health supervision (and of illness care also) lies in the pediatrician's ability to influence the parents to follow the advice and prescriptions given them. Professional competence is of little use if parental compliance is not obtained. The level of compliance is positively correlated with satisfaction, and satisfaction with effective communication between the parent and the physician, nurse, or other health professional. These interactions are extremely complex and, in part, relate to addressing the parent's concerns and expectations and the need to understand the rationale for recommendations made. The degree of satisfaction and compliance achieved depends on the extent to which these needs are acknowledged and met and on the parent's perception of the physician's empathy and view of him or her as a person (reflexive self-concept). These perceptions are formed very rapidly, often in the first moments of communication. The means by which communication and maternal compliance are enhanced are discussed in detail in Chapter 12.

There is reason to believe, on the basis of observation of individual practitioners, that health professionals are doing a good job in meeting the objectives of child health supervision for *some* of their patients and their families. However, this is not the case for most of the children in the country. Studies of the levels of child health care achieved for specific population groups demonstrate that, for most children, practitioners fall far short of their goals. These data show that in poor urban and rural areas, less than 5% of children receive levels of well-child care consistent with the AAP's recommendations, and even in relatively affluent suburban and rural communities only one third to two fifths of children receive care at that level.

There are indications that practitioners are not meeting the objectives of well-child care for the vast majority of children whose parents seek such care for them.

Time-motion studies of pediatricians conducting well-child care have shown that very little time is spent on well-child visits—12 minutes on average. This has been true for private as well as clinic patients. One must question whether the objectives of well-child care can be reached in such a short period of time. These studies show that pediatric nurse practitioners working in the same practices spend considerably more time on well-child care (30 minutes) than do their physician colleagues.

Very few studies have assessed the content of well-child visits in terms of the amount of time pediatricians and parents spend discussing psychosocial issues and concerns. Reisinger and Bires[8] demonstrated that anticipatory guidance constituted only about 8.4% of the total time pediatricians spent in well-child visits. The researchers averaged 52 seconds in providing such guidance, with a high of 97 seconds for visits involving infants 5 months of age or younger and a low of 7 seconds for patients 13 to 18 years of age.

The AAP's guidelines for health supervision are controversial because of concerns that (1) there have been no data to indicate the need for so many visits or the value of what is done during them, save administering immunizations; and (2) there are not nor will there ever be enough health care professionals (pediatricians, family medicine practitioners, nurse practitioners, or physician's assistants) to deliver such care to all or even a significant portion of our children.[2,7] Others are concerned that adhering to these guidelines ensures that the maldistribution of pediatricians (too many in suburban areas and not enough in inner city, urban, and rural areas) will continue, denying access by underserved children (Medicaid recipients) to all facets of child health care.[5]

During the past 30 years many investigators have reviewed the overall effectiveness of child health supervision; these reviews were incorporated in a 1988 report by a study group of the Office of Technology Assessment (OTA) of the U.S. Congress. The report was an in-depth study of preventive child health services, including well-child care.[9] The study group's conclusions ranged from strongly negative to strongly positive, based on its opinion regarding intervening or process outcomes the group viewed as bad (high costs, uneven personnel distribution, overdependence of parents on health care providers) or as good (parent and provider satisfaction, improved parental compliance with provider instructions, better acute care through establishment of an informed and trusting relationship). However, the study group was unable to base its conclusions on any prospective studies that meet Elinson's accepted criteria.[4] These criteria require that studies be prospective, involve some planned intervention (such as child health supervision as recommended by the AAP) designed to achieve specific end points (such as improved child health in terms of decreased mortality and morbidity), and include control as well as experimental groups. Meeting Elinson's criteria presents some difficulties in evaluating the effectiveness of child health supervision.

In its 1977 report, the AAP's Ad Hoc Committee on the Value of Preventive Child Health Care[6] stated, in applying Elinson's criteria to child health supervision, that preventive child health care is a process applied throughout infancy and childhood and would require study over many years if its overall value were to be proven. This creates problems in maintaining sample and investigator continuity, because patient mobility and academic permanency (a condition affecting potential researchers) is, in general, short lived. Overcoming patient mobility could be counteracted by appropriately increasing the size of the initial experimental and control groups to allow for losses. Maintaining investigator continuity would require personal commitment and good health over time; these requisites, particularly that of continuity, are not always assured for academicians, who are most likely to be chosen for principal investigator positions in studies of this type.

The end points chosen could include indexes of health and illness, school performance, or psychosocial adjustment. New instruments for the measurement of indexes in any of these areas, however, would have to be developed, particularly to maintain uniformity throughout the samples. Large samples would be required, because there would be multiple intervening independent variables, and the differences in the end points would most likely be small. A multicenter study design would be required to overcome geographic, economic, and cultural population variables; this would compound the investigator-continuity problems and create difficulties in standardization.

Any long-range study carries the risk of process and measurement obsolescence. For example, new preventive care procedures could become operative at midpoint and distort planned end-point measures; or end points considered significant at the beginning of the study may no longer be significant at the end of the study through interim social, political, educational, or medical changes.

The costs of conducting a study of this type would be extremely high, and the prospects for assured, continued funding, even with sanction and direction from the AAP, might not be bright.

Another consideration is the ethical issue of withholding from children in the control group methods of medical management considered valuable. This could be addressed through a passive relationship with the control group and an aggressive promotion of the AAP's preventive care recommendations with the experimental group. A retrospective approach could be used with the control group consisting of children who had received no or few preventive health care services.

The Ad Hoc Committee on the Value of Preventive Child Health Care recognized that the task it recommended is complex and will require considerable time and effort to complete. Nevertheless, it must be done, and the necessary steps must be taken to ensure that these recommendations are carried out.

The OTA study group[9] added to these limitations of studying the overall effectiveness of child health supervision the observation that, "The health status of children in particular (and the population in general) is far more strongly determined by social and economic factors than by the nature of medical care; hence, the contribution that well-child care can make to health outcomes is likely to be modest, and studies to detect these modest contributions must be based on very large samples. Few available studies of the effectiveness of child health care have had very large samples. None of them directly address the question of the overall effectiveness of well-child care."

The OTA study group's review of the literature evaluating the effectiveness of well-child care as a whole concludes that well-child care as now performed (other than immunization) has no overall effect on childhood mortality or morbidity and exerts little influence on developmental and social functioning outcomes. Despite this, child health supervision will remain the basis upon which most pediatric practices are built, because it provides parental and physician satisfaction and reassurance (in some cases conviction) that well-child visits keep children well and prevent serious illnesses.

ALTERATION OF STANDARDS

If society accepts the premises that large segments of the child population are not receiving what practitioners feel to be optimal health care and that good health care is an inherent right of all citizens and not simply a privilege available to those who can afford it, it becomes obvious that practitioners must compromise their standards of adequate well-child care, the methods of delivering that care, or both.

In regard to altering the standards of child health supervision, practitioners must consider that there is some substantiation that a reduction in the frequency of visits, at least for infants who have been identified as being at low risk, does not alter the outcomes in terms of their physical health. Thus, decreasing the number of visits by 50% could be accomplished without compromising one aspect of the quality of care. Practitioners must consider that some children may require only minimal health supervision other than completion of immunization schedules, whereas others will require much, much more.

Another alternative would be the use of persons other than physicians to provide child health care. Pediatricians have, for the most part, been reluctant to do this for a variety of reasons, not the least of which is their concern that quality of child health supervision would be reduced in these circumstances. There is, however, good evidence that the use of nonphysicians, particularly the pediatric nurse practitioner, for most elements of well-child care does not reduce the quality of child care. Studies performed in private practices, prepaid group practices, and university hospital clinics have demonstrated that pediatric nurse practitioners are entirely competent to provide well-child care and that the care they render does not result in altered health outcomes, increased utilization, decreased compliance, or decreased parental satisfaction. Equally important, this model is less expensive than that in which the physician provides all elements of well-child care.

Consideration of the costs of care must include (1) use of physician time that might be more effectively applied to other health problems; (2) the extent to which taxes should be used to support activities that have so few proved beneficial outcomes; and (3) a family's ability to afford the fees charged, the expenditures for transportation and baby-sitting services while the parent is away from the home, and the loss of income for working parents who must comply with daytime private practice, clinic, and health center visit schedules.

DISCUSSION

Studies of pediatric practices carried out from the early 1930s through the early 1980s have consistently shown that one third to one half of visits made to pediatricians are for child health supervision and that as much as 50% of the time pediatricians spend in their offices is spent in this activity. In adhering to the AAP's guidelines, pediatricians would limit the number of children they can care for who have other health and illness care needs that are currently unmet. It seems that practitioners must either explore further the evidence at hand to determine if they can reduce the frequency of well-child visits or employ others to conduct them. Practitioners need to alter their perspectives on traditional professional roles and methods and focus on the goal of meeting the health supervision needs of all children.

REFERENCES

1. American Academy of Pediatrics: Guidelines for health supervision II, Elk Grove Village, Ill, 1988, The Academy.
2. Chamberlin RW, Schiff DW, and Rogers KD: Are routine periodic child health visits beneficial? In Smith DH and Hoekelman RA, editors: Controversies in child health and pediatric practice, New York, 1981, McGraw-Hill Book Co.
3. Committee on Child Health: Health supervision of young children, New York, 1955, American Public Health Association.
4. Elinson J: Effectiveness of social action programs in health and welfare. Assessing the Effectiveness of Children's Health Services. Report of the fifty-sixth Ross Conference on Pediatric Research, Columbus, Ohio, 1967, Ross Laboratories.
5. Fossett JW and Peterson JA: Physician supply and Medicaid participation, Med Care 27:386, 1989.
6. Hoekelman RA and Thompson HC: Value of preventive child health care, Evanston, Ill, 1977, American Academy of Pediatrics.
7. Hoekelman RA: Well-child visits revisited, Am J Dis Child 137:17, 1983.
8. Reisinger KS and Bires JA: Anticipatory guidance in pediatric practice, Pediatrics 66:889, 1980.
9. US Congress, Office of Technology Assessment: Healthy children: investing in the future, Pub No OTA-H-345, Washington, DC, 1988, US Government Printing Office.

SUGGESTED READING

Hoekelman RA: An appraisal of the effectiveness of child health supervision, Curr Opinion Pediatr 1:146, 1989.

4

Legal Aspects of Pediatric Medicine

Richard E. Cuskar, M. Aileen Brown, and Judith M. Norman

OVERVIEW

In addition to diagnosing and treating a variety of patients of varying ages and providing an ever-increasing number of medical services, pediatricians frequently must deal with legal issues and questions that arise in the course of their practice. Although this chapter is not intended to provide definitive answers to these legal questions, many of the issues are addressed to alert practitioners to the situations that can give rise to legal concerns.

"The law," as it may be referred to, is actually a compilation created from a variety of sources. First, there are statutes, which are enacted by both the states and the federal government. Next, there are regulations, which are promulgated by either a governmental entity or an administrative agency and which generally supplement and explain the statutes in greater detail. Finally, there is *case* law, which is the judicial interpretation of the written law as presented in various situations. In addition, a practitioner's actions may be affected by the bylaws of various health care entities, such as hospitals, which regulate those individuals who work and practice therein.

Because the body of law is constantly changing and evolving, and because the statutes, regulations, and case results often vary greatly from state to state, it would be impossible for this chapter to provide conclusive answers to every legal question that might come up in a pediatric practice. In addition, new medical-legal issues often arise that require legislative action in an area where none existed before, such as the many statutes recently enacted regarding acquired immune deficiency syndrome (AIDS). Hence, what follows contains only general statements of law that may be helpful in creating a conceptual knowledge of legal principles relevant in a pediatrician's daily practice. When specific legal questions occur in particular medical situations, a physician should not hesitate to consult an attorney knowledgeable in this field for more definitive answers and guidance.

Right to Treatment

Although people often assume that everyone has an absolute right to medical treatment, no such constitutional or legislative endowment actually exists. Since the fourteenth century, an accepted principle of English and American common law has obligated each person to pay for provision of "necessaries" for himself or herself and spouse and dependents. Among these necessaries, which include food, shelter, and clothing, are medical services.

A burgeoning area for granting an absolute right to treatment is emergencies. In some states, court decisions or statutes now require that health care providers furnish the care necessary to alleviate an emergency, and one may be held civilly or criminally liable if such care is not rendered. Although some believe that these rules apply primarily to public institutions, many more locales have made it illegal for health care providers generally to refuse emergency treatment, regardless of the patient's ability to pay.

There are also situations in which individuals must be treated regardless of payment source. For example, participants in the Medicare system cannot be denied treatment by facilities or by practitioners who participate in the Medicare program. The same is true in many state systems of medical reimbursement, such as Medicaid. Licensed health care facilities must not discriminate in providing treatment. This protection is based on the Fourteenth Amendment's equal protection clause and on Medicare and Medicaid regulations governing participation.

Private physicians, however, operate under different circumstances. Physicians in most states can refuse to treat any private patient for any reason. Although they are ethically bound to refer appropriately a patient who has been refused treatment, there is usually no legal requirement to do so. A physician who has already initiated care, however, is legally obligated to continue such care or, if this proves impossible, to effect a referral. This follows the common law theory of negligence that an individual is not required to assist another person in need; however, particularly in a medical practitioner's case, once care is provided, it cannot be terminated if harm might come to the patient. Termination at such point can be deemed patient abandonment, which can be grounds for disciplinary, civil, and possibly criminal action. Therefore, to terminate the relationship with a private patient, the physician should give sufficient notice and assistance so as not to jeopardize the individual's medical condition.

Parent-Child Relationship

With respect to children, their right to treatment is governed to a certain extent by the actions of their parents or guardians, who are generally vested with the authority to consent to medical treatment for children. Common law required a parent to be responsible for both the care and the acts of his offspring. Historically, a child had no legal existence outside

Portions of this chapter were written by Jeffrey M. Alexander, J.D. and appeared in the first edition of this book as "Legal Issues in Child Health."

that of his father. Were the father a noble, a free man, or a serf, so was the child. No concept of the child having rights independent of the parent existed. The child lived totally under parental tyranny, for better or for worse. If the parent kept a child out of school, denied a child medical treatment, or whipped or starved a child to death, this was considered a family matter of no concern to the state.

Such control, however, creates obligations for parents nowadays. Under modern law parents must act in the child's best interest. Unlike common law, there exist today numerous child protection statutes, ranging from the child labor restrictions and school attendance requirements of the last century to today's child abuse and neglect statutes. The parent who does not care for his or her child, mistreats the child, or fails to protect the child's best interest and welfare can be removed from his or her natural role by the state. Although the law naturally prefers allowing parents to raise their own children, this century has also introduced the legal theory of *parens patriae*.

Parens patriae means "parent of the country" and originates in ancient common law, whereby the king possessed a royal prerogative to act as the guardian of all disabled persons, such as infants and mentally and physically disabled. If the child's natural parent does not fulfill his or her parental obligations, the state can act *in loco parentis,* in place of the parent, and fulfill the parent's duties and responsibilities. Evidence of the state's *parens patriae* power is common today, from child welfare and child protective statutes to enforcement of school attendance laws and the mandating of specific health care for certain children.

All states in this country now possess some mechanism to remove a child from parental physical, emotional, or sexual abuse. The state acts *in loco parentis* in such cases, with authority to place the child in a state institution or with foster parents; if the home situation is sufficiently severe, the state can even allow the child to be adopted.

To some degree, however, the concept of absolute parental control still exists. A child's legal interests generally must be represented by the parents or legal guardians, who also remain to this day responsible for the child's support and most aspects of his or her physical, spiritual, and intellectual upbringing. This responsibility vests the parent or guardian with considerable power in making medical decisions for the child, as will be discussed in more detail later in the chapter.

Definition of Minority

In order to determine whether a child has the legal capacity to consent to or contract for medical services, a physician must determine whether under state law the child is a minor without legal capacity to consent or whether the child has reached an age where he or she is presumed to have the capacity to consent to and contract for such medical services. All states have statutes that provide an age at which a child is assumed to be an adult for legal purposes, at which time the child is said to have reached the *age of majority*. Typically, the statute is brief and states something to the effect that all persons of the age of 18 years or more, who are under no legal disability, are capable of contracting and are of full age for all purposes.[1]

Before attaining the age of majority, a child is limited both in ability to contract for the provision of medical services and in ability to consent to the provision of such services. Generally, unless a minor is emancipated, the only instances when a minor can consent to the provision of medical services are those situations in which a statute or regulation has expressly made provisions for the child's consent. Aside from such statutory provisions, parents are given a great deal of authority with respect to their children. One Georgia statute, in fact, specifically provides that until reaching the age of majority, a child "shall remain under the control of his parents, who are entitled to his services and the proceeds of his labor."[2]

CONSENT ISSUES IN PEDIATRICS

Doctrine of Informed Consent

The concept of *informed consent* has its roots in common law. Common law required a patient to have a *fiduciary relationship* with the physician; that is, the patient placed a "special trust or confidence" in the physician, who was required to act in good faith and in the patient's best interest. Because of the physician's special knowledge and training and "the ignorance and helplessness of the patient regarding his own physical condition," the physician has a duty to disclose to the patient all pertinent facts regarding the patient's condition and the recommended treatment.[3]

Informed consent concerns the patient's right of self-determination of medical treatment. Legally competent adults or emancipated minors (those who are under 18 years of age and married, parents of their own offspring, or self-sufficiently living away from the family domicile with parental consent) have the right to accept or reject treatment by a physician. Medical treatment cannot be forced on them should they decide to decline its possible benefits. As Justice Benjamin Cardozo stated in a landmark informed consent decision,

> Every human being of adult years and sound mind has a right to determine what shall be done with his own body; and a surgeon who performs an operation without his patient's consent commits an assault, for which he is liable in damages.[4]

Elements of Informed Consent

The physician's obligation is "to explain the procedure to the patient and to warn him of any material risks or dangers inherent in or collateral to the therapy, so as to enable the patient to make an intelligent and informed choice about whether or not to undergo such treatment."[5] Courts generally require that the patient be told, in language that he or she can comprehend, the diagnosis, the nature and purpose of the proposed procedure, the risks and benefits of such treatment, the prognosis if the proposed treatment is declined, and any alternative methods of treatment as well as the risks and consequences of the same, if any.

Obviously these concepts often are beyond the comprehension of pediatric patients, and disclosure to them would serve no useful purpose. In such a case the disclosure should be made to the competent adult responsible for the child's medical needs. Parents may consent for their minor children, or a legal guardian may consent for his or her ward, as is discussed more fully below.

The question often arises as to what risks need be revealed to a patient or the parents and which ones are so insignificant as not to require revelation. As one court has stated, "what is a reasonable disclosure in one instance may not be reasonable in another."[6]

The general rule is that if a procedure presents even a *remote* possibility of *serious* harm, then the patient must be informed. However, *known* side effects of even an extremely dangerous procedure (e.g., surgical incisions are painful) need not be revealed. There is a greater obligation to inform patients of relatively remote risks when alternative procedures exist that present less risk, with lesser or greater probabilities of success. Of course, the physician need not disclose a risk of which he or she is unaware *if* the physician's ignorance is not itself a violation of the duty of due care.

Informed consent, although possibly a burdensome process, can be the physician's best friend. The discussion regarding informed consent creates better rapport and confidence between patients and practitioners. A properly informed patient (or the parents in the case of a minor) may be less likely to bring legal action if the discussed complications do arise. Informed consent should not cause problems when discussions with the patient are adequately documented, even if the patient has forgotten. The informed consent conversation should lessen legal claims based on misunderstandings or unrealistic expectations.

The physician should take responsibility for discussing the proposed treatment with the patient. The physician should note in the medical record that the informed consent process was completed and should ensure that the required form has been placed in the record after having been signed by the patient or, if the patient cannot consent, by a relative. The consent form should indicate the condition to be treated, all the requirements of informed consent (risk, consequences of other treatment, possible alternatives), and the reasons the condition must be treated. If for some reason the patient is not informed of the risks of the procedure, this information should be stringently documented in the patient's chart.

Statutory Requirements

In most states the matter of informed consent is regulated by statute. Generally, a physician is required to disclose any information that a reasonable physician would have disclosed under similar circumstances. Some states, however, look to what a reasonable person in the patient's position should know. In New York, the patient has a medical malpractice cause of action if the required disclosures—alternative treatment and reasonably foreseeable risks and benefits of the proposed treatment, which a reasonable medical practitioner in similar circumstances would have disclosed "in a manner permitting the patient to make a knowledgeable evaluation"—are not made.[7]

Generally, informed consent is not required if (1) the risk is commonly known, (2) an emergency exists, and attempts to obtain consent would delay treatment and result in increased risk to the patient's life or health, (3) the patient has knowingly refused to be informed of any of the possible consequences or has made it clear that he or she would undergo any treatment, procedure, or diagnosis regardless of the risk, or (4) the patient's condition is such that the physician believes that informing him or her of certain information would have a substantial adverse effect (referred to as the *therapeutic privilege*).[8] This last exception, however, is of very limited application.

Consent for Treatment of Minors

In most states consent for treating minors can be given by either parent, even if the parents are legally separated, except in certain divorce situations in which the custody decree gives one parent exclusive control over the child's medical care.

Such consent should be obtained from the parent, documented in the chart, and supported by a signed consent form. The best consent is that received in person. If in an emergency consent cannot be received in person, a recorded telephone call, a call with a witness on the line, or a call that is later documented in the chart, in that order, may suffice. A letter or, if time is crucial, an exchange of telegrams can act as even better documentation until other arrangements are made.

A Massachusetts statute that is common elsewhere states that no physician, dentist, or hospital will be held liable for failure to obtain the consent of a parent or guardian to emergency examination or treatment if delay in treatment would endanger the life, limb, or mental well-being of the patient.[9] In addition, consent usually does not have to be obtained for routine, low-risk, nonsurgical care. For example, should the child have a cut finger, application of antiseptic and a bandage does not require consent. Similarly, a child brought by a parent into a physician's office or a hospital for treatment can be given basic care (e.g., have blood drawn, temperature taken, intravenous line inserted, medication prescribed) through a theory of *implied consent*—that is, a parent would not have brought the child into the office or hospital if he or she did not want the child to receive medical attention.

When a child is residing away from the parents, a physician cannot automatically assume that the party with whom the child is residing has the authority to consent to the child's medical treatment. Children residing with relatives or family friends, as well as children in institutions and foster homes, may or may not still require parental, as opposed to surrogate parental, consent.

Although foster homes, social service agencies, and juvenile facilities may have custody of the child's body, even they may not be empowered to consent to the child's medical care. Most states have statutory provisions allowing social service agencies to consent to medical care and treatment for children within their custody, although some do not. Although the child is living away from the parental abode, in many instances parental consent still is necessary and may be obtained from parents before placing the child in a foster home or protective custody. This can be difficult, however, when the parents have disappeared or are uncooperative.

In a possible or clear emergency, the assumption always should be on the side of treating the child. Arizona specifically allows that any person, standing in place of the parents, can acquiesce to a minor's emergency treatment when the parents of the child cannot be located for the purposes of consenting to the treatment.[10] When there is no emergency and a real question about elective treatment exists, in many localities it is possible to apply for court resolution of a minor's guardianship or for the appointment of a temporary guardian whose sole action would be to consent to the recommended treatment.

Minor's Consent to Treatment

In virtually all the states an individual is legally a minor and is incapable of consenting to treatment until he or she has reached the age of 18. Minors are presumed in most situations to lack the capacity to comprehend the impact of their decisions fully when they are requested to consent to medical treatment. In such situations therefore a parent or guardian is legally authorized to make such determinations.

At times, however, a physician may accept a minor's own consent to treatment without parental concurrence. States recognize that minors who have been emancipated by marriage, parenthood, military service, consent of their parents, or judicial decree may consent to medical treatment. Some states have taken the concept of the emancipated minor one step further and have allowed minors of a certain age (commonly 16) who have not lived at home for a specific period of time (commonly 6 months) to seek a judicial determination of emancipation. Parental permission to live away from home and financial self-support are not necessary ingredients for this status.

Other states have statutes that specifically allow minors of a certain age (typically 15 or 16) to consent to medical or surgical care without their parents' consent. Furthermore, many state statutes dealing with conditions such as venereal disease and pregnancy allow treatment of all minors, regardless of whether they have been emancipated, when there is a possibility of harm resulting from delay or nontreatment because of the minor's fear of telling his or her parents.

The minor's consent is generally not required if a parent or guardian consents; however, the practitioner, particularly with older, more mature minors, may find cooperation much easier if the patient can be involved in the decision regarding treatment. Should a minor be of sufficient "maturity" to take part in making a treatment decision, the pediatrician may approach the parents and suggest that the child be involved in this discussion.

If consent to medical treatment has been obtained from a minor, courts generally have held that such consent is binding upon the minor and may not be disaffirmed when the minor reaches the age of majority. In one case a minor who consented to a nonemergency surgical operation later attempted to disaffirm her consent upon reaching the age of majority so as to bring a malpractice action. The court refused to disaffirm her consent, because she had reached the age of discretion when she consented, and there was nothing to indicate that she was under any physical or mental disability at that time.[11]

Parental Refusal to Consent

If medical treatment is necessary and the parents for any reason refuse to consent (e.g., on religious grounds), the courts may ignore the parental objections and order the necessary procedure. This may even occur in the case of a pregnant mother who refuses treatment that may aid her unborn child. Frequently, courts will order the pregnant mother, a competent adult who ordinarily would have the exclusive right to refuse treatment, to accept medical care for her unborn child's benefit.

Often state laws and the courts ensure the child's right to receive proper health care. There are many cases in which courts have required blood transfusions for the children of Jehovah's Witnesses when the parents refused such transfusions on religious grounds. Courts have held that although a competent adult, who will leave no dependents who will become wards of the state, has a total right to make decisions regarding his or her own medical treatment, even if such a decision surely will lead to death, a parent does not have that power over a child's life. As with other types of parental decisions with respect to children, the courts have been unwilling to stand by and allow parents to make a martyr of their child.[12]

In its role of *parens patriae,* the state is often empowered by the courts to take over the parental function for a specific purpose, such as consenting to a blood transfusion. In one case a father who was a member and lay minister of a religious sect that believed that God is "all curing" refused to allow his 12-year-old daughter, who was suffering from cancer, to receive treatment. A Tennessee court took the child away from her father and ordered the state Human Services director to consent to and seek chemotherapy and radiation treatments for the child until her parents agreed to provide her with this care.[13]

The problem may be more difficult when the child shares the parents' religious or other beliefs or for other reasons concurs in the refusal of treatment. Courts may uphold the minor's right to refuse treatment whether the parents agree or disagree. In one case a court ruled that a lower court decision mandating a blood transfusion for a child of Jehovah's Witnesses should be remanded to determine the child's opinion.[14] In a later decision the court noted that the child had expressed a desire not to have the operation that would have necessitated the blood transfusion, and therefore dismissed the petition that requested the transfusion.[15]

Treatment of Handicapped Newborns

Another question that has caused considerable controversy is whether a parent has the right to refuse possible lifesaving medical or surgical treatment for a profoundly disabled newborn infant. The federal government, through section 504 of the Rehabilitation Act of 1973,[16] had sought in several cases to intercede in hospital decisions concerning the treatment of seriously ill newborns. Section 504 provides that no qualified handicapped individual "shall, solely by reason of his handicap, be excluded from the participation in, be denied the benefits of, or be subjected to discrimination under any program or activity receiving federal financial assistance. . . . "

The hospitals that were fighting the government's interpretation argued that section 504 was not applicable to decisions of medical treatment involving *severely* impaired newborns and that by trying to make it applicable, the federal government was usurping traditional state review of health care. A federal Circuit Court of Appeals agreed with the hospitals and held that handicapped newborns did not fall within section 504's definition and that there was no indication that Congress, in enacting that section, intended to allow the federal government to regulate a traditional state concern (health care).[17]

This issue was later addressed by the U.S. Supreme Court, which upheld the earlier decision that the discrimination statutes are an inadequate basis for the U.S. Department of Health and Human Service's regulations concerning treatment of newborns. Federal law was held not to require hospitals to treat severely handicapped infants without parental consent, nor to require parents to give such consent.[18]

Despite the Supreme Court's rejection of the use of discrimination statutes as a basis for regulating the care given to handicapped newborns, other federal and state statutes still raise issues concerning treatment of handicapped newborns. For example, after courts rejected the application of the discrimination statutes, similar provisions governing care of handicapped newborns were included in the federal Child Abuse Amendments of 1984. Pursuant to these regulations, each state must have procedures within its child protective service system for the purpose of responding to reports that medically indicated treatment is being withheld from disabled infants with life-threatening conditions. Without such procedures, a state may fail to qualify for federal child abuse and neglect protection funds.

Generally, these regulations prohibit the withholding of medically indicated treatment from a disabled infant with a life-threatening condition.[19] This includes a hospital's failure to provide appropriate nutrition, hydration, and medication that in the treating physician's medical judgment would be most effective in ameliorating or correcting all of a disabled infant's conditions.[20] These regulations do not apply in limited circumstances, such as when the infant is irreversibly comatose or when providing such treatment would prolong dying and would be virtually futile in terms of the infant's survival.

Several of the states have also enacted statutes that govern the medical care provided to handicapped infants. Louisiana, for example, provides that:

> (1) No infant born alive shall be denied or deprived of food or nutrients, water, or oxygen by any person whomsoever with the intent to cause or allow the death of the child for any reason, including but not limited to the following:
> (a) The child was born with physical or mental handicapping conditions that, in the opinion of the parent or parents of the child, the physician, or other persons, diminishes the quality of the child's life. . . .[21]

Similarly, Rhode Island requires that a child abuse report be filed in any instance "where parents of an infant have requested deprivation of nutrition that is necessary to sustain life and/or who have requested deprivation of medical or surgical intervention that is necessary to remedy or ameliorate a life-threatening medical condition" if the nutrition or medical or surgical intervention is of the type generally provided to infants regardless of whether they are handicapped.[22]

Do Not Resuscitate Orders

An important corollary to the right to refuse medical treatment is the do not resuscitate (DNR) order, particularly in cases involving patients who have terminal illnesses. Generally, when adults have the capacity to consent, they are given the option, by statute in some states, to consent to the issuance of an order not to resuscitate in the event cardiopulmonary resuscitation becomes necessary. If an adult is found to be lacking the capacity to consent to such an order, a surrogate may be appointed for him or her in some instances.[23]

In New York a minor child may also be involved in the decision-making with respect to a DNR order, provided an attending physician, in consultation with the minor's parent or legal guardian, determines that the minor has the capacity to make a decision regarding resuscitation.[24] If a minor is determined to have the capacity to consent, the minor's consent and the consent of his or her parent or legal guardian must both be obtained before a DNR order is issued.

The New York statute, however, limits instances in which DNR orders can be issued to cases in which the minor has a terminal condition, the minor is permanently unconscious, resuscitation would be medically futile, or resuscitation would impose an extraordinary burden on the minor in light of the child's medical condition and the expected outcome of resuscitation.[25] The statute also provides that when parents are making a decision regarding cardiopulmonary resuscitation, they shall consider the minor's wishes and religious and moral beliefs.

CONFIDENTIALITY ISSUES IN PEDIATRICS

The Right to Privacy

Under common law and as codified in many state statutes, a physician-patient confidentiality privilege exists, requiring a physician to retain as completely confidential all information regarding the patient's medical status received in the course of treatment. This is an important patient right that may not be waived by the physician. The privilege belongs to the patient, and waiver thereof is entirely the patient's prerogative.

Privileged information generally may only be exchanged among professionals involved in the patient's care—nurses, other physicians, social workers, residents, medical students, and the like—or in situations of medical urgency, making release of information imperative, in the patient's best interest, and necessary for provision of care to the patient (e.g., the patient is in another care facility, and the physician's privileged knowledge of the patient's medical history is pertinent and necessary for his or her current treatment).

Breach of the physician-patient privilege by the physician is unethical and in many states can lead to disciplinary action or civil liability. In some states, however, statutes permit providers to release medical information without an authorization to certain specified individuals or entities. Generally, release is allowed pursuant to court order, subpoena, or search warrant; in those situations in which information is being provided to other health care facilities or providers for purposes of diagnosis or treatment of the patient; and to any insurer, governmental entity, or other third party payor to allow responsibility for payment to be determined and payment to be made.[26] However, unless a physician is authorized by statute or receives permission from the patient or direction from a court, disclosure of confidential medical information to any other source may subject the physician to civil liability and damages.

On the other hand, it should be understood that the right of privacy is not absolute. Most insurance companies, health maintenance organizations, and governmental payors require participants to sign a release of their records to the payors. In addition, the physician may be permitted to disclose confidential information in cases in which the patient places his or her medical condition in issue (e.g., accident cases in which the patient is hurt and the physician is subpoenaed by the other side) or in situations in which the physician has sued the patient, or vice versa (e.g., when a bill is not paid and the physician must prove what services were rendered, or in malpractice cases).

Many states have laws that require physicians to report the incidence of certain diseases, births, deaths, and other vital statistics. Criminal codes in many states require reporting gunshot and stab wounds, incidents of rape, and most commonly, incidents of child abuse. In fact in many states health practitioners must report child abuse if they have reasonable cause to suspect that a child whom they have seen in their professional capacity has been abused.[27] Court orders, summonses, and subpoenas in some states also can require the physician to breach the patient's right to privacy.

Access to Medical Records

The rules regarding patients' access to their own medical records differ from state to state. In some states patients have total and complete access to their medical records and limited access to psychiatric records. In others the patient's right to his or her own medical records is not so defined, leaving much more to the physician's or hospital's discretion. Some states modify these two limitations by not specifically defining the patient's right to his or her records but by requiring that the records be forwarded upon a patient's authorization, either to any party the patient directs or to parties specifically enumerated (other physicians, attorneys, and the like).

Parents usually have access rights to their children's medical records, except for certain confidential treatments discussed later in this chapter. Minors' rights to their own records, however, are not so clear. Although in some states minors are allowed the same access to their confidential medical records as adults, in other states they are allowed none. Some states have taken an intermediate approach, allowing minors access only to those medical records pertaining to health care of the type that the minor is lawfully entitled to consent (i.e., drug or alcohol abuse treatment and pregnancy or birth control treatment, depending on state law).[28] Furthermore, in most states minors have absolutely no right of access to their own psychiatric records. Children, of course, may need access to their medical records later in life, but minors may find on reaching majority that their medical records have been sealed or destroyed. Adoptive children, in addition, may have no access to medical information about their natural parents and may not have sufficient information on which to make important health care decisions about themselves as adults.

Similarly, it is generally the parent, not the minor, who is authorized to release the minor's medical information to others. Although parents are responsible for ensuring that the forwarding of confidential information to whatever source is in the child's best interest, the medical facility, provider, or governmental agency may not be so obligated to inform the parent or child of a request for medical records or of the information's release.

The patient's bill of rights that has been codified in several states ensures confidentiality of patients' hospital records and in some areas creates a cause of action for patients when this confidentiality is breached by one of the authorities mentioned previously. When dealing with schools, clubs, or other groups that request health information about minors, physicians are well advised to request written authorization from the minor's parents and if possible and feasible also from the minor, if he or she is mature, before releasing any of the minor's confidential medical records.

The patient's right of access to hospital records varies from state to state. There is case law in some states holding that hospital records are the property of the hospital and that therefore the patient does not have an unqualified right to access. With physicians' records, this property right has rarely been held so absolute. Practitioner records often are considered shared property with the patient, although few of the statutes speak of minors specifically. Under modifications of the law, when minors seek their own medical care they possess the same access rights as adults.

ISSUES CONCERNING SCHOOL-AGE CHILDREN

Very often the legal issues facing minors arise in the context of either their school activities or relationships that develop in the school environment. As young children grow into their teenage years, they go through periods of both physical growth and emotional development, and many new issues can arise in both the medical and legal context. In this section we'll discuss some issues concerning younger schoolchildren; in the next section we'll focus on some issues that concern older children.

Immunization Requirements

One of the first legal requirements that affect a child of school age is the requirement that certain immunizations be obtained before the child attends school. Virtually all states require these immunizations to prevent epidemics of easily transmitted contagious diseases such as measles. Massachusetts, for example, provides in part that:

> No child shall, except as hereinafter provided, be admitted to school except upon presentation of a physician's certificate that the child has been successfully immunized against diphtheria, pertussis, tetanus, measles and poliomyelitis and such other communicable diseases as may be specified from time to time by the department of public health. . . .[29]

In some situations, however, states will acquiesce to parents' refusal to consent to immunizations of their children if such refusal is based on the religious beliefs of the family, provided no medical exigency exists. In Connecticut, for example, children are exempt from the requirement that they be immunized before attending school if the immunization would violate the religious beliefs of the family.[30]

If a child receiving mandatory immunizations is injured, compensation may be available pursuant to federal law. In 1986 a National Vaccine Injury Compensation program was established to provide compensation for vaccine-related injuries or death.[31] The program provides that vaccine administrators cannot be made a party to civil actions for damages in an amount greater than $1,000 for an injury or death associated with the administration of a vaccine. Instead, the statute establishes a procedure whereby once an affidavit and supporting document are filed indicating that the injury or death occurred within a certain period after administration of the vaccine, the U.S. Claims Court determines if compensation is proper and awards such compensation from a fund established to provide payment in such situations.[32] Pediatricians whose patients are injured by the administration of a vaccine might alert and assist parents in making appropriate claims for compensation under this statute.

AIDS and Exclusion from School

One medical phenomenon that has had an increasingly significant impact on school-age children has been the disease AIDS and related infections. Although AIDS is transmitted in a variety of ways among adults, children usually acquire the disease either by receiving contaminated blood or blood products or by perinatal transmission from a mother afflicted with AIDS or a related infection. As the number of children with AIDS has increased, school districts, parents, and courts have begun to consider the issue of whether a child with AIDS or AIDS-related complex (commonly known as ARC) can be excluded from school, day care, or foster care because of the affliction.

Several organizations, including the federal Centers for Disease Control (CDC) and the American Academy of Pediatrics (AAP), have considered the issue of whether children infected with the human immune deficiency virus (HIV) antibody should be permitted to attend school. The CDC's recommendations essentially state that decisions concerning the type of educational and care settings for infected children should be based on the behavior, neurologic development, and physical condition of the child and on the expected interaction with others in that setting.[33] This determination should be made by a team comprising the child's parent, the physician, and public health and educational personnel. It is anticipated that most school-age children will be able to participate in school or day care and can be placed in foster care.

The situations in which a child should be cared for in a restricted setting, according to the CDC, are those involving preschool-age children, neurologically handicapped children who lack control of their bodily secretions or who display behavior such as biting, and children who have uncoverable, oozing lesions.[34] In its June 1988 update, the CDC stated that these universal precautions do not apply to feces, nasal secretions, sputum, sweat, tears, urine, or vomitus unless they contain visible blood. The CDC states that the risk of transmitting the HIV antibody through these fluids and materials is extremely low or nonexistent unless blood is visible. In general, however, the CDC does not recommend mandatory screening as a condition for school entry. Similarly, the AAP recommends that most infected school-age children and adolescents be allowed to attend school without restrictions, on approval of the child's physician, assuming that the child is not displaying biting behavior and that he or she does not have exudative skin sores that cannot be covered.[35]

In addition to these guidelines, several court cases have examined the issue of whether a school district can automatically exclude children with AIDS from school. In New York, following the issuance of a joint statement by the mayor of New York City, the New York City school chancellor, and the health commissioner that provided for a case-by-case review of children with AIDS to determine if they could attend school in an unrestricted setting, a group brought suit seeking to have all children with AIDS automatically excluded from attending normal classroom instruction. The court denied the request, holding that the school could not automatically exclude all children with AIDS and finding that the case-by-case review was appropriate.[36]

Similarly, other courts that have considered the issue have held that a child may not be excluded from attending school in an unrestricted setting merely because he or she has AIDS. Rather, the courts will examine the following factors, based on reasonable medical judgment and the state of medical knowledge: the nature of the risk of another child contracting the disease, the duration of the risk, the severity of the harm, and the probability of transmission of the disease. There must be some indication of a significant risk of transmission to other students, a risk of disease transmission from the other students to the AIDS-afflicted student, or an indication that the afflicted child cannot perform in a typical educational setting because of his or her physical limitations, before the AIDS-affected child should be excluded from the classroom.[37]

Finally, a variety of state statutes may apply to children with AIDS in the educational context. For example, an Illinois statute requires that whenever a child of school age is reported to the health department as having a diagnosis of AIDS or ARC or as having been exposed to the virus, the Health Department shall give prompt and confidential notice to the principal of the school in which the child is enrolled.[38] Other states require that all students in public schools be provided instruction in the prevention of AIDS[39] or that students be instructed in the prevention of AIDS to graduate from high school.[40] Thus legal involvement on the part of the state and local authorities with regard to both educating children with AIDS and educating children *about* AIDS are areas that seem to be expanding rapidly.

ISSUES CONCERNING OLDER CHILDREN

Drug and Alcohol Abuse

One increasingly prevalent problem confronting older children is drug and alcohol abuse, which has affected a large number of minors because of the easy availability of drugs and alcohol. Legal issues may arise when practitioners seek to provide services and resources to minors who have been abusing drugs or alcohol. More than half the states now have specific laws that allow minors to obtain aid for drug and alcohol abuse without their parents' consent. For example, in New Jersey if a minor believes he or she is suffering from the use of drugs or is drug dependent, a statute provides that the minor's "consent to treatment under the supervision of a physician licensed to practice medicine shall be valid and binding as if the minor had achieved his or her majority."[41] Pursuant to this law the consent of no other person, including a spouse, parent, custodian, or guardian, is necessary to authorize such medical care and treatment.

States also have taken other steps to ensure treatment for drug use among minors. In Georgia a new statute requires in part that:

> Any person exercising *in loco parentis* control over a child under the age of 18 years who has reasonable cause to believe that the child is habitually using in an unlawful manner any controlled substance or marijuana . . . is encouraged to report such information to the child's parents and a child welfare agency providing protective services, as designated by the Department of Human Resources.[42]

This law provides that staff members of schools, social agencies, or similar facilities that are exercising *in loco parentis* control over a child shall notify the person in charge of the facility, and that individual shall make the required report. The statute provides that an oral report shall be made by telephone as soon as possible and be followed up with a written report detailing the child's name and address and those of the parents, the child's age, and the nature and extent of the child's controlled substance or marijuana abuse history, if known.

When the reporting person or official has actual knowledge that a child under 18 years of age has unlawfully consumed or otherwise used any controlled substance or marijuana, the child welfare agency is also required by the statute to forward a copy of all reports to the Juvenile Court.[43]

Most states also have statutes that allow minors to consent to treatment for alcohol abuse. A typical statutory provision, such as the one in Illinois, provides that when a minor 12 years of age or older may be determined to be an alcoholic or an intoxicated person, he or she may give consent to the furnishing of medical care or counseling relating to the diagnosis or treatment of the disease.[44] The consent of the parent or legal guardian of the minor is not required. The statute does provide, however, that if a minor over 12 years of age is being treated for alcohol use, the person furnishing the treatment shall notify the parent or the guardian of the minor following the second treatment, unless the person furnishing the treatment believes that notification would jeopardize the course of treatment being pursued. In no case, however, is a period of 3 months to elapse without the parent or guardian of the minor being notified of the treatment that is being given.[45]

Use of Anabolic Steroids

Another increasingly prevalent problem among teenagers, particularly males, has been the use of anabolic steroids to increase body mass and enhance physical performance.[46] As more and more information has come to light regarding the long-term physical effects of anabolic steroids and the resulting health problems they cause, states have begun to treat steroids as dangerous drugs and controlled substances and to enact a variety of statutory measures governing their use.

First, some states have adopted criminal statutes regulating the possession and distribution of steroids. These provisions vary in scope. Generally, however, the statutes impose penalties for possession of anabolic steroids without a prescription. For example, an Indiana law states that it is unlawful for a person to possess or use an anabolic steroid without a valid prescription,[47] whereas a Louisiana statute states that it is unlawful for any person to furnish or sell an anabolic steroid except upon prescription by a licensed physician, dentist, or veterinarian.[48]

Second, prescription of steroids to teenagers for nontherapeutic purposes may give rise to criminal sanctions against practitioners. Indiana law, for example, states:

> It is unlawful for a practitioner to prescribe, order, distribute, supply, or sell an anabolic steroid for:
> (1) Enhancing performance in an exercise, sport, or game; or
> (2) Hormonal manipulation intended to increase muscle mass, strength, or weight, without a medical necessity.[49]

Third, several states have included provisions regarding the unnecessary prescription of steroids in their definitions of professional misconduct by physicians, thus raising the potential of disciplinary action. Arizona includes the following within its definition of unprofessional conduct: "[p]rescribing, dispensing, or administering anabolic androgenic steroids for other than therapeutic purposes."[50] Similarly, a Colorado statute defines unprofessional conduct as including the acts of "dispensing, injecting, or prescribing an anabolic steroid . . . for the purpose of the hormonal manipulation that is intended to increase muscle mass, strength, or weight without a medical necessity to do so or for the intended purpose of improving performance in any form of exercise, sport, or game."[51]

Because of the apparent increase in steroid use by adolescents, it is probable that states will increasingly take steps to curtail steroid use and to educate minors regarding the health problems that can result from this use. In California schools are encouraged to include a lesson on the effects of anabolic steroids in science, health, or physical education programs for students in grades 7 through 12.[52] In addition any time athletic facilities are leased or rented for instruction, training, or assistance in various sports such as football, wrestling, weight lifting, baseball, basketball, or track and field, a warning statement must be posted in every locker room of the athletic facility that states:

> WARNING: CALIFORNIA LAW PROVIDES THAT IT IS ILLEGAL TO AID OR ABET IN THE UNLAWFUL SALE, USE, OR EXCHANGE OF ANABOLIC STEROIDS, TESTOSTERONE, AND HUMAN GROWTH HORMONE.[53]

With the addition of such statutes regulating the use of steroids, expansion of educational programs, and careful prescription by practitioners, the states are hoping that steroid use by adolescents and its devastating effects can be substantially reduced.

Treatment for Venereal Disease

As in the case of treatment for drugs or alcohol abuse, most states now have laws that allow minors to obtain treatment for venereal disease without parental consent or fear of later parental involvement.

Michigan, for example, provides that a minor who "is or professes to be infected with a venereal disease or HIV" may consent to the provision of medical or surgical care, treatment, or services by a hospital, clinic, or physician. The consent of the minor is binding, and the physician need not also obtain the consent of any other person, including a spouse, parent, guardian, or person *in loco parentis*.[54]

The state laws generally stipulate a minimum age, usually between 12 and 14, for this protection. In some states, including Michigan and Hawaii, physicians and other health providers may at their discretion advise a minor's parents, guardian, or spouse if venereal disease is found on examination. In Michigan the consent of the minor is not required before this information is given to the persons indicated, and the information may be provided to these individuals notwithstanding the minor's express refusal to have it given to them.[55]

Access to Contraceptives

Minors in most areas of the country may now obtain contraceptive services without parental consent. Some state laws refer to "services related to pregnancy" or services related to "the prevention, diagnosis, and treatment of pregnancy," specifically delineating the services that may be provided without parental consent. Although the U.S. Supreme Court overturned a New York statute prohibiting minors from purchasing contraceptives,[56] a few jurisdictions still attempt to enforce prohibitions on minors purchasing prophylactics. Planned Parenthood and other groups make these services available to individuals of any age and have been very active in challenging laws that require parental consent or require that parents be notified when contraceptive services or information is provided to minors.

The U.S. Department of Health and Human Services' regulations on allocation of Title XIX and Title XX funds, some of which are used in pregnancy prevention and family planning education programs, prohibit discrimination on the basis of age or marital status. In the past the Department of Health and Human Services has attempted to limit federal funding to family planning programs that mandate parental notification, despite arguments that such a limitation would have a chilling effect on the physician-patient relationship and on the ability of these programs to disseminate information to individuals recognized as the most needy—children under 18 years of age. In *Doe v. Irwin,*[57] however, the court ruled that a publicly operated family planning clinic's practice of distributing contraceptives to unemancipated minors without notice to their parents did not infringe upon a constitutional right of the parents. Likewise, as will be discussed later in regard to abortions, the U.S. Supreme Court has ruled that parental consent is not required for a minor's abortion. Presumably this reasoning can be extrapolated and applied to the minor's receipt of contraceptive services.

Pregnancy and Abortion Issues

Many states permit minors to receive confidential services for diagnosis and treatment of possible pregnancy. The benefits of early prenatal care, particularly to young mothers and to the unborn child, are held to be overriding. This treatment is consistent with the Supreme Court's abortion decisions, discussed later on, which greatly limit the requirement of parental consent. In fact many of the pertinent issues with respect to a minor's right to access for contraceptive, pregnancy, and abortion services are governed by the U.S. Supreme Court decisions with respect to what has become known as the constitutional right to privacy.

In the landmark case of *Griswold v. Connecticut,*[58] the U.S. Supreme Court first recognized the constitutional right to privacy. This decision overturned a Connecticut statute prohibiting the sale of contraceptives, even to married couples, by prescription or otherwise. The court determined that these matters are best left to the privacy of the physician-patient relationship or of the marital domicile. Governmental involvement was held to violate the individual's right to privacy.

The court later expanded this right to privacy by applying it to a woman's abortion rights. In *Roe v. Wade* the court held a woman's right to an abortion to be a protected privacy interest which, as in *Griswold,* is protected from state scrutiny and the necessity of state approval.[59] *Roe v. Wade* led to a plethora of privacy cases on both the federal and state levels. Interestingly, many of these cases deal with the relationship between the physician and the patient. For example, the Supreme Court has determined that at the time a woman receives an abortion and other health care, a state may not require the consent of her husband before the abortion is performed.[60] A state may not require a waiting period before a woman may receive an abortion,[61] nor may a state place a blanket prohibition denying minors the right to an abortion.[62] All of these are held to be health care decisions; thus all are governed by the patient's right to privacy.

In *Roe v. Wade,*[63] the Court determined:

> For the stage prior to approximately the end of the first trimester, the abortion decision and its effectuation must be left to the medical judgment of the pregnant woman's attending physician. For the stage subsequent to approximately the end of the first trimester the state, in promoting its interests in the health of the mother, may, if it chooses, regulate the abortion procedure in ways that are reasonably related to maternal health.

Even with such definitive opinions, very few states followed *Roe v. Wade* with statutes that allowed minors to obtain abortions without parental consent.

Parental Consent Laws. The controversy over parental consent laws was resolved to some degree in *Planned Parenthood of Central Missouri v. Danforth,*[64] in which the U.S. Supreme Court ruled that minor girls may receive elective abortions without parental or judicial consent. However, the court later limited this decision in *Bellotti v. Baird.*[65] The court reemphasized that a state may not allow a parent or guardian an absolute veto over a minor's abortion decision but concluded that a state may require either parental consent or judicial determination before an abortion can be performed on an "immature minor." In such states the determination of maturity is to be made at a court hearing. If the judge determines that the abortion is in the child's best interest, even if the child is immature, the judge may allow the abortion to proceed.[66] To date the court has consistently held that a state must provide an alternative procedure whereby a pregnant minor may demonstrate that she is sufficiently mature to make the abortion decision by herself, or that despite her immaturity an abortion would be in her best interests.[67]

Parental Notification Laws. In *H.L. v. Matheson,*[68] the Supreme Court first considered the issue of the constitutionality of a parental notification (as opposed to parental consent) statute. The court upheld a Utah statute that required physicians to notify "if possible" parents of minors who plan to have abortions, under the stipulation that parents are not empowered to "veto" an abortion. The court found that the Utah statute protected family integrity, safeguarded minors, and allowed parents to aid the child emotionally.

The issue of parental notification in the abortion context, however, is one that continues to be litigated. In June 1989, the Supreme Court agreed to consider a case, *Akron Center for Reproductive Health v. Slaby,*[69] which involves an Ohio statute requiring parental notification. The statute in question requires the person who seeks to perform the abortion on an unmarried, unemancipated minor to notify the minor's parent or parents or a guardian or, in the alternative, requires the minor to submit to a judicial bypass procedure. The judicial bypass procedure requires the minor to prove by clear and convincing evidence that she is entitled to proceed without notification. The issues to be presented to the Supreme Court include whether the judicial bypass procedure is a constitutionally required component for the parental notification statute, whether the Ohio statute provides a constitutionally sufficient framework for ensuring the due process rights of minors seeking abortions, and whether Ohio can constitutionally require physicians to notify a parent or other individual authorized to receive notice.

In addition the Supreme Court agreed to consider the constitutionality of a Minnesota statute that requires a minor to inform both parents at least 48 hours before obtaining an abortion or submit to a judicial bypass procedure in which a court may authorize the abortion without notification if the minor is mature and capable of giving informed consent or if notification is not in the minor's best interests.[70]

MENTAL HEALTH ISSUES IN PEDIATRICS

Treatment and Confidentiality

Allowing minors to receive psychiatric help on their own consent has also been allowed in several states for some time, the theory being that it is better for the child to receive treatment in some form than to be held on a possibly destructive course by a nonconsenting parent. Often parental abuse, be it mental, physical, or both, causes the child's problem, and state legislatures have felt that the minor should have an avenue of treatment beyond parental control. As with pregnancy, drug, and alcohol treatment, the benefits of early treatment for mental and emotional problems are felt to outweigh this loss of parental control.

In New York minors may voluntarily commit themselves for mental observation, possessing rights beyond their parents' in areas of both treatment and release. Likewise New York allows mental health practitioners to provide outpatient services to minors voluntarily seeking such services without parental or guardian consent. The practitioner must determine that (1) the minor knowingly and voluntarily seeks treatment, (2) the provision of services is clinically indicated and necessary to the minor's well-being, and (3) parental or guardian consent or involvement would have a detrimental effect on the course of the minor's treatment or that the parent or guardian has refused to give such consent and a physician determines that treatment is necessary and in the minor's best interest. The initial interview with the minor always can be held without parental or guardian involvement if its purpose is to determine whether nonconsensual treatment criteria are met.[71]

Civil Commitment of Minors

Although mental health care is often desired by the patient, the parents, and the practitioner, at times a physician may be confronted with a situation in which the parents of a minor believe that the minor is in need of mental health counseling or treatment, whereas the minor is actively resisting such treatment. Although, as stated previously, parents can generally consent to medical treatment for their children, problems may arise in the context of mental health treatment when the child is rebellious or if the parents are in conflict with the child, raising the question of whether civil commitment of the child is appropriate.

Voluntary Civil Commitment

In general the law recognizes that commitment of any individual, whether an adult or a minor, to a mental institution necessarily entails a massive curtailment of liberty and inevitably affects fundamental rights held by the individual. Thus any type of commitment of a minor should be examined to determine both if it is medically necessary and if a less restrictive alternative is available. For some time, however, the question of whether a judicial or administrative hearing was required in cases in which a parent had consented to the commitment of a child was unresolved.

In *Parham v. J.R.*[72] the Supreme Court considered the question of whether an adversary proceeding is required either before or after the commitment of a minor child when the parents seek to institutionalize the child for mental health care. The case concerned a child in Georgia whose parents had committed him to a mental hospital because they were unable to control him at home or in school. The court determined that a judicial or agency hearing was not required.[73]

The conclusion of the Supreme Court in *Parham* was that a child's rights were adequately protected as long as some kind of inquiry is made by a "neutral fact finder" to ensure that no error was made in the parental decision to have the child institutionalized. The inquiry must include an interview with the child and an examination of the child's background using all available sources, including parents, schools, and social agencies. The decision-maker must then have the authority to refuse to admit any child who does not satisfy the medical standards for admission, and the child's continuing need for commitment must be reviewed periodically by an independent individual.[74]

Therefore, although states are free to enact statutes that require hearings when minors are being committed, if a state does not have such a statute, all that is required is that a neutral fact finder conduct an inquiry into the child's background. If it is determined that the child is mentally ill and that he or she can benefit from the type of treatment provided by the state, then the child may be committed without a hearing, upon the parent's consent.

In some states, however, statutes exist that specifically provide for hearings for mentally ill children committed to a state hospital or mental health facility. In Connecticut a hospital may admit any child for diagnosis and treatment of a mental disorder upon the written request of the child's parent.[75] However, if the child is 14 years of age or older, he or she may request in writing, or may have a representative request, a hearing to review his or her status as a voluntary patient. If such a hearing is requested, it must be held within 3 business days. At the hearing the child has the right to be present, to cross-examine all witnesses testifying, and to be represented by counsel. At the conclusion of the hearing, unless the court finds there is clear and convincing evidence to conclude that the child suffers from a mental disorder, that the child needs hospitalization, that such treatment is available, and that there is no less restrictive alternative available, the court will order the release of the child from the hospital.[76]

In addition the Connecticut statute requires that children be informed in writing of their rights under the statute either upon admission to the hospital or shortly after they reach the age of 14. If the child is hospitalized for a period of 1 year, the court will appoint a psychiatrist to examine the child and determine whether the child needs continued hospitalization.[77]

Some states also have procedures whereby the parents can consent to the child's commitment as a voluntary patient, but the consent of the parents is not required for the child's release. In New York a parent, legal guardian, or next-of-kin of the patient may request the patient's voluntary admission; however, if the patient is under 18 years of age, the patient can request at any time that he or she be discharged.[78] The consent of the individual who requested the child's admission is not necessary when the child himself or herself has requested the discharge. Thus both commitment procedures for children and the procedures whereby children may be discharged from mental health care facilities depend on state law, which may vary to a great degree from one state to another.

Involuntary Civil Commitment

As with adult patients, there are some situations wherein emergency involuntary civil commitment of a child may be required. Again, although mental health laws vary from state to state, many states do have specific statutes that govern the involuntary civil commitment of minors.

In California, when a minor, as a result of a mental disorder, is a danger to himself or herself or others or is gravely disabled and authorization for voluntary treatment is unavailable, then various individuals such as peace officers, members of the attending staff of a designated evaluation facility, or designated members of a mobile crisis team may place the minor in a designated facility for 72 hours of evaluation and treatment.[79] If a child is taken into custody for evaluation and treatment, the treatment facility is required to attempt to notify the minor's parent or legal guardian as soon as possible.

Once the child has been detained, the facility must make a clinical evaluation of the minor's medical, psychological, developmental, educational, legal, and other relevant conditions. If it is determined that the minor needs additional mental health treatment, the California statute requires that a treatment plan be written, upon consultation with the family or legal guardian of the minor, that identifies the least restrictive placement alternative in which the minor can receive the necessary treatment.[80] Once a treatment plan has been formulated, the consent of a parent or legal guardian is not required if the child is gravely disabled or is a danger to himself or herself or others. Thus, depending on the particular state statute that governs, the situations in which a minor can be involuntarily committed may differ.

OTHER LEGAL ISSUES IN PEDIATRICS

Rape and Statutory Rape

Although rape is never an easy subject with which to deal, it becomes even more difficult when it involves minors. The countervailing priorities of parental autonomy versus child abuse reporting obligations may need to be considered. Except in emergencies and in certain other situations previously discussed, parental consent is generally required for medical treatment of a child. However, this right must be weighed against modern child abuse statutes, which in many states require health care practitioners to report child abuse, including rape, if they have reasonable cause to suspect a child has been abused.

Often modern child abuse statutes that require reporting of suspected physical, mental, and sexual abuse of minors can be interpreted to require the physician not only to report a minor's rape but also to treat him or her. Fortunately, these statutes have taken the old "family right of privacy" argument away from abusive parents by making such reporting and treatment mandatory.

In addition some states have enacted laws that specifically allow a minor to consent to treatment when he or she has been sexually assaulted or abused. These statutes typically provide that when a minor is the victim of criminal sexual assault or criminal sexual abuse, the consent of the minor's parent or legal guradian need not be obtained to authorize a hospital, physician, or other medical personnel to furnish medical care or counseling related to the diagnosis or treatment of any disease or injury arising from the offense. The minor may consent to the diagnosis, treatment, or counseling as if he or she had reached the age of majority.[81]

The American College of Obstetricians and Gynecologists has adopted guidelines for physicians treating rape victims. In addition to notifying the child welfare, child protective, or police authorities where required, the physician may also be required to wait until a police surgeon or other authorized medical person arrives before examining the patient. The physician should document the details of the examination, including any observations or tests performed, in the appropriate medical report or form.

Clothing, photographs, and other potential evidence should also be identified and retained. In New York a regulation requires that hospitals retain all rape evidence for at least 96 hours from the time that the patient is treated. During that time no evidence (including personal belongings such as clothing or the like) may be returned to the patient.[82]

The physician should take the customary steps to check for the presence of secretions so as to facilitate chemical analysis. In addition a culture should be collected to check for exposure to venereal disease. To check for pregnancy, the physician should also monitor the patient with respect to her next menstrual period. Finally, the physician, as an individual in close contact with the patient following the attack, will frequently be called upon to provide emotional and psychological counseling and support to the patient.

Statutory Rape

All states have laws stipulating that both male and female minors below a certain age cannot be held to have consented to sexual intercourse no matter how willing a partner. The difference between this type of rape and others is its statutory mandate. That is, even should the sexual contact be consensual, the defendant may nonetheless be tried for rape simply because of the child's young age. This results from a societal determination that sexual intercourse with young, unknowledgeable persons should be illegal.

In the case of statutory rape, evidence of forceful, nonconsensual penetration or other physical contact plays a lesser role. The mere fact that an individual has had coitus with a minor (as defined by the statute) is all the evidence of the crime that is necessary. The statutory rape age limitation varies from state to state: In Tennessee and New Jersey, for example, minors 13 or older may consent to sexual intercourse.[83] In the majority of states, however, the age limitation is between 16 and 18. It may also constitute some form of criminal offense if an individual over the age of majority has intercourse with a minor.[84]

Although rape statutes may not specifically require physicians to report incidents of statutory rape, the practitioner may be so required under the state child abuse statute. Therefore physcians should be sensitive to identifying instances of consensual intercourse when the victim was under the age of majority and the defendent was over the age of majority, to the extent this situation constitutes statutory rape in many states. As with all child abuse, when the physician suspects that sexual interplay is by force or coercion or is suspect in any other manner, then he or she may be obligated under a state statute to report it as child abuse, regardless of its consensual or nonconsensual nature.

The question of whether a physician is required to report consensual sexual activity involving two minors, however, again depends on state law. In California, for example, a health care practitioner need not report consensual sexual activity as child abuse, even that resulting in pregnancy or a sexually transmitted disease, if the activity is between two minors of a similar age and no force or coercion is involved.[85] However, if the sexual activity is between one minor and an individual over the age of majority, the practitioner or health care clinic must report such sexual activity as child abuse, even if the minor consented to engaging in the sexual conduct and no force or coercion was present.[86] This result is based in part on the fact that such activity between a minor under 14 years of age and an individual over the age of majority constitutes a crime in California.

Sterilization of Minors

Sterilization of minors because of sexual promiscuity or for other reasons has been a matter of considerable legal debate. Some states (North Carolina and Georgia among them) specify that all persons must be 18 years of age or legally married if under the age of 18 in order for a sterilization to be legally performed. Although the parent's right to consent to medical treatment comes into play, the future impairment to the minor and to his or her ability to procreate may outweigh these parental rights, as with abortion and mental health care. In one case a woman won a judgment against her mother, who had requested sterilization for her daughter, and against the physician who had performed the procedure on the daughter while she was a minor, at a time when she was sexually promiscuous.[87]

Sterilization of mentally defective minors was an acceptable practice for many years. The laws of many states even mandated that these individuals be sterilized. The criteria for involuntarily sterilizing mentally ill or retarded individuals historically have been (1) the unlikelihood of improvement in the disabling condition, (2) sexual activity with the capacity to conceive and thus a high probability that the offspring would inherit the disease or defect, (3) an inability to care for the children produced, (4) an inability to use other forms of birth control, and (5) minimal risk from the procedure to the person's health.

In recent years, however, serious concerns have been raised over this practice and over protecting the individual's rights. Current Department of Health and Human Services guidelines prohibit use of federal funds for the sterilization of anyone under 21 years of age, regardless of the situation. This restriction was upheld in *Peck v. Califano*[88] and *Voe v. Califano*.[89] Courts have become more reluctant to order sterilizations of young, retarded individuals on grounds (upheld in several civil actions) that these individuals have a right to procreate.

The courts have not completely abandoned the converse, however. In a New Jersey case in which the parents of a 24-year-old woman with Down syndrome were seeking to have her sterilized, the decision of a trial court that allowed the sterilization was overturned by the state's Supreme Court. However, the Supreme Court stated that sterilization of an incompetent may be allowed in such case where the trial court, after examination of various factors, is persuaded by clear and convincing evidence that sterilization is in the incompetent individual's best interests.[90] In other cases parents have sometimes been allowed to have abortions performed on mentally impaired female children who had been sexually exploited and subsequently became pregnant.

Minors as Organ Donors

Living minors generally are not allowed to serve as organ donors except in actual emergencies when no other alternative exists for saving the life of the intended recipient—for example, in the case of identical twins or siblings, when the proper tissue match is unavailable from any other source. The courts have been hesitant to allow such procedures except with the fully informed consent of both the parents and the involved children and when the effect on the donor child has been determined not to be permanently disfiguring or hazardous, emotionally or physically.

Rules for obtaining permission for the use of organs from deceased minors for transplantation, research, education, or any other purpose do not differ greatly from those applied to adults. The proper consent is required, in this case parental, and the proper procedures must be followed. A minor, unlike an adult, generally cannot bequeath his or her body or individual organs for scientific purposes or transplantation. If such is done and a parent or guardian objects to the bequest upon the child's death, then the wishes of the parent or guardian usually are followed.

In New York the anatomic gift statute provides that organ donation requests must be made in every medically appropriate hospital death. That is, the deceased's family must be asked, by anyone but the physician who declares the individual dead, to donate body organs and tissues for transplantation, research, or education, unless the hospital has actual notice of the deceased's or the family's objection.[91] When the request is made, a Department of Health form must be completed and attached to the individual's death certificate. As elsewhere, in the case of a minor's death, the request must be made of the parents or of the legal guardian.[92]

Minors as Research Subjects

There is a general rule in research protocols that neither minors nor their parents may consent to any research or human experimentation, even if beneficial to others, if the research or experimentation poses a possible serious risk for the child. Protocols must ensure that minor subjects are well protected and that their well-being will not be compromised. Before minors are used in a research program, the investigator should be prepared for a higher degree of scrutiny than in any similar adult program.

Generally, state laws dealing with research protocols have more stringent informed consent requirements than those detailed previously (*see* Informed Consent, pp. 9 to 18). New York, for example, requires (1) a fair explanation to the individual of the procedures to be followed and their purposes, including identification of any procedures that are experimental; (2) a description of any attendant discomfort and risks reasonably to be expected; (3) a description of any benefits reasonably to be expected; (4) a disclosure of any appropriate alternative procedures that might be advantageous for the individual; (5) an offer to answer any inquiry by the individual concerning the procedure; and (6) an instruction that the individual is free to withdraw his or her consent and to discontinue participation in the human research at any time without prejudice to the individual. "No such voluntary informed consent shall include any language through which the human subject waives, or appears to waive, any of his legal rights, including any release of any individual, institution or agency, or any agents thereof, from liability for negligence."[93]

The National Commission for the Protection of Human Subjects of Biomedical and Behavioral Research was created by Congress in 1974 in response to unauthorized and unnecessary experiments performed in part on mentally disabled children at Willowbrook State Hospital in Staten Island, New York. The commission's recommendations were codified by the Department of Health and Human Services in 1983. These regulations impose serious responsibility on Institutional Review Boards (IRBs), which must determine the degree of risk involved in procedures performed on children.

The regulations define children as persons who have not obtained the legal age under state law for consent to the treatment procedures. Permission must be obtained from the parent or the guardian before the child can participate in the research. Assent to participation in the research must be affirmative; it cannot merely be a failure to object.[94] Research involving greater than minimal risk but presenting the prospect of direct benefit to the involved children requires the IRB to find that (1) the risk is justified by the anticipated benefit to the subjects, (2) the risk is at least equal to the available alternative treatment, and (3) the children's assent and parental permission have been obtained.[95]

In research that involves a greater-than-minimal risk and has no prospect of direct benefit to individual subjects, there must be a strong possibility of aiding knowledge about a subject's disorder or condition. In addition the risk to the child must be a minor increase over minimal risk. The research should not create different medical, dental, psychological, social, or educational situations than those that the patient would be expected to encounter in the course of the disease.[96]

For research that generally would not be approved, the IRB may consider whether the research may reasonably lead to further understanding, prevention, or alleviation of a serious childhood problem. In addition the secretary of Health and Human Services, after consultation with a panel of experts "in pertinent disciplines" and after public review, must determine that the research both meets the aforementioned conditions and will be conducted in accordance with sound ethical principles.[97]

In determining whether a child is capable of assenting, the IRB must consider the age, maturity, and psychological state of the child. This judgment may be made for all involved children or for each child individually. If the IRB determines that the child cannot assent, the IRB can waive the requirement of consent if the research, intervention, or procedure may directly benefit his or her health or well-being. When the research presents a prospect of direct benefit to the individual subject, the IRB may allow the research to proceed with the consent of only one parent. Otherwise, permission must be obtained from both parents unless one is deceased, unknown, incompetent, or not reasonably available, or unless one parent has total legal responsibility for the child's care and custody.[98]

If the IRB determines that a research protocol is designed for a subject population not requiring parental consent (e.g., neglected or abused children), it may waive the consent requirements. Children who are wards of the state or of any agency, institute, or entity can be included in research related to their status as wards or in research conducted in schools, camps, hospitals, institutions, or similar settings where other children are involved, with the appointment of an advocate for each ward.[99]

TORTS, NEGLIGENCE, AND MALPRACTICE LAW

Negligence is one of the "newer" torts, first used by courts during the Industrial Revolution under theories of fault and carelessness. The four elements of negligence, on which medical malpractice actions are usually based, are fairly universal: (1) a duty or obligation recognized by the law, requiring a person to conform to a certain standard of conduct, to protect others against unreasonable risks; (2) a failure by a person to conform to the societal standard required—a breach of the necessary and understood duty; (3) a reasonably close causal connection between the conduct and the resulting injury—this is what is commonly known as "proximate cause"; and (4) actual loss or damage resulting to the interest of another.

Statutes of Limitations

A statute of limitations sets a time within which a party must commence a legal action based on specific, timed occurrences, after which this right will no longer exist. For example, if a certain type of tort has a 4-year statute of limitations and party A commits that tort on party B on October 1, 1990, then party B has until October 1, 1994, to sue party A. After October 1, 1994, party B will be forever barred from enforcing this right to possible compensation.

In most states the statute of limitations does not apply to individuals still in minority. Therefore minors usually have until they reach the age of majority (usually 18 years of age) plus the time of the original statute of limitations (4 years in our example) to bring legal action. Thus in the above situation, if party A were 14 years old when the tort was committed, he would have 8 years, until his twenty-second birthday (4 years until party A reaches the age of majority plus the 4-year statute of limitations), to bring the action.

For pediatricians this can be an onerous burden. An infant injured negligently at birth could wait 22 years (using the above-noted statute of limitations) to bring legal action. Consequently, some jurisdictions have revised their malpractice statutes of limitations as follows: The time to bring such actions has been arbitrarily set at a fixed number of years (say 10) from the time that the malpractice was or should have been discovered. For example, a 7-year-old whose parents know of his being negligently treated would have until his seventeenth birthday (7 plus 10) to bring legal action.

However, lawsuits may also be brought past the time limit set by the statute of limitations in certain tort actions, such as medical malpractice or product liability, where the damage is held not to have occurred until the injured party knows of the damage or should have known of it. This "discovery rule," unfortunately, may leave the defendant open to suit indefinitely after the event occurred. For example, a surgical sponge left in a patient in 1980 but not discovered until 1995 would be fresh for legal action on its discovery. The statute of limitations runs from when the sponge was or should have been discovered, not from when it was implanted.

Medical Malpractice

Medical malpractice is a form of negligence whereby a physician breaches his or her duty to the patient by providing care that is less than the standard of care that generally would be provided by a reasonably prudent physician with the same or similar background in the field. Generally, a physician has the duty of (1) possessing a reasonable degree of learning and skill that is ordinarily possessed by physicians in the locality where he or she practices, (2) applying such knowledge with reasonable care, and (3) keeping abreast of approved methods in general use and exercising his or her best judgment.

In addition some states apply a geographic standard. Under a strict locality rule, the physician is measured by the practice in the community where the alleged malpractice occurred. If the physician is from a rural area with limited access to various equipment and other items available to physicians in large cities, he or she will be held only to the standard of other physicians in that locale. In some instances, however, a physician may be liable for failure to refer a patient to a specialist, if a reasonably prudent physician would have done so.

Other states subscribe to the same or similar community standard, whereby a physician can be held to the standard of care of a physician in a community of similar size with approximately the same access to technology and continuing education. Finally, some states have adopted a national standard, particularly for specialists, that is premised upon the idea that national licensing examinations have decreased the potential for significant variances in the knowledge and skill required of specialists.

Generally, as transportation and communication improve, the geographic area in which the physician practices may be of less significance in the malpractice determination. Hence a physician generally should be concerned only with providing patients with the best care he or she is able to provide. The physician should be diligent and always use his or her best medical judgment, letting it control treatment actions rather than worrying about the potential for a malpractice suit with respect to every patient. If a physician provides the patient with the proper information to make an informed decision, avoids making decisions based on emotion more than on reason, and does not provide treatment alternatives or procedures beyond his or her ability, then even should a malpractice action be brought, the physician will be as protected as humanly possible.

SUMMARY

Obviously no physician can be expected to be an expert with regard to all the legal issues that may arise in the course of a pediatrics practice. In fact as new developments expand the frontiers of technology and medicine, many questions may be presented for which there are no definite answers or legal precedent on which to rely. In general a pediatrician should be guided in his or her actions by the best interests of the child, providing the minor patient with the best possible care and treatment that can be provided in the particular circumstances.

When two or more conflicting interests are presented in a situation, it need not be the physician's responsibility alone to choose one interest over another. Legal advice may be available from an attorney for the facility or the physician's own attorney, or in appropriate cases from a judge through the court system. In any event the pediatrician should be aware of some of the legal principles that may apply in the pediatric practice.

REFERENCES

1. Ohio Rev. Code Ann. § 3109.01.
2. Official Ga. Code Ann. § 19-7-1.
3. *Miller v. Kennedy,* 522 P2d 852, 860 (Wash. Ct. App. 1974); *aff'd per curium,* 530 P2d 334 (Wash. 1975). *See also, Natanson v. Kline,* 350 P2d 1093, 1101-1102 (Kan. 1960).
4. *Schloendorff v. Society of the New York Hospital,* 105 NE 92, 93 (N.Y. 1914).
5. *Sard v. Hardy,* 379 A2d 1014, 1020 (Md. 1977).
6. *Wilkinson v. Vesey,* 295 A2d 676, 688 (R.I. 1972).
7. N.Y. Pub. Health Law § 2805(d).
8. In a situation such as no. 4, discussion should first be held with the patient's family, legal advocate, or guardian.
9. Mass. Gen. Laws Ann. ch. 112, § 12F.
10. Ariz. Rev. Stat. Ann. § 43-133.
11. *Bach v. Long Island Jewish Hospital,* 49 Misc2d 207 (N.Y. S.Ct. 1966).
12. *Prince v. Massachusetts,* 321 US 158 (1943).
13. *Matter of Hamilton,* 657 SW2d 425 (Tenn. App. 1983).
14. *In re Green,* 292 A2d 387 (Pa. 1972).
15. *In re Green,* 307 A2d 279 (Pa. 1973).
16. 29 U.S.C. § 794.
17. *United States v. University Hospital, State University of New York at Stony Brook,* 729 F2d 144 (2d Cir. 1984).
18. *Bowen v. American Hospital Association,* 476 US 610 (1986).
19. 45 CFR § 1340.15(b).
20. 45 CFR § 1340.15(b)(2).
21. La. Rev. Stat. Ann. § 40:1299.36.1.
22. R.I. Gen. Laws § 40-11-3.
23. N.Y. Pub. Health Law § 2965.
24. N.Y. Pub. Health Law § 2967.
25. N.Y. Pub. Health Law §§ 2965, 2967.
26. Cal. Civ. Code Ann. § 56.10.
27. N.Y. Soc. Services Law § 413.
28. Cal. Health & Safety Code Ann. § 1795.12.
29. Mass. Gen. Laws Ann. ch. 76, § 15.
30. Conn. Gen. Stat. § 10-204a.
31. 42 U.S.C. § 300aa-10, et seq.
32. 42 U.S.C. §§ 300aa-12, 300aa-13.
33. Centers for Disease Control Recommendations for the Education and Foster Care of AIDS Infected Children, August 1985.
34. *Id.*
35. Report of the Committe on Infectious Diseases, American Academy of Pediatrics, 1986, 1988.
36. *Matter of District 27 Community School Board v. Board of Educ. of City of New York,* 130 Misc2d 398 (Sup. Ct. Queens Cty. 1986).
37. *See, Martinez v. School Bd. of Hillsborough County, Fla.,* 711 F Supp 1066 (M.D. Fla. 1989); *Doe v. Belleville Public School Dist. No. 118,* 672 F Supp 342 (S.D. Ill. 1987); *Ray v. The School District of DeSoto County,* 666 F Supp 1524 (M.D. Fla. 1987).
38. Ill. Rev. Stat. ch 111 ½, § 22.12a
39. N.C. Gen. Stat. § 115C-8.
40. Fla. Stat. Ann. § 232.246.
41. N.J. Stat. Ann. § 17A-4.
42. Ga. Code Ann. § 19-7-6(b).
43. Ga. Code Ann. § 19-7-6(h).
44. Ill. Ann. Stat. ch. 111, § 4504.
45. *Id.*
46. *See,* Johnson, et al., *Anabolic Steroid Use by Male Adolescents;* Pediatrics, Vol. 83(921), June 1989.
47. Ind. Stat. Ann. § 16-6-8-3.
48. La. Stat. Ann. § 1239.
49. Ind. Stat. Ann. § 16-6-8-12(b)(1), (2).
50. Ariz. Rev. Stat. Ann. §§ 32-2922, 32-1401.
51. Colo. Rev. Stat. § 12-36-117.
52. Cal. Educ. Code Ann. § 51262.
53. Cal. Civ. Code Ann. § 1812.97.
54. Mich. Comp. Laws Ann. § 333.5127.
55. *Id.*
56. *Carey v. Population Services International,* 431 US 678 (1977).
57. 615 F2d 1162 (6th Cir. 1980), *cert. denied,* 449 US 829 (1980).
58. 381 US 479 (1965).
59. 410 US 113 (1973).
60. *Planned Parenthood of Central Missouri v. Danforth,* 428 US 52 (1976).
61. *City of Akron v. Akron Center for Reproductive Health, Inc.,* 462 US 416 (1983).
62. *Planned Parenthood of Central Missouri v. Danforth,* 428 US 52 (1976).
63. 410 US 113, 163 (1973), *see also, Doe v. Bolton,* 410 US 179 (1973).
64. 428 US 52 (1976).
65. 443 US 622 (1979).
66. *Planned Parenthood Ass'n of Kansas City, Missouri, Inc. v. Ashcroft,* 462 US 476 (1983).
67. *City of Akron v. Akron Center for Reproductive Health,* 462 US 416, 439-440 (1983).
68. 450 US 398 (1981).
69. 854 F2d 852 (6th Cir. 1988), *probable juris. noted,* 109 SCt 3239 (U.S., July 3, 1989) (No. 88-805).
70. *Hodgson v. Minnesota,* 853 F2d 1452 (8th Cir. 1988), *cert. granted,*, 109 S.Ct. 3240 (U.S., July 3, 1989) (No. 88-1125).
71. N.Y. Mental Hyg. Law § 33.21.
72. 442 US 584 (1984).
73. *Parham,* at 601-606.
74. *Parham,* at 606-607.
75. Conn. Gen. Stat. § 17-205f.
76. *Id.*
77. Conn. Gen. Stat. § 17-205g.
78. N.Y. Mental Hyg. Law § 9.13.
79. Cal. Welf. & Inst. Code § 5585.
80. Cal. Welf. & Inst. Code § 5585.53.
81. Ill. Ann. Stat. ch. 111, § 4503.
82. 10 NYCRR 405.9(c).
83. Tenn. Code Ann. § 39-13-506 (1989 Supp); N.J. Stat. Ann. § 2C:14-2 (1989 Cumul. Ann. Pocket Part).
84. N.Y. Penal Law § 130.25.
85. *Planned Parenthood Affiliates v. Van de Kamp,* 181 Cal. App. 3d 245, 226 Cal. Rptr. 361 (Cal. App. 1st Dist. 1986).
86. *People v. Stockton Pregnancy Control Med. Clinic,* 203 Cal. App. 3d 225, 249 Cal. Rptr. 762 (Cal. App. 3rd Dist. 1988).
87. *Wade v. Bethesda Hospital,* 356 F Supp 380 (S.D. Ohio 1973).
88. 454 F Supp 484 (D. Utah 1977).
89. 434 F Supp 1058 (D. Conn 1977).
90. *In re Grady,* 405 A2d 851 (N.J. Super., 1979), *vacated,* 426 A2d 467 (1981).
91. N.Y. Pub. Health Law § 4351.
92. N.Y. Pub. Health Law § 4351.
93. N.Y. Pub. Health Law § 2442.
94. 45 CFR § 46.402, (a), (b).
95. 45 CFR § 46.405.
96. 45 CFR § 46.406.
97. 45 CFR § 46.407.
98. 45 CFR § 46.408.
99. 45 CFR §§ 46.408, 46.409.

SUGGESTED READINGS

American Academy of Pediatrics, Task Force on Medical Liability: An introduction to medical liability for pediatricians, Evanston, Ill, 1975, The Academy.

American College of Physicians: Health care needs of the adolescent (position paper), Ann Intern Med 110:930, 1989.

American Psychological Association, Task Force on Pediatric AIDS: Pediatric AIDS and human immunodeficiency virus infection: psychological issues, Am Psychol 44:258, 1989.

Appelbaum PS: Admitting children to psychiatric hospitals: a controversy revived, Hosp Community Psychiatry 49:334, 1989.

Brent DA: Suicide and suicidal behavior in children and adolescents, Pediatrics in Review 10:269, 1989.

Gibofsky A and Laurence JC: AIDS: current medical and scientific aspects, J Leg Med (Chicago) 9:497, 1988.

Holder, AR: Disclosure and consent problems in pediatrics; Law, Medicine & Health Care 16:219, 1988.

Johnson MD et al: Anabolic steroid use by male adolescents, Pediatrics 83:921, 1989.

Leikin SL: Medical progress: minors' assent or dissent to medical treatment, J Pediatr 102:169, 1983.

Nivet H: Harvesting organs for paediatric transplantation: medical features, Intensive Care Med 15(suppl 1):S64, 1989.

Otte JB et al: Organ procurement in children: surgical, anaesthetic and logistic aspects, Intensive Care Med 15(suppl 1):S67, 1989.

Trautman PD and Shaffer D: Pediatric management of suicidal behavior, Pediatr Ann 18:134, 1989.

5

Community-Wide Approaches to Promoting the Health and Development of Families and Children

Robert W. Chamberlin

Many of our major child health and developmental problems, such as low-birth-weight babies, sudden infant deaths, child abuse and neglect, and school failure are related to poor family functioning.[3] Before the child is born, family dysfunction manifests itself in the physician's office as poor health habits that affect the outcome of the pregnancy, such as inadequate prenatal care, poor nutrition, too closely spaced pregnancies, and cigarettes, alcohol, and drug use. After the child is born, family dysfunction shows up as poor parenting skills, such as lack of or inappropriate developmental stimulation, abuse and neglect, exposure to hazardous environments, and inadequate use of preventive services.

Currently American families are trying to function under increasingly heavy stress at a time when traditional family and community support systems have eroded.[6,8] Common risk factors for family dysfunction include being a single parent; working for companies without paid pregnancy and child care leave or flexible hours; lack of access to affordable, high-quality day care; not having enough income to meet the basic expenses of food, clothing, medical care, and housing; being young and inexperienced in child rearing without grandparents available nearby and willing to help out; living in isolated circumstances because of lack of transportation or unsafe neighborhoods; or having a difficult-to-care-for child or too many children for one's coping capacity.

Families that face these risk factors are now in all our communities because of high divorce rates and out-of-wedlock births; teenage pregnancies; geographic mobility and residence in "mega" suburbs or inner city ghettoes that have lost their sense of cohesiveness; a shifting economy that has replaced high-paying manufacturing jobs with lower paying service jobs; and increasing costs of housing, medical care, food, and transportation.

Although the physician can provide some education and support during individual office visits, he or she must combine forces with other community providers and leaders to see that the basic community support systems are in place for all parents and children.

Most state government and local community responses to these changes are latent and come into play only after some crisis has affected a family or child, such as a low-birth-weight baby who needs intensive care, abuse or neglect, failure in school, or becoming homeless.[2,9] However, public health experience has taught us that when risk factors are widespread throughout all levels of the population and risk scores assume a bell-shaped distribution curve with most of the population falling in the medium-risk range, a community-wide approach is more effective because primary prevention works best by preventing low- and medium-risk families from becoming high-risk families. This is because there are many more medium-risk families that will become high risk as their life circumstances change than there are high-risk families that will be cured by some kind of intervention[12,13] (Fig. 5-1).

For example, we no longer try to prevent heart disease by paying attention only to those who have had heart attacks. Instead we try to reduce the risk of the population at large by helping people improve health habits related to heart disease such as lack of exercise, high-cholesterol diets, and cigarette smoking. A similiar argument can be made for families. In the long run, reducing family stress and helping families cope are more effective in preventing all the above-mentioned problems than trying to rescue families after they have become severely dysfunctional.

The problem with this approach, however, is that community-wide efforts are difficult to carry out and take time to become effective. They require interagency collaboration at the state and local levels; the development of an array of parent education and support programs; social marketing, advocacy, and fund raising; and the training of community leaders in primary prevention. Fortunately, we have examples from this country and abroad of how this can be done.

IMPLEMENTING COMMUNITY-WIDE APPROACHES

At a 1987 conference sponsored by the National Center for Education in Maternal and Child Health, a number of successful community-wide preventive and promotive programs used in this country and abroad were studied, and the basic

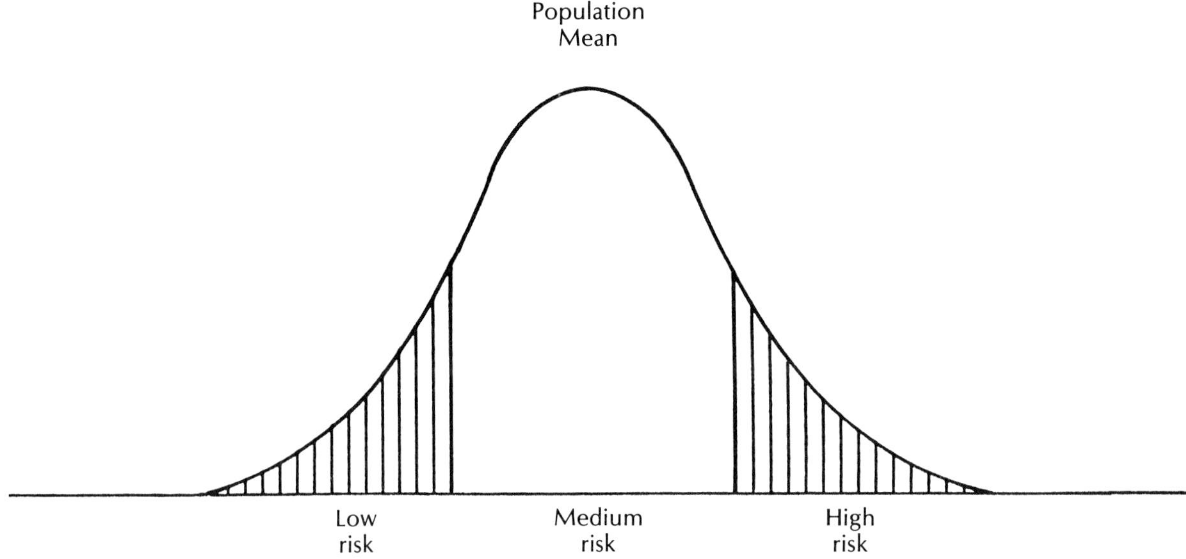

Fig. 5-1 Distribution of risk scores for family dysfunction.

design elements common to all were identified.[3] These elements included:

1. A geographic catchment area to be covered was defined.
2. A broad-based constituency of area leaders was developed to establish a data base for needs, assessing and monitoring program effects over time; to develop a framework to guide program development and coordination; and to identify priorities for filling in missing pieces.
3. A comprehensive, coordinated array of programs was set up to meet the needs of different families at different times in their lives. These programs would be those of proven value, such as home visits to new mothers and families with special needs; parent-child drop-in centers to promote parental competence and self-esteem and to provide peer support; early childhood programs to promote the social, emotional, and cognitive skills of young children; worksite and school-site parenting programs; and wellness programs for prenatal and well-child care.
4. Social marketing techniques were used to educate the public about the need for parent education and support and early childhood programs.
5. Stable, long-term funding was established, a task often accomplished through local and state-wide advocacy groups set up to promote partial funding through legislation and private and public collaboration.

The consensus at the conference was that communities must have local control over priorities and over running the programs on a day-to-day basis, but the state or some other regional body can help by providing start-up money and technical assistance and by developing standards to ensure the quality of the programs.

Stanford Heart Disease Prevention Project

One of the best examples of how to implement a community-wide preventive and promotive program is the Stanford Heart Disease Prevention Project, which developed a three-part ecologic framework to guide program development and coordination.[7] (See box p. 51.)

The column on the right shows the status indicators followed to monitor the success of the project, in this case the frequency of various types of cardiovascular disease. For families, the status indicators might be the rates for low-weight births, child abuse, school readiness, and dropping out of school.

The middle column shows factors that influence individual risk factors related to the occurrence of the condition or disease. These influencing factors include knowledge about risk factors and what to do to decrease one's susceptibility to them, attitudes and beliefs about one's susceptibility to the condition in question, and the effectiveness of the proposed preventive strategies. This column also identifies specific individual habits and skills related to the occurrence of preventable problems. For heart disease these include diet and exercise and how to resist peer pressure to smoke. For child health and developmental outcomes, examples would be health habits of the mother related to pregnancy outcome and parenting skills related to promoting the health and development of the child at various times.

The column on the left identifies all those social context factors that influence individual knowledge and behavior. Among these are immediate social level variables such as family traditions and local peer culture. Next come organizational level variables such as school health curricula, practices of health care providers, and worksite programs and policies. At the community level are variables such as what is reflected in the mass media, what local and state policies and regulations affect individual behavior and attitudes, and whether residents feel a sense of community where they live.

By using this overall framework, one can identify where a particular community is on any one of these variables and set priorities for adding, altering, or coordinating programs and services.

The Stanford group has also worked out a sophisticated

Stanford Model for Prevention of Heart Disease

Community Health Education Program	Factors that Influence Individual Risk of Disease	Rates of Coronary Heart Disease
SOCIAL LEVEL VARIABLES Parental behaviors Peer pressure Social-cultural norms **ORGANIZATIONAL LEVEL VARIABLES** School health curricula Worksite facilities and policies Grocery store labeling **COMMUNITY LEVEL VARIABLES** Mass media Labeling laws Social trends for smoking, exercise, and diet	**AWARENESS AND KNOWLEDGE ABOUT** Cardiovascular risk factors Community resources **ATTITUDES AND BELIEFS ABOUT** One's probability of developing heart disease **SKILLS** Resisting peer pressure Label reading **BEHAVIORS** Diet and nutrition Physical activity **DEMOGRAPHY** Socioeconomic status Age Gender	**CHRONIC DISEASE** Angina pectoris Myocardial infarction **PREMATURE DEATH** Heart attack Stroke

From Stanford Heart Disease Prevention Program

approach to social marketing,[4] including how to identify different segments of the population to reach, how to develop messages and activities that will be understood and followed, and how often and by what method to deliver this information. Finally, the group has developed a number of skills for building a broad-based constituency to support preventive programs. Much of this technology can be adopted to promote healthy families and children.

The Brookline Early Education Program

An example of a successful neighborhood-based, community-wide preventive program for families and children is the Brookline Early Education Program, implemented as a demonstration project in Brookline, Massachusetts, in the 1970s. This project, based in a school district, consisted of four components: a home visitor program, a parent drop-in center, a center-based early childhood program, and periodic health and development screening. The home visits and parent groups focused on understanding normal child development, on developing networks of people who cared about and assisted each other, and on developing a sense of community, a sense of belonging to the town. Any new parent living in the area was eligible to participate. The outcome measures were the effects of the program on parents and on children's school functioning.

The Brookline program found no one component to be crucial for all families. Rather, validating for the role of the parent was found to be the essence of any component, and different parents found this in different ways, such as from their child's teacher, from the pediatrician or nurse, from the psychologist after the examinations, from the home visitor, and from "networking" with other parents. The program also taught parents the importance of understanding and appreciating their child as a unique and important individual; of understanding the rate of their child's development, including the wide range of normal development; and of realizing that no child is perfect. The program also fostered friendships among the children. Even by the end of second grade, several of these children said that their closest friendships were those they had formed early on through the program. Parents whose children are now in the eight or ninth grade have said that their children still maintain those friendships, even with some children who have moved.

The children who participated in the program were found to be more socially competent on entering school and to have significantly fewer reading problems at the end of second grade. One of the most important findings of the study was that families under the heaviest stress needed more intensive outreach services such as home visits in order for their children to show significant gains in reading achievement. The need for more intensive services for families at higher risk for family dysfunction was also a central finding in the review of successful health, education, and support programs described by Schorr.[14]

The Brookline program has provided a model for the implementation of state-wide, school-based parent education and support programs in Minnesota and Missouri.[11]

The Addison County Parent/Child Center

An example of a community-wide approach to promoting the health and development of families and children in a more rural setting comes from Addison County, Vermont.[10] The Addison County Parent/Child Center, located in Middlebury, the state's largest town, has programs involving 1500 families in 23 towns in a county with a total population of about 32,000. This program has evolved over 10 years. The basic principles of the program are building the self-esteem of parents and children, developing communication skills, and building a sense of community where people live.

Center-based activities include providing affordable child care of high quality; training child care workers; providing an early intervention program for children with disabilities; and providing support groups for persons undergoing a variety of life crises and transitions. Parental self-esteem is promoted through a variety of opportunitiies for learning and skill building, including learning to drive and repair cars, to cook and sew, to read and to get a high-school equivalency diploma, learning about child care and parenting, and learning skills such as typing and word processing.

Outreach activities include holding toddler play groups weekly in nine towns throughout the county. There is a home visitor program for first-time parents and for families with special needs. Programs are held in schools on such topics as family life, being a teenage parent, and how to develop communication skills and resist peer pressure for participation in sex or use of cigarettes, drugs, and alcohol. Community building is fostered by holding spaghetti dinners and promoting events such as family fairs and toddler Olympics. Transportation is provided to all activities.

A recent evaluation of the program by the University of Vermont has shown a considerable decrease in teenage pregnancy, as well as in births of low-weight babies, infant mortality, child abuse, and dropping out of school for county residents.

This program has been so successful that parent-child centers have been started in all Vermont counties, and the legislature funds about 25% of each center's budget through an annual line-item appropriation. Vermont has also developed a strong state-wide advocacy group called the Children's Forum, which has successfully turned out a large number of parents to lobby on its behalf when funding decisions are being made by the legislature. Other states, such as Connecticut and Maryland, are also starting networks of parent-child centers.[15]

THE ROLE OF THE PRIMARY HEALTH CARE PROVIDER

Some physicians have responded to altered family conditions by employing a social worker or psychologist to work directly with families in the practice and by holding group meetings for parents.

A partnership in Norway, Maine, has combined a traditional fee for service practice with a variety of programs serving a greater geographic catchment area of about 10,000 residents.[1] These additional programs include an early intervention program for children with developmental delays and an associated nursery school that provides "mainstreaming" experiences. A parent drop-in center was added later that offers information, referral services, and exercise classes, as well as other informal activities for parents and children. To qualify for funds from state agencies and other sources, the practice has been established as a nonprofit health and service agency called the Child Health Center of Norway, Maine. This broader orientation has resulted in a close relationship with other community services that refer families to the center, such as the area public health nurses, the local child abuse prevention councils, and the local school systems.

Pediatric departments in hospitals and medical schools have also become more community oriented. The University of Rochester in Rochester, New York, has a program that pioneered in this direction.[5] The Martin Luther King–Drew Medical Center's Department of Pediatrics serves the Watts area in inner city Los Angeles.[14] This group operates on the principle that the health care of children can only be addressed in the context of their surroundings. Thus the department has been instrumental in establishing a model child care center, a family day care network, a Head Start program, a training program for child care workers, and a consortium of community early childhood centers. Members of the department have also become involved in a program for teenage mothers at the local high school and have helped develop a magnet high school for the health professions, in which students from all over Los Angeles combine high school classes with apprenticeships in the King–Drew Medical Center laboratories.

SUMMARY

Primary prevention works by preventing low- and medium-risk families from becoming high-risk families. Because of the widespread distribution of risk factors for family dysfunction in all segments of our communities and the bell-shaped distribution curve of family risk scores, it will be necessary to develop comprehensive, coordinated, non-deficit-oriented community-wide approaches to promoting healthy families and children if we hope to reduce significantly the incidence of such problems as low-birth-weight babies, child abuse, and failure in school.

We know what basic programs are needed, and most of the technology for developing community-wide approaches has been worked out and is available. However, to get these basic programs, pediatricians and other primary health care providers must become advocates for families and children and must educate legislators and public officials on the penny-wise, pound-foolish nature of the current practices that tend to wait until a family or child is severely dysfunctional before providing services.

REFERENCES

1. Bauer S: Report of the Maine delegation: the Norway, Maine, Child Health Center. In Chamberlin RW, editor: Beyond individual risk assessment: community-wide approaches to promoting the health and development of families and children, Washington, DC, 1988, National Center for Education in Maternal and Child Health.
2. Bronfenbrenner U and Weiss HB: Beyond policies without people: an ecologic perspective on child and family policy. In Zigler E, Kagan SL,

and Klugman E, editors: Children, families, and government, Cambridge, England, 1983, Cambridge University Press.

3. Chamberlin RW, editor: Beyond individual risk assessment: community-wide approaches to promoting the health and development of families and children, Washington, DC, 1988, National Center for Education in Maternal and Child Health.
4. Farquhar J, Maccoby N, and Wood P: Education and communication studies. In Holland W, Deters R, and Knox G, editors: Oxford textbook of public health, vol 3, Oxford, England, 1985, Oxford University Press, Inc.
5. Haggerty R, Roghmann K, and Pless I, editors: Child health and the community, New York, 1975, John Wiley & Sons, Inc.
6. Hobbs N et al: Strengthening families, San Francisco, 1984, Jossey-Bass, Inc, Publishers.
7. Jackson C: A community-based approach to preventing heart disease: the Stanford experience. In Chamberlin RW, editor: Beyond individual risk assessment: community-wide approaches to promoting the health and development of families and children, Washington, DC, 1988, National Center for Education in Maternal and Child Health.
8. Kagan S et al, editors: Family support programs, New Haven, Conn, 1987, Yale University Press.
9. Kozol J: Rachel and her children: homeless families in America, New York, 1988, Fawcett.
10. Mitchell C: Report of the Vermont delegation: the Addison County Parent/Child Center. In Chamberlin RW, editor: Beyond individual risk assessment: community-wide approaches to promoting the health and development of families and children, Washington, DC, 1988, National Center for Education in Maternal and Child Health.
11. Pierson D: A school system–based approach to promoting healthy families and children. In Chamberlin RW, editor: Beyond individual risk assessment: community-wide approaches to promoting the health and development of families and children, Washington, DC, 1988, National Center for Education in Maternal and Child Health.
12. Rose G: Sick individuals and sick populations, Int J Epidemiol 114:32, 1985.
13. Rose G: Environmental factors and disease: the manmade environment, Br Med J 294:963, 1987.
14. Schorr L: Within our reach: breaking the cycle of disadvantage, New York, 1988, Anchor Doubleday.
15. Weiss H: State family support and education programs: lessons from the pioneers, Am J Orthopsychiatry 59:32, 1989.

SUGGESTED READING

Olds D et al: Improving the life-course development of socially disadvantaged mothers: a randomized trial of nurse-home visitation, Am J Public Health 78:1436, 1988.

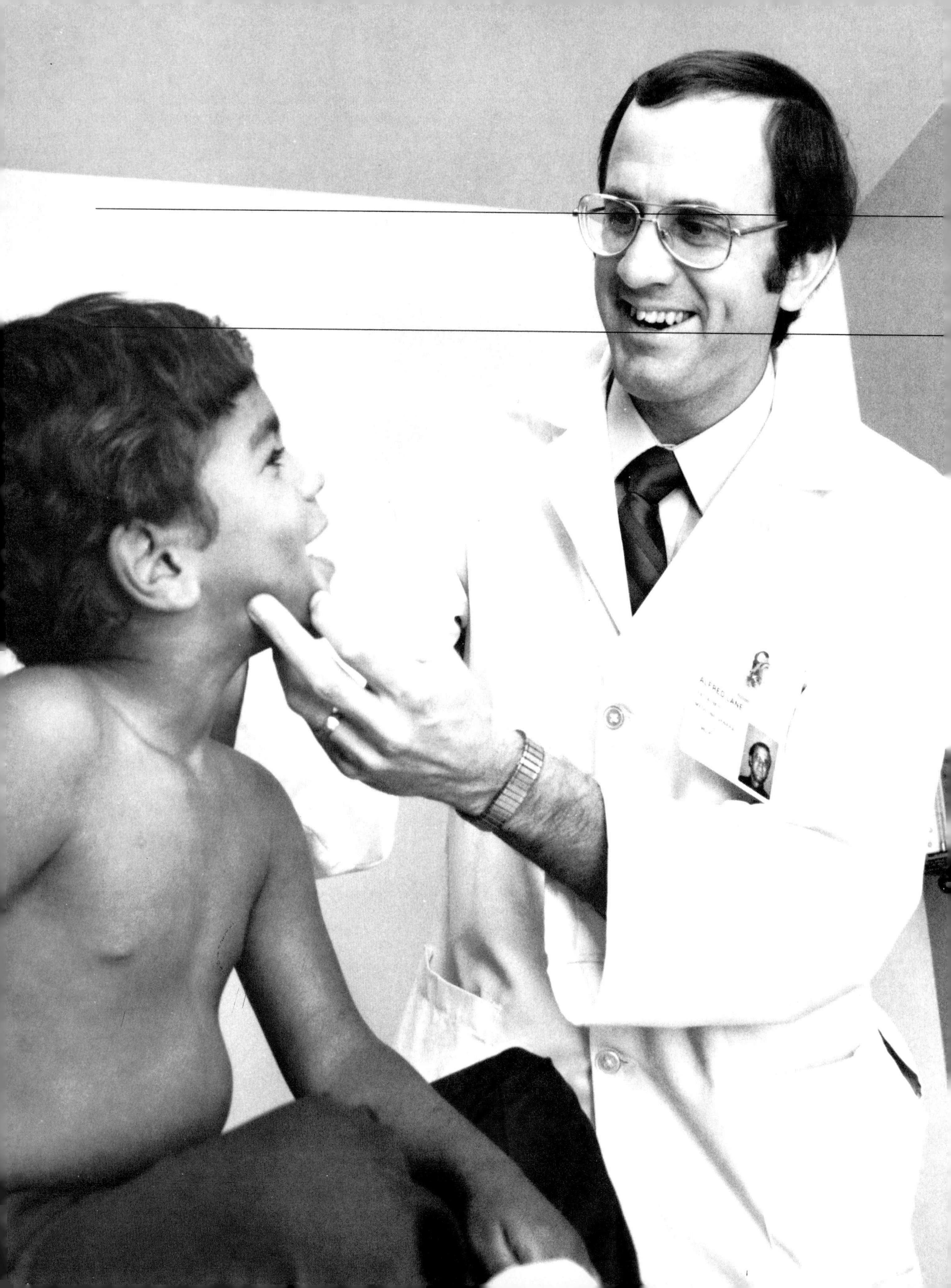

Part Two

Evaluation and Communication

6

The Pediatric History

William E. Boyle, Jr., and Robert A. Hoekelman

A good history carefully obtained from an intelligent mother . . . puts the physician in possession of a fund of information about the patient which is of greatest value, not only in arriving at a diagnosis in the illness for which he is consulted, but is exceedingly helpful in the future management of the child.

***L. Emmett Holt, 1908*[1]**

Perhaps in no other medical field is a history as important as it is in pediatrics. For early detection of problems related to health (including growth, development, and nutrition) and for prevention of future difficulties, the practitioner must have a thorough knowledge of the child and the family, their lifestyle, and their environment. Unlike other areas of medicine, the pediatric history is usually given by someone other than the patient. Thus a certain amount of subjectivity and objectivity is lost. Signs and symptoms are filtered through parental perspectives before emerging as historical data and are therefore influenced by parental hopes and fears. A pediatric history is a compilation of information gathered in a variety of ways—through interviews, direct observations, questionnaire results, and medical records—that usually provides a concise record of the child and the child's family.

Traditionally training in interviewing and history-taking took place in an acute illness situation in which the concern or complaint was readily stated or easily viewed. Today, however, children are treated for an increasing number of psychosocial problems, usually in an outpatient setting. These problems may include learning difficulties, chronic or handicapping conditions, or developmental problems—all of which require sensitive and insightful listening. Thus the pediatrician must have a thorough knowledge of the child's health status, developmental stage, and cognitive level, as well as of the family's functional characteristics, belief systems, and socioeconomic circumstances.

Much of pediatrics has to do with vague questions or concerns, such as "Why does she cry so much?" "Why is he so thin?" or "Is that cough serious?" These concerns must be answered and expectations dealt with if the encounter is to be fruitful. If the physician and parent or patient have different perceptions of the problem, the physician must attempt to "tease out" and understand the patient's or parents' concerns.

Much transpires during the initial interview between a practitioner and a family other than the gathering of historical facts. The tone of all future encounters is established, and ideally the family begins to develop a trusting, confident relationship with the practitioner. Just as the practitioner is trying to assess the problem at hand, so too are the parents (and child) "sizing up" the practitioner and trying to feel comfortable with him or her. A warm, friendly, nonjudgmental, courteous manner certainly facilitates this.

History-taking requires some degree of decision-making on the part of the interviewer as to what is relevant. It is not merely the gathering of a list of all symptoms and pertinent historical "negatives"; it also involves the synthesis of various facts, attitudes, and observations. To do this well requires experience, tact, and some degree of intuition. It is a difficult task. Compiling a history can be accomplished best if, for each visit, the practitioner can obtain the answers to three questions: "Why did you come today?"; "What are you worried about most?"; and "Why does that worry you?" Not only will the answers direct further inquiry, but also they will provide clues to parent and patient concerns that need to be allayed or dealt with directly during the visit and perhaps thereafter. For example, the parent who brings his or her child to a physician because of swollen cervical lymph nodes may be worried that they represent the first signs of malignancy, because an aunt who died of Hodgkin disease had the same problem. Parents, older children, and adolescents need to be told what symptoms and signs do *not* represent, as well as what they do represent, especially if the parents and patient are worried that the symptoms and signs indicate a serious or fatal illness.

SETTING AND AMBIENCE

Although pediatric histories are taken in a variety of locations, a comfortable environment should be used to enhance communication. If the practitioner projects courtesy, interest, and a desire to help, a trusting, positive relationship is likely to develop. Patients and parents are acutely aware of *what the physician thinks of them* or what they perceive the physician's opinion to be—the *reflexive self-concept*. ("The doctor thinks I'm a good parent.") If the reflexive self-concept is high, parent (or patient) satisfaction and compliance with management recommendations are more likely to be high. Some questions to consider are: Does the practitioner imply disinterest in the patient by allowing constant interruptions by others during the history-taking? Is privacy ensured? Are children made comfortable? Is there a place for clothing and belongings (other than a lap)? Obviously, seating should be available for all, and the history-taker should remain seated for the session. Parents or guardians should be called by their formal names (Mrs. Williams, Mr. Adams), unless a personal relationship has been established that enables the use of first names, rather than "Mother," "Dad," or "Grandma." Children should be referred to by their first names, for example, "Chris" or "Jane," rather than "he," "she," or "the baby." Notes can be taken so long as this does not distract from the continuity or spontaneity of the interview. Most parents find coping with more than one child disruptive and distracting, so seeing more than one child at a time or having others in the room should be discouraged. Formula and toys should be available to help quiet infants and toddlers if necessary.

Clothing and appearance may affect the ease with which a relationship is established. Parents and children view a visit to the pediatrician as a special occasion and frequently dress accordingly. They hope their practitioner will view the visit in the same manner. The practitioner's dress should be appropriate to the population served and consistent with local values. Most pediatricians refrain from wearing a white coat because it may evoke fearful memories for the child, although this has never been substantiated.

TYPES OF INTERVIEWS

The pediatric history is obtained in a variety of settings and for a variety of reasons. The initial history may be taken during an interview with the parents before their baby's birth, in the hospital following birth, in the physician's office during the first visit for whatever reason, in an emergency room at the time of an acute illness, or in a hospital room following an admission for a specific illness or elective surgery. The time devoted to the initial interview and the amount of information gathered will depend on the circumstances. Likewise, subsequent history-taking will vary in depth and breadth, depending on the reason for the visit and the amount of time that has elapsed since the last visit.

This chapter focuses on the information to be gathered and the techniques used in obtaining the comprehensive pediatric history, which is usually accomplished in a single sitting. Circumstances may preclude the completion of this exercise during the initial visit, however, and much of the information will have to be gathered at subsequent visits. For example, the initial history obtained for a child with acute otitis media who is "squeezed in" during fully scheduled office hours will be brief and directed primarily to the chief complaint. The rest of the history can be obtained during a scheduled follow-up visit when adequate time is allotted for this purpose.

Prenatal Interview

Ideally, the first encounter that parents have with a pediatrician should occur before their baby is born. To many, the idea of bringing a baby in utero to the pediatrician seems strange, but much information can be gathered at this time, and a strong, understanding relationship between the parents and the pediatrician can be fostered. In addition, problems can be identified and intervention instituted then rather than waiting until the frantic, unsettled postpartum period. An example is the isolated, deprived, pregnant girl who should be identified before she delivers, so that appropriate social and psychological support can be provided.

Pregnancy is much more than a period of gestation, growth, and development of a fetus. During this time the mother must adapt to profound psychobiologic changes. A life grows within her, distorting her self-image and causing nausea and then fatigue and disequilibrium. She feels obese and uncomfortable. After quickening, she begins to identify this life within her as a separate individual and to fantasize about its sex, size, and soundness. Frequently she becomes introspective and withdrawn, which may stress her marital relationship. As term approaches, she wants the discomfort of pregnancy to end, yet views the work of labor and delivery with some trepidation. All this is hard work for both her body and her psyche.

Many women have spent high school and college years preparing for careers, and approaching motherhood frequently means temporarily relinquishing a rewarding and prestigious job. It means embarking on a new "career" without much training and frequently without much status. In addition, our society is mobile. There are fewer extended families and thus fewer experiences and less advice such families can bring to the task of child rearing. Most young couples live alone and are often far removed from parents and siblings. These couples seldom have a wide range of friends on whom they can rely for help and support. Because of these societal changes, young couples usually find coping with the stresses of parenthood difficult and often turn to professionals for support and assistance.

Ideally, the person who has cared for the woman throughout her pregnancy and delivery and who understands her needs should be the person who will help her understand her new role as a mother. In many communities this is not done. Obstetricians traditionally care for women only throughout pregnancy and the immediate postpartum period. Pediatricians traditionally assume care of the infant at birth. Many women find it difficult to leave someone who has supported them through a difficult psychobiologic change and to develop a new relationship while they learn the new role of motherhood. Thus a prenatal interview can greatly assist in this transition.

Prenatal interviews do not need to be long or detailed; 20 to 30 minutes should suffice. In addition to gathering facts, the pediatrician should set a tone for future encounters. Husband and wife should be interviewed together, if possible, both to air parental concerns and to help them be supportive of each other. All parents are anxious about their adequacy and the health of their unborn infant, and a supportive attitude and tacit acknowledgment that these fears are understandable can be most helpful.

Taking a thorough family history is *one* way of evidencing concern, not just for the child but for the entire family. Parents should understand the physician's interest in them as individuals and not merely as Craig's or Ann's mother and father.

During a typical prenatal interview, plans for labor and delivery should be discussed, as well as a program of childbirth education and the type of infant feeding that is contemplated. Plans about circumcision should be discussed. It is also helpful to point out to the parents that they obviously have imagined a variety of circumstances for their child, which the practitioner can understand and will help with if they arise. It should be noted whether one or both parents desire a child of a particular sex, which may affect their abilities as parents.

The mother's blood type, medications taken, and rubella status (if known) should be elicited. Genetic information should be gathered about both sets of grandparents. In addition to searching for inherited disorders and birth defects, familial tendencies such as obesity, hypertension, and short stature should be investigated. It is also wise to ask what the couple's own parents were like, since parenting techniques and styles are frequently passed from one generation to the next.

After dealing with the family history, the practitioner needs to acquire some information concerning other supportive individuals. Who will help out when the baby comes home? Will the husband have a paternity leave of some sort? Grandparents traditionally visit shortly after delivery, and the pediatrician should point this out and ask if they will be helpful or another burden. He or she should also inquire if transportation and a telephone are readily available. The physician should be alert at all times for evidence of undue stress, isolation, and prior deprivation, as these factors are know to be predictors of poor parenting. Parents will want to know when the pediatrician will see the baby in the hospital, what the appointment schedule will be, and how the pediatrician can be reached. Fees for visits can also be discussed at this time.

Parents should be allowed to ask questions about their concerns. It is best to support their instincts rather than to direct and show one's own personal bias. The pediatrician should anticipate certain normal variations such as sleepy babies, the postpartum "blues," and the physiologic slump that lasts from 6 to 8 weeks after birth. Parental questions may seem trivial (skin care, type of diapers), but all evolve around the question, "Will we be good parents?" Strong reassurance that their instincts are good serves to reinforce and strengthen their tendencies toward good parenting and leads to a confident beginning as parents.

At the conclusion of the interview the practitioner should have an idea of the life-style and coping mechanisms of the parents, and they should feel reassured that they have a supportive person who will help them enter parenthood.

As prenatal interviewing has become more widespread, interview requests for second or subsequent pregnancies have become more common. These are generally not quite so formal and can take place during the routine health maintenance visits of an older child. Parental concerns deal not only with the health and soundness of the unborn, but also with coping with another child. "Will I be able to divide myself and still survive?" The mother finds herself torn between her baby in utero and her baby at home, and this issue must be addressed. She may have her child attempt, inappropriately, new developmental tasks such as toilet-training, so that in essence she will have only one baby. She may also force a child to "grow up" and relinquish a crib, stroller, or high chair. All these efforts should be discouraged.

Separation at the time of delivery can be a problem for a sibling, who must be told that mother will depart for a while and then return. This should be done shortly before the expected confinement. The mother's departure can be made easier by having the child help the mother pack for her hospital stay. The separation will also stress the supports the family has developed, and the practitioner should review these at this time. It is also important to recount the previous birth experience to identify conflicts or problems and thus avoid them a second time. The mother should be assured that she will be able to cope and that support will be available.

Comprehensive Pediatric History Interview

Traditionally history-taking has been a stepwise delineation of the events that led to the practitioner-patient encounter. Most practitioners learned this technique while dealing with hospitalized or acutely ill children, where the problem was frequently visible or obvious. Fortunately a great deal of history-taking now takes place outside of hospitals and frequently does not involve illness. Therefore the discussion should focus on the *pediatric interview*, of which historical data are merely a part. The interview should include observations of behavior and family interactions. Essentially a history is a narrative about an encounter between practitioner and parent and child that includes subjective and objective data and omits some details considered irrelevant.

The accompanying boxed material is a suggested outline for components of a *comprehensive pediatric history*. In certain settings some of the data will have already been gathered, but a thorough knowledge of each component of the history is essential. Obviously, under certain circumstances it may be necessary to gather other information; the boxed material merely suggests a general format.

Usually the interview begins with the parents stating the concerns that led to the present encounter—the *chief complaint*. Parents should then be allowed, with as little interruption as possible, to relate the history as they recall it. Certain areas may be amplified and clarified, but direct or challenging questions should be avoided.

After eliciting the chief complaint, the practitioner should enumerate the events associated with it in an orderly sequence *(present illness)*. In addition to facts, parental concerns and feelings about these symptoms should be elicited. The parents should be asked to speculate on what they think is causing the complaint or symptom. This information can be valuable in several respects. First, it demonstrates the level of parental concern, which may influence subsequent care and treatment. Thus the parents who equate nosebleeds with leukemia will need more than simple reassurance. Second, parental concerns about causation may color the history a great deal; for example, their concern about developmental delay can influence the information they supply about achievement of early milestones.

It is always important to discover how the present illness affects the rest of the family. This information will help the physician to better understand the family's concerns about and responses to a given symptom or illness and what, if any, secondary gain exists for the child.

Although the chief complaint must remain the central focus of the interview, it is frequently obvious that it is not the main problem. This is especially true when dealing with very young children. Tired, anxious, or frightened parents often perceive their reactions to an infant as being abnormal in some way; they then project this as something being wrong with the baby. This makes seeking help acceptable. Once the practitioner recognizes this, he or she should try to create an atmosphere that will allow the parents to express all their concerns. Questions such as "Are there any other problems with Kathy you would like to discuss?" or "Is there anything else bothering you about Teddy?" might facilitate communication.

After the present illness has been defined and elaborated, certain significant events should be enumerated *(past medical history)*. Much of this material is factual and can be obtained by using a direct question-and-answer format. Significant events such as operations, serious injuries, and hospitalizations should be verified by obtaining and reviewing appropriate hospital records.

When obtaining the patient's early history, the practitioner should elicit medically significant facts from conception to the onset of the present illness. All areas delineated in the box on pp. 60-62 should be touched on to some degree. The amount of information obtained may vary, but prenatal problems such as bleeding, eclampsia, or infection should be noted, and birth weight, type of delivery, and neonatal problems, if any, must be described. Information about nutrition can reveal a great deal about family dynamics and parental perceptions and expectations. "Tell me how Jennifer eats" frequently brings forth a torrent of information, but its value, nutritionally speaking, may be limited. "Good eaters" and "picky eaters" frequently weigh the same, and those who "hardly eat a thing" are often overweight.

In dealing with issues of development it is frequently best to ask an indirect question such as "Tell me what Harold did during his first (or second) year." This usually elicits much more information than do direct questions about motor milestones. The practitioner should seek information concerning the level of skill rather than the age of achievement; for example, it is more important to know that the child could make simple wants known at age 2 than the age when the first word was uttered. Some information concerning social adaptability and temperament should be obtained (see Chapter 71, "Interviewing Children," and Chapter 102, "Interviewing Adolescents").

Previous health care is important, and the immunization status of the child is a significant part of the early history. The practitioner should record all immunizations, skin tests, and pertinent screening information on a separate sheet that is readily accessible and retrievable. Filling out a few history forms later on camp or preschool entry will prove the value of this record.

Allergies and allergic reactions are also an important part of the early history. Specific allergic reactions should be described in as much detail as possible to clarify the reaction. For example, it is known that ampicillin can cause a variety of cutaneous and gastrointestinal reactions, but only urticaria is a true allergic response to the medication. Idiosyncratic reactions to drugs such as phenothiazides should also be described.

The *family history* contains variable information but is often difficult to construct. An attempt should be made to trace back at least two generations on each side of the family, and any data obtained should be appropriately recorded. Fig. 6-1 demonstrates one method of recording such data. The names, birth dates, and health of the three generations concerned are usually listed below the pedigree (although not shown here), using a number indicating each person. As more data such as births, deaths, and disease become available, they can be easily added.

Consanguinity of parents should be specifically investi-

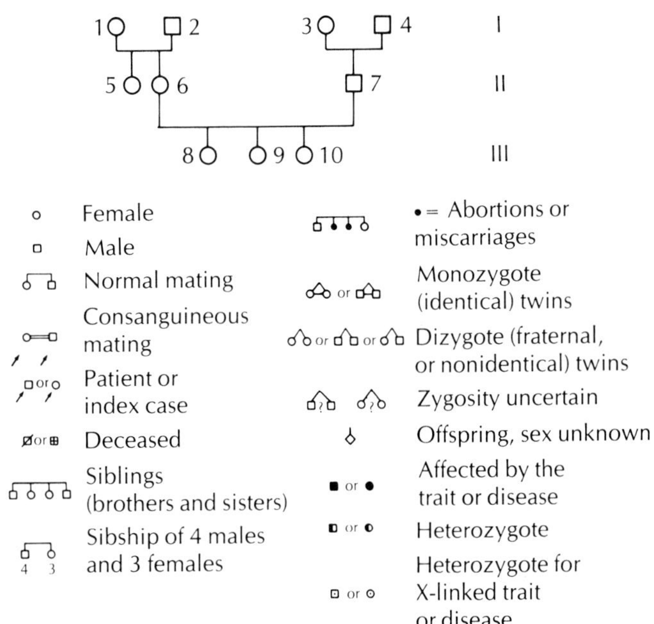

Fig. 6-1 Chart and symbols used to construct a family history, or family pedigree. Roman numerals indicate generations.

Comprehensive Pediatric History

The following comprehensive pediatric history is exhaustive and obviously not meant to be used in its entirety on all patients. However, depending on the patient's age and sex and on the nature of the chief complaint and present illness, the interviewer will need to explore in depth some or all of the subjects listed. In most instances common sense must be used in deciding how little or how much information should be gathered.

DATE OF INTERVIEW

IDENTIFYING DATA

Include date and place of birth, sex, race, religious preference, nickname (particularly for those between 2 and 10 years of age), first names of parents (and last names of each, if different), and where they can be reached during work hours.

SOURCE OF AND REASON FOR REFERRAL

SOURCE OF HISTORY

This may be the parents, the patient, or sometimes a relative or friend, coupled with the practitioner's judgment of the validity of his or her reporting. Other possible sources include the patient's medical record or a letter from the referring physician.

CHIEF COMPLAINTS

When possible, quote the parents or .he patient. Clarify whether these are concerns of the patient, the parents, or both. In some instances it may be a third party, such as a schoolteacher, who has expressed concerns about the child.

PRESENT ILLNESS

This is a clear, chronologic narrative account of the problems for which the patient is seeking care. It should include the onset of the problem, the setting in which it developed, its manifestations and treatments, its impact on the patient's life, and its meaning to the patient, parents, or both. The principal symptoms should be described in terms of their (1) location, (2) quality, (3) quantity or severity, (4) timing (i.e., onset, duration, and frequency), (5) setting, (6) factors that have aggravated or relieved these symptoms, and (7) associated manifestations. Relevant data from the patient's chart, such as laboratory reports, also belong in the present illness report, as do significant negatives (i.e., the absence of certain symptoms that will aid in differential diagnosis). Include how each member of the family responds to the patient's symptoms, their concerns about them, and whether the patient achieves any secondary gains from them.

Modified from Bates B and Hoekelman RA: Interviewing and the health history. In Bates B, editor: A guide to physical examination and history taking, ed 5, Philadelphia, 1991, JB Lippincott Co.

PAST MEDICAL HISTORY

General State of Health

Birth History

This is particularly important during the first 2 years of life and when dealing with neurologic and developmental problems. Hospital records should be reviewed if preliminary information from the parents indicates significant difficulties before, during, or after delivery.

Prenatal History. Determine maternal health before and during pregnancy, including nutritional patterns and specific illnesses related to or complicated by pregnancy; doses and duration of all drugs taken during pregnancy; weight gain; vaginal bleeding; duration of pregnancy; and parental attitudes concerning the pregnancy and parenthood in general and for this child in particular.

Natal History. Determine the nature of labor and delivery, including degree of difficulty, analgesia used, and complications encountered; birth order if a multiple birth; and birth weight.

Neonatal History. Determine the onset of respirations; resuscitation efforts; Apgar scores and estimation of gestational age; specific problems with feeding, respiratory distress, cyanosis, jaundice, anemia, convulsions, congenital anomalies, or infection; mother's health after delivery; separation of mother and infant and reasons for this; initial maternal reactions to her baby and the nature of bonding; and patterns of crying and sleeping and of urination and defecation.

Feeding History

This is particularly important during the first 2 years of life and in dealing with problems of undernutrition and overnutrition.

Infancy. *Breast-feeding*—frequency and duration of feeds, use of complementary or supplementary artificial feedings, difficulties encountered, and timing and method of weaning. *Artificial feeding*—type, concentration, amount, and frequency of feeds; difficulties (regurgitation, colic, diarrhea) encountered; and timing and method of weaning. *Vitamin and iron supplements*—type, amount given, frequency, and duration. *Solid foods*—types and amounts of baby foods given, when introduced, infant's response, introduction of junior and table foods, self-feeding, and maternal and infant responses to feeding process.

Childhood. *Eating habits*—likes and dislikes, specific types and amounts of food eaten, parental attitudes toward eating in general and toward

Comprehensive Pediatric History—cont'd

this child's undereating or overeating, and parental response to any feeding problems. A diet diary kept over a 7- to 14-day period may be required for an accurate assessment of food intake in childhood feeding problems.

Growth and Development History

This is particularly important during infancy and childhood and in dealing with problems of delayed physical growth, psychomotor and intellectual retardation, and behavioral disturbances.

Physical Growth. Determine the actual (or approximate) weight and height at birth and at 1, 2, 5, and 10 years; history of any slow or rapid gains or losses; and tooth eruption and loss pattern.

Developmental Milestones. Ages at which patient held up head while prone; rolled over from front to back and back to front; sat with support and alone; stood with support and alone; walked with support and alone; said first word, combinations of words, and sentences; tied own shoes; and dressed without help.

Social Development. *Sleep*—amount and patterns during day and at night; bedtime routines; type and location of bed; and nightmares, terrors, and somnambulation. *Toileting*—methods of training used, when bladder and bowel control attained, occurrence of accidents or of enuresis or encopresis, parental attitudes, and terms used within the family for urination and defecation (important to know when a young child is admitted to hospital). *Speech*—hesitation, stuttering, baby talk, lisping, and estimate of number of words in vocabulary. *Habits*—bed-rocking, head-banging, tics, thumb-sucking, nail-biting, pica, ritualistic behavior, and use of tobacco, alcohol, or drugs. *Discipline*—parental assessment of child's temperament and response to discipline, methods used and their success or failure, negativism, temper tantrums, withdrawal, and aggressive behavior. *Schooling*—experience with day care, nursery school, and kindergarten; age and adjustment on entry; current parental and child satisfaction; academic achievement; and school's concerns. *Sexuality*—relations with members of opposite sex; inquisitiveness regarding conception, pregnancy, and girl-boy differences; parental responses to child's questions and the sex education they have offered regarding masturbation, menstruation, nocturnal emissions, development of secondary sexual characteristics, and sexual urges; and dating patterns. *Personality*—degree of independence; relationship with parents, siblings, and peers; group and independent activities and interests; congeniality; special friends (real or imaginary); major assets and skills; and self-image.

Childhood Illness

This should include specific illnesses experienced, such as rubeola, rubella, chickenpox, or mumps, and any recent exposures to communicable childhood diseases.

Immunizations

Specific dates of the administration of each vaccine should be recorded so that an ongoing booster program can be maintained throughout childhood and adolescence. Any untoward reactions to specific vaccines should also be recorded.

Screening Procedures

The dates and results of any screening tests performed should be recorded. For all children tests included would be vision, hearing, tuberculin tests, urinalysis, hematocrit, and phenylketonuria, galactosemia, and other genetic-metabolic disorders and for certain high-risk populations, sickle cell, human immune deficiency virus (HIV), blood lead, alpha-1-antitrypsin deficiency, and others that may be indicated.

Operations, Injuries, and Hospitalizations

Details of these events and the reactions of the child and his or her parents should be elicited.

Allergies

Particular attention should be given to those allergies that are more prevalent during infancy and childhood—eczema, urticaria, perennial allergic rhinitis, asthma, and insect hypersensitivity.

Current Medications

Include home remedies, nonprescription drugs, and medicine borrowed from family or friends. When it seems a patient might be taking one or more medications, survey one 24-hour period in detail: "Take yesterday, for example. Starting from when he woke up, what was the first medicine Scott took? How much? How often during the day did he take it? What is he taking it for? What other medications. . . ?"

Family History

The education attained, job history, emotional health, and family background of each parent or parent substitute; the family's socioeconomic circumstances, including income, type of dwelling, and neighborhood in which they live; parental work schedules; family cohesiveness and interdependence; support available from relatives, friends, and neighbors; the ethnic and cultural milieu in which the family lives; and parental expectations of the patient and attitudes toward him or her in relation to siblings. (All or portions of this information can be recorded in the pres-

Continued.

Comprehensive Pediatric History—cont'd

ent illness section, if pertinent to it, or under psychosocial history.)

The age and health or age and cause of death of each immediate family member, including parents, should be recorded (see Fig. 6-1).

The occurrence within the family of any of the following conditions should be noted: diabetes, tuberculosis, heart disease, high blood pressure, stroke, kidney disease, cancer, arthritis, anemia, headaches, mental illness, or symptoms like those of the patient.

Psychosocial History

This is an outline or narrative description that captures the important and relevant information about the patient as a person:

The patient's life-style, home situation, and "significant others"

A typical day—how the patient spends his or her time from when he or she gets up to when he or she goes to bed

Religious and health beliefs of the family relevant to perceptions of wellness, illness, and treatment

The patient's outlook on the future

REVIEW OF SYSTEMS

General. Usual weight, recent weight change, weakness, fatigue, fever, pallor.

Skin. Rashes, lumps, itching, dryness, color change, changes in hair or nails.

Head. Headache, head injury.

Eyes. Vision, glasses or contact lenses, last eye examination, pain, redness, excessive tearing, double vision.

Ears. Hearing, tinnitus, vertigo, earaches, infection, discharge.

Nose and Sinuses. Frequent colds, nasal stuffiness, hay fever, nosebleeds, sinus trouble.

Mouth and Throat. Condition of teeth and gums, bleeding gums, last dental examination, frequent sore throats, hoarseness.

Neck. Lumps in neck, swollen glands, goiter, pain in neck.

Breasts. Lumps, pain, nipple discharge.

Respiratory. Cough, sputum (color, quantity), hemoptysis, wheezing, asthma, bronchitis, pneumonia, tuberculosis, pleurisy; results of last chest roentgenogram.

Cardiac. High blood pressure, rheumatic fever, heart murmurs; dyspnea, cyanosis, edema; chest pain, palpitations; results of past electrocardiograms or other heart tests.

Gastrointestinal. Trouble swallowing, loss of appetite, nausea, vomiting, vomiting of blood, indigestion; frequency of bowel movements, change in bowel habits, rectal bleeding or black tarry stools, constipation, diarrhea; abdominal pain, food intolerance, excessive passing of gas; jaundice, hepatitis.

Urinary. Frequency of urination; polyuria; nocturia; dysuria; hematuria; urgency; hesitancy; incontinence; urinary infections.

Genitoreproductive

Male. Discharge from or sores on penis; history of venereal disease and its treatment; hernias; testicular pain or masses; frequency of intercourse; libido; sexual difficulties.

Female. Age at menarche; regularity, frequency, and duration of periods; amount of bleeding, bleeding between periods, last menstrual period; dysmenorrhea; discharge, itching, venereal disease and its treatment; number of pregnancies, number of deliveries, number of abortions (spontaneous and induced); complications of pregnancy; birth control methods; frequency of intercourse; libido; sexual difficulties.

Musculoskeletal. Joint pains or stiffness, arthritis, backache; if present, describe location and symptoms (e.g., swelling, redness, pain, stiffness, weakness, limitation of motion or activity); muscle pains or cramps.

Neurologic. Fainting, blackouts, seizures, paralysis, local weakness, numbness, tingling, tremors, memory loss.

Psychiatric. Nervousness, tension, moodiness, depression.

Endocrine. Thyroid trouble, heat or cold intolerance, excessive sweating, diabetes, and excessive thirst, hunger, or urination.

Hematologic. Anemia, easy bruising or bleeding, and past transfusions and possible reactions to them.

gated by asking if parents are related by blood. In addition to seeking known inherited diseases such as diabetes, hemophilia, or neuromuscular disorders, the practitioner should note familial tendencies such as obesity, short stature, early heart disease, and hypertension. Sometimes it is also appropriate to inquire about the parenting techniques of forebears. It has been shown that abusive parents frequently were deprived or abused as children. It is also important to ask specifically about the health of parental brothers or sisters, since they are often overlooked during an interview.

The *psychosocial history* describes the child in his or her present milieu and relationships with family, peers, school, and community. This should include information about the physical setting (e.g., housing), environment, and degree of isolation. Determining how children spend the day, who cares for them, what they like to do, and what their hobbies are is important. Inquiry should be made about the support system within the family—for example, the nature of an extended family, their supportive or conflicting roles, the elements of stress that exist for this child, and how the child and family cope with them.

The psychosocial history should also touch on parental attitudes toward discipline and expectations about achievement. When appropriate, the practitioner should determine how the parents compare this child to his or her siblings or to other children. It is also appropriate at this time to ask the parents to describe the child's temperament (e.g., "mellow," "fiesty," "lazy") and also to describe what they see as his or her strengths.

The *review of systems* should be detailed completely to obtain a baseline evaluation of all systems and their level of function. Children change over time, and various systems may be the target of stress or disease processes. Therefore the practitioner should periodically reassess all organ systems and record their apparent level of function.

INTERVIEWING TECHNIQUES

Although most interviews are direct and straightforward, difficulties are occasionally encountered. Certain pitfalls can be avoided by changing the interview format or adapting particular strategies. Clarification of certain terms is always essential. For example, *diarrhea* and *flu* mean different things to different people, and no true communication can occur until such terms are defined. The temporal nature of complaints must also be carefully assessed. Children who are "always sick" may have recurrent infections that clear in 5 to 7 days, or a perpetually runny nose, which is seen in some children with allergies.

If the patient has been seen before, the medical record should be reviewed before the visit to refresh the memory on past health and illnesses that may relate to the reason for the current visit. Consultants should review the letter of referral and the reason for and goals of the visit before interviewing the parents and patient.

Many parents see their skills as parents being challenged during the pediatric interview: "After all, if we did things right, we wouldn't need to see the doctor." They become defensive and may answer questions "ideally." At the same time, they want to share fears and worries with a caring, empathetic practitioner. The practitioner must strive to develop this trusting relationship. By being facilitative, the practitioner enables parents to ventilate fears and frustrations and sort out thoughts. Statements such as "That must have worried you" or "I bet that's upsetting" let parents know the practitioner is concerned with much more than the facts in the interview. On the other hand, statements that suggest the parents have not managed their child's illness properly, such as "You should have brought Gretchen in sooner." "It would have been better not to have fed Clifford," or "Why did you do *that?*" should always be avoided.

The techniques used in obtaining a complete and accurate history vary with the situation and the person being interviewed.

Types of Questions Asked

In emergencies only direct questions (non-open-ended) that will quickly elicit the important facts needed to make decisions regarding management should be used. In nonemergencies, where time is not a factor, direct questions should be used to obtain identifying data and information about pregnancy, birth, growth and development, feeding, immunizations, screening tests, previous illnesses, injuries and hospitalizations, family history, and review of systems.

Direct questions should be asked one at a time. Rapid-order, direct questions such as "Has Karl ever had eczema, hay fever, asthma, or allergic reactions to drugs?" are logical to the questioner, but are likely to confuse the respondent and lead to an overall "no" answer when a "yes" answer would be appropriate for one or more of the elements of the question.

Indirect (open-ended) questions are extremely useful in eliciting the present illness and psychosocial history. The extreme type of open-ended question—"How does Bonnie spend a typical day?"—is discussed below. The answers to open-ended questions often provide clues to underlying, unstated problems and cues for pursuing specific elements of the patient's illness. However, the use of open-ended questions may have to be curtailed because of time limitations, the parents' verbosity, or the parents' inability to focus on the information sought.

Direct questions also are important in eliciting the details of the present illness and the psychosocial history. For example, if a cough is mentioned as a symptom in the patient's illness, the following sequence of direct questions is appropriate: "How long has Bobbie had the cough?"; "When does he have it?"; "Does it wake him up at night?"; "What does it sound like?"; "Does he cough up any phlegm?"; "How much?"; "What does it look like?" Thus open-ended questions identify the direction for further inquiry, and direct questions help to determine the importance of the symptoms or signs identified.

Leading direct questions—such as "Does Bethany do well in school?"—should be avoided, since they are more likely to result in "expected," affirmative answers than are non-leading direct questions such as "What kinds of grades does Bethany get in school?"

Helping the Parent or Patient Communicate

Throughout the interview the parents or patient should be assisted in several ways to relate all necessary information fully. The practitioner should use medical terminology understood by the parents or patient. Words such as *tinnitus*, *palpitation*, and *incontinence* may have little meaning to the parents or patient, who will often be too embarrassed to ask for a definition and may simply answer "no" when asked if those signs and symptoms are present.

The interview process is one of interaction between the practitioner and the parents or patient. The person providing information should do most of the talking and the practitioner most of the listening. However, the parents or patient can be encouraged by the practitioner to communicate their story through the use of the following seven techniques.

1. *Facilitation*. This is designed to convey interest in what the parent or patient is saying. Maintaining eye contact, leaning forward, nodding in affirmation, and saying "yes," "uh huh," "I see," etc., all convey interest and encourage the parent or patient to continue.
2. *Reflection*. Repetition of words that the parent or patient has said encourages him or her to provide more detail, as demonstrated in the following example:

Parent: Kara woke up in the middle of the night breathing hard.

Interviewer: Breathing hard?

Parent: Yes, she seemed to be breathing fast and making a wheezing noise.

Interviewer: A wheezing noise?

Parent: Yes, in and out—a musical wheezing sound.

By using reflection, the interviewer was able to elicit the nature of the child's breathing difficulty without influencing its description or diverting the parent's thoughts.

3. *Clarification*. It is often necessary for the interviewer to clarify what the parent or patient has said—for example, "What do you mean by 'Rob wasn't acting right'?"
4. *Empathy*. Recognizing and responding to a parent's or a patient's feelings of concern, fear, or embarrassment show understanding and acceptance and encourage continued expression of the emotion. "I can understand why that upset you" or "That must have been difficult to deal with" is an empathetic expression that tells the parent or patient that the practitioner appreciates what he or she has been experiencing and is sympathetic. The practitioner can also ask the parent or patient how he or she feels or felt about a particular situation that has been related. This displays an interest in the parent's or patient's feelings as well as in the medical facts.
5. *Confrontation*. This technique is used to clarify what seems to be a contradiction between the parent's or patient's feelings and actions: "You say Sally loves school but misses a lot because she has an upset stomach most mornings." Although clarification is sought with confrontation, it may also lead to interpretation of the meaning of the contradiction.
6. *Interpretation*. This technique is used to move beyond clarification to an inference to be made from the circumstances presented. Thus the above example might lead to the following statement and questions by the practitioner: "Maybe there is some relationship between Sally's upset stomach and her wanting or not wanting to go to school. Do you think that's possible?"
7. *Recapitulation*. This technique is especially useful when a long and complicated or an unusual history is presented. The practitioner summarizes to the parent or patient the history as he or she (the practitioner) understands it. This may be done at more than one point during the interview and serves to confirm the validity of the history. It also allows for possible changes.

Hindrances to Communication

Although a calm, reserved, interested demeanor is important to enhance communication, the practitioner must guard against appearing casual. Constant eye contact with the parent, interrupted by glances at the child (if present), should be maintained. Evidence of boredom or impatience—looking away from the parents or patient, tapping the fingers or a pencil on a tabletop, or rushing through the interview—must be avoided. Inappropriate smiling or laughter also hinders a good communication. The parents or patient should always feel they have the practitioner's undivided attention. If time is short, the parents or patient should be informed and another appointment made for completing the interview.

Interviewing the Child

A great deal of information can be gained by interviewing the child directly (see Chapter 71). Many children will interact spontaneously with the pediatrician and readily answer direct questions. Frequently only the child can reveal the severity of the pain or the extent of the symptoms. Sometimes it is better to approach children indirectly, encouraging them to talk about their symptoms rather than seeking direct answers. For example, "Tell me about your cold, Gordon" is preferable to "Do you cough?" The pediatrician should always support the child's "own story." It should be taken seriously, and confidences should not be violated except in unusual circumstances.

With chronic problems such as constipation or enuresis it is helpful to review with patients their knowledge of the complaint. Patients can be asked what they were told before coming to the physician's office, how they feel about the visit, how their symptoms affect them and alter their lifestyle, and whether they are able to attend school and carry out all their regular activities. It is also important to ask children what they think is causing their symptoms, what they are worried about, and why it worries them.

Interviewing the child also provides another opportunity to assess parent-child interaction. Many parents cannot let their child speak without addition, interruption, or correction. A school-age child who clings to a parent's lap and cannot be coaxed to make eye contact with the practitioner or interact in any way is probably overly shy and dependent. As adolescence approaches, parent-child conflicts become more intense. Given the chance, many adolescents will make this obvious. Under these circumstances, separate interviews are probably preferable (see Chapter 102, "Interviewing Adolescents").

"Typical Day" Technique

In many situations, information about a child's typical day can be very helpful and informative, and most parents can readily relate this information. In addition to concrete material (e.g., sleep patterns and feeding activities), much can be learned about areas of stress and harmony within a family. As with other aspects of the history, such information should be obtained as objectively as possible. Parents frequently find it difficult to discuss situations without seeking approval, even if tacit, of their own actions. Mothers who are confused or unsure of themselves frequently may ask advice on a particular aspect of their child's behavior as it is presented in the description of the child's typical day; however, it is best to defer answers until the description of the entire day has been completed.

Discussion can begin with an introduction, such as "In order to find out more about Kim, I am going to ask you to tell me how she spends a typical day." The practitioner should then begin by asking what time the patient arises and what happens. Some parents will launch into vivid descriptions and will require little direction, whereas others must be encouraged. Details can be elicited by asking some simple questions such as "What is her mood on awakening?", "Who takes care of her?", and "What does she usually eat for breakfast?" Discussion can include likes and dislikes of foods, skill in eating, and conduct at the table. The practitioner can also learn about the child's activities, habits, and television-viewing practices. The subject of discipline might come up during this discussion, and the parents' beliefs about prohibitions and punishments can be ascertained.

Lunchtime, afternoon rest periods, and activities are reviewed in much the same way. Descriptions of trips to the market or to other stores can provide information about behavior with others and reactions to new experiences.

The evening meal is often stressful in many families, and knowing how this proceeds can give many clues to family dynamics. For example, the practitioner should find out when the parents arrive home, whether the child eats with the parents, and if so, what types of interactions occur. Information about the events surrounding preparation for sleep, bedtime rituals, and sleeping patterns is also important.

At the end of such an interview it should be possible to assess not only the style and temperament of the child but also the strengths of the family. This information is essential for providing advice to parents of children who are experiencing developmental and maturational problems.

RECORDING HISTORICAL INFORMATION

There are two main goals in recording the historical data gained in an interview. First, the patient's symptoms and medical history, which will help in formulating a diagnosis and therapeutic plan, should be documented. This document serves as a legal record of the practitioner-patient encounter. Second, a reasonable account of the patient's medical status will be available to others who are also involved in the care of the patient and to the person who initially gathered the information.

The historical data base should contain all the medically significant facts in the life of the child. The recorded history is a synthesis of material and observations gained during the interview, compiled in a legible, retrievable form (see Chapter 9, "The Pediatric Record and Clinical Decision-Making").

The present illness needs to be recorded clearly and concisely. Consistency is paramount, especially when dealing with events in time. Events must be recorded using either of these methods: "Scott developed a cough on March 17" or "Scott developed a cough 5 days before our interview on March 23." "Tuesdays" and "Fridays" are difficult to identify 2 weeks after an interview.

There are a variety of ways to record data obtained during an interview, ranging from tape-recording the entire session, a method often used by psychiatrists, to merely noting "Dx—acute otitis media; Rx—amoxicillin × 10 days" on an index card. Records should be legible, and much of the data should be retrievable without having to pore over voluminous sheets of paper. This requires some foresight and planning so that different parts of the history can be separated for later use. Ideally the historical data base should be standard and uniform. However, certain problems (hip clicks, birthmarks) change with time and vary by age and sex of the patient (menstrual irregularities), by type of population served, and by geographic locale.

A variety of questionnaires have been developed to facilitate development of the data base. These are designed to be age appropriate and can be filled out by the parent, a nurse, physician assistant, or other office personnel. Such questionnaires can be used to gather a large amount of data quickly, thoroughly, and concisely. However, they also present several drawbacks. First, questions tend to be answered in an idealized way, since parents usually have a skewed opinion of their children. Second, all logical sequencing of information gathering is lost, and degrees of concern are not readily expressed. Third, unless the data base is frequently updated by subsequent questionnaires, much of the information soon becomes irrelevant.

Gathering and recording a history and communicating compassionately and courteously with patients and their families are difficult tasks. These are not innate skills but rather require work, insight, perseverance, and practice. The work is hard, but the rewards are great.

REFERENCE

1. Holt LE: The diseases of infancy and childhood, New York, 1908, Appleton-Century-Crofts.

SUGGESTED READINGS

Bates B and Hoekelman RA: Interviewing and the health history. In Bates B, editor: A guide to physical examination and history taking, ed 5, Philadelphia, 1991, JB Lippincott Co.

Cassell EJ: Talking with patients, vol 2, Clinical technique, Cambridge, Mass, 1985, The MIT Press.

Feinstein AR: Clinical judgment, Baltimore, 1967, Williams & Wilkins.

Klaus MH and Kennell JH: Parent-infant bonding, ed 2, St Louis, 1982, The CV Mosby Co.

Thornton SM and Frankenburg WK, editors: Child health care communications, Johnson & Johnson Pediatric Round Table No 8, 1983.

Wessel MA: The prenatal pediatric visit, Pediatrics 32:826, 1963.

7

The Pediatric Physical Examination

John H. Gundy

The examination of an infant or child by a physician or nurse practitioner has the potential of accomplishing several goals simultaneously. With children, as opposed to adults, the physical examination is often the first direct contact between the examiner and the patient, the history having been obtained primarily from a parent. Therefore one of the crucial outcomes of the examination is the relationship that will be initiated and continued between the physician and the child. The quality and quantity of care plans and future attitudes of the child in medical settings will depend in part on this relationship. This chapter emphasizes approaches to examining children of different ages that will enhance the physician-child relationship.

The physician-*parent* relationship, which is initiated during history taking, can be further enhanced during the physical examination by a relaxed and gentle approach to the child and, no less important, by a thorough examination of the child appropriate to the setting and the chief complaint. Parents develop trust in physicians in a number of ways, not the least of which is the consideration the physician shows for the child's fears and the parents' concern about a particular symptom or sign. For each organ system discussed in this chapter, common symptoms for which physicians are consulted are linked to a suggested level of "completeness" in performing a physical examination.

The physician must be sensitive to the potential for iatrogenic concerns initiated by his or her comments during the examination and should anticipate the child's wondering, "What's wrong with me?" and the parent's worrying, "What did I do wrong?" Reactions such as these are very common. A thorough grounding in the normal stages of growth and development of the organ systems and the body as a whole allows the examining physician to respond to such questions by emphasizing the normal physical findings, as well as by interpreting abnormal findings in the context of normal developmental patterns. The description of each organ system in this chapter begins with important stages of growth and development, particularly those steps that can be monitored by serial physical examinations. The characteristics of common physical abnormalities will be linked whenever possible to the child's age and stage of growth.

The physical examination has limited value as a screening mechanism for occult disease (see Chapter 18, Two, "The Physical Examination as a Screening Test") and has been shown to be much less productive in detecting problems in schoolchildren, for instance, than does a comprehensive history. In general, the physical examination of children confirms abnormalities suggested by the history, as well as normal growth and development. For children examined in the presence of their parent(s) the physical examination can provide strong clues about the strength and characteristics of the parent-child relationship.

Each portion of the physical examination is discussed according to the special characteristics of each of five age groups: newborn, infancy (ages 1 week to 12 months), early childhood (ages 1 to 5 years), late childhood (ages 6 to 12 years), and adolescence (ages 12 to 18 years).

APPROACH TO THE PATIENT

Newborn

The newborn infant is routinely examined on three or more separate occasions while in the hospital. At least one of these examinations should be accomplished in the presence of the parent(s) to facilitate both evaluation of the parent-infant relationship and attention to the parents' questions about their baby. The newborn infant is examined immediately after birth to assess adequacy of pulmonary ventilation and integrity of the cardiovascular and central nervous systems. While assessing the need for resuscitation, the examiner should minimize the exposure of the wet infant to cool ambient air and conduct the examination with the infant under a warming device. Recovery from the birth process is measured by the use of the Apgar scale, with scores of 0, 1, or 2 given for degree of cyanosis, respiratory rate, heart rate, reflex irritability (reaction to a soft catheter introduced into the external nares), and muscle tone (Table 7-1). The infant is scored at 1 and 5 minutes following birth; total scores of less than 7 or 8 at 1 minute usually indicate some degree of central nervous system depression, and scores of less than 3 or 4 indicate severe depression requiring resuscitation. If the Apgar score is 8 or more at 5 minutes and the baby's airway is clear, the remainder of the body is surveyed briefly to identify gross congenital abnormalities and to estimate gestational age. After the baby is weighed, the weight–gestational age category is determined by use of a standard gestational age growth chart (see Fig. 35-4), which predicts certain risks for each group (hypoglycemia and congenital anomalies in babies small for gestational age, hypoglycemia and infant of a diabetic mother in babies large for gestational age). The neuromuscular part of the gestational age determination ideally is postponed until the infant is fully stabilized (12 to 48 hours after birth) as shown in Fig. 36-8.

Table 7-1 *The Apgar Score*

SIGN	SCORE 0	1	2
Heart rate	Absent	<100	>100
Respiratory effort	Absent	Weak, irregular	Good, crying
Muscle tone	Flaccid	Some flexion of extremities	Well flexed
Reflex irritability (catheter in nose)	No response	Grimace	Cough or sneeze
Color	Blue, pale	Body pink; extremities blue	Completely pink

From Klaus MH and Fanaroff AA: Care of the high-risk neonate, ed 3, Philadelphia, 1986, WB Saunders Co.

In many hospitals a second, more thorough, examination is performed within 12 hours after birth to assess degree of recovery from the birth process, presence or absence of signs of respiratory distress, and readiness to begin routine feedings. This examination can be a safety check before transferring the baby from the "transition" nursery to the "routine" nursery. It should take place in a warmed environment with the baby undressed to allow careful observation of the respiratory rate, the degree of respiratory effort as evidenced by intercostal retractions, the color, and spontaneous activity. Often quiet babies can arouse themselves with a "startle," or Moro, response that can interfere with the examination. Giving the baby something to suck on (rubber nipple, examiner's finger, or baby's fist) will help keep the infant as relaxed as possible; examination several hours after a feeding is ideal. Although it is important to assess the intensity and pitch of the cry, as much of the painless parts of the examination as possible should be performed before fully arousing the baby. Therefore, with the baby supine, and following general observations, many examiners begin by listening to the heart and lungs, then palpating the abdomen before examining the remaining systems, leaving the usually discomforting abduction of the hips until last.

Examination of the undressed baby with the parents present just before discharge affords the opportunity to point out normal findings, answer questions about perceived imperfections (and sometimes allow both parents a first look at their baby's entire body), and observe the quality of the parent-infant attachment while the baby is being held or fed. Holding the baby in an *en face* position (where the mother's face is rotated such that her eyes and those of the infant meet fully in the same vertical plane of rotation as shown in Fig. 7-1), smiling at the baby, responding to signs of hunger or satiation, and talking about the baby positively and confidently are all signs that strong parent-infant bonds are being formed and have been enhanced by the hospital experience.

Infancy

Infants between the ages of 1 and 6 months are almost always a pleasure to examine because of their responsiveness to the examiner's face and their increasing interest in environmental objects such as tongue depressors and penlights. At this age infants can be examined successfully on the examination table, with the parent usually standing close beside the table. With the infant's clothes removed except for the diaper, spontaneous activity, state of alertness, and responsiveness to both the examiner and the parent may be observed. The order of the examination varies. If the infant is asleep in the parent's lap or held upright at the breast or shoulder, the heart and respiratory rates can be obtained, and the heart, lungs, and even the abdomen can be examined without waking the baby. Again, the relatively uncomfortable abducting of the hips and speculum examination of the tympanic membranes are best left until last. Prolonged or painful procedures, such as deep palpation of the abdomen or a rectal examination, are best done while the baby is being fed. The infant should be examined as if physically attached to the parent, and the parent's response, especially to painful procedures, should be noted. Sometimes the parent may appropriately thank the examiner for removing an irritable, crying baby to the examining table (or to another room if on a house call), but the physician must never be lulled into thinking that the isolated examination of the infant is a complete examination. With a chronically hospitalized baby, a continuous-care nurse may substitute for an absent parent during the examination.

Infants 6 to 12 months of age are increasingly difficult to examine because of their normally developing anxiety toward faces of those other than their parents and perceived separation from the parent. Offering interesting objects or allowing infants to sit and reach for objects or to walk or crawl around the office can help distract them. Direct eye contact with the strange face of the examiner can be especially frightening to the baby. Examination at these ages is usually easier with the baby held in the parent's arms or on the parent's lap. In many clinical situations direct observation of a breast-feeding or a bottle-feeding is extremely useful and can identify problems such as improper feeding techniques, weak sucking movements, and dysfunctional swallowing.

Early Childhood

With children in this age group the most effective initial approach is to form a supportive relationship with the parent or older sibling, who, it is hoped, will become the physician's ally in examining the child. This alliance is aided by identifying the parent's emotional state and anxiety level during the history and then "tuning in" nonjudgmentally. For instance, if the parent appears both anxious about the child's symptoms and guilty about having had to bother the physi-

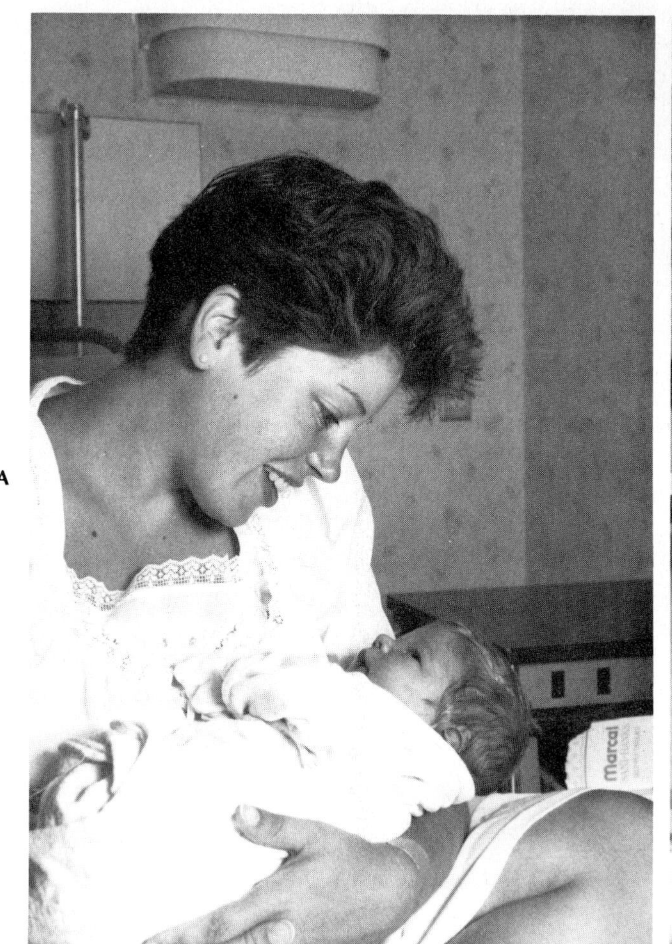

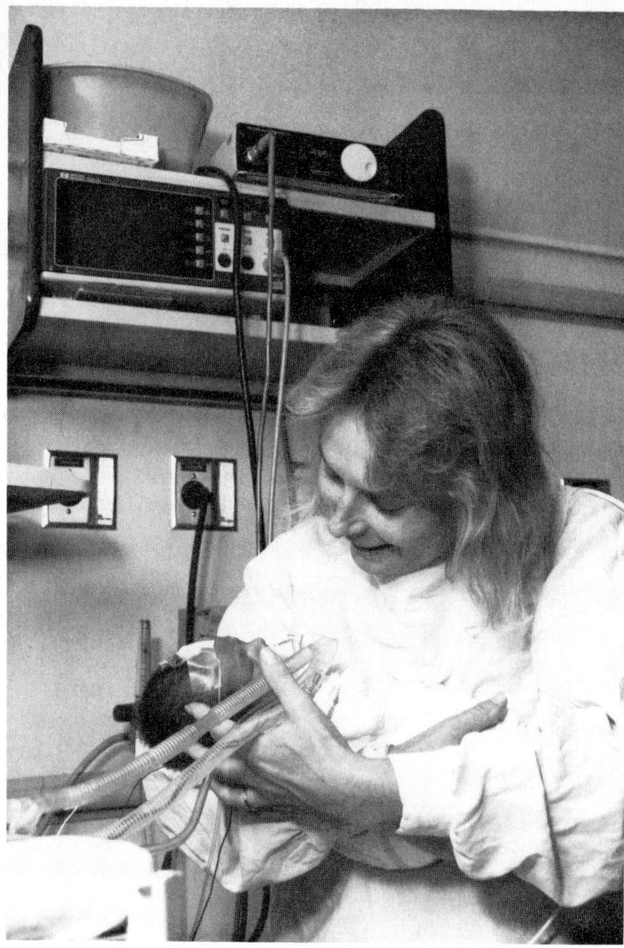

Fig. 7-1 A, Full-term 1-day-old infant looking "en face" eye-to-eye with his mother. **B,** The mother of a 2-day-old, 31-week, 1400 g premature infant on a ventilator positions herself so she can look eye-to-eye with her son.
Courtesy Ruth A. Lawrence, M.D.

cian, the physician might say, "I know it can be frightening to hear a baby cough like that, and I'm glad you brought him in to be examined." A parent who appears angry sometimes can be "defused" by a remark such as, "I know how aggravating it must be to have to bring your child in for so many ear infections." Tired, worn-out parents will work with the physician who is sympathetic, but they can be distracting and even disruptive if they receive nonverbal and verbal messages that they are improperly dressed, somewhat less than adequate as parents, or a general nuisance to those who practice medicine.

In most situations children 1 to 5 years of age are easiest to examine while being held by the parent, a position that is also comforting to the child when the history is initiated. A few toys and books on a low table, colorful photographs and children's drawings on the walls, and the absence of a white coat on the examiner often will lead children to relax and encourage them to leave the parent and explore the office. It can be helpful to offer the child a piece of examining equipment such as a stethoscope or percussion hammer to handle while the history is being taken. The examiner often can alleviate fear by showing the child what an otoscope is and demonstrating its use before using it on the child. Observing the child's handling of objects and interest and confidence in exploring a new environment, as well as the parent's reaction to the child's curiosity or fear, gives the examiner information important to understanding the child's developmental status and anticipating the parent's ability to cope with any problems that the child may have.

In general, older children in this age group are increasingly able to communicate verbally with the examiner. A conversation that starts about the child's pet cat or siblings can then lead to a description of what is about to be done. Continuing to describe what is being done ("I am now listening to your heart beating") can soothe even the child who starts off by screaming and kicking. With a frightened child, prolonged silence on the part of the examiner can be interpreted by the parent as disgust or anger with the child or parent. A continuing conversation with the parent and the child during the examination also signals to the child that the examiner is on the parent's side, and this may increase the child's confidence that nothing too drastic will be done.

It is optimal to have the child remain dressed until just before the examination, and portions of an examination can be accomplished by only partially removing pieces of clothing. Even before having the parent undress the child, important general observations about the child can be made, such as the activity level, gross and fine motor coordination, receptive and expressive language function, skin color, respiratory rate, and ability to cope with a foreign environment. Some specific portions of a developmental assessment, such as throwing and catching a ball or drawing a circle, often can break the ice and help the child into a gamelike atmosphere that can be continued throughout the examination.

Again, the order of the examination should be flexible; painful (ears, throat) and frightening (anything that requires lying down) procedures should be postponed until last. A steady pace, coupled with gentle but firm anticipatory statements ("Now I'm going to have you lie down so I can listen to your tummy"), will enhance a relatively brief encounter, which in turn will keep the parent on your side.

Restraining is often necessary—for instance, for an adequate examination of the tympanic membranes—and can be done in a number of ways, all enhanced by continuing the descriptions and discussions in a calm voice. The parent is usually the best assistant. The child can be restrained by holding the outstretched arms against the child's head or against the child's abdomen while the examiner's body and one elbow immobilize the lower half of the child's body. The parents should be reassured that struggling is a normal response to an examination in this age group, especially if the child is berated or threatened by them. The examiner's goal should be to evaluate the health and illness of the child adequately and at the same time maintain the trust and confidence of both the child and parent. Achieving this goal requires long hours of practice, the flexibility to ask other professionals for help when the examiner's (or the parent's) patience is about to run out, and most important, an enjoyment of the diversity, unpredictability, and spontaneity of children.

Late Childhood

Children in this age group usually are a pleasure to examine and rarely present any problems. A key ingredient to the successful examination is a relaxed conversation with the child about subjects such as school, hobbies, or favorite friends, interspersed with brief comments about the examination itself. Occasionally, a child who as an infant had an unpleasant experience with a physician will need more time for the preparatory description of the examination. School-age children usually prefer wearing a simple drape over their underpants and also prefer siblings of the opposite sex being absent, particularly when the genitalia are examined. The order of the examination can be the same as in adults (vital signs, then head to foot), with care taken to anticipate any painful manipulations or procedures. As in examining younger children, the examiner can make the following critical observations without the actual "laying on of hands": the activity level, ability to follow simple directions, ability to read passages of varying difficulty and to write, clarity of

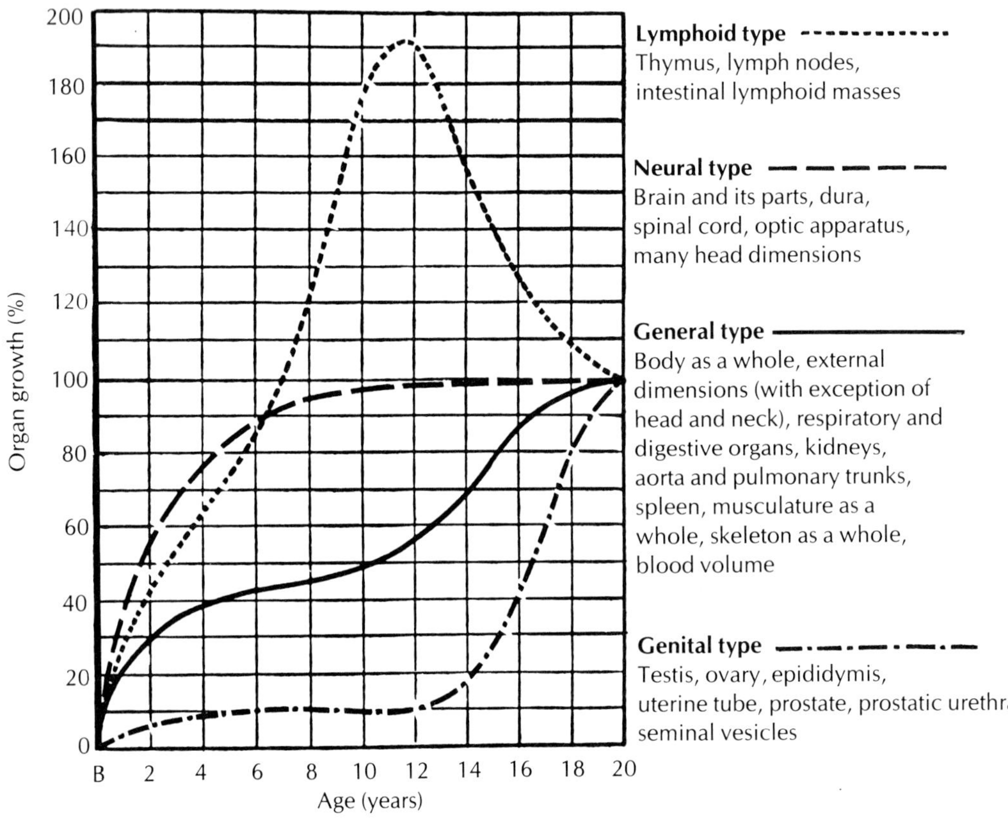

Fig. 7-2 Differential organ growth curves.
From Harris JA et al: The measurement of man, Minneapolis, 1930, University of Minnesota Press.

articulation, mood, level of neuromaturational functioning as tested by tasks such as hopping on one foot and rapidly alternating hand movements, and the relationship with the parent.

Adolescence

Adolescents can be examined successfully in the absence of their parents, but the value to anxious parents of seeing their teenager cope successfully with an examination should not be overlooked. Most adolescents respect a straightforward, uncondescending approach, and parents usually respect the examiner who approaches adolescents as though they were adults. Decisions about who will be present when the patient is examined should be discussed openly with both the parent and the adolescent. If the parent elects to step away during the examination, the examiner is afforded an opportunity to review pertinent history or concerns directly with the adolescent. Most pubertal boys and girls have concerns about what is happening to their bodies, and a physical examination allows the examiner to illuminate and try to answer these concerns. Some special clinics for adolescents use brief, self-administered questionnaires so that the examiner can more quickly tune in to the present concerns of the adolescent. While performing the examination, the examiner can reassure the pubertal child about normal developmental stages such as unilateral gynecomastia in boys, rapidly enlarging feet, the beginning of acne, and the interrelationships of the adolescent growth spurt and sexual development. The examiner's ability to approach the child's emerging sexuality factually or nonanxiously will help adolescents view themselves, at least briefly, with objectivity.

VITAL SIGNS AND EVALUATION OF SOMATIC GROWTH

Just as general observations of a child's behavior can give important clues about the child's general level of functioning, the measuring of vital signs and characteristics of somatic growth often provides the basis for decisions concerning the overall health or illness of the child. An abnormal vital sign or physical measurement often is the only outward indication of a problem in a child. Interpretation of vital signs and physical measurements depends on a knowledge of the normal biologic changes of the growing infant, child, and adolescent. One principal characteristic of human growth is that different organ systems mature according to different rates and timing throughout fetal life, infancy, and childhood. Fig. 7-2 compares the longitudinal growth of the body as a whole with three component tissues: lymphoid, neural, and genital.

Temperature

Body temperature usually is measured rectally in infants and children up to the age of 6 or 7 years and orally in older children who can understand directions about retaining the thermometer. Axillary temperature sometimes is measured, especially in infants with excoriated bottoms or in small premature infants, and generally is 2° F lower than the rectal and 1° F lower than the oral temperature. The rectal temperature usually is measured with the infant or child held prone on the parent's lap (Fig. 7-3), the buttocks separated, and the lubricated thermometer inserted through the anal sphincter at an angle of about 20 degrees toward the table for a distance of 1½ inches. The thermometer is held in place for approximately 1 minute, either by the examiner or by the parent. Because of the relative thermal instability of newborns, especially prematurely born babies, the ambient temperature often is measured and recorded at the same time and sometimes can explain an abnormally elevated or depressed rectal temperature. Temperatures of newborns normally are higher than temperatures of older children, averaging approximately 99.5° F (37.5° C) during the first 6 months of life, falling below 99° F (37.2° C) after 3 years of age, and reaching 98° F (36.7° C) by age 11 years. A circadian rhythm of body temperature is observable by age 2 years and is well developed by age 5 years, with increasingly higher temperatures during the daylight hours and a fall in temperature during the night (Fig. 7-4). In infants and children there often is little relationship between the degree of temperature elevation and the severity of illness. In fact, hypothermia sometimes develops in infants with profound infection, and children can have rectal temperatures as high as 101° F (38.3° C) after vigorous activity. It is not uncommon for children with elective hospital admissions to have elevated temperatures initially, probably because of transient anxiety.

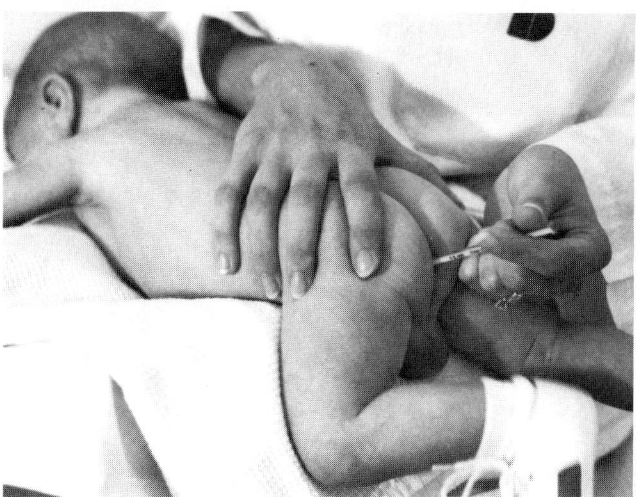

Fig. 7-3 Temperature measurement in infants.
Photograph by P. Ruben.

Pulse

The heart rate is measured by palpating the peripheral pulse (femoral, radial, or carotid arteries), by observing the pulsating anterior fontanelle, or by directly palpating or auscultating the heart. The pulse can be increased significantly in normal infants and children by anxiety, fever, and exercise before or during the examination, as well as by inflammatory illnesses, shock, and congestive heart failure. There are major changes in resting heart rate with increasing age, probably reflecting increasing functional control by the vagus nerve

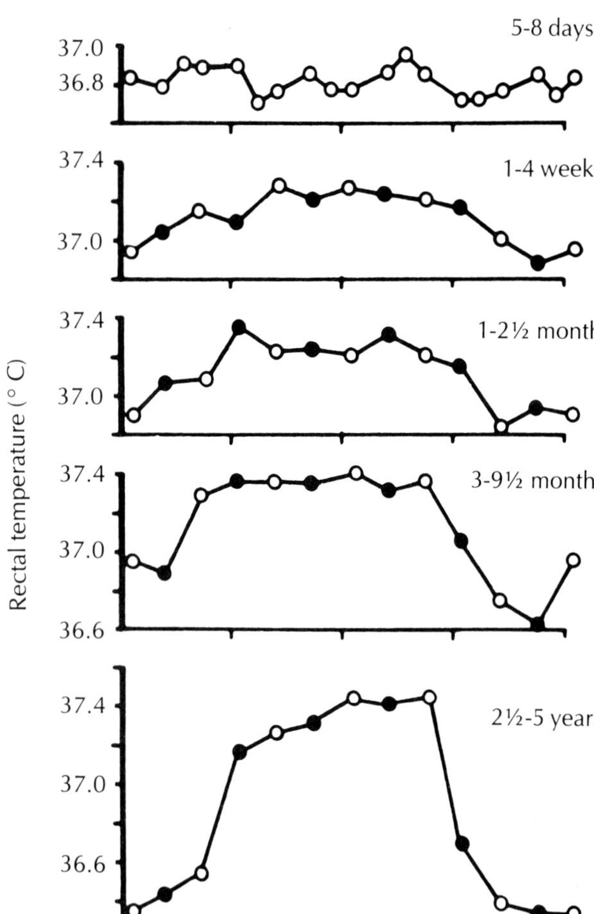

Fig. 7-4 Mean rectal temperature at different hours in groups of infants at different ages. Except in the youngest group, measurements were made every 4 hours. The hollow and solid circles represent different groups of 3 to 18 infants observed over 2 to 11 days. *MN*, Midnight.

From Davis JA and Dobbing J: Scientific foundations of pediatrics, ed 2, Baltimore, Md, 1981, University Park Press.

(Table 7-2). A circadian rhythm in the heart rate is observed by 2 years of age with a fall of 10 to 20 beats/min during sleep; an absence of this rate slowing with sleep can be helpful in diagnosing acute rheumatic fever or thyrotoxicosis.

The rhythm of the heartbeat is assessed; equal spacing between consecutive beats is recorded as regular sinus rhythm (RSR). The cardiac rhythm is more commonly irregular than regular, especially in early and late childhood, reflecting sinus arrhythmia and increasing vagal control. Extrasystoles, appearing as irregularly spaced beats with or without a compensatory pause, are common in healthy children, can usually be abolished by exercise, and rarely occur as the only physical finding of underlying heart disease. Heart rates greater than 180 beats/min (especially if rigidly regular) in infants beyond the neonatal period may indicate atrial *tachycardia*. Other arrhythmias in children are rare and occur mostly in those with underlying heart disease (e.g., congenital heart disease, rheumatic fever, and Kawasaki disease). Tachycardia with shock in infants and children usually is associated with a weak pulse and cold, sweaty extremities. Tachycardia caused by congestive heart failure usually coexists with significant tachypnea, with or without hepatic enlargement. Heart block can occur in children with Lyme disease who have myocardial involvement.

Table 7-2 *Average Heart Rate for Infants and Children at Rest*

AGE	AVERAGE RATE	TWO STANDARD DEVIATIONS
Birth	140	50
First month	130	45
1-6 mo	130	45
6-12 mo	115	40
1-2 yr	110	40
2-4 yr	105	35
6-10 yr	95	30
10-14 yr	85	30
14-18 yr	82	25

Reproduced with permission from Lowrey GH: Growth and development of children, ed 8. Copyright © 1986 by Year Book Medical Publishers, Inc., Chicago.

Respirations

Observations of the rate, depth, and ease of respiration begin at the first encounter with the child. The rate of respiration, like the heart rate, is significantly influenced by emotion and exercise, making it necessary to wait in some instances until a resting state is reached or to count the rate immediately if the infant or child is first encountered asleep. The rate may be counted by observing abdominal excursion in infants and thoracic excursion in children, ideally at a moment when the child is not paying attention to the examiner. In a sleeping infant the respiratory sounds may be counted with the bell of the stethoscope held just in front of the nose. The respiratory rate varies with age, reflecting variables such as aspirated amniotic fluid in the newborn and increasing numbers of alveoli and increasing lung compliance with postnatal growth. Rates vary between 30 and 80 breaths/min in the newborn, 20 and 40 during infancy and early childhood, and 15 and 25 during late childhood; adult levels of 15 to 20 are reached by age 15. Because changes in respiratory rate are common over short periods, the rate should be counted for at least 1 minute, especially in crying or excited infants. Observation of the respiratory rate is necessary for several minutes in newborn babies, especially in premature babies of less than 2 kg and 36 weeks of gestational age, to discover apneic episodes (absent respirations for 20 seconds or more) and periodic breathing (apneic periods of between 5 and 10 seconds). In early and late childhood irregular respirations such as Cheyne-Stokes breathing are seen only in severely ill children, such as those with overwhelming infection or severe head trauma.

Depth of respiration is determined subjectively and compared with norms observed for that age group; deep breathing may be observed in states of metabolic acidosis, and shallow breathing in severe obstructive states such as asthma. Ease of respiration is in part a subjective determination, as in estimating degree of dyspnea, and is discussed in the section of this chapter on the chest and lungs.

Blood Pressure

In recent years there has been an interest in the possibility of identifying individuals with essential hypertension before health supervision visits. In addition, as intensive care techniques have improved, blood pressure determinations in hospitalized infants and children are more regularly obtained. It is essential to measure the blood pressure in evaluating all children with suspected congenital heart disease and suspected chronic renal disease and in unconscious patients. Blood pressure measurements in healthy ambulatory patients are compared with standard norms (see Figs. 141-1, 141-2, and 141-3).

The auscultatory method of determining blood pressure is useful and practiced in children beyond age 5 or 6 years; between ages 2 and 5 some children are cooperative, but others remain agitated and anxious. It is helpful to remember that blood pressures of hospitalized chidren, especially those admitted for elective reasons, are higher during the first 1 or 2 days and then tend to plateau at lower levels; the blood pressure of sick hospitalized children tends to remain constant throughout the hospitalization. Several determinations may be required to obtain values unaffected by anxiety. Having children "watch the silver column rise" and warning them that the balloon will gently squeeze their arm usually decrease anxiety.

The size of the cuff is important because cuffs that are too small will cause falsely elevated values. The optimal cuff size is one that covers two thirds of the distance between the antecubital fossa and the shoulder or between the popliteal fossa and the hip. The rubber bag inside the cuff should completely encircle the extremity. At every site used for examining infants and children, there should be cuffs varying from 1 to 4 inches in width.

In the auscultation method the point at which the sounds are first heard is recorded as the systolic pressure, and the point at which the sounds disappear is recorded as the diastolic pressure. When the pulse sounds cannot be auscultated, a distal artery (radial, popliteal, or dorsalis pedis) can be palpated, and the point at which the first pulsation is felt is about 10 mm Hg lower than the auscultated systolic pressure. The flush method can be used in infants and young children. The elevated extremity, with the uninflated cuff in place, is stroked and "milked" from the hand to the elbow. The cuff is then inflated to a point above the estimated systolic pressure, and the pressure is slowly released. A sudden flush or reddening of the extremity, compared with the color of the opposite extremity, will occur at a point approximately halfway between the systolic and diastolic pressures. Normally, the systolic pressure is higher in the lower extremities, and the diastolic pressure is the same in the arms and legs.

Somatic Growth

Assessing somatic growth is a crucial part of every evaluation of an infant or a child because growth is the central characteristic of normal children and deviations from the child's norm provide an early warning of pathologic processes. Several tools exist to aid in this evaluation; the most important are growth charts constructed either by longitudinal, serial measurements of a single cohort of children or by measurements of large numbers of children of different ages over a brief period of time. Although physical measurements of a child at a single point in time will give some useful clinical information, serial measurements over months or years provide an accurate record of the infant's or child's overall general pattern of growth, with deviations from the subject's norm indicating some intrinsic defect or environmental insult. The physical measurements most often used in assessing children are height and weight and, in infants and young children, the head circumference as well. To be clinically useful, all these measurements should be made with care and with the use of a consistent technique.

Of the different growth charts currently available, the most recent were published by the National Center for Health Statistics and include the following: length-for-age or stature-for-age, weight-for-age, head circumference-for-age (to 36 months), and weight-for-length or weight-for-stature from birth to puberty. There are separate charts for boys and girls of two age groups: birth to 36 months and 2 to 18 years (Figs. 7-5 to 7-16). The percentile lines on these charts indicate the number of normal children expected to fall above and below the index child's measurement. For instance, a 2-year-old girl whose length is 34 inches is in the 50th percentile for length; 50% of all normal 2-year-old girls will be expected to be taller, and 50% shorter.

Other growth charts indicate the mean and standard deviations from the mean by chronologic age. Standard deviations (SD) are defined mathematically, such as 1 SD above and below the mean includes about 67% of the measurements, and 2 SD above and below the mean includes about 95% of the measurements.

Velocity growth curves (Fig. 7-17) are used to measure differential rates of growth at different ages. Although not generally used in clinical settings, they illustrate the two periods of rapid growth—infancy and puberty—and the differences by sex at puberty.

Height. Standing height can be measured fairly accurately in children older than 2 or 3 years of age. Some growth charts, such as Stuart's, use standing height measurements beginning at age 6; others, such as new National Center for Health Statistics charts, plot standing heights beginning at age 2 years. Stand-up scales with attachments for measuring height generally are inaccurate. Short of buying an expensive wall-mounted apparatus (Stadiometer), accurate measurements can be made by attaching a graduated tape or ruler to a wall and placing a flat surface on top of the head to determine the height (Fig. 7-18). This measurement should be made with the child standing in stockings or bare feet with the heels back and shoulders just touching the wall.

Length of infants is most accurately measured by the use of flat boards placed across and perpendicular to the examining table in contact with the vertex of the head and the soles of the feet and reading the measurement from a scale attached to the surface of the table (Fig. 7-19); care must be taken, in newborns particularly, to extend the hips and knees fully.

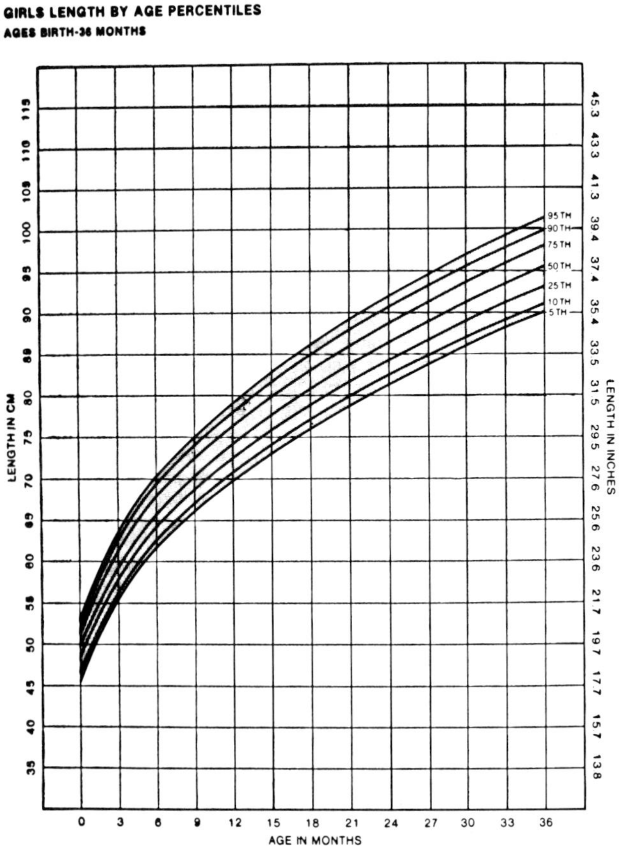

GIRLS LENGTH BY AGE PERCENTILES
AGES BIRTH-36 MONTHS

LENGTH IN CM

LENGTH IN INCHES

AGE IN MONTHS

95TH
90TH
75TH
50TH
25TH
10TH
5TH

Fig. 7-5 Girls from birth to 36 months: length by age.

Modified from Hamill VV, Drizd TA, Johnson CL et al: Physical growth: National Center for Health Statistics percentiles, Am J Clin Nutr 32:607, 1979.

GIRLS WEIGHT BY AGE PERCENTILES
AGES BIRTH-36 MONTHS

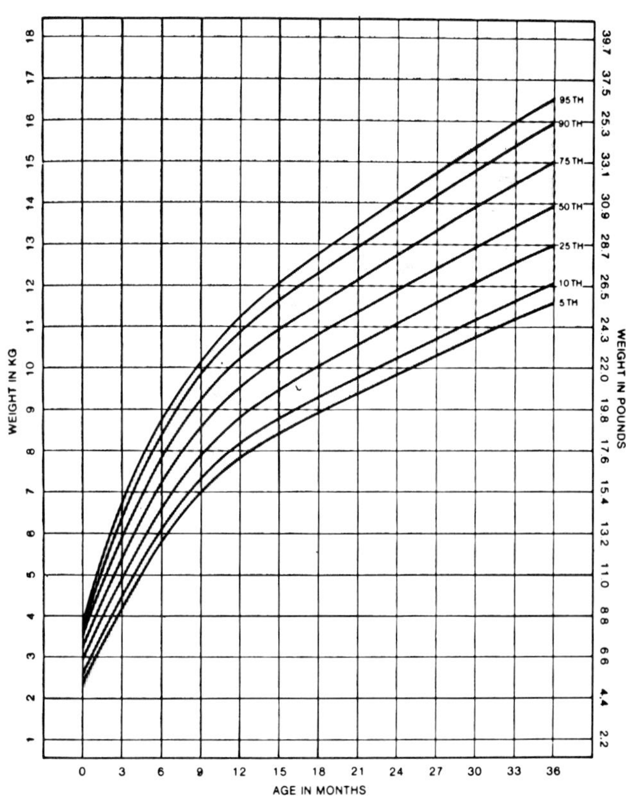

Fig. 7-6 Girls from birth to 36 months: weight by age.

Modified from Hamill VV, Drizd TA, Johnson CL et al: Physical growth: National Center for Health Statistics percentiles, Am J Clin Nutr 32:607, 1979.

GIRLS HEAD CIRCUMFERENCE BY AGE PERCENTILES
AGES BIRTH-36 MONTHS

AGE IN MONTHS

HEAD CIRCUMFERENCE IN CM

WEIGHT IN KG

LENGHT IN CM

GIRLS WEIGHT BY LENGTH PERCENTILES
AGES BIRTH-36 MONTHS

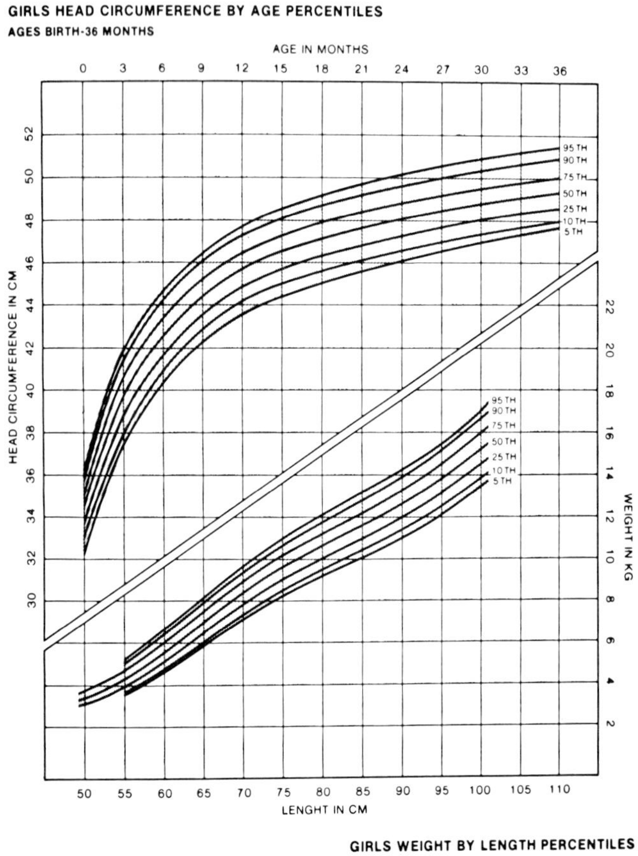

Fig. 7-7 Girls from birth to 36 months: head circumference by age and weight by length.

Modified from Hamill VV, Drizd TA, Johnson CL et al: Physical growth: National Center for Health Statistics percentiles, Am J Clin Nutr 32:607, 1979.

GIRLS STATURE BY AGE PERCENTILES
AGES 2-18 YEARS

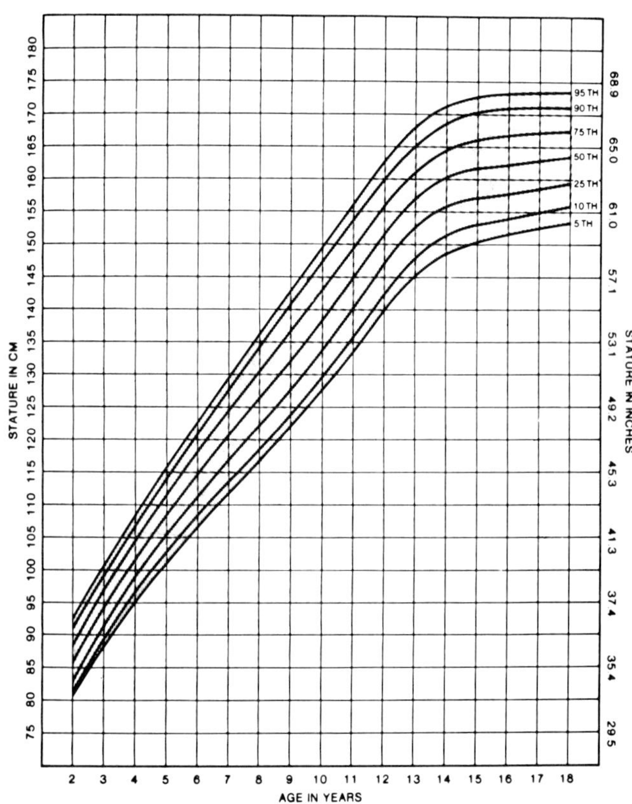

Fig. 7-8 Girls from 2 to 18 years: stature by age.

Modified from Hamill VV, Drizd TA, Johnson CL et al: Physical growth: National Center for Health Statistics percentiles, Am J Clin Nutr 32:607, 1979.

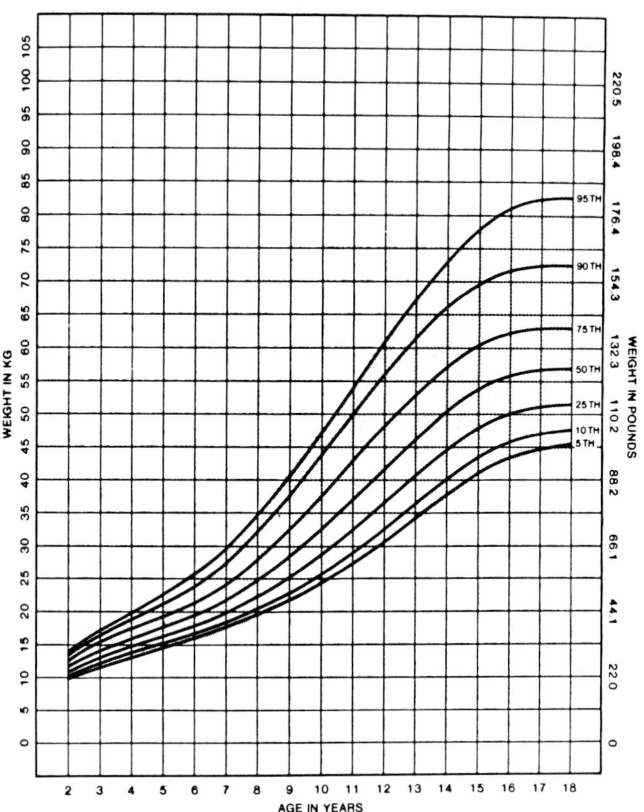

Fig. 7-9 Girls from 2 to 18 years: weight by age.

Modified from Hamill VV, Drizd TA, Johnson CL et al: Physical growth: National Center for Health Statistics percentiles, Am J Clin Nutr 32:607, 1979.

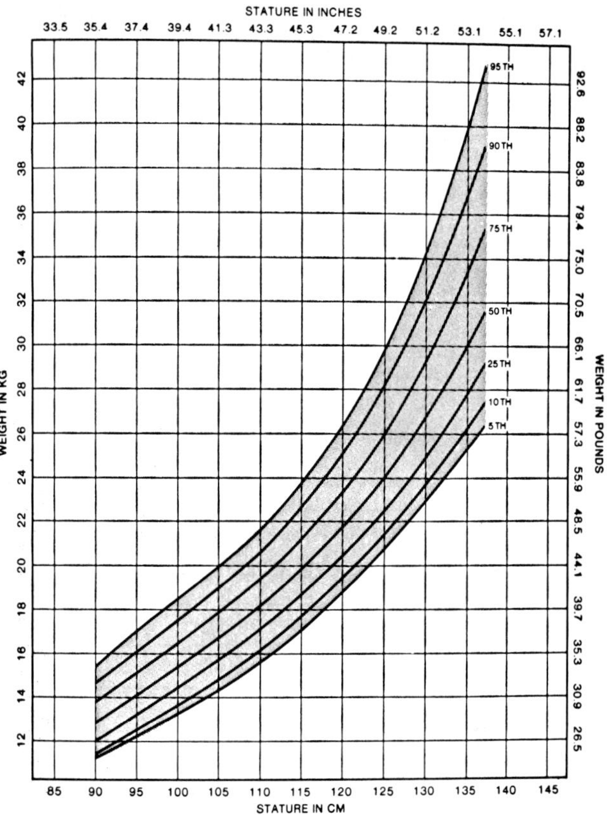

Fig. 7-10 Prepubertal girls: weight by stature.

Modified from Hamill VV, Drizd TA, Johnson CL et al: Physical growth: National Center for Health Statistics percentiles, Am J Clin Nutr 32:607, 1979.

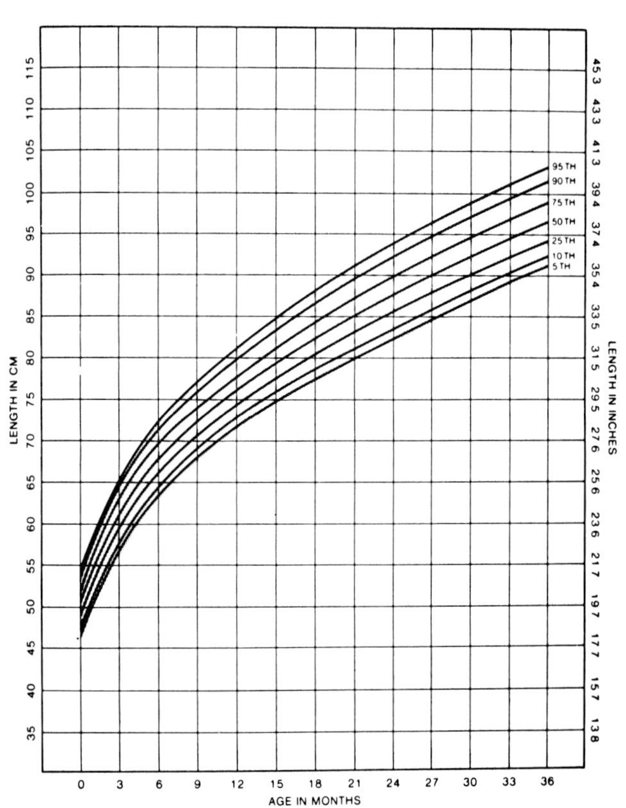

Fig. 7-11 Boys from birth to 36 months: length by age.

Modified from Hamill VV, Drizd TA, Johnson CL et al: Physical growth: National Center for Health Statistics percentiles, Am J Clin Nutr 32:607, 1979.

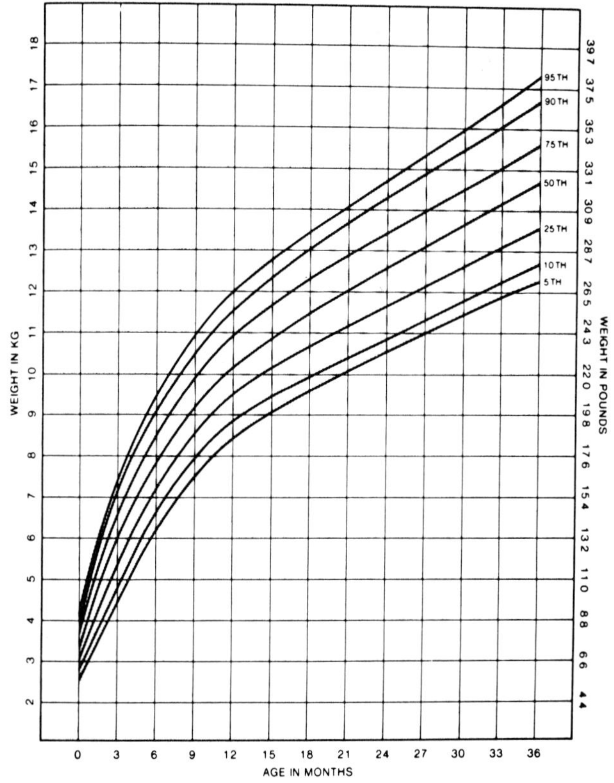

Fig. 7-12 Boys from birth to 36 months: weight by age.

Modified from Hamill VV, Drizd TA, Johnson CL et al: Physical growth: National Center for Health Statistics percentiles, Am J Clin Nutr 32:607, 1979.

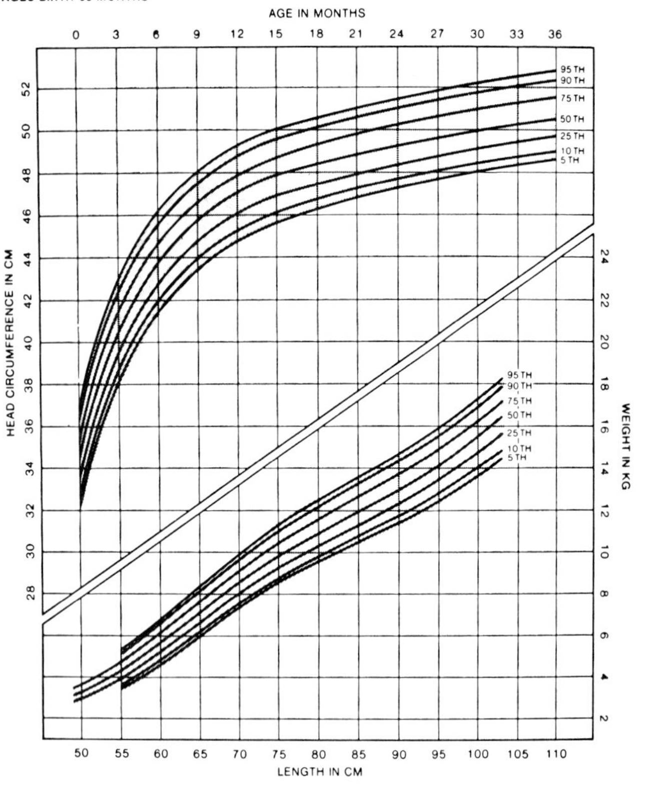

Fig. 7-13 Boys from birth to 36 months: head circumference by age and weight by length.

Modified from Hamill VV, Drizd TA, Johnson CL et al: Physical growth: National Center for Health Statistics percentiles, Am J Clin Nutr 32:607, 1979.

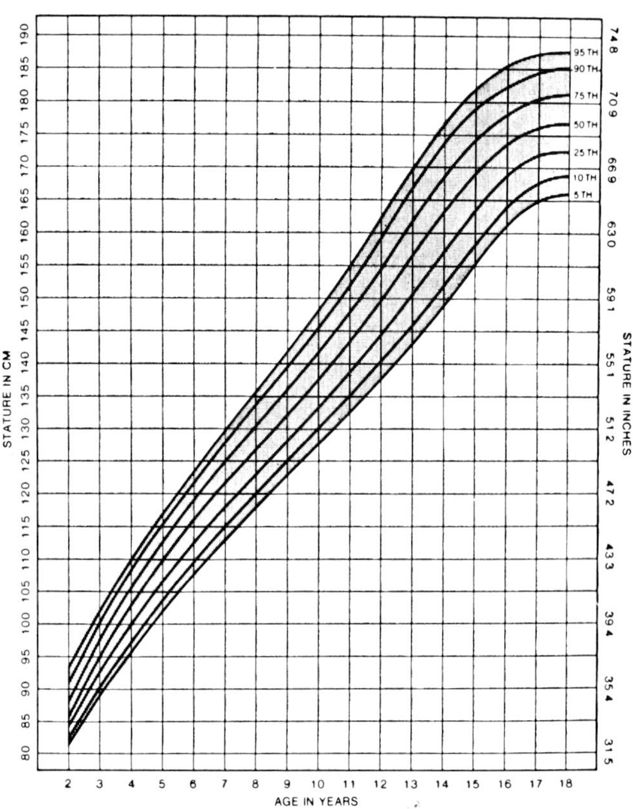

Fig. 7-14 Boys from 2 to 18 years: stature by age.

Modified from Hamill VV, Drizd TA, Johnson CL et al: Physical growth: National Center for Health Statistics percentiles, Am J Clin Nutr 32:607, 1979.

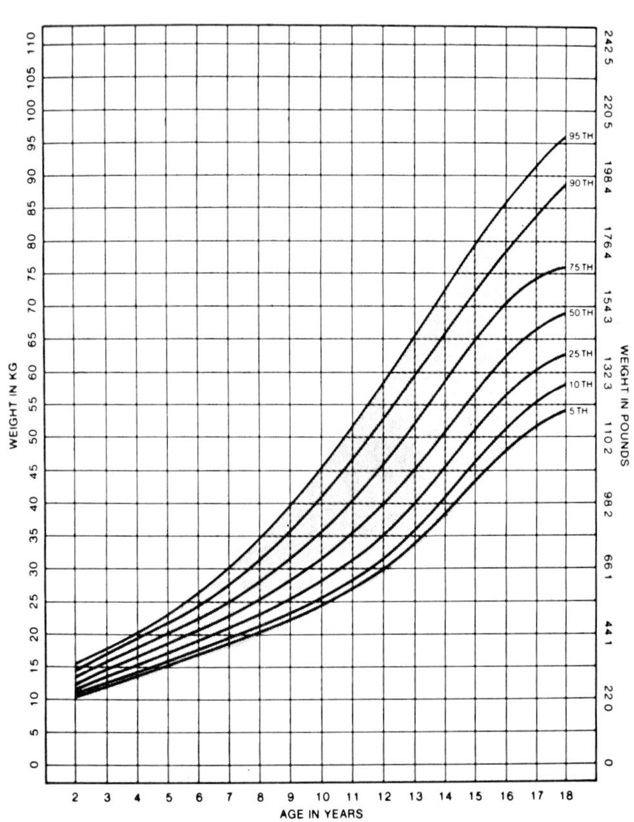

Fig. 7-15 Boys from 2 to 18 years: weight by age.

Modified from Hamill VV, Drizd TA, Johnson CL et al: Physical growth: National Center for Health Statistics percentiles, Am J Clin Nutr 32:607, 1979.

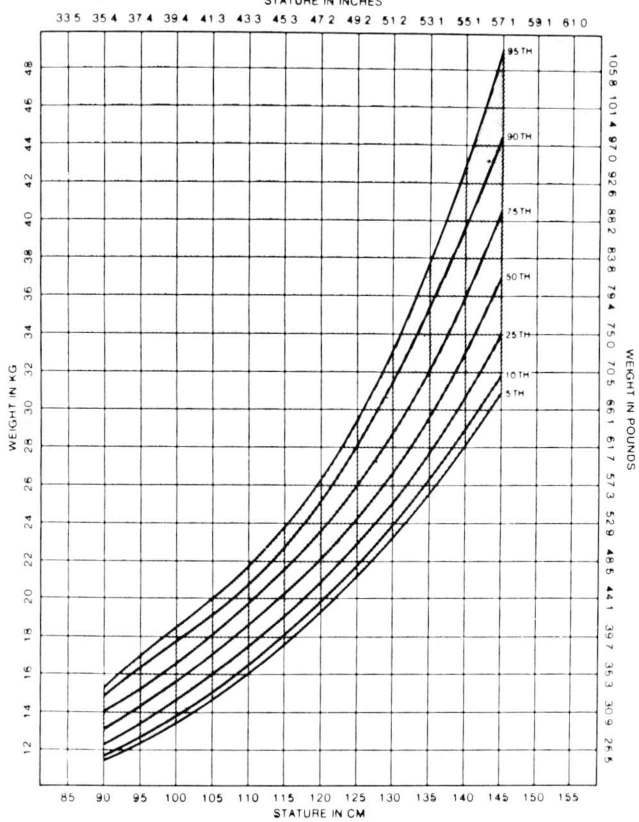

Fig. 7-16 Prepubertal boys: weight by stature.

Modified from Hamill VV, Drizd TA, Johnson CL et al: Physical growth: National Center for Health Statistics percentiles, Am J Clin Nutr 32:607, 1979.

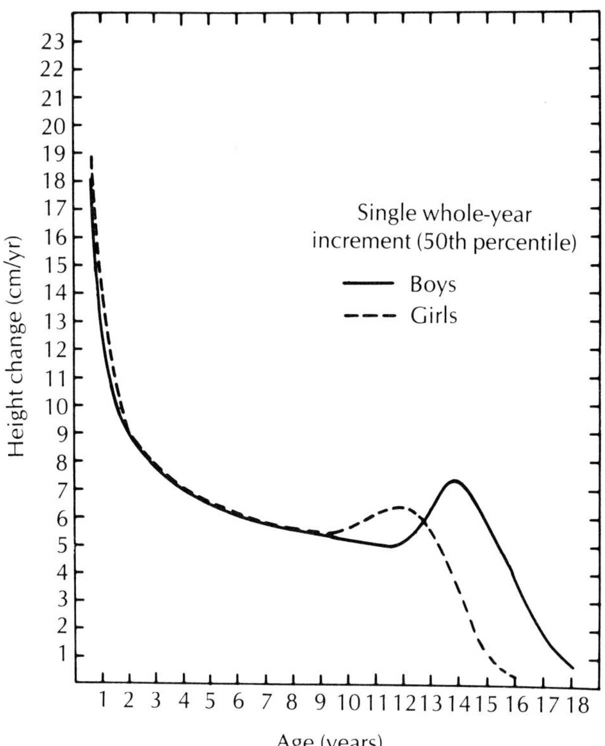

Fig. 7-17 Velocity curves for length and height for boys and girls based on intervals of 1 year.

Reproduced by permission from Lowrey GH: Growth and development of children, 8th edition. Copyright © 1986 by Year Book Medical Publishers, Inc., Chicago.

Weight. Infants are weighed on infant scales, with the infant clothed only in a diaper. Children old enough to stand are weighed in their underpants on stand-up scales. Stand-up scales, because of their usually wobbly base, may be frightening to children 1 to 3 years old, and it sometimes is necessary to weigh the child by subtracting the parent's weight from the combined parent-child weight. Ideally, serial measurements are made using the same scale. In most normally growing children the height and weight measurements, when plotted on growth charts, fall within two standard percentile lines of each other (e.g., the 3rd, 10th, 25th, 50th, 75th, 90th, and 97th percentiles). Children with measurements either above the 97th or below the 3rd percentile require further evaluation, as do children whose height and weight differ by more than two percentile lines or categories.

Head Circumference. The head circumference is measured and plotted on a standard growth chart during each health maintenance examination from birth to 2 years, the period of maximum rate of brain growth. Head circumference measurements on children older than 2 years are obtained on initial examination of any child and when any component of the growth curve has been abnormal.

The measurement is made by placing a cloth tape measure around the maximum occipitofrontal circumference, taking three separate readings and selecting the largest value. In measuring the heads of infants it is usually necessary to have the infant supine with the arms held firmly against the body by the parent or nurse; with children the examiner can improve cooperation by first demonstrating the use of the measuring tape on himself or herself.

Chest and Other Measurements. In newborns the chest circumference is compared with the head circumference, the head having a larger circumference. The chest circumference normally equals and then exceeds the head circumference during the first year of life. Chest circumference is measured at the level of the nipples midway between expiration and inspiration. Another chest measurement sometimes used in following up children with chronic pulmonary disease is the thoracic index, obtained by dividing the anteroposterior by the transverse chest diameters. This index normally decreases from 0.85 at birth to 0.74 at age 6 years, because of the more rapid growth of the transverse diameter. The transverse (side-to-side) and anteroposterior (sternum-to-vertebrae spinous

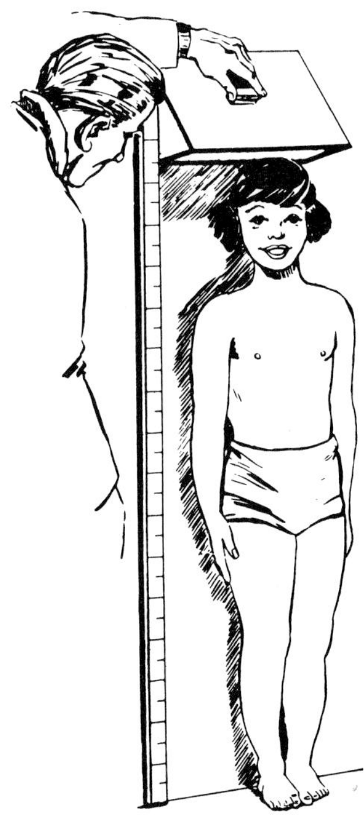

Fig. 7-18 Measurement of height.

From Evaluation of body size and physical growth of children, 1976, Rockville, Md, The Maternal and Child Health Program, US Department of Health, Education and Welfare.

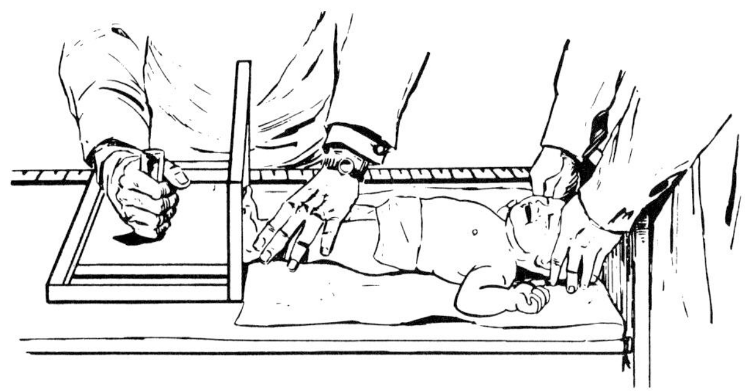

Fig. 7-19 Measurement of length in the infant.

From Evaluation of body size and physical growth of children, 1976, Rockville, Md., The Maternal and Child Health Program, US Department of Health, Education and Welfare.

process) diameters are most accurately measured at the level of the nipples with special calipers.

Additional somatic measurements can be useful in the evaluation of children with abnormal somatic growth. The ratio of the upper to the lower half of the body is obtained by measuring the distance from crown to symphysis pubis and then from symphysis pubis to the floor (or to the heel in an infant) in the standing position. This ratio changes from 1.7:1 in the newborn to 1:1 in the adult. The arm span, normally equal to the standing height, is measured from fingertip to fingertip of the third fingers with the arms outstretched. Norms for these measurements by age and by height are available in pediatric endocrinology textbooks.

ORGAN SYSTEMS

Skin

During the development of the fetus, neural crest cells, or melanoblasts, with the potential for producing melanin, migrate from the dorsal region of the developing embryo. Under genetic control and mediated by tyrosinase, the melanoblasts produce varying amounts and shades of melanin, which make up the pigment of the skin, the hair, and the iris. Midline, ventral areas of defective pigmentation, such as piebaldism, can result from several developmental causes and sometimes are associated with defects in the development of the neural crest cells that give rise to the bipolar cells of the auditory nerve. Individuals with absent tyrosinase lack pigmentation and have albinism. Localized areas of depigmentation shaped like a leaf are seen in tuberous sclerosis.

The periderm is a superficial layer of epidermis with absorption properties that normally is shed before birth; persistence of the periderm is seen in the "collodion baby" and in forms of congenital ichthyosis. Hair follicles begin developing during the third fetal month, and skin keratinization first occurs at their openings. Sebaceous glands, whose secretions contribute to the formation of vernix caseosa, are active starting in the latter months of pregnancy; then, following birth, they are relatively inactive until puberty. Apocrine glands are formed in the fetus but are not fully developed until puberty. Sweat glands, growing most rapidly between the twenty-second and twenty-fourth fetal weeks, are inactive in the fetus. They become active after several weeks in the newborn, reaching a maximal rate of activity by age 2 years. Sweat gland secretion may be under some degree of cortical control, possibly explaining the increased tendency of children to sweat at all times and the tendency of adults to sweat more while asleep.

Adipose tissue begins to develop during fetal life and constitutes 28% of the body weight at term. The number of fat cells increases especially rapidly during the first year of life, adipose tissue constituting from 40% to 70% of the body weight at 4 months of age. Cell numbers increase at a slower rate until puberty, when there is a second growth spurt. In adults, adipose tissue constitutes 15% to 40% of body weight in men, and 25% to 50% in women. The fat content of adipose tissue in the nonobese individual increases from 40% at birth to 80% in the adult.

Examination of the skin often yields important clues to both normal and pathologic systemic processes. For instance, the characteristics of the newborn's skin reflect in part the length of gestation, and such observations as the opacity of the skin and the distribution of body hair can help determine the gestational age. The onset, distribution, and characteristics of some exanthems are specific for certain infectious diseases of children, and a few lesions are associated with abnormalities of other organ systems, especially the central nervous system (the phakomatoses). The skin should be thoroughly examined, therefore, in each newborn, each acutely ill or febrile child, and each child with suspected congenital anomalies. A thorough examination of the skin includes observations of the skin color, consistency, and turgor; distribution and type of lesions; and characteristics of sweat and sebaceous glands, of body and scalp hair, and of the nails.

Newborn. During the first minutes following birth, the newborn's Apgar score is partially determined by assessment for the presence and distribution of cyanosis. The normal, nonchilled newborn usually progresses from generalized cyanosis to generalized pinkness while normal respirations are established during the first 5 to 10 minutes of extrauterine life. Acrocyanosis, especially on exposure to a cool environment, is commonly seen in newborns for several weeks after birth, as is mottling of the skin, a lattice-like pattern of pale and dark areas appearing especially on the extremities. Severe cold stress can cause generalized cyanosis. Transient cyanosis of an entire half of the baby (harlequin color change) or of one or more extremities is noted occasionally in newborns; presumably this is caused by temporary vascular instability. Persistent generalized cyanosis is usually a sign of depression from maternal drugs or anesthesia, primary pulmonary disease, congenital heart disease, overwhelming infection, or hypoglycemia. Plethora in newborns may indicate high levels of hemoglobin, seen for instance in the twin-to-twin transfusion syndrome, and pallor in newborns may be a sign of anemia, cold stress, or less commonly, congestive heart failure or shock.

The skin of newborns is covered by varying amounts of white, greasy, vernix caseosa, with larger amounts being present in preterm babies. Skin color in the newborn is determined in part by the amount of subcutaneous fat present. Premature babies have lesser amounts of subcutaneous fat and generally appear redder than full-term babies; they also have more transparent skin and therefore more visible subcutaneous blood vessels. Yellow staining of the vernix by meconium suggests that birth was preceded by acute fetal distress; with more prolonged fetal distress, as in the postmature baby with placental insufficiency, the yellow (or yellow-green) staining can involve the umbilicus and nails. The skin tends to progress from being smooth to scaly with varying amounts of desquamation and fissuring as the gestation progresses from preterm to postterm. This latter condition usually changes to normal, smooth skin without specific treatment within 1 to 2 weeks. Nonspecific edema, especially of the hands and feet, is less prominent as the gestational age approaches term. Generalized or localized petechiae, ecchymoses of the scalp or face, lacerations of the external ears, and diffuse or localized scalp edema can all be caused by physical trauma sustained during birth.

Jaundice can be expected to appear in at least 50% of

normal term babies and in a higher percentage of preterm babies in the third or fourth day of life, usually indicating the presence of physiologic jaundice. However, jaundice appearing at any time during the neonatal period may be an early sign of infection or of metabolic or primary hepatic disease. The early onset of jaundice also raises the question of blood group incompatibility and erythroblastosis. Clinically apparent jaundice usually indicates a serum bilirubin of at least 6 mg/dl, although the lack of subcutaneous fat in premature infants may delay its detection. Because of the variable lighting in many newborn nurseries and maternity units, clinical estimation of the bilirubin level is notoriously inaccurate, although some experienced neonatologists find that jaundice tends to progress from the head to the proximal and then distal extremities with increasing serum concentrations of bilirubin. The most consistent observations can be made by examining the skin in direct daylight. The presence of jaundice is best appreciated after pressure is applied to an area of skin over the forehead or sternum with the flat surface of a glass slide to empty the capillary bed.

The amount of melanin in the skin is variable at birth. Babies of black parents may demonstrate very little as neonates. Pigmented areas over the lumbar region and buttocks, known as mongolian spots, are commonly present in black, darker-complexioned white, and Oriental babies at birth. They become less prominent and eventually disappear during childhood. A number of other spots can be seen on healthy newborn babies' skin, including the common telangiectasias (nevus flammeus) on the eyelids, bridge of the nose, upper lip, and nape of the neck, which usually disappear during infancy; red or purple strawberry hemangiomas or more deep-seated, cavernous hemangiomas; tiny white papules on the nose, cheeks, forehead, and occasionally the trunk caused by plugging of the sebaceous glands (milia); pinpoint vesicles with or without surrounding erythema caused by plugging of the sweat glands (miliaria); erythematous flares with central pinpoint white vesicles or papules, known as erythema toxicum, which may appear and disappear over several hours during the first week of life; and areas of either decreased or increased pigmentation, café-au-lait spots being one example, which may occur in isolation or be associated with generalized disease such as neurofibromatosis.

The newborn's skin often is covered with fine lanugo hair, more prominently seen in premature infants, which is lost after several weeks of life. Scalp hair at birth, which is variable in amount, commonly is shed and replaced by permanent hair of a different degree of pigmentation. Fingernails may be long in postmature babies, and their color can be influenced by amniotic fluid staining and melanin pigmentation of the nail beds. Incurving of the lateral margins of toenails is common and can be associated with local inflammation.

Examination of the fingerprint and palmar crease patterns in newborns sometimes is useful because of the association of abnormal dermatoglyphics with certain chromosomal abnormalities and intrauterine infections. Magnification is essential in determining the fingerprint pattern on the distal phalanges and the position of the axial triradius of the palm. A single transverse palmar crease (simian line) can occur in normal individuals but more commonly is associated with chromosomal abnormalities such as Down syndrome.

The newborn's skin should be carefully checked for defects and sinus tracts, especially over the entire length of the spine and the midline of the head from the nape of the neck to the bridge of the nose. Sinus tracts sometimes communicate with intracranial and intraspinal spaces or masses, as with dermoid cysts and encephaloceles. Preauricular sinuses may or may not communicate with a persistent brachial cleft space. A more common minor abnormality of the preauricular area is the skin tag, which usually has a cartilaginous core.

Infancy. Careful inspection of the completely undressed infant during health maintenance checks often will detect minor abnormalities such as cradle cap and diaper dermatitis, the sometimes chronic lesions of infantile acne that first appear at 3 to 4 months of age, and, less commonly, scattered ecchymoses of varying ages that can signal child abuse. Palpation of the skin, preferably over the lateral abdominal wall, allows qualitative measurement of subcutaneous adipose tissue during infancy and also observation of the skin turgor (the rate of return to resting position after the skin is lifted and released), which is decreased in dehydration.

Early and Late Childhood. For all children, evaluation of acute or chronic rashes is greatly helped by a careful description of their major characteristics (macular, papular, pustular, vesicular, petechial, ecchymotic, oozing, scaly, exfoliative, abraded, erythematous, or pigmented), their location (trunk, face, extremities, intertriginous, or hairy areas), their developmental history, and their temporal association with other signs and symptoms. In fact, most infectious exanthems of children are diagnosed by certain constellations of these factors. One recently described infectious disease, Lyme disease, is diagnosed in its early stages solely by a rash (expanding, red, macular rash with or without a central mark from a tick bite) (see Chapter 225).

Adolescence. Examination of the skin of adolescents allows the monitoring of important pubertal changes such as areolar pigmentation, pigmentation of the external genitalia, development of pubic and axillary hair, increased functioning of sweat and apocrine glands, and an increase in subcutaneous fat. The prominent signs of acne vulgaris on the face and trunk can be anticipated in many adolescents.

Head and Face

The rapid rate of brain growth during infancy and childhood explains the increased size of the head relative to body length in newborns and infants as contrasted with that of adults. The facial contours and dimensions change considerably during the first 10 years of life, reflecting the downward and forward growth of the mandible and vertical growth of the maxilla and nasal bones. These changing proportions are best summarized by the proportion of cranium to face volumes at different ages: 8:1 at birth, 5:1 at age 2, and 2:1 by age 18. A thorough examination of the head includes measuring the head circumference and plotting the value on a standard growth chart, observing the shape and symmetry, and palpating the sutures and fontanelles; occasionally percussion, auscultation, and transillumination are needed. The head should be thoroughly examined in clinical situations in which there is growth or developmental failure, suspected trauma, a seizure disorder, or fever in an infant and as part of every health maintenance examination from birth to age 2 years.

Newborn. The newborn skull is composed of partially calcified bony plates that interface with each other at predictably located suture lines. The major sutures palpable at birth are the coronal, lambdoid, sagittal, and metopic (Fig. 7-20). Because of overriding of one cranial bone on another after molding of the skull during descent through the birth canal, the newborn's sutures often feel like ridges. The anterior fontanelle is located at the junction of the sagittal and coronal sutures and varies considerably in size in normal infants; it usually measures about 1 inch at its greatest diameter and is diamond shaped. The posterior fontanelle, found at the junction of the sagittal and lambdoid sutures, only occasionally is palpable at birth. Vascular pulsations, transmitted by the cerebrospinal fluid (CSF), normally can be seen over the anterior fontanelle. With normal CSF pressure, and with the infant in an upright position and not crying, the anterior fontanelle is soft and flat to palpation. A bulging fontanelle is a sign of increased intracranial pressure, whereas a depressed fontanelle is a sign of decreased intravascular volume, as in dehydration.

At birth it is common to palpate localized edema over one or more areas of the head. A palpable swelling, particularly over the vertex, that recedes after 1 or 2 days represents subcutaneous edema and is called *caput succedaneum*. Swollen areas whose margins are limited to suture lines and that often require weeks to recede represent subperiosteal hemorrhage and are called *cephalhematomas*. These resolve partially by calcification, which initially may feel like a mass with a heaped-up bony rim and a soft center. Other commonly seen effects of the birth process include linear or curved abraded or lacerated areas, especially over the zygomatic arches and preauricular areas, resulting from use of obstetric forceps. The infant's face may be asymmetric at birth because of intrauterine positioning with the chin touching one shoulder. Facial palsy manifested by a drooping corner of the mouth during crying usually is caused by obstetric forceps exerting pressure over the facial nerve in the preauricular area.

The cranial bones normally become firmer to palpation with increasing gestational age. One exception occurs when the sutural edges of the cranial bones are pliable and "springy," a condition known as *craniotabes*, which is found

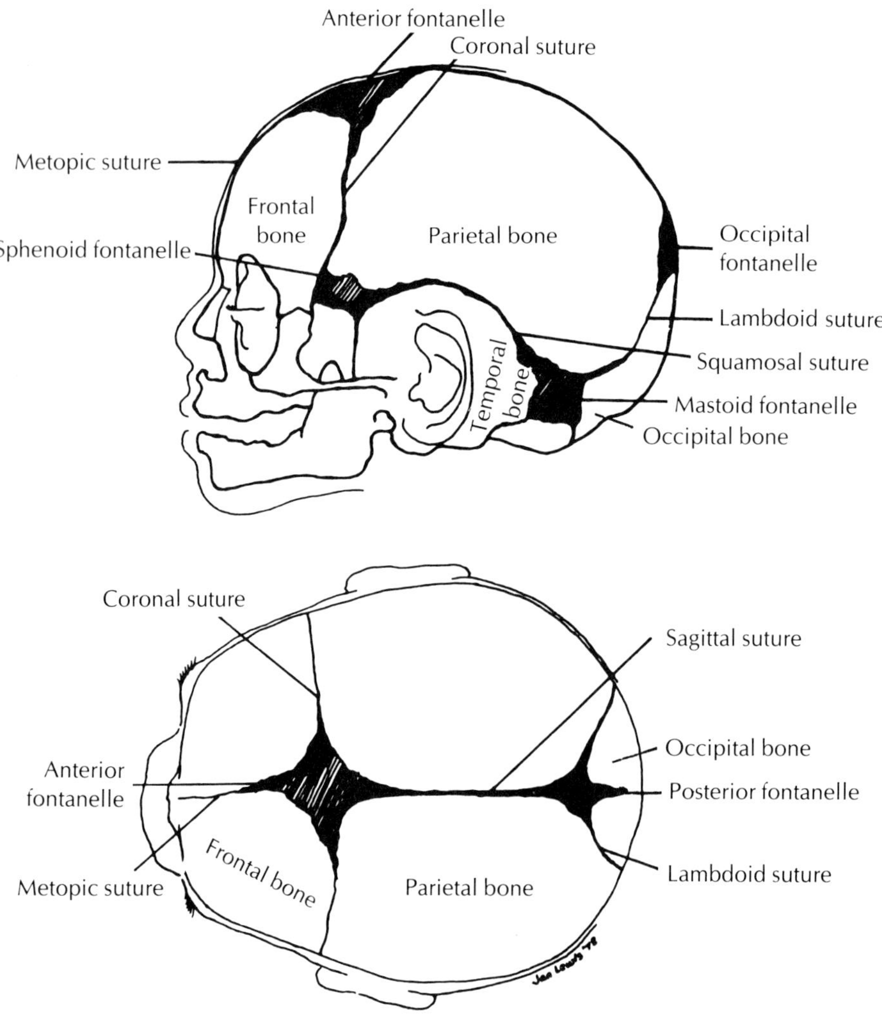

Fig. 7-20 Two views of the neonatal skull showing clinically important fontanelles and sutures.

From Scanlon JW et al: A system of newborn physical examination, Baltimore, 1979, University Park Press. Reprinted with permission of Aspen Publishers, Inc.

in many normal infants and rarely is a sign of rickets. A disproportionately large head at birth may indicate hydrocephalus or intrauterine growth retardation in which overall brain growth is often relatively normal.

Transillumination of the newborn and infant head is a procedure that is useful in evaluating asymmetric or disproportionately large heads as well as unexplained neurologic signs and symptoms. The procedure is accomplished in a completely darkened room by use of a bright light source, such as a three-battery flashlight or a special high-intensity light. If a flashlight is used, it should be fitted with a soft foam rubber collar and held against the head tangentially in such a way as to allow uniform intensity of illumination of the head around the full circumference of the light. Localized bright spots may indicate acquired problems, such as subdural effusions, or congenital defects, such as porencephalic cysts. The entire head will "light up" in the presence of hydranencephaly.

Infancy, Childhood, and Adolescence. By measuring and plotting serial occipitofrontal head circumferences, the examiner monitors the normal growth of the brain within the normally yielding cranial bones, which are separated from each other by suture lines that remain patent until brain growth is complete. A head circumference that is increasing at an abnormally slow rate may indicate either a slowly growing brain (intrinsic or acquired defect) or cranial sutures that have closed too soon (craniosynostosis). The normally proportioned small head is termed *microcephaly*, and a small head associated with premature suture closure is termed according to the shape distortion caused by the suture involved (scaphocephaly, plagiocephaly, acrocephaly). Craniosynostosis, a diagnosis that requires confirmation by roentgenography, often is associated with prominence or ridging of the involved suture line. A head that is growing too rapidly when compared with the rate of height and weight gain always should be evaluated for hydrocephalus and subdural effusions. Sometimes the head is asymmetric with a normally increasing head circumference; this can suggest either intrauterine or extrauterine positional effects, such as the flat occiput seen in babies who are left to lie for long periods and the flattening of one occipital bone and the opposite frontal bone sometimes associated with torticollis (cranioscoliosis). Prominent frontal bone bossing, with or without associated saddle-nose deformity, may be a sign of the developing osteomyelitis associated with congenital syphilis. The anterior fontanelle is normally not palpable beyond 18 months of age and may disappear as early as 3 months of age.

Percussion of the head by directly tapping with the middle finger normally elicits a flat sound. A "cracked-pot" sound may be heard in infants with an open fontanelle or in infants with closed fontanelles with increased intracranial pressure, as is seen with hydrocephalus. Auscultation of the head for localized bruits, indicating vascular anomalies, is included in the evaluation of children with seizures or other neurologic abnormalities. Up to the age of 5 years, however, systolic or continuous bruits may be heard over the temporal areas in normal children.

Examination of the face begins with an overall impression, which occasionally gives important diagnostic clues. Examples include the dull, immobile face associated with hypothyroidism; the open-mouthed expression of the child with chronic nasopharyngeal obstruction caused by hypertrophied adenoids; the multiply bruised face of the battered child; and the small nose, open mouth, and prominent epicanthal skin folds of the child with Down syndrome. Facial puffiness, or edema, especially involving the eyelids, can be an early sign of fluid retention secondary to acute or chronic renal disease or congestive heart failure. The distance between the eyes, usually measured as the interpupillary distance, can be increased as well as decreased in a number of syndromes of chromosomal origin and with other developmental anomalies.

The Chvostek sign, elicited by tapping the cheek just under the zygoma and causing unilateral facial grimacing, sometimes is a helpful diagnostic sign of hypocalcemia or hyperventilation tetany in older children; it also can be present in normal infants and young children.

Parotid gland swelling often is difficult to distinguish from cervical adenitis. The swollen parotid gland lies mainly anterior to the angle of the mandible and often pushes the ear pinna away from the side of the head, which can be seen when the patient is viewed from behind. Swelling and tenderness below a line drawn from the angle of the mandible to the mastoid process is caused by cervical adenitis. Nonobstructive parotitis usually is viral: when acute, it usually is caused by the mumps; when recurrent or chronic, human immunodeficiency virus should be considered (see Chapters 178 and 194).

Eyes

Studies of the process of mother-infant bonding during the neonatal period highlight the functional importance of an intact visual system in babies from the first minutes after birth.[4] Although examination of the eye is important in picking up clues to congenital and acquired systemic abnormalities, the overriding goal of examining the eye in infants and children is to ascertain that normal functioning is taking place and that potentially remediable processes affecting visual acuity are detected early.

At birth the eye is almost full grown compared with the other organs and the body. By this time the retina is completely developed except for the central foveal region, which is fully developed by 4 months of age, as is myelination of the central optic radiations and differentiation of the optic cortex. The cornea increases in diameter from 10 mm at birth to the final adult size of 11.5 mm. The lens doubles in weight between the time of birth and age 20 years, but then continues to increase another 50% by age 80. The pupillary reflex to light is functioning by 29 to 31 weeks of gestation. At birth the globe tends to be short in relation to the focusing ability of the lens and cornea (hypermetropia), and up until age 12 to 14 years there is a gradual lengthening of the globe with a resulting tendency for visual images to be focused in front of the retina (myopia). At birth babies can respond to faces and to colored as well as black and white objects. The fixed focal length of the newborn's eyes (20 cm), along with the aforementioned factors and distracting influences (startle reflex, hunger, temperature changes), limit the newborn's ability to respond visually for more than brief moments.

The ability to accommodate is present by 4 months of age,

and the ability to follow a moving light through different planes at various angles from the face is fully developed by age 6 months.

Examination of the eye is an important part of every examination of an infant or child. The completeness of the examination may vary according to the reason for the visit (health maintenance versus emergency head trauma) and chief complaint (headaches versus sprained knee). A thorough examination of the eye includes observation of the lids, including eyelashes, tear ducts, and glands; the conjunctiva; the sclera and cornea; the pupils, including reaction to light and accommodation; and the lens. A qualitative estimate of globe size and intraocular pressure should be made, and the extraocular movements should be tested to note presence or absence of nystagmus or strabismus. Examination of the fundus includes assessment of the optic disk, macula, retina, and central vessels; this should be accomplished in every child who is examined because of headache, head trauma, or other suspected intracranial lesion. Assessment of visual acuity should be part of every health maintenance examination.

Newborn. Several attempts may be required to complete the examination of the newborn's eyes because of transient edema of the eyelids caused by the birth process or by the conjunctivitis induced by silver nitrate instillation soon after birth. The upper eyelid may have a midline notch from incomplete fusion of its embryonic medial and lateral portions. The eyelids normally are fused until the eighth month of gestation. The lids often are slippery with vernix caseosa and conjunctival exudate, which can be gently removed with a dry cloth, allowing separation of the lids with a finger placed on each lid. Occasionally, one or both eyelids will be everted after birth. Episcleral and subconjunctival hemorrhages, either focal or diffuse, commonly are present after birth and can be expected to recede spontaneously. Less commonly, hyphema (blood in the anterior chamber) can be present. Cloudiness of the cornea can be caused by congenital glaucoma and requires ophthalmologic consultation. Opaque particles or strands in the lens may be cataracts or remnants of the artery that supplies the lens in its early stages of development (hyaloid artery). This iris often is less pigmented at birth. Its final color develops during the first year of life. Although a ring of white specks around the periphery of the iris is present in some normal infants, it is more prominent and common in children with Down syndrome (Brushfield spots). Defects in the iris, particularly in the ventral aspect, can be associated with parallel defects in the lens and retina (colobomas) and represent incomplete closure of the embryonic optic fissure.

A careful examination of the newborn's retina is difficult without the use of mydriatics. The appearance of a "red reflex" seen when the ophthalmoscope is held 10 to 12 inches in front of the eye ascertains that there are no major obstructions in light between the cornea and retina, such as corneal opacities, cataracts, and retinal tumors. Funduscopic examination of the newborn is indicated in babies in whom the red reflex is absent, in babies who have been given supplemental oxygen, and in babies in whom central nervous system trauma or septicemia is suspected. In some newborn nurseries every newborn is given a funduscopic examination. With the ophthalmoscope, the cornea usually can be seen at +20 diopters, the lens at +15 diopters, and the fundus at 0 diopters. The fundus is examined 30 minutes after the instillation of a drop of 2.5% phenylephrine (Neo-Synephrine) ophthalmic solution in each eye, optimally with the assistance of another person who can offer the baby a sugar nipple. The physician notes size and color of the optic disk and macula and any areas of hemorrhage or increased or decreased pigmentation of the retina. In newborns and in infants the optic disk is paler than in older children, the peripheral retina vessels are not well developed, and the foveal light reflection is absent. Papilledema rarely occurs before age 3 years because of the ability of the fontanelles and open sutures to absorb increases in intracranial pressure.

Perhaps the most productive method for observing both structure and function of the newborn's eyes is for the examiner to hold the infant upright, in which position the infant often will spontaneously open his or her eyes. Abnormalities in the size of the eyes should be noted, inasmuch as microphthalmia is a part of several rare congenital defect syndromes. Any upward or downward slanting of the axis of the eyelids (palpebral fissures) also should be noted; the presence of upward slanting is characteristic of children with Down syndrome. Although inner epicanthal folds can occur in normal infants, they are common in children with Down syndrome and in those with other chromosomal abnormalities. The setting-sun sign—a portion of the white sclera is seen between the upper lid margin and the iris—occurs in some normal premature and full-term infants, but persistence suggests the possibility of hydrocephalus.

When the baby is held at arm's length and turned slowly in one direction (Fig. 7-21), the eyes turn toward that direction. When rotation stops, the eyes turn toward the opposite direction after a few quick, unsustained, nystagmoid movements. More sustained nystagmus with this maneuver or at rest may indicate blindness or other central nervous system problems. When just the head of the baby is slowly moved through its full range of motion, the eyes do not move but remain in their original position (doll's eye reflex). This ma-

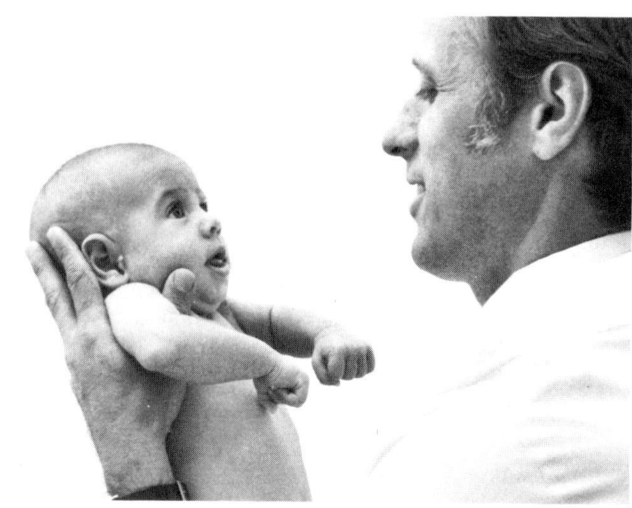

Fig. 7-21 Vestibular function testing in the infant.
Photograph by P. Ruben.

neuver can demonstrate paresis of the lateral rectus muscle. Strabismus, the condition in which the visual axes of both eyes in fixing a distal point are not parallel, is commonly seen as an intermittent phenomenon in normal newborns and may persist up to 6 months of age. The infant should be carefully examined for inward deviation of the eye, or esotropia, and outward deviation, or exotropia—whether alternating, fixed, or transient. Prominent epicanthal folds sometimes can give the erroneous impression that strabismus is present. Any fixed divergence of the eyes and any transient outward divergence in the newborn require immediate neurologic and ophthalmologic consultation.

Visual acuity in the newborn is assessed indirectly by means of visual reflexes such as consensual pupillary constriction in response to a bright light; blinking in response to a bright light and to an object moved quickly toward the eyes; and opticokinetic nystagmus, which the normal infant demonstrates when a cylinder with alternating vertical black and white lines is rotated at specified distances from the eyes.

Infancy. In addition to the findings on the examination described for the newborn, a few additional common problems particularly affect young infants. Tears are often not present at birth but are produced by 4 months of age. The nasolacrimal duct, however, sometimes is not patent until 6 months of age, leading to a chronically tearing eye with or without purulent discharge. Pressure over the nasolacrimal sac on the medial edge of the lower eyelid will confirm the diagnosis of nasolacrimal duct obstruction by yielding mucoid or purulent fluid. There usually is minimal to no conjunctival inflammation, and ophthalmologic consultation is not indicated unless the tearing and discharge persist beyond 6 months of age.

Although acute conjunctival inflammation with purulent exudate in neonates sometimes occurs in reaction to the routine instillation of silver nitrate drops, other causes that must be considered include infection by *Neisseria gonorrhoeae*, *Staphylococcus aureus*, or *Chlamydia trachomatis*. The last-named infection can be diagnosed by the presence of cytoplasmic material in the epithelial cells of conjunctival scrapings. An acutely red, tearing eye in infants often is caused by corneal abrasions inflicted by the infant's own fingernails; this diagnosis can be confirmed by placing a damp fluorescein strip in the corner of the eye and observing the green staining of the abraded corneal epithelium.

Unilateral or bilateral ptosis of the lids may be better appreciated after the immediate postbirth period and can be familial, part of a syndrome of congenital anomalies, or caused by oculomotor nerve palsy. Unilateral exophthalmos, or protrusion of the eye, can result from retroorbital tumor or abscess.

Childhood and Adolescence. Beyond the neonatal period and up until the ages of 3 to 5 years, visual acuity continues to be determined by qualitative observations of the parents and the examiner. By 4 weeks of age the infant is able to fixate on an object; by 6 weeks coordinated movements in following an object are seen. By 3 months the infant can follow an object moving across his or her midline, and convergence of the eyes is present. Beginning at 4 to 5 months the infant can reach for and grasp objects. Increasing recognition of familiar objects and faces by 5 to 6 months of age confirms normally developing cortical as well as visual systems. Between the ages of 1 and 3 years the infant's response to and use of brightly colored toys and children's books and the ability to circumnavigate the examiner's office can be observed. Standardized tests of visual acuity for children younger than 3 years of age have been developed and require that the child "match" a toy or ball with small test objects that the examiner holds. These tests, which are not widely known or used at present, may offer the child health worker a useful screening tool.

Infants and children who fail to perform according to the tests outlined here should be further examined for blindness or mental retardation. Besides those instances of blindness that are genetically determined or caused by perinatal insults, amblyopia (or decreased visual acuity) results from suppression of one or two unequal images in the visual cortex. Its importance is that it can be reversed only if diagnosed early enough, by 6 years of age at the latest, to allow treatment of the underlying cause. There are two major categories of causes of amblyopia: obstructive amblyopia secondary to a cataract, corneal opacity, or severe ptosis and amblyopia ex anopsia secondary to uniocular squint (strabismus) or refractive (anisometropia) error. Strabismus is detected by use of the pupillary light reflex and the cover tests. The symmetry of the pupillary light reflex is observed while the child focuses on a penlight 12 inches from the eyes; asymmetry indicates esotropia or exotropia. In the cover test, with the child focusing on the penlight, the visual axis of one eye is interrupted by the examiner's hand; any movement of the uncovered eye indicates strabismus.

Loss of visual acuity in one eye determined during a screening evaluation often is the first indication of amblyopia. Vision is screened by use of the Snellen illiterate E chart for children between the ages of 3 and 5 and the Snellen E chart for children 5 years of age and older (see Chapter 18, Ten, Vision Screening).

The most common abnormalities of the eyes of children seen in an ambulatory setting are swelling and redness of the eyelids and the red, tearing eye. Swelling and redness of the eyelids occur with obstruction of the nasolacrimal duct, blepharitis, hordeolum, and chalazion. Edema, tenderness, and warmth of the eyelid, usually indicative of periorbital cellulitis, can be caused by infection as a result of local trauma or insect bites, or they can be associated with upper respiratory tract infections and otitis media. Orbital cellulitis is characterized by marked lid edema, proptosis, chemosis, reduced vision, and decreased motility with pain on movement of the globe (see Chapter 241). The red, tearing eye can be caused by acute conjunctivitis, subconjunctival hemorrhage, keratitis, acute iridocyclitis, and acute glaucoma. Conjunctivitis characterized by prominence of the conjunctival blood vessels is one of the signs of Kawasaki disease. Evaluation of children with head trauma or suspected overwhelming infection necessitates careful, repeated testing of the extraocular movements in the six cardinal fields of gaze and the pupillary light reflex and observation of the conjunctivae and fundi, looking for unilateral abnormalities, hemorrhage, and papilledema. For example, lateral rectus muscle palsy often is the earliest sign of increased intracranial pressure (see Chapter 282).

Ears

The inner ear develops early in the first trimester of pregnancy, and response to sound can be shown in the twenty-sixth fetal week. At birth the cochlea and vestibule are anatomically mature.

Successful examination of the ears in infants and children, a skill that requires years of practice to develop, is extremely important because of the high incidence of middle-ear abnormalities in children. The student should approach the use of the otoscope and the almost universal presence of ceruminous impediments to visualization of the external auditory canal in children with patience and a willingness to ask for confirmation of findings as often as needed. A thorough examination of the ear, noting the characteristics of the external ear, external canal, and tympanic membrane and assessing hearing acuity, should be included in every physical examination.

Newborn. The external ear is flat and shapeless up until 34 weeks of gestation; once folded, it may remain so unless placed back in the flat position. Between 34 and 40 weeks of gestation an incurving of the periphery of the pinna develops along with an increasing ability to return spontaneously from the folded to the flat position. Minor anomalies in the shape of the external ear should be noted, including the occasional preauricular skin tags or preauricular sinuses. The position of the upper attachment of the external ears should be noted in relation to a line drawn connecting the inner and outer canthus of the eye. Attachments that fall below this line sometimes are associated with other congenital abnormalities, particularly renal agenesis. The patency of the external auditory canals can be determined by direct observation after pulling the pinna away from the side of the head. The tympanic membrane is coated with vernix caseosa for several days after birth and usually cannot be visualized.

Auditory screening in the neonate begins with identifying individuals at risk for hearing loss, such as those with a familial hearing disorder, intrauterine viral infection, hyperbilirubinemia with bilirubin levels greater than 20 mg/dl, prior receipt of an oxtotoxic drug such as gentamycin, and defects of the ear, nose, or throat. These infants at risk should be screened in the neonatal period for hearing loss. Their subsequent language should be closely monitored, and referral should be made to an audiologist for any signs suggesting hearing loss (see Chapter 18, Nine, Auditory and Speech Screening).

Infancy and Childhood. Visualization of the tympanic membrane is aided by several techniques. The infant's head should be stabilized to prevent painful jamming of the speculum into the ear canal. This sometimes can be accomplished by the parent or nurse holding the infant against the chest with the infant's head on one and then the opposite shoulder. The best stabilization of the head usually is achieved by having the infant lie supine on the examining table with the arms held against the body or in an extended position on either side of the head by the parent or nurse. If the positioning of the infant is accompanied by some form of visual distraction and verbal reassurances, the examiner usually is afforded a brief struggle-free period in which to accomplish the otoscopic examination. Varying amounts of resistance, however, are almost universal, and a rapid examination is desirable for the infant, the parents, and the examiner. One hand is used to grasp the ear pinna and gently pull it laterally and posteriorly to straighten the lumen of the external canal. The external canal in infants tends to be perpendicular to the temporal bone, with a slight upward angle; further growth of the skull results in a slightly anterior and downward direction of the canal. If the otoscope is held upside down, the infant's head can be further stabilized by the hand holding the ear pinna and the ulnar surface of the hand holding the otoscope (Fig. 7-22).

The examiner can further stabilize the infant's body by leaning across the chest and abdomen. The ear speculum is then introduced into the external canal and gently advanced to the point where the bony portion of the canal prevents further entry. Cerumen, which can be soft, firm, or flaky and varies from white to dark brown, may have to be removed. A flexible wire loop ear curette removes soft cerumen in small to moderate amounts with less risk of abrading the canal wall or tympanic membrane than with a rigid curette. Curetting is most safely done through the otoscopic head. Larger amounts of hard, inspissated cerumen may require irrigation with warm water and sometimes prior treatment with softening agents such as hydrogen peroxide. An ear canal filled with purulent exudate usually reflects acute otitis media with perforation or otitis externa, the latter being accompanied by pain when the pinna is moved; irrigation usually is unsuccessful and may be dangerous, especially with tympanic membrane perforation. Several sizes of specula should be tried to find the largest size that fits into the ear canal, thus allowing visualization of the largest area of tympanic membrane; a rotating motion of the otoscope usually is necessary to view all the important landmarks.

The normal tympanic membrane (Fig. 7-23) is semitransparent, roughly cone shaped, and slanted away from the examiner. The light reflex in the anteroinferior quadrant often is the first landmark seen, with its origin at the central umbo. The examiner, moving the light superiorly from the umbo, can see the long process of the malleus through the membrane, which ends in a bony protuberance that marks the junction

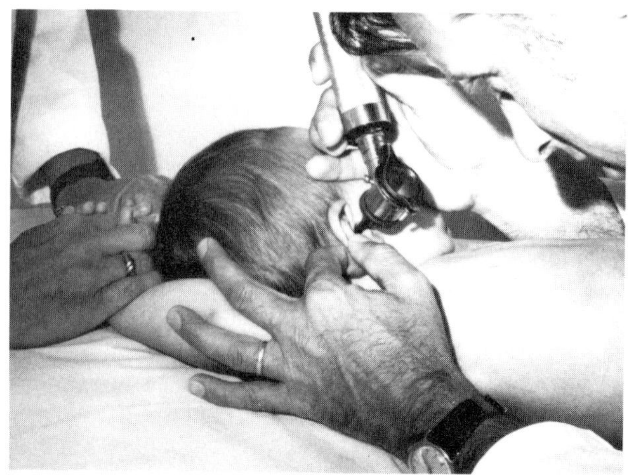

Fig. 7-22 Otoscopic examination of the child.
Photograph by P. Ruben.

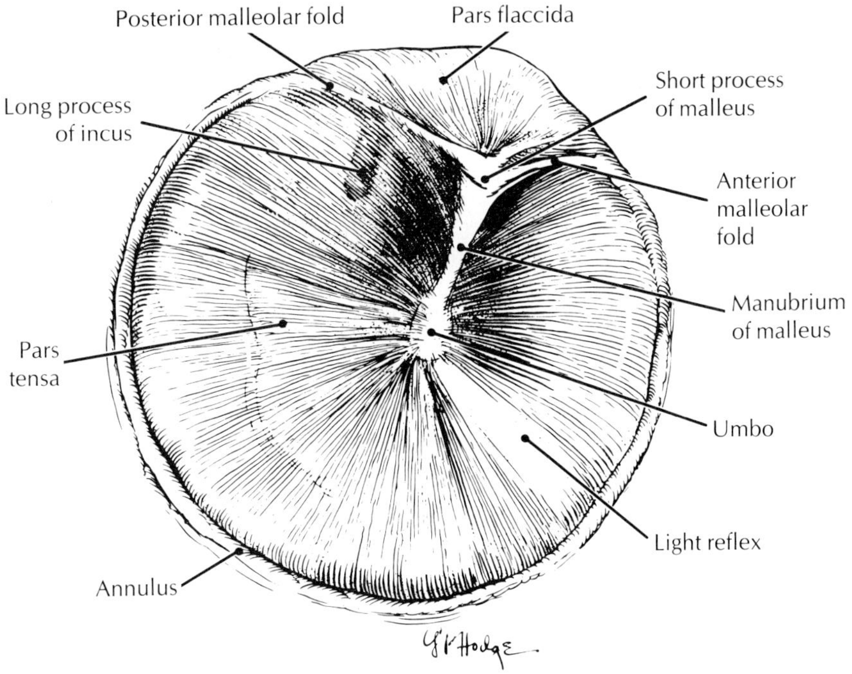

Fig. 7-23 Anatomy of the tympanic membrane.
From Strome M, editor: Differential diagnosis in pediatric otolaryngology, Boston, 1975, Little, Brown & Co.

of the pars tensa inferiorly and pars flaccida superiorly. Vague outlines of the incus sometimes can be seen in the posterosuperior quadrant. Air insufflation by means of a diagnostic otoscopic head fitted with a mouth tube or small bulb permits direct observation of the movement of the eardrum as both positive and negative pressures are gently applied (pneumatoscopy).

During the development of acute otitis media the tympanic membrane becomes increasingly opaque and erythematous, usually progressing superiorly to inferiorly, with progressive outward bulging and eventual loss of the outlines of the malleus and of the light reflex. Air insufflation will demonstrate decreasing mobility and sometimes the changing menisci of fluid levels within the middle ear. With healing of acute otitis media these changes resolve inferiorly to superiorly, with final resolution of opacity, limited motion, and fluid levels sometimes requiring several months.

Bullous myringitis appears as a bubblelike swelling that can almost fill the bony portion of the external ear canal. Blood behind the eardrum, either red or purple, is a sign of basilar skull fracture and should be looked for in children who have suffered head trauma. White plaques on the eardrum represent scars from old infections. A white mass in the posterosuperior quadrant may be a cholesteatoma, which is present with chronic obstructive middle-ear disease. In the examination of acutely ill children with suspected middle-ear infection the mastoid process should be inspected for overlying swelling and erythema and palpated for tenderness—signs of acute mastoiditis.

Screening for auditory acuity in infants is performed directly and indirectly. The indirect method relies on the effect of normal hearing on language development. Normal infants make cooing sounds (semipurposeful vocalization of vowel sounds) by 6 weeks of age, laugh out loud by 3 months, babble (repetitive sounds like "baabaa") by 6 months, echo sounds made in their presence by 9 months, and say their first meaningful word between 12 and 15 months. An infant who fails to progress beyond any of these developmental stages or who regresses should be further examined for hearing loss, as well as for mental retardation. Hearing can be assessed qualitatively by noting the infant's response to a nearby sound, made without visually distracting the infant or producing vibrations of the air or of the surface on which the infant is lying. Responses often are difficult to interpret but include blinking of the eyes in a neonate, momentary ceasing of body movements at 1 to 2 months, and turning the head toward the sound by 3 to 4 months of age. The test sounds can be made by a snap of the fingers or a bell. For older infants, tongue clucking produces a test sound with the frequencies of normal speech (500 to 2000 Hz). Asking the parents about the infant's responses to sounds may be as reliable as simple office screening.

In children 1 to 5 years of age, normal hearing is necessary for language development beyond the one-word stage. Qualitative hearing screening can be accomplished by whispering, as softly as possible, a number into the child's ear and asking the child to repeat it, or by asking whether the child can hear a ticking watch held a few inches from either ear.

Audiometric testing is indicated for any infant or child who fails any of these qualitative tests. In addition, formal testing should be a routine procedure for every child before starting school. Because of the high incidence of middle-ear infections in infants and preschool children, hearing screening is a routine procedure in many offices and well-child clinics, both in following up known infections and as an annual procedure (see Chapter 18).

Late Childhood and Adolescence. Examination of the tympanic membrane in this age group usually can be performed without resistance, with the child sitting. For the child who has experienced a previous painful examination or who has ear pain, the supine position will make head stabilization easier. A qualitative hearing test for children of these ages is with the use of tuning forks, particularly with frequencies in the human voice range of 500 to 2000 Hz. The examiner's own acuity, presuming it is normal, can be compared with the child's. Comparing bone and air conduction (Rinne test) and testing for lateralization of bone conduction with the handle of the tuning fork held against the midforehead (Weber test) can qualitatively distinguish between conductive and nerve hearing loss; with conductive loss, air conduction is less than bone conduction, and there is lateralization to the affected ear. Audiometric screening for this age group is routine in many schools. Some children with chronic middle-ear disease have fluctuating hearing loss that can be missed on a single puretone screening. In such cases, pneumatoscopy and impedance audiometry are relied on for a definitive diagnosis.

Nose

The relative size and shape of the nose normally are influenced by the downward and forward growth of the maxillary bones and to a lesser extent by the increase in the bizygomatic width during childhood. The bony orbits are nearer adult size in the newborn than are the other facial bones, and the palate grows most rapidly during the first year of postnatal life. The paranasal sinuses are represented only by the centrally placed ethmoid sinuses at birth; the maxillary sinuses develop from birth and usually are apparent on roentgenograms by the fourth year and the sphenoid sinuses by the sixth year. The frontal sinuses usually have reached the level of the roof of the orbits by 6 to 7 years. The nose functions to humidify incoming air and to trap bacteria and noxious materials in its continuous mucous blanket, which are moved toward the pharynx by ciliary action. Olfactory function appears to be present at birth and to increase with age.

A thorough examination of the nose includes inspection of its external form, the condition of the external nares, the mucous membranes of the septum, the turbinates and floor of the nose, and a description of any exudate present. The nose should be examined in all newborns and in all children with upper respiratory tract symptoms, noisy breathing, epistaxis, head trauma, headache, and fever.

Newborn. In examining the newborn's nose, it is important to rule out the presence of unilateral or bilateral choanal atresia, which can produce severe respiratory distress, inasmuch as most newborns are unable to breathe easily through their mouths. This examination is performed by introducing a soft No. 8 feeding tube into each external naris and advancing the catheter to the pharynx. Advancing the feeding tube farther into the stomach rules out esophageal obstructions such as atresia and allows aspiration of the amniotic fluid from the stomach. A simpler technique for testing choanal patency is to close one and then the other nostril while holding the mouth closed. Obstructed nasal breathing in the newborn sometimes is seen briefly after birth because of inhaled blood and amniotic debris, which can cause moderate to severe distress, especially in those few infants with congenitally narrow nasal cavities. A profuse purulent nasal discharge in the neonatal period could suggest the presence of congenital syphilis.

Infancy, Childhood, and Adolescence. With elevation of the tip of the child's nose and use of a nasal speculum, the membranes covering the nasal septum, floor of the nose, and inferior, middle, and superior turbinates in the lateral nasal wall can be inspected for signs of inflammation and bleeding points. The nasal septum occasionally is deviated to one side, sometimes obstructing breathing on that side. The fairly common occurrence of intranasal foreign bodies should be anticipated in the examination of any child with chronic nasal discharge, with or without associated bleeding. Epithelial polyps of the nasal mucosa are rare in children and usually indicate underlying cystic fibrosis or chronic allergic rhinitis. A pale, swollen, boggy nasal mucosa indicates allergic rhinitis, whereas with viral rhinitis the nasal membranes are red and bleed easily. Sinusitis should be suspected whenever purulent exudate appears from beneath any of the three nasal turbinates, especially in a child with a history of chronic nasal congestion, chronic tracheobronchitis, recurrent otitis media, and fever. Transillumination of the paranasal sinuses in younger children is of limited value to physicians other than otorhinolaryngologists because of the variable development of the sinuses before ages 8 and 10. Beyond 10 years of age the frontal sinuses can be transilluminated in a darkened room by holding a bright light source (transilluminator attachment for an otoscope-ophthalmoscope handle) against the superomedial aspect of the orbit, and the maxillary sinuses can be transilluminated by holding the light against the lateral aspects of the hard palate within the closed mouth.

Clear fluid draining from the nose after head trauma should be tested for sugar, which is present with a cerebrospinal fluid leak. In the child with a history of epistaxis the anteroinferior portion of the septum is a common location of prominent blood vessels that bleed easily, especially when aggravated by local inflammation and self-inflicted abrasions.

Swelling about the bridge of the nose can be caused by a cavernous hemangioma or less commonly by a nasal encephalocele. Erythematous swelling that involves the lateral portion of the bridge of the nose and adjacent eyelids can be a sign of orbital or periorbital cellulitis, which requires immediate intensive investigation and treatment.

The primary care physician often is called to examine a child who has suffered trauma to the nose. Children with bleeding from the nose after injury, evidence of a septal hematoma, or any question of depression of the base of the nose or of deviation from the normal straight-line vertical axis of the nose require immediate subspecialty consultation.

Mouth and Pharynx

The size and shape of the mouth and pharynx change during infancy and childhood with further growth of the hard palate during the first year and also of the mandible, which expands on all surfaces through the second year, extending downward and forward as a result of mandibular condylar growth. The most useful clinical evidence of growth about the mouth is the eruption, further growth, and shedding of the 20 primary (deciduous) teeth, with subsequent eruption of the 32 secondary (permanent) teeth. Intrauterine tooth growth begins during the second fetal month. Eruption of the deciduous teeth usually begins by 6 months of extrauterine life, and further tooth eruption continues roughly with one new tooth for each month after 6 months of age, with eruption of all deciduous teeth by 28 months of age. Table 7-3 summarizes the chronology of eruption and shedding of teeth in the growing human. Shedding of the deciduous teeth and eruption of the permanent teeth normally begin at 5 years of age in boys and 5½ years in girls and continue through age 14, with permanent tooth eruption completed by age 20.

The pharyngeal tonsils steadily increase in size during childhood and then begin to recede during puberty, a pattern of growth shared with adenoidal lymphoid tissue and peripheral lymph nodes.

The mouth and pharynx should be examined carefully during all visits for health maintenance and in all children with respiratory symptoms, fever of unknown origin, and ear or

Table 7-3 *Most Common Pattern of Dental Development*

DENTAL AGE (YEARS)	ERUPTING* (upper, left half)	ERUPTING* (upper, right half)	ERUPTING* (lower, left half)	ERUPTING* (lower, right half)	EXFOLIATING (upper, left half)	EXFOLIATING (upper, right half)	EXFOLIATING (lower, left half)	EXFOLIATING (lower, right half)
0-1	b a	a b	b a	a b				
1-2	c	c d	d c	c d				
2-3	e	e	e	e				
3-4								
4-5								
5-6	6	6	6 1	1 6			a	a
6-7	1	1	2	2	a	a	b	b
7-8	2	2			b	b		
8-9								
9-10								
10-11	4	4	4 3	3 4	d	d	d c	c d
11-12	5 3	3 5	5	5	e c	c e	e	e
12-13	7	7	7	7				
16-24	8	8	8	8				

From Barkin RM and Rosen P: Emergency pediatrics, ed 3, St Louis, 1990, The CV Mosby Co.

*a-e, Primary teeth; *1-8*, secondary teeth.

facial pain. A complete examination includes inspection and palpation of the lips, buccal mucosa, gingiva, hard palate, and mandible, plus inspection of the teeth, tongue, soft palate, tonsillar pillars, tonsils, and posterior pharyngeal wall.

Newborn. The initial examination of the newborn's mouth often is performed by means of the sucking reflex, with the examiner's finger inside the baby's mouth. This can quiet the baby and expedite other parts of the examination. The relative size of the mandible is noted, small mandibles sometimes being associated with underdevelopment of other facial bones as part of a generalized or genetic disorder. Clefts of the upper lip may be unilateral, bilateral, or midline and may be associated with palatal clefts. A common normal variant is a prominent mucosal fold connecting the inner midline of the upper lip to the posterior portion of the upper gum, leaving a deep notch in the midline of the gum. The upper and lower gums have finely serrated borders. Occasionally, small white retention cysts, which may be mistaken for teeth, are present. White retention cysts at the midline of the posterior border of the hard palate are known as Epstein pearls. Both types of mucus-retention cysts disappear spontaneously within a few months. Filmy, patchy white membranes over the gingiva and inner lips that cannot be removed by scraping and that sometimes overlie an erythematous base can be seen in some healthy newborns and represent monilial stomatitis, or thrush.

A prominent tongue, which may protrude from the mouth, is seen in congenital hypothyroidism and in Down syndrome. A frenulum attaches to the tongue's inferior surface and may extend almost to the tip. When this is thickened and shortened, protrusion of the tongue is limited. Although a source of concern to the parents, such "tongue-tie" rarely interferes with speech and requires no treatment. Salivation is relatively scanty in the normal newborn; therefore excess collection of saliva and mucus in the mouth should lead one to investigate for esophageal atresia.

The pharynx of the newborn is difficult to visualize except during crying because of the strong gag reflex induced by the tongue blade, which may cause the pharynx to fill with stomach contents. Tonsillar tissue is not visible in the newborn.

The quality of the infant's cry should be noted. A strong, lusty cry indicates a healthy baby with normally functioning airways and lungs; expiratory grunting is associated with respiratory distress; inspiratory stridor is caused by a number of lesions obstructing internal and external airways; a high-pitched cry suggests intracranial diseases, either congenital or acquired; a hoarse cry suggests hypocalcemic tetany or cretinism; and absence of a cry suggests severe illness or mental retardation.

Infancy, Childhood, and Adolescence. It is usually difficult to examine the mouth and pharynx of preschool children; therefore these attempts are best saved until the end of the examination. Some manner of restraint usually is required; in one of the most effective methods the infant is seated on the mother's lap with the head held stationary by the mother's hand (Fig. 7-24). Some infants and toddlers will permit a brief period of "looking at the teeth" with the tongue depressor being used gently to retract the lips and buccal mucosa. The crying infant usually gives the examiner struggle-free glimpses of the mouth and pharynx without the need for manipulation. The closed-mouthed, frightened infant or child can be examined, while adequately restrained, by slipping the tongue depressor between the teeth and onto the tongue: in older children, firm pressure on the anterior half of the tongue, with the tongue not protruded, will suffice; in infants it usually is necessary to induce the gag reflex by slipping the tongue depressor onto the posterior half of the tongue. In general, children who are sick or who have respiratory tract infections are the most reluctant to have their mouths peered into. Healthy children, on the other hand, can sometimes be persuaded to say "aaah," with prior description and even demonstration on a favorite doll or toy animal.

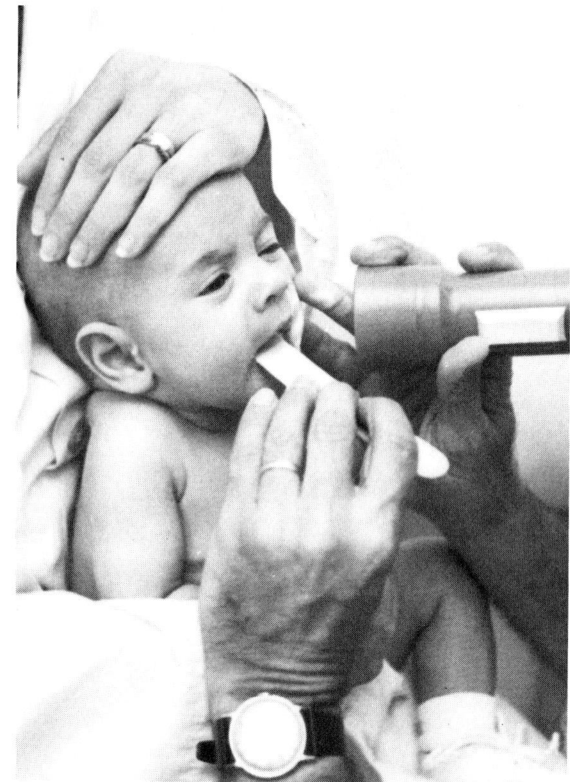

Fig. 7-24 Examination of the pharynx in the infant.
Photograph by P. Ruben.

Salivation normally increases to full capacity during the third month of life, the age when salivary drooling first is observed because of the infant's limited ability to swallow and the lack of lower front teeth to serve as a dam. Increased salivation that is associated with respiratory distress and fever usually suggests herpes simplex stomatitis or epiglottitis. Salivation also may be increased temporarily with the eruption of new teeth. During the winter months the lips can be dry and cracked, especially at the corners of the mouth. Deeper fissures at the corner of the mouth, cheilosis, occur in several nutritional deficiency states.

The gingivae should be inspected for localized as well as diffuse inflammatory lesions. Shallow, white-based ulcers with surrounding erythema can be seen, usually singly, on the gingivae in association with upper respiratory tract infections. Numerous gingival ulcers with concomitant involvement of the tongue and lips associated with increased salivation, fever, and pain usually result from primary herpes simplex infection, which is most common during the first years of life. Recurrent herpes simplex stomatitis or "cold sores" involving the lips can occur after the primary bout of stomatitis. Localized or diffuse gingival inflammation is most often associated with dental disease, particularly plaque buildup of the gingival borders because of inadequate tooth brushing. Dental abscesses sometimes exhibit an erythematous soft tissue mass that exudes pus opposite the root of the involved tooth. Easy bleeding of the gingivae most often reflects poor mouth hygiene and irritation by bacterial plaque, but it can, albeit rarely, be a sign of blood dyscrasia, a clotting deficit, or vitamin C deficiency (scurvy).

The buccal mucosa can be involved with nonspecific ulcerative processes, but occasionally it is the site of important signs of specific infectious diseases. In measles, on the second or third day of the illness, before the onset of the generalized rash, Koplik spots can be seen on the buccal mucosa; these are white pinpoint spots appearing at the level of the lower teeth. In parotitis, usually caused by the mumps virus but occasionally by other organisms, Stensen duct openings, found at the level of the upper molars, are red, swollen, and tender. Scattered white ulcers of varying size can occur on the buccal mucosa in chickenpox. In Kawasaki disease several abnormalities can be seen, including cracked and fissured lips and diffuse redness of the pharynx. Chronic thrush can be an early sign of human immunodeficiency virus (HIV) infection in infants and children (see Chapter 178).

The teeth are counted with the expectation that the infant has, on the average, one tooth for each month of age past 6 months up to 26 to 30 months, when the full complement of primary teeth will have erupted. Delayed tooth eruption can accompany serious chronic disease or may accompany generalized developmental delay. The individual teeth are examined in the infant for localized or generalized enamel hypoplasia, which reflects a variety of causes, including hereditary enamel hypoplasia, intrauterine insults such as infections, and prematurity (Fig. 7-25). Staining of the infant's teeth can occur after use of tetracyclines either during pregnancy or after birth, causing a permanent yellow, gray, or brown discoloration; mottled, pitted teeth with lusterless, opaque enamel can be caused by excessive fluoride intake. Oral iron preparations can stain the teeth green, as can elevated bilirubin levels during the neonatal period.

The spacing of the teeth should be observed, with special attention paid to teeth that are too close together or too far apart, both of which may cause spacing problems later on. Dental occlusion can be checked by having the child bite down and then observing for maxillary protrusion (overbite) or mandibular protrusion (underbite). Malocclusion has numerous causes, including chronic mouth breathing caused by nasal or nasopharyngeal obstruction, the rare instances of mandibular overgrowth secondary to temporomandibular arthritis in juvenile rheumatoid arthritis, and maxillary overgrowth in untreated hereditary hemolytic anemias, such as Cooley anemia.

The texture and appearance of the tongue may indicate specific diseases. Dryness, with or without coating, may be seen in chronic mouth breathing or in states of dehydration. The strawberry tongue, a result of the prominence of the papillae, is seen during the course of scarlet fever and in Kawasaki disease. Thrush and herpes simplex, previously described, can involve the tongue. Geographic tongue, in which the surface has the appearance of a relief map, may be nonspecific or associated with underlying allergic disease. Deep furrows in the tongue (scrotal tongue) have no significance. Fine and gross tremor of the tongue, including fasciculations and fibrillations, can be seen in both central nervous system disease (such as Sydenham chorea) and in peripheral nerve and neuromuscular junction diseases (Werdnig-Hoffmann disease).

Petechiae sometimes are present on the hard and soft palates in association with pharyngitis, especially streptococcal pharyngitis. The upward motion of the uvula and soft palate should be confirmed during phonation and with the gag reflex to rule out paralysis. A bifid uvula (Fig. 7-26) should be recognized because it can be associated with a submucous cleft of the soft palate. In this condition the soft palate is relatively short and does not reach the posterior pharyngeal wall. Palatal closure against the posterior pharyngeal wall, essential for normal articulation and voice resonance, can be aided in this condition by the presence of hypertrophied na-

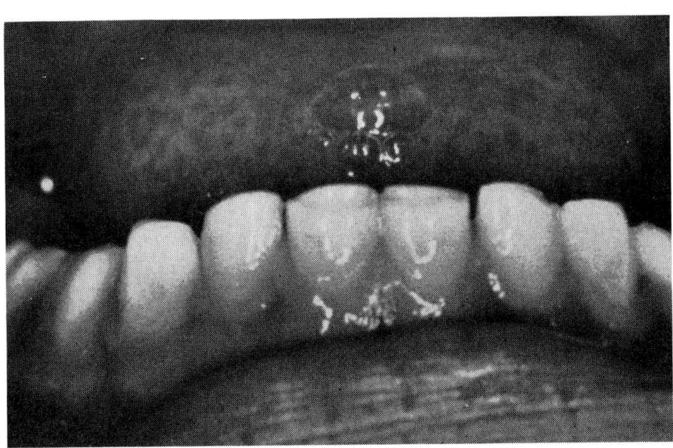

Fig. 7-25 Enamel hypoplasia in a premature child.

From McDonald RE and Avery DR: Dentistry for the child and adolescent, ed 5, St Louis, 1987, The CV Mosby Co.

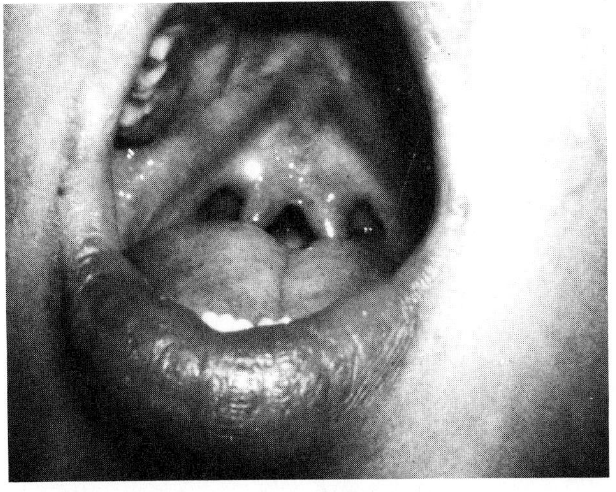

Fig. 7-26 Submucosal cleft palate with bifid uvula.

sopharyngeal lymphoid tissue. Therefore in the preoperative examination of children scheduled for adenoidectomy, the presence of submucous cleft of the palate should be looked for because it may affect the decision to operate (see Chapter 260).

The anterior and posterior pillars that border the tonsils are difficult to distinguish in most infants. The tonsils (palatal tonsils) are proportionately larger in preschool and school-age children than in adults. Tonsillar size is arbitrarily estimated on a scale of 1 to 4+, 1+ indicating easy visibility and 4+ indicating that the tonsils meet in the midline. The tonsils normally appear more prominent during gagging or crying, and their relative size can be assessed accurately only with the infant or child at rest. The tonsillar crypts normally contain variable amounts of desquamated cells, which appear as white spots on the surface. True tonsillar exudate, however, is usually less localized to the crypts and extends over greater portions of the surface. Some examiners try to distinguish the color of the exudate—yellow being more common with streptococcal infection, white with viral infections, and gray with diphtheria. The only reliable way to determine cause, at least for the presence or absence of group A beta-hemolytic streptococci, is to obtain a throat culture, especially of the tonsillar exudate in children older than 2 to 3 years of age. Tonsillar erythema and edema which also should be noted, are particularly conspicuous with streptococcal infection.

Shallow, white-based ulcers with erythematous edges, which may involve the adjacent pillars and posterior pharynx, suggest herpangina, caused by coxsackievirus A, and can be distinguished from the more anterior location of the herpes simplex ulcers. The diphtheritic membrane may be confluent over the tonsils, pharynx, and uvula, and bleeding ensues when the membrane is pulled away. In infants a diffusely red pharynx and tonsillar area, with or without exudate, is most likely of viral origin. A peritonsillar abscess is suggested by asymmetric enlargement of the tonsils, often associated with lateral displacement of the uvula.

The posterior pharyngeal wall should be inspected for evidence of lymphoid hyperplasia, which has a "cobblestone" appearance and indicates chronic postnasal drainage, as seen in chronic allergic rhinitis or bacterial sinusitis. Postnasal drainage into the pharynx is to be expected in infants and children with upper respiratory tract infections, and the characteristics of the mucus suggest various causes. Clear mucus is present in allergic rhinitis or in the early stages of acute rhinitis, whereas purulent mucus appears in the late stages of a viral rhinitis or with chronic bacterial sinusitis.

The presence and size of the adenoidal lymphoid tissue can be estimated indirectly by noting the amount of mouth breathing at rest, by observing the ease of breathing through the nostrils, and by noting any nasality to the voice. Direct palpation of the adenoids with a finger introduced through the mouth and around the soft palate is uncomfortable and difficult for all involved. Use of the nasopharyngeal mirror for this purpose is most helpful to those who use it every day, such as otolaryngologists.

The epiglottis sometimes is visualized by chance when the throat of a child with an upper respiratory tract infection is being examined. In children with croupy cough, especially if of sudden onset and associated with high fever, drooling, and signs of upper-airway obstruction, the epiglottis must be visualized to rule out acute bacteral epiglottitis, a true emergency in children. The epiglottis may be swollen several times its usual size and is cherry red. Because of the danger of complete airway obstruction and of cardiac arrest during this examination, endotracheal tubes, a tracheotomy set, and an oxygen source should be at hand. Some primary care physicians choose to rely on a lateral neck roentgenogram initially to evaluate the size of the epiglottis and postpone direct visualization until a surgeon is present.

Neck

The neck is relatively short in infants and lengthens during childhood as a result of vertebral growth. Consequently the epiglottis descends from the level of the first cervical vertebral body at birth to the lower third of the third cervical vertebral body by adulthood. The larynx is one third the adult size at birth. It grows rapidly until age 3 years, becoming wider as well as longer, and then grows slowly until puberty, when there is another rapid increase in all dimensions, especially in boys. The trachea at birth is approximately one third the adult length, and both the anteroposterior and lateral diameters of the trachea increase by nearly 300% from birth to puberty. The thyroid gland increases approximately 10 times in weight from birth through puberty, with most growth occurring during puberty. Cervical lymph nodes, a few of which may be palpable at birth, increase in size, following the growth curve for the body's lymphatic tissues in general, and therefore those of less than 1 cm are commonly present in most normal children.

A thorough examination of the neck should be performed periodically on healthy infants and children and on all those with respiratory or febrile illnesses. It includes observation of the neck's overall dimensions; resistance to passive motion; size and location of lymph nodes, thyroid gland, and other masses; status of neck vessels; and palpation of the trachea.

Newborn. The relatively short neck of the newborn should be inspected for position and overall size. Torticollis, a condition in which the head is tilted to one side with the chin rotated toward the opposite shoulder, usually is associated with a palpable hematoma of the involved sternocleidomastoid muscle. It is believed to arise from a birth injury and may require physical therapy. Opisthotonos, in which the neck and back are held in extreme extension, is an ominous sign that indicates either meningeal irritation or, in the infant with jaundice, kernicterus. In infants, frequent opisthotonic positioning associated with a relative paucity of trunk flexion movements may be an early sign of the spasticity of cerebral palsy. An unusually short neck may indicate cervical spine anomalies (Klippel-Feil syndrome), and a webbed neck is seen in Turner syndrome. The newborn clavicles should be palpated routinely to rule out clavicular fractures, which usually occur at the junction of the middle and outer thirds of the bone and can occur during birth. Palpable neck masses in the newborn include the midline thyroglossal duct cyst, the supraclavicular cystic hygroma, which transilluminates, and brachial cleft cysts with or without associated skin tags and fistulas along the anterior border of the sternocleidomastoid muscle. Palpable cervical lymph nodes in normal newborns usually are less than 5 mm in diameter. A crackly sensation to palpation in the supraclavicular areas usually indicates pneumomediastinum.

Infancy, Childhood, and Adolescence. When palpably enlarged lymph nodes are found, the examiner should note their location, size and number, consistency, tenderness, mobility, and attachment to other structures. Anterior cervical lymph nodes commonly enlarge in association with upper respiratory tract infections, dental infections, and stomatitis and less commonly with mycobacterial infection. Posterior cervical node enlargement is common secondary to otitis media and insect bites or inflammatory lesions of the scalp. Generalized cervical lymph node enlargement is present with many viral syndromes, especially rubella, measles, and infectious mononucleosis. Enlarged lymph nodes because of an inflammation usually return to normal size days or weeks after subsidence of the primary infection. Enlarged lymph nodes are combined with other signs in Kawasaki disease. Lymph nodes that are enlarging in the absence of signs of infection raise the suspicion of Hodgkin disease and other lymphomas. Generalized chronically enlarged lymph nodes throughout the body can be present in HIV infection (see Chapter 178).

Every infant and child with acute illness should be checked for nuchal rigidity, an important sign of meningeal irritation from meningitis. Ideally the infant or child should be quiet and relaxed, lying supine as the examiner gently lifts the head from the examining table with a hand at either side of the infant's head and notes the degree of suppleness and any resistance to flexion. Flexion of the thighs associated with neck flexion (Brudzinski sign) and flexion of the extended lower extremity while its opposite is fully extended and flexed 90 degrees at the hip (Kernig sign) are less often present in infants with meningitis than in older children and adolescents. The child with nuchal rigidity is unable to touch the chin to the chest and assumes a tripod position when asked to sit up—that is, rests backward on extended arms while the legs are extended on the examining table.

The thyroid gland is normally difficult to palpate, if palpable at all, before puberty; it should be palpated, as should the trachea, from both in front of and behind the child. An enlarged thyroid in children can occur with euthyroid, hypothyroid, or hyperthyroid states and can be caused by iodine deficiency as well as iodine excess (from iodine-containing cough medicines), congenital or familial blocks in thyroxine synthesis, thyroiditis, diffuse or nodular hyperplasia, and, rarely, carcinoma. Normally the trachea is slightly deviated to the right; deviation from this norm indicates mediastinal shift as may occur with foreign body–induced atelectasis and pneumothorax. Neck venous pulsations and distention, which usually are difficult to determine in infants because of their relatively short necks, can give clues to heart disease and congestive heart failure in older children.

Children with painful or limited neck motion should be checked for a full range of flexion, extension, lateral rotation, and lateral flexion. A fairly common cause of limited head motion is wryneck, or torticollis, that can occur after a play injury or sometimes a respiratory tract infection. The head is tilted to one side, with the sternocleidomastoid tenderness on the long or stretched side (as distinguished from neonatal torticollis, in which the involved sternocleidomastoid muscle is on the short side); the underlying cause of wryneck is a rotary subluxation of the first two cervical vertebrae.

Chest and Lungs

The chest wall in the fetus and newborn is round; with further growth there is a gradual flattening of its shape, with the lateral diameter exceeding the anteroposterior diameter. Serial measurements of thoracic index (transverse/anteroposterior diameter) are made in some clinics that treat children with chronic obstructive lung disease, such as cystic fibrosis, as a means of monitoring the degree of formation of a "barrel chest." The infant's chest wall is relatively thin compared with the adult's; therefore heart and lung sounds are more clearly transmitted. Respirations are predominantly abdominal in infants, reflecting the greater role of the diaphragm; by age 6 years they are predominantly thoracic, reflecting the increased role of the thoracic musculature in normal breathing.

By 16 weeks of gestation the bronchial tree is fully developed, with the adult number of segments and subsegments. Alveoli, in comparison, are just forming by the time of birth, with only 8% of the average adult number present. The number of alveoli increases until 8 years of age, after which they primarily increase in size rather than in number until adulthood. Pulmonary blood vessels develop parallel to the developing bronchial tree and alveoli, with the appearance of increasing amounts of muscle in the walls of the more distal arterioles over time. By 28 weeks of gestation the airway and blood vessel development usually is adequate for gas transfer. By 34 to 36 weeks of gestation sufficient amounts of a surface-active lipid are present within the alveoli to maintain them in a partially expanded position, rather than remaining collapsed at the end of each expiration. As noted previously, the respiratory rate decreases with age, in part because of further postnatal development of the alveoli, with a resulting increase in lung volume.

The breasts of many normal male and female infants are transiently hypertrophied at birth, sometimes producing small amounts of clear or white fluid called *witch's milk*. This breast hypertrophy normally disappears by 2 to 3 months of age. Many pubertal males have transient unilateral or bilateral firm, sometimes painful, subareolar masses that disappear within a year of onset. Female pubertal breast development often is asymmetric and proceeds through several stages, starting with an increase in the areolar diameter between ages 8 and 13, and is completed between ages 12 and 19 (Fig. 7-27).

The chest and lungs should be thoroughly examined in every child with any respiratory symptoms, fever, abdominal pain, or chest pain. The examination should include notation of the size, symmetry, movement with respirations, localized tenderness or masses, and breast characteristics. The three goals in the examination of the lungs by observation, percussion, and auscultation are determination of (1) the nature of respiration, including the rate, depth, and ease, (2) the adequacy of gas exchange, as indicated by signs of hypoxia or hypercapnia, and (3) localization of disease. The examiner should use and become familiar with the sound characteristics of one stethoscope. Except for auscultating the chest of the small premature baby, an adult-sized stethoscope with both a bell and diaphragm generally is effective in examining infants and children of all ages.

Newborn. During the few moments following birth the adequacy of the developing lungs for gas exchange, which is influenced by factors such as maternal anesthesia, birth trauma, and the normality of the infant's central nervous and cardiovascular systems, is grossly assessed by the Apgar score, which includes observations about the color and initiation of respirations. Once normal respirations have been established, the baby's chest is inspected for deformities, such as a markedly bulging or markedly concave sternum (pectus carinatum or excavatum); asymmetry caused by an uneven chest expansion, absent or deformed ribs, or absence of the pectoral muscle; and overall size, inasmuch as small thoracic

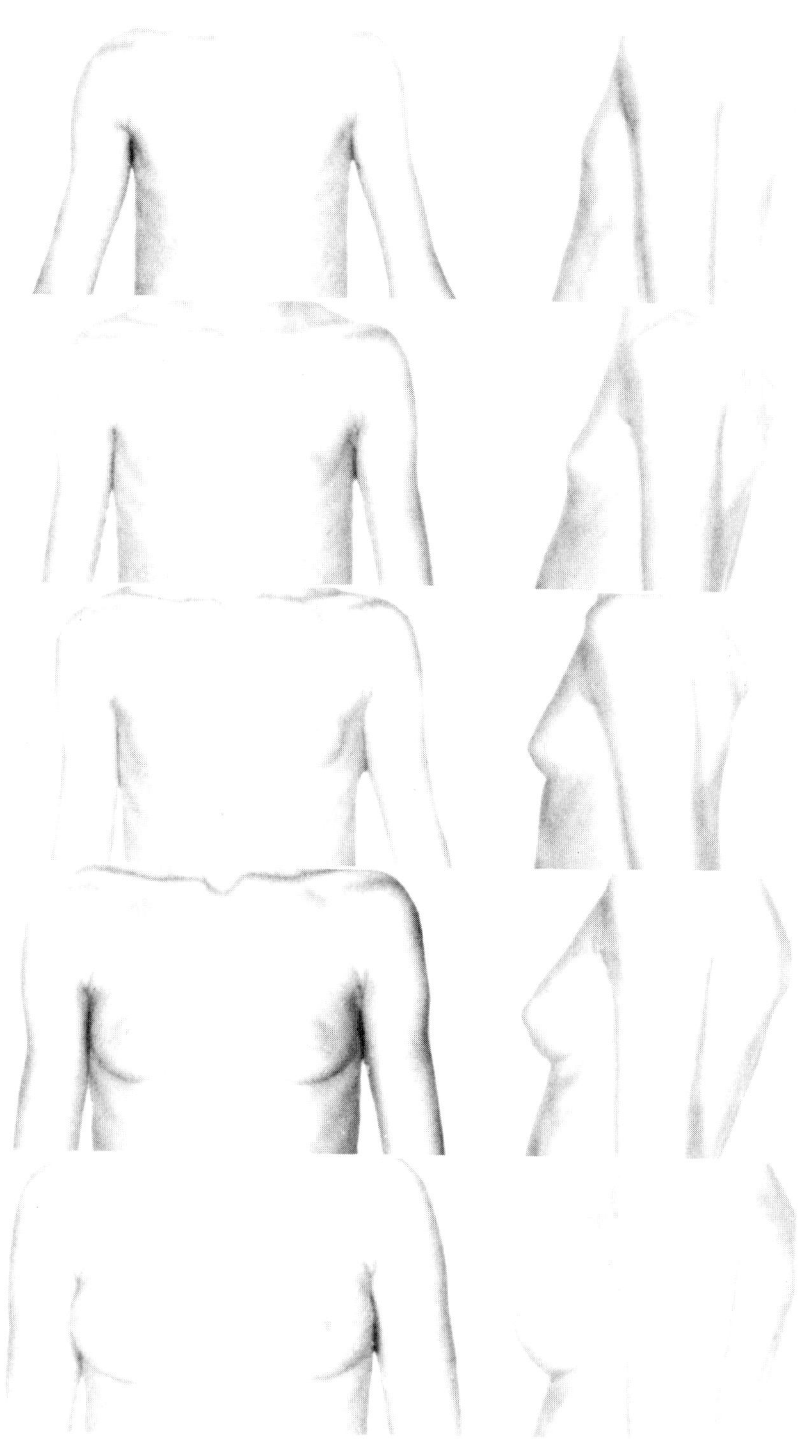

Fig. 7-27 Stages of development of the female breast.

From Tanner JM: Growth at adolescence, ed 2, Oxford, 1962, Blackwell Scientific Publications, Ltd.

cages are part of several congenital anomalies. The respiratory rate normally falls from as high as 60/min immediately after birth to 30 to 40/min by several hours of age. In the normal newborn the auscultated breath sounds are easily heard and are of higher pitch than are those in the older child and adult.

The newborn with respiratory distress from any cause will exhibit some or all of the following signs: tachypnea, cyanosis, expiratory grunting, intercostal retractions (also possible are subcostal, substernal, and supraclavicular retractions), and decreased air entry as measured by decreased breath sounds. A useful clinical tool for serially monitoring the severity of newborn respiratory distress, particularly that caused by hyaline membrane disease, is the Downes score (Table 7-4). Persistent scores of 5 or more usually indicate the need for respiratory assistance. Simple auscultation of the newborn with respiratory distress should aid in the diagnosis of (1) unilateral lesions such as aspiration pneumonia, congenital diaphragmatic hernia, congenital hypoplastic segments or emphysema, and unilateral pneumothorax and (2) congenital heart disease and heart murmurs.

The respiratory rate of newborns, particularly premature newborns, can be quite irregular during the first few days of life and sometimes can slow to the point of apnea. Two patterns should be differentiated in premature infants. *Periodic breathing* is associated with relatively brief periods of apnea lasting 5 to 10 seconds, usually without secondary bradycardia. It occurs more commonly when the baby is awake and is uncommon before 5 days of age. True apneic spells, on the other hand, last more than 20 seconds, are associated with bradycardia, can be associated with pulmonary disease, and are more common in infants weighing less than 1250 g.

Infancy, Childhood, and Adolescence. For this age group, auscultation and percussion, along with observation of breathing patterns, are particularly useful techniques in evaluating the chest and lungs. Auscultation often is most successfully accomplished with the infant or child only minimally aware of being examined—for example, while asleep, being fed, or being held up to the parent's shoulder. When preschool children are asked to "take a deep breath," they often hold their breath. It is easier to start by auscultating while the child breathes at a resting level. If the child is crying, the inspiratory phase can be thoroughly auscultated, but predominantly expiratory adventitous sounds, such as wheezes, can be missed. After the examiner listens to breath sounds at rest or during crying, a useful technique for accentuating adventitious sounds, particularly during the expiratory phase, is inducing forced expiration. The examiner may accomplish this by holding the hands on opposing anterior and posterior sides of the chest, with the stethoscope in one hand held against the chest, and gently squeezing the hands together as expiration is ending.

Breath sounds in infants and children tend to be audible during both inspiration and expiration—that is, bronchovesicular—and are more clearly heard than in adults. Secretions in any part of the respiratory tree usually are loudly audible throughout the chest, and the examiner should repeat his or her observations to rule out transmitted sounds from the nose or pharynx. It is tempting for inexperienced examiners to suspect pneumonia in most children evaluated for acute respiratory illnesses because of the fairly usual occurrence of tracheal and bronchial inflammation with common viral infections. The more or less generalized coarse rhonchi (continuous, low-pitched sounds) from bronchial secretions and the wheezes (higher pitched, predominantly expiratory) from bronchiolar secretions should be distinguished from the much less common, usually localized, crackling rales caused by alveolar fluid or exudate heard best at the end of inspiration. Pneumonia in infants and young children is almost always accompanied by fever and tachypnea, whereas rales, bronchial breath sounds, dullness to percussion, and a productive cough are less constant findings than in adults.

There are several objective signs of respiratory distress in infants and children. Orthopnea occurs in children with asthma or congestive heart failure. The maximal use of accessory muscles of respiration causes several useful physical signs. These include head bobbing, seen especially in infants, with the head bobbing forward in synchrony with each inspiration, and flaring of the nasal alae, resulting from contraction of the anterior and posterior dilator naris muscles. These signs indicate increased work of breathing, or inspiratory efforts shortened by pain, as occurs in pleuritis or thoracic trauma. Intercostal retractions, an exaggerated inspiratory sinking in of intercostal and sometimes supraclavicular soft tissue, indicate increased inspiratory effort and reflect airway obstruction and lung stiffness. Intercostal space bulging during expiration occurs in situations of increased expiratory effort such as asthma, bronchiolitis, and cystic fibrosis. Subcostal retractions, seen anteriorly at the lower costal margins, reflect flattening of the diaphragm and occur in conditions with diffuse lower-airway obstruction. Substernal retractions can be seen in children with severe upper-airway obstruction and in newborns, especially premature infants, with various pulmonary diseases. Audible wheezes

Table 7-4 *Downes Score: A Method for Monitoring Respiratory Distress*

SCORE	0	1	2
Respiratory rate (breaths/min)	60	60-80	>80 or apneic episode
Cyanosis	None	In air	In 40% oxygen
Retractions	None	Mild	Moderate to severe
Grunting	None	Audible with stethoscope	Audible without stethoscope
Air entry (crying)	Clear	Delayed or decreased	Barely audible

From Downes JJ: Respiratory distress in newborn infants, Clin Pediatr 9:326, 1970.

usually indicate obstruction of the larger airways, and grunting can be associated with pneumonia, chest pain, and the respiratory distress syndrome in neonates. A "thud" may be heard on inspiration in children with a tracheal foreign body as it moves in response to air flow.

The adequacy of gas exchange is judged primarily by seeking signs of hypoxia. Cyanosis, which results from more than 5 g of reduced hemoglobin in the capillaries, is either peripheral, as with exposure to a cold environment, or central (seen as blue mucous membranes), which can be of pulmonary or cardiac origin. Tachycardia, dyspnea on exertion, and central nervous system depression are additional signs of hypoxia that can be critical in following up a child with marginally adequate gas exchange, as in severe croup. Progressive signs of hypercapnia in acute respiratory illnesses include hot hands, small pupils, engorged fundal veins, muscular twitching, coma, and papilledema.

Localization of intrathoracic lesions in children is aided by palpating for tracheal deviation and observing for unequal respiratory movements of one half of the chest, localized areas of dull or flat percussion notes, and the presence of tactile fremitus. Percussion also can be used to delineate the lung boundaries in inspiration and expiration.

Heart

The major anatomic characteristics of the heart have been formed long before birth, as have most congenital heart defects. In the normal newborn's heart the right ventricle has a muscle mass equal to that of the left ventricle, reflecting the fetal circulation when both ventricles pump blood into the systemic circulation, the right through the ductus arteriosus. After birth the left ventricle gains weight relative to the right ventricle, reaching the adult weight ratio of approximately 2:1 by age 1 year, reflecting the major changes in postnatal circulation. At birth, or shortly thereafter, the ductus arteriosus normally closes, and the flap of the foramen ovale is held closely by the rise in pressure in the left atrium. Up to 50% of newborns have transient murmurs during the first 24 to 48 hours of life, some of which are caused by a late-closing ductus arteriosus.

Congenital heart defects can be classified according to the embryonic stages of development during which an abnormality arises: position anomalies (dextrocardia with or without situs inversus), anomalous growth of the atrial chambers (atrioventricular canal, ostium primum defect, persistent foramen ovale), anomalous bulboventricular growth and septation (ventricular septal defect, tetralogy of Fallot, double-outlet right ventricle, transposition of the great vessels), and maldevelopment of the truncus (truncus arteriosus, patent ductus arteriosus, coarctation of the aorta).

The significant and normal changes in pulse and blood pressure that occur with age in infants and children have been described earlier in this chapter. The examiner is reminded that optimal auscultation of the heart requires the use of a stethoscope with both a bell and a diaphragm, the bell picking up lower-pitched sounds and the diaphragm picking up higher-pitched sounds. Proper use of the bell involves holding it lightly against the chest while the diaphragm is pressed firmly to the chest. Stethoscope tubing should be no more than 10 to 12 inches in length. During auscultation, gentle traction on the earpiece end of the stethoscope will enhance the audibility of heart sounds by making a tighter seal between the earpiece and the examiner's external auditory canal. Because infants have relatively rapid heart rates, detecting abnormalities in their heart sounds demands that each of the two major heart sounds be listened to in isolation, with attention given to each interval between these sounds. As in adults, auscultation of the heart is performed initially over the four cardinal areas (apex, or *mitral area*; lower left sternal border, or *tricuspid area*; second left intercostal space at the sternal margin, or *pulmonary area*; and second right intercostal space, or *aortic area*). Auscultation then proceeds to the remainder of the precordium and chest, including the infraclavicular and supraclavicular area, the axillae, the back, and the neck.

A thorough examination of the heart should be part of all physical examinations of infants and children and includes notation of the heart rate and rhythm, heart size, and characteristics of the first and second heart sounds, especially in the second left interspace. The following information should be recorded about murmurs: timing in the cardiac cycle (early, late, or pansystolic; protodiastolic, middiastolic, or presystolic), quality (blowing, harsh, rumbling, musical, and others), grade of maximal intensity (on a scale of I to VI, with V and VI being associated with a palpable thrill), duration, point of maximal intensity, and transmission. In all infants and children whose findings suggest congenital heart disease, palpation of peripheral pulses is especially important to determine if the pulses in the lower extremities are diminished and those in the upper extremities increased, as occurs with coarctation of the aorta. Blood pressure is obtained as described earlier in this chapter.

Newborn and Infant. The general appearance of the infant can provide clues to underlying heart disease and may mandate a more sophisticated cardiac examination. Examples of conditions frequently associated with congenital heart disease are Down syndrome (endocardial cushion defect), Turner syndrome (coarctation of the aorta), trisomy 13, trisomy 18, and congenital rubella syndrome (patent ductus arteriosus, pulmonary stenosis). Important clinical signs of significant heart disease include cyanosis, growth failure, and lethargy. The most prominent signs of congestive heart failure in infants are tachypnea, tachycardia, and liver enlargement. Peripheral edema and pulmonary rales are late findings and therefore not as helpful as in adults. Visible chest pulsations can indicate a hyperdynamic state caused by an increased metabolic rate or an inefficient pumping action from valvular or septal incompetency or other defect. Dextrocardia is suggested by a right-sided cardiac impulse and may be associated with abdominal situs inversus (reversal of the position of the liver, spleen, and intestines).

The apical impulse in infants normally is palpated in the fourth left interspace just outside the midclavicular line; after age 7 it is in the adult position of the fifth left interspace in the midclavicular line. The point of maximal impulse of the heart can suggest individual ventricular enlargement. An impulse at the xiphoid process or lower left sternal border suggests right ventricular hypertrophy, whereas an impulse maximal at the apex suggests left ventricular hypertrophy.

The heart sounds of infants often are difficult to differentiate from their breath sounds because the pitches and rates of each can be similar. Watching the abdominal excursions with respiration and palpating a peripheral pulse while auscultating the chest can aid in this differentiation. The examiner should be prepared to spend at least several minutes listening to the precordial area, at which time the heart and respiratory rates and rhythms can be determined. For each heart sound the intensity, point of maximal intensity, and degrees of splitting should be noted. Normally the second heart sound is louder than the first in the second left interspace and often is split (reflecting the pulmonary valve closing after the aortic valve); the split often widens with inspiration. Examples of abnormalities of the heart sounds are the loud first sound heard at the apex in mitral stenosis, the loud second sound in the pulmonary area indicating pulmonary hypertension, and the fixed, split second sound in the pulmonary area with atrial septal defect. A third heart sound can be heard at the apex of normal children and should be distinguished from the higher intensity, third-sound gallop that occurs with tachycardia and indicates congestive heart failure.

Heart murmurs are more difficult to localize in infants than in children and adolescents because in infants they are often so well transmitted and heard throughout the chest. Gross anatomic localization can be helpful, however, as illustrated by (1) the prominence over the back of the murmurs of coarctation of the aorta and some cases of patent ductus arteriosus, (2) the precordial systolic murmur of ventricular septal defect growing louder as one descends the left sternal border to the xiphoid, and (3) the murmur(s) of peripheral pulmonary artery stenosis becoming louder as one moves the stethoscope laterally from the precordium. On the other hand, the typical to-and-fro continuous murmur of patent ductus arteriosus described in older children can be absent in affected infants and represented only by a precordial systolic murmur.

Childhood and Adolescence. The cardiac examination of children and adolescents follows the outline already given and is different from the examination of infants largely because of the need to distinguish organic murmurs from the "innocent" murmur, which occurs in as many as 50% of normal children. Innocent murmurs are unassociated with any symptomatic, radiographic, or electrocardiographic evidence of heart disease, and the three types have several characteristics in common. They usually are low pitched and therefore heard best with the bell. They are musical or vibratory as distinguished from the more complex range of frequencies of "significant" murmurs and are illustrated phonocardiographically in Fig. 7-28. Their intensity usually is no greater than I or II/VI, and both their presence and their intensity vary with change in the child's position or respiratory phase. Innocent murmurs are heard most commonly either at the second left interspace or halfway between the lower left sternal border and the apex. At these sites the murmurs are of short duration and early in systole. A third common location is above or beneath either clavicle, where the murmur is called a *venous hum*. This is an impressive-sounding murmur, often continuous throughout systole; it is heard best with the child sitting and does not occur in the supine position.

In contrast to the innocent murmurs, significant murmurs are usually, but not always, of greater intensity, less localized,

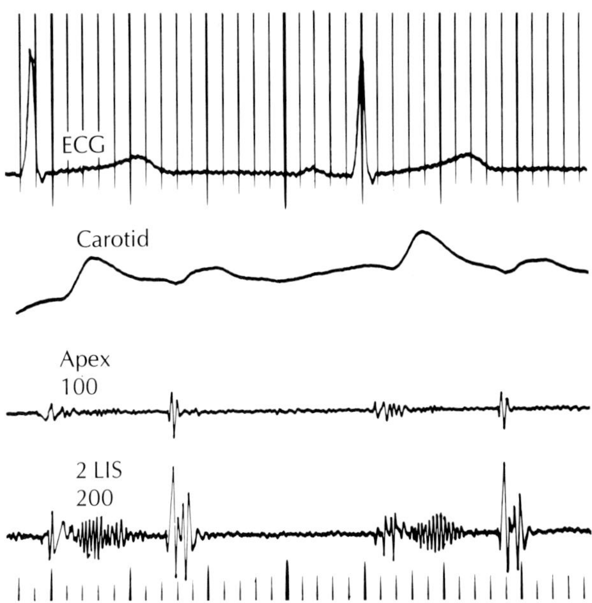

Fig. 7-28 An innocent murmur: phonocardiogram. Note the even harmonic quality of a stringlike murmur. *2 LIS*, Second left interspace.

From Nadas AS and Fyler DC: Pediatric cardiology, ed 3, Philadelphia, 1972, WB Saunders Co.

and more likely to radiate over parts of the chest and usually do not change in loudness with a change in the child's position or respiratory phase. Systolic murmurs can be classified as *stenotic*, *regurgitant*, and *uneven*. Stenotic systolic murmurs are associated with a pressure gradient across the aortic or pulmonary valve and are of high frequency, diamond shaped, and transmitted to the neck. Soft systolic murmurs heard in the pulmonary area and associated not with a valvular pressure gradient but with increased flow, are present with an atrial septal defect. Atrioventricular valve regurgitant murmurs begin immediately with the first sound, are either decreased or pansystolic, are blowing in character, and are best heard at the lower left sternal border or at the apex, with radiation to the axilla and back. The murmur of mitral insufficiency, which is heard at the apex in a large percentage of children with acute rheumatic fever, can be transient and soft; its discovery can be aided by auscultating over the apex with the supine child rotated partly onto the left side. The systolic murmur along the left sternal border heard with a ventricular septal defect usually is pansystolic but is of harsher quality than the atrioventricular valve regurgitant murmurs and is transmitted less well to the axilla, neck, and back. An uneven systolic murmur is heard with patent ductus arteriosus along the upper left sternal border. Although pansystolic with or without a diastolic component, the sound of the murmur varies in pitch and intensity from beat to beat.

Most diastolic murmurs are caused by three types of cardiac abnormalities. Protodiastolic murmurs of high pitch with a crescendo-decrescendo pattern are heard with aortic or pulmonary valve regurgitation. Middiastolic murmurs, which are low pitched, rumbling, often crescendo in pattern, and preceded by an opening snap and followed by an accentuated first sound, are heard with mitral (and, rarely, tricuspid) stenosis. Diastolic flow murmurs, occurring with all large left-to-right shunts and with acute rheumatic fever with mitral regurgitation, are caused by increased flow through a normal-size atrioventricular orifice and are of low frequency, are early or middiastolic in timing, and are associated with a loud third heart sound.

Continuous murmurs—that is, murmurs that extend through systole into diastole—are heard most commonly with patent ductus arteriosus and are sometimes called "machinery" murmurs. These murmurs are usually loud, high pitched, and heard along the left upper sternal border, with radiation to the neck and back.

The most common presenting signs of congestive heart failure in children, as in infants, are tachypnea, orthopnea, liver enlargement, and sometimes increased sweating. Peripheral edema and pulmonary rales tend to be late findings. In children the appearance of facial edema more commonly indicates either an allergic reaction or renal disease such as acute glomerulonephritis. Swelling and redness of the hands and feet are features of Kawasaki disease, as in congestive heart failure (and in a small number, myocardial infarction). Heart failure in children occurs most often with acute or chronic myocarditis (especially acute rheumatic fever), in some children with congenital heart disease, in overwhelming infections, and in hypovolemic states.

Hypertension in children usually is found to be of renal origin, once anxiety has been ruled out. The types of underlying renal disease include acute illnesses such as acute poststreptococcal glomerulonephritis and acute pyelonephritis, end stages of various chronic renal diseases (glomerulonephropathies, chronic obstruction or infection, developmental renal anomalies), kidney tumors such as Wilms tumor, and renal vessel thrombosis and anomalies. Other causes of hypertension include those related to the central nervous system (poliomyelitis, encephalitis, increasing intracranial pressure of many causes), cardiovascular disease (coarctation of the aorta and aortic runoffs as with patent ductus arteriosus, anemia, and thyrotoxicosis), endocrine-metabolic disturbances (cortisone therapy, pheochromocytoma, Cushing disease, congenital adrenal hyperplasia, primary aldosteronism, and porphyria), lead and mercury poisoning, and essential hypertension in which none of these conditions exists. Increasing experience in the routine measurement of blood pressure in children and adolescents suggests that essential hypertension may be more prevalent among adolescents than was previously believed.

The physical findings of heart disease in infants and children only begin to define the nature of the etiology of the disease. Chest roentgenography and electrocardiography, as well as echocardiography, phonocardiography, and cardiac catheterization, are used to further define the basic lesion. Thus physical examination of the heart is an important step in cardiac diagnosis but is only the first of many steps that require interpretation by a qualified cardiologist.

Abdomen

The size and shape of the abdomen change with age, reflecting, in part, changes in the intraabdominal and intrathoracic organs. During the neonatal period the abdomen is relatively protuberant because of (1) the intrathoracic expansion of the lungs with downward movement of the diaphragm and (2) the relatively large liver caused by intrauterine extramedullary hematopoiesis. The first meconium stool usually is passed within 24 hours of birth, and intestinal gas is visible by roentgenogram throughout the normal bowel by 48 hours of age. The horizontal position of the stomach within the abdomen in infancy accounts for the increased postprandial protuberance of the epigastric area. The more vertical, adult position of the stomach is developed slowly throughout childhood. The stomach capacity increases rapidly during the first years of life, from an average of 30 to 90 ml at birth to 210 to 360 ml at 1 year of age, 500 ml at 2 years, then increasing slowly to the adult capacity of 750 to 900 ml. Abdominal protuberance in preschool children is caused by a transient and normal lumbar lordosis. The abdominal musculature is relatively hypotonic at birth, allowing deep palpation. Midline defects include the relatively common and usually transient diastasis recti, the fairly common umbilical hernia, and the rare omphalocele.

A thorough examination of the abdomen should be performed during all health maintenance examinations and in children with gastrointestinal symptoms, fever, cough, and any other evidence of acute illness. It includes inspection of the abdominal contour and size; palpation for tenderness, enlarged liver, spleen, kidneys, or masses; percussion; and auscultation of bowel sounds. An examination of the rectum is indicated in all children with evidence of intraabdominal or pelvic disorders, with fecal elimination problems, or with rectal bleeding.

Newborn and Infant. Absence of the normal prominence of the abdomen in a newborn should lead to further investigation for diaphragmatic hernia or high intestinal atresia. Subcutaneous abdominal wall blood vessels are easily visible in most infants because of their relatively small amounts of subcutaneous fat. Abdominal movement is due to the prominent role of the diaphragm in breathing and, in addition, to intestinal peristalsis. Visible peristaltic waves can be observed over any quadrant of the abdomen, especially in premature babies with relatively thin abdominal walls. Prominent gastric peristaltic waves moving from left to right across the upper portion of the abdomen are present with congenital pyloric stenosis, which usually manifests by 4 to 6 weeks of age.

The umbilical stump is inspected at birth for meconium (yellow) staining, a sign associated with chronic fetal distress. The normal umbilicus contains two ventrally placed, thick-walled, smaller arteries, and one dorsally placed, thin-walled, larger vein. In the past, infants with a single umbilical artery were believed to have a higher than normal incidence of congenital malformations, but this finding recently has been shown to have no significance if it is an isolated anomaly. The umbilical stump, if left uncovered after birth, shrinks to a relatively hard, dark brown eschar, which normally separates from the abdomen by 1 to 2 weeks after birth. The central core area of the umbilicus usually is covered with skin no later than 3 to 4 weeks of age, a process that sometimes is delayed by growth of pink granulation tissue (umbilical granuloma). Transient spotty bleeding of the umbilical area after separation of the umbilical eschar is common and usually lasts no longer than a few days. Chronic drainage of clear fluid from the umbilicus suggests the presence of persistently patent urachus, a urachal cyst, or a communicating

Meckel diverticulum or omphalomesenteric duct. Erythema of the periumbilical skin with or without purulent or foul-smelling discharge suggests omphalitis, a local infection that can rapidly spread to the bloodstream and meninges. Umbilical hernias may be associated with palpable abdominal wall defects that vary from 0.5 to 5 or 6 cm in diameter and that protrude equally as far, especially when crying and straining occur.

A light touch of the examining fingers against the infant's abdominal wall usually contacts the liver edge, 1 to 2 cm below the right costal margin. A spleen tip may or may not be palpated in normal infants at the left costal margin. Midline structures such as the enlarged pylorus of infants with pyloric stenosis sometimes are difficult to palpate because of the contraction of the rectus muscles. Holding the infant's thighs in a flexed position and palpating while the infant is sucking will usually permit deep, midline palpation. The kidneys are accessible to palpation, especially at birth, by the technique of ballottement. One hand is held with the fingers in the costovertebral angle while the other hand presses downward from the anterior costal margin. The posterior hand then "flips" the kidney toward the anterior hand, which usually can "catch" the lower pole of the kidney. It also can be felt as it drops back against the posterior hand. In this manner, symmetry of kidney size can be determined. A unilaterally large kidney occurs with a multicystic kidney, unilateral hydronephrosis, Wilms tumor, invasive neuroblastoma, or renal vein thrombosis. Other palpable abdominal masses include the dilated bladder secondary to urethral obstruction, the bilateral flank masses of hydronephrosis and polycystic kidney disease, duplications of the bowel, and rare primary hepatic tumors. Palpable masses associated with signs of intestinal obstruction (vomiting, abdominal distention, and failure to pass stool) include the meconium masses associated with imperforate anus, Hirschsprung disease, meconium plug syndrome, and meconium ileus; midgut volvulus associated with intestinal malrotation; and the sausage-shaped, usually right lower-quadrant abdominal mass of intussusception associated with bloody or currant-jelly stools. Infants with signs of intestinal obstruction and no palpable mass need immediate further evaluation for congenital atresia or stenosis of any portion of the bowel, peritonitis, and in premature infants, necrotizing enterocolitis.

Percussion of the abdomen of infants can be helpful in determining the size of organs or masses and also will outline the relatively large area of the upper portion of the abdomen filled by the stomach. Ascites may accompany peritonitis, liver or kidney disease, and lymphangiomas of the small bowel mesentery. Bowel sounds (peristaltic sounds) are metallic tinkling sounds heard normally every 10 to 30 seconds. They occur more frequently with intestinal obstruction or gastroenteritis and are diminished with ileus, which can accompany almost any infectious process in infants, especially pneumonitis or gastroenteritis.

The rectal examination performed with the fifth finger can be useful in differentiating bladder from sacral masses, in palpating the uterus, and in detecting the absence of rectal feces in some infants with Hirschsprung disease. In examining the rectum of infants, some examiners prefer to use the index finger because of its greater length, flexibility, sensitivity, and mobility.

Childhood and Adolescence. The shape of the abdomen becomes increasingly scaphoid in school-age children, with the exception of children with exogenous obesity. Frightened, uncomfortable, or ticklish children can be successfully examined if the thighs are held in partial flexion and the abdomen is approached first with the stethoscope. As one listens for bowel sounds, the stethoscope can be pushed gently into the abdomen and areas of rigidity or tenderness noted. The examiner's hands should be warm, and in older children, deep breathing will enhance abdominal palpation. Another useful technique is placing the child's hand between the abdominal wall and the examiner's hand. It can be especially difficult to detect rigidity or tenderness in the crying or nonverbal child. The examiner can watch for facial grimacing and can attempt to "catch" the brief instant of relative relaxation of the abdomen at the end of expiration. The protuberant abdomen of the child with hyperexpanded lungs, forceful abdominal muscle contractions on expiration, and sore abdominal muscles—present, for instance, in status asthmaticus—can be especially difficult to examine for the presence of intraabdominal abnormalities. Asking such a child to raise the head from the supine position usually will lessen intraabdominal pain but will increase abdominal muscle soreness.

Abdominal tenderness in children can be localized by the responses to direct palpation, by referred pain on rebound tenderness, by shake tenderness in which the child's pelvis is gently lifted off the examining table and gently shaken, by pain accompanying hyperextension of the hips (psoas sign) or flexion and external rotation of the hip with the knee held in flexion (obturator sign), and by the palpation of a finger in the rectum against the posterior pelvic wall. The tenderness from an inflamed appendix usually is maximal in the right lower quadrant. Diffuse tenderness can accompany paralytic ileus secondary to extraabdominal or intraabdominal infection, as well as the more serious peritonitis or ruptured abdominal organ or viscus. Midline tenderness especially in the lower portion of the abdomen can be elicited by palpating the abdominal aorta or a full bladder.

With a soft abdomen the cecum and the sigmoid colon often can be rolled between the examining fingers and the adjacent iliac crest. The entire colon is sometimes palpable when filled with feces in association with functional fecal retention. The spleen tip and liver edge may be palpable, especially on deep inspiration, in normal children. The spleen commonly enlarges in association with a number of acute infectious diseases and with a number of blood dyscrasias. Liver enlargement can occur with heart failure, hepatitis, septicemia, metastatic tumor, blood dyscrasia, and various storage diseases. Upper quadrant direct tenderness or shock tenderness (elicited by gently pounding the lower anterior rib cage) as signs of liver or splenic bleeding or rupture should be investigated in all children who have sustained trauma to the abdomen.

Genitalia

By the end of the third fetal month the undifferentiated fetal gonad has developed into an ovary or, under the influence of the XY chromosome, into a testis. With production of testosterone by the fetal testis (the medulla of the fetal gonad), the wolffian duct system further develops into the epididymis, ductus deferens, and seminal vesicles, and development of the müllerian duct system is inhibited by an as yet unidentified factor. The testes descend into the scrotum between the seventh and eighth months of gestation, followed by a sleeve of parietal peritoneum, the processus vaginalis, which closes off in most babies by the time of birth. At the time of birth one or more testes are undescended in 3% to 4% of male babies. Most of these descend by 3 months of age, leaving 1% of babies by age 1 year with unilateral or bilateral undescended testes. The processus vaginalis can remain patent and retain its connection with the peritoneal cavity, causing an inguinal hernia that usually is apparent within a few months following birth. A fluid-filled segment of the processus vaginalis within the scrotum, a hydrocele, is present in 10% of male babies and can be associated with an inguinal hernia. Many hydroceles apparent at birth disappear spontaneously within the first few months of life.

In the absence of fetal testosterone and another undetermined factor, the müllerian duct system develops into fallopian tubes, uterus, and upper vagina. Following birth, as a result of withdrawal of maternal estrogen, the uterus decreases in size and then grows slowly back to its birth size by age 5 years. By 10 years of age the corpus of the uterus has grown to a size equal to that of the uterine cervix. The cervix grows rapidly again in the premenarcheal years, followed by further growth of the uterine corpus.

The development of secondary sex characteristics during puberty varies considerably as to time of onset, duration, and sequential timing in both boys and girls (Figs. 7-29 and 7-30). In girls, breast development begins between the ages of 8 and 13 and is completed between the ages of 12 and 19. Pubic hair develops roughly in parallel with breast development. Peak velocity of growth in height occurs on the average of 1 year after onset of breast development, whereas menarche occurs approximately 2 years after onset of breast development. The duration of puberty in girls varies between 1½ and 6 years.

In boys, testicular enlargement precedes development of pubic hair, processes that begin between 9½ and 13½ years. An increase in the size of the penis parallels an increase in testicular size, following an initial lag phase. The peak velocity of growth in height occurs later in boys than it does in girls, commencing at an average age of 14 years. The duration of puberty in boys varies between 1.8 and 4.7 years.

Stages of development of pubic hair in boys and girls are illustrated in Figs. 7-31 and 7-32. Sequential recording of a given child's progress can be used both to diagnose abnormal development and to reassure the worried normal adolescent.

A thorough examination of the external genitalia is mandatory immediately following birth to allow rapid evaluation of babies with ambiguous genitalia. The external genitalia are examined during all health maintenance examinations and in all children seeking medical attention for abdominal pain. The penis, testes, and external inguinal rings should be examined in boys. In girls, the clitoris, labia majora and minora, vaginal orifice, urethral orifice, and external inguinal rings should be examined. Internal inspection of the vagina and cervix and bimanual palpation of the internal genitalia are not part of the routine examination of children; they are, however, performed in the evaluation of problems such as vaginal discharge or bleeding (see following discussion).

When the primary care physician evaluates an infant, a child, or an adolescent for suspected sexual abuse, the child and parent must be prepared with patience and with attention to their fears and concerns. The child must have some control over the position, draping, and pace of the examination and should not be restrained. The examination can proceed with the child supine in the mother's lap, supine on the examining table in a frog-leg position, in a lateral decubitus position with the knees drawn up to the chest, or in a knee-chest position. The examiner should explain and answer concerns both before and during each step. After the body as a whole is inspected for signs of trauma, the external genitalia and anus are observed for old or new abrasions or lacerations

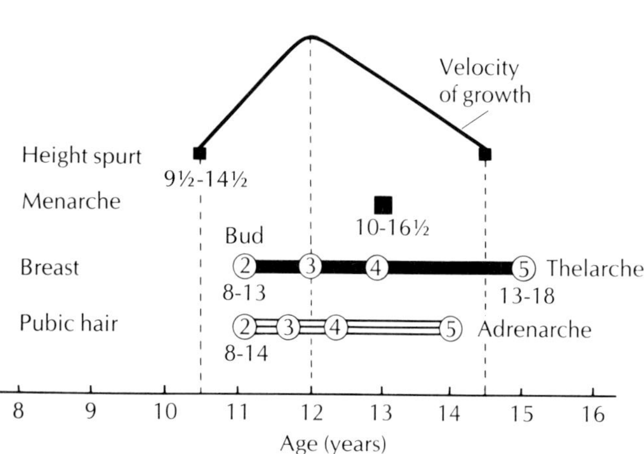

Fig. 7-29 Sequence of events in adolescent girls. An average girl is represented; the range of ages within which some of the events may occur is given by the figures placed directly below the bars.

From Marshall WA and Tanner JM: Variation in the pattern of pubertal changes in boys, Arch Dis Child 45:13, 1970.

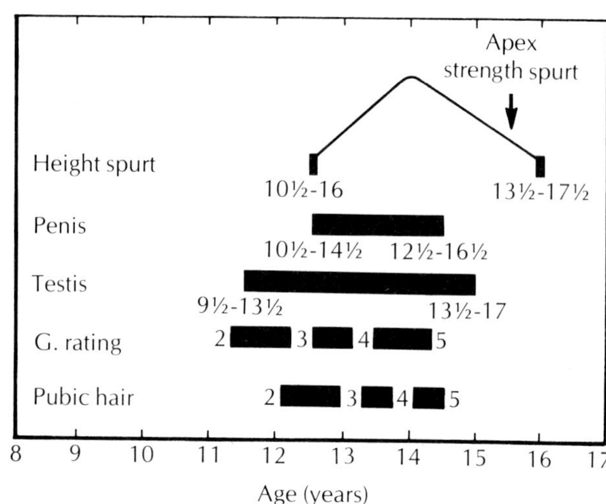

Fig. 7-30 Sequence of events in adolescent boys. An average boy is represented; the range of ages within which some of the events may occur is given by the figures placed directly below the bars.

From Marshall WA and Tanner JM: Variation in the pattern of pubertal changes in boys, Arch Dis Child 45:13, 1970.

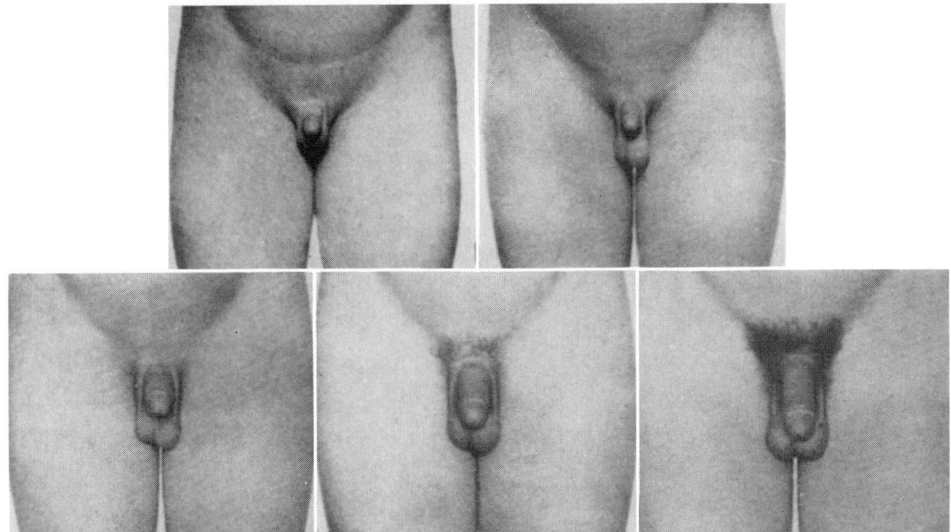

Fig. 7-31 Standards for genitalia maturity ratings in boys.

From Tanner JM: Growth at adolescence, ed 2, Oxford, 1962, Blackwell Scientific Publications, Ltd.

(facilitated by prior application of toluidine blue dye), scars, hyperpigmentation, verrucae, and enlarged orifices. The hymen is inspected for stretching, injury, or thickening; a vaginal orifice of greater than 4 mm in prepubertal children has been correlated with prior vaginal penetration. All findings should be recorded clearly, with diagrams if necessary for possible use in future child protective custody hearings. Culture specimens of perineal tissue and/or exudate are routinely obtained to ascertain the presence of *Neisseria gonorrhoeae* and, when suspected, *Chlamydia trachomatis*, herpes simplex virus, and *Trichomonas* and *Gardnerella* organisms. Venereal warts (condyloma acuminatum) can be seen in their earliest stages after application of 3% to 5% acetic acid solution to perineal tissues; their presence only suggests sexual molestation.

Newborn. At birth the appearance of the external genitalia provides information that is useful in assessing gestational age. In the male the testes are undescended before the thirtieth week of gestation, are high in the inguinal canal between the thirtieth and thirty-sixth weeks, and normally are completely descended into the scrotum by 40 weeks. The scrotal rugae appear, progressing inferiorly to superiorly, between the thirtieth and fortieth weeks. In the female the labia majora are widely separated and the clitoris is prominent up to the thirty-sixth week; by 40 weeks the labia majora completely cover the labia minora and clitoris.

A white vaginal discharge, occasionally mixed with blood, can be seen for several days following birth and results from withdrawal from the relatively high levels of maternally derived estrogen. Maternal estrogen also can cause a transient hypertrophy of the labia majora as seen at birth. The urethral and vaginal orifices can be visualized by downward and lateral traction on each side of the perineum (Fig. 7-33). The hymen varies in thickness and size, the central orifice usually measuring 4 mm or less in diameter in infants. Rarely is the hymen imperforate at birth.

The foreskin of the penis usually is nonretractable at birth, a condition that can persist for up to 1 year. Ordinarily, sufficient retraction is possible to allow visualization of the external urethral meatus at the tip of the glans penis. Inspection of the ventral surface of the penis for hypospadias (an abnormal position of the external urethral meatus located anywhere between the midline scrotum to the tip of the glans) is necessary at birth because its presence is a contraindication to circumcision. Hypospadias may be accompanied by chordee, a fixed downward bowing of the penis. Rarely, the urethral meatus is located on the dorsal surface of the penis,

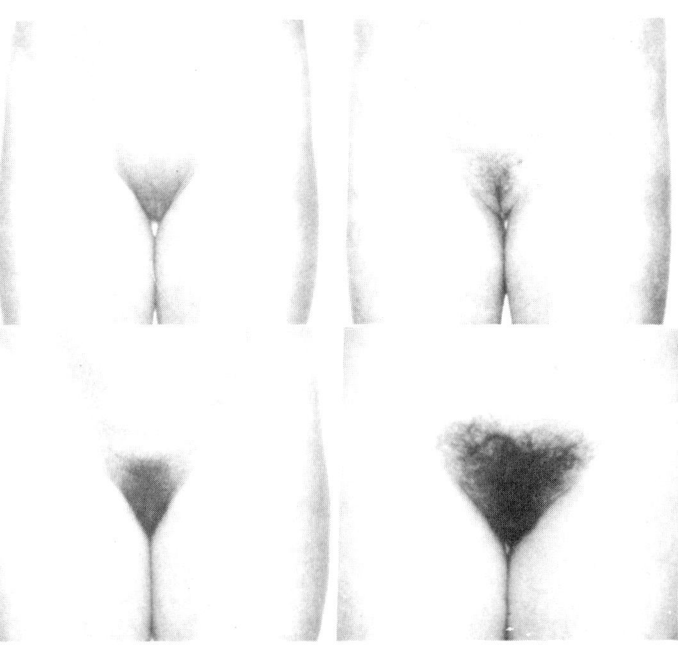

Fig. 7-32 Stages of development of pubic hair in girls. Stage 1 is not shown; there is no pubic hair.

From Tanner JM: Growth at adolescence, ed 2, Oxford, 1962, Blackwell Scientific Publications, Ltd.

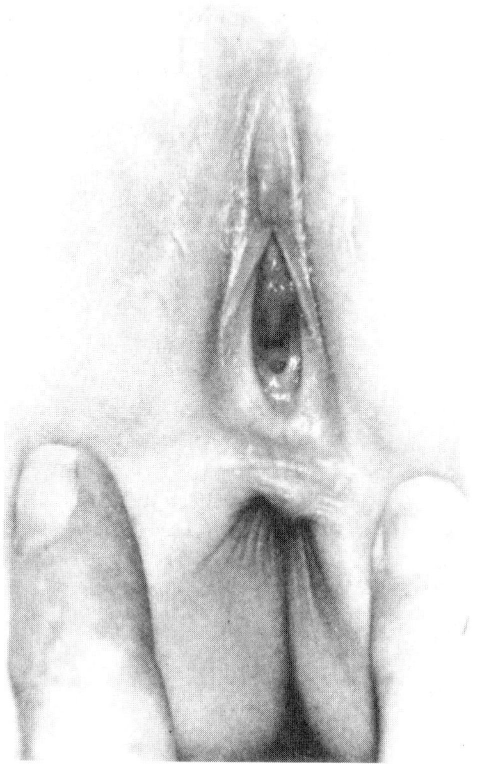

Fig. 7-33 Inspection of the infant vulva.

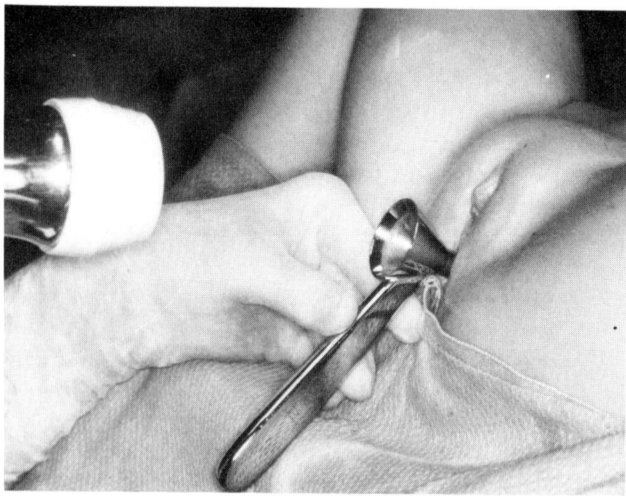

Fig. 7-34 Inspection of the vagina by use of a children's vaginoscope and simple illumination with a flashlight.

known as epispadias. After circumcision the glans penis and the remaining lip of foreskin are swollen and erythematous for several days.

Palpation of the testes should proceed downward from the external inguinal ring to the scrotum to counteract the active cremasteric reflex in infants. This technique is important in accurately diagnosing the undescended testis. Inguinal hernias in infants occur as unilateral or bilateral inguinal and scrotal bulges that usually are reducible and may appear only with crying or straining. Hydroceles are scrotal and sometimes inguinal masses that often are attached to the testes and are nonreducible, nontender, and transilluminate.

Rarely, the appearance of the external genitalia may present difficulties in the determination of gender. For instance, there may be a midline phallus with apparent scrotal hypospadias and partially fused scrotal-appearing skin with no palpable scrotal masses. In this situation careful inspection and in some cases probing of the midline of the perineum for a vaginal orifice is an important first step in making a diagnosis of ambiguous external genitalia in a female baby, as is rectal examination to palpate for the presence of a uterus.

Infancy and Early Childhood. Several minor physical abnormalities are common during the first years of life. Ammoniacal dermatitis involving the perineum (diaper rash) in both the circumcised and uncircumcised infant can cause balanitis, an acute inflammation of the glans penis, sometimes associated with purulent exudate. After an episode of balanitis the external urethral meatus can become stenotic, causing a narrow urinary stream and prolonged duration of bladder emptying. Balanitis in the uncircumcised boy can leave adhesions between the glans penis and foreskin, preventing retraction of the foreskin.

It is important to diagnose accurately the undescended testis because corrective surgery can protect the functioning of a normal, undescended testis only if performed during the first few years of life. The acutely tender testis may represent torsion of the testis, or orchitis, a complication of mumps that occurs commonly in young men.

In female infants, paper-thin adhesions between the labia minora are commonly seen during the first few years of life, sometimes completely covering the vulvar vestibule, with a small opening through which urine escapes. These vulvar adhesions sometimes can be parted by applying gentle pressure laterally on the labia majora. They also will disappear after application of an estrogen-containing cream for several weeks.

Vulvovaginal discharge in preschool-age girls is most commonly caused by vaginal foreign bodies, usually bits of toilet paper; occasionally a specific bacterial organism can be cultured or pinworms discovered. Cultures that are positive for *Neisseria gonorrhoeae* and *Chlamydia trachomatis* almost always indicate sexual abuse. Making these diagnoses occasionally requires vaginoscopy with a special instrument such as the Huffman vaginoscope or a nasal speculum (Fig. 7-34). Vaginal specimens for smears and cultures are most painlessly obtained by first instilling a small amount of sterile nutrient broth into the vagina with a medicine dropper.

Although digital examination of the vagina usually is not possible in prepubertal girls, the uterus can be palpated for size, shape, and tenderness with one hand placed over the lower portion of the abdomen and a finger of the other hand inserted into the rectum.

During the performance of a rectal examination in a girl, the cervix is the predominant part of the uterus that is palpable; the ovaries normally are not felt. Examination of the rectum in both boys and girls usually is helped by telling the child that "this will be just like having your temperature taken" and by talking with the child in a relaxed manner while doing the examination.

Late Childhood. Children usually begin to have uncomfortable feelings about being undressed in front of adults by the time they reach 5 or 6 years of age. Examination of school-age children can be enhanced by soliciting reassurances from the parent and by the use of drapes or gowns.

Occasionally, secondary sexual characteristics begin to develop in children in this age group. Evaluation of such children must distinguish among premature thelarche, premature menarche, and precocious puberty.

One method for examining normally retractile testes is to palpate the scrotum with the boy squatting; the examiner begins to palpate over the inguinal areas and works downward onto the scrotum. This technique is especially helpful in the examination of boys with exogenous obesity, whose external genitalia can be "engulfed" in excess peripubic and perineal adipose tissue. Palpation for an inguinal hernia over the external inguinal ring while the boy coughs, with the examining finger inserted into the scrotal tissue and slid upward into the inguinal canal, usually is possible by the age of 4 years. Tender acute swelling of the scrotum can be caused by torsion of the testes, epididymitis, orchitis (often caused by mumps), or an incarcerated inguinal hernia.

Adolescence. Examination of the adolescent's genitalia affords an opportunity for reassurance about the normal progression of the stages of puberty. The examiner should be aware of an adolescent's excellent ability to deny real concerns and worries and should be especially sensitive to questions that might relate to a concern about venereal disease, pregnancy, or even cancer. Honest and direct answers to the adolescent's questions, coupled with a careful description of the examination before it is performed, will help to establish a trusting relationship.

Bimanual palpation of the uterus, as just described, usually is adequate in examining prepubertal and virginal pubertal girls. A complete pelvic examination is indicated in any adolescent with vaginal discharge, dysuria, pyuria, lower abdominal pain, irregular vaginal bleeding, or amenorrhea and in the sexually active adolescent. This examination is aided by proper instruments, including a vaginoscope or small speculum, culture media, glass slides, and a cytology fixative. The physician should be patient and gentle and should avoid painful procedures and embarrassment for the patient. After inspection of the external genitalia and examination with the speculum or vaginoscope, the uterus and ovaries are palpated by means of the bimanual technique; normally the ovaries are not palpable. Specimens should be obtained periodically in sexually active adolescents to culture for *Neisseria gonorrhoeae*.

Musculoskeletal System

The changes in the musculoskeletal system of infants, children, and adolescents over time give the examiner the most visible evidence of human growth. A child whose sequential measurements of height fall within the norms of a standard growth curve presents strong evidence not only that bone growth is normal but also that the numerous factors necessary for normal growth are operating appropriately. In addition, because of its visibility, the musculoskeletal system is most often the source of questions from parents concerning possible deviations from normal, including the possible effects of trauma, a leading cause of morbidity and mortality in children.

The outward manifestations of growth of the trunk and extremities reflect primarily growth of bone, muscle, and adipose tissue. Bone grows in the fetus starting with cartilage, then from the primary centers of ossification, primarily in the long bones. Postnatally, new bone formation occurs in secondary centers of ossification at the ends of long bones and the vertebral bodies and in the membranes of the flat bones of the cranium and clavicle. In addition to longitudinal growth of long bones and vertebral bodies, internal remodeling takes place throughout infancy and childhood, resulting in less dense bone, a changing thickness of the bone cortex, and changing amounts of red marrow and fat within the diaphyses of bone. In addition to hormonal factors, bone remodeling is influenced by mechanical forces caused by muscle attachments and gravity. Bone growth is completed with ossification of the growth cartilage and union of the epiphyses and diaphyses of long bones by 25 years of age. The roentgenographic appearance of the onset, size, and shape of secondary ossification centers can be compared with established norms in determining the bone age, a measurement that, despite its variability, can be helpful in assessing children with suspected abnormal growth.

Growth in stature predominates in the lower extremities before puberty and in the trunk during puberty. The distal extremities reach adult size before the proximal extremities, thus the common complaint of preadolescent children that their feet are too big.

Muscle growth, resulting from increases in number, size, and length of cells, proceeds throughout childhood according to the following increasing proportions of muscle mass to body weight: 1:5 to 1:4 at birth, 1:3 in early adolescence, and 2:5 in early maturity. There is a rapid spurt in the increase in muscle cell numbers at 2 years of age and a maximal increase between the ages of 10 and 16. Muscle cell size increases more rapidly in girls than in boys between the ages of 3 and 10, with both the number and size of muscle cells in boys surpassing that of girls after 14 years of age. An increase in the number of muscle fibers progresses slowly until the fifth decade of life.

A thorough evaluation of the musculoskeletal system should be part of every newborn examination, every child health maintenance examination, and the examination of any child with an abnormality of growth, stature, or gait. It includes an appraisal of (1) posture, position, and gross deformities, (2) skin color, temperature, and tenderness, (3) bone or joint tenderness, (4) range of joint motion, (5) muscle size, symmetry, and strength, and (6) the configuration and motility of the back.

Newborn. The position and appearance of the extremities at birth can reflect intrauterine position. The folded position of the lower extremities on the abdomen in the fetus results in the common appearance in newborns of externally rotated, somewhat bowed, lower extremities with everted feet. The baby born after a breech presentation often has markedly flexed hips and extended knees. Traction on the brachial plexus during delivery can cause what is usually a temporary paresis of the proximal upper extremity muscles (Erb palsy), usually appearing as an asymmetric Moro reflex (see p. 107). Another common cause of an asymmetric Moro reflex resulting from a birth injury is a fractured clavicle, which can be confirmed by palpating an area of crepitance, usually over the distal third of the clavicle.

Gross deformities should be recognized at birth, both for early treatment and for possible clues to generalized genetic or metabolic diseases. Relatively common deformities include short or absent extremities, absence of one bone in an extremity, hypertrophy of one bone in an extremity or of an entire half of the body (hemihypertrophy), extra fingers or toes (polydactyly), webbed or fused fingers or toes (syndactyly), and annular constricting bands around a portion of an extremity with or without distal amputation or lack of development. The ratio of extremity length to body length should be noted. In the normal newborn the ratio of the upper to the lower segment of the body (above and below the symphysis pubis) is approximately 1.7:1. In various types of dwarfism the extremities alone may be short, as in achondroplasia, or both extremities and trunk may be shortened, as in Morquio disease. The entire length of the vertebral column should be examined and palpated for bony defects with or without overlying skin defects.

The joints are tested for range of motion, noting any asymmetry, undue tightness, or contractures, as well as the muscle tone. A floppy or hypotonic baby may have central nervous system disease, a metabolic disturbance, primary muscle disease, or anterior horn cell disease. Limited unilateral joint motion with or without associated bone or joint tenderness and fever should be vigorously evaluated as a possible sign of osteomyelitis.

Perhaps the most important part of the examination of the newborn's extremities is of the lower extremities, with special attention to the hips and feet. The hips are examined particularly to rule out congenital dislocation, a condition that is relatively easily treated and has good results only if treatment is started early. The examiner tests for an unstable or actually dislocated femoral head by abducting one hip at a time and feeling for a click when the femoral head passes back into the acetabulum. The amount of hip abduction required for this maneuver usually is 70 to 80 degrees. Downward pressure over the hips transmitted through the flexed knee can be used to attempt to produce posterior dislocation of the femoral head (Fig. 7-35). The click or clunk of the reducing femoral head should be distinguished from the clicks felt with rotation of the hip and the click felt with simultaneous movement of the knee. Beyond the newborn period the hip click (Ortolani sign) with congenitally dislocated hips disappears, and other signs become helpful in making this diagnosis. The thigh may appear shorter on the affected side, the thigh skin folds may be asymmetric (although this does occur in some normal babies), and the hip has limited abduction on the affected side. Tight hip abductors in the neonatal period are not a sign of congenital hip dislocation.

The feet of the newborn and infant often appear flat because of a plantar fat pad that gradually disappears during the first year or two of life. The most severe foot deformity at birth is the equinovarus deformity, or clubfoot. True clubfoot deformities cannot be passively corrected, nor do they correct with stroking of the foot's lateral side. This deformity includes fixed forefoot adduction, fixed inversion especially of the hindfoot, equinus position, internal tibial torsion, and small calf muscles.

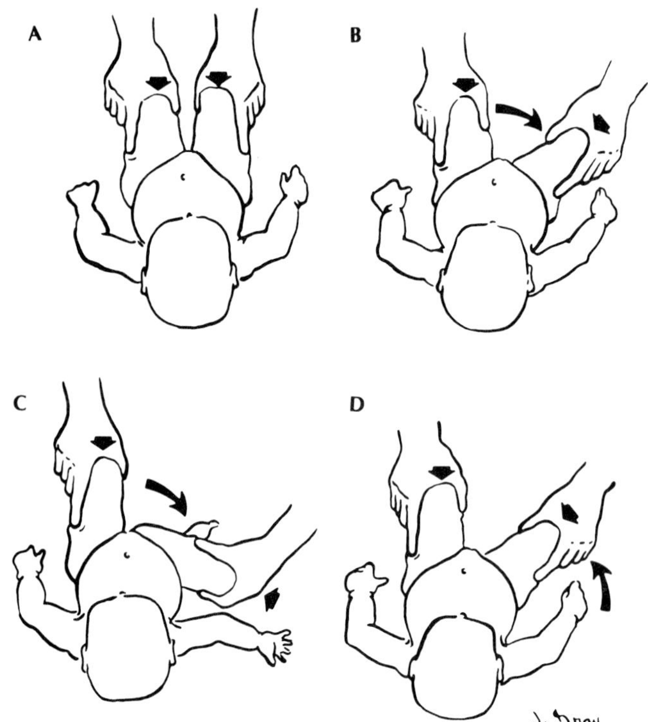

Fig. 7-35 Examination for congenital dislocation of the hip. **A,** Downward pressure on the hips to produce posterior dislocation. **B,** The hip to be examined is then abducted. **C** and **D,** A positive Ortolani sign is elicited by feeling the head reenter the acetabulum with a click. Examiner's finger is on baby's greater trochanter during all phases of examination.

From Stanisavljevic S: Diagnosis and treatment of congenital hip pathology in the newborn. © 1964, The Williams & Wilkins Co, Baltimore.

Viewing the sole of the resting foot (not spontaneously inverted or everted) allows observation for the normal single anteroposterior plantar axis. In metatarsus varus deformity the forefoot is adducted in relation to the hindfoot, thus describing two anteroposterior axes, and this position is not correctable by stroking the foot's lateral border. In calcaneovalgus deformity the foot is dorsiflexed and everted.

One way to examine the alignment of the lower extremity is shown in Fig. 7-36. With the infant supine, draw an imaginary line connecting the anterior superior "iliac" spine with the midpatella and continue down to the foot; if the line falls medial to the first toe, external tibial torsion is present; if it falls lateral to the second toe, internal tibial torsion is present. See Chapter 133 for a complete discussion of developmental orthopedic variations of the lower extremities.

Infancy and Early Childhood. The infant's lower extremities often remain bowlegged with externally rotated feet for the first year or two of life. With ambulation the feet gradually assume the straight-ahead position, and the knock-knee, or genu valgum, position normally is seen between the ages of 2 and 6 years or longer.

Severe bowing of the legs raises the question of rickets or epiphyseal damage from inflammation or trauma (Blount disease). The infant with toeing-in should be examined for metatarsus varus, internal tibial torsion, or femoral anteversion. Flatfeet, or feet with an absent longitudinal arch, are com-

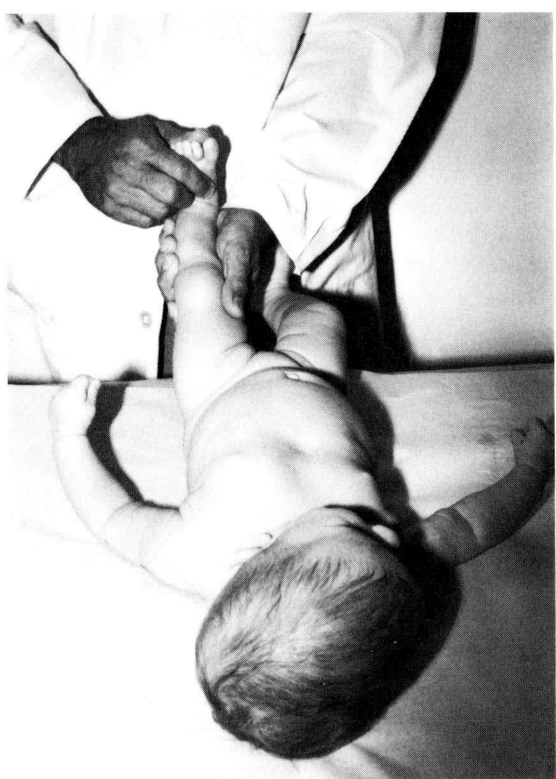

Fig. 7-36 Examination of the lower extremities.
Photograph by P. Ruben.

monly seen, especially in children with generalized ligamentous laxity.

The examination of the lower extremities of toddlers is best accomplished by first observing the spontaneous gait with the infant undressed. The normal gait usually is wide based and somewhat unstable, with prominent lumbar lordosis. Then, especially if positional deformities are noted, a careful examination in the supine position of the hips, knees, legs, ankles, and feet can confirm the presence of any fixed deformity. The child with a limp should be carefully examined for signs of trauma; localized bone or joint tenderness from fracture or infection; joint effusions with limited range of motion from trauma, infection, or noninfectious arthritis; peripheral muscle weakness; unilateral or bilateral spasticity, especially manifested by a tight Achilles tendon; and proximal muscle weakness, particularly weakness resulting from unrecognized hip disease such as congenital dislocated hip or coxa vara. The last-named condition can be tested by having the child raise one foot while standing. This normally produces an elevation in the contralateral hip. The inability of the hip abductors to elevate the contralateral hip is considered a positive Trendelenburg sign (Fig. 7-37).

Child abuse should be suspected in all cases of trauma if the history of the injury is inconsistent with its severity; if there are signs of multiple blunt trauma to the extremities, trunk (especially the buttocks), and face; if trauma is recurrent; and if there is a significant delay between the episode of injury and the seeking of medical attention.

The infant with a tender elbow held in pronation, usually after a pulling episode (nursemaid elbow), suffers from subluxation of the radial head, which can be easily reduced by supinating the arm while applying pressure to the radial head.

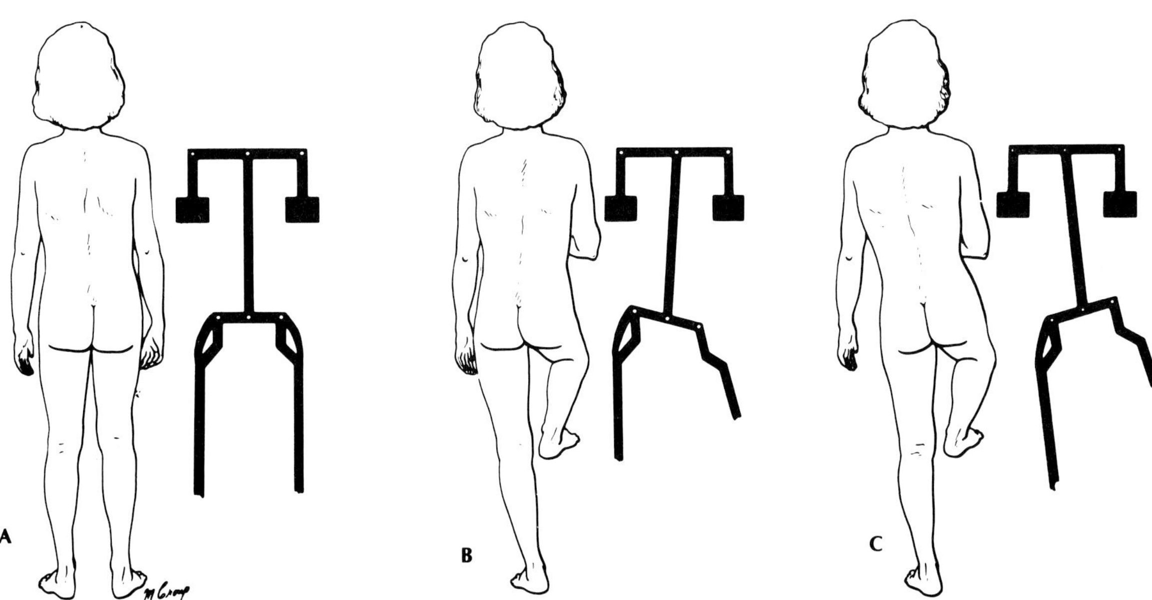

Fig. 7-37 Trendelenburg sign, showing weakness of the gluteus medius muscle. **A,** Normal standing. **B,** Dropping of pelvis of contralateral side when standing on affected leg. **C,** Compensation for weakness when walking by shifting center of gravity of trunk to elevate pelvis on opposite side.
From Ferguson Am Jr: Orthopaedic surgery in infancy and childhood, ed 5. © 1981, the Williams & Wilkins Co, Baltimore.

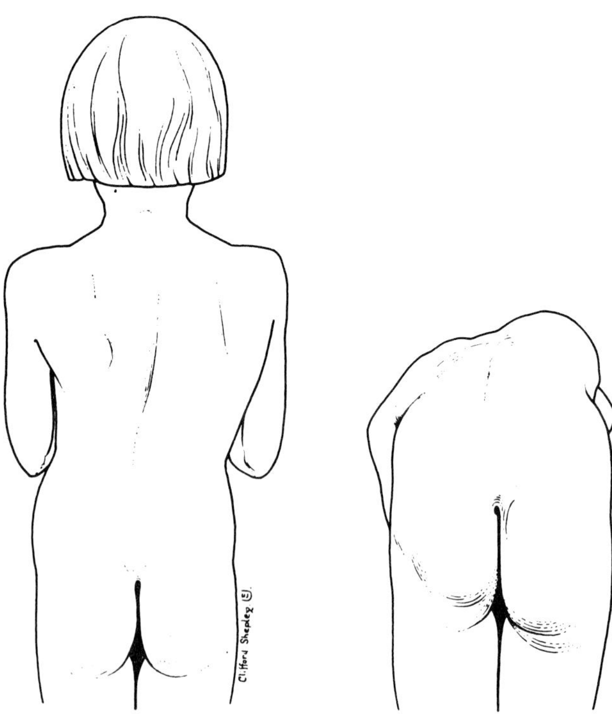

Fig. 7-38 Examination for scoliosis.
From James JIP: Scoliosis, Edinburgh, 1976, E & S Livingstone, Ltd.

Late Childhood and Adolescence. A limp in the child between the ages of 4 and 8, especially if accompanied by knee pain, raises the possibility of Legg-Calvé-Perthes disease, as well as the conditions previously mentioned. The same symptoms in the child of 9 to 12 years may be caused by slipped femoral capital epiphysis. Tenderness over the tibial tubercle may be a sign of Osgood-Schlatter disease. Painful heels can be caused by partial evulsion of the Achilles tendon.

Examination of an injured knee should include testing the medial and lateral collateral ligaments by abducting and adducting the tibia on the femur; the cruciate ligaments by pulling the tibia forward, then pushing it backward with the knee flexed; the medial and lateral menisci by extending the knee with the foot held in eversion and then inversion; the patella by pushing it posteriorly against the femur; and the joint space for effusion by pressing over the suprapatellar bursa and then attempting ballottement of the patella.

School-age children and adolescents should be examined for scoliosis, or lateral curvature of the vertebral column. Before the appearance of spinal curvature with the child standing in an erect position, lesser degrees of curvature can be observed by having the child bend forward approximately 50 degrees, letting the shoulders droop forward and the arms hang freely. The examiner then looks for a unilateral elevation of the lower thoracic ribs and flank that accompanies the rotational deformity of scoliosis (Fig. 7-38).

Nervous System

The manifestations of growth of the nervous system as contrasted with other organ systems in infants and children are the most dynamic. Therefore the definitions of normality for any sign that reflects the state of the nervous system or one of its parts are critically age dependent. These norms also demonstrate wide variation among individuals, as well as within a single individual on different days and under variable conditions. There are two ways to assess the growth and integrity of the growing nervous system. One is to describe the changes in a child's abilities in various behavioral areas over time, in reference to established norms; this is developmental assessment and is discussed in Chapter 18, Eleven, Developmental Assessment. The other is neurologic assessment, in which often-changing physical signs that reflect the state of subsystems of the nervous system are described over time. The developmental stage depends in part on the neurologic stage but also is influenced greatly by the child's environmental experiences. The major goal of neurologic assessment in children is to monitor the maturation of the nervous system, although the methods described for localizing nervous system lesions in adults are useful in evaluating certain problems in children.

The nervous system grows most rapidly during fetal and early postnatal life, reaching approximately one fourth the adult size at birth, one half by age 1, four fifths by age 3, and nine tenths by age 7. At the cellular level there are two distinct peaks of growth rate. The first involves multiplication of neuroblasts, which occurs between 10 and 18 weeks of fetal life, beyond which time there is probably little increase in neuronal cell numbers. The second and more striking spurt of brain growth occurs between midgestation and approximately 18 months of age and reflects multiplication of glial cells, production of myelin by the glial cells, and development of dendrites and synaptic connections. Myelination continues at a relatively rapid rate until age 4, after which there is a gradual increase to adult levels.

The growth of the spinal cord, after fusion of the neural folds cranially and caudally, is initially most rapid in the lumbar and cervical regions, with the thoracic region developing most rapidly during the third trimester of pregnancy. Because during the third fetal month the rate of growth of the developing vertebral column becomes more rapid than that of the spinal cord, the cordal end of the spinal cord moves cranially from the level of the fourth lumbar vertebra in the fifth month to the adult level of the first or second lumbar vertebra by the second postnatal month. Myelination of the cord proceeds cephalocaudad.

Spontaneous and reflexive motor activity, reflecting developing muscular innervation and spinal reflex arcs, begins during the tenth week of fetal life. At 12 weeks of fetal age a primitive rooting and grasp response can be seen; withdrawal of the lower extremities in response to stimulation of the feet and the gastrocnemius stretch reflex are seen at 16 weeks, and by 19 weeks, regular respiratory movements are seen in response to hypoxia. Tonic myotactic reflexes, responsible for the recoil of an extended extremity, are well developed in the term infant. Rhythmic motor neuron activity responsible for jerky repetitive movements with activity (e.g., the jerking jaw movements accompanying crying) develops increased rhythmicity with increasing gestational age. At term, stretch reflexes, such as the knee jerk, are diminished by sleep, whereas exteroceptive reflexes (superficial abdominal and Babinski) are not.

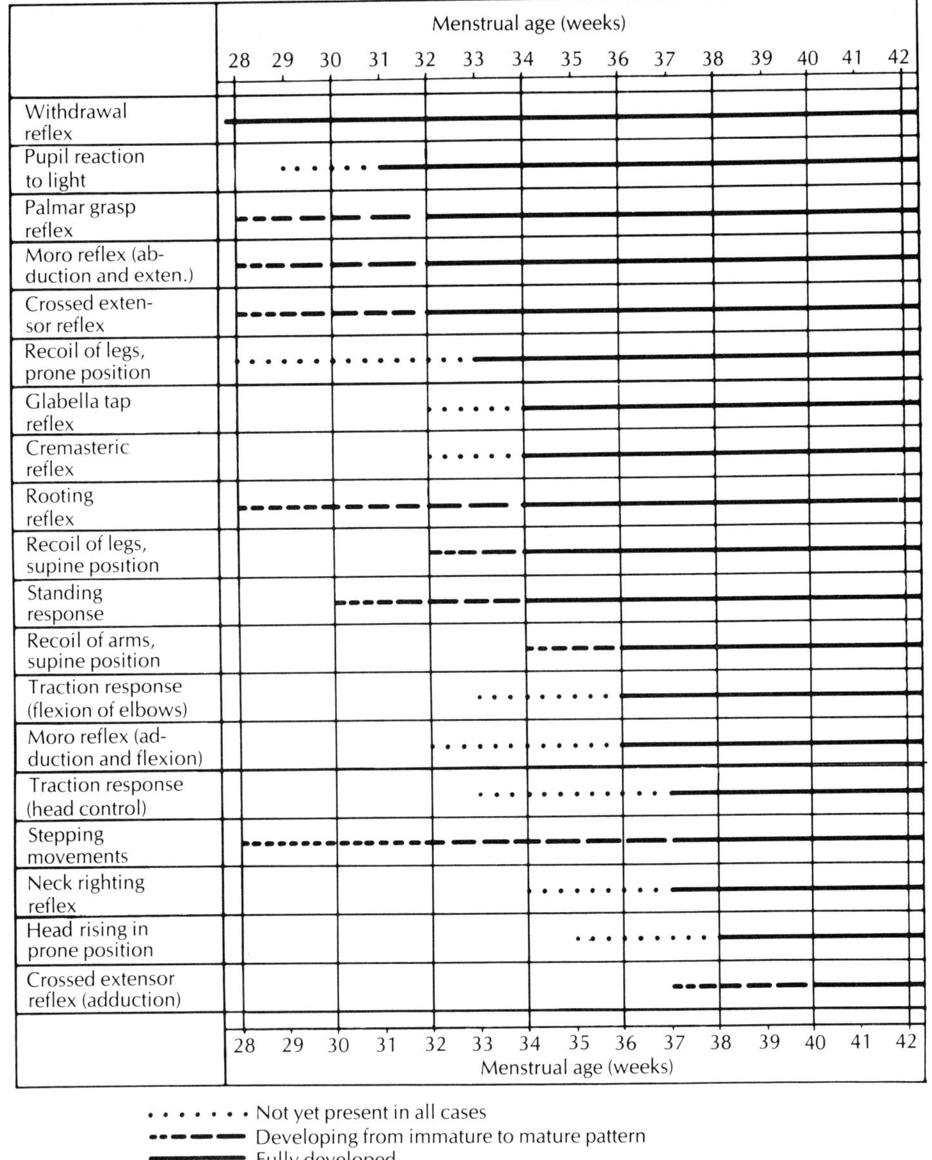

Fig. 7-39 Developmental sequence of various reflexes and motor automatisms.

From Davis JA and Dobbing J, editors: Scientific foundations of paediatrics, ed 2, Baltimore, Md, 1981, University Park Press.

The normal sequence of changes in the infant's posture, muscle tone, and reflexes with increasing gestational age from 28 to 40 weeks has been described by several observers and, despite their differences, can be used in assessing a neonate's gestational age (Fig. 7-39). Similarly, the persistence and eventual cessation of certain characteristics of the infant's posture, tone, and reflexes follow a defined pattern with age (Table 7-5). Changes in the infant's and child's developmental abilities (see Chapter 18, Eleven, Developmental Assessment) also are based on the continuing maturation of the nervous system.

An additional behavioral characteristic of the maturing nervous system is the change in sleep-wake cycles with age. The neonate's sleep-wake cycle usually is quite irregular, but it becomes regular by 15 weeks of age. Rapid eye movement (REM) sleep occurs during a greater proportion of sleeping time in infants than in adults. A small number of neonates are found to have irregular respirations during sleep, sometimes to the point of apnea, a condition that has been discarded as a precursor of the sudden infant death syndrome.

A neurologic examination should be performed on every neonate and on infants and preschool children during health maintenance visits. Other indications for a careful neurologic assessment include developmental delay, school failure, abnormal social behavior, headache, head trauma, seizures, sensory disturbances, changes in states of consciousness, abnormal gait, recent personality change, and fever of unknown origin. Structural and functional abnormalities of the nervous system of infants and children can produce delays in the normal maturational sequences and localizing signs. Therefore the neurologic assessment must include observations of spontaneous and elicited activity that reflect brain maturation, as well as the ordered sequence of the neurologic examination as described for adults. Suggested organizations for the neu-

Table 7-5 *Normal Values for Appearance and Dissolution of Neurologic Items According to Different Authors*

RESPONSE	TAFT-COHEN	DiLEO	VASSELLA	MITCHELL
Sucking	Persists			
Rooting	3-4 mo	12 mo	4 mo	
Palmar grasp	5-6 mo	4-5 mo	3-4 mo	
Plantar grasp	9-12 mo	Walking age	End baby age	
Crossed extension	Persists			
Asymmetric tonic neck	6-7 mo	4 mo	4-5 mo	
Neck-righting	9-12 mo		4 mo	
Moro	4-6 mo	4-5 mo	4-5 mo	3-5 mo
Stepping	3-4 mo	1½ mo	1 mo	
Tactile foot placement	1 yr			
Galant	2-3 mo			
Babinski	12-18 mo	During 2nd yr	6 mo to walking	
Positive supporting	Variable, 2-3 mo		3 mo	
Landau	3 mo*→2nd yr†		4 mo*	3 mo*→1 yr†
Parachute (prone)	7-9 mo*		5 mo*	
Lateral supporting	5-7 mo*		7 mo*	

From Touwen BCL: The neurological development of the infant. In Davis JA and Dobbing J, editors: Scientific foundations of paediatrics, ed 2, Baltimore, Md, 1981, University Park Press, p 835.

NOTE: Most data are averages or average ranges; only Paine's are full ranges.

*Time of appearance.

†Time of dissolution.

rologic examinations of neonates are described by Prechtl and Beintema,[5] for infants during the first year of life by Amiel-Tison,[1] and for children with behavioral or learning disabilities by Touwen and Prechtl.[6] A method for organizing the data of a neurologic examination that includes parts of these age-specific evaluations with the standard adult neurologic examination is shown in the accompanying box. Various components of this summary are discussed in other chapters in this text. The following sections will highlight the approach to the neurologic examination of children of different age groups, including major areas of emphasis for each group.

Newborn and Infancy. Careful observation is the most important tool in the neurologic examination of the newborn and infant, taking into account the optimal environmental conditions previously described. Even when the infant is asleep and dressed, the examiner can note the posture, especially the degree of flexion of the extremities; any hyperextension of the neck, including overt opisthotonos; the symmetry of the position of the extremities; and the amount, quality, and symmetry of spontaneous movements, including tonic or clonic convulsions. Holding the thumb curled under the flexed fingers is a sign present with many abnormalities of the brain (cerebral thumb). In normal premature infants, continuous athetoid movements are common (such as simultaneous flexion of the elbow and rotation of the upper portion of the arm). Athetoid postures also are common in normal term infants. Tremor with or without crying is seen in many healthy newborns during the first days of life. Spontaneous assumption of the tonic neck position (extension of the ipsilateral extremities after rotation of the head to one side) may occur in normal infants, but an obligatory tonic neck reflex (one that is always present) is abnormal. The face is observed for expression (alert, bland, fussing, crying); symmetry of eye closure after a tap on the glabella (glabella

Scheme for Organization of the Pediatric Neurologic Examination

- Conditions under which the examination is conducted
  - Behavioral state of child
  - Environmental conditions
- Mental status
  - State of consciousness
  - Language—receptive and expressive
  - Cognitive functioning
  - Mood
  - Social and self-awareness
- Station and gait
- Head
  - Skull
  - Cranial nerves I to XII
- Motor
  - Muscle size, symmetry, contractures, tone, and strength
  - Spontaneous activity when prone, supine, sitting, standing, walking, including both fine and gross motor abilities
  - Resistance to passive stretch
  - Coordination
  - Involuntary movements, including fasciculations, tremor, chorea, athetosis, dystonia, and myotonic jerks
- Sensory
- Reflexes
  - Neonatal
  - Deep tendon reflexes, including plantar response
  - Abdominal, cremasteric, and anal reflexes
  - Clonus
- Autonomic nervous system
  - Cardiac and respiratory rate, bladder functioning, temperature control

DEKABAN	MILANI-COMPARETTI	ILLINGWORTH	ST. ANNE-DARGASSIES	PAINE ET AL.
End 1st yr				
End 1st yr				
3-4 mo	3½ mo		3 mo	After 2 mo
	9 mo		12 mo	After 2 mo
		6 mo		
3-6 mo	4 mo	4 mo		1-6 mo
8 mo*→3-5 yr†				1-10 mo*
3-6 mo	4 mo	6 mo		1-5 mo
2-6 mo			3-6 mo	Early months
				1 yr
1 yr				1 yr
1-2 mo		2 mo	3-6 mo	1-9 mo
10 mo*-28 mo†			3 mo*→7 mo†	1-2 mo*→7 mo†
6 mo*	4 mo*		7-9 mo*	7-12 mo*
	6 mo*		7-9 mo*	

reflex); and symmetry of position and movement of the eyes, including presence of symmetry and pupillary constriction and blinking of the eyelids in response to a hand clap approximately 12 inches from the infant's face.

With the baby now undressed, resistance to passive stretch is tested in the extremities, trunk, and neck, noting particularly any symmetric and asymmetric increase or decrease. Many infants in whom spasticity develops later are hypotonic during the neonatal period. Symmetry of the biceps, patellar, superficial abdominal, cremasteric, and anal reflexes is noted, and an attempt is made to elicit ankle clonus, recording the number of beats obtained. The palmar and plantar grasps are tested (Fig. 7-40) for differences of intensity between the two sides (unilaterally decreased in Erb palsy, for instance) or bilateral absence, as with cord lesions. As Fig. 7-40 shows, it is important to press the infant's palm from the ulnar side, with the infant's head in the midline position. The Babinski reflex (with a flexor response and fanning of the toes) expected in normal newborns is tested for symmetry, as is the withdrawal reflex of the lower extremities.

The rooting response is elicited while the baby's hands are held against the chest (Fig. 7-41). In addition to the response shown, with stimulation of the upper lip, the mouth is opened and the head is retroflexed; with stimulation of the lower lip, the mouth opens and the jaw drops. This reflex is absent in depressed infants: the sucking response to the examiner's fingers placed into the infant's mouth is decreased in strength, frequency of sucks, and duration.

In the traction response test (Fig. 7-42) the supine infant is pulled into a sitting position, and the examiner notes the degree of resistance to extension of the arms at the elbow and the degree to which the head is held in the upright position. In the normal term infant some degree of flexion of the elbow is maintained, and head control is relatively weak, with neither head flexors nor extensors predominating.

The Moro response is a critically important sign of an intact nervous system, particularly during the neonatal period. It is best elicited, as shown in Fig. 7-43, by supporting the infant's body in one hand, then suddenly allowing the head to drop a few centimeters with the other hand during a moment when the head is in the midline position and the neck muscles are relaxed. A complete Moro response consists of symmetric abduction of the upper extremity at the shoulder, extension of the forearm at the elbow, and extension of the fingers, all followed by abduction of the arm at the shoulder. The Moro response also can be elicited by holding the baby supine and then suddenly lowering the entire body about 12 inches and by producing a sudden loud noise.

The infant in the prone position is observed for spontaneous head movements (brief lifting or turning from side to side), spontaneous crawling movements, and the incurvation, or Galant, reflex (lateral curvation of the trunk after stimulation with a finger or pin along a paravertebral line from the shoulder to the buttocks about 3 cm from the midline). The infant is then held in the air in the prone position with the examiner's hands around the chest. The normal newborn is somewhat flaccid during this maneuver, but the hypertonic or opisthotonic baby will show varying degrees of lifting of the head and extension of the lower extremities. With the infant still upright, the placing and stepping responses are noted. In the placing response the dorsum of one foot is allowed to brush against the undersurface of a tabletop edge and is followed normally by simultaneous flexion of the knees and hips and placement of the stimulated foot on the table. In the stepping response the soles of the feet are allowed to touch the surface of the table, which elicits alternating stepping movements with both legs.

Throughout the neurologic examination the quality and

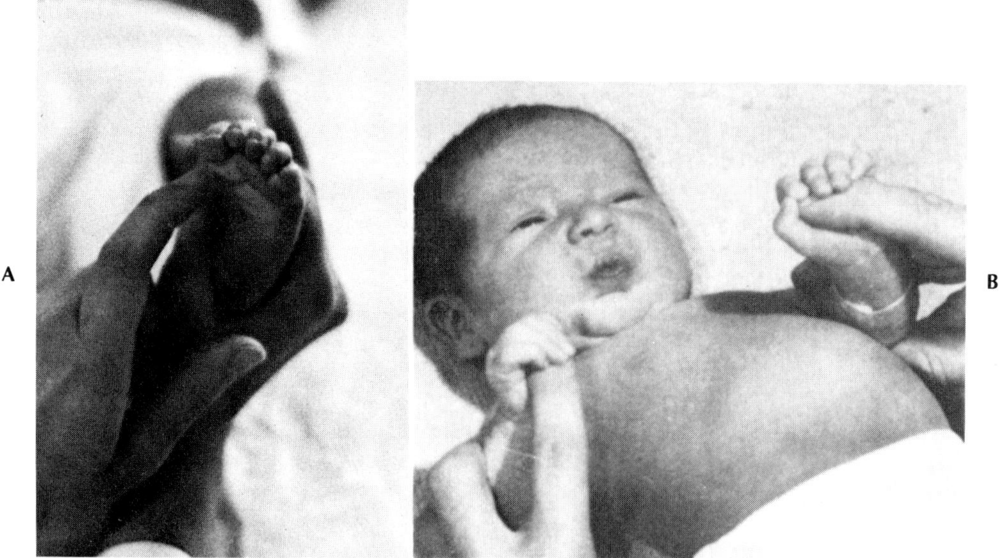

Fig. 7-40 A, Plantar grasp. **B,** Palmar grasp.

A from Whaley LF and Wong DL: Nursing care of infants and children, ed 4, St Louis, 1991, The CV Mosby Co; **B** from Prechtl, HFR: The neurological examination of the full-term newborn infant, ed 2, London, 1977, S.I.M.P. with Heinemann Medical; Philadelphia, Lippincott.

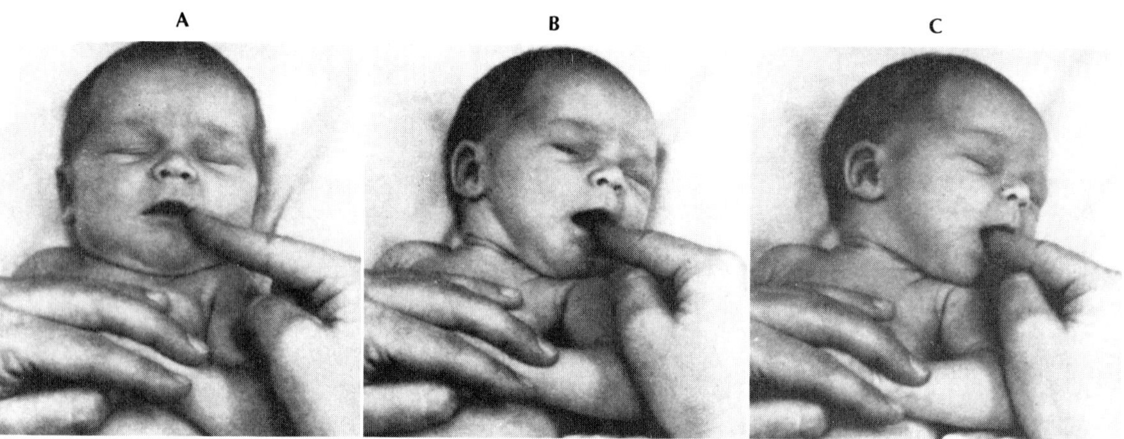

Fig. 7-41 Rooting response. **A,** Stimulation. **B,** Head turning. **C,** Grasping with the mouth.

From Prechtl HFR: The neurological examination of the full-term newborn infant, ed 2, London, 1977, S.I.M.P. with Heinemann Medical; Philadelphia, Lippincott.

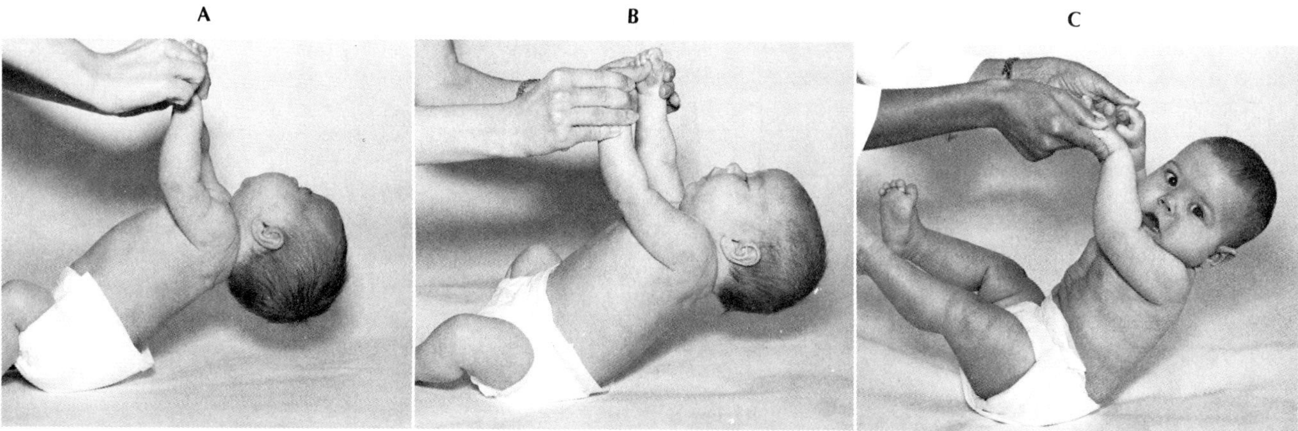

Fig. 7-42 Sitting development. **A,** First 4 weeks or so—complete head lag when being pulled into sitting position. **B,** About 2 months—considerable head lag when being pulled into sitting position, but lag is not complete. **C,** Four months—no head lag when being pulled into sitting position.

From Whaley LF and Wong DL: Nursing care of infants and children, ed 2, St Louis, 1983, The CV Mosby Co.

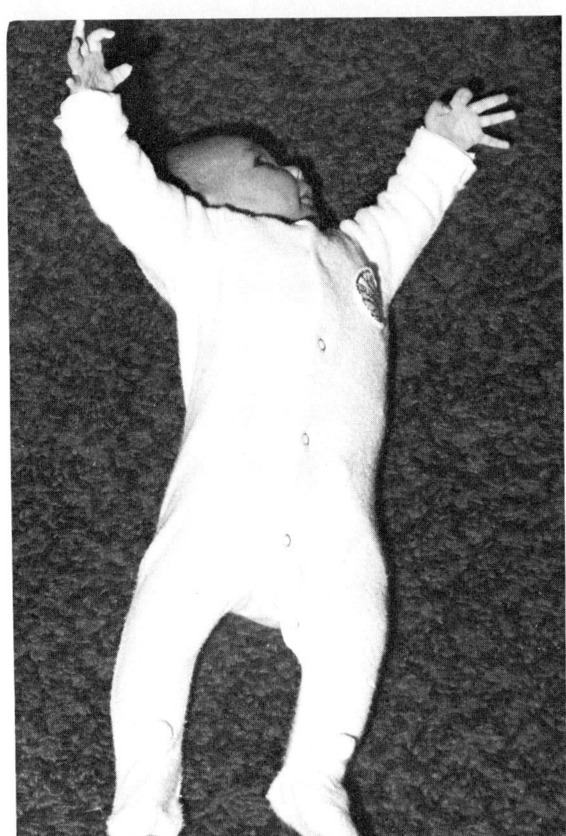

Fig. 7-43 Moro response.

From Whaley LF and Wong DL: Nursing care of infants and children, ed 4, St Louis, 1991, The CV Mosby Co.

duration of the infant's cry are noted, and the high-pitched, excessive, or weak cries that can accompany brain lesions are listened for. Completion of cranial nerve testing is accomplished by testing the corneal and jaw jerk reflexes (fifth cranial nerve); the response during rotation of the upright infant's eyes to turning in the same direction the infant is moved (vestibular eighth cranial nerve); the gag reflex, symmetric elevation of the palate and swallowing movements (ninth and tenth cranial nerves); and by observing for torticollis (eleventh cranial nerve) and the symmetry of the tongue, including observation for fasciculations (twelfth cranial nerve).

The results of all these maneuvers occasionally indicate a localized brain lesion such as hemiparesis secondary to intracranial bleeding. More often, however, the general state of the infant's nervous system will be determined to be normal, hyperexcitable, apathetic, or comatose. The physician must then decide what further diagnostic tests are indicated and on the frequency of follow-up examinations.

As the infant matures, many of the neonatal reflexes disappear (see Table 7-5). Persistence of neonatal reflexes beyond these age-appropriate norms usually indicates nervous system abnormality. Some of the techniques for examining neonates are continued during the first year to ascertain further development of strength and coordination. For instance, the normal 3-month-old infant no longer demonstrates head lag when pulled to a sitting position; the 5-month-old infant lifts the head from the supine position when about to be pulled up; and sitting without support takes place between 5 and 8 months of age. Walking without support occurs normally between 12 and 18 months. The development of hand coordination is important to monitor. The normal infant can reach and grasp objects by 5 months of age, transfer objects from hand to hand by 7 months, and pick up a raisin using a pincer grasp by 10 months (Fig. 7-44). Beyond 8 months the normal infant demonstrates symmetric parachute and lateral propping reactions. The parachute reflex occurs after a flinging motion toward the examination table of the ventrally suspended infant, eliciting an extension of the arms. In the lateral propping reaction the sitting infant is pushed to one side, the arms extended to prevent falling. During these maneuvers the examiner looks for asymmetric movement.

Early and Late Childhood. Further growth of the infant and child's nervous system is monitored by observing walking, the development of speech and language abilities, inter-

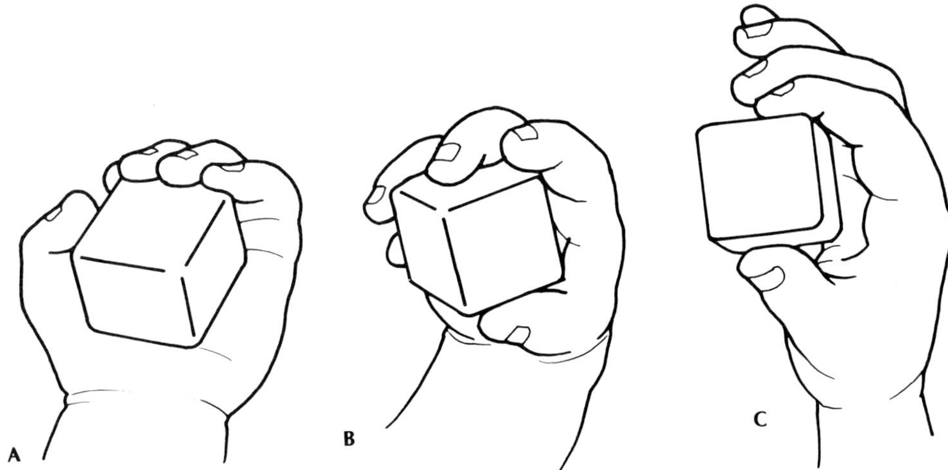

Fig. 7-44 Manipulation. **A,** Six months—immature palmar grasp of a cube. **B,** Eight months—grasp at the intermediate stage. **C,** One year—mature grasp of a cube.

action with parents, and abilities to manipulate small objects, use pencils and crayons, climb and run, throw and catch a ball, and follow simple directions. Muscle strength in the lower extremities is best tested by observing gait, heel and toe walking, standing and hopping on one leg, and the ability to rise from the floor from a supine position. Coordination can be observed in all these maneuvers, as well as in heel-to-shin, finger-to-nose pointing, and tandem walking. In the child with delayed development or a history of school failure, further tests of neurophysiologic maturation, as described in Chapter 18, Eleven, Developmental Assessment, can aid in defining both abilities and areas needing special teaching methods.

As with infants, the neurologic examination of school-age children with nervous system abnormalities usually defines some degree of maturational delay. The presence of localizing neurologic signs is less common, occurring in children most often as a result of traumatic intracranial bleeding and brain tumors and after central nervous system infection.

Adolescence. Although reading ability and comprehension, improved coordination, and increased strength can all be used to monitor further neuromuscular maturation in adolescents, the neurologic examination in this age group is similar to the adult examination. While evaluating the mental status, the examiner should anticipate the variable mood swings, confused thinking, and resistance to authority of many normal adolescents.

REFERENCES

1. Amiel-Tison C: A method for neurological evaluation within the first year of life, Curr Probl Pediatr 8(1):1976.
2. Chadwick DL et al: Color atlas of child sexual abuse, Chicago, 1989, Year Book Medical Publishers, Inc.
3. Herman-Giddens ME and Frothingham TE: Prepubertal female genitalia: examination for evidence of sexual abuse, Pediatrics 80(2):1987.
4. Klaus MH and Kennell JH: Bonding: the beginnings of parent-infant attachment, St Louis, 1983, The CV Mosby Co.
5. Prechtl H and Beintema D: The neurological examination of the full term new born infant, London, 1964, Heinemann.
6. Touwen BCL and Prechtl H: The neurological examination of the child with minor nervous dysfunction, London, 1970, Heinemann.

SUGGESTED READINGS

American Academy of Pediatrics, Joint Committee on Infant Hearing: Position statement 1982, Pediatrics 70:496, 1982.

Davis JA and Dobbing J: Scientific foundations of paediatrics, ed 2, Baltimore, Md, 1981, University Park Press.

Ferguson AB: Orthopaedic surgery in infancy and childhood, ed 4, Baltimore, 1975, Williams & Wilkins.

Gammon JA: Visual system screening in infants and young children, Pediatr Rev 4:71, 1982.

Hoekelman RA: The pediatric physical examination and history taking. In Bates B, editor: A guide to physical examination, ed 5, Philadelphia, 1986, JB Lippincott Co.

James JIP: Scoliosis, Edinburgh, 1976, E & S Livingstone.

Lowrey GH: Growth and development of children, ed 8, Chicago, 1986, Year Book Medical Publishers, Inc.

Lynch A: Use of health history in upgrading school health care. Paper presented at the annual meeting of the New Orleans American Public Health Association, 1974.

McDowell F and Wolff HG: Handbook of neurological diagnostic methods, Baltimore, 1960, Williams & Wilkins.

Nadas AS and Fyler DC: Pediatric cardiology, ed 3, Philadelphia, 1972, WB Saunders Co.

Smith TF, O'Day D, and Wright PF: Clinical implications of preseptal (periorbital) cellulitis in childhood, Pediatrics 62:1006, 1978.

Stanisavljevic S: Diagnosis and treatment of congenital hip pathology in the newborn, Baltimore, 1964, Williams & Wilkins.

Wilkin L: The diagnosis and treatment of endocrine disorders in childhood and adolescence, ed 3, Springfield, Ill, 1965, Charles C Thomas, Publisher.

8

Structural and Functional Analysis of Body Systems

Nicholas M. Nelson

The essential task of the physician, perhaps more than the surgeon, is that of problem delineation. To be sure, the medical practitioner is involved in the solution of problems, once defined, but these solutions tend to emphasize the enhancement of normal and the suppression of abnormal physiologic responses, often by pharmacologic means, rather than by the surgeon's direct attack upon an anatomic structure that has been altered by disease or development.

The symptoms of which the patient complains and the signs that the physician elicits serve to suggest involvement of one or more organ systems, so that the patient's history and physical examination may be viewed as what applied mathematicians and statisticians call *exploratory data analysis*. It is in this earliest phase of clinical problem-solving that the physician assembles the differential diagnosis, then orders that list in descending likelihood, based on his or her knowledge of the epidemiology and, particularly, the natural history of the diseases in question.

This chapter is concerned with a succeeding phase of clinical investigation—the work-up, or *confirmatory data analysis*, wherein the physician's suspicions, intuitions, and knowledge of the location and extent of the patient's condition are confirmed or denied. Of course, many of the problems encountered in primary care are self-evident or otherwise sufficiently familiar as not to require investigation beyond the history or physical examination; yet no primary care practitioner is likely to see very many patients without recourse to the clinical laboratory and radiologic or other consultative support of his or her effort to define the patient's problem. During this effort the practitioner must increasingly bear in mind the cost-benefit ratio of the investigations proposed—"cost" to include not only the fiscal but also the morbid and even mortal risks of the procedures under consideration, as constantly displayed against the benefits likely to be returned in the form of useful or definitive diagnostic information. A sequence of investigations should be planned that is pertinent to the organ system or systems whose involvement has been suggested by the exploratory analysis of the clinical data gathered and that is coordinated with the current differential diagnosis. This list should begin with those procedures that are inexpensive, noninvasive, and of high sensitivity to many diseases ("coarse focus") but of low specificity for any single disease ("fine focus").

Table 8-1 *Assessment of Growth*

EXAMINATION	
BASIC	SPECIALIZED
General	
Growth charts	Cell size (RNA)
Cross-sectional	Cell number (DNA)
Premature infant	
Lubchenko, Usher (weight, length, head)[2,5,10]	
Infant and child	
NCHS (weight, length, head)[7]	
Nellhaus (head)[8]	
Longitudinal	
Premature infant	
Bellevue (weight)[3]	
Babson, Marks (weight, length, head)[1,6]	
Infant and child	
Tanner (weight, length)[9]	
Chemical	
Alkaline phosphatase	N_2-balance
	K-balance
Bone age—hand, wrist, and:	
Knee (newborn)	
Body fat	
Skinfold thickness	Underwater weight
Harpenden calipers	Total body water
	40_k distribution

GENERAL ASSESSMENT

The quintessence of pediatrics, in contrast to other clinical disciplines, is its constant concern with change over time, with the growth and development of its patients. The child seriously involved with disease usually announces the intensity of that involvement by primary or secondary disruptions of somatic growth and psychomotor development, almost regardless of precise etiology. These aspects are treated in much greater depth elsewhere in this volume, but Tables 8-1 and 8-2 set out some of the more important benchmarks against which the pediatrician measures the patient's progress in these areas.

The Lubchenko, Bellevue, and Babson charts help the neonatologist assess the growth of premature infants, just as the National Center for Health Statistics charts (which have largely displaced the older "Harvard" or "Iowa" or

Table 8-2 *Developmental Assessment*

	SOCIAL ADAPTATION	LANGUAGE	COGNITION AND INTELLECT	PERCEPTION AND MOTOR	EMOTION AND PROJECTIVE	ACADEMIC ACHIEVEMENT
Screening tests						
Premature[4]						
Dubowitz				X		
Infant						
Brazelton	X			X		
Child						
Denver	X	X	X	X		
Portage	X	X	X	X		
Slosson		X	X	X		
Peabody		X	X			
Goodenough			X	X	X	
School		X	X			X
Psychometric tests						
Infant						
Cattell	X	X	X	X		
Bayley	X	X	X	X		
Child	Alpern-Boll	Illinois	Stanford-Binet	Bender-Gestalt	Rorschach	Woodcock Johnson
			WISC-R	SCSIT	Thematic Apperception	
				Frostig		

Brazelton, Neonatal Behavioral Assessment Scale
Denver, Denver Developmental Screening Test
Portage, Portage Project Checklist
Slosson, Slosson Intelligence Test
Peabody, Peabody Picture Vocabulary Test
Goodenough, Goodenough-Harris ("Draw-a-Man") Test
School, School Readiness Survey
Cattell, Cattell Infant Intelligence Scale
Bayley, Bayley Scales of Infant Development
Alpern-Boll, Alpern-Boll Developmental Test
Illinois, Illinois Test of Psycholinguistic Abilities
WISC-R, Wechsler Intelligence Scale for Children-Revised
SCSIT, Southern California Sensory Integration Tests
Frostig, Frostig Developmental Test of Visual Perception
(See also Chapter 18, part II, "Developmental Assessment" and Appendix D.)

"Wetzel grid" standards of an earlier era) serve those who are concerned with the growth of children from term birth through adolescence. The Dubowitz examination inverts the usual approach to developmental assessment by using established age norms of physical and neuromotor characteristics to estimate gestational age; it assumes that the child being assessed is normally developed for his or her gestational age (which is to be estimated), in contrast to the more typical process of referring the assessed stage of growth and development to the child's (known) age.

The available tools for developmental assessment of the young infant necessarily emphasize motor over cognitive phenomena, and many feel that cognition is best estimated by the adaptive and language components of the various screening instruments. The alleged cultural "loading" of most of the formal psychometric estimators of intelligence (Table 8-2) has brought them under political and scientific critical fire—yet, whatever their "fairness," their position as reliable predictors of school performance has not been challenged.

The screening tests noted in Table 8-2 are sufficiently simple and brief to administer, after reasonable practice, as to merit consideration for inclusion in a primary care practice, either as a routine assessment or as a preliminary to formal psychometric testing upon symptomatic indication.

ORGAN IMAGING

The past two decades have witnessed such rapid and fundamental changes in organ imaging, as scintigraphic, sonographic, magnetic, and computer technologies have intermarried with that of radiation, that some departments of radiology have seriously considered changing their names to departments of "medical imaging." In some areas the field is also shifting from one in which the technician occupies the major portion of the patient's experience to one in which the radiologist (imagist?) dominates, especially in the techniques of angiointervention and ultrasound.

Throughout the development of the field, the goals of optimum resolution of the tissue of interest and its optimum differentiation from neighboring tissues of noninterest have come in constant conflict with the restraints of cumulative radiation dosage and the desire to minimize invasiveness. Great strides have recently been made in diminishing risk while increasing definition, but at such an increase in cost of the technology as to raise serious question regarding the relative contribution of these techniques toward establishing and maintaining the public health. Before dismissing technologic advance in medicine on grounds of cost alone, however, physicians, if not politicians, might well reflect upon the "costs" of the modern computed tomographic or magnetic resonance documentation of a posterior fossa tumor in a 4-year-old (and in 40 minutes!) versus the "lesser costs" of an obsolete evaluation extracted through the pain and risk of a pneumonencephalogram, a ventriculogram, or cerebral angiography (with luck, in 5 days!).

Table 8-3 offers a survey of current imaging techniques and their ability to contribute to our understanding of the patient.

Table 8-3 *Imaging Techniques**

MODALITY	USEFULNESS FOR DELINEATION OF STATIC STRUCTURE	DYNAMIC MOTION	METABOLIC FUNCTION	IMAGING CRITERION
Ultrasound	++	+++	0	Acoustic impedance
Magnetic resonance imaging (MRI)				
Hydrogen	++	+	0	Water content
Phosphorus	+	0	++	Energy metabolism
Radionuclide	+	+	++	Gamma emission
Positron emission tomography (PET)	+	0	++	Positron emission (metabolic activity)
Roentgenography				
Standard roentgenogram	+++	0	0	Roentgen ray density
Computed tomography (CT)	++	+	0	(enhanced spectrum)
Angiography				
Standard	+++	0	0	
Cine/video	++	+++	0	
Digital subtraction	++	0	0	(reduced background)
Fluoroscopy	++	+++	0	

*In approximate ascending order of energizing radiation sustained by the patient.

Roentgenography

Still the "gold standard" against which to measure the resolving power of any imaging technique, classic roentgenography has nevertheless rarely been able to differentiate the soft tissues of interest within a body region unless abetted by natural (air) or artificial (barium, iodine, or other radiopaque compound) increases in contrast. This is because the transmission of roentgen rays through body tissues is a function of their radioabsorption—mineral and bone being the most opaque, water and air being the least. Water, blood, and muscle are, unfortunately, so similar in radiopacity as to render most difficult the precise appreciation of anything more than gross organ dimension within the abdomen, for instance. Angiography, urography, bronchography, and other techniques for instilling contrast agents are very valuable, but all require some level of invasiveness, and many require local or general anesthesia. Moreover, the contrast agents themselves are not benign—for example, they may produce anaphylaxis or hemiplegia after cerebral angiography or myocardial ischemia after coronary angiography. Digital subtraction techniques in venous or arterial angiography can improve differentiation from confusing background structures and even diminish the dose of contrast agent required, but not the necessity for invading the vascular tree.

Radionuclide Imaging

One of the happier aspects of the nuclear age has been the discovery or development of a vast array of radioactive and nonradioactive isotopic tracer elements without which most of modern biochemistry and even archaeology and paleontology could not have proceeded. Nuclear medicine has emphasized the attachment of a radioactive label with requisite physical characteristics to a biologically active carrier molecule, which is concentrated by natural body processes into the area or organ of interest, there to emit gamma radiation, which is then recorded, typically by a scintillation camera. This concentration in normal tissues means that diseased areas are usually revealed as silent areas of absent radioactivity, because of loss of microvasculature and replacement of normal tissue. Occasionally, areas of abnormal increases in blood flow are displayed by inflamed tissues or tumors.

Because these synthetic radiopharmaceuticals reside and radiate within the body, they must either have a short half-life ($t_{1/2}$) for radiation or be rapidly excreted, or both. On the other hand, the $t_{1/2}$ must be long enough to allow for transport from the site of preparation to that of instillation into the patient. Technetium (Tc) is an element that naturally (without carrier) concentrates especially well in the choroid plexus, the salivary and thyroid glands, and the stomach, but the basic reasons for its prominence as a label in Table 8-4 are its relative ease of preparation, its $t_{1/2}$ of 6 hours, and gamma emission at energy levels (140 Kv) that prevent absorption by the body (up to 20 Kv), yet are below those levels (above 600 Kv) where radiation scatter becomes so gross as to render organ delineation hopeless. Indeed, the poor resolving power of most radionuclide techniques has in many instances led to their gradual displacement by equally noninvasive ultrasound or computed tomography (CT), wherever the issue has been only that of delineating organ structure.

The carrier molecules for certain radionuclide techniques, however, are specific examiners of an organ's function (e.g., ^{99m}Tc DTPA in the assessment of glomerular filtration, or ^{99m}Tc sulfur colloid, which is phagocytosed by Kuppfer cells) and can therefore challenge nuclear magnetic resonance imaging (MRI) and positron emission tomography (PET) on the grounds of informed functional analysis of certain organs. Few sights, for instance, are more rewarding to the pediatric surgeon, faced with a child who has massive rectal bleeding, than a positive "Meckel diverticulum scan," where the pertechnetate label has concentrated in the parietal cells of ectopic gastric tissue and thus narrowed the surgeon's otherwise unguided search throughout the intestine for an attackable bleeding site.

Table 8-4 *Radionuclide Scans*

ORGAN	LABEL	CARRIER	CONCENTRATION MECHANISM
Liver	^{99m}Tc	Sulfur colloid	Phagocytosis (Kuppfer cells)
	^{131}I	Rose bengal	Active transport (biliary polygonal cells)
	^{99m}Tc	HIDA	Active transport (extrahepatic cells)
	^{99m}Tc	PIPIDA	Active transport (biliary cells)
Kidneys	$^{99m}TcO_4$	None	Flow diffusion
	^{99m}Tc	DTPA	Active transport (glomerulus)
	^{125}I	Thalamate	Active transport (glomerulus)
	^{131}I	Hippuran	Active transport (tubule)
Lungs	^{133}Xe	None	Active transport (alveolar gas)
	^{99m}Tc	HSA (macroaggregated)	Capillary blockade
Heart	$^{99m}TcO_4$	None	Flow diffusion
Blood pool	^{99m}Tc	HSA	Compartmentation
	^{99m}Tc	RBC	Compartmentation
Spleen	^{99m}Tc	Sulfur colloid	Phagocytosis (Kuppfer cells)
RE system	^{99m}Tc	RBC	Sequestration
Gut	$^{99m}TcO_4$	None	Active transport (parietal cells)
Abscess, tumor	^{67}Gallium	None	? Transport (inflammatory cells)
			? Diffusion (tumor cells)
Bone	^{99m}Tc	Diphosphonate	Active transport
Thyroid	$^{99m}TcO_4$	None	Flow diffusion
	^{131}I	None	Active transport (thyroid cells)
Adrenal	^{131}I	Cholesterol	Active transport (cortical cells)
	^{125}I		
CSF	^{99m}Tc	HSA	Compartmentation
Brain	$^{99m}TcO_4$	None	Active transport (choroid plexus)

Abbreviations: HIDA, hepatoimidodiacetic acid; PIPIDA, paraisopropylimidodiacetic acid; DTPA, diethylenetriamine pentaacetic acid; HSA, human serum albumin; RBC, red blood cells; RE, reticuloendothelial; CSF, cerebrospinal fluid

Ultrasonography

The precocious infancy of this technology is just now maturing into an adolescence in which it has already become the fundamental means for assessment of fetal growth and development, as well as for neonatal and infant intracranial examination, not to mention its earlier and continuing contributions in cardiology (echocardiography) and in the examination of the abdominal viscera. Although to the untrained eye the current interpretation of ultrasonic scans may seem to approach the mystic, image quality is nonetheless vastly superior to that of radionuclide imaging. There is no ionizing radiation, and the sound energy levels used are as yet believed to be far below the threshold for tissue damage.

The critical factor for tissue differentiation is acoustic impedance (analogous to radiodensity), but the range of values displayed by various tissues is much wider than that for radiation. Hence blood or water in the ultrasonogram (in contrast to the unenhanced roentgenogram) is easily distinguished from connective tissue and muscle; on this fact rests modern echocardiography. Bone, however, is near totally opaque to ultrasound, so that the cranial and thoracic contents can only be examined through the sonic "windows" offered by the open anterior fontanelle, an intercostal space, the subxiphoid region, or the suprasternal notch.

M (for motion) -mode ultrasonography, videorecorded in "real time," and two-dimensional "sector scanning" (B-mode) form the sonic dynamic equivalents of classic fluoroscopy or cineangiography. That is, the motions of the heart and its valves, the fetus, or the lungs can be viewed, reviewed, and analyzed, often by the same analytic formulae originally developed and substantiated through the more invasive techniques of angiography.

To the advantages of relative safety, high image quality, and the dynamic, as well as static, recording afforded by ultrasonography can be added the highest degree of portability of all the imaging techniques—the equipment is easily brought to the bedside on vehicles substantially smaller and lighter than the usual "portable" roentgenography machine. However, imaging still requires a high degree of patience, experience, and artistry on the part of the examiner wielding the sonic transducer, so that interpretability of recordings is much more in direct proportion to the expertise of the physician or technician at the bedside than is the case in, say, roentgenography.

Computed Tomography (CT)

Computed tomography is derived from the earlier methods of plain tomography, wherein either the roentgen ray tube or the film cassette (or both) are rotated during exposure so as to blur all tissues except those at the axis of rotation. With CT, a computer enhancement of the digitally analyzed "grey scale" of received roentgen ray transmission vastly widens the scale of appreciable radiodensity differences among tissues beyond that of the "mineral-bone-water-air scale" of classic roentgenography. The body is thus viewable as a sequence of axial planar "cuts," reminiscent of the frozen whole-body sections of gross anatomy. However, the technique is relatively slow to complete a "cut," usually requires

Table 8-5 *Heart and Circulation*

	EXAMINATION	
	BASIC	SPECIALIZED
Structure	Chest roentgenogram Fluorography	Radionuclide scan Echocardiogram Angiography
Function		
Hemodynamics Preload Contractility Afterload Distribution of flow	Auscultation Sphygmomanometry Electrocardiogram Oximetry Blood gases	Phonocardiogram Vectorcardiogram Echocardiogram Radionuclide scan Cardiac catheterization Thermodilution Dye dilution Venography
Microcirculation	Exercise test Maximum O_2 consumption	

contrast enhancement, and is distinctly static, quite expensive, and most certainly nonportable. Nonetheless it has revolutionized clinical neurology and has essentially destroyed the need for pneumoencephalography and ventriculography, while relegating cerebral angiography to the status of a strictly preoperative procedure.

Positron Emission Tomography (PET)

Related to CT scanning in that tomography is used to produce a tissue "slice," PET scans view the positrons emitted by appropriately excited body tissues, rather than roentgen rays. If the excitation is produced by isotopes of metabolically active molecules and compounds (e.g., oxygen, glucose), it then becomes possible to examine sites of metabolic activity (and blood flow to them). The concept is similar to, but much more rapidly and accurately defined than, radionuclide scans. However, the equipment is vastly expensive, totally nonportable, and must be tied rather closely in geographic proximity to the cyclotron or other heavy nuclear gear that must produce the short-lived isotopes for its examination. PET scanning is thus currently much more a research tool than a practical one for clinical management.

Magnetic Resonance Imaging (MRI)

MRI is the newest and in some ways the most promising (but hardly the least expensive) imaging technique for general future usefulness. It is just now beginning to blossom and assume its place in the diagnostic imaging armamentarium. It also is noninvasive (and nonportable) and is based on the phenomenon of the magnetic resonance of uniform spin, induced in the atomic particles of all tissues placed in a strong magnetic field and then struck by a radiofrequency pulse delivered at the natural vibrational frequency of the atom in question (e.g., hydrogen). As the imposed radiofrequency pulse subsides, the atomic particles "relax" into their natural random spin orientation and emit a recordable electromagnetic pulse whose density scale is a function of the density of that atom in the tissue so bombarded.

If the imposed radiofrequency pulse is "tuned" (like a radio or TV receiver) to resonate in hydrogen nuclei (protons), then the emitted electromagnetic pulse reflects the varying water (i.e., hydrogen proton) content of those tissues. If, on the other hand, the pulse is tuned to the phosphorus atom, intimately involved in most of the body's energy-transforming biochemical reactions, then the recorded image (as in PET scanning) tends to reflect metabolic activity within the tissues examined. Although the image quality of MRI hydrogen scanning already compares favorably with or exceeds that of CT and PET scanning, it is as yet too early to specify whether the promise of bloodless biochemical biopsy through MRI (phosphorus or other atom) can be realized in practical terms.

SYSTEMIC EVALUATION

The assessment of structure and function of the organ systems within the body involves both biochemical and biophysical means for tracing the effectiveness with which an organ performs its tasks. Disruptions of gross structure need not impair function (e.g., hepatic metastases), and disruptions of function need not impair gross structure (e.g., renal tubular acidosis); thus evaluation of both is often necessary to rule out disease, especially in those organs that have multiple functions, such as the liver and kidneys.

The functional evaluation of the heart and circulation, the respiratory tract, the neuromotor system, the skin, the eyes, and the ears is largely accomplished by the physician during the physical examination. In contrast, physiologic assessment of the hematopoietic, immune, and endocrine systems, the kidneys and the urinary tract, as well as the liver and intestinal tract, depends heavily on laboratory tests. In all, however, a careful medical history designed to test, by system-oriented symptomatic questioning, the presence or absence of normal organ function should direct the exploration of the patient's problem and contribute most to its solution.

Heart and Circulation

Appropriate indicators for investigation of this system (Table 8-5) may range from a presumably innocent cardiac murmur to cyanosis and frank heart failure. The increasing sophisti-

Table 8-6 *Lungs and Respiratory Tract*

	EXAMINATION	
	BASIC	SPECIALIZED
Structure		
Overall	Chest roentgenogram Fluoroscopy Sinus roentgenograms Barium swallow Sputum Analysis Culture	Nasopharyngoscopy Bronchoscopy Laryngoscopy
Lung volumes	Spirometry Pneumotachometry Tomograms	Gas dilution (N_2, H_2) Body plethysmography Bronchography Angiography Puncture Biopsy
Function		
Ventilation	Spirometry Flow rates	Gas washout (N_2, H_2) Flow-volume loops Occluded breath-mouth pressure Radionuclide scan Body plethysmography
Perfusion		Radionuclide scan Gas absorption (N_2O, acetylene)
Diffusion		Diffusing capacity (CO,O_2)
Gas exchange	Oximetry Transcutaneous blood gases Arterial blood gases	Alveolar-arterial (O_2,CO_2,N_2) gas gradients
Mechanics		Body plethysmography Compliance Resistance
Stress	Exercise Cold air breathing	

cation of echocardiography has served to place formal catheterization largely in the category of a preoperative and postoperative procedure in which accurate measurement of chamber pressures and pulmonary and systemic flow ratios may be demanded. Phonocardiograms and vectorcardiograms are used mostly in confirmation of clinical auscultation and scalar electrocardiography, respectively.

The hemodynamic stress placed on the heart by excessive venous return (preload) or excessive outflow resistance (afterload) tends to produce dilation or hypertrophy, respectively, of the chamber so loaded. Preload may be estimated clinically by measurement of venous pressure, detection of "flow" murmurs, roentgenographic assessment of pulmonary vasculature and the like, whereas the more difficult judgment of afterload depends on the site or sites of vascular resistance—at the outflow tract (stenotic semilunar valves), in the great vessels (coarctation), or at the level of the resistance vessels themselves (diastolic hypertension). A sense of chamber wall thickness may be derived from chest fluoroscopy or roentgenography, and electrocardiography-vectorcardiography may reflect (in the amplitude of QRS deflections) the relative ventricular thicknesses; but the echocardiogram has become the modern gold standard for measurement of chamber diameters and wall and valve dimensions. Moreover, cardiovascular shunts may be traced during the echocardiogram by simple saline injections or (color) Doppler echocardiography, whereas chamber hemodynamics (ejection fraction, circumferential shortening velocity, systolic time intervals) may be accurately and repeatedly measured as clinical indices of myocardial contractility.

The invasive procedures (cardiac catheterization, angiography, venography) are generally reserved for those situations requiring precise anatomic detail in anticipation or documentation of surgical repair.

Lungs and Respiratory Tract

The patient with symptoms referable to the respiratory tract (e.g., cough, hyperpnea) may be suffering from more global disease (allergy, diabetic ketoacidosis), but those children with signs of impending or actual respiratory failure (dyspnea, cyanosis) usually are found to have significant disruption of lung tissue, most often the airways.

The overall aim and usual result of pulmonary function testing (Table 8-6) is the classification of the child's problem as either "obstructive" or "restrictive." Obstructive disease of the airways (asthma or other bronchospastic disease, cystic fibrosis) slows flow rates and alters gaseous outflow curves and flow-volume loops, often producing secondary increases in residual lung volume and functional residual capacity. Restrictive lung disease (pneumonia, hyaline membrane disease, neurologic disease, or other conditions that impair the thoracic "bellows") encompasses those processes that restrict or replace alveolar volume and ventilation.

Unfortunately, most of the apparatus and maneuvers developed to assess pulmonary function require a level of un-

Table 8-7 *Kidneys and Urinary Tract*

	EXAMINATION	
	BASIC	SPECIALIZED
Structure	Ultrasound Intravenous urography CT scan ^{99m}Tc DTPA scan	^{131}I hippuran scan Angiography Retrograde cystourethrography Cystoscopy Biopsy
Function		
Urinary tract	Urinalysis	Voiding cystourethrogram Cystometrics Lasix-stimulated Diethylene Triamine Pentacetic Acid (DTPA) scan
Glomerulus	BUN Creatinine Urine flow Creatinine clearance	^{125}I thalamate scan Inulin clearance
Tubule	Fluid restriction test Phosphate clearance Urine and serum electrolytes	Vasopressin test Para-amino hippurate (PAH) clearance NH_4Cl loading test

derstanding and cooperation on the part of the patient that is beyond the capabilities of most children under about 5 to 7 years of age unless they are swaddled and satiated (i.e., essentially "thalamic") newborn infants. Hence in practical terms the clinical assessment of pulmonary function in most cases reduces to simple flow studies (e.g., Wright peak flowmeter) and estimates of gas exchange (oximetry, transcutaneous, or arterial blood gases).

Kidneys and Urinary Tract

Critical disruption of renal function (Table 8-7) can be notoriously subtle and insidious, evoking no detectable symptoms until far advanced. Hence the cautious physician usually includes a urinalysis and determinations of blood urea nitrogen (BUN) and creatinine in the evaluation of any child whose growth or general health is at all in question, even in the presence of a normal urinalysis. The younger child's announcement of renal disease is often in the form of an abdominal mass (hydronephrosis, Wilms' tumor, cystic disease), delineation of which is the special and spectacular province of the ultrasonogram; indeed, these renal lesions are currently being detected during careful *fetal* ultrasound examination. Hence urography is now only rarely used to assess extrarenal retroperitoneal involvement and is more circumscribed to evaluation of the renal pelvis and ureter per se, complementary to the ultrasound examination and CT scan.

Intestinal Tract

The modes for investigation of the gastrointestinal tract (endoscopy excepted) have changed less in the last generation, perhaps, than those of any other organ system (Table 8-8); the development of flexible fiberoptic instrumentation has placed nearly the entire alimentary canal under direct scrutiny by endoscopic procedures that, if unpleasant and requiring sedation or anesthesia, are nonetheless accurate and repeatable. In contrast to the older child and adult, fundamental gastrointestinal disease in the younger child more frequently involves malformations than chronic inflammation (e.g., enteritis, colitis), despite the prominence of acute gastrointestinal intercurrent infectious illness in any primary pediatric practice.

Liver

Beyond the newborn period, in which hyperbilirubinemia is a daily concern, primary liver disease other than hepatitis is relatively rare among children. However, the liver is frequently yet secondarily involved in multisystemic disease (vascular congestion and obstructions, abscess, storage disease) because of its strategic vascular location and global metabolic activity. The omnipresent, multimembered "liver panels" much beloved by younger house officers often produce information redundant to the usually sufficient items shown in Table 8-9. The assessment of bile flow in the jaundiced but acholic young infant continues to frustrate the pediatrician attempting to distinguish biliary atresia from "neonatal hepatitis" by such fallible means as ^{131}I rose bengal liver excretion or red cell peroxidation (as an index of gastrointestinal bile–assisted vitamin E absorption), but improvements in the safety of direct (endoscopic or transhepatic) cholangiography have served to diminish delay in selecting candidates for hepatic portoenterostomy (Kasai procedure) or, more recently, liver transplantation.

Nervous and Neuromuscular Systems

Perhaps more than in any other organ system, functional assessment of the nervous and neuromuscular systems is principally accomplished during the performance of a careful neurologic examination, especially in the older child, for whom communication is not a barrier. The evaluation of no other system, however, has been as revolutionized by the development of CT and MRI (Table 8-10), which has all but obliterated the need for invasive "air studies" (pneumoencephalography, ventriculography). Moreover, the various evoked response tests have placed the assessment of the visual and auditory apparatus of the young infant on more secure ground than did the traditional bedside maneuvers. Yet true

Table 8-8 *Intestinal Tract*

	EXAMINATION	
	BASIC	SPECIALIZED
Structure	Abdominal plain roentgenogram	Computed tomography
	Flat	
	Upright	Radionuclide scan
	Contrast/fluoroscopy	
	Barium esophagogram	
	Upper GI series	Endoscopy
	Barium enema	Esophagoscopy
	Ultrasound scan	Gastroduodenoscopy
		Cholangiopancreatography
		Colonoscopy
		Biopsy
Function		
Peristalsis	Contrast fluoroscopy	Manometry
Secretion	Gastric pH	Duodenal aspiration
		Enzymes
		Bile
Absorption	Fecal analysis	Hydrogen excretion
	Reducing sugar	
	Fat	^{51}CrCl excretion
	Trypsin	
	α1-Antitrypsin	Mucosal enzymes (biopsy)
	Loading (tolerance) tests	
	Oral glucose	
	D-xylose	
	Serum carotene	

Table 8-9 *Liver*

	EXAMINATION	
	BASIC	SPECIALIZED
Structure	Ultrasound	Computed tomography
	Radionuclide scan	
	^{131}I rose bengal	
	^{99m}Tc PIPIDA	Endoscopy
		Cholangiopancreatography
		Transhepatic/operative cholangiography
		Biopsy
		Splenoportography
Function		
Protein synthesis	Serum albumin	
	Prothrombin time	
	Gamma globulin	Electrophoresis
Biotransformation	SGOT	5′-Nucleotidase
	SGPT	Gamma-glutamyltransferase
		Leucine aminopeptidase
Conjugation	Bilirubin (direct/total)	
Excretion	Alkaline phosphatase	
Bile flow	Duodenal intubation	^{131}I rose bengal
		Red cell peroxidation
		^{99m}Tc IDA
Special		NH_3
		α1-Antitrypsin
		Ceruloplasmin

Abbreviations: PIPIDA, paraisopropylimidodiacetic acid
IDA, imidodiacetic acid
SGOT, serum glutamic-oxaloacetic transaminase
SGPT, serum glutamic-pyruvic transaminase

Table 8-10 *Neuromuscular and Central Nervous Systems*

	EXAMINATION	
	BASIC	SPECIALIZED
Structure	Plain skull roentgenograms Ultrasound	
		CT, MRI scans Radionuclide (^{99m}Tm) scan PET scan Myelography Cerebral angiography Biopsy Muscle Nerve Brain
Function		
Sensory	Neurologic exam	
Vision	Vision testing	VER, ERG, EOG, FPL
Hearing	Perimetry	BAER
Cutaneous	Audiometry	SER
	EEG	
Motor	Neurologic exam	EMG
	EEG	EOG
	CPK	Nerve conduction study
Integrated	Developmental testing	Psychometric evaluation
Global	CSF	Subdural tap
		Ventricular tap

Abbreviations: PET, positron emission tomography; VER, visual evoked responses; ERG, electroretinography; EOG, electrooculogram; FPL, forced preferential looking; BAER, brainstem auditory evoked responses; SER, somatosensory evoked responses; EEG, electroencephalogram; EMG, electromyogram; CPK, creatine phosphokinase; CSF, cerebrospinal fluid

vision and hearing require integrated processing of the signals documented (by evoked potentials, say) as being received and sent along the optic and acoustic nerves, so that the possibility of "cortical" blindness or deafness is still best investigated by the behavioral responses of an alert and cooperative patient.

Eye and Ear

The primary care pediatrician's involvement with these organs is properly limited to first aid and functional screening, despite the prominence of conjunctivitis, and otitis media and externa in any such practice. His or her role, then, is largely that of prevention and limitation of disease by referral of those patients whose response to relatively straightforward treatment of upper respiratory and ocular problems is unsatisfactory. The development of practical impedance tympanometry has served to sharpen the indications for such referral. Tables 8-11 and 8-12 set out some of those procedures by which the ophthalmologist and otolaryngologist seek to define the finer aspects of structure and function. Both disciplines have now developed a number of individuals who confine their practice to children.

Skeleton

Pertinent modalities for assessment of the body's bony support are set out in Table 8-13, the radionuclide scans being particularly valuable in the investigation of infectious or metastatic involvement of bone. Radioimmunoassay procedures have brought measurement of the hormones pertinent to bone metabolism (parathyroid hormone, calcitonin, the vitamin D system) out of the research laboratory and into clinical medicine.

Skin and Appendages

Functional disruptions of cutaneous function are certainly much less frequent causes for presenting complaint than are the itches, rashes, and eruptions that consume much of the pediatrician's day, but such disruptions most often reflect general systemic disease, usually of infectious or iatrogenic origin. The hand lens is perhaps the technologic support most frequently used by the inspecting dermatologist, yet exudates, scrapings, and cuttings occasionally require detailed analysis, as indicated in Table 8-14.

Endocrine System

Confirmatory data analysis in this system is almost exclusively functional in nature and dependent on the radioimmunoassay laboratory (Table 8-15), whether the fluid examined is blood or urine, the latter being viewed as an "integrating averager" of hormone secretion (which in blood often displays diurnal rhythms). To be sure, roentgenographic, ultrasound, angiographic, and radionuclide tech-

Table 8-11 *Eye*

	EXAMINATION	
	BASIC	SPECIALIZED
Structure		
Media	Direct ophthalmoscopy	Indirect ophthalmoscopy
Retina	Fluorescein dye (conjunctivae)	Slitlamp biomicroscopy
		Ophthalmic ultrasound
		Fluorescein angiography
Function		
Intraocular pressure		Indentation (Schiötz) tonometry
		Applanation tonometry (Perkins)
Visual response	Startle reflex	Optokinetic nystagmus
	Fixation	Electrooculogram
		Electroretinogram
		Visual evoked responses
Ocular alignment	Corneal light reflex (Hirschberg's method)	
	Alternate cover tests	
Ocular motility	Conjugate eye movements	
Visual acuity	Snellen charts	Refraction
	Illiterate "E" charts	Retinoscopy
		Forced preferential looking
Visual fields	Confrontation	Perimetry
	Attraction	Scotometry
Color vision	Pseudoisochromatic test (Ishihara test)	Farnsworth-Munsell D-100 color test

Table 8-12 *Ear*

	EXAMINATION	
	BASIC	SPECIALIZED
Structure	Head light and mirror	Microscopic otoscopy
	Pneumatic otoscopy	Computed tomography
	Plain roentgenography	Magnetic resonance imaging
Function		
Hearing	Visual response	BAER*
	Play response	Central auditory processing
	Speech response	Cochleography
	Impedance audiometry	
	Conventional audiometry	
Vestibular	Bárány chair (or equivalent)	Electronystamography
	Caloric stimulation	Posturography
Eustachian tube		Pressure-flow study
Sound conduction	Impedance tympanometry	
	Acoustic reflexes	

*Brainstem auditory evoked responses.

Table 8-13 *Bone*

	EXAMINATION	
	BASIC	SPECIALIZED
Structure	Physical examination	Radionuclide scan
	Plain roentgenograms	^{99m}Tc polyphosphate
	CT scan	^{67}Gallium citrate
		Roentgen-ray absorptiometry
		Arthrocentesis
		Bone biopsy
Function	Alkaline phosphatase	Parathyroid hormone
	Ca, P	Calcitonin
		Vitamin D_3
		25-OH-D_3
		1 , 25-$(OH)_2$-D_3

Table 8-14 *Skin and Appendages*

	EXAMINATION	
	BASIC	SPECIALIZED
Structure	Inspection	
	Direct (hand lens)	Dark field
	Wood's lamp	Biopsy
		Immunofluorescent studies
	Exudates	
	Smear	
	Culture	
	Scrapings	
	Direct oil	
	KOH	
	Tzanck smear	
		Cuttings (chemical analyses)
		Hair
		Nails
Function		
Vasoreactivity		Catechol iontophoresis
		Skin blood flow
Sweating	Starch-iodine examination	
	Pilocarpine iontophoresis	

Table 8-15 *Endocrine System*

END-ORGAN HORMONES	INTERMEDIARIES	RELEASERS
Adrenal cortex	ACTH (corticotropin)	CRH (corticotropin-releasing hormone)
Cortisol		
Aldosterone	Angiotensin II (kidneys)	
Dehydroepiandrosterone		
Adrenal medulla		
Epinephrine		
Norepinephrine		
Dopamine		
Gonads		
Testosterone	FSH (follicle-stimulating hormone)	LH-RH (luteinizing hormone–releasing hormone)
Estradiol	LH (luteinizing hormone)	
Progesterone		
Thyroid		
Triiodothyronine (T_3)	TSH (thyroid-stimulating hormone [thyrotropin])	TRH (thyroid-releasing hormone)
Thyroxine (T_4)		
Parafollicular cells		
Calcitonin		
Parathyroid		
Parathyroid hormone	Vitamin D	
Growth		
Somatomedin action	GH (growth hormone, somatotropin)	GHRH (growth hormone–releasing hormone)
Lactation		
Direct action	PRL (prolactin)	PRH (prolactin-inhibiting hormone)
Melanocyte	MSH (melanocyte-stimulating hormone)	MRF (melanocyte-releasing factor)
Direct action		
Distal renal tubule		
Direct action	ADH (arginine vasopressin)	
Uterus		
Direct action	Oxytocin	

Table 8-16 *Blood and Hematopoietic System*

	EXAMINATION	
	BASIC	SPECIALIZED

Structure	Hemoglobin
	Hematocrit
	Reticulocyte count
	Cell counts
	  Red cell
	  White cell
	  Platelet
	Peripheral smear
	Marrow aspiration
		Marrow biopsy
		Marrow culture

Function		
Neutrophil		
Chemotaxis	Rebuck skin window technique	Boyden chamber
Phagocytosis		Vital staining (myeloperoxidase)
Bacterial killing	Nitroblue tetrazolium test	Chemiluminescence
Red cell		
Gas transport	Hemoglobin electrophoresis	Po_2 at 50% saturation; 2,3-diphosphoglycerate
Membrane stability	Osmotic fragility	Peroxidation NADPH* generation
Glycolysis		
Hemostasis		
Total	Clotting time	
Vascular phase	Tourniquet test	
Platelet phase	Bleeding time Clot retraction	Platelet aggregation
Phase III	Thrombin time	Fibrinogen, factor XIII
Phase II	Prothrombin time (PT)	Prothrombin, factors V, VII, and X
Phase I	Partial thromboplastin time (PTT) Prothrombin consumption	Thromboplastin generation Factors VII, VIII, IX, XI, and XII

*NADPH, nicotinamide adenine dinucleotide phosphate.

niques are often used for a rather gross overview of endocrine organ outlines (sella turcica, adrenal cortex, thyroid), but picogram quantities of hormones and small clusters of specialized cells are beyond the powers even of histologic techniques for resolution of structure. In most cases in Table 8-15, a "negative feedback axis" is involved that shuts down the hypothalamic activation of the pituitary gland's stimulation of end-organ hormone production. An increased end-organ hormonal level in the blood is the (negative) signal that impedes further trophic hormone release—analagous to the increased heat that shuts off the living room thermostat.

The suspicion of end-organ malfunction and even the measurement of some of the pertinent hormones (especially adrenal and thyroid) are in the province of the primary pediatrician, but detailed assessment of the pituitary and hypothalamic feedback loops by various evocative tests (see Table 8-15) is normally under the proper jurisdiction of the pediatric endocrinologist.

Blood

Although structural assessment of at least the circulating elements in the hematopoietic system is part of the armamentarium of any physician, the hematologist should be called on to examine those aspects of hemostasis whose disruption may be suggested by the various screening tests of clotting function (Table 8-16). Yet the pediatrician's most frequent contact with this system is probably in tracing its involvement with disease of nutritional, infectious, or cancerous origin.

Immune System

The body's immunologic defenses constitute an elaborate system that has evolved over eons of assault by "non self" invaders, potential or real. The developmental costs of this system to the species have been the very common occurrence of those atopic individuals who overreact to the antigens in their environment (with reactions of eczema, asthma, rhinitis), the much rarer occurrence of individuals who, by confusing self with nonself, develop "autoimmune" disease (e.g., myasthenia gravis, rheumatic fever, glomerulonephritis, and possibly diabetes), and those unfortunates whose normal immune defenses have been naturally impaired (through infection with the human immune deficiency virus [HIV]) or whose immune defenses must be artificially crippled to improve the likelihood of successful transplantation of foreign tissues and organs.

The frustrating frequency with which parents and pediatricians deal with infections contracted by the "immunologic virgins" who are their children has often led to fruitless attempts to document immunologic incompetence. Most often, however, quiet epidemiologic reflection will indicate that recurrent infections among otherwise healthy young American children are usually caused by a plethora of microbial invaders rather than by a paucity of defenses. Relatively simple screening tests of immediate and delayed hypersensitivity, as well as antibody level, are usually sufficient to dispel doubt.

The availability of radioallergosorbent tests (RAST) (Table 8-17) for specific antigen-associated IgE has considerably

Table 8-17 *Immune System*

	EXAMINATION	
	BASIC	SPECIALIZED
Structure		
Lymphocytes		
Overall	Lymphocyte count	Biopsy (node, thymus, spleen, gut)
T cells	Lateral chest roentgenogram	
	Rosette formation (sheep RBC)	Monoclonal markers (helper, suppressor)
B cells	Serum IgG, IgM levels	IgM cell markers
	Serum isohemagglutin levels	
Complement system	Total hemolytic complement level	Specific complement protein levels (C3,C4)
Allergen system	Total IgE (radioimmunoassay)	
Function		
T cell	Skin tests (tuberculin, *Candida*)	Stimulated lymphocyte culture
B cell	Skin tests (Schick test)	Stimulated lymphocyte culture
Allergen	Eosinophils	Provocative testing (airways)
	Skin testing	Prausnitz-Küstner passive transfer
	Specific radioallergosorbent tests (RAST)	Leukocyte histamine release

simplified, not to mention humanized, the allergic evaluation of the symptomatic child under consideration for desensitization therapy; however, it should never replace a carefully chronologic and historical review of the onset and offset of those symptoms.

ETIOLOGIC DELINEATION

It is a sweet irony that a textbook of pediatrics, such as this volume, can now afford a relative neglect of nutritional and infectious disease on the ground that, at least in developed countries, social, sanitary, economic, and medical advances have diminished the prominence of the serious nutritional (apart from obesity) and infectious diseases that brought the clinical discipline that is pediatrics into being. A concurrent and corollary emphasis on problems of early development (perinatology, neonatology, congenital anomalies) and behavior (a principal focus of this volume) will likely characterize the pediatrics of the next 100 years. Hence, of the usual etiologic classification of disease (see the box below), we will here consider only briefly and broadly those of genetic or infectious origin. Discussions of psychogenic disease are found throughout this volume, whereas the possibility of iatrogenic disease lurks in every contact between child and primary pediatrician, particularly when the latter is oriented to treatment rather than to *thinking* and reflecting on the fact that the vast majority of his or her sick patients are dealing with self-limited, intercurrent illnesses that usually require only sympathetic support and symptomatic treatment. The pediatrician's therapeutic zeal is better reserved for those few life-threatening emergencies discussed elsewhere in this book.

Etiologic Classification of Disease Origin

- Genetic and developmental
- Nutritional
- Infectious
- Neoplastic
- Traumatic and physical agents
- Hypersensitivity
- Psychogenic
- Unknown or unclassified

Genetic Disease

It could be argued that hemolytic disease of the newborn and the prevention of those cases caused by the D-antigen represents a model approach to genetic disease. Few if any other known genetic diseases, however, result in an individual who is phenotypically normal but thrust into the genetically inhospitable environment of a "foreign" amniotic sac (although who now could specify that such is not the mechanism for production of some "multifactorial" congenital anomalies?).

A classification of the mechanisms of birth defects is offered in the box on p. 125, along with some pertinent examples. Current approaches to the prevention of birth defects (actually, prevention of birth for those who are defective) is shown in the box on p. 125. Although crude, this scheme can be effective—yet, apart from advanced maternal age (as an index of risk for nondisjunction during meiosis), entry into such a system is by definition purchased at the price of a previous genetic disaster. Genetic engineering for gene replacement or alteration of established genetic disease is as yet, analagously speaking, somewhere between Isaac Newton's discovery of the Law of Universal Gravitation and human arrival on the surface of the moon—that is, much engineering remains to be done.

The pediatrician is called upon now, however, to be aware of and deal with the genetic disease already established in the patient. He or she must attempt to clarify the clinical presentation, always suspicious of the possibility of an inborn error of metabolism, particularly among those infants who are phenotypically normal, yet give a history of vomiting, dysphagia, and neurologic catastrophe (severe alterations in muscle tone, seizures, coma) after exposure to ingested sugars or protein. A scheme for screening infants with regard to the

Table 8-18 *Genetic Screening*

EXAMINATIONS	
BASIC	SPECIALIZED
Newborn (nonselective mass screening)	
Blood bacterial inhibition assay (Guthrie test)	
Phenylalanine (phenylketonuria)	
Leucine (maple syrup urine disease)	
Methionine (homocystinuria)	
Tyrosine (tyrosinemia)	
Fluorescent spot test (Beutler)	
Galactose (galactosemia)	
Radioimmunoassay	
Thyroxine (hypothyroidism)	
Infant (symptomatic)	
Blood	
Ca, Mg, electrolytes	
pH, sugar, ketone, NH_3	
Urine	
Odor	
Sugar	
Ketones	
Amino acids	
Direct reagent spot test	Amino acids
$FeCl_3$	High-pressure liquid chromatography
Dinitrophenylhydrazine	Organic acids
Ketoacids	Gas chromatographic mass spectroscopy
Nitrosonaphthol	
Tyrosine	
Cyanide/nitroprusside	
Cystine	
Homocystine	
Paper or thin-layer chromatography	
Carbohydrates	
Benedict solution (Clinitest)	
Reducing sugar	
Glucose oxidase (Labstix)	
Glucose	
Toluidine blue	
Mucopolysaccharides	

Table 8-19 *Assessment of Genetic Disease*

EXAMINATIONS	
BASIC	SPECIALIZED
Pedigree	Genotype
	Karyotype (cultured)
Proband	Amniotic cells
Phenotype	Leukocytes
Dysmorphologic	Bone marrow
Dermatoglyphic	Genome mapping
	Specific protein product
	Enzyme
	Skin fibroblast culture
	Red cells
	Substrate/metabolic product
	Urine
	Blood
	Tissue culture

more common (although all are relatively rare) inborn errors of metabolism is displayed in Table 8-18.

In those infants who are phenotypically abnormal, the pediatrician must strive to identify the dysmorphologic pattern presented, often in consultation with an appropriate atlas of known defects or a clinical geneticist. The painstaking work of establishing the family pedigree (often a severe challenge in this nation of mobile immigrants) must be undertaken to provide the essential groundwork for genetic counseling.

The genotype must be established, where possible (Table 8-19), and biochemical efforts to assay the putative missing enzyme, abnormal substrate (e.g., the glucocerebroside in Gaucher's disease), or deficient protein product (e.g., factor VIII in hemophilia) undertaken to identify the affected biochemical pathway.

Prompt detection of some inborn errors (phenylketonuria, maple syrup urine disease) can lead to a rewarding plan for prevention of mental retardation. Some families (those with trisomy 21 syndrome) will require consistent, sympathetic support over a long period of time; others (those with trisomy 13 or 18) may require more intensive support

Mechanisms of Birth Defects

SINGLE MUTANT GENE

Autosomal dominant (e.g., achondroplasia, neurofibromatosis, polycystic kidney)
Autosomal recessive (e.g., adrenogenital syndrome, cystic fibrosis, sickle cell disease)
X-linked (e.g., chronic granulomatous disease, glucose 6-phosphate dehydrogenase [G6PD] deficiency, hemophilia A)

CHROMOSOMAL DISORDERS

Aneuploidy

Monosomy

XO: Turner's syndrome

Trisomies

13: Patau's syndrome
18: Edwards' syndrome
21: Down syndrome
XXY: Klinefelter's syndrome
XYY
XXX

Structural changes

Translocations (balanced, unbalanced)

Robertsonian
Reciprocal

Deletions

Chromosome 5: cri-du-chat syndrome

Breakage

Multifactorial (gene-environment interaction)

Single congenital

Cardiac defects
Cleft lip or palate
Meningomyelocele

Age related

Diabetes
Schizophrenia

Prenatal Diagnostic Screening for Birth Defects

INDICATIONS

Advanced maternal age
Known "carrier"
  Balanced translocation
  X-linked
Previous affected child
  Trisomy
  Neural tube defect

PROCEDURES

Radiography
Ultrasound
Chorionic villus sampling
Amniocentesis
Amniography
Fetoscopy

AMNIOTIC FLUID ANALYSIS

Fluid (secretory products)
  Alpha-fetoprotein
Cultured cells
  Karyotype
  Enzymatic analysis
  Genome (DNA)
    Molecular hybridization
    Restriction endonucleases

Table 8-20 *Assessment of Infectious Diseases*

EXAMINATIONS	
BASIC	SPECIALIZED
Epidemiology	
Body fluids/exudates/tissues	
Direct examination	
Method	
Saline suspension	Special stains
Potassium hydroxide preparation	Dyes
Gram stain	Fluorescent antibodies
Tzanck preparation	Electron microscopy
Light microscopy	
Laboratory culture	
Appropriate selective media	
Typing	
Antibiotic sensitivity	Typing
Enzymatic screening	Phage
	Serologic
	Specific antibody responses
	Complement fixing
	Neutralizing
	Hemagglutination inhibiting
	Precipitating
	Special serologic assays
	Monospot
	Venereal Disease Research Laboratory (VDRL)
	Fluorescent antibodies
	Radioimmunoassay (RIA)
	Enzyme-linked immunosorbent assay (ELISA)

Table 8-21 *Perinatal Infections (relative North American incidence)*

COMMON	RARE	"RETIRED"
Viral		
Cytomegalovirus		Rubella
Hepatitis B	Varicella	
Herpes	Coxsackie	
Bacterial		
Streptococcus B	*Staphylococcus aureus*	Streptococcus A
Escherichia coli (especially K1)	*Pseudomonas*	Syphilis
Listeria	*Klebsiella-Enterobacter*	Gonorrhea
	Proteus	
	Pneumococcus	
	Pertussis	
	Haemophilus influenzae	
Other		
Chlamydia		
Mycoplasma		
Toxoplasma		

Table 8-22 *Respiratory and Pharyngeal Infections (relative North American incidence)*

COMMON	RARE	"RETIRED"
Viral		
Respiratory syncytial virus	Coxsackievirus	Measles
Parainfluenza	Epstein-Barr virus	
Influenza	Herpesvirus	
Rhinovirus	Coronavirus	
Adenovirus		
Bacterial		
Streptococcus A	*Staphylococcus aureus*	Tuberculosis
Pneumococcus	*Legionella*	Diphtheria
Haemophilus influenzae		Pertussis
Other		
Mycoplasma		
Chlamydia		

Table 8-23 *Gastrointestinal and Diarrheal Infections (relative North American incidence)*

COMMON	RARE	"RETIRED"
Viral		
Rotavirus	Norwalk virus	Poliovirus
Echovirus		
Coxsackievirus		
Adenovirus		
Bacterial		
Escherichia coli	*Yersinia*	Cholera
Enteropathogenic	*Salmonella*	Typhoid
Enterovirulent	*Shigella*	
Enteroinvasive	*Campylobacter*	
Other		
Giardia	Tapeworm	
	Amebiasis	

Table 8-24 *Other Significant Infectious-Disease Agents (relative North American incidence)*

COMMON	RARE	"RETIRED"
Bacteria		
Staphylococcus aureus	*Yersinia*	Tetanus
Haemophilus influenzae	*Campylobacter*	
	Brucella	
	Meningococcus	
	Clostridium difficile	
	Leptospira	
	Actinomycosis	
	Nocardiosis	
Viruses		
Hepatitis A, B	Arthropod borne (arbovirus)	Mumps
Varicella-zoster		Rabies
		Smallpox
		Rubella
Rickettsiae	Spotted fever	Typhus
Fungi/Yeast		
Tinea	Coccidioidomycosis	
Candida	*Cryptococcus*	
	Aspergillosis	
	Histoplasmosis	
Protozoa	Amebiasis	Malaria
	Sporozoea	
	Pneumocystis carinii	
Helminths		
Ascaris	*Toxocara caris*	Hookworm
Enterobius		Trichinella

Table 8-25 *Opportunistic Infections*

Agents

Many
- Low virulence
- Unusual pathogens

Opportunities

Natural

Development
- Anatomic defects of the skin
- Premature infant (small inoculum)
- Term infant (large inoculum)
- Immune defect

Disease
- Cystic fibrosis
- Diabetes
- Malignancy
- Nephrotic syndrome
- Sickle cell disease

Acquired

Acquired immune deficiency syndrome (AIDS)
Burns
Malnutrition
Trauma

Iatrogenic

Anatomic invasion
- Surgical procedures
- Dental procedures
- Indwelling catheters and shunts
  - Urinary
  - Vascular
  - Peritoneal
  - Ventricular

Ecologic disruption
- Antibiotics
- Inhalation therapy

Immune interference
- Suppression
  - Malignancy
  - Transplantation
- Splenectomy

over a shorter period of time. It is the pediatrician's duty early to decide which type of problem the patient represents.

Infectious Disease

The prior claims to possession of the planet anciently established by the one-celled organisms, the evolution of host defenses by "higher forms" to deal with those microbes by whom they are threatened, and the genetic ingenuity regularly displayed by such organisms in rapidly developing resistance to human antimicrobials all suggest that infectious diseases will forever remain a fundamental concern for all primary care practitioners, most especially pediatricians. Although most of the great scourges have subsided (for now) in developed countries (e.g., "summer diarrhea," polio, and smallpox) good fortune in genetically driven "antigenic shifts" (e.g., influenza and staphylococcal and streptococcal diseases) has apparently played at least as important a role as clean water, good housing, antimicrobials, and vaccines. Yet every young child with intact host defenses can, in any society, be overwhelmed by too large an inoculum in the process of developing immunity first-hand.

The basic diagnostic approaches to the infected child are outlined in Table 8-20, the most powerful tool being the practitioner's constant epidemiologic awareness of the endemic or invasive infectious disease currently prevalent in his or her community. A selected microbial demography of common pediatric infectious diseases is set out in Tables 8-21, 8-22, 8-23, and 8-24. Of increasing concern are the many opportunistic infections (Table 8-25) that complicate the course of those patients already suffering from serious primary disease, whose host defenses have been assaulted and diminished by human or natural intervention.

REFERENCES

1. Babson SG: Growth of low-birth weight infants, J Pediatr 77:11, 1970.
2. Battaglia FC and Lubchenco LO: A practical classification of newborn infants by weight and gestational age, J Pediatr 71:161, 1967.
3. Dancis J, O'Connell JR, and Holt LE: A grid for recording the weight of premature infants, J Pediatr 33:570, 1948.
4. Dubowitz L, Dubowitz V, and Goldberg C: Clinical assessment of gestational age in the newborn infant, J Pediatr 77:1, 1970.
5. Lubchenco LO, Hansman C, and Boyd E: Intrauterine growth in length and head circumference as estimated from live births at gestational ages from 26 to 42 weeks, Pediatrics 37:403, 1966.
6. Marks KH et al: Head growth in sick premature infants: a longitudinal study, J Pediatr 94:282, 1979.
7. Hamill PV et al: Physical growth: National Center for Health Statistics Percentiles, Am J Clin Nutr 32:607-629, 1979.
8. Nellhaus G: Head circumference from birth to eighteen years: practical composite international and interracial graphs, Pediatrics 41:106, 1968.
9. Tanner JM and Whitehouse RH: Clinical longitudinal standards for height, weight, height velocity, weight velocity, and stages of puberty, Arch Dis Child 51:170, 1976.
10. Usher R and McLean F: Intrauterine growth of live-born Caucasian infants at sea level: standards obtained from measurements in 7 dimensions of infants born between 25 and 44 weeks of gestation, J Pediatr 74:901, 1969.

SUGGESTED READINGS

Frankenburg WK and Camp BW: Pediatric screening test, Springfield 1975, CC Thomas.

Thorpe HS and Werner EE: Developmental screening of preschool children, Pediatrics 53:362, 1974.

9

The Pediatric Record and Clinical Decision-Making

James R. Campbell

Clinical decision-making involves delineating a clinical problem and formulating a plan for that problem. These are termed, respectively, diagnostic decision-making and management decision-making.

This chapter describes the cognitive process underlying diagnostic decision-making and presents a structure for the recording of problems. The pediatric record facilitates management decision-making. The last section of the chapter describes management decision-making.

DIAGNOSTIC DECISION-MAKING

The purpose of diagnostic decision-making is to determine a diagnosis or problem. The cognitive process presented by Feinstein[4,5] moves from effect to cause and consists of multiple stations (Fig. 9-1), which are defined in the next section.

The Structure of Diagnostic Decision-Making

The diagnostic process begins with the presentation of an abnormality, or *manifestation*. This manifestation could be a symptom, a sign, an abnormal laboratory value, or roentgenographic finding for which an explanation is sought.

Once a manifestation is recognized, its structural or functional source is identified; this is the *domain*. A domain can be an organ, an anatomic region (e.g., head, mediastinum, abdomen), a group of sequential structures (e.g., genitourinary tract, digestive tract), or a functional system (e.g., hematopoietic system, endocrine system).

Often a domain encompasses many anatomic or functional structures; therefore it is necessary to define further the source of the manifestation within the domain. This source is the *focus*. If the torso is the defined domain of abdominal pain, for instance, it is necessary to identify a focus, such as the gallbladder, lungs, fallopian tubes, or appendix. In some cases further specification will not be required, such as the eye with ocular pain.

The next station is a *disorder*. A disorder is a gross abnormality in the structure or function of a domain or focus. A disorder can be an anatomic lesion (e.g., hypertrophy, consolidation, herniation) or a physiologic dysfunction (e.g., malabsorption, tachycardia, hemolysis).

A *derangement* is a pathologic process responsible for the disorder. It differs from a disorder in that it is identifiable microscopically or chemically rather than grossly. Glucose-6-phosphate dehydrogenase deficiency, a derangement, can cause the disorder of hemolysis. Splenomegaly is a disorder that can be caused by many derangements, such as inflammation, congestion, or neoplastic infiltration. Other pathologic processes that are derangements include fibrosis, congenital anomalies, infarction, trauma, and degeneration. A disorder can be caused by one or more derangements.

A *pathoanatomic entity* is a specific morphologic or topographic abnormality that may lead to or constitute a disorder or derangement. Examples include atrial septal defect, pneumonia of the right upper lobe, slipped femoral epiphysis, and cholelithiasis. Because a morphologic abnormality is not present in all diagnoses, this station is not always involved.

A *pathogenetic entity* is the circumstance or agent that causes, provokes, or predisposes to the disorder, derangement, or pathoanatomic entity. This entity includes microbial, immunologic, and biochemical abnormalities. The mutant gene that causes the valine substitution for glutamic acid in β-hemoglobin is the pathogenetic entity in sickle cell anemia.

The Process of Diagnostic Reasoning

Diagnostic reasoning begins with consideration of one or more manifestations for which a clinician seeks a diagnosis. The first decision involves the selection of a domain and focus of the manifestation. Although these stations are seldom stated, their proper identification is imperative; domain and focus specify a location and direct the diagnostician to consider disorders, derangements, and pathogenetic entities that may occur in that location. Thus, to prevent inadvertent exclusion of possible diagnoses, it is prudent not to limit the list of domains. In the evaluation of abdominal pain, for example, it is important to recall that a pathologic condition in the thorax can cause pain in the abdomen; if the diagnostic domain is limited to abdominal anatomy, a misdiagnosis may result.

Conversely, manifestations may allow the diagnostician to be explicit in anatomic localization. A patient with jaundice and pain in the right upper quadrant of the abdomen, for example, is unlikely to have a pathologic condition of the pelvis with pain referred to the abdomen.

In summary, a diagnostician should be as explicit in localization as the data allow, but not more so.[1]

A disorder (the next station in the sequence) of diagnostic reasoning, is identified or suggested by the history and physical examination. It is often useful at this point to confirm the disorder by means of laboratory tests, roentgenograms,

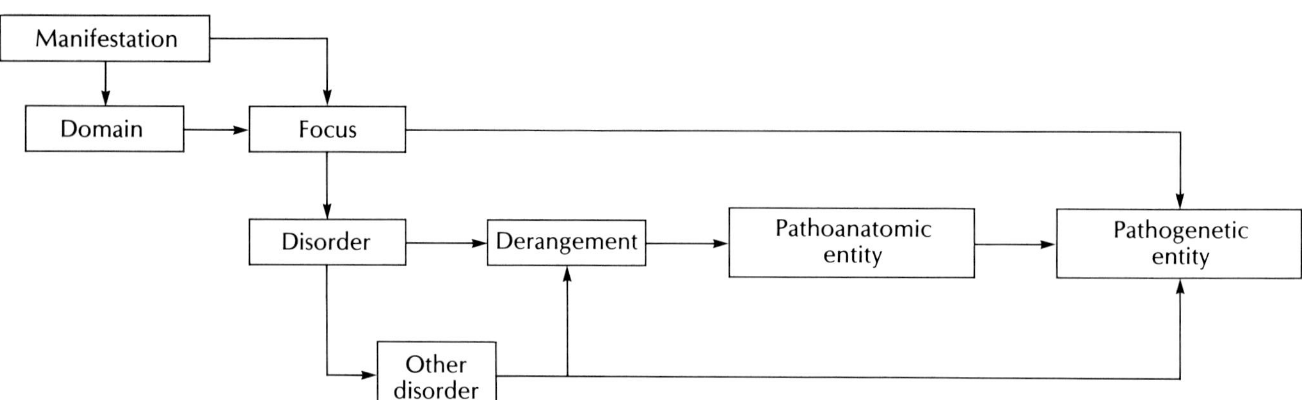

Fig. 9-1 Sequential stations in the intellectual pathway of diagnostic reasoning.
From Feinstein AR: Yale J Biol Med 46:212, 1973.

or other auxiliary examinations. This verification assists in preventing erroneous diagnostic decisions and the expense of a nondiscriminatory battery of tests.[4,9] Once a disorder is confirmed, the remaining reasoning process seeks to explain *it* rather than the manifestation.

In some cases, especially for emergent conditions, a disorder may indicate the type of therapy. For example, transfusion of packed red blood cells for acute blood loss is a therapeutic end point. A disorder also may be the final diagnosis in conditions in which the derangement, pathoanatomic entity, and pathogenetic entity (also stations within the sequence of diagnostic reasoning) are unknown or inconsequential. Examples include depression, schizophrenia, and "fever without focus" in a febrile but otherwise normal toddler.

A diagnostician identifies the subsequent station to explain a previous one. In this process the diagnostician can list candidates (a differential diagnosis) in considering possible derangements, pathoanatomic entities, or pathogenetic entities. Errors may result if possible candidates are not included in the listing; thus the actual diagnosis may not be considered. To keep the list manageable,[1] however, it is useful to concentrate on the most specific manifestations. If a patient has fatigue, fever, and jaundice, for example, it is more efficient to list a differential diagnosis based on the jaundice rather than on the nonspecific manifestation of fatigue. The listing of candidates is, of course, facilitated by knowledge and experience; texts are available to aid the clinician.[11]

Once a list has been written, the diagnostician then must exclude unlikely candidates. It is expedient to consider the most common candidates first.[6] It also is important, however, to consider those candidates, regardless of their prevalence, for which effective treatment is available and in which failure to treat would lead to serious consequences.[3] For example, a diagnostician should consider the rare but treatable condition of Wilson disease in a teenager with neurologic symptoms and hepatitis.

Examples of Diagnostic Reasoning

Example No. 1. A 24-month-old child with Down syndrome has fever. This manifestation can arise from anywhere; therefore the body is the domain. A focus now needs to be defined. The history from the mother does not identify other symptoms; the child has been playful and eating well. The physical examination reveals a red, bulging tympanic membrane in the right ear; the remainder of the examination shows normal findings. The focus is the right middle ear, and the disorder is the bulging tympanic membrane. The redness of the tympanic membrane and fever suggest the derangement of inflammation. A Gram stain of fluid from a tympanocentesis reveals many neutrophils, which confirms the derangement of inflammation. A culture of this fluid grows *Streptococcus pneumoniae,* which identifies the pathogenetic entity. Because the child has Down syndrome, the probable pathoanatomic entity is poor drainage of the middle ear.

Example No. 2. A 10-year-old child has bilateral periorbital swelling. On physical examination a resident identifies pretibial pitting edema and presumptively defines the domain as the kidney, the focus as the glomeruli, and the disorder as increased glomerular protein loss. Results of tests for protein in a urine sample, however, are negative. The resident then performs a more thorough physical examination; she identifies a rapid heart rate, an S3 heart sound, a displaced apical impulse, fever, and hepatomegaly. The domain is redefined as the cardiovascular system, with the focus as the heart. One disorder, according to the second physical examination, is cardiomegaly. Another disorder is hepatomegaly, and a third disorder is tachycardia. A chest roentgenogram confirms the clinical impression of cardiomegaly. The resident reassesses these multiple disorders and combines them into a single, unifying disorder: congestive heart failure, which a cardiologist confirms. The resident then seeks the derangement of this disorder. With the presence of fever, she presumes the derangement to be due to inflammation; this is further suggested by an elevated erythrocyte sedimentation rate. The resident then seeks to identify inflammatory conditions that cause congestive heart failure. She considers systemic lupus erythematosus, but laboratory evaluation is nonconfirmatory. She then considers rheumatic heart fever; the antistreptolysin titer is elevated. This test confirms an antecedent streptococcal infection and identifies the pathogenetic entity. An echocardiogram identifies mitral stenosis, which is the pathoanatomic entity.

The Problems of Diagnostic Decision-Making

A common difficulty in diagnostic decision-making is dealing with inaccurate data. Nearly all information with which the clinician deals is subject to error. If manifestations are erroneously interpreted or overlooked, the final diagnosis may be incorrect. Thus all manifestations, whether they are symptoms, physical signs, or laboratory values, need to be precisely reviewed. Patients, however, may be forgetful or may intentionally omit embarrassing yet vital information; clinicians may neglect to ask pertinent questions or examine important regions. Some of these errors can be eliminated by conscientious investigation, yet many potential errors are inherent in the diagnostic process. To compensate for these deficiencies, the concepts of sensitivity, specificity, and predictive value for each diagnostic test were developed; several texts describe these concepts.[7,10] Yet even with the knowledge of these test parameters, a diagnostician needs to remember that errors occur and that it is necessary to reevaluate original data when inconsistencies arise in decision-making.

A second common difficulty is deciding when it is appropriate to cluster manifestations to assist in the decision process, as was illustrated in the second example above. This skill improves with knowledge and experience. A few guidelines are as follows: (1) younger patients are more likely to have single conditions that explain multiple manifestations than are older patients, (2) signs and symptoms that occur temporally are more likely to be related to a single condition, and (3) signs and symptoms identifiable with a single organ system are more likely to be related to a single condition.[1]

THE PEDIATRIC RECORD

Once a problem is defined, it must be recorded; however, a record-keeping system should not simply document information. Because clinicians can fail to find recorded information, a good medical record also should minimize the oversight of pertinent information and allow rapid retrieval of data.

A pediatric record also should enhance communication among practitioners, facilitate documentation, simplify quality assurance, and show how problems were assessed, what plans were made, and how the patient responded. The problem-oriented system was designed to achieve these ends.[8,12] Its general structure and dynamics are described in the next section.

The Structure of the Problem-Oriented System

The problem-oriented system consists of (1) a data base, (2) a problem list, (3) a plan for management, and (4) progress notes of patient encounters.

The *data base* in the medical record is the recorded information pertinent to the patient's problems. The basic components of the pediatric data base are the medical history, physical examination, growth charts, developmental flow sheets, screening tests, laboratory data, and problem-specific flow sheets.

The content of the data base will vary with the patient's age, life-style, and environment.[2] Teenagers who develop normally, for example, do not require continued developmental assessment. Similarly, marathoners need periodic assessment for anemia secondary to occult gastrointestinal bleeding, and their data base should indicate this medically relevant activity.

The medical history includes past medical problems, allergies, previous surgeries, medication history, previous hospitalizations, family history, social history, and occupational history. Flow sheets—forms for the documentation of data for patients with particular problems—can be used for health care maintenance. An example of a problem-specific flow sheet for asthma is illustrated in Fig. 9-2. These flow sheets allow a clinician to review a long and complex history quickly.

The *problem list* is a list of anything that requires management or diagnostic work-up. It consists not only of diagnoses but any medical, social, developmental, psychological, economic, or environmental problem identified from the data base. Therefore any sign, symptom, abnormal laboratory test result, family history of disease, or psychosocial dysfunction should be noted.

The *plan for management* is an explicit description of the actions to be taken on each problem. It should contain information related to (1) diagnosis, (2) treatment, (3) patient education, and (4) follow-up. A description of management decision-making, which details how plans are to be implemented, is presented in the last section.

If the listed problem is a sign or symptom, the differential diagnosis that is considered and the diagnostic work-up should be written as part of the management plan. If treatment has been instituted and drugs prescribed, therapeutic end points and contingency plans need to be explicitly stated. Follow-up plans can include the protocol to be followed and the time for reappointment.

A *progress note* documents each patient encounter. It can follow the SOAP format (subjective, objective, assessment, plan). Under the "subjective" heading the course of symptoms is documented; the "objective" heading specifies the course of criteria observable to the clinician, such as physical signs or laboratory tests. The "assessment" is not necessarily synonymous with diagnosis; it summarizes the course of the previously diagnosed condition. The "plan" is a statement of specific actions that result from the patient-clinician encounter; it may simply be a reiteration of any part of the management plan.

The Dynamics of the Problem-Oriented System

The problem-oriented system begins with a data base. The various components of the data base are collected by the physician, nurse, or technician and entered in the chart. For completeness, data may be obtained by means of standardized questionnaires.[8] As problems are identified from the data base, they are entered on the problem list and assigned a number that is used consistently in the chart.

Each problem on the problem list should be substantiated by objective information so that the decision-making process

Asthma Follow-up

GUIDELINES	VISIT INFORMATION—FOR ALL VISITS TO CLINIC				
	VISIT	VISIT	VISIT	VISIT	VISIT
Health Supervision & "Tune-up" Visits Minimum q 6 mo.	Date ____ Tune-up ____ Float ____	Date ____ Tune-up ____ Float ____	Date ____ Tune-up ____ Float ____	Date ____ Tune-up ____ Float ____	Date ____ Tune-up ____ Float ____
Current Meds: Record: dose/frequency/chronic/prn	*Regimen Dose/Freq/Dur*	*Regimen Dose/Freq/Dur*	*Regimen Dose/Freq/Dur*	*Regimen Dose/Freq/Dur*	*Regimen Dose/Freq/Dur*
A) Cromolyn					
B) Theophylline					
C) Liquid Alupent/Albuterol					
D) Inhal Alupent/Albuterol					
E) Home Nebulizer					
F) Prednisone					
G) Other ____					
Labs:	DATE/RESULT	DATE/RESULT	DATE/RESULT	DATE/RESULT	DATE/RESULT
A) Theophylline Level q 6 mo (if on chronic Theoph)					
B) Influenza Vaccine (date) Give in Oct-Dec.					
Referrals: If Needed	RECORD THE DATE OF THE INITIAL REFERRAL				
A) Pulmonary					
B) PFTs					
C) Allergy					
D) Other ____					
Disease Status:	RECORD YOUR RESULTS				
A) Wheezing Attacks 1. Frequency? (q day, q wk) 2. Severity? 1-mild, 2-mod., 3-severe 3. Triggered By?					
B) Interim Hospitalization Yes (date, duration); No					
C) Interim ER Visit Yes (date, reason); No					
D) Schl Absence From Asthma # days last month? # days last 6 months?					
Side Effects: (if on chronic meds)	RECORD YOUR RESULTS				
A) GI Y/N					
B) Behavior Y/N					
C) Other ____					

Fig. 9-2 Sample of problem-specific flow sheet.

is not diverted from the true diagnosis.[2] If a patient has headaches with left arm weakness, for example, it is better to list "headaches with left arm weakness" rather than "rule out intracranial mass," even though the latter is in the differential diagnosis. In this way other possible etiologic factors, such as complex migraines, will less likely be overlooked. (The cognitive process underlying differential diagnosis is discussed in Diagnostic Decision-Making at the beginning of this chapter.)

It is helpful to list self-limited problems (e.g., upper

Problem List

Name: ***Janet Doe***
DOB: ***11/16/74***

ENTRY DATE	#	ACTIVE PROBLEMS	DATE RESOLVED	INACTIVE PROBLEMS
	1	Well-Child Care		
9/12/89	2	Acne Vulgaris		
10/15/89 10/16/89	3	Headaches and diplopia → Pseudotumor cerebri		

Temporary Problem List

NO.	PROBLEM	ONSET: RESOLUTION						
1	Upper Respiratory Tract Infection	6/12-6/14						
2	Gastroenteritis	4/12-4/14						

Fig. 9-3 Sample problem list.

respiratory tract infections) on a "temporary list" to prevent the problem list from becoming unmanageably long. If a particular problem on this list recurs or becomes chronic (e.g., otitis media), it could then be listed on the problem list. As problems are resolved, this should be indicated on the problem list along with the date of resolution (Fig. 9-3).

Listed problems that indicate abnormal signs, symptoms, or laboratory test results will, ideally, be further defined. This information can be indicated on the problem list, for example, "headaches and diplopia" on a teenager's problem list. After initial evaluation the diagnosis may be pseudotumor cerebri; an arrow can be drawn from the initial problem to the final diagnosis. A date is written over the arrow whenever a problem is updated (see Fig. 9-3). When managed in this way, the problem list will encourage logical rather than intuitive thinking.

A plan for each problem is formulated and stated in the management plan (see Management Decision-Making). The progress notes document the ongoing management of these problems and collects further information. Any pertinent information identified in an encounter also should be documented in the data base.

The Shortcomings of the Problem-Oriented System

A shortcoming in the use of the problem-oriented system is the failure to update the data base. Information that warrants ready retrievability may become lost among multiple pages of progress notes. One approach to alleviate this problem is to update the data base with a short entry and refer the reader to the progress note for details. For instance, if the parents of a patient separate, this could be recorded in the social history section of the data base as "parental separation — see progress note, 10/3/90." The indicated progress note then would detail the problem.

Another difficulty is in the generation of the problem list. A clinician may list related signs and symptoms separately and therefore not integrate the data into a single diagnosis. This problem, however, is related to improper clustering of manifestations in diagnostic decision-making (see The Problems of Diagnostic-Decision Making). Experience in diagnosis, of course, improves this skill and the resultant problem list.

A third shortcoming is the tendency for the problem list to include unnecessary problems and therefore to become too long. Problem lists should contain items that may have long-term significance. A toddler, for example, is admitted to the hospital with pneumococcal meningitis; his course is complicated by an ampicillin reaction and a minor infiltration of an intravenous infusion site. Although each detail is a problem, the child's permanent problem list should include only pneumococcal meningitis and ampicillin reaction.

Even if strict criteria are followed, the problem list may become lengthy and cumbersome. Thus it is realistic for the primary clinician to revise the problem list periodically.

MANAGEMENT DECISION-MAKING

The previous sections describe how diagnoses are formulated; however, diseases are not the only problems that clinicians need to manage. Divorce and school failure also threaten a child. Thus identifying and managing these social and emotional problems are as appropriate as dealing with organic diseases.

Diagnostic decision-making determines why manifestations are present. Management decision-making, on the other hand, incorporates a patient's emotional and social components into its framework and determines how plans will be implemented.

The Structure of Management Decision-Making

Management decision-making seeks to set a course by defining objectives for identified problems. These objectives then guide the formulation of plans.

General objectives that can be applied to ill children for successful adaptation of medical problems are (1) to provide optimal medical intervention, (2) to promote the ability of the patient's family and community to provide the most supportive environment possible, (3) to enhance the patient's self-esteem and self-image as a competent, independent person, and (4) to coordinate, evaluate, and revise patient care strategies.

The successful achievement of these objectives requires that clinicians be specific in their description. Consider the case of a 3-year-old boy with classic hemophilia. An objective for his care could be stated thus: "to minimize the complications of hemophilia through optimal medical management." This objective, however, lacks specificity. A better objective would be "to minimize the frequency of hemarthrosis to no more than three episodes per month." The latter is more exact and would facilitate any revision of management decisions.

Once objectives are defined, specific plans for their implementation can be stated. Family and societal assets, resources, and risk factors need to be carefully considered in formulating the methods by which objectives are to be met. To achieve the aforementioned objective, the clinician could specify the following: (1) Institute a home infusion program for factor VIII through Home Infusion Services, Inc. and (2) teach time-out techniques to the parents so that they can effectively set limits on potentially dangerous activities such as standing on chairs.

REFERENCES

1. Bates B: A guide to physical examination and history taking, ed 5, Philadelphia, 1991, JB Lippincott Co.
2. Behrman RE, Vaughan VC III, and Nelson WE: Nelson's textbook of pediatrics, ed 13, 1987, WB Saunders Co.
3. Cook CD: Assuming quality out-patient care for children, New York, 1988, Oxford University Press.
4. Feinstein AR: An analysis of diagnostic reasoning. I. The domains and disorders of clinical macrobiology, Yale J Biol Med 46:212, 1973.
5. Feinstein AR: An analysis of diagnostic reasoning. II. The strategy of intermediate decision, Yale J Biol Med 46:264, 1973.
6. Fulginiti VA: Pediatric clinical problem solving, Baltimore, 1981, Williams & Wilkins.
7. Hennekens CH: Epidemiology in medicine, Boston, 1987, Little, Brown & Co.
8. Margolis CG: The pediatric problem-oriented record. A manual for implementation, Pleasantville, NY, 1977, Docent Corp.
9. Ober KP: Uncle Remus and the cascade effect in clinical medicine: Brer Rabbit kicks the tar-baby, Am J Med 82:1009, 1987.
10. Riegelman RK: Studying a study and testing a test: how to read the medical literature, ed 1, Boston, 1981, Little, Brown & Co.
11. Tunnessen WW: Signs and symptoms in pediatrics, ed 2, Philadelphia, 1988, JP Lippincott Co.
12. Walker HK, Hurst JW, and Woody MF, editors: Applying the problem-oriented system, New York, 1973, MEDCOM Press.

10

Communication with Parents and Patients

Ruth Messinger, Philip N. Davidson, and Robert A. Hoekelman

One important goal of any diagnostic procedure is to facilitate choice of treatment and shed light on the prognosis. An extremely important component of this goal is conveying pertinent information to the parents or advocates of the child or to the child. In most clinical circumstances in which the illness is minor or carries an excellent prognosis, such information is presented straightforwardly by the diagnostician to the patient or the advocates. In those cases, however, that involve gravely ill, severely handicapped, mentally retarded, learning disabled, or emotionally disturbed children, the situation becomes far more complex for clinicians, patients, and parents. The interpretive presentation must become part of a broader counseling session that deals with feelings and emotions, as well as facts, to ensure understanding of the information being shared.

This chapter focuses on the process of information sharing with parents or patient as an extension of the diagnostic process itself. The goal of interpreting diagnostic findings is more than merely announcing technical information. The real objective in providing that information is to establish a partnership between the provider and parents that will enhance the parents' capacity to respond appropriately to their child's illness and to comply with the recommended treatment.

Recent legislative changes that mandate participation by parents in decisions about their children with special needs and that emphasize family-centered, coordinated, case-managed care make this partnership even more crucial. The Education of All Handicapped Children Act Amendment of 1987 (Public Law #99-457), for example, specifically mandates parental participation in planning the education of their offspring with disabilities.

There is no one blueprint for building the very important relationship between clinician and parents; however, interpretation of the physician's findings to parents, without unnecessary delay, is an essential part of case management, as is the need to attend to the family's expectations and questions initially and over time.

Kirkpatrick and colleagues[3] provide an in-depth analysis of the development of trust and the complicated trust-doubt-anger triangle that occurs when parents are confronted with distressing information. This triangle may be further complicated when clinicians become frustrated by their inability to cure or "save" the child, when they know there are no local resources to deal with the child's problem, or when the parents ask questions that the clinician cannot answer.

A professional-parent relationship based on the posture, "I have the information and I know what's best for your child," represents a basic misinterpretation of the kind of relationship between parent and clinician that is necessary when information about a complex and threatening illness has to be shared. Whereas diagnosis and treatment are biomedical, psychosocial, or educational matters, their presentation to parents is decidedly nonmedical—such presentation is itself a psychosocial process of interpersonal communication. It is inappropriate to assume that simply "having the information" or knowledge about "what's best" for the child is sufficient for communicating diagnostic, therapeutic, and prognostic information to the parents.

Myers[5] cautions that to communicate effectively, clinicians must maintain a flow of information between parents and themselves; simply telling parents the facts of an evaluation does not guarantee that they will hear or understand. Fuller and Geis[1], Lynch and Staloch[4], and Triggs and Perrin[6] agree that clinicians must communicate with the parents, and the parents with them, for an understanding to be achieved. Such communication can be described in general terms, but its effective implementation depends on careful individual planning and a reasonable investment of time.

The box on p. 136 outlines a method for conducting an interpretive conference. The format outlines four major steps, each equally important, that are essential for an effective outcome. It is applicable when the child is evaluated by the clinician alone (physician, nurse, psychologist, social worker, or educational specialist) or when several professionals have been involved as members of an interdisciplinary team in the diagnostic evaluation.

PREPARATION FOR AN INTERPRETIVE CONFERENCE

The interpretive conference must be planned beforehand, to ensure that the conference will achieve its purpose. The conference should occur as soon as possible after the examination and testing of the patient. The clinician who conducts the conference is best prepared, both emotionally and cognitively, immediately after the last visit or staffing conference, and parents are anxious to hear about the outcome of the evaluation as soon as possible.

If more than one professional is involved in the conference, the basic aim should be to establish maximum communication

Interpretive Conference Format Outline

I. Entry pattern
  A. Review of evaluation procedures conducted
  B. Parents' and child's perceptions
  C. Restatement of parental concerns
    1. Main worry
    2. Additional concerns
II. Presentation of findings
  A. Encapsulation: brief overview
  B. Reaction by parents and patient
  C. Detailed findings
    1. Reactions to normal test results
    2. Reactions to abnormal test results
III. Recommendations—only after time has been allowed for reactions
  A. Restatement of concerns with both parents
  B. Recommendations—one at a time
  C. Reactions after each recommendation
  D. Sharing with the child
IV. Summary
  A. Repetition of findings, in varied wording if possible
  B. Restatement by parents or patient
  C. Planning for future contacts

between parents and professionals while this expertise is available to ensure that most parental questions can be effectively answered. With certain conditions, such as mental retardation and learning or emotional disorders, the physician may not be included in the conference or may not be the primary spokesperson. In these circumstances the psychologist, special educator, or social work clinician might serve that role.

There are instances in which the physician is viewed by the parents as an authority figure. The implication of this perception is that the credibility of a team that does not include the physician may be impaired. On the other hand, the physician need not automatically be cast in the role of leader at an interpretive conference unless the bulk of the information to be discussed is biomedical. In no case should the interpretation of technical material to parents be left in the hands of nonprofessionals or professionals whose lack of expertise could lead to parental misunderstanding. Also, the information should not be revealed by someone who did not participate in the diagnostic work-up.

Once the team members have been selected, they should meet long enough to organize the conference, following the outline in the box to the left. This planning session should allow enough time to ensure that all the team members agree on the major information to be shared with the parents and that all terminology is understood. Team members should also select a leader who will structure the conference. This is of paramount importance because organization of the conference is the key to satisfactory communication. The leader's responsibility is to control the flow of information from professionals to parents, and vice versa to ensure two-way communication. *Control* implies not only organization but also a certain empathic sensitivity for the parents' feelings and reactions, so that emotional highs and lows can be adequately recognized, permitted, and dealt with, without the purpose of the conference being disrupted.

The clinician who is to present the information alone also should plan the presentation, following the same procedures recommended for the team. Preparation is especially important for individual presentations because the individual has a more difficult task of control than does the group once the conference has begun. In this circumstance the clinician must continuously play the role of spokesperson, without having the chance to listen to another professional present information while organizing his or her own thoughts or "picking up" on points that others have not made clear or have not made at all.

CONDUCTING THE CONFERENCE

Entry Pattern

The beginning of the interview often sets the tone for what follows. It is assumed that planning has included those physical requirements that create an empathic climate, privacy, and freedom from interruption.

A review of what has been done diagnostically should be shared with a minimum of technical jargon so that parents will not be intimidated when asked to discuss their "main worry." During such a discussion a "hidden agenda" often surfaces, related either to the cause of the problem or to the problem itself. Therefore, before the information is presented to the parents, the parents' perception of the child and the child's current situation should be sought. For example, the practitioner might ask both parents, "How do you see Mary's problem today?" Even if both parents have accompanied their child throughout the evaluation, each may have different knowledge about and reactions to what is happening. This also is an appropriate time to ask what they already have been told of their child's condition by others.

Presentation of Findings

Dwelling on technical data that do little to enhance the parents' understanding of their child's disorder accomplishes nothing and may interfere with establishing good professional-parent communication. Such data only serve to confuse, rather than clarify, the parents' concerns. When several different tests have been done in a lengthy, technical evaluation, it is especially helpful for parents to understand that the data presented summarize the results of all those tests.

Some parents need a name for their child's illness or problem. If labels have not already been used by others, they may well be in the future. Most parents want honest appraisals and will resent ambiguous assurances that border on deception. For example, if a child has leukemia, the parents should be told that that is the diagnosis rather than given vague terms such as blood dyscrasia or bone marrow dysfunction to explain their child's illness.

The practitioner(s) should focus on the parents' own perceptions of their child when explaining findings, particularly as these may relate to their experiences with other children. Age or grade equivalents rather than ratio scores are useful when it is necessary to convey the presence of developmental delay or immaturity. For example, the clinician should say, "Your daughter seems in many ways to behave more like a 10-year-old than a 15-year-old," instead of saying, "Your daughter has an IQ of 55." It is clearer to say, "Susan can read single words as well as most of the children in her fifth grade class, but she has difficulty storing and then applying her math facts; in math, she works more like a first grader," rather than, "Susan's test scores show scatter."

It often is said that after the parents hear the bad news, they hear very little else. For this reason the actual presentation should begin with areas of strength or normality. Abnormal findings, stated frankly but gently, should be restated more than once, and by using different words to convey the same findings. Indeed, Gesell and Armatruda[2], in emphasizing the relationship between empathy and honesty, have stated: "No one can impart a grave diagnosis properly who cannot imagine the nature of the sorrow involved." Parents should be encouraged to react to the diagnosis of the problem, and their feelings, including the anger that is often directed at the clinician, should be accepted. Responses that reflect shock, guilt, bereavement, and inadequacy frequently are seen in various intensities and combinations. Communication at this level also is influenced by any sociocultural and educational differences between the professionals and the parents.

Recommendations

Specific information should be shared at a pace that can be handled emotionally and cognitively. Parents seldom feel comfortable asking for clarification, but if they are asked to restate their "main worry" and other worries, the practitioner's recommendations can be made meaningful and relevant. Parents usually find it helpful to receive recommendations that include, among other things, communication with other parents with a similar problem and referral elsewhere for help.

Recommendations are not complete until the interpreter and both parents are able to decide what will be communicated to the child and who will do it. Parents' wishes and the cognitive and emotional development of the child are important considerations in this very important issue.

SUMMARY

After recommendations have been shared and before termination of the session, findings should be highlighted once again. One successful method for obtaining feedback is to ask parents to restate what they heard and what decisions were made. This provides the professional with the parents' perception and understanding of the problem and allows for further clarification if necessary.

Often more than one interpretive session is indicated. This can be planned by arranging for parents to contact the clinician by telephone (at a definite time) when they have had time to think about and react to the information that was shared or when further questions and concerns arise. The session should be terminated only after the clinician has stated a willingness and an ability to participate in a therapeutic alliance with the parents.

Discussion of diagnostic findings is a dynamic process that is an initial step in building a therapeutic milieu. The model presented here organizes a typically complex, often unwieldy, process that can easily end in a disastrous interaction between the professional and the parents and decrease chances for successful therapeutic intervention with the patient. If the clinical findings, diagnosis, and prognosis are clearly presented during the conference, two-way communication will be facilitated because both the professional and the parents can identify the limits of the situation and focus on the problems that can be dealt with successfully. This method of imparting information enhances the professional-parent relationship and facilitates immediate and future communication and compliance with recommendations.

REFERENCES

1. Fuller R and Geis S: Communicating with the grieving family, J Fam Prac 21:139, 1985.
2. Gesell A and Armatruda C: Parent counseling in developmental disabilities. In Knobloch H and Pasamanick B, editors: Developmental diagnosis, Hagerstown, Md, 1974, Harper & Row, Publishers, Inc.
3. Kirkpatrick K, Hoffman I, and Futterman EH: Dilemma of trust: relationship between medical care givers and parents of fatally ill children, Pediatrics 54:169, 1974.
4. Lynch EG and Staloch NH: Parental perceptions of physicians' communication in the informing process, Ment Retard 26:77, 1988.
5. Myers B: The informing interview, Am J Dis Child 137:572, 1983.
6. Triggs EG and Perrin E: Improving communication about behavior and development, Clin Pediatr 28:185, 1989.

SUGGESTED READINGS

Able-Boone H, Dopecki PR, and Smith MS: Parent and health care provider communication and decision making in the intensive care nursery, Child Health Care 18:133, 1989.

Fletcher AB and Saren AV: Communicating with parents of high-risk infants, Pediatr Annal 17:477, 1988.

Greenberg LW et al: Giving information for a life-threatening diagnosis, Am J Dis Child 138:649, 1984.

Johnson SH: Ten ways to help the families of a critically ill patient, Nursing 1:50, 1986.

Stone D: A parent speaks. Professional perceptions of parental adaptation to a child with special needs, Child Health Care 18:174, 1989.

Turnbull AP and Turnbull HR, editors: Parents speak out: Then and now, Columbus, OH, 1985, Merrill.

11

Cultural Issues in Primary Pediatric Care

Karen Olness

You are a resident at a Children's Hospital in the United States. A 2-year-old Lao child (recently arrived in the United States) is hospitalized for treatment of meningitis. Each morning you see sharp knives sticking out between crib slats. Nursing staff are very concerned. They remove the knives repeatedly and speak to the parents about the accident hazard, but each time the knives are replaced within hours.

• • •

You are a middle-aged pediatrician working in the outpatient department of a large county hospital. A Hmong child is brought in with a cold and fever. You conduct a thorough examination, including otoscopy, and diagnose otitis media. Through the interpreter you prescribe amoxicillin and arrange for a follow-up appointment. Two days later the child, who is still febrile, returns in the company of 10 adult relatives and the interpreter. You begin an examination. However, when you reach for the otoscope, the interpreter says that the family requests that you not use it.

• • •

You are working in a small group practice and have many Mexican-American families as clients. One of the nurse assistants is Mexican-American, and she brings her children to the practice for well-child care. She is well-liked by families and colleagues within the practice. One day she mentions that her 4-year-old son is ill and asks to leave early. You offer to see him, and she replies that he has "empacho," a gastrointestinal illness, and that she is taking him to see a healer in the family. She says that "empacho" cannot be cured by conventional medical treatment.

Ways to Develop Cultural Sensitivity

1. Recognize that cultural diversity exists.
2. Demonstrate respect for people as unique individuals, with culture as one factor that contributes to their uniqueness.
3. Respect the unfamiliar.
4. Identify and examine your own cultural beliefs.
5. Recognize that some cultural groups have definitions of health and illness as well as practices that attempt to promote health and cure illness, which may differ from the provider's.
6. Be willing to modify health care delivery in keeping with the patient's cultural background.
7. Do not expect all members of one cultural group to behave in exactly the same way.
8. Appreciate that each person's cultural values are ingrained and therefore very difficult to change.

Modified from Stulc DM: The family as a bearer of culture. JN Cookfair: Nursing process and practice in the community, St Louis, 1990, Mosby–Year Book, Inc.

The above examples represent the types of cross-cultural situations encountered by pediatricians. As they become familiar with the particular belief guiding the placement of knives or the use of an otoscope or the diagnosis of "empacho," they learn how to cope with these situations. More complex cross-cultural issues are those never manifested overtly by clients; they can result in noncompliance, the seeking of another physician, or misinterpretation of the diagnosis and treatment. The goal of transcultural medicine, now taught in many medical schools, is not to familiarize physicians with all cultural issues related to medicine, but rather to sensitize physicians to different cultural beliefs (see box). It is hoped that they may take into account different expectations regarding their roles and different explanations for disease that evolve from varying cultural beliefs.

American child health professionals have more cross-cultural issues to consider than child health professionals in any other country, and they receive less guidance and preparation for these issues than many of their foreign colleagues. American child health providers encounter cross-cultural issues when diagnosing and treating families who are newcomers to the United States,[11] whose cultural heritages related to parents or grandparents who immigrated to the United States, and who have a tendency to change practice locales. In the future it is likely that the services of American child health experts will be required increasingly in Third World areas[6,9] where 87% of the world's babies are born. It is also likely that cross-cultural issues will become more important.

DEFINITIONS

Americans living in urban areas encounter cultural differences every day and may be unaware of them as they work, shop, and play. Culture, cultural norms, and one's perception of social self all play a part in the way reality is defined. The term *social self* is the way individuals perceive or present themselves to others. It includes whether individuals accept all or part of the culture or subculture they are in and how they project that acceptance or rejection to those around them. The term *culture* is defined as a way of life for a group of people—how they work; how they relax; their values, prejudices, and biases; and the way they interact with one another. This involves ethical and moral or traditional principles of a given society—termed *cultural norms*. Cultural norms are usually unwritten but, nevertheless, are understood as the rules by which a culture functions. People are expected to abide by these unwritten rules or norms. When they violate these, they may be criticized or ostracized by others within the culture. Cultural norms include unwritten definitions about what is health and what is sickness, what is abnormal, and what is not.

Culture of the Workplace

A popular current phrase is "the culture of the workplace." Managers use this phrase often; yet those within a work environment are not provided with guidelines for assessing one's own cultural norms and how they may fit or conflict with the culture of a workplace. It is possible for a pediatrician to feel comfortable in a children's hospital (i.e., workplace), whether that pediatrician is American or French or Ethiopian, but to feel distinctly out of place in social, recreational, or political aspects of that society. The workplace culture often becomes the principal and most comfortable culture for health professionals regardless of their own ethnic background, age, sex, or linguistic abilities.

Cross-cultural discomforts in the pediatric workplace may arise from efforts to communicate with families who have different cultural norms.[5,13] The child health professional may feel uncomfortable in spite of efforts to be nonjudgmental, because cultural norms are powerful determinants of our perceptions. Furthermore, medical training itself is an enculturating process leading one to hold the same values as one's medical peers.

Explanations of Disease: Cultural Variations

Namboze noted that cultural beliefs about disease causation in Ganda society fall under the following categories: magical, supernatural, infectious, and hereditary.[20] She notes that some of these beliefs are beneficial and can be included in health teaching. Others are harmless and best left alone by child health professionals; some cultural practices, however, are harmful.

It is well-known that many ethnic groups within the United States bring their ill children to both pediatricians and traditional healers within the community.[14,21] Special ceremonies, herbal remedies, chanting, and prayer are often prescribed by the latter. It is unusual for the family to share this information with their pediatricians unless the pediatrician is of the same ethnic group, speaks the same language, or has a long-standing, trusting relationship with the family. It should be noted that well-educated American parents may purchase vitamins, minerals, and food supplements at health food stores or consult chiropractors for their children and also may not inform their pediatricians about all treatments being used.

CULTURAL ASSESSMENT

Appraising a patient or parent's cultural beliefs, values, and customs is an essential part of health assessment[24] (Table 11-1). In Leininger's opinion, a cultural assessment is as important as a physical or psychological assessment.[15] Cultural assessments can be used to understand behavior that could be interpreted as negative or noncompliant, as in the case of the Laotian family placing knives between the crib slats.

It is important to remain sensitive to individual differences within the cultural groups while gathering information concerning a particular family: it is important not to make assumptions from the stereotypes. Problems arise when a negative attitude comes from these erroneous assumptions. For example, although alcoholism is prevalent in many Native American tribes, it would be a poor assumption to believe that any Native American treated is an alcoholic.

Developing a false sense of cultural knowledge can impede the practitioner from learning specific aspects about a particular culture. An accurate understanding of several cultures would certainly take an anthropologist years of study. The best recommendation is to review the available literature and interview colleagues who are members of a specific cultural group. Observation and interview are two useful tools when assessing cultural background.[24] Tripp-Reimer, Brink, and Saunders present several aspects to the cultural assessment that involve:[30]

1. Ethnic group affiliation and racial background
2. Major values and beliefs
3. Health beliefs and practices
4. Religious influences or special rituals
5. Language barriers and communication styles
6. Parenting styles and role of the family
7. Dietary practices

Ethnic Group Affiliation and Racial Background

Racial background refers to specific physical and structural characteristics. These characteristics, which are transmitted genetically, distinguish one group from another. Some diseases are more prevalent for genetic reasons in certain racial or ethnic groups, such as sickle cell anemia in African Americans and Tay-Sachs disease in families of Ashkenazi Jewish origin. It is also important to note that many ethnic minority groups are overrepresented in the lower socioeconomic class in American society.[2] This unfortunate fact makes it difficult to differentiate between cultural and poverty-related behaviors. Increased vulnerability to disease because of overcrowded conditions and poor nutrition contribute to this situation.[24]

Major Values and Beliefs

Values, present in all cultures, describe views on how members of a particular group should think, act, and behave.

Table 11-1 *Characteristics of Culturally Diverse Families**

ORIGIN	ETHNIC AFFILIATION/RACIAL BACKGROUND	MAJOR VALUES/BELIEFS	HEALTH BELIEFS/PRACTICES
Eastern Asian	Pacific Islands, Japan, China, Phillipines, Korea, Vietnam, Laos Characteristics include Mongolian spots or irregular areas of deep-blue pigmentation, commonly seen in sacral/gluteal regions. Lactase deficiency is common.[4] Sensitive to alcohol, characterized by hypotension, tachycardia, and bronchial constriction in Japanese.[8]	Dignity paramount; important to "save face." Emotions should be controlled to think logically and to judge objectively. *Tendency to keep problems to themselves.*	Disease is caused by imbalance between opposing forces of yin and yang. Disharmony results from improper care of body or unhappiness with oneself or society; can result in disease. *Balance is disrupted by blood being drawn for tests. Therefore, there is a reluctance to cooperate. Problem: when herbal medicines are taken along with prescribed medications, effects are unknown but patients should be warned that one might weaken the other.*
Hispanic	Puerto Rican, Cuban, Mexican, and South and Central American. Ancestry can be Aztec and Mayan, Spanish, and African blacks. *Although some pride themselves on "mixed" descent, others do not.*	Loyalty to family is more important than individual needs. Belief: humans have very little control over their future; they stress the "will of God."	Health is considered a gift from God; illness is punishment for wrongdoing. Cure is sought from *curanderos* (folk healers) who use prayer, ritual, and laying on of the hands. Less common disorders are will of God. *Health is considered a balance among the four humors of the body* (blood, phlegm, black bile, and yellow bile). "Hot" diseases require "cold" treatment and vice versa. For example: Penicillin is considered "hot" and may not be taken if patient has fever. *Noncompliance results.*
Native American	400 Indian tribes in United States and Canada; more than 280 reservations. No one language or style of dress.	Respect for harmony between humans and nature, generosity, sharing of possessions, personal integrity and bravery, brotherhood, compassion for others. Competitive behavior discouraged.	Health is a state of harmony between humans and nature. Illness is caused by witchcraft, violation of taboos, possession by spirits, loss of soul, disease or object intrusion into the body.[31] Prevention may involve wearing a talisman or carrying a special sack of herbs.
African American	Heterogeneous group, the majority of whom are descendents of people from West Africa (formerly Ivory Coast). *Sickle cell anemia is common in blacks, along with glucose-6-phosphate dehydrogenase (G6PD) deficiency.*	Orientation toward the present rather than the future, *implications for preventive health maintenance.* Orientation to time is flexible in terms of schedules and appointments. Needs of family are valued over punctuality.	Health beliefs for low-income black Americans are described as a blend of elements from Africa, folk medicine, selected aspects of modern scientific medicine, with others of Christianity, voodoo, and magic. Southern communities use roots, herb potions, oils, powders, tokens, rituals, and ceremonies. Prayer is used as a method of treatment because illness is a punishment for failure to abide by God's rules.

*It is very important to use this chart as a guideline for information concerning culturally diversified families rather than as a set of restrictions and rules. Suggested readings and references along with patient/family interviews will be helpful in obtaining more information about a particular group of people. Potential problems are set in italics.

Data from Stulc DM: The family as a bearer of culture. In Cookfair JM: nursing process and practice in the community, St Louis, 1991, Mosby–Year Book, Inc.

Table 11-1 *Characteristics of Culturally Diverse Families—cont'd*

RELIGIOUS INFLUENCES	LANGUAGE BARRIERS/COMMUNICATIONS STYLES	PARENTING STYLES/ROLE OF THE FAMILY	DIETARY PRACTICES
Eastern Asian			
Families may practice Buddhism, Confucianism, Taoism, or "Western" religions (Judaism or Christianity). Confucianism stresses duty toward others. Taoism self-realization through harmony, which influences followers to avoid conflict. Buddists believe their present lives predetermine their destiny. Death is accepted as a natural part of the life cycle. Many prefer to die in their own home. Belief: a person who dies outside of the home will become a wandering soul with no place to rest.)	May smile or laugh to mask emotions or nod "yes" even when they disagree. To question authority figures or to look directly into eyes is considered sign of disrespect. Eastern Asians may wait silently rather than ask questions because they believe the health care provider will know best. *Use of touch through handshaking is uncomfortable;* should be avoided unless the patient offers first. Needs permission before touching head. (Belief: head is sacred part of body). Disrespectful to point toe in someone's direction or show bottom of shoes, while crossing legs. (Belief: foot is the lowliest part of the body.) Many Eastern Asians will offer food or drink; it is disrespectful not to accept. Wait until patient partakes first.	Extended family may live together. In more traditional families, the father is the authority figure. Early childhood parenting is permissive. Infants seldom cry. Feed on demand. Weaning takes place later than in Anglo-American infants. Parents may allow children to sleep with them. At age 5 or 6, sterner discipline in which obedience is stressed begins. Physical and nonphysical disciplinary techniques (scolding and shaming) are implemented. Aggression (fighting) is disapproved of and admonished. The mother is the primary disciplinarian and plays the major role in child-rearing.[26]	Rice is the main starch. Milk is not readily consumed because a taste for it has not been acquired. *Possible lactose intolerance. Calcium acquired through soybeans, small bony fish, sesame seeds, and tofu.*
Hispanic			
Approximately 85% to 90% are Catholic.[18] Priest plays important role as spiritual leader and adviser.	Spanish is the predominant language. *Translators should be same sex as patient because modesty is valued and may make sexual discussion uncomfortable.* Touch is an acceptable form of expression and may be used among friends and family through hugging, kissing, and holding hands.	Strong sense of family exists. Many live in extended families. Communities are paternalistic, so men must be considered in all decisions; however, they are minimally involved in child care. Children are highly valued. Parents provide much physical attention. Independence is encouraged in boys; girls are protected. *Respect for authority figures may cause adults to feign agreement or understanding.* Attitude that "problems" should stay within family.	Basic staples: rice and beans, along with corn, fruits such as green bananas, and chilis. Diet is high in vegetable protein, carbohydrates, smaller amounts of animal protein and calcium.[18] *Hispanics see fat babies as a sign of good health.* Putting additional cereal in bottle is a common practice. *Consider "hot" and "cold" foods in diet is a part of treatment.* Believe that "hot" foods are more easily digested than "cold."[7] (Chili peppers, grains, kidney beans, alcoholic beverages, beef, lamb.)

Continued.

Table 11-1 *Characteristics of Culturally Diverse Families—cont'd*

RELIGIOUS INFLUENCES	LANGUAGE BARRIERS/COMMUNICATIONS STYLES	PARENTING STYLES/ROLE OF THE FAMILY	
Native American			
Religion plays an integral part. Mountains, rivers, and all geographical features considered sacred.	Many different languages exist. Many tribes value nonverbal language. Periods of silence might mean one is becoming sensitive to environment or gathering thoughts for greater impact when speaking. Do not value individuals who hurry speech, interrupt, and interject. Sensitive to nervous mannerisms. Appreciate hand shake and eye contact. Unwavering eye gaze should be avoided because it is viewed as insulting.	Clan membership is inherited through the mother. Elders are respected. Parents value children highly. Children are seldom disciplined by the raising of the voice or by use of physical force. Parents instill respect not only for elders but also for worthy objects within nature.	Foods may be used in ceremonies to ward off illness or to regain health. Delaware Indians prohibit eating meat during a febrile illness. One restriction, such as cow's milk, is based on prevalent lactose intolerance.[35] Corn, squash, and beans are typical staples.
African American			
After the Civil War, religion provided support for struggle with poverty, unemployment, and overcrowded living. Leadership often attained through church roles. Ministers play an important role in community and provide support during stress.	Health care providers from dominant white cultures create barriers and prevent effective communication. Attempts to imitate stereotypical and stylized "black English" may be perceived as mockery and should be avoided.	Close-knit circle of relatives and family is the norm; all participate in child rearing. Thus structure is seen as buffer from stress.[28] Socialization of black children can pose special challenges.[1,34] "To raise a black child without any notion that he is viewed differently because of race would be disastrous."[34] The child's individuality is highly valued. First-born children tend to receive more mothering. Adolescent girls are encouraged to accept more responsibilities; teenage boys are given freedom from responsibility.	Salt pork as a seasoning is common and greens such as collard, mustard, chard, and kale are common. Vinegar and hot peppers are condiments. Boiling and frying are the main method of preparation. *Hypertension and strokes cause high mortality among black Americans, with men 15.5 times more affected than their white counterparts.*[29]

Variation in these values is thought to be one of the most important differences among cultures.[10]

Health Beliefs and Practices

Viewpoints on health and healing vary from group to group. The basic definition of illness stems from a dominant American culture and is based on Western scientific thought, which views illness as a breakdown in a body part because of invasion by an organism.[24] Extreme effort is necessary to see illness and healing from a different perspective. Sensitivity is important because a lack of it can affect patient safety. The issue of pain is dealt with in Zborowski's classic study. While the dominant American culture values stoicism and nonemotional expressions of pain, other cultures may express pain through screaming, moaning, and verbal complaining.[36] An understanding of these differences is essential in treatment.

Religious Influences or Special Rituals

The dominant culture has separated "church and state" for so many years that it is quite common to separate those entities in health care as well. However, for many cultures, religion still holds a strong influence on beliefs concerning health and illness, death, and treatment. It is important to assess the role of significant religious persons during those times while dealing with culturally diverse families. More important for the pediatrician, the child may neither adhere to nor fully understand all the implications behind these decisions and beliefs; thus it is important to deal with the family as a whole and to integrate their religious beliefs when dealing with these issues.

Language Barriers and Communication Styles

Determining which language is spoken at home is essential in assessing the culture.[24] Also important is the knowledge that although the family and child may speak English, their words and understanding, especially of cognitive expression, may be limited. It is recommended that an interpreter accompany the primary caregiver when explaining potentially complex topics. Assessing a family's ability to read and write in English is also important.

Nonverbal communication may have different meanings in different cultures. Many Eastern–Asian–Americans nod out of respect, not necessarily out of understanding. Some behaviors can lead to alienation and eventually withdrawal; thus, their meanings are essential in keeping communication open. In Bulgaria, one nods the head to mean "no" and moves the head back and forth to denote "yes" (the opposite of Westerners)!

Parenting Styles and Role of Family

Understanding that "parenting is neither good nor bad in any culture, simply different," is the basis of acknowledging differing cultures' attitudes toward the family.[3] It is inaccurate to assume that the dominant American culture has all the answers when it comes to parenting. While the dominant American culture may value independence in children, another culture may value submissiveness.[24] Attitudes toward family members vary with each culture. Culture will address how different members' advice is held and whether those members are involved in decisions. Culture will also affect the value held on children, family structure, and gender.

Dietary Practices

Diet is an integral part of a person's culture. Dietary practices can include not only preferences and dislikes of particular foods but also food preparation, consumption, frequency, time of eating, and utensils used. When a prescribed diet is part of a patient's treatment, it is essential to assess the cultural influences involved. Consulting a nutritionist, a cultural informant, or colleagues of various ethnic backgrounds can be helpful.

In Table 11-1, four different cultures are outlined according to seven points of assessment. There is a tendency to assume that all members of a similar cultural background share commonalities, such as language, religion, and viewpoints.[27] Knowing the differences of the backgrounds within the different cultures is essential to becoming sensitive to cultural assessments.

HOW PEOPLE INTERACT: EXPECTATIONS FOR APPROPRIATE BEHAVIOR

Perhaps, in a century, all people of the world will share a common culture with respect to appropriate interactions. The U.S. population has scores of views regarding appropriate interpersonal interactions.[16] More than common language is required to develop a consensus regarding, for example, eye contact, touching, personal space or territory, appearance, gestures, use of the voice, greetings, partings, and facial expressions. Even responses to pain vary among different cultural groups, including subcultures in the United States.[12] Most humans tend to use the rules (regarding these interactions) developed from childhood cultural experiences. Complicating this within the United States is that chaotic living situations for children may not provide models for appropriate interpersonal interactions. Young children who watch television a great deal and who are unable to distinguish what is real from what isn't (acting) often imitate unusual or inappropriate interpersonal interactions.

In diplomatic circles there are norms, some of them written, with respect to communication. Diplomats are encouraged to learn about cultural norms within their host country—for example, who can shake hands, how close to another one stands at a reception, and how much eye contact is allowed. Yet diplomats make mistakes and are, therefore, misinterpreted. American child health professionals who interact with peers from other cultures should study cultural norms before working with foreign colleagues, whether in this country or theirs. Visitors from East Africa and Southeast Asia often complain that they find American friendliness superficial. The immediate pleasant friendliness of Americans would represent a more advanced stage of personal intimacy and friendship in their cultures, and they are offended when they discover that it does not necessarily reflect depth. They also find it difficult to accept gifts from Americans because, in many cultures, gifts are only in exchange for something or to acquire an advantage. Direct expression of feelings is inappropriate and considered bizarre in many cultures. In Thailand, for example, one turns anger toward another object, either animate or inanimate, called "prachot." This is done consciously to alert the person (who is the object of one's displeasure and annoyance) to how the injured party feels. In Southeast Asia, avoiding confrontation is considered positive and expressing anger, hatred, and annoyance overtly is considered negative.

There are a number of training programs to increase sensitivity among people toward varying cultural norms and values. Pediatricians who plan to work in other cultures may benefit from a game ("Bafa-bafa") in which participants are divided into two groups and provided with values, expectations, and customs of a new culture.[23]

PERCEPTUAL DIFFERENCES AMONG CULTURES

Perceptual differences among various groups of humans relate not only to group beliefs, customs, and experiences but also to differences in sensory systems that may have evolved in response to the need for individual survival or to society's needs. These are well-documented differences in auditory, visual, musical, and tactile skills and may relate to differences in eye-hand coordination, information processing, and language and spatial perceptions.

Some of the differences may be genetic, but others reflect the emphasis, focus, and practice of a skill within a culture. For example, an infant's perceptual abilities are modified by listening to a particular language. Syllables, words, and sentences used in all human languages are formed from a set of speech sounds called phones. Only part of the phones are used in any particular language. Young infants can discriminate nearly every phonetic contrast, but this broad-based sensitivity declines by 1 year of age.[32] Adults have difficulty discriminating phones that do not connote meaning in their own native language and thus are handicapped when learning a new language. English-speaking natives have difficulty in perceiving the difference between two "k" phonemes used in Thai. Japanese speaking adults have difficulty distinguishing between the English /ra/ and /la/. Adults who learn another language early but who do not practice the language as they mature may lose their ability to differentiate among its phones.

Learning the language of another culture is essential to understanding that culture. Dependency on bilingual translators or interpreters is fraught with the likelihood of misunderstanding, especially in medical situations. In some cultures, the status of the interpreter will affect what information is provided by the patient and how it is prepared for the ears of the foreign health professional. If the patient is of "higher" status than the interpreter, an awkward situation can result for the interpreter. If the interpreter has little specific knowledge regarding health and medical matters, translation is less than ideal. Furthermore, abstract concepts may not translate well from English to other languages. For example, it is much more difficult to express abstract concepts in Norwegian or in Russian than in English. Many words from Western languages do not exist in Asian languages; therefore, the concepts do not exist. Similarly, some Asian concepts cannot be expressed in English. The Lao language, for example, is richer in terms of words related to family relationships than is the English language.

Many studies have demonstrated that information processing differs among cultures. For example, a study of university students from four cultures demonstrated culturally dependent differences in processing information that affected choices of color dominance.[15] Numerous studies have demonstrated cultural differences in children's preferences for colors and shapes. For example, one study demonstrated that African children clearly prefer color to form right into their adolescence.[25] Euro-American children, however, selected form over color from kindergarten age into adulthood. Language structure may determine perceptual preference with respect to form or color. For example, Navajo children demonstrate form preferences, and the Navajo language uses different labels for the same objects in different tenses. How often do child health professionals consider how information processing or preferences by a child or his or her parent may depend on the original language or cultural background? Morely has noted that information processing styles, preferences for forms and colors, and educational background must be considered in preparing health education materials for use in developing countries.[19]

ETHICAL ISSUES IN CROSS-CULTURAL MEDICINE

There are many ethical issues operative in making transcultural diagnostic and treatment decisions. These relate to communication barriers, varying explanations for disease, and different expectations regarding what is honest or valuable.

Can an American pediatrician truly explain a surgical consent form to newly arrived parents of a Southeast Asian baby?

When newly arrived refugees fear they will be returned and therefore sign anything or do anything to gain favor, is it ethical to ask them to sign a consent form to have blood drawn for clinical research?

Mental illness is defined very differently among cultures.[14,33] Is it ethical to use psychotherapy when therapist and patient are ethically unmatched?

REVERSE CULTURE SHOCK

Child health professionals who spend substantial time working in different cultures may find the culture shock when returning to the United States to be as noticeable as the shock when arriving in the new culture. In fact, a benefit of cross-cultural travel (if it goes beyond Western hotels and into indigenous communities) is that one becomes more sensitized to cultural norms. We may recognize idiosyncracies of our own cultures such as loud voices, frenetic days, instant breakfasts, direct expression of feelings, pampered pets, or written invitations to social events. We may be uncomfortable in our forays to department stores that provide too many choices.

SUMMARY

Cross-cultural issues in pediatrics affect communication, expectations, and medical explanations. Pediatricians, while enculturated by their specialty training, also have individual ethnic norms, which affect their beliefs and values. It is therefore helpful for child health professionals to learn about beliefs of their colleagues and patients.[16] Wherever there may be a strong belief in a folk explanation for the cause of an illness, pediatricians are likely to be most successful if they acknowledge the belief and attempt to work with it. When simultaneous use of a traditional and Western medical regimen is possible, and will do no harm, it is likely to facilitate long-term, trusting relationships. Awareness of cultural evolution, perceptual differences related to cultural background, and implications for decision making with respect to children is essential for child health professionals throughout the world.

REFERENCES

1. Billingsley A: Black families in white America, Englewood Cliffs, NJ, 1968, Prentice-Hall.
2. Bloch B: Bloch's assessment guide for ethnic/cultural variations. In Orque M, Bloch B, and Monrroy I, editors: Ethnic nursing care: a multicultural approach. St Louis, 1983, The CV Mosby Co.
3. Brink P: An anthropological perspective on parenting. In Horowitz J, Hughes C, and Perdue B, editors: parenting reassessed: a nursing perspective Englewood Cliffs, NJ, 1982, Prentice-Hall.
4. Chen-Louie T: Nursing care of Chinese American patients. In Orque M, Bloch B, and Monrroy I, editors: Ethnic nursing care: a multicultural approach. St. Louis, 1983, The CV Mosby Co.
5. Clark MM: Cultural context of medical practice, West J Med 139:2, 1983.
6. Colehan JL: Navajo Indian medicine: implications for healing, J Fam Prac 10:55, 1980.
7. Currier R: The hot-cold syndrome and symbolic balance in Mexican and Spanish folk medicine. In Martinez R, editor: Hispanic culture and health care: Fact, fiction, and folklore, St. Louis, 1978, The CV Mosby Co.
8. Hashizume S and Takano J: Nursing care of the Japanese American patient. In Orque M, Bloch B, and Monrroy L, editors: ethnic nursing care: a multicultural approach. St. Louis, 1983, The CV Mosby Co.
9. Jelliffe DB and Bennett FJ: Indigenous medical systems and child health, J Pediatr 57:248, 1960.
10. Kluckhohn F: Dominant and variant value orientation. In Brink P, editor: Transcultural nursing: a book of readings. Engelwood Cliffs, NJ, 1976, Prentice-Hall.
11. Knoll T: Becoming Americans, Asian sojourners, immigrants, and refugees in the western United States, Portland, Ore., 1982, Coast to Coast Books.
12. Konner M: Minding the pain, The Sciences 30:6, 1990.
13. Korbin JE and Johnston M: Steps toward resolving cultural conflict in a pediatric hospital, Clin Pediatr 21:259, 1982.
14. Krener PG and Sabin C: Indochinese immigrant children problems in psychiatric diagnosis, J Amer Acad Child Psych 24:453, 1985.
15. Leininger, M: Transcultural nursing: Concepts, theories, and practices, New York, 1978, Wiley and Sons, Inc.
16. Marsh P: Eye to eye: how people interact, Topsfield, Mass., 1988, Salem House Publishers.
17. Miller N: Social work services to urban Indians. In Green J, editor: Cultural awareness in the human services. Engelwood Cliffs, NJ, 1982, Prentice-Hall.
18. Monrroy D, Bloch B, and Orque MS: Ethnic nursing care: a multicultural approach. St. Louis, 1983, The CV Mosby Co.
19. Morley D: Beliefs and attitudes to child-rearing and disease. In Morley D, editor: Paediatric priorities in the developing world, London, 1973, Butterworths.
20. Namboze JM: Health and culture in an African society, Soc Sci Med 17:2041, 1983.
21. Olness KN: Cultural aspects in working in Lao refugees, Minn Med 62:871, 1979.
22. Schkade LL, Ramani S, and Masakazu J: Human information processing and environmental complexity—an experiment in four cultures, ASCI J of Management 8:56, 1978.
23. Shirts RG and Bafa'Ba Fa': A cross cultural simulation, Del Mar, Calif, 1977, Simile Publications II.
24. Stulc DM: The family as a bearer of culture. In Cookfair JM: Nursing process and practice in the community, St. Louis, 1991, Mosby-Year Book, Inc.
25. Suchman RG: Cultural differences in children's color and form preferences, J Social Psych 70:3, 1966.
26. Suzuki, B: The Asian American family. In Fantini M and Cardenas R, editors: Parenting in a multicultural society, New York, Longman.
27. Theirderman S: Workshops in cross-cultural health care: The challenge of "ethnographic dynamite." Journal of Continuing Education in Nursing 19(1), 25-27, 1988.
28. Thomas D: Black American patient care. In Henderson G and Primeaux M, editors: Transcultural health care. Lopec, Calif, 1981, Addison-Wesley.
29. Thompson D: Hypertension: implications of comparisons among blacks and whites. Urban Health 9, 31-33, 1980.
30. Tripp-Reimer T, Brink P, and Saunders J: Cultural assessment: content and process. Nursing Outlook, 32(2), 78-82, 1984.
31. Vogel V: American Indian medicine. In Henderson G and Primeaux M, editors: Transcultural health care. Menlo Park, Calif, 1981, Addison-Wesley.
32. Werker JF: Becoming a native listener, Amer Scientist 77:54, 1989.
33. Westermeyer J: Poppies, pipes, and people: opium and its use in Laos, Berkeley, Calif, 1982, University of California Press.
34. Williams J: The color of their skin. Parenting 3, 48-53, 1988.
35. Wilson U: Nursing care of American Indian patients. In Orque M, Bloch B, and Monrroy L, editors: Ethnic nursing care: a multicultural approach. St. Louis, 1983, The CV Mosby Co.
36. Zborowski M: Cultural components in response to pain. Journal of Social Issues 8, 16-30, 1952.

SUGGESTED READINGS

Chesney AP et al: Mexican-American folk medicine: implications for the family physician, J Fam Prac 11:567, 1980.

Fabrega H and Tyma S: Language and cultural influences in the description of pain, Br J Med Psychol 49:349, 1976.

Grouse LD: The far-away look, JAMA 244:2053, 1980.

Henderson G and Primeaux M: Transcultural health care. Menlo Park, Calif 1981, Addison-Wesley.

Klausner W: Conflict or communication, Bangkok, 1978, Business in Thailand Publications.

Lin TV: Psychiatry and Chinese culture, West J Med 139:58, 1983.

Logan B and Semmes C: Culture and ethnicity. In Logan B and Dawkin C, editors: Family-centered nursing in the community. Menlo Park, Calif, 1986, Addison-Wesley.

Lozoff B, Kamath KR, and Feldman RA: Infection and disease in South Indian families beliefs about childhood diarrhea, Human Organization 34:353, 1975.

Maduro R: Curanderismo and Latino views of disease and curing, West J Med 139:64, 1983.

Mattson S: The need for cultural concepts in nursing curriculum. J Nurs Educ 26, 206-208, 1987.

Olness KN: On "Reflections on caring for Indochinese children and youths" commentary, J Dev Behav Pediatr 7:129, 1986.

Ornstein R and Ehrlich P: New World New Mind, New York, 1989, Doubleday.

Vogel V: American Indian medicine. In Henderson G and Primeaux M, editors: Transcultural health care. Menlo Park, Calif, 1981, Addison-Wesley.

Waddell WH, Pierre-Leoni RG, and Suter E: International health perspectives, New York, 1977, Springer Publishing Company, Inc.

Westermeyer J, Tanner R, and Smelker J: Changes in health care services for Indian Americans, Minn Med 57:732, 1974.

12

Compliance with Pediatric Health Care Recommendations

Lois A. Maiman and Lance E. Rodewald

The success of outpatient therapy depends on (1) the physician's ability to diagnose the illness correctly and to offer efficacious treatment and (2) the patient's compliance with the therapeutic plan. Although the physician's role in successful therapy has been emphasized in theory, factors that influence patient cooperation are not an integral aspect of medical education. The consequences of noncompliance are seen in everyday pediatric practice, for example, wheezing children with asthma whose blood shows no detectable theophylline and children with diabetes who have repeated episodes of ketoacidosis and highly elevated hemoglobin A1c levels. Although not all therapeutic failures are due to noncompliance, the differential diagnosis in a child unresponsive to therapy should include a compliance-oriented history that indicates whether the child has taken the medication. This chapter addresses practical steps the pediatrician can take to enhance patient compliance.

Many studies have documented low rates of compliance by parents with prescribed regimens for their children. Although the rates of noncompliance vary with the characteristics of the condition, treatment, and patient, an extensive review of the literature by Sackett[42] reveals that at least 33% of the subjects in most studies fail to follow the practitioner's advice. Moreover, when the recommended action is for prevention or requires sustained behavior, as in chronic illnesses, only about 50% of patients are compliant. As Haynes[22] notes, "In an era when efficacious therapies exist or are being developed at a rapid rate, it is truly discouraging that one-half of the patients for whom appropriate therapy is prescribed fail to receive full benefits through inadequate adherence to treatment."

Dramatic evidence of noncompliance exists with regard to 10-day antibiotic regimens for otitis media and streptococcal pharyngitis. Studies[6,17,19,21] show that 40% to 80% of children do not receive the entire course of treatment; moreover, compliance is less than 50% by the fifth day of treatment.[2] Similar low rates of compliance are found in the self-management of chronic conditions such as diabetes. The importance of participation by the patient and family in the management of juvenile diabetes is widely recognized; the therapeutic regimen necessitates a continuous process of both prescriptive (e.g., administration of insulin or urine testing) and proscriptive (e.g., management of diet or exercise) behaviors. Complex regimens of long duration that require the alteration of existing behavior patterns usually are associated with inadequate levels of patient compliance, which is certainly the case with juvenile diabetes.

In reviewing the determinants of compliance, Becker and Maiman[5] describe how poor compliance creates significant barriers to effective delivery of medical care. Noncompliance weakens or invalidates the potential benefits of the prescribed regimen, and it frequently exposes the patient to additional medical tests or alternative therapies that may be duplicative or unnecessary (and that may result in iatrogenically poor outcomes). It also interferes with the pediatrician-parent relationship (e.g., dissatisfaction about poor medical outcomes resulting from noncompliance; negative reactions by pediatricians to "problem" patients), and it prevents accurate evaluations of the treatment's efficacy.

Unfortunately, research studies (many of which have focused on pediatric patients[23]) show that there are no readily observable characteristics of poorly compliant patients that might permit easy identification nor do individuals reveal their noncompliance without specific efforts by the pediatrician to assess levels of adherence. Moreover, physicians appear unable to predict their patients' likely compliance any more accurately than one could by chance.[10,15] Practitioners overestimate the compliance rates of their own patients and underestimate the compliance rates of their colleagues' patients. Furthermore, practitioners are inclined to blame noncompliance on the patient's personality, and in general they express little desire to understand the problem and little sympathy for the uncooperative patient. Studies of medical students show that their compliance-related attitudes and behaviors resemble those of patients in general.[7]

Numerous studies have shown that sociodemographic characteristics (mother's age, race, education, income, marital status) do not predict compliance. One consistent exception is the association of noncompliance with the extremes of age, possibly because young children are more resistant to taking bad-tasting medicine and elderly persons may be forgetful. Research on personality traits of the patient (e.g., illness dependency, authoritarianism, and frustration tolerance) has not found significant associations between these factors and compliance. Therefore the pediatrician must view every mother as a potential noncomplier.

STRATEGIES FOR IMPROVING PATIENT COMPLIANCE

Given the dramatic rates of noncompliance and the difficulty it causes, pediatricians need to learn about the causes of noncompliance and its cure. Although no all-purpose solution has been discovered, careful research during the past two decades has yielded substantial practical knowledge and techniques for increasing compliance in pediatric practices. This chapter discusses some major factors that contribute to noncompliance and describes steps pediatricians can take to help reduce the problem.

Providing Information

A logical starting point for influencing the likelihood of adherence to therapy is the pediatrician's instructions. Some parents will not really understand (i.e., know) what is expected of them after the visit.

Knowledge affects compliance in several ways: (1) knowledge about certain details of prescribed therapy (e.g., the duration of the regimen, dosage, and frequency of administration) is essential for correct compliance; (2) parents frequently do not possess all the information they need to follow the regimen; and (3) provision of the necessary information rarely is sufficient to produce adequate patient cooperation because of the other variables, such as poor recall or insufficient motivation on the part of the patient.

Studies by Ley and co-workers[31,32] show that patient recall declines rapidly; about 50% of the information given to patients is forgotten 15 minutes after meeting with the physician. Patients remember best what occurred during the first one third of the visit and remember more about the diagnosis than about the details of the prescribed therapy. In a study of communication between pediatricians and mothers, Korsch and co-workers[29] demonstrated inadequate maternal comprehension of terms such as "incubation period" (interpreted as instructions to stay in bed) and "lumbar puncture" (identified as draining of the lungs). Considerable variation in understanding has even been shown for terms such as "evening" and "with meals" applied to directions for administrating medications. This confusion suggests the need either to explain many of the most common medical terms or to provide substitute terms.

These findings point to several strategies for modifying features of physician-patient communication. The pediatrician should provide the parent with individualized, written instructions (preferably written in the parent's presence). The best results are obtained when the pediatrician describes the details of the regimen orally, writes them down, and reviews the written instructions. Second, the physician should emphasize the important details of the regimen and avoid causing "information overload"; general information about the disease and about the specific action of the medication is unlikely to increase compliance. Finally, detailed therapeutic instructions should be presented early in the discussion about treatment.

Changing Characteristics of the Regimen

Compliance is reduced when the regimen is complex, inconvenient, or expensive; is of long duration; or requires an alteration of the patient's life-style.[24,28,30,39] Although a particular regimen may not be modifiable, the pediatrician should consider several methods to improve compliance. The regimen can be simplified by reducing the number of medications prescribed and the number of doses given per day (if clinically appropriate) and by administering doses simultaneously when more than one medication is required. Other effective approaches include avoiding the prescription of medications that are not essential to the treatment (such as use of a decongestant with the antibiotic prescribed for otitis media) and minimizing both inconvenience and forgetfulness by matching the regimen to the parent's and child's regular daily activities.

The duration of the regimen may not be modifiable, but we suggest using the shortest regimen consistent with good medical practice. In long-term therapy, strategies for inducing a feeling of shorter regimen duration include scheduling follow-up visits in quick succession to demonstrate progress and telephoning the parent 3 to 4 days after the visit to check on progress or problems with the regimen. If life-style (e.g., diet and exercise) must be modified, Dunbar and Stunkard[16] suggest that changes be introduced one at a time, that whatever compliance is achieved be reinforced, and that the next therapeutic task be added. Finally, the physician may be able to reduce the cost of the treatment by prescribing generic drugs, refraining from prescribing unnecessary drugs, and encouraging shopping for the most economical prescription rates.

Altering Health-Related Beliefs

Current medical training does not emphasize ways to encourage patient education and motivation. Few schools attempt to teach the medical student how to identify conditions under which patients will follow advice, the methods most likely to generate effective communication with patients, or interviewing skills that will determine what the patient is concerned about, knows, or believes.

Patients' beliefs about their health, illness, and its treatment strongly influence the probability of compliance. Evidence[5] supports a health belief model, which hypothesizes that whether an individual will follow a practitioner's advice often depends on four factors: (1) *health motivation*—degree of interest in and concern about health matters in general, (2) *susceptibility*—perceptions of vulnerability to the particular illness (or to its sequelae), including acceptance of the practitioner's diagnosis, (3) *severity*—perceptions concerning the probable seriousness of the consequences, on both bodily and social dimensions, of contracting the illness or of leaving it untreated, and (4) *benefits and costs*—an evaluation of the advocated health behavior concerning its probable effectiveness in preventing or treating the condition, weighed against estimates of various barriers that might be involved in undertaking the recommended action (e.g., financial expense, physical or emotional discomfort, inconvenience, or possibility of adverse side effects).

Data emphasizing the importance of these health benefits in pediatric settings are available from studies[12,20,26] of cooperation with many different types of recommended therapies. These studies ranged from participation in screening programs to compliance with various short- and long-term medication regimens. A study by Becker and co-workers[3] indicates that mothers who are concerned about their child's illness, feel their child is vulnerable to otitis media and perceive it as a threat to the child, believe in the accuracy of the diagnosis, and have confidence in the benefits of the medication are more likely to comply with a 10-day antibiotic regimen for otitis media than mothers who don't have these traits.

These findings, including the successful role of health beliefs in compliance by adults with their own regimens, together with research results[28] demonstrating that health attitudes and perceptions can be altered, support the recommendation by Podell[39] that more attention should be paid to monitoring and motivating the patient or parents along health belief dimensions. Matthews and Hingson[36] suggest that a compliance-oriented history of health beliefs should be a routine part of the patient or parent interview. For example, the practitioner should determine whether the mother shows appropriate concern about the child's health problem, agrees with the diagnosis, perceives the child's illness as serious, believes the recommended therapy will work, fears medication side effects, or feels the regimen will be too hard to follow.

Giving attention to health beliefs during the diagnostic phase of the visit helps the practitioner determine what beliefs might cause noncompliance and what content should be emphasized in teaching. In developing a strategy for effective persuasion, the practitioner should know that simply providing the correct facts is sometimes sufficient; at other times more extensive discussion or motive-arousing appeals, such as fear, parental or family responsibility, or pride, may be required. In other instances recommendations by sources of information viewed as being credible, such as other patients (or their parents) for whom the same treatment was successful, may be beneficial. The pediatrician should encourage parents to discuss their concerns about the diagnosis or the treatment plan and to disclose *all* their worries about their child's illness and treatment.

The positive effects of practitioner awareness on patient compliance have been illustrated in controlled trials.[25,34] A recent study was designed to increase pediatrician knowledge about compliance-enhancing strategies, to increase the use of these strategies by pediatricians and to improve mothers' compliance with an antibiotic regimen for their child's otitis media.[34] One of three groups of randomly assigned pediatricians was given special 5-hour tutorials, with accompanying printed materials that emphasized the difficulties experienced by parents in complying with their child's treatment plans and possible strategies for enhancing compliance (including modifying parents' health beliefs). The second group received only the printed materials; the third, the control group, received nothing. Both educational formats produced increases in pediatrician knowledge about compliance-enhancing techniques. Mothers of children whose pediatricians were in the study group used the prescribed antibiotic regimen more correctly and consistently than did mothers of control-group pediatricians. The positive influence of physician education on patient compliance suggests that health care organizations should provide training for all staff members in compliance-oriented history-taking and other compliance-related techniques.

Improving Practitioner-Patient Interaction

Numerous aspects of practitioner-patient interaction, such as impersonality and brevity of encounter,[11,27] negatively affect patient behavior. Lack of communication, particularly communication of an emotional nature, usually is the problem. According to Davis,[15] patterns of communication that deviate from the patient's expectations of the practitioner-patient relationship are associated with a patient's failure to comply with a practitioner's advice. Such deviations include interactions in which tension is not released and in which the practitioner is formal, rejecting, or controlling, as well as interactions in which the practitioner disagrees completely with the patient or interviews the patient at length without giving subsequent feedback.

Many investigations* have shown that good pediatrician-mother interaction is associated with positive outcomes for children, including appointment keeping, problem resolution, and compliance. Frances and co-workers[20] report that a mother's compliance with a regimen prescribed for her child and her own satisfaction are increased when the affective elements of the communication are enhanced (e.g., when she feels the practitioner is friendly and understands the complaint, when her expectations from the medical visit are met, and when she receives an explanation of the diagnosis and cause of the child's illness). In another study of pediatrician-mother interaction, by Liptak and co-workers,[33] the extent of a pediatrician's awareness of maternal concerns, and the adequacy of communication, were directly related to two outcomes in well-child care: mother-child adaptation and maternal satisfaction with medical care.

How this interaction may affect compliance and parental concerns is suggested by studies of otitis media and asthma. When communication between the practitioner and parents includes agreement on the child's diagnosis and the need for follow-up visits and an explanation of the details of the regimen, compliance with administering a 10-day antibiotic regimen for otitis media and keeping the follow-up appointments was increased.[2] Further, a descriptive study by Clark and co-workers[13] of problems confronting parents of children with asthma showed that practitioner-patient communication often is inadequate. Major concerns of almost 50% of the parents were lack of information from the child's physician, difficulty in comprehending responses to questions, and lack of discussion on preventive measures.

Increasing Patient Supervision

Another important dimension of the practitioner-patient interaction concerns the amount of supervision. A variety of "before-and-after" studies[22,40] have shown increased patient cooperation when outpatient visits are increased, home visits are added, patients receive negative feedback concerning their noncompliance, and patients receive continuity of care. Methods of continually monitoring compliance include calling the parents to remind them of the regimen or the follow-up visit, requesting that empty bottles or those containing unused pills be brought to the next visit, and instructing the parents or patient to keep a record of the time and dose of daily medication administration. Monitoring blood levels of medications taken on a continuing basis, such as anticonvulsants and theophylline, also helps detect noncompliance. When techniques to measure blood levels are unavailable for a specific medication, indirect measures can be used (e.g., ascer-

*See references 2, 18, 29, 43, and 44.

taining appropriate suppression as a result of the prednisone regimen by obtaining a cortisol level in a steroid-dependent child with asthma).

A development that attempts to capitalize on and in some ways improve the relationship between practitioner and patient is the *therapeutic contract*. Lewis and Michnich[30] describe the technique by which both parties set forth a treatment goal, decide the specific obligations of each party in attempting to achieve that goal, and then set a time limit for its achievement. Studies of juvenile diabetic patients, pediatric dialysis patients, and overweight adolescents support the practitioner-patient contract as a tool for increasing patient compliance in pediatrics.

Enlisting Family Support

Members of the patient's family can remind, assist, encourage, and reinforce the patient or parent in following medical advice. A supportive family is associated with greater compliance and is especially important in long-term treatment that requires continual self-management.

For example, in studies[8,41] of weight control, investigators found that persons who were assisted by another family member in the reinforcement of proper eating behavior were more likely to lose weight and to maintain that weight loss. Similar outcomes have been noted concerning the family's influence on compliance with recommendations for obtaining immunizations and other preventive measures and for taking medications. Many studies[1,4,37,38] of family-level variables have documented relationships between the extent of patient compliance and a family's own health beliefs and the family's evaluation of the patient's illness and recommended treatment. Compliance also can be increased if the family assumes responsibility for the sick member's care and provides sympathy, support, and encouragement. Compliance is enhanced when the normal roles and patterns of the family are compatible with the patient's illness or when family members are willing to incorporate changes in their lives and environment to accommodate the demands of the illness.

However, the family also can negatively affect a member's willingness to initiate or continue care. Therefore the practitioner should carefully evaluate the role of family members in the patient's therapy and attempt to maximize their potential constructive contributions and minimize their possible destructive influences.

Using Other Health Care Providers

The physician can benefit from the compliance-oriented interventions of other health care practitioners, who can provide additional assessment, instruction, clarification, and reinforcement. Marston[35] contends that nurses, by virtue of their numbers and amount of patient contact, have the greatest potential of any group of health professionals for affecting patient health behavior. Important nursing compliance-related activities are developing patient contracts, instituting behavior modification, diagnosing or monitoring adherence levels, using health education to clarify the regimen, developing strategies to change health attitudes, and enlisting support of the patient's family and other significant persons.

A review of investigations by Canada[9] emphasizes the potential role of the pharmacist in enhancing patient compliance. Consultation with the pharmacist before hospital discharge led to a 75% reduction in a high baseline rate of deviation from prescribed drug regimens. In the case of outpatients, counseling by pharmacists (including written reinforcement of counseling information and telephone or mailed reminders when the patient's supply of medication was scheduled to run out) increased the percentage of prescriptions refilled on time and decreased the proportion of nonrefills. Suggestions for pharmacist involvement include actions to be taken if the patient fails to pick up the original prescription, written instructions on special precautions to be taken with various types of drugs, and maintenance of a patient medication profile. Implementation of these suggestions could aid in preventing overdose, allergic reactions, and adverse drug interactions, and they also could serve as a mechanism to monitor compliance.

SUMMARY

This chapter summarizes the results of a variety of studies about the problem and determinants of patient compliance. Despite Osler's observation[14] that "the desire to take medicine is perhaps the greatest feature which distinguishes man from animals," the practitioner's problem in delivering efficacious care often is not selecting a treatment regimen but rather obtaining patient—and with the child patient, parent,—cooperation with the recommended therapy.

We suggest a multifactorial approach to understanding and increasing compliance and encourage the practitioner concerned with increasing cooperation with therapies (1) to try to improve the patient's or parents' knowledge of the specifics of the regimen, reinforce essential points with review, discussion, and clearly written instructions, and emphasize the importance of the therapeutic plan, (2) to take appropriate steps to reduce the cost, complexity, duration, and amount of behavioral change required by the regimen and to increase the convenience of the regimen, (3) to obtain a compliance-oriented history of previous experiences and present health beliefs and, when it is necessary, employ strategies to modify the patient's or parents' perceptions that might inhibit compliance, (4) to improve levels of satisfaction, particularly with the practitioner-patient relationship, and encourage questions concerning the diagnosis and proposed therapy, (5) to arrange for continued monitoring of subsequent compliance to treatment (e.g., establish specific follow-up appointments and telephone reminders), (6) to enlist family support for the therapeutic regimen, and (7) to use other members of the health care team.

REFERENCES

1. Baric L: Conjugal roles as indicators of family influence on health-directed action, Int J Health Educ 13:58, 1970.
2. Becker MH, Drachman RH, and Kirscht JP: Predicting mothers' compliance with pediatric medical regimens, J Pediatr 81:843, 1972.
3. Becker MH, Drachman RH, and Kirscht JP: A new approach to explaning sick-role behavior in low-income populations, Am J Public Health 64:205, 1974.

4. Becker MH and Green LW: A family approach to compliance with medical treatment: a selective review of the literature, Int J Health Educ 18:173, 1975.
5. Becker MH and Maiman LA: Sociobehavioral determinants of compliance with health and medical care recommendations, Med Care 13:10, 1975.
6. Bergman AB and Werner RJ: Failure of children to receive penicillin by mouth, N Engl J Med 268:1334, 1963.
7. Blackwell B, Griffin B, Magill M et al: Teaching medical students about treatment compliance, J Med Educ 53:672, 1978.
8. Brownell KD et al: The effect of couples training and partner cooperativeness in the behavioral treatment of obesity, Behav Res Ther 16:323, 1978.
9. Canada AT: The pharmacist and drug compliance. In Jackett DL and Haynes RB, editors: Compliance with therapeutic regimens, Baltimore, 1976, Johns Hopkins University Press.
10. Caron HS and Roth HP: Patients' cooperation with a medical regimen, JAMA 203:922, 1968.
11. Charney E: Patient-doctor communication, Pediatr Clin North Am 19:263, 1972.
12. Charney E et al: How well do patients take oral penicillin? A collaborative study in private practice, Pediatrics 40:188, 1967.
13. Clark NM et al: Developing education for children with asthma through study of self-management behavior, Health Educ Q 7:278, 1980.
14. Cushing H: The life of Sir William Osler, vol 1, New York, 1925, Oxford University Press.
15. Davis MA: Variations in patients' compliance with doctors' orders: analysis of congruence between survey responses and results of empirical investigation, J Med Educ 41:1037, 1966.
16. Dunbar JM and Stunkard AJ: Adherence to diet and drug regimen. In Levy R et al, editors: Nutrition, lipids, and coronary heart disease, New York, 1979, Raven Press.
17. Elling R, Whittemore R, and Green M: Patient participation in a pediatric program, J Health Hum Behav 1:183, 1960.
18. Falvo D, Woehlke P, and Deichmann J: Relationship of physician behavior to patient compliance, Patient Counsel Health Educ 2:185, 1980.
19. Feinstein AR et al: A controlled study of three methods of prophylaxis against streptococcal infection in a population of rheumatic children, N Engl J Med 260:697, 1959.
20. Frances V, Korsch BM, and Morris MJ: Gaps in doctor-patient communication: patients' response to medical advice, N Engl J Med 280:535, 1969.
21. Gordis L, Markowitz M, and Lilienfeld AM: Studies in the epidemiology and preventability of rheumatic fever, IV. A quantitative determination of compliance in children on oral penicillin prophylaxis, Pediatrics 43:173, 1969.
22. Haynes RB: A critical review of the "determinants" of patient compliance with therapeutic regimens. In Sackett DL and Haynes RB, editors: Compliance with therapeutic regimens, Baltimore, 1976, Johns Hopkins University Press.
23. Haynes RB, Taylor DW, and Sackett DL: Compliance in health care, Baltimore, 1979, Johns Hopkins University Press.
24. Hellmuth GA, Johannsen WJ, and Sorauf T: Psychological factors in cardiac patients, Arch Environ Health 12:771, 1966.
25. Inui TS, Yourtee EL, and Williamson JW: Improved outcomes in hypertension after physician tutorials: a controlled trial, Ann Intern Med 84:646, 1976.
26. Johnson AJ et al: Epidemiology of polio vaccine acceptance: a social and psychological analysis, Monograph Series No. 3, Jacksonville, 1962, Florida State Board of Health.
27. Joyce CRB et al: Quantitative study of doctor-patient communication, Q J Med 38:183, 1969.
28. Kirscht JP: Research related to modification of health beliefs, Health Educ Monogr 2:455, 1974.
29. Korsch BM, Gozzi EK, and Francis V: Gaps in doctor-patient communication. I. Doctor-patient interaction and patient satisfaction, Pediatrics 42:855, 1968.
30. Lewis CE and Michnich M: Contracts as a means of improving patient compliance. In Barofsky I, editor: Medication compliance: a behavioral management approach, Thorofare, NJ, 1977, Charles B Slack, Inc.
31. Ley P: Primacy, rated importance, and the recall of medical statements, J Health Soc Behav 13:311, 1972.
32. Ley P et al: A method for increasing patients' recall of information presented by doctors, Psychol Med 3:217, 1973.
33. Liptak GS, Hulka BS, and Cassel JC: Effectiveness of physician-mother interaction during infancy, Pediatrics 60:186, 1977.
34. Maiman LA et al: Improving pediatricians' compliance-enhancing practices: a randomized trial, Am J Dis Child 142:773, 1988.
35. Marston M: Compliance with medical regimens: a review of the literature, Nurs Res 19:312, 1970.
36. Matthews D and Hingson R: Improving patient compliance: a guide for physicians, Med Clin North Am 61:879, 1977.
37. Oakes TW et al: Family expectations and arthritis patient compliance to a hand-resting splint regimen, J Chronic Dis 22:757, 1970.
38. Picken B and Ireland G: Family patterns of medical care utilization: possible influences of family size, role and social class on illness behavior, J Chronic Dis 22:181, 1969.
39. Podell RN: Physician's guide to compliance in hypertension, West Point, Penn, 1975, Merck & Co.
40. Rokart JF and Hofmann PB: Physician and patient behavior under different scheduling systems in a hospital outpatient department, Med Care 7:463, 1969.
41. Saccone AJ and Israel AC: Effects of experimenter versus significant other controlled reinforcement and choice of target behavior on weight loss, Behav Ther 9:271, 1978.
42. Sackett DL: The magnitude of compliance and non-compliance. In Sackett DL and Haynes RB, editors: Compliance with therapeutic regimens, Balitmore, 1976, Johns Hopkins University Press.
43. Starfield B et al: Patient-doctor agreement about problems needing follow-up visit, JAMA 242:344, 1979.
44. Starfield B et al: The influence of patient-practitioner agreement on outcome of care, Am J Public Health 71:127, 1981.

13

The Art of Consultation

Henry M. Seidel

The major purpose of consultation is to obtain assistance in the diagnosis, treatment, or management of a patient's problem, as well as to reassure the patient and family. Indeed, a practitioner often wants similar reassurance, sometimes for legal purposes. Unfortunately some insecure practitioners may hesitate to ask for consultation for fear of appearing incompetent. This is intolerable because the welfare of the patient cannot be compromised.

Trust is essential in the relationship between the practitioner and patient and family; it is not undermined by appropriate consultation. In fact the relationship usually is reinforced. Patients and parents appreciate and respond to a practitioner's candor in defining the areas of his or her expertise and in stating limitations. Sound communication maintains trust, whatever the consultant contributes, and it requires that the role of each participant in the process be clearly defined. These fundamental principles apply whatever the practice arrangement of the referring physician and the consultant, a health maintenance organization, a large group practice, or a fee-for-service setting.

It is necessary to distinguish between a consultation and a referral. The physician who requests a consultation is not seeking to transfer care to another physician or to share care with another physician. In some circumstances, however, the transfer of care may be appropriate or, more often, the sharing of care serves the best interests of the patient.

PRIMARY CARE PROVIDERS

The primary care provider is responsible for arranging a consultation whenever it is in the patient's best interest. The ultimate value of a consultation depends in large part on how skillfully it is managed by the primary care practitioner. The need for a consultation often arises during the stress of an acute illness, a time when the family and patient may react to the suggestion with increased anxiety about the gravity of the illness. This anxiety can be tempered by acknowledging it and by putting any underlying fears in appropriate and honest context. In addition, problems can be anticipated in choosing a consultant if there is frank discussion of skills, personalities, and cost.

The information given to the consultant by the referring physician provides the basis for a successful consultation. Any behavioral, emotional, social, and economic factors that can influence decision-making should be made clear to the consultant. Problems must be concisely stated, and individual responsibilities for the patient's continuing care should be delegated according to the competence, knowledge, and persuasive skills of the referring and consulting physicians. The primary care provider orchestrates the entire process and must be available to keep all participants fully informed in order to maintain their optimal contributions. The consultant must clearly understand the goals of the interaction and that the primary care provider's role in the decision-making process is not abdicated.

The time at which the patient returns to the referring physician must be clearly defined. The consultant may need to continue contact with the patient, however, and these visits often may parallel visits to the referring physician. When the relationship with the consultant ends, the referring physician must ensure follow-up care.

NONPHYSICIAN HEALTH PROFESSIONALS

Over the past three decades the work of the primary pediatrician has been increasingly complemented by that of nonphysician health professionals. The team of health workers that provides varied services to a significant number of patients includes nurses, nurse practitioners, and physician assistants; physical, occupational, and speech therapists; educational, developmental, and clinical psychologists; audiologists; social workers; and nutritionists. The pediatrician is responsible for understanding the resources provided by these professionals, referring patients to them when indicated, and maintaining effective communication among all involved.

The rules for communication are the same as those that govern consultation with a physician. Three-way interaction is essential when the patient needs a service that is not within the competence of the pediatrician or that requires time that the pediatrician does not have. The nonphysician health professional takes on all the responsibilities of any consultant, including that of maintaining open and respectful communication.

CONSULTANTS

The patient and family usually are anxious about the unresolved problem presented to the consultant. Concerns about illness and practical considerations of cost must be understood. The consultant should avoid demeaning the referring practitioner, because any suggestion of incompetence or error, whether verbal or nonverbal, can destroy trust among all participants. Sometimes hindsight, new information, or superior knowledge might prompt a criticism of past management. This must be constructive and also discussed, without hesitancy, with the referring physician in private. Health care decision-making should tolerate disagreement, however, because two or more valid approaches to a problem are often possible. On occasion, evidence of the referring physician's incompetence, for a variety of reasons, does surface. In such cases the needs of the patient always come first. It is a circumstance that demands honesty and delicacy but also at times requires a difficult step—the provision of information to responsible authorities in hospitals, medical societies, and licensing boards.

The consultant cannot rely solely on the observations of others. Information should be obtained independently, because the answer to a puzzle may lie in a retaken history, a discriminating observation during the physical examination, or a reevaluation of laboratory data. Reconstruction, reinterpretation, and careful attention to detail are critical.

The consultant must give prompt recommendations, either in person or by telephone. Documentation of findings and recommendations must be included on the hospital chart or in the consultant's office file and also in a letter to the referring practitioner. Information that has not been made available to the primary physician should not be shared with the patient and family. If the patient and family circumvent the primary physician and seek additional advice without his or her knowledge, an awkward or threatening situation for the primary care provider could result. The consultant must be sensitive to this while still holding the patient's needs paramount.

The pediatrician who is asked to be a consultant should be aware that many physicians who ask for consultation may not have the necessary education and training for continuing management of a given child's problem. One should be sensitive to this possibility and to the delicate issue that arises from a perception of competition between pediatricians and family practitioners. The reality here is far less than the supposition; nevertheless, it cannot be ignored. Again, the patient's needs, however, remain paramount, and the consulting pediatrician must be prepared to share care and to accept a transfer of responsibility without usurping that responsibility inappropriately.

Cost Containment

Second opinions have been suggested, particularly when surgery is being considered, as a means of ensuring an appropriate and perhaps cost-saving decision. Ideally only necessary surgery will be performed, and the expectation is that a second opinion will ensure this. Empiric evidence seems to prove the validity of this theory. There is no certainty, however, that the second opinion is more valid than the first. An obvious absurdity can ensue if the patient is subjected to the whim of an uneven number of experts on a panel to avoid a tie vote. This absurdity can be avoided if the rules of consultation are scrupulously observed and if the consultant is objective. Referring physicians should take care that no conflict of interest exists between them and the clinicians they consult. Further opinions rarely are necessary when a primary physician and a consultant communicate well with each other and, above all, keep the patient fully and appropriately informed.

Recommendations made by the consultant are not binding and may be rejected by the patient and family and referring physician. They all retain the privilege of being involved in the final decision. The consultation process does lose value if it is diluted by too many opinions, and the referring physician must see that balance is maintained. Thus optimal patient care requires the orchestrating hand of the primary pediatrician while a variety of individuals contribute their special skills to understanding and solving the patient's problems.

The accompanying boxes outline situations in which a practitioner may decide that a consultation would be in the best interests of the patient and family.

Reasons for Consultation with Physicians and Nonphysicians in a Variety of Health and Medical Disciplines

1. Uncertainty in diagnosis
2. Confirmation of diagnosis
3. Specific skill required for diagnostic process, for example:
   a. Pediatric subspecialist—to perform a variety of diagnostic techniques
   b. Radiologist to consider all the "imaging" modalities and to select them appropriately
   c. Endoscopist—to see a lesion and perform a biopsy
   d. Surgeon—to explore and remove a lesion, to obtain a biopsy specimen, or to correct problem
   e. Pathologist—to interpret the nature of the tissue removed
   f. Psychologist, psychiatrist, and mental health counselor—to search for more subjective insights
   g. Teacher and social worker—to discover aspects of patient and family life unknown to the referring physician
4. Uncertainty as to appropriate management or therapy, or both
5. Specific skill required for therapy or management, or both, for example, the variety of surgical disciplines
6. Reassurance for the patient and family or the primary pediatrician, for example:
   a. Reassurance as to the diagnosis (even in the face of certainty)
   b. Reassurance as to a suggested course of action
7. Assistance in long-term follow-up and management of chronic illness, for example:
   a. Physical therapist
   b. Occupational therapist
   c. Rehabilitationist
   d. Schoolteacher

Guidelines for Requesting a Consultation

- Be precise in stating your goals for the consultation and the information you need.
- Be aware of uncertainty in the patient and family and in yourself, and be prepared to take every step necessary to resolve it.
- Keep the needs of patient and family sharply in mind, and keep them well-informed and active in the decision-making process.
- Clarify the extent to which you want only to consult or to which you want to refer and share in the care of the patient; do not abdicate your role in decision-making.
- Do not abdicate your responsibilities for keeping informed, coordinating information, and maintaining continuity and communication with all the persons involved; this, of course, requires precise and detailed record keeping.

Guidelines for Providing a Consultation

- Be precise and prompt in providing information, using language appropriate to each of the persons involved; different professionals have different jargon, but patients have variable understanding of jargon, most often none at all.
- Keep the patient and family informed but not without parallel or prior information to the referring physician.
- Be available for sharing, but not usurping, the privilege of care for a child who is referred by someone more specifically experienced in the care of adults.
- Keep thorough records, and always provide the referring physician with a detailed consultation note; do not rely solely on spoken communication, whether in person or on the telephone.
- Define information with your own observations; accept the word of others only in rare circumstances.
- Be wary of "off-the-cuff" corridor or telephone consultation; when there is the least uncertainty, see the patient.

SUGGESTED READINGS

Balint M: The doctor, his patient, and the illness, New York, 1972, International Universities Press, Inc.

Bursztajn H et al: Medical chances: how patients' families and physicians can cope with uncertainty, New York, 1981, Delacorte Press/Seymour Lawrence, Inc.

Committee on Standards of Child Health Care: Communication with nonphysician health personnel, Evanston, Ill, April 1979, American Academy of Pediatrics.

Editorial Note: Contrasts in academic consultation, Ann Intern Med 94:537, 1981.

Stickler GB: The pediatrician as a consultant, Am J Dis Child 143:73, 1989.

Stickler GB: Telephone etiquette, Am J Dis Child 143:520, 1989.

Symposium: When the pediatrician is the consultant, Contemp Pediatr 5:96,137, 1988.

Tumulty PA: The effective clinician, Philadelphia, 1973, WB Saunders Co.

14

Assessing the Medical Literature

S. Michael Plaut

In 1974 the *New England Journal of Medicine* reported two studies of the relationship between the smoking of marijuana and levels of testosterone in young adult men.[4,5] One study reported a statistically significant dose-related relationship between these two variables, whereas the other could find no relationship at all. What is a practitioner to make of this discrepency in results? Perhaps the answer lies in the methods used in these two studies. The first study used retrospective self-reports of marijuana smoking in the subjects' normal life environment. In the second study testosterone levels were measured before, during, and after the smoking of standardized government-issued "joints" in a controlled institutional environment. Can either of these methods be considered inherently better than the other? Each study included the use of certain screening devices to minimize suspected extraneous factors that might affect the results. But were all such factors accounted for? In dealing with a value-laden topic about which the reader might have some prejudices, the interpreter must honestly ask whether personal feelings might color his or her interpretation of the data. Thus a number of factors, including logistic and methodologic limitations, the possibility of human bias, and a practitioner's knowledge of the field and its technology, are involved in the appropriate interpretation of a scientific study.

IMPORTANCE OF CRITICAL EVALUATION

"The physician," writes Dykes,[3] "will be equipped to allow the public access to high quality medical care only to the extent that he has been able to keep up with and to grasp the import of advances in the science of medicine." For a practitioner to maintain currency in his or her field requires a level of dissatisfaction with the status quo in clinical medicine and a commitment to the idea that science itself "depends for its vitality on a milieu that fosters vigorous, open dissent."[3] Beveridge[1] wrote, "Nothing could be more damaging to science than abandonment of the critical attitude and its replacement by too ready acceptance of hypotheses put forward on slender evidence." This chapter discusses factors important to the critical evaluation of research data and provides specific guidelines that may be useful in the interpretation of papers and presentations.

Limitations of Individual Studies

No matter how well conceived and designed a study may be, and regardless of how effectively it is communicated, certain necessary limitations must be taken into account in interpreting its value. Such limitations are explored in the following discussion.

Scope and Feasibility. As implied by the discussion of the two studies in the introductory paragraph, certain decisions must be made in designing a study that eventually define the nature and extent of its usefulness. The investigator may opt for the natural conditions of a field study or may choose the higher level of control afforded by a laboratory or institutional setting. Although a heterogeneous subject population allows greater generalizability of results, a homogeneous sample tends to reduce variability in the data, thus requiring fewer subjects for conclusive results. Although an investigator may wish to observe many aspects of a phenomenon, the number of variables that can be accounted for will be limited by factors such as the investigator's breadth of expertise, the amount of blood or tissue that can be feasibly collected, a subject's ability to concentrate for long periods in completing questionnaires, or the possibility that the measurement of one variable might influence the reliability of another variable.

Relevance and Application. Because an investigator must set limits with regard to the design of a study, these limits must necessarily extend to the interpretation of data and their applicability. For example, although human studies may be considered more relevant than animal studies for clinical purposes, animal studies have the advantage of allowing a measure of manipulation and control that only rarely is possible with human subjects. Any one study can investigate only a relatively small facet of the larger conceptual problem it attempts to address. Thus the ultimate value of any study depends on the replication of findings in different research settings and the synthesis of these findings into a comprehensive picture of the field of study.

Medium of Presentation. Review papers and books are the best source of comprehensive summaries of research findings. However, although such sources have the advantage of a longer perspective on a field of study, they do not provide the currency of the journal article or meeting presentation. In addition to being current, the journal paper possesses the additional advantages of procedural detail and peer review before publication. Although information presented at a scientific meeting or in a professional "throwaway" publication has a shorter time lag, it often has not undergone thorough peer review. Thus the source of a practitioner's scientific information also must be considered in evaluating its scientific merit or its practical relevance.

Human Element in Research

A second major consideration in the assessment of scientific literature is the individual contribution that each participant brings to the research process. As suggested in the aforementioned marijuana studies, cultural or personal value systems will probably color one's approach to a research area. In addition, researchers may respond to real or implied institutional pressures to produce a certain quantity of research output. Such pressures may affect many aspects of the research process, from the choice of a research question based on expediency, to excessive haste in the publication of results. An investigator's emotional investment in his or her research may be especially high in areas that might be considered "faddish" or controversial or that reflect a strong theoretic or cultural bias. Recent examples in developmental research include the areas of mother-infant bonding, hyperactivity, and intelligence testing. Even at best the knowledge of a researcher, reviewer, or reader is finite, and this limitation may become most apparent in dealing with multidisciplinary issues. As Dykes[3] has written, "Physicians must recognize the fallibility of even our species' greatest intellects . . . . The biases of eminent men are still biases."

Subjective factors may influence the evaluation of research in many ways. A few common examples are given here.

Dichotomous Thinking. Practitioners often tend to oversimplify their thinking about natural phenomena by placing the phenomena in categories rather than on continua. Thus mental illness has either a behavioral or a biologic origin, adult traits are determined either genetically or environmentally, and diseases are either physical or psychosomatic. A practitioner may be prone to think of research subjects as being either normal or abnormal, depending on the issue in question. Although such categorizations often are useful or even necessary, few biologic questions can be answered in a simplistic all-or-nothing manner. It usually is more fruitful to think in terms of the degree to which each of several factors may interact to influence a phenomenon, rather than attempting to attribute cause exclusively to one or another factor.

Overemphasis on Results and Applications. An author's interest in publication or a reader's interest in application may often lead him or her to be data oriented in conducting or evaluating research. The value of a study, however, can be determined only by examining the methods used to gather the data. Factors such as the validity of operational definitions, the appropriate use of controls, the choice of subject population, and the use of appropriate methods and procedures for collecting and analyzing data are all critical to the appropriate interpretation of results.

Conformance to Expectations. Claude Bernard (cited by Beveridge[1]) once said that "men who have excessive faith in their theories or ideas are not only ill-prepared for making discoveries; they also make poor observations." Although research papers often are written as though the results obtained were exactly as predicted in the introduction, this rarely is the case. Many scientific discoveries are made by the alert, open-minded observer of an unexpected finding. Bernard further admonishes the scientist to forget his or her hypothesis once the study begins, and the reader of a paper should do the same. As mentioned earlier, it is only by challenging one's expectations and assumptions that any scientific field can be advanced.

Assumed Attributes of Design. Readers of research papers sometimes assume that certain attributes of scientific studies are universally desirable. Such attributes include the use of control or comparison groups of subjects, the randomization of procedures, and the use of large numbers of subjects. None of these procedures, however, is necessarily of service to the research question being asked. For example, a hypothesis regarding the relationship between two characteristics (e.g., nutritional status and school performance) of a given subject population does not need a control group to be adequately tested, *unless* the prediction is that the relationship between those characteristics is not of the same magnitude in another subpopulation, as defined by age, race, sex, or whatever qualities are relevant. The absence of a control group also means, however, that the group studied cannot necessarily be considered *distinctive* on the basis of a single study. The fact that nutritional status is found to be related to school performance in a group of diabetic children cannot be considered uniquely characteristic of such children unless nondiabetic children are studied in a similar way.

Faith in Technical Complexity. Studies often appear to be more credible when highly technical procedures are described in detail. However, the fact that a standardized questionnaire or test was used to measure some aspect of social interaction or that a computer was used to analyze the data does not necessarily mean that the methods used were appropriate to the research question being asked or that the data derived from these procedures led to valid conclusions.

Practice of More Objective Appraisal. The realization that human frailties and technical limitations are a real part of the research process can sometimes tend to make a practitioner *hyper*critical of all research results. It should be apparent, however, that the cause of biomedical science would not be served by either total acceptance or rejection of all scientific endeavor. A spirit of openness, curiosity, and a healthy skepticism regarding scientific thinking are necessary no matter whose work the practitioner evaluates. This kind of attitude can make science both exciting and productive.

Role of Socially Validated Standards. It also is important to realize that many of the practices of science are determined, at least in part, by social standards within the broad community of scientists or within society itself. Thus what is now considered unethical scientific practice might not have been so 30 or 40 years ago. Other socially validated standards include authorship practices, expectations for publication frequency, levels of statistical significance that define the reliability of data, and even the use of statistical criteria for the interpretation of data. These practices not only vary with the passage of time and social events but also differ among various scientific specialities.

USEFUL KNOWLEDGE AND SKILLS

The preceding section of this chapter has emphasized the attitudinal aspects of effective research critique. In addition, certain knowledge and skills are extremely useful in the effective evaluation of research results.

Content and Methods

An important characteristic of research is that it builds on the thinking and findings of the past. Therefore some knowledge of the literature of the field in question will help determine whether the rationale behind a given study and the techniques and procedures used in conducting the study are based on current practices, controversies, or interpretations.

Minimizing Bias and "Confounds". Probably the greatest number of errors made in the interpretation of data derive from a poor understanding of the importance of instituting good operational definitions and control procedures and accounting for confounded variables in conducting any research. For example, in the study by Kolodny and coworkers[4] mentioned earlier, any statement made about differences in testosterone levels between users and nonusers of marijuana had to account for the possibility that users and nonusers of marijuana may have used other substances to a different extent than did nonusers of marijuana, inasmuch as such substances also might alter levels of testosterone. Without accounting for this possible *confound,* it would be difficult to attribute any difference between the groups to marijuana use per se. Thus by taking a good history, the investigator can control for the possible effect of substance use other than the substance of interest to the study. In addition, because this study was based on reported use of "street variety" marijuana, the *operational definition* of marijuana necessarily includes any impurities that might be contained in the joints smoked by the study subjects.

Data Presentation and Analysis. Another frequent impediment to the interpretation of scientific findings is the difficulty in understanding and interpreting statistical terms and test results. For example, the concept of *variance* is basic to the understanding of the quantitative expression of data but often is overlooked in their interpretation. Yet, as illustrated in Fig. 14-1, a practitioner's interpretation of the difference between two means must depend on the spread of individual data points around those means. The more dispersed the data are around the mean, the less certain the practitioner can be about the distinction between groups of subjects. Beveridge[1] has suggested that practitioners should try to learn at least enough about statistical methods to maintain some respect for them and to know when to consult someone else on a statistical issue. A course in basic statistics, coupled with hands-on problem-solving experience, will help the practitioner feel more at ease with these concepts and methods.

Literature Search Techniques. For some clinicians the review of scientific literature will involve reading the journals to which they subscribe and attending professional meetings. If, however, a clinician wishes to pursue any area of research in greater depth, he or she should have some knowledge of the most advanced techniques for keeping up with and researching specialized literature. In addition to a number of publications available in medical libraries or by subscription, such as *Current Contents, Index Medicus,* and *Science Citation Index,* there are an increasing number of computer search services, which can be invaluable for either gaining

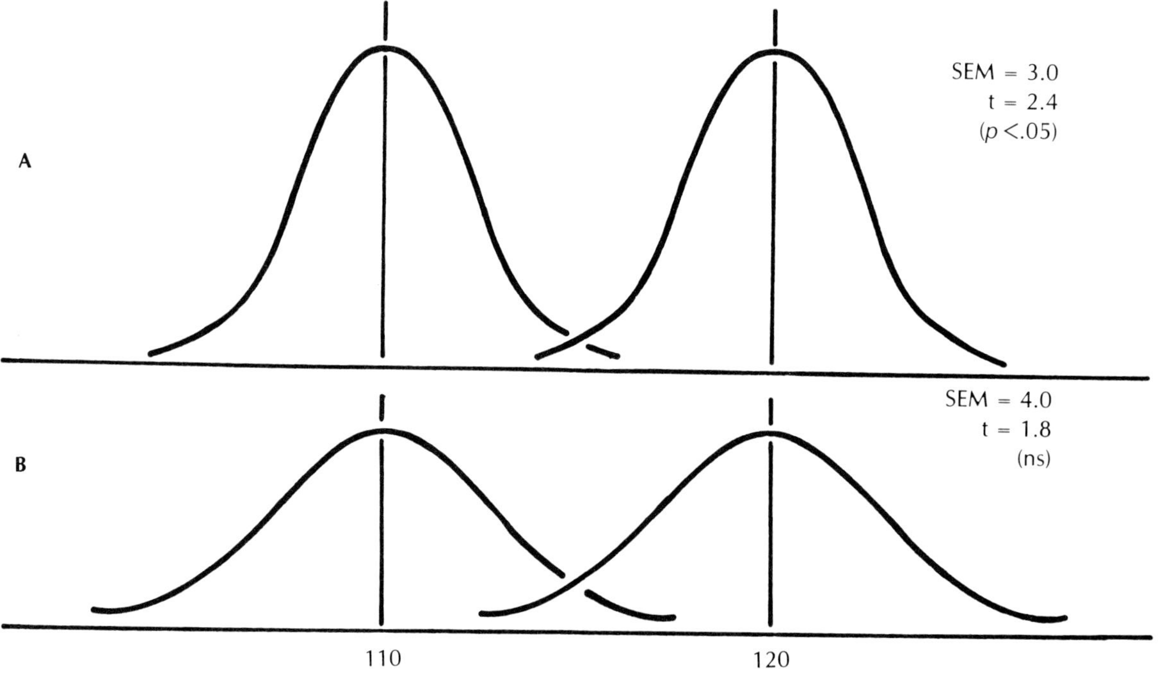

Fig. 14-1 Importance of variance in determining significance of a difference between means using the *t* test. Once *t* is computed, a table is consulted to determine whether it meets the criterion for significance. **A,** The smaller variance or standard error of the mean (SEM) leads to a larger *t* value and thus to the conclusion that a difference between means of that magnitude could have occurred by chance less than once in 20 times *($p < .05$)*. This is not the case in **B,** even though the means are the same, since the variances (SEMs) are too large. Thus the difference is considered not significant *(ns)*.

From Plant SM: Psychosocial aspects of scientific investigation. In Balis GU, Wurmser L, McDaniel E, and Grenell RG, editors: The psychiatric foundations of medicine: dimensions of behavior, London, 1978, Butterworth & Co.

a historical perspective or maintaining a current awareness in any field.

Scientific Communication. It is easier to assess the value of a paper or presentation realistically if the practitioner has some appreciation for the processes by which scientific data are disseminated. Learning how to prepare a good paper or presentation can be helpful in assessing the quality of the work of others. It also is useful to have some knowledge of the screening processes involved in the selection of research reports for presentation or publication. For example, journals typically submit their papers to a more rigorous peer review process than do meeting program committees, and there is some variability in the extent of peer review to which a report is subjected even within those two spheres.

Nature of the Research Process. Finally, intensive involvement with a research project can go a long way toward acquainting the clinician with both the technical and the human aspects of the research process. The value of supervised research training early in a career cannot be overemphasized. If such an experience is not possible, participation in a research methodology course or journal club can provide some guided experience in the critical evaluation of research reports. A third but less effective alternative would involve reading in some of the aforementioned areas.

EVALUATION GUIDELINES

A research study should be timely, reflecting a knowledge of current developments in its field of interest and using methodology that is up to current standards as well. It usually is not important for the author to provide a comprehensive review of the literature. Rather the author should demonstrate that he or she has accounted for relevant knowledge, issues, and controversies related to the topic of interest.

Method

A logical consistency should exist among the stated purpose of the study, the definitions of variables and terms, the methods and procedures used, the reporting of data, and the interpretation of results. Using the marijuana studies as an example, one study was based on the use of street marijuana, which could have contained impurities, preventing the investigator from conclusively attributing any effects to marijuana per se. The other study used joints that were manufactured and standardized specifically for the study, resulting in a more specific operational definition of the independent variable *marijuana*. If a practitioner wishes to apply the results of these studies, he or she must consider which of these two operational definitions is more relevant to his or her purpose. Which is relevant: whether the smoking of marijuana itself affects testosterone levels in a controlled, institutional setting, or whether the experience of using marijuana in more customary life situations is related to levels of this hormone? Each of these questions will be more relevant for certain readers and for certain purposes of application or further investigation.

An important and often stated rule of thumb for writing the method section of a paper is that it should "provide enough detail that a competent worker can repeat the experiments . . . . The cornerstone of the scientific method," writes Day,[2] "*requires* that your results, to be of scientific merit, must be reproducible; and, for the results to be adjudged reproducible, you must provide the basis for repetition of the experiments by others." A complete presentation also will make it easier to evaluate the timeliness, relevance, and effectiveness of the methods and procedures used.

Results

Authors sometimes tend to present only the results of statistical tests, as though the only intent of the study were to report the difference between two groups of subjects or a relationship between two variables. It is important that sufficient descriptive data be presented so that the reader can see the data on which these statistical tests were performed. However, journal space limitations require that the author make some judgments as to which data are best presented in graphs, tables, text, or not at all. The primary concern of the practitioner should be that the questions addressed by the study are appropriately reflected in the data presented and that any interpretation of results is supported by the actual presentation of relevant data. At times there may be relatively subtle aspects of data presentation that the reader should consider. For example, if an author reports relative changes in the scores of two groups of subjects over time as the percentage of an initial value, the practitioner should expect that the author also will provide some information about the initial values themselves. If a group of children performed extremely well on an achievement test, it might not be appropriate to expect that an experimental training program would improve their scores on that particular test.

Statistical Analysis

Three factors, which are presented next, should be considered in evaluating the use of statistical methods.

Relevance to the Research Question. The statistical methods used should reflect the nature of the question asked by the study. For example, if an author were to predict a systematic relationship between body weight and blood pressure in a group of young adolescents, dividing the children into two discrete groups of body weight and comparing the mean blood pressures by use of a t test would not provide the most sensitive method for exploring this question. A correlational technique that takes into account the individual weights of the children would be a more sensitive and appropriate way to proceed.

Conformance to Underlying Assumptions. The appropriate use of any statistical test is based on making certain assumptions about the data. For example, certain tests require that the data approximate a normal or gaussian distribution, that the number of observations exceeds a certain level, or that two groups of data being compared be independently acquired. If a test that is used to analyze a body of data does not adequately meet its underlying assumptions, inappropriate conclusions may result.

Use of Appropriate Documentation. If the statistical tests used are not as widely known as, for example, the chi-square, t test, or Pearson correlation, the author should provide a reference to the source of the test used. The fact that a particular computer was used for data analysis is not acceptable documentation. The work of a computer will be no more effective than the program it is asked to follow, and the program itself must reflect an appropriate statistical method. Finally, the reader should expect that all tests used be identified and, in most cases, that actual test results be reported. The simple assertion that "the difference was significant ($p < .05$)" does not allow the reader to address the statistical issues outlined here.

Discussion

The reader should determine whether the interpretation of results is consistent with and limited to the data presented. Were conclusions based on data that were either not presented or ambiguous? Does the author generalize inappropriately to populations with different characteristics from those of the one observed? Sound data and clear thinking usually result in a logical, concise interpretation.

As mentioned previously, the effectiveness of a scientist often is related to his or her alertness to the unexpected finding and to his or her willingness to consider various alternative explanations for a phenomenon. Whether the author of a paper considers such alternatives, it certainly is a useful exercise for the reader to be as alert to what the discussion section does not contain as to what it does contain. As Beveridge[1] has said, "The most difficult mental act of all is to rearrange a familiar bundle of data, to look at it differently and escape from the prevailing doctrine."

SUMMARY

In assessing medical literature, the practitioner must keep in mind that the value of any study is limited by certain technical considerations and that every aspect of research is somewhat affected by the psychosocial milieu of both researcher and audience. Good scientific pursuit and effective critique depend on an understanding of these facts, plus a conscious effort to look at relationships in new and unexpected ways, as well as a certain level of technical knowledge in the area of research methodology. A conscientious, competent evaluation of research serves not only the clinician and his or her patients; ultimately it will enhance the quality of published research as well.

REFERENCES

1. Beveridge WIB: The art of scientific investigation, ed 3, New York, 1957, Vintage.
2. Day RA: How to write and publish a scientific paper, ed 3, Phoenix, 1988, Oryx Press.
3. Dykes MHM: The physician: the key to the clinical application of scientific information, JAMA 237:239, 1977.
4. Kolodny RC et al: Depression of plasma testosterone levels after chronic intensive marihuana use, N Engl J Med 290:872, 1974.
5. Mendelson JH, Plasma testosterone levels before, during and after chronic marihuana smoking, N Engl J Med 291:1051, 1974.

SUGGESTED READINGS

Feinstein AR: Clinical epidemiology: the architecture of clinical research, Philadelphia, 1985, WB Saunders Co.

Fletcher RW, Fletcher SW, and Wagner EH: Clinical epidemiology—the essentials, Baltimore, 1982, Williams & Wilkins.

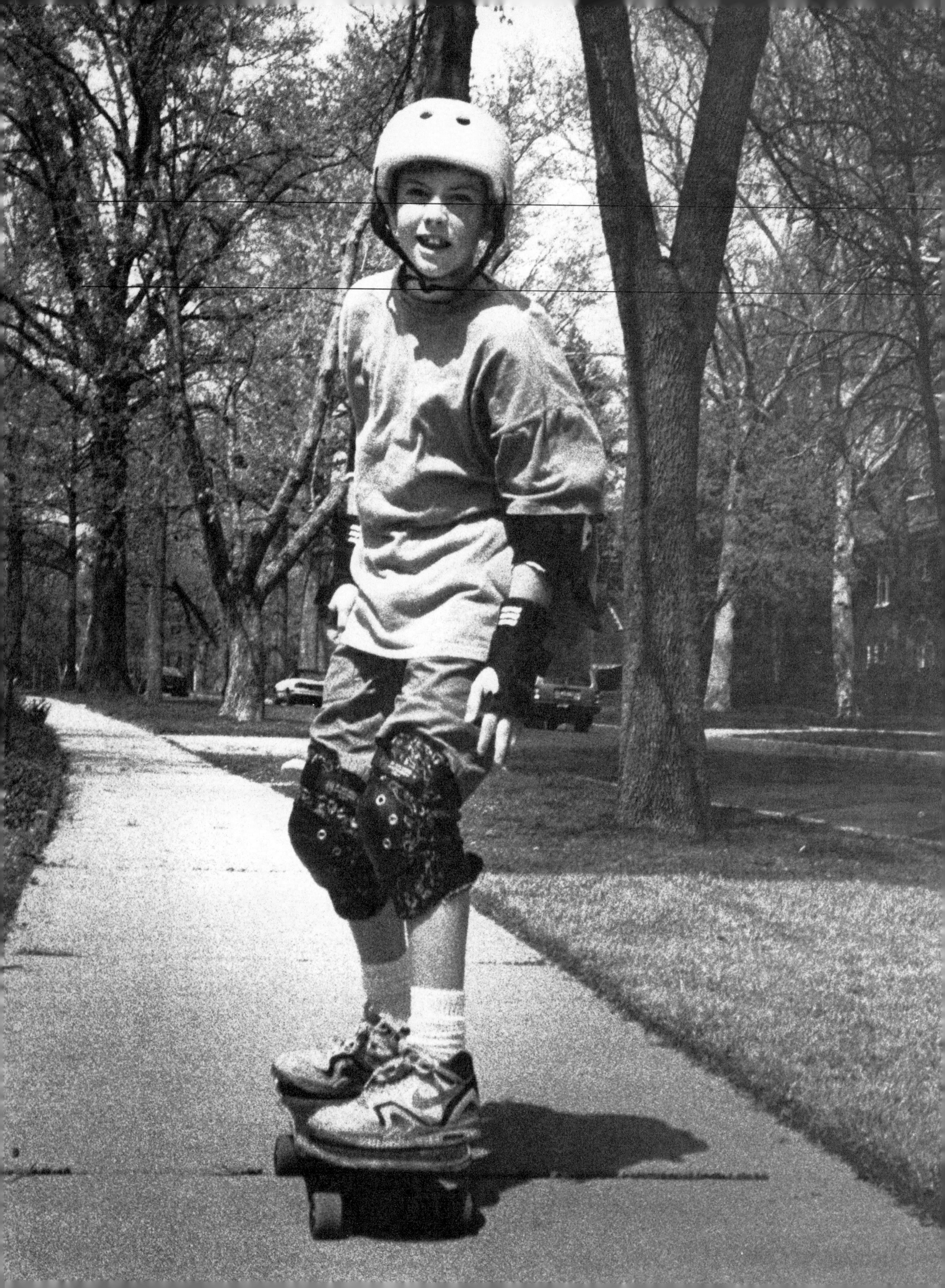

Part Three

Principles of Patient Care

Section One: Prevention of Disease

Section Two: Treatment of Disease

15

Anticipatory Guidance

Howard R. Foye, Jr.

Anticipatory guidance is the key to achieving the primary pediatric care goals of health promotion and disease prevention. It is a challenge to provide anticipatory guidance in primary care because of the range and complexity of appropriate issues, the enormous individual differences among normal children and their families, and the limited time available in health supervision visits. Other than time constraints involved, these challenges can be the greatest source of interesting variety and rewarding physician-patient interactions in the practice of primary pediatric care.

Three major activities are involved in anticipatory guidance: (1) gathering information, (2) establishing a therapeutic alliance, and (3) providing education and guidance.

Many discussions of anticipatory guidance focus only on the third activity. Without the first two, however, education and guidance often will be misguided or ineffective.

GATHERING INFORMATION AND ESTABLISHING A THERAPEUTIC ALLIANCE

Gathering information through careful history taking and observation is a prerequisite if the physician is to understand and respect the unique qualities of the child and family. Effective anticipatory guidance, like any teaching, should begin with an understanding of the student's knowledge base, preconceptions, and motivation. It will be effective to the extent that it is targeted to the individual.

A therapeutic alliance between the parents and the physician, based on mutual trust and respect, is another prerequisite for effective anticipatory guidance. In addition to enhancing the effectiveness of teaching, the therapeutic alliance can be a powerful source of emotional support. By listening respectfully, sympathizing with the parents' frustrations, and positively reinforcing effective parenting, the physician can help the parents gain a sense of competence and confidence in their parenting. As the child develops, it also is of increasing importance to establish a therapeutic alliance directly with the child. This relationship is important for support and anticipatory guidance as the child becomes more independent.

The accompanying box outlines information that should be gathered before anticipatory guidance is provided. The two major categories are information about the *child* and information about the *child's environment*. Traditional pediatric health care focuses on the child, particularly on issues of physical health promotion, disease prevention, detection and treatment, and developmental milestones. More recently, pediatric health care has broadened its focus to include issues of behavior and the environment in which the child is developing. The list is imposing, particularly given the time limitations of primary care visits, but at least brief attention to these areas is necessary to target anticipatory guidance appropriately. Prior knowledge of the child and family will obviate the need to survey all these topics at each visit, although frequent updates are important.

Some fundamental principles about the prerequisites for anticipatory guidance need to be highlighted:

1. Give the parents and child the opportunity to express their concerns at the beginning of every visit; your agenda for the visit will not get their attention until you have addressed *their* agenda.

Pertinent Information for Anticipatory Guidance

A. Information about the *child*
   1. *Concerns:* expressed by parent or child
   2. *Health:* current status and follow-up of past problems
   3. *Routine care:* feeding, sleep, and elimination
   4. *Development:* evaluated by school performance or with standardized tests (e.g., Denver Developmental Screening Test,[6] Early Language Milestone Scale [3])
   5. *Behavior:* temperament and interaction with family, peers, and others

B. Information about the child's *environment*
   1. *Family composition* (at home)
   2. *Caregiving schedule:* who and when
   3. *Family stresses:* e.g., work, finances, illness, death, move, marital, and other relationships
   4. *Family supports:* relatives, friends, organizations, material resources
   5. *Stimulation* in the home
   6. *Stimulation/activities* outside the home, e.g., preschool/school, peers, organizations
   7. *Safety*

2. Because it is important to develop a good relationship with the child as well as the parents, interact warmly with children at each visit. Even if only briefly, greet, talk, and play with them before proceeding to more threatening interactions such as the physical examination and immunizations.
3. Always inquire about how things are going for the parents. Particularly in our society of fragmented families, parenting can be a lonely, demanding job. To be a good nurturer, one needs to be nurtured. Take advantage of every opportunity to compliment the parents. Encourage them to save time for themselves and each other. By supporting parents and helping them support each other, you can indirectly help the parents nurture their child.

Some questions that are worth frequent repeating include the following:

What do you and your child enjoy doing together?

Is there enough time for spontaneity—for listening to your child and for doing what the child wants to do with you?

PROVIDING EDUCATION AND GUIDANCE

With the information outlined on p. 162, the physician is in a position to provide individualized anticipatory guidance. This is particularly important because time does not permit

Table 15-1 *Anticipatory Guidance Topics*

Prenatal and newborn

Prenatal visit

1. *Health:* pregnancy course, worries, tobacco, alcohol, drug use, hospital and pediatric office procedures
2. *Safety:* infant car seat, crib safety
3. *Nutrition:* planned feeding method
4. *Child care:* help after birth, later arrangements
5. *Family:* changes in relationships (spouse, siblings), supports, stresses, return to work

Newborn visits

1. *Health:* jaundice, umbilical cord care, circumcision, other common problems, when to call the physician's office
2. *Safety:* infant car seat, smoke detector, choking, keeping tap water temperature below 120° F
3. *Nutrition:* feeding, normal weight loss, spitting, vitamin and fluoride supplements
4. *Development/behavior:* individuality, "consolability," visual and auditory responsiveness
5. *Child care:* importance of interaction, parenting books, support for primary caregiver
6. *Family:* postpartum adjustments, fatigue, "blues," special time for siblings

First year

Up to 6 months

1. *Health:* immunizations, exposure to infections
2. *Safety:* falls, aspiration of small objects or powder, entanglement in mobiles with long strings
3. *Nutrition:* supplementation of breast milk or formula, introduction of solids, iron
4. *Development/behavior:* crying/colic, irregular schedules (eating, sleeping, eliminating), responding to infant cues, reciprocity, interactive games, beginning eye-hand coordination
5. *Child care:* responsive and affectionate care, caregiving schedule
6. *Family:* return to work, the nurturing of all family relationships (spouse and siblings)

6-12 months

1. *Safety:* locks for household poisons and medications, gates for stairs, ipecac, poison center telephone number; outlet safety covers; avoid dangling cords or tablecloths; safety devices for windows/screens, toddler car seat at 20 pounds; avoid toys with small detachable pieces; supervise child in tub or near water
2. *Nutrition:* discourage use of bottle as a pacifier or while in bed; offer cup and soft finger foods (with supervision); introduce new foods one at a time
3. *Development/behavior:* attachment, basic trust versus mistrust, stranger awareness, night waking, separation anxiety, bedtime routine, transitional object
4. *Child care:* prohibitions few but firm and consistent across caregiving settings; discipline defined as "learning" (not punishment)
5. *Family:* spacing of children

Second year

1-2 years

1. *Health:* immunizations
2. *Safety:* climbing and falls common; supervise outdoor play; ensure safety caps on medicine bottles; note dangers of plastic bags, pan handles hanging over stove, and space heaters
3. *Nutrition:* avoid feeding conflicts (decreased appetite common); period of self-feeding, weaning from breast or bottle; avoid sweet or salty snacks
4. *Development/behavior:* autonomy versus shame/doubt, ambivalence (independence/dependence), tantrums, negativism, getting into everything, night fears, readiness for toilet training, self-comforting behaviors (thumb sucking, masturbation), speech, imaginative play, no sharing in play, positive reinforcement for desired behavior
5. *Child care:* freedom to explore in safe place; day care; home a safer place to vent frustrations; needs show of affection, language stimulation through reading and conversation
6. *Family:* sibling relationships

Continued.

Table 15-1 *Anticipatory Guidance Topics—cont'd*

Preschool
2 to 5 years
1. *Health:* tooth brushing, first dental visit
2. *Safety:* needs close supervision near water or street; home safety factors include padding of sharp furniture corners, fire escape plan for home, and locking up power tools; should have car lap belt at 40 pounds and bike helmet; should know (a) name, address and telephone number, (b) not to provoke dogs, and (c) to say "no" to strangers
3. *Nutrition:* balanced diet; avoid sweet or salty snacks; child should participate in conversation at meals
4. *Development/behavior:* initiative versus guilt; difficulty with impulse control and sharing; developing interest in peers, high activity level; speaking in sentences by age 3; speech mostly intelligible to stranger by age 3, reading books; curiosity about body parts; magical thinking, egocentrism
5. *Child care/preschool:* needs daily special time with parent(s), bedtime routine; talk about day in day-care; limit TV and watch with child, reprimand privately, answer questions factually and simply; adjustment to preschool, kindergarten readiness
6. *Family:* chores, responsibilities

Middle childhood
5 to 10 years
1. *Health:* appropriate weight; regular exercise; somatic complaints (limb and abdominal pain, headaches); alcohol, tobacco, and drug use; sexual development; physician and child dealings (more direct)
2. *Safety:* bike helmets and street safety; car seat belts; swimming lessons; use of matches, firearms, and power tools; fire escape plan for home; saying "no" to strangers
3. *Nutrition:* balanced diet, daily breakfast, limited sweet and salty snacks, moderate fatty foods
4. *Development/behavior:* industry versus inferiority, need for successes, peer interactions, adequate sleep
5. *School:* school performance, homework, parent interest
6. *Family:* more time away but continuing need for family support, approval, affection, time together, and communication; family rules about bedtime, chores, and responsibilities; guidance in using money; parent(s) should encourage reading; limit TV watching and discuss programs seen together
7. *Other activities:* organized sports, religious groups, other organizations, use of spare time

Adolescence
Discuss with adolescent
1. *Health:* alcohol, tobacco, and drug use, dental care, physical activity, immunizations
2. *Safety:* bike and skateboard helmet and safety, car seat belts, driving while intoxicated, water safety, hitchhiking, risk-taking
3. *Nutrition:* balanced diet, appropriate weight, avoidance of junk foods
4. *Sexuality:* physical changes, sex education, peer pressure for sexual activity, sense of responsibility for self and partner, OK to say no, prevention of pregnancy and sexually transmitted diseases, breast and testes self-examination
5. *Development/relationships:* identity versus role confusion, family, peers, dating, independence, trying different roles
6. *School:* academics, homework
7. *Other activities:* sports, hobbies, organizations, jobs
8. *Future plans:* school, work, relationships with others

Discuss with parent
1. *Communication:* let adolescent participate in discussion and development of family rules; needs frequent praise and affection, time together, interest in adolescent's activities
2. *Independence:* parent and child ambivalence about independence; expect periods of estrangement; promote self-responsibility and independence; still needs supervision
3. *Role model:* actions speak louder than words—parents provide model of responsible, reasonable, and compassionate behavior

guidance on all potentially important topics. Table 15-1 suggests topics for anticipatory guidance by age. For general categories, some discussion, education, or guidance is warranted at each health supervision visit. Examples of more specific topics that are likely to be relevant at specific ages are listed after the headings.

Many potentially important topics may be overlooked if anticipatory guidance is limited to topics linked to specific ages. Topics that may be among the most important at any age and therefore always worthy of consideration include the following:

1. *Family stresses*, for example, single parenthood, divorce, separation, move, illness, death, unemployment
2. *Temperament*[8]
3. *Hurried children*[4]—tight schedules and pressures to achieve and grow up fast
4. *Self-esteem*—development of a sense of competence[9]

The lists in Table 15-1 should not limit the physician's scope but merely serve as examples and reminders. Much anticipatory guidance will follow from information gathered at the beginning of the visit, including new concerns of the parent or child and follow-up of old problems. The following sections supplement information in Table 15-1 by listing the major developmental tasks of each period and briefly discussing related anticipatory guidance issues.

Prenatal Visit

The family's developmental tasks in the period before delivery involve planning and preparing for the birth and early care of the infant. The main goal of the prenatal visit is to begin the development of a therapeutic alliance with the family. Specific objectives include learning about the family's health and social history and discussing its plans and concerns about the remainder of the pregnancy, labor, delivery, and early child care. Other objectives include a discussion of the nature of the physician's working relationship with the family and details about how the practice functions. Anticipatory guidance topics are listed in Table 15-1.

Newborn Visits

During the newborn period the major developmental tasks for infants involve the transition to the extrauterine environment. The major tasks for parents include bonding and learning to respond appropriately to the emotional and physical needs of their infant. Objectives of newborn pediatric care include the assessment of the infant's physical status, behavioral individuality, and caregiving environment at home; the management of health problems; and the promotion of bonding and parenting competence and confidence. Anticipatory guidance topics are listed in Table 15-1.

Up to 6 Months

The major developmental tasks in the first six months include socioemotional development—caregiver-infant reciprocity[2]; cognitive development—attention to events in the external environment; and physical development—rapid growth and visually guided manipulation with the hands.

Reciprocity is a term used to describe the achievement of mutually satisfying and predictable interactions between an infant and a caregiver. The development of reciprocity is influenced by the clarity and predictability of the cues provided by the infant, as well as by the sensitivity, responsiveness, and predictability of the caregiver. This is an important period of learning for all participants in these interactions. Learning is more difficult when the infant is irritable or unpredictable or when the caregiver's responsiveness is hindered by fatigue, depression, or distractions because of family stress. The following anticipatory guidance may be helpful: (1) anticipatory teaching about the normal unpredictability of feeding and sleeping schedules and the frequent occurrence of unexplained episodes of crying in the first few months, (2) discussion of the parenting of infants with various temperaments, and (3) discussion and counseling about issues that may be interfering with the caregiver's ability to provide a responsive environment for the infant.

The major cognitive developmental task for the infant in this period involves a shift from activities centered on the body (e.g., sucking) to greater interest in the external environment. At first this is manifested by increasing visual and auditory attention to external events. Then from 4 to 6 months there is rapid progress in the infant's ability to visually guide the grasp and to manipulate objects.

Table 15-1 provides anticipatory guidance topics for this age-group.

6 to 12 Months

The major developmental tasks of the infant 6 to 12 months old include socioemotional development—attachment,[1] basic trust versus mistrust[5]; cognitive development—object permanence, early means-end relationships[7]; and physical development—mobility.

The concepts of attachment and basic trust are similar. Basic trust develops in the first year to the extent that an infant learns that the caregiver is a predictable and reliable provider of essential physical and emotional needs. Trust in this most important aspect of the external environment, the primary caregiver, is believed to result in more confident exploration of the wider environment during the second year, when autonomy becomes the major socioemotional issue. Attachment theorists refer to this as exploration from a secure base. An infant who is insecurely attached (who mistrusts more than trusts) because of unpredictable or unreliable caregiving in the first year will more likely be inhibited in exploring the environment. The insecurely attached infant also is more likely to be clinging and demanding as a result of insecurity about the caregiver's availability. These behaviors may lead to the erroneous conclusion that the infant is too "attached" to its caregiver. It is important to remember, however, that most infants go through a period of separation anxiety toward the end of the first year when clinging behavior will be increased. Also, some infants who are temperamentally more timid or socially withdrawn may have an extended period of "clinginess."

Object permanence means that the infant now understands that objects continue to exist even when they are not present in the immediate physical environment. Calls for an absent primary caregiver often are the earliest evidence that the infant has developed this cognitive ability. Separation anxiety and night waking also may be manifestations of this new achievement. A budding understanding of means-end relationships is apparent in the infant's ability to remove a barrier or to use a second object to retrieve a toy that is out of reach. Another manifestation may be the infant's association of the coat closet with Mommy's departure and therefore the bitter protests that occur when the mother approaches the closet.

Increasing mobility has many implications for anticipatory guidance, particularly regarding safety issues. (See Table 15-1 for anticipatory guidance topics for the 6- to 12-month old.)

1 to 2 Years

The major developmental tasks of the 1- to 2-year-old include socioemotional development—autonomy versus shame and doubt[5]; ambivalence regarding dependence and independence; cognitive development—exploration, early language, "pretend" play; physical development—ambulation and slower growth.

The issue of autonomy is at the heart of "the terrible twos," which actually start during the second year of life. This period is characterized by frustrating, dramatic behavioral shifts from stubborn independence ("I want to do it myself" and "no" to most parental requests) to infantile clinging and dependence. Parents often wish that their child were both more independent and less independent at the same time. The wild fluctuations are related to the child's newly acquired walking and climbing skills, as well as eagerness to explore, often outstripping the cognitive ability to anticipate danger or surprise. The brazen explorer can quickly be reduced to a tearful clinger to Mommy's skirt.

The second year is a very exciting time for cognitive development. The developing ability to understand and to use language is a manifestation of the child's cognitive ability to use symbols for objects. By 2 years of age the child's play becomes a theater for imitating past events and demonstrating a budding ability to think symbolically and creatively.

Decreased growth rate in the second year is the cause of one of the most frequent parental concerns in this period: "He eats like a bird." Education about normal growth and intake usually is reassuring.

Table 15-1 presents anticipatory guidance topics for the second year.

Preschool: 2 to 5 Years

The major developmental tasks of the preschool period include socioemotional development—initiative versus guilt,[5] mastery (e.g., toilet training), and peer interactions with true sharing; cognitive development—speech, deferred imitation, and imagination; and physical development—steady growth and increasing coordination.

The initiative that characterizes this period is demonstrated in widening interactions with the physical environment and with people outside the family. Good parenting involves giving the child opportunities to exercise initiative and to experience mastery over new challenges, while ensuring close supervision to provide necessary support and encouragement and to prevent harm. An overprotective or restrictive caregiving environment may result in fear or guilt and the inhibition of initiative and the developing sense of self-mastery. A caregiving environment that pushes the child too hard toward "independence" may not provide enough supervision and support to allow the child to master the developmental tasks of this period.

During the preschool period, language develops so remarkably that it is easy to forget that the preschooler's thinking often is still illogical. It is characterized by an egocentrism that cannot comprehend a perspective other than the child's own and assumes that other people have seen and experienced exactly what the child has. It also is characterized by magical thinking—the blurring of fantasy and reality; wishes, dreams, and actual events are not clearly distinguished. These logical limitations may help explain the common occurrence of irrational fears and exasperating misunderstandings between parent and child. A wish that a new sibling would go away may be a frightening source of guilt and self-blame when the new infant is hospitalized. The child may think that wishing made it happen. Careless comments by a parent also may be a source of anxiety for a child who cannot distinguish a threat from reality.

Table 15-1 lists anticipatory guidance topics for the preschool child.

Middle Childhood: 5 to 10 Years

The major developmental tasks of middle childhood include socioemotional development—industry versus inferiority[5]; cognitive development—concrete logical thinking,[7] basic functions of mathematics and classification of objects; and physical development—preadolescence.

This is the period when the physician should increasingly engage the child directly in discussions and anticipatory guidance. By the end of this period some physicians already are spending part of each visit alone with the child.

Middle childhood is the period when critical appraisal of a child's abilities begins in earnest. Although preschool children (and their parents) frequently compare themselves with their age mates, comparisons become much more quantitative and official in middle childhood. Tests and opportunities for public humiliation in school are unending. Even when teachers are careful to avoid overt comparisons, the children know how they measure up. After-school activities, particularly sports, often are highly competitive. It is easy to understand how a child may develop a sense of inferiority, particularly in a culture that so emphasizes being number one, as if anything else is not good enough.

The socioemotional task of industry (i.e., motivation to succeed through work) requires that the child experience successes. Lack of successes leads to a feeling of inferiority, discouragement, and giving up. This is an important issue for anticipatory guidance, because parents also may have accepted the notion that the child is not good at anything. Some creative thinking must take place to provide successful experiences for each child so that lack of motivation does not rob the child of his or her potential.

Table 15-1 lists anticipatory guidance topics for middle childhood.

Adolescence

The major developmental tasks of adolescence include socioemotional development—identity versus role confusion[4]; cognitive development—abstract and hypothetical thinking[5]; and physical development—puberty.

Adolescence frequently is described in terms of three stages. Early adolescence (roughly from 10 to 13 years) is the period of most rapid physical growth and sexual development. Because of the rapid changes, many children are preoccupied with their bodies and comparing themselves with their peers. In addition, they begin to separate from their parents, frequently challenging parental authority. During middle adolescence (roughly from 14 to 17 years) there is less preoccupation with physical changes. This period is characterized by intense involvement with peers, conflicts over independence with parents, and, often, sexual exploration. Late adolescence (roughly from 18 years) is characterized by increased concern over future plans, including college studies and career plans. Social skills are more advanced, and many adolescents are involved in committed, intimate relationships.

Table 15-1 lists anticipatory guidance topics for adolescence.

LITERATURE FOR PARENTS AND CHILDREN

Parent literature and children's books frequently can provide valuable supplementation to discussions with the physician about anticipatory guidance topics. Often physicians lack sufficient time to discuss an issue in depth in the office. One alternative is to begin a discussion in the time available and then suggest a pertinent reference. Literature references for parent and child are listed at the end of the chapter; however, follow-up is crucial. Perhaps the next regular visit is soon enough, but it is always appropriate to invite the family to call or to make an appointment if family members wish to discuss further questions sooner. Of course, there are times when a definite follow-up visit or referral should be scheduled immediately.

A note of caution about book recommendations is warranted. Some parents have a tendency to overintellectualize parenting—to place too much reliance on specific "expert" advice that is not individualized to their family. Good parent literature points out that specific advice needs to be tailored to the unique qualities of the child, the parents, and the environment in which they live. Good parenting involves more than general knowledge about children and behavior management. It also involves sensitivity and responsiveness to the special qualities of each child and self-awareness about how the parent's feelings and events in the environment influence interactions with the child. Written advice alone therefore is not sufficient. The parents must interpret and modify the advice to fit their situation. Some can do this themselves; many will benefit by anticipatory guidance from their physician.

Most parents will want to have at least one of the following books:

Brazelton TB: *Working and caring,* Reading, Mass, 1984, Addison-Wesley Publishing Co., Inc. A wonderful book for parents trying to balance working and child care—honest and positive.

Hoekelman R, MacDonald N, and Baum D: *The new American encyclopedia of children's health,* New York, 1989, New American Library Publishing Co., Inc. A handy A to Z guide written especially for parents; addresses their common concerns.

Leach P: *Your baby and child from birth to age five,* New York, 1986, Alfred A Knopf, Inc. Another superb wide-ranging reference with an emphasis on child development.

Spock B and Rothenberg M: *Dr. Spock's baby and child care,* New York, 1985, Pocket Books. This updated classic is still an invaluable, enjoyable, wide-ranging book for parents.

The following professional texts contain extensive, annotated bibliographies of parent and child literature on a wide variety of topics (health and development):

Dixon S and Stein M: *Encounters with children: pediatric behavior and development,* Chicago, 1987, Year Book Medical Publishers, Inc.

Sahler OJ and McAnarney E: *The child from three to eighteen,* St Louis, 1981, The CV Mosby Co.

REFERENCES

1. Bowlby J: Attachment, ed 2, New York, 1983, Basic Books, Inc., Publishers.
2. Brazelton TB, Koslowski B, and Main M: The origins of reciprocity: the early mother-infant interaction. In Lewis M and Rosenblum L, editors: The effect of the infant on its caregiver, New York, 1974, John Wiley & Sons, Inc.
3. Coplan J: Evaluation of the child with delayed speech or language, Pediatr Ann 14:203, 1985.
4. Elkind D: The hurried child: growing up too fast too soon, Reading, Mass, 1981, Addison-Wesley Publishing Co., Inc.
5. Erikson E: Childhood and society (35th anniversary ed), New York, 1986, WW Norton & Co., Inc.
6. Frankenburg W, Sciarillo W, and Burgess D. The newly abbreviated and revised Denver Developmental Screening Test, J Pediatr 99:995, 1981.
7. Ginsburg H and Opper S: Piaget's theory of intellectual development, ed 3, Englewood Cliffs, NJ, 1988, Prentice-Hall, Inc.
8. Thomas A, Chess S, and Birch H: Temperament and behavior disorders in children, New York, 1968, New York University Press.
9. White R: Motivation reconsidered: the concept of competence, Psychol Rev 66:297, 1959.

SUGGESTED READINGS

Brazelton TB: Anticipatory guidance, Pediatr Clin North Am 22:533, 1975.

Casey P, Sharp M, and Loda F: Child-health supervision for children under 2 years of age: a review of its content and effectiveness, J Pediatr 95:1, 1979.

Chamberlin R, Szumowski E, and Zastowny T: An evaluation of efforts to educate mothers about child development in pediatric office practices. Am J Public Health 69:875, 1979.

Committee on Psychosocial Aspects of Child and Family Health: Guidelines for health supervision II, Elk Grove Village, Ill, 1988, American Academy of Pediatrics.

Telzrow R: Anticipatory guidance in pediatric practice, Journal of Clinical and Experimental Pediatrics, p. 14, July 1978.

16

Nutrition

One

Nutritional Requirements

Gilbert B. Forbes

To live, to grow, and to thrive, human beings must take in nutrients from their environment. Before birth these are supplied by the mother, but thereafter they must be ingested. If too little is provided, the infant or child will not grow and may become ill, and too much may lead to toxicity or obesity. Nutritionists have tried for decades to define the optimum intakes for various nutrients; a few are known, yet for the majority the only data available are in the form of educated guesses. In an attempt to cover the maximum conceivable need (individuals do vary in size, and there may be individual differences in requirements), quasi-official bodies such as the National Academy of Sciences have recommended generous allowances of most nutrients. Although this would provide for the upper extremes of need, in effect it advises most of the population to eat more than they need. Therefore dietary surveys among healthy individuals show that the diets of many do not satisfy the listed recommended dietary allowances. Perhaps this is just as well, inasmuch as overnutrition is now a greater problem in this country than is undernutrition, and there is concern over the possibility that the former may be a factor in longevity.

Nutritional requirements can be considered on the basis of several considerations: age, body size, growth rate, physiologic losses (as in menstruation and lactation), and caloric intake. The following discussion deals primarily with the normal child; for the most part, those situations that call for special nutritional advice are dealt with in other chapters.

Note should be taken of the contribution of food technology to the modern nutritional scene: the pasteurization of milk, the addition of certain vitamins and minerals to some foods, alterations in milk composition to serve better the needs of young infants, hypoallergenic formulas, and the special formulas for infants with certain inborn errors of metabolism (such as phenylketonuria). All this has made it possible to feed the majority of infants in a most satisfactory manner. The only undesirable consequence has been a decline in breast-feeding; although of minor nutritional importance in Western society, this decline may be disadvantageous in poor countries and in depressed areas where sanitation is inadequate and there is a meager supply of animal protein. However, there has been a resurgence of interest in breast-feeding in recent years in all societies.

ENERGY

Energy Metabolism

Energy is being continuously expended by the body in the form of heat and work. Body temperature must be maintained, physical activity provided for, and the processes of digestion, cellular transport, and tissue synthesis supported. The unit of energy generally employed in metabolism is the kilocalorie (kcal),* usually designated simply as a *calorie* (Cal). Foodstuffs have approximately the following energy equivalents when burned in the body:

1 g protein = 4 calories (protein is 16% nitrogen)
1 g carbohydrate = 4 calories
1 g fat = 9 calories

It is axiomatic that the body cannot exist on only one or even two of these sources of energy, so it is fortunate that nature has provided a mixture of the three in many foodstuffs. Diets found to be satisfactory and palatable for infants and children (and adults, too) provide 8% to 15% of total calories from protein and 30% to 50% each from fat and carbohydrate.

There are five broad uses to which energy intake is put.

1. *Basal metabolism.* This term refers to energy expenditure at rest in the fasting state. On a body weight basis the basal metabolic rate (BMR) is higher in infants than in adults, primarily because (a) infants' surface area–to–weight ratio is higher, (b) in infants a certain amount of "basal" energy is being used for growth, and (c) the relative size of the viscera and brain (the most metabolically active organs in the body) is considerably greater in infants. During the first year of life the BMR is about 55 Cal/kg/day; afterward this value diminishes gradually to the adult level of about 25 to 30 Cal/kg/day. Because adipose tissue has a low metabolic rate, the BMR *per kilogram of body weight* will be lower in obese than in thin individuals and in women

*A kilocalorie is the amount of heat required to raise the temperature of 1 kg of water by 1° C (from 14.5° to 15.5° C) and equals 1000 small calories. Some desire to replace this by another unit of energy, the *joule* (equivalent to 10^7 ergs), which is in common use by physical scientists. One kilojoule (kJ) equals 0.239 kcal; to convert kilocalories to kilojoules, multiply by 4.18.

as compared with men. However, BMR bears a linear relationship to *lean weight* in adolescents and adults.

2. *Requirement for growth.* The synthesis of tissue obviously requires energy. The exact amount required is not known, but studies of young children recovering from malnutrition and studies of intentionally overfed adults show that 4 to 10 extra calories are required for each gram of weight gain. During the first 4 months of life, one third of the total caloric intake is used for growth. By the end of the second year of life this has dropped to 1% to 2% of calories.
3. *Energy lost in excreta.* Some nitrogen is excreted in the urine, and feces contain both protein and fat. It is estimated that such losses constitute about 10% of the energy intake of usual diets.
4. *Specific dynamic action.* Resting metabolism rises somewhat after a meal, especially after a generous intake of protein, and may not return to the baseline for several hours. The amount of energy dissipated in this manner is estimated to be 5% to 10% of total calories ingested.
5. *Requirement for physical activity.* Studies of adults show that sedentary men require about 2700 Cal/day and very active men 4000; for women, these values are 2000 and 3000 Cal/day, respectively. Thus very active people need 1½ times more food. Although estimates of this sort are not available for infants and children, casual observation confirms that variations in physical activity do occur. Some infants are more restless than others, and there is an obvious difference in energy expenditure by high school athletes and their spectator friends. Because a major portion of the total energy expenditure is directly proportional to body weight, large persons expend more energy in a given task and at rest.

Table 16-1 lists energy expenditures for adults (these values would apply to late adolescence as well) for various activities.

The total daily energy requirement as a function of age and sex is depicted in Fig. 16-1. These data are based on reports by the Food and Nutrition Board of the National Academy of Sciences and the World Health Organization. The diagram shows the estimated average requirement. Note the sex difference both in total calories and calories per kilogram during adolescence. This is due to (1) the greater lean weight of boys and (2) their greater physical activity. The values for persons aged 19 to 20 years equal those for young adults.

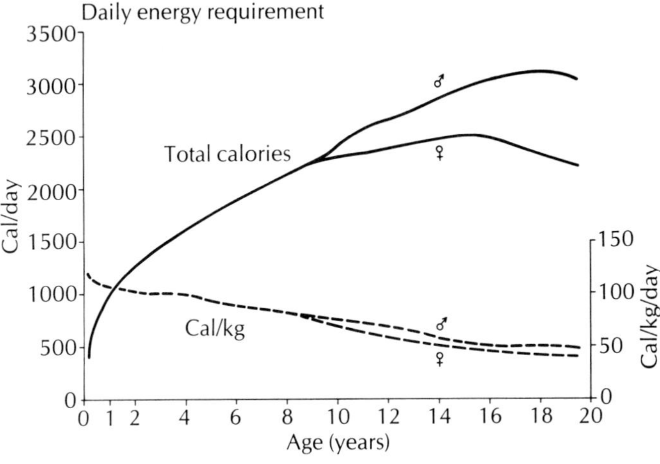

Fig. 16-1 Daily energy requirement as a function of age and sex.

In this context it is instructive to consider the growth of the lean body mass (LBM) inasmuch as this represents the bulk of the metabolically active tissue of the body, whereas the adipose tissue component is relatively inert. The data shown in Fig. 16-2 are based on total body potassium measurements.* Note that the growth curve of the LBM differs from that of total body weight, because the latter includes a variable proportion of fat. The adolescent growth spurt in LBM is considerably greater for boys than for girls. It should be obvious that the adolescent boy has a greater need for calories and for many nutrients, particularly calcium and nitrogen. Indeed, in the midst of his adolescent growth spurt, a boy's need for iron to provide growth of blood volume and muscle mass may equal that of a postmenarcheal girl.

Fig. 16-1 shows the *average* energy requirement. Larger individuals will need more calories both for maintenance and for a given degree of physical activity; smaller persons will need less. In normal circumstances, appetite is a good indication of caloric need. In situations of abnormal growth, either too little or too much, reference to this chart will help in determining whether the stated intake of food is appropriate and thus whether food intake could be a contributing factor.

Low-birth-weight-neonates need a generous intake of calories (i.e., 130-150 Cal/kg/day) to provide for "catch-up" growth, and their inadequate fat stores demand that feeding be started as soon after birth as possible.

One additional point is worthy of note: if calories are being obtained from a variety of foods, an adequate intake of calories usually will ensure an adequate intake of essential nutrients. Therefore calories should be the first item to be evaluated in assessing a dietary history.

Table 16-1 *Calories (kcal) Expended per Hour by Adults*

	CALORIES	
ACTIVITY	MEN	WOMEN
Sleeping	65	54
Sitting quietly	83	69
Walking (3 miles/hr)	220	180
Swimming, tennis	400	300
Rowing	450+	360+

*One of the naturally occurring isotopes of potassium (^{40}K) is radioactive, and there is enough of this isotope in the body to permit its measurement by specially designed scintillation counters. Because potassium is found only in lean tissue, an estimate of LBM can be made.

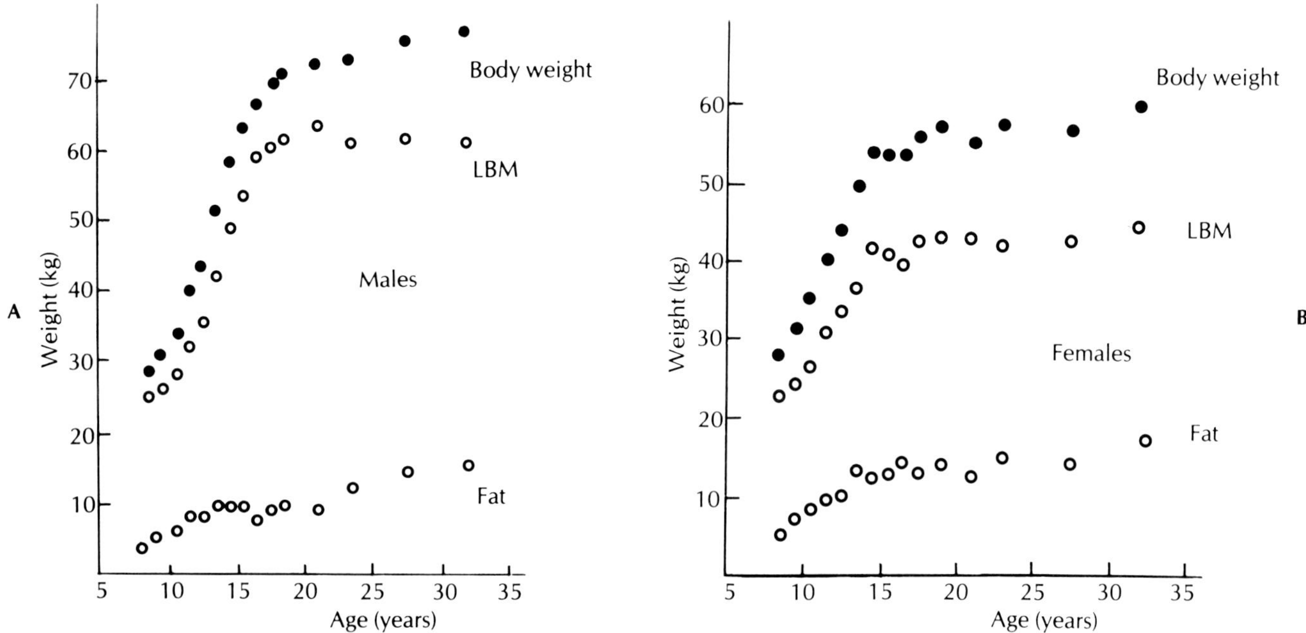

Fig. 16-2 Mean body weight and estimated lean body mass *(LBM)* and fat by ^{40}K counting for 604 males **(A)** and 467 females **(B)** aged 8 to 35 years.

Pregnancy and Lactation

The recent increase in the number of teenage pregnancies demands that pediatricians and child health personnel be aware of the extra energy requirements for pregnancy and lactation. Studies of chronically undernourished poverty groups have shown that the birth weight and chances for infant survival can be improved by providing additional calories during pregnancy; it is now generally admitted that a weight gain of 10 to 13 kg is desirable. Weight gain during pregnancy, as well as prepregnancy weight, has an influence on birth weight. The extra energy cost to the mother is estimated at 150 to 300 Cal/day throughout pregnancy, depending on the degree to which physical activity is curtailed. Although based on adults, these figures should pertain equally well to the pregnant teenager.

Lactation requires even more energy. Each deciliter of milk produced contains 72 calories, and milk production is said to be 80% efficient; thus 90 extra calories must be ingested by the mother for each deciliter of milk produced. The total milk production of 850 ml/day thus requires an extra 760 calories. The underweight mother should be urged to take more than this, whereas the well-nourished mother needs less—perhaps an extra 500 Cal/day—because she can draw on her generous fat stores.

PROTEIN

Proteins are high-molecular-weight polypeptides that serve many functions in the body. Enzymes are proteins, as are antibodies and some hormones; hemoglobin, plasma albumin, and the contractile elements of muscle are also proteins. All proteins are composed of some 20 amino acids, in varying proportions; the function of a particular protein is governed by the sequence of amino acids within the molecule. Of these amino acids, nine cannot be synthesized by the body; therefore they are known as *essential amino acids*. They are histidine, isoleucine, leucine, lysine, methionine, phenylalanine, threonine, tryptophan, and valine, and there are indications that cystine and taurine may be essential for the low-birth-weight infant. These essential amino acids must be supplied in food.

As is the case for energy, the body needs a constant supply of protein: during growth, new tissue must be synthesized because *all* tissues (even bone and adipose tissue) contain protein; even during adult life there is a constant turnover of protein, with some nitrogen being lost in the urine even on a protein-free diet and during fasting. There is a requirement for growth and for maintenance, and this is an unremitting requirement because there is no storage site for protein within the body. An inadequate supply results in a slowing of growth, compromise of many body functions, and the wasting of muscle; in severe deprivation, impaired resistance to infection, reduced mentality, and even death may result.

Ingested protein first must undergo hydrolysis, a process that is begun in the stomach and carried to partial completion in the upper small intestine, principally by pancreatic enzymes. The resultant amino acids and small peptides are then transported by specific metabolic processes (which themselves involve special proteins) into the interior of the intestinal mucosal cells (the peptide bonds having been split at the brush border), and the amino acids are absorbed into the portal blood.

The end products of protein metabolism appear in the urine mainly as urea, the deaminated amino acids being either converted to carbohydrate and fat or burned to carbon dioxide and water.

Biologic Quality

The variable amino acid composition of food proteins leads to variations in the efficiency with which they supply the body's needs. The methods for estimating the biologic quality of a given protein include tests on animals, observations of growth of children on differing diets, nitrogen balance studies on adult volunteers, and a chemical score based on the amino acid content. Although these do not always yield the same result, there is general agreement on the biologic quality of the proteins in various food groups. In Table 16-2, the highest two are arbitrarily assigned a score of 100.

Simply stated, a child must ingest more of a low-quality protein to achieve proper nutrition and the desired rate of growth. The low quality of vegetable proteins is due to relative deficiencies of one or more essential amino acids. For example, wheat is low in lysine, corn is low in lysine and tryptophan, rice is low in lysine and threonine, and beans are low in methionine. Commercial formulas based on processed soy flour have been found to be satisfactory for infants. Some vegetables are so low in protein (e.g., cassava has only 0.35 g of protein per 100 Cal) that it becomes impossible to eat enough to meet the protein need. However, a judicious mixture of vegetables can yield a most satisfactory result. Strict vegetarians have survived in apparent health for many years, and tests of suitable vegetable mixtures have shown good results in the treatment of protein malnutrition.

Generally speaking, it is wise to include some animal protein in the diet; even if only a third of the total protein intake comes from this source, the risk of a specific amino acid deficit becomes negligible.

Requirement

There are many problems in estimating the precise requirement for protein at any age; these include variations in growth rate, size of the LBM, and protein quality, and finally and most important, the difficulties, both technical and ethical, in carrying out the necessary experiments on human beings. Indeed, estimates for the early months of life are based on average intakes of human milk of infants who appear to be thriving. Fig. 16-3 represents a composite of estimates by the National Academy of Sciences (NAS) and the World Health Organization (WHO). It should be noted that the usual American diet, which includes 12% to 15% of calories from protein (human milk is an exception: 8%) and an average per capita consumption of 100 g, provides protein well in excess of actual need.

It is important to note that the protein requirements (per kilogram of weight) of the young infant are relatively high compared with those of the older child or the adult. High-quality protein is important for the young infant, and this is ensured by a reasonable intake of milk. There is, however, no particular advantage to providing protein in excess of actual need, inasmuch as the excess cannot be stored and therefore is metabolized as an energy source to appear in the urine as urea and amino acids. Studies of infants recovering from severe malnutrition have shown that satisfactory recovery can be achieved at protein intakes as low as 2.5 g/kg. In fact, there is serious doubt that really high protein diets are needed under any circumstances save those associated with abnormal protein losses (as in extensive burns and chronic renal or gastrointestinal disease).

Several groups require special consideration. The rapid growth rate of the low-birth-weight newborn demands a protein intake of 3 to 4 g/kg during the early months of life. Lactating women need an extra supply: 850 ml of human milk contains 10 g of protein; under the assumption that protein utilization is only 60% efficient, the mother should receive an extra 17 g of protein daily. The extra demand for protein during pregnancy is appreciable but not great; the body of the term newborn contains about 400 g of protein, to which should be added the 500 g contained in the placenta, gravid uterus, and breasts and in the expanded blood volume. Most of this increase occurs during the latter half of pregnancy, when it averages 6 g/day.

Excessive quantities of protein (5g/kg or more) can lead to toxicity. The concentration of blood urea nitrogen rises, the urine may contain albumin and casts, and if water intake is low, the excessive renal solute load leads to an increase in obligatory renal water excretion and to dehydration; that plus the increased specific dynamic action can result in fever, the so-called protein fever.

Table 16-2 *Relative Biologic Quality of Food Protein*

FOOD	SCORE
Human milk	100
Whole egg	100
Cow milk	95+
Meat	80+
Processed soy flour	80+
Vegetable proteins	50-70

FAT

Fat is a constituent of all body tissues. This term is applied to a heterogeneous group of low-molecular-weight compounds that contain fatty acids and that have in common the property of being soluble in solvents such as chloroform and ether. Neutral fats, or triglycerides, are fatty acid esters of glycerol. They serve the functions of energy storage and insulation against cold, and they provide a cushion for internal organs. This depot fat accounts for about 14% of body weight in term newborns and 10% to 30% in adults. Fig. 16-2 shows that body fat content varies with age and sex. Obese individuals may have as much as 50% fat.

The high energy content of adipose tissue (composed of fat-laden adipocytes and a connective tissue stroma) is due to two factors: the high caloric value of fat itself (it has the energy equivalent of gasoline) and the fact that fat deposition is not, as is the case with protein and carbohydrate, accompanied by an increase in tissue water content. This makes for efficient energy storage; indeed a moderately thin adult can survive fasting for at least a month, and the very obese have survived for as long as 250 days. Newborn animals, including

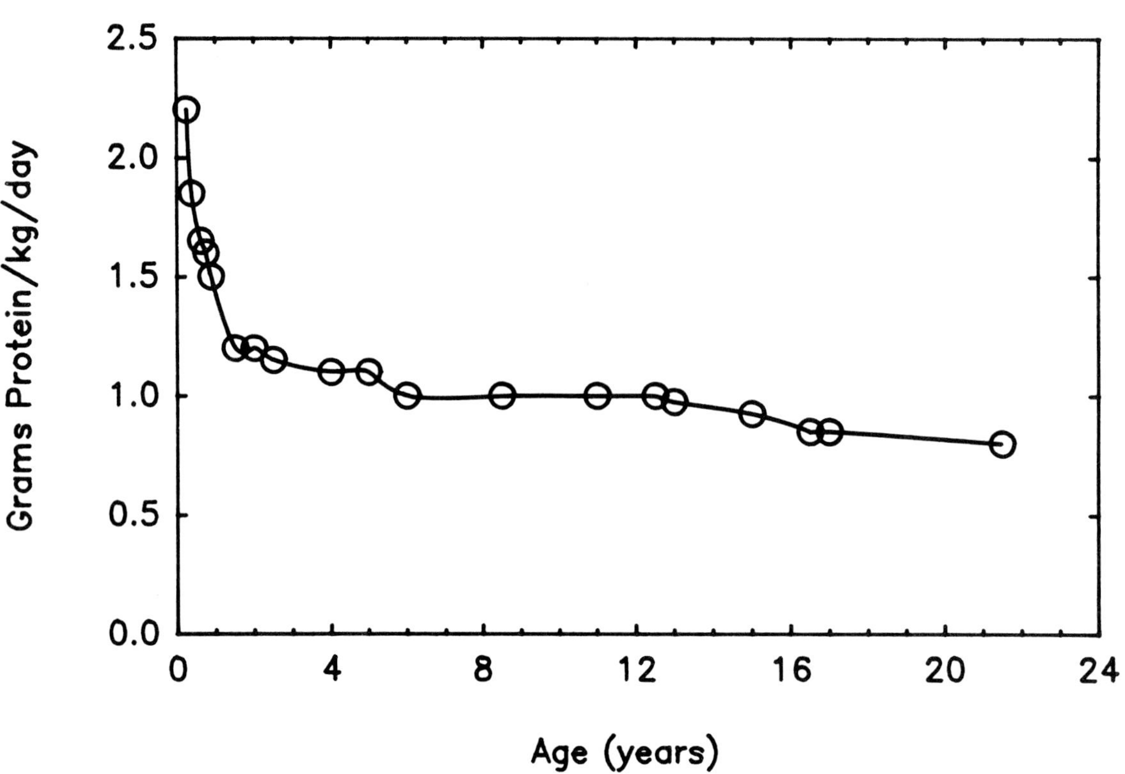

Fig. 16-3 Estimates of protein requirements as a function of age.

humans, and adult hibernators have a special adipose organ—brown fat—for the purpose of quickly supplying energy in response to cold.

Fatty acids are classified according to the number of double bonds in the hydrocarbon chain. *Saturated fat* contains a relatively small percentage of fatty acids with double bonds, and *polyunsaturated fat* contains a high percentage of fatty acids with such bonds. Generally, the former have higher melting points and thus a firmer consistency at room temperature (compare lard and corn oil). Fats of vegetable origin tend to be more unsaturated than those of animal origin (an exception is human milk fat, which is less saturated than cow milk fat).

In addition to neutral fats, there are other fats. Some contain phosphorus or galactose, which are essential components of tissue. Some—the lipoproteins—are linked to protein; these contribute to the stability of cell membranes and serve in combination with proteins and polysaccharides as structural components of cells (lysozymes and myelin sheaths are examples).

With the exception of linoleic, linolenic, and arachidonic acids, the multitude of fats found in the body can be formed from protein or carbohydrate precursors. Although symptoms and signs of essential fatty acid deficiency (dermatitis, impaired growth, and impaired lipid transport) have been observed under experimental conditions and in patients fed parenterally for long periods, the requirement is low, only 1% to 2% of total calories, so that such deficiencies have not been described under natural circumstances. Essential fatty acids are precursors of an important series of compounds, the prostaglandins.

Cholesterol, which is a sterol and not a fat in the true sense, has an important role in metabolism. It is a precursor of bile acids, vitamin D, adrenocortical steroids, and sex hormones. It is synthesized in the body and is thus present in foods of animal origin, and its absorption by the intestine is facilitated by a high fat diet. Diets high in fat and cholesterol are thought to accelerate the process of atherosclerosis.

Fat digestion occurs in the upper small intestine by the action of pancreatic and intestinal lipases, which split off two fatty acids from glycerol. The 2-monoacyl glycerol residue combines with bile salts to form micelles (which, incidentally, incorporate fat-soluble vitamins and cholesterol), which act to dissolve the free fatty acids and are taken up by the mucosal cells. Here the triglycerides are reconstituted and released into the lymph as chylomicrons. Short- and medium-chain fats (12-carbon chains or less) are handled differently; these are hydrolyzed by the brush border of mucosal cell, and the resultant fatty acids are released into the portal vein.

Fat exists in several forms in plasma: triglycerides, free fatty acids, lipoproteins, and phospholipids. Fatty acids are used as a source of energy by muscle, and they can be esterified by adipocytes to form depot fat; they also can be synthesized in liver and adipose tissue from dietary carbohydrate precursors.

Unsaturated fatty acids with a double bond at the third carbon from the methyl terminal (alpha-linolenic acid is one such omega-3 fatty acid) are present in significant amounts in marine fish oils. These fatty acids and their derivatives reduce platelet aggregation and appear to retard the progress of atherosclerosis. Fish-eating populations have less atheroslerotic disease and also have slightly longer bleeding times.

CARBOHYDRATES

As the name implies, carbohydrates are a series of compounds composed of carbon, hydrogen, and oxygen. They generally are classified into three groups: monosaccharides, containing five or six carbon atoms (glucose and fructose are examples); disaccharides, containing 12 carbon atoms (sucrose and lactose are examples); and polysaccharides, which are high-molecular-weight polymers (glycogen and starch are examples). Their main function is to supply energy, although certain specialized forms are involved in antigen-antibody reactions. Deoxyribonucleic acid (DNA) and ribonucleic acid (RNA) both contain a five-carbon sugar (deoxyribose and ribose, respectively); glucose and galactose are essential constituents of tissues such as collagen and cerebrosides; and the various glycoproteins serve specialized functions.

Some tissues, such as muscle, can use fatty acids as a prime source of energy, but the brain derives most of its energy from glucose. In theory the body can exist without dietary carbohydrate (CHO) because it can be formed from protein and fat; however, very low–CHO diets (less than 5% of calories) quickly lead to excessive combustion of fat and a rise in fatty acid and ketone body levels in the blood, and thus to acidosis. This is what occurs when a ketogenic diet is used in the treatment of epilepsy.

Monosaccharides require no digestion. Disaccharides are hydrolyzed in the upper small intestine by specific enzymes. Starch digestion begins in the mouth (salivary amylase) and is carried to completion in the intestine by the action of pancreatic amylase and specific disaccharidases in the brush border of the jejunal epithelial cells. The resultant mixture of simple sugars, principally glucose, is taken into the mucosal cells and then into the portal circulation. In the liver, fructose and galactose are converted to glucose; some glucose is released to the general circulation, and some is stored as glycogen. The entry of glucose into cells of all types, save brain cells, is facilitated by the action of insulin. The level of blood glucose is maintained by the combined action of pituitary and adrenal as well as pancreatic hormones.

Diets very high in monosaccharides or disaccharides may cause diarrhea, and if these sugars (particularly sucrose) are present in a physical form that adheres to teeth, dental caries is promoted.

Generally, the proportions of protein, CHO, and fat in the diet can vary considerably without metabolic or nutritional risk. The limits are rather wide: protein, 8% to 20% of calories; CHO, 15% to 60% of calories; and fat, 25% to 60% of calories. Contrary to widespread belief, obesity is *not* the result of an abnormal distribution of calories among these three dietary components (e.g., starches are no more "fattening" than fat); rather it is the *total* caloric intake that is at fault. There is evidence that high fat diets, particularly those that provide large amounts of saturated fats and cholesterol, can be detrimental to health; however, excess total calories together with a sedentary life-style also are important in this regard.

WATER

All tissues contain water (dental enamel has 1% to 2%), and for most tissues this is the principal constituent. Most chemical reactions take place only in an aqueous medium, and the rate of water turnover in the body is relatively high. Thus it is no accident that most edible foods contain large amounts of this dietary essential.

Water is continuously lost from the body by a number of routes. There is an obligatory loss in urine, resulting from the kidney having a limited capacity to produce a concentrated urine. In children and adults this limit is about 1400 mOsm/L,* corresponding to a specific gravity of about 1.040. Diets high in solutes, which are largely excreted in the urine (nitrogen, sodium, phosphorus), thus call for a large urine volume. It should be noted that very young infants are able to achieve a urine concentration of only 700 mOsm/L.

Water also is being continuously lost from lungs and skin in the absence of sweating, the so-called insensible water loss, the amount of which is roughly proportional to the BMR. Such losses amount to about 10 ml/kg/day in the adult and 30 ml/kg/day in the infant. Losses of water as a result of sweating vary with environmental temperature and humidity and with physical activity. Under extreme conditions an adult can lose 500 ml/hr from sweating.

Daily fecal losses of water amount to about 150 ml in the adult and 10 ml/kg in the infant.

In addition to food and drink, there is a source of water within the body. The burning of fat and CHO produces carbon dioxide and water, the so-called water of oxidation (100 gm fat yields 107 ml H_2O, 100 gm glucose yields 60 ml H_2O). For the adult this amounts to about 300 ml/day and for the infant, about 90 ml/day.

Fig. 16-4 depicts the overall water economy for the average infant and the average adult. It is apparent that the former is at greater risk from water deprivation inasmuch as water turnover is much larger—about 16% of total body water each day compared with about 6% per day in adults. Likewise, the infant is at greater risk from conditions that accelerate water loss, such as vomiting and diarrhea, from heat stress, and from diets that provide excessive amounts of solute for urinary excretion (high protein, high salt). It is no accident that human milk has a high ratio of water to solute.

MINERALS

The diet must provide the minerals that are essential components of body tissues. Deficiency of these leads to diminished growth and to disease, and excessive intakes may result in toxicity. Table 16-3 provides information on function, dietary sources, and requirements for the minerals whose requirements have been estimated.

With the exceptions of iron and fluoride, a well-balanced diet provides a satisfactory intake of minerals. Iron deficiency

*An osmole is the molecular weight in grams of an osmotically active particle, whether it be a nonionized compound such as glucose or urea, or an ion such as Na^+ or Cl^-. A milliosmole (mOsm) is one thousandth of an osmole.

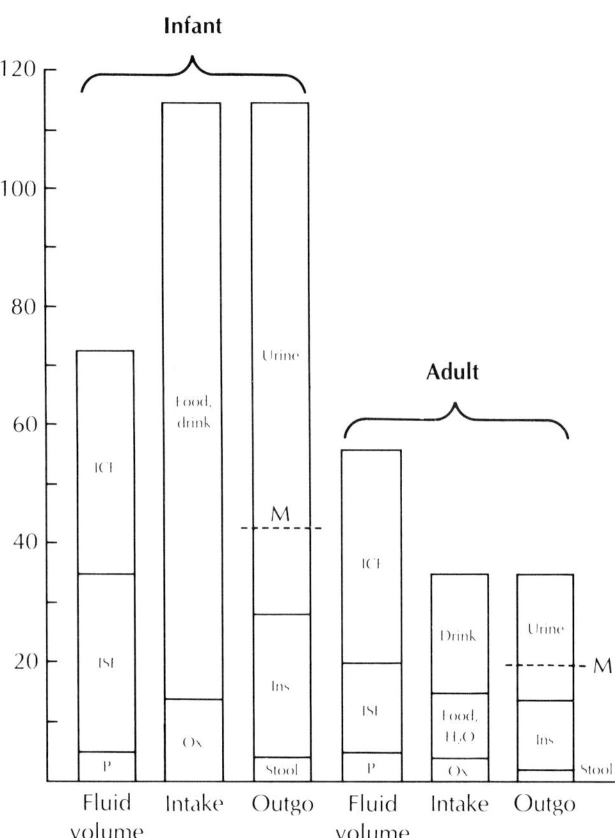

Fig. 16-4 Comparisons of body fluid volumes (percent of body weight) and of daily intake and outgo of water (ml/kg) for infant and adult. The values shown are averages and vary somewhat with the method used and with the fat content of the subject. *Dashed line (M),* Value for minimal water expenditure; *P,* plasma volume; *ISF,* interstitial fluid volume; *ICF,* intracellular fluid volume; *Ox,* water of oxidation; *Ins,* insensible water loss.

From Farmer T, editor: Pediatric neurology, ed. 3, New York, 1983, Harper & Row, Publishers, Inc.

is now the most common nutritional deficiency in this country. Attempts to improve this situation have been made through fortification of cereal products and infant formulas. Fluoride is added to the drinking water in many communities, as well as to toothpastes.

It should be mentioned here that the average U.S. diet provides a generous amount of salt, to the point that some nutritionists are concerned about this as a possible factor in the pathogenesis of hypertension.

There are, in addition to those listed in Table 16-3, a number of minerals known to be essential for animals and presumably for humans. These are chloride, chromium, manganese, molybdenum, nickel, silicon, tin, and vanadium. Deficiencies of these are unlikely to occur except with protracted parenteral feeding or, in the case of chloride, with excessive vomiting.

VITAMINS

As the word itself implies, vitamins are necessary for proper tissue function and thus for growth. These compounds function as cofactors for a number of enzymes. Most cannot be synthesized in the body and so must be supplied in the diet. Exceptions to this rule include vitamin D (activation of skin sterols by sunlight) and vitamin K (synthesized by intestinal bacteria); small amounts of vitamin B_{12} are manufactured by intestinal bacteria and some niacin by conversion from tryptophan, but not in quantities sufficient to meet requirements. Vitamin deficiencies result in disease, and excessive intakes may lead to toxicity. The story of the discovery of the relationship of certain diseases to dietary inadequacies, of the presence of certain "vital amines" in trace amounts of food, and of the elucidation of their chemical structures and metabolic functions is a fascinating one, intimately associated with the development of modern nutritional science.

Table 16-4 lists those vitamins known to be important for humans, including chemical name, function, estimated dietary requirement, dietary sources, and toxicity.

It should be noted that certain foods are fortified with vitamins. Addition of vitamin D to milk is mandated by law; vitamins now are added to many commercial infant formulas, to certain cereal products, to some breads, to fruit substitute drinks, and to other foods; and vitamin products are widely sold. The result of all this activity is that overt vitamin deficiencies are now rare in the United States. Nevertheless, it should be kept in mind that the infant and the child are at greater risk than the adult because their requirements are proportionally greater, so that dietary deficiency will more quickly result in disease.

Recent claims have been made that massive intakes of vitamin C and the B complex will protect against respiratory tract infection and atherosclerosis and will ameliorate abnormal behavior and poor school performance. Terms such as *megavitamin therapy* and *orthomolecular treatment* now appear in the lay literature and in a few scientific publications. There is no proof for such claims.

NUTRITIONAL SCENE IN THE UNITED STATES TODAY

Of the many factors that bear on today's nutritional scene, none has had a greater impact than *food technology* and *sanitation*. These modern developments have resulted from combined actions by government, industry, nutritional scientists, and physicians.

Before the turn of the century the greatest hazards to infant health were infection and improper food. The whole history of infant nutrition is one of attempts to devise a satisfactory milk for those babies who could not be fed at the breast. It was the realization in the past that raw cow milk was not a satisfactory food for young infants that led the fortunate few to employ wet nurses for their young.

The following features of raw cow milk render it less than suitable for young infants. *Bacterial contamination* arises from several sources: the cow herself (tubercle bacilli, streptococci [mastitis is common in high producing herds], and *Brucella* organisms) and the various humans who handle the milk, any one of whom may add bacteria to the milk from respiratory or cutaneous foci. Lack of suitable refrigeration facilities in former days (or in some areas still) accentuated the problem.

Text continued on p. 180

Table 16-3 *Nutritionally Important Minerals*

MINERAL	FUNCTION	PHYSIOLOGY	EFFECTS OF DEFICIENCY	EFFECTS OF EXCESS	DAILY REQUIREMENT	SOURCES
Calcium	Structure of bone, ion transport across cell membranes, neuromuscular excitability, blood coagulation	Absorption aided by vitamin D and parathyroid hormone (PTH), hindered by phosphate; PTH facilitates release from bone, thyrocalcitonin inhibits; gravity and muscle tension needed for skeletal stability	Osteoporosis only with severe deficiency, muscle paralysis, or malabsorption	Hypercalcuria with excessive vitamin D, and immobilization	Infants—400-600 mg Adolescents—600-700 mg Pregnancy (latter half), lactation—1000-1200 mg	Milk, cheese, green leafy vegetables, beans, canned salmon
Copper	Cofactor for certain enzymes, cross-linking of collagen	Plasma level 110 µg/dl, mostly as ceruloplasmin; intestinal absorption hindered by excessive zinc	Anemia, osteoporosis, defective myelination	None, except with massive ingestion	0.5-2 mg	Liver, meats, grains
Fluoride	Bone and tooth structure, caries resistance	Deposited in bone as fluorapatite	Tendency to dental caries	4-8 mg/day—mottled teeth 20+ mg/day for long periods—osteosclerosis Large doses—acute poisoning	1 mg/L in drinking water	Seafoods, many municipal water supplies
Iodine	Constituent of thyroid hormone	Concentrated in thyroid gland	Simple goiter, endemic cretinism	Iodism	40-150 µg	Seafoods, iodized salt
Iron	Constituent of hemoglobin, myoglobulin, enzymes	Absorption regulated by gastrointestinal mucosa, level of blood hemoglobin; menstrual loss averages 0.7 mg/day	Anemia; if severe, cardiac failure, poor growth, lethargy	Hemosiderosis, poisoning by medicinal iron	Infants—1 mg/kg Adolescents—10-18 mg	Liver, whole grains, egg, legumes, meat

Table 16-3 *Nutritionally Important Minerals—cont'd*

MINERAL	FUNCTION	PHYSIOLOGY	EFFECTS OF DEFICIENCY	EFFECTS OF EXCESS	DAILY REQUIREMENT	SOURCES
Magnesium	Cofactor for enzymes, neuromuscular excitability	Principal cation of intracellular fluid	Tetany, hypocalcemia	Poisoning from medicinal magnesium (intravenous or intramuscular)	Infants—4 mg/kg	Meat, cereals, milk
Phosphorus	Constituent of phospholipids, ATP, nucleic acids; intermediary metabolism	Absorption regulated by vitamin D, dietary calcium, PTH; latter affects renal excretion	Muscle weakness; dysethesia; rickets in premature infants	In newborn, hypocalcemia	Infants—two thirds of calcium requirement All others—same as calcium requirement	Most foods
Potassium	Cellular transport, CHO and protein metabolism, membrane potential in muscle and nerve	Principal cation of intracellular fluid; regulation by adrenocortical steroids	Muscle weakness, abdominal distention, cardiac failure, alkalosis	Cardiac failure	1.5-2 mEq/kg	All foods
Selenium	Constituent of glutathione peroxidase	Interaction with vitamin E, heavy metals	Cardiomyopathy; muscle degeneration (animals)	Animals—"blind staggers"	Adults—50-200 μg	Seafood, liver, meat
Sodium	Osmotic pressure, cellular transport, extracellular fluid volume	Principal cation of extracellular fluid; regulation by adrenocortical hormones	Weakness, dehydration	Edema; CNS irritability if severe	2 mEq/kg	Most foods
Zinc	Constituent of enzymes	Absorption impaired by diet high in calcium, fiber	Growth failure, hypogonadism, reduced taste acuity	None, except with massive ingestion	Children—6 mg Adults—15 mg	Meat, especially pork, whole grains, nuts, cheese

Table 16-4 *Nutritionally Important Vitamins*

VITAMIN	CHARACTERISTICS	BIOCHEMICAL ACTION	EFFECTS OF DEFICIENCY	EFFECTS OF EXCESS	DAILY REQUIREMENT	FOOD SOURCES
Vitamin A (retinol); 1 IU = 0.3 μg retinol	Fat soluble, heat stable; bile necessary for absorption, specific binding protein in plasma; stored in liver	Component of visual purple; integrity of epithelial tissues, bone cell function	Night blindness, xerophthalmia, keratomalacia, poor growth, impaired resistance to infection	Hyperostosis, hepatomegaly, alopecia, increased cerebrospinal fluid pressure	Infants—300 μg Adolescents—750 μg Lactation—1200 μg	Milk fat, egg, liver
Provitamin A (beta-carotene); one sixth the activity of retinol	Converted to retinol in liver, intestinal mucosa			Carotenemia		Dark green vegetables, yellow fruits and vegetables, tomatoes
Biotin	Water soluble; synthesized by intestinal bacteria; deficiency with large intake of egg *white*, total parenteral nutrition	Coenzyme	Dermatitis, anorexia, muscle pain, pallor	Unknown	Unknown	Liver, egg yolk, peanuts
Cobalamin (vitamin B_{12})	Slightly soluble in water, heat stable only at neutral pH, light sensitive; absorption (ileum) dependent on gastric intrinsic factor; cobalt a part of the molecule	Coenzyme component; red blood cell maturation; CNS metabolism	Pernicious anemia, neurologic deterioration	Unknown	1-2 μg	Animal foods only; meat, milk, egg
Folacin (group of compounds containing pteridine ring, *p*-aminobenzoic and glutamic acids)	Slightly soluble in water, light sensitive, heat stable; some production by intestinal bacteria; ascorbic acid involved in interconversions; interference from oral contraceptives, anticonvulsants	Tetrahydrofolic acid (the active form): synthesis of purines and pyrimidines, and methylation reactions	Megaloblastic anemia	Only in patients with pernicious anemia not receiving cobalamin	Infants—60 μg Adolescents—200 μg Pregnancy—400 μg	Liver, green vegetables, cereals, oranges

Continued.

Table 16-4 *Nutritionally Important Vitamins—cont'd*

VITAMIN	CHARACTERISTICS	BIOCHEMICAL ACTION	EFFECTS OF DEFICIENCY	EFFECTS OF EXCESS	DAILY REQUIREMENT	FOOD SOURCES
Niacin (nicotinic acid, nicotinamide)	Water soluble, heat and light stable; availability from corn enhanced by alkali; synthesized in the body from tryptophan (60:1), some by intestinal bacteria	Component of coenzymes I and II (NAD, NADP); many enzymatic reactions	Pellagra: dermatitis, diarrhea, dementia	Nicotinic acid (not the amide): flushing, pruritus	6.6 mg/1000 Cal	Meat, fish, whole grains, green vegetables
Pantothenic acid	Water soluble, heat stable	Component of coenzyme A; many enzymatic reactions	Observed only with use of antagonists; depression, hypotension, muscle weakness, abdominal pain	Unknown	Unknown—estimated at 5-10 mg	Most foods
Vitamin B_5 (pyridoxine, pyridoxal, pyridoxamine)	Water soluble, heat and light labile; interference from isoniazid; pyridoxal is the active form	Cofactor for many enzymes	Dermatitis, glossitis, cheilosis, peripheral neuritis; infants—irritability, convulsions, anemia	Polyneuropathy	Infants—0.2-0.3 mg Adults—1-2 mg	Liver, meat, whole grains, corn, soybeans
Riboflavin	Water soluble, light labile, heat stable; synthesis by intestinal bacteria (?)	Cofactor for many enzymes	Photophobia, cheilosis, glossitis, corneal vascularization, poor growth	Unknown	0.6 mg/1000 Cal	Meat, milk, egg, green vegetables, whole grains
Thiamine (vitamin B_1)	Heat labile; absorption impaired by alcohol; requirement a function of CHO intake; synthesis by intestinal bacteria	Coenzyme for decarboxylation, other reactions	Beriberi; neuritis, edema, cardiac failure; hoarseness, anorexia, restlessness, aphonia	Unknown	0.4 mg/1000 Cal	Liver, meat, milk, whole grains, legumes
Ascorbic acid (vitamin C)	Easily oxidized, especially in presence of copper, iron, high pH; absorption by simple diffusion	Exact mechanism unknown; functions in folacin metabolism, collagen biosynthesis, iron absorption and transport, tyrosine metabolism	Scurvy	Massive doses may lead to temporary increase in requirement	Infants—10-20 mg Adolescents—30 mg	Citrus fruits, tomatoes, cabbage, potatoes, human milk

Continued.

Table 16-4 *Nutritionally Important Vitamins—cont'd*

VITAMIN	CHARACTERISTICS	BIOCHEMICAL ACTION	EFFECTS OF DEFICIENCY	EFFECTS OF EXCESS	DAILY REQUIREMENT	FOOD SOURCES
Vitamin D (D_2—activated calciferol; D_3—activated dehydrocholesterol); 1 IU = 0.025 μg	D_2 from diet, D_3 from action of ultraviolet light on skin; hydroxylated sequentially in liver and kidney to form 1,25-dihydroxycholecalciferol, the active compound; regulated by dietary calcium and PTH; now called a hormone; anticonvulsant drugs interfere with metabolism	Formation of calcium transport protein in duodenal mucosa; facilitates bone resorption and phosphorus absorption	Rickets, osteomalacia	Hypercalcemia, azotemia, poor growth, vomiting, nephrocalcinosis	Infants—10 μg (400 IU) Others—2.5-10 μg (100-400 IU)	Fortified milk, fish liver, salmon, sardines, mackerel, egg yolk, sunlight; human milk not an adequate source
Vitamin E; 1 IU = 1 mg alpha-tocopherol acetate	Stored in adipose tissue, transported with beta-lipoproteins; absorption dependent on pancreatic juice and bile (iron may interfere); requirement increased by large amounts of polyunsaturated fats	Antioxidant; role in red blood cell fragility	Hemolytic anemia in premature infants; otherwise, no clear-cut deficiency syndrome in humans	Unknown	Infants—4 mg Adolescents—15 mg	Cereal seed oils, peanuts, soybeans, milk fat, turnip greens
Vitamin K (naphthoquinones)	Fat soluble, bile necessary for absorption, synthesis by intestinal bacteria	Blood coagulation: factors II, VII, IX, X	Hemorrhagic manifestations	Water soluble analogs only: hyperbilirubinemia	Newborn—single dose of 1 mg; thereafter 5 μg/day Older infants and children—unknown	Cow milk, green leafy vegetables, pork liver

Cow milk contains about three times as much protein as human milk, and it is this high protein content (a large fraction of which is casein) that accounts for the formation of tough, voluminous curds on gastric acidification and thus leads to *impaired digestibility*. According to casual observation, formula-fed infants have larger stool volumes than do breast-fed babies.

The sum total of solutes available for renal excretion is 2½ times higher in cow milk than in human milk, and this *high solute load* calls for a higher obligatory urine volume; thus the infant is at greater risk from hot weather. For the newborn the high phosphorus content of cow milk is one factor in the pathogenesis of neonatal hypocalcemia.

Raw cow milk supplies barely enough *ascorbic acid* (21 mg/L) to prevent scurvy, and unfortunately the process of pasteurization destroys about half the vitamin present. A few infants are *allergic* to cow milk protein and will suffer gastrointestinal disturbances or eczema as a result.

Modern technology has overcome these difficulties. Pasteurization, combined with mandated refrigeration, has virtually eliminated bacterial contamination, and evaporated milk is sterile and keeps well without refrigeration. Heat treatment also improves digestibility, and diluting the milk with water and adding carbohydrate to restore the caloric content reduces the solute load.

Industry also has modified modern cow milk formulas in many respects: addition of ascorbic acid, vitamin D, and iron; reduction in phosphorus content; development of hypoallergenic milks based on soybean and meat protein; reduction in sodium and protein content; and substitution of vegetable fat for milk fat. Some commercial infant formulas contain added vitamin E and B complex, some are free of lactose (this sugar might not be tolerated by babies with gastrointestinal disorders), and others contain hydrolyzed casein as a source of nitrogen. This wide variety of infant formula products makes it possible to feed satisfactorily every baby by formula from nonhuman sources. Modern technology has wrought a change of unprecedented magnitude in infant welfare.

However, there are two disadvantages. These are cost and the decline in breast-feeding. The former is important to the poor of our country and a major stumbling block to the exportation of our food technology to the poverty-striken nations of the world. Moreover, the more advanced the technology, the higher is the cost. For example, the mother who nurses her 2- to 3-month-old infant needs only an extra pint of pasteurized milk each day to satisfy the additional calcium and protein requirements, plus an extra two slices of bread and one potato (or 10 g of butter) to complete the caloric need, together with vitamin D drops for the baby. The feeding of an evaporated milk–water–Karo syrup formula is also inexpensive (additional vitamin C is needed), whereas the cost of a commercial ready-to-feed formula complete with added vitamins is considerably greater.

The ease and convenience of formula feeding have led inevitably to a decline in breast-feeding in our society and even in some nonindustrial societies. There is some evidence of an immunologic advantage in human milk and for better iron, zinc, and fat absorption; furthermore, the lack of contamination and the psychological benefit that may accrue with nursing are clear advantages. It is appropriate therefore to encourage breast-feeding in situations in which sanitation is poor, refrigeration is lacking, and cost is critical. It is encouraging to note that many more mothers have chosen to nurse their babies in recent years. It should be remembered that human milk has inadequate amounts of vitamin D; thus nurslings must be given this vitamin, and mothers should be advised to eat a well-balanced diet.

Governmental regulations, public health activities, and governmental assistance are of the utmost importance to the modern nutritional scene. Municipal water supplies are now pure and pasteurization is a uniform requirement for the sale of cow milk commercially. Dairy cattle are tested for tuberculosis and brucellosis, and those with mastitis are removed from production. Other measures include inspection of food handlers and of meats, inspection of restaurant kitchens, codes for infant formulas shipped from one state to another, and codes for commercially canned foods. The result is that diseases such as typhoid fever, bovine tuberculosis, trichinosis, botulism, and staphylococcal food poisoning are now rare.

Many studies have shown the deleterious effects of severe infection, particularly gastroenteritis, on nutrition (vitamin turnover increases, and nitrogen balance becomes negative). The high prevalence of infantile malnutrition in nonindustrialized societies is due in part to the occurrence of repeated infections. The Food and Drug Administration (FDA) was formed in 1938; this agency has the authority to regulate, among other things, food quality, food labeling, use of food additives, and vitamin fortification. The Federal Trade Commission monitors advertising claims. These measures have resulted in better, cleaner, and more wholesome food. One of the most dramatic improvements was effected by the mandatory addition of vitamin D to milk, which has led to the virtual elimination of deficiency rickets in this country.

Food assistance programs are now fairly widespread. These include school lunch programs, the food stamp program, the program for women, infants, and children (WIC), and, in reality, the farm subsidy program. As a result, families with limited financial means can augment their otherwise meager food supply. Many millions of persons are receiving food stamps, and 600,000 are enrolled in the WIC program.

Finally, there is the important role of local, state, and federal governments in providing free or low-cost health care for poor people and salaries for school and public health nutritionists and for helping to defray the cost of special foods for children with certain diseases, such as phenylketonuria.

The result of these efforts, both industrial and governmental, is that with but one exception (iron-deficiency anemia), overt nutritional deficiency now is uncommon in the United States, and we are now left with obesity and dental caries as the most prevalent "nutritional" conditions.

Two quasi-official organizations have published recommendations for nutritional allowances (not requirements!): the Food and Nutrition Board of the National Academy of Sciences–National Research Council and the Food and Agricultural Organization of the United Nations. The former organization publishes a series of pamphlets at roughly 5-year intervals, the most recent one in 1989, which include a listing of recommended dietary allowances (RDAs) for persons of all ages. These are based on present knowledge of actual requirements, to which is added a generous "safety factor" to account for the supposed individual variation in requirements and for variations in food quality. Except for calories, the "recommended" amounts all are in excess of actual need for the average individual; therefore it is not surprising that dietary surveys reveal that a sizable proportion of the population consumes less of many nutrients than the NAS recommends. The Food and Agricultural Organization (FAO) recommendations are closer to actual requirements for protein, calcium, and a number of vitamins (see WHO *Handbook*), but unfortunately this list of nutrients is not as complete as the one published by NAS.

POSSIBLE ROLE OF INFANT AND CHILD NUTRITION IN ADULT HEALTH

Generally, the nutritional status of infants and children today is reasonably good. There are some who say that our biggest challenge is the adults—namely, whether current infant feeding practices are compromising their health and longevity.

Several facts have been established. An intake of fluoride in early life, at a time when dental enamel is forming, results in a long-term diminution of the dental caries rate. It is known that a high intake of sucrose, particularly in solid sticky foods, predisposes a person to dental caries, so that the early acquisition of food habits that minimize the consumption of such foods should be beneficial.* It is known that childhood obesity tends to persist into adult life and that obesity shortens the life span; attempts to prevent childhood obesity are therefore important. Severe malnutrition in *early life* may impair intellectual performance† and should be avoided through procedures such as early feeding of premature infants, use of intravenous alimentation in certain critical situations, and early seeking of medical advice and treatment for diseases that compromise nutrition during infancy.

The most challenging question relates to atherosclerosis and its cardiac and cerebral consequences. (Omitted from the discussion here is consideration of the inherited abnormalities of lipoprotein metabolism associated with early onset arterial disease.) It is known that arterial changes (the fatty streaks) appear in childhood and that by age 20 an appreciable percentage of men already have atherosclerotic plaques. The dietary components that have been considered as possible factors in initiating or intensifying this aging process are total calories, animal protein, saturated fats, and cholesterol. Cross-cultural surveys of adult autopsies reveal that any one or all of these factors may be at fault; there is also some evidence that "postcoronary" adults who limit their intake of calories, saturated fat, and cholesterol have a better prognosis. The possible preventive role of fish has been mentioned earlier; however, certain species now are contaminated with mercury and polychlorinated hydrocarbons.

Experiments conducted many years ago showed that rats fed (from weaning) an amount of food equal to about two thirds of their usual intake lived much longer and had less arterial disease and fewer tumors that those fed ad libitum. These results have subsequently been confirmed by Ross,[2] who states, "The effects of chronic restriction in food intake on laboratory animals have been so apparent that it is difficult to avoid concluding that no environmental factor so decisively reduces the rate or expression of the aging process" and "The mechanisms through which nutrition influences the aging processes are already operative during the *youthful stage* of life [italics mine]." If dietary restriction is postponed until maturity, the benefits are not as great.

Recent surveys show that the average protein intake by citizens in the United States is at least twice the estimated requirement, that average milk consumption is about a pint a day, that solid food supplements are offered at a very early age, and that obesity is prevalent; thus the results of the animal experiments are worth serious consideration. Berry[1] makes this cogent comment: "Throughout the world the State does not accept the responsibility to protect its individuals from overnutrition." It is of interest that strict vegetarians are leaner and have lower levels of serum lipids and lower blood pressures than do nonvegetarians.

Some students of nutrition claim that there is evidence for a deleterious effect of modern refined foods, in that their consumption favors the incidence of diverticulosis and colonic tumors. They advocate a diet that has a higher fiber content, such as whole grain cereals, bran, and raw vegetables. Others caution against excesses of dietary fiber because this may interfere with the absorption of certain minerals.

Committees of the U.S. Senate and of the American Heart Association suggest that it would be advantageous for everyone to reduce intakes of saturated fats, refined sugar, salt, and cholesterol, while proportionally increasing the amount of complex carbohydrates, and to balance energy intake with energy expenditure. These "dietary goals" should apply to children (but not infants!) as well as to adults.

THE "WELL-BALANCED" DIET

The consumption of a variety of foods is the best protection against nutritional deficiency. Except for the first few months of life, when milk is the principal if not the sole food, the daily diet should include items from each of the following general food groups, known in nutritional circles as "the basic four":

1. Meat, fish, poultry, eggs
2. Dairy products—milk, cheese, and milk products
3. Fruits and vegetables
4. Cereal grains, potatoes, rice

Today one frequently hears the term *junk foods* in reference to prepared foods high in refined carbohydrate and low in protein and vitamins, full of so-called empty calories. These foods do supply energy, and one cannot help thinking of the simpler life of previous generations when foods of similar

*Statements by manufacturers reveal a generous consumption of sucrose: for the United States, this amounts to about 50 kg per capita per year, equivalent to 125 g, or 500 calories, per day. Furthermore, this figure has remained fairly constant during the past 50 years.

†There is reasonable evidence for such an effect when malnutrition occurs in the early months of life, and particularly when it is prolonged. In late infancy and childhood the effect has not been clearly demonstrated, probably because brain maturation is well on its way to completion. Nor has nutritional deprivation during pregnancy been shown to impair intellectual performance of the offspring. The effect of malnutrition per se is very difficult to study because it is almost always accompanied by cultural or emotional disadvantages.

composition, such as apple pie, cake with thick frosting, jellied preserves, and home canned fruits, were consumed freely, without opprobrium, their production being considered the hallmark of the successful housewife.

Vegans, the colloquial term for strict vegetarians, should be counseled by a nutritionist because their diet is devoid of vitamin B_{12} and is likely to be low in calcium. The choice of grains and vegetables must be such as to include all the essential amino acids.

All persons consuming "fad diets" of one sort or another and those who voluntarily limit food intake in an effort to lose weight should also receive nutritional guidance, inasmuch as such diets may be lacking in one or more essential nutrients. There are now reports of growth failure in adolescents who consume low-fat diets.

Two
The Feeding of Infants and Children

Marvin S. Eiger

Infant nutrition should be considered a holistic enterprise. After the initial physical examination and the pronouncement of normality of her new offspring, the mother's primary concern is how she will nourish her baby. During pregnancy, maternal good health, a carefully supervised dietary intake, and adequate rest all ensure proper nutrition of the fetus. This symbiotic union persists once infant and mother become two separate beings, and adequate nutrition for the infant then becomes a more purposeful procedure, the details of which usurp much of the mother's time and energies during the first 6 to 12 months of the infant's life. This is the period of most rapid extrauterine growth, during which infants double their birth weight in the first 5 months and triple it by the twelfth month. Food during this period satisfies both physical and emotional growth, and the milieu in which it is provided is of paramount importance to the infant, whose oral orientation translates food into ego satisfaction. Thus the practice of infant feeding cannot be based solely on what *type of milk* the infant should receive. Numerous other factors must be considered.

Most infants appear to grow normally and maintain a satisfactory state of health in spite of variations in nutritional management. The goal of infant nutrition is to produce an adequately (but not overly) nourished child whose diet is readily digestible, with all the essential nutrients being provided through a reasonable distribution of calories derived from protein, fat, and carbohydrate. Because the pattern and content of feeding in infancy will strongly affect dietary habits later in life, much care must be given to constructing the early dietary milieu.

Based on studies of nutritional requirements in infancy, reasonable recommendations for full-term infants are that 7% to 16% of calories be derived from protein, 30% to 55% from fat, and the remainder from carbohydrate.[4] Human milk provides approximately 7% of calories from protein, 55% from fat, and 38% from lactose. Most commercially prepared formulas in the United States are modeled after human milk and provide 9% to 15% of calories from protein, 45% to 50% from fat, and the remainder from carbohydrate, usually lactose.

With the exceptions of vitamin D, iron, and fluoride, the infant fed breast milk from a healthy mother apparently receives more than adequate nutrition without further supplementation for at least the first 6 months of life. Thus, from a physiologic and teleologic point of view, the maxims of "breast is best" and "human milk is for humans, cow milk is for cows" are unchallengeable. Only in the past 50 years or so has there been any question as to whether a mother would breast-feed her baby. With the advent of pasteurization, dependable refrigeration, and production of formulas from cow milk, alternatives have been provided. Thus the decision to breast-feed depends on a multiplicity of factors: the customs of the community; attitudes of the obstetrician, pediatrician, and family; life-style; and the personality of the mother. In 1980 the American Academy of Pediatrics, in its strongest statement ever, advised pediatricians and other health providers for children of the importance of and the need to recommend breast-feeding over formula feeding. The pediatrician must be aware of the advantages of human milk over cow milk for infant feeding and encourage mothers to breast-feed. However, the pediatrician must remain sensitive to the new mother's own feelings and needs.

COMPARISON OF HUMAN MILK AND COW MILK

Milk is the primary source for satisfying nutritional needs during the entire first year of life. Solid foods are unnecessary for most infants until 4 to 6 months of age. Therefore it is essential that the physician be knowledgeable about the composition of human milk and cow milk. The manufacturers of infant formulas constantly attempt to modify cow milk to produce a product comparable to human milk. It is of interest that growth rates of the human infant and the calf are different. An infant takes two to three times longer than a calf to double its birth weight. Inasmuch as cow milk contains 3.5 g of protein per deciliter to human milk's 1.1 g, a ratio of 3:1, the symmetry of nature is satisfied. (See Table 16-5 and Appendix C, Tables C-10 and C-11, for comparisons of human milk and various cow milk formulas.)

In addition to the larger amount of protein in cow milk than in human milk, there are qualitative differences in the protein in the two milks. The percentage of casein, as compared with whey proteins (lactalbumin and lactoglobulins), is higher in cow milk. Both proteins are of high biologic value, but casein causes higher curd tension in the infant's stomach and thus must be treated by homogenization, heating, and acidification for better digestion.

Table 16-5 *Comparison of Nutrients in Formulas and Mature Human Milk*

COMPONENT (per dl)	RECOMMENDED DAILY DIETARY ALLOWANCES (0-6 MONTHS)	HUMAN MILK—VALUES VARIABLE	"HUMANIZED" FORMULAS			EVAPORATED MILK, 1:1 DILUTION	EVAPORATED MILK 13 OZ, WATER 19 OZ, CARBOHYDRATE 1 OZ	WHOLE MILK 3.5% FAT
			ENFAMIL WITH IRON	SIMILAC WITH IRON	SMA			
Calories (kcal)	117 kcal/kg	67-75	67	68	67	69	67	66
Protein (g)	2.2 g/kg	1.1	1.5	1.6	1.5	3.5	2.8	3.5
Fat, total (g)	Not listed	4.5	3.7	3.6	3.6	3.8	3.0	3.5-3.7
Saturated		2.2	1.2	1.4	1.6	2.4	1.9	2.2
Unsaturated		2.3	2.5	2.2	2.0	1.4	1.1	1.3
Cholesterol (mg)	Not listed	7-47	1.4	1.6	3.3	10-34	8-28	10-35
Carbohydrate (g)	Not listed	6.8 lactose	7 lactose	7.1 lactose	7.2 lactose	4.8 lactose	7.0 lactose sucrose	4.9 lactose
Calcium (mg)	360	34	55	58	44	126	100	118
Phosphorus (mg)	240	14	46	43	33	102	81	92
Sodium (mg)	Not listed	16	28	25	16	60	48	50
Potassium (mg)	Not listed	51	69	75	56	152	122	137
Magnesium (mg)	60	4	4	4	5	12	10	12
Iron (mg)	10	0.05	1.2	1.2	1.3	0.05	0.04	0.05
Copper (μg)	Not listed	40	60	40	50	Estimate 30	Estimate 20	30
Zinc (mg)	3	0.3-0.5	0.4	0.5	0.4	0.3-0.5	0.2-0.4	0.3-0.5
Iodine (μg)	35	3	7	10	7	5	4	5
Vitamin A (IU)	1400	200	170	250	264	185	150	140
Thiamine (mg)	0.3	0.016	0.05	0.07	0.07	0.03	0.02	0.17
Riboflavin (mg)	0.4	0.036	0.06	0.1	0.1	0.19	0.16	0.17
Niacin (mg)	5	0.1	0.8	0.7	0.7	0.1	0.1	0.1
Pyridoxine (mg)	0.3	0.01	0.04	0.04	0.04	0.04	0.03	0.06
Folacin (mg)	0.05	0.005	0.01	0.005	0.005	0.005	0.004	0.005
Vitamin B_{12} (μg)	0.3	0.03	0.2	0.2	0.1	0.08	0.06	0.4
Vitamin C (mg)	35	4	5	6	6	0.5	0.4	1
Vitamin D (IU)	400	2	42	40	42	Fortified 40	Fortified 32	Fortified 42
Vitamin E (IU)	4	0.2	1.3	1.5	1	0.04	0.03	0.04
Vitamin K (μg)	Not listed	1.5	6	9	5.8	Estimate 6	Estimate 5	6

Modified from Fomon SJ: Infant nutrition, ed 2, Philadelphia, 1980, WB Saunders Co; and Committee on Dietary Allowances. Recommended dietary allowance, ed 9, rev ed, Washington DC, 1980, National Academy of Sciences.

The fat of cow milk (butterfat) contains, predominantly, saturated fatty acids and is less well digested by infants than is the fat of human milk, which contains, predominantly, monounsaturated fatty acids such as oleic acid and adequate amounts of polyunsaturated fatty acids such as essential linoleic acid. The fat composition in human milk allows for excellent fat and calcium absorption and ensures that all essential fatty acids are provided. Human milk, in contrast to cow milk, is rich in lipase, which, added to intestinal lipase, aids in the rapid splitting of free fatty acids from triglycerides to ensure their rapid absorption. It has been shown that free fatty acids are the most important sources of energy for the young infant, and the lipase in human milk makes these free fatty acids available rapidly, even before digestion with intestinal lipase commences.

Lactose is present in higher concentrations in human milk than in the milk of any other mammal. Lactose is split into glucose and galactose. Galactose is synthesized into galactolipid, which is an essential component of the central nervous system in mammals. In most commercial formulas, lactose is provided as the carbohydrate in a percentage similar to that found in human milk.

The total ash content of human milk (0.2%) is less than one third that of cow milk (0.7%), thus providing a greater margin of safety for renal excretion during illness in early infancy.

*BREAST-FEEDING VERSUS ARTIFICIAL FEEDING**

Many studies indicate that fewer gastrointestinal infections, respiratory illnesses, and allergic reactions develop in breast-fed than in artifically fed infants.[5,8] These differences are most striking in the developing countries, where poor sanitary practices prevail. However, a large degree of protection against illness is afforded to the breast-fed infant in the developed countries of the world as well. Protection is based on the presence of secretory antibodies in colostrum; the bifidus factor in human milk, which promotes the development of the characteristic intestinal microflora of *Lactobacillus bifidus;* and other defense factors (Table 16-6). Each year, researchers add other defensive factors against disease found in breast milk to this list of properties. Maximum protection against infection is afforded the infant if breast milk alone, without solid foods, is offered until 6 months of life.

The breast-fed infant has been shown to have a lower incidence of allergic diseases when foreign food antigens are avoided for the first 6 months of life.[3] In one study of more than 20,000 infants, those who were fed artificially were seven times as likely to develop eczema as those who were completely breast-fed.[6] The first 6 months is the period in which infants' passively acquired transplacental antibodies are being replaced with their own; thus lack of exposure to foreign food antigens presumably results in a reduced frequency of allergic reactions. Infants are never allergic to their mother's milk, whereas allergy to cow milk does occur.

An infant can digest human milk much more easily than the milk of other mammalian species. Breast milk forms softer curds in the infant's stomach than does cow milk and is more rapidly assimilated. Although it contains less protein than cow milk, virtually all the protein in breast milk is used by the infant, whereas about half the protein in cow milk is passed in the stool. The breast-fed infant rarely gets diarrhea and rarely becomes constipated because breast milk does not form hard stools in the intestinal tract.

There are no synthetic compounds, no preservatives, and no artificial ingredients in breast milk. It always is available at the right temperature and the right consistency. Sucking at the breast is good for the infant's tooth and jaw development. Nursing is technically different from artifical feeding in that the bottle-fed infant does not have to exercise the jaws so energetically inasmuch as light sucking alone produces a rapid flow of milk. Bottle-fed infants use their tongue in a manner quite opposite that of the breast-fed baby; the flow of milk through the rubber nipple is produced by a tongue-thrusting motion with each suck while the infant's lips create a negative pressure in the oral cavity, thus suctioning milk from the bottle.

The breast-fed baby places the tongue over the lower jaw, where it remains throughout the nursing session, and draws the nipple by suction well into the mouth, elongating it to three times its normal length and extending it to the junction between the hard and the soft palates. The elongated nipple rests in a trough formed by the U-shaped tongue. As each suckling cycle is initiated, the infant's jaws compress the milk sinuses just under and proximal to the areola, pinching off a bolus of milk and propelling it toward the posterior pharynx by a reverse peristaltic, wavelike motion. This rollerlike movement, beginning at the anterior tip of the tongue and progressing toward its base, effectively strips the milk bolus from the base of the nipple out toward its tip where it exits into the infant's mouth and is swallowed (Fig. 16-5). The jaw muscles are thus strenuously exercised, encouraging

Table 16-6 *Host Resistance Factors in Human Milk*

COMPONENTS	PROPOSED MODE OF ACTION
Growth factor of *L. bifidus*	*L. bifidus* interferes with intestinal colonization of enteric pathogens
Antistaphylococcal factor	Inhibits staphylococci
Secretory IgA and other immunoglobulins	Protective antibodies for the gut and respiratory tract
C4 and C3	C3 fragments have opsonic, chemotactic, and anaphylatoxic activities
Lysozyme	Lysis of bacterial cell wall
Lactoperoxidase-H_2O_2-thiocyanate	Killing of streptococci
Lactoferrin	Kills microorganisms by chelating iron
Leukocytes	Phagocytosis
	Cell-mediated immunity—production of IgA, C4, C3, lysozyme, and lactoferrin

*See Chapter 36, Four, Adjustment Period, for additional discussion of breast-feeding.

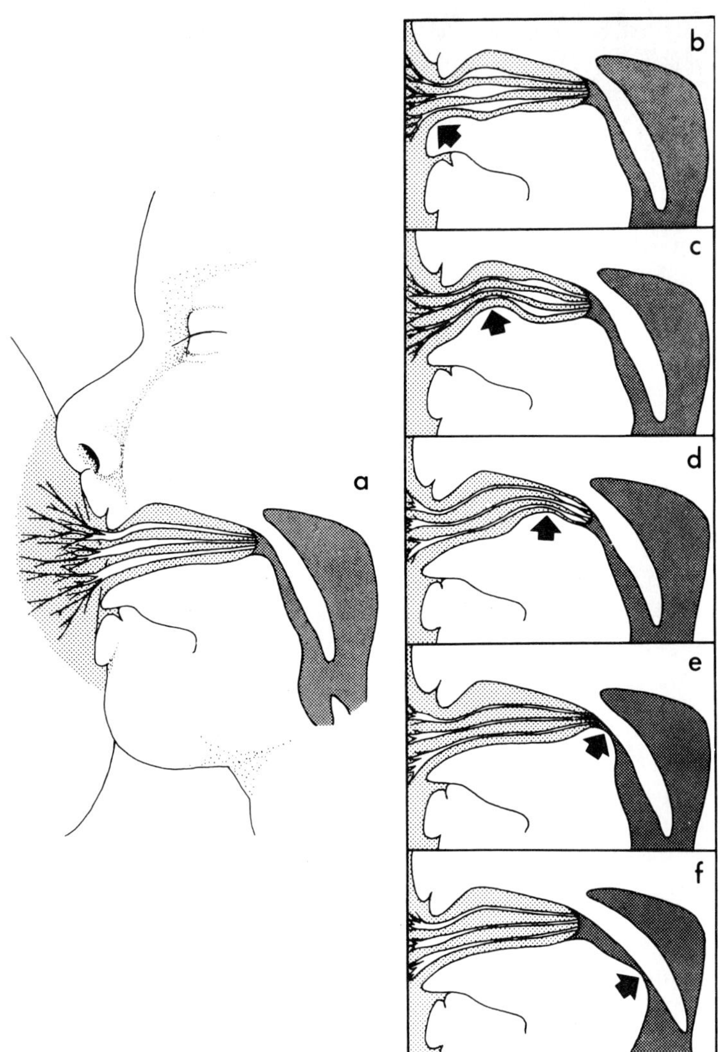

Fig. 16-5 Complete "suck" cycle. (A), infant's jaws compress sinuses, nipple drawn into mouth with tip at junction of hard and soft palates, tongue cradling nipple; (B), lower jaw constricts nipple base and thus pinching off milk bolus, anterior tip of tongue begins wavelike motion; (C), roller-like tongue action moves milk posteriorly; (D&E), wave of compression pushes milk into oropharynx where it is swallowed; (F), jaw lowers allowing milk to flow into nipple base again as the next "suck" cycle begins.

From the *"Anatomy" of Infant Sucking*, Midwifery, 2, p. 166, 1986, Woolridge, M.W.

the development of well-formed jaws and straight, healthy teeth.[14]

Perhaps most important, although most nebulous, are the psychological benefits the infant derives from breast-feeding.[1] Factors such as the more intimate interaction between the breast-feeding mother and child and the more immediate satisfaction of the nursing baby's hunger seem to augur healthier mental development. The infant does gain a sense of security from the warmth and closeness of the mother's body. Breast-feeding eliminates the practice of bottle propping; the infant, of necessity, must be drawn close at each feeding. Although the bottle-feeding mother also can show her love for her baby by holding and cuddling the baby at feeding times, in actual practice she may do less of this, and, of course, she cannot duplicate the *unique* skin-to-skin contact between the nursing mother and her infant. Montagu[11] states, "The breast feeding relationship constitutes the foundation for the development of all human social relationships, and the communications the infant receives through the warmth of the mother's skin constitute the first of the socializing experiences of his life." Babies gain a sense of well-being from secure handling, and mothers who nurse their infants successfully often seem more confident in their management of them. Whether the woman who is sure of her maternal abilities is more likely to breast-feed—or whether the experience itself infuses her with self-confidence—is difficult to determine. Mothers who nurse may be better able to soothe their babies when they are upset, perhaps because the very act of putting them to the breast is such a comfort to them that the mothers do not have to search for other ways of reassuring the babies.

There are distinct benefits of breast-feeding for the mother. These include (1) stimulation, by sucking, of oxytocin secretions, which fosters uterine contractions and hastens postpartum uterine involution, (2) convenience, obviating the need for formula preparation, nipple and bottle sterilization, and refrigeration of formula when traveling, (3) economy,

(4) esthetics—breast-fed infants smell better because the odor of both bowel movements and spit-up milk is less offensive than that of bottle-fed infants, (5) possible decreased risk of postpartum thromboembolism and breast cancer in women who have nursed their children, and (6) emotional satisfaction and sense of fulfillment gained from breast-feeding. The "nursing couple," mother and baby, forge an especially close and interdependent relationship. The baby depends on the mother for sustenance and comfort, and the mother looks forward to feeding times to gain a pleasurable sense of comfort with her infant and a period of rest and relaxation during her busy day. Because of this unique relationship, many women consider the nursing months among the most fulfilling times of their lives.

A mother should not breast-feed unless she is fully convinced that she wants to. In most instances the wishes of the baby's father affect the decision to breast-feed inasmuch as he, because of the replacement of the extended family by the nuclear family, has become the nursing mother's chief support system. For most women, nursing is easily accomplished; however, if for any reason the desire to breast-feed is lacking or poorly supported, initiating or continuing nursing may be difficult and may produce emotional strains that could disrupt the mother-child-father relationships. Physicians should support the mother completely whether her decision is to nurse, not to nurse, or to discontinue nursing, regardless of their personal opinions on the matter.

Breast-feeding may be difficult for the working mother because of the time she is away from the home and because of physical fatigue. However, a sympathetic family and physician and access to various support systems will help the working mother to continue nursing.[12] Fatigue also may be a contributing factor in the mother who is physically ill.

BREAST-FEEDING

Basis of Lactation

Successful breast-feeding depends on a strongly motivated mother, a healthy infant with a strong sucking impulse, and a physician who is confident and competent in his or her knowledge of the anatomy of the mammary gland and physiology of the lactation process.

Directly beneath and behind the areola is a group of milk pools, or lactiferous sinuses, that, with proper latch-on, the nursing infant's jaws will compress and squeeze milk into and along the pores of the nipple. The nipple itself is merely a spout through which the milk is conducted into the infant's mouth and should not itself be traumatized by the infant's jaws. The sinuses are widened parts of the lactiferous ducts, of which there are 15 to 20, each emptying into the nipple. At their proximal ends within the breast, the ducts branch off into smaller canals called *ductules*. At the end of each ductule is a grapelike structure composed of a cluster of tiny rounded saclike alveoli, in which the milk is made. The ducts and the alveoli are lined with myoepithelial cells that contract (in response to oxytocin) to squeeze the milk into and through the entire duct system, finally ending up in the sinuses. Clusters of alveoli compose the lobules, which are bound together by connective tissue, richly interwoven with blood vessels and lymphatics into the 15 to 20 lobes in each breast. Each lobe is connected to one duct, each duct emptying into one opening on the nipple (Fig. 16-6).

Physiology of Lactation

Successful lactation is a simple process, the result of reflex interactions between the nursing couple; it is based on the

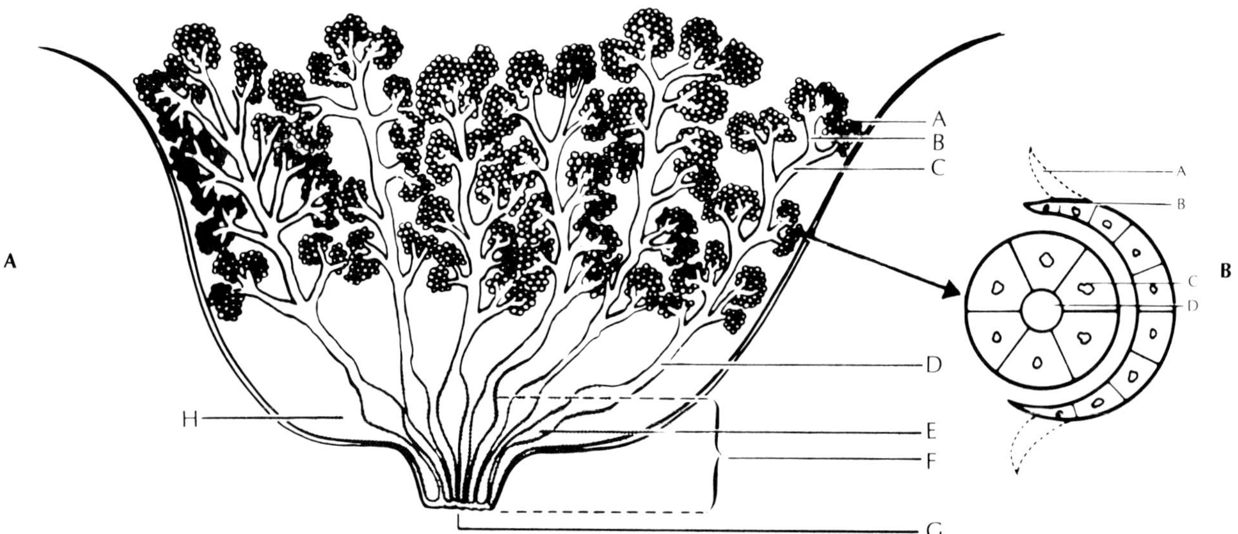

Fig. 16-6 A, Diagram of the breast as a "forest of trees." With full development of the uterine-menstrual cycle, groups of gland-secreting cells (alveoli) bud from the small ducts (ductules). The alveoli secrete milk under the influence of prolactin, a hormone of the pituitary gland. *A*, Alveolus; *B*, ductule; *C*, duct; *D*, lactiferous duct; *E*, lactiferous sinus; *F*, ampulla; *G*, nipple pore; *H*, areolar margin. **B,** Diagram of an alveolus. Gland-secreting cells are arranged in a circle about the ductule opening. About the alveolus is a contractile cell. When sucking begins, this cell, under the influence of oxytocin from the pituitary gland, contracts and squeezes the milk into the duct system. This reflex is called letdown. *A*, Uncontracted myoepithelial cell; *B*, contracted myoepithelial cell; *C*, gland-secreting cell; *D*, ductule opening.

From Applebaum RM: The modern management of successful breast feeding, Pediatr Clin North Am 17(1):205, 1970.

superimposition of two reflex triangles, the *prolactin* (or milk secretion) *reflex* and the *letdown* (or milk ejection) *reflex*.

Prolactin Reflex. The infant suckling on the breast stimulates the maternal anterior pituitary gland via the vagus nerve and the hypothalamus to secrete the hormone prolactin, which then acts on the breast alveoli to produce milk. Prolactin secretion is determined by the frequency of stimulation of nipple and areola by the infant. Until the milk supply is well established, which normally takes 3 to 6 weeks of total breast-feeding without supplementation with either water or formula, the breasts will require stimulation on an average of 8 to 12 times each 24-hour period.

Let-down Reflex. This was originally a dairy term, referring to the ability of the cow to "let down" her milk. It is essential for getting the milk to the baby and can be inhibited by anxiety, illness, breast engorgement, pain, emotional tension, and fatigue. *Maternal confidence* and reassurance are required for its efficient action. After the infant has been nursing for 2 to 3 minutes, the posterior pituitary gland releases oxytocin, another hormone that, traveling through the bloodstream to the breast, contracts the myoepithelial cells surrounding the alveoli and milk ducts, thus ejecting milk toward the lactiferous sinuses (Fig. 16-7). The cell membranes of the secretory cells rupture during this process so that larger and more concentrated fatty globules and protein particles are added to the milk. This high-calorie fatty milk is named "hindmilk"; it constitutes the final two thirds of the volume of milk and is added to the previous one third of "foremilk" produced during the height of the earlier prolactin secretion. A vigorous let-down reflex thus increases the caloric content of the milk and, by forceful ejection refills the milk sinuses with the rich, creamy "hindmilk" that, when obtained regularly by the infant, ensures a rapid weight gain. The securing of adequate drainage of milk by means of an all effective let-down reflex prevents engorgement and is essential for successful lactation.

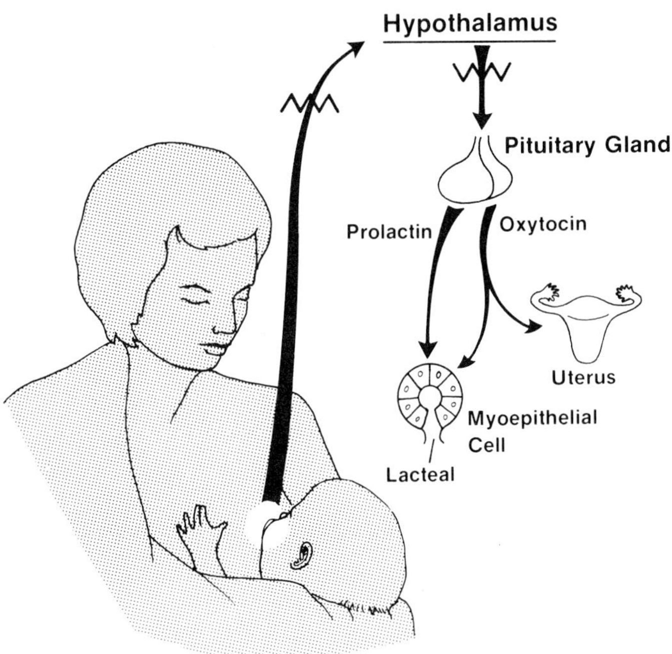

Fig. 16-7 Diagrammatic outline of ejection reflex arc. When the infant suckles a breast, he stimulates mechanoreceptors in the nipple and areola that send stimulus along nerve pathways to hypothalamus, which stimulates the posterior pituitary to release oxytocin. It is carried via bloodstream to breast and uterus. Oxytocin stimulates myoepithelial cell in breast to contract and eject milk from alveolus. Prolactin is responsible for milk production in alveolus. It is secreted by anterior pituitary gland in response to suckling. Stress such as pain and anxiety can inhibit letdown reflex. The sight or cry of infant can stimulate it.

From Lawrence RA: Breastfeeding: a guide for the medical profession, ed. 2, St. Louis, 1985, The C.V. Mosby Co.

Technique of Nursing

Early stimulation by frequent nursing will encourage milk flow and provide an adequate milk supply rapidly. The infant should be placed on the mother's abdomen and put to the breast in the delivery room or, if this is not possible, soon after the initial newborn physical examination. In many hospitals one or two feedings of sterile water precede the first milk feeding to rule out esophageal anomalies. In most normal-appearing full-term infants, this is not necessary.

The breast will produce colostrum in the first few days after delivery. Colostrum is a high-fat, high-protein substance and therefore calorically excellent. It sustains the newborn until the "real milk" comes in on approximately the third to the sixth day. The breast-fed baby is a hungry baby who cries often to be fed. This s a normal response and occurs at 2- to 3-hour intervals in the first 4 to 6 weeks of life. Because breast milk is more digestible than cow milk, the emptying time of the breast-fed infant's stomach is shorter. The breast-fed baby will therefore require feeding more often than does the bottle baby (8 to 12 feedings in 24 hours versus 6 for the bottle baby).

Optimal breast-feeding is *demand feeding*. Maximal milk production is provided when engorgement is reduced and the *breast is emptied frequently* by the infant. A breast emptied of milk will *quickly* produce more, and a natural state of equilibrium is established between the mother and the infant.

Successful breast-feeding can be thwarted by overrigid hospital administrators' concern for a germ-free environment and tight nursing and medical staff regulations, which can be extremely inconvenient for the nursing couple. The optimal physical and emotional health of mothers and infants sometimes demands certain changes in many traditional hospital procedures. Demand feeding of the breast-fed infant is ideally effected by a complete rooming-in program. The infant should be allowed to be with the mother for as long as possible to allow the mother to become acquainted with her new infant and to get used to the baby's natural eating and sleeping rhythms.

A comfortable position, either sitting or lying, is essential for successful nursing. The *cradle* position, the most commonly employed hold, is best accomplished with the mother sitting in an armless chair, the leg on the side on which she is nursing resting on a footstool, and a pillow on her lap supporting the forearm on which her baby is resting. Her infant should be facing her directly, his stomach against hers, his head in line with his body, his neck in the bend of her elbow, with her hand on his buttocks so he is pulled up close, with his face almost touching the breast. The mother's free hand then will grasp the breast in the C-hold, thumb on top and well behind the areola, index finger opposite, below, and again well behind the areola, with the other three fingers supporting the breast from underneath. The infant's mouth in this position directly opposes the nipple, which should then be stroked patiently against the infant's lower lip (rooting reflex) until the mouth opens quite wide to accept the nipple, at which point the mother then pulls the baby's head firmly onto the breast, inserting the nipple deep into his mouth, and allowing the infant to close his jaws over the base of the nipple for proper and effective *latch-on* (Fig. 16-8). When feeding on the first side is complete, the mother breaks the suction by placing her fifth finger into the corner of the infant's mouth before transferring him to the other breast.

An effective latch-on, or attachment of baby to breast, is essential for the efficient and painless initiation of lactation. Although breast-feeding is a natural process, it is the result of the transmission to the new mother of a generationally accumulated experience that is to a great extent lacking in our modern, technologically oriented Western society, where the extended family has been replaced by its inadequate nuclear counterpart and wherein the central hospital nursery severely interferes with the necessary interaction between mother and infant.[10] The latch-on is not instinctual, and the new mother must be taught by trained, knowledgeable personnel in the immediate postpartum hours how to perform it properly. Breast-feeding should not be painful, even at the beginning, and with correct latch-on technique it will be comfortable for the mother, thus allowing an effective let-down and the early and rapid establishing of a rhythm of frequent draining and filling of the breasts, which is essential to building a dependable milk supply.

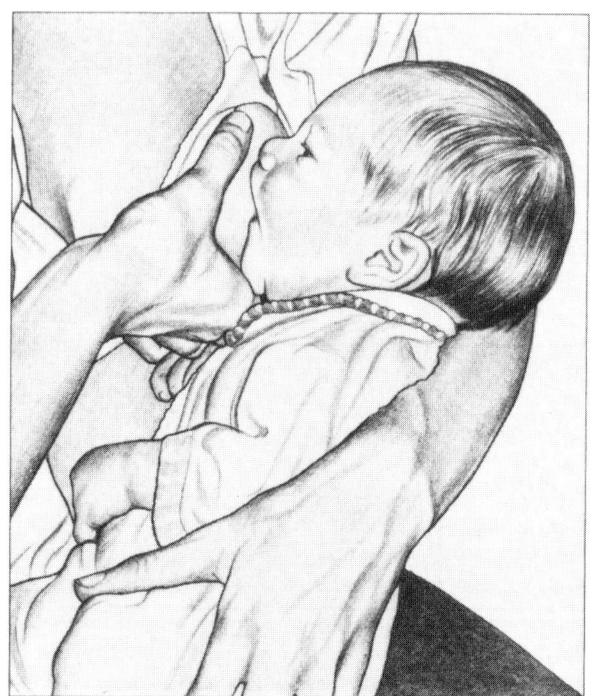

Fig. 16-8 Correct latch-on position with baby's head, in line with body, resting in crook of mother's arm with her free hand supporting breast using C-hold.

From Eiger MS and Olds SW, *The Complete Book of Breastfeeding*, Rev. Ed. 1987, Workman, Bantam.

There should be no imposed time limit to nursing on each breast, even in the early days, because the infant's jaws will not traumatize the nipple when the mother employs correct latch-on technique.[9] In the first few weeks, however, the baby should be encouraged to stimulate both breasts at each nursing session, and the breast used last at the previous feeding should be used first at the next feeding. The mother should be taught to listen for her infant's swallowing sounds (short, sighing-like noises), rather than observing the suckling, as an indication that her baby is removing milk from her breast. The ideal ratio is no more than one to two sucks per swallow. After the first few weeks, when the milk supply is adequate, the older, thriving infant may desire to remain on one breast throughout the entire feeding to obtain the benefits of the rich, satiety-producing hindmilk, and the mother should be told that this is acceptable so long as the breasts are alternated at ensuing feeding sessions.[13]

Breast-fed babies may lose up to 10% of their birth weight, but the initial weight loss can be markedly decreased by the immediate initiation of nursing in the delivery suite, by frequent unrestricted demand feeding sessions with mother and baby rooming-in together, by avoidance of supplementation of either water or formula, and with the constant support of trained medical and nursing personnel. Attention must be given in the early weeks to the adequacy of maternal milk supply build-up. The young infant *(younger than 1 month)* who is ingesting sufficient mother's milk, is *never* constipated and should be having at least four or more stools per 24-hour day. Fewer than that number, even if the infant is wetting frequently, represents a danger sign, and intervention is necessary. Bottle supplementation in the early weeks should rarely be employed because of the physiologic differences in suckling and the consequent risk of nipple confusion. Many new and exciting techniques have been developed to increase an insufficient milk supply, and formula supplementation at the breast with nursing supplementers is available to tide the infant over, without undermining the development of the sucking mechanism until the mother's milk supply increases.

Drugs in Breast Milk

All drugs ingested by the lactating woman appear in the breast milk, usually in amounts that approximate in concentration the mother's plasma levels. The total amount excreted into the milk after a single maternal dose is a function of time and nursing frequency, and for most drugs the amount is less than 1% to 2% of the amount taken by the mother.[1] Reasonable concern exists regarding the effect on the nursing infant of substances ingested by the mother. The effect on the infant is determined by the volume of milk ingested, the amount absorbed from the intestine, the activity of the drug, the sensitivity and tolerance of the infant to the specific substance, the chronicity of therapy with the particular drug to avoid accumulation, and the size and maturity of the infant. Maternal dosing immediately after a nursing session will minimize the entry of the substance into the milk at the next feeding, inasmuch as the peak maternal plasma level will follow the curve of peak milk production. Short-acting preparations should be prescribed, if possible, rather than long-acting dosage forms. Data are rapidly becoming available to guide practitioners' recommendations to mothers regarding the drugs they may ingest without fear of adversely affecting their babies.[2]

The factors that affect the appearance of a drug in breast milk are its lipid solubility, its pK_a, its protein-binding ability, and the pH of the milk. Unionized drugs with high lipid solubility will be transported better than ionized ones. The concentration of a drug in breast milk depends on the volume of mammary alveoli cells and the concentration of unbound drug in the plasma of the mother. Drugs usually pass through membranes by passive diffusion dependent on the concentration gradient and their lipid solubility. Breast milk has a pH of approximately 7.0 and plasma one of approximately 7.4; therefore weak acids usually have low milk/plasma ratios, whereas weak bases are likely to have high ratios. Most drugs for which specific information is available can be grouped into categories relating to their potential effect on the nursing infant (Table 16-7). Steroids, when taken in large doses over time by the mother, can suppress growth and interfere with endogenous steroid production in the infant. Infants with a G6PD deficiency may suffer hemolysis from ingestion of nalidixic acid, sulfonamides, and other oxidant drugs in breast milk. Chronic salicylate ingestion by the mother can produce hemorrhagic problems in her breast-feeding infant.

Antibiotics do not usually produce acute adverse effects in infants who are being breast-fed (see Chapter 28). However, continuous ingestion of the aminoglycosides may alter

Table 16-7 *Drugs in Breast Milk*

DRUG	REPORTED SIGN OR SYMPTOM IN INFANT OR EFFECT ON LACTATION
Contraindicated in nursing mothers	
Bromocriptine	Suppresses lactation
Cyclophosphamide	Possible immune suppression; unknown effect on growth or association with carcinogenesis; neutropenia
Cyclosporine	Possible immune suppression; unknown effect on growth or association with carcinogenesis
Ergotamine	Vomiting, diarrhea, convulsions (doses used in migraine medications)
Lithium	⅓ to ½ therapeutic blood concentration in infants
Methotrexate	Possible immunosuppression; unknown effect on growth or association with carcinogenesis; neutropenia
Phenindione	Anticoagulant: caused prothrombin and partial prothromboplastin time in one infant; not used in the United States
Drugs of abuse*	
Amphetamine	Irritability, poor sleeping pattern
Cocaine	Cocaine intoxication
Heroin	Heroin intoxication
Marijuana	Only one report in literature; no effect mentioned
Nicotine (smoking)	Shock, vomiting, diarrhea, rapid heart rate, restlessness; decreased milk production
Phencylidine (PCP)	Potent hallucinogen
Requires temporary cessation of breast-feeding	
Radiopharmaceutical agents	Radioactivity present in milk; consult nuclear medicine physician before performing diagnostic study so that radionuclide that has shortest excretion time in breast milk can be used; before study the mother should pump her breast and store enough milk in freezer for feeding the infant; after study the mother should pump her breast to maintain milk production but discard all milk pumped for the period of time that radioactivity is present in milk.
Require caution in administering to nursing mothers	
psychotropic drugs†	
Diazepam	None
Amitriptyline	None
Desipramine	None
Imipramine	None
Chlorpromazine	Galactorrhea in adult; drowsiness and lethargy in infant
Haloperidol	None
Chloramphenicol	Possible idiosyncratic bone marrow suppression
Metoclopramide	None described; potent central nervous system drug
Metronidazole	In vitro mutagen; may discontinue breast-feeding 12-24 hr to allow excretion of dose therapy given to mother
Salicylates	Metabolic acidosis (dose related); may affect platelet function; rash
Clemastine	Drowsiness, irritability, refusal to feed, high-pitched cry, neck stiffness (one case)
Phenobarbital	Sedation; infantile spasms after weaning from milk containing phenobarbital, methemoglobinemia (one case)
Primidone	Sedation, feeding problems
Sulfasalazine	Bloody diarrhea in one infant

*The American Academy of Pediatrics Committee on Drugs believes strongly that nursing mothers should not ingest any of these compounds. They are not only hazardous to the nursing infant but some are detrimental to the physical and/or emotional health of the mother.

†These drugs are of special concern when given to nursing mothers for long periods of time.

Modified from American Academy of Pediatrics Committee on Drugs: Transfer of drugs and other chemicals into human milk, Pediatrics 84:824, 1989.

the intestinal flora of an infant, affect some immune mechanisms, and predispose him or her to hypersensitivity. Tetracycline ingestion via breast milk has not been reported to cause mottled teeth in breast-fed infants, even when tetracyclines are found in high concentrations in breast milk, probably because the calcium complexing of tetracyclines in milk interferes with their absorption by the infant.

Lactating mothers always must be aware that anything they ingest may have an undesirable effect on their infant by passage into their milk. Physicians, dentists, and paramedical personnel responsible for prescribing drugs should be informed that the mother is breast-feeding so that care can be exerted in prescribing a drug compatible with the nursing baby. Should it be necessary to prescribe a medication that is incompatible with breast-feeding, a reasonable and safe alternative almost always can be substituted. Nursing should never arbitrarily be terminated because of the need for maternal therapy. Should a temporary cessation of breast-feeding become necessary, a breast-pumping regimen to maintain maternal milk supply, in addition to the continuous support of family and sympathetic medical personnel, will allow for its successful resumption. Over-the-counter medications, taken for the short-term, rarely present problems for the nursing baby, but caution should be exerted in their administration as well.

Complications of Breast-Feeding

The complications of nursing usually pertain to difficulties experienced by the mother, but occasionally an infant will become seriously ill for a prolonged period and will be unable to nurse adequately. During brief illnesses in which feeding at the breast is not possible, the breast can be emptied periodically during maternal-infant separation with an electric breast pump and the infant fed the expressed breast milk via a nursing supplementer or a bottle, depending on the baby's age and maturity.

Sore, cracked nipples need not occur if careful attention is paid to correct latch-on techniques, proper positioning, and prevention of engorgement. Pain on latch-on is a signal that the baby must be removed from the breast and a correction must immediately be instituted. Mothers should be aware that breast-feeding is a pleasurable experience and the adage that "if it hurts, then it is wrong" is valid. If nipple trauma does occur, treatment consists of nipple exposure, relief of engorgement by frequent feeding or mechanical pumping, *avoidance* of any creams or ointments because the nipple pores are easily blocked, and application of the mother's own expressed breast milk, coupled with instruction in proper positioning and latch-on.

Incomplete emptying of a portion of the breast can easily lead to a plugged duct in that area. Nursing mothers should palpate their breasts regularly to become aware of the appearance of full areas, which when found should be treated with breast massage and by specific positioning of the infant on that breast to empty the area under suspicion frequently and effectively.

Breast engorgement and plugged ducts, when unattended, can rapidly lead to mastitis, which is *not* a contraindication to continuing nursing. If fever and breast tenderness and erythema develop, there is ample evidence that administering antibiotics and continuing nursing—because it relieves engorgement and thus secures drainage of the affected areas of the breast— will prevent many cases of mastitis from progressing to breast abscesses, which then may require surgical incision. The infant who nurses on the infected breast does *not* become ill and is in *no* danger. Feeding from the affected breast may be temporarily discontinued just after surgical drainage, but breast-feeding may be effectively resumed from that breast after the wound has healed.

Concomitant with the resurgence of breast-feeding in the 1980s, there has been a rapid expansion of knowledge in the field of lactation, and a new specialist, the lactation counselor, armed with innovative intervention techniques, has emerged to aid the physician in diagnosing and treating problems of the nursing couple. The lactation counselor has clarified the

Preparation and Terminal Sterilization of Infant Formula

PREPARATION OF FORMULA

1. Measure the prescribed number of ounces of hot water into a clean quart pitcher.
2. Stir in the carbohydrate. Measure powdered sugar with a standard-size tablespoon and level each spoonful with a table knife.
3. Add the prescribed number of ounces of milk to the formula and stir to mix well.
4. Pour the formula into clean nursing bottles.
5. Put nipples and caps on the bottles, leaving the caps loose.

STERILIZATION OF FORMULA

1. Put the bottles of formula on a rack in the sterilizer or deep kettle. Caps should be loose, not screwed on tightly. Put about 3 inches of water in the sterilizer, and cover.
2. Bring the water to a boil over moderate heat, then allow to boil gently (with the sterilizer still covered) for 25 minutes.
3. Remove the sterilizer from the heat. Leave it closed (do not even lift the lid) until the side of the sterilizer has cooled enough so that you can touch it with the palm of your hand.
4. Open the sterilizer. Then cool the bottles gradually, adding a small amount of cool water to the hot water in the sterilizer. (Gradual cooling prevents "skimming," which frequently causes nipple clogging.)
5. Remove the cooled bottles and screw the caps tight.
6. Store the bottles of formula in the refrigerator.

concept of "insufficient milk syndrome"—that it actually is a composite of multiple maternal and infant etiologic factors that usually are correctable with supportive professional management.

ARTIFICIAL FEEDING

When bottle feeding is chosen, or if breast-feeding is not feasible or successful, the infant will thrive on an artificially prepared formula. Commercially prepared formulas for normal infants are modifications of whole cow milk that approximate the composition of human milk as closely as possible. Thus the "humanized" formulas compare favorably with breast milk in their content of protein, carbohydrate (lactose), and saturated and unsaturated fats. Special formulas are available for the milk-intolerant infant and for those infants with specific malabsorptive problems (see Appendix C).

Feeding Schedule

When bottle feeding is employed, a demand schedule should be encouraged, as with the breast-fed infant. Bottle-fed babies should be fed only as much as they desire, although maternal pressure may subtly urge them to empty the bottle. This should be discouraged inasmuch as overfeeding at this age may establish a pattern of eating that will result in eventual obesity. Because bottle-fed babies' gastric emptying time is longer, they will require less frequent feedings than do their breast-fed counterparts. The artifically fed infant usually has a greater weight gain than the breast-fed infant. There is no evidence that this increased weight gain is desirable; indeed it probably is not.

Whether breast- or bottle-fed, the infant who is fed on demand will adjust intake to needs for growth. The following patterns, with some variation, usually are established:

Age (mo)	Number of Feedings per 24 Hours
0-1	6-8
2-6	4-5
7-10	3-4
11-12	3

Age (mo)	Ounces per Feeding
1	2-4
2	5
3	5-6
4	6-7
5-12	8

It should be noted that during the second or third month of life, most infants eliminate the night feeding.

Preparation of Formula

In most instances in the United States, artificial feeding with cow milk is accomplished with proprietary formulas prepared commercially and supplied as "ready-to-feed" or "easy-to-mix" in presterilized bottles and cans. The ready-to-feed formulas are supplied with attached nipples in 4-, 6-, and 8-ounce bottles that are disposable and in 1-quart cans. Ready-to-feed formulas offer convenience to mothers who must travel with their infants and often are used as complementary and supplementary feedings for breast-fed babies but are too expensive for everyday use for most families. Easy-to-mix, concentrated formulas are supplied in 13-ounce cans of liquid that is mixed with equal amounts of water and in 6-ounce cans of powder that is mixed with appropriate amounts of water, usually in a 1:2 ratio.

The calculation of the ingredients required to prepare an infant formula from whole cow milk (20 Cal/oz) or evaporated milk (44 Cal/oz) is based on four principles: (1) all formulas should contain milk, water, and carbohydrate with an energy content that approximates 20 Cal/oz; (2) full-term infants require 110 to 120 Cal/kg and 150 to 180 ml of fluid per kilogram each day; (3) 2 ounces of evaporated milk (EM) or 4 ounces of whole milk (WM) per kilogram are required each day; and (4) most infants require feeding five or six times in every 24 hours. According to these principles, a 24-hour supply of formula for a 10-pound (4.5 kg) baby would consist of approximately 500 calories and 750 ml. The amount of EM required would be 10 ounces (300 ml),* which would provide 440 calories. The balance of fluid required (450 ml) would be made up with water, and the balance of 60 calories would be supplied with carbohydrates (table sugar = 60 Cal/tbsp; Karo = 60 Cal/tbsp; and Dextri-Maltose = 30 Cal/tbsp). The formula, then, would consist of 10 ounces of evaporated milk, 15 ounces of water, and 1 to 2 tablespoons of carbohydrate (depending on the kind used). The 25 ounces of formula would contain 500 calories, or 20 Cal/oz, and would be divided into five or six bottles, each containing 4 to 5 ounces. When larger amounts of formula are needed or when whole milk is used, the four formula principles can be met with either of the following mixtures: 13 ounces of EM, 19 ounces of water, and 120 calories (2 to 4 tablespoons) of carbohydrates; 23 ounces of WM, 9 ounces of water, and 180 calories (3 to 6 tablespoons) of carbohydrates. These formulas would meet the needs of a baby weighing 6 kg or more. A fifth principle of artificial feeding is that babies rarely require more than 1 quart of formula per 24 hours.

The method of mixing formulas described here implies that a full 24-hour supply will be prepared. Single 8-ounce feedings can be mixed (3 ounces EM, 5 ounces water, and 30 calories of carbohydrate), or fractions thereof, depending on the amount the baby usually takes.

It is reasonable to instruct the mother to prepare her infant's formula under aseptic conditions or to use terminal sterilization because milk is a rich culture medium and significant contamination may result if one of these methods is not used in an area where the water supply is not dependable. However, in most urban areas with safe water systems, sterilization is unnecessary. The box on p. 190 outlines a method of preparation and sterilization of infant formula, which should be applied when well water is used and when organism counts in tap water are too high. Aseptic methods for preparation of single or 24-hour formulas also can be used under these circumstances. They require boiling of water, bottles, nipples, and utensils beforehand. Refrigeration of prepared

*For ease of calculation, 1 ounce is considered to contain 30 ml.

formula reduces the number of bacteria found in contaminated bottles. Realistically, as Kendall and colleagues[7] and others have shown, fewer than 50% of mothers are able to prepare a sterile formula using either method. Therefore, when the physician suspects that a mother is not likely to follow aseptic or terminal sterilization techniques, a presterilized proprietary formula or single feeding mixtures should be used. It probably is wise to use some form of sterile formula preparation during the first 4 months of life.

Although most mothers warm their infants' bottles before feeding, there is no evidence to indicate that babies prefer their milk warmed. Parents should be cautioned to avoid warming baby bottles in microwave ovens, which can result in overheating of the formula and can cause esophageal burns on ingestion. In addition, steam can form inside the bottle, resulting in an explosion.

VITAMIN SUPPLEMENTS

At birth, most infants have adequate vitamin stores, with the exception of vitamin K, until rapid postnatal growth ensues at 10 to 14 days of life. At that time vitamin supplementation should begin. Most of the commercially prepared formulas contain adequate vitamin content; therefore, except for special needs, no added vitamins need be given to infants nourished with them. Although human milk may be expected to satisfy the requirements advisable for vitamins A, C, and E and the B vitamins, the day-to-day variability in content and demand makes it advisable to provide a preparation containing the minimum daily requirement of vitamins A, C, and D to the breast-fed infant. In addition, all infants living in areas that lack fluoridation of the water supply should receive 0.5 mg of fluoride daily because it has been effectively demonstrated that this amount of fluoride does inhibit the development of dental caries (Table 16-8 and 16-9). For infants fed on whole-milk and evaporated-milk formulas, the same vitamin supplements should be provided until they are 18 to 24 months of age, or longer if they are poor eaters.

IRON SUPPLEMENTATION IN INFANCY

The Committee on Nutrition of the American Academy of Pediatrics recommends that infants during their first year of life receive an iron intake of 1 mg/kg/day to a maximum of 15 mg/day for at least the first year of life to prevent the development of iron deficiency anemia. Milk, both human and cow, is deficient in iron. Commercial formulas are supplemented with 8 to 12 mg iron/liter. Breast-fed infants need not receive this amount of iron with their vitamin supplements because the small amount of iron in breast milk is almost completely bioavailable to the nursing infant; thus breast milk provides sufficient iron until the sixth month of life.

Table 16-8 *Public Health Service–Recommended Fluoride Control Limits*

ANNUAL AVERAGE OF MAXIMUM DAILY AIR TEMPERATURES (°F)*	OPTIMUM FLUORIDE CONCENTRATIONS (mg/L, ppm)
50.0-53.7	1.2
53.8-58.3	1.1
58.4-63.8	1.0
63.9-70.6	0.9
70.7-79.2	0.8
79.3-90.5	0.7

From US Public Health Service.
*Based on temperature data obtained for a minimum of 5 years.

WEANING

Weaning customs vary considerably around the world. In many countries, babies are routinely nursed well into the second and sometimes the third year of life. In the United States and some other Western countries, mothers plan to wean their babies from the breast at sometime between 6 and 15 months of life. By 6 months, babies in an industrialized society can meet their nutritional needs through cow milk formula and a wide variety of solid foods because of the maturation of their gastrointestinal tract and the development of their digestive ability to handle foreign proteins. Breast milk no longer is as important to them as when it provided their only source of nourishment. After 9 months a nursing mother usually produces less milk and her let-down reflex becomes sluggish. However, the emotional benefits that a mother and baby derive from breast-feeding are just as great at 9 months or at a year or even later.

The age at which an infant is weaned from the breast should be decided by the mother. If the baby is younger than 12 months of age, weaning to a bottle formula is usually advisable. The older infant may be weaned directly to whole milk from a bottle or a cup.

The process of weaning should be gradual and should begin with substitution of one breast-feeding with a bottle or cup feeding, usually at the midday feeding. Once the bottle or cup is accepted, other breast-feedings are similarly eliminated and replaced gradually over a 1- to 4-week period. The maternal milk supply will diminish during this time because the stimulus of regular emptying of the breast is removed. Some mothers, however, are able to continue one or two breast-feedings over several months should they so choose.

Occasionally, because of an illness in the mother or the infant or the development of a complication of nursing, it is necessary to discontinue breast-feeding abruptly. To diminish the mother's discomfort, she should be instructed to wear a tight breast binder, diminish her fluid intake, and apply ice packs to her breasts. The administration of 20 mg of stilbestrol orally each day for 3 days is also effective in reducing her discomfort and in " drying up" her milk supply but is seldom necessary.

Whenever possible, weaning should not be instituted during very warm weather because some babies will initially refuse any feeding other than breast milk for as long as 24 to 48 hours.

The formula-fed infant can appropriately be weaned from a bottle to whole cow milk from a cup by 9 to 12 months in the same manner already outlined.

Skim milk should not be given to infants until at least 1 year of age because, at a time when milk serves as a major source of food, skim milk would provide too few calories,

Table 16-9 *Recommended Daily Oral Fluoride Dosage Schedule*

AGE	FLUORIDE CONTENT OF WATER (mg/L, ppm)			
	0-0.25	0.25-0.50	0.50-0.75	0.75+
0-12 mo	0.25	0.0	0.0	0.0
1-4 yr	0.50	0.25	0.0	0.0
4-8 yr	0.75	0.50	0.25	0.0
8-12 yr	1.00	0.75	0.50	0.0

an excessive protein intake, and an inadequate intake of essential fatty acids.

FEEDING OF SOLID FOODS

Introduction to Solid Foods

From a developmental view there are cogent reasons why solids should not be added to the infant diet before 4 to 6 months of life. When a solid object like a spoon or a tongue depressor is introduced between the lips of the young baby, he purses his lips, raises his tongue, and pushes against the object vigorously (extrusion reflex). By 4 to 6 months the behavior changes so that when a spoon is inserted between the lips, they part, the tongue depresses, and food placed in the mouth is drawn to the back of the pharynx and swallowed. Thus the physiologically appropriate time to begin feeding solids is somewhere between 4 and 6 months. Somewhat later, at about 7 to 9 months, rhythmic biting movements begin even in the absence of teeth, and at this time foods requiring some chewing may be added to the diet.

Schedule of Solid Foods

An appropriate regimen for introduction of solid foods begins with the grains and fruits. Rice cereal appears to be the least allergenic of the cereals and thus should be offered first. Progression through vegetables, meats, and eggs can be accomplished in the following manner:

5-6 mo	Cereals and fruits
6-7 mo	Meats and vegetables
7-8 mo	Egg yolk
8-9 mo	Egg white

To ensure an adequate amount of protein, fat, and carbohydrate during the sixth to twelfth months, infants should be offered and should consume no more than an average of 28 ounces of milk each day in addition to their quota of solids. An example of an infant diet in this age-group follows:

Breakfast	Cereal and milk
Midmorning snack	Cup of orange juice
Lunch	Meat, yellow or green vegetables, fruit, milk
Midafternoon snack	Cup of orange juice or milk
Dinner	Cottage cheese or yogurt, egg, vegetable, fruit, and milk
Bedtime	Milk

When solid foods are introduced to the infant, they may be easily prepared in the home from fresh ingredients and pureed by use of a food grinder and blender, or commercially prepared baby foods may be used.

In late infancy and particularly during the toddler period (12 to 30 months), the normal physiologic decrease in appetite, paralleling the decrease in growth rate, occurs. The parent should be made aware of the normal decrease in interest in food, particularly at mealtimes, and also the concomitant reduction in milk intake, which may drop to 16 ounces per day by 24 to 36 months of life. By 4 to 7 years the appetite normally increases, as does the growth rate. The intake of *total* calories increases rapidly during the first year of life, then less rapidly to about 4 years, then increases rapidly again. That is, the average full-term infant by 7 to 10 days of life will consume approximately 300 calories; thereafter the first-year increment is nearly 600 Cal/day, the second-year increment nearly 275 Cal/day, the third- and fourth-year increments nearly 100 Cal/day, and the fifth- to seventh-year increments nearly 130 to 140 Cal/day.

Thus, despite a decrease in appetite, the actual *intake of calories* does not decrease during the preschool period and patterns of growth remain satisfactory.

THE PRUDENT DIET OF THE SCHOOL-AGE CHILD AND THE ADOLESCENT

The diet of the school-age child and the adolescent should be similar to that of the active adult; however, the extra caloric needs necessitated by the period of rapid growth should be taken into account. Dietary habits and food preferences are closely linked with early associations and family influences. *Children will eat what they see their families eat.* Parents must be told that their infants and young toddlers will crave salt and sugar in their foods as older children and adults if that is what they have been accustomed to in early life. Basically, the preparation of foods without additives for infants and young children will provide adequate nutrition and lay the basis for sound eating habits in later life.

The pediatrician is in a position to educate entire families in how to eat more healthful foods in an attempt to prevent obesity and atherosclerosis. Physicians need to know facts about good nutrition if they are to effect changes in the lifetime habits of families toward consuming fewer calories and less fat, salt, and refined sugars.

The American Health Association has endorsed a prudent diet for the child and adolescent, which in simplified form has the following requirements:

A high-quality protein with every meal
Milk, preferably skimmed, and other low-fat dairy products
Vegetables high in vitamin A
Fruits for vitamin C
Whole grain or enriched breads or cereals
Vegetable oils high in polyunsaturated fats
Meat—4 servings per week of 4 ounces each
Fish (a good source of polyunsaturated fats)—1 to 2 times a week
Poultry (low fat)—1 to 2 times a week
Dark green, leafy, or deep yellow vegetables—at least 4 times weekly, preferably once a day
Eggs—a maximum of 4 per week

The prudent diet thus limits excessive use of fatty meats, high-fat dairy products, eggs, and hydrogenated shortenings and recommends consuming more fish and substituting polyunsaturated vegetable oils and margarines for butter, lard, and other saturated fats.

Three

Obesity*

Gilbert B. Forbes

Obesity is the most common "nutritional" disorder of Western society today, far outranking the classic deficiency states whose descriptions occupy so much space in nutrition texts. It is not a new disorder—there are corpulent statues dating from antiquity, and Captain Cook reported seeing fat natives on his voyages to the South Sea Islands. We have no information as to whether obesity is more or less common today than in former times, inasmuch as systematic surveys of body size are a recent innovation. We do know, however, that there has been a change in mean body weight and height of children over the past century and that this secular change has occurred in all countries for which comparative data are available. For example, the average 15-year-old American boy in 1960 was almost 15 kg heavier and 13 cm taller than his 1880 counterpart. The cause(s) of this secular change is not known; possibilities include improved nutrition, relative decline in chronic disease, and the phenomenon of hybrid vigor.

The prevalence of obesity today, the fact that so many obese youngsters are refractory to treatment and thus tend to remain obese as adults, and the general opinion that obesity, at least in the adult, constitutes a health hazard (diabetes, hypertension, cerebrovascular disease) strongly point to the need for prevention.

ETIOLOGY

Preventive measures must perforce be based on etiologic concepts. As far as the usual type of human obesity is concerned, there are two aspects to be considered: proximate cause and contributing factors.

The *proximate cause* is, quite simply, relative hyperphagia. Energy is consumed in excess of need, and the energy excess is stored as fat because adipose tissue is the only organ available for this purpose on such a large scale. Either energy intake is too high, energy expenditure is too low, or both: the laws of thermodynamics are not to be denied. Thus obesity is a form of overnutrition, a concept that is confirmed by the fact that obese children tend to be a little taller than average,[3] to have a larger lean body mass as well as excess body fat,[5] to have a slightly advanced bone age, to mature a bit earlier, and to have higher hemoglobin values. It often is claimed that obese individuals eat less than their thin brethren, and some dietary surveys indicate that such is the case. The careful study of individuals, however, reveals that obese persons have higher basal metabolic rates and higher levels of total energy expenditure than do those who are thin.[4] When tested under controlled observation, obese individuals invariably lose weight on low energy diets. Mann[7] speaks to those who continue to invoke a metabolic cause: "There is an old and treasured notion that obesity is caused by a metabolic defect, whether acquired or inherited, and this makes obesity a kind of act of God. It removes all blame and postpones successful management, at least until the biochemical lesion is well understood."

Now let us consider *contributing factors*. Most persons are successful in balancing energy intake and outgo, so that body weight (or, in children, growth in weight) remains relatively constant over long periods. What is it that leads some to ingest more food than they need? Although not all the considerations that follow can be blamed for instances of massive obesity, when viewed in concert they do conspire to produce overweight citizens and to facilitate true obesity.

Food Supply and Food Technology

The United States produces an abundance of food, and it is food of high biologic quality, attractively advertised, and widely available. In terms of real wages, food is cheaper than ever before. Food technology has made it possible to feed infants high-calorie formulas, and modern foods are easily masticated and digested. Today may well be the very first time in the history of the human race that so many people in Western society have had so much to eat.

Nutritional Attitudes

Perception of Health. Parents want their children to grow well. Mothers compare weights of their infants: a plump baby is regarded as a healthy baby—one even sees evidence of this in Renaissance paintings. Food and feeding are integral

*Excluded from this discussion are those rare conditions, such as hypothalamic lesions, the Prader-Willi syndrome, and hyperadrenal states, that are associated with obesity.

parts of motherhood, and a "well-filled out" infant or child is solid evidence of maternal success. The current megavitamin craze is an example of this phenomenon carried to an extreme.

Attitudes of Nutritionists. The optimal requirement, or even the minimal requirement, of many nutrients for infants and children is not known. Nutritionists respond by making an educated guess and then add a generous "margin of safety." The result is what the National Research Council calls recommended dietary allowances, which, if adhered to, lead to overconsumption of several nutrients.

Socioeconomic Status. Studies of children and adults show that the incidence of obesity is inversely related to social class. It should be noted, however, that this inverse relationship does not consistently apply to families whose incomes are below the poverty level: here it turns out that preadolescent children are relatively thinner, thus proving that poor children are not well fed. On the other hand, adolescent girls and women are fatter, whereas boys and men tend to remain thin. These trends hold for both blacks and whites.

Sex

Girls and women suffer from obesity more frequently than do boys and men.

Emotional Factors

Some people find solace in eating when depressed or frustrated, when they perceive that life's problems are too difficult to cope with. Bruch[2] is of the opinion that such individuals have been conditioned from early life to view food as a pacifier and eventually develop a disturbed hunger awareness, which culminates in the use of food as a pseudosolution for life's conflicts and problems. Eating to excess may be viewed as a form of coping behavior (analogous to the use of alcohol or tobacco) that provides some perceived benefit to the affected individual, which is why obesity is so resistant to treatment.

Physical Exercise

Modern life-styles offer relatively little opportunity for adequate energy expenditure: suburban living with its dependence on the automobile; single-story houses with multiple telephones; paucity of sidewalks; heavy traffic, which frightens mothers into proscribing bicycles; labor-saving devices of all sorts; high-heeled shoes for women; the fascination of television (American children watch an average of 3 hours daily); school buses; power lawn mowers; undue emphasis on varsity sports to the detriment of intramural contests; and the decline in walking as a pastime. It is no surprise that more weight is likely to be gained in winter than in summer and that many modern citizens are truly sedentary individuals. Casual observation confirms the deliberate movements and the relative inactivity of many obese persons.

Heredity

The majority of obese children have at least one obese parent. Studies of twins and of adopted children confirm the presence of a hereditary factor(s). However, the relative magnitude of the genetic and environmental influences has not been established; nor has the mechanism that is inherited been elucidated.

PREVENTION

On the basis of the aforementioned data, one can define the population at greatest risk for obesity: (1) those born to obese parents, (2) those who gain weight rapidly in infancy, (3) individuals of low socioeconomic status, and (4) those whose mothers use food as a means of controlling behavior.

Once established, obesity tends to persist; the majority of obese children become obese adults, and recent data show that the same is true of large babies. Thus, preventive measures should be aimed at the young.

Bruch[1], a veteran and perceptive student of childhood obesity, offers a simple prescription: "If a child is fed when hungry, played with when needing attention, and encouraged to be active when restless, he or she is not likely to grow up inhibited and passive, or overstuffed and helpless, unable to control eating because every discomfort is misinterpreted as a need to eat."

A list of reasonable, although admittedly untested, measures includes those that follow.

Encouraging Breast-Feeding

"Nursing is a useful way both to restore energy balance in the (often overweight) mother and to prevent obesity in the baby."[7] The supply of breast milk is, after all, limited, which usually is not true of infant formulas.

Postponing Introduction of Solid Foods

A recent compilation[6] shows that by age 3 months, solid foods supply almost one third of total calories, the result of a headlong race in recent decades to see who can entice infants into taking solids at an earlier age. On purely nutritional grounds, solid food supplements are not needed before age 4 to 5 months.

Avoiding High-Calorie Foods

With the exception of certain low-birth-weight infants, formula concentration should not exceed 67 to 70 Cal/dl. The usual dessert foods should be used sparingly; an "anti-sweet tooth" also can be acquired. High fiber-low energy foods should be offered in moderate amounts.

Monitoring Infant Weight Gain

As stated earlier, the infant who gains weight rapidly is more likely to be an overweight adult. The weight record can be used to reassure mothers who are concerned about what is perceived as a poor appetite during the second and third years.

Encouraging Physical Exercise

Children (and adults!) should walk to destinations whenever possible. Twice- or thrice-weekly gym sessions in school do not fill the need for exercise. Weekend sports should take precedence over television.

Reviewing Family Eating Habits and Life-Style

The ritual of mealtime should include family togetherness as well as food itself. Parents should be taught to distinguish between hunger and restlessness and to emphasize noncaloric rewards, and they should cooperate in devising a regular mealtime pattern, a discipline of eating behavior. Children should not be treated as circus dogs whose every act is rewarded by a coveted biscuit.

The type of food consumed is of secondary importance. So-called junk foods are no more fattening than others. Calorie for calorie, there is relatively little difference in energy contribution. However, one should advise against the use of skim milk for young infants because the solute-to-calorie ratio is too high. Diets low in carbohydrates may produce ketosis, and their only real advantage is novelty.

Developing a Sense of Identity and Purpose in Life

Bruch[2] has found that the behavior of obese children reflects their underlying sense of insecurity, which results from an unrealistic upbringing that includes the expectation that they compensate for the frustrations and unfulfilled ambitions of their parents' lives. Perhaps the American culture, with its dream of success for everyone, plays a role here. As a people, our level of expectation is high, unrealistically high for the majority, and this design fosters frustration.

One must recognize that obesity is not a metabolic disease, but rather a disorder of *appetite* that is distinct from physiologic *hunger*. One of the most promising treatments for established obesity is behavioral modification, with its features of contingency and environmental management and of self-monitoring. Perhaps these same principles could be applied to prevention.

REFERENCES

Nutritional Requirements

1. Berry WTC: Nutrition in a health service. In McLaren DS and Burman, D, editors: Textbook of paediatric nutrition, New York, 1976, Churchill Livingstone, Inc.
2. Ross MH: Nutrition and longevity in experimental animals. In Winick M, editor: Nutrition and aging, New York, 1976, John Wiley & Sons, Inc.

The Feeding of Infants and Children

1. Berlin CM: Drugs and chemicals in breast milk, Personal communication, June 26, 1989.
2. Committee on Drugs, American Academy of Pediatrics: The transfer of drugs and other chemicals into human milk, revised 1989.
3. Eiger MS and Olds SW: The complete book of breastfeeding, rev ed, New York, 1987, Workman Publishing Co., Inc.
4. Fomon SJ: Infant nutrition, ed 2, Philadelphia, 1974, WB Saunders Co.
5. Goldman AS and Smith CW: Host resistance factors in human milk, J Pediatr 82:1082, 1973.
6. Grulee and Sanford HN: The influence of breast and artificial feeding on infantile eczema, J Pediatr 9:223, 1936.
7. Kendall N, Vaughn VC, and Kusakcioglu A: Study of preparation of infant formulas, Am J Dis Child 122:215, 1971.
8. Lawrence RA: Breastfeeding: a guide for the medical profession, ed 3, St Louis, 1989, The CV Mosby Co.
9. L'Esperance C and Frantz K: Time limitation for early breastfeeding, J Obstet Gynecol Neonatal Nurs 14(2):114, 1985.
10. Lozoff B et al: The Mother-newborn relationship: limits of adaptability, J Pediatrics 91:1, 1977.
11. Montagu A: Touching: the human significance of the skin, New York, 1971, Harper & Row, Publishers, Inc.
12. Olds SW: The working parents' survival guide, New York, 1983, Bantam Books, Inc.
13. Woolridge MW: Colic, "overfeeding", and symptoms of lactose malabsorption in the breast-fed baby: a possible artifact of feed management? Lancet, vol. 2, p. 382, August 13, 1988.
14. Woolridge MW: The anatomy of infant sucking, Midwifery 2:164, 1986.

Obesity

1. Bruch H: Eating disorders: obesity, anorexia nervosa, and the person within, New York, 1973, Basic Books, Inc, Publishers.
2. Bruch H: The importance of overweight. In Collipp PJ, editor: Childhood obesity, Acton, Mass, 1975, Publishing Sciences Group, Inc.
3. Forbes GB: Nutrition and growth, J Pediatr 91:40, 1977.
4. Forbes GB: Maintenance energy needs for women as a function of body size and composition, Am J Clin Nutr 50:404, 1989.
5. Forbes GB and Welle SL: Lean body mass in obesity, Int J Obesity 7:99, 1983.
6. Forbes GB and Woodruff CW, editors: Pediatric nutrition handbook, ed 2, Elk Grove Village, Ill, 1985, American Academy of Pediatrics.
7. Mann GV: The influence of obesity on health, N Engl J Med 291:175, 1974.

SUGGESTED READINGS

Nutritional Requirements

American Psychiatric Association Task Force: Megavitamins and orthomolecular therapy in psychiatry, Washington, DC, 1973, The Association.

Burkitt DP, Walker ARP, and Painter NS: Dietary fiber and disease, JAMA 229:1068, 1974.

Fomon SJ: Infant nutrition, ed 2, Philadelphia, 1974, WB Saunders Co.

Food and Nutrition Board, National Academy of Sciences: Recommended dietary allowances, ed 10, Washington, DC, 1989, The Academy.

Forbes GB: Food fads: safe feeding of children, Pediatr Rev 1:207, 1980.

Forbes GB and Woodruff CW, editors: Pediatric nutrition handbook, ed 2, Elk Grove Village, Ill, 1985, American Academy of Pediatrics.

Grand RJ, Sutphen JL, and Dietz WH, editors: Pediatric nutrition, Boston, 1987, Butterworth Publishers, Inc.

Hytten FE and Leitch I: Physiology of human pregnancy, ed 2, Oxford, 1971, Blackwell Scientific Publications, Ltd.

Klein PS, Forbes GB, and Nader PR: Effects of starvation in infancy (pyloric stenosis) on subsequent learning abilities, J Pediatr 87:8, 1975.

Leaf A and Weber PC: Cardiovascular effects of *n*-3 fatty acids, N Engl J Med 318:549, 1988.

Lechtig A et al: Maternal nutrition and fetal growth in developing countries, Am J Dis Child 129:553, 1975.

McCann ML, and Schwartz R: The effects of milk solute on urinary cast excretion in premature infants, Pediatrics 38:555, 1966.

McKigney JI and Munro HN, editors: Nutrient requirements in adolescence, Cambridge, Mass, 1976, The MIT Press.

Mertz W: The essential trace elements, Science 213:1332, 1981.

Pike RL and Brown ML: Nutrition: an integrated approach, ed 2, New York, 1975, John Wiley & Sons, Inc.

Rush D, Davis H, and Susser M: Antecedents of low birth weight in Harlem, New York City, Int J Epidemiol 1:393, 1972.

Sacks FM et al: Plasma lipids and lipoproteins in vegetarians and controls, N Engl J Med 292:1148, 1975.

Stein Z et al: Famine and human development, New York, 1975, Oxford University Press.

Tsang RC and Nichols BL, editors: Nutrition during infancy, Philadelphia, 1988, Hanley & Belfus, Inc.

Walker WA and Watkins JB, editors: Nutrition in pediatrics, Boston, 1985, Little, Brown & Co.

Waterlow JC and Alleyne GAO: Protein malnutrition in children. In Anfinsen CB Jr, Edsall JT, and Richards FM, editors: Advances in protein chemistry, vol 25, New York, 1971, Academic Press, Inc.

World Health Organization: Energy and protein requirements. Report of a Joint FAO/WHO/UNU expert consultation, Tech Rep Series 724, Geneva, 1985, WHO.

The Feeding of Infants and Children

Applebaum RM: The modern management of successful breast feeding, Pediatr Clin North Am 17:1, 1970.

Bakwin H: Feeding program for infants, I. Fed Proc 23:1, 1964.

Beal VA: On the acceptance of solid foods and other food patterns of infants and children, Pediatrics 20:448, 1957.

Bennett I and Simon M: The prudent diet, Port Washington, NY, 1973, David White, Inc.

Briggs G, Freeman R, and Yaffe S: Drugs in pregnancy and lactation, ed 2, Baltimore, Md, Williams & Wilkins, 1986.

Eiger MS, Rausen AR, and Silverio J: Morbidity of breast-fed vs bottle-fed infants, Clin Pediatr 23:9, 1984.

Gerard JW: Breastfeeding: second thoughts, Pediatrics 54:6, 1974.

Grulee CG and Sanford HN: The influence of breast and artificial feeding on infantile eczema, Journal of Pediatrics 9:223, 1936.

Kendall N, Vaughn VC, and Kusakcioglu A: Study of preparation of infant formulas, Am J Dis Child 122:215, 1971.

Lawson D and Conlon J: Superbaby cookbook, New York, 1974, Macmillan, Inc.

Minchin M: Breastfeeding matters, Australia, 1985, Alma Publications.

Oseid BJ: Breastfeeding and infant health, Clin Obstet Gynecol 18:149, 1975.

Reina D: Infant nutrition, Clin Perinatol 2:373, 1975.

The uniqueness of human milk, symposium, Am J Clin Nutr 24:968, 1971.

Winikoff B and Baer EC: The obstetrician's opportunity: translating "breast is best" from theory to practice, Am J Obstet Gynecol 138:105, 1980.

Obesity

Charney E et al: The childhood antecedents of adult obesity: do chubby infants become obese adults? N Engl J Med 295:6, 1976.

Stunkard AJ, editor: Obesity, Philadelphia, 1980, WB Saunders Co.

17

Immunizations

John H. Dossett

BASIC CONCEPTS

General Immunity

General immunity, sometimes called *natural immunity*, refers to a general and immunologically mediated resistance to infection caused by microbial organisms of low virulence. Infection with such organisms may be inhibited by (1) broadly cross-reacting or nonspecific antibodies, (2) antibodies plus complement, (3) complement alone, or (4) phagocytosis, which is mediated by general rather than specific opsonins. Most microbes are in this category. Thus human beings with normal host resistance can live and grow in a physical environment that is teeming with microbes. Water, food, soil, and air are all alive with microbial organisms, and yet humans are not constantly infected.

Specific Immunity

In contrast to the interaction of organisms of low virulence and general immunity, there are hundreds of highly virulent microbes that possess specific characteristics which allow them to produce human disease. Moreover, specific immunologically mediated responses of the host are required to rid or protect humans from infection with such organisms. Such a specific immunity is an *acquired immunity* that may be either actively or passively acquired.

Active Immunity. Active immunity refers to the endogenous development of specific immunity in response to contact with microbial antigens. This immunity occurs within the host; it may be either humoral or cellular immunity but usually is both. The microbial antigens responsible for active immunity may be derived either from intact living microbial organisms or from nonliving microbial antigens.

Living Microbial Antigens. Most active immunity is spontaneously acquired in that it results from random community-acquired infections. These usually are infections with wild-strain microbes, and they may or may not be associated with a clinical illness. Examples of such immunity include the protection against subsequent episodes of chickenpox, mumps, and polio, for example, conferred by having contracted the natural disease. Moreover, some persons are protected from such diseases as the result of an unrecognized infection. In contrast to such spontaneously acquired immunity, and commonly associated with significant morbidity and mortality, is the notion of *electively induced immunity*, the principal subject of this discussion.

Intrinsically associated with electively induced immunity is the ideal of prevention of illness, including that caused by community-acquired infections and by the actual immunizing agent. Fortunately, these dual goals have been largely accomplished for many infectious diseases, and the scientific and human interest stories of the research, development, and implementation of these several triumphs constitute some of the greatest dramas of the twentieth century.

Immunoprophylaxis. Immunoprophylaxis (electively induced immunity) may be accomplished with the antigens of either living or nonliving microbes. There are advantages and disadvantages to both (see box below). The use of live vaccines brings about a "controlled infection"; the objective

Advantages and Disadvantages of Live Attenuated and Killed Vaccines

LIVE ATTENUATED VACCINES

Advantages

1. Produce controlled infections that emulate natural immunity
2. More likely to provide long-lasting or permanent immunity than are killed vaccines

Disadvantages

1. Risk of vaccine-induced disease in recipient
2. Risk of spreading vaccine strain to secondary host

KILLED VACCINES

Advantages

1. No risk of vaccine-induced infection
2. May use purified antigens
3. Safe for immunocompromised hosts
4. Safe for pregnant hosts

Disadvantages

1. Immunity unlikely to be prolonged or permanent
2. Less likely to induce protective immunity than are live attenuated vaccines

is to induce a protective immunity without producing significant clinical illness. The control is sought by managing (1) the virulence of the infectious agent, (2) the inoculum size, and (3) the site of infection. Examples of *attenuated live vaccines* (possessing diminished virulence) include polio (Sabin), measles, rubella, and mumps virus vaccines.

Immunity also may be induced by giving controlled amounts of *killed microbial antigens*. This principle uses the administration of specific microbial components or killed whole microbes to stimulate endogenous production of protective immunity. Examples of killed whole microbe vaccines include pertussis, influenza, and polio (Salk) vaccines. Examples of specific microbial component vaccines include tetanus, diphtheria, pneumococcal, meningococcal, and hepatitis B vaccines.

Passive Immunity. The major remaining means for acquiring protective immunity is through acquisition by the host of *preformed host-defense factors* (humoral antibodies, transfer factor, or competent cells) from an exogenous source. Examples of such passive immunity include (1) the placental transfer of maternal IgG to newborn infants, (2) the administration of immune serum globulin to protect against hepatitis A and measles, and (3) the administration of varicella-zoster immunoglobulin (VZIG) or hepatitis B immunoglobulin (HBIG) to protect against chickenpox or hepatitis B. In general, passive immunity is used to supply a measure of protection to persons who have already been exposed to a virulent infectious agent or to those who are at high risk of being exposed to such an agent to which they have no active immunity. The relative strengths and limitations of active and passive immunoprophylaxis are shown in the box below.

Advantages and Limitations of Active and Passive Immunoprophylaxis

ACTIVE IMMUNITY

Advantages

Prolonged or permanent protection

Limitations

1. Protection delayed
2. Risks related to the use of live organisms
3. Difficulty getting vaccine to at-risk populations
4. Only weak immune response produced in some young hosts

PASSIVE IMMUNITY

Advantages

Immediate protection

Limitations

1. Protection only brief
2. Risk of serum sickness
3. Active immune response to some vaccines inhibited
4. Protection frequently given too late

Epidemic Control and Prevention

The use of immunoprophylaxis to prevent the epidemic spread of infections may be divided into three major control strategies. These include the notions of spot control, herd control, and selective control.

Spot Control. Immunization of known and potential contacts of cases to prevent further spread of disease is considered spot control. Application of this principle requires that infected persons be readily identifiable so that they can be isolated and their contacts immunized. Clearly, communicable diseases marked by significant subclinical infection do not lend themselves to this method. Smallpox is a good example of a disease in which use of this method has been successful. Conversely, poliomyelitis (polio) is an example of a disease with a high incidence of subclinical infection unsuited to the application of spot control methods.

Herd Control. When the number of persons susceptible to a given communicable disease can be reduced to the point that it becomes impossible for disease to spread in epidemic proportions, the principle of herd control is in effect. Control of polio is a good example of the application of this principle: even though isolated clinical and subclinical cases occur, they cannot reach epidemic proportions because most of the population is not at risk, by virtue of previous immunization. Application of this principle also has been remarkably successful in preventing epidemics of rubella and rubeola. It will be even more successful when a larger majority of the population than at present is removed from the "at-risk" category through effective immunization.

Selective Control. The principle of selective control assumes that specific groups of persons are at significant epidemiologic risk for certain communicable diseases. It further implies that the rest of the population is at low risk for such infection. Thus only the specific groups at risk are selected for immunization. For example, hemodialysis patients and male homosexuals are at great risk for infection with hepatitis B virus and are therefore selectively chosen as groups for whom hepatitis B vaccine is recommended.

Vaccine Limitations

Clearly, the goal of public health agencies and of workers in infectious disease is to develop methods for prevention of all infectious disease. Some important communicable diseases, however, have not succumbed either to environmental or to immunologic control with vaccines. For instance, vaccine made from group A streptococci can produce rheumatic fever. In addition, a number of vaccines produce excellent immune response among older children and adults but poor immune response among young children. For example, pneumococcal vaccine is ineffective in its major target population, in that *Streptococcus pneumoniae* strains cause frequent and severe diseases in young children, but children younger than 2 years do not make protective antibodies on being vaccinated. Similarly, *Haemophilus influenzae* type b is the leading cause of childhood meningitis, but the first vaccines produced from these bacteria induced only a poor antibody response in the target population (again, those younger than 2 years of age). Fortunately, the *H. influenzae* type b polysaccarides have now been successfully linked with proteins that render these conjugate vaccines immunogenic in young infants.

The ultimate criterion regarding the effectiveness of any vaccine is whether the vaccinated person is protected against the target disease. Unfortunately, there are no reliable and inexpensive laboratory tests to indicate the level of protection a given person has acquired. Specifically, it would be prohibitively expensive to test every person after each vaccination to determine antibody titers. Field studies, however, have determined the dosage of vaccine and the number of doses that will result in a vaccine being 90% to 95% protective. For example, a single dose of measles vaccine given after age 1 year results in greater than 95% of infants being protected. In contrast, approximately 70% of infants are protected after a single dose of pertussis vaccine; only after three doses is 85% protection approached.

The laboratory criteria for protection have been rather arbitrarily established for some diseases. Regarding rubella, for example, it is recommended that any woman in the child-bearing years whose rubella antibody titer is lower than 10 be vaccinated, irrespective of whether she has been vaccinated previously. Certainly some women with titers lower than 10 are protected, but the consequences of gestational rubella justify this arbitrary recommendation.

PRACTICE OF IMMUNIZATION

With a few exceptions, it is clear that all children should be immunized with vaccines that are safe and effective. However, *no vaccine is perfectly safe and always effective*. Consequently, one weighs the risk of infection—morbidity and mortality—against the risks and benefits of the corresponding vaccination.

It is good practice to discuss these issues with parents and guardians. They are entitled to know the risks of infection (incidence, morbidity, and mortality) and the benefits and risks of the corresponding vaccinations. Although vaccination for several of the common childhood infections is mandated by law as a condition for school attendance, parents need accurate information so that they can be informed participants in decisions regarding immunization of their children.

Many of the current practices in immunization have evolved from attempts to minimize the cost, inconvenience, and discomfort of vaccine administration without compromising efficacy or safety. Consequently many vaccines have been combined (e.g., diphtheria, tetanus, pertussis [DTP] and mumps, measles, rubella [MMR]) to meet these goals. It is expected that in 1991, DPT and Hib will be combined.

In addition, the recommended schedule for administration of vaccines is rather arbitrarily selected to synchronize with a reasonable schedule for health supervision during infancy. *There is certainly nothing sacred about a primary schedule for immunization at ages 2, 4, and 6 months*. It is important, however, to monitor the growth and development of children in their first year of life at these intervals, and such a schedule is conveniently meshed with effective immunization.

The schedule generally recommended has been endorsed by the Advisory Committee on Immunization Practices (ACIP) of the U.S. Public Health Service and by the Committee on Infectious Diseases of the American Academy of Pediatrics (Table 17-1).

Interrupted Schedule

Contrary to common notions, interruption of the recommended schedule does not require restarting the entire immunization schedule. Immunization of preschool children should proceed from the point at which it was interrupted, regardless of the interval since the last dose was given (Table 17-2).

Table 17-1 *Recommended Schedule for Active Immunization of Normal Infants and Children*

RECOMMENDED AGE*	VACCINE(S)†	COMMENTS
2 mo	DTP-1§, OPV-1‖, Hib-1‡	Can be given earlier in areas of high endemicity
4 mo	DTP-2, OPV-2, Hib-2	6-8 wk interval desired between OPV doses to avoid interference
6 mo	DTP-3, Hib-3	Additional dose of OPV at this time optional for use in areas with a high risk of polio exposure
15 mo#	MMR-1**, Hib-4	
18 mo#	DTP-4, OPV-3	Completion of primary series
4-6 yr††	DTP-5, OPV-4, MMR-2	Preferably at or before school entry
14-16 yr	Td‡‡	Repeat every 10 years throughout life

*Recommended ages should not be construed as absolute (e.g., 2 mo can be 6-10 wk).

†For all products used, consult manufacturer's package enclosure for instructions on storage, handling, and administration. Immunobiologic agents prepared by different manufacturers may vary, and those of the same manufacturer may change from time to time. The package insert should be followed for a specific product. These schedules are those recommended by the USPHS Advisory Committee on Immunization Practices (ACIP) and the Committee on Infectious Diseases of the American Academy of Pediatrics.

‡Hib, *Haemophilus influenza,* type b polysaccharide/protein conjugate.

§*DTP,* Diphtheria and tetanus toxoids and pertussis vaccine.

‖*OPV,* Oral, attenuated poliovirus vaccine contains poliovirus types 1, 2, and 3.

#Simultaneous administration of MMR, DTP, OPV, and Hib is appropriate for patients whose compliance with medical care recommendations cannot be ensured.

***MMR,* Live measles, mumps, and rubella viruses in a combined vaccine.

††Up to the seventh birthday.

‡‡*Td,* Adult tetanus toxoid and diphtheria toxoid in combination, which contains the same dose of tetanus toxoid as DTP or DT and a reduced dose of diphtheria toxoid.

Unimmunized Children

Children not immunized in the first year of life may be started on a course of primary immunization any time before the age of 7 years. The schedule should be modified for these children so that they are properly protected against as many of the communicable diseases as possible. Thus it is recommended that they receive MMR, DTP, Hib, and oral polio vaccine (OPV) initially and that they receive subsequent DTP, OPV, and Hib at 8-week intervals. This should be continued until the child has received three doses each of DTP and OPV and zero to three more of Hib, depending on the child's age. Except in measles epidemics, MMR vaccine should not be given until the child is 15 months old. A second MMR should be given at the time the child starts to school. For children starting or continuing vaccinations after age 7 years, pertussis vaccine should be deleted (Tables 17-2 and 17-3).

Vaccine Interference

Some physicians believe that active response to one vaccine may interfere with the host response to another vaccine, but large field studies have demonstrated that this notion is not true; for instance, DTP and MMR give good responses to each of the components in these combined vaccines. Moreover, all these combinations (DTP, OPV, Hib, and MMR) may be given simultaneously without interfering with each other.

Intercurrent Illnesses and Vaccination

The presence of mild upper respiratory tract infections or a mild episode of diarrhea should not preclude routine vaccination. However, *children with febrile illnesses should have their vaccinations deferred until the illness is resolved*. Rather

Table 17-2 *Recommended Immunization Schedule to the Seventh Birthday of Children Not Immunized at the Recommended Time in Early Infancy**

TIMING	VACCINE(S)	COMMENTS
First visit	DTP-1,† OPV-1,‡ Hib-1, Hib‖, and if child is at least 15 mo old, MMR-1¶	DTP, OPV, Hib, and MMR can be administered simultaneously to children at least 15 mo old
2 mo after first dose of DTP, OPV, Hib	DTP-2, OPV-2, Hib	Second, third, and fourth doses of Hib are given only to infants beginning their immunizations at 3 to 6 months of age. Those beginning between 7 and 14 months of age receive fewer doses.
2 mo after second dose of DTP, Hib	DTP-3, Hib-3	Additional dose of OPV at this time optional for use in areas with a high risk of polio exposure
6-12 mo after third dose of DTP, Hib	DTP-4, OPV-3	
Preschool# (4-6 yr)	DTP-5, OPV-4, MMR-2	Preferably at or before school entry
14-16 yr	Td**	Repeat every 10 yr throughout life

*If initiated in the first year of life, give DTP-1, 2, and 3 and OPV-1 and 2 according to this schedule, and give MMR when the child is 15 mo old.
†*DTP,* Diphtheria and tetanus toxoids and pertussis vaccine. DTP may be used up to the seventh birthday.
‡*OPV,* Oral, attenuated poliovirus vaccine contains poliovirus types 1, 2, and 3.
§Hib, *Haemophilus influenzae,* type b polysaccharide/protein conjugate.
‖*Hib, H. influenzae* type b polysaccharide/protein conjugate.
¶*MMR,* Live measles, mumps, and rubella viruses in a combined vaccine.
#The preschool dose is not necessary if the fourth dose of DTP and third dose of OPV are administered after the fourth birthday.
***Td,* Adult tetanus toxoid and diphtheria toxoid in combination, which contains the same dose of tetanus toxoid as DTP or DT and a reduced dose of diphtheria toxoid.
These schedules are those recommended by the USDHS Advisory Committee on Immunization Practices (ACIP) and the Committee of Infectious Diseases of the American Academy of Pediatrics (AAP).

Table 17-3 *Recommended Immunization Schedule for Persons 7 Years of Age or Older**

TIMING	VACCINE(S)	COMMENTS
First visit	Td-1†, OPV-1‡, and MMR§	OPV not routinely administered to those aged 18 yr or older
2 mo after first dose of Td, OPV	Td-2, OPV-2	
6-12 mo after second dose of Td, OPV	Td-3, OPV-3	OPV-3 may be given as soon as 6 wk after OPV-2
10 yr after dose of Td-3	Td	Repeat every 10 yr throughout life

*See individual U.S. Public Health Services Advisory Committee on Immunization Practices recommendations for details.
†*Td,* Tetanus and diphtheria toxoids (adult type) are used after the seventh birthday. The DTP doses given to children younger than age 7 who remain incompletely immunized at age 7 or older should be counted as prior exposure to tetanus and diphtheria toxoids (e.g., a child who previously received two doses of DTP only needs one dose of Td to complete primary series).
‡*OPV,* Oral, attenuated poliovirus vaccine contains poliovirus types 1, 2, and 3. When polio vaccine is given to individuals 18 yr or older, inactivated polio vaccine (IPV) is preferred. (See ACIP statement on polio vaccine for immunization schedule for IPV.)
§*MMR,* Live measles, mumps, and rubella in a combined vaccine. Persons born before 1957 generally can be considered immune to measles and mumps and need not be immunized. Rubella vaccine may be given to persons of any age, particularly to women of childbearing age. MMR may be used because administration of vaccine to persons already immune is not deleterious. (See text for discussion of single versus combination vaccines.)

than implying a danger, this precaution is mainly intended to avoid confusion and the likely difficult interpretation of symptoms when fever caused by vaccination is superimposed on that of the intercurrent illness.

Barriers to Use of Immunoprophylaxis

Despite the long record of safety and success of the established vaccines, there remain many people in the United States who are susceptible to preventable infectious illnesses. Unfortunately, this susceptibility is not caused by vaccine failures but by neglect of vaccination for significant numbers of children and adolescents.

This *neglect of vaccination results from a general ignorance of the target diseases and a fear of or hostility toward the vaccines*. The present (and subsequent) generation of young parents has had no experience with the ravages of polio, measles, diphtheria, pertussis, or tetanus; consequently, they have no experiential reason to fear these diseases, as did previous generations. Frequently, even young physicians have never seen these diseases, which makes it difficult for them to convey to parents the urgency of immunization.

The general lack of knowledge regarding these once common and devastating diseases is so widespread that formal instruction regarding their history and control might profitably become part of the core curriculum in high school. Surely such information is as important to them and to society as driver's or sex education.

Vaccine Efficacy

Vaccine efficacy is the efficiency with which a given vaccine protects vaccinees against disease in settings in which virtually all persons are uniformly exposed to the infectious agent. It is calculated with the standard formula:

$$\text{VE}\ (\%) = \frac{\text{ARU} - \text{ARV}}{\text{ARU}} \times 100$$

where ARU and ARV are attack rates in the unvaccinated and vaccinated subjects, respectively.

International Travel

Several communicable diseases that no longer are a threat in North America remain endemic to other parts of the world. For specific information regarding the risks of infections in the various countries, the Centers for Disease Control (CDC) annually publishes *Health Information for International Travel*. This always current resource provides appropriate recommendations regarding yellow fever, typhus, cholera, plague, malaria, typhoid fever, and hepatitis A and B.

SPECIFIC IMMUNIZATIONS

Diphtheria Immunization

Fifty years ago diphtheria was a common respiratory illness with fatalities in the range of 5% to 10%. In the past 5 to 6 years, fewer than 100 cases have been reported annually, but some case fatalities continue each year.

Vaccine. Diphtheria vaccine is a toxoid produced from virulent bacterial toxin in toxigenic strains of *Corynebacterium diphtheriae*. It is a good antigen that induces excellent antitoxin titers.

Administration. Diptheria toxoid generally is given to infants in combination with tetanus and pertussis (DTP) or just tetanus (DT). Because diphtheria toxoid is more likely to cause adverse reactions (e.g., fever and local tenderness) in adults, an adult vaccine (Td) is recommended for this population. Td contains the standard amount of tetanus toxoid but only 20% of the diphtheria toxoid supplied by DTP or DT.

Adverse Reactions. Diphtheria toxoid is a safe vaccine with a low incidence of fever and local pain at the site of injection.

Efficacy. The primary series of DTP is greater than 90% effective in preventing serious diphtheria infections. However, it does not prevent carriage of *C. diphtheriae* on the skin or in the nasopharynx. It is believed to be protective for at least 10 years and perhaps for much longer.

Target Population. Young children are particularly susceptible to the myocarditis and neuritis of *C. diphtheriae* infection. Most cases occur in unimmunized children and adults.

Table 17-4 *Guide to Tetanus Prophylaxis in Wound Management*

HISTORY OF TETANUS IMMUNIZATION	TYPE OF WOUND AND TYPE OF IMMUNIZATION GIVEN: CLEAN MINOR WOUND	MODERATELY TETANUS PRONE	VERY TETANUS PRONE
Incomplete or uncertain	Td	Td + TIG-H* (250 U)	Td + TIG-H (500 U)
Fully immunized but >10 yr since last dose of Td	Td	Td	Td
Fully immunized but 5-10 yr since last dose of Td	None	Td	Td
Fully immunized but <5 yr since last dose of Td	None	None	None

NOTE: 1. Children younger than age 7 yr should have DTP rather than Td.
2. Persons are considered to have had a full primary series if they have had two doses of tetanus toxoid separated by 2 mo's time and have had a booster at least 6 mo after the second dose.

**TIG-H,* Tetanus immunoglobulin–human, a specific tetanus antitoxin collected from human volunteers.
†*Td,* Tetanus and diphtheria toxoids (adult type).
This schedule is recommended by the USPHS Advisory Committee on Immunization Practices

Tetanus Immunization

The general use of tetanus toxoid has resulted in a dramatic decrease in the number of cases of tetanus seen in the United States. However, approximately 100 cases per year continue to be reported. In recent years more than 50% of these cases have occurred in persons older than 50 years of age who were either unimmunized or partially immunized or whose immunization status was unknown.

Vaccine. The vaccine is a toxoid made from the virulent neurotoxin of *Clostridium tetani*.

Administration. Tetanus toxoid usually is administered in combination with diphtheria and pertussis vaccine (DTP) in preschool children and with a lesser amount of diphtheria in older children and adults (Td).

Adverse Reactions. Tetanus toxoid is associated with a low incidence of mild fever and mild local tenderness at the injection site.

Efficacy. Tetanus toxoid is remarkably effective and generally induces protective antitoxin levels that persist at least 10 years after full immunization.

Target Population. Because there is little natural immunity to tetanus toxin and because strains of *C. tetani* are found everywhere, all persons of all ages should be immunized with tetanus toxoid.

Wound Management. Wounds are particularly prone to tetanus contamination if they are more than 24 hours old, contain devitalized tissue, or are heavily contaminated with bacteria. Such wounds include farm machinery injuries, gunshot wounds to the abdomen, and certain crush injuries sustained in automobile and motorcycle accidents.

Wounds are moderately prone to tetanus if there is moderate bacterial contamination, extension into muscle, crushing of tissue, or a puncture. Wounds that are not tetanus prone are clean, are usually fewer than 24 hours old, are not associated with crushing or puncture, and do not extend into muscle (Table 17-4).

Pertussis Immunization

During the 1930s and 1940s pertussis was a leading cause of infectious mortality and morbidity among children. The general use of pertussis vaccine has brought about a remarkable reduction in deaths from pertussis. However, there continues to be an unacceptably high incidence of pertussis—approximately 2500 cases per year. Among these cases is a mortality of 0.4% and an encephalopathy rate of 0.4%. *Since the 1950s all deaths and serious complications have occurred in children younger than 1 year.*

Vaccine. Pertussis vaccine is a crude vaccine prepared from killed whole organisms. The essential antigen or antigens in this vaccine are still unknown.

Administration. The vaccine usually is given in combination with tetanus and diphtheria toxoids (DTP). Because the greatest mortality and morbidity of pertussis occur in young children, the vaccine should be started at age 2 months; however, it is not routinely recommended for children older than age 7 years.

Adverse Reactions. Pertussis vaccine is associated with a higher incidence of reactions and complications than are most other vaccines. More than 50% of the children have temporary local tenderness at the site of the DTP injection, and approximately 50% have mild and brief systemic signs such as fever, irritability, or lethargy. More serious reactions, such as convulsions and hypotonic hyporesponsiveness, occur in approximately 1 of 2000 of those children vaccinated. Virtually all these children recover quickly and without sequelae.

Grave complications are much less frequent. Encephalopathy occurs in approximately 1 of 100,000 vaccinees, and permanent neurologic sequelae occur in approximately 1 of 300,000 vaccinees. Recent data, however, indicate quite clearly that pertussis immunization cannot be statistically linked to encephalopathy, neurological damage, or death. Clearly, *children who have had seizures, have been unresponsive, or have had prolonged high fever after receiving DTP should not receive further pertussis vaccine.*

Efficacy. Pertussis is highly communicable with attack rates as high as 90% in unimmunized household contacts; however, the vaccine is highly effective in preventing or attenuating disease so that serious complications are prevented. Its calculated efficacy is 80% to 85%.

Target Population. All children except those with an evolving neurologic illness should be immunized. Children with stable neurologic deficits should be immunized just as any other child.

Risk/Benefit. In recent years there has been great popular concern about the safety of pertussis vaccine; much of this concern has resulted from the propagation of wrong information regarding the incidence of encephalopathy and permanent neurologic sequelae. Such misinformation has caused many parents to resist immunization of their infants with pertussis vaccine.

Although the vaccine does have risks, the risk of death or encephalopathy from pertussis infection in the unimmunized child is much greater. The recent experience in Great Britain and Japan has shown that when the rate of pertussis immunization dropped from 80% to 30%, large epidemics of pertussis in both countries followed.

Projections from the experience in these recent epidemics indicate that *the risk of pertussis-related death is 10 times greater in an unimmunized population than in an immunized population* of children. With a cohort of 3.5 million births per year, the projected number of deaths from pertussis and pertussis vaccination is 44 per year. The same group without vaccination is projected to have 457 deaths. A similar tenfold greater incidence is projected for frequency of hospitalization, encephalitis episodes, and cost in an unimmunized cohort of children.[2]

Most experts expect that within the next few years a more highly purified pertussis vaccine will be developed—one that will be more effective in preventing disease and less likely to cause local and systemic reactions in children and adults than the current whole-cell vaccine.

Polio Immunization

Before the introduction of inactivated polio vaccine (IPV) in 1955, more than 18,000 cases of paralytic polio were reported in epidemic years. In one of the most dramatic of public health success stories, the general use of polio vaccine has almost eradicated paralytic polio from highly developed countries. However, 5 to 15 cases are still reported in the United

States each year, usually among unimmunized persons who are illegal aliens or other groups who have for various reasons refused or not sought immunization.

Vaccine. The first vaccine licensed (1955) was the IPV. After a primary series of immunizations, it protected the child against paralytic disease but not against polio *infection*. In 1963 the oral polio vaccine (OPV) was licensed. It is a live, attenuated poliovirus given orally. All three serotypes of poliovirus have been combined into a highly effective trivalent vaccine that gives gastrointestinal mucosal immunity to infection. Moreover, the vaccine virus may spread via the fecal-oral route, much like the spread of wild virus. This has the added advantage of immunizing secondary and tertiary contacts.

Administration. OPV is given by mouth and should be started at the 2- or 4-month visit. Second and third doses of OPV are recommended at ages 4 and 6 months. Booster doses are recommended at approximately age 18 months and again when the child starts school. It may be given at the same time as DTP and MMR, if the primary immunizations have been delayed beyond the first birthday. It has been shown that *breast milk with antibodies to polio is capable of neutralizing the vaccine but does not interfere with development of immunity;* therefore breast-fed babies also should be immunized according to the routine recommended schedule.

Adverse Reactions. OPV is remarkably safe with virtually no minor reactions. A few cases of vaccine-associated paralytic disease have been reported—the risk in primary vaccinees is approximately 1 of 19 million cases. If paralytic disease among close contacts of vaccinees also is counted, then the risk is approximately 1 of 4 million. Whichever the case, the benefit of polio vaccination remains overwhelming.

Efficacy. Polio is highly communicable and spreads rapidly through immunized populations, as witnessed in a recent epidemic in Taiwan. Calculations from recent experiences have estimated vaccine efficacy to be 82% after one dose, 96% after two doses, and 98% after three doses.

Target Population. Trivalent oral polio vaccine should be given to all children, except those with immunodeficiency syndromes and the household contacts of children with immunodeficiency syndromes.

Measles Immunization

Until the 1960s approximately 500,000 cases of measles were reported in the United States each year. Because of underreporting, the actual number may have been five times that many or more. The major complications of measles are encephalitis and bronchopneumonia, with approximately one case of encephalitis or pneumonia in every 1000 cases of measles, resulting in death or neurologic sequelae of varying severity. Large epidemics of measles occurring before the 1960s caused the deaths of up to 1 in 15 children affected.

Vaccine. Live measles virus vaccine is prepared in chick embryo cells from the Edmonston-B strain, which has been further attenuated. It is used primarily in combination with mumps and rubella vaccines (MMR). However, it is available in a monovalent form or in combination with rubella (MR).

Administration. It is recommended that measles vaccine be given at age 15 months along with rubella and mumps (MMR) inasmuch as *children immunized before age 1 year are less likely to make protective antibodies because of neutralization of the vaccine by maternal antibodies.* It may be given at the same time as other vaccines if the child has not been immunized according to the recommended schedule. A second dose of MMR should be given at the time children enter school. It is most important that the vaccine be handled properly; to prevent inactivation, it should be transported and stored at 35.5° to 50° F (2° to 10° C) and should be protected from light.

Adverse Reactions. Measles vaccine has an outstanding safety record. Fever that may last up to 5 days develops in approximately 5% of vaccinees between the sixth and tenth day after vaccination. Usually no other symptoms occur, although transient rashes have been reported in 3% to 5% of vaccinees.

Persons who have received the killed measles vaccine are more likely to experience fever and local tenderness when revaccinated with live measles vaccine. However, this risk is far less than their risk of severe atypical measles on exposure to wild measles virus.

Efficacy. The development of measles antibodies protects at least 95% of measles vaccinees from clinical measles. A single dose at approximately age 15 months protects for at least 15 years and probably for a lifetime. General use of the vaccine has resulted in a 99% reduction in the number of reported cases of measles.

Target Population. All persons who have not had measles infection or measles immunization are at risk for infection. Persons born before 1957 are likely to have had measles; those born after 1957 should be immunized unless they have had physician-diagnosed measles, serologic evidence of measles immunity, or documented measles immunization subsequent to their first birthday. In the decade of the 1980s, more than 50% of the cases of measles occurred in adolescents and young adults. Clearly, greater emphasis must be placed on immunizing persons of high school and college age. Most states have now passed legislation that requires evidence of measles immunity to attend school, and many colleges require measles revaccination before matriculation. Preschool children remain at risk and should be immunized promptly at 15 months.

Revaccination. Through the 1980s many epidemics of measles occurred in teenagers and young adults. This appeared to be, in part, the result of waning immunity in persons who were vaccinated at 15 months. Consequently, it is now recommended that all young persons (5 to 21 years of age) have a second measles vaccination. This second dose is preferably given at the time of school entry; however, those persons who haven't received a second dose should receive it at whatever age they are identified. In the decade of 1990s, middle school, high school, and college-aged youth should be specifically targeted for revaccination.

Contraindications. As with all live virus vaccines, there is a theoretic risk of fetal infection if pregnant women are vaccinated. However, no direct experiences with any of the common vaccines (MMR and OPV) have confirmed this fear. Mild upper respiratory tract infections should not be cause for postponing MMR vaccination. Persons with febrile illnesses, however, should not receive MMR vaccination because diagnostic confusion could result.

Children who have experienced anaphylactic reactions to eggs should not be immunized; such children are so rare, however, that this risk will hardly ever preclude measles immunization. Immunocompromised children such as those with leukemia, lymphoma, disseminated malignancy, or immunodeficiency or those receiving steroid therapy should consult a specialist in the field before receiving live virus vaccines. There is general agreement that children infected with human immunodeficiency virus (HIV) should receive MMR vaccine but that enhanced inactivated poliovirus (EIPV) rather than live poliovirus vaccine should be used.

Mumps Immunization

Mumps generally is a benign infection commonly characterized by fever and parotitis. At least 30% of cases are subclinical, and about 15% of affected patients have meningeal signs but recover without sequelae. Rare *nerve deafness* is the primary serious permanent sequel. Since mumps vaccine was introduced in 1967, its general use has resulted in a 98% reduction in the number of cases of mumps reported annually.

Vaccine. Mumps vaccine is an attenuated live virus prepared in chick embryo cultures. It produces a subclinical infection that has virtually no side effects. It is most often combined with measles and rubella vaccines to reduce the cost and discomfort of injections.

Administration. It is recommended that mumps vaccine be given to all generally healthy children at age 15 months. It should be given with measles and rubella vaccine (MMR). Like measles vaccine, it should be transported and stored at 35.5° to 50° F (2° to 10° C) and protected from light. A single dose of mumps vaccine can be expected to provide durable immunity, probably lifelong.

Adverse Reactions. There are rare reports of fever and rash temporally related to mumps vaccination. Reports of seizures and encephalitis are rare; the frequency of these is even lower than the incidence of central nervous system dysfunction expected in the general population.

Efficacy. Vaccine efficacy, calculated in several studies, ranges from 80% to 90%. Measurable antibodies develop in more than 90% of vaccinees.

Target Population. Because of interference from maternally transported antibodies, protective antibodies are less likely to develop in children immunized before age 1 year. However, all children and young adults who have not been immunized or have not had clinical mumps would benefit from the vaccine. There is no additional risk to persons who actually may have had preceding subclinical mumps or to those whose immunization status is uncertain. The cost/benefit ratio of mumps vaccine has been clearly documented. Because adolescents and young adults born since 1967 are less likely to have been immunized by natural infection, special emphasis should be placed on immunizing this group.

Rubella Immunization

Rubella is one of the common childhood exanthems usually manifested by brief low-grade fever, suboccipital and postauricular lymphadenopathy, and mild arthralgia. It produces transient arthritis in infected adolescent and young adult women. Before the general use of rubella vaccine, the disease occurred in epidemic form approximately every 7 years. Infection of pregnant women is complicated by a high incidence of fetal infection. Fetal infection results in a high incidence of deaths, malformations, and neurologic sequelae and constitutes the major public health problem posed by rubella. Since 1980 more than 75% of rubella cases have occurred in young adults older than 15 years of age.

Vaccine. Live rubella vaccine is an attenuated rubella virus prepared in human diploid cell culture. It is produced as a monovalent vaccine and in combination with measles (MR) or with mumps and measles (MMR) vaccine. The vaccine produces subclinical infection in vaccinees but does not spread to susceptible contacts.

Administration and Target Population. All children, adolescents, and young adults who do not have serologic evidence of rubella immunity should be vaccinated. It is recommended that infants receive the vaccine in combination with measles and mumps vaccine at age 15 months. Because most adolescents and young adults who have not received rubella vaccine have also not received measles or mumps vaccines, they too should receive MMR vaccine.

Although general immunization of young children has successfully prevented large statewide epidemics, small epidemics still occur regularly in high schools, colleges, military bases, and businesses that employ many young people. These groups constitute a major priority for targeting because they are in their peak childbearing years. *All women who attend prenatal clinics should be screened for rubella immunity* so that those who are susceptible can be immunized immediately following birth. *A history of rubella is not reliable and should not be accepted in lieu of vaccination.*

Adverse Reactions. A significant number of vaccinees (30%) may have transient rash, lymphadenopathy, or arthralgia. Approximately 1% have self-limited arthritis; this reaction occurs more often in women than in children.

The primary concerns regarding rubella vaccine have been that (1) young women in their first trimester of pregnancy might inadvertently be vaccinated and (2) the vaccine virus might be as teratogenic as is the wild virus. The first concern has been confirmed in that at least 1000 pregnant women have inadvertently received rubella vaccine. However, in none of these women has congenital rubella syndrome been diagnosed. A few of the infants also were infected, but they had no illness attributable to the vaccine virus. Even so, *it is recommended that women known to be pregnant not be vaccinated with rubella vaccine or with any other live virus vaccine.* If, however, such vaccination inadvertently occurs, there is no reason to recommend that the pregnancy be terminated.

Efficacy. Protective antibodies develop in approximately 95% of susceptible persons who are older than age 1 year and who receive a single dose of rubella vaccine. Their immunity is long-term and probably protects them against viremia and clinical illnesses for life.

Hepatitis B Immunization

Hepatitis B virus infects approximately 200,000 persons per year in the United States and results in about 10,000 hospitalizations and 250 acute deaths. Many more deaths result from later complications such as cirrhosis or hepatoma. Risk of infection is concentrated in certain groups such as male homosexuals, institutionalized retarded children, certain health care personnel, and household contacts of infected persons.

Vaccine. There are two effective hepatitis B vaccines. The first is hepatitis B surface antigen (HB_sAg) that has been harvested from the plasma of stable human carriers of the hepatitis B virus (HBV). It is purified by a series of ultracentrifugation steps and then inactivated by treatment with pepsin, urea, and formalin. Any one of these last steps inactivates all known human viruses. The vaccine is then absorbed with alum to increase potency. It is best stored at 39° F (4° C) but should be protected from freezing. The other is a recombinant hepatitis B vaccine released in the late 1980s. In this vaccine the HBgAg is harvested from yeast that has the gene coding for hepatitis B surface antigen incorporated into its DNA. This vaccine has no connection to blood or any other mammalian tissue.

Administration. The dose for adults is 10 μg (1.0 ml) and is reduced to 5 μg (0.5 ml) for children younger than 9 years. Three doses are needed to raise protective antibodies. The first two doses are given 1 month apart; the third dose is given 6 months after the first. These are all given intramuscularly.

Adverse Reactions. Approximately 15% of vaccine recipients have mild local tenderness at the site of injection.

Efficacy. Protective antibodies develop in more than 90% of healthy adults after three intramuscular doses of HBV vaccine. Up to 95% of susceptible vaccinees in field trials have been protected against hepatitis.

Target Population. The high cost of the vaccine and the low risk for most pediatric patients combine to make recommendation for vaccination of any but the most highly targeted groups impractical. For instance, each institution for the mentally retarded should develop its own immunization strategy on the basis of the prevelance of hepatitis B antibodies and the presence of heaptitis B carriers in its population. These strategies should be revised as more experience with the vaccine is accumulated and the costs of screening and vaccinating susceptible persons are modified.[3]

Pediatricians will encounter infants born to mothers with HB_sAg positivity, as well as children who live in households with chronic hepatitis B virus carriers. Babies born to mothers with HB_sAg positivity are particularly vulnerable; they should receive hepatitis B immunoglobulin (HBIG) *and* HBV vaccine. Follow-up serologic testing (anti HB_sAg) should be performed when the infant is 12 to 15 months of age to determine the vaccine response. It is recommended that children from households with chronic carriers receive the vaccine only. Perinatal transmission of hepatitis B virus can be prevented by prenatal screening of all pregnant women for HB_sAg and administering HBIG and HBV vaccine to the newborn infants of mothers who are HBV carriers. Some states require universal prenatal screening for HB_sAg.

Influenza Immunization

Infection with influenza virus produces an illness generally manifested by fever, cough, paratracheal pain, and myalgia. Its primary morbidity and mortality are among elderly persons and the chronically ill.

Influenza infections occur every winter, but large epidemics occur when there are major shifts in the antigenic structure of the prevalent strains. Influenza A viruses are classified on the basis of their hemagglutinin and neuraminidase antigens. Three subtypes of hemagglutinin ($H_1H_2H_3$) and two subtypes of neuraminidase (N_1N_2) have been recognized in those strains that cause human disease. Immunity to a specific hemagglutinin protects against infections and serious disease. *Because influenza A virus antigens are always changing, a reliable vaccine for protection of susceptible populations is particularly difficult to develop.*

Vaccine Strategy. Each summer the ACIP attempts to predict the subtypes of influenza virus likely to be prevalent in the coming respiratory virus season. This prediction is based upon analysis of the strains most prevalent at the end of the previous season. On the basis of these predictions, vaccine is prepared and distributed in the late summer and fall of each year.

Vaccine. The vaccines are either whole virus or split virus preparations that have been grown on chick embryo cells. In recent years the vaccines have been purified of vir-

Perinatal Hepatitis B Prophylaxis

1. Infants born to mothers with hepatitis B antigen positivity have a great probability of being infected.
   a. HB_sAg positive, 25% probability
   b. HB_eAg positive, 85% probability
   c. Infection may occur anytime in the first year after birth
2. Infants who are infected with HBV have a 90% probability of becoming chronic HBV carriers.
3. Perinatal administration of HBIG is 75% effective in preventing chronic infection.
4. Perinatal administration of HBIG and HBV vaccine is 90% effective in preventing chronic infection.
5. Both HBIG and HBV vaccine are recommended.

	Perinatal exposure	Household contact
HBIG		
Dose	0.5 ml IM	None
Timing	Within 12 hr of birth	
HBV vaccine		
Dose	0.5 ml IM	0.5 ml IM
Timing	Within 2 mo of birth, repeated at age 1 mo and 6 mo after the initial dose (may be given at same time as HBIG and at the same time as other childhood immunizations)	When contact is identified; repeat after 1 mo and 6 mo

tually all egg protein, and the antigen concentration has been stabilized.

Administration and Target Population. Recommendations regarding the number of doses and target population vary from year to year, but current CDC recommendations are published in a number of readily available sources each summer; *Morbidity and Mortality Weekly Reports* is a good source.[1]

Children with chronic illness are at greater risk for serious complications and are the only ones who should be vaccinated. Children with the following conditions warrant protection with influenza vaccine:

1. Chronic pulmonary disease, such as cystic fibrosis, asthma, severe scoliosis, bronchopulmonary dysplasia, and neuromotor diseases resulting in compromised ventilation
2. Heart disease with altered circulatory dynamics
3. Chronic renal disease with azotemia
4. Diabetes mellitus and other metabolic diseases
5. Immunocompromised conditions
6. Severe chronic anemias

Adverse Reactions. A mild local induration at the site of injection develops in approximately one third of vaccinees. Systemic reactions of fever, malaise, or myalgia are infrequent. In 1976 a temporal association was noted between administration of the "swine" influenza vaccine and Guillain-Barré syndrome (GBS) in adults. No increase in GBS has been seen after influenza vaccinations since 1978.

Rabies Prevention

Rabies has been almost eliminated from humans in the United States. This is largely the result of compulsory rabies vaccination of dogs. Even so, thousands of people are injured annually by rabid or potentially rabid animals. Now that rabies has largely been controlled among domestic animals, *wild animals (especially skunks, foxes, raccoons, and bats) account for approximately 75% of animal rabies.* Because it is such a lethal disease, all persons exposed to the risk of rabies infection need to be immunized.

Vaccine. The currently recommended rabies vaccine is a human diploid cell rabies vaccine (HDCV). It is an inactivated virus vaccine that produces good antibody responses with only mild side effects. This HDCV has now replaced the duck embryo vaccine (DEV), which requires four times as many injections, has more side effects, and results in much lower antibody titers.

Human rabies immune globulin (RIG) is prepared from the plasma of hyperimmunized human donors. It is standardized to contain 150 IU of rabies-neutralizing antibodies per milliliter.

Administration and Target Population. Children who are bitten or scratched by animals should be regarded as having been exposed to rabies, and decisions for rabies prophylaxis should be based on knowledge of the (1) circumstances of the bite, (2) species of animal, (3) health of the animal (when possible), and (4) type of exposure.

Circumstances of Biting Incident—Provoked or Unprovoked. An unprovoked attack is more likely to indicate that the animal is rabid. Bites or scratch injuries to a person attempting to feed, pet, or handle an apparently healthy animal generally should be regarded as provoked injuries.

Species of Biting Animal. A few species of animals are more likely to be infected with rabies virus than are others. In the United States since 1960, these animals have included skunks, raccoons, foxes, bats, coyotes, and bobcats. Any possible rabies exposure (bite or nonbite) to these animals mandates postexposure prophylaxis, unless the animal is tested and shown to be free of rabies.

Rodents such as squirrels, chipmunks, rats, mice, hamsters, guinea pigs, and gerbils and also rabbits are only rarely infected and have not been known to cause human rabies in the United States. Consequently, bites by such animals are almost never an indication for rabies prophylaxis.

Type of Exposure—Bite and Nonbite. Rabies is transmitted by introducing the virus into cuts and wounds or through contamination of mucous membranes. A *bite* is defined as any penetration of the skin by the animal's teeth. Nonbite exposure includes scratches, cuts, open wounds, or mucous membranes contaminated by animal saliva or other potentially infected materials.

Health of the Implicated Animal. *Any healthy domestic dog or cat that bites a child should be confined and observed for 10 days.* If during the confinement the animal shows any signs of illness, it should be evaluated by a veterinarian. If signs suggestive of rabies develop, the animal should be humanely killed and the head submitted to a qualified laboratory for rabies examination. Any stray domestic dog or cat that bites a person should be killed immediately and its head submitted for examination.

Signs of rabies in wild animals cannot be reliably interpreted; therefore any wild animal that bites or scratches a person should be killed if possible and submitted for examination. If fluorescent antibody examination of the brain tissue of any animal (domestic or wild) is shown to be negative for rabies, the injured person does not need to be treated.

Postexposure Prophylaxis. Immediate and thorough washing with soap and water of all bite and nonbite wounds is as important to the prevention of rabies as is immunization. The decision to administer rabies prophylaxis should never be taken lightly, because it requires multiple injections, considerable expense, and some risk of side effects. (See Table 17-5 for postexposure antirabies treatment guidelines.) Rabies prophylaxis should always include HDCV and RIG.

RIG is given only once—at the beginning of treatment. The dose is 20 IU/kg. If possible, half the dose should be infiltrated around the site of exposure and the rest given intramuscularly. Next, five 1 ml doses of HDCV are given intramuscularly on days 1, 3, 7, 14, and 28. A serum specimen for rabies antibody testing should be collected 2 to 3 weeks after the last injection. Testing for rabies antibodies can be arranged through a state health department laboratory. If antibody response is not confirmed, the patient should receive a booster dose of the vaccine.

Adverse Reactions. Approximately 25% of persons receiving HDCV report local reactions, such as pain or swelling at the site of injection. Mild systemic reactions, such as headache, dizziness, and muscle aches, occur in 20% of recipients. The occurrence of these mild adverse reactions should not result in discontinuing rabies prophylaxis, because the reactions usually can be managed with aspirin or other antiinflammatory agents.

Table 17-5 *Postexposure Antirabies Treatment Guide**

SPECIES OF ANIMAL	CONDITION OF ANIMAL AT TIME OF ATTACK	TREATMENT OF EXPOSED HUMAN
Wild skunk, fox, coyote, raccoon, and bat	Regard as rabid	RIG§ and HDCV#†
Domestic dog and cat	Healthy	None‡
	Unknown (escaped)	Call public health official
	Rabid or suspected to be rabid	RIG and HDCV‡
Other	Consider individually	

Modified from Report of the Committee on Infectious Disease: Red book, ed 19, Evanston, Ill, 1982, American Academy of Pediatrics, p. 213.
*These recommendations are only a guide. They should be applied in conjunction with knowledge of the animal species involved, circumstances of the bite or other exposure, vaccination status of the animal, and presence of rabies in the region.
†Discontinue vaccine if fluorescent antibody tests of animal killed at time of attack show negative results.
‡Begin RIG and HDCV at first sign of rabies in biting dog or cat during holding period (10 days).
§Human rabies immune globulin
#Human diploid cell (rabies) vaccine

Efficacy. This regimen has been used in more than 150 persons who were bitten by animals known to be rabid. There were no resultant cases of rabies.

Smallpox Immunization

There has been no case of smallpox in the United States since 1947. The last community-acquired cases of smallpox in the world were in the fall of 1979. Consequently, the risk of complications from the vaccinia vaccine far outweighs any risk of acquiring smallpox. Therefore routine smallpox immunization no longer is recommended. Vaccination is now indicated only for those laboratory workers directly involved with smallpox or closely related viruses. Vaccination is not indicated for international travel.

Pneumococcal Vaccination

Virulent strains of *Streptococcus pneumoniae* are a major cause of morbidity and mortality in the very young, elderly persons, and certain patients with deficiencies of host defense. Several controlled trials over three decades have demonstrated that polyvalent pneumococcal vaccines can significantly reduce the incidence and mortality of pneumococcal disease caused by those specific strains that were incorporated in the vaccine. Within the first 2 years of life otitis media caused by pneumococci develops in about 20% of all children; 50% of the cases of pneumococcal meningitis occur in young children. However, this major pediatric target population, unfortunately, does not respond to pneumococcal vaccination with protective antibody titers. The recent highly successful development of *H. influenzae* type B polysaccharide/protein conjugate, which is immunogenic in young children, provides encouragement that similar techniques can be applied to pneumococcal vaccines.

Vaccine. The current vaccine is polyvalent and contains the polysaccharides of 23 common pneumococcal strains, which account for 85% of the *S. pneumoniae* isolates. Each 0.5 ml dose of vaccine contains 25 mg of purified polysaccharide from each of the 23 strains.

Administration. The vaccine (0.5 ml) should be given intramuscularly or subcutaneously in the thigh or deltoid muscle. Intradermal injections have been associated with severe local reactions.

Adverse Reactions. Local erythema and mild soreness occur in approximately 50% of vaccinees. Severe adverse reactions have been quite rare. When adults have been given a second immunization, more severe local and systemic reactions have been common. Therefore booster doses or repeat immunizations are contraindicated in adults. The safety of second doses in children has not been determined.

Efficacy. In persons older than 2 years, there is about an 80% reduction in type-specific pneumococcal diseases after immunization. This reduction includes pneumococcal bacteremia, pneumonia, and otitis media.

Target Population. The vaccine is recommended for all persons older than 50 years of age. Younger persons with increased risk of pneumococcal disease and death also should be immunized, for example, those persons with congenital and traumatic asplenia, sickle cell disease, nephrotic syndrome, or other immunodeficiency syndromes. Patients with Hodgkin disease should be immunized before beginning therapy. It is recommended that pneumococcal vaccine be given *in addition to* penicillin prophylaxis in those patients for whom a valid indication for chronic penicillin prophylaxis exists.

Haemophilus Influenzae Type b Immunization

H. influenzae type b meningitis occurs in 15,000 to 20,000 children per year in the United States, making it a leading cause of acquired mental retardation. These risks are coupled with many other serious infections such as epiglottitis, pericarditis, pneumonia, orbital cellulitis, and bone and joint infection. More than 75% of these infections occur in children younger than age 2 years.

In the late 1980s, several vaccines were developed that linked *H. influenzae* type b polyribose ribosyl phosphate (PRP) to various protein antigens such as diphtheria toxoid (PRP-D), tetanus toxoid (PRP-T), and outer membrane protein complex (PRP-OMPC) of *Neisseria meningitidis*. Another vaccine with exciting potential was produced with *H. influenzae* type b oligosaccharide conjugated to cross-reacting material (^{197}CRM or HbOC, a nontoxic mutant diptheria toxin.)

Three of these conjugate vaccines have induced excellent anti-PRP titers in young infants. Moreover, small trials indicate that these conjugate vaccines are effective in preventing *H. influenzae* disease in infants 6 months old or younger. On October 4, 1990, the Food and Drug Administration (FDA) approved the use of the HbOC (Lederle-Praxis Biologicals' Hibtiter[R]) vaccine for administration to infants beginning at 2 months of age. Prior to this, Hibtiter[R] and two other licensed Hib protein-conjugate vaccines, PRP-D (Connaught Laboratories' Pro Hibit[R]) and PRP-OMPC (Merck, Sharp, and Dohme Laboratories' Pedvax HIB[TM]) had been approved for infants ages 15 months and older. The approval of a vaccine for use beginning at 2 months of age is important because the peak incidence of Hib infections occurs between 6 and 12 months of age, with more than 5,000 cases reported in this age group annually. Equally important, earlier immunization is more effective in preventing Hib infections in older infants and children. Overall, one of every 200 children in the United States suffers a Hib infection before age 5.

It is estimated that each year 800 of these infants and children die and another 3,500 suffer neurological sequelae, including paralysis, blindness, hearing loss, mental retardation, and speech and learning problems. The overall costs of Hib infections amount to $2.5 billion annually.

The Kaiser Permanente Vaccine Study Center reported to the FDA that 98% of infants who received Hibtiter[R] at 2, 4, and 6 months of age had protective Hib antibody titers (≥ 1 μg/mL) approximately 1 month after receiving the third dose and that the efficacy of the vaccine between the second and third doses was 100%.[1]

The American Academy of Pediatrics' Committee on Infectious Diseases responded to the FDA licensing of Hibtiter[R] with the recommendations for immunizing infants and children shown in tables 17-1 and 17-2.

Side Effects. Approximately half the vaccinees have mild fever and mild local reaction at the vaccination site. Significant fever occurs in only 1% of the vaccinees. When this vaccine has been given simultaneously with DTP, the incidence of reactions is no greater than with DTP alone.

Meningococcal Vaccine

Meningitis and bacteremia caused by *N. meningitidis* continue to result in significant morbidity and mortality in children. The secondary attack rate among household contacts is about 0.3%. However, in epidemics the secondary attack rate among household contacts can increase at least tenfold (3% to 10%); these epidemics have dictated the need for an effective vaccine. Purified polysaccharide vaccines to serotypes A, B, and C have been tested. The A and C vaccines are safe and effective, but the type B vaccine is a weak antigen that results in poor antibody responses. This has particular significance in that, during the past decade, most meningococcal disease in the United States has been caused by group B strains.

Vaccine. Four vaccine preparations currently are available. These include monovalent group A and group C vaccines, a divalent vaccine that contains both group A and group C polysaccharides, and a four-valence vaccine that includes group A, group C, group Y, and group W135 polysaccharides.

Efficacy. Under epidemic conditions the group A vaccine has been effective in children older than 6 months of age. In epidemic conditions the group C vaccine was highly effective in children older than age 2 years but less protective for younger children. In its failure to protect very young children, the group C vaccine is thus similar to pneumococcal vaccine and *H. influenzae* type B vaccine.

Target Population. Meningococcal vaccine currently is recommended for use in epidemic outbreaks of group A or group C disease. Clearly, persons should be immunized when they travel to a city or country in which an epidemic is ongoing. Local epidemics should be defined in conjunction with state health departments and the CDC before large-scale vaccination is implemented.

Vaccination should be considered for household contacts, day care center contacts, and selected hospital contacts when the index case in found to be infected with a group A or group C strain of *N. meningitidis*.

Varicella Vaccination

Varicella (chickenpox) generally is a self-limited infection with only moderate morbidity and infrequent long-term sequelae among healthy persons. However, recent advances in intensive care and in cancer chemotherapy have resulted in a much larger number of immunocompromised children who are at risk for serious disease and death from varicella infection. The additions of Reye syndrome and neonatal varicella to the list of established varicella complications have sparked interest in the development of appropriate vaccines.

Vaccine. The *OKA and KMcC strains have both been tested and found safe and immunogenic in children.* Moreover, significant antibody titers have persisted for more than 5 years, and the vaccinated children have been protected when exposed to active chickenpox.

Administration and Target Population. Specific recommendations regarding the use of these vaccines have not yet been developed by the Immunization Practice Committees of either the CDC or the American Academy of Pediatrics. However, specific groups of children will surely benefit in the near future from the selective use of these vaccines.

Tuberculosis Vaccination

Tuberculosis continues to decline in the United States. Recently, the prevalence of children entering school with positive reactions to purified protein derivative (PPD) was less than 0.2%. Therefore the strategy for control of tuberculosis in the United States has been to identify and treat the cases and to follow up their contacts with close surveillance. Vaccination has been reserved only for selected groups.

Vaccine. Bacille Calmette-Guérin (BCG) is an attenuated strain of *Mycobacterium bovis*. All current vaccines are derived from the original strain.

Administration. BCG is given intradermally. Newborn infants receive 0.05 ml, whereas older infants and children receive 0.1 ml. The vaccine should be given 2 to 3 months before the anticipated exposure, and the tuberculin skin test is repeated 2 to 3 months after the vaccination. If the skin test shows a negative reaction, the BCG vaccination should be repeated.

Efficacy. *BCG has been shown to be effective in preventing clinical tuberculosis among selected infants at great risk for becoming infected with the tubercle bacillus.* It also is protective in those developing countries in which tuberculosis is still prevalent.

Target Population. Infants born to mothers with active (sputum-positive) tuberculosis are at significant risk for the development of disseminated tuberculosis. BCG should be given to any such infant, who should be separated from the mother until she has had adequate treatment. A diligent effort should be made to identify any other infected persons in the infant's environment so that they also may be "separated" and treated. The vaccinated infant should remain separated from any infected person until the patient's sputum is negative for the tubercle bacillus or until the infant's tuberculin skin test (PPD) shows an antibody response.

Persons whose PPD test results are negative and who are likely to enter areas where they will have repeated exposure to untreated tuberculosis are candidates for BCG vaccine. Such persons would include Peace Corps families, some military families, some missionary families, and health care professionals in selected sites of the world.

Contraindications. BCG should not be given to persons using isoniazid because this antibiotic prevents vaccine replication and thus inhibits immunization. BCG should not be given to immunocompromised persons. Pregnancy, burns, and skin infections also are specific contraindications to BCG immunization.

The duration of tuberculin skin test positivity after BCG vaccination is unknown. Consequently, a positive reaction to PPD after BCG vaccination may be confusing. If a BCG-vaccinated person has a large skin reaction that is compatible with tuberculosis exposure it should be interpreted as being disease related and should not be attributed to the BCG vaccination.

Typhoid Vaccination

The remarkable decline in the incidence of typhoid fever in the United States is the result of general public health measures such as good plumbing and is not attributable to the typhoid vaccine.

Vaccine. Killed typhoid vaccines result in significant antibody titers in 70% to 80% of immunized persons. These antibody titers are protective against a small inoculum of *Salmonella typhi,* but a large inoculum can easily overcome the resistance of immunized persons. Moreover, the vaccines regularly produce local pain, regional adenopathy, and systemic reactions of significant fever and malaise.

Target Population. *Because of its limited protection and frequent untoward side effects, typhoid vaccine is rarely recommended.* It may be used in community or institutional outbreaks of typhoid fever and in persons with intimate exposure to typhoid carriers.

Cholera Vaccination

The risk of cholera to persons who travel to endemic areas is small. Even so, the best protection is in avoiding any potentially contaminated water or foods, the *currently available vaccines are not very effective.*

Target Population. The vaccine is recommended only for those persons who are required to show evidence of cholera vaccination to gain entrance to a specific country. A single primary immunization (0.2 ml for children ages 1 to 5 years, 0.3 ml for those ages 5 to 10 years, and 0.5 ml for those older than 10 years) is sufficient to satisfy regulations.

REFERENCES

1. Centers for Disease Control: Inactivated hepatitis B virus vaccine, MMWR 31:317, 1982.
2. Hinmann AR and Koplan JP: Pertussis and pertussis vaccine—reanalysis of benefits, risks, and costs, JAMA 251:3109, 1984.
3. Mann JM, Kane MA, and Hull HF: Hepatitis B, hepatitis B vaccine, and education for the handicapped, Pediatr Infect Dis 2:273, 1983.

SUGGESTED READINGS

Current status of *Haemophilus influenzae* type b vaccines, Pediatrics 85 (suppl): 631, 1990.

Madore DV et al: Safety and immunologic response to *Haemophilus influenzae* type b oligosaccharide–CRM_{197}, conjugate vaccine in 1 to 6 month old infants, Pediatrics 85:331, 1990.

18

Screening

One

General Considerations

William K. Frankenburg
Susan M. Thornton

During the past decade, health providers have witnessed a vast increase in the list of conditions for which screening is recommended or even mandated. In some cases large-scale screening programs have been undertaken without preliminary consideration of the ethical issues involved. Such hasty programming all too often has resulted in inaccurate findings, expensive duplication, omission of services, and in some cases even harm to the public at large. If certain principles in screening had been considered before the implementation of such screening programs, these problems could have been avoided. Thirteen principles are briefly presented here to assist the health provider in making decisions about what to screen for, whom to screen, when to screen, how to screen, and which screening tests to use.

1. *Screen only for conditions that can be diagnosed with certainty.* If you cannot diagnose a condition with certainty after evaluation by the best-trained experts using the most sophisticated procedures, do not attempt to screen for it with simple procedures in the hands of less-trained personnel. One condition that sometimes presents difficulty in diagnosis is child abuse. In some cases it is exceedingly difficult for diagnosticians to achieve unanimity about whether trauma suffered by a child is due to willful abuse or an accident. At this time screening procedures to predict child abuse are being developed.

2. *Obtain parental consent before screening children.* Too often, children have been subjected to screening procedures without prior parental approval. This practice is common among neonatal screening procedures such as those designed to detect phenylketonuria (PKU) and congenital hearing losses. Parents whose children have initial positive screening findings are urged to have their children evaluated further.

When prior consent has not been obtained and the parents have not been informed about the screening programs, the parents often become alarmed when asked to have their children so evaluated. In view of the potential false-positive and false-negative findings, the often unfruitful but expensive follow-up work that must be borne by the parents, and the undue anxiety, one must condemn screening without prior parental approval. Such approval is particularly important in regard to screening for genetic disorders such as Tay-Sachs disease and sickle cell disease, inasmuch as the findings may be stigmatizing. Screening without parental approval may be interpreted as an invasion of privacy.

3. *Screen only for conditions that will benefit from early diagnosis and treatment.* If such benefits are not realized, one must question the value of the screening effort. Juvenile diabetes mellitus and cystic fibrosis are examples. As yet there is no consensus that early diagnosis and treatment of these disorders alter their morbidity. If this is true, how can one justify screening the general population for these conditions?

4. *Use only screening tests and procedures that are known to be highly accurate.* Although rigorous standards of accuracy are required for routine laboratory determinations, such standards often are overlooked in behavioral screening procedures such as those employed to detect developmental, speech and language, and school learning disorders. Sometimes screeners administer only a few test items of their own choosing or develop their own methods of scoring, and then they are inappropriately critical of the test for yielding inaccurate results. Failure to administer and score a test correctly yields only the tester's subjective opinion.

5. *Begin screening only after the staff has become highly proficient in test administration and interpretation.* In the hands of improperly trained personnel, even the most accurate test will yield inaccurate results.

6. *Be certain that positive screening findings are followed by appropriate diagnostic evaluations and treatment.* One of the major criticisms of the Early Periodic Screening, Diagnosis and Treatment (EPSDT) component of Medicaid has been the failure to ensure that all children with suspect screening findings receive appropriate diagnostic and treatment services. Screening without concomitant diagnosis and treatment is not likely to benefit the patient.

7. *Develop procedures to protect the confidentiality of screening results.* One of the criticisms leveled against the screening for sickle cell anemia is that there has been a failure to protect the confidentiality of screening findings. Therefore it is possible for insurance companies and potential employers who learn of screening results to discriminate against a person found to have sickle cell disease.

8. *Monitor the screening to ensure that each of the previously mentioned safeguards is maintained.* For instance, there is a continuous need to monitor screening procedures for accuracy. Over time even well-trained screeners may become careless or begin taking shortcuts. Thus it is necessary for program administrators to monitor screening carefully, including periodic observation of screeners' procedures and evaluation of the rate of false-positive and false-negative results.

9. *Take steps to avoid a potential conflict of interest when large-scale screening is undertaken outside the offices of the primary health care provider.* This situation has occurred more than once when civic-minded persons have offered to provide not only screening but also follow-up diagnosis and treatment. Thus cost in these cases is not a factor, which sometimes results in overreferrals for diagnostic and treatment procedures. The result is that the patient is treated unnecessarily. Such excessive treatment is unethical, expensive, and in some cases even dangerous.

10. *In the selection of a screening test, ensure—whether practitioner or program director—that the test is designed to measure what is being screened for.* For example, the Denver Developmental Screening Test (DDST) was criticized in one study for failure to identify children with articulation errors and problems in syntax—even though the test was not designed to measure either. In screening for anemia one would not use a test designed to screen for PKU; similar care should be taken in the selection of an appropriate developmental screening test.

11. *Do not attempt to predict later developmental status from a developmental screening test.* A common mistake is assuming that a developmental screening test identifies all children who later will be "normal" and all those who later will have delays in development. The professional should be aware that a developmental screening test evaluates the child's development only at the current time. For one thing, it is far more difficult to determine the intactness of complex developmental functions in a young child than in a child of school age. For another, attempting to predict later normal development on the basis of the results of a development screen is perilous because many environmental and medical factors may subsequently intervene to cause developmental problems. (Conversely, however, if a child has major developmental delays early in life, prediction of later problems can be made with a somewhat greater degree of confidence.)

12. *Ensure that the screening test is valid for the population to be screened.* If, for example, a program is being designed to screen the general population of children for possible delays in development, the screening test should have been validated by use of children drawn from the general population. In the past, some test developers used an aberrant "convenience sample" of children (e.g., children referred for evaluation of possible developmental problems) and then erroneously claimed very high rates of accuracy in identifying children with delays in the population at large. Thus it is important for the professional to examine the evaluation sample on which a test's claims for validity are based.

13. *Weigh the overall cost of the screening, diagnosis, and treatment against the human and financial costs of detecting the disease at a later stage.* In weighing the pros and cons of screening for each condition, one must consider the following points.

The benefit of early detection and treatment will depend on the natural course of the disease and the stage in that process when treatment is begun. For conditions that progress relatively rapidly from onset through the critical period for treatment, the maximum benefit from early treatment may be achieved only during a short period. For example, if brain damage and neurologic impairment are to be avoided in PKU, most children with this condition will require initial treatment during the first month of life. Treatment begun after this time generally is less beneficial.

The benefit of correct identification of disease-free children may be permanent, as in screening for genetic disorders such as sickle cell disease; however, there may be less benefit in screening for conditions that may not begin until a later age. For instance, a child screened for the presence of tuberculosis or hearing loss will require later rescreening, even though the initial findings were negative.

The cost or implication of a false-positive result also depends on the particular disease. The factors to be considered are undue parental anxiety, the resources available to perform the follow-up work, and the monetary cost of the follow-up work. If only limited resources are available and the cost is high, few false-positive results can be tolerated.

The cost of a false-negative result, once again, depends on the disease in question. For conditions with no one critical time after which treatment is less effective, a false-negative result is not so costly, because the condition may be detected through rescreening at a later stage in the disease process. Examples of such conditions are developmental problems and refractive errors.

By assigning a relative value to each of these conditions (true positive, true negative, false positive, false negative) and knowing the sensitivity and specificity* of the procedure for a given population, one can determine the relative value of the screening process. This relative value can subsequently be compared (a) for various times (or ages) at which a given screening procedure is performed, (b) for different screening procedures, and (c) for different diseases. Through such comparisons, one can determine the timing and method that yield the highest cost/benefit ratio.

• • •

In weighing the ethics of clinical investigation, Illingworth[1] suggested that three questions be asked: (1) What good may it do? (2) What harm may be done by not doing it? and (3) What harm may it do? These questions also can be applied to the question of screening.

**Sensitivity* is defined as the ability of a procedure to identify correctly *all* those who have the disease. *Specificity* is defined as the ability of a procedure to correctly identify all those free of the disease in question.

Two
The Physical Examination as a Screening Test

Robert A. Hoekelman

The physical examination is a composite of individual screening tests that assess the structure and, in part, the function of the human body. It includes a series of specific measurements, as well as many objective observations, that the examiner makes by using the senses of sight, smell, hearing, touch, and occasionally taste. Judgments as to the normality or abnormality of these measurements and observations are then made on the basis of predetermined standards. The methodology for conducting the physical examination and some of the standards of normality are discussed in Chapter 7.

When performed on a healthy child as part of a well visit, the physical examination is more of a screening test than it is when it is performed as one aspect of the evaluation of a specific complaint. The physical examination is an extremely sensitive and specific screening test for some conditions (e.g., strabismus, umbilical hernia, and dental caries), but not for most others. The yield from all or parts of the physical examination varies with the prevalence of abnormal conditions in the population screened. Thus, for infants and children, tonometric and proctoscopic examinations are not performed except under unusual circumstances, whereas auscultation of the heart and lungs and otoscopic examination are performed routinely.

In the screening of healthy children, certain parts of the physical examination ordinarily need to be performed only once to determine the presence or absence of a specific condition (e.g., undescended testicle, choanal atresia, or color blindness). Once height, weight, head circumference, and blood pressure have been initially determined to be in the normal range for the infant's or child's age, they are highly unlikely to become abnormal without specific signs or symptoms that bring the child to the physician's attention.

Other procedures, however, require repeated performance inasmuch as illnesses are acquired and many congenital or genetically determined conditions may not be evident on examinations performed early in life (e.g., pyloric stenosis, scoliosis, patent ductus arteriosus, and Marfan syndrome). Indeed, a normal finding may be only an assurance of normality for very brief periods (e.g., absence of an abdominal mass, presence of normal mobility of the tympanic membrane, or normal skin turgor).

There is a yield from the physical examination beyond the determination of normality or abnormality. Certain benefits accrue "a laying on of hands" in terms of strengthening the physician-patient-parent relationship. The thoroughness, deftness, gentleness, and consideration shown to the patient by the physician in conducting the examination can be as reassuring as the results of the examination itself.

Pronouncement by the physician that the examination results show no negative findings and the child is normal may lead the parents to sense that all is well even though many aspects of health and normality have not been confirmed simply by the child's "passing" a physical examination. Periodic examinations also may lead the parents to cease using their own powers of observation and judgment regarding their children's health and often to delay seeking care for observed deviations from normal because the examination is scheduled for performance in the near future.

On the other hand, parents may misinterpret the meaning of variations in normal findings discovered in the routine physical examination (e.g., the innocent heart murmur), which can cause undue alarm and far-reaching consequences.

The actual yield of abnormal findings (not known to be present beforehand) on routine, periodic physical examinations of presumably well children is extremely small (1.5% in infants during their first year,[1] 2.5% in preschool children,[5] and 4% in primary schoolchildren[10] and high school students[9]). Because most of these findings can be detected by other means, periodic, routine physical examinations of well children is considered to be an inefficient use of medical personnel and of little value from a case-finding (screening) point of view.[3,6]

Many of the elements of the physical examination—specifically, determination of height, weight, head circumference, vital signs, and hearing and visual acuity—involve measurements that physicians usually delegate to others. These are apt to yield more in terms of early detection of disease than are the remaining elements of the physical examination. There are, however, specific conditions that at certain ages might go unrecognized by parents or teachers or might remain undiscovered through routine screening measures but that are detectable on the physical examination:

Cataract	Glaucoma
Congenital dislocation of the hip	Lymphadenopathy
Congenital heart disease	Scoliosis
Cryptorchism	Strabismus
Genetic syndromes	Tumors (benign and malignant)

Screening is generally believed to be important in two of these conditions: congenital dislocation of the hip (CDH) during infancy and scoliosis during late childhood and early adolescence.

However, a recent study conducted in Birmingham, England, casts serious doubts on the effectiveness of screening for CDH in terms of reducing the frequency of late discovery and poor outcome of the anomaly; it suggests that the screening tests used (the Barlow and Ortolani maneuvers) and early management of "unstable" hips by holding them in an extended and flexed position may in themselves cause CDH.[7] Studies of ultrasound screening for CDH in newborns with repeat ultrasonographic examination throughout infancy indicate that the Barlow and Ortolani maneuvers can lead to false-negative results and that positive ultrasound results in the neonatal period are not highly predictive of eventual CDH requiring treatment.[2]

Although screening for scoliosis has a low yield—2 in 100 children require follow-up and 2 in 1000 require active treatment[8]—it generally is regarded as a cost-effective screening test despite the large numbers of children who are referred, on the basis of screening, for radiographic assessment and orthopedic consultation. The use of Moiré topography (a photographic technique that defines the body contours) as a secondary screening procedure may reduce the number of these referrals.[4]

In relation to the 10 diagnoses listed above and the amount of medical time spent on the physical examination, we need to ask two questions. First, in which of these 10 conditions will waiting until signs and symptoms of the disease become evident to the parents, with the ensuing delay in making the diagnosis, change the outcome? Second, can those elements of the physical examination that must be performed to detect these conditions be taught adequately to persons other than physicians—that is, in a way that ensures a sufficiently high degree of sensitivity and specificity?

The frequency with which physical examinations for purposes of screening need to be performed in infants and children should reflect the risk of abnormality that each child runs. That risk is determined by a number of variables that must be assessed by the physician. The risk is not the same for all children; therefore the scheduling of physical examinations for the purpose of screening depends on the patient. For the well child at low risk, "screening" physical examinations probably need to be performed only at birth, 1 and 6 months, and 1, 2, 5, 10, and 14 years of age.

Three
Screening for Genetic-Metabolic Disorders

Neil A. Holtzman

In the presence of suspicious clinical findings, simple, rapid, inexpensive tests can help to indicate whether the presence of genetic-metabolic disorders is likely (Table 18-1). The use of such tests in the presence of symptoms is not, however, *screening*. That term is reserved for tests applied to *apparently healthy populations*. Some of the tests used in the diagnosis of symptomatic conditions also are used in screening populations.

The distinction is important because the circumstances under which the test is performed influence the significance of a positive result. In patients with symptoms a positive test result is highly suggestive of disease. More refined tests are needed primarily to pinpoint the diagnosis, but the diagnosis should seldom, if ever, be based on a single test result. In apparently healthy populations the prevalence of disease is low. Consequently the ratio of false-positive to true-positive

Table 18-1 *Readily Available Urine Tests for Genetic-Metabolic Diseases and Indications for Their Use**

TYPE OF COMPOUND DETECTED†	TEST	SOME INDICATIONS
Reducing substances (including glucose, galactose, fructose, lactose)	Clinitest‡ Benedict test Chromatography	1-7§
Keto acids (including acetone and acetoacetic acid [ketone bodies], branched-chain keto acids, other alpha-keto acids)	Acetest‡ (ketone bodies only) Dinitrophenylhydrazine‡ Chromatography	1, 2, 4, 6-8
Methylmalonic acid	Chromatography	1, 7, 9
Some amino acid metabolites (including phenylpyruvic acid, imidazole pyruvic acid, and branched-chain ketoaciduria)	Ferric chloride‡	1, 2, 4, 7-9
Sulfhydryl compounds (including cysteine, homocysteine)	Nitroprusside‡	8, 10-13
Tyrosine and some of its metabolites	Nitrosonaphthol‡	2, 4, 14
Amino acids	Chromatography Electrophoresis	1-14
Mucopolysaccharides	Acid albumin turbidity Cetyltrimethylammonium bromide Toluidine blue	15-19
Oligosaccharides (accumulate in some lysosomal glycoprotein disorders)	Chromatography	8, 15-24
Oxalic acid	Titration of calcium oxalate	10, 25

*Most of the methods can be found in Thomas GH and Howell RR: Selected screening tests for genetic metabolic diseases, Chicago, 1973, Year Book Medical Publishers, Inc. The oligosaccharide method was reported by Humbel R and Collant M: Oligosaccharides in urine of patients with glycoprotein storage diseases, Clin Chim Acta 60:143, 1975. All the tests are performed in the Genetic Laboratory, John F. Kennedy Institute, Johns Hopkins University School of Medicine.
†Compounds other than those that may be elevated in genetic-metabolic diseases also can give positive reactions with some of the tests. They are not shown.
‡Test readily performed by a practitioner.
§*1*, Vomiting, lethargy, poor feeding in early infancy; *2*, jaundice in early infancy; *3*, malabsorption; *4*, unexplained liver disease; *5*, renal tubular dysfunction; *6*, suspicion of diabetes mellitus; *7*, respiratory distress (metabolic acidosis); *8*, mental retardation; *9*, unexplained ketoaciduria; *10*, renal stone or renal colic; *11*, lens dislocation; *12*, vascular thrombosis; *13*, tall stature, long extremities; *14*, vitamin D–resistant rickets; *15*, growth retardation; *16*, skeletal abnormalities; *17*, cloudy cornea; *18*, hepatosplenomegaly; *19*, coarse facies; *20*, seizures; *21*, developmental regression; *22*, loss of vision, *23*, cherry-red macula; *24*, vacuolated lymphocytes; *25*, chronic renal disease.

results will be higher than it is in patients with *clinical* indications of the disease; follow-up studies are almost always necessary to ensure that unaffected individuals will not be mislabeled as affected. Of course false-negative test results can occur both in patients with symptoms and in populations that are screened. Reasons for false-negative results, including sophisticated as well as simple tests, are shown in the box below.

WHY SCREEN?

For some disorders, such as PKU, the initiation of treatment before symptoms appear is the only way that irreversible damage can be prevented. Screening of newborns permits the diagnosis to be made in time for effective treatment.

Infants with other disorders, such as galactosemia and branched-chain ketoaciduria, will show symptoms soon after milk feedings are started. Because of their nonspecific nature—most prominently, vomiting, lethargy, and poor feeding—these symptoms may not lead to prompt clinical diagnosis. Provided that blood specimens are processed rapidly and abnormal results are immediately reported and followed up, routine screening of all newborns for these conditions can accelerate the diagnosis and lead to treatment before death or irreversible damage occurs.

Screening of older persons for genetic susceptibilities may enable some to avoid drugs or foods harmful to them. Screening for carriers of severe autosomal recessive conditions permits parents to avoid the conception or birth of infants with such conditions. Pregnancy screening for some chromosome abnormalities and neural tube defects also allows parents to avoid the birth of affected offspring if they so choose.

ROLE OF PRIMARY CARE PROVIDERS

In some cases the primary health care provider advises patients whether to be screened. In others, he or she does the screening or at least collects the specimen; in still others, he or she is involved in follow-up, treatment, or counseling. Thus some knowledge of the indications for screening, of the interpretation of results, and of subsequent actions to be taken will enhance the provider's contribution to the reduction of morbidity and mortality.

Each of the following sections describes currently available screening procedures. It must be emphasized that the field is changing rapidly and that no textbook can keep the provider abreast of new developments.

NEWBORN PERIOD

Screening tests for PKU, galactosemia, branched-chain ketoaciduria (BCK, or maple syrup urine disease), hypothyroidism, and sickle cell anemia (and other hemoglobinopathies) are performed in many states today. Because states differ in the tests that are required, it is incumbent on health care providers to be familiar with the policies in their own state. Tests for several other disorders are being pilot tested for such conditions as cystic fibrosis, biotinidase deficiency, and congenital adrenal hyperplasia. All these tests can be performed from the few drops of blood obtained from a heel prick and collected on filter paper.

With the less than perfect sensitivity of many screening tests, practitioners should not place undue faith in a negative result. A repeat test, or a more definitive one, should be obtained in infants with suspicious findings. Nor should treatment be started simply on the basis of one positive screening test result. Consultation with someone experienced in the evaluation of metabolic disorders is highly recommended. Not every infant with an abnormal screening test result requires treatment; false-positive reactions and variant abnormalities do occur. When treatment is indicated, the response may vary; careful monitoring and expert evaluation are needed. Furthermore, consultation is reassuring to the family.

Screening for PKU and hypothyroidism is cost effective. The addition of other tests from which infants will benefit usually involves only marginal cost increments. Centraliza-

Some Reasons for False-Negative Test Results

1. Reagents out of date (e.g., Dextrostix, Phenistix)
2. Specimen too old; substance unstable (e.g., only fresh PKU urine gives positive ferric chloride test results; tests for mucopolysaccharides require fresh urine)
3. Ingestion inadequate (e.g., galactosemic patient placed on intravenous fluids before urine specimen for reducing substance obtained)
4. Syndrome intermittent (e.g., variant form of branched-chain ketoaciduria)
5. Newborns
   a. Accumulation of substance inadequate (e.g., screening for homocystinuria and histidinemia in first week of life results in many false negatives)
   b. Deficiency not yet evident (e.g., thyroxine [T_4] may be present in hypothyroid infants in the first few days of life, resulting in false negatives)
   c. Enzyme system immature (e.g., delayed maturation of transaminase results in false negative ferric chloride tests in young infants with PKU)
6. Substances interfere (e.g., purple color from aspirin in ferric chloride test masks presence of other metabolites; phosphates inhibit ferric chloride color)
7. Urine too dilute (e.g., any unsensitive spot test [mucopolysaccharides])
8. Test improperly performed or interpreted
9. Test does not detect variant forms of the disorder

tion of laboratories and more stringent regulations for quality control will reduce laboratory error as well as dollar costs to the patient and will increase cost effectiveness.

When newborn screening for genetic disorders began in the early 1960s, the only way to reduce the risk of giving birth to additional affected children was to forego having any additional children; prenatal diagnosis of genetic disorders had not even been attempted, and abortion was illegal in most states. With the advent of midtrimester amniocentesis in prenatal diagnosis in the late 1960s, only a few single gene disorders could be detected by enzyme assays in cultured amniotic fluid cells. Most of the disorders such as PKU for which newborn screening was possible were not among those that could be detected prenatally. The picture changed with the application of recombinant deoxyribonucleic acid (DNA) technology to the elucidation of genetic disorders. Prenatal diagnosis—with the option of aborting affected fetuses—is now possible for most of the single-gene disorders for which neonatal screening is conducted, including PKU, sickle cell anemia, and cystic fibrosis; theoretically it is possible for all of them. Advances in reproductive technology have provided parents with additional options for avoiding the conception of affected infants. Intrauterine therapy of a few single-gene disorders also is possible. The availability of these options is another justification for identifying couples at risk through newborn screening.

In contrast to newborn screening as a means of identifying couples at risk, carrier screening can do so before a couple has had an affected offspring. For couples who elect not to terminate an affected pregnancy, carrier screening also facilitates the detection and early treatment of affected newborns. For conditions for which extensive carrier screening will be conducted, only the newborns of couples at risk need to be tested.

Phenylketonuria

In the United States most babies are screened for PKU before they leave the nursery. As many as 16% of infants with PKU could be missed by screening on the first day of life. This proportion falls to about 2% on the second day and to 0.3% on the third day. The American Academy of Pediatrics recommends that every infant be screened before discharge from the nursery but that infants initially screened before 24 hours of age should be rescreened before the third week of life. Premature and sick infants should be screened by the seventh day. Assays for blood phenylalanine (fluormetric or bacterial inhibition) are the preferred screening methods. The ferric chloride test, at any age, is less sensitive than are tests for blood phenylalanine, and the latter always should be used in screening symptom-free infants. Because infants with PKU may have only minimal elevations of blood phenylalanine at the time they are screened, the screening detection level must be set low enough (4 mg/dl) so that as many as 10 to 20 normal infants will have positive test results (false positives) for every infant with PKU who has a positive test (true positive) result. Thus no infant should be started on treatment until a confirmatory test has been obtained. Follow-up of positive test results should be performed promptly to permit the initiation of dietary therapy as soon as possible but no later than the third week of life. There is good evidence that intellectual performance correlates with the age at which treatment is started.

In addition to the predominant phenylalanine hydroxylase deficiency, defects in the synthesis or regeneration of biopterin cofactors for the conversion of phenylalanine to tyrosine also result in positive screening test results and clinical disease. Dietary restriction of phenylalanine is insufficient to prevent mental deterioration in these infants, but the use of biopterin compounds or neurotransmitter precursors offers hope of improving the outcome. Infants with these disorders will be discovered by neonatal screening for PKU; they represent fewer than 3% of all infants in whom elevations of phenylalanine persist. Tests for these variant forms should be performed in any infant with persistently elevated blood phenylalanine levels. These biopterin-deficient forms may be present in infants with blood phenylalanine levels in the 10 to 20 mg/dl range who are receiving a normal diet.

Branched-Chain Ketoaciduria and Galactosemia

Infants with either BCK or galactosemia usually show symptoms within 2 weeks of birth. The course can be fulminant and rapidly fatal, but early treatment is often effective. It is not known whether every infant affected with either condition can be identified by screening in the first few days of life. Consequently, if unexplained lethargy, poor feeding, or vomiting develops in infants with negative test results, tests should be repeated and the specimen rapidly processed. Sometimes confirmation of a diagnosis of BCK or galactosemia in these infants can be accelerated by contacting the laboratory responsible for performing newborn screening; a positive result may already have been obtained. Often the laboratory can process the specimen quickly on the basis of a special request.

Hypothyroidism

Screening for hypothyroidism is now widespread in the United States. A low thyroxine (T_4) level as well as an elevated thyroid-stimulating hormone (TSH) level, both of which can be assayed on the drop of blood obtained from the neonate for screening, should be present and confirmed before treatment is started. Most infants who have persistently low T_4 levels, but who have normal TSH levels, will prove on further study to have normal free T_4 concentrations and thyroid-binding globulin deficiency; they do not require treatment. Benign thyroid-binding globulin deficiency is a much more frequent cause of low T_4 and normal TSH levels than is hypothyroidism caused by hypopituitary failure. Occasionally an infant with initial low T_4 and normal TSH levels will have a delayed rise in TSH level and symptoms of hypothyroidism. The TSH value of an infant with an initial low T_4 level and a normal TSH level should be retested if symptoms occur.

The need for long-term thyroid replacement can be assumed if scans or other studies reveal absent or ectopic thyroid or goiter caused by an enzyme defect. In the absence of these findings but when low T_4 and elevated TSH levels indicate the need for early treatment, therapy should be discontinued for 30 days when the child is between 3 and 4 years of age. At that time serum should be obtained for T_4 and TSH assays.

If findings are normal, no further treatment is needed. Such transient cases usually are those in which the TSH level was only moderately elevated (20 to 100 μU/ml).

Sickle Cell Anemia

Because of a randomized controlled trial demonstrating that penicillin prophylaxis reduces the incidence of pneumococcal infections in symptom-free sickle cell anemia, several states have added sickle cell screening to their newborn screening programs. Before screening was initiated, approximately 10% of infants in the United States with sickle cell disease died by 10 years of age. The effectiveness of screening to reduce morbidity and mortality depends on ensuring that infants detected by screening are referred to a continuing source of care from which parents can receive penicillin and learn how to reduce the chance that their children will suffer sickle cell crises. Parents also must administer the penicillin faithfully. As yet there is no specific treatment for sickle cell anemia.

The screening test, hemoglobin electrophoresis, will discover hemoglobinopathies in addition to sickle cell anemia, not all of which will result in symptoms. The test also identifies infants with sickle trait who will remain healthy. However, a couple that delivers an infant with "trait" may be at risk for having an infant with sickle cell anemia if both partners are carriers of the sickle cell gene. A screening program will have 40 times more carriers to notify than parents of infants with sickle cell anemia, raising the costs of the program. The purpose of notifying the parents of a trait would be to determine whether they are at risk for having an affected offspring and, if they are, to offer them prenatal diagnosis and selective abortion of affected fetuses.

Homocystinuria

Some forms of homocystinuria are easily and effectively treated. However, screening tests, which detect elevated blood methionine levels, will not detect all the forms. Moreover, the screening tests are less sensitive in the first few days of life than later. Tests that measure blood or urine homocystine after the first week of life may prove more sensitive than neonatal tests for hypermethioninemia. In view of the rarity of the disorder (1/50,000 to 1/100,000) such testing is hard to justify.

Histidinemia

Many infants with histidinemia are missed by screening in the first week of life. However, it is doubtful that treatment for this condition is necessary; consequently routine screening cannot be justified.

Cystic Fibrosis

Immunoreactive trypsin (IRT) is elevated in the blood of most newborns with cystic fibrosis (CF). Colorado and Wisconsin currently are performing the test. In Wisconsin a long-term randomized controlled trial is being conducted to determine whether neonatal detection improves the health of children with this disorder. There is no treatment yet available that prevents the clinical manifestations, but earlier therapy may ameliorate the condition. Infants with meconium ileus often have false-negative IRT results, as may 3% to 10% of other infants with the disorder. Approximately 1 in 300 infants without CF will have false-positive IRT results.

Congenital Adrenal Hyperplasia

In 21-hydroxylase deficiency, which accounts for more than 90% of those with congenital adrenal hyperplasia (CAH), cortisol production is impaired. The disorder has an incidence of about 1 in 12,000. As a result of the deficiency, feedback inhibition of adrenocorticotropic hormone (ACTH) is lacking, and cortisol precursors, including those with androgenic activity, are overproduced. 17-Hydroxyprogesterone (17-OHP) is increased in the blood and is the basis of the screening test, which currently is performed on the PKU blood spot in the state of Washington. In girls, ambiguous genitalia should permit clinical diagnosis in the neonatal period, obviating the need for screening. Because the diagnosis is not always made, screening would lead to prompt recognition of the infant who could be more readily raised as a female. More than 50% of infants with 21-hydroxylase deficiency are salt "losers"; they may suffer severe dehydration and vascular collapse accompanied by hyponatremia during the first 2 weeks after birth. By establishing the diagnosis and leading to prompt mineralocorticoid therapy, screening could prevent these sometimes fatal episodes. Salt-losing crises, however, often can occur before the results of screening are known. The common practice of collecting serum electrolytes helps establish a clinical diagnosis. In the absence of salt loss, boys with CAH are difficult to diagnose in the neonatal period. Screening offers an advantage to them; steroid therapy will prevent virilization, rapid early growth, and premature closure of the epiphyses with resultant short adult stature. At the present time the sensitivity of screening is estimated at more than 95%. False-positive test results occur in approximately 0.2% of full-term infants but in a much higher percentage of very low–birth-weight infants.

Symptom-free adults with genetic variant forms of 21-hydroxylase deficiency have been identified. The possibility arises therefore that clinical problems will not develop in all symptom-free infants with confirmed deficiency and unambiguous genitalia.

Biotinidase Deficiency

Biotin is a cofactor of a number of carboxylases. Its availability through recycling is reduced in inherited deficiencies of biotinidase. Pilot screening indicates the incidence of this disorder to average about 1 in 70,000, making it one of the most rare disorders for which screening is available. At least nine states are screening for biotinidase deficiency.

The manifestations and age of onset of biotinidase deficiency vary, possibly because of differences in the completeness of the deficiency and the amount of biotin available to the infant. In reported cases, first symptoms have occurred between 2 weeks and 3 years. Ataxia, alopecia, hearing loss, decreased vision, optic atrophy, and seizures have been observed. It is not yet known whether the infants with the disorder could remain free of symptoms or how many of the infants detected so far would develop symptoms if left untreated. The treatment—providing supplemental biotin—is simple and inexpensive. Although biotin reverses some of the symptoms after they appear, this is not always true for the hearing and visual impairments and developmental delay. Moreover, it is by no means clear that clinical diagnosis always will be made promptly. Infants treated as a result of screening have so far remained symptom-free.

Tyrosinemia

Familial tyrosinemia and tyrosinosis are rare disorders in the United States. (Tyrosinosis has a high incidence in the Chicoutimi–Lac St. Jean region of Quebec because of mutation many generations ago in a relatively closed population.) Approximately 1% of all newborns have transient tyrosine elevations. Thus the ratio of false-positive to true-positive reactions is very high, which means that the cost of follow-up to identify one case of the inherited disorder also is very high. Prematurity, high-protein feedings, and lack of vitamin C contribute to the transient elevations. Impairments revealed by psychological testing have been reported in some children with transient neonatal tyrosinemia. In view of its high frequency and the ease of lowering serum tyrosine levels by moderate protein intakes and vitamin C, routine use of this regimen in newborns, which is now widespread, seems more appropriate than screening.

The determination of tyrosine levels from specimens in which the phenylalanine levels are elevated could be useful in establishing priorities for follow-up; infants with only phenylalanine elevation should be reevaluated before those in whom both amino acids are elevated.

POSTNEONATAL PERIOD

Although screening for aminoacidurias and methylmalonic aciduria (MMA) on urine specimens collected on filter paper and mailed by parents to a central laboratory is feasible, it is not widely employed. Not all forms of MMA or the aminoacidurias discovered by urine testing are treatable.

Screening for genetically determined drug sensitivities in infancy or childhood would enable parents and health providers to avoid the administration of harmful medicines. Approximately 10% of American black males have glucose 6-phosphate dehydrogenase deficiency and are predisposed to hemolytic anemia from a variety of drugs administered anytime in life.

LATE CHILDHOOD AND ADOLESCENCE

Hypercholesterolemia

Screening all children for hypercholesterolemia is controversial. Premature coronary artery disease (CAD) develops in fewer than one third of middle aged men with serum cholesterol values in the highest quintile. There is no evidence to suggest that the proportion would be higher in children with elevated cholesterol levels. Nor is there yet definitive evidence that dietary changes designed to lower cholesterol levels will be effective in preventing or delaying CAD when these changes are started in childhood. The poor reliability of cholesterol testing, particularly those results obtained in the laboratories of physicians' offices, as well as the lack of validity of a single cholesterol determination is reason to oppose routine cholesterol screening of children. On the other hand, screening may identify children at risk, and the initiation of dietary changes may help lower their risk, but this has not been proved. Even if proof is obtained, many children not at risk will be labeled as being at risk. The consequences of such labeling have not been adequately studied. Labeling can be avoided and a population-wide reduction of CAD still can be accomplished by the adoption of a diet lower in saturated fats and cholesterol by everyone older than 2 years of age. However, severe dietary restrictions of these foods can lead to poor nutrition.

The chance of a false-positive hypercholesterolemia finding is much lower among children who are tested because at least one of their parents has premature CAD. An effective way to screen for CAD—and other diseases as well—is obtaining a complete family history. This procedure can be systematized by the use of a pedigree (family tree) diagram. When the family history shows premature CAD, the children can be tested. Several inherited disorders of lipid metabolism are associated with premature CAD. Measurement of high-density lipoprotein (HDL) and low-density lipoprotein (LDL) cholesterol values should be used to follow up elevations in total cholesterol levels. Tests for LDL receptor defects, which account for about 5% of premature, hyperlipidemic CAD, should soon be available.

Alpha-1-Antitrypsin Deficiency

It may be possible to reduce the occurrence of pulmonary emphysema in children with inherited deficiencies of alpha-1-antitrypsin, which affects about 1 in 2000 individuals. They should not smoke, and they should minimize their contact with respiratory irritants (including tobacco smoke exhaled by others). Although tests suitable for screening are available, screening is not performed in the United States routinely.

CARRIER SCREENING

The identification of a person as a carrier for a gene that is only deleterious when present in a double dose (homozygote) influences decisions that the person makes as an adult, not as a child. Therefore such screening should be delayed until the person being screened can appreciate its significance. Carrier screening programs have been launched for Tay-Sachs disease in Jewish communities, for sickle cell disease in black communities, and for thalassemia in Greek and Italian communities.

School-based screening programs for sickle cell and Tay-Sachs carriers probably reach a much higher proportion of the at-risk population than do community programs or office or clinic screening programs. However, they may lead to the stigmatization of students identified as carriers unless all those being screened understand the reasons for the screening and the significance of the results. As a minimum indication of understanding, *informed* consent should be obtained. In addition, all results must be handled confidentially. Although human genetics deserves greater emphasis in primary and secondary school curricula so that students can better evaluate the need for genetic screening, regular providers of care, such as pediatricians and family physicians, are more appropriate sources of screening than the schools. The problem, then, is to reach the target population.

The extent to which individuals identified through carrier screening programs make decisions that will reduce the incidence of the homozygous condition in the next generation is not yet known. The severity of the condition, the options available—which may include prenatal diagnosis and abortion, artificial insemination, adoption, or the avoidance of reproduction with another carrier—and their acceptability will influence the decisions that are made.

If prenatal diagnosis of a condition is available and abortion of an affected fetus acceptable, there is less reason to offer screening before mating. Couples could be screened before the woman becomes pregnant or even early in pregnancy. (The screening test for Tay-Sachs carriers cannot be used reliably in pregnant women; a more expensive leukocyte assay can be performed, however). If both partners are found to be carriers for an autosomal recessive condition, prenatal diagnosis should be offered.

Carrier screening has resulted in a significant decrease in Tay-Sachs disease in many Jewish communities and in thalassemia in a number of Mediterranean countries. Most couples found to be at risk have elected prenatal diagnosis and abortion of affected fetuses.

With the discovery of the genes for cystic fibrosis, Duchenne muscular dystrophy, and hemophilia, intensive efforts to develop carrier tests may soon bear fruit, permitting population-wide screening of young adults. Although screening in pregnancy would be possible, it would have to be performed early enough to permit prenatal diagnosis.

PREGNANCY

Practitioners who provide care to the young usually do not have primary responsibility for managing pregnancy. However, they often will have prior contact with the mother and the father and can contribute to the parents' understanding of the indications for screening in pregnancy. They also may be contacted by obstetricians to assist in counseling or in anticipation of high-risk newborns.

Until recently, amniocentesis at 15 to 20 weeks was the only means of obtaining fetal cells for prenatal diagnosis. Now, however, chorionic villus sampling at 9 to 12 weeks has been demonstrated to be as effective as amniocentesis in prenatal diagnosis, although it results in a somewhat higher risk of unintended fetal loss. Abortion earlier in pregnancy is safer to the pregnant woman than is midtrimester amniocentesis. Preliminary data suggest that amniocentesis also may be safe and effective when performed between 12 and 14 weeks of gestation.

Neural Tube Defects

Elevation of serum alpha-fetoprotein (AFP) levels in pregnant women between the sixteenth and eighteenth weeks of pregnancy increases the likelihood of a fetus with open spina bifida or with anencephaly. The test is not specific; for every true positive reaction, approximately 30 women without affected fetuses will have false-positive results. In women with confirmed elevations of maternal serum AFP, sonographic examination is needed to determine the accuracy of the gestational age estimate; the normal maternal serum AFP concentration is highly dependent on gestational age. If sonography fails to explain the elevation, amniotic fluid AFP and acetylcholinesterase determinations are needed. This screening approach is widely used in the United Kingdom, where the incidence of neural tube defects is considerably higher than in the United States. At the present time its use in the United States should be limited to well-coordinated programs in which the appropriate follow-up tests and counseling of women with AFP elevations can be ensured.

Screening for neural tube defects is increasing rapidly in the United States. California requires that physicians offer AFP screening to all pregnant women but that informed consent be obtained before the test is performed. California also limits the number of laboratories performing AFP testing and ensures that counseling is available to women with positive AFP test results.

Down Syndrome

Until recently, prenatal diagnosis for Down syndrome (DS) was offered routinely only to pregnant women 35 years and older. The lower incidence in younger women, as well as the risk and costs of obtaining fetal cells on which karyotypes could be performed, made it difficult to justify testing all pregnant women. Nevertheless, most infants with DS are born to women younger than 35 years of age. In recent years an association between low concentrations of AFP in the sera of pregnant women of all ages at 16 to 20 weeks of gestation and DS has become evident. The association is far from perfect; most women with low serum AFP levels will not be carrying affected fetuses, and as many as 75% of women younger than 35 years carrying fetuses with DS will not have low serum AFP levels. Because of the large number of false-positive reactions, amniocentesis to obtain fetal cells for karyotyping is needed in younger women with low AFP levels to make a correct diagnosis of DS. A number of centers are systematically following up women with low AFP levels. The Food and Drug Administration has not approved maternal serum AFP kits for DS screening, and many laboratories may not be qualified to provide the test. The kits currently used have been refined to detect elevations rather than reductions of AFP.

Tay-Sachs Disease, Sickle Cell Disease, and Thalassemia

Prenatal diagnosis by enzyme assay is widely available for Tay-Sachs disease. Restriction enzyme analysis of DNA has been successfully employed for the prenatal diagnosis of sickle cell anemia and many forms of thalassemia. Thus, if prenatal diagnosis and abortion are acceptable options to couples in whom the risk of these disorders is high (because of their ethnic or racial background), they should be offered carrier screening. There is little point in establishing carrier status if the woman is already beyond the sixteenth week of pregnancy, because it is doubtful that prenatal diagnosis could be completed in time to abort an affected fetus. In most matings, carrier testing of either the mother or the father will suffice. The other mate need be tested only when the first is shown to be a carrier.

If prenatal diagnosis of the hemoglobinopathies is not available or is not acceptable to the parents, then knowledge of the mother's carrier status determines whether her newborn will need testing; only infants of mothers who are carriers need to be tested.

Rh Screening

Screening of all pregnant women for Rh-negative genotypes is probably the oldest, most widely accepted genetic screening procedure. With the demonstrated efficacy of anti-Rh immunoglobulin (RhIg) in preventing Rh sensitization, it is imperative that every Rh-negative unsensitized mother who delivers an Rh-positive infant receive RhIg at least once during pregnancy and within 24 hours of delivery. All unsensitized Rh-negative women undergoing amniocentesis or abortion also should receive RhIg.

AVAILABILITY OF SCREENING TESTS

Health departments usually can provide information about newborn screening and hemoglobinopathy screening. Centers that offer a multitude of services for genetic disease and counseling are listed by the March of Dimes. The National Center for Education in Maternal and Child Health publishes a list of centers for metabolic disorders. Community groups for sickle cell anemia, thalassemia, Tay-Sachs disease, and cystic fibrosis often know where screening for these conditions can be obtained. The Alliance of Genetic Support Groups (Washington, D.C.) also can provide information.

FUTURE OF GENETIC SCREENING

With the advent of recombinant DNA technology, it will be possible to screen for genetic predispositions to several common conditions. In addition, carrier tests for other conditions such as cystic fibrosis will be available, offering opportunities for avoiding the birth of affected offspring. Such programs will involve a large proportion of the population and considerable expenditures. If the cost of these screening programs is less than the cost of not screening—that is, of caring for those with conditions that could have been avoided or whose manifestations could have been prevented—resources are more likely to be allocated to the screening programs. To maximize benefits, such programs should reach all those in the target population. It is possible, however, that people will not come to be screened or will not act to prevent the birth of offspring with severe disease. Such responses reduce the cost savings of the program and could lead either to their abandonment or to compulsory participation. Mandatory screening of newborns for PKU might be tolerable (it is already the law in most states), but mandatory sterilization of carriers for certain conditions or abortion of affected fetuses, regardless of the wishes of the parents, surely is not. Increased public understanding and voluntary acceptance of such programs provide safeguards against these and other hazards of genetic screening. Health care providers have a major responsibility to contribute to this educational process.

Four
Tuberculin Skin Testing

Ciro V. Sumaya

The tuberculin test is one of the most valuable procedures available for the control of tuberculosis. It may surprise physicians to learn that veterinarians were the first to use tuberculin testing—for the control of tuberculosis in cattle.

ANTIGENS

Two preparations of tuberculin antigens, old tuberculin (OT) and purified protein derivative (PPD), are extensively used at present. PPD is preferred because its strength is standardized. The addition of antiadsorbent polysorbate 60 (Tween 80) to PPD has provided a more stable preparation, which circumvents the previous problem of antigenic absorption to the glass or plastic vial or syringe. All tuberculins should be kept away from sunlight and should be refrigerated when possible.

Awareness in the late 1970s of the lack of appropriate standardization of several commercially available tuberculin skin tests brought about implementation of more scientific methods to demonstrate the effectiveness of these products in human beings.

The availability of antigens to prototype strains of atypical mycobacteria, groups I through IV, has been curtailed because of problems with specificity and standardization.

TECHNIQUES

Two techniques for tuberculin tests are currently used: the intradermal (Mantoux) and the multiple-puncture (Tine, Heaf, Sterneedle, Mono-Vacc, Aplitest, Sclavotest) methods. The patch test (Vollmer) no longer is recommended. The Mantoux is the most definitive technique, and multiple-puncture methods are useful for survey and screening purposes. If the latter test method elicits positive results, the Mantoux test should be applied for confirmation. Exceptions should be made when there is extensive induration or vesiculation from the multiple-puncture test or when *Mycobacterium tuberculosis* has been recovered from the patient.

DOSES

The standard dose of PPD tuberculin is 5 tuberculin units (TU) in 0.1 ml of solution, commonly called "intermediate-strength" PPD. Other commercially available doses exist, such as 1 TU and 250 TU, but they have limited value. The 1 TU PPD dose may be appropriate in children with hypersensitivity manifestations—such as erythema nodosum and, possibly, pleural effusion—as part of their initial tuberculous presentation. If the 1 TU dose gives a negative result in such patients, one may proceed with 5 TU PPD test. The 250 TU dose, also called "second strength," may be applied to individuals who fail to react to a previous injection of 5 TU; it is known, however, that the 250 TU dose may elicit nonspecific sensitivity to any mycobacterial antigen and has given a negative result even in proved cases of tuberculosis.

INTERPRETATION OF REACTIONS

In interpreting the test, one should consider only induration. Reading of tests by recipients or their parents should be discouraged unless there are overwhelming reasons why a trained person cannot evaluate the test.

Mantoux Method

With the standard test dose applied by the Mantoux method, an induration of 15 mm or more at 48 to 72 hours is considered a positive reaction for children with no known risk factors. This is interpreted as positive for past or present infection with *M. tuberculosis*. A positive result is in itself sufficient justification for chemoprophylaxis in children. When there are clinical symptoms or signs consistent with tuberculosis, a positive reaction strongly supports the diagnosis.

Induration of 10 to 14 mm is interpreted as a positive reaction in children who (1) were born in Asia, Africa, or Latin America (high-prevalence regions), (2) suffer a chronic illness, such as diabetes and Hodgkin disease, that increases susceptibility to tuberculosis, (3) live in institutions or shelters for the homeless, or (4) are intravenous drug abusers.

Induration of 5 to 9 mm constitutes a doubtful reaction. Reactions in this range reflect sensitivity to either atypical mycobacteria or *M. tuberculosis*. A doubtful reaction may signify infection with *M. tuberculosis* in the presence of (1) x-ray evidence of pulmonary tuberculosis, (2) known exposure to a person with active pulmonary tuberculosis, and (3) underlying human immunodeficiency virus infection (see Chapter 178). In selected persons, an intradermal test with an atypical mycobacterial antigen might be performed.

An induration of 0 to 4 mm is a negative reaction. This reflects a lack of tuberculin sensitivity or a low-grade sensitivity that probably is not caused by *M. tuberculosis* infection. Another skin test is not needed unless there is enough clinical or epidemiologic evidence of tuberculosis.

A large erythematous reaction without induration may indicate that the injection was made too deeply. Retesting is then indicated.

Multiple-Puncture Technique

In determining the amount of induration, one should measure the diameter of the largest single reaction. If the reaction consists of discrete papules, the diameters of the separate areas of induration should not be added. Induration of 5 mm or more or vesiculation is considered a positive reaction; induration of 2 to 4 mm, a doubtful reaction; and induration of less than 2 mm, a negative reaction. A positive reaction, or in some cases a doubtful reaction, especially if there is suspicion of tuberculosis, should be confirmed by a Mantoux test. If vesiculation or extensive induration has occurred with the multiple-puncture technique, a subsequent Mantoux test need not be performed to confirm the reaction.

SCREENING

In patients in whom the diagnosis of tuberculosis is considered, or in high-risk populations, the Mantoux test rather than multiple-puncture tests should be applied. Screening procedures such as the multipuncture tests, which apply a less precise amount of tuberculin antigen than is used in the Mantoux procedure, are indicated in other types of populations. Clinicians should be aware that false-negative, as well as false-positive, reactions are much more common with the multipuncture techniques (1% to 11% and 20%, respectively).

As the incidence of tuberculosis declined in the early 1980s, the use of tuberculin skin testing as a screening control measure in children was reevaluated by various national health bodies. Some believed that routine tuberculin testing for schoolchildren, as well as similar programs, should be abandoned if the yield of positive skin reactions reached very low levels, such as less than 1%. Committees within the American Academy of Pediatrics, however, firmly believed that this approach would leave undetected some children, albeit few, with unsuspected infection, who would then be in danger of developing serious illness. The pediatricians pointed out that children with uncomplicated primary tuberculosis rarely have symptoms and can be identified only by means of the tuberculin test.

The Report of the American Academy of Pediatrics' Committee on Infectious Diseases[1] (i.e., the Red Book) currently recommends annual tuberculin testing, preferably by the Mantoux technique, for children at high risk. Those at high risk include American Indian and Alaskan native children; children living in neighborhoods in which the case rate is higher than the national average; children from or whose parents have immigrated from Asia, Africa, the Middle East, Latin America, or the Caribbean; and children in households with one or more cases of tuberculosis.

In low-risk groups, tuberculin testing could be performed at three stages: (1) 12 to 15 months of age, (2) before school entry (4 to 6 years of age); and (3) at adolescence (14 to 16 years of age).

Close surveillance of the prevalence of tuberculosis is important, because increases in disease rates, such as those noted recently—related to the influx of high-risk immigrants and patients with underlying human immunodeficiency virus infections—will alter routine tuberculin skin testing recommendations.

PROBLEMS IN INTERPRETATION

Like any diagnostic test, the result must be considered in context. The antigens used, methods of administration, and condition of the child tested are all of consequence to the reaction. The following discussion considers only the Mantoux test, with PPD tuberculin at a dose of 5 TU and Tween 80 adsorbent added. It is known that lower doses increase the likelihood of false-negative results, and higher doses increase the likelihood of false-positive results. Methods other than Mantoux usually deliver varying doses of tuberculin and thereby cause significant numbers of false reactions.

Most of the usual mistakes with the technique of administering the tuberculin test lead to smaller reactions. Even the antigen with Tween 80 should be used as quickly as possible after being placed in a syringe. This will prevent any adsorption that could still take place. If leakage from the syringe occurs or tuberculin is not injected intradermally but into deeper layers, the test should be repeated in another area. Carelessness in measuring a tuberculin reaction may result in false-negative or false-positive reactions. A caliper is ideal for measuring induration. Tuberculin sensitivity may decrease or disappear temporarily (1) during any severe or febrile illness, measles, or other viral diseases, (2) on administration of live viral vaccines, (3) during overwhelming tuberculosis, or (4) after administration of immunosuppressive drugs. Some investigators have noted that tuberculin sensitivity may decrease or disappear if tuberculosis is treated in its earlier stages.

Tuberculin sensitivity also may wane with age. If tuberculin sensitivity has not been challenged for many years, the PPD test results may become negative or doubtful. The placement of the skin test, however, boosts the individual's immunity, so that a repeat tuberculin skin test soon afterward may show a positive reaction. The booster phenomenon, incorrectly thought to be "conversion," is predominantly a problem in adults older than 55 years of age.

COMMENT

It is apparent that a child-centered program to prevent tuberculosis must include not only the use of tuberculin skin tests but a search for sources of infection among contacts of those children who have primary tuberculosis, a prompt evaluation and preventive treatment for contacts of active cases or other high-risk groups, and adequate follow-up care of adult active cases and their contacts, especially children. (See also Chapter 263.)

Five

Screening for Anemia

Sergio Piomelli

Pediatricians screen for anemia to uncover correctable nutritional anemias such as iron deficiency and to identify other anemias that are genetically determined or secondary to generalized disorders. Detection is only the first step: anemia itself is not a disease but an indication of some underlying disorder; therefore, once anemia is detected, it becomes necessary to search for its cause. For example, iron deficiency may reflect a nutritional defect, but it also can result from bleeding.

In pediatrics the two most common causes of anemia are iron deficiency and thalassemia trait. Both are microcytic anemias identified readily by means of electronic cell counters, which indicate the presence of a low mean corpuscular volume (MCV). It must be noted, in fact, that of all hematologic parameters, the MCV is the one measured with the greatest precision by the electronic counters. Unfortunately, these instruments are not capable of further differentiating thalassemia trait. Therefore, although the electronic counter can diagnose microcytosis accurately, the differentiation between iron deficiency and thalassemia trait must rest on additional evidence. The simplest differentiation is provided by the measurement of erythrocyte porphyrins (EP), whose levels are elevated only in cases of iron deficiency anemia. It must be noted that measurement of both hemoglobin and EP from samples collected on filter paper provides at the same time a diagnosis of anemia and a differential diagnosis of iron deficiency at little cost.

Children should be screened for anemia at 6 months of age, when the majority of congenital anemias become apparent, and then again at 12 to 18 months, the period in life when the possibility of iron deficiency is high. For children who have been tested and whose results are normal at 18 months of age, later screening is unnecessary until adolescence, when there is an increased incidence of iron deficiency anemia.

Three techniques are available to screen for anemia: (1) measurement of microhematocrit, (2) measurement of hemoglobin, and (3) measurement of multiple hematologic parameters with an electronic counter.

The microhematocrit is by far the simplest, cheapest, and most reliable measure. The blood is collected by finger puncture in a small capillary tube; this is sealed with modeling clay and centrifuged for 4 minutes in a special, relatively inexpensive, small centrifuge. The microhematocrit is almost a foolproof technique, with essentially no source of error, if care is taken to collect free-flowing blood from the puncture. The only negative aspect of the method is that the centrifuge is quite noisy, a problem in a small office.

Measurement of hemoglobin provides the most physiologically relevant measure of anemia. Although theoretically a fairly simple test, this is, in practice, subject to several sources of error and therefore may be quite unreliable. The measurement of hemoglobin is more expensive than that of the microhematocrit, because it requires more expensive capillary pipettes, standards, and a photometer. Yet this technique is more commonly used in the physician's office because of its apparent (but deceiving) simplicity and, in part, because of tradition. A technique has been developed for collecting samples for hemoglobin measurement on filter paper; the paper is then mailed to a central laboratory, where the measurement is obtained under more controlled and accurate conditions. This technique can be most effective in large-scale screening because it allows samples to be collected by completely untrained personnel. It also can be combined with measurement of EP for lead poisoning screening and can be conveniently used in the physician's office.

Electronic counters are among the latest products of automated technology. These instruments are expensive and impressive with their many dials and flickering lights. They are fast and analyze several hematologic parameters simultaneously. The results they provide, however, are less accurate than their complex and sophisticated appearance would lead one to expect. As their name indicates, these instruments are cell counters. Of all the parameters that they provide, only the numbers of red and white cells, the MCV, and the hemoglobin concentration actually are measured; all others are derived indirectly by computation, with formulas that are not precise for extreme values. Moreover, because all measurements are obtained from a single initial dilution, any error will be reflected equally in all parameters. For these reasons it is good practice at least to check the hematocrit manually on a separate sample, particularly when, as in pediatrics, the initial dilution has been obtained by finger puncture. The cost/benefit ratio of electronic counters is high because of their enormous initial cost and their expensive reagents. Very few pathologists, however, even in small hospitals, can resist the temptation to purchase at least one of these instruments. When an electronic counter is available, it can be advantageous because it not only identifies an anemia but also provides some clues to its type and nature.

When anemia is detected, it becomes necessary to clarify its cause. When anemia is minimal and due to genetic problems, such as in the case of thalassemia trait, reassurance and counseling are all that is needed. On the other hand, iron deficiency anemia, even if modest, should be carefully investigated, because it may reflect other more complex problems, such as gastrointestinal bleeding and/or parasites. As already mentioned, in cases of microcytic anemias it is important to differentiate iron deficiency from thalassemia, but it is also important to remember that these conditions can coexist.

Six

Screening for Lead Poisoning

Sergio Piomelli

The clinical symptoms of lead (Pb) poisoning in children may be vague and ill defined until frank neurologic disturbances develop. Neurologic toxicity may not be preceded by any premonitory signs; however, once neurologic damage occurs, it often is irreversible, and permanent sequelae may remain even after adequate prolonged therapy. Subtle neurologic and intellectual damage results from an excessive body burden of Pb, even in the absence of overt clinical symptoms. For these reasons it is important that symptom-free children be screened periodically for evidence of increased body burden of Pb from potentially deleterious exposure and to prevent neurologic toxicity.

Because Pb poisoning occurs most frequently between the ages of 18 months and 5 years, screening should be concentrated in these age groups. In areas with many homes built before World War II and thus with Pb-containing paint, efforts at screening should be more intensive. Screening should be conducted every 6 months for children between 18 and 36 months of age and every year thereafter. It must be remembered that a screening test indicates the status of Pb intoxication in a particular child at a given moment. Severe Pb poisoning may develop in a period of 2 to 3 months; thus, in the presence of suspicious symptoms, testing should be repeated despite a history of normal findings.

Screening for Pb poisoning can be based on evidence of increased Pb absorption, provided by measurements of blood Pb, or on evidence of its metabolic effects provided by measurements of erythrocyte porphyrins (EP) levels. The measurement of blood Pb is difficult and expensive; moreover, when the blood sample is obtained by finger puncture, contamination by ubiquitous environmental Pb quite frequently results in spuriously elevated values. Measurement of EP, on the other hand, has none of these shortcomings: It is simple, reliable, inexpensive, and not subject to environmental contamination; therefore it is preferred as a primary screening test for Pb poisoning. It must be noted, however, that even though an elevated EP value provides a great index of suspicion for Pb poisoning, it does not establish a diagnosis. Elevation of the EP level may result not only from Pb poisoning but also from Fe deficiency anemia and, rarely, from the genetic disorder erythropoietic protoporthyria, often asymptomatic in childhood. The EP test therefore is useful for determining rapidly and economically, from a large population of children, those with the greatest index of suspicion and bringing them to medical attention. In this way a more expensive workup need be required only for a small group. From a public health standpoint, the capacity of the EP test to identify children with marked iron deficiency also appears to be an important advantage. Thus, measurement of EP is worthwhile in children between 18 months and 5 years of age every time a blood sample is obtained for any reason.

Three alternatives are available for screening by the EP test: (1) immediate measurement of EP with one of the several commercially available hematofluorometers, (2) collection of blood samples in a microcapillary tube, and (3) collection of blood samples on filter paper for mailing to the laboratory. The first alternative is the obvious choice for large pediatric clinics; the result is obtained instantly, and immediate investigations may be initiated in all "positive" children without need for recalls. These should include sampling for blood Pb by venipuncture. The second and third alternatives are the choices when only a small number of children is tested and recall of suspected cases is relatively easy. It may be convenient in some circumstances to collect samples for both EP and blood Pb at the same time but to instruct the laboratory to measure blood Pb levels only in those cases in which the EP value is high. This approach, however, has two inherent difficulties. First, it is necessary to scrub the finger carefully with citric acid and ethanol and then apply a thin film of collodion to obtain the sample for blood Pb measurements. The precautions are both cumbersome and time-consuming and are not necessary for measuring only the EP level. Second, despite all precautions, falsely elevated blood Pb values resulting from contamination are seen with great frequency. Thus for capillary blood samples only a low blood Pb value is significant; a high value is suspicious and needs to be confirmed on a venous blood sample. An elevated capillary blood Pb level with a normal EP value is obviously an error; an elevated capillary blood Pb level with an elevated EP value can still be a false-positive result in a child with iron deficiency. These tests identify all children with EP positivity because of excess Pb exposure, as well as the majority of those in whom the positive EP result is due to iron deficiency; only those children with an elevated EP value and a high microsample blood Pb level need recalling for confirmation.

The cost/benefit ratios of the various approaches are directly related to the cost of recalling patients. When a sufficient number of patients are tested and recalls are difficult and costly (as in a large pediatric clinic), screening with hematofluorometer and immediate venous blood sampling for confirmation offers the best cost/benefit ratio. In such a situation the relatively high cost of the hematofluorometer is rapidly amortized. When few patients are seen and recalls are relatively inexpensive, the best cost/benefit ratio is obtained by screening with the EP test only. The analysis can be performed at a central laboratory, using blood collected in a capillary tube or on filter paper. Individuals with a positive result should be recalled for further detailed investigation. The collection of the blood sample on filter paper is eminently suited for use in the pediatrician's office. In programs in which many samples are collected each day but at several different locations (such as in cities with several screening centers at many public health stations), the best cost/benefit ratio may be effected by collecting on filter paper the samples for both EP and blood Pb measurements. In such cases the savings obtained by the use of a central laboratory are obvious. An example of this is the screening program in New York City, where approximately 250,000 children per year are screened by this technique in nearly 100 different stations, each of which collects 2 to 10 samples a day.

In recent years, it has become obvious from the work of our laboratory and that of others that adverse effects of Pb occur at BPb levels well below ≥25 μg/dl. These effects, while not demonstrable in the individual child, are obvious at an epidemiological level. For these reasons, the concept of screening has been changed by the CDC, and an additional task has been included: the detection of communities with a larger than normal percentage of children with higher than "acceptable" BPb levels (this is now redefined as ≥10 μg/dl). The new scheme of population screening differs from the old approach, as it does not utilize EP for diagnostic purposes. In fact, EP is not useful in detecting children with very low BPb level, since at a BPb level of 35 μg/dl, 50% of children are EP negative.

The new scheme, based solely on measurements of BPb, now includes the category of children with a BPb level of 10 to 19 μg/dl. These will not be referred to medical attention, but will be used as *living detectors* of excessive exposure to Pb in their community. For children with a BPb of 15 to 19 μg/dl, educational and dietary advice are recommended. For children with a BPb of 20 to 25 μg/dl, an environmental analysis to ascertain the source of Pb, including home visits, is recommended. At BPb ≥ 25 μg/dl, the current recommendation for the management of asymptomatic children is similar to prior ones:

For all children with a BPb ≥25 μg/dl:	environmental scrutiny for removal of Pb source.
In addition, *for children with:*	
1) *BPb 25 to 54 μg/dl:*	decision to chelate based on the EDTA provocation test.
2) *BPb 55 to 69 μg/dl:*	treatment with CaNaEDTA alone.
3) *BPb ≥70 μg/dl:*	emergency hospitalization; treatment with BAL/CaNaEDTA.

The above guidelines are meant to set priorities for environmental and medical intervention and do not represent a diagnostic scheme. It cannot be emphasized enough that this scheme should not be used as a rigid set of slots, but must be tempered by appropriate medical judgment. For instance, a 13-month-old child with a BPb level of 26 μg/dl is at much greater risk than an 8-year-old child with a BPb level of 29 μg/dl; yet both cases would fit into the same category by rigid criteria.

The impact of the new screening regulations is going to be profound. It is estimated that with the continuing phase-down of Pb in gasoline, the national average BPb level in the United States is currently decreased to 5 to 6 μg/dl. Still, approximately 4 to 5 million children in the United States have BPb levels 10 to 19 μg/dl. Testing all these children is going to be formidable. Screening will have to be universal, not just targeted to "at risk" groups. A major additional problem is that, at this low BPb level, the accuracy of the current technology is not quite adequate to the task. Certainly if such a massive effort is set in motion without funding for education and cleanup, it will not be very effective.

Seven
Screening for Drugs

S. Kenneth Schonberg

Improved methods now allow, with a high degree of accuracy, for the detection of drugs in body fluids. As a result of these advances, screening pregnant women, newborns, and adolescents has been a subject of much controversy and debate in pediatric circles. Much would be gained by the early detection of substance abuse at either end of the pediatric patient–care spectrum; however, both ethical and practical considerations would suggest caution about imposing drug screening on unwilling patients or parents.

METHODS

A variety of techniques are available to detect the metabolites of drugs of abuse in urine and other body fluids. In general, the less expensive and less complex methods generate a greater incidence of false-positive and false-negative results than do their counterparts. Such methods range from simple litmus spot tests, which can be performed in the physician's office, to gas chromatography–mass spectrometry (GC-MS) tests, which require highly technical and expensive equipment. The most commonly employed drug screening used in clinical practice is the enzyme multiplication immunoassay technique (EMIT). This test is available at most laboratories and is reasonably accurate and affordable. False-positive tests do occur; thus positive results should be confirmed with more sophisticated techniques (GC-MS). The length of time since the last drug use that test results will remain positive varies with the drug, the extent of its abuse, and the sensitivity of the test employed. With the EMIT system, most drugs can be detected for at least 2 to 3 days after their last use. The metabolites of phencyclidine (PCP), however, may be detected for up to 1 week, and cannabinoids can be found for up to 3 to 4 weeks in heavy users.[2]

The major issues concerning drug screening do not relate to the expense of the testing, the accuracy of the results, or the number of days that testing will show a positive reaction. Rather the controversies regarding drug screening have focused on the ethical and practical implications of such screening procedures. Seeking evidence of substance abuse differs greatly from other screening procedures in which patient and physician share a mutual concern in detecting a condition previously unknown to either.

PERINATAL ISSUES

It is estimated that more than 300,000 infants are born each year to women who are abusing crack/cocaine,[4] an additional 10,000 to mothers abusing opiates,[5] and a greater, unknown number to mothers abusing alcohol, marijuana, and other drugs. Although there is reason for concern regarding any perinatal drug abuse because most of these, including alcohol and marijuana, have been associated with teratogenetic effects and sociologic implications, the greatest anxieties relate to the abuse of the "harder" drugs, crack/cocaine and opiates in particular. Part of this concern is directed toward toxicity in the fetus, neonatal addiction and abstinence syndromes, and potential long-term, adverse cognitive and behavioral sequelae. Part of the concern is directed toward continuing parental drug abuse, which has been associated with (1) an increased frequency of physical abuse in their infants, (2) diversion of their limited family resources and their involvement in criminal activity to enable them to buy drugs, and (3) their high risk for mental and physical illness.[3] Thus the desire to use all means to detect parental drug abuse is most understandable; however, the use of maternal or neonatal drug screening for such detection raises a series of ethical and practical concerns.

Mandatory or coerced testing of pregnant women stands in contrast to traditional adherence to ethical principles of informed voluntary consent for all physician-patient interactions. Similarly, testing a neonate for the presence of drugs is, in fact, an assessment of maternal drug use. Thus many find it difficult to justify ethically testing of either the baby or the mother without appropriate consent. Identical concerns have been raised regarding testing for human immunodeficiency virus, and most jurisdictions forbid such testing without informed parental consent.

A second concern is that the practice of screening mothers for drugs will cause pregnant women to delay or to avoid prenatal care. Although this avoidance of care because of fear of detection remains unproved, it is not illogical to expect that pregnant women who use drugs would not want this known for social and legal reasons.

Finally, there are concerns regarding how to best use the information gathered from drug screening. There would be little concern if it was used only to provide support services to families in difficulty and to facilitate drug abuse treatment. Unfortunately, this is not the case in many areas of the country, particularly in those communities in which drug abuse is most common. Often the mandatory or voluntary reporting of positive findings to child protective agencies results only in punitive actions that, although motivated by the presumed best interest of the infant, cause separation of the mother and her newborn and other interventions that do not well serve the needs of the family or the child in all instances.

Screening should be performed on infants born to mothers who have clinical indicators of drug use; social indicators such as low income, race, and ethnic origin are not sufficient reasons for selective screening. When clinical indicators are present and the screening test results are positive, caretakers have the opportunity to intervene positively for the benefit of the family and the infant. These interventions include the following:

1. Exercising influence for early enrollment of the mother and/or father in local drug treatment centers
2. Observing the infant carefully for signs of drug withdrawal and initiating early treatment or on occurrence of symptoms

3. Discouraging breast-feeding, which can cause further toxicity in the infant
4. Monitoring the infant for signs of central nervous system and renal dysfunction, including the use of central nervous system and renal ultrasound testing, when indicated

Guidelines for newborn urine drug screening currently in effect at the University of Rochester Strong Memorial Hospital Medical Center, Rochester, New York, are shown in the accompanying box.

Screening for drug abuse with informed voluntary consent or when clinically indicated in a particular newborn (with parental or court-ordered consent) is not at issue. However, the *routine* screening of *all* newborns or their mothers without consent *is*, and it must be viewed as ethically questionable because of its unproved benefits and its potential to affect adversely other aspects of perinatal care.

ADOLESCENT ISSUES

More than 90% of high school seniors have had some experience with alcohol; two thirds report use during the previous month, and nearly 5% are drinking daily. Approximately 20% of these adolescents use marijuana at least once per month; smaller numbers abuse opiates, cocaine/crack, and other drugs.[6] Such substance use and abuse emerges as a leading cause of death among adolescents; it is also a cause of major morbidity and social and educational disruption.

There may be a great temptation to screen all youths for substance abuse, both to intercede on their behalf and to diminish the effects of the presence of drug abusers on society. Despite such arguments, there are ethical and practical concerns regarding routine, nonconsensual drug screening of adolescents.[1]

Although parental consent most often is sufficient for performing any procedure in the younger child who lacks the capacity to make informed judgments, parental permission alone is not sufficient for performing diagnostic or therapeutic procedures on competent adolescents. Despite the temptation to apply a different ethical standard to adolescents in the search for drug abuse, there is great danger in a policy of adherence to principles of informed consent only because such adherence is convenient or expedient.

Beyond ethical issues are concerns regarding the impact

Guidelines for Newborn Urine Drug Screening

I. Infants whose mothers have any of the following:
   A. History of drug abuse in present or previous pregnancies
   B. Limited prenatal care (less than five prenatal visits)
   C. History of hepatitis B, AIDS, syphilis, gonorrhea, prostitution
   D. Unexplained placental abruption
   E. Unexplained premature labor

II. Infants who have any of the following:
   A. Unexplained neurologic complications (e.g., intracranial hemorrhage or infarction, seizures)
   B. Evidence of possible drug withdrawal (e.g., hypertonia, irritability, seizures, tremulousness, muscle rigidity, decreased or increased stooling)
   C. Unexplained intrauterine growth retardation

If any of these criteria are met:
1. Nurses will automatically place a urine collection bag on the infant.
2. The urine screen will not be sent *until* a physician writes the order.

If a urine screen is sent, the physician writing the order must:
1. Notify the infant's attending physician (if not the same) that the screen is being sent
2. Document the indication for the screen in the infant's hospital chart

If a urine screen is sent, the physician writing the order or the infant's attending physician (if not the same) must:
1. Notify the infant's mother and tell her the indication for the screen
2. Notify the mother's obstetrician that the screen is being sent
3. Notify social services that the screen is being sent. If social service had not been previously consulted because there were no other concerns, personnel will simply review the chart and talk only to the mother after discussion with her obstetricianand/or the infant's physician.

If the newborn drug screen results are positive:
1. The physician of the newborn is responsible for notifying the mother of the results of the screen.
2. Social services will evaluate the mother, her resources, home situation, and associated problems and will assist the mother with rehabilitation programs, parenting courses, parent support groups, home health aides, public health nurses, and medical/mental health referrals as necessary, as well as inform the local child protection services office.
3. HIV and hepatitis B status should be established in the mother, and appropriate care of the infant should follow.
4. The infant should have close neurodevelopmental follow-up.
5. Performance of a head and renal ultrasound should be considered.
6. Breast-feeding should be discouraged.

Reproduced with permission from the Pediatric Service of the University of Rochester Strong Memorial Hospital Medical Center.

on the physician-adolescent relationship inherent in the practice of nonconsensual (and even secret) screening for drugs. Such a practice would not remain secret for long. The major concerns are that (1) adolescents who use drugs know they are using drugs and, wishing to keep that behavior a secret from their physician, would not seek care if involuntary screening was a part of that care; (2) adolescents would abstain from drug use for the few days necessary to produce a clean and deceptively reassuring urine specimen; (3) pediatricians would not be willing to collect urine specimens under direct observation to prevent the adulteration or substitution techniques available to knowledgeable young drug abusers; and (4) the information gained from such involuntary screening would not sufficiently add to the knowledge acquired from interview to justify the risk of establishing an adversarial relationship with the teenager.

Certainly requisites for consent and voluntary screening may be waived when there is reason to doubt competency or when information gathered by interview of the parent or adolescent suggests that the adolescent is out of control or at high risk to self and others. However, both ethical and practical questions strongly indicate that routine involuntary screening of all adolescents to detect drug abuse is not essential. The advancing technology of drug screening should be applied selectively to monitoring the therapeutic progress of known drug abusers and to testing young persons who have been identified to be at special risk for drug abuse.

Eight

Use of Urinalysis and the Urine Culture in Screening

Edward J. Ruley
J. Ramon Ongkingco

Examination of the urine is a simple office procedure that may provide clues to specific urinary abnormalities or more generalized diseases. For the results to be meaningful, a clean-caught, midstream specimen should be examined as soon as possible after it is obtained.

Urinalyses and urine cultures have been used to screen children and adolescents for proteinuria, hematuria, glucosuria, and bacteriuria. Investigations of large populations have defined the prevalence of urinary abnormalities in symptom-free children and determined the cost effectiveness of early detection and treatment. The prevalence of urine abnormalities in any population depends on (1) the definition of the amount and frequency of urine aberration that is considered abnormal, (2) the presence of concomitant clinical factors that may increase the number of false-positive results, and (3) the age and sex distribution of the study population. The cost effectiveness of mass urine screening depends on the total monetary and psychosocial cost of performing the screening test compared with the value of early detection in ameliorating or preventing subsequent progression of the disease. Of significance is a study by Dodge and associates,[1] who determined a cumulative occurrence of bacteriuria, proteinuria, and hematuria (i.e., having one or more of these findings) to be 6475 cases per 100,000 children aged 6 to 12 years. This occurrence exceeds the number of persons expected to have significant morbidity from progressive renal disease and is much greater than the predicted number of deaths resulting from renal disease in the United States (28 per 1 million population per year). Such a finding reflects the high degree of sensitivity and the lack of specificity of current urine tests in detecting significant renal or urinary tract disease in symptom-free children. In contrast, in a more recent report, extensive urine screening of symptom-free schoolchildren in Japan detected a small number who were then shown to have biopsy-proved glomerular disease.[4] Although the early discovery of a symptom-free child with renal disease may prove to be important, the cost effectiveness to society of mass screening remains unproved. In otherwise healthy children, a single complete urinalysis performed before school entry should be sufficient screening for health maintenance purposes. The American Academy of Pediatrics, however, recommends that a complete urinalysis be performed during infancy (the first year of life), during early childhood (1 through 4 years), during late childhood (5 through 12 years), and during adolescence (see Chapter 3).

PROTEINURIA

Proteinuria is most easily detected by the dipstick method, which makes use of a paper or plastic strip to which is affixed the indicator, tetrabromophenol blue. The presence of protein causes a change in color from yellow to blue-green that is proportional to the amount of protein present. False-positive findings can occur in highly alkaline urine (pH > 6.5) or in urine contaminated by skin antiseptics such as chlorhexidine or benzalkonium chloride. The small quantity of protein that healthy persons excrete normally usually is not detected by this method, although the reading may show a "trace" amount if the urine is concentrated (specific gravity > 1.025). In contrast, the presence of a trace amount of protein in a dilute urine may reflect significant losses and should be investigated. Detection of protein by acid precipitation with sulfosalicylic acid is more specific and can be used for urine with an alkaline pH. The clinical approach to children with proteinuria is discussed in Chapter 157.

The prevalence rate for proteinuria in the symptom-free pediatric population varies, depending on the degree and frequency of proteinuria that is considered abnormal. Gutgesell[2] found the prevalence of proteinuria to be 6.3% in 2309 children with and without symptoms who made their first visits to a neighborhood clinic in which screening was performed by use of a 1+ or greater on a single urine specimen measured by a dip-and-read strip as the criterion for proteinuria. When Silverberg[6,7] applied a more stringent criterion for proteinuria (2+ or greater on two urinalyses) to more than 50,000 schoolchildren, he found the prevalence to be only 0.45% for boys and 1.6% for girls. Several investigators have noted a direct relationship of proteinuria to age during childhood, the incidence peaking at adolescence and then rapidly declining only to rise progressively thereafter into adulthood. Furthermore, proteinuria is more common at each age in girls during childhood, with the occurrence rates in boys lagging 3 to 5 years behind. It has been hypothesized that these sex differences are due to the earlier onset of adolescence in girls. No differences in prevalence have been noted by ethnic group or socioeconomic level. From Silverberg's data it is not surprising that the highest prevalence was found in the adolescent population (14.8%) when less rigorous criteria for screening were used. The prevalence of proteinuria (alone or in combination with glucosuria or hematuria) determined by urinalysis on routine hospital admission has been reported to be 2.5%. This value is similar to values in outpatient studies. When the criterion was made more stringent by requiring two consecutive abnormal urinalysis results, the prevalence decreased to 2%. Finally, if the number of false-positive results was minimized by collecting samples only from patients who were afebrile and not menstruating, the prevalence decreased to 0.6%. The influence of such clinical factors must be taken into account when any data on the prevalence of proteinuria are considered.

Although screening for proteinuria as part of well-child health care has become a hallowed tradition for many practitioners, there is no evidence that this procedure benefits the population being screened. At least 75% of symptom-free patients found to have protein in a single urinalysis will be free of it on repeat testing. Furthermore, of those having several positive random urinalysis results, 60% will have orthostatic proteinuria. The transient form of orthostatic proteinuria resolves before adulthood and does not recur. The fixed and reproducible form of orthostatic proteinuria often persists into adulthood but is not considered to be a harbinger of clinically significant renal disease. In one 10-year follow-up study of young men with persistent orthostatic proteinuria, none developed renal insufficiency, including the 53% who had nonspecific glomerular abnormalities on renal biopsy.[8] Regular follow-up, however, remains important for these children so that any changes in the pattern of protein excretion can be detected and appropriately investigated.

Follow-up care of children determined by screening tests to have proteinuria has shown an incidence of identifiable renal disease in only 1 child per 1000 children screened. Furthermore, large studies have shown that children who have been identified as having renal disease by screening usually (1) are already known to have renal disease by their parents and physicians (e.g., nephrotic syndrome), (2) have an abnormality that requires no additional management (e.g., a hypoplastic kidney), or (3) have a renal disease for which no specific treatment is available (e.g., membranoproliferative glomerulonephritis). Even in urinary tract infections, the urinary abnormality most amenable to treatment—proteinuria—often is not present in the symptom-free child. It is important to note that most children with significant renal disease will have other signs and symptoms (e.g., edema, poor weight gain, or hypertension) that will cause them to seek medical care and thus to be identified even in the absence of screening programs.

Besides the lack of a positive effect on the population, screening can have a negative effect in producing undue anxiety in patients and parents and in serving as an impetus for the practitioner to perform more invasive testing, which often provides no new information. Such factors may detract from the overall well-being of the population.

In our current state of knowledge there is no indication for mass screening for proteinuria in symptom-free children, although this may change as new tests are developed. The nonproductiveness of screening symptom-free patients, however, does not apply to children with symptoms. Urinalysis is an important tool in evaluating the child with renal symptoms and should even by employed in patients with vague symptoms, such as failure to thrive, or with recurrent diarrhea, inasmuch as some renal disease may manifest with such nonspecific symptoms.

HEMATURIA

Hematuria can be detected by chemical tests for blood or by microscopic examination for erythrocytes in urine specimens. The commercially available dipstick tests depend on the color change that results from the oxidation of orthotolidine and cumene hydroperoxide, which is catalyzed by the presence of hemoglobin (or myoglobin) in the urine. False-positive tests for blood in the urine may result from the presence of contaminating oxidizing cleansing agents such as povidone-iodine or hypochlorite or microbial peroxidases. False-negative tests result from the presence of ascorbic acid in the urine from orally ingested vitamin C preparations. A positive dipstick result for blood does not discriminate between hemoglobin and myoglobin; differentiation requires spectrophotometric analysis. Furthermore, the dipstick test will not differentiate hemoglobinuria from hematuria or give clues to whether the blood originates from the upper or lower urinary tracts. For these questions the microscopic examination of the centrifuged urine sediment is necessary (see Chapter 137).

The number of erythrocytes per high-power field in a centrifuged urine sediment that is abnormal is variable. This variability occurs because the concentration of erythrocytes in the centrifuged sediment depends primarily on the volume of urine centrifuged and the amount of supernatant decanted from the centrifuge tube before microscopic examination. The results are affected to a lesser degree by the centrifuge speed and duration. Another source of variation is the practice of reporting the average number of erythrocytes in each field inasmuch as few observers take the time to count each cell in several fields and then average them. Meticulous technique minimizes these methodologic problems but significantly increases the labor intensiveness of the urinalysis. Dodge and associates[1] have suggested that five or more erythrocytes per high-power field in at least two or three consecutive urine specimens be considered abnormal.

The prevalence of microscopic hematuria in an ambulatory setting varies from 4% if a single urinalysis is abnormal to

0.07% if two urinalyses are abnormal. As with proteinuria, the point prevalence (number of existing cases) of hematuria increases with age among children of both sexes and is greater at each age for girls than for boys, although one recent study failed to find such differences. Whereas one study found no differences in prevalence among ethnic groups or socioeconomic classes, another found a higher prevalence among white and Oriental children than among black and Mexican-American children. The prevalence of hematuria (alone or in combination with glucosuria or proteinuria) in children admitted to the hospital for medical illnesses was 5.3%. When sources of false positivity (fever or menstruation) were eliminated and the criteria were made more stringent by requiring two consecutive abnormal specimens, the prevalence decreased to 2.2%.

Few of the children detected in screening programs to have hematuria are found to have significant renal or urologic disease. Thus, for much the same reasons as those advanced for proteinuria, it has been suggested that there is no justification for mass screening for hematuria.

GLUCOSURIA

Screening for glucosuria can be performed by use of the highly specific glucose oxidase–impregnated dipsticks. Normally, 99% of the glucose in the glomerular ultrafiltrate is reabsorbed by the proximal tubules. Glucosuria may occur (1) at high blood glucose levels when the glucose concentration in the ultrafiltrate exceeds the capacity of the proximal tubular reabsorptive mechanism or (2) at normal blood glucose levels when there is tubular reabsorptive dysfunction. Measurement of blood glucose will differentiate these two mechanisms. Rarely will early diabetes mellitus or Fanconi syndrome will be detected in a child by means of urinalysis. The cost effectiveness, however, is so low that routine screening of well children for glucosuria is not recommended.

BACTERIURIA

In the past it was considered to be cost effective to screen symptom-free girls for bacteriuria, ostensibly (1) to prevent the morbidity and complications of symptomatic infection and (2) to identify individuals in whom urologic investigation to prevent renal parenchymal damage is indicated. Subsequent studies showed that nontreatment did not increase the frequency of pyelonephritis, interfere with renal growth, or cause renal insufficiency.[5,9] Moreover, the incidence of significant structural abnormalities was remarkable low.[3] Furthermore, recent studies suggest that treatment of asymptomatic bacteriuria may be associated with a greater risk for pyelonephritis because of the development of resistant organisms. Therefore, because most current research suggests that children with asymptomatic bacteriuria do not have a high frequency of associated urinary structural abnormalities and treatment of asymptomatic bacteriuria is contraindicated, there is no reason to screen the pediatric population for its occurrence. It must be emphasized that these caveats apply only to children who are overtly healthy; they do not apply to children who are sick, even those with poorly defined symptoms, in whom a renal evaluation may be indicated.

Nine

Auditory Screening

David R. Cunningham

JUSTIFICATION

Routine screening for hearing loss or otopathology might be justified on the basis of the number of infants and older children known to have these disorders. Surveys of neonatal screening programs indicate that 1 in every 2000 infants will have severe congenital hearing loss at birth. (Compare this with the 1 in 14,000 who have PKU at birth.) By 2 years of age, 1 in 25 children will have a mild to moderate (20 to 50 dB) hearing loss resulting from ear disease. Studies indicate that nearly 20% of the public schoolchildren in disadvantaged neighborhoods fail auditory screening tests. Perhaps the most important rationale for beginning or continuing an auditory screening program is the consequence of not doing so. Overwhelming evidence indicates that the first 18 months of life are critical for the acquisition of normal speech and language skills. Undetected, severe hearing loss in this period may lead to irreparable communicative and learning disorders. Early intervention in the form of amplification, parental counseling, and special education is crucial in these cases. Regular hearing screening for the older infant and the school-aged child is important not only because of the seriousness of the medical sequelae of active middle-ear disease but also because of the implications that even mild (15 to 20 dB) hearing loss (either conductive or sensorineural) has for language growth, academic success, and even behavioral development.

GOALS

The goal of auditory screening is essentially the same for each age-group: to identify hearing loss regardless of degree. The methods of achieving this goal differ from one age-group to another. In the neonatal and infant periods the aim is to discover severe (70 dB or greater) congenital sensorineural hearing losses. Because the first 18 months of life are so critical to language acquisition, however, it also is necessary to seek out those milder hearing losses known to inhibit normal speech and language development. In the preschool period the screening technology should be adjusted to detect ear disease and even milder hearing losses, as well as yet unnoticed sensorineural hearing loss. Routine screening of the school-aged child is designed to maintain educationally adequate hearing. In this group practitioners also must be alert to those academic underachievers who suffer little or no peripheral hearing loss but who exhibit signs of specific auditory learning disabilities. What follows here is a discussion of feasible and economical screening techniques for children in these three age-groups.

NEONATAL AND EARLY INFANT PERIOD

Screening of infants in newborn nurseries for hearing loss has been virtually abandoned in the United States because it is costly and produces unacceptable levels of false-positive and false-negative results.

Guidelines developed by the American Speech-Language Hearing Association (ASHA) Committee on Infant Hearing in 1982 recommended that infants with one or more of the following risk factors be considered at risk for hearing impairment and should receive brainstem auditory evoked response (BAER) screening:

1. A family history of childhood hearing impairment
2. Congenital perinatal infection (e.g., cytomegalovirus [CMV], herpes, rubella, toxoplasmosis, and syphilis)
3. Birth weight <1500 g
4. Hyperbilirubinemia at levels exceeding indications for exchange transfusion
5. Bacterial meningitis (especially *Haemophilus influenzae*)
6. Severe asphyxia, which may include infants with Apgar scores 0 to 3 who fail to initiate spontaneous respiration by 10 minutes and those with hypotonia persisting for the first 2 hours of life
7. Anatomic malformation involving the head or neck (e.g., branchial arch syndromes, cleft palate, submucous cleft of the palate, and malformed, absent, or low-set pinna

Some evidence suggests that infants with other problems be screened as well. These factors, which have not been universally endorsed, but may be included in future recommendations, are (1) parent consanguinity, (2) severe neonatal sepsis, (3) persistent pulmonary hypertension in the newborn, (4) aminoglycoside therapy, or (5) *any* admission to the neonatal intensive care nursery.[1]

Ideally, all children at risk should be included in a wide risk registry and follow-up scheme. In several states the risk criteria are included on the birth certificate. Long-term tracking and follow-up are facilitated when a single state agency (e.g., commission for handicapped children or public health department) manages the high-risk registry. These mechanisms organize the data base, aid in the notification of the primary care physician or clinic, and are useful for monitoring the sensitivity and specificity of the pass/fail risk criteria.

All high-risk infants should be screened audiologically *before* discharge from the hospital. When this is impossible, the audiologic screening must be completed in the first 3 or 4 months of life. Within the time frame of the hospitalization and screening, the parents/caregivers should be given information about (1) the screening and follow-up process, (2) milestones in normal auditory and speech/language development, and (3) the importance of obtaining a complete audiologic evaluation should it become necessary on the basis of the screening results.

The ASHA recommends BAER as the screening technique for all at-risk infants.[1] "Passing" the BAER screening requires a repeatable response from both ears at intensity levels of 40 dB or less referenced to the normal hearing level (nHL), that is, 40 dB nHL. It should be understood, however, that passing the BAER screening does not completely rule out the presence of a very mild hearing loss, the existence of a central auditory "processing" disorder, which may manifest later in childhood, or the possibility of a progressive hearing impairment. Those infants who pass the screening but are at risk for progressive hearing loss should be monitored carefully by all caregivers for signs of poor speech/language development. Those etiologic factors known to be associated with progressive hearing loss in children include (1) CMV, (2) family history of progressive hearing loss, and (3) persistent fetal circulation (PFC).[2-4] Infants who "fail" the BAER screening should be referred for a more exhaustive audiologic evaluation. The full-range audiologic examination may include a comprehensive BAER threshold determination, behavioral observation, audiometric examination, acoustic reflex threshold measurement, and tympanometric examination. These tests should be repeated, as necessary, to rule out hearing loss or to document the extent of the auditory deficit (Table 18-2).

During infancy and early childhood the acuteness of hearing is indirectly screened through parental and physician observations of the child's response to vocal and environmental sounds and through the monitoring of speech and language development. Parental suspicions that their baby cannot hear should be taken seriously and should prompt complete audiologic testing.

Table 18-2 *Use of Impedance Audiometry to Help Confirm Audiometric Impressions in the Evaluation of Young Children*

TYMPANOMETRY	STATIC COMPLIANCE	ACOUSTIC REFLEX	CONFIRM BEHAVIORAL AUDIOMETRIC IMPRESSION
Type A bilaterally	Within normal range, bilaterally	Normal bilaterally	Bilateral normal hearing or bilateral mild to moderate sensorineural hearing loss or unilateral mild to moderate sensorineural hearing loss
Type A in one ear; type B or C in other ear	Normal in A ear; low in B or C ear	Absent bilaterally	Unilateral conductive loss
Type B or C bilaterally	Low bilaterally	Absent bilaterally	Bilateral conductive loss

From Northern J and Downs M: Hearing in children, ed. 2. © 1978, The Williams & Wilkins Co, Baltimore.

PRESCHOOL PERIOD

Well-baby visits should routinely include an examination of the child's ears and a gross assessment of hearing. The goal is to detect otologic (middle ear) disease and adventitious sensorineural hearing losses. Beginning at age 4 years, children should be given standard, pure-tone screening audiometric tests. An inexpensive, calibrated screening audiometer should be standard equipment in the physician's office. The stimulus should include pure tones at frequencies of 1, 2, 4, and 6 kHz; the intensity should be adjusted to 25 dB at each frequency. Failure to hear the stimulus at two frequencies in one ear is grounds for referral to an audiologist. One must bear in mind that "passing" this simple hearing screening test does not necessarily indicate that the child is free of active middle ear disease. Because of this, the preschool screening protocol also should include tympanometric examination.

Substantial evidence supports the use of tympanometry for the early detection of middle ear disorders in preschool and school-aged populations. It provides accurate information about the integrity of the tympanic membrane (e.g., the presence of perforations and the patency of tympanostomy tubes), the pressure contained in the middle ear space, the patency of the eustachian tube, and the mobility of the tympanic membrane–ossicular chain complex. This inexpensive technologic procedure produces objective data about middle ear function that compare favorably with the results obtained by pneumootoscopic examination performed by a skilled clinician. The test is essentially noninvasive, quickly administered, and does not require the absolute cooperation of the child.

Fig. 18-1 shows the five classical tympanogram types. *Type A* is found in normal ears, *type* A_D in ears with hypercompliant tympanic membrane–ossicular systems, *type* A_S in hypocompliant middle ears, *type B* in noncompliant systems (e.g., otitis media with effusion), and *type C* with negative middle ear pressure (e.g., possible eustachian tube dysfunction). Table 18-3 provides a basic scheme for relating audiometric and tympanometric findings in the detection of hearing loss and/or middle ear disease.

SCHOOL-AGE POPULATION

The primary goal of screening school-aged children is the maintenance of educationally adequate hearing. The secondary goal is the detection of remediable ear disease. Under the most ideal circumstances these goals will be met best by a three-pronged approach: pure-tone "sweep" audiometric examination, acoustic-impedance measurement, and pneumo-otoscopic examination. The implication is that pure-tone screening by itself is not especially sensitive to subtle but important middle ear disease, which might predispose a child to fluctuating hearing levels. Such a child might barely pass a hearing screening test with thresholds in the 20 to 25 dB range one day and then suffer from the frustration of listening with a 40 dB hearing loss for weeks at a time. In cases like these, evidence of reduced tympanic-membrane compliance, significant negative middle ear pressure, absence of stapedial

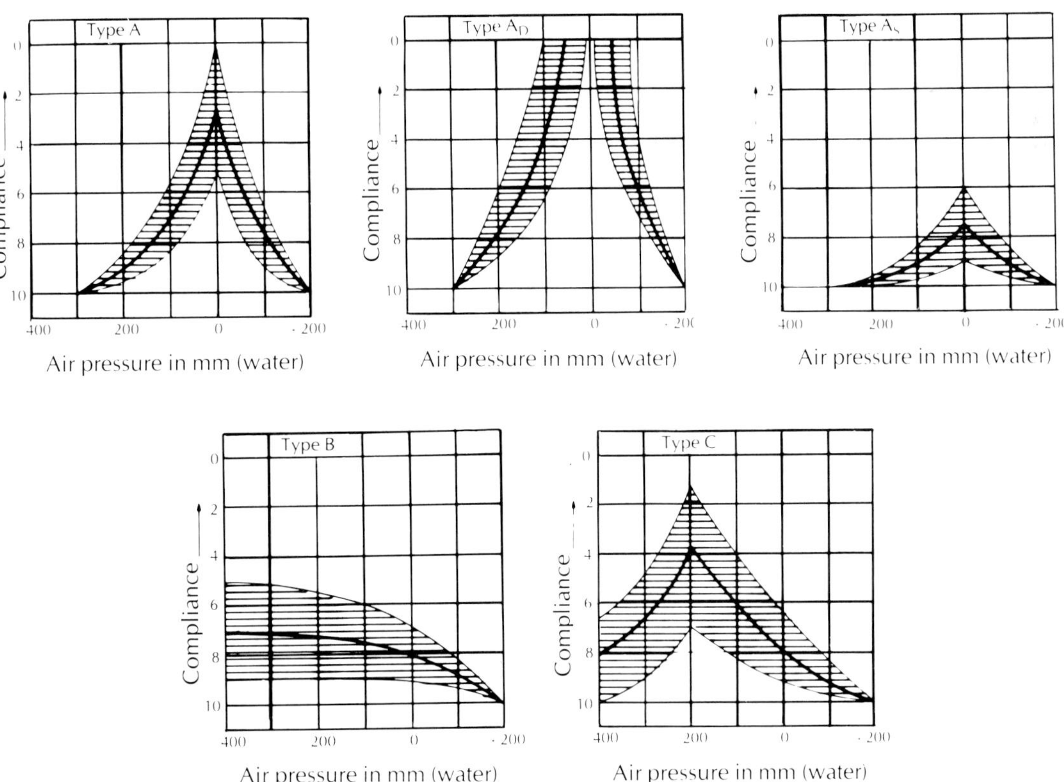

Fig. 18-1 Classification of tympanograms. Lined areas of tympanograms represent range of results; solid lines represent average tympanogram of each pattern. See text for clinical significance of each type of tympanogram.

From Northern J and Downs M: Hearing in children, ed. 2. © 1978, the Williams & Wilkins Co., Baltimore.

Table 18-3 *Recommended Guidelines for Combining Results from Hearing Screening and Impedance Measures*

POSSIBLE OUTCOME (SEE EXPLANATION BELOW)	SEVERITY TYPE	FOLLOW-UP	DISPOSITION AFTER FOLLOW-UP
1. T: peak normal§* R: present‖† H: pass¶‡	I	None—pass	A. Change to type I—pass
2. T: peak normal R: absent H: pass	II	Retest in 2 to 6 wk	B. No change or other type II—at risk—retest C. Change to type III—refer for audiological testing D. Change to type IV—medical referral
3. T: peak normal R: absent H: fail	III	Retest in 2 to 6 wk	A. Change to type I—pass B. Change to type II—at risk—retest C. No change or other type III—refer for audiological testing D. Change to type IV—medical referral
4. T: peak normal R: present H: fail	III	Retest in 2 to 6 wk	A. Change to type I—pass B. Change to type II—at risk—retest C. No change or other type III—refer for audiological testing D. Change to type IV—medical referral
5. T: no peak or rounded R: present H: pass	II	Not a likely finding—check equipment; retest if confirmed	A. Change to type I—pass B. No change or other type II—at risk—retest C. Change to type III—refer for audiological testing D. Change to type IV—medical referral
6. T: no peak or rounded R: absent H: pass	IV	Immediate medical referral	
7. T: no peak or rounded R: absent H: fail	IV	Immediate medical referral	
8. T: no peak or rounded R: present H: fail	IV	Not a likely finding—check equipment; immediate medical referral if confirmed	
9. T: abnormal peak§ R: present H: pass	II	Retest in 2 to 6 wk	A. Change to type I—pass B. No change or other type II—at risk—retest C. Change to type III—refer for audiological testing D. Change to type IV—medical referral
10. T: abnormal peak R: absent H: pass	II	Retest in 2 to 6 wk	A. Change to type I—pass B. No change or other type II—at risk—retest C. Change to type III—refer for audiological testing D. Change to type IV—medical referral
11. T: abnormal peak R: absent H: fail	III	Retest in 2 to 6 wk	A. Change to type I—pass B. Change to type II—at risk—retest C. No change or other type III—refer for audiological testing D. Change to type IV—medical referral
12. T: abnormal peak R: present H: fail	III	Retest in 2 to 6 wk	A. Change to type I—pass B. Change to type II—at risk—retest C. No change or other type III—refer for audiological testing D. Change to type IV—medical referral

From Roeser RJ and Northern JL: Screening for hearing loss and middle ear disorders. In Roeser RJ and Downs M, editors: Auditory disorders in schoolchildren, New York, 1981, Thieme-Stratton, Inc, pp 143-144.

T, Tympanogram; *R*, reflex; *H*, Hearing screening.

*+59 to −200 mm H_2O.

†1000 Hz contralateral tone at 100 dB HL.

‡Failure to respond to 1000 or 2000 Hz at 20 dB HL or 4000 Hz at 25 dB HL in either ear.

§Greater than +50 mm H_2O or more negative than −2000 mm H_2O.

reflexes, or otoscopic abnormalities would alert the examiner to the presence of middle ear disease and the possibility of fluctuating hearing levels. Roeser and Northern[5] offer a detailed description of recommended guidelines for combining the results from hearing screening and impedance screening measures. Table 18-3 lists the possible outcomes, severity type (an indicator of the need for medical referral), follow-up, and disposition for all combinations of screening results. These guidelines should serve as the basis of a rational approach to the screening of older preschool and school-aged children.

When insufficient resources prevent the implementation of the "ideal" program, an alternative is available. This is the auditory screening program carried out by the majority of the school systems. Under this plan all children in kindergarten and first, third, fifth, and seventh grades are tested. All transfer students and all pupils who have had protracted illness should be screened on entry into school, and all students with known histories of ear disease or hearing loss and students in speech therapy and special classrooms should be screened annually. The hearing level of the calibrated screening audiometer should be set at 25 dB (as recommended by the American National Standards Institute). The test frequencies should be 1, 2, 3, and 4 or 6 kHz. Students who fail to respond to 1 or 2 kHz or who fail to respond to two out of the three higher frequencies should be referred to a qualified audiologist for complete, standard audiologic assessment and impedance measurements. The audiologist will refer the child to the pediatrician or otolaryngologist if there is evidence of hearing loss or ear disease.

Particular attention should be paid to the acoustics of the test environment and the training of the screening personnel. Volunteers can be taught the auditory screening technique. They should be supervised closely by an audiologist, school nurse–teacher, or public health clinician.

Central Auditory Dysfunction

The pediatrician should be alert to the subtle but significant learning problems of the child with central auditory dysfunction. These children generally have normal peripheral hearing sensitivity, although they may have a history of early middle ear disease. They usually are academic underachievers. Most are boys. Teachers and parents report that these children respond inconsistently to auditory stimuli; they are inattentive and easily distracted from their work. Such children often have difficulty remembering and following verbal directions. Many have problems with spelling, reading, and language. Some exhibit either gross or fine motor incoordination, including speech articulation errors. Because of their frustrations with learning, they may either withdraw from activities or behave aggressively. Children with one or more of these characteristics should be referred to the audiology clinic for extensive central auditory tests and recommendations for remediation.

PERSONNEL AND EQUIPMENT

Because most of the screening techniques described can be mastered by paraprofessionals or volunteers, the costs per patient or student can be very low, perhaps a few cents per child. In major screening programs, part of a supervisor's salary must be considered a direct cost. Initial setup expenses include the costs of equipment and paper supplies and the fee paid to the consultant. The consultant should be expected to train the personnel, conduct an awareness campaign, draft letters of notification, choose appropriate equipment and calibrate it, make sound-level measurements of the test sites, and interpret the screening data. A simple portable screening audiometer costs about $900. A screening impedance bridge is priced between $1500 and $2500. BAER equipment for screening is priced between $7000 and $12,000. These pieces of equipment are durable, maintain calibration well, and can be used for literally thousands of tests over several years.

Ten
Vision Screening

Ellen R. Strahlman

Vision screening is an important aspect of preventive pediatrics, inasmuch as vision defects are among the more common handicapping conditions of childhood. The primary purpose of vision screening in children is to detect potentially blinding diseases or vision impairments that might interfere with the development and education of the child. Reduced visual acuity may indicate (1) eye diseases that could lead to blindness, (2) associated systemic disease, (3) a space-occupying lesion or other disorder of the central nervous system, or (4) refractive errors that might be correctable. An important reason for early vision screening is the detection of amblyopia, because further loss of vision in the "unused" eye can be prevented. Vision screening may be performed by a nurse, a physician's aide, or a properly trained layperson.

All children should be screened at birth, again during the first year of life, and then every 2 or 3 years thereafter. Vision testing in young children requires examiner patience and skill. A repeat examination may be necessary to verify suspected visual defects. Several techniques are used to determine visual acuity. The method used will depend, to a large extent, on the age and cooperation of the child. For children younger than 3 years of age, visual acuity is best estimated by fixation pattern. Preschool children may be tested with the Snellen Illiterate E chart. The Snellen chart with standard letters of the alphabet usually is employed for older children.

Estimation of visual acuity by fixation pattern is the method of choice for children younger than 3 years of age, the mentally retarded, and those with severe brain damage. The technique also is effective for determining the visual acuity of children with strabismus. The examiner has the child fixate on an object such as a toy, picture, or cartoon. The examiner then covers one eye and has the child look steadily at the fixation target, making sure that the direction of gaze is roughly in the target's direction. The examiner then uncovers the first eye, covers the other one, and follows the same procedure. Covering the "good" eye of a child who has deep amblyopia in the other eye will precipitate anxiety and avoidance maneuvers, because the child is severely handicapped by occlusion of the better eye. Thus a patient with strabismus and amblyopia in one eye will strongly prefer his or her better eye and will switch fixation to that eye during the test.

The vision of preschool children is most often tested by use of the Snellen Illiterate E chart (the so-called Tumbling E game). The patient is placed at a specific distance (usually 20 feet) from a well-illuminated chart (satisfactory illumination can be obtained from a gooseneck lamp with a 100-watt bulb). The lamp should be placed just to one side of the chart. Glasses should be worn if they are normally used for distance vision. The child may be told that the configurations on the chart are pictures of a table and instructed to point in the direction the "legs of the table" are pointing. The child or parent then covers each eye separately, and the child points in the direction of the "legs" of the various Es indicated by the examiner pointing at the chart. The smallest line of figures correctly identified indicates the child's level of visual acuity. With some patients it may be advantageous for the parent and child to practice the procedure at home before examination by the physician.

For older children the Snellen chart with letters of the alphabet is used, and the procedure followed is the same as already described for the Illiterate E chart. The patient's visual acuity is indicated by the smallest line in which more than half the letters can be seen. If the largest letter is not seen, the patient should be moved a specific distance closer to the chart; the visual acuity is recorded according to that distance. For example, if the patient sees the 20/200 letter at a distance of 4 feet, the visual acuity would be 4/200. If visual acuity is less than 20/40 in either eye, or if there is a difference of more than two Snellen lines between eyes, referral to an ophthalmologist is advisable. It must be emphasized that testing for problems with near vision in young children is not satisfactory because of the wide range of accommodation normally present in this age-group.

The vision tests described thus far test each eye separately for visual function. Another group of tests examines the child's ability to use both eyes together to assess binocularity. Examples of these tests include the Titmus Fly Test and the Random Dot E Stereogram. The examiner gives the child a special pair of spectacles to wear during the testing, and the child is instructed to look at the test device and describe certain features of the three-dimensional images produced by wearing the glasses. Because such tests generally are more complicated than fixation testing or Snellen visual acuity testing, they are not suitable for children younger than 4 years of age.

Each of the aforementioned visual acuity tests is *subjective*—that is, the examiner depends on the patient to relate what is seen. The patient's motivation and understanding of what is expected, as well as the actual degree of visual acuity, can influence the results obtained. Although newer *objective* techniques for determining visual acuity in young children are being developed, these methods are not yet available for widespread use.

Children 4 years of age or older can be screened for color blindness. The most common type of color blindness is a red-green defect, which is sex-linked. This condition, easily detected by means of standard color plates, does not cause loss of central vision and remains stable throughout life.

Machines for testing vision are available and are widely used in health department screening programs, in schools, and in some private offices. Although they are helpful for detecting reduced visual acuity, strabismus, color defects, and problems with near vision, they most often are used to test school-aged children. Because the correctable features of many childhood vision defects are best managed before the age of 6 years, vision screening in the pediatrician's office is essential to the detection and prevention of visual disability in children.

Eleven
Developmental Assessment

Rune J. Simeonsson
Nancy E. Simeonsson

Even though the importance of early intervention for children with developmental problems is widely recognized, the identification of children who need intervention, particularly those with subtle deficits, has been fraught with complications. At issue has been the need for identification procedures that are sufficiently sensitive to detect significant variations in development and yet are usable in clinical contexts without extensive effort. Screening tests have constituted the major identification approach, but concerns recently have been raised about limitations of this approach. Drawing on alternate perspectives from Europe and Great Britain, Dworkin[3] has advocated developmental surveillance, defined as a "flexible, continuous process that is broader in scope than screening, whereby knowledgeable professionals perform skilled observations of children throughout all encounters during child health care." This approach is comprehensive and encompasses monitoring, identification, and assessment. As such it is very much in keeping with the American Academy of Pediatrics recommendation[1] for continuity of comprehensive care as embodied in the monitoring guidelines for preventive pediatric health care (see Chapter 3).

Two aspects of these guidelines are particularly relevant to developmental surveillance. First, the importance of the early years is evident in the recommendation for six visits in the first year of life and five from 1 through 4 years of age.[8] Second, integration of effort can be promoted by attention to monitoring the domains of history, sensory screening, and developmental and behavioral guidance for both parents and child. In this context developmental surveillance and assessment are seen as clinical skills that require familiarity with developmental processes and that capitalize on opportunities for observation in all encounters with children. Such skills can yield diagnostic information for the practitioner, provide a basis for parent counseling, and result in referral or habilitation prescriptions when appropriate. Developmental assessment also may have value in the documentation and monitoring of interventions for children.

DEVELOPMENTAL PERSPECTIVE

Valid assessment of children requires a perspective that encompasses quantitative as well as qualitative changes of developmental processes. A common perspective views development as a sequence of milestones normally achieved at specific ages. Development also can be seen as a series of critical tasks to be mastered within certain stages of life, such as infancy, early childhood, and adolescence. Other developmental perspectives can be derived from stage-based theories, such as Freud's theory of psychosexual stages or Piaget's stages of cognitive growth.

A brief integration of ages, tasks, and Piaget's cognitive stages reveals infancy as a period in which the physical and social environment is understood and mastered through sensation and motor activity. This is expressed in a sequence of stages leading to independent mobility as well as the control involved in feeding, elimination, exploration, and primitive symbol use in gestures and speech. These characteristics of infancy change in the toddler and preschool period to increasingly sophisticated language obstruction, coordination of gross and fine motor movements for games and play, and increased awareness and conformity to peer and adult demands. The child's awareness of physical and social reality, however, is constrained by intuitive and idiosyncratic perceptions. As the child reaches school age, a qualitative cognitive shift occurs, in which understanding no longer remains unidimensional and personally focused but can adequately integrate several dimensions and alternative perspectives. This is reflected in the child's ability to reason logically and to classify and perform numerical operations skills necessary for academic tasks. The qualitative nature of abstract hypothetic thought, however, usually does not become evident until the prepubertal and adolescent periods. Formal education covering a wide range of scientific, artistic, cultural, and vocational issues contributes to the adolescent's cognitive social and emotional growth.

FOCUS ON THE PRESCHOOL YEARS

The importance of developmental assessment is based on the conviction that patterns of development observed in the earliest years of life are sequential and therefore predictable. Biologic maturation stimulates, as well as reflects, developmental changes in interaction with the environment. Although current developmental status can be assessed sensitively, predicting ultimate intellectual competence is hazardous and should be avoided. Individual variations from developmental norms may be transient and, initially, simply should indicate the need for more comprehensive evaluation. The primary care practitioner's role in developmental assessment is, perhaps, more critical in the preschool years than in any other period because (1) growth and development are particularly rapid, (2) the pediatrician has a central role with children of this age, and (3) qualitative developmental indexes such as language and socialization serve as "markers" for school readiness.

PRINCIPLES OF DEVELOPMENTAL ASSESSMENT

Assessment of development should be effectively integrated into the pediatric examination; it involves (1) a good history, (2) knowledge of environmental influences, (3) familiarity with normal development, and (4) awareness of the relative significance of developmental indicators.

Particularly relevant here is a recognition of the collaborative role of parents and other professionals in developmental assessment and intervention. This recognition is evident in Hutchison and Nicoll's[8] recommendation for parental partnership and interprofessional cooperation, concepts similar to the emphasis on parent involvement and multidisciplinary approach in Public Law 99-457.

Obtaining a good history begins with a review of the family history, with particular attention to disorders of development. Details of the pregnancy, delivery, and perinatal period contribute indexes to identify children at risk. Understanding the influence of the environment on development, which includes nutrition, illness, and medication history as well as social and psychologic variables, is important in developmental assessment. More specifically, the characteristics of the parent-child interaction, the nature and availability of developmental stimulation, and the makeup of the social environment in terms of siblings, parents, or extended caretakers need to be considered.

Valid developmental assessment requires an awareness of the relative importance of developmental areas. Speech, social and emotional behavior (such as smiling), and fine motor coordination, particularly in a young child, have greater prognostic significance than more traditionally accepted indexes of development, such as acquisition of gross motor skills and mastery of toileting. The times at which speech and language skills develop are perhaps the most useful clues in the determination of normality. Second in importance, and closely related to speech, are appropriate social behaviors. Delayed or atypical communication and socialization behaviors are highly significant in identifying children at risk in terms of development.

A final consideration is an emphasis on *rate as a principle* in developmental surveillance. Observations and assessments should be made on two or more occasions to determine developmental rate. This is particularly necessary in ruling out transient deficits resulting from normal variation or from the influence of illness or fatigue. The use of systematic procedures for developmental assessment can be helpful in this regard. For example, studies of parents participating in behavioral management of their children have demonstrated that they are capable of making valid and reliable observations. Asking parents to document the frequency, duration, and pattern of a particular problem (e.g., enuresis or temper tantrums) can provide a rich base of information for developmental assessment. A variety of useful observation techniques (e.g., diary, interval and time sampling) can be used by parents in this regard.

SELECTED SCREENING TESTS

The crux of developmental assessment is to differentiate the child with a significant developmental problem from the one who manifests variations within a normal pattern. Appropriate measures can assist a clinician to identify developmental problems in infancy, and the preschool physical examination provides an excellent opportunity to make a developmental assesment of value in predicting school performance. A valid and efficient assessment can be made of the developmental status of most preschool children by use of the physical examination and selected screening instruments. (See Table 18-4).

Although the Denver Developmental Screening Test (DDST) has been widely used and meets the criteria for specificity, it has been criticized for low sensitivity in that underreferrals are likely. This problem has led Meisels[9-11] to recommend that it be used in clinical contexts and that only tests that meet both specificity and sensitivity criteria be used in general screening efforts. This situation underscores the importance of attending to the larger issue of quality control in the purpose and method of screening. This is particularly significant for children whose at-risk condition may be confounded by poverty conditions or minority status. As Frankenburg et al.[6] have cautioned, any screening measure is subject to misuse; thus care needs to be taken to ensure that common pitfalls are avoided in screening and assessment of development. This assessment should encompass vision screening, hearing screening, and expressive and receptive language reflecting cognitive development, school readiness, self-awareness, and social awareness. Several screening instruments are available for these purposes and can be incorporated in the pediatric visit. Meisels[11] has recommended three screening measures that have both high specificity and sensitivity: the Minnesota Child Development Inventory (MCDI), the Early Screening Inventory (ESI), and the Minnesota Preschool Screening Inventory (MPSI). The Peabody Picture Vocabulary Test (PPVT) assesses receptive language in terms of a mental age and an intelligence quotient (IQ) and correlates well with more general measures of intellectual development. The Goodenough-Harris Drawing Test assesses general development and provides an index of self-awareness and social awareness. The DDST provides an overall assessment of development as well as specific data on personal-social, fine motor, language, and gross motor status. The School Readiness Survey is a simple screening technique that can be used by practitioners or parents to assess school readiness.

The various available screening instruments that focus on the preschool period and can facilitate identification of developmental delays are listed in Table 18-4. For more technical information (validity, specificity) on screening instruments, see Frankenburg and Camp,[5] Meisels,[10] and Meisels and Provence[12] (see also Appendix D).

Table 18-4 *Selected Screening Instruments*

INSTRUMENT	AGE (YR)
Denver Developmental Screening Test	0-6
Minnesota Child Developmental Inventory (MCDI)	6 mo-6
Peabody Picture Vocabulary Test (PPVT)[2]	2-adult
Early Screening Inventory (ESI)	3-6
Minnesota Preschool Screening Inventory (MPSI)	3½-5½
Goodenough-Harris Drawing Test	3-15
School Readiness Survey	4-6

The DDST, in its original and revised (DDST-R) recording forms, underwent major revisions and a restandardization in 1989. The new test, the Denver II shown in Fig. 18-2, differs from the DDST in items included (increased from 105 to 125 and changed to include more language items), the test form (the age scale conforms to the American Academy of Pediatrics Health Supervision Visit Schedule, the norms are updated and restandardized, and ratings of behavioral characteristics are included), and the interpretation (includes only the child's current developmental status). The Denver II also enables identification of significant subpopulation differences attributable to race, sex, maternal education, and place of residence (rural, semirural, urban).

The DDST is easy to administer (see sample test materials, Fig. 18-3), covers the age range of birth to 6 years, is highly reliable, and has concurrent and predictive validity. Only a few test items are needed, and instructions for administration of items, shown in Fig. 18-4, are printed on the back of the test form (Fig. 18-2). More detailed administration and scoring instructions are given in the DDST manual, which must be used to ensure accurate administration of the test.

The Denver Prescreening Developmental Questionnaire (PDQ) and its revised form (R-PDQ)[7] are questionnaires to be completed by parents and that can be interpreted in a few minutes. The R-PDQ includes all the DDST items and uses the same titles, which allows a comparison of a child's achievement with that of the standardization sample. Questions are arranged age-appropriately so that parents can see their child's developmental status. Given that the PDQ and the R-PDQ represent parental perception, verification of the information should be obtained by administering the DDST either in full or in part during the physical examination.*

CRITERIA FOR REFERRAL

The practitioner who is not sufficiently familiar with developmental diagnosis or management to be comfortable with independent handling of the case should make a referral to allied health professionals. Because of the complex needs of many children with developmental problems, it is highly desirable that assessment and management be integrated into an overall plan for the child's care.

Such an overall plan is implicit in the requirements of the Individualized Education Plan (IEP) for preschool and school-aged children and in the Individualized Family Service Plan (IFSP) defined in Public Law 99-457. Particularly important is establishing lines of communication and accountability on behalf of the family having a child with special needs. Given that the family may have contacts with many medical and nonmedical professionals, it is essential that someone serve as the coordinator of all services rendered (case manager).

*Testing kits, test forms, and reference manuals for the Denver Developmental Screening Test and Denver Prescreening Developmental Questionnaire may be ordered from the Denver Developmental Materials, Inc., P.O. Box 6919, Denver, CO 80206-0919.

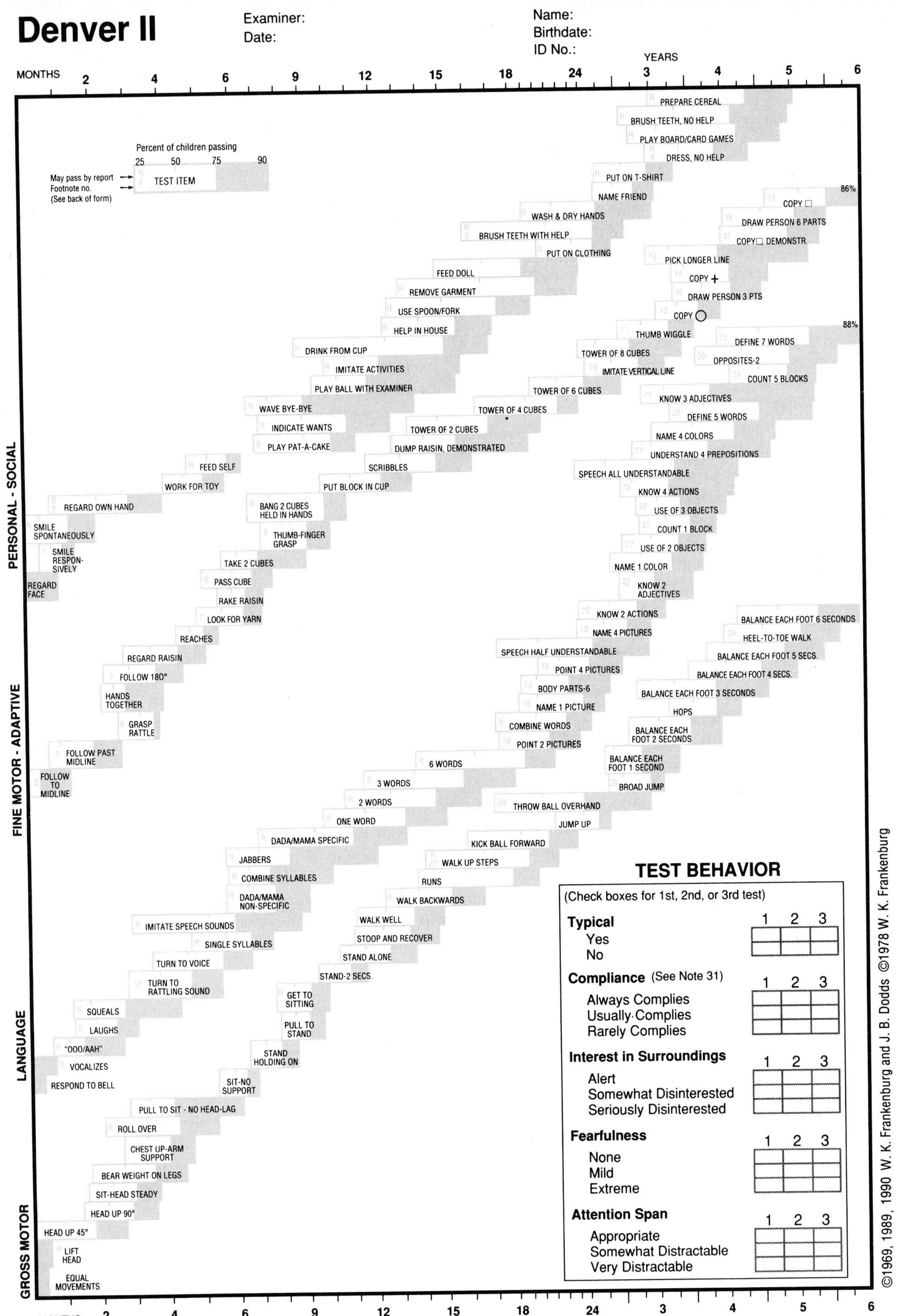

Fig. 18-2 Testing kits, test forms, and reference manuals (which must be used to ensure accuracy in administration of the test) for the DDST may be ordered from Denver Developmental Materials Incorporated, P.O. Box 6919, Denver, CO 80206-0919.

Reprinted with permission from William K. Frankenburg, M.D.

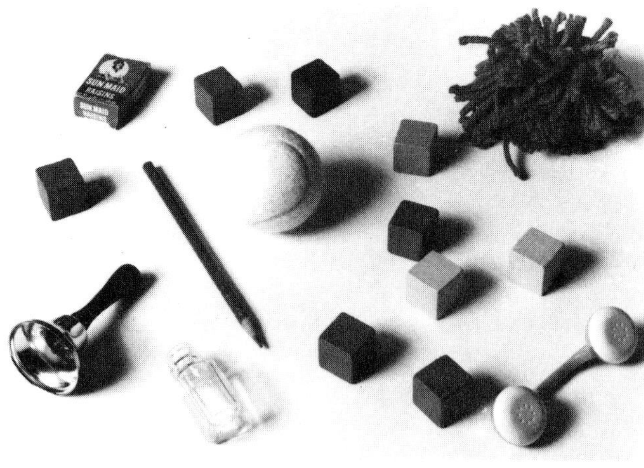

Fig. 18-3 Testing materials used in administering the Denver Developmental Screening Test.

The following categories of findings may serve as the basis for referrals for further services.

Delayed Development

When a child is at least one third below the expected age level in mental or motor development on the basis of developmental assessment or screening, referral to a psychologist or a physical therapist may be appropriate. The Denver Developmental Screening Test (DDST), the Peabody Picture Vocabulary Test (PPVT), the Minnesota Child Development Inventory (MCDI), the Minnesota Preschool Screening Inventory (MPSI), and the Early Screening Inventory (ESI) (see Table 18-4) may be useful for documenting such delays. The conditions most often associated with such delays are mild to moderate mental retardation and mild forms of cerebral palsy.

Abnormal or Atypical Development

Screening for emotional and behavioral problems is difficult in that the defining characteristics of atypical behavior vary as a function of sociocultural and developmental factors. Behavior considered inappropriate and deviant in a middle-class setting might not evoke concern in a lower-class environment.

Identifying psychological problems in young children is not without difficulty. Caregiver-completed questionnaires and checklists, as well as interview responses, may not be accurate, particularly when there may be reluctance to reveal a problem. The reading level of some instruments may be inappropriate for many parents, yielding questionable results. The use of psychological tests and formal observation may not be an assessment option for most practitioners, given the need for specialized training and administration time.

Presented with these difficulties, the physician who wishes to screen for psychological problems adequately should work with mental health professionals to identify effective and efficient methods. To this end, research findings suggest that the Behavior Screening Questionnaire[4] and the Pediatric Examination of Educational Readiness[9] may potentially be useful screening instruments for the pediatrician.

The presence of echolalia; repetitive, stereotypic mannerisms; withdrawn, uncontrollable, self-destructive, or abusive behavior; or poor or absent eye contact and social communication suggests the need for referral to a psychologist or a psychiatrist. Alone or in combination, these may reflect a variety of emotional and behavioral disturbances, ranging from acting out and testing of limits to expressions of psychopathologic conditions.

Erratic or Discrepant Development

Some children demonstrate wide gaps in developmental skills. Most notably, they may experience difficulty with fine or gross motor coordination, understanding or producing language, and encoding or decoding letters and numbers. The child's developmental profile may reflect a wide range of skills that include some average abilities. A modality or functional deficit is suggested when a discrepancy of one third or more is observed in developmental skills between one area and others; such a discrepancy should be the basis for referring for further assessment and possible intervention by developmental specialists. These discrepancies may signal sensory problems, perceptual or learning disabilities, or minimal brain dysfunction. In one screening study, for example, Morrison[13] and colleagues found an association between reading failure and behavior problems in children, indicating the need for focused diagnostic workups.

A key outcome of referral is the establishment of a diagnosis. This is particularly important in the area of parental counseling and acceptance of the child's problem and may indicate the need for genetic counseling. If speech, occupational, or physical therapy is required, referral can afford parents and health care providers a realistic assessment of the child's abilities and the development of specific plans for habilitation. Referral to the psychologist can result in more formal evaluation of both intellectual and personal-social functioning. Such information is a valuable base for parental understanding and involvement in interventions for the child.

One must not lose sight of how necessary the primary care practitioner's advocacy role is when referral is made. To avoid potential problems in the referral process, the information and interventions desired from the consultant should be clearly defined. When the pediatrician receives a referral—for example, from teachers or parents—pertaining to a child's inappropriate behavior, medication to effect behavioral change may be considered; when medication is indicated, it should be carefully monitored. Sensitivity to environmental or situational factors is particularly significant in monitoring the course of treatment for the so-called hyperactive child. Finally, referral for evaluation and diagnosis should be predicted on knowledge that intervention services and resources are available. Although schools are typical providers of special services for children with developmental problems, other resources exist at private, community, county, and state levels. Familiarity with available specialized resources for the treatment of handicapped children is essential if a comprehensive management plan is to be developed and implemented.

DIRECTIONS FOR ADMINISTRATION

1. Try to get child to smile by smiling, talking or waving. Do not touch him/her.
2. Child must stare at hand several seconds.
3. Parent may help guide toothbrush and put toothpaste on brush.
4. Child does not have to be able to tie shoes or button/zip in the back.
5. Move yarn slowly in an arc from one side to the other, about 8" above child's face.
6. Pass if child grasps rattle when it is touched to the backs or tips of fingers.
7. Pass if child tries to see where yarn went. Yarn should be dropped quickly from sight from tester's hand without arm movement.
8. Child must transfer cube from hand to hand without help of body, mouth, or table.
9. Pass if child picks up raisin with any part of thumb and finger.
10. Line can vary only 30 degrees or less from tester's line.
11. Make a fist with thumb pointing upward and wiggle only the thumb. Pass if child imitates and does not move any fingers other than the thumb.

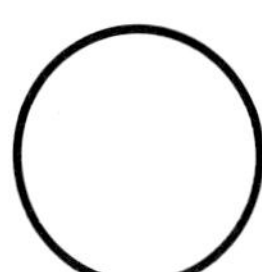

12. Pass any enclosed form. Fail continuous round motions.

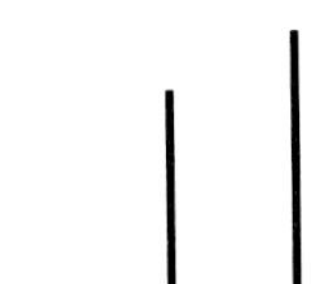

13. Which line is longer? (Not bigger.) Turn paper upside down and repeat. (pass 3 of 3 or 5 of 6)

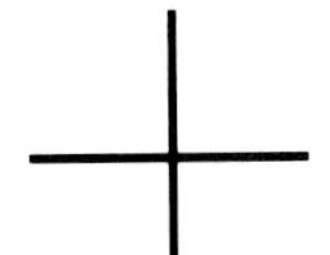

14. Pass any lines crossing near midpoint.

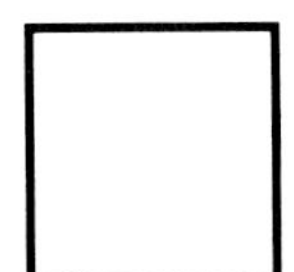

15. Have child copy first. If failed, demonstrate.

When giving items 12, 14, and 15, do not name the forms. Do not demonstrate 12 and 14.

16. When scoring, each pair (2 arms, 2 legs, etc.) counts as one part.
17. Place one cube in cup and shake gently near child's ear, but out of sight. Repeat for other ear.
18. Point to picture and have child name it. (No credit is given for sounds only.) If less than 4 pictures are named correctly, have child point to picture as each is named by tester.

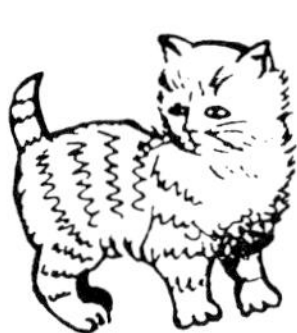
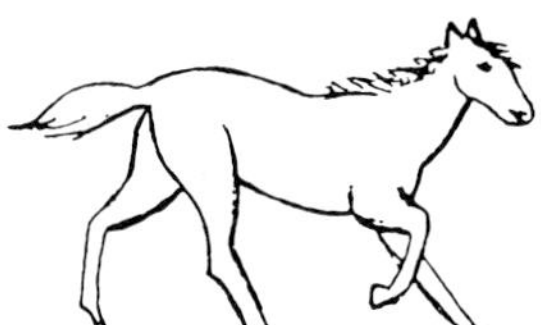
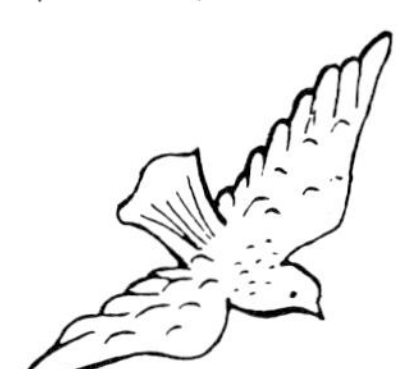
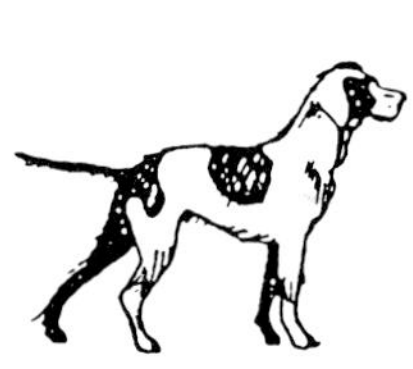
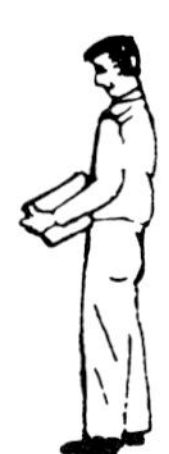

19. Using doll, tell child: Show me the nose, eyes, ears, mouth, hands, feet, tummy, hair. Pass 6 of 8.
20. Using pictures, ask child: Which one flies?... says meow?... talks?... barks?... gallops? Pass 2 of 5, 4 of 5.
21. Ask child: What do you do when you are cold?... tired?... hungry? Pass 2 of 3, 3 of 3.
22. Ask child: What do you do with a cup? What is a chair used for? What is a pencil used for? Action words must be included in answers.
23. Pass if child correctly places and says how many blocks are on paper. (1, 5).
24. Tell child: Put block **on** table; **under** table; **in front of** me, **behind** me. Pass 4 of 4. (Do not help child by pointing, moving head or eyes.)
25. Ask child: What is a ball?... lake?... desk?... house?... banana?... curtain?... fence?... ceiling? Pass if defined in terms of use, shape, what it is made of, or general category (such as banana is fruit, not just yellow). Pass 5 of 8, 7 of 8.
26. Ask child: If a horse is big, a mouse is __? If fire is hot, ice is __? If the sun shines during the day, the moon shines during the __? Pass 2 of 3.
27. Child may use wall or rail only, not person. May not crawl.
28. Child must throw ball overhand 3 feet to within arm's reach of tester.
29. Child must perform standing broad jump over width of test sheet (8 1/2 inches).
30. Tell child to walk forward, heel within 1 inch of toe. Tester may demonstrate. Child must walk 4 consecutive steps.
31. In the second year, half of normal children are non-compliant.

OBSERVATIONS:

Fig. 18-4 Instructions printed on the back of the DDST form for administering some of the items contained in the Denver Developmental Screening Test.

Reprinted with permission from William K. Frankenburg, M.D.

Twelve
Sickle Cell Conditions

Charles F. Whitten

There are two distinctly different types of sickle cell conditions: (1) sickle cell disease (primarily sickle cell anemia, sickle cell–hemoglobin C disease, and sickle cell–beta thalassemia disease) and (2) sickle cell trait. As for all health problems, screening for sickle cell conditions is justifiable only if those whose screening test results are positive receive some beneficial service. Beneficial services and methods for providing them are available for both types of sickle cell conditions.

Screening is of value with respect to the sickle cell diseases, although they are incurable and there are no established procedures for preventing the episodic complications or the progressive damage to tissues. Because of splenic dysfunction, children with sickle cell disease are prone to the development of bacterial infections, particularly by *Streptococcus pneumoniae,* which can proceed to septicemia and death ("sudden death") in a matter of hours. The level of fetal hemoglobin is high enough for the first several months to prevent intravascular sickling and the resultant manifestations of sickle cell disease. After that time, although intravascular sickling is present, overwhelming bacterial infections that lead to death can occur before the onset of characteristic symptoms that result in the diagnosis of sickle cell disease. A study conducted by the National Institutes of Health (NIH)[2] has clearly demonstrated the value of twice-daily oral administration of penicillin in preventing pneumococcal infections and death in young children with a sickle cell condition. On the basis of results of that study, participants in an NIH consensus conference[1] recommended that all newborns be screened for hemoglobinopathies and that penicillin be given for the first 5 years of life to those who have a sickle cell disease.

APPROACH TO SCREENING

Given the scope of the problem, the consensus conference participants further recommended that state governments mandate newborn screening for hemoglobinopathies and that there be established effective follow-up service programs.

For screening to be an effective factor in reducing morbidity and mortality from infections, several services must accompany screening of the newborn:

1. A repeat test must be performed after the first month or two because the newborn test results are only presumptive, unless it is known that both parents have sickle cell trait. There is a possibility that the fetal and sickle hemoglobin (FS) pattern, which is present if the newborn has sickle cell anemia, is also found if the newborn has another condition—that is, sickle cell hereditary persistence of fetal hemoglobin. Also, when an FS pattern is detected, it is possible that a small amount of normal adult hemoglobin (hemoglobin A) is present but not detected. The presence of small amounts of normal adult hemoglobin with FS hemoglobin is characteristic of sickle cell–beta thalassemia disease at birth.
2. Parents must be taught the manifestations of sickle cell disease.
3. Parents must be told of the need for penicillin prophylaxis and instructed how they should respond if the early signs and symptoms of infection or acute splenic sequestration (another cause of "sudden death") should occur. Symptoms include nasal congestion, cough, fever, lassitude, anorexia, pallor, and enlargement of the spleen.
4. Emergency rooms must be prepared to respond appropriately when a child with sickle cell disease has the aforementioned signs and symptoms. For example, in addition to receiving appropriate emergent medical care, which consists of antibiotics and/or transfusions, they must be seen immediately. Children with pneumococcal septicemia have died in emergency rooms while waiting to be seen by a physician.
5. Efforts must be made to ensure that potential barriers to the maintenance of penicillin prophylaxis (e.g., transportation and paying for penicillin) are removed.
6. The maintenance of penicillin prophylaxis must be monitored.

In many communities voluntary sickle cell organizations have trained counselors and social workers to assist in the provision of the necessary services—some of which are difficult or impossible for private physicians to provide.

In those states that do not mandate hemoglobinopathy screening during the newborn period, it is incumbent on physicians to screen all their infants who are at risk for sickle cell disease by the third month of age, thus enabling affected infants to be started on penicillin prophylaxis by the fourth month.

The recommendation of penicillin prophylaxis, of course, is not restricted to children whose disease is detected through newborn screening. All children younger than the age of 6 years who are diagnosed as having sickle cell disease should be placed on penicillin prophylaxis immediately.

There are other benefits to the identification of sickle cell disease in the newborn period. A high percentage of adults with sickle cell disease are not economically self-sufficient—that is, they depend on public assistance or their parents for support despite the only limitations with respect to employment being heavy manual labor and the potential for frequent attacks of pain that result in a high level of absenteeism that is incompatible with the employer's expectations. There is considerable evidence that the discrepancy between the potential for a person to be employed and that person's ability to gain and retain employment is the result of poor adjustment to the disease. Thus the early identification of sickle cell disease provides an opportunity for health care providers to begin to work with parents during their child's infancy to help them and their child make appropriate life-style adjustments to the disease. This attitude might be stated simplistically that children with a sickle cell disease are to be treated as being ill *only* when they are experiencing a manifestation of the disease; at all other times they are to be treated as though they are well.

With respect to the second sickle condition, sickle cell trait, it needs to be recognized that individuals who have this condition rarely have related health problems and thus usually do not discover their sickle cell trait other than through screening. These persons, however, have the potential (25% chance in each pregnancy) for having a child with one of the sickle cell diseases if their mate has a gene for one of the hemoglobinopathies. Unless they are made aware of this potential, they may have children with a sickle cell disease whom they might have chosen not to have, or they may suffer emotional and adjustment problems through lack of preparation for handling the difficulties associated with these illnesses. Thus the purpose of screening for sickle cell trait is to provide counseling that will enable those counseled to make informed decisions that they believe are in their best interest with respect to marriage and childbearing.

Screening for sickle cell trait therefore is only of benefit to children who are approaching childbearing age—a time at which information regarding marriage and reproduction is relevant. At that time the services consist of providing substantive information on the nature of sickle cell conditions, the risk of having a child with sickle cell disease, and the available reproductive options.[3] Traditionally this is termed *counseling,* but the process is really one of education, because persons should not be advised of what they should do but simply informed of consequences and the options available to them.

The physician should present a balanced picture of sickle cell anemia in counseling individuals who have sickle cell trait. Presentations that underplay the potential severity can influence persons to take the chance of having a child with sickle cell anemia whom they would not have had if they had been accurately informed. Presentations that fail to indicate the spectrum of severity and the potential for individuals with sickle cell anemia to live satisfying lives can influence potential parents not to take the risk despite strong wishes and needs to have children.

The physician should not assume that the differences between sickle cell trait and sickle cell anemia are understood among the laity. There is still a great deal of confusion about the nature of these conditions, their genetic origins, and the health status of persons who suffer from them. Thus, when some individuals are told that they have sickle cell trait, they may believe that their health status is threatened—a belief that can generate severe anxiety and depression.

The physician should not depict sickle cell trait as a disease. Other than the rare occurrence of hematuria, it has not been documented that sickle cell trait has any influence on health status under usual physiologic circumstances. Although there is a theoretic risk of intravascular sickling if sufficient oxygen deprivation occurs during surgery, there is no reason to assume that the competent surgeon and anesthesiologist would handle an oxygen-deprived person with sickle cell trait differently from one with normal hemoglobin patterns.

As indicated, the optimum time for sickle cell testing is at birth, a procedure that, if universally practiced, would lead to a population that would not require testing at any other time. However, because an at-risk population exists—which to a large extent has not been screened for sickle cell conditions either through mandatory newborn testing programs or testing by health care providers—it is important to decide when sickle cell testing/screening should occur for the unscreened.

For sickle cell trait, inasmuch as the sole purpose of screening is to enable personal marriage and reproductive decisions, the procedure should be deferred until just before the childbearing age is reached. It is of no value, for example, for an 8-year-old to be tested for sickle cell trait.

For sickle cell diseases, because the purpose is to provide comprehensive care, there is no need to screen the population after the age of 5 years because by that age manifestations of the disease invariably will have led to the diagnosis.

Although from a programatic standpoint the optimal timing for screening for sickle cell diseases and sickle cell trait is different, all screening methods identify both types of conditions. Thus, in screening newborns for sickle cell disease, newborns with sickle trait are identified. This is potentially advantageous because it means that at least one and possibly both parents have sickle cell trait, which results in a highly cost-beneficial detection of couples with sickle cell trait at a time when they are having children. Among the black population of the United States, the incidence of couples with sickle cell trait is approximately 1 in 144, whereas if a newborn has sickle cell trait, the probability of both parents having sickle cell trait is 1 in 12.

In addition to implementing service programs that achieve the benefits of screening, it is equally important to institute policies, procedures, and practices that avoid potential harmful outcomes. One of these is the exposure of nonpaternity. Instances in which the putative father is not the biologic father will be discovered in genetics counseling in all racial groups, and this information can traumatize and even destroy previously stable families.

It can be assumed that when a father is told that the child he thought was his is not, it is highly likely that this information will have a negative impact on his relationship with his partner and the child, particularly when the child has a chronic illness. The impaired relationship with the child might extend throughout a lifetime. To a large extent, this situation can be avoided through newborn screening programs. Unless it is absolutely essential for the treatment of the child or for providing reproductive counseling, the parents need not be tested when the child has a sickle cell disease. In most instances the diagnosis is clear and the parents can be told which genes they collectively have; the service providers do not need to know whether one or both parents carry the gene. Obviously, if the parents request testing, it should be performed. By the same token, if the newborn has one of the hemoglobinopathy traits transmitted by a single recessive gene, the mother should be tested for the purposes of reproductive counseling. If the mother does not have the trait (gene) in question, she can be told that the baby's father does. There is absolutely no need for the service providers to seek confirmation by testing the alleged father. On the other hand, if the mother has the trait, the father can then be tested with impunity (to determine the potential for the couple having a child with the disease) inasmuch as a source of the child's single, recessive gene (the mother) has been identified. If the providers in a given program feel morally compelled to give all fathers their test results (which means that in some cases fathers will become aware that they are not the father of the baby in question), they must implement informed consent procedures that give mothers sufficient information for them to decide whether they wish to take the risk of disclosing nonpaternity when they agree to parental testing.

Newborn screening for sickle cell conditions with current methods also detects the presence of other hemoglobinopathies that generally do not require immediate intervention because of morbidity or mortality. Given that the racial mix and thus the incidence of the various hemoglobinopathies vary from state to state, each state must determine how this information will be handled.

SCREENING TESTS

Several methods currently are used to screen newborns for sickle cell disease, including hemoglobin electrophoresis (cellulose acetate followed by citrate agar), ion exchange chromatography, isoelectric focusing, and high-performance liquid chromatography. The method to be used in central laboratories for statewide programs should be selected after careful consideration of the advantages and disadvantages of each.

In the past the solubility test has been used in screening programs conducted by voluntary sickle cell organizations and by individual physicians. It is simple and inexpensive to perform but should not be used alone for primary screening. Although the solubility test accurately identifies all who have inherited one or more sickle hemoglobin genes, it is not the screening procedure of choice. It will not detect individuals who have inherited the gene for hemoglobin C. Hemoglobin C occurs in about 2% of the black population and gives a negative solubility test result, leading persons screened by this procedure to assume that they cannot have a child with sickle cell disease. However, a black person with hemoglobin C trait who marries a black person has approximately an 8% chance of having married a person with sickle cell trait. Should this occur, there is a 25% chance in each pregnancy for the child to have sickle cell–hemoglobin C disease, a condition that is accompanied by the same symptoms found in sickle cell anemia, although it tends to be a milder disorder. Screening programs therefore should use a test that will detect hemoglobin C trait, as well as hemoglobin C disease. Persons with hemoglobin C disease may have a mild hemolytic anemia.

The primary screening test for small programs should be cellulose acetate electrophoresis. In such instances the solubility test can play an important role because it differentiates between hemoglobin S and hemoglobin D, which are not differentiated by cellulose acetate electrophoresis. The alternative is to follow cellulose acetate electrophoresis with citrate agar electrophoresis, which is far more expensive.

Thirteen

Programmatic Considerations in Initiating and Maintaining a Community Screening Program

William K. Frankenburg

It is ironic that the federal government does not permit the sale of new vaccines until extensive field trials have been undertaken and that the same government launches large-scale screening programs, such as the Early and Pediatric Screening, Diagnosis and Treatment (EPSDT) program, which services more than 12 million persons at a cost of many millions of dollars, without a single previous field trial. The EPSDT undertaking has resulted in programs of predictably uneven quality, expensive duplication of services, and lack of follow-through. Experience to date has demonstrated that proper community-based planning will do much to avoid such costly mismanagement. It is the purpose of this section to review the essential planning components needed to ensure a smoothly coordinated, efficient, and economical screening process.

In a community "child-find" effort, the most effective manner of ensuring that the program runs efficiently is to organize a steering committee comprising representatives of many sectors of the community. For instance, private physicians, nurses, welfare workers, teachers, psychologists, and specialists in audiology and speech pathology might represent the provider groups. Representation by locally elected officials, community leaders, and parents of the target population can assist greatly in the planning and execution of the project. Generally, such a committee could have the following functions:

1. To develop scientifically sound and efficient plans
2. To obtain full cooperation of various community and lay groups
3. To ensure that the plans make maximum use of community resources and that each phase of the program is fully coordinated

Another important step is to define the population that is to be screened. In doing so it is necessary to determine the geographic location of the people, their transportation needs, their ages, and their eligibility requirements.

Having defined the population, the committee is in a position to develop a list of health problems and handicapping conditions that are either known to or may afflict the population in question. Next the committee should consider each of the 13 principles of screening for each of the conditions listed (see Section One, General Considerations of this chapter, p. 211). By applying these principles, it can determine which diseases qualify and how and at what ages to screen. It also must consider who will carry out the actual screening and whether training or retraining of personnel will be required. The purchase of equipment may be necessary, and when and where children will be screened must be considered.

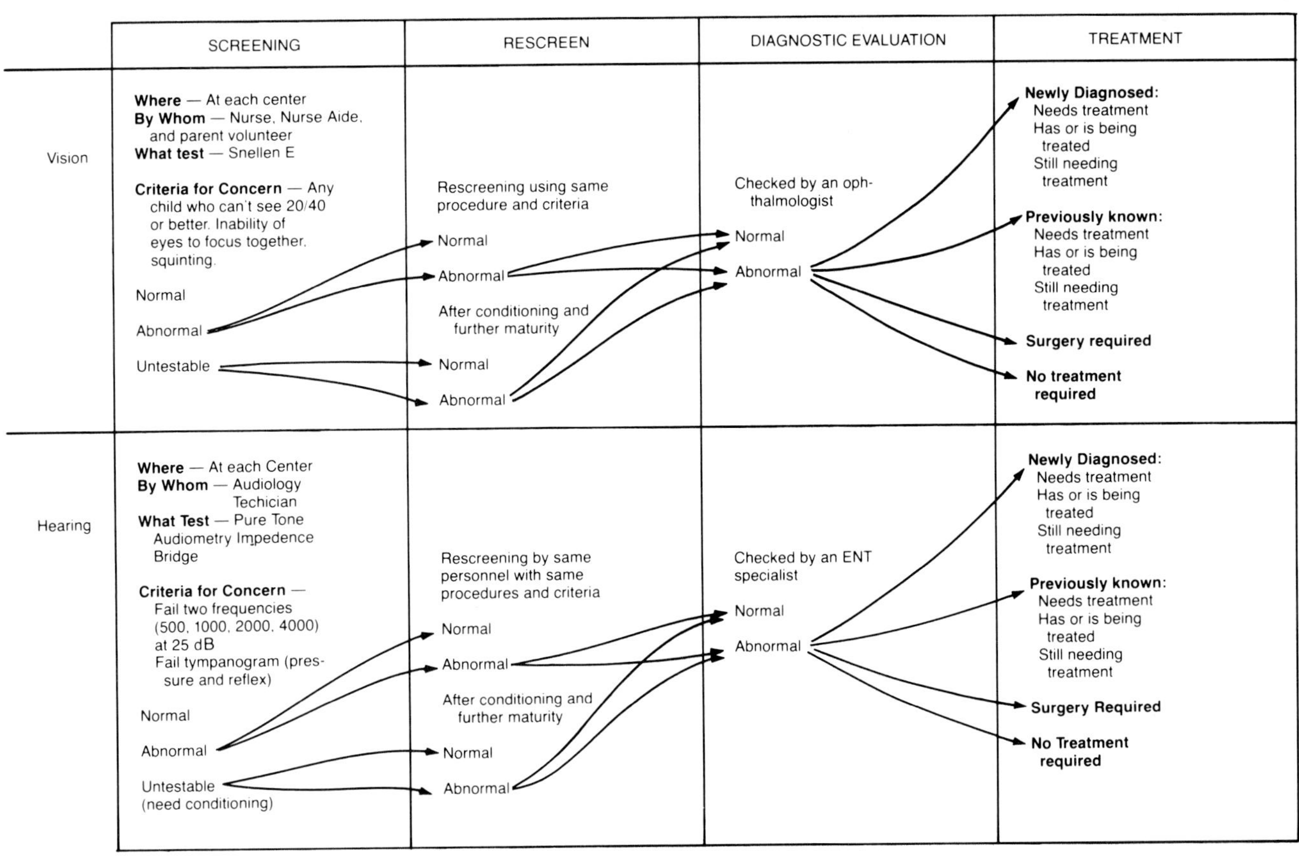

Fig. 18-5 Sample flowchart of screening, diagnosis, and treatment activities.

In general, it is ideal to ensure that all children with suspect findings are further evaluated and, when indicated, treated. Possible sites for screening include the primary health care setting, schools, public buildings, churches, and even the children's own homes.

In planning the follow-up of patients, it is helpful first to compile a list of the existing services in the community. While this is being done, gaps in services become readily apparent. Another consideration is the setting of priorities for diagnostic follow-up and treatment, because financial constraints sometimes preclude the treatment of minor problems.

The steering committee also must develop a flowchart of activities for coordinating the screening, diagnosis, and treatment of each condition with those of all the conditions. A sample flowchart is shown in Fig. 18-5. Through horizontal and vertical integration of services, the committee can minimize the trips to screening sites and to the physician.

Someone should be identified who is responsible for coordinating the entire program and monitoring the progress of individual children.

Assuming that all the foregoing has been accomplished, preparations must be made to inform the population of the program and to register all the children to be screened. In some cases, "outreach" workers must be used to find hard-to-contact parents and to provide transportation. Home visits for the actual testing may be necessary in some cases, even though they are extremely expensive. As parents have their children registered, the process should be explained to them, risks should be identified, and informed consent should be obtained. The last is particularly important in screening for genetic disorders.

An effective record-keeping system must be established to identify potential problems within the program and to facilitate the tracking of individual children. Adequate safeguards must be developed to ensure the confidentiality of findings.

The final consideration is the cost of each of the previously cited steps and the sources of necessary funds.

In short, a "child-find" project involves far more than screening. Rather, it is a community-wide effort to identify accurately and treat health hazards at minimum cost and effort and, at the same time, to protect the public from the many hazards of such an endeavor.

REFERENCES

General Considerations

1. Illingworth RS: The development of the infant and young child, ed 9, New York, 1987, Churchill Livingstone.

The Physical Examination as a Screening Test

1. Anderson FP: Evaluation of the routine physical examination of infants in the first year of life, Pediatrics 45:950, 1970.
2. Castelein RM and Sauter AJM: Ultrasound screening for congenital dysplasia of the hip in newborns: its value, J Pediatr Orthop 8:666, 1988.
3. Del Mar CB and Miller IS: Are child surveillance clinics worthwhile? Lancet 2:1334, 1987.
4. Editorial: School screening for scoliosis, Lancet 2:378, 1988.

5. Hoekelman RA: A summer Head Start medical program, Rochester, N.Y., 1969: implications for change, JAMA 219:730, 1972.
6. Kennedy FD: Have school-entry medicals had their day? Arch Dis Child 63:1261, 1988.
7. Knox EG and Lancashire RJ: Effectiveness of screening for congenital dislocation of the hip, J Epidemiol Community Health 41:283, 1987.
8. Renshaw TS: Screening school children for scoliosis, Clin Orthop 229:26, 1988.
9. Rogers KD and Reese G: Health studies—presumably normal high school students. I. Physical appraisal, Am J Dis Child 108:572, 1964.
10. Yankauer A and Lawrence R: A study of periodic school medical examinations. II, The annual increment of new "defects," Am J Public Health 46:1553, 1956.

Tuberculin Skin Testing

1. American Academy of Pediatrics: Report of the Committee on Infectious Diseases, ed 24, Evanston, Ill, 1990, The Academy.

Screening for Drugs

1. American Academy of Pediatrics: Screening for drugs of abuse in children and adolescents, Pediatrics 84:396, 1989.
2. American Medical Association, Council on Scientific Affairs: Scientific issues in drug testing, JAMA 257:3110, 1987.
3. Bays J: Substance abuse and child abuse, Pediatr Clin North Am 37:881, 1990.
4. Chasnoff IJ: Drug use and women: establishing a standard of care, Ann NY Acad Sci 562:208, 1989.
5. Hans SL: Developmental consequences of prenatal exposure to methadone, Ann NY Acad Sci 562:195, 1989.
6. Johnson LD, O'Malley PM, and Bachman JG: Drug use by high school seniors—the class of 1986, US Department of Health and Human Services Pub No (ADM) 87-1535, Rockville, Md, 1987.

Use of Urinalysis and the Urine Culture in Screening

1. Dodge WF et al: Proteinuria and hematuria in schoolchildren: epidemiology and natural history, J Pediatr 88:329, 1976.
2. Gutgesell M: Practicality of screening urinalysis in asymptomatic children in a primary care setting, Pediatrics 62:103, 1978.
3. Hansson S et al: Untreated bacteriuria in asymptomatic girls with renal scarring, Pediatrics 84:964, 1989.
4. Kitagawa T: Screening for renal disease in school children: experience in Japan, Indian J Pediatr 55:481, 1988.
5. Newcastle Covert Bacteriuria Research Group: Covert bacteriuria in schoolgirls in Newcastle upon Tyne: a 5-year follow-up, Arch Dis Child 56:585, 1981.
6. Silverberg DS: City-wide screening for urinary abnormalities in schoolgirls, Can Med Assoc J 109:981, 1973.
7. Silverberg DS: City-wide screening for urinary abnormalities in schoolboys, Can Med Assoc J 111:410, 1974.
8. Thompson AL et al: Fixed and reproducible orthostatic proteinuria. VI. Results of a 10-year follow-up evaluation, Ann Intern Med 73:235, 1970.
9. Verier Jones K et al: Glomerular filtration rate in schoolgirls with covert bacteriuria, Br Med J 285:1307, 1982.

Auditory Screening

1. American Speech-Language-Hearing Association: Audiologic screening of newborn infants who are at risk for hearing impairment, ASHA 31:89, 1989.
2. Dahle AJ et al: Progressive hearing impairment in children with congenital cytomegalovirus infection. J Speech and Hear Dis 44:220, 1979.
3. Konigsmark BW and Gorlin RJ: Genetic and metabolic deafness, Saunders, Philadelphia, 1976.
4. Naulty CM, Weiss IP, and Herez GR: Progressive sensorineural hearing loss in survivors of persistent fetal circulation, Ear and Hearing 7:74, 1986.
5. Roeser RJ and Northern JL: Screening for hearing loss and middle ear disorders. In Roeser RJ and Downs M, editors: Auditory disorders in school children, New York, 1981, Thieme-Stratton, Inc.

Developmental Assessment

1. American Academy of Pediatrics: Recommendations for preventive pediatric health care, Pediatrics 81:466, 1988.
2. Dunn LM: Manual for the Peabody Picture Vocabulary Test–Revised, Circle Pines, Minn, 1981, American Guidance Service.
3. Dworkin PH: Developmental screening—expecting the impossible? Pediatrics 84:619, 1989.
4. Earls F et al: Concurrent validation of a behavior problems scale for use with 3-year-olds, J Am Acad Child Adol Psychiatry 21:47, 1982.
5. Frankenburg WK and Camp BW, editors: Pediatric screening tests, Springfield, Ill, 1975, Charles C Thomas, Publisher.
6. Frankenburg WK, Chen J, and Thornton SM: Common pitfalls in the evaluation of developmental screening tests, J Pediatr 113:1110, 1988.
7. Frankenburg WK, Fandal AW, and Thornton SM: The revised prescreening developmental questionnaire.
8. Hutchinson T and Nicoll A: Developmental screening and surveillance, Br J Hosp Med 39:22, 1988.
9. Levine M et al: The pediatric examination of educational readiness: validation of an extended observation procedure, Pediatrics 66:341, 1980.
10. Meisels SJ: Developmental screening in early childhood: the interaction of research and social policy, Annu Rev Public Health 9:527, 1988.
11. Meisels SJ: Can developmental screening tests identify children who are developmentally at risk? Pediatrics 83:578, 1989.
12. Meisels SJ and Provence S: Screening and assessment: guidelines for identifying young disabled and developmentally vulnerable children and their families, Washington, DC, 1989, National Center for Clinical Infant Programs.
13. Morrison D, Mantizicopoulos P, and Cart E: Preacademic screening for learning and behavior problems, J Am Acad Child Adolesc Psychiatry, 28:101, 1985.

Sickle Cell Conditions

1. Consensus conference: Newborn screening for sickle cell disease and other hemoglobinopathies, JAMA 254:1205, 1987.
2. Gaston MD et al: Prophylaxis with oral penicillin in children with sickle cell anemia, N Engl J Med 314:1593, 1986.
3. Whitten CF, Thomas J, and Nishiura EN: Sickle cell trait counseling: evaluation of counselors and counselees, Am J Hum Genet 33:802, 1981.

SUGGESTED READINGS

General Considerations

American Academy of Pediatrics, Committee on Practice and Ambulatory Medicine: Recommendations for preventative pediatric health care, Pediatrics 81:466, 1988.

Dworkin PH: British and American recommendations for developmental monitoring—the role of surveillance, Pediatrics 84:1000, 1989.

Klaucke DN et al: Guidelines for evaluating surveillance systems, MMWR 37(suppl):May 6, 1988.

Screening for Genetic-Metabolic Disorders

American Academy of Pediatrics Committee on Genetics: New issues in newborn screening for phenylketonuria and congenital hypothyroidism, Pediatrics 69:104, 1982.

American Academy of Pediatrics Committee on Genetics: Newborn screening fact sheets, Pediatrics 83:449, 1989.

American Academy of Pediatrics Committee on Genetics and American Thyroid Association: Newborn screening for congenital hypothyroidism: recommended guidelines, Pediatrics 80:745, 1987.

American Academy of Pediatrics Committee on Nutrition: Indications for cholesterol testing in children, Pediatrics 83:141, 1989.

Consensus conference: Newborn screening for sickle cell disease and other hemoglobinopathies, JAMA 258:1205, 1987.

Holtzman NA: Proceed with caution: predicting genetic risks in the recombinant DNA era, Baltimore, 1989, The Johns Hopkins University Press.

Holtzman NA, Leonard CO, and Farfel MR: Issues in antenatal and neonatal screening and surveillance for hereditary and congenital disorders, Annu Rev Public Health 2:219, 1981.

March of Dimes Birth Defects Foundation: International directory of genetic services, White Plains, NY, 1986, The Foundation.

National Center for Education in Maternal and Child Health: State treatment centers for metabolic disorders, Washington, DC, 1986, The Center.

New England Regional Genetics Group Prenatal Collaborative Study of Down Syndrome Screening: Combining maternal serum alpha-fetoprotein measurements and age to screen for Down syndrome in pregnant women under age 35, Am J Obstet Gynecol 160:575, 1989.

Rhoads GG et al: The safety and efficacy of chorionic villus sampling for early prenatal diagnosis of cytogenetic abnormalities, N Engl J Med 320:609, 1989.

Scriver CR et al: The metabolic basis of inherited disease, ed 6, New York, 1989, McGraw Hill, Inc.

Tuberculin Skin Testing

American Thoracic Society: Statement by the Committee on Diagnostic Skin Testing, Am Rev Respir Dis 102:466, 1971.

Brickman HF, Beaudry PH, and Marks MI: The timing of tuberculin tests in relation to immunization with live viral vaccines, Pediatrics 55:392, 1975.

Gantz NM: Tuberculin skin testing: when and how to use it, Hosp Pract 21:25, 1986.

Inselman LS: Tuberculosis in children: an unsettling forecast, Contemp Pediatr 7:110, 1990.

Kraut JR et al: Assessment of tuberculin screening in an urban pediatric clinic, Pediatrics 64:856, 1979.

MacLean RA: Tuberculin testing antigens and techniques, Chest 68(suppl):455, 1975.

Skin test antigens: An evaluation whose time has come, Am Rev Respir Dis 118:1, 1978 (editorial).

Sokal JE: Measurement of delayed skin test responses, N Engl J Med 293:501, 1975.

Screening for Anemia

Piomelli S: Diagnostic approach to anemia, Pediatr Clin North Am 18:3, 1971.

Piomelli S, Brickman A, and Carlos E: Rapid diagnosis of Fe deficiency by measurement of free erythrocyte porphyrins (FEP) and hemoglobin: the FEP/hemoglobin ratio, Pediatrics 57:136, 1976.

Screening for Lead Poisoning

U.S. Centers for Disease Control. Strategic plan for eradicating childhood lead poisoning in the 1990s, 1991

Screening for Drugs

Amaro H, Zuckerman B, and Cabral H: Drug use among adolescent mothers: profile of risk, Pediatrics 84:144, 1989.

Chávez GF, Mulinare J, and Cordero JF: Maternal cocaine use during early pregnancy as a risk factor for congenital urogenital anomalies, JAMA 262:795, 1989.

Frank DA et al: Cocaine use during pregnancy: prevalence and correlates, Pediatrics 82:888, 1988.

Hadeed AJ and Siegel SR: Maternal cocaine use during pregnancy: effect on the newborn infant, Pediatrics 84:205, 1989.

Matera C et al: Prevalence of use of cocaine and other substances in an obstetric population, Am J Obstet Gynecol 163:797, 1990.

Tennant F and Shannon J: Quantitative urine testing: a new tool for diagnosing and treating cocaine use, Postgrad Med 86(3):107, 1989.

Zuckerman B, Amaro H, and Cabral H: Validity of self-reporting of marijuana and cocaine use among pregnant adolescents, J Pediatr 115:812, 1989.

Zuckerman B et al: Effects of maternal marijuana and cocaine use on fetal growth, N Engl J Med 320:762, 1989.

Use of Urinalysis and the Urine Culture in Screening

Bee DE, James GP, and Paul KL: Hemoglobinuria and hematuria: accuracy and precision of laboratory diagnosis, Clin Chem 25:1696, 1979.

Corman LI et al: Simplified urinary microscopy to detect significant bacteriuria, Pediatrics 70:133, 1982.

Glassock RJ: Postural proteinuria: no cause for concern, N Engl J Med 305:639, 1981.

Hermansen MC and Blodgett FM: Prospective evaluation of routine admission urinalyses, Am J Dis Child 135:126, 1981.

Jaffe RM et al: Inhibition by ascorbic acid (vitamin C) of chemical detection of blood in urine, Am J Clin Pathol 72:468, 1979.

Jodal U: The natural history of bacteriuria in childhood, Infect Dis Clin North Am 1:713, 1987.

Kiel DP and Moskowitz MA: The urinalysis: a critical approach, Med Clin North Am 71:607, 1987.

Norman ME: An office approach to hematuria and proteinuria, Pediatr Clin North Am 34:545, 1987.

Rytand DA and Spreiter S: Prognosis in postural (orthostatic) proteinuria, N Engl J Med 305:618, 1981.

Vehaskari VM and Rapola J: Isolated proteinuria: analysis of a school-age population, J Pediatr 101:661, 1982.

Auditory Screening

Jerger J, editor: Handbook of clinical impedance audiometry, Dobbs Ferry, NY, 1975, American Electromedics Corp.

Galambos R, Hicks GE, and Wilson MJ: Identification audiometry in neonates: a reply to Simmons, Ear Hear 3:189, 1972.

McCandless G and Thomas G: Impedance as a screening procedure for middle ear disease, Trans Am Acad Ophthalmol Otolaryngol 78:98, 1974.

Northern JL and Downs M: Hearing in children, ed 3, Baltimore, 1984, The Williams & Wilkins Co.

Simmons BF: Comment on hearing loss in graduates of a tertiary intensive care nursery, Ear Hear 3:188, 1982.

Simmons BF: Identification of hearing loss in children, Otolaryngol Clin North Am 11:19, 1978.

Developmental Assessment

Beery KE: Developmental test of visual-motor integration: administration and scoring manual, Chicago, 1967, Follett Educational Corp.

Earls F et al: Concurrent validation of a behavior problems scale for use with 3-year-olds, J Am Acad Child Adolesc Psychiatry 21:47, 1982.

Frankenburg WK, Sciarillo W, and Burgess D: The newly abbreviated and revised Denver Developmental Screening Test, J Pediatr 99:995, 1981.

Jordan FL and Massey J: School readiness survey, Palo Alto, Calif, 1967, Consulting Psychologists Press.

Levine M et al: The pediatric examination of educational readiness: validation of an extended observation procedure, Pediatrics 66:341, 1980.

19

Physical Fitness in Children

R. Joseph Jopling

Health-related fitness is not necessarily associated with athletic ability or physical appearance; rather, it represents a number of life-style decisions that allow individuals to maximize their inherent genetic potential for a healthy life.[8] The decline of health-related fitness parameters among children in the United States is well documented,[20] and the relationship of those parameters to preventable diseases of adulthood has been strongly suggested if not proven.[12,13,24] The problem is pervasive and has certainly seemed refractory to change. This chapter suggests how primary care pediatricians might discuss the problem with their patients and then help them devise a health-related fitness program.

HEALTH-RELATED FITNESS PARAMETERS AND PREVENTABLE DISEASES

Cardiovascular diseases (myocardial infarctions, hypertension, and stroke), obesity, and some cancers (such as lung and colon cancer) are not only major sources of morbidity and mortality but are also thought to be preventable at least in part by changes in life-style.[15,17] Because life-styles are begun and largely learned in childhood, it would seem logical that risk factors present in childhood will be present in adulthood. Life-styles tend to become more difficult to change as individuals become older. Therefore the younger the patient, the more likely that changes in life-style will help prevent or at least reduce the effects later in life of these major diseases, and the more easily these changes in life-style can be made. It might be easier and more cost effective to prevent inherently active children from becoming sedentary as adults than it would be to try to change these habits after they reach adulthood.

Most experts agree that poor health-related fitness parameters correlate directly with an increase in cardiovascular disease risk factors such as obesity, hypertension, elevated serum cholesterol levels, and physical inactivity. Sixty percent of adults are overweight, and more than 25% are obese (more than 20 pounds overweight). Twelve percent of prepubertal children and 16% of adolescents are considered to be overweight. Worse yet, the number of overweight children is increasing.[6] Among adults, 10% to 20% have high serum cholesterol levels; however, increased serum lipids is not just a disease of adulthood; the problem begins in childhood. Atherosclerotic fatty streaks have been found in children as young as 3 years of age. By 22 years of age, from 45% to 77% of individuals may have evidence of atherosclerosis. Ten percent of adults and 5% of children are considered hypertensive. Most cigarette smokers begin smoking by 20 years of age. Psychosocial stress is more intense and more prevalent at earlier ages than ever before. In an epidemiologic review study conducted by the Centers for Disease Control, physical inactivity was shown to be as strong a risk factor in coronary heart disease as the traditional risk factors of smoking, hypertension, and high serum cholesterol levels.[16] Even more important, physical inactivity was shown to be three to six times more prevalent than any other risk factor. Only 20% of adults exercise adequately, and 60% are completely inactive. Only 36% of children have daily physical education classes. According to the 1984 National Children and Youth Fitness Study, only 66% of children 10 to 17 years of age were participating in physical activity at the recommended level (three or more times per week, 20 minutes or longer per session, in an activity that was likely to be done as an adult, that required 60% or more of cardiorespiratory capacity, and that involved large muscle groups in dynamic contraction).

Clearly the U.S. Public Health Service's 1990 goal of greater than 90% participation has not been met, and with budgetary constraints squeezing educational systems across the country, there is a definite risk of the proportion of children participating even declining, much less rising. Even when physical education classes are offered, many of the classes emphasize team sports instead of individual lifelong activities (e.g., aerobic exercises that can be done alone, such as walking, swimming, or cycling). Adding to the inactivity problem is the fact that American children average 25 hours a week sitting in front of the television set, frequently consuming some type of snack food while doing so.

Contrary to what one might think, this is not a recently identified issue. As early as the 1940s, Kraus and Webber recognized a health-related physical fitness problem.[9,10,24] Comparison of their findings in American children to those in European children showed that American children were woefully less fit than their European counterparts. That fact helped lead to the formation of the President's Council on Youth Fitness (known today as the President's Council on Physical Fitness and Sports).

Recently, fewer than half of the children taking the fitness test of the President's Council on Physical Fitness and Sports passed it. Only 60% of boys 6 to 12 years of age and only 30% of girls 6 to 17 years of age could do more than one chin-up. Similarly, only 64% of boys and 50% of girls 6 to 12 years of age could run or walk a mile in less than 10 minutes. In 1984 only 2% of all children taking the "President's Challenge" could qualify for the award that required them to do well uniformly in chin-ups, sit-ups, flexibility, a 1-mile run or walk, and a shuttle run.

Again, almost all experts agree that the best way to try to

reverse these problems is to change life-styles. One of the best ways to accomplish changes in life-style is through implementing health-related fitness programs. Such programs promote cardiovascular endurance, large muscle strength and endurance, flexibility, a healthy percent of body fat for age and sex, a healthy diet, and acquisition of stress management techniques (see box below).

CARDIOVASCULAR ENDURANCE

Cardiovascular endurance (cardiovascular fitness) is achieved by performing aerobic exercise for a minimum of 30 minutes at a time while maintaining the heart rate at 60% to 80% of a calculated maximum. Initially, the minimum exercise time thought to be needed for an aerobic effect was 15 and then 20 minutes; now it is 30 minutes. An inactive person would be best off starting at whatever level and duration of continuous activity can be tolerated safely and gradually working up to 30 minutes.

Recommendations for an intensity level have also gone through several changes. Initially, exercise physiologists proposed that reaching a target heart rate is necessary for achieving an aerobic exercise threshold that leads to improvement in aerobic fitness. Now most exercise physiologists and cardiologists feel that unless an individual is already relatively fit, it is a mistake even to discuss target heart rates. Instead, they would initially stress increasing one's level of physical activity.[1] Borg has proposed a "perceived exertion" scale as an adequate measure of one's heart rate.[2] A common rule of thumb that can be used to gauge proper intensity is to exercise at least enough to perspire while maintaining the ability to carry on a conversation. Specifically, a person who has been relatively inactive should aim for the 60% target range when first starting an aerobic exercise program. People who are already active and want more specific information should consult published guidelines for heart rates during exercise (Table 19-1). It cannot be overemphasized that these numbers are based on *suggestions* for training athletes and should not be thought of as hard-and-fast rules.

Overuse syndromes and undue pressure on children from well-intentioned adults must be mentioned when discussing intensity. Exercising to the point of pain should be discouraged, for it eventually leads to injury. The advice "slow but sure" most often prevails in trying to achieve long-term changes. It is always wise to suggest that adults over 40 years of age or those who have a family history of cardiovascular disease see their physician before starting any type of exercise program.

Components of Health-Related Fitness

CARDIORESPIRATORY ENDURANCE

This is achieved through performing any one of a number of aerobic exercises while maintaining heart rate at 60%-80% of a calculated maximum for a minimum of 30 minutes at a time, at least three times per week, for a minimum of 6 consecutive months.

MUSCULAR STRENGTH

Leg muscle strength is related to the ability to perform aerobic exercise. Abdominal muscle strength aids in proper breathing technique and helps to protect the lower back. Upper body strength is important to overall muscle balance and aids in many everyday activities.

FLEXIBILITY

Flexibility helps prevent musculoskeletal injuries and can make one feel more spry. Without warm-up and cool-down stretching periods, an exercise program can lead to a loss of flexibility.

PROPER DIET

A diet composed of a balance of the four basic food groups, high in carbohydrates, low to moderate in proteins, low in fats, and moderate in total calories is essential to any fitness program.

BODY COMPOSITION

Baseline and follow-up measurement of percentage of body fat is one of the best indicators of progress in health-related fitness. Following body weight or height-to-weight ratio can be misleading in assessing fitness level.

Modified from Jopling RJ: Health-related fitness as preventive medicine, Pediatr Rev 10:141, 1988.

Table 19-1 *Suggested Training Heart Rates**

AGE (YR)	HEART RATE (BEATS/MIN) MAXIMUM	80%	60%
5-8	220	176	132
10	210	168	126
11	209	167	125
12	208	166	125
13	207	165	124
14	206	165	123
15	205	164	123
16	204	163	122
17	203	162	122
18	202	162	121
19	201	161	121
20	200	160	120
22	198	158	118
24	196	157	117
26	194	155	116
28	192	154	115
30	190	152	114
32	189	151	113
34	187	150	112
36	186	149	111
38	184	147	110
40	182	146	109
45	179	143	107
50	175	140	105
55	171	137	102
60	160	128	96
65	150	120	90

*These numbers are taken from a variety of sources and are suggested guidelines initially developed for training athletes. Individuals will vary. If the target heart rate seems too hard to maintain, then a lower one should be accepted; conversely, if the target heart rate does not seem high enough to produce a sweat, the individual should work harder. (From Jopling RJ: Health-related fitness as preventive medicine, Pediatr Rev 10:141, 1988.)

Gradual warm-up and cool-down periods help to ensure a safe workout by allowing muscles, joints, and the cardiovascular system to adapt to the changes of exercise. Just after the warm-up and cool-down periods are also the optimum times to stretch to help maintain flexibility.

Exercising a minimum of three times per week helps to maintain an aerobic fitness level; exercising five times a week usually ensures an increase in one's aerobic fitness level. These training guidelines are well established for adults, and although there is less documentation for children, these guidelines have been applied by some to children as young as 6 years of age.

Most people need a commitment of at least 6 months (and some more than 12 months) to any exercise program to see any significant changes in the parameters of their health-related fitness. The reverse is also true in that the positive changes gained from a health-related fitness program are lost if the program is not maintained. A review of some of the benefits and risks of physical activity is found in Table 19-2.

Numerous activities can qualify as aerobic (see box below). Brisk walking deserves special mention, because it is an aerobic activity that can be done by almost everyone right from the beginning of any fitness program. Few exercises enable a family to exercise as a unit and at the same time allow all of the members to achieve an aerobic intensity level, but walking at a brisk pace can usually be done aerobically at the same time by all, or at least by most, family members. It can be done around the neighborhood for convenience or as a hike for variation. If inclement weather pre-

Table 19-2 *Benefits and Risks of Physical Activity**

SYSTEM AND BENEFIT	SURETY RATING	RISK	SURETY RATING
Cardiovascular			
Blood pressure	2+	Cardiac arrest	2+
Improved serum lipid profile	1+		
Smoking cessation/prevention	0+		
Weight control	2+		
Independent effect	2+		
Psychological			
Improved affect	1+	Exercise addiction	1+
Increased self-esteem	2+		
Positive personality change	0		
Improved cognition	0		
Musculoskeletal: Prevention of postmenopausal bone loss	2+	Amenorrhea/bone loss	2+
		Trauma	2+
Central nervous system: Improved sleep	0		
Endocrine: Decreased risk of type II diabetes	0	Decreased libido	0
Gastrointestinal tract: Increased colonic motility	0	Diarrhea	1+

*The surety rating is derived from a review of the literature and is a subjective judgment of Dr. Phelps. 0, The current literature presents mixed data claiming benefit or risk; 1+, most but not all data in the literature support the claim; 2+, data in the current literature establish the benefit of risk. (From Phelps JR: Physical activity and health maintenance: exactly what is known? West J Med 146:200, 1987.)

Suggestions for Fitness Activities (minimum of 30 minutes daily)

- Brisk walk
- 5K walk/run
- Cycling
- Swimming
- Aerobic exercise class
- Dance
- Basketball
- Tumbling
- Skating
- Playground activities
- Cross-country skiing
- Racquet sports
- Jogging
- Hiking
- Soccer
- Jump rope
- Strength training
- Volleyball
- Stretching
- Martial arts
- Tag games
- Other ________

NOTE:

Stretch before and after every activity.
For a more balanced fitness program, include activities for stomach muscles (modified sit-ups) and for upper body muscles (push-ups/pull-ups).

From the Governor's Family FUN Award Program, Utah Governor's Council on Health and Physical Fitness, Salt Lake City, Utah.

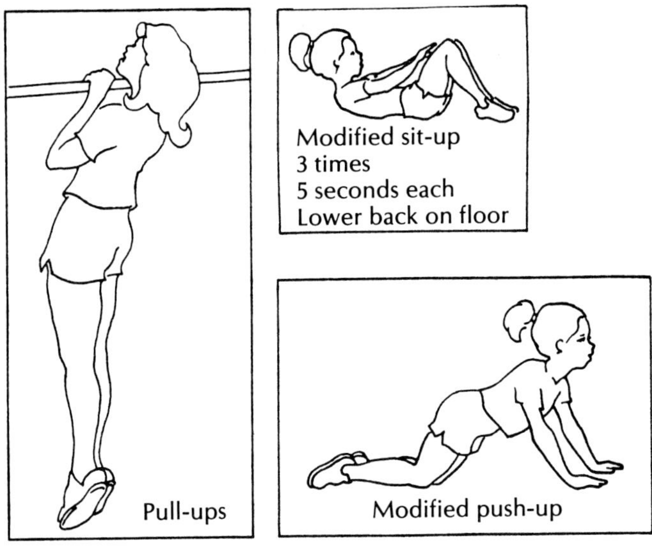

Fig. 19-1 Suggested exercises for muscular strength.
From "Youth Fitness," an educational handout from Ross Laboratories.

sents a problem, walking can be done inside a shopping mall or gym.

Stationary bicycles, cross-country ski machines, and rowing machines are reasonable investments to ensure family access to aerobic exercise day or night. With a little insistence, one of these activities could replace snacking as the activity that most frequently accompanies TV viewing.

LARGE MUSCLE STRENGTH

Large muscle strength and endurance are related to aerobic exercise for two reasons. Larger muscle groups are usually the ones used in aerobic activities, and a large muscle relaxation-contraction cycle repeated for a sufficient length of time results in an increased mitochondrial mass of the muscle tissue and therefore in increased aerobic enzymes per unit of tissue mass. Muscle contraction tends to occlude local circulation when the muscle is contracting at more than 30% of maximum capacity. As muscles become stronger, they can perform more work before interfering with local circulation and therefore stay aerobic longer whether they are performing intense or everyday activities.

Abdominal muscles help in breathing and protecting the lower back muscles. The safest way to strengthen the abdominal muscles is to increase gradually the number of modified sit-ups one can do. Modified sit-ups are done with the knees flexed and the feet on the ground or with the lower legs resting on a chair while maintaining the lumbar spine in contact with the floor during the sit-up (Fig. 19-1).

Upper body strength is also important, because it is helpful in everyday activities and makes for more of a balance in overall fitness. Push-ups or modified push-ups and pull-ups (or flexed-arm hangs) are easy ways to improve upper body strength (Fig. 19-1). If free weights or weight machines are used to strengthen muscles, relatively low weights and a high number of repetitions (20 or more) are most helpful, since they develop muscle endurance and strength rather than muscle bulk.

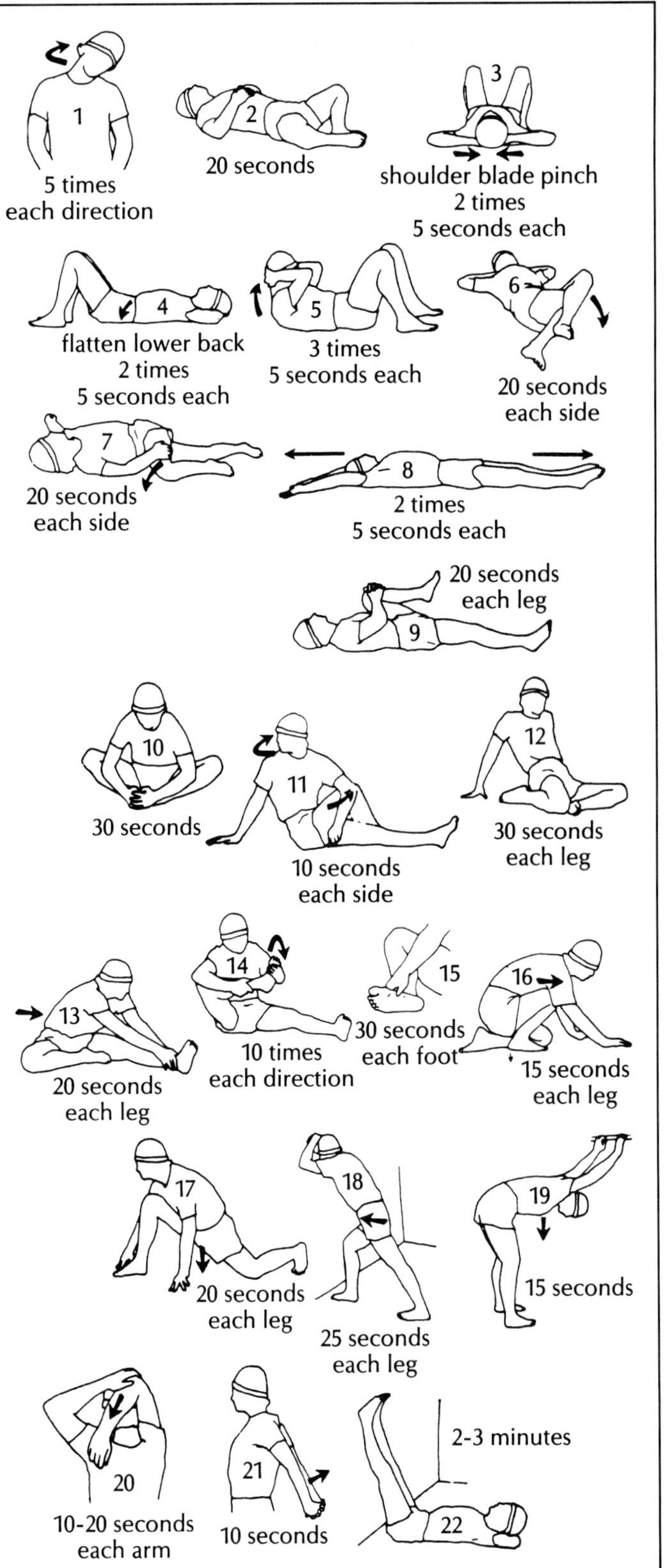

Fig. 19-2 Everyday stretches—approximately 10 to 15 minutes. Use these stretches every day to fine-tune your muscles. This is a general routine that emphasizes stretching and relaxing muscles more frequently used during normal day-to-day activities. In simple tasks of everyday living, we often use our bodies in strained or awkward ways, creating stress and tension. A kind of muscular rigor mortis sets in. If you can set aside 10 to 15 minutes every day for stretching, you will offset this accumulated tension so you can use your body with greater ease.
From Anderson B: Stretching, Bolinas, CA, 1980, Shelter Publications, Inc.

FLEXIBILITY

Flexibility helps in preventing musculoskeletal injuries and in making one feel more spry. Stretching after the warm-up period can help prevent injury during exercise. Stretching after the cool-down period can help prevent muscles from tightening up after exercise, which would decrease flexibility and increase muscle soreness.

Static stretching involves stretching a muscle group to the point where a sense of tightness is first felt, holding the stretch for 20 to 30 seconds, then releasing the stretch. This is repeated several times for each muscle group being stretched. Ballistic stretching, which involves bouncing during the stretch, is potentially dangerous, since it can lead to muscle or tendon damage.

Stretching, by Bob Anderson (see Additional Readings), is an excellent resource on the subject of stretching. It has numerous illustrations of the techniques of everyday stretches and of sport-specific stretches, all of which could be used as patient education handouts. Examples of everyday stretches are shown in Fig. 19-2.

BODY COMPOSITION

A percent of body fat measurement should be performed at the start of a health-related fitness program and should be repeated at regular intervals to help assess progress. A body composition appraisal is a significantly more accurate reflection of health-related fitness than are weight and height percentile comparisons. Growth chart weight and height percentile comparisons do not take body habitus into consideration. A muscular or large-framed person with a low percent of body fat may still have a weight percentile greater than the height percentile.

When first starting a fitness program a person may actually gain weight, although the percentage of body fat will be the same or even lower. This phenomenon is explained by the fact that muscle is more dense than fat; as a person starts to exercise, muscle may be added faster than fat is lost, which would make for an overall weight gain. This seems to be especially true for individuals who have not been very active before starting an exercise program.

Hydrostatic, or underwater, weighing is considered the most accurate way to measure body composition; it has a 1% to 3% factor for error. It is also the most inconvenient method to use. With practice, the use of skin calipers can reach a 3% to 5% error factor, and skin calipers are much more convenient.

The use of electrical impedance is also becoming more reliable and may in time become the most commonly used method of measuring percent of body fat. Whatever method is used, the final numbers are most helpful when comparing a person's individual progress over time, much as growth charts or blood pressure charts are used, and are less helpful when looking at any one point in time.

When skin calipers are used, the more skin sights measured, the more accurate the final determination of percent body fat. The triceps and calf sites are the most common sites used by school systems when doing mass testing and for that reason should be used if only two sites are selected. Proper techniques for using skin calipers can be found in many references. A graph of suggested ranges of percent body fat can be found in Fig. 19-3.

DIETARY EDUCATION

Proper diet and physical activity are equally important in achieving improved health-related fitness. Sustaining weight loss and improving health-related fitness parameters are difficult if not impossible to achieve without making use of both a proper diet and routine exercise.[3] Crash diets and ketogenic diets are essentially starvation diets, which lead to loss of muscle tissue while sparing fat tissue. Obviously this does not improve health.

A proper diet is actually fairly simple. When trying to lose weight, the most important point is to make the total caloric intake for 1 day be less than the total caloric output for that day. Consuming fewer calories or less fatty foods per day is a good place to start. Even when the total number of calories is unchanged, eating the largest meal of the day at breakfast instead of at night has been shown to help people lose weight. The total number of calories recommended per day according to age is listed in Table 19-3.

Carbohydrates should be the main source of calories. Current recommendations for the proportion of carbohydrates needed in relation to total daily calories range from 55% to 70%. Complex carbohydrates such as those found in fruits, vegetables, legumes, and whole-grain cereals are preferable to the refined carbohydrates found in candy. For adults and children over 2 years of age, it is recommended that 30% or less of the total number of calories come from fats, with vegetable fats (except palm oil and coconut oil) recommended over animal fats.[11] There is some controversy concerning how much fat is appropriate for the diet of a child under 2 years of age. The American Academy of Pediatrics currently recommends 30% to 40%, to ensure adequate fat for myelination of the nervous system.[12] Protein should make up the remaining 15% to 20% of the total daily caloric intake. Because fish and poultry have a lower percentage of fat than do beef and pork, they are considered safer from a cardiovascular standpoint. Other dietary recommendations include using low-fat dairy products, increasing dietary fiber, and decreasing the use of salt. Some specific suggestions for improving dietary habits are listed in the box on p. 252.

The role of cholesterol in the diet is intriguing and has produced a heated debate. In a detailed review by Kwiterovich, most scientific studies showed a cause-and-effect relationship between elevated cholesterol, low-density lipoproteins, and atherosclerosis.[11] In 1985, the National Institutes of Health Consensus Conference on Lowering Blood Cholesterol to Prevent Heart Disease gave specific recommendations for screening and blood testing in children from 2 to 20 years of age (see box on p. 253). The recommendations included using a positive family history as a basis for obtaining a serum cholesterol level for people under 20 years of age.[4] For those over 20 years of age, obtaining a baseline serum cholesterol level is recommended, to be followed by obtaining a repeat serum cholesterol level once every 5 years. Suggestions are now being proposed for mass cholesterol screening for all children entering school for the first time.[5]

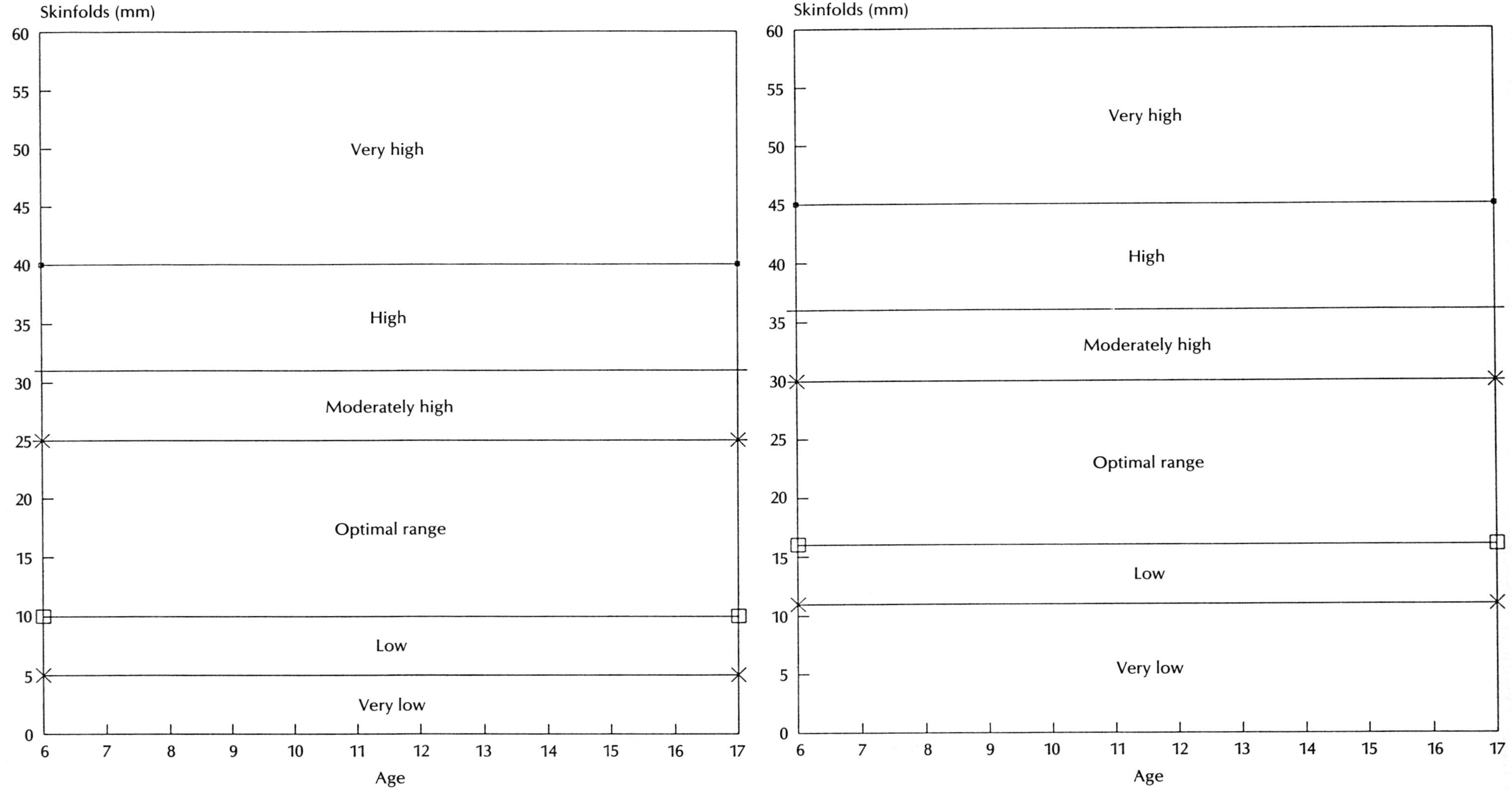

Fig. 19-3 Skinfold measurement ranges for the triceps and calf combination.

Adapted from Lohman TG. In Coaches guide to nutrition and weight control, Eisenman PA, Johnson SC, and Benson JE (eds), Salt Lake City, Utah, 1990, Human Kinetics, Champaign, Ill.

Table 19-3 *Recommended Total Daily Calories* (Moderate Activity Level)*

GROUP AND AGE (YR)	WT (KG [LB])	HEIGHT (CM [IN])	ENERGY NEEDS (KCAL [RANGE])
Children			
1-3	13 (29)	90 (35)	1,300 (900-1,800)
4-6	20 (44)	112 (44)	1,800 (1,300-2,300)
7-10	28 (62)	132 (52)	2,000 (1,650-3,300)
Males			
11-14	45 (99)	157 (62)	2,500 (2,000-3,700)
15-18	66 (145)	176 (69)	3,000 (2,100-3,900)
19-22	70 (154)	177 (70)	2,900 (2,500-3,300)
23-50	70 (154)	178 (70)	2,900 (2,300-3,100)
51-75	70 (154)	178 (70)	2,300 (2,000-2,800)
76+	70 (154)	178 (70)	2,050 (1,650-2,450)
Females			
11-14	46 (101)	157 (62)	2,200 (1,500-3,000)
15-18	55 (120)	163 (64)	2,200 (1,200-3,000)
19-22	55 (120)	163 (64)	2,200 (1,700-2,500)
23-50	55 (120)	163 (64)	2,200 (1,600-2,400)
51-75	55 (120)	163 (64)	1,900 (1,400-2,200)
76+	55 (120)	163 (64)	1,600 (1,200-2,000)

*These recommendations may vary significantly up or down in specific sports and in very active children and adolescents. (Modified From Food and Nutrition Board: Recommended Dietary Allowances, ed 10, Washington, DC, 1989, National Academy of Sciences, National Research Council.)

Suggestions for Practicing Good Nutrition

Develop a weekly meal plan
Eat a balanced meal from the four food groups
Bake, boil, or broil rather than fry
Reduce sugar intake
Eat fruit for a snack
Use high-fiber cereals, grains, and breads
Use low-fat dairy products
Eat more chicken and fish
Eat a low-fat meal
Cut use of butter and gravies in half
Don't add salt to food
Don't add sugar to food
Eat more raw and fresh fruits and vegetables
Drink more water

Modified from the Governor's Family FUN Award Program, Utah Governor's Council on Health and Physical Fitness, Salt Lake City, Utah.

Guidelines for interpreting serum cholesterol levels in children and young people under 20 years of age can be found in Table 19-4. However, many say that cholesterol screening should not be done in children at all for the following reasons:

1. It is not known if lowering the cholesterol level by diet or medication will prevent coronary heart disease early in life.
2. Compliance with a cholesterol-lowering regimen over many years cannot be effected in most instances.
3. Low-fat diets and cholesterol-lowering drugs can cause significant side effects.
4. Serious psychological consequences may result in children labeled "at risk" for an early death.
5. "Labeling" can affect insurability and employment opportunities.[7]

These conflicting opinions are disturbing and need to be resolved before imposing cholesterol screening on patients. However, many pediatricians already have implemented such screening, either for all their patients or for those with a family history that places them at high risk.

In the adult literature, whenever a positive relationship between exercise and the lowering of the serum cholesterol level was found, the more vigorous and the more sustained the exercise, the greater the impact of the exercise.[6]

PSYCHOLOGICAL ASPECTS

Learning stress management techniques and the use of behavior modification to help with compliance represent the psychological components of most health-related fitness programs. Pediatricians have been presenting aspects of stress management and behavior modification for years, as when they discuss anticipatory guidance with parents during well-baby visits.

Stress management is incorporated because many of the diseases targeted for prevention are related to psychological stress in various ways. Common examples of stress management strategies and techniques, including deep breathing, ascending muscle relaxation, body awareness, positive mental imagery, meditation, priority setting, and time management, are well known to many physicians. Examples of some family activities that can aid in stress management can be found in the box on p. 254. For an extensive reference on stress management, refer to the *Handbook of Stress: Theoretical and Clinical Aspects* (see Suggested Readings).

An integral factor, if not the most important one, in the ultimate success or failure of all fitness programs is compliance. The keys to compliance are education and motivation. Martin and Coates have put some salient points on helping patients change behavior into a concise package.[14] These include setting goals, modifying the environment, developing new experiences, and making incremental changes.

Educating the patient or the family about the problem may be motivation enough for starting a health-related fitness pro-

Summary of National Institutes of Health Guidelines for Healthy Children Over 2 Years of Age

1. "It is desirable to begin prevention in childhood because patterns of life-style are developed in childhood. The moderate-fat and moderate-cholesterol diets recommended for the population at large in this report should be suitable for all family members, including healthy children older than 2 years. For children, the diets should provide all nutrients in quantities adequate to growth and development and meet energy requirements. Excessive gain in weight should be avoided."

2. "*Children at 'high risk' should be identified primarily by carefully obtained family histories rather than routine screening.* The history should include parents, grandparents, and all first-degree relatives. A family history of hypercholesterolemia or premature coronary heart disease should alert the physician to obtain at least two blood cholesterol determinations."

3. "If the blood cholesterol level in such 'high-risk' children is above the 75th percentile (approximately 170 mg/dl for children aged 2 to 19 years), total and HDL [high-density lipoprotein] cholesterol measurements should be obtained. Those children with blood cholesterol levels between the 75th and 90th percentile (170 to 185 mg/dl) should be counseled regarding diet and other cardiovascular risk factors and then followed up at one-year intervals. Those with levels above the 90th percentile (>185 mg/dl) require special dietary instruction and close supervision with evaluation of other risk factors. A child with a blood cholesterol level above the 95th percentile (>200 mg/dl) on two occasions is in a special category and may have one of the hereditary hypercholesterolemias. Strict dietary intervention is indicated and will be sufficient for many children. Nonresponders should be considered for treatment with a lipid-lowering agent, a bile-acid sequestrant (such as cholestyramine). All family members should be screened."

4. "Dietary management of children with elevated blood cholesterol levels should be part of total management that includes regular exercise programs, maintenance of ideal weight, avoidance of excess salt, and avoidance of cigarette smoking."

From National Institutes of Health Consensus Conference: Lowering blood cholesterol to prevent heart disease, JAMA 253:2080, 1985.

gram. Long-term compliance, however, is a more difficult matter. When the physical and mental benefits of the program start becoming noticeable, they may provide a self-sustaining motivation. It is in the gap between starting a program and reaching a certain plateau where the benefits are tangible (by as early as the third month or as late as the twelfth month) that the greatest drop-out rate occurs. The average drop-out rate within the first 6 to 12 months of starting a fitness program is usually 50% or more.[19] As stated earlier, the beneficial

Table 19-4 *Normal Plasma Lipid Concentrations Before 20 Years of Age**

	CHOLESTEROL (MG/DL)											
	HIGH-DENSITY LIPOPROTEIN (PERCENTILE)				LOW-DENSITY LIPOPROTEIN (PERCENTILE)				VERY-LOW-DENSITY LIPOPROTEIN (PERCENTILE)			
AGE (YR) AND SEX	NO.	5TH	50TH	95TH	NO.	5TH	50TH	95TH	NO.	5TH	50TH	95TH
5-9												
M	145	38	56	75	132	63	93	129	132	0	8	18
F	127	36	53	73	114	68	100	140	113	1	10	24
10-14												
M	298	37	55	74	288	64	97	133	288	1	10	22
F	248	37	52	70	245	68	97	136	245	2	11	23
15-19												
M	300	30	46	63	298	62	94	130	297	2	13	26
F	297	35	52	74	295	59	96	137	295	2	12	24

*Data are from the *Lipid Research Clinic Data Book.* Lipoproteins were determined on plasma from 1,415 fasting, white subjects (743 boys, 672 girls) who were studied in seven North American Lipid Research Clinics, by use of common protocols and laboratory methodology. (From Kwiterovich PO Jr: Biochemical, clinical, epidemiologic, genetic, and pathologic data in the pediatric age group relevant to the cholesterol hypothesis, Pediatrics 78:349, 1986.

Suggested Family Activities for Stress Management

Keep a family calendar
Keep a family job list
Hold a family meeting
Have a family game night
Attend a health fair
Read together
Keep a stress diary
Get involved in service projects
Set aside meditation and quiet time
Prepare a meal together
Keep a journal
Engage in family outdoor adventures
Have a family picnic
Get adequate sleep
Cut television time in half
Discuss family budgeting
Attend cultural events
Play new games together

Modified from the Governor's Family FUN Award Program, Utah Governor's Council on Health and Physical Fitness, Salt Lake City, Utah.

changes achieved through any health-related fitness program are not sustained if the program is discontinued. That is why the concept of a life-style change is important for the family to comprehend.

Many factors have been addressed in trying to solve this problem. Some of the important findings in an adult survey included scheduling the time, gaining access to facilities, the weather, the time of year, and the presence of an interested friend or family member.[18] In a survey of diabetic children and adolescents who participated in an exercise program, the most important factors affecting compliance were enthusiastic leadership, individual attention, and parental support. For children therefore a motivated and involved adult is essential. The most likely person to fill that role is usually one of the parents, or both. (The next most likely individual may be a schoolteacher or an organization leader in Scouts, YMCA or YWCA, or a church group.)

Instructing a patient to keep a daily log of his or her fitness program and to bring it back in a month can be an incentive to comply and a basis for discussion at the follow-up visit.

Use of age-appropriate and time-appropriate rewards is essential. Some examples would be taking the family out for frozen yogurt (instead of ice cream) if 1 week's goal is met, allowing each family member to buy a desired article of clothing if 1 month's goal is met, and taking a family vacation to a favorite spot if a 6- or 12-month goal is met. Each family member should be allowed to help decide what reward is important.

Varying the selection of exercise activities makes for a more interesting exercise program and helps prevent overuse injuries, which aids in compliance. For example, a person could walk twice a week and hike on a family outing once a week.

For many individuals as well as families, a lack of time to begin or to maintain a fitness program is one of the major obstacles to be overcome. A good starting point is to divide the day into 30-minute increments, then make the program a priority to be worked into one of those increments. Specific suggestions for getting in the desired exercise time include getting up 30 minutes earlier in the morning, using 30 minutes of a lunch break, or allotting 30 minutes after dinner.

EATING DISORDERS AND EXERCISE

The pediatrician should always keep in mind that some patients may have the hidden agenda of an eating disorder when they come to the practitioner for information on diet and exercise. Adolescents and older children who seem involved in unusual amounts of exercise or unusual diets may be at risk for or may have already started the bulimia-anorexia process. Gymnasts, wrestlers, long-distance runners, dancers, drill-team members, and cheerleaders are in activities in which weight loss is not only encouraged but may actually be demanded by adult sponsors, parents, or peers. If a patient is psychologically susceptible to the bulimia-anorexia process, then adult prodding or peer pressure may help precipitate the syndrome. If in doubt, a psychological evaluation can help determine whether a patient is indeed at risk. (See Additional Readings for Newman and Halverson's *Anorexia Nervosa and Bulimia: A Handbook for Counselors and Therapists,* which has an extensive reference section on this topic.)

SPECIFIC FITNESS PROGRAMS

Although health-related fitness should be based first on family fitness programs, it is better when supplemented by a school fitness program. There is also the very real possibility that the school fitness program will be the only fitness program that any one child may be exposed to. Health-related fitness programs for schools and families are already available in a variety of forms. In the past many physical education classes consisted mainly of competitive sports, and for many people who were less athletically inclined, they fostered negative connotations about exercise. Although everyone needs motivation and encouragement to stay with any health-related fitness program, this is easier to achieve if the program is fun to do. This is important for adults, but it is critical for children. A list of programs is in the box on p. 255. This list is not meant to be all encompassing, nor does it constitute an endorsement of the programs mentioned.

POTENTIAL OPPORTUNITIES FOR DISCUSSING HEALTH-RELATED FITNESS

One of the best times to broach the topic of health-related fitness is at a consultation for a specific problem (e.g., obesity, reactive airway disease). It is then that the parent or patient may be especially receptive to advice concerning specific therapeutic or preventive measures.[21,22] Preventive health care visits such as well-child check-ups, camp physicals, and sports preparticipation physicals are some of the other visits during which health-related fitness could be discussed. The kindergarten check-up is frequently the last time a pediatrician can uniformly count on seeing patients for a preventive health care visit, and it is probably the earliest age at which a pro-

Examples of Health-Related Fitness Programs

SCHOOL PROGRAMS

1. "Feeling Good"
   This program appears to be the most extensive in depth (covering all of the areas mentioned in this article and more) and in breadth (books available for children, kindergarten through high school levels, for parents, and for administrators). The emphasis in the exercise time is on noncompetitive cardiovascular movement through "fun" games. It has a "homework" segment to help involve families. Contact: Charles Kuntzleman, Ph.D, Fitness Finders, 133 Teft Road, Spring Arbor, MI 49283-0507.
2. The Governor's Golden Sneaker Awards Program
   This is a basic aerobic exercise program that only requires an enthusiastic teacher. Points are awarded on a basis of time units of aerobic activities done at school and/or at home. Awards are given to the student from the governor's office upon completion of the program, depending on the total number of points earned. The best points of this program are that it is simple and inexpensive. Contact: The Utah Governor's Council on Health and Physical Fitness, % Primary Children's Medical Center, 100 N. Medical Drive, Salt Lake City, UT 84113, (801) 588-2000.
3. "Know Your Body"
   This program was developed as a school-based program that focuses on teaching decision-making skills in the areas of nutrition, exercise, and preventing cigarette smoking. It has been used in all socioeconomic settings. Contact: The American Health Foundation, 320 East 43rd St, NY, NY 10017.
4. "Growing Healthy"
   This is a comprehensive school-based program that covers many areas, including exercise and nutrition. Contact: The National Center for Health, 30 East 29th St, NY, NY 10016.

PERSONAL AND FAMILY PROGRAMS

1. The Body Shop
   This program was originally developed at Methodist Hospital in St Louis Park, Minnesota, and now is marketed to other hospitals. It calls for intense, direct adult supervision by hospital personnel to lead children aged 8-18 years and their parents through 10 weeks of behavior modification and experiential skill building, which will allow them to take control of their eating and exercise behaviors and to improve their self-esteem. Contact: The Body Shop, Methodist Hospital, 6500 Excelsior Boulevard, St Louis Park, MN 55426.
2. Utah Governor's Council on Health and Physical Fitness Family F.U.N. Award Program
   This program was developed as a free-standing, eight-page fold-up brochure that introduces families to health-related fitness over a suggested 6-month period. The F.U.N. stands for fitness (to include cardiorespiratory endurance, large muscle strength, and flexibility), unity (family stress management), and nutrition. Suggestions for starting and maintaining a family fitness program are included. At this time brochures are free for Utah residents and physicians from any state, but nonphysician residents of states other than Utah can obtain a brochure for 30 cents. Contact: The Utah Governor's Council on Health and Physical Fitness, % Primary Children's Medical Center, 100 N. Medical Dr., Salt Lake City, UT 84113, (801) 588-2000.
3. The Reader's Digest Guide to Family Fitness
   This is a program developed for *The Readers Digest* by several nationally recognized experts. It includes an introduction, information on testing a family's fitness level, and suggestions about how to start a family exercise program. It does not include diet or stress management. Contact: Reprint Editor, Reader's Digest, Pleasantville, NY 10570.
4. The Well Family Book
   This book was written by Charles T. Kuntzleman, PhD. It is a good resource for specific examples of family fitness, family nutrition, and family stress management. Contact: Fitness Finders, 133 Teft Road, Spring Arbor, MI 49283-0507.

Modified from Jopling RJ: Health-related fitness as preventive medicine, Pediatr Rev 10:141, 1988.

gram including exercise recommendations can be introduced. For those reasons it should be strongly considered as a time to discuss family fitness.

At any of the above-mentioned visits, the patient's height, weight, and blood pressure can easily be measured and plotted on an age- and sex-appropriate graph before the child sees the physician. After a little practice, skin caliper measurements can be done with relative ease and proficiency by the nurse or examining physician. This information can then be compared with age- and sex-appropriate graphs to be used as a baseline for future reference and can be the basis for introducing this topic to the patient and the parents.

A practitioner frequently cannot impart all of the information needed to start a new family fitness program in the 20 or 30 minutes that is generally scheduled for preventive health care visits (most such visits are much shorter—10 to 15 minutes). Important keys to remember are: (1) introduce the topics of discussion by quickly going over the major points that are already listed in a brochure or handout that the patient or parent can take home, (2) make some specific suggestions to get the family started (e.g., writing in a daily log on the family calender for each area being worked on—exercise,

*Specific Programs for Developing a Health-Related Fitness Profile**

1. Physical Best program of the American Alliance for Health, Physical Education, Recreation and Dance (AAHPERD), 1900 Association Drive, Reston, VA 22091.
2. President's Physical Fitness Award Program of the President's Council on Physical Fitness and Sports, Washington, DC 20001.
3. The Fitness Gram of the Institute for Aerobics Research, the Aerobics Center, 12330 Preston Road, Dallas, TX 75230.

*These programs apply national standards according to age and sex.

stress management, and nutrition), and (3) schedule a follow-up visit for 2 to 4 weeks later. At the follow-up visit the daily log can be reviewed, repeat measurements can be obtained, and the program can be reinforced and clarified.

Primary care pediatricians should try to collaborate with the local school system to compile a "health-related fitness profile" for all of the children in that particular school system.[23] The school can test the students in the areas of cardiovascular endurance capacity (run 1 mile), muscle strength and endurance (do flexed-arm hangs and pull-ups for 1 minute, then sit-ups for 1 minute), and flexibility (sit on floor and reach as far as possible past feet). The individual's physician or the school could measure body composition (triceps and calf skin caliper measurements), height, weight, and blood pressure. When the child's test results are known, the child's physician or a physician appointed by the school could work with the parents and teachers to improve the individual's deficient areas. For details on specific programs already available, refer to the box above.

With all of the problems facing medicine today, is all this important enough to take up the time of the primary care pediatrician? Can we financially afford to educate our patient population, to fight for insurance reimbursement, and to encourage schools to include this topic in their curriculum? Some feel that the answer awaits longitudinal studies yet to be done. However, most professionals in the interrelated areas of health, nutrition, and exercise believe that health-related fitness can enhance the quality and duration of life within the framework of a person's genetic potential for health.

REFERENCES

1. Blair SN and Kohl HW: Physical activity or physical fitness: which is more important for health? Med Sci Sports Exerc 20(suppl):88, 1988.
2. Borg GAV: A category-ratio perceived exertion scale: relationship to blood and muscle lactates and heart rate, Med Sci Sports Exerc 15:523, 1983.
3. Brownell KD and Nelson Steen S: Modern methods for weight control: the physiology and psychology of dieting, Physician Sports Med 15:122, 1987.
4. Garcia RE and Moodie DS: A case for routine cholesterol surveillence in childhood, Pediatrics 84:751, 1989.
5. Geitmaker SL and Dietz WH: Increasing pediatric obesity in the United States, Am J Dis Child 141:535, 1987.
6. Hoekelman RA: A pediatrician's view, Pediatr Ann 19:229, 1990 (editorial).
7. Jopling RJ: Health-related fitness as preventive medicine, Pediatr Rev 10:141, 1988.
8. Kraus H: Unfit kids: a call to action, Contemp Pediatr 5:18, 1988.
9. Kraus H and Hirschland RP: Minimum muscular fitness tests in school children, Res Q 25:178, 1954.
10. Kwiterovich PO Jr: Biochemical, clinical, epidemiologic, genetic, and pathologic data in the pediatric age group relevant to the cholesterol hypothesis, Pediatrics 78:349, 1986.
11. LaRosa J and Finberg L: Preliminary report from a conference entitled "Prevention of adult atherosclerosis during childhood," J Pediatr 112:317, 1988.
12. Lauer RM and Clarke WR: Childhood risk factors for high blood pressure, Pediatrics 84 (4):633, 1989.
13. Martin AR and Coates TJ: A clinician's guide to helping patients change behavior, West J Med 146:751, 1987.
14. National Institutes of Health Consensus Conference: Lowering blood cholesterol to prevent heart disease, JAMA 253:2080, 1985.
15. Phelps JR: Physical activity and health maintenance: exactly what is known? West J Med 146:200, 1987.
16. Powell KE et al: Physical activity and the incidence of coronary heart disease, Annu Rev Public Health 8:253, 1987.
17. Rippe JM: The health benefits of exercise, Physician Sports Med 15:115, 1987.
18. Shepard RJ: Motivation: the key to fitness compliance, Physician Sports Med 13:88, 1985.
19. Song TK, Shepard RJ, and Cox M: Absenteeism, employee turnover, and sustained exercise participation, J Sports Med Phys Fitness 22:392, 1983.
20. Status of the 1990 physical fitness and exercise objectives, MMWR 34:521, 1985.
21. Strong WB: You are a preventive cardiologist: the scope of pediatric preventive cardiology, Am J Dis Child 143:1145, 1989.
22. Strong WB and Dennison BA: Pediatric preventive cardiology: atherosclerosis and coronary heart disease, Pediatr Rev 9:303, 1988.
23. Strong WB and Wilmore JH: Unfit kids: an office-based approach to physical fitness, Contemp Pediatr 5:33, 1988.
24. Webber LS et al: Cardiovascular risk factors from birth to 7 years of age: the Bogalusa heart study, Pediatrics 80:767, 1987.

SUGGESTED READINGS

Anderson B: Stretching, Bolinas, Calif, 1980, Shelter Publications, Inc (Random House, Inc).

Dishman RK: Exercise adherence, its impact on public health, Champaign, Ill, 1990, Human Kinetics Publishers, Inc.

Eisenman PA, Johnson SC, and Benson JE: Coaches' guide to nutrition and weight control, Champaign, Ill, 1990, Human Kinetics Publishers, Inc.

Fish HT, Fish RB, and Golding LA: Starting out well, a parents' guide to physical activity and nutrition, Champaign, Ill, 1989, Human Kinetics Publishers, Inc.

Goldberger L and Breznitz S: Handbook of stress: theoretical and clinical aspects, New York, 1982, The Free Press (Macmillan Publishing Co).

Linder CW and DuRant RH: Exercise, serum lipids, and cardiovascular disease: risk factors in children, Pediatr Clin North Am 29:1341, 1982.

Newman P and Halverson P: Anorexia nervosa and bulimia: a handbook for counselors and therapists, New York, 1983, Van Nostrand Reinhold Co, Inc.

Rowland TW: Exercise and children's health, Champaign, Ill, 1990, Human Kinetics Publishers, Inc.

Suskind RM and Varna RN: Assessment of the nutritional status of children, Pediatr Rev 5:195, 1984.

Vartabedian RE and Matthews K: Nutripoints: the breakthrough point system for optimal nutrition, New York, 1990, Harper & Row, Publishers, Inc.

Wilmore JH: Sensible fitness, Champaign, Ill, 1986, Leisure Press (Human Kinetics Publishers, Inc).

20

Preventive Aspects of Dental Care

Donald J. Forrester

Because pediatricians provide care to children from birth, they are in a unique position to influence the establishment and maintenance of a child's dental health. While providing comprehensive health care for an infant, the pediatrician also should examine the soft and hard tissues of the infant's mouth. It should be remembered that primary teeth begin erupting into the oral cavity when the child is approximately 6 months of age; usually all have erupted by the age of 2 years (Table 20-1).

All infants should be referred to a pedodontist (pediatric dentist) no later than 12 months of age for a dental examination and oral health counseling, even if significant problems are not evident.[5] Early referral will enable the pediatric dentist to institute a preventive dental health care program in a pleasant, trauma-free environment before prolonged or extensive dental care is needed. Early dental referral is especially desirable for the medically compromised child as well as the physically or mentally handicapped child.

Table 20-1 *Abbreviated Chronology of Human Dentition*

TOOTH	HARD TISSUE FORMATION BEGINS	ERUPTION	EXFOLIATION (YR)
Primary dentition			
Maxillary	**Mo in utero**		
Central incisor	3½	7½ mo	6-7
Lateral incisor	4	9 mo	7-8
Cuspid	4½	18 mo	10-11
First molar	4	14 mo	9-11
Second molar	4½	24 mo	10-12
Mandibular			
Central incisor	3½	6 mo	6-7
Lateral incisor	4	7 mo	7-8
Cuspid	4½	16 mo	9-12
First molar	4	12 mo	9-11
Second molar	4½	20 mo	10-12
Permanent dentition			
Maxillary			
Central incisor	3-4 mo	7-8 yr	
Lateral incisor	10-12 mo	8-9 yr	
Cuspid	4-5 mo	11-12 yr	
First bicuspid	1½-1¾ mo	10-11 yr	
Second bicuspid	2-2¼ mo	10-12 yr	
First molar	At birth	6-7 yr	
Second molar	2½-3 yr	12-13 yr	
Third molar	7-9 yr	17-21 yr	
Mandibular			
Central incisor	3-4 mo	6-7 yr	
Lateral incisor	3-4 mo	7-8 yr	
Cuspid	4-5 mo	9-10 yr	
First bicuspid	1¾-2 yr	10-12 yr	
Second bicuspid	2¼-2½ yr	11-12 yr	
First molar	At birth	6-7 yr	
Second molar	2½-3 yr	11-13 yr	
Third molar	8-10 yr	17-21 yr	

Modified from American Dental Association: J Am Dent Assoc 20:379, 1933.

Fluoridation

The fluoridation of public water supplies repeatedly has been proved to be the most economical, safe, convenient, and effective measure available to prevent dental caries.[7] Studies have shown that the cost of dental care in a fluoridated area can be less than one half that for a fluoride-deficient area.[4] During the period of tooth formation and eruption, the ingestion of water that contains the optimum concentration of fluoride has consistently resulted in a 40% to 60% reduction in dental caries.[8] The optimum concentration of fluoride in community water supplies depends on the annual average maximum daily air temperature in the individual community.[12] The U.S. Public Health Service recommends the concentrations shown in Table 20-2.

Determining the fluoride content in drinking water is a service provided by all local health departments in the United States. Accordingly, a fluoride analysis should be performed for any child who consumes well water or water from public supplies that are unfluoridated. Fluoride supplementation should be recommended for all children consuming water with a fluoride content less than 0.7 parts per million (ppm). The regular administration of dietary fluoride supplements provides a reduction in dental caries almost equal to that furnished by regularly drinking fluoridated water.[7] The American Dental Association and the American Academy of Pediatrics jointly developed a supplemental fluoride dosage schedule (Table 20-3) that reflects the amount of fluoride that should be part of a child's dietary intake.

Fluoride Supplementation

Administration of fluoride supplements should begin soon after birth and continue until all permanent teeth, excluding third molars, have erupted. In most children the eruption of permanent teeth, except for third molars, will near completion between the ages of 12 and 14 years (Table 20-1). Fluoride supplements can be dispensed as drops, mouth rinses, tablets, lozenges, or vitamin and fluoride combination preparations. Studies have shown that lozenge or mouth rinse supplements maximize potential benefits because they provide both topical benefits before being swallowed and systemic effects in preventing dental caries.[1] An increasing number of studies have consistently reported reductions of 35% to 40% in the incidence of dental decay among school-age children who use 0.05% fluoride rinses daily, which now are available without a prescription.[2] Consequently, children should be urged to use fluoride rinses. Successful results from fluoride supplementation depend mostly on parents' ensuring that their children receive their daily dose. Therefore the pediatrician must clearly instruct and frequently reinforce the need for daily ingestion of fluoride supplements.

Prenatal Administration

Available data differ greatly regarding the benefits of prenatal administration of fluoride. Because of the equivocal results of these studies, the United States Food and Drug Administration has concluded that sufficient evidence does not exist to support efficacy claims of prenatal fluoride supplements, although their safety is not in question.[3]

Toothbrushing

A wide variety of toothbrush designs are available for consumer use. Numerous studies agree that the preferred toothbrush for children has a small, straight brush head with soft-textured multitufted nylon bristles.[13] Clinical studies indicate that electrically powered toothbrushes also are effective, especially on the teeth of handicapped children who have difficulty cleaning their teeth.

Because the toothbrush has a beneficial effect on a child's gingival health and oral hygiene, parents should be informed that by the age of 2 years each child should own a toothbrush. There are numerous techniques of tooth brushing, but most are too complex for a child's use. Because of its simplicity, the use of short, horizontal, scrubbing strokes (the scrub brush technique) is a desirable method that can be readily mastered by both the child and parents.[13] Preschool-age children cannot be expected to develop a conscientious and effective toothbrushing habit; thus parents must be informed of their responsibility to clean their child's teeth and gums at least once a day, preferably at bedtime because of a normally occurring decrease in saliva flow and increased salivary viscosity during a child's sleep.

According to studies by Head Start programs and elementary schools, children usually do not clean their teeth effectively without supervision before the age of 8 years.[10] Therefore parents should be informed of the necessity to closely supervise their child's oral hygiene habits until this age.

Table 20-2 *PHS-Recommended Fluoride Control Limits*

ANNUAL AVERAGE OF MAXIMUM DAILY AIR TEMPERATURES (° F)*	OPTIMUM FLUORIDE CONCENTRATIONS IN DRINKING WATER (mg/L, ppm)
50.0-53.7	1.2
53.8-58.3	1.1
58.4-63.8	1.0
63.9-70.6	0.9
70.7-79.2	0.8
79.3-90.5	0.7

From US Public Health Service.

*Based on temperature data obtained for a minimum of 5 yr.

Table 20-3 *Supplemental Fluoride Dosage Schedule (mg/day*) According to Fluoride Concentration in Drinking Water*

	CONCENTRATION OF FLUORIDE IN DRINKING WATER (ppm)		
AGE (YR)	<0.3	0.3-0.7	>0.7
Birth to 2	0.25	0	0
2 to 3	0.50	0.25	0
3 to 13	1.00	0.50	0

From Council on Dental Therapeutics: Accepted dental therapies, ed 39, Chicago, 1982, American Dental Association.

*2.2 mg sodium fluoride contain 1 mg fluoride.

Dental Floss

Although dental floss has proved to be an effective mechanical agent for interproximal tooth cleaning, its use by children is not practical because of the digital skill required for its proper use.

Nutrition

Diet significantly influences oral health. The pediatrician should be alert for the sign of nursing bottle caries,[6] which is manifested by the rapid development of extensive dental caries on maxillary anterior teeth in children between the ages of 1 and 2 years. This serious, painful, and premature form of dental caries is easily prevented by ensuring that the infant does not go to sleep with a bottle that contains any refined carbohydrate.

Carbohydrates have repeatedly proved to be of major importance in the formation of caries because of two aspects: their physical character and the frequency of ingestion. Thus the pediatrician can contribute to a child's dental health by recommending that parents limit their child's eating of sticky-sweet desserts to mealtime. Suitable between-meal snacks are readily cleared fermentable carbohydrates that have a low caries potential index, such as fresh fruits and vegetables, juices, and soft drinks.

Sealants

The application of plastic sealants to caries-susceptible pits and fissures of posterior teeth is a recent advancement in the prevention of dental caries. Because fluoride exerts its maximum effect on smooth enamel surfaces, it still is necessary to protect developmental faults from invasion and colonization by decay-producing bacteria. The rationale for successful plastic application is based on the principle of micromechanical retention. A mild acidic solution is used to etch the upper 10 to 20 μm of enamel and selectively dissolve the inorganic elements of enamel rod cores. After the etched surface is thoroughly washed and dried, a thin layer of plastic is applied to the tooth. The plastic penetrates enamel tags created by the etching process. The basic chemicals used are bisphenol A and glycidyl methacrylate, which are combined and applied as a light polymerized liquid plastic. The most significant feature of this preventive method is the conservation of tooth structure. Only micrometers of enamel are dissolved during the application, and anesthesia is not necessary for placement.

Numerous studies have been conducted to determine the relationship between caries prevention and sealant retention. Depending on the material tested and methods employed, most studies have reported 50% to 80% retention and 40% to 80% caries reduction between the ages of 1 and 7 years, when compared with a contralateral untreated susceptible tooth.[9] Evidence indicates that sealants remain within the enamel surface long after they are clinically detectable. Because of this observation, differences exist in reported caries prevention and in reported sealant retention. Reapplication of sealant may be necessary approximately every 2 years, although studies report that at least 50% of sealant applications retain their effectiveness for longer periods.[9] In spite of more than 20 years of research findings that prove sealants to be safe, effective, and economical in preventing tooth decay, a recent National Institute of Dental Research survey revealed that fewer than 8% of American schoolchildren have dental sealants on their teeth.[11] Consequently, the physician's key role as a health provider places him or her in a position to strongly recommend this proved caries preventive procedure.

REFERENCES

1. Driscoll WS, Heifetz SB, and Korts, DC: Effect of chewable fluoride tablets on dental caries in schoolchildren: results after six years of use, J Am Dent Assoc 97:820, 1976.
2. Driscoll, WS et al: Caries-preventive effects of daily and weekly fluoride mouthrinsing in a fluoridated community: final results after 30 months, J Am Dent Assoc 105:1010, 1982.
3. Food and Drug Administration: Statement of general policy or interpretation, oral prenatal drugs containing fluorides for human use, Federal Register, Oct 20, 1966.
4. Horowitz HS: The assessment of cost-effectiveness of caries preventive agents and procedures. In Final technical report: dental caries studies of the Commission on Oral Health, Federation Dentaire Internationale, Research and Epidemiology, 1980.
5. American Academy of Pediatric Dentistry: Infant oral health care, recommended standard revised May 1989.
6. McIlveen LP: Chronology and development of the dentition, pediatric basics, No 53, Winter 1990, Gerber Medical Services.
7. Mellberg JR, Ripa LW, and Leske GS: Fluoride in preventive dentistry, Chicago, 1983, Quintessence Publishing Co.
8. Newbrun E: Effectiveness of water fluoridation, J Public Health Dentistry 49(5) (special issue):279, 1989.
9. Ripa LW: The current status of pit and fissure sealants, a review, J Can Dent Assoc 51:367, 1985.
10. Rugg-Gunn AJ and MacGregor IDM: A survey of toothbrushing behavior in children and young adults, J Periodont Res 13:382, 1978.
11. Sealant Use Low, Am Dent Assoc News 20:24, April 3, 1989.
12. Public Health Service drinking water standards, Pub US Public Health Service No 956, Washington, DC, 1962, US Government Printing Office.
13. Wei SHY: Mechanical and chemical plaque control in pediatric dentistry: total patient care, Philadelphia, 1988, Lea & Febiger.

21

Accident Prevention

Howard C. Mofenson and Joseph Greensher

CASUALTIES, CAUSES, AND CURES[42]

This chapter updates the challenge laid down to pediatricians by Dietrich in 1954[15] that "accident prevention in childhood is your problem, too." In the past, accidents have been regarded as product-related or behavioral problems rather than public health problems. As will be evident from the National Safety Council (NSC) statistics cited here, the casualty count in both lives lost and children maimed is significant enough to warrant the concerted action of primary care physicians. There has been considerable progress made in understanding the environmental situations and circumstances that contribute to the occurrence of accidents. A better knowledge of the causal factors will give a more rational approach toward the solution of this problem.

The first organized effort to secure information on product-related injuries in children began with the establishment of the Accident Prevention Committee of the American Academy of Pediatrics in 1952. This has been the basis for continued activities in cooperation with many other organizations, manufacturers, and government to improve the safety of products, which has resulted in safety education, identification of environmental hazards, voluntary compliance, and legislation of safety standards.

Casualties

Accidents are the leading cause of death among all persons from 1 to 44 years of age. The 1987 accident death total was approximately 44,000. Disability injuries numbered about 8.8 million, including 350,000 resulting in some degree of permanent impairment. Accident costs amounted to about $133.2 billion.

In children and youth between the ages of 1 to 24 years, accidents accounted for almost 50% of the 54,207 total deaths in 1985. This disproportion is dramatically illustrated in the years of potential life lost by each death that occurs before age 65 years. The aggregate loss to society is staggering. Of 62.4 million victims injured in 1986, about 45% were younger than 25 years of age.

Accidents account for more deaths in the age-group 1 through 14 than the next six most commonly reported causes: cancer, congenital anomalies, pneumonia, heart disease, homicide, and cerebrovascular diseases. Although no accurate statistics are available, child abuse also represents a significant cause of death in children.

It is estimated that 40,000 to 50,000 children are permanently injured each year, and a minimum of 1 million seek medical care because of injuries from accidents. An accurate gathering of statistics is hampered by the practice of listing only those accidents that cause high numbers of fatalities. The kind of accidents that produce fatalities are not necessarily the type that cause a large number of nonfatal injuries.

Accidental injury in the past three decades became the leading cause of death in children. This can be attributed indirectly to the medical profession and in no small part to pediatricians, whose work in public health, medical practice, and research has sharply reduced the incidence and consequences of many formerly fatal diseases. It is through this decline in other causes of death that accidents achieved this dubious distinction. In 1920 only 10% of childhood deaths were caused by accidental injury; by 1987, however, the figure had risen to 40%.

The statistical breakdown for the various types of accidents is presented under their individual discussions.

Causes[26,33,38]

The word *accidents* has proved a barrier to elucidating their causes. This word implies that they are "bad breaks" or "acts of God" not understandable in terms of the usual causes of disease, and people often attribute their avoidance to "sheer luck" or "a miracle." The terms *injury* or *injury control* are preferable. Through research and experience in injury control many of those at risk for particular kinds of injuries have been identified, as have preventive strategies that can be put into practice to save lives, health, and resources.

Three facets of injuries warrant investigation: the host (who is affected), the agent (the object that is the direct cause), and the environment (where and when it happened).

The importance of the *host* as a factor in causing injuries is evident from the difference in incidence at various ages. The preschool child is endangered by poisonings, the school-age child by drowning and firearm accidents. The immobile child younger than 1 year of age faces different hazards on becoming a toddler. These factors are important in planning prevention.

Some children are more susceptible, and boys generally are more likely to be injured than are girls; the male death rate from injury is twice that of the female. A child who has had a poisoning episode is more likely to have a second than is a matched control to have a first.

The identification of *agents* involved—for example, flammable fabrics and refrigerators (entrapment)—has allowed some preventive measures to be taken, but it will prove impossible to control injuries completely by abolishing the agents.

The physical and social *environments* play important roles in causing injuries; they are the settings in which the host and agent interact. Time of year, time of day, the child's health, relocation, and frequent injuries in other family members are all factors associated with the occurrence of accidents.

A Boston study[27] showed that injuries occur when additional stress is present. The stressful situations found included:

1. Hunger or fatigue. Injuries occurred more frequently during the hour before a scheduled meal, in the late afternoon, or before bedtime. Maternal tension probably is an important factor at these times.
2. Hyperactivity.
3. Maternal illness.
4. Recent change in the caretaker of the child.
5. Illness or death of other family members.
6. A tense relationship between the child's parents.
7. Sudden changes in environment, such as those that occur when relocating or at vacation time.
8. Maternal preoccupation—rushed or too busy. Saturday was found to be the worst accident day, and 3 to 6 PM were the worst hours.

Another study has suggested that childhood accidents are recurring symptoms of maladjustments to environment or family. Poor housing, marital disharmony, and physical or mental ill health in family members were found in significant number in the study. With the use of poisoning as an example of childhood accidents, it was found that repetitive poisoning was not related to environmental hazards or lack of supervision but rather to marital tension and a tense and distant parent-child relationship.[49]

Understanding various concepts that have been used in the literature and research on accidents is essential.

Injury proneness implies personality characteristics that predispose an individual to accidents. This implication tends to exclude further investigation of the environment. The concept of injury proneness is skeptically regarded by researchers.

Injury repetitiveness is an observed pattern of behavior that lasts for varying periods of time.

Injury liability views the individual in relation to the environment. In children this implies that not only the child but also the family and the environment are involved in accidents. Liability results from personality characteristics as well as from many other factors, such as exposure to hazards; sensory, motor, and neural functioning; capacity to make judgments; degree of experience and training; and exposure to social and other stresses.

Certain behavioral characteristics have been found to increase exposure to accident liability or to reduce a child's ability to cope with hazards. Most of these features are present at 1 year of age and may be useful in identifying the child at risk.

The child with increased exposure (1) is very active, daring, curious, and happy-go-lucky, (2) mimics the behavior of older people, and (3) has exaggerated oral tendencies.

The child with reduced ability to cope with hazards (1) is high-strung, hot-headed, stubborn, and easily irritated or frustrated, (2) is careless in play, (3) lacks self-control, (4) is aggressive, and (5) has poor concentration or ability to pay attention.

Family life-style also has been found to be a factor in accidents. Men with dull jobs appear to have a greater need for instant gratification. They seek recreational thrills and surround themselves with more dangerous devices. The children in their families have been noted to have more accidents.

Hospitalization that requires separation of infants from parents has been correlated with an increase in the incidence of childhood accidents and child abuse. Child abuse or neglect may be a significant cause of accidents; estimates vary from 10% to 50% (see Chapter 46).

Any child with two or more significant accidents in a 12-month period needs an in-depth investigation of the circumstances.

Cures

In 1970 Sobel[49] stated that if any progress was to be made in accident prevention, practitioners must broaden their perspective to include consideration of parental mental health and capacity to provide a milieu in which the child's needs are met. It is not unreasonable to believe that a profile of the family and child at risk can be developed to aid in identification of individuals in need of behavior modification and other techniques to reduce accidents.

Parents are more likely to perform one-time or occasional efforts necessary for injury prevention (e.g., acquiring a smoke detector); these actions, therefore, lend themselves to effective counseling.

The physician can gain insight into potential problems by obtaining a history of the family that includes parental occupation, education, and income; attitudes toward the children and each other; use of medication, alcohol, and tobacco; television-watching patterns; and previous automobile accidents. A clue to the family life-style may be indicated by family recreational activities and hobbies.

Medical personnel can attempt to gain insight into parent-child rapport. The following observation by Levy[35] can be useful: he found that when something complimentary was said about a baby while the mother was holding him or her, the average mother would look down at the baby. If she failed to do this, there often was a lack of good rapport. Observations of the way the parent stands beside the infant who is on the examining table also may indicate an awareness of the baby's safety and comfort.

Parents, particularly mothers, should be made aware of the signals of increased accident risk and should take extra precautions during stressful times, simplifying family life and doing only those things necessary to maintain health and comfort.

THE ROLE OF PHYSICIANS IN THE PROMOTION OF CHILD SAFETY

What can physicians do in their offices to help prevent childhood injuries? Recognition that injuries are the foremost public health problem that affects children already has spurred a great deal of activity to identify accidents as amenable to study and prevention. Too many parents, however, continue to believe that drugs and kidnapping, for example, are the greatest risk to the life of their developing child. Preventive counseling by pediatricians and emphasizing a developmental approach have been strongly advocated; until recently, however, no system was available to inform the practitioner on the content needed and to make available materials for parent education.

Responding to the need for an office-based, pediatrician-initiated counseling program to use in reducing the risk of injuries through *influencing* behavior, the American Academy of Pediatrics, in cooperation with government and private industry, developed the Injury Prevention Program (TIPP). Its executive board policy statement on injury prevention states: "Anticipatory guidance for injury prevention should be an integral part of the medical care provided for all infants and children." Initially the program focused on children from birth to the age of 5 years, emphasizing the use of car restraints, smoke detectors, safe hot water temperature, window and stairway guards/gates, and the availability of syrup of ipecac. TIPP has been extended to cover children to the age of 12 years and now includes a strong emphasis on bicycle, pedestrian, and water and sports safety for older children. The program offers a structured approach to both advocacy and education, roles that should be uniquely suited to physicians who care for children.*

Table 21-1 *Safety Counseling for Parents, Children, and Adolescents*

PERIOD	TOPICS
Perinatal	Cribs, other furniture, faucets, smoke detectors, infant car seats
1-4 mo	Furniture, falls, toy safety
4-7 mo	Ingestions, scalds, aspirations
7 mo–1 yr	Syrup of ipecac, poison control telephone number, safety packaging, poison proofing
1-3 yr	Car seats, mimicking adult behavior
3-5 yr	Supervised play; water, street, and yard safety
5-10 yr	Car seat belts, water and bicycle safety, fire and burn prevention
10-14 yr	Motor vehicle, water, fire, and firearm safety
Adolescents	Drugs, alcohol, cigarettes, sports safety, cardiopulmonary resuscitation

THE VICTIMS

The stages of childhood development can serve as a guide for accident-prevention education. A Boston study[27] found a lack of understanding of developmental expectations to be present in 87% of the parents whose children had accidents. The physician should understand and be able to give a general view of the developmental stages, hazards common to each, and precautions that can be taken to prevent typical accidents. Table 21-1 is a useful guide to the safety counseling necessary at the various stages of development.

The Infant from Birth to 4 Months

These infants can wiggle and squirm but are completely helpless. Instruction is needed to prevent drowning, burns, falls, and aspiration hazards; to promote crib safety; and to avoid the dangers of pillows, filmy plastics, and harnesses. Proper automotive restraints and flame-retardant garments should be purchased and used.

The Infant from 4 to 7 Months

These infants are becoming more active and learning to reach, to roll over, and to sit. The parents need advice on infant furniture and toy safety. The crib or playpen is the safest area for this age-group. Proper automotive restraints and flame-retardant garments continue to be necessary.

The Infant from 7 Months to 1 Year

These mobile infants are in increasing danger of falling as they begin to crawl, stand, and walk. Parents must be made aware that as children pull themselves erect, they pull everything down. There is danger from hanging tablecloths, hot foods on the stove, dangling electric cords, electric sockets, unguarded staircases, and reachable dangerous household products and medicines. Flame-retardant clothing and proper automotive restraints are essential.

The infant younger than 1 year of age needs 100% protection. The major accidents to be prevented are mechanical suffocation, ingestion or inhalation of food or foreign objects, motor vehicle injuries, fire and burn injuries, and falls. Mechanical suffocation has been listed as the leading cause of death in this age-group, but this category is suspect because it also may include cases of sudden infant death syndrome and infection.

The Toddler 1 to 2 Years of Age

Parents should be alerted to this curious investigator, who opens doors, windows, and drawers. Toddlers' climbing ability is excellent; they like to play in water and to take everything apart. They can stoop and recover; can mimic behavior of adults and older children; can push, pull, lift, and carry; and have no sense of danger. Parents must be aware of thermal and electric hazards and the perils of water. Safe toys should be purchased and play supervised. Syrup of ipecac should be available in the home for emergency treatment of poisonous ingestions. The safest area for this age-group is the playpen or a blocked-off play area, with free periods of supervised house roaming.

*A complete presentation of the TIPP program entitled *A Guide to Safety Counseling in Office Practice* is available from the American Academy of Pediatrics, Department of Publications, 141 Northwest Point Blvd., P.O. Box 927, Elk Grove Village, IL 60009.

The 2- and 3-Year-Old Child

This hurrying child is lightning fast and runs much of the time. The same precautions as for the toddler must still be continued.

The 3- to 5-Year-Old Child

Children of this age are teachable and should be taught their full names, traffic safety, obedience, and responsibility. Children at this age begin to develop skills and can throw objects, ride tricycles, climb trees, and explore the neighborhood. Parents should supervise the areas where their children play and also remove dangerous hazards. The children should not be relied on to protect themselves; supervised play is advised until the age of 5 years.

The major accidents to be prevented in 1- to 5-year-olds are motor vehicle accidents, fire and burn injuries, drownings, and poisonings.

The 5- to 10-Year-Old Child

Daring and adventurous activity characterizes children in this age-group. These children often are part of a group and will "try anything." They should be taught water safety, bicycle safety, and fire and burn prevention. Appropriate care should be taken if firearms are in the home. Care of pets and animal-bite prevention can be taught. By age 6, the safety of this age-group will depend on their own judgment and action 90% of the time.

The 10- to 14-Year-Old Child

Strenuous physical activity marks those in this age-group. Supervised recreational facilities should be available. Good examples should be set in preparation for automobile driving.

The major accidents in this age-group are motor vehicle accidents, drownings, and fire, burn, and firearm injuries.

ANIMAL BITES[40]

The pet population has kept pace with our own. Since 1945 the number of pet animals has more than tripled. It is estimated that there are more than 110 million cats and dogs, 20 million birds, and many more exotic pets in the United States. As the number of pets grows, so does human contact with them, which increases the potential of animal-produced injuries.

Every year there are approximately 1 million Americans who require medical attention for animal bites. Of these, 75% are children. More than 60,000 of these bites result in loss of sight, facial disfigurement, or other serious physical or psychological problems.

To reduce the number of persons bitten by animals, all members of the community must become actively involved in a program of prevention. The community must establish laws; the veterinarian must treat the animal and advise the owner; the physician must educate the parent; and the parent must educate the child.

The Community's Role

All pet dogs should be licensed and leashed or confined. Routine vaccination and immunization, along with the elimination of the reservoir of rabies—particularly bats, skunks, and foxes—should be carried out. Homeless or stray animals must be confined or destroyed.

The Veterinarian's Role

The immunization of pets should be accomplished and kept current. New animal owners should be educated about bite prevention and zoonoses (diseases communicable from animals to humans). Facilities should be available for the care of "veterinarian indigent" pets.

Cooperative Efforts

The veterinarian and the physician can work together and accomplish a great deal in a prevention program. They can advise on pet ownership, educate owners on how to prevent bites and zoonoses, encourage immunization of all animals, and provide instruction on the reporting of bites to proper authorities. Parents must be made aware that the greatest portion of responsibility for the care of pets—walking, bathing, feeding, and nursing—is theirs.

The child's maturity is another very important factor. Can the child differentiate between the animal as a live being and a toy? Does the child know that the animal's tail is not a "leash" by which the animal is pulled? It must be realized that some parents and children should never have pets.

Prospective owners should be informed that most animal bites occur when the pet is young. Therefore a more mature and placid animal is better for a child. Zoonoses also are more common with young animals.

A thorough understanding of animal behavior and an honest respect for all animals will go a long way in preventing animal bites. It is imperative that animal owners, and especially all children, be apprised of how to treat animals and how to react to them (see boxes, pp. 264 and 265).

Animal bites are further addressed in Chapter 180, and the issue of rabies associated with animal bites is discussed in Chapter 17.

ASPIRATION ACCIDENTS

Aspiration is a common cause of home accidental death in children younger than 4 years of age. Originally, safety pins were most frequently involved in aspiration by infants from birth to 1 year of age, with coins and peanuts more common in the 2- to 4-year age-group. The NSC reported approximately 3200 deaths in 1987 as a result of suffocation caused by ingested foreign objects; 180 of these episodes occurred in children younger than 5 years of age. Jackson and Jackson's review[32] of more than 3000 incidents of foreign bodies in the air and food passages noted a frequent history of eating too rapidly, chewing improperly, laughing, running with food in the mouth, or just holding a foreign body in the mouth, such as a pin, nail, nut, or small toy. Peanuts and peanut candy were very common offenders.

How to Have Safe Contact with Animals

1. Avoid all strange animals, especially wild, sick, or injured ones. The same techniques employed in teaching children not to talk to strangers should be used to teach them not to approach strange animals.
2. Notify the health department or police of any wild, sick, or injured animals.
3. Never permit a child to break up an animal fight, even when his or her own pet is involved. Use a rake, broom, or garden hose to separate the animals.
4. Become aware, and make children aware, of the danger of mistreating or teasing pets. Never pull the tail of an animal or take away food, a bone, or a toy with which an animal is playing. Pets are not toys, but living creatures that will bite if mauled, annoyed, or frightened.
5. Alert children to dangerous and nervous animals in the neighborhood, and do not permit children to enter yards or houses that harbor them.
6. Stress to children the importance of avoiding routes, when riding bicycles or tricycles, where dogs are known to chase vehicles.
7. Have children make friends, under adult supervision, with pets with which the children will be in contact in the immediate neighborhood.
8. Do not allow children to disturb an animal that is eating or sleeping. Set a good example by your own behavior.
9. Do not let pets come into indiscriminate contact with other animals.
10. Do not purchase or obtain a pet for children until they demonstrate their maturity and ability to handle and care for the pet. This ability is rare in a child younger than 4 years of age and unusual in a child younger than 6. Factors to be considered at any age are the maturity and disposition of the child and of the animal. Some people never develop this maturity.
11. Teach children that each animal has the right to a free existence and freedom from human-inflicted pain. Set a good example by your own behavior.
12. Never hold your face or allow the child to hold his or her face close to an animal.
13. Do not permit a child to lead a large dog.
14. Do not run, ride a bicycle, or skate in front of a dog. It will startle the animal.
15. Do not touch a dog that is asleep or unaware of your presence. Always speak to any dog that has not seen you approach so that the dog becomes aware of your presence and will not be startled.
16. Do not overexcite an animal, even in play.
17. Do not keep an animal confined with short ropes or chains. This may make the animal aggressive and vicious, especially if teased.
18. Have children avoid a dog raised in a home without children. Such an animal may resent children.
19. Do not allow an inexperienced child or adult to feed a dog. Such a person may pull back when the animal moves to take the food, frightening the animal. This practice is dangerous.

Predisposing factors to aspiration exist in conditions that decrease the gag or cough reflex. Drugs, alcohol intoxication, seizures, anesthesia, head trauma with unconsciousness, and uncommon conditions such as familial dysautonomia or certain types of cerebral palsy may be factors that facilitate aspiration.

Because foreign body aspiration is a common hazard in young children, physicians involved in their care should emphasize the dangers (see accompanying box on p. 265).

The treatment of foreign body aspiration is determined by the location of the object. Upper airway foreign bodies are life threatening and require immediate treatment when the child is choking.

"Blind sweeps" of the forefinger in the posterior pharynx should be avoided in young children to prevent pushing the foreign body posteriorly, causing greater obstruction. If a foreign body can be seen, it can be removed with a finger. If the child can speak or breathe and is coughing, the foreign object may dislodge spontaneously; therefore first aid action is unnecessary and potentially dangerous. Immediate relief is required for partial obstruction with poor air exchange or with cyanosis, as well as for complete obstruction.

In children the abdominal thrust (Heimlich maneuver) is recommended as the single procedure to be performed.[29] In infants younger than 1 year of age a combination of back blows and chest thrusts continues to be recommended to produce an increase in pressure in the blocked respiratory passages to expel the foreign body.

An infant should be held face down with the head lower than the trunk. The four back blows are delivered with the heel of the hand. The four chest thrusts are delivered as for external cardiac compression. Physicians, health professionals, and the general public should familiarize themselves with recommended resuscitation techniques.

If these emergency first aid measures fail, the victim must be transported immediately and rapidly to a medical facility.

AUTOMOTIVE INJURIES[14,44]

In 1987, 20.8 million accidents occurred among the 186 million motor vehicles registered in this country; 1.8 million Americans, or more than 1 in 100, suffered a disabling injury, and 48,700 died.

The staggering death toll was actually a significant reduc-

Safety Rules for Meeting a Strange Dog

Meeting a strange dog can be a very frightening and potentially dangerous situation. It is important to try to remain calm and, if possible, follow these suggestions:

1. Stop, stand still, and speak softly.
2. Wait and see what the dog is going to do.
3. Look for the signs of the unsafe dog: rigid body; stiff tail at "half mast"; shrill, hysterical bark; crouching or slinking position, with head lowered and nose close to ground; staring expression and an attempt to circle behind you.
4. Pivot slowly if the dog tries to circle behind you. Wait until the dog stops moving, then move slowly; stop when the dog moves again.
5. Never turn your back on a dog moving toward you.
6. Never touch a strange dog.
7. Never strike, kick, or make any threatening gesture.
8. Do not hand a person a package or shake hands when the person's dog is nearby. The dog may misinterpret the move.
9. Do not make the first overture of friendship with a dog. Allow the dog to do this, which he will not do until he smells you.

tion from the 1972 high of 56,278 fatalities. This is thought to be attributable in part to the energy crisis that began in the spring of 1973, resulting in a lowering of the speed limit to 55 mi/hr on main roads and concomitant changes in driving habits. The number of fatalities for children from birth to 14 years of age was 3500 in 1987; children were passengers in 2050 and pedestrians in 1450 of these deaths. Approximately 145,000 children are injured yearly while passengers in vehicles.

Safety belts are now available for nearly all passenger-car occupants. It is estimated that 12,000 lives could be saved annually if all passengers used belts at all times and that an additional 6000 to 9000 lives could be saved if air-cushion restraint systems were installed in all passenger cars.

A study in Victoria, Australia, attributed a 14% reduction in driver deaths to increased seat belt usage. Scherz[45] reported the effectiveness of seat belts in reducing morbidity and mortality in the state of Washington, as shown in Table 21-2. Other studies have demonstrated that restraining devices could reduce fatalities by 45% and prevent many injuries.

Infants are especially vulnerable to fatal injuries in motor vehicle accidents. In one study,[4] infants younger than 6 months had the highest occupant death rate: 9.1/100,000, compared with 4.8/100,000 for children 6 months through 12 years of age. Infants who are held on the laps of passengers are particularly vulnerable to serious injury. As a response the American Academy of Pediatrics (AAP) initiated "The First Ride . . . A Safe Ride" campaign in October 1980 to involve pediatricians in educating the public in the use of safety seats.

How to Prevent Aspiration

1. Young children should not be allowed to play with small objects. As a guide, the government has proposed a small-parts standard that requires toys for children younger than 3 years old to be a minimum size of 1¼ inches in diameter and not fit into a truncated circular cylinder 2¼ inches long. This standard is under review; an increase in the dimensions of the small parts covered under the regulations is being considered. "Testing" tubes are often available to parents through mail-order toy catalogs.
2. Older children should be taught not to hold foreign bodies in their mouths.
3. Hard, smooth vegetable-type foods (e.g., peanuts) or smooth, round foods (e.g., hot dogs and grapes) that require a grinding motion should be avoided as foods for children. The chewing habit is not well established until the age of 4 years. Therefore chewable tablets should not be given until that time.
4. Children should not be given coins as rewards or play items.
5. Infants and toddlers should not put large pieces of food in their mouths. Cut and break food into bite-size pieces, and encourage children to chew thoroughly.
6. Children should be kept quiet while eating food or candy. Excitement or activity, such as running and walking, predisposes them to inhalation of food. Speaking when eating should be forbidden.
7. Safety pins should be kept closed and pinned into the caretaker's clothing to keep this very serious aspiration or ingestion hazard out of the child's reach.
8. An uninflated balloon is an aspiration hazard and may be sucked into the posterior pharynx or even the larynx or trachea. Thirteen of 21 death certificates related to toy aspirations reviewed by the U.S. Consumer Products Safety Commission revealed balloons as a cause of death.
9. The dry cleaner's plastic bag is not a true aspiration hazard, but can cause suffocation when it clings to the face of a small child or infant.

Table 21-2 *Fatalities of Children from Birth to 4 Years as Passengers in Motor Vehicles (Washington, 1970-1980)*

	NUMBER KILLED	TOTAL NUMBER OF PASSENGERS	RATIO KILLED/PASSENGERS
Unrestrained	146	33,200	1/227
Restrained	2	6,300	1/3150

From Scherz RG: Auto safety: "The first ride . . . A safe ride" campaign. In Bergman AB, editor: Preventing childhood injuries. Reprinted with permission of Ross Laboratories, Columbus, OH 43216, from report of the twelfth Ross Roundtable on Critical Approaches to Common Pediatric Problems, © 1982, Ross Laboratories.

Encouraged by the 1978 passage of a child passenger protection law in Tennessee and the positive effect of an educational and police enforcement campaign in reducing fatalities and injuries, all the states had passed child restraint laws by 1985.

Standard safety belts usually should not be worn by small children because they cause abdominal injuries in a collision. To protect children younger than 4 to 5 years of age, it is necessary to provide them with special restraining devices.[48]

AUTOMOTIVE RESTRAINTS FOR INFANTS AND SMALL CHILDREN

The Federal Standard for Automotive Restraining Devices in Children went into effect in April 1971, under the Motor Vehicle Safety Standard No. 213, Child Seating Systems. Unfortunately, the standard was based on static rather than dynamic testing.

To provide effective protection, restraining devices must distribute deceleration forces over a large area of the body and be secured to the vehicle by means of a standard lap belt or by anchoring the device itself. They should be of strong, energy-absorbing material and be free of potentially injury-producing components.

It should be emphasized that the previously used child restraint seats that merely hooked over the back of the car seat or harnesses that were secured by looping a strap around the back of the car seat were *not* designed to protect in a collision.

In January 1981 a new regulation, Federal Standard No. 213-80, replaced static testing with 20 and 30 mi/hr dynamic testing that more closely represented car crashes. The regulation covers all types of systems used to restrain children in motor vehicles, such as infant carriers, child seats, harnesses, and car beds.

The dynamic testing standard prohibits restraints from collapsing and requires the retention of a test dummy within the confines of the restraint during the testing. It requires a minimum level of safety performance for restraints equipped with top tether straps or arm rests, even if the top tether is not used or the arm rest is in place but the child restraint system's belts are not buckled (the arm rest must function as a protective barrier). The new standard also specifies padding requirements for restraints used by children who weigh less than 20 pounds and limits the force exerted on the head and chest of a test dummy during testing of restraints for children who weigh more than 20 pounds. This regulation also specifies the force needed to open buckles on the restraint belts so that young children cannot unbuckle them but adults can easily do so. Proper instructions for use are required to be posted on the child restraints.

Periodically, the AAP publishes a list of the crash-tested devices available (as shown in the box on pp. 267 and 268). Proper installation is vitally important.

Children 4 to 5 years of age or those who weigh more than 40 pounds may, if necessary, use a standard lap belt. The child should be placed on a firm cushion and should sit up straight against the seat back. The belt should then be adjusted snugly to fit across the hips; it must not be permitted to ride up across the stomach. Abdominal injuries can result from improperly adjusted belts. A lap/shoulder belt combination provides better protection than a lap belt alone. The shoulder belt should fit across the shoulder and should not cross the face and neck. If it crosses the face and neck, it should be placed behind the child's back.

Children under 55 inches in height should *not* use a shoulder strap, and no one should use a shoulder strap without a lap belt.

The Insurance Institute for Highway Safety[19] studied 8893 children younger than 10 years old in 5050 cars and found only 7% to be properly restrained against possible crash injuries; other studies report higher percentages of use, but at least 75% of these children were not adequately protected.

Parents fail to use seat belts and restraints for children for the following reasons:

1. Inconvenience or discomfort for the child
2. Prohibitive cost
3. Fear of entrapment
4. Faulty reasoning: "It just can't happen to me"
5. Belief that it is safer to hold a child on one's lap
6. Belief that restraints are needed only on long trips or express highways
7. Forgetfulness

Failure of physicians to counsel about child automotive safety devices may result from a lack of knowledge about the proper restraining devices available and where to buy them. There also is the lack of gratification in not actually seeing improvement in the health status of the community as a result of advice given.

Bass and Wilson[9] demonstrated that personal contact in a pediatric practice, followed by letters, produced a considerable increase in seat-belt use, whereas a saturation campaign of television commercials urging seat-belt use had no effect.

Schemes that may be adopted by physicians and health

Available Crash-Treated Restraints Meeting or Exceeding Current Federal Safety Standard No. 213-80:1989

The infant, convertible, and booster seats on this list have been certified by the manufacturer as meeting this standard.

The 3-point harness consists of two shoulder straps that connect to a crotch strap. The 5-point harness consists of two shoulder straps, two hip straps, and a crotch strap. A harness-shield consists of two shoulder straps attached to a body pad or shelf-type shield with a crotch strap. Strap positions refer to shoulder strap height adjustments available to fit growing children properly.

INFANT SAFETY SEATS
Birth to approximately 20 pounds
Semi-reclined for rear-facing use only

Century 570 Infant Car Seat. 3 Pt harness 2 strap positions
Retail price $25-30

Century 580 Infant Car Seat Deluxe. 3 Pt harness/2 strap positions/"stay-in-car" base
Retail price $40-60

Century Infant Love Seat. 3 Pt harness/ 2 strap positions
Retail price $30-40

Cosco First Ride. 3 Pt harness w/one-step adjustment/1 strap position/2 recline positions
Retail price $35-50

Cosco TLC. 3 Pt harness w/one-step adjustment/2 strap positions
Retail price $25-45

Evenflo Dyn-O-Mite. 3 Pt harness/2 strap positions/ 4 recline positions
Retail price $24-26

Evenflo Infant Seat. 3 Pt harness/2 strap positions/ 2 recline positions
Retail price $32-35

Evenflo Joy Ride. 3 Pt harness/2 strap positions
Retail price $29-47

Fisher-Price Infant Car Seat. Harness-shield/2 strap positions/locks into shopping cart
Retail price $49-95

Kolcraft Rock 'N Ride. 3 Pt harness/1 strap position
Retail price $35-45

CONVERTIBLE SAFETY SEATS
Birth to approximately 40 pounds
Infants: Rear-facing
Toddlers: Forward-facing
(2 strap positions unless noted)

Babyhood Wonda Chair 810. 5 Pt harness
Retail price $79-95

Century 1000 STE. 5 Pt harness w/one-step adjustment/3 strap positions
Retail price $50-70

Century 2000, 3000 & 5000 STE. Harness-shield w/ one-step adjustment/3 strap positions
Retail price $70-130

Cosco AutoTrac. Harness-shield/adjustable harness retractor
Retail price $80-90

Cosco Communter. Harness-shield
Retail price $70-100

Cosco Communter 5-Pt. 5 Pt harness/shoulder harness repositioned w/o rethreading
Retail price $55-70

Evenflo Convertible. 5 Pt harness/sold to institutions only
Retail price .... N/A

Evenflo One-Step. Harness-shield
Retail price $58-69

Evenflo Seven Year Car Seat. Harness-shield/converts to booster seat
Retail price $90-96

Evenflo Ultara I & II. Harness-shield/3 strap positions
Retail price $62-82

Fisher-Price Car Seat. Harness-shield/automatic locking retractor
Retail price $88

Gerry Guardian. Harness-shield/3 strap positions/ emergency locking retractor
Retail price $60-90

Kolcraft Dial-A-Fit. Harness-shield w/one-step adjustment/3 strap positions
Retail price $65-85

Nissan Infant/Child Safety Seat. Harness-shield/ emergency locking retractor
Retail price $99

Strolee GT 2000 & 3000. 5 Pt harness or harness-shield
Retail price $60-90

Strolee Wee Care Car Seats. 5 Pt harness or harness-shield
Retail price $39-200

Virco/Pride Trimble Pride Ride. 5 Pt harness/removable shield
Retail price $65-140

Volvo Child Safety Seat. 5 Pt harness/fits Volvo and other cars
Retail price $200

Modified from 1989 family shopping guide to infant/child safety seats, Elk Grove Village, IL, 1989, American Academy of Pediatrics.

Continued.

Available Crash-Treated Restraints Meeting or Exceeding Current Federal Safety Standard No. 213-80:1989—cont'd

BOOSTER SEATS
30-60 pounds
Forward-facing
(All have shields unless noted)

Century Commander. Multi-position shield/opens to the side
Retail price $20-30

Century CR-3. Shield removes for use w/lap-shoulder belt
Retail price $20-35

Cosco Explorer 1. Multi-position shield/2 seating heights/opens to the side
Retail price $25-35

Evenflo Booster. Adjustable split-shield/opens upward/crotch strap
Retail price $36-41

Evenflo Sightseer. Adjustable shield/opens to the side
Retail price $21-25

Evenflo Wings. Adjustable split-shield/opens upward
Retail price $30-40

Ford Tot Guard. Extra-large shield/2 seat heights
Retail price $65

Gerry DoubleGuard. Shield removes for use w/lap-shoulder belt/opens from either side/lap belt secures base
Retail price $40-50

Gerry Voyager. Adjustable shield/opens upward/lap belt secures base
Retail price $35-45

Kolcraft Flip 'N Go II & Quik Step. Adjustable shield/opens downward
Retail price $20-45

Strolee Quick Click Booster. Adjustable shield/opens to the side
Retail price $25-45

Virco/Pride Trimble Click 'N Go. Adjustable shield/opens upward
Retail price $31-41

SPECIAL NEEDS SEATS
Designed for premature infants and physically or neurologically handicapped children.
A tether strap attaches to the safety seat back and is bolted to the rear window shelf or vehicle floor. Tethers are an added safety feature and should be used when available.

Columbia Orthopedic Positioning Seat. 5 Pt harness/up to 65 lbs/fits stroller base
Retail price $429

E-Z-On Vest. 4 Pt harness/supports child upright/up to 164 lbs./tether
Retail price $53-57

E-Z-On Modified Vest. 3 Pt harness/to transport children in "lying-down" position
Retail price $40

Fabrication Enterprises Britax Special Seat. 5 Pt harness/4 adjustable shoulder and hip straps/20-105 lbs./up to 5 ft./fits stroller base/tether
Retail price $425

Fabrication Enterprises Swinger Infant Car Bed/Carry-Cot. To transport infants/"lying-down" position/up to 20 lbs./26 inches
Retail price $275

Gunnell Kidster KI & KP. 5 Pt harness/custom fit/up to 50 lbs./reclining/roller base/optional safety harness/tether
Retail price $1,078-1,349

Koziatek Low Birthweight Bunting. Must be used w/Swinger Infant Car Bed (listed above)/4¾-7 lbs.
Retail price $35

Koziatek Spelcast. 5 Pt harness/used w/spica or body casts/up to 40 lbs./tether
Retail price $130

Ortho-Kinetics Travel Chair. Adaptive one-piece chair/2 widths/12 and 15-inches/lap-shoulder belt and additional lap belt required (not supplied)/tether
Retail price $698-765

Safety Rehab Systems 501, 502 & 900 Series. 5 Pt harness/adaptive travel chair/1 year through young adult/removable seat and base/optional bases and support pads/tether
Retail price $850-1,213

Snug Seat. 5 Pt harness/positioning chair and car seat/up to 35 lbs./fits stroller or trolley base/tether
Retail price $599

Tumble Forms Carrie Pre-School Seat. 4 Pt tether/20-40 lbs./30-38 inches/removable footrest and tray*
Retail price $675

Tumble Forms Carrie Elementary Seat. 4 Pt tether/30-60 lbs./38-48 inches/removable footrest and tray*
Retail price $685

Tumble Forms Carrie Jr. Seat. 4 Pt tether/50-100 lbs./48-58 inches/removable footrest & tray*
Retail price $785

*Fits Rover stroller frame.

care personnel to increase the use of automotive restraining devices can include a combination of the following:

1. List it as an immunization on the child's record.
2. Explain to parents the danger of holding an infant in the event of an emergency stop or collision: the weight of the infant times the speed of the car is the weight that must be restrained by the person holding the child.
3. Explain to parents that studies have shown better behavior by children traveling in car seats than by those sitting unrestrained; they cannot stand up or climb around, and they do not cry or fuss as much as unrestrained children.
4. Arrange for physicians and hospitals to encourage parents of newborns to take their infants home in a safe restraining device.
5. Establish a lending or swapping scheme for the devices as infants and children outgrow them.

Temporary measures for children as passengers should include the following:

1. Children are safer if restrained in adult seat belts when riding in the back seat (which is recommended for children older than 5 years) than if allowed to ride unrestrained. The lap belt should be worn across the hips, not the abdomen. A pillow will help to elevate the child to the proper position.
2. Children are safer in the back seat of the car standing on the floor and holding onto the back of the front seat than sitting in a front seat.

Children as Pedestrians

A pedestrian injury is twice as likely as a passenger injury to be fatal. It essentially is an urban problem, with two thirds of the fatalities occurring between sunset and dawn. More than 1000 children are killed annually as a result of nighttime pedestrian injuries. Fatalities are highest in the 5- to 9-year-old age-group; in the older of these children they often result from darting out into traffic. Children younger than 6 years of age have difficulty distinguishing right from left, and their peripheral vision is not as well developed as that of adults.

Pedestrian safety education programs for children that address midblock "dart-outs" and intersection dashes have been developed by the National Highway Traffic Safety Association for primary school use; their use should be encouraged.

Retroflective material* should be worn by children exposed to the danger of roadways at night. It may be purchased as an integral part of garments to be worn at night, as strips of tape that require sewing on, or as an adhesive tape. The concept of "reflecting" pedestrians and bicycle-riding children has the support of the Accident Prevention Committee of the AAP and deserves implementation.

Driveway Injuries

Pedestrian fatalities in children younger than 5 years of age are most likely to result from parents backing over a child in the driveway. The hazard of allowing children to play in driveways should be emphasized, and parents should be alert to this potential danger. The following are *safe family driving hints*:

1. Before the car moves:
   a. All seat belts should be fastened and all restraining devices secured.
   b. All doors should be locked.
   c. All children not in approved restraining devices should be in the back seat.
   d. No heavy or sharp objects should be placed on the same seat with children. Groceries should be put in the trunk.
2. Nothing should be carried on the shelf under the back window.
3. Children should never be left alone in the car and should never be allowed to play in one.
4. Rules for behavior while in the car should be made to prevent distracting the driver. Take something along to keep children quietly occupied.
5. Children should not be permitted to hang arms, legs, or heads out of the window.
6. If the driveway is the only play area for your children, a car can be parked at the entrance in case cars pull in quickly without noticing children (i.e., cars turning around or parent coming home).

Drinking and Driving

It is estimated that half of all automobile fatalities are related to ethanol consumption. Although ethanol is not a stimulant, it may appear to have such action because it relaxes the individual by depressing the central nervous system's higher centers, resulting in uninhibited behavior but depression of those vital reflexes needed in driving.

Although ethanol reactions vary depending on the rate of consumption, the presence of food in the stomach, and the person's mood at the time of consumption, guidelines may be used to convey to drivers the dangers of ethanol consumption and driving (Table 21-3). At blood ethanol levels of 80 mg/dl (now the legal limit in many states), the chance of a fatal crash increases dramatically; at levels of 100 mg/dl, the probability of such a crash is 5 to 12 times that for the nondrinking driver.

Ethanol is metabolized at 12 to 20 mg/dl/hr; drinking coffee, taking a cold shower, or exercising will not increase this rate or decrease the ethanol impairment or depression resulting from consumption. Before driving it is wise to wait at least an hour for each drink consumed. Driver education programs in schools have not succeeded in reducing injury rates. Collisions occur two and one-half times as frequently in drivers younger than 18 years of age as in those above this age. Drinking may play a role.

BICYCLE INJURIES[11,25,53]

The bicycle leads the Consumer Product Safety Commission's National Electronic Injury Surveillance System (NEISS) list of hazardous products in the United States. NEISS projects 1 million bicycle-related injuries yearly and predicts that 372,000 of these will be seen in hospital emergency rooms.

*Retroreflective material is produced by the 3M Company and is available from many retailers, such as the JC Penney Co.

Table 21-3 *Alcoholic Drinks Consumed in Terms of Blood Ethanol Level, Resulting Symptoms, and Hours Needed to Metabolize*

BLOOD ETHANOL LEVEL (mg/dl)	SYMPTOMS	AMOUNT CONSUMED			HOURS NEEDED TO METABOLIZE
		COCKTAIL, 1.5 OZ (50% ETHANOL)	BEER, 12 OZ (5% ETHANOL)	WINE, 5 OZ (12% ETHANOL)	
20	Feel good	1.0	1.0	1.0	1-2
50	Relaxed	1.5	1.5	1.5	2-3
100	Impaired (legal definition)	3.0	3.0	3.0	5-7
150	Intoxicated	4.0	4.5	4.5	7-10
300	Drunk	8.0	9.0	9.0	15-20
500	Dead	14.0	15.0	15.0	—

In 1987, 111 million bicycles were in use in the United States. Of 1400 deaths reported in association with their use, 31% occurred in the birth to 14-year-old age-group.[46] The proportion of deaths occurring in children younger than 14 years of age has steadily decreased from 78% in 1960 to 31% in 1987, reflecting a change in use and ownership of bicycles. Little comfort should be taken from this inasmuch as the total number of deaths has risen because of the greater number of bicycles in use. Approximately 90% of bicycle deaths result from collisions with motor vehicles.

Estimates of the annual total number of bicycle injuries requiring medical attention or causing one or more days of restricted activity have ranged from 180,000 to as high as 1 million; the largest proportion of those injured are children. The accident rate for young riders 5 to 12 years of age averages 2% annually, with an estimated 20% of the accidents resulting in fractures and an estimated 5% in concussions.

In a series of 107 injuries to children,[25] 20% resulting from collision with an automobile, trauma to the head was the most common injury found. This led the authors to suggest passage of laws requiring mandatory use of helmets (similar to those required for motorcycle riders) for bicycle riders. National children's safety advocates are strongly urging that bicycle helmets become standard equipment for every ride, and they advise the purchase of a helmet along with the bike. Lightweight helmets approved by the American National Standards Institute or the Snell Memorial Foundation are available for children at reasonable prices. With the increased use of motorized bicycles (mopeds), physicians can expect an accident incidence even greater than that for nonmotorized bicycles.

Factors in Bicycle Injuries

The following three factors account for most injuries:

1. *Horseplay* accounts for a large number of the accidents. Daredevil feats by young boys imitating Evel Knievel's exploits have led to an increase in injuries.

2. *Riding double* with a passenger on the handlebars, the crossbar of the frame, or the rear fender with no support for the feet produces large numbers of "bicycle spoke" injuries, which deserve special mention.

In the "bicycle spoke" injury, the tissue is lacerated from the knifelike action of the spokes, the foot is crushed from being caught between the wheel and frame, and the foot sustains a shearing injury from a combination of these two forces. Full recognition of the injury may not be apparent on initial examination because damage to the underlying structures can take several hours to appear. This injury needs careful observation as with wringer arm injuries.[31]

3. *Poor-fitting bicycles* are overrepresented in accidents involving a motor vehicle and bicycle collision. The bicycle seat should be no higher than the rider's hips so that the feet can touch the ground without causing the bicycle to lean.

Remedies to Reduce Injuries

Bicycles need design changes in the wheels (e.g., shields to prevent contact with the spokes), flat surfaces where the handlebars join the fork to prevent loosening, and professional assembly rather than do-it-yourself kits. Use of reflective paint would make the entire bicycle more visible at night.

Proof of rider proficiency through examination and licensing before being allowed on public roads should be considered, with children younger than 9 years of age excluded from use of public highways. Mandatory helmet-use regulations would reduce the number and severity of head injuries.

The Consumer Product Safety Commission (CPSC) has set bicycle safety standards for brakes, seats, tires, reflectors, front fork frames, and steering systems and recommends a predelivery road test.

Safe Bicycling

Bicycle riders require education and training to avoid accidents. Loss of control by the rider has been found to be a factor in 63% of injuries. Violating traffic rules—such as turning across the path of a car, disregarding signals and signs, riding against traffic, and riding into a car's path from a driveway, alley, or intersection—play a part in 80% of injuries.

A composite of safety suggestions from the AAP and the CPSC is listed in the box on p. 271.

MINIBIKE, MOPED, MOTORCYCLE, AND ALL-TERRAIN VEHICLE INJURIES[5]

The CPSC estimated there to be 75,000 *minibike* injuries in 1973. Approximately 63,000 minibike-related injuries are treated in hospital emergency rooms annually. Nearly half these injuries happen to children 10 to 15 years old and another fifth to persons 15 to 20 years old. Males incur four fifths of the injuries. The leg was the most frequent body part

Suggestions for Safe Bicycling

1. Always wear a helmet when riding a bicycle.
2. Learn and obey all traffic rules, signs, and signals.
3. Use bicycle paths when possible. Do not ride on streets that have heavy automobile traffic. When riding on the sidewalk, give pedestrians the right of way. Until age 7 years, ride with adult supervision and off the street.
4. If it is necessary to ride in the street, ride on the right side with the flow of traffic, not against it.
5. Walk, do not ride, the bicycle across busy intersections and around left-turn corners. Avoid riding in wet weather.
6. Do not ride double. Balancing is difficult, and vision may be blocked. Spoke injuries to the foot and leg are common in passengers.
7. Do not ride barefoot; wear rubber-soled shoes and keep both feet on the pedals while riding. Avoid plastic pedals; use rubber-treated or metal pedals with serrated edges.
8. Use retroflective tape on all bikes, front and rear. For night riding, a headlight and a taillight or a red reflector on the rear are necessary, and the rider should wear light-colored clothing. Retroflective tape (white in front and red in rear) and retroflective clothing also will help the rider to be seen at night.
9. Choose carrier seats for children older than 9 months of age with foot rests, foot guards, foot straps, and seat belts to prevent injuries.
10. Keep the bicycle in good condition. Check and be familiar with the brakes. Regular expert maintenance is essential for safe riding. Complicated work should be done by an experienced repairman.
11. Carefully choose bicycles to suit the child's size and age. The bicycle seat should be no higher than the rider's hips, the feet should reach the pedals without the use of blocks, and the handlebars should be within easy reach. When sitting on the seat with hands on the handlebars, the child must be able to place the balls of both feet on the ground. Straddling the center bar, the child should be able to keep both feet flat on the ground with 1 inch of clearance between crotch and bar. Younger children's bicycles should have coaster brakes; hand brakes require too much strength and coordination for beginners.

injured (52%), followed by the arm (19%) and the head (18%).

Minibikes are particularly dangerous because of poor handling, resulting from a short wheelbase and small tires, insufficient acceleration, inadequate brakes, and small size, which decrease visibility and give inadequate protection to drivers in collisions. Life-threatening injuries to the larynx by cables and fence wire have been reported.[2] Lack of safety devices or defective and poorly constructed components were involved in a third of 21 in-depth investigations made by the CPSC.

The AAP Joint Committee of Physical Fitness, Recreation, and Sports Medicine has urged parents to refuse to allow their children to own or operate minibikes.

Mopeds (from *mo*tor plus *ped*als) are low-speed, lightweight motorcycles that share the operating characteristics of bicycles and motorcycles. Mopeds are commonplace in Europe, and their popularity grew in the United States when fuel became scarce and expensive; an estimated 150,000 mopeds were sold in 1977. With little horsepower the acceleration of a moped often is inadequate for mixing with city traffic and thus creates dangerous situations. Because of its low speed, it also is inappropriate (and often illegal) for use on arterial highways and bridges and in many tunnels.

According to 1980 data from the Kentucky Department of Public Safety and the Ohio Department of Highway Safety, 83% of the accidents involving mopeds caused injuries, 16% caused property damage, and 1% were fatal. Injury patterns reveal that head and lower extremity injuries are those most usually serious. Helmets protect the head but do not alter the incidence or severity of neck injuries. When driving on streets, moped operators can be expected to encounter the same hazards as motorcycle operators.

Most European countries now require that moped operators wear safety helmets. Both Great Britain and France, which have helmet laws, have reported a one-third reduction in serious head injuries. This parallels experience with helmet use by motorcycle drivers in the United States. Most states and the District of Columbia have a variety of laws governing moped use or banning them from the road. Few states, however, require the operator to wear a helmet.

There were 5,148,000 *motorcycles* in use in 1987; 4200 fatalities and 460,000 injuries were associated with their use. The death rate for motorcycle riders was estimated at about 43 deaths per 100 million miles of motorcycle travel compared with the overall motor vehicle death rate of 2.55. Accidents involving motorcycles tend to occur during the warm months, on weekends, and between noon and 4 PM and 6 and 11 PM. About 90% of the operators are males, 60% of whom are younger than 25 years of age.

As a result of a federal requirement, all but three states had mandatory helmet-use laws for motorcyclists by 1975. When the federal requirement was repealed in 1976, there began a steady repeal of state laws. In 1982 there were 9 states with no helmet laws and 22 with amended laws, requiring helmets only for teenage drivers. Between 1976 and 1980, deaths from motorcycle accidents increased by 49%; more than 30% of the fatal accidents occurred to persons younger than 20 years of age. The protective effect of helmets has been shown at all levels of injury severity. A nonhelmeted rider is twice as likely to acquire a minor head injury and five times as likely to acquire a severe or critical injury as is a helmeted rider.[13]

All-terrain vehicles (ATVs) are three- or four-wheel recreational vehicles intended for off-the-road use on rough terrain; they were originally promoted for use by children and adolescents. With more than 2.5 million in use they have become linked to more than 1000 deaths since 1982 and are associated with approximately 86,000 injuries yearly. The AAP found these vehicles to be a major hazard to children and backed demands for a sales ban and recall of the three-wheeled vehicles. In 1983 an agreement was reached by the U.S. Justice Department and manufacturers, which banned the sale of all three-wheeled vehicles and restricted the purchase of four-wheeled vehicles to riders older than 16 years of age.[24] However, these bans are often not enforced.

BURNS[6,7,10,18,22,51]

Burn injuries cause 1.75 million Americans to seek medical attention annually; 40% of these are children younger than 15 years of age. At least 5500 persons die annually from burns, and a fifth of these are children younger than 14 years old. House fires cause 75% of all burn-related deaths, with young children and elderly persons at highest risk. About 50% of all fires involve cigarettes, frequently with associated alcohol use.

Burn deaths rank second behind motor vehicle deaths in the 1- to 4-year age-group and third behind motor vehicle and drowning fatalities in the 5- to 14-year age-group. The annual death rate from fire in the United States is 4 per 100,000 population, exceeding that of every other industrialized nation.

The vectors of burn injury have been classified as combustible materials, hot substances, electric sources, and chemical compounds.

According to Galveston Shriner's Burn Institute,[10,22] combustible substances such as flammable fabrics are the leading cause of major burn injuries. Flammable fabrics, usually cotton dresses or nightgowns, have been incriminated in 54% and flammable liquids in 35% of burns. A Duke University study[12] classified the causes of burns as 55% resulting from clothing ignition, 25% from direct contact with fires, 15% from gasoline or kerosene, and 5% from scalds.

Elderly persons and the very young are the most thin-skinned people, and what might produce only a second-degree burn in a hairy young man may well produce a third-degree burn in them. The young (under 10 years) and the elderly (over 65 years) were injured in one out of seven burn incidents in which they were involved, but the 11- to 65-year age-group was injured in only 1 out of 25 such incidents.

Flammable Fabrics[7]

In 1975 the CPSC estimated that each year 3000 to 5000 deaths and 150,000 to 250,000 injuries were associated with flammable fabrics. The importance of these burns lies in their severity. The mortality in the event of clothing ignition burns was four times as high, the surface area burned twice as large, the hospital stay was 50% longer, and the medical expenses were twice those of nonclothing ignition burns.

The flammable-fabric burn problem was like the smoldering fire that bursts into flames periodically. In 1945 cowboy chaps caused an epidemic of clothing ignition fires. In 1951 the incendiary "torch" sweater caused another flash of insight into clothing burn injuries before it was banned.

The most common igniters of these combustibles were space heaters (usually gas) 19%, matches 16%, outdoor fires 16%, gas hot-water heaters 8%, and kitchen stoves 4%.

In 1953 the first Flammable Fabric Act was passed and was infamous in allowing 99% of all fabrics marketed in this country to pass its standards. Its main focus was on clothing that came into contact with the skin while the vast majority of flammable fabrics were overlooked. England has had a Fabrics Act since 1913 and a Children's Nightdress Regulation since 1964.

In 1967 an amended fabric act was passed to include all wearing apparel and home furnishings, but the unsatisfactory standards test was retained. In 1972 the act was further amended to improve the testing of flame-retardant materials and to ban the sale of children's sleepwear up to size 6X (6-year-old size) that did not meet the standards. In 1975 this regulation was extended to include children's sleepwear up to size 14X (14-year-old size). This new regulation stipulated that the garment remain flame retardant for at least 50 washings.

On April 7, 1977, CPSC banned the sale of any children's clothing treated with the flame-retardant chemical *Tris* (2,3-dibromopropyl phosphate). The ban resulted after a 2-year rat-feeding study showed the presence of cancer in test animals. The CPSC feared that Tris could be absorbed through the skin or by "mouthing," but there have been no instances reported of cancer in humans from Tris.

A Guide to Flame-Retardant Fabrics Used in Children's Sleepwear

FIBERS POSSIBLY TREATED WITH TRIS

Acetate
Acetate blends
Triacetates
Triacetate blends

FIBERS INHERENTLY FLAME RESISTANT, NOT REQUIRING ADDITION OF CHEMICALS

Modacrylic (Verel, SEF, Kanecaron)
Modacrylic blends
Matrix (Cordelan)
Matrix blends
Vinyon (Leavil)
Vinyon blends

FIBERS TREATED WITH CHEMICAL OTHER THAN TRIS

Cotton, 100%
Nylon

At first it was believed that washing Tris-treated garments three or more times would substantially reduce the risk of exposure; however, tests suggested that 10% of the Tris may remain even after 10 washings. Thus Tris-treated garments should be avoided, but substitute flame-retardant clothing is available. See the box on p. 272 for a guide to flame-retardant fabrics used in children's sleepwear.

As a result of flammable fabric legislation and a change in the style and fabrics used for sleepwear and children's clothing, the incidence of clothing ignitions that cause significant burns in children has been reduced markedly. This is one of the success stories in injury prevention. However, parents should continue to be reminded that the risk of burns remains much greater without flame-retardant clothing.

Useful hints for the prevention of burn injuries are presented in the box on p. 274.

The majority of fire-related deaths occur at night and result from the inhalation of smoke or toxic gas. Smoke detectors, effective in saving lives, should be installed on each floor and particularly in furnace and sleeping areas. Occupants should take no more than 4 minutes to get outside the home after the alarm sounds.

Scalds

Scalds are a frequent cause of children being hospitalized with burns. The majority of these are caused by spilled coffee or tea, tipped-over stove pots, splattered hot grease, and other hot foods. Prevention of these scalding burns depends predominantly on informed parents and adequate supervision of children. Turning pot handles so that they cannot be reached is part of burn prevention.

Each year 2000 to 3000 people require emergency room treatment for tap water scalds. The most frequent victims are infants and toddlers, and the severity of the burns results in a high incidence of hospitalization, scarring, and death. At 150° F (65° C) deep second- or third-degree burns occur within 2 seconds.

Tap water temperature is related to the burn hazard, which rises sharply with water temperatures above 130° F (55° C). The CPSC has developed a voluntary *new* tub and shower installation standard that requires antiscald devices that limit water flow at temperatures above 120° F (49° C); existing plumbing fixtures cannot be so equipped. One fourth of the tap water burns, however, do not occur in the bathtub or shower.[6,51]

The CPSC has been petitioned to enact requirements limiting new home water heaters to a maximum temperature of 130° F (55° C). Physicians should recommend to families with infants and toddlers that they set their water heater thermostat between 120° and 130° F (49° and 55° C).

Electric Burns and Injuries[52]

There were 984 accidental deaths attributed to electric current in 1978. A 1972 analysis by the Department of Health, Education and Welfare of 212 electric injuries revealed 103 cases (48.6%) of burns, 19 cases of electric shock, and the remainder of mechanical injuries; 122 cases (57.5%) involved children younger than 14 years of age.

Injury in young children most frequently results from the mouthing of a plugged-in extension cord's recipient end; the second most frequent cause of injury is from chewing on a poorly insulated wire. In a series of 54 cases reported by Gifford and colleagues,[21] plastic surgical revision of the burns was necessary in 83%. High-voltage injuries occur most commonly in boys between the ages of 7 and 16 years and frequently involve risky activities.

The number of fatal accidents that involve electricity begins to rise in the late spring and attains its peak in the summer months, with more than 40% occurring from June to August. It is believed that perspiration, which occurs more in the warmer weather, increases the body's conduction of electric energy. More than 25% of electric current deaths occur inside the home.

Prevention. The following precautions can help prevent electric burns and injuries:

1. An extension cord not in use should never be left plugged into a socket.
2. Plastic caps should cover all unused electric outlets.
3. Periodic inspection of wiring should be undertaken and broken plugs or poorly insulated wires replaced.
4. Older children should be taught about electric current hazards, particularly their association with wetness.
5. Place all holiday lights out of the reach of toddlers, who are prone to bite them.

Treatment. The unique feature of electric mouth burns is the serious bleeding that can occur from the erosion of the labial artery in the first 3 weeks after the injury (25% of the cases). This features demands very careful observation, preferably in a hospital, to avoid exsanguinating hemorrhage. Suture ligatures may be needed to control the bleeding.[21,52]

EYE INJURIES[3,30,36]

It is estimated that 50,000 needless eye injuries occur annually; home, recreation, and automobile accidents pose the greatest danger. Of all ocular injuries, 66% occur in persons 16 years of age or younger. The first decade of life yields more lost eyes than does any subsequent decade, with a third of these losses resulting from injuries that are largely preventable.

In 1972 the government mandated protection for the 100 million Americans who wear prescription glasses and the many millions more who wear sunglasses. The Food and Drug Administration (FDA) issued a regulation requiring all eyeglass and sunglass lenses manufactured after January 1972 to be impact resistant. A lens is considered impact resistant if it passes the "drop-ball test," which consists of dropping a ⅝-inch steel ball weighing approximately 0.5 ounce on the lens from a height of 50 inches.

The physician can give important guidance in this accident-conducive area. Safety programs that need implementation include requiring the wearing and proper use of safety glasses in school chemistry and industrial laboratories; advising hobby shops not to sell hobby products that can cause eye injury unless safety glasses are sold also; and permitting sunlamps to be sold only with protective glasses.

Program planning can include meetings with ophthalmologists, optometrists, school authorities, school nurses, and

Prevention of Burn Injuries

1. "Fireproof" all children. Clothes are guaranteed not to fade, shrink, or wrinkle and should also be guaranteed *not to burn.* Ask parents: "How safe are the clothes your children wear?" "How safe are the fabrics on the furniture and floors in your home?"
2. Encourage parents to buy flame-retardant garments for their children.
3. Emphasize that those likely to get burned—the very young, the handicapped, and the elderly—must be protected.
4. Emphasize the fabric most often involved in clothing ignitions (cotton) and the likeliest time (3 to 9 PM), season (winter), and place (kitchen) for burns to occur.
5. Evaluate for situations that make certain children more vulnerable (e.g., hyperactivity, separated or divorced parents, a large family, a working mother, crowded living conditions). Obese boys are reported to be more vulnerable to severe burns than are nonobese ones.
6. Modify igniters of combustibles. Household appliances are a major source in two thirds of 5.6 million fires.

Hazard	**Modification**
Matches	Design child-proof containers and striking surfaces.
Gasoline	Store safely; educate public to use appropriately and sensibly.
Space heaters	Guard, vent, maintain, and locate safely.
Water heaters	Locate where the ignition of flammable liquids is unlikely.
Scalding tap water	Design thermostats so that scalding tap water temperatures cannot be reached. Keep water heater temperature between 120° and 130° F (49° and 55° C).
Stoves	Recess burners so that pots will be stable; locate burners near the back of the range so that (1) pan handles do not overhang and (2) reaching across lighted burners is unnecessary.
Clothing and furnishings	Design and market flame-retardant fabrics for those of all ages.

7. Store and use flammable materials properly. Never use flammable liquids near a source of flame. In starting a charcoal fire, use only labeled charcoal starters and ensure good ventilation. Do not store gasoline in the trunk of a car. Buy minimal amounts of flammable liquids, keep tightly capped and never in glass containers, and store out of reach of children.
8. Inspect electric equipment periodically for defective wiring.
9. Educate adults that smoking in bed and that improper disposal of ashes or butts are dangerous to children sleeping in adjacent rooms, who may be trapped in case of fire.
10. Advise against the use of defective heating equipment or improper cooking utensils.
11. Caution about use of steam vaporizers or pots, which if overturned can cause severe burns. Hot steam vaporizers heat the water to 176° F (80° C). The cool vaporizer, which contains a central core that serves to heat only a small volume of water, is safer but must be kept very clean to avoid water-borne bacterial spread.
12. Keep cords out of reach. Pulling over percolators, skillets, and other electric equipment by their cords is a frequent cause of burns in children.
13. Never leave children younger than 10 years of age alone in the house, because they are helpless victims. An adequate fire escape plan should be part of safety education in every home.
14. Never leave children alone in bathtubs, which pose a drowning hazard and are a source of scalding burns.
15. Avoid drinking hot beverages while caring for or holding a baby.
16. Be sure that camping tents are of flame-retardant material.
17. Install *smoke detectors* in each sleeping area and at the head of each stairway.

Eye Injuries: Prevention and First Aid

PREVENTION

1. Safety glasses should be worn when working or performing recreational activities that may be hazardous to the eyes, particularly in school laboratories and shops and in certain sports. Special protective glasses are particularly needed during arc welding and metal hammering and on exposure to (a) sunlight and sun lamps for tanning and (b) snow-reflected sunlight.
2. Children and parents should be warned about the dangers of pointed sticks, pellet guns, bows and arrows, BB guns and air rifles, slingshots, and fireworks. Children should be instructed not to throw or point things at each other.
3. Children's glasses of all types, including those worn for recreation (such as sunglasses), should have safety lenses and frames.
4. Children should be warned against sun gazing. An eclipse is especially dangerous because the sunspot blocks out the visible rays, which usually deter them from watching, but does not eliminate the infrared rays, which are still as damaging. Proper viewing techniques should be publicized each time the phenomenon occurs. News media publicizing of this hazard has resulted in a reduction of retinal burns in children and adults.
5. Parents should be warned against placing young babies in direct sunlight.
6. Proper instruction should be given for handling hazardous equipment, including lawn mowers and glass doors.
7. Proper emergency first aid therapy of common eye injuries should be publicized.

FIRST AID

1. Avoid topical anesthetics, which may delay healing. If a topical anesthetic is used, warn the patient about loss of the protective reflex (blinking).
2. Evaluate vision routinely in all eye injuries after first aid is given.
3. Always refer patients with abnormalities of the pupil to an ophthalmologist.
4. Advise that corneal injury is serious. Fluorescein staining often is needed to delineate the extent of the injury.
5. Use fluorescein strips instead of bottles of fluorescein dye, which may provide a desirable culture medium for bacterial growth.
6. Chemical burns to the eye require immediate irrigation with copious amounts of tap water or normal saline over a period of 15 minutes to 1 hour. Ophthalmologic consultation should be sought.

representatives from the National Society for Prevention of Blindness. At these programs speakers can distribute educational pamphlets; suggest safety modification of potentially dangerous products; seek the banning of specific hazards, such as fireworks; and advance good first aid treatment of eye injuries in the home, emergency room, and physician's office (see box above).

FALLS AND INFANT AND JUVENILE FURNITURE INJURIES[34,47]

The National Safety Coucil reported 11,300 deaths to have resulted from falls in 1987. Of these, 160 occurred in children younger than 14 years of age. Falls rank as the second highest cause of accidental death for the general population and the sixth highest cause in children.

In infancy, falls most commonly begin to occur at the age of 7 to 7½ months, when infants begin to roll from a prone to a supine position, to sit up, to pull themselves to a standing position, and to climb.

A study of 536 infants showed an incidence of 47.5% falls in the first year of life. If this incidence were found in the national population, about 1,750,000 infants could be expected to sustain at least one fall during the first year of life. The most common preventable fall occurred when a baby climbed out of a crib.[34]

Crib Injuries and Prevention

The CPSC estimates that more than 100 infants die every year of injuries involving nursery equipment. About 40,000 infants are injured so seriously that they need hospital emergency room treatment. Most of these accidents occur when infants fall while climbing out of their cribs. Others occur as a result of poor crib design (see box on p. 276). Nearly all fatalities result from strangulation occurring when the baby's head and neck become wedged between crib slats.

An infant should never be left in the crib with the side rails down. The mattress should be lowered before the baby can sit unassisted and set at its lowest position as soon as the infant can stand. No toys or other articles that can be used as steps in climbing out should be left in the crib.

There should be no hanging crib toys within reach in which the child could get tangled, and the infant should not wear necklaces of any type. The crib should not be used as a playpen, and the child should be removed from the crib once the height of the side rail is less than three fourths of the child's height or when the child is 35 inches tall.

Other Furniture Safety

It is important to be aware of hazards and safety features of juvenile furnishings other than the crib.

Recommendations for Crib Safety

1. Cribs should have at least 12 slats to a side, no more than 2⅜ inches apart. There should be no crossbars or toe-holds on the sides; when fully lowered, the sides shold be 4 inches above the mattress. The sides should be operated with a locking hand-operated latch, which must be safe and secure from accidental release. Many of these recommendations were enacted into law on February 1, 1974. Corner posts (finials) should be less than ⅝ inch high. Choose a new crib that has a label indicating that it meets federal crib standards.
2. The mattress should fit snugly; if more than two fingers fit between it and the sides, the mattress is too small. The minimum rail height should be 22 inches from the top of the railing to the mattress.
3. The wood surfaces should be free of splinters and cracks, and no lead paint should be used anywhere. Any metal on the crib must be safe and have no rough edges. There should be no plastic bells or balls used as ornaments. There should be no cut-out spaces that would permit limb or head entrapment.
4. Bumper pads should be used around the entire crib until the baby starts to pull up to a standing position, at which time they can be removed. These bumpers should have at least six straps.
5. Parents should be advised to purchase a crib with the largest distance between the top of the side rail and mattress. If extenders are used, they should not be taller than the end panels, should not have easily removable nuts or bolts, and should have narrowly spaced slats.
6. Cribs should be placed far enough away from windows so that infants cannot reach venetian blinds or drapery pull cords.

Bunk Bed Selection and Safe Use. Bunk beds should have rounded edges, tight-fitting mattresses, a ladder that grips the frame firmly without slipping, and a secured guardrail without open spaces. The beds should be placed in a corner of the room, so that there are walls on two of the four sides, the guardrails should be in place at all times, and the ladder should always be used.

Younger children should use the lower bunk; rough play should be prohibited; and a low-wattage night light should be kept on to allow the ladder to be seen.

Dressing Tables. Stable concave dressing tables with guardrails are preferred.

High Chairs. According to the CPSC, most of the estimated 7000 victims of falls from high chairs who were treated in hospital emergency rooms in 1974 were younger than 4 years of age, and 25% were younger than 1 year old.

A high chair should not be easily pushed or tipped over and should not fold up while the child is in the chair. The child should be properly and securely strapped and not allowed to stand. Children should not be left unattended, and older siblings should not climb on the high chair. The chair should not be kept near counters and tables from which the child can push and tip the high chair.

Infant Carriers (Plastic-Type Seat). The carrier must be stable with a wide base and a nonskid surface on the bottom. It should be wide enough to allow separation of the infant's thighs. It should never be placed on a chair, counter, or table or be used as a car seat. The belts or restraining devices provided should be used, and the infant should never be left unattended. It is recommended that the carrier bear a label warning about leaving the set on an elevated surface and also specifying the maximum weight and age for its use.

NOTE: A young infant is safest in the parent's arms except when traveling in a vehicle. Mothers have been known to fall and completely protect the baby in their arms, whereas they have thrown the inanimate seat (to protect themselves), forgetting the baby was in it.

Jumpers and Walkers. More than 55% of infants in the United States are placed in walkers before they begin to walk. However, walkers have not been shown to enhance walking, and the risk of injury associated with their use has been significant. An estimated 23,900 injuries requiring treatment resulted from baby walkers in 1980; most of the victims were younger than 2 years of age. Fifty percent of the infants who used walkers experienced at least one accident involving a tip-over, a fall down stairs, or finger entrapment. In one 15-month observation period, coil spring–activated devices were reported to have caused 21 amputations or near amputations of fingers.

In view of the risks posed, the use of walkers should not be recommended. If used, walkers should be selected that have covered coil springs and locking devices that prevent collapse. The wheelbase should be longer and wider than the frame, and walkers should be used only on flat surfaces away from carpets, door thresholds, and stairways.

Safety Gates. The installation of safety gates firmly attached and permanently mounted at the top and bottom of all stairways to thwart toddlers from dangerous explorations is recommended. However, accordion-style gates or expandable enclosures with large V-shaped openings along the top edge or diamond-shaped openings within are dangerous and should never be used so that head entrapment will not occur.

Falls from Windows. Falls from heights accounted for 20% of the accidental deaths of children in New York City during 1966; 67% of the children were younger than 5 years of age. During the period 1965 to 1969, 125 children younger than 15 years of age died falling from windows. Of these, 113 were younger than 5 years of age.[47] To prevent these falls, all screens should be secure but should not be depended on. Handles should be removed from windows. Windows should be opened only from the top or 4 to 5 inches from the bottom and secured at the desired height with a window "burglar lock" obtainable at any hardware store. Window guards are the most effective tools. New York City's 1970 ordinance requiring window guard installation in apartments housing children younger than 10 years of age resulted in a marked decline of deaths as a result of falls from windows. A recent resurgence of falls, however, indicates a need for compliance surveillance.

A child's bed, crib, or other furniture should never be placed next to or under a window. Balconies and fire escapes should be secured.

FIREARM INJURIES

In the United States in 1987, 1400 persons were accidentally killed by firearms. Of these, 280 were children younger than 15 years of age, and an additional 850 were in the 15- to 24-year age-group. Firearms injure 8000 children and teenagers annually, leaving 25% permanently disabled. Prevention programs for firearm accidents often emphasize the hazard to the hunter, but fewer than 600 of the deaths were in this category: 700 of the deaths occurred at home—many while children were cleaning or playing with guns.

An in-depth analysis of gunshot injuries involving children in Detroit suggested a dramatic increase since 1967. In the 80 cases analyzed, 10 children died, and 23 were left with permanent disability; 14 of the children were younger than 5 years of age, and 16 were between 6 and 10 years of age. The victims were mostly black males from a low socioeconomic group. The long gun was the weapon most often involved, and most accidents occurred when the children were playing with the firearms unsupervised. The majority of the guns came from questionable sources and were purchased for protection against crime or violence. The children were, for the most part, innocent victims of gun availability.

The prevention of firearm accidents should not have to wait for shameful events such as the assassination or attempted assassination of a president to highlight the carnage occurring daily; firearm accidents often involve the vital organs, leaving the victim little chance of survival.

Home Safety Precautions

All guns should be kept unloaded under lock and key and equipped with a trigger lock. They should be stored out of sight of casual visitors and away from children's play areas. All ammunition should be stored under lock in a location separate from the firearms.

During handling, guns always should be carefully checked to make sure they are unloaded, and the muzzle always should be pointed in a safe direction. Horseplay with firearms should be strictly forbidden.

Gas, air, and spring-operated guns also represent hazards to children.

Air Rifle Injuries

Air guns used by children are potentially lethal. Regulations are ineffective and parents are ignorant regarding these weapons. Multiple-pump air rifles have muzzle velocities far exceeding the power of the old BB gun.

More than 85,000 cases of injuries resulting from air guns were reported to the CPSC in 1980; 10 deaths were recorded between 1972 and 1980. Those injured usually are boys between 5 and 19 years of age.

The classic Daisy single-lever action (spring compression type) has an average muzzle velocity of 83.8 to 106.7 ft/sec, which limits serious injury to the eye. On the other hand, the multiple-pump action rifles introduced in 1972 can attain compression muzzle velocities of more than 650 ft/sec.

Most of the deaths have come from intracranial injury that results from penetration of the orbit or the child's thin frontal bone. Penetrations of the thorax and other anatomic areas also have caused death.

The multiple-pump air rifle must be regarded as a lethal weapon and should not be used by children without direct supervision. Stricter regulations of sale to and use by children are needed.

FIREWORKS INJURIES

During 1985 there were seven deaths and 9800 injuries associated with fireworks. More than half the injuries were burns or lacerations, and many occurred to children younger than 15 years of age. The most frequently injured part of the body was the arm, including the hand and fingers. Some injuries were quite severe, involving loss of hearing, sight, or a limb.

The AAP has been on record since 1972 in support of the petition by the National Association for the Prevention of Blindness to ban all fireworks except for those used for public displays. This ban should include the popular sparkler, which often is erroneously considered a safe alternative to fireworks. The ignited sparkler can reach a searing temperature of 1800° F (982° C) and has caused 6% of the fireworks injuries.

SLED, SNOW DISK, AND SNOWMOBILE INJURIES

An estimated 23,000 persons require hospital emergency room treatment for sled injuries annually, and snow disks cause an additional 1200 injuries. As many as 300 children are killed each year because of sledding accidents, and many more are seriously injured.

The accidents are associated with problems of mechanical and structural design, such as poor or no steering devices and flimsy materials, coupled with poor riding conditions, loss of control, and collision without protection with automobiles, other sleds, or stationary objects.

The first snowfall often brings with it an influx of injured people to the hospital emergency room and the physician's office. Plans for safe sledding should be made before the snow appears, along with plans for snow removal (see box on p. 278).

In 1985 the CPSC recorded 12,687 injuries related to snowmobile use; 2200 occurred to children younger than 14 years of age. Collisions with fixed objects and other moving vehicles and drownings were the most common causes of fatalities. In nonfatal injuries the most frequent causes were collisions and "overturns." Head injuries are the major cause of fatalities, with drowning a close second. Frostbite also is a major risk of this activity.

Safety features that have been suggested to reduce accidents and the extent of injuries include wearing a helmet, face shield, snowmobile suit, and ear protection against noise. The snowmobile should be prohibited on highways, and there should be a minimum age for drivers. Paradoxically, the accident rate appears to increase with the driver's experience.

Prevention of Sledding Injuries

1. Sleds should be sturdy and have no sharp, jagged edges or rivets. They should have a protective guard or bumper, a good steering mechanism, and rounded runners without sharp end hooks.
2. Communities should make available supervised areas reserved for sledding. If special areas are not available, parents should be encouraged to select safe locations for sledding, free of holes, large rocks, stumps, trees, fences, or posts, and should not permit their children to sled on streets, driveways, or highways.
3. A safe time should be selected for sledding.
4. Children should be taught how to handle a sled. Both arms and legs should be on the sled. Knowing how to stop is essential—this can be accomplished by dragging the feet, dropping a hat under the runner, rolling off the sled onto the ground while cradling the face and head, steering into a snowbank, or making a sharp right turn.
5. When using sled runs, the child should keep to the right, wait for a clear path before starting, and move quickly off the slope and out of the path of others.
6. Sleds should be kept in good condition by drying them before storing, rubbing the runners and metal parts with candle wax, and lubricating metal bolts with oil.
7. Sleds should never be used near or with automobiles. Hitching rides on automobiles should be a legal violation.
8. No sledding should be allowed on ice ponds.

TOY INJURIES[37,50]

The CPSC estimated that in 1986, 113,000 persons required emergency room treatment for injuries associated with toys. Toy injuries, however, produce only 1% of accident fatalities.

The CPSC has legislative authority to ban hazardous toys, including those with the potential for electrical, mechanical, or thermal injury. The law has been updated to state that a toy or article intended for use by children can be a hazard if it presents an unreasonable risk of personal injury or illness in normal use or when it is subjected to reasonably foreseeable damage or abuse.

Despite the laws and volunteer consumer deputies who regularly canvass the marketplace, especially during each Christmas season, the responsibility for choosing safe toys remains with parents. The Toy Manufacturers Association (TMA) has been working with the government to establish toy safety standards, but there are 1500 toy manufacturers (many do not belong to the TMA), 150,000 different kinds of toys, 5000 new toys produced each year, and 83,000 toys imported annually.

The physician can advise patients to buy toys appropriate to the child's age, sex, development, and temperament and not to buy impulsively what the persuasive television advertisements peddle. Parents usually consider their child's chronologic age, but maturity also must be considered[37] (see box on p. 279).

The toys that adults buy should have the least potential for misuse. The instructions and labels should be carefully read, and the packaging should contain the minimum age for use. Play should be supervised according to the situation, particularly in children younger than 5 years of age. Children should be taught to play safely by the parents setting a good example. Children should be taught to store toys in their proper places to avoid tripping over them. The toys of older children will be available to younger ones in the family, who should be protected from potentially dangerous toys. Periodic inspection should be carried out, including the repair or discarding of broken toys (see box on p. 280).

PLAYGROUND EQUIPMENT INJURIES

It is estimated that more than 200,000 persons receive hospital emergency room treatment for injuries associated with public and home playground equipment. Most of the injured children are between the ages of 5 to 10 years. About 25% of the injuries occur at school and another 25% at other public playgrounds; the remainder occur predominantly at home. Twenty thousand preschool children are injured while in day care; 72% of the emergency room visits involve falls to the ground.

An in-depth analysis by the National Electronic Injury Surveillance System of 61 reports of injuries to children younger than 15 years of age revealed seven cases that required hospital admission and two deaths. Nearly 40% of the injuries occurred between 5 and 7 PM, more than 40% included fractures, and another 33% included lacerations. The face and head were involved in 43% of the cases. Horizontal bars and jungle gyms were involved in a higher proportion of the more serious injuries.

Parents contemplating buying playground equipment should be counseled to consider stability and absence of protrusions such as screws or bolts unless capped or taped over. No equipment should have open-ended S hooks, moving parts that can pinch or crush fingers, sharp edges, or rough surfaces. Rings should be more than 5 but less than 10 inches in diameter to avoid head entrapment.

Equipment should be installed at least 6 feet from fences, walls, and other obstructions and not on a concrete or other hard surface unless covered by a resilient surface. The equipment should be checked every 2 weeks for wear, and necessary repairs should be made. Children should be taught that rough play, twisting swing chains, and swinging empty seats will not be allowed.

WRINGER INJURIES[20,39]

Wringer accidents occur predominantly in young children, with 65% being reported in children younger than 10 years of age and 51% in children younger than the age of 5 years. A wringer injury is due to a twisting force to an extremity which crushes the soft tissues.

This type of injury has been reduced with the decreased

Toys Appropriate for Various Age-Groups

Infants need toys that produce *sensory stimulation*—visual, auditory, and tactile:
- Bright moving objects suspended over the baby (out of reach)
- Cradle gym
- Rattles (doughnuts, dumbbells)
- Soft balls
- Soft washable dolls and animals
- Floating bath toys
- Music boxes or animals
- Small plastic or wooden blocks
- Pots and pans

Toddlers (1 to 2 years) use toys for *investigation:*
- Cloth, plastic books (illustrations of familiar objects, preferably one to a page)
- Nested blocks and cups of soft plastic or wood
- Kiddy car
- Push-and-pull toys
- Toy telephone
- Dolls (beware of eyes or nose that can detach)
- Musical top
- Pots and pans

Preschoolers (2 to 5 years) should have toys that *imitate* parents' and older children's activities and that are *experimental* in nature:
- Record players, nursery rhymes
- Large wooden beads for stringing
- Housekeeping toys
- Transportation toys (tricycles, trucks, cars, wagons)
- Building blocks
- Floor trains
- Blackboards and chalk
- Easels and brushes
- Clay, crayons, fingerpaints (must be nontoxic)
- Outdoor toys (sandbox, swing, small slide)
- Hammers and peg benches
- Drums and bells
- Books (short stories, action stories)

Kindergarten and first-grade children (5 to 6 years) are in a phase of *creativity* and *skill:*
- Blocks
- Dolls
- Housekeeping toys
- Dress-up clothes, eating utensils
- Medical kits
- Outdoor toys
- Easels, blackboards, paints
- Doll houses
- Blunt scissors, simple sewing sets, paste, colored paper
- Simple puzzles
- Matching card games
- Hand puppets
- Small trucks
- Books, records

Older children (6 to 9 years) have greater *dexterity* with their hands:
- Paper dolls
- Table games
- Electric trains
- Crafts
- Bicycles
- Workbenches, with good tools and materials
- Puppets and marionettes
- Books (for reading alone)

Middle childhood (9 to 12 years) is the period for starting *hobbies* and *scientific activities:*
- Hobby collections
- Model cars, boats, planes
- Microscopes
- Table and board games
- Sewing, knitting, needlework
- Outdoor sports
- Checkers, chess, dominoes

use of wringer attachments to the old-style washing machine. An identical injury can be produced by the spinning wheel of a vehicle, such as the spoke injury in bicycle accidents, or from a fan belt. Severe spinning injuries have been reported from spin clothes dryers. Estimates of the number of antiquated wringers still being used and capable of producing injury vary from 9 to 17 million.

Clinical Signs

The degree of the injury is related to the speed and tightness of the roller and the amount of time that the extremity remains trapped. Because the roller often gets stuck at the elbow or axilla, these areas receive the most serious injury.

In the initial few hours, most cases may exhibit only abrasions and ecchymoses, without significant external signs despite severe soft tissue injury and closed-space compression. All wringer injuries should be considered severe until proved otherwise with the passage of time.

The analysis by Allen and colleagues[1] in Table 21-4 illustrates the surgical procedures required in 32 patients with wringer injuries. Other series have reported lacerations in 20%; fractures, usually of the phalanges, in 3%; the need for grafting in 10%; and some degree of motion limitation in 7%.

Treatment

Most authorities recommend hospital admission and close observation until the natural course of the injury is determined. Others recommend outpatient observation with close follow-up. The following are symptoms to look for in wringer-type injuries:

1. Edema that may become massive after the first 4 to 6 hours
2. Hemorrhage and discolored abrasions
3. Avulsion of the skin with a distally based flap
4. Pain

Thirteen Toy Hazards

1. *Aspiration or ingestion.* Toys should not be too small, come apart, or be easily shattered. They should be larger than 1¼ inches in diameter and not fit into a truncated circular cylinder 2¼ inches long.
2. *Burns.* Toys should not be made of flammable materials or be a thermal hazard with surfaces that can reach high temperatures. Hobby items, such as wood-burning kits, are *not* recommended for children younger than 12 years of age.
3. *"Catch" injuries.* Toys should not have exposed gears, springs, or hinged parts that can pinch fingers or catch clothes or hair.
4. *Crumple or collapse injuries.* Children have fallen on rubber and plastic toys with metal axles that have penetrated their skulls. This type of accident would be less likely to occur if toys were made so that the chassis would not collapse or so that the axle would collapse.
5. *Electric shock.* Battery-operated toys are preferred. Electric plug-in toys with heating elements should not be purchased for children younger than 8 years old. The minimum age recommendation always should be checked.

   Electric toys require supervision and instruction in their proper use. Children should be taught to disconnect an electric appliance by grasping the plug, *not* by pulling the cord. Parents should use the toy a few times together with the child to make sure the child understands how the toy should be used. These toys should have the electric wires checked monthly for wear.

   Electric toys should bear the *UL label.* However, this label ensures only that the cord and the electric device are engineered to electric safety standards for any household equipment. It does *not* indicate that the toy is safe for use by the child or is safe against misuse.
6. *Explosion injuries.* Chemistry sets and rocket-fuel kits must be selected for the appropriate age levels, usually for the over-12 age-group. Dry ice in a stoppered bottle, match heads in a pipe or bottle, or weed killer mixed with sugar can explode. One should be alert for unsupervised scientific activity in the attic or basement.
7. *Lacerations.* Toys should not contain sharp edges, glass, or rigid plastic that will shatter.
8. *Poisoning.* Toys that contain toxic material or those made of poisonous material should *not* be bought.
9. *Eye injuries.* Projectile-type toys can injure the eyes; thus they should be used under adult supervision.
10. *Strangling.* Ropes or loops can cause strangling. Strings on pull toys should be less than 10 inches long. Cradle gyms should be removed when the infant is able to sit.
11. *Abrasions.* These can be caused by rough surfaces.
12. *Punctures.* Because sharp points can cause punctures, suction tips covering such points must not be removable.
13. *Hearing damage.* Toys should not produce sound levels that can damage the hearing; the noise level should be under 100 dB. The label on toy-gun caps now states that they should not be used indoors or closer to the ear than 1 foot.

N.B. Displaying these toy hazards on a bulletin board in the waiting room will serve as a reminder to parents of these dangers.

5. Anesthesia of the skin
6. Absent pulses in fingers or major arteries

The extent of necrosis or edema cannot be predicted from the initial appearance.

In the event of wringer-type injuries, the following should be done:

1. Observe and record at least every ½ to 1 hour the pulses of the arteries, pallor of the extremity, pain, paresthesias (numbness and cold), and paralysis.
2. Débride all wounds and treat the skin as in a thermal burn, with topical antimicrobials such as silver sulfadiazine and povidone-iodine antiseptic.

Controvery exists over the application of a standard compression dressing or a bulky loose dressing; in either case

Table 21-4 *Type of Surgical Procedure Required for Wringer Injuries (n = 32)*

INJURY REPAIR	NUMBER
Laceration repair	17
Hematoma drainage	7
Débridement	11
Skin graft	13
Scar excision	10
Nerve repair	2
Fasciotomy (with early elevation and compression dressing)	0

From Allen JE, Beck AR, and Jewett TC Jr: Wringer injuries in children, Arch Surg 97:194, 1968.

the extremity should be elevated and the distal portion left exposed for inspection. The dressing should be changed in 24 hours.

Edema begins in 4 to 6 hours and in rare cases may require a fasciotomy to relieve pressure on nerves and blood vessels.

The primary physician should realize that this type of injury is potentially serious and requires close observation and experienced care.

MISCELLANEOUS INJURIES

The following are hazards that may not be recognized as such by the parent or by a casual observer.

Baby Powder Aspiration

Both talc and zinc preparations have been implicated in severe and occasionally fatal inhalation episodes from containers that are deceptively similar to nursing bottles; the "look-alike" appearance is an invitation to trouble. Medicated powders containing calcium undecylenate also may be toxic if aspirated. Baby powders must be considered potentially harmful if aspirated. Their use should be discouraged until a drastic change is made in the appearance of the containers and a safety cap is developed that prevents accidental spillage.

Digit Tourniquets

Hairs or thin fibers can become tightly wrapped around digits or the penis, resulting in gangrene and amputations. There also have been reports of leotard garments causing tourniquet-like constriction of digits. Any infant with uncontrollable crying should have the digits, and in boys the penis, examined for a possible tourniquet accident. The long hair of mothers or others should be tied up when dressing or bathing babies.

Glass Door Injuries

It is estimated that more than 190,000 persons require hospital emergency room treatment yearly for injuries associated with glass doors and windows. Of these, 50% of the victims are children. Thirty states have passed laws requiring installation of safety glass in all new homes. There are four types of safety glass: tempered, laminated, wired, and rigid plastic. Ideally, all regular glass doors should be replaced with safety glass. If this cannot be done, then precautions, such as those mentioned below, should be instituted.[17]

Furniture or planters can be placed in front of doors opening to the exterior. Decals or colored tape will show the presence of glass, and a safety bar at handle level will prevent contact. The area in front of glass doors should be clear of loose rugs, toys, and other materials that can cause a person to trip or fall. In bathrooms, nonskid mats should be used. Unmounted glass should not be left unprotected.

Lawn Mower Injuries

More than 30 million lawn mowers are in use in the United States, causing an estimated 60,000 injuries a year. Four of five seriously injured children have fallen into the path of a lawn mower. Injuries also can occur from objects hurled by the blades. Improvements in design must be worked toward, and the cautious use of these tools must be stressed.[23]

Cotton Swab Injuries

Cotton applicators should not be used in or around the auditory canal of infants or children. Older children can cause themselves severe auditory injury using swabs.[8]

Refrigerator Entrapment

From 1946 to 1962 there were 237 reported suffocations with 35 fatalities. More than two thirds of the 1962 fatalities involved appliances that were out of service. With support of the AAP Committee on Accident Prevention, Public Law 930 was enacted in 1956 and went into effect in 1958, mandating inside safety releases for refrigerator doors. There have been no fatalities involving a refrigerator with the prescribed release, but some of the old types are still in use and can cause suffocation. If a refrigerator or freezer is discarded, the door should be completely removed or padlocked shut.

Skateboard Injuries

In the late 1970s skateboard riding had a resurgence of popularity among children. In 1975 the CPSC reported an incidence of 27,500 injuries that required hospital emergency room treatment.[16] The Hawaii chapter of the AAP reported an alarming increase in severe injuries during 1975 and one death in early 1976.[28] Injuries in 1977 reached 140,000, and 25 deaths were reported in a 30-month period from February 1975 to July 1977. An analysis of accidental injury involving skateboards revealed structural problems (e.g., improper modifications and repair and excessive wobbliness), poor skateboarding surface, inexperience, and skateboarding in traffic as contributors to severe injury.

Parents and retailers of skateboards must be made aware that riders younger than 13 years of age may not have adequate muscle coordination to maintain balance and sufficient maturity to exercise judgment about types of maneuvers to attempt.

Proper and safe use of skateboards must be taught, protective equipment—helmet, gloves, elbow and knee pads—worn, and supervised areas made available for skateboard use to avoid the high toll of injury associated with this sport. Unpredictably, a decrease in popularity of this activity occurred, which dramatically reduced the use of skateboards and the associated injuries. In 1982 only 14,700 injuries were reported, and it appeared that skateboarding was just a fad. However, the movie *Back to the Future* resurrected the glamour of daring skateboard use, which resulted in its resurgence. In 1986 the CPSC reported 81,000 skateboard injuries.

Boys, during late childhood, are often fascinated with ropes, ties, shoelaces, and belts as instruments to play "hanging" games. Parents should be aware of this and should warn their children of the dangers involved in playing such "games."

Toilet Seat Trauma

The penis of a small boy can be injured by the dropping of an elevated toilet seat. This trauma can be avoided by the presence of high rubber washers under the toilet seat.[41]

SAFETY IN THE PHYSICIAN'S OFFICE, CLINIC, AND EMERGENCY ROOM

If physicians hope to instruct parents to set good examples for their children, then offices and clinics should be models of safety.

1. Is a *fire extinguisher* nearby?
2. Are *toxic agents* properly identified and kept out of the reach of small children?
3. Are *syringes and needles* disposed of safely?
4. Are "patient pleasers" safe for children, even if misused?
5. Are "harmful" *instruments* stored safely?
6. Is the *lighting* adequate?
7. Are *drug samples* disposed of safely?
8. Are the *electric circuits* and *electric equipment* safe?
9. Is a member of the staff assigned the task of *checking for safety*?
10. Are *stools* available to reach high places?
11. Are *rugs* kept in good condition? Are there nonskid preparations used on highly waxed *floors*?
12. Do the nurse and aide instruct the parents to *stand close* while their children are on elevated surfaces and to *hold* onto them?
13. Are parents instructed to *supervise* their toddlers and preschool children during waiting time?

It really comes down to safe storage, safe disposal, periodic checks on furniture and equipment to be sure there are no sharp corners or edges, and supervision of children.

EMERGENCY MEDICAL SERVICES: TRAUMA CENTERS[43]

Trauma is a national problem of huge magnitude. It is essential to have not only programs for prevention of trauma but also systems of local emergency medical services to provide optimum prehospital and prompt, effective in-hospital care. Regional categorization of hospitals, based on capabilities to receive and render treatment for the critically injured, has been proposed, and regional trauma centers already have been developed.

The Emergency Medical Service Systems Act of 1973 added a section to the Public Health Services Act of 1944 "to provide assistance and encouragement for the development of comprehensive area-wide emergency medical systems." The provisions of this law have effected profound changes in the handling of trauma cases.

Data are necessary to identify problems and review performance of emergency facilities. A trauma registry was developed at the Children's Regional Trauma Unit at the Johns Hopkins University School of Medicine to gather objective data on children with major injuries. The registry was designed to include events that occur during management from the scene of the accident, through resuscitation, and throughout in-hospital care. Problems highlighted by the data from studies such as this determined the most efficient transportation, the level of training needed by personnel, the number of centers needed in a region, and the type of back-up facilities required in a regional trauma center.

It became obvious that the traumatized child has special needs. Blunt-impact trauma accounts for 80% of multiple injuries; head injuries are extremely common. Physicians need patience, experience, and sensitivity when dealing with pediatric trauma to lessen the impact of these experiences.

Because children are different from adults, resources and skills must be available to meet their needs. Consideration should be given to the following essential resources:

1. Rescue personnel with special training, protocols, and equipment to care for pediatric patients
2. Emergency rooms designed to meet the needs of pediatric injury victims
3. A community-designated pediatric trauma center or centers identified to provide care for the severely injured child
4. An interhospital transport system with established protocols to minimize delay

Pediatricians should help organize community resources and responses to the needs of injured children.

FIRST AID MEASURES

The basic principles of treating traumatic injury are easily remembered with the mnemonic ICE: I—immobilize (do not use or move the injured area), C—compress (apply pressure to stop bleeding and cool compresses to stop swelling), E—elevate (raise the injured area to stop bleeding and decrease swelling). Remove any ring, bracelet, or constricting garment before any swelling occurs.

Equipment that primary care physicians may need for management of pediatric emergencies is listed in the box on p. 283.

To facilitate the rendering of first aid and to ensure proper care for their patients, physicians should require that a Medic Alert bracelet* be obtained and worn by all persons with any medical condition that cannot be seen, such as an allergy, diabetes, epilepsy, or a heart condition.

Parents should be advised to have telephone numbers of their physician, poison control center, police, fire department, ambulance or taxi service, and hospital easily accessible. These should be readily available to babysitters, as should a first-aid kit. Parents should be advised to employ babysitters who are trained in first-aid and who know what to do in the event of an emergency. "Latch-key" children should be given specific instructions on what they can and cannot do when they are left alone, as well as what to do in emergencies (see Chapter 54: "Latch-Key Kids.")

*These can be obtained from the Medic Alert Foundation, P.O. Box 1009, Turlock, CA 95380.

*Equipment for Pediatric Emergencies**

Physicians and personnel should be familiar with the equipment chosen and should maintain it in good working order.

RESPIRATORY EQUIPMENT

Manual resuscitator with self-filling bag and masks, various sizes
Oxygen supply with a flowmeter
Oral pharyngeal airways, various sizes
Endotracheal tubes and adapter, various sizes
Laryngoscope and blades, various sizes for infants, children, and adults (straight preferred in children)
Suction machine and suction catheters, various sizes

CIRCULATORY EQUIPMENT

Syringes and adapter to fit catheter, sizes 2, 5, 10, 20, 50 ml
Needles, sizes 25, 21, 19, 15, 13 (with short bevel); butterfly needles, sizes 19, 21, 23, 25, 27
Intraosseous needles
Sphygmomanometer with pediatric cuffs
Vasopressors: epinephrine 1:1000 and 1:10,000; norepinephrine
IV solutions—normal saline, 5% glucose in saline, lactated Ringer
IV tubing with microdrop setup
Polyethylene tubing, sterile, various sizes, cutdown tray
Blood administration set

MEDICATION†

Activated charcoal, 500 g
Aminophylline, 0.5 g/20 ml ampules
Antibiotics
Atropine sulfate injection, 0.1 mg/ml ampules
Barbiturate (phenobarbital) for IV and IM use
Calcium chloride or gluconate
Dextrose injection, 50%, 50 ml/vial
Diazepam, 5 mg/ml
Digoxin, 0.25 mg/ml
Dimercaprol, 100 mg/ml
Diphenhydramine injection, 50 mg/ml
Dopamine
DT, DPT, tetanus
Furosemide, 20 mg/2 ml
Glucagon
Hydrocortisone sodium succinate
Insulin, regular and NPH
Isoproterenol (Isuprel), 0.2 mg/ml
Lidocaine, 1%, 2%
Lilly Cyanide Kit M-76, sodium nitrite, sodium thiosulfate
Mannitol, 10%, 20%, 25%
Morphine sulfate and meperidine
Naloxone, 0.4 mg/ml
Normal saline solution, 30 ml/ampule
Novocain or lidocaine (Xylocaine) 1%
Sodium bicarbonate ampules, 50 mg (1 ml = 1 mEq)
Syrup of ipecac
Water for injection, 30 ml/ampule

INSTRUMENTS AND DRESSINGS

Adhesive tape, sizes ½, 1, 2 inch
Alcohol (70%) or other disinfectant
Antiseptic soap
Applicator sticks
Bandage scissors
Blankets
Catheters, sterile, sizes 8 Fr, 10 Fr, 12 Fr, 20 Fr
Compresses, sterile
Culture tubes
Cutdown tray with various sized tubing
Dextrostix for rough glucose estimation
Emergency tags and pencils
Emesis basins
Eyelid retractors
Fluorescein strips for eyes
Gauze pads, sterile, 2 × 2 and 4 × 4 inches
Instrument set (scissors, hemostat, forceps, scalpel, blades)
Kling bandages, various sizes
Lubricant
Muslin roller bandage, 6 × 6 inches
Roller bandages, 1 inch × 5 yards; 2 inches × 5 yards
Safety pins and sheets for restraint
Specimen bottles
Splints, triangular slings, cervical collars, various sizes
Stethoscope, otoscope, ophthalmoscope, flashlight
Surgical gloves
Sutures, sizes 2-0, 3-0, 4-0, 5-0, 6-0
Test tubes, sterile, with and without oxalate
Thermometers, oral and rectal
Tongue depressors
Tourniquets
Tracheotomy set with tubes, various sizes
Tubes for gastric lavage with adapters, various sizes

*The extent of equipment needed in the physician's bag, office, or emergency room on the hospital floor depends on the distance from available intensive care facilities.
†Generally, no drug should be administered to patients in shock. If medication is given, the name, dose, and method of administration should be placed on an emergency tag attached to the patient.

REFERENCES

1. Allen JE, Beck AR, and Jewett TC Jr: Wringer injuries in children, Arch Surg 97:194, 1968.
2. Alonso WA: Minibike accidents lead to severe neck injury, JAMA 224:1344, 1973.
3. American Academy of Pediatrics, Committee on Accident Prevention: Ocular hazards in injury control for children and youth, Elk Grove Village, Ill, 1987, The Academy.
4. Baker SP: Motor vehicle occupant deaths in young children, Pediatrics 64:860, 1979.
5. Balcerak JC, Pancione KL, and States JD: Moped, minibike, and motorcycle accidents: associated injury problems, NY State J Med 78:628, 1978.
6. Baptiste MS and Feck G: Preventing tap water burns, Am J Public Health 70:727, 1980.
7. Barnako D: Flammable fabrics, JAMA 221:189, 1972.
8. Barton RT: Q-Tip otalgia, JAMA 220:1619, 1972.
9. Bass LW and Wilson TR: The pediatrician's influence in private practice measured by a controlled seat belt study, Pediatrics 56:271, 1975.
10. Berman W Jr et al: Childhood burn injuries and deaths, Pediatrics 51:1069, 1973.
11. Bicycle-related injuries: data from the National Electronic Injury Surveillance System, MMWR 36:269, 1987.
12. Black EE: Causes of burns in children, JAMA 158:100, 1955.
13. Carr WP, Brandt D, and Swanson K: Injury patterns and helmet effectiveness among hospitalized motorcyclists, Minn Med 64:521, 1981.
14. Charles S and Shelness A: Children as passengers in automobiles: the neglected minority on the nation's highways, Pediatrics 56:271, 1975.
15. Dietrich HF: Accident prevention in childhood is your problem, too, Pediatr Clin North Am, p. 759, Nov 1954.
16. Fact Sheet: Roller skates, ice skates, and skateboards, US Consumer Product Safety Commission No. 84, Washington, DC, 1976, US Government Printing Office.
17. Feinberg SN: Storm door hazards, Pediatrics 46:936, 1070.
18. Feldman KW: Prevention of childhood accidents: recent progress, Pediatr Rev 2:75, 1980.
19. Few children protected in cars, Insurance Institute for Highway Safety 10(10):1, May 12, 1985.
20. Galasko CS: Spin dryer injuries, Br Med J 4:646, 1972.
21. Gifford GH Jr, Marty AT, and MacCollum DW: The management of electrical mouth burns in children, Pediatrics 47:113, 1971.
22. Goldman AS, Larson DL, and Abston S: The silent epidemic, JAMA 221:403, 1972.
23. Graham WP III, DeMuth WE Jr, and Gordon SL: A summer warning: lawnmowers can maim, JAMA 225:355, 1973.
24. Greensher J: Recent advances in injury prevention, Pediatr Rev 10:171, 1988.
25. Guichon DMP and Miles ST: Bicycle injuries: one year sample in Calgary, J Trauma 15:504, 1975.
26. Haddon W Jr, Suchman EA, and Klein D: Accident research: methods and approaches, New York, 1964, Harper & Row, Publishers, Inc.
27. Haggerty RJ: Emotions and childhood accidents, Mod Med, p 58, March 1963.
28. Hawaii Chapter, AAP: The hazards of skateboard-riding, Pediatrics 46:793, 1976.
29. Heimlich HJ: A life saving maneuver to prevent food choking, JAMA 234:398, 1975.
30. Helveston EM: Eye trauma in childhood, Pediatr Clin North Am 22:501, 1975.
31. Izant RJ Jr, Rothmann BF, and Frankel VH: Bicycle spoke injuries of the foot and ankle in children: an underestimated "minor" injury, J Pediatr Surg 4:654, 1969.
32. Jackson C and Jackson CL: Diseases of the air and food passages of foreign body origin, Philadelphia, 1907, WB Saunders Co.
33. Klein D: The influence of societal values on rates of death and injury, J Safety Res 3:1, 1971.
34. Kravitz H et al: Accidental falls from elevated surfaces in infants from birth to one year of age, Pediatrics 44(suppl):869, 1969.
35. Levy D: Observations of attitudes and behavior in the child health center, Am J Public Health 41:182, 1951.
36. Low MB: The significance of vision problems of children and youth: eye safety in pediatric practice, J Pediatr Ophthalmol 6:223, 1969.
37. Lund DH: Choosing toys for children of all ages, New York, 1972, American Toy Institute.
38. Matheny AP, Brown AM, and Wilson RS: Assessment of children's behavioral characteristics: a tool in accident prevention, Clin Pediatr 11:437, 1972.
39. McCulloch JH, Boswick JA Jr, and Jonas R: Household wringer injuries: a three year review, J Trauma 13:1, 1973.
40. Mofenson HC and Greensher J: How to avoid animal bites, Med Times 100:92, 1972.
41. Mofenson HC and Greensher J: Penile trauma, JAMA 225:1038, 1973.
42. National Committee for Injury Prevention and Control: Injury prevention: meeting the challenge, Am J Prev Med 5(suppl):1, 1989.
43. National Committee for Injury Prevention and Control: Injury prevention: meeting the challenge. Trauma care systems, Am J Prev Med 5(suppl):271, 1989.
44. Pless IB, Roghmann K, and Algranati P: The prevention of injuries to children in automobiles, Pediatrics 49:420, 1972.
45. Scherz RG: Auto safety: "The first ride . . . a safe ride" campaign. In Bergman AB, editor: Preventing childhood injuries. Report of the twelfth Ross Roundtable on Critical Approaches to Common Pediatric Problems, Columbus, Ohio, 1982, Ross Laboratories.
46. Selbst S, Alexander D, and Ruddy R: Bicycle-related injuries, Am J Dis Child 141:140, 1987.
47. Sieben RL, Leavitt JD, and French JH: Falls as childhood accidents: an increasing urban risk, Pediatrics 47:886, 1971.
48. Snyder RG and O'Neill B: Are 1974-1975 automotive belt systems hazardous to children? Am J Dis Child 129:946, 1975.
49. Sobel R: The psychiatric implications of accidental poisoning in childhood, Pediatr Clin North Am 17:653, 1970.
50. Swartz EM: Toys that don't care, Boston, 1971, Gambit.
51. Thomson HG: Bathtub burn: pediatric disaster, Can J Surg 14:399, 1971.
52. Thomson HG, Juckes AW, and Farmer AW: Electric burns to the mouth in children, Plast Reconstr Surg 35:466, 1965.
53. Weiss BD: Bicycle helmet use by children, Pediatrics 77:677, 1986.

SUGGESTED READING

Rodriguez JG: Childhood Injuries in the United States, Am J Dis Child 144:625, June 1990.

22

The Ill Child

Marianne E. Felice and Stanford B. Friedman

Although great strides have been made in the prevention, diagnosis, and treatment of childhood illnesses in the past 60 years, children continue to become ill. Illnesses today, however, are different from those of former years and to a great extent represent chronic illnesses that in the past were fatal.[10] Therefore sick children and their families continue to consume a major portion of the pediatrician's time, talents, and energy. It is important that the specific knowledge and skills of pediatricians reflect the changing patterns of childhood disease.

A discussion of the management of the ill child must encompass a variety of topics, including the degree and duration of illness, hospitalization and the medical delivery system, family support systems, the emotional components of physical illness, and, finally, the plight of the dying child.

THE ACUTELY ILL CHILD

Treatment at Home

Whenever possible, the acutely ill child should be treated at home surrounded by a familiar environment and tended by a responsible, caring adult who knows the child well. Fortunately this is the usual case, rather than the exception, because most youngsters are only mildly to moderately ill for a brief period and have their parents, extended family members, or reliable, familiar baby-sitters to tend to them. The pediatrician, however, should not always presume that adults are in attendance. When deciding whether to treat a child at home, the physician should specifically seek answers to the following questions: Who will assume responsibility for the child during the illness? Is a telephone easily available? Are medical facilities relatively nearby? Above all, do the parents understand the nature of the child's illness and the instructions that have been given? The answer to the last question should be verified by having one or both parents repeat the instructions to the physician.

In two-parent households, fathers should be encouraged to participate actively in their children's health care. Often mothers assume full responsibility for the children's health and fathers are ignored; thus fathers cannot support either the mother or the child. This leaves the mother in the difficult position of having not only to tend to the child but also to repeat the physician's explanations and directions to her husband, a situation that can be the source of misunderstanding, misinterpretation, and resentment for both parents. When a child has a significant illness, the pediatrician should encourage *both* parents to bring the child to the physician whenever possible, and the physician should relate directions and explanations to both parents simultaneously. In this way parents can share the task of caring for their sick child and support each other.

Not all families are established two-parent households, and currently, more women are employed outside the home than in previous years, including nearly 50% of mothers with preschool children.[36] Consequently physicians always should be aware of and sensitive to the household composition and problems, particularly in giving directions concerning at-home care. For example, single-parent fathers may be new to the primary caretaker role; surrounded by experienced mothers in the pediatrician's office, they may feel uncomfortable. They may be unsure of details concerning the child's birth or immunizations. This parent may need more detailed information than do other parents about the treatment of an acute illness. Working mothers may feel caught between the demands of their jobs and the demands of their sick child and feel guilty about asking the physician for advice. In fact, it has been shown that at least some pediatricians are biased against working mothers.[12] Physicians will best serve the child's needs by being attuned to these psychosocial and societal issues.

Treating an ill child at home offers an opportunity for the pediatrician to teach parents about medications. If a drug is prescribed, the physician should explain the name of the drug, why it is being given, and the common side effects that should be anticipated. Antibiotic therapy frequently results in low compliance; parents begin to give antibiotics to their child and then stop when the child starts to feel better, usually after 24 to 48 hours of treatment. Parents may need to be told that many types of infections require a full course of antibiotic therapy. When a medication is discontinued by a physician before all the liquid, pills, or capsules are finished, the parents should be advised about what to do with the unused portion. For example, those medications that decompose with time, such as tetracycline, should be discarded; other medications, such as antihistamines, may be used again at a later date. Parents also should be taught which over-the-counter drugs they should have available, such as acetaminophen for children and ipecac syrup, and how to use them. Physicians can also educate parents by teaching them the proper administration of medications. The familiar "1 teaspoon 4 times a day" may result in varied quantities of medicine being administered if careful directions are not given. Some parents may need practical hints for helping a child to take an unpalatable medicine—for example, crushing a tablet in applesauce.

In most families there is a tradition of myths and home remedies for common acute illnesses, and parents often turn to these ideas when their children are ill. Again, this provides the opportune time for parent education. For example, when talking to the parents of a child with an upper respiratory tract infection, the physician can explain that the youngster did not "catch cold" because of failure to wear galoshes in the rain. In explaining the management of fever, a physician may wish to emphasize certain *do nots* in an effort to dispel misconceptions; *do not* give enemas to bring down fever; *do not* give cold baths to bring down fever (see Chapter 23, "Management of Fever"). Some myths and home remedies are peculiar to certain communities and cultures, and each pediatrician should become familiar with the traditions of the locality (see Chapter 11, "Cultural Issues in Primary Pediatric Care").

In this age of widespread immunization programs, issues of contagion often are neglected. Parents should be informed of the infectious nature of certain childhood illnesses in order to protect other siblings, pregnant relatives, and elderly persons. The most common examples are protecting pregnant relatives from German measles or warning those taking steroids or immunosuppressive drugs to avoid contact with children who have chickenpox.

Acutely ill children at home often pose problems for the parents caring for them. Parents unaccustomed to seeing their normally active toddler listless may feel compelled to entertain the child without realizing that the child may need rest and may not be in the mood for entertainment. On the other hand, many parents may try to restrain a child and insist on bed rest when the child feels well enough to play. Parents need to be reminded that children restrict their own activity when they are ill. Parents also have a tendency to overfeed a sick child, and they must be reassured that if a child drinks appropriate fluids, this is sufficient intake during a brief illness.

It is natural for parents to become anxious when their children are ill, and this anxiety may result in frequent telephone calls to the pediatrician. The pediatrician may perceive such calls as unneeded and annoying without appreciating how frightened parents may be. New parents in particular require support during their child's illnesses, and the pediatrician should patiently teach parents when it is appropriate to call and when it is not. The pediatrician should not frighten parents into not calling and reporting on their child's progress. When a physician decides to treat a child at home, arrangements should be made for a follow-up check, either in terms of a telephone conversation or another office visit, and the importance of such follow-up visits should be explained and emphasized to the parents.

Indications for Hospitalization

It is not always feasible or safe to treat an acutely ill child at home; hospitalization may become necessary. *Whom* to hospitalize and *when* to hospitalize are not always clear-cut issues.[24] Children who are critically or seriously ill are obvious candidates for inpatient care. Children who are not seriously ill also must be considered for hospitalization if the circumstances at home are such that the child will not receive adequate care. Some hospitalizations, however, can be averted by tapping available community resources such as public health nurses, homemaker services, and medical home care programs. Such alternate arrangements not only may be far more economical but also allow the child and parents to remain in their home.[16]

In teaching hospitals, children with unusual diseases at times may be admitted to the hospital for the purpose of teaching or research, in addition to receiving specific therapy. This situation can result in a child receiving more than the customary services and laboratory tests. Even though a child usually receives excellent medical care at a teaching hospital, physicians should carefully weigh the advantages of medical research and medical education against the psychological trauma a youngster may experience and any added expense to parents.

It is sometimes necessary to hospitalize children for diagnostic workups. Most diagnostic procedures can be accomplished on an outpatient basis and should be done so as often as possible. Occasionally children require numerous or complicated tests or clinical observation, and it may be more efficient to admit them for a few days for evaluation. When this is necessary, the pediatrician should schedule the admission carefully, keeping the hospital stay as short as possible; the pediatrician, for example, should postpone an admission from Friday to Monday if no tests or only a few tests can be performed over the weekend.

Some children require elective surgical procedures. In recent years the pediatric literature has reflected an emphasis on the timing of these procedures based on the observation that between the ages of 4 and 7 years children seem to be dramatically concerned about body integrity. Psychiatrists refer to this as *mutilation anxiety* or *castration anxiety*. Some authorities have recommended that elective surgery not be done during these particular years of psychosocial development. In actual clinical practice, however, it usually is not feasible to postpone surgical procedures for 3 to 4 years. An alternative approach is to delay surgery only long enough to explain to the child what is going to happen to him or her. This explanation should be given gradually, using age-appropriate language, and the parents should be the primary supportive resources.[6,35]

Unfortunately, children sometimes are admitted to the hospital primarily for the convenience of the physician. After receiving a call from the parents late at night, the pediatrician may have the child admitted at a later hour and attended by a pediatric house officer on call, thus avoiding having to examine the child at that time. The pediatrician should look into the "real" reason for ordering the hospitalization and avoid doing so for personal convenience.

Care of the Child in the Hospital

When a child is admitted to the hospital, the child and the family become enmeshed in an unfamiliar and often frightening web known as the *medical delivery system*. To the lay person, hospital activities are unpredictable, and families lack control over this environment. In such a milieu both the child and the parents may express their fear in several ways. For instance, the child may cry and be uncooperative. The child is afraid of separation from the parents, of pain, of the unfamiliar environment and strange people, and of the unknown. Parents may become hostile or agitated or may constantly question the health team. They realize that their child's care is being usurped from them, and they fear that they no longer can care for or protect their child. They too are afraid of the strange people and the unknown environment.

There may be no facilities for parents on the pediatric floor, not even a waiting area. Nevertheless, the supportive role of the parents in helping their child get well must be emphasized, and the parents should be assured that they are needed and welcomed on the pediatric floor. It has been demonstrated that parental involvement in the lives of hospitalized children is beneficial to the child.[5] Furthermore, in the complicated network of hospital personnel who encounter the youngster, the parents should have one person consistently available to them for communication concerning their child's care. This person, usually the primary care physician, should report at least daily to the parents and more often if the child is critically ill. Whenever possible, information should be given to both parents at the same time. They then have the opportunity to ask questions, and neither parent needs to interpret the physician's remarks to the other.

In this age of specialization it is common for a youngster to have one or even multiple consultants during hospitalization. It is vital that the child and the parents be notified that a consultation has been requested and the reasons for it explained. Communication between the pediatrician and the consultant should be made clear before the consultant sees the child so that the parents do not receive conflicting or confusing reports. The following case vignette illustrates the confusion that can occur in the process of consultation:

> Gary was an obese 10-year-old admitted to the hospital for a diagnostic workup of recent "spells" consisting of dizziness and falling down. The degree of consciousness after each episode was unclear. On the day of hospital admission, Gary appeared to vacillate between a state of near coma and insensitivity to pain and aggressive fighting behavior. The physical examination disclosed no abnormal findings. All study results were negative except those of an equivocal electroencephalogram. Neurologic consultation was requested without Gary's or his parents' knowledge. The neurologist told the mother that Gary probably had a form of seizure disorder and that medication would be recommended to the pediatrician.
>
> The nurses noted that Gary seemed quiet and did not play with other children, and a child psychiatric consultation was requested. Because the pediatrician feared the mother would object to psychiatry, she was simply told that "another doctor" would be talking to her son. The child psychiatrist arrived on the ward and introduced himself to the mother as a psychiatrist. The mother said that she was confused. While the psychiatrist talked to Gary, the mother was told to wait in the hall until the interview was over. A few minutes later the mother went to the nurses' station and demanded to see her son's pediatrician, who was paged but did not answer. The child psychiatrist returned to the mother and said that Gary appeared to be depressed and that he would return the following day to take the boy to the playroom to complete the evaluation. The mother began shouting at the nurses about the quality of care in the hospital.

This vignette illustrates the importance of good communication between the primary care physician and the consultant.[25] Such problems can be easily avoided if, before the consultant sees the patient, the primary care physician and the consultant decide together who will discuss the consultant's findings with the child and the family (Fig. 22-1).

Just as it is important for the pediatrician to communicate with parents, it is necessary for the pediatrician to communicate with the child, no matter what the child's age, in a developmentally appropriate manner.[28] This communication may take the form of actions rather than words. For example, it is more comforting for a toddler to be held for reassurance than to hear words of reassurance. When speaking to a child, the pediatrician should remember to sit down at the child's eye level and use age-appropriate words to ensure that the child understands what is to be done and to allow the child an opportunity to ask questions. To help the youngster trust hospital personnel, procedures should be explained honestly: if a child is to have blood drawn, for instance, and asks whether it will hurt, the pediatrician should admit that it will hurt for a few moments. All painful procedures should be performed as quickly and gently as possible. Often it is appropriate to perform any painful procedures in a special treatment room so that the ward or hospital room is not associated with unpleasant experiences.

Children who must undergo surgery should have the surgical procedure explained to them.[6,35] The physician can use a doll and a bandage to show where the patient's bandage will be. Children should be told where they will be when they awaken and who will be there. If a child is expected to be returned to an intensive care unit after major surgery, the nurses from that unit should visit the child before the surgery so the child will feel more at ease in the new surroundings after surgery.

In preparation for anesthesia the child should be forewarned about the anesthesia mask and the odor of the gas. Many physicians find that the presence of parents during the induction and recovery phases of anesthesia helps to alleviate much of the fear and fantasy for both parents and child.

It generally is accepted that children admitted to hospitals should be placed in pediatric units especially designed for children and staffed by personnel trained to care for children. In large children's centers children may be assigned to wards by age and type of medical problem. In community hospitals children usually are assigned to wards according to age alone, and in smaller hospitals children of all ages may be assigned to one pediatric ward. Any of these arrangements is appropriate. Many hospitals have no facilities for adolescent pa-

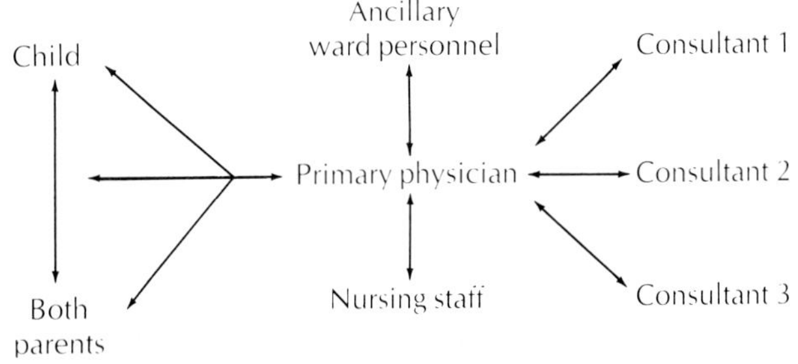

Fig. 22-1 Relationship between the primary care physician and all consultants.

tients, and teenagers are admitted to the adult wards. For a few older adolescents this may be acceptable, but for younger adolescents and some older ones such an arrangement may be detrimental to their emotional health. Whenever possible, adolescents should be placed together in a setting designed for their needs.

For young children in particular, separation from their parents is painful.[22] In these instances rooming-in arrangements are strongly recommended until the child adjusts to the hospitalization. In fact, rooming-in may result in a shorter hospital stay for the child[34] and lower anxiety for both child and parents.[1]

The issues of visiting hours and who may visit are important in pediatrics. Policies regarding these issues should be based on what is best for the child and the family and not on what is most convenient for the hospital personnel.

The question of whether it is more beneficial for a child to have a private room than to be with other children is often raised. The answer depends on the patient's particular needs and illness. Parents often believe that their child will receive better care if placed in a private room; if this is not true, the pediatrician should communicate this to the parents. As a general rule, children should have as much contact with other children as is medically feasible.

When hospitalized, children often regress in development, commonly in toilet training. Parents need reassurance that this phenomenon may occur because of the strange and frightening hospital environment. Neither children nor adolescents are accustomed to medical terminology to describe urination and defecation, and they may hesitate to express these needs to nurses. Parents can be invaluable in clarifying these terms to their children. It is important to respect a child's or an adolescent's need for privacy in completing his or her toilette, in dressing or undressing, or in being examined. Hospital personnel should be sensitive to a child's embarrassment and pull curtains around the bed when the child is undressing or draw a sheet over the child's naked genitalia when the abdomen is being examined in full view of the hall.

Although isolation may be medically necessary, pediatric personnel must remember that it does affect the child.[26] Children in isolation receive fewer visits from the nurses, may rarely see their physician, and spend less time with their parents. When someone does come into the room, the visitor is gowned and often masked. This can be frightening, stressful, and depressing. One such youngster portrayed his feelings in a drawing (Fig. 22-2). Isolation should be kept to as brief a time as medically feasible, and the physician in charge should ensure that all steps have been completed to avoid unnecessary days in isolation—for example, obtaining proper specimens for cultures and checking culture reports frequently. Parents of children in isolation may also need additional support during those days their child is in isolation.[15,26]

When a child is hospitalized, siblings should not be neglected by the parents.[19] Some children resent the attention being paid to the hospitalized child and begin to misbehave at home. Other children, particularly those of school age, are confused by their brother's or sister's absence from home and may even fantasize that they caused the hospitalization in some way. Parents may need to be reminded that *all* the

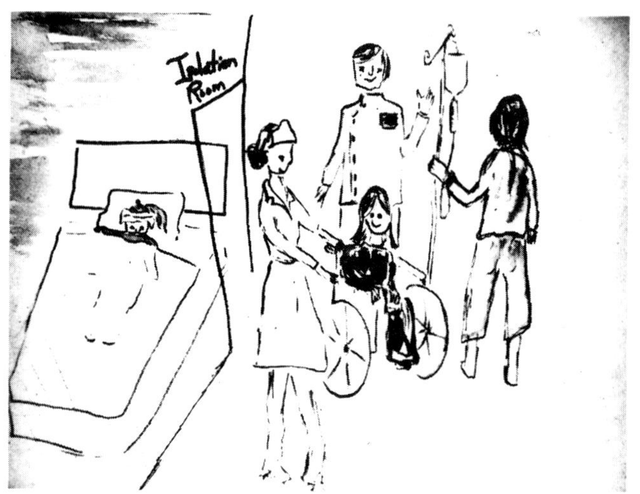

Fig. 22-2 Drawing by a 13-year-old boy in isolation.

children should be informed of their sibling's hospitalization and told the reason for it. It sometimes helps the children at home feel included and needed if each one has a special chore to do for the hospitalized youngster—for example, feeding the patient's goldfish or painting a picture to decorate the hospital room. Whenever practical, the nonhospitalized siblings should speak to their hospitalized brother or sister by telephone and be encouraged to visit the hospital. Siblings told that the hospitalized child has a minor problem (e.g., anemia or the flu) when indeed the medical situation is serious or potentially fatal may be psychologically vulnerable in later life when they have these same minor medical problems.

A major component of a child's life is school. School-age children admitted to the hospital miss their usual classroom instruction. Obviously, children who are critically or seriously ill cannot be expected to study, but children who are convalescing should be given as much schooling as possible to prevent their falling too far behind their peers. If a child is hospitalized for a short time (e.g., 7 to 10 days), the parents can serve as liaison between the classroom and the child and can work with the child's teacher to ensure that the youngster keeps abreast of classes. Children whose anticipated hospitalization is for a longer period should receive instruction through the school system by a hospital or home tutor as soon as possible. In many school systems hospital instruction cannot be requested until the child has been out of school for 6 weeks or more. This is too much time for a child to miss schoolwork, and whenever possible the physician should protest such a policy.

Another valuable component to any child's life is play. For the hospitalized child, play is also important, and most pediatric floors are well stocked with age-appropriate toys and games. A structured activities program is now common in most pediatric wards and is known by various names in different hospitals, for example, the child life program, play program, or children's activities program. Physicians should make use of a child life program in caring for their patients and welcome the observations made of the child at play. Such observations often can add insight to a child's progress or lack of progress in the hospital. Children should be encouraged to act out or "draw out" their feelings about their illness or hospitalization.[22] Where there are structured activities, as many children as possible should participate. Youngsters with intravenous lines should have the tubing anchored in such a way that walking is possible. Children in traction or restricted to bed can often have their beds moved to the playroom so that they too can take part in the activities.

While recuperating from a long illness in the hospital, children should be able to receive "leave" or passes. Pediatric health care personnel sometimes neglect the importance of children attending significant and meaningful events in their lives, such as a school occasion or a family celebration. Often a child can be allowed to leave the hospital for a few hours without detriment to his or her health, particularly for the adolescent struggling to maintain peer group acceptance during the illness.[14]

Patients, parents, and members of a hospital staff are partners in the healing process. Each has rights and responsibilities (see accompanying box). The primary care physician, as the patient's advocate and a member of the hospital staff,

Rights of Patients and Parents

1. Patients have the right to receive treatment without discrimination as to age, sex, religion, race, color, national origin, disability, sexual orientation, or source of payment.
2. Patients have the right to receive emergency care if needed.
3. Patients and parents have the right to receive considerate and respectful care in a clean and safe environment free of unnecessary restraints.
4. Patients and parents have the right to have the names and functions of all persons concerned with their care explained to them.
5. Patients and parents have the right to privacy during the hospitalization period.
6. Patients and parents have the right to complete and current information concerning their diagnosis, treatment, and prognosis, as well as administrative and financial policies affecting them, in terms the patients or parents can reasonably be expected to understand. They should be involved whenever possible in all decisions related to their care and should understand their responsibility to be as informative as possible to all concerned with their care.
7. Patients and parents have the right to receive all information necessary to give informed consent for an order not to resuscitate and to designate an individual to give this consent if the patient or parent is unable to do so.
8. Patients and parents have the right to confidentiality of all information and records regarding their care. Medical center staff members may use medical records for research projects without disclosing the patient's identity.
9. Patients and parents have the right to receive all the information necessary to give informed consent for any proposed treatment or procedure. This information should include the reasons for the procedure, the reasonably foreseeable discomforts and risks, and some indication of medically significant alternatives.
10. Patients and parents have the right to refuse treatment, examination, or observation to the extent permitted by law and to be informed of the medical consequences of such refusal.
11. Patients and parents have the right to review the patient's medical record without charge and to obtain a copy of the record, for which the hospital can charge a reasonable fee.
12. Patients and parents have the right to explanations of the nature and the risks of any clinical investigations in which they are asked to participate. They can refuse to take part in research. Furthermore, patients and parents have the right to withdraw from any study at any time without prejudicing their medical care.
13. Patients and parents have the right to (a) participate in all decisions regarding their treatment and discharge from the hospital and (b) receive a written discharge plan and description of how the plan can be reversed by the patient or parent.
14. Patients and parents have the right to receive an itemized bill and explanation of all charges.
15. Patients and parents have the right to the name and position of the physician in charge of their care in the hospital.
16. Patients and parents have the right to a no-smoking room.
17. Patients and parents have the right to complain without fear or reprisals about the care and services and to have the hospital respond, if requested, in writing. If not satisfied with this response, the patient or parent can complain to the state health department. The hospital must provide the patient and/or parent with the telephone number of the health department in most states.

Modified from University of Rochester Strong Memorial Hospital Medical Center: Statement on patients' rights, Rochester, NY, December 1988.

should ensure that all concerned understand and respect these rights and responsibilities.[23]

NOTE: A common practice in teaching hospitals is to rotate all medical students through the pediatric service. All students, regardless of their career interests, are then taught pediatric procedures (e.g., starting IVs, drawing blood, and performing spinal taps and bone marrow aspirations) by practicing on young patients. Although students interested in pediatrics must learn these procedures, they will have ample opportunity to do so as first-year house officers. Pediatric teaching programs should be reevaluated to determine whether *all* students need to master pediatric procedures and if alternative methods are available to acquire these skills, such as the use of mannequins and animal models. Current New York State Department of Health regulations severely limit medical student involvement in performing these procedures. It is likely that other states will follow suit.

Indications for Discharge from the Hospital

It sometimes is as difficult to decide when to discharge children from the hospital as it is to decide when to admit them. Children should not be kept in the hospital unnecessarily, but what constitutes an unnecessary length of time is not always clear. Fortunately most children are admitted for a given symptom, diagnosed, treated, and then sent home within a brief period. Some children require extended convalescence with minimal nursing care; for these children, alternatives to traditional hospitalization should be sought, such as convalescent homes for children, chronic illness hospitals, and visiting nurse programs. If parents are expected to perform nursing tasks for the child at home, such as injections, gavage, or dressing changes, they should be taught the procedure gradually, and the child should be discharged only when the parents and physician both feel comfortable that proper care can be given at home. Again, public health nurses can be invaluable in helping such families.[18]

Often children are admitted to the hospital with suspected primary psychosocial problems, such as those caused by child abuse. In these cases social work consultation should be requested as early as possible so that the child will not spend extra days in the hospital while such a consultation and disposition are implemented. Pediatric health care personnel must be innovative and imaginative to minimize the length of hospitalization and to encourage comprehensive rehabilitation of the child.

THE CHRONICALLY ILL CHILD

Chronically ill children pose many issues for pediatric health care personnel.[23] Sometimes these youngsters have complex medical problems and thus require the services of several physicians or clinics. These children may have significant psychosocial problems concomitant with or as a result of their illness.[25] They often require frequent checkups and characteristically have thick, illegible medical records. Their families need and deserve much support, understanding, and guidance concerning the disease and its effect on the total family. Finally, children with chronic disease evoke a vast array of feelings in the staff members who work with them. These feelings often are ignored, suppressed, or displaced.

The number of children with chronic illnesses is rapidly increasing as advances in technology are enabling physicians to change the natural history of many diseases and prolong life.[10,25] This advancement, however, has resulted in some new problems. For example, before the era of antibiotics, children with cystic fibrosis usually died before adolescence; now these patients frequently live to young adulthood. When adolescents, they usually depend on several medications simultaneously and may resent this dependence. Boys with cystic fibrosis are sterile; adolescent girls with cystic fibrosis must grapple with their fears of having children when their own life expectancy is so uncertain. Therefore physicians must now focus on the psychosocial and psychosexual problems related to these issues of sterility and pregnancy.

Effect of Chronic Illness on the Child's Development

How a chronic illness influences a child's development is contingent on several questions: Was the child born with the illness? Is the illness an inherited disorder, or was it acquired? How old was the child when the illness was acquired or when it was diagnosed? The importance of these answers relates to children's beginning development of a body image even in infancy. Five-month-old infants explore their own bodies, including their fingers, toes, genitalia, and faces, and they incorporate their findings into their developing self-images. By the age of 2 or 3 years, these youngsters have some concept of their own bodies that they identify as "mine." If in their exploration they discover that an arm or a leg is absent or that they have some other abnormality, they incorporate that abnormality into their self-image. Later, at age 3, 4, or 5 years, they begin to compare their body with other children's bodies and recognize that they are different from other children. The child growing up with an abnormality appears to be better adjusted and more accepting of his or her self-image than the child who acquires a disability during later years.[3]

After children with a chronic illness or physical deformity have accepted their self-image, they must learn to cope with their peers' perceptions.[32] Young children are adaptive and generally will play with other children to the best of their abilities in spite of their deformities. Although youngsters can be cruel and tease one another about their differences, usually children accept other children, particularly if the disabled children accept themselves. Parents, however, often become anxious about their disabled or chronically ill children being in the presence of "normal" children and may try to shield them from their peers. Physicians should reassure and support the parents so that the child is given the opportunity to relate to normal peers. See Chapter 66, "Chronically Ill and Disabled Children in School."

Children with visible disabilities often receive more attention and support than do children with "hidden" ones. For example, the child with rheumatoid arthritis who has visibly swollen joints and difficulty moving often will evoke much support from family, teachers, and friends. On the other hand, the child with juvenile diabetes, whose disability is not visible, often will not receive similar support.

A major problem for children with chronic illnesses is the difficulty that physicians and parents have in allowing them to develop independence.[20,37] Parents tend to overprotect their handicapped child, and physicians contribute to that overprotectiveness by emphasizing restrictions. It is helpful to both parents and child if the physician lists those activities the child *should* do and those activities the child *should not* do.

When treating a chronically ill child over several years, the physician can attend to vocational planning for the youngster, either personally or through staff members. Each child should be encouraged to develop socially and intellectually as completely as possible, but the physician also must recognize a child's limitations and encourage realistic aspirations.

One problem peculiar to pediatricians is their reluctance to terminate the physician-patient relationship when a youngster reaches adulthood, particularly if the pediatrician has followed up the child from infancy. Whenever possible, chronically ill children, on reaching adulthood, should be transferred to internists or family practitioners; such a transfer supports the patient's striving for independence. The patient should be prepared for this change over several visits.

Effects of Chronic Illness on the Family

The parents of chronically ill children often feel guilty about their child's illness. If a child has an inherited disorder, both parents may scrutinize their family backgrounds to see how the disease was inherited. If the illness is acquired, the parents may feel that they did not adequately protect their child from getting the disease. If an infant is born with a congenital but not inherited disorder, the mother may become obsessed about her prenatal activities and wonder if some action of hers caused the disorder.

Guilt often leads to anger (Fig. 22-3). Guilt feelings cause discomfort, and the parents become angry at feeling uncomfortable.[20] This anger may be directed toward the physician who initially diagnosed the child's illness, toward each other, toward themselves, and even toward the afflicted child.

The marital relationship between parents of a chronically ill child either remarkably improves or drastically disintegrates shortly after the illness is diagnosed. Being told that one's youngster has a chronic illness is a crisis and imposes stress on most marriages. If the marriage is stable and the parents are mutually supportive, the marital bonds grow stronger. If the marriage is unstable, the child's illness serves as a final stress that may sever marital ties.

To the family, the monetary cost of having a child with a chronic illness may be astounding, in which case the parents will need help finding financial aid. Most families are not able to carry the financial burden of their child's illness alone, but they may be too proud to ask for help. Physicians should be sensitive to these needs and offer their help or the services of their staff whenever possible.

To society, the cost of children who are chronically ill can be immeasurable. These children often require expensive medications and repeated hospitalizations, and some require long-term institutional care. Often the physician can help by educating the local community concerning chronic illnesses and by working with various agencies to improve their services to chronically ill children and their families.[25]

The siblings of children with chronic illness deserve some attention.[19] Siblings often worry about whether they will have

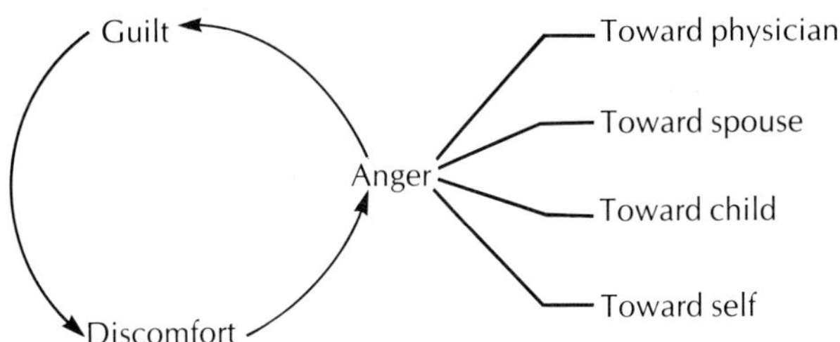

Fig. 22-3 Parental guilt over a child's chronic illness often leads to anger.

the same disease if it is congenital or inherited. If the disorder is inherited and they have been spared, they often feel guilty. If the disease is acquired, these children may think or fantasize that their brother or sister did something to deserve the illness. Often in sibling rivalry a child may wish that the brother or sister were dead. When that brother or sister acquires an illness, the sibling may then feel tremendous guilt and responsibility for "causing" the illness. The primary physician caring for the child with a chronic illness should always inquire as to the health, well-being, and psychological state of the youngster's siblings and may be able to provide insight to the parents concerning the siblings' behavior.

The Medical Delivery System

Children with chronic illnesses often receive fragmented health care.[25] Frequently a primary care physician suspects an illness and requests a consultation at a children's hospital or service, where the child is taken, a workup is completed, and a diagnosis is made. The child is then assigned to a specialty clinic, returning regularly for care. Usually this clinic is attended by full-time staff specialists, but at each visit the child is seen by a different house officer who does not know or recognize either the child or the family. The contribution to the overall care by the primary care physician who originally referred the child often is ignored.

There may be controversy over whether a child with a chronic illness should receive care from specialty clinics or from a primary care physician. Often a child can be seen once or twice a year at the specialty clinic and have other checkups through the regular pediatrician. This arrangement is suitable if communication is good between the specialist and the primary care physician. During adolescence children with chronic illnesses often continue to be treated in pediatric clinics, where they now feel uncomfortable, and their dependency is reinforced. Whenever possible, adolescents should be treated in a setting designed for teens.[14] If this is not possible, it may be appropriate to have adolescents treated by adult medical groups if those physicians are sensitive to the issues of development.

When to hospitalize the chronically ill child is a difficult question to answer.[24] Usually the parents are able to cope with innumerable medical problems at home simply through years of experience. Hospitalization often takes on special meaning to the child who is a regular visitor to the physician or hospital; the child may view hospitalization as being followed by death if the reasons for hospitalization are not carefully explained.

Pediatricians and their staff must be aware of their own emotional responses to the chronically ill child. This child, more than any other youngster, is able to evoke mixed feelings and frustration in the staff. The staff members often are angry while caring for the child; they are frustrated because their patient does not get better. Often the care of a chronically ill child involves several consultants, and each consultant may give different messages to the child and the family. Complicated cases, especially those involving mental retardation, often are rejected by all members of the medical delivery system. When such children are hospitalized, they and their families frequently spend much time in the admissions office while house officers and administrative clerks decide where the children belong. The 15-year-old mentally retarded patient with cerebral palsy may be rejected by the staff responsible for adolescent care because the patient looks like an 8-year-old child; the same patient may be rejected by the ward for school-age children because the child "is really an adolescent."

Counseling

Chronically ill children and adolescents and their parents should have opportunities to receive counseling. Usually parents need this help early in the disease, shortly after the diagnosis is made. Youngsters generally need this assistance as they approach adolescence. Not all chronically ill children and their parents will require counseling, but all should be given this option.

Usually the counseling can be provided by a sensitive and understanding physician willing to take time with the family. Social workers and psychologists also are capable of handling these problems and can work closely with the physician who cares for the child. A group of adolescents with similar problems may wish to meet regularly with an interested physician or staff member to share their common problems. In many areas parents of chronically ill children meet to support one another.

Role of the School

As mentioned earlier, an important component of any child's life is school. Children with chronic illnesses frequently are absent from school because of their illness, clinic or physician visits, or hospitalization.[9] Absence from school should be minimized. In some communities children with chronic illnesses attend special schools, particularly when they are severely handicapped. However, many children with moderately severe chronic illnesses attend regular schools. According to Public Law 94-142, children must receive (1) education in the least restricted environment that is compatible with their condition and (2) related services to facilitate their education. In either situation the school should be made aware of the children's medical problems.

Teachers may be helpful as objective observers of a child's condition. When medications are changed, teachers can be instructed to look for untoward side effects. With the parent's and child's permission, a physician may contact the school and notify the teacher, principal, or school nurse of changes in a youngster's illness. Often parents prefer to communicate this information themselves. Not all teachers are medically knowledgeable, and they may welcome information the medical profession can given them about a youngster in their classroom. In this way the school system and the medical system can collaborate to benefit the chronically ill youngster.

THE DYING CHILD

To care for the dying child properly, the physician must recognize that children have different concepts concerning death that depend on many factors, including chronologic age, cognitive development, other experience with death, and religious and cultural beliefs. All these factors should be considered when caring for the dying child.

Developmental Aspects of Death

To understand a child's concept of death, it is useful to apply Piaget's theory of sequential cognitive development[30] (Table 22-1). Infants and toddlers (2 years of age or younger) are in the *sensorimotor* stage of cognitive development. They learn through their senses (seeing, hearing, touching, and tasting) and they use their advancing motor skills to find new objects and experiences to see, hear, touch, or taste. Although young infants are in the process of language development, they are essentially preverbal, and the word *death* has no meaning for them. As they realize differences in individuals around them, however, infants can experience separation from loved ones (parents) and "know" the feelings of separation anxiety.

The next stage of cognitive development, described as *preoperational,* is characteristic of most children between 2 and 6 years of age. In this stage of development children have verbal skills but cannot yet think logically. Thus the preschooler has a very limited concept of death. By age 2 to 6 years youngsters generally have had some contact with death; a pet or a grandparent may have died. It is believed that these young children consider death a reversible phenomenon, as demonstrated in movies and television. For example, it is common to see a cartoon character flattened like a pancake with a steamroller and the next moment up and about and racing down the road. Such activity is completely plausible in the mind of the preschooler.

The school-age child 6 to 12 years old usually is in the *concrete operational* stage, when logical thought about the physical world is developed. Children's concepts of death undergo many changes during this time. For example, by the age of 6 to 8 years, the youngster often views death as a prolongation of sleep: dead people's eyes are closed as though they were asleep; therefore they must be asleep, and they simply do not wake up. After accepting the concept of irreversibility, the child who views death as a prolongation of sleep generally asks questions such as: What happens when you die and you get put in the ground? Who does Jackie play with? Doesn't he need some cookies and milk? Won't he get cold? Isn't it dark down there? How can somebody be in the ground and heaven at the same time? Later, when 8 to 10 years old, the youngster may see death personified, usually as a monster who sneaks in at night and kills the living. This fantasy is often "substantiated" by movies and television.

Table 22-1 *Development of the Concept of Death*

RANGE (YEARS)	PIAGETIAN DEVELOPMENTAL STAGE	CONCEPT OF DEATH	APPROXIMATE AGE
0-2	Sensorimotor *Preverbal* Reflex activity Purposeful activity Rudimentary thought	Expresses discomfort with separation	Infancy
2-6	Preoperational *Prelogical*	Uses word *dead* but only to distinguish "not alive"	3 yr
	Development of representational or symbolic language	Limited notion; may express no personal emotion but may associate death with sorrow of others	4 yr
	Initial reasoning	Avoids dead things; imagines death as a personified being; believes he or she will always live, only other people (especially older ones) die	5 yr
		Associates death with "old age"; may be violent and emotional about death, including representations (e.g., magazine pictures), or may display intense curiosity about dead things	6 yr
6-12	Concrete operational *Logical*	Morbid interest in details (e.g., graveyards, coffins, possible causes); seeks answers through observation of decomposition, etc.; suspects he himself may die	7 yr
	Problem-solving restricted to physically present, real objects that can be manipulated	Less morbid, more expansive; interested in what happens after death; accepts, without emotion, that he too will die	8 yr
	Development of logical functions (e.g., classification of objects)	Understands logical and biologic (e.g., absence of pulse) essentials of death; can accept full and rational explanation of death process	9-10 yr
12+	Formal operational *Abstract* Comprehension of purely abstract or symbolic content Development of advanced logical functions (e.g., complex analogy, deduction)	Meaning of death appreciated, but reality of personal death not accepted	Adolescence

From Sahler OJZ and Friedman SB: The dying child, Pediatr Rev 3:160, Nov 1981. Reproduced by permission of *Pediatrics,* copyright 1981.

The final stage of cognitive development, known as *formal operational,* is marked by the ability to understand abstract concepts and to verbalize those concepts. Sometime during adolescence, usually by the midpoint, the teenager is able to perceive the concept of death as an irreversible phenomenon.[11] This recognition may occur at the same time that most adolescents begin to deal with various philosophies, such as those concerning the purpose of life and the meaning of existence. Sometime in late adolescence or early adulthood most people begin to grapple with the concept of their own death.[17]

Children, as well as adults, have fears concerning death; frequently physicians do not recognize or acknowledge these fears. Dying children, whose concept of death is poorly defined, exhibit a fear of abandonment and are concerned that while they are dying their parents will leave them alone. The child who is terminally ill and has experienced innumerable medical tests and studies is usually more afraid of bodily harm than of death. How much children know about their impending death is not completely understood.

A comparative study[31] of chronically ill school-age children who were not terminally ill and children with leukemia who were terminally ill but in remission revealed much higher anxiety levels in the children with leukemia. This study suggests that school-age children are more aware of the seriousness of their illnesses than physicians previously believed.

In managing the care of the dying child, medical personnel and parents must be aware that in addition to the normal developmental concepts of death, a child's perceptions can be affected by other experiences with death: the death of a sibling, a parent, or a grandparent. How the family reacted to the death of another family member may be reflected in the dying child's behavior. The child who has seen a torturous death of a very sick grandparent or sibling may be more frightened of the pain or bodily harm associated with dying than of death itself. Children from religious families also will be influenced by the family's religious attitude toward death.

The Family of the Dying Child

Parents of terminally ill children typically react to the information that their child has a fatal illness with initial disbelief and shock, which may take days or several weeks to subside. This disbelief may not necessarily be intellectual denial. The parents usually can accept the diagnosis intellectually but cannot absorb the full emotional impact. Parents may desire a second opinion, as a result of denial or in the hope that the diagnosis is incorrect. They can be warned that these feelings may occur.

After the initial disbelief and shock, the parents frequently experience anger.[17] The anger may be directed toward the physician who made the diagnosis, toward staff members caring for the child, toward each other, or toward themselves for not having protected their child from contracting the terminal illness. After anger, parents may experience the "bargaining" stage when they say to themselves, "If I give up such and such, perhaps my child will be cured." After going through the bargaining stage, parents generally feel depressed and only then perhaps begin to deal with their feelings about the illness. Some parents actually grieve over the loss while their child is still alive, particularly if they are parents of children with leukemia at the terminal stages of the disease.

As part of their "anticipatory grieving," some parents have experienced what may be described as the *Lazarus syndrome*. A child is expected to die and is quite ill, and the parents actually grieve as though the death had already taken place, psychologically preparing themselves for it. The child then recovers unexpectedly and the parents are not always psychologically equipped to deal with the child. The physician can help the parents deal with their feelings at this time.

The marriage of parents who have a terminally ill or dying child often is stressful.[13] In traditional two-parent families it may be typical for the husband to support his wife emotionally early in the course of their child's illness and to make the important family decisions, thus allowing his wife to experience more emotion than he. In fact the husband may truly feel the impact of the diagnosis only some days or weeks later, when his wife no longer needs such intensive support. In some instances, of course, these roles are reversed. Parents' supporting each other is extremely important for the child, for the parents themselves, and for the other siblings. When children are hospitalized, mothers may be more comfortable than are fathers in caring for them. Because of their inexperience in caring for a child and their work schedules, fathers may spend significantly less time with the child in the ward and have little contact with the physician. The mother then has to tell the father what the physician has said. Also, both parents may work. In estranged families, one parent may shoulder major responsibility for the child and feel little support from the other parent, or the other parent may feel "left out" of the decision-making process and resent the former spouse or the physician, or both. To avoid such a situation, the physician should inform both parents about their child's condition, preferably at the same time.

The siblings of the dying child often are ignored by the parents and the physician. To decide what to tell siblings and how to tell them, parents must take into account their children's ages, development, and past experiences. They should be told that their brother or sister is dying, but with words and in a manner that is comfortable for the family. They should be made to feel that they are still part of the family and can help deal with this family crisis. If the siblings are old enough, issues such as heredity or contagion should be brought up to reassure them that they themselves do not have the same illness.

The parents also may ask for help coping with extended family members and deciding what to tell grandparents, aunts, and uncles. What information parents give depends on the relationship with family members and how close they feel to them. All family members, however, should be told the same thing so that they do not hear conflicting information. Parents also should be warned that extended family members and neighbors may unintentionally add more stress to their lives. Relatives may say things such as "Johnny can't have leukemia, he looks too healthy," or they may send newspaper and magazine articles that contradict what the physician has told the family. Well-meaning grandparents or relatives may not allow the parents to lead normal lives when their child is terminally ill or shortly after their child's death. They may make statements such as "How can you have a party when one of your children is dying?" or "How can you go away on a trip when your son just died a few months ago?" If parents are forewarned of these possibilities, they may be better equipped to deal with them.

The role of religion in helping families deal with a dying child also must be considered. Ministers, priests, and rabbis can be greatly supportive to the parents and the dying child, and religious families often contact their pastor for help. In some hospitals there is a ministry devoted to dying patients and their families, and even though these clergy may not be of the same faith as the family, they can be of help to them.

Most studies and written discussions to date concerning terminally ill children have been about parents of children whose deaths followed a terminal illness. Parents who lose a child suddenly or unexpectedly may not respond to the child's death in the same manner as parents who have had time to prepare themselves psychologically for the loss.[8,29] They often experience disbelief that may last for several weeks. Parents may deny the death of the child for some time and often dream of the deceased youngster. Parents who endure the sudden, unexpected loss of a child experience intense, disruptive, and at times almost intolerable grief reactions.

Death by accident deserves special attention because the parents or an older sibling may feel indirectly responsible for the death. The resulting guilt may persist, particularly if the accident might have been prevented by better judgment or supervision by the parent or sibling responsible for the child's safety. Guilt arising under such circumstances often is not resolved by the usual grief process.

The Medical Delivery System

Open communication should be maintained among the staff members caring for the dying child to determine ahead of time who will be responsible for telling the parents that the child is dying or has died. When a child has multiple consultants, the physician with the closest rapport with the family and the child should inform the parents of the death.[4] This responsibility should be shouldered by the primary care physician and not left to an unfamiliar intern.

How to tell parents that their child has died is another issue of concern. In talking about the diagnosis of terminal illness or about death, privacy for the parents and the physician is needed. Most physicians are sensitive to parents' needs, yet often parents are told about the diagnosis or the death in the hallways and in the presence of other people. By *sitting down* with the parents, the physician assures the parents that he or she plans to spend some time with them and is not eager to leave as soon as possible.

In talking to the parents about the terminal illness or about their child's impending death, the physician should keep explanations as simple as possible. Parents often complain that they do not understand the medical situation. What they primarily want is only enough information to comprehend the situation, to understand the recommendations of the physician, and to know what is expected of them as parents.

The parents should be spoken to every day, and the same information usually should be repeated several times, because they may not hear what the physician says the first time. The various details of the illness should be conveyed in a series of discussions rather than all at once. During these discussions the parents can be forewarned about the questions they may be asked by relatives and friends, and they can also be told to anticipate the desire to shift to a different hospital or a different physician. Then if and when they actually have these feelings, they will be relieved to know that this is what their physician had expected.

Staff members who care for a dying child often are depressed, and the morale of the nurses, house staff, and medical students suffers. On "losing" a child, the staff may experience feelings of failure and loss, and often it is desirable for them to meet to discuss a child's death as soon as possible after the event. Blame should not be placed by one group of professionals on another; rather a supportive attitude should be maintained by those in charge. Staff members in intensive care nurseries and other intensive care units are particularly susceptible to feelings of depression and low morale. To be constantly in the presence of severely ill children and to cope with the reactions of strained parents is stressful; therefore the programs of such units should always include outlets for emotional release and discussion of feelings concerning the death of infants and youngsters.[2]

Whenever medically appropriate, permission for a postmortem examination should be obtained. This request should come from the physician who has the closest rapport with the family, and the responsibility should not be shifted from attending physician to house staff to student. Ideally it would be best not to ask for the autopsy at the same time that the physician is informing the parents of their child's death. Unfortunately the postmortem examination must be done within a brief time after death, and the time the parents first learn of their child's death may be the only chance that the physician has to ask the parents. Regardless of when the subject is broached, the physician should be as frank as possible, explain the reasons for the postmortem examination, and reassure the parents that mutilation and maiming will not result.

Follow-Up After Death

The physician should try to contact the parents about 6 weeks after the child's death and offer to talk with them,[4,7,13,29] giving the parents an opportunity to ask the physician those questions they did not ask earlier. Parents often relive the illness and ask questions they had asked previously to assure themselves that their understanding of the child's disease was correct. As one mother said, "Talking later put a period on the whole episode." The physician also has the opportunity to see how the parents and siblings are adjusting and to inform them about the postmortem examination. Such actions assure the parents that the physician still cares about them and their adaptation to the stress of their child's death.

A family naturally grieves after a child has died, and the physician should support the grief reaction.[17] Lindemann[21] describes the process of mourning in detail, distinguishing features of acute grief such as frequent sighing respirations, waves of somatic distress, exhaustion, and digestive symptoms. The period of mourning cannot be sharply defined because there are marked differences among individuals. In general, however, feelings related to the loss are intense for 3 to 4 months after the death of a child. Birthdays, the date of the child's death, and holiday seasons all may remind parents of their loss and even years later may be associated with renewed periods of grieving. In the normal mourning process, however, parents return more or less to their previous level of psychological and social functioning approximately 4 to 6 months after their child's death.

After parents have lost a child through death, they may wonder whether they should have another child. After discussing this possibility with the parents, the physician generally can recommend that they have another child but should also forewarn them that the new baby is not to be a replacement. A phenomenon known as the *replacement child syndrome* occasionally occurs in which parents attempt to have another child as soon as possible after the death of a child and to make the new child into the one who has died.[27,33] In some extreme cases the same name is given to the second child. A sensitive physician who maintains contact with the parents can help them avoid this potential problem and realize that no child can truly replace another and that a subsequent child might be emotionally damaged in the attempt.

Everyone involved finds dealing with dying children difficult and painful. The parents and siblings of these children need support from the physician during the terminal illness as well as after the death, and pediatric staff members, particularly nurses and house staff members, need opportunities to express their feelings of failure and loss when an infant or child dies.

REFERENCES

1. Alexander D et al: Anxiety levels of rooming-in and non-rooming-in parents of young hospitalized children, Matern Child Nurs J 17:79, 1988.
2. Berman S and Villarreal S: Use of a seminar as an aid in helping interns care for dying children and their families, Clin Pediatr 22:175, 1983.
3. Bibace R and Walsh ME: Development of children's concepts of illness, Pediatrics 66:912, 1980.
4. Brent DA: A death in the family: the pediatrician's role, Pediatrics 72:645, 1983.
5. Cleary J et al: Parental involvement in the lives of children in hospital, Arch Dis Child 61:779, 1986.
6. Edwinson M, Arnbjornsson E, and Erkman R: Psychologic preparation program for children undergoing acute appendectomy, Pediatrics 82:30, 1988.
7. Fischoff J and O'Brien N: After the child dies, J Pediatr 88:140, 1976.
8. Friedman SB: Psychological aspects of unexpected death in infants and children, Pediatr Clin North Am 21:103, 1974.
9. Fowler MG, Johnson MP, and Atkinson SS: School achievement and absence in children with chronic health conditions, J Pediatr 106:683, 1985.
10. Green M and Haggerty RJ: Ambulatory pediatrics II, Philadelphia, 1977, WB Saunders Co.
11. Hankoff LD: Adolescence and the crisis of dying, Adolescence 10:373, 1975.
12. Heins M et al: Attitudes of pediatricians toward maternal employment, Pediatrics 72:283, 1983.
13. Johnson-Soderberg S: Parents who have lost a child by death. In Hoekelman RA, editor: Minimizing high-risk parenting, Media, Penn, 1983, Harwal Publishing Co.
14. Kellerman J et al: Psychological effects of illness in adolescence. I. Anxiety, self-esteem, and perception of control, J Pediatr 97:126, 1980.
15. Kirkpatrick J, Hoffman I, and Futterman EH: Dilemma of trust: relationship between medical care givers and parents of fatally ill children, Pediatrics 54:169, 1974.
16. Kreger BE and Restuccia JO: Assessing the need to hospitalize children: pediatric appropriateness evaluation protocol, Pediatrics 84:242, 1989.
17. Kübler-Ross E: On death and dying, New York, 1969, Macmillan Publishing Co, Inc.
18. Lauer ME and Camitta BM: Home care for dying children: a nursing model, J Pediatr 97:1032, 1980.
19. Lavigne JV and Ryan M: Psychologic adjustment of siblings of children with chronic illness, Pediatrics 63:616, 1979.
20. Leightman SR and Friedman SB: Social and psychological development of adolescents and the relationship to chronic illness, Med Clin North Am 59:1319, 1975.
21. Lindemann E: Symptomatology and management of acute grief, Am J Psychiatry 101:141, 1944.
22. Mason EA: The hospitalized child: his emotional needs, N Engl J Med 272:406, 1965.
23. Moore TD, editor: Care of children with chronic illnesses, Report of the Sixty-seventh Conference of Pediatric Research, Columbus, Ohio, 1975.
24. North AF Jr: When should a child be in the hospital? Pediatrics 57:540, 1976.
25. Pless IB, Satterwhite B, and VanVechten D: Chronic illness in childhood: a regional survey of care, Pediatrics 58:37, 1976.
26. Powazek M et al: Emotional reactions of children to isolation in a cancer hospital, J Pediatr 92:834, 1978.
27. Poznanski EO: The "replacement child": a saga of unresolved parental grief, J Pediatr 81:1190, 1972.
28. Rasnake KL and Linscheid TR: Anxiety reduction in children receiving medical care: developmental considerations, J Dev Behav Pediatr 10:169, 1989.
29. Rowe J et al: Follow-up of families who experience a perinatal death, Pediatrics 62:166, 1978.
30. Sahler OJZ and Friedman SB: The dying child, Pediatr Rev 3:159, 1981.
31. Spinetta JJ and Maloney LJ: Death anxiety in the outpatient leukemic child, Pediatrics 56:1034, 1975.
32. Steinhaver PD: Psychological aspects of chronic illness, Pediatr Clin North Am 21:825, 1974.
33. Szybist C: The subsequent child, 1976, US Department of Health, Education and Welfare, Pub No (HSA) 76-5145, Rockville, Md, 1976, Bureau of Community Health Services.
34. Taylor MR and O'Connor P: Resident parents and shorter hospital stay, Arch Dis Child 64:274, 1989.
35. Wolfer JA and Visintainer MA: Prehospital psychological preparation for tonsillectomy patients: effects on children's and parents' adjustment, Pediatrics 64:646, 1979.
36. US Department of Labor: Facts on women workers, Washington, DC, 1980, Office of the Secretary, Women's Bureau.
37. Zeltzer L et al: Psychologic effects of illness in adolescence. II. Impact of illness in adolescents—crucial issues and coping styles, J Pediatr 97:132, 1980.

23

Management of Fever

Louis C. Littlefield

THERMOREGULATION AND PATHOGENESIS OF FEVER

Under normal conditions, body temperature is maintained around a specific set-point temperature by neuronal regulatory mechanisms within the hypothalamus that produce a balance between heat production and heat dissipation.[5] The preoptic area of the hypothalamus and adjacent regions of the anterior hypothalamus contain the neurons that are capable of altering body functions to increase heat loss and decrease heat production when the body temperature is elevated. Similarly, when the hypothalamic temperature control center receives signals from cold receptors via the posterior hypothalamus, body functions are altered to increase heat production and reduce heat dissipation.

Although the terms *fever* and *hyperthermia* sometimes are used interchangeably, each is a distinct pathophysiologic entity.[23] *Fever* is an elevated thermoregulatory set-point that alters physiologic processes to increase body temperature. *Hyperthermia* is a condition wherein the body's thermoregulatory set-point may be normal, but abnormal physiologic processes exist to produce an elevated body temperature.

An example of hyperthermia is heat stroke, in which overexertion in an excessively hot and humid environment results in increased heat production under conditions that do not permit heat dissipation.[28] Exercising children are particularly susceptible to hyperthermia because they do not adapt to temperature extremes as effectively as do adults.[9] Children have a greater surface area/mass ratio than do adults, which results in a greater heat transfer between the environment and the body. Walking and running produce more metabolic heat per mass unit in adults than in children, who also have a decreased capacity to sweat and to convect heat from the body core to the skin during exercise. All these factors contribute to a greater risk of serious hyperthermia in children who exercise in an environmental temperature that exceeds their skin temperature.

Hyperthermia attributable to an increased metabolic rate may accompany endocrinologic disorders such as thyrotoxicosis and pheochromocytoma.[36] Hypothalamic lesions caused by stroke, neurosurgical procedures, or tumors may impair thermoregulatory mechanisms. Several drugs are associated with hyperthermia when they are ingested in toxic doses. Examples include lysergic acid diethylamide (LSD), cocaine, amphetamines, salicylates, anticholinergics, and tricyclic antidepressants. Another drug-induced alteration of thermoregulatory function has been reported in a few patients receiving inhalation anesthetics and muscle relaxants during surgery.[6] The term *malignant hyperthermia* is used to describe this pharmacogenetic myopathy, which usually begins with sinus tachycardia, increased blood pressure, and tachypnea. Sustained contraction of skeletal muscles is accompanied by metabolic and respiratory acidosis, increased oxygen consumption, and a rapid rise in body temperature.[35]

In most cases, fever probably results from a pyrogen-mediated elevation in the set-point temperature, which causes alterations in physiologic functions in an attempt to decrease heat dissipation and to increase heat production. Heat conservation may be achieved by cutaneous vasoconstriction, which prevents the conduction of body heat from internal body compartments to the skin. The cutaneous vasoconstriction generally results from increased posterior hypothalamic sympathetic activity. Another method of conserving heat is decreased sweating, which usually accompanies febrile states. Increased heat production may be manifested as shivering. A primary motor center for shivering is located in the posterior hypothalamus; it can transmit impulses to anterior motor neurons in response to an elevated set-point temperature. These impulses increase skeletal muscle tone throughout the body. Although significant increases in body temperature can occur without shivering, when muscle tone exceeds a critical level, shivering ensues and heat production can increase to as high as five times normal.

Augmented cellular metabolism induced by sympathetic stimulation and circulating catecholamine is a second method of increasing heat production. This method may be particularly significant in newborns. The production capability of this method is believed to be related to the amount of mitochondrion-rich brown fat present in body tissue. Because newborns have a small amount of brown fat stores, heat production may be increased by as much as 100% through stimulation of alternate metabolic pathways.[21]

Although exogenous pyrogens, such as a gram-negative endotoxin or an antigen-antibody complex, may act directly to elevate body temperature, most experimental evidence[11] supports the concept that body substances produced in response to exogenous pyrogens act directly on the hypothalamic thermoregulatory center. In the past the term *endoge-*

nous pyrogen was used to describe the substances released by phagocytic cells that produced an increase in body temperature. More recently there have been several investigations[2,12] to prove that infections, inflammation, and immunologic reactions can induce a series of reactions collectively termed the *acute phase response*. The components of this response are stimulated by hormonelike mediators produced by macrophages and cells of the reticuloendothelial system. These mediators are believed (1) to increase the central nervous system production of prostaglandin E_2, which acts to increase the hypothalamic set-point temperature, (2) to stimulate neutrophil release from the bone marrow, (3) to produce decreases in serum iron and zinc, (4) to alter hepatic protein production, and (5) to stimulate T lymphocyte proliferation. One substance that appears to be common in all these pathways is a large-molecular-weight protein, interleukin-1, which is produced by activated monocytes.[13]

Although fever in children generally results from acute viral and bacterial illnesses, other causes must be examined to avoid inappropriate treatment. Dehydration, regardless of whether it results from an infection, can elevate body temperature.[3] In such instances the favored treatment is restoring intravascular volume rather than introducing specific antipyretic therapy. Traumatic brain injury or congenital central nervous system malformations can cause recurrent, transient temperature elevations that usually do not require specific antipyretic therapy. Other noninfectious causes of fever include heavy blankets and overdressing, thrombophlebitis caused by intravenous catheters and irritating fluids, and endocrine disorders.

Drugs also can produce fever through several mechanisms.[40,44] A fever caused by drugs themselves (*drug fever*) may be a manifestation of a hypersensitivity reaction resulting from administration of any one of several drugs, particularly antibiotics. In such cases the fever might be accompanied by signs and symptoms of a systemic allergic reaction. If an unexplained fever develops in a patient who shows clinical improvement after receiving drugs known to produce febrile reactions 7 to 10 days after their institution, the physician should consider drugs as the cause. Similarly, drugs that increase heat production by stimulating the basal metabolic rate or by increasing skeletal muscle activity, and those that decrease cutaneous blood flow, may produce an elevated body temperature that becomes normal on discontinuation of the drug.

DEFINITION OF FEVER AND TEMPERATURE MEASUREMENTS

The accepted clinical definition of *fever* is a rectal temperature above 100.4° F (38° C), an oral temperature above 100° F (37.8° C), or an axillary temperature above 99° F (37.2° C).[33] Although the accepted average oral temperature is 98.6° F (37° C), the normal range may vary anywhere from 97.7° to 99.5° F (36° to 37° C) in older children and adults and may be higher in infants.[10] One reason for higher temperatures in infants may be a reduced capacity of the newborn to sweat in response to increased environmental temperatures. Also, excessive bundling or clothing on the newborn may contribute significantly to an elevation in body temperature. In contrast, the newborn is highly susceptible to environmentally induced hypothermia caused by decreased autonomic control of peripheral blood flow. Although it is an important consideration in the assessment of every patient, the influence of environmental temperature and conditions on body temperature must be evaluated carefully in interpreting newborn body temperature recordings.

A diurnal temperature variation exists in all normal persons. The zenith of this variation occurs in the later afternoon or early evening, and the nadir occurs in the early morning between 3 and 5 AM.[4] This 2° and 3° F variation appears to be independent of sleep habits and eating and working patterns.

Body temperature can best be determined by measuring rectal temperature, although care must be taken to ensure accurate recordings, especially in young children; measuring oral temperature may be a better method for the child who is fully cooperative and does not have a respiratory illness. Axillary temperatures may be less accurate than rectal recordings[25] but they are easier to measure in young infants. Another consideration in recording body temperature is the accuracy or inaccuracy of the recording device.

An accepted procedure for recording rectal temperatures is to position the child face down, lubricate the tip of the thermometer with petrolatum to minimize rectal discomfort and resistance, and insert the thermometer to a depth of 1 inch for 3 minutes. Obtaining an accurate oral temperature generally takes about 5 minutes, whereas axillary temperatures can be recorded in 3 to 5 minutes. The pediatrician should remind parents not to take their child's oral temperature just after the mouth has been artificially cooled or heated with food or beverages, because spurious recordings may be obtained. Similarly, the patient should not breathe through the mouth while the oral temperature is being recorded inasmuch as a falsely low value may be obtained, particularly in the patient with tachypnea.[42] In spite of adequate precautionary efforts, thermometers may break. Because only small, nontoxic amounts of mercury could be ingested, however, glass particles constitute the chief hazard.

FACTORS AFFECTING TREATMENT DECISIONS

Perhaps the most important factor that affects diagnostic and therapeutic decisions is the age of the febrile child. Usually the younger the child, the more subtle are the clinical manifestations of life-threatening infections. In the newborn, immature immune responses increase the risk of disseminated infections accompanied by minimal localizing signs or alterations in fever patterns. Therefore, although the pediatrician can appropriately offer reassurance and conservative therapy to a parent of a 3-year-old febrile child with mild symptoms, he or she must regard fever in an infant from birth to 2 to 3 months old as a sign of illness and proceed with rigorous diagnostic evaluation and aggressive therapeutic intervention, concurrent with close monitoring.

With a febrile child, one decision the physician must make is whether the child's body temperature needs to be reduced. It is not well established whether fever is an essential host defense mechanism or a normal, but insignificant, biologic response to infection. The possible beneficial role of fever in host responses to infection has been a subject of debate. Some evidence exists to support the concept that fever enhances specific resistance mechanisms under certain clinical and experimental conditions.[26,38] A second and perhaps more practical consideration is whether the febrile course should be allowed to continue for purposes of diagnostic and therapeutic follow-up care.

Before instituting therapy, the pediatrician also must weigh the relative risks of available treatments against potential benefits derived from lowering the body temperature. There is little risk of serious complications until body temperature exceeds 106° F (41° C), which is uncommon. Most parents do not appreciate this fact and may become anxious if their child's body temperature exceeds 102° F (39° C).[32] Although fever-triggered seizures remain a concern of the pediatrician, this risk in an otherwise normal patient is extremely low until the body temperature exceeds 104° to 106° F (40° to 41° C). In Tomlinson's review[45] of high fevers among 101 pediatric patients without a history of seizures, convulsions occurred in only 12 of 108 episodes of fever greater than 104° F (40° C). Because the majority of febrile seizures reported in nonepileptic patients occur before a decision regarding antipyretic therapy can be made, it appears that only a relatively small percentage of patients will benefit from aggressive antipyretic therapy. Patients with a history of repeated febrile seizures are best treated with chronic anticonvulsant therapy, as well as aggressive antipyretic therapy.

A serious concern relative to the risk of antipyretic therapy is the reported epidemiologic association between aspirin administration and Reye syndrome.[46] Although such an association does not prove causation, the Food and Drug Administration (FDA),[41] the Centers for Disease Control,[39] and the American Academy of Pediatrics[8] have issued statements warning people to avoid the use of salicylates in children with suspected influenza or chickenpox and, in general, in all children who are febrile. Although several factors can affect the selection of antipyretics in children, studies[1,31] have clearly shown a decrease in the use of aspirin and an increase in the use of acetaminophen between 1980 and 1985. During this same period the incidence of Reye syndrome decreased, providing additional support for the possible role of aspirin as an etiologic factor. A recent report[15] suggested that acetaminophen may slow scabbing and that, compared with placebo, it does not relieve pruritus. These findings support the American Academy of Pediatrics' recommendation of caution with respect to the use of any antipyretic in children with viral illnesses.

THERAPEUTIC APPROACHES TO TREATMENT OF FEVER

Once the decision has been made to treat the febrile child, the pediatrician's next important decision is the selection of an appropriate therapy. The need for specific antipyretic therapy in the patient with fever often can be reduced by employing general supportive measures. Particularly in the young infant, removing blankets and heavy clothing, maintaining a relatively normal room temperature, and increasing air circulation within the room may be sufficient to adequately reduce body temperature. Obtaining maximal heat dissipation is based on maintaining adequate cutaneous blood flow. Therefore restoring intravascular volume in a dehydrated patient and maintaining an adequate state of hydration in a febrile patient are essential components of general antipyretic therapy. If these maneuvers are unsuccessful, then more specific antipyretic therapy may be necessary.

Specific antipyretic therapy includes oral antipyretics and topical sponging. Although some physicians prefer intermittent sponging with tepid water, this usually does not produce a sustained reduction in body temperature. Sponging is most effective when a centrally acting antipyretic is given first; otherwise the hypothalamic thermoregulatory center will continue to alter physiologic processes to maintain body temperature at the elevated set-point temperature. In addition, caution should be exercised in using tepid-water sponging routinely on more critically ill patients with possible intravascular volume contraction. In such patients, sponging may further increase the degree of peripheral vasoconstriction, thereby increasing heat retention. Although hydroalcoholic solutions and ice water can be used to reduce body temperature more rapidly, such measures are associated with increased patient discomfort and also may be associated with increased risk of serious complications. There are several reports[18,27,34] of severe hypoglycemic episodes and comas associated with the excessive use of sponging with hydroalcoholic solutions.

If tepid-water sponging has failed to reduce body temperature adequately, or if more aggressive antipyretic therapy is appropriate, then an oral antipyretic can be considered. In selecting and recommending an oral antipyretic agent, the physician should consider each of the following factors: cost, convenience of available dosage forms, relative effectiveness, toxic potential, and the patient's concurrent illness or conditions. Aspirin, acetaminophen, and more recently, ibuprofen have been thoroughly investigated with respect to their antipyretic effects in pediatric patients.[24] Nonsteroidal antiinflammatory drugs other than ibuprofen may possess antipyretic activity but have undergone only limited investigations in pediatric patients. The three drugs (aspirin, acetaminophen, and ibuprofen) are believed to act by inhibiting the action of interleukin-1 on hypothalamic thermoregulatory centers. In addition, aspirin acts on vascular smooth muscle to produce peripheral vasodilation, which also increases heat dissipation. This additional effect may be undesirable in a patient with moderate to severe dehydration accompanied by intravascular volume depletion. However, the combined analgesic, antipyretic, and antiinflammatory properties of aspirin can be advantageous in those patients with febrile episodes associated with acute symptoms of inflammatory diseases. Although acetaminophen may act to inhibit prostaglandin synthetase, its lack of antiinflammatory actions probably reflects minimal peripheral prostaglandin synthetase inhibition.

The antipyretic effectiveness of aspirin, acetaminophen, and ibuprofen has been studied in a number of well-designed clinical investigations.[7,16,43,47] In general, these studies have shown that aspirin and acetaminophen are comparable in onset, peak, and duration of antipyretic action when administered in equal doses, whereas ibuprofen appears to have a longer duration of effect, usually lasting up to 8 hours. Acetaminophen, because of its increased water solubility, is marketed in a greater number of dosage forms convenient for administration to pediatric patients. However, the large number of acetaminophen liquid dosage forms may sometimes result in confusion regarding specific doses to be administered to children. Parents should be discouraged from constantly changing from a liquid, syrup, or elixir to the pediatric drops because the variation in concentration of active ingredients alters the dosage amount. Ibuprofen is marketed in a pediatric suspension (100 mg/5 ml) and several tablet strengths, whereas aspirin, the least expensive of the three drugs, is available only in solid and chewable oral dosages.

Therapeutic doses of acetaminophen, in contrast to ibuprofen and aspirin, are remarkably free from adverse effects. Even mild overdoses of acetaminophen result in virtually no clinical manifestations. In contrast, the early signs and symptoms of mild salicylism (nausea, vomiting, irritability, hyperpnea, and hyperthermia) can closely resemble the clinical manifestations of the disease that necessitated the administration of aspirin. Therefore, parents, not knowing this, may tend to continue aspirin administration that can result in therapeutic intoxication. After acute ingestions a fatal dose of acetaminophen has been reported to be as low as 0.2 g/kg, whereas that of aspirin is reported to be 0.4 g/kg. Hepatocellular destruction is the primary acute toxic effect of acetaminophen, whereas the salicylates involve multiple organ systems. Therefore, although acetaminophen may possess fewer side effects than aspirin at therapeutic doses, it appears to possess a greater toxic potential after ingestion of large single doses.

In certain patients the pharmacologic and toxicologic properties of aspirin and ibuprofen may be so potentially serious that the drugs should be avoided altogether. For example, the effects of aspirin and, to a lesser extent, ibuprofen on decreasing platelet adhesiveness and its interference with prothrombin synthesis contraindicate their use in patients with bleeding disorders or patients receiving anticoagulants. Although earlier studies suggested that aspirin be avoided in patients with glucose 6-phosphate dehydrogenase deficiencies, more recent literature[19] indicates that short-term administration of antipyretic-analgesic doses does not result in red blood cell hemolysis. Because the administration of aspirin and ibuprofen may result in epigastric distress, nausea, and vomiting, they are generally less desirable than acetaminophen for patients with concurrent gastrointestinal illnesses. Studies[17,30] of adult and pediatric patients with asthma have revealed that approximately 20% of these patients exhibit a significant deterioration of pulmonary function after administration of a single aspirin dose.

A variety of pediatric dosage schedules for orally administered aspirin and acetaminophen based on age, body surface area, and body weight appear in pediatric literature. Regardless of the method of administration, clinical studies[43,48] have shown that the effective antipyretic dose for each of these two agents is similar. Calculating body surface area provides a method of obtaining a reliable dosage estimate up through 10 years of age, but often it is impractical to calculate this area accurately. Age provides a more convenient means by which to estimate antipyretic doses; however, the physician always must exercise care when a patient's weight is disproportionately heavy or light for his or her age. The revised FDA aspirin dosage schedule for children uses age as the criterion for labeling aspirin products. A review[14] of aspirin dosage recommendations suggests that body weight provides an effective and consistent criterion for calculating pediatric antipyretic doses.

Either aspirin or acetaminophen can be administered in oral antipyretic dosages of 50 to 65 mg/kg/day, given in divided doses every 4 to 6 hours. Usually the oral route of administration is preferred. Despite the lack of information regarding adequate bioavailability and clinical response, there has been a persistent interest in the use of aspirin suppositories for patients who cannot tolerate oral medications. Evidence[29] suggests that both the amount absorbed and the rate of absorption after rectal administration may result in unpredictable therapeutic outcomes. Therefore adequate hydration and sponging may be the best therapeutic approaches to lower body temperature in patients with severe gastroenteritis who cannot tolerate oral dosage forms.

According to published reports of single-dose[20,47] and multiple-dose[24] studies, ibuprofen 30 mg/kg/day, given in three divided doses, appears to be a safe and effective regimen for children older than 6 months of age. Because of the lack of published data, use of ibuprofen in young children for more than 24 hours is not advisable except under very close medical supervision.

Alternating the use of aspirin and acetaminophen has become increasingly popular, although controlled studies that demonstrate any therapeutic advantage of this regimen have not been performed. A single-dose study reported by Steele and associates[37] did show that the simultaneous administration of aspirin and acetaminophen produced a more sustained antipyretic effect than either agent alone, but these results cannot be used to establish the safety and efficacy of multiple-dose alternating regimens.

The best treatment for fever in the neonate is sponging with tepid water rather than administering aspirin, ibuprofen, or acetaminophen. The primary support for this theory is the decreased ability of the neonate to eliminate these drugs. Newborns can have a significantly reduced salicylate elimination capacity because of decreased hepatic metabolism and decreased renal excretion. The resultant salicylate elimination half-life may be increased 1½ to 4 times that reported for adults. Although acetaminophen is eliminated almost totally by hepatic metabolism and does not show as great an accumulation potential as aspirin, its elimination half-life may be increased by 5% to 75% in the neonate.

REFERENCES

1. Arrowsmith JB et al: National patterns of aspirin use and Reye syndrome reporting, United States, 1980 to 1985, Pediatrics 79:858, 1987.
2. Atkins E: Fever—new perspectives on an old phenomenon, N Engl J Med 308:958, 1983.
3. Aynsley-Green A and Pickering D: Use of central and peripheral temperature measurements in care of the critically ill child, Arch Dis Child 49:477, 1974.
4. Bayley N and Stolz HR: Maturational changes in rectal temperatures of 61 infants from 1 to 36 months, Child Dev 8:195, 1937.
5. Benzinger TH: Clinical temperature: new physiological basis, JAMA 209:1200, 1969.
6. Britt BA: Etiology and pathophysiology of malignant hyperthermia, Fed Proc 38:44, 1979.

7. Colgan MT and Mintz AA: The comparative antipyretic effect of N-acetyl-P-aminophenol and acetylsalicylic acid, J Pediatr 50:552, 1957.
8. Committee on Infectious Diseases, American Academy of Pediatrics: Special report: aspirin and Reye syndrome, Pediatrics 69:810, 1982.
9. Committee on Sports Medicine, American Academy of Pediatrics: Climatic heat stress and the exercising child, Pediatrics 69:808, 1982.
10. Cone TJ: Diagnosis and treatment: children with fevers, Pediatrics 43:290, 1969.
11. Dinarello CA and Wolff SM: Pathogenesis of fever in man, N Engl J Med 298:607, 1978.
12. Dinarello CA and Wolff SM: Molecular basis of fever in humans, Am J Med 72:799, 1982.
13. Dinarello CA: Interleukin-1 and the pathogenesis of the acute-phase response, N Engl J Med 311:1413, 1984.
14. Done AK, Yaffe SJ, and Clayton JM: Aspirin dosage for infants and children, J Pediatr 95:617, 1979.
15. Doran TF et al: Acetaminophen: more harm than good for chickenpox? J Pediatr 114:1045, 1989.
16. Eden AN and Kaufman A: Clinical comparison of three antipyretic agents, Am J Dis Child 114:284, 1967.
17. Fischer TJ et al: Adverse pulmonary responses to aspirin and acetaminophen in chronic childhood asthma, Pediatrics 71:313, 1983.
18. Garrison RF: Acute poisoning from use of isopropyl alcohol in tepid sponging, JAMA 152:317, 1958.
19. Glader NE: Evaluation of the hemolytic role of aspirin in glucose-6-phosphate dehydrogenase deficiency, J Pediatr 89:1027, 1976.
20. Heremens G et al: A single-blind parallel group study investigating the antipyretic properties of ibuprofen syrup versus acetylsalicylic acid syrup in febrile children, Br J Clin Pract 42:245, 1988.
21. Hull D: Temperature regulation and disturbance in the newborn infant, Clin Endocrinol Metab 5:39, 1976.
22. Hurwitz ES et al: Public Health Service study of Reye's syndrome and medications: report of the main study, JAMA 257:1905, 1987.
23. Kluger MJ: Fever, Pediatrics 66:720, 1980.
24. Kotob A: A comparative study of two dosage levels of ibuprofen syrup in children with pyrexia, J Int Med Res 13:122, 1985.
25. Kresch MJ: Axillary temperature as a screening test for fever in children, J Pediatr 104:596, 1984.
26. Mackowiak PA: Direct effects of hyperthermia on pathogenic microorganisms: teleologic implications with regard to fever, Rev Infect Dis 3:508, 1981.
27. McFadden SW and Haddow JE: Coma produced by topical application of isopropanol, Pediatrics 43:622, 1969.
28. Musacchia XJ: Fever and hyperthermia, Fed Proc 38:27, 1979.
29. Nowak MM, Brundhofer B, and Gibaldi M: Rectal absorption from aspirin suppositories in children and adults, Pediatrics 54:23, 1974.
30. Rachelefsky GS et al: Aspirin intolerance in chronic childhood asthma: detected by oral challenge, Pediatrics 56:443, 1975.
31. Rahwan GL and Rahwan RG: Aspirin and Reye's syndrome: the change in prescribing habits of health professionals, Drug Intell Clin Pharm 20:143, 1986.
32. Schmitt BD: Fever phobia: misconceptions of parents about fevers, Am J Dis Child 134:176, 1980.
33. Schmitt BD: Fever in childhood, Pediatrics 74(suppl):929, 1984.
34. Senz EH and Goldfarb DL: Coma in a child following use of isopropyl alcohol in sponging, J Pediatr 53:322, 1958.
35. Sessler DI: Malignant hyperthermia, J Pediatr 109:9, 1986.
36. Sitt JT: Fever versus hyperthermia, Fed Proc 38:39, 1979.
37. Steele RW et al: Oral antipyretic therapy: evaluation of aspirin-acetaminophen combination, Am J Dis Child 1234:204, 1972.
38. Stern RC: Pathophysiologic basis for symptomatic treatment of fever, Pediatrics 59:92, 1977.
39. Surgeon General's advisory on the use of salicylates and Reye syndrome, MMWR 31:289, 1982.
40. Tabor PA: Drug-induced fever, Drug Intell Clin Pharm 20:413, 1986.
41. Take two aspirin? FDA Consumer 14:17, 1980-81.
42. Tandberg D and Sklar D: Effect of tachypnea on the estimation of body temperature by an oral thermometer, N Engl J Med 308:945, 1983.
43. Tarlin L et al: A comparison of the antipyretic effect of acetaminophen and aspirin: another approach to poison prevention, Am J Dis Child 124:880, 1972.
44. Tierney L: Drug fever, West J Med 129:321, 1978.
45. Tomlinson WA: High fever: experience in private practice, Am J Dis Child 129:693, 1975.
46. Waldman RJ et al: Aspirin as a risk factor in Reye's syndrome, JAMA 247:3089, 1982.
47. Walson PD et al: Ibuprofen, acetaminophen, and placebo treatment of febrile children, Clin Pharmacol Ther 46:9, 1989.
48. Wilson JT et al: Efficacy, disposition and pharmacodynamics of aspirin, acetaminophen and choline salicylate in young febrile children, Ther Drug Monit 4:147, 1982.

24

The Management of Acute Pain in Children

Myron Yaster and Lynne G. Maxwell

I will use my power to help the sick to the best of my ability and judgement; I will abstain from harming or wronging any man by it.

Hippocrates

Even when their pain is obvious, children frequently receive no treatment or inadequate treatment for pain or for painful procedures.[4,17,27] The common "wisdom" that children neither respond to, nor remember, painful experiences to the same degree that adults do is simply not true.* Unfortunately, even when physicians decide to treat children in pain, they rarely prescribe potent analgesics or adequate doses because of their overriding concern that children may be harmed by the use of these drugs.[2,25,27] This is not at all surprising because physicians are taught throughout their training that opiates cause respiratory depression, cardiovascular collapse, depressed levels of consciousness, vomiting, and, with repeated use, addiction. Rarely, if ever, are the appropriate therapeutic uses of these drugs, or rational dosing regimens, discussed. Indeed, it is difficult to find pain and its medical management in any of the current textbooks of pediatric medicine and surgery.[36]

Nurses are taught to be wary of physicians' orders (and patients' requests) as well. The most common prescription order for potent analgesics, "to give as needed" (pro re nata ["prn"]) has come to mean "to give as infrequently as possible." The prn order also means that either the patient must ask for pain medication or the nurse must identify when a patient is in pain. This is particularly difficult in dealing with children because it may be impossible for the very young to articulate when or where they hurt. Many children will withdraw or will deny their pain in an attempt to avoid yet another terrifying and painful experience—the intramuscular injection or "shot." Finally, several studies have documented the inability of nurses and physicians to identify and treat pain correctly even postoperatively in pediatric patients.

NEUROPHYSIOLOGY OF PAIN

The physiology of pain is complex; it involves more than the transmission of nociceptive input from peripheral pain receptors (nociceptors) to the brain. It probably is best understood in terms of Wall and Melzack's "gate theory of pain," which can be summarized as follows.[33] After an injury, peripheral pain receptors transmit sensory information to the spinal cord via relatively small-diameter sensory nerves (A-delta and C) whose cell bodies are located within the dorsal root ganglia. A-delta fibers are associated with sharp, well localized pain, whereas C fibers are associated with dull, burning, diffusely localized pain. The C fibers also include efferent sympathetic nerve fibers, which increase the sensitivity of peripheral nociceptors to pain. At the site of injury, local release of prostaglandins, serotonin, bradykinin, norepinephrine, hydrogen ion, potassium ion, and substance P, a peripheral pain transmitter, can increase the responsiveness of the peripheral nociceptors to painful stimuli (Fig. 24-1). Pharmacologic manipulations of these local factors by prostaglandin inhibitors (e.g., aspirin, acetaminophen, or ibuprofen) can thereby blunt pain transmission.

The nociceptive impulse is transmitted to the dorsal horn of the spinal cord where diverse synapses occur with essentially all incoming sensory input.[3,33] In the dorsal horn of the spinal cord, interneurons are activated, releasing substance P, an 11-amino acid peptide pain transmitter that facilitates nociceptive transmission. It is of interest that substance P is depleted by capsaicin, a substance commonly found in hot chili and paprika, which may explain the taste bud "anesthesia" that follows the initial burning sensation of Mexican or Hungarian food. Alternatively, the nociceptive impulse may be inhibited or completely blocked at the interneurons of the dorsal horn if the interneurons are overwhelmed by innocuous, nonpainful information from other peripheral nerve fibers. Stimulation of large-diameter peripheral nerve fibers can thereby effectively block nociceptive information from the site of injury. This principle underlies the use of transcutaneous electrical nerve stimulation (TENS).[3,33] Descending fibers also synapse at the interneurons to inhibit or to modulate sensory input from the site of injury as well, via the release of the neuropeptides. Of these neuropeptides the opioid peptides such as endorphins and enkephalins are the best known and most extensively studied. Indeed, the identification of mu, kappa, and to a lesser degree delta, opioid receptors in the dorsal horn of the spinal cord, explains the effects of intrathecal and epidural opioid administration in the management of pain.[3,7,33]

If unblocked, nonciceptive input is transmitted to the brain

*See references 2, 4, 17, 27, and 36.

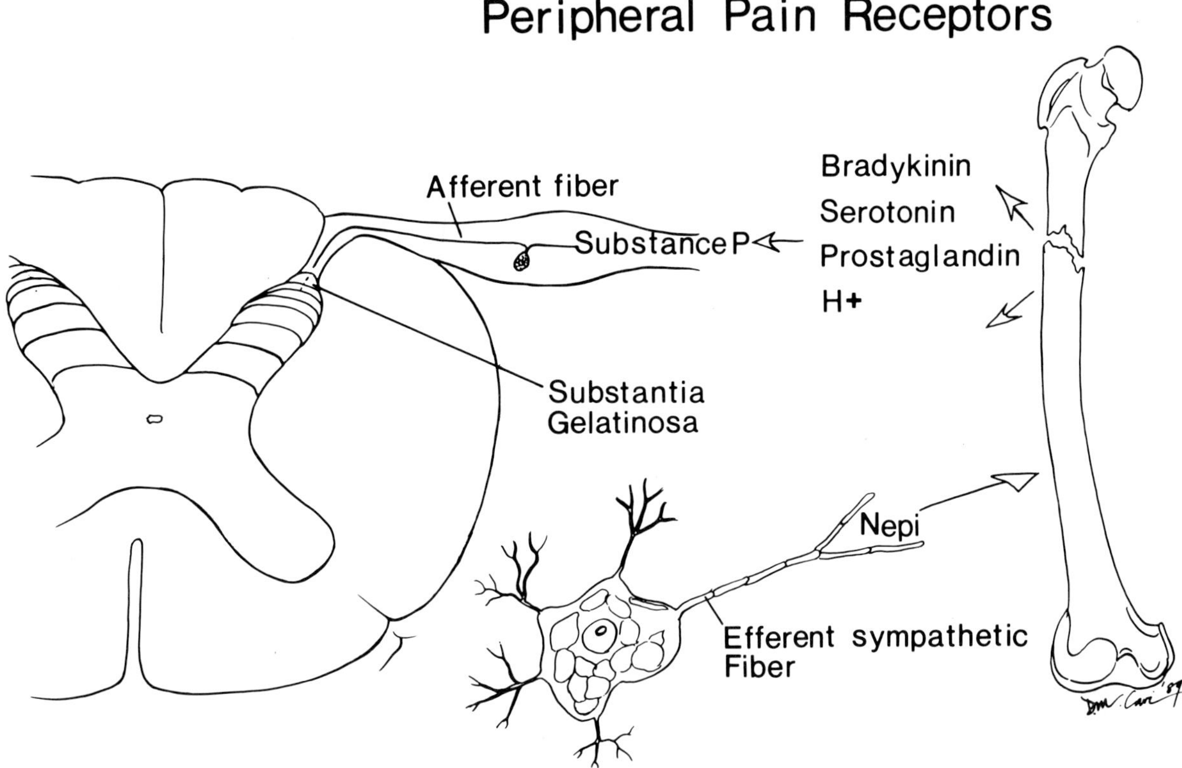

Fig. 24-1 Peripheral pain receptors and modulation of their activity are depicted. Note that physical stimuli, (e.g., a bone fracture), the chemical environment (pH), adrenergic tone (serotonin level), and mediator (bradykinin, prostaglandin, etc.) release modify peripheral receptor (afferent fiber) activity. Substance P is the probable peripheral pain transmitter.

via the classic spinothalamic and spinoreticular nerve pathways. Several areas within the brain may further modulate or abolish pain transmission, including the brain stem's medial and lateral reticular formations, the nuclei of the medullary median raphe, the periaqueductal gray matter, the thalamus and the cerebral cortex. Binding of either endogenous or pharmacologically administered opiates to receptors in these central locations initiates the modulation of pain transmission.[3,33] The gate theory therefore depends not only on peripheral stimulation and transmission but also on modulation of the transmission within the spinal cord and higher structures.

Thus pain or the transmission of nociceptive impulses requires intact neuroanatomic pathways from the peripheral pain receptors to the central nervous system. These pathways and receptors develop in early fetal life and are essentially mature and completely developed by birth.[2] The development of descending inhibition pathways of nonciceptive neurons and interneurons in the dorsal horn of the spinal cord and within the brain stem occurs during the final three months of gestation and is completed during infancy and early childhood.

Pain management therefore can best be understood or designed in terms of afferent pain pathways and descending pain modulation. Pain can be relieved (1) by reducing the sensory input from damaged tissue (by administration of prostaglandin inhibitors or local anesthetics); (2) by modulating the transmission of the nociceptive input through the central nervous system (by TENS, pharmacologic opioid administration, or the administration of local anesthetics); and (3) by altering the patient's emotional responses to such actual or perceived sensory input (by administration of antidepressant, hypnotic, or amnestic agents). Before pain can be effectively treated, however, one must be able to measure and assess pain accurately and have full knowledge of the therapies used in treating it.

PAIN ASSESSMENT

The International Association for the Study of Pain (IASP) defines pain as "an unpleasant and emotional experience associated with actual or potential tissue damage, or described in terms of such damage."[19] Pain is a subjective experience; It can be defined operationally as "what the patient says hurts" and exists "when the patient says it does." Infants, preverbal children, and children between the ages of 2 and 7 years (Piaget's "preoperational thought stage") may be unable to describe their pain or their subjective experiences. This inability has led many to conclude that children do not experience pain in the same way that adults do. Clearly, children do not have to know or be able to express the meaning of an experience in order to have the experience. On the other hand, because pain is essentially a subjective experience, it is becoming increasingly clear that the child's perspective of pain is an indispensable facet of pediatric pain management and an essential element in the specialized study of childhood pain. Indeed, pain assessment and management are interdependent; one is essentially useless without the other. The goal of pain assessment is to provide accurate data about the location and intensity of pain, as well as the effectiveness of measures used to reduce or abolish it.

Validated, reliable instruments currently exist to measure and assess pain in children older than 3 years of age.[5] These instruments, which measure the quality and intensity of pain, are "self-report measures" and use pictures or descriptive words to describe pain. Pain intensity or severity can be measured in chidlren as young as 3 years of age by the use of either (1) the Oucher scale, a two part scale with a vertical numerical scale (0-100) on one side and six photographs of a young child on the other, depicting various levels of pain, (2) a visual linear scale, or (3) a 10-cm line with a smiling face on one end and a distraught, crying face on the other (Fig. 24-2). In addition, color, word-graphic rating scales, and poker chips have been used to assess the intensity of pain in children. In infants and newborns, pain has been assessed by measuring physiologic responses to a nociceptive stimuli, such as blood pressure and heart rate changes, or by measuring levels of adrenal stress hormones.[5,12,16] Alternatively, behavioral approaches have utilized facial expression, body movements, and the intensity and quality of crying as indexes of response to nociceptive stimuli. Finally, it is important to define the location of pain accurately. This is readily accomplished by the use of either dolls, action figures, or drawings of body outlines, both front and back.

NONOPIOID (OR "WEAKER") ANALGESIC AGENTS

The "weaker" or "milder" analgesics, of which acetaminophen (Tylenol) and salicylates (aspirin) are the classic ex-

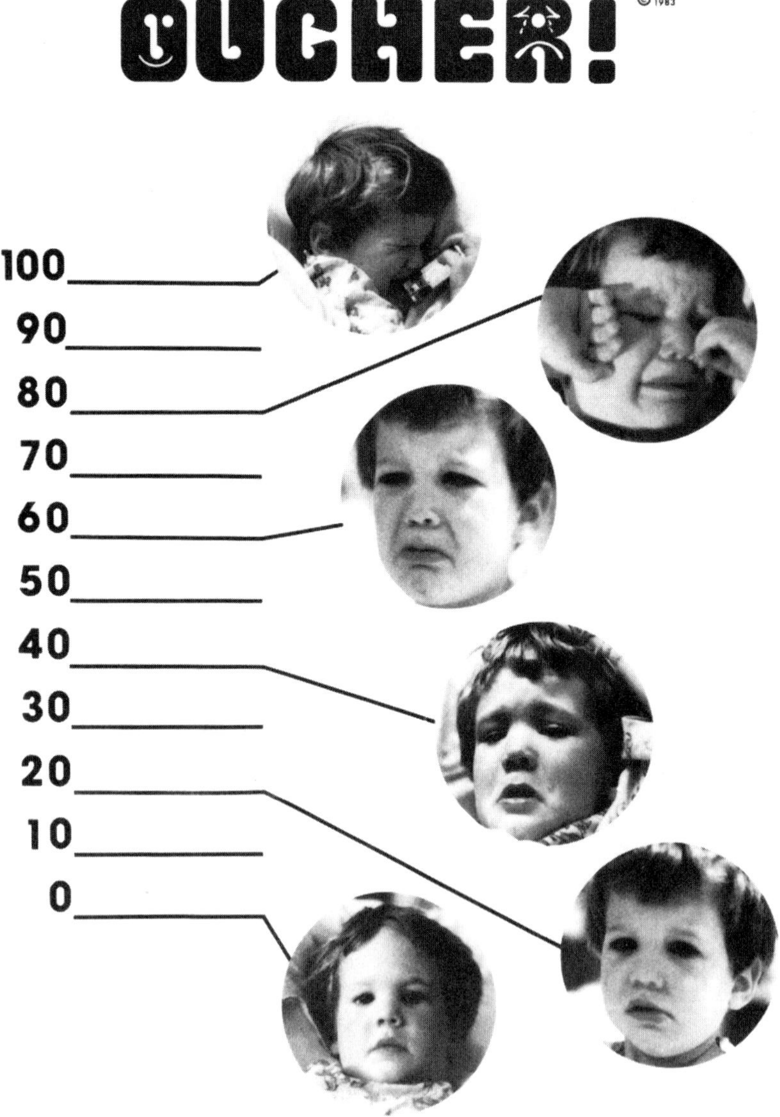

Fig. 24-2, A The Oucher scale is a visual analog scale used in pain assessment in children. Note that the higher the score, the greater the child's pain. It was developed and copyrighted by Judith E. Beyer, RN, PhD, 1983. For more information, contact Dr. Beyer at the University of Colorado Health Sciences Center School of Nursing, Denver. The Oucher scale is reprinted with permission from its author.

amples, comprise a heterogenous group of nonsteroidal anti-inflammatory drugs (NSAIDs) that provide analgesia primarily by blocking peripheral prostaglandin production (see Fig. 24-1).[36,38] These agents are administered enterally via the oral or, on occasion, the rectal route and are particularly useful for inflammatory, bony, or rheumatic pain. They are the preferred analgesics prescribed by pediatricians because they are relatively safe, have few cardiopulmonary side effects, and are nonaddictive. Unfortunately, regardless of dose, they reach a "ceiling effect" above which pain cannot be relieved by these drugs alone (Table 24-1). Consequently, nonopioid analgesics often are administered in combination with other, more potent agents such as codeine.

There is very little information in the pediatric literature on the use of the newer NSAIDs, such as ibuprofen, naproxen, tolmetin, or indomethacin. Furthermore, because of its possible role in causing Reye syndrome, aspirin has been largely abandoned in pediatric practice. Fortunately, acetaminophen is equally effective and potent as aspirin in the treatment of pain. When administered in normal doses, it has very few serious side effects. Acute overdosage or poisoning may produce fulminant hepatic failure and death. Fortunately, timely emergency management with acetylcysteine, administered via the oral or parenteral route, can prevent the occurrence of these dire consequences.

LOCAL ANESTHETIC AGENTS

Pharmacology and Pharmacokinetics of Local Anesthetics

The local anesthetics, which are tertiary amines, are of two types: either esters such as tetracaine (Pontocaine), procaine (Novocain), chloroprocaine (Nesacaine), and cocaine or amides such as lidocaine (Xylocaine), prilocaine (Citanest), bupivacaine (Marcaine, Sensorcaine) (Table 24-2).[9,32] Both the ester and amide local anesthetics are weak bases that block nerve conduction primarily at the sodium channel when they are in their ionized (cation) form. To reach the sodium channel the local anesthetic must cross the nerve membrane, and it is only the nonionized (base) form of the drug that can do this. How much drug is available to cross the nerve membrane depends on the pKa of the drug and the pH of the fluid surrounding the nerve. Thus the lower the pKa of the drug, the more nonionized drug is available to cross the nerve membrane at the physiologic pH. For example, 28% of li-

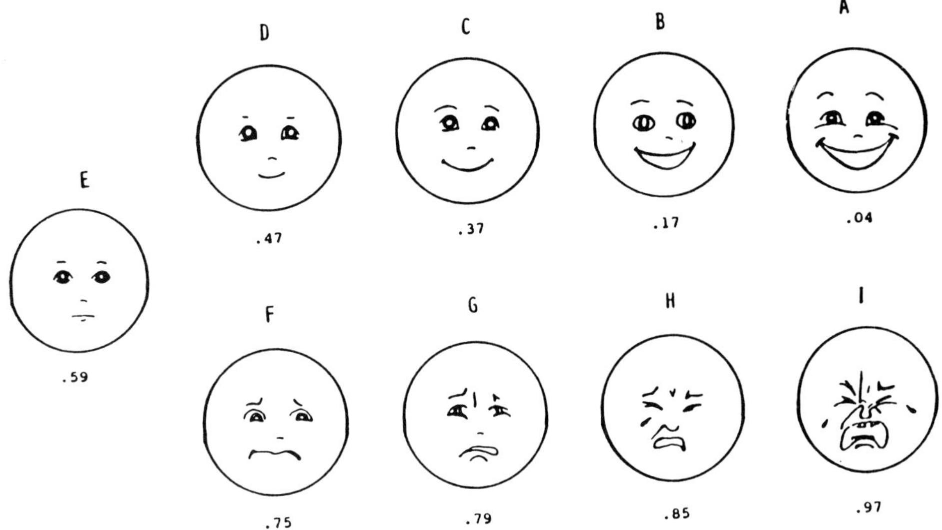

Fig. 24-2, B A nine face linear scale developed by Patricia A. McGrath, PhD and is reprinted with permission.

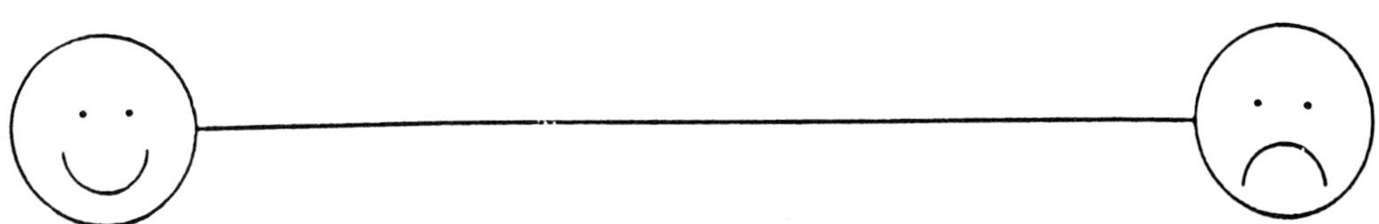

Fig. 24-2, C A 10 centimeter linear scale developed by James W. Varni, PhD. Reprinted with permission from Thompson KL and Varni JW: A developmental cognitive biobehavioral approach to pediatric pain assessment, Pain 25:283, 1986.

Table 24-1 *Nonsteroidal Antiinflammatory Drugs for Use in Children*

GENERIC NAME	TRADE NAME	DOSAGE (mg/kg/day)	DOSE INTERVAL
Aspirin	Aspirin*,†	60-80	q4-6h
Acetaminophen	Tylenol*,†,‡ Panadol*,‡	60-80	q4-6h
Ibuprofen	Motrin, Advil	30-40	q6-8h
Indomethacin	Indocin§	1-2.5	q6-8h
Naproxen	Naprosyn*,‡	10-20	q12h
Tolmetin	Tolectin*	20-30	q6-8h

*Approved by FDA for use in children.
†Approved as rectal suppository.
‡Available in liquid form.
§Approved only for neonatal use.

Table 24-2 *Suggested Maximum Doses of Local Anesthetics*

DRUG	DOSAGE OF LOCAL ANESTHETIC (mg/kg)	DURATION OF ACTION (hr)	COMMENTS
Peripheral nerve block* OR *local infiltration			
Lidocaine	5-7†	1-1.5†	Higher dose and duration when epinephrine added†
Bupivacaine	2-3†	2-6†	Higher dose and duration when epinephrine added†
Topical application			
Tetracaine, adrenaline, cocaine (TAC)	3ml	1-1.5	Formulation (mg/ml): tetracaine (5), adrenaline (0.5), cocaine (118)
Cocaine	1 mg/kg	0.5-1	For topical nasal anesthesia; highest abuse potential
EMLA cream (eutectic mixture of local anesthesics)	2 ml	1	Formulation: lidocaine (25 mg/ml) and prilocaine (25 mg/ml); requires occlusive dressing for 60 min before procedure

†These are suggested, safe upper limits for local anesthetic administration; accidental intravenous or intraarterial injection of even a fraction of these amounts may result in toxicity.

docaine exists in the base form at pH 7.4 compared with only 2.5% for chloroprocaine because the pKa of these drugs are 7.9 and 9.0, respectively. Acidosis and hypercapnia, by significantly affecting tissue drug uptake, also increase the toxicity of local anesthetics. Indeed, studies in rats have shown that both hypercapnia and acidosis drastically lower the convulsive threshold of local anesthetics and elevate total plasma and tissue concentrations of drug.

The standard of local anesthetic potency is the minimum concentration (C_m) of local anesthetic necessary to block impulse conduction along a given nerve fiber. A variety of factors affect C_m, including fiber size and degree of myelination of the nerve to be blocked, pH, local calcium concentration, and the rate at which a nerve is stimulated. Relatively unmyelinated fibers, such as the A-delta and C fibers carry nociceptive information and have a lower C_m than do heavily myelinated fibers that control muscle contraction. Because of the lower C_m, less local anesthetic is necessary to block the transmission of pain than is required to produce muscle paralysis. Thus by the use of dilute concentrations of local anesthetics, it is possible to block pain sensation and not motor function. In fact, concentrated local anesthetic solutions (e.g., 2% lidocaine versus 1.0%) increase the quality of sensory blockade only minimally. On the other hand, a concentrated local anesthetic will increase the incidence of motor blockade and systemic toxicity. (Concentrated solutions of local anesthetics can be diluted with *preservative-free* normal saline.) Furthermore, because the process of myelinization of the central nervous system is not completed until approximately 18 months following birth, C_m may be reduced in younger children.[37] Thus with the use of even dilute concentrations of local anesthetics, complete analgesia and even motor blockade can occur in newborns and infants.

Other factors also influence the quality and duration of a nerve block, such as the addition of a vasoconstrictor to the anesthetic mixture, the use of mixtures of local anesthetics, and the site of drug administration. Vasoconstrictors, particularly epinephrine, frequently are added to local anesthetic solutions. Epinephrine decreases the rate of vascular reabsorption of local anesthetic from the site of administration and thereby lengthens the duration of sensory blockade. By causing local vasoconstriction, epinephrine also reduces bleeding at sites of injury. It is of interest that epinephrine also improves the intensity of anesthesia achieved and increases the effectiveness of dilute concentration of local anesthetics. *Epinephrine-containing solutions should never be injected into areas supplied by end arteries, such as the penis or digits.* Injection of an epinephrine-containing solution into these areas may lead to tissue ischemia or necrosis. Finally, epinephrine is most commonly added to local anesthetic solutions in concentrations of 0.005 mg/ml (1:200,000).

The onset and duration of a local anesthetic also is affected by the use of combinations of local anesthetics, as well as by the site of injection. Mixtures of local anesthetics allow the practitioner to combine drugs with rapid onset but short duration of action, such as chloroprocaine or lidocaine, with drugs with longer latencies and duration of action, such as bupivacaine. The combination of lidocaine and bupivacaine is used occasionally in peripheral nerve blocks (e.g., the femoral or brachial plexus nerve block). The site of an injection also alters the duration of a nerve block in terms of the nerve's anatomy, differences in the rate of drug absorption, and the amount of drug deposited. Bupivacaine, for example, has a 4-hour duration when injected epidurally but a 10-hour duration when injected into the brachial plexus.

Toxicity

The systemic effects of local anesthetics are determined by the total dose of drug administered and by the rapidity of absorption into the blood. This belies the idea of accepted "maximum" doses of these drugs, since even small fractions of the accepted "maximum" doses of local anesthetics will produce toxic systemic effects if the local anesthetic is injected intraarterially, intravenously or into any highly vascular location. In general, peak absorption of local anesthetic depends on the site of the block. The order of absorption from highest to lowest is as follows:[9,32]

Intercostal, intratracheal > caudal/epidural > brachial plexus > distal peripheral > subcutaneous.

Peak local anesthetic blood levels are directly related to the dose of drug administered, regardless of the injection site or the solution volume used. Thus the most dilute concentration of a local anesthetic should be used.

At recommended clinical doses (see Table 24-2), plasma levels usually remain well below recognized toxic concentrations. A continuum of toxic effects exists and depends on the rapidity of rise and the total plasma concentration achieved after drug administration. Mild side effects such as tinnitus, lightheadedness, visual and auditory disturbances, restlessness, and muscular twitching occur at low plasma concentration and severe side effects (seizures, arrhythmias, coma, cardiovascular collapse, respiratory arrest) occur as plasma levels increase. Cardiovascular and central nervous system toxicity rarely have been observed in children after local anesthetic administration. The hemodynamic response to regional anesthesia, even after fairly extensive epidural blockade (cutaneous analgesia below T4-T5), is minimal in children compared with adults. Convulsions rarely are noted; either they are masked or the seizure threshold may be increased by the use of sedatives, particularly the benzodiazepines. Alternatively, children may be less sensitive to the toxic effects of local anesthetics than are adults, which is unlikely, inasmuch as several animal studies that compared sensitivity to the toxic effects of local anesthetics in newborn and adult animals demonstrated the absence of significant differences between the two groups.

The treatment of toxic responses to local anesthetics is the same as for any emergency namely, maintaining a patent *a*irway, ensuring adequate *b*reathing, and supporting *c*irculation; that is, the ABC's of resuscitation. Patients in whom seizures occur for even brief periods of time have acidosis and ineffective ventilation. Thus emergency airway and resuscitative equipment must be available for immediate use before the administration of any local anesthetic agent (see the accompanying box).[1] Finally, bupivacaine as a cause of

Emergency Drugs and Equipment Required for Sedation and Local Anesthetic Administration

I. Personnel
  A. The practitioner performing the procedure
  B. A qualified person to monitor and administer drugs
    1. training in basic life support (CPR)
    2. knowledge of emergency cart inventory
II. Equipment for intravenous access
  A. Catheters (various sizes)
  B. Administration sets
  C. Fluids
    1. Ringer's lactate
    2. D_5W + NaCl (0.2, 0.45, 0.9%)
III. Emergency cart
  A. Suction (large-bore device, e.g., Yankauer suction device)
  B. Oxygen and oxygen delivery system
  C. Airway
    1. oral airways (various sizes)
    2. masks (various sizes)
    3. laryngoscope and appropriate size blades
    4. endotracheal tubes (various sizes)
    5. stylets
  D. Drugs
    1. Epinephrine
    2. Bicarbonate
    3. Atropine
    4. Lidocaine, bretylium
    5. Calcium
    6. Glucose
    7. Naloxone, physostigmine
    8. Anticonvulsants (thiopental, diazepam, or midazolam)
IV. Monitoring equipment*
  A. Electrocardiograph
  B. Sphygmomanometer
  C. Pulse oximeter

Modified from the American Academy of Pediatrics, Committee on Drugs Section on Anesthesiology: Guidelines for the elective use of conscious sedation, deep sedation, and general anesthesia in pediatric anesthesia, Pediatrics 76:317, 1985.

*Monitoring equipment should be available, particularly if the child is being sedated for a procedure.

arrhythmias and cardiovascular collapse is particularly worrisome because it has been relatively refractory to treatment. The ventricular arrhythmias that precede cardiovascular collapse seen after bupivacaine toxicity are more responsive to treatment with intravenous bretylium than with lidocaine.

Although drug allergy is uncommon with the use of amide local anesthetics, it occurs with the ester family of drugs. Usually there is a previous history of allergies to local anesthetics or to suntan lotions that contain para amino benzoic acid (PABA). Local anesthetic allergy is, however, rare; adverse experiences that occur during dental anesthesia are often mistaken for true allergy. In the dentist's office many patients experience tachycardia and a sense of flushing and dizziness after nerve root infiltration with procaine and epinephrine. This reaction usually is caused by direct intravascular injection of epinephrine and does not mean that the patient is allergic to local anesthetics.

Pharmacokinetics

The ester local anesthetics are metabolized by plasma cholinesterase. Neonates and infants up to 6 months of age have less than half the adult levels of this plasma enzyme. Clearance thereby may be reduced and the effects of ester local anesthetics prolonged. Amides, on the other hand, are metabolized in the liver and bound by plasma proteins. Neonates and young infants (younger than 3 months of age) have reduced liver blood flow and immature metabolic degradation pathways. Thus larger fractions of local anesthetics are unmetabolized and remain more active in the infant's plasma than in the adult's. More local anesthetic is excreted in the urine unchanged. Further more, neonates and infants may be at increased risk for the toxic effects of amide local anesthetics because of lower levels of albumin and alpha-1 acid glycoproteins which are essential for drug binding. This deficiency leads to increased concentrations of free drug and potential toxicity, particularly with bupivacaine. On the other hand, the larger volume of distribution at steady state seen in the neonate for these and other drugs may confer some clinical protection by lowering plasma drug levels.

The metabolism of the amide local anesthetic prilocaine is unique in that it results in the production of oxidants that can lead to the development of methemoglobinemia. This occurs in adults with doses of prilocaine greater than 600 mg. Because premature and full-term infants have decreased levels of methemoglobin reductase, they are more susceptible to the development of methemoglobinemia. An additional factor that increases their susceptibility is the relative ease by which fetal hemoglobin is oxidized compared with adult hemoglobin. Thus prilocaine cannot be recommended for use in neonates.

Finholt et al[10] found that the volume of distribution, clearance, and elimination half-life of an intravenous bolus of lidocaine, 1 to 2 mg/kg, used to facilitate tracheal intubation or to treat arrhythmias is similar in children older than 6 months of age and in adults. They recommend that lidocaine doses need not be altered on the basis of age alone when it is administered intravenously. The elimination half-life of intravenously administered lidocaine in infants younger than 6 months of age is prolonged, however. Because protein binding is reduced in neonates multiple doses of lidocaine may predispose them to the development of toxic concentrations of drug. The routine administration of intravenous lidocaine in children with right-to-left intracardiac shunts may produce systemic toxicity.[6] Normally, approximately 60% to 80% of an intravenous lidocaine bolus is absorbed on the first pass through the lungs, then subsequently released over time. In patients with right-to-left intracardiac shunts, venous blood enters directly into the systemic circulation through the intracardiac defect, bypassing the lungs. Peak arterial concentrations of lidocaine would be expected to be higher and occur more rapidly. In fact, in lambs with right-to-left intracardiac shunts, lidocaine levels were double those of normal control subjects.[6]

REGIONAL ANESTHETIC TECHNIQUES

Subcutaneous Injection

Subcutaneous infiltration of the skin with a local anesthetic solution is the most commonly performed regional ("local") anesthetic technique in pediatric practice. To minimize procedure-related pain, local anesthetics, particularly lidocaine, are commonly injected subcutaneously before the performance of many painful medical and surgical procedures. Examples of procedures that benefit from prior local anesthetic infiltration include repair of minor surgical wounds (traumatic lacerations or deliberate incisions, e.g., before a cutdown for venous access), insertion of an arterial or an intravenous catheter (e.g., routine percutaneous intravenous access or cardiac catheterization), bone marrow aspiration, thoracostomy tube placement, and lumbar puncture. When used in this way, the local anesthetic agent blocks nerve conduction at the most terminal branches of the sensory nerves.

Local anesthetic infiltration of traumatic lacerations requires special attention. Commonly the wound is dirty and requires extensive scrubbing and irrigation. One needs to consider whether the local anesthetic should be administered before the cleansing, which would make it painless, or afterwards, to avoid introducing dirt and bacteria into the surrounding tissue. It is reasonable to inject the local anesthetic through intact skin adjacent to the wound before the wound is cleaned. Alternatively, the peripheral nerve supplying the injured area can be blocked more proximally because smaller amounts of local anesthetic are used and fewer injections are required.

Because local anesthetics are manufactured at a pH of 4 to 5 and are administered by injection, they are in and of themselves painful. This pain can be minimized by the use of buffered anesthetic solutions and small needles. Buffering a local anesthetic solution, such as lidocaine, with sodium bicarbonate (9 ml lidocaine combined with 1 ml bicarbonate, a 10:1 solution) may make the injection painless and shorten the time to onset of analgesia.[18] Local anesthetics are not manufactured with buffer because the buffering affects the shelf life of the drug. Obviously, the use of small-gauge needles also affects the amount of pain produced during the infiltration of local anesthetics. Either 26- or 30-gauge needles can be used, with the local anesthetic immediately injected as the needle punctures the skin. *It is not necessary to aspirate first* because the amount of local anesthetic injected is so small (0.1-0.2 ml) that even an intravascular injection would be inconsequential. Consequently, local anesthetics can be injected as the needle is advanced forward.

TOPICAL ANESTHETICS

TAC Solution

Topical local anesthetics such as *t*etracaine, *a*drenaline, and *c*ocaine solution (TAC) or a cream eutectic mixture of local anesthetics (EMLA) can be used. TAC solution is an innovative method of topical anesthesia that avoids the use of a local anesthetic injection altogether.[26] TAC is a solution of tetracaine 0.5%, epinephreine 1:2000, and cocaine 11.8% (see Table 24-2) that is applied directly to a laceration. The clear solution is made in the hospital pharmacy by mixing 60 ml of 2% tetracaine with 120 ml 1:1000 epinephrine, and 28.32 g cocaine; normal saline is added to bring the total voume to 240 ml. Because it is applied topically, it eliminates the need for an injection into the dirty wound edge and achieves anesthesia for both wound cleaning and suturing. It is most effective when used on lacerations of the face and scalp and less effective when used on lacerations of an extremity.

Because TAC contains epinephrine and cocaine, the only local anesthetic that is a vasoconstrictor, it cannot be used in areas of the body that are supplied by end arteries, such as the digits, pinna, or nose. Furthermore, because of its cocaine content, inadvertent ingestion of the solution by patients can be catastrophic. Similarly, inasmuch as cocaine is readily absorbed through mucosal surfaces, the use of TAC solution near mucous membranes should be avoided. Indeed, seizures have been reported even in children in whom the solution was applied properly to wound edges without a mucosal surface. Unfortunately, cocaine cannot be eliminated from the solution because solutions that contain only tetracaine and adrenaline are much less effective in producing analgesia than are solutions that contain cocaine.[26]

Before administration, a history should be obtained to rule out allergy to PABA-containing suntan lotion or to local anesthetics because both tetracaine and cocaine are the ester-type of local anesthetic agents. Typically, a 3-ml solution of TAC provides analgesia for a laceration of approximately 3 cm in length. Half the solution is instilled directly into the wound, and the other half is applied to a gauze pad held on the wound surface for 10 to 15 minutes. Failure to keep the TAC solution in contact with the wound surface for the requisite number of minutes accounts for most inadequate blocks. In the 10% to 25% of patients in whom TAC is not completely effective, the subsequent injection of lidocaine is much less painful. Use of this topical preparation also avoids the swelling and distortion of the wound edges that may be caused by injected local anesthetics.

TAC solutions are best provided as unit doses and kept in the narcotics cabinet in the emergency room or office. Indeed, much of the hesitancy in using TAC relates to the addiction potential of cocaine. Many responsible health care professionals believe that the presence of a cocaine-containing solution is a temptation to staff members who must administer it. Finally, gloves must be worn by all personnel coming into contact with TAC solution because it can cause vasoconstriction even in intact skin.

EMLA Cream

EMLA (eutectic mixture of local anesthetics) cream, a topical emulsion composed of prilocaine and lidocaine, produces complete anesthesia of intact skin after application (see Table 24-2).[30] Unfortunately, for best effect, EMLA cream must be applied and covered with an occlusive dressing (such as plastic wrap) for 60 minutes before a procedure is performed. This delay limits its use in the emergency room or office unless the site is prepared well in advance of anticipated use. Furthermore, if the procedure is a venipuncture, multiple sites must be prepared in the event the initial attempt is unsuccessful.

Unfortunately, the effectiveness of EMLA cream (like all other methods) at reducing pain depends on who makes the assessment. Soliman et al[30] studied the efficacy of EMLA cream compared with injected lidocaine in reducing the pain associated with venipuncture. Both an observer and a physician performing the procedure judged pain relief to be virtually complete with both techniques. The children involved in the study were less sanguine; they were equally dissatisfied with both methods, particularly if the needle used for venipuncture was visible to them. Thus even though two observers believed that the child was pain free, the child's cooperation with venipuncture did not improve. Therefore it is not clear whether the delay involved in the use of EMLA (60-minute wait for effect) is justified. On the other hand, EMLA may be more effective in children accustomed to frequent medical procedures (e.g., oncology patients) or for procedures in which the child cannot see the needle, such as lumbar puncture or bone marrow aspiration.

PERIPHERAL NERVE BLOCKS

As mentioned previously, emergency airway and resuscitative equipment, as well as personnel trained in using it, must be available for use before the performance of a peripheral nerve block.[1] Additionally, if a patient is to be sedated during the performance of a nerve block, one member of the health care team must be responsible for his or her overall well-being. This person is responsible for monitoring vital signs, assessing the adequacy of the airway, and alerting other members of the health care team if a problem is occurring.[1]

Digital Nerve Blocks

The digital nerve block provides excellent anesthesia for surgery performed on either the fingers or toes. It is particularly useful for incising and draining an abscess (paronychia). The alternative, local anesthetic infiltration, may fail because the acidic pH of infected tissue may not allow the active (nonionized base) form of the local anesthetic to reach the nerve membrane.

Performance of the Digital Nerve Block

Digital nerve block is performed similarly for both fingers and toes. Each digit is supplied by two pairs of nerves (dorsal and ventral) that travel on either side of that digit (Fig. 24-3). ½ to 1 ml *epinephrine-free* local anesthetic is injected between the metacarpal (metatarsal) heads on either side of the digit. The 25-gauge needle is kept perpendicular to the plane of the hand or foot and advanced from the dorsal to the palmar surface. Local anesthetic is injected continuously. Aspiration before injection is unnecessary because the volume of local anesthetic is small.

Complications are few. Obviously, the digital nerve block should never be performed when there is any question of the digit's blood supply. Indeed, even when epinephrine is not used, the most serious complication of this block is caused by the use of too large a volume of local anesthetic. A large volume within a closed fascial space may result in vascular compression (compartment syndrome).

Penile Nerve Block

Although routine circumcision of newborns has been condemned by various groups, it remains a common practice. (See Chapter 26, Establishment of Equilibrium.) Active campaigns by pediatricians and obstetricians to discourage the procedure in the newborn has resulted in increasingly large numbers of older children undergoing this surgery, who then, obviously, require general anesthesia. In both the newborn and the older child the penile nerve block can be used either for complete anesthesia or for postoperative pain relief.[16] The efficacy and safety of the penile nerve block for newborn circumcision have been demonstrated in several studies. In both the older child and the newborn, profound postoperative analgesia also can be provided by the topical application of 2% lidocaine jelly.[31]

Performance of the Penile Nerve Block

In the newborn, 0.8 ml of 1% lidocaine and in older children from 1 to 3 ml 0.25% bupivacaine is used. Peak plasma lidocaine levels in the newborn average less than 0.6 mcg/ml. In either case, it is vital that *epinephrine-free solution* be used because the artery supplying the penis is an end artery, and vasconstriction by epinephrine can cause catastrophic consequences. The dorsal nerves of the penis (Fig. 24-4) lie on either side of its dorsal artery and vein. They are deep to Buck's fascia but are superficial with respect to the skin at the penile base. After aseptic preparation of the skin, two injections of local anesthetic solution are done with either a 25- or 26-gauge needle. The anesthetic solution is injected at the 10:30- and 1:30-o'clock positions at the penile base just beneath Buck's fascia. This fascia is approximately 3 to

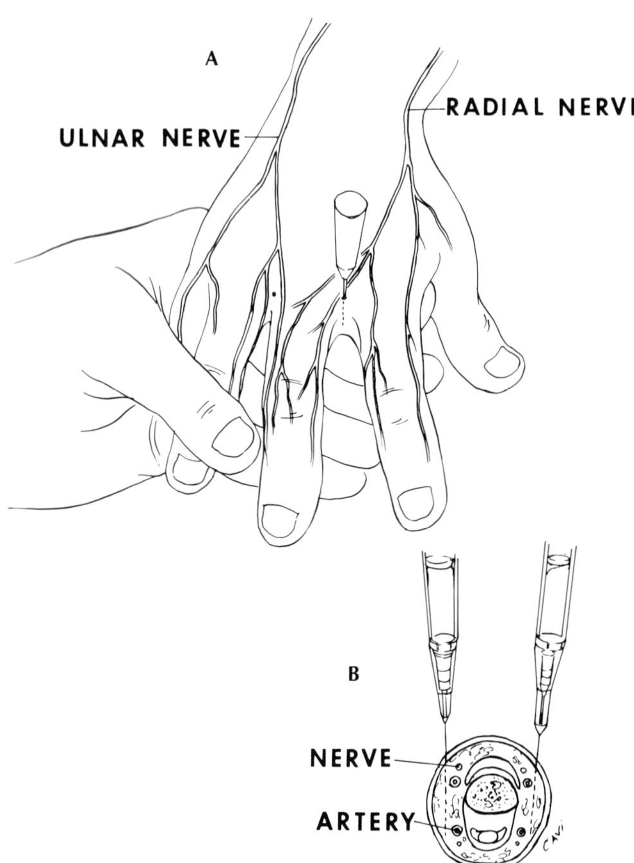

Fig. 24-3 The digital nerve block is depicted. **A,** A 25-gauge needle is inserted between the heads of the metacarpals (metatarsals) on either side of the digit to be anesthetized. Both dorsal and ventral branches are blocked by continuously injecting local anesthetic during advancement of the needle from the dorsal surface to the ventral surface. **B,** The anatomic relationship of the digital nerves and arteries is depicted in this cross section at the level of the metacarpal head.

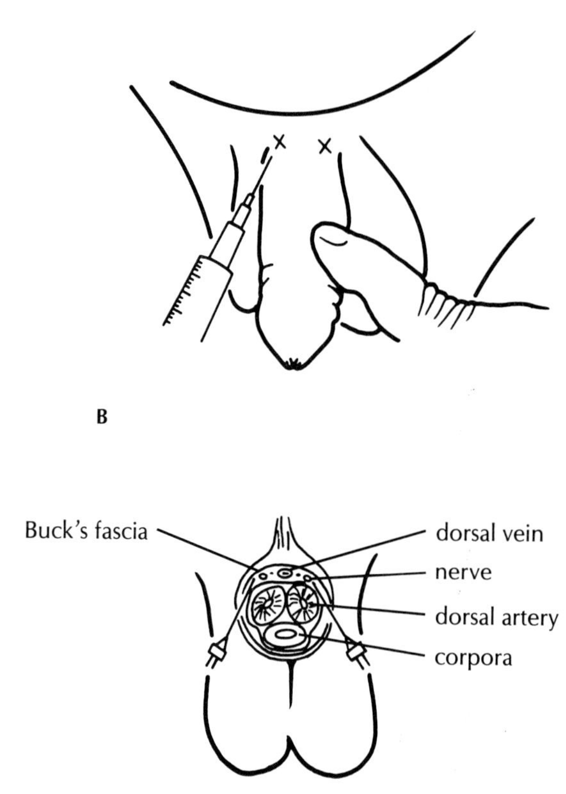

Fig. 24-4 The penile nerve block is demonstrated. **A,** A 25-gauge needle is inserted at the 10:30 and 1:30 o'clock positions at the penile base. The fascia is entered approximately 3 to 5 mm below the skin surface. **B,** One can see the dorsal vein of the penis, the two dorsal arteries, and the two nerves lying in Buck's fascia. Directly below this fascia, one can see the corpora of the penis. Reprinted with permission.

From Maxwell L et al: Obstet Gynecol 70:415, 1987.

5 mm below the skin surface. Alternatively, a single midline injection can be used. In this technique the needle is advanced to the lower surface of the pubic symphysis in the midline. Local anesthetic (approximately 1 to 3 ml) is injected slowly as the needle is withdrawn. As the needle passes through Buck's fascia, the local anesthetic is spread to both sides, anesthetizing the nerves. Complications are rare and clinically insignificant.

Axillary Block

The axillary nerve block is an ideal block for upper extremity procedures and, because of its simplicity, is the preferred approach to the brachial plexus. It carries little risk of pneumothorax, phrenic nerve block, or subarachnoid injection. It is particularly useful for fracture reductions and repair of lacerations of the hand and forearm. Because the axillary artery lies within the fascial sheath of the brachial plexus and the spread of local anesthetic solutions within a fascial sheath results in nerve block, local anesthetic solutions deposited anywhere near the axillary artery usually produce an adequate nerve block.[35]

Performance of the Axillary Nerve Block. The patient's arm is abducted at a right angle, with the forearm and hand supinated; the elbow is flexed with the hand under the head or in a "saluting position." The axillary artery and brachial plexus are very superficial and the artery is used as the landmark. After aseptic preparation of the skin, the physician's nonoperative hand is positioned so that the middle finger lies directly over the artery and compresses it and the brachial plexus against the humerus. A wheal of local anesthetic is deposited directly over the pulsating artery. By use of a 25-gauge needle, local anesthetic is deposited on each side of the artery, staying as close as possible to the border of the axillary artery. On the initial pass on each side of the artery, the needle is inserted at a depth of approximately ½ inch, aspirating constantly. As the needle is withdrawn, 1 ml local anesthetic is injected. Then, in a fanlike manner, 1 ml local anesthetic is injected on each sweep away from the artery. Typically 5 ml local anesthetic (either 1% lidocaine with 1:200,000 epinephrine or 0.25% bupivacaine with 1:200,000 epinephrine) is used on each side of the artery for a total dose of 10 ml. An alternative approach is a modification of the Winnie block in which the axillary artery is deliberately transfixed with the needle.[35] The drug is injected deep and superficial to the artery at the point where active blood return, as demonstrated by aspiration through the needle, ceases.

Femoral Nerve Block

The femoral nerve block (L2 - L4) is the quickest, easiest, and most effective technique for relieving the pain of a femoral shaft fracture. When bupivacaine without epinephrine is used in a femoral nerve block, such patients are provided adequate anesthesia for the application of traction, as well as for the necessary (and usually painful) manipulations that occur during radiologic examinations. The duration of analgesia is approximately 3 hours.

Performance of the Block. Following aseptic preparation of the skin, a 25-gauge needle is inserted perpendicularly, approximately 3 to 5 mm lateral to the pulsation of the femoral artery at the level of the inguinal ligament (Fig. 24-5). The needle is inserted to a depth clearly deeper than the artery. The sensation of puncturing the fascia over the nerve (a distinct "pop") helps one judge the depth of penetration. After aspiration for blood yields negative results, 5 to 10 ml of local anesthetic solution (0.25% bupivacaine with 1:200,000 epinephrine) is injected. Local anesthetic solution then is injected, fanlike, lateral and deep to the femoral artery. The maximum dose of 0.25% bupivacaine used is 1 ml/kg.

OPIOIDS

Terminology

The terminology used to describe potent analgesic drugs is constantly changing. These drugs commonly are referred to as narcotics (from the Greek *narco* - to deaden), opiates (from the Greek *opion* - poppy juice, for drugs derived from the poppy plant), opioids (for all drugs with morphinelike effects, whether synthetic or naturally occurring), or euphemistically as "strong analgesics" (when the physician is reluctant to tell the patient or the patient's family that narcotics are being used). Furthermore, the discovery of endogenous endorphins and opioid receptors has necessitated the reclassification of these drugs into agonists, antagonists, and mixed agonist-antagonists on the basis of their receptor binding properties.[20,29]

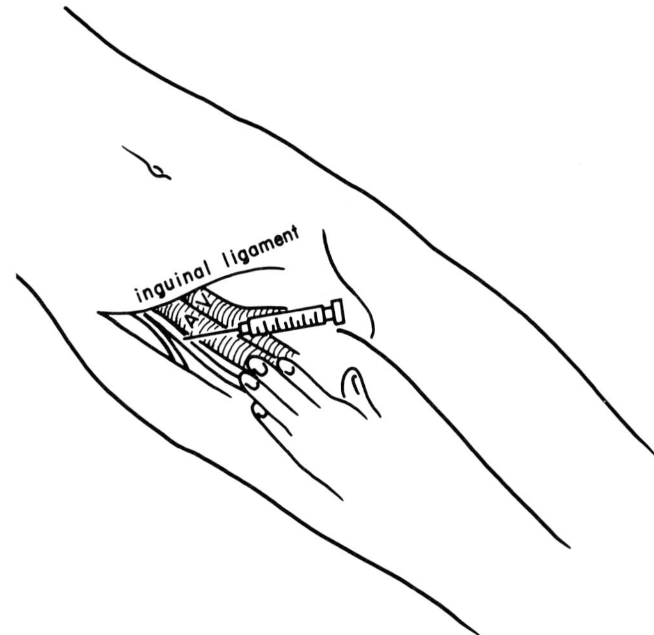

Fig. 24-5 The femoral nerve block is depicted. After placing a skin wheal, the physician's nonoperative hand compresses the femoral artery and nerve against the underlying tissue and bone immediately below the inguinal ligament. A 22- or 25-gauge needle is then inserted perpendicularly, approximately 0.5 to 1 cm lateral to the pulsation of the femoral artery into the perineural fascia of the femoral nerve. Reprinted with permission.

From Yaster M and Maxwell L: Anesthesiology 70:324, 1989.

The differentiation of agonists and antagonists is fundamental to pharmacology. A neurotransmitter is defined as having agonist activity, whereas a drug that blocks the action of the neurotransmitter is an antagonist. By definition, receptor recognition of an agonist is "translated" into other cellular alterations, whereas an antagonist occupies the receptor without initiating the transduction step.[20,29] Morphine and related opiates are agonists and drugs that block the effects of opiates, such as naloxone, are designated antagonists.

Narcotics interact with specific receptors that are widely distributed throughout the central nervous system. Different effects, sensitivities, and anatomical localization have been ascribed to these various receptors. Although there are as many as eight different opioid receptors, four are of major importance in terms of pain management. These are designated as the mu, delta, kappa, and sigma receptors (Table 24-4). The mu receptor and its subspecies and the delta receptor are related to analgesia, respiratory depression, euphoria, and physical dependence. Morphine is fifty to one hundred times weaker at the delta than at the mu receptor. By contrast, the endogenous opiate-like neurotransmitter peptides known as enkephalins tend to be more potent at delta than mu receptors. The kappa receptor, located primarily in the spinal cord, is related to spinal analgesia, miosis, and sedation. The sigma receptor is responsible for the psychotomimetic effects observed with some opiate drugs, particularly the mixed agonist-antagonist drugs. These effects include dysphoria and hallucinations.

A number of studies suggest that the respiratory depression and analgesia produced by opiates involve different receptor subtypes. These receptors change in number in an age-related fashion and can be blocked by naloxone. Pasternak et al, working with newborn rats, showed that 14-day-old rats are 40 times more sensitive to morphine analgesia than 2-day-old rats.[24] Nevertheless, morphine depresses the respiratory rate in 2-day-old rats to a greater degree than in 14-day-old rats. Thus, the newborn is particularly sensitive to the respiratory depressant effects of the opioids in what may be an age-related receptor phenomenon. Obviously this has important clinical implications for the use of narcotics in the newborn (see below).

Myths and Misconceptions Concerning Opioids

Despite the confusion of terminology and the plethora of available drugs, it is essential to realize that at *equipotent* analgesic doses, all commonly used opioids produce similar degrees of respiratory depression, sedation, euphoria, nausea, biliary tract spasm, and constipation. Mixed agonist-antagonist drugs such as pentazocine (Talwin), nalbuphine (Nubain), and butorphanol (Stadol) produce significantly less respiratory depression and biliary spasm than do pure agonist drugs such as morphine. However, they also are significantly less potent analgesics than the pure agonists and reach a "ceiling" above which no further analgesia can be achieved. Furthermore, they reverse previously induced narcotic analgesia and should never be used in patients who chronically use (or are addicted to) opioids. Although an enormous number of opioids are available for clinical use, each with some purported advantage (typically "more effective," or cause "less respiratory depression", or have "less addiction" potential) the drugs listed in Tables 24-3 and 24-4 are the most commonly used.

Opioids usually are administered at fixed intervals despite enormous variability in patient response. It is not uncommon for physicians to order doses that are too small and at intervals that are too long for individual patient needs. Furthermore, nurses often delay administering narcotics because of lack of recognition of the child's pain symptoms, demand of other

Table 24-3 *Commonly Used Opioids**

NAME		EQUIPOTENT DOSE				
GENERIC	TRADE	PARENTERAL (mg/kg)	ORAL (mg/kg)	PARENTERAL: ORAL RATIO	DURATION OF EFFECTIVENESS (hr)	COMMENTS
Morphine		0.1	0.5	1:5	3-4	Vasodilator (avoid in shock); causes seizures at high doses, long-acting oral form available
Fentanyl	Sublimaze	0.001	NA	NA	0.5-1	Side effects: chest wall rigidity, bradycardia
Meperidine	Demerol	1.0	2.0	1:2-3.0	3-4	Side effects: tachycardia, seizures, catastrophic interactions with MAO inhibitors
Codeine		1.0	1.5	1:1.5	4	Oral bioavailability 60%
Methadone	Dolophine	0.1	0.1-0.15	1:1.2	4-12	Potential use as a long-acting analgesic

*When administered intravenously, titration of opioid doses always is recommended to minimize complications. MAO, Monamine oxidase; NA, not applicable.

Table 24-4 *Practical Guide to Pediatric Opioid Dosage**

DRUG	ORAL	INTRAMUSCULAR	IV BOLUS	IV CONTINUOUS INFUSION
Morphine	0.5 mg/kg/dose q6h	0.2 mg/kg	0.05-0.1 mg/kg	0.01-0.05 mg/kg/hr
Fentanyl		1-2 μg/kg	1-2 μg/kg	1-3 μg/kg/hr
Codeine	0.5-1.0 mg/kg/dose to 60 mg/dose q4h	1 mg/kg	Not recommended	—
Meperidine	1 mg/kg/dose to 100 mg/dose q4h	1 mg/kg	0.5-1.0 mg/kg	0.1-0.5 mg/kg/hr
Methadone	0.1-0.2 mg/kg/dose q8-12h	0.2 mg/kg	0.05-0.1 mg/kg	—

*When administered intravenously, titration of opioid doses always is recommended to minimize complications. The suggested IV bolus dose is a starting point. Individual patients may require more or less than the suggested dose.

patients, fear of addiction and difficulty in finding keys to the locked narcotic cabinet. As Cousins and Phillips stated, "Rational use of opioids requires a flexible, patient-oriented approach to allow for variability in individual pain experience and tolerance, as well as both the beneficial and adverse effects of the particular drug being used."[8]

Morphine

Morphine (from Morpheus, the Greek God of Sleep) is the standard for analgesia against which all other opioids are compared. When small intravenous or intramuscular doses, 0.1 mg/kg, are administered to otherwise unmedicated patients in pain, analgesia usually occurs without loss of consciousness. The relief of tension, anxiety and pain usually results in drowsiness and sleep as well. A sense of well being and/or euphoria usually follows morphine administration in older patients suffering from discomfort and pain. When morphine is given to pain-free adults, however, they may show the opposite effect, namely, dysphoria and increased fear and anxiety. Mental clouding, drowsiness, lethargy, and an inability to concentrate may occur after morphine administration even in the absence of pain. Less advantageous central nervous system effects of morphine include nausea and vomiting, miosis, and at high doses, seizures. Seizures are a particular problem in the newborn because they may occur at commonly prescribed doses (0.1 mg/kg).[14] The nausea and vomiting that occur with morphine administration are due to stimulation of the chemoreceptor trigger zone in the brainstem.

Morphine (as well as all other opioids at equipotent doses) depresses respiration, principally by reducing the sensitivity of the brainstem respiratory centers to arterial carbon dioxide content. Infants younger than 1 to 2 months of age are particularly sensitive to this depression.[13] Indeed, this is of such great concern that *the use of any narcotic in children younger than 2 months of age must be limited to a monitored, intensive care unit setting*. Possible explanations for this increased sensitivity include differences in opiate receptors (see preceding discussion), the blood-brain barrier, and pharmacokinetics.

Way et al[34] suggested that an incomplete blood-brain barrier (as demonstrated in newborn rats) allows greater penetration of morphine to central nervous system receptor sites. Presumably this would allow more drug to enter the central nervous system and produce a more profound effect. Several studies have demonstrated a prolonged elimination half life (6.8 versus 2.9 hours) and decreased morphine clearance (6.3 versus 23.8 ml/min/kg) of morphine in infants younger than 1 month of age when compared with older infants and adults. Nevertheless, the half-life of elimination and clearance of morphine in children older than 1 month of age is similar to adult values. Thus infants younger than 1 month of age will attain higher serum levels that will decline more slowly than in older children and adults and may account for the increased respiratory depression seen in this age group. On the other hand, on the basis of its relatively short half-life (2.9 hours), one would expect older children and adults to require morphine supplementation every 2 to 3 hours when being treated for pain, particularly if the morphine is administered intravenously. This has led to the recent use of continuous infusion regimens of morphine and patient-controlled analgesia (see discussion that follows), which maximize pain-free periods.

Although morphine produces peripheral vasodilation and venous pooling it has minimal hemodynamic effects in normal, normovolemic, supine patients. The vasodilation associated with morphine is due primarily to its histamine-releasing effects. Significant hypotension may occur if sedatives such as diazepam are administered concurrently with morphine. Otherwise, it produces virtually no cardiovascular effects when used alone. It causes significant hypotension in patients with hypovolemia; its use in trauma is therefore limited.

Morphine (and all other narcotics at equipotent doses) inhibits intestinal smooth muscle motility. This decrease in peristalsis and increase in sphincter tone explains the historic use of opioids in the treatment of diarrhea as well as their side-effect in the treatment of chronic pain, namely, constipation. In fact, laxatives are routinely prescribed for patients expected to be treated with narcotics for more than 2 or 3 days. Obviously, morphine (and all mu agonists, including meperidine) will potentiate biliary colic by causing spasm of Oddi's sphincter and should be used with caution in patients with, or at risk for, cholelithiasis (e.g., sickle cell disease). Finally, to minimize the complications associated with intravenously administered morphine (or any opioid), *titration of the dose at the bedside* is recommended until the desired level of analgesia is achieved.

Fentanyl

Because of its rapid onset and brief duration of action, fentanyl has become a favored analgesic for short procedures, such as bone marrow aspirations, fracture reductions, suturing lacerations, endoscopy, and dental procedures. Fentanyl is approximately 100 times more potent than morphine (the equianalgesic dose is 0.001 mg/kg, Table 24-3) and is largely devoid of hypnotic or sedative activity. Its ability to block nociceptive stimuli with concomitant hemodynamic stability is excellent and makes it the drug of choice for patients in trauma, cardiac, or intensive care units. In addition to its ability to block the systemic and pulmonary hemodynamic responses to pain, fentanyl also prevents the biochemical and endocrine stress (catabolic) response to painful stimuli that can be highly detrimental to the seriously ill patient. Fentanyl does have a serious side effect, namely, the development of chest wall rigidity after rapid infusions of 0.005 mg/kg or greater. This effect can make ventilation difficult or impossible. Chest wall rigidity can be reversed with either muscle relaxants, such as succinylcholine or pancuronium, or naloxone.

Fentanyl is a highly lipophilic drug and rapidly penetrates all membranes including the blood brain barrier. It is rapidly eliminated from plasma as the result of its extensive uptake by body tissues. Fentanyl pharmacokinetics differ among newborn infants, children, and adults. The total body clearance of fentanyl is greater in infants 3 to 12 months of age than in children older than 1 year of age or than in adults, and the half-life of elimination is longer. The prolonged elimination half-life of fentanyl from plasma has important clinical implications. Repeated doses of fentanyl for maintenance of analgesic effects will lead to its accumulation and its ventilatory depressant effects. Very large doses (0.05-0.10 mg/kg, as used in anesthesia) may be expected to induce long-lasting effects because during the distribution phases, plasma fentanyl levels will not fall below the threshold level at which spontaneous breathing occurs. On the other hand, the greater clearance of fentanyl in infants older than 3 months of age produces lower plasma concentrations of the drug and may allow these children to tolerate more drug without respiratory depression.

Meperidine

Meperidine (Demerol) is a synthetic narcotic that is used most commonly in children either as a preanesthesia sedative or for treating postoperative pain. It is a potent analgesic with pharmacokinetic properties similar to those of morphine. Meperidine is a narcotic agonist that binds to opioid receptors in the central nervous system and can produce analgesia, sedation, euphoria, dysphoria, miosis, and respiratory depression. At equipotent doses (See Tables 24-3 and 24-4), there is little quantitative difference between meperidine and morphine in producing these effects. Both stimulate the chemoreceptor trigger zone in the brain stem to the same degree and thereby may produce either nausea or vomiting, or both. Meperidine differs from morphine in that large doses (toxic levels) may produce slow waves on the electroencephalogram. Additionally, high levels of meperidine's principal metabolite, normeperidine, may produce tremors, muscle twitches, hyperactive reflexes and convulsions. Because of the accumulation of this toxic metabolite, the prolonged use of meperidine or its use as a continuous intravenous infusion should be discouraged, if not avoided completely.

At equipotent doses (See Tables 24-3 and 24-4), meperidine's effects on respiration and gastrointestinal motility are similar to those of the other opioid analgesics. Meperidine is a potent respiratory depressant and antitussive. Unlike morphine, meperidine depresses minute ventilation through a primary reduction in tidal volume rather than a reduction in respiratory rate. It depresses intestinal smooth muscle motility and exerts a spasmogenic effect on those muscles. Thus gastric motility is decreased, and the gastric emptying time of the stomach is increased. Some studies suggest that meperidine exerts less of an effect on the biliary tract, including the common bile duct, than does morphine. Specifically, at equipotent doses, biliary tract pressure may increase to a lesser extent after meperidine than morphine administration, the significance of which is more anecdotal than real. Finally, meperidine, unlike the other opioids, produces a tachycardia when administered intravenously.

Meperidine is effective whether administered orally or parenterally. The drug is extremely well absorbed from the gastrointestinal tract and has a bioavailability of approximately 50%, making it among the most popularly prescribed oral narcotics. It is available in both liquid (syrup) and tablet form, and is given in doses of 1 to 2 mg/kg every 3 to 4 hours. Typically, it can exert analgesic effects within 15 to 30 minutes of oral administration and achieves peak plasma concentrations within 1 to 2 hours of ingestion. Intramuscular injection provides a more rapid onset of analgesia (approximately 10 minutes) and reaches a peak effect within 60 minutes of administration. Obviously, plasma concentrations may show marked variability after intramuscular injection on the basis of an individual patient's state of peripheral perfusion.

Meperidine is nearly completely metabolized in the liver with a plasma half-life of elimination of approximately 3 hours. Its principal metabolic pathways are hydrolysis and *N*-demethylation. The latter process produces normeperidine which is principally responsible for meperidine's sedative and convulsive effects. Normeperidine is about one half as active as meperidine as an analgesic but twice as active as a convulsant. The levels of normeperidine may be increased by ingestion of large doses or because of enzyme induction. Urinary excretion of the metabolites is responsible for final elimination of the drug.

Meperidine commonly is administered intramuscularly for moderate to severe pain or as part of a lytic (sedative) cocktail (meperidine, promethazine, and chlorpromazine). Intramuscular administration of analgesics is not recommended in children, nor is the use of the lytic cocktail. In fact, the lytic cocktail is an archaic and dangerous sedative combination. It is mentioned *only to condemn its use!* Although an intramuscular injection results in higher sustained plasma levels of meperidine and lengthens the patient's pain-free intervals, it is clear that children often will suffer in silence to avoid yet another pain, namely, the "shot." When administered intravenously (1 mg/kg), meperidine offers few advantages over morphine and must be given cautiously. Alternatives to the intramuscular injection of meperidine is the use of continuous intravenous infusions of an opioid such as morphine which does not have a toxic metabolite. Alternatively, a narcotic with a longer plasma half-life, such as methadone, may be used.[11]

Methadone

Primarily considered a drug to treat narcotic-addicted patients, methadone is being used increasingly for postoperative pain relief and for the treatment of intractable pain.[11] It is noted for its slow elimination, very long duration of effective analgesia, and high oral bioavailability.

Methadone has the longest elimination half-life ($t_{1/2}$ beta) of any of the commonly available opiates and provides 12 to 36 hours of analgesia after intravenous injection. In children 1 to 18 years of age, the half-life of methadone averages 19.2 hours and its clearance averages 5.4 ml/min/kg. Thus, methadone's pharmacokinetic characteristics are indistinguishable in children and adults. Because the use of methadone as an analgesic is a relatively recent practice, very little is known of the influence of pathophysiology on its pharmacokinetics and pharmacodynamics. Methadone is extremely well absorbed from the gastrointestinal tract and has a bioavailability of 80% to 90%. Therefore, it is extremely easy to convert intravenous dosing regimens to oral ones.

Because a single dose of methadone can achieve and sustain a high drug plasma level, it is a convenient way to provide prolonged analgesia without requiring an intramuscular injection. Indeed, when administered either orally or intravenously, it may be viewed as a "poor man's" alternative to the use of continuous intravenous opioid infusions. Typically patients receive an initial dose of 0.1 to 0.2 mg/kg administered intravenously. If this dose is insufficient to produce adequate analgesia, additional amounts in doses of 0.05 mg/kg can be given to control pain. Subsequent doses of 0.05 to 0.1 mg/kg are given every 6 to 12 hours as needed.

Codeine

Codeine is an opiate that frequently is used to treat pain in children and adults. Although effective when administered either orally or parenterally, it is most commonly administered orally, usually in combination with acetaminophen. In equipotent doses (See Tables 24-3 and 24-4), codeine's efficacy as an analgesic and respiratory depressant approaches that of morphine. In addition, codeine shares with morphine and the other narcotics common effects on the central nervous system, including sedation and respiratory depression, and stimulation of the chemoreceptor trigger zone in the brain stem. It also delays gastric emptying and can increase biliary tract pressure. Finally, it has potent antitussive properties that are similar to all other opioids and is commonly prescribed for this effect.

Codeine has a bioavailability of approximately 60% after oral ingestion. The analgesic effects occur as early as 20 minutes after ingestion and reach a maximum at 60 to 120 minutes. The plasma half-life of elimination is 2.5 to 3 hours. Codeine undergoes nearly complete metabolism in the liver before its final excretion in urine.

Although conventional pediatric teaching is to prescribe single agent drugs, this is not the case with codeine, because codeine as a single agent is not ordinarily available in liquid form at most pharmacies and if available is almost twice as expensive as in its combined form. Furthermore, acetaminophen potentiates the analgesia produced by codeine and allows the practitioner to use less narcotic and yet achieve satisfactory analgesia. Progressive increases in dose are associated with greater degrees of respiratory depression, delayed gastric emptying, nausea, and constipation, as with other opioid drugs. Although it is an effective analgesic when administered parenterally, intramuscular codeine has no advantage over morphine or meperidine. Intravenous administration of codeine is associated with serious complications, including apnea and severe hypotension, probably secondary to histamine release. Therefore, the intravenous administration of this drug is not recommended in children. In summary, codeine is used for the treatment of mild to moderate pain (or cough), usually in an outpatient setting. Typically, it is prescribed in a dose of 0.5 to 1 mg/kg along with 10 mg/kg of acetaminophen.

Opioid Antagonists

A discussion of narcotic analgesics would be incomplete without mentioning the opioid antagonists. As noted previously, a drug that blocks the action of a neurotransmitter is an antagonist. By definition, receptor recognition of an agonist is "translated" into other cellular alterations, whereas an antagonist occupies the receptor without initiating the transduction step.[29] Naloxone is a pure opioid antagonist with virtually no agonist activity. It antagonizes the effects of the pure agonist drugs, such as morphine, as well as the mixed agonist-antagonist drugs, such as butorphanol. In fact, it is the most commonly used opioid antagonist in clinical practice today. Naloxone is extremely potent and nonselective in its opioid reversal effects. It reverses not only the undesirable sedation, respiratory depression, and gastrointestinal effects of the opioid agonists but the analgesia as well. Indeed, the antagonism of opioid agonist effects must be accomplished with great caution, particularly in patients who have been receiving prolonged opioid therapy, who exhibit opioid dependence, or who are in extreme pain because the use of these antagonists may be accompanied by overt narcotic withdrawal symptoms. Occasionally a life-threatening "overshoot" phenomenon may occur in patients given these drugs, with the development of tachypnea, tachycardia, hypertension, nausea and vomiting, and sudden death. In healthy young adults this phenomenon may be accompanied by the onset of pulmonary edema. Indeed, mechanical ventilation is a safer treatment for narcotic-induced respiratory depression in dependent patients or patients in severe pain. Obviously, the magnitude of the withdrawal syndrome depends on the dose of naloxone administered, as well as on the degree of the patient's physical dependence on the opioid and on his or her pain-control needs. On the other hand, when naloxone is administered to patients who have not received opioids, it produces little or no effect (except in patients in shock; see following discussion) and does not induce physical dependence or tolerance.

Naloxone is rapidly metabolized through conjugation with glucuronic acid in the liver and is best given parenterally because of its rapid first-pass extraction through the liver when it is given orally. After intravenous administration, it reverses opioid effects virtually instantaneously. Unfortunately, it has a plasma elimination half-life of only 60 minutes and a duration of action that is shorter than the opioid agonists whose action it is used to reverse. Therefore, when naloxone is used to reverse opioid-induced respiratory depression, patients must be monitored in terms of the half-life of the opioid agonist for return of the depression. Repeated intravenous doses, intramuscular (depot) injection or a continuous intravenous infusion may be required to prevent recurrence of the symptoms of opioid overdose.

Naloxone is supplied as a parenteral solution (0.4 mg/kg or 0.02 mg/kg). The usual initial dose in children and adults is 0.01 mg/kg given intravenously. Doses as low as 0.001 to 0.002 mg/kg may be effective in reversing opioid-induced respiratory depression (or other unwanted side effects such as pruritus or biliary spasm) without reversing analgesia. If the initial dose of naloxone does not result in the desired degree of clinical improvement, a subsequent dose of 0.02, 0.04, 0.08, or 0.1 mg/kg may be administered stepwise. When used to reverse neonatal respiratory depression (from narcotics administered to the mother in labor) the usual initial dose is the same as that used in older children (0.01 mg/kg). If an intravenous route is unavailable, naloxone may be administered intramuscularly or subcutaneously.

Theoretically, the action of naloxone on opioid receptors of the central nervous system also may prove beneficial in the amelioration of septic and anaphylactic shock states. It is possible that endorphin release induced by anaphylaxis or endotoxemia may mediate the systemic hypotension observed in these situations. Reversal of the central opioid receptor activation produced by these substances should theoretically reverse or improve the state of shock. If this can be substantiated by animal and human studies, naloxone therapy may prove to be clinically useful in the treatment of shock.

NEWER MODES OF OPIOID THERAPY

Patient Controlled Analgesia

The method of opioid administration may be as important as the drug selected to treat pain. On the basis of pharmacokinetics of the opioids, it should be clear that intravenous boluses of morphine or meperidine need to be given at intervals of 1 to 2 hours to avoid marked fluctuations in plasma drug levels. Continuous intravenous infusions can provide steady analgesic levels and are preferable to intramuscular injections. Unfortunately, the perception of pain is not constant. To give patients some measure of control over their pain therapy, demand analgesia or patient controlled analgesia (PCA) devices have been developed.[22,23] Indeed, this treatment modality may be particularly suitable for adolescent patients and patients with sickle cell anemia who have vaso-occlusive crisis. Demand analgesia devices allow patients to administer small amounts of an analgesic whenever they feel a need for more pain relief. An upper limit per time interval is preprogrammed into the equipment by the physician so that the patient cannot self-administer an excessive dose. Many units use low "background" continuous infusions in addition to self-administered boluses. Difficulties with PCA include its inflexibility in terms of differing agents and dosing regimens, its limitation to children older than 6 to 8 years of age, and its increased equipment cost.

Intrathecal/Epidural Opioid Analgesia

The presence of high concentrations of opioid receptors in the spinal cord makes it possible to achieve analgesia with small doses of narcotics administered in either the subarachnoid or epidural spaces.[7] Intrathecal/epidural opioids produce more profound and prolonged analgesia than do comparable narcotic doses administered parenterally and are capable of relieving both visceral and somatic pain. Even when administered caudally, epidural morphine has been shown to be an efficacious postoperative analgesic for abdominal, thoracic, and cardiac surgery.[15] Recently, intrathecal morphine has been administered intraoperatively to children having craniofacial procedures, especially when placement of a lumbar cerebrospinal fluid drain was required to withdraw CSF to reduce intracranial pressure. The intrathecal morphine provides excellent quality intraoperative analgesia and prolonged postoperative trigeminal nerve analgesia with minimal side effects.

Side effects that accompany intrathecal/epidural narcotic administration include facial pruritus, urinary retention, nausea and vomiting, and respiratory depression. These side effects occur with greater frequency with intrathecal than with epidural administration. Except for urinary retention, reversal of adverse side effects, with maintenance of adequate analgesia, can be achieved with the use of a low dose (0.001-0.002 mg/kg) intravenous naloxone infusion. Urinary retention has not been a reported complication in children because in the pediatric population studied to date, all patients have had bladder catheters as part of their postoperative management regimen.

Although rare, respiratory depression is a major risk in the use of intrathecal/epidural opioids. Indeed, the ventilatory response to carbon dioxide is depressed for as long as 22 hours after the epidural administration 0.05 mg/kg of morphine. Clinical respiratory depression usually occurs within the first 6 hours after the administration of epidural or intrathecal morphine, but late respiratory depression (up to 18 hours) has been reported.[21] This has been most common when intravenous or intramuscular narcotics have been administered to supplement the intrathecal opioid. The risk of respiratory depression can be minimized with the use of smaller doses of supplemental narcotics, or epidural use of shorter-acting, more lipid-soluble agents (such as fentanyl and sufentanil). Nevertheless, respiratory depression is so grave a complication and experience in children so limited that the use of spinal opioids should be confined to patients admitted to intensive care units.

REFERENCES

1. American Academy of Pediatrics Committee on Drugs Section on Anesthesiology: Guidelines for the elective use of conscious sedation, deep sedation, and general anesthesia in pediatric anesthesia, Pediatrics 76:317-321, 1985.
2. Anand KJ and Hickey PR: Pain and its effects in the human neonate and fetus, N Engl J Med 317:1321-1329, 1987.
3. Behbehani M: Physiology of pain. In Raj PP, editors: Practical management of pain, Chicago, 1986, Year Book Medical Publishers.
4. Beyer JE and Bournaki MC: Assessment and management of postoperative pain in children, Pediatrician 16:30-38, 1989.
5. Beyer JE and Wells N: The assessment of pain in children, Pediatr Clin North Am 36:837-854, 1989.
6. Bokesch PM et al: The influence of a right-to-left cardiac shunt on lidocaine pharmacokinetics, Anesthesiology 67:739-744, 1987.
7. Cousin MJ and Mather LE: Intrathecal and epidural administration of opioids, Anesthesiology 61:276-310, 1984.
8. Cousin MJ, Cherry DA, and Gourlay GK. Acute and chronic pain: use of spinal opioids. In Cousins MJ and Bridenbaugh PO, editors: Neural blockade in clinical anesthesia and management of pain, Philadelphia, 1988, J.B. Lippincott Co.
9. Covino BG: Clinical pharmacology of local anesthetic agents. In Cousins MJ and Bridenbaugh PO, editors: Neural blockade in clinical anesthesia and management of pain. Philadelphia: J.B. Lippincott Company 111-114, 1988.
10. Finholt DA et al: Lidocaine pharmocokinetics in children during general anesthesia, Anesth Analg 65:279-282, 1986.
11. Gourlay GK, Wilson PR, and Glynn CJ: Pharmacodynamics and pharmocokinetics of methadone during the perioperative period, Anesthesiology 57:458-467, 1982.
12. Grunau RV and Craig KD: Pain expression in neonates: facial action and cry, Pain 28:395-410, 1987.
13. Hertzka RE et al: Fentanyl-induced ventilatory depression: effects of age, Anesthesiology 70:213-218, 1989.
14. Koren G et al: Postoperative morphine infusion in newborn infants: assessment of disposition characteristics and safety, J Pediatr 107:963-967, 1985.
15. Krane EJ, Tyler DC, and Jacobson LE: The dose response of caudal morphine in children, Anesthesiology 71:48-52, 1989.
16. Maxwell LG et al: Penile nerve block for newborn circumcision, Obstet Gynecol 70:415-419, 1987.
17. McGrath PJ and Unruh AM: Pain in children and adolescents, Amsterdam, 1987, Elsevier.
18. McKay W, Morris R, and Mushlin P: Sodium bicarbonate attenuates pain on skin infiltration with lidocaine, with or without epinephrine, Anesth Analg 66:572-574, 1987.
19. Mersky H: Pain terms: A list with definitions and notes on usage. Recommended by the IASP subcommittee on taxonomy, Pain 6:249-252, 1979.
20. Millan MJ: Multiple opioid systems and pain, Pain 27:303-347, 1986.
21. Nichols DG et al: Disposition and respiratory effects of intrathecal morphine in children, Anesthesiology 73(suppl):A1135, 1990.
22. Owen H et al: Variables of patient-controlled analgesia, 1. Bolus size, Anaesthesia 44:7-10, 1989.
23. Owen H et al: Variables of patient-controlled analgesia. 2. Concurrent infusion, Anaesthesia 44:11-13, 1989.
24. Pasternak GW, Zhang AZ, and Tecott L: Developmental differences between high and low affinity opiate binding sites: their relationship to analgesia and respiratory depression, Life Sci 27:1185-1190, 1980.
25. Phillips GD and Cousins MJ: Neurological mechanisms of pain and the relationship of pain, anxiety, and sleep. In Cousins MJ, Phillips GD, editors: Acute pain management, New York, 1986, Churchill Livingstone.
26. Schaffer DJ: Clinical comparison of TAC anesthetic solutions with and without cocaine, Ann Emerg Med 14:1077-1086, 1985.
27. Schechter NL: The undertreatment of pain in children: an overview, Pediatr Clin North Am 36:781-794, 1989.
28. Shannon M and Berde CB: Pharmacologic management of pain in children and adolescents, Pediatr Clin North Am 36:855-871, 1989.
29. Snyder SH: Drug and neurotransmitter receptors in the brain, Science 224:22-31, 1984.
30. Soliman IE, et al: Comparison of the analgesic effects of EMLA (eutectic mixture of local anesthetics) to intradermal lidocaine infiltration prior to venous cannulation in unpremedicated children, Anesthesiology 68:804-806, 1988.
31. Tree-Trakarn T and Pirayavaraporn S: Postoperative pain relief for circumcision in children: Comparison among morphine, nerve block, and topical analgesia, Anesthesiology 62:519-522, 1985.
32. Tucker GT: Pharmacokinetics of local anaesthetics, Br J Anaesth 58:717-731, 1986.
33. Wall PD and Melzack R, editors: Management of pain, New York, 1985, Churchill Livingstone.
34. Way WL, Costley EC, and Way EL: Respiratory sensitivity of the newborn infant to meperidine and morphine, Clin Pharmacol Ther 6:454-461, 1965.
35. Winnie AP et al: Factors influencing distribution of local anesthetic injected into the brachial plexus sheath, Anesth Analg 58:225-234, 1979.
36. Yaster M and Dishpande JK: Management of pediatric pain with opioid analgesics, J Pediatr 113:421-429, 1988.
37. Yaster M and Maxwell LG: Pediatric regional anesthesia, Anesthesiology 70:324-338, 1989.
38. Yaster M, Deshpande JK, and Maxwell LG: The pharmacologic management of pain in children, Compr Ther 15:14-26, 1989.

25

Fluid Therapy

Alice D. Ackerman

Regulation of body water, solute concentration, and acid-base parameters is important to the preservation of health in humans. Almost every disease process faced by the clinician results in some alteration of input, output, or need for water or solute; therefore, a thorough understanding of these aspects of physiology is mandatory to enable physicians to take a rational approach to the care of their patients.

This chapter reviews some basic homeostatic mechanisms that enable the human body to maintain relative stability despite large fluctuations of intake, metabolism, and excretion. Specific instances in which those mechanisms are inadequate and the physiologic responses that occur to meet the challenge of alterations in body fluid chemistry are also addressed. Finally, ways to correct various derangements are examined, and specific and unusual situations concerning fluid administration are discussed.

One

Theory: Body Fluid, Electrolyte Concentration, and Acid-Base Composition

BODY FLUID COMPARTMENTS

The entire body mass comprises total body water (TBW) and body solids (fat, skeletal muscle, and cellular solids). Traditionally, TBW has been viewed as a composite of intracellular fluid (ICF) and extracellular fluid (ECF). ECF is composed of intravascular fluid (plasma) and interstitial fluid (ISF). Although further subdivisions of extravascular fluid have been devised, it is sufficient for the purposes of most clinical situations to view the body fluid compartments as depicted in Fig. 25-1.

Essential in the clinical approach to fluid management is the knowledge that the size of the body's fluid compartments changes significantly with age. Fig. 25-2 shows that TBW makes up nearly 75% of the newborn's weight but only 60% of an adult man's weight. By about 1 year of age, the proportionate distribution of body water begins to approximate that of the adult, and only minor changes occur thereafter. At puberty characteristic sex differences become apparent. Males have more body water because females have a larger proportion of fat. Plasma volume remains nearly unchanged throughout the growth process, although this is not specifically noted in Fig. 25-2.

Another fluid compartment not explicitly represented in Figs. 25-1 or 25-2 is transcellular fluid, which is secreted by cells surrounding certain body spaces. This includes fluids within the gastrointestinal, pleural, peritoneal, joint, ocular, cerebrospinal, and pericardial spaces. Even though transcellular fluid in the healthy body accounts for only 2% to 3% of TBW, in certain disease processes it can increase dramatically (e.g., ascites secondary to portal hypertension or pleural and pericardial effusions caused by inflammatory processes in those areas).

SOLUTE CONCENTRATIONS

Clinically, the only available measurements of solute concentration involve quantitating the various electrolyte concentrations and other solute particles found in the plasma. Most solutes are electrically charged particles. In plasma, sodium is the major cationic (positively charged) particle, with smaller concentrations of calcium, magnesium, and potassium present. To maintain electroneutrality, there also must be an equal number of anionic (negatively charged) particles. These are primarily chloride, bicarbonate, and protein. However, there are also the unmeasured anions that constitute the "anion gap"—phosphate, sulfate, and various organic acids. Fig. 25-3 depicts a "Gamble-gram," in which solute concentrations are presented in milliequivalents per liter of water. For each body fluid compartment, the cations are on the left and the anions on the right. As seen in Fig. 25-3, the major difference between plasma and ISF is the protein component, because the two compartments are separated by a capillary membrane that is permeable to all except the largest of the charged particles (i.e., proteins).

However, ICF has a composition different from that of ISF and plasma. Potassium is the major intracellular cation, followed by magnesium and a relatively small amount of sodium. The anions are led by inorganic phosphates and proteins, with smaller concentrations of bicarbonate and sulfate. The exact composition of intracellular contents is difficult to determine accurately and probably varies substantially from one tissue type to another.

As depicted in Fig. 25-3, there is a large concentration gradient for sodium, potassium, and chloride between the ICF and ECF. These gradients are maintained by active transport mechanisms essential for the preservation of cellular integrity.

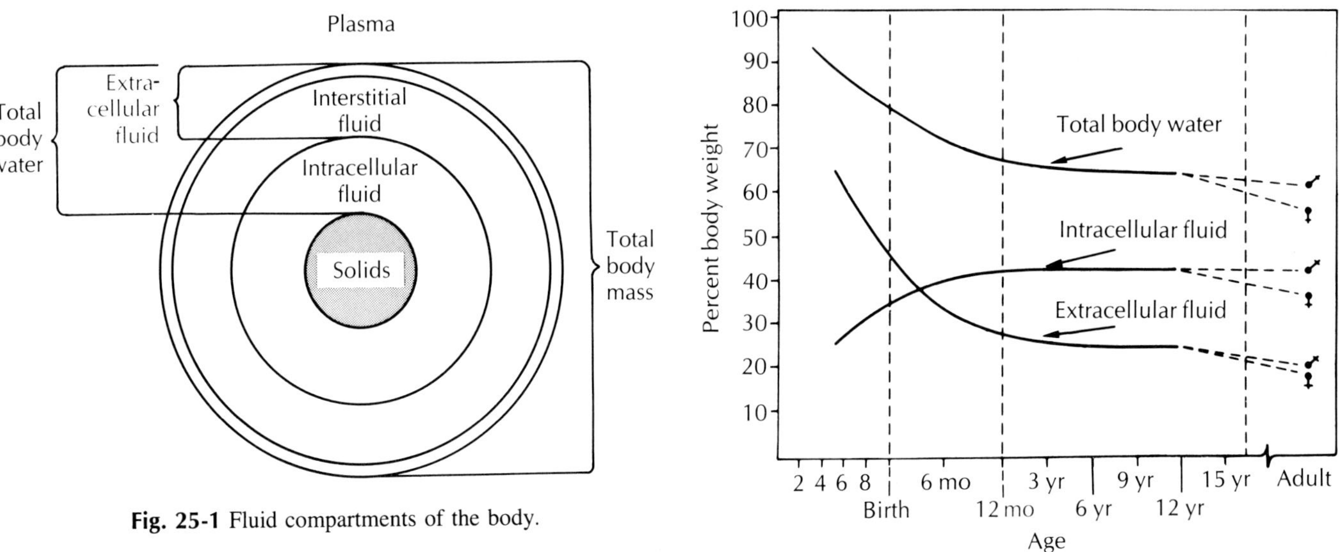

Fig. 25-1 Fluid compartments of the body.

Fig. 25-2 Changes in body fluid compartments with age. Total body water remains relatively stable after 1 year of age, with the exception of changes that occur at puberty.

From Winters RW, editor: The body fluids in pediatrics, Boston, 1973, Little, Brown & Co.

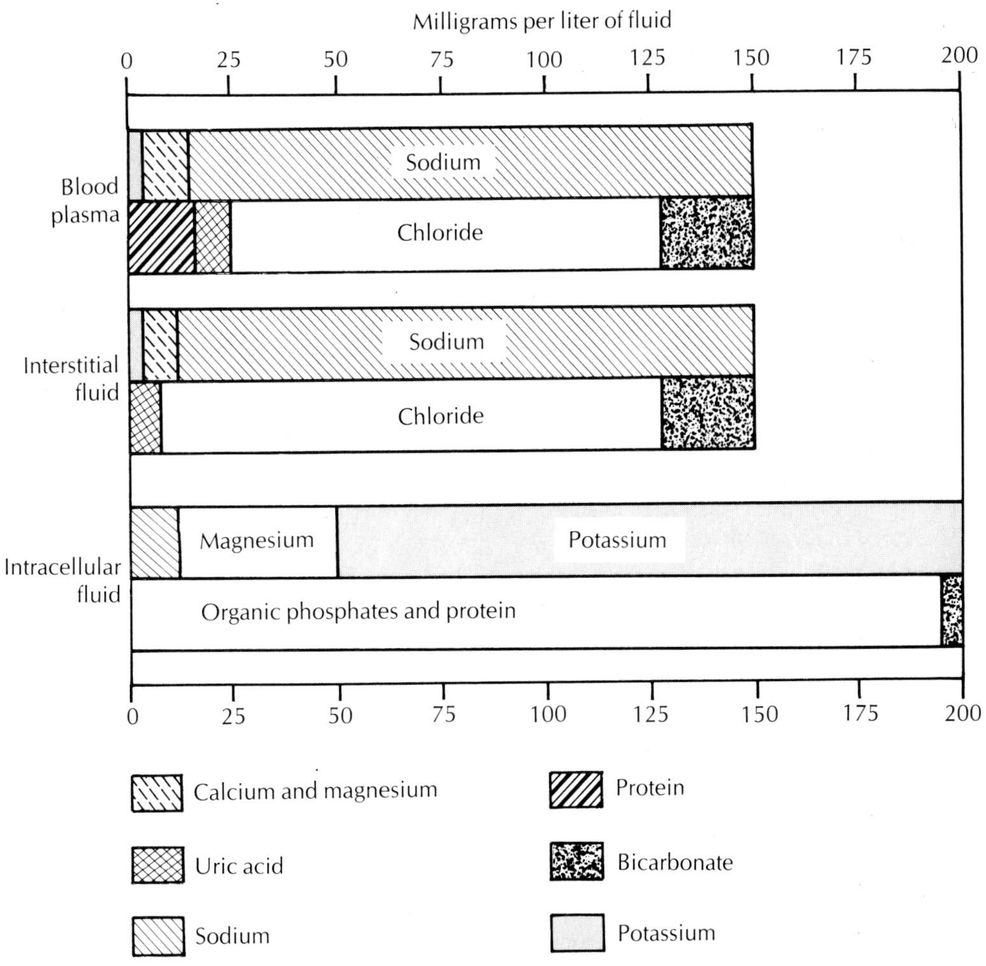

Fig. 25-3 "Gamble-gram" showing the various body fluid compartments and their electrolyte makeup.

Modified from Winters RW, editor: The body fluids in pediatrics, Boston, 1973, Little, Brown & Co.

Although the solute concentrations present in plasma are readily measured, the values reported by the clinical laboratory are in milliequivalents per volume of *plasma,* not water. The total volume of plasma includes any suspended solids such as lipids or proteins, which usually constitute about 7% of the total volume. If the concentrations of these substances are abnormally elevated, the resultant measured electrolyte values will fall relatively, although their actual concentration in plasma *water* will remain essentially unchanged. Because of its predominance in ECF, the plasma solute most commonly affected is sodium, and the expected reduction of its concentration can be calculated easily if the concentration of the offending serum solid is known. In the presence of hyperlipidemia, multiplying the plasma lipid concentration (expressed in milligrams per deciliter) by 0.002 will yield the reduction (in milliequivalents per liter) of serum sodium as a result of displacement by this solid. The same information (milliequivalents per liter reduction in serum sodium) resulting from hyperproteinemia can be obtained by dividing the plasma protein concentration in excess of 8 mg/dl by 4. For example, if the serum total protein concentration is 12, the measured sodium concentration will be 1 mEq lower than its actual concentration in plasma water:

$$\frac{12 - 8}{4} = 1$$

OSMOLALITY AND OSMOTIC PRESSURE

The osmolality of any aqueous solution is a function of the total number of solute particles within it, regardless of their size or charge. When two solutions of different osmolality are separated by a membrane permeable only to water, movement of water through that membrane occurs to equalize the osmolality or tonicity of the two solutions. The force enabling this water movement (osmotic pressure) is proportional to the difference in osmolality between the two solutions. The resultant measured *hydrostatic* pressure of water in each compartment reflects the osmotic pressure of the particles that resulted in the transmembrane movement of water. The portion of osmotic pressure exerted by the plasma proteins represents the *oncotic* pressure present in the intravascular space.

Clinically, it is simpler to look directly at the osmolality (number of particles per kilogram of water) or osmolarity (number of particles per liter of fluid) by actual measurement (most laboratories use freezing point depression) or by calculation rather than by measurement of hydrostatic pressure. The unit of osmolality most commonly used is the milliosmol, which is defined by:

$$\text{Milliosmol} = \text{Millimol} \times \text{n}$$

where *n* equals the number of particles produced by dissociation of a millimol of a given solute. Therefore, because it does not dissociate, a millimol of glucose would represent 1 mOsm. The number of particles for sodium chloride would be 2, for calcium chloride 3, and so on.

By far the most substantial contribution to normal plasma osmolality is made by sodium and its associated anions. Under most circumstances, the plasma osmolality is approximately equivalent to twice the concentration of plasma sodium. However, under unusual circumstances or for precision, the osmolality can be calculated via the following formula:

$$\text{Osmolality (mOsm/kg body water)} = 2\,[\text{Na}^+]\ \text{mEq/L} + \frac{[\text{Glucose}]\ \text{mg/dl}}{18} + \frac{[\text{BUN}]\ \text{mg/dl}}{28}$$

Normally, osmolality is maintained between 286 and 294 mOsm/kg of body water. The measurement of plasma osmolality is a fairly good estimate of the osmolality of other body fluids. However, plasma osmolality is slightly higher than that of the ISF, since plasma contains a slightly greater concentration of nondiffusible protein. This difference accounts for 1 to 1.5 mOsm/kg water, but it exerts a pressure known as *plasma protein osmotic pressure,* which is between 20 and 30 mm Hg.

To understand the control of the flow of fluid across capillary membranes, it is necessary to consider the three Starling forces that determine fluid movement. *Hydrostatic pressure*—the pressure exerted by the water of plasma—is determined both by the force with which it is being pumped (mean arterial pressure) and by the distensibility of the vessel. Therefore plasma hydrostatic pressure changes from arteriole to capillary to venule, but in general it favors the movement of plasma fluid into the interstitial space. Hydrostatic pressure is opposed by *ISF pressure* and *plasma osmotic pressure,* both of which tend to move fluid into the intravascular space. Although in health these bulk fluid movements are small and remain in equilibrium, they become more significant in several pathologic situations, most notably in peripheral edema formation and other processes described below.

CONTROL OF BODY FLUID VOLUME AND OSMOLALITY

The remarkable consistency of plasma osmolality has been mentioned already, yet it is important to reiterate that both plasma volume and osmolality remain nearly constant despite wide variations of water and solute intake. Control of osmolality and volume can be viewed as two separate but related mechanisms that are involved in a thirst-regulating hypothalamus-pituitary-kidney feedback system that works to adjust intake or output of water rapidly in response to changes, however minor, in plasma osmolality. The feedback mechanism hinges on the action (or lack thereof) of antidiuretic hormone (ADH) on the kidney's distal and collecting tubules to increase renal reabsorption of water.

Thirst and Antidiuretic Hormone

Thirst is regulated by body osmolality. Normal adults begin to experience thirst at plasma osmolality levels of 290 mOsm/kg, with profoundly increasing intensity as the osmolality reaches 300 to 305 mOsm/kg. At this point the person consumes large amounts of water (assuming free access, which is not the case with infants and young children) until plasma osmolality is brought back below the threshold level. Secretion of ADH occurs at a lower threshold than that for thirst and is initiated (thus inhibiting renal water loss) at a plasma osmolality level above 280. With rising osmolality, ADH secretion increases, so that changes in osmolality as small as 2.9 mOsm/kg effect a measurable increase in ADH release. Maximum antidiuresis usually occurs at around the same osmolality level responsible for initiation of the thirst mechanism just described. The ADH mechanism is far more sensitive than that of thirst, but drinking is the only physiologic way to replace large losses of fluid. When osmolality levels fall below 280, ADH secretion is inhibited, enabling the kidney to secrete a high volume of dilute urine. The thirst mechanism is simultaneously repressed.

Many factors may alter the usual response of the ADH-thirst system. These include individual (genetically determined) variations, pregnancy, various drugs, and the nature of the osmolar load. However, the most important variable is the hemodynamic status of the patient. Regardless of the plasma osmolality level, any short-term reduction of blood volume or arterial pressure of at least 10% increases ADH secretion, whereas similar increases in volume or pressure have the opposite effect, thereby altering the threshold or set point but not disrupting the previously described reactions to osmolar changes.

TOTAL BODY FLUID HOMEOSTASIS

In addition to the primary factors regulating water intake and output, there are other organs that contribute to fluid gain or loss, and they must be considered when trying to understand TBW homeostasis. In health, these organs or systems work together to preserve the integrity of the child; in disease, however, any or all systems may either malfunction individually or lose the ability to compensate for the instability of another system.

The gastrointestinal (GI) tract is responsible for the digestion and absorption of nutrients—calories (in the form of fat, carbohydrate, and protein), vitamins, minerals, and water—and the excretion of food-derived waste products, including water. Numerous diseases may inhibit adequate intake or stimulate large losses.

The evaporative water loss of sweat makes the skin the major organ of temperature regulation. The lungs also excrete some water and may provide some component of temperature control. In addition to responding to alterations in ADH release, the kidneys adjust their water output to meet the requirements of the solutes they secrete. Finally, the exocrine glands contribute to water needs and excretion by altering the metabolic rate or the systemic blood pressure, among other means.

CONTROL OF INDIVIDUAL SOLUTE CONCENTRATIONS

Sodium

As stated in the earlier section on osmolality, sodium is the major osmotically active cation in plasma. The total body content of sodium approximates 60 mEq/kg, but almost 43% of this is contained in bone, most of which plays almost no role in daily regulation of sodium concentration. Of the remainder, the majority is concentrated in the interstitial and plasma fractions with only a small amount in the intracellular space.

Sodium homeostasis results from the balance of sodium intake and excretion. Intake is controlled by dietary habits and cultural customs, and although there may be some higher central regulation for sodium intake, as there is for thirst (many patients who lose salt seem to develop a craving for sodium), it appears to be poorly developed and has not yet been localized. The typical American adult's diet contains 100 to 170 mEq of sodium per day; the amount of sodium in the infant's diet varies according to the formula he or she receives. Most of the dietary sodium is actively absorbed in the jejunum. Aldosterone secretion increases gastrointestinal sodium absorption.

Sodium excretion is controlled primarily by the kidneys but is also accomplished by the GI tract and skin. Although a large amount of sodium is presented to the kidneys during glomerular filtration, almost 99% of it is reabsorbed in the kidney tubules. In conditions of severe sodium depletion, volume depletion, or both, this amount may increase to nearly 100%; in cases of sodium and water overload, it may decrease to approximately 90%. The renin-angiotensin-aldosterone system, when stimulated by decreased renal blood flow, facilitates a greater degree of sodium reabsorption in the distal convoluted tubules and collecting ducts through the action of aldosterone at those sites.

Hypernatremia and hyponatremia are conditions usually closely tied to changes in the extracellular volume and are fully discussed in the clinical sections on dehydration and fluid overload. However, a brief overview of associated conditions is included here.

Hypernatremia (serum sodium ≥150 mEq/L) may follow dehydration if there is a greater loss of water than sodium. These losses may occur through the lungs, skin, stool, or urine (especially in the presence of diabetes insipidus). Another important although infrequent cause of hypernatremia in young children is the overuse of commercial enema preparations containing high concentrations of phosphate and sodium. Signs and symptoms of hypernatremic dehydration may be difficult to interpret accurately, and the severity of dehydration may not be apparent on the basis of a physical examination alone. ECF volume remains relatively well preserved. Therefore shock is unlikely even with marked loss of body water, and skin turgor and perfusion may remain close to normal. Notable hypernatremia results in marked changes in central nervous system (CNS) function, especially if the electrolyte disturbance occurred rapidly (a few hours), which is common in small children. Affected infants exhibit marked irritability alternating with severe lethargy—the hallmark of acute hypernatremia. Seizures may occur and may be followed by coma if the condition is not diagnosed and adequate therapy is not initiated. In addition, elevation of the serum sodium concentration may lead to skeletal muscle rigidity and hyperactive deep tendon reflexes. In small children one may observe fever, emesis, and respiratory distress when the onset is acute.

Hyponatremia (serum sodium <130 mEq/L) occurs whenever body sodium stores are diluted or depleted. It is more often related to failure to excrete adequate amounts of water than to simple overhydration, although in small infants, intake of hypotonic formulas may result in substantial lowering of the plasma sodium concentration.

Although less common than isotonic or hypernatremic dehydration, hyponatremic dehydration occurs with diarrhea in approximately 10% of cases and is most often encountered because large stool losses are replaced with solutions containing little or no sodium. Any situation creating increased secretion of ADH may be associated with low serum sodium concentrations. This is seen in patients with the syndrome of inappropriate antidiuretic hormone secretion (SIADH) resulting from CNS disease or postoperative water intoxication. Addison disease and congenital adrenal hyperplasia are associated with excessive loss of sodium in the urine and retention of potassium. Children with obstructive uropathy and progressive renal failure are less able to reabsorb sodium from their renal tubules. Therefore they sustain large sodium losses and may exhibit mild dehydration with a borderline or low serum sodium concentration. The administration of enemas low in saline concentration may also result in hyponatremia. An excessive loss of sodium and water occurs in individuals suffering from heat-related illnesses. Also, as previously mentioned, the serum sodium concentration reported by the laboratory may be artificially low in the presence of marked hyperlipidemia and hyperglycemia. Highly elevated concentrations of blood glucose (as in diabetic ketoacidosis) are associated with real and apparent hyponatremia.

Signs and symptoms of hyponatremia are related as much to the duration of the lowered serum sodium concentration and to the plasma volume status as to the degree of hyponatremia present. Hyponatremia associated with diminished plasma volume results in anorexia, muscle cramps, lethargy, and shortness of breath when exercising. With further decreases in sodium concentration, nausea, emesis, and muscle weakness ensue, which may proceed to delirium and seizures. Hyponatremia associated with acute water intoxication is more likely to result in seizures and coma than in conditions in which the plasma volume remains unchanged.

Potassium

In contrast to sodium, only a small fraction of total body potassium is present in the intravascular and extracellular spaces. The total potassium content is approximately 50 mEq/kg body weight, with concentrations of intracellular and extracellular potassium of 145 mEq/L and 4 to 5 mEq/L, respectively.

The majority of potassium absorption occurs in the proximal portions of the GI tract. It is excreted in the colon in exchange for sodium. Increased potassium loss results from diarrhea or overuse of laxatives. Elevated levels of plasma aldosterone also increase potassium excretion from the GI tract, the skin (losses here are relatively minimal), and the kidneys. Urinary excretion of potassium results from tubular secretion rather than glomerular filtration. Aldosterone acts at the level of the distal tubule to foster sodium reabsorption and potassium secretion. There are frequent shifts of potassium between the intracellular and extracellular spaces, mediated mostly by alterations in the serum acid-base status. An increase in extracellular potassium concentration occurs with systemic acidosis. Alkalosis results in movement of potassium into the cell.

Cardiac toxicity is the most significant effect of hyperkalemia. Electrocardiographic changes may be seen, such as elevation and peaking of T waves, depression of ST segments, disappearance of P waves, heart block, and asystole. The most severe effects are not seen until the serum potassium concentration is greater than 8 mEq/L. Most frequently, the clinical findings in hypokalemia include muscle weakness and ileus. There may also be cardiac effects exhibited on the electrocardiogram by low voltage, flattening of the T waves, depression of ST segments, prominence of U waves, arrhythmias, and asystole. However, these effects are not usually seen until the serum potassium concentration falls below 2.0 mEq/L. Hypokalemia may also lead to an inhibition of renal concentrating ability and a worsening of any existing hypochloremic alkalosis.

Calcium

The total body calcium content ranges from 400 to 950 mEq/kg body weight, increasing with advancing age. Almost all of it (99%) is contained in bone, and nearly 50% of the remainder is protein bound. Of the entire mass of calcium, only about nine tenths of 1% exists in the noncomplexed free state. This is the physiologically significant ionized fraction of body calcium. The concentration of ionized calcium is pH dependent, increasing with acidosis and decreasing with alkalosis.

Calcium homeostasis is controlled mostly through the action of 1,25-dihydroxycholecalciferol (the metabolically active form of vitamin D), which increases the intestinal absorption of calcium (1) in the presence of an elevated serum parathyroid hormone level, (2) during pregnancy, (3) when calcium intake is low, and (4) when vitamin D is ingested. Excretion of calcium through the kidney is minimal except under certain circumstances, such as with prolonged bed rest, during protracted fasting, following the administration of diuretic drugs, and in the presence of metabolic acidosis.

The other major mechanism for control of serum calcium concentration is the balance that exists between ionized calcium and bone calcium, which is influenced by parathyroid hormone (parathyroid hormone increases resorption of calcium from bone). This regulatory mechanism may produce wide variations in the ionized fraction of serum calcium, while the total serum calcium concentration remains nearly constant.

Hypercalcemia usually results from the inability of the kidneys to increase excretion adequately when calcium delivery to the ECF is increased. This may occur with hyperparathyroidism, immobilization, vitamin D intoxication, various endocrine disorders, sarcoidosis, malignancies, thiazide administration, milk alkali syndrome, and familial hypocalciuric hypercalcemia. Signs and symptoms of hypercalcemia may be negligible if the condition is mild or short-lived. However, severe short-term elevations of ionized serum calcium concentration may result in acute hypercalcemic intoxication, a rare syndrome characterized by acute renal insufficiency, lethargy with progressive coma and death, and sometimes ventricular tachyarrhythmias. Less critical but more common symptoms of hypercalcemia may be renal lithiasis, nausea, anorexia, constipation, polyuria, and polydipsia. In addition, rapid infusions of intravenous calcium solutions may result in bradycardia and cardiac arrest. The classic electrocardiographic findings are shortening of the QT interval, followed by widening of the T wave as the serum calcium concentration increases. With prolonged, markedly elevated serum calcium concentrations, the urine becomes hypotonic.

Vitamin D deficiency, hypoalbuminemia, hyperphosphatemia, and hypoparathyroidism produce hypocalcemia. It is also seen in some premature infants and in neonates with polycythemia or hypoglycemia. The ionized fraction of serum calcium may decrease with alkalosis. The major clinical manifestation of hypocalcemia is tetany. In children, a grand mal seizure is often the presenting symptom. There may be muscle weakness, mental confusion, decreased myocardial contractility, and sometimes congestive heart failure. Classically, the QT interval is prolonged on the electrocardiogram.

Magnesium

As an intracellular cation, magnesium is second in concentration only to potassium. About 50% of all magnesium is contained in bone. The majority of the remainder is found in muscle. Approximately 70% of plasma magnesium is in the free or ionized form; the rest is protein bound.

Although the details are poorly understood, magnesium homeostasis is accomplished mostly in the kidneys. Excretion is 5% to 10% of the amount filtered through the glomerulus. This amount increases with elevated plasma magnesium concentrations, volume overload, hypercalcemia, and the administration of diuretics. Tubular reabsorption is enhanced by both dietary magnesium restriction and parathyroid hormone secretion, though the effects of the latter may be overshadowed by the changes it causes in the serum calcium concentration. There is little regulation of gastrointestinal magnesium absorption. Between 25% and 60% of ingested magnesium is absorbed, primarily in the ileum. This does not appear to be under hormonal control.

Hypermagnesemia is most often an iatrogenic disease, related to the use of antacids and enemas that contain magnesium or to the intravenous administration of magnesium sulfate for treatment of toxemia of pregnancy. Symptoms and signs are rarely observed at a serum concentration of less than 4 to 5 mEq/L. They include diminution of deep tendon reflexes, drowsiness, coma, hypotension, and respiratory depression. Prolongation of the PR interval, sometimes progressing to complete heart block and cardiac arrest, can be seen on electrocardiogram.

Conversely, hypomagnesemia is common and is related to a myriad of clinical situations, although it is most commonly associated with malabsorption, hypoparathyroidism, prolonged laxative abuse, and chronic alcoholism. Symptoms may mimic those of hypocalcemia, which include tetany, muscle weakness, seizures, and changes in mental status.

Phosphorus

Phosphorus is involved in a wide variety of essential physiologic functions. In adults the total body phosphorus content is 700 to 800 g, 15% of which is in the soft tissues and the remainder in the bones. Available phosphorus is predominantly intracellular. It is a major constituent of phospholipid bilayer cell membranes, intramitochondrial nucleic acids, and phosphoproteins. Although its most important function is as the source of high-energy bonds in adenosine triphosphate (ATP), it is also critical to the control of 2,3-diphosphoroglycerate (2,3-DPG) synthesis in the red cell (which regulates oxygen delivery to tissues) and to numerous other hormonal functions.

Approximately 80% of ingested phosphate is absorbed in the jejunum. The kidneys regulate most of phosphate homeostasis by tubular resorption of 85% to 90% of the amount filtered through the glomerulus under normal circumstances. Tubular resorption is increased by the influences of thyroxine and growth hormone and is decreased by the actions of parathyroid hormone and vitamin D_3.

The level of serum phosphate may vary significantly throughout the day, reflecting shifts from cells to plasma. The levels in children may normally be considerably higher than those in adults.

Hypophosphatemia most often reflects movement from plasma into muscle, liver, or fat but may represent total body phosphate depletion. These shifts may occur in diabetic ketoacidosis; in association with severe burns; and with respiratory, and to a lesser extent, metabolic alkalosis. The transfer of phosphate into muscle and liver cells is enhanced by glucose and insulin infusions, which decrease its uptake by erythrocytes. This causes diminished levels of 2,3-DPG and shifts the oxyhemoglobin dissociation curve to the left, potentially creating tissue anoxia because of enhanced hemoglobin affinity for oxygen. In metabolic alkalosis, there is a fall in intracellular hydrogen ion concentration; this stimulates glycolysis, which results in the rapid uptake of phosphate by cells because of their increased need to produce phosphorylated compounds. Clinical situations in which total body phosphate depletion exists include mostly those leading to excessive losses of phosphate through the kidney, such as the Fanconi syndrome, Wilson disease, heavy metal poisoning, and vitamin D–resistant rickets. Although rare, nutritional deprivation (usually resulting from malabsorption or vomiting) may result in clinically notable hypophosphatemia.

Symptoms of phosphate deficiency are protean and are easily correlated with two of its most important functions: maintenance of energy stores via ATP and adequate oxygen delivery via 2,3-DPG. Muscular weakness, anorexia, general malaise, decreased myocardial contractility, and ventilatory insufficiency occur with phosphate deficiency. The patient may also experience seizures or become comatose. Deficient oxygen delivery to the tissues may result in hemolysis and myolysis. There may also be adverse effects on leukocyte and platelet function.

Chloride

Chloride is the predominant extracellular anion; it accounts for approximately 60% of the negatively charged ions in plasma. Although small amounts of chloride can be found in bone, connective tissue, and red blood cells, over 50% of it is found in the ECF spaces. Total body chloride has been estimated at between 30 and 50 mEq/kg body weight, being slightly higher in infancy than in adulthood.

Homeostasis of the chloride ion is related directly to sodium metabolism, and in most situations movement of chloride ions from one body compartment to another is thought to be a passive accompaniment to that of sodium ions. However, this may be reversed in portions of the renal tubule and in some other situations. Concentrations of the chloride ion also vary with changes in acid-base status.

Dietary chloride is readily absorbed in the jejunum, but over 90% is excreted, mainly in the urine. Although the usual dietary source is table salt, it is also found in most commonly eaten foods, especially eggs, milk, and red meats.

Hypochloremic conditions are generally associated with alkalosis and may result from increased gastrointestinal losses because of excessive vomiting or excretion of intestinal fluids rich in chloride.

Children with Cushing syndrome usually manifest a hypochloremic, hypokalemic metabolic alkalosis associated with normal serum sodium levels and accelerated urinary excretion of chloride and potassium. Any situation resulting in hyperaldosteronism, such as hypovolemia, excessive licorice ingestion, or Bartter syndrome, is usually accompanied by hypochloremia and a metabolic alkalosis with potassium wasting. Chloride's major physiologic role appears to be to enable the kidneys to excrete bicarbonate. Therefore chloride ion must be replaced to allow renal correction of alkalosis, especially when alkalosis is associated with hypokalemia.

Hyperchloremia occurs in the presence of metabolic acidosis not associated with elevated unmeasured anions (anion gap) and may result from acute expansion of the extracellular space with infused fluids that contain chloride. The specific physiologic effects of chloride excess are unknown.

Hydrogen Ion and Bicarbonate (Acid-Base Parameters)

Disturbances in plasma hydrogen ion and bicarbonate concentration lead to alterations of blood pH levels and the development of alkalosis or acidosis and are important clinically because of the extreme sensitivity of all essential physiologic functions to changes in the body's acid-base balance. When the blood pH level is outside the normal range (7.35 to 7.45), detrimental effects occur in the central nervous, respiratory, gastrointestinal, musculoskeletal, renal, and cardiovascular systems. The outside limits of pH levels compatible with life are 6.8 and 8.0. The body can tolerate marked deviations approaching these limits only under optimum conditions and for short periods of time.

The concentration of free hydrogen ion in ECF is lower (average 40 mEq/L) than in water (100 mEq/L). Thus ECF is more alkaline than water and has a relative "base excess." Acidosis and alkalosis can be viewed respectively as conditions in which there is a negative or a positive base excess.

Acid-base homeostasis is accomplished through a complicated set of buffering systems and by more definitive mechanisms for removal or excretion of excess hydrogen and bicarbonate ions. A *buffer* is defined as a weak acid plus its salt, or conjugate base. The acid-base pair is in equilibrium, so that when any acid or base is added to the system, the resultant change in pH level is minimized. Physiologically the most important (though not the only) buffer is that formed by the bicarbonate ion–carbonic acid pair. The Henderson-Hasselbalch equation, which defines the relation between an acid and its conjugate base, is as follows:

$$1.\ \mathrm{pH} = \mathrm{pK} + \mathrm{Log}\,\frac{[\mathrm{Base}]}{[\mathrm{Acid}]}$$

where *pK* represents the dissociation constant of the acid, and the brackets indicate concentration. This equation promotes understanding of the relation between bicarbonate (HCO_3^-) and carbonic acid (H_2CO_3) as they exist in the equilibrium expressed by the following:

$$2.\ [H^+] + [HCO_3^-] \rightleftharpoons H_2CO_3 \rightleftharpoons CO_2 + H_2O$$

This relation can be expressed in several ways. Substituting the acid-base pair into equation 1 gives the following:

$$3.\ \mathrm{pH} = \mathrm{pK} + \mathrm{Log}\,\frac{[HCO_3^-]}{[H_2CO_3]}$$

Because carbonic acid accumulation is short-lived, and its concentration is difficult to measure, the next equation is derived by knowing that the concentration of carbonic acid is equal to the product of the partial pressure of carbon dioxide in arterial blood ($P\text{CO}_2$) and its solubility coefficient (a):

$$4.\ \mathrm{pH} = \mathrm{pK} + \mathrm{Log}\,\frac{[HCO_3^-]}{[a \times P\text{CO}_2]}$$

Under usual physiologic conditions, pK = 6.1, a = 0.03, $[HCO_3^-]$ = 24, and $P\text{CO}_2$ = 40; therefore the following substitutions can be made:

$$5.\ \mathrm{pH} = 6.1 + \mathrm{Log}\,\frac{24}{0.03 \times 40}$$

$$\mathrm{pH} = 6.1 + \mathrm{Log}\,\frac{24}{1.2}$$

$$\mathrm{pH} = 6.1 + \mathrm{Log}\ 20$$

$$\mathrm{pH} = 6.1 + 1.3$$

$$\mathrm{pH} = 7.4$$

To maintain the ratio of bicarbonate to carbonic acid at 20:1 and therefore the pH level at 7.4, with any change of either the bicarbonate or the carbonic acid concentration, there must be a corresponding change in the other parameter. Understanding the equations as they relate to the bicarbonate buffering system is essential to appreciating the classification of acid-base disturbances. For any buffering system to maintain blood pH levels effectively, a mechanism must exist to enable excretion of excess acid (hydrogen ion) or base (bicarbonate ion and carbon dioxide). In the bicarbonate system, this happens via the lungs (carbon dioxide) and kidneys (bicarbonate and hydrogen ions). Regardless of any compensatory mechanisms, blood pH levels rarely return to normal until the underlying problem is resolved.

Of the non-bicarbonate-related buffers, the major system is the hemoglobin-oxyhemoglobin pair. Buffering is also accomplished by small amounts of organic and inorganic phosphates and plasma proteins. A complete discussion of these systems is beyond the scope of this chapter, which focuses on further exploration of acid-base physiology as it applies to bicarbonate and its related compounds.

Traditionally, acid-base disturbances have been classified as "metabolic" or "respiratory," describing abnormalities that primarily involve the kidneys or lungs, respectively. The major mechanism used to compensate for bicarbonate alterations is renal and that for carbonic acid alterations, respiratory (via carbon dioxide exchange); the terms *metabolic* and *respiratory* can be further related to the numerator and denominator of the Henderson-Hasselbalch equation (4), respectively.

Acidemia and *alkalemia* indicate absolute alterations of blood pH levels below or above the normal range. *Acidosis* and *alkalosis*, more commonly used terms, actually refer to the relative gain or loss of each acid-base parameter (H^+, HCO_3^-, CO_2) that results in a change of pH level or a *tendency* toward such a change.

Acidosis and alkalosis are also classified as primary, secondary (compensatory), or mixed disturbances. In general, compensation for respiratory alkalosis or acidosis occurs via renal mechanisms, whereas the lungs may compensate for metabolic aberrations. All parameters return to baseline levels only when the underlying disorder is resolved.

Before making a specific etiologic diagnosis, it is important to classify acid-base disorders as just described. This is easily accomplished by measuring blood pH and P_{CO_2} levels in the clinical laboratory, where a reflection of bicarbonate is expressed as the calculated value for total carbon dioxide. Once any two of the values have been generated, the third may be estimated by using one of the readily available nomograms, thereby defining the disorder. The magnitude of expected compensatory mechanisms for any primary disorder must be known in order to determine whether a mixed disturbance is present (Table 25-1). Examination of the patient may often provide the best clues to the nature of the problem, and one should not mistakenly rely totally on laboratory data. It is also important to remember that acid-base disturbances rarely occur alone but are generally associated with changes in the concentration of potassium or other electrolyte concentrates. Therefore obtaining measurements of those parameters is helpful in making the definitive diagnosis or in finding an appropriate therapy.

Metabolic Acidosis. Primary metabolic acidosis (pH usually less than 7.35, P_{CO_2} less than 35 mm Hg) occurs with the accelerated loss of bicarbonate ion, increased production of hydrogen ion, or inadequate excretion of the normal acid by-products of metabolism. Clinical classification of such disorders usually separates those that result in an elevated concentration of unmeasured anions (negatively charged ions other than bicarbonate and chloride) from those disorders in which there is no such elevation and thus a normal "anion gap." The anion gap is easily calculated by subtracting the sum of the serum chloride and bicarbonate concentrations from the serum sodium concentration; the serum potassium concentration is usually ignored in this calculation. The normal plasma concentration of unmeasured anions ranges between 10 and 15 mEq/L. Thus an elevated anion gap occurs when such concentrations exceed 15 mEq/L.

Elevation of the anion gap indicates an acidosis related to (1) accumulation of organic acids such as ketone bodies, which occurs in diabetic ketoacidosis or starvation; (2) increased lactic acid production because of diminished tissue perfusion and oxygenation, which occurs in shock, sepsis, congestive heart failure, or pulmonary insufficiency; (3) ingestion of various toxins, including salicylates and ethanol, whose metabolism results in elevated levels of various organic acids; and (4) retention of abnormally high levels of sulfates and phosphates, as occurs in profound renal failure.

Metabolic acidosis with a normal anion gap occurs whenever there is loss of bicarbonate ion through the GI tract (as in profound diarrhea) or the kidneys (as in proximal or distal renal acidosis). Distal renal tubular acidosis is associated with failure to excrete the filtered acid load appropriately or with the use of carbonic acid inhibitors that block proximal tubular resorption of bicarbonate. Metabolic acidosis may also be seen with administration of an exogenous acid load and with amino acid infusions during total parenteral nutrition. Usually the decreased bicarbonate concentration is accompanied by elevation of serum chloride, thus maintaining the anion gap at a normal level. Therefore these situations are sometimes referred to as the *hyperchloremic metabolic acidoses*. Most

Table 25-1 *Primary Acid-Base Abnormalities and Their Expected Compensatory Changes*

DISORDER	PRIMARY ABNORMALITY	ASSOCIATED ABNORMALITIES	EXPECTED COMPENSATORY CHANGES IF SIMPLE DISORDER EXISTS
Metabolic acidosis	Elevation in hydrogen ion concentration (↓ pH)	↓ Bicarbonate concentration and total CO_2; negative base excess	P_{CO_2} will fall by 1.5 times the fall in bicarbonate concentration (maximum change is 10 mm Hg)
Respiratory acidosis	Elevation in P_{CO_2}	↑ Hydrogen ion concentration and total CO_2; ↓ pH	Bicarbonate concentration rises by 3.5-4 mEq/L for each 10 mm Hg rise in P_{CO_2} (cannot be above 30 mEq/L if the problem is short term, 45 if long term)
Metabolic alkalosis	Decreased hydrogen ion concentration (↑ pH)	↑ Bicarbonate concentration and total CO_2; positive base excess	P_{CO_2} rises by 0.5-1 mm Hg for every 1 mEq rise in bicarbonate concentration (to a maximum of 55 mm Hg)
Respiratory alkalosis	Decreased P_{CO_2}	↓ Hydrogen ion concentration and total CO_2; ↑ pH	Bicarbonate concentration falls by 2.5-5 mEq/L for each 10 mm Hg fall in P_{CO_2} (lower limit is 18 mEq/L if short term, 12-15 mEq/L if long term)

of these disorders are also associated with hypokalemia. A normal or an elevated serum potassium concentration signals early renal failure, exogenous acid ingestion, or hyperaldosteronism as possible causes of the metabolic acidosis.

If the plasma pH is less than 7.2 in a short-term situation, treatment of metabolic acidosis should be considered. A level of 6.9 or lower is a medical emergency. Sodium bicarbonate should be administered, *but only if the body is able to excrete the generated carbon dioxide via the lungs*. The most common complications of this therapy are hypernatremia (hyperosmolality) with volume overload and hypokalemia. Because of improved protein binding of calcium when the acidosis is corrected, tetany may result from a sudden fall in the ionized portion of the serum calcium. Too rapid correction of the body pH level may result in an "overshoot" alkalosis or in paradoxical CNS acidosis associated with cerebral edema. Although it is necessary to be aware of these potential complications and to be appropriately cautious, they should not impede adequate therapy of life-threatening acidosis.

Respiratory Acidosis. Respiratory acidosis is always related to failure of the lungs to excrete accumulated carbon dioxide. With initial elevation in the serum P_{CO_2} level (hypercapnia), excess hydrogen ion is buffered within 10 to 15 minutes and leads to an increase in blood bicarbonate concentration. In the first few hours of continued respiratory insufficiency, bicarbonate may rise as much as 1 mEq/L for each 10 mm Hg rise in P_{CO_2}. However, after several days of hypercapnia, bicarbonate concentration rises even more as the kidneys respond to the lowered pH level by increasing their excretion of acid. Under these circumstances, bicarbonate concentration increases as much as 4 mEq/L for each 10 mm Hg rise in P_{CO_2}. Therefore, by observing the degree of bicarbonate elevation, one may be able to estimate the duration of an observed respiratory acidosis.

The severity of clinical manifestations of respiratory acidosis may also be related to its duration. Although the major manifestation of hypercapnia is lethargy with a diminished sensorium, it is more profound earlier rather than later in its course.

Dysfunction of both the pulmonary and central nervous systems must be considered in determining the cause of hypercapnia. Substantial hypercapnia is never related simply to an increased production of carbon dioxide. If the brain and lungs are functioning normally, accelerated production of carbon dioxide simply results in increased alveolar ventilation (increased rate and depth of breathing).

Probably the most common disorder leading to retention of carbon dioxide in children is severe status asthmaticus. Other pulmonary causes include multilobar pneumonia, abnormalities of the chest wall, and neuromuscular disorders that affect the muscles of respiration. Chronic obstructive lung disease is the most common cause of respiratory acidosis in adults but is seen infrequently in children except in those with advanced cystic fibrosis or bronchopulmonary dysplasia. In a previously healthy child with an acute rise in P_{CO_2}, one should always consider the presence of a compression lung injury such as hemothorax or pneumothorax or the presence of a large pleural effusion.

CNS conditions that relate to hypercapnia involve inhibition of the respiratory drive and include (1) severe diffuse CNS infections such as encephalitis or meningitis, (2) trauma to the CNS resulting in elevated cerebral pressure or vascular compromise (hemorrhage or thrombosis), and (3) ingestion of drugs known to depress the CNS (such as barbiturates, narcotics, and sedatives).

Treatment should always address the underlying pathophysiology and should increase alveolar ventilation to allow appropriate excretion of carbon dioxide. With a rapidly rising P_{CO_2}, intubation with assisted ventilation may be necessary. Conversely, well-compensated respiratory acidosis can usually be treated conservatively by correcting the fundamental abnormality, unless the patient is on the verge of respiratory failure or is exhibiting substantial neurologic dysfunction.

Because the kidneys continue to excrete acid for several days after correction of lowered pH levels caused by retention of carbon dioxide, one may see a notable metabolic alkalosis for as long as 36 hours after correction. This condition is self-limited and resolves without intervention.

Chronic respiratory acidosis usually does not require short-term therapy but rather a conservative approach aimed at improving air exchange. Bronchodilators to relieve airway obstruction, judicious use of oxygen (some of these patients require some hypoxia to stimulate respiration), and measures to decrease excess lung water may all be helpful. Implementation of vigorous pulmonary toileting (postural drainage and percussion) helps to relieve airway obstruction caused by inspissated secretions.

Metabolic Alkalosis. In contrast to the urgency with which one must approach metabolic and respiratory acidosis, alkalosis or alkalemia is seldom of sufficient magnitude to cause alarm. A loss of hydrochloric acid or gain of bicarbonate or other forms of alkali may result in the elevation of blood pH levels. Uncommonly seen alone, these disturbances are usually accompanied by altered plasma concentrations of potassium and chloride. Therefore the clinical diseases generally have been divided into two categories related to those that do and do not respond to the administration of fluids that contain chloride as the major therapeutic intervention.

Chloride-sensitive conditions generally result from ongoing losses of hydrochloric acid via the GI tract, skin, or kidneys, and although the hypochloremia is associated with hypokalemia and elevated bicarbonate concentration, neither pH level nor potassium ion abnormalities can be corrected by administration of potassium if salts that contain chloride are withheld. The kidneys secrete additional bicarbonate in an attempt to return the blood pH level to normal, and with deficits of sodium and hydrogen ions, they selectively secrete potassium to maintain electroneutrality.

The most common pediatric problem associated with hypochloremic, hypokalemic metabolic alkalosis is excessive vomiting, such as is seen with pyloric stenosis; however, it may also occur in cystic fibrosis (electrolyte and acid-base imbalance may infrequently be the initial presentation of this genetically acquired disease). Treatment with potent diuretic compounds, such as the thiazides and furosemide, causes urinary losses of potassium chloride and sodium in excess of bicarbonate losses. This also generates a hypochloremic, metabolic alkalosis usually associated with hyponatremia.

Of the chloride-resistant pediatric conditions, the one most frequently encountered is excessive mineralocorticoid activity, as seen with the adrenogenital syndrome, Bartter syndrome, Cushing disease, and excessive licorice ingestion.

Contraction of the blood volume and profound potassium depletion may also lead to metabolic alkalosis and remain resistant to all measures except correction of the underlying abnormalities.

The symptoms and signs of marked alkalosis include neuromuscular irritability with muscle cramps, weakness, paresthesias, and tetany. Seizures and hyperreflexia usually precede cardiac arrhythmias, which are more common in the presence of hypocalcemia (low Ca^{++} concentration often accompanies metabolic alkalosis). Treatment almost never requires addition of acidic compounds but is usually directed at the underlying diseases and restoration of normal electrolyte and fluid status.

Respiratory Alkalosis. Primary disorders that lead to lower arterial P_{CO_2} involve an increase in alveolar ventilation, but the stimulus for such hyperventilation may stem from the CNS, the lungs, drugs, or other factors that stimulate breathing. In the pediatric age group, respiratory alkalosis is most commonly observed in the *hyperventilation syndrome,* which is usually a response to anxiety and is associated with tachypnea, numbness and tingling of the extremities, and other symptoms that may mimic more serious disorders. Another central cause of respiratory alkalosis is elevation of intracranial pressure; this may be seen in space-occupying lesions, head trauma, or infection. In young children and infants, hyperthermia may be sufficient to induce hyperpnea, alkalosis, and even tetany.

Pulmonary stimuli of ventilation are most frequently associated with hypoxemia. In an attempt to compensate for hypoxemia, the child increases the rate and depth of breathing, thus creating a pure respiratory alkalosis. Any type of pneumonia, pulmonary inflammation, or pulmonary edema may lead to alkalosis. Severe anemia with a resultant decrease in oxygen-carrying capacity also leads to hyperventilation and respiratory alkalosis.

Specific drugs that have been implicated in respiratory alkalosis include salicylates, paraldehyde, amphetamines, and progestational agents. Ammonia is a respiratory stimulant, and accumulation of this compound in the body tissues also leads to respiratory alkalosis (as in children with urea cycle defects or Reye syndrome).

Signs and symptoms of respiratory alkalosis are nonspecific. Treatment is based on the underlying problem; appropriate attention must be paid to associated electrolyte disturbances.

Mixed Disturbances. In clinical practice one is often faced with a combination of acid-base disturbances, and determining the primary defect or defects may not be as straightforward as the previous descriptions have made it seem. In these situations one must continually return to the basics of good medical practice and rely heavily on obtaining an adequate history and performing a thorough physical examination. Armed with these primary tools, the clinician may be able to predict acid-base abnormalities and gain valuable insight into possible causative mechanisms and then use the laboratory data to confirm or reject the proposed diagnosis. At this point in the diagnostic process, it is helpful to compare available acid-base results (pH, P_{CO_2}) with any of the nomograms mentioned previously. One may consult a chart, such as Table 25-1, to look at expected compensatory mechanisms and then decide whether the numbers "fit" into a simple disturbance. However, there are two rules that can be invaluable in evaluating simple versus mixed acid-base disturbances:

1. In a simple acid-base disturbance, the bicarbonate abnormality is *always* in the same direction as the P_{CO_2}.
2. Under most circumstances the body does not *over*compensate.

Common sense and a lot of thinking about physiology and expected changes in acid-base disorders enable the clinician to diagnose most of these problems accurately without relying on cumbersome formulas and nomograms, which are sometimes inaccessible.

Two

Fluids and Electrolytes in Clinical Practice

MAINTENANCE REQUIREMENTS

As described in previous sections, the body's numerous homeostatic mechanisms combine to orchestrate a complex balance between gains of water and electrolytes (ingested, administered, or internally generated) and obligatory losses (via kidneys, lungs, skin, and GI tract). Fortunately, the human organism is adaptable and in health can adjust easily to most conditions of excess and can tolerate limitations to a point. However, to support vital functions, maintain health, and encourage adequate growth, the body must be supplied with at least minimum amounts of water, electrolytes, nutrients, and vitamins. This chapter deals predominantly with water and solute requirements; other nutritional necessities for health maintenance are discussed in Chapter 16, One, "Nutritional Requirements."

Knowledge of fluid and salt needs is helpful in everyday pediatric practice but becomes most important in situations in which the physician is responsible for the child's intake. Notably, these situations occur when parenteral fluids are administered to a child who is unable to drink or who has experienced major losses in addition to his or her usual excretion of water and solutes.

Furthermore, familiarity with basic requirements is important when physicians attempt to determine why a child loses weight or "fails to thrive." Before one can approach the fluid therapy for any of the previously described circumstances, it is essential to understand the child's needs under usual conditions and then adjust the intervention to meet his or her altered requirements.

Water

Traditionally, the foundation for calculating water requirements has been by one of three methods: body weight, body surface area, or metabolic rate. Water need per unit of body weight changes dramatically with age and size and therefore is not very useful. Body surface area was once thought to correlate well with both metabolic expenditure and fluid needs, but this has subsequently been shown not to be the case, especially in small babies during the newborn period and in children between 6 months and 3 years of age. Additionally, surface area is determined by comparing height and weight with a nomogram, which is cumbersome and depends on accurate measurements (height is notoriously difficult to measure in young children and infants). Use of the metabolic rate to calculate fluid requirements is attractive because it is based on physiologic principles and is a constant number: approximately 100 ml (1 deciliter [dl]) of water is needed for every 100 calories consumed.

Bedside methods of measuring caloric expenditures in children have been developed. These methods are cumbersome and are not often used in clinical practice. Fortunately, adequate estimates exist to allow one to predict the caloric expenditure of a *hospitalized patient who is receiving only parenteral fluid therapy*. These values rest nearly midway between those of a normally active, healthy individual and those of a child with a basal metabolic rate (Fig. 25-4). The middle curve can be divided into three sections and caloric expenditure related to weight as follows: from 2 to 10 kg, 100 Cal/kg; from 10 to 20 kg, 50 calories for each kilogram over 10; and beyond 20 kg, 20 Cal/kg. Thus a child weighing 17 kg (hospitalized and confined to bed) would require 1350 Cal/day ([10 × 100] + [7 × 50]), and an adult weighing 70 kg would require 2500 Cal/day ([10 × 100] + [10 × 50] + [50 × 20]). It is easy to memorize these relationships, and they are useful in determining caloric needs and fluid requirements in the appropriate hospitalized patients, assuming there are no unusual heat or fluid losses and there is no net increase or loss of water, calories, or solutes.

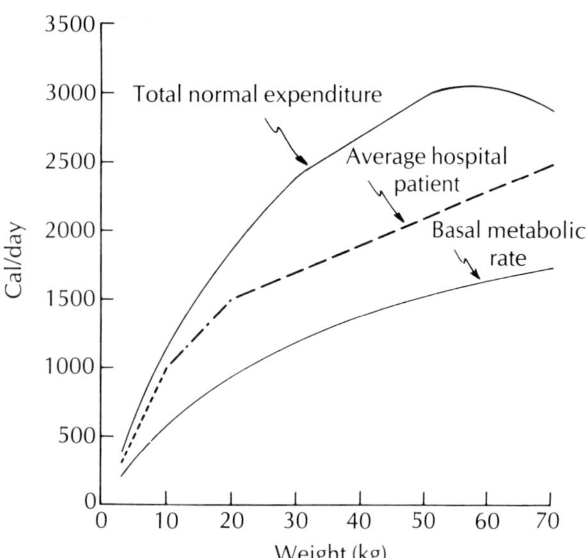

Fig. 25-4 Metabolic requirements of the average hospitalized patient. The center line represents calculated caloric requirements for average hospitalized patients. See text for explanation of the three sections of the curve.

From Winters RW, editor: The body fluids in pediatrics, Boston, 1973, Little, Brown & Co. Modified from Segar WE: Pediatrics 19:823, 1957.

The next step is to consider the usual modes of fluid and solute loss and to calculate the magnitude of these losses, relating the results to units of caloric expenditure. Fluid is lost through the kidneys along with solute, through the lungs and skin as insensible water loss, through the skin as sweat, and in stool (negligible in a hospitalized child who is receiving only parenteral fluids). Although the human kidney can excrete a relatively concentrated urine (1500 mOsm/kg water), the aim of maintenance fluid therapy is to provide enough water to allow excretion of the renal solute load (electrolytes and urea) without unduly taxing renal concentrating ability. Therefore the aim is to excrete a urine with a concentration of between 200 and 400 mOsm/kg water, which is equivalent to a specific gravity of 1.010 to 1.015. To excrete the usual renal solute load of 12 to 20 mOsm/100 Cal of expended energy at a reasonable concentration, a urine volume of between 45 and 65 ml/100 Cal, or approximately 55 ml/100 Cal, is required.

Nearly 15 ml of water is lost via the lungs for every 100 calories expended. In addition, insensible loss through the skin amounts to about 30 ml/100 Cal. Specific water loss caused by sweating varies with ambient temperature and in most cases equals less than 20 ml/100 Cal. As mentioned, stool losses can generally be ignored because, except under unusual circumstances, stool water losses rarely exceed 5 to 10 ml/100 Cal.

As the various obligatory water losses are tallied, it must be remembered that the metabolism of calories to heat and energy produces carbon dioxide and water. This "hidden" water intake is approximately 12 ml/100 Cal. Therefore, if we ignore stool losses and add fluid requirements for urine excretion (55 ml/100 Cal), insensible loss (45 ml/100 Cal), and sweat (10 to 20 ml/100 Cal), then subtract the unseen water intake (12 ml/100 Cal), the usual maintenance water requirement is approximately 1 dl for every 100 calories of energy expended.

Electrolytes

When determining maintenance solute requirements (sodium, chloride, and potassium primarily), the aim is to provide more than absolute minimum requirements but not to present the child with so much as to tax the body's excretory abilities. Because the diet of infants varies widely with respect to electrolyte concentration, the figures suggested for specific solutes represent average numbers based on usual intakes that allow optimum functioning of the organism. As with water requirements, these maintenance values can be expressed as milliequivalents per kilogram of body weight or of body surface area. However, caloric expenditure is continually used as the base of reference in this chapter.

The maintenance requirement of sodium for the average

infant is between 2 and 3 mEq/100 Cal; potassium is closer to 2 mEq/100 Cal. Because sodium and potassium are routinely supplied in the form of chloride salt, the infant or child receives between 4 and 5 mEq/100 Cal of chloride ion, although the absolute chloride requirement is probably very small. Conversely, renal excretory ability is such that this amount does not present any particular hardship under normal conditions.

Calories

In the section of this chapter dealing with total parenteral nutrition, alternatives for providing adequate calories for patients with limited oral intake are considered. For short-term administration of parenteral fluids, little consideration is usually given to trying to replace caloric expenditure, calorie per calorie. Rather, the reason for adding calories in the form of dextrose to parenteral fluids is to prevent ketosis and the breakdown of endogenous protein. In the average hospitalized patient, this requires that approximately 25% of caloric expenditure be provided with an intravenous solution that contains glucose. Therefore, the aim should be 25 Cal/100 Cal expended energy. Because each gram of dextrose provides 4 calories, this equates to 5.1 g of dextrose per 100 calories expended. For infants and small children, the absolute glucose requirement to prevent ketosis and overt hypoglycemia is between 4 and 6 mg per kg per minute.

COMPOSITION OF MAINTENANCE FLUID FOR PARENTERAL USE

To summarize the previous sections on maintenance requirements and to determine the composition of a parenteral fluid that can be administered *under normal circumstances* to hospitalized patients for a *short period* (up to several days), it should be understood that for every 100 calories expended, it is necessary to provide 1 dl water, 2 to 3 mEq sodium, 2 mEq potassium, and 5 g glucose.

Because prepared intravenous fluids are formulated on the basis of 1 liter bottles, the composition of a suitable fluid for maintenance therapy would be (values expressed per liter) 20 to 30 mEq sodium, 20 mEq potassium, and 50 g glucose.

Values of sodium in parenteral fluids are usually expressed as a fraction of "normal saline solution." Normal saline (NS) is a 0.9% solution of sodium chloride that provides 154 mEq of sodium per liter of solution. Therefore, the most commonly available prepared solutions contain either "half-normal" saline (77 mEq of sodium per liter) or "quarter-normal" saline (38 mEq of sodium per liter). Because of the body's ability to excrete any excess sodium, a solution containing quarter-normal (or 0.225%) saline is an acceptable preparation. This is usually formulated with 5% glucose (50 g/L), and to each liter one can add 20 mEq of potassium, yielding a solution that is slightly hypertonic (compared with plasma), with an osmolarity of 386 mOsm/L, but that is hypotonic with respect to sodium. It is possible to add sodium in any desired concentration to a liter of 5% dextrose in water if the need arises, but usually this is unnecessarily time consuming and expensive.

ADMINISTRATION

Once the appropriate concentration of each solute in the parenteral fluid has been determined, the solution is administered at a rate of 100 ml/100 Cal of expected energy expenditure via a peripheral vein (extremity or scalp). Procedures for gaining vascular access in children are well described in Appendix B. Although not a new method, the technique of administering fluids and medications into the bone marrow (intraosseous infusion) has recently been demonstrated to be safe and effective in providing volume replacement and resuscitation drugs in an *emergency*. It may be used in infants and children up to 3 years of age when intravenous access cannot be rapidly obtained. Techniques for performing this procedure are also found in Appendix B.

WHEN MAINTENANCE IS NOT ADEQUATE

In the preceding sections, a rational approach was developed for supplying children with maintenance fluids. Based on the physiology of his or her illness, the needs of any given child may differ considerably from these "maintenance" requirements. However, the calculations presented remain valid over a wide range of situations if used as a base to which unusual losses are added. Any and all of the organs normally involved in water homeostasis may be included: water lost through the GI tract in the form of diarrhea; massive renal excretion of water in diabetes mellitus or diabetes insipidus or following the administration of osmotic or other diuretics; excessive sweating caused by autonomic instability, fever, or high ambient temperature; and an increased loss of lung water with hyperpnea from any cause, including hyperpyrexia. Processes that do not normally contribute to water loss may also be involved, such as massive vomiting, losses via a nasogastric tube, and acute blood loss. In addition, increased demands for fluids also exist in various conditions of elevated metabolic rate (e.g., thyrotoxicosis), in situations that create large shifts in the body's fluid compartments (usually of the vascular space), and in many perioperative conditions (third spacing) that if uncorrected may produce shock.

Persistence of any of these abnormal conditions in the absence of adequate fluid intake leads to water or electrolyte deficits or both. The purpose of replacement fluid therapy is to determine a rational approach to body water and electrolyte restoration. Additionally, the fluid administration scheme so devised has to take into consideration the ongoing losses that persist beyond the institution of parenteral fluid therapy and provide appropriate replacement of these lost fluids.

There are situations in which fluids need to be supplied in amounts *below* those estimated for the average hospitalized patient. Any child with a diminished urine output because of renal failure does not require as much free water as his or her normal counterpart. Children who are placed in mist tents or maintained on ventilators lose less water through their lungs and should have a lower estimate made of insensible water loss. Children with activity levels below those predicted for most bedridden patients (e.g., those in coma or with paralysis) expend fewer calories and therefore require less water (see Fig. 25-4; water requirement is closer to that for the basal metabolic rate).

ESTIMATION AND CORRECTION OF DEFICITS AND ONGOING LOSSES

The best way to estimate fluid and electrolyte deficits is to determine how much fluid has been lost from each body compartment, the electrolyte concentration of the lost fluid, and the period of time over which such losses have occurred. In most short-term situations therapy must be initiated before all of these data can be collected. In addition, volumes of diarrheal or emetic losses may be extremely difficult to measure.

The first step in evaluating any child is to determine the severity and acuteness of the problem. For children who have a history of abnormal losses, the clinician's first priority must be to assess the *adequacy of the intravascular volume*. This is accomplished by evaluating the child's overall condition: Is he or she alert and awake, or has he or she suffered an alteration in CNS functioning (perhaps from diminished cerebral perfusion or electrolyte abnormalities, discussed later)? Are the pulses strong and full, or "thready," weak, and rapid? Is there normal blood flow to the skin or is the perfusion decreased and the skin cool and clammy? What is the quality of the skin turgor; is it normally firm and moist or has it become dry and loose, with a doughy feeling to the abdomen and "tenting" of the overlying skin when pinched lightly between the fingers? If any of these indications of impending circulatory collapse exists, it is essential to begin parenteral fluid therapy *without delay*. An intravenous line should be placed and a bolus of fluid administered (20 ml/kg of expected body weight of a solution containing approximately 150 mEq/L of sodium) as rapidly as feasible while the physician completes his or her evaluation. Once the lifesaving therapy is in progress, or if the child's vital functions appear satisfactory, the child's parent or guardian should be questioned to obtain details of the history, and a thorough physical examination (including weight and length) should be performed. It is helpful to inquire about the child's last known weight, for example, at the latest visit to his or her pediatrician. If recent, this information can help the physician decide on the degree of dehydration or volume depletion by using the following formula:

$$\text{Percent dehydration} = \frac{(\text{Expected or recent weight}) - (\text{Current weight})}{\text{Expected weight}} \times 100$$

For example, a 3-year-old child who weighed 15 kg at a well-child visit to the pediatrician 2 weeks ago and who now weighs 12 kg after 3 days of vomiting and diarrhea has lost 20% of his or her body weight:

$$\frac{(15 - 12)}{15} = \frac{3}{15} = 0.2 \times 100 = 20\%$$

When an accurate recent weight is unavailable, one may substitute predicted (average) weight for age, assuming the child is of average stature and physique (Table 25-2).

Initial evaluation of the dehydrated child should also include laboratory evaluation of the serum electrolyte concentrations and measurement of the ions contained in whatever fluid is being lost. While waiting for these laboratory results, however, it is feasible to use estimates based on the known average concentration of solutes in various body fluids (Table 25-3).

Table 25-2 *Average Weight by Age*

AGE	WEIGHT (kg) GIRL	WEIGHT (kg) BOY	CONVENIENT WEIGHT TO REMEMBER (kg)
Newborn	3.4	3.2	3
3 mo	6.0	5.9	6
6 mo	8.5	7.7	
9 mo	9.6	9.0	9
1 yr	10.8	10.0	10
2 yr	13.3	12.5	
3 yr	15.2	14.8	15
4 yr	17.3	16.9	
5 yr	19.5	19.2	20
8 yr	29.4	29.9	30
10 yr	34.9	35.5	35
15 yr	60.1	57.5	60

The approach to definitive therapy is based on the magnitude of dehydration and the estimated solute deficit. Table 25-4 describes the expected findings at various degrees of dehydration. It is important to remember that the clinical signs relate mostly to extracellular (especially *intravascular*) volume status and may not always reflect total body fluid loss accurately.

Because in many situations loss of either water or solute may predominate, the resultant dehydration may be either hypertonic or hypotonic. In hypertonic (hypernatremic) conditions, water moves out of cells and into the extracellular spaces, thus preventing (to some extent) skin turgor abnormalities and many of the other parameters that determine the clinical severity of dehydration. Therefore, to exhibit the same signs of dehydration when plasma is hypertonic, one must have lost more total fluid than when isotonic or hypotonic dehydration is present. This means that clinical assessment usually *underestimates* the magnitude of dehydration in a child who is hypernatremic. Conversely, symptoms and signs generally appear more severe in hypotonic dehydration. Therefore the table should be used to judge severity only in patients with isotonic dehydration, and adjustments should be made depending on the value of the serum sodium.

As noted previously, rehydration is accomplished in stages. Step 1 has already been mentioned: the restoration of effective circulatory volume by rapid infusion of an isotonic salt solution (normal saline or lactated Ringer solution), 20 ml/kg, if systemic blood pressure is low or if tissue perfusion is inadequate. In less severe situations one may begin with a bolus of 10 ml/kg. If this step is ineffective in improving vital signs and CNS responses, it may be repeated. Assuming that step 1 is successful, the next step is to restore ECF volume over the succeeding 24 hours. Attempts are generally made to replace 50% of the calculated deficit in the first 8 hours of this period, to restore the remaining 50% over the following 16 hours, and to continue to supply fluid for maintenance and ongoing losses. A positive response is appreciated by noting return of body weight to near baseline and gradual normalization of all the other signs, symptoms, and laboratory data.

Table 25-3 *Usual Electrolyte Composition of Abnormal Gastrointestinal Fluids*

	ELECTROLYTES (mEq/L)		
SOURCE	SODIUM	POTASSIUM	CHLORIDE
Stomach	20-80	5-20	100-150
Small intestine	100-140	5-15	90-130
Colon	10-90	10-80	10-110

Table 25-4 *Signs and Symptoms Related to Degree of Dehydration**

	DEGREE OF DEHYDRATION		
PARAMETER	MILD	MODERATE	SEVERE
Weight loss (%)†	3-5 (2-3)	10 (7)	15 (9-12)
Skin color	Pale	Gray	Mottled
Skin turgor	May be normal	Decreased	Tenting
Mucous membranes	Slightly dry	Dry	Dry, parched, collapse of sublingual veins
Eyes	Probably normal	Decreased tears	Sunken, absence of tears, soft globes
CNS	Normal	Irritable	Lethargic
Pulse			
Quality	Strong	Somewhat decreased	Distal pulse not palpable
Rate	Probably normal	Somewhat increased (orthostatic changes)	Markedly tachycardic
Capillary refill	Normal (>2 seconds)	2-4 seconds	> 4 seconds
Blood pressure	No change	Orthostatic decrease	Decreased while supine
Urine	Probably normal or slightly decreased volume	Elevated specific gravity, decreased volume	Less than 0.5 ml/kg/hr over past 12-24 hr; may be anuric

*Table is most useful for situations involving isotonic dehydration. (See text for adjustments needed for other forms of dehydration.)
†Percentage of weight loss listed applies to infants younger than 1 year of age. In older children and adults, dehydration becomes more notable with smaller losses of water (these values are listed in parentheses).

Over the following days to weeks, the third step is accomplished—replacement of intracellular potassium stores and restoration of the child's nutritional status.

At this juncture it is helpful to consider a case of isotonic dehydration (the special issues of hyponatremia and hypernatremia are discussed later).

Linda is a 4-year-old girl with no underlying health problems, who is brought to the emergency department with a 2-day history of vomiting and diarrhea. During this time she has been able to tolerate only small amounts of fluids by mouth. Her mother states that she has urinated only twice in the past 18 hours. She is irritable, but when she cries, her mother has noticed that she produces no tears. Her most recent weight, almost a year ago at her last well-child visit, was 14.5 kg. On examination she has a pulse of 140 beats/min; a systolic blood pressure of 65 mm Hg; skin that does not tent, is dry, and is pale; dry mucous membranes; and ocular globes that are not soft. Her weight is 15.8 kg. Laboratory data reveal normal sodium and potassium levels. Her blood urea nitrogen level is 36 mg/dl, and her urine specific gravity is 1.035.

This child has signs and symptoms of moderate dehydration. Although her recent weight was unknown, her weight 1 year ago was close to the average for her age; thus it may be assumed that her current weight should be close to 17 kg. This would indicate dehydration close to 7%, which correlates well with the clinical impression of moderate dehydration.

Step 1. Restoration of intravascular volume. The child is not in shock, but it would still be reasonable to administer a bolus of isotonic fluid over the first 20 to 30 minutes (10 ml/kg of ideal weight = 170 ml of normal saline solution).

Step 2. Replacement of ECF volume over the next 24 hours (to include maintenance and ongoing losses). First, the 24-hour maintenance water requirement (1 dl/100 Cal) is calculated, based on an expected caloric expenditure of:

$$(100\ \text{Cal/kg} \times 10\ \text{kg}) + (50\ \text{Cal/kg} \times 7\ \text{kg}) = 1350\ \text{Cal/day}$$

Therefore, the maintenance fluid requirement is 1350 ml/day, which is equivalent to a rate of 56 ml/hr.

Step 3. Calculation of the deficit:

$$7\%\ \text{of}\ 17\ \text{kg} = 1.19\ \text{kg}$$

which is equivalent to 1190 ml of volume lost. However, 170 ml has been already replaced, which leaves 1020 ml of deficit to be replaced over the next 24 hours. Ideally, half of the total amount should be replaced in the first 8 hours (510 ÷ 8 hr = 64 ml/hr).

Step 4. Next, addition of the maintenance rate (56 ml/hr) *to the deficit rate* (64 ml/hr) *and administration of the in-*

travenous solution at this rate (120 ml/hr) *over the next 8 hours*. Then the rate is changed so that the remainder of the solution is delivered at a rate of 88 ml/hr over the following 16 hours. Rates can be rounded to even numbers. One must monitor ongoing losses and replace those as needed, volume for volume. The child needs glucose in her fluids, since severe vomiting prohibits any oral intake initially. Therefore, although she should have a solution close in concentration to isotonic saline, a hypertonic solution is not advisable; thus, her intravenous solution should be changed from normal saline to 5% dextrose in water (D_5W), containing 77 mEq/L of sodium chloride (half-normal saline solution), and it should be given at the rate determined. *Potassium should not be added until an adequate urine output is certain*. Serum electrolytes, urine output, and vital signs need to be determined at regular intervals, and the fluid therapy (content and rate of administration) should be adjusted as necessary. The volume and electrolyte content of any parenteral medications administered should be considered in these calculations (many pharmaceutical preparations, especially antibiotics, have a high concentration of either potassium or sodium).

In general, two approaches to replacement therapy exist: one is to calculate the water deficit and assume isotonic losses (except in the case of extreme hypernatremia) as in the example just given; the second is to calculate specific solute needs and determine a precise formula for rehydration and repletion of electrolyte concentrations.

Solute deficit is determined by calculating the total numbers of milliequivalents required and is accomplished through the use of a formula into which one must substitute values for patient weight, current electrolyte concentrations, and a plasma "distribution factor" (fraction of the body water in which the substance is distributed). However, these measurements and calculations are only helpful when dealing with predominantly extracellular electrolyte particles; they are useless in determining potassium deficiency. Table 25-5 lists normal values, distribution factors, and the desired concentration most commonly used in estimating the deficits (these usually correspond to the lower end of normal values).

The formula used to calculate solute deficit is:

$$\text{Deficit (mEq)} = \text{Body weight (kg)} \times [\text{Desired concentration (mEq/L)} - \text{Actual concentration (mEq/L)}] \times \text{Distribution factor}$$

For example, the total sodium deficit in a 10 kg child with a serum sodium concentration of 123 mEq/L is 10 kg × (12 mEq/L) × (0.6) = 72 mEq of sodium, which should be replaced similarly to water—half the deficit in the first 8 hours and the remainder in the following 16 hours.

Similar calculations can be performed for bicarbonate and chloride, and a final fluid and electrolyte prescription can be written. Only half the calculated bicarbonate deficit is replaced during the first 24 hours as a precaution against too rapid a correction, which might lead to alkalosis.

The case of dehydration presented earlier should be reconsidered and the following information added: the serum sodium concentration (125 mEq/L) and the serum bicarbonate (12 mEq/L). With this formula, the child's electrolyte deficits can be calculated as follows:

$$\text{Sodium deficit} = 17\text{ kg} \times (135\text{ mEq/L} - 125\text{ mEq/L}) \times 0.6 = 102\text{ mEq}$$

However, we gave 26 mEq of sodium in our initial bolus of saline solution, leaving a residual deficit of 76 mEq.

$$\text{Bicarbonate deficit} = 17\text{ kg} \times (15\text{ mEq/L} - 12\text{ mEq/L}) \times 0.5 = 25\text{ mEq}$$

The water deficit is unchanged from the previous calculation. Therefore, in the first 8 hours she needs to receive 960 ml of water—half her deficit (510 ml) plus one-third daily maintenance (450 ml)—in which are dissolved 38 mEq of sodium and 12 mEq of bicarbonate (one-half deficit) with additional sodium to equal one third of the maintenance requirements (approximately 3 mEq/kg/day), or 17 mEq. The formula would then call for mixing 1 liter of D_5W with 43 mEq of sodium chloride and 12 mEq of sodium bicarbonate and administering this solution at the previously described rate.

Toward the end of the first 8 hours of rehydration therapy a recalculation of solute deficit must be performed, based on the current values of electrolyte concentrations. It is particularly important to remember that bicarbonate deficits are often corrected much more quickly than predicted. Therefore, to avoid producing an "overshoot" alkalosis when administering bicarbonate, its serum concentration must be carefully monitored.

THERAPEUTIC APPROACH TO SPECIAL SITUATIONS

Shock

Severe plasma volume deficit, with actual or impending cardiovascular collapse, is a life-threatening pediatric emergency, requiring *immediate* action; initial therapy is as above, replacing the intravascular volume depletion with *whatever appropriate solution is most available*. In most hospitals this

Table 25-5 *Values Required to Calculate Solute Deficits in Children*

SOLUTE	NORMAL CONCENTRATION RANGE (mEq/L)	DESIRED CORRECTED CONCENTRATION (mEq/L)	DISTRIBUTION FACTOR
Sodium	135-145	135	0.5-0.7
Chloride	100-106	100	0.2-0.3
Bicarbonate	24-30 20-26 (neonates)	15	0.4-0.5

would be either a normal saline or lactated Ringer solution; the latter formulation contains small amounts of potassium and calcium as well as base in the form of lactate. The utility of the lactate requires the liver to be able to convert it to bicarbonate. In the presence of severe lactic acidosis, which may accompany hypoxia and markedly diminished tissue perfusion, the administration of lactate may be harmful and actually worsen the metabolic acidosis. Hemorrhagic shock, which must be considered with any history of trauma or any possible internal source of bleeding (e.g., a known peptic ulcer or other gastrointestinal disease that might lead to acute blood loss), must be treated with administration of packed red blood cells. This is because administering additional electrolyte solutions to a patient with an already diminished hematocrit further decreases oxygen-carrying capacity and may result in irreversible damage to vital organs (especially the heart and brain). Therefore most hospital blood banks keep a fairly ready supply of type O blood, which should be infused as rapidly as possible once the diagnosis of hemorrhagic shock has been considered. A sample of the patient's blood (obtained *before* transfusion) should be sent to the blood bank so that a properly matched unit of donor blood can be obtained without delay in case it is needed for further therapy. Also, if the patient's blood type is known, one may administer type-specific noncross-matched blood, which carries less risk than the use of O noncross-matched blood. While awaiting the arrival of blood from the blood bank, normal saline or lactated Ringer solution should be given as noted previously. The use of colloid-containing plasma expanders such as albumin or dextran remains controversial and probably provides no benefit over the use of a crystalloid solution unless shock is on the basis of protein loss. Additionally, if shock is cardiogenic, administration of albumin may worsen pulmonary edema. In sepsis, where volume depletion is caused by leaky capillaries and exudation of plasma into extravascular spaces, fresh-frozen plasma may be useful (since it also replaces many clotting factors) and is sometimes used in combination with other fluids.

Shock in babies and small children is almost invariably associated with depletion of glycogen stores. Thus hypoglycemia may often complicate the picture. Administration of 2 to 4 ml/kg of a 25% dextrose solution will correct hypoglycemia and improve the results of further resuscitation efforts. For this reason, rapid bedside determination of blood glucose concentration should always be part of the initial evaluation of the infant or child in shock (current or impending).

Serious Electrolyte Abnormalities

Sodium. The most commonly encountered pediatric electrolyte aberrations relate to sodium balance, and they ordinarily occur with dehydration. However, there is a wide range of possibilities to be considered. It is probably most convenient to consider the clinical conditions of hyponatremia and hypernatremia, for they pertain to both the patient's volume status and plasma osmolality.

Hyponatremia. Hyponatremia is usually associated with hypotonicity. When it is not, the clinician must suspect either artifactual lowering of the serum sodium such as with hyperlipidemia and hyperproteinemia as described earlier or the presence of an osmotically active substance such as glucose or mannitol. These compounds cause a shift of intracellular water into the extracellular space to restore osmotic neutrality, thereby lowering effective serum sodium by 1.6 mEq/L for every 100 mg/dl rise in serum glucose or mannitol concentration. Such situations are almost universally associated with preservation of intravascular volume (except in some extreme cases of diabetic ketoacidosis) and are often apparent from the history, physical examination, or a few simple laboratory tests.

The most common clinical situation leading to hyponatremia is volume loss, usually caused by diarrhea, in which the child has lost fluid with a sodium concentration higher than that of the serum. If ongoing diarrheal losses are replaced with hypotonic fluids, hyponatremia will develop, even if the volume deficit is not great. Sodium-rich fluid is also lost from the intravascular space when ascites or other abnormal accumulations of fluid occupy a body cavity. This phenomenon is known as *third spacing* and is discussed fully in this chapter in a later section on perioperative fluid management.

When volume status is normal, one must consider situations that lead to a combination of sodium loss with water intake sufficient to maintain usual hydration. Such negative sodium balance can result from severe restriction of sodium intake or profound loss of sodium via the skin, GI tract, or kidneys (salt-losing nephropathy or diuretic use).

Mild hyponatremia (serum sodium 128 to 134 mEq/dl) with normovolemia or hypovolemia can be managed by providing isotonic sodium solutions with adequate fluid administration, thereby allowing excretion of water at an appropriate rate. It is important in these circumstances to replace ongoing losses with the correct solution (i.e., measure electrolyte concentration of the fluid lost and infuse fluid of that concentration milliliter for milliliter) so that the patient's sodium concentration returns to normal. When there are simultaneous large deficits of both water and saline solution, it is important to replace both effectively; the usual normal saline solution is sufficient at the outset.

Severe potassium depletion, sometimes overlooked, may lead to persistent hyponatremia. Because potassium is the major intracellular cation, sodium ions enter the cells to replace potassium ions to provide electric neutrality; therefore, the concentration of sodium in the extracellular space may fall. Potassium must then be supplied to allow the restoration of normal sodium balance.

More rapid correction of the sodium deficit is necessary with serious symptoms (seizures), which may accompany a large or precipitous decline in serum sodium concentration. This can be achieved through the administration of 3% saline solution (containing 500 mEq of sodium per liter), which allows rapid replacement of sodium without infusing a large volume of water.

The sodium deficit is calculated as detailed previously, but half the calculated deficit should be administered rapidly to try to resolve the seizure activity. *Once the seizures have abated, the infusion should be stopped.* If seizures continue for 10 or 15 minutes beyond the end of the initial infusion, a second serum sodium value should be determined and the remainder of the deficit replaced (without necessarily knowing what the repeat value is before administering the rest of the sodium solution). It is presumed that this rapid infusion of hypertonic saline solution eases convulsions by reversing the cerebral edema that developed when, because of extracellular hyponatremia, water moved into the brain cells in an attempt to restore osmotic neutrality. Osmotic equilibrium is rapidly established once intravascular tonicity is restored, because sodium is distributed quickly throughout all body fluid compartments. Intravenous administration of hypertonic sodium chloride solutions is not without risk to the patient, however, especially one with cardiac or renal disease. Such infusions cause a rapid shift of water into the intravascular space and may lead to acute volume overload. Such therapy must therefore be reserved for potentially life-threatening situations.

When hyponatremia exists with expanded vascular volume, the most likely cause is excessive secretion of ADH, which may occur because of increased intracranial pressure, severe pneumonia, or the stress of certain surgical procedures. The diagnosis of SIADH is made on the basis of laboratory and physical examination data and requires the presence of hyponatremia with normal or increased intravascular volume (the diagnosis *cannot* be made if the patient has an adequate intravascular volume) and a urine osmolality that is less than maximally dilute. Sodium excretion in the urine is variable but is usually higher than expected for the level of serum sodium concentration. Treatment of this disorder, whatever the cause, consists of *fluid restriction* and not sodium administration unless the patient is convulsing. Some authors have urged the simultaneous use of a potent diuretic such as furosemide, which is expected to induce the loss of more water than sodium. In most cases, however, fluid restriction remains the safest and most efficacious mode of therapy. Once the sodium concentration returns to near normal, moderate fluid restriction (generally to two thirds of maintenance requirements) may need to be continued, usually for at least 24 hours, but sometimes for as long as the underlying disorder continues.

Hypernatremia. As with decreased serum sodium concentration, hypernatremia may occur with overhydration, dehydration, or normal hydration. However, unlike hyponatremia, an elevated serum sodium level is *always* associated with hypertonicity.

Hypernatremia associated with overhydration is generally an iatrogenic problem created by (1) administering intravenous or oral solutions with high salt content and (2) not providing the requisite free water. Patients treated with large amounts of sodium bicarbonate for metabolic acidosis are also at risk of developing marked hypernatremia (there is approximately 1 mEq of sodium for every milliliter of bicarbonate solution administered). Occasionally, when infant formulas are being mixed, mistakes occur that result in markedly hypertonic solutions that may induce particularly severe hypernatremias. These patients are all at risk of developing obvious signs of plasma volume overload, including hypertension, congestive heart failure, and pulmonary edema.

Under such circumstances, administration of additional fluid is risky and may prove to be fatal. The most rational approach is to limit sodium and water input and attempt to induce sodium loss to a greater extent than water. This may be accomplished by the use of a potent loop diuretic such as furosemide, which will induce a net sodium loss if the child's renal function is adequate. One must concurrently watch closely for the development of dehydration, as it is impossible to predict precisely how much water and sodium will be lost. Generally, some portions of the induced urine output (50% to 75%) should be replaced with intravenous fluid that is slightly hypotonic (i.e., 66% or 75% normal saline solution) until normal hydration and tonicity have been achieved. In patients with *severe* hypernatremia (ordinarily considered as a serum sodium value over 155 or 160 mEq/L), severe complications may occur if the sodium concentration falls too rapidly. This action produces marked shifts of extracellular water to the intracellular space and results in cellular swelling. This is most worrisome in the CNS because cerebral edema may occur, which may lead to seizures, coma, or death. Therefore, when the serum sodium value is high and is accompanied by overhydration, the preferred therapeutic approach is to restrict sodium and water, thus permitting a spontaneous diuresis to occur. Serum electrolyte values must be monitored every few hours. If the patient has substantially decreased renal function, hemodialysis or peritoneal dialysis should be considered, especially in the presence of hypertension or pulmonary edema.

Hypernatremia associated with decreased plasma volume is encountered frequently in pediatric practice. It is caused most commonly by acute gastroenteritis that induces relatively larger losses of water than sodium. Although these children may have severe hypernatremia, their total body sodium content is usually depleted; they therefore present quite a therapeutic challenge.

Evaluation of patients with this condition requires careful attention to detail. The physician must consider all the aspects of dehydration previously discussed but must remember that because ECF volume is relatively well preserved, he or she may seriously underestimate the severity of the plasma volume loss. Even with *significant* fluid losses, these children rarely have signs of incipient vascular collapse. When using the signs and symptoms of dehydration shown in Table 25-4 to determine the degree of dehydration, if the serum sodium concentration is over 155 mEq/L, another 3% to 5% should be added to the predicted degree of dehydration.

Fluid therapy of hypernatremia dehydration is not nearly as straightforward as for other types of dehydration, since the risk of creating major fluid shifts and cerebral edema is great. One cannot simply try to remove sodium, since a decrease in the plasma tonicity without an increase in plasma water may induce circulatory collapse. Therefore, a cautious rehydration scheme must be developed.

Instead of being rehydrated over a 24-hour period, as with isonatremic or hyponatremic dehydration, the child with a serum sodium over 155 mEq/L should have his or her fluid deficit replaced over 48 to 72 hours. It is *not* possible to calculate the actual amount of sodium lost. The physician should estimate the water deficit (based on weight and clinical signs) and plan to replace that volume evenly over 48 to 72 hours. The solution used should be *slightly hyponatremic* (containing 100 to 120 mEq of sodium per liter). Glucose should be added so that the solution is not hypotonic. As soon as the urine output is judged to be adequate, potassium should be added to the intravenous solution to correct the potassium deficit and to preserve the intracellular osmolality, thus helping to prevent intracellular edema. It is particularly important to monitor serum electrolyte concentrations, serum osmolality, and urine output and osmolality as frequently as possible. Although one needs to avoid a persistent elevation of the serum sodium concentration, it is also important to ensure a slow, steady decline in the serum sodium and osmolality levels. Decreases in serum tonicity should be limited to a rate of 5 mOsm/hr. In many cases it is possible to add up to 40 mEq of potassium per liter to the infused solution and thereby reduce its sodium concentration to 50 mEq/L.

Sometimes, no matter how carefully hypernatremia is handled, seizures ensue during the rehydration period. They can usually be managed successfully by infusing a solution slightly more hypertonic than the one being given (i.e., normal saline or lactated Ringer solution). If the seizures are particularly severe, or if there is evidence of brain herniation, the use of a hypertonic agent such as mannitol may be required. Unfortunately, the diuresis induced by mannitol may substantially worsen the dehydration. Also, mannitol should *not* be used if urine output has not been established.

A relatively uncommon cause of hypernatremia is diabetes insipidus, which usually is evident as hypernatremia with a normal plasma volume. This presupposes an intact thirst mechanism and that the patient has access to the large volume of water required to replace renal losses. Such is not the case for small babies and certain other patients with diabetes insipidus who have hypernatremic dehydration. Large renal losses of free water may occur because of deficient ADH (central or pituitary diabetes insipidus) or impairment of the normal renal response to the hormone (nephrogenic diabetes insipidus).

In infants and children the most common cause of central diabetes insipidus is a brain tumor, such as a craniopharyngioma. The syndrome may also follow intracranial surgical procedures or trauma. Other causes include CNS diseases of vascular, infectious, or granulomatous origin or histiocytosis. The familial form of central diabetes insipidus accounts for fewer than 1% of all cases. Probably 50% of adult patients with diabetes insipidus remain classified as *idiopathic;* that percentage is much lower in children.

Nephrogenic diabetes insipidus may be evident as a congenital disorder, but more commonly it is secondary to renal failure (particularly that caused by obstructive uropathy) or to electrolyte disorders, drug ingestions, or sickle cell disease. Laboratory findings in diabetes insipidus usually include a moderate to marked hypernatremia (depending on how adequately the lost fluid volume has been replaced) and dilute urine, usually produced in large volumes. Clinically these patients exhibit a tremendous thirst (often craving ice-cold water) and, as already mentioned, usually show signs of normal hydration. The laboratory differentiation between central and nephrogenic diabetes insipidus is unnecessary when the cause is apparent (e.g., after surgical removal of a craniopharyngioma) but in other situations is essential to help guide the therapeutic approach. This determination is generally accomplished by performing a "water deprivation test." Water is withheld from the patient until approximately 3% of the body weight has been lost, until three consecutive hourly urine samples show no further increase in osmolality, or until the serum osmolality reaches 295 mOsm. Although in the adult patient the desired effects may take 10 to 12 hours to become manifest, a child with complete central diabetes insipidus may become notably dehydrated in just a few hours. Therefore, throughout the period of water deprivation, the child must be watched carefully with (1) frequent monitoring of vital signs, (2) hourly monitoring of urine volume and osmolality, and (3) measurement of serum electrolyte concentrations and osmolality every 1 to 2 hours.

When the end point is reached, a normal person exhibits maximum urinary concentration with a marked fall of urinary output but little change in the serum sodium concentration. A patient with either total central diabetes insipidus or nephrogenic diabetes insipidus exhibits little change in urinary concentration or flow but develops an elevated serum sodium concentration and a high serum osmolality. A slight increase in urine concentrating ability that stabilizes at a fairly low level (but substantially higher than when the patient is well hydrated) indicates probable incomplete central diabetes insipidus. If further resolution of the problem is necessary, subcutaneous injection of aqueous vasopressin (5 units in adults) is performed, and the urine output and concentration are followed hourly. No further change is seen in normal individuals who had previously concentrated their urine maximally (i.e., already had high circulating levels of ADH). Also, patients with nephrogenic diabetes insipidus show no decrease in urine volume or elevation of urine osmolality following the vasopressin injection because the defect lies in the kidneys' inability to respond to ADH. Patients with complete or partial central diabetes insipidus respond with a dramatic rise in their renal concentrating function. It cannot be overly stressed that *although the water deprivation test is useful, it is also dangerous and requires the utmost care, with close observation of the patient and knowledge of resuscitation maneuvers. The advice and supervision of a pediatric endocrinologist should be sought if there are any concerns.*

Treatment of diabetes insipidus requires an accurate diagnosis and the ability to monitor the patient carefully. Postoperative central diabetes insipidus may be transient and can therefore be treated by replacing urinary losses of water and sodium. If the volume needed exceeds the physician's ability to replace it (mostly an intravenous access problem), if the condition continues for more than several days, or if the patient had signs of diabetes insipidus preoperatively, the most rational approach is hormonal replacement. In the past this was accomplished by using intramuscular vasopressin tannate in oil (a difficult product to deal with and one with an unreliably predictable half-life) or subcutaneous aqueous vasopressin (Pitressin), but this has a short half-life and needs to be repeated every 2 to 3 hours. The most recent development in ADH replacement therapy has been the production of a synthetic analog of vasopressin—1-desamino-8-D-arginine-vasopressin (DDAVP)—that can be administered intranasally or intravenously. It has a long half-life and reaches peak activity within the first 30 minutes. The dose and schedule are adapted to the patient's response. The recommended starting dose is 0.3 μg/kg intravenously or 0.05 to 0.3 ml (5 to 30 μg) intranasally administered once or twice daily. The intranasal preparation can be used as easily in the hospital as in the home and is relatively free of side effects. It is effective for both partial and complete central diabetes insipidus.

Nephrogenic diabetes insipidus is more difficult to treat and generally requires chronic provision of adequate fluid volume, unless the underlying abnormality can be corrected. This is usually not a problem as long as the patient has an intact thirst mechanism and fluid is readily available. Some success has been achieved with diuretic therapy in association with low sodium intake to prevent hypernatremia. Also, prostaglandins may be useful in reducing the urine volume.

Potassium

Hypokalemia. Symptoms of hypokalemia were discussed in the sections on solute homeostasis. A low serum potassium concentration seldom represents an emergency unless cardiac effects are seen, and this does not typically occur until the concentration is less than 2 mEq/L. In patients receiving digitalis preparations, however, a combined cardiac toxicity may ensue, and the typical T wave changes and arrhythmias of hypokalemia may occur at serum potassium levels closer to normal. Other patients at risk of exhibiting an exaggerated response to mild hypokalemia include those with an acid-base disturbance or other ionic aberration that may create a cardiac conduction disturbance by substantially altering the flux of ions between the intracellular and extracellular spaces. At particular risk of developing such alterations are children receiving long-term diuretic therapy. Hypokalemia may occur following large losses of potassium from the GI tract during treatment for diabetic ketoacidosis and as a manifestation of hyperaldosteronism.

When emergency therapy for hypokalemia is necessary (in the situations just mentioned and in the *preoperative patient with a serum potassium concentration less than 3.5 mEq/L*), intravenous potassium repletion should be implemented. This is accomplished either by increasing the concentration of potassium ion in the fluids given intravenously (maximum of 80 mEq/L) or by administering a bolus of potassium into a central vein. The maximum amount of potassium that may be given is 1 mEq/kg over a 1-hour period (with the physician at the bedside and continuous electrocardiographic monitoring), but it is generally safer to deliver only 20% or 25% of that amount and to repeat the dose as necessary to raise the concentration to a safe level.

Hyperkalemia. Substantial elevations of serum potassium concentration are most frequently encountered with renal failure or systemic acidosis, combined with an increased intake of potassium or a rapid breakdown of tissue or blood products.

When the potassium concentration reaches 8 mEq/L or more, the child is in grave danger of cardiac toxicity. Such a patient should have continuous electrocardiographic monitoring, and immediate steps should be taken to *protect the heart from the effects of severe hyperkalemia*. The first priority is the infusion of intravenous calcium, 0.2 ml/kg of 10% calcium chloride given over 2 to 5 minutes. This should be followed by the administration of sodium bicarbonate (2 to 3 mEq/kg given within a 30-minute period) to raise the serum pH level and help move the potassium into cells, thereby decreasing (transiently) the intravascular potassium concentration. Simultaneously, or immediately following the above steps, one should infuse a mixture of glucose and insulin, which also induces movement of potassium ions from the extracellular to the intracellular spaces. This accelerates the usual process by which glucose moves into the cells and is converted to glycogen. A dose of 2 ml/kg of a 25% glucose solution is given along with 1 U/kg of regular insulin. This solution may be administered over 30 minutes and repeated as necessary.

Once these lifesaving measures have been instituted, attention must be given to removing potassium from the body. One of the most effective means of accomplishing this is with hemodialysis or peritoneal dialysis. One or the other should be initiated without delay in patients with hyperkalemia accompanied by congestive heart failure and volume overload. The other commonly used mechanism for removing potassium from the body is to bind potassium in the GI tract by using an exchange resin such as sodium polystyrene sulfonate (Kayexalate). This is usually introduced through a retention enema containing sorbitol. One can expect a decline in serum potassium of 1 mEq/g of resin introduced. The dose is calculated on the basis of the severity of the hyperkalemia, but the usual adult dose does not exceed 60 g. Caution should be used in patients with renal failure, because sodium is absorbed as potassium is excreted and each gram of resin contains 4.1 mEq of sodium. Therefore, hypernatremia and hypervolemia may result. Additionally, one must monitor the patient for the development of hypocalcemia and hypomagnesemia. Metabolic alkalosis may result from repeated polystyrene sulfonate enemas. When hyperkalemia becomes a chronic but not life-threatening problem, the best approach is concomitantly to restrict dietary potassium and administer potassium-losing diuretics.

Calcium

Hypercalcemia. A serum calcium concentration over 15 mg/dl constitutes a medical emergency but is rarely seen in pediatric patients. Signs and symptoms of acute hypercalcemia intoxication were reviewed earlier in this chapter. Therapy should be aimed at bringing the total calcium concentration below 12 mg/dl. If urine output is adequate, one should rapidly administer intravenous normal saline solution at a rate of 20 to 30 ml/kg over several hours. This may be combined with the use of thiazide diuretics, which increase calcium excretion through the kidneys. In addition, it is essential to eliminate as much calcium from the diet as is feasible and to restrict the gastrointestinal absorption of calcium by administering a corticosteroid preparation. Patients unresponsive to these procedures may benefit from rectal administration of a Fleet enema that contains phosphorus. In children with substantially impaired renal function, hemodialysis may be the only solution.

Hypocalcemia. When hypocalcemia is symptomatic, it requires immediate treatment with the intravenous administration of a calcium salt. The most commonly used preparations are calcium gluceptate and calcium gluconate. The solution chosen should be given in a dose of 0.5 mEq/kg or 10 mg of elemental calcium per kilogram (approximately 1 ml/kg of calcium gluconate). *Whenever calcium is provided intravenously, the cardiac rate and rhythm must be continuously monitored, since notable bradycardia may occur with an abrupt rise of the ionized fraction of calcium.*

Sick neonates may benefit from the continuous administration of intravenous calcium to prevent substantial declines in the calcium concentration. This should be provided at a rate of 2 to 4 mEq/kg/day. The intravenous access site must be checked frequently because extravasated calcium causes striking necrosis of the subcutaneous tissues.

THERAPY OF CLINICAL ACID-BASE DISORDERS

Metabolic Acidosis

Previous sections have touched on the approach to the life-threatening problem of metabolic acidosis, but its importance demands reconsideration. As already described, a pH level lower than 7.2 requires immediate therapy. This task has traditionally been accomplished by calculating a bicarbonate deficit as

$$\text{Weight in kilograms} \times (\text{Desired concentration} - \text{Actual concentration}) \times \text{Volume of distribution}$$

where the desired concentration is 15 mEq/L and the volume of distribution is between 0.4 and 0.6 (0.5 is used mostly for younger children, 0.4 for those over 1 year of age). As noted in the section on dehydration, only half the calculated deficit is administered, and the acid-base status is reevaluated several hours later because in the absence of persistent acid production, the deficit is usually overestimated if this formula is used.

The most important element to remember in bicarbonate replacement is that *it is essential to follow serial electrolyte values and adjust the therapy accordingly*. Again, the complications of bicarbonate therapy include hypokalemia (with a lessening of acid environment, potassium is shifted back into the cells); hyponatremia; volume overload; and, occasionally, tetany (caused by improved binding of calcium to protein, with a subsequent decline of the ionized fraction of calcium). As mentioned previously, overly rapid correction of the blood pH level may result in CNS acidosis and cerebral edema. Although it may not always be possible to prevent such iatrogenic developments, the clinician must remain aware that even well-intentioned therapy may include undesirable results. Therefore, such therapy should never be undertaken lightly or when the patient cannot be adequately observed and emergency measures taken if indicated.

There are some occasions when bicarbonate administration is contraindicated. Patients suffering from congestive heart failure may not be able to tolerate the rapid expansion of intravascular volume that accompanies the administration of sodium bicarbonate. Bicarbonate infusion in children with ventilatory insufficiency may actually cause a decline in the level of plasma pH. Neonates may be adversely affected by the elevation of plasma osmolality. Such patients may benefit from an organic amine buffer, tris-(hydroxymethyl)aminomethane (THAM), also known as TRIS, or tromethamine. It induces a rapid decline of P_{CO_2} by metabolizing carbonic acid to bicarbonate.

THAM is available as a 3.6% solution with a pH level of 10. The total dose in milliliters to be administered is the base deficit multiplied by the weight in kilograms. This dose should be spread over 1 or more hours, with 25% administered in the initial few minutes and the remainder given slowly with ongoing monitoring of serum pH levels and electrolyte concentrations. Important and possibly fatal complications associated with the use of THAM include hypoglycemia, induction of a marked diuresis, and apnea from a sudden decline of P_{CO_2}. Therefore, these parameters must be monitored frequently throughout the period of therapy. It is recommended that THAM be used only in situations where administration of sodium bicarbonate is clearly contraindicated.

Respiratory Acidosis

When respiratory acidosis is severe (pH level less than 7 and/or P_{CO_2} greater than 55), the best mode of therapy is intubation and hyperventilation, unless the patient suffers from chronic respiratory failure, in which the effects of an elevated P_{CO_2} are well compensated for by an increased serum bicarbonate level, resulting in a normal or nearly normal pH. The use of bicarbonate should be avoided until adequate excretion of the generated carbon dioxide is ensured. Formulas and mechanisms to determine appropriate ventilator settings are beyond the scope of this text. When treating acidosis with assisted ventilation, it is essential to observe the patient's preintubation rate and depth of breathing. The use of standard rates and tidal volumes may seriously compromise the patient and be less efficient than no such intervention. Once an artificial airway and assisted ventilation are established, arterial blood gases must be determined within 15 minutes.

Because respirator-provided air is humidified, the patient's water maintenance requirements need adjustment. As described earlier, the typical hospitalized child loses up to 15 ml/100 Cal/day via the respiratory tract. Because specific amounts of water delivered by the ventilator vary in different systems and mucosal absorption varies according to the nature of the child's illness, it is impossible to predict accurately the magnitude of the reduction in water maintenance required. Therefore, it is reasonable to reduce fluid administration by approximately 10%, assuming *all other variables remain the same*, but to follow the patient's weight and serum electrolyte levels closely. In rare cases, in very small babies and in those persons with severe inflammatory disease of the airways, there may actually be a *net gain* of water through respiratory tract absorption, which may lead to water intoxication and hyponatremia.

Metabolic and Respiratory Alkalosis

As already mentioned, metabolic and respiratory alkaloses generally do not require specific therapy but respond to treatment of the underlying abnormalities. Most important in the clinical approach to alkalosis is the recognition of concomitant electrolyte aberrations such as hypokalemia, hypocalcemia, and hypochloremia.

CLINICAL FLUID PROBLEMS INVOLVING GLUCOSE METABOLISM

The serum glucose should be measured in all seriously ill children, especially youngsters less than 1 year of age, who are particularly prone to hypoglycemia. Because this topic is covered in detail in Chapter 281, "Hypoglycemia," specific issues of diagnosis and therapy are not considered here. To be successful in fluid management, baseline caloric needs (to prevent ketosis) must be provided. The requirements of a patient who needs long periods of maintenance fluid therapy are discussed later in this chapter in the section on parenteral nutrition.

Diabetic ketoacidosis, with notable hyperglycemia, is associated with a myriad of other fluid and solute abnormalities. The diagnosis must always be considered with a child who is in coma of undetermined cause. The approach to this complicated problem is also presented in Chapter 271, "Diabetic Ketoacidosis."

PERIOPERATIVE FLUID MANAGEMENT AND THE CONCEPT OF THIRD SPACING

The outcome of a surgical procedure depends on intraoperative events and the nature of the child's illness. Also of major importance is the preoperative status of the patient. Recognized only within the last half century is the concept that the presence of hypovolemia or hypervolemia in the preoperative patient may adversely affect outcome.

Any child having routine elective surgery should have his or her fluid status evaluated 12 to 24 hours before the scheduled surgery. Most healthy children have intravascular volume and electrolyte concentrations at the proper levels. However, the preoperative assessment should always include an estimation of hydration status on physical examination and measurement of urine specific gravity. It is imperative to obtain an accurate preoperative weight for calculating maintenance fluid requirements and drug dosages and for helping in the assessment of postoperative changes in fluid balance. Any child who has had vomiting, diarrhea, or a substantial limitation of oral intake in the 72-hour period preceding surgery will benefit from the measurement of serum electrolyte concentrations. Young babies (especially neonates) should have their glucose and calcium concentrations measured preoperatively. If a substantially abnormal balance of water or solute is discovered, the operative procedure should be delayed until the identified problem has been corrected. Preoperative hypovolemia induced by a prolonged period of restricted fluid intake may cause a small child to exhibit notable difficulties following surgery. The neonate or young infant who must remain without oral intake for longer than 4 to 6 hours should have an intravenous line placed and maintenance fluids administered.

A more complicated situation exists when an ill child requires immediate surgery. In such cases, initial steps should be taken to restore normal fluid status before inducing anesthesia. Fluid balance restoration should continue during the intraoperative and postoperative periods. Optimum care depends on frequent and detailed communication among pediatrician, surgeon, and anesthesiologist.

In some cases fluid losses are relatively easy to estimate (e.g., gastric outlet obstruction with subsequent vomiting). However, in any situation in which third spacing is likely to occur, losses from the intravascular space may be grossly underestimated. *Third spacing* is the term given to any situation in which there is movement of intravascular fluid into any of the potential or real spaces of the body. It may occur in all conditions associated with tissue injury that result in the formation of edema, a collection of extracellular, extravascular fluid having the electrolyte composition of plasma. Third space losses may be particularly marked in patients suffering from peritonitis, bowel obstruction, tissue ischemia or necrosis, perforation of an intraabdominal viscus, major crush injuries of the extremities, or ascites. Some degree of third spacing accompanies even simple uncomplicated surgical procedures. Generally, movement of fluid into tissues is preceded by movement of plasma proteins, blood, or pus. Therefore fluid is retained in the extravascular space because of the elevation of tissue oncotic pressure. As healing occurs, extravascular oncotic pressure diminishes, capillary integrity is restored, and fluid returns to the intravascular space. This generally occurs between 48 and 72 hours following the injury.

The initial evaluation of a child at risk of developing notable third space losses must include consideration of the specific disease entity involved and the duration of the problem before fluid therapy is initiated. If the child is adequately hydrated when first seen, fluids can be administered at a rate of one and one-half to two times the maintenance requirement. If the underlying process has been ongoing for several hours or more, the patient will almost certainly be volume depleted and may require large amounts of a physiologic electrolyte solution (normal saline or lactated Ringer solution). Occasionally such children also require administration of albumin or plasma to restore intravascular oncotic pressure. Failure to provide an adequate circulating fluid volume preoperatively may result in profound shock once anesthesia is induced.

Preoperative assessment in particularly severe cases may require the use of invasive monitoring techniques. Central venous pressures may help determine the adequacy of preload while enabling large volumes of fluid to be administered rapidly when necessary. An indwelling arterial line permits continuous monitoring of the blood pressure while permitting easy access for frequent arterial blood gas determination. A balloon-tipped, flow-directed pulmonary artery (Swan-Ganz) catheter permits evaluation of the patient's cardiac output and calculation of oxygen consumption, which is of paramount importance in the child with significant shock. The use of any of these monitoring modalities generally requires placement of the patient in an intensive care unit.

Intraoperative control of the child's fluid volume status is generally the responsibility of the anesthesiologist, who must also ensure for the patient adequate ventilation, oxygenation, temperature control, analgesia, immobility, and muscle relaxation. Decisions regarding fluid needs made during surgery depend on many complex variables, the discussion of which is beyond the scope of this chapter. Paramount are the adjustments required to maintain vital signs and urine output within the normal range. Blood losses should be replaced if they constitute 5% or more of the patient's calculated blood volume. If tissue perfusion or oxygenation is diminished, a transfusion may be necessary even if blood losses are minimal.

Postoperatively, communication between the surgeon and the pediatrician becomes essential because the postoperative fluid management depends on both the events that transpired in the operating room and an estimation of expected ongoing losses. Those depend to a great degree on the nature of the surgery and the intraoperative findings. Prediction of third space losses is based primarily on experience and on knowledge of the anatomy and physiology of the tissues involved.

Where possible, external losses should be accurately measured and replaced with suitable solutions. The frequency with which such measurements are made depends on the child's size, general health, and volume of fluid lost.

In the immediate postoperative period, the goal is to stabilize the vital signs and avoid or correct any major fluid, electrolyte, or acid-base derangement. General monitoring in this situation relies on the principles previously discussed. In evaluating the child's general condition, there is no substitute for a thorough physical examination. Likewise, careful monitoring of laboratory data (serum electrolytes, blood gases, blood glucose, and hematocrit) is essential. This needs to be coupled with close attention to the patient's vital signs, mental status, urine output, and weight. Placement of a central venous pressure or a Swan-Ganz catheter may be necessary for children with substantial cardiac, renal, or respiratory dysfunction.

The child who has had a relatively straightforward surgical procedure that has not been accompanied by ongoing tissue damage caused by a persistent infection or leakage of intraabdominal contents may be expected to begin diuresis on the third postoperative day. Third spacing generally stops by that time, and the extravasated fluid returns to the intravascular space. To avoid fluid overload and its cardiorespiratory and renal effects, the pediatrician must watch for the onset of such diuresis and alter fluid therapy accordingly. If the anticipated rise of urine output does not occur at this time, one must suspect a perioperative complication. The appropriate studies to exclude infection and hyponatremia should be performed in consultation with the surgical team.

Pain, anxiety, and the stress of surgery can lead to an accelerated secretion of ADH. Before considering the diagnosis of postoperative SIADH, however, it is essential to correct any underlying hypovolemia. Some authors assert that the additional secretion of ADH is appropriate with the intravascular volume depletion associated with third spacing, as already discussed. If the syndrome does occur in the postoperative period, its duration is usually short, and fluid restriction is not often required. Its presence, however, may make using urine output to help judge volume status unreliable.

Surgery places a person in negative nitrogen balance. If the operation is simple and if oral intake can be resumed within several days, clear fluids may be used for hydration. After several days, however, it becomes imperative to establish a positive nitrogen balance to aid wound healing and the return of normal function. Provision of adequate calories, protein, vitamins, and essential fats is more important in children than in adults because of the need for continued growth and development in children. These goals can be achieved through the use of parenteral nutrition when oral intake is not possible. A later section deals with the indications for and the composition and administration of such fluids. A significant infection in the postoperative period adds to the patient's metabolic requirements and must be considered in the physician's treatment plan if healing is to continue and metabolic acidosis is to be avoided.

CLINICAL APPROACH TO FLUID MANAGEMENT OF BURNS

Despite recent advances in legislation and education aimed at fire prevention, burn injuries to children remain a serious problem in our society. Estimates of numbers of affected children vary widely, but as many as 150,000 youngsters are moderately to severely burned each year. Of the close to 8000 deaths per year in the United States attributed to burns or smoke inhalation, nearly 30% occur in children younger than 15 years of age.

As mentioned before, the skin, as the body's largest organ, serves a variety of physiologic functions. Most important, it serves as a barrier that prevents large losses of body fluids and prohibits invasion by microorganisms. Its sweat glands are important in temperature regulation, and it is the organ of sensation and of vitamin D metabolism. The epidermis is a thin outer layer of dead cornified cells that serves as a tough and protective shell; the dermis or corium is the thicker area that lies beneath the epidermis and contains all the cutaneous nerves, blood vessels, hair follicles, and sweat glands. The dermis may be only half as thick in children as in adults.

The physiologic effects of a burn depend on the depth to which tissue has been destroyed (i.e., just epidermis or all or part of the dermis) and the area of the body that is burned. Although burns traditionally have been classified as first, second, and third degree, this distinction is not always apparent on initial evaluation. It is probably more reasonable from a functional standpoint to classify a burn as being of partial thickness (which although it may be severe, heals with time) or full thickness (which usually requires grafting).

Simple first-degree burns involve only the epidermis and are characterized by pain and redness that last up to 72 hours, followed in 5 to 10 days by peeling of the involved area. Superficial second-degree burns involve all the epidermis and variable parts of the dermis. They are characterized by pain, erythema, and blisters that enlarge for several hours following exposure. These burns also, in the absence of infection, usually heal without scarring. A deep second-degree burn injury extends far into the dermis. The injured skin looks tough and is usually red but blanches with pressure. Although there is no permanent anesthesia, pain sensation may be lost for the first 48 hours. Healing is slow and occurs by the epithelium of the sweat glands and hair follicles regenerating. Generally the patient is left with deep scars. These burns can become full-thickness burns if infection occurs. Third-degree burns are full-thickness burns, with complete necrosis of the skin and all of its elements. The color is usually brown, tan, black, or white. Occasionally the burned skin looks red, but it does not blanch with pressure.

The size of a burn is generally described in terms of percentage of body surface area (BSA) affected. The rule of 9s, sometimes employed in adults, is not helpful in small children, in which the most useful determination is made with the use of a burn chart. If not available, one can assume that the skin overlying the patient's closed fist represents 1% of his or her BSA, as does the skin of the perineum. Table 25-6 presents the percentage of BSA of various body parts as a function of age.

Generally the first question to be considered in evaluating

Table 25-6 *Percentage of Body Surface Area (BSA) in Relation to Age*

BODY PART	PERCENT BSA BY AGE				
	INFANT	1-4 YEARS	5-9 YEARS	10-14 YEARS	ADULT
Parts that change with age					
Head	19	17	13	11	7
Each thigh	5.5	6.5	8	8.5	9.5
Each leg	5	5	5.5	6	7
Parts that do not change with age					
Neck	2				
Anterior trunk	13				
Posterior trunk	13				
Buttocks	5				
Genitalia	1				
Both arms	14				
Both hands	5				
Both feet	7				

the burned child is whether hospitalization is required and, if so, whether admission to a specialized burn center or to a community hospital is more appropriate. Outpatient management of a child may be considered if (1) superficial, second-degree burns involving no more than 10% of the BSA or (2) third-degree burns of less than 2%, but not involving the hands or face, are present. Second-degree burns involving 10% to 20% of the BSA may be managed in a community hospital if fluid and electrolyte support can be provided. Most full-thickness burns and all partial-thickness burns greater than 30% of the BSA, as well as any substantial burns of the face, perineum, hands, or feet, are best referred to a specialized burn center. Additionally, any child with evidence of inhalation injury complicating the burn (respiratory distress, wheezing, stridor, sooty oral or nasal secretions, deteriorating blood gas values, or any abnormality seen on a chest roentgenogram) needs specialized care, as does any youngster with a notable, underlying medical problem. Most burn experts also agree that the burn center's intensive care unit is the proper place for the child who is younger than 2 years of age and for most electrical and chemical burns. Any situation in which the physician suspects child abuse or neglect is an indication for hospitalization.

Outpatient therapy of minor burns requires observation of the wound at least every other day to ensure that adequate healing occurs and that infection is avoided. A 1% silver sulfadiazine cream is applied to the burned area, which is wrapped with a gauze dressing (susceptible patients should be screened for glucose 6-phosphate dehydrogenase deficiency). Fresh applications of the cream should be made every 24 to 48 hours until adequate healing has taken place.

Optimum initial fluid therapy for critical burns is essential in reducing mortality and must begin immediately, even when there are plans to transfer the patient to a tertiary care facility. Large amounts of fluid may be required in the first several days following the thermal injury. Markedly increased capillary permeability occurs in the layers of tissue immediately beneath the burned skin, with concomitant losses of water and protein. Although normal intact skin excludes up to 15 ml/hr/m^2, the patient with a partial- or full-thickness burn may lose up to 3 dl/hr/m^2 of burned skin. These losses are accompanied by elevated oxygen and calorie consumption with profound loss of heat. There are also chemical mediators at work in the damaged areas that further increase capillary permeability—not only in the affected places but also systemically. In general, fluid losses are at their maximum immediately after the injury, and by 24 to 48 hours after the burn has occurred, capillary permeability approaches normal, and the extravasated fluid begins to resorb.

General resuscitative efforts should commence as soon as possible. As with any other acute injury, the first step is to evaluate the adequacy of the child's airway and assess the possibility of an accompanying inhalation injury. This possibility is suspected in cases of a fire within an enclosed space, of thermal injuries on the upper torso or face, and when the physical findings previously listed are present. If smoke inhalation is suspected, humidified oxygen should be administered by mask, and blood gases and a carboxyhemoglobin level should be measured (to evaluate the possibility of carbon monoxide poisoning). If the child is dyspneic or critically ill, intubation should be accomplished as soon as possible; increasing airway edema makes the procedure more difficult later. As soon as the airway is ensured, the circulatory status of the patient should be assessed and the depth and severity of the burn evaluated. In a severe or large burn, at least two large-bore intravenous lines should be established (if possible, one should be a central line or Swan-Ganz catheter) and a Foley catheter inserted.

Over the years, multiple regimens have been developed to guide fluid and electrolyte replacement, but the most important aspect of fluid therapy in the measurement of burn injuries is *monitoring* the patient's vital signs and other important physiologic parameters.

As a helpful starting point, however, the most favored regimen uses the Parkland formula. This requires the administration of 4 ml of fluid per kilogram per percentage of BSA burned during the first 24 hours, giving 50% of the total in the first 8 hours. A balanced salt solution such as Ringer lactate solution should be used. *Glucose should not be given.* Severe burns induce a marked outpouring of catecholamines and steroids, which raises the serum glucose concentration and renders the child relatively resistant to insulin. Exogenously administered glucose concentrates in the burned area, increasing the likelihood of infection. The need for glucose is best determined by measuring the blood glucose frequently, especially in young children.

Although the initial rate of intravenous fluid administration is guided by the Parkland formula, one should ensure that sufficient fluid is given to maintain a urine output of 0.5 to 2.0 ml/kg/hr. In this situation, more *is not better,* since too much fluid worsens peripheral edema, delays healing, and may lead to heart failure when the extravasated liquid begins to resorb. The best indicator of optimum fluid therapy is a normal cardiac output. However, placement of a pulmonary artery catheter is required to measure cardiac output accurately. Blood pressure, heart rate, and weight measurement may be helpful in measuring cardiac output indirectly, but each of these can be affected by a number of other factors. In children with burns of less than 30% BSA and in all infants maintenance requirements should be added to the daily fluids suggested by the Parkland formula.

Colloid (such as plasma or albumin) is generally withheld until 24 hours after the burn has occurred, but because with children there is some evidence of earlier healing of the capillary bed, it may be useful at 12 to 18 hours. The usual dosage is 0.5 ml/kg/% of burned BSA given over 24 hours, with D_5W added to reach a total of approximately 50% of the previous day's requirement. Measuring electrolyte concentrations carefully and frequently (especially potassium, because with burns there can be massive losses of this ion through the kidneys) determines whether and how much electrolyte solution is necessary.

Care of the burn wound may require excision, escharotomy, or eventual grafting and is best left in the hands of an experienced surgical team. Tetanus prophylaxis should be administered. Low-dose penicillin therapy is usually employed but has become controversial. There are effective arguments on both sides; the majority of authorities, however, suggest that penicillin be used prophylactically against wound infection.

After the first several days, a fluid rate of an amount close to maintenance may be sufficient (at approximately 72 hours maximum resorption of edema has taken place). If the burn is of major proportions, parenteral nutrition should be initiated once the electrolyte balance is stable. Needless to say, attention must also be paid to the social and psychological needs of the child and the family. Recovery from a major burn injury is slow, is fraught with complications, and leaves substantial scars. If the child's emotional well-being is not adequately tended to, the psychological scars may outweigh any physical disability that results.

PARENTERAL NUTRITION

In previous sections of this chapter many situations have been noted in which provision of maintenance fluid and electrolyte concentrations in the standard glucose solutions is insufficient to meet caloric or nutritional requirements. Such situations occur whenever oral intake is limited or impossible for prolonged periods of time (over 1 week in older children, 2 to 3 days in the infant or neonate) or the body's metabolic demands exceed those that can be supplied orally. The accompanying box lists some of the major indications for parenteral nutrition in the pediatric population.

Major Pediatric Indications for Use of Parenteral Nutrition

- Gastrointestinal lesions preventing adequate oral intake
  - Congenital: anterior abdominal wall defects, intestinal atresia
  - Acquired: necrotizing enterocolitis, chronic fistulas, intestinal obstruction
- Gastrointestinal lesions precluding adequate absorption
  - Status after bowel resections, chronic diarrhea, inflammatory bowel disease
- Severe hypermetabolic or catabolic conditions
  - Multiple trauma, malignancies, major burns, extensive surgery
- Severely undernourished patients
  - Malnutrition, anorexia nervosa
- Acute and chronic renal failure
- Small premature infants

Intravenous provision of nutrients and calories may be in the form of total parenteral nutrition (TPN) or partial parenteral nutrition. For the majority of children who are able to tolerate at least small amounts of oral intake, partial parenteral nutrition is preferred. The choice between TPN and partial parenteral nutrition depends on the nature of the child's illness and the length of time nutritional support is required. Parenteral nutrition fluids consist of the following components.

Calories

The basic goal of parenteral nutrition is the prevention of protein breakdown. In long-term pediatric users, an additional goal is the promotion of normal growth and development. Caloric needs vary with age. The neonate requires 130 to 140 Cal/kg/day; the 1-year-old child, 100 Cal/kg/day; and the adult, 30 Cal/kg/day. Between 1 year of age and adulthood, the drop in caloric requirements is approximately 10 Cal/kg/day for each 3-year increment. After 10 years of age, girls require fewer calories than boys. It is impossible to predict the precise caloric requirements of an individual patient. Preexisting nutritional deprivation, recent weight loss, and hypermetabolic conditions increase caloric needs.

Calories may be supplied as carbohydrate (usually dextrose), as protein (amino acid mixtures), or as fat (usually an isotonic soybean emulsion). Calories derived from different sources are not equivalent in their ability to generate a positive nitrogen balance. Amino acids are generally incorporated into the lean body mass unless a positive nitrogen balance already exists, in which case they yield 4 Cal/g administered. In the calorically deprived patient, carbohydrate exerts a much better protein-sparing effect than does fat on a calorie-for-calorie basis. Studies have shown that nitrogen balance is best preserved under these circumstances when at least 80% of the administered calories consist of carbohydrate. On the other hand, because the metabolism of glucose results in thermogenesis and increases the metabolic rate, providing such a high percentage of the calories as carbohydrate may lead to an elevation of the respiratory quotient and potentiate existing or imminent respiratory failure. High glucose loads also increase circulating levels of endogenous catecholamines, and patients may become insulin resistant. Therefore, glucose administration should be limited to no more than one half the total calories, when feasible.

Protein

Children beyond the neonatal period require between 1 and 3 g of protein per kilogram per day. This is usually supplied as a mixture of amino acids in which the final concentration of protein is between 1.7% and 2.75%. Whatever solution is used should provide adequate amounts of the essential amino acids—lysine, threonine, tryptophan, phenylalanine, methionine, leucine, isoleucine, and valine. Most solutions also contain the nonessential amino acids. Protein is administered primarily to provide adequate material for the repair of tissues and the synthesis of new cells, *not* to provide calories per se. In general, at least 30 calories should be provided for every gram of protein delivered in a 24-hour period.

Because the majority of nitrogen losses occur via the urinary tract, the child with marginal or failing renal function usually requires an adjustment in the type and amount of protein given to avoid worsening azotemia.

Carbohydrate

Carbohydrate in the form of glucose is the major source of calories in standard parenteral nutrition solutions. Although carbohydrates ordinarily provide 4 Cal/g, most parenteral nutrition solutions contain hydrated glucose, which provides only 3.4 Cal/g. Glucose concentration depends primarily on the *method* of administration. Although concentrated glucose solutions (20% or 25%) provide a large number of calories, they present a high osmotic load (1120 and 1400 mOsm/kg, respectively) and cannot be administered through a peripheral vein because of problems with phlebitis and thrombosis. To deliver such glucose solutions, the placement of a central venous catheter is necessary. The catheter should be placed so that the tip is near the junction of the superior vena cava and right atrium. Intraatrial placement should be avoided because of the risk of the catheter perforating the atrial wall.

Central venous catheters are difficult to place in small children. For this reason and for long-term use, most pediatric centers are using a soft Silastic catheter placed in the operating room and tunneled several centimeters beneath the skin. The Hickman and Broviac catheters are specifically designed for this purpose. Each has a Dacron cuff that, when placed in the skin tunnel, allows growth of fibrous tissue, thus fixing them in place and obviating the need for sutures. Such lines may remain in place for a year or longer, provided they are cared for properly.

If a central line cannot be placed or is deemed unnecessary, glucose and amino acid solutions may be infused through a peripheral vein. The glucose concentration of solutions used in this situation is generally limited to 10% to 12%. The caloric content is limited by the volume of fluid the child can tolerate. In the majority of cases, adequate calories cannot be provided by such glucose–amino acid mixtures alone.

Fat

Currently, the lipid solutions used are derived from an emulsion of soybean oil in water to which egg yolk–phospholipid and glycerol are added, resulting in an isotonic solution containing linoleic, oleic, palmitic, and linolenic acids. The most widely used fatty acid mixture (Intralipid) is available in 10% and 20% solutions, containing 1.1 Cal/ml and 2.2 Cal/ml, respectively. Daily administration of Intralipid provides an isotonic solution high in calories, which can be presented through a peripheral vein, thereby improving the usefulness of peripheral parenteral nutrition. The maximum tolerance for fat given in this way is 4 g/kg/day; in no case should the fat administered exceed 60% of the daily caloric intake.

Children receiving large doses of lipid may have difficulty "clearing" the emulsion from their serum. This may result in deposition of fat droplets within pulmonary capillaries, with a concomitant decrease in pulmonary diffusion capacity. Another consequence of lipid administration is the binding of free fatty acids to albumin, in competition with bilirubin. This is therefore considered hazardous in infants with total bilirubin concentrations greater than 8 to 10 mg/dl. Long-term administration of fat emulsions also leads to deposition of an unusual pigment within the reticuloendothelial cells of bone marrow, lymph nodes, liver, and spleen. The significance of this pigment is unknown, but no disruption of normal function has been documented.

Essential fatty acid requirements can be met by providing between 4% and 10% of the child's caloric needs as lipid. However, because of the above-noted problems from too much glucose administration and because of amino acid tolerance limitations, 30% to 60% of the total calories are generally delivered in the form of fat.

Electrolyte Concentrations

The electrolyte content of each solution varies according to the source of amino acids. The sodium content, for example, ranges from less than 10 to more than 50 mEq/L, with other common minerals varying just as widely. Electrolyte concentrations may be added to each solution so that daily requirements are met.

Trace Minerals

Trace elements known to be essential for pediatric growth and development include copper, zinc, chromium, manganese, selenium, iodine, and iron. The first four are available as a premixed pediatric trace element additive. When needed, selenium and iron can be added separately. Iodine is not generally administered enterally, as it is absorbed through the skin during the process of dressing the catheter site.

Vitamins

A standard mixture of vitamin supplements is available for addition to TPN solutions in infants and children (M.V.I.* Pediatric). The product comes as a powder; after reconstitution with sterile water, each 5 ml contains the following:

*Multivitamin infusion.

Vitamin A (retinol)	0.7 mg (2300 USP units)
Vitamin C (ascorbic acid)	80 mg
Vitamin D (ergocalciferol)	10 μg (400 USP units)
Vitamin E (alpha-tocopheroyl acetate)	7 mg (7 USP units)
Vitamin B_1 (thiamine)	1.2 mg
Vitamin B_2 (riboflavin)	1.4 mg
Vitamin B_6 (pyridoxine)	1 mg
Vitamin B_{12} (cyanocobalamin)	1 μg
Vitamin K_1 (phytonadione)	200 μg
Biotin	20 μg
Dexpanthenol	5 mg
Folic acid	140 μg
Niacinamide	17 mg

For children under 11 years of age who weigh more than 3 kg, the entire 5 ml should be administered (dissolved in the TPN solution). Infants weighing between 1 and 3 kg receive 3.25 ml, and neonates weighing less than 1 kg receive 1.5 ml of the reconstituted solution. It is no longer necessary to administer vitamins K or B_{12} as weekly intramuscular injections, as was the case until recently.

Parenteral Nutrition in Clinical Practice

It is cumbersome and expensive to fully personalize the parenteral solution administered to each patient. Therefore most hospitals have devised standard solutions of protein, glucose, electrolyte concentrations, and minerals. Generally these determinations are made by a group of professionals (physician, nurse, pharmacist, nutrition specialist) who have a special interest and expertise in parenteral nutrition. In some hospitals, the duties of such a team may be assumed by a single person (physician or pharmacist). Such specialists are available for consultation regarding the best mode of parenteral nutrition, the delivery systems, and the makeup of solutions to be used.

The use of parenteral nutrition requires careful monitoring of the patient's blood glucose levels, serum protein and electrolyte values, hematocrit, liver enzyme levels, and renal function. Results of laboratory determinations should be maintained on a flow sheet, which also lists the daily weight, urine output, and fluid administered (including the type and glucose content of each). Some major centers with large nutritional support teams are able to manage chronically ill patients on a home parenteral nutrition program.

FLUID THERAPY OF THE NEONATE

The provision of adequate fluid replacement therapy for newborn infants depends on perinatal alterations in body composition and the infant's size and gestational age. Hydration of sick premature babies who weigh less than 1500 g is beyond the scope of this chapter. Specific issues relating to the health of the neonate are presented in Part Five.

TBW content decreases progressively throughout gestation and the first year of postnatal life. This is accompanied by increases in the body's content of protein and fat. Shrinkage of the ECF compartment accounts largely for the decrease in TBW. In the first few days of extrauterine life, both term and premature babies normally lose up to 10% of their body weight. Although this is considered a physiologic reduction, failure to replace such losses may lead to substantial dehydration.

All newborns show a progressive increase in their metabolic rate. The metabolic rate for full-term infants approximates 32 Cal/kg/day at birth and reaches close to 43 Cal/kg/day within 3 days. Following this, there is a slow, steady increase over the first 2 weeks of life. Premature infants maintain a higher metabolic rate than full-term babies, even when they achieve a similar weight.

In addition to the baseline metabolic expenditure of calories, newborns use energy with cold, stress, and muscular activity. The growth rate is rapid during this period, and the average newborn requires 25 to 35 Cal/kg/day for growth. Therefore the total caloric need of an infant over 3 days of age is between 100 and 125 Cal/kg/day.

Water requirements are governed by losses via the skin, respiratory tract, and kidneys. Evaporative losses through the skin generally average 20 to 30 ml/kg/day, whereas respiratory losses account for approximately 15 ml/kg/day. Both parameters are affected by ambient humidity, and respiratory losses may actually be reduced by 50% with provision of high humidity to the baby's immediate environment.

The newborn's kidneys are limited in their ability to concentrate urine because of the relative shortness of the loops of Henle and the absence of a notable concentration gradient. Thus they are at best able to excrete urine with an osmolality that approaches 300 mOsm/kg. As the solute load increases, the free water requirement rises, so that for a formula-fed infant, urinary water loss may be as high as 120 ml/kg/day. However, the average range is probably closer to 60 to 75 ml/kg/day.

Electrolyte requirements for infants have not been fully established, but they seem to tolerate a fairly wide range of electrolyte provisions. Fluids that have been used successfully yield between 1 and 3 mEq of sodium per 100 calories per day, and this has become the recommended starting range for maintenance fluid therapy.

When preparing a maintenance parenteral fluid formula for newborns, it is important to ensure adequate monitoring, which will indicate whether fluid estimates have been adequate. It is also important, especially with the sick neonate, to record weights once or twice a day and to frequently record intake, output, vital signs, urinary osmolality, electrolyte concentrations, and other indications of optimum cardiac and respiratory homeostasis. Frequent changes may be needed; therefore the physician must never become "locked into" a particular formula but rather must apply the basic rules of fluid therapy to the situation logically and be ready to compensate for failing systems or increasing losses when necessary.

HYDRATION OF THE AMBULATORY PATIENT: ALTERNATIVES TO PARENTERAL FLUID THERAPY

It is fairly common practice for pediatricians in the United States to recommend oral fluids for young patients with mild diarrhea or vomiting. Such therapy has been suggested for many years on totally empiric grounds, and most physicians have urged the use of a dilute solution that contains sodium and potassium in concentrations of 30 and 20 mEq/L, respectively, and 5% to 7% glucose. When diarrhea leads to moderate or severe dehydration, or if substantial emesis accompanies the illness, the standard teaching had dictated hospitalization of such children and "resting" the GI tract with the use of parenteral therapy, as outlined in previous sections.

Through the efforts of scientists working with the World Health Organization (WHO) in an effort to curb the large diarrhea-associated mortality seen in underdeveloped countries, many data concerning gastrointestinal function in diarrhea have been accumulated.

Sodium absorption in the small intestine depends on the presence of glucose or small neutral amino acids such as glycine or alanine. Likewise, the absorption of glucose is enhanced by the presence of sodium salts. Movement of salt and glucose across the mucosal border is accompanied by an influx of water and other electrolyte concentrations. Maximum rates of absorption are achieved when (1) sodium and glucose are present in a 1 : 1 to 1 : 2 molecular ratio, (2) glucose concentration is between 110 and 140 mmol (2% to 2.5% solution), and (3) sodium concentration is not substantially less than that of normal jejunal fluid.

Based on this and other information, WHO derived a formula for use with all patients suffering from diarrheal illness regardless of its cause. It contains 90 mmol of sodium, 20 mmol of potassium, 30 mmol of bicarbonate, 80 mmol of chloride, and 111 mmol of glucose per liter. This formulation provides a solution that has an osmolality of 331. When given ad lib to patients with diarrhea, it corrects dehydration rapidly and can return electrolyte concentrations to the normal range regardless of the presence of hyponatremia or hypernatremia on initial evaluation. Large field studies have documented its successful use in patients who have ongoing emesis. There has been no evidence to suggest that the use of such fluid prolongs the duration of diarrhea; just the reverse appears to be the case. In addition, children given this oral rehydration therapy (ORT) seem to tolerate resumption of a regular diet earlier than those treated solely with intravenous fluids.

In 1985, the American Academy of Pediatrics (AAP) Committee on Nutrition published recommendations for the use of the WHO solution or similar solutions in developed countries. The committee concluded that the WHO oral rehydration solution (WHO-ORS) is appropriate for use in the initial phases of rehydration and should be used for the first 6 hours to replace acute volume loss. After this time, the committee recommends that the solution be replaced with one containing 40 to 60 mEq of sodium per liter, for maintenance of hydration in the child who continues to have stool losses, or as the only solution administered to a child who is not acutely dehydrated. Alternatively as used in the developing countries in the maintenance phase, children may be given the ORS on a 1 : 1 basis with fluid low in sodium content, such as breast milk or water, to avoid potential hypernatremia.

There are commercially available preparations that meet WHO and AAP guidelines, as indicated above. Because such preparations are available in ready-to-use form, the bicarbonate found in the WHO powder has been replaced with citrate. Studies have documented equivalent efficacy of the two bases in correcting the mild acidosis that accompanies mild-to-moderate diarrhea. Most of the large-scale evaluations that have been performed in the United States have excluded the use of ORS in patients in shock who are treated initially with intravenous fluids.

In summary, oral rehydration therapy provides a cost-efficient approach to the problem of childhood diarrhea for the patient who is able to drink, is not in shock, and has a relative or other responsible person who can understand the instructions for using the ORT formula. Such a therapeutic approach avoids the hospitalization of a child and the consequent disruption in the lives of the family members. More important, this treatment approach eliminates the potential complications of intravenous therapy.

SUGGESTED READINGS

American Academy of Pediatrics Committee on Nutrition: Use of intravenous fat emulsions in pediatric patients, Pediatrics 68:738, 1981.

American Academy of Pediatrics Committee on Nutrition: Use of oral fluid therapy and posttreatment feeding following enteritis in children in a developed country, Pediatrics 75:358, 1985.

Cochran EB, Phelps SJ, and Helms RA: Parenteral nutrition in pediatric patients, Clin Pharm 7:351, 1988.

Friis-Hansen B: Body water compartments in children: changes during growth and related changes in body composition, Pediatrics 28:169, 1961.

Hazard P and Griffin J: Calculation of sodium bicarbonate requirements in metabolic acidosis, Am J Med Sci 283:18, 1982.

Hirschhorn N: Oral rehydration therapy for diarrhea in children—a basic primer, Nutr Rev 40:97, 1982.

Holliday MA and Segar WE: The maintenance need for water in parenteral fluid therapy, Pediatrics 19:823, 1957.

Kohler M et al: Comparative study of intranasal, subcutaneous, and intravenous administration of desamino-D-arginine vasopressin (DDAVP), Thromb Haemost 55:108, 1986.

McDonald JA et al: Treatment of the young child with postoperative central diabetes insipidus, Am J Dis Child 143:201, 1989.

Poole GV, Meredith JW, and Pennell T: Comparison of colloids and crystalloids in resuscitation from hemorrhagic shock, Surg Gynecol Obstet 154:577, 1982.

Salazar-Lindo E et al: Bicarbonate versus citrate in oral rehydration therapy in infants with watery diarrhea: a controlled clinical trial, J Pediatr 108:55, 1986.

Santosham M et al: Oral rehydration therapy for acute diarrhea in ambulatory children in the United States: a double-blind comparison of four different solutions, Pediatrics 76:159, 1985.

Santosham M, Daum RS, and Dillman L: Oral rehydration therapy of infantile diarrhea, N Engl J Med 306:1070, 1982.

Tamer AM et al: Oral rehydration of infants in a large urban U.S. medical center, J Pediatr 107:14, 1985.

Winters RW, editor: The body fluids in pediatrics, Boston, 1973, Little, Brown & Co.

26

Blood Products and Their Uses

Thomas E. Williams

Blood and its components are limited resources requiring judicious use. The principal guide to the transfusion of blood or any of its derivatives is to administer only that component that is needed. Since transfusions may carry significant risks, the decision to transfuse should never be made lightly.[3,6] For example, elective surgery should be delayed in the anemic patient if the hemoglobin concentration can be corrected medically. Equally important is to administer only the amount that will correct the physiologic derangement that requires transfusion. For example, it is seldom necessary to correct the hematocrit or platelet count to normal values in order to correct metabolic abnormalities secondary to anemia or to stop thrombocytopenic bleeding. The treatment of most hematologic deficiencies seldom depends on transfusions but rather on specific therapy for the underlying condition. Table 26-1 outlines the blood products commonly used in pediatric patients.

HAZARDS OF TRANSFUSION[1,2]

Infections

The greatest risk associated with transfusion is the possibility of transmitting an infectious agent. Although bacterial and malarial infections are uncommon, the transmission of viral infections remains difficult to prevent. It should be noted, however, that significant progress has been made recently in the immunologic screening of blood for hepatitis B, human immune deficiency virus (HIV), cytomegalovirus (CMV), and hepatitis C. Equally important in lowering the risk of transfusion-associated infections has been the policy of deferring payment for blood donations, thus avoiding many high-risk donors. Moreover, new techniques of processing concentrates of pooled plasma have decreased the risk of transfusion-acquired hepatitis and acquired immune deficiency syndrome (AIDS). Nonetheless, the risk of infection increases with the number of transfusions given from various donors; therefore, patients given multiple transfusions should receive adequate follow-up in the form of liver function studies to detect both clinical and subclinical cases of posttransfusion infection. Special care must be taken for the CMV-seronegative immunocompromised recipient, such as patients receiving transplants, premature neonates, and patients with AIDS. The use of CMV-seronegative donors has greatly decreased the risk of cytomegalovirus infections in these patients.

Hypervolemia

When a transfusion is being given to a child with a stable vascular volume, the volume of blood component administered should not exceed 10% of the blood volume and should be administered *at an even rate* over a 3-hour period. In most instances this means that the volume should not exceed 10 ml/kg. Persons responsible for the administration of the transfusion should be specifically instructed regarding the rate of administration and should not be allowed to exceed that rate. Special care in selecting transfusion volume and rate should be exercised with children having cardiac anomalies and with chronically anemic children, who often have an expanded plasma volume. The cardiopulmonary status of these patients should be carefully evaluated throughout the transfusion.

Tranfusion Reactions

Immediate reactions to a blood transfusion may include fever spikes caused by bacterial contamination, leukoagglutinins, and/or histamine. If the patient has not experienced febrile reactions to blood or blood products in the past, it is advisable to discontinue the transfusions and to culture the transfusate as well as the patient's own blood. Febrile reactions to leukoagglutinins may be eliminated by filters designed specifically to remove leukocytes. Hemolytic transfusion reactions result from the reaction of preformed (natural) antibodies to antigens on the donor erythrocytes. Fever, nausea, vomiting, abdominal and back pain, hemoglobinuria, and oliguria may ensue, and they require immediate discontinuance of the transfusion. The blood being transfused and samples of the patient's blood and urine (if obtainable) should be sent to the blood bank to determine if there has been a mistake in the cross-match. Most instances of hemolytic transfusion reactions, however, result from (1) errors in labeling the patient's blood used in the cross-match and (2) administration of the transfusion to the wrong recipient. Allergic reactions to blood products may be associated with fever, urticaria, and asthma and are not predicted by the Coombs test performed during the cross-match. This is a particularly recurrent problem for patients with hemophilia who require repeated transfusions with cryoprecipitate, fresh-frozen plasma, and plasma concentrates. Special care should be taken with patients who have had previous transfusions, for they may have developed

Table 26-1 *Blood Products and Their Uses*

SPECIFIC BLOOD PRODUCT	INDICATIONS	ROUTE, VOLUME, AND RATE OF ADMINISTRATION
Whole blood	Acute blood loss Exchange transfusion Extracorporeal oxygenator	IV—rates and volume depend on clinical severity of bleeding
Packed red cells	Anemia that is not associated with signs and symptoms of acute blood loss	IV—volume not to exceed 10% of blood volume at even rate over 3 hr
Platelet-rich plasma	Thrombocytopenia secondary to decreased platelet production when the risk of hypervolemia is not a major concern	IV—volume not to exceed 10% of blood volume at even rate over 3 hr
Platelet concentrate	Thrombocytopenia secondary to decreased platelet production when the risk of hypervolemia is a major concern	IV—usual volume of 20 ml/U; given slowly by push
Granulocytes	Temporary increase in circulating granulocytes for treatment of bacterial infections	IV—volume depends on method of preparation
Fresh-frozen plasma	Correction of plasma coagulation deficiences of stable factors and of labile factors when the risk of hypervolemia is small	IV—volume of 20 ml/kg body weight given over 2 to 3 hr
Cryoprecipitate	Hemophilia A, congenital or acquired hypofibrinogenemia, von Willebrand disease	IV—small volume usually given by push
Antihemophilic Factor VIII Hemofil M (Hyland) Humate P (Armour) Monoclate Factor VIII:C Koate-HS (Miles-Cutter) Koate-HT (Miles-Cutter) Monoclate (Alpha Therapeutic) Profilate HP (Alpha Therapeutic) Profilate SD (Alpha Therapeutic)	Hemophilia A	IV—small volume usually given by push
Factor IX complex Konyne-HT (Miles-Cutter) Proplex T (Hyland) Profilnine heat-treated (Alpha Therapeutic)	Hemophilia B	IV—small volume usually given by push
Antiinhibitor coagulant Complex Autoplex T (Hyland)	Hemophilia A with inhibitor	IV—small volume usually given by push
Albumin	See text	IV—1 g/kg body weight
Hyperimmune gamma globulin	See text	IM—volume depends on clinical indication for use
Globulin, immune Gammar (Armour) Gamimune N (Miles-Cutter) Gammagard (Hyland) Sandoglobulin (Sandoz) Venoglobulin-I (Alpha Therapeutic)	See text	IV—see manufacturer's instructions

immunoglobulin A (IgA) deficiency as a result of having acquired antibody directed against IgA. Although these patients may not have a febrile response to transfusions, they may develop prolonged hypotension.

Delayed transfusion reactions usually result from isoimmunizations by any of the three major cellular components of blood. Because no attempt is usually made to match platelets, platelet isoimmunization is inherent in platelet transfusions from multiple random donors. Consequently, the effectiveness of platelet transfusions lessens after 10 or more separate units are administered. Erythrocyte isoimmunization cannot always be detected by the usual cross-matching procedures. Red cell types A, B, and O and the Rh antigens are routinely determined, but there are more than 30 other antigens on human erythrocytes capable of causing sensitization. Thus with subsequent transfusion of the same antigenic type, a transfusion reaction may occur. This may be a delayed or an anamnestic reaction.

Specific Hazards Pertaining to an Exchange Transfusion

An exchange transfusion is commonly used either to accomplish a rapid increase in circulating erythrocytes, for which sedimented erythrocytes are preferred, or for the removal of a noxious agent (bilirubin, drugs, or chemicals), for which whole blood is best. A two-volume exchange is usually tolerated well by the neonate. Specific hazards include (1) inaccurate increments of exchange that leave the infant with a deficit or an excess of blood volume at the end of the exchange, (2) hypocalcemia induced by the citrated anticoagulant of the transfused blood, and (3) hyperkalemia induced by hemolysis of red cells secondary to improper warming of the blood, prolonged storage, and injudicious admixture of the blood with hypotonic solutions. Most of these risks can be avoided by (1) frequent measurement of the venous pressure during the exchange transfusion to ensure that it does not exceed 10 cm of water; (2) administration of 1 ml of 10% calcium gluconate slowly over 10 minutes after each deciliter of exchange, with careful cardiac monitoring to ensure that the cardiac rate does not fall below 100 beats/min; and (3) use of blood no less than 3 days old that is allowed to come to room temperature without warming devices and that is administered without dilution in hypotonic intravenous solutions.

Other Risks of Transfusions

Children with chronic and refractory anemias, such as sickle cell anemia, thalassemia, Fanconi pancytopenia, and congenital hypoplastic anemia (Blackfan-Diamond syndrome), may require repeated transfusions, which result in transfusion hemosiderosis. Chelation therapy with deferoxamine may hold promise for these patients. Because on storage blood loses its labile factors I, II, V, and VIII and its platelets, rapid and massive transfusions of whole blood may result in hemostatic defects.

Special Considerations for the Potential Transplant Recipient

Care should be taken to avoid presensitization of the potential bone marrow transplant recipient by cellular antigens of the prospective donor. Therefore it is advisable to avoid blood transfusions from relatives before transplantations. Particular attention should be given to the patient with severe aplastic anemia. Bone marrow transplantation is the therapy of choice if the patient has a histocompatible relative, usually a sibling. It has been repeatedly observed that graft rejection is more common among patients who are multiply transfused before transplantation than among those who are not.

Transfusion-Associated Graft Versus Host Disease

Immunologically compromised patients such as bone marrow transplant recipients and patients with certain types of congenital immune deficiency are at risk of graft versus host disease when immunocompetent lymphocytes are present in the transfusate. This has also been observed in neonates, particularly premature infants, and in "normal" recipients who receive fresh whole blood. It may be prevented by the routine irradiation of all cellular blood components.

CELLULAR COMPONENTS

Erythrocyte Transfusions

Sedimented erythrocytes (packed red cells) are the preferred blood components for the correction of anemia in the child whose anemia is not caused by active acute blood loss and whose vascular volume is stabilized and is expected to remain so. The goal of transfusion in this situation is simply to increase the intravascular red cell mass. This can be accomplished more expeditiously with packed cells than with whole blood, because the same mass of red cells can be administered in approximately half the volume. This becomes particularly important in the small child, whose risk of volume overload is great.

The decision to transfuse requires sound clinical judgment by the practitioner. Among the questions to be answered are whether the anemia is amenable to medical therapy or whether it is likely to worsen before medical management is effective. For example, the anemia of a patient with newly diagnosed acute lymphocytic leukemia is likely to worsen during the first 3 to 4 weeks of induction therapy, so that the decision to transfuse may be made before there are physiologic aberrations of anemia, such as dizziness, headache, and orthostatic hypotension. Children with iron deficiency anemia, however, may respond to adequate nutrition or ferrous sulfate treatment within 4 to 6 weeks and may have few or no symptoms in the interim. The volume of packed cells required to raise the hematocrit or hemoglobin concentration can be easily ascertained by (1) calculating the total-body hematocrit, using known and reasonably accurate estimates of blood volume, and (2) making certain assumptions concerning the hematocrit of the transfusate. Remembering that the correction of physiologic derangement is the goal of transfusion therapy, one usually can determine the need for further transfusion by simply observing the patient's symptoms and measuring the hematocrit. It must be emphasized that the arbitrary correction of the hematocrit by transfusion alone to normal levels is seldom necessary and exposes the child to the added risk of unnecessary transfusion.

Platelet Transfusions

Platelet transfusions can be administered as platelet-rich plasma or platelet concentrates. Although the platelet yield of a unit of platelet concentrates is less than that of a unit of platelet-rich plasma, the volume of administration is only approximately one tenth that of platelet-rich plasma. In most situations involving pediatric patients, therefore, platelet concentrates are preferred because of the lower risk of hypervolemia.[4] Platelet concentrates may be prepared either by double plasmapheresis of the donor or by continuous flow centrifugation, using a cell separator. The former method is most widely used, resulting in approximately 7.5×10^9

platelets concentrated into 20 ml of plasma. In the adult the observed rise in the peripheral platelet count following transfusion of 1 U of platelet concentration is approximately 12,000 mm^3, which loosely extrapolates to an increment of 20,000 mm^3 for a child with a body surface area of 1 m^2.

In thrombocytopenic states, the risk of severe, life-threatening bleeding is low until the platelet count falls below 20,000 mm^3. In those conditions caused by a primary failure in platelet production, a reasonable goal is to raise the platelet count at least above 20,000 mm^3; it is seldom necessary to maintain the platelet count above 50,000 mm^3. The following formula provides a rough estimate of the number of units of platelet concentrates required to obtain the desired peripheral platelet count:

$$\frac{\text{Desired platelet count} - \text{Patient's platelet count}}{20{,}000} \times \text{Patient's body surface area } (m^2) = \text{Number of units of platelet concentrates}$$

For instance, a child with a body surface area of 0.7 m^2 and whose peripheral platelet count is 5000 would require 1.6 U to raise the peripheral platelet count to 50,000, whereas a child of 1.5 m^2 would require 3.4 U. It must be emphasized that this is a very rough estimate based on the assumptions that (1) the donor has a normal platelet count, (2) the platelet yield is approximately 70%, (3) the platelets are stored at room temperature in a volume of 20 ml, and (4) the platelets are used within 24 hours. Platelet transfusions appear to be relatively useless, however, in thrombocytopenic conditions associated with shortened platelet survival, such as immunologic thrombocytopenia and hypersplenism.

It is commonly observed that repeated platelet transfusions from random donors result in a refractory state caused by the development of platelet antibodies. This may be circumvented by using platelets from human lymphocyte antigen (HLA)-matched siblings.

Granulocyte Transfusions

The risk of severe infection is greatest when the absolute neutrophil count (ANC) falls below 500 mm^3 and is markedly reduced if the ANC can be maintained about 1500 mm^3. To raise the peripheral ANC by an increment of 1000 mm^3 in the adult requires on the order of 10^{10} granulocytes, an amount that cannot be easily obtained from the normal donor by plasmapheresis. However, using the cell separator, normal donors can give 5×10^9 granulocytes, enough to raise the peripheral granulocyte count by an increment of 300 mm^3.

Lymphocyte Products

Although the transfusion of lymphocytes currently has no known indication, the administration of transfer factor, a product of lymphocyte dialysis, has been shown to confer immunologic reactivity, such as delayed hypersensitivity to tuberculin, in previously unsensitized persons. Interferon may be produced from human lymphocytes or from lymphocytes in culture. Lymphocytes cultured during exposure to interleukin-2 may prove useful in the future for selected malignancies.

TRANSFUSION THERAPY WITH PLASMA COMPONENTS

Fresh-Frozen Plasma

The major use of fresh-frozen plasma is in those conditions in which labile coagulation factors are deficient. However, like whole blood its usefulness is limited by the large volumes that must be administered to raise the coagulation factor levels commensurate with normal hemostasis. Nevertheless it remains the only product that contains every plasma coagulation factor, and it is often used in an emergency when time is too short to perform the diagnostic studies needed to delineate the specific factor or factors that are lacking.

Cryoprecipitate

The technique of Pool and Shannon,[5] whereby concentrates of factor VIII may be prepared by precipitates formed during freezing and thawing of plasma, revolutionized the care of the classic hemophiliac patient and made the therapy of some acquired disorders of factor VIII deficiency more readily treatable by providing a convenient source of large amounts of factor VIII in a relatively small volume. However, only approximately 50% of the factor VIII activity of the original plasma was recoverable in the cryoprecipitate. The other major disadvantages of cryoprecipitate are that (1) the factor VIII activity in each bag may vary widely, since the donor's level may range from 60% to 160%; (2) it must be stored in a freezer at −20° C; and (3) the potential risk of transfusion-related infection exists. A bag of cryoprecipitate prepared from 1 U of plasma contains approximately 200 mg of fibrinogen and is preferable to fibrinogen concentrates made from pooled plasma as a source of fibrinogen for the uncommon situations in which isolated fibrinogen deficiency must be corrected.

Commercial Concentrates

Commercially prepared plasma concentrate products have several advantages compared with cryoprecipitate. They are lyophilized and can be stored in an ordinary refrigerator (4° C). They are assayed by the manufacturer; therefore the number of units (equivalent to the activity of 1 ml of fresh plasma) in each vial is known. Until recently, the convenience of these products had to be weighed against the risk of hepatitis and AIDS (since they are pooled plasma products) and against their greater cost in relation to that of cryoprecipitate. However, recent improvements have decreased these risks markedly. Heat-treated commercial concentrates carry little, if any, risk of AIDS. Detergent treatment markedly decreases the risk of HIV and hepatitis virus transmission. Plasma concentrates purified by monoclonal antibody absorption techniques and heat treated appear to have virtually eliminated the risks of hepatitis and AIDS. Pasteurization also appears to eliminate HIV and hepatitis virus transmission risks.

Fibrinogen Concentrates

There are two major disadvantages to the use of fibrinogen concentrates: The risk of hepatitis is extremely great, and the risk of a thrombotic crisis is accentuated in the presence of even low-grade intravascular coagulation. These concentrates appear to have little usefulness in pediatric patients.

Gamma Globulin

Patients with congenital forms of hypogammaglobulinemia, such as Bruton agammaglobulinemia, may benefit from monthly prophylactic injections of pooled gamma globulin, which can now be administered intravenously. Intravenously administered gamma globulin preparations have also been found useful in the therapy of isoimmune thrombocytopenic purpura. So-called hyperimmune gamma globulin obtained from patients convalescing from the natural disease has been prepared for varicella, pertussis, and tetanus. Pooled gamma globulin may help in the prophylaxis of measles, rubella, and infectious hepatitis, but its usefulness depends on the concentration of specific antibodies in the preparation, a concentration that varies.

Albumin

Albumin is indicated in the treatment of hypoalbuminemia of chronic liver disease and preceding exchange transfusion to bind unconjugated bilirubin, thus effecting its more efficient removal. When used for hypoalbuminemia of nephrosis, the benefit is temporary.

WHOLE BLOOD

Whole blood is best reserved for those times when acute blood loss is associated with signs and symptoms of hypovolemia. It is important to remember that acute blood loss may not be associated with a decrease in hematocrit or hemoglobin levels, since a finite period of time must elapse following control of the hemorrhage when vascular volume is partially corrected by shifts of interstitial fluid. Only then will the true extent of hemorrhage be mirrored in concentration measurements. The volume of whole blood and the rate of its administration depend on the severity of the hemorrhage. Unlike the child who is anemic but has a stable vascular volume, the child with acute blood loss may receive any volume of blood and at any rate that may be necessary to reestablish the vascular volume rapidly.

REFERENCES

1. College of American Pathologists Conference XIV on Safety in Transfusion Practices, Arch Pathol Lab Med 113:213, 1989.
2. Kasprisin DO and Luban NLC, editors: Pediatric transfusion medicine, vols 1 and 2, Boca Raton, Fla, 1987, CRC Press.
3. Mollison FL: Blood transfusion in clinical medicine, ed 5, Philadelphia, 1972, JB Lippincott Co.
4. Murphy S: Platelet transfusion. In Speat TH, editor: Progress in hemostasis and thrombosis, vol 3, New York, 1976, Grune & Stratton, Inc.
5. Pool JG and Shannon AE: Products of high potency concentration of anti-hemophilic globulin in a closed bag system, N Engl J Med 273:1443, 1965.
6. Smit Sibinga CTH, Das PC, and Forfar JO, editors: Paediatrics and blood transfusion, The Hague, Netherlands, 1982, Martin Nijhoff.

27

Clinical Pharmacology

Therese K. Schmalbach

Pharmacology is the field of science concerned with the physiologic effects of xenobiotics. This discipline encompasses the design, testing, clinical application, and biochemistry of drugs, as well as their metabolism, excretion, and toxicity and the methods for monitoring drug levels in patients. Pediatric pharmacology applies these scientific principles to the pediatric patient.

The recognition of pharmacologic differences in the pediatric population was dramatized by several tragedies in the 1950s. Administration of accepted doses of chloramphenicol to premature infants resulted in vascular collapse—the "gray-baby syndrome." Subsequent investigation revealed that because of their incompletely developed renal and hepatic systems, newborns, especially premature infants, are unable to metabolize and excrete chloramphenicol as rapidly as adults. Thus the use of modified adult dose regimens resulted in the accumulation of lethal levels of the drug.[21] Similarly, the treatment of suspected neonatal sepsis with sulfisoxazole caused death from kernicterus, because this drug binds to albumin, displacing bilirubin.[16] The epidemic of phocomelia following the widespread use of thalidomide emphasized the risk maternal drug use poses to the developing fetus.

One consequence of these disasters is the extensive preclinical and clinical drug testing regulations currently enforced by the U.S. Food and Drug Administration (FDA). The FDA regulations require data demonstrating the safety and efficacy of a medication before approval of its use; however, federal regulations do not routinely require information regarding the use of a new drug in children. Only drugs specifically labeled for use in the pediatric population must have a thorough investigation of their effects in infants and children. The complex ethical and medicolegal issues of experimentation on children have hindered pedatric experimentation and the development of new pediatric drug regimens.[20] Theoretically, this results in restricting potentially efficacious therapy. It has been estimated that 75% of the drugs marketed in the United States do not carry the FDA indication for pediatric use.[3] In actuality, children are receiving medication that is not labeled for pediatric use; one study revealed that 7% of the drugs prescribed for pediatric inpatients during a single 19-day period were not specifically designated for use in the pediatric population.[18] The hazards of this situation are recognized. The American Academy of Pediatrics has published guidelines for the ethical conduct of drug studies in children and encourages such investigation.[3]

These pharmacologic investigations will result in safer and more efficacious drug therapy, both by increasing pediatricians' armamentarium of drugs and by clarifying proper doses and dosing regimens for our patients. As the chloramphenicol experience illustrated, adult drug doses cannot be extrapolated to children. Average pediatric doses are most accurately calculated based on the child's body surface area or weight, and drug doses may frequently need to be adjusted to the individual's unique response and medical condition. Thus individualization of drug doses is often required to achieve the desired therapeutic response. An understanding of the basic principles of pharmacology is therefore imperative for safe and effective pediatric prescribing practices.

DRUG DISPOSITION

The production of a physiologic response requires that a therapeutic concentration of a drug or its active metabolite be present at its site of action. Physiochemical characteristics of the drug, such as lipid solubility, the degree of ionization at physiologic pH, the molecular weight (i.e., size) of the drug, and the affinity to biologic proteins, will affect the movement of the drug through body membranes. However, these are properties of the drug itself and will not vary significantly among patients.

Pharmacokinetic parameters play an integral role in the therapeutic or toxic effects of drugs; growth and maturation are associated with numerous physiologic changes that influence drug handling. Thus the pediatrician is confronted with a variety of patients with differing physiologic capabilities and medicinal needs. An understanding of basic pharmacokinetics will optimize drug therapy and increase the safety with which drugs are used. Four pharmacokinetic factors—absorption, distribution, metabolism, and excretion—can be used to describe the movement of a drug through the body.

ABSORPTION

One primary consideration of drug therapy is absorption, the translocation of a drug from its site of administration into the circulation. This process depends on the physical and chemical properties of the individual drug, as previously mentioned, and on the route of administration. The term *bioavailability* refers to the rate and extent of absorption of a drug. Because it is a measure of the amount of the drug that is actually absorbed and available to interact with drug receptors, this concept allows comparison of different pharmaceutical formulations and dosages of the active compound. The peak plasma concentration of a drug depends on the rate and extent of absorption. The time required to reach this peak concentration depends only on the rate of absorption.[8]

A drug's route of administration will affect its bioavailability. Commonly, the intravenous (IV) route is used for efficient and controlled (e.g., either rapid or slow) delivery of a medication directly into the circulation. This method eliminates the absorptive process common to other methods of drug administration. However, other factors may affect the bioavailability of drugs administered intravenously. The absorption of medication onto filter surfaces of the infusion apparatus may decrease the dose the patient receives. The IV flow rate and the volume of drug suspension will affect blood levels of the drug. This can be especially problematic with pediatric patients, for whom IV fluid rates on the order of a few milliliters per hour are common. For example, injection of a drug at a site in the infusion line somewhat removed from the patient may result in approximately 5 to 10 ml of intervening fluid volume. At an infusion rate of 3 ml/hr, it takes approximately 1.7 to 3.3 hours before the drug actually begins to reach the patient. A quick bolus injection followed by a "flush" will rapidly deliver the entire dose to the patient, resulting in higher peak blood levels. Typically, the larger the volume of the drug solution, the longer the administration time. In a fluid-restricted patient or in an infant receiving minimal fluids, administration of numerous medications, each of which is suspended in a certain volume of fluid, may provide for the total daily fluid requirement.[9] Thus intravenous administration of drugs circumvents the absorptive process, but the bioavailability of a drug may still be affected by the rate of infusion and the quantity of drug actually delivered to the patient.[10,13]

The pediatric age groups receive many drugs orally. Although the stomach is not the major site of drug absorption, the rich blood supply, the potential for prolonged contact of a drug with the gastric epithelium, and the relatively large epithelial surface facilitate the entry of drugs into the circulation. The changing pattern of gastric acidity, the relatively slow gastric emptying time seen in neonates and premature infants, and the nearly continuous presence of milk in the stomach of formula-fed babies all affect the gastric absorption of medication.[10,12]

The major site of drug absorption is the small intestine. This is because of the large surface area and the presence of specialized absorptive cells within this organ. The intestinal motility, enzymatic activity, permeability and maturation of the mucosal membrane, the ileal bile salt pool, bacterial flora, and the presence and type of food in the gastrointestinal (GI) tract play a role in drug absorption and may alter the dose requirement, efficacy, and toxicity of the drug. In addition, certain common childhood diseases such as diarrhea of viral, bacterial, or genetic origins (e.g., cystic fibrosis or celiac disease) affect the intestinal absorption of drugs.[5,10]

Intramuscular absorption in neonates, infants, and young children may be unpredictable because of vasomotor instability, decreased muscle tone and contraction, and diminished muscle oxygenation.[1,12] The absorption of a topically applied medication is inversely related to the thickness of the stratum corneum and directly related to hydration of the skin and therefore is increased in the newborn and young infant.[12] The ratio of surface area to body weight in the full-term neonate is much greater than that of an adult. If a newborn received the same percutaneous dose of a medication as an adult, the systemic availability per kilogram of body weight would be approximately 2.7 times greater in the neonate.[1] Tissue perfusion is also an important variable affecting the absorption of a medication applied subcutaneously, intramuscularly, or topically; absorption from these sites may be decreased because of circulatory insufficiency.

Medication administered per rectum (PR) may be absorbed very rapidly, depending on the formulation of the compound. This has been clinically exploited in several instances, such as in the use of diazepam PR to suppress seizure activity rapidly or in the administration of antiemetics to patients with nausea and vomiting. The disadvantages of this method of administration include a lack of patient acceptability, an interruption of absorption by defecation, and the much smaller absorptive surface area of the rectum compared with the small intestine.[4]

It should be noted that not all medications require absorption for activity. Some drugs, such as cholestyramine or bulk laxatives, are specifically formulated to remain within the GI tract with little or none of the drug entering the general circulation.

DISTRIBUTION

After absorption into the bloodstream, drugs are distributed to the body tissues. The specific distribution of a drug within the body can only be determined by direct tissue analysis. However, a useful concept relating the concentration of the drug in the plasma to its concentration in the remaining areas of the body (the volume of distribution [V_d]) provides some insight into drug distribution. The V_d is the hypothetical fluid space needed to contain the total body store of a drug if the concentration throughout the whole body equals that measured in the plasma. V_d is calculated by dividing the total amount of drug in the body by the plasma concentration that would exist, assuming instant equilibration, at time zero following a bolus intravenous injection (Fig. 27-1).

$$V_d \text{ (liters)} = \frac{\text{Total drug in body (mg)}}{\text{Plasma concentration (mg/L)}}$$

Because the V_d often exceeds the plasma volume, it is also referred to as the *apparent volume of distribution*. The larger the V_d, the greater the tissue concentration of the drug.[1,5] The concept of the V_d is useful in calculating drug doses (see further discussion under "Drug Dosing Regimens" below) and in comparing different age groups or disease states in which intrinsic patient variables alter the distribution of drug.

One variable that affects drug distribution is the change in the relative volumes of the water constituting the body mass (see Fig. 27-1). Neonates have a much higher proportion of body mass in the form of water (85% in premature infants, 75% in full-term infants) than the older child (59% at 1 year of age) or adult (55%). The ratio of extracellular water to intracellular water is also higher in neonates, infants, and children. Total body water declines rapidly during the first year of life, and adult levels are reached by 12 years of age.[5] Higher doses of drugs, on a per kilogram of body weight

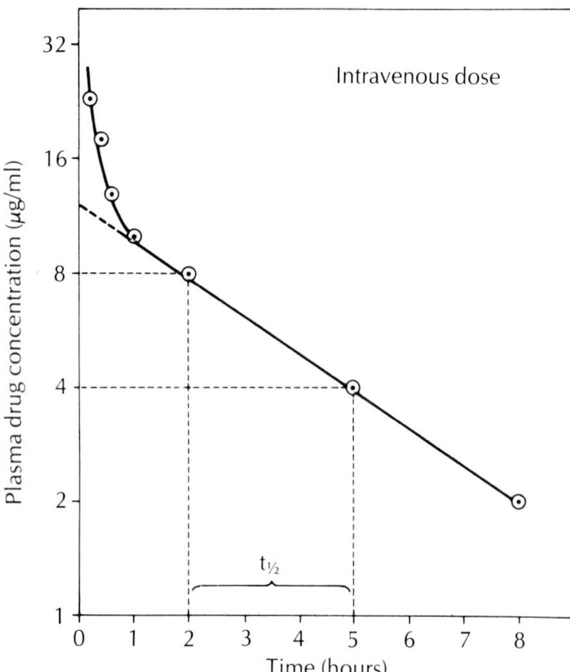

Fig. 27-1 Fundamental pharmacokinetic relationships for single doses of drugs. A drug (500 mg) is administered intravenously, and plasma samples are obtained for determination of drug concentration. The concentration falls rapidly initially, as distribution occurs. First-order elimination kinetics follows. Extrapolation of this line indicates a hypothetical plasma concentration of 12 μg/ml at zero time. The volume of distribution (V_d) is thus 500/0.012, or 41.7 L. The half-time of drug elimination (when the plasma concentration is 6 μg/ml) is estimated to be 3 hours.

Modified from Goodman LS and Gilman A: The pharmacological basis of therapeutics, ed 6, New York, 1980, Macmillan Publishing Co, Inc.

basis, that distribute into the extracellular fluid must be given to infants and children to achieve plasma and tissue concentrations comparable to adult concentrations.[1]

The relative amount of adipose tissue also fluctuates during growth. At birth adipose tissue makes up 10% to 15% of the total body mass and at 1 year of age accounts for 20% to 25% of body weight. This percentage declines between 1 and 2 years of age with the onset of walking and development of greater muscle mass and remains unchanged until puberty. In girls there is a rather sudden increase in adipose tissue at puberty, whereas the increase is less prominent in boys, in whom growth of muscle and skeletal mass predominate.[10]

Another factor affecting the V_d of a drug is the affinity of the drug for plasma proteins. The degree of protein binding is inversely related to the V_d because the large protein-drug complexes do not leave the vascular compartment readily. Renal clearance of the drug is decreased because only free drug is filtered at the glomerulus. Protein binding also increases the half-life of the drug (i.e., the time required for the concentration of drug in the plasma to decline to half the original level). The bound complexes slowly dissociate, resulting in the prolonged release of free drug into the circulation.[10]

Albumin is the protein primarily responsible for binding acidic drugs (e.g., salicylate, phenobarbital), and basic drugs are bound by a variety of plasma proteins such as lipoproteins, alpha-1-acid glycoproteins, and beta-globulins. In addition to diminished levels, neonatal albumin also exhibits a decreased affinity for many drugs (e.g., phenytoin). The full plasma-protein levels are not reached until approximately the end of the first year of life.[5]

One additional variable affecting protein binding is competition of endogenous molecules for binding sites. Endogenous molecules may displace drugs from binding sites, creating a transient rise in free drug and intensifying the pharmacologic response. This effect is transient because the free drug undergoes renal excretion, restoring a steady-state level. Alternatively, the drug may displace an endogenous molecule.[1] In the case of sulfisoxazole, bilirubin is displaced, increasing the risk of kernicterus.[16]

Cardiac output, blood flow to individual organs and tissues, variations in pH, and the acid-base balance all influence the distribution of drugs within the body. These factors are variable during the first days of life and may also vary depending on the medical condition of the patient.[12]

In summary, the V_d is influenced by the blood volume, the tissue volume and perfusion, the fraction of unbound drug in the blood, and the fraction of unbound drug in body tissues. For example, the aminoglycoside antibiotics are highly water soluble, exhibit poor penetration of lipid membranes, and have minimum tissue and protein-binding. The mean V_d is 0.25 to 0.45 L/kg for children and 0.50 L/kg in neonates, reflecting the extracellular fluid (ECF) volume. Disease states that increase the ECF volume (e.g., ascites) increase the distribution of these drugs. In contrast, theophylline is partially lipid and water soluble and is approximately 60% protein bound. Theophylline's V_d is greater in newborns, because of decreased protein binding and increased total body water, than in children or adults (0.6 to 0.9 L/kg versus 0.3 to 0.7 L/kg, respectively).[8]

DRUG METABOLISM

Metabolism and excretion are the primary mechanisms of drug elimination. The relatively high lipophilicity of most drugs inhibits their elimination in the unchanged form because intestinal and renal reabsorption are very efficient for lipid-soluble compounds. Renal excretion is facilitated by biotransformation of drugs into more water-soluble metabolites. Lipophilic compounds are generally less toxic, although also usually less pharmacologically active, so metabolism has also been described as drug detoxification.[10] However, biotransformation reactions can often activate a xenobiotic, initiating or potentiating physiologic responses to the compound.

The liver is quantitatively the most important organ for drug metabolism, although the kidneys, gut, and skin possess a variety of drug-metabolizing functions.[10] Uptake of the drug is the first step in hepatic biotransformation. Drugs are delivered to the liver via the portal vein following gastric or intestinal absorption. A drug that is exposed to hepatic metabolism before reaching the general circulation is subject to substantial hepatic biotransformation, and the resulting moiety that enters the systemic circulation may be predominantly in the form of inactive metabolites. Thus this initial "pass" through the liver may result in a drug that is substantially inactivated, causing a significant decrease in the pharmacologically active species. This process is known as the *first-pass effect*. Lidocaine, propranolol, meperidine, and morphine are drugs subject to substantial first-pass effects.[11]

Following delivery to the liver, carrier proteins transport the drug into the hepatic cell. The neonate has a lower concentration of transport proteins than does the adult.[1,5,10] For example, the level of ligandin, a basic protein that binds organic anions and bilirubin, is low at birth but reaches adult levels by 5 to 10 days of age.[1]

Once the drug is within the cell, it may be biotransformed by one or more of the phase I reactions, which may in turn be followed by a phase II reaction. Phase I reactions change a drug into a more active metabolite (e.g., chloramphenicol succinate to chloramphenicol), or into an equally active, less active, or inactive metabolite; phase II reactions generally result in inactive products. Biotransformation may also result in the transformation of a drug into a metabolite whose activity qualitatively differs from that of the parent compound.[1,10] For example, theophylline in neonates is methylated to caffeine; in older children and adults, this elimination pathway is insignificant.

Phase I reactions include oxidation, reduction, hydrolysis, and hydroxylation. The chemical structure, configuration, and presence of functional groups determine the type of reaction a particular drug undergoes. The hepatic mixed-function oxidases (cytochrome P-450 and NADPH-cytochrome C reductase) are responsible for most of the phase I reactions catalyzed by the human liver. Low levels of these enzymes are also present in the kidneys and lungs. Most phase I enzymes at gestation are present at low levels and remain low at birth, but the oxidative enzymes exhibit rapid postnatal maturation. At birth hepatic clearance of drugs is reduced, but within the first several weeks of life hepatic clearance equals or exceeds adult rates.[1] Drugs administered to the mother, either prepartum or during labor, may induce hepatic enzyme activity in the fetus or neonate. Examples of such drugs include phenytoin, phenobarbital, diazepam, and tricyclic antidepressants.[10]

Phase II reactions involve the combination of the drug with an endogenous molecule, thereby rendering the drug more water soluble and facilitating renal excretion. A relatively small number of such synthetic reactions are known in human beings. They include *conjugation* with glucuronide, glycine, glutathione, and sulfate, as well as *methylation* and *acetylation*.[1,10] Glucuronidation is depressed at birth and reaches adult levels by 3 years of age. Thus agents that are eliminated almost entirely by this pathway are potential toxins in neonates and infants, because alternate pathways of metabolism are not available. In contrast, sulfate conjugation is more efficient in neonates than in adults. In children, acetaminophen is excreted predominantly via sulfate conjugation, whereas in adults the glucuronide conjugate is the major metabolite.

Variations in biotransformation should not be assumed to always result in impaired drug elimination. Oral quinidine, for example, is cleared significantly faster by pediatric patients than by adults.[5]

EXCRETION

There are a variety of routes through which xenobiotics can be eliminated. Drugs may be excreted in the bile, feces, urine, or via exhalation through the lungs.[11]

Most drugs and their metabolites are excreted from the body by the kidneys. In the newborn, the ratio of the kidney weight to body mass is approximately twofold higher than that of adults. However, the organ is anatomically and functionally immature, and all aspects of renal function are reduced.[12]

Renal excretion depends on glomerular filtration, tubular reabsorption, and tubular secretion. At birth the glomerular filtration rate (GFR) is directly proportional to gestational age, and adult GFRs are not reached until 2.5 to 5 months of age.[1,5] This increase is most likely the result of the combination of increased cardiac output, decreased peripheral vascular resistance, increased mean arterial pressure, increased surface area for filtration, and increased membrane pore size.[1] In the preterm infant, the GFR is further reduced, and the rate of increase in renal function lags behind that observed in the full-term neonate. Low clearance rates for aminoglycoside antibiotics and indomethacin, both of which depend on glomerular filtration for excretion, are common. For example, the administration of gentamicin according to guidelines established for full-term newborns resulted in extremely high plasma concentrations in premature neonates. Digoxin is another drug primarily eliminated via glomerular filtration. Renal clearance of digoxin is low in the neonate and increases progressively until reaching adult levels by the first year of life.[5]

However, glomerular function is more advanced than tubular function. This imbalance may persist until 6 months of age and is reflected in functional differences of secretion in the proximal tubular cells. Many drugs rely on either the organic anion or cation transport systems present in the proximal tubule for renal excretion (e.g., penicillins, sulfonamides, and furosemide).[1] Elimination of these drugs exhibits

Table 27-1 *Factors That May Contribute to Variations in Pharmacokinetics in Infants and Children*

PARAMETER	NEWBORNS	OLDER CHILDREN
Absorption	↓ Intestinal motility ↓ Gastric acidity Delayed intestinal enzyme development	
Distribution	Relative fat content, blood flow Alteration in body water compartments ↓ Serum albumin Variations in albumin drug-binding capacity	Relative fat content, blood flow Alteration in body water compartments
Metabolism	Enzyme immaturity	
Excretion	↓ Glomerular filtration rate ↓ Tubular function	

an age-related alteration, and adjustments in drug doses are essential to prevent toxicity.

Some factors that contribute to alterations in pharmacokinetics in infants and children are summarized in Table 27-1.

KINETICS OF DRUG ELIMINATION

Following drug administration, plasma levels are determined by the pharmacokinetic characteristics of the drug. The drug is absorbed and distributed into various tissues, and the amount of drug remaining in the body is determined by the rate of elimination. Clearance refers to the overall rate of drug removal and thus is the sum of the clearance of drug by various routes, including the liver, kidneys, lungs, and skin.[11] The total body clearance (TBC) is the volume of body fluid from which a drug is removed per unit time; it may be calculated by:

$$TBC = K(V_d)$$

where V_d is the volume of distribution and K is the elimination rate constant for a given drug.

It is simpler to consider drug disappearance following intravenous injection because other drug delivery modes may have prolonged absorption times.[7] Initially there is a rapid decrease in the plasma concentration as the drug distributes throughout the body (Fig. 27-2). As the drug is cleared, a slower decline ensues, reflecting the elimination of drug from the body. Most drugs are eliminated from the body following first-order kinetics—that is, a constant fraction of the drug in the plasma is eliminated per unit time. This implies that the amount of drug eliminated per unit time is proportional to the plasma drug concentration and gradually declines as the plasma concentration decreases.

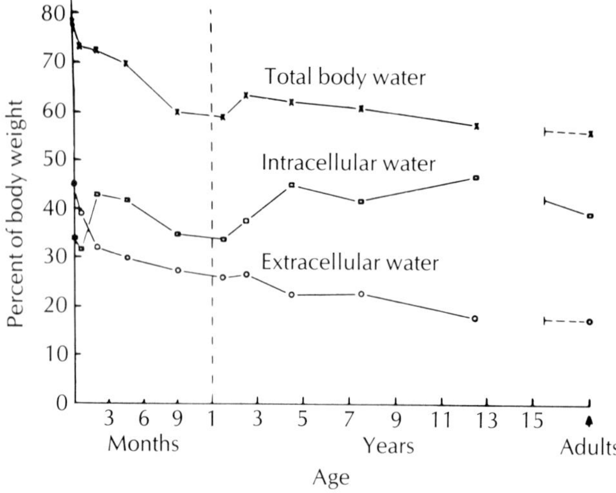

Fig. 27-2 Developmental changes in total body water, intracellular water, and extracellular water in infants and children. The changes are expressed as percentages of body weight.

From Rane A and Wilson JT: Clinical pharmacokinetics in infants and children, Clin Pharmacokinet 1:2, 1976; data from Friis-Hansen B: Body water compartments in children: changes during growth and related changes in body composition, Pediatrics 28:169, 1961.

This relationship is graphically depicted in Fig. 27-3, *A*. Note that the rate of elimination of the drug (represented by the tangent to the curve) varies continuously depending on its concentration at any given time. The decline in plasma concentration is exponential, and the results are usually plotted on a semilogarithmic scale (Fig. 27-3, *B*). This representation demonstrates that a constant fraction of the drug in the plasma is eliminated per unit time.[7]

Further analysis of the semilogarithmic graph yields useful information about the biologic half-life, represented by $t½$. The half-life is the time required for the concentration of drug in the plasma to decline to half its original level. Note that a constant fraction—that is, 50%—of the drug is eliminated per unit time regardless of the plasma concentration. Half-life can be calculated as :

$$t_{1/2} = \frac{0.693(V_d)}{\text{Plasma clearance}}$$

The half-life reflects the efficiency of drug removal and is determined by the clearance as well as the volume of distribution. A change in half-life may not necessarily reflect a change in clearance. For example, the clearance of kanamycin by neonates is approximately half that observed in adults. The half-life, however, is four times longer, reflecting the approximately twofold increase in the V_d in neonates.[11] Both parameters must be considered for proper dosing.

Some drugs are eliminated following zero-order kinetics. For these drugs, elimination occurs at a constant rate regardless of the plasma concentration; a constant amount (as opposed to a fraction, as with first-order kinetics) of the drug is eliminated per unit time (see Fig. 27-4). The half-life, then, depends on the plasma concentration of the drug.

In some instances the elimination may follow zero-order kinetics because of saturation of the elimination processes. This is significant, because ingestion or absorption of a drug at a rate exceeding the elimination can raise plasma drug concentrations, increasing the risk of toxicity. Ethanol, aspirin, and phenytoin all exhibit this phenomenon. At low doses, elimination proceeds according to first-order kinetics. At high doses, saturation of renal transport occurs, and elimination follows zero-order kinetics. Once saturation occurs, continued intake of the drug at a rate exceeding elimination will raise plasma concentrations to potentially toxic levels. The threshold at which first-order kinetics changes to zero-order kinetics varies in each individual. Once this threshold has been exceeded, small changes in drug dose may cause unanticipated increases in the plasma concentration.[7]

Drugs may enter organs or other body tissues in addition to distributing within the general circulation. These other areas are referred to as *compartments*, and the presence of drugs within these various compartments alters the kinetics of elimination. For example, the concentration of a drug within the plasma equilibrates with the concentration of drug in the second compartment. As elimination from the plasma occurs, the drug moves from the second compartment back into the plasma (from a higher concentration to a lower concentration). The rate of elimination is determined by the concentration of drug within the plasma, but the presence of drug within the second compartment provides a reservoir that

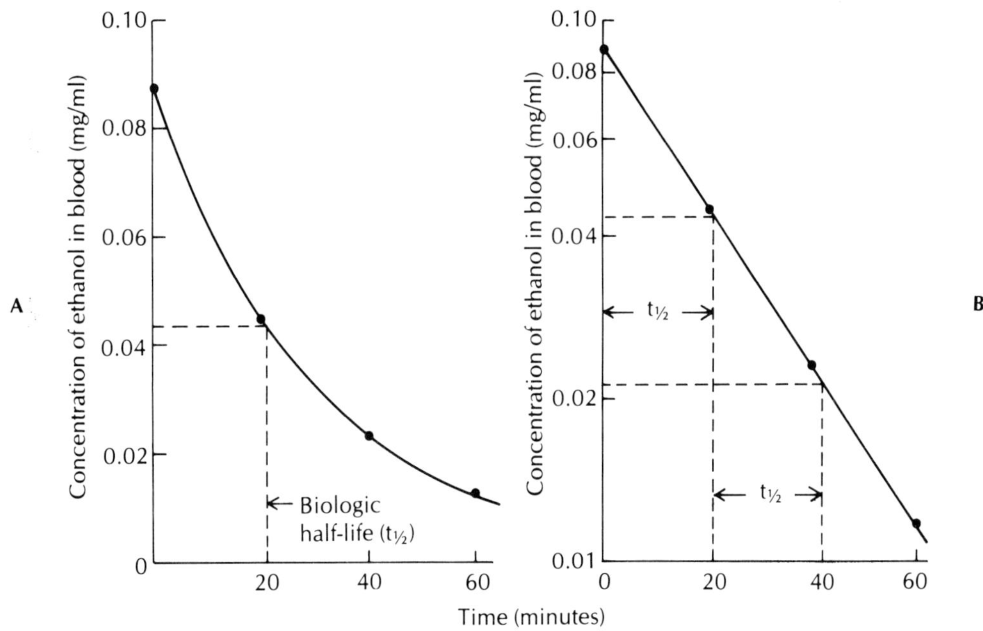

Fig. 27-3 First-order rate of elimination. Decline of ethanol content in blood following IV administration of a *small* dose to a dog. The ordinate reflects the concentration of ethanol in blood (mg/ml) on an arithmetic scale (**A**) and on a logarithmic scale (**B**). Biologic half-time ($t_{1/2}$) is about 20 minutes on both scales.

Modified from Marshall EK Jr and Frity WF: The metabolism of ethyl alcohol, J Pharmacol Exp Ther 109:431, 1953.

maintains plasma levels of the drug, thereby prolonging elimination. To complicate matters further, reentry of the drug into the plasma may occur slowly, thus extending the half-life of the drug.[2] These factors affect the dose and frequency of drug administration.

PHARMACODYNAMICS

The term *pharmacodynamics* describes the action of drugs within the living system. At the cellular level, xenobiotics may function outside of the cell membrane, at the cell membrane, or at an intracellular organelle such as the nucleus.

Generally, drugs that act outside the cell membrane react with some constituent of the extracellular fluid or within the gastrointestinal or renal tubular lumen. For example, antacids such as sodium bicarbonate act outside the cell by directly neutralizing gastric acidity. The chelators penicillamine and desferrioxamine are also effective without cellular interaction. Developmental differences are evident with the latter two drugs. Lead is deposited in the bone of children to a greater extent than in adults. Thus chelation of the lead in circulation may produce a greater efflux of lead from bone in children, aggravating the symptoms of plumbism.[10]

The volatile general anesthetics are examples of drugs that interact with cell membranes. There is evidence that these compounds act at specific areas of membranes and produce conformational changes in membrane proteins and lipids. Similarly, the osmotic diuretics function by establishing an osmotic gradient between the two sides of a cell or cell membrane.[10]

The most common interaction between drugs and body tissues involves the reaction with a cellular receptor. The important features of a drug-receptor interaction include the specificity and affinity of a drug for certain receptors, the reversibility of the interaction, and the proximity of the drug to the receptor.

The affinity and concentration of receptors are not static but can be modulated by the ligand. The affinity of insulin for its receptor varies inversely with the number of receptors occupied, a process known as negative cooperativity. Hyperinsulinemia may decrease, or "down regulate," the receptor concentration at the cell surface. Down regulation of receptors may explain tachyphylaxis, the phenomenon of a decreased physiologic response to a drug over time. "Up regulation" of receptors occurs when the receptor concentration increases in the presence of low levels of ligand.[10]

Most of the developmental studies of receptor levels and function have been performed in animals, and careful interpretation of these data is necessary. However, age-related modulation of receptor sites has been reported. The binding of insulin has been observed to be greater in neonates than in adults. The larger digoxin doses required by neonates can be partially explained by receptor differences. Digoxin receptor sites are twice as numerous in the neonate per unit of tissue as in the adult, but the receptor affinity for digoxin is less in the neonate. Thus higher doses of digoxin are required to achieve physiologic effects comparable to those in adults.[5,10]

Pharmacologic effects of drugs can be altered by the interaction between two or more drugs. Pharmaceutical incompatibility is one of the simpler types of drug interactions. Physicochemical properties of two or more drugs (or their excipients) or of a drug and the infusion fluid may result in a diminished or absent therapeutic effect. Some incompatibilities are obvious, such as the precipitation of a compound in the infusion fluid (e.g., mixing amphotericin B with ami-

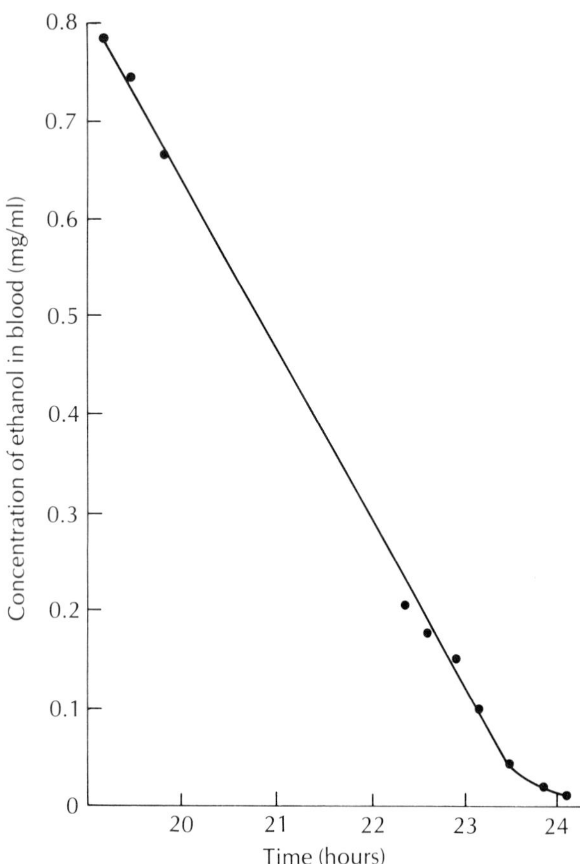

Fig. 27-4 Zero-order of elimination. Curve illustrating decline of ethanol content in blood following IV administration of a *large* dose to a dog. The ordinate is concentration of ethanol in the blood (mg/ml) on an *arithmetic* scale. The plotted data show the change from zero-order to first-order kinetics when low concentrations are reached between 23 and 24 hours after administration.

From Marshall EK Jr and Frity WF: The metabolism of ethyl alcohol, J Pharmacol Exp Ther 109:431, 1953.

kacin sulfate). Others may not be easily visualized, such as the decomposition of ampicillin and gentamicin sulfate when combined.[22]

Drug interactions can alter absorption by altering either the amount of drug absorbed or the relative rates of absorption. Antacids containing polyvalent cations chelate tetracyclines, forming an insoluble, inactive, and nonabsorbable complex. Alterations in the pH, typically by antacids, can also affect drug delivery. The concomitant administration of an antacid with an enteric-coated preparation can cause undesired side effects; the enteric-coated drug begins to dissolve in the elevated gastric pH produced by the antacid.[19,22]

Administration of two or more drugs that compete for protein-binding sites may increase, decrease, or have no effect on the amount of drug at the receptor site. The concomitant administration of methotrexate with either aspirin or sulfisoxazole, which increases the displacement of methotrexate from its binding site, can significantly potentiate toxicity because of elevated levels of methotrexate.[22]

Interactions of drugs at receptor sites are another area of clinical significance. Administration of diuretics can cause hypokalemia, which in turn may induce digitalis toxicity. It is proposed that digitalis acts by inhibiting the enzyme regulating the sodium potassium pump. If extracellular potassium is decreased, more digitalis binds to this enzyme, lowering the amount of potassium entering the myocardial cell. Myocardial contractility is therefore increased, and arrhythmias can occur.[22]

The induction or inhibition of metabolic enzymes by one drug can significantly affect concomitantly administered drugs. A toxic reaction to phenytoin has been reported as a result of the inhibition of metabolism by isoniazid. The induction of hepatic enzymes has been exploited by clinicians, as previously mentioned, to speed excretion.[10,22]

Renal excretion of drugs depends on the net effect of glomerular filtration, tubular secretion, and tubular reabsorption. Glomerular filtration is not markedly altered by other drugs. Tubular secretion can be altered by drug interactions, a fact that has been used to therapeutic advantage. The use of probenecid to inhibit tubular secretion of penicillin is well known. Manipulating tubular reabsorption also has clinical significance. For example, alkalinizing the urine prevents the reabsorption of weak acids, such as phenobarbital and aspirin, and has been used in the treatment of overdoses with these medications.[19,22]

Drug interactions can be potentially hazardous *or* can increase the therapeutic efficacy of drugs. The number of possible drug interactions has resulted in the publication of lists of potentially hazardous drug combinations. More recently, computer programs exist that can perform similar functions. Drug interactions are less common in the pediatric population, because few patients receive several drugs, but such interactions still pose a risk that is easily avoided by the informed physician.

PHARMACOGENETICS

Pharmacogenetics identifies the part that heredity contributes to clinically significant variations in drug response. Most of the pharmacogenetic disorders that have been characterized are at the level of drug metabolism. For the clinician, pharmacogenetic variation in the elimination of drugs is usually handled by recognizing that such variation exists and by the use of therapeutic drug monitoring. In practical terms, the cause of the variation is not often important, but the appropriate individualization of the drug dose is imperative. The example of succinylcholine sensitivity, however, exemplifies one extreme genetic variability. Shortly after use of this drug became widespread, extreme sensitivity to succinylcholine was observed in some patients, and several deaths associated with its use were reported. The rapid hydrolysis of succinylcholine by pseudocholinesterase typically limits the duration of action of this drug to 2 to 3 minutes. However, genetically inherited variants of this enzyme are responsible for prolonging the half-life of succinylcholine, thereby increasing the pharmacologic action of the drug. Several drugs can induce hemolysis of red blood cells in patients with glucose 6-phosphate dehydrogenase deficiency, one of the commonest hereditary enzymatic abnormalitities.[10,22]

DRUG-DOSING REGIMENS

The goal of drug therapy is to produce the desired pharmacologic response. This requires administration of the proper type and amount of drug at an appropriate frequency. In many cases there is a need to individualize therapy by altering the amount of drug administered, the frequency of doses, and the route of administration. For most drugs there is a plasma concentration below which subtherapeutic responses occur. Higher concentrations of the drug elicit the desired therapeutic effect, and still higher concentrations may result in adverse side effects. The goal of drug-dosing regimens is to maintain the plasma concentration of the drug within the therapeutic range.[10]

Several factors must be considered in selecting the appropriate drug dose. The condition being treated and any other potentially complicating medical conditions are of foremost importance. As previously discussed, other drugs that the patient may be taking can influence the current therapy. The child's age, size, and development, as well as the status of organs responsible for drug elimination, are important in the pharmacokinetics of the medication.

Many empirical rules and formulas have been published for pediatric drug dosing, reflecting the complexity of prescribing. The most acceptable general guide to drug dosing in children is based on the child's body surface area. Nomograms are available in several references along with tables of recommended drug doses.[6,10,14,17]

In some situations the observed response is readily utilized as a therapeutic end point (e.g., as with antihypertensives and diuretics), but for other drugs such an objective response is not readily available. Monitoring drug plasma levels may facilitate the modification of therapeutic regimens.[11] This therapeutic monitoring can be very useful if a strong correlation exists between the plasma concentration of a drug and the pharmacologic effect. That is, a therapeutic level can be determined within which the majority of patients will have the desired therapeutic response without sustaining undesired side effects. Above this range the risk of adverse reactions increases, and below the range the optimum therapy is not achieved.[10] The method of drug analysis must be reliable and relatively rapid for effective drug monitoring. Typically, therapeutic monitoring is used with drugs that exhibit a low therapeutic index—that is, the ratio of the plasma concentration providing therapeutic effects and that causing toxicity is low.

To use this method of determining an effective drug dose, peak plasma drug concentrations are obtained shortly after infusion of the medication. However, pharmacokinetic parameters of the individual drug must be considered when obtaining drug levels. If the peak plasma level is subtherapeutic, the dose is increased. Trough levels (or minimum plasma concentrations) typically occur immediately before the subsequent dose.[10] Low trough levels signal a need either to increase the dose, increase the frequency of drug administration, or both in order to maintain the plasma concentration within the therapeutic range.

Many clinical situations require continuous drug administration over a period of time. In this situation plasma drug levels are determined by the efficiency, rather than rate, of drug elimination. Administration of a drug either by continuous infusion, which provides a smooth plasma level–time curve, or by intermittent dosing, which yields a sawtooth profile, results in drug accumulation until a steady-state level is reached (Fig. 27-5). The ultimate average steady-state con-

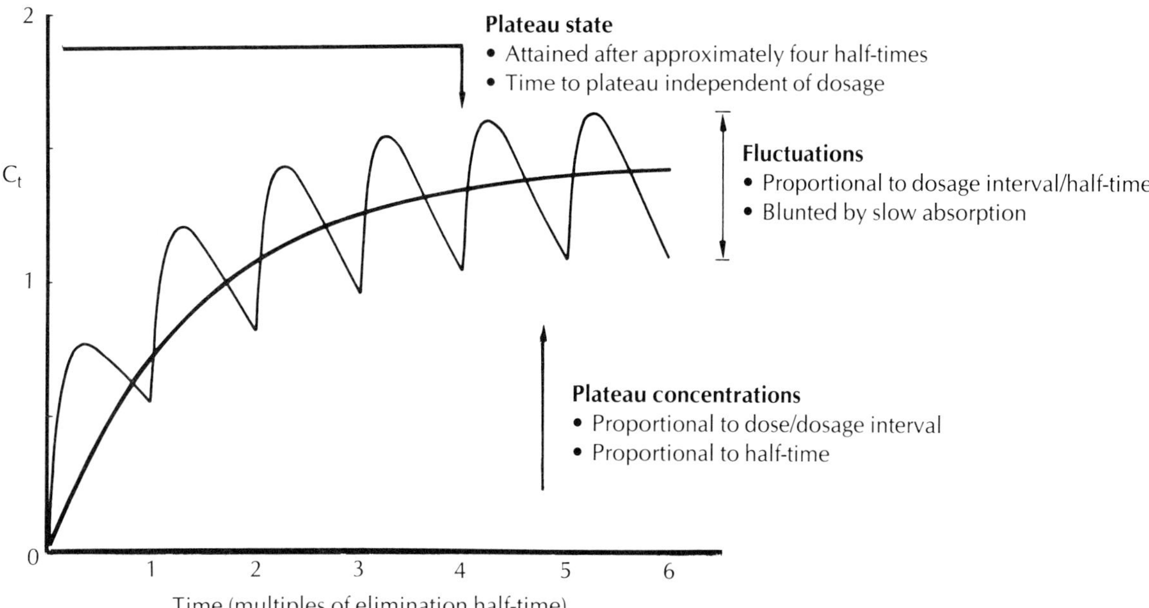

Fig. 27-5 Fundamental pharmacokinetic relationships for repeated administration of drugs. The light fluctuating line represents the pattern of drug accumulation during repeated administration of a drug as intervals equal to its elimination half-time. The heavy nonfluctuating line depicts the pattern during administration of equivalent dosage by continuous IV infusion. C_t, Concentration of a drug in plasma at time t.

From Goodman LS and Gilman A: The pharmacological basis of therapeutics, ed 6, New York, 1980, Macmillan Publishing Co, Inc.

centration achieved with either dosing pattern is directly proportional to the dosage rate (D/τ, where D = dose and τ = time) and inversely related to the efficiency of the systemic clearance (i.e., the drug removal from the plasma). Thus

$$\text{Concentration steady state} = \frac{\text{Dosage rate}}{\text{Plasma clearance}} = \frac{D/\tau}{\text{Systemic clearance}}$$

Individual variability in systemic clearance requires modification of the dosing rate to provide the desired steady-state plasma level. Therefore if systemic clearance is altered because of disease or developmental maturation, an inversely proportional change in the steady-state level results. For example, the faster elimination of theophylline observed in children necessitates more frequent dosing.[10]

Although the plasma elimination half-life is not useful in individualizing therapy, it is important in determining the length of time required to achieve steady state or to change from one steady-state level to another. Approximately four to five half-lives are required to attain a steady-state condition after beginning or altering the dose rate. The half-life is also used in determining the frequency of drug administration following an intermittent, repetitive regimen. For any given steady-state plasma level, the fluctuations between the peak and trough levels depend on the ratio of the half-life to the dosage interval. The smaller the dosage interval relative to the half-life, the smaller the fluctuations. Large doses given at greater intervals cause greater fluctuations in the plasma level and increase the risk of potentially toxic drug levels occurring soon after drug administration. Subtherapeutic levels may occur at the end of these long dosing intervals.[10]

In some therapeutic situations it may be undesirable to wait for drug accumulation to reach therapeutic levels, especially if the drug's half-life is prolonged. In this case a loading dose may be administered in order to achieve the desired plasma level and pharmacologic response immediately. The loading dose is larger than the usual maintenance dose and hence carries a risk of toxicity. The loading dose may be divided and given as multiple doses over a short period of time to avoid this risk. The size of the loading dose depends on the desired plasma level and the volume of distribution of the drug.

$$\text{Loading dose (mg/kg)} = V_d \text{ (L/kg)} \times \text{Desired drug concentration (mg/L)}$$

Maintenance doses are then instituted to keep the plasma level within the therapeutic range. The maintenance dose interval is determined primarily by the drug's half-life, as previously discussed.[10]

The plasma concentration of drugs, and therefore the therapeutic efficacy, can be affected by the drug formulation, time of sampling, absorption, metabolism, and patient compliance. Compliance can adversely affect even the most optimum drug regimen. It is estimated that the noncompliance rate in the pediatric clinic population is approximately 50%, with a range from 20% to 80%[22]; noncompliance rates in private practices are slightly lower.[15] Compliance can be improved by minimizing the number of drugs prescribed, by prescribing a palatable form of the drug that is easy to administer, and by simplifying drug regimens. Whenever possible the frequency of drug administration should be amenable to the family's regular schedule. In addition, careful instructions to the patient and parent and a positive interaction among the health care providers and the parents and patient increase compliance.[15] Sufficient amounts of the medication should be prescribed for treatment so that there will be no significant amount left after therapy is completed, and parents should be instructed to discard any surplus medication. Parent and patient perception of the therapy, method, and goals of treatment critically affect the outcome, and the time the pediatrician spends understanding these perceptions and educating the parents and patient will be amply rewarded. (See Chapter 12 for further discussions of compliance.)

SPECIAL CONDITIONS

Almost every drug is capable of eliciting an adverse reaction if sufficient quantities are administered. Idiosyncratic toxicity may be caused by an altered response to or metabolism of a drug or its metabolic products. A variety of drugs can induce hemolytic anemia in patients with glucose 6-phosphate dehydrogenase deficiency. Drug metabolites can act as haptens, inducing secondary immunologic responses. Often a detailed family history will reveal a pattern of toxicity to a particular class of drugs, thus guiding therapeutic choices.[10]

In a growing child additional considerations about drug toxicity arise because some medications interfere with the normal growth process. Corticosteroid therapy, for example, can halt growth, particularly linear growth. Tetracyclines interfere with calcium metabolism; in growing children, enamel hypoplasia can result in permanent dental staining in addition to a temporary inhibition of bone growth.[7]

Breast milk represents one potential source of drugs for the newborn. Drug passage into breast milk is favored if the drug has a low molecular weight, is present in an unionized (lipid-soluble) form, and has low affinity for plasma proteins.[10] Social drug use, including nicotine and ethanol, should be considered in addition to the mother's use of prescription medication. Although the use of drugs that are absolutely contraindicated for the breast-feeding mother is short and the relative concentration of a given drug within the breast milk may be so low that adverse effects for the infant are unlikely, it is prudent to minimize maternal drug exposure.[10,22] If maternal medication is unavoidable, drug exposure for the nursing child can be minimized by scheduling maternal drug dosing around nursing times. For most medications this can be achieved by instructing the mother to ingest the medication just after nursing or at least 4 hours before the next nursing period.[22] (See Chapter 16 for further information about drugs in breast milk.)

PRACTICAL APPLICATION OF PHARMACOLOGIC PRINCIPLES

From the preceding discussion it is clear that significant differences exist between children and adults, and these differences determine optimum medical therapy. The overview of the use of theophylline in the pediatric patient[22] provided below highlights many of the pharmacologic parameters previously discussed in this chapter and exemplifies a systematic approach to optimizing one drug regimen.

Absorption

Theophylline is rapidly, completely, and consistently absorbed when it is administered in liquid or uncoated tablets. Enteric-coated tablets and rectal suppositories have been associated with slow and incomplete absorption. Although sustained-release formulations may exhibit variable bioavailability, this limitation may be superseded by their therapeutic advantage in children in whom elimination is rapid and fluctuations in the plasma concentration between doses can be excessive.

Distribution

Once absorbed, theophylline is rapidly distributed throughout the body water; plasma levels equilibrate with interstitial fluids within 1 hour following IV injection. The apparent volume of distribution shows age-dependent changes. The V_d in a newborn is approximately 0.6 L/kg, reflecting the newborn's larger fraction of extracellular fluid; in children and adults the V_d is approximately 0.45 L/kg. Protein binding of the drug varies as well, with approximately 40% of the absorbed drug bound in the neonate versus approximately 60% in older children. Theophylline passes freely into breast milk, where the concentration approaches that of the plasma, and crosses the placenta. However, no serious consequences have been reported resulting from the transplacental passage of therapeutic theophylline levels or ingestion of breast milk containing theophylline.

Elimination

Renal excretion accounts for 10% of the drug clearance, and theophylline appears in unchanged form in the urine. The majority of the drug is metabolized in the liver via oxidation and demethylation reactions. Demethylation varies among individuals, and because the enzyme has a limited capacity, increasing plasma concentrations of theophylline results in a decreasing fraction of the drug being eliminated by this pathway. Thus changes in the drug dose may result in disproportionately large changes in the plasma concentration. The variability in clearance of theophylline, therefore, is a function of the rate of biotransformation, which is influenced by age, physiologic abnormalities of the patient, and concomitant use of other medications.

Clinical Use and Dosing

The bronchodilatory effect of theophylline has been shown to be proportional to the log of the plasma concentration over the range of 5 to 20 μg of theophylline per milliliter of plasma. Similarly, symptoms associated with chronic asthma have been prevented when plasma theophylline levels are maintained within 10 to 20 μg/ml. The potential for serious toxicity also correlates well with increasing plasma concentration. These observations have prompted monitoring of theophylline plasma concentrations to provide safe and optimum drug-dosing regimens.

When theophylline is used as an acute bronchodilator, the therapeutic goal is to relieve symptoms as rapidly as possible. A therapeutic concentration can be achieved quickly by administering an initial or loading dose of the drug in a form that provides rapid and reliable absorption (e.g., intravenous or oral preparation). Because of theophylline's rapid absorption and distribution, the resulting plasma concentration is more closely related to the V_d than to the rate of elimination. The plasma concentration (C) subsequently approaches a value equal to the administered dose (D) divided by the volume of distribution, $C = D/V_d$. Assuming a V_d of approximately 0.5 L/kg, each 1 mg of theophylline administered in rapidly absorbable form results in a 2 μg/ml increase in the plasma concentration. For example, a 7.5 mg/kg dose would be expected to result in a peak plasma theophylline concentration of approximately 15 μg/ml, assuming the patient has had no other medication containing theophylline. If a patient has an initial theophylline level of 10 μg/ml and the desired concentration is 15 μg/ml, the loading dose can be estimated as follows:

$$D = C \times V_d \text{ therefore,}$$

$$\text{Estimated loading dose} = (15\ \mu g/ml - 10\ \mu g/ml)(500\ ml/kg) = 2500\ \mu g/kg = 2.5\ mg/kg$$

Excessively rapid intravenous administration will result in transiently higher-than-predicted plasma concentrations, because a finite period of time is required for distribution of the drug. Delayed gastric emptying (e.g., as a result of food in the stomach) may result in lower peak plasma levels because of slower absorption of the medication. During this lag period, elimination of the drug begins and the expected peak levels may not be achieved. Interpatient variability in the V_d will also cause variation in peak plasma concentrations; therefore, aiming for initial peak levels of approximately 15 μg/ml should result in safe, therapeutic drug levels for most patients.

The therapeutic level of theophylline achieved with the loading dose is maintained by administering a continuous IV infusion at a rate that matches the patient's rate of drug elimination. This infusion rate is based on the age and clinical condition of the patient. Monitoring plasma theophylline levels will help determine the appropriate infusion parameters. This maintenance dose can then be used to determine the appropriate oral dose for the patient. The same total daily dose, in milligrams administered per 24-hour period, is divided by the desired dosing interval to determine the intermittent medication regimen. The dosing interval is a function of the absorption rate of the particular theophylline preparation used and the individual patient's rate of elimination.

If theophylline is started on an outpatient basis, and therefore no IV infusion is planned, the dose titration can be followed by periodic measurement of the plasma theophylline concentration. Reevaluation of therapy is important, because children tend to "outgrow" their doses, and frequent reassessment of therapeutic regimens is necessary during periods of rapid growth.

Trough levels may not provide essential therapeutic information. For example, if trough levels are low but the patient is symptom free, no adjustment of dose is needed. If the patient is symptomatic before the next drug dose, the peak-trough differential may be too great. This can be reduced by giving the same total daily dose at shorter intervals or by changing to a more slowly absorbed preparation.

SUMMARY

An appreciation of the numerous physiologic changes that occur during the development and maturation of the human body creates the unique challenges faced by the pediatrician. Clinical pharmacology has a unique role in the physician's daily practice. It is through an understanding of basic pharmacologic principles that these challenges are successfully met and optimum therapy is provided to the patient.

REFERENCES

1. Besunder JB, Reed MD, and Blumer JL: Principles of drug biodistribution in the neonate, Clin Pharmacokinet 14:189, 1988.
2. Clark B and Smith DA: An introduction to pharmacokinetics, Oxford, 1981, Blackwell Scientific Publications, Inc.
3. American Academy of Pediatrics Committee on Drugs: Guidelines for the ethical conduct of studies to evaluate drugs in pediatric populations, Pediatrics 60:91, 1977.
4. de Boer AG et al: Rectal drug administration: clinical pharmacokinetic considerations, Clin Pharmacokinet 7:285, 1982.
5. Evans WE and Jusko WJ, editors: Applied pharmacokinetics: principles of therapeutic drug monitoring, Spokane, Wash, 1986, Applied Therapeutics, Inc.
6. Gellis SS and Kagan BM, editors: Current pediatric therapy, vol 12, Philadelphia, 1986, WB Saunders Co.
7. Gilmar AG et al, editors: The pharmacological basis of therapeutics, ed 7, New York, 1985, Macmillan Publishing Co.
8. Kelly HW: Pharmacotherapy of pediatric lung disease: differences between children and adults, Chest Med 8: 681, 1987.
9. Leff RD and Roberts RJ: Problems in drug therapy for pediatric patients, Am J Hosp Pharm 44:865, 1987.
10. MacLeod SM and Radde IC, editors: Textbook of pediatric clinical pharmacology, Littleton, Mass., 1985, PSG-Wright Publishing Co., Inc.
11. Mirkin BL, editor: Clinical pharmacology and therapeutics: a pediatric perspective, Chicago, 1978, Year Book Medical Publishers, Inc.
12. Morselli PL, Franco-Morselli R, and Bossi L: Clinical pharmacokinetics in newborns and infants, Clin Pharmacokinet 5:485, 1980.
13. Roberts RJ: Intravenous administration of medication in pediatric patients: problems and solutions, Pediatr Clin North Am 28:23, 1981.
14. Rowe PC: The Harriet Lane handbook: a manual for pediatric house officers, Chicago, 1987, Year Book Medical Publishers, Inc.
15. Shope JT: Medication compliance, Pediatr Clin North Am 28:5, 1981.
16. Silverman WA et al: A difference in mortality rate and incidence of kernicterus among premature infants allotted to two prophylactic antibacterial regimens, Pediatrics 18:614, 1956.
17. Tendler C, Grossman S, and Tenenbaum J: Medication dosages during pediatric emergencies: a simple and comprehensive guide, Pediatrics 84:731, 1989.
18. Thompson DF and Heflin NR: Frequency and appropriateness of drug prescribing for unlabeled uses in pediatric patients, Am J Hosp Pharm 44:792, 1987.
19. Valman HB, editor: Pediatric therapeutics, Oxford, 1979, Blackwell Scientific Publications.
20. Ward RM and Green TP: Developmental pharmacology and toxicology: principles of study design and problems of methodology, Pharmacol Ther 36:309, 1988.
21. Weiss CF, Glazko AJ, and Weston JK: Chloramphenicol in the newborn infant, N Engl J Med 262:187, 1960.
22. Yaffe SJ, editor: Pediatric pharmacology: therapeutic principles in practice, New York, 1980, Grune & Stratton, Inc.

28

Antimicrobial Therapy

Keith R. Powell

The use of antimicrobial agents to treat diseases caused by bacteria is part of the day-to-day practice of pediatrics. At the same time, antimicrobial therapy has advanced and continues to advance at a rate unparalleled in medicine. It is difficult even for experts on infectious diseases to stay abreast of new agents and their pharmacology and pharmacodynamics. Developing a rationale for the use of antimicrobial agents should help prevent overuse and make it possible to evaluate consistently the merits and drawbacks of new antimicrobial agents. It is more important for the practitioner to know how to use a limited number of antimicrobial agents well than to have a meager knowledge of many.

APPROACH TO ANTIMICROBIAL THERAPY

Three important questions should be answered before beginning antimicrobial therapy: (1) where is the infection (anatomic site)?; (2) what pathogens usually cause infections at this site?; and (3) which antimicrobial agents, given by which route of administration, will achieve effective concentrations at that site? The answers to the first two questions are usually critically addressed by the practitioner. However, selection of an antimicrobial agent is more likely to be based on a "bug-drug" relationship than on knowledge about the ability to achieve an effective concentration at the site of infection.

The anatomic site of the majority of bacterial infections can be identified by a combination of historical information and findings on physical examination. When the site of infection is more obscure, diagnostic studies such as roentgenograms, radionucleotide scans, computed tomography scans, magnetic resonance imaging, and ultrasound evaluation are often helpful.

Based on the site of infection, the patient's age, habitat, history of exposures, and clinical signs and symptoms, it is usually possible to develop a list of potential bacterial pathogens. Knowing the site of infection and possible causative agents helps the clinician to decide what (if any) specimens should be cultured for bacteria, as well as whether the laboratory should be alerted to use special culture media or techniques. Selecting an antimicrobial agent based on its ability to achieve effective concentrations at the site of infection requires a working concept of what an effective concentration is. In order to define an "effective concentration," it is first necessary to review some of the basic pharmacodynamics of antimicrobial agents.

PHARMACODYNAMICS

The term *pharmacodynamics* describes the relationship between antimicrobial activity and the pharmacokinetics of an antimicrobial agent.

Minimum Inhibitory and Bactericidal Concentration

The activity of an antimicrobial agent against a particular bacterium in vitro is expressed as the agent's minimal inhibitory concentration (MIC) or minimal bactericidal concentration (MBC). To determine the MIC, bacteria are grown in broth to a concentration of 100,000 (10^5) microorganisms per milliliter. The broth containing bacteria, which is clear to the naked eye, is placed in a series of test tubes. To each test tube is added a decreasing amount of antibiotic. The broth containing bacteria and antibiotic is incubated overnight and then examined for visible turbidity. Turbidity represents bacterial growth. The test tube containing the smallest amount of antibiotic that remains clear to the naked eye is the MIC. To determine whether the antibiotic is bactericidal, the tubes that remained clear are quantitatively subcultured onto agar plates. After overnight incubation, bacterial colonies are counted. Each colony represents one bacterium that survived, or one colony-forming unit (CFU). The smallest amount of antibiotic that results in the death of 99,900 (99.9%) of the original 100,000 microorganisms per milliliter inoculum (a 1000-fold reduction) is the MBC. MIC and MBC results are reported in micrograms of antibiotic per milliliter of broth required to inhibit or kill, respectively.

Serum Inhibitory and Bactericidal Titers

An approximation of antimicrobial activity in vivo can be made by determining inhibitory or bactericidal titers. Although the test is usually performed using serum, it can be done with most body fluids that are clear, with the exception of urine. The test is performed by growing organisms to 10^5 CFU/ml of broth, as for determination of the MIC. However, instead of adding known concentrations of antibiotic to each test tube, serial twofold dilutions of serum (or other body fluids) are added to sequential tubes (i.e., undiluted serum is added to the first tube, serum diluted 1:2 to the second tube, 1:4 to the third, and so on). After incubation overnight, the tubes are examined for visible turbidity; the most dilute sample with no visible turbidity is the serum inhibitory titer. To determine if the bacteria are being killed, the broth is quantitatively cultured as for the MBC, and the most dilute specimen that results in the death of 99.9% of the original inoculum is the serum bactericidal titer.

The outcome of bacterial infections is usually associated with the peak serum bactericidal titer. In general, a peak serum bactericidal titer at a 1:8 dilution correlates with a clinical and microbiologic cure. In order to measure peak activity, it is necessary to time blood sampling based on when the drug is given, the route by which it is given, and the time after administration that peak serum concentrations are reached. The times that peak serum concentrations are reached with selected antimicrobial agents are listed in Table 28-1.

Tolerance

Tolerance to an antimicrobial agent describes the situation in which organisms are inhibited by usual concentrations of a bactericidal agent but require much higher concentrations of the agent to achieve a bactericidal effect. The clinical significance of tolerance is still controversial, but it appears that for infections that require bactericidal activity to effect a cure, this phenomenon may be important.[5]

Bacteriostatic Versus Bactericidal

A bactericidal antimicrobial agent is not required to treat the majority of infections in normal children. In general, bactericidal agents are necessary to treat bacterial endocarditis, meningitis, and osteomyelitis optimally. The effectiveness of bacteriostatic agents depends on the host's ability to opsonize and phagocytize bacteria that have been inhibited. Therefore, bactericidal agents are usually necessary to treat bacterial infections in the neutropenic host.

Pharmacokinetics

Because blood samples are easily obtained, the pharmacokinetics of antimicrobial agents are usually described as serum concentrations over time. Once administered to a patient, an antimicrobial agent is initially distributed throughout the intravascular volume and the extracellular fluid of those tissues with high perfusion rates. Entry into tissues that are not highly perfused occurs at a slower rate. Some antimicrobial agents, such as the beta-lactams, are distributed only in extracellular fluid, whereas others distribute intracellularly as well (rifampin, trimethoprim-sulfamethoxazole).

The pharmacokinetic parameter that best correlates with microbiologic cure is the amount of time that the serum concentration of the antimicrobial agent exceeds the minimal inhibitory concentration (MIC). Thus it is important to know not only the specific activity of the antimicrobial agent against the infecting organism, but also the serum concentrations above this activity that can be reached (peak serum concentration) and how long the activity will be sustained (serum half-life). The peak serum concentration that can be achieved is determined by both the rate of absorption and the rate of excretion of the antimicrobic agent. Higher peak serum concentrations are achieved with antibiotics that are absorbed readily and excreted slowly. When an administered agent is given intravenously, absorption does not play a role in peak serum concentrations. Some of the relationships between pharmacokinetics and antimicrobial activity are illustrated in Fig. 28-1.

The route by which an antibiotic is administered depends on the condition of the patient and the pharmacokinetics of the antimicrobial agent being considered. For some antibiotics, such as chloramphenicol and trimethoprim-sulfamethoxazole, peak serum concentrations after oral (PO) and intravenous (IV) administration are equivalent. For others, such as ampicillin, peak serum concentrations are 100-fold higher after intravenous administration. Any time oral antimicrobial

Table 28-1 *Times That Peak Serum Concentrations Are Reached After Administration of Antimicrobial Agents*

	ROUTE OF ADMINISTRATION*	TIME OF PEAK CONCENTRATION
Penicillins	IV	5 minutes†
Cephalosporins	IV	5 minutes
Penicillin V	PO	½-1 hr
Amoxicillin	PO	2 hr
Cephalexin	PO	1 hr
Aminoglycosides	IV	½ hr
	IM	1 hr
Trimethoprim-sulfamethoxazole	PO	1-2 hr
Sulfisoxazole	PO	2-3 hr
Erythromycin (estolate or ethylsuccinate)	PO	2 hr
Clindamycin	PO	1-2 hr
Chloramphenicol	PO/IV	2 hr
Vancomycin	IV	2 hr
Rifampin	PO	2 hr

*Abbreviations: IV, intravenous; PO, oral; IM, intramuscular.
†For drugs given intravenously, the time of peak serum concentrations is stated in minutes or hours after *completion* of the infusion.

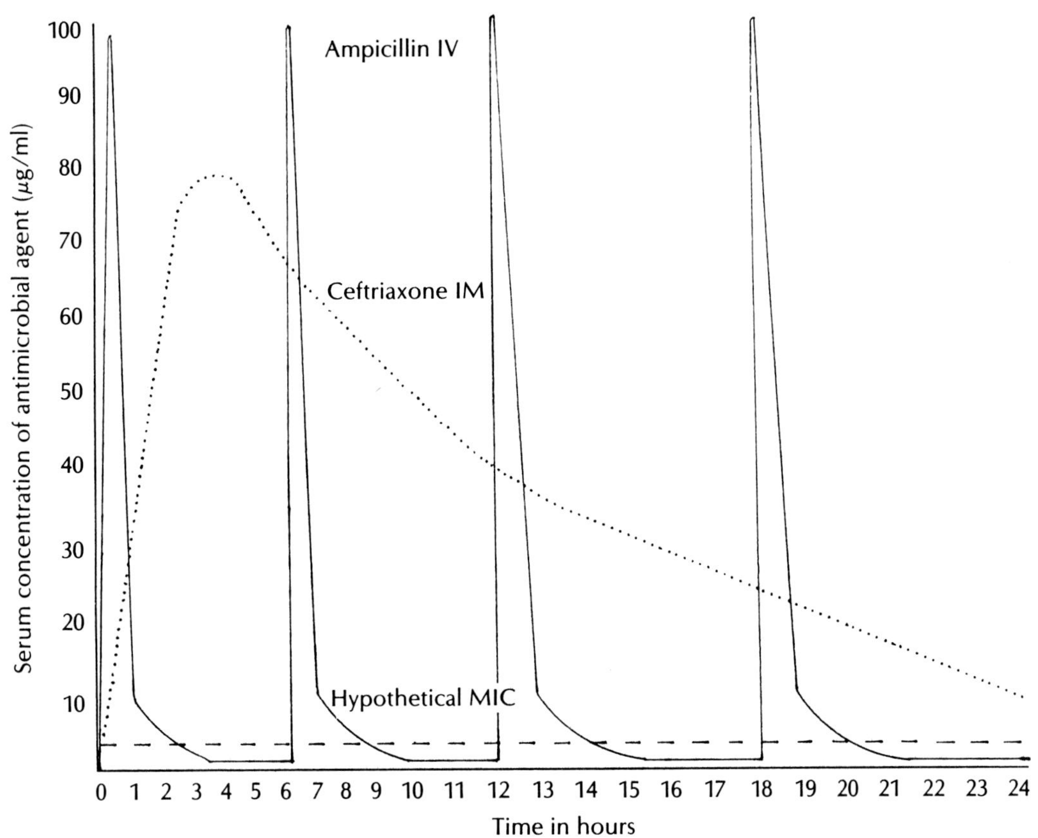

Fig. 28-1 The solid line represents serum concentrations of an antibiotic with a short serum half-life (e.g., ampicillin), given by rapid intravenous infusion. The peak serum concentration is achieved during the infusion; then concentrations fall rapidly. The length of time the serum concentration remains above the MIC depends on the actual value of the MIC. The dotted line represents serum concentrations of an antibiotic with a long half-life, given by the intramuscular route (e.g., ceftriaxone). It takes longer to reach the peak serum concentration after intramuscular administration because the antimicrobial agent must be absorbed from the muscle before it can be excreted. Because of slow excretion, serum concentrations remain above the MIC of susceptible organisms for a longer period of time. When a rapidly excreted antibiotic (like ampicillin) is given intramuscularly, peak serum concentrations are not very high because the drug is excreted almost as rapidly as it is absorbed.

therapy is considered, the ability of the patient to take, retain, and absorb the drug must be considered.

Inhibitory Quotient

One way to express the relationship between antimicrobial activity and pharmacokinetics is the inhibitory quotient (IQ). The IQ is derived by dividing the concentration of antimicrobial agent that can be achieved at the site of infection by the MIC of the agent required for the causative bacteria.[3]

$$IQ = \frac{\text{Concentration of antimicrobial agent}}{\text{MIC for causative bacteria}}$$

If the concentration of the antimicrobial agent at the site of infection exceeds the MIC by a factor of 10, the outcome is likely to be clinical and microbiologic cure. For the treatment of infections in well-perfused tissues, a favorable outcome can be expected when the peak serum concentration exceeds the MIC tenfold. For infections in sites such as the central nervous system (CNS), it is necessary to know how well antimicrobial agents reach these sites.

Role of the Laboratory in Antimicrobial Therapy

For the vast majority of bacterial infections treated in the ambulatory setting, little or no laboratory testing is necessary to use antimicrobial agents rationally. For example, otitis media is the most common infection of children treated with antibiotics in the ambulatory setting. The site of infection is determined by physical examination. The bacterial pathogens that cause otitis media have been well established, and several antimicrobial agents have been shown to result in a clinical and microbiologic cure when administered orally. It is not until empiric therapy has failed that it is necessary to perform a tympanocentesis to obtain a specimen for the isolation of bacteria and susceptibility testing. Likewise, by knowing the usual pathogens and their susceptibility to antimicrobial agents, it is possible to manage common infections such as impetigo, cellulitis, cervical adenitis, local abscesses, and conjunctivitis without obtaining specimens for culture.

Culture and Susceptibility

When usual therapy fails, when the patient is more seriously ill or is immunocompromised, or when the clinical situation is unusual, the first step is to obtain appropriate specimens to culture for bacterial pathogens. When bacterial pathogens are isolated from a usually sterile specimen, antimicrobial susceptibility testing is performed.

Susceptibility testing is performed by either determining the MIC as described previously or by using the disk diffusion method. The disk diffusion method is performed by first inoculating a culture plate with the bacteria to be tested. Paper disks that contain standardized concentrations of antimicrobial agents are then placed on the surface of the culture medium. The culture plates are incubated, and the moisture from the medium allows the antimicrobial agents to diffuse out of the paper disks. The farther away from the disk, the lower the concentration of antimicrobial agent. If the bacteria are inhibited by the antimicrobial agent, there will be a zone around the disk in which the bacteria do not grow. The zone of inhibition is measured after overnight incubation and, based on the diameter of the zone of inhibition, the organism is determined to be "susceptible" or "resistant." A report of "intermediate" or "indeterminant" should be interpreted to mean that the microorganism is resistant or that the MIC should be determined. The diameter of the zone of inhibition has been correlated to MIC determinations so that "susceptible" actually means that the MIC will be equal to or less than a certain concentration of the antimicrobial agent. When an organism is reported to be susceptible by disk, it means that 95% of strains of this bacteria are *inhibited* by concentrations of the antimicrobial agent that can be achieved in the *serum* if the antimicrobial agent is given at the usual dose by the usual route of administration for an infection with that organism. This concentration is termed the MIC_{95}. The MIC_{95} of selected antimicrobial agents for bacteria reported as susceptible by disk are listed in Table 28-2. Thus it is important to consider the site of infection, the activity of the antimicrobial agent against the pathogen, and the concentration of antimicrobial agent that can be achieved at the site of infection.

For example, "susceptible to ampicillin" has very different meanings, depending on the organism that is being tested. When gram-negative organisms or enterococci are reported as susceptible to ampicillin, it means that 95% of these organisms are inhibited by 8 μg/ml or less of ampicillin.[7] For gram-positive cocci, susceptible means that 95% are inhibited by 0.2 μg/ml or less, or 40 times less ampicillin than it takes to inhibit gram-negative enterics.[7] For *Haemophilus influenzae*, susceptible means that it takes 2 μg/ml or less to inhibit 95% of all strains.[7] Unless the MIC has been determined for the individual isolate, the clinician must assume that it will be necessary to achieve the MIC_{95} at the site of infection in order to inhibit the isolate. Thus to treat pyelonephritis caused by *Escherichia coli* with ampicillin, the practitioner would ideally like to achieve concentrations of ampicillin 10 times the MIC in renal parenchymal cells. Since susceptible means that 95% of *E. coli* are inhibited by ≤8 μg/ml, the concentration of ampicillin required in renal parenchymal cells should be assumed to be 80 μg/ml (IQ = $^{80}/_{8}$ = 10) unless the actual MIC for the isolate is known.

SPECIFIC ANTIBACTERIAL AGENTS

Because a large number of antimicrobial agents are currently available, there are usually several that are equally effective for a given infectious disease. The antimicrobial agents preferred by a practitioner reflect the drugs' cost and availability as well as the physician's training and local practices. In general, it is far better to know how to use a small number of antimicrobial agents well than to know all of the possible alternatives. The antimicrobial agents that physicians use most frequently and selected pharmacologic and pharmacodynamic information concerning them are presented in Table 28-2. This table is intended to serve as an example of the information that a practitioner should have at hand when using antimicrobial agents; the specific antibiotics that should be used for selected infections are discussed later in this chapter, after some general information about classes of antibiotics.

Penicillins

Mechanism of Action. Although the general mechanism of action of penicillins is to inhibit cell wall synthesis, precisely how penicillins do this is not known. Current evidence points to the inhibition of transpeptidation as the mechanism of action. Most bacteria have penicillin-binding proteins (PBP) in their cell membranes. There are a number of penicillin-binding proteins, and the number and type vary from bacteria to bacteria. The activity of penicillins generally correlates with the number of high-affinity PBPs the organism has.

Resistance of Bacteria to Penicillins. Resistance to penicillins can be based on several factors. Bacteria that lack appropriate PBP will be resistant. However, in order for penicillins to reach the PBP, they must first pass through the protein layers on the outer surface of the organism's membrane. Some bacteria are resistant because, as a result of shape or electronic charge, the penicillin is not able to reach the binding sites. The most important mechanism of resistance is bacterial production of beta-lactamases. These enzymes hydrolyze the beta-lactam structure, rendering the penicillin inactive. There are also some organisms that bind penicillin and are inhibited but do not undergo autolysis and death. These organisms are penicillin tolerant.

Classification of Penicillins. Penicillins can be loosely classified based on their specific antibacterial activity into (1) natural, (2) penicillinase resistant, (3) amino-, (4) antipseudomonas, and (5) extended-spectrum penicillins. The practitioner should be well versed in the use of one penicillin from each class, as presented below under "Use of Selected Penicillins."

Pharmacologic Properties. Penicillins vary greatly in absorption after oral administration, with penicillin V, amoxicillin, cloxacillin, and dicloxacillin having the greatest absorption. Food decreases the absorption of oxacillin and dicloxacillin but not of penicillin V or amoxicillin. Procaine penicillin G and benzathine penicillin G are slowly absorbed after intramuscular injections and are given every 12 to 24

Table 28-2 *Dosage, Peak Serum Concentrations, and MIC_{95} for Selected Antimicrobial Agents*

ANTIMICROBIAL AGENT	ROUTE OF ADMINISTRATION	AGE: UNDER 1 WEEK* (UNDER 2000 G) MG/KG/DOSE/INTERVAL	AGE: 1 WEEK TO 1 MONTH* (UNDER 2000 G) MG/KG/DOSE/INTERVAL	AGE: OVER 1 MONTH MG/KG/DOSE/INTERVAL	AGE: ADULT DOSE† MG/KG/DOSE/INTERVAL	PEAK SERUM CONCENTRATION μG/ML	SUSCEPTIBLE (MIC_{95}) μG/ML
Penicillin G	IV	50,000 U q8h (50,000 U q12h)	50,000 U q6h (50,000 U q8h)	25,000- 50,000 U q4-6h	25,000- 50,000 U q4-6h	400 U	≤0.1 *Listeria monocytogenes* ≤2
Procaine	IM	50,000 U q24h (50,000 U q24h)	50,000 U q24h (50,000 U q24h)	25,000-50,000 U q12-24h	25,000-50,000 U q12-24h	1 U	≤0.1
Benzathine	IM	50,000 U; 1 dose (50,000 U; 1 dose)	50,000 U; 1 dose (50,000 U; 1 dose)	50,000 U 1 dose	50,000 U 1 dose	0.12 U	≤0.1
Penicillin V	PO	NR‡	NR	6.25-12.5 q6h	0.25-0.5 q6h	3-5	≤0.1
Ampicillin	IV IM	25-50 q8h (25-50 q12h)	25-50 q6h (25-50 q8h)	25-75 q4-6h	1-2 q4-6h	40 8	Gram negative ≤8 Streptococci ≤0.1 *H. influenzae* ≤2
Amoxicillin	PO	NR	NR	10-15 q8h	0.25-0.5 q8h	4.7-7.5	As for ampicillin
Nafcillin	IV	17 q8h (25 q12h)	18.75 q6h (25 q8h)	25-50 q6h	0.5-1.5 q4-6h	11	≤1
Methicillin§	IV	25-50 q8h (25-50 q12h)	25-50 q6h (25-50 q8h)	—	—	—	—
Dicloxacillin	PO	NR	NR	3.125-6.25	0.25-0.5 q6h	15-18	≤1
Mezlocillin	IV IM	75 q12h (75 q12h)	75 q8h (75 q8h)	50-75 q4-6h	3 q4h or 4 q6h	200-300 15	≤64
Cefazolin	IV IM	20 q12h (20 q12h)	20 q8h (20 q12h)	8.3-25 q6-8h	0.5-1.5 q6-8h	188	≤8
Cephalexin	PO	NR	NR	6.25-12.5 q6h	0.25-1 q6h	8-40	≤8
Cefoxitin	IV IM	NR	NR	20-26.6 q4-q6h	1-2 q4-q6h or 3 q8h	110-125	≤8
Cefotaxime	IV	50 q12h (50 q12h)	50 q8h (50 q8h)	25-50 q6h	1-2 q4-q6h	1 g 40 2 g 80-90	≤8
Ceftriaxone	IV IM	50 q24h (50 q24h)	50-80 q24h (50 q24h)	50 q24h CNS: 80 q24h	0.5-2 q24h	1 g 150 1 g 50	≤8
Ceftazidime	IV IM	30 q12h (30 q12h)	30 q8h (30 q8h)	25-50 q6h	0.5-2 q8-12h	1 g 85 1 g 34	≤8
Amikacin	IV IM	10 q12h (7.5 q12h)	10 q8h (7.5 q8h)	5 q8h or 7.5 q12h	.005 q8h or q12h	20-40 20	≤16
Gentamicin	IV IM	2.5 q12h (2.5 q12h)	2.5 q8h (2.5 q8h)	1-2.5 q8h		4-10 7	≤4

Continued.

Table 28-2 *Dosage, Peak Serum Concentrations, and MIC_{95} for Selected Antimicrobial Agents—cont'd*

ANTIMICROBIAL AGENT	ROUTE OF ADMINISTRATION	MG/KG/DOSE/INTERVAL, BY AGE: UNDER 1 WEEK* (UNDER 2000 G)	1 WEEK TO 1 MONTH* (UNDER 2000 G)	OVER 1 MONTH	ADULT DOSE† (G)	PEAK SERUM CONCENTRATION µG/ML	SUSCEPTIBLE (MIC_{95}) µG/ML
Tobramycin	IV IM	2 q12h (2 q12h)	2 q8h (2 q8h)	2-2.5 q8h	1-1.7 **mg/kg** q8h	4-14 4	≤4
Trimethoprim (TMP)-sulfa-methoxazole (SMX)	PO IV	NR	NR	3-6 TMP/15-30 SMX q12h 5 TMP/25 SMX q6h for *Pneu-mocystis*	0.16 TMP/0.8 SMX q12h	2-4/80-100	≤2/38
Sulfisoxazole	PO	NR	NR	37.5 q6h	0.5-1 q6h	40-50	≤100 (urinary tract in-fection only)
Erythromycin estolate	PO	10 q12h (10 q12h)	10-12.5 q8h (10 q8h)	10 q8h or 15 q12h	0.25-0.5 q6h	4.2	≤0.5
Erythromycin ethylsuccinate	PO	10 q12h (10 q12h)	10 q8h (10 q8h)	10 q6h	0.25-0.5 q6h	1.5	≤0.5
Clindamycin	PO IV	5 q8h (5 q12h)	5 q6h (5 q8h)	2.5-7.5 q6h	0.15-.45 q6h	2.5-3.6	≤0.5
Chloram-phenicol	IV PO	25 q12h (25 q24h)	25 q24h (25 q24h)	12.5-18.75 q6h 18.75-25 q6h (meningitis)	12.5-25 **mg/kg** q6h	19 25	*H. influen-zae* ≤4 Others ≤12.5
Tetracycline	IV PO	NR	NR	Children >8 yr 6-25-12.5 q6h	0.25-0.5 q6h	8 4	≤4
Vancomycin	IV	15 q12h (15 q12h)	15 q8h (15 q8h)	10-15 q6h	15 **mg/kg** q12h or 6.5-8 **mg/kg** q6h	30-40	≤5
Metronidazole	PO IV	7.5 q12h (7.5 q12h)	15 q12h (7.5 q12h)	5-12 q8h 7.5 q6h	7.5 **mg/kg** q6h	11.5 20-25	≤4
Rifampin	PO	NR	NR	10-20 q24h	0.6 q24h	7	≤1

*Doses and intervals for infants less than 1 week of age and 1 week to 1 month of age are indicated without parentheses for infants with a birth weight of 2000 g or more; the doses and intervals for infants with a birth weight of less than 2000 g are given in parentheses.

†Maximum recommended doses; units other than grams are *boldfaced*.

‡NR Not recommended.

§Methicillin is preferred for newborns when kernicterus is a concern.

hours and every 15 to 20 days, respectively. Penicillins are excreted by renal tubular cells and have a very short half-life, ranging from less than 30 minutes to slightly over 1 hour. Penicillins are distributed to most areas of the body if inflammation is present. However, they are poorly lipid soluble and do not enter the central nervous system well even in the presence of inflammation. Penicillins do not enter cells well. Passage of penicillins from the serum of a pregnant woman to her fetus depends on the degree of protein binding present, with little of highly protein-bound penicillins reaching the fetus.

Side Effects of Penicillins. The most important adverse reactions to penicillins are caused by hypersensitivity; they range from skin rashes to anaphylaxis. Anaphylactic reactions to penicillin are IgE mediated and occur in about two of every 1000 courses of treatment; about one of every 100,000 courses results in a fatality. The morbilliform rashes seen during therapy with penicillins are probably IgM mediated and often disappear even when therapy is continued. Less common reactions include serum sickness, exfoliative dermatitis, and Stevens-Johnson syndrome.

Penicillin Desensitization. When it is deemed important to use penicillin in a patient in whom an anaphylactic reaction is feared, immunotolerance to penicillin can be achieved by starting with very small doses. An effective protocol is to administer 5 U of penicillin G intracutaneously in the forearm and then at 60- to 90-minute intervals, increase the dose to 10, 100, 1000, 10,000, and 50,000 U. If the intradermal doses are tolerated, intravenous penicillin can be instituted.

Use of Selected Penicillins (Table 28-2). The natural penicillins listed in Table 28-2 are penicillin G (aqueous, procaine, and benzathine) and penicillin V. These antimicrobial agents are most active against both aerobic and anaerobic gram-positive cocci, *Neisseria meningitidis, Neisseria gonorrhoeae, Fusobacterium* species, *Eikenella* species, *Listeria monocytogenes,* and *Borrelia burgdorferi*. Penicillins remain the mainstay of therapy for infections caused by group A beta-hemolytic streptococci, group B streptococci, *Streptococcus pneumoniae, N. meningitidis,* and *L. monocytogenes*. Penicillin is also the drug of choice for acute infections with *B. burgdorferi* (Lyme disease) in children and infections caused by anaerobes that are normally found in the mouth.

The potassium salt of penicillin G is usually used and is given almost exclusively intravenously. When given intramuscularly, aqueous penicillin G is excreted very rapidly; when given by mouth, it is poorly absorbed. For intramuscular administration, either procaine or benzathine preparations are used. It must be remembered, however, that very low serum concentrations are achieved with these preparations, and they can only be used for exquisitely sensitive organisms and generally should not be used to treat central nervous system infections. Procaine penicillin can be used in the newborn to treat neurosyphilis. Penicillin V is well absorbed from the gastrointestinal tract and therefore is preferred for oral administration. Peak serum concentrations and MIC_{95} equivalents for susceptibility by disk are listed for individual penicillins in Table 28-2.

Ampicillin has the same general activity of penicillin but is also active against *Escherichia coli, Proteus mirabilis, Salmonella* species, and *Shigella* species and more active against group D streptococci and *L. monocytogenes*. Amoxicillin differs in its molecular composition from ampicillin only by the presence of a hydroxyl group. It is absorbed much better than ampicillin so that peak serum concentrations of amoxicillin after oral administration are equal to those achieved with an equivalent dose of ampicillin given intramuscularly. The antimicrobial activity of amoxicillin is virtually identical to that of ampicillin except that it is not useful in the treatment of shigellosis.

Clavulanic acid is a beta-lactamase inhibitor that is available in a fixed combination with amoxicillin and marketed as Augmentin. The beta-lactamase inhibitor extends the activity of amoxicillin to include organisms that produce beta-lactamases. The MIC of Augmentin for beta-lactamase–producing *Staphylococcus aureus, Haemophilus influenzae, N. gonorrhoeae,* and *Moraxella catarrhalis* is 2 μg/ml, and its MIC for *E. coli, Klebsiella, Proteus,* and *Bacteroides fragilis* ranges from 8 to 16 μg/ml.

Nafcillin is one of several penicillinase-resistant penicillins that are used primarily to treat infections caused by *S. aureus*. Most strains of *S. aureus* are inhibited by concentrations of 2 to 3 μg/ml. Because nafcillin is highly protein bound, methicillin is preferred for newborns when the possibility of kernicterus is a concern. Absorption of nafcillin from the gastrointestinal tract is erratic; it should not be given orally. Dicloxacillin is absorbed from the gastrointestinal tract more consistently than is nafcillin and is a good oral agent for the treatment of *S. aureus* infections. The oral suspension of dicloxacillin has a very bitter taste, which can create problems with compliance.

Several antipseudomonas and extended-activity penicillins currently are available. In general, pseudomonas infections should be treated with a combination of one of these agents plus an aminoglycoside both for synergy and to decrease the emergence of resistant bacteria. Mezlocillin has the antipseudomonal activity of carbenicillin and ticarcillin, plus it is more active against enterococci, *Klebsiella* species, *H. influenzae,* and *B. fragilis*. It is important to remember that a report of "susceptible to mezlocillin" means that it will take concentrations of as much as 64 μg/ml to inhibit 95% of the strains tested. This is compensated for by the high serum concentrations achieved when the drug is given intravenously (peak serum concentration equals 300 μg/ml after a dose of 4 g).

Cephalosporins

Mechanism of Action. Like penicillins, cephalosporins are beta-lactam antibiotics that interfere with cell wall synthesis. However, the precise mechanism is not known, and the effects of cephalosporins on bacteria range from lysis of the organism to production of bacteria with unusual morphologies.

Resistance of Bacteria to Cephalosporins. Resistance to cephalosporins can result from their inactivation by beta-lactamases, their inability to reach antibiotic binding proteins, the absence of appropriate binding sites on the bacteria, or tolerance (see penicillins above).

Classification of Cephalosporins. More new cephalosporins have been introduced for general use in the past decade than any other type of antimicrobial agent. The usual classification system is based on antibacterial activity and refers to first, second, and third generation cephalosporins. In general the first generation cephalosporins have good activity against gram-positive cocci except enterococci, coagulase-negative staphylococcal species, and methicillin-resistant *S. aureus;* they have limited activity against gram-negative organisms except *E. coli, Klebsiella pneumoniae,* and *P. mirabilis*. The second generation cephalosporins have the general activity of the first generation but are somewhat more active against gram-negative organisms, including *H. influenzae*. The third generation cephalosporins are more active against gram-negative organisms than are the second generation but are less active against gram-positive organisms than the first generation drugs.

Pharmacologic Properties. Because of the number of cephalosporins and the wide variations in pharmacology, each drug should be considered individually.

Side Effects of Cephalosporins. The side effects seen with cephalosporins are generally those seen with penicillins. Hypersensitivity reactions are the most common side effects. Although immunologic studies have shown about 20% cross-reactivity between penicillins and cephalosporins, in practice only 5% to 10% of those who have hypersensitivity reactions to penicillins have them with cephalosporins. In general, if patients have had only a nonurticarial rash as the manifestation of penicillin hypersensitivity, it is safe to use cephalosporins. In patients who have had urticaria or an anaphylactic reaction to penicillins, cephalosporins should be used with great caution or not at all. Less common side effects seen with cephalosporins are nephrotoxicity (avoid cephaloridine), diarrhea, alcohol intolerance, and bleeding.

Use of Selected Cephalosporins

First Generation Cephalosporins. First generation cephalosporins are useful to treat infections with gram-positive cocci when penicillin cannot be used, to treat infections caused by methicillin-sensitive *S. aureus,* and to provide coverage against *E. coli, K. pneumoniae,* and *P. mirabilis*. Cefazolin is preferable to cephalothin because it has greater activity against *E. coli* and *Klebsiella* species, achieves higher peak serum concentrations, and has a longer half-life. Peak serum concentrations of cefazolin after a dose of 1 g given intravenously are 188 μg/ml; the serum half-life is 1½ to 2 hours. Susceptible by disk means that 95% of the bacteria tested are inhibited by 8 μg/ml or less. Cephalexin (Keflex) is a first generation cephalosporin that can be given orally. A peak serum concentration of 16 μg/ml can be achieved with a dose of 0.5 g. The antibacterial activity of cephalexin is similar to that of cefazolin.

Second Generation Cephalosporins. Although several second generation cephalosporins enjoy widespread use, there is usually a penicillin or a first or third generation cephalosporin that will have advantages in either cost or specific activity. The most useful exception is cefoxitin. Cefoxitin is highly resistant to beta-lactamases and is more active against anaerobes, especially *B. fragilis,* than other cephalosporins. It is not as active as other second generation cephalosporins against *H. influenzae* and Enterobacteriaceae, nor is it as active against gram-positive cocci as are first generation cephalosporins. Because of its activity against anaerobes plus some gram-positive and gram-negative aerobes, cefoxitin has proved useful in the treatment of pelvic inflammatory disease and lung abscesses. The peak serum concentration after a dose of 1 g given intravenously is about 22 μg/ml, and the serum half-life is about 50 minutes. Susceptible by disk means that the MIC_{95} for the organism will be 8 μg/ml or less.

Cefuroxime is the only second generation cephalosporin that achieves therapeutic concentrations in cerebrospinal fluid (CSF). For a period of time cefuroxime was advocated as single drug therapy for bacterial meningitis in infants and children over 2 months of age. However, cefuroxime does not sterilize the CSF as rapidly as ampicillin plus chloramphenicol or selected third generation cephalosporins and should not be used to treat meningitis. Cefuroxime can be used when parenteral coverage for both *S. aureus* and *H. influenzae* is desirable in a patient without central nervous system (CNS) infection.

Third Generation Cephalosporins. Third generation cephalosporins can be thought of as those having a role in treating *Pseudomonas* infections and those that do not. Cefotaxime was the first third generation cephalosporin to be widely used in the United States and continues to be clinically useful. Ceftriaxone is very similar to cefotaxime in antibacterial activity but has a much longer half-life. Both cefotaxime and ceftriaxone are active against most gram-positive aerobes except enterococci and *L. monocytogenes*. Neither is active against methicillin-resistant *S. aureus* or coagulase-negative staphylococci. Both are active against most gram-negative aerobic bacteria, with the exception of *Pseudomonas* species. The disacetyl breakdown product of cefotaxime also has a broad range of activity, but specific activity is less than that of cefotaxime itself. The peak serum concentration after 1 g of cefotaxime given intravenously is about 40 μg/ml, compared with 150 μg/ml for ceftriaxone. The serum half-life of cefotaxime is about 1 hour, compared with 8 hours for ceftriaxone. Because ceftriaxone is excreted slowly, a peak serum concentration of 50 μg/ml is achieved after an intramuscular dose of 0.5 g in adults. Susceptible by disk means that the MIC of either drug for the bacteria tested is 8 μg/ml or less.

Third generation cephalosporins with good antipseudomonal activity include cefoperazone and ceftazidime. Ceftazidime is more active than cefoperazone against *Pseudomonas* in vitro but is less active than cefotaxime against gram-positive organisms. Whether ceftazidime should be used as a single agent to treat *Pseudomonas* infections is still controversial. The peak serum concentration of ceftazidime after 1 g is given intravenously in adults is 85 μg/ml; the serum half-life is about 1.8 hours. About 90% of *Pseudomonas* isolates are inhibited by 8 μg/ml or less of ceftazidime.

Other Beta-Lactam Antibiotics

Other beta-lactam antibiotics that currently have a limited role in the treatment of bacterial infections in children include imipenem and aztreonam. Imipenem has an extremely broad spectrum of activity that includes most gram-positive organisms—enterococci, *Listeria* species, and methicillin-susceptible staphylococci, including coagulase-negative staphylococci. Imipenem also inhibits most Enterobacteriaceae, *Pseudomonas aeruginosa,* and *Pseudomonas maltophilia,* as well as most anaerobic bacteria. Imipenem is rapidly destroyed by a renal peptidase; to prevent this, it is supplied in a fixed combination with a dehydropeptidase inhibitor called cilastatin. Peak serum concentrations after a dose of 500 mg of imipenem with cilastatin is given intravenously in adults average 33 μg/ml, and the serum half-life is about 1 hour. The MIC_{95} to imipenim of bacteria reported as susceptible by disk is 4 μg/ml or less. Imipenem's broad spectrum of antimicrobial activity is seldom required in clinical practice.

Aztreonam is a monobactam that has little activity against gram-positive or anaerobic bacteria. This is so because these bacteria have little penicillin-binding protein 3, which is the primary binding site for aztreonam. On the other hand, aztreonam is very active against Enterobacteriaceae (MIC, 0.5 μg/ml or less) and moderately active against *P. aeruginosa* (MIC, 16 μg/ml or less). One gram of aztreonam given intravenously in adults results in a peak serum concentration of about 125 μg/ml, and the serum half-life is 1.7 hours. Susceptible by disk means that the MIC_{95} will be 8 μg/ml or less. There is very little experience with the use of aztreonam in children.

Aminoglycosides

Mechanisms of Action. It is known that aminoglycosides inhibit bacterial protein synthesis, but it appears that a second mechanism is necessary to explain bacterial killing. The second mechanism is not yet known. The inhibition of protein synthesis occurs through interaction with bacterial ribosomes at the interface between the smaller and larger ribosome subunits.

Resistance of Bacteria to Aminoglycosides. There are three known mechanisms of resistance to aminoglycosides. The first, ribosomal resistance, is known only to occur with streptomycin where alteration in the protein of the smaller ribosomal subunit results in the inability to bind streptomycin. The most common mechanism of resistance is the production of enzymes that inactivate the aminoglycosides. Because aminoglycosides are similar in structure, certain enzymes can inactivate more than one aminoglycoside. The capacity to produce aminoglycoside-inactivating enzymes is inherent among gram-negative anaerobic bacteria and seldom occurs by induction. The number and types of enzymes vary among places and populations. As an aminoglycoside is more widely used, bacteria that produce inactivating enzymes become more prevalent. The ability to produce inactivating enzymes can be carried by plasmids and transferred among gram-negative bacteria. The third mechanism of resistance is impermeability of bacteria to aminoglycosides. This mechanism is not very common, and it has been observed that permeability mutants are generally not very virulent. When an organism is susceptible to tobramycin, gentamicin, or both but is resistant to amikacin, the amikacin resistance must be based on the inability of amikacin to enter the organism. This has to be the case because the only enzyme produced by gram-negative organisms that inhibits amikacin also inhibits tobramycin and gentamicin.

Pharmacologic Properties. Aminoglycosides are absorbed poorly or not at all after oral administration. Absorption after intramuscular administration is excellent, with peak serum concentrations occurring 30 to 90 minutes after administration. Serum concentrations after intravenous administration over 20 to 30 minutes are about the same as after intramuscular administration. Aminoglycosides do not cross cell membranes well and therefore achieve poor concentrations inside most cells except renal tubular cells, which actively transport these agents. In general, only low concentrations of aminoglycosides are achieved in the CNS, eye, biliary tract, or prostatic fluid. Aminoglycosides do enter synovial fluid well.

Aminoglycosides are excreted by glomerular filtration, and care must be taken to adjust doses in renal failure. After filtration some aminoglycoside is reabsorbed by the proximal renal tubular cell, which probably plays a role in nephrotoxicity. By convention, peak serum concentrations are measured ½ hour after infusion of the drug over ½ hour is completed. Peak serum concentrations are measured 1 hour after intramuscular administration. Because the therapeutic-to-toxic index is very low for aminoglycosides, serum concentrations should be monitored.

Side Effects of Aminoglycosides. The two most common toxicities of aminoglycosides are ototoxicity and nephrotoxicity. Ototoxicity is caused by destruction of the outer hair cells in the organ of Corti and is possibly related to the concentration of aminoglycoside in the endolymph or perilymph that bathes these cells. Transient elevations in aminoglycoside concentrations probably do not affect hearing. Nephrotoxicity results in a decrease in the glomerular filtration rate. Both ototoxicity and nephrotoxicity seem to occur less often in children than in adults. Nonetheless, it is important to measure serum concentrations to make sure they are both safe and therapeutic.

Aminoglycosides can also produce neuromuscular paralysis, particularly with curare-like drugs, in the presence of botulinus toxin, and in patients with myasthenia gravis. Neuromuscular paralysis usually does not occur if aminoglycosides are given intramuscularly or if they are infused over 30 minutes. If neuromuscular paralysis occurs, it can be treated by giving calcium.

Use of Selected Aminoglycosides. Streptomycin, the first aminoglycoside used clinically, is currently used almost exclusively for the treatment of tuberculosis, but it is also used to treat tularemia, plague, and brucellosis. Neomycin is used primarily to reduce the number of bacteria in the large bowel. Neomycin is given by mouth, and very little reaches the bloodstream.

The three aminoglycosides currently used systemically to treat serious infections caused by gram-negative aerobic bacteria are gentamicin, tobramycin, and amikacin. In general there is no evidence that one of these aminoglycosides is clinically superior to another in the treatment of susceptible bacteria. Tobramycin is more active against *P. aeruginosa* than is gentamicin or amikacin, but differences in clinical effectiveness have not been observed. Tobramycin and amikacin are somewhat less nephrotoxic than gentamicin. Amikacin is susceptible to inactivation by one aminoglycoside-inactivating enzyme, whereas tobramycin and gentamicin are inactivated by at least six enzymes. Thus organisms are less likely to be resistant to amikacin than to either tobramycin or gentamicin. Because amikacin is less toxic on a weight basis, larger doses are given and higher peak serum concentrations are achieved. With a dose of 7.5 mg/kg of amikacin given intravenously, the peak serum concentration averages 38 μg/ml. At a dose of 2 mg/kg of tobramycin or gentamicin, peak serum concentrations range from 3 to 12 μg/ml. All three drugs have a serum half-life of 2 to 2½ hours. The MIC_{95} of amikacin for bacteria reported susceptible by disk is 16 μg/ml or less; the MIC_{95} of gentamicin or tobramycin is 4 μg/ml or less.

Sulfonamides and Trimethoprim

Mechanisms of Action. Sulfonamides inhibit bacterial growth by decreasing bacterial folic acid synthesis, which results in decreased bacterial nucleotides. Trimethoprim inhibits bacterial dihydrofolate reductase, which is the step in folic acid synthesis that follows the one inhibited by sulfonamides. The combination of trimethoprim and sulfamethoxazole results in a sequential blockage of folic acid, which is synergistic.

Resistance of Bacteria to Sulfonamides and Trimethoprim. Resistance to sulfonamides can be based on overproduction of substrate by the bacteria or a change in enzyme structure to one with reduced sulfonamide binding. Trimethoprim resistance may also be caused by the bacteria's decreased capacity to bind the drug or to a change in dihydrofolate reductase. Resistance to both drugs can result from decreased permeability of organisms to the drugs. Resistance occurs less frequently when the combination of trimethoprim-sulfamethoxazole is used.

Pharmacologic Properties. The sulfonamides currently used in the United States, either alone or in combination with trimethoprim, are sulfisoxazole (Gantricin), sulfamethoxazole, and sulfadiazine. Sulfonamides are usually given orally, but intravenous preparations of sulfadiazine and sulfisoxazole are available. Absorption of these sulfonamides from the stomach and small intestine is rapid and complete. These sulfonamides are distributed throughout the body, including the CSF. Sulfonamides readily cross the placenta and are found in fetal blood. Sulfonamides are partially metabolized in the liver, and free drug metabolites are excreted by glomerular filtration.

Trimethoprim is also usually given orally and is readily absorbed. It is well distributed throughout the body, with CSF concentrations reaching about 40% of serum concentrations. Excretion is primarily by renal tubular secretion.

Side Effects of Sulfonamides and Trimethoprim. A wide range of toxicities are associated with sulfonamides, ranging from gastrointestinal upset, headache, and rash to serum sickness and hepatic necrosis. Severe hypersensitivity reactions, including toxic epidermal necrolysis, Stevens-Johnson syndrome, erythema nodosum, vasculitis, and anaphylaxis, can occur. Blood cell disorders, including aplastic anemia, granulocytopenia, thrombocytopenia, and leukopenia, have been attributed to sulfonamides. Patients with glucose 6-phosphate dehydrogenase deficiency are at risk for aplastic anemia. Sulfonamides should be avoided during the last month of pregnancy, since they cross the placenta and compete for bilirubin-binding sites, thus increasing the risk for kernicterus. All the side effects associated with sulfonamides can occur with trimethoprim as well, the most common being gastrointestinal upset and hypersensitivity reactions. With prolonged use trimethoprim can interfere with folate metabolism and result in a megaloblastic anemia. This can be prevented by the administration of folinic acid.

Use of Trimethoprim-Sulfamethoxazole and Selected Sulfonamides. The combination of trimethoprim and sulfamethoxazole was initially introduced to treat urinary tract infections. However, because of its wide range of antibacterial activity, trimethoprim-sulfamethoxazole has proved useful in a number of bacterial infections. Gram-positive organisms susceptible to trimethoprim-sulfamethoxazole include both coagulase-positive and coagulase-negative staphylococci, *S. pneumoniae*, enterococci, *Listeria* species, and *S. pyogenes*. However, trimethoprim-sulfamethoxazole is not as effective as penicillin in the treatment of *S. pyogenes*. Trimethoprim-sulfamethoxazole is also inhibitory for a wide range of gram-negative aerobic organisms, including *E. coli*, *Klebsiella* species, *Salmonella* species, *Shigella* species, *H. influenzae*, and *N. meningitidis*.

Trimethoprim-sulfamethoxazole is useful in the treatment of acute urinary tract infections, long-term suppression in patients with chronic or recurrent urinary tract infections, respiratory tract infections, otitis media, sinusitis, prostatitis, orchitis, and epididymitis. Trimethoprim-sulfamethoxazole is the drug of choice for the treatment of *P. carinii* infections and has been shown to be effective in preventing *P. carinii* in children with malignancies. Many adults with human immunodeficiency virus (HIV) infection do not tolerate trimethoprim-sulfamethoxazole well. To date, however, this has not been a major problem in HIV-infected infants. Peak serum concentrations for both drugs are reached about 2 hours after an oral dose and average 2 μg/ml for trimethoprim and 60 μg/ml for sulfamethoxazole. After repeated doses the peak serum concentration of trimethoprim will approach 9 μg/ml. The MIC_{95} for bacteria susceptible to the combination is 2 μg/ml or less for trimethoprim and 38 μg/ml or less for sulfamethoxazole. However, the combination is usually synergistic in vivo.

Sulfisoxazole is primarily used for the treatment of acute urinary tract infections or long-term suppression in patients with chronic or recurrent urinary tract infections. Sulfadiazine is effective prophylaxis for close contacts of patients with *N. meningitidis* infections if the strain is known to be susceptible (see Meningococcemia, Chapter 283). Peak serum concentrations after an oral dose of 2 g range from 30 to 60 μg/ml for sulfadiazine, 40 to 50 μg/ml for sulfisoxazole, and 80 to 100 μg/ml for sulfamethoxazole.

Topical sulfonamides are used primarily in two settings. Ophthalmic preparations of sulfacetamide are used in the treatment of acute conjunctivitis and as adjunctive therapy in the treatment of trachoma. Silver sulfadiazine is used in the topical treatment of burns. In this combination the sulfadiazine serves principally as a vehicle for the release of silver ions, which have an antibacterial effect.

Erythromycin

Mechanism of Action. Erythromycin inhibits RNA-dependent protein synthesis at the step of chain elongation.

Resistance of Bacteria to Erythromycin. Bacteria that lack the appropriate binding site are resistant to erythromycin, as are bacteria that exhibit decreased permeability to the drug.

Pharmacologic Properties. A number of erythromycin preparations are available for oral administration. Erythromycin base is destroyed by gastric acid and therefore is useful only when given as an enteric-coated tablet. Pediatric preparations utilize the ester or ester salt derivatives of erythromycin because they are acid stable, soluble, and tasteless. Preparations vary in their rate and degree of absorption from the gastrointestinal tract. The best absorbed is the estolate ester, which results in peak serum concentrations of about 4 μg/ml. The ethylsuccinate and stearate preparations result in peak serum concentrations that range from 0.4 to 1.9 μg/ml when given at a dose equivalent to the estolate.

Erythromycin is distributed throughout the body and persists in tissue longer than in the blood. Therapeutic concentrations are reached in middle ear fluid, paranasal sinuses, tonsils, and pleural fluid. Therapeutic concentrations of erythromycin do not enter the CSF even when the meninges are inflamed. Limited data suggest that entry of erythromycin into synovial fluid is poor.

Erythromycin's route of elimination is not clear. A small percentage of a dose of erythromycin can be found in the urine, and erythromycin is known to be concentrated in and excreted with bile. However, most of an administered dose of erythromycin cannot be recovered.

Side Effects of Erythromycin. The most common side effect of erythromycin is gastrointestinal upset. Allergic reactions occur but are relatively uncommon. Cholestatic hepatitis has been reported following treatment with the estolate ester. This side effect has primarily been seen in adults. The better absorption characteristics of the estolate probably outweigh the slight risk of cholestatic hepatitis in children.

Use of Erythromycin. Erythromycin has a broad range of antibacterial activity and is the drug of choice for infections caused by *Mycoplasma pneumoniae, Legionella* species, *C. diphtheriae, Bordetella pertussis, Chlamydia trachomatis,* and *Campylobacter jejuni*. Erythromycin is an alternative drug for the treatment of streptococcal staphylococcal infections, and as prophylaxis for syphilis, urinary tract infections, rheumatic fever, and bacterial endocarditis. The MIC_{95} of erythromycin required to inhibit bacteria reported as susceptible by disk is 0.5 μg/ml or less. Lactobionate and gluceptate preparations are available for parenteral administration but are not frequently used. The peak serum concentration after intravenous administration is about equal to that achieved when estolate is given by mouth.

Clindamycin

Mechanism of Action. Clindamycin shares binding sites with erythromycin and chloramphenicol on the 50S ribosomal subunit and interferes with protein synthesis by inhibiting the transpeptidation reaction. Mechanisms of resistance are the same as those for erythromycin.

Pharmacologic Properties. Clindamycin is usually given orally, but preparations for intramuscular and intravenous administration are available. About 90% of a dose of clindamycin is absorbed after oral administration, and peak serum concentrations are reached in 1 hour and are dose dependent. Clindamycin palmitate (oral suspension) and clindamycin phosphate (preparation for intravenous administration) are inactive but are rapidly hydrolyzed in vivo to the active free base. Clindamycin is well distributed throughout the body except for the CSF. Clindamycin is one of the few antibiotics that is concentrated in polymorphonuclear neutrophils. The serum half-life of clindamycin is about 2.4 hours. Most clindamycin is metabolized in the liver to products with variable antibacterial activity. Antibacterial activity in the bile and gastrointestinal tract is very high and results in a dramatic decrease in sensitive bowel flora.

Side Effects of Clindamycin. The most highly publicized side effect of clindamycin is the occurrence of colitis secondary to the toxin of *Clostridium difficile* (pseudomembranous colitis). This complication has now been associated with many other antibiotics and seems to occur less frequently in children than in adults. Other side effects include allergic reactions, rashes, and minor elevations in transaminase concentrations.

Use of Clindamycin. Clindamycin is highly active against most gram-positive aerobic bacteria and most anaerobic bacteria. The major clinical use of clindamycin is in the treatment of anaerobic infections. Clindamycin is routinely used when intraabdominal spillage of fecal material has occurred and in the treatment of anaerobic bronchopulmonary infections. Clindamycin is also used as alternative therapy for groups A and B streptococcal infections and as oral therapy to complete a course of antibiotics for *S. aureus* osteomyelitis. Clindamycin does not enter the CSF in useful concentrations. Peak serum concentrations of 2.5 to 3.6 μg/ml are achieved about 1 hour after oral administration, and concentrations of 6 to 9 μg/ml can be reached after intravenous infusion. The MIC_{95} of clindamycin for bacteria reported as susceptible by disk is 0.5 μg/ml or less.

Chloramphenicol

Mechanism of Action. Like erythromycin and clindamycin, chloramphenicol binds to 50S ribosomal subunit and inhibits protein synthesis.

Resistance of Bacteria to Chloramphenicol. Mechanisms of resistance include (1) bacterial production of an acetyltransferase that inactivates chloramphenicol and (2) the inability of chloramphenicol to enter bacteria.

Pharmacologic Properties. Chloramphenicol can be given orally as the free base or as chloramphenicol palmitate, which is hydrolyzed in the intestine to free base. Because chloramphenicol is extremely bitter, oral palmitate suspension is given to patients who cannot take capsules containing free base. The intravenous preparation is chloramphenicol succinate, which is also hydrolyzed to free base. Because the palmitate is more completely hydrolyzed than the succinate, peak serum concentrations are generally higher after oral administration. Chloramphenicol distributes well throughout the body, including the brain and CSF. Chloramphenicol is conjugated by the liver and excreted in an inactive form in urine.

Side Effects of Chloramphenicol. The major side effects of chloramphenicol are dose-related bone marrow suppression, which is reversible, aplastic anemia, which is idiosyncratic and usually fatal, and gray-baby syndrome. Gray-baby syndrome was first described and most commonly occurs in infants but has been reported in all age groups. The syndrome is characterized by cyanosis, circulatory collapse, and death and occurs when chloramphenicol concentrations get very high.

Use of Chloramphenicol. The importance of chloramphenicol in the treatment of infectious diseases has waxed and waned since its introduction in the late 1940s. Because of the side effects associated with the use of chloramphenicol, practitioners have tended to use alternative antimicrobial agents whenever possible. However, because of its antibacterial and pharmacologic properties, it has frequently been necessary to include chloramphenicol to optimize treatment. With the introduction of the third generation cephalosporins, the use of chloramphenicol in the United States is again on the decline. Some experts on infectious diseases still maintain that chloramphenicol is the drug of choice for the treatment of brain abscesses, bacterial meningitis in infants and children over 2 months of age, typhoid fever, and salmonellosis. Others prefer metronidazole for anaerobic coverage in brain abscesses, ceftriaxone for bacterial meningitis, and either trimethoprim-sulfamethoxazole or ceftriaxone to treat typhoid fever and salmonellosis. Chloramphenicol remains the drug of choice for rickettsial infections in children under 8 years of age in whom the side effects of tetracycline preclude its use.

When it is necessary to use chloramphenicol, the peak serum concentration should be measured after four or five doses to ensure that concentrations are safe and therapeutic and that the drug is not accumulating in the patient. A complete blood count and differential count should be determined twice a week while the patient is receiving chloramphenicol to check for dose-related bone marrow suppression. Peak serum concentrations are reached between 1 and 2 hours after oral or intravenous administration and average 25 μg/ml and 19 μg/ml, respectively.[10] The serum half-life of chloramphenicol is about 4 hours. The MIC_{95} of chloramphenicol for bacteria reported as susceptible by disk is 4 μg/ml or less for *H. influenzae* and 12.5 μg/ml or less for other organisms. Although chloramphenicol is bactericidal for *H. influenzae*, *S. pneumoniae*, and *N. meningitidis*, it is bacteriostatic for most other bacteria. When it is used in combination with a beta-lactam to treat organisms that are only inhibited by chloramphenicol, antagonism may occur.[2]

Tetracycline

Mechanism of Action. Tetracyclines bind to the 30S ribosomal subunit and block aminoacyl-tRNA binding to the receptor site; this action inhibits protein synthesis.

Resistance of Bacteria to Tetracycline. Entry of tetracycline into bacterial cells is an energy-dependent process, and resistance is usually based on interference with entry into the cell. In general, tetracyclines are not altered by resistant bacteria.

Pharmacologic Properties. A number of analogs of tetracyclines have been produced, but the range of antibacterial activity is similar for each. The semisynthetic analogs, minocycline and deoxycycline, are the most active tetracyclines but are used less commonly than other tetracyclines because they are considerably more expensive.

Tetracyclines have a broad spectrum of activity that includes inhibition of *Streptococcus* species, *Neisseria* species, *E. coli*, and many common anaerobic bacteria. Tetracyclines are well absorbed from the intestinal tract, and peak serum concentrations are achieved 1 to 3 hours after oral administration. Tetracyclines distribute in varying concentrations throughout most of the body, with concentrations in synovial fluid, urine, and the maxillary sinuses approaching serum concentrations, whereas CSF concentrations reach only 10% to 20% of serum concentrations.

Side Effects of Tetracyclines. The side effects of tetracyclines essentially preclude their use in children under 8 years of age and in pregnant women. Tetracyclines cause a permanent gray-brown to yellowish discoloration of teeth and can be associated with hypoplasia of the enamel. Skeletal growth depression can occur when premature infants are given tetracycline. Although bone and tooth defects are associated with the total dose of tetracycline given and occur more often after repeated courses, it is safest to avoid use during pregnancy and in young children. Other side effects of tetracycline include allergic reactions and skin toxicity.

Use of Tetracyclines. For individuals over 8 years of age, tetracycline is considered the drug of choice for brucellosis, chlamydial infections, lymphogranuloma venereum, epididymitis, granuloma inguinale, infections with spirochetes (Lyme disease, relapsing fever, leptospirosis), pelvic inflammatory disease, plague, prostatitis, and rickettsial infections. Tetracycline is also an effective alternative therapy for many other infectious diseases.

Peak serum concentrations following the oral administration of 500 mg of tetracycline or 200 mg of doxycycline or minocycline in adults are 4 μg/ml, 2.5 μg/ml, and 2.5 μg/ml respectively. Peak serum concentrations are reached 1 to 3 hours after administration. The serum half-life of tetracycline is 8 hours, compared with 16 hours for minocycline and 18 hours for doxycycline. Intravenous administration of tetracyclines results in peak serum concentrations about twice those achieved when the same dose is given by mouth. The MIC_{95} of tetracycline for bacteria reported as susceptible by disk is 4 μg/ml or less.

Vancomycin

Mechanism of Action. Vancomycin inhibits cell wall synthesis and alters the permeability of the cytoplasmic membrane of protoplasts.

Resistance of Bacteria to Vancomycin. To date, no cross-resistance between vancomycin and other antimicrobial agents has been observed. Organisms susceptible to vancomycin have not been observed to become resistant to vancomycin during therapy.

Pharmacologic Properties. Vancomycin is minimally absorbed after oral administration and is given orally only to treat pseudomembranous colitis caused by the toxin of *C. difficile*. After intravenous administration, vancomycin is distributed throughout the body with the exception of the aqueous humor of the eye and the CSF when the meninges are not inflamed. Bactericidal concentrations can be achieved in the CSF in cases of meningitis caused by susceptible organisms. Sometimes it is necessary to administer vancomycin intraventricularly to treat meningitis with or without ventriculitis adequately. Vancomycin is excreted unchanged in the urine by glomerular filtration. It is therefore important to monitor serum concentrations and adjust doses based on renal function.

Side Effects of Vancomycin. When vancomycin initially became available for clinical use, commercial preparations contained as much as 20% of another substance, and its use was limited by toxicity. Currently available preparations are more highly purified and less toxic. The most common side effects are fever, chills, and pain at the injection site or, less frequently, flushing and tingling of the face, neck, and thorax (red-neck syndrome). These side effects are largely avoided by infusing vancomycin slowly in a large volume of fluid. Auditory nerve damage is common when serum concentrations exceed 80 μg/ml but is uncommon if serum concentrations are kept less than 30 to 40 μg/ml. Nephrotoxicity occurs infrequently with current preparations of vancomycin, but a high incidence of nephrotoxicity has been reported when vancomycin and an aminoglycoside are both given to a patient.

Uses of Vancomycin. In recent years infections caused by methicillin-resistant *S. aureus* and coagulase-negative staphylococci (such as *S. epidermidis*) have become major clinical problems for which vancomycin is the drug of choice. Vancomycin is active against most aerobic gram-positive cocci, including most *Streptococcus* species and *L. monocytogenes*, and is synergistic in combination with streptomycin or gentamicin against enterococci. Many anaerobic streptococci are also susceptible to vancomycin, whereas most gram-negative bacteria are resistant. Some methicillin-resistant staphylococci have demonstrated tolerance to vancomycin killing, and rifampin or trimethoprim-sulfamethoxazole must be added to achieve bacterial killing. Vancomycin is the drug of choice to treat serious infections with methicillin-resistant staphylococci or coagulase-negative staphylococci and to treat enterococcal endocarditis in patients who are allergic to penicillin. The initial dose of vancomycin should be a full therapeutic dose even in patients with renal failure. Subsequent doses and intervals should be adjusted to achieve peak serum concentrations of 30 to 40 μg/ml. The MIC_{95} of vancomycin for bacteria reported as susceptible by disk is 5 μg/ml or less.

Metronidazole

Mechanism of Action. After being taken up by bacteria, metronidazole is reduced to intermediate products that are toxic to the bacteria; inactive end products are then released by the organism.

Resistance of Bacteria to Metronidazole. Resistance to metronidazole develops only infrequently and has been associated with decreased entry of the drug into bacteria and a decreased rate of reduction once in the cells.

Pharmacologic Properties. Metronidazole is active against most anaerobic bacteria, *T. pallidum, Campylobacter fetus,* and *Trichomonas vaginalis,* as well as certain parasites. After oral administration, metronidazole is absorbed rapidly and completely, with peak serum concentrations being proportional to the dose administered. Metronidazole is distributed well throughout the body, including the CNS and the aqueous humor of the eye. The serum half-life of metronidazole is about 8 hours; after being metabolized, metronidazole is excreted primarily in the urine.

Side Effects of Metronidazole. The most common side effect of metronidazole is gastrointestinal upset. Metronidazole has also been associated with CNS dysfunction (seizures, encephalopathy, ataxia) and peripheral neuropathy. Metronidazole can also potentiate the effects of warfarin and can cause a disulfiram reaction when alcohol is consumed. A major concern over the use of metronidazole has been its carcinogenic potential. Although rats and mice that have received metronidazole for a long period of time have shown an increase in neoplasms, mutagenicity for human cells has not been demonstrated in vitro, and follow-up studies on women who have received metronidazole for the treatment of trichomonas have shown that they did not have an increased frequency of tumors up to 10 years later.

Use of Metronidazole. Originally introduced for the treatment of *T. vaginalis,* metronidazole has also been effective in the treatment of amebiasis and giardiasis. More recently it has gained widespread use in the treatment of anaerobic bacterial infections; it is not effective in the treatment of actinomycosis or *Propionibacterium acnes* infections. Metronidazole is also not optimally effective in the treatment of anerobic lower respiratory tract infections. This may be because of the presence of aerobic bacteria, and the outcome is generally good if penicillin or ampicillin is given concomitantly.

The peak serum concentration achieved in adults after 0.5 g of metronidazole is given orally averages 11.5 μg/ml; after an intravenous dose of 0.5 g, serum concentrations range from 20 to 25 μg/ml. The MIC_{95} of metronidazole for susceptible bacteria is usually 4 μg/ml or less. Most diagnostic microbiology laboratories do not routinely test anaerobic bacteria for susceptibility.

Rifampin

Mechanism of Action. Rifampin works by inhibiting DNA-dependent RNA polymerase at the B subunit. This prevents chain initiation but not elongation.

Resistance of Bacteria to Rifampin. Resistance to rifampin occurs rapidly by mutation of the DNA-dependent RNA polymerase. Rates of mutation are so high that they preclude the use of rifampin as monotherapy except for very short courses of prophylaxis.

Pharmacologic Properties. Rifampin is administered orally and is completely and rapidly absorbed, with peak serum concentrations being achieved 1 to 4 hours after ingestion. Rifampin is distributed throughout the body, deacetylated by the liver, and excreted in the bile. The serum half-life is 2 to 5 hours early in therapy but decreases over time because of increased biliary excretion. Rifampin is also able to enter phagocytes and kill viable intracellular organisms. This may explain why rifampin is better able to enter and sterilize abscesses than are other antimicrobial agents.

Table 28-3 *Initial Empiric Therapy for Selected Infections**

CLINICAL DIAGNOSIS	MOST LIKELY OFFENDING ORGANISMS	ANTIMICROBIAL AGENT(S)
Meningitis	Neonate—group B streptococci, *Listeria monocytogenes, Escherichia coli*	Ampicillin and cefotaxime (or ceftriaxone)
	Child—*Haemophilus influenzae* type b, *Streptococcus pneumoniae, Neisseria meningitidis*	Ceftriaxone or cefotaxime or ampicillin plus chloramphenicol
Brain abscess	Streptococcal species, anaerobes, *Staphylococcus aureus*	Penicillin and metronidazole (add nafcillin if suspect *S. aureus*)
Orbital cellulitis	*H. influenzae* type b, streptococcal species, *S. aureus*	Ceftriaxone or cefotaxime
Epiglottitis	*H. influenzae* type b	Ceftriaxone or cefotaxime
Pneumonia (lobar or segmental)	Neonate—group B streptococci, *S. aureus*, gram-negative organisms	Ampicillin and amikacin
	Child—*S. pneumoniae, H. influenzae* type b, *S. aureus, Streptococcus pyogenes, Mycoplasma pneumoniae*	Penicillin, nafcillin, or erythromycin
Infective endocarditis	*Streptococcus viridans, S. aureus*	Nafcillin and an aminoglycoside
Acute diarrhea (fecal WBC present)	*Campylobacter, Salmonella, Shigella* species	Trimethoprim-sulfamethoxazole (TMP-SMX) or ampicillin
Abdominal sepsis	Anaerobes, aerobic enterics, enterococci	Clindamycin, amikacin, and ampicillin
Urinary tract infection	Acute—*E. coli, Klebsiella* species	Ampicillin or sulfisoxazole
	Chronic—*E. coli, Proteus* species, *Pseudomonas* species	Await culture and sensitivity results
Osteomyelitis	Neonate—group B streptococci, *S. aureus, S. pyogenes, S. pneumoniae*	Nafcillin and amikacin
	Child—*S. aureus, S. pyogenes, H. influenzae* type b	Ceftriaxone or cefotaxime (test MIC for *S. aureus*) plus nafcillin
Pyogenic arthritis	Neonate—*S. aureus, S. pyogenes, H. influenzae* type b, *N. gonorrhoeae*, group B streptococci	Nafcillin and amikacin
	Child—*H. influenzae* type b (<5 yr old), *S. aureus, S. pyogenes, N. gonorrhoeae*	Ceftriaxone or cefotaxime (test MIC for *S. aureus*) plus nafcillin
Suspected sepsis	Neonate—group B streptococci, *L. monocytogenes*, gram-negative enteric organisms	Ampicillin plus amikacin
	Infant 1-6 weeks—as for neonate plus as for child	Ampicillin plus ceftriaxone
	Child—*S. pneumoniae, H. influenzae* type b, *N. meningitidis*	Ceftriaxone
Compromised host		
Fever only	*S. aureus, E. coli, Pseudomonas* species	Amikacin (or ceftazidime) and mezlocillin
Pneumonia	As under pneumonia above, and *Pneumocystis carinii, Candida albicans*, other fungi	TMP-SMX; if patient's condition deteriorates, lung biopsy or aspirate data needed to direct therapy
Shock (sepsis without source)	Neonate—group B streptococci, enterics	Ampicillin and amikacin (or cefotaxime)
	Child—*N. meningitidis, H. influenzae* type b	Ceftriaxone or cefotaxime or chloramphenicol plus penicillin

*For most clinical diagnoses an acceptable alternative choice of antibiotics could be proposed.

Side Effects of Rifampin. The most common side effects of rifampin when given daily are a mild self-limited rash and mild gastrointestinal complaints. When rifampin is used intermittently at high individual doses, a flulike syndrome with fever, aches, and chills develops in up to 20% of patients. Rifampin crosses the placenta, and teratogenic effects have been observed in rodents. Therefore rifampin should not be used during pregnancy except in severe cases of tuberculosis. Patients or parents should be warned that urine, feces, saliva, and tears may turn a red-orange color while they are taking the drug. Contact lenses should not be worn, as they can be permanently discolored.

Use of Rifampin. Rifampin is extremely active against a wide range of organisms. Most strains of *S. aureus* and coagulase-negative staphylococci are exquisitely sensitive to rifampin, and rifampin is also active against most other gram-positive cocci. *H. influenzae, N. meningitidis,* and *N. gonorrhoeae* are exquisitely susceptible to rifampin, but other aerobic gram-negative pathogens are less susceptible. Rifampin is also active against *Legionella* species and *M. tuberculosis*.

Despite its widespread use for the treatment of tuberculosis and prophylaxis for *N. meningitidis* and *H. influenzae*, no pediatric preparation of rifampin is available. Instructions for preparing a suspension for pediatric use are detailed in the *Physicians' Desk Reference*.[9] Internationally, the greatest use of rifampin is for the treatment of tuberculosis and leprosy. Rifampin is also recommended for the prophylaxis of close contacts of patients with meningococcal disease and for household contacts of children with systemic *H. influenzae*

Table 28-4 *Antimicrobial Prophylaxis Against Specific Pathogenic Agents*

PATHOGEN	DISEASE TO BE PREVENTED	ANTIMICROBIAL AGENT	DOSE, DURATION OF THERAPY	
Bacteria				
Haemophilus influenzae type b	Secondary cases of systemic infection in close contacts <4 yr	Rifampin	≤1 mo: 10-20 mg/kg >1 mo: 20/mg/kg Maximum: 600 mg	Give once a day for 4 days
Mycobacterium tuberculosis	Overt pulmonary or metastatic infection	Isoniazid	10-20 mg/kg	Once daily (not to exceed 300 mg) for 9 months
Neisseria meningitidis	Meningococcemia in exposed susceptible persons	Rifampin	≤1 mo: 5-10 mg/kg >1 mo: 10 mg/kg Maximum: 600 mg	Give every 12 hours for 4 doses
Neisseria gonorrhoeae	Gonococcal infection in exposed persons; ophthalmia neonatorum	Ceftriaxone	250 mg—one dose	
Streptococcus pneumoniae	Fulminant pneumococcal infection in those with asplenia or sickle cell disease	Penicillin V	125 mg	Twice daily (throughout life)
Group A streptococcus	Recurrent rheumatic fever	Benzathine penicillin **or** penicillin V **or** sulfadiazine	1.2 million U every 4 weeks 125-250 mg twice daily 1 g once a day if >60 lb and 0.5 g <60 lb (throughout life)	
Group B streptococcus	Neonatal infection	Ampicillin	Intrapartum to mother 2 g IV followed by 1 g q4h until delivery Infants: 50 mg/kg given IM q12h for 2 days	
Vibrio cholerae	Cholera in close contacts of a case	Tetracycline; trimethoprim-sulfamethoxazole	250 mg q6h for 3-5 days (patients >8 yr) May be effective in children	
Treponema pallidum	Syphilis in exposed persons	Benzathine penicillin	2.4 million U IM at a single session	
Plasmodium species (malaria)	Overt infection in endemic areas	Chloroquine	5 mg/kg base once a week (maximum dose: 300 mg base), beginning 2 weeks before entering, while in, and 6 weeks after leaving endemic area	
Pneumocystis carinii	Pneumonia in compromised host	Trimethoprim-sulfamethoxazole	5 mg trimethoprim/25 mg sulfamethoxazole once daily while on chemotherapy	
Viruses				
Influenza A	Influenza in those at risk of complications	Amantadine	1-9 yr: 2-4.4 mg/kg q12h (maximum: 150 mg/day) >9 yr: 100 mg q12h Duration of an influenza outbreak	

Modified from Peter G et al, editors: Report of the Committee on Infectious Diseases: 1988 Red Book, ed 21, Elk Grove Village, Ill, 1988, The American Academy of Pediatrics.

type b disease. When rifampin is added with another antimicrobial agent for the last 4 days of therapy of group A beta-hemolytic streptococcal infections, the microbiologic failure rate falls to almost zero. Rifampin in combination with other antistaphylococcal agents has been used to treat severe staphylococcal infections such as *S. aureus* endocarditis, osteomyelitis, and CSF shunt infections caused by coagulase-negative staphylococci.

The peak serum concentration of rifampin after oral administration of 600 mg to an adult or 10 mg/kg to a child averages 7 μg/ml. Because of the long half-life of rifampin, the peak serum concentrations and bioavailability are better when it is given once a day. The MIC_{95} of bacteria reported as susceptible by disk to rifampin is 1 μg/ml or less.

INITIAL THERAPY OF SELECTED ACUTE INFECTIONS

In most clinical situations the physician must decide which antimicrobial agent or agents to use before the offending organism has been positively identified through culture results, serologic tests, or microscopic examination of material obtained from the infected site. The following considerations must be taken into account before treatment is instituted:

1. Patient's age and immune status
2. Presence of concomitant disease
3. History of exposure to infectious agents
4. Administration of antimicrobial agents currently or recently
5. Findings on physical examination

Table 28-5 *Clinical Situations in which Prophylaxis with Antimicrobial Agents Has Been Shown to Be Effective*

BODY SITE	INFECTION TO BE PREVENTED	AGENTS	RECOMMENDED DOSAGE
Conjunctivae	Neonatal gonococcal ophthalmia	1% silver nitrate, 0.5% erythromycin, 1% tetracycline, penicillin	Applied topically once shortly after delivery
Abnormal heart valve	Bacterial endocarditis (e.g., following dental extraction)	Penicillin, ampicillin	For standard-risk patients, oral procedures: penicillin V, 2 g orally, then 1 g 6 hours later; For high-risk patients, dental or all patients, GU or GI tract procedures: ampicillin, 2 g IM or IV plus gentamicin, 1.5-2 mg/kg ½ hour before and 8 hours after procedure
Surgical wound	Serious postoperative wound infection	Appropriate for expected contaminants	See Kaiser AB: Antimicrobial prophylaxis in surgery, N Engl J Med 315:1129, 1986.[4]
Middle ear	Recurrent otitis media	Amoxicillin, sulfisoxazole	5-10 mg/kg given q12h 40-50 mg/kg given q12h (given during winter and spring)
Urinary tract	Recurrent urinary infection	Trimethoprim-sulfamethoxazole, nitrofurantoin	2 mg TMP and 10 mg SMX/kg once daily 1-2 mg/kg once daily Duration: months to years, depending on clinical situation

Modified from Peter G et al, editors: Report of the Committee on Infectious Diseases: ed 21, Elk Grove Village, Ill, 1988, The American Academy of Pediatrics.

Table 28-6 *Antiviral Drugs*

DRUG: GENERIC (TRADE)	INDICATIONS	USUAL RECOMMENDED DOSAGE
Acyclovir (Zovirax)	Genital herpes simplex infection (HSV), first episode	Oral: 200 mg, 5 times/day for 5-10 days Topical: 5% ointment, 4-6 times/day (localized lesions only), for 7 days IV: 15 mg/kg/day in 3 divided doses for 7 days
	Frequent recurrent episodes (1 or more episodes per month) of genital herpes simplex infection; chronic suppressive therapy; intermittent therapy	 Oral: 200 mg, 2-5 times/day for 6-12 mo Oral: 200 mg, 5 times/day for 5 days
	HSV in immunocompromised host (localized, progressive, or disseminated*)	IV: 15-30 mg/kg/day in 3 divided doses for 7-14 days Oral: 200 mg, 5 times/day for 7-14 days
	HSV encephalitis†	IV: 30 mg/kg/day in 3 divided doses for 10-14 days
	Neonatal HSV*	IV: 30 mg/kg/day in 3 divided doses for 10-14 days
	Varicella or zoster in immunocompromised host	IV: 30 mg/kg/day in 3 divided doses Duration: 5-10 days
	Zoster in immunocompetent host	IV: 30 mg/kg/day in 3 divided doses Duration: 5-10 days
Amantadine (Symmetrel)	Influenza A: treatment or prophylaxis	Oral: 1-9 yr: 4.4-8.8 mg/kg/day in 2 doses (maximum: 150 mg) >9 yr: 200 mg/day in 2 doses
Ribavirin (Virazole)	Treatment of respiratory syncytial virus (RSV) infection; treatment of influenza*	By aerosol using a small particle generator, in a solution containing 20 mg/ml, for 12-18 hr/day for 3-7 days; longer treatment may be necessary in some patients
Zidovudine (Retrovir, formerly termed azidothymidine [AZT])	Human immunodeficiency virus (HIV)	Oral: 180 mg/m²/dose given q6h; duration is indeterminant

*Drug is not licensed for this indication as of August, 1990.
†Studies have demonstrated the superiority of acyclovir to vidarabine for this indication.
Modified from Peter G et al, editors: Report of the Committee on Infectious Diseases: ed 21, Elk Grove Village, Ill, 1988, The American Academy of Pediatrics.

Appropriate specimens for bacterial and viral cultures and specimens for serologic tests and microscopic examinations should be obtained before starting antimicrobial therapy, and specific adjunctive, supportive therapy should be instituted concomitantly. Table 28-3 lists the most likely offending organisms and antimicrobial agent or agents that could be used empirically for various diagnoses under these circumstances. Local susceptibility patterns and other special situations should always be considered.

PROPHYLAXIS

Antimicrobial agents can be given to prevent colonization, to eradicate carriage, to prevent bacteria that colonize one body site from causing disease at a usually sterile site, or to prevent bacteria that have been introduced into a usually sterile site from causing disease.[4] In general, an antimicrobial agent with the narrowest spectrum that is effective against the most likely pathogen or pathogens should be used at the lowest dose and for the shortest period of time that will prevent infection. Prophylaxis should also be restricted to situations in which prophylaxis is known to be effective and the risk of infection exceeds the potential risks of the antimicrobial agent or the emergence of resistant bacteria. Specific bacterial pathogens for which prophylaxis has been shown effective are summarized in Table 28-4, and clinical situations in which prophylactic antimicrobial agents might be effective are listed in Table 28-5. The reader is referred to the *Red Book* (Report of the Committee on Infectious Diseases, American Academy of Pediatrics) for regularly updated recommendations for prophylaxis in specific situations—for example in the prevention of bacterial endocarditis.[1]

ANTIMICROBIAL THERAPY FOR VIRAL, FUNGAL, AND PARASITIC INFECTIONS

There are currently a limited number of agents available and a limited number of indications for systemic therapy for viral, fungal, and parastic infections in the United States. For this reason it is unlikely that many practitioners will be familiar with the use of these agents. Therefore it is recommended that a specialist in pediatric infectious diseases be consulted before using these agents. Currently available antiviral agents and their indications and doses are listed in Table 28-6. Antifungal drugs and their doses and adverse reactions are listed in Table 28-7. The treatment of parasitic infections is discussed in the appropriate chapters in this text, in the Red Book,[1] *The Pocketbook of Pediatric Antimicrobial Therapy,*[8] or the *Medical Letter Handbook of Antimicrobial Therapy.*[6] The use of topical antifungal and antiviral agents is also discussed in the appropriate chapters in this text.

Table 28-7 *Recommended Doses of Parenteral and Oral Antifungal Drugs*

DRUG	ROUTE	DOSE (PER DAY)	ADVERSE REACTIONS
Amphotericin B	IV	0.25 mg/kg (following test dose*) initially, increase as tolerated to 0.5 to 1 mg/kg; infuse as single dose during 1-4 hr	Fever, chills, phlebitis, renal dysfunction, hypokalemia, anemia, cardiac arrhythmias, anaphylactoid reaction, hematologic abnormalities
	IT	0.025 mg, increase to 0.1 to 0.5 mg twice weekly	Radiculitis, sensory loss, and foot drop
Clotrimazole troches	PO	10 mg tablet 6 times daily; let dissolve slowly in mouth	Nausea, vomiting, and increase in serum transaminase
Flucytosine	PO	100 to 150 mg/kg in 4 doses at 6-hr intervals	Bone marrow suppression; renal dysfunction can lead to drug accumulation; nausea, vomiting, increase in transaminases, BUN, and creatinine
Griseofulvin	PO	Ultramicrosize: 7.3 mg/kg, single dose; maximum dose, 375 to 750 mg Microsize: 10-12 mg/kg; maximum dose, 500-1000 mg	Rash, leukopenia, proteinuria, paresthesias, gastrointestinal symptoms, and mental confusion
Ketoconazole	PO	Children: 3.3 to 6.6 mg/kg, single dose† Adult: 200-400 mg, single dose	Rash, anaphylaxis, nausea, vomiting, abdominal pain, fever, gynecomastia, thrombocytopenia, hepatotoxicity, and depression of endocrine function (dose dependent, reversible)
Miconazole	IV	20 to 40 mg/kg, divided into 3 infusions 8 hr apart; never exceed 15 mg/kg per infusion Infuse over 30-60 min	Phlebitis, rash, fever, nausea, anemia, hyponatremia, thrombocytopenia, and hyperlipema
	IT	20 mg per dose for 3 to 7 days	
Nystatin	PO	Infants: 200,000 U 4 times daily Children and adults: 400,000 to 600,000 U 4 times daily	Nausea, vomiting, and diarrhea

Abbreviations: IV, intravenous; IT, intrathecal; PO, oral.
*Test dose is 0.1 mg/kg, with maximum dose of 1 mg/kg given during 3- to 4-hour period.
†The daily dose has not been established for children 2 years of age or younger.
From Peter G et al, editors: Report of the Committee on Infectious Diseases: ed 21, Elk Grove Village, Ill, 1988, The American Academy of Pediatrics.

REFERENCES

1. Peter G et al, editors: Report of the Committee on Infectious Diseases: 1988 Red Book, ed 21, Elk Grove Village, Ill, 1988, The American Academy of Pediatrics.
2. Asmar BI and Dajani S: Ampicillin-chloramphenicol interaction against enteric gram-negative organisms, Pediatr Infect Dis J 2:39, 1983.
3. Ellner PD and New HC: The inhibitory quotient: a method of interpreting minimum inhibitory concentration data, JAMA 246:1575, 1981.
4. Kaiser AB: Antimicrobial prophylaxis in surgery, N Engl J Med 315:1129, 1986.
5. Kim KS: Clinical perspectives on penicillin tolerance, J Pediatr 112:509, 1988.
6. Abramaowicz M, editor: The medical letter handbook of antimicrobial therapy, New Rochelle, New York, 1990, The Medical Letter, Inc.
7. National Committee for Clinical Laboratory Standards: Performance standards for antimicrobial disk susceptibility tests, ed 3, 1984.*

*771 East Lancaster Ave, Villanova, Pa 19085.

8. Nelson JD: 1987-1988 Pocketbook of pediatric antimicrobial therapy. Brown CL, Napora L (Eds.), Baltimore, 1987, Williams & Wilkins.
9. Physicians' Desk Reference, ed 44, Oradell, NJ, 1990, Medical Economics Co.
10. Tuomanen EI et al: Oral chloramphenicol in the treatment of *Haemophilus influenzae* meningitis, J Pediatr 99:968, 1981.

SUGGESTED READINGS

Donowitz GR and Mandell GL: Beta-lactam antibiotics, N Engl J Med 318:419, 1988, and 318:490, 1988.

Kucers A and Bennett N: The use of antibiotics, ed 4, Philadelphia, 1987, JB Lippincott Co.

Mandell GL, Douglas RG Jr, and Bennett JE, editors: Principles and practice of infectious diseases, ed 2, New York, 1985, John Wiley & Sons, Inc.

Moellering RC, editor: Antibacterial agents: pharmacodynamics, pharmacology, new agents. Infectious disease clinics of North America, vol 3, Philadelphia, 1989, WB Saunder Co.

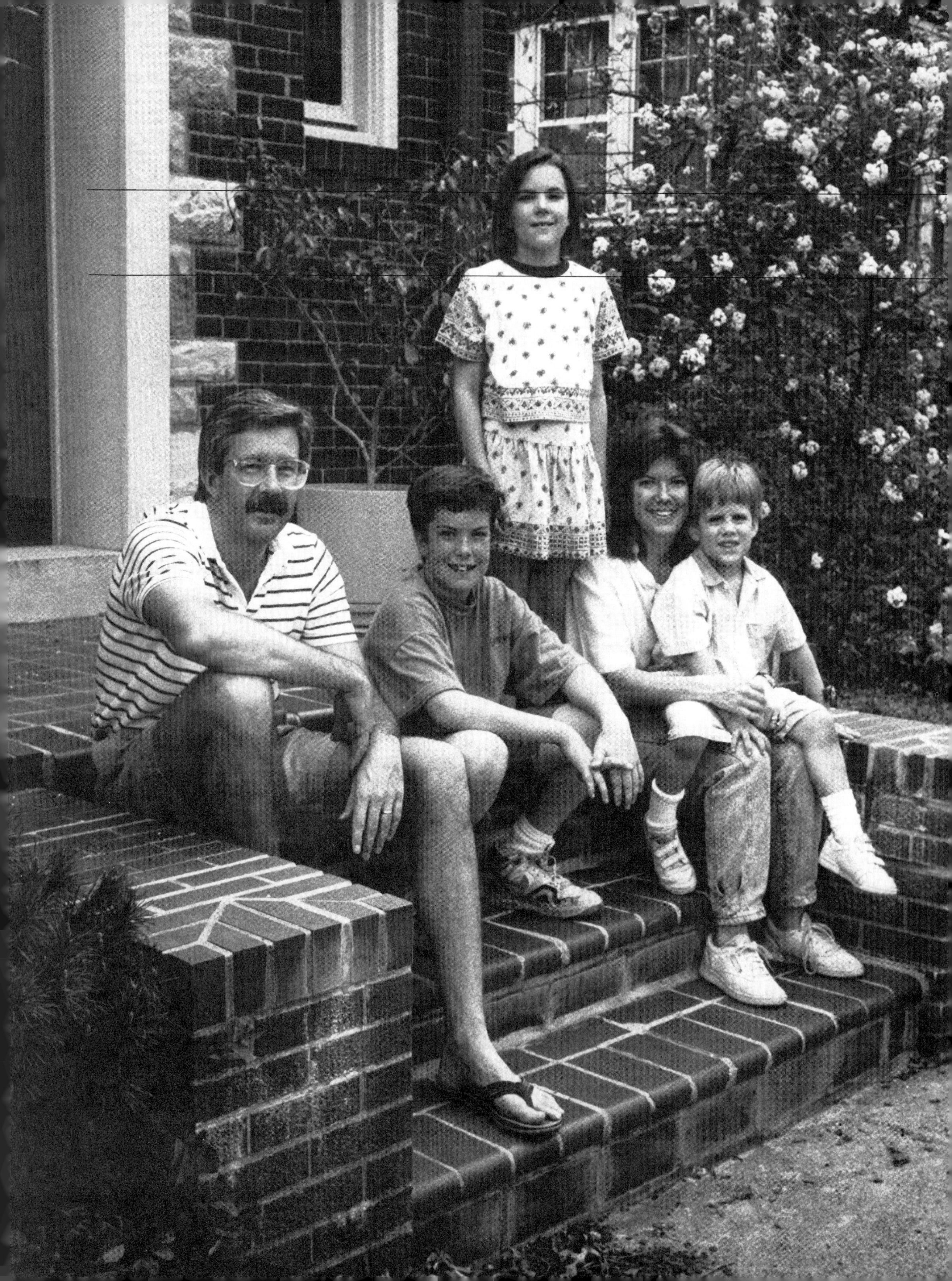

Part Four

The Reproductive Process

Section One

Antepartum Considerations

Section Two

Perinatal Medicine

29

Genetic Diseases

Marvin E. Miller

Physicians who care for children need to be aware of how genetic diseases and congenital malformations can be diagnosed, which individuals are at increased risk for these disorders, and the availability of various laboratory tests for the diagnosis of these disorders. For almost 30 years chromosome analysis has made possible the accurate diagnosis of most chromosomal disorders. More recently, the application of molecular genetics has resulted in remarkable advances in the diagnosis of common genetic diseases. The alpha and beta hemoglobin genes, the cystic fibrosis gene, and the dystrophin gene have been cloned and sequenced, which permits molecular diagnosis of the various hemoglobinopathies, cystic fibrosis, and Duchenne muscular dystrophy. Significant advances also have been made in the prenatal diagnosis of congenital malformations and genetic disease through amniocentesis, chorionic villus sampling, maternal serum alphafetoprotein screening, and ultrasound. In spite of all these scientific and technologic advances, the taking of a family history and understanding the types of genetic diseases and their inheritance patterns still provide the foundation for the diagnosis of genetic disease.

TYPES OF GENETIC DISEASE

The human genome consists of 23 pairs of chromosomes: 22 pairs of autosomes that are the same for males and females and a sex chromosome pair that is different in the two sexes. Females have two X chromosomes (XX); males have one X chromosome and one Y chromosome (XY). There are about 50,000 genetic loci in the human genome. The X chromosome contains several thousand loci and thus is similar to the autosomal chromosomes. The Y chromosome, however, contains only one or perhaps only a few genetic loci that determine male gonadal differentiation.

The 24 different chromosomes (22 autosomes, X, and Y) can be readily distinguished from each other by their size, centromere location, and banding pattern. Each of the 22 autosomes is designated by a number. Chromosomal disorders can be diagnosed by a karyotype, which is a photographic enlargement of the chromosomes arranged by their numbered pairs.

One chromosome of each chromosomal pair is inherited from the father; the other chromosome of that pair is inherited from the mother. Thus at each genetic locus an individual has two genes that are more properly called *alleles*.

There are four categories of genetic disorders:

1. Chromosomal disorders in which there is an excess or a deficiency of chromosomal material
2. Mendelian disorders in which there is an abnormality (mutation) at a single genetic locus in one or both of the alleles at that locus
3. Polygenic disorders in which there are mutations at two or more genetic loci
4. Multifactorial disorders in which there are mutations at one or more genetic loci that interact with an environmental factor such as exposure to a drug, an infectious agent, or a xenobiotic.

Chromosomal Disorders

Chromosome abnormalities occur in 0.5% of newborns; almost all arise from meiotic nondisjunction (i.e., abnormal splitting of homologous chromosomes so that one daughter cell receives both and the other receives none) in one of the parental gametes (sperm and egg). This produces a fertilized egg with a chromosomal number that is different from the normal diploid number of 46 chromosomes and is called aneuploidy (i.e, any numerical deviation from the normal 46 chromosome human karyotype). Most aneuploidy abnormalities have 47 chromosomes such as trisomy 13, 18, and 21. Although the etiology of nondisjunctions is unclear, there is an association with advanced maternal age in some chromosomal disorders such as the autosomal trisomies. This association is the reason that prenatal diagnosis with amniocentesis is offered to pregnant women 35 years of age and older. The recurrence risk for aneuploidy abnormalities is small—1% or less.

The karyotypes of parents who have had an offspring with an aneuploidy abnormality are normal and thus need not be obtained. However, parents who have had offspring with an unbalanced karyotype, in which there are 46 chromosomes but additional material is attached to another chromosome (duplication) or is deleted from one chromosome (deletion), should have their karyotypes determined. In these situations one of the parents could be a balanced carrier and at increased risk for having another offspring with a chromosome abnormality.

Mendelian Disorders

There are four Mendelian, or single-gene, inheritance patterns: autosomal dominant, autosomal recessive, X-linked recessive, and X-linked dominant (Table 29-1). Determination of the pattern involved is based on whether (1) the genetic locus is on an autosome or on the X chromosome and (2) a single dose of the mutant allele causes the disease (dominant); or whether a double dose of the mutant allele causes the disease (recessive). There are no known Y-linked human diseases.

Autosomal Dominant Inheritance. Persons with an autosomal dominant disorder have one normal (N) and one abnormal (A) or mutant allele at the genetic locus in question. An affected individual thus has the genotype of NA and has a 50% chance of passing the N allele and a 50% chance of passing the A allele to each offspring. Because an affected person's mate almost always has two normal alleles (NN) at the same locus, there is a 50% chance that the offspring will inherit the A allele and thus have the disorder.

Pedigrees of autosomal dominant disorders often show successive generations of affected individuals in which affected offspring have an affected parent. An individual with an autosomal dominant condition, however, sometimes can have normal parents who do not have the condition, which illustrates the concept of a new mutation. In this situation the risk of the normal parents to have another affected offspring is negligible, whereas the risk of the person who has the new mutation to have an affected offspring is 50%.

Achondroplasia is a well-documented autosomal dominant condition that most likely represents new mutations; 90% of affected persons are born to parents of normal stature. Advanced paternal age has been associated with new mutations in a number of autosomal dominant conditions, including, achondroplasia, Apert syndrome, and myositis ossificans.

On average, equal numbers of males and females are affected, and male to male transmission also occurs. These two characteristics help distinguish autosomal dominant inheritance from X-linked recessive inheritance. In X-linked inheritance, females almost never are affected and male to male transmission cannot occur.

Variable expressivity is another feature of some autosomal dominant disorders in which there can be a spectrum of clinical manifestations in affected individuals. This principle is illustrated in the autosomal dominant condition of Marfan syndrome, in which any combination of the following can occur: musculoskeletal abnormalities, including long, thin fingers, high arched palate, pectus excavatum, and scoliosis; the eye abnormality of dislocated lenses; and cardiac abnormalities, including mitral valve prolapse and a dilated aortic root.

Autosomal Recessive Inheritance. Individuals with an autosomal recessive disorder have two mutant alleles at the genetic locus in question; thus they have the genotype AA and are homozygous for the mutant allele. Most individuals at this locus, however, are homozygous for the normal allele (NN), although the frequency of the heterozygote or carrier (NA) can be as high as 5% for some common autosomal recessive disorders such as cystic fibrosis. Persons who have the NA genotype are entirely normal and show no evidence of the disease in question.

Couples who have had an offspring with an autosomal recessive condition are both carriers (NA) of one abnormal allele; the other allele is normal. Each parent has a 50% chance of passing the A allele to subsequent offspring. Thus the probability that both will pass on the A allele to produce

Table 29-1 *Characteristics of Mendelian Inheritance Patterns*

	AUTOSOMAL DOMINANT	AUTOSOMAL RECESSIVE	X-LINKED RECESSIVE	X-LINKED DOMINANT
Sex	M = F	M = F	Only M	F > M (2:1)
Genotype of affected individual	AN	AA	X^A Y	X^A Y; X^A X^N
Generations affected	Successive	Single	Successive; through carrier females	Successive
Recurrence risk for parents with affected child	50% if parent affected; negligible if parents unaffected	25%	25% if mother is carrier; negligible if new mutation	If M affected, all daughters affected; no sons affected. If F affected, 50% offspring affected
Male-to-male transmission	Yes	NA	No	No
Other features	Advanced paternal age with new mutations in some disorders; variable expressivity	Consanguinity sometimes found	—	Rare inheritance pattern

A, Abnormal allele on autosomal chromosome; *F*, female; *M*, male; *N*, normal allele on autosomal chromosome A; *NA*, not applicable, *X*, abnormal allele on X chromosome.

an affected offspring is 50% × 50%, which is 25%. On average, equal numbers of males and females are affected. Pedigrees almost always show the disease confined to one sibship without transmission of the disease from generation to generation. The probability that an affected individual will have an affected offspring is negligible because the mate of this individual also would have to be a carrier of the same abnormal allele, which is relatively unlikely. Consanguinity sometimes is found in pedigrees of autosomal recessive diseases, especially very rare conditions, because inbreeding increases the likelihood of two individuals having the same mutant allele at a genetic locus that they can pass on to their offspring.

X-Linked Recessive Inheritance. X-linked recessive disorders are caused by a mutation at a genetic locus on the X chromosome. Because females have two X chromosomes, it is highly unlikely that they will have mutant alleles at a given locus on both X chromosomes. Males, however, have only one X chromosome; if they inherit an X chromosome from their mother with a mutation at a disease-associated locus, then they will have the disease. Thus females rarely are affected with X-linked recessive disorders; for all practical purposes they affect only males. Males can inherit an X-linked disorder from a carrier female, or the X chromosome that the mother passes on can undergo mutation and thus give rise to the disorder.

Male to male transmission in X-linked recessive inheritance never occurs because the genetic locus is on the X chromosome and a male has to pass the Y chromosome, not the X chromosome, to his male offspring. The sons of carrier females have a 50% chance of being affected with an X-linked recessive disorder; the daughters of carrier females have a 50% chance of being carriers. In those X-linked conditions in which males can reproduce, such as hemophilia, none of the male offspring of affected fathers will be affected, but all female offspring will be carriers.

X-Linked Dominant Inheritance. X-linked dominant is a rare inheritance pattern; twice as many females are affected as males, there is no male to male transmission, and all female offspring of affected males are affected.

Polygenic and Multifactorial Inheritance

Because it is difficult to distinguish between multifactorial and polygenic inheritance in human genetic diseases, they will be discussed together. These disorders are characterized by a recurrence risk that is greater for the development of the disorder than the general population's risk but that is clearly lower than that of the 25% autosomal recessive or 50% autosomal dominant mendelian disorders. Table 29-2 lists some of these disorders, with general population frequency and recurrence risk if a couple already has had an affected child. These disorders are important in pediatrics because they are common and because many are associated with significant morbidity and mortality. It has been difficult to define the specific genetic loci and environmental factors that cause these disorders. Etiologic heterogeneity is one explanation for the observation of an intermediate risk after a couple has an affected child. This means that there could be distinctly different causes of the same clinical phenotype. For example, some cases of congenital heart disease may result from an environmental cause such as a congenital infection, whereas others may result from a single gene disorder such as the Holt-Oram syndrome. Thus the recurrence risk for each is clearly different. In the former, the risk would be negligible, whereas in the latter, which is an autosomal dominant disorder, it would be 50% if there is an affected parent.

FAMILY HISTORY

A family history should be part of the medical record of every pediatric patient. It should consist of a three-generation pedigree that shows the age and state of health of all living individuals and the age and cause of death of all deceased individuals. Spontaneous and induced abortions should be listed, as well as stillbirths. The ethnic backgrounds of both sides of the family should be noted, as should consanguinity, if present.

As shown in Table 29-3, certain ethnic groups have an increased frequency of disease-associated alleles and thus are at increased risk for some genetic diseases. Consanguinity increases the risk that an offspring will be homozygous for a disease-associated allele and thus for autosomal recessive diseases. For example, first-cousin matings have a twofold greater risk (4% to 6%) for a congenital disorder, compared with the background risk of unrelated matings (2% to 3%).

PRENATAL SCREENING

Amniocentesis

Amniocentesis is the removal of amniotic fluid from the amniotic cavity by a needle puncture through the abdominal wall and anterior portion of the uterus. It is a safe procedure that typically is performed at about 16 weeks of gestation although it can be done as early as 12 to 13 weeks of gestation. The amniotic fluid contains fetal cells that can be karyotyped or used for biochemical and DNA analysis.

The most common indication for amniocentesis is advanced maternal age, because older mothers are at increased

Table 29-2 *Polygenic/Multifactorial Diseases*

DISORDER	GENERAL POPULATION FREQUENCY (%)	RECURRENCE RISK AFTER ONE AFFECTED CHILD (%)
Neural tube defects	0.1	4
Congenital heart disease	0.6	3
Cleft lip ± palate	0.1	4
Juvenile diabetes	0.1	4

risk for chromosomal disorders. Pregnant women 35 years of age and older are offered amniocentesis with fetal chromosome analysis as part of their prenatal care. Couples with an offspring who has a chromosomal abnormality or who are balanced translocation carriers also are offered amniocentesis with fetal karyotyping.

Couples who have had a child with a genetic disease may choose to have amniocentesis if the condition can be diagnosed by enzyme analysis of fetal cells or by biochemical analysis of amniotic fluid. For example, Hurler syndrome is an autosomal recessive disorder with a 25% recurrence risk that causes severe mental retardation; most affected children die by adolescence. The disease is caused by a lack of production of the enzyme iduronidase. The disorder can be diagnosed by determination of the iduronidase activity in fetal cells obtained by amniocentesis.

Molecular genetics has paved the way for the prenatal diagnosis of some of the more common and severe genetic disorders. DNA analysis of fetal cells obtained from amniocentesis can be used for the diagnosis of cystic fibrosis, Duchenne muscular dystrophy, sickle cell anemia, β-thalassemia, and α-thalassemia. Couples with an offspring with one of these disorders have a 25% risk of having another affected child. Because DNA diagnosis is highly accurate, many couples with an affected child choose to have amniocentesis and DNA analysis in subsequent pregnancies.

Amniotic fluid also can be analyzed for alpha-fetoprotein, which is significantly elevated in neural tube defects. The alpha-fetoprotein concentration is usually determined when an amniocentesis is performed for advanced maternal age. Couples who are at increased risk for having a baby with a neural tube defect may choose to have amniocentesis, including the determination of alpha-fetoprotein, as well as fetal ultrasound. At increased risk for having a baby with a neural tube defect are couples with an offspring who has this defect; additional risks are maternal diabetes and maternal use of valproic acid during pregnancy.

Chorionic Villus Sampling

Chorionic villus sampling (CVS) is another technique to procure fetal tissue that can be used for chromosomal, biochemical, or DNA analysis. Fetal tissue is obtained transcervically by means of a catheter that can retrieve small pieces of chorionic villus. The procedure is relatively safe, although there is not as much experience with CVS as there is with amniocentesis. Because CVS can be performed at an earlier time in pregnancy, couples who are extremely anxious about having a child with a particular condition may choose to have CVS rather than amniocentesis for this reason.

Ultrasound

Significant advances in fetal ultrasound have resulted in the diagnosis of many congenital abnormalities during pregnancy. These conditions include major central nervous system abnormalities such as hydrocephalus, anencephaly, myelomeningocele, and holoprosencephaly; gastrointestinal abnormalities such as duodenal atresia and diaphragmatic hernia; many types of congenital heart disease; genitourinary abnormalities such as polycystic kidney disease and hydronephrosis; and many types of skeletal disorders. Ultrasound has been helpful to couples who have had children with congenital abnormalities and who want reassurance that subsequent offspring will be unaffected.

Maternal Serum Alpha-fetoprotein Screening

Because elevated levels of alpha-fetoprotein are associated with an increased risk for neural tube defects, pregnant women are now being offered maternal serum alpha-fetoprotein screening (MSAFP). Although the test is not as accurate as amniotic alpha-fetoprotein determination, it requires only a maternal blood specimen. If the levels are high, then ultrasound or amniocentesis with amniotic alpha-fetoprotein analysis can be considered. Recently, low levels of MSAFP have been associated with Down syndrome; however, this association is weak and the test was not designed to detect Down syndrome. Couples whose MSAFP reveals low levels of alpha-fetoprotein may consider having an amniocentesis with fetal karyotyping to detect the presence of Down syndrome.

It should be noted that prenatal screening for genetic diseases is designed to provide accurate information about the likelihood of an offspring being affected with one of these diseases. Parents are advised of the consequences of such an outcome so that they may make an informed decision as to whether they wish to continue the pregnancy.

NEWBORN SCREENING

All states have mandatory newborn screening programs. Although the tests vary from state to state, all states test for phenylketonuria and congenital hypothyroidism because they are relatively common, easily treated, and clearly cost effective. Some states mandate testing for maple syrup urine dis-

Table 29-3 *Populations at Increased Risk for Specific Genetic Diseases*

POPULATION	DISEASE	DISEASE FREQUENCY/ 10,000 BIRTHS
African American	Sickle cell	20
Ashkenazi Jew	Tay-Sachs	3
Mediterranean	β-Thalassemia	20
Southeast Asian	α-Thalassemia	20
Caucasian	Cystic fibrosis	5
Eskimo	Congenital adrenal hyperplasia	20

Table 29-4 *Common Genetic Disorders*

DISORDER	MANIFESTATION	FREQUENCY/ 10,000 BIRTHS
Chromosomal		
Trisomy 21	Congenital heart disease, Brushfield spots, short hands, clinodactyly, simian crease, hypotonia, dysmorphic facies	16
Trisomy 18	Congenital heart disease, SGA, clenched fist, rocker-bottom foot, dysmorphic facies	3
Trisomy 13	Congenital heart disease, SGA, polydactyly, holoprosencephaly, dysmorphic facies	2
XO	Congenital peripheral edema, webbed neck, short stature, primary amenorrhea	3
XXY	Behavior problems, small testes, infertility, clinodactyly	5
Autosomal recessive		
Sickle cell disease	Anemia, infection	20 (African American)
β-Thalassemia	Anemia	20 (Mediterranean)
Cystic fibrosis	Failure to thrive, malabsorption, cough, recurrent pneumonia	5 Caucasian
Autosomal dominant		
Familial hypercholesterolemia	Family history of early coronary artery disease	20
Neurofibromatosis	Café au lait spots	3
X-Linked recessive		
Fragile X	Mental retardation, large testes, dysmorphic facies	5
Duchenne muscular dystrophy	Muscle weakness, pseudohypertrophy of calf	1

SGA, Small for gestational age.

ease, homocystinuria, cystic fibrosis, hemoglobinopathies, biotinidase deficiency, congenital adrenal hyperplasia, and galactosemia. The results of newborn screening tests usually are available 1 to 2 weeks after an infant's discharge from the hospital; the pediatrician always should ascertain that the newborn screening test has been performed and is normal. Obviously, any abnormal values should be investigated further.

DIAGNOSIS OF PEDIATRIC GENETIC DISORDERS

It is beyond the intent of this chapter to describe in any detail the numerous genetic diseases that exist. Table 29-4 lists some of the more common genetic diseases in children. The pediatrician should be aware of two excellent references that may be of most help in establishing a genetic diagnosis or a dysmorphology syndrome: Jones' *Smith's Recognizable Patterns of Human Malformation*[1] and McKusick's *Mendelian Inheritance in Man.*[2]

REFERENCES

1. Jones KL: Smith's recognizable patterns of human malformation, ed 4, Philadelphia, 1988, WB Saunders Co.
2. McKusick VA: Mendelian inheritance in man, ed 8, Baltimore, 1988, Johns Hopkins University Press.

SUGGESTED READINGS

Kelly TE: Clinical genetics and genetic counseling, ed 2, Chicago, 1986, Year Book Medical Publishers, Inc.

Sutton HE: An introduction to human genetics, ed 4, New York, 1988, Harcourt Brace Jovanovich, Inc.

Thompson MW: Genetics in medicine, ed 4, Philadelphia, 1986, WB Saunders Co.

30

Contraception

Eric A. Schaff

In industrialized countries before the twentieth century—and in many undeveloped countries today—family size was dictated largely by famine, infectious diseases, war, and abortion. Fortunately, contraception now provides a choice: whether to have children and when to have them. The use of contraception also can help to decrease the medical and social morbidity associated with unplanned, premature pregnancy in teenagers.

Many American teenagers are in need of comprehensive health care, especially contraceptive services. National studies have indicated that almost 50% of 15- to 19-year-old teenage women are sexually active, ranging from 20% of 15-year-olds to over 70% of 19-year-olds. The rates among teenage males are higher. Whereas one quarter of teenage women seek family planning services before or at the time of becoming sexually active, three fourths wait an average of almost 2 years before a family planning health visit.[4] Approximately 1 million teenagers become pregnant each year; the majority of these pregnancies are unintended. Two thirds of these young women have a child, and one third have abortions. The increase in sexually transmitted diseases (STD) in this age-group also is a growing concern, especially with the advent of the human immunodeficiency virus (HIV).

The pediatrician is in a unique position to provide anticipatory guidance to parents, preteens, and sexually active and nonsexually active teenagers regarding puberty, peer pressure, reproduction, contraception, and the risks of STD. Pediatricians must assure the teenager of confidentiality, must develop a nonjudgmental approach in obtaining a sexual history, and must provide straightforward information. Pediatricians also can provide family planning services, as well as screening for and treatment of STD. All physicians should be aware of community family planning services available to teenagers regardless of their financial status.

The ideal contraceptive for the sexually active teenager is (1) 100% effective at preventing pregnancy and STD, (2) easy to use, (3) associated with no side effects, and (4) reversible. Barring abstinence, there is no contraceptive method that fits this ideal.

The effectiveness of different contraceptive methods should be presented without bias. Theoretic and actual effectiveness rates should not be confused. For example, if oral contraceptives are used correctly and consistently, their *theoretic effectiveness* (0.1% accidental pregnancies during the first year of use) compares favorably with that of both condoms and diaphragms (3% accidental pregnancies). The *actual effectiveness* of oral contraceptives in a teenage population that stops using them, frequently because of minor side effects, is similar to the actual effectiveness of condoms and diaphragms (80% to 90%). The message is clear: it does not matter what method one uses as long as one uses it correctly. The use of two methods simultaneously and the availability of a back-up method significantly decrease the likelihood of an unintended pregnancy.

Teenagers have had legal access to family planning services since the Supreme Court decision in the case of *Belotti v. Baird* in 1976. Confidential care also can be inferred from Public Law 7896 regarding confidential treatment of STD and "related services." Required parental notification or consent laws place an additional barrier to health services for teenagers who are unable or unwilling to involve their parents.

Several birth control methods, including oral contraceptives, the "morning-after" pill, and the intrauterine device, are opposed by antiabortion groups who claim these methods are abortifacients. Other groups claim that these methods decrease the need for abortion.

CONDOMS

In the 1990s condoms must be recommended very highly to sexually active teenagers because of their effectiveness at preventing pregnancy (if used consistently and correctly) and because they are the most effective contraceptive method in decreasing the spread of all STDs, including HIV. Teenagers who prefer another method for pregnancy prevention also should be strongly encouraged to use condoms for additional disease prevention. Further, condoms are (1) inexpensive, (2) available over-the-counter, (3) involve male responsibility, (4) lubricated and thus help to prevent dyspareunia, (5) associated with no side effects, (6) simple to use, (7) remediable if broken by the use of the morning-after pill (discussed in the next section) or possibly the insertion of spermicidal foam, (8) protective against infertility and cervical cancer by reducing STD, and (9) a possible prevention for premature ejaculation.

Condoms, however, can decrease genital sensation for both males and females. They also are not entirely protective against STD because external genitalia lesions and vaginal secretions on the pubic area and on the hands and mouth can lead to infection.

For optimal compliance the following information should be offered to teenagers verbally and, ideally, in writing:

1. Condoms are highly effective at preventing pregnancy when used consistently and correctly.
2. Condoms are highly effective at preventing sexually

transmitted diseases and the virus that causes acquired immunodeficiency syndrome (AIDS).
3. Latex condoms with spermicidal lubricant offer the best protection. "Natural" condoms (made from caecum of lamb intestine) provide significantly less protection because of greater permeability (to viruses) and are not recommended.
4. Condoms should be placed on the erect penis just before insertion into the vagina.
5. To prevent condom breakage, (a) avoid storing them in warm places, such as in a wallet, for long periods of time, (b) avoid petroleum-based lubricants such as Vaseline, (c) use prelubricated condoms, (d) allow for room at the condom's end for ejaculate fluid, and (e) do not reuse them.
6. To avoid accidental spillage, remove the penis shortly after ejaculation while holding the rim of the condom on the penis.
7. If spillage occurs or a condom breaks, insert spermicidal vaginal foam, which may help, or consult your physician regarding the morning-after pill.

ORAL CONTRACEPTIVES

Oral contraceptives are one of the most studied pharmacologic agents. As newer and lower dose preparations become available, the reports continue to show fewer serious health problems[3] and more beneficial side effects from their use. Oral contraceptives consist of an estrogen and progestin compound. All currently used low-dose pills contain only ethinyl estradiol as the estrogen component, and multiple progestational agents are available that are metabolized either to norethindrone or to levonorgestrel. Although levonorgestrel is 10 to 20 times more potent than norethindrone, it is proportionately reduced. The small doses now used reduce the potential for adverse side effects.

The combination pill is prescribed on a 28-day cycle: 21 days of taking active ingredients and 7 days of taking either inert pills or no pills at all. The estrogen and progestin compounds in the pill can be fixed or, most recently, the concentrations may vary during the 21-day period (multiphasic pills). The low-dose estrogen preparations, 30 to 35 μg, have been as effective as the higher-dose estrogen pills, 50 μg, at preventing pregnancy. The advantage of the multiphasic pills over most fixed combination pills is the lowering of the total amount of hormone administered during each cycle.

In most cases, oral contraceptives suppress luteinizing- and follicle-stimulating hormones, thereby inhibiting ovulation. They also thicken cervical mucus, making it less penetrable by sperm, and alter the endometrium, making it less receptive for implantation of a fertilized ovum.

Complications

The most serious complications of oral contraceptives are thromboembolic disorders: thrombophlebitis, pulmonary embolism, and cerebral vascular occlusion. These disorders are proportional to the amount of the estrogen component; for this reason all women should be started on the low-dose, 30 to 35 μg, estrogen pills.

To reduce these rare but major complications significantly, oral contraceptives should not be prescribed to teenagers with a history of thromboembolic events or to those at risk for these problems because of diabetes, sickle cell disease, and collagen vascular diseases. Relative contraindications to the prescribing of birth control pills include thromboembolic and cardiovascular risk factors such as heavy cigarette smoking, high blood pressure, severe obesity, migraines, and a family history of early cardiovascular disease or hyperlipidemia.

Gallbladder disease is another rare complication of oral contraceptive use. To avoid exacerbating a current condition, the prescription of oral contraceptives is contraindicated in cases of active liver disease, undiagnosed uterine bleeding, estrogen-dependent tumors, and suspected pregnancy.

Recent studies[2] have shown an association between the use of oral contraceptives and breast cancer; this finding needs further verification. In the meantime the use of the lower hormone doses is likely to lower any risk from the use of oral contraceptives.

Side Effects

Some teenagers ascribe to oral contraceptives side effects that are likely to resolve but that will cause them to abandon contraceptive use. Common minor side effects include breast tenderness, nausea, breakthrough vaginal bleeding, weight gain, and mood changes, which often abate after the first several cycles. Amenorrhea is common with low-dose pills after the first several months and patients should be forewarned. Changing to another low-dose pill or using a 50 μg estrogen pill for two cycles may eliminate the problem.

A more detailed listing of side effects and their management can be found in the two additional readings noted at the end of this chapter.

Beneficial Effects

Oral contraceptives are prescribed for the treatment of anovulatory uterine bleeding and dysmenorrhea. Pill users also have less iron deficiency anemia, benign breast disease, ovarian cysts, and ectopic pregnancies. Recent studies also have indicated a protective effect against ovarian[6] and endometrial cancer.[1]

Prescribing

Healthy female teenagers who have or who anticipate having regular sexual intercourse are excellent candidates for the use of oral contraceptives. Before prescribing, the pediatrician should obtain a medical history and perform a complete physical examination, including a pelvic examination. A Pap test should be performed. Vaginal secretions should be examined and cervical secretions cultured for STD. Obtaining a hematocrit value is recommended because of the high prevalence of iron deficiency anemia in this age-group. Those without documented rubella and rubeola immunizations should receive them after informed consent is obtained and they are advised that pregnancy should be avoided for 3 months. A yearly serologic test for syphilis is indicated if the prevalence in the community is high. A lipid profile may be indicated for a teenager with a family history of early coronary artery disease.

In the very young sexually active teenager, the pediatrician must weigh the theoretic risks of hormonal contraception on future growth and fertility versus the medical and social risks of a premature pregnancy. Currently there is no evidence that early use of oral contraceptives either limits growth or affects future fertility.

The pediatrician may prescribe any of the many low-dose (30 to 35 μg) estrogen pills. There is no clinical difference in effectiveness among these pills; therefore cost should be the deciding factor. The recent release of generic low-dose oral contraceptives has significantly decreased the cost. The lowest-dose preparation is a fixed combination of ethinyl estradiol, 35 μg, and norethindrone, 0.4 mg (Ovcon-35).

For a multitude of reasons, many teenagers will stop using oral contraceptives during the initial cycles. Teenagers should have a return appointment in 1 to 3 months to reinforce compliance and to measure the blood pressure. Follow-up appointments can then be scheduled every 6 to 12 months or, if clinically indicated, more frequently.

Pediatricians will rarely need to prescribe progestin-only pills, also called "mini-pills." They usually are recommended for women in whom estrogen use is contraindicated.

Compliance

To maximize compliance with an oral contraceptive regimen, the pediatrician should provide the following anticipatory guidance verbally and, ideally, in writing:

1. Oral contraceptive pills should be started on day 5 after the onset of menses to ensure that the patient is not pregnant.
2. Oral contraceptives, taken daily, should effectively inhibit ovulation after 1 week of medication, but reliance on an additional contraceptive method is essential in the first week and is advisable during the first cycle.
3. Pills should be taken the same time each day for 21 days and then either omitted for 7 days or the seven placebo pills in the 28-day pill package should be taken. Withdrawal bleeding usually occurs on day 2 or 3 after the last hormonal pill has been taken.
4. Ovulation and therefore pregnancy is possible if a pill is missed, particularly during the first 7 days. Therefore, taking the missed pill on the following day to "catch up" and using an additional contraceptive method during that cycle are recommended for that cycle.
5. Mild side effects such as vaginal bleeding (spotting), nausea, bloating, and irritability are likely to resolve after several months of an oral contraceptive regimen. If not, the prescription can be changed.
6. Menses usually become lighter and occasionally are absent while oral contraceptive pills are taken. If there are no menses, the pills should be continued but a pregnancy test should be performed for reassurance and to determine if the rare possibility of pregnancy has occurred.
7. The major side effect of oral contraceptives is thrombosis. This is significantly more likely to occur in women older than 40 years of age, women older than 35 years who smoke, and women with additional risk factors for thrombosis such as hypertension, diabetes, hypercholesterolemia, and obesity. Warning signs requiring medical consultation include severe head, chest, or leg pain. The risks to a healthy teenager are extremely low.
8. The major disadvantage of oral contraceptives is the lack of protection against STD, including the AIDS virus. Condoms are strongly encouraged to prevent STD.
9. Oral contraceptives are less effective when taken with certain medications such as antibiotics (e.g., amoxicillin and doxycycline) and certain anticonvulsants (e.g., phenobarbital and phenytoin). The simultaneous use of condoms or other barrier methods provides additional protection.

"MORNING-AFTER" PILLS

This method of contraception is helpful when other methods fail, when no form of contraception was used, or when rape occurred. Attention should be given to the time during the menstrual cycle when ovulation occurs and conception is possible. There may be no need for this method if conception is unlikely. The treatment regimen consists of two tablets of a combination of ethinyl estradiol (50 μg) and norgestrel (0.5 mg) (Ovral-Rx) followed by two more tablets 12 hours later. It should be used as soon after intercourse as possible but no later than 72 hours afterward. Medication for nausea may be necessary. Menses should occur 2 to 3 weeks later. If this does not occur, the patient should be instructed to return for a pregnancy test. The mechanism of action is suspected to be related to luteal phase dysfunction, endometrial changes that make implantation less likely, and fallopian tube mobility alterations that adversely affect the movement of the fertilized ovum to the uterus.

Although the "morning-after" pill is not approved by the Food and Drug Administration, it has been extensively used in Europe and for rape victims in the United States.

IMPLANTABLE CONTRACEPTIVES

Levonorgestrel subdermal implants have recently been approved by the Federal Drug Administration. Their advantages include (1) 99% effectiveness, (2) ease of compliance, (3) effective for as long as 5 years, and (4) reversibility. The disadvantages include (1) the technical skills required for insertion, (2) the current costs (around $300), and (3) the side effects—menstrual irregularities, headaches, and nausea.

Teenagers who have difficulty with contraceptive compliance may be excellent candidates for this method. Unfortunately, these teenagers also frequently change their minds, making implants an impractical option.

DIAPHRAGM AND CERVICAL CAP

The diaphragm is an excellent contraceptive method that offers some protection from STD and has minimal side effects. It is a thin rubber dome that, when inserted into the vagina, blocks sperm from entering the cervix. It must be used with spermicidal contraceptive jelly whose active ingredient is nonoxynol 9. The diaphragm's failure rate varies from 2% to 16%. Occasionally it is chosen by the older, more motivated teenager. The disadvantages of the diaphragm for the patient include (1) the technical skill needed for correct placement, (2) the need to leave it in place 6 hours after intercourse, (3) the need for a second application of spermicidal jelly if intercourse is repeated, and (4) the association with vaginitis, urinary tract infections, and rarely, toxic shock syndrome.

Disadvantages for the pediatrician include the necessity of keeping a set of diaphragm rings for sizing and the maintenance of the skill required for fitting one when the number of requests is likely to be few.

The cervical cap is a thimble-shaped latex device that fits over the cervix and can be left in place up to 48 hours. Its advantages and effectiveness rates are similar to those of the diaphragm. Disadvantages include (1) the skill needed for insertion and removal (significantly more than that for the diaphragm), (2) the association of cervical dysplasia in the early months of use, and (3) the inability to fit the cervixes of some women.

SPERMICIDALS: VAGINAL SPONGE, VAGINAL FOAM, AND VAGINAL SUPPOSITORY

The vaginal sponge, vaginal foam, and vaginal suppository all use the spermicidal agent nonoxynol 9, which has in vitro and in vivo properties against some STD. All are relatively simple, effective, and inexpensive methods that require no prescription. They are slightly less effective at preventing pregnancies than is the diaphragm, and they tend to have similar actions, advantages, and disadvantages. The spermicidals are excellent complementary methods (1) when used with condoms, (2) when intercourse is intermittent, and (3) when used as a backup for other birth control methods.

After the vaginal sponge is moistened with water, it can be inserted several hours before intercourse; it remains effective for 24 hours. Vaginal suppositories must be left in place 10 to 30 minutes before intercourse to allow them to dissolve.

NATURAL FAMILY PLANNING

Natural family planning methods include (1) calendar charting of menstrual cycles, (2) recording of basal body temperatures, and (3) cervical mucus monitoring to determine when ovulation occurs. Few teenagers rely solely on these methods. Advantages include the lack of side effects, acceptance by religious groups opposed to other medical and mechanical methods, and the knowledge gained about reproductive physiology. Disadvantages for teenagers include their irregular menstrual cycles and the high degree of motivation required for effective use.

INTRAUTERINE DEVICE

How the intrauterine device (IUD) works is not known. It probably causes the endometrium to become unsuitable for implantation of a fertilized egg. However, the IUD has become relatively contraindicated in the healthy teenager because of the increased risk of pelvic inflammatory disease and its associated risk of infertility. A marked decline in IUD availability is due to its increased cost as a result of the expenses incurred by pharmaceutical companies in defending the large number of lawsuits related to IUD use. The major advantage of an IUD is that once in place, it requires no effort for continued effectiveness.

COITUS INTERRUPTUS

Coitus interruptus is the withdrawal of the penis from the vagina before ejaculation. Its disadvantages are that preejaculatory penile secretions can contain sperm, that the penis commonly is not withdrawn in time, and that coital gratification is lessened. The only advantage of this method is that it is significantly better than no method at all.

ABSTINENCE

Teenagers who choose abstinence should be offered support and encouragement, as well as contraceptive information if and when they choose to have intercourse.

SUMMARY

Many teenagers are sexually active. Unintended pregnancies are common and associated with adverse social and medical outcomes for the teenager and her child. One third of pregnant teenagers seek abortions.

Pediatricians must ensure that teenagers are receiving appropriate sex education from their families and schools and that all sexually active teenagers have ready access to safe, effective contraceptive services.

REFERENCES

1. Cancer and steroid hormone study: combination oral contraceptive use and the risk of endometrial cancer, JAMA 257:796, 1987.
2. Oral contraceptive use and breast cancer risk in young women. UK National Case-Control Study Group, Lancet, p 973, May 6, 1989.
3. Hofferth SL, Kahn JR, Baldwin W: Premarital sexual activity among U.S. teenage women over the past three decades, Fam Plann Perspect 19(2),46-53, 1987.
4. Mosher WD, Horn MC: First family planning visits by young women, Fam Plann Persp 20(1):33-40, 1988.
5. Stampfer MJ, Willett WC, Colditz GA, Speizer FE, Hennekens CH: A prospective study of past use of oral contraceptive agents and risk of cardiovascular diseases, N Engl J Med, 319(20):1313-1317, 1988.
6. Vessey M et al: Ovarian neoplasms, functional ovarian cysts and oral contraceptives, Br Med J 294:1518, 1987.
7. Yuzpe AA, Percival-Smith R, Rademaker AW: A multicenter clinical investigation employing ethinyestradiol combined with dl-norgestrel as a postcoital contraceptive agent, Fertil Steril 37:508, 1982.

SUGGESTED READINGS

Dickey RP: Managing contraceptive pill patients, ed 5, Durant, Okla, 1987, Creative Informatics, Inc.

Hatcher RA et al: Contraceptive technology 1988-89, ed 14, New York, 1988, Irvington Publishers, Inc.

31

The Fetus at Risk

George A. Little

The fetus is a future patient of the student or practitioner of pediatrics as well as a present responsibility. In past decades pediatricians usually first saw their perinatal patients in the nursery, where a philosophy to intervene as little as possible with sick infants often dominated. Today, pediatricians should assist in fetal risk identification and clinical decisions and then be present at delivery to assume primary responsibility for the newly born infant.

A basic appreciation of fetal health includes the interaction of the fetus with mother, family, health professional, and society. The pediatrician also requires knowledge of fetal medicine for genetic counseling, neonatology, and the care of adolescent mothers. Although major strides in morphologic and physiologic sciences have made available a broader understanding of fetal well-being, the fund of knowledge is still inadequate.

Prospective parents and professionals have good reason to be concerned about the immediate and long-term effect of agents or processes on the fetus. There are too many well-documented examples of negative impact and increasing evidence of ability to prevent or treat to allow denial of the value of fetal assessment as part of prenatal care. Infections such as rubella can result in fetal loss or multisystem disease. The magnitude and seriousness of manifestations of maternal alcohol consumption or use of cocaine and its derivatives during pregnancy may be evident in physical appearance or behavior at the time of birth. Diethylstilbestrol (DES) given to mothers for threatened abortion may not manifest until the appearance of clear cell–carcinoma of the vagina in female offspring 10 to 20 years later; this is a reminder of the other extreme of the time span.

Growth and development are as much a key to fetal medicine as to pediatrics. One must regard human growth and development as a continuum beginning with conception. This section depicts some of the normal physical and interactive aspects of fetal existence, followed by a discussion of selected pathophysiologic states that may adversely affect that existence.

FETAL LIFE SPAN

The human product of conception *technically becomes a fetus at the end of the eighth week* after fertilization and remains so until birth. The normal human pregnancy lasts 36 to 40 weeks from fertilization or 38 to 42 weeks from the last menstrual period (by menstrual dating). Fetal development begins at fertilization, when a sperm combines with an ovum to form a zygote. The fetal life span is defined here in the broad sense to include the entire gestational interval (Fig. 31-1).

The process from conception to birth has three periods: (1) the dividing zygote, (2) the embryo, and (3) the fetus. The conceptus, or product of conception, is made up of all structures that develop from the zygote, both embryonic and extraembryonic (i.e., the embryo or fetus and the membranes, including the placenta).

The *period of the dividing zygote* begins with the complicated process of fertilization, wherein a single sperm enzymatically penetrates the ovum and enters the cytoplasm. Genetic material from the two haploid cells intermingles and produces a diploid cell with 46 chromosomes. A full complement of genetic material of biparental origin is thus assured. Fertilization usually takes place in the ampulla of the fallopian tube.

During the next 72 hours, rapid mitotic divisions occur as the zygote is propelled down the fallopian tube. This results in a solid 16-cell ball called the morula. Subsequently, a cavity forms in the morula, resulting in a blastocyst, which adheres to the maternal endometrial epithelium on the sixth day. An inner cell mass, or embryoblast, becomes the first embryonic germ layer to develop, while an outer layer of cells, the trophoblast, develops on the surface and begins the process resulting in the formation of the placenta.

During the second week, the last week of the period of the dividing zygote, very rapid changes occur and the blastocyst becomes more deeply implanted in the endometrium. A bilaminar embryonic disk consisting of ectoderm and endoderm evolves at the same time that extraembryonic mesoderm enters the blastocyst cavity. All this development takes place before the first missed menstrual period.

The embryonic period encompasses approximately weeks 3 to 8 and is characterized by the differentiation of all major organs that will be present in the fetus, the newborn, and the adult. Near the beginning of this interval, the woman usually becomes aware of cessation of menstruation. Laboratory tests are available that can confirm pregnancy by this time.

The importance of rapid development of the major organ systems cannot be overstressed. During the zygotic period, adverse conditions may cause the death of the products of conception. This often occurs just before the time when a menstrual period would have been expected. *Adverse influences during the embryonic period can cause major and se-*

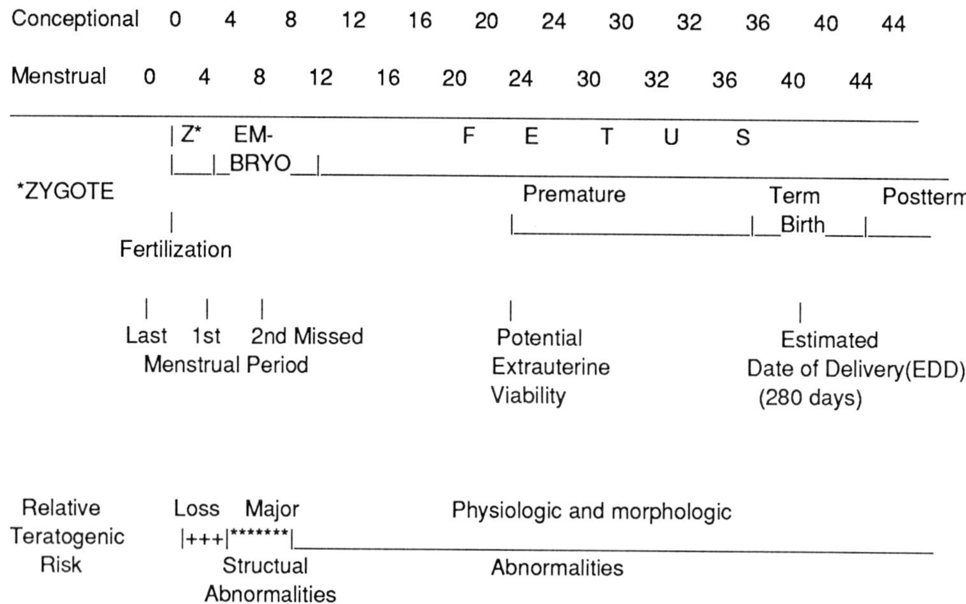

Fig. 31-1 Pregnancy dating and relative teratogenic risk by weeks.

vere interruptions in the pattern of system development, resulting in major congenital anomalies in a surviving fetus. The embryo is recognizable as humanoid toward the end of this period; and malformations, such as those of the limbs, resulting, for example, from maternal ingestion of thalidomide, are readily identifiable.

The *fetal period,* the longest of the three periods of the fetal life span, ends with delivery. Growth in size is the most apparent change during this interval, but maturation of organ systems and bodily processes is equally important. The high incidence and problems of premature birth make the degree of organ and enzyme systems maturation of compelling interest to the pediatrician. *The development of pulmonary surfactant is probably the single most important maturational process directly affecting survival in premature infants.*

The late fetal period is the focus of increasingly sophisticated diagnostic techniques. Ultrasonography not only is providing real-time images of the fetus but also is facilitating invasive procedures, such as amniocentesis, with the result that specimens of amniotic fluid or fetal cells can be obtained with little risk. The pediatrician needs to keep pace with developments in this area, such as intrauterine transfusion and, eventually, the addition or modification of genetic material.

INTRAUTERINE GROWTH AND NUTRITION

The physician dealing with the newborn must have a firm conceptual framework of intrauterine growth in order to evaluate and effectively treat the normal and abnormal newborn. In particular, the common clinical problem of prematurity can be more appropriately managed if one appreciates growth patterns as they relate to gestational age.

The growth rate of the fetus is especially noteworthy during the period from 12 to 16 weeks and again during the final months. Both rapid growth phases are associated with events of immediate concern for the practitioner. By the end of the sixteenth week after fertilization, the size and activity of the fetus have reached a point that both multiparous and primiparous women are able to feel fetal motion. This event, known as *quickening,* is a valuable tool in assessing fetal age and well-being. The late growth phase can be monitored by several means, including physical examination or the measurement of the height of the fundus above the symphysis.

The period from 8 to 12 weeks after fertilization begins with a fetus whose head makes up almost half of the total length. By 12 weeks, the total length has doubled, but the head represents a smaller proportion. The 12- to 16-week interval is characterized by extremely rapid growth in length. In the 17- to 20-week interval, growth slows somewhat, but extremities assume their relative proportions. The 21- to 25-week interval after fertilization is characterized by both significant length and weight gains.

Twenty-one weeks after fertilization, or 23 weeks from the last menstrual period, represents an extremely important milestone. Studies from several centers have shown that *the point of potential extrauterine viability is reached at approximately 23 weeks* (by menstrual gestational dating).

Many studies have attempted to quantify fetal growth through the use of postnatal data. Such growth curves derived from measuring live-born infants can give an approximation of intrauterine growth, but they have shortcomings. The fact is that the baseline population is by definition abnormal, since the babies were born before term. In addition, the population of live births is very difficult to standardize for factors such as race, parity, socioeconomic level, and maternal smoking and disease states.

In spite of all this, intrauterine growth curves derived from postnatal data can be of great conceptual and clinical assistance. The *Colorado Intrauterine Growth Curves* depicted in Fig. 31-2 are among the better known. Percentiles of intra-

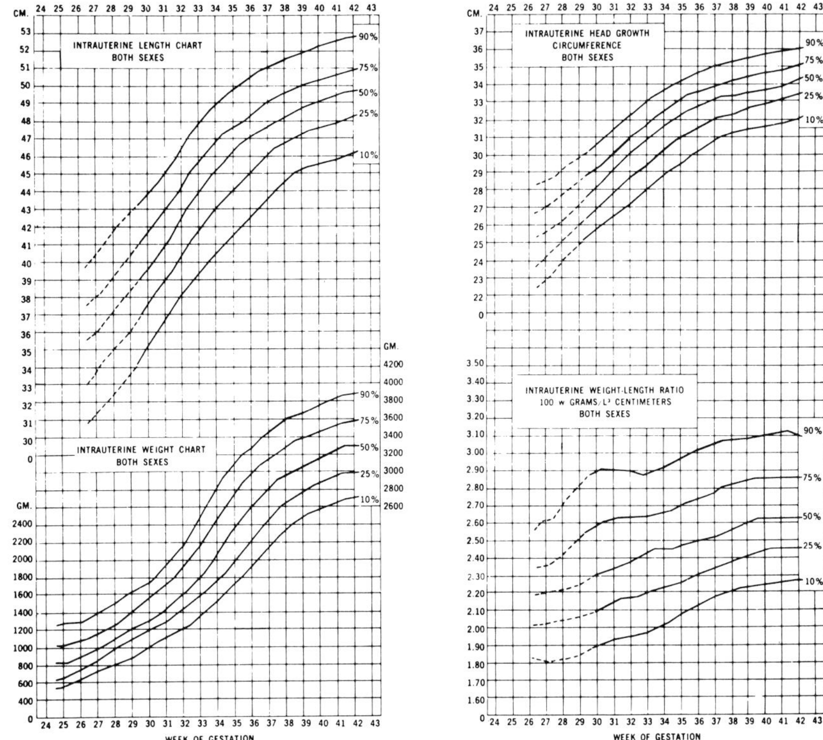

Fig. 31-2 Colorado intrauterine growth charts.

From Lubchenco LO et al: Intrauterine growth in length and head circumference as estimated from live births at gestational ages from 26 to 42 weeks, Pediatrics 37:403, 1966. Reproduced by permission of *Pediatrics,* copyright 1966.

uterine growth for weight, length, and head circumference are given. In addition, a weight/length ratio is shown. From weight and length data a *ponderal index* can be derived to depict proportionality. The growth curves in Fig. 31-2 were derived from a population of inborn and outborn infants with mixed racial backgrounds living at an altitude of 5000 feet. Intrauterine growth curves derived from live births from different populations show significantly different values, particularly at some of the higher percentiles. However, the basic sigmoid shape of the curve persists.

Intrauterine growth curves for the last trimester of pregnancy can be very helpful in both fetal and neonatal medicine. One cannot assume without reservation that intrauterine growth is a steady process; it is conceivable that growth occurs in bursts of undetermined length. However, monitoring individual fetuses for growth against a baseline of an intrauterine growth scale can be helpful. These graphs are also used widely for risk identification in the immediate neonatal period.

Fetal nutrition is a subject of great importance when the growth rate and rapid change in composition of the products of conception are considered. The relative increase in proportion of intracellular to extracellular water reflects a continued increase in the proportion of weight represented by cellular matter. Before 20 weeks of gestation, 90% or more of the composition of the fetus is water with little or no fat present. By term, the total body water, although still high in comparison with the adult, is about 76% and the amount of fat is approximately 16%.

Historically, glucose has been considered to be the main or even sole metabolite of the fetus. Evidence suggests, however, that the fetus also utilizes amino acids. The fetal pancreas produces insulin, and in certain pathologic states (most notably that of the infant of the diabetic mother), fetal growth often is accelerated. Apparently, insulin is integrated into the fetal growth regulation system.

The clinician dealing with newborns should consider the prior fetal nutritional state. Infusions of glucose have been shown to be very important in establishing homeostasis in stressed newborns. Glycogen stores are present in liver and muscle at birth but are rapidly depleted, especially if the fetal life span has been shortened by prematurity or if the fetus was malnourished in utero. Difficulties with glucose regulation after birth can alert the clinician to possible aberrations in insulin levels. Amino acids are used in clinical situations as part of parenteral alimentation regimens, but knowledge of fetal and neonatal requirements is incomplete. As fetal nutritional processes are better understood, neonatal nutritional efforts will be improved, especially for the very premature or immature infant.

FETAL SYSTEM FORMATION AND MALFORMATION

Teratology is the study of the etiology, development, structure, and classification of fetal abnormalities. It is very important that physicians understand the teratologic process as clearly as possible. The several organ systems have recognizable completeness of their component parts by 12 weeks after conception or 14 weeks by menstrual history. However, abnormalities in structure or function still can arise thereafter as a result of disruption of growth, differentiation, or maturation.

There are three major ways in which system formation can be affected. First, genetic factors can be operative, resulting in frank changes in chromosome complements with resultant morphologic abnormalities. These *genetic factors,* which have their origin in the parental cell lines or in aberrations of initial cellular division after fertilization, are discussed in Chapter 29, "Genetic Diseases." Second, *intrauterine factors,* such as amniotic bands, can lead to morphologic changes in the fetus. Such isolated intrauterine factors without a contribution from outside the uterine cavity are unusual. Third, *physical agents or forces* can affect the fetus during growth and development. Agents such as alcohol crossing the placenta, irradiation, or infectious diseases are examples of situations that can lead to pathologic changes. One must recognize that the degree of expression may be influenced by other factors, such as genetic predisposition or gestational age at the time of the insult.

Central Nervous System

The central nervous system starts from an ectodermal origin at day 18 of gestation, and development continues through delivery and long after birth. It is susceptible to teratogenic factors throughout the embryonic and fetal periods and is most susceptible during the first half to two thirds of the embryonic period.

The original neural plate develops into a neural tube with cranial and caudal ends. The neural tube walls develop to become the brain and spinal cord; the inner part evolves into the ventricles of the brain and the central canal of the spinal cord. Brain development is very complex and passes through stages of a forebrain, midbrain, and hindbrain, with subsequent development of the cerebrum, midbrain structures, pons and cerebellum. Cells that originally separated from the neural plate and became the neural crest develop into cranial, spinal, and autonomic ganglia, as well as the autonomic nervous system and chromaffin tissue, especially the adrenal medulla.

Malformations of the central nervous system frequently confront the clinican. Some of these defects are among the most grotesque, such as the *anencephalic* baby or infants with very large *encephaloceles*. Other anomalies, such as *microcephaly* or cystic lesions in the brain, may be compatible with life for variable lengths of time but carry extremely bleak prognoses.

Congenital malformations of the spinal column, especially those with defects in overlying tissue, can pose major moral and ethical dilemmas to parents and health professionals, when potentially treatable complications are superimposed on a poor prognosis. Some central nervous system lesions are of known origin, but others, such as *meningomyelocele,* may be the result of interactions between genetic predisposition and extrinsic factors.

Of major concern is the evidence that intrauterine exposure of the developing nervous system to substances such as "crack" cocaine, or alcohol results in permanent functional morbidity, as well as structural changes. Although morphologic and behavioral changes often appear together, which invites the postulation of cause and effect, there is no reason to think that the two are always related. Theoretically, there may be long-term effects on higher cerebral function and behavior without morphologic effects, and vice versa.

Cardiovascular System

The cardiovascular system is the first to function, with a rudimentary blood circulation beginning in the third week. Initially two tubes fuse to form a single tube that evolves into the four-chambered heart and great vessels. By the end of the fourth or fifth week, partitioning of the chambers is completed, with two atria and two ventricles. Equally complex is the initial formation of a truncus arteriosus, aortic sac, and aortic arches, which evolve by the eighth week into a fetal circulatory pattern. This system undergoes changes in flow patterns during adjustment to extrauterine existence.

Schematic representations of the process whereby the initial pair of tubes forms a single tube with subsequent twisting and formation of chambers and very complex vascular structures—some of which become atretic whereas others become dominant—can be helpful in understanding spatial relationships and the reasons why specific lesions develop. The lymphatic system develops in a similar time frame, although initially seen somewhat later than is the cardiovascular system. The lymphatics have connections with the venous side of the developing cardiovascular system.

Malformations of the cardiovascular system occur in approximately 7.5 of 1000 live births. The critical period for teratogenic effects is over relatively early in the intrauterine period, but the process of formation is so complex that a multitude of possibilities for maldevelopment exists. The degree of severity varies considerably.

Some structural malformations, such as the patent foramen ovale type of *atrial septal defect,* may be functional only when another pathologic condition exists. The *patent ductus arteriosus* as a pathologic entity occurs when involution fails after birth. Early malrotation of the fused cardiac tubes can result in *dextrocardia*. This can occur with an otherwise normal heart and great vessel structures and may not be a clinical problem if complete situs inversus of the viscera is also present. Dextrocardia without situs inversus is often a major problem because of a tendency for associated complex intrinsic abnormalities.

Intracardiac malformations, such as *septal defects,* are very common, especially in the ventricle. Complex problems, with formation of the great vessels evolving from an inappropriate partitioning of the *truncus arteriosus,* are also fairly common. *Coarctation of the aortic arch* is an example of a malformation that may be some distance from the heart itself. Manifestations of malformations can occur in utero and are believed in some instances to result in large-for-gestational-age infants (Fig. 31-3). In severe and relatively rare instances they can produce a form of hydrops fetalis.

The pediatrician, pediatric cardiologist, and neonatologist are becoming increasingly involved with cardiac dysfunction before birth. The evaluation of fetal well-being includes that of cardiac status, with the result that problems such as cardiac arrhythmia or cardiac failure can be detected prenatally. Maternal digitalization for fetal cardiac arrhythmia is being at-

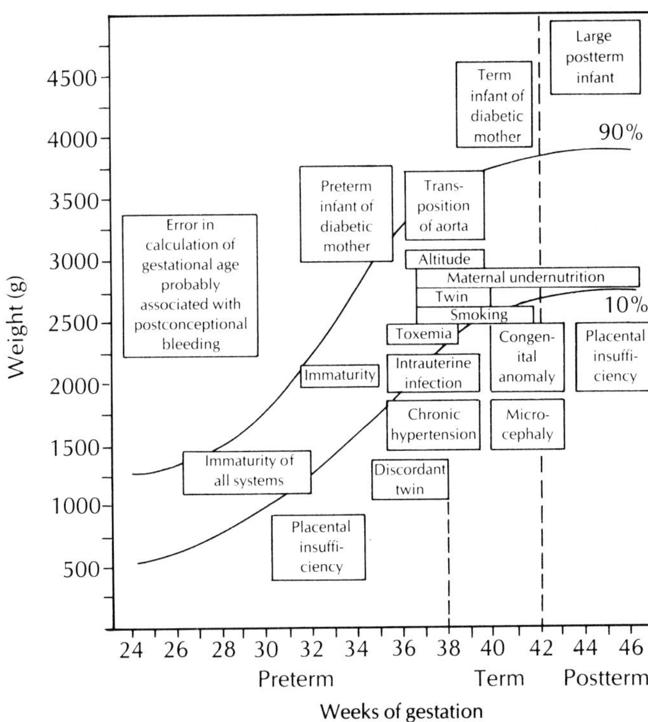

Fig. 31-3 Birth weight and gestational age groupings of selected neonates affected by intrauterine pathophysiologic processes.

From Lubchenco LO: Major problems in clinical pediatrics. XIV: The high risk infant, Philadelphia, 1976, WB Saunders Co.

tempted in some of these cases. Fetal echocardiography can now detect specific structural defects.

Musculoskeletal System

Formation of the musculoskeletal structures becomes grossly apparent in the embryo at least by the fourth week, when limb buds—first the upper and subsequently the lower—become obvious. Bone evolves from mesoderm that undergoes a process of chondrification. Muscle structures originate from mesoderm, much of which arises directly from the somites. Cardiac muscle and other smooth muscles have a different origin in the splanchnic mesoderm of the primitive gastrointestinal tract. The origin of some muscles, such as those of the iris and extrinsic eye, is unclear. The limb buds elongate while forming bone and large-muscle masses. A process of rotation and growth, in which upper and lower extremities rotate in different directions, results in the muscle groupings and dermatome patterns of the child and adult.

Malformations of the limbs are relatively common; otherwise skeletal and muscular abnormalities are rare. The health professional providing newborn care often is struck by the significant attention paid by parents to the extremities, particularly the hands of newborns. For this reason, relatively minor defects can have major emotional import. *Polydactyly* or *syndactyly* are among the more common human malformations.

Many limb abnormalities are genetic in origin, but some malformations result from genetic predisposition interacting with environmental factors. The thalidomide deformities are a specific and perhaps relatively isolated example of limb teratogenesis.

Gastrointestinal System

The alimentary tract, developing from a primitive anlage seen initially at the fourth week, has three main divisions: foregut, midgut, and hindgut. Each of these has its own specific blood supply in the celiac, superior mesenteric, and inferior mesenteric arteries. Because development of each tract can be traced, abnormalities of the individual divisions are seen. The *foregut,* from the pharynx to the insertion of the common bile duct, develops into various structures, including the intestine and the liver and pancreas. *Midgut* structures include all the small intestines (with the exception of the duodenum before the insertion of the common bile duct) plus the cecum, appendix, ascending colon, and about two thirds of the proximal transverse colon. The midgut structures go through a complex rotation during development, whereby an initial loop develops outside the fetal abdomen and rotates approximately 90 degrees at that time. At approximately the tenth week, these midgut intestinal structures return to the abdomen and go through a further complex rotation of 180 degrees, leading to the final anatomic relationships of the intestine. *Hindgut* structures include the transverse, descending, and sigmoid colon and rectum through the final portion of the anal canal, which develops from an anal pit. The cloaca, or early expanded end of the hindgut, and tissues of other origin lead to the perineal structures.

Alimentary tract malformations are fairly common and are often associated with other anomalies. The foregut has an initial tracheoesophageal common origin, with subsequent separation. *Tracheoesophageal fistulas* resulting from errors in formation of the tracheoesophageal septum occur in four basic patterns; early detection is important to avoid extensive aspiration pneumonitis.

Errors of midgut development and malrotation lead to many problems, the most spectacular of which is the lack of return of the bowel to the abdominal cavity, with a resultant *omphalocele*. Other malrotation presentations include acute intestinal obstruction and ischemia in utero or at varying lengths of time after birth, often after initial feedings. Malformations of the intestinal tube in the form of *stenosis, duplication, or atresia* are of unclear origin but may result from problems with recanalization or from a compromised vascular supply.

Hindgut malformations most commonly occur at the most distal portion, resulting in lack of continuity or *imperforate anus,* stenosis, or membranous conditions. Many other intestinal malformations can be seen. Of special interest is *Meckel diverticulum* (an outpouching in the ileum), representing the remnant of the yolk stalk.

Respiratory System

Respiratory system formation is noteworthy for development that begins at approximately 26 days and goes on long after birth. Initial cell lines arise on the floor of the primitive pharynx and produce a laryngotracheal tube. Endoderm of this tube becomes the lining and glands of the lower respiratory system; connective tissue and cartilage of the respiratory system arise from splanchnic mesoderm.

Further growth of the endotracheal tube results in two lung buds that divide further into two sections on the left and three on the right; these correspond to the adult lobes. Branching continues after this point from the pulmonary segment system. At approximately 5 to 7 weeks after fertilization, a pseudoglandular period exists during which there is major growth of the bronchi and terminal bronchioles.

During an overlapping canalicular period beginning at 13 weeks and continuing to approximately 25 weeks, bronchioles and alveolar ducts, as well as significant vascularization, develop. From 24 weeks until birth, terminal sacs arise and become alveoli. These initially are lined by a cuboidal epithelium, which changes to a squamous form at about 26 weeks of gestation. Alveolar development continues through early childhood.

The enzymatic maturation of systems leading to the production of surfactant does not take place until alveoli are formed. Complex cell types lining the alveoli have been described. A vacuolated cell, the type II pneumocyte, appears to have a secretory function and involvement in alveolar stabilization through surfactant elaboration.

Anatomic malformations of the respiratory system are unusual, but include many dysplastic and cystic abnormalities. The clinician often is confronted with functional problems related closely to the formative status of the lung. For example, an immature lung that is not well into the stage of alveolar formation may only be able to support life for a period of hours until the immature infant dies from pulmonary insufficiency refractory to present-day treatment. *Respiratory distress syndrome* is related to the absence of surfactant and often can be treated successfully.

Abnormalities in development of the diaphragm, the most common of which is *diaphragmatic hernia,* are most common on the left and often are associated with severe restriction of lung development on one or both sides; detection and management of this condition require speed and sophistication.

Hematopoietic System

Initial red cell formation is seen as early as day 14 after conception, when cells containing embryonic hemoglobin arise from the endothelium of primitive vessels of the yolk sac. Hematopoiesis within the embryo begins in the liver at approximately the sixth week. The liver is the most active site of hematopoiesis for the early part of the fetal life span. The bone marrow assumes the primary role at about the sixth month, and other sites, especially the spleen and lymph nodes, play a contributory role.

Fetal hemoglobin (Hb F) predominates for much of intrauterine existence and under normal circumstances is seen to a small degree in early infancy. Beginning at about the third month, some hemoglobin A (Hb A) (5% to 10%) is present, and the proportion of Hb A to Hb F increases rapidly from about 35 weeks to term, when blood is approximately 50% to 65% Hb F. Hb F has an increased oxygen affinity compared with Hb A; this is probably the result of a differing action of 2,3-diphosphoglycerate (2,3-DPG), which facilitates oxygen saturation in the intrauterine environment. Blood group antigens are familial in their determination and can be identified as early as the second month of fetal life. Platelets are also seen at approximately the second month.

The presence of hematopoietic abnormalities is important for the clinician to recognize. In the first place, certain *hemoglobinopathies* may result in intrauterine disease. Alphathalassemia results in hemoglobin Bart (tetrameric gamma chains), which has a very high oxygen affinity, resulting in intrauterine distress and nonhemolytic hydrops fetalis.

Other hemoglobinopathies, such as homozygous thalassemia and sickle cell disease, can be diagnosed antenatally through analysis of fetal blood. Hemolytic anemia secondary to *maternal-fetal blood group incompatibilities* and transplacental passage of antibody is an immune disease; however, it has a marked effect on hematopoiesis, resulting in erythroblastosis fetalis, an extensive proliferation of hematopoietic tissue. Fetal *thrombocytopenia* may be primarily of fetal origin, or it may be associated with some form of extrinsic agent or process, such as immune antibody of maternal origin or intrauterine infection. Many fetal intrauterine hematologic manifestations are part of disease processes involving other systems.

Percutaneous umbilical blood sampling (see p. 401) is clinically useful in many fetal hematologic disorders.

Immune System

Immune system components function very early in fetal life, with some parts present as early as the eighth week and with a total rudimentary system capability by the twelfth. Activation usually does not occur before birth. The cellular immune system originates in liver or spleen stem cells that migrate to the thymus at about the eighth week. These "T" cells enter the bloodstream and are distributed to the body, mainly to lymph nodes and spleen. The antibody immune system generates IgM in lymphoid tissues as early as the eleventh week and IgG at about the twelfth week. IgA, IgD, and IgE are seen in the fetus in small amounts toward the end of pregnancy. Current thinking suggests that specific immunoglobulin synthesis occurs in a stem or B cell. Passive transfer of maternal antibody has been demonstrated very early in fetal life. Maternal IgG is detectable as early as the fortieth day, and practically all cord IgG is maternal in origin, arising from both passive and active enzymatic transplacental passage. IgM is not passively transferred. The complement system has some fractions present during the embryonic period at the eighth week, and by 12 to 14 weeks of gestation a considerable complement fraction is present.

Malformations of the fetal immune system, either of familial or developmental origin, have been described and have contributed to an understanding of the adult system. Abnormalities are believed to exist in all parts of the immune system, and it is important that the clinician understand the basic possibilities because of fetal and neonatal diseases that result. *Fetal graft-versus-host reactions* have been documented after intrauterine transfusions. Congenital infections activate the immune system, with an elevated cord IgM level being possible evidence of such infections. Transplacental antibody passage with effects on the fetus, as seen in isoimmunization (Rh disease), is one of the more common forms of fetal immune system disease.

Urogenital System

A close interrelationship exists between the development of two basic systems: the urinary (or excretory) system and the genital (or reproductive) system. There are three separate excretory organs in the human embryo: the pronephros, the mesonephros, and the metanephros. The metanephros appears at approximately the fifth week after fertilization, functions 2 to 3 weeks later, and remains as the permanent kidneys. The other two systems involute, with the mesonephros remaining as a few ducts in the male genital tract and as a vestigial remnant in the female. There are two main divisions in the final excretory system. The entire collecting system from the kidney to the bladder originates from the ureteric bud; nephrons arise from the mesodermic-metanephric mass. The kidney tissue appears originally in the early pelvic region and ascends into the abdomen. The bladder develops from the urogenital sinus and splanchnic mesenchyme. Excretory system function is present by approximately the ninth week, and, theoretically, contributions to amniotic fluid become possible at this time and are definitely a major component later in gestation.

The prospective phenotype of the genital system is determined at fertilization. However, there is an indifferent stage of genital development ending at approximately the seventh week, with the gonads showing specific sexual characteristics. By the twelfth week after fertilization, genitalia are distinctly male or female. The Y chromosome appears to be responsible for the differentiation of testes. Masculinizing hormones from the testes stimulate development of mesonephric ducts into genital components and result in the external genitalia forming a penis and scrotum. Feminization of the external genitalia seemingly occurs in the absence of androgens. Gonadal tissue has its origin in the lateral abdominal wall, with the testes descending into the scrotum late in fetal life.

Malformations of the urogenital system are relatively common and result in a myriad of morphologic and microscopic manifestations. Some entities, such as *renal agenesis,* result in intrauterine manifestations, including oligohydramnios, and in morphologic changes in the fetus. Other manifestations may occur in the immediate neonatal period. For example, renal abnormalities that result in cystic lesions of the kidneys initially may be detected in the newborn period as abdominal masses found on physical examination, or abnormalities in renal function. Malformations in the vascular supply to the kidneys or the collecting system result in congenital anomalies that predispose the person to renal disease that manifests in infancy and childhood. Malformations arising from problems of formation of the urogenital sinus and urachus may be severe, as in *exstrophy of the bladder* or, less obvious, as in fistulae between perineal structures.

Malformations of the genitalia also can be complex in origin. Those resulting from errors in the sex-determining mechanism can result in *hermaphrodites,* but such errors are rare. Errors in sexual differentiation, producing *pseudohermaphrodites,* are somewhat more common. The presence of neonatal ambiguous genitalia is a true medical emergency; the *adrenogenital syndrome,* with fetal adrenal androgen excess resulting in masculinization of a female genotype, is one cause of ambiguous genitalia.

Special Considerations

Certain situations of fetal formation and malformation deserve special mention. The special senses, specifically those of *the eyes and ears, are very sensitive to teratogenic activity* and result in profound effects on the developing infant and child. Eye formation begins at the fourth week and proceeds very rapidly, especially through the sixth week. Malformations of the eye and ear may be associated with errors in genetic material; some syndromic conditions have readily identifiable eye and ear malformation patterns. Intrauterine infections, particularly rubella, can affect the eye and inner ear. The external ear migrates up to its final location on the head; errors in position or morphology often are associated with other malformations.

Malformations of the face and palate are of major concern. These have their origin in the embryonic branchial apparatus from which the face, pharynx, and attendant structures develop. Cleft lip often is associated with cleft palate but arises from distinctly different origins. Difficulties in these areas are probably of mixed genetic and environmental causation. The branchial arch merging in the formation of palate structures is most susceptible to teratogenic factors between 6 and 10 weeks of gestation.

FETUS, MOTHER, AND FAMILY

The fetus influences both the mother and the family. Expectations regarding conception and childbearing vary, but the overall viewpoint should be positive. Psychological factors involved in the decision to become pregnant are extremely complex and heavily influenced by the reproductive instinct. *Psychosocial situations with a negative "set" before conception should be interpreted as the beginning of potential fetal risk.* There are many maternal and familial situations of unfortunate familiarity to the physician that provide such a negative start for the fetus. A common example is pregnancy in the younger adolescent, who is both physically and emotionally immature and who may not have a stable interpersonal relationship with her male partner. Preconceptual factors interact once fertilization occurs, with a progression of biochemical, physical, and emotional changes that influence mother, father, and family.

These changes, some subtle and some not, result in an alteration of the previous life situation. New situations demand behavioral adaptations and a process of coping. If this coping process is successful, then major developmental progress has been made, especially by the mother; this is usually true to a lesser extent in the father and to varying degrees in people further removed. But, if attitudes and the coping process are unsatisfactory, then in certain situations abortion might be considered.

The first missed menstrual period, an overt sign of change to many women, does not occur until after the period of the dividing zygote is essentially complete. By the time of the second missed menstrual period, the embryonic period is half over. Apparently the *zygotic period is relatively unaffected by teratogens, but the embryonic period is one of very high risk.* Maternal and familial habits potentially injurious to the fetus are difficult to alter under any circumstances and are even more so when the mother does not yet realize that she is pregnant. Confirmation of pregnancy often does not take place in the present medical system until after the second missed menstrual period.

The *first trimester* may be the most important phase of adjustment to the fetal presence. Many physical symptoms such as fatigue, nausea, headache, and changes in emotional status may be reflections of emotional tension. However, there also are complex interactions of psychological stress and physiologic change that can involve the autonomic nervous system and produce discomfort. These can result in alterations in prior life-style and, if very disruptive, might produce untoward effects, because the fetus, at this early time, has the potential of establishing a very negative set within its future family.

Biochemical relationships among the fetus, its placenta, and the mother are of major interest to the clinician. They form the basis for many tests confirming pregnancy and assessing fetal well-being. The placenta, a fetal organ, plays a very active metabolic role. Theoretically, placental hormones can supply much of the endocrine support that ordinarily originates in the woman's pituitary glands, adrenal cortex, and ovaries. The rare appearance of panhypopituitarism in the postpartum period supports this phenomenon.

Many of these endocrinologic processes are of major practical interest to the clinician. *Human chorionic gonadotropin* is produced by trophoblastic cells within a few days of implantation. Concentrations of this substance in maternal blood and urine are highest during the first trimester and decrease through the remainder of pregnancy. Most current early pregnancy tests take advantage of this phenomenon. *Human placental lactogen,* a polypeptide also produced by trophoblastic cells, appears in the serum of pregnant women about the sixth week of gestation and is present throughout pregnancy. The placenta plays a very active role in the synthesis and metabolism of progesterone and estrogen. End products of estrogen metabolism in the form of maternal *estriol* are the basis for an important test of fetal well-being.

The *second trimester* usually is marked by less overt signs of physical and emotional adjustment. System development of the fetus is basically complete, and major growth is occurring. This leads to the phenomenon of quickening, when a woman feels fetal movements for the first time. This usually occurs at about week 18 in the primigravida; in the multigravida such movement may be felt 1 to 2 weeks earlier. Quickening undoubtedly represents a major milestone in the relationship between a mother and her fetus. This is the first overt or direct sign of independent fetal activity. Quickening can provide important information about fetal or gestational age. For some women it also may serve as a milestone after which abortion is a less acceptable alternative.

The *third trimester* is marked by an acceleration of the fetal alteration of life-style. Maternal physical activity, previously easily undertaken, may become increasingly difficult. Sexual activity between parents may be subject to changes or even cessation. Preparation for delivery becomes more of a part of everyday life; childbirth education, financial planning, and other aspects of preparation and emotional adjustment should be in progress. Initially in the third trimester the maternal emotional state is largely oriented toward the fetus; however, as labor and delivery approach, a mother's concern, and very often the father's, tends to become more centered on maternal well-being.

FETUS, HEALTH PROFESSIONAL, AND SOCIETY

There is great concern about the influence of factors such as smoking, alcohol consumption, radiation, and pesticides, and researchers continue to develop an objective data base. Societies that advocate menstrual registration and the introduction of special employment, nutritional, and life-style changes for women as soon as they miss a period (or even before conception) may be the most enlightened in terms of fetal advocacy.

Amniocentesis (chorionic villus and percutaneous umbilical cord sampling see p. 401) represent procedures of major interest to individuals and society because they enable physicians to detect conditions incompatible with what is considered normal human existence. Moral and ethical concerns over these procedures are related to those associated with a terminating abortion. The debate over abortion and its legalization has brought to the fore concerns about the legal and interpersonal status of the fetus. Health professionals are embroiled in this debate, and arguments continue over whether a practitioner of perinatal medicine can personally oppose abortion.

Viability, or the capability of a fetus to assume an independent extrauterine existence, is a concept that demands attention and thought. We do know that 23 to 24 weeks from the last menstrual period is the time at which a few fetuses, if born, survive. Neonatal intensive care has increased the chance for survival of the very premature and low-birth-weight infant, but survival is still essentially impossible before 23 to 24 weeks of gestation.

The clinician must be aware of the close approximation of potential viability and legal gestation limits on legal abortion and the worrisome, significant variations in estimates of fetal age; under *Roe v. Wade,* abortion can be performed legally until 24 weeks, the beginning of viability, but it is not unusual for maternal and physician joint appraisals of gestational age to be erroneous by as much as 4 weeks. This is more likely to occur in patients who receive little prenatal care or who have menstrual irregularity because of youth or other factors.

THE IDENTIFICATION AND MANAGEMENT OF FETAL AND MATERNAL RISK

Any factor that increases the possibility of an adverse outcome for a pregnancy contributes to risk. Medical risk includes physiologic, nutritional, obstetric, and genetic factors. Psychosocial risk includes psychological, social, environmental, or behavioral factors and personal habits. These two broad categories of risk often act concurrently, and individual risks may overlap, accompany, or follow each other.[1] The relationship between risk factors and adverse outcome may be obvious, as with a specific toxic agent such as mercury; more often, however, risk is subtle and cumulative.

Preconception Care

Health before pregnancy is being increasingly recognized as an important determinant of pregnancy outcome. Preparation for pregnancy should begin before conception, including assessment of risk and preventive or therapeutic intervention. The accompanying box illustrates the general categories and some specific problems that should be included in preconceptional care.

The concept of care before conception is related to, but not exactly the same as, family planning. More is involved than the spacing of pregnancies. Wider acceptance of this concept within society may have a major impact on the outcome of pregnancy in specific populations such as adolescents.

Preconception Care Inventory

FAMILY HISTORY

Diabetes
Hypertension
Epilepsy
Multiple pregnancies

GENETIC HISTORY

Disease related to ethnic background (e.g., Tay-Sachs)
Muscular dystrophy
Hemophilia
Cystic fibrosis
Birth defects
Mental retardation

PARENTAL MEDICAL HISTORY

Diabetes, hypertension, epilepsy
Anemia
Rubella
Specific medical and surgical problems
Possible exposure to sexually transmitted diseases, including AIDS
Immunizations
Allergies
Medications, including over-the-counter
Substance use and abuse
- Alcohol
- Caffeine
- Smoking
- Drugs

NUTRITION

ENVIRONMENTAL

Occupational exposures
Pets

Modified from American Academy of Pediatrics, American College of Obstetricians: Guidelines for perinatal care (Appendix B), ed 2, Elk Grove Village, Ill, 1988, The Academy.

Prenatal Care

A report entitled *Caring for Our Future: The Content of Prenatal Care* published by the U.S. Department of Health and Human Services (HHS) in 1989 defines the three basic components of prenatal care as (1) early and continuing risk assessment, (2) health promotion, and (3) medical and psychosocial interventions and follow-up.[1]

Previous discussion has emphasized that during the prenatal period the fetus is undergoing rapid and continual growth and development. Anything that jeopardizes that process must be recognized as a fetal risk factor and subjected to assessment. Major contributors to fetal risk are listed in the box on p. 400.

There is little doubt that prenatal care results in healthier babies and mothers. Much of the original interest and emphasis in prenatal care involved pregnancy-induced hypertension (PIH) and the use of periodic blood pressure determinations. Standardized schedules (with details such as number and timing of visits, procedures, and studies) are available. In addition, the aforementioned HHS report offers suggestions, including the addition of preconception care to traditional prenatal care.

Assessing Fetal Status Before Labor

The clinician is obligated to make every effort to identify risk processes and to practice *expectant fetal medicine*. Pediatricians must be familiar with the basic principles of techniques used to gather information concerning high-risk pregnancies and deliveries in which they are involved as members of the perinatal care team. Fetal history, structure and growth, heart rate, and amniotic fluid and fetal blood analyses provide the basis for the majority of these methods. Some are noninvasive; they have been included in obstetric practice for years and provide statistically valid information—for example, history taking and uterine-size measurement. They are employed as screening procedures that may indicate a need for other investigative techniques, such as those discussed next.

Fetal Activity. Quickening, which is defined as the point at which the mother first perceives fetal activity, can be valuable in confirming length of pregnancy. *The duration, amplitude, and frequency of fetal movement after quickening and in the third trimester can provide important information about fetal well-being*. An inactive fetus may be chronically compromised. Rapid onset of inactivity in a previously active fetus can be ominous. Assessment of fetal activity lacks standardization and specificity for cause but is of clinical value.

Fetal Heart Rate. The normal fetal heart rate (FHR) settles in the 120 to 160 beats/min range by the last trimester and is easily monitored by use of a stethoscope (fetoscope) or an electronically amplified device. FHR monitoring is most commonly used for evaluation of fetal status during labor but can be helpful in prenatal assessment (see stress test below).

Bradycardia, especially less than 100 beats/min, is of concern because of an association with acute or chronic distress. Explanation for its presence must be sought. The list of possible causes is long and includes many with a poor outcome, such as placental insufficiency. An intrinsic fetal cause, heart block, is not as ominous. *Tachycardia* usually occurs as an autonomic response to stimulation and can in-

Major Contributors to Fetal Risk

- Genetic
  - Chromosome abnormalities
  - Inherited traits
- Maternal-familial environment and life-style
  - Socioeconomic status
  - Social environment
  - Physical environment
    - Radiation
    - Teratogens
  - Nutrition
  - Smoking or secondary exposure to smoke
  - Drugs or alcohol abuse
  - Lack of prenatal care
- Maternal reproductive capability and health
  - Age, weight, height
  - Reproductive tract abnormalities
  - Maternal medical disorders
    - Cardiac
    - Respiratory
    - Renal
    - Hematologic (e.g., sickle cell disease)
    - Metabolic (e.g., diabetes, thyroid disorders, phenylketonuria)
    - Epilepsy
  - Emotional status
- Placenta and membrane disorders
  - Implantation (abdominal, tubal, previa)
  - Vessel and cord complications
  - Abruption
  - Premature rupture of membranes (PROM) and infection
- Maternal-fetal unit
  - Multiple gestation
  - Obstetric complications
    - Malposition and malpresentation
    - Cephalopelvic disproportion
  - Abnormal fetal growth and gestation
  - Isoimmunization (erythroblastosis fetalis)
  - Intrauterine infections
  - Pregnancy-induced hypertension

dicate fetal normality. It may be associated with a maternal condition, such as pyrexia. Intrinsic fetal arrhythmias, such as supraventricular tachycardia, can result in secondary manifestations, including hydrops fetalis.

Uterine Size. The uterus and the products of conception are monitored closely during prenatal care. Measurements of fundal height above the symphysis are obtained and plotted. The umbilicus is reached at 20 to 22 weeks. Deviations from the expected curve may indicate a number of abnormal and high-risk states.

Fundal height at a level greater than expected may be due to miscalculation of dates, with the pregnancy further along than anticipated. Another relatively straightforward cause of unexpectedly large uterine size is multiple pregnancy. Conversely, fetal causes of smaller than expected uterine size include pregnancy less advanced than anticipated and many problems that lead to *intrauterine growth retardation* (IUGR) (see also p. 405).

Amniotic fluid volume deviations in the form of oligohydramnios or polyhydramnios may be detected initially by abnormal uterine size or fundal height. Confirmation and further study by ultrasonography should follow, because imaging by ultrasound can estimate the volume of fluid present and can assess fetal structures.

Under normal circumstances amniotic fluid volume increases until 40 weeks and then decreases. *Oligohydramnios* thus can be associated with postterm and postmature pregnancies. The pediatrician also needs to be alert to situations in preterm pregnancies in which oligohydramnios occurs, inasmuch as this may be associated with a number of disease processes, including IUGR and renal abnormalities. If renal function is severely compromised due to renal agenesis or dysplasia, structural (Potter syndrome) and functional (pulmonary insufficiency) neonatal problems may become evident after birth.

Polyhydramnios may result from maternal problems such as eclampsia or diabetes. The pediatrician should immediately suspect fetal and neonatal abnormalities of the gastrointestinal tract that lead to disorders of fetal swallowing or obstruction. Normal circulation of amniotic fluid is interrupted on the absorptive side of the loop. Many other conditions can be associated with this state, such as fetal cardiac disease.

Ultrasonography. Clinical ultrasound has had a profound effect on all aspects of perinatal medicine. A transducer, acoustically linked to the skin surface, transmits ultrasonic vibrations, and the returning sound echoes are electronically processed to produce a two-dimensional pictorial "slice" of the organs being imaged.

Types of ultrasound used in obstetrics are listed in Table 31-1. B-scan systems with their pulsed cross-sectional images of tissue are assuming remarkable clarity. When images are presented sequentially faster than the flicker rate of the eye, then real-time "movie" imaging occurs, which documents motion. "Doppler" ultrasound usually is used clinically to monitor fetal heart rate.

All areas of reproductive medicine have been directly influenced by ultrasound technology. *Fetal growth and development* can be monitored for *structural abnormalities* and growth rate. Structural normality of maternal reproductive organs can be documented, as can placental site. In fact, the potential uses and benefits of ultrasound in pregnancy are so extensive that many individual authorities and some European health care systems advocate routine screening in all pregnancies. However, safety has been and remains a concern. There have been no clinically significant untoward effects documented in humans. Biologic effects might be structural (morphologic) or functional. At the energy levels used in most clinical imaging, the possibility of risk cannot be eliminated. Doppler ultrasound theoretically has greater potential for harm because of the continuous, rather than pulsed, wave and the amount of time such devices may be used.

Indications for use of diagnostic ultrasound imaging in pregnancy were addressed by a National Institute of Health Consensus Development Conference in 1984.[3] The panel concluded that, when there is an accepted medical indication, ultrasound improves pregnancy management and outcome. A large number of specific clinical situations were mentioned. Routine screening, identification of fetal sex, or educational

Table 31-1 *Types of Obstetric Ultrasound*

TYPE	WAVE	USE
A-scan	Unidirectional	Historical interest; displays distance (e.g., fetal biparietal diameter)
B-scan	Cross sectional, pulsed	Displays composite image (e.g., fetal skull or placenta)
Real-time imaging	As in B-scan	Displays continuous changes in spatial configuration (i.e., fetal motion)
Doppler	Usually continuous	Detects and measures blood flow or heart rate; energy input may be high with prolonged use

purposes were not considered appropriate reasons for imaging because risk should not be discounted at this time. There are, however, advocates for just such routine screening.

Amniocentesis. Amniotic fluid bathes the fetus, is swallowed by the fetus, and contains fetal cells, urine, and other substances. The technique for obtaining a specimen of this fluid by percutaneous aspiration has been made safer and more successful by the use of real-time ultrasonography.

Diagnostic amniocentesis at 14 to 15 weeks of gestation in conjunction with ultrasonography provides placental localization, fetal size, and gestational age confirmation in addition to information obtained from fluid analysis. Evaluation of fetal cells through *karyotyping* can detect chromosome abnormalities before potential extrauterine viability, and abortion can be considered. Metabolic disorders can be subject to the same diagnostic approach through *cell culture;* at least 150 such problems can now be diagnosed. Neural tube defects can be diagnosed by evaluation of maternal serum and amniotic fluid *alpha-fetoprotein.*

Chorionic Villus Sampling (CVS). This technique involves ultrasound-directed aspiration of trophoblastic tissue surrounding the gestational sac during the first trimester. The approach can be transcervical, vaginal, or abdominal. Transcervical sampling commonly is done at 9 to 12 completed gestational weeks.

A study[7] of the safety and efficacy of transcervical CVS for early prenatal diagnosis of cytogenetic abnormalities concluded that it may have a somewhat higher risk of procedure failure, maternal complication, and fetal loss than does amniocentesis. There are, however, major advantages (e.g., *rapid karyotyping*) to first versus second trimester diagnosis if intervention is contemplated. Furthermore, the additional risk associated with CVS is seemingly small and may decrease as experience with the technique expands.

Percutaneous Umbilical Blood Sampling (PUBS). Direct aspiration of fetal blood by means of a needle placed transabdominally through maternal skin and into a fetal blood vessel is another technique facilitated by ultrasound that has significantly improved fetal diagnosis and therapy. Sampling is possible from about 17 weeks to term with greater apparent safety than with other techniques. *Fetoscopy* has a complication rate of 4% to 5%, *fetal scalp sampling* requires labor and cervical dilation, and placental aspiration results in contamination with maternal blood in more than 50% of attempts.

The most common diagnostic indications for PUBS are the need for *rapid fetal karyotype* and evaluation of fetal isoimmune hemolytic disease. The main treatment is *transfusion for fetal anemia.* The list of indications (Table 31-2) undoubtedly will expand if safety and efficacy are further delineated and complications prove to be limited. At present, this is a specialized technique that requires sophisticated technology and expertise.

Nonstress and Contraction Stress Tests. The pediatrician or other provider of newborn care frequently is confronted with information obtained during evaluation of fetal well-being (p. 399). Tests that record FHR and the presence, absence, or temporal sequence of uterine contractions are used extensively. The FHR is driven by neurogenic reflex mechanisms similar to those seen in newborns.

The nonstress test (NST) is used when a pregnant patient is not in labor. The interrelationship between FHR and movement or spontaneous uterine contractions is observed. Such testing can begin at 26 to 28 weeks, but usually is performed closer to term and if a risk factor has been identified. This simple, easily repeated test can provide valuable information. A normal or reactive NST has two or more accelerations of the FHR in 10 to 20 minutes along with normal baseline rate and variability (120 to 160 beats/min, 5 to 15 beats/min). A nonreactive or abnormal NST is defined as one that does not meet standardized criteria and that may show decelerations.

The *contraction stress test (CST),* or oxytocin challenge test (OCT), uses oxytocin-stimulated uterine contractions and FHR response. The NST is now used more commonly, with the CST employed by some physicians only after a nonreactive (abnormal) NST result. The presence of repeated late decelerations is considered problematic. Interpretations can be difficult and there are relative and absolute contraindications for performing CST, along with an appreciable high false positive rate. Interpretation requires experience. Nipple stimulation rather than oxytocin challenge is used by some practitioners to induce uterine contractions.

Fetal Biophysical Profile. Fetal well-being can be assessed through the use of multiple parameters collated in a standardized fashion. Items such as muscle tone, body movement, breathing movement, amniotic fluid volume, and results of the NST can be identified, and a score can be derived in a fashion similar to that for determining an Apgar score. The use of multiple noninvasive procedures to assess fetal status is being constantly refined.

Fetoscopy. This technique involves introduction of a small optical viewing instrument into the amniotic cavity, using real-time ultrasound to assist the physician in the procedure. Fetoscopy is difficult, and its place in clinical medicine presently is diminishing as other techniques prove efficacious.

Table 31-2 *Ultrasound-Directed Methods for Obtaining Fetal Specimens*

SPECIMEN	TECHNIQUE	EXAMPLE OF USE
Trophoblastic tissue	CVS	Genetic diagnosis in first trimester (9-12 wk)
Amniotic fluid	Amniocentesis	Genetic diagnosis in second trimester (14-16 wk)
		Diagnosis of fetal disease (isoimmune)
		Evaluation of fetal maturity (L/S ratio)
Fetal blood	PUBS	Rapid genetic diagnosis (late second trimester)
		Diagnosis of fetal disease (thrombocytopenia)
		Evaluation of fetal well-being (blood gas or acid-base)

CVS, Chorionic villus sampling; *L/S*, lecithin/sphingomyelin; *PUBS*, percutaneous umbilical blood sampling.

Maternal and Familial Environment and Life-Style

Many authorities have pointed to socioeconomic status and social environment as causal factors in fetal risk. Delineation of specific influences is difficult, but *poverty* is undoubtedly important, as are *nutrition* and *hygiene*. Intrauterine infection is frequent in mothers of lower socioeconomic status. Emotional influences on fetal wastage have been discussed, and the possibility that medical disenfranchisement contributes cannot be discounted.

Environmental factors, such as radiation, chemicals, and drugs, affect all socioeconomic classes. *Radiation* exposure in mammals causes fetal death, growth retardation, and congenital malformation, with the central nervous system commonly affected. The relationship between embryonic or fetal irradiation and carcinogenesis is unclear. Effects are both dose- and rate-related. Death during the preimplantation period, malformation during early organogenesis, and cell deletion and hypoplasia during fetal life form a general pattern in animal studies. There are guidelines for limiting radiation to the embryo and fetus during occupational exposure or elective diagnostic techniques; however, dilemmas often arise as a result of lack of foreknowledge about pregnancy, nonelective medical evaluations, and emotional factors. Whenever possible, a radiation therapist should be consulted.

Chemicals in the environment are of natural and synthetic origin, with the latter being of greater concern. Certain substances, such as pesticides and mercury, have received publicity, but a hidden teratogenic potential exists that needs further elucidation. Many agents are potentially more toxic to the embryo, fetus, and neonate than to older children and adults. *Drugs* are a problem in legitimate nonprescription and prescription use, as well as in situations of fraud abuse, and a considerable amount of literature documents actual and hypothetical fetal effects. Alcohol abuse has been documented to cause a morphologically distinctive fetal syndrome. (See also Chapter 33 on noxious substances crossing the placenta and Chapter 229, "Neonatal Abstinence Syndrome").

Fetal pathology secondary to *maternal nutrition* is not well understood. Studies of the human placenta and animal models cause concern. Stigmata may persist into childhood and adulthood in spite of adequate nutrition after birth. Clinical application of available information includes rejection of the former practice of weight gain restriction in pregnancy and acceptance of that of enhanced nutritional support for women during pregnancy and the postpartum period.

Women who *smoke*, have smoked, or who take up smoking after their babies are conceived give birth to babies smaller than the average (by 100 to 300 g). In addition, their babies are at risk for a high incidence of prematurity and perinatal mortality. Although the nicotine, carbon monoxide, and cyanide in smoke may have direct fetal effects, maternal physiologic predispositions could be the determining factors.

Identification of environmental and life-style risk relies largely on the maternal medical history. When specific factors such as radiation or chemical exposure are detected, then assessment of fetal well-being, especially growth and morphology, might be helpful. In many situations, however, decisions to continue, interrupt, or enhance pregnancies are made on the basis of nebulous possible fetal effects. Thus may the art be extrapolated from the science of fetal medicine!

Maternal Reproductive Capability and Health

Certain maternal factors result in risk to the fetus regardless of the nature of the products of conception. Pregnancy can produce physiologic changes in the mother that may adversely affect preexisting maternal conditions, thereby jeopardizing the fetus.

Maternal biologic factors such as age, weight, height, race, parity, and previous obstetric history directly affect fetal risk. *Age* in particular has been clearly demonstrated to relate to perinatal mortality, with minimal risk occurring between 20 and 30 years of age. *Weight and height* are related to maternal nutrition, socioeconomic status, and other variables; they may jeopardize the fetus by increasing the incidence of prematurity or intrapartum complications. *Race* is complex with socioeconomic determinants; some congenital anomalies and medical conditions may have a racial predisposition. Maternal *reproductive tract abnormalities*, such as congenital malformations, frequently are associated with fetal wastage by spontaneous abortion or prematurity. *Cervical incompetence* occurs in 1 of 500 to 600 pregnancies and results in premature delivery.

Maternal medical disorders in pregnancy carry a significant risk to fetus and mother. Cyanotic congenital heart disease in a mother has a clear relationship to fetal problems, with intrauterine growth retardation and premature delivery frequently resulting. Elective abortion is a consideration if maternal cardiac decompensation later in pregnancy is anticipated. Asthma in pregnancy can threaten mother and fetus.

Tuberculosis demands aggressive management of maternal disease and potential fetal exposure to drugs. Pregnancy in women with cystic fibrosis is being seen more frequently, with the fetus being exposed to medications, maternal pulmonary insufficiency, and atypical labor and delivery.

Renal disease is a frequent occurrence in pregnancy. When infection or hypertension is present, fetal risk increases markedly. Hypertension can result in placental changes and in intrauterine growth retardation. Fetal mortality and morbidity resulting from second-trimester abortion and prematurity are associated with urinary tract infections. The risk to the fetus in the event of renal transplantation is not clear; many do very well even in the presence of maternal treatment with corticosteroids.

Hematologic maternal problems are very common. In developing countries, *anemia* has been demonstrated to correlate with low birth weight; the effect on the fetus of moderate maternal iron and folic acid deficiency is unclear. Some hemoglobinopathies can profoundly increase fetal mortality and morbidity, either as a result of maternal state of health or of fetal disease. Pregnant patients with sickle cell disease have a fetal wastage of one in three. Sensitization problems (Rh, ABO) are discussed in Chapter 40.

Maternal metabolic disorders can be significant to the fetus. The interaction of mother and fetus seems limitless; compounds are actively metabolized on both sides of the placenta. In addition, fetal organogenesis and development may be affected, and end organs may respond to maternal abnormalities. Two conditions, diabetes and thyroid disorder, deserve special mention.

Diabetes in pregnancy causes a myriad of fetal complications, including death (stillbirth), increased frequency of congenital anomalies, macrosomia (a large-for-gestational-age state characterized by an increase in fat, but not total body water), and conversely, growth retardation in a small number of infants whose mothers develop renal complications. Recent evidence suggests that fetal pulmonary and neurologic maturity may be delayed in these pregnancies. In addition, obstetric problems, including preeclampsia, hydramnios, and intrapartum complications resulting from excessive size, further increase risk. As discussed previously, glucose is a primary metabolite of the fetus. Pregnancies complicated by diabetes probably result in fluctuations of maternal-fetal glucose and potential fetal hyperinsulinism and hypoglycemia. These fetuses have an increase in pancreatic islet tissue. Fetal hyperinsulinism may have a growth hormone effect that results in macrosomia. More severe degrees of maternal diabetes may result in smaller fetuses because of placental insufficiency and fetal nutritional deficit rather than macrosomia. Close control of maternal diabetes results in a better overall perinatal outcome.

Maternal thyroid disease is much less common than diabetes but also has profound fetal effects. Fetal thyroid function appears by 12 weeks of gestation; thyroxine and triiodothyronine can probably cross the placenta in small amounts in either direction. The effect of maternal hypothyroidism on the fetus is unclear, but evidence suggests that fetal nervous system development may be negatively affected; IQs in offspring are also lower. Abortions, stillbirths, anomalies, and prematurity are definitely associated with hypothyroidism. Hyperthyroidism, when untreated, increases fetal wastage. In addition, treatment carries a definite fetal risk because antithyroid drugs may affect the fetal thyroid, and surgical intervention carries an operative risk to fetus and mother. Postoperative treatment with thyroid-replacement therapy may minimize fetal complications.

Although *seizure disorders* are common, their course during pregnancy is difficult to predict with certainty. The status of approximately half those affected is unchanged, and of the remaining number, half improve and half become worse. Destabilizing seizure manifestations, as in status epilepticus, are an emergency for the mother and fetus. Unfortunately, there appears to be an increased incidence of congenital anomalies among infants of mothers with seizure disorders, even with cessation of an anticonvulsant regimen. Some anticonvulsants, such as trimethadione and valproic acid, seem clearly teratogenic. Phenytoin has been linked with a fetal hydantoin syndrome, but controversy over the actual incidence continues.[8] Phenobarbital, carbamazepine, and other medications may increase risk because of their possible broad-based impact on fetal enzymatic systems.

Seizures that appear de novo in pregnancy must be evaluated thoroughly. *Eclampsia* usually manifests with other signs and symptoms but is associated with a high incidence of fetal and neonatal complications (see Pregnancy-Induced Hypertension, p. 407).

Maternal emotional status has too complex an involvment with changes in physical states and with familial status, as previously mentioned, to be used to identify a specific fetal risk in many situations. Whether maternal emotional illness, not related to pregnancy, can directly affect the fetus is unclear. Pregnancy-caused or pregnancy-aggravated crises leading to abortion, drug abuse, or poor maternal nutrition can have obvious fetal consequences. *Hyperemesis gravidarum*, an entity of unclear but perhaps emotional origin, can result in profound fetal growth retardation.

Placenta and Membrane Disorders

Pathologic conditions of the gestational products—outside of the fetus itself—on which the fetus depends for respiration, nutrition, protection, and other functions are major contributors to fetal disease. Manifestations of disease in the fetus are diverse and severe and include fetal death, distress, hypoxia, shock, anemia, polycythemia, infection, congenital anomalies, and neoplasia.

The *implantation site* is normally in the upper uterus but may be in the lower uterus, in the tubes, or independently in the abdominal cavity. Maternal anatomic factors may contribute to abnormal implantations. Abdominal and tubal (ectopic) pregnancies are potential disasters for both mother and fetus; with the exception of a rare surviving abdominal fetus, fetal wastage is nearly uniform and maternal mortality and morbidity are common.

Placenta previa is associated with multiparity and places the fetus at risk in the event of hemorrhage; premature delivery, often by cesarean section, is necessary. *Abruption of the placenta* often is associated with maternal problems, including toxemia, hypertension, renal disease, and multiparity. Sudden fetal demise may occur in severe separation, with lesser degrees resulting in hypoxia and acute fetal stress. Bleeding in placenta previa and abruption usually is maternal, but it can be fetal in a minority of cases and sufficient to cause fetal hypovolemia and anemia.

Cord abnormalities are unusual but may be severe in consequence. A short umbilical cord may be complicated by abruption. True knots are present in 2% of deliveries and increase perinatal losses twofold. *Vasa previa, velamentous insertion, or circumvallate placenta* are difficult to identify before labor and can result in fetal exsanguination. Vascular abnormalities within the main placental structure occur rarely; fetal risk in monozygous multiple pregnancy includes the possibility of *twin-to-twin transfusion syndrome,* in which vascular anastomoses may result in exchange of blood between fetuses and in severe circulatory problems for one or both.

Vascular abnormality of the cord itself is frequently observed (1% of pregnancies) as a two-vessel cord with a single umbilical artery. Fetal risk is higher when this occurs because of associated congenital anomalies. In most situations the cord anomaly is probably not the cause; contrary to prior opinion, some current thought suggests that, in fact, no particular fetal abnormalities are involved in a two-vessel cord.

Premature, or prolonged, rupture of membranes (PROM) is a major contributor to perinatal mortality and morbidity. It is often defined as rupture that occurs an hour or more before onset of labor; it may be spontaneous, accidental during an examination, or artificial for induction of labor. Regardless of classification, the perinatal care team must be aware that an inevitable process of increased fetal risk begins soon after rupture and that prospective treatment protocols are desirable. Most protocols stipulate evaluation and treatment in relation to intervals since rupture. Many authorities consider 24 hours after rupture of membranes to be the beginning of accelerated risk.

The primary cause of fetal and maternal morbidity and mortality in PROM is sepsis. At term, labor occurs within 24 hours of rupture in 80% of pregnancies; in preterm pregnancies labor begins within 24 hours in less than 50%. Prolonged rupture of membranes with 24 hours or more elapsed before delivery, is much more common in preterm pregnancies. The cause of spontaneous rupture often is not clear, and with the exception of entities such as incompetent cervix, statistical correlation and prior risk identification are unsuccessful. Some conditions, including breech presentation and prolapse, are associated with PROM. *Chorioamnionitis* may be an important cause.

The frequency and degree of inflammation of membranes, cord, or fetus vary directly with time and onset of labor. Infection apparently ascends to the fetus via the cervix, with labor accelerating the process. Antibiotics are of questionable effectiveness before delivery.

A dilemma in fetal risk assessment occurs in the PROM pregnancy that is significantly preterm. The fetus in this situation is at risk not only from infection but also from premature birth and its complications, especially respiratory distress syndrome (RDS). On the other hand, there is an unresolved debate about whether PROM results in acceleration of fetal lung maturity and therefore decreased RDS. The clinician has available prepartum agents (corticosteroids) that seem to accelerate pulmonary maturity in certain situations and improve postpartum status overall in certain populations. Fetal risk can be minimized if the proper choice of therapeutic modalities is employed.

Maternal-Fetal Unit

Fetal risk frequently is associated with pathophysiologic processes in which both mother and fetus play an integral role. Major causality in situations in which the basic process is well understood often cannot be directed to one party, as in, for example, isoimmunization. There are also situations such as toxemia in which causality is not yet understood.

Premature Birth. Prematurity and its complications are prime contributors to perinatal mortality and morbidity.[4] Only birth asphyxia challenges this entity in total demand for prompt skilled intervention by providers of newborn care. These providers must clearly understand the relationship between prematurity (gestational age) and low birth weight. The problems of prematurity and low birth weight are similar but not identical (see Intrauterine Growth and Nutrition and Assessment of Gestational Age in Chapter 36, Three, Recovery Period).

Prevention of premature birth has been and remains a primary objective of perinatal care providers. Causality is probably multifactorial and remains uncertain inasmuch as the precise mechanisms that cause labor have yet to be elucidated. Many of the factors mentioned on p. 400 as contributors to fetal risk precipitate adverse outcomes directly or indirectly through premature birth.

Pharmacologic Intervention. Tocolysis, or inhibition of uterine activity, is therapy directed at preventing premature birth, once labor has begun. Pharmacologic agents have been employed with this intent for some time but with limited or minimal success. Progesterone and ethanol once were used extensively but have now been replaced by more promising agents.

The theoretic basis for the use of *beta-mimetic drugs* as tocolytics is their inhibitory effect on uterine contractions through activation of beta-adrenergic receptors. Alpha-receptor stimulation causes uterine contractions. Beta-receptors are subdivided into beta-one and beta-two groups, with the latter dominant in blood vessels and uterus.

Isoxsuprine hydrochloride, a derivative of catecholamine, *ritodrine* hydrochloride, and *terbutaline* sulfate have been used and are believed to be effective in depressing uterine contractions. Other agents are available, but a beta-mimetic that has a narrow impact on only the uterus has yet to become available. Thus maternal and fetal or neonatal side effects do occur, with cardiovascular, pulmonary, and metabolic complications documented. For example, neonatal hypoglycemia is a recognized complication of isoxsuprine therapy.

Calcium antagonists may have usefulness in the future but as yet are unproved. Magnesium sulfate is no more effective than other agents. Prostaglandin synthetase inhibitors may have a future role, but their use at present cannot be recommended because of their potential vasoactive effect on the fetus, especially on the ductus arteriosus.

Tocolytic therapy continues to be controversial; however, such intervention appears beneficial in some preterm labors.

Analysis of neonatal and maternal care suggests that in certain situations, especially between 26 and 33 weeks of gestation, such therapy is cost effective when one calculates cost of maternal and neonatal intensive care.[5]

Prevention of Prematurity. Certain authorities, in particular Papiernik and colleagues[6] in France and Creasy and Resnick[2] in the United States, have aggressively documented and promoted comprehensive programs to *prevent prematurity through alteration of patient and professional behavior.* Key to such efforts is identification of the risk factors associated with prematurity. Subsequent intervention to alter risk might be medical, but social and behavioral interventions may be equally important. Unfortunately, studies of such intervention have had, at best, mixed results.

Health professionals such as nurse coordinators can play a major role in programs because they ensure that the need for intervention is documented and that intervention occurs. In addition to management of problems such as elevated blood pressure, there may need to be alterations in life-style, work environment, and behavior patterns. Good prenatal care and early work leave may be very important. Countries such as Sweden, where such policies exist, have low prematurity rates.

Multiple Gestation. Multiple gestation is relatively common (twins occur in 1 in 80 births and triplets in 1 in 902) and increases risk to the point where only a singleton gestation can be considered normal. This results from a host of complications ranging from those that are placental in origin, such as twin-to-twin transfusion, to fetal malformations that can be obscure and spectacular, as in compound twins; to much more frequent problems, such as prematurity and obstetric complications. Multiple gestation is one of the three most common causes of prematurity. Complications of labor and delivery markedly increase the risk of hypoxia or trauma, with the second-born twin more susceptible than the first.

Obstetric Complications. Obstetric complications jeopardize the fetus, with the most overt manifestation being intrapartum fetal demise. Even the most ideally healthy fetus is at increased risk during labor and delivery. Stress to the fetus may be documented retrospectively by low Apgar scores, poor recovery after birth, and subsequent complications. A fetus already influenced by adverse factors, such as diabetes in pregnancy, is at even greater risk when obstetric problems arise. New means for fetal monitoring are currently documenting fetal distress and furthering rational application of obstetric techniques that can alleviate stress and decrease risk.

Abnormal presentations, such as breech and transverse lie, greatly increase fetal risk, as does cephalopelvic disproportion (a mismatch between the maternal pelvis and the fetal head). Malproportion can be predominantly fetal, as in congenital hydrocephalus, or maternal when congenital pelvic bone abnormalities exist.

Abnormal Growth and Gestation. Abnormal fetal growth and gestation often are manifestations of an underlying disease process but may occur without apparent cause. A general discussion of intrauterine growth and nutrition, including growth curves, was introduced earlier (see Fig. 31-2). Regardless of cause, discrepancies in growth and gestation often can result in such severe risk to the fetus as to be of essentially greater consequence than the underlying problem itself. Prematurity is considered to be the leading cause of perinatal mortality and morbidity and is the outcome of a number of abnormal processes. Postmaturity occurs much less frequently but presents a greatly increased risk. Little or no growth occurs in the human fetus after term, and many postterm fetuses and infants are, in fact, dysmature and tolerate the stress of labor and delivery poorly. They have a significantly increased chance of neonatal problems such as hypoglycemia and aspiration pneumonia.

The combination of deviations of growth and gestation can be cumulative for fetal risk. The premature infant who is affected by intrauterine growth retardation tolerates intrauterine stress poorly, may manifest RDS or gestationally related apnea after birth, and is at risk for the development of hypoglycemia. The clinician should appreciate that evaluation of the fetus or newborn by combined birth weight and gestational age can provide specific information that facilitates diagnosis and treatment (see Fig. 31-3).

Isoimmunization. Isoimmunization is a disease of the maternal-fetal unit. Passage into the maternal circulation of fetal red cells, which possess antigens not present in the mother, stimulates the production of antibodies. Maternal antibodies of the IgG class cross the placenta, resulting in a hemolytic process in the fetus that can be severe. Variations on this basic theme occur. The initial isoimmunization can occur with blood transfusions, with an abortion, or with the first or subsequent pregnancy. Small amounts of antigen on amounts of blood of 1 ml or less, especially if repeated, can cause antibody response even in normal pregnancies. Sensitization incidence is increased by complications such as toxemia or cesarean section.

Rh incompatibility is associated with a variable but often severe sensitization that can cause stillbirth, massive fetal erythropoiesis or erythroblastosis, anemia, hydrops fetalis (a syndrome with edema and anasarca), and other systemic manifestations. Hyperbilirubinemia occurs in the newborn and to a lesser degree in utero, where the placenta clears bilirubin.

The incidence of Rh disease varies with the prevalence of Rh negativity. Rh negativity rarely occurs in Orientals and American Indians. However, it occurs in 15% of American whites, resulting in the possibility of approximately 9% of their pregnancies involving an Rh-negative woman carrying an Rh-positive fetus.

Since the delineation of the cause of RH-sensitization, a wide range of diagnostic and therapeutic methods has become available, to make Rh treatment a paradigm for intensive perinatal care. Routine procedures for the disease today include initial screening for possible "setups"; maternal serum and amniotic fluid analyses for severity of sensitization; intrauterine fetal transfusions when indicated; planned delivery, taking into consideration fetal well-being and maturity; and aggressive neonatal intensive care, including exchange transfusions and cardiopulmonary support. Behind all this effort is an ongoing program of prevention, utilizing Rh_o globulin (RhoGAM).

Complicating the Rh story is the fact that the major Rh antigen group, or D antigen, is but one of several causes for isoimmunuzation: C and E genes also exist, but at much lower frequencies. Most clinical tests and screening efforts involve the D antigen.

Incompatibilities of the ABO system result from the presence of maternal anti-A or anti-B when the fetus' blood type is group A or B and the mother's group O. Severe hemolysis is less common even though ABO incompatibility is potentially present in about 20% of pregnancies. Fetal erythrocytes appear to have fewer antigenic loci, and maternal antibody appears as IgA, IgM, and IgG, with only the latter crossing the placenta. These facts may explain why ABO isoimmunization usually is of greater concern in the newborn than in the fetus. Stillbirths and hydrops fetalis are rare, but prolonged neonatal hyperbilirubinemia occurs frequently. Other incompatibilities, such as *anti-Kell sensitization,* are of low frequency (less than 1% of newborn hemolytic disease) but do on rare occasions present significant fetal and newborn risks.

Intrauterine Infections. Intrauterine infections with fetal involvement are a major and diverse cause of fetal mortality and morbidity. Expression ranges from spontaneous abortion and stillbirth through very severe teratogenic manifestations to subtle manifestations of the central nervous system not detected until later in childhood. Agents include viruses, bacteria, spirochetes, and protozoa. The route of infection varies with the agent and includes transplacental, transcervical ascending (usually in the presence of ruptured membranes), and direct contact with the fetus during passage through the birth canal.

The scope of the problem of intrauterine infections and their fetal effects has been broadened considerably in recent years but is probably far from completely delineated. Chronic infections may be more prevalent than currently appreciated. Three viruses—rubella, cytomegalovirus, and herpes simplex—are recognized teratogens, and the potential for others exists. An acronym helpful in remembering common agents is depicted in Table 31-3. A more detailed discussion of a few specific infections follows.

Rubella. Rubella virus is recognized as a potent teratogen. Infections during the first trimester result in approximately 20% of fetuses being severely damaged or malformed, with second trimester involvement damaging 10%. Third-trimester infection has presented few clinical problems. Manifestations of first-trimester fetal disease can be severe (e.g., abortion, stillbirth, and the findings of severe rubella syndrome). Severe rubella syndrome includes growth retardation; eye defects, including cataracts and microphthalmia; congenital cardiac defects; deafness; thrombocytopenic purpura; hepatosplenomegaly; bone lesions; pneumonitis; and cerebral defects, including microcephaly, encephalitis, mental retardation, and spastic quadriparesis. Infections in the second trimester are more variable and tend to be less severe. It now is apparent that the classic fetal presentation, with the severe manifestations listed above, is at one end of a spectrum that extends to documented infection with little or no apparent disease and that the expression of rubella syndrome is variable and unpredictable. The 1964 rubella epidemic affected thousands of infants.

The high fetal risk and potentially devastating consequences of intrauterine rubella have stimulated aggressive preventive and pregnancy termination efforts. Congenital rubella is a reportable disease. Vaccination of children between the ages of 1 and 12 years is routine, but administration to women of childbearing age has been controversial because of potential teratogenic effects of the vaccine virus on the fetus. *Antibody screening can establish whether an individual woman is among the 85% who are immune.* Obstetricians should monitor their patients for risk of rubella infection. When probable rubella infection occurs in early pregnancy, abortion is an alternative considered and frequently employed.

Cytomegalovirus (CMV) Infections. The cytomegaloviruses may be the most common cause of congenital infections, occurring in somewhat less than 1% of births. This group of viruses is widespread and produces various apparent and inapparent infections in the general population. Among pregnant women, 3% to 5% have this virus in their cervix or urine. Fetal infection usually occurs transplacentally, although intrauterine transfusion as a cause has been documented.

The fetal disease has been called cytomegalic inclusion disease (CID) because of the large inclusion-bearing cells found in urine and many organs. Severe CID includes, hepatosplenomegaly, microcephaly, cerebral calcifications, mental and motor manifestations, and chorioretinitis. Reviews suggest that expression of intrauterine infections is quite variable and that full recognition of incidence is yet to come. Serologic tests for CMV are available and can provide presumptive evidence for infection; however, reliability is not as good as with rubella titers, and a vaccine is not available.

Table 31-3 *Maternal-Fetal Infections: The TORCH Acronym*

INFECTION	AGENT	COMMENT
T—Toxoplasmosis	Protozoa	Transplacental passage; mild maternal illness, variable fetal or neonatal manifestations; maternal antibody test available
O—Other	Virus, bacteria, parasite	HIV, *Listeria,* syphilis, gonococcus, group B streptococcus, varicella-zoster, malaria
R—Rubella	Virus	Prototype for transplacental viral infections; severe and chronic fetal or neonatal disease; antibody test and immunization available
C—Cytomegalovirus	Virus	Transplacental passage, ubiquitous agent; broad spectrum of fetal or infant manifestations
H—Herpes simplex	Virus	Rare transplacental passage, usual intrapartum transmission from maternal genitalia; severe neonatal disease; antiviral treatment available

Modified with permission from Nahmias AJ: The Torch complex, Hosp Pract 9:5, 1974.

Herpes Simplex Virus Infections. Herpes simplex virus (HSV) infections in humans are from two strains, types 1 and 2, with distinct serotypes but some cross-reactivity. *Perinatal disease usually is associated with type 2,* although type 1 is more common in the general population. Type 2 produces genital lesions and is venereally transmitted in most instances. Herpetic disease in the fetus or newborn is relatively rare but devastating. Transmission occurs by direct contact at birth or by ascending transcervical infection after rupture of membranes. Transplacental infection early in pregnancy with fetal manifestations similar to those of CMV infection has been documented in at least one case. Whether transplacental transmission is a frequent problem is unclear, as is the severity of manifestations.

Newborn manifestations of intrapartum contact are well known. They range from vesicular lesions of the skin to encephalitis and severe systemic disease with a mortality rate of more than 90% and severe central nervous system morbidity in those who survive. Expression probably is linked to primary versus recurrent maternal disease, being more intense in the latter form.

A major recent development is the *success of antiviral agents* in the treatment of systemic herpes infection and, in particular, encephalitis. Early diagnosis and treatment are essential. Prevention is desirable and possible. (See discussion of venereal diseases in Chapter 255 and of herpes infections in Chapter 212.)

Present recommended management for a pregnant mother with genital lesions is a *cesarean section* to prevent fetal inoculation by contact. This should be done within 4 hours of rupture of the membranes.

Toxoplasmosis. Toxoplasmosis is caused by an intracellular protozoan parasite, *Toxoplasma gondii.* Infection is widespread, is congenital or acquired, and varies in expression from almost asymptomatic to generalized and fatal. The fetus is at risk for death when the infection occurs early in pregnancy or may be born with fully developed disease indicative of a long intrauterine course. *Chorioretinitis, cerebral calcification, hydrocephalus or microcephaly, hepatosplenomegaly, and a host of systemic manifestations* are observed. Long-term sequelae, especially involving the central nervous system, are present in the majority of infants with severe infection who survive.

It is believed that pregnant women become infected through exposure to cat feces or incompletely cooked meat. Incidence of the perinatal disease is higher in certain locales. Antibody detection by means of the Sabin-Feldman dye test and a complement-fixing test can document the onset of infection, but antibodies remain high for several years. Thus high initial titers without subsequent change do not necessarily indicate current fetal infection. Children born to mothers with a prior congenitally affected child are rarely, if ever, infected. Prospective antibody studies on children for disappearance of transplacentally acquired dye antibody at 4 months of age can help to rule out congenital infection. Congenital infection may be inapparent at birth and produce central nervous system signs late in infancy.

Human immunodeficiency virus (HIV) can infect the fetus transplacentally. The actual risk of congenital or perinatal transmission from an HIV-infected mother to her fetus or newborn is difficult to quantify but may range from 30% to 50%. Factors responsible for transmission have not been identified. Acquired immunodeficiency syndrome (AIDS) usually does not manifest for a varying interval after birth, making actual time of infection, intrauterine or peripartum, difficult to pinpoint. When AIDS does occur, it usually is in the first year after birth.

Other Intrauterine Infections. Fetal *syphilis* is caused by transplacental passage of *Treponema pallidum.* Fetal infection has been thought not to occur before the eighteenth week of gestation, but this may be subject to dispute. Pregnancy in a woman with primary- or secondary-stage disease may terminate in stillbirth. Other manifestations vary from presentation in the newborn to those appearing in the first 2 years of life or later. In general, the earlier the infection, the more severe are the lesions. Severe fetal infection manifests in early infancy by osteochondritis and periostitis, rhinitis (snuffles), rash, and mucosal fissures or patches. Premarital and prenatal screening for syphilis, in conjunction with antibiotic treatment, has effectively decreased the incidence of intrauterine disease, especially that with the more severe or classic manifestations. Unfortunately, somewhat of a resurgence may be occurring. Recently trained clinicians have not had the experience in recognizing congenital syphilis that many of their older compatriots have had, sometimes resulting in a delayed diagnosis.

Listeria monocytogenes is a gram-positive bacillus that probably plays an important role in overall fetal wastage. Incidence varies widely. Fetal death may occur after a relatively mild systemic maternal disease. Neonatal manifestations include systemic disease at birth or a delayed appearance as meningitis in the second to fifth week of life, with a characteristic monocellular cerebrospinal fluid manifestation.

Group B streptococcal disease has many similarities in presentation to that of the *Listeria* organisms and is a more common problem. A fulminant hemorrhagic pneumonitis in the first hours of life and a delayed meningitis cause very high mortality. Fetal infection probably occurs in the intrapartum period from organisms in the birth canal. Maternal immune status may play a role. An effective protocol involving prenatal detection and treatment is needed.

Other known intrauterine infections include agents of all classes, and undoubtedly many others will be discovered. Many viruses can cause fetal infection or manifestations, including varicella, coxsackievirus, mumps, rubeola, echovirus, hepatitis, and others. *Mycoplasma* may be an important perinatal agent, and malaria is a significant fetal threat in many areas of the world.

Assessment of fetal well-being in suspected intrauterine infection follows the precepts set out above, plus other attempts to document infections. Serologic tests have been alluded to in the discussion of individual entities and may be helpful, as in rubella. Unfortunately, although diagnostic certainty often is quite satisfactory for the newborn, it is less reliable for the fetus.

Pregnancy-Induced Hypertension. Hypertension of pregnancy is a major contributor to fetal risk. A group of diseases seen only in pregnancy and presenting with acute and chronic manifestations of hypertension, edema, and proteinuria may be lumped together in this category. *Preeclamp-*

sia is another term for the basic process, which can be severe; when convulsions or coma occurs, *eclampsia* is present. Chronic hypertensive vascular disease with pregnancy is believed by many to be a separate disease state that can have superimposed toxemic manifestations.

Spontaneous labor occurs frequently in all hypertensive gestations (for unclear reasons), leading to a risk of premature birth, which is increased further in incidence because early delivery is frequently employed. As the severity of the disease increases and particularly when eclampsia intervenes, stillbirth and maternal death become much more frequent. Intrauterine growth retardation is seen in a third of perinatal deaths associated with toxemia. From the fetal viewpoint, this disease process presents a bleak perspective; prenatal stress is significant, labor and delivery often are premature and timed for maternal rather than fetal well-being, and neonatal complications are many and severe.

Risk identification and evaluation in hypertension rely heavily on prenatal detection. When the process is discovered, intensive perinatal care may be necessary, with sedatives and anticonvulsants, especially magnesium sulfate, a mainstay of therapy. Fetal well-being and maturity can be assessed by regular observation of fetal heart rate, uterine growth, estriols, and ultrasound and by amniotic fluid parameters. Oxytocin for stress testing or induction may cause fluid retention. The physician responsible for the infant may be confronted by unfavorable test results of fetal well-being and maturity plus the need for imminent delivery. In addition, medication such as magnesium sulfate used before delivery may complicate neonatal management, adding to risk.

REFERENCES

1. Caring for our future: the content of prenatal care, Report of the Public Health Service Expert Panel on the Content of Prenatal Care, US Public Health Service, Washington, DC, 1989, Department of Health and Human Services.
2. Creasy RK and Resnik R, editors: Maternal-fetal medicine: principles and practice, ed 2, Philadelphia, 1989, WB Saunders Co.
3. Diagnostic ultrasound imaging in pregnancy, Report of a Consensus Development Conference, Feb 6-8, 1984, NIH Pub No 84-667, Washington, DC, 1984, Department of Health and Human Services.
4. Fuchs F and Stubblefield PG, editors: Preterm birth: causes, prevention and management, New York, 1984, Macmillan Publishing Co, Inc.
5. Korenbrot CC, Alto LH, and Laros RK Jr: The cost effectiveness of stopping labor with beta-adrenergic treatment, N Engl J Med 310:691, 1984.
6. Papiernik E et al: Prevention of preterm births: a perinatal study in Haguenau, France, Pediatrics 76:154, 1985.
7. Rhoads GC et al: The safety and efficacy of chorionic villus sampling for early prenatal diagnosis of cytogenetic abnormalities, N Engl J Med 320:10, 1989.
8. Smith DW: Recognizable patterns of human malformation, major problems in clinical pediatrics, ed 3, Philadelphia, 1982, WB Saunders Co.

SUGGESTED READINGS

Avery ME, Fletcher BD, and Williams RG, editors: Major problems in clinical pediatrics, vol 1, The lung and its disorders in the newborn infant, ed 4, Philadelphia, 1981, WB Saunders Co.

Beckman DA and Brent RL: Mechanisms of known environmental teratogens: drugs and chemicals. Clin Perinatol 13:649-687, 1986.

Cefalo RC and Moos M-K: Preconceptional health promotion: a practical guide, Rockville, Md, 1988, Aspen Publishers, Inc.

Chalmers I, Enkin M, and Keirse M, editors: Effective care in pregnancy and childbirth, Oxford, 1989, Oxford University Press.

Dorris M: The broken cord, New York, 1989, Harper & Row, Publishers, Inc.

Frigoletto FD and Little GA, editors: Guidelines for perinatal care, ed 2, American Academy of Pediatrics, American College of Obstetricians and Gynecologists, Elk Grove Village, Ill, 1988, The Academy.

Hobbins JC et al: Percutaneous umbilical blood sampling, Am J Obstet Gynecol 152:1, 1985.

Jones KL: Teratogens: what we know and don't know about them. In Kaback M, editor: Genetic issues in pediatric and obstetric practice, Chicago, 1981, Year Book Medical Publishers, Inc.

Jones KL: Smith's recognizable patterns of human malformation, ed 4, Philadelphia, 1988, WB Saunders Co.

Lubchenco LO: Major problems in clinical pediatrics, vol 14, The high-risk infant, Philadelphia, 1976, WB Saunders Co.

Milunsky A: Current concepts in genetics: prenatal diagnosis of genetic disorders, N Engl J Med 295:277, 1976.

Moore KL: The developing human: clinically oriented embryology, ed 4, Philadelphia, 1988, WB Saunders Co.

Nahmias AS: The TORCH complex, Hosp Pract 9:65, 1974.

Shepard TJ: Detection of human teratogenic agents, J Pediatr 101:5:810, 1982.

Stiehm ER: Fetal defense mechanisms, Am J Dis Child 129:438, 1975.

Warshaw JB: Fetal disease, Clin Perinatol 6:2, 1979.

32

Maternal Nutritional Status and Fetal Growth

Pedro Rosso

Nutritional disorders are caused by an imbalance between nutrient availability and needs. Individuals can suffer from either nutrient deficiencies or an excess of nutrients. Traditionally, nutrient deficiencies have been classified into two types: those caused by energy-protein deficiency and those involving single nutrients such as vitamins and minerals, also called *specific deficiencies*. This is a rather schematic classification because most malnourished persons have combined energy-protein and specific deficiencies.

During postnatal life both deficiencies and excessive intake of nutrients have a direct impact on the growth and development of a child. Signs of nutritional disorders include weight loss, growth retardation, obesity, anemia, behavioral abnormalities, and a variety of other changes.

During prenatal life the nutritional disorders that affect the conceptus always result from maternal disorders; consequently, their impact will depend on a variety of factors, including the nature of the problem, the maternal capacity to adapt to the disorder, and the time of gestation when the disorder takes place.

In the past, misconceptions about maternal-fetal exchange of nutrients—that is, the idea that the fetus is a maternal parasite—led to a great deal of confusion concerning the fetal consequences of maternal nutritional disorders. Similarly, the erroneous idea that maternal dietary changes would directly influence fetal growth created false expectations about the efficacy of nutritional interventions in pregnant women. These misconceptions, fostered by studies that judged by present standards are fraught with methodologic errors, have greatly contributed to the prevailing skepticism concerning the role of nutrition in fetal growth and well-being. A detailed discussion of each of the controversies surrounding this area is beyond the scope of the present chapter. The information presented here is limited to well-established facts and potentially relevant new evidence. Together they constitute a body of knowledge that strongly supports the concept that maternal nutritional status is an important determinant of prenatal growth.

MATERNAL NUTRITIONAL DISORDERS AND PRENATAL GROWTH

The nutritional disorders known to affect prenatal growth and those that are presently suspected of being capable of affecting prenatal growth are listed in Table 32-1.

Energy

Maternal energy deficiency causes a reduced prenatal body weight for height and/or a reduced weight gain during pregnancy. Both situations lead to fetal growth retardation that is more severe when these two conditions are combined with an underweight mother who fails to gain adequate weight during gestation.

Chronic energy deficiency can be easily recognized by assessing the adequacy of maternal weight for height relative to standard weight.[16] Women whose prepregnancy weight for height is less than 90% of the standard are considered to be underweight. Women who are underweight early in pregnancy tend to deliver lighter than average babies unless during pregnancy they gain more than average weight. Ideally, they should recover from their initial weight deficit and gain the recommended weight, which is equivalent to 20% of their standard weight.[16] In absolute values this may represent weight gains in excess of 15 to 17 kg (Table 32-2).

Although it is not uncommon for underweight mothers to deliver infants of average size, the mean birth weight of babies of underweight or nonobese mothers who gain little weight during pregnancy is considerably below average (Table

Table 32-1 *Maternal Nutritional Disorders and Fetal Growth*

MATERNAL DEFICIENCIES	FETAL CONSEQUENCES
Energy	***Growth retardation***
Vitamins	
Folic acid	Neural tube defects?
Vitamin D	Neonatal hypocalcemia, congenital rickets
Thiamin	Congenital beriberi
Vitamin B_{12}	Low vitamin B_{12} stores
Minerals	
Iron	Low iron stores
Zinc	Neural tube defects? Growth retardation?
Iodine	Congenital cretinism
Manganese	Congenital malformations
MATERNAL EXCESSES	*FETAL CONSEQUENCES*
Obesity	Macrosomia
Vitamin A	Congenital malformations

Table 32-2 *Effect of Pregnancy Weight Gain on Birth Weight in Women with Different Prepregnancy Weight/Height Standards*

PREPREGNANCY WEIGHT/HEIGHT (as % of standard)	PREGNANCY WEIGHT GAIN AND BIRTH WEIGHT*		
	<7 kg	7-14 kg	>14 kg
<90%	2731 ± 302	3093 ± 363	3387 ± 382
90-110%	3029 ± 341	3281 ± 379	3490 ± 429
>110%	3473 ± 423	3561 ± 434	3515 ± 473

Modified from Rosso P: Am J Clin Nutr 41:644, 1985.
*Mean birth weight in grams ± standard deviation.

Table 32-3 *Influence of Maternal Iron Status on the Infant at Birth and at 6 Months of Age*

MATERNAL IRON STATUS* (at delivery)	NEWBORN INFANT		INFANT (6 mo)	
	FERRITIN† (μg/L)	HEMOGLOBIN (g/dL)	FERRITIN† (μg/L)	HEMOGLOBIN (g/dL)
Low maternal iron stores	222 (107-459)‡	14.7 ± 1.1	99 (49-199)‡	11.9 ± 1.0
Normal maternal iron stores	324 (168-625)	15.7 ± 1.2	150 (81-275)	11.8 ± 0.9

Modified from Puolakka J, Janne D, Vihko R: Acta Obstet Gynecol Scand (Suppl) 95:53, 1980.
*Low iron stores: mean ferritin values, <28 μg/L; normal maternal iron stores: mean ferritin values, >102 μg/L.
†Geometric value ±1 SD in parentheses.
‡Significantly lower ($p < 0.05$).

32-2). This shift to the left of the birth weight distribution curve determines a higher percentage of small-for-gestational age babies in these women.

The opposite situation is observed in women who are overweight and obese before pregnancy (Table 32-2). Mean birth weight for infants of these mothers is higher than average and increases even more when weight gain during pregnancy is greater than 20% of standard weight. The greater mean birth weight is associated with a higher frequency of macrosomic infants, which in turn determines a greater risk of intrapartum complications and the need for cesarean section.

Vitamins

Maternal folic acid deficiency has been linked to congenital malformations, including neural tube defects. The strongest evidence supporting this possibility stems from supplementation trials with mothers at risk of delivering infants with neural tube defects because of having previously delivered such an infant.[7,21] In one of these studies[21] a multivitamin preparation was used whereas in the other only folic acid was given. In both trials the use of the vitamin supplements was associated with a significant reduction in the frequency of neural tube defects compared with mothers of similar background who did not receive supplementation. These results cannot be considered conclusive because neither randomization of subjects nor a control group was employed. Further research is needed to dispel these doubts.

Vitamin D deficiency reduces the availability of calcium for both the mother and the fetus. Although most mothers with vitamin D deficiency remain free of symptoms, the fetus may have manifestations of calcium deficiency, ranging from neonatal hypocalcemia to congenital rickets.[13,14,17,25] Most of the cases reported in the literature relate to immigrants from India and Pakistan living in England.

Thiamin deficiency, which in decades past was endemic, is becoming increasingly rare in a rice-consuming population. The infants of mothers with thiamin deficiency are at high risk for the development of one of the various forms of congenital beriberi. In the most severe cases symptoms start during the first week of life, and heart failure, as a result of myocardial injury, is the most serious complication.[5] This type of heart failure does not respond to digitalis and diuretics and is fatal unless thiamin is given promptly.

Vitamin B_{12} deficiency has been noted in mothers who are strict vegetarians. Although this deficiency does not alter fetal growth, the infant is born with reduced vitamin B_{12} stores. Because the milk of mothers with this deficiency is poor in vitamin B_{12}, breast-fed infants may become severely depleted during the first 6 months of life. Early symptoms include retarded psychomotor development, irritability, and anorexia. In more advanced stages severe megaloblastic anemia, loss of consciousness, and hyperpigmentation of the extremities have been described.[3,6]

Excessive intake of vitamin A or vitamin A analogs during the periconceptional period may cause severe congenital malformations. The cases reported in the literature include women who self-prescribed vitamin A in large doses (more than 25,000 IU daily), as well as users of antiacne preparations containing synthetic derivatives of retinoic acid.[15]

Minerals

Iron deficiency is the most common specific nutrient deficiency worldwide. Maternal iron deficiency, even when severe enough to cause anemia, does not affect fetal growth.

However, the reduced maternal serum iron levels cause a reduced placental transfer of this mineral and, consequently, low iron stores in the newborn. In turn, this would make the infant more susceptible to the development of iron deficiency during the first year of life unless iron-fortified foods are provided.

The idea that maternal iron deficiency may lead to the sequence of events described here is not universally accepted. Because fetal cord hemoglobin concentration is normal even in severely anemic mothers, many still believe that the fetus is a parasite of maternal iron. However, strong evidence counters the possibility of fetal parasitism. Newborns of anemic mothers apparently maintain a normal hemoglobin concentration because their total blood volume and red cell mass are reduced.[20] A positive correlation between serum ferritin concentration in maternal and cord blood has been demonstrated.[4,8] Furthermore, the infants of mothers with lower serum ferritin concentrations at delivery also have lower serum ferritin concentrations at 6 months of age[12] (Table 32-3).

Maternal zinc deficiency has been linked to a higher risk of congenital malformations, including neural tube defects and fetal growth retardation.[22,23] Although the evidence supporting a causal role of marginal zinc deficiency in neural tube defects indicates alternative explanations, the data linking zinc deficiency and fetal growth retardation are more convincing. Women who deliver infants small for gestational age were found to have lower leukocyte zinc concentrations than were mothers giving birth to fully grown babies.[10,19] Similarly, zinc concentrations were lower in cord blood leukocytes of infants small for gestational age than in those infants of normal size.[9] However, these results are in apparent contrast with other studies that have failed to find correlations between birth weight and maternal zinc status.[1,24] The problem is complex because zinc measurements are difficult to obtain, and there are no well-established clinical or biochemical criteria to diagnose marginal zinc deficiency. This area remains the focus of active research; new information available in the near future may help to clarify present doubts.

Iodine deficiency manifested by endemic goiter continues to be a problem in certain areas of the world. Women affected by iodine deficiency may deliver infants with cretinism.[11] Newborns with endemic cretinism show growth retardation and exhibit delayed neurologic development[2] (see Chapter 215).

Manganese deficiency has been associated with congenital malformations such as cleft palate, digital aplasia, hermaphroditism, and neural tube defects in a Turkish population.[18] In the hair of malformed infants and their mothers, manganese concentrations were 50% and 75% lower, respectively, than in control infants and mothers. This observation has not yet been duplicated.

REFERENCES

1. Campbell-Brown M et al: Zinc and copper in Asian pregnancies—is there evidence for a nutritional deficiency? Br J Obstet Gynaecol 92:875, 1985.
2. Hetzel BS and Querido A: Iodine deficiency, thyroid function and brain development. In Stanbury JB and Hetzel BS, editors: Endemic goiter and endemic cretinism, New York, 1980, John Wiley & Sons, Inc.
3. Higginbotton MC, Sweetman L, and Nyhan WL: A syndrome of methylmalonic aciduria, homocystinuria, megaloblastic anemia and neurologic abnormalities in a vitamin B_{12}-deficient breast-fed infant of a strict vegetarian, N Engl J Med 299:317, 1978.
4. Kaneshige F: Serum ferritin as an assessment of iron stores and other hematological parameters during pregnancy, Obstet Gynecol 57:238, 1981.
5. King EQ: Acute cardiac failure in the newborn due to thiamin deficiency, Exp Med Surg 25:173, 1967.
6. Lampkin BC and Saunders EF: Nutritional vitamin B_{12} deficiency in an infant, J Pediatr 75:1053, 1969.
7. Laurence KM et al: Double-blind randomized controlled trial of folate treatment before conception to prevent recurrence of neural tube defects, Br Med J (Clin Res) 282:1509, 1981.
8. MacPhail AP et al: The relationship between maternal and infant iron status, Scand J Haematol 25:141, 1980.
9. Meadows N et al: Peripheral blood leukocyte zinc depletion in babies with intrauterine growth retardation, Arch Dis Child 58:807, 1983.
10. Meadows NJ et al: Zinc and small babies, Lancet 2:1135, 1981.
11. Pharoah P et al: Endemic cretinism. In Stanbury JB and Hetzel BS, editors: Endemic goiter and endemic cretinism, New York, 1980, John Wiley & Sons, Inc.
12. Puolakka J, Janne O, and Vihko R: Evaluation by serum ferritin assay of the influence of maternal iron stores on the iron status of newborns and infants, Acta Obstet Gynecol Scand (Suppl) 95:53, 1980.
13. Purvis RJ et al: Enamel hypoplasia of the teeth associated with neonatal tetany: a manifestation of maternal vitamin D deficiency, Lancet 3:811, 1973.
14. Roberts SA, Cohen MD, and Forfar JD: Antenatal factors associated with neonatal hypocalcaemic convulsions, Lancet 2:809, 1973.
15. Rosa FW, Wilk AL, and Kelsey FO: Teratogen update: vitamin A congeners, Teratology 33:355, 1986.
16. Rosso P: A new chart to monitor weight gain during pregnancy, Am J Clin Nutr 41:644, 1985.
17. Russell JGB and Hill LF: True fetal rickets, Br J Radiol 47:732, 1974.
18. Saner G, Dagöglù T, and Ozden T: Hair manganese concentrations in newborns and their mothers, Am J Clin Nutr 41:1042, 1985.
19. Simmer K and Thompson RPH: Maternal zinc and intrauterine growth retardation, Clin Sci 68:395, 1985.
20. Sisson TRC and Lund CJ: The influence of maternal iron deficiency on the newborn, Am J Clin Nutr 6:376, 1958.
21. Smithells RW et al: Possible prevention of neural tube defects by periconceptional vitamin supplementation, Lancet 1:339, 1980.
22. Solomons NW, Helitzer-Allen DL, and Villar J: Zinc needs during pregnancy, Clin Nutr 5:63, 1986.
23. Swanson CA and King JC: Zinc and pregnancy outcome, Am J Clin Nutr 46:763, 1987.
24. Tuttle S et al: Zinc and copper nutrition in human nutrition pregnancy: a longitudinal study in normal primigravidas and in primigravidae at risk of delivering a growth retarded baby, Am J Clin Nutr 41:1032, 1985.
25. Watney PJM et al: Maternal factors in neonatal hypocalcemia: a study in three ethnic groups, Br Med J 2:432, 1971.

33

The Effects of Drugs and Other Substances on the Fetus

Jonathan M. Davis and Charles E. Mercier

The concept of the placenta as an effective barrier that separates the maternal and fetal circulations has been discarded.[4] Any drug administered to the mother can cross the placenta to a certain extent and thus can affect the fetus. Despite this fact, recent studies have shown that drug use during pregnancy is increasing.[2] This exposure to drugs is partially responsible for the large number of congenital anomalies seen in newborn infants (Table 33-1).

Experiments with a variety of animal species have yielded valuable information concerning the potential teratogenicity of many drugs. Many of these findings in animals, however, cannot be extrapolated to apply to human beings. Before its use in humans, thalidomide had been studied in several animal species and had not been found to be teratogenic. Thalidomide then was administered to pregnant women for several years, resulting in the birth of thousands of infants with characteristic phocomelia and facial defects before a strong relationship was established. This result demonstrates the difficulty in establishing a definite causal relationship between drugs administered during pregnancy and congenital anomalies occurring in the newborn. Now, virtually all drugs are considered to be potentially teratogenic, and most obstetricians advise women to abstain from all drug ingestion during pregnancy. If a drug must be used, the therapeutic benefits to the mother and potential risk to the fetus must be carefully weighed by the physician.

It is the purpose of this chapter to review current knowledge of drugs to which women are most likely to be exposed during pregnancy. First, general principles regarding the passage of drugs from the maternal circulation to the fetal circulation via the placenta will be discussed.

Table 33-1 *Etiology of Major Malformations Among 18,155 Newborns, 1972 to 1975*

CAUSE	INCIDENCE (%)*
Genetic abnormalities	1.1
Uterine factors	0.1
Drugs taken by mother	0.01
Maternal conditions	0.1
Unknown etiology	1.1

Reproduced with permission from Holmes LB: Congenital malformations. In Cloherty J and Stark A, editors: Manual of neonatal care, ed 2, Boston, 1985, Little, Brown & Co, p 127.
* Incidence would be expected to be higher today.

MATERNAL-FETAL PHARMACOLOGY

The passage of a drug across the placenta occurs primarily by simple diffusion (Fig. 33-1). Transfer by facilitated diffusion (requiring a specific carrier) and active transport (requiring energy) occur to a lesser degree.[12] Diffusion of a drug is proportional to the chemical properties of the drug (small, nonionic, lipid-soluble drugs diffuse best) and the concentration gradient.[1] Any drug in the maternal circulation eventually will cross the placenta and enter the fetal circulation, especially if the drug is used for prolonged periods. The placenta actually can biotransform some drugs by oxidation, reduction, dealkylation, and conjugation, which can make the drugs either more or less active.[12]

Drugs crossing the placenta can reach fetal concentrations of 10% to 100% of maternal serum concentrations. Timing and duration of drug exposure are critical. Drugs taken in the first trimester may influence organogenesis and contribute to physical defects. Drugs taken later in pregnancy may affect the growth and development of the fetus, especially the brain.[9] The fetus is particularly sensitive to the effects of drugs because serum proteins are lower in the fetus than in the adult; thus more free drug will circulate. In addition, enzymatic detoxification, which primarily occurs in the liver, is significantly less active. Renal excretion of drugs also can be delayed in the fetus, and drugs excreted in the amniotic fluid can be swallowed, absorbed, and reenter the fetal circulation.[12]

SOCIALLY ABUSED DRUGS

Alcohol

Fetal alcohol syndrome (FAS) describes a specific group of congenital malformations occurring in infants born to mothers who drink heavily throughout pregnancy.[6,7] FAS was first described in 1973 and includes (1) prenatal and postnatal growth retardation, (2) craniofacial defects (microcephaly, short palpebral fissures, ptosis, smooth philtrum, thin upper vermilion border, cleft lip/palate), (3) developmental delay (mental retardation, fine motor problems), (4) skeletal anomalies (joint contractures, dislocations), and (5) cardiac defects (atrial and ventricular septal defects). The incidence of FAS varies between 1/300 and 1/2000 live births, and 30% to 50% of infants born to mothers who drink more than 3 oz of pure alcohol per day will show features consistent with FAS. Some features of FAS have been seen with lesser amounts of alcohol intake. The effect of alcohol on the fetus significantly correlates with exposure during the first 2 months of the first trimester. Alcohol, or one of its metabolites (i.e., acetaldehyde) may disrupt protein synthesis and cellular function, which will result in FAS. Pregnant patients should be strongly discouraged from drinking any alcohol, especially during the first trimester, although FAS has not been described when absolute alcohol consumption is maintained at less than 1 to 2 oz per day.

Cigarettes

Studies performed since the 1950s have shown consistently that cigarette smoking during pregnancy results in infants born on average 200 g lighter than infants born to nonsmoking mothers.[5] Decreased birth length also has been described. Women who do not smoke but who are exposed to passive cigarette smoke for more than 2 hours per day also may be at greater risk for delivering a growth-retarded infant. In addition, maternal smoking increases the risk of spontaneous abortion, placenta previa, abruptio placentae, and premature rupture of membranes. Nicotine is a potently addictive drug and acts as a placental vasoconstrictor; carbon monoxide exposure increases fetal thiocyanate levels, which can lead to the decreased growth. Long-term neurodevelopmental effects are controversial; some studies demonstrate decreased reading, mathematics, and other cognitive abilities in children between 7 and 11 years of age, whereas other studies have not confirmed these findings.

Women should be strongly advised to stop smoking during pregnancy, but if they are unable to quit, they should limit their smoking to fewer than five cigarettes per day.

Cocaine

Cocaine and its derivative "crack" are the most addictive and abused street drugs currently in use. Cocaine acts as a potent vasoconstrictor and, when administered to pregnant sheep, caused significant dose-dependent increases in maternal blood pressure, uterine vascular resistance, and decreased uterine blood flow.[5] These responses were accompanied by severe fetal hypoxemia, hypertension, and tachycardia.

Cocaine's addictive properties are explained in part by the unique manner in which addicts use the drug. Unlike heroin (see next section), which is titrated by the addict to maintain a uniform sense of well-being, cocaine is taken in large quantities over short periods of time. Although the "high" of cocaine results from an initial accumulation of certain neurotransmitters in the brain, this process ultimately leads to neurotransmitter depletion, depression, and psychosis. The addict needs to use larger doses of cocaine more frequently to avoid these adverse side effects.

Several recent studies have suggested that mothers who

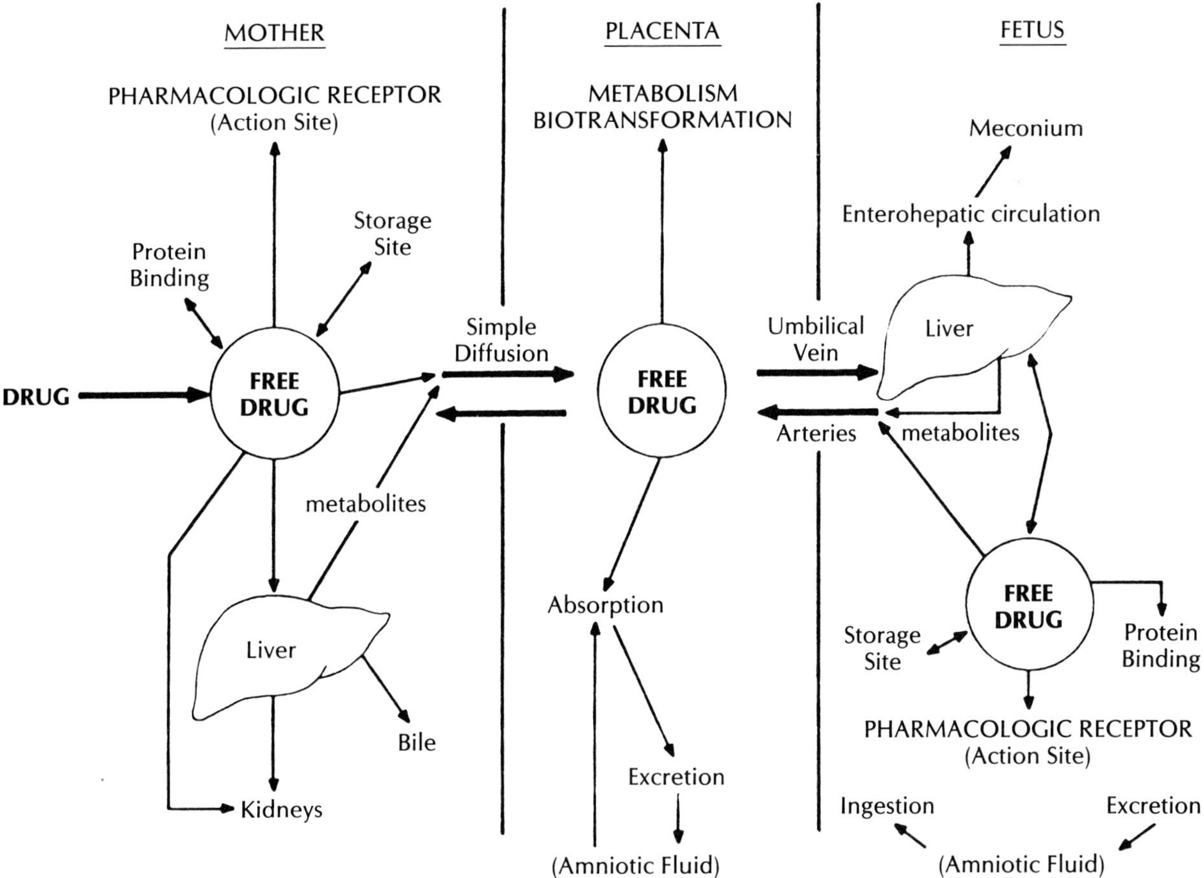

Fig. 33-1 Schematic diagram of movement of drugs between maternal and fetal circulations.

From Rayburn WF and Anderson BD: Principles of perinatal pharmacology. In Rayburn WF and Zuspan FP, editors: Drug therapy in obstetrics and gynecology, Norwalk, Conn, 1982, Appleton-Century-Crofts.

use cocaine during pregnancy have premature deliveries, abruptio placentae, and spontaneous abortions more frequently than do nondrug users.[5] Infants are at risk for congenital urogenital anomalies, microcephaly, bony defects, intracranial hemorrhage and infarcts, and intrauterine growth retardation. Symptoms consistent with acute drug withdrawal that requires treatment can occur in 10% to 15% of infants prenatally exposed to cocaine, and Brazelton Neurodevelopmental Assessments may show depressed interactive behavior and poor response to external stimuli. Mothers who use cocaine also may use alcohol, cigarettes, and other drugs that may act synergistically on the fetus. The long-term effects of cocaine on infants are largely unknown, and any outcome studies will be complicated by multiple confounding social and environmental variables.

Heroin and Methadone

Women who use heroin during pregnancy tend to receive little or no prenatal care, have a poor diet, and use alcohol, cigarettes, and several other drugs.[5,9] Significant fetal concentrations of heroin can be found within 1 hour of administration to the mother. Acute withdrawal in the mother may be associated with simultaneous withdrawal in the fetus, which can be related to an increased incidence of stillbirth and neonatal deaths.

A number of studies have reported increased rates of congenital anomalies in women who use heroin during pregnancy.[2] These anomalies are multiple and exhibit no specific pattern. Infants tend to be of low birth weight and small for gestational age. Withdrawal can occur in 20% to 90% of infants in the first 24 to 72 hours of life and can be acutely precipitated if infants receive naloxone at birth for treatment of respiratory depression. Long-term effects of heroin on growth and behavioral development have been described.[9]

Methadone is used to treat heroin addiction during pregnancy. Increases in congenital anomalies as a result of methadone use have not been described, but manifestation of severe neonatal narcotic withdrawal has been observed in 60% to 90% of infants. The risk of severe withdrawal that requires treatment is decreased if mothers can be maintained on a regimen of 20 mg or less per day.[9] Withdrawal can occur soon after birth or can be delayed up to 14 days. Impaired fetal growth that occurs with heroin addiction can be partially reversed with methadone therapy.

Marijuana

Marijuana use by women in their late teens and early twenties has been reported to be as high as 31%, which has important implications to young, pregnant women.[6] The drug is fat soluble, easily crosses the placenta, and a single exposure may take up to 30 days to be completely excreted by the fetus. Smoking marijuana can cause significant increases in fetal carbon monoxide levels. These effects have been linked to significant impairments in fetal growth. In addition, although marijuana has not been associated with specific congenital anomalies, mothers who use marijuana during pregnancy may deliver infants with features consistent with fetal alcohol syndrome.[5] Although heavy marijuana use (more than five cigarettes/week) is associated with transient neonatal neurologic abnormalities, long-term neurodevelopmental defects have not been described.

THERAPEUTIC AGENTS

Pregnant women take prescribed medications for two specific reasons. Many women are taking a particular medication early in pregnancy before they recognize that they are pregnant. This may be important because organogenesis typically occurs in the fetus within the first 3 to 9 weeks of gestation. Medications also may need to be initiated and continued during a known pregnancy for specific medical indications (e.g., anticonvulsants prescribed for epilepsy). If this is the case, then a medication that will have the greatest therapeutic benefit/risk ratio should be used if possible. This section provides a general review of many classes of therapeutic agents, with a description of known or suspected side effects on the fetus. It is impossible to review every drug and its potential impact on the fetus. The reader is referred to further, in-depth evaluations if detailed information on a specific drug is necessary.

Nonnarcotic Analgesics

Nonnarcotic analgesics represent a heterogeneous group of chemically unrelated compounds that have certain therapeutic actions and side effects in common. The reason for this similarity depends largely on the ability of these agents to inhibit specific reactions in the biosynthetic pathway of prostaglandins.

Aspirin is a salicylic acid derivative that possesses analgesic, antipyretic, and antiinflammatory actions. It is one of the most frequently used drugs during pregnancy, and it readily crosses the placenta. Maternal effects of aspirin consumption include anemia, antepartum or postpartum hemorrhage, prolonged gestation, and prolonged labor. The risk of hemorrhage is presumably secondary to disturbed platelet function. Disruption of platelet function occurs because aspirin prevents formation of thromboxane A_2, a potent aggregating agent. Gestation and labor are prolonged when aspirin disrupts uterine biosynthesis of prostaglandins, which normally initiates uterine contractions.

The use of aspirin in pregnancy has not been associated with specific congenital anomalies.[2] There are, however, fetal and newborn effects that are well documented. These effects include increased perinatal mortality, intrauterine growth retardation, and depressed albumin-binding capacity. Congenital salicylate intoxication has been reported in infants exposed to high doses of aspirin before delivery. Withdrawal consists of hypertonia, increased reflex irritability, agitation, and a high-pitched cry. The clotting ability of the newborn also is affected by maternal aspirin ingestion around the time of delivery. Decreased platelet aggregation and factor XII activity leading to increased bleeding time has been reported. An increased incidence of intracranial hemorrhage also has been reported in premature, very low-birth-weight ($<$1500 g) infants with maternal use of aspirin near delivery.[13] In conclusion, the use of high doses of aspirin during pregnancy should be avoided; even low doses are not recommended near term.

Acetaminophen has analgesic and antipyretic effects but little antiinflammatory action. Acetaminophen is metabolized mainly in the liver and readily crosses the placenta. Maternal overdosage occurring in the third trimester has not been reported to cause damage to the fetal liver if acetylcysteine has been promptly administered.[3] Maternal ingestion of acetaminophen has been associated with congenital dislocation of the hip and clubfoot, and it may be related to the development of cataracts. Causal relationships have not been definitely confirmed in these cases.[4]

Ibuprofen is a nonsteroidal antiinflammatory agent. No reports have associated its use with congenital malformations. As a prostaglandin synthetase inhibitor, however, ibuprofen could inhibit the onset of labor and prolong pregnancy. The use of indomethacin as a labor suppressant may be associated with premature closure of the ductus arteriosus in the fetus, with resulting persistent pulmonary hypertension in the newborn.

Narcotic Analgesics

Narcotics and their related synthetic compounds typically are grouped as to their agonist and agonist-antagonist properties. For example, morphine, codeine, hydromorphone (Dilaudid), meperidine (Demerol), and propoxyphene (Darvon) stimulate opioid receptors in the central nervous system. Others such as butorphanol (Stadol), nalbuphine (Nubain), and pentazocine (Talwin) are mixed agonist-antagonists. They act as an agonist at one type of opiate receptor and as a competitive antagonist at another. All classes of narcotics rapidly cross the placenta. Although no large categories of major or minor malformations have been linked to the *therapeutic* use of these agents, neonatal withdrawal symptoms after illicit use have been well documented.

Use of narcotic analgesics for managing pain during labor has been most extensively studied with the use of meperidine. Decreased beat-to-beat variability of the fetal heart and decreased respiratory effort have been reported. Neonatal respiratory depression is uncommon, usually mild, and transient unless delivery occurs 2 to 3 hours after administration. Naloxone (Narcan) administered to the newborn reverses respiratory depression from narcotics use by acting as a narcotics antagonist.

Anesthetic Agents

Local anesthetics play a role in the management of pain during labor. Direct fetal effects may occur after maternal injection of a local anesthetic into highly vascular spaces.[12] Paracervical blocks during labor may place the fetus at greater risk compared with epidural blocks. Lidocaine or mepivacaine (Carbocaine), which are used routinely in these blocks, may cause transient hypotonia of the newborn. Fetal asphyxia and acidosis also may potentiate the central nervous system effects of local anesthetics.

General anesthesia may be necessary for some deliveries by cesarean section and other operative procedures. Typically the risks of central nervous system and respiratory depression are related to the dose of the agent and length of exposure. Prolonged induction to delivery time is associated with a greater chance of acidosis and respiratory depression in the newborn.[9]

Anesthetic inhalation agents include nitrous oxide, methoxyflurane (Penthrane), and halothane. No increase in anomalies has been reported with the use of nitrous oxide during pregnancy, and no adverse effects on neonatal neurobehavior have been seen with its use in labor. Methoxyflurane and halothane are halogenated agents. Their use has not been shown to be directly associated with malformations. Both agents produce uterine relaxation, which is positively correlated with the dose, and may increase uterine bleeding. Transient fetal central nervous system and respiratory depression, proportional to the depth and duration of maternal anesthesia, also may occur.

Adjuncts to inhaled anesthetic agents are skeletal muscle relaxants. These agents cross the placenta in small amounts despite a high degree of ionization; it is possible that they will affect the fetus.[12]

Atropine, a commonly used anesthetic premedication, crosses the placenta rapidly, and there is significant fetal uptake. A direct effect on fetal heart rate may be seen 5 minutes after maternal administration; this effect may last for 1 hour or more.

Antimicrobial Agents

Antimicrobials are most frequently used during pregnancy for treatment of urinary tract or gynecologic infections. The penicillins are among the first line of choice for the majority of anaerobic organisms causing these infections, with the exception of *Bacteroides fragilis*. These drugs are also the least toxic of available antimicrobials. No adverse effects have been reported with their use throughout pregnancy.[2] Penicillins cross the placenta, and in the case of ampicillin, fetal levels will exceed maternal plasma levels shortly after maternal administration. Cephalosporins are similar to penicillins in structure, mechanism of action, and general antimicrobial activity. Like penicillins, no adverse effects have been reported with their use at any time during pregnancy. Although they also cross the placenta, no consistent relationship has been described between maternal and fetal levels.

Aminoglycosides are used for their bactericidal activity over a wide range of gram-positive and gram-negative organisms. Aminoglycosides readily cross the placenta, but the fetal serum level generally will be lower than the maternal level. The concern with administration of aminoglycosides during pregnancy is ototoxicity as a result of eighth cranial nerve damage.[2] Such toxicity has been well documented after fetal exposure to kanamycin and streptomycin but not with maternal administration of gentamicin, amikacin, or tobramycin. There have been no reports associating the maternal administration of aminoglycosides with congenital malformations in the newborn.

Other antibiotics that may be commonly used during pregnancy include chloramphenicol, clindamycin, erythromycin, miconazole, and nitrofurantoin. All these agents cross the placenta, but no congenital malformations have been associated with their use. Nitrofurantoin (Macrodantin) may precipitate hemolysis in infants with glucose-6-phosphate dehydrogenase deficiency.[11]

Tetracyclines and sulfa drugs represent two classes of antimicrobials that have been demonstrated to have adverse fetal effects. Tetracycline use during the first trimester has resulted in bone fluorescence and cataracts in the newborn. Tetracyclines also have been shown to chelate calcium in fetal teeth, resulting in tooth discoloration. Although significant tetracycline concentrations in the bones also would be expected, newborn growth and development have not been shown to be affected. There is a suggested relationship between tetracycline use during pregnancy and minor malformations in the newborn, including hypospadias, inguinal hernias, and partial limb hypoplasia.[2] Confirmation with additional studies is necessary.

Sulfa drugs readily cross the placenta at all stages of gestation. Toxicities that may be observed in the newborn include jaundice and hemolytic anemia. Kernicterus, however, has not been reported to occur in the newborn after in utero sulfonamide exposure. Sulfonamide exposure has not been associated with congenital malformations in the newborn.

Anticoagulant Agents

Medical management of primary disorders of coagulation during pregnancy necessitates the use of anticoagulant agents. Such management must account for changes in coagulation factors during pregnancy, namely increased levels of factors VII, VIII, and X; platelets; and fibrinolytic activity and decreased levels of factors XI and XIII.

Two agents principally used are heparin and warfarin. Heparin potentiates the action of antithrombin III, which inhibits thrombin-induced platelet aggregation. Heparin does not cross the placenta, and there have been no reports of associated congenital defects.

Conversely, warfarin, a coumarin derivative, has been demonstrated to cause significant problems in the fetus and newborn.[7] The use of warfarin during the first trimester may result in significant anomalies in up to 30% of the exposed cases. The fetal warfarin syndrome classically includes facial abnormalities and stippling of the axial skeleton epiphyses. Other features that may be present include mild hypoplasia of the nails, shortened fingers, low birth weight, and central nervous system and eye abnormalities. Scoliosis and congenital heart defects also have been reported. Recent prospective studies suggest that exposure to warfarin during the second and third trimesters will not cause central nervous system or eye abnormalities in newborns.[7]

Anticonvulsant Agents

The objective of anticonvulsant therapy during pregnancy is to minimize the severity and frequency of seizures in the mother and to decrease the risk to the fetus. Unfortunately, data on teratogenicity for many anticonvulsant agents are difficult to interpret because poorly controlled seizures with resulting hypoxia in both the mother and fetus may act as a confounding variable.

Phenobarbital is an anticonvulsant used in the treatment of grand mal and focal motor-seizure disorders. Use of phenobarbital has been linked to facial defects and mild to moderate growth retardation. Newborn coagulation defects that may result in severe hemorrhage immediately after birth also have been described.[2] The exact mechanism is unknown but may involve fetal vitamin K depletion and suppression of vitamin K–dependent coagulation factors. Additional vitamin K and fresh frozen plasma can be given for treatment. Neonatal withdrawal and hypocalcemia also have been observed in infants exposed to phenobarbital in utero.

Phenytoin (Dilantin) is another anticonvulsant used in the treatment of grand mal, focal-motor, and psychomotor seizures and status epilepticus during pregnancy. Fetal hydantoin syndrome is caused by phenytoin exposure and includes mild to moderate growth retardation, mild cognitive and motor delays, and craniofacial and limb abnormalities.[7] No safe dose of phenytoin during pregnancy has been found. As with phenobarbital, newborn coagulation defects with phenytoin use have been observed. These defects occur despite vitamin K administration at birth.

Primidone (Mysoline) is an anticonvulsant often used to treat psychomotor seizures. Although a number of anomalies have been reported, none appear to be consistently associated with its use.[2] These include dysmorphic facies, phalangeal hypoplasia, growth retardation, microcephaly, and cardiac defects. These anomalies are similar to those observed with phenytoin or phenobarbital use, which is not unusual because phenobarbital is a normal metabolite of primidone. The exposed infant, therefore, is also at risk for hemorrhagic disease and withdrawal.

Ethosuximide (Zarontin) is an anticonvulsant used to control petit mal seizures. Specific information relating ethosuximide to congenital defects does not exist. Trimethadione (Tridione) is another anticonvulsant that may be used to treat petit mal epilepsy. It has been associated, however, with increased fetal loss when used during pregnancy. A fetal trimethadione syndrome of congenital malformations also has been described.[7] This syndrome consists of mental and growth deficiencies and craniofacial, cardiovascular, and genitourinary anomalies. The use of agents other than trimethadione during pregnancy is recommended.

Valproic acid (Depakene) is an anticonvulsant often used as adjunct therapy to control a variety of seizure disorders. In animal studies it has been noted to be a potent teratogen. In humans, malformations similar to the fetal hydantoin syndrome have been reported. Valproic acid should be used with caution during pregnancy.

In summary, the use of anticonvulsants during pregnancy presents risks to the fetus that must be weighed against the risks of poorly controlled seizures. Studies investigating the teratogenic potential of various agents have been hampered by the necessary use of multiple drug therapies. The American Academy of Pediatrics' Committee on Drugs recommends that therapy with phenobarbital or phenytoin during pregnancy should not be changed in favor of other anticonvulsants.[9]

Asthma Medications

Although there are no reports linking beta-sympathomimetic agents (i.e., isoproterenol, albuterol, and terbutaline) to congenital anomalies, direct effects on the fetus have been demonstrated at birth. One effect is transient fetal hyperglycemia followed by an increase in serum insulin and subsequent fetal hypoglycemia. Adverse cardiovascular effects, including maternal and fetal tachycardia and hypotension, have been reported. Fetal distress after such episodes of hypotension has not been reported. Finally, beta-mimetics are known to decrease the severity of neonatal respiratory distress syndrome by stimulating production and secretion of surfactant.

No reports associate aminophylline or theophylline with congenital defects.[2] Theophylline readily crosses the placenta in amounts comparable with that in maternal serum. Transient tachycardia, jitteriness, irritability, and vomiting have been reported in newborns when maternal serum levels have been in the high therapeutic range at the time of delivery. There have been reports of neonatal theophylline withdrawal characterized by episodes of apnea, which resolve with theophylline treatment.

Cardiovascular Medications

There is no evidence demonstrating an association between cardiac glycosides and congenital defects. Digitalis and its metabolites do cross the placenta, with higher fetal concentrations for a given dose being achieved later in pregnancy. For this reason some fetal tachyarrhythmias have been treated with maternal digoxin administration. Methyldopa (Aldomet) also crosses the placenta, and similar concentrations appear in fetal and maternal serum.[12] The newborn infant will excrete the drug slowly after delivery. Fetal serum levels may be sufficient to lower systolic blood pressure in the first days of life. No reports associate the maternal use of methyldopa with major malformations.

The maternal use of quinidine, an antiarrhythmic drug, has not been associated with congenital anomalies in the newborn. Neonatal thrombocytopenia has been reported with maternal use. Procainamide (Pronestyl), an antiarrhythmic agent with actions similar to quinidine, also is not associated with congenital anomalies. Fetal tachyarrhythmias have been successfully treated with maternal administration.

Diuretics are commonly used drugs in the management of hypertension and cardiovascular disease. They are not indicated in the treatment of hypertension associated with preeclampsia because they are ineffective and actually may decrease placental perfusion. Furosemide (Lasix) is a potent diuretic that readily crosses the placenta and can result in increased fetal urine production. Furosemide may further elevate serum uric acid levels already increased in toxemia. No fetal anomalies have been associated with its use. Thiazide diuretics (i.e., hydrochlorothiazide) readily cross the placenta and have not been shown to be associated with congenital malformations when used in the second and third trimester.[2] Data on first trimester use are limited. There has been associated neonatal thrombocytopenia with the use of thiazide diuretics near term. Spironolactone (Aldactone), a potassium-conserving diuretic often used as adjunct therapy with thiazide diuretics, has not been associated with congenital defects. The known antiandrogenic effects of spironolactone, however, may be a relative contraindication for use during pregnancy.

Chemotherapeutic Agents

Chemotherapy is the mainstay of treatment for disseminated neoplastic disease. Chemotherapeutic agents administered during pregnancy need special consideration.[2] However, evaluation of pregnancies during which chemotherapy was given—that is, evaluation of their outcomes—is limited by the small number of cases. Multiple drug regimens and concurrent use of radiation therapy make evaluations of specific agents extremely difficult.

Alkylating agents represent the single most commonly used group of chemotherapeutic agents. Their mechanism of cytotoxicity is not well understood. Cyclophosphamide (Cytoxan) has been reported to be associated with congenital malformations after first trimester use. These include a flattened nasal bridge, anomalous extremities, single coronary artery, inguinal hernias, imperforate anus, and growth retardation. Exposure to cyclophosphamide during the second and third trimesters does not appear to increase risk for congenital malformations. Nitrogen mustard is another alkylating agent that has been used during the first trimester in a limited number of cases and that has not been associated with congenital malformations.

The data for cytosine arabinoside, an antimetabolite, are less straightforward. Although normal outcomes have been reported after use during the first trimester, congenital and chromosomal anomalies also have been reported. These include anomalies of the extremities and atretic external auditory canals. Fluorouracil is a pyrimidine analogue that also has been reported to cause malformations after first trimester use, although experience with this agent is limited. Thioguanine is a purine analogue that has been associated with malformations and chromosomal anomalies. Mercaptopurine is associated with infant stillbirth and prematurity. Methotrexate, an antimetabolite that antagonizes folic acid, has been reported to result in normal pregnancies and in anomalies such as cranial malformations and digital defects. The vinca alkaloids are antimitotic chemotherapeutic agents. Use of vincristine during the first trimester has been limited, but there is one report of an association with small malpositioned kidneys.[10]

Finally, daunorubicin, an anthracycline antibiotic, has been studied mostly after use in later pregnancy. There have been no observed congenital defects. Doxorubicin (Adriamycin), another anthracycline antibiotic, similarly has been reported to be free from association with congenital defects.

Obstetric Drugs

Many of the drugs used during the course of obstetric practice are discussed elsewhere (see discussion of narcotic analgesics and hormonal agents). Magnesium sulfate is a commonly used tocolytic agent for treatment of premature labor. Magnesium readily crosses the placenta, resulting in elevated fetal serum levels that may remain elevated, because of a rather long elimination half-life, for up to 7 days after delivery. Reports associate maternal administration of magnesium sulfate with neurologic depression of the neonate. Respiratory depression, muscle weakness, gastrointestinal disturbances, and loss of reflexes also may occur. Interaction with aminoglycoside antibiotics has been reported to potentiate respiratory depression.[8]

Oxytocin (Pitocin) is a pharmacologic agent used to induce or augment labor at term. Its use has been associated to some degree with hyperbilirubinemia in the neonate.[14]

Psychoactive Agents. Diazepam (Valium) is a commonly used sedative and antianxiety agent. It rapidly crosses the placenta to equilibrate with maternal serum levels. First trimester use of this type of agent has been associated with inguinal hernias, cardiac defects, and pyloric stenosis. Second trimester use is associated with hemangiomas and cardiac defects. Adverse effects are seen in the neonate with use of diazepam at high doses or for extended periods around the time of delivery. These include hypertonia, lethargy, and feeding difficulties. Characteristics of withdrawal —namely tremors, irritability and hypertonicity, diarrhea, and vomiting—also have been observed.

Haloperidol (Haldol) is an antipsychotic drug that has not been associated with congenital malformations.

Tricyclic antidepressants are agents that block norepinephrine and serotonin uptake. They include amitriptyline (Elavil), desipramine (Norpramin), imipramine (Tofranil), and nortriptyline (Aventyl). In general, neonatal withdrawal after in utero exposure can be expected, and urinary retention may occur in some infants. Although there is no definite correlation between these agents and congenital malformations, case reports suggest a possible association with limb reduction anomalies, craniofacial anomalies, adrenal hypoplasia, and diaphragmatic hernias.[2]

Lithium, an antimanic agent, has been definitely related to congenital anomalies of the cardiovascular system after maternal use in the first trimester.[2] The most frequent cardiovascular defect is the Ebstein anomaly. When lithium is used near term, symptoms of toxicity in the newborn have been reported. These include cyanosis, hypotonia, bradycardia, thyroid depression, cardiac arrhythmias, gastrointestinal bleeding, diabetes insipidus, and shock.

Phenothiazines, as typified by promethazine (Phenergan) and chlorpromazine, readily cross the placenta. Neonatal depression characterized by hypotonia and lethargy has been noted when excessive doses are ingested around term. In addition, extrapyramidal side effects have been observed in term infants delivered soon after maternal ingestion. These effects may persist for months after delivery. No evidence of an association between chlorpromazine and congenital malformations has been noted.

Hormonal Agents

The classic case of a hormonal agent adversely affecting the fetus is diethylstilbestrol (DES). DES has been implicated as a causal agent of multiple types of reproductive anomalies, including carcinoma of the cervix, which occurs in female infants born to mothers who used this agent during pregnancy.[2] Male infants may show genital anomalies as well.

The use of estrogens during pregnancy, such as continued use of birth control medications, has been linked to masculinization of female infants. The use of these agents with progesterone activity also has been shown to result in female virilization. Further, ambiguous genitalia of males has been reported with progesterone exposure. Hypospadias is reported to be associated with estrogen exposure.

Dexamethasone is a corticosteroid often used to promote the maturation of the fetal respiratory system in cases of premature labor and delivery. No reports associate dexamethasone use at any time during gestation with congenital malformations.

Clomiphene (Clomid) is an agent used to promote ovulation in infertile women. It is contraindicated once ovulation and fertilization have occurred. Use of clomiphene after fertilization has been demonstrated to cause a high rate of malformations. Reported malformations include cleft lip, hypospadias, imperforate anus, polydactyly, Down syndrome, congenital heart defects, and anencephaly.[2]

The use of antithyroid agents during pregnancy has been associated with fetal hypothyroidism, growth retardation, and other congenital malformations. The incidence of these anomalies depends on which antithyroid agent is used. Propylthiouracil now is considered the agent of choice in the management of maternal hyperthyroidism during pregnancy.

As one might expect, radioactive iodine is contraindicated in pregnancy because of its simultaneous ablation of the maternal as well as the fetal thyroid gland. In fact, the use of providone-iodine before delivery has been reported to cause transient hypothyroidism in some newborns.

Toxin Exposure

Mercury poisoning demonstrated in the Minamata disease series and the Iraqi experience has heightened awareness of the potentially devastating effects of environmental toxins. Methylmercury is a teratogen, especially in the developing brain.[6] It may result in abortion, stillbirth, neonatal death, microcephaly, cerebral palsy, deafness, blindness, and growth deficiency. Polychlorinated biphenyl (PCB) exposure also may adversely affect the fetus. The effects include growth retardation and altered immune function. A particular constellation of symptoms, including dark skin, eye disease, severe acne, and growth retardation, also has been reported in offspring exposed in utero. However, the relationship between maternal dose and fetal complications remains unclear.

REFERENCES

1. Aranda JV, Hales BF, and Gibbs J: Perinatal pharmacology. In Fanaroff AA and Martin RJ, editors: Neonatal-perinatal medicine, ed 4, St Louis, 1987, The CV Mosby Co.
2. Briggs GG, Freeman RK, and Yaffe SJ: Drugs in pregnancy and lactation, ed 2, Baltimore, 1986, Williams & Wilkins.
3. Byer AJ, Taylor TR, and Semmer JR: Acetaminophen overdose in the third trimester of pregnancy, JAMA 247:3114, 1982.
4. Heinonen OP, Sone D, and Shapiro S: Birth defects and drugs in pregnancy, Littleton, Mass, 1977, Publishing Sciences Group.
5. Hutchings DE, editor: Prenatal abuse of licit and illicit drugs, New York, 1989, Annals of the New York Academy of Sciences.
6. Jones KL: Effects of chemical and environmental agents. In Creasy RK and Resnik R, editors: Maternal-fetal medicine: principles and practice, ed 2, Philadelphia, 1989, WB Saunders Co.
7. Jones KL: Smiths' recognizable patterns of human malformation, ed 4, Philadelphia, 1988, WB Saunders Co.
8. L'Hommedien CS, et al: Potentiation of magnesium sulfate-induced neuromuscular weakness by gentamicin, tobramycin and amikacin, J Pediatr 102:629, 1983.
9. Marx CM: Effect of drugs on the fetus. In Cloherty J and Stark A, editors: Manual of neonatal care, ed 2, Boston, 1985, Little, Brown & Co.
10. Mennati MT, Shepard TH, and Mellman WS: Fetal renal malformation following treatment of Hodgkin's disease during pregnancy, Obstet Gynecol 46:194, 1975.
11. Powell RD, DeGowin RL, and Alving AS: Nitrofuzantoin-induced hemolysis, J Lab Clin Med 62:1002, 1963.
12. Rayburn WF and Zuspan FP: Drug therapy in obstetrics and gynecology, Norwalk, Conn, 1982, Appleton-Century-Crofts.
13. Rumack CM, et al: Neonatal intracranial hemorrhage and maternal use of aspirin, Obstet Gynecol 58(suppl):525, 1981.
14. Singhi S and Singh M: Pathogenesis of oxytocin-induced neonatal hyperbilirubinaemia, Arch Dis Child 54:100, 1979.

34

Abortion

Eric A. Schaff

An induced abortion is a purposeful termination of a pregnancy before extrauterine viability. Women always have relied on abortions as a last means to control their family size. Only when contraceptive services become universally available to all sexually active persons will the need for abortion be significantly reduced.

In the United States before 1973 each state had regulations regarding the criteria for a legal abortion. Epidemiologic surveillance studies on abortion in the United States and Europe demonstrated that legal abortion had a beneficial effect on the health of women with an unintended pregnancy by offering a safer option than an illegal abortion or carrying a pregnancy to term.

In 1973 the Supreme Court set the following guidelines in the well-known case, *Roe v. Wade:*

1. In the first trimester (up to 13 weeks from the onset of the last menstrual period), a woman in consultation with her physician is free to choose an abortion.
2. In the second trimester (from 13 to 24 weeks gestation) the state can regulate the abortion procedure to promote the health of the pregnant woman.
3. After viability the state has interests in promoting fetal life and can regulate or ban the abortion procedure except to preserve the life or health of a pregnant woman.

Approximately 1.3 million abortions are performed annually in the United States, a ratio of one abortion to every three live births. About 26% of abortions are performed on women 19 years of age or younger; 67% of the women are white, 80% are unmarried, and more than 50% have not been pregnant previously.[1]

A brief review of legal decisions regarding teenagers and abortion is included to help pediatricians understand issues of parental consent and notification laws.

In 1976, in *Planned Parenthood of Central Missouri v. Danforth,* the Supreme Court decided that a teenager has a legal right to abortion in consultation with her physician and without parental consent.

In 1979, in *Belloti v. Baird,* the Supreme Court reaffirmed a minor's right to an abortion and found that a Massachusetts parental consent law was unconstitutional. The Court left open the possibility that parental consent might be permissible if a judicial or an administrative bypass was an option for the minor to demonstrate her maturity or to serve her best interests by means of a confidential abortion.

In 1986, in *Hodgson v. Minnesota,* a district court struck down a parental consent law with a judicial bypass because it was unduly burdensome, requiring both parents to consent and a mandatory waiting period that was too long. The court also found that the law failed to protect minors and did not promote or improve parent-child communication.

In 1988 a federal court overruled the *Hodgson v. Minnesota* decision, claiming that the two-parent consent and a waiting period were constitutional. The Supreme Court will likely rule on these issues in the near future.

In caring for adolescent patients it is important to keep pregnancy high on the differential diagnosis list because it can accompany vague symptoms. Denial of the possibility of pregnancy is common. Many pregnancy tests are readily available and are rapid, simple, and inexpensive to perform in the office. Positive blood and urine pregnancy test results generally are reliable 10 days after conception. A negative pregnancy test result should be repeated every 2 weeks until menses occur or the test result becomes positive.

The medical evaluation of a pregnant teenager should include a complete pelvic examination to estimate uterine size and to obtain routine cultures for the presence of gonorrhea and chlamydia. Early dating of the pregnancy and detection and treatment of diseases are important regardless of the outcome of the pregnancy. In case of doubt about the dates of a pregnancy, ultrasound, which has a high degree of accuracy, can be used. The possibility of rape or incest should be considered, particularly for very young teenagers.

When contemplating her pregnancy alternatives, each teenager must consider many facets of her life, such as her age, marital status, health, education, financial situation, religious upbringing, family support, and future plans, as well as the medical prognosis for her fetus. Pregnant teenagers need to know their options, including carrying the pregnancy to term and keeping the infant, adoption, and abortion. They should be encouraged to make this decision by considering the entire perspective of their lives.

The pediatrician should provide nonjudgmental support and explore whether the youth can involve family members or other potential sources of counsel such as relatives, siblings, clergy, teachers, counselors, and boyfriend. Some teenagers are unable to involve their parents in a discussion of their pregnancy. Some effort should be made to assess the boyfriend's emotional involvement.

Pediatricians should be aware of state laws regarding public funding for abortion through Medicaid and parental notification or consent requirements. If the teenager chooses an abortion, the pediatrician should provide information about the procedure, the risks, and the alternatives. Pediatricians who are morally unable to support an abortion decision should refer their patient to a colleague who can.

FIRST TRIMESTER AND EARLY SECOND TRIMESTER ABORTIONS

Suction curettage initially was used only in first trimester pregnancies. With additional experience, gynecologists have successfully used this procedure for the first 20 weeks of gestation. This procedure requires the insertion of cervical plugs for predilation softening 6 to 24 hours before the procedure, local cervical anesthesia (rarely general anesthesia), dilation of the cervix with metal dilators, and the introduction of various sizes of cannula tips to suction fetal and placental parts. A very early abortion, sometimes called a *menstrual extraction,* can be accomplished in one visit with a thin suction cannula and without dilation of the cervix.

Products of conception should be identified and examined microscopically by a pathologist. In early second trimester abortions, a curette and/or a forceps may be used to ensure that the uterine cavity is empty. Suction or curettage were used in almost 98% of all abortions performed in 1985.

Approximately 90% of all abortions occur in the first trimester. The maternal mortality rate for early abortions is 0.5 to 0.7/100,000 procedures.[1] Occasionally infections, bleeding, retained products of conception, and "missed" abortion occur; uterine perforation occurs rarely.

LATE SECOND TRIMESTER ABORTIONS

Later abortions involve the injection of hypertonic saline, hypertonic urea, or prostaglandin, often in combination with cervical plug insertion and oxytocin to augment contractions. Later abortions are more dangerous, with a mortality rate of about 3/100,000. In 1985 fewer than 2% of abortions were performed by these methods. Complications include those seen with earlier abortions, as well as embolism, hypernatremia, disseminated intravascular coagulation, and cervical laceration.

All women with Rh negativity should receive an injection of Rh immunoglobulin. Contraceptive methods should be discussed and prescribed if appropriate. Oral contraceptive pills can be started in the first week after abortion. In 2 to 3 weeks the teenager should return to receive follow-up counseling and should be reexamined when the uterus is almost back to normal size.

The majority of studies on abortion conclude that there is no evidence that infertility, spontaneous miscarriages, or a propensity to deliver babies prematurely are late sequelae. Neither is there evidence that psychiatric problems after abortion are more common than those after childbirth.

RU 486

RU 486, Mifepristone, is an antiprogestin agent that has been studied in France and has been found to be 95% effective as an early abortifacient.[2] It is taken orally or vaginally up to 7 weeks after the last menses in conjunction with a prostaglandin. It is not an invasive procedure, and therefore there is no risk of infection or perforation. Reported side effects include mild gastrointestinal problems and prolonged uterine bleeding. A small percentage of women require instrumentation to complete the abortion. RU 486 also is being tested in the treatment of Cushing syndrome, breast cancer, endometriosis, and glaucoma.

Presently RU 486 is unavailable in the United States. Although abortion continues to be a divisive issue, if RU 486 proves to be safer than surgical abortion, then it should be made available to all women who choose abortion.

REFERENCES

1. Abortion surveillance, United States, 1984-85, MMWR 39(SS-2):11, 1989.
2. Couzinet B et al: Termination of early pregnancy by the progesterone antagonist RU 486 (Mifepristone), N Engl J Med 315:1565, 1986.

35

Perinatal Medicine

One

Overview

Nicholas M. Nelson

PERINATAL MEDICINE

The sharper inflection of the general and continuing downward trend in neonatal mortality in the United States beginning around 1970 (Fig. 35-1) has engendered much discussion because it is chronologically coincident with the rise of modern perinatal-neonatal medicine. This field has been characterized by a level of intense obstetric and pediatric collaboration on the needs of the fetus and newborn that was unknown a generation ago.

Fig. 35-2 shows that much of this progress has been achieved through better management of the obstetric aspects of the perinatal period, particularly near or at term gestation. This has been associated with a reciprocal rise to prominence

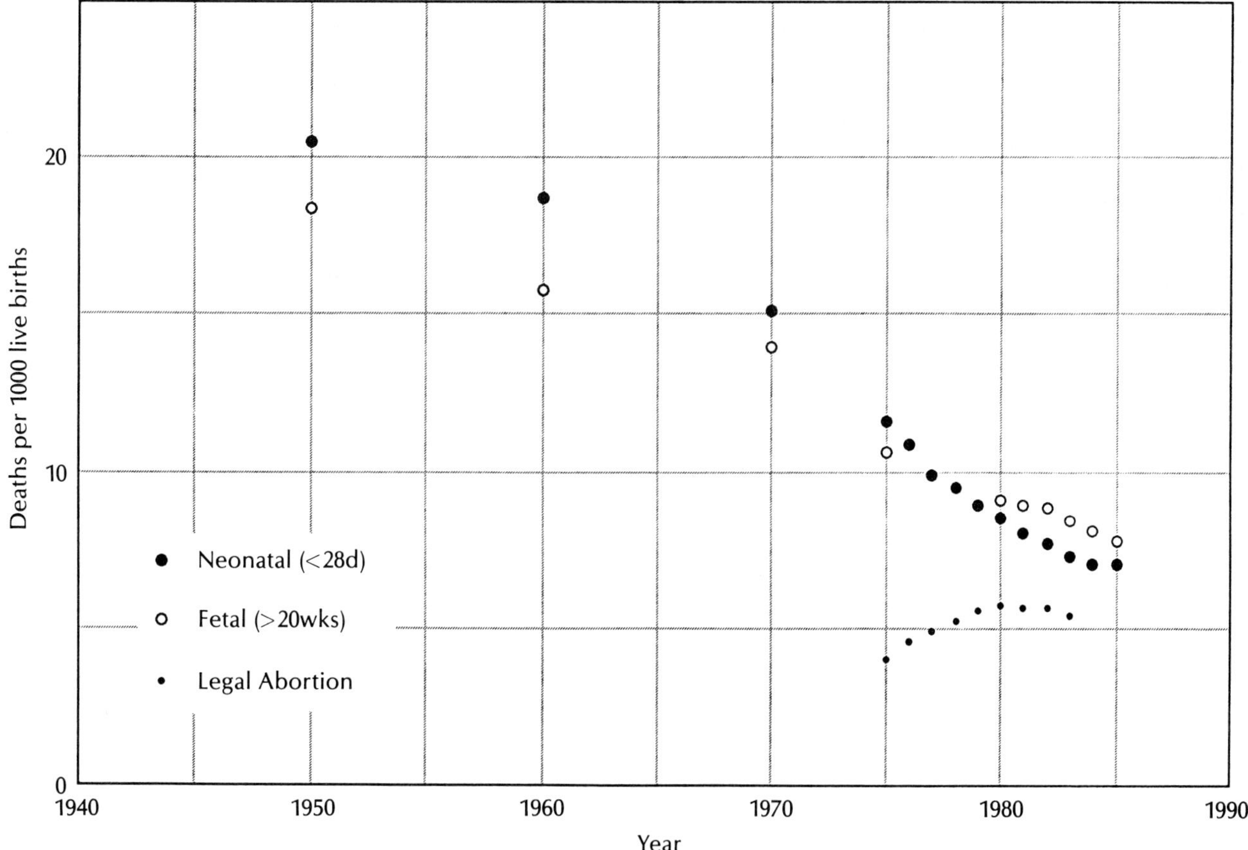

Fig. 35-1 Fetal and neonatal mortality in the United States.

Data from Health, United States, 1987. U.S. Department of Health and Human Services—Public Health Service, Centers for Diseases Control, National Center for Health Statistics, Hyattsville, Maryland, 1988, DHHS Publication No. (PHS) 88-1232.

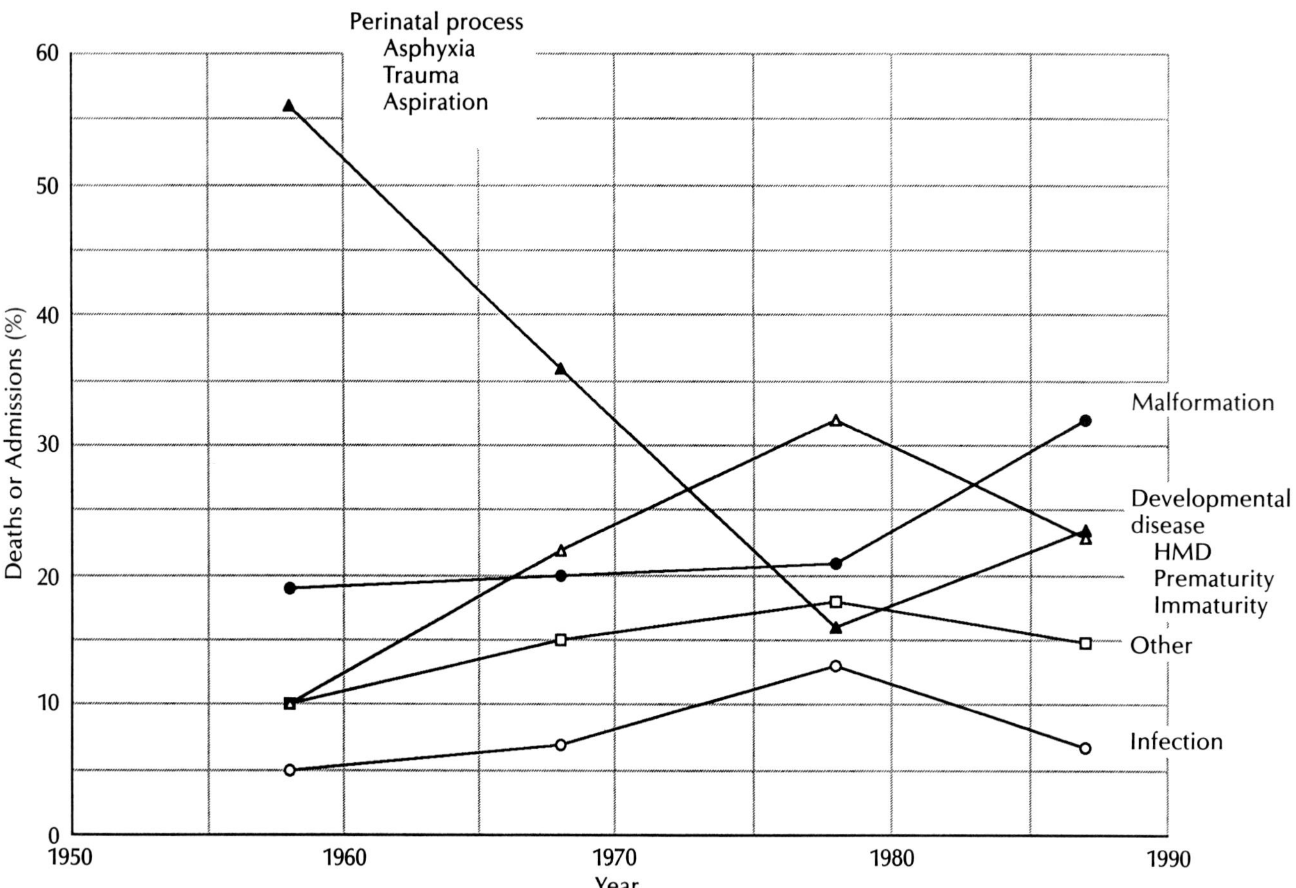

Fig. 35-2 Incidence and fatality rates of certain perinatal conditions. Experience at Milton S Hershey Medical Center, Hershey, Penn (1973-1987) and the United Kingdom. *HMD,* Hyaline membrane disease.

Modified from Vuilliamy DG: The newborn child, ed 2, Boston, 1967, Little, Brown, & Co.

of premature labor (which precipitates immature but genetically sound fetuses) as the major unyielding problem of modern obstetrics. If that issue were resolved, most neonatologists could retire from active duty and instead observe and support the progress of geneticists, teratologists, and others in addressing the bedrock problems of congenital malformations and heritable diseases.

Scientific and technologic advances (Table 35-1) have formed a necessary, but not sufficient, foundation for this achievement. Just as the entrepreneur must have channels for the distribution of his or her product from factory through dealership to consumer, neonatal and perinatal care providers must establish ways of identifying the high-risk target population likely to need such care and then bringing that population to the site for their provision, inasmuch as multidisciplinary human services are not as easily distributed as are products.

Meeting this requirement has necessitated assessing the risk of perinatal morbidity or mortality as far in advance of the anticipated risk event as possible (Table 35-2). Pregnant women identified as being at risk of having a complicated pregnancy, labor, or delivery (about 15% of the total) are best managed under the supervision of a perinatologist, typically in their own community hospital (level I), where about 50% may deliver safely, the remainder being referred to a facility of broader capabilities (level II). Nearly 1 in 15 of these moderate-risk patients probably will have an unanticipated stillbirth; of the 80% of pregnant women initially identified as being at low risk, however, about 1 in 30 will develop an unanticipated problem in pregnancy (e.g., toxemia, vaginal bleeding, or premature labor) and require referral. The delivered infant may also develop unanticipated problems requiring referral, but Table 35-3 shows that most neonatal morbidity and mortality risk factors (e.g., maternal age, diabetes, abortion, gestational age, or birth weight) can be anticipated well before delivery.

Although the perinatologist (the only physician who always attends two patients) who has accepted the responsibility for safeguarding the health of the mother and fetus is first concerned with the mother, the near-total conquest of maternal mortality in developed countries has allowed him or her to focus at least equal attention on fetal health—both prepartum and intrapartum (Tables 35-4 and 35-5).

Fetal growth, and therefore accurate gestational age, is monitored by abdominal ultrasound techniques with considerable accuracy (even to the point of identifying "catch up" growth in some growth-retarded fetuses) by measuring the fetal crown-rump length (at 6 to 14 weeks) and later the biparietal diameter (at 17 to 26 weeks). Total intrauterine volume also can be estimated and the frequency and intensity

Table 35-1 *Advances in Perinatal-Neonatal Medicine*

YEARS	MORTALITY/1000 LIVE BIRTHS		BASIC SCIENCE	OBSTETRICS	ANESTHESIA	PEDIATRICS
	FETAL	NEONATAL				
1940-1950	18	21	Blood grouping, antibiotics	Elimination of maternal mortality		Umbilical venous catheterization, exchange transfusion
1950-1960	16	18	Human karyotyping, surfactant, blood gas measurements, pulmonary function tests	Elimination of mid forceps and high forceps	Apgar score, local anesthesia	Phototherapy
1960-1970	15	15	Lecithin/sphingomyelin ratio, shake test, ultrasound	Liberalized abortion practices, RhoGAM, fetal heart rate monitoring		Umbilical artery catheterization, regionalization of care
1970-1980	10	10	Rubella vaccine, steroid induction of surfactant	Liberal use of cesarean section, deferred labor, regionalization of care, stress testing	Constant positive airway pressure, positive end-expiratory pressure	Total parenteral nutrition
1980-1990	6 (?)	6 (?)	Prostglandins cause of onset of labor (?)	Fetal ultrasound	High-frequency ventilation	Neonatal ultrasound, surfactant replacement
1990-2000	(?)	(?)		Arrest premature labor (?)	(?)	(?)

Table 35-2 *Prenatal Risk Factors*

	MAJOR	MODERATE	MINOR
Fetal	Premature (Hx*)		
	Postmature (Hx)	Infant >10 lb (Hx)	Congenital malformation (Hx)
	Stillbirth (Hx)	Intrauterine growth retardation (Hx)	
	Neonatal death (Hx)		
	Exchange transfusion (Hx)	Rh sensitization	
Obstetric	Uterine malformation	Small pelvis	
		Infertility	
	Abnormal cytologic findings	Vaginal spotting	
	Incompetent cervix	Habitual aborter (Hx)	
	Multiple pregnancy	Grand multiparity (>5)	
	Abnormal presentation	Cesarean birth (Hx)	
	Polyhydramnios	Uterine dystocia	
	Toxemia, moderate to severe	Toxemia, mild	Toxemia (Hx)
		Eclampsia (Hx)	
Medical	Endocrine ablation (Hx)	Thyroid disease	Small stature (<60 in)
	Sickle cell disease	Hemoglobin <9 g/dl	Hemoglobin 9-10.9 g/dl
	Heart disease, severe (II-IV)	Heart disease, moderate (I)	
	Renal disease, moderate to severe	Pyelitis (present or Hx)	Cystitis (present or Hx)
	Hypertension, chronic diabetes (≥class A-II)	Prediabetes (Class A-I)	Diabetes (family Hx)
		Viral disease	
		"Flu" syndrome, severe	
		Pulmonary disease	
		Positive tuberculosis skin test (Hx)	
		Epilepsy (Hx)	
Psychosocial		≤15 yr, ≥35 yr age	
		<100 lb, >200 lb	Emotional problems
		Uneducated	
		Unmarried	
		Unregistered (prenatal care)	
		Medically indigent	
		Drug abuse (including alcohol)	Moderate alcohol use
			Smoker

From Hobel CJ et al: Prenatal and intrapartum high-risk screening, Am J Obstet Gynecol 117:1, 1973.
**Hx*, History of.

of fetal breathing movements observed as indexes of fetal well-being. The perinatologist uses either a Doppler-shift measuring device or a filtered electrocardiograph to assess fetal heart rate patterns when seeking evidence of healthy variability in the basal fetal heart rate in association with normal fetal movements (nonstress test).

If such variability is lacking (nonreactive nonstress test), or if there is evidence of fetal growth failure or a failing pregnancy (e.g., low maternal urinary estriol, indicating fetoplacental endocrine failure), then the perinatologist may want to stress the fetoplacental unit by mimicking labor, using sufficient oxytocin to produce at least three uterine contractions within 10 minutes. A positive test result, indicating uteroplacental insufficiency, is one in which each induced contraction is followed by a late (10-second delay) deceleration of the fetal heart rate (Table 35-5). This evidence is then weighed against that of fetal pulmonary maturity and the availability of neonatal special care, among other factors, in deciding whether to continue or terminate the pregnancy.

When assessing fetal health, many practitioners also wisely consult the mother regarding fetal activity. Indeed, some have incorporated her observations into a simple and effective plan for surveillance, despite an acknowledged lack of reproducibility of such observations.

NEONATAL MEDICINE

The major problems currently faced in neonatal special care units are indicated in the typical experiences shown in Table 35-6. Overall survival is exquisitely sensitive to gestational age (Fig. 35-3), and hyaline membrane disease of the newborn often imposes an added burden that can be fatal.

The major intellectual advance in neonatal medicine in the last generation probably has been the description of the appropriately grown (or inappropriately grown) infant (Fig. 35-4). Once grasped, this concept enhances the practitioner's approach to the newborn patient by focusing attention on those problems most likely to be encountered in the patient experiencing normal growth, undergrowth, or (more rarely) overgrowth. This approach depends critically on accurately assessing gestational age; in this assessment the fetal sonographic data, physical examination, and the mother's opinion should all be accorded approximately equal importance. Note also, in Fig. 35-4, that overall *mortality decreases by approximately 50% with each biweekly advance in gestation* beyond the onset of viability (currently around 25 weeks of gestation).

Some have questioned the wisdom and even the morality of investing precious societal resources in the effort to achieve

Table 35-3 *Neonatal Morbidity Risk**

RISK	PERCENT AFFECTED
Birth weight (g)	
≤1500	61.7
1501-2000	55.0
2001-2500	15.8
2501-3500	4.3
>3500	5.0
Gestational age (wk)	
≤27	21.6
28-31	18.4
32-33	15.0
34-35	9.0
36-37	3.8
≥38	1.1
Unknown	2.7
Maternal age (yr)	
<15	7.4
15-19	1.9
20-34	0
≥35	3.9
Perinatal asphyxia	
Absent (Apgar 8-10)	0
Moderate (Apgar 5-7)	3.1
Severe (Apgar 0-4)	11.0
Pregnancy	
Diabetes	34.7
Habitual aborter (≥3)	10.4
Premature rupture (≥24 hr)	6.3
Toxemia	4.5
Labor	
Complicated: e.g., induction, dystocia, hemorrhage	4.1
Delivery	
Abnormal presentation	6.4
Local anesthesia	2.4
Resuscitation	
Stimulants	11.8
Positive pressure	6.4
Male infant	4.1

*Experience at Milton S Hershey Medical Center, Hershey, Penn (1973-1989). The figures denote the percent of infants with a given descriptor who died or suffered severe illness.

survival in infants weighing less than 1500 or 1000 g at birth, in whom the incidence of chronic and crippling diseases (e.g., necrotizing enterocolitis and bronchopulmonary dysplasia) and crushing disappointments (e.g., intraventricular hemorrhage and the attendant neurologic catastrophe) begins to rise dramatically. These critics should study the data in Table 35-7 and be challenged to present 28% to 54% *normal* survivors of comparably devastating illnesses occurring at any other stage in life. Similarly criticized in 1913 regarding his efforts on behalf of marasmic infants in New York City's foundling hospitals, Dr. L. Emmet Holt, Sr., insisted, "These infants are *not* unfit, they are merely unfortunate!" Nonetheless, it would currently appear that 25 weeks of gestation and 700 g birth weight is the absolute floor for fetal viability.

REGIONALIZATION OF CARE

The advent of neonatal intensive care around 1960 presaged and somewhat catalyzed similar developments in obstetrics in such a manner that, around 1975, neonatally oriented pediatricians and fetally oriented obstetricians began engaging in close daily therapeutic collaboration over the needs of their patients. This and other forces led to the development of subspecialty boards of examiners in each discipline and culminated in the joint production in 1983 (by the American Academy of Pediatrics [AAP] and the American College of Obstetricians and Gynecologists [ACOG]) of *Guidelines for Perinatal Care,*[1] supplanting the AAP's preceding 5-yearly revisions of *Standards and Recommendations for Hospital Care of Newborn Infants*. This publication properly celebrates recent achievement in diminishing perinatal mortality (see Figs. 35-1 to 35-4), particularly in the under–1500 g birth weight group, and codifies many of the means that have brought it about, especially the process of regionalization in perinatal health care. This process is defined as a systems approach in which program components in a geographic area are defined and coordinated.

The phrase *defined and coordinated* implies more centralized planning than was historically the case. Rather, pioneering efforts in improving neonatal mortality were spontaneously and separately undertaken in Montreal, Toronto, New York, Denver, San Francisco, Boston, and many other sites beginning around 1960. These efforts attracted the attention of obstetricians, pediatricians, primary care physicians, parents, medical equipment developers, and, later, hos-

Table 35-4 *Assessment of Fetal Health—Prepartum*

	BIOCHEMICAL	BIOPHYSICAL
Genome	Karyotype by chorionic villus sampling*	
Well-being	Maternal urinary estriol determination Fetal blood sampling from cord vessels*	Electronic monitoring of fetal heart rate Nonstress test Oxytocin challenge test Ultrasound monitoring of fetal breathing
Maturity	Renal and muscular by amniotic creatinine* Pulmonary by amniotic lecithin/sphingomyelin ratio,* shake test*	Ultrasound monitoring of crown-rump length (early) and fetal biparietal diameter (late)
Semiqualitative		Maternal notation of fetal activity

*Invasive procedure.

pital boards of trustees, partly because they were glamorous, but mostly because they were successful. In a process of healthy and natural self-selection, hospitals began to identify themselves as providing what has come to be known as (level I, II, or III) perinatal-neonatal care. Given the size, demographics, and medical history of North America, a certain amount of natural geographic coalescence was inevitable. Also given the tendency for medical personnel to congregate in attractive urban and suburban environments, compounded by a certain amount of entrepreneurial spirit, some conflict over turf and duplication of services was equally inevitable—especially under a system of unlimited reimbursement in the United States that automatically paid back to hospitals nearly every dollar expended *(cost reimbursement)*. The *prospective hospital payment* system (diagnosis-related group [DRG]) inaugurated in the United States in July 1984 has not so far reversed unnecessary proliferation of perinatal services, despite the fact that they are expensive and many of the most needful consumers lack medical insurance.

Table 35-5 *Assessment of Fetal Health—Intrapartum*

OBSERVATION	SIGNIFICANCE
Monitoring of fetal heart rate during and after uterine contractions (stages I, II)	
Early deceleration	Compression of fetal head
Variable deceleration	Compression of umbilical cord
Late deceleration	Uteroplacental insufficiency
Sampling of fetal scalp pH (stage II)	Anticipate postpartum difficulties if pH <7.25

Nevertheless, regionalization of perinatal services has been remarkably effective in reducing perinatal mortality and, as important, has now been officially embraced as policy by the two most pertinent professional groups (AAP and ACOG).

How the concept develops in a given geographic area begins with the definition by her primary care provider of the pregnant patient's status and needs as she enters the health care system. That definition, once displayed against local availability of the requisite services, helps her physician determine the level of the institution that can best serve her needs.

To the physician in a given local community who would contend that the infant with respiratory distress or the laboring woman with ineffectual contractions is "within my level of competence," the proper response is "Agreed, but is the problem within your level of *availability?" A patient's medical outcome is not affected by the expertise of the physician who is not present*. The particular medical and surgical skills most frequently employed by the perinatologist and neonatologist were learned by nearly every general pediatrician or obstetrician during his or her residency. However, the neonatologist and perinatologist are hospital-based and *have no medical commitment other* than the high-risk pregnant mother or sick newborn, and these attentions of *time* (as well as expertise) have been the most important factors in reducing perinatal mortality.

Thus, based on the presumption that appropriate expertise is constantly available at each institutional level, the AAP-ACOG *Guidelines*[1] for institutional responsibility are shown

Table 35-6 *Discharge Diagnosis from Neonatal Intensive Care Unit, 3339 Admissions (1973-1980)**

DIAGNOSES	INFANTS AFFECTED (%)	TOTAL ADMISSIONS (%)
Developmental disease—1125 admissions		34
Hyaline membrane disease	70	
Immaturity, prematurity	16	
Other	14	
TOTAL	100	
Malformations—694 admissions		21
Cardiac	34	
Gastrointestinal	24	
Multiple	12	
Neurologic	10	
Other	20	
TOTAL	100	
Perinatal process—496 admissions		15
Transient tachypnea	45	
Perinatal asphyxia	34	
Aspiration syndromes	15	
Other	6	
TOTAL	100	
Infection—442 admissions		13
Congenital pneumonia	53	
Sepsis	36	
Acquired pneumonia	6	
Intrauterine infection	5	
TOTAL	100	
Other disease—582 admissions		17
Hematologic	31	
Metabolic	21	
Gastrointestinal	18	
Respiratory	8	
Renal	2	
Other	20	
TOTAL	100	
GRAND TOTAL		100

*Experience at Milton S Hershey Medical Center, Hershey, Penn.

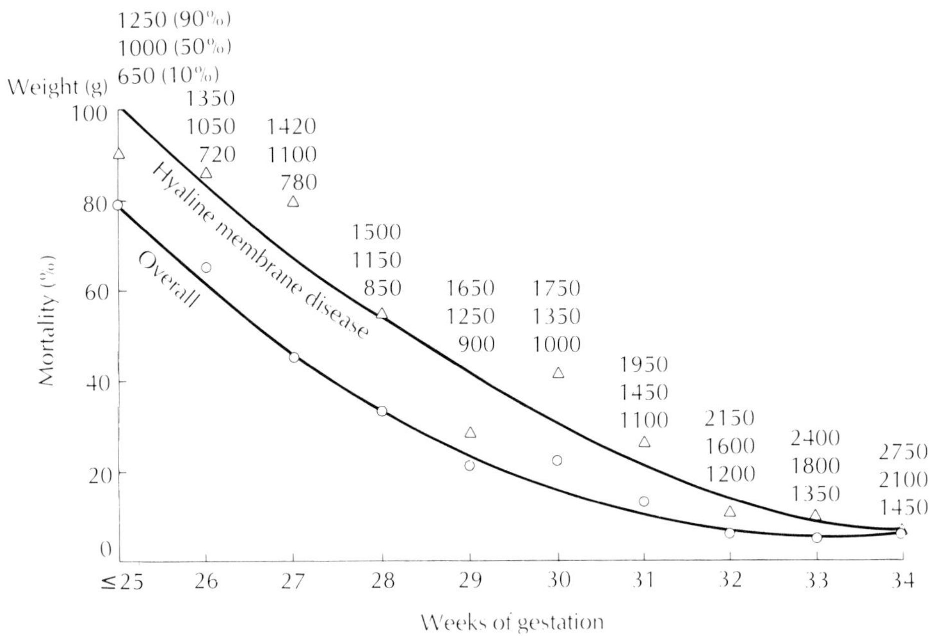

Fig. 35-3 Neonatal mortality in 1114 admissions at Milton S. Hershey Medical Center (1976-1980), caused by haline membrane disease and overall factors. The 90th, 50th, and 10th percentiles for grams birth weight at each week of gestation are taken from the Denver data.

From Battalgia FC and Lubchenco LO: A practical classification of newborn infants by weight and gestational age, J Pediatr 71:159, 1967.

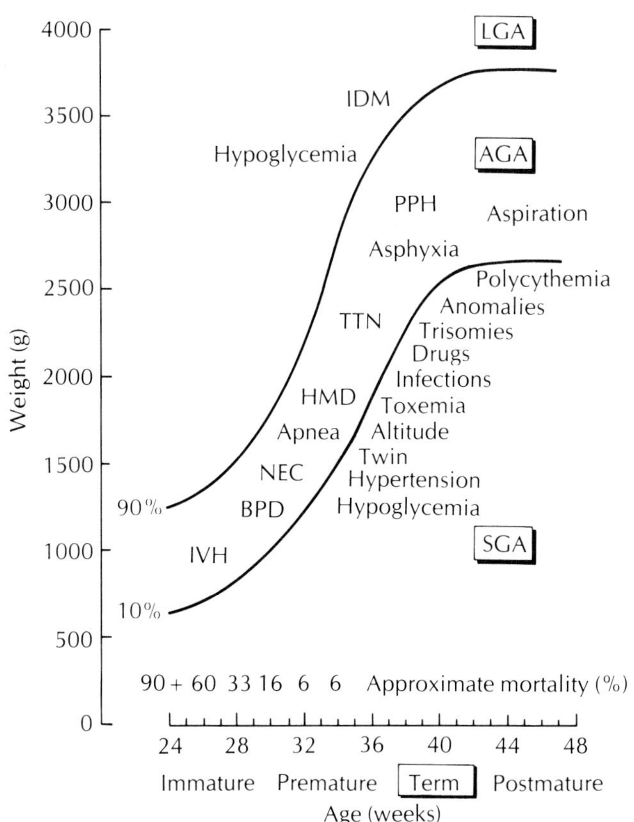

Fig. 35-4 Specific perinatal clinical entities frequently encountered in the three major developmental channels: (1) large for gestational age *(LGA)*; (2) appropriate for gestational age *(AGA)*; (3) small for gestational age *(SGA)*. Expected approximate overall mortality (Fig. 36-3) is superimposed on the abscissa. *IDM*, Infant of a diabetic mother; *IVH*, intraventricular hemorrhage; *BPD*, bronchopulmonary dysplasia; *NEC*, necrotizing enterocolitis; *HMD*, hyaline membrane disease; *TTN*, transient tachypnea of the newborn; *PPH*, persistent pulmonary hypertension or persistent fetal circulation.

From Battaglia FC and Lubchenco LO: A practical classification of newborn infants by weight and gestational age, J Pediatr 71:159, 1967.

Table 35-7 *Neurologic Outcome Among Very Low–Birth-Weight Infants: Results from a 2-Year Follow-Up Study*

OUTCOME	90 INFANTS, 501-1000 g (%)	201 INFANTS, 1001-1500 g (%)
Normal	27.8	53.7
Impaired	7.8	10.0
Died	60.0	23.9
Lost to follow-up care	4.4	12.4

From Hack M, Fanaroff AA, and Merrkatz IR: The low-birth-weight infant—evaluation of a changing outlook, N Engl J Med 301:1162, 1979.

in Tables 35-8 to 35-10. These guidelines imply and demand a high level of bidirectional and tridirectional communication, education, and, where necessary, transportation (including return transportation of the infant to his or her hospital of birth, once the need for intensive care has subsided). *Education and communication frequently diminish the need for transportation of the infant.*

Some primary care practitioners may feel that taking responsibility for a level I unit provides insufficient professional gratification or challenge. They should inspect the experience, set out in Table 35-11, from a large and unselected maternal population and note how many of the problems listed they are likely to encounter in their own primary care practice. They also should note how many of these conditions they

Table 35-8 *Perinatal Care Programs—Ancillary Services**

SERVICES	LEVEL I	LEVEL II	LEVEL III
Laboratory (microtechnique for neonates)			
Within 15 min	Hematocrit		
Within 1 hr	Glucose, BUN, creatinine, blood gases, routine urinalysis	Blood gases, blood type, and Rh, electrolytes, coagulation studies, blood available from type and screen program	Special blood and amniotic fluid tests (creatinine, lecithin/sphingomyelin ratio, shake, karyotype)
Within 1-6 hr	CBC, platelet appearance on smear, blood chemistries, blood type and cross-match, Coombs' test, bacterial smear	Coagulation studies, magnesium, urine, electrolytes, and chemistries	
Within 24-28 hr	Bacterial cultures and antibiotic sensitivity	Level I plus liver function tests, metabolic screening	
Within hospital or facilities available	Viral cultures		All laboratory facilities available
Radiography and ultrasound	Technicians on call 24 hr/day available in 30 min Technicians experienced in performing abdominal, pelvic, and obstetric ultrasound examinations Professional interpretation available on 24-hr basis Portable x-ray and ultrasound equipment available to labor and delivery rooms and nurseries	Experienced radiology technicians immediately available in hospital (ultrasound on call) Professional interpretation immediately available Portable x-ray equipment Ultrasound equipment may be in labor and delivery or nursery areas Sophisticated equipment for emergency GI, GU, or CNS studies available 24 hr/day	Computed tomography Magnetic resonance imaging
Blood bank	Technicians on call 24 hr/day, available in 30 min, for routine blood banking procedures	Experienced technicians immediately available in hospital for blood banking procedures and identification of irregular antibodies Blood component therapy readily available	Resource center for network Direct line communication to labor and delivery area and nurseries

*All ancillary services listed for level I nurseries should be available at level II and III nurseries, and those listed for level II nurseries should be available at level III nurseries.

Table 35-9 *Levels of Program Development (I, II, III)*

LEVELS OF BASIC PERINATAL NETWORK	FUNCTIONAL ACTIVITIES	USUAL LOCATIONS	USUAL PHYSICIAN LEADERSHIP (PRACTICE AND STYLE)
I	Usual focus of patient entry into system Assess risk Carry out uncomplicated perinatal care Stabilize unexpected problems Initiate maternal, neonatal transport Accept return neonatal transport Collect data Sponsor local education	Community hospital or colocated at level II, III facilities	Primary care physician or specialist (solo practitioner)
II	Initiate and receive maternal, neonatal transport Initiate return neonatal transport Diagnose and treat selected high-risk pregnancies and neonatal problems Educate part of network	Large community hospital with many support services or colocated at level III facility	Specialist or subspecialist (monodisciplinary group practice)
III	Receive maternal, neonatal transport Initiate return neonatal transport Diagnose and treat most perinatal problems Research and outcome surveillance Educate regionally Administer regionally	Large academic medical centers with comprehensive residency programs	Subspecialist (multidisciplinary team practice)

Table 35-10 *Perinatal Care Programs—Medical Personnel*

PERSONNEL	LEVEL I	LEVEL II	LEVEL III
Chief of service	One general physician responsible for perinatal care (or codirectors from obstetrics and pediatrics)	Ob: Board-certified obstetrician with subcertification, special interest, experience, or training in maternal-fetal medicine Ped: Board-certified pediatrician with subcertification, special interest, experience, or training in neonatology	Ob: Full-time obstetrician board-certified in maternal-fetal medicine Ped: Full-time pediatrician board-certified in neonatal-perinatal medicine
Other physicians	Physician (or certified nurse-midwife) at all deliveries Anesthesia services Physician care for neonates	Board-certified director of anesthesia services Medical, surgical, radiologic, pathologic consultation	Anesthesiologists with special training or experience in perinatal and pediatric anesthesia Obstetric, pediatric, surgical subspecialists
Supervisory nurse	RN in charge of perinatal facilities	Ob: Supervisory RN with education and experience in normal and high-risk pregnancy Ped: Supervisory RN with neonatal specialist certification or equivalent experience	Supervisor of perinatal services with advanced skills Separate head nurses for maternal-fetal and neonatal services, master's degree level certification
Staff nurse/patient ratio	Normal labor—1:2 Delivery in second stage—1:1 Oxytocin induction—1:2 Cesarean delivery—2:1 Normal nursery—1:6-8	Complicated labor, delivery—1:1 Intermediate nursery—1:3-4	Intensive neonatal care—1:1-2 Critical care of unstable neonate—2:1
Other personnel	LPN, assistants under direction of head nurse	Social service, respiratory therapy, biomedical laboratory as needed	Designated full-time social service, respiratory therapy, biomedical engineering, laboratory technician Nurse-clinician and specialists Nurse program and education coordinators

Ob, Obstetrician; *Ped*, pediatrician.

Table 35-11 *Morbidity Among Premature Infants**

CAUSES	PERCENT AFFECTED
Metabolic	
Acidosis	43
Glucose (outside 40-150 mg/dl range)	26
Calcium (<7 mg/dl)	24
Body temperature on admission (<96° F [<36° C])	24
Sodium (outside 130-150 mEq/L range)	15
TOTAL	132†
Cardiorespiratory	
Asphyxia at birth (Apgar 0-6)	54
Apnea	29
Respiratory distress syndrome	20
Patent ductus arteriosus	19
Bronchopulmonary dysplasia, air leak	10
TOTAL	132
Hematologic	
Hemoglobin (outside 10-21 g/dl range)	64
Platelets (<100,000/mm^3)	11
TOTAL	75
Infection	
Premature rupture of membranes	25
Localized systemic	16
Sepsis	5
TOTAL	46
Gastrointestinal	
Hyperbilirubinemia (>12 mg/dl)	12
Necrotizing enterocolitis	11
Cholestatic jaundice	10
TOTAL	33
Neurologic—Convulsions	5

Data from Usher RH: The special problems of the premature infant. In Avery GB, editor: Neonatology, ed 3, Philadelphia, 1987, JB Lippincott Co.
*Data from 110 preterm infants (<34 weeks of gestation) from an unselected maternal population.
†Cumulative frequencies may exceed 100% because of multiple occurrences.

alone have the first opportunity to prevent or correct. Indeed, many feel the major portion of the recent reduction in perinatal mortality is attributable solely to improved monitoring of the fetus, better timing of the termination of the threatened pregnancy, and careful attention to the oxygen, thermal, and nutritional needs of the "large" 1500 to 2500 g infant.

Two
Perinatal Transport

George A. Little

HISTORICAL PERSPECTIVE

The early literature regarding perinatal transport describes the transfer of stable, pregnant women to hospitals, but little mention is given to critically ill newborns. With the development of regional centers for the care of premature infants and the improvement in mortality and morbidity rates at these centers, transfer of neonatal patients became increasingly important. Early transport services were primitive by today's standards, involving the use of equipment such as wood or tin boxes heated with hot water bottles. In 1948 the New York City Department of Health and Hospitals instituted a service staffed by five nurses to transport infants to centers caring for premature infants. Denver instituted a similar program at about the same time.

PRESENT STATUS

There are three types of perinatal transport: maternal-fetal transport, neonatal transport, and return transport of the neonate. Maternal-fetal transport is initiated for an identified high-risk condition in the mother (e.g., poorly controlled diabetes, preeclampsia) or for fetal risk (e.g., premature rupture of membranes at less than 34 weeks of gestation). The concept of maternal-fetal transport has tended to evolve more slowly than that of neonatal transport. Issues in the establishment of maternal-fetal transport have included uncertainty about the level of risk, cost containment, and the reluctance of local physicians to refer patients. With increasing documentation favoring the maternal-fetal transport system, many neonatal intensive care units (NICUs) now receive the majority of their neonates in utero.

Maternal-fetal transports are accomplished by use of local ambulances. Patients should be accompanied by the referring physician and a nurse-midwife or an obstetric nurse. A complicated delivery or the birth of a high-risk infant en route is thus anticipated and the risks minimized. Maternal-fetal and neonatal transports that originate at a community hospital and do not involve the center transport team are known as *one-way transports*. These transports can shorten the time it takes for the patient to arrive at the regional center. In less acute situations, when little or no risk of delivery en route is involved, the pregnant patient may be transported in a private vehicle. In all situations direct communication between the referring physician and the physician who will be responsible for the patient's care at the center is mandatory before departure.

Neonatal transports are initiated by the referring physician. Most often the physician calls the regional center to ask for transport when a problem is identified after birth; however, the request may be made before the birth. For example, if a woman who is at 28 weeks of gestation arrives at the hospital in active labor and delivery is imminent, this should prompt nurses and physicians to consider requesting the regional center's transport team to be present for the delivery or to arrive soon thereafter. These *two-way transports,* in which an ambulance and team from the regional center travel to the community hospital to pick up the neonate, are the most common means of neonatal transport. Yet, increasing numbers of community hospitals now have the equipment and personnel necessary for one-way transports to their regional center.

The request for a neonatal transfer to the regional center should prompt the initiation of an established protocol that immediately alerts the provider of the transport vehicle, the transport personnel, and the responsible neonatologist. Telephone communication with the referring physician enables the regional center's neonatologist to define a plan for stabilizing and meeting the immediate needs of the infant. Depending on the capabilities of the local hospital, this plan may include placing an arterial or a venous catheter, expanding fluid volume, determining serum electrolytes and blood gases, and obtaining appropriate roentgenograms. Communication should be continuous to allow for management changes according to a neonate's needs. The regional center's transport team usually assumes responsibility for care of the infant on their arrival at the community hospital but works closely with the referring physician, who should be present when the team arrives. Samples of maternal and umbilical cord blood, roentgenograms, and copies of records should accompany the newborn to the regional center. The physician should obtain the placenta for examination.

Optimal transport of a newborn is best achieved when stabilization of the newborn is as complete as possible before departure to the referral NICU. *The neonate's stable condition is more important than a quick return to the regional center.*

Parents should have the opportunity to see, to touch, and, if possible, to hold their newborn before transport and to receive information from the transport team members about the best means for communication with regional center personnel. A brochure listing names of center personnel and telephone numbers can be helpful. A photograph of the newborn taken before transport can be a comfort for the parents during the stressful period of separation from their infant. A telephone call from the transport team to the parents and the referring physician is important to bring them up-to-date on the neonate's status on completion of the transport. Center personnel should make subsequent contact with the parents or the referring physician at least daily and more frequently if the neonate's condition is critical.

It is often possible to transfer the mother to the postpartum floor of the tertiary center so that she can be close to her newborn. Parents should be encouraged to visit the NICU at any hour to see, touch, and hold their baby and to participate in his or her care as soon as possible. Perinatal care providers should be aware that parental grief and stress reactions develop when a pregnancy does not complete its anticipated normal course, and parents may variably express their grief verbally or behaviorally.

Return transport is indicated as soon as the infant can be treated appropriately at the community hospital and the services of a regional center are no longer needed. The infant may be growing well but still require gavage feedings and monitoring for occasional apneic episodes. The timing of the return depends on the facilities and the capabilities of the staff of the local hospital. Communication between the staffs of the community hospital and the regional center, and with the parents, regarding plans for return transport must be established well before the return is scheduled. A NICU nurse who can discuss the neonate's problems and needs with the nursing staff of the community hospital should accompany the neonate on the return transport to ensure the greatest continuity of care. A return transport places the infant in his or her own community near the parents and frees space and resources at the regional center for treatment of other critically ill newborns. A significant factor in this system is the return of direct responsibility for the infant's care to the primary care physician.

MECHANISM OF TRANSPORTATION

Specially equipped ambulances ensure optimal care for sick neonates during transit and are adequate for distances up to 80 to 100 miles. For longer distances fixed-wing aircraft are often more efficient than ground vehicles. Pressurized aircraft may be necessary for lengthy transport at higher altitudes. Helicopters are used for intermediate distances or to reach neonates in areas of difficult terrain. Ground transportation by ambulance from the community hospital to the airport or heloport and from these sites to the NICU is necessary. The transport team should stabilize the infant at the community hospital and accompany him or her through each phase of the journey.

PERSONNEL

The quality of the care rendered before and during transport depends critically on the capabilities of the transport team. Traditionally the team consists of an experienced physician and a neonatal nurse. More recently, some centers have used specially trained neonatal nurse clinicians as the primary transport specialist. An emergency care nurse, a respiratory therapist, or an emergency medical technician also may be a member of the team.

A NICU nurse, preferably the newborn's primary care nurse, usually accompanies the newborn on the return transport to communicate the neonate's current status, including the feeding routine, the presence of apneic episodes, and any special family problems, to the receiving nurse at the community hospital.

The importance of primary care physicians in the care of the neonate cannot be overemphasized. The identification of the newborn at risk, the initial resuscitation and stabilization of the newborn, the communication with the regional center before transport and thereafter, and the management of the neonate on return from the regional center are their special responsibilities (Table 35-12).

Table 35-12 *Physician Responsibility in Perinatal Transport*

PHYSICIAN BASE	MATERNAL-FETAL TRANSPORT (MFT)	NEONATAL TRANSPORT	RETURN NEONATAL TRANSPORT
Community	Understand benefits of MFT. Identify high-risk situations at earliest moment. Communicate with regional center. Transport properly and accompany the patient to regional center. Assume care of the patient on return to the community.	Understand benefits of neonatal transport. Identify problems and initiate communication with regional center. Initiate stabilization of the infant and provide appropriate therapy until transport team arrives; then assist the transport until departure. Provide appropriate documentation, including hospital record, maternal and cord blood, and roentgenograms. Participate in case discussion at follow-up conferences.	Assess local resources and provide optimal neonatal care at community hospital. Accept the infant in transfer as soon as medically indicated. Understand importance and support of continuity of care, including parental participation.
Center	Educate regional physicians about benefits of MFT. Establish and maintain a 24-hour telephone consultation and referral system. Establish and maintain data collection for evaluation and educational purposes. Provide tertiary care for the mother and the fetus. Maintain communication with community health care providers. Discuss the case with local physicians at all stages, including a follow-up conference and case-based transport conferences.	Educate regional physicians on benefits of neonatal transport. Establish and maintain a 24-hour telephone consultation referral system. Ensure immediate availability of an experienced transport team. Assess responsibility for the infant at community hospital, and direct the continuing stabilization process before transport. Communicate with the family and their physicians at all stages of care. Discuss case with local physicians in a follow-up conference and case-based transport conferences.	Maintain knowledge of local hospital capabilities. Communicate with local physicians, nurses, and parents in anticipation of transfer. Provide documentation, including a written discharge summary to accompany the patient.

EQUIPMENT

Neonatal transport equipment should be adequate to provide full intensive care and should include a transport incubator, a portable ventilator, an oxygen mixing and measuring system, a cardiorespiratory monitor, blood pressure monitors, infusion pumps, and essential drugs and supplies such as chest tubes. All electrically powered equipment should have "stand alone" capability with batteries as an alternate power source. Batteries must have sufficient longevity for the duration of the transport, should electricity not be available. Critical care equipment should be adaptable to 12- and 24-volt DC and 110-volt AC power for use in a hospital or an ambulance in order to avoid excessive use of batteries.

EDUCATION

The responsibility of the regional perinatal center does not end with the successful transport and treatment of the patient. Most *referral centers assume direct responsibility for the continuing education of perinatal care professionals in their region.* These activities should include didactic presentations and the distribution of related printed materials.

Case-based transport conferences at the community hospital can be educationally effective. These conferences also should involve physicians and nurses from the regional center to promote interaction with referring community hospital staff members. Open discussion of all aspects of care, including management at the community and center levels, is important. Such discussion facilitates development of improved clinical skills, decision-making, and continuity of care.

REFERENCE
Overview and Regionalization

1. American Academy of Pediatrics and the American College of Obstetricians and Gynecologists: Guidelines for perinatal care, ed 2, Elk Grove Village, Ill, 1988, The Academy.

SUGGESTED READINGS
Overview and Regionalization

Avery GB, editor: Neonatology—pathophysiology and management of the newborn, ed 3, Philadelphia, 1987, JB Lippincott Co.

Avery ME and Taeusch HW: Intrauterine growth retardation. In Avery ME and Taeusch HW, editors: Schaffer's diseases of the newborn, ed 5, Philadelphia, 1984, WB Saunders Co.

Benedetti T, Platt L, and Druzin M: Vaginal delivery after previous cesarean section for a nonrecurrent cause, Am J Obstet Gynecol 142:358, 1982.

Budin P: The nursling—the feeding and hygiene of premature and full-term infants, London, 1907, CEEPI, Ltd (Translated by WJ Maloney).

Cassady G: The small-for-date infant. In Avery G, editor: Neonatology: pathophysiology and management of the newborn, ed 3, Philadelphia, 1987, JB Lippincott Co.

Clifford SH: Postmaturity with placental dysfunction; clinical syndrome and pathological findings, J Pediatr 44:1, 1954.

Curran JS: Birth-associated injury, Clin Perinatol 8:111, 1981.

Davis JA and Dobbing J, editors: Scientific foundations of pediatrics, ed 2, Baltimore, 1982, University Park Press.

DeVore GR and Hobbins JC: Diagnosis of structural abnormalities in the fetus, Clin Perinatol 6:293, 1979.

Fanaroff AA and Martin RJ, editors: Behrman's neonatal-perinatal medicine: diseases of the fetus and infant, ed 4, St Louis, 1987, The CV Mosby Co.

Fitzhardinge PM and Steven EM: The small-for-date infant. I. Later growth patterns, Pediatrics 49:671, 1971.

Fitzhardinge PM and Steven EM: The small-for-date infant. II. Neurological and intellectual sequelae, Pediatrics 50:50, 1972.

Goodlin RC: Fetal monitoring, Semin Perinatol 5(suppl 2), 1981.

Gordon M et al: The immediate and long-term outcome of obstetric birth trauma. I. Brachial plexus paralysis, Am J Obstet Gynecol 117:51, 1973.

Gruenwald P: Infants of low birth weight among 5,000 deliveries, Pediatrics 34:157, 1964.

Klaus MH and Fanaroff AA, editors: Care of the high-risk neonate, ed 3, Philadelphia, 1986, WB Saunders Co.

Ledger WJ: Bacterial infections complicating pregnancy, Clin Obstet Gynecol 21:455, 1978.

Lubchenco LO: The high risk infant, Philadelphia, 1976, WB Saunders Co.

Lubchenco LO: Assessment of weight and gestational age. In Avery GB, editor: Neonatology: pathophysiology and management of the newborn, ed 3, Philadelphia, 1987, JB Lippincott Co.

Lubchenco LO et al: Intrauterine growth as estimated from liveborn birthweight data at 24 to 42 weeks gestation, Pediatrics 32:793, 1963.

Monheit AG and Resnik R: Cesarean section: current trends and perspectives, Clin Perinatol 8:101, 1982.

Painter MJ and Bergman I: Obstetrical trauma to the neonatal central and peripheral nervous system, Semin Perinatol 6:89, 1982.

Parmalee AH: Management of the newborn, ed 2, Chicago, 1959, Year Book Medical Publishers, Inc.

Quilligan EJ, Nochimson DJ, and Freeman RK: Management of the high-risk pregnancy. In Avery GB, editor: Neonatology: pathophysiology and management of the newborn, ed 3, Philadelphia, 1987, JB Lippincott Co.

Sweet AY: Classification of the low-birth-weight infant. In Klaus MH and Fanaroff AA, editors: Care of the high-risk neonate, ed 3, Philadelphia, 1986, WB Saunders Co.

von Reuss AR: The diseases of the newborn, New York, 1922, William Wood.

Vulliamy DG: The newborn child, ed 2, Boston, 1967, Little, Brown & Co.

Perinatal Transport

Boehm FH and Haire MF: One-way maternal transport: an evolving concept in patient services, Am J Obstet Gynecol 134:484, 1979.

Ferrara A and Harin A: Emergency transfer of the high-risk neonate: a working manual for medical, nursing, and administrative personnel, St Louis, 1980, The CV Mosby Co.

Harris TB, Isamen J, and Giles HR: Improved neonatal survival through maternal transport, Obstet Gynecol 52:294, 1978.

Segal S, editor: Manual for the transport of high-risk newborn infants: principles, policies, equipment, techniques, Vancouver, BC, 1972, Canadian Pediatric Society.

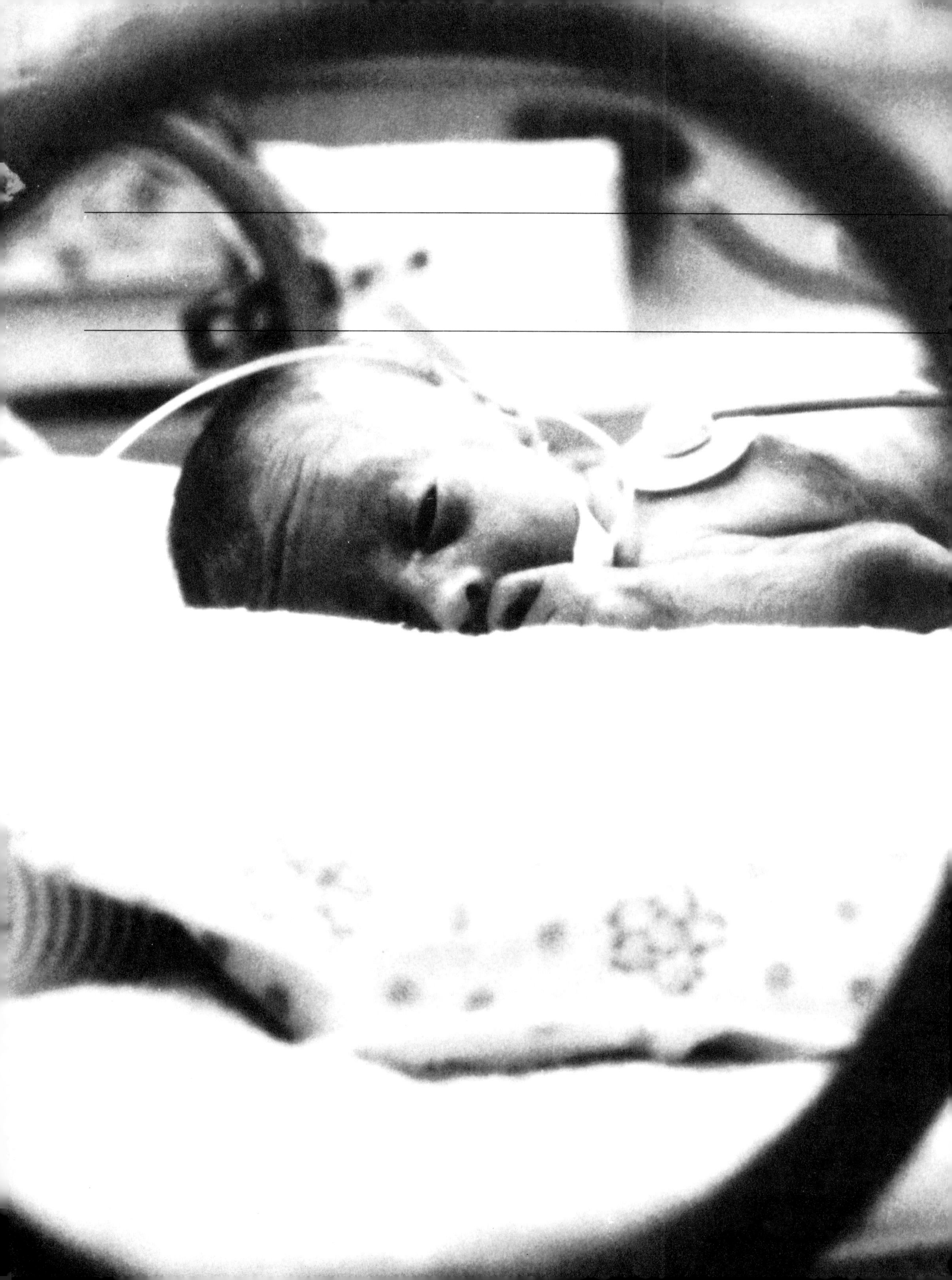

Part Five

The Newborn

36

Neonatal Adaptations

The component of pediatric practice that concerns neonatal adaptations has as its fundamental objective the healthy transition of the fetus from intrauterine to extrauterine life. The most effective strategy for achieving this objective is the enlistment by the physician of the parents (and their extended family) in a continuous collaboration designed to stimulate, form, and enhance their developing parenting skills.

It has often accurately been noted that no human activity of comparable magnitude in responsibility is more frequently undertaken with so little preparation or training than that of parenthood. Humans, as a species, appear to have lost, somewhere in past millennia, many of those instinctual elements of parenting behavior so clearly designed to foster thriving survival of the young that we observe daily, for example, in the parenting of house pets. The possible role of the health professions in contributing to this loss of skills is a matter outside the scope of this chapter, but evidence will be found throughout this book (e.g., failure to thrive and the abused child) to support the contention that many pediatric problems stem from the misfortune of the child who is unwelcome on arrival. Conversely, there are few better guarantees for the health of a child or even optimal adjustment to ill health than that his or her birth be happily and lovingly anticipated by both parents—a blessing that far outweighs any material supports, public or private. The obstetrician and pediatrician are equally blessed who have the good fortune to work with parents motivated by such love to seek and sustain health for their child.

The best tactic to optimize parenting skills is a staged approach to anticipatory guidance and problem management, marked by continuing obstetric-pediatric collaboration extending throughout gestation and the puerperium (Table 36-1). Each stage is pursued in a (typically) different site, is addressed to different processes, pursues different objectives, requires different observations, and may indicate different interventions.

One
Peripartum Considerations

M. Jeffrey Maisels
Nicholas M. Nelson

The performance sites for the peripartum stage of management of the newborn (from 0 to 40 weeks of gestation) include principally the obstetrician's office but also the community hospital's prenatal, labor, and birth classes and its high-risk pregnancy clinics. The main biologic processes being supervised are organogenesis in the first trimester, then maternal and fetal nutrition in the second and third trimester, with more strictly obstetric concerns focused on in the latter. The embryo is largely unavailable for scrutiny in the first trimester but, chiefly through the techniques of amniocentesis and ultrasound, becomes so during the second trimester, where its activity, breathing, growth, and general well-being are observed. A considerable capability has been developed to diagnose structural defects, particularly during the last trimester—a capability nearly as sophisticated as that used to diagnose genetic defects in the second trimester. However, present abilities for specific repair in utero of genotypic or phenotypic defects are still rudimentary, and the fundamental decision to be made concerning a pregnancy so threatened is whether it should be terminated well before the threshold of viability (currently around 25 weeks' gestation) or as far beyond that threshold as is consonant with reasonable fetal health.

Increasingly frequent is the decision that the fetus threatened by conditions such as intrauterine growth retardation, uteroplacental insufficiency, hemolytic disease, maternal diabetes, hydronephrosis, hydrocephalus, and ileal atresia is offered a better chance for effective intervention by early delivery and management in a neonatal intensive care unit than by continuing in utero much beyond the stage of fetal pulmonary maturation (about 32 weeks).

In developed nations for the past 50 years, birth has taken place nearly exclusively in the hospital, to which is attributed by most the near total conquest of maternal death. However, benefits for the term infant, the mother-infant pair, and the nuclear family have been called into increasing question, as overly rigid hospital "routines," erected under the banner of safeguarding the mother and infant (and often serving only to maximize hospital efficiency and staff convenience), decreased the "lying-in" period from 2 weeks to 2 days, placed fishbowl glass between infant and parents (with occasional excursions to the breast of that relatively rare mother who bravely defied hospital pressures to the contrary), and generally depersonalized the central human event that is birth.

The inevitable counterrevolution of the last generation has

Table 36-1 *Management of the Newborn**

STAGE	AGE	OBSTETRICS	PEDIATRICS
Prenatal	0-40 wk	*****	*
Birth	0-1 hr	****	**
Recovery	1-8 hr	***	***
Adjustment	8-48 hr	**	****
Establishment	48 hr-6 wk	*	*****

*Asterisks indicate degree of involvement in management decisions for obstetricians and pediatricians.

seen the medical profession yield significantly on its more pompous stances regarding the management of the birth process to the extent that fathers in labor classes and labor and delivery rooms, infant and mother rooming-in together (both enjoying visits from siblings), breast-feeding (replete with hospital support), and "birthing rooms" (née delivery rooms) have become happy commonplaces. These advances are still almost exclusively in the hospital (although it is more home-like), and maternal mortality remains near zero, with perinatal (fetal plus neonatal) mortality approaching the zero level, provided gestation has proceeded beyond about 36 weeks. The major current dinosaurs in this evolution are the unsolved problems of premature labor and whether the rapidly rising incidence of electronic fetal monitoring and cesarean birth (now more than 20% of all deliveries in some hospitals) should be properly regarded as merely the present medical means for dehumanization of the birth process or rather as instruments for fetal salvation.

CONVERSION FROM PLACENTAL TO PULMONARY RESPIRATION

The biologic processes concerned at this stage are the non-negotiable demands placed upon the fetus for rapid and successful conversion from placental to pulmonary respiration and the ability to support its metabolic needs (to defend body temperature and create new tissue) through its own, rather than the mother's, organs of digestion and excretion.

The first breaths (the fetus has actually been "panting" in utero for some weeks) are taken in response to many stimuli—sound (beyond the maternal souffle), light, chilling (from 98.6° to 71.6° F [37° to 22° C]), pressure, and probably pain. This "sensory overload" has been compared with that of weightless astronauts returning from orbit and modulates the fundamental respiratory regulation by the chemoreceptors of the carotid and aortic bodies and by the medullary centers.

Every normal labor is, to a degree, an asphyxiating event, since each uterine contraction interrupts umbilical venous flow. This brief and intermittent asphyxia is often reflected in simultaneous and brief slowing of the fetal heart rate. Indeed, many infants at cesarean delivery not preceded by labor are notably slow to take their first breath until submitted to that ultimate asphyxiating event, the clamping (or natural constriction) of the umbilical cord vessels. If excessive prenatal asphyxia (as from placental infarction) or intranatal asphyxia (as from a "nuchal," or knotted, umbilical cord) occurs, agonal or preagonal responses may well lead to meconium passage, aspiration, and inspissation in utero.

As the fetal thorax is compressed by passage through the birth canal and the head emerges on the perineum, a certain amount of fetal lung liquid may be expressed through the airways to the exterior. As the chest wall recoils to its natural proportions after emergence of the thorax, some small amount of air may then be drawn into the airways, thus establishing an air-liquid interface. Next, the first breaths and cries are taken, and the airless (but liquid-filled) alveoli begin to establish air-liquid interfaces under the counterforces of increased surface tension tending toward atelectatic collapse. It is the special function of the alveolar phospholipoprotein complex (pulmonary surfactant, produced by alveolar pneumocytes) to diminish surface tension at the air-liquid interface, thus promoting alveolar stability. Once the lung is expanded, usually within one or two breaths, its vascular resistance (as high as the systemic resistance in utero) begins to decline rapidly, as pericapillary alveolar pressure diminishes and arteriolar resistance relaxes under the influence of the rapid rise in Pa_{O_2} from the normal fetal level of about 25 torr to that of the newborn (about 80 torr). With this done, pulmonary blood flow (only about 5% of total cardiac output in utero) increases vastly, such that the left atrium, receiving increased pulmonary venous return, begins to distend its walls to their compliant limits and left atrial pressure rises to exceed that of the right (which is decreasing with diminishing umbilical venous return); thus the foramen ovale (basically a one-way flutter valve barring egress from the left atrium) closes. Meanwhile, the placental circulation (formerly a low-resistance shunt during fetal life) shuts down, as its vessels are either naturally constricted or artificially clamped.

Thus, birth converts the systemic circulation to one of higher total vascular resistance than that of the pulmonary circulation; blood returning to the right side of the heart from the superior and inferior venae cavae now preferentially flows through the pulmonary circulation, whereas in fetal life the right ventricular output had largely bypassed the high-resistance pulmonary artery by flowing through the ductus arteriosus directly into the aorta, which bathes the coronary and carotid vessels with the best-oxygenated blood available to the fetus—that from the umbilical vein, which crosses the liver via the ductus venosus, coursing to the inferior cava and the right atrium. Two thirds of this fetal blood directly crosses the foramen ovale into the left atrium, and the remainder passes through the right ventricle and ductus arteriosus (from the right to the left circulations) to the aortic isthmus. However, as these respective circulations' vascular resistances reverse after birth, blood returning from the lungs to the left atrium is pumped by the left ventricle to the aortic root where again it confronts an open ductus arteriosus and a now higher systemic than pulmonary resistance; thus it preferentially passes through the ductus (from left to right) to *recirculate* through the lungs. At this stage of life (within the first 1 or 2 hours after birth) the circulation is "transitional," in that the foramen ovale is functionally closed, while the ductus arteriosus is still open and is recirculating blood from the left to the right circulatory systems through the lungs. Moreover, during this period the volume and pressure load on the left ventricle nearly triples compared with fetal life, during which the right ventricle was dominant in both load and size and both ventricles worked "in parallel," connected by the foramen ovale and the ductus arteriosus.

The terminal phase in conversion of the fetal to the neonatal circulatory patterns is marked by closure of the ductus arteriosus in a process of interaction between the increasing oxygen content of the blood coursing through it and decreasing levels of circulating or local tissue prostaglandins. This usually occurs somewhere in the second 12 hours of the first day of life when early systolic murmurs at the base of the heart may often be heard, presumably related to the process.

OBSERVATIONS DURING LABOR AND DELIVERY AND IMMEDIATELY THEREAFTER

Observations during the perinatal period should be directed to ensuring that the fetus remains well-oxygenated, the chief evidence for which is sought during labor through monitoring of the fetal heart rate by either acoustic or electronic means. Meconium staining of the amniotic fluid (in vertex deliveries) is taken as evidence of significant fetal hypoxia, acute or chronic, and should alert the attending physician to the potential need for aspiration of meconium from the nasopharynx and trachea before the infant has the opportunity to aspirate and inspissate that viscous material into the airways with the first few breaths.

After full cervical dilation, the fetal scalp becomes available for microsampling of fetal blood gases; the pH is a more reliable indicator of hypoxia than is oxygen tension under these circumstances. At delivery the cord blood becomes available for the same purpose.

However, immediately after delivery, the entire infant is assessed to establish the success of oxygenation throughout labor by means of the Apgar score (see Chapter 7, Table 7-1), which includes a grading of neuromuscular reactivity (muscle tone and reflex irritability), as well as heart rate, respiration, and color. The 1-minute assessment has not nearly the overall prognostic power of the 5-minute score, but most serious decisions for resuscitative intervention are or should be made for the child whose respiratory effort is absent or failing at 1 minute after birth and certainly if the heart rate is decreasing.

PHYSICAL EXAMINATION

The responsibility for the delivery room examination of the newborn will most often fall, in the case of the uncomplicated delivery of a low-risk fetus, to the person performing the delivery. At high-risk deliveries, resuscitation, if required, and initial delivery room assessment are normally in the hands of the pediatrician in attendance. Whether an elective cesarean birth at term constitutes a high-risk delivery requiring the attendance of a pediatrician is more a matter of individual circumstance and local custom than actual likelihood of resuscitative intervention.

Once the decision can be made that active resuscitation from birth asphyxia is unnecessary, or after its successful completion, the infant should receive a brief and directed physical examination in the delivery room (if possible, before formal introduction to the parents) under circumstances promoting maximum visibility while avoiding chilling (an overhead radiant warmer or floodlight illumination is simple and effective). The principal objectives of this examination are to seek evidence of obstetric trauma, particularly in the instance of a "difficult delivery" (e.g., shoulder dystocia, aftercoming head of the breech delivery, and any operative delivery more challenging than simple "outlet forceps") and unanticipated gross congenital anomalies (many of these are now detected by ultrasound in utero) and to assess gestational age.

Most of the important information at this stage is gathered by careful observation, along with brief palpation and auscultation, with an emphasis on the points listed in the accompanying box. Obstetric situations in which to be especially wary of possible delivery trauma are indicated in Table 36-2.

The infant who displays good flexor muscle tone, who is properly reactive to tactile stimuli, who is unarguably "pink" in midface and trunk (as opposed to the often still blue extremities) by about 5 minutes of age, who has a perforate anus, whose genitalia are unambiguous, and whose neural tube and palate are closed can be presented to his or her parents as "normal," after auscultation of the chest and palpation of the abdomen (see description of the physical examination in the next section, "Physiologic Status of the Healthy Infant").

Infants who are tachycardic or who have grunting expirations and flaring alae nasi at about 10 minutes of age may be regarded with some suspicion but not yet alarm, since there is much fetal lung fluid (about 20 ml/kg) to be absorbed into the circulation. If air entry into the lungs is satisfactory, the outlook may well be sanguine. The heart examination may reveal an early systolic murmur that merits continuing observation. The second sound is usually single until increasing pulmonary blood flow leads to its normal splitting some hours later.

The more detailed physical examination can safely wait until after the infant's admission to the "recovery room" (nursery), where prophylactic eye ointment and vitamin K may also be given. Apart from sharing in the parents' joy and relief, the primary physician's remaining time in the delivery room might more profitably be devoted to study of the placenta, which is usually available for inspection about the time the initial examination of the infant is completed. It should be searched for gross areas of infarction, marginal separation, velamentous insertion of vessels, meconium staining, and purulence, as clues to the infant who may be pallid (from occult blood loss) or subsequently septic. The cord vessels (two arteries and one vein) should also be confirmed as normal, since there appears to be an association (of arguable

Delivery Room Assessment

A. General
  1. Whole
    a. Proportions
    b. Symmetry
    c. Facies
    d. Gestational age (approximate)
  2. Skin—color, subcutaneous tissue, and imperfections—bands and birthmarks
  3. Neuromuscular
    a. Movements
    b. Responses
    c. Tone (flexor)
B. Head and neck
  1. Head
    a. Shape
    b. Circumference
    c. Molding
    d. Swellings
    e. Depressions
    f. Occipital overhang
  2. Fontanelles, sutures
    a. Size
    b. Tension
  3. Eyes
    a. Size
    b. Separation
    c. Cataracts
    d. Colobomas
  4. Ears
    a. Placement
    b. Complexity
    c. Preauricular tags or sinuses
  5. Mouth
    a. Symmetry
    b. Size
    c. Clefts
  6. Neck
    a. Swellings
    b. Fistulas
C. Lungs and respiration
  1. Retraction
  2. Grunt
  3. Air entry (breath sounds)
D. Heart and circulation
  1. Rate
  2. Rhythm
  3. Murmurs
  4. Sounds
E. Abdomen
  1. Musculature
  2. Bowel sounds
  3. Cord vessels
  4. Distention
  5. Scaphoid shape
  6. Masses
F. Genitalia and anus
  1. Placement
  2. Testes
  3. Labia
  4. Phallus
G. Extremities
  1. Bands
  2. Digits (number and overlapping)
H. Spine
  1. Symmetry
  2. Scoliosis
  3. Sinuses

validity) between the presence of a single umbilical artery and other anomalies.

INTERVENTIONS AT BIRTH

Placental Transfusions

Even before the infant's attendant has had an opportunity to wipe away the greasy vernix, the initial intervention (or decision not to intervene) has been taken by the obstetrician. Some clamp the umbilical cord immediately, some wait until the pulsations have ceased, and others prefer to wait until the infant has breathed and cried *or* placental artery pulsations have ceased (whichever is later), with the infant kept below the introitus and thus ensured of the maximal "placental transfusion" of blood (nearly 150 ml in term deliveries) within about 2 minutes.

Perinatal scientists have yet to achieve a consensus on the proper management of the placental transfusion, since it is not yet clear whether the "extra" blood presents an intended advantage or whether the documented increase in blood pressure and cardiac load presented by such transfusion presents a significant cardiopulmonary disadvantage. Recollection that the primeval delivery posture probably placed the mother on her knees or in a squatting position, so as better to attend the infant and afterbirth *before* the cord was cut, may suggest nature's (as opposed to medicine's) intent in the matter.

Resuscitation from Asphyxia

Perinatal asphyxia is the most frequent example of acute respiratory failure in the neonatal period. It occurs in the delivery room when the infant fails to initiate adequate respiration or when respirations are simply insufficient to provide adequate gas exchange. It arises nearly always as the result of intrauterine asphyxia, during which the fetus becomes hypoxic and hypercarbic and may develop metabolic acidosis. The sine qua non of its management is to provide immediate ventilatory assistance.

Planning for Resuscitation. Obstetric events usually herald the arrival of an asphyxiated infant in sufficient time to allow for preparation. However, ongoing organization and preplanning are essential to ensure appropriate care for the unanticipated problem. The "disaster plan" for delivery room resuscitation should be the primary responsibility of a physician and should be periodically reviewed. The delivery room

Table 36-2 *Obstetric Situations in Which Delivery Trauma May Occur*

TYPE OF INJURY	NORMAL VERTEX	CESAREAN	PREMATURE	PRECIPITATE	DIFFICULT		
					BREECH EXTRACTION	LARGE INFANT	HIGH MIDFORCEPS
Hemorrhage							
Cerebral							
Subdural							X
Subarachnoid				X	X	X	X
Intraventricular			X				
Abdominal							
Liver					X	X	
Spleen					X	X	
Adrenal gland					X	X	
Cutaneous, presenting part	X				X		
Conjunctival	X						
Fracture or dislocation							
Clavicle						X	
Humerus					X		
Femur					X		
Skull							X
Nerve injury							
Brachial plexus						X	
Spinal cord					X		
Facial	X						
Laceration		X					

staff should have on permanent and prominent display a list of maternal and fetal complications that require the presence in the delivery room of a professional who is specifically qualified in newborn resuscitation (see box).

Equipment Required. All equipment should be checked regularly (as well as before any delivery) for readiness and appropriate function. Is the laryngoscope light bright? Does the bag and mask ventilation system provide adequate flow? Is it free of leaks? A list of suggested equipment is provided in the box on p. 441.

Personnel. Proper resuscitation cannot be performed alone. Two people (e.g., physician and nurse) must be solely responsible for the infant's care directly after birth, undistracted by the needs of the mother.

Apgar Score. The Apgar score should be determined 1 and 5 minutes after birth (see Table 7-1). If the 5-minute score is less than 7, then additional scores should be obtained every 5 minutes up to 20 minutes, unless and until two successive scores are 8 or greater. Ideally, the Apgar score should be assigned by a person not directly involved in the resuscitation (e.g., a nurse).

Resuscitation Procedure. Fig. 36-1 outlines the initial steps.

1. *Temperature control*. Immediately after delivery, the infant should be placed under a previously heated radiant warmer and completely dried with prewarmed towels to avoid excessive evaporative heat loss.
2. *Suctioning*. Suctioning is not essential in all infants; however, if necessary, it should be gentle. In particular, vigorous suctioning of the posterior pharynx must be avoided, since this frequently produces significant bradycardia. If the amniotic fluid is meconium-stained, the mouth and pharynx should be suctioned thoroughly with a De Lee trap before the delivery of the shoulders to prevent meconium aspiration. In the presence of thick or particulate meconium, the larynx should be visualized and direct suction applied by means of an endotracheal tube. This procedure should be repeated as often as necessary to remove as much material as possible. Guidelines for endotracheal tube sizes and suction catheters are provided in Table 36-3.
3. *Establishing respiration*. The normal infant should breathe within a few seconds of delivery and establish regular, effective respiration by 1 minute of life. An infant who at any age is not breathing spontaneously and whose heart rate is less than 100 beats/min requires immediate ventilation without recourse to a precise Apgar score. Fig. 36-2 provides a flowchart for positive pressure ventilation.

With few exceptions, bag and mask ventilation, correctly performed, will provide adequate ventilation for most infants. The few infants in whom it should not be used include those with meconium-stained amniotic fluid and those who have a diaphragmatic hernia. In addition, it may be very difficult to achieve adequate lung expansion with bag and mask ventilation in small premature infants with noncompliant lungs. These *exceptional cases require endotracheal intubation*.

Critical to the success of bag and mask ventilation are a good facial seal and a nonobstructed airway, obtained by positioning the infant with his or her neck slightly extended and by lifting the infant's face to the mask by using the fingers of the left hand (Fig. 36-3). The little finger should actually elevate the angle of the jaw, thus bringing the tongue forward and opening the airway. Pushing the mask into the baby's face pushes the tongue back to obstruct the airway. The neck must *not* be hyperextended—this narrows the airway.

Some Perinatal Conditions That Increase the Risk of Neonatal Asphyxia

ANTEPARTUM CONDITIONS

1. Diabetes
2. Toxemia
3. Hypertension
4. Rh sensitization
5. Previous stillbirth or neonatal death
6. Third trimester bleeding
7. Maternal infection
8. Polyhydramnios
9. Oligohydramnios
10. Postterm gestation
11. Multiple gestation
12. Intrauterine growth retardation

INTRAPARTUM CONDITIONS

1. Operative delivery
   a. Cesarean section
   b. Midforceps delivery
2. Breech or other abnormal presentation
3. Premature labor
4. Chorioamnionitis
   a. Maternal fever, tachycardia, or both
   b. Ruptured membranes (>24 hours)
   c. Tender uterus
   d. Foul-smelling amniotic fluid
5. Prolonged labor (>24 hours)
6. Fetal distress
   a. Fetal tachycardia (>160 beats/min)
   b. Fetal bradycardia (<120 beats/min)
   c. Persistent late decelerations
   d. Severe variable decelerations without baseline variability
   e. Scalp pH ≤7.25
   f. Meconium-stained amniotic fluid
   g. Cord prolapse
7. General anesthesia
8. Narcotics administered during labor
9. Abruptio placentae
10. Placenta previa

Equipment Required for Resuscitation

VENTILATION

1. Oxygen source—oxygen, preferably warmed and humidified
2. Suction—De Lee suction trap, wall suction with adjustable pressure gauge; suction catheters; sizes 6, 8, 10, 12 Fr
3. Ventilation bag—500 cc self-inflating type with reservoir (capable of delivering 100% O_2); 500 cc anesthesia type
4. Face masks—infant sizes, premature and term
5. Laryngoscope—blade sizes 0 and 1, spare batteries, and bulbs
6. Endotracheal tubes—sizes 2.5, 3.0, and 3.5 mm with plastic adapters attached
7. Soft metal stylets
8. Stethoscope
9. Feeding tube—8 Fr tubes to evacuate stomach contents

TEMPERATURE CONTROL

1. Evaporation—warm towels
2. Conduction—mattress covered with prewarmed towels
3. Convection—turn down air conditioning; delivery room temperature 75° F (23.9° C) minimum
4. Radiation—radiant warmer

CIRCULATION AND BIOCHEMICAL RESUSCITATION

1. Umbilical catheterization tray
2. Drugs and volume expanders

OTHER

50 cc syringe with three-way stopcock and 21-gauge butterfly needle for evacuation for pneumothorax

There are two kinds of bags: (1) the open-ended *anesthesia bag* that requires continual gas flow for inflation and (2) the *self-expanding (Ambu) bag* that remains inflated with or without gas flow. The latter is the more convenient to use, particularly for less experienced resuscitators, and several models are available. However, these bags must be fitted with an oxygen reservoir to deliver high concentrations of oxygen. The absence of a reservoir limits oxygen delivery to only 40% to 50%, a level grossly inadequate for delivery room resuscitation. Note also that the valve assembly in most self-inflating bags permits oxygen flow *only when the bag is being compressed*. Thus, these bags cannot be used to provide free-flowing oxygen to the baby's face.

With successful ventilation, the chest should rise and fall while the infant's heart rate and color rapidly improve. If this does not occur, the seal between mask and face must be checked; continued inability to obtain adequate chest movement by bag and mask ventilation mandates endotracheal intubation.

Whether ventilation is provided via mask or endotracheal tube, *the appropriate inflating pressure is that which is required to expand the chest and improve gas exchange*. It is not to be determined solely by reference to a manometer. If the manometer indicates that high pressures are necessary to expand the chest, then the possibilities of airway obstruction, severe hyaline membrane disease, and hypoplastic lungs should be considered. Although overinflation entails a risk of producing a pneumothorax, this is relatively rare. On the other hand, underventilation is a far more frequent occurrence that usually results from the unwise choice of a predetermined pressure limit, as shown by a manometer rather than by observation of the chest wall.

Effective assisted ventilation is the *only* intervention required in the overwhelming majority of severely asphyxiated neonates. With few exceptions, asphyxiated infants respond promptly to adequate ventilation.

The infant's heart rate should be monitored continuously by an assistant during the resuscitation procedure because this

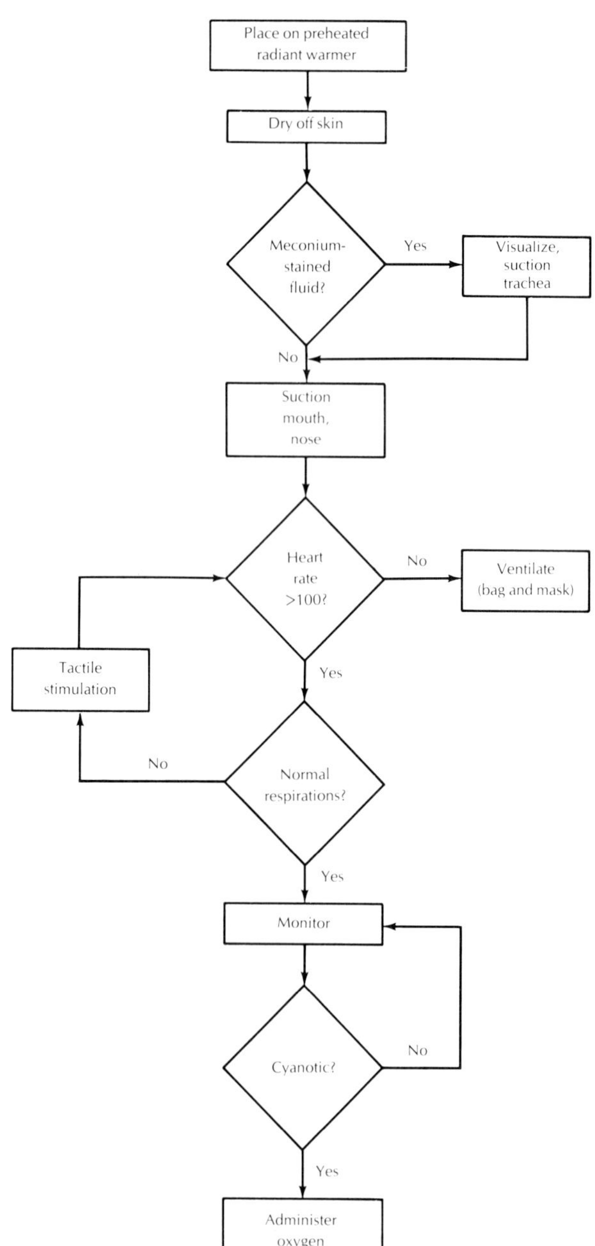

Fig. 36-1 Protocol for initial steps in an infant's resuscitation in the delivery room.

Modified from Klaus MH and Fanaroff AA: Care of the high-risk neonate, ed 2, Philadelphia, 1979, WB Saunders Co.

is the most useful and readily measurable criterion of the effectiveness of resuscitation. After intubation, the chest should be observed to ensure that it expands well and symmetrically and that equal breath sounds are heard in both axillae (not over the apices). Improvement in heart rate, color, and muscle tone confirms that ventilation is adequate. If any doubt exists regarding the position of the endotracheal tube, it should be checked by direct visualization of the larynx with a laryngoscope.

Meconium Aspiration

If thick particulate meconium is present in the amniotic fluid, the nose and pharynx should then be suctioned by the obstetrician using a De Lee catheter as soon as the head is delivered. If possible, the physician who resuscitates should suction the baby's larynx before spontaneous breathing occurs. Whether or not the baby has breathed, the larynx should be visualized, and meconium should be directly removed by suction through an endotracheal tube. The process is repeated until the larynx is clear. If bradycardia has occurred, it may be necessary to ventilate the infant between suctioning.

External Cardiac Massage

If the heart rate does not increase above 80 beats/min after effective ventilation with oxygen, external cardiac heart massage should then be instituted immediately while ventilation is continued; the technique is shown in Fig. 36-3. The thumbs should be positioned over the midportion of the sternum, the chest encircled with both hands, and the sternum compressed ½ to ¾ inch (1.5 to 2 cm) 120 times per minute. Ventilation should continue while cardiac massage is administered. The actual timing of ventilation during cardiac massage is probably not critical, although some authorities recommend that a breath be provided after every third compression. If cardiac massage does not produce rapid improvement in the heart rate, appropriate drug therapy and volume expansion (if indicated) should then be initiated.

Drugs

Drugs are rarely necessary for resuscitation in the delivery room. They should certainly never be administered until after adequate ventilation has first been established. If possible, drugs should be administered via the umbilical vein; however, if these routes are unavailable, epinephrine and naloxone can

Table 36-3 *Guidelines for Endotracheal Tubes and Suction Catheters*

WEIGHT (kg)	ENDOTRACHEAL TUBE ID* (mm)	DEPTH OF INSERTION FROM UPPER LIP (cm)	SUCTION CATHETER SIZE (Fr)
1	2.5	7	5
2	3.0	8	6
3	3.5	9	8

**ID*, Internal diameter.

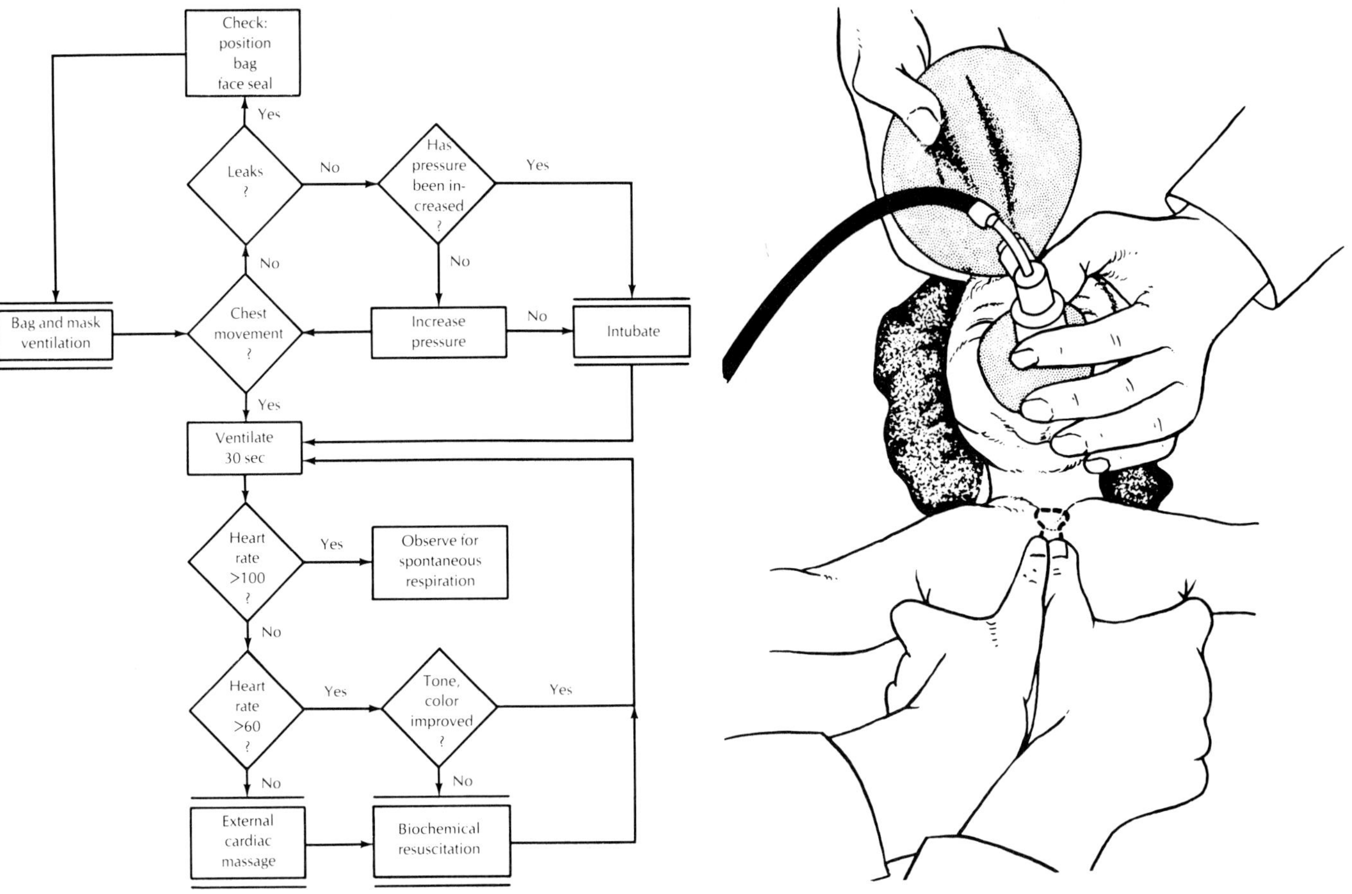

Fig. 36-2 Protocol for positive pressure ventilation for an infant's resuscitation in the delivery room.

Modified from Klaus MH and Fanaroff AA: Care of the high-risk neonate, ed 2, Philadelphia, 1979, WB Saunders Co.

Fig. 36-3 Technique for bag and mask ventilation, as well as external cardiac massage.

From American Academy of Pediatrics and the American College of Obstetricians and Gynecologists: Guidelines for perinatal care, Washington, DC, 1983, p. 72. Reproduced by permission of *Pediatrics*, copyright 1983.

Table 36-4 *Indications for Drugs in Resuscitation of the Newborn*

INDICATION	DRUG	DOSE
Metabolic acidosis	Sodium bicarbonate	2 mEq/kg initially
Bradycardia	Epinephrine hydrochloride	0.1 ml/kg of 1:10,000 solution
Low blood volume	Albumin, human (Albumisol)	10 ml/kg of 5% solution
	Ringer lactate	10 ml/kg
Respiratory depression secondary to narcotics	Naloxone	0.1 mg/kg

be administered via the endotracheal tube. A list of drugs and appropriate doses is provided in Tables 36-4 and 41-2.

Asphyxiated infants usually have a combined metabolic and respiratory acidosis, the proper treatment of which is correction of the cause. Therefore, respiratory acidosis, the result of hypoventilation, is treated by intermittent positive pressure ventilation. Some experimental evidence indicates that metabolic acidosis has a specific detrimental effect on myocardial function in the hypoxic heart, but it has also been shown that the performance of the ischemic heart is more closely related to tissue P_{CO_2} than to the pH and that non-ischemic cardiac muscle performance is also depressed by increases in P_{CO_2}. Thus these observations further emphasize the primary role of ventilation in acid-base adjustments during resuscitation—adequate ventilation is the sine qua non, but if bradycardia or poor perfusion persists despite adequate ventilation, then 2 mEq/kg sodium bicarbonate may be given as a last resort. It should be diluted 1:1 with sterile water to a concentration of 0.5 mEq/ml and infused at a rate no greater than 1 to 2 mEq/min.

Hypovolemia

Most asphyxiated neonates are not hypovolemic. Moreover, it is important to recognize that there are potential hazards (e.g., intracranial hemorrhage) to overzealous volume expansion. On the other hand, there are certain conditions, such as vasa previa or fetal-maternal bleeding, that may produce significant hemorrhage from the fetoplacental unit. Compression of the umbilical cord during labor, compounded by failure to allow for the normal placental transfusion, may also be associated with hypovolemia. If significant hypovolemia is suspected (clinical signs of shock are not usually apparent until 20% to 25% of the blood volume has been lost), then small infusions of volume expanders (5 to 10 ml/kg) may be given (Table 36-4). The infant's response should be assessed after each infusion, and volume expansion should be discontinued as soon as tissue perfusion is adequate.

Respiratory Depression Caused by Narcotics

Respiratory depression caused by narcotics can be managed by assisted ventilation alone; however, if respiratory depression persists despite adequate assisted ventilation, naloxone (0.1 mg/kg) may then be given.

Two
Physiologic Status of the Healthy Infant

Nicholas M. Nelson

Throughout fetal life the placenta is at once the necessary and sufficient organ for respiration, nutrition, metabolism, excretion, and immune defense, whereas certain endocrine functions (likely including growth itself), as well as the events of parturition, require more active fetal effort. The fetal lung, gut, liver, kidney, thymus, and even the brain have no functional assignment, other than to grow, differentiate, and be ready to assume function at birth. Thus it is perfectly possible for nature to carry many of her human "experiments" to term with no kidneys, gut, liver, lungs, or brain. However, a fetal circulatory system, comprising pump and "exchange" vessels (capillaries), is necessary very early in gestation for all placental mammals, although a single ventricle will do.

CIRCULATORY SYSTEM

The major cardiorespiratory events that attend birth (discussed previously) serve to sever the *parallel* connections of the greater (systemic) and lesser (pulmonary) circulations through the foramen ovale and ductus arteriosus, resulting in a *serial* circulatory pathway from right ventricle to pulmonary circulation to left ventricle to systemic circulation and guaranteeing that 100% of cardiac output (rather than about 5%, as in the fetus) passes through the lungs. This, perhaps paradoxically, results in a decrease in load on the right ventricle because pulmonary vascular resistance decreases, concomitant with an increase in left ventricular load, as the low-resistance placental shunt is removed by birth, which simultaneously converts a low-flow, high-resistance circuit (the pulmonary) to its inverse and a higher-flow, lesser-resistance circuit (the systemic) to its inverse. The result is that the right ventricular preponderance characteristic of fetal and early neonatal life begins to give way to the left ventricular dominance of later life, with these events most obvious in the changing QRS and T vectors on an electrocardiogram of the developing infant's heart. All these alterations in hemodynamics serve to set the conditions that place the two ventricles (especially the left) high on their respective function curves-that is, producing relatively high cardiac outputs, but with little further reserve for emergencies.

It appears that the infant myocardium is less able than that of the adult to *sustain* tension against the loads imposed by high-volume ("preload") or high-pressure ("afterload") work loads. This possibly results from a level of sympathetic innervation that is as yet incomplete, even by term gestation, so that myocardial "beta"-receptors are insufficiently stimulated. In any case, and especially in the premature newborn, there appears to be a parasympathetic/sympathetic innervational imbalance with parasympathetic dominance and frequent bradycardia, which is often responsive to atropine.

Moreover, the pulmonary arterioles retain for a time their thick fetal musculature, which renders them supersensitive to any vasoconstrictive stimuli, such as hypoxia. The condition known as persistent pulmonary hypertension of the newborn (also as "persistent *fetal* circulation"), is characterized by such vasoconstriction, which forces blood right to left across the still-open (anatomically) shunts of the foramen ovale and ductus arteriosus to produce cyanosis and a general clinical picture quite difficult to distinguish clinically from true cyanotic congenital heart disease.

HEMATOPOIETIC SYSTEM

Certainly the earliest fetal organ function to become established, hematopoiesis (and later hemostasis), is sited first in the yolk sac (0 to 2 months), then the liver (2 to 6 months), and, finally, the bone marrow (6 to 9 months).

The ontogeny of the hemoglobin chains is such that at birth fetal hemoglobin (hemoglobin F) is dominant. During the chronic hypoxic insult that is fetal life (with an average oxygen tension of perhaps 35 mm Hg), renal production of erythropoietin is stimulated; this, in turn, stimulates production of red cells to maximize oxygen-carrying capacity such that at birth the red cell mass is at a maximum (hematocrit level of 55% to 65%), beyond which increasing blood viscosity would so impede blood flow as to actually decrease oxygen transfer. With birth these largely young red cells (abetted by an extra supply provided by a "placental transfusion" of up to 150 ml of whole blood, where the infant has been kept below the vaginal introitus and the cord left unclamped until after the first breath) rapidly begin to be torn down to add to the infant's bilirubin load. Oxygen transfer from placenta to red cell in the relatively hypoxic fetus is aided by hemoglobin F, which displays greater affinity for oxygen than does adult hemoglobin and a decreased affinity for its reciprocally binding coenzyme, 2,3-diphosphoglycerate (DPG). Immediately after birth the concentration of DPG rises sharply, and the oxygen affinity of the infant's blood falls conveniently because, now after birth, the infant is operating at an oxygen pressure of about 100 mm Hg (rather than at 30 mm Hg) and needs not so much to be able to snatch precious oxygen molecules from a "hypoxic" placenta into the death grip of fetal hemoglobin as to be able graciously to give up the oxygen so carried to the harder working peripheral tissues of his or her newly born and better oxygenated body.

The several components of reliable hemostasis (blood vessels that can constrict, aggregatable platelets, and a functioning coagulation cascade of clotting proteins) appear largely intact in the term newborn, with the likely exception of the vitamin K–dependent factors (II, VII, IX, and X). These are present, but at levels of 50% or less than those of adults, which may descend even further to as low as 5% to 20% of adult levels and risk hemorrhagic disease, unless vitamin K is given.

RESPIRATORY SYSTEM

During fetal life the infant's respiratory system, made up of gas-exchanging alveoli and air-conducting pathways, prepares developmentally to take on, following very rapidly on ligation of the cord, the awesome responsibility for gaseous metabolism previously assumed by the placenta.

From about 25 to 35 weeks of gestation, the alveoli, complete with their integrated perfusing blood supply, develop from "glandular" to more acinar structures. Concomitantly, the alveolar pneumocytes (type II cells) elaborate the complex of phospholipids and protein known as *pulmonary surfactant* and store it against the moment of the first breaths of life, when surfactant is spread in a thin layer over the alveolar epithelium, there to stabilize the alveoli by diminishing the surface tension established at the air-liquid interface. A somewhat leisurely process of absorption of fetal lung liquid occurs during the first hour of life (principally through the lymphatics), after full expansion of the lung and after the vast initial decrease in pulmonary vascular resistance and reciprocal increase in pulmonary blood flow (described in the previous section) takes place. Disruptions in this process of liquid resorption are thought to play a role in the condition called *transient tachypnea of the newborn*.

By the time of birth at term, the neuromuscular and skeletal apparatus that constitutes the thoracic bellows (ribs, intercostal muscles, and diaphragm) has had considerable intrauterine practice at breathing through a paroxysmal form of rapid "panting" (oscillatory movement of only very small amounts of amniotic fluid in the airways). These paroxysms (at least in fetal sheep) temporally coincide with episodes of "active sleep" (see Three, "Recovery Period"). The only significant inefficiency of the thoracic bellows occurs during active sleep, when there is a widespread inhibition of motor neurons, particularly those responsible for ongoing intercostal muscle tone. As a consequence, the chest wall becomes rather less fixed and stiff (i.e., more "compliant," like a loose-fitting glove); thus the tendency of the underlying stretched lung to collapse is less opposed by a firm chest wall than is the case in quiet sleep; the descending diaphragm is able to pull the lower rib cage counterproductively *inward* during inspiration ("paradoxical" respiration). Therefore, the mechanical situation for the infant's lung is a bit more tenuous than is the case for the adult—specifically, the infant's lung tends to operate at a level rather close to its "collapse volume"; this tendency must be counteracted by increasing inspiratory muscle tone, as well as laryngeal tone, during expiration.

Nonetheless, the newborn's ability to ventilate and perfuse his or her alveoli, and thereby permit exchange of carbon dioxide for oxygen within them, is (relative to his or her metabolic needs) quite on a par with that of an Olympic runner. Indeed, the reason for the characteristic mild hypoxemia (arterial Po_2 of 70 to 85 torr) of the newborn is not that arterialization of venous blood within the lung is imperfect, but rather that a certain amount of right-to-left "fetal" shunting of desaturated venous blood continues to occur across the foramen ovale and ductus arteriosus until such time as vascular resistance and pressure within the pulmonary circulation decrease more nearly to adult levels. It remains uncertain whether the mild hypocapnia typical of neonatal life (arterial Pco_2 of 35 torr) results from a progesterone-mediated lowering of the respiratory center's threshold for carbon dioxide, or whether it simply reflects the result, in the form of a lowered serum and cerebrospinal bicarbonate level, of the prolonged fluid volume expansion of fetal life.

RENAL FUNCTION

It has been suggested of the perinatal kidney that it emerges at birth from a primeval, water-rich swamp out onto an extrauterine desert because the fetus and newly born infant behave in many ways as does a chronically volume-expanded subject with decreased tubular resorption of water and sodium (leading to "wasting" into the fetal urine), as well as bicarbonate, glucose, and phosphate. The teleologic and metaphysical question arises whether the fetus sustains such polyuria in order to maintain amniotic fluid volume. This question is not yet answered, but certainly the fetus with renal agenesis (Potter syndrome) exists on a dry intrauterine desert (called *amnion nodosum* to describe profound oligohydramnios).

Renal vascular resistance, like that of the lung, is increased in the fetus and also decreases after birth, although not so rapidly and possibly under the influence of the prostaglandins. Partly because of this, glomerular filtration and renal plasma flow are reduced relative to what they will shortly become. The interim effect is an infant who can easily be overloaded with water despite his or her difficulty conserving it. However, these problems seem strikingly to occur at the hands of physicians, not mothers.

DIGESTIVE SYSTEM

The newborn at term is neuromuscularly equipped to create the successively caudad sequence of intraluminal pressure gradients that constitute a sufficient peristalsis for movement of an ingested bolus from mouth to anus. These pressure gradients begin at the mouth in the form of the primeval act of deglutition, which requires a cooperative intermingling of motor and sensory effectiveness throughout the hindbrain (ninth, tenth, and twelfth cranial nerves) working in concert with the midbrain (fifth and seventh cranial nerves). Although gastrointestinal motility immediately postpartum may appear uncoordinated by adult standards, it is nevertheless extremely effective in moving swallowed air from mouth to rectum by 2 to 4 hours of age.

By histologic criteria, all the requisite structures (e.g., microvilli) for efficient absorption from the small bowel would appear to be in place by the time of term birth. The biochemical necessities for absorption would also appear to be satisfied for digestion of carbohydrates (amylase, lactase, and other disaccharidases) and proteins (gastric acid and pepsin, trypsin, and other pancreatic peptidases).

On the other hand, fat absorption is more tenuous. Lipase and bile salts are present by term; their rate of functional appearance is a linear function of gestational age. However, some significant doubt has long surrounded the question of which form of exogenous nutritional fat is the best to offer a newborn infant. The best current answer to this appears to be that the optimum ratio of unsaturated to saturated fatty acids and the optimum distribution of carbon chain lengths of saturated fatty acids are provided each species by its own *mother's milk*.

The microbiologic sterility of the newborn gut at birth *(gnotobiosis)* begins to change immediately after birth through invasion of the mouth and anus by ambient microorganisms. This is a necessary act of matriculation as a human (or other terrestrial) being, which will be best handled by the newborn's unhurried introduction only to those benign microbial species that will dominate the intestinal tract and eventually aid in producing vitamin K and reducing the likelihood of contracting hemorrhagic disease of the newborn.

HEPATIC FUNCTION

During fetal life most hepatic duties are assumed by the maternal liver via the placenta. Indeed, most fetal blood flow returning from the placenta is actually shunted through the liver via the ductus venosus, which collapses after birth (as umbilical and placental venous return collapses), thus forcing perfusion of the liver by the portal circulation.

The liver's stores of glycogen are rapidly depleted after birth to supply energy until effective oral feeding is established. Stored fat is used next, after the supply of liver glycogen becomes depleted. Liver and cardiac glycogen and the energy these stores contain are the likely basis for the greater resistance of the newborn to hypoxia.

However, the major lifetime job of the liver is the production of proteins—the plasma proteins (albumin and globulins), enzymes, and clotting factors, and it is in this area that the neonatal liver appears most immature for reasons not yet clear. Many drug or other detoxifying reactions under enzymatic control are slow in infants, leading to prolonged half-lives for many drugs compared with those in adults.

The best known example of this enzymatic torpor in the newborn is the conjugation of free bilirubin (lipid soluble) with glucuronic acid to form excretable (water-soluble) bilirubin diglucuronide. The reaction is under the control of glucuronyl transferase, an enzyme whose activity is diminished at birth (which helps account for the frequency of jaundice in newborns) but rises rapidly to adult levels thereafter.

IMMUNE SYSTEM

B-cell functions (the production of antibody) develop relatively late in fetal life. Moreover, the bacteriologically sterile fetus receives no stimulus from foreign antigen to produce antibodies. Why maternal cells leaking into this system are apparently not soon rejected as immunologic invaders is one of the great mysteries of reproductive biology. In any case, the only significant antibody level mounted at birth is that of IgG, passively obtained transplacentally from the mother, but the infant will (or should) shortly receive a good deal of IgA and macrophages from the mother's colostrum and breast milk. Diagnostic use can be made of these facts, in that elevations of cord blood IgM may be taken as evidence for preexisting (long enough to mount an antibody response) intrauterine infection.

Cellular immunity (T-cell function) is largely intact in newborns and is, along with the borrowed maternal IgG, the bedrock of their immune competence; phagocytosis is depressed, however, and, in the face of large bacterial inocula, sometimes critically so. The problem is that although the infant's macrophages and neutrophils are quite capable of ingestion and digestion, the particles and bacteria to be attacked are insufficiently opsonized by the low serum complement levels of the newborn. Thus although the infant must inevitably learn to deal with microorganisms through exposure, it would be most prudent to arrange that all such exposures be in moderation.

ENDOCRINE SYSTEM

The *thyroid* gland is operative early in fetal life and by term has stored sufficient T_3 and T_4 to sustain the infant's metabolism against thermal and nutritional stress, by virtue of a miniature thyroid storm (in this case "rush") precipitated by his or her eviction from the womb.

The *parathyroid* gland is similarly functional, but perhaps not robustly so. The relatively high serum calcium level of fetal life drops rapidly at birth from about 11 to 8.5 mg/dl, as phosphorus rises, and yet apparently does not elicit a reactive resorption of bone to defend serum calcium or an enhanced excretion of phosphorus. Precise explanations are not at hand but may deal in part with a high ingested phosphorus load, especially in the infant who is fed cow milk–based formula.

The *adrenal cortex* of the normal infant is quite capable of mounting a suitable glucocorticoid and mineralocorticoid response to stress. On the other hand, the *adrenal medulla* (and the paraspinal chromaffin organ of Zuckerkandl) is almost totally devoted to the production of norepinephrine (an alpha-agonist) rather than to epinephrine (an alpha- and beta-agonist). Perhaps these organs are aware that the heart is at the peak of its function curve and may not be able to respond to further beta-stimulation without decompensation. In addition, norepinephrine is the facilitator of thermogenesis within dark adipose tissue ("brown fat"), an important factor in helping infants maintain their body temperature after birth.

The hormones of the pancreatic islet cells, *insulin* and *glucagon*—and, just as important, their receptors in the body's tissues—are functional at birth, although (in the case of insulin) somewhat sluggishly released.

NEUROLOGIC SYSTEM

Through most of the last half of fetal life, glial and neuronal cells differentiate in the paraventricular germinal matrix, with the neuronal axons developing dendrites that, through a prolonged process of arborization, develop many thousands of synapses. The process of neuronal migration distributes these neurons throughout the neuraxis (cord, hindbrain, midbrain, forebrain) in the form of compact nuclei or looser reticular formations or the laminated sheets (six in all) of the cerebral gray matter.

The axonal pathways are formed when neurons and glial cells are combined and become myelinated, but differentially (caudad to cephalad), so that at birth the forebrain and midbrain are still largely unmyelinated. Although unmyelinated pathways have slower conduction times, the shorter interneuronal and neuromuscular distances to be traveled in the newborn result in reflex arcs not much different in duration of action from those of adults.

The behavior of reflexes is much influenced by the (behavioral) state of consciousness. Proprioceptive reflexes, which generate postural body tonus, are abolished during active (rapid eye movement) sleep, which strongly inhibits motor neurons. Similarly, quiet sleep diminishes the exteroceptive reflexes whose efferent arcs come from skin, retinal, and aural receptors, rather than from the muscle stretch receptors of proprioception.

The higher cortical functions are just now being investigated by both biophysical and psychologic techniques. It already appears that newborn humans are a great deal more involved with and occasionally manipulative of their environment and caregivers than was previously supposed.

Three
Recovery Period

Nicholas M. Nelson

The most major of modern surgical procedures is unlikely to equal the physiologic strains on the infant of a normal birth—massive head trauma, asphyxiation, massive blood transfusion with cardiopulmonary bypass, and often resuscitation, all followed by major hypothermic insult—no wonder the infant cries! Clement Smith[1] has called this "the Valley of the Shadow of Birth," but it is a normal event experienced by every human being (just as is death) and may be regarded as the disease from which *nearly* everyone recovers. However, where should the "recovery room" be located?

Important observations need to be made in these first few hours, and it is not easy in either home or hospital (however homelike) to make them without untoward medical intrusion on what many would wish were more of a private family affair. The solution is to begin early in pregnancy to build toward extending the parents' "family" to include the hospital's perinatal personnel to the point that it becomes almost immaterial whether these observations are made in the mother's room or in a contiguous recovery room (observation nursery).

CONVERSION FROM PLACENTAL TO ORAL ENERGY ASSIMILATION

The eviction from the womb that is birth may be compared, metabolically speaking, with forceful ejection from one's warm and friendly neighborhood "pub" into the cold, midwinter streets—naked and without a free lunch. The sober adult in such circumstances would immediately seek clothing not out of civilized modesty but out of primal necessity to prevent excessive loss of body heat through convection by surrounding the skin with layers of insulating dead air. He would simultaneously vasoconstrict his skin ("blue with cold"—acrocyanosis), shiver to produce muscular heat, and begin to generate an increased amount of chemical heat by releasing thyroxin (to energize all cells) and catecholamines (to release the energy stored in fat by its lipolysis into glycerol and free fatty acids). The newborn child does precisely the same (but does not shiver) and with at least as great efficiency (Fig. 36-4).

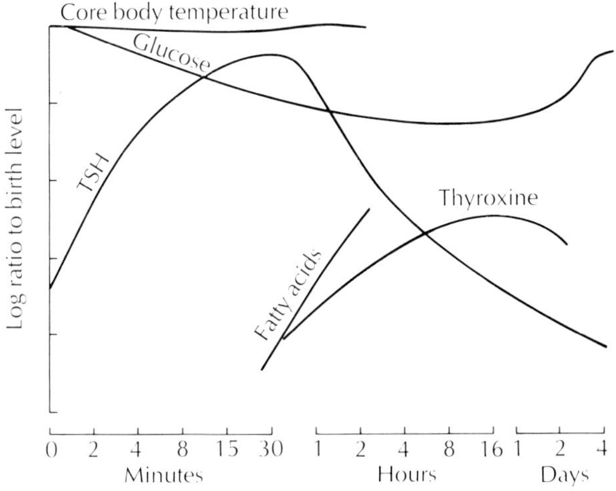

Fig. 36-4 Metabolic changes at birth. Data are shown as the approximate log [(Value at time)/(Value at birth)], which ranges from zero *(bottom tic)* to one *(top tic)*.

From data of Smith CA and Nelson NM: The physiology of the newborn infant, ed 4, Springfield, Ill, 1976, Charles C Thomas, Publisher.

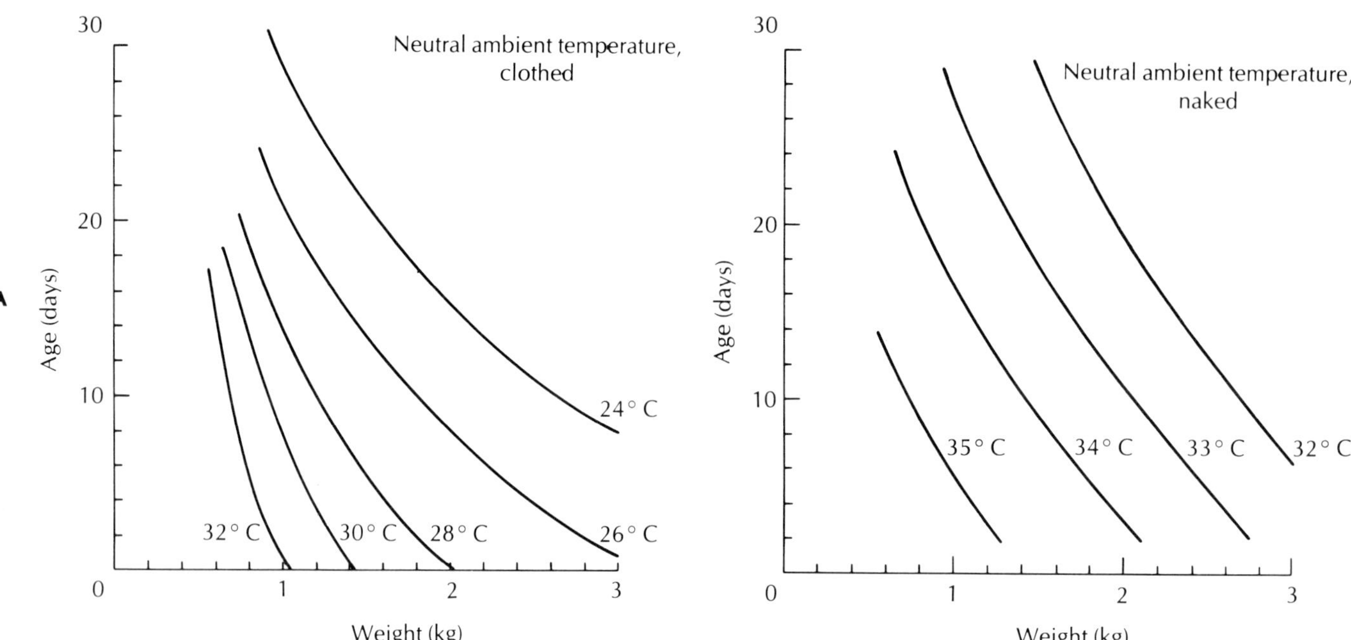

Fig. 36-5 Neutral ambient temperature for clothed **(A)** and naked **(B)** infants of varying postpartum age and weight. The neutral temperature is that ambient temperature at which energy expenditure to maintain body temperature is minimal (e.g., a naked 1-kg infant at age 10 days requires an ambient temperature of about 34.5° C for minimal energy expenditure to defend body temperature).

From data of Scopes JW and Ahmed I: Range of critical temperatures in sick and premature newborn babies, Arch Dis Child 41:417, 1966.

Thoughtful medical attendants to that child will supply warm clothing or warmth by radiant warmer, incubator, or other thermal device and arrange the ambient temperature so that minimal thermal energy demands (the "neutral temperature," Fig. 36-5) are made of the infant, who must concentrate most of his or her stored energy investment into the principal continuing task of growth and development, at least until ingestion, digestion, and excretion are well established.

TRANSITION AND ESTABLISHMENT OF VITAL FUNCTION

The initial hours of recovery have been clinically characterized as *alert* (0 to 30 minutes), then *unresponsive* (30 minutes to 2 hours), and finally *reactive* (2 to 8 hours), as shown in Fig. 36-6, during which time the infant displays signs of general sympathetic (tachycardia, tachypnea, and vasomotion) and then parasympathetic (peristalsis) discharge, probably in response to the sensory overload that attends birth, particularly chilling. The onset of peristalsis heralds the first defecation and micturition, the timing of which should be carefully noted, since untoward delay in either (Fig. 36-7) may signal significant gastrointestinal or genitourinary abnormalities.

In the event of normal birth, the pediatrician is likely to make first physical acquaintance with the newborn in the nursery rather than in the delivery room. Therefore, after a period of observation by the nursery ("recovery room") staff, those elements calling for special surveillance (Table 36-5) need to be gleaned from the obstetric history and communicated to the pediatrician as a confirmation of previous alerts from the obstetric staff.

Even in the absence of such obstetric markers of high risk for neonatal morbidity, *observers in the nursery should always assume that every infant harbors clinically occult congenital anomalies or birth trauma* that may have escaped detection in the initial (delivery room) or subsequent detailed (nursery) physical examination until the passage of time gradually documents the establishment of certain vital functions without error (Table 36-6).

During this period of stabilization for the newborn infant, the following are most closely observed: body temperature, skin color, heart rate, blood pressure, peripheral circulation, respiratory rate and type of effort, muscle tone, body activity, and apparent behavioral state.

MATURATIONAL, BEHAVIORAL, PHYSICAL, AND NEUROLOGIC EXAMINATIONS

As in all of pediatrics, the components of a physician's thinking about a normal or abnormal infant are very much structured around the baby's growth and development in comparison with accepted norms. In later infancy and childhood, the required time dimension (the *x* axis of growth charts) is measured in months or years, and the origin is fixed with certainty (date of birth). The practice of these principles is more difficult in the perinatal period because time is measured in weeks and the date of conception cannot be fixed with any real certainty. Nonetheless, fetal and neonatal examinations of many infants of many different populations by many observers have now produced a number of acceptable norms and have standardized the assessment of gestational age.

Assessment of Gestational Age

The combined assessment of neuromuscular maturity (see box on p. 450) and certain physical features of genitalia, ears, skin, breast, plantar creases, and hair has proved to be a

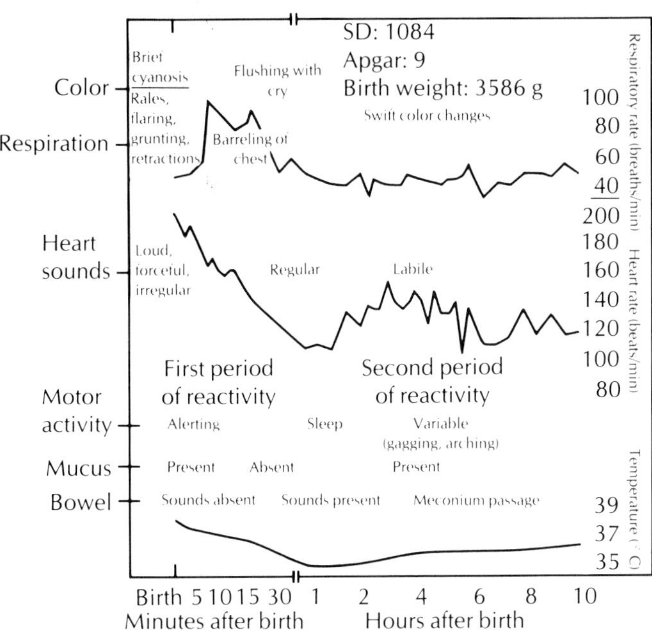

Fig. 36-6 Autonomic changes during the period of transition after birth. *SD,* Subject designation.

From Desmond MM, Rudolph AJ, and Phitaksphraiwan P: The transitional care nursery: a mechanism for preventive medicine in the newborn, Pediatr Clin North Am 13:656, 1966.

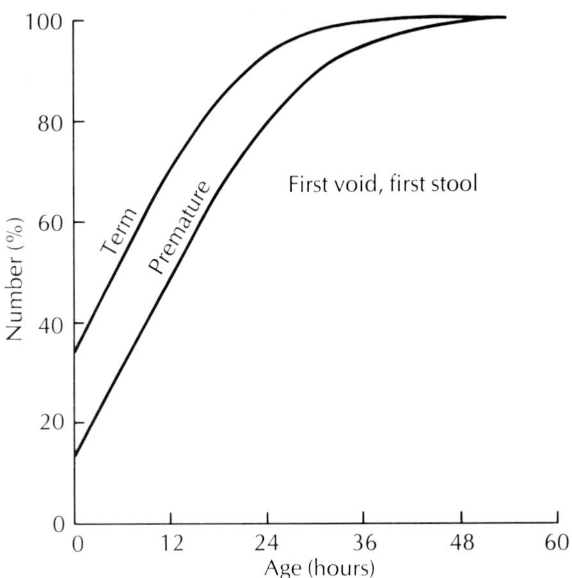

Fig. 36-7 First stool and void after birth: age by which the indicated cumulative percentage of infants have stooled and voided.

From data of Sherry SN and Kramer I: The time of passage of the first stool and the first urine by the newborn infant, J Pediatr 46:158, 1955; and Kramer I and Sherry SN: The time of passage of the first stool and urine by the premature infant. J Pediatr 51:373, 1957.

Table 36-5 *Levels of Surveillance of the Newborn Based on the Obstetric History*

	LEVEL OF SURVEILLANCE		
HISTORY	NORMAL	ALERT	ALARM
Pregnancy			
Surveillance	Registered during first trimester	Unregistered during second trimester	Unregistered and in labor
Genetic disease	None known	In family	In sibling of fetus
Uterine volume		Polyhydramnios	Oligohydramnios
Fetal movement		Increased	Decreased
Biochemical		Decreased estriol levels	
Biophysical		Positive oxytocin challenge test	Uterine ultrasound abnormality
Maternal disease		Diabetes and hypertension	Active tuberculosis
Rupture of membranes		<36 wk	
Labor	36-42 wk	<36, >42 wk	<34 wk
Delivery			
Vaginal		"Difficult" breech	
Cesarean	Elective (repeat)	Elective (initial)	Emergency
Fetus	Apgar 8-10	Apgar 4-7, visible congenital anomaly	Asphyxia (Apgar <4) and hydrops fetalis

reliable means for estimating gestational age (Fig. 36-8). Further corroboration may be sought by examining the vascularity in the anterior capsule of the lens (Fig. 36-9). Thus armed with a working knowledge of gestational age in comparison with birth weight against established norms (e.g., the Colorado interuterine growth charts), the examiner should next judge whether the infant is large, appropriate, or small for his or her gestational age (LGA, AGA, and SGA, respectively) and thus become appropriately alerted to diagnostic possibilities (see Fig. 35-4). Specific characteristics of premature, postmature, SGA, and LGA infants are discussed in a later section of this chapter, under "Stages of Maturation."

Behavioral Assessment

Although not often part of the routine surveillance of the normal newborn infant, a Brazelton score awarded by a skilled observer of newborn behavior has proved to be a

Table 36-6 *Levels of Surveillance of the Newborn Based on Vital Functions*

VITAL FUNCTION	LEVEL OF SURVEILLANCE		
	NORMAL	ALERT	ALARM
Respiration	Paradoxical	Periodic tachypnea or retractions	Apnea, bradycardia, grunting, or gasping
Circulation	Acrocyanosis and heart rate 110-165 beats/min	Tachycardia, hypertension, or cardiac murmur	Central cyanosis, bradycardia, hypotension, enlarged heart, or pallor
Metabolism	Body temperature of 95.9° to 99.5° F (35.5° to 37.5° C)	Hyperthermia	Hypothermia
Digestion	Drooling or "transitional" stools	Spitting	Vomiting or diarrhea
Excretion		No voiding (>24 hr) and no stooling (>24 hr)	Dribbling stream
Behavior	Alert, unresponsive, reactive, startle, or sneeze	Hyperactive, jittery, or yawning	Coma or convulsions

Techniques for Assessment of Neuromuscular Maturity

POSTURE

With the infant supine and quiet, score as follows:

- Arms and legs extended = 0
- Slight or moderate flexion of hips and knees = 1
- Moderate to strong flexion of hips and knees = 2
- Legs flexed and abducted, arms slightly flexed = 3
- Full flexion of arms and legs = 4

SQUARE WINDOW

Flex the hand at the wrist; exert pressure sufficient to get as much flexion as possible. The angle between the hypothenar eminence and the anterior aspect of the forearm is measured and scored according to Fig. 36-8. Do not rotate the wrist.

ARM RECOIL

With the infant supine, fully flex the forearm for 5 seconds, then fully extend by pulling the hands and releasing. Score the reaction according to the following:

- Remains extended or random movements = 0
- Incomplete or partial flexion = 1
- Brisk return to full flexion = 2

POPLITEAL ANGLE

With the infant supine and the pelvis flat on the examining surface, the leg is flexed on the thigh and the thigh is fully flexed with the use of one hand. With the other hand the leg is then extended, and the angle attained is scored as in Fig. 36-8.

SCARF SIGN

With the infant supine, take the infant's hand and draw it across the neck and as far across the opposite shoulder as possible. Assistance to the elbow is permissible by lifting it across the body. Score according to the location of the elbow:

- Elbow reaches beyond the opposite anterior axillary line = 0
- Elbow reaches to the opposite anterior axillary line = 1
- Elbow is between opposite anterior axillary line and midline of thorax = 2
- Elbow is at midline of thorax = 3
- Elbow does not reach midline of thorax = 4

HEEL-TO-EAR MANEUVER

With the infant supine, hold the infant's foot with one hand and move it as near to the head as possible without forcing it. Keep the pelvis flat on the examining surface. Score as in Fig. 36-8.

From Amiel-Tison C: Neurological evaluation of the maturity of newborn infants, Arch Dis Child 43:89, 1968; Dubowitz LMS, Dubowitz V, and Goldberg C: Clinical assessment of gestational age in the newborn infant, J Pediatr 77:1, 1970.

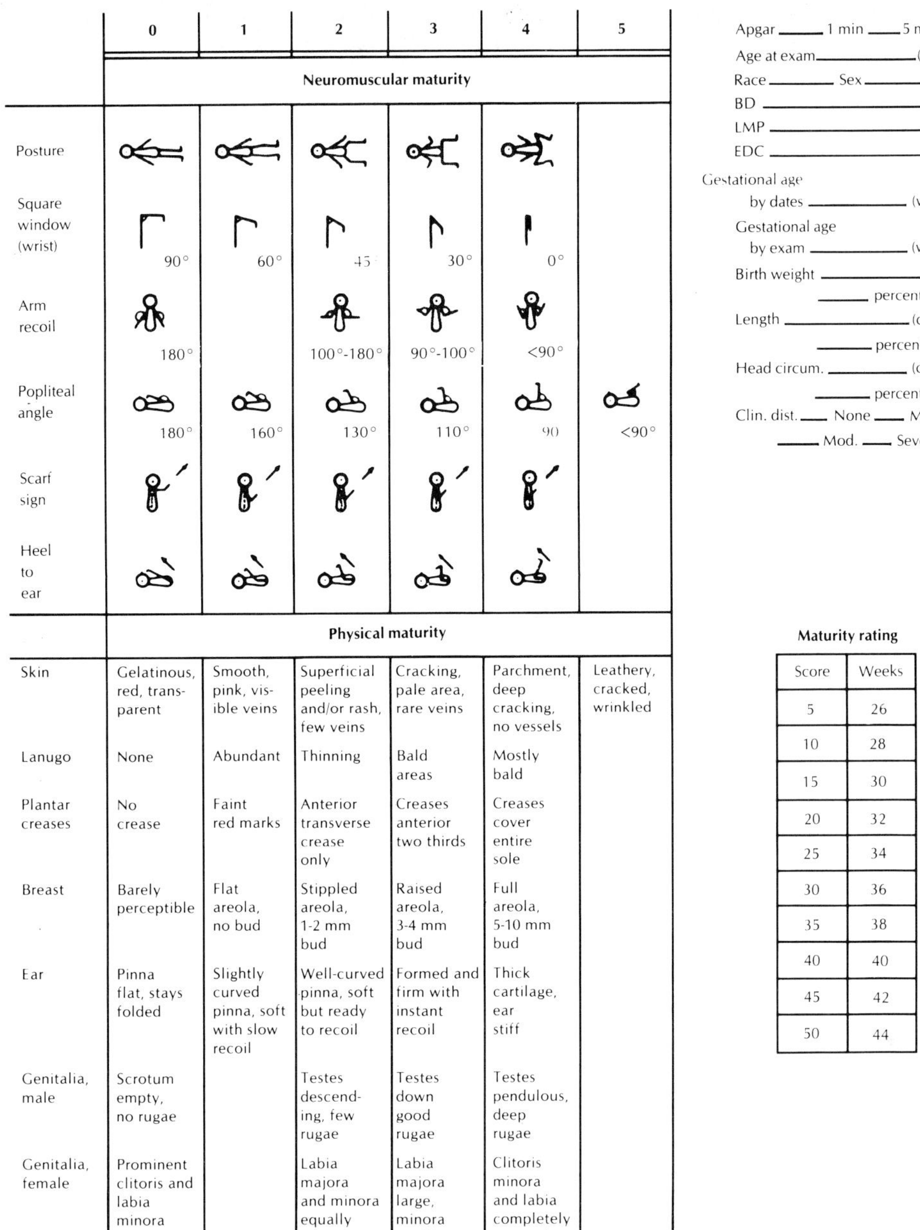

	0	1	2	3	4	5
Neuromuscular maturity						
Posture						
Square window (wrist)	90°	60°	45°	30°	0°	
Arm recoil	180°		100°-180°	90°-100°	<90°	
Popliteal angle	180°	160°	130°	110°	90°	<90°
Scarf sign						
Heel to ear						
Physical maturity						
Skin	Gelatinous, red, transparent	Smooth, pink, visible veins	Superficial peeling and/or rash, few veins	Cracking, pale area, rare veins	Parchment, deep cracking, no vessels	Leathery, cracked, wrinkled
Lanugo	None	Abundant	Thinning	Bald areas	Mostly bald	
Plantar creases	No crease	Faint red marks	Anterior transverse crease only	Creases anterior two thirds	Creases cover entire sole	
Breast	Barely perceptible	Flat areola, no bud	Stippled areola, 1-2 mm bud	Raised areola, 3-4 mm bud	Full areola, 5-10 mm bud	
Ear	Pinna flat, stays folded	Slightly curved pinna, soft with slow recoil	Well-curved pinna, soft but ready to recoil	Formed and firm with instant recoil	Thick cartilage, ear stiff	
Genitalia, male	Scrotum empty, no rugae		Testes descending, few rugae	Testes down good rugae	Testes pendulous, deep rugae	
Genitalia, female	Prominent clitoris and labia minora		Labia majora and minora equally prominent	Labia majora large, minora small	Clitoris minora and labia completely covered	

Apgar ___ 1 min ___ 5 min
Age at exam ___ (hr)
Race ___ Sex ___
BD ___
LMP ___
EDC ___
Gestational age by dates ___ (wk)
Gestational age by exam ___ (wk)
Birth weight ___ (g)
___ percentile
Length ___ (cm)
___ percentile
Head circum. ___ (cm)
___ percentile
Clin. dist. ___ None ___ Mild
___ Mod. ___ Severe

Maturity rating

Score	Weeks
5	26
10	28
15	30
20	32
25	34
30	36
35	38
40	40
45	42
50	44

Fig. 36-8 Assessment of gestational age in weeks, using neuromuscular and physical maturity criteria combined. The box at left describes methods used to assess neuromuscular maturity. The assessment is quickly and easily performed because the box includes measures of physical maturity and measures of passive but not active tone. Physical maturity is most accurately assessed in the minutes or hour or so following birth. The score for each item is indicated at the top of the vertical column. However, neuromuscular maturity may be spuriously retarded in the asphyxiated neonate or the neonate obtunded by anesthetic agents or drugs. Thus the neuromuscular maturity rating should be repeated after a day or two. The sum of scores on all the items of physical and neuromuscular maturity provides an estimate of maturity in weeks *(see lower right)*.

From American Academy of Pediatrics and the American College of Obstetricians and Gynecologists: Guidelines for perinatal care, Washington, DC, 1983, p. 83. Reproduced by permission of *Pediatrics*, copyright 1983.

reproducible and valid means for evaluating infant behavior (see box on p. 453) and detecting behavioral changes imposed by birth injury or maternal analgesics.

Through this and other means, it has recently become apparent that term newborns regularly indulge in considerably more environmental interaction and even manipulation than heretofore suspected: they prefer human faces to other faces, listen to high-pitched voices, and respond to speech cadences; they are soothed by resumption of the intrauterine "position of comfort"; and they can smell their mother's milk.

How much of this behavioral display may be available for viewing depends on the infant's behavioral "state," which includes several states of sleep, variously graded on a scale of 4 points (awake, active sleep, indeterminate sleep, and

POINTS	0	1	2	3	4
BREAST SIZE		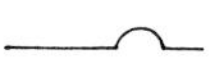 < .5 cm	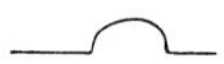 > .5 cm < 1 cm	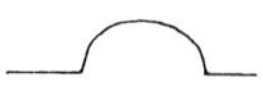 > 1 cm	
FOOT CREASES	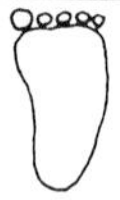	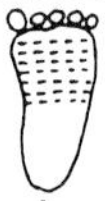 faint red marks ant. half	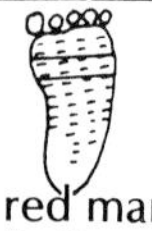 faint red marks >ant half indent. <ant $1/3$	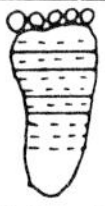 indent >ant. $1/3$	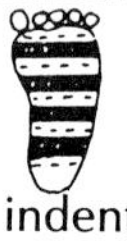 deep indent. >ant $1/3$
EAR FIRMNESS	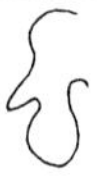 soft easily folded no recoil	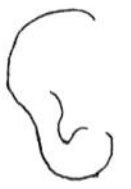 soft easily folded slow recoil	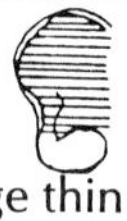 cartilage thin in places ready recoil	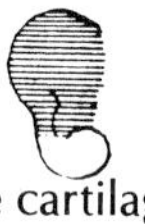 definite cartilage extend. to periph. immediate recoil	
LENS	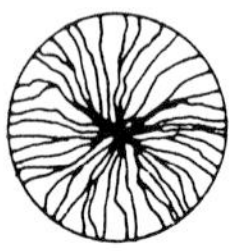	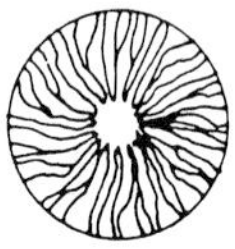	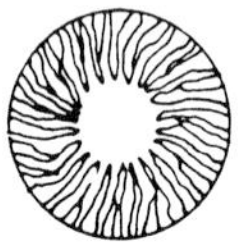	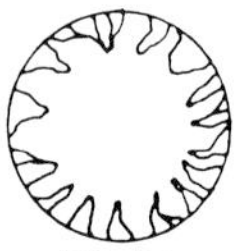	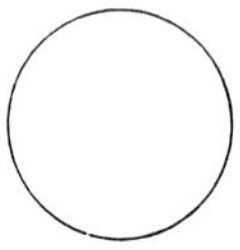
wks	27-28	29-30	31-32	33-34	>35

Total Score	Gestational Age Weeks
1	28
2	29
3	29½
4	30½
5	31

GESTATIONAL AGE

For scores >5: Score + 26 = weeks gestational age (example: score = 6 (+ 26) = 32 weeks gestational age).

BREAST SIZE—measured by picking up the breast tissue between finger and thumb.
0 = no breast tissue palpable.
1 = breast tissue palpable on one or both sides, neither being more than 0.5cm in diameter.
2 = breast tissue palpable on both sides, one or both being 0.5 to 1cm in diameter.
3 = breast tissue palpable on both sides, one or both being more than 1 cm in diameter.

PLANTAR SKIN CREASES—assessed by noting the creases which persist when the skin of the sole is stretched from toes to heel.
0 = no skin creases present.
1 = skin creases are faint red marks over the anterior half of the sole.
2 = creases are definite red marks over more than the anterior half of the sole, and indentation is present over no more than the anterior third.
3 = as (2) but the indentation is present over more than the anterior third of the sole.
4 = deep indentations present > ant ⅓ of sole

EAR FIRMNESS—tested by palpation and folding of the upper pinna between finger and thumb.
0 = pinna feels soft, and is easily folded into bizzare positions without springing back into position spontaneously.
1 = pinna feels soft along the edge and is easily folded, but returns slowly to the correct position spontaneously.
2 = cartilage can be felt to the edge of the pinna, though it is thin in places, and the pinna springs back readily after being folded.
3 = pinna firm, with definite cartilage extending to the periphery, and springs back into position immediately after being folded.

LENS—tested by examination of the anterior vascular capsule of the lens[2].
0 = vessels completely covering the lens.
1 = small area of clearing, the diameter of which is less than one fourth that of the lens.
2 = larger area of clearing, the diameter of which is one fourth of one half that of the lens.
3 = small loops at the periphery with diameter of the area of clearing more than one half that of the lens.
4 = lens completely clear or having only an occasional strand or faint loop.

Adapted from personal communication of Palmor C from data of:

1. Narayanan I, et al. Pediatrics 69(1):27, 1982
2. Hittner HM et al. J Pediatr 91:456, 1977

Fig. 36-9 Rapid assessment of gestational age.[1]

Brazelton Behavioral Scale

ENVIRONMENTAL INTERACTIONS
Alertness
Consolability
Cuddliness
Orientation

STRESS RESPONSES
Skin color lability
Startle reaction
Tremulousness

MOTOR PROCESSES
Activity
Defensive reactions
Hand-to-mouth movement
Maturity
Reflex
Tone

PHYSIOLOGIC STATE
Habituation to stimuli
Self-quieting

quiet sleep) or 6 points (awake-crying, awake-active, quiet-alert, drowsy, rapid-eye-movement [REM] sleep, and deep sleep). They are at their most behaviorally competent in the quiet-alert state and at their most physiologically interesting in REM sleep (Fig. 36-10). During REM sleep, for instance, breathing becomes irregular and "paradoxical," as intercostal muscle tone collapses (thus weakening the chest wall) to allow the diaphragm to pull the thorax inward during its inspiratory descent.

General Physical Examination

As is implicit from the preceding discussion, the newborn infant's first formal and complete physical examination (Fig. 36-11) occurs during the period of transition in a setting of continuous and intense scrutiny by both the delivery room and nursery staffs, not to mention the parents. Moreover, there is considerable overlap of observations and interventions during the nursery stay.

The vital signs are observed by the nursing staff (Fig. 36-12). These have not traditionally included *blood pressure* because of the difficulty in auscultating Korotkoff sounds, but the increasing availability of oscillometers and Doppler devices should now make this important measurement routine.

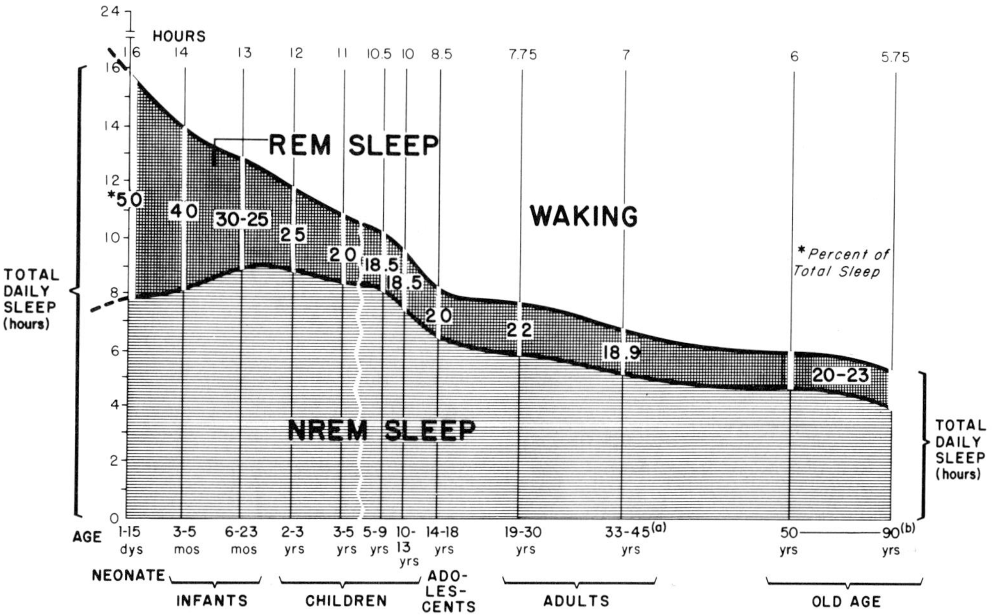

Fig. 36-10 Graph showing changes (with age) in total amounts of daily sleep, daily rapid eye movement *(REM)* sleep, and percentage of REM sleep. Note sharp diminution of REM sleep in the early years. REM sleep falls from 8 hours at birth to less than 1 hour in old age. The amount of nonrapid eye movement *(NREM)* sleep throughout life remains more constant, falling from 8 hours to 5 hours. In contrast to the steep decline of REM sleep, the quantity of NREM sleep is undiminished for many years. Although total daily REM sleep falls steadily during life, the percentage rises slightly in adolescence and early adulthood. This rise does not reflect an increase in amount; it is caused by the fact that REM sleep does not diminish as quickly as total sleep.

From Roffwarg HP, Muzio JN, and Dement WC: Ontogenetic development of the human sleep-dream cycle, Science 152:604-619, 1966. Copyright 1966 by the American Association for the Advancement of Science. (Revised since publication.)

NEONATAL RECORD (2)—NURSERY

BIRTH

BORN AT HOSPITAL	CITY	STATE
TIME	DATE	REFERRING PHYSICIAN M.D.

LMP	EDC	GESTATIONAL AGE WKS	VIT K_1 GIVEN AT HRS OF AGE

INTERVAL HISTORY

NURSERY EXAMINATION

DATE	TIME	AGE HRS	WGT GMS	SEX	RACE

LENGTH CMS	BIP CMS	SKULL CMS	CHEST CMS	ABDOMEN CMS

[KEY ✓= NORMAL, 0 = ABSENT, X = ABNORMAL]	EFFECTS OF FETAL POSTURE	GENERAL APPEARANCE

SKIN	SC TISSUE	FACIES	MASSES	SPLEEN	HIPS
VERNIX	EDEMA	EYES	THORAX	KIDNEYS	CNS-REFLEXES
PALLOR	NODES	EARS	BREATHING	CORD	CRY
ICTERUS	HEAD	NARES	LUNGS	ANUS	TONE
CYANOSIS	FONTANELLES	MOUTH	HEART	GENITALIA	PARALYSIS
BIRTHMARKS	SUTURES	NECK	ABDOMEN	SKELETON	MORO
BRUISING	CPHLHMTOMA	THYROID	LIVER	CLAVICLES	GRASP

GESTATIONAL AGE ASSESSMENT = WEEKS

ABNORMAL FINDINGS

IMPRESSION

SIGNED M.D.

Fig. 36-11 Data relevant to the neonatal physical examination.

NEWBORN NURSING ASSESSMENT

Admission: Date _____ Time _____ Birth: Date _____ Time _____ Weight _____ Length _____ Head _____

Gestation: By Dates _____ By Dubowitz _____ AGA/LGA/SGA _____

Relevant OB History

Ears & Eyes — $AgNO_3$ 1% Crede 2 gtts each eye ☐

Nose — Nares Patent: By occlusion ☐ catheter ☐

Mouth

Skin

Head

Chest

Abdomen, Umbilical Vessels

Genitals — Anus Patent: By appearance ☐ catheter ☐

Extremities, Skeleton

Nervous System

Activity

Transitional TPR

Time		Comments	Initials

General Comments

Signature: _____

Six Hour Assessment

Skin _____

Chest _____

Abdomen _____

Nervous System _____

Activity _____

Comments:

Signature: _____

Fig. 36-12 Nursing surveillance of the normal newborn infant.

The most cooperative infant will be one who is 1 to 2 hours postprandial, in the quiet-alert *behavioral state,* and examined under thermal conditions not too far from his or her neutral thermal environment (see Fig. 36-5). The infant's *general appearance* will have been noted during the assessment of gestational age, but particular attention should now be redirected to his or her apparent *nutritional state* (especially subcutaneous tissue and muscle mass) and *postural tone.* The more mature the infant, the greater is the flexor tone displayed as part of the resting posture.

The most productive physical (and neurologic) examination is one conducted on an infant who is 1 to 2 hours postprandial, at a reasonably normal ambient temperature, and in a quiet-alert state of consciousness.

Much of the normal (or normal variant) findings of the newborn infant's physical examination are presented in Chapter 7, "The Pediatric Physical Examination." Here we will focus on those aspects that should raise the suspicion of abnormality. Nevertheless, those portions of Chapter 7 dealing with the physical examination of each of the organ systems under the heading of the "Newborn" should also be consulted.

The Skin and Its Appendages (Table 36-7). The naked infant should be most carefully observed regarding skin color; *pallor, jaundice,* and *cyanosis* may each become an indication for alarm, depending on time of onset, duration, and intensity. *Excoriations* of the epidermis can easily be a normal result of long fingernails but, when observed in a yawning or "jittery" baby, may also indicate neonatal abstinence (withdrawal from maternal narcotics) syndrome (see Chapter 229, "Neonatal Abstinence Syndrome"). A *lumbosacral tuft* of hair may point to pilonidal sinus, diastematomyelia, or teratoma. One needs reassurance that a *scalp defect* is not accompanied by other signs of trisomy 13 (see Chapter 29, "Genetic Diseases"). The skin's texture is normally soft and moist ("as a baby's bottom") at term, but it lacks fullness of subcutaneous tissue in the preterm infant and becomes dry, cracked, or peeling in the vernix-deprived postmature or undergrown infant. It is grotesquely thickened and crusted ("collodion baby") in various rare types of *ichthyosis.* An apparently normal phenomenon of vascular reactivity is the mottled ("marbled") vascular pattern of dilated venules in the (usually chilled) newborn. When persistent, this mottled *cutis marmorata* may be an associate of trisomy 18 (see Chapter 29) or trisomy 21 (see Chapter 199, "Down Syndrome"). A phenomenon of the late neonatal period (1 month) is *acne* (true comedo), seen mostly over the cheeks and chin as tiny, coalescing erythematous papules that usually disappear over a few weeks.

The clay-colored greasy *vernix caseosa* that covers the healthy term newborn at birth almost magically evaporates within hours after birth and is sparse to absent in the postmature infant, whose superficial epidermal layers are soon cracked and *peeling.* However, this is quite different from the full-thickness denudation that marks the *scalded skin syndrome* (toxic epidermal necrolysis) of staphylococcal sepsis.

As what are probably the most common tumors of all

Table 36-7 *Levels of Surveillance of the Newborn Based on the Examination of the Skin and its Appendages*

CHARACTERISTIC	LEVEL OF SURVEILLANCE NORMAL	ALERT	ALARM
Color (age of occurrence)			
Cyanosis	Acrocyanosis (<12 hr)	Central (<1 hr)	Central (>1 hr)
Jaundice	>24 hr	18-24 hr	<18 hr
Pallor			>30 min
Epidermis	Dermatoglyphics	Excoriations	Sloughing
Hair	Lanugo	Lumbosacral tuft and scalp defect	
Texture	Soft and moist	Dry and scaling	Thickened and crusting
Vascular pattern	Harlequin, mottling (cold)	Persistent mottling	
Cysts	Milia and Epstein pearls		
Papules	Acne and miliaria		
Desquamation	Delicate scaling (>2 days)	Peeling (<2 days)	Denuded sheets (anytime)
Hemangiomas	Telangiectatic (forehead, lids, lips, and nape)	Telangiectatic (trigeminal) and angiomatous (few)	Angiomatous (multiple)
Hemorrhage	Petechiae (head or upper body)	Petechiae (elsewhere)	Ecchymoses and purpura
Macules	Mongolian spots	Café-au-lait spots (<6 spots)	Café-au-lait spots (>5 spots) and "mountain ash" leaf
Pustules	Erythema toxicum		Large and dermal
Vesicles			Any
Nodules		Subcutaneous fat necrosis	Sclerema

humans (or, certainly, infants), hemangiomas range from the telangiectatic ("capillary") nevi or "salmon patch," so common on the lids, forehead, and nape ("stork bite") of the newborn, to the multiple or massive and often grotesque angiomatous ("cavernous") variety (see Chapter 37, "Skin Lesions of the Neonate"). Diffuse neonatal *hemangiomatosis* is the rare but fatal maximum expression of this spectrum, often marked by cardiac failure to manage the vast volume overload presented by these multiple arteriovenous fistulas, often in major organs (liver, brain, etc.). Between these extremes may reside *Sturge-Weber syndrome* (venous angiomatosis of leptomeninges, atrophic cerebral cortex, buphthalmos, seizures, hemiparesis, and mental retardation), suggested by an ipsilateral facial port-wine stain in the trigeminal distribution. However, the linkage of cerebral and cutaneous venous angiomatosis is not firm, since many patients with a *port-wine stain* have perfectly normal cerebral function.

A cutaneous *hemorrhage* in any form is justifiable cause for concern that some form of bleeding diathesis may be at hand. Yet some *petechiae* (and *subconjunctival hemorrhage*) may well be observed within the superior vena caval drainage system after a normal vertex delivery, as an expression of the significant pressure differentials to which the fetus is subject on rupture of the forewaters.

The very common, completely mysterious, and completely benign perifollicular eruption that is *erythema toxicum* ("flea-bite dermatitis") appears on the second or third day of life as 1 to 3 mm white or pale yellow papules or pustules on a small erythematous but uninflamed base. They can become much larger and even confluent, to risk confusion with bacterial pyoderma; however, smears of the sterile contents of these lesions reveal eosinophils rather than neutrophils. The infants are well, and the pustules resolve simultaneously within hours to days.

Vesicles may be associated with benign conditions (e.g., transient neonatal pustular melanosis) but must always raise concern that the infant is involved with a serious disease, whether infectious (e.g., herpes, syphilis, toxic epidermal necrolysis) or inherited (e.g., epidermolysis bullosa or incontinentia pigmenti). Therefore these lesions demand expert consultation.

Nodules are perhaps the least frequent primary cutaneous lesion to be seen in the newborn. *Subcutaneous fat necrosis* (pseudosclerema) appears in the first few days as localized areas of induration over buttocks, cheeks, or the back, with blotchy and reddened overlying skin. Its definitive cause is unknown, but it is attributed to poor perfusion caused by cold stress or asphyxia, and it spontaneously resolves over weeks

Table 36-8 *Levels of Surveillance of the Newborn Based on the Head and Neck Examination*

LOCATION	LEVEL OF SURVEILLANCE		
	NORMAL	ALERT	ALARM
Skull	Caput succedaneum molding, or occipital overhang	Cephalohematoma, craniotabes, large fontanelle, or forceps mark	Craniosynostosis, transillumination, or bruit
Facies		Hypoplasia or palsy	
Eyes		Mongoloid slant	Aniridia and enlarged cornea
Nose		Nasal obstruction	
Mouth		High-arched palate or macroglossia	Cleft palate and/or lip or micrognathia
Ears		"Simple" structure or low set	
Neck	Rotation ±90 degrees	Dimple or webbing	

to months. *Sclerema neonatorum* is a presumably related process of induration in adipose tissue, formerly seen in hypothermic and usually moribund premature infants.

The Head and Neck (Table 36-8). *Caput succedaneum* is subcutaneous edema over the presenting part of the head; it is far more common than is cephalohematoma, is usually situated over the occiput, and crosses suture lines. Caput tends to feel soft and lacks a well-defined outline but is not fluctuant like a cephalohematoma. The edema is most pronounced at birth and subsides within 2 or 3 days. It is particularly common after delivery by vacuum extraction.

On the other hand, *cephalohematoma* is a subperiosteal collection of blood and as such is bounded by suture lines. It occurs in full-term healthy babies, most often in the parietal region. Cephalohematoma may not be obvious at birth but increases in size over the first few hours or days of life, giving rise to a firm mass with a well-defined edge. The center of the swelling may liquify, giving a feel of fluctuance or an erroneous impression of a depressed skull fracture. The mass occasionally calcifies and persists for weeks to months. Complications include hyperbilirubinemia and underlying skull fracture, the latter being associated with about 20% of cephalohematomas.

A *subgaleal hemorrhage* is sometimes mistaken for cephalohematoma. However, the subgaleal space is not limited by suture lines, and the blood tends to collect in dependent positions. Moreover, the space is large; thus a newborn may lose a large amount of blood, leading to hyperbilirubinemia and anemia or even shock.

Molding refers to the overriding of sagittal, coronal, or lambdoid sutures in a normal newborn delivered vaginally from the vertex position. Molding serves as benign testimony to the forces of labor, not shared by the infant delivered by cesarean section or from the breech position; the latter is often characterized by a pronounced occipital "overhang" in the skull contour. The head is often irregular in shape, with the parietooccipital region prominent; the forehead tends to slope backward. Molding is especially likely to be seen in first babies, in a large infant after prolonged labor, or where there is an element of cephalopelvic disproportion. The abnormal skull features usually return to normal by 5 or 6 days after birth.

A *large anterior fontanelle* should alert the examiner to the possibility of a defect in membranous bone formation (e.g., achondroplasia, hypophosphatasia, or cretinism) or increased intracranial pressure. *Small or absent fontanelles*, if associated with a pronouncedly misshapen skull or facies, may indicate a number of cosmetically threatening but treatable bony abnormalities, such as Crouzon disease or craniosynostosis, although the latter is usually not evident in the immediate neonatal period. The uninformed observer is often too willing to attribute a unilateral *facial palsy* to "misapplied" forceps, which often leaves their blade mark temporarily over the eye or cheek. Most such infants have a shoulder that neatly tucks under the ear (and into the stylomastoid foramen) of the palsied side. In any case, these palsies tend to resolve quickly after birth. Two of the most threatening observations to be made of the skull are also two of the most subtle: (1) a *bruit* must be specifically listened for and may indicate a cerebral arteriovenous fistula, and (2) positive *transillumination* ("candling") of the head (by flashlight in a darkened room or by high-intensity "Chun gun" beam in a lighted room) may be the only clinical indication of hydranencephaly—massive liquefaction of cerebral tissue (see Fig. 7-12).

After noting the presence of a retinal *red reflex* and palpebral fissures of normal size, the examiner should also ensure that there is no *mongoloid slant* (as in Down syndrome) and that the iris is present, since there is a high association of Wilm tumor and aniridia. An *enlarged or cloudy cornea* may be the only visual indication of *congenital glaucoma*.

The *high-arched palate*, described as a frequent accompaniment of many complex malformation syndromes, usually is simply short and hypoplastic. The observation of *macroglossia* should stimulate the search for other signs of cretinism or Beckwith-Wiedemann syndrome, whereas *micrognathia* suggests, among others, Treacher Collins and Pierre Robin syndromes. Although *cleft lip or palate* may occur singly, the examiner should determine whether other signs of trisomy 13 (i.e., low-set or malformed ears, webbing of the neck, scalp defects, microphthalmia, and micrognathia) are present. Similarly, any ear that is apparently low-set (i.e., whose upper attachment to the scalp is below an imaginary line connecting the inner and outer canthi and extended to the occiput), particularly if the foldings of pinna and tragus appear "simpli-

Table 36-9 *Levels of Surveillance of the Newborn Based on the Chest Examination*

	LEVEL OF SURVEILLANCE		
CHARACTERISTIC	NORMAL	ALERT	ALARM
Respiration		Paradoxical, periodic, or retractions	Apnea, expiratory grunt, or flaring alae nasii
Auscultation		Decreased air entry	Bowel sounds
Chest roentgenogram		Enlarged heart	Oligemia or plethora
Cardiac			
Impulse	Tapping	Heaving, lifting	
Pulses	Full	Decreased	Absent (femoral) and lag (cardiac-radial)
Rate and rhythm	110-165, sinus arrhythmia	Sinus bradycardia	Persistent sinus tachycardia
Sounds	"Tic-toc"	S_2 widely split	S_2 fixed split
Murmurs	Systolic (<24 hr)	Systolic (>24 hr)	Diastolic
Electrocardiograph (QRS)			
Vector	+35 to +180 degrees		0 to −90 degrees; −90 to −180 degrees
Amplitude			
V_1	Rs	Rs	rS
V_6	qrS	qRs	qRs

fied," should prompt a search for bilateral renal agenesis (Potter syndrome) and other markers of genetic disease (e.g., webbed neck, "rocker-bottom" feet, and hypoplastic and incurved fifth digit).

The neck should be freely rotatable and free of dimples or masses, which could suggest a *thyroglossal duct* cyst (midline) or *branchial cleft* cyst (anterolateral).

The Chest (Table 36-9). Apart from inspection of the newborn's breasts and their potential engorgement or discharge, the thoracic wall is most closely observed in the attempt to characterize respiration. *Paradoxical respirations* are those in which inspiratory efforts are accompanied by protuberance of the abdomen and a sinking in of the lower ribs as the diaphragm descends, unopposed by adequate intercostal muscle tone. Although this phenomenon is characteristic of normal active (REM) sleep in the newborn, it can also signify abnormal respiration. Inspiratory *retractions* of the lower sternum and intercostal spaces, particularly if accompanied by the use of accessory respiratory muscles (alae nasii and sternocleidomastoids), imply a decrease in lung compliance (stiffening), often caused by atelectasis or accumulation of fluid within the lung. Expiratory *grunting* (actually, an explosive Valsalva maneuver) is the hallmark of loss of alveolar volume and is most frequently displayed in pediatric experience by the small premature infant whose lungs are atelectatic shortly after birth because of insufficient amounts of stabilizing pulmonary surfactant (i.e., hyaline membrane disease). However, other causes of respiratory distress (e.g., transient tachypnea, meconium aspiration, and congenital pneumonia) may be impossible to distinguish clinically, on the basis of the physical characteristics alone.

Decreased auscultatable *air entry* on inspiration is difficult to evaluate during quiet breathing. However, when observed in situations in which greater respiratory effort is seen yet not heard, this means that the tidal volume of air flow is decreased, potentially caused by atelectasis and airway obstruction.

When *bowel sounds* are clearly audible within the chest, especially the left hemithorax and particularly when accompanied by a displacement of heart sounds to the right, a diaphragmatic hernia must be ruled out (by chest roentgenogram) instantly, whether or not there is obvious respiratory distress.

Indeed, although its use cannot be routinely advocated for newborns without symptoms, the *chest roentgenogram should be the diagnostic supplement of first resort* to the physical examination (especially of the chest and abdomen) of the ill infant. If it is used, the maximum advantage should be extracted from it, particularly by inspecting last those areas of prime interest; this policy will avert many embarrassing omissions of such "incidental" findings as a fractured clavicle or rib, a hemivertebra or spina bifida, or a paralyzed diaphragm. The character of the lung parenchyma should be noted, as well as the presence or absence of fluid or effusion, an "air bronchogram," or a distinct cardiac border (an indistinct border signifying lack of alveolar air). In those infants with any cardiovascular symptoms, the examiner should be especially careful to estimate the cardiac size and determine if the vascularity of the lung fields is oligemic, normal, or plethoric.

The physician should be concerned by a *cardiac impulse* that lifts rather than taps at the examining palm or fingertips, since this implies a more generously developed left ventricle than should be the case at the immediate conclusion of fetal life, during which the right ventricle is dominant in both pressure and volume work. Any diminishment of *peripheral pulses* (especially femoral) is evidence of impeded left ventricular outflow (e.g., coarctation of the aorta) and demands blood pressure determination in all four extremities. Sinus *bradycardia* may be precipitated, presumably by vagal reflex, during suctioning or other stimulations of the nasopharynx. Some immature infants may sustain alarming but transient episodes of bradycardia with no apparent stimulus (or symptoms, including apnea), but bradycardia is seen most frequently during the episodes of prolonged apnea so common in the premature newborn. Indeed, many authorities believe that cardiac (rather than cardio*respiratory*) monitoring is a perfectly adequate means for monitoring vital signs in the newborn special care unit. Unameliorated paroxysmal auricular *tachycardia* can lead to cardiac exhaustion and failure.

The normal tic-toc quality of the *heart sounds* results from the near-equal duration of systole and diastole. The high (but subsiding) pulmonary vascular resistance of the first hours and days of life normally accentuates the intensity of the pulmonary component of S_2, at first difficult to distinguish from the preceding aortic component. However, as pulmonary vascular resistance decreases (hence, pulmonary flow increases), the "splitting" of S_2 widens, since pulmonary valve closure is delayed by the longer time required to eject the increased right-sided stroke volume. Similarly, the widened and "fixed split" in the S_2 of critical pulmonary stenosis denotes the increased time required to force blood past the obstructed outflow tract of the right ventricle.

The acute and undistracted ear may often (about 20% to 30% of the time) hear transient *systolic ejection murmurs* at the base of the heart during the first day, presumably associated with flow through the closing ductus arteriosus. Later developing murmurs are of more significance, because the increasing resistance (and pressure) differential between the pulmonary and systemic circulations allows the expression of murmurs caused by increasing flow across abnormal connections (e.g., septal defects) between the two circulations. Systolic ejection murmurs heard early (even in fetal life) and that persist throughout the neonatal period may well result from flow across a stenotic valve (i.e., pulmonary or aortic stenosis). *Diastolic murmurs* should alarm the examiner whenever heard, but they are rarely solitary.

Apart from specific diagnostic aid regarding the type and likely origin of an arrhythmia, the electrocardiogram, like the chest roentgenogram, is a helpful supplement to the physical examination in assessing the volume (*preload*) and pressure (*afterload*) loads presented to the ventricles. Indeed, knowledge of three major data points alone—whether the right or left ventricle is electrically dominant, whether there is plethora or oligemia of the pulmonary vasculature seen on a chest roentgenogram, and whether cyanosis is clinically present or absent—with application of a suitable diagnostic algorithm ("recipe" for systematic assessment of clinical data), can narrow the likely cardiac diagnosis to two or three entities before echocardiographic or catheter confirmation and without reference to murmurs. For instance, the "adult progression" of *precordial QRS complexes* (rS in V_1, qRs in V_6) suggests an abnormally dominant left ventricle (or abnormally diminished right ventricle). Combined with cyanosis and oligemic lung fields, these data might well suggest pulmonary atresia.

The Abdomen (Table 36-10). A significantly *distended* abdomen is usually distinctly tense and accompanied by signs of obstruction (no stool, vomiting). The traditional f *scaphoid* (empty) abdomen of a diaphragmatic hernia is perhaps more the exception than the rule, depending on the amount of intestinal gas. Generally, the normal infant abdomen is pleasingly round, soft, and full in the flanks. It often appears to lack a muscular wall, until it becomes rigid during the expiratory phase of crying (or, less fortunately, it displays the "prune belly" appearance of truly absent abdominal musculature).

Although the drainage of clear liquid from the navel can accompany a simple (and cauterizable) *umbilical granuloma*, the examiner must be careful not to miss a *urachal fistula*. The grosser umbilical malformations (*omphalocele* and *gastroschisis*) are impossible to miss and demand immediate intervention. Any sign of inflammation must be closely watched; however, the use of "triple dye" for cord care may so discolor the skin (while exerting bacteriostatic action) as to render its inspection quite difficult. Finding less than the normal complement of one large-diameter, thin-walled central vein and two smaller-diameter, thicker-walled arteries at about the 4-o'clock and 8-o'clock positions (facing the infant) in the freshly cut surface of the umbilical cord (best done in the delivery room) should alert one to the likelihood of other developmental anomalies, especially genitourinary.

The detection of true enlargement of either the *liver* or *spleen* must be regarded with suspicion. However, the upper borders of both organs should be located by percussion before conclusions are drawn about enlargement, since they are easily displaced downward by the diaphragm under a lung often distended during the early hours after birth by the "wet lung" conditions (e.g., transient tachypnea).

Table 36-10 *Levels of Surveillance of the Newborn Based on Examination of the Abdomen*

	LEVEL OF SURVEILLANCE		
CHARACTERISTIC	NORMAL	ALERT	ALARM
Shape	Cylindric	Scaphoid	Distended
Muscular wall	Diastasis recti		Absent
Umbilicus	Amniotic navel or cutaneous navel	Exudation or leakage, granuloma, hernia, inflammation, or less than 3 cord vessels	Gastroschisis, omphalitis, or omphalocele
Liver	Smooth edge		Enlarged
Spleen	Nonpalpable	Palpable	Enlarged
Kidneys	Lobulated or palpable (lower poles)	Horseshoe	Enlarged

The *kidneys* are easier to evaluate at this time than perhaps at any subsequent period in life, since the infant abdomen offers little resistance to a gentle yet deep bimanual paraspinal exploration, which should easily yield the impression of at least the (often lobulated) lower poles of the kidneys.

Any apparent malformation or enlargement should immediately be confirmed by ultrasonographic examination, as should any frank intraabdominal mass.

The Perineum (Table 36-11). This examination is straightforward and mainly involves ensuring that the *anus* is patent and puckers, that the male *phallus* is well formed and accompanied by palpable gonads, and that the female *vaginal vault* is patent and contains no extraneous tissues. An incorrect assignment of sex is extremely difficult to retract; therefore any initial ambiguities must be carefully and courageously faced with the parents while the ambiguities are being definitively explored.

The Musculoskeletal System (Table 36-12). All late fetuses spend considerable periods of time (when not kicking their mothers) in one rather cramped *position of "comfort,"* which can easily and visibly be restored during the nursery examination by enfolding feet, tibias, and femurs with gentle pressure placed on the soles of the feet. Everything then seems to fall magically into place as it was in utero, and the infant becomes soothed (and the origin of the *tibial torsion* of infancy becomes obvious). Given current obstetric trends away from the vaginal delivery of the breech presentation, the splayed and extended legs (and hematomas and edema of the buttocks and perineal parts) of the frank breech delivery are increasingly rare. Although a dominantly extensor posture of the extremities is characteristic of the premature infant (and a fundamental part of gestational age assessment by physical examination), its appearance in a newborn at term should suggest significant neuromuscular abnormality.

A certain amount of digital webbing can be familial and normal, but true *syndactyly* and *polydactyly* are frequent items in many complex congenital syndromes of malformation; they also occur singly. Similarly, although normal infants frequently (but transiently) manipulate their digits into strange positions, a persistent and almost obligatory grasping of the

Table 36-11 *Levels of Surveillance of the Newborn Based on Examination of the Perineum*

	LEVEL OF SURVEILLANCE		
LOCATION	NORMAL	ALERT	ALARM
Anus		Coccygeal dimple	Imperforate, fistula, patulous
Female			
Clitoris		Enlarged, hooded	
Vulva	Bloody secretion, edema, gaping labia, or hymenal tags		Hydrometrocolpos
Male			
Gonad	Edema, hydrocele	Bifid scrotum, cryptorchidism, inguinal hernia	
Phallus	Phimosis	Chordee, hypospadias	Microphallus

Table 36-12 *Levels of Surveillance of the Newborn Based on Examination of the Musculoskeletal System*

	LEVEL OF SURVEILLANCE		
CHARACTERISTIC	NORMAL	ALERT	ALARM
Fetal posture	Flexor, position of comfort	Frank breech	Extensor
Hand	Webbing	Cortical thumb, overlapping fingers, short, incurved little finger	Polydactyly, syndactyly
Foot	Dorsiflex 90 degrees, plantar flex 90 degrees, abduct or adduct forefoot 45 degrees, invert or evert ankle 45 degrees	Decreased range of motion	Fixed
Extremities	Tibial bowing		Constriction bands, amputations
Neck	Rotate ±90 degrees		
Joints		Reluctance to use	Subluxation (hips), contracture

thumb within the "fisted" fingers suggests the *cortical thumb* of corticospinal tract malformation. A shortened and curved little finger (*clinodactyly*) can be, just as a "simple" ear, a general marker of genetic disease. The foot that can pass the normal range of motion outlined in Table 36-12 cannot be a *clubfoot*, whereas one more restrained may be. General joint contractures (*arthrogryposis*) suggest neuromuscular disease, but the infant's reluctance to use a normal-appearing joint should suggest trauma. However, subluxated hips are congenital and should be treated forthwith.

The Nervous System. Recent discoveries regarding the behavior of newborns, particularly their responses to visual and auditory stimuli, have made it clear that it is no longer appropriate to consider them, at least in their quiet-alert state, as "thalamic" animals. The *exteroceptive reflexes* (rooting, grasping, plantar, and superficial abdominal), involving touch receptors, are emphasized in the quiet-alert state, whereas the *proprioceptive reflexes* (deep tendon, Moro, and ankle clonus) are accentuated during quiet sleep.

Depressive changes in mental status, if occurring early (less than 1 to 2 days of life), are most often related to the birth process (oxygenation, trauma, or drugs); if occurring later, then metabolic processes are likely involved. For instance, the infant who is normal at birth but days later (after digestion of milk and assimilation of its protein and carbohydrate) develops lethargy, stupor, coma, or convulsions (and may have a peculiar odor of, say, maple syrup) might very well harbor an *inborn error of metabolism*.

The less flexor and symmetric the posture, the less wise it is to accept a term infant as neurologically normal. Distinguishing between *neuro*muscular tone and neuro*muscular* strength as being responsible for the *floppy baby* who slides between one's opposing palms in upright suspension or who droops over one's uplifting palm in ventral suspension can be difficult. Beyond the purely neuromuscular causes of hypotonia (hypoxic, metabolic, or genetic encephalopathies; traumatic, toxic, and infectious myelopathies and neuropathies; and congenital, structural, and metabolic myopathies) can lurk a bewildering and poorly understood array of connective tissue, endocrine, and totally idiopathic causes of floppiness.

The jittery, tremulous baby is a common sight in nurseries, and such movements occasionally raise concern that the infant may be sustaining a convulsion. However, unlike "jitters," the true *seizure* tends to be asymmetric and stimulus insensitive. The tremors of *jitteriness* are most often precipitated by noise or motion and can usually be obliterated, unlike the seizure, by the examiner's manual restraint of the involved limb.

The most useful and diagnostically informative *reflexes* to be elicited from the newborn are listed in Table 36-13. As in most other aspects of the neurologic examination, the reflex responses are normally symmetric and tend to diminish in intensity (habituate) on repetition. Because of slow *nerve conduction*, relative to the adult, sensory responses can be quite slow in the newborn. Yet a definite response to a pinprick, and certainly to more noxious stimuli, must be elicitable from all areas of the body.

Table 36-14 should make clear that all the cranial nerves, possibly excluding the olfactory, are easily tested in the newborn. The visual and auditory responses require the most patience and equipment (including, if necessary, formal evaluation of evoked electroencephalographic potentials); yet one dealing with a seeing and hearing infant can gain considerable confidence in the baby's possession of those abilities by presenting a red ball or human face to determine his or her ability to fix and follow, and a human voice or loud noise to assess aural attention. The "Crib-O-Gram" is, in fact, a commercial but increasingly respected device for standardizing the presented auditory stimulus and recording the behavioral response (chiefly a suspension of or a change in motion).

Table 36-13 *Levels of Surveillance of the Newborn Based on Examination of the Nervous System*

	LEVEL OF SURVEILLANCE		
CHARACTERISTIC	NORMAL	ALERT	ALARM
State	Awake: crying, active, quiet alert Asleep: active, indeterminate, quiet	Hyperalert, lethargic	Stupor, coma
Motor			
Posture	Flexor, symmetric	Extensor, asymmetric	Obligatory, decerebrate
Tone	Obtuse popliteal angle	Limp in upright suspension	Limp in ventral suspension
Movement	All extremities, nonrepetitive, random, symmetric	Jitteriness, tremor	Seizures
Reflexes	Deep tendon, grasp, Moro, placing and stepping, sucking, tonic neck	Asymmetric, do not habituate	Absent
Sensory	Pinprick response slow (2-3 sec)	Pinprick response equivocal	No response

Table 36-14 *Levels of Surveillance of the Newborn Based on Examination of the Cranial Nerves*

	LEVEL OF SURVEILLANCE		
CRANIAL NERVES	NORMAL	ALERT	ALARM
Forebrain: II	Fix and follow (visual-evoked potential)	Equivocal (arc <60 degrees)	No response
Midbrain: III, IV, VI, and VIII	Pupillary response, doll's eye response	Unequal, disconjugate, nystagmus	Absent, fixed position
Hindbrain			
VIII	Crib-O-Gram (auditory-evoked potentials)	Diminished	No response
V, VII, and XII	Sucking	Weak	Unequal
IX and X	Swallowing	Uncoordinated	
XI	Sternocleidomastoid muscles	Weak	

Initial Care of the Newborn Designed to Detect or Avert Difficulties During the Neonatal Period

AT DELIVERY

Cord blood—*saved* for possible ABO typing, Rh typing, or Coombs test
Identification of infant as belonging to mother

AT NURSERY ADMISSION

If not previously done in the delivery room, then perform:
- Eye care—1% silver nitrate drops or 1% tetracycline or 0.5% erythromycin ointments
- Hemorrhagic prophylaxis—0.5 to 1.0 mg vitamin K_1 oxide (phytonadione [Pholloquinone]), parenteral

SUBSEQUENT CARE

Skin care—"dry" (after initial cleansing with sterile water and cotton sponges)
Cord care—triple dye or bacitracin ointment

DIAGNOSTIC CARE

If indicated by:
- Premature rupture of membranes
- Temperature instability
- Small or large for gestational age
- Pallor

Then:
- Search for leukocytes and bacteria in gastric aspirate and ear secretions
- Perform blood glucose screen
- Obtain hemogram (hemoglobin, hematocrit, red blood cell count)

Interventions: Measures to Ensure the Integrity of the Newborn Infant

These are enumerated in the box above and are quite straightforward. Although effective for the prophylaxis of gonorrheal ophthalmitis, 1% silver nitrate uniformly produces a brief *chemical conjunctivitis* (which may distress uninformed parents), and any drops spilled on the skin will temporarily discolor it. For these reasons, the antibiotic ointments have gained favor as prophylactic agents.

Apart from strictly cosmetic issues, skin and cord care is addressed to controlling the rate at which and the microorganisms with which the gnotobiotic infant's skin is to become colonized, as it inevitably must. Previous efforts to prevent establishment of a staphylococcal flora by use of hexachlorophene baths and the like were doomed to failure. The current emphasis is on permitting controlled colonization with what one hopes are benign bacterial strains. This is complemented by rigid exclusion of any staphylococcal "carriers" from contact with the newborn and by minimal handling of the infant by all involved in his or her care. However, since it affords a direct route to the bloodstream, excessive infestation of the cord stump is discouraged with the application of some form of bacteriostatic agent.

Premature rupture of the membranes places the fetus at risk for ascending *amnionitis* and the physician in a quandary as to just how aggressively to approach prevention or treatment of what may often turn out not to be a problem. Many find it helpful to be guided by the presence of leukocytes or bacteria (usually dead or otherwise nonculturable) in the gastric aspirate or ear canal.

Hypoglycemia is sufficiently frequent and threatening that it must be aggressively sought out and treated. *Occult hemorrhage* is certainly less frequent, but failure to detect and treat it can be instantly tragic.

Four
Adjustment Period

Kathleen L. Gifford
M. Jeffrey Maisels
Nicholas M. Nelson

The next sequential but overlapping stage in management of the newborn is replacing the maternal-fetal unit with the mother-infant pair; this pairing encompasses both the tactile and emotional with the biologic and nutritional. Beyond this and as important as the obvious processes of feeding, stooling, burping, and weighing are the mystical, magical, and arguable processes of "bonding" and extending the family to include father, siblings, and grandparents, as well as medical personnel. Much of this will already have been achieved during a properly managed pregnancy, but reinforcement is always in order.

ONSET OF ORAL NUTRITIONAL INTAKE AND PARENTING

These next few days (or hours in those hospitals practicing early discharge) will largely be devoted to mutual patterning by mother and child, as their mutual schedules for sleeping, eating, relaxing, and playing begin to mesh. This prolonged and productive process seems easier and certainly more natural if managed in a rooming-in setting, whether at home or in the hospital.

As the new or experienced mother establishes or refines her skills at mothering during this period, she should expect and certainly receive from hospital personnel nothing but the warmest, most enthusiastic support, regardless of how many tiresome and routine deliveries were managed that day without morbidity or death. In teaching hospitals these personnel will often include young pediatric house officers who typically are terrified by (and therefore avoid) the daily duty of confidently answering the normal questions of normal mothers about their normal infants—the place to learn this aspect of the art of medicine is not in a book but rather in the mother's room.

OBSERVATIONS AND EXAMINATION

Although in the absence of specific symptoms no particular examination of the infant is called for, the processes of feeding, growing, and excreting are monitored with particular care—the amount (of formula) ingested, the amount regurgitated, the quality and strength of sucking, the frequency and type of stooling and voiding, and the daily weight gain or loss.

One expects a loss of 6% to 8% of birth weight over the first 3 or 4 days, which is largely the result of normal fluid shifts but is also occasioned by the decreased oral (as opposed to placental) fluid and nutritional intake in the first days of life. Therefore this weight loss tends to be somewhat more pronounced and prolonged in the nursing infant. Weight usually begins to increase after the fourth day, and birth weight should be regained by 1 to 2 weeks of age; however, the outline offered here is purposefully vague, since there is much normal variation.

FEEDING

The decision for breast- or bottle-feeding will have best been made by the unpressured mother well before her delivery (see Chapter 16). That decision should be supported without undue proselytizing in either direction. On the other hand, the mother who is frankly undecided can without prejudice or commitment be apprised of the advantages of nursing (simplicity, certainty, safety, nutritional equality, and immunologic and economic superiority).

A strictly biochemical comparison of breast and formula feeding is presented in Table 16-5, wherein it is noted that breast milk is lower in protein and higher in fat, lower in calcium and much lower in phosphorus. The various commercial formulas have been fortified with vitamins (particularly vitamin D), and the nursing infant should probably receive vitamin supplementation. Although the well-mothered, well-fed normal infant in North American society can certainly expect to receive adequate nutritional iron by the appropriate age (4 to 6 months) as his or her diet expands to include fortified cereals, meats, and egg yolks, it is still an unhappy fact that not all infants are so fortunate. In addition, many if not most of these latter babies are probably not currently breast-fed. In any case, the recommendation has been made and implemented that all infant formulas be supplemented with iron as a means for improving infant health (similar to the fluoridation of water). There seems to be little question that both forms of supplementation have been effective passive health supports. Iron supplementation for the nursing infant is optional but probably wise.

ESTABLISHMENT OF LACTATION

Human milk is the ideal food for human infants, and breastfeeding is the most natural and practical way to feed a baby. It is emotionally satisfying, provides the closest possible contact between mother and infant, and should produce a sense of fulfillment that is unique. Unfortunately, breast-feeding in the Western world is no longer instinctive, and mothers desiring to nurse their infants require guidance and emotional support. At no time is this more important or the mother more receptive than in the immediate postpartum period. However, the psychologic and physical preparation for nursing should begin well before delivery, with information about nursing and a detailed discussion of its benefits.

Given an uncomplicated delivery and a vigorous infant, the baby should be nursed within the first hour of life during the first stage of transition, when he or she is alert and shows an interest in sucking. "Test feeds" of water are unnecessary, since patency of the esophagus can be confirmed on examination in the nursery. Babies should be nursed on demand and no less than eight times a day to ensure the establishment of adequate lactation; some will require nursing as often as every 2 hours. This is normal and thus to be encouraged. Frequent nursing (more than eight times a day) has been shown to reduce serum bilirubin levels in the newborn, produce good "letdown," and help prevent breast engorgement.

A schedule of 5 minutes on each breast the first day, 5 to 10 minutes on each breast the second day, and 10 to 15 minutes on each breast for each feeding thereafter is said to prevent nipple soreness, although satisfactory data to support this contention are lacking. However, it has been shown that most infants can empty a breast in about 7 minutes, so that additional sucking, however pleasant for either or both parties, is nonnutritive and may lead to sore nipples. These time limits are *not* sacrosanct, and mothers should be encouraged not to nurse "by the clock." To ensure adequate emptying and stimulation of both breasts, the mother should be instructed to alternate the breast with which she begins each feeding.

Good technique includes hand washing, a comfortable position and support, use of the rooting reflex (placing the infant's cheek against the warm, naked breast, which stimulates him or her to turn the face into the breast) to encourage the baby's grasp of the entire nipple and areola, and use of a finger placed in the corner of the baby's mouth to break suction.

An explanation of the anatomy and physiology of lactation and suckling helps the mother respond naturally to the process and avoid complications. Hormonal changes immediately after delivery enhance the process that provides colostrum. The production of milk occurs secondary to the release of prolactin and oxytocin in response to a number of stimuli, including the tactile stimulus of the suckling infant. In fact, the milk ejection (letdown) reflex and the release of oxytocin occur in most women before actual suckling begins, and further release of oxytocin follows in response to the sucking. Oxytocin produces contraction of smooth muscle cells around the alveolar cells (milk glands), leading to a release of milk, which flows via the ducts into the lactiferous sinuses (milk pools) situated behind the areola. The release of oxytocin is readily affected by the mother's emotional state and her ability to relax before and during nursing.

The letdown reflex is of utmost importance because its failure can lead to congestion, engorgement, decrease in milk supply, and a hungry baby. Mothers recognize the letdown when they feel a tingling sensation in the breasts or start to leak milk from the unused breast. To encourage letdown, mothers should practice relaxing in a quiet room and should feed their infant on demand. Warm showers, warm compresses, and warm beverages may also be helpful.

Technique

When the infant grasps the nipple, he or she uses the tongue to pull it into the mouth and press it against the palate. This brings the lactiferous sinuses into a position where they are accessible to pressure from the gums and facial muscles. It is the baby's pressure on these sinuses and *not* the sucking that squeezes milk from the breast and is necessary for adequate emptying.

Establishment of a good nursing pattern should be the major goal during the first few weeks; supplementation with formula or water, which disrupts this pattern, should be avoided. Offering a bottle confuses the infant, diminishes his or her desire to suckle, and may cause the mother concern about her ability to provide adequate nutrition. Contrary to popular belief, water supplementation does not lower serum bilirubin levels in the breast-fed baby.

Common Complications

Sometime during the first 24 hours, the mother is likely to complain of a "lazy" baby who refuses to suck. She can be reassured that the baby does not require large amounts during the first day. Despite lack of vigorous sucking, each session at the breast provides experience in position and technique for both mother and child. By the second day the baby's appetite and technique should begin to improve.

Mothers often develop sore nipples when the baby begins to suck with vigor, but this can be prevented or minimized by feeding the baby on demand and by good technique (see box).

Sometime between 48 and 96 hours postpartum, when true (i.e., noncolostrum) milk production occurs, most mothers experience some degree of engorgement caused by venous and lymphatic stasis in the breast tissue and the presence of milk in the alveolar cells (and therefore merit congratulatory reassurance that milk production has begun). This lasts for several days and decreases as the breast adjusts to the nursing pattern. Frequent suckling is the most effective means for the prevention and treatment of engorgement and helps ameliorate discomfort by relieving pressure from the presence of milk. A badly engorged breast prevents the baby from drawing the nipple well into the mouth and makes it difficult for him or her to nurse. Manual or mechanical expression of a little milk before nursing, sufficient to soften the breast and extend the nipple, will allow the infant to grasp it easily.

Aids to Sore Nipples

1. Air-dry nipples after each feeding.
2. Change bra and breast pads when they become moist.
3. Clean nipples with water only. Excessive soap dries the nipples.
4. Nurse every 2 hours, but for only 5 to 7 minutes on each breast, and offer the least sore nipple first.
5. Apply a small amount of breast cream, anhydrous lanolin, or hydrophilic ointment to the nipples after each feeding. (The efficacy of this therapy is questionable.)
6. Change the baby's nursing position to alter the mouth-to-nipple pressure points.
7. As a last resort, use a nipple shield for 24 to 48 hours to allow for healing before commencing the toughening process again.

Special Situations

Inverted Nipples. Nongraspable or nonprotractile nipples may be manipulated in the prenatal or postpartum periods to loosen adhesions and improve protractility. A breast pump, stretching techniques, milk cups, and nipple shields will draw the nipples out so that the infant can grasp them.

Cesarean Section. The processes of postoperative recovery provoke only slight variations in the initial breast-feeding routine. Comfort techniques, analgesics, and appropriate position help improve the nursing experience.

Twins. Mothers are able to produce sufficient milk for twins and sometimes for triplets. The babies may be fed either simultaneously or separately. Various positions are possible.

Jaundice. Breast-feeding has been associated with an increased incidence of jaundice in the first week of life. The increased levels of bilirubin are generally small and of no clinical importance. Frequent nursing (at least eight times per day) may ameliorate this problem. If bilirubin levels approach 20 mg/dl ("true" breast-milk jaundice syndrome), nursing should be interrupted for 24 to 48 hours, the mother pumping her breasts in the interim. Invariably this will produce a decline in serum bilirubin levels so that breast-feeding can be resumed. Positive support and reinforcement should be provided to assure the mother that it is desirable and safe for her to continue nursing. After resumption of breast-feeding, a slight rise in the bilirubin level may occur but rarely to the previous concentration.

Prematurity. Recent experience shows that premature infants thrive on breast milk and can suckle adequately at the breast by about 34 weeks of gestation. Expressed breast milk can be given to the more premature infant. To succeed, the mother needs instruction in breast pumping and milk collection, accompanied by continued support and, obviously, a strong personal motivation. The milk from the mother of a premature infant has a higher protein content than that from the mother of a full-term infant. Thus the infant's own mother's milk is more desirable than either pooled or "banked" breast milk.

Cleft Lip and Palate. Difficulty in nursing may occur when a cleft in the lip or palate prevents the infant from maintaining sufficient suction to seal the nipple in the mouth. If the infant has a cleft lip but intact palate, the mother's soft breast tissue should help to occlude the cleft and improve the seal, but a palatal cleft complicates the infant's attempt to press the nipple against the palate and "milk" it. In the case of a unilateral cleft, placement of the nipple may avoid this problem. Highly motivated mothers have been successful in maintaining breast-feeding by holding the nipple in place, by manual expression directly into the infant's mouth, or by pumping her breasts and then bottle-feeding the expressed milk.

Additional Concerns

Additional concerns about breast-feeding include the following:

1. Leakage of milk may occur for several months and, if embarrassing, can be controlled by pressure to the nipple and absorbent breast pads (not plastic).
2. During the first weeks, engorgement diminishes as the baby's demands increase. This may lead the mother to be concerned about a lack of milk. Reassurance, a discussion of supply and demand, and an explanation of physiology will help.
3. The baby is "getting enough" when six or seven moderately wet diapers must be changed each day.
4. A periodic replacement bottle may be offered after the first 2 to 3 weeks, but only after consistent feeding patterns and a steady milk supply have been established.
5. A plugged milk duct is seen as a small, tender lump in the breast that persists after a feeding. Massage, frequent feedings, and cleansing of caked milk from the nipple will usually resolve the problem.
6. Mastitis has flulike symptoms and a reddened, tender area on one or both breasts. It should be treated with rest, warm compresses to the affected breast, frequent nursing to prevent stasis, and antibiotics (if symptoms persist). Left untreated, mastitis can progress to a breast abscess requiring surgical drainage and discontinuation of feeding at the affected breast until healing occurs.

Vitamins, Iron, and Fluoride

The need to supplement the diet of breast-fed infants with vitamins, iron, and fluoride is controversial. However, on the basis of estimated needs of growing infants, many feel it wise to provide additional vitamin D and iron. The fluoride content of breast milk is low, so that fully breast-fed infants also require supplemental fluoride.

Maternal Medication and Diet

Almost all drugs ingested by the mother are excreted in breast milk, but very few in amounts large enough to be hazardous to the infant (Table 16-7). To minimize risk, however, maternal drugs should be avoided whenever possible. If maternal medication is absolutely necessary, the infant should be nursed before each dose.

The mother requires a well-balanced diet during pregnancy, plus approximately 200 additional calories in high-protein food while breast-feeding. The nursing period is no time for "crash" or fad dieting.

Five
Establishment of Equilibrium

Nicholas M. Nelson
Dennis M. Super

In this final phase of management of the newborn, one pursues the twin objectives of completing the infant's perinatal adjustments and integrating the mother-infant pair into an ongoing program for their health supervision. Precisely where this begins or is implemented (hospital, home, private office, or clinic) will vary with local facilities, resources, and expectations, but the principal expectation to be instilled before discharge is that continuing health supervision is the best guarantee for maintaining the healthy process already begun.

In these later days of the infant's hospital course, *jaundice* is especially sought out and, if excessive (more than 10 to 12 mg/dl total bilirubin), investigated. The various requirements for statewide screening programs (e.g., phenylketonuria and hypothyroidism) need to be fulfilled and a decision reached (not imposed) concerning the *circumcision* of a male infant.

The benefits of neonatal circumcision remain controversial in North America. In the United States, over 70% of male infants are circumcised, whereas in Europe, neonatal circumcision is rare.[7] Proponents state that neonatal circumcision reduces the risk of penile carcinoma; prevents balanoposthitis, phimosis, and paraphimosis; has a lower anesthetic risk than does circumcision performed later in life; and eliminates the need for penile hygiene. Opponents state that it subjects the neonate to additional stress and that the procedure has a definite complication rate. They also argue that proper penile hygiene will prevent phimosis, paraphimosis, balanoposthitis, and penile cancer and that the foreskin protects the delicate urethral meatus from the irritation of solid diapers. In 1989, the American Academy of Pediatrics Task Force on Circumcision stated that neonatal circumcision has potential medical benefits as well as disadvantages and risks.[4]

An association between urinary tract infections and the uncircumcised neonate has been noted in numerous retrospective studies.[7] A possible explanation for this association may be because the urethra of an uncircumcised neonate is readily colonized with uropathogenic organisms in contrast to the urethra of a circumcised infant.[8]

An alternative to circumcision in preventing infantile urinary tract infections may be to foster more natural colonization of the infant's urethra by promoting strict rooming in of the mother and baby or by active colonization of the baby with the mother's nonpathogenic, anaerobic gut flora.[6] Future studies are needed to determine which of these interventions may best prevent urinary tract infections.

In 1976 the risks of a neonatal circumcision were reviewed by Gee and Ansell.[1] In their study of 5882 male births at the University of Washington from 1963 to 1972, 5521 (94%) infants were circumcised. Almost 2% had a complication of the procedure, including hemorrhage (1%), postcircumcision infection (0.4%), wound dehiscence (0.16%), strangulation of the glans from a tight plastic bell (0.13%), and circumcision in children with hypospadias (0.15%, or 36% of all children with hypospadias). The percentage of severe complications was 0.2%, which included life-threatening hemorrhage (one case), systemic infection (four cases), circumcision of a child with hypospadias (eight cases), and denudation of the shaft of the penis (one case). The only significant difference between the complication rates of the Gomco and the Plastibell techniques was a lower incidence of wound infection with the Gomco technique. Other complications are urethral cutaneous fistula, penile amputation, recurrent pneumothorax, transient hypoxia, penile lacerations, postcircumcision phimosis, and death.[2] The contraindications of a neonatal circumcision are (1) any type of congenital anomaly (especially hypospadias), (2) bleeding diathesis, (3) prematurity, and (4) any neonatal illness.

The physician should perform a circumcision only after a complete physical examination has been carried out and after the child has urinated. Circumcision should be delayed until after the first day of life because the infant may not have fully recovered from the stress of delivery. Also, some illnesses may take some time to become clinically evident during the neonatal period.

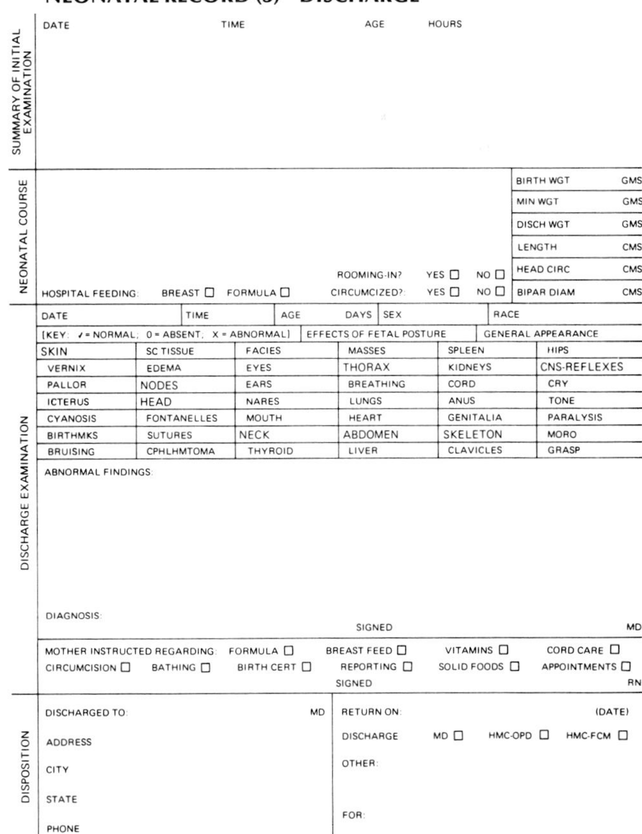

NEONATAL RECORD (3)—DISCHARGE

SUMMARY OF INITIAL EXAMINATION

DATE TIME AGE HOURS

NEONATAL COURSE

HOSPITAL FEEDING: BREAST ☐ FORMULA ☐

ROOMING-IN? YES ☐ NO ☐

CIRCUMCIZED?: YES ☐ NO ☐

BIRTH WGT	GMS
MIN WGT	GMS
DISCH WGT	GMS
LENGTH	CMS
HEAD CIRC	CMS
BIPAR DIAM	CMS

DISCHARGE EXAMINATION

DATE | TIME | AGE DAYS | SEX | RACE

[KEY: ✓ = NORMAL; 0 = ABSENT; X = ABNORMAL] | EFFECTS OF FETAL POSTURE | GENERAL APPEARANCE

SKIN	SC TISSUE	FACIES	MASSES	SPLEEN	HIPS
VERNIX	EDEMA	EYES	THORAX	KIDNEYS	CNS-REFLEXES
PALLOR	NODES	EARS	BREATHING	CORD	CRY
ICTERUS	HEAD	NARES	LUNGS	ANUS	TONE
CYANOSIS	FONTANELLES	MOUTH	HEART	GENITALIA	PARALYSIS
BIRTHMKS	SUTURES	NECK	ABDOMEN	SKELETON	MORO
BRUISING	CPHLHMTOMA	THYROID	LIVER	CLAVICLES	GRASP

ABNORMAL FINDINGS:

DIAGNOSIS:

SIGNED MD

MOTHER INSTRUCTED REGARDING: FORMULA ☐ BREAST FEED ☐ VITAMINS ☐ CORD CARE ☐
CIRCUMCISION ☐ BATHING ☐ BIRTH CERT ☐ REPORTING ☐ SOLID FOODS ☐ APPOINTMENTS ☐

SIGNED RN

DISPOSITION

DISCHARGED TO: MD
ADDRESS
CITY
STATE
PHONE

RETURN ON: (DATE)
DISCHARGE MD ☐ HMC-OPD ☐ HMC-FCM ☐
OTHER:
FOR:

Fig. 36-13 Data relevant to the entire neonatal course to be conveyed from the hospital of birth to the physician assuming responsibility for continuing health supervision.

The parent's desire for their son to be circumcised should be discussed during a prenatal visit during which they can calmly and rationally reflect on the risks and benefits of the procedure.[4] If they decide against circumcision, the physician should include proper foreskin hygiene in their anticipatory guidance during subsequent health maintenance visits. Once the foreskin is easily retracted, the parents should be instructed to gently retract it each day, to wash the glans and foreskin with soapy water, and to dry the area thoroughly.[3]

Perhaps no wiser words have ever been spoken on the subject of infant circumcision than the following[5]:

> My dear C.,
>
> Your patient C.D., at age 7 months, has the prepuce with which he was born. You ask me, with a note of persuasion in your question, if it should be excised. Am I to make this decision on scientific grounds, or am I to acquiesce in a ritual which took its origin at the behest of that arch-sanitarian Moses?
>
> If you can show good reason why a ritual designed to ease the penalties of concupiscence amidst the sand and flies of the Syrian deserts should be continued in this England of clean bed-linen and lesser opportunity, I shall listen to your argument, but if you base your argument on anatomical faults, then I must refute it.
>
> The anatomists have never studied the form and evolution of the preputial orifice. They do not understand that Nature does not intend it to be stretched and retracted in the Temples of the Welfare Centres or ritually removed in the precincts of the operating theatres. Retract the prepuce and you see a pin-point opening, but draw it forward and you see a channel wide enough for all the purposes for which the infant needs the organ at that early age. What looks like a pin-point opening at 7 months will become a wide channel of communication at 17.
>
> Nature is a possessive mistress, and whatever mistakes she makes about the structure of the less essential organs such as the brain and stomach, in which she is not much interested, you can be sure that she knows best about the genital organs.

Despite such wisdom and its frequent reiteration, many parents expect, some insist on, and not a few physicians and hospitals seem too anxious to support the continuing North American medical rituals of circumcision and (later) tonsillectomy.

On the day of discharge a careful physical examination needs to be repeated, particularly emphasizing the baby's behavioral state, the appearance (or disappearance) of any cardiac murmurs, and a close inspection of the cord. These findings and a recapitulation of the infant's progress since birth need to be recorded in a form (Fig. 36-13) easily transmissible to that physician or facility assuming responsibility for the infant's continuing care.

Although the first follow-up visit of the mother-infant pair may not be necessary strictly on medical grounds until 6 weeks after birth, a great deal of information useful to the family, as well as to the physician who serves it, can be pleasantly gathered from a relaxed house call 2 or 3 weeks after delivery.

By this time weight gain should be well-established, the mother's breast milk abundantly flowing, the father back to work, and the infant's real impact on the household readily apparent. There could not be any more sincere expression, in an era of no house calls, of the physician's interest in his or her patient.

REFERENCES

Recovery Period

1. Smith CA: The valley of the shadow at birth, Am J Dis Child 82:171, 1951.

Establishment of Equilibrium

1. Gee WF and Ansell JS: Neonatal circumcision. A 10-year overview: with comparison of the Gomco clamp and the Plastibell device, Pediatrics 58:824, 1976.
2. Kaplan GW: Complications of circumcision, Urol Clin North Am 10(3):543, 1983.
3. Osborn LM, Metcalf TL, and Mariani EM: Hygienic care in uncircumcised infants, Pediatrics 67:365, 1981.
4. Schoen EJ et al: Report of the Task Force on Circumcision, Pediatrics 84(4):388, 1989.
5. Spence J: Letter of 1950 to a general practitioner, Lancet 2:902, 1964.
6. Winberg J et al: The prepuce: a mistake of nature? Lancet 598, (1)598-599, March 18, 1989.
7. Wiswell TE et al: Declining frequency of circumcision: implications for changes in the absolute incidence and male to female sex ratio of urinary tract infections in early infancy, Pediatrics 79(3):338, 1987.
8. Wiswell TE et al: Effect of circumcision status on periurethral bacterial flora during the first year of life, J Pediatr 113(3):442, 1988.

SUGGESTED READINGS

American Academy of Pediatrics and The American College of Obstetricians and Gynecologists: Guidelines for perinatal care, ed 2, Washington, DC, 1988.

Amiel-Tison C: A method for neurologic evaluation within the first year of life, Curr Probl Pediatr 7(1):3, 1976.

Anisfeld E and Lipper E: Effects of perinatal events on mother-infant bonding, Paper presented at the Society for Research in Child Development Biennial Meeting, April 3, 1981.

Avery GB, editor: Neonatology—pathophysiology and management of the newborn, ed 3, Philadelphia, 1987, JB Lippincott Co.

Avery ME, Fletcher BD, and Williams RG: The lung and its disorders in the newborn infant, ed 4, Philadelphia, 1981, WB Saunders Co.

Avery ME and Taeusch HW: Intrauterine growth retardation. In Avery ME and Taeusch HW, editors: Schaffer's diseases of the newborn, ed 5, Philadelphia, 1984, WB Saunders Co.

Aylward GP: Fourth week full-term and pre-term neurologic differences. In Lipsett LD and Field TM, editors: Infant behavior and development: perinatal risk and newborn behavior, Norwood, NJ, 1982, Ablex Publishing Corp.

Ballard J, Kazmaier K, and Driver M: A simplified assessment of gestational age, Pediatr Res 11:374, 1977.

Bland RD, McMillan DD, Bressack MA, et al: Clearance of liquid from lungs of newborn rabbits, J Appl Physiol 49:171, 1980.

Bolande RP: Ritualistic surgery—circumcision and tonsillectomy, N Engl J Med 280:591, 1969.

Brazelton TB: The neonatal behavioural assessment scale, Clin Devel Med Ser, vol. 50, London, 1973, Spastics International.

Budin P: The nursling—the feeding and hygiene of premature and full-term infants, London, 1907, Caxton Publishing Co, Ltd. (Translated by W.J. Maloney.)

Cassady G: The small-for-date infant. In Avery GB, editor: Neonatology, ed 3, Philadelphia, 1987, JB Lippincott Co.

Clifford SH: Postmaturity with placental dysfunction: clinical syndrome and pathological findings, J Pediatr 44:1, 1954.

Curran JS: Birth-associated injury, Clin Perinatol 8:111, 1981.

Davis JA and Dobbing J, editors: Scientific foundations of pediatrics, ed 2, Baltimore, 1982, University Park Press.

DeCarvalho M, Klaus MH, and Merkatz R: The effects of frequency and duration of breast feeding on serum bilirubin, weight gain and milk output, Pediatr Res 15:530, 1981.

Dubowitz L, Dubowitz V, and Goldberg C: Clinical assessment of gestational age in the newborn infant, J Pediatr 77:1, 1970.

Eavey RD, Stool SE, Peckham GJ, et al: How to examine the ear of the neonate, Clin Pediatr 15:338, 1976.

Fanaroff AA and Martin RJ, editors: Neonatal-perinatal medicine, ed 4, St Louis, 1987, The CV Mosby Co.

Fenichel GM: The newborn with poor muscle tone, Semin Perinatol 6:68, 1982.

Fitzhardinge PM and Steven EM: The small-for-date infant I. Later growth patterns, Pediatrics 49:671, 1971.

Fitzhardinge PM and Steven EM: The small-for-date infant II. Neurological and intellectual sequelae, Pediatrics 50:50, 1972.

Gruenwald P: Infants of low birth weight among 5,000 deliveries, Pediatrics 34:157, 1964.

Gryboski J: The colon, rectum, and anus. In Gryboski J, editor: Gastrointestinal problems in the infant, Philadelphia, 1975, WB Saunders Co.

Hittner H, Hirsch N, and Rudolph AJ: Assessment of gestational age by examination of the anterior capsule of the lens, J Pediatr 91:455, 1977.

Hodes ME, Cole J, Palmer CG, et al: Clinical experience with trisomies 18 and 13, J Med Genet 15:48, 1978.

Jones KL and Smith S: Recognizable patterns of human malformation, ed 3, Philadelphia, 1982, WB Saunders Co.

Klaus MH and Fanaroff AA, editors: Care of the high-risk neonate, ed 3, Philadelphia, 1986, WB Saunders Co.

Lubchenco LO: The high risk infant, Philadelphia, 1976, WB Saunders Co.

Lubchenco LO: Assessment of weight and gestational age. In Avery GB, editor: Neonatology, ed 3, Philadelphia, 1987, JB Lippincott Co.

Lubchenco LO, Hansman C, Dressler M, et al: Intrauterine growth as estimated from liveborn birth-weight data at 24 to 42 weeks gestation, Pediatrics 32:793, 1963.

Lugo G and Cassady G: Intrauterine growth retardation: clinicopathologic findings in 233 consecutive infants, Am J Obstet Gynecol 109:615, 1971.

Mangurten HH, Slade CI, and Reidl CJ: First stool in the preterm, low-birth-weight infant, J Pediatr 82:1033, 1973.

Miller HC and Hassanein K: Fetal malnutrition in white newborn infants: maternal factors, Pediatrics 52:504, 1973.

Miller FC, Sacks DA, Yeh SY, et al: Significance of meconium during labor, Am J Obstet Gynecol 122:573, 1975.

Narayanan I, Dua K, Gujral VV, et al: A simple method of assessment of gestational age in newborn infants, Pediatrics 69:27, 1982.

Nelson KB and Eng GD: Congenital hypoplasia of the depressor anguli oris muscle: differentiation from congenital facial palsy, J Pediatr 81:16, 1972.

Painter MJ and Bergman I: Obstetrical trauma to the neonatal central and peripheral nervous system, Semin Perinatol 6:89, 1982.

Parmalee AH: Management of the newborn, ed 2, Chicago, 1959, Year Book Medical Publishers, Inc.

Phibbs RH: Delivery room management of the newborn. In Avery GB, editor: Neonatology, ed 3, Philadelphia, 1987, JB Lippincott Co.

Prechtl HFR: Assessment and significance of behavioral states. In Berenberg SR, editor: Brain, fetal and infant: current research on normal and abnormal development, The Hague, 1977, Martinus Nijhoff.

Prechtl H and Beintema D: The neurological examination of the full-term infant. In Lavenham L, editor: Little club clinics in developmental medicine, no. 12, London, 1964, William Heinemann.

Smith CA and Nelson NM, editors: The physiology of the newborn infant, ed 4, Springfield, Ill, 1976, Charles C Thomas, Publisher.

Sweet AY: Classification of the low-birth-weight infant. In Klaus MH and Fanaroff AA, editors: Care of the high-risk neonate, ed 3, Philadelphia, 1986, WB Saunders Co.

Volpe JJ: Neurology of the newborn, ed 2, Philadelphia, 1982, WB Saunders Co.

von Reuss AR: The diseases of the newborn, New York, 1922, William Wood.

Vulliamy DG: The newborn child, ed 2, Boston, 1967, Little, Brown & Co., Inc.

Wesenberg RL: The newborn chest, Hagerstown, Md, 1973, Harper & Row, Publishers, Inc.

37

Skin Lesions of the Neonate

Marvin Elliott Miller

Birthmarks are common, and many babies will exhibit some type of skin lesion in the newborn period that may arouse parental concern. Fortunately, the overwhelming majority of these skin lesions are benign. It is important for the practicing physician who evaluates newborns to be familiar with these benign birthmarks and also to recognize the much less common birthmarks that may indicate a significant underlying condition. This section reviews skin lesions from this perspective. Listed in Table 37-1 are the birthmarks that will be discussed and their approximate frequency in newborns.

SKIN LESIONS

Transient Lesions[2,5,7]

Several common, transient skin abnormalities occur in the newborn. Since they are self-limited, no medical treatment is indicated.

Milia. Milia are multiple, small (1 to 2 mm) pearly white papules that are found on the forehead, cheeks, and nose. When found on the oral mucosa, they are called Epstein pearls. Milia are found in about 50% of newborns and represent cystic inclusions of keratin and sebaceous material in the pilosebaceous apparatus. They spontaneously disappear during the first month of life and require no treatment.

Miliaria. Miliaria, or neonatal prickly heat, are clear, thin-walled vesicles 1 to 2 mm in diameter that are filled with fluid. They are very fragile and will rupture when light pressure is applied. Miliaria result from eccrine duct occlusion and sweat retention. These lesions occur when an infant is placed in a warm and humid environment; they will disappear when a dry and cooler environment is provided or the infant is dressed in lighter clothing. Topical medications should not be used, since they often exacerbate these lesions.

Erythema Toxicum. Erythema toxicum consists of yellow-white papulopustules surrounded by erythema. Erythema toxicum is seen in 50% of full-term newborns but only rarely in premature babies. The lesions can be seen on any part of the body except the palms and soles. They usually appear at 1 to 2 days of age and are rarely present at birth or after 5 days of life. The lesions persist for several hours to as long as a few days. Smears of the papular contents show numerous eosinophils but no organisms. The cause of erythema toxicum is unknown. These babies are well while they have the lesions, and no treatment is necessary.

Transient Neonatal Pustular Melanosis. The lesions of transient neonatal pustular melanosis are present at birth and consist of superficial vesiculopustules that are easily ruptured to leave a collarette of white scales around a central pinhead-sized macule of hyperpigmentation. This hyperpigmentation remains for several weeks to several months. The clusters of lesions are most often seen on the forehead, under the chin, on the back of the neck, on the lower back, and on the shins.

The pustules last from 1 to 2 days, but cultures of the lesions are sterile and smears of the pustules show cellular debris with variable numbers of neutrophils. Small numbers of eosinophils are sometimes present, but never in such abundance as in erythema toxicum. Babies who have transient neonatal pustular melanosis are healthy, and no treatment is needed. This condition is less common than the other transient lesions and is found in 4% of black newborns and 0.3% of white newborns.

Table 37-1 *Birthmarks and Their Frequency*[1,5,7]

BIRTHMARK	FREQUENCY
Transient lesions	
Milia	50%
Miliaria	Common
Erythema toxicum	50%
Transient neonatal pustular melanosis	Uncommon
Nevi	
Vascular nevi	
Salmon patch	40%
Flat hemangiomas	0.3%
Raised hemangiomas	3%
Hemangiomas associated with malformation syndromes	Rare
Lymphangiomas	Uncommon
Hyperpigmented lesions	
Café-au-lait spots	Common*
Pigmented nevi	Common*
Mongolian spots	Common*
Hypopigmented lesions	Uncommon
Epidermal nevi	Uncommon
Miscellaneous	
Cutis marmorata	Common
Birthmarks from delivery trauma	Common
Cutis aplasia	Rare
Purpura	Rare

*There is a significant difference in the frequency of hyperpigmented lesions between black and white newborns: the frequency of café-au-lait spots, 12% versus 0.3%; pigmented nevi, 20% versus 2%; and Mongolian spots, 90% versus 10%, respectively.

Nevi [1-4,7]

Nevi constitute a group of common birthmarks that result from the local proliferation of any of the following three major cell types that make up the skin:

1. **Cells that line the vascular channels** of either capillaries (hemangiomas) or lymph vessels (lymphangiomas)
2. **Cells that produce pigment** (pigmented nevi)
3. **Cells from the epidermis** (epidermal nevi), including those which make keratin or those that compose the epidermal appendages

Vascular Nevi

Salmon Patch (Nevus Simplex, Telangiectatic Nevus). The salmon patch is the most common vascular lesion of infancy and is found in about 40% of all newborns. This lesion is flat and light pink, with poorly defined borders; it is commonly seen on the nape of the neck, glabella, forehead, upper eyelids, or the nasolabial region. The salmon patch is not a true nevus because there is not an actual proliferation of vascular elements, which is seen in the flat hemangiomas. Histopathologic examination of the salmon patch reveals distended dermal capillaries, representing a persistent, localized fetal capillary bed that usually matures over time into the normal vasculature.

Ninety-five percent of salmon patches fade within the first year of life although portions can persist, particularly those found on the nape of the neck. Salmon patches are not associated with any malformation syndromes. No treatment is necessary, and parents can be reassured that the salmon patch is a benign lesion that will almost always fade and disappear.

Flat Hemangiomas (Nevus Flammeus). The flat hemangioma, or *port wine stain,* is similar in appearance to the salmon patch but is darker and has a deep red or purplish red hue. Port wine stains usually involve the face or the extremities and are usually, but not always, unilateral. These stains are commonly present at birth and grow in proportion to the child's growth. Microscopic examination shows proliferation of dilated dermal capillaries. Flat hemangiomas usually do not fade completely or involute. Various treatments such as cryosurgery and Ganz rays have not been very successful. In cosmetically sensitive areas a tinted opaque waterproof cream (such as Covermark) may be helpful in masking the hemangiomas.

Raised Hemangiomas. The raised hemangiomas, also called *strawberry hemangiomas,* can be histologically divided into capillary hemangiomas and cavernous hemangiomas, although the distinction has no important clinical relevance. The cavernous hemangioma consists of larger capillaries that empty into sinusoidal blood spaces; the capillary hemangiomas merely show capillary proliferation. Strawberry hemangiomas may be present at birth but more commonly become apparent within the first weeks of life; 90% are noted by 1 month of age. They usually begin as a circumscribed area of grayish white discoloration, grow rapidly, and develop into red, raised, well-defined lesions that are lobulated and compressible, although they usually do not blanch. Strawberry hemangiomas can occur on any part of the body; about 38% occur on the head and neck and 29% on the trunk (80% of affected individuals have an isolated lesion; 20% have more than one). Strawberry hemangiomas grow rapidly during the first 6 months of life and then begin to show signs of involution by 15 months of age. Most strawberry hemangiomas grow to 3 to 4 cm in diameter, with some as small as a few millimeters and others as large as 20 cm. At least 90% of strawberry hemangiomas will resolve by 9 years of age without treatment. Although various modes of treatment have been used to remove strawberry hemangiomas, the rational approach is to let these lesions regress on their own, since the cosmetic appearance is much better than those treated by surgery or radiotherapy. Parents should be reassured that time is the best treatment for the majority of these lesions.

Laser therapy has recently been shown to be very effective in treating selected hemangiomas, with no significant side effects. *Flat hemangiomas that are cosmetically displeasing and raised hemangiomas that compromise vital functions should be considered for laser therapy.*[6]

There are several malformation syndromes in which flat or raised hemangiomas are seen; the features of these syndromes are listed in Table 37-2. The vast majority of hemangiomas are not associated with any other malformations.

Lymphangiomas. Lymphangiomas are much less common than hemangiomas; sometimes elements of both are found in one lesion. Lymphangiomas usually present as (1) a cluster of circumscribed gelatinous papules of 2 to 4 mm in diameter containing clear lymph fluid (lymphangioma circumscription), (2) a larger cavernous nodule (cavernous lymphangioma), or (3) a large mass (cystic hygroma). There is no satisfactory treatment. Surgical removal can be attempted, but recurrences are common.

Hyperpigmented Nevi. There are several common hyperpigmented lesions present at or shortly after birth. As

Table 37-2 *Malformation Syndromes Associated with Congenital Hemangiomas*[2,3]

CONDITION	NATURE OF HEMANGIOMA	OTHER FEATURES
Sturge-Weber syndrome	Large, flat hemangioma over face; usually involves ophthalmic branch of trigeminal nerve; usually unilateral	Seizures Glaucoma Mental deficiency
Kasabach-Merritt syndrome	Usually large cavernous hemangiomas, although small ones have been reported	Thrombocytopenia from platelet sequestration
Klippel-Trenaunay-Weber syndrome	Large flat hemangioma on an extremity	Hemangioma overlies area of soft tissue and bone overgrowth Macrocephaly
Diffuse neonatal hemangiomatosis	Multiple hemangiomas that can involve skin and internal organs	High output cardiac failure poor prognosis

shown in Table 37-1 and demonstrated in the following discussions, black newborns have a greater frequency of each of the three common hyperpigmented lesions than do white newborns.

Café-au-Lait Spots. Café-au-lait spots are flat, sharply bordered, uniformly light brown, pigmented lesions that are of varying shape and are usually less than several centimeters in their greatest dimension at birth. An isolated café-au-lait spot has no medical implications. However, the presence of multiple café-au-lait spots with smooth (rather than ragged) borders is diagnostic of neurofibromatosis, and such individuals are susceptible to the complications of this genetic condition. A striking difference has been noted in the frequency of café-au-lait spots in white versus black newborns. Only 0.3% of white newborns will have one café-au-lait spot as opposed to 12% of black newborns; 1.8% of black newborns will have three or more café-au-lait spots without evidence of neurofibromatosis on follow-up care and by family history. Thus the finding of several café-au-lait spots in a black newborn is not in itself indicative of neurofibromatosis.

Café-au-lait spots are not always present at birth and may appear during infancy. Histologically, café-au-lait spots result from increased melanogenesis in a group of melanocytes and thus are not true nevi. In adults, more than six café-au-lait spots greater than 1.5 cm in diameter are diagnostic of neurofibromatosis. In children with neurofibromatosis, however, the café-au-lait spots may be fewer in number and smaller in size, since the spots increase in number and size over time. Thus, in children under 5 years of age, the finding of five café-au-lait spots greater than 0.5 cm in diameter is strongly suggestive of neurofibromatosis. Café-au-lait spots can also be seen in McCune-Albright syndrome (polyostotic fibrous dysplasia and pubertal precocity), but the café-au-lait spots in this condition are larger and have irregular borders.

Pigmented Nevi (Pigmented Moles, Melanocytic Nevi, Neurocellular Nevi). Pigmented nevi are very common in adults (most adults have an average of 30 lesions), and many people call them birthmarks because they believe they were born with them. However, such is usually not the case, since almost all pigmented nevi are acquired and do not appear until later in infancy; some do not appear until adolescence. Only 1% of white newborns and 18% of black newborns are born with pigmented nevi. These congenital, pigmented moles are flat, dark brown or black, irregularly pigmented, and sharply demarcated. They tend to be larger than the acquired moles, and the major concern about congenital pigmented moles is their potential for malignant transformation, which is significantly greater than that of acquired moles. There are no firm guidelines as to when a congenital pigmented mole should be removed, although the large congenital pigmented moles ("bathing trunk nevus" or "garment nevus") are usually surgically removed.

Mongolian Spots. Mongolian spots are large, flat, diffuse, and poorly circumscribed areas of hyperpigmentation that are blue, black, or slate colored and are located over the buttocks or lumbosacral area. Once again, there is a striking ethnic difference in the frequency of this hyperpigmented lesion. Although it is noted in over 80% of Oriental, American Indian, and black newborns, it is seen in less than 10% of white newborns. The natural history of Mongolian spots is benign, with most disappearing by late childhood. They result from pigment-producing cells in the dermis. When a similar appearing lesion is seen in the periorbital region, it is called an *Ota nevus;* when seen on one side of the neck and shoulder, it is referred to as an *Ito nevus.*

Hypopigmented Lesions. Hypopigmented lesions are uncommon in newborns, and their presence may be the first sign of a more serious condition. There are two important neurocutaneous conditions (phacomatoses) in which hypopigmented areas that appear at birth or in early infancy are usually found—tuberous sclerosis and hypomelanosis of Ito. It is important for the physician to recognize these conditions because of the likelihood of some neurologic dysfunction.

Almost 90% of individuals with *tuberous sclerosis* will have multiple white macules present at birth or in early infancy. These white macules are usually 1 to 3 cm in diameter and have irregular leaf-shaped margins. They are almost always the first manifestation of tuberous sclerosis, other features of which include developmental delay, seizures, cutaneous angiofibromas, and intracranial calcifications.

Hypomelanosis of Ito (incontinentia pigmenti achromiens) is a recently described and poorly understood condition in which irregular swirls and whorls of hypopigmentation appear at birth or in infancy. Like tuberous sclerosis there is a high association with neurologic abnormalities such as developmental delay and seizures. In addition, ocular and musculoskeletal abnormalities can be seen.

Epidermal Nevi. Epidermal nevi are skin lesions appearing at birth or in the first few weeks of life. They are composed of aggregates of epithelial cells (keratinocytes) or cells of any of the epidermal appendages (apocrine, eccrine, sebaceous gland, or hair follicle). Although lesions of mixed histology are common, there is usually one predominant cellular element.

The verrucose nevus represents a proliferation of the epidermal cells and their product, keratin. These lesions are raised, yellow-brown, velvety or rough and warty, and often pigmented. They are usually found as a cluster of lesions; they are frequently arranged in a linear fashion when seen on the limbs. Surgical excision is indicated for cosmetic reasons, and the tendency for malignant degeneration is small.

Sebaceous nevi are found on the face and scalp and are elevated, granular, waxy, orange plaques. Surgical excision is the treatment of choice, since these nevi can develop into basal cell carcinomas during adulthood.

Miscellaneous Lesions[2,7]

There are several other congenital skin abnormalities with which the physician should be familiar.

Cutis Marmorata. Cutis marmorata is a reticulated bluish mottling of the skin, which is the normal newborn response to chilling. When the infant is warmed, the cutis marmorata disappears. The tendency may persist for several months, and there is usually no medical significance. However, cutis marmorata may be a persistent feature in the dysmorphic conditions of de Lange syndrome, congenital hypothyroidism, or in Klippel-Trenaunay-Weber syndrome.

Birthmarks from Delivery Trauma. Birthmarks from the mechanical trauma of forceps or suction are common. Ecchymoses of the face where forceps have been placed are often distressing to parents. The marks themselves will disappear, but when they are present, the physician should be certain that no neurologic deficit in ocular or facial muscle function is present. Suction marks on the vertex of the scalp are almost always seen when suction is used to augment delivery. These are benign, they indicate no underlying brain lesions, and the parents should be reassured that they will disappear.

Cutis Aplasia. Cutis aplasia is a congenital absence of skin that most commonly occurs on the vertex of the scalp. The lesion appears as a punched-out ulcer that may be weeping or covered by a thin membrane. Management is directed at prevention of infection until healing is complete. Cutis aplasia can be seen in any one of several settings. First, it can be transmitted as an autosomal dominant condition with variable expression, thus a family history is important. Second, it can be an isolated lesion with an unremarkable family history. Third, it can be seen in association with other birth defects such as brain malformation, limb anomalies, and gastrointestinal defects. In this group, a vascular origin is likely. Scalp defects can also be seen in infants with trisomy 13.

Purpura. Purpura are flat bluish purple lesions of variable size that represent subcutaneous bleeding and can be present at birth. If they are very small, they are called petechiae; if large areas are involved, they are called ecchymoses. The differential diagnosis of neonatal purpura includes congenital infection, coagulation defects, autoimmune disorders, and hemangioma with platelet trapping.

REFERENCES

1. Alper J, Holmes LB, and Mihm MC Jr: Birthmarks with serious medical significance: nevocellular nevi, sebaceous nevi, and multiple café-au-lait spots, J Pediatr 95:696, 1979.
2. Hurwitz S: Clinical pediatric dermatology, Philadelphia, 1981, WB Saunders Co.
3. Jacobs AH: Birthmarks. 1. Vascular nevi, Pediatr Rev 1:21, 1979.
4. Jacobs AH: Birthmarks. 2. Melanocytic and epidermal nevi, Pediatr Rev 1:47, 1979.
5. Jacobs AH and Walton RG: The incidence of birthmarks in the neonate, Pediatrics 58:218, 1976.
6. Tan OT and Gilchrest BA: Laser therapy for selected cutaneous vascular lesions in the pediatric population: a review, Pediatrics 82:652-662, 1988.
7. Weinberg S and Hoekelman RA: Pediatric dermatology for the primary care practitioner, New York, 1978, McGraw-Hill Book Co.

38

Pediatric Support for Parents

John H. Kennell and Marshall H. Klaus

Experiences during pregnancy, labor, and delivery and events shortly after birth may greatly affect the later development of an infant. We explore here what is known about this period in the life of the infant, the parents, and the family and emphasize what interventions may aid the maturation of the family.

It has been difficult to assess which factors determine the parenting behavior of human beings and how pediatric support can alter the process. Parents' actions and responses toward their infant derive from a complex combination of their own genetic endowment, the way the baby responds to them, the long history of interpersonal relations within their own families and with each other, their experiences in this or previous pregnancies, the practices and values of their respective cultures, and—probably most importantly—how each was raised by his or her own mother and father. The mothering or fathering behavior of each woman and man, their ability to tolerate stress, and their need for support may differ greatly and will depend on a mixture of all these factors.

Fig. 38-1 presents our present conception of the major influences on parenting behavior and the resulting disturbances that we postulate as arising from them. Included under parental background are the following:

1. Parent's care by his or her own mother
2. Endowment or genetics of parents
3. Practices of the culture
4. Experiences with previous pregnancies
5. Planning, course, and events during pregnancy

Although the effects of these particular determinants were once thought to be fixed and unchangeable, it has been observed that their impact may be altered, both favorably and unfavorably, during the experience of birth. Parenting behavior and the parent-child relationship may also be significantly influenced by factors such as the parents' observation of attitudes, statements, and practices of the nurses and physicians in the hospital; whether the mother is alone for short periods during her labor; whether there is separation from the infant in the first few days of life; the nature and temperament of the infant; and whether the infant is healthy, sick, or malformed.

Included under parenting disorders are the following:

1. Child abuse and neglect
2. Nonorganic failure to thrive
3. Vulnerable child syndrome
4. Disturbed parent-child relationship
5. Some developmental and emotional problems in high-risk infants

The following questions provide a helpful focus on the special needs of each mother:

1. How long have you lived in this area and where do most of your own family live?
2. How often do you see your mother and other close relatives?
3. Has anything happened to you in the past (or do you currently have any condition) that causes you to worry about the pregnancy or the baby?
4. What was your husband's reaction to your becoming pregnant?
5. What other responsibilities do you have outside the family?

It is important to inquire about how the pregnant woman herself was mothered: did she have a neglected and deprived infancy and childhood, or did she grow up in a warm and intact family?

In addition to those who received inadequate or disturbed mothering in their own early life, other mothers with special needs include single, young, or adoptive parents. We will consider the needs of all these women who have healthy full-term newborns, together with those of healthy parents from "normal" backgrounds.

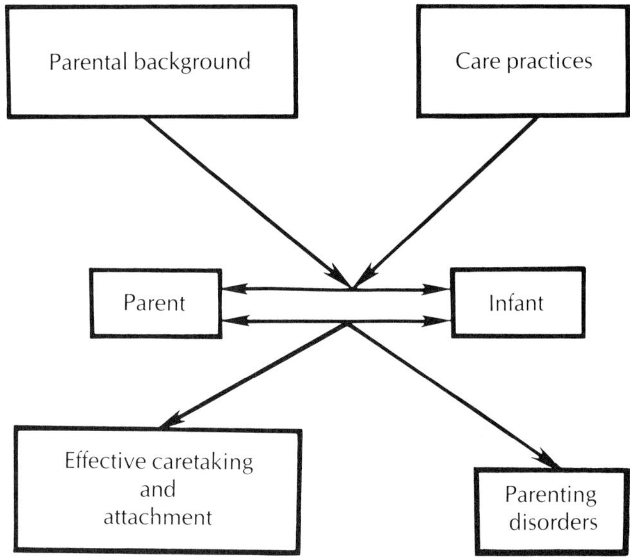

Fig. 38-1 The major influences on parent-infant attachment and the resulting outcomes.

From Klaus MH and Kennell JH: Parent-infant bonding, ed 2, St Louis, 1982, The CV Mosby Co.

INFANT STATE

For parents to begin to understand and meet their infant's needs, it is important that they understand the differing states of consciousness of the infant. The "state" or "pattern" of behavior refers to the infant's overall level of functioning at any given time—ranging from deep sleep to wakefulness, activity, or crying.

Wolff[44] originally designed the descriptive scale for rating the state of the full-term infant. He defined six states, but Prechtl and Beintema[31] omitted the "drowsy" state, regarding it as a transition between states, thus defining five states (Table 38-1). These states can be differentiated by recording physiologic measurements, including respiration, heart rate, eye movements, and electromyelography, as well as by behavioral observation.

These states appear to form a continuum that differs qualitatively and with distinct types of organizations. They are relatively stable and recur in regular cycles during day and night. Practically every behavior and body function of the newborn depends on his or her state and on the stability and control of this state. Cognitive functions in the newborn period, for instance, can best be assessed in the quiet alert state. However, in a sick newborn the state of quiet alertness cannot always be achieved.

STUDIES OF A SENSITIVE PERIOD

The question of whether additional time for close contact between the mother and her full-term infant in the first minutes and hours of life can alter the quality of the mother-infant bonding over time has been the subject of numerous studies and extensive debate. Because hospital practices have recently been altered on the basis of these studies, it is essential to explore their design, ecology, and outcome measures.

Thirteen separate studies have looked at the effect of additional mother-infant contact in the first hour of life, with contact after this period being similar in both the experimental and the control groups.* In 9 of the 13 studies, differences in the behavior of both mother and infant were noted in the experimental group.

In six of those nine studies, breast-feeding continued for a significantly longer period for those mothers who had contact that involved suckling their babies in the first hour after birth than for those whose suckling occurred later. It is difficult to know whether it was the early contact per se or, more specifically, the early suckling that altered the length of time that these mothers continued to breast-feed. It may be argued that the length of breast-feeding is not a valid assessment of the strength of the mother-infant bond, since bonding is culture determined to a great extent.

*References 1, 4, 5, 11, 12, 14, 15, 22, 25, 37, 39, 40.

It is useful to compare the study of O'Connor and associates[29] with that of Siegel and colleagues[34] (Table 38-2). In the two groups he studied, Siegel noted no differences in parenting disorders, child abuse, neglect, abandonment, or nonorganic failure to thrive. O'Connor, on the other hand, noted that infants of mothers who were allowed 12 additional hours of contact in the first 2 days had significantly lower hospital admission rates for parenting disorders, as well as fewer accidents and poisonings. Thus there is disagreement over whether additional early contact prevents or alters parenting failures.

Because of the relatively small number of patients studied, the negative finding by Siegel and co-workers does not answer the important question of whether extended contact for all mothers in the United States would prevent child abuse in some of the 100,000 infants presently abused each year. It can be calculated that a study of about 1600 patients would be needed to detect a reduction in child abuse from 3% to 1.5% eighty percent of the time, performance criteria that have not yet been met. Thus, although the majority of studies of additional early or extended contact do show changes in maternal and paternal behavior in the first days and weeks of life, the question remains concerning the clinical significance of the long-term effects.*

Feelings of love for the infant are not necessarily instantaneous with initial contact. Many mothers have shared with us their distress and disappointment that they did not experience the feelings of love for their baby in the first minutes or hours after birth. It should be reassuring for them to learn of the following study of normal, healthy mothers in England. MacFarlane and associates[26] asked 97 Oxford mothers, "When did you first feel love for your baby?" The replies were as follows: during pregnancy, 41%; at birth, 24%; first week, 27%; and after the first week, 8%.

A review of a representative ethnographic sample shows that 183 of 186 nonindustrial societies expect mothers and babies to "nest" together for days or weeks after delivery (a rooming-in equivalent) and virtually none permit the degree of separation that has been routine in many "developed" maternity hospitals. This early rooming-in is usually followed by extensive mother-infant contact and prolonged, frequent

*References 1, 5, 11, 12, 14, 22, 23, 25, 30, 32, 33, 34, 37, 38.

Table 38-1 *Levels of Functioning for Infants*

PRECHTL AND BEINTEMA[31]	WOLFF[44]
1. Deep sleep: eyes closed, regular respiration, no movements	1. Same
2. Active sleep (REM): eyes closed, irregular respiration, small movements	2. Same
3. Quiet alert: eyes open, no movements	3. Drowsy
4. Active alert: eyes open, gross movements, no crying	4. Quiet alert: no movements
5. Crying (vocalization): eyes open	5. Active alert: gross movements, no crying
—	6. Crying (vocalization)

Table 38-2 *Relationship Between Extended Early Mother-Infant Contact and Child Abuse and Neglect*

STUDY	NUMBER OF SUBJECTS	NUMBER OF CASES
O'Connor et al[29] (1980)		
Extended contact	134	2
Control	143	10*
Seigel et al[34] (1980)		
Extended contact	97	7
Control	105	10

Modified from Klaus MH and Kennell JH: Parent-infant bonding, St Louis, 1982, The CV Mosby Co.
*$p<0.05$.

breast-feeding during the early months. This almost universal practice of protecting and supporting the mother-infant pair together in the first weeks has evolved over thousands of years. Does it have significance for the industrialized societies of today, particularly in view of a recent widespread shift to early hospital discharge and the absence of legislated maternity or paternity leave in the United States?

In 1957 Winnicott[43] made remarkably perceptive observations that appear to describe what we call the sensitive period. He proposed that a healthy mother goes through a period of "primary maternal preoccupation," which "gradually develops and becomes a state of heightened sensitivity during, and especially toward the end of, the pregnancy. It lasts for a few weeks after the birth of the child." According to Winnicott, "The mother who develops this state . . . provides a setting for the infant's constitution to begin to make itself evident . . . and for the infant to . . . become the owner of the sensations that are appropriate to this early phase of life." He notes further that this is true only if a mother is sensitized in the way described and can identify with her baby's needs and thus is better able to meet them. As a result of recent changes in American society and modified expectations of young parents, some might consider the roles of the father and the mother as increasingly indistinguishable in relation to their newborn. We, however, tend to agree with Winnicott that each parent has a separate and unique role. He noted that fathers "can provide a space in which the woman has elbow room." When so protected, the mother does not have to deal with her surroundings just at the time that she wants to be "concerned with the inside of the circle she can make with her arms, in the center of which is the baby." This period does not last long, but "the mother's bond with the baby is very powerful at the beginning, and we must do all we can to enable her to be preoccupied with her baby at this time—the natural time."

Several studies[6,30,42] have shown that when the father is more supportive of the mother, she evaluates her maternal skills more positively and is more effective in feeding her baby. But it might also be the case that competent mothers generally elicit more positive evaluation and support from their husbands; therefore it is important to avoid fitting the data to expectations. However, the facts seem to indicate that increased paternal contact and involvement at the time of early infancy can provide important benefits to the newborn, to the mother, and to the father himself.[45] For this reason it seems particularly important to provide support and encouragement to both parents during labor, delivery, and the postpartum period. It is also beneficial to provide for early and extended mother-infant contact, especially for single and teenaged parents.

Anisfeld and Lipper[2] have reported that mothers with poor social supports (i.e., two or more of the following: unmarried, on public assistance, not a high school graduate, no father or other support person in the delivery room) showed greatly reduced affectionate interaction with their infants when they received routine care that separated mother and infant after delivery. On the other hand, mothers from the same background who were given their infants for the first hour showed a high level of affectionate interaction, even higher than mothers with better social supports. At the 3-month checkup, 69% of the low social support mothers with early contact returned with their infants for the scheduled appointment, in contrast to 26% in the group that had received only routine care.

There are no extant studies that have specifically considered the effects of early or delayed contact between infants and adoptive parents. Most adoptive parents do, of course, achieve a satisfactory attachment to their infant, but this may take extra time, effort, patience, and motivation. On the basis of the evidence now available, we believe that parents and adoptive infants should be brought together as soon as possible after birth and that the parents should be encouraged to take over full responsibility for care and planning for the infant, just as do other parents.

In summary, although there is increasing evidence from many studies* of a sensitive period that is helpful in parenting, this does not imply that every mother and father develop a close tie to their infant within a few minutes of the first contact.[24] Parents do not react in a standard or predictable manner to the complex environmental influences that occur in this brief period. However, rather than considering this to be evidence against the concept of a sensitive period, we think that it represents only the multiple individual differences among mothers and fathers generally.

LABOR, DELIVERY, AND THE FIRST DAYS FOR PARENTS OF NORMAL FULL-TERM INFANTS

In 1959 Bibring[3] wrote, "What was once a crisis with carefully worked-out traditional customs of giving support to the woman passing through this crisis period has become at this time a crisis with no mechanisms within the society for helping the woman involved in this profound change of conflict-solutions and adjustive tasks." This deficiency may account for the recent development of the many support systems in our society, such as the wide assortment of childbirth classes.

A review of ethnographic material has recently shown that in 127 of 128 representative, nonindustrialized societies, another woman was present with the mother during labor—in only one society did the mother labor alone. The significance of this almost universal custom of support has been revealed in three randomized controlled studies, which have shown that the presence of a supportive woman companion (a

*References 1, 5, 11, 12, 14-17, 22, 23, 25, 29, 32, 34, 37, 38.

"doula") during labor and delivery resulted in a significant decrease in cesarean deliveries, less use of anesthesia, and shorter labors when compared to women laboring alone.[18,19] In one study, mothers who had received doula support were awake most of the time, were with their newborns after delivery, and showed more affectionate interaction with their babies. Interestingly, fewer infants born after a doula-supported labor in the United States had a prolonged hospital course.

We feel that supportive management of labor and delivery should adhere to the following principles:

1. The less anxiety the mother experiences during delivery, the better will be her immediate relation with her baby. Thus she and her husband (or other support person) should visit the maternity unit to see where labor and delivery will take place and to learn about delivery routines. What will happen should be presented in detail, realistically but tactfully, if not previously covered in the childbirth class. For example, one of four mothers will have a cesarean delivery.
2. The mother ought to have one person for guidance and reassurance (husband, mother, friend, midwife, nurse, or obstetrician) continuously present at her side throughout labor and birth.[36] *No woman should ever labor alone.*
3. Once delivery has been completed, it is important for her to have a few seconds to regain her composure before she proceeds to the next task. It is best not to present her with her baby before briefly examining the infant to confirm that he or she is completely normal or before the mother indicates that she is ready to take her baby; it should be her decision.
4. It is valuable for the mother, father, and infant to be together for at least 1 hour. The mother and father usually never forget this significant and stimulating, shared experience. It helps some parents to begin the process of attaching themselves to the real infant. We wish to emphasize that this should be a private, "executive" session and that many normal parents take many days to fall in love with their infants.
5. The mother and father should stay together continuously or have long periods together in the days after the birth. The postpartum period should be a time when the mother interacts with her infant, becoming acquainted and gaining confidence in her own abilities. It is suggested that the infant stay in a small bassinet at the mother's side for a minimum of 5 hours per day (Fig. 38-2). After a cesarean delivery it will be painful for the mother to pick up, feed, and manage her infant without assistance. The father or another family member should be encouraged to stay with the new mother throughout the day to provide this assistance.
6. It is essential that parents be involved in the many decisions associated with labor and birth.
7. Whenever possible, infants who require additional heat in an incubator should be allowed to remain with the mother, and phototherapy for hyperbilirubinemia should take place in the mother's room. A mother may become extremely anxious about the health of her baby when they are apart and is reassured by the baby's presence. This is a common example of Winnicott's proposal of primary maternal preoccupation.[43]
8. Breast-feeding mothers should be encouraged to feed their babies on demand. This can mean between 8 and 18 feedings in a 24-hour period. Studies by de Carvalho[8-10] reveal that women who feed this frequently in the first 14 days have a larger milk output at 2 weeks, minimum nipple soreness, and infants with significantly lower bilirubin levels than do those women who nurse fewer than eight times a day in the first 2 weeks.
9. The mother needs the emotional support of close contact with her husband or chosen companion, as well as with any other of her children during this period, especially those under 3 years of age. Even under a policy of early discharge, sadness on separation from husband and children may compel a woman to leave the hospital before she is physically ready. The first few days at home usually go more smoothly for the siblings and mother if they have had daily visits during the hospitalization.

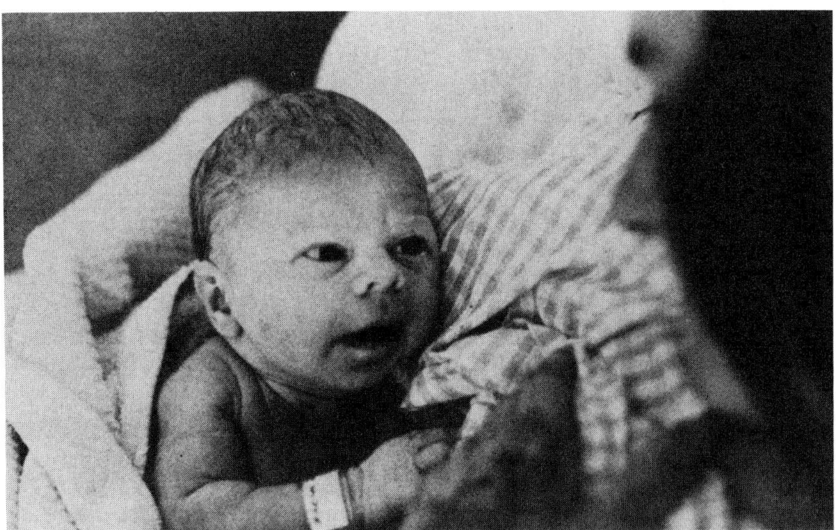

Fig. 38-2 What the mother sometimes sees.

From Klaus MH and Kennell JH: Parent-infant bonding, ed 2, St Louis, 1982, The CV Mosby Co.

10. We strongly recommend that nurses, physicians, and other maternity staff be consistently optimistic and avoid criticism in their interaction with the new mothers. In the postpartum period even a perfectly normal woman may be extremely sensitive to opinions and statements expressed by doctors and nurses.
11. If the baby must be moved to an intensive care unit, whether near or distant, it is helpful to give the mother a chance to see, touch, and hold her infant before departure and to have the father travel with the infant and report back to the mother once or twice a day.

THE PARENTS OF A SICK, PREMATURE, OR HIGH-RISK INFANT

When talking to the parents of an infant in the neonatal intensive care unit (NICU) or to the mother before her first NICU visit, it is best to describe what the infant looks like and how the infant will appear physically to the mother. Rather than talking about chances of survival, rates, or percentages, we stress that most babies survive despite early and often worrisome problems. There is no need to emphasize problems that may occur in the future; however, we do try to anticipate common developments (e.g., the need for bilirubin reduction lights for jaundice in small premature infants). The following guidelines may be helpful:

1. A mother's room arrangements should be adjusted to her needs . . . does she or does she not wish to be with other mothers who have healthy, full-term infants?
2. If at all possible, mother and infant should be kept near each other, and the mother should be able to visit whenever she wishes.
3. It is best to talk with the mother and father together, whenever possible. At least once a day, discuss with the parents how the infant is doing; talk with them at least twice a day if the baby is critically ill. It is necessary to find out what the mother believes is going to happen and what she has read about the problem. Any discussion should move at her pace.
4. The physician should not relieve his or her own anxiety by unburdening to the parents; once mentioned, for instance, the thought of death or brain damage can never be completely erased.
5. During the mother's first NICU visit, a chair should always be nearby so that she can sit down. A nurse can stay at her side during most of the visits, describing in detail the procedures being carried out.
6. It is important to remember the feelings of love for the baby are often elicited through eye-to-eye contact. Therefore the lights should be turned off and the eye patches removed from an infant under bilirubin lights, so that mother and infant can see each other.
7. It may be possible to enhance normal attachment behavior as late as several days or weeks following birth by permitting a special "nesting" period of 2 or more days and nights of close physical contact, with privacy and virtual isolation during which the mother provides complete care for her small infant, with help and nursing support readily available nearby.[21] Maternal attachment is enhanced by providing care, so it is desirable to involve the mother in tasks appropriate for the infant's condition as early as possible (e.g., stroking the baby's extremities to decrease apnea, changing the diaper, or assisting with nasogastric feedings).

Minde and colleagues[28] have reported a randomized trial in which parents of premature infants who participated in self-help groups rated themselves as being more competent on infant care measures; visiting their infants more often; and more often touching, talking to, and looking at their infants "en face." This interest in the infant persisted at home until at least 3 months after discharge.

At the Ramon Sarda Mother and Infant Hospital in Buenos Aires, Argentina, an exemplary program has been developed, based on extensive research of premature infants and their parents. The program applies those features that have been shown to enhance the attachment of mothers to sick and premature infants and decreases or removes factors, such as mother-infant separation, that interfere with it. Mothers are invited to stay at the Residence for Mothers when discharged from the obstetric unit. The poorer mother usually stays until her baby is discharged. Beds and meals are provided. The mothers rest and are well fed, and collectively they make up a community with common concerns—their children's premature birth or illness. There are formal and informal group meetings to develop maternal abilities and to teach mothers how to care for special infants. At the human milk bank, a mother extracts colostrum and breast milk to be given to her infant. The mother has access to the neonatal intensive care unit, with no time restrictions. She is involved actively in the care of her infant, usually from the time of admission. She learns from experience by sharing ideas and by "imitating" within the group of resident mothers.

In contrast to most neonatal intensive care centers, the poor mothers living in the residence usually develop a solid relationship with their infants and the hospital (Fig. 38-3). This is shown by the excellent rate of breast-feeding, continuous attendance at follow-up evaluations, and the disappearance of preventable diseases or problems such as malnutrition and diarrhea, child abuse, neglect, or desertion of children.

A STILLBORN OR NEONATAL DEATH

When the diagnosis of stillbirth is established in utero, both parents should be fully informed and the events surrounding labor and delivery explained thoroughly. As much as possible, an atmosphere of understanding and mutual support should be established between the bereaved parents and the medical staff.

Many have emphasized the importance of establishing the stillborn infant's identity. A death without a body that has been seen by a family member seems unreal. Grief following stillbirth is susceptible to distortion, since there are no postpartum experiences with the baby to remember, and the infant is often perceived as someone who did not exist, a person without a name. This sense of nonexistence is exaggerated in women who are heavily sedated or anesthetized during delivery and thereby deprived of the memories necessary for normal grief. The infant's identity can best be established if the bereaved parents are encouraged to look at, touch, and hold their child.

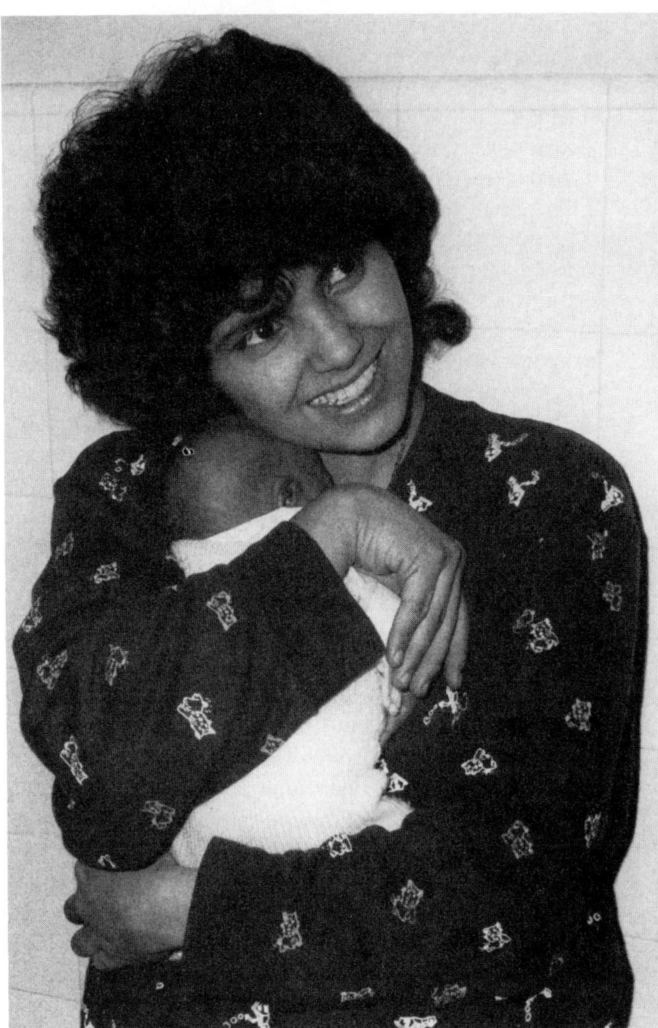

Fig. 38-3 A mother who has lived in the Residence for Mothers and cared for her premature infant from birth.

From Klaus MH and Kennell JH: Parent-infant bonding, ed 2, St Louis, 1982, The CV Mosby Co.

The parents may sometimes find the idea of holding a dead baby abhorrent at first, but once the baby is dead, there is no need to rush. We have found that parents will frequently change their minds; to facilitate this, we may keep the baby on the delivery floor for a few hours. Parents who have held their stillborn infant or dead neonate report that this was a meaningful experience they "never would have wanted to miss."

We have gradually come to appreciate that almost no baby is so deformed that the parents will not benefit from viewing the infant—if they so wish. It is often possible to present such babies (e.g., a baby with anencephaly) to parents, using receiving blankets in such a way to minimize any shock that might arise on seeing the malformation.

If a mother loses an infant anytime after she has felt movement, she usually goes through a long period of intense mourning. To help with the mourning process after a neonatal death or stillbirth, mothers should be encouraged to see and handle the infant after death, in privacy, if they desire. Some parents choose to hold the dying baby when intensive resuscitation efforts are no longer appropriate. Some mothers have cleaned, diapered, and dressed their dead baby. At first one might think that it is only good to remember the baby as a normal, active infant, but it is important for parents to see the dead infant, so that they have clear, visual proof that the baby really died. Also, if the baby had been rushed away right after birth, it is particularly valuable for the mother and father to see that they really did produce a baby that was normal in most respects. Many mothers report having lost a baby in the past and wishing for years that they could have seen, touched, handled, or even just seen a picture of the baby before he or she was taken away. Most have had none of these opportunities. If the mother is still confined in another hospital, there should be no reason that the infant's body cannot be held until the mother is discharged and ready to see the baby and participate in the funeral.

The experience of seeing and holding a stillborn infant may temporarily deepen the sadness of both parents, but it provides concrete memories that will facilitate normal mourning. It is highly desirable to obtain a photograph of every stillborn infant or live-born infant who dies, even if the parents do not wish to see it at the time.

Our general plan is to meet with the parents at least three times after a neonatal death or stillbirth. The first time is right after the death. At this moment they are so overwhelmed that they are unable to hear or retain anything other than the event of death. However, we do describe the details of the mourning process in simple terms. For example, we explain that they may have physical symptoms, such as chest pains. Waves of sadness may come on them intensely for the first few weeks, then gradually diminish up to 6 months and cease after 1 year. At times they may find themselves angry with each other and their friends and feel guilty about the death of their infant, believing that actions they could have taken would have saved the infant or prevented the illness in the first place. At times they may imagine that they see their baby alive and hence believe they are going crazy.

We meet with both parents together for a second time (sometimes with their own parents), usually within the first 3 days but at least within the first week. At this meeting it is much easier to review the grieving process. It is helpful for them to understand what the usual reactions are, so that they will not worry that they are ill. The most important action is to listen and listen again. We stress that the parents meet with us together to maintain rapport and communication.

The third meeting with the parents occurs 3 to 6 months after the death. We meet with them to ensure that their grieving is progressing normally and that there is no persistently high level of mourning or other sign of pathologic grief. If such symptoms are noted during the interview, referral to a psychiatrist should be made.

Our attendance over two decades at monthly meetings of parents who have experienced a perinatal loss has shown the great value of parents supporting, understanding, and listening to other parents who have experienced a similar loss. This little monthly window into the lives of bereaved parents has progressively broadened our own view of what is the "normal" range and duration of mourning reactions.

Helping parents through these experiences is, to be sure, taxing and difficult; it is important, however, and this essence of "physicianship" can be quite rewarding.

THE PARENTS OF AN INFANT WITH A CONGENITAL ANOMALY

Although previous investigators[7,13,27,41] agree that the birth of an infant with a congenital malformation often precipitates major family stress, Solnit and Stark's conceptualization[35] of parental reactions is most valuable. They note that the malformed infant is a distortion of the ideal infant that was dreamed of and planned for. The parents must first mourn the loss of the normal child they had expected before they can become fully attached to their living and defective infant. This significant aspect of adaptation may take many months. Parental reactions to the birth of a child with a congenital malformation appear to follow a predictable course (Fig. 38-4). Most parents experience initial shock, disbelief, and a period of intense emotional upset (including sadness, anger, guilt, and anxiety), followed by a period of gradual adaptation that is marked by a lessening of intense anxiety and emotional reaction. This adaptation is characterized by an increased satisfaction with and ability to care for the baby.

These stages in parental reactions are similar to those reported in other crises, such as having a terminally ill child. The intense emotional turmoil described by parents who have produced a child with a congenital malformation is a period of crisis (defined as an "upset in a state of equilibrium caused by a hazardous event which creates a threat, a loss, or a challenge for the individual"[13]). During such crises, a person is at least temporarily unable to respond with his or her usual problem-solving activities.

The sequence of parental reactions to the birth of a baby with a malformation differs from that following the death of a child in one important respect: the mother must become attached to her living but damaged child. The task of becoming attached to the malformed infant and providing for his or her ongoing physical care can be overwhelming to parents at just the time around birth when they are physiologically and psychologically depleted. The mother's initiation of the relationship with her child is a major step in the reduction of anxiety and emotional upset associated with the trauma of birth.

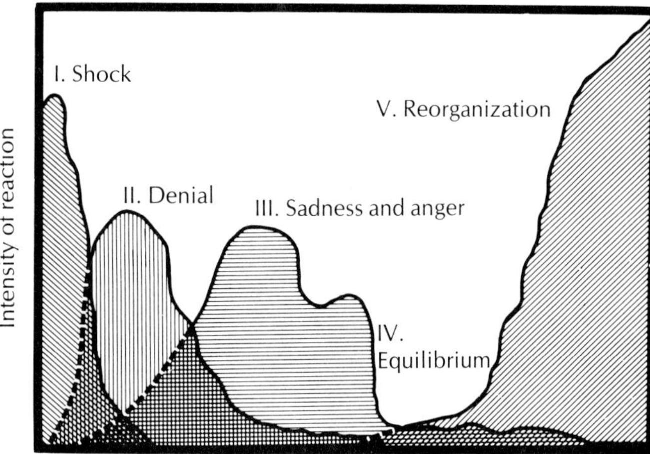

Fig. 38-4 Hypothetical model of the sequence of normal parental reactions to the birth of a child with congenital malformations.

From Drotar D, Baskiewicz A, Irvin N, et al: The adaptation of parents to the birth of an infant with a congenital malformation: a hypothetical model. Reproduced by permission of *Pediatrics*, vol 56, p 710, copyright 1975.

1. The parents' mental picture of the anomaly may often be far more severe and distorted than is merited by the actual defect. Any delay in seeing and touching the baby greatly heightens their anxiety. Therefore, we suggest bringing the baby to both parents when they are together as soon after delivery as possible.
2. Parents should not be given tranquilizers, which tend to blunt responses and slow adaptation to the problem.
3. Parents who become very involved by trying to find out what the best corrective procedures are and who ask many questions about the care of their baby and his or her abnormality can sometimes be annoying but often adapt best in the end. It is important to be more concerned about those parents who ask few questions and who appear stunned or overwhelmed by the problem.
4. It is best to move at the parents' pace. If we move too quickly, we run the risk of losing the parents along the way. It is beneficial to ask parents how they view their infant. We try to show parents one problem at a time (or wait until several can be put together in a logically related set).
5. Each parent moves through the process of shock, denial, anger, guilt, and adaptation at his or her own pace. If they are unable to talk with one another about the baby, their own relationship may be disrupted. During our discussions with parents we ask the mother how she is doing, how she feels her husband is doing, and how he feels about the infant. We then reverse the questions and ask the father how he is doing and how he thinks his wife is progressing. Thus they start to think not only about each other but also about their own adaptation. Often communication between the parents improves after one or two of these sessions. Some couples who did not seem to be close previously may move closer together over the next weeks and months. As with any painful experience, the parents may emerge much stronger after they have gone through the ordeal together.

REFERENCES

1. Ali Z and Lowry M: Early maternal-child contact: effects on later behaviour, Dev Med Child Neurol 23:337, 1981.
2. Anisfeld E and Lipper E: Effects of perinatal events on mother-infant bonding. Paper presented at biennial meeting of the Society for Research in Child Development, Boston, April 3, 1981.
3. Bibring GL: Some considerations of the psychological processes in pregnancy, Psychoanal Study Child 14:113, 1959.
4. Campbell SBG and Taylor PM: Bonding and attachment: theoretical issues, Semin Perinatol 3:3, 1979.
5. Carlsson SG et al: Effects of various amounts of contact between mother and child on the mother's nursing behavior: a follow-up study, Infant Behav Dev 2:209, 1979.
6. Curry MA: Contact during the first hour with the wrapped or naked newborn: effect on maternal attachment behaviors at 36 hours and 3 months, Birth Fam J 6:227, 1979.
7. Daniels LL and Berg GM: The crisis of birth and adaptive patterns of amputee children, Clin Proc Child Hosp DC 24:108, 1968.

8. de Carvalho M, Klaus MH, and Merkatz RB: Frequency of breast-feeding and serum bilirubin concentration, Am J Dis Child 136:737, 1982.
9. de Carvalho M et al: Effect of frequent breast-feeding on early milk production and infant weight gain, Pediatrics 72:307, 1983.
10. de Carvalho M et al: Milk intake and frequency of feeding in breast-fed infants, Early Hum Dev 7:155, 1982.
11. De Chateau P and Wiberg B: Long-term effect on mother-infant behaviour of extra contact during the first hour post partum. I. First observations at 36 hours, Acta Paediatr Scand 66:137, 1977.
12. De Chateau P and Wiberg B: Long-term effect on mother-infant behaviour of extra contact during the first hour post partum. II. Follow-up at three months, Acta Paediatr Scand 66:145, 1977.
13. Drotar D et al: The adaptation of parents to the birth of an infant with a congenital malformation: a hypothetical model, Pediatrics 56:710, 1975.
14. Hales DJ et al: Defining the limits of the maternal sensitive period, Dev Med Child Neurol 19:454, 1977.
15. Johnson NW: Breast-feeding at one hour of age, Am J Matern Child Nurs 1:12, 1976.
16. Keller WD, Hildebrandt KA, and Richards M: Effects of extended father-infant contact during the newborn period, Infant Behav Devel 8:337, 1985.
17. Kennell JH et al: Maternal behavior one year after early and extended post-partum contact, Dev Med Child Neurol 16:172, 1974.
18. Kennell JH et al: Medical intervention: the effect of social support during labor, Pediatr Res 23:211, 801, 1988.
19. Kennell JH et al: Labor support: what's good for mother is good for baby, Pediatr Res 25:15, 1989.
20. Kennell JH and Klaus MH: The perinatal paradigm: Is it time for a change? Clin Perinatol 15:801, 1988.
21. Klaus MH and Kennell JH: Interventions in the premature nursery: impact on development, Pediatr Clin North Am 29:(1263) 1982.
22. Klaus MH, Trause MA, and Kennell JH: Does human maternal behaviour after delivery show a characteristic pattern? In Parent-infant interaction, Ciba Foundation Symposium 33, Amsterdam, 1975, Elsevier Publishing Co.
23. Klaus MH et al: Maternal attachment: importance of the first post-partum days, N Engl J Med 286:460, 1972.
24. Klaus MH and Kennell JH: Parent-infant bonding, St Louis, 1982, The CV Mosby Co.
25. Kontos D: A study of the effects of extended mother-infant contact on maternal behavior at one and three months, Birth Fam J 5:133, 1978.
26. MacFarlane JA, Smith DM, and Garrow DH: The relationship between mother and neonate. In Kitzinger S and Davis JA, editors: The place of birth, New York, 1978, Oxford University Press.
27. Miller LG: Toward a greater understanding of the parents of the mentally retarded child, J Pediatr 73:699, 1968.
28. Minde K et al: Self-help groups in a premature nursery: a controlled evaluation, J Pediatr 96:933, 1980.
29. O'Connor S et al: Reduced incidence of parenting inadequacy following rooming-in, Pediatrics 66:176, 1980.
30. Pedersen FA: Mother, father and infant as an interactive system. Paper presented at the annual convention of the American Psychological Association, Chicago, Sept 1975.
31. Prechtl H and Beintema D: The neurological examination of the full-term newborn infant. In Lavenham L, editor: Little club clinics in developmental medicine, No 12, London, 1964, William Heinemann.
32. Ringler NM et al: Mother-to-child speech at 2 years—effects of early postnatal contact, J Pediatr 86:141, 1975.
33. Rodholm M: Effects of father-infant postpartum contact on their interaction 3 months after birth, Early Hum Dev 5:79, 1981.
34. Siegel E et al: Hospital and home support during infancy: impact on maternal attachment, child abuse and neglect, and health care utilization, Pediatrics 66:183, 1980.
35. Solnit AJ and Stark MH: Mourning and the birth of a defective child, Psychoanal Study Child 16:523, 1961.
36. Sosa R et al: The effect of a supportive companion on perinatal problems, length of labor, and mother-infant interaction, N Engl J Med 303:597, 1980.
37. Sosa R et al: The effect of early mother-infant contact on breast-feeding, infection and growth. In Breast-feeding and the mother, Ciba Foundation Symposium 45 (new series), Amsterdam, 1976, Elsevier Publishing Co.
38. Sousa PLR et al: Attachment and lactation. Proceedings of the Fifteenth International Congress of Pediatrics, Buenos Aires, Oct 3, 1974.
39. Svejda MJ, Campos JJ, and Emde RN: Mother-infant bonding: failure to generalize, Child Dev 51:775, 1980.
40. Thomson ME, Hartsock TG, and Larson C: The importance of immediate postnatal contact: its effect on breastfeeding, Can Fam Physician 25:1374, 1979.
41. Voysey M: Impression management by parents with disabled children, J Health Soc Behav 13:80, 1972.
42. Westbrook MT: The reactions to child-bearing and early maternal experience of women with differing marital relationships, Br J Med Psychol 51:191, 1978.
43. Winnicott DW: The child, the family, and the outside world, New York, 1964, Penguin Books.
44. Wolff PH: Observations on newborn infants, Psychosom Med 21:110, 1959.
45. Yogman MW: Development of the father-infant relationship. In Fitzgerald HE, Lester BM, and Yogman MW, editors: Theory and research in behavioral pediatrics, vol 1, New York, 1980, Plenum Press.

39

Signs and Symptoms of Neonatal Illness

Keith J. Gallaher

The term *clinical signs* refers to objective evidence of disease, whereas the term *symptoms* refers primarily to subjective descriptions. The infant, although unable to verbalize complaints, is able to relay information in ways that are equally informative to the astute clinician. The recognition of neonatal illness therefore relies primarily on the correct interpretation of objective findings. The clinical assessment of newborn infants provides an excellent opportunity to go back to the basic skills of assessment. Much of the information relevant to evaluating the health of an infant can be obtained simply by looking, without palpation or auscultation. The determination of vital signs and growth parameters provides further clues to health status. Although it is not possible to get a history directly from the newborn infant, one must not underestimate the diagnostic value (and courtesy) of speaking with the parents and reviewing the maternal chart.

In this chapter signs commonly noted in full-term newborns are described and correlated with more specific clinical diagnoses. In most cases, more information related to specific diagnoses can be found in subsequent chapters. The material is organized in the fashion by which most infants are actually monitored in the normal newborn nursery.

VITAL SIGNS

Heart Rate

Abnormalities of the heart rate (HR) or rhythm are quite common in the newborn period and, if isolated, are usually benign. In some instances the abnormalities may first be noted prenatally or during labor and delivery. For the first few days of life, the normal heart rate is 130 plus or minus 20 beats per minute. Abnormalities of rate fall into two main groups: tachycardia (HR over 170 beats per minute) or bradycardia (HR under 90 beats per minute). The initial evaluation of heart rate or rhythm abnormalities includes a 12-lead electrocardiogram and "rhythm strip."

Tachycardia

Sinus Tachycardia. The differential diagnosis of a narrow QRS complex tachycardia with a P wave preceding each QRS complex is between sinus tachycardia and paroxysmal supraventricular tachycardia (SVT). Sinus tachycardia can usually be differentiated from SVT on the following basis: (1) the heart rate is usually less than 200 beats per minute; (2) the beat-to-beat interval varies; and (3) vagal stimulation slows the heart rate gradually. Sinus tachycardia is a common manifestation of a wide variety of both physiologic and pathologic factors. It may be caused by an elevated temperature and thus be an early warning of infection or inappropriate environmental heart regulation. It may also be a sign of the infant's physiologic attempts to increase cardiac output, such as is seen in situations of severe anemia, congestive heart failure, or shock.

Supraventricular Tachycardia (SVT). SVT (also referred to as paroxysmal atrial tachycardia, or PAT) is usually associated with a more rapid heart rate (220 to 320 beats per minute) than is seen with sinus tachycardia. Often no P waves are visible preceding the narrow QRS complexes. Infants tolerate this rate for variable periods of time but often have associated irritability, poor feeding, tachypnea, and poor perfusion. Although SVT is associated with structural anomalies less than 20% of the time, infants with SVT need an echocardiographic assessment of this possibility. Other etiologies include underlying abnormalities of the conducting system, such as Wolff-Parkinson-White syndrome (WPW), and conditions that increase myocardial irritability, such as infectious or metabolic cardiomyopathies.

Ventricular Tachycardia. Ventricular tachycardia is an unusual problem in the newborn period. When seen, it is usually associated with severe underlying electrolyte disturbances or structural heart disease. The ECG manifestation is usually one of wide-complex tachycardia. By definition, it is abnormal and potentially life threatening.

Bradycardia

Sinus Bradycardia. Sinus bradycardia is the most common form of slow heart rate seen in the neonatal period. The heart rate is usually less than 90 beats per minute with a well-formed P wave preceding each QRS complex. The episodes are usually transient and associated with feeding or sleeping. The heart rate speeds up readily with stimulation. Persistent bradycardia not responding to stimulation should be evaluated further. Abnormalities occasionally associated with persistent sinus bradycardia include increased intracranial pressure, hypoxemia, and hypothyroidism.

Congenital Heart Block. Congenital heart block, on the other hand, is diagnosed by varying degrees of incoordination between atrial and ventricular depolarizations. The most serious form of congenital heart block is third-degree block (complete atrioventricular [A-V] dissociation). Approximately 30% of infants with complete A-V dissociation will have underlying structural heart disease (e.g., atrial septal defect, corrected transposition). In addition, it is closely associated with and often precedes the diagnosis of connective tissue disorders in the mother. The heart rate is usually in the range of 50 to 80 beats per minute, and infants are usually asymptomatic. Symptomatic infants usually have rates of 30 to 50 beats per minute.

Irregular Heart Rate. The most common cause of irregular heart rate in the newborn is an extrasystolic arrhythmia, such as premature atrial or ventricular contractions. Both are usually considered benign in the absence of underlying heart disease and if they disappear with increasing heart rate originating from the sinus node (i.e., upon stimulation of the infant). They usually disappear entirely within a few days or weeks. Infants with frequent extra beats or extra beats associated with cardiopulmonary symptoms deserve further evaluation to rule out electrolyte abnormalities or cardiomyopathies.

Blood Pressure

It is unusual to have blood pressure (BP) abnormalities as isolated findings in neonatal illness. Low blood pressure (systolic pressure less than 65 mm Hg for a full-term infant) is most often associated with tachycardia and signs of poor cardiac output. Hypertension (systolic BP greater than 90 mm Hg, diastolic BP greater than 60 mm Hg) is also unusual in the otherwise healthy newborn infant. Coarctation of the aorta is often diagnosed by the combination of increased blood pressure in the upper extremities with low blood pressure and/or poor pulses in the lower extremities. Renovascular occlusion may also manifest initially as persistently elevated blood pressure. This should especially be considered if the infant has had umbilical artery catheterization. Determination of serum electrolytes as well as evaluation of renal structure and perfusion are often helpful in evaluating the infant with persistently elevated blood pressure.

Temperature

Meticulous attention to the thermal status of the newly born infant is a hallmark of good newborn care. The increased surface area-to-volume relation characteristic of newborns makes them extremely sensitive to environmental conditions, especially when they are wet after delivery. The infant should be carefully dried and placed in a heat-gaining environment until stabilized. Infants should not be bathed until thermal stability is assured. Term infants should be dressed and blanketed, and the room temperature should be 24° C to 26.5° C in the normal newborn nursery.

Variations of body temperature (T) are more common than stable pyrexia in the sick infant. Thus persistent hyperthermia (T higher than 37.5° C axillary) is usually a manifestation of poor environmental heat control. One clue to whether a fever is disease related is the core temperature (rectal) to leg temperature (midthigh) gradient. A gradient of more than 1.7° C (core greater than thigh) suggests a disease-related fever.

Hypothermia is a prominent finding in neonatal illness, especially sepsis. Hypothermia, on an environmental basis, increases the metabolic demands on the infant and can be disastrous in terms of metabolic acidosis, pulmonary hypertension, and hypoxemia.

Respiration

Given the dramatic physiologic changes associated with the conversion from the aqueous fetal environs to the free-breathing newborn state, it is not surprising that respiratory compromise is a prominent finding in the newborn period. Abnormalities in respiratory rate, as well as in the quality of respiratory effort, are both often associated with neonatal illness. The normal respiratory rate of the term infant is approximately 40 breaths per minute.

Tachypnea. Although it may be difficult for infants to increase their tidal volume, it is not uncommon for them to attempt to increase their minute ventilation through increases in respiratory rate. Tachypnea is described as a respiratory rate of more than 60 breaths per minute. A primary pulmonary etiology of tachypnea is suggested by other signs of respiratory distress, including expiratory grunting, nasal flaring, inspiratory crackles, or rales. Evaluation of neonatal respiratory distress includes chest roentgenography, which in this instance can be considered part of the physical examination. This study can eliminate from consideration congenital malformations such as diaphragmatic hernia or cystic adenomatoid malformation as being the underlying etiology. The diagnosis of tracheoesophageal fistula with a proximal esophageal pouch and a distal fistula should be suspected when copious oral secretions and tachypnea are associated with the presence of a nasogastric tube coiled in the proximal esophagus.

Pneumonia. The most worrisome cause of tachypnea is infection, and concerns over this possibility have largely dictated our approach to all infants with evidence of respiratory compromise. Congenital pneumonia is an ominous cause of respiratory distress in the infant, and group B beta-hemolytic streptococcus is probably the best-known pathogen. Often the clues to the diagnosis are subtle, and if the pathogen is not treated promptly, death can result.

Transient Tachypnea. Transient tachypnea of the newborn probably represents delayed clearing of the normal fetal lung fluid, resulting in lungs that are somewhat stiff. The onset is at birth; typically, gradual improvement with time is noted. The physical findings are not so distinctive, however, as to preclude further evaluation if the signs persist for longer than a few hours.

Aspiration Syndrome. Aspiration syndromes are also relatively common. This category includes both blood and amniotic fluid aspirations. Infants with aspiration pneumonitis typically have a barrel-shaped, hyperexpanded chest and rapid, shallow respirations. If the aspirated amniotic fluid is meconium stained, clinical management may become especially problematic. In addition, pulmonary "airleaks" (e.g., pneumothorax) often accompany aspiration pneumonitis. In the case of suspected meconium aspiration, in addition to managing the acute respiratory problem, attention should focus on determining why the infant passed meconium in the first place. Often the answer to this question has a greater bearing on the long-term outcome than does the aspiration itself. Again, one worries about asphyxial insults or infection.

Spontaneous Pneumothorax. Spontaneous pneumothoraces are relatively common occurrences in otherwise healthy infants and may also initially manifest as tachypnea. Usually auscultation of the lungs helps in the clinical diagnosis, because decreased breath sounds over the involved lung may be noted. In addition, the chest is often hyperresonant to percussion on the side of the air leak. The diagnosis is confirmed by chest roentgenogram. Treatment options are dictated by the degree of cardiopulmonary compromise.

Metabolic Acidosis. Metabolic acidosis may elicit an increase in respiratory rate in the attempt to provide respiratory compensation. An arterial blood gas will assist in the recognition of this possibility. The differential diagnosis of metabolic acidosis is extensive and can be broadly divided into two groups: bicarbonate wasting (most commonly in the urine) or acid gain. Lactic acidosis signifies either *tissue hypoxia* (most commonly) or an *inborn error of metabolism*. Other circulating acids (e.g., pyruvic or methylmalonic acid) may cause a metabolic acidosis as a sign of an inborn error of metabolism.

Apnea. In direct contrast to breathing too rapidly, some ill infants may breathe too slowly or not at all. Apnea is defined as the cessation of air flow and may result from decreased respiratory drive, airway obstruction, or a combination of the two (mixed apnea). Symptomatic (prolonged) apnea is defined as apnea lasting for 20 seconds or longer or as shorter periods of apnea associated with cyanosis, marked pallor, hypotonia, or bradycardia. There are a wide variety of disorders that display the common sign of apnea. Pathologic apnea is never a normal finding in the term or near-term (over 35 weeks' gestation) infant. Perhaps the most ominous etiology is *infection*; however, any *metabolic disturbance* or *airway anomaly* may result in apnea. Certain drugs administered to the mother may also predispose the infant to inadequate respiratory drive, especially *narcotics* and *magnesium sulfate*. This sign deserves a meticulous search for an etiology. Although specific antidotes may be available in certain instances (e.g., naloxone for narcotic depression), the first treatment is to assure adequate ventilation.

Periodic Breathing. Periodic breathing is a breathing pattern in which there are three or more respiratory pauses lasting longer than 3 seconds with less than 20 seconds of respiration between pauses. Most commonly, periodic breathing is a normal event, especially in infants born prematurely. However, it may also be a manifestation of instability of the brainstem respiratory control center, a condition induced by disease.

GROWTH

Body Weight

One of the first questions asked by new parents is, "How much does my baby weigh?" The answer to this question may give the clinician valuable clues to the health of the infant. Abnormalities in growth may reflect effects of fetal nutrition, environmental toxins, systemic infections, chromosomal or syndromic influences, or family heritage. The adequacy of growth is usually assessed by comparing an infant's measurements with normal values obtained from published standards. This involves accurate determination of gestational age so that the appropriate standards can be used. The "gold standard" for determination of gestational age is good obstetrical dating. Examination of the infant systematically may provide confirmation.

Macrosomia. The term macrosomia refers to infants whose weight places them above the 90th percentile compared with other infants of similar gestational age. Infants born to mothers with diabetes are often macrosomic. This is believed to represent the effects of increased fetal insulin levels, which result from exposure to a chronically elevated blood glucose. This syndrome is associated with an increased incidence of congenital anomalies. Acute complications may also include hypoglycemia, hyperbilirubinemia, hypocalcemia, and polycythemia. Macrosomia may also result from intrinsic hyperinsulinemia. These are unusual problems characterized by early onset of hypoglycemia and elevated glucose requirements. The best-known disorder (but still uncommon) is Beckwith-Wiedemann syndrome. Infants with this problem also have macroglossia and omphalocele. Macrosomic infants may be difficult to deliver and thus may be predisposed to birth trauma.

Microsomia. Microsomia (intrauterine growth retardation), on the other hand, is most often defined as a birth weight below the 10th percentile compared with other infants of the same gestation. Other growth parameters, such as length or head circumference, may or may not be similarly affected. Discordant growth retardation (underweight for length and head circumference) often suggests that the problem occurred relatively recently, whereas symmetric growth retardation often (but not always) suggests either a long-lasting etiology or a problem intrinsic to the infant such as congenital viral infection or chromosomal abnormality. Of note is that certain ethnic groups (e.g., East Asian) have infants who "plot" as being small compared with normal American standards, whereas these infants are appropriate relative to other infants of their heritage. Microsomic infants may have hypoglycemia, because glycogen stores are often very minimal. Therefore close attention must be directed at maintaining adequate blood glucose levels.

Head Growth

Macrocephaly. Infants whose head circumference exceeds two standard deviations above the mean, or the 97th percentile, are said to be macrocephalic. It is critical to evaluate for evidence of neurologic impairment. Macrocephaly may be caused by volume increases in any of the normal components of the cranial vault, namely brain, blood, or cerebrospinal fluid. Increases in the cerebrospinal fluid compartment, either intraventricular or external to the ventricles around the surfaces of the brain, are referred to as hydrocephalus. This finding is often associated with a rapid rate of increase in the head circumference. The shape of the cranium may give clues as to whether fluid collections are intraventricular (frontal bossing) or external to the brain (biparietal enlargement). Hydrocephalus may or may not be a progressive finding and is relatively easily diagnosed by cranial ultrasonography or computed tomography.

Increases in brain volume may also be noted. This may represent either normal brain (as in benign familial megalencephaly), accumulation of abnormal metabolic products (e.g., lipidoses, mucopolysaccharidoses), a generalized growth disorder (e.g., achondroplasia) or, in rare cases, tumors.

Blood collections either in or around the brain may result in macrocephaly. Intracranial hemorrhage is an unusual primary etiology of increased head size, but is a common etiology of hydrocephalus.

Microcephaly. Microcephaly refers to a head circumference of less than two standard deviations below the mean, or less than the 3rd percentile. It is an ominous finding, often indicating a severe underlying abnormality of brain growth or development or both, caused by either primary brain dysgenesis or secondary insults such as teratogens, infection, or hypoxic-ischemic encephalopathy.

Body Length

Abnormally short or long infants usually fit into the classification of the connective tissue or skeletal disorders. Unfortunately, this measurement is notoriously one of the most inaccurate measurements made in the nursery. If there is some suspicion about the inappropriate length of an infant, further measurements such as long bone or upper-to-lower segment ratios may be beneficial along with a skeletal survey.

TONE, POSTURE, AND ACTIVITY

The normal term infant assumes a flexed posture of all limbs and when awake is active when gently stimulated. Limbs often move in an alternating fashion. When pulled to sit, the head should be held in the same plane as the rest of the body for several seconds. Muscle tone is best evaluated by passive limb manipulation.

Hypertonia

Hypertonia can be a prominent manifestation of hypoxic-ischemic brain injury, meningitis, or intracranial hemorrhage. Arching of the back (opisthotonos) is a manifestation of extensor hypertonia.

Hypotonia

Hypotonia is perhaps the most common motor abnormality noted in the neonatal period. Any acutely ill infant may demonstrate some degree of mild hypotonia. Most often hypotonia is associated with at least some degree of weakness, although significant disproportionality may be noted. The hypotonic infant often assumes a "spread-eagle" posture, with little to no resting limb flexion. Certain patterns of tone and weakness are associated with specific disorders.

Increased Activity

Increased activity is clearly a subjective finding based to a great extent on the past clinical experiences of the observer. Unfortunately, an important etiology in today's society is neonatal abstinence syndrome (drug withdrawal). The importance of recognizing this syndrome cannot be overemphasized. Diagnosis is made usually by the demonstration of illicit drugs in the infant's urine or stool.

Decreased Activity

Decreased activity may represent the effects of pharmacologic agents administered in the peripartum period, such as narcotics or magnesium sulfate. Both of these agents may also result in transient but significant respiratory depression. Once again, sepsis remains a possibility in any infant who has persistently decreased activity. Underlying neurologic abnormality also needs to be considered.

Jitteriness

"Jitteriness" is defined as rhythmic tremors of equal amplitude and is probably the most common involuntary movement of the healthy infant. The movements of jitteriness (or tremors) are usually provoked easily in susceptible neonates by external stimuli such as handling or loud noise and can be stopped by simply holding the affected extremity gently. Although they usually occur in healthy infants, seizures and jitteriness share similar etiologies, including hypoglycemia, hypocalcemia, and perinatal asphyxia. In addition, neonatal jitteriness is seen in association with maternal use of marijuana, cocaine, and narcotics.

Seizures

Only rarely will newborns with seizures have dramatic, well-organized, symmetric, generalized tonic/clonic episodes. More frequently, seizure episodes appear as focal abnormalities or as subtle findings, including staring, blinking, or sucking movements. Seizures in the newborn represent relative medical emergencies, since they are usually a sign of an underlying abnormality, including primary central nervous system disease, systemic illness, or metabolic abnormality. It is important to diagnose and treat neonatal seizures and their etiologies expeditiously.

COLOR

Cyanosis

Peripheral cyanosis involving the hands and feet (acrocyanosis) is a common normal finding in the first 1 to 2 days of life. In contrast, persistent central cyanosis is always abnormal. The ability to detect it, however, depends on the skill of the observer. Its presence suggests an abnormality in blood oxygen content resulting in 3 to 5 g of unoxygenated hemoglobin. If a respiratory etiology is involved, cyanosis is rarely if ever the only manifestation. Cyanosis without respiratory distress often suggests an anatomic right-to-left shunt caused by congenital cardiac anomaly. This right-to-left shunt can be confirmed by a minimum increase in pO_2 (pO_2 less than 100) with administration of 100% oxygen. In rare instances cyanosis may be caused by abnormal hemoglobin such as methemoglobin.

Jaundice

Visible jaundice in the first 24 hours of life usually suggests an increase in red blood cell turnover and resulting rapid production of bilirubin. Hemolysis, on an immune or an infectious basis, is the most frequent etiology. Inherited red cell membrane defects are less common problems that are often difficult to diagnose in the first few days of life. Aggressive treatment aimed at keeping levels of indirect bilirubin from climbing too rapidly is important in avoiding the central nervous system complications of hyperbilirubinemia. Although some degree of jaundice may be normal in healthy newborns, direct or conjugated hyperbilirubinemia is not. Levels of direct bilirubin persistently above 1.5 mg/dl require further evaluation, including but not limited to assessments of liver function.

Petechiae/Purpura

Petechiae are pinpoint hemorrhages into the skin that don't blanch with pressure, whereas purpura are larger, nonblanching areas of bleeding into the skin. Petechiae may normally appear at the presenting part for a vaginal delivery and do not signify underlying abnormalities. Extensive, generalized petechiae, on the other hand, may be the initial manifestation of an underlying platelet abnormality. The differential diagnosis includes infectious, immunologic, hematologic, and other miscellaneous causes.

Pallor

The term pallor, or paleness, describes a decrease in the normal rosy skin color of the Caucasian newborn. It may result from anemia or a generalized vasoconstriction.

Anemia. Anemia that appears in the newborn (hematocrit under 45) may have multiple etiologies, which can be subdivided into two main categories—excessive losses of red blood cells (e.g., acute or chronic hemorrhage, hemolysis) and inadequate production (red cell hypoplasia). The first group is much more common than the latter. Diagnostic evaluation includes assessment of cardiovascular stability, because hypotension, tachycardia, and delayed capillary refill may be seen in cases of acute blood loss. Determination of central hematocrit, red blood cell indexes, indexes of red blood cell production, and quantity of other blood cell lines (white blood cells, platelets) may give other clues. The detection of acid-stable hemoglobin in maternal blood (Betke-Kleihauer test) is diagnostic of fetal bleeding into the maternal circulation (fetomaternal hemorrhage). Anemia in the newborn is discussed more thoroughly in Chapter 112, "Anemia and Pallor."

Vasoconstriction. Pallor caused by vasoconstriction may represent the normal physiologic response to cold stress and thus respond simply to thermoregulatory management. On the other hand, this finding may be a clue to underlying hemodynamic compromise most commonly related to hypovolemia or cardiac dysfunction. In this case pallor often accompanies tachycardia, weak pulse, and low blood pressure. A history of blood loss during delivery may provide an additional clue to the diagnosis of hypovolemia; a therapeutic response to volume expansion confirms this diagnosis. If cardiac dysfunction is the underlying etiology, then other physical findings may be present, including a gallop heart rhythm, pulmonary rales, and hepatomegaly. In this situation volume expansion may actually exacerbate the problem.

Plethora

Plethora is usually caused by polycythemia, and a venous hematocrit reading of greater than 65% confirms the diagnosis. Polycythemia is noted with increasing frequency among infants who are *postmature*, who demonstrate *intrauterine growth retardation*, or who are born to *mothers who smoke or have diabetes or preeclampsia. Twin-to-twin transfusion* and chromosomal anomalies (e.g., *trisomies 13, 18, and 21*) are other etiologies. The main clinical concern related to polycythemia is that a high hematocrit is often associated with an elevated blood viscosity, which may impede tissue blood flow. Therefore, a wide variety of clinical signs may also be associated with plethora, including respiratory distress and cyanosis, central nervous system (CNS) signs, poor feeding, hypoglycemia, and many others. The treatment for symptomatic polycythemia is a partial exchange transfusion aimed at decreasing the hematocrit to approximately 50 and thus eliminating hyperviscosity.

SOUNDS

Cry

Abnormalities of the infant's cry have long been recognized as markers for a variety of neonatal disorders. More recently, advances in electronics have enabled investigators to characterize individual cry patterns. High-pitched cries may herald *CNS abnormalities*, whereas hoarse or low-pitched cries can be associated with *upper airway* abnormalities.

Breathing

Noisy breathing is often a clue to underlying airway problems and is associated with clinical evidence of increased work of breathing. Inspiratory stridors implicate extrathoracic airway obstructions, which include anomalies such as laryngomalacia, laryngeal web, and vocal cord paralysis. Accurate diagnosis is usually achieved by direct visualization by someone trained in airway management of the newborn. Less invasive methods of evaluation include fluoroscopy or measurement of air flow-volume loops. Expiratory grunting is often noted in infants with poorly compliant lungs and represents a compensatory maneuver that increases end-expiratory lung volume. Expiratory stridors and wheezing implicate intra thoracic obstruction involving the small and midsize airways.

ODORS

The astute clinician uses all his or her senses in the evaluation of newborns, including the sense of smell. Inborn errors of metabolism are often associated with unusual odors of the urine or of the infant itself. Although individual inborn errors of metabolism are relatively uncommon, as a group they are not rare. Unusual odors have been described, for example, as mustiness (phenylketonuria), sweaty feet (isovaleric acidemia), and maple syrup (maple syrup urine disease). Screening of urine and plasma for specific metabolic compounds will provide an initial step toward diagnosis.

BODY HABITUS

Abdominal Distention

Although mild gastric distention can be a normal finding, moderate distention that persists or is associated with other systemic signs of illness should be evaluated. Abdominal distention can result from gas, fluid, or abdominal mass.

Gaseous Distention. Gaseous distention can be diagnosed by hyperresonance to percussion. Functional decreases in bowel motility (*ileus*) can accompany a wide variety of systemic illnesses in the neonate. Usually there is no associated tenderness. Mechanical *bowel obstruction* is often associated with bilious emesis and delayed passage of stools. Free intraabdominal air resulting from perforated viscus is usually accompanied by signs of *peritonitis*, which include erythema of the abdominal wall, marked tenderness to palpation, and absence of bowel sounds.

Fluid Distention. Intraabdominal fluid is diagnosed by a fluid wave on palpation or by shifting dullness to percussion. *Hemoperitoneum* is occasionally noted after a difficult delivery or in association with disorders characterized by massive splenomegaly (e.g., erythroblastosis). Urinary ascites is occasionally noted in association with *obstructive uropathy*. The most common cause of fluid distention (*ascites*) is transudation. Conditions associated with this include hemolytic disease, congestive heart failure, or nonimmune hydrops.

Distention Caused By Abdominal Mass

Urogenital. Most abdominal masses in the newborn are urogenital in origin. Palpation of the abdomen may give clues as to location and consistency; however, the diagnostic modality of choice is an abdominal ultrasound examination. Flank masses (either unilateral or bilateral) usually are caused by *cystic dysplasia of the kidneys* or by *hydronephrosis*. *Cystic* ovary may appear as a lower abdominal mass in female infants.

Hepatomegaly. Hepatomegaly may also appear as an enlargement of the abdomen. The liver may normally be palpable 2 cm below the right costal margin with the upper border typically percussed at the fifth intercostal space. Liver enlargement can be seen with a wide variety of systemic illnesses, including infections, primary hepatic disease, congestive heart failure, hematologic disorders, storage disorders, trauma, and in rare cases, tumors.

Splenomegaly. The tip of the spleen may occasionally be palpable in normal infants during the first days of life. A prominent spleen may be associated with *congenital viral infection*, *inborn errors of metabolism*, or more commonly in association with the increased extramedullary hematopoiesis noted with *hemolytic disease*.

Adrenal Hemorrhage. Massive adrenal hemorrhage may manifest as a flank mass in a stressed infant after a *difficult delivery*. Risk factors include macrosomia, breech presentation, and perinatal asphyxia.

Gastrointestinal. Enteric *duplication cysts* may be palpable and can lead to bowel obstruction. An olive-size mass in the epigastrium can be caused by the hypertrophied pylorus of *pyloric stenosis*.

Tumor. *Wilms' tumor*, *neuroblastoma*, and congenital *mesoblastic* nephromas are uncommon; however, their usual presenting sign is abdominal swelling or a palpable abdominal mass.

INTAKE AND OUTPUT

Feeding Problems

Oral feeding, although often taken for granted, represents a very complicated neuromotor process involving coordination of sucking, swallowing, and breathing. Disinterest in feeding may also be noted in conjunction with other systemic illnesses. As a result, difficulties in feeding are seen in association with a wide variety of disorders. Although this group of disorders is nonspecific, it is commonly seen in *infants born prematurely* or in infants with *CNS and neuromuscular disorders*. Less commonly, the etiology may be anatomic abnormalities such as *tracheoesophageal fistula*.

Oliguria

Most infants (more than 90%) void by 24 hours of age and 99% do so by 48 hours; they will maintain adequate output thereafter (more than 1 ml/kg/hr). Failure to pass urine by 48 hours thereafter suggests either *primary renal dysfunction* or *obstructive uropathy*.

Polyuria

Polyuria is uncommon in the newborn. It is considered pathologic when the infant is unable to achieve normal total body water and electrolytes because of persistent passage of unconcentrated urine. Most commonly this represents *renal tubular dysfunction*, as can be seen after acute tubular necrosis or in association with a partial obstruction of the renal collecting system. A less common etiology would be *inadequate antidiuretic hormone response*.

Hematuria/Hemoglobinuria

Red urine usually indicates hematuria; however, other possible etiologies include the presence of hemoglobin, uric acid, or porphyrins. Examination of a freshly voided urine will aid in the diagnosis. If intact red blood cells are detected, *extraurinary sources* (e.g., rectal bleeding) must be excluded.

If associated with the presence of red cell or other types of renal casts, then *parenchymal kidney disease* is the likely etiology. The differential diagnosis of hematuria in the newborn includes asphyxial kidney injury (e.g., acute tubular necrosis, cortical necrosis), renovascular accident (e.g., renal vein thrombosis), obstructive uropathy, cystitis, nephritis, or underlying coagulopathy.

Hemoglobinuria is most commonly seen in association with intravascular hemolysis. Urate crystals may give a reddish-orange cast to the urine in infants who are otherwise healthy.

Proteinuria

A small amount of protein may normally be detected in the urine of healthy infants; however, most term infants excrete less than 25 mg in 24 hours. If excessive proteinuria is suspected, then a timed urine collection should be obtained. Proteinuria may be seen in association with nearly any form of renal disease.

Constipation

Most term infants (94%) pass their first meconium stool by 24 hours of age; 99% pass meconium by 48 hours. Delays in passage may represent significant underlying bowel pathology, including Hirschsprung's disease, atresias, and meconium ileus.

Melena/Hematochezia

A common source of blood in the newborn infant's stool is maternal blood swallowed at delivery. These infants typically are not ill. This etiology can be diagnosed quickly at the bedside by the Apt-Downey test for adult hemoglobin. Gastrointestinal hemorrhage may be acute and life threatening or may be detected only in trace amounts by stool heme testing. Gastrointestinal (GI) hemorrhage may be the presenting sign of a generalized bleeding disorder such as vitamin K deficiency, disseminated intravascular coagulation, thrombocytopenia, or hereditary coagulopathy. Upper GI trauma such as from vigorous suctioning or placement of a nasogastric tube usually results only in occult bleeding, whereas bleeding caused by primary lower GI pathology is typically more pronounced. The differential diagnosis includes but is not limited to peptic ulcers, necrotizing enterocolitis, malrotation and volvulus, Meckel's diverticulum, and intussusception. Hematochezia with mucus may result from infectious enteritis, which can be diagnosed by appropriate cultures.

Vomiting

Although the "spitting up" ("posseting" in British infants) of small amounts of formula occurs frequently in otherwise healthy newborns, a large volume of or persistent vomiting may be an early warning of underlying pathology. Vomiting of non-bile-stained fluid usually represents anatomic or functional obstruction at or above the first portion of the duodenum. Etiologies include esophageal atresia, gastric web, and pyloric stenosis. Severe gastroesophageal reflux (GER) may also show up as vomiting. However, it is still important to rule out an anatomic obstruction before linking the diagnosis of vomiting to GER alone. Obstruction below the opening of the bile duct may result in bilious vomiting. This may be a functional ileus caused by systemic illness, metabolic derangements such as in hypokalemia, adrenal hyperplasia or elevated intracranial hemorrhage, or a structural problem (e.g., malrotation and volvulus, atresia). Diagnostic tests start with anteroposterior and horizontal beam abdominal roentgenograms.

Diarrhea

Diarrhea is the passage of frequent stools. Newborn infants may have up to five or six stools per day, especially if breastfed. Persistent passage of watery stools, however, is abnormal and may be a sign of enteric or systemic function.

Gastroenteritis. Bacterial gastroenteritis is unusual in the newborn period; however, nursery epidemics, as well as isolated cases, do occur. The diagnosis is suggested by the presence of blood and mucus in the stools and is confirmed by appropriate cultures. Viral gastroenteritis, especially that caused by rotavirus, has been described in newborns.

Lactose Intolerance. Lactose intolerance is a very common cause of diarrhea in the newborn. Stools are watery and test positive for reducing sugar. The diagnosis is further suggested when these findings resolve after a lactose-free formula is begun. Most commonly this represents a transient lactose deficiency.

Other Causes. Other less common etiologies include phototherapy, neonatal abstinence syndrome, thyrotoxicosis, and other specific malabsorption syndromes such as cystic fibrosis.

OTHER FINDINGS ON EXAMINATION

Leukokoria

Leukokoria literally means white pupil and is not a normal finding in the newborn. The observation of a white pupil requires immediate, further evaluation by an ophthalmologist experienced in examining newborns. The most common etiology is a cataract, of which nearly 50% have diagnosable and potentially treatable causes. Other etiologies include persistent hyperplastic primary vitreous, cicatricial retinopathy of prematurity, retinal dysplasia, tumor (retinoblastoma), glaucoma, and numerous other causes.

Red Eye

Ophthalmia neonatorum, or neonatal conjunctivitis, often manifests as a red eye with exudate (see Chapter 162, "The Red Eye"). The cause is chemical (silver nitrate), bacterial, viral, or chlamydial in nature. All cases should be examined thoroughly with appropriate cultures performed and appropriate therapy instituted promptly, especially with marked swelling of the eyelids and a purulent discharge, which is most likely caused by infection with *Neisseria gonorrhoeae*.

Heart Murmur

A large number of normal, healthy infants have a soft, short systolic murmur in the first few days of life. The absence of a murmur, on the other hand, does not eliminate the diagnosis of serious cardiac anomaly. Falling pulmonary vascular resistance over the first few days of life also affects the presence and the quality of the murmur. A significant murmur heard on the first day of life is more likely to be caused by an obstructive lesion such as aortic stenosis, pulmonic stenosis, or coarctation, whereas a murmur heard later suggests a shunt lesion such as a patent ductus arteriosus or ventricular septal defect. Loud, persistent systolic murmurs, especially if accompanied by other cardiopulmonary findings, require further evaluation.

SUGGESTED READINGS

Baylen BG and Emmanouilides GC: Neonatal cardiopulmonary distress, Chicago, 1988, Year Book Medical Publishers, Inc.

Catalano DJ: Leukokoria: the differential diagnosis of a white pupil, Pediatr Ann 12:498, 1983.

Fanaroff AA and Martin RJ: Neonatal-perinatal medicine, St Louis, 1987, The CV Mosby Co.

Jones KL: Smith's recognizable patterns of human malformation, ed 4, Philadelphia, 1988, WB Saunders Co.

Klaus MH and Fanaroff AA: Care of the high-risk neonate, Philadelphia, 1986, WB Saunders Co.

Nelson NM, editor: Current therapy in neonatal-perinatal medicine-2, Philadelphia, 1990, BC Decker, Inc.

Parker S et al: Jitteriness in full-term neonates: prevalence and correlates, Pediatrics 85:17, 1990.

Volpe JJ: Neurology of the newborn, Philadelphia, 1987, WB Saunders Co.

40

Common Neonatal Illnesses

Charles Palmer

APNEA

Irregularity in the pattern of breathing is common in newborn infants. The preterm infant responds to a fall in inspired oxygen concentration with a transient increase in ventilation, only to be followed by a sustained depression of ventilation. In addition, infants at fewer than 33 weeks of gestation exhibit reduced ventilatory responses to inspired carbon dioxide. A similar response has been observed in the term infant during the first week of life, when a progressive decrease in inspired oxygen concentration results in reduced carbon dioxide responsiveness.

Apnea is defined as a cessation of respiratory air flow. The respiratory pause may be central (i.e., no respiratory effort), obstructive, or mixed. Short (<15 seconds) central apnea can be normal at all ages. *Periodic breathing* is commonly seen in premature infants and is defined as a breathing pattern in which there are three or more respiratory pauses of more than 3 seconds' duration with <20 seconds of respiration between pauses. *Pathologic apnea* is defined as a respiratory pause that is prolonged (>20 seconds) or a shorter period associated with cyanosis, marked pallor, hypotonia, or bradycardia.[5] *Apnea of prematurity* is defined as periodic breathing with pathologic apnea in a premature infant.

Apnea of prematurity is more frequent during rapid eye movement sleep than during quiet sleep. It usually starts after the first day of life and resolves by 37 weeks of gestation but occasionally persists to several weeks postterm. It is a common finding in preterm infants and, if the apneic periods are prolonged, can lead to hypoxemia and bradycardia.

Although uncomplicated apnea of prematurity is common, apnea may be symptomatic of an underlying disorder even in the preterm infant. Specific causes for apnea include (1) septicemia (e.g., meningitis or necrotizing enterocolitis); (2) impaired oxygenation, hypoxemia, severe anemia, and shock or marked systemic to pulmonary circulatory shunt (e.g., patent ductus arteriosus); (3) metabolic disorders (e.g., hypoglycemia, hypercalcemia, hyponatremia, hypernatremia, and hyperammonemia); (4) drugs (e.g., narcotics or central nervous system depressants taken by the mother); (5) central nervous system disorders (e.g., intracranial hemorrhage, seizures, or malformations of the brain); and (6) thermal instability (i.e., a rapid increase or decrease of temperature).

Investigation for an underlying cause should be pursued vigorously if one of the following conditions obtains: (1) apnea occurring within 24 hours of delivery, (2) apnea occurring after 36 weeks of gestation, (3) apnea requiring vigorous resuscitation, (4) apnea associated with cyanosis, and (5) an increase in the severity of existing apneic episodes.

The preterm infant should be monitored for apnea and, because bradycardia usually follows within 30 seconds of obstructive apnea, heart rate monitoring also should be included. This is important because obstructive apnea (in which breathing effort continues but air flow ceases because of obstruction in the upper airways) will not trigger the usual form of respiratory monitor, which relies on changes in the chest wall electrical impedance. Convenient monitors of both respiration and heart rate are available.

Treatment of neonatal apnea should address its underlying cause. Several treatments are available for apnea of prematurity, including the following:

1. Tactile stimulation. Gentle tapping on the infant's heel usually suffices. A pulsating waterbed sometimes is used for recurrent episodes.
2. Pharmacologic intervention with methylxanthines (theophylline or caffeine). A loading dose of theophylline (5 mg/kg) is followed by maintenance at 1 to 2 mg/kg/dose (twice a day). Caffeine usually is given as 20 mg/kg loading dose orally, followed by 5 mg/kg/day.
3. Continuous positive airway pressure by nasal prongs.
4. Small increases in inspired oxygen from 21% to 25% with monitoring of the response to maintain the arterial oxygen pressure (Pa_{O_2}) between 50 and 90 mm Hg.
5. Endotracheal intubation with positive end-expiratory pressure may be required for a short period in some cases.

When pharmacologic therapy is used, age-related variations in theophylline metabolism necessitate monitoring the plasma theophylline concentration. The concentration required for apnea is less than that required for bronchodilation; thus levels should be maintained between 6 and 13 μg/ml. Because caffeine, in contrast, has a broad therapeutic index, its concentration usually does not need to be monitored if given in the prescribed dose. Physicians who administer methylxanthines should be aware that the hepatic metabolism of these drugs is slowed by macrolide antibiotics, such as erythromycin, and by intercurrent viral illnesses. The toxicity of theophylline is related to its serum level; clinical manifestations usually begin with tachycardia, followed by jitteriness, irritability, and signs of gastrointestinal dysfunction. Occasionally, if apnea of prematurity does not cease by 37 weeks, the infant may be discharged home with an apnea monitor. In these cases the parents are expected to be skilled in cardiopulmonary resuscitation and the use of the monitor.

The term *apnea of infancy* applies to the occasional infant who has an unexplained respiratory pause for at least 20 seconds, or a shorter respiratory pause associated with bradycardia, cyanosis, pallor, and/or marked hypotonia. The term generally refers to infants with fewer than 37 weeks of gestation at the onset of pathologic apnea. An *apparent life-threatening event* is an episode that is frightening to the observer and characterized by some combination of apnea (central or obstructive), color change (cyanosis or pallor), marked change in muscle tone (usually marked limpness), choking, or gagging. In some cases the observer fears that the infant has died. These incidents should be investigated for an underlying cause, especially gastroesophageal reflux and possible seizures. When the diagnosis of such apnea is in question, the simultaneous recording of respiratory electrical impedance and the electrocardiogram for prolonged periods ("pneumograms") can be used to document the occurrence of apnea and bradycardia.

The outcome of apnea of prematurity usually is good, provided appropriate monitoring and treatment are ensured to prevent long periods of hypoxia. Survivors of apnea of infancy, in which the apneas have been severe enough to require resuscitation, are at increased risk for sudden infant death syndrome. Unfortunately, pneumograms cannot predict which infants will die during a subsequent event or which will require resuscitation to terminate a subsequent apneic spell. When compared with a control group, however, infants with apnea of infancy have significantly higher respiratory and heart rates. Thus, although the pneumogram does not predict the risk of an adverse outcome in a population of infants with severe apnea of infancy, it can reveal subtle cardiorespiratory differences.

HYPERBILIRUBINEMIA

Hyperbilirubinemia occurs commonly during the first week of life. It is usually physiologic, and appropriate management includes reassurance, with avoidance of unnecessary investigations and maternal-infant separation. Occasionally, hyperbilirubinemia is symptomatic of an underlying pathologic condition. These cases need identification and etiologic work-up. Select cases may require specific management to prevent the harmful effects of excessive unconjugated bilirubin on the central nervous system.

Physiologic Jaundice

Clinical jaundice is visible at serum bilirubin levels of approximately 5 to 7 mg/dl (85 to 120 μM/l. Approximately 50% of all normal newborns and a higher percentage of premature infants appear jaundiced during the first week of life. Nearly all newborns will have some degree of mild hyperbilirubinemia that disappears after a few days; this transient hyperbilirubinemia has been called physiologic jaundice. Mechanisms involved in producing physiologic jaundice include an interaction between an increased load of bilirubin (from the high fetal hematocrit) and a decreased ability of the newborn liver to clear bilirubin. The clinician can recognize the presence of physiologic jaundice by certain criteria. It is clinically evident *after* the first 24 hours of life. It peaks between days 3 and 5, and in normal full-term infants it does not rise higher than 12.7 to 12.9 mg/dl.[4] The bilirubin is almost all unconjugated. Jaundice usually is not detectable after 10 days. Deviation from this physiologic pattern generally signifies a pathologic process and requires special investigations to define a cause.

Breast-feeding and Jaundice

Breast-feeding has been associated with increased levels of bilirubin and prolongation of hyperbilirubinemia. The association between breast-feeding and jaundice in the healthy, full-term newborn can be considered in terms of two categories: (1) the jaundice that is *associated* with breast-feeding and (2) true breast-milk jaundice.

Breast-feeding–Associated Jaundice. Prolonged hyperbilirubinemia in association with breast-feeding occurs in about 30% of breast-fed babies. There is some indication that frequent feeding may reduce the incidence of hyperbilirubinemia and that breast-feeding should not be withheld. An association between decreased frequency of nursing and higher bilirubin levels has been found. Hence, breast-feeding mothers should be encouraged to nurse their infants as frequently as possible. If it appears that the bilirubin concentration will rise above 20 mg/dl, feeding should be temporarily stopped for 48 hours and then resumed.

True Breast-Milk Jaundice. The syndrome of true breast-milk jaundice in which the bilirubin concentration rises progressively from the fourth day of life, reaching a maximum of 10 to 30 mg/dl (171-153 μM/l) by 10 to 15 days, develops in approximately 1% to 2% of breast-fed neonates. If breast-feeding continues, the bilirubin may continue to rise before declining after about 4 to 10 days to reach normal levels by 3 to 12 weeks of age. Finally, if breast-feeding is interrupted at any stage, the bilirubin concentration declines markedly within 48 hours. With resumption of nursing, bilirubin concentrations may rise moderately by 1 to 3 mg/dl but usually do not reach the previous level.

If breast-feeding needs to be withheld temporarily, mothers should be given enthusiastic support and encouraged to resume breast-feeding after a 48-hour interruption. They also should be encouraged to maintain lactation by breast pump or manual expression.

Pathologic Jaundice

Pathologic jaundice refers to a pattern of hyperbilirubinemia that falls outside the limits defined for physiologic jaundice. It may occur earlier, last longer, or reach higher levels. In these cases, jaundice should be regarded as symptomatic of an underlying pathologic condition. The following criteria, modified from Maisels,[4] help identify pathologic hyperbilirubinemia:

1. Clinical jaundice in the first 24 hours of life
2. Total serum bilirubin concentrations increasing by more than 5 mg/dl (85 μM/l/day)
3. Total serum bilirubin concentrations exceeding 12.9 mg/dl (221 μM/l) in full-term infants or 15 mg/dl (257 μm/L) in premature infants
4. Direct (conjugated) serum bilirubin concentration exceeding 1.5-2 mg/dl (26-34 μM/l)

5. Clinical jaundice persisting for more than 1 week in full-term infants or 2 weeks in premature infants

Deviations from these guidelines should be investigated.

In patients physiologic jaundice will reach levels above 12.9 mg/dl, and a higher level may be tolerated before special investigations are initiated. In a recent study[6] only 6% of infants admitted to a well-baby nursery had serum bilirubin levels that exceeded 12.9 mg/dl. Serum bilirubin levels above 12.9 mg/dl were significantly associated with breast-feeding, maternal diabetes, oxytocin-induced labor, prematurity, Oriental race, and male sex. Appreciation of these factors permits a more rational approach to the level of bilirubin at which to initiate special studies. In these patients a peak bilirubin level of 15 mg/dl can be tolerated as the upper range of normal before investigation is warranted. In the absence of these factors, values higher than 12 mg/dl should be used as the level at which jaundice should be investigated.[6]

Causes of Pathologic Jaundice in the Neonate. The newborn with jaundice should have a total and direct (conjugated) bilirubin estimation made as soon as jaundice is diagnosed. Jaundice is clinically first evident after 48 hours. That occurring during the first 24 hours usually is caused by an excessive load of bilirubin, resulting from hemolysis caused by maternal antibodies against fetal red cell ABO or Rh antigens. Nonimmune causes of hemolysis also should be considered, including hereditary spherocytosis and deficiency of glucose-6-phosphate dehydrogenase.

Infants of mothers with diabetes are prone to increased bilirubin production, as are patients with increased intrahepatic circulation of bilirubin secondary to small or large bowel obstruction. Decreased clearance of bilirubin also can occur in premature infants, with breast-feeding, and with certain inborn errors of metabolism such as hypothyroidism. Essential investigations for nonphysiologic jaundice include (1) serum bilirubin concentration, both direct and total, (2) peripheral blood smear for red cell morphology and reticulocyte count, (3) blood typing of both mother and infant, (4) direct Coombs test on the infant, and (5) hematocrit level. An increased direct bilirubin level exceeding 1.5 to 2 mg/dl (or one third of the total serum bilirubin) requires diagnostic evaluation. This should proceed rapidly because patients with biliary atresia require early surgical intervention for optimal outcome.

The presence of pathologic jaundice should provoke a review of the maternal and infant history and a thorough examination of the infant. A family history of jaundice and liver disease and a maternal history of illness, diabetes, or drug ingestion during pregnancy should be sought. The history of labor and delivery should be reviewed for documentation of oxytocin administration, delayed cord clamping, and vacuum extraction, because all may lead to increased red cell mass, and thus serum bilirubin level from hemolysis. The maternal history should be further evaluated for evidence of bacterial or viral infection (fever, premature rupture of membranes), and the mother's blood needs to be analyzed for ABO and Rh blood groups and the presence of isoantibodies. Any maternal history of hepatitis and family history of anemia or glucose-6-phosphate dehydrogenase deficiency should be noted.

The infant with nonphysiologic (pathologic) jaundice (especially if jaundice is prolonged or associated with an elevated direct fraction) should be examined carefully for signs of sepsis such as lethargy, temperature instability, a change in feeding pattern, cutaneous petechiae, and poor capillary perfusion. Signs of extramedullary hematopoiesis, including hematosplenomegaly, may reflect a congenital infection. The presence of a hematoma, extensive bruising, plethora, polycythemia, or ingested maternal blood provides an additional hemoglobin source and thus may lead to an elevated serum bilirubin level.

Conjugated Hyperbilirubinemia. An increase in direct (conjugated) bilirubin greater than 1.5 to 2 mg/dl (or more than 33% of the total serum bilirubin concentration) is almost always pathologic. Causes include liver inflammation and/or obstruction to bile flow. Hepatitis can be caused by sepsis, intrauterine infections, and inborn errors of metabolism such as alpha[1]-antitrypsin deficiency, galactosemia, and pyloric stenosis. Inflammation of the liver and cholestasis can be produced by prolonged parenteral nutrition.

Cholestasis in the infant also can be caused by biliary atresia, either intrahepatic or extrahepatic, a choledochal cyst, or inspissated bile. The presence of bile pigment in the stool or duodenal aspirate excludes complete biliary atresia. Such patients should be carefully examined for the signs of hepatosplenomegaly (which would support a congenital infection), and the urine should be cultured to exclude a urinary tract infection; blood cultures should be drawn to exclude septicemia. An ultrasound examination of the liver can demonstrate the presence of a choledochal cyst and dilated biliary structures. Bile flow also can be evaluated with radioisotopes excreted by the hepatobiliary system. Finally, a liver biopsy and a cholangiogram may be necessary to determine specific pathology.

Patients with conjugated hyperbilirubinemia should be investigated at a referral center where facilities permit full investigation of this disorder. The Kasai procedure of hepatic enterostomy (portoenterostomy) can improve bile drainage for patients with extrahepatic biliary atresia; the earlier the procedure is performed, the better the results. Thus every effort should be made to arrive at a diagnosis and to begin appropriate intervention early.

Treatment of Neonatal Hyperbilirubinemia

Observations made some 30 years ago established a strong association between severe (hemolytic) hyperbilirubinemia and the clinical syndrome of kernicterus in patients with erythroblastosis fetalis. Kernicterus refers to the autopsy findings of yellow discoloration and neuronal degeneration of the brain, particularly the basal ganglia, hippocampus, and cerebellum. Survivors often manifest severe neuropathologic sequelae, including athetoid cerebral palsy, deafness, and failure of the upward gaze. Kernicterus was not seen in full-term infants if the serum bilirubin concentration was maintained below 20 mg/dl (342 μm/L). Despite the absence of randomized clinical trials, a serum unconjugated bilirubin level of 20 mg/dl has been widely adopted as the maximum acceptable for full-term infants *with hemolytic jaundice*. Levels above this are lowered by performing an exchange transfusion; this practice dramatically diminished the incidence of kernicterus.

The precise mechanism of bilirubin neurotoxicity is not known, although animal and human experiments demonstrate that hyperbilirubinemia can disrupt neurotransmission, producing lethargy, cry disturbances, and impairment of the brainstem auditory-evoked response at levels of serum bilirubin below 20 mg/dl. These changes, however, are reversible and may not reflect permanent neuronal injury. Theoretically, bilirubin must be "free" (from binding with albumin) to cross the blood-brain barrier. Animal studies have shown that when the normal blood-brain barrier is disrupted by exposure to hyperbilirubinemia, then both bound and unbound bilirubin can cross it. Recent studies have shown that, in addition to imparting a yellow color to the brain tissue, disruption of the blood-brain barrier in the presence of hyperbilirubinemia also can impair cellular energy metabolism. Other experiments indicate that acidosis further exacerbates bilirubin toxicity.

Although both exchange transfusion and phototherapy can effectively lower serum bilirubin, the indications for their use remain hotly debated. With the exception of the infant with hemolytic jaundice, most current recommendations for use of these therapies have not yet been validated by properly designed studies.

Phototherapy. Phototherapy is effective in lowering serum bilirubin levels and may reduce but not eliminate the need for exchange transfusion in patients with ABO and Rh hemolytic disease. It is especially useful for achieving prolonged reduction of bilirubin in infants with nonhemolytic jaundice. Bilirubin absorbs light maximally in the wavelengths near 460 nm, which can be found in the blue-green part of the visible light spectrum. During phototherapy the bilirubin molecule undergoes isomerization. These photoisomers are hydrophilic and are directly excreted in bile.

Although blue light delivers the optimal wavelength for phototherapy, it also obscures the infant's skin color and can induce headaches and nausea among nursing staff. This problem can be alleviated by combining three or four blue lamps (Westinghouse 20W F2OT12BB) with daylight lamps placed on the outside of the phototherapy unit. The response to phototherapy increases with irradiance until a saturation point is reached at an irradiance level of approximately 25 to 30 $\mu W/cm^2/nm$ in the blue spectrum. For optimal effect the infant can be surrounded by more than one bank of lights. Furthermore, because irradiance is inversely proportional to the square of the distance from the light source, free-standing phototherapy units should be no further than 35 to 40 cm from the infant. When such a unit is used to its maximum, a 40% to 50% decline in the serum bilirubin level generally can be obtained during the first 24 hours.

As a general guideline, phototherapy is often started at a bilirubin level 5 mg/dl lower than that used as the indication for exchange transfusion. The Fetus and Newborn Committee of the Canadian Pediatric Society recommends that "an otherwise healthy newborn with non-hemolytic jaundice should not receive phototherapy unless bilirubin levels are >255 μM/l (15 mg/dl) and rising."[3] They also alert against the routine use of phototherapy in infants identified by cord blood screening as having ABO incompatibility, since severe hyperbilirubinemia develops in only a minority of these infants, even when the Coombs test shows a positive reaction.

Some authorities base their management of hemolytic disease, whether a result of Rh or ABO incompatibility, on the rate of serum bilirubin rise. Phototherapy is started when there is a rapid rise in bilirubin, as defined by an increase of 1 mg/dl/hr or more. An exchange transfusion is performed if the shape of the bilirubin curve (of concentration versus time) indicates that it will exceed 20 mg/dl.

Whenever phototherapy is used serum bilirubin measurements must be followed, because the skin is bleached by phototherapy, making it an unreliable indicator of the degree of jaundice. Side effects of phototherapy include increased insensible water loss, frequent loose stools, occasional abdominal distention, lethargy, and skin erythema. The skin irritation can be reduced by placing an acrylic plastic shield between the patient and the light source. This is used to filter out damaging ultraviolet and infrared rays. Patients with an elevated conjugated bilirubin level who receive phototherapy develop a dark green-brown skin discoloration. Because retinal damage has been reported to occur in animals during phototherapy, the infant's eyes must be shielded with opaque eye patches. These patches need constant supervision to ensure that they do not obstruct the nares and cause apnea. No long-term harmful sequelae of phototherapy have been identified.

Much concern has been expressed regarding the risk of kernicterus in sick, low-birth-weight infants. Yellow-stained brain tissue has been reported at autopsy among premature neonates in whom the serum bilirubin concentrations were below 10 mg/dl; in premature infants, then, serum bilirubin levels alone do not accurately predict kernicterus. Thus decisions regarding the initiation of phototherapy and an exchange transfusion should include consideration of possible risk factors predisposing to bilirubin neurotoxicity such as acidosis, impairment of the blood-brain barrier, or displacement of bilirubin from albumin.

In their guidelines for perinatal care, the American Academy of Pediatrics and the American College of Obstetrics and Gynecology comment as follows:

> Many physicians currently use published guidelines that recommend aggressive treatment of jaundice in low-birthweight neonates, initiating phototherapy early and performing exchange transfusion in certain neonates with very low bilirubin concentrations (less than 10 mg/dl). Nevertheless, this approach will not prevent kernicterus consistently. Some pediatricians prefer to adopt a more conservative therapeutic stance and allow serum bilirubin concentrations to approach 15-20 mg/dl (257-342 μM/l) even in low-birthweight neonates, before considering an exchange transfusion. At present, both of these approaches to treatment should be considered rational.[2]

Thus far the association between increasing levels of serum bilirubin concentration below 20 mg/dl and developmental outcome in both full-term and preterm infants remains unresolved. A recent report,[6] in which the published literature regarding hyperbilirubinemia and its neurologic effects was reviewed, concluded that *at levels below 25 mg/dl in full-term infants without hemolysis,* there was good evidence that *hyperbilirubinemia does not cause significant cognitive, neurologic, or hearing impairment.*

Home Phototherapy. Equipment designed for delivering phototherapy in the home has become available in the past few years. This service was developed to reduce costs of hospitalization and to prevent separation of the mother and infant. The service is especially appreciated by lactating mothers because it facilitates continuation of breast-feeding. A physician should limit the use of home phototherapy to infants with the following characteristics (as amended from the recommendations outlined by the Committee on Fetus and Newborn of the American Academy of Pediatrics)[1]:

1. Term infants older than 48 hours who are otherwise healthy
2. Serum bilirubin concentrations greater than 14 mg/dl but less than 18 mg/dl
3. No elevation in direct reacting (conjugated) bilirubin
4. No pathologic causes of hyperbilirubinemia

A candidate for home phototherapy should have caretakers who can follow instructions regarding use of the equipment, correct application of eye patches, and provision of adequate hydration. Therapy should be under the supervision of a physician who should contact the caretakers daily and ensure that arrangements are made for serum bilirubin to be measured at least every 12 to 24 hours. The committee suggests that the infant should be removed from phototherapy during feedings and diaper changes and when the parents are asleep. Phototherapy should be discontinued once the serum bilirubin concentration falls below 14 mg/dl. The serum bilirubin concentration should be remeasured 12 to 24 hours after cessation of phototherapy, because a rebound in bilirubin concentration may occur.

THE INFANT OF THE MOTHER WITH DIABETES

Maternal diabetes during pregnancy encompasses a range of metabolic disturbances involving carbohydrate intolerance with an elevation in serum glucose levels. Included is the mother who manifests glucose intolerance only during pregnancy (gestational diabetes), as well as one with long-standing insulin-dependent diabetes.

Maternal hyperglycemia imposes a continuous glucose load on the fetus because glucose readily crosses the placenta. In the face of continuing hyperglycemia the fetal pancreatic islet cells undergo hypertrophy and hyperplasia, and the fetus produces large amounts of insulin from about 12 to 14 weeks of gestation. This hyperinsulinemia stimulates the intracellular transport of glucose and is the main mechanism of the diabetic fetopathy that produces infants with enlarged and immature organs. The reported incidence of gestational diabetes varies from 0.15% to 12.3%. The highest prevalence rates are found among young black women. It is now recognized that all pregnant women should be screened for gestational diabetes at least once during the course of their pregnancy. The screening procedure consists of a 50-g glucose load that is administered orally and an assessment of venous plasma glucose made 1 hour later. A serum glucose level ≥140 mg/dl (7.8 mmol/L) is considered a positive finding. This screening procedure has a sensitivity of 79% and a specificity of 11% for all pregnant women. A positive screening test result is followed by the oral glucose tolerance test.

Control of maternal diabetes is important to outcome for the fetus. Mothers with diabetes who have good metabolic control before conception have a spontaneous abortion rate approximating that of the general population, whereas women with poorly controlled diabetes have a significantly higher rate of pregnancy loss at all stages of gestation. Pregnancy loss correlates with the degree of hyperglycemia and with glycosylated hemoglobin levels in the first trimester. When adequate control of diabetes is not achieved, the pediatrician often must deal with complications among infants of affected mothers. These complications include congenital malformations, birth injury, neonatal asphyxia, hypoglycemia, respiratory distress, polycythemia, hyperbilirubinemia, hypocalcemia, and renal vein thrombosis.

Structural Abnormalities

At birth the infant of a diabetic mother (IDM) may have the classic appearance of being large-for-gestational-age and lethargic. The head appears small because adipose tissue is concentrated around the trunk. Occasionally the infant is appropriately grown or even small for gestational age and is at great risk for teratogenesis with major organ system malformation. The major defects occur within four systems: central nervous, cardiovascular, urinary tract, and gastrointestinal.

The caudal regression syndrome comprises the classic central nervous system abnormality. This syndrome consists of absence or maldevelopment of the sacrum and coccyx, with hypoplastic femurs, dislocated hips, and defects in the tibias or fibulas. It occurs in 0.5% of diabetic pregnancies. Neural tube defects, as well as hydrocephaly and microcephaly, also are reported more frequently in diabetic pregnancies.

The incidence of congenital heart disease in IDMs is five times that of the general population. The most common malformations are septal defects, transposition of the great vessels, coarctation of the aorta, and situs inversus. The IDM also is susceptible to a cardiomyopathy secondary to asymmetric septal hypertrophy from glycogen deposition in the myocardium. Hypertrophic changes may occur in the ventricular septum or in the subaortic valve area to produce a self-limiting idiopathic hypertrophic subaortic stenosis. Treatment with digoxin or other inotropic agents worsens the obstruction, but a decrease in myocardial wall tension can be achieved with propranolol. Cardiomegaly with or without congestive heart failure can be seen on chest roentgenogram and may reflect prior hypoxia, hyperglycemia, hypocalcemia, or current hypertrophic cardiac disease.

Management

The pediatrician should be prepared to resuscitate the IDM, especially because delivery may be complicated by vigorous attempts to deliver a large infant vaginally. Thus birth injury commonly is encountered in the macrosomic infant; this takes the form of shoulder dystocia and associated fracture of the clavicle or humerus, or brachial plexus injury. As polycythemia and hyperviscosity are common complications in the IDM, the umbilical cord should be clamped early to prevent an excessive placental transfusion.

Hypoglycemia. The hypoglycemia that occurs in the IDM is largely related to fetal hyperinsulinemia and can be aggravated by maternal hyperglycemia immediately before delivery. Hypoglycemia in the infant usually occurs within the first 1 to 3 hours of age, and the diagnosis is based on a blood glucose determination below 30 mg/dl (1.7 mmol/L) in term infants or below 20 mg/dl (1.1 mmol/L) in preterm infants. Hypoglycemia often manifests no symptoms because newborns have the capability to utilize alternative substrates, such as ketone bodies. Blood glucose screening should begin within the first hour of delivery and continue at least hourly for 6 hours; if the baby is stable, the screening is continued less frequently for the first 3 days. Glucose levels can be monitored by use of drops of whole blood obtained from heel pricks and a glucose oxidase enzyme method (Chemstrip or Dextrostix). If the infant shows symptoms or if the glucose screen shows a level of less than 45 mg/dl, the blood glucose should be measured directly.

Expectant management of the IDM should include an intravenous glucose infusion begun as early as possible, despite lack of symptoms. These infants, apart from having hyperinsulinemia, are unable to produce glucose because they lack the normal neonatal surge in circulating free fatty acids and they also have depressed glucagon levels. They should receive an infusion of glucose via peripheral vein at a dose of 4 to 6 mg/kg/min to bring and maintain the blood glucose levels to normal. Because it can be difficult to cannulate peripheral veins, the umbilical vein may provide convenient access, provided that the catheter is placed within the ductus venosus or in the inferior vena cava (with radiologic confirmation). Symptomatic hypoglycemia can be prevented by this management, and early feeding should be initiated within the first 2 to 6 hours of life if the cardiorespiratory status allows it. Small feedings, starting with 5% glucose in water followed by advancement to milk formula or breast milk, can be provided every 2 hours, and the intravenous infusion of glucose can be tapered once feeding is established and the patient's condition is stable. Symptomatic hypoglycemia can have a wide range of clinical manifestations that include jitteriness, tremors, seizures, apathy, apnea, difficulty in feeding, and an abnormal cry. Because these symptoms may be caused by other life-threatening conditions, such as sepsis and asphyxia, it is imperative that the diagnosis of symptomatic hypoglycemia be confirmed by a blood glucose estimation and that the symptoms promptly disappear after parenteral glucose administration. Symptomatic hypoglycemia warrants immediate treatment with an intravenous infusion of 10% to 12.5% glucose that delivers 6 mg/kg/min. The response to treatment should be monitored every 15 minutes until the blood glucose level has normalized. Treatment should *not* be instituted with a rapid infusion of 25% to 50% glucose because of its high osmolality and because it also stimulates insulin secretion, resulting in "rebound" hypoglycemia. If hypoglycemia persists despite glucose infusion of 12 mg/kg/min, then glucagon administered intramuscularly (0.3 mg/kg) will generally maintain the blood glucose at normal levels for 2 to 3 hours. Refractory hypoglycemia can be treated with hydrocortisone (5 mg/kg/day divided into three doses), which usually will stabilize the glucose level. The physician should ensure that hypoglycemia has not been induced by inappropriate treatment with hypertonic glucose infusion and that an umbilical arterial catheter does not deliver glucose above the level of the diaphragm because this circumstance may stimulate pancreatic insulin secretion. In rare cases, refractory hypoglycemia may be caused by hyperinsulinism accompanying disorders of the pancreas.

The IDM is at increased risk for several other neonatal problems. Among these is respiratory distress syndrome, which may be caused by an inhibition of surfactant production secondary to fetal hyperinsulinemia. The synthesis of phosphatidylcholine and phosphatidylglycerol (PG) is inhibited in the IDM. Monitoring of fetal lung maturity during the diabetic pregnancy calls for the assessment of both the amniotic fluid lecithin/sphingomyelin (L/S) ratio and the amniotic PG. An L/S ratio of less than 2:1 indicates a high potential risk for respiratory distress syndrome. Because of the delay in the appearance of PG among IDMs, the usually adequate L/S ratio of 2:1 does not completely ensure a low risk for respiratory distress syndrome, because low PG itself also is associated with respiratory distress syndrome, despite a normal L/S ratio. An amniotic PG measurement thus should also be obtained, in addition to the L/S ratio; in the absence of a biochemical assay for PG, an L/S ratio greater than 3.1 generally correlates with an adequate PG level.

The IDM also is prone to respiratory distress from causes other than surfactant deficiency (hyaline membrane disease). The infant is at increased risk for transient tachypnea of the newborn, which can be related to such conditions as asphyxia, hyperglycemia, retained lung fluid, congestive heart failure, and polycythemia. There is an increased incidence of physiologic hyperbilirubinemia in the IDM (see previous section). Management should include the usual modalities of phototherapy and exchange transfusion.

Chronic intrauterine hypoxia often occurs in the IDM. This stimulates erythropoietin production, resulting in an increased incidence of polycythemia (central hematocrit >65) and hyperviscosity. In addition, the IDM is susceptible to an excessive placental transfusion at delivery. Because this adds to the polycythemia, the cord should be clamped immediately after delivery of the body to minimize further postnatal placental transfusion.

The appropriate treatment for polycythemia and hyperviscosity is a partial exchange transfusion. This consists of the removal of the patient's blood and its isovolemic replacement with a volume expander, usually 5% albumin or saline. Most authors agree that such treatment of polycythemia should be begun only when signs become detectable. These include arterial and venous thromboses, pulmonary hemorrhage, apnea, lethargy, transient tachypnea (with evidence of interlobar fluid on chest roentgenogram), jitteriness, and hypoglycemia. There also may be signs of impending congestive heart failure and necrotizing enterocolitis. Patients with central hematocrit values in excess of 65% who display the foregoing symptoms should receive a partial exchange transfusion. The indications for treatment in symptom-free patients with hematocrit values *below* 65% to 70% are not pressing. When the hematocrit level is above 70% to 75% at less than 12 hours after birth, it is also best to treat with a partial exchange transfusion, even in the absence of symptoms.

TRANSIENT TACHYPNEA OF THE NEWBORN

Transient tachypnea of the newborn (TTN) refers to one of the commonest causes of respiratory distress in the neonatal period. It is believed to be caused by a delay in the absorption of the normal fetal lung fluid. Between 2 and 6 hours after birth, tachypnea, grunting, chest wall retractions, and cyanosis in room air develop. Typically the symptoms are mild and resolve within 72 hours after birth. The terms *wet lung* and *transient tachypnea* refer to the same condition.

The fetal lung secretes fluid that fills the airways. During vaginal delivery some of this fluid is squeezed out of the major airways, but the remainder takes between 2 and 6 hours to be reabsorbed from the alveoli. This fluid passes into the interstitial space and then into the perivascular lymphatics and venules. According to hypothesis (the Starling equilibrium), this resorption can be impeded by (1) decreased capillary or lymphatic oncotic pressure (e.g., low serum protein, often found in premature infants), (2) increased capillary or lymphatic hydrostatic pressure (e.g., hypervolemia and polycythemia, which may occur with delayed cord clamping), (3) increased alveolar or interstitial fluid osmotic pressure, or (4) decreased alveolar or interstitial fluid hydrostatic pressure.

Thus, as normal lung fluid is being absorbed during the first 4 hours of life, mild respiratory symptoms may be accepted as a variant of normal; the diagnosis of TTN should not be made unless symptoms persist or progress beyond 4 hours. Infants born by cesarean section are not subjected to a thoracic squeeze and the resultant expulsion of lung fluid that occurs during passage through the birth canal. Consequently, with increased lung fluid present, they commonly manifest mild transient tachypnea. Birth asphyxia and premature labor also predispose to TTN.

Transient tachypnea (wet lung syndrome) usually occurs in the more mature preterm infant (34 to 37 weeks) and in term infants born by cesarean section. Tachypnea usually persists beyond the first few hours, peaks by 6 to 36 hours, and resolves in 5 or 6 days. The clinical picture is characterized by signs of air trapping with widening of the anteroposterior diameter of the chest. The liver often is palpable well below the right costal margin because it is pushed down by pulmonary hyperaeration. Tachypnea shortly after birth in the full-term or more mature preterm infant must be differentiated from pneumonitis (e.g., meconium aspiration and bacterial infection), air leak (e.g., pneumothorax and pneumomediastinum), pulmonary vascular congestion resulting from congestive heart failure or polycythemia, and the respiratory restriction imposed by congenital diaphragmatic hernia or cystic adenomatoid malformation of the lung. Last, tachypnea in the face of a normal-appearing chest roentgenogram may be symptomatic of a central nervous system disorder (such as drug withdrawal) or a metabolic derangement (such as acidosis, hyperthermia, or hypoglycemia).

Infants with mild TTN usually do not need more than 40% oxygen to maintain adequate oxygenation (PaO_2 of 50 to 70 mm Hg), but the severity may vary and rarely may require intermittent positive pressure ventilation for respiratory failure. TTN is nonprogressive, and supplemental oxygen usually is not necessary for longer than 1 to 3 days. Treatment of the excess lung water is not required. Because bacterial pneumonia cannot practically be excluded from the initial diagnostic presentation as a primary cause or secondary complication, antibiotics should be given after blood cultures have been obtained. Oral feedings should be suspended, because the ability to suck and swallow feedings may be impaired by the respiratory difficulty. Intravenous fluids should be minimized to equal only insensible fluid losses and to maintain serum glucose concentration.

The radiologic changes of transient tachypnea are characteristic and help to differentiate it from hyaline membrane disease. According to Wesenberg:

> The earliest films usually are taken at age 2-6 hours, when the tachypnea becomes evident clinically. In infants having the most lung fluid, the initial films show a pattern of diffuse bilateral alveolar edema with concomitant hyperaeration of the lungs, sternal retraction, and an air bronchogram effect. In the next 8-10 hours, there is progressive clearing of the alveoli, with some patients developing a bilateral granular or miliary pattern suggestive of hyaline membrane disease. This is a transitory stage, usually lasting only several hours. The lung fields remain hyperaerated. The pulmonary vascularity becomes prominent during this stage. This then progresses to complete clearing of the alveoli with congestive pulmonary vascularity secondary to interstitial edema, engorged perivascular lymphatics and the standard pulmonary capillaries. Occasionally, a small amount of pleural fluid is present. The lower lobes are last to clear. The clearing pattern of the lung fluid is thus from peripheral to central and upper to lower lung fields. By 48-72 hours, the chest films are within normal limits.[7]

Occasionally the fetus will inhale a small amount of amniotic fluid into the already fluid-filled upper airway. Amniotic fluid has more protein than does fetal lung fluid, and the increased protein concentration lowers the oncotic gradient between the alveoli and the pulmonary lymphatics. Amniotic fluid also contains desquamated cellular debris and lanugo. After delivery, this debris is transported into the alveoli and may produce a syndrome indistinguishable from TTN. Such aspiration of amniotic fluid occurs more frequently in breech deliveries, because the thoracic squeeze occurs while the head is still within the uterine cavity and the cord is compressed between the infant and the pelvic brim. These asphyxiated infants are more likely to gasp in utero and inhale their amniotic fluid. If the fetus has passed meconium, it also will be inhaled into the upper airway. Such *aspiration of meconium must be prevented* because it can cause a life-threatening pneumonitis, usually accompanied by severe pulmonary air trapping, respiratory failure, and pulmonary hypertension. Therefore, when delivery is imminent and thick (particulate) meconium is present in the amniotic fluid, attendants should prepare to suction the oropharynx of the infant as soon as the head delivers and before the first breath; immediately after delivery of the infant the trachea should be suctioned via an endotracheal tube to clear the meconium.

Intrauterine passage of meconium increases with advancing gestation to a frequency as high as 30% by 42 weeks In addition to meconium aspiration, postmature infants (older than 42 weeks of gestation) are at risk for hypoglycemia and intrauterine asphyxia as a result of uteroplacental insufficiency. These three potential problems should be anticipated in postmature infants. Hyperaeration may persist for 4 to 5 days in infants who aspirate clear amniotic fluid.

LOW BIRTH WEIGHT

The commonest causes of low birth weight are prematurity and intrauterine growth retardation.

Prematurity

Accurate assessment of gestational age is critical to the appropriate care of the mild to moderately premature infant, because knowledge of gestational age guides management, helps one to anticipate potential problems, and provides a standard by which to assess developmental changes related to postconceptional age (gestational age at birth plus postnatal age). Traditionally many problems of the premature infant have been related to the more easily and accurately measured birth weight rather than to gestational age because for a large population of appropriately grown infants, the two are closely related. In the individual patient, however, the use of birth weight alone may lead to overestimating or underestimating potential problems often related to immaturity. Considering only infants who are appropriately grown for gestational age (AGA), a birth weight of 1700 g may be associated with a gestational age of 30 to 35 weeks; yet a baby who weighs 2500 g at birth may have a gestational age of 33.5 to 39 weeks. Thus the infant born weighing more than 1700 or even more than 2500 g still may be at significant risk for perinatal problems that relate to prematurity, not size.

Standard criteria have been developed to assess gestational age in the first 3 days after birth. Physicians who care for newborn infants must become skilled in the use of these methods, because maternal dates may not be accurate and birth weight per se may not accurately reflect the perinatal problems likely in the individual patient; the frequency of most neonatal problems decreases as gestational age increases.

Premature Infant: Birth Weight 1700 g or More. Despite the major physiologic differences between infants of equal birth weight but of different gestational age, most countries maintain neonatal mortality statistics according to birth weight. Thus, in what follows, we consider the gestational age of the infant who weighs 1700 g or more. For the fetus whose gestation has progressed 32 to 38 weeks, a small risk remains for development of severe neonatal problems related to prematurity (e.g., hyaline membrane disease, persistent patent ductus arteriosus, necrotizing enterocolitis, sepsis and pneumonia, symptomatic apnea, and intracranial hemorrhage). Fortunately, however, the problems of the premature infant beyond 32 to 33 weeks of gestation and weighing more than 1700 g are most often not severe or life-threatening and are limited mainly to simple apnea, hyperbilirubinemia, and an inability to feed orally or to maintain body temperature outside an incubator. Management of these infants is ordinarily well within the competence of most primary care facilities (e.g., level I or level II nurseries). Nonetheless, physicians who accept responsibility for the care of these infants must be aware of the signs of more serious disorders that should be recognized promptly if they are to be optimally managed.

The cause of premature onset of labor should be determined, inasmuch as a small portion of cases may occur because of placental abruption, a multiple gestation, or a uterine abnormality. Spontaneous and premature rupture of membranes has been associated with an increased incidence of neonatal infection. Whether the infection leads to the early rupture or the early rupture leads to the infection is still debated. The risk of neonatal septicemia increases when membranes have been ruptured for longer than 24 hours.

Obstetric management of the preterm fetus with premature rupture of membranes can be assisted by daily fetal biophysical profile assessment. The first manifestations of impending fetal infection are usually a nonreactive, nonstress test result and the absence of fetal breathing movements. Loss of fetal movements and fetal tone are later and more ominous signs of fetal infection. A poor fetal biophysical profile in patients with premature rupture of membranes may be an early predictor of fetal infection and can help determine obstetric management.

Management of infants born after prolonged rupture of membranes should include careful observation for such subtle signs of infection as lethargy, poor feeding, hyperthermia, hypothermia, early hyperbilirubinemia, jitteriness, poor skin perfusion, diarrhea, or abdominal distention as a result of ileus. Prematurity may mask some signs of the nonspecific origin of sepsis.

Examination of placentas from a large group of premature infants frequently reveals evidence of chorioamnionitis. Therefore clinical signs of amnionitis, such as uterine tenderness or maternal fever, indicate the need to obtain a culture specimen from the neonate and to initiate antibiotic treatment. Prophylactic antibiotics administered to the mother before delivery will not effectively treat fetal infection and actually may impair accurate cultures of the newborn (false negative culture results). Any clinical sign of infection in a premature infant warrants cultures of blood and cerebrospinal fluid, followed by treatment with appropriate antibiotics. It is the usual practice to culture blood, cerebrospinal fluid, and urine specimens and treat with ampicillin and gentamicin for 3 to 4 days while definitive culture results are pending. Significant systemic signs of infection, such as pneumonia, seizures, apnea, or shock, may mandate active treatment of sepsis for 7 to 10 days, even in the absence of positive culture results.

Certain laboratory tests are helpful in the diagnosis of chorioamnionitis. A Gram stain of a gastric aspirate taken before the first feed, showing more than five cells per high-powered field and the presence of organisms, indicates chorioamnionitis, but not necessarily fetal infection. Histopathologic examination of the placenta is the definitive method of diagnosis.

Management. For infants whose birth weight is between 1700 and 1900 g (less than 36 weeks), respiration and heart rate should be monitored during the first 10 days at least, because there is some risk of apnea. Until consistent weight gain is established, these infants should remain in incubators kept at the "neutral temperature" to maintain body heat and to prevent excessive caloric expenditure. Some infants of very low birth weight in this weight range may grow rapidly in a bassinet, but they are exceptions to the rule.

Management of feedings and fluids is the most important aspect of care for the healthy, mildly to moderately premature infant. Feedings can be initiated within the first 24 hours after birth in the infant who is stable and without preceding perinatal distress or birth asphyxia (which may have compromised intestinal perfusion). During the first 8 hours of life, little is to be gained by initiating feeds with sterile water. Breast milk or dilute proprietary formula may be given orally or via gastric tube in an initial volume of 2 to 4 ml/kg every 3 hours. Infants whose gestational age is less than 34 weeks are initially fed by nasogastric tube. Proprietary formulas with a 60:40 whey:casein ratio more closely resemble human milk and are better suited for the preterm infant. Unmodified cow milk is not suitable for the preterm newborn, because its predominant casein content is not well tolerated.

Breast milk may be fed to any preterm infant whose mother wishes to do so and who can supply it. The milk is individually collected into a sterile container after careful washing of the breast and nipple. When possible, the milk is given immediately to the infant. Otherwise it is refrigerated for up to 24 hours and either used or immediately frozen. Once full-volume feedings are well tolerated, breast milk needs to be fortified with carbohydrate, protein, and essential minerals to provide optimal nutrition for the growing premature infant. Special powdered preparations for breast milk fortification are available, which when added to breast milk bring up the caloric density to that of standard premature formulas (80 cal/dl).

If feeding must be delayed or is not well tolerated, 10% dextrose in 25% normal saline should be infused intravenously. Fluid and caloric intake should be calculated daily, and growth parameters of length, weight, and head circumference should be plotted weekly to assess adequacy of caloric intake. Feeding volumes should be increased slowly from 60 to 80 ml/kg/day and only if tolerated without emesis or increasing gastric residual volumes of formula before feedings. A total fluid volume of 150 to 180 ml/kg/day or 100 to 120 kcal/kg/day should be reached by 7 days of age. Fluid requirements depend largely on environmental conditions. The infant receiving phototherapy, for instance, may well require increased fluid.

When the infant is ready to progress from tube to oral feeding, the tube may be used for an extra 12 to 24 hours to measure gastric residual. A residual of more than 3 to 4 ml immediately before the next feeding suggests intolerance; this situation may require a reduction in the feeding volume after systemic illness is carefully considered and excluded. Abdominal distention or bile-stained gastric drainage from a properly positioned gastric tube (not in the duodenum) warrants immediate cessation of feedings and evaluation of the intestinal tract. Examination of the stool for macroscopic and microscopic blood should be performed. Microscopic blood (positive occult blood test result) may not in itself suggest a pathologic condition unless it becomes more severe or represents a recent change.

Although coordination of sucking and swallowing develops around 33 to 34 weeks of gestation, the care of each infant should be managed individually and cooperatively between physician and nurse. The nurse experienced at feeding premature infants can provide helpful guidance concerning the infant's tolerance of the workload imposed by oral feeding. No more than 30 minutes should ordinarily be spent coaxing an infant to take a feeding if he or she lacks sufficient endurance to persist in sucking. Infants should be cuddled comfortably and securely in the feeder's lap: there is great benefit to be derived from cuddling and close body contact during feeding. The bottle should be held so that air rises in the upturned bottle and the infant sucks in milk and not air through the nipple. The bottle should never be propped unattended for a young infant.

Patients are discharged from the hospital when they can maintain body temperature in a bassinet, can feed sufficiently on demand, and can show evidence of normal growth.

The overall prognosis for the premature infant between 33 and 38 weeks of gestation is good because of an inherently lower incidence and a better tolerance of severe neonatal problems. For the healthy premature infant weighing more than 1700 g, survival and outcome approach those of full-term infants. Intellectual function generally is normal.

The Infant Who is Small for Gestational Age

The infant whose birth weight is at or below the tenth percentile for gestational age is considered small for gestational age (SGA). Poor fetal weight gain results from aberrant maternal, placental, or fetal circumstances that restrain growth. Other categories in which these infants may be placed include *light-for-date, intrauterine growth retardation,* and *dysmaturity.* These infants show an increase in perinatal mortality (both fetal and neonatal) that is four to eight times that of the appropriately grown infant of equal gestational age.

Early diagnosis is difficult, and most patients are diagnosed after birth. A high index of suspicion, accompanied by serial physical examinations, during which progressive growth of the uterine fundus is palpated through the abdominal wall, aids early diagnosis. A fundal height less than 4 cm or less than that for the estimated gestational age suggests poor intrauterine growth. This clinical impression can be confirmed by careful fetal ultrasound examination. Ideally, serial ultrasound measurements of fetal growth parameters should be obtained. The head/abdominal ratio (as defined by the head circumference divided by the abdominal circumference) is used to detect asymmetric (abdomen undergrown relative to head) forms of intrauterine growth retardation. The normal ratio is approximately 1 from 32 to 36 weeks and less than 1 from 36 weeks to term.

Etiologic Factors. Growth of the fetus is determined by genetic, nutritional, and environmental factors. Fetal factors that can compromise growth potential include (1) congenital abnormalities, (2) congenital infections—for example, toxoplasmosis, rubella, cytomegalovirus, herpes, and syphilis TORCHES, (3) chromosomal defects, and (4) inborn errors of metabolism. Inherent fetal conditions usually result in early growth retardation and an actual reduction in the number of fetal cells. These patients appear symmetrically growth retarded (head and abdomen equally undergrown). Maternal factors include low maternal weight (less than 50 kg), poor weight gain during pregnancy, and chronic maternal disease, especially conditions that produce hypoxemia or reduce placental blood flow (e.g., chronic hypertension, preeclampsia, toxemia, cyanotic congenital heart disease, and sickle cell disease). Drug ingestion, including alcohol, cigarette smoke, and heroin, can affect the quality of fetal growth adversely. Phenylketonuria often results in decreased fetal growth and microcephaly; thus the maternal diet must be strictly controlled during pregnancy.

During the third trimester, less than adequate maternal-placental transport becomes the major growth-limiting factor, despite normal fetal growth potential. Optimal fetal growth depends on the placenta for nutrient and gaseous exchange. The placenta promotes fetal growth by actively transporting amino acids and synthesizing chorionic somatomammotropin, which is responsible for mobilizing maternal substrate for the fetus. Diminished placental function thus will adversely affect total nutrient and gaseous transfer, resulting in fetal growth retardation. Placental insufficiency is classically associated with postmaturity; therefore it is understandable that placental abnormalities, such as chronic abruption, infarction, single umbilical artery, and multiple fetuses, directly affect the transfer of fetal nutrients during the third trimester. The box below lists factors associated with poor intrauterine growth.

Factors Associated with Poor Intrauterine Growth

MATERNAL

1. Prepregnancy weight <50 kg
2. Poor nutrition; poor weight gain during pregnancy; socioeconomic factors
3. Maternal illness:
   a. Associated with uterine ischemia: hypertensive vascular disease, preeclampsia, diabetes mellitus, sickle cell anemia, autoimmune vasculitis
   b. Associated with chronic hypoxia: cyanotic congenital heart disease, high altitude
4. Drug ingestion:
   a. Drugs that affect fetal growth directly, e.g., ethanol, methadone, heroin
   b. Drugs that inhibit placental blood flow (nicotine)
5. Multiple gestation, primiparity, grand multiparity

PLACENTAL

1. Villitis associated with congenital infections (TORCHES)
2. Ischemic villous necrosis or infarction
3. Chronic separation (abruptio placentae)
4. Diffuse fibrinosis
5. Abnormal insertion
6. Umbilical vascular thrombosis

FETAL

1. Syndromes associated with diminished birth weight; e.g., Cornelia de Lange syndrome, Potter disease, anencephaly, and dwarfism
2. Metabolic disorders (inborn errors of metabolism)
3. Chromosomal disorders: trisomies 13, 18, 21; XO
4. Congenital infections: TORCHES, malaria, varicella

Clinical Presentation. The SGA infant may be "symmetrically" growth retarded in some cases; in others birth weight may be reduced relatively more than length and head circumference. Fetuses subjected to third trimester "starvation" may have a normal length but appear wasted. The skin is parchmentlike, and the head appears too large for the body. These infants are often termed *asymmetrically growth retarded*. These various presentations offer some insight into etiologic factors because symmetric growth retardation usually implies a more chronic problem—for example, chromosomal or congenital infection.

If based on physical criteria alone, gestational age assessment of the SGA infant may be misleading. Because there is less vernix production in these infants, the skin is continuously exposed to amniotic fluid and will begin to desquamate after birth. Sole creases are more mature and breast tissue markedly reduced as a result of the diminished estriol levels. Ear cartilage also may be diminished. In contrast, neurologic criteria are less affected by intrauterine growth retardation than are physical criteria, inasmuch as organ maturation continues despite diminished somatic growth. Moreover, stress in utero may even promote the maturation of some organ systems, such as the lung. This may explain why respiratory distress syndrome is less frequent in SGA infants.

Because the SGA infant is prone to perinatal asphyxia and its sequelae, optimal management should begin with antenatal assessment. Expert resuscitation must be provided for these infants in the delivery room, with strict attention to the prevention of possible meconium aspiration, because decreased placental reserve and decreased cardiac glycogen stores put the fetus at risk for perinatal asphyxia. The infant should be delivered if at or near term, but even earlier if tests of placental function, such as stress and nonstress monitoring, indicate fetal compromise. When gestational age is not known, the risks of preterm birth can be better defined by assessing pulmonary maturity by use of amniocentesis (lecithin/sphingomyelin ratio). Occasionally, maternal disease will necessitate delivery of a preterm, growth-retarded infant who will be prone to all the complications of both immaturity and growth retardation (see the box on p. 498).

The SGA newborn, especially when showing evidence of third trimester wasting with low ponderal index, is more prone to fasting hypoglycemia because of decreased glycogen stores and impaired gluconeogenesis. Thus, frequent determinations of blood glucose values must be made in the first few days of birth. Hourly recordings are recommended in the first 4 hours of life. Thereafter, if the infant is stable, measurement of blood glucose levels can be more widely spaced. If asymptomatic hypoglycemia occurs (whole blood glucose concentrations less than 30 mg/dl during the first 3 days in term or 20 mg/dl in preterm infants), a glucose infusion of 4 to 8 mg/kg/min should be started. If symptomatic hypoglycemia—especially concomitant with seizure activity—has occurred, an intravenous bolus of 10% dextrose in water at 200 mg/kg (2 ml/kg) should be given, followed by constant glucose infusion. As a consequence of their increased metabolic rate, these infants often need a higher caloric intake.

Attention to thermoregulation is required because decreased subcutaneous fat stores impair conservation of body heat. This is important in delivery room management where these patients frequently are compromised by perinatal as-

Neonatal Problems in Infants of Low Birth Weight

PRETERM
Respiratory distress syndrome
Patent ductus arteriosus
Retinopathy of prematurity
Hyperbilirubinemia
Necrotizing enterocolitis

SMALL FOR GESTATIONAL AGE
Perinatal asphyxia
Meconium aspiration
Polycythemia

COMMON TO BOTH GROUPS
Fasting hypoglycemia
Temperature instability
Hypocalcemia

phyxia. Radiant heat and warm dry towels will help to maintain the infant's body temperature during neonatal resuscitation.

A thorough examination for clinical stigmata of congenital infection is indicated in all SGA babies, as well as appropriate screening for intrauterine infection. This should include estimation of total IgM and a urine culture for cytomegalovirus. A urine (and especially stool) screen for illicit drugs may provide evidence of maternal drug exposure otherwise denied. Because chronic fetal hypoxia stimulates erythropoietin production, polycythemia and hyperviscosity also should be excluded.

Prognosis. The growth and developmental outcome for the SGA infant depend on the cause of the growth failure. The prognosis is poorest for infants with congenital infections, chromosomal disorders, and severe congenital abnormalities. Intellectual development in the remaining infants depends on the presence or absence of adverse perinatal events, in addition to the specific etiologic factors of the growth retardation. Even when perinatal problems are minimal, the SGA infant may have developmental handicaps. Developmental problems should be looked for beyond infancy and may become manifest only at 2 to 5 years of age or even later. Term SGA infants may exhibit little difference in developmental quotient during infancy, but their school performance is poor, in part because of behavioral and learning disabilities. SGA infants who demonstrate decreased fetal head growth earlier than 26 weeks of gestation have diminished developmental quotients in infancy. SGA infants, however, are a heterogeneous group; in some follow-up studies of both term and preterm SGA infants, they have compared well with appropriate-for-gestational-age (AGA) infants. Perhaps this discrepancy in outcome reporting depends on obstetric and early neonatal management and the quality of home care and parental involvement.

With regard to postnatal growth, the cause of the intrauterine growth retardation and the time of its onset during gestation will dictate the infant's growth potential. Newborns with early-onset intrauterine growth retardation (because of an intrauterine infection, teratogen, or chromosomal abnormality) will remain small throughout life. Those with late-onset third trimester intrauterine growth retardation, however, may show evidence of catch-up growth in the first 6 months postnatally and usually catch up to their AGA counterparts.

REFERENCES

1. American Academy of Pediatrics, Committee on Fetus and Newborn: home phototherapy, Pediatrics 76:136, 1985.
2. Guidelines for perinatal care (2nd Ed.) Elk Grove Village, Ill: American Academy of Pediatrics; Washington, DC: American College of Obstetricians and Gynecologists, 1988.
3. Canadian Pediatric Society, Fetus and Newborn Committee: Use of phototherapy for neonatal hyperbilirubinemia, Can Med Assoc J 134:1237, 1986.
4. Maisels MJ: Jaundice in the newborn, Pediatr Rev 3:305, 1982.
5. National Institutes of Health Consensus Development Conference on Infantile Apnea and Home Monitoring, Sept 29 to Oct 1, 1986. Pediatrics, 79:292, 1987.
6. Newman TB: How much cognitive, neurologic or hearing impairment does hyperbilirubinemia cause in well babies without hemolysis? Pediatr Res 27:250, 1990 (abstract).
7. Wesenberg RL: Wet lung disease and aspiration of clear amniotic fluid. In Wesenberg RL, editor: The newborn chest, Hagerstown, Md, 1973, Harper & Row, Publishers, Inc.

SUGGESTED READINGS

Cornblath M: Hypoglycemia. In Nelson NM, editor: Current therapy in neonatal-perinatal medicine, vol 2, Canada, 1990, Brian C Decker, Publishers.

Dickinson JE and Palmer SM: Gestational diabetes: pathophysiology and diagnosis, Semin Perinatol 14:2, 1990.

Kliegman RM and Hulman SE: Intrauterine growth retardation: determinants of aberrant fetal growth. In Fanaroff AA and Martin RJ, editors; Neonatal-perinatal medicine: disease of the fetus and infant, ed 4, St Louis, 1987, The CV Mosby Co.

Lawrence S, Yeomans ER, and Rosenfeld CR: Intrauterine growth retardation: pediatric aspects. In Nelson NM, editor: Current therapy in neonatal-perinatal medicine, vol 2, Canada, 1990, Brian C Decker, Publishers.

Maisels MJ: Hyperbilirubinemia. In Nelson NM, editor: Current therapy in neonatal-perinatal medicine, vol 2, Philadelphia, 1990, Brian C Decker, Publishers.

Meyer BA and Palmer SM: Pregestational diabetes, Semin Perinatol 14:12, 1990.

Vintzileos AM, Campbell WA, and Nochimson DJ: Premature rupture of the membranes. In Nelson NM, editor: Current therapy in neonatal-perinatal medicine, vol 2, Canada, 1990, Brian C Decker, Publishers.

41

Critical Neonatal Illnesses

Keith H. Marks and M. Jeffrey Maisels

It is important for the physician who is called on to treat the newborn in a critical situation to be able to make a diagnosis, institute immediate management, and plan for appropriate continuing consultation in caring for the patient. Errors or omissions may result in the infant's permanent damage or death, so that recognition and immediate resuscitation of a baby in distress require an organized plan for the actions of immediately available and qualified personnel, supported by the proper equipment.

The emergence throughout the Western world of regionalized systems for neonatal care has played a crucial role in the general improvement in neonatal outcome and has made it possible, as well as desirable, for almost all critically ill infants to be cared for in a tertiary care neonatal center. Assuming that most primary care physicians embrace this approach, the following discussion deals mainly with those conditions that require recognition, management, and stabilization preceding the transport of infants to such centers.

Safe and efficient transport of an infant requires an organized approach.* Here we deal specifically with the preparation and stabilization of the infant before transport. In doing so, we will cover those critical situations with which the primary care physician must deal immediately.

The resources available at the hospital of birth will determine the need for transport. In general, therefore, transport should be considered when those resources immediately available (equipment, support services, expertise, and available *time* of the attending physician) are inadequate to deal with the infant's current or anticipated medical and surgical problems. Note, however, that the decision to transfer a newborn should be made only *after* consultation with the neonatologist at the receiving hospital, so that bed availability can be confirmed and preparations undertaken.

STABILIZATION

Certain basic laboratory investigations should be performed on every critically ill infant (see box); every hospital must be capable of performing these tests *instantly*. The information so gained frequently will provide an accurate diagnosis (e.g., the chest roentgenogram reveals evidence of hyaline membrane disease or of cardiomegaly; the hematocrit reading indicates polycythemia as the cause of respiratory distress) and lead to appropriate intervention.

*Discussed in detail in American Academy of Pediatrics and the American College of Obstetricians and Gynecologists: Guidelines for perinatal care, Elk Grove Village, Ill, 1988, The Academy.

By far the most frequent reason for referral of an infant to a neonatal intensive care facility (ICU) is the onset of respiratory distress soon after birth. Such infants most often demonstrate tachypnea, retractions, expiratory grunting, nasal flaring, and, frequently, cyanosis. However, they may show only apnea or shock. An approach to the differential diagnosis of respiratory distress is shown in the box on p. 500.

In some cases the suddenness and severity of the distress make it apparent that immediate referral to an ICU is necessary. In others, the major challenge to the primary care physician is to separate those infants whose respiratory distress or cyanosis may be only transient, and likely to improve, from those whose condition will almost certainly deteriorate to require further investigation and intervention.

Changes in clinical status can occur with frightening rapidity, so that constant vigilance is necessary to anticipate and prevent potentially disastrous deterioration. Infants with respiratory failure require immediate referral to a neonatal center.

Respiratory failure can be anticipated as imminent or actual when any of the following signs is present:

- Increasing tachypnea, retractions, and grunting
- Persistent tachycardia with minimal variability in heart rate
- Poor peripheral perfusion (shock)
- Congestive heart failure
- Cyanosis unresponsive to the administration of oxygen at 40% or greater concentrations
- Apnea
- Rising $Paco_2$, falling pH, and falling Pao_2

Laboratory Investigations to Be Performed on All Acutely Ill Newborn Infants

- Hematocrit reading
- Dextrostix* (or Chemstrip) or quantitative laboratory blood glucose determination
- Portable chest roentgenogram
- Arterial (or arterialized capillary†) Po_2, Pco_2, and pH
- White cell count and differential
- Blood culture
- Response of infant's Pao_2, $Paco_2$, and pH† to breathing oxygen

*Ames Division, Miles Laboratories, Inc, Elkhart, Ind.
†These measurements are unreliable in the presence of shock or when the Pao_2 exceeds 50 to 60 mm Hg.

Causes of Respiratory Distress in the Newborn

PULMONARY CAUSES	NONPULMONARY CAUSES
Common	**Cerebral**
Hyaline membrane disease	Hemorrhage
Transient tachypnea of the newborn (TTN)	Edema
Meconium aspiration	
Primary pulmonary hypertension	**Metabolic**
	Acidosis
Occasional	Hypoglycemia
Pulmonary hemorrhage	Hypothermia
Pneumonia	
Pneumothorax	**Hematologic**
Pulmonary dysmaturity	Hypovolemia
	Acute blood loss
Rare	Twin-to-twin transfusion
Airway obstruction	Hyperviscosity
Choanal atresia	
Space-occupying lesion	
Diaphragmatic hernia	
Cysts	
Tumors	

Any infant who is cyanotic and does not respond to the administration of oxygen requires immediate attention. Central cyanosis (as opposed to acrocyanosis) should never be disregarded in the hope that it will disappear. Such infants inevitably get worse, and their cyanosis requires urgent investigation and treatment. Many cyanotic infants also have significant respiratory distress, so that their referral tends to be effectively mandated; others, however, may merely appear "dusky" and not suffer from respiratory distress, thus inviting an unwise expectant temporization before eventual emergent transfer.

By definition, cyanosis reflects the presence in the circulation of at least 3 g of reduced (desaturated) hemoglobin. *Central* cyanosis (as opposed to *peripheral* acrocyanosis) implies cyanosis of the lips, tongue, and oral mucous membranes. Because cyanosis is produced by a definitive amount (not relative concentration) of desaturated hemoglobin, it may be detected even at high arterial oxygen saturations, should the total hemoglobin concentration be sufficiently elevated (polycythemia). In other words, polycythemic infants may actually have normal PaO_2 levels, yet be clinically cyanotic. Conversely, when the hemoglobin concentration is low, as in severe anemia, significant central cyanosis may not be visually apparent, despite substantial arterial desaturation.

The *immediate investigations required in all cyanotic infants* are as follows:

Chest roentgenogram
Measurement of O_2 saturation by pulse oximetry
Measurement of arterial PO_2, PCO_2, pH
Response of the PaO_2 or O_2 saturation to breathing 100% oxygen
Hematocrit, blood glucose determinations
Electrocardiogram

Any infant who is cyanotic and whose PaO_2 does not respond promptly to the administration of 100% oxygen should be referred immediately to an appropriate center for treatment. Such infants are likely to have *cyanotic congenital heart disease, persistent pulmonary hypertension* (persistent fetal circulation), or *severe respiratory disease*.

The approach to all critical situations is similar—namely, to establish and maintain vital functions. Thus the *maintenance of oxygenation, perfusion, blood glucose, and body temperature is the cornerstone of successful initial management*.

Ventilation

The first thing always to be considered is that *oxygen should be provided in whatever concentration (including 100%) is necessary to keep the baby pink*. This point cannot be overemphasized! The legacy of the alleged association between hyperoxia and retrolental fibroplasia (RLF—renamed as retinopathy of prematurity) remains to haunt us, with the fear of litigation subverting reasoned judgment, but the fact is that no clear relation between *brief* periods (several hours) of hyperoxia (PaO_2 levels >150 mm Hg) and RLF has *ever* been documented. In fact, documentation of *any* relation between the magnitude of elevated PaO_2 (as opposed to the duration of oxygen administration) and RLF is extremely limited. Moreover, recent data suggest that there may be an association of RLF with episodes of *hypoxemia* (PaO_2 <40 mm Hg). Thus, although historically emphasis has been placed on the necessity for avoiding hyperoxia, it may be equally if not more important to avoid periods of hypoxia, as well as of compromised perfusion.

Degrees of "pinkness" cannot be used to estimate PaO_2 levels reliably; therefore actual measurements of arterial blood gases or oxygen saturation by pulse oximetry are necessary for optimal management. The wide availability of pulse oximetry has removed much of the guesswork from the assessment of oxygenation. Pulse oximetry is simpler and more reliable than capillary blood gas measurement. Supplemental oxygen should be given sufficient to maintain the baby's Pa_{O_2} within the range of the normal newborn (50 to 100 mm Hg) or the oxygen saturation (Sa_{O_2}) $> 90\%$. Oxygen should be warmed, humidified, and delivered via an oxygen hood. If, despite breathing 100% oxygen, the baby remains cyanotic, or if the Pa_{O_2} is less than 50 mm Hg, or the Sa_{O_2} is less than 90%, then the infant should receive artificial ventilation.

Assisted ventilation also is indicated if respiratory failure is evidenced by recurrent apnea, a Pa_{CO_2} greater than 50 to 60 mm Hg (and rising), and a pH of less than 7.25, with a rising Pa_{CO_2} or Pa_{O_2} of less than 50 mm Hg in 70% to 100% oxygen. Infants meeting these criteria should receive ventilation, preferably via an endotracheal tube. Should someone skilled in infant intubation not be immediately available, then bag and mask ventilation must be used.* The bag used must be capable of delivering 100% oxygen (see section on delivery room management in Chapter 36, Neonatal Adaptation, and Fig. 36-7) for the technique of bag and mask ventilation. An orogastric tube should be in place to avoid gastric distention.

The correct management of respiratory acidosis is *ventilation*, not "buffering" with intravenous (IV) sodium bicarbonate. Among infants with severe hyaline membrane disease, it is invariably necessary to perform endotracheal intubation (see Appendix B, "Special Procedures" for technique to be used) to ensure adequate ventilation. Intubation also allows the application of positive end-expiratory pressure (PEEP), which is critical to maintaining adequate oxygenation by overcoming atelectasis.

Perfusion

Infants who are in shock have a low effective circulating blood volume and show all the *signs of poor perfusion: paleness, mottled skin, and poor capillary filling*. Adequate capillary filling is present when normal pink color returns to the toes within 3 seconds after squeezing. The infant in shock also frequently has cyanosis, tachycardia, and acidosis but may or may not have low blood pressure. The blood pressure should be determined by the oscillometric technique (e.g., DynaMap. Table 41-1 shows normal systolic and diastolic levels for newborns at various birth weights. This method, used carefully, is quite accurate for the noninvasive determination of arterial blood pressure, but two important conditions must be met: (1) the width of the cuff must be at least 50% to 60% of the limb circumference and (2) the infant must be quite still during the measurement to avoid motion artifact in the readings. The physician should note, however, that *many infants, despite severe underperfusion, may maintain normal blood pressure by means of vasoconstriction. Thus a normal blood pressure by no means rules out the diagnosis of shock* (hypoperfusion of the peripheral tissues).

Hypovolemia is the single most important cause of shock and should always be considered when metabolic acidosis exists. Shock is treated by expanding the circulating blood volume by use of 10 to 20 ml/kg of whole blood or, if blood is not available, plasma or a 5% albumin solution.

Metabolism

Blood glucose concentration should be determined on all sick infants by a semiquantitative screening technique (Dextrostix or Chemstrip). If the screening test indicates a blood glucose level of less than 45 mg/dl, then quantitative laboratory analysis of blood glucose should be performed. If hypoglycemia is thus documented as present (quantitative blood glucose level of <40 mg/dl), it is treated by administration of a continuous IV infusion of 10% dextrose in water solution. An initial bolus of 3 to 4 ml/kg should be given slowly over about 5 minutes and the infusion then continued at a rate of 5 ml/kg/hr (this provides 8 mg/kg/min of glucose). Another Dextrostix test should be performed within 15 minutes. If the blood glucose level remains persistently low, then 15% glucose in water solution should be infused. If there is still no response, hydrocortisone (5 mg/kg) should be given every 12 hours. (See also p. 503.)

All sick infants, and particularly those of very low birth weight, require meticulous attention to thermoregulation. The body temperature should be maintained in the neutral thermal environment (see Fig. 36-5), for which purpose it is useful to swaddle these babies in plastic wrap or similar insulating material.

Most sick infants have some degree of ileus and should not be fed by mouth. All require IV fluids. An appropriate IV solution is 0.2% saline in 10% dextrose in water administered initially at a rate of 50 to 60 ml/kg/day. Adjustments to this rate of fluid administration may be required if the infant has hypoglycemia or evidence of gastrointestinal obstruction, when large amounts of fluid may be lost into the bowel lumen.

Metabolic acidosis occurs when organic acids accumulate in tissues that are hypoxemic or underperfused. Other causes are loss of bicarbonate (which does not occur in the first hours or days of life) and some rare inborn errors of metabolism. The proper treatment of metabolic acidosis is directed to its cause rather than to its effect (i.e., adequate oxygenation and perfusion should be provided rather than bicarbonate given). The administration of sodium bicarbonate should be limited

Table 41-1 *Blood Pressure in Newborns*

BIRTH WEIGHT (g)	SYSTOLIC (mm Hg)		DIASTOLIC (mm Hg)	
	5%	95%	5%	95%
1000	35	58	16	36
1500	40	62	19	39
2000	43	67	22	41
2500	48	70	25	43
3000	50	73	28	48
3500	54	78	30	49
4000	58	81	31	51

Data from Versmold HT et al: Aortic blood pressure during the first 12 hours of life in infants with birth weight 610 to 4,220 grams, Pediatrics 67:607, 1981.

*Diaphragmatic hernia is one situation in which bag and mask ventilation should not be used (see p. 502).

to those very few infants in whom metabolic acidosis is not self-corrected by the time the Po_2 is normal and adequate perfusion has been ensured. Respiratory acidosis is, by definition, an elevation of the $Paco_2$ and can therefore be treated only by the use of assisted ventilation; bicarbonate administration is not indicated in this situation.

SPECIFIC CONDITIONS

Abstinence Syndrome

Infants born to mothers who are users of narcotics will have withdrawal symptoms in the first days of life. When the symptoms include *severe irritability and tremors* (which prevent normal feeding), *vomiting and diarrhea, seizures, hypothermia or hyperthermia, or severe tachypnea,* then treatment is indicated. Phenobarbital, paregoric, diazepam, and methadone have all been used to treat neonatal narcotic withdrawal. Paregoric is a useful and easy drug to use and is administered orally in a dosage of four to six drops every 4 to 6 hours. If there is no improvement, the dose is increased by two drops per dose until clinical improvement is apparent (see Chapter 229).

Ambiguous Genitalia

The finding of ambiguous genitalia must raise the suspicion of congenital adrenal hyperplasia, which can produce convincing masculinization of the female external genitalia, leading to unfortunate (and difficult to retract) *misassignment of sex* in the delivery room. Some of these infants have a salt-losing syndrome and develop *profound hyponatremia with vascular collapse*. Congenital adrenal hyperplasia should therefore be suspected in all infants with ambiguous genitalia, as well as in all those with *vomiting, dehydration, or failure to thrive in the first weeks of life*. Treatment involves expansion of the circulating volume with isotonic saline, and subsequently, the administration of glucocorticoids. Diagnosis is confirmed by serum and urinary electrolyte patterns, hormonal measurements, and occasionally, karyotyping.

Diaphragmatic Hernia

Diaphragmatic hernia occurs in 1 in 2200 live births and is almost always (90%) found on the left side. The infant *may show very little respiratory distress or may be profoundly distressed with severe cyanosis that is unresponsive to ventilation*. The diagnosis should be suspected if the infant has a *flat or scaphoid abdomen* or if *bowel sounds are heard in the chest*. Because the hernia usually is on the left, the *heart sounds may be displaced to the right*. The diagnosis is confirmed by a chest roentgenogram. All these infants should be placed in 100% oxygen and a large-bore (10 or 12 Fr) orogastric tube should be inserted into the stomach, to which intermittent suction at low pressure is applied. If there is significant respiratory distress, endotracheal intubation and intermittent positive pressure ventilation must be performed. This is one of the few situations in which bag and mask ventilation is contraindicated because such ventilation will force gas into the intestinal tract, thus increasing distention of the intestine that lies within the thorax and further compromising pulmonary function.

Gastroschisis or Omphalocele

Infants with gastroschisis or omphalocele may suffer from severe evaporative fluid loss and hypothermia. They are best managed by placing the entire body below the shoulders in a bowel bag (a clear sterile plastic bag). A drawstring permits the bag to be tightened at the level of the axillae, preventing both heat and fluid loss. A large-bore (10 to 12 Fr) orogastric tube should be inserted and intermittent suction applied to decrease intestinal distention. IV fluids should be administered at a rate of 8 to 10 ml/kg/hr while the baby is transported to a tertiary care pediatric facility where definitive corrective surgery can be performed.

Hydrops Fetalis

The care of women likely to deliver infants with severe erythroblastosis should be managed exclusively in perinatal centers capable of the full range of obstetric and neonatal intensive care. The successful management of these previously doomed infants demands a comprehensive team approach that includes intensive monitoring and vigorous treatment of asphyxia, acidosis, hypoglycemia, and hypothermia. Assisted ventilation frequently is required.

Hypoglycemia

The maintenance of a normal blood glucose concentration in the newborn is important because glucose is the primary energy substrate for the brain. Thus hypoglycemia may result in central nervous system (CNS) damage. Newborns have brain weights that are greater in relation to body weight than is the case in adults and are thus at greater risk from the effects of hypoglycemia. Long-term follow-up studies regarding the neurologic impairment of infants who have had symptomatic hypoglycemia in the newborn period indicate that hypoglycemia represents a critical situation for the newborn. This requires that all nurseries have a plan to screen newborns for hypoglycemia and to institute immediate therapy when it is diagnosed.

We recommend that any infant, term or preterm, with a Dextrostix determination of blood glucose of 45 mg/dl or less have an immediate quantitative blood glucose level (glucose oxidase method) determined in the laboratory. The following glucose levels require immediate intervention and subsequent glucose monitoring: a whole blood glucose level of less than 35 mg/dl in the first 24 hours or 40 mg/dl thereafter; a plasma glucose level of less than 40 mg/dl in the first 24 hours or 45 mg/dl thereafter.

Transient Neonatal Hypoglycemia. CNS abnormalities—for example, septooptic dysplasia associated with agenesis of the septum pellucidum, malformation of the optic chiasma, agenesis of the corpus callosum, and growth hormone deficiency—can all cause transient neonatal hypoglycemia. Other causes include asphyxia, anoxia, respiratory distress syndrome, sepsis, cold injury, prolonged starvation, and abrupt cessation of IV hypotonic glucose solution. Infants of diabetic mothers (IDMs), as well as those whose mothers have been given certain drugs (e.g., propranolol) and those with erythroblastosis fetalis also are prone to develop symptomatic transient hypoglycemia of the newborn. Finally, this difficulty may develop in some infants without apparent predisposing causes.

Persistent Neonatal Hypoglycemia. Any of the following conditions can give rise to persistent hypoglycemia in the newborn: (1) pancreatic defects (hyperinsulinism, nesidioblastosis, islet cell adenoma, focal adenomatosis, microadenomatosis, beta-cell hyperplasia, Beckwith-Wiedemann syndrome, idiopathic leucine sensitivity); (2) hereditary defects of carbohydrate metabolism (glycogen storage diseases, deficiencies of enzymes important to gluconeogenesis, other enzyme defects such as galactosemia and hereditary fructose intolerance); (3) hereditary defects in amino acid and organic acid metabolism (maple syrup urine disease, propionic acidemia, methylmalonic aciduria, tyrosinosis, 3-hydroxy-3-methylglutaric aciduria, glutaric aciduria type II); (4) hereditary defects of fat metabolism (systemic carnitine deficiency, carnitine palmitoyl transferase deficiency); and (5) hormone deficiencies (congenital hypopituitarism or hypothalamic abnormalities that lead to diminished production of growth hormone, cortisol, adrenocorticotropic hormone [ACTH], glucagon, thyroid hormone, and catecholamines).

Although the clinical manifestations of neonatal hypoglycemia are varied, they may include episodes of *tremor (jitteriness), apnea, cyanosis, irregular respirations, limpness, twitching, sweating, hypothermia, weak cry, refusal to feed, eye rolling, and convulsions.*

In infants at risk for hypoglycemia it is common practice to estimate the plasma glucose concentration by Dextrostix as soon as possible after birth, at 2 hours, and again at 4 to 6 hours of age. In all infants at increased risk for hypoglycemia, including small-for-gestational-age babies and IDMs, it is advisable to monitor blood glucose levels more frequently until the plasma glucose is stable within the normal range and oral milk feedings have been well established. In the event of a confirmed blood glucose reading of less than 45 mg/dl, the infant should be started immediately on a feeding of 5% glucose, followed by standard formula feedings at intervals of 2 to 3 hours. The blood glucose level should be monitored before each feeding. Adequate glucose concentrations usually can be maintained by this regimen; however, if plasma glucose values remain below 40 mg/dl, an IV infusion of 10% glucose should be started to provide 5 to 8 mg/kg/min of glucose. On rare occasions when hypoglycemia persists despite such an infusion of glucose, cortisone acetate may need to be administered intravenously or intramuscularly at intervals of 8 hours to a total dose of 5 mg/kg body weight/day. On this regimen the blood glucose level in most infants should stabilize rapidly. The IV infusion of glucose can be tapered after 48 hours and the cortisone therapy gradually eliminated during the subsequent 4 to 5 days. Should the hypoglycemia persist for more than 72 hours on this regimen, other causes must be sought (see Chapter 281).

Meningitis

For a discussion of meningitis, see Chapter 227.

Pneumothorax

Spontaneous pneumothorax occurs in 0.5% to 2% of all newborns but with much greater frequency among infants with severe hyaline membrane disease or aspiration pneumonia. The clinical diagnosis may be entertained when an infant shows signs of *respiratory distress with breath sounds that are decreased on one side*. This physical sign, however, may be very difficult to elicit, particularly in the small premature infant; a more reliable technique therefore is to transilluminate the chest with a high-intensity fiberoptic light. Increased lucency on one side of the chest suggests the presence of a pneumothorax. Ultimately, however, the "gold standard" for diagnosis is the chest roentgenogram, which reveals lucency in one hemithorax, partial collapse of the lung, and displacement of the mediastinum to the opposite side of the chest. Indeed, a roentgenogram of the chest should be part of the routine assessment of all ill newborns.

A small pneumothorax in a full-term infant, which produces only mild distress, may well require no therapy other than observation. On the other hand, in an infant who is severely distressed and has cyanosis or bradycardia (as signs of cardiovascular compromise by a tension pneumothorax), immediate evacuation of the accumulated intrathoracic air is essential. This is performed by inserting a No. 21 scalp vein needle through the chest wall, usually at the superior edge of the third or fourth rib, in the anterior axillary line. The needle is connected to an airtight stopcock and a 50-ml syringe. As the needle is advanced into the chest, negative pressure is applied to the syringe until air enters it. This procedure, which may at first appear intimidating, actually is remarkably simple and relatively safe; because the intercostal blood vessels course along the inferior border of the rib, there is no danger of producing a hemorrhage by inserting the needle over its superior rim. Furthermore, the presence of the pneumothorax tends to prevent inadvertent puncture of the lung. Even if a lung puncture or a hemorrhage does occur, rarely is either severe.

Persistence of a significant pneumothorax requires insertion of a chest tube, although an Intracath may be used as a temporary device for transporting the baby to a neonatal ICU. If an Intracath or a chest tube is left in place, it should be connected to underwater drainage. If no underwater seal is available, a one-way Heimlich flutter valve may be used (Bard-Parker No. 3460).

Respiratory Distress

For a discussion of respiratory distress, see Chapters 39 and 40.

Seizures

For a complete discussion of neonatal seizures, see Chapter 253.

Shock, Including Sepsis

Shock may be defined as an acute hemodynamic disturbance that causes significant and generalized reduction of capillary blood flow throughout the body, with consequent decreased tissue perfusion and anoxia, which, if prolonged, leads to a generalized impairment of cellular function. The major causes of shock in the newborn are hypovolemia, sepsis, severe congestive heart failure with low cardiac output (e.g., the hypoplastic left heart syndrome), and, rarely, endocrine failure (hypoadrenocorticism). (See also Chapter 288.)

Hypovolemic Shock. Shock caused by hypovolemia is most often attributable to (1) hemorrhage associated with obstetric accidents or malformations of the placenta and cord, (2) occult hemorrhage from the fetus into the maternal circulation or into a twin fetus, and (3) internal hemorrhages (e.g., ruptured liver or spleen, intracranial hemorrhage, or adrenal hemorrhage—see box on p. 505).

Loss of plasma (rather than whole blood) from the circulatory system sometimes can be severe enough to cause hypovolemic shock (e.g., the exudation of severe extensive peritonitis, necrotizing enterocolitis, or gastroschisis).

Loss of fluid and electrolytes also may cause dehydration sufficient to reduce the circulating blood volume and result in hypovolemic shock similar to that caused by actual hemorrhage. Causes in the newborn include fluid losses in severe diarrhea or vomiting, inadequate intake of fluid and electrolytes (particularly with the use of potent diuretics), or inadequate replacement of large insensible water losses from the very premature infant.

The relation between cardiac output and hypovolemia depends not only on the amount of blood or fluid lost but also on the rate of that loss; during slow bleeding, compensatory mechanisms come into play for which there is insufficient time if the bleeding is acute. Clinical signs of shock may not become apparent until 10% to 25% of the blood volume has been lost, if that loss is sufficiently slow. *The immediate reaction of the body to oligemia from acute, unreplaced blood loss is to maintain circulation to vital areas (brain, heart, and lungs) by sacrifice of perfusion (vasoconstriction) of less vital vessels in the skin, muscles, and splanchnic bed.* Initiated by powerful sympathetic reflexes that stimulate the release of circulating epinephrine, this compensatory mechanism increases the peripheral resistance and raises the blood pressure but decreases the tissue perfusion. This emergency increase in peripheral sympathetic activity is manifested clinically by tachycardia and by rapid, shallow, and irregular respirations, as well as by a pale and cold skin that frequently appears mottled because capillary filling is slow. The low peripheral venous pressure also manifests clinically by empty peripheral veins; thus it may be difficult to introduce a transfusion needle.

Reflexes from pressure receptors initially maintain total body perfusion to some extent in the early shock state by increasing cardiac output. When blood loss exceeds this compensation, however, shock ensues. With the decrease in venous return to the heart and consequent poor cardiac filling, poor cardiac output results eventually in a further drop in blood pressure. Ischemic damage to the myocardium then may produce myocardial failure, which further reduces cardiac output and aggravates the fall of arterial blood pressure. At this state the infant usually will display *gasping respirations and an altered state of consciousness*. The peripheral pulses are weak and the blood pressure is low or unobtainable.

When the blood volume lost is more than that which can be compensated, blood pressure falls to produce what is known as *uncompensated oligemic shock*. If the oligemia is not severe, circulating blood volume may be partially restored by absorption of fluid from interstitial tissues and gradual replacement of red cells, so that blood pressure is reasonably well maintained; this is known as *compensated oligemic shock*.

Diagnosis. In the evaluation of acute blood loss from the fetus at the time of delivery, the bleeding site, appearance of the blood, signs of blood loss, and evidence for disordered hemostasis should all be considered. The sites and common causes of bleeding are listed in the box on p. 505.

It is mandatory as part of the diagnosis to examine the placenta and cord carefully in an attempt to ascertain the site of blood loss. Factors in the obstetric history that should arouse suspicion of hemorrhage include placenta previa, abruptio placentae, and antepartum hemorrhage occurring in the third trimester. A traumatic delivery should arouse suspicion of possible internal bleeding (e.g., intracranial hemorrhage, ruptured liver or spleen, and hemorrhage into the retroperitoneal space). Hemorrhage into the adrenal glands may manifest as enlarging abdominal masses. This may also occur with subcapsular hematoma of the liver or spleen.

The appearance and intensity of signs and symptoms depend on the amount and rate of bleeding. The blood pressure may be normal, whether indirectly measured by the oscillometric technique or by a pressure transducer connected directly to an umbilical artery catheter. The hemoglobin concentration and hematocrit reading often are initially normal but may be low if measured immediately after hemorrhage. It must be emphasized that if the infant is in shock, *capillary hemoglobin and hematocrit levels may be misleadingly high* because of peripheral sludging and stasis, so that hemoglobin and hematocrit determinations should be performed only on central venous blood samples obtained as blood is drawn for cross-matching. If the hemoglobin level is initially high, the determination should then be repeated and followed closely during the next 12 to 24 hours of life to observe the fall expected as hemodilution occurs.

The diagnosis of fetomaternal hemorrhage is made by demonstrating the presence of fetal red cells in the maternal circulation (Kleihauer-Betke test). A twin-to-twin transfusion should be suspected when a hemoglobin difference greater than 5 g/dl exists between identical twins. Hemoglobin and hematocrit determinations should be performed on venous blood to avoid sampling errors that might lead to misinterpretation of results.

The metabolic response to acute blood loss also depends on the degree of the hemorrhage. *If recruitment of extracellular fluid and contraction of the great veins are sufficient to compensate for the loss of circulating blood volume, then the metabolic response will be slight and signs and symptoms transient.* With further blood loss the increased glycolysis and lipolysis are manifested by increased blood glucose, fatty acid, and lactate levels in the blood. A ventilatory alkalosis can be detected in the arterial blood gas levels, and decreased urinary sodium and volume are noted. With more severe blood loss a severe lactic acidosis occurs, and severe oliguria is noted.

Types of Hemorrhage in the Newborn

OBSTETRIC ACCIDENTS AND MALFORMATION OF THE PLACENTA AND CORD

Rupture of a normal umbilical cord
- Precipitous delivery
- Entanglement

Hematoma of the cord or placenta
Rupture of an abnormal umbilical cord
- Varices
- Aneurysm

Rupture of anomalous vessels
- Aberrant vessel
- Velamentous insertion
- Communicating vessels in multilobed placenta

Incision of placenta during cesarean section
Placenta previa
Abruptio placentae

OCCULT HEMORRHAGE BEFORE BIRTH

Fetoplacental
- Tight nuchal cord
- Cesarean section
- Placental hematoma

Fetomaternal
- Traumatic amniocentesis
- Following external cephalic version, manual removal of placenta, or use of oxytocin
- Spontaneous
- Chorioangioma of the placenta
- Choriocarcinoma of the placenta

Twin-to-twin transfusion
- Chronic
- Acute

INTERNAL HEMORRHAGE

Intracranial
Giant cephalohematoma, subgaleal, or caput succedaneum
Adrenal
Retroperitoneal
Ruptured liver, ruptured spleen
Pulmonary

IATROGENIC BLOOD LOSS

Blood sampling

Modified from Oski FA and Naiman JL: Hematologic problems in the newborn, ed 3, Philadelphia, 1982, WB Saunders Co.

Optimal treatment has but four goals:

1. *Ensure adequate ventilation and oxygenation.* Poor tissue perfusion results in anoxia and anaerobic metabolism with metabolic acidosis, which may be aggravated in the presence of hypoxia. Therefore oxygen should be administered, and an adequate airway must be ensured. An endotracheal tube may be necessary for intermittent positive pressure ventilation.

2. *Stop the hemorrhage.* An infant with a ruptured liver generally appears to be well for 24 to 48 hours and then suddenly goes into shock, coinciding with that time when the gradually increasing hematoma finally ruptures the hepatic capsule and hemoperitoneum occurs. Splenic rupture also may occur after a difficult delivery, particularly if the spleen is already enlarged as a result of severe erythroblastosis. Both these situations may require an operation after adequate resuscitation by blood transfusion.

3. *Restore the circulating blood volume by transfusion.* Treatment should be directed toward restoration of cardiac output and tissue perfusion to prevent the ongoing effects of continuing anoxia. If significant hypovolemia is suspected, it should be treated with repeated small infusions of volume expanders given over 5 to 10 minutes (5 to 10 ml/kg). The neonate's response should be assessed after each infusion. Therapy is stopped only when tissue perfusion is judged adequate (improved mental state, urinary output, skin color, and temperature). Group O, Rh-negative packed red cells cross-matched against the mother's blood are best to use but may not be available. For unanticipated shock, the infant's own heparinized placental blood may be used in an emergency. This is obtained from the umbilical cord after sterilization with a solution of 1% iodine and 70% alcohol. Blood is withdrawn into a 20-ml syringe containing 1 ml of 50 U/ml heparin and administered by use of the filter from an IV blood administration set. Alternatively, 5% albumin, Ringer's lactate, or normal saline may be used.

The amount of blood, plasma, or Ringer lactate solution that should be infused must be judged by the response of the infant to a satisfactory circulatory blood volume: the pulse rate should come down; the skin should become pink, warm, and dry; the urinary volume should increase; the central venous pressure should rise to normal; and the blood pressure should rise. Note that the estimation of hemoglobin should be used only with caution in assessing the amount of blood to be transfused, particularly if whole blood is administered, inasmuch as normal transfused blood has a low hematocrit reading, and any attempt to restore a neonate's hemoglobin level to normal with transfused blood may result in overtransfusion; total blood volume (not red cell mass) is the critical datum here.

4. *Improve cardiac function with external cardiac massage and appropriate drugs when indicated.** If the heart rate is less than 100 beats/min and does not increase to normal with ventilation, then closed-chest cardiac massage should be instituted at a rate of 120 chest compressions per minute (see Appendix A). Drug therapy rarely is necessary for resusci-

*This is discussed in detail in American Academy of Pediatrics: Textbook of neonatal resuscitation, Dallas, 1989, American Heart Association.

tation of the infant in the delivery room. When cardiotonic agents are needed, they should not be administered until adequate ventilation has been established. The preferred route for administration is the umbilical vein. Epinephrine and naloxone also can be administered via the endotracheal tube (Table 41-2).

The immediate and obvious effects of hemorrhage are on the general circulation, but virtually all vital organs (lungs, kidneys, liver, gut, muscle) are likely to display evidence of impaired perfusion. Less frequently considered, but often altered, are body chemical composition, the hormonal settings that control fluid, fuel, and electrolyte balance, neurologic function, circulating inflammatory mediators, and the antibacterial defense systems.

After resuscitation the infant may become irritable and have involuntary muscular movements, often resulting from electrolyte abnormalities. Many of these infants have hypoglycemia, hypokalemia, and hypocalcemia in the first days after birth. They often require 10% glucose administered intravenously to keep blood glucose levels above 45 mg/dl, as well as additional calcium gluconate (200 to 400 mg/kg/24 hr).

Increased pulmonary capillary permeability often persists, even after perfusion pressure is restored to normal, so that transient pulmonary edema with worsening respiratory distress should be anticipated by frequent monitoring of arterial blood gases. The patient may suffer from increased susceptibility to pulmonary infection after a major hemorrhage, which increases pulmonary insufficiency. The effect of severe hemorrhage on the gastrointestinal tract also is significant: small ulcerations may occur in the stomach and progress to necrotic ulcers; alterations in the distribution of blood flow combined with the general decrease in blood flow, producing ischemic injury to the mucosa, can result in enterocolitis. The liver often is damaged by severe hemorrhage; jaundice with an elevation of liver enzymes is a frequent finding, and centrilobular necrosis with fatty infiltration of the liver is found at autopsy. Disorders of hemostasis with bleeding are common after hemorrhagic shock and generally are associated with a deficiency of coagulation products secondary to disseminated intravascular coagulation.

Septic Shock. A complex form of shock can result from bacterial infection. The most common bacteria that cause septic shock in neonates include *group B streptococci* and gram-negative *Escherichia coli* (which may produce endotoxic shock). The physician should suspect overwhelming herpesvirus infection in those infants in whom an acute shocklike state develops within a week to 10 days after delivery, particularly when there is a history of genital herpesvirus infection in the mother.

Septic ("hot") shock is characterized by vasodilation of peripheral vessels with the loss of peripheral resistance, a drop in the blood pressure, poor tissue perfusion, diminished venous return, and reduced cardiac output. Damage to the capillary endothelium results in an increase in capillary permeability, edema, and loss of fluid from the intravascular space into the extravascular tissues, resulting in hypovolemia and a shocklike state. A direct toxic effect on the heart with cardiac failure may occur, as well as the toxic effects in other vital organs noted above.

The onset of respiratory distress or apnea together with shock in full-term or preterm infants ominously heralds group B streptococcal disease. Signs include a low blood pressure, congested mottled skin, and the effects of the toxin on other vital organs. The underlying illness, such as peritonitis or necrotizing enterocolitis, may modify the vascular response because of superimposed hypovolemia.

The diagnosis of neonatal septicemia ultimately depends on a positive blood culture, but cerebrospinal fluid and urine cultures also should be obtained. Indirect evidence of the presumptive diagnosis of overwhelming sepsis includes abnormally elevated or depressed neutrophil band counts with thrombocytopenia. Disseminated intravascular coagulation with generalized bleeding may complicate the shock.

Treatment for presumed neonatal septicemia must be instituted immediately after appropriate diagnostic studies have been performed, including a blood culture, spinal tap, and urine culture. Antibiotics must be administered before final or even initial identification of the responsible microorganism. The choice of antibiotic will depend on the location of the infection, as well as on the timing of the onset of septic shock. When the presumed septicemia occurs within the first 48 to 72 hours of life *(perinatal infection)*, antibiotic coverage with ampicillin and gentamicin (or cefotaxime) is most often used. In late septicemia, secondary to hospital-acquired infection, a penicillinase-resistant penicillin, such as nafcillin, should be given in combination with an aminoglycoside. Once the specific pathogen has been identified, the best combination of drugs is selected on the basis of susceptibility of the organism in vitro.

Although correct antibiotic therapy is the key to successful management of neonatal septic shock, competent supportive measures also are essential. These include increasing the circulating blood volume by transfusion of packed red cells, plasma, or Ringer lactate, as necessary. An attempt to improve cardiac function and vasomotor tone with use of cardiotonic drugs should be considered. Careful monitoring of fluid balance is necessary, with intake and output measurements while monitoring fluid and electrolyte status. Gastric dilation, increased gastric secretion, and ileus are common; decompression of the stomach and bowel should be instituted to avoid aspiration. In severe, overwhelming sepsis the use of an exchange transfusion and infusion of granulocytes may prove to be useful, although more knowledge needs to be gained in this area (see also Chapter 132).

Cardiogenic Shock. Cardiogenic shock usually is associated with underlying severe congestive heart failure, with low cardiac output states secondary to an obstructive lesion of the left ventricular outflow tract such as severe coarctation of the aorta or hypoplastic left heart syndrome. Because there is no output from the left ventricle, the venous blood returning to the left atrium must pass through the atrial septum to the right atrium. The smaller the atrial opening, the greater the pulmonary venous hypertension and congestion—hence the earlier the appearance of symptoms. These infants generally have poor pulses (although they may be normal early in life), mild to moderate cyanosis, characteristic mottling of the skin, and hepatomegaly. Diagnosis is made by clinical, radiographic, electrocardiographic, and especially echocardiographic procedures, followed rapidly by cardiac catheterization

Table 41-2 *Medications for Neonatal Resuscitation*

MEDICATION	CONCENTRATION TO ADMINISTER	PREPARATION	DOSAGE/ ROUTE*	TOTAL DOSE/INFANT			RATE/PRECAUTIONS
Epinephrine	1 : 10,000	1 mL	0.1-0.3 mL/kg I.V. or I.T.	**weight** 1 kg 2 kg 3 kg 4 kg	**total mL's** 0.1-0.3 mL 0.2-0.6 mL 0.3-0.9 mL 0.4-1.2 mL		Give rapidly
Volume expanders	Whole blood 5% Albumin Normal saline Ringer lactate	40 mL	10 mL/kg I.V.	**weight** 1 kg 2 kg 3 kg 4 kg	**total mL's** 10 mL 20 mL 30 mL 40 mL		Give over 5—10 min
Sodium bicarbonate	0.5 mEq/mL (4.2% solution)	20 mL or two 10-mL prefilled syringes	2 mEq/kg I.V.	**weight** 1 kg 2 kg 3 kg 4 kg	**total dose** 2 mEq 4 mEq 6 mEq 8 mEq	**total mL's** 4 mL 8 mL 12 mL 16 mL	Give *slowly,* over at least 2 min Give only if infant being effectively ventilated
Naloxone	0.4 mg/mL	1 mL	0.25 mL/kg I.V., I.M., S.Q., I.T.	**weight** 1 kg 2 kg 3 kg 4 kg	**total mL's** 0.25 mL 0.50 mL 0.75 mL 1.00 mL		Give rapidly
	1.0 mg/mL	1 mL	0.1 mL/kg I.V., I.M., S.Q., I.T.	1 kg 2 kg 3 kg 4 kg	0.1 mL 0.2 mL 0.3 mL 0.4 mL		
Dopamine	$\frac{6 \times \text{weight (kg)} \times \text{desired dose (mcg/kg/min)}}{\text{desired fluid (mL/hr)}} = $ mg of dopamine per 100 mL of solution		Begin at 5 mcg/kg/min (may increase to 20 mcg/kg/min if necessary) I.V.	**weight** 1 kg 2 kg 3 kg 4 kg	**total mcg/min** 5-20 mcg/min 10-40 mcg/min 15-60 mcg/min 20-80 mcg/min		Give as a continuous infusion using an infusion pump Monitor HR and BP closely Seek consultation

*I.M.—intramuscular; I.T.—intratracheal; I.V.—intravenous; S.Q.—subcutaneous and surgery in selected infants. An infusion of prostaglandin E_1 (0.05 μg/kg/min IV) should be started to maintain the patency of the ductus arteriosus (to bypass the obstructed left ventricular outflow) before surgical correction of the lesion.

Shock Resulting from Hypoadrenocorticism. In the neonatal period, bilateral adrenal hemorrhage after a traumatic delivery can lead to shock from blood loss and adrenal insufficiency. A mass may be palpable in each flank and visible on abdominal ultrasound examination. The disorder occurs most often in large infants who have had a traumatic delivery, and it must be differentiated from renal vein thrombosis. The latter is associated with gross hematuria, whereas in an adrenal hemorrhage the hematuria usually is microscopic. Infants with unilateral adrenal hemorrhage do not have symptoms of adrenal insufficiency, but they may experience shock from blood loss.

Congenital adrenal hyperplasia is a group of inherited autosomal recessive disorders caused by the absence of essential enzymes in the pathways for synthesis of cortisol and aldosterone. The interruption of the normal negative-feedback systems stimulates excessive release of ACTH and overactivity in the biosynthetic steps preceding the block, with a resultant accumulation of androgenic steroids. The most common variety is 21-hydroxylase deficiency, which may be seen in affected females as virilization at birth, including clitoral hypertrophy and variable fusion of the labia minora. *These masculinized girls may, tragically, be confused with males with hypospadias and cryptorchism.* Prompt recognition of this problem is less easy in males, who may not easily be diagnosed before an adrenal crisis, which usually occurs in the second week of life. The crisis often is preceded by vomiting and poor weight gain and is biochemically characterized by low serum sodium and high serum potassium levels.

A salt-losing crisis demands urgent therapy with IV saline, glucose, and hydrocortisone, whereas the aim of long-term management must be to suppress the hyperplastic adrenal glands and provide replacement hydrocortisone and a salt-retaining steroid such as fluorocortisone. Elevation of the plasma 17-hydroxyprogesterone level confirms the diagnosis of 21-hydroxylase deficiency, and cortisol is the drug of choice for replacement of glucocorticoid action in adrenal insufficiency. Acutely, the use of desoxycorticosterone (Doca) (1 mg intramuscularly) is indicated and will not interfere with the measurement of the 17-hydroxyprogesterone. Hydrocortisone (Solu-Cortef) is given intravenously as a 50-mg bolus, with an additional 25 mg placed in the IV maintenance solution. Should the patient show further decompensation, then plasma (10 ml/kg) instead of isotonic saline should be given. The use of morphine, barbiturates, or other sedatives is contraindicated. Potassium should not be added to any of the IV fluids. A prompt and complete endocrinologic workup and maintenance therapy are required for these infants.

Tracheoesophageal Fistula or Esophageal Atresia

The diagnosis of tracheoesophageal fistula or esophageal atresia is to be suspected whenever there is a history of *polyhydramnios* during the pregnancy. As many as 85% of these infants have a blind proximal esophageal pouch and a fistulous connection from the distal esophagus to the trachea. The infant is unable to swallow secretions, giving rise to the clinical presentation of excessive oral secretions, with or without aspiration pneumonia soon after birth. The diagnosis is suspected when a nasogastric tube cannot be passed into the stomach and the contents aspirated. It is confirmed by a roentgenogram of a radiopaque tube curled up in the short, blind esophageal pouch. These infants should be kept with the head up (45-degree angle), a Replogle tube inserted into the upper esophageal pouch, and constant suction maintained. If a Replogle tube is not available, a large-bore (10 to 12 Fr) catheter will suffice. Immediate transfer to a regional neonatal ICU is mandatory (for definitive diagnostic testing and surgical correction of the defect).

SUGGESTED READINGS

American Academy of Pediatrics: Textbook of neonatal resuscitation, Dallas, 1989, American Heart Association.

American Academy of Pediatrics and American College of Obstetricians and Gynecologists: Guidelines for perinatal care, ed 2, Evanston, Ill, 1988, The Academy.

Avery ME, Fletcher BD, and Williams RG: The lung and its disorders in the newborn infant, ed 4, Philadelphia, 1981, WB Saunders Co.

Avery ME, Gatewood OB, and Brumley G: Transient tachypnea of the newborn, Am J Dis Child 111:380, 1966.

Boyle RJ et al: Early identification of sepsis in infants with respiratory distress, Pediatrics 62:744, 1978.

Collins JA: The pathophysiology of hemorrhage shock. In Collins JA, Murawski K, and Shafer AW, editors: Massive transfusion in surgery and trauma, New York, 1982, Alan R Liss, Inc.

Cornblath M and Schwartz R: Infants of the diabetic mother. In Disorders of carbohydrate metabolism in infancy, ed 2, Philadelphia, 1976, WB Saunders Co.

Fletcher AB: The infant of the diabetic mother. In Avery GB, editor: Neonatology, ed 2, Philadephia, 1981, JB Lippincott Co.

Halliday HL, McClure C, and Reid M: Transient tachypnoea of the newborn: two distinct clinical entities? Arch Dis Child 56:322, 1981.

Klaus MH and Fanaroff AA, editors: Care of the high-risk neonate, ed 3, Philadelphia, 1986, WB Saunders Co.

Klein JO: Bacterial infections of the respiratory tract. In Remington JS and Klein JO: Infectious disease of the fetus and newborn infant, Philadelphia, 1983, WB Saunders Co.

Oski FA and Naiman JL: Hematologic problems in the newborn, ed 3, Philadelphia, 1982, WB Saunders Co.

Painter MJ and Bergman I: Obstetrical trauma to the neonatal central and peripheral nervous system, Semin Perinatol 6:89, 1982.

Phibbs RH: Delivery room management of the newborn. In Avery GB, editor: Neonatology, pathophysiology and management of the newborn, ed 2, Philadelphia, 1981, JB Lippincott Co.

Pildes RS and Lilien LD: Carbohydrate metabolism in the fetus and neonate. In Fanaroff AA and Martin RJ, editors: Neonatal-perinatal medicine, ed 4, St Louis, 1987, The CV Mosby Co.

Rowe RD et al: The neonate with congenital heart disease, Philadelphia, 1981, WB Saunders Co.

Sabata V et al: The effect of glucose in the prenatal treatment of small-for-date fetuses, Biol Neonate 22:78, 1973.

Shires GT, Carrico CJ, and Canizaro PC: Shock, vol. 13. Major problems in clinical surgery, Philadelphia, 1973, WB Saunders Co.

Sundell H, Garrott J, and Blankenship WJ: Studies on infants with type II respiratory distress syndrome, J Pediatr 78:754, 1971.

Volpe JJ: Neurology of the newborn, ed 2, Philadelphia, 1987, WB Saunders Co.

42

High-Risk Follow-Up

Dennis J. Mujsce and Nicholas M. Nelson

Discharge from the neonatal intensive care unit (NICU) does not terminate the problems of high-risk infants, their families, medical care providers, or society. Although the special needs of seriously ill neonates usually lessen during the course of hospitalization, their follow-up home care remains formidable. These survivors have markedly higher rates of serious illness, rehospitalization, and death in the first years of life than do infants not requiring neonatal intensive care. Their high risk is reflected in a persistently high postdischarge infant mortality rate, which is five to nine times greater than the postneonatal mortality rate of other infants.[1,20] Once home, these infants demand large amounts of time, energy, and financial resources, but many are discharged to severely disadvantaged homes poorly equipped to manage a normal infant, much less one subjected to such stresses.

CHARACTERISTICS OF HIGH-RISK INFANTS

The term *high risk* can be appropriately applied to any infant who experiences an unusual perinatal course, has a greater than normal likelihood of morbidity or mortality, or requires other than standard newborn care. Recognizing the high-risk status of a patient is an important first step toward anticipation of defined problems and rendering optimal care.

Population

Premature Neonates. The cornucopia for high-risk infants is the premature population, in which remarkable reductions in mortality related to birth weight has occurred during the past three decades.[17] The mortality rates for those infants delivered in 1960 with birth weights less than 1500 g or less than 1000 g were roughly 70% and 90%, respectively, whereas by 1985 these figures had nearly been halved to 30% and 50%.[27] Unfortunately, the advances in neonatal care responsible for these improved survival rates have not eradicated many of the serious sequelae that continue to handicap 5% to 10% of current NICU survivors. Thus, larger numbers of both well and handicapped infants are being seen today in the follow-up clinics for this high-risk population.

Other Neonates. Although prematurity and its attendant complications contribute most heavily to the high-risk pool, numerous other causes of neonatal morbidity and mortality (see the accompanying box) are now being treated in NICUs. Indeed, expanded diagnostic and therapeutic capabilities (see the box on p. 510) allow for aggressive management of a growing number of disorders, some of which were once considered fatal. Survivors of these newborn conditions may well have follow-up needs that equal or exceed those of the tiniest premature infants.

Special Needs

Each high-risk infant is an individual who brings a unique mix of problems and needs to the health care system. All these patients require standard well-baby care, but few will move smoothly and quickly through a pediatric office or clinic, because they represent extraordinary medical illnesses, treatments, sequelae, and altered family dynamics that de-

Some Major Neonatal Illnesses Treated in Contemporary NICUs

- Altered growth and gestation
  - Infants of extremely low birth weight (<750 g)
  - Severe intrauterine growth retardation
- Pulmonary disorders
  - Hyaline membrane disease (respiratory distress syndrome)
  - Meconium aspiration syndrome
  - Pneumonia
  - Pulmonary hemorrhage
- Cardiovascular disorders
  - Acyanotic heart diseases (e.g., hypoplastic left-heart syndrome)
  - Arrhythmias and heart blocks
  - Cyanotic heart disease (e.g., transposition, pulmonary atresia)
  - Persistent fetal circulation
- Renal/genitourinary disorders
  - Obstructive uropathy
  - Renal dysplasias
- Gastrointestinal disorders
  - Biliary atresia
  - Diaphragmatic hernia
  - Malformations (e.g., gastroschisis, omphalocele, bowel atresias)
- Central nervous system disorders
  - Developmental anomalies (e.g., hydrocephalus, Arnold-Chiari malformation, neural tube defect)
  - Hypoxic-ischemic encephalopathy
  - Intracranial hemorrhage
- Inborn errors of metabolism
- Genetic and chromosomal disorders

Expanding Repertoire of NICU Treatment Options

DIAGNOSTIC MODALITIES

Cardiac catheterization and angiography (heart, blood vessels)
Computed tomography (brain, abdomen, body)
Magnetic resonance imaging (brain)
Nuclear medicine scans (renal, hepatobiliary)
Positron emission tomography (brain)
Real-time and Doppler ultrasonography (brain, heart, abdomen)

THERAPEUTIC INTERVENTIONS

Medical managements
- Continuous prostaglandin E_1 infusion (to maintain ductus arteriosus patency)
- Conventional and high-frequency ventilation (respiratory failure)
- Exogenous surfactant administration (hyaline membrane disease)
- Immunoglobulin and antibiotic therapy (infection)
- Steroid therapy (bronchopulmonary dysplasia)

Surgical managements
- Cardiopulmonary bypass, hypothermic circulatory arrest (cardiac repair)
- Dialysis and hemofiltration (renal failure)
- Extracorporeal membrane oxygenation (diaphragmatic hernia)
- Neurosurgical procedures (to correct anomalies of central nervous system)
- Organ transplantation (biliary atresia)

mand considerable time and attention. Physicians who care for high-risk infants therefore must be prepared to allocate a disproportionate amount of effort toward this minority of patients.

Comprehensive care for these infants often is best accomplished as a team effort between the follow-up group of the tertiary care center and the infant's own primary care physician. To remain effective members of the high-risk follow-up team, however, all health care providers need to achieve and maintain familiarity with treatments that originally were confined to hospital settings: supplemental oxygen, ventilator support, tracheostomy care, gastrostomy tube feedings, intravenous hyperalimentation, peritoneal dialysis, and home apnea monitoring. In addition to such technical forms of therapy, physicians also are called upon to stay abreast of the wide range of medications and services now incorporated into the outpatient care of high-risk infants. In addition, the disease processes themselves must be understood so that serious changes or deteriorations in an infant's condition can be detected and addressed promptly.

Perhaps most important, the primary health care provider must appreciate subtle impairments of motor development, cognition, and behavior that can manifest late, yet adversely affect the high-risk infant's quality of life.

DISCHARGE PLANNING

Follow-up care begins with discharge planning, one of the least dramatic, but most important, aspects of neonatal intensive care. The continued success of even the most spectacular NICU story requires a comprehensive plan at discharge that had, in fact, been continuously developed throughout the infant's course of hospitalization.

The first step is the identification of those infants who will benefit from high-risk follow-up. Opinions vary, but the box on p. 511 lists some conditions that most agree warrant special attention after discharge. In addition to these infants who can best be followed up by primary care practitioners cooperatively with high-risk clinics, many neonates with specific problems (e.g., imperforate anus, congenital heart defects, ventriculoperitoneal shunts) require services now available only in certain subspecialty clinics. Follow-up care for these babies proceeds best through collaboration of the primary care physician and the appropriate subspecialists.

Development of a discharge plan early in the infant's hospitalization helps to ensure that discharge occurs at the appropriate time, that all the infant's needs will be met, and that parental anxiety is kept to a minimum. Parents require a great deal of time and repetition of explanations and instructions to assimilate all the necessary information. Logistic barriers to information exchange, such as early discharge of the mother and large distances separating the family from the infant in the tertiary care center, make early communication imperative. A truly multidisciplinary plan must be formulated, one that is based on the opinions of parents, nurses, social workers, neonatologists, subspecialists, and the infant's primary care physician.

A primary goal of discharge planning is to provide a smooth transition of the infant's care from the highly staffed, specialized NICU environment to a home setting in which adequate support mechanisms are in place. A successful discharge plan must outline the support network clearly, match infant needs with appropriate resources, and precisely define the responsibilities of all follow-up participants. An effective plan is kept as simple as possible, while ensuring that there are no delays, duplications, absences, or fragmentation of necessary services. Furthermore, sound discharge planning must provide for ongoing reevaluation of the plan itself and for alternative steps to be taken in the event of unforeseen emergencies. The timing of the actual discharge will depend on the readiness of the infant, the family, the home, and the follow-up team. Thus each must be thoroughly assessed before discharge.

Many contemporary neonatal staffs no longer insist on achievement of a minimum body weight for discharge, provided the infant's medical problems have stabilized and the infant can competently maintain body temperature while in a bassinette; feed regularly by mouth (or gastrostomy tube in selected cases); maintain consistent growth; and breathe regularly without frequent or severe apnea.[6] It is essential that any high-risk infant's discharge be preceded by documentation of caretaker competency and adequacy of the home environment.

Most NICU patients are discharged directly into the care of their parents. However, stable high-risk infants are in-

Entry Criteria for Neonatal High-Risk Follow-Up Programs

Birth weight ≤1500 g
Bronchopulmonary dysplasia
Hydrocephalus/microcephaly
Hyperbilirubinemia requiring exchange transfusion
Intracranial hemorrhage/periventricular leukomalacia
Meningitis and sepsis
Persistent fetal circulation
Severe intrauterine growth retardation (<5%)
Severe meconium aspiration syndrome
Symptomatic hypoglycemia
Symptomatic perinatal asphyxia

creasingly being transferred from distant tertiary care centers to "level II" NICUs or lower-level nurseries for further management nearer their homes, before actually being sent to their own home. These internursery transfers reduce health care costs and open NICU beds for new acutely ill patients. The receiving health care providers thus must share responsibility for discharge planning with the referring NICU staff.

GOALS OF HIGH-RISK FOLLOW-UP

Longitudinal studies of high-risk patients are the "gold standard" source for information to guide and gauge the effectiveness of NICU care. Educators, politicians, and policy makers at all levels require such follow-up data to allocate funds and resources on the basis of the special medical and educational needs of NICU graduates. Parents, of course, need the best information available to understand what may lie in store for their child and family and to plan their lives accordingly. Although short-term neonatal mortality and morbidity can be estimated from acute NICU statistics, many effects of neonatal intensive care are appreciated only through the data gathered in long-term follow-up studies—e.g., later mortality and health problems, incidence of rehospitalization, neurodevelopmental outcome, academic achievement, quality of life, effects on family and society, costs, and resource usage. It is now known, for example, that the incidence of neurologic abnormalities in very-low-birth-weight (VLBW) infants jumps from 10%-30% to 30%-60% if learning disabilities are added to the list of sequelae (such as cerebral palsy, developmental delay, and seizures) that are classically identified at an earlier age.[22] In addition, the incidence of severe handicaps in infants does not appear to differ significantly from that of older children, but this may be misleading, because the same child can be classified as having differing handicaps at different ages.[19]

Parents often are reluctant to return with their infants to high-risk follow-up programs for a variety of real or perceived reasons. Some of these include extra cost, inconvenience, time away from the job, distance between the home and clinic, prior unpleasant NICU experiences, fear of uncovering new abnormalities, and the conviction that the clinic benefits more from the visit than does the infant or family. Primary care physicians, concentrating on immediate infant care issues, may unintentionally reinforce the belief that there is little to be gained from return visits to the follow-up clinic. Such "dropouts" can seriously skew outcome figures. One report[30] found that only 4.4% of "easy to review" patients were severely disabled, whereas the percentage within the "hard to review" group was 35%!

Most medical students and pediatric residents learn about the management of acute neonatal problems within the NICU, but few receive sufficient exposure to a structured high-risk follow-up clinic to realize that each critically ill infant is indeed a person who is part of a family and that most of them will ultimately improve. The majority of recently graduated pediatricians regard their residency training as their primary source of information concerning the care of high-risk infants.[9] Therefore a residency curriculum that provides its house staff with encouragement and guidance in a high-risk clinic should produce better prepared pediatricians.

Return visits to the follow-up clinic by thriving high-risk infants can rejuvenate the morale of NICU personnel who spend long, stressful hours attending sick infants whose outcome is uncertain. This forum is a good opportunity to review information, dispel misconceptions, and address the new questions that parents invariably think of, once their high-risk infant is home.

ORGANIZATION OF HIGH-RISK FOLLOW-UP

In some clinics the neonatologists who cared for the infants in the NICU maintain a strong presence, whereas other programs turn over the outpatients to teams that specialize in high-risk follow-up. Yet other infants are discharged from NICUs (lacking an organized neonatal follow-up program) directly to the infant's primary physician. There are several public health, community, and ancillary health services (see box on p. 512) of which these physicians in particular should be aware and should utilize to the benefit of their high-risk patients.

Several common threads run through all successful strategies for high-risk follow-up. First, each infant requires an individual discharge plan that is specifically tailored to provide routine pediatric care while simultaneously attending to his or her particular needs. Second, there must be continuity of care as the infant is discharged home, when different people assume new roles in patient management. Finally, communication must exist among all follow-up participants, and it must be made clear who holds coordinating responsibility for the infant's care.

The Neonatal Intensive Care Unit

The NICU staff has weeks or months to become familiar with the infants it manages. It generally is in the best position to identify patient needs, initiate discharge planning, and ensure that the required components of the follow-up team are in place. Responsibility for identifying high-risk infants is assumed by the infant's primary nurse, the neonatologist, or a neonatal follow-up coordinator, who might be either a nurse

Some Resources Available to Families of High-Risk Infants

ANCILLARY HEALTH CARE SERVICES

Dietitians and nutrition specialists
Home health equipment and services vendors
Home nursing services
Physical, occupational, and hearing and speech therapy
Social services

COMMUNITY RESOURCES

Churches and religious organizations
Community health nurses
Departments of public health
County and state financial-support programs
Early intervention programs
Hospice and respite services
Parental support groups
Schools and special educational programs
Specialized foster care parents

FAMILY SUPPORT NETWORK

Extended family
Significant friends

or a physician. High-risk infants are identified as quickly as possible, their parents are notified, and an immediate attempt is made to enroll the patient into the comprehensive follow-up program. Early discussion with the parents is essential inasmuch as it allows them to contribute to and understand the objectives of the follow-up plan. Neonatal staff members must ensure that all the infant's needs will be met after discharge by a system that has been designed to avoid complexity, duplication, fragmentation, and omission of services.

As the day of discharge from the NICU approaches, neonatal staff members must be satisfied that the infant's condition is stable and that the family is capable of assuming his or her care. Any major medical problems should either have been resolved or stabilized. Medication regimens should be rechecked to determine that each has been simplified to the extent possible, that all dosages are correct, that appropriate blood levels have been obtained, and that adverse reactions or side effects have been explained. The final days of hospitalization also provide the opportunity to ensure that all necessary testing has been completed (e.g., hematocrit levels, hearing screening, an ophthalmology examination for retinopathy of prematurity, head ultrasonography, or echocardiography). The infant's medical history is reviewed with family members, their questions answered, and their residual concerns addressed and, if possible, assuaged.

Unfortunately, evidence persists that (1) many infants leave the NICU without their parents having a good understanding of what has transpired or what they can expect and that (2) the primary care physician has not even been notified of the discharge via a formal narrative summary of the infant's hospital course, much less been included in the discharge planning by a simple telephone call from the neonatologist. Despite the barrier posed by a busy practitioner's even busier telephone line, it can be a powerful tool for the exchange of information; such a call allows each party to discuss issues of concern, provides an opportunity for the primary physician to be updated about new treatment modalities, fosters a feeling of collaboration, and encourages future discussion. Despite the availability of such avenues of communication, as many as 55% of pediatricians in one survey[18] believed that they had been inadequately informed about the NICU discharge status of their high-risk infants before the first office visit.

High-Risk Follow-Up Programs

High-risk neonatal follow-up clinics are not meant to provide primary care or in any way to replace the community physician. Indeed, most high-risk clinics prefer to work in conjunction with the infant's primary physician, assisting wherever possible and offering supplemental services. A typical neonatal high-risk follow-up schedule calls for an initial visit 2 to 6 weeks after the infant's discharge, followed by visits at 6 months, 1 year, and 2 years of age.

The strengths of a neonatal high-risk clinic include its multidisciplinary composition and its linkages to other health care resources. During a clinic visit an infant may be evaluated by any combination of the following personnel: neonatologists, nurses, physical therapists, social workers, developmental specialists, and child psychologists. This team of experts, coupled with adequate time, permits a look beyond the child's more immediate medical problems to focus on such long-range issues as infant development and behavior, family stresses, and financial problems.

Subspecialty Clinics

Among the services neonatal patients and their illnesses attract into the NICU are cardiology, endocrinology, genetics, hematology, surgery, orthopedics, urology, cardiothoracic surgery, neurosurgery, and ophthalmology. Dietitians, physical therapists, audiologists, nurses specializing in wound care, and many others also participate in the care of NICU patients. The neonatal high-risk follow-up clinic is the natural coordinating center for the continuing efforts of these individuals and their communciation with the primary care physician.

Ancillary Health Services

A number of nonphysician personnel can considerably enhance the care given to high-risk infants in the NICU and in their homes.

Neonatal nurses, who bond with the infants they care for day after day, develop relationships with the families that persist beyond the day of discharge. Social workers are consulted with great frequency in the NICU, for families of high-risk infants frequently are themselves at high risk—single-parent households, young and uneducated parents, inadequate home environment, unemployment and financial stress, child abuse and neglect, drug abuse, and other difficulties that all have major implications for the well-being of discharged infants. These problems often are magnified during the hospital course in the NICU. Physical, occupational, and speech therapists strengthen follow-up and enhance the quality of life for high-risk infants. Physicians, also, rely on them to perform serial assessments of gross and fine motor development, reflexes, muscle tone, strength, range of motion, posture, ambulation, sensory perception, feeding abilities, phonation, and adaptational skills. After a thorough evaluation, these therapists are able to counsel parents and physicians, suggest management strategies, and instruct parents in the execution of specific therapies. As therapy proceeds, they should participate in the reevaluation of both the patient and the therapeutic plan.

Commercial home health care service companies are now burgeoning, and all physicians need to be familiar with and utilize them, because they supply a wide range of services and home health care equipment that are especially applicable to discharged high-risk infants—home oxygen, ventilators, pulse oximeters, apnea monitors, and suction machines. The equipment supplied is backed up by 24-hour maintenance and service, in addition to professionals with pediatric experience who can go into the home and conduct teaching or physical assessments at the direction of the physician. These companies rely on physician referrals, and they usually are conscientious about reporting problems within the home or changes in the infant's condition. Thus they can serve as an essential local link of expertise between the high-risk follow-up staff and the primary care physician.

Community Resources and Public Health Services

A comprehensive review of all community resources and public health services is not possible here, but knowledge of regionally available programs will greatly assist the physician in the management of high-risk infants: visits from community health nurses or special services for children, special educational programs, early intervention programs with evaluation and rehabilitation, specialized foster care, parental support groups, respite or hospice care, and financial assistance for food, supplies, and medical needs. In considering community resources, one should not neglect friends, relatives, and persons with religious or social significance to the family. Physicians should learn to take advantage of these types of resources because they can have significant impact on the immediate health and long-term development of their patients.

Parents of High-Risk Infants

By necessity, the parents of a high-risk infant become immediate members of the follow-up team. These are the persons with the heaviest emotional investment in their baby, and ultimately they will assume the greatest share of the caretaking responsibilities. A major prerequisite for adequate parenting (sadly, not always satisfied!) is that the parents have a genuine interest in the infant and his or her well-being. Once it is established that this basic requirement has been fulfilled, the neonatal staff must begin the rigorous preparation that these parents need most.

During the hospitalization the parents should have developed a reasonable idea of their infant's illnesses, symptoms, treatments, and prognoses. This information provides the groundwork for the observational skills the parents will use in the home to monitor the medical condition of their infant. Because they will have the most extensive contact with the baby, the parents must be capable of detecting deteriorations or significant alterations in their infant's health and bringing these findings to medical attention. Parents who will be expected to administer medications must demonstrate understanding and competence regarding dosages, timing, routes of administration, adverse effects, and precautions. Parents of infants who are discharged with special equipment (e.g., nasal cannula oxygen, intravenous hyperalimentation, home apnea monitors) must be completely and explicitly schooled in its use. They also must understand what to do, and whom to notify when malfunctions occur.

Parents often must be required to learn certain basic or even "high-tech" nursing functions, such as cardiopulmonary resuscitation. Nonetheless, time spent demonstrating how to feed, bathe, dress, and simply enjoy their baby will enhance the quality of care rendered and boost parental self-esteem. The neonatal team also should ascertain that the parents can procure food, clothing, a car seat, and a crib for their infant, as well as have access to a telephone and transportation.

Although it is mandatory to establish that these requirements have been fulfilled before an infant's discharge from the NICU, it is equally important to ensure that circumstances do not subsequently deteriorate. The primary care physican must assume principal responsibility for monitoring these aspects of the infant's family and home.

The Primary Care Physician

The distribution of high-risk infant survivors is such that any primary care practitioner today can expect to be called on to care for them (approximately 5 to 10 such infants per year in the average primary care practice). Whether that involvement occurs during or subsequent to the NICU stay is very much a function of local custom, as well as the practitioner's interest, training, available time and, particularly, geography relative to the NICU.

The practitioner's fundamental role, however, is to serve as the family's principal assimilator and translator of the onslaught of often-confusing information presented by a deluge of nurses, neonatologists, cardiologists, gastroenterologists, neurologists, surgeons, dietitians and technologists, and, often, medical and nursing students, all encountered during the NICU stay or subsequent visits to the high-risk follow-up clinic. As the only person in this vast array who will have known the family before and after the added stress of its high-risk infant, the primary care physician is the natural "case manager" for this child. In this setting it is no more necessary that the practitioner be possessed of personal expertise in perinatal/neonatal care than that the manager of the Cincinnati Reds need be a .400 hitter; however, it *is* required that the practitioner be prepared to provide a link between the family and the NICU and its follow-up staff.

MEDICAL MANAGEMENT OF HIGH-RISK INFANTS

A comprehensive catalog of common and critical neonatal illnesses and treatments is provided in chapters 40 and 41; the review presented here concentrates on VLBW infants—

those weighing <1500 g at birth—and those of their diverse problems with which the primary care practitioner necessarily becomes involved.

Primary Health Care Considerations

In addition to monitoring the identified medical problems of high-risk infants, primary care physicians also must promote normal growth and development, anticipate normal age-appropriate problems, and educate parents about routine pediatric issues, just as they do with their low-risk patients. For example, anticipatory counseling about injury prevention is indicated, even though parents may not initially realize that their NICU graduate eventually will encounter the same hazards as other children. Likewise, pediatricians need to emphasize that infants be adequately secured whenever traveling by automobile; all states now enforce seat belt legislation meant to prevent the 500 annual deaths and 53,000 annual injuries that occur in the United States in children younger than 4 years old, whether or not they be high risk. Parents taking VLBW infants home must realize that most infant-restraint systems are marketed for babies who weigh more than 7 pounds. Some of these systems may be inappropriate for tiny infants, because they do not provide enough support to prevent airway compromise with decreases in arterial oxygen saturation when the infant is seated upright. Any medical equipment also must be secured and, if an apnea monitor has been recommended for the infant, it should be functioning properly during any automobile travel. Helpful guidelines are available from the American Academy of Pediatrics' Committee on Accident and Poison Prevention.

Growth

Growth, an exquisitely sensitive marker of health, must be monitored and documented frequently. Weight, length, and head circumference must be measured and plotted against "corrected age" (postnatal age in weeks less the number of weeks by which the infant was prematurely born) on appropriate growth curves. Although specific growth charts exist for sick, tiny premature infants while in the NICU, these generally are not required after an infant's discharge; standard growth charts are suitable. Weight should be plotted against the infant's corrected age until 24 months of age, after which time premature infants generally follow the same weight curves as do children who were born at term. Significant deviations from expected weight gain may indicate excess fluid retention or inadequate caloric intake relative to metabolic demands. Length should similarly be corrected for prematurity until the infant is 3.5 years of age, whereas head circumference (as an indicator of brain growth) should be plotted against corrected age until 18 months of age. Although not entirely predictive, correlations do exist between growth failure and neurodevelopmental delays.[29] Conversely, the achievement of a normal head circumference by 8 months is a predictor of normal psychosocial development at 3 years of age.[16]

Many premature infants at discharge are smaller than the third growth percentiles for corrected age, either because of intrauterine growth retardation or because of serious neonatal illness. "Catch-up growth" should be expected and promoted in most of these infants in the first year of life. Generally, head circumference reaches a normal percentile first, followed next by length and, finally, by weight. Catch-up growth is maximal between 36 to 44 postnatal weeks; most infants will begin to grow along their new growth curve by 6 to 12 months. If a premature infant of birth weight appropriate for gestational age does not achieve at least the third percentile by 3 years of age, future catch-up growth cannot be anticipated. Premature infants with severe intrauterine growth retardation usually do not achieve normal values postnatally.

Nutrition

The American Academy of Pediatrics recommends breast milk as the feeding of choice for infants, including those who are premature. Before their attainment of 1800 to 2000 g of body weight, premature infants require either calorically dense "premature formula" or mother's breast milk, fortified by calories, minerals, and vitamins. The Academy's Committee on Infant Nutrition suggests that, after a weight of 2000 g is achieved, breast milk alone is a practical, nutritionally adequate feeding with immunologic properties that may decrease the incidence of respiratory and gastrointestinal infections. Mothers who opt not to breast-feed may use any standard infant formula after the infant's weight reaches 2000 g. Breast-fed infants who are well enough to be discharged from the NICU should receive standard amounts of vitamins A, D, and C, with fluoride added, if the family's water supply is fluoride-deficient. The need for vitamin E supplementation usually diminishes after 6 to 8 weeks of postnatal age, by which time the risk of hemolytic anemia has passed. Despite the osteopenia common to acutely ill premature infants, most can manage normal bone development on the usual amounts of calcium and phosphorus found in standard lactose-based infant formulas. Finally, formula-fed premature infants should receive 2 to 3 mg/kg/day of supplemental elemental iron from 6 to 8 weeks of postnatal age until approximately 6 months of age. Some believe that infants of birth weight less than 1000 g may benefit from supplementary doses of iron approaching 4 mg/kg/day until they are 1 year old. Finally, dietary advances in premature infants should be based on their actual, rather than "corrected," postnatal age.

The feeding of high-risk infants should be normalized to the extent possible, but there are many qualifying conditions in this population of patients that deserve consideration. In some infants, such as those with intrauterine growth retardation or bronchopulmonary dysplasia, their high metabolic rates demand at least 120 to 150 calories/kg/day for sustained growth. Ironically, many infants with the highest caloric requirements have the misfortune also to require fluid restriction. In others, a structural or functional short bowel syndrome (secondary to conditions such as necrotizing enterocolitis, gastroschisis, bowel atresia, malrotation, meconium ileus or Hirschsprung disease) can seriously limit enteral nutrition. Loss of gastrointestinal surface area because of such diseases, or their surgical treatment, also can limit absorption of other important nutrients, such as vitamins and minerals. The amount and composition of the infant's feedings will require ongoing alteration and reevaluation in many of these instances. Protein, fat, and carbohydrate can be added to breast milk for formula to provide a more calorically dense feeding. Caloric densities of 30 calories/oz can be achieved, but care must be taken to avoid unwanted gastrointestinal or renal effects as a result of inordinate amounts of any one source of calories. In those patients whose enteral caloric intake will not be sufficient for acceptable growth, intravenous total parenteral nutrition should be instituted. This route for nutrition is quite demanding and requires profound parental commitment, a central venous catheter, many monitoring laboratory determinations, and a qualified team responsible for designing and monitoring the nutritional strategy and working with the primary care physician.

Aside from monitoring growth variables, the primary care physician also should review details of the infant's feeding habits, such as schedules, amount and type of feeding, signs of gastroesophageal reflux, or other feeding difficulties. Graduates of the unnatural NICU environment who have experienced insufficient amounts of nonnutritive sucking and prolonged periods of nasogastric or endotracheal intubation can be notoriously difficult feeders. Parents often will need much reassurance, coaching, and support in this regard; referral to a qualified feeding specialist occasionally is indicated. The physician also should inquire about stooling and voiding patterns. These may be clues to underlying conditions, such as malabsorption or colonic stricture (secondary to previous episodes of necrotizing enterocolitis).

Immunizations

In general, immunization schedules for high-risk premature infants do not differ from those recommended by the American Academy of Pediatrics' Committee on Infectious Disease for term infants. Dosages should not be reduced, divided, or delayed to correct for prematurity. Moreover, these recommendations are continuously being updated; thus primary care practitioners must stay abreast of revisions as they occur.

Pediatricians who care for high-risk infants also must be aware of two other vaccines: hepatitis B and influenza. Hepatitis B frequently is encountered in high-risk pregnancies, and any infant born to a mother who is seropositive for hepatitis B surface antigen is a candidate for prophylactic therapy. Such infants should receive 0.5 ml of hepatitis B immunoglobulin intramuscularly within the first 12 hours of life, followed by 0.5 ml of hepatitis B vaccine (10 μg) intramuscularly within the first week, at 1 month, and again at 6 months.

Certain chronically ill high-risk infants, such as patients with bronchopulmonary dysplasia or congestive heart failure, should be vaccinated annually against influenza. Infants generally are given two doses (0.25 ml) of split-virus vaccine intramuscularly at least 4 weeks apart, in the fall before the influenza season begins.

Other Primary Care Issues

As with any other children, pediatricians should screen their NICU graduates for such common problems as anemia, lead intoxication, and tuberculosis. Issues of infant behavior, development, sleep patterns, and parental bonding frequently are areas of intense concern and stress for parents of high-risk infants who have completed a lengthy stay in a NICU. Finally, all health care providers must guard against the chronic environmental insults of malnutrition, poor hygiene, abuse, and neglect.

Rehospitalization

The path back to the hospital will be well-worn during the first year or two following discharge of the VLBW child from the NICU: between one fourth to one third of these infants will require rehospitalization, principally for exacerbations of those developmental problems that derive from their prematurity—postnecrotizing enterocolitis, postligation for patent ductus arteriosus, herniorrhaphies, and revisions of ventriculoperitoneal (or other) shunts for posthemorrhagic hydrocephalus.[23,25] Especially wearing can be the rehospitalizations of the child receiving home oxygen therapy for residual bronchopulmonary dysplasia during the winter season for respiratory infectious disease (particularly respiratory syncytial virus).

All these assaults can easily weaken the resolve and decimate the morale of even the most robust of family networks, but they are infinitely more oppressive for the frequently dysfunctional non-families in which many of these infants are deposited. An uneducated, drug-abusing, single, teenaged child-mother (with or without the support of her unemployed boyfriend), recently thrown out of the house of her alcoholic parents (to maximize the social pathology!) is among the more severe tests that modern society can throw at the medical establishment, with demands for instant resolution. It is gratifyingly remarkable what often can be accomplished in such a setting by a primary physician/social worker team knowledgeable about the mother and her community and easily conversant with the pertinent NICU's high-risk follow-up staff.

Specific Neonatal Problems

Hearing. The situation of the high-risk infant is fraught with opportunities to sustain significant sensorineural hearing loss: asphyxia, hyperbilirubinemia, and both nosocomial (meningitis) and congenital (cytomegalovirus, rubella, herpes, toxoplasmosis, syphilis) infection, as well as frequent exposure to aminoglycoside antibiotics. Moderate to profound hearing loss is two to five times more likely to develop in the high-risk infant than in the general population of children, whereas the VLBW child is at even greater risk for severe hearing loss. The usual behavioral-observational pace of ascertaining whether a child hears is simply too slow to be of much help in this assessment, so that the recent development of fairly reliable early screening methods—the Crib-O-Gram and the brainstem auditory evoked response (BAER), an electroencephalographic technique—has been most welcome, especially in meeting the challenge of the infant younger than 6 months of age.[3,26] These screenings usually are performed before discharge from the NICU, but regular reassessment often is necessary.

Retinopathy of Prematurity. The renaming of retrolental fibroplasia (RLF) to retinopathy of prematurity (ROP) has served to emphasize that it is much more a developmental than an iatrogenic phenomenon. Indeed, as VLBW infants increasingly survive, their risk for the development of ROP is nearly 50% (if <1000 g birth weight), regardless of the oxygen environment sustained. This risk falls to less than 3% as birth weight advances to >1500 g, so that the so-called second epidemic (of RLF since the original episode of the 1950s) is attributable to the increasing survival of the "tiny premature" at maximum developmental risk for ROP.[13] The principal risk factors remain: immaturity of retinal vascularization and oxygen, increased levels of the latter still being necessary to allow the infant to undertake that risk by surviving.

The present approach toward minimization of that risk is principally one of increased ophthalmologic surveillance (indirect ophthalmoscopic examination under pupillary dilation by the pediatric ophthalmologist) and early intervention (by cryotherapy) if disease threatens to advance beyond the reversible early stages to irreversible, cicatricial disease. Fortunately, even some cicatricial disease eventually may resolve. The prevention of ROP by administration of vitamin E is not as yet well-established.[28]

Cryotherapy, wherein the affected retina is actually frozen at multiple points, apparently arrests the continual excessive retinal vascularization characteristic of ROP.[5,8]

Bronchopulmonary Dysplasia (BPD). This condition is the frustrating outcome for nearly 20% of the VLBW survivors of hyaline membrane disease. The necessary ingredients in its causation are pulmonary immaturity (including surfactant deficiency), increased alveolar oxygen concentration, and the "barotrauma" imposed by long periods of artificial ventilation at high airway pressures. It will likely be impossible to separate these factors completely. The pathophysiologic behavior of BPD is similar to that of the chronic obstructive lung disease (COLD) seen in later life. These behavioral features include (1) "reactive" small airway disease, characterized by increased resistance to gaseous flow through the airways, as well as increased vascular resistance (and right-sided heart strain) and (2) consequent "air trapping" and mismatching of deoxygenated pulmonary blood flow with deoxygenated, rather than fresh, alveolar gas. Just as in adult emphysema, the gas-exchanging hallmark is one of hypercapnia and hypoxemia. The former usually is compensated by bicarbonate, and the latter can be palliated with an enriched oxygen environment. Treatment is similar to that of other reactive airway diseases (e.g., asthma) and currently features bronchodilators, diuretics, physiotherapy, and, increasingly, steroids. The primary care practitioner assisting in the home care of these infants needs to help the family deal with home oxygen therapy (chiefly by nasal cannula), apnea monitoring (usually by pulsed oxygen saturation or impedance monitoring) during the 4 to 6 months usually required for improvement (probably through remodeling of the growing and differentiating lung). Experience appears to indicate that oxygen saturation maintained at greater than 92% will support adequate growth and activity. During this trying period, the infant can be expected to be particularly susceptible to respiratory infections (especially respiratory syncytial virus), so that exposure to such infections should be minimized wherever possible and rehospitalization quickly entertained for possible respiratory support, should such prevention not succeed. Such attentions eventually are rewarded by normalization of the chest roentgenogram at about 2 years of age; yet abnormal small airways are detectable by certain pulmonary function tests well into adolescence, evidently more related to the fact of prematurity than to artificial ventilation therapy.[9,12,14]

Developmental Delays. Despite the frequently multiple episodes of apnea and bradycardia that characterize premature infants during their NICU stay, a happy developmental outcome for most (at least those VLBW infants >1000 g at birth) has been the gratifying norm. However, it is intraventricular hemorrhage, rather than asphyxia, that is the principal contributor to poor, even devastating, neurodevelopmental outcome[15]; this and the other developmental scars of premature birth (such as patent ductus arteriosus, surfactant deficiency, and necrotizing enterocolitis) increase in frequency with decreasing gestational age. The current biologic threshold for reasonable expectation of a *healthy* viability appears to be about 25 weeks of gestation and 750 g birth weight, if the infant is appropriately grown for gestational age.[17] Major handicaps (mental retardation, cerebral palsy, hydrocephalus, seizure disorders, sensorineural impairments) can be expected in about 30% of surviving infants below this threshold.[10,22]

The screening and more definitive tools available for assessing the extent and impact of such disabilities in these infants are the same as those developed for the general evaluation of gross and fine motor function, language skills, and social adaptation (see Chapter 18, Eleven), in addition to the more technologically based sensorineural testing procedures for touch, vision, and hearing.

Even the more horrendous developmental disabilities, once sustained, tend to be stable, rather than progressive. Infants with hydrocephalus who have shunts in place are, however, susceptible to shunt malfunction and infection. These events are so common that the neurosurgeon necessarily shares with the primary care physician the role of maintaining the shunt. Indeed, the ongoing management of shunts in these children is a paradigm for the multidisciplinary approach required to best serve all multiply handicapped children.

The government also plays a role in the multidisciplinary approach. Public Law 94-142 (Education for All Handicapped Children, 1975) stipulated the provision of special education within the school system for handicapped children and was extended by Public Law 99-457 (1986) to include infants and preschool children. It thus supports the extension of appropriate early intervention services directly to NICU graduates as they are enrolled in high-risk follow-up clinics.

Apnea/Bradycardia. Prolonged apnea has been operationally defined as a cessation of breathing for at least 20 seconds, or as a briefer episode of apnea that is associated with bradycardia, cyanosis, or pallor. Briefer episodes, as well as frank periodic breathing (similar to Cheyne-Stokes respiration), are normal features of preterm, air-breathing infants, especially those born at less than 37 weeks of gestation. Many otherwise thriving prematures are now discharged from NICUs to their homes to continue the same sort of cardiorespiratory monitoring that characterized their NICU stay (simple cardiac rate, impedance pneumography, or pulse oximetry) until their respiratory function matures (at around 40 gestational weeks of age or after about 8 alarmless weeks of monitoring, whichever comes first). Impedance pneumography is the most common (but least reliable) of these several modes, with frequent false alarms being related simply to poor electrode-skin contact.

Much emotion, but little information, has, for some years now, swirled around the presumption that infantile apnea (long or short) is related to the sudden infant death syndrome (SIDS). Parents (but not their physicians) may be excused for confusing a very large population of normal premature infants with immature respiratory systems from the (probably) very different population of infants at true risk for SIDS. These latter infants include the siblings of infants dead of SIDS, as well as babies who have suffered an acute life-threatening event (ALTE) of sudden apnea, pallor or cyanosis, limpness, and unconsciousness, and those who suffer from severe bronchopulmonary dysplasia.

The infant with an ALTE merits particular investigation to rule out gastroesophageal reflux, upper airway obstruction, seizure disorder, anemia, or other remedial disorders, before being automatically placed on a regimen of home apnea monitoring. More than a decade of such monitoring efforts have not appeared to have prevented many SIDS deaths; however, many lesser episodes of apnea may have been ameliorated.[2,21]

SUMMARY

As difficult as the VLBW infant may have been to care for within the protective shell of the NICU, the challenge presented to the family does not quickly slacken after discharge. These children are more expensive, more temperamentally "difficult,"[25] and often perceived as more vulnerable than a child of term birth. The emotional and fiscal burdens that they present often are unloaded on a shaky family structure. Simple tools for examining this structure—the Pediatric Review and Observation of Children's Environmental Support and Stimulation (PROCESS) inventory; and the Home Observation for Measurement of the Environment (HOME) inventory[7] or its office equivalent, Home Screening Questionnaire (HSQ)[11]—recently have become available to assess and follow the success of the interventional strategies used to maximize the full development of each infant's potential.[4]

The happy photographic "rogue's gallery" of NICU graduates that adorns the entrance to most such units bears smiling testimony to the level of success that can be anticipated to reward this effort.

REFERENCES

1. Allen DM et al: Mortality in infants discharged from neonatal intensive care units in Georgia, JAMA 261:1763, 1989.
2. American Academy of Pediatrics' Committee Statement: Task Force on Prolonged Infantile Apnea, Prolonged infantile apnea: 1985, Pediatrics 76:129, 1985.
3. American Academy of Pediatrics' Joint Committee on Infant Hearing: Position statement 1982, Pediatrics 70:496, 1982.
4. Barrera ME, Cunningham CE, and Rosenbaum PL: Low birth weight and home intervention strategies: preterm infants, J Dev Behav Pediatr 7:361, 1986.
5. Ben Sira I, Nissenkorn I, and Kremer I: Retinopathy of prematurity. Surv Ophthalmol 33:1, 1988.
6. Brooten D et al: A randomized clinical trial of early hospital discharge and home follow-up of very-low-birth-weight infants, N Engl J Med 315:934, 1986.
7. Casey PH et al: The clinical assessment of a child's social and physical environment during health visits, J Dev Behav Pediatr 9:333, 1988.
8. Cryotherapy for Retinopathy of Prematurity Cooperative Group: Multicenter trial of cryotherapy for retinopathy of prematurity: preliminary results, Pediatrics 81:697, 1988.
9. Fiascone JM et al: Bronchopulmonary dysplasia: review for the pediatrician, Curr Probl Pediatr 19:169, 1989.
10. Field TM et al: Teenage, lower-class, black mothers and their preterm infants: an intervention and developmental follow-up, Child Dev 51:426, 1980.
11. Frankenburg WK and Coons CE: Home Screening Questionnaire: its validity in assessing home environment, J Pediatr 108:624, 1986.
12. Galdès-Sebaldt M et al: Prematurity is associated with abnormal airway function in childhood, Pediatr Pulmonol 7:259, 1989.
13. Gibson DL et al: Retinopathy of prematurity-induced blindness: birth weight–specific survival and the new epidemic, Pediatrics 86:405, 1990.
14. Goldson E: Severe bronchopulmonary dysplasia in the very low birth weight infant: its relationship to developmental outcome, J Dev Behav Pediatr 5:165, 1984.
15. Guzzetta F et al: Periventricular intraparenchymal echodensities in the premature newborn: critical determinant of neurologic outcome, Pediatrics 78:995, 1986.
16. Hack M and Breslau N: Very low birth weight infants: effects of brain growth during infancy on intelligence quotient at 3 years of age, Pediatrics 77:196, 1986.
17. Hack M and Fanaroff AA: Outcomes of extremely-low-birth-weight infants between 1982 and 1988, N Engl J Med 321:1642, 1989.
18. Hurt H: Continuing care of the high-risk infant, Clin Perinatol 11:3, 1984.
19. Kitchen WH et al: Children of birthweight <1000 g: changing outcome between 2 and 5 years, J Pediatr 110:283, 1987.
20. Kulkarni P et al: Postneonatal infant mortality in infants admitted to a neonatal intensive care unit, Pediatrics 62:178, 1978.
21. Light MJ and Sheridan MS: Home monitoring in Hawaii: the first 1,000 patients, Hawaii Med J, 48:304, 1989.
22. McCormick MC: Long-term follow-up of infants discharged from neonatal intensive care units. JAMA 261:1767, 1989.
23. McCormick MC, Shapiro S, and Starfield BH: Rehospitalization in the first year of life for high-risk survivors, Pediatrics 66:991, 1980.
24. Medoff-Cooper B: Temperament in very low birth weight infants, Nurs Res 35:139, 1986.
25. Mutch L et al: Secular rehospitalization of very low birth weight infants, Pediatrics 78:164, 1986.
26. Nield TA et al. Unexpected hearing loss in high-risk infants, Pediatrics 78:417, 1986.
27. Office of Technology Assessment: Neonatal Care for low birthweight infants: costs and effectiveness, Health Technology Case Study 38, Pub No OTA-HCS-38, Washington, DC, 1987, US Government Printing Office.
28. Phelps DL et al: Tocopherol efficacy and safety for preventing retinopathy of prematurity: a randomized, controlled, double-masked trial, Pediatrics 79:489, 1987.
29. Saigal S et al: Follow-up of infants 501 to 1,500 gm birth weight delivered to residents of a geographically defined region with perinatal intensive care facilities, J Pediatr 100:606, 1982.
30. Wariyar UK and Sam R: Morbidity and preterm delivery: importance of 100% followup, Lancet 1:387, 1989.

SUGGESTED READINGS

Hurt H: Continuing care of the high-risk infant, Clin Perinatol 11(1), 1984.

Taeusch HW and Yogman MW: Follow-up management of the high-risk infant, Boston, 1987, Little, Brown & Co.

Section One: Psychological Development

Section Two: The Family

Section Three: School Health

Part Six

Psychosocial Issues in Child Health Care

Section Four: Childhood Behavioral Problems

Section Five: Adolescent Behavioral Problems

Section One *Psychological Development*

43

Theories and Concepts of Development As They Relate to Pediatric Practice

Olle Jane Z. Sahler

This chapter focuses on the psychological development of the child from fetal life through adolescence. For the purposes of this discussion, *psychology* is defined as that branch of science devoted to the study of emotion, cognition, and social conduct. Because the individual is part of a larger psychosocial-biologic system, the chapter incorporates discussions of heredity, environmental influences, and biologic maturation on development. Finally, two specific issues, the development of moral judgment and the development of gender identity, are examined.

There is no one unified developmental theory that, by itself, explains or defines all of the behaviors that can be observed in any particular child. Thus several theories are presented that, taken collectively, allow us to understand and interpret behaviors common to a particular developmental age. With this framework it becomes possible to devise treatment strategies that can help children and their families cope with common stressful situations effectively.

The ever-developing personality style and cognitive functioning of the pediatric patient add the burden of constant reevaluation and renegotiation to any treatment regimen, regardless of whether a child's problem is physical or a combination of physical and emotional elements. However, this very fluidity and malleability often make substantive intervention possible with the pediatric patient when it would be impossible with the adult. The ability of the practitioner to help rechannel and refocus the child's emotional energy along more constructive paths, before undesirable habits or other maladaptive behaviors become fixed, is one of the rewards of working with children. Primary prevention is a realistic goal. Conversely, the child's relatively unformed and fragile sense of self is particularly vulnerable to outside influences that might have little or no effect on the adult. Thus the practitioner has an obligation to evaluate the social network surrounding the child to identify and help eliminate impediments to the child's realization of his or her fullest potential. In this context, the practitioner as developmentalist can become a knowledgeable and effective advocate for someone who is too young, too inexperienced, and too politically naive to speak as an independent individual.

FORCES THAT INFLUENCE PSYCHOLOGICAL DEVELOPMENT

It is still unclear how much of what a child becomes as an adult is predetermined by innate capacities (heredity) and how much is the result of indoctrination and training (environment). In recent years, developmentalists have become more moderate in the nature-versus-nurture controversy; most have adopted an interactional model,[22] whereby some action of the individual or some event in the environment sets up a chain of reactions that influences and changes both the person and his or her surroundings. This interactional model helps to explain the observation that individuals evolve by successive changes that seem to be related to experience. It also permits the individual to identify desired goals with the hope that these actually can be achieved through modifying behavior.

Heredity

Temperament. Although genetic composition determines an almost infinite variety of individual characteristics, only a few, such as sex and race, have traditionally been scrutinized by psychologists. More recently, however, investigators such as Thomas and Chess[26] have identified a complex system of idiosyncratic differences in responsiveness of infants and young children that appear to be innate personality characteristics and that are persistent features of a child's behavior at least throughout the first few years of life. This collection of personal attributes has been termed *temperament,* and the following nine elements have been found to be useful descriptors of how a child behaves: (1) activity level, (2) rhythmicity, (3) approach and/or withdrawal from a new stimulus, (4) adaptability, (5) intensity of reaction,(6) threshold of responsiveness, (7) mood, (8) distractibility, and (9) attention span and persistence. It appears that most infants tend to be regular, highly adaptable, and usually positive in mood; furthermore, these traits tend to be maintained over time.

Temperamental traits give rise to parental perceptions that a particular child is "easygoing" or "difficult." Such judgments are based on the parents' observations of how the child responds to various environmental stimuli and the degree to which the child is self-sufficient in meeting his or her own needs for contentment.

Gender and birth order. Gender and position in the family have been associated with certain behavior patterns in infants. For example, in general infant boys are more irritable and become calm less easily than infant girls, and first-born boys tend to be more irritable than second-born boys. The nature-nurture interactional model of development provides an interesting explanation for these findings: the greater neurologic maturity of the girl at birth[23] (nature) may result in less spontaneous random activity, distractibility, and intensity of reaction and greater attentiveness, persistence, and rhythmicity in baseline behavior; parental response (nurture) may then reinforce some of these behaviors in accord with culturally defined gender-specific expectations (see the section on gender identity in Chapter 78, "Cross-Sex Behavior"). In other words, quiet, demure, compliant girls and alert, aggressive, intense boys may be rewarded with parental attention. Indeed, parents have been observed to treat their male and female offspring differently from birth, usually being more physically active with boys.[16,20] Thus, over time, the behavioral characteristics evident at birth may be positively reinforced by the environment to the extent that they eventually become an integral part of the child's usual way of responding to others. Fortunately, most children are seen by their parents as adaptable and regular in their responses even at birth; such positive parental perceptions of their infants facilitate their mutual interactions and help ensure that the infants receive nurturant caregiving.

Intelligence. The capacity to perceive and understand facts and to reason about them is, in large measure, genetically determined. *Intelligence* as defined in our culture is a composite of specific abilities, including verbal ability (use of language), quantitative ability (use of numbers), spatial ability (discrimination of objects in space), disembedding (separation of an element from its background), analytic ability (problem-solving), reasoning (formulation and testing of hypotheses), and mastery of concepts. Individuals are not born with all these skills, nor are they all learned during infancy. Rather, there is a gradual acquisition of skills that extends into adolescence and even into adulthood. Thus the concept of the intelligence quotient (IQ) or ratio of the cognitive maturational age (MA) to the chronologic age (CA) of the individual ($IQ = MA/CA \times 100$) has become a popular device for comparing the abilities of a given child with those of other children at a similar age. Although test interpretations vary somewhat, IQs in the range of 90 to 110 are usually considered average.

Studies[19] of the contribution of inherited or genetic factors to intelligence have focused primarily on sex and racial differences uncovered in responses to standardized tests. Although there are no consistent sex differences in total IQ scores on tests that present a balanced contribution from all the skill groups, there are sex differences in certain specific ability areas, beginning in adolescence. Thus females in general have greater verbal ability than males; conversely, males have greater visual-spatial and quantitative abilities than females. Studies[4,12,13] of children and adolescents reared in single-parent homes have shown that boys raised in father-absent homes may have more "female" cognitive traits and girls raised in mother-absent homes may have more "male" cognitive traits than sex-matched controls raised in traditional two-parent families. This finding is somewhat inconsistent and appears to depend on the child's age at the time of separation and the degree to which the same-sex parent or a replacement figure interacts with the child. However, the finding that these changes may occur even to a limited extent is important, because it points to the role of the environment in modifying what were once thought to be inherited sex-specific traits and further highlights the interaction between nature and nurture in psychological development.

Racial differences in intelligence testing have been found. Results of international studies have shown that members of Oriental populations originating in Japan and China and white populations originating in Northern Europe tend to score highest on IQ tests. These findings should be interpreted with caution. Although "global" intelligence tests have been designed to equalize the relative contributions of each of the specific skill areas in which scores vary by sex, psychologists have been less successful in devising "culture-fair" tests that can measure mental ability separately from learned cognitive skills and independently of social or economic effects. Thus it is still arguable whether differences in test scores among various population groups obtained to date reflect true superior racial ability or merely greater cultural emphasis on training in the particular skills being measured.

Environment

Although various physical, economic, and environmental conditions, including climate, nutrition, available educational opportunities, and general standard of living undoubtedly influence psychological development, they are not discussed here. However, three social environments—the family of origin, the school, and the peer group—are particularly important to the development of children and adolescents and deserve special attention here, because they are entities that can be influenced by the pediatrician in promoting the well-being of the child.

The Family. The family is the first social unit to which a child belongs. Membership in a family helps to ensure that the child is physically and emotionally nurtured. In addition, the cultural biases and beliefs of the family are transmitted to the child. The ultimate goal of the family is to produce an autonomous individual who can separate physically and emotionally from it to begin another family unit. The family as a dynamic unit of complex intergenerational relationships is discussed in Chapter 52.

The School. The two basic functions of the school are education and socialization. For some children, the first regular and routine experiences outside the home are provided by attending school.

In its role as an agent of socialization, school provides a graded transition from the circumscribed environment of the home to the world at large. This role is less well defined but equally as important as cognitive instruction. The most crucial social goals of early schooling are separation from the family, subordination of gross motor activity to decorum in the class-

Text continued on p. 526.

Table 43-1 *Psychological Development from Infancy to Young Adulthood*

	PSYCHOSEXUAL				
PERIOD	STAGE	EROGENOUS ZONE	SOURCE OF LIBIDINAL PLEASURE	CONFLICT	RESOLUTION
Infancy	Oral	Mouth	Touch; incorporation; biting	Weaning	Independence; emergence of the ego
	Anal	Anus	Expulsion; retention	Toilet-training	Self-control
Toddlerhood, preschool	Phallic	Genitalia	Masturbation	Oedipal complex	Identification with same sex parent; emergence of superego

* Modified from Erikson EH: Childhood and society, ed 2, New York, 1963, WW Norton Co.

PSYCHOSOCIAL		COGNITIVE		SOCIAL LEARNING	
STAGE	DESCRIPTION*	STAGE	DISTINGUISHING CHARACTERISTICS OF COGNITIVE FUNCTIONING	PHASE	DESCRIPTION
I Basic trust vs. basic mistrust	"Trust . . . implies not only that one has learned to rely on the sameness and continuity of the outer providers, but also that one may trust oneself. . . ."	Sensorimotor	Preverbal Reflexive activity to purposeful activity Development of object permanence and rudimentary thought	I Rudimentary behavior: initial behavioral learning	Basic need requirements met by parents Positive reinforcement is primary socializing agent
II Autonomy vs. shame and doubt	"From a sense of self-control without loss of self-esteem comes a lasting sense of good will and pride. . . ."				
III Initiative vs. guilt	". . . the child is . . . ready . . . to become bigger in the sense of sharing obligation and performance . . . (he moves) toward the possible and the tangible, which permits the dreams of early childhood to be attached to the goals of an active adult life."	Preoperational	Prelogical Inability to deal with several aspects of a problem simultaneously Development of representational language and use of symbols	II Secondary motivational systems: family-centered learning	Socialization within larger family environment Negative reinforcement introduced as socializing agent

Continued.

Table 43-1 *Psychological Development from Infancy to Young Adulthood—cont'd*

	PSYCHOSEXUAL				
PERIOD	STAGE	EROGENOUS ZONE	SOURCE OF LIBIDINAL PLEASURE	CONFLICT	RESOLUTION
School age	Latency	—	—	—	—
Adolescence/ adulthood	Genital	Genitalia	Sexual stimulation	Incest taboo; frustration of genital impulses	Selection of a hetero-sexual partner

PSYCHOSOCIAL		COGNITIVE		SOCIAL LEARNING	
STAGE	DESCRIPTION*	STAGE	DISTINGUISHING CHARACTERISTICS OF COGNITIVE FUNCTIONING	PHASE	DESCRIPTION
IV Industry vs. inferiority	". . . he now learns to win recognition by producing things."	Concrete operational	Logical Problem-solving restricted to physically present or real objects and imagery Development of logical operations (e.g., classification, conservation)	III Secondary motivational systems: extrafamilial learning	Social penetration into neighborhood and beyond Controls universally defined and internally enforced
V Identity vs. role confusion	"The sense of ego identity, then, is the accrued confidence that the inner sameness and continuity prepared in the past are matched by the sameness and continuity of one's meaning for others, as evidenced in the tangible promise of a career."	Formal operational	Abstract Comprehension of purely abstract or symbolic content Development of advanced logical operations (e.g., complex analogy, induction, deduction, higher mathematics)		
VI Intimacy vs. isolation	". . . the young adult, emerging from the search for and the insistence on identity, is eager and willing to fuse his identity with that of others. He is ready for intimacy. . . ."				

room, mastery of those fine motor skills that are prerequisites to learning to read and write, and initiation of certain habits that are important to the educational process, such as cooperation, successful completion of tasks, and respect for others.

By the late elementary grades, competition and achievement become prominent aspects of school life. Differences in innate ability and degree of motivation (derived both from self and the environment) determine a student's achievement level. Problems that can arise as a consequence of each of these psychosocial challenges, their effects on learning, and possible solutions are discussed in detail in the section on "School Health."

The Peer Group. Although the family of origin has the greatest influence on development of the individual as a person who relates to others, and the school has the greatest influence on how an individual handles setting and attaining goals, the peer group is the major ongoing source of influence on overt behavior throughout life beyond infancy. Peers model behavior, help determine value systems, and provide the security of group identity not only for the school-age child and adolescent but for the adult as well.

The earliest peer group is the sibling subsystem of the family; unlike later associations, membership in this group is immutable despite those occasional conflicts that are of such magnitude that they would sever ties of mere friendship. The earliest peer interactions occur at about 6 months of age, when infants placed together look at and may approach and explore one another for a few seconds.[11] These interactions increase in duration and complexity. Complementary and reciprocal social play emerges by about 1 year; social pretend play appears at about 2 years; and most children have developed a characteristic way of relating to their peers, independently seeking friendships and engaging in social activities, by about 3 years of age. Most early friendships are based on proximity (the child next door). Later, the classroom is the source of many friends. Finally, friendships become defined by mutual interests.

As might be expected, friendships become more enduring as children grow older. For example, it is common for friendships of older school-age children to remain stable over the course of a school year.[3] Those friendships perceived as intimate are most likely to endure, and good friends tend to be of similar age and peer status. The key determinants of friendship formation include common interests and the clarity of the intent of both verbal and nonverbal communication. Self-disclosure of feelings and of private thoughts, especially among girls, contributes to the bond between friends. Children also come to value mutual respect and loyalty. Whereas younger friends, especially boys, tend to be competitive with one another, older friends seek equality through sharing.

During adolescence the peer group becomes more influential than the family with regard to social activity and the development of value systems. In some instances adolescents deliberately choose a peer group with social values that are antithetical to those of the parents, so that through the process of strong group identification, they can separate from the family—a major goal of late adolescence. This period is conflict ridden, and some of the habits adopted by youth can be antisocial and self-destructive (see Chapter 95).

THEORIES OF DEVELOPMENT

Even seemingly bizarre behavior can become understandable when we know why a child acts as he or she does. Because there is no single theory that explains all aspects of psychological (emotional, cognitive, and social) development, it has become customary to examine behavior from the perspective of several viewpoints. Although cumbersome at times, this approach is analogous to that of physiologic systems, in which an observable process occurs as a result of, for example, a combination of biochemical and anatomic events. Each can be explained but only in terms defined by its own particular basic science.

In psychology, there are many schools of thought (basic sciences) regarding development. However, we will focus only on three major theoretic frameworks: psychodynamic theory (Freud and psychosexual development, Erikson and psychosocial development), cognitive-intellectual theory (Piaget), and learning theory (Skinner and conditioning, Sears and social learning). Each approaches human development from different perspectives (psychodynamic: relationship and motivation; cognitive-intellectual: thought process and content; learning theory: observable behavior). Each approach has its own vocabulary and set of processes. Interestingly, each of these theories relies on the presence of certain primitive instinctual behaviors that are operative at birth and later modified by the environment. Given our original definition of psychology as the study of emotion, cognition, and social conduct, we immediately see that each theory is incomplete; taken collectively, however, they complement each other. Table 43-1 provides a summary of psychological development from these perspectives from childhood through young adulthood.

Psychodynamic Theory

Freud and Psychosexual Development. The theory of psychosexual development is derived from Freud's in-depth examination and retrospective analysis of childhood behaviors he thought might have contributed to the neuroses for which his patients, as adults, were seeking treatment. Based on the contents of memories supplied by his patients, Freud theorized that personality formation results from those intrapsychic struggles between polar forces experienced by an individual as he or she matures. This particular approach and the theoretic framework derived from it are limited in that (1) objective observations of current behavior are lacking and (2) heavy focus is placed on explanations for the development of undesirable adult behaviors rather than on behaviors in general. Despite these shortcomings, Freud and his work have had a formidable influence on generations of developmental psychologists.

The family triad of mother-father-child and, in particular, the early mother-child dyad were central to Freud's investigation, interpretation, and explanation of later adult behaviors. Although pediatric psychology currently focuses largely on the individual in relation to a broader social unit than the family and on coping mechanisms (positive management strategies in stressful situations) rather than on defense mechanisms (often interpreted as negative management strategies), elements of freudian theory are represented in or are the foundation of a variety of other major developmental theories. Similarly, Freud's discussions of both conscious and unconscious factors that motivate observable behavior provide a unique framework for understanding otherwise apparently inexplicable conduct.

The total personality as conceived by Freud consists of three parts or motivating forces—the id, the ego, and the superego. The *id* is the foundation of the personality; its aim is to avoid pain, find satisfaction or pleasure, and maintain constancy in the midst of internal or external disturbance.

The *ego*, that part of the personality most visible to the external world, is the intermediary system between the id and reality; it provides the individual with an accurate perception of what exists in the environment. On some occasions, fulfillment of pleasure as desired by the id may be temporarily suspended by the ego in acknowledgment of reality.

The *superego* is the moral function of the personality; it is concerned with strivings for perfection rather than for pleasure or for responses to reality. Freud further divided the superego into the *ego ideal*, the conception of what is morally good, and *conscience*, the conception of what is morally bad. To the superego, thought is synonymous with action; therefore feelings of guilt or satisfaction may be experienced merely by thinking something "bad" or "good." Clinically, this has relevance to psychosomatic illness, which is considered by psychoanalysts to be an example of pain or dysfunction resulting from the superego's displeasure with the individual.

Although behavior can be motivated by the drive to fulfill a variety of needs (e.g., food, sleep), the major motivational system according to the psychosexual theory of development is libido, or the instinctual (sexual) drive to preserve the species. Satisfaction of the sexual instinct is derived from stimulation or manipulation of both genital and nongenital body regions that have been termed *erogenous zones*. Three primary erogenous zones, each with its associated vital need and presented in the order in which each gains prominence, are (1) the mouth and eating, (2) the anus and elimination, and (3) the genitalia and reproduction. According to Freud, the action an individual takes to reduce tension (derive pleasure) in an erogenous zone may or may not actually fufill the vital need associated with that area (e.g., both eating and nonnutrient thumb-sucking may produce pleasure in the oral area).

Activities involving the erogenous zones may bring the child into conflict with the parents. The resulting frustrations and anxieties associated with these conflicts lead to the development of a number of adaptive maneuvers or defense mechanisms such as repression, regression, denial, projection, intellectualization, and sublimation. Resolution of the conflict associated with a given stage allows the individual to progress onto the next (higher) developmental stage. Freud conceptualized five psychosexual stages: oral, anal, phallic, latency, and genital. Full maturation of psychosexual development is thought to occur in late adolescence or early adulthood with the establishment of a stable heterosexual relationship.

Erikson and Psychosocial Development. Whereas Freud focused on the intrinsic development of the individual, especially as it is shaped by the triadic relationship of the child with his or her parents, Erikson focused on the development of the individual within the wider context of his or her historical-cultural-social milieu. For Erikson, unconscious motivation (id) exists, but it is the process of socialization that facilitates development and determines an individual's outcome. Unlike Freud, Erikson studied individuals and their families within the spheres of their everyday lives and at a particular moment in their cultural history. Also, unlike freudian theory, Erikson's theory focuses with optimism on an individual's potential for mastery by successfully resolving developmental crises rather than with pessimism on the potential for dysfunction from persistent psychological conflict.

Two assumptions underlie Erikson's construction[7] of the theory of psychosocial development:

> (1) That the human personality . . . develops according to steps predetermined in the growing person's readiness to be driven toward, to be aware of, and to interact with a widening social radius; and (2) that society . . . tends to be so constituted as to meet and invite this succession of potentialities for interaction and attempts to safeguard and to encourage the proper rate and the proper sequence of their unfolding.

Thus Erikson postulates a close, sequentially patterned mutual relationship between individual capabilities and environmental demands. An individual cannot develop outside of or beyond the readiness of his or her social context, nor can society progress independent of the individual.

Erikson conceived eight ages in human life; these represent a reformulation and extension of Freud's five psychosexual stages of development. However, whereas psychosexual theory postulates that the individual attains full developmental maturity at entry into the genital stage, which begins during adolescence or young adulthood, psychosocial theory postulates the continuation of substantial developmental change throughout all of life. The first six Eriksonian ages are easily associated with their corresponding freudian stages: basic trust versus basic mistrust (oral), autonomy versus shame and doubt (anal), initiative versus guilt (phallic), industry versus inferiority (latency), and identity versus role confusion and intimacy versus isolation (genital). The last two ages, generativity versus stagnation and ego integrity versus despair, have no one-to-one correspondence in freudian theory and deal with specific developmental crises of middle and old age.

Cognitive-Intellectual Theory

Piaget and Cognitive Development. Cognition is the means by which an individual accumulates organized knowledge about of the world and uses that knowledge to solve problems and modify behavior. Whereas the psychodynamic schools of developmental theory are concerned primarily with issues of motivation as a force for change, the cognitive-intellectual theory is centered almost exclusively on the process of acquiring and using knowledge. Piaget, although influenced by Freud and tacitly subscribing to the notion that why a child learns is a valid question, did not (himself) critically investigate this issue. Rather, his research largely ignores emotion and motivation and concentrates instead on the organizational structure of cognitive functioning and how it influences understanding and therefore behavior.

According to piagetian theory, cognitive development is the result of neurophysiologic maturation, environmental stimulation, experience, and constant internal cognitive reorganization. Two major principles form the framework for Piaget's theory: (1) there is a tendency for all species to *organize* or order their activities in a hierarchical fashion and (2) there is a tendency for all species to *adapt* through assimilation (incorporating new information or unfamiliar objects into an already existing idea about the world) and accommodation (changing ideas about the world and behavior in response to new knowledge or situations). For example, if an infant is handed a set of small blocks for the first time, he or she may bite or shake them (assimilation). Once being shown or discovering that they can be used to build a tower, the child changes his or her behavior and builds towers each time blocks are presented (accommodation).

As is true of all developmentally based psychological theories, Piaget's theory is premised on a stepwise, ordered sequence of learning in response to experience. He defined four discrete stages of cognitive development between birth and adulthood: sensorimotor, preoperational, concrete operational, and formal operational. The exact chronologic age at which certain abilities are attained depends on factors such as individual differences in physiologic functioning, experience, and environment. Transitional periods, during which children exhibit some, but not all, characteristics of the next higher stage of thinking exist between developmental phases. Teaching during these times may result in the rapid acquisition of new cognitive skills. Although the concept of transitional periods is not unique to piagetian theory, the nature of Piaget's particular investigational techniques for studying concept mastery is better defined than those which can be employed to test, for example, the psychoanalytic theories; thus they lend themselves to more precise analysis and staging.

Learning Theory

Learning theory is an outgrowth of behaviorism, or stimulus-response psychology. The following are several basic principles of learning theory:

1. Behavior is learned; however, genetic factors and innate, involuntary reflexive behaviors influence this learning.
2. All types, patterns, and combinations of behavior can be learned as long as they are not physically incompatible.
3. Behavior can be conditioned.
4. Behavior can be shaped.
5. Behavior is learned through reinforcement, which may be internal or external and positive or negative.
6. Learning results from many independent processes, including observation and imitation.

There are two ways in which behavior can be conditioned. In the process of classical conditioning, usually associated with the Russian physiologist Pavlov, a reflex response associated in nature with one stimulus can be modified in such a way that it can be evoked by another stimulus. In Pavlov's original experiment, reflexive salivation in a dog at the sight of food could be induced eventually merely by the sound of a ringing bell, which over a period of time had been "paired" with eating. (Interestingly, the saliva evoked by the ringing bell differed slightly in chemical content from naturally occurring saliva.)

In the process of instrumental conditioning, a nonreflexive behavior is learned because it is positively reinforced. For example, in an experiment, a rat in a cage might, by chance, depress a lever. If a pellet of food is released each time this occurs, the rat will "learn" to depress the lever and will do so with increasing frequency, especially when hungry.

There are several features of conditioned behavior that are important from a clinical point of view. Conditioned behavior can be *extinguished,* or undone, by repeatedly failing to reinforce it; it can be *inhibited,* or counteracted, by the individual to avoid punishment; it can be *partially reinforced* by inconsistent or random responses; it can be *generalized* so that a variety of similar stimuli will elicit the same response; and it can be made *discriminatory* so that by selective reinforcement only one (or a few) specific stimuli elicit the response.

Reinforcement is a key element in learning behavior theory. According to the theoretic framework, the individual is motivated to perform a certain behavior because of the positive effect (reward) derived from it or to not perform a certain behavior either because of the negative effect derived from it (punishment) or because some other behavior gives more benefit. Thus giving a neutral response (not reinforcing, ignoring) or negatively reinforcing a behavior leads ultimately to the behavior's being extinguished. A consistent response, whether it is positively or negatively reinforcing, leads to the most rapid learning.

Shaping is the process of molding a given behavior to be more like a desired behavior. This is accomplished by positively reinforcing successive approximations of the desired behavior. A classic example of this has been described by Baldwin[2] in his recounting of the work of B.F. Skinner:

> When Skinner wants to teach a pigeon to hit a ping pong ball through a pair of goal posts by pecking at it, he can't wait until the pigeon just happens to do so. He begins by reinforcing the pigeon whenever it is within a certain distance of the ball. The pigeon gradually learns to stay close to the ball. The experimenter now reinforces the pigeon only when he is close to the ball and looking in its direction, thus teaching the pigeon to keep his eye on the ball. In the next stage, the experimenter requires the pigeon to peck at the ball to receive a reinforcement. Finally, the pigeon must peck the ball in the right direction.

In the strictest sense, learning theory, in and of itself, is not a developmental theory because there is no intrinsic sequential order or hierarchical staging to learning behavior as long as the individual has the neurophysiologic maturation to be physically able to perform the desired task. However, a group of early workers in the field sought to incorporate psychoanalytic hypotheses (both psychosexual and psychosocial) into explanations for certain observable behaviors. This group became known as the *school of social learning theory.*

An important aspect of social learning theory is its attention to the dyadic nature of human behavior. Thus the child is in constant interaction with his or her environment and other individuals in that environment. The child's response to an environmental stimulus acts as a stimulus itself, thus evoking a response from the environment, and so on. In turn, the child's development of new levels of functioning depends on the ability of the environment to shape the child's behavior so that it conforms with increasing regularity to what will eventually be expected from him or her as an adult. This transactional scheme is in keeping with current general psychological theories that highlight the interactional quality of developmental processes, and the individual-society dyad is highly reminiscent of Erikson's psychosocial theory.

In the foregoing discussion of learning theory, desired behaviors were viewed as being obtained through some direct effect on the performer. Learning also occurs indirectly through observation and imitation. In *observational learning* the individual watches others and modifies his or her behavior in accord with the rewards and punishments others receive. *Imitative learning* is rooted in the process of identification (Freud). The child acts like (i.e., copies) a desired model (e.g., mother or father) and is positively reinforced with rewards that are either internal (being proud of oneself) or external (being praised by others). Both observational and imitative learning are particularly common in social groups.

THE RELATION BETWEEN PHYSIOLOGIC AND PSYCHOLOGICAL DEVELOPMENT

In this section we examine the child at different chronologic ages, beginning with parental response to pregnancy and its potential effects on the child's later psychological development.

Because the basic premise of the developmental theories presented is that innate, involuntary reflexive behavior is the foundation on which all future behaviors are built, psychological development is heavily dependent on physiologic (especially neurologic and sexual) maturation. Thus the physical capacities of an individual at any point in time help to determine the extent of interaction he or she will have with the environment.

Several important principles of physical development that bear directly on psychological development can be summarized as follows:

1. Development is a continuous process that begins at conception. Birth is merely an event in the natural course of development, although it signals the beginning of the individual's ability to cope independently with the environment.
2. The sequence of development of the individual as a whole and of each of the organ systems is unchanging, although the rate at which development occurs is highly variable and maturation may occur at various times in different systems.
3. Development of both involuntary (autonomic) and voluntary activity is intimately related to the maturation of the nervous systems.
4. Certain primitive reflexes (stepping, grasping) must be "lost" before the corresponding voluntary (learned) movement is acquired.
5. Development occurs in a cephalocaudal direction.

Pregnancy

The bonds of attachment that will eventually be formed between the infant and its caregivers are initiated during pregnancy. According to Mary Ainsworth,[1] attachment is an emotional tie that one person has with another that persists even when they are apart and that lasts over time. By this definition, one can be attached to more than one person but not to many people at one time. In addition, attachment implies emotion. Although the emotions of attachment are complex and vary from time to time, in general, positive feelings toward the other person predominate, and attachment is thought of as implying feelings of affection or love.

"Precursors of attachment" are physical and psychosocial changes that occur in couples anticipating and preparing for the birth of their child. These changes have been better researched in pregnant women, but recent studies[27] suggest that expectant fathers also experience emotional change and psychological readjustment and share many of the same feelings as expectant mothers.

For those who have difficulty conceiving, unconscious expectations may begin well in advance of conception and be heightened by family and social factors. More commonly, however, anticipatory or expectant behavior begins, at least consciously, at the time the pregnancy first becomes known. Examples of such behavior include changes in social patterns associated with the physical demands of pregnancy, alterations in the family's economic planning, and preparation for the child by the accumulation of various material goods. On another level, many expectant parents report a heightened sense of responsibility to keep the mother (and therefore the fetus) well and fit (such as abstaining from tobacco, drugs, or alcohol) and to protect the father (such as increasing use of seat belts while riding in a car). Planning for the future of someone else who will be totally dependent on them becomes a major preoccupation of the pregnant couple.

During pregnancy, a woman concurrently experiences two types of developmental change: physical and emotional changes within herself and the growth of the fetus. Two adaptive tasks face the pregnant woman: acceptance of the pregnancy and perception of the fetus as an individual.

Most women report strong emotional swings that vary from positive to negative anticipation; frequently they feel ambivalent about the pregnancy. Perceiving the fetus as an individual usually commences with quickening. If the original reaction to the pregnancy was predominantly negative (unplanned, unwanted), many women report heightened acceptance and noticeable changes in attitude when fetal movement is first felt. After quickening, women usually begin to have fantasies about the infant, including those of physical and personality characteristics they hope the child will have.[14]

Most likely every couple has some kind of fantasy, regardless of how vehemently they may deny it or how carefully they attempt to avoid it. Sex preference is probably the most common; but inherent in all individuals is the wish to have progeny who will be a credit to them, carry on tradition, excel in some activity, and be attractive, good, and healthy. As the time of delivery approaches, this last concern, to have a healthy baby, appears to increase in importance. Thus, should a child be born with a congenital defect, life threatening or not, the parents actually suffer the loss of their "expected" child, and an extended period of time may pass before they can reorganize their expectations and accept their child.

The Birthing Process

Data relating to the birthing process suggest that mothers who are relaxed during labor and who have a supportive person (whether family, friend, or a lay volunteer helper) assisting them are more likely to have a shorter period of labor and to be more alert and interactive with (stroke, smile, talk to) their infant on first sight.[24] Unconsciousness during birth does not seem to lead to rejection of the infant, although systematic studies in this important area are lacking. What is known, however, is that the more difficult the labor, the less likely the mother is to breast-feed.

Various delivery procedures and anesthetics also appear to have an impact on both the mother and child at birth. An infant who is in a physiologically depressed state because of administration of a narcotic agent to the mother just before or during delivery is more likely to respond poorly on initial contact or during feedings and thus is less stimulating to the mother.

Research[9] on the behavior of fathers toward the newborn has shown that engrossment, absorption, and preoccupation with the infant occur in men as well as in women. A sense of increased self-esteem also has been reported among new fathers.[9]

The Immediate Postpartum Period

The time immediately after birth has been termed the *maternal sensitive period.*[14] Mother-infant interaction is truly reciprocal. The mother supplies touch, eye-to-eye (en face) contact, high-pitched voice, heat, and odor; the infant supplies eye-to-eye contact, odor, entertainment, and, if nursing at the breast, stimulation of maternal production of prolactin and oxytocin.

The mother's behaviors match certain infant needs. For example, the female voice is naturally high pitched and consciously made more so by the mother. This fits the infant's sensitive auditory perception and attraction to speech in the high-frequency range. The odor of the mother also appears to affect the infant. It has been found that infants can discriminate their own mother's axillary odor[5] and the smell of their own mother's breast milk from those of other women.

The infant's reflexive behaviors (crying, sucking, following, and clinging) are care-eliciting behaviors; that is, they serve the function of ensuring the survival of the individual by bringing the caregiver closer to the child and helping to maintain physical and emotional contact between them by mutual reinforcement. Thus parental reinforcement behaviors (feeding, fondling) in response to the child's care-eliciting behaviors lead to further sucking, following, and clinging. In this way, the infant's innate behaviors and the responses they generate in the caregiver form the basis of that special relationship that eventually becomes true attachment.

Certain factors can impede the development of attachment. For example, the provocative stimulus of the young infant's intense gaze is missing if the child is blind. Variations of normal behavior, such as an infant who does not cling but rather stiffens on being held, may be a response to anxiety in the caregiver or a demonstration of a particular temperament type. A psychological impediment to attachment is the tendency of some parents to identify their own or another's undesirable traits in the infant, thus hindering bond formation through the mechanism of projective identification.

Infancy

The period of infancy, which extends from birth to 24 months of age, is most logically divided at 12 months. The first year is marked by tremendous physical growth and the development of rudimentary skills, culminating in the ability to walk several steps unassisted and to speak about three to six intelligible words.

The second year is characterized by skill refinement to the point where some children can pedal a tricycle and speak in relatively complete, although syntactically poor, sentences. Infants also learn that other individuals inhabit their world and that these individuals, most notably family members, come and go and return again. Lastly, they learn that they have a will and can purposefully manipulate their environment rather than be merely its captive.

Intricately interwoven with somatic growth is the differentiation and beginning emotional maturation of the individual. Of the many events taking place, two principal psychological tasks are mastered within the period of infancy: attachment (first year) and separation (second year).

Attachment is not dependent on the infant's perceiving the attachment figure as separate from self and actually is facilitated by the newborn's earliest perception of the caregiver as an extension of self. Indeed, *bonding,* an early manifestation of attachment, is usually discussed with reference to mother-child interactions in the newborn period. Thus, recognition of potential impediments to bonding (use of anesthesia or narcotics, separation of mother and infant) have led to major changes in obstetric and newborn care. However, true attachment is such an important element for successful growth and development that it is "overdetermined"; that is, many opportunities, over time, are available to facilitate and cement formation, not only with the mother but with other significant caregivers as well. Attachment to the father, for example, is thought to occur at about 7 months of age. Interestingly, the infant's expectations for the father's behavior are different from those expected of the mother; and fathers do, in fact, act differently, providing less predictable and rhythmic and more exciting physical and auditory stimulation than do mothers.[17,18] Despite these differences, however, as well as despite the smaller amount of time fathers typically spend with infants, attachment between the infant and any caregiver takes place and is strengthened by continued mutual reinforcement.

If we assume that object permanence (out of sight but not out of mind) is a prerequisite for the formation of true attachment, attachment between the infant and caregiver probably does not occur before 6 to 8 months of age. At this age, the infant and caregiver can continually derive enough positive reinforcement from each other so that periods of negative feedback do not interrupt the essential tie; that is, true attachment has not taken place if it remains tenuous and dependent on constant positive reinforcement.

Separation is a direct extension of attachment because without attachment there is no separation; rather, there is merely movement from one more or less contiguous relationship to another. Just as positive affect usually is associated with attachment, negative affect usually is associated with separation.

Separation anxiety occurs after the child becomes able to recognize and discriminate among individuals. It is manifested by various degrees of crying and withdrawal when the attachment figure is not present. Closely allied with separation anxiety is *stranger anxiety*—that is, fear of someone unfamiliar to or not closely associated with the infant regularly or daily. A stranger, however, is reasonably well tolerated when a familiar caregiver who apparently is viewed by the infant as providing protection and security also is present.

Psychosexual Development: Oral and Anal Stages. In freudian or psychosexual terms, the child younger than 12 months of age is considered to be in the *oral phase* of development, so termed because the mouth is the primary source of tension and pleasure. Satisfaction of hunger, as well as many of the comforting maneuvers provided by both the child and the caregiver (such as finger-sucking and object-sucking), center around stimulation of the mouth.

The mouth has at least five primary modes of functioning that, in analytic theory, are prototypes for certain later personality types: (1) taking in (acquisitiveness), (2) holding on (tenacity), (3) biting (destructiveness), (4) spitting out (rejection), and (5) closing (negativism). Whether any of these traits actually become part of the mature personality is thought to depend on the amount of anxiety or frustration the individual experiences in his or her original encounter with a particular function. For example, abrupt weaning may lead to a strong tendency to hold onto things; or a child who is oral-aggressive and bites with his or her teeth may become an adult who is oral-aggressive and "bites" with sarcasm.

The infant depends on someone else, usually the mother, for relief from oral distress and fulfillment of oral pleasure. The mother can control the infant's conduct by giving or withholding food. Typically, food becomes equated with love and approval of the mother. Weaning from the breast or bottle, a natural developmental stage, is also a point of conflict because it can be experienced by the infant as rejection or disapproval by the mother. In psychoanalytic theory, successful resolution of this conflict occurs when the infant, developing a sense of separate individuality, learns to satisfy needs through his or her own personal effort. This is in contrast to the so-called oral-dependent character style, which can arise when this conflict is not adequately resolved; it is typified by the person who expects others to provide things when he or she is good and withhold or take away things when he or she is bad.

During the second year of life the infant moves into the *anal stage* of psychosexual development. Tensions arise in the anal region as the result of the accumulation of fecal material. Expulsion brings relief. It is hypothesized that as a consequence of experiencing a pleasant reduction in tension from elimination, the infant may use this action to reduce tensions arising in other parts of the body. Expulsive elimination is thus considered the prototype for emotional outbursts, temper tantrums, rages, and other primitive discharge reactions.

Usually, during the second to fourth year of life, involuntary expulsive reflexes are brought under voluntary control through a set of experiences known as toilet-training. This is usually the first crucial experience the child has with discipline and external authority. It represents a conflict between instinct and an external barrier.

The methods employed by caregivers in training the child and their attitudes about defecation, cleanliness, control, and responsibility are thought to leave indelible imprints on the forming personality structure. For example, if the method of training is strict and punitive, the child may react by soiling intentionally. When older, the child may react to authority figures by being messy, disorderly, or irresponsible. Because there is pleasure in both retention and expulsion, psychoanalysts have postulated that those who derive pleasure from holding back feces and become fixated on this form of erotic pleasure may develop interests in collecting objects. Those who derive pleasure from expulsion may feel impelled to give objects away.

Psychosocial Development: Basic Trust Versus Basic Mistrust and Autonomy Versus Shame and Guilt. In psychosocial or eriksonian terms, the infant faces the tasks of the first two of the eight stages of human development. The first task, occurring during the first year, is *developing a sense of basic trust and overcoming a sense of mistrust*. According to Erikson, to do this the young infant needs to experience a mutually satisfying relationship based on familiarity, regularity, and predictability. The development of trust initially requires a feeling of physical comfort, which then promotes emotional comfort. If this feeling of comfort is achieved, the infant will become trusting even in new situations because of confidence that the environment will be supportive and helpful in meeting new challenges. If, however, the infant experiences physical discomfort or is uncertain about whether needs will be met (because responses elicited from the environment are unpredictable), new experiences will be faced with apprehension or mistrust. Thus developing a sense of confidence in the well-intentioned motives of others (motives that he or she also eventually learns to emulate) is the foundation for success in future relationships and endeavors.

Basic trust is mutual and, according to Erikson[7]:

> implies not only that one has learned to rely on the sameness and continuity of the outer providers, but also that one may trust oneself and the capacity of one's own organs to cope with urges; and that one is able to consider oneself trustworthy enough so that the providers will not need to be on guard lest they be nipped.

Thus unlike the emphasis placed on food and physical nurturance by Freud, Erickson emphasizes the sense of trust that the child develops. Such a sense of trust depends on the overall physical and emotional quality of the maternal or, more broadly, caregiving relationship that the infant has with the total environment.

Basic trust is the foundation of true attachment, and basic trust cannot be complete until there has been significant and sufficient testing. Erikson[7] describes this vividly: "The constant tasting and testing of the relationship . . . meets its crucial test during the rages of the biting stage, when the teeth cause pain from within and when outer friends either prove of no avail or withdraw from the only action which promises relief: biting."

The second eriksonian stage of psychosocial development, *autonomy versus shame and doubt,* is analogous to the anal stage of freudian psychology. It begins in infancy but is not fully realized until toddlerhood. Erikson notes that muscular maturation during this time is an important element for experimentation with two simultaneous sets of social modalities: holding on and letting go.

With increasing control over both self and the environment, the child begins to experiment with manipulation and control. At times the child is successful and at other times not. The manner in which successes and failures are met by caregivers becomes decisive in the early formation of freedom of self-expression and its suppression. "From a sense of self-control without loss of self-esteem comes a lasting sense of good will and pride; from a sense of loss of self-control and of foreign overcontrol comes a lasting propensity for doubt and shame."[7]

Cognitive Development: Sensorimotor Period. According to piagetian theory, the child from birth to approximately 2 years of age is in the *sensorimotor stage,* manifested by sensory exploration, the attainment of purposeful movement, repetition of activities, manipulation of the environment, and imitation. Although the infant is largely preverbal throughout this period, the development of instrumental language (the use of words to indicate wants or needs or to identify objects) occurs toward the end of this phase.

The sensorimotor period can be divided into six stages: stage 1—the infant initially depends heavily on reflex activity, which is modified by experience (e.g., rooting evolves into active searching for the nipple); stage 2—the infant can anticipate (e.g., make sucking movements at the sight of the bottle); stage 3—the infant attempts to imitate familiar behavior (e.g., clapping hands in imitation of the mother); stage 4—the infant can act purposefully (e.g., remove an obstacle to a goal); stage 5—the infant is interested in producing novel behaviors (e.g., trying new methods to remove an obstacle to a goal); and stage 6 (transition phase)—the infant or child begins to think about problems, to imitate an absent model from memory, and to use words to designate ongoing events, immediate desires, or objects that are present. In addition, the child has a fully developed sense of object permanence; that is, he or she will look for a vanished object even if it has been displaced. Thus the child appears to understand that things exist independently of the self.

Social Learning Development: Rudimentary Behavior Phase. The social learning theorists describe infancy as the period during which basic needs are met and initial learning takes place within the intimate environment of the home. Positive reinforcement in the form of attention (feeding, comforting) is the predominant mode used by the family to shape the infant's behavior. Reflexive activities (grasping in response to a parental finger in the infant's palm) are rewarded (parent plays with the infant's hand, talks, and coos; i.e., gives attention). In time, true grasp is learned and is followed by lifting the arms as a signal to be played with or to be held. Thus a naturally occurring primitive reflex evolves into a purposeful activity. A further step takes place during later infancy when the child begins to be able to modify behavior in response to signals that are not directly or immediately physically rewarding (e.g., a smile rather than actually being held). Sensitivity to nonphysical as well as physical cues is the foundation for the social component of human learning. In freudian and eriksonian terms, such responsiveness to the environment and acknowledgment that we are only part of it mark the *development of the ego.*

Toddlerhood and Preschool Age (2 to 5 Years)

During the toddler stage, the growth rate slows, personality develops further, and important strides are made in cognitive ability. Bowel and bladder control usually occurs during the third year, although the range extends from 15 months to 4 years and sometimes beyond.

Many interactions among the various aspects of development take place during this period. For example, what the child can physically do influences perception of self, which in turn influences social development and independence. The positive feedback loop of testing leading to success, leading to confidence, leading to further testing is particularly significant in this stage of rapid achievement of milestones.

Psychosexual Development: Phallic Stage. According to Freud, during the late preschool period the child is preoccupied with his or her genitalia as a body area from which pleasure is derived through self-stimulation. This masturbatory drive is different from the sexual drive of the later genital stage characteristic of adolescence and adulthood, even though the same erogenous zone is involved. The basic innocence of this behavior in both boys and girls deserves repeated emphasis, especially to parents who may be unduly concerned or disturbed by it.

According to Freud, during the *phallic stage* both boys and girls experience a period of intense attachment to the parent of the opposite sex and hostility toward the same-sex parent. This situation has been termed the *oedipal complex* after the mythologic Greek character who killed his father and married his mother. The sex-specific rivalries are the oedipal conflict (males) and the Electra conflict (females).

Before the phallic stage the mother is the primary love object for both boys and girls. During the phallic stage the boy develops a more intense relationship with his mother and becomes jealous of and rivalrous with his father for his mother's attention. Conversely, the girl begins to pursue her father, relying on him to be her ally against the mother. Such behavior can produce consternation within the family unit if the parents do not appreciate the reason for—indeed, the universality of—such alliances. Conflict resolution begins when the child recognizes the futility of his or her desires and, instead of wishing to take the place of the same-sex parent, moves in the direction of trying to become more like him or her. This process, by which boys desire to become more like men in their self-concept and girls desire to become more like women, has been termed *identification.* It includes the incorporation of many of the same-sex parent's qualities into the child's own personality. Resolution of this stage is complete when incorporation of parental qualities (internalization of parental controls) is sufficient for what Freud has termed *superego formation,* or the development of conscience. That is, the child develops a rudimentary sense of right and wrong based on instruction by and modeling of the parent.

Freud assumed that all people are constitutionally bisexual and that the tendencies of both sexes are inherited by each child. Furthermore, he also hypothesized that a child experiences some degree of identification with each parent. Ultimately, the degree of masculinity or femininity that the child will display in later life depends on the relative strengths of his or her innate masculine or feminine tendencies, the degree to which these tendencies are rewarded or inhibited, and the strength of identification he or she has with each parent.

Psychosocial Development: Initiative Versus Guilt. Erikson perceived children in the *initiative versus guilt stage* to be moving into a larger social environment in which they are able to initiate new activities. Occasionally, the sense of personal autonomy they had developed previously is challenged or frustrated by the autonomous activity of others. The ensuing conflict may lead to a sense of guilt for having gone too far in striving for initiative. This sense of guilt is overcome by learning self-modulation through the development of a conscience that reflects parental and therefore social values. Thus, without denegrating themselves, children begin to learn to put personal and social needs into perspective and to modify the one to be in concert with the other.

Cognitive Development: Preoperational Period. Extending from 2 to 7 years of age, the *preoperational period,* as defined by Piaget, is distinguished by the appearance of representational language and rudimentary reasoning. Problem-solving during this period is intuitive rather than logical, and the child cannot explain his or her reasoning strategies.

The thought processes of the preoperational child are limited by centration (the inability to consider several aspects or dimensions of a situation simultaneously), syncretism (the tendency to group several apparently unrelated things or events together into a confused whole), juxtaposition (the failure to perceive the real connection among several things or events), irreversibility (the inability to understand successive changes or transformations), egocentrism (perception of the world only from his or her own point of view or the belief that he or she is the origin of all actions in the world), and magical thinking (the equation of thought and fantasy with action; i.e., feeling that a wish can cause some external event).

The thought content of the preoperational child is influenced by animism (the belief that inanimate objects are alive as people are alive), artificialism (the belief that all things are made for a purpose), and participation (the belief that there is some continuing connection or interaction between human actions and natural processes).

Social Learning Development: Phase of Secondary Motivational Systems; Family-Centered Learning. As the child becomes able to move within a larger environment, a greater number of individuals are available to serve as models and reinforcers of behavior. In addition, negative reinforcement (punishment) is introduced as an agent for modifying the child's behavior. Discipline that is either too prescriptive or too indulgent can produce a child who has no internal sense of responsibility for personal actions. In the first instance, the child relies on the environment to provide all cues about what is or is not acceptable. In the latter instance, excessive indulgence provides such insufficient cueing that the child does not learn to distinguish right from wrong.

It is at this age that negative attention-seeking behaviors become common. These are most often seen in situations in which the child, who has become accustomed to reinforcement as a method of guiding behavior, becomes frustrated by persistent nonreinforcement (such as might occur if a new infant is born into the family, diverting much of the parents' time and attention away from the preschooler). Frustration at lack of positive reinforcement for good behavior may lead to bad behavior that demands attention, negative though it is. The child may learn, in time, to use even violent behavior to meet needs for attention, despite the attention elicited being disapproving, deprecating, or punitive. Although some children may fear the punishment they receive for their behavior, such punishment may seem preferable to feeling neglected, unimportant, or even nonexistent in their parents' lives.

School Age (6 to 12 Years)

The developmental stage between the end of toddlerhood and the onset of adolescence was termed *latency* by Freud to describe the relatively quiescent period of sexual activity between the resolution of the oedipal conflict and the emergence of the sexual drives of adolescence. Actually, the child is not really latent (present but not visible or active; i.e., dormant) at all. Nor, as we shall see, is sexual drive absent; it is, however, channeled differently.

The first major task of the latency-age child is to enter into school and achieve independence from the strict confines of home. Teachers, who are at first parent surrogates and then independent role models and authority figures, become important resources for the developing child. Teachers join with parents in setting expectations and goals for behavior and achievement.

The child of 6 years of age has the ability to perform most gross and fine motor tasks rudimentarily. Thus latency is the time when skills are refined. Progress, then, is tested not so much by the acquisition of new skills as by the rapidity and accuracy with which old skills are performed.

Skill plays an important part in the development of the emerging personality. For the child for whom physical activity is easy and therefore filled with positive reinforcement, playing games and being a member of the team bring pleasure and friendship. For the child for whom physical activity does not come easily, there is less, if any, positive reinforcement from these activities, and the individual looks for other areas in which strengths may lie. Some children who are not good with their hands can turn to books and receive the praise of their parents and teachers. However, it should be noted that peer group emphasis, especially in boys, is on athletic prowess, and academic distinction is less prized, especially in early latency. There is tremendous pressure on the 8-year-old boy to play sports well; if clumsy, he can be at a decided disadvantage in making and retaining friends.

The child who cannot do anything well, sports or schoolwork, presents a special problem and becomes a prime candidate for acting-out behavior. For this child, like the toddler who is displaced by a new baby in the family, attention (usually reprimand) comes primarily from negative attention-seeking devices, and true approbation comes from a peer group that either baits him or joins him in these activities, marveling at his prowess at getting into trouble and his apparent lack of concern about inviting punishment.

Girls usually fall into one of two groups during latency. Some girls demonstrate characteristics known as *tomboyism.* These girls tend to be athletically aggressive, and because of their slightly greater physical maturity as contrasted with boys of the same age, they can be as skilled or more skilled than their male counterparts in physical activities. On the other hand, there is another group of girls that displays little proclivity toward athletics. During latency, these girls tend to enjoy activities and games that are much more gender-specific in the traditional sense and revolve around playing house and other more strictly "feminine" activities.

As social roles have become less restrictive for both boys and girls, there has been a move toward less competition and more cooperation, resulting in greater acceptance of all individuals into any given activity. In addition, a new value system for social roles has emerged that encourages both athleticism in girls and home-centered interests in boys.

During latency there is no qualitative change in the external genitalia, which retain their infantile appearance. In general, the hypothalamus and pituitary gland are highly sensitive participants in a negative feedback system that results in suppression of any gonadal activity. At the point of late latency and early adolescence, the sensitivity of the hypothalamus and pituitary gland declines, permitting increased synthesis of luteinizing hormone and follicle-stimulating hormone. With higher circulating levels of these hormones, the physical changes of sexual development begin. Enlargement of the breasts and rounding of the contours of the hips are the first discernible changes in girls. Increasing size of the testes and penis with the appearance of pubic hair at the base of the penis are the first changes noted in boys. Although these changes can occur as early as 8 years of age in girls and 10 years in boys, the average age of onset of adolescence is usually 10 and 12 years, respectively.

Lack of outward physical change and diminution of sexually oriented drives do not mean that children are uninterested in sex, especially sex differences. Curiosity is common among 5- to 7-year-old boys and girls. Because children have been taught (sometimes through shaming) to keep themselves clothed in the presence of others, especially members of the opposite sex, "playing doctor" becomes a relatively socially acceptable way of satisfying natural curiosity. Girls and boys of middle latency often "kiss and run"; snapping the bra strap of a more mature member of the group is common in late latency. "Crushes," often intense and frequently focused on some unattainable hero or idol, occur with regularity. Parents sometimes need reassurance that these practices are widespread and represent normal behavior.

Psychosexual Development: Latency. Freud has described the *latency stage* as that period of development when the previously active libidinal and aggressive drives of the oedipal stage become latent, and a truce ensues between the id and the ego until the emergence of the true sexual drive in the genital stage. At the beginning of latency, the superego (conscience) becomes more firmly internalized. The child derives comfort from the representations of parental values and outlooks contained within his or her own being, as embodied in the superego. These internalized parental values not only have resolved the otherwise intolerable oedipal conflict from within but also continue to offer definite answers to troublesome moral and ethical problems from without. The outlook of the latency-age child is fairly black and white; notions about good and bad are clear and absolute and follow the guidelines set by the family.

Psychosocial Development: Industry Versus Inferiority. Erikson[7] has termed the latency period the *age of industry versus inferiority,* stating that the child

> has mastered the ambulatory field and the organ modes. He has experienced a sense of finality regarding the fact that there is no workable future within the womb of his family, and thus becomes ready to apply himself to given skills and tasks, which go far beyond the mere playful expression of his organ modes or the pleasure in the function of his limbs. He develops a sense of industry—i.e., he adjusts himself to the inorganic laws of the tool world. He can become an eager and absorbed unit of a productive situation. To bring a productive situation to completion is an aim which gradually supercedes the whims and wishes of play.

The issue of the status of one's self and one's possessions has its beginning in latency and intensifies during the period of strong peer group identity of adolescence. According to Erikson, the potential danger to the child at this stage lies in acquiring a sense of inadequacy or inferiority. If the child does not feel that he or she has adequate tools or skills, it may not be possible to become a successful member of the group. Failure to become a member of the group may result in withdrawal into the family and social isolation.

Systematic instruction occurs in all cultures during this time, although not all learning takes place within the confines of school. Much is learned about the world through experience and manipulation rather than by explanation; perhaps the greatest amount is learned from older children, who are perceived as "touchable" heroes. Society's contribution to the successful navigation of this stage is support for questing, gentle guidance, and perhaps most important, praise for achievements, even if small.

Cognitive Development: Concrete Operational Stage. The cognitive processes in the latency-age child have been characterized by Piaget as *concrete operational.* The child is able to view the world from an external point of view; logic and objectivity are increased over previous stages. Thinking becomes dynamic, decentralized, and reversible. It becomes possible to understand the intermediate steps between two states. It also becomes possible to "conserve." In Piaget's classic experiment about conservation, a clay ball is rolled into (i.e., becomes) a clay sausage. If the child can think about the transformation in such a way that there is an appreciation that shape does not alter quantity, he or she is described as able to conserve, or to recognize that certain changes (e.g., physical rearrangement) do not necessarily alter other properties (e.g., quantity) of a substance. Conservation is the result of the child's ability to focus on several aspects of a problem or situation at one time and relate them. Thus as exemplified in the ball-sausage experiment, the child who can *conserve* mass can understand the reciprocity of length and width in the problem presented.

A child in the early concrete operational period can solve a problem only if the elements of the problem are physically present, and often they must actually be manipulated for full understanding. By the late concrete operational period, the child can solve problems of space and time; can conserve substance, quantity, weight, and volume; and can classify objects into hierarchical systems. Physical manipulation remains helpful but is not essential to problem-solving.

Social Learning Development: Secondary Motivational Systems; Extrafamilial Learning. Beginning with entrance into school and extending throughout the remainder of life, individuals are increasingly influenced by the social values and customs of those outside their family. The dependency on family that the child has developed must be unlearned; instead, he or she must learn to act independently and in compliance with expectations made by nonfamily members of the larger social group. The child's identification with models among adults or peers in school or in the community provides initial instruction through imitative or observational learning. Reinforcement, such as admiration or approval, serves to perpetuate socially acceptable behaviors. If desirable behaviors are not consistently reinforced or if the only attention the child receives is through participation in socially unacceptable behaviors, undesirable behaviors will be learned at this stage just as they were at earlier ages within the confines of the home. Thus the basic principles of learning are invariant and independent of the individual's age and setting.

Adolescence and Young Adulthood

The term *adolescence* is derived from the Latin, *adolescere* (to grow up), and refers to the psychological, biologic, and sociologic aspects of development that occur during the second decade of life. *Puberty* refers to the condition of becoming sexually mature and being capable of sexual reproduction.

The age of onset of puberty has varied considerably over the centuries, a phenomenon known as the *secular trend.*[25] Earlier maturation was noted over a period of 150 years during the nineteenth and early twentieth centuries, but reached a plateau in American teenagers beginning in the 1960s. Reasons for such changes have been related to a variety of factors such as nutrition and global temperature cycles.

Adolescence is usually divided into three stages: early, middle, and late. During early adolescence the majority of the individual's physical and emotional energy is centered on physical change and its consequences; during middle adolescence on separation from parents; and during late adolescence on preparation for an adult identity.

Important sex-specific differences exist in both the timing of growth and final adult size. The female growth spurt occurs about 2 years earlier than the male growth spurt, but the final adult height of women is less than that of men because of the shorter growth period. Muscle growth appears to be primarily influenced by androgenic stimulation. Thus there is greater muscle mass and strength in the mature man than in the mature woman.

Increase in body size and maturation of neuronal pathways contribute to the child's and adolescent's increasing ability to perform complex motor tasks. Large muscles develop before small muscles. Therefore younger children are more skillful in activities involving gross motor movements than they are in activities requiring fine motor coordination. In early adolescence differential bone and muscle growth can result in transient increases in awkwardness, particularly in gross motor functioning. During middle and late adolescence, the diminution in growth rate over time leads to greater stability in body proportions; motor awkwardness gradually decreases.

Throughout infancy and childhood, circulating levels of pituitary follicle-stimulating hormone and luteinizing hormone are low. Although growth of both the internal and external genitalia parallels increases in body size, the genitalia retain their infantile appearance and function until the onset of pubertal change.

Pubertal change can be divided into three stages. During the first, prepubescence (prepuberty), the gonadotropin and sex steroid levels remain low; however, secondary sexual characteristics begin to appear. In girls, the earliest sign of the initiation of sexual maturation is often pelvic girdle widening. This is followed by breast and pubic hair development and the onset of the height spurt. In boys, testicular growth precedes penile growth, development of pubic hair, and the onset of the height spurt.

For reasons that are not completely clear but may be related to critical body weight, the hypothalamus begins to become less sensitive to negative feedback from circulating gonadotropin levels. Luteinizing hormone–releasing factor is produced and gonadotropin secretion is enhanced, rising progressively toward adult levels.

During the second stage, pubescence (puberty), the reproductive organs (primary sexual characteristics) become functional, and the secondary sexual characteristics become more evident. The last stage, postpubescence (postpuberty), includes a 1- to 2-year period of relative reproductive infertility. During this time skeletal growth is completed.

Psychosexual Development: The Genital Stage. According to freudian theory, sexual impulses reemerge during adolescence, marking the onset of the *genital stage*. Whereas pleasure-seeking through oral, anal, and genital stimulation was the aim of the infantile form of sexuality, during puberty another sexual aim arises: reproduction, through a mature heterosexual relationship with a love object.

During early adolescence there is thought to be a partial recrudescence of the oedipal complex or a regression to the psychosexual stage characteristic of the preschool child. This may occur because the adolescent feels safer expressing some of his or her new and confusing sexual feelings within the familiar environment of the family. However, the adolescent recognizes that emotional closeness to the parent of the opposite sex is both unrealistic and unacceptable. The adolescent has also learned from experiences during the phallic stage that real competition with the same-sex parent is hopeless.

In addition to whatever sexual overtones may be associated with movement into the genital stage, the process of renewed competition with the same-sex parent also stirs in the adolescent a questioning of the behavior, values, and judgments of the parent. Recall that resolution of the oedipal phase in early childhood brought with it acceptance of the parental value system and a desire to be like the parent. The value system that was accepted, however, was primitive and rudimentary, because the child was not cognitively capable of full understanding; for example, the preoperational child cannot comprehend that although modifications of behavior sometimes occur depending on the situation, such modifications do not necessarily impair the basic underlying value system. That is, for the young child, judgments are black and white and very little, if any, gray area exists. But, as we shall see as we discuss cognitive growth during adolescence, the ability to understand hypothetical situations and to argue both for and against certain points of view renders the teenager's previous value system inadequate to deal with larger moral and philosophic issues. However, rather than turn to the parent for explanation and clarification, the adolescent assumes that the parents' value system is exactly as he or she conceived of it as a young child (recall how often parents of adolescents comment, "My teenager thinks I don't know anything."); thus, the adolescent turns to peers or adults outside the family, looking for a new, expanded set of values and at least to some extent rejecting the values of the parents. Eventually, the adolescent seeks independence from both parents, not just the same-sex parent. In some cases a period of alienation from the family may be necessary to attain sufficient distance for independence to be truly attained. During the resolution of the parent-child conflict of the genital stage, the boy completes his (adult) identification with his father by choosing a female partner. Similarly, the girl completes her (adult) identification with her mother by seeking a male partner. Thus full sexual maturity, in freudian terms, is attained when feelings directed toward a parent of the opposite sex are successfully transferred to a love object that is not taboo. Homosexual alliances, because they do not fulfill the reproductive aim that is a characteristic of the genital stage as defined by Freud, have traditionally been considered by psychoanalysts to be deviant and immature forms of sexual love.

The genital stage is the longest phase in the psychosexual developmental framework, lasting from adolescence to senility, when regression to the pregenital stage is thought to be common. Attainment of the genital stage does not necessarily preclude continuing to derive pleasure from satisfaction of pregenital as well as genital drives. In addition, the personality constructs and defense mechanisms developed during the pregenital stages continue as part of the individual's permanent character structure and are manifested throughout life.

Psychosocial Development: Identity Versus Role Confusion and Intimacy Versus Isolation. Identity formation is thought by many to involve answering three questions: Who am I as a physical being? Who am I as a vocational being? And, who am I as a sexual being? However, Erikson considers the major focus of this phase of development to be the task of choosing an occupational identity (i.e., selecting a role to play within the adult community, including investment in the choice of work and the work itself and involvement in the community for the community's sake).

The process of general identity formation begins in early adolescence. The individual becomes determined to be the same as other members of his or her peer group, which usually is composed of same-sex members and is often an extension or continuation of a latency age "chum" group. Often cruel in its exclusion of others, the "in" group attempts to establish its identity as a separate social unit in and of itself. The security of the small group permits individual members to clarify their particular roles within the group and thus eventually to move toward a sense of personal identity as members of society as a whole.

Cliques, because of the rigidity of their structure and customs, serve the useful purpose of guarding the individual from a sense of confusion about role. Thus, as the adolescent moves out of the known environment of family into the world, he or she passes through a transitional phase as a member of a closely knit peer group. This group, in much the same way as parents did, helps to define acceptable and unacceptable behavior. However, to facilitate separation from family, the rules and values of the group the adolescent chooses are often different from if not antithetical to those of the family. In this way teenagers try to demonstrate that they are their own persons, doing their "own thing."

Part of developing identity is (1) recognizing specific personal strengths and weaknesses, (2) aspiring to goals that are realistic and attainable, and (3) seeking after those goals. The potential danger is never achieving clarity of role; closely allied is having too many nebulous or halfhearted roles (identity diffusion) or choosing a role without sufficiently exploring options (identity foreclosure).

Some adolescents may choose a negative identity (i.e., an identity counter to that suggested by society) because they see conformity as the route to being a nonentity. The role of the individual with a negative identity can be social change. In such situations, even though overcoming the inertia of the status quo requires energy and commitment, the result of such deviancy can have such a major effect on social mores that the effort is perceived as worthwhile by the individual. For example, many of the characteristics of the hippie of the late 1960s could be found in conventional youth by the mid-1970s; similarly, the antiwar sentiments of young people who were ostracized in the 1970s became common in the 1980s. For those who advocated such changes, assuming an identity outside the mainstream may have appeared to be the only option for changing the system. The danger of assuming a counterculture identity, however, is permanent ostracism: never achieving sufficient reintegration to effect desired change or to derive a satisfying sense of self from society.

During late adolescence and young adulthood, the individual moves into the stage of *intimacy versus isolation*. Once personal identity becomes established, the young adult is eager to fuse his or her identity with that of another—to develop intimacy or the capacity to commit oneself to a partnership, despite personal sacrifice and compromise. Although often thought of in sexual terms, intimacy includes close friendships, inspiring teacher-student relationships, and other affiliations in which personal vulnerability and true glimpses of the self are permitted. The antithesis of intimacy, in eriksonian terms, is the state of *distantiation*—isolation from or the destruction of those who appear to be a danger to oneself or to one's intimate relations (i.e., prejudices against those who are unfamiliar or foreign and thus threatening).

True genitality, a term borrowed from Freud, develops during this phase. Erikson states that to be of lasting social significance, true genitality should include a heterosexual love relationship that ultimately produces children.

The danger of this adolescent and young adult phase is selection of an inappropriate "permanent" partner for reasons of expediency rather than for complementary elaboration or fulfillment of mutual purposes.

Cognitive Development: Formal Operational Period. Beginning in early adolescence and extending throughout adulthood, the period of *formal operations* is distinguished by the ability to use abstract thought. Characteristics of formal operational thought include flexibility, complex reasoning, and hypothesis formation.

Not all adolescents or all adults apply formal operational thinking to all aspects of reality, nor are they "formal operational" under all conditions and circumstances. Instead, the use of formal operations is often restricted to cognitive functioning in areas of particular personal interest or professional concern and is most productively applied at times of low stress and anxiety. In addition, sex-specific differences exist; thus females are more likely than males to apply formal operations to interpersonal matters; males are more likely to apply formal operations to scientific matters.

The development of formal operational or abstract thought allows the adolescent to understand certain moral, political, and philosophic ideas and values for the first time. With the emergence of the ability to deal with concepts such as liberty and justice, adolescents become preoccupied with social, religious, and political issues. Because they can conceive of the ideal, be it society, religion, or family, they become aware of the contradictions, falsehoods, and shortcomings embedded in their previously accepted beliefs.

Adolescents can think about thinking; they understand the thought processes of others and wonder how individuals see them and what these individuals really think about them. A belief that others may dwell on or constantly evaluate their appearance and behaviors results in the egocentrism or self-centeredness particularly characteristic of the early and middle adolescent. Self-consciousness is a direct reflection of this self-centeredness. As formal operational thinking becomes better established (in middle to late adolescence), the individual begins to distinguish between personal preoccupation and the thoughts of others. Once this distinction can be made, the adolescent can enter into an intimate emotional relationship with others.

Stress, such as illness, can have a profound influence on the individual's ability to use higher order cognitive skills in solving a problem. The general physical and emotional regression seen in the hospitalized child, regardless of his or her usual functional ability, is often also accompanied by a cognitive regression. Such phenomena as magical thinking (my wish equals action) or egocentrism (my action caused some external unrelated event) are commonly seen. The ability to think futuristically when considering the potential consequences of current actions can be impaired. Conversely, long-term illness in some individuals results in increased learning and adultlike understanding about related issues. Because this can occur in children of all ages, it is not unusual for children with long-term, fatal malignancies, for example, to have an understanding of body function or a conception of death that is surprisingly mature. This finding is in keeping with Piaget's premise that cognitive functioning is highly dependent on and molded by experience.

Social Learning Development: Secondary Motivational Systems; Extrafamilial Learning. As the individual matures, the nature and scope of interactions with others are broadened. Reinforcement of particular behaviors becomes less critical because participation in the large class of socially acceptable behaviors has become habitual. Rewards and punishments are largely based on internal rather than external controls. Thus the adolescent is able to enter into relationships based on the mutuality of needs of two or more independent persons.

SPECIFIC DEVELOPMENTAL ISSUES

Research that has focused on the development of the child's understanding of certain concepts has provided the opportunity for pragmatic application of certain developmental theories. The development of moral judgment provides an excellent example.

Development of Moral Judgment

Although studies in the area of experimental honesty have generally failed to show a consistent increase in "resistance to temptation" in children between ages 4 and 14 years, it is apparent that the moral judgments of children differ qualitatively from those of adults. Pioneering work in this field has been done by Kohlberg,[15] who based his model on the cognitive-intellectual principles described by Piaget. Thus this model is restricted to a description of moral thought processes rather than of moral behavior; the theory can help explain how and why a child might arrive at a particular moral decision, although it does not provide a basis for altering actual behavior. By extension, however, application of freudian and eriksonian theories can help provide an understanding of the mechanism by which behaviors come about or might be changed.

According to Kohlberg's theory, thinking about moral issues proceeds through a fixed series of psychological conditions that are dependent on and representative of the individual's general cognitive stage. In addition, he suggests that there is a "cultural universality" to the sequencing of moral development, although the chronologic ages at which certain stages appear may be different in various cultures—and within a culture, they may depend on particular social experiences.

In Kohlberg's scheme there are three overall levels of moral judgment: *preconventional* (premoral), *conventional*, and *postconventional* (principled). Each level is subdivided into stages.

Level I. The preconventional level is characteristic of children in the sensorimotor and preoperational periods of cognitive piagetian development. Judgments about right and wrong are determined by the external physical consequences of the actions; that is, whether the actions elicit punishment or rewards.

Stage 1 moral judgment is clearly based on the principle of punishment and obedience. Stage 2 behavior is instrumental and relativistic. This stage is exemplified by the child who acts to satisfy his or her own needs and only occasionally the needs of others. Fairness, reciprocity, and sharing are pragmatic ("I help you; you help me") rather than based on an understanding of loyalty or gratitude.

These stages are analogous to the oral and anal stages of freudian psychology and the trust versus mistrust and autonomy versus shame and doubt stages elaborated by Erikson. In stage 1, the child depends entirely on the external cues of the caregiver for decisions about right and wrong behavior, and compliance is motivated by a desire to obtain love and nurturance. In stage 2, the child is able to take some responsibility for satisfying personal needs but behaves out of a sense of pleasing him or herself primarily and others only secondarily.

In the early premoral stage, behavior is first conditioned and then shaped (in learning theory terms) by rewarding desirable behaviors through positive reinforcement and punishing undesirable behaviors through nonreinforcement (withholding attention). Late in this stage, punishment through negative reinforcement is introduced. Because the child lacks experience to make judgments that might have lasting negative consequences, punishment (such as loud verbal cues and spanking) is used to denote other, more serious outcomes that could occur if the child persisted in the behavior. Restraint and redirection are other tactics often used to change behavior.

Level II. At the conventional level, moral judgments are based on wanting to perform a desired role (and thus fulfilling the expectations of others in anticipation of praise) and wanting to maintain order. Unlike judgments characteristic of level I, those characteristic of level II are based on a consideration of the desires of others, regardless of the actual physical consequences of the action.

Stage 3 behavior is that which pleases or helps others, who then show their approval by designating the child a "good boy" or a "nice girl." Stage 4 behavior, based on the principles of "law and order," is determined by respect for authority and the fixed rules of the social group, which are seen as unchangeable. That is, rules are fixed and independent of circumstance or situation.

In freudian and eriksonian terms, this is the stage that develops in concert with resolution of the oedipal conflict and during the stages of initiative versus guilt and industry versus inferiority.[10] Thus the child is learning to sublimate his or her own immediate aims and desires and incorporate the values of others into his or her personal goal system (through the process of identification as defined by Freud). Desire to be like the parent drives the child to internalize parental qualities that please others. With this process comes the emergence of the superego, or conscience. Similarly, in accord with the eriksonian stages, the child modulates both wishes and behavior to please others. Part of pleasing others is to construct products, attend to learning, and refine skills—in other words, to become an industrious person as perceived by society.

According to social learning theory, the child is moving into the community and learning through observation and imitation of an increasingly large pool of individuals outside the family who act as models. Conformity to rules and respect for authority are particularly important attributes for successful participation in large group activities and therefore are strongly reinforced as socially acceptable behaviors.

Level III. At this stage, moral judgments are based on personal conformity to principles that are valid apart from social authority and convention. This level of reasoning requires full formal operational thinking.

Stage 5, sometimes known as the social contract or legalistic stage, recognizes that individual rights and standards exist and that personal values and opinions are relative. Procedural rules for reaching consensus are exercised; laws are recognized as changeable to meet the needs of the common good rather than as rigid and inflexible. Stage 6 judgments are based on broad abstract moral principles (e.g., the Golden Rule) rather than on concrete moral imperatives (e.g., the Ten Commandments). Universal principles of justice, reciprocity, equality of human rights, and respect for human dignity are applied to moral decision-making.

Again, the analogy to the genital stage of freudian psychology and the identity versus role confusion stage of eriksonian psychology can be made. Knowledge of and respect for oneself as an individual allow the adolescent or young adult to engage in mutual and totally reciprocal relationships with other people, the basis of "true genitality."

In social learning theory terms, participation in broad extrafamilial learning systems in which the motivations for behavior are secondary and derived from nonimmediate reinforcement permits the individual to obtain satisfaction from behavior that is beneficial to obtaining some higher social goal even though it may be personally unsatisfying in the short term.

In keeping with other general developmental theorists, Kohlberg[15] states that individuals who have attained certain levels of moral judgment reasoning still have available to them, and use on occasion, lower levels of judgment. He has termed this regression a *judgment of ease* as opposed to a *judgment of preference* because he assumes that an individual would, under all circumstances, prefer to use the highest level of moral reasoning available to him or her. Kohlberg also suggests that the motivation for a given behavior may not always be clear from the behavior itself. For example, if the driver of a car decelerates to the speed limit when a police car appears ahead on the road, such behavior may represent a judgment of ease based on stage 1 (obedience and punishment) reasoning or higher order stage 4 (law and order) reasoning. (Interestingly, it is possible that someone operating at stages 5 and 6 might not slow down at all if traffic were light and the driving conditions excellent, arguing that speed limits are arbitrary and the spirit of the law [safe driving] and not the letter of the law [55 mile-per-hour speed limit] is the more valid ethic on which to base behavior.)

Although the Kohlberg model provides a reasonable framework for understanding moral development in general, its applicability is limited by its reliance on boys and men as the major subject pool from which his observations were drawn. Gilligan[8] and others who have studied girls and women have questioned whether the intense focus on competitiveness and following rules is as crucial in the development of moral reasoning and judgment in females as it may be in males. Indeed, it has been suggested that compared with boys, girls are more pragmatic about rules, more willing to make exceptions especially when such exceptions will promote harmony among the group, and more adaptable to innovation. This is thought to reflect society's traditional tendency to socialize girls so that they will view "playing of the game" as subordinate to keeping friends—a tradition that has placed them at substantial disadvantage when seeking the time-honored version of corporate success. The trend in current

American society is toward less sex-role stereotyping; how this will influence both male and female moral judgments remains to be seen.

Development of Gender Identity

The relationship between physiologic and psychological growth and development is particularly well illustrated by the development of gender identity, or the individual's own self-concept of being either male, female, or ambivalent. The final expression of adult gender identity is preceded by a series of events, some biologic and others social or psychological in nature.

Initial biologic differentiation is determined on the basis of chromosomal composition, which directs primordial gonadal development. Although most families are unaware of the gender of the fetus, conscious or unconscious expectations, wishes, and anxieties of the parents play a role in their developing attachment to the unborn child.

The morphology of the newborn's external genitalia has an immediate psychological effect on the family that persists for the remainder of the individual's life. On first contact with the infant after birth and determination of the child's gender, a set of cultural expectations influences all communication to and about the child, including choice of the child's name and the kinds of external reinforcers that are employed (blue versus pink clothes, types of toys). Subtle differences in parental voice inflection and handling of the infant occur, depending on the gender of the child and of the particular parent. In addition, different temperamental characteristics in the infant are reinforced, depending on gender. Thus clinging by female infants and active play by male infants may be selectively reinforced from the time of birth. This is consistent with the biases of most cultures, which designate aggressive, assertive behavior as masculine and dependent and socially compliant behavior as feminine.[21]

Sex Role Behaviors

As the child matures, both the behavior of others and the child's image of his or her physical self in comparison with others serve as cues about how to internalize a concept of self as a sexual being. Thus, for boys, behaviors that are culturally masculine and those that are culturally feminine are available to him through observation and imitation. Interestingly, however, he generally does not adopt behaviors that are specific for the female gender role. Instead, he incorporates behaviors that are masculine into his behavioral repertoire. In learning theory terms, it can be hypothesized that "appropriate" role behaviors are being reinforced and "inappropriate" role behaviors are being inhibited. In a study[6] of children attending a day care center that deemphasized sex role stereotyping in play, it was found that even when given free selection, boys still are likely to choose traditionally masculine toys (cars, trucks) and girls still are likely to choose traditionally feminine toys (baby dolls, cooking utensils). Interestingly, the stereotypically determined selection rate for girls tends to be less pronounced than that for boys. This finding suggests that cues about sexual behaviors are highly pervasive in our society and that, to date, Western culture has been more successful in providing latitude in the definition of acceptable behavior for girls than it has for boys.

Children between 2 and 4 years of age can identify themselves as boys or girls (although they may not yet be able to identify the sex of other people correctly). Although certain personality characteristics already may have developed in a given child because of selected sex-specific reinforcement, actual behavior is less stereotyped than it may become later. Much imitative behavior in children of both sexes revolves around housework, which is usually (but not always) modeled by the mother, the first "identificatory" object, as defined by Freud. As children experience and resolve the oedipal conflict and more strongly identify with the same-sex parent, they adopt an increasing number of what they perceive to be specific gender-role behaviors appropriate to their biologic sex ("When I grow up, I want to do 'man things,' like Daddy"). Later the peer group defines acceptable and unacceptable behaviors and becomes a more potent force than the family for many older children and adolescents.

Sexual Behavior

As children mature, they undergo somatic and pubertal changes that directly affect their psychological development. However, cultural tradition prescribes how they will express their sexuality, and this behavior is highly age dependent. *Sexual behavior* is a broad term and ranges from the sex-related activities of the infant and young child to the truly genital behaviors of the adolescent and adult. Most of the behavior occurs because it satisfies curiosity and is pleasurable although not necessarily erotic. However, it is behavior that to some degree is an expression of masculinity or femininity. Sexual behavior is an integral part of the developmental process, and certain types of behaviors are particularly common at certain ages.

Penile erections have been noted on ultrasonography of the developing male fetus. Vaginal lubrication occurs at least from birth. During the first year of life, boys become aware of their penis and girls become aware of their clitoris as sources of pleasurable and painful sensations. Masturbation is common among children between 2 and 5 years of age.

Natural inquisitiveness about their bodies leads young children to touch not only themselves but their parents and siblings as well. Older children "play doctor" or "family" with their peers, games that often entail some undressing and mutual touching.

By early school age, humor or conversation involving "dirty" words and giggled references to body functions is used as a way of coping with parental admonitions about modesty and what constitutes socially acceptable behavior. In some children, modesty is taken so literally that it can lead to such a strong generalized sense of privacy that even a physical examination by a physician is vigorously opposed. This extreme desire for personal physical privacy can extend into adolescence unless parental guidance is available to help the child learn to judge those circumstances under which the definition of modesty is appropriately and necessarily subject to modification.

Many children express their sexuality through a reemergence of masturbatory behavior in early adolescence. Many also engage in homosexual behaviors. These modalities of sexual expression appear to occur because they are perceived as less threatening than heterosexual behavior. Actually, homosexual experimentation, especially in the early genital stage, is common enough to be considered a normal developmental phase rather than neccesarily a sign of fixed homosexual orientation.

Once heterosexual encounters begin, they necessarily follow a common but not invariable pattern. They initially occur within the context of group dating with little or no actual boy-girl pairing, progress through a transitional stage of double dating, and then finally enter into a phase of individual dating, in time with an exclusive partner. The earliest sexual activity during adolescence is holding hands. This is followed, usually in order, by kissing, petting, and finally, coitus.

In summary, boys and girls appear to be reared differently from the moment their particular morphologic sex is assigned at birth, if not before through the conscious or unconscious expectations of their parents during pregnancy. Children develop a sense of their own gender identity through selective environmental inhibition or reinforcement of certain kinds of behaviors that have been deemed by their culture to be consistent with the expression of male or female roles. Gender identity, the objective perception of oneself as male or female, is the sum total of one's feelings and behaviors. It is displayed in a variety of ways in daily living, beginning in earliest childhood. The most intimate expression of gender identity is mature sexual activity within the confines of a stable mutual relationship.

SOME FINAL THOUGHTS ON "IT'S JUST A STAGE"

Although, theoretically, children and adolescents achieve biopsychosocial maturity in a predictable specific fashion, in reality, human variability and dissonance between growth and development make predictions about a given individual difficult, frustrating, and challenging. When reassurance can be given about the temporary nature of a particular undesirable or anxiety-provoking stage of development, children and their families often are better able to cope, knowing that minor changes in parenting expectations or interpersonal relationships will result in a smoother adjustment and transition to the next stage.

Although the spectrum of variability is broad, not all deviations from average expected development are normal. The greatest challenge to the practitioner is to distinguish between adequate, although not necessarily perfect, development and true dysfunction. Passing a situation off as merely a "stage" is only justified when the true limits of acceptable behavior for that stage are clearly understood, the reasons for the behavior can be explained in such a way that the parents and/or child can understand what they are experiencing and why, and appropriate guidance to help them master the stage is provided.

REFERENCES

1. Ainsworth MDS: Object relations, dependency and attachment: a theoretical review of the infant-mother relationship, Child Dev 40:969, 1969.
2. Baldwin AL: Theories of child development, New York, 1967, John Wiley & Sons, Inc.
3. Berndt TJ, Hawkins JA, and Hoyle SG: Changes in friendship during a school year, Child Dev 57:1284, 1986.
4. Biller HB: Father absence and the personality development of the child, Dev Psychol 2:181, 1970.
5. Cernoch JM and Porter RH: Recognition of maternal axillary odor by infants, Child Dev 56:1593, 1985.
6. Cole HJ, Zucker KJ, and Bradley SJ: Patterns of gender-role behavior in children attending traditional and non-traditional day care centers, Can J Psychiatry 27:410, 1982.
7. Erikson EH: Childhood and society, ed 2, New York, 1963, WW Norton & Co, Inc.
8. Gilligan C: In a different voice: psychological theory and women's development, Cambridge, Mass, 1982, Harvard University Press.
9. Greenberg M and Morris N: Engrossment: the newborn's impact upon the father, Am J Orthopsychiatry 44:520, 1974.
10. Hall CS: A primer of freudian psychology, New York, 1954, World.
11. Hay D, Nash A, and Pedersen J: Interactions between six-month-old peers, Child Dev 54:557, 1983.
12. Hetherington EM: Effects of natural absence in sex-typed behaviors in negro and white preadolescent males, J Pers Soc Psychol 14:87, 1966.
13. Kestenbaum CJ and Stone MH: The effects of fatherless homes upon daughters: clinical impressions regarding paternal deprivation, J Am Acad Psychoanal 4:171, 1976.
14. Klaus MH and Kennell JH: Parent-infant bonding, ed 2, St Louis, 1982, The CV Mosby Co.
15. Kohlberg L: Moral development. In Sills DL, editor: International encyclopedia of the social sciences, New York, 1968, Macmillan Publishing Co.
16. Korner AF: The effect of the infant's state level of arousal, sex, and ontogenetic stage on the caregivers. In Lewis M and Rosenblum LA, editors: The effect of the infant on its caregiver, New York, 1974, John Wiley & Sons, Inc.
17. Lamb ME: Father-infant and mother-infant interaction in the first year of life, Child Dev 48:167, 1977.
18. Lamb ME: The role of the father: an overview. In Lamb ME, editor: The role of the father in child development, New York, 1981, John Wiley & Sons, Inc.
19. Osborne RT, Noble CE, and Weyl N: Human variation: the biopsychology of age, race and sex, Orlando, Fla, 1978, Academic Press, Inc.
20. Parke RD: Perspectives on father-infant interaction. In Osofsky, JD, editor: Handbook of infant development, New York, 1979, John Wiley & Sons, Inc.
21. Rubin JZ, Provenzano FJ, and Luria Z: The eye of the beholder: parents' views on sex of newborns, Am J Orthopsychiatry 44:512, 1974.
22. Sameroff AJ: Early influences in development: fact or fantasy? Merrill-Palmer Q 21:267, 1975.
23. Sears RR: A theoretical framework for personality and social behavior, Am Psychol 6:476, 1951.
24. Sosa R et al: The effect of a supportive companion on perinatal problems, length of labor, and mother-infant interaction, N Engl J Med 303:597, 1980.
25. Tanner JM: Fetus into man: physical growth from conception to maturity, Cambridge, Mass, 1978, Harvard University Press.
26. Thomas A and Chess S: Temperament and development, New York, 1977, Brunner/Mazel, Inc.
27. Yogman MW: Development of the father-infant relationship. In Fitzgerald H et al, editors: Theory and research in behavioral pediatrics, New York, 1980, Plenum Publishing Corp.

SUGGESTED READINGS

Bandura A: Principles of behavior modification, New York, 1969, Holt, Rinehart & Winston General Book.

Bell RQ and Harper LV: Child effects on adults, Hillsdale, NJ, 1977, Lawrence Erlbaum Associates, Inc.

Bowlby J: Attachment, New York, 1969, Basic Books.

Elkind D: The child and society, New York, 1979, Oxford University Press, Inc.

Freud A: Adolescence, Psychoanal Study Child 13:255, 1958.

Freud A: Normality and pathology in childhood, New York, 1965, International Universities Press, Inc.

Ginsberg H and Opper S: Piaget's theory of intellectual development, ed 2, Englewood Cliffs, NJ, 1979, Prentice-Hall, Inc.

Inhelder B and Piaget J: The early growth of logic in childhood, New York, 1964, WW Norton & Co, Inc.

Lamb ME: The role of the father in child development, New York, 1976, John Wiley & Sons, Inc.

Maccoby EE and Jacklin CN: The psychology of sex differences, Stanford, Calif, 1974, Stanford University Press.

Miller NE and Dollard J: Social learning and imitation, New Haven, Conn, 1941, Yale University Press.

Money J and Ehrhardt AA: Man and woman, boy and girl: the differentiation and dimorphism of gender identity from conception to maturity, Baltimore, 1972, Johns Hopkins University Press.

Moss HA: Early sex differences and mother-infant interaction. In Friedman RC, Richart RM, and VandeWiele RL, editors: Sex differences in behaviors, New York, 1973, John Wiley & Sons, Inc.

Mowrer OH: Learning theory and behavior, New York, 1960, John Wiley & Sons, Inc.

Phillips JL: The origins of intellect: Piaget's theory, New York, 1975, WH Freeman & Co, Publishers.

Rest J, Turiel E, and Kohlberg L: Level of moral development as a determinant of preference and comprehension of moral judgments of others, J Pers 37:225, 1969.

Rutter M: Normal psychosexual development. In Chess S and Thomas A, editors: Annual progress in child psychiatry and child development, New York, 1972, Brunner/Mazel, Inc.

44

Adoption and Foster Care

Steven L. Nickman

Adoption and foster care are the two major forms of substitute care. They resemble each other in some respects, but in other ways are quite different; some health care providers are not clear on the differences. Foster care is intended to be temporary and in the majority of cases lasts from weeks to months; children in care longer than this are the exception. Adoption is a permanent commitment and means the child becomes a legal member of a family, even if he or she was well past infancy when adopted. Physicians should understand these differences; foster parents should not be expected to have detailed developmental information, for example, and adoptive parents should not be treated as though they were temporary caretakers.

ADOPTION

Adoption is defined as the assumption of permanent social and legal responsibility for a minor child by a couple or individual other than the biologic parents. Demographic studies[16,20] indicate that approximately 1.6% of children in the United States are adopted by people to whom they have no blood relationship; another 1% are adopted by relatives other than parents or by a stepparent while they continue to live with one biologic parent (after loss of the other parent by death or divorce). Adoption for the second group—sometimes referred to as "intrafamilial" adoptees, as opposed to "extrafamilial" or "nonrelative" adoptees—does not usually carry the same depth or quality of psychological meaning as it does for the first group. The issues of intrafamilial adoptees are primarily those of parental divorce, remarriage, and the creation of a stepfamily, whereas unrelated adoptees must contend with a special set of circumstances, including loss of the original parents (before or after meaningful ties were formed) and a relative or absolute lack of knowledge about those parents. This chapter therefore addresses itself to extrafamilial adoption.

History of Adoption

Present-day adoption has evolved over the last century, in occidental countries, to meet the needs of unwanted children for a family and infertile married couples for a child. The changing nature of adoption, however, requires that this brief description be qualified. Not all children placed for adoption are unwanted; some have been removed from their homes, against parents' wishes, following neglect or abuse. And not all adoptive parents are infertile. Though a majority adopt for this reason, numerous couples and single individuals apply to adopt a child—particularly an older child or one with special needs—because they feel a desire or special capability to do so, even if they already have biologic children. Additionally, there has been a shift in the atmosphere of adoptive practice over the last 15 years, from finding the child to suit the family to finding a family to suit the child.

Adoption exists in many preliterate societies. It was also practiced in many centers of ancient civilization, including Rome, Greece, China, India, and Babylonia. Its role in these societies included the functions ascribed above to contemporary adoption, but its preeminent purposes were social and economic: it provided continuity for a family line or ancestor-worshipping cult or for the agricultural or commercial holdings of a given lineage. In some cultures (particularly Polynesia and Central Africa) it afforded a medium of exchange between adults who had a certain kinship relation with one another. The extreme of this latter situation is represented by certain Pacific islands in which as many as a third of the population is adopted by mutual consent between biologic parents and adopters.

In medieval Europe, abandonment of children was common,[1] as was the sale of children. Abandonment was generally not on lonely hillsides, but rather in the marketplace or in front of the church; it was expected that the child would be saved, and tokens were left with the child to signify the abandoning family's social status and to identify the child in case of a subsequent attempt to regain custody. Such attempts were sometimes litigated, and court records are reminiscent of contemporary custody struggles. The status of such children was between that of contemporary adoptees and foster children, but some of them were raised as slaves.

The first modern adoption laws were passed in certain states in the United States and parts of the British Empire in the last half of the nineteenth century. The major motives for such legislation were to legitimize existing ties, make inheritance possible by adoptees, and remove from adoptees the lifelong stigma of being officially illegitimate.

After World War I the social pressure for adoption laws increased, particularly in Great Britain, because of the large numbers of children who had lost their fathers and whose mothers were unable to cope. In the early years of this century, adoption policies began to be influenced by social workers who initially were untrained members of the upper classes, but who by the 1940s had acquired a strong professional identity that was based on training and was unassociated with social class. Their emphasis was largely on infant placement and the matching of infants with parents to the greatest degree possible.

The humane treatment of unmarried mothers (e.g., in special homes) coexisted with a degree of prejudice against them. There was a strong societal belief in the correlation between intellectual inferiority and unacceptable social behavior, and as a consequence it became a standard professional belief that these young women tended to have blunted emotional responses. It was assumed, therefore, that they should have minimum or no contact with their infants and that they would soon forget the emotional pain of giving birth to an infant and immediately relinquishing it.

Since the 1950s there has been a growing trend to make adoption a social institution more representative of society as a whole than it was during the second quarter of this century. Attempts at matching infants to parents—taking into account the predicted intelligence (risky at best), coloration, and physical stature of the child—are seen as decreasingly relevant to changing social realities. Healthy infants with the same characteristics as the prospective parents are far less available because of improved birth-control methods, availability of abortion, and increased social acceptability of raising a child as a single parent.

Transracial adoption, adoption of children from war-torn and economically deprived countries, and the adoption of physically or mentally handicapped children or older children who may fit into one or more of these categories have all become common in recent years. Some of these—particularly transracial placements and emergency procedures such as the Vietnam "baby-lift"—have been the object of controversy with regard to ethical issues that some people consider to have been raised by such placements.

For a large number of adopting families, because of the child's color, lack of fluency in English, or age, it is impossible to pretend that their new child was born to them, as some adopters of infants tried to do in the past. This relatively new situation forces adopters to confront their inability to mold these children in their own image; many of the children have had years of life's experiences before being adopted. This new situation also influences those who adopt infants by helping them to realize that children, even if adopted in the earliest weeks of life, deserve some dialogue with their parents about their origins and biologic forebears.[11,19,25]

Beginning in the 1940s, and increasingly in the past 20 years, the literature of child psychiatry and pediatrics[23] has reflected a somewhat greater incidence of adjustment problems and psychopathology in adoptees than would be expected from their numeric representation in the child population. Although existing studies are not free from error, the validity of this observation is generally accepted. Just what the pathogenic factors are, however, is not completely understood. When adequate prospective studies with matched controls are done, it seems likely that many factors will be shown to contribute to these problems. Most writers are of the opinion that the establishment of a bond between child and parents, and the maintenance of good family relations in spite of the differences within the family that adoption introduces, are probably the most important ways to prevent future problems. Clinicians who have worked with many adoptees and studied the developmental issues involved generally agree that environmental factors are preeminent in the causation of problems. When heredity plays a part, it most commonly takes the form of parents not taking into account that, for a multiplicity of reasons, their child will grow up to be *different* from but not necessarily worse than themselves. A related concern is when parents have too-high expectations of an adoptee who has already been damaged by his or her environment before placement with the family. The remainder of this chapter focuses on chronologic stages of the adoptive process, with particular attention given to vulnerabilities of the adoptive bond that may predispose the parent-child relationship to later difficulty. Remember that this chapter primarily deals with nonrelative adoptions.

The Adoptive Process

The majority of adoptions are arranged by public or private adoption agencies, and those that are not actually arranged by agencies are subject to agency approval. In recent years, many states that had already outlawed black market adoptions—the commerce in babies, often at exorbitant profit, and without legal protection for anyone—also outlawed the so-called gray market adoptions. These were arranged by a qualified intermediary—usually a doctor, clergyman, or attorney—but even these adoptions were found excessively vulnerable to disruption, as more lawsuits arose over babies whose mothers initially signed consents for adoption and subsequently withdrew their consent.

The law in most states now requires that a certified child-placing agency either do a home study and place a child in the home, or (in the case of children adopted from abroad or those whose birth parents and adopters find each other "through channels," which is happening increasingly) that the agency do the home study during the time of the placement and supervise the adoption until the probate or family court renders it legal, 6 to 12 months later. In "identified adoption," a growing trend, adoptees and birth mothers are in contact with each other, sometimes through an intermediary that can be an individual or an agency. Birth mothers are now sometimes able to choose the family in which their child will grow up. The role of birth mothers in the adoptive process has changed in the direction of greater empowerment, but their continuing involvement with the children in various degrees of what is known as *open adoption* is controversial.

Would-be adopters must be more resourceful and diligent and must be prepared to wait longer than was necessary 20 years ago. At that time virtually all adoption agencies handled only infants and a few toddlers; older, ill, and handicapped children were for the most part regarded as unadoptable. The adoption process was geared toward "consumerism" on the part of adopters, who virtually always wanted a healthy infant of the same racial group as themselves. For various reasons the climate has changed in the direction of wider opportunities for both parents and children: more kinds of children are seen as adoptable, and more kinds of parents are seen as potential adopters. Such parents—often older, sometimes single, and at times different in outlook from "typical" adoptive parents—might not have been accepted as adopters years ago. However many actually have an uncommon degree of resilience and resourcefulness. Many child-placing organizations have mottos, such as, "All children grow better in families," and "There's a family for any child if you look hard enough," to emphasize recent changes in attitudes regarding placement.

Many of the older adoption agencies have switched over to special needs adoption, and new agencies have arisen to handle the changing circumstances surrounding infant adoption. Some of these specialize in international adoptions, whereas others deal with "identified adoption," which corresponds roughly with what used to be called "private" or gray market adoption. State laws vary with respect to the legality of nonagency "middle-man" operations. A black market in infants still exists in some areas, and parents should be warned against any individual or organization that advertises the availability of easy, "no questions asked" adoptive placements. (In case of doubt, inquiry should be directed to the state child-protection agency or another licensed adoption agency.)

What families need to know before adopting, and what supports they need before, during, and after placement, depend on the nature of the family and of the child. A brief list can include the following:

1. Have we come to terms with our infertility (or other reason for adopting) to the extent that we will not need to have him or her be just like us or just like a child we lost? Can we instead encourage our child to keep memories of the past or to have fantasies about his or her unknown parents?
2. How much do we want to know about the child's past history or about the birth parents, and how much is available to us? (Usually when parents do not want to know details of the child's heritage, it is a sign that there is a part of the child they cannot accept. This augurs poorly for the eventual development of a strong emotional bond.)
3. Do we have an adequate medical and social history? (This should be insisted on insofar as the agency has the data. In some cases, however, especially with international adoptions, the data are scant or nonexistent.)
4. Have we been given enough information about the birth parents and their physical characteristics, interests, and reasons for placing the child so that we can answer our child's questions when they arise? (In cases of neglect or abuse, adopters sometimes question how much should be shared with children, and this is often not easy to answer.)
5. Have we been given full and detailed information about health or emotional problems we are likely to encounter in our child?
6. Has the agency offered postplacement support services? These are particularly important with older, traumatized, or disabled children but can also be extremely useful in international and infant adoptions when thoughtful parents have questions about how to handle issues of "telling," abandonment, the child's appearance differing from that of the adopters, and related questions.

Most adoptive parents have suffered both the psychological insult of infertility and the probing questions of social workers. They have already lived through a prolonged period of stress by the time a child is placed with them and have a natural tendency to assume that matters will go well once the placement occurs. This optimism is warranted in most instances and serves the useful function of protecting all concerned from excessive worry, which could interfere with the formation of emotional ties.

Forming emotional ties, or *bonding*, is critically important, and many adoptive placements have subsequently been disrupted because it did not occur to an adequate degree. The adoption of a young infant is undeniably different from bearing, or fathering, a biologic child, and taking a 3-, 5-, or 10-year-old child into one's home is very different from what most people imagine that becoming a parent is like. The many recent studies of early parent-child bonding, as well as earlier work by Spitz,[26] Bowlby,[3] and Rutter,[22] raise questions about the ultimate effects of removal from a caretaking adult—even in the earliest weeks—on the formation of a child's personality.

Bonding is such a complex matter that it is crucial for professionals who deal with adoptive families to remain optimistic and to attempt catalyzing bond formation and reducing parent-child misunderstandings whenever possible. Kennell and co-workers[10] found substantial differences between school-age children who had been placed on their mothers' abdomens in the newborn nursery and those who had not. But no study has sufficiently addressed the question, "Given that very early parent-child attachments take place, does this necessarily mean that a change in mothering figures either early in infancy or later on is detrimental to a child's development?" Too literal a reading of Kennell's findings[10] may effect a fatalistic approach on the physician's part, which is unwarranted given the present state of knowledge, and can deprive parents of needed encouragement. The positive, connection-seeking, receptive parts of the child's and parents' personalities need to be recognized and given every opportunity to emerge and develop. The vicissitudes of the infant's reattachment to a new caretaker and of adoptive parents' attachment to a child not born to them deserve continuing study, but the positive outcomes of the great majority of adoptions give pause to anyone counseling pessimism.

Later-placed children whose early attachments were unsuccessful or disappointing may indeed be unable to relate warmly to their new parents or attach to them. This is one of the many problems that used to be thought of as making a child categorically unfit for adoption. However, there are degrees of severity in a child's ability to attach to new parents, and there are many adopting parents who are willing to accept this challenge.

A way of conceptualizing the difficulties early in a placement is that of "mutual misunderstanding." An example of overcoming misunderstandings with very young children was given by two adoptive mothers of Oriental infants.[5] Their babies had both shown excessive irritability as well as sleep disturbance. By traveling to Korea and meeting her daughter's former foster mother, one of the mothers learned that both children were probably accustomed to being carried around much more than is common in the United States. She also learned details of the typical Korean infant diet that she and her friend had not known. After putting their newly acquired knowledge into practice, the mothers found that their babies became calmer, as did the lives of both families.

The Period of Placement

Early Childhood. A major question faced by parents who adopt infants or very young children is when and how to tell their children about the adoption. Opinions among professionals are far from unanimous on this point. The arguments for "early telling" (i.e., gradual introduction of the word *adopted* and related ideas from earliest times and presentation of the facts of adoption by 4 or 5 years of age) and for "later telling" (i.e., during the latency, or school-age, period, between 6 and 10 years) are as follows:

1. One should tell a child early because he or she might hear the news from someone else, be hurt, and lose trust in the parents. Beyond that, there is nothing shameful in being adopted; to learn about it later would make the child wonder why he or she had not been told before. In any event, circumstances often make it impossible to keep adoption a secret, especially when there is a racial difference or a large talkative family or social circle. And even if parents try to keep it secret, the child will guess and be more troubled by the secrecy than the facts.

   Recent studies[4] indicate that even children told early about their being adopted undergo a mourning period around 7, 8, or 9 years of age, when the growth of their cognitive capacities leads them to reassess their knowledge of all sorts of relationships, including the sadness of having been "given away" by their natural parents. This can be used to argue against later disclosure, because if later telling does not spare children such sadness, then their hearing about their adoptive status from someone other then their adoptive parents will only add to it.
2. The opposite position—held by a minority these days—favors telling a child at the end of the oedipal period or early in latency—approximately between 6 and 9 years of age. It is argued that a child in the preschool years is attempting to find his or her place in the family. This task is complex enough without introducing the ideas that the child (1) did not originally belong with the parents and (2) was actually abandoned by another set of parents. "Adoption trauma" is real and can be demonstrated in the histories of many children in psychotherapy; the confusion and intermingling of abandonment and rescue with oral, anal, and phallic themes in these patients' analytic material argues convincingly for leaving these discussions until a time when a child is better able to understand adoption as resulting from a complicated social transaction between mature people, rather than as a rejection of oneself because one is worthless.

It is possible that some of the adopted children who had trouble with early telling had been subjected to additional stresses, particularly an overemphasis by the parents on the adoption story, which made the children feel rejected. On balance, it is probably best to initiate the process early—bearing in mind that it is a process and not a one-time event—mainly because the longer one waits, the harder it becomes to justify choosing any particular moment as the moment for disclosure; this moment, then, begins to take on a kind of dramatic importance in the parents' minds, which may undermine their ability to create a relaxed atmosphere for conversation.

The most important aspect of the "when to tell" debate, that disclosure will inevitably cause pain to the child, is one that is often left out of the discussion. Learning that one is adopted leads to confusion, disappointment, and anger in the initial stages and represents the beginning of a long developmental trajectory that may take the child some distance away from typical, average experiences and behavior before he or she returns to what is expected. (This refers especially to adolescents.) Parents may be forgiven for sensing that this is the case and wanting either to delay it as long as possible or to begin it as soon as possible in the magical hope that this will obviate the need for the knowledge to be processed over a long period of time. Parents need to view "telling" as a painful but necessary process, and the quality most necessary for them is the ability to inflict necessary pain with understanding and compassion but without so much empathy for the child that the task remains undone. These are the same parental qualities that are needed for successful extraction of a splinter—but it takes a lot longer!

The question thus becomes less "when the child is ready" and more "when the parents are ready." In general, beginning the process before the first grade might be used as a guideline; in this way one at least knows that a child's major negotiations with family have already been carried out or set in motion before his or her main sphere of activity switches from home to the peer group in school; one knows, too, that at this time there are no major surprises that lie in wait for the child and might make it necessary for him or her to call a moratorium on academic and social life in order to deal with feelings of betrayal or shock.

Children placed after 3 or 4 years of age need their adopters to talk with them at intervals about their past lives to foster continuity in the children's sense of self. Some adopters of children who have been neglected or abused are reluctant to talk with the children about their past lives; such parents need to realize that if they completely blockout their child's past, this will probably lead the child to feel that there is a part of him or her—the early years—that they do not value.

Children placed as toddlers present a more complex management question with respect to disclosure and dialogue. Many will have preverbal memories or memories encoded in language. Sensitive adopters will be alert to moments when these children seem to be reacting to internal or external stimuli with thoughtful silence or some puzzling emotional reaction. Parents can then tell the child, "Maybe you're remembering something" and promote further conversation. If a scrapbook exists with photographs of previous homes and caretakers, this is a boon to parents helping toddler- and older-placed children to make sense of their lives.[19]

Pediatricians should be alert to dogmatic approaches to adoptive issues on the part of parents, which include unrealistic expectations, fears of "bad heredity" leading to future misconduct, and refusal to enter into a dialogue about what adoption means to the child. Finding such attitudes should prompt the physician to gently call the parents' attention to what he or she has observed, ask if the observation is a valid description of their beliefs, and offer to discuss the issues with them if they so desire. Important preventive work can be done in this way.

School Age. The following statements are both accurate but seem paradoxical when taken together: "There is nothing really special or different about an adopted child"; "Adopted kids almost always think a great deal about their origins at various times during their growing up; they wonder why they were given up and whether being adopted is equivalent to being worthless." Often adoptive parents are made to feel estranged from their children, who unconsciously reject the adoptive parents as a way of getting back at the rejecting biologic parents. Adopted children sometimes underachieve in school and may be socially immature; such symptoms are related to problems of low self-esteem or absorption in fantasy about their original parents. Such difficulties may require psychiatric referral, and generally, when adopted children are referred to a psychiatrist, adoptive issues are prominent among the matters that are bothering them. Yet it should be stressed that the majority of adopted children do well in school, socially, and within their families.

Adolescence. Early adolescence is a period of turbulence and is even more so for adoptees. Ideas about searching for original parents are entertained cautiously as the child comes to appreciate his or her increased physical and cognitive powers and greater mobility. The fact of adoption may be seen by the adolescent as a basic injustice that can be undone by means of a successful search. When such feelings are intense, they may be motivated in part by poor relationships within the adoptive family. However, it should be recognized that being adopted does constitute a real deprivation of lineage and a blow to self-esteem. Consequently, an adolescent adoptee's searching (whether fantasized or actually carried out) is often psychologically complex. It represents the adoptee's particular brand of normal adolescent rebellion against parents and, in addition, a protest against the loss of his or her roots. Parents need to know that such feelings are usually normal in adoptees and rarely if ever result in loss of their child's loyalty, even if the biologic parent is actually found.

Successful searches are rarely carried out by individuals younger than 21, and parents should not take an active stance to encourage searching before that age; the possibilities of rejection or complicated postreunion relationships are such that an adult level of maturity is advisable in a searcher. Many adoptees never search in reality, although they may do so in imagination. The developmental task of adoptees in middle to late adolescence is perhaps best conceptualized as a process of deciding whether one wants to search in the near future. Such decision-making helps a person to feel more in control of his or her own life—whether the decision is to search or not to search at a given moment in time. There may be some pressure on the adoptee, who wonders how much time is left and whether the birth parents are alive or in good health. Professionals can best help such adoptees by encouraging them to look at the pros and cons of searching. Referral to an adoptees search-and-support group may be helpful, particularly if the physician is familiar with individuals in the group and has confidence that they will not precipitate the adoptee into a premature search. Such advisors are often expert at helping people look at the various personal issues involved.

The teenager also can prepare by reading some of the available age-appropriate literature[6,12,14,18] and talking to adopted friends. This way, the adoptee can learn more about what an intense experience searching can be and come to an informed decision about whether this is something he or she wants to undertake.

Adolescent adoptees sometimes engage in a variety of highly provoking behaviors, and how seriously these should be regarded depends on the severity of the behavior and the quality of relationships within the family. Referral for psychotherapy is often appropriate.

It is not uncommon for severe stress to occur within adoptive families during the adoptee's adolescence, particularly if the placement was made after infancy. Parents may question whether they can continue to parent an acting-out adolescent, or the adolescent may express a desire to leave the family. Health care and social service providers, faced with such an emergency, may be impressed with the extent of family pathology they observe and may support the idea that the teenager cannot "make it" in that particular family. The truth is usually more complicated, however, and it is essential to look for the positive aspects of the child's relationship with the family and conserve these as far as possible. Temporary placements according to the clinical need (brief, respite foster care, hospitalization, boarding school, or residential treatment) are generally preferable to the adolescent's entering the social service system and going into regular foster care, since in most cases the teenager already has a loving family and the difficulty is not primarily in the family, but in the adolescent's inability to make use of them at that particular time. "Disrupted adoptions" do occur, but probably fewer disruptions would take place if the particularly dramatic manifestations that can occur in adolescence were better understood.

Transcultural Adoptions

Adopting a child who spent the first months or years of life in another country, and (if old enough) speaks another language, puts a premium on parents' ability to do two things. The first is the ability to allow the child time to get acclimated to new customs, a new language, new foods, and even new ways of being held or rocked. The second is the ability to live with the sense of being seen as different from other families, even at times stigmatized. (This holds even more for parents who adopt developmentally delayed children.) A solid relationship between the spouses is important; also, parents must have high enough self-esteem as individuals so that they do not need to have their children grow up as "carbon copies" of themselves (or what is more to the point, carbon copies of the individuals the parents wish they were). It is not the duty of children, whether they enter a family biologically or by adoption, to validate the self-worth of a parent with low self-esteem.

Many adopters plan to take their foreign-born children, at

some point during their growing up, to their country of origin. The parents are often also advised to take their children to restaurants serving food indigenous to that country and otherwise expose them to their hereditary cultural roots. It is difficult to generalize about the wisdom of such procedures. Parents should remember that they must navigate between two extremes: on the one hand, making the child feel they ignore or devalue his or her heritage (and by extension himself or herself); and on the other, placing so much emphasis on the child's differentness that he or she feels less than fully accepted as a family member. Usually the child's own degree of interest in pursuing such experiences is the parents' best guide.

Coping with Ambiguity and Social Change

From a social structure in which the adoptee was stigmatized, society is evolving toward more openness and variety in family organization. Meanwhile, the very structure of language reflects society's past ambivalence toward substitute parental arrangements. Adoptees, like foster children, are sometimes at a disadvantage in the use of words denoting family relationships and must often resort to qualifying adjectives such as *adoptive, biologic,* and *real.* Birth records for the most part are still sealed. Society is going through a period of questioning about the rights of biologic parents, adoptees, and adoptive parents and about the ways in which the rights of these groups may sometimes overlap and sometimes conflict with respect to the "right to know" and the "right to anonymity."

Pediatric Perspectives

Pediatricians have several opportunities to help both adoptive parents and children:

1. Pediatricians can contribute a great deal on the individual level by counseling children and their parents as they attempt to deal with various special aspects of the adoptive situation (as outlined in several of the preceding sections) and by being alert to potential future trouble in the family because of parents' unresolved feelings about adoption.[23,28]

   Families do not deal with adoption by means of one or two conversations. Rather, the acceptance of oneself as an adoptive parent or as an adoptee occurs gradually over the course of a child's growing up within the family. Virtually every common developmental stage or maturational crisis has a special twist for adoptive families, and the successful negotiation of each such crisis is a step on the way to mature acceptance of adoptive status.

   Separations, losses, and arrivals of new siblings all tend to stimulate adoption-related feelings and fantasies in a child; by the same token, negativism, rebellious behavior, and rejecting attitudes toward parents are often much more difficult for adopters to cope with in their child than for other parents. Pediatricians should remember that many parent-child conflicts in adoptive families can be alleviated by improved dialogue within the family—often, dialogue about adoption itself. The physician is in an excellent position to point this out. There are a number of useful books available to would-be adopters,[8,13] adoptive parents,[15,17,18] and adopted children[6,9,12,18,21-27] and adolescents[6,12,14,18,21] that can be recommended when appropriate.

2. Pediatricians are often asked to provide an opinion on the health of a newborn or older infant with respect to the child's adoptability. In the past, any questions about normal development meant prolonged waiting periods of months or even years, lasting until the physician could feel comfortable assuring the agency that it could "guarantee" the adopters a normal baby.

   More recently much pressure has come to bear for early decisions in this regard, so that the child can be placed and the bonding process can begin. When real doubt exists, this must be conveyed to the agency, which in turn has the responsibility to explore with the potential adopters how well they could accept a child who might later have some degree of intellectual or physical disability. The onus for decisions about adoptability has shifted for the most part, however, from physician to agency. The physician can consider his or her job well done if observations have been reported fully and a prognosis that is as accurate as possible has been made.

3. Before an older child's adoption, pediatricians may be asked by agencies to make an overall health assessment, which will be shared with the adopters. Adoptive parents may ask their own pediatrician to perform such an evaluation soon after placement. It is important in such situations not only to report whatever problems may be found, but also to comment on healthy or appealing aspects of the child. A hopeful, reassuring attitude should be conveyed as much as possible to the adopters, who are undoubtedly experiencing some anxiety in this new situation. If the pediatrician has uncovered some serious defect that was previously unsuspected, a rare occurrence, he or she should report the findings and give the prospective adoptive parents time to react and to process this new information thoroughly before committing themselves to the child. Some pediatricians may discover prejudices in themselves; they may find it hard to understand why parents would want to adopt children with certain types of problems. In such a case, if the parents themselves already have a fairly good understanding of what is involved, it would be an error for the physician to convey by word or attitude his or her disapproval of what they are about to undertake. The parents, after all, are entering the situation with their eyes open. However, such parents need specific, ongoing guidance about the management of any chronic health problem borne by the child.

4. Referral to a child psychiatrist or other child mental health professional is important when adoptive families are trying to cope with adjustment problems of more than transient duration. The pediatrician's experience may indicate that some mental health providers are more familiar than others with adoption-related concerns. Obviously, not all emotional difficulties in adop-

tees are connected with adoption, but if there is a therapist skilled in adoption issues in the community, it may be advisable to refer adoptive families there in case the problem turns out to be adoption related.

5. On the level of social policy, pediatricians who so desire can lend their influence to the various groups that are working toward greater openness in the adoptive process. Pediatricians can also support legislation that proposes opening birth records to adoptees on reaching the age of 18 years. They can sometimes be of help to adults who wish to set up an open adoption, in which the original parents and the child have some continuing access to each other. A solid sense of identity is as much a child's right as good nutrition, and there is evidence[27] that adoptees will be at a disadvantage until open-records legislation becomes general and until society ceases to attach a stigma, whether overt or subtle, to the process of adoption. (Whether "openness" in the form of actual contact between birth parents and adoptive families is in the children's interest remains to be seen.)

FOSTER CARE

Approximately 400,000 American children, or 5 per 1000 children, are unable to live with their families for varying periods of time; of these, 75% live with foster families and 25% are in group living situations. (Adopted children are considered to be living with their own families.) Informal fostering arrangements, not initiated or supervised by any agency, add an additional unknown figure to the total.

According to Geiser,[7] the following reasons account for foster placements: physical illness of a parent or other adult caretaker, approximately 30%; mental illness of the mother, 15%; emotional or behavioral problems in the child, 15%; abuse by parents or other caretakers, 10%; and various other family problems, 30%. "These figures," writes Geiser, "like many social statistics, oversimplify what is a complex and multidetermined event."

In contrast to adoption, foster care is temporary by intent. The discrepancy between the intent and the reality constitutes the most serious problem in the foster care system.

History of Foster Care

Foster care is an ancient institution.[2] The history of foster care in the United States[7] began with indenture, or "binding out." In prerevolutionary days, most work was done either within the home or nearby. Children whose parents had died or could not care for them were placed, either voluntarily or at the behest of the town authorities, in homes where they were to act as general servants or learn a specific trade. The practice was regulated by law to protect the interests of the child (e.g., he or she was to be given a certain number of years of schooling) and also of the master or mistress. The dividing line between indenture and apprenticeship is difficult to draw. Other forms of care for dependent children in early days included placement in almshouses (generally an unhealthy and unsatisfactory arrangement) and "outdoor relief," which was the provision of public funds for the support of a child within his or her home (and was also the precursor of today's Aid to Dependent Children).

Through the first half of the nineteenth century, charitable institutions sprang up in response to public indignation about poor conditions in the almshouses and abusive treatment of indentured children. Both indenture and institutional care, however, came under attack in the third quarter of the century, and the alternative of foster or adoptive homes was promoted. (The distinction between the two was not nearly so clear then as it is today.) Foster homes were seen as able to provide more loving care and a religious upbringing similar to what the child would find in his or her own background, whereas indenture and institutions were considered lacking in those respects; in addition, foster care was cheaper for the public treasury than maintaining a child in an institution. Dogmatic positions were sometimes taken, then as now, in the public debate about care of dependent children.

In the last 50 years the tendency has been toward more foster home placement and away from large group settings. Although this trend was influenced by Spitz's demonstration[26] of marasmus in young children in group settings, group homes have never been proven dangerous to older children in such a dramatic way. Yet the formation of character tends to proceed more normally within the confines of a family. In general, children are usually placed in foster homes when an expectation exists that the child's family will be able to care for him or her in the foreseeable future. Correspondingly, children are usually placed for adoption when such a hope does not exist. Group care facilities are used for children who may or may not be under the legal guardianship of their parents but who are unable, because of their poor emotional development, to make use of a family and contribute to family life. Some such homes are truly therapeutic, whereas others are little better than warehouses for the storage of children.

Adoptive homes are increasingly being provided for those children whose parents show little promise of being able to care for them. This tendency springs from the wishes of would-be adopters for a child and from the presumed deficiencies of both institutional facilities and of life in a series of foster homes.

This interface between adoption and foster care is an important current social issue, because when a child is adopted, this often means the severing of ties with parents who may have been maintaining some degree of emotionally meaningful contact with the child. The exception is when open adoption takes place. Open adoption is controversial but is increasingly favored by some family court judges as an alternative that is better than terminating parental rights.

Placement of a child outside the home is ordered by a juvenile or probate court judge after consideration of all aspects of the case. The actual placement is carried out and supervised by a public agency, usually the state department of public welfare. Other children enter foster care by a voluntary agreement between parents and the placing agency, without involvement by the court.

Foster Parents

The selection of foster parents is a heavy responsibility for child welfare agencies. Ideally, couples or individuals who serve in this capacity have the ability to provide a warm home life for the child, to understand the irregularities of the child's behavior as stemming from past experiences, and to help the child mature, while at the same time not becoming so attached that they make difficult any future placement with the original or adoptive parents.

In past years some state agencies even had a deliberate policy of moving foster children from one home to another every year or two so that they did not become too emotionally attached. This policy had predictably disastrous results for many children's subsequent adjustment.

Since people who aspire to foster parent status may do so from a variety of motives, it is not surprising that the complex task required of them is sometimes not very well performed. Still, the majority of foster parents are dedicated people who see themselves, and deserve to be seen, as paraprofessionals.[7] They require specialized training and ongoing support, which have often been inadequate because of lack of governmental insight, funds, or both. In addition, it has been recognized more and more that the fostering process by its very nature leads to bond formation.

Rather than being advised to keep an optimum level of emotional distance from a child, what foster parents need is a more active role assigned by the placing agency. Are the natural parents likely to regain custody? If so, the foster parents could facilitate visits and reintegration of the family. Is the child likely to be placed for adoption? If so, the foster parents (if the placement is proceeding well) should be consulted regarding their possible wish and capacity to adopt the child themselves.

Lack of public funding and interest has led to a situation in which children placed in foster homes often receive only minimum supervision by the placing agency, the foster parents receive little guidance, and the original family is not helped in a substantive way to resume parental functions. Foster parents, through ignorance, may occasionally perpetuate the idea that the original parents were bad or inadequate. They may even say, "Your parents didn't love you; if they did you wouldn't be here." Such denigration of parents by foster parents is extremely damaging, since love is hard to define and cannot be equated with the day-to-day ability to care for a child. Even worse, statistics indicate that although a majority of foster placements are planned as short-term arrangements, relatively few foster children rejoin their families permanently. The majority move from one placement to another until late adolescence, at which time they enter the world poorly equipped to meet its demands or make a useful contribution.

Foster Children

In contrast to most adopted children, a foster child is usually placed at an age when he or she retains many vivid memories of his or her biologic family and, in a majority of cases, feels a strong desire to return to them. Such children suffer from long-standing anxiety about a number of questions: What happened to my parents? Did I do something bad to be taken from them? I have been shunted from one place to another; will there ever be a permanent home for me? Does anyone really love me? Am I of real value as a human being? Why did all this happen to me? Will I be given the affection, controls, and guidance I need to begin my adult life on a competitive level with others of my age? The effect of these unanswered questions is seen in a 12-year-old boy who had spent his life alternating between a foster home and his mother's home and was asked about his friends, He replied, "I hang around with a lot of kids, but I don't really talk to anybody. If I did, it would come out that I don't live with my family, and I have a social worker, and then everybody would know it. I'd rather keep that stuff to myself." The stigmatized aspect of being a foster child is often overlooked by adults.

Pediatric Perspectives

Pediatricians are in a position to help foster children in a number of ways:

1. They can be alert to the child's foster status and inquire casually how the placement is working out and what contacts, if any, the child is having with his or her original family. Ideally, before making such inquiries, the pediatrician should speak to the child's social worker to ask what the existing service plan for the child is, including the agency's expectations about whether the child will eventually return home and the frequency of parent visitation and rationale for same.

   A pediatrician who has developed a relationship with a child in foster care should feel free to ask the foster parent how the child seems to be doing (and in that process form an impression of the quality of foster care); even more important, the pediatrician should feel free to ask the child questions addressed to his or her general sense of well-being. Though such questions are always pertinent in a pediatric evaluation, they have particular importance for foster children, since sometimes no other adult whom the child perceives as friendly and wise is asking such questions. Even when the child has a good relationship with the foster parents and the social worker, these individuals may be perceived by the child as having a vested interest in where he or she is placed, whereas this is rarely true of a child's attitude toward the pediatrician.

   Such an approach, based in reality, has the potential for reassuring the child that his or her situation is understood. Avoidance of the subject would not be actively harmful but might deprive a troubled or worried child of an opportunity to ventilate feelings and discover a new source of adult interest and support.
2. Pediatricians should perform thorough physical examinations, including visual and auditory screening tests, whenever possible. A majority of foster children have slipped through the cracks of the health care system and suffer from at least one kind of chronic medical or dental complaint as a result of inadequate care.[24]
3. Pediatricians can be alert to chronic anxiety states and depressions; such conditions are often manifested by hyperactive behavior, aggressiveness, and poor school performance. In particular, prescribing stimulants for a presumed attention deficit disorder in such children should be considered only after ruling out the existence

of a disorder that is primarily emotional in nature. Referral to a child psychiatrist or other expert trained in child mental health is often an important part of medical management: the consultant may recommend regular psychotherapy; case management in the form of less-than-weekly visits; or psychotropic medications when indicated.

Although it is true that the best psychotherapy for a child in a disturbed social environment is to improve the environment substantially, such a step is often not humanly possible. Child psychotherapists, whether they be psychiatrists, psychologists, or social workers, can often help a child through a period of intense self-doubt or anger at the world and also help him or her keep a focus on realistic goals.

4. Finally, pediatricians can be advocates for these children by communicating with social workers, teachers, probation officers, judges, and other professionals involved with a particular child. By investing a little extra time in such a case, the pediatrician is often surprised to find how much his or her interest is appreciated by such "teammates" and how much influence it can have on the fate of the child.

REFERENCES

1. Bolles EB: The Penguin adoption handbook, New York, 1984, Penguin Books.
2. Boswell J: The kindness of strangers: the abandonment of children in Western Europe from late antiquity to the Renaissance, New York, 1988, Pantheon Books, Inc.
3. Bowlby J: Child care and the growth of love, Baltimore, 1953, Penguin Books.
4. Brodzinsky DM et al: Psychological and academic adjustment in adopted children, J Consult Clin Psychol 53:582, 1984.
5. Coyne A and Flynn L: The importance of other parents in adoption, Child Today 9:7, 1980.
6. DuPrau J: Adoption: the facts, feelings and issues of a double heritage, New York, 1981, Julian Messner.
7. Geiser RL: The illusion of caring: children in foster care, Boston, 1973, Beacon Press.
8. Gilman L: The adoption resource book, New York, 1984, Harper & Row, Publishers, Inc.
9. Gordon S: The boy who wanted a family, New York, 1980, Dell Yearling Books.
10. Kennell JH et al: The effect of early mother-infant separation on later maternal performance, Pediatr Res 4:473, 1970.
11. Kirk HD: Shared fate: a theory of adoption and mental health, New York, 1964, Free Press.
12. Krementz J: How it feels to be adopted, New York, 1983, Alfred A Knopf, Inc (photo-essays).
13. Lasnik RS: A parent's guide to adoption, New York, 1979, Sterling Publishing Co, Inc.
14. Lifton BJ: I'm still me, New York, 1982, Bantam Books.
15. Lifton BJ: Lost and found: the adoption experience, New York, 1979, Dial Press.
16. Maza P: Child Welfare League of America, Washington, DC, 1984 (personal communication).
17. Melina LR: Raising adopted children: a manual for adoptive parents, New York, 1986, Harper & Row, Publishers, Inc.
18. Nickman SL: The adoption experience: stories and commentaries, New York, 1985, Julian Messner.
19. Nickman SL: Loss in adoption: the need for dialogue, Psychoanal Study Child 40:365, 1985.
20. Peterson JJ: Child Trends, Inc, Washington, DC, 1986 (personal communication).
21. Powledge F: So you're adopted, New York, 1982, Scribner Book Co, Inc.
22. Rutter M: Maternal deprivation reassessed, ed 2, New York, 1981, Penguin Books.
23. Schechter MD and Holter FR: Adopted children in their adoptive families, Pediatr Clin North Am 22:653, 1975.
24. Schor EL: The foster care system and health status of foster children, Pediatrics 69:521, 1982.
25. Sorosky AD, Baran A, and Pannor B: The adoption triangle, Garden City, NY, 1979, Anchor Books.
26. Spitz RA: Anaclitic depression, Psychoanal Study Child 2:313, 1946.
27. Stein SB: The adopted one: an open family book for parents and children together, New York, 1979, Walker & Co.
28. US Department of Health and Human Services: Adoption disruptions, DHHS Pub No (OHDS) 81-30319, Washington, DC, 1981.

SUGGESTED READING

Backrach CA et al: Adoption in the 1980's: advance data from vital and health statistics, No 181, 1989, Hyattsville, Md, National Center for Health Statistics.

45

Changing American Families

Shirley A. Smoyak

Pediatrics is best practiced with a solid groundwork in the family, including its biologic, cultural, socioeconomic, and demographic dimensions. The family contexts in which infants, children, and adolescents are raised set the patterns for response to illness and the expectations of caregivers. Families' beliefs about health and illness, what is preventable, what is treatable, what is natural, what is good, and what is to be avoided are communicated to upcoming generations in subtle and direct ways. Although it is true that physical and mental illnesses can be complex, vary greatly in each patient's case, and need to be considered within a context of many intervening variables, the complexity and variability of families is such that physical illnesses in comparison with mental illnesses.

Scientists who attempt to study the family are faced with a peculiar dilemma. Something very familiar to all of us growing up in a family somehow eludes the grasp of the scientific method. Because most of us have experienced childhood and adolescence in some type of family setting, and because most of us, as adults, create families of our own, the temptation is great to view our experiences as normal and to use them as a standard for understanding others. This ethnocentric tendency leads to assumptions that the familiar must be the correct or better way and that other styles or patterns at best are strange and at worst are wrong or deviant. The "family" is an elusive concept; its shape, character, and functions have been interpreted very differently by historians, sociologists, psychologists, and anthropologists. Economists cannot even agree on what to name and how to describe a family economic unit; instead they focus on individuals and study the changes over time as individuals move in and out of family settings and relationships.

Privacy about matters of family life has produced what sociologists call *pluralistic ignorance*. Each of us knows what goes on in our own bedrooms and bathrooms, and how we handle a sassy 2-year-old at bedtime or an adolescent who comes home drunk or smelling of pot, but we really do not know how the neighbors do it. Systematic, rigorous research on the intimacies of family life is in its infancy, although the study of marriage and the family can be traced back several centuries.

Until recently most family research was conducted by academicians who saw the family as one specialization among several that they pursued. Thus the research literature on the family developed slowly.[11] In the last three decades, scientists who have a primary interest in the family have emerged in large numbers. Research productivity has expanded, even though there has been far less federal or private-sector financial support for family research than for biomedical endeavors. On the other hand, the family field received former President Jimmy Carter's strong support. In the official White House announcement of the 1980 White House Conference on Families, he stated, "Families are both the foundation of American society and its most important institution. In a world becoming more complex every day, our families remain the most lasting influence on our lives." Families fared less well during the Reagan administration, and it is too soon to determine what support they will receive with President George Bush in office. Despite the less than adequate funding for research on the family, the literature growth has been voluminous. Today there are nearly two dozen professional journals that deal with the family, some specializing in theory and research, some on family issues and policy matters, and many on clinical and therapeutic concerns. Family agendas are addressed at conferences convened by prominent professional associations in the major social science disciplines, and the field is not lacking in newsletters, monographs, audiotapes and videotapes, and books.

This chapter provides an overview of changing patterns of family structure and the associated changes in functions. It attempts to explode some cherished myths about what "the American family" is and to provide clinicians who treat sick, injured, or well children with a more realistic understanding about families. In this chapter a family will be viewed as a married couple or other group of adult kinsfolk who cooperate economically and psychosocially in bringing up children and sharing a common dwelling.

FAMILY ORIGINS

According to Gough,[5] "The trouble with the origin of the family is that no one knows." She provides evidence that it is not known *when* the family originated (probably between 2 million and 100,000 years ago) nor whether some kind of embryonic family came before, with, or after the origin of language. Although varying a great deal in terms of structures and functions, some kind of family exists in all known human societies. "Family" implies several universals: (1) that sexual relations between close relatives are forbidden, (2) that men and women cooperate through a division of labor based on gender, and (3) that marriage is a durable although not necessarily a lifelong arrangement. Another universal, that men in general have higher status and authority than the women in their families, has generated much controversy between feminist scholars and other historians. Although feminist writers have persuasively demonstrated the long-standing, erroneous bias of earlier male "scholars," they disagree among themselves about the exact nature of past relationships among men and women in families.

The exact nature of family structure and gender relationships is shrouded in many layers of conjecture and scientific guesswork. Since the beginning of recorded history, no fixed pattern across cultures has been found.[6] Culture, not biology, determines the rules of organization within families. In most primitive, nomadic, communal societies, family descent was traced through the mothers, possibly because maternity could be verified, whereas paternity was many times a mystery. Roughly 5000 years ago, when the development of agriculture so drastically changed how people lived and organized themselves, patrilineal groups emerged. As the concept of private property developed, the transfer of such property from father to son influenced not only economic but social patterns.

Historians of the family, notably Aries,[1] have taught us that much of what we take as familiar and commonplace is a relatively recent invention. Childhood as a concept to us is real; Aries maintains that it did not exist, as an idea, before the Middle Ages. In medieval days, as soon as a child could live without the constant attention of its mother, he or she was accorded adult status. According to Sagan, no institution has been changed so remarkably by modernization as has the family. Until the late eighteenth century, families were primarily economic units.[10] Marriages were arranged for the purpose of preserving property, and children were a cheap source of labor or a hedge against poverty in old age.

Historically, all the work needed for safety and survival was done within family units. Within the boundaries of the family, functions performed were educating the young, ensuring safety from invaders, praying to God or a superior being, providing nurturance, clothing, and shelter, and caring for the sick, infirm, young, or disabled. Every family textbook includes a discussion of the "erosion of family functions," and it has been popular from time to time to predict the eventual demise of the family as we know it, because all the reasons for its existence have been reassigned to institutions outside the family, such as schools, hospitals, welfare boards, and churches. There actually have been several experiments in alternative forms of living in human groups, but none have survived. Although there is no general societal law that people must live in families, most do.

A historical perspective aids in understanding social contexts and institutions. Present patterns, when the observer can see their roots, make more sense. More important, such understanding eliminates or dampens the tendency toward emotionality over issues of intimacy, closeness, and human relationships. Perceptions of American family life are full of myths, such as the belief that a three-generational household is and was the norm. Such beliefs generate a false nostalgia—a longing for what never was. Norman Rockwell, in popularizing a picture of the American family as three generations in one household, actually did a disservice to the American public. Folks looking at the lovely families on the covers of the *Saturday Evening Post* often negatively compared their own families, who fell short of that standard. Such negative comparisons, founded on inaccurate data, lead to unnecessary agonizing about one's own shortcomings. Such nostalgic beliefs also led to conclusions about generalized family breakdown, which is not the case at all. Recently, researchers studying the family in preindustrial America have dispelled the myths about the existence of ideal three-generational families. There had never been a time when three generations living in one household was typical. Given the short life span (an expected 49 years at the turn of the century), most parents could not have expected to live with their grandchildren. Although the three-generation family of the past was largely mythic, today more grandparents are alive than ever before. In 1920 the chance of a 10-year-old having two living grandparents was 40%; today it is 75%. In 1920 the chance of a 10-year-old having four living grandparents was 1.7%; today, it is 8%.[13] For the first time in history there are families with four or five generations alive. Children today may have not only living grandparents but great-grandparents and great-great grandparents as well. This increased longevity poses problems for families that they have never faced before.[13] On a simple level there is the question of what the "layers" of grandparents should be called by their grandchildren. On a more serious level there is great economic and psychosocial concern facing middle-aged persons who see their retirement years not as golden but as burdened by financial and social support of several elder generations.

There are two major reasons for the difficulty in tracing accurate patterns and structures for families. First, upper-class or high-status families were grossly overrepresented in the literature. Second, until about the last 60 years, writers tended to describe families as they *should* be, rather than as they really were. This led to what Goode has so aptly labeled "the classical extended family of Western nostalgia."[4] For instance, some accounts of colonial families in America are so steeped in nostalgia that the reader concludes that those times were not so rough at all and that if they were, the close, warm family ties healed all wounds.

Families have turned over many of their previous functions, already noted, to institutions, organizations, and professionals outside the family. Yet they have maintained the functions of childbearing, primary socialization of the children, and psychosocial validation or "refueling" for all their members. This last function, the provision of psychosocial verification, worth, and meaning, is probably the most important. Standards for its performance have increased tremendously in recent years, with the popular press reporting all types of help available to meet increased expectations, from individual psychotherapy and counseling to retreats and renewals, self-help books and groups, and high-priced encounters with marriage and family specialists. At the turn of this century the only interpersonal, behavioral requirement between husbands and wives was that they be civil to one another. The new requirement is that they love one another and continue to express this love unfailingly, even into their elder years. An associated new requirement is for increased intimacy through sexuality. The current high rate of divorce is an indicator that marriage, as only an economic arrangement, is definitely past.

"THE AMERICAN FAMILY"

Everyone knows (even non-Americans) what "the American family" is. It is thought to be a white, middle-class mother and father living together in a suburban home with their boy child and girl child (and an optional third child of either sex). The father leaves for work daily and is successful in his career; the mother transforms the house into a home and is not expected to work full time until the last child is in school.

Although this stereotype is rapidly changing, it is to a great extent still thought to be true, even among minorities or those who live in dual-career families or single-parent families. The stereotype excludes more than half the population in the United States today. It is a tribute to American advertising to realize how pervasive this "ideal type" of picture is, although census data provide contradictory evidence. The 1990 census probably will show a growth in the number of households comprised of other than the biologic father and mother and their children.

One of the most difficult tasks facing researchers is to design ways to capture the changing structures of modern families. The old notions of family life span are dysfunctional, when so many families change their structures repeatedly by marriage, divorce, and remarriage, interspersed with varying lengths of time alone or as single-parent families. For instance, in precontemporary literature the sequence described was courtship, marriage, childbearing and rearing, empty nest, retirement, and death of one or both spouses. Today any reader can detail many departures from this sequence. Among alternative family forms are unmarried couples living together (with or without children); homosexual couples (with or without children); deliberately childless couples, married or not; single-parent families with either a father or a mother as the parent; middle-aged couples whose divorced adult children return home with their young children; middle-aged couples living in very crowded situations because of the former pattern and, in addition, their elderly parent or parents living with them; various types of blended families, created by divorced or widowed parents remarrying, and group families, in which several unrelated families share a large space. Within each of these varied structures the rules of organization for carrying out daily living chores differ widely.

For pediatricians, the relevance of these different structural arrangements and rules of organization is that children being raised within them are experiencing very different levels of support and nurturance and are being socialized to value challenge or to reject it, to expect the worst of the world or better, and so on. Children's basic approaches to life make them more resilient or more vulnerable to life's stresses. Knowledge about the family in which the child lives and how he or she views the world provides as valuable information as do the results of physiologic tests.

Although it is not possible to turn pediatricians into sociologists, enticing them toward embracing a sociologic perspective would expand their thinking and encourage them to hypothesize about the most relevant variables of any given case. They also would be less likely to continue to hold mythic or stereotypic views of the families of the children they care for and treat.

One trend in American families, of which most physicians certainly are aware, is that families are smaller. They may not, however, be aware that the number of children in families is related to their general physical and mental health. The obvious inverse correlation of the more "kids," the fewer resources for each reveals some surprises when social class is added. Infant and childhood mortality rates fell for both upper and lower classes when fewer children were born into the families. Young children of large families continue to have more infections, more accidents, and a higher overall mortality rate than do the children of small families, regardless of social class.[10] Sagan, quoting a 1971 study by Columbia University sociologist Joe Wray, notes that the effects of family size can outweigh those of social class. An only child in a poor family has about the same chance of surviving the first year of life as a child who is born into a professional family but who has four or more siblings.

Small families, however, are more prone to violence. One possibility for the increased likelihood of violence in small families is that when a crisis or trouble occurs, there are fewer resources to call upon. For instance, in a family with a single mother and two children younger than 5 years old, if the parent becomes ill, she is likely to be less tolerant of noise or even simple demands of the children. If they do not sleep, or even if they remain relatively quiet when she is trying to rest, they are more likely to be hit or punished. Divorced fathers, trying to make every moment of their visits count, often lose their tempers and end up verbally or physically abusing their children. Spouse abuse also is more common in smaller than in larger families.

Although it is unlikely that pediatricians have the proclivity to examine the findings of family researchers in any great detail or depth, they certainly would find it useful to know more about the specific families in their practices. Studying the trends in one-parent families, or dual-career families, or how urban poor families handle stress compared with suburban families would be a less pragmatic use of their time than learning some new techniques to assess their patients and their families quickly. The genogram is a family assessment device being used in a wide variety of clinical settings.

THE GENOGRAM

The genogram provides a succinct picture of family structures and relationships that includes all family members and shows their generational context.[12,13] It can be drawn quickly with the use of only plain white paper and a pencil; recently there have been attempts to produce computerized versions.[3] There has been increasing interest among clinicians in ways to assess and use psychosocial data in diagnosis and treatment. Articles in journals on family medicine, primary care, and pediatrics repeat the message regarding the importance of psychosocial and family information; yet they usually are not clear about how the clinician is to do this. Like and colleagues[7] note: "How family information should be used appropriately in problem definition and management in everyday clinical encounters, however, has not been made explicit or specific." They make the point that genograms are diagnostic tests and suggest that diagnosis is more than just the process of labeling: "It is the elucidation of the contributing causes of the patient's distress or complaints in such as manner that the clinician will be able to understand more about the way in which a patient is ill, the mechanisms by which the illness is produced, and the reasons why the patient is ill at this particular time so that an appropriate therapeutic intervention can be initiated."[7]

Rogers and Durkin[9] suggest that most physicians would

agree on the importance of taking a family history yet note the general lack of information about the relative utility of different methods of collecting this information. They conducted a study to test the efficacy of genogram use compared with informal interviews during first visits of patients to a university family practice center. The average time for the construction of the genogram was 20 minutes, and it resulted in four times as much information being gathered.

There is a growing body of evidence supporting the long-held notion of seasoned practicing physicians that family function is related to patterns of illness: how a family functions is tied to the physical and emotional well-being of its members. An ill family member does not exist in a vacuum but rather clearly influences those around him or her and is influenced by them. Family dynamics, as causal, contributory, or simply correlational, also have been examined. For example, family stresses have been related to the frequency of a variety of illnesses, as well as to the severity and duration of respiratory illnesses in children.[2]

The construction of a genogram benefits both clinicians and families beyond the data gathered. This creative data-gathering device shows the family that the clinician is interested in them, and establishes a firmer rapport. Families are likely to remember contributory events more clearly and to become more involved in discovering relevant factors and historical events. Because simple paper and pencil are used, the families do not feel subjected to the sometimes frightening "high-tech" machinery and materials now associated with scientific medicine. They can see what is being drawn and understand what the physician is trying to discover. Physicians can teach as they draw, pointing out areas for further inquiry and asking more focused questions. For example, if a child has been seen repeatedly for upper respiratory infections or asthma, the smokers in the family could be highlighted on the genogram in color, thus illustrating more graphically the family's role in the child's illness. This approach is more likely to demonstrate the physician's concern and less apt to induce guilt or to communicate disapproval. Admonitions to "quit smoking" in the absence of graphic portrayal of the effects probably are ineffective.

Rogers and Durkin list another potential use of genograms—as aids in practicing preventive medicine.[9] If pediatricians hold the view that they should see their patients as populations at risk, then the genograms could be used to assess the risk of familial disease and future illness. For example, an obese child in an Italian family in which one parent and two of the four grandparents have diabetes needs more careful monitoring and preventive strategies.

Drawing the Genogram

The clinician should sit so that the family members can watch what is being drawn. At the outset it is useful to tell the family that this is a diagnostic device, much like blood work or an X-ray examination. It also helps to allay anxiety by pointing out that this is not the kind of "test" one encounters in school and that the eraser is handy and almost always is used, because most people remember more accurately and see the need to make corrections as the figure is being developed.

Males are placed on the genogram in boxes, and females in circles. Marriages are indicated by a straight horizontal line connecting the male and female, with the husband on the left and the wife on the right. Dotted horizontal lines indicate cohabitation without marriage; these lines also can be used to connect members of a homosexual couple. Children are drawn by suspending them on a sibling line, which is a horizontal line below the parents, connected by a vertical line. Boxes for boys and circles for girls are drawn, with the oldest to the left. Nonparous pregnancies are indicated as triangles in the appropriate place on the sibling line. If there is only one child, or in case of a first pregnancy, then only the vertical line from the parent's (marriage) line is drawn. Adoptions are shown by use of a dotted line drawn vertically to the marriage line. Divorces and separations are noted by drawing parallel slashes in the middle of the marriage line, where *m* for the date of marriage is shown; *d* indicates divorce and *s* separation. Persons who are not family members but are closely involved in family life can be shown on the genogram and connected by dotted lines where appropriate. For instance, a female au pair would be represented by a circle connected by a dotted line to the parent(s). Companions, home health aides, and very frequent visitors can be shown similarly, as needed.

Genograms can contain only basic data about a family, or data can be added to suit the goals of the clinician, such as prevention or hypothesis testing. For most purposes the following data should be noted for each person on the genogram:

1. The birthdate, preceded by *b* and noted under the box or circle
2. Education, noted by whatever shorthand system the clinician likes to use (e.g., hs, 4th gr., MS)
3. Occupation (e.g., acc't., stu.)
4. If someone dies, a slash is drawn across the box or circle and the death date placed below the birthdate.

The ethnic/religious origin of the oldest generational level is noted above the oldest person in that generation; a shorthand system can be used (e.g., Irish RC, Russ. Jew). Additional information that may be noted includes health and illness status, risk factors, or geographic location of the members.

A practical technique is to copy the genogram on a photocopier, reproducing the darkest image available. The family can have a copy, and clinicians can use their copy to circle currently ill family members or to design hypothetic drawings of alliances, cutoffs, or problems. Color coding can be used to track illnesses such as diabetes or depression. For example, in one family in which three adolescents were seriously overweight, the family designed a color code to indicate exactly how overweight each family member was, including other generations.

Fig. 45-1 illustrates a basic genogram constructed in a pediatrician's office by the pediatric nurse practitioner, who had learned about genograms in a family course. Bobby, age 10, had repeatedly been brought to the office for upper respiratory infections and stomachaches, usually occurring on a Monday morning. His grandmother, who worked as a nurse in an associate's office, was able to bring him for visits more easily than was his mother, also a nurse, who was working nearly 15 hours a day at two full-time jobs. On his fourth visit to the pediatrician in less than a month, he pointed to

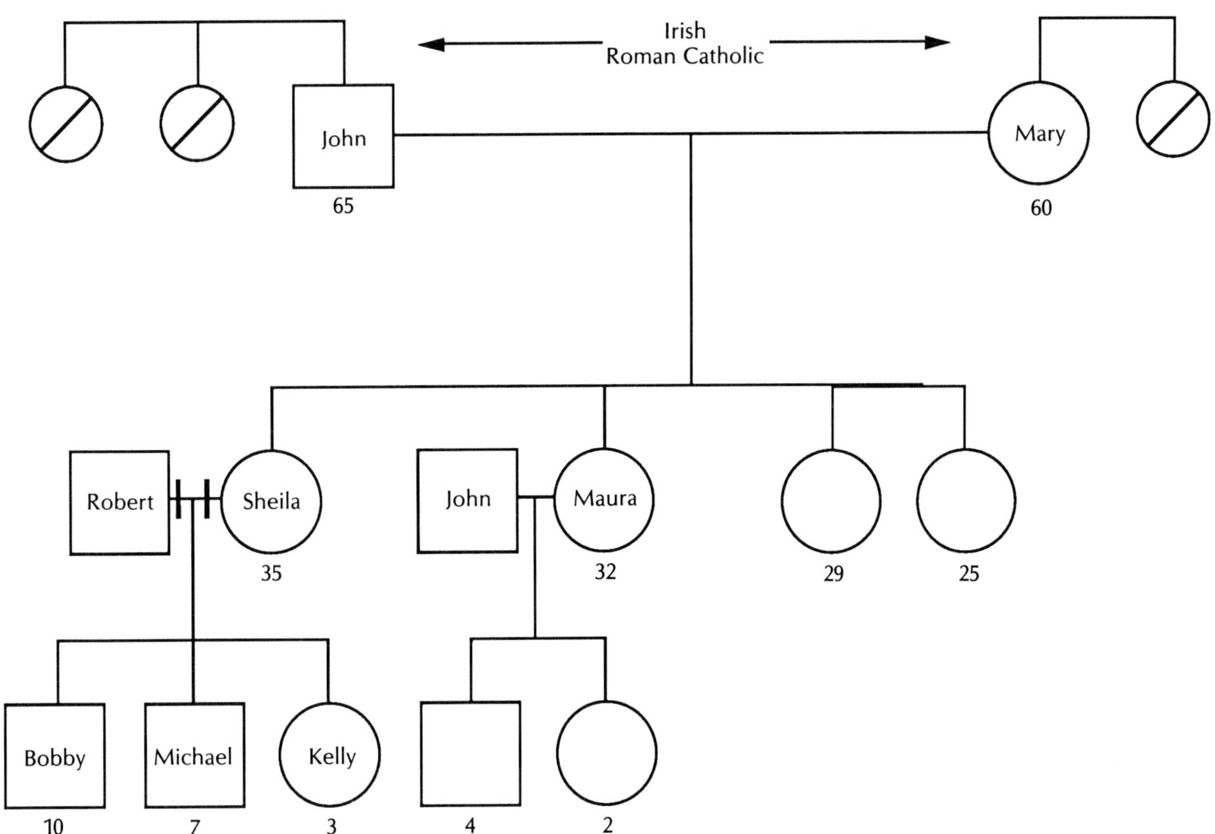

Fig. 45-1 The Flanagan family.

the "Please—lungs at work!! Don't smoke" sign in the waiting room and asked the nurse if he could have one to take home. That opened a discussion of how upset he was with his grandfather's smoking. Mary, the grandmother, and Bobby provided the data shown on the abbreviated genogram.

The Flanagans, John age 65 and Mary age 60, had been planning for many years for their retirement, looking forward to increased leisure and travel. Their four daughters, ranging in age from 25 to 35 years, had not been living at home for the last 5 years. Mary planned to retire at age 62. John had retired at 62 and was spending his time doing all the long-neglected household repairs and watching their daughter Maura's preschoolers while she finished graduate school. John and Mary lived 10 miles from Maura in central New Jersey. The two younger daughters were in California; Sheila, the oldest, was in Washington, D.C., with her political-scientist husband, Michael, and three children.

As Mary describes their family, "We were a typical family, fun-loving, family-centered Irish—not big on expression, but happy. We were atypical only in that no one had any serious drinking problems. Then the bomb struck."

The "bomb" was Sheila's telephone call, announcing that Michael had telephoned her from his assignment in Japan and told her that he was not coming home from the business trip as planned because he was in love with another woman, a Japanese business associate. He said there was no need for hysteria and that his mind was made up and settled. When Sheila consulted a lawyer and began to assess her financial status, she discovered that Michael had remortgaged their home and that the second mortgage was 3 months in arrears. Further financial problems and debts also were discovered. Sheila asked her parents to allow her and the children to come home "temporarily" while she sorted out her life and found a good job. Now John and Mary have a six-person household, plus Maura's two children, most of the week.

John had quit smoking 10 years earlier after a mild stroke but resumed the habit with the increased stress from his expanded family. He quickly went back to smoking nearly three packs a day. Maura, who also smokes, spends more time at her parents, trying to be helpful. Mary's gastric ulcer is bothering her, but she is trying to keep things under control by liberal use of liquid and tablet antacids. Mary reported that Sheila "runs on coffee and cigarettes": two gallons and two packs get her through the day. Bobby had had some asthma attacks as a toddler but none until this current stress. He was the vocal one in the family, expressing sadness and fear; the others were more typical—stalwart, silent Irish—in their coping. His obvious distress was unsettling to his mother and grandparents; their fears were that he was not strong enough and might "turn into a wimp." He was negatively compared with Michael, who was doing well in second grade, and Kelly, whose easy smile and pleasant ways earned her many positive responses.

These data were recorded, along with the genogram, in psychosocial notes. Referral to a mental health center for help with the family distress was rejected. The family agreed only to one family session with a pediatric resident to discuss possible strategies for dealing with Bobby's symptoms. Acknowledgment of the relatedness of Bobby's respiratory problems to his smoke-filled home came only after family members read proffered articles and saw a documentary program on public television. The family believed that Bobby had inherited his grandmother's "weak stomach'" and that nothing much could be done about it. The pediatric staff was frustrated but not demoralized, recognizing that timing differs in families' acceptance of new ideas. Six months after the first visit, Bobby reported spending more time at school and finding friends nearby. He continued his antismoking campaign at home and won an art contest at school for a poster on the dangers of smoking.

FAMILY THEORY AND RESEARCH

Voluminous additions to family literature have been made in recent decades; however, clinical theory about dysfunctional families has not kept pace with the dramatic changes that have occurred in family structures and associated functions and ways of living. As Walsh[15] points out, "Most clinical theory explicitly or implicitly upholds the ideal model of the family as intact, with father as primary wage-earner and instrumental leader and mother as primary parent, homemaker, and socioemotional caretaker." However, fewer than 20% of American families fit this pattern. Still, deviation from this standard is regarded in much of the literature as unquestionably pathogenic. Current textbooks used in clinical training virtually ignore alternative arrangements as possibly more normative. Even when divorce or separation are acknowledged as occurring in half the marriages, the normal sequence of dissolution of ties, emotional upset, management of stress, and adaptations to community demands are not given appropriate consideration.

Clinicians, according to Walsh, thus lack knowledge about what is and is not normal in family life.[15] She describes two types of errors frequently made: the first is to mistakenly identify as pathologic a family pattern that is normal; the second is to assume normality because of failure to recognize a dysfunctional pattern. An example of the first error is the reaction of a clinician, reared in a family in which adults did not openly demonstrate affection and children were supposed to follow the directions of adults, who encounters a family that is noisy, affectionate, and open in expressions of joy and anguish. This clinician, seeing the solicitous concern of a mother for her child—to the point of her bringing in homemade lasagna for her hospitalized child—might view this behavior as enmeshment or symbiosis instead of normal caring. Of course, clinicians do not always assume that what they experienced at home was normal. Some instead see their own upbringing as departing from normal and then apply this view to the families they see; when they encounter one like their own, they view it suspiciously and diagnose the behavior as pathologic.

An example of Walsh's second error is acceptance of the myth that healthy families are free of conflict. Such a view would preclude the clinician from exploring further an assertion by a couple that they have not disagreed in 20 years of marriage. What is common also may be accepted as normal. For instance, noncustodial fathers are so frequently cut off from their children after a divorce that clinicians may fall into the trap of seeing this as normal and thus fail to explore ways that the father and his children might be together.

Pediatricians who feel uncomfortable about exploring the psychosocial aspects of their patients' families miss opportunities to suggest repairs and to help families rethink destructive relationships. Recent research findings demonstrate a positive association between continued supportive contact with the noncustodial parent and long-term adjustment of children. Such contact also affects the custodial mothers positively. Even when previous contact had negative consequences, continuing paternal detachment produces poorer functioning and more symptomatic behavior, especially with boys. Fathers who had negative relationships with their children before divorce have been able in many cases to develop improved relationships after divorce. Walsh, citing several long-term studies, concludes that a clinical imperative in cases of nonparticipating parents is to assess and build the coparenting alliance in postdivorce families.

The degree to which pediatricians feel comfortable in adding psychosocial exploration to their "intakes" or ongoing assessments of treatment or monitoring depends on the messages they received from their mentors or subsequent pushes to change practice habits, which might come from colleagues or the families themselves. Some are reluctant to suggest that psychiatric consultation be sought, even when there is clear evidence either in the child or in the parent of the need. Some are reluctant to discuss behavior that is willful or that reflects a life-style rather than an illness. Drug and alcohol abuse are examples of problems that, even when noticed, are not mentioned by many clinicians.

Early research in family behavior tended to overrepresent white, Anglo-Saxon, Protestant, middle-class families. Comparative studies[8] have included the differences in structures and styles of relating among varied ethnic groups. Other recent studies focus on alternate family forms, such as single-parent and blended family systems. Wallerstein[14] has contributed an insightful and clinically relevant study of the children of divorce, following up families 5 and 10 years after breakup.

An emergent theme is that no single pattern distinguishes well-functioning families from pathologic ones. Something that looks like intrusiveness to a less-than-careful observer may simply be caring, expressed in a particular ethnic style. Also, no single family structure is healthier than other arrangements. If the stresses and the available resources are more or less equivalent, children in single-parent families or children raised by a homosexual couple can do just as well as those in families in which two biologic parents are present.

Walsh[16] cautions that "too often, families with the same presenting problem are presumed to have a similar dysfunctional style, when research, albeit limited to date, reveals a good deal of diversity among families with similarly diagnosed members." Clinicians need to remind themselves that there is no one-to-one correspondence between symptom and system. In the past, rigid application of theories, unsubstantiated by adequate research, created additional strains for families who were already burdened by caring for a sick child. For instance, about 35 years ago, a fairly popular idea was to remove children with asthma from their families as a therapeutic strategy; this was called a "parentectomy," the reasoning being that overinvolved, enmeshed, emotionality between parent (mostly mothers) and child precipitated attacks. Just as there is no single pattern that clearly demarcates a normal family, families cannot be typed by the diagnosis of a family member, whether that is asthma or alcoholism or cancer. Keeping in mind that families are tremendously complex and that a wide array of variables is operative at any moment prevents premature jumping to faulty conclusions. A better stance is forming tentative hypotheses and then engaging the family in their mutual exploration.

CHANGING SOCIALIZATION NORMS

As functions formerly performed by families were transferred to agencies and institutions outside the home, the remaining functions of childbearing, child rearing, and primary socialization assumed more importance. Generations ago, parents simply bore and raised children, with almost no input from strangers and generally little, depending on ethnicity, from extended family members. Today there are specialists for every dimension of these functions, from how to be healthy in pregnancy to how to respond to an adolescent's bad manners.

Americans are generally the greatest consumers of advice on children and health in the world. Parents, depending on their social class and culture, choose different authorities to consult. The appropriate resource for parents' questions is very much determined by their social group, their level of education, and their general sense of assuredness about parenting. Most parents measure the advice not against a standard of good research but rather against a more pragmatic one of whether the advice giver is trustworthy or has a track record of sensible prior advice. All of us, parents or not, tend to hear and believe what we *want* to hear and believe.

Fifty years ago, no profession identified as one of its functions how to teach parents to be parents. Parents were supposed to know how to be good parents either intuitively or because they learned it from growing up in large, extended families. Today, advice, counseling, and teaching about parenting are considered part of the work of pediatricians, pediatric nurse practitioners, child study specialists, health educators, child psychologists, and behavior modifiers. Courses on effective parenting can be found in high school, college, and graduate school curricula, as well as on public television. Socialization failure might be treated by an educational course or by a stay at a psychiatric hospital; some parents still see the military as a solution for offspring who fail to adopt parental values and norms. When a younger child behaves badly in the classroom or resists going to school entirely, the tendency now is to treat this as a "system" difficulty and to use a range of strategies to involve the parents in some type of parenting program. There are even programs for parents whose teenagers abuse drugs or alcohol and for other comparable sibling support groups.

Children do not become well-adjusted adults unless nurtured in some type of close, continuing social unit in which norms are clearly set, self-esteem is fostered, and issues of separateness and connectedness are pursued openly and directly. The most important work of parents as socializing agents is to motivate each succeeding generation to want to go on: In one way or another parents have to help their children become "hooked" on the idea of continuity. Simply put, they have to make it pleasant to be alive and to suggest that one's "debt" for such pleasure is to pass it on to the next person or the next generation. Warmth and tenderness must be experienced before they can be valued and shared with others. Too many people have had traumatic experiences with love turned to hate, warmth to cold, and tenderness to hostility. They fear being vulnerable and fear trusting others.

A large dimension of parenting is to protect children from distrust and hostility and to predispose them to enjoy working and to appreciate tenderness. In other words, parents must convince children that they live in a just world. Otherwise, "behaving," achieving, and going on would make no sense.

More children today are being reared androgynously; they are being invited to explore the dimensions of experience previously totally sex-linked. Boys in nursery school cuddle baby dolls or offer to do the cooking; girls learn how to operate dump trucks. Boys in junior high learn how to sew; girls take woodworking. Most gym classes are no longer sex-segregated; each child is challenged to perform to his or her physical potential. Doomsayers see this as producing mass confusion over sex identity in the next generation. Optimists rejoice at the creation of more fully human persons.

FAMILY TIES

Sagan has suggested that the real reason we live longer is directly related to changes in how children are treated within families rather than to advances in medicine and science.[10] It is well known that life expectancy has risen dramatically in most societies over the past few centuries. As noted earlier, as recently as 1900 the typical American lived only 49 years and one child in five died in infancy. Today, the life expectancy for Americans is 75 years, and infant mortality has declined to one in every 100 births. Both physicians and the public credit modern medicine for these bold achievements, assuming, almost reflexively, that people who lack expert medical care die earlier and that providing more care is the key to longer life. Sagan's plea is that we look more carefully at these assumptions, which are largely unfounded. He provides compelling data for our rethinking of the assumptions we tend to make about the relationship between our efforts at health care on the one hand and our actual health on the other. He shows that although Americans spend more on health care than does any other nation in the world, in many respects we are not actually healthier. He does not deny that modern medicine has accomplished much that is of great value, such as alleviating suffering and developing useful surgical treatments for illnesses or trauma. Yet he clearly shows that neither saving individual lives nor alleviating suffering has contributed to overall life expectancy. Most therapy is not aimed directly at prolonging life, nor do the vast majority of missed physician's appointments endanger life. He reminds the reader that too often what physicians do is not necessary or is based on poor research or no research and that the medicines they prescribe are too many, often without justification for their use.

Having described many compelling instances of how medicine has saved or improved individual lives, Sagan concludes that it has had little effect on the overall health of large populations.[10] What remains is a need for an explanation of why life expectancy has increased spectacularly during the nineteenth and twentieth centuries. There is no question that sanitation and nutrition, the other factors most often cited, have been beneficial. Neither of these, however, accounts fully for the leaps in longevity. Sagan attributes family ties as the key variable in longevity: "It is, in a word, impossible to trace the hardiness of modern people directly to improvements in medicine, sanitation, or diet. There is an alternative explanation for our increased life expectancy, however—one that has less to do with these developments than with changes in our psychological environment."[10]

According to Sagan, growing up and living surrounded by scarcity and ignorance and constant loss is to endure a special misery, that which is a consequence of forces beyond one's control. By extension, a kind of personal powerlessness prevails, in which one's best efforts are not enough to ward off disaster. There is ample evidence that such a sense of helplessness often is associated with apathy, depression, and death—whether in laboratory animals or in prisoners of war. The reader is reminded of Martin Seligman's classic experiments with dogs, which resulted in the concept of learned helplessness as an explanation for why animals and human beings give up, endure pain, or die, rather than take actions to avoid pain and death. People in poverty now share a feature of most premodern societies. Modernization, with its associated community supports such as fire departments, building codes, social insurance, and emergency medical care, cushions most of us from physical, psychic, and economic disaster. These supports have created circumstances in which few of us feel utterly powerless or unable to take control over our lives. We generally feel like the masters of our own destinies, "and that, in itself, leaves us better equipped to fight off disease."[10]

Sagan directly connects the sources of such a sense of personal efficacy and self-esteem to the changed family. Until the late eighteenth century, families were primarily economic units. Marriages were arranged for the purpose of preserving property and children were cheap labor, as noted earlier in this chapter. Beating and whipping were commonplace, even among royalty, as approved tools to teach or extract conformity and obedience. Then, during the Enlightenment, the standards and goals of child rearing began to change. Philosophers argued, eloquently and at length, that if children were to survive in a disorderly and unpredictable world, they could not rely passively on traditional authority. They needed reasoned judgment. To develop such judgment, children needed affection and guidance, not harsh unreasoned discipline and brute force. Gradually, as these ideas took hold, childhood came to be recognized as a special stage of life.[1] Affection and nurturing replaced obligation and duty as the cohesive elements among family members.

Childhood mortality rates fell as a direct consequence of families having fewer children. Families, starting with the upper classes, came to see that children had needs of their own and did not exist to serve the family. This totally new idea resulted in curtailing the numbers of births. Children were seen as individuals in their own right, to be paid attention to and nurtured rather than always to do for others. As lower classes also had fewer children, mortality rates fell among them also. Family size is an excellent predictor of childhood survival, even today. Children in small families are strengthened by the extra nurturance and resources available to them; several studies of infants in institutions, during World War II and after, demonstrated that infants who receive only physical care do not survive.

The new field of psychoneuroimmunology is pursuing the connections between emotional and physical health. Whatever the mechanism that produces greater physical health during periods of emotional well-being needs to be understood. Affection and security may be thought of as natural vaccines. Children who receive consistent love and attention—who grow up in situations in which self-reliance and optimism are nurtured and expected—are better survivors.

THE FUTURE

The future of the family cannot be predicted without placing it squarely in its social context. The trends toward equality of the sexes within families and the larger society certainly have increased self-esteem for women but may cause new stress for men. Careful watching of morbidity and mortality trends will give us a clue to the impact of this important social movement. Divorce rates have leveled, and marriage is again gaining in popularity. The number of dual-career or dual-job marriages and unions is growing each year. Although such arrangements improve the family's economic assets, child care becomes a complex and costly issue, especially in the preschool years.

Considering recent "trend" analyses and surveys, it seems likely that the following future directions for American families might be possible:

1. There will continue to be increasing value placed on human potential, tenderness and warmth, and psychosocial needs being met, rather than on material pursuits as a primary goal for families.
2. The trend toward decreasing numbers of children per family will continue. This will result in greater attention being paid to parent-child relationships and an increased use of professionals as parenting advisers.
3. Neighborhoods will be reinvented, along with community support centers.
4. Extended families will gain the attention of researchers, as will grandparent-grandchild relationships.
5. The new American ideal—strength without domination—will gain impetus and influence in family socialization patterns.

The challenge for pediatricians in this new day will be to keep abreast of changes in family patterns and dynamics and to use this knowledge in providing humanistically oriented and enlightened patient care. The expanded dimension of practice will include the consultant role in the area of parenting. Pediatric practices would do well to invite investigators to use office and hospital visits as opportunities for exploring the areas described here.

REFERENCES

1. Aries P: Centuries of childhood, New York, 1962, Random House, Inc.
2. Boyce T et al: The influence of life events and family routines on childhood respiratory infections, Pediatrics 60:609, 1977.
3. Chan D et al: A microcomputer-based computerized medical record system for a general practice teaching clinic, J Fam Pract 24:537, 1987.
4. Goode WJ: World revolution and family patterns, New York, 1963, The Free Press.
5. Gough K: The origin of the family. In Skolnick A and Skolnick J: Family in transition: rethinking marriage, sexuality, child rearing and family organization, Boston, 1986, Little, Brown & Co.
6. Hareven T: American families in transition: historical perspectives on change. In Walsh F, editor: Normal family processes, New York, 1982, The Guilford Press.
7. Like R, Rogers J, and McGoldrick M: Reading and interpreting genograms: a systematic approach, J Fam Pract 26:407, 1988.
8. McGoldrick M, Pearce J, and Giordano J, editors: Ethnicity and family therapy, New York, 1982, The Guilford Press.
9. Rogers J and Durkin M: The semi-structured genogram interview. I. Protocol. II. Evaluation, Fam Systems Med 2:176, 1984.
10. Sagan L: Family ties: the real reason that people are living longer. In Annual editions: health, '89/'90, Guilford, Conn, 1989, Dushkin Press.
11. Spanier G: The changing profile of the American family, J Fam Pract 13:61, 1981.
12. Smoyak S: Family systems: use of genograms as an assessment tool. In Clements I and Buchanan D, editors: Family therapy in perspective, New York, 1982, John Wiley & Sons, Inc.
13. Smoyak S: Assessing aging caretakers and their families. In Wright L and Leahey M: Families and chronic illness, Springhouse, Penn, 1987, Springhouse Corp.
14. Wallerstein J: Second chances: men, women and children a decade after divorce, New York, 1989, Ticknor & Fields.
15. Walsh F: The clinical utility of normal family research, Psychotherapy 24:496, 1987.

46

Child Abuse and Neglect

Harold P. Martin

Adults sometimes get angry and hit their children; perhaps most do this on occasion. Other adults attack and kill their children. Most parents do not beat up their children, but some do. Most parents at times yell or scream at their children. A few parents regularly disparage, insult, and verbally attack their children. All parents fail on occasion to provide and meet the needs of their infants and children. A minority of parents regularly fail to attend to their children's basic needs for nutrition, health care, stimulation, and emotional nurturance. Although it is common for a parent to respond to the physical attractiveness of their child, a few parents act on their sexual arousal and perform sexual acts on a son or a daughter.

What is child abuse or neglect? In most instances it is clear when an injury to a child falls outside of what we would agree is the result of normal parenting. In a few instances the diagnosis falls into a gray area. The mistreatment of children spans a wide range spectrum of phenomena. No one expects or asks parents to be perfect. Yet we all have some idea of what constitutes a minimally acceptable environment. The concept of "good enough" parenting serves us well in this regard. The "good enough" parent does not break bones or cause burns, bruises, or lacerations by physical punishment or attack. The average acceptable environment provides adequate nutrition, medical care for illness, and intellectual and emotional respect for children.

Child abuse and neglect have been defined in various ways. The essence of all definitions is to identify those child-rearing behaviors and patterns that fall outside the community's standards for adequate or "good enough" parenting. One national definition, a good standard, is that child abuse is the physical or mental injury, sexual abuse, negligent treatment, or maltreatment of a child younger than the age of 18 years by a person who is responsible for the child's welfare under circumstances indicating that the child's health or welfare is harmed or threatened thereby.

The injury or negligence or maltreatment need not stem from malice or necessarily be deliberate. Rather it may arise from ignorance, thoughtlessness, or unavoidable social circumstances. The real essence of the concept is that the child is not safe. Regardless of the reasons, if and when the child's health or welfare is in jeopardy, something needs to be done to protect that child.

The frequency of abuse and neglect can only be estimated. Estimates vary and change as reporting rates change and accuracy of identification improves. Whenever public education and awareness of this syndrome increase, so does the rate of reported cases of abuse. It is said, for example, that sexual abuse tripled in the 1980s, and the incidence of physical abuse rose by more than 75% in that same period. It is not clear whether the actual incidence changed or whether awareness and reporting became more accurate. It was estimated that 1.5 million children were abused or neglected in 1986. Homicide is the leading cause of mortality from injuries in children younger than 1 year of age and accounts for 5% of all deaths in children. Some studies estimate abuse to occur in 1% of all children, whereas others have found that more than 10% of children are physically assaulted each year.

HISTORY AND PATHOGENESIS

Parents have been mistreating their children for centuries. We have been increasingly aware of and concerned about the problem for the past 40 years. If there are any heroes in this saga, they are two. The first is the radiologist John Caffey who in the late 1940s was the first to recognize this syndrome. He noticed some unusual radiologic findings in healing fractures of differing ages and speculated that they might be serially inflicted injuries rather than some arcane metabolic disorder.[1] The second hero was actually a team of clinicians headed by a pediatrician, C. Henry Kempe. In a 1962 article this team called national attention to what they termed "the battered child syndrome."[2] These two events brought to public awareness the physical abuse and mistreatment of children. Reports of child abuse and studies on the subject proliferated after the publication of the 1962 article. All 50 states now have laws mandating the reporting of suspected abuse or neglect. Child protection agencies are over-burdened by identification and treatment of abused children and their families. Newspaper articles regularly report on dramatic or bizarre accountings of child abuse. In the 1970s the number of workshops and conferences on child abuse and neglect grew dramatically.

The question clearly arises: how does this syndrome come about? Why would parents and caretakers mistreat their young? There is no single or simple answer. A great deal, however, is known about the pathogenesis of this disorder. Three interacting factors increase the risk of abuse or neglect: the characteristics of the mistreating adult, the characteristics of the child that may place him or her at increased risk of abuse, and the social context that increases risk of maltreatment.

THE ADULT

Most, but not all, abusive adults were mistreated themselves as children. It is not uncommon to identify families in which abuse or neglect can be seen reaching over several generations. Why might this be so? First, the adult in this situation has learned an abusive style of parenting. We all learn how to parent from our own experiences in being parented as children. Thus the abusive adult may have grown up internalizing mistreatment of children as an expectable, common, and normal way that parents deal with their children. Just as important, mistreated children may grow up with flaws and psychological weaknesses in their characters that lead to abuse of their own children.

Certain personality flaws or weaknesses lead to violence. Abusive parents usually do not deal well with emotions, especially anger, frustration, or humiliation. Further, adults who cannot easily tolerate these feelings may have a pattern of responding to them through physical action, for example, yelling, hitting, and having tantrums. An additional weakness involves a limited repertoire of self-soothing behaviors. All adults get upset or "out of sorts" at times. We all have adaptive mechanisms that help restore our psychological equilibrium. Some of these mechanisms are healthy, some are not. Individuals may isolate themselves, talk to friends, go for a walk, read a book, have too much to drink, go shopping, or escape into the world of television. Abusive adults have limited ways to overcome stress and make themselves feel better. One of their few coping strategies is to strike out at others, either verbally or physically. Abusive adults are also often emotionally labile—that is, they get upset or angry more easily than do most adults. Small, rather insignificant events may move them quickly from a state of emotional equilibrium to rage. Most adults have a spectrum of emotions. A specific event may result in the adult feeling mildly upset, miffed, irritated, moderately angry, annoyed, incensed, or enraged. The abusive adult may move quickly to the most extreme of these feelings with little ability to stop along the way at a less intense level.

Consequently when an adult gets angry easily, cannot tolerate feeling strong emotions, has few self-soothing behaviors, and tends to react to upset by verbally or physically attacking people or things, the presence of an infant or young child in the home leads to a volatile situation.

Further, most abusing adults are lonely and dependent persons who feel unloved and unworthy and who have low self-esteem. They may turn to their child for their quotient of love. They may fantasize and assume that when they have a child, there finally will be someone who will unconditionally love them and make them feel good about themselves. Obviously it does not work that way. Infants and children do not always love their parents or fulfill their needs. Infants and children often act in ways that do not make the parent feel proud of the child, and therefore proud of themselves, but rather make them feel dismayed at having had a "bad child." The disillusionment and disappointment may be too much to bear.

Turning to one's child for love and nurturance in the extreme is a behavior termed *role reversal,* which involves the child taking responsibility for the parent in concrete physical ways or in psychological areas. However, the limited capacity of the child to perform these functions inevitably results in failure and frustration. When a parent's ability to feel good about himself or herself is predicated by and dependent on loving and good behavior from a child, the child is in for a world of trouble.

Some abusive adults are uncompromising taskmasters with rigid ideas of what is right and wrong. They see life in black and white terms. Things are right or wrong; behaviors are good or bad. These persons have minimal capacity for empathy. If others behave in ways they do not approve, they are quick to judge and condemn them. Such adults are not able to appreciate what life is like for an infant or young child. They find it impossible to think and feel from the child's point of view and to imagine why, for example, the child might misbehave. Abusive adults of this type may have found the rigid structure of a military career or a judgmental fundamentalist religious group comforting and in tune with their personality. Such adults frequently justify their abusive behavior by stating that they were only trying to teach the child how to be good and well behaved.

We all have those occasional impulses to quit a job, sock someone, "rear-end" an offending fellow driver, or tell someone off. Most of us hold those impulses in check. We weigh whether the behavior is wise, just, right, or judicious. We can contain our impulses and see that what we imagine doing is wrong or self-defeating or dangerous. Abusive parents, on the other hand, have impaired or tenuous impulse control. It must be emphasized that alcohol and other mind-altering drugs significantly impair impulse control. Anyone, and especially the abuse-prone adult, is at increased risk for getting angry and violent when drunk or impaired from drugs such as amphetamines, heroin, or cocaine. The role of substance abuse in precipitating child abuse is significant.

A small percentage of abusive adults are mentally disturbed or psychotic. The diagnosis of this condition is important because of the need for specific treatment approaches. Most abusive adults, however, are *not* suffering from such disorders.

In summary, it is clear that all adults have the potential to mistreat other adults or children; most of us, however, do not carry out such abusive or neglectful acts. All abusive adults are not the same. They range from drug-abusing sociopaths to pathetic, lonely, isolated, depressed, poor mothers to respectable, uptight professionals who cannot tolerate misbehavior or control the anger that it generates. The aforementioned characteristics that are likely to be found in abusive and neglectful parents suggest treatment and intervention strategies to ameliorate their destructive behavior. Such strategies are addressed later in this chapter.

THE CHILD

It should be made very clear that the victim of mistreatment is not to be assigned responsibility or blame for the behavior of the abusing adult. However, certain behaviors, stages, and characteristics of children place them at increased risk for mistreatment. If the abusive adult cannot tolerate stress or turbulence in his or her life, it stands to reason that children who are "difficult" may trigger mistreatment.

When the child does not meet the expectations of the abuse-prone adult, the risk of mistreatment rises. This may be as simple a matter as the child being of the wrong gender, or it may be more complex. The parent may be unrealistic about developmental levels, expecting the infant not to cry and the 1 year old to be toilet trained. When the child is not quiet, polite, loving, or "good," the abuse-prone adult with unrealistic expectations of such behaviors often will explode and abuse the child.

Some normal children are more difficult to care for than others. The baby who is colicky, overactive, or difficult to feed or soothe is vulnerable if the parent has an increased propensity to be abusive. There should be special concern for the infant or young child who is hyperactive. Because these children are not usually identified as abnormal or special, normal and usual expectations are held for their behavior. When such a child is unconsolable, molds poorly to the shoulder when being held, takes a long time to feed, and later is hyperactive and has a poor attention span, he or she is apt to be upsetting to any parent.

The child's specific developmental stage may be especially stressful to an individual parent. All adults have certain preferences for developmental stages that they especially enjoy and certain stages that they find stressful or ungratifying. Some of us love dependent infants; others do not find infancy a particularly enjoyable stage. Some adults take great joy in the active, talkative, creative preschool-aged child; others find this developmental stage unpleasant and stressful. Although the incidence of abuse is highest in infants, some children fare well until they are of preschool age or until latency or early adolescence occurs; then abuse starts.

The mentally, physically, or medically disabled child may be at increased risk of mistreatment. The child with these problems has not met the expectations of the parents and, further, may be more difficult to care for. Clearly the child with a disability may be less able to give to the parent and/or make the parent feel proud. Additionally, the child with a developmental or medical disorder places serious economic stress on the family. There are data showing that an unduly large percentage of mentally retarded children have been physically abused. Physical or emotional neglect and deprivation may result from the parents' distancing themselves from the child who has special medical or developmental needs.

When there has been a significant impediment to bonding and attachment in the immediate newborn period, it is believed the risks of abuse and neglect increase. In some cohorts of mistreated children, there is an increase in prenatal and perinatal complications. These complications may result in impairments in bonding. The clinician should be alert to increased risk of mistreatment in parent-infant dyads in which difficulties in bonding and attachment have occurred.

THE SOCIAL CONTEXT

Adults from all economic, education, and social strata abuse their children. Economic stress, however, increases the incidence of abuse. Unemployment, poverty, poor housing, and large numbers of children in conjunction with limited resources are clearly associated with increasing incidences of substance abuse, spouse abuse, and child abuse. Certainly most families who are poor, disadvantaged, or poorly educated raise their children quite adequately. One does not need money, education, or social status to be a good parent. The point is that social, economic, or psychological stressors may trigger abuse by adults who are at increased risk of mistreating others. This suggests that the clinician should ask the parent of a child with an injury whether there have been changes in their lives recently. Has the adult lost a job, been evicted from home, lost a friend or lover or spouse, or had other life changes that may account for child neglect or for venting anger and frustration on a child.

IDENTIFICATION AND DIAGNOSIS

Abuse should be suspected when any of the following are identified:

1. The child has injuries of different stages of healing. This suggests repeated or serial physical abuse.
2. The history the parents give keeps changing, is vague, or does not readily explain the type or nature of the injury. For instance, when a child falls, there typically will not be injuries both to the front and back sides of the child nor in the axillae. Rolling from a sofa to the floor is unlikely to result in a skull fracture.
3. There may be pathognomic signs on physical examination, for example, bite marks, cigarette burns, or belt buckle marks.
4. When a child has injuries, suspicion rises when the parents have delayed seeking medical attention or when parents are upset with the child and unsympathetic with the child's pain and fear.
5. Abuse is suspected when there are signs of neglect such as undernutrition, poor hygiene, or untreated medical illness. About one third of abused children are also neglected.

Evaluation of the child should include the following:

1. A complete physical examination is required. It is especially important to look inside the mouth, inspect the genitals and the anal area, examine the fundi for retinal hemorrhages, and to look for signs of previous injuries.
2. When abuse is suspected in children younger than 4 years of age or when an injured child is comatose, the clinician should consider obtaining a skeletal survey (roentgenograms of skull, long bones, and vertebrae) to check for old, healing fractures.
3. Detailed description of injuries, including exact measurements, must be recorded in the chart. Photographs of injuries are especially helpful in documenting them.
4. When abuse is suspected, a "screening" battery of tests for bleeding disorders should be considered to rule out a bleeding or clotting disorder in the child with multiple bruises.
5. The physician who suspects abuse or neglect is legally mandated to report his or her suspicions to the appropriate agency within 24 hours, if not immediately. The agency to contact is usually the county or municipal child protection service agency or the local police. The parents need to be informed that the clinician is making such a report. The physician is obligated to report not only absolutely proved mistreatment but *suspicion* of abuse or neglect. Unverifiable reports will, unfortunately, occur on occasion, but if the report

is made in good faith, the reporter is protected by law.

6. At some later point the siblings of the injured patient should be seen and examined for possible neglect or abuse.

7. After the initial examination, when time and the condition of the child allow, developmental screening of the child must be performed. Developmental delays are found in a large percentage of abused children younger than 5 years of age.

8. The physician must make an immediate decision as to whether the child needs to be hospitalized for medical reasons and whether is is safe for the child to leave the hospital with the caretaker(s). This possibility requires a prompt judgment concerning the child's departure from the office or the emergency room. If the parents do not agree to hospitalization, immediate help from hospital security personnel, the police, a child protective service agency, or a local judge may be needed.

Child protective services are charged with the task of evaluating the family, the child, and the total situation. At this point the decisions about the disposition of the child are taken over by agents of the community—that is, the child protective agency, the courts, or the police. It is their responsibility to determine if the child will be safe at home, whether there is probable cause to assume physical abuse or neglect, where the child shall reside, and what treatments and interventions are necessary and mandated for family and child. The observations and judgments of the physician and nurses will help significantly in these decisions. Although a clinician may be reluctant to turn over such evaluation and decision making to others, those public agencies are legally given that responsibility and their personnel are well trained to carry out those tasks.

TREATMENT

Treatment for the parents may be required by the courts or may be suggested and recommended by the physician, social worker, or others. The kinds of treatment that have been found to be helpful include the following:

1. Parenting classes that provide information and education about children, appropriate developmental expectations, and assistance in learning how to teach and discipline children.

2. Individual or group psychotherapy for most abusers. As previously noted, abusing adults often have character or personality flaws and weaknesses that require professional attention. Parents need to learn how to deal with stress, how to discharge their anger safely, how to identify high-risk times for their child, and how to enlarge their repertoire of self-soothing behaviors.

3. Support groups, such as Parents Anonymous. As with other conditions, it is helpful to know others who have the same problem. Empathic support and constructive help often are accepted more readily from peers than from professionals.

4. In some communities, the assignment of a lay therapist. Lay therapists are nonprofessionals who have been trained and supervised to work with abusing adults. Their work combines the roles of friend, surrogate parent, and big sister or big brother. They make home visits and help the abuser cope with emotional difficulties and everyday problems. They help identify social resources for the abuser to contact and use.

5. Social support. This may include job training, help with accessing social and economic resources, finding child care, and intervening with landlords, employers, or relatives of either parent.

6. Alcohol or drug abuse treatment if appropriate.

7. Couples therapy.

Treatment for the child may involve any or all of the following:

1. Attention to the immediate medical injuries takes first priority.

2. Concomitant treatment of medical problems.

3. A place of safety for the child. Most mistreated children can return home with their parents, if not immediately, within a reasonable time.

4. Consultation from a mental health professional if the primary physician or nurse cannot adequately manage a psychological crisis in the child that may have been precipitated by an inflicted injury.

5. Long-term treatment for the abused child.

Short- or long-term foster care may be required, which is arranged by child protective services. The foster parents will need information from the physician about the medical, psychological, and developmental needs of the child. Day care or preschool placements are helpful treatment strategies for the child who is living with his or her parents. This affords the parents respite and distance from the child, and it provides the child normal and appropriate adult role models. Preschools offer developmental stimulation, peer contact, and assistance with emotional issues created in the home.

Specific treatment may be necessary for developmental delays. This may involve speech therapy, special educational programs, physical therapy, or other specific programs. The mistreated child also may need individual psychotherapy. By the time the problem is identified, behavior problems, depression, difficulties relating to other people, or maladaptive ways of coping with their abusing family have developed in most of these children.

SEQUELAE

In addition to the physical injuries and the medical complications of neglect, a large percentage of mistreated children will have significant neurologic, developmental, or emotional problems. This necessitates careful neurologic examination, developmental screening or more extensive testing, and evaluation of the child's personality traits and interpersonal skills. This screening may be performed by the child's primary physician, or depending on the time, interests, and skills of the physician in question, consultation can be obtained.

Approximately one third of abused or neglected children will have some neurodevelopmental delay. Multiple studies have shown the developmental or intellectual abilities of mistreated children to be lower than those of comparison groups. A few will show significant mental retardation, sometimes from neurologic damage from injuries. It must be emphasized, however, that even without neurologic damage the abusive or neglectful home environment leads to developmental delays. Further, cognition, speech and language development, and perceptual-motor coordination may be delayed as a result of environmental deprivation.

Most mistreated children with developmental delays will show considerable improvement when alternative home care and developmental stimulation are provided or when improvement in the home occurs. One must not necessarily assume that the developmentally delayed abused child is slow because of central nervous system damage. Considerable if not complete rehabilitation is possible with most of these children.

Mistreated children older than 5 years of age may have learning disorders, with or without attention-deficit hyperactivity disorder. Special help through the schools is required to help these children catch up and adapt to a formal learning environment (see Chapter 63).

The psychological problems of abused children tend to be at one end or the other of the spectrum of most psychological parameters. For example, some will be quite fearful and cautious around strangers. Just as many, however, will be indiscriminately friendly with anyone they meet. Some will be hyperactive and have behavior problems; just as many will be quite polite and obsequious people pleasers. Some will be careless, disorganized, and fearless and will always be getting into dangerous situations; others will be unduly cautious and timid.

Children who have been repeatedly abused show deficiencies in their ability to trust others. They cannot trust people or situations; nor can they trust their own ability to predict what will happen to them next. They will be wary and fearful of further mistreatment. The abused are not able to express their anger at being mistreated for fear of further abuse. The most common description of mistreated children is that they are unhappy. These psychological injuries may heal partially when changes in the parents and environment occur. Alternatively, they may require mental health treatment for adequate healing to take place.

PREVENTION

The prevention of abuse and neglect involves social, economic, and political policies and programs. The following comments, however, focus on what the individual health professional can do to prevent child abuse and neglect.

Well-child examinations provide an ideal opportunity to identify families in which there are high-risk factors that increase the chances of abuse occurring. Observations of the parent-child interaction are necessary during routine well-child visits. One can note the parent who is disinterested in the child or, more important, who has unduly high and unrealistic developmental expectations. The physician or nurse may observe parents who turn inappropriately to their child for gratification and fulfillment of their own needs. The use of alcohol or illegal substances should be determined. When marital, economic, or personal stress is high, the risk for substance abuse increases. The clinician should be on the lookout for the aforementioned abnormal personality features in the parents. When the bonding process between parent and newborn has been disrupted or the child is a disappointment to the parents, the outlook is one of high-risk potential.

The key to prevention then is to identify families at increased risk for abuse. At that point, special help and attention may promote prevention of abuse or neglect. Education about child development and discipline should be introduced, and parenting classes can be recommended. It is important to aid the family in developing social networks to which it can during times of crisis. Day care or some sort of alternate care, as well as preschool for the older child, can help defuse a volatile family situation. High-risk parents need to learn ways to solve problems and to prevent and resolve crises. If the physician cannot provide this assistance, then mental health clinics, child protection agencies, psychotherapists, and groups such as Parents Anonymous can do so.

The ultimate prevention of child abuse will occur through providing extensive and adequate treatment to mistreated children so that they will not grow up to repeat the pattern of child maltreatment with their children.

SEXUAL ABUSE

The key to the diagnosis of sexual abuse of infants and young children is maintaining a high index of suspicion. Most health care providers usually do not think of sexual exploitation of very young children. Included in the differential diagnosis whenever there are symptoms or signs related to the anal or genital areas of either boys or girls should be sexual abuse. The physician whose index of suspicion is low or whose reaction is denial may attribute problems as obvious as venereal disease to nongenital contact.

Few children lie or make up stories about sexual behavior. If the child tells of sexual contact, or if his or her behavior suggests unusual preoccupation with sexuality, then an evaluation for sexual abuse must be included in the workup. Most sexual abuse of children is perpetrated by family members or by friends of the family, including parents and grandparents. The sexually abusing adult may not be neglectful or have the personality traits of physically abusive parents.

The child can be more emotionally traumatized by poor management of the incident than by the original sexual abuse. The pelvic examination, or any examination of the genitalia, must be performed with privacy and a great respect for the fearfulness, embarrassment, and shame of the child. It is quite common for sexual victims to be held culpable for their own victimization. It is absolutely essential that no one imply that the child is responsible for the exploitive acts of the abusing adult. When sexual molestation of a young girl is identified, the common response is to move her out of the home. Taking her away from her home, siblings, neighbors, and playmates commonly is interpreted by the child as punishment for something she has done. Careful and empathic explanations are required so that the child does not make that assumption.

When a girl reports sexual mistreatment from her father, she often is the target of anger and resentment from her mother and siblings. It is because of her that Dad is in trouble, may lose his job, or may go to jail. Although that reaction may be understandable, it is essential that counseling for the girl and the entire family be initiated. This may be necessary to prevent the sexually abused girl from paying the additional emotional price of guilt, enmity from the family, and erroneously assumed culpability.

SUMMARY

It is difficult for health professionals to recognize and manage child abuse. To suspect or diagnose child abuse forces one to acknowledge that such behavior happens and is a potential problem in any family. It is easy to become judgmental or emotionally overinvolved in working with a physically or sexually abused child. It is especially difficult to recognize abuse in parents whose educational or social background is similar to that of the health professional. It may be helpful to remember that most abusing adults are ashamed of their behavior and desire to stop. The clinician can help the parent by identifying and reporting suspected abuse and by becoming active in treatment planning. It is through this process that subsequent injury to the child can be prevented, that the chances of the family regaining functional status can be maximized, and that the integrity of the family can be reinstituted.

REFERENCES

1. Caffey JP: Pediatric x-ray diagnosis: a textbook for students and practitioners of pediatrics, surgery and radiology, ed 2, Chicago, 1950, Year Book Medical Publishers, Inc.
2. Kempe CH et al: The battered-child syndrome, JAMA 181:17, 1962.

SUGGESTED READINGS

Berkowitz C: Sexual abuse of children and adolescents, Arch Pediatr 34:275, 1987.

Garbarino J: Preventing childhood injury: developmental and mental health issues, Am J Orthopsychiatry 58:25, 1988.

Garbarino J, Guttman J, Seeley J: The psychologically battered child, San Francisco, 1986, Josey-Bass, Inc, Publishers.

Levine MI: a pediatrician's view, Pediatr Ann 18:467, 1989 (editorial).

Martin HP: The abused child: a multidisciplinary approach to developmental issues and treatment, Cambridge Mass, 1976, Ballinger Publishing Co.

Olds DL, Henderson CR, and Chamberlin R: Preventing child abuse and neglect: a randomized trial of nurse home visitation, Pediatrics 78:65, 1986.

Strauss MA and Gelles RJ: Societal change and change in family violence from 1975-1985 as revealed by two national surveys, J Marriage Fam 45:465, 1986.

47

Child Custody

Alice G. Dvoskin

Child custody has only recently become an issue for contest in the courts. Under Roman law, the father had absolute control over his wife and children; the mother, chattel herself, had no rights. Subsequently, Roman law was adopted as common law in feudal England. By the end of the eighteenth century, however, English courts were becoming more aware of the need to protect the welfare of children, a development reflected in a famous 1817 decision in which the poet Percy Bysshe Shelley lost custody of his children after the suicide of their mother because the court rejected his moral standards and life-style. The English courts exercised their jurisdiction over the welfare of children under the doctrine of *parens patriae*. The Lord Talfourd Acts of 1839 applied *parens patriae* specifically to children under 7 years of age and thus became known as the Tender Years Doctrine. It was believed that children in this age group were in need of their mothers. The Guardianship of Infants Act of 1925 clearly announced the woman's equal right to the child.

The history of custody determination in the United States has closely paralleled that of England. However, once the Tender Years Doctrine became accepted in the United States, a clear preference for awarding custody to the mother emerged in the majority of cases, regardless of the child's age, thus constituting a maternal presumption. The Tender Years Doctrine and the maternal presumption then became factors to be considered by courts in applying the current criterion of "best interests of the child."

Increased divorce rates and parental mobility, combined with a change in socially acceptable gender role definitions, have necessitated reevaluation of current custody policies. Statistics, which have remained relatively constant over the past 20 years, indicate that mothers now receive custody in roughly 90% of all cases. Although the majority of divorcing couples agree on custody arrangements out of court and only about 20% of custody adjudications are contests before a judge, societal debate about child custody appears to be growing in magnitude and intensity. The civil rights and women's movements have drawn attention to discriminatory policies based on sex. In the past, maternal unfitness had to be proven for a father to overcome the presumption that the child was better off with his or her mother. Previous guidelines based on beliefs that fitness is related to past misconduct, maternal employment, religious conviction, or cohabitation without wedlock are currently being strongly challenged. Also challenged are biases with regard to sexual preference of the parent and psychiatric history. The custody arena is further complicated by efforts by grandparents and other major caretakers for the child to obtain either custody or visitation privileges. The concept of "psychological parent," first proposed by Goldstein, Freud, and Solnit in their landmark book, *Beyond the Best Interests of the Child*,[2] has been cited by courts in awarding custody to a caretaker other than the natural parent.

An increasing body of literature on fathering must also be considered in any discussion of child custody policies. As cases such as the Salk decision (in which the father was awarded custody of his children based on his superior ability to serve their emotional and cultural needs despite clearly determined maternal fitness) receive publicity, more fathers will be encouraged to seek custody. The same societal changes that apparently are leading to an increased number of custody cases reaching the courts are also questioning the guidelines that judges have traditionally used in custody decisions. The paucity of meaningful and updated guidelines often leaves judges in an uncomfortable position, forcing them to make critical decisions in the absence of conventions or proven methods of evaluating evidence. And the evidence itself may be varied and complex. In addition to the testimony of the parents, evidence may be derived from the testimony of the child. The court also may request custody reports from a state social services agency and recommendations from health professionals and may consider results of private investigations solicited by the litigants. In recognition of the child's rights and privileges in the light of an often bloody battle between the parents, courts in many jurisdictions have seen fit to appoint an attorney for the child in contested custody matters. It may be within the role of this individual, sometimes known as a guardian *ad litem*, to solicit information from professionals familiar with the child for assistance in decision-making. The child's attorney also might be asked to screen out testimony before the court that may be harmful to the child or otherwise violate his or her confidentiality privilege.

CUSTODY EVALUATION CRITERIA

All parties to custody litigation pay lip service to their paramount concern for the best interests of the child. This "concern," however, is meaningless without specific criteria for evaluating the motivation and capacity of each parent to provide for the healthy physical, emotional, and social development of the child. Because the courts are increasingly calling on health and mental health professionals to testify regarding such issues, it has become necessary for these experts to develop more systematic criteria for evaluation.

To date, the most comprehensive set of criteria defining the best interests of the child is that set forth by the Michigan Progressive Child Custody Act of 1970:

1. The love, affection, and other emotional ties existing between competing parents and the child.
2. The capacity and disposition of competing parents to give the child love, affection, and guidance and to continue educating and raising the child in his or her religion or creed, if any.
3. The capacity and disposition of competing parents to provide the child with food, clothing, medical care, or other remedial care recognized and permitted under the laws of the child's home state.
4. The length of time the child has lived in a stable, satisfactory environment and the desirability of maintaining continuity.
5. The permanence of the family unit in the existing or proposed custodial home.
6. The moral fitness of the competing parents.
7. The mental and physical health of the competing parents.
8. The child's record of home, school, and community functioning.
9. The reasonable preference of the child if the court deems the child to be of sufficient age to express a preference.
10. Any other factor considered by the court to be relevant to a particular child custody dispute.

An important consideration frequently added to this list is that custody be awarded to the parent who will most facilitate the child's visitation with the noncustodial parent.

The above criteria clearly imply that simply interviewing a parent and assessing parental fitness is insufficient. Decision-makers need data about the child's entire environment. It is therefore likely that either the court or the mental health professional asked to offer a recommendation to the court will request reports from school personnel, pediatricians, and community health facilities, and other relevant social agencies.

The Child Custody Evaluation

Because custody decision-making involves highly complex issues of family and child processes and engenders considerable emotion and self-interest in the principals, the input of an impartial expert schooled in child development and family dynamics is increasingly relied upon. Child psychologists and psychiatrists often are asked to perform an evaluation and make custody recommendations. Social workers and counselors may be asked to visit the home and observe the child's living arrangement.

The foremost consideration for the mental health professional is to maintain objectivity. Ideally the evaluator should be appointed by the court, but in practice he or she often is solicited by an attorney representing one of the adult parties to the dispute. In order to make a creditable recommendation with regard to child custody, the evaluator must first ensure the cooperation of all parties to the dispute, have free access to the child in the company of both parents, and be granted access to all relevant documents and reports. Interviews should include individual clinical interviews with each parent, stepparents when present, and each child. Observations of the child with each parent, especially when evaluating a very young child, are most helpful. Psychological testing can be helpful in corroborating clinical impressions. Although projective personality testing is useful with both adults and children, the legal system is more likely to comprehend and give greater weight to objective measures. Information from significant others in the child's life, such as grandparents and baby-sitters, should be used. Many evaluators also recommend home and school visits.

An issue of increasing concern appearing in the course of evaluation is the allegation, by one or the other parties to the dispute, of abuse, either physical or sexual, directed toward the child. Such an allegation may necessitate medical examination of the child and the involvement of a child protective community service agency. Such an allegation may require the evaluator to be trained in specialized interviewing skills and to use special equipment such as anatomically correct dolls, to generate the evidence.

DYNAMICS OF CHILD CUSTODY DISPUTES

Divorce represents the inability of two people to fulfill the reciprocal roles of husband, wife, and lover. They may enter court in a custody battle to exonerate themselves through the child; each parent often has a strong need to establish, in the public forum of the court, that the other parent is at fault and is incompetent. Parents may project their own hurt and rejection into statements about the child's ill treatment by the other spouse. The child often becomes the vehicle for the fulfillment of a parent's emotional needs left unmet after separation. In addition to these issues of parental self-esteem, the practical issue of support can provide another motive for seeking custody: Some fathers may seek custody to avoid child support payments to the ex-wife; custody would thus return to the father control over the child's life and control over the money he spends on the child. Often parents are prodded into custody battles by grandparents. This occurs more frequently when one or both of the parents (and child) have lived with one set of grandparents, who thus have had an opportunity to become more attached to the child.

Divorce resulting from marital infidelity is often accompanied by significant rage. One outlet for a vindictive response is to demand custody to protect the child from the influence of this "immoral" person. It must not be forgotten that a custody battle in court necessitates continued contact between warring parents. Parents who are legally but not yet emotionally divorced may unconsciously seek to keep their relationship alive by this means.

On the other hand, hostility and the need for retribution are not always the grounds for pursuing a custody suit. Parents often act out of the sincere conviction that they can best provide for their children's physical, social, and emotional development. To this end they may demonstrate a willingness to make significant personal, financial, and professional sacrifices.

Whatever the motives for requesting custody, the process is further complicated by current divorce litigation procedures, which define custody of children as a bargaining chip in the settlement. For example, recent divorce reform legislation in some states has awarded continued residence in the family home to the parent retaining custody. The possibilities for abuse during custody disputes have been sadly evident in the increased number of child-snatching cases, a problem that requires changes in federal laws regarding moving such children across state lines before it can be resolved.

TYPES OF CUSTODY ARRANGEMENTS

There are now a number of recommended custody and visitation arrangements. In an attempt to reduce the adversarial nature of the process, many jurisdictions have begun to refer to parenting arrangements rather than custody. *Sole custody* is the traditional arrangement, whereby one parent is awarded custody and is expected to assume responsibility for major decisions regarding the child. This may be the best alternative when parents have clearly demonstrated their inability to cooperate. *Split custody* refers to a situation in which the parents each assume custody of one or more of their children. This alternative is rarely used, since there are compelling arguments for keeping children together, the most important being that they often provide one another with mutual support and with the only consistency in their environment.

Joint custody is an increasingly popular alternative that implies shared responsibility as well as shared time spent in the care of the child. The exact amount of time spent with each parent may vary among families, but the basic assumption remains that both parents will continue to share equally in the rights and responsibilities implicit in child rearing. Arguments in favor of joint custody include the assurance to the child of unbroken contact with both parents as well as protection for parents against the sense of loss and ultimate distance that often develops for the noncustodial parent. Advocates of joint custody state that it encourages parental participation and lessens the responsibility of the sole custodial parent. They also tout it as promoting overall cooperation and decreasing postdivorce litigation. However, joint custody is not a panacea, and the risks should be recognized: Children may be thrust into the role of "spy" or "messenger" if parents are unable to communicate and cooperate; such an arrangement requires parents to live in close physical proximity so that the children's school and social needs are not disrupted; and joint custody may prove more expensive, since each parent must maintain full facilities for the children. Thus joint custody has been characterized as an alternative for the middle to upper socioeconomic classes. Finally, critics of joint custody brand it an easy way out for judges who find sole custody decisions to be agonizing.

To date, studies attempting to assess the long-term effects of custody alternatives remain inconclusive. Unbiased, empirical research would require a longitudinal study of families randomly assigned to the different custody arrangements; such a format is obviously impossible. Nevertheless, legal and mental health experts agree that joint custody or shared parenting has as a prerequisite open communication and cooperation between parents, since it concerns their children. Thus custody questions before the court must still be determined case by case.

Child Custody Mediation

Mediation and conciliation have long been techniques of conflict resolution in a variety of cultures. Typical examples include the Quakers in the United States, who commonly use mediation and arbitration, and the Peoples Conciliation Committees of China. In the past, before social change dislodged the structure of the large extended family, matriarchs and patriarchs served as mediators of disputes within the family.

Changes in divorce legislation, specifically no-fault divorce laws, acknowledge the shift from the courts to the parties involved with regard to responsibility for determining whether the divorce is warranted. Nevertheless, when the issue is children or parenting, the adversarial system is typically used, with its characterizations of plaintiff and defendant, winner and loser.

Studies by mental health professionals of the family and communication systems within the family (in conjunction with legal precedents of arbitration and negotiation) have provided an alternative to the adversarial system. The potential now exists to help divorcing families through the psychological aspects of the divorce and to assist them in understanding the contractual definitions of individual and shared responsibilities for meeting the needs of the children.

Originally the goal of promoting reconciliation between separating couples motivated California, in 1939, to establish court-connected conciliation services. Recognizing a great need, conciliators began offering mediation services, specifically custody mediation, for couples unwilling to reconcile.

The theory behind custody mediation is essentially that primary emphasis be placed on the responsibility of the participants to make decisions that will affect their own lives and those of their children. The process of mediation consists of systematically isolating the points of agreement and disagreement, developing options, and considering compromise through the use of an impartial third party (mediator). The mediator acts as a facilitator of communication as well as an individual who may help the parties define issues and promote settlement. Recognizing the extent of emotions associated with divorce, the mediator attempts to educate the spouses about each other's needs and those of the children. Unique and personal approaches to dispute resolution are developed for use at the time of the divorce and for the future when circumstances, of necessity, will change. Mediation is typically private and confidential and frequently restricted to the principals only (i.e., without their lawyers).

Mediation offers the advantage of being expeditious. That is, individuals need not be delayed by a crowded court docket. Mediation may be considerably less costly than the traditional adversarial method; it is also procedurally more reasonable and comprehensible. Perhaps most important, mediation teaches and promotes skills of negotiation and cooperation that hopefully can be used by parents for dispute resolution over the lifetime of their children.

The practice of mediation may be court based, either mandated by the judge or entered into voluntarily. Such programs have become increasingly widespread as judges recognize the dysfunctional effects of the adversarial process on families of divorce. Mediation also may be obtained through a private practice, fee for service model. Finally, community mental health agencies or clinics may offer mediation services from a position of child advocacy.

Although a viable alternative to litigation, mediation is not for everyone. It is generally believed that mediation is inappropriate in matters in which there has been allegation or evidence of child abuse or neglect or in matters with a history of any domestic violence. Likewise, mediation is not recommended in cases involving considerable postdivorce conflict that resulted in frequent court appearances. Finally, mediation is not recommended when either member of the couple has a history of mental retardation, serious psychiatric illness, or antisocial acting out.

The increasing use of mediation as an alternative to litigation has created an urgent need for the determination of professional qualifications for mediators and some form of regulatory control over the practice.

THE PEDIATRICIAN'S ROLE

A child's pediatrician may become involved in the custody adjudication process at the evaluative stage, the implementation stage, or both. While a case is being evaluated for custody and visitation recommendations, the pediatrician might participate at several points. The minimum involvement may require only an awareness of the evaluation and a sensitivity to the needs of the child and parents. Or the pediatrician may be asked to file a report or be interviewed by an attorney or investigating mental health professional. Finally, the pediatrician may be subpoenaed to appear and testify in court regarding his or her evaluation and recommendations.

The pediatrician also may play a role in the implementation of the postdivorce custody and visitation process. Again, the extent of involvement may range from being sensitive to the emotional adjustments required of the child, to being a supportive ally of the child and parents, to participating in the contractual arrangement as child advocate. The pediatrician should be aware of how easily he or she, as a concerned community professional, can be swept into the parental struggles, as illustrated in the following example:

> In one divorced family, the children, an 11-year-old boy and a 16-year-old girl, remained in their mother's custody; the father lived out of town. The father's visits with the children had only recently resumed after a 4-year hiatus and required considerable advance planning. However, as the date of the visit approached, the son would become asthmatic and his mother would claim that he was too ill to see his father. Since the father had to travel 1600 miles for each visit, considerable friction developed between the mother and father. The father believed that his ex-wife was exaggerating their son's symptoms to sabotage the visits. Eventually the parents agreed to accept the opinion of the pediatrician as to the child's physical ability to have the father visit at the appointed time.

Although such an arrangement appears equitable, it can prove burdensome and time consuming to physicians, particularly when they find themselves caught in the middle.

Recognizing the emotionally charged nature of custody and visitation negotiations, the pediatrician may sometimes find it necessary to refer the family for mediation or psychological counseling. Also, it is not unusual for attorneys to transcend their role of providing legal advice to parents by offering further advice regarding which custody arrangements would be in the best interest of the child. Such advice may be based on intuitive or even mistaken notions about child development. In such situations a telephone or office conference with one or both attorneys (with or without the parents) can help clarify the appropriate division of professional expertise and responsibility in the case. The pediatrician should not hesitate to advise parents or their lawyers on specific parenting issues that might come about as a result of separation and divorce. Having specialized knowledge of the child in question, as well as developmental issues in general, the pediatrician is equipped to provide guidelines on issues of parental contact or age-appropriate sleeping or health care arrangements. More concretely, the age and personality of a specific child may warrant daily scheduled phone contact with the noncustodial parent as opposed to spontaneous contact. Similarly, the pediatrician may recommend fewer but extended visits rather than frequent, brief visits so as to reduce painful transitions for a younger or otherwise more vulnerable child. A publication by the American Psychiatric Association, "Child Custody Consultation," provides useful information and guidelines on such matters as custody evaluation methods and preparation for court appearances. It is highly recommended to the pediatrician who becomes involved in this difficult area. Professional and community resources and books for children, parents, and other family members that can be of help in sorting out the difficulties that attend divorce and custody arrangements are discussed in Chapter 48, "Children of Divorce."

REFERENCES

1. American Psychiatric Association Task Force on Clinical Assessment in Child Custody: Child custody consultation, American Psychiatric Association, 1400 K Street, NW, Washington, DC, 20005.
2. Goldstein J, Freud A, and Solnit AJ: Beyond the best interests of the child, New York, 1973, The Free Press.

SUGGESTED READINGS

Bernstein JE: Books to help children cope with separation and loss, New York, 1977, RR Bowker Co.

Emery RE: Interparental conflict and the children of discord and divorce, Psychol Bull 92:310, 1982.

Folberg J and Miene A, editors: Divorce mediation theory and practice, New York, 1988, The Guilford Press.

Kappelman MM and Black J: Children of divorce: the pediatrician's responsibility, Pediatr Ann 9:50, 1980.

Keller WG and Bloom LJ: Child custody evaluation practices: a survey of experienced professionals, Professional Psychology: Research and Practice 17:338, 1986.

Lamb ME: The role of the father in child development, New York, 1981, John Wiley & Sons, Inc.

Wallerstein JS and Kelly JB: Surviving the breakup: how children and parents cope with divorce, New York, 1980, Basic Books, Inc, Publishers.

48

Children of Divorce

Muki W. Fairchild and Bradley H. Zebal

The past two decades have been marked by increasing societal concern about the impact of marital separation, divorce, and child custody arrangements on the family. Similarly, remarriage and the subsequent difficulties involved in stepfamilies are also receiving greater attention. These concerns have been reflected in both the popular media and the professional literature; indeed, after years of relative neglect, the study of divorce and related phenomena is now a rapidly growing area of scientific investigation. Given the striking increase in divorce rates in the United States in recent years, it is clear that a significant number of children and adolescents being seen by pediatricians are from families involved in marital and family disruption.

Each step in this process poses unique challenges to the coping abilities of the parents and children involved, and the process as a whole is difficult and painful for even the healthiest families. Because the pediatrician will probably have continual contact with family members throughout the separation and divorce, he or she has a unique opportunity to support all family members and to act as an advocate for the children when required. Fortunately, the pediatrician is aided in this effort by a growing body of increasingly sophisticated research. Early studies focused on whether divorce really affects children negatively and if so, what the negative consequences are. More recent studies have begun to delineate what specifically about divorce is stressful to which children under which conditions, in the short term as well as the long run.

INCIDENCE

It has become customary to begin discussions about divorce with a recitation of dramatic statistics concerning its increasing prevalence in the United States. Although a number of sources confirm the rising divorce rate, the frequently offered statistic that there is currently one divorce for every two marriages in the United States must be interpreted with caution; such figures include *all* marriages, and the divorce rate for subsequent marriages is higher than that for first marriages.

Nevertheless, the figures are sobering. The divorce rate in 1984 (4.9 per 1000 population) was nearly double that in 1966 (2.5 per 1000 population), and it is estimated that more than 60% of divorces now involve families with children under 18 years of age.[4] Roughly 350,000 children were involved in divorces in 1956; the current annual figure is well in excess of 1 million. An even greater number of children are likely to be affected in the future. It has been suggested that 38% of all white children and 75% of all black children born to married parents will experience a parental divorce before 18 years of age. When children born to unmarried parents are included with those separated from their parents through divorce, the figures are even higher. Recent projections suggest that for children born in the late 1970s and early 1980s, at least 50% and possibly up to 75% will spend some time in a single-parent family.[4,6] Since most divorced parents do remarry, it seems likely that between one third and one half of all children born around 1980 will also live in a stepparent family at some point in their childhood. Because 55% of remarriages are expected to end within 10 years, about 35% of these children will undergo a second divorce and family disruption. Another divorce statistic bears mentioning. Because of an increased incidence of divorce in young adults, the average length of marriage before a legal divorce is now only 6.6 years. Thus most children of divorce experience the divorce during their preschool years.[4,15]

STAGES OF DIVORCE

Divorce is best understood as a lengthy process with multiple stages that unfolds over many years rather than as a single discrete event. All family members are called upon to make a series of adjustments over time.[9,16,19] It begins with a period of marital unhappiness culminating in a decision to separate. This decision, only seldom mutually wished for, ushers in the acute stage, which may last up to 2 years after the actual legal divorce has taken place. The acute stage is frequently marked by extraordinary stress for the entire family, as conflict escalates and parents act in ways that may be markedly different from their usual behavior. During this period of great turmoil, children suffer not only from the disintegration of the family structure as they have known it but also from diminished parenting, because their parents are preoccupied with their own troubles.

The transitional phase is characterized by a general settling, as the new single-parent family attempts to rebuild and create a new and, it is hoped, better life. Although change and some instability continue to be important features as new relationships and life decisions are made, tried, and sometimes rejected, this period is characterized for children by greater participation in the events of the family. Visitation patterns tend to become more stable, although there is some evidence that a general shift toward a decline in visitation with the noncustodial parent over time takes place.

The final phase is the postdivorce stage, which is reached when a fairly stable single-parent household has been achieved. Since 75% of all divorced women and 80% of divorced men do remarry,[7] the change into a remarried household may still occur and entail yet another period of destabilization and adjustment, made more complicated by the ghosts of the failed marriage and the reactions of children, grandparents, and ex-spouses on all sides.

NATURE OF THE EXPERIENCE

To appreciate fully the impact of a divorce on children, it is helpful to understand some of the ways in which a divorce is unique and different from other traumas and losses, such as the death of a parent. First and foremost, divorce is a process perceived and experienced differently by children and adults. Divorce is a choice, a hoped-for solution to a problem in the lives of the adults; children rarely wish for such a rupture and rarely are glad when it has occurred. On the contrary, reconciliation wishes are persistent and enduring, despite remarriages and the passage of time. The nature of a divorce in and of itself poses a dilemma for the child. Under normal circumstances, children view their parents as sources of comfort when problems arise. It may be difficult for a child to turn for solace to the very creators of the problem. Indeed, the angry feelings that the parents' "choice" of a divorce has engendered may well add to the child's inability to use his or her parents' concern and support. Another major difference between the child whose parents have divorced and the child who has lost a parent through death is the lack of social supports. At a time when diminished parenting typically occurs, there are few societal supports or rituals to fill the void or ease the pain. Whereas the death of a parent or a natural catastrophe such as a hurricane tends to mobilize the family and community, divorce all too often results in increased isolation and loss.

The child of divorce may sustain numerous losses, some less obvious than others. For most children the greatest and most immediate loss is that of one parent, typically the father. Despite the growing availability of joint custody, 90% of all children are in sole custody arrangements with their mothers.[4,20] A marked decline in visitation with the noncustodial parent over time is not unusual; 50% of the children in one nationally representative survey had not seen their fathers in 1 year or longer.[4] Surprisingly, there has been no correlation between the predivorce and postdivorce relationships; fathers who were close and invested in the lives of their children before the divorce became aloof and uninvolved in later years, and vice versa.[4,19]

The loss of the family structure has profound economic implications. Initially, there is a drop in both men's and women's predivorce levels of income; 5 years later, men's income has increased 23% above and women's has decreased 30% below predivorce levels.[4] Child support payments are poorly enforced. One 1981 study found that only 47% of divorced women get full child support, 25% get partial child support, and the remaining 28% receive no support.[4] These economic changes may force women to work more and longer hours, further decreasing the time and energy available for parenting. Another possible associated loss is a geographic move. Hetherington, Cox, and Cox found that children of divorce undergo more negative life changes than do children in nondivorced families.[11] A change of residence can lead to a change of neighborhood, school, church, clubs, and friends.

If the divorce has been acrimonious and if the extended family takes sides in the conflict, the child may also lose access to one set of grandparents. Grandparents have long been acknowledged to be important figures in the lives of their grandchildren, and they have responded by turning increasingly to the courts and obtaining legal support for visitation rights of their own.

Although most children remain in the physical custody of their mothers, many of them nonetheless lose the predivorce relationship they once had with her. Custodial mothers have been found to spend less time with their children, to be less sensitive to their needs, and to provide less discipline after a divorce.[10,15,19] Their parenting is characterized by increased order and decreased warmth, which results in a vicious cycle in which the child becomes increasingly oppositional and the mothers even less warm. Mothers and sons appear to be at particular risk for developing this kind of relationship, and although improvement has been noted 2 years after the divorce, it is still not as good as the nondivorced mother-son relationship. This pattern is of particular concern because of research suggesting that the most important protective factor in psychological development of children after divorce may be the custodial mother's mental health and quality of parenting.[12,15,16,19] In fact, it appears that children can be buffered from divorce-engendered stresses, including the pernicious effects of decreased economic resources, hostility from an ex-spouse, and the increased burden of single parenting, if a loving, effective mother-child relationship is able to continue. A comparison has been drawn between the children of divorce and the children of the London blitz.[12] Despite physical destruction and danger, economic hardship, and the absence of their fathers, the children who remained with their mothers during the German bombing raids on London in World War II did better emotionally than the children who were removed from their homes and sent to physical safety in the countryside.

EFFECTS OF DIVORCE

There appears to be an emerging consensus among clinicians and researchers alike that most children experience their parents' divorce as painful and stressful. During the first 2 years after divorce, disruptions in functioning and acute emotional distress are likely. However, many children do improve if the divorce is not compounded by additional trauma or continued stress. Two longitudinal studies, the California Children of Divorce Project[15-19] and the Virginia Longitudinal Study of Divorce and Remarriage,[7,10,11] have provided extensive information on the impact of children's adjustment to divorce.

The pioneering work of Wallerstein and Kelly began in 1971 with a longitudinal study of 131 children in northern California, divided almost equally between boys and girls, who were 2 to 18 years of age at the time of separation. These children, who came from middle-class backgrounds and had no history of emotional disturbance or developmental delays, were studied at the time of separation and then 18 months, 5 years, and 10 years later. Extensive clinical interviews have provided a wealth of data about and from these families.

Wallerstein and Kelly found that characteristic initial responses in children were largely influenced by the age and developmental level of the child. Preschool children, 2 to 5 years of age at the time of the divorce, were initially highly symptomatic. Regressive, clinging, and demanding behavior as well as acute separation fears and sleep disturbances were common. The children appeared angry, sad, and forlorn. Intense yearning for the departed parent was observed, as well as increased aggression toward adults and children. Fantasies of abandonment, blame, and guilt for the divorce were more likely in this age group than with the older children. Overall, Wallerstein and Kelly were struck by the intense emotional neediness that characterized these young children.

Early school-age children, 5 to 8 years of age, responded to the divorce with open grief, pervasive sadness, and loneliness. These children were simultaneously concerned and worried about the absent parent and themselves, fearing rejection and replacement. Half of the children in this group suffered a sharp drop in school performance. Whereas only a few of these children felt personally responsible for the divorce, more were at risk for experiencing conflicts of loyalty.

In the older school-age children 9 to 12 years of age, the most pervasive response seemed to be intense anger at one or both parents. Compared with those in the younger age groups, these children demonstrated more successful adaptive responses and outwardly appeared to cope better. However, youngsters of this age tend to view the world in black and white terms and thus were prone to intense albeit shifting loyalties. They were easily "co-opted" in parental battles. Half of the children in this group suffered a decline in school performance and peer relationships.

For the adolescents, the experience of divorce appeared particularly difficult, as the normal adolescent developmental process was disrupted and reversed. High levels of anxiety, acute depression, and intense anger were seen. These children felt abandoned at a critical time; instead of their leaving, they were being left. Worries about the future, their own identities, and intimate relationships were common. Although some of these adolescents became symptomatic, delinquent, or both, a significant number were able to master the divorce experience and demonstrate an impressive capacity to grow in maturity and independence. Compared with the younger children, these adolescents were able to disengage themselves from conflicts of loyalty more successfully and increase their emotional investment in peer and other activities.

At the 18-month follow-up, sex differences were evident. Although boys and girls did not differ markedly in their overall psychological adjustment at the time of the divorce, 18 months later the adjustment of the boys had deteriorated significantly, whereas that of the girls had improved. Improvement was also seen in children separated from a disturbed parent. By the 5-year mark, the age and sex of the child were less critical. Instead, a strong connection was apparent between the overall quality of life within the family and the adjustment of the children. One third of the children manifested moderate to severe depression. Even when symptomatology had abated, feelings about the divorce continued to be intense. And even when visitation was irregular or nonexistent, the psychological importance of the noncustodial father remained undiminished. The 10-year follow-up provided some surprising results. No significant gender differences in overall psychological adjustment were found at the 10-year mark. The once highly symptomatic preschool group now seemed least burdened by the unhappy memories of the divorce and most hopeful and optimistic about the future. A delayed, or "sleeper," effect was observed among one third of the young adult women. The emergence of intense anxieties around their relationships with men appeared to complicate heterosexual relationships significantly. Perhaps the most sobering finding of this study is the youngsters' own perception—that for most of them, the experience of divorce had been the central disorganizing event of their childhoods. The researchers concluded that the consequences of a divorce are potentially serious and long lasting.

Despite the hazards posed by a parental divorce, some children did continue to flourish in their overall development. Wallerstein and Kelly identified a number of factors related to good outcome: (1) the extent to which the parents were able to put aside conflict and anger, (2) the resumption of good parenting by the custodial parent and an ongoing, good relationship with the noncustodial parent, (3) the dilution of a predivorce pathologic parent-child relationship, (4) the age, sex, and predivorce personality strengths and weaknesses of the child as well as the postdivorce absence of chronic anger and depression, and (5) the availability of a support system that the child had the ability to use.

The Virginia Longitudinal Study of Divorce and Remarriage examined 144 middle-class white children and their parents. Unlike with the California study, a control group was included: 50% of the children were from divorced mother-custody families and the other 50% from nondivorced families. Within each group, 50% of the children were boys and 50% were girls. One child who was 4 years of age at the time of the divorce was selected for study at 2 months, 1 year, 2 years, and 6 years following divorce. A new group of families was added to the original sample at the 6-year follow-up in order to create three groups—a nonremarried mother-custody group, a nondivorced group, and a remarried mother-stepfather group.

As was true in the California study, Hetherington, Cox, and Cox found that in the 2 years after divorce, most children and their families experienced significant emotional distress, psychological health and behavior problems, disruptions in family functioning, and problems in adjusting to the life changes. Gender differences were again apparent. Boys from divorced families tended to show more antisocial and acting out behaviors as well as difficulties in peer relationships and school achievement. A drop in cognitive performance, especially problem-solving skills, was noted. This group of preschool boys was noted to be anxious, unhappy, and more aggressive, even during free play. Girls, although initially whiny and dependent, were functioning better and had more positive relationships with their custodial mothers than did the boys. Even 6 years after divorce, boys continued to show more problematic behavior than either boys in nondivorced families or girls in divorced families. However, when a custodial mother remarried, girls began to act out, leading researchers to hypothesize that remarriage is more disruptive for girls. In an earlier study, Hetherington had already found differences in heterosexual relationships between adolescent daughters of divorced mothers and those of widowed mothers.[8] Children in divorced families were also found to undergo more negative life changes than children in nondivorced families, which was again associated with behavior problems at the 6-year mark.

In Hetherington's view, children of divorce can ultimately turn out to be survivors, winners, or losers, with the outcome dependent not only on the age, gender, and temperament of the child but also on the available resources and subsequent life experiences and relationships.

Other studies, including large-scale survey studies and national surveys using representative samples,[5,14] have confirmed that children of divorce do less well than children from intact families for several years after the divorce. Children of intact but high-conflict families are an exception; they exhibit similar behavioral problems.[4] This would suggest that interparental conflict is a key variable in child behavioral problems. In fact, the prognosis for children from separated yet relatively low-conflict families is better than for children who are exposed to continued high marital conflict in intact families. This finding also underscores the importance of the postdivorce relationship between the parents. Camara and Resnick[1] found that the quality rather than quantity of conflict between divorced parents was the predictive factor. Poorer child adjustment was associated with verbal attacks, physically violent behavior, or total avoidance of the other parent. Parents who used negotiation and compromise when disagreement occurred were more likely to have better-adjusted children.

The finding that boys are more adversely affected by divorce than girls has also been corroborated. In an extensive review of the literature, Zaslow[21,22] found that boys do indeed respond more negatively to parental divorce in the short and long term if they are living with a custodial nonremarried mother. However, girls fared worse in families where the mother had remarried or there was father custody. This would suggest not that boys show greater vulnerability to family stress, but that there are specific postdivorce family forms that are more likely to be stressful or buffering for boys and girls. In general, researchers have tended to look at the effects of divorce on white, school-age, middle-class populations. The effects of parental divorce on nonwhite, lower socioeconomic groups as well as on very young children and adolescents are areas that need considerable further study.

ROLE OF THE PEDIATRICIAN

With the protracted nature of the divorce process come multiple opportunities for the pediatrician to intervene. Just as divorce can be broken down into identifiable stages, Wallerstein and Blakeslee[16] have outlined the crucial psychological tasks for parents and children to accomplish along the way. These are helpful guideposts in determining how well a particular child and family are mastering a divorce. For children, these psychological tasks are:

1. Understanding the divorce, both the immediate concrete consequences and, at a later date, the reasons for the divorce
2. Resuming the usual activities of childhood and getting on with their lives; that is, strategic withdrawal
3. Dealing with loss, especially the loss of the departing parent and overcoming the intense feelings these losses have engendered
4. Dealing with anger and forgiving their parents
5. Working out guilt—feelings of responsibility and guilty ties
6. Accepting the permanence of divorce
7. Taking a chance on love; being able to love and be loved, the central task for adolescents and young adults

These are tasks in addition to the normal developmental tasks associated with growing up and may be reworked at different developmental stages with further mastery. For both parents and children, these tasks may be worked on simultaneously as well as sequentially. For parents, the psychological tasks are:

1. Ending the marriage in as civilized a way as possible, because the way in which a separation happens sets the stage for future family relationships
2. Acknowledging the loss of the marriage and adequately mourning its end in order to be able to move on
3. Establishing a new sense of self and identity—a third step in being able to give up the marriage
4. Containing passions or feelings in order to prevent being dominated by the failed marriage and divorce in subsequent years
5. Venturing forth again and finding the courage to try again—new relationships, new roles, and new solutions
6. Rebuilding one's life by mastering all of the previous tasks in order to create a new and, it is hoped, better life—one that can coexist peacefully with the past
7. Helping the children navigate through the divorce and the adjustment to the subsequent transitions

The greatest challenge for divorcing parents is learning to separate the parental and marital roles. This requires that parents make long-lasting commitments to their children at the same time that they are ending their commitment to each other. It means learning to negotiate conflict and differences but without any of the rewards or satisfactions of the marital relationship. It means being able to separate parents' feelings and needs from those of the child. These are difficult tasks for the parents in even the most amicable divorce.

Although the pediatrician's primary concern may be the last task—helping the parents help the children—the parents' ability to negotiate the other six successfully will profoundly affect the children and may therefore be considered appropriate areas for intervention. Many children and parents benefit from sympathetic inquiries and brief counseling during routine office visits. Providing information and anticipatory guidance for parents contemplating a marital separation can be critical. Areas of particular concern to parents are likely to be (1) the possible reactions of and effect on the children, (2) how and when to tell the children about the separation, (3) custody arrangements, (4) visitation and the role of the noncustodial parent, and (5) decisions about the future—when to start working, make a move, or begin new adult relationships. A number of articles are available to help the pediatrician address these very important issues.[2,13,20]

In working with separating or divorced parents, the pediatrician should make every effort whenever possible to speak with each parent. Because of the nature of divorce and the intense emotions it arouses, it can be a grave error to base one's entire assessment and interventions on information obtained from only one source.

Based on his review of the literature, Emery offers four suggestions for preventing further adverse effects during the divorce.[3] First, parents should work toward the difficult goal of keeping their children out of their angry disagreements, lest the children learn that differences are resolved by yelling, fighting, or hitting. Second, parents should attempt to agree in front of the child about at least one important topic—discipline. Third, parents should make a special effort to maintain their individual relationship with each child to help buffer the child from the interparental conflict. And finally, all parents need to be aware that conflicts between them can affect their children negatively. Parents need to be sensitive to how their children react to marital turmoil and prepare to seek outside help if these reactions are prolonged.

RESOURCES FOR FAMILIES

Professional and Community Resources

Many communities have a broad range of services available for families undergoing divorce. These services can range from professional services such as family therapy, divorce counseling, and divorce mediation to mutual support groups for single parents, fathers seeking child custody, and stepfamilies. School-based support groups for children have become increasingly available. Depending on the community, these services may be found in diverse settings such as schools, social service agencies, community mental health centers, religious organizations, and the courts. Sources of information about such services include mental health workers at community agencies and announcements in newspapers.

Books for Family Members

A growing body of lay literature is available to help family members master the diverse conflicts, reactions, and emotions accompanying divorce. Literature appropriate for children, adolescents, or adults can provide a useful frame of reference and perspective for the reader. In addition, reading about the experiences of others can help reduce the sense of isolation that many family members experience as a result of divorce. In fact, parents may gain insight into their children's experiences by reading children's literature. Finally, when parents and children read a story together, they may be more comfortable sharing their own experiences and feelings. Physicians may want to recommend the following books:

Parents

Lansky V: Vicki Lansky's divorce book for parents: helping your children cope with divorce and its aftermath, New York, 1981, New American Library. (Includes an excellent bibliography for books on divorce for parents and children of all ages.)

Resci I: Mom's house, Dad's house: making shared custody work, New York, 1980, Macmillan Publishing Co.

Salk L: What every child would like parents to know about divorce, New York, 1978, Harper & Row, Publishers, Inc.

Wallerstein K and Blakeslee S: Second chances: men, women, and children a decade after divorce, New York, 1989, Ticknor & Fields.

Adolescents

Blume J: It's not the end of the world, Scarsdale, NY, 1972, Bradbury Press.

Richards A and Willis I: How to get it together when your parents are coming apart, New York, 1976, David McKay Co, Inc.

Children

Gardner RA: Boys and girls book about divorce, New York, 1970, Jason Aronson, Inc.

Goff B: Where is Daddy? The story of a divorce, Boston, 1969, Beacon Press.

REFERENCES

1. Camara A and Resnick G: Styles of conflict resolution and cooperation between divorced parents: effects on child behavior and adjustment, Am J Orthopsychiatry 59:560, 1989.
2. Derdeyn A: Children of divorce: interventions in the phase of separation, Pediatrics 60:20, 1977.
3. Emery RE: Interparental conflict and the children of discord and divorce, Psychol Bull 92:310, 1982.
4. Emery RE: Marriage, divorce, and children's adjustment, Newbury Park, Calif, 1988, Sage Publications, Inc.
5. Guidubaldi J and Perry JD: Divorce and mental health sequelae for children: a two-year follow-up of a nationwide sample, J Am Acad Child Adolesc Psychiatry 24:531, 1985.
6. Hernandez DJ: Demographic trends and the living arrangements of children. In Hetherington EM and Arasteh JD, editors: Impact of divorce, single parenting, and stepparenting on children, Hillsdale, NJ, 1988, Lawrence Erlbaum Associates.
7. Hetherington EM: Coping with family transitions: winners, losers, and survivors, Child Dev 60:1, 1989.
8. Hetherington EM: Effects of fathers' absence on personality development in adolescent daughters, Developmental Psychol 7:313, 1972.
9. Hetherington EM, Arnett JD, and Hollier EA: Adjustment of parents and children to remarriage. In Wolchik SA and Karoly P, editors: Children of divorce: empirical perspectives on adjustment, New York, 1988, Gardner Press, Inc.
10. Hetherington EM, Cox M, and Cox R: Effects of divorce on parents and children. In Lamb M, editor: Nontraditional families: parenting and child development, Hillsdale, NJ, 1982, Lawrence Erlbaum Associates.
11. Hetherington EM, Cox M, and Cox R: Long-term effects of divorce and remarriage on the adjustment of children, J Am Acad Child Adolesc Psychiatry 24:518, 1985.
12. Kalter N et al: Predicators of children's postdivorce adjustment, Am J Orthopsychiatry 59:605, 1989.
13. Kappelman MM and Black J: Children of divorce: the pediatrician's responsibility, Pediatr Ann 9:48, 1980.
14. Peterson JL and Zill N: Marital disruption, parent-child relationships, and behavior problems in children, J Marriage and the Family, 48:295, 1986.
15. Wallerstein JS: Children of divorce: emerging trends, Psychiatr Clin North Am 8:837, 1985.
16. Wallerstein JS and Blakeslee S: Second chances: men, women, and children a decade after divorce, New York, 1989, Ticknor & Fields.
17. Wallerstein JS and Corbin SB: Daughters of divorce: report from a ten-year follow-up, Am J Orthopsychiatry 59:593, 1989.
18. Wallerstein JS, Corbin SB, and Lewis JM: Children of divorce: a 10-year study. In Hetherington EM and Arasteh JD, editors: Impact of divorce, single parenting, and stepparenting on children, Hillsdale, NJ, 1988, Lawrence Erlbaum Associates.
19. Wallerstein JS and Kelly JB: Surviving the breakup: how parents and children cope with divorce, New York, 1980, Basic Books, Inc, Publishers.
20. Weitzman M and Adair R: Divorce and children, Pediatr Clin North Am 35:1313, 1988.
21. Zaslow MJ: Sex difference in children's response to parental divorce. I. Research methodology and postdivorce family forms, Am J Orthopsychiatry 58:355, 1988.
22. Zaslow MJ: Sex differences in children's response to parental divorce. II. Samples, variables, ages, and sources, Am J Orthopsychiatry 59:118, 1989.

49

Day Care and Preschool Programs

William R. Beardslee and Julius B. Richmond

Major changes in the structure of the American family have made day care and preschool programs increasingly important in the life and growth of the young child. Consequently, issues concerning programs for the care of infants and young children, especially various forms of day care, are coming to the attention of pediatricians more often. There are more requests by parents for such programs for their children than ever before. Unfortunately, the need for adequate services far outstrips the available resources.

In 1985 the U.S. Department of Health, Education and Welfare reported about 1.7 million children in all licensed day care centers, 0.4 million in Head Start programs, and 5.5 million in approved family day care homes. During that same year, 9 million of the 21 million children under age 6 in the United States lived in families in which the mother worked.

Day care and other programs for the care of young children are designed to help families rear their children. This chapter discusses only those defined as *developmental* day care or preschool programs. *Custodial* programs are generally substandard and do not serve the best interests of children and parents. There is sufficient knowledge concerning desirable environments for children to justify this elimination of custodial care.[7] Unfortunately, far too many day care programs represent custodial care. Major new initiatives, particularly in the specification of standards for day care centers and adequate staff-to-children ratios, will be needed to bring the high quality of care and education offered in developmental day care and preschool programs to all children. We believe that where custodial care exists, efforts should be made to improve it to the point where it is comparable to a developmentally oriented program.

A developmental day care or preschool program is one that provides care for the child during the day; is not located in the child's home; is comprehensive in its approach, including giving attention to the physical, cognitive, and emotional development of the child; and provides for significant involvement of the parents in the program. The financial support for a day care center or preschool program may come from government, private philanthropic organizations, industries, the collection of fees from parents, or a combination of these sources. Generally, *day care* refers to care for the child from birth to age 3 years and *preschool* to care for the child from age 3 to 6 years. Although the developmental needs of children vary according to their age, day care and preschool programs will be discussed together. The issues facing the pediatrician are similar across the age range, and the pediatrician's concern is not primarily with details of these centers' curricula, but rather with their appropriateness and the quality of care provided.

Until recently, day care and preschool programs were usually custodial. In 1854 the first nursery in the United States was established by a philanthropic woman's organization to care for the children of poor working mothers.[5] After the Civil War, public taxes financed kindergartens and day nurseries to take care of the children of war widows looking for work. The federal government provided day care centers for children during World War I, the Depression, and World War II. When World War II ended, federally supported centers were closed, with the exception of those in California, which were primarily custodial and were sustained because of the demand from women in the labor force, rather than from a desire to meet the needs of children.

It was not until the 1960s, with the funding of Head Start and the Great Society program, that the federal government again became active in care for young children. The pattern of government involvement in day care and preschool programs in the United States is in curious contrast to that in many other countries as diverse as Israel, Denmark, and Hungary, which make day care and preschool programs more available to families. Such centers form an integral part of the health care and education systems of these countries, although there are certainly major differences in the ways these programs are run.

Recent changes in the structure of the American family demonstrate the need for readily available day care and preschool educational programs of quality. In 1988, 65% of all women with children under age 18 years, 73.3% of mothers with school-age children 6 to 17 years, 56.1% of women with preschool children, and 51.1% of mothers with infants under age 1 were in the labor force. The majority of mothers were working out of economic necessity. Younger mothers, under age 25, are more likely to return to work than older mothers. In addition, a much larger proportion of children are being raised in single-parent families. Between 1959 and 1985 the number of female-headed households with children more than tripled. Approximately 25% of America's children live in single-parent families, and the poverty rate for children in these families exceeds 50%. The amount of time spent in poverty is much longer in single-parent, female-headed families than in two-parent families. A large proportion of these single-parent families are not part of an extended family.[15]

Single-parent families occur much more frequently in lower income groups: 67% of families with incomes under $7000 a year have only one parent, and single parenthood is especially prevalent in young families.

As the possibility of adequate care within the family for the young child becomes increasingly limited, and as the family structure continues to change, families are seeking alternatives to home child care during the daytime.

ROLE OF PEDIATRICIANS

Pediatricians are involved with day care and preschool programs in many ways. First, the pediatrician may be consulted by parents about placing their child in a day care or preschool program. Through a comprehensive approach to the child, which integrates knowledge of the biology of health, disease, and development, awareness of emotional needs, and an understanding of the family within the larger social context, the pediatrician is in a favorable position to provide guidance. In addition to working with individual families, many pediatricians provide screening examinations for the early detection of developmental deviations and illness to children in centers and also give specific advice to centers about nutrition, safety, lighting, the control of infectious disease, and other health-related matters—particularly the health and qualifications of staff members. Many pediatricians also serve as consultants to programs, facilitating the psychosocial development of children through guidance to the staff on the structure, curriculum, and administrative organization of the centers. Finally, some pediatricians are involved in establishing the standards by which a day care or preschool program should be run and in insisting on adherence to these standards.

Discussions with parents about day care or preschool programs provide pediatricians with an excellent opportunity to share their approach to child rearing with the parents. A full discussion of this is important in establishing the pediatrician's future rapport and relationship with the parents. The pediatrician should review what is known about developmental day care or preschool programs, help them think through what their child's needs are, and provide them with an opportunity to voice their feelings and ask questions. Such a discussion can help parents learn how to conceptualize the needs of their children, which are relevant not just to a decision about a preschool program, but also to many other decisions parents will make concerning child rearing.

It is useful to place such a discussion in the context of the child's general developmental needs. It is important that the pediatrician be aware of parent-child attachment and separation patterns. The pediatrician could find it worthwhile to review with the parent the child's needs for (1) intimacy and nurturance in human interactions, (2) regularity and predictability in the environment, (3) adequate nutrition, and (4) a setting that is physically safe and cognitively stimulating and that encourages exploration and mastery. Parents should consider these needs as they evaluate day care centers or other alternatives for daytime care.

When parents have decided to place a child in a day care program, the pediatrician should discuss the separation of parents and child and their feelings about it. For many children, going to a day care center will be their first major separation from the parents. Although the evidence does not support this conclusion, parents may fear that they soon will be replaced in the child's affection. Parents should be aware that the child may show some initial signs of anxiety. Parents may also have difficulty in letting the child go and may need help and support to do so. In a well-conducted day care or preschool program, the professional staff is generally helpful in facilitating this process of separation for both parents and child. Professionals in the day care or preschool center can observe the child and give appropriate guidance to the family concerning the separation process.

The pediatrician's meeting with the parents should also allow discussion of the parent's or parents' reasons for seeking high-quality day care. Common experiences of parents are worry and guilt about going back to work. Parents often experience tension between the reasons for working and concern for their child's welfare. Reassurance to parents can be offered; furthermore, clear exploration of the reasons for care will help in the decision of what center under what condition should be chosen.

CHOOSING A PROGRAM

Parents should be encouraged to visit and observe various centers when choosing a program. In communities where there are no choices, the parents and pediatrician must judge whether the only available facility is a developmental or a custodial day care center. Once a child is enrolled, it is appropriate and helpful for the parents to be actively involved in the program.

Parents often ask if there is an increased risk of illness among children who attend day care or preschool programs. Although there may be an increased risk of some minor illnesses, especially to younger children, there is no evidence to suggest that such a risk is a contraindication to day care or that children cannot be safely cared for from a medical standpoint in a day care or preschool program if adequate medical support and consultation are available to the center. The available evidence does not indicate that serious impairing illnesses are more likely because of attendance at a day care center, although there may be a slightly higher rate of certain highly infectious, easily transmitted childhood diseases through more frequent contact with other children in day care. Of particular concern, of course, is AIDS. Regulations change rapidly and need to be reviewed in the particular state and city in which the child resides and the pediatrician practices. At present, for example, it is recommended in Massachusetts that children with AIDS in day care not be segregated from other children. It it likely that this will become a generally accepted policy.[6]

A key question in the minds of most parents is whether day care or preschool education is safe, or whether placing their child in day care is likely to harm the child. Naturally, the answer to this question can only be given after complete evaluation of the individual child and family. In general, it is fair to conclude that evidence does *not* indicate that developmental day care or preschool education programs of high quality are harmful. Moreover, there is evidence that such an experience is beneficial for many children.

Effects of Day Care and Preschool Programs

After a major review of the studies of the effects on children of having mothers who work, Rutter[8] concludes that such children are not more likely than other children to become psychologically ill or delinquent. He also says there is no evidence that the children have difficulties caused by being in the care of several mother figures, as long as the care is of high quality. Finally, he asserts that there are no data to support the view that day care nurseries inevitably cause psychologic damage. In the past, considerable professional concern has been expressed about these matters, based on some evidence from studies of custodial centers.

Bronfenbrenner[2-4] has examined the carefully controlled studies that have compared good day care with good care at home. He reports that these studies show no significant differential effects on children's intelligence quotients (IQ), although there was relatively little sustained longitudinal evidence. The existing evidence did not justify regarding day care as an emotionally harmful experience. Bronfenbrenner also stresses that more research in this area is needed.

It is important to realize that these studies compared two sites of high-quality care. Many homes, because of economic or other adversity, cannot offer care of high quality during the day. Moreover, many children, because of their special needs, can especially benefit from day dare and preschool programs.

It is useful at this point to review what has been learned about the development of disadvantaged children. Without any sort of enrichment program, a *general* downward drift in developmental performance is seen over a period of years in children of low-income families; this does not apply, of course, to every child in this situation. This is the trend that Head Start and other early childhood day care and preschool programs sought to reverse.

There is a sound conceptual base and empiric data for trying to reverse this developmental decline. The conceptual base is that the environment does have considerable impact on later development. Empiric data demonstrate that enrichment programs such as Head Start do make a significant difference and that the developmental attrition so often observed in unfavorable environmental circumstances can be prevented through such programs. Moreover, it is clear that not only children from disadvantaged areas, but also those with disabilities such as mental retardation, sensory deficits, or cerebral palsy, benefit significantly from such programs. Although there had been some conflicting studies on how long the IQ gains that children make in Head Start and similar programs last, it is now clear that permanent gains are made by many children enrolled in these programs.

The importance of Head Start and other programs is increased because there has been a dramatic increase in the number of children growing up in poverty. There was a decline from the mid 1960s of the number of children in poverty, which reached a low of 14.4% in 1974. Beginning in the early 1980s the rate of children in poverty rose, reaching a high of 22% in 1983. This increase is clearly related to the earlier-mentioned rapid growth of single-parent families, of female-headed households, of erratic child support from fathers, to a decline in public assistance to families with children, and to the gradual decline in general of earnings of families with children. Disparity in poverty rates between blacks, Hispanics, and white children is particularly clear. Furthermore, children in poverty often have inadequate access to health care, which compounds the problem. In light of the changes in the American family and particularly the increase in poverty, the day care center will play a larger role in the lives of many families. Head Start and similar programs attempt to correct these negative impacts. Programs for these children, as for all children, must meet the standards for developmental day care; custodial day care is not a desirable option. The nation cannot afford the developmental attrition that is an outcome of poor child care.

The importance of the parents' involvement in day care and preschool programs is emphasized by a review of longitudinal evaluations of preschool programs. It has been demonstrated in several studies that intervention including both parent and child had a major impact on the child, leading to substantial, lasting gains, and that there were also benefits for other children in the family and for the parent involved. Further, Head Start and other similar programs have benefited their participants in many ways beyond those measured by cognitive testing. Early detection and treatment of illness, more adequate nutrition, and general gains in emotional well-being and motivation for learning are but four examples of these additional benefits. Finally, there is evidence that the presence of the centers themselves has had beneficial effects on the communities in which they are located.

Pediatricians will find it useful to visit centers and observe their operation. Many pediatricians, in fact, work as consultants to such centers. The American Academy of Pediatrics[1] has published information on the operation of day care centers and preschool programs that is relevant for pediatricians, especially in their role as consultants. The guidelines detail how to review the administrative organization of the center, the center's progress, and the health needs of the children in terms of screening and ongoing care. The U.S. Department of Health and Human Services has a resource guide available that is also useful in advising centers. In assessing the quality of care in day care or preschool programs, the pediatrician should pay special attention to the ratio of staff to children enrolled, the professional training and orientation of the staff, and the typical daily experience for a child in the center.

Family difficulties may first appear to be evident to members of the day care staff. For example, cases of abuse are often first identified in day care, as are cases of inadequate immunization or other health-related concerns. The pediatrician may well be called upon to assess and assist in these matters.

In many ways, the most rewarding part of involvement with a day care center is being there when it is in operation. A well-run day care center is an excellent place to observe healthy children at different ages and stages of development. Working with a day care center can be an important part of pediatricians' training because it gives them a unique opportunity to observe children who are not under the stress of illness or hospitalization. It is a refreshing change and a rewarding experience for busy practitioners. Day care and preschool programs provide pediatricians with an opportunity to help bring about creative solutions to the problems posed by the evolving changes in family structure. Many day care centers provide essential education and support for children with disabilities and for the parents of these children. The centers also provide the beginnings of a way out of the cycle of poverty and despair that has limited so many young children in low-income neighborhoods. Especially with the changes in family structure, the day care or preschool center also serves as an organizer and source of friends and social support for parents of young children. Thus the center is a vital component of the community, and involvement in its operation is a unique opportunity for the pediatrician to contribute to its success.

REFERENCES

1. American Academy of Pediatrics: Health and Day Care, Elk Grove Village, Ill, 1987.
2. Bronfenbrenner U: Is early intervention effective? In A report on longitudinal evaluations of preschool programs, vol. 2, Washington, D.C., 1974, U.S. Office of Human Development.
3. Bronfenbrenner U: Appendix A, Research on the effects of day care on child development. In Advisory Committee on Child Development of the National Research Council: Toward a national policy for children and families, Washington, D.C., 1976, National Academy of Sciences.
4. Bronfenbrenner U: Who cares for America's children? In Vaughan VC III and Brazelton TB, editors: The family—can it be saved? Chicago, 1976, Year Book Medical Publishers, Inc.
5. Fein G and Stewart OD: Day care in context, New York, 1973, John Wiley & Sons, Inc.
6. HIV Infection/AIDS & Early Childhood Settings: Information for Caregivers and Parents. Department of Public Health, 1989, Commonwealth of Massachusetts.
7. Hoskins R and Kotch J: Day care and illness: evidence, costs, and public policy. *Pediatrics,* 77(6, 2):951-982.
8. Rutter M: Parent-child separation: psychological effects on the children, J Child Psychol Psychiatry 12:233, 1971.

SUGGESTED READINGS

Berrueta-Clement J, Schweinhart L, Barnett W et al: Changed Lives: the Effects of the Perry Preschool Program on Youths through Age 19. Ypsilanti, MI, 1985, High/Scope Press.

Lazar I and Darlington R: Lasting effects of early education: a report from the consortium for longitudinal studies, Monographs of the Society for Research in Child Development, vol. 47, no. 195, 1982.

Richmond JB: Disadvantaged children: what have they compelled us to learn? Yale J Biol Med 43:127, 1970.

Richmond JB, Zigler E, and Stipek D: Head Start: the first decade, Washington, D.C., 1977, U.S. Office of Child Development.

Schweinhart LJ and Weikart DP: Young children grow up: the effects of the Perry Preschool Program on Youths Through Age 15, Ypsilanti, Mich., 1980, High/Scope Educational Research Foundation.

Vanderpool NA and Richmond JB: Child Health: Prospects for the 1990s. Annual Review of Public Health, 1990, vol. 2, 185-205.

Zigler E and Valentine J, editors: Project Head Start: a legacy of the war on poverty, New York, 1979, Free Press.

50

Family Interactions: Children with Unexplained Physical Symptoms

John Sargent

Illness and physical symptoms are physical, psychological, and social events. The family, as the child's primary social context, is significantly affected by a child's physical condition; in turn the family affects both the child's physical status and psychological well-being.[7] The family, in collaboration with health care providers, is responsible for managing appropriate treatment and promoting the child's psychosocial adaptation. Because of the importance of the family, the investigation and treatment of unexplained physical symptoms should include the interaction between the family and the child.

CHARACTERISTICS OF FAMILIES WITH CHILDREN WITH PSYCHOSOMATIC DISORDERS

Liebman and others[2] and Minuchin and colleagues[3,4] investigated the influence of a child's family in maintaining the symptoms of chronic illness and functional physical symptoms. Their work involved children with recurrent diabetic ketoacidosis and intractable asthma and adolescents with anorexia nervosa. They studied the patterns of interaction of these families and identified five specific characteristics of family interaction that typified their daily responses and manner of reacting to the child's physical symptoms: (1) enmeshment, (2) overprotection, (3) rigidity, (4) lack of resolution of family conflict, and (5) involvement of the symptomatic child in unresolved parental conflict.

Enmeshment refers to an extremely high degree of involvement and responsiveness among family members. Members are exquisitely sensitive to one another, and minor upsets of one individual may lead to rapid attempts of another to restore calm. Relationships can be overly close to the point that individuation and autonomy are sacrificed. Family members report that they feel for one another and that they know what other family members are thinking. Where parents and infants are concerned, enmeshment is an appropriate and necessary quality. However, as a child grows and develops, more distance in family relationships and independence for the child are required. Pathologic enmeshment always entails excessive parental involvement for the child's developmental stage. Enmeshment between parents and child also interferes with the child's development of problem-solving skills, since the parents rapidly act to relieve the child's distress rather than require that the child individually respond to stressful situations. Family members also excessively accommodate viewpoints of others, even when they disagree. Therefore family cohesion is based on submerged and denied family conflict rather than on negotiation, compromise, and agreement.

A child with a chronic illness, such as diabetes, may become angry about the need for medical treatment and dietary discretion. Parents in "adaptive" families learn to allow the child to become upset while continuing to require necessary adherence to the treatment regimen. In the pathologically enmeshed family, the parents become upset when the child attempts to deny his or her disease and need to comply with its treatment regimens, and the parents attempt to rationalize the restrictions of the illness and its treatment.[1] The parents may also carry out illness management tasks that the child can perform. Finally, one or both parents may become so involved with the ill child that they recognize the symptoms before the child does. In sum, these family responses seriously inhibit the child's acceptance of the illness and autonomy in learning to manage and control his or her body.

The *overprotectiveness* seen in these families refers to an overly high degree of concern of all family members for one another. Although the ill child is the most obviously vulnerable member of the family, all members are perceived as vulnerable and in need of protection. Evidence of distress in anyone induces protective responses from the rest of the family. The father may be perceived as explosive and in need of calming, the mother as depressed, incompetent, and in need of paternalistic treatment, and the ill child as sick and weak and in need of care and attention. Immature behavior on the child's part is allowed, and any difficulties that the child might experience at school or with peers lead to pity and excuses from the parents. The parents may try to shield the child from unpleasant events, such as medical procedures, even to the child's physical detriment.

The *rigidity* of these families is demonstrated in their attempts to deny family problems and repeat the same ineffective solutions over and over and in their desire to maintain fixed relationships among one another, even when development or stress requires change. Each family member steadfastly states that he or she cannot alter how he or she or others behave, regardless of the need for change. A mother will report that she cannot bring her husband to the doctor's office or hospital no matter how ill the child is. A father will insist that he cannot assist his wife in following through with illness treatment for their child (e.g., giving insulin injections by himself). The child will state that he cannot help his parents understand his feelings about his chronic illness. These protestations of incompetence persist, thereby increasing the overall family stress and leading to a deterioration in the child's condition and further ineffective family responses, resulting in a circular pattern. These families appear to be in a tenuous balance, with any change seen as highly threatening.

Disagreement and conflict exist in all families. However, in those families in which a member has a psychosomatic disorder, to maintain these rigid patterns of extreme closeness and protectiveness, *conflict is denied* and therefore unresolved. Family members contradict themselves to maintain a facade of agreement, and an immediate consensus develops concerning even small issues of disagreement. If a consensus cannot be achieved immediately, distractions occur that dissipate the conflict, or the disagreeing family members avoid one another until the situation calms. There is an air of chronic tension in the family, which is reinforced by avoidance, denial, or outright capitulation by one member. These unresolved disagreements may involve any aspect of family life; however, the physician should note in particular that the parents do not resolve differences of opinion about the ill child and management of his or her disease.[1]

Finally, when conflict occurs between the parents, the *ill child becomes involved in the disagreement,* distracting attention to himself or herself and thus significantly reducing the disagreement. The balance of harmony and consensus is then restored. The child is often asked to mediate between the parents; at times he or she sides with one parent against the other; at other times the parents unite (leaving their disagreement) either to protect and nurture the sick child or to attack the child and blame him or her for all family troubles. Chronic marital strife is reinforced as more and more disagreements remain unresolved. Yet often because of the child's illness or symptoms, neither parent leaves the family. The ill child remains highly vigilant to future family disagreements and experiences increasing stress as family tension persists. It is precisely at the point of parental disagreement and personal stress that the child becomes symptomatic, requiring medical care and hospitalization. The cycle then begins again.

Thus the child's participation in parental conflict reduces physical and psychological distress in the parents but induces symptoms in the labile child. The family's patterns of interaction induce symptoms in the child, while the child's symptoms assist the family in maintaining stability. Minuchin and colleagues[3,4] found that all these family characteristics occurred in families with children with unexplained (functional) physical symptoms, regardless of the child's primary diagnosis. Although all families engage in enmeshed, protective, and conflict-avoiding interactions, those families engage in these patterns to an inordinate amount, even when such patterns are unproductive. This does not mean that the family causes the insulin deficiency of diabetes or the reactive airway diathesis of asthma. The physiologic differences in these children are specific vulnerabilities that are affected by the family and other factors to become repeatedly symptomatic. Thus functional or unexplained symptoms become a circular process, reinforcing and reinforced by the child's vulnerability and the family's characteristic patterns of interaction.

IMPLICATIONS FOR THE PEDIATRICIAN

Diagnosis

Assessment of the family, including both parents, is essential in evaluating situations in which a child's illness becomes repeatedly symptomatic at home and yet is controlled easily in the hospital.[6,8] The pediatrician should note how family members behave with one another and should directly question each member about his or her impressions of the causes of the child's frequent symptoms. The pediatrician can suggest to family members that they discuss the problem together and can observe their nonverbal responses when other members are talking. The pediatrician will need to attend to the process of family interaction, as well as to the content of their statements.

These families are typically well informed about their child's medical condition, and they understand and carry out treatment plans. However, they often appear helpless and defeated and relate to the physician in a dependent and frequently demanding fashion. Parental overprotectiveness is common, and the enmeshment within the family is demonstrated as parent and child constantly maintain eye contact, speak for one another, and sit very close together. Therefore the physician will often find it difficult to develop an independent relationship with the child. The father also may be devalued and thus may appear disinterested and unsympathetic. The parents may present differing views of the situation, and when asked to reconcile these different perceptions, they are unable to do so. The child is often immature or pseudomature and frequently clings to one parent. He or she usually has limited peer relationships and is the primary focus of parental attention because of the symptoms. The child's lack of insight and general sense of incompetence and helplessness are often striking. Finally, both family and symptomatic child readily deny psychological difficulties, and all maintain a strongly somatic orientation.

Pediatric Interventions

When caring for an ill child, the pediatrician, noting parental overinvolvement and overprotectiveness, can help the parents require more independent responsibility from their child. If the physician determines that the parents disagree about how to accomplish this and are thus rendered ineffective, he or she can stress the need for them to act cooperatively. The pediatrician can also ensure that the child is participating in school and in activities with peers. Regular follow-up will be necessary to determine if the parents can cooperate and act to encourage more maturity from their child and also if that maturity leads to improvements in the child's physical condition.[5] If the child improves, the pediatrician will need to watch for signs of marital distress in the parents. He or she can then discuss with the parents the need to resolve their differences either independently or through psychotherapy. Three principles should guide the pediatrician's efforts: (1) attend first to the physical and psychological difficulties of the ill child before making any attempts to address stress in the marriage directly; (2) in working with the family, develop and maintain an attitude that places responsibility on them to act to ensure their child's physical and psychosocial adjustment; and (3) pursue regular follow-up care with the family to ensure that progress is maintained.

Referral for family psychotherapy is indicated in situations in which the ill child demonstrates serious emotional and behavioral immaturity or in which his illness is so labile that he is hospitalized repeatedly, which leads to school absence, further social isolation, and worsening parental concern.[5,6] Referral is also indicated when the parents are unable to decrease overinvolvement and overprotectiveness with the physician's assistance or to develop and carry out cooperative methods of dealing with the ill child. Before referral, the pediatrician must accurately identify the child's physical condition and outline appropriate medical treatment. All physicians involved in the child's care must agree on the diagnosis, treatment, and recommendation for family therapy. The therapist should be familiar and comfortable with family-oriented treatment of serious physical and emotional disorders in children.[8] In the treatment of these disorders, the physician and family therapist collaborate in the treatment. The therapist can best be introduced to the family as a professional who will help them manage their child's illness or symptoms more effectively and assist them in reducing the stressful effects of the child's symptoms on both child and family. The physician can further state that therapy is a highly important part of treatment and that without therapy the physician will continue to be ineffective in reducing the symptoms. The family should not perceive the referral for therapy as implying blame for their problems. Rather, it can be described as an opportunity for the family and the physician to improve the child's condition.

Pediatrician-Therapist Collaboration

The pediatrician actively assists the course of therapy by directly answering the medical questions of the family and by informing the family of the improvements that should be achieved through their work with the therapist. Both professionals will need to support each other's efforts and encourage the family to resolve differences straightforwardly with each of them. The physician should avoid answering psychological questions that the family raises and should inform the family that these issues will need to be addressed with the therapist. This support enables the family to work directly with the therapist and resolve any disagreements they may have with him or her straightforwardly. It also prevents the family from pitting the therapist against the physician during treatment. The therapist in turn refers any medical questions the family raises to the physician.

During the initial phases of family treatment, the child's medical condition may worsen, and short-term emergencies may develop at stressful points during the therapy. Both the therapist and the physician will need to be available to the family at these times. By maintaining a mutually supportive relationship and open communication, the pediatrician and the family therapist can assist one another through difficult phases of treatment. Working together, pediatrician, therapist, and the family can dramatically improve the child's physical and psychological condition.

REFERENCES

1. Baker L et al: Psychosomatic aspects of juvenile diabetes mellitus: a progress report, Mod Probl Paediatr 12:332, 1975.
2. Liebman R, Minuchin S, and Baker L: The use of structural family therapy in the treatment of intractible asthma, Am J Psychiatry 131:535, 1974.
3. Minuchin S et al: A conceptual model of psychosomatic illness in childhood, Arch Gen Psychiatry 32:1031, 1975.
4. Minuchin S, Rosman BL, and Baker L: Psychosomatic families: anorexia nervosa in context, Cambridge, Mass, 1978, Harvard University Press.
5. Sargent J: Physician-family therapist collaboration: children with medical problems, Family Systems Medicine 3:454, 1985.
6. Sargent J: The family and childhood psychosomatic disorders, Gen Hosp Psychiatry 5:41, 1983.
7. Sargent J: The sick child: family complications, J Behav and Devel Pediat 4:50, 1983.
8. Sargent J and Liebman R: Childhood chronic illness: issues for psychotherapists, Community Ment Health J 21:294, 1985.

51

Family Systems Intervention in Pediatric Practice

Herb Klar

FAMILY THEORY: DEVELOPMENTAL CONSIDERATIONS

Pediatricians are often asked for advice when parents are troubled by their children's behavior, even when it is clear that those problems have no medical basis. The child's ability to sleep through the night or toilet train, to separate from the family to start day care or school, and to make the transition from elementary school to junior and senior high school are often worrisome for parents. So is the onset of their child's puberty. Each of these represents milestones in the child's individuation—his or her growing up and moving away from parents. Each of these developmental steps tests the family's capacity to support the child's individuation. Problematic manifestations of these phases are often related to the family's circumstances. The pediatrician who wishes to understand the child's behavior will do well to remember the role of the child in the family system and the relationship of the child's development to the family life cycle.

Family systems theory sees the child and the family as mutually involved. The birth of the child moves his or her parents forward one generation, defines them as caretakers, and imposes a host of new responsibilities to be shared and negotiated. The growing child's developmental milestones occur in the context of a family system that itself is changing and developing in response to each member's evolving needs and the impact of external conditions.

The parents must at the same time care for the child, adjust to the changing needs of their own development, and address their responsibilities to their extended family, their friends, and their jobs at a time of immense social change. The interrelated phenomena of a lower birth rate, longer life expectancy, the changing role of women, the postponement of marriage and childbearing, and the increased divorce and remarriage rates represent increasingly frequent challenges to family life. On any given pediatric office day, the majority of parents attending a child's visit may be addressing a number of issues: the demands of work versus the responsibilities of parenthood, the needs of offspring versus increasing responsibility for aging parents, and the problems associated with divorce, single parenthood, or remarriages.

Pediatricians should routinely ask how their patients are doing in school, in other activities, and with friends. The pediatrician who sees the child as part of a family system that both shapes and adjusts to the child's development will routinely invite discussion concerning changes and losses in the family, their effect on the child, and the impact of the child's development on other members of the family.

ROLE OF THE PEDIATRICIAN: CASE EXAMPLE

> A first-time mother, a young woman in her early thirties, tells her pediatrician that her otherwise healthy infant daughter wakes up in the middle of the night and cries unconsolably unless she gets up and holds the baby until she falls asleep. The child gives no evidence of any medical problem by history or physical examination, and the pediatrician advises, "Don't worry. She's only going through a phase; she'll grow out of it."

The advice is sound but ineffective. The pediatrician's inquiry focuses exclusively on the child and the medically inconsequential ramifications of her behavior. It does not consider the impact of the child's care on her parents and their need to adjust their relationship to meet a host of unfamiliar and stressful responsibilities. The pediatrician does not ask if the father shares wake-up call responsibility and is not told that the couple disagrees strongly on how to respond. He or she does not know that the mother resumed work 3 months after delivery in an executive position with a new employer and that the job requires 10- to 12-hour workdays, leaving weekends and the infant's nocturnal wake-ups as the only time for the mother and child to spend together. The answer, "It's only a phase," may be less helpful than intended because it ignores the powerful impact that commonplace developmental milestones often have on families and the ways in which peripheral circumstances undermine parental cooperation and competence. Although such problems often resolve benignly with time, many are imprinted in family relationships permanently in ways that obstruct coping on the child's and the parents' part. This often leads to a pattern of repeated crises, to family strife, and even to dissolution.

Pediatricians who dismiss parental concerns over other similarly phase-related, nonmedical issues miss an important opportunity. As a caregiver who develops long-lasting relationships with children and their parents via routine contacts through the illnesses and milestones of the child's development, the pediatrician is equally familiar with the family's strengths and deficits. Parents often seek help when transitional stages in their child's development upset established relationships and ways of coping. The pediatrician is uniquely positioned to address these kinds of disruptions before they become a permanent part of the way in which family members interact. The stakes are particularly high for families of young children, a staple of pediatric practice, because the highest rate of divorce involves parents at this stage of the family life cycle.

FAMILY THEORY: STRUCTURAL CONSIDERATION

Family systems theorists do not regard normal family life as problem free. Change is often disruptive. The normal family experiences growing pains. Children develop and have different needs of their parents at different stages of development. Parents arrange their priorities according to their place in their own life cycles.

Dealing with the problems and adjustments that come with change is an important aspect of family life. What differentiates functional from dysfunctional families is the way in which they organize themselves to adjust to change.

In working with children in the context of the family system, four concepts drawn from structural family therapy are particularly useful: structure, subsystems, boundaries, and triangulation. *Structure* describes the tendency of family members to interact in predictable patterns and sequences. Such patterns are so repeated and pervasive that they become the structure around which the family's life is organized.

For example, when a child's father tells him that he cannot watch television until he finishes his homework, but the boy gets permission from his mother before completing his work on evenings when the father works, a pattern of interaction begins to develop. Repeated often enough, it becomes a structure that defines family roles and the emotional distance between members. The father is the disciplinarian. The mother is permissive; she enjoys a "close" relationship with the boy. The father is seen as "distant." In the meantime the boy's school performance declines, and his mother and father argue about the appropriate response.

A second concept, *subsystems,* refers to the subgroups into which individual members organize and align. Although subsystems may be organized by gender or common interest, the most important subsystems in families with children are generational.

Virtually all schools of family therapy see family structure as hierarchical, with parents having more authority than children. The focus of that authority and the ways in which it is conveyed, shared, or delegated change as the child develops—a crucial adjustment for parents.

Because children require a basically consistent, predictable set of parental limits and expectations, it is important for parents to support one another's authority. In structural family therapy terms, it is essential that parent and child subsystems be well differentiated. *Boundaries* within the family regulate the degree of differentiation between subsystems.

In the example cited previously, the child's school problems result from diffuse boundaries between parent and child subsystems. Angry at her husband's absences, the mother engages her son in a covert alliance against the father's rules. Instead of a parent-parent subsystem articulating and supporting mutually agreeable rules, the family structure is organized around a parent-child subsystem that undermines them. The boy's school problems distract his parents from the real issue: their disagreement over the father's time at work.

Structural family therapists define a family *triangle* as an alliance between two family members from different generations against a third family member. When a child is "triangulated" in this way, he or she may develop behavioral problems symptomatic of breakdowns in family structure. The pediatrician who focuses exclusively on the child and his or her behavior without considering the family process that produces it risks missing the real problem.

Such structural problems occur intermittently in even the most functional families as they adjust to change. Shifts in career or job status and geographic moves impose changes on the family structure from outside. Separation, divorce, and remarriage are potentially major disruptions. The birth of a new child or sibling and the passage of individual members through the key milestones of each one's life cycle represent potentially unsettling normative transitions.

INTERVENTION

The onset of behavioral problems or medically ambiguous symptoms on a child's part is often a sign that family structure has not adjusted to a change, transition, or crisis. As the first caregivers from whom parents often seek advice, pediatricians can help families by doing the following:

1. Be aware of changes that impinge on the family. Educate and sensitize the family about the impact such changes have on family structure and the ways they relate to the health and behavior of children.
2. Raise questions about the child's problems in ways that suggest their possible connection to disruptions in family structure. For example, asking a mother if she believes her son's behavior problems are related to any problems in the family risks sounding like blaming the family. Rather, asking her how she and the boy's father decide on a response to the boy's resistance to homework connects the child's behavior to the family issue in a nonthreatening way.
3. If the family is not adjusting to any external change, consider the impact of recent transitions in the child's development. For example, parents who raise concerns about their youngest child's withdrawn, angry attitude may themselves be dealing with his upcoming high school graduation and the loss it represents. Raising questions gently about their plans after the boy leaves home will provide useful information about the family's prospective adjustment to the "empty nest" phase of their family's life cycle.
4. When working with children whose presenting problems point to difficult family transitions, involve both parents in the discussion. Pediatricians who involve fathers in such instances support the importance of shared responsibility and the integrity of the parental hierarchy. The outright refusal of one or the other parent to be involved in such a discussion often indicates deeper family problems.

5. Remember that breakdown in family structure affects each family member. Inquiring about the status of siblings at a time when the pediatrician knows the family is going through changes or crises addresses the needs of each child. It also shifts focus from the problematic child to the family system. While it is important to convey interest in and respect for each member of the family, this should not be done in a way that undermines parental responsibility.
6. Give credit where it is due, supporting examples of success and parental competence. Reframe or rephrase problems in such a way that functional processes are supported and reinforced.

REFERRAL

Many families have chronic or deep-seated problems that require more intensive intervention. When working with family systems, the pediatrician should proceed selectively. If he or she feels uncomfortable addressing family issues or feels that they are beyond his or her expertise, referral for family therapy is strongly recommended. The following types of families should be considered for referral:

1. Families beset by past, sudden, or unresolved changes or losses
2. Chronically dysfunctional families
3. Families in which there is an intense degree of marital conflict or violence
4. Substance-abusing families
5. Families that seem bent on blaming or making the misbehaving child a scapegoat
6. Families in which children are victimized by emotional, physical, or sexual abuse

SUGGESTED READINGS

Camp H: Structural family therapy: an outsider's perspective, Fam Process 12(3):269, 1973.

Camp H: Structural family therapy. Family therapy, concepts and methods, New York, 1984, Gardner Press, Inc.

Carter B and McGoldrick M: Overview: the changing family life cycle: a framework for family therapy. In Carter B and McGoldrick M, editors: The family life cycle: a framework for family therapy, New York, 1980, Gardner Press, Inc.

Framo J: Symptoms from a family transactional viewpoint. In Ackerman NW, Leib J, and Pierce JK, editors: Family therapy in transition, Boston, 1970, Little, Brown & Co.

Napier AY and Whitaker C: Problems of the beginning family therapist. In Block D, editor: Techniques of family psychotherapy: a primer, New York, 1973, Grune & Stratton, Inc.

Walsh F: Conceptualizations of normal family functioning. In Walsh F, editor: Normal family process, New York, 1982, The Guilford Press.

Wells KC: Family therapy. In Wells KC and Forehand R, editors: Conduct disorders, primary pediatric care, St Louis, Mosby–Year Book, Inc. (in press).

52

Health Care Management of the Family: The Family as the Focus of Treatment in Pediatrics

Bayard W. Allmond, Jr.

CLINICAL ILLUSTRATION

It is not unusual for parents to ask the pediatrician for assistance with their toddler who is not sleeping through the night. Such a complaint is one of many that are common issues in pediatrics, well within the pediatrician's realm of expertise. One mother, for example, asked for help with just this problem: getting her 20-month-old daughter to sleep through the night. Medically, the pediatrician noted that the child appeared well, except that she was overweight, somewhat pasty looking, and pale, possessing many of the hallmarks of a "milk baby." This finding was consistent with the child's nightly demand for large quantities of cow's milk—a demand uncontested by her parents through the many months of sleepless nights.

The likely presence of iron-deficiency anemia secondary to excessive milk intake was one facet of the disturbed sleep pattern with direct consequences for the child herself. However, it represented just the tip of the iceberg. Other dimensions included the following:

1. The mother was exhausted; she no longer slept with her husband. In fact, she no longer slept at all except when she and her daughter lay down together after an ever-lengthening nightly ritual that included rocking, holding, stories, songs, food, protests, threats, and pleading. She had left her part-time job to devote all her energies to her daughter's complaint.
2. The father was frustrated and furious at this disruption to family routine; he slept badly. His punctuality and efficiency during the day had slipped considerably.
3. Major disputes between the parents over appropriate management of this phenomenon had occurred and were an integral part of the family's nocturnal behavior. The mother saw her husband as unsupportive of her and unreasonably harsh; the father felt disregarded and disqualified in his parenting attempts.
4. A 7-year-old sibling had been hearing these parental disputes at night from her own bed. She experienced recurring abdominal pain at these times, but her parents appeared to have little time or energy for her and her stomachaches. She resented her sister and her nighttime behavior immensely. This common issue in pediatrics was having significant implications for everyone in the household. Such issues usually do.

Family members, in or out of a pediatrician's office, behave much like the individual pieces of a mobile—that is, each is capable of independent behavior, but each is connected to another; therefore any movement by a single member influences and changes the movement of the group as a whole. Visualize a mobile with four or five pieces suspended from the ceiling, gently moving in the air. The whole is in balance, steady yet moving. Some pieces are moving rapidly; others are almost stationary. Some are heavier and appear to hold more influence over the ultimate direction of the mobile's movement; others seem to go along for the ride. A breeze catching only one piece of the mobile immediately influences movement of every piece (some more than others), and the pace picks up with some pieces unbalancing themselves and moving about chaotically for a time. Gradually the whole exerts its influence on the errant piece(s) and balance is reestablished, but not before a decided change in the direction of the whole may have taken place.

Notice also the changeability regarding closeness and distance among the pieces—the result of actual contact of one with another—and the importance of vertical hierarchy. Coalitions of movement may be observed between two pieces, or one piece may persistently appear isolated from the others; yet its position of isolation is essential to the balance of the entire system. The parallels hold at all levels; they describe the behavior and relationships among individuals in a family as well as the behavior and relationships among individual pieces in a mobile. This analogy has been noted abundantly in the work of many family systems theorists and practitioners.[4] The concept of homeostatic balance within a system is most important here—balance and movement, movement and balance, a group of elements in dynamic equilibrium.

FAMILY HOMEOSTASIS

Pediatric practitioners are indebted to their mental health colleagues for the concept of applying homeostatic balance to families; family homeostasis was one of the early building blocks in the development of family systems theory, family interviewing, and family therapy. In 1957 Jackson[2] noted that family members were moving constantly to maintain a precarious balance in their individual relationships with one another. In his psychiatric work with the individual treatment of a schizophrenic patient, he observed:

> Other family members interfered with, tried to become a part of, or sabotaged the individual treatment of the "sick" member, as though the family had a stake in his sickness. The hospitalized . . . patient often got worse or regressed after a visit from family members, as though family interaction had a direct bearing on his symptoms. Other family members got worse as the patient got better, as though sickness in one of the family members was essential to the family's way of operating.

Following these observations, Jackson coined the term *family homeostasis*. This formulation called for a treatment process that would include all parts of the family mobile. The treatment of the family together in one room, *conjoint family therapy,* arose in part from this basic observation about the behavior of individuals within a family.[3]

The notion of homeostasis as applied to families, however, transcends psychiatric conditions. Family homeostasis is as observable in pediatrics as in psychiatry, and the pediatrician will benefit from enlarging his or her frame of reference to include all of the family in order to understand better a family's relationship to and participation in the child's problem. The focus for both diagnosis and treatment in pediatrics will shift as a result; it is no longer on a single individual. Nor, if the family includes others, is it limited to one parent and one child; rather, the unit of treatment is the family.[1]

Application in Pediatric Practice

The 20-month-old girl mentioned earlier illustrates this point. She had developed a discrete set of signs and symptoms that could be grouped under the pediatric label of *sleep disturbance*. Her symptoms seemed to precipitate a variety of difficulties among other family members, including exhaustion, frustration, marital discord, psychosomatic complaints, and sibling rivalry. A linear cause-and-effect view is easily constructed: the child's symptoms are causing disruption and consequences for each family member and for the family as a whole. This etiologic hypothesis suggests a straightforward treatment approach—focus on the child, remove the offending problem (the child's disturbed sleep pattern), and the child and her family will be restored to health.

Before agreeing with such a course of action, it is wise to reverse the traditional cause-and-effect view just postulated. Isn't it equally possible that the mother's exhaustion, father's frustration, marital discord, sibling rivalry, and sister's psychosomatic pain might have preceded the toddler's sleeplessness and even stimulated the initial appearance of her symptoms? Such was actually the case here. Isn't it also possible that the maintenance of the child's symptoms might have become strongly linked with the factors cited, that is, the mother's exhaustion, father's frustration, continuing marital discord, and so forth? Again, the answer in this situation was "yes."

Therefore a simple linear view fails to address the complexities of the situation, and treatment based on such a view may also fail. Cause-and-effect relationships become hopelessly tangled if a practitioner insists on such a linear perspective. Clarity may be achieved by the simple conceptualization of the child and family as an interrelating, dynamic, balanced system, in which single elements influence and are influenced by all others simultaneously.

Such a homeostatic appraisal of children and their families carries many implications for the form and style of treatment in pediatric practice. But focusing on the family constellation surrounding a child is hardly a new idea. It is a time-honored tradition in pediatrics to obtain a complete family history when undertaking the medical care of a child. Indeed, pediatricians seem to be particularly family oriented in their views of children and children's health care. No pediatrician finishes training without realizing that he or she is almost always working with at least two "patients" simultaneously—a child and a parent. So in this sense, pediatricians are already committed to the idea that working with a child means working with others (usually the mother) in a child's family.

I am suggesting, however, something beyond the general consensus that families are important and that a thorough family history should be obtained by talking with one parent. Since pediatrics is a family-oriented discipline, and since children usually cannot be managed or treated apart from their family context, pediatricians can consider the treatment unit quite often and quite literally to be the family. In the case cited, this would mean that the pediatrician must pay explicit attention to the mother's exhaustion, the father's frustration, their marital difficulties, and their older child's stomachaches when formulating any specific directives for enhancing the toddler's capacity for sleeping through the night. A child-only focus with a well-intentioned suggestion to "let her cry it out" without attending to the other pieces of the family's mobile may cause some disruptive transient shaking of the family's equilibrium; ultimately, however, the balancing forces within the system will tend to return the family to its previously balanced, albeit painful, state.

There is a myriad of pediatric conditions and complaints in which such a view of the family as a homeostatic system is useful. This frame of reference can be used in conceptualizing the presenting problem and, even more importantly, in determining the appropriate course of treatment and management. Among those conditions are:

- School phobia
- Eating disorders, including anorexia nervosa
- Enuresis
- Encopresis
- Sleep disorders
- Behavioral aspects of psychosomatic conditions, such as recurrent abdominal pain and headaches
- Juvenile diabetes mellitus
- Short stature
- Acting-out behavior
- Psychosocial complications of chronic illnesses, including asthma, seizure disorders, cystic fibrosis, and hemophilia
- Awesome psychosocial aspects of fatal diseases, such as leukemia and solid tumors
- Difficulties associated with a wide variety of developmental disorders, from specific learning disabilities to mental retardation

Coping problems accompanying physical handicaps

Multitudinous behavioral problems associated with no particular disease, for which anxious parents often first consult physicians

Of course there are more, and practitioners may compile their own lists. In fact, they probably should do so. The conclusion is unmistakable: In modern pediatrics, the family is the patient.

REFERENCES

1. Allmond BW, Buckman W, and Gofman HF: The family is the patient: an approach to behavioral pediatrics for the clinician, St Louis, 1979, The CV Mosby Co.
2. Jackson D: The question of family homeostatis, Psychiatr Q 31(suppl):79, 1957.
3. Satir V: Conjoint family therapy: a guide to theory and technique, Palo Alto, Calif, 1974, Science & Behavior Books.
4. Satir V: Peoplemaking, Palo Alto, Calif, 1972, Science & Behavior Books.

SUGGESTED READINGS

Haley J: The family life cycle. In Uncommon therapy: the psychiatric techniques of Milton H Erikson, New York, 1977, WW Norton & Co, Inc.

Zuk G: Family therapy: a triadic-based approach, New York, 1981, Behavioral Books.

53

Health Needs of Parents

Henry M. Seidel

The health needs of parents, like those of children, are determined by physical, social, and emotional factors. Because pediatric practitioners are basically advocates of the child, they do not as a rule view the parent in isolation—that is, as an individual with needs that may not always include the child as a prime factor. However, it is still essential to the care of the child to understand the differing characteristics of the various groupings possible within a family.

For example, given a family of three—mother, father, and child—the various "units" include each of them as individuals, the group of three, and the three dyads—mother-father, mother-child, father-child—a total of seven combinations. Thus a family of four would have 13 such units. The characteristic of a given unit varies with an infinite subtlety, depending on the particular combination and the basis of the interaction in which it may be involved at any given time. Thus appropriate care of the child requires an understanding of the parent and that parent's own health needs.

Although the physical, social, and emotional needs of the parent may be evident, primary care practitioners are most likely to become involved with the emotional needs. Within their individual practices and in the broader public arena, pediatricians have often acted as "experts," suggesting "principles" to parents regarding their relationship with their children and their life-styles. One effect of this advice in recent decades has been a diminution in the self-confidence of parents, a loss of their ability to resort to common sense, and a consequent breach in their composure and naturalness. In the latter part of the twentieth century, their sense of direction has often been confused by the dizzying impact of the audiovisual media and the disruption in the extended family.

The care of children might be improved if we, as a society, took greater advantage of the resources inherent in the intelligence, humor, and judgment of parents. To advise parents, pediatricians must work to exploit just these resources, putting aside value judgments and the occasional impulse to preach. Perhaps their major contribution to the health needs of parents can be to make available an objective listening ear and provide the opportunity to work together to achieve a balanced viewpoint.

There is a problem in determining the extent to which pediatricians should become involved with the health needs of parents. For example, should pediatric practitioners take care of the sore throat of a child but not of that child's parent? Is it appropriate, when both are in the office, to send the older person off to another setting at the cost of convenience, dollars, and delay? Much of the response will depend on the following:

1. An objective assessment of one's experience and competency. There may be much in primary care that requires a technical sophistication that a practitioner cannot invoke with appropriate confidence. On the other hand, one often possesses the relevant skills.
2. The circumstance of the particular family and the individual parent's access to care. The burdens of additional cost or an unreasonable wait for care elsewhere should be alleviated if possible. Often transportation may be a problem.
3. The equipment and the physical setting available. One is not likely to diagnose and treat a vaginal discharge in a parent if the appropriate adult examining table is not at hand.
4. The practitioner's concern over the possibility of a malpractice action. The risk is greater if the boundaries of one's specialty are extended.

It is practical to limit involvement to those aspects of parental health that are immediately relevant to the child. A gray area exists in which there is an unspoken constraint on going beyond the limits of one's certified area of competence—the constraint imposed by the manner in which medical responsibilities and economic rewards have been apportioned to the various health care specialties. Thus one is left to judge the parent's need and decide accordingly. Such a judgment is easier in the following instances.

THE ADOLESCENT PARENT

The adolescent parent has needs that require total care from a professional with a sound perspective on the young. A poignant example is that of the teenage, unmarried mother who elects to raise her child and who sees and treats that child as a "baby doll." The professional can provide a sensitive understanding of the interdependencies of that dyad and a ready availability (1) to the mother when she needs reassurance about her own self-worth when her baby does not behave perfectly and (2) to the baby when the mother acts out in frustration.

THE ABUSED PARENT OF THE BATTERED CHILD

The origins of child abuse are most often set in the socially disorganized childhood experience of the parent. To end the abuse and preserve the family, the parent must be included within the caring and the curing efforts of the professional involved. The parent should be "gathered in" rather than "referred out" as much as possible. Fragmentation of service to the individuals concerned, with the consequent requirement of a difficult to achieve, sensitive communication among too many persons, can only endanger the potential of successful outcomes.

THE PARENTS OF FIRSTBORNS

Anticipatory guidance is a major responsibility of primary care practitioners and reflects a common need in parents, especially those who are parents for the first time. For example, the emotionally nourishing interdependence of the man-woman dyad before the birth of a child may easily be threatened by that new child when care is left to the mother and when she may then have diminishing ability to attend to the care and feeding of the father. Resentment and a strain on the bond between the parents may develop.

THE SICK OR POTENTIALLY SICK PARENT

There are many instances in which pediatricians can extend caring and curing to parents as a result of their involvement with the child. Depression in the parent is a good example. If depression can be described as an inner feeling of helplessness resulting from a wide gap between one's perception of who one is and who one should be, then it is easy to understand the stress imposed by child rearing and the role of the pediatrician in reacting sensitively to parental symptoms such as anorexia, fatigue, crying spells, or insomnia, all of which are associated with depression.

Although the day of the house call is largely past, it is still possible in the office or clinic, without observing the home environment, to sense the presence of alcoholism or inappropriate dependency on drugs as a problem within some families. In addition, illness detected in the child should alert one to the possibility of a related condition in the parent. Obviously, for genetically determined diseases, access to genetic counseling and discussions aimed at resolving parental guilt must be available. In fact the awareness of the potential of parental guilt must be a common denominator in the development of a management plan for all childhood illness. An expression of physical abnormality in the child should initiate appropriate screening for a similar expression in the parent. Obvious environmental and genetic examples are tuberculosis, venereal disease, streptococcal disease, lead poisoning, and hearing loss. The less obvious circumstance includes the increased susceptibility to major psychic disturbance in the relatives of children with phenylketonuria and the increased likelihood of glucose 6-phosphate dehydrogenase deficiency in a family in which an index finding appears in a child.

PARENTS INVOLVED IN MARITAL CONFLICT OR DIVORCE

Marital conflict is a major source of "morbidity" among children today. Statistically, each year there is nearly one divorce for every two marriages. There is, on average, one child per divorce; therefore, many children have divorce as a factor in their lives. Moreover, because the median duration of marriage is slightly more than 7 years, most divorces affect young children. Ninety percent of the time the father becomes the noncustodial parent; however, the tendency in this direction is shifting somewhat, and there are currently arrangements in which parents attempt to share the care of the child equally.

We must remember that divorce is a process and not a discrete pathologic entity to which psychological disturbances in children can be neatly ascribed. It is in the precursors of divorce that one finds the psychopathologic root in the child and the parents. There are obviously competing priorities for the attention of health professionals, who must walk a fine line, recognizing the priority of the child and the imperative that in serving that priority, they do not take "sides" with one or the other parent. They cannot ignore the parental need, and they must try to preserve the integrity of the family unit; failing this, they must then attempt an arrangement that might provide optimum nurturance for the child and appropriate support for each parent.

Thus the potential responsibilities that the pediatric practitioner has to the health needs of parents are numerous and recurrent. The degree of need and the practitioner's consequent involvement may result in a judgment based not only on the variables already mentioned but also on an assessment of the psychosocial competence of the parents involved. In fact there may at times be a competition for loyalties. It is likely that most practitioners will choose in favor of the child. However, lest this be considered too simplistic, it is well to ponder, for example, the development of a therapeutic plan for the child born with a meningomyelocele, or the content of testimony in a divorce action when there is legal representation for each adult but none for the child, or that the rights to due process are not fully extended to children in our society. There is a point, then, when the pediatric practitioner must refer the parent elsewhere for medical assistance and emotional support, if for no other reasons than the requirement of technical skills or the priority of child advocacy.

SUGGESTED READINGS

Annual summary of births, deaths, marriages and divorces, United States, July, 1988. Monthly Vital Statistics Report, National Center for Health Statistics, vol 37, no 7, Oct 15, 1988.

Wegman ME: Annual summary of vital statistics—1989, Pediatrics 86:835, 1990.

54

Latchkey Children: Children in Self-Care

Rickey L. Williams

An estimated 8 to 10 million American children younger than 18 years of age are in self-care before or after school. Two to five million of these "latchkey" children are grade schoolers 6 to 13 years of age.[2] Even greater numbers of children are cared for by older siblings.

In this era of single parent families and families with two employed parents, many children must return to an empty home after school. In many communities, affordable, conveniently located care programs are unavailable or have long waiting lists; parents in such communities may leave a child in self-care because they have no alternative. Some parents may simply be unwilling to pay for child care or feel that self-care arrangements are acceptable. In addition, many parents fear that baby-sitters or program personnel may abuse their children; they may feel more comfortable leaving their child home alone than at a center or with a baby-sitter. Of course, there will never be enough centers and personnel to permit every child to be adequately supervised in a program.

Even if adequate child care is arranged, children might at times be in self-care, especially during minor illnesses. Working parents may find it difficult to leave their jobs for each mild communicable illness that their children acquire; day care centers frequently exclude children with fever, vomiting, diarrhea, and other communicable diseases.[8]

Pediatricians may not be familiar with self-care. In a publication for pediatricians on the effects on child development when both parents work, child care arrangements were discussed, but no mention was made of self-care.[5] In contrast to the amount of attention and research focused on day care centers, virtually no research has been carried out on the various informal care arrangements for school-age children, even though there are far more children in such arrangements.[7]

Research on children in self-care is difficult because the self-care status of a particular child may not remain stable over time, due to several factors, including parental employment, economic necessity, and the availability of other types of care. Students or parents involved in surveys of children in self-care may not be willing to admit that children are or were in self-care.[2]

The effects of self-care on children are unknown and depend on many factors, including the child's age and maturity level, the circumstances surrounding the reason for the child being in self-care, and the community in which the child lives. Hypothesized benefits of self-care include increased maturity, self-reliance, decision-making, freedom, and responsibility.[4] Negative aspects of self-care include feeling or actually being neglected, in danger, isolated, or at medical risk.[2] One report suggests that many children in self-care fear attack from intruders and from other children, particularly siblings.[6] Some children in self-care will thrive, some will just manage to cope, and others will actually be harmed in some way.[1]

Studies of academic achievement and school adjustment in children in self-care have yielded mixed results. Some[12] studies reported lower academic achievement and social problems in children in self-care compared with other children of working mothers who had adult supervision; other studies[3,7,10] found no differences in academic achievement, self-competence, or school adjustment between those children in self-care versus those in adult care. One study[9] found that the less directly supervised children were, the more susceptible they were to peer pressure.

Are children in self-care less physically fit or less healthy than those in adult care? One can postulate that children in self-care are at especially high risk for obesity, since they are less likely to be permitted to play outside after school than are children in adult care or sibling care.[6] However, a recent study[11] found no differences in weight or body mass index between children in self-care and those in adult care. In addition, there were no differences between the two groups of children in the number of school days missed or in the number of visits to the school health office.

Parents of children in self-care might be made to feel guilty that they are leaving their children in self-care, and articles in the lay press suggest that being in self-care has negative consequences. For example, results of a recent Lewis Harris and Associates, Inc., poll were published by the Associated Press and stated that a majority of parents and teachers believe that students would perform better in the classroom if adults did not leave the youngsters by themselves so much after school (Tucson Citizen, September 3, 1987, p. 7A).

Pediatric health professionals cannot reverse maternal employment and child care trends. They can, however, advocate for children through counseling of individual parents about self-care of their children and by supporting the establishment of affordable, after-school care programs of quality in their communities.

REFERENCES

1. Coolsen P, Seligson M, and Garbarino J: When school's out and nobody's home. Chicago, National Committee for Prevention of Child Abuse, 1985.
2. Fosarelli PD: Latchkey children, J Dev Behav Pediatr 5:173-177, 1984.
3. Galambos NL and Garbarino J: Identifying the missing links in the study of latchkey children, Child Today 12(5):2-4, 40-41, 1983.
4. Garbarino J: Latchkey children: getting the short end of the stick, Vital Issues 30(3):1-4, 1980.
5. Lerner JV: When both parents work: effects on the development of children. Children are different: behavioral development monogram series: number 12. Columbus, Ohio, Ross Laboratories, 1985.
6. Long T and Long L: Latchkey children: the child's view of self care, ERIC Doc ED 211229, 1981.
7. Rodman H, Pratto DJ, and Nelson RS: Child care arrangements and children's functioning: a comparison of self-care and adult-care children, Dev Psychol 21:413-418, 1985.
8. Shapiro ED: Exclusion of ill children from day-care centers: policy and practice in New Haven, Connecticut, Clin Pediatr 23:689-691, 1984.
9. Steinberg L: Latchkey children and susceptibility to peer pressure: an ecological analysis, Dev Psychol 22:433-439, 1986.
10. Vandell DL and Corasaniti MA: The relation between third graders' after-school care and social, academic, and emotional functioning, Child Development 59:868-875, 1988.
11. Williams RL and Boyce WT: Health status of children in self-care, Am J Dis Child 143:112-115, 1989.
12. Woods M: The unsupervised child of the working mother, Dev Psychol 6:14-25, 1972.

55

Mental Health of the Young

An Overview

Julius B. Richmond and William R. Beardslee

Advances in knowledge of child development, gained through the in-depth study of healthy infants and children as well as through observations of deviations or delays in development, have provided the pediatrician with the conceptual framework needed to deal effectively with the mental health needs of children. Recent advances within child psychiatry have also contributed substantially, including, for example, the development of reliable, standardized interview instruments, a criterion-based diagnostic system (Diagnostic and Statistical Manual-III-Revised of the American Psychiatric Association), more effective pharmacologic treatments for affective and attention deficit disorders, and the description of the epidemiology of a number of childhood mental disorders. A more sophisticated understanding of the prevalence and nature of neurodevelopmental and neuropsychiatric difficulties has also substantially expanded the information available to the pediatrician. A broadening knowledge base in the neurosciences, including genetics, will undoubtedly in the years to come lead to major advances in clinical pediatric practice.

Advances in the development of preventive and therapeutic agents over the past 40 years have brought about major reductions in infant mortality and childhood morbidity and mortality. No longer is the practicing pediatrician's time consumed by rickets, scurvy, or the acute infectious diseases such as measles, pertussis, diphtheria, and poliomyelitis. Rather, more time and energy are available to focus on the prevention of disease and the early detection and care of children with chronic disorders, including developmental disabilities.

In addition, the past decade has been characterized by an increasing awareness by organized consumers of the desirability of high-quality child health and child care services. Pressure from communities for improved child health services has increased, a concern reflected in the development of such programs as Head Start; maternal and infant care (M&I); children and youth (C&Y) early periodic screening, diagnosis, and treatment (EPSDT) for Medicaid-eligible children; and community mental health centers. The new approaches to more comprehensive services for the handicapped also reflect intensified community sophistication, such as the Education for All Handicapped Children Act (Public Law 94-142), which emphasizes the need to "mainstream" such children. Public Law 99-457 has mandated adequate services for younger handicapped children. There is continued interest in more comprehensive health insurance for children, which also will have a significant impact.

The increasing interest in child health will undoubtedly result in an effort to reorganize services and generate local initiatives to reflect local needs and priorities. The emphasis will be increasingly on the enhancement of health and the prevention of disease. Thus competence in the assessment and guidance of growth and development needs to be among the pediatrician's clinical skills.

Knowing the cultural and psychological background of a child's family is important for understanding the mental health needs of that child. The emotional climate in which a child is reared reflects the personality development of the parents or parent substitutes. Therefore the pediatrician must know about the developmental background of each parent and the immediate environmental factors that are significant in the child's life. Since different families impose different roles on children, it is important for the pediatrician to know how the child fits into the family constellation. Just as the physiologic structure and function of an infant have determinants that antedate birth, the practices and attitudes that determine how the child will be cared for have comparable antecedents. The pediatrician may develop an understanding of these factors as they become apparent during the prenatal period or after birth as he or she comes to know the family as a unit.

The pediatrician can regard the family as carrying the "chromosomes" that perpetuate the culture and that also form the cornerstone of emotional development. Cultural influences are like a mainstream with many tributaries: each varies from time to time in depth, rate of flow, and course; the mainstream is modified by its tributaries, but also influences them.

In the United States many variations exist in cultural patterns relating to childbearing attitudes and practices. These are determined in part by geographic, religious, educational, social, and economic backgrounds. For example, in some communities a great premium is placed on the first child being male. Religious backgrounds definitely tend to influence the size of families. Higher educational backgrounds of parents have been correlated with a later childbearing age and with limitation in family size.

The relative rapidity of social movement tends to confuse young parents in terms of their basic group identification. Also, increasing educational opportunities usually generate upward social mobility for many young parents. The pediatrician should know how much parents identify with their old and how much with their new social grouping and its culture. Either of these identifications (usually some of both) involves some reintegration on the part of the parents, who may require professional assistance. Moreover, changes in the structure of the American family have led to a large increase in the number of single-parent families and to a marked decrease in the availability of the extended family for assistance in child care. Therefore parents are relying more and more on pediatricians and other practitioners for guidance.

The pediatrician should learn to adjust his or her cultural background and attitudes toward childbearing and child rearing with the cultural backgrounds and attitudes of parents who seek advice. It then becomes easier to understand that there is no "right" attitude or practice. A certain practice may be effective for one family and yet its objectives fail with another. Thus the pediatrician can help by being objective rather than judgmental in viewing the family. This requires the capacity to observe, listen, and, as a consequence, understand.

The pediatrician can develop an objective attitude by remembering that it is the culture and not the physician that, within certain limits, defines mental health. For example, Erikson[2] and others have pointed out that children brought up in one Native American culture might not be considered capable of performing the developmental tasks required of children in another tribe living in a different climate with significantly different cultural demands. Many similar cross-cultural comparisons can be made. Although the pediatrician generally deals with more subtle contrasts, they are nevertheless real and significant for each family. In a country of people with such varied origins and so much educational, social, economic, and geographic movement, it is unlikely that any one stable tradition of child-rearing practices will emerge in the next several decades. Therefore the objective in each instance is to help each family attain its goal in child rearing in its unique and most effective manner.

To assist in reaching this goal, the pediatrician must have a firm grasp of the child development field. Piaget's work[3] provides the most useful framework within the cognitive sphere because of its emphasis on the child's actions as necessary for the acquisition of knowledge and on the predictable sequence of stages through which a child passes in developing intelligence. Skinner's work[6] in the area of behavior modification and its applications have proved valuable both in helping children to learn and in suggesting ways to manage difficult or troublesome symptoms. Several workers in the area of early infant and child behavior, including Thomas, Chess, and Birch,[7] have helped to focus attention on the importance of temperament as an early influence.

Psychoanalytic theory and formulations have contributed to our understanding of all aspects of the development of the child.[6,7]

The work of Erikson[2] probably provides the best integrative framework through which pediatricians can understand the different factors shaping the mental health of the child and then best meet the needs of their patients. Erikson stresses the importance of all three major factors—biologic, intrapsychic, and cultural—in the child's mental health. He sees the child as going through a series of stages in development and formulates the essential task or critical area to be mastered for each stage. Thus, as one example, the dilemma for the very young infant is basic trust versus mistrust, and firm patterns for the solution of this dilemma must be successfully established for the infant to develop in a healthy way. As another example, the dilemma for the adolescent is identity versus role diffusion. Youths in this stage must come to understand their own physical endowments, experiences, and opportunities in a way that allows them to function in the world and have a sense of certainty about themselves. Specifically, youths must come to grips with three areas: (1) relationships with others, both sexual and nonsexual, (2) independence from family, and (3) choice of work or career. Familiarity with each stage, both with its task and the signs of its successful resolution, provides the pediatrician with knowledge of the principles of child mental health.

Common to a series of recent investigations of youngsters at risk because of poverty or parental mental illness or other stressors is the finding that no matter how great the risk, a significant number of children turn out to do well and, indeed, function very effectively. Rutter[5] has indicated a variety of conceptual areas to be reviewed in studying the sources of resiliency and looking for explanations. These include genetic effects, individual differences, particularly the role of temperament, inner psychological processes, and the role of influences outside of the home, especially the schools. The presence of close confiding relationships that provide support and direction has been found crucial in all of the studies of resilient individuals. Of particular relevance to pediatric practice are a number of studies of resilient individuals that have emphasized the importance of the way these individuals understand themselves and what they have accomplished—their self-understanding.[1] This self-understanding involves adequate appraisal of the stresses to be dealt with, realistic assessment of the capacity to act, and actions congruent with the assessment and has characterized people in such diverse circumstances as survivors of cancer, civil rights workers, and children of parents with an affective disorder. The recognition and characterization of resilient behavior in pediatric practice in high-risk families is important and emphasizes the need to assess a child or family's strengths and capacities to adapt in addition to identifying a pathologic condition.[4]

Schools, families, child care centers, and hospitals are all concerned with the mental health of children. The pediatrician can combine medical findings with observations of children within their families and perceptions of larger cultural influences to evaluate and meet the mental health needs of children. The evaluation of psychological health is a vital part of the comprehensive pediatric assessment of children. Such evaluations provide the basis for helping parents become more effective in rearing their children through helping them to articulate and realize their own goals for them. Because of the increasing numbers of health professionals and disciplines that work with children, the pediatrician's role has become even more integrative: he or she is the one who brings together the different disciplines and different kinds of knowledge—biologic, psychological, and social—in a comprehensive understanding of the treatment program for the child.

When the pediatrician approaches the management of illness as one aspect of the total care of the child and is interested in the interpersonal relations between the pediatrician and family, each child can provide an intriguing study. The pediatrician also has the opportunity to help foster the psychological development of the child. In this regard, and in dealing with the child and parents, the pediatrician's attitudes, interest, and curiosity about human behavior and relations are important, probably more so than formal knowledge in this area. The pediatrician's receptivity and alertness in recognizing psychologically charged situations will extend, condition, or limit his or her effectiveness in the care of many children.

Assuming the primary responsibility for all physical and medical care of the child also provides pediatricians with responsibility and opportunity to learn about and care for the psychological and mental health needs of children. Pediatricians who wish to provide total care should be interested in children not only in intellectual terms but also in emotional terms. Those pediatricians are in a favorable and unique position from which to encourage wholesome attitudes of child rearing during each contact with the family. Concomitantly, they can detect unwholesome attitudes and disturbances early in a child's life and endeavor to provide a more favorable setting for the child through interviews and counseling with the parents. In situations of severe distress, the pediatrician may decide that more extensive psychological treatment through psychotherapy or other means is needed and make a referral for psychiatric consultation. But fundamentally, he or she remains the key professional that evaluates comprehensively the overall health of the child, including the child's mental health, while serving as the central person in the parents' eyes for counseling and guidance.

REFERENCES

1. Beardslee WR: The role of self-understanding in resilient individuals: the development of a perspective, Am J Orthopsychiatry 59:266, 1989.
2. Erikson EH: Childhood and society, ed 2, New York, 1963, WW Norton & Co, Inc.
3. Piaget J: The origins of intelligence in children, New York, 1963, WW Norton & Co, Inc.
4. Richmond JB and Beardslee WR: Resiliency: research and practical implications for pediatricians, J Dev Behav Pediatr 9:157, 1988.
5. Rutter M: Meyerian psychobiology, personality development, and the role of life experiences, Am J Psychiatry 143:1077, 1986.
6. Skinner BF: Science and human behavior, New York, 1953, Macmillan.
7. Thomas A, Chess S, and Birch H: Temperament and behavior disorders in children, New York, 1968, New York University Press.

SUGGESTED READINGS

Richmond JB: Child development: a basic science for pediatrics, Pediatrics 39:649, 1967.

Richmond JB: An idea whose time has arrived, Pediatr Clin North Am 22:517, 1975.

56

Parenting Skills and Discipline

John L. Green

It is difficult to be an effective parent in today's society and to raise one's children to be freethinking, self-assured, agreeable, and ready to face adulthood with confidence and maturity. Parents are bombarded with advice on child rearing from multiple sources and often end up confused. Yet parents can be responsible and effective in child rearing through a combination of acquired skills and management techniques, good common sense, even temperament, and courage to overcome the fear of making mistakes. Pediatricians can and should be involved in helping parents advance these skills beyond the traditional well child-care visits. As the American Academy of Pediatrics (AAP)[1] states, "Preventive pediatrics is the core of quality medical care for children" and "discussing and counseling is the most important element of current child health care."

Every well-child care visit should include an evaluation of that child's behavior and actions and, when appropriate, guidelines for anticipatory guidance and management. Practicing pediatricians are involved daily with the emotional interactions of patients and their families and therefore are in a powerful position to provide guidance and support routinely through the formative years. Pediatricians should spend time teaching and helping parents to enjoy their children more. To gain a sense of self and security and the ability to cope with life, children must have love, consistency, and security in their lives. A lack of such nurturance will lead to anxious, insecure children with resulting maladaptive behavior.

PARENTING SKILLS

Parents cannot change a child's personality, temperament, or emotional experiences, but they *can* change the child's behavior. Temperament is believed to be largely biologically determined. The work of Chess and associates[4] superbly defines nine characteristics of behavior that are relatively stable across time and that are most helpful in our learning to understand children. Parents must accept a child's temperamental qualities and concentrate their efforts and energies not on trying to alter that temperament or challenging their child's feelings or emotions but on molding acceptable behavior by praising appropriate positive interactions and extinguishing negative and manipulative behavior.

Health care providers should promote parental competency by teaching parents to interact with their children in affectionate, consistent, and cognitively stimulating ways. Parenting skills needed for this task include (1) listening and communicating with children, (2) praising and reinforcing acceptable, positive behavior, (3) limiting and not reinforcing unacceptable, negative behavior, (4) encouraging mutual respect, (5) interacting consistently, (6) setting appropriate limits, and (7) responding effectively when limits are exceeded.

Communicating

Communication is the key to all family interactions, and good communications with children requires listening and exchanging both words and feelings. Techniques outlined by Baruch[2] and Ginott[8] effectively encourage parents to be sensitive to the meanings behind children's words and actions. Parents must be trained to listen carefully and to think before responding to their children, especially with negative expressions. What makes a child produce "bad" behavior is usually bad feelings, and most misbehavior occurs when children are feeling hurt, angry, frightened, and lonely. To understand the child's behavior, the parent should first try to recognize those underlying feelings and help the child find safe and appropriate ways of expressing them. Parents must not be hasty to criticize, ridicule, or scold when bad feelings lead to bad behavior; rather they should quietly verbalize, reflect, and discuss their thoughts and feelings with their children. For a parent to state, "I know how upset and angry you must be," or "I know how scary and frightening this is," can lead to far more enlightening and effective communication with a child of preschool or school age than to say, "What's bugging you today?" or "What in the world do you mean by stomping around and throwing things like that?" Children must be permitted to express their feelings in safety and without judgment. The cardinal message of the disciplinary dialogue should be "your feelings are accepted and respected; only your actions and behavior are judged."[12] Being understanding goes a long way in gaining the child's cooperation, which is vital to effective, consistent parenting.

Reinforcing Positive Behavior

Techniques and procedures that increase or reinforce positive behavior and decrease or extinguish negative behavior form the basis of most behavior modification techniques in use today. Parents condition or influence children's behavior in three basic ways: (1) by shaping or teaching the child new behavior, (2) by strengthening and positively reinforcing satisfactory behavior, and (3) by extinguishing or punishing undesirable behavior.

To *reinforce* positively is to praise and reward behavior that the parent wishes to encourage and strengthen. Ideally, most of the day should be spent in positive interaction with one's children, such as using continual verbal reinforcers (e.g., words of praise and gestures of warmth and admiration) and spending time in pleasant activities.

Unfortunately, most of a parent's day may well be spent in negative interactions with his or her children. Such interaction should be altered. Children "tune out" their parents if they are "on their case" all day. Although parents must be negative at times, they should make such comments infrequently and only when previously set limits are exceeded. The emphasis should be shifted from negative comments such as "no, don't do that" or shrieks of "get away from there," to positive comments such as "come, let's do this" or "you've been quiet and well-behaved, so Mommy will read to you now." Parents should give positive attention, time, and praise to their children when they are behaving appropriately so that they will be motivated to maintain their behavior. This concept is difficult for parents to master inasmuch as many parents tend to ignore their children when they are behaving well. Instead, parents increase their interactions with their children at times when they misbehave because that is when they "need it" and seem to be asking for it. Such "negative attention" actually may reinforce misbehavior and thus should be avoided.

Positive feedback includes physical actions, such as a hug, a pat on the head or shoulders, a smile, a kiss, a "thumbs up" sign, a wink, an affectionate rubbing of hair, or an arm around the shoulders. It also consists of verbal feedback about specific actions, such as "I like it when the table is cleared," "great," "good job," "I'm pleased when you come the first time I call," "thanks for getting ready for bed," "Mom will sure be pleased when I tell her how well you helped me."

Limiting Negative Behavior

To extinguish is to limit unacceptable behavior by turning away, withdrawing, and ignoring the behavior that the parent wishes to discourage. To eliminate such behavior it is far preferable to use extinction rather than punishment; when unacceptable behavior is not reinforced, it is likely to decrease in frequency and strength and eventually disappear.[7] For example, when a parent is with a child at home and the child misbehaves, the parent should simply turn away from the child and attend to something else in the room. If the misbehavior continues or escalates, then the parent should leave the room if possible, return later, and interact positively with the child when he or she is behaving more appropriately. With parental consistency the child will learn that good behavior elicits praise and loving interaction from parents and misbehavior achieves only separation and avoidance.

This behavior modification technique is far more effective than punishment, which usually involves negative parent-child interaction, evokes fear, and is counterproductive to learning. Such negative interaction is to be avoided whenever possible in dealing with undesirable behavior. Rather the goal should be to consistently ignore or disapprove of undesirable behavior; otherwise that behavior will likely become stronger. To give in to a child's tantrum either at home or away will likely only increase the magnitude of the tantrums at other times and make that behavior harder and harder to eliminate. Consistently and repetitively ignoring negative and inappropriate behavior should decrease and eventually extinguish that behavior.[10]

Encouraging Mutual Respect

If a child's behavior is interfering with the basic rights of other human beings and the mutual respect between that child and others is broken, then some consistent, immediate, meaningful, and effective response is required. Mutual respect in parent-child relationships means respecting the rights and dignity of another to live, enjoy, and function without excessive negative interactions. For a parent it means trying to understand and respect what a child is feeling when he or she carries out an action or verbalizes a thought. It means respecting the rights of children to think all kinds of thoughts; one cannot expect a child not to have worrisome thoughts any more than one can expect him not to breathe, jump, or be happy or sad. For a child it means gaining the understanding that others have feelings, desires, and rights and that they too should be respected as human beings—a difficult chore for young children because of their egocentric nature.

Children act for the moment, and they need guidance. They are not goal oriented but instead act on impulse. They must have free time to grow, experiment, and play—time to be just children without constantly trying to please parents by living up to their expectations. If parents remain reasonable, unruffled, and loving and are consistent and fair in their interactions with their children, then mutual respect should follow and become rooted in their children's everyday lives.

Interacting Consistently

Overpermissive and overauthoritarian methods are two extremes to be avoided; worse yet are inconsistency and variation in day-to-day management of children. Parents should agree on their approach to child-rearing practices and strive daily for consistent interactions so that their children cannot play one parent against the other or manipulate parental responses from one day to another. Children feel comfortable and secure when they know and can reasonably predict what is going to happen. When children who misbehave are uncertain of what response will be forthcoming, they become frightened, confused, and unsure, and their actions show it. With regular and predictable discipline, children may not like the expected and known response, but they will still respect the one who disciplines, especially if that parent accepts the child's right not to like what is happening.

Such external consistency and structure will both help parents to relax and gain a sense of security and control and help the child to develop an internal sense of stability and self-control.

Interactions at their best build children's self-esteem. The famous children's television personality, Captain Kangaroo (Bob Keeshan), believes that self-esteem is the most critical part of personality development for children 6 years old and younger and that if we develop other parts of the child's character and skip self-esteem, we have failed the child.

Limit-Setting and Discipline

Parents are role models for their children; as such, they should teach their children positive values while trying hard not to be negative in their daily living. Spanking, hitting, or other forms of corporal punishment and abuse in response to children's behavior is not only ineffective but also confusing to a child. It teaches only that "might makes right" and conveys the message that, when older, he or she is entitled to inflict such punishment on younger or smaller individuals. Spanking signifies a loss of adult control and should not be condoned. Christophersen[5] notes that in the absence of some type of positive feedback regarding more appropriate behavior, physical punishment has at best only a limited or temporary effect and little lasting educational value. That temporary effect often is no more than a reduction of the undesirable behavior in the presence of the punishing parent; unfortunately, that behavior can persist or even increase as soon as the parent is not present.

Verbal shrieking and abuse—shaming and cajoling, nagging and scolding—also are not beneficial and in fact serve to model negative behavior. If parents shriek and verbally abuse their children either as an emotional outlet or as a method of punishment, then children likely will adopt this behavior and be verbal, loud, and overactive in their communications with others as they grow. To tease or to shame only confuses the child, who cannot comprehend why loved and trusted adults are attacking him or her with disrespectful words or tone of voice.

When parents use physical force, verbal threats, or excessive punishment, the result is to make children feel frightened and helpless; the children may provoke further confrontations if only to prove they still have feelings and worth and some vestige of autonomy.[14] Children copy and mirror their parents, and if parents "blow up" and lose control in their family interactions, their children are likely to do so, too. Parents always should strive to be role models, expressing their own angry feelings reasonably rather than resorting to hitting, yelling, or profanity; again, they always should direct their anger toward the child's actions and the effects and consequences of those actions rather than toward the child's personality and temperament.[13]

What forms of "discipline" then, should parents use to guide and direct their children to appropriate behavior? This is best accomplished through positive limit-setting and consistency in parental response when previously set rules and standards are exceeded. Parents who do not teach their children that there are limits to acceptable behavior run the risk of raising a truly spoiled child who is unable to control his or her behavior or to respect the rights and possessions of others.[11]

Discipline without love can be as useless and harmful as love without discipline. It is acceptable not to like an action that a child performs and to say so, but it is a mistake to tell a child that he or she is not loved because of something he or she has said or done. Despite their misbehavior, children must be told repeatedly that they are loved.

To repeat, the key function of discipline is to encourage appropriate behavior and discourage or limit unacceptable behavior. Clearly, discipline should not be focused on punishment (negative) but should be oriented toward teaching the child (positive) to reach the desired goal of acceptable, approvable behavior. To do this, parents must set rules or limits because without them children will waver, flounder, lack self-esteem, and almost certainly become manipulative. These rules or limits should be clearly defined and positively implemented with regular, consistent parental responses to violations of these rules. Parents who have clear and definite values, who set appropriate age-related limits to their children's behavior, and who treat their children with firmness, consistency, and respect for their feelings are more likely to rear children with high respect for themselves and for others. Such children will be far more likely to achieve with pride and to get along well with others. Clearly, one must be content and comfortable with oneself before one can be happy and content with others.

However unfortunate, it is the nature of children to test their parents constantly over set limits and to try to alter those limits if possible. Parents must recognize this early and formulate effective ways to counteract inevitable manipulative actions. To be meaningful, limits should be as few in number as possible. If an excessive number of limits are placed on a child's everyday behavior, the child will tend to ignore them all. To give a child a sense of achievement, parents must be certain not to overload him or her with countless commands. An effective approach is to ask parents to jot down carefully over a 2- to 3-day period the demands and prohibitions that they convey to their child throughout the day. They usually are surprised by the number. By reviewing this list, parents are then better able to reduce the number of set limits.

A key limit is that a child is not to interfere with the rights and dignity of another human being, that is, hitting or taunting a sibling, destroying others' toys or property, or manipulating parents. On the other hand, nuisance behavior (behavior that parents do not necessarily approve of but that really does not interfere with the rights of others) should be ignored whenever possible rather than be included in limits.

Furthermore, the limits set must be consistent and approved by both parents and then discussed with the child, if the child is old enough to understand. Children must know what constitutes a limit, what is encouraged, and what is to be avoided. They must be taught that if a limit is ignored or violated, a response will be forthcoming, and that the response will be the same regardless of what caregiver is present at that time. Ideally, of course, the plan also should include grandparents and baby-sitters. The response must be meaningful enough so that children will be encouraged not to exceed the set limit and receive the expected response but rather to alter their behavior and experience more positive responses and pleasanter interactions.

A concrete example illustrates this principle. The parents set a limit or rule that bedtime is 8 PM each night. The child will be most likely to follow that rule only if he or she (1) knows specifically what the rule is, (2) knows why the rule has been made (the child is tired by then and needs sleep to be fresh and happy the next day), (3) knows what the consequences will be for not following that rule (e.g., going to bed 15 minutes earlier the next night), and (4) knows that there is no chance to get away with violating the rule. After the explanation is given, the child has the right to have a say, and the parents must recognize the child's right not to "like" the rule. However, a rule is to be followed in *every* circumstance. With this approach the child is not only being disciplined but also in effect learning self-discipline.[15]

Responding Effectively

The best researched and most frequently used alternative to verbal or physical punishment in responding to children's exceeding set limits is the use of isolation or separation—"time-out" procedures. Christophersen[6] discusses the use of time-out for behavioral problems in a guideline for parents that can be easily incorporated in everyday child care. For example, time-out involves placing the child on a chair for a short period of time after an occurrence of unacceptable behavior. This procedure has been effective in reducing problem behaviors such as tantrums, hitting, biting, failure to follow directions, leaving the yard without permission, and others. Parents have found that time-out is more effective than spanking, yelling, or threatening their children. It is most appropriate for children from 18 months of age through 10 years.

After carefully describing the steps of preparation, practice, and actual use of time-out, Christophersen[6] summarizes rules for parents, children, and siblings:

1. Deciding ahead of time about behaviors for which time-out will apply and discussing these with the child.

2. Not leaving the child in time-out for unduly long periods or forgetting about him. The child needs to remain in time-out only until two criteria are met: a quiet period is accomplished with the child seated in a chair and the period has been long enough to be uncomfortable and unpleasant for the child. This time period will vary with the age of the child and may be only a few minutes for children 2 to 4 years to 10 to 15 minutes for children 6 to 10 years. In any case the child should *not* be allowed to leave the chair until quiet, however long that might be.

3. Not nagging, scolding, or talking to the child in time-out. All siblings and family members must follow this rule.

4. Allowing the child to start with a "clean slate" after finishing a time-out period. Within 5 minutes after time-out, parents should look for and praise good behavior, remembering to "catch them being good" and to positively reinforce such behavior. This serves several purposes. First, it prevents the parent from carrying a grudge; second, and more important, it teaches the child that the parent is no longer angry and is willing to praise good behavior. From this the child learns that it is the behavior that gets praise or penalty—that is, it is the child's *choice* of behavior that causes the choice of consequences, praise or penalty. This also ensures that the parent is never punishing more than praising the child.

5. Remaining calm, particularly when the child is being testy. Parents should always try to use a firm voice and firm arm and hand gestures and should try *not* to lose control of their voice or emotions. This is extremely difficult to do with testy children, and becoming angry is human. Nevertheless, anger should always be directed to the child's action and deeds and not to the child's negative emotional qualities and judgments.

It is helpful for parents to use this temporary separation to cool off and think quietly by themselves. Such isolation-separation averts the impulsive forcing of compliance by upset parents, which invariably leads to frustration for both parent and child and accomplishes little. If parents want to discuss feelings and behavior with their children, and by all means they should, such discussion best occurs when all concerned are quiet and relaxed rather than in the midst of turmoil or when either parent or child is threatened.

Behavior modification techniques and the use of penalties for exceeding set limits and rules are used to encourage acceptable behavior rather than to make the child suffer undue punishment. Time-out usually is successful precisely because it is not a severe punishment and does not attack a child's self-esteem or personality. Rather it is only a penalty for a limit-exceeding unacceptable behavior, not an attack on the child's basic feelings. It is the consistency of the punishment, not its severity, that helps the child to learn and comply with the rules.[11]

As children grow older, the old-fashioned technique of rewards and penalties becomes an effective tool. Children and adolescents should be taught over the years that good behavior will be rewarded and that unacceptable behavior will be penalized by loss of privileges. Such loss works best when a fair penalty is imposed quickly after the offense occurs. Furthermore, the parent must be firm and matter-of-fact about the penalty and should not become engaged in lengthy arguments with the child. If the penalty—that is, loss of privileges—has been previously set and mutually understood by all, and if parents are consistent in applying the penalty, then this technique becomes an excellent motivator to promote appropriate judgment and direction for the child.

With older children this technique often works best by means of a written contract with the child in which he or she has a say in the imposed penalty. When the child or adolescent has been involved in the decision-making and feels that the penalty is appropriate and fair, then he or she has a stake in making that contract work, and everyone is more apt to "win." Such contracting helps eliminate arguing because the participants have agreed on the terms before the specific action takes place.

With this technique, parents must be careful not to engage in overkill. The penalty should be for a limited time and should be strictly adhered to. Consequences and penalties should always be clearly related to the nonacceptable, limit-exceeding behavior. They should be neither overly harsh nor given in retribution but rather fair consequences for actions.

Effective examples of loss of privileges include (1) "grounding" for a few days, to go nowhere but school and home, (2) being unable to watch television or listen to the stereo for a week, (3) not using the telephone to communicate with friends for several days or a week, (4) being unable to have friends over to play or visit for several days to a week, and (5) not using the car for a weekend or evenings for a week. School privileges and special school activities, including athletics, plays, or dances, should not be taken away because this deprivation can be detrimental to a child's self-esteem. Rather, only home-based privileges should be restricted.

COUNSELING PARENTS

When parents discuss their children's behavioral problems together, misunderstandings often escalate as each tries to promote and defend his or her opinions without effectively listening to the other. A respected third person whose knowledge includes not only children's behavior in general but also the involved family's style of living and personalities can alter each parent's communications and help each to listen to the other's feelings and desires. Both parents then may cooperate more effectively in further discussion and implementation plans in joint sessions with that respected physician. Perhaps the most important theme to emerge from such counseling sessions should be that establishing a pattern of love, trust, and mutual understanding of acceptable predetermined limits within each family is what really counts—rather than numerous technical details of implementation.[3]

Such counseling sessions should be scheduled at a time when the physician is not rushed or pressed with everyday office or hospital concerns. Time can be set aside specifically for such sessions, such as during regular but off-peak office hours, evening hours, or on weekends, when the physician can comfortably listen and counsel without the pressures and restrictions of time.[9]

REFERRALS

Situations always occur that should prompt early referral to more specialized professional or community resources if available. These circumstances include not only specific patient or family indicators but also physician discomfort or lack of experience or training in the assessment and management of certain problems.

Specific referral indicators generally include chronic or severe emotional disorders; suicide gestures or attempts; significant alcoholism or drug abuse; severe acting-out behavior; significant depression in child or parent; marital problems, including physical abuse of one of the family members; and a continuation or increased intensity of behavioral problems, even after several counseling sessions. Before referral the physician should strive for some personal contact with the referring social worker, specialist, or agency to expedite appropriate follow-up and feedback regarding the management of the problem. This knowledge may be useful when the practitioner is confronted with similar cases in the future.

REFERENCES

1. American Academy of Pediatrics: Standards of child health care, ed 3, Evanston, Ill, 1977, The Academy.
2. Baruch D: How to discipline your children, New York Public Affairs Pamphlet No 154, New York, 1949, Public Affairs Committee.
3. Brophy B: Dr. Spock had it right, US News and World Report, p. 49, Aug 7, 1989.
4. Chess S, Thomas A, and Birch H: Your child is a person: a psychological approach to parenthood without guilt, New York, 1965, Viking Press.
5. Christophersen ER: The pediatrician and parental discipline, Pediatrics 66:641, 1980.
6. Christophersen ER: Incorporating behavioral pediatrics into primary care, Pediatr Clin North Am 29:261, 1982.
7. Drabman RS and Jarvie G: Counseling parents of children with behavior problems: the use of extinction and time-out techniques, Pediatrics 51:78, 1977.
8. Ginott HG: Between parent and child, New York, 1965, Macmillan, Inc.
9. Haran J and Friedman SB: Managing emotional problems of children and adolescents, Pediatr Ann 9:24, 1980.
10. Madsen C Jr and Stephens J: Behavioral discipline. In Dorr D, Zax M, and Bonner J III, editors: The psychology of discipline, New York, 1983, International Universities Press, Inc.
11. McIntosh BJ: Spoiled child syndrome, Pediatrics 83:114, 1989.
12. Orgel A: Haim Girott's approach to discipline. In Dorr D, Zax M, and Bonner J III, editors: The psychology of discipline, New York, 1983, International Universities Press, Inc.
13. Salk L: How to deal with temper tantrums, Bottom Line, p. 13, Nov 30, 1986.
14. Samalyn N and Tablow MM: Loving your child is not enough: positive discipline that works, New York, 1988, Viking Penguin, Inc.
15. Waters V: The rational-emotive point of view of discipline. In Dorr D, Zax M and Bonner J III, editors: The psychology of discipline, New York, 1983, International Universities Press, Inc.

57

Sexual Abuse of Children

Alvin Rosenfeld and Richard M. Sarles

In the late 1960s, child abuse laws in many states were broadened to include sexual abuse. Since that time, child protection agencies have been perplexed and disturbed by the increasing numbers of cases reported to them. Children referred to these agencies represent all ages from infancy through adolescence. The sexual activities reported include rape, molestation, and confrontation by an exhibitionist. Those children involved in prostitution and pornography may not come to the attention of these agencies.

Because the inappropriate sexual activities between children and adults are so varied, Brant and Tisza[2] coined the term *sexual misuse* as a more accurate description of the spectrum. They defined it as "exposure of a child within a given social-cultural context to sexual stimulation inappropriate for the child's age and level of development." This term seems more useful from a psychological perspective, inasmuch as it includes not only overt acts but also sexual seductiveness by an adult. Such covert sexual inappropriateness causes symptoms in the child, such as enuresis or nightmares, even though there is no actual physical contact between adult and child.

Because a rapist forces a woman or a man or boy or girl to have sex, rape should be considered physical rather than sexual abuse. In contrast to the violence experienced by raped children, most prepubertal children having sexual contact with adults are involved in genital activities that can be termed *immature gratification;* these behaviors consist of looking, touching, feeling, or kissing and do not involve intercourse.

Child abuse statutes have conceptualized *sexual abuse* as sharing traits of both physical abuse and rape. Sexual relationships between adults and children are seen as interactions between victims and perpetrators, with the adult forcing his or her will on a person too young to have the ability to give informed consent. Like the rape victim, the child is thought of as being forced into sexual activities either by physical force or through irresistible deception and manipulation by the adult.

This definition is accurate for all rape cases and many molestations and is necessary in a legal context in which culpability must rest with the adult. In a psychological sense, however, the victim-perpetrator model inaccurately portrays an important subgroup of sexual abuse cases—those cases in which the child has in some psychological way participated, however ambivalently, in the activity. This subgroup is important because it may be the one in which the greatest psychiatric morbidity is found.

Professionals have been debating for years whether some children who are sexually involved with adults desire or participate in the activity. Some have argued that every molested child is the innocent victim of a troubled and deranged adult. Others consider this conceptualization naive because some molested children are deprived and seem to desire contact that turns out to include sexual activity. In the past, some authors[9] even suggested that molested children had some inborn defect that made them more desirous of early sexual contact. Others[10,11] have also contended that those children who seek out or do not object strongly to sexual contact do so to obtain emotional nurturance because their home environment is otherwise depriving. Although there probably is some truth in each position, it remains difficult to assess whether and to what extent a child participated in a sexual activity with an adult, particularly since a child can never give informed consent.

ACCIDENTAL AND PARTICIPANT VICTIMS OF SEXUAL ABUSE

Weiss et al.[16] delineated two types of sexual involvement between adults and children—*accidental* and *participant*. In the accidental involvement, children were the unwary victims of a truly abusive situation, whereas in the participant involvement, children seemed to be active participants in or initiators of a relationship with an adult. Although participant victims were far more common in the sample cited by Weiss et al., subsequent survey research in which larger, unselected populations were studied suggests that this may have been a result of the types of cases reported. Thus participant victims come to the attention of authorities more commonly, whereas accidental cases, which appear to be far more frequent, do not usually come to professional attention.

Accidental Victims

Accidental victims usually are approached by an exhibitionist or fondled by a stranger on a single occasion. Because these children trust their parents and realize that they are available as protective adults, accidental victims usually tell a parent relatively soon after the molestation. If the parents are psychologically capable of supporting the child, they will discuss the event with the child and provide reassurance. When the child has not been physically injured, long-term psychological sequelae seem unlikely.

Portions of this chapter were modified from Rosenfeld AA: Sexual abuse of children: personal and professional responses. In Newberger E, editor: Child abuse, Boston, 1982, Little, Brown & Co.

Participant Victims

Participant victims often are involved over long periods with a person they know well. There are several possible reasons why the parent rarely is informed of the relationship. In some cases the child has learned that the parent does not wish to know and, if informed, will accuse the child of fabrication. In other cases the child has become aware that the parent's ability to be protective is impaired. This may result from a lack of parental commitment and concern about the child, debilitating parental depression, preoccupation with personal matters, or abnormal patterns of child rearing. Clinical experience suggests that in a large proportion of cases, the parent's impaired ability is associated (in an as yet unclear way) with the same-sex parent having had a similar sexual experience in the formative years, often when that parent was the same age as the child is at present. Research studies[5] support clinical impressions in that both sexually and physically abusive parents are significantly more likely than the control subjects to have been sexually abused as children.

Participant victims can be divided into two major subgroups—victims of incest and victims of molestation. In some families a child actually is raped by a parent or a person who stands in the psychological position of parent. Like other cases of actual rape, these should be considered acts of physical abuse and should be handled accordingly. In most cases of incest, however, either the charge is not rape or the accusation that a rape took place is contrary to the term's usual definitions, inasmuch as the rape turns out to be a relationship that has lasted for years, and these children seem to have been to one degree or another participants in the relationship.

Participant Victims of Incest

Incest refers to sexual relationships between persons too closely related to marry. These relationships can mean an overt action by one partner with a sexual intent ranging from physical fondling to genital contact or intercourse. This definition of incest is broadened in many localities to include adopted children and stepchildren. Although this definition technically includes prepubertal sex play between siblings, clear-cut evidence of exploitative, victimizing sexual intent is lacking, and curiosity generally appears to be the motivating factor in the preadolescent age-group.

Incest is one of the few universal taboos found in almost every culture, yet its occurrence is amply recorded throughout history. Although the exact incidence of incest is not known and may never be known, estimates range from one case per million to 5000 cases per million population. Professionals interested in the area of sexual abuse and incest generally agree that accurate statistics are difficult to obtain and that available figures reflect gross underreporting. Some professionals believe that the true incidence of cases of incest must be at least 10 times higher than available figures show. This conjecture is supported by some studies indicating that only 10% to 30% of incest cases are ever reported. The underreporting of incest is thought to be influenced by professionals' lack of awareness of the magnitude of sexual abuse and incest, their own denial that such behavior could and does occur, and their reluctance to become involved in such a difficult and uncomfortable psychosocial issue. Reporting also is influenced by the abusing family's and the abused individual's need to keep incest a secret because of the strong sociocultural prohibition against such behavior. It is of interest, however, that in certain rural areas of the United States, incestuous behavior is not looked on with great disdain.

Father-daughter incest, including stepfather-stepdaughter incest, constitutes approximately 80% of all reported cases. There are indications that brother-sister incest is far more common but does not come to the attention of the authorities. Prepubertal sex play among siblings should not be considered incestuous. When there is an appreciable age difference between the siblings (e.g., a teenage brother and his prepubertal sister) and when there is clear exploitation and victimization, the label of incest is correct. Mother-son incest is uncommon. Little is known concerning other unusual types of incestuous behaviors, which include multiple family member groupings and father-son and mother-daughter incestuous relationships.

A striking feature of many incestuous relationships is that their existence often is common knowledge to most family members. Such a relationship may continue for several years and may even be passed in succession from oldest to youngest daughter. Children who participate in incest over long periods come from grossly dysfunctional families. Although this is immediately obvious in some cases, it may take several interviews to appreciate in others. Many scholars now think of actual incest as a symptom of defective family functioning. Generational boundaries that once supported distinct social and psychological roles for parents and children have been obliterated. Thus, in father-daughter incest, the mother often has abrogated the duties appropriate to her traditional role (cooking, cleaning, and rearing the younger children) to one daughter. Both parents often have experienced multiple losses, both actual and psychological, early in life. The marriage often is strife torn; the father and mother are sexually estranged. In some cases of father-daughter incest, the fathers believe that adultery is more reprehensible than incest. In addition, whereas adultery threatens to break up the family, incest may serve a tension-reducing function that keeps the family intact. To quote Lustig and co-workers,[8] "The family members appear uniformly frightened of family dissolution, and the function of incest to the family unit as a whole appears to be its preservation as an ongoing system."

Many incest cases, particularly those that last for years, must be viewed as a relationship among at least three people: the two participants and the nonparticipating parent (usually the mother), who often denies any knowledge of the incest and who may even act as the martyred victim. Even when the nonparticipating mother is fully aware of the relationship, she may ignore it because she fears losing her husband's income through incarceration more than she fears the social disapproval of incest. On occasion, the mother is relieved to be freed of her coital "chores."

In most cases the child becomes aware that the nonparticipating parent will not serve as a protective adult. Therefore the adult participant often can easily intimidate the child into silence. In other cases, however, the child does not see the relationship as entirely bad. In a setting of emotional deprivation the incestuous relationship may provide the child with a sense of attention and warmth, albeit in a highly inappropriate and anxiety-arousing fashion. The positive aspects of some children's experience in participant relationships and their sense of responsibility for the involvement make them reluctant to report the relationships even in the absence of threats. Although incest is a sexual activity, its psychological meaning usually is more elementary, embodying a search for the safety, comfort, and nurturance of a good protective parent that neither parents nor children ever had. In this way, sexuality is used as a substitute for nonsexual closeness, and pleasure is found in spending intimate time together.

Participant Victims of Molestation

Some children who are molested by someone other than an immediate relative may in some way participate in the activity. Anecdotal reports and clinical experiences[12] suggest that these children often have a same-sex parent who was misused in an almost identical fashion at the same age. In these families parents often disagree significantly, particularly over sexual matters. Furthermore, the children are in some way included in, or privy to, the parental sexual discord. In some cases the disagreement may be manifested in arguments between the parents about proper ways to educate children about sexuality. A child may get two incompatible messages about appropriate sexual behavior and, because of anxiety and internal discomfort, externalize the conflict by acting out the parental disagreement. In other families the children frequently witness parental squabbling about whether one or another sexual activity will be performed. Whether through overstimulation, seduction, or excessive warnings about the evils of sexuality, both parents may inadvertently focus the young child's attention on sexuality and foster an excessive curiosity, confusion, or excitement that culminates in inappropriate sexual activity.

PROSTITUTION AND PORNOGRAPHY

Female Prostitution

Teenage female prostitution is common and flourishing, although an accurate estimate of the number of adolescents engaged in prostitution is unavailable. The difficulty in obtaining accurate statistics is caused partially by the fact that prostitution provides these girls with a means of survival and by the fear of violent retribution from the pimp if the girls seek help. In addition, it appears that the psychopathology of these girls compels them to pursue repeated degradation and exploitation with little personal conflict and thus little desire to seek help.

Most adolescent prostitutes are runaways. Their use of alcohol and street drugs and a family history of conflict, marital discord, divorce, alcoholism, and physical or sexual abuse are common. Increasingly, they run the risk of acquiring the human immunodeficiency virus (HIV). There are indications that up to 75% of these prostitutes have experienced incestuous relationships or have been sexually abused as children or adolescents. Although these girls characteristically do not demonstrate psychotic thinking, they usually suffer from a poor self-image, low self-esteem, and lack of intimate relationships with family members or boyfriends. They probably quit school out of boredom, believing education has no relevance to their future, and they are unable or unwilling to hold "legitimate" employment because of its lack of glamor or insufficient financial remuneration. They often express no desire to have children or a family of their own.

Many adolescent female prostitutes continue as adult prostitutes, some graduate to become sophisticated call girls, and some reform and enter legitimate occupations or marry. The long-term sequelae and outcome of teenage prostitution, however, are unknown and unclear.

Male Prostitution

Male adolescent prostitution is less well publicized, less easily recognized than its female counterpart, seldom prosecuted by legal authorities, and generally not acknowledged to be as significant a problem by public or professional groups. Adolescent male prostitution, however, thrives as a major industry in every large city in the world. There are indications that in the adolescent age-group, male prostitution may equal or exceed female prostitution in magnitude.

These boys share several common characteristics with their female counterparts. They often come from emotionally impoverished families in which divorce, marital strife, alcoholism, and physical or sexual abuse are common. In contrast to the female prostitute's pimp, men who befriend some of these boys generally are not interested in force, violence, or rape. These adults often feed and clothe the boys, take them to sporting events, and allow the boys to live with them in a protective fashion. The boys not only provide sexual favors for their benefactor but also engage in prostitution in the community. Being a "kept" boy is highly desired by many male prostitutes. This relatively stable commitment is seen by the boys as a sign of being desirable, loved, and accepted.

Street hustlers, in contrast, represent the most common form of male prostitution and are lowest in the social hierarchy of this subculture. They generally are self-employed entrepreneurs who rely on a large volume of customers. These boys may live at home and commute to the city or reside with a group of boys who also are prostitutes.

The majority of male prostitutes do not regard themselves as homosexuals, and only a small percent enter the gay community as they grow older. Most male prostitutes view their prostitution purely as an economic venture that enables them to make easy money while retaining their male pride in being capable of succeeding in the world.

As with its female counterpart, the long-term consequences of adolescent male prostitution are unknown. It does appear, however, that the career of male prostitutes is shorter than that of females, inasmuch as it is limited to late adolescence and early adulthood because their boyish adolescent physique, appearance, and mannerisms, which are highly desired by their customers, then mature into adult male physical characteristics. What effect the acquired immunodeficiency syndrome (AIDS) epidemic will have on male prostitution remains to be seen.

Pornography

Child and adolescent pornography represents a multimillion dollar international business. Adult bookstores in all large cities display numerous publications dedicated to child pornography, and ample selections of movie films and videotapes are available. Types of sexual behavior illustrated in the pornographic material encompass every form and permutation of sexuality known. A more subtle form of pornography results from the current trend of commercial filmmakers to exploit children and pubescent adolescents in films such as *Pretty Baby* or in advertisements that show young children in erotic poses.

It is not uncommon for a young male or female prostitute also to engage in pornography, and it is suspected that most of the children and adolescents who are used in the pornographic industry are sexually abused.

Unfortunately, there is virtually no literature available as to the psychiatric consequences for those children and adolescents who are involved in the pornographic subculture; therefore the effects of participation in child and adolescent pornography are presently unknown. Because of the close association of pornography with sexual abuse and prostitution, what is known about these children is similar to the family backgrounds, personality patterns, and the exploitative history of children involved in sexual abuse, incest, and prostitution. The effects may be similar to those associated with other forms of sexual abuse and exploitation. However, only careful scientific, sociologic, and psychiatric study will help to clarify this belief.

SIGNS AND SYMPTOMS OF SEXUAL MISUSE

When an adult brings a child to the emergency room because the child has been molested, the technical approach is straightforward, unless the physician or other emergency room personnel do not believe the adult or the child. However, most cases of sexual abuse or incest are harder to identify. In these the adult brings a child complaining of a common childhood illness or difficulty; abuse is detected only because something arouses the physician's suspicion. The signs and symptoms of these types of cases can be divided into four categories: genital complaints, common behavioral and psychosomatic childhood problems, alterations in behavior, and acting-out behavior.

Genital Complaints

Genital injuries, irritations, or discharges may indicate abuse. Nonetheless, even if the symptoms are glaring, some physicians dismiss these cases as being "of unknown cause." The genital abrasion or inflammation may be treated topically.

However, no physician can overlook venereal disease in a child. The incidence of gonorrhea in children aged 1 to 9 years is increasing. Venereal disease in children must be seen as evidence of sexual abuse unless proved otherwise. Although some cases in the literature have been ascribed to transmission by fomites, this unlikely origin should be considered last rather than first in a differential diagnosis.

Any sexually transmitted disease that is detected in prepubertal children, especially gonococcal infection, mandates a thorough investigation of the possibility of sexual misuse. Nonvenereal urethritis and nonvenereal vaginitis may indicate urethral trauma or irritation as a result of excessive penile manipulation, urethral instrumentation, vulval manipulation, or vaginal penetration.

Physicians should be alert to the possibility of sexual misuse when a pregnant teenager refuses to divulge, or claims ignorance of, the identity of the father of her child. Pregnancy in the pubertal adolescent also should raise the question of incest.

On occasion, children and adolescents who have been involved in incestuous relationships may turn to a trusted friend or adult to question if overt sexual behavior is normal between parent and child or even openly declare that incestuous behavior has occurred or is occurring. Such accusations must always be taken seriously and investigated. Although the question of children falsifying reports of incest has been raised, there has been little indication that such accusations are any more likely to be falsified than the reporting of any type of emotionally charged event.

Although children do not usually fabricate molestation, some authorities believe that very young children, because their language and cognitive abilities are limited, may accuse the wrong person of the molestation, perhaps a father instead of the adult male who actually is guilty. Only a few cases of this sort have been reported. We do not know of cases in which children older than 9 or 10 years have made these mistakes.

In some recent cases of contested custody, a mother has accused the father of molestation, hoping that she will generate enough alarm to convince a judge to terminate the father's visitation rights. In some of these cases there may be truth to the accusation. According to anecdotal reports, however, in others there has been no clear-cut evidence that any molestation has occurred.

Children who have been sexually misused may dress or act in a provocative, sexual fashion. For example, one girl consistently tried to stroke the neck or inner thigh of any man with whom she had to interact, such as her teacher and physician. Another girl exhibited precocious sexual behavior by dressing in a pseudomature seductive manner, by making constant sexual comments to her peers, and by asking intimate sexual questions of her neighbors and teachers.

Professionals should be alerted if a parent consistently requests a thorough examination of a child's genitalia and especially if a history is elicited of repeated examination of the child's genitalia by one or both parents at home.

Childhood masturbation is normal, not pathologic. Spitz[14] found that almost all very young children reared in good family homes but only a tiny percent of children raised in an institution could be observed playing with their genitalia. He considered such genital play a sign of good mothering and a precursor of good interpersonal relationships in the future. Compulsive constant (as opposed to usual childhood) masturbation, however, may indicate sexual abuse of a child, although it also may indicate a central nervous system disease or an attempt by a neglected child to obtain some needed stimulation.

Common Behavioral and Psychosomatic Childhood Problems

Most cases of sexual abuse that come to medical attention first appear during treatment of other problems. The parents may complain that the child is "antisocial"; has problems making friends; is a poor student; is hyperactive; or has asthma, anorexia nervosa, bulimia, enuresis, or encopresis. The list of possibilities is endless.

However, pediatricians sometimes encounter somatic symptoms for which no organic cause can be found. A child may have recurrent abdominal pain or an anal or genital itch. Although children frequently have psychomatic complaints for many reasons, in some cases the physical symptom is an attempt to communicate that a sexual abuse has occurred. Hysterical seizures frequently are caused by sexual abuse, as are other somatizations. Only careful attention to what the child does and says enables the pediatrician to separate those symptoms that reflect abuse from those that arise from other conflictive situations.

Obviously, most complaints of childhood physical and behavioral problems do not involve sexual abuse. The challenge is to recognize those cases that do, without suspecting everyone. The task is not easy, but the physician who is open to the possibility and asks a question or two that might uncover molestation will create an atmosphere in which an accurate diagnosis of sexual abuse is possible.[13]

Recent Alterations in Behavior

Abrupt changes in behavior may be a child's response to molestation. The symptoms may express feelings that the child cannot put into words. Any sudden appearance of symptoms mentioned in the preceding section on childhood problems may be the traumatic effect of molestation and of the child's fear or inability to talk about it. Some examples are the child who abruptly develops a school phobia or whose grades precipitously decline; an open, warm child who suddenly becomes extremely shy, withdrawn, or afraid of going outside; a previously pleasant child who suddenly turns acutely hostile and nasty; a well-behaved child who begins to steal; or a child who starts to develop persistent stomachaches or conversion reactions.[13] Obviously, sexual abuse accounts for only a fraction of all such cases; however, if the physician sets the child at ease and includes sexual abuse in the differential diagnosis by asking questions, such as whether the child has been touched in a sexual manner, an accurate diagnosis of sexual abuse is more likely to be made.

Acting-Out Behaviors

Children and adults occasionally act out because they cannot tolerate the intense pain, anger, or sadness they feel. Sometimes desperation may never be expressed, but the person will begin frantic activity to hide from these feelings. One common mode of acting out is through sexuality.

Childhood promiscuity, teenage pregnancy, running away, drug abuse, and suicide attempts, as well as fears of any sexual activity, have all been associated with sexual abuse in the home. Studies[4] in psychiatric hospitals, juvenile detention homes, and programs for substance abusers and teenage prostitutes have indicated that girls who act out often have been molested in their homes. Therefore any pediatrician who is a consultant for a facility concerned with children and adolescents who have been in serious legal or social difficulty should include in the differential diagnosis questions about the possibility of molestation. However, the pediatrician should not limit his or her thinking to simple cause-and-effect relationships, because the families of acting-out adolescents may be generally chaotic and depriving. These parents maltreat their children in many ways besides sexual maltreatment.

MANAGEMENT

Inasmuch as sexual misuse encompasses so many different behaviors, it has no typical presentation. Parents may try to hide this misuse out of a sense of shame or because of allegiance to another family member. In these cases only a careful history and a willingness to ask about and hear about sexual involvements of a child will lead to a more complete understanding of the situation.

Cases of sexual misuse arouse a multiplicity of strong feelings, ranging from outrage to curiosity over the details of the events. Because these feelings are uncomfortable, a physician can begin to act in ill-chosen ways. For instance, a pediatrician may overlook ongoing misuse to avoid facing unpleasant realities. In this situation, repeated vaginal rashes in a 6-year-old girl may be described as "nonspecific" with the cause "unknown." In other cases, when a clear-cut case of long-term participant misuse is seen, the physician might begin to cry rape and to act in an alarmed, outraged fashion. Thus a careful assessment may not be made because of the physician's intense moral indignation. A conscientious staff often has a personal, naturally protective attitude toward children and can find it difficult to accept that a child might have participated in and perhaps enjoyed the attention and even the sexual excitement that went along with the sexual misuse. Sometimes, out of anxiety, the pediatrician or physician may quickly pass the case on to a psychiatrist, psychologist, or social worker before completing a careful assessment.

The proper approach in all cases of sexual misuse is to remain calm and thoughtful. All family members should be interviewed; each should have an opportunity to see the evaluator separately. An interrogatory style of interviewing usually alienates the family and creates resistance to professional intervention. Although the physician has to ascertain the realities, the families often are reluctant to provide information because they are suspicious, frightened, or embarrassed, a situation exacerbated by the physician's mandatory obligation to report the case. Although the physician must inform the family of this obligation, he or she also should let them know that his or her goal is to assist the family.

This stance maximizes the chance that the physician will receive the information needed to help in the child's medical care. Having proceeded in this fashion, the physician also can complete the medical record and gather the necessary evidence without feeling that he or she has tricked or entrapped the family into confessing. The physician may be surprised to find that some families are relieved that the secret is revealed and hope that help will be forthcoming. It also helps if the physician has a sober attitude and conveys the impression that, like all human predicaments, this one is manageable.

It is important to discover whether the child is an accidental or participant victim, because reassuring the parents of accidental victims who did not suffer physical trauma usually will enable the parents to support the child and thus avoid long-term ill effects. Clues to the accidental or participant involvement of the child are provided by answers to the following questions: (1) Was the relationship prolonged? (2) Has the child been involved with more than one adult? (3) Did the child accept gifts or remuneration? (4) Did the child know the adult? (5) Did the child immediately tell the parent of the event? Of course, these distinctions are not absolute or easy to make. In one recent case a 15-year-old girl was hospitalized because of severe conversion symptoms and a repeatedly expressed wish that she were dead. After some time in the hospital, she confided to a female nurse that her symptoms began when her brother's friend raped her. Although she knew that her parents would have been protective and supportive, she had been too frightened to tell them because she feared that her father would kill her brother's friend.

Accidental Victims

Although supportive parents can ameliorate the effects of molestation, not all parents have that capacity. Lewis and Sarrell[7] emphasize that in accidental cases, if parents overreact or try to deal with their guilt feelings by vociferous attempts to punish or attack the offending adult, "the child observes the reaction of rage in the parents and develops a revulsion against all future sexual feelings and experience."

The physician should try to help the parents be more supportive in their reaction by being supportive of them. If the parents appear to have insufficient personal resources to deal with the situation, they should be referred for more intensive counseling.

In our experience, despite parents' natural worry that they had failed in the task of protecting their child from harm, most parents in this type of case have reared their child well, as their ability to support and protect the child through this crisis demonstrates. Because life unfortunately can be dangerous, no parent can protect a child from everything; to try to do so would be smothering and stifling.

Parents of an accidental victim who come to an emergency room and are able to support their child psychologically help prevent long-term psychological sequelae. Because the emergency room physician comes into contact with the family at a critical juncture, he or she also can play an important role. The parents are worried that their child has been damaged, and they are concerned that they have failed. Their feelings are natural. By listening carefully to the parents' words and to the concerns that those words reflect, the physician can tailor comments directly to the parents' concerns and fears.

Many parents of accidental victims need more than straightforward and respectful treatment; they need reassurance that their child is not permanently harmed and that they need not build moats around him or her in the future. By strengthening the parents (on whom the child has always been able to depend for solace), the physician can minimize any damaging effects of the accidental molestation.

If the accidental victim has been physically forced, as in rape, or hurt, as in intercourse with a 4-year-old, he or she will be troubled. A serious strain has been placed on the child's personality because a sexual encounter has been fused with fear and pain. The emergency room physician or a team member should follow the child's case over the next several months. In some hospitals these cases are referred to a crisis intervention team. In all cases of this sort we believe that the parents should be offered the opportunity to have a child psychiatric assessment made if their child becomes phobic or counterphobic or shows any other symptoms after the first few weeks.

Participant Victims

The participant victim cases present different problems. Physicians often are perplexed about why a case has come to professional attention after so many years of misuse. Sometimes the reason has to do with biologic or psychological changes in the child. As the child becomes pubertal, he or she sees the relationship in the context of the intense sexual stirrings of that age. This new, sexual perception of the relationship may lead the adolescent to demand that the molestation end. In other cases the adolescent becomes aware of the social condemnation of incest, feels ashamed, and stops the relationship. An adolescent who is striving to form a sexual relationship with a peer may call in the authorities because an incestuous sexual relationship stands in the way. In still other cases the relationship may be reported by the child as a way of punishing a parent for some other matter totally unrelated to the sexual relationship.

Participant victims differ from accidental ones in several regards. The adult is not a stranger; he or she often is a person with whom the child is amicable—a parent, a relative, a neighbor, a friend, or an authority figure. The sexual relationship lasts for months or years. One woman we treated was involved with her biologic father for 18 years. The notion of trauma caused by shock and pain does not fit such a situation because the situation could never persist for so long if the molestation were so overwhelming an experience that the person could not adapt in some way. The child would have shown symptoms or told someone much sooner.

After the initial evaluation in a participant case, the physician should seek consultation from or referral to those professionals interested in behavioral issues of childhood and adolescence such as child psychiatrists, child psychologists, behavioral pediatricians, and social workers. The consultant is expected to perform a thorough psychosocial evaluation of the family and the involved child and to recommend an appropriate treatment plan. Treatment often is difficult in cases of participant incest. Removal of the parent or the child from the home provides only temporary relief, and incarceration of the parent offers little hope for rehabilitation and may deprive the family of financial support. Group or individual psychotherapy for the child can help reduce feelings of intense rage, anger, guilt, and shame and help to refocus his or her sexual behavior toward more appropriate partners outside the home. Direct supportive counseling for the nonparticipating parent often has a powerful effect in restructuring the family because it helps that parent set appropriate limits and boundaries for himself or herself, the participating parent, and the child. In other cases more drastic interventions, including placing the child in a foster home or residential treatment setting, are necessary.

In many states, sexual misuse cases are grouped with child abuse cases in legislation that mandates protective services for children. Therefore pediatricians should be familiar with the laws and mandatory reporting requirements in their states. When the offender is not a parent, the physician or consultant may be expected to assess and report whether the adult represents a threat to other young children, thus providing information the agency or court needs when deciding what action is necessary. In cases of incest the evaluator should determine whether therapeutic intervention promises to improve the situation enough to make incarceration of the offender unnecessary.

Prosecution is invariably upsetting to children, although some localities try to reduce the stress by having the child testify in the judge's chambers rather than in an open courtroom. Forty percent of all cases are dismissed outright.[4] During prosecuted cases, children often are required to tell their story over and over again and may be subjected to strenuous cross-examination. Therefore, if prosecution is planned, the child must be prepared for and supported through this trying experience.[3]

Practical Issues

It was stated earlier that cases of sexual misuse can arouse strong and uncomfortable feelings in the physician. However, these feelings must not distract the practitioner from helping the child. The physician also should avoid adopting a condescending manner in speaking with the child. A child's ability to understand complex terms is limited, but he or she is an intelligent human and, like everyone else, should be treated respectfully.

Rather than using technical medical terminology, the physician should use words with which the child is familiar. He or she can ask the parent what words the child uses for body parts. These words, such as *tush, bottom, poo-pee* and *pee-pee,* may not be formal English terminology, but they are familiar and descriptive, and children (as well as most adults) know what they mean. Other children have been brought up to use accurate anatomic terms; with these children, *penis* and *vagina* are the right words to use.

Before adolescence, children think concretely and literally. For instance, a 5-year-old who is told that babies start as eggs that grow inside the mother may want to listen to her stomach. Why? To hear the chicken clucking. Or the child may ask the mother not to eat so that food is not splattered on the baby's head. Therefore the physician should choose words carefully. He or she should not be abstract or rely on a child's understanding of nuance to be correctly understood. Young children do not understand nuances.

Black[1] gives a marvelous illustration. No one could understand why a young boy said that, when people die, their feet are cut off and sent to heaven. Finally, he told someone that he had heard the fact on the radio. What *exactly* did the radio say, he was asked. He answered that when people die, their souls go to heaven. He understood *soul* as *sole,* the underside of the foot; hence his idea. The use of simple terms is best. Many children are too embarrassed to admit that they do not understand a word. If the physician thinks that a child is trying to cover up ignorance, he or she can explain the meaning a second time; then, if still uncertain whether the child understood, the physician can rephrase what was said.

A child who must be examined should be prepared for it. If it is possible, invite a familiar adult whom the child likes into the examining room. The examination should be performed in a sensitive manner with consideration given to the child's fear, weakness, and insecurity.

One way to conceptualize a sensitive examination is to imagine giving the child the same respect the physician would give to a valued senior colleague on whom he or she had to perform a gynecologic examination. Genital examinations should be performed in privacy with the drapes shut. The nurse, chaperone, or physician should give the child a sheet with which to cover himself or herself. The child should be told in simple language what will be done. Children sometimes are calmed when they can examine the instruments; they usually are calmed when their questions are answered forthrightly.

Medical Issues

The medical issues that the physician should watch for in both participant and accident cases are (1) risk of pregnancy; (2) risk of venereal disease; (3) physical trauma, especially in children who were raped; and (4) psychological trauma.

Pregnancy. Tilelli and colleagues[15] believe that the risk of pregnancy is low in both participant and accidental cases. Because difficulties have been reported with the use of diethylstilbestrol, they recommend that it be used only when there is a clearly documented ovulatory cycle and ejaculation during a rape has occurred in the middle of a woman's menstrual cycle. Because of possible effects on victim and fetus, informed consent should be obtained before this drug is used.

Venereal Disease. Although experts differ in their estimates of how frequently abused children contract gonorrhea, antibiotics obviously are indicated if serial cultures and serologic data indicate infection.

Physical Trauma. In their study Tilelli and associates[15] reported a significant incidence of physical trauma, with cases ranging from mild to severe. If present, this trauma should be noted with accurate detail in the medical record and treated appropriately.

Psychological Sequelae. The major cause of symptoms among sexually abused children is psychological trauma. Because its management varies with the type of case, the physician should try to determine whether a case of molestation is accidental or participant. The presence of guilt does not help separate the two types of molestation because, when psychological trauma is apparent, most parents *express* guilt about their failure to prevent the abuse.

Intervention for the Adult

As stated earlier, in the absence of gross physical trauma, if the physician provides a supportive, empathic environment for the parents of accidental victims, they will be able to protect their child as always. Some professionals believe that older adolescents who have been abused sexually are helped by peer counselors or support groups outside the family.

In participant molestations and incest cases, a thorough psychiatric evaluation of the adult is imperative. Psychiatric treatment not only of the victim but also of the whole family may be necessary. The details of that evaluation, however, are a subject for psychiatric literature, as is the debate over whether individual or group or family psychotherapy is the treatment of choice. Unfortunately, the tone of those discussions sometimes has not been that of a scholarly debate; all too often it has seemed more suited to a religious war.

Although many physicians are keenly aware of the child's needs and try to provide for them in the emergency room setting, they often overlook the needs of the offending adult. The physician should remember that parents who have been involved in incest may feel enormously guilty. When incest has occurred or has come to light, the participating parent may become psychotic or suicidal. When incest has been detected and reported, the risk of psychosis or suicide increases. Yet because the problem has been revealed, appropriate medical interventions become possible.

SEXUAL MISUSE AND THE LAW

Legal Reports

All suspected cases of sexual misuse, whether participant or accidental, must be reported to the authorities. As stated earlier, it is important for the physician to discuss the process with the family. By the time a case of long-term sexual abuse has come to professional attention, one or more family members may welcome the court's help in enforcing its end. In some localities, reporting can be combined with a mandated treatment program, which is said to benefit the family greatly. However, reliable data to test this assertion have yet to be gathered. We question the validity of some of the supposed measures used in past studies. For instance, it is not clear to us that, after incest has been reported to the police, recidivism is a major problem. Many times the case is reported because one family member has decided to put an end to the incest. Under these circumstances, is a low recidivism rate the result of treatment? Is the reconstitution of an incestuous family equivalent to a good outcome? The children in many incestuous families may be better off if they are raised elsewhere and the families are never reconstituted. Yet the solution to finding new environments for children, other than foster homes that all too often resemble storage bins, is expensive and unlikely.

Physicians should learn exactly what services are available in their communities and support the provision of them to incestuous families; without these services the physician's reporting the case to authorities may increase the suffering of all family members with little ultimate benefit. Recommending these services is especially important if the state's remedy is to incarcerate, castrate, or execute the offending adult, thereby possibly causing the child to withdraw the complaint to avoid seeing the parent punished that severely or to comply with the family's pressure to deny the accusations.

In some cases the family regards the problem as belonging to the child, not the incestuous parent. The following example illustrates this point:

> Louise, an adolescent girl, reported her father to authorities. He had for years fondled her genitalia. Once Louise's menses began, her father stopped fondling her and initiated a relationship with her younger sister. When he gave the younger sister a gift and refused to give Louise the transistor radio she wanted, she reported him to the police. The entire family supported the father and was angry at Louise for being so "selfish."

Evidence

We concur with the method of collection of evidence brought out by Kempe and Helfer[6]:

> If a crime has been committed (that is not for the medical team to determine), the ability of the prosecutor to make a charge and obtain a conviction may depend upon the evidence collected and whether or not it is admissible in court.
>
> A search should be made of the patient's clothing for any material that may be needed as evidence. The clothing may also be considered as evidence. Follow instructions in the "Rape Kit" on the type of evidence to be collected and the method of collecting evidence.
>
> The "Rape Kit" consists of a sealed manila envelope with the necessary material for collecting evidence. The envelope should have the name of the examiner, date, and statement of time the seal was broken. All specimens should be collected, labeled with the initials of the examiner, and placed in the manila envelope. The examiner's name or initials should be retained as part of the evidence. Individual pieces of clothing should be placed in clean paper bags, sealed, and initialed by the examiner. All evidence should be placed in a cardboard box and sealed with tape. The name or initials of the examiner should be written over the seal. The box should be given to the investigating police officer.
>
> The following data should be recorded, lab tests obtained, and treatment initiated, if the pelvic examination is completed:
>
> 1. Record evidence of torn clothing, bruises, blood, or semen stains on body or undergarments, and evidence of vaginal or anal penetration
> 2. Save any garments which are torn or stained, label such with name of patient and date, and give to on-call hospital administrator or the police officer for secure storage in cases of criminal prosecution of alleged rapists
> 3. Depending on history, obtain specimens of vagina, rectum, and pharynx for:
>   a. cultures for gonorrhea (to be obtained by examining physician)
>   b. wet prep to examine for motile sperm (to be performed by examining physician) from vagina and/or rectum
> 4. Obtain a serological test for syphilis (VDRL) and urine for pregnancy test in pubertal females

Prosecution

In almost all cases, whether accidental or participant, prosecution appears to be a difficult experience for children. Some experts believe that the legal process causes more harm than the molestation itself. Legal practice will now sometimes allow a videotape made of the child's statement to replace live testimony in court. Although these tapes would reduce the child's trauma by ending the need for repeated testimony, it remains to be seen whether eliminating the opportunity for cross-examination will be ruled constitutional.

Under current courtroom procedures, some parents elect not to press charges because they fear that the process of prosecution might prove harmful to the child. This attitude is especially prevalent in cases of accidental molestation by a stranger and is difficult to contest. Although some legal authorities assert that the stance of these parents is hazardous because molesters go on to commit even more serious crimes against other children, we know of no scientific study that supports this claim.

Prosecution is clearly indicated when (1) the child wants

to testify against the offending adult, (2) serious violence has accompanied the molestation, and the offender is a clear threat to all children, including the one already victimized, or (3) it appears that treatment promises to be effective only under court order. Whether court-mandated treatment can be effective has been the topic of vigorous debate. We have serious doubts that it does more than ameliorate symptoms or reduce the patient's willingness to report sexual improprieties to the court-sponsored therapist.

SUMMARY

Many physicians choose not to become involved in incest and sexual misuse cases because they are messy, time-consuming, and potentially emotionally draining. It is important that more physicians become alert to the possibility of molestation and use thoughtful, empathic intervention techniques. Because of the power and authority vested in the physician's role, these evaluations should be supervised by a physician. Yet for emotional problems to remain a medical concern, medical schools will have to train physicians more thoroughly. Medical students will have to learn more about and become sensitive to the social and emotional aspects of illness and medical care, as well as become empathic and skilled in interviewing techniques and in psychiatric approaches. Funds to train nonmedical personnel and to treat victims of all forms of abuse and their families also are clearly needed.

Furthermore, if practitioners are ever to be able to make interventions (in sexual misuse cases) that are based on knowledge rather than on blindness, state governments will have to make available funds to sponsor scientific research that is free of the political bias and rhetoric that pervades so much of the current literature in this field.

REFERENCES

1. Black D: Personal communication, 1982.
2. Brant RS and Tisza VB: The sexually misused child, Am J Orthopsychiatry 47:80, 1977.
3. DeFrancis V: Protecting child victims of sex crimes committed by adults (booklet), Denver, 1969, American Human Association of Denver.
4. Emslie G and Rosenfeld A: Incest reported by children and adolescents hospitalized for severe psychiatric problems, Am J Psychiatry 140:708, 1983.
5. Goodwin J, McCarthy T, and Divasto P: Prior incest in mothers of abnormal children, Child Abuse Negl 5:87, 1981.
6. Kempe CH and Helfer RE, editors: Helping the battered child and his family, Philadelphia, 1973, JB Lippincott Co.
7. Lewis M and Sarrell M: Some psychological aspects of seduction, incest and rape in childhood, J Am Acad Child Psychiatry 8:609, 1969.
8. Lustig N et al: Incest, Arch Gen Psychiatry 14:31, 1966.
9. Notman N and Nadelson CC: Psychodynamic and life stage considerations in the response to rape. In McComie S, editor: Rape crisis intervention handbook, New York, 1980, Plenum Publishing Corp.
10. Rosenfeld AA: Endogamic incest and the victim-perpetrator model, Am J Dis Child 133:406, 1979.
11. Rosenfeld AA, Nadelson CC, and Krieger MJ: Fantasy versus reality in patient reports of incest, Am J Clin Psychiatry 40:159, 1979.
12. Rosenfeld AA et al: Incest and sexual abuse of children, J Am Acad Child Psychiatry 16:327, 1977.
13. Shapiro EG and Rosenfeld AA: The somatizing child, New York, 1987, Springer-Verlag, Inc.
14. Spitz R: Autoeroticism re-examined, Psychoanal Study Child 17:283, 1962.
15. Tilelli JA, Turck D, and Jaffe AC: Sexual abuse of children, N Engl J Med 302:319, 1980.
16. Weiss T et al: A study of girl sex victims, Psychiatr Q 29:1, 1955.

SUGGESTED READINGS

Galdston R: Dysfunctions of parenting, the battered child, the exploited child. In Howells JG, editor: Modern perspectives in international child psychiatry, vol 3, New York, 1971, Brunner/Mazel, Inc.

Kempe CH, Silverman FN, and Steele PF: The battered child syndrome, JAMA 181(1):17, 1962.

Mohr J, Turner R, and Jerry N: Pedophilia and exhibitionism, Toronto, 1964, University of Toronto Press.

Rosenfeld AA: Sexual abuse of children, JAMA 240:43, 1978.

Rosenfeld AA: Sexual abuse of children: personal and professional responses. In Newberger E, editor: Child abuse, Boston, 1982, Little, Brown & Co.

Sarles RM: Incest, Pediatr Rev 2:51, 1980.

Sarles RM: Sexual abuse in the adolescent. In Moss AJ, editor: Pediatric update: review for physicians, New York, 1981, Elsevier Science Publishing Co, Inc.

Schetky DH and Green AH: Child sexual abuse: a handbook for health care and legal professionals, New York, 1988, Brunner/Mazel, Inc.

Spitz RA: Autoeroticism: some empirical findings and hypotheses on three of its manifestations in the first year of life. In Eissler RS et al, editors: The psychoanalytic study of the child, vols. 3 and 4, New York, 1945, International Universities Press, Inc.

Wald M: State intervention on behalf of "neglected" children: a search for realistic standards, Stanford Law Rev 27:985, 1975.

Weinberg LK: Incest behavior, Secaucus, NJ, 1955, Citadel Press.

58

Television and the Family

Joyce Sprafkin

The television set in the average American household is on for 7 to 8 hours a day. Most children are exposed to commercial television by the time they are 6 months old and have become purposeful viewers with favorite shows by the time they are 3 years old. Viewing time generally increases during the preschool and elementary school years and reaches an average of almost 4 hours daily during early adolescence. Viewing then levels off in the later teens at 2 to 3 hours a day, which is the amount watched by the typical adult. These estimates do not include time spent viewing VCR tapes.

Thus today's children are getting a far heavier dose of TV entertainment than their grandparents got out of comic books, movies, and phonograph records combined. A fair amount of the shows children see on TV are considered *children's programming* (or *kidvid)* and usually are aired on Saturday and Sunday mornings. However, most of the programs children watch are designed for adult or family audiences.

TELEVISION VIOLENCE

As early as 1954, Senator Estes Kefauver, then Chairman of the Senate Subcommittee on Juvenile Delinquency, questioned the need for violent content in TV entertainment. Network representatives claimed at that time that research on how children were affected by viewing violence was inconclusive, although they admitted that some risk existed. There has been much research in this area in the ensuing years. Through the 1960s individual psychologists investigated the possible effects of TV violence on youth, and most suggested that such content stimulated overt aggressive behavior in some youngsters. By the late 1960s public concern had reached the point where a national investigation was warranted, culminating in the 1972 surgeon general's report on TV violence.[8] Based on more than 60 specially commissioned studies and the collaboration of several hundred scientists, the report tentatively concluded that exposure to TV violence could lead to increased aggression. In 1982 an update of the surgeon general's 1972 report was issued by the National Institute of Mental Health[9]:

> The convergence of findings supports the conclusion of a causal relationship between televised violence and later aggressive behavior. The evidence now is drawn from a large body of literature. Adherents to this convergence approach agree that the conclusions reached in the Surgeon General's program have been significantly strengthened by more recent research.

In a 1986 metaanalysis of 230 studies on the effects of television on behavior, Hearold[5] concluded the following:

1. The effects of TV violence on physical aggression are about the same for girls and boys up until about age 10. Thereafter the effect increases for boys but decreases for girls.
2. Seeing violence that appears justified and realistic has a greater aggression-instigating effect than seeing violence that appears unjustified and/or that brings negative consequences to the aggressor.
3. TV violence can have an effect even when the observer is not aroused, but either frustration or provocation will increase its aggression-producing effects.

In addition to behavioral effects, there is evidence that viewing of TV violence can cultivate antisocial attitudes and persuade viewers to aggressive behavior as an appropriate way of dealing with others. Excessive exposure to violent portrayals can produce a heightened sense of danger in a "mean" world[4] and make children apathetic to aggression in others.

TELEVISION ADVERTISING

There is no doubt that the nation's TV habits make the medium an attractive place to advertise. Because of graphics, camera work, and old-fashioned cleverness, the TV commercial is a potent way of advertising, especially to the credulous young child. In fact, a children's TV commercial is carefully written, designed, and usually musically scored with the help of private research agencies to maximize its impact on young viewers.

Many concerns have been expressed about TV advertising aimed at children, most notably from the parent group Action for Children's Television (ACT). After pressing its case for 10 years, ACT finally succeeded in 1979 in forcing the Federal Trade Commission (FTC) to engage in a full-scale inquiry involving testimony from specialists in developmental psychology and communications, as well as representatives from the advertising, broadcasting, and manufacturing industries. The FTC's final statement follows[3]:

> The record developed during the rulemaking proceeding adequately supports the following conclusions regarding child-oriented television advertising and young children six years and under: (1) they place indiscriminate trust in televised advertising messages; (2) they do not understand the persuasive bias in television advertising; and (3) the techniques, focus and themes used in child-oriented television advertising enhance the appeal of the advertising message and the advertised product. Consequently, young children do not possess the cognitive ability to evaluate adequately child-oriented television advertising. Despite the fact that these conclusions can be drawn from the evidence, the record establishes that the only effective remedy would be a ban on all advertisements oriented toward young children, and such a ban, as a practical matter, cannot be implemented.

Even before the FTC staff report was released, Robert Choate,[1] the child advocate and founder of the Center for Children, Media, and Merchandising, sensed that regulatory action was unlikely and that parents would have to assume the responsibility of protecting their children against the abuses of advertisement manipulation. He warned, "The handwriting on the wall is clear: Parents must help their children to comprehend the totality of the message in the more than 20,000 commercials per year they view." Work in this direction has begun. An active interest has emerged in developing critical viewing skills in children to make them less vulnerable to the persuasive techniques used in TV advertising and potential adverse effects of programming.[10]

TV RACE AND SEX STEREOTYPING

The cultivation of children's attitudes through the stories they are told originated with the earliest fairy tale. Concern now focuses on race and sex stereotyping and the portrayal of sexuality on TV. Research has shown that children's social attitudes and perceptions regarding race and sex are significantly influenced by what they see on television. For example, women and minorities tend to be placed in restricted and relatively powerless roles on TV, and this pattern is repeated in the attitudes of youngsters who view a lot of television.[6]

TV has only recently been accused of being pornographic, and no doubt this is because sexuality was considered taboo by broadcasters until the mid-1970s. Content analyses show that there has been an increasing emphasis on sexual themes over the past decade (causing critics to hiss that the networks responded to the surgeon general's report by trading violence for sex).[6] Research suggests that teenagers understand a fair amount of televised sexual innuendos, but virtually nothing is known about children's reactions to such content, let alone the effects of viewing it. The potential impact of televised portrayals of sexuality, however, is suggested by the results of a recent survey[7] in which adolescents ranked entertainment TV as fourth as a source of sex information (after friends, parents, and courses at school). About 50% believed that TV dealt realistically with such topics as pregnancy, the personal consequences of sex, and the likelihood of contracting a sexually transmitted disease. This is alarming to groups such as Planned Parenthood that point to the virtual absence of discussion of birth control or sexually transmitted diseases on entertainment TV as a source of misinformation for teens.

HARNESSING TELEVISION'S POTENTIAL

Interest in harnessing TV's potential to benefit children and society in general can be traced to the earliest days of the medium. Crude educational television in the 1950s was transformed by the Corporation for Public Broadcasting and other organizations into a network of public television stations that broadcast quality programs for a wide audience, as well as specialized programs for children. *Sesame Street,* an exemplary example of such children's programs, is proved to have some academic and instructional value but probably has its greatest influence on advantaged children, who are the ones most likely to watch it.

Stimulated in part by the goal of harnessing TV's potential more effectively, researchers in the 1970s began to investigate how to use TV as an active force in the socialization of children.[9] Rooted in early laboratory experiments using simulated TV programs (which showed that TV models could increase children's generosity and self-control), researchers looked for instances of prosocial behavior in regular programs and then demonstrated that exposure to shows naturally rich in such examples had discernible effects on child audiences. Of greater significance, perhaps, social scientists and producers collaborated on creating children's TV programming that was to have specific social effects on the attitudes and behavior of the child audience. Moreover, once made, these programs with a social message were tested during production (formative research) and after broadcast (summative research) to ensure that the desired effects were occurring while guarding against possible side effects (e.g., inadvertently triggering a child's aggression or creating an inaccurate stereotype[6]). The results must be considered encouraging. Although it is doubtful that any one program can have a dramative or even lasting effect on many children, it does appear that heavily saturating entertainment TV with models who reflect a consistent set of values could greatly influence children. Whether this is progressive education or a chilling new form of brainwashing and what, if anything, will be done with TV's great potential power over the young have become the great unanswered questions.

Practical Suggestions

Given the enormous significance of television in the lives of children, parents should capitalize on TV's potential and minimize its undesirable effects by the following measures:

1. Restricting overall TV viewing. Excessive amounts of TV viewing may indicate that the child has other problems. For example, many children who are troubled by peer or family conflicts use TV as an escape. There also is evidence that heavy TV use is associated with obesity in children.[2]
2. Forbidding the viewing of programs with excessive violence.[4] Aside from possible behavioral effects, exposure to an aggression-saturated TV diet can adversely impact social attitudes and values.
3. Viewing TV with the child, generating discussions about what is seen in programs and commercials, and taking every opportunity to convey reactions to the content. It is particularly important to point out how the TV portrayals depart from reality. For example, programs often underestimate the consequences of violent action, and commercials often overestimate the attributes of advertised products.

REFERENCES

1. Choate RB: The politics of change. In Palmer EL and Dorr A, editors: Children and the faces of television. Orlando, Fla, 1980, Academic Press, Inc.
2. Dietz W and Gortmaker S: Do we fatten our children at the television set? Obesity and television viewing in children and adolescents, Pediatrics 75:807, 1985.

3. Federal Trade Commission: FTC final staff report and recommendation, Federal Review, No 17967, 1981.
4. Gerbner G et al: Television's mean world: violence profile No 14-15, Philadelphia, 1986, University of Pennsylvania, Annenberg School of Communications.
5. Hearold S: A synthesis of 1043 effects of television on social behavior. In Comstock G, editor: Public communications and behavior, vol 1, New York, 1986, Academic Press, Inc.
6. Liebert RM and Spratkin J: The early window: effects of television on children and youth, Elmsford, NY, 1988, Pergamon Press, Inc.
7. Louis Harris & Associates: American teens speak: sex, myths, TV, and birth control, New York, 1986, Planned Parenthood Federation of America.
8. National Institute of Mental Health: Television and growing up: impact of televised violence, Washington, DC, 1972, US Government Printing Office.
9. National Institute of Mental Health: Television and behavior: ten years of scientific progress and implications for the eighties, Washington, DC, 1982, US Government Printing Office.
10. Singer DG, Singer JL, and Zuckerman DM: Getting the most out of TV, Santa Monica, Calif, 1981, Goodyear Publishing Co, Inc.

59

Overview of School Health

Philip R. Nader, Bill S. Caldwell, and Guy S. Parcel

Almost every school in the nation has some notion of what is included in the term *school health.* Yet many educators and health care providers differ in their ideas of and goals for a school health program. To accomplish such goals, however, agreement first must be reached by all those concerned about a definition of school health.

The health program in a school traditionally was considered to comprise health services (often limited to services provided by nursing and medical staff), health education (often limited to a health instruction curriculum), and health environment (often limited to the physical environment and safety).

More recently the health program has begun to be considered as part of all aspects of the total school program that might influence or be influenced by a child's health. In this sense, then, it includes services not only from health and health-related personnel, such as physicians, nurses, social workers, psychologists, aides, and volunteers, but also from educators and counselors. In this broader definition, all school staff members have a responsibility and a recognized role.

This chapter examines the clinical issues of school readiness, school absenteeism, and school refusal problems faced by the school-aged child and family. Other common problems involving schools include learning and language problems, attention deficit syndromes, and children with chronic handicapping conditions and chronic illnesses such as asthma, diabetes, and seizure disorders. These topics are covered elsewhere in this text. Thus the relationship of primary health care providers to schools is examined here.

SCHOOL READINESS AND THE PRIMARY CARE PROVIDER

Primary care physicians often are the most critical persons concerned with school readiness because they are the first professionals who see a child of preschool age. They have the opportunity not only of securing key data in evaluating readiness but also of identifying problem areas and arranging for remediation long before the child enters school.

Primary care physicians may be called on to perform a physical examination required for school entry. If only a cursory physical examination is performed and nothing more, clinicians are missing an opportunity to have a significant voice in the overall planning for the child.

It has been increasingly clear from studies of preschool examinations by physicians that they overlook a significant number of abnormalities in carrying out such examinations. However, school personnel also can overlook deficiencies. If the school conceives of readiness as a score on a standardized readiness test, and if the primary care provider thinks of readiness only according to physical clearance, then the child with special needs may be lost in those gray areas that have been the concern of neither. On the other hand, a physician's expression of concern for the "entire" child, in school and out, reassures the parent that he or she will be a resource for a variety of school-related problems.

DEFINITION OF READINESS

Readiness is a term used frequently by educators and others who work with young children. One hears of readiness tests, readiness tasks, and readiness skills. These terms imply that children are being examined to determine whether they are ready for something and that their status will be measured against a fixed goal. Usually this goal is entry into school.

The skilled primary care provider conceptualizes school readiness in terms broad enough to include both the exceptional and the typical child and to take into account all the variables that influence school progress. Readiness should not be equated with fixed standards of performance for all children. Many handicapped children never will reach fixed standards, and normal children will vary greatly in their abilities to handle readiness tasks. Thus it is as important to think in terms of whether parents and the school are ready for the child as it is to think of whether the child is ready for school.

Many children are ready for school who do not meet fixed standards, whether these are established by group norms, developmental specialists, or curriculum guides. The physician should be acutely aware of the rate at which a child is developing, the child's level of functioning, the demands that the parents impose, and the expectations held by the local school for beginning pupils. Therefore school readiness should mean the degree of "fit" between the variables that characterize the child and family and those that characterize the school system (Fig. 59-1).

ASSESSMENT OF SCHOOL READINESS

Because most preschool children cannot read and do not engage in most types of abstract thinking, assessment of school

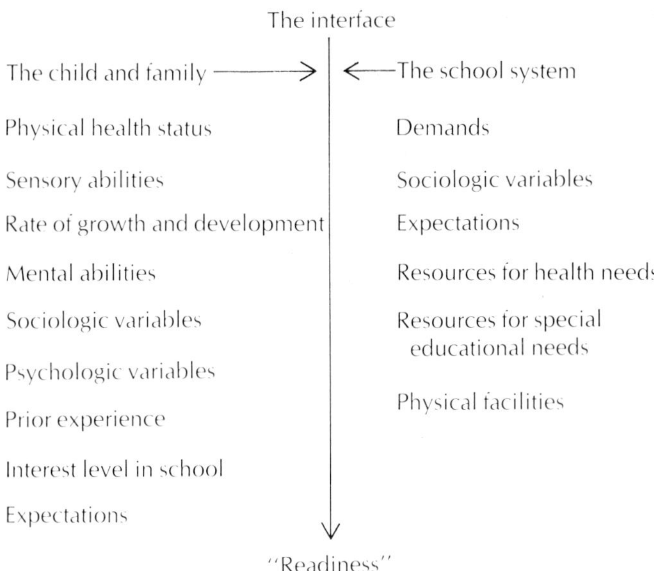

Fig. 59-1 School readiness variables characterizing the child and family and those characterizing the school. These variables must be weighed when assessing whether a given child is ready to begin school. It is equally important to assess whether the school and parents are ready to offer the child the optimal learning situation.

readiness is not merely a matter of determining whether a child can pass a given test. All phases of screening, testing, and evaluating data critically depend on a solid knowledge of how and why children grow and develop. The norms for typical children, which are based on studies conducted over several years, should become as fixed in the physician's memory as certain other bits of knowledge used daily. It is important to distinguish school readiness testing from routine developmental screening. Readiness tests focus on skills the child has already acquired, but they generally give no information on the child's potential to learn or his or her developmental status.

No test, assessment technique, or short-term observation can replace a carefully elicited, closely analyzed history.[2] A test score is a sample of behavior on a given day for certain specified tasks. By contrast, good history adds perspective, time, and breadth in determining school readiness. The history taken in preparation for a discussion with the parents of their child's school readiness should include questions relative to knowledge and skills that are considered important by the schools in the community in which the child lives. If possible, both parents should be involved in their child's evaluation for readiness. The physician may use an established parent questionnaire or may devise one to facilitate the history-taking.

The history should include not only the usual questions concerning developmental stages, illnesses, accidents, and hospitalizations but also questions concerning the child's cognitive development. The physician should attempt to elicit from the parent the way in which the child approaches a problem, how defeat is handled in attempts to learn, whether the child imitates others in solving new situations, whether curiosity is displayed, the extent of exposure to and participation in reading activities, and manifestations of imagination. Many physicians find that a standardized measurement, such as that provided by the Vineland Scale of Adaptive Behavior, is a good framework for gathering information about social development, supplemented by additional questions. Other excellent examples of questionnaires include those developed by Caldwell.[1] Because parental perceptions of a child are critical to the child's progress, it is extremely helpful to have a standardized measure of these perceptions. One of the most useful instruments is the Minnesota Child Development Inventory, which is completed by a parent. Although it is rather lengthy, it can be filled out in a waiting room or it can be completed at home and returned.

As the history is taken, the physician must be alert to inconsistent data and must be exacting in securing information from the parents regarding whether a child can perform a certain task and how the task is performed, the ease with which it is accomplished, and whether this skill is an isolated one or part of a continuing activity. One child may, with much effort, be able to cut with a pair of scissors when asked to do so and given paper and scissors. A second child may pick up a pair of scissors while making something, use the scissors appropriately, and proceed with the job at hand. Parental responses to questions can help the physician distinguish between these two types of children.

In securing a history, it is advisable to ask the parent to describe the child's behavior and accomplishments rather than to ask the parent to evaluate the behavior. It is better to ask, "What happens when Steven is with his friends?" than to ask, "Does Steven get along with other children?" In the latter case, a simple "yes" leaves little room for further discussion. The skillful physician uses many questions that require descriptions of behavior: "Tell me, how does . . .?"; "Describe Mary Lou's afternoons when . . ."; "And then what happens?"; and "What would Jerry do if . . .?"

A useful technique in gathering data about a child and his or her place in the family is to say to the parent, "What words would you use to describe . . .?" Additional information can be obtained by extensions of this question: "And what words would describe his (mental abilities, physical health, relationships with others) . . .?" Information also can be obtained by asking, "Do you think Jimmy is more like you or your wife (husband)?" Follow the response with "Why?" if necessary.

As the physician gains knowledge about the child, he or she also assesses the parents' readiness for their child's entry into school. The physician finds out, by direct questioning if necessary, the parents' expectations for their child, their concepts of the child's school and what it can provide, and the degree to which they believe their child will adjust to and succeed in school in both academic progress and psychosocial adjustment.

When a careful history has been obtained, the physician will have learned about some of the child's personal characteristics, likes and dislikes, and strengths and weaknesses and will be ready to examine the child. The examination includes both a physical examination and readiness (developmental) tests. With many children it is best to carry out the "games" of developmental testing first, leaving the physical examination until last.

It is certainly appropriate for primary care physicians to

Appropriate Abilities at Various Ages

TWO-YEAR-OLDS

Walks downstairs alone, holding rail, both feet on each step
Imitates a vertical line
Identifies self in mirror
Lifts and drinks from cup
Uses "me" and "you" and refers to self by name
Follows simple instructions

THREE-YEAR-OLDS

Chooses the longer of two lines
Can point to teeth and chin on request
Cuts with scissors
Makes three-cube pyramid in approximately 15 seconds
Copies a circle
Jumps with feet together
Identifies six body parts by pointing at pictures

FOUR-YEAR-OLDS

Goes up and down stairs one foot per step
Copies a cross
Washes hands unaided
When shown two circles, can tell "how many"
Completes "A hat goes on your head, shoes on your ________"
Can button
Takes care of self at toilet

FIVE-YEAR-OLDS

Dresses self except tying shoes
Copies a square
Can count six objects when asked, "How many?"
Can correctly answer "What is a chair (dress, shoes) made of?"

SIX-YEAR-OLDS

Tells how crayon and pencil are the same and different
Can tell how many pieces there are if something is cut in half
Can tell the difference between common objects: dog and bird, shirt and coat, milk and water
Can complete "A lemon is sour; sugar is ________"
Can tell what a forest is made of

use developmental tests, provided they understand the tests' weaknesses and restrictions. The best readiness assessment will be carried out by the physician who is most knowledgeable about specific age-appropriate behaviors. A collection of such behaviors taken from the most popular tests for young children includes age-appropriate abilities at 2, 3, 4, 5, and 6 years of age (see accompanying box).

The primary care physician does not need to become a psychologist but does need to know how to administer simple screening tests. If skilled in the use of the Denver Developmental Screening Test, the Draw-a-Person Test, and the drawing of geometric figures exercise, the physician can secure an immense amount of data. Each of these tests should be used in a standardized way and scored by an exact method. It is a waste of time to use such tests unless they are administered correctly and the results used appropriately. Any screening test is simply a sample of behavior. Even without a standardized test, a physician can develop a repertoire of test items that, if used objectively, can give a good estimate of a child's cognitive abilities.

INTERPRETATION OF READINESS

In assessing school readiness, the primary care provider is concerned with a child's physical, mental, and psychosocial characteristics. Data are used from an expanded history, from indications of functional levels shown by developmental and readiness tests, and from data emerging as the result of a thorough physical examination. Such a battery of assessment techniques is time-consuming, but it should be remembered that the child is entering a critical time of his or her life. The degree to which the physician can develop an accurate profile of the "whole child" may determine success or failure in school.

Perhaps the greatest danger in assessing school readiness is a tendency to "overinterpret" findings. Readiness is affected by some physical and mental variables whose characteristics allow us to predict whether they will or will not continue to influence the individual. This is true with certain sensory deficits and certain metabolic and genetic conditions. When a person is assessing cognitive abilities and personality variables, however, only the novice or fool will make definite predictions.

In most instances in describing the child, the physician should include strengths and deficits according to age-related behavior. For example, "Mary has no physical deficits; in most areas she has the knowledge, skills, and emotional behavior of most children her age. However, her ability to handle paper and pencil tasks seems more like that of a 4-year-old." The physician should not be content to make a few checkmarks on a sheet of paper to indicate readiness status. The child should be described to the parents according to the data obtained from the various evaluation procedures, and this description should be compared with the parents' own description and their expectations of the child.

REFERRAL AFTER THE READINESS EVALUATION

If the primary care provider cannot reach a decision relative to a child's physical, mental, and psychosocial status, a consultation or referral should then be considered. Most important, a decision must be made regarding whether the primary care provider should continue the overall management of this child. Information from a consultant may be needed before making this decision. Parents should be told exactly why a consultation or referral is appropriate. If this is not done, misconception of the severity of the problem could be unknowingly implanted, and the parents could react to their child adversely.

When the advice of another professional is being sought, it is helpful if one provides the following information: specific reasons the consultation is requested, exact questions that are to be answered, and how the information obtained will be used. Criteria for referral are not finite and specific. In general, however, a primary care provider should refer for consultation in the following instances:

1. If there are questions regarding the sensory status of the child
2. If examination reveals a physical defect that is unfamiliar or one that requires a special treatment
3. If there is evidence that the child is 25% or more behind in relation to age-appropriate skills and knowledge, that is, if the child's age and corresponding performance level fall into any of the following categories:

Chronologic Age (Yr)	Performance Level
6	4 yr—6 mo or less
5	3 yr—9 mo or less
4	3 yr or less
3	2 yr—3 mo or less

4. If the child has a physical, mental, or emotional handicap that will require the services of a specialist (physical therapist, speech therapist, psychologist, or special educator)

The primary care practitioner provides continuing care for most children. Therefore information obtained from consultations should be integrated with other data so that the parents will receive a comprehensive, understandable explanation of their child's status. It may be necessary to reinterpret what has been told the parents by someone else. This comprehensive explanation is a very important part of school readiness visits to the primary care provider.

By using information concerning the child and knowledge of local school programs and by becoming acquainted with available resources, the primary care provider will determine to a large degree whether the parents understand the concept of readiness and act according to this understanding. A broader concept of school readiness on the primary care provider's part, greater attention to the many areas that determine readiness, and more judicious use of consultants and referral sources will ensure a good start for more children when they enter school.

ROLES AND RESPONSIBILITIES OF THE PHYSICIAN

The previous sections of this chapter and other portions of this text have dealt with specific developmental or clinical problems in relation to the school-aged child. Over and over again, interaction and communication among the health care provider, the school, and those in the home have been emphasized. Intervention is required for these three to interact to benefit the child. The physician or other primary health care provider is the necessary ingredient to catalyze such interactions. The efforts of others also will be required, but without support and action from physicians, it is unlikely that much in the way of cooperative programs between the health and education professions will be achieved.

Physicians potentially have numerous roles and interests in schools—as parents, school board members, community leaders, and providers of care to children. Some also may have formal full- or part-time consulting arrangements with schools for sports or athletic programs and with school districts, nurses, and health educators. As the compulsory education law broadens to include younger and older groups and the severely physically and mentally handicapped, physicians will be mandated by law to assess such persons and to see that such children are placed in school.

Medical training does not routinely equip a physician to consult or work with school personnel, but the physician trained in child health brings deep knowledge of and experience with child development, how to deal with families, and follow-up case management skills that are valuable in the school. These same skills, which equip physicians for a unique role with an individual patient or family, may work against them when they encounter another area, such as the school. Here the physician is not necessarily asked for an opinion, and if one is offered, it is not necessarily accepted. Thus the professional often becomes an educator and persuader rather than a final decision-maker. Teamwork when one is not captain of the team can be difficult for a physician.

Increasing numbers of residencies, fellowships, and medical schools have begun to offer exposure to school health, but most physicians have little prepractice experience in dealing with the school-related problems of children. The interested physician will become equipped by reading and consulting with others who are experienced. A willingness to become involved and time for mutual trust to develop are prerequisites for successful school consultation. However, these are necessary but not sufficient activities. Physicians should be informed about community resources and those of the school system, the major child health needs within the community, and community concerns about them. They should learn who the key personnel are and what the crucial administrative relationships are and have some notion of what a school health program might include.

GETTING STARTED IN SCHOOL HEALTH

Not all physicians can or will become involved in school health. Those who do will do so in a variety of ways and to different degrees, inasmuch as there is no single model. Involvement depends on interest, available time, and receptivity of school personnel. Getting started is probably the most difficult task.

Some time commitment is necessary. Because most health care providers are unable to devote large blocks of time without compensation, a few hours a week may have to be sacrificed to initiate interest on the part of school authorities before a formal relationship can be worked out.

One possible starting point is for the physician to talk to parents and schoolchildren. The physician probably has more direct contact with children and their parents than any other professional. He or she should find out the following from patients and parents: what they perceive as important health education and health service activities, what activities they are already participating in within school programs, their perceptions regarding the value of these activities, and what additional activities they think the schools should conduct.

Next the physician should visit the schools to learn what is actually going on. He or she should avoid the role of the medical expert and express a sincere interest in learning about the school's activities concerned with health. A key administrator often can facilitate entry into the system. This could be a health education coordinator (if there is one), a curriculum coordinator, a nursing services coordinator, or the school superintendent. The physician should express interest in child development and child health and ask for an opportunity to talk to teachers, nurses, and students and to observe health education and service activities.

In visiting the school, the physician should always make contact first with the key person—the school principal. Some principals will be very interested in helping the physician visit people in the school, and some principals will be so puzzled by why a physician would visit a school that they will not know how to be of assistance. Regardless of the reception by the principal, the physician should *never* go into a school without contacting the principal.

Informal conversations with the teachers sometimes are more successful than organized meetings. It should be remembered that extra meetings usually are not very popular with teachers after they have spent a full day working with children. The teachers' lounge and the cafeteria are excellent settings in which to talk with teachers. Conversation over a cup of coffee provides the physician with a conducive atmosphere in which to learn about health-related activities and the teacher's perception of the children's health needs.

The school nurse is a key member of the school health team whom the physician should visit as soon as possible and whose views and knowledge of health-related activities and needs should be heeded. The physician should also talk to other members of the health team—the school psychologist, counselor, and special education teachers; they are good resources for learning about the types of problems that occur in that particular school.

At this point, the physician might see obvious opportunities to help with health services and education programs or have some constructive suggestions regarding what could be done. However, the physician should first attempt to find out what school personnel perceive as an important area in which to assist. The physician also should try to help meet their needs even if it may not be highest on his or her list of priorities. It may be as simple as helping persuade parents to turn out for a Parent-Teacher Association meeting. This would be a service to the school, and school personnel will be able to see evidence of the physician's interest in meeting their needs.

When that is accomplished, the physician is *in* the school system and in a better position to work as a team member to develop, plan, and conduct health-related activities.

REFERENCES

1. Caldwell BM: Cooperative preschool inventory, rev ed, Berkeley, Calif, 1970, Educational Testing Services.
2. Nader PR: School entry. In Stein M and Dixon D: Handbook of developmental and behavioral pediatrics, Chicago, 1986, Year Book Medical Publishers, Inc.

SUGGESTED READINGS

Boder E and Jarrico S: A diagnostic screening test for subtypes of reading disability, New York, 1982, Grune & Stratton, Inc.

Dworkin PH: School readiness. In learning and behavior problems of school children, Philadelphia, 1985, WB Saunders Co.

Thorpe HS and Werner EE: Developmental screening of preschool children: a critical review of inventories used in health and education programs, Pediatrics 53:3, 1974.

Welch MM, Saulsbury FT, and Kesler RW: The value of the preschool examination in screening for health problems, J Pediatr 100:232, 1982.

60

School Health Program Goals

Philip R. Nader

A unique and essential ingredient often is overlooked in planning and operating school health programs: the interaction among three groups—the child and the family, school personnel and the education system, and health care providers working in the systems of health care delivery. Each group has different perceptions, priorities, and values that influence the child's health and development. These differences form barriers that frequently keep the groups from interacting effectively. They also present a challenge to develop ways to enhance the interaction of these groups in working toward the total health of the child.

School health is the arena in which these three groups can come together. Examination of their interaction and their perceptions, priorities, and values in relation to health is a prerequisite for approaching the development of a school health program.

THE HOME AND THE FAMILY

Constraints Placed on Children

The target of most school health efforts is those children who for the most part remain passive recipients of program activities. Both the school and home place this constraint on children. Health care providers often reinforce this passive role and rely on parents to initiate and maintain desired behaviors for their children. The opportunity for children to practice skills in relation to their own health could be available and reinforced in the school. The family, however, remains the major unit that provides the social learning that will lead to independent or self-directed health-related behavior.

School health programs should help children become active participants in and decision-makers regarding their health care. More knowledge, however, is needed about children's concepts and perceptions of health and illness. We also need to find ways to help children learn how to promote and maintain their health. The school remains that institution in society charged with instruction of children. Information gradually is accumulating indicating that the development of both health concepts and health behaviors is related to the child's cognitive development and social learning. The extent of the constraint placed on children in relation to health decision-making is most pronounced when high school students are permitted to drive a car but need special permission to go to the school nurse. This is one constraint that school health programs could attempt to overcome.

Family Stress and Child Health

Mechanic[2] studied the health and illness behaviors of fourth and eighth graders—350 mother-child pairs. Although the overall results indicate little maternal influence in determining children's patterns of illness behavior, it was found that family stress made mothers more likely to report their own and their children's symptoms. They also were more likely to contact the physician concerning their children's health. The work of Roghmann and Haggerty[6] documents the influence of family stress on coping patterns. Stress was found to increase health care use via that portion of the health care system that is more responsive to demands of access, namely, telephone calls and emergency room visits. The family stress surrounding a chronically ill child is increased by lack of knowledge. For children with asthma, Pless and Roghmann[5] found that the better the parents' knowledge and understanding of the child's illness, the better the child's adjustment: "Only 27% of children whose parents had 'excellent' knowledge of their illnesses had low adjustment scores, compared with 43% of those with parents having 'poor' understanding."

A school health program with appropriate outreach and parental involvement can respond more quickly to families' and children's stress. Over an extended period it also may be possible to alter the coping styles and strengths that families and children have available to deal with stress when it inevitably appears.

THE SCHOOL

Adult Attitudes and Expectations

Adult attitudes and beliefs directly affect the children who are the recipients of school programs. Both parent-child and teacher-child interactions are based on knowledge, beliefs, and experiences that often do not allow them to respond most effectively to children's health or developmental needs. Previous experiences with health care systems may cause inappropriate fear, lack of understanding, and unrealistic expectations of the seemingly magical intervention of health professionals. Common examples include teachers (1) being concerned about showing moving pictures to epileptic students for fear of precipitating a seizure, (2) ascribing chewing on pencils and other forms of pica to mineral or other dietary deficiencies, and (3) paying excessive attention to children subject to attacks of asthma. Other unrealistic expectations commonly encountered include the value of a brain wave or medication in solving a difficult behavioral and educational problem.

School health programs have an obligation to attempt to overcome these knowledge and attitudinal barriers through education. Teachers generally are enthusiastic regarding joint in-service efforts to address some of these health-related areas, if administrators can be convinced of their value over more pressing educational priorities. The support of parents can be critical in establishing the priority for such efforts. Parents also may be valuable in recruiting health care professionals from the community to serve as resources for such seminars. Health care providers will gain insight into the problems faced by educators through mutual participation in such health-related seminars.

Priority for Health in Education

Health education and promotion of health often are of low priority in the educational curriculum. Seminars such as the ones mentioned previously may stimulate interest. Another avenue may be to develop health education programs outside the formal curriculum that are specifically focused on children with specialized educational needs or those who suffer the consequences of a health or developmental problem. Examples include children with physical disabilities or chronic illnesses. The following outcomes should be predicted and measured: improved educational performance; better social adjustment and improved school attendance; better understanding of the nature of the problem; and improved coping skills for the child, parents, and teachers. School health programing that takes into account the needs of each system has a better chance of overcoming the inherent obstacles previously mentioned.

THE HEALTH CARE SYSTEM

The "New Morbidity"

For today's school-aged children and adolescents, the "new morbidity" and major unmet health needs are dental, emotional, and learning problems and problems associated with alcohol and drug use. Making decisions about sexual behavior and coping with chronic handicapping conditions are areas that also have received too little attention. These needs clearly stand out as striking, even in areas in which more traditional health problems are prevalent. Therefore it becomes necessary to develop school health programs and activities with these needs in mind. Health care providers (as well as parents and teachers), however, are hampered by their lack of knowledge and experience in dealing with these health concerns. Difficulties also may result from working in an environment that traditionally has emphasized disease and episodic illness care more often than health maintenance, comprehensive primary health, or preventive medicine. The disease orientation and training of many health care providers may ill equip them to learn firsthand about the numerous physical and mental health problems that are to be found undetected and untreated in a community. This environment also inhibits the development of health care providers' roles in the prevention and early detection of these problems.

Preventive School Health

It has been suggested[3] that a modification of Caplan's preventive health model[1] be adapted by primary health care providers working in collaboration with school systems. Primary preventive activities are those that improve the school environment. Secondary preventive activities are those that relate to early detection of conditions inimical to a child's sound physical, social, or educational growth. Tertiary preventive activities are those dealing with individual illnesses. The goal is to overcome existing problems and to help children with a handicapping condition to reach their optimal level of function.

For example, a practicing pediatrician in a group practice caring for most students in the schools in a given geographic area is retained by that district as a school medical consultant. In the area of primary prevention, a portion of the physician's time is spent with teachers in in-service teaching sessions on developmental variations normally observed in young elementary schoolchildren. This service can improve the general milieu of the school environment, and teachers learn that normal variation may be observed without unnecessary labeling of children as "deviant" or "problems." This interaction also benefits the physician who desires an opportunity to practice preventive medicine and sees service as a school consultant as potentially affecting a large number of children influenced by a small group of teachers, compared with the relatively small number of children on whom the physician could have an impact in the office, seeing individual children and adolescents.

In secondary and tertiary preventive areas, health care providers, by interacting with school personnel concerned with pupil learning and with adjustment problems, can widen their horizons. They discover important information related to the future health or development of patients—information that might not otherwise have been brought to their attention by the parent. Through this kind of interaction, school personnel also will benefit by not feeling isolated in attempting to deal with the problems and by having support from a professional who may be highly respected by parents.

In all areas the family and child should benefit from the increased communication that naturally occurs among concerned professionals.

Access to Health Care

Adequate access to health care requires joint efforts among those in the home, the source of care, and the school. When health care systems are not used, providers often blame the family for "poor" attituides or their lack of motivation or knowledge rather than pay enough attention to issues of trust and confidence in their physician and health priorities that persons must consider and decide on before participating in curative or preventive health services. The school health service offers a natural setting to assist in this process of providing smooth and adequate access to health care.[4] Those in a school health program have the opportunity to interact with the child in his or her role as a student rather than as a patient. This emphasis is especially attractive to many who view school health as a possible vehicle for overcoming some of the actual or perceived barriers that block adequate access to a health care system.[3] This goal may necessitate going beyond the usual home visit that occurs after a written notification of a child's health problem is sent to the parent. In some instances it may even entail placing direct services (such as a dental clinic) in the school. Access may be enhanced by providing school health nurses with additional skills in problem assessment and management (e.g., school nurse practitioners). It may include providing outreach workers who can become familiar with both families and services. It also may mean (1) developing more formal relations between individual schools and specific sources of health care for children and (2) training physicians more adequately to handle school health consultative services.[7]

The following general goals are suggested for groups considering establishing a modification of community school health programs:

1. A school health program should provide ways to enhance the health and learning environment of children:
   a. Through protection against disease and disability and through guidance for optimal health (primary prevention)
   b. Through early identification of health problems and remediation to limit them (secondary prevention)
   c. Through prevention of complications and rehabilitation when health problems are fixed (tertiary prevention)
2. A school health program should provide a bridge between school health services and health care providers in a community:
   a. By using a simple referral procedure between the school and the health care provider
   b. By maintaining, improving, or developing communication between school personnel and health care providers
   c. By using, improving, or developing adequate communication among those in the home, the school, and the health care systems in the community
3. A school health program should assist children and their parents in becoming more responsible and assertive about their health:
   a. By determining critical skills for different developmental age-groups and specific skills for groups of children with special health needs
   b. By designing activities (both content and process) to facilitate the development of specific skills
   c. By providing opportunities for the practice of the particular skills
4. A school health program should use health resources effectively and efficiently in enhancing the health and learning environment of children:
   a. Through the use of all members of the educational team
   b. Through consultation
   c. Through training programs
   d. Through sharing responsibilities in the school with the health care provider
   e. Through sharing responsibilities in the school with the home
5. A school health program should periodically assess the effectiveness of health services provided in the school and the community:
   a. Through the collection of data to determine the type of program change or implementation that is needed ("needs assessment")
   b. Through the description of roles and processes involved in the implementation of program activities
   c. Through the comparison of stated objectives and outcome of the program activities

REFERENCES

1. Caplan G: Principles of preventative psychiatry, New York, 1964, Basic Books, Inc.
2. Mechanic D: Influences on children's health attitudes and behavior, Pediatrics 33:3, 1966.
3. Nader PR: The school health service: making primary care effective, Pediatr Clin North Am 21:1, 1974.
4. Nader PR, Gilman S, and Bee D: Factors influencing access to primary health care via school health services, Pediatrics 65:3, 1980.
5. Pless IB and Roghmann KH: Chronic illness and its consequences: observations based on three epidemiologic surveys, J Pediatr 79:351, 1971.
6. Roghmann K and Haggerty RJ: The stress model for illness behavior. In Haggerty RJ, Roghmann KJ, and Pless IB, editors: Child health and the community, New York, 1975, John Wiley & Sons, Inc.
7. Wright GF and Vanderpool NA: School and the pediatrician, Pediatr Clin North Am 28:643, 1981.

SUGGESTED READING

Nader PR: School health services. In Wallace HM, Ryan G, and Oglesby A, editors: Maternal and child health practices, ed 3, Oakland, Calif, 1988, Third Party Publishing Co.

61

School Health Education

Guy S. Parcel

Public health measures and medical advances such as immunizations, sanitation, and antibiotics have contributed considerably to altering the nature of major health problems. What people do for themselves regarding their health may be more important than what others do for them. An increased awareness of the limitations inherent in the curative aspects of health care has made for greater emphasis on the importance of health maintenance and preventive medicine. Through the years the process of health education has been used to assist people in preventing illness and maintaining levels of health. The underlying assumption has been that an informed public is better prepared to make decisions that will promote health.

Within this framework health education in the schools has become particularly attractive. Almost all children go to school and while in school constitute a captive audience; because schools have become the major institution for learning, they have been suggested as the logical place for children to learn about health and to develop the abilities that are needed to make effective decisions about health-related behavior. That schools can meet this objective has yet to be demonstrated. As the search for improving the effectiveness of school health education continues, there is an increasing awareness that success must involve a cooperative effort between educational personnel and child health care personnel. For example, the pediatrician's knowledge of child health and child development is much greater than that of most educational personnel in the schools. Thus the child heath care professional has an essential role and an important contribution to make in school health education programs. On the other hand, most educational personnel have more refined and effective skills in teaching and an opportunity to reach more children than does the pediatrician.

Inasmuch as most health care providers have limited contact and experience in working with schools and probably were last in a school as students or parents, the following background information concerning school health education may be helpful.

The inclusion of health education as part of the instructional program in schools is by no means a new concept. Traditionally health education has been found within the school program in two distinct areas. Through the involvement of a school nurse or school physician, health education activities have been included as a part of health services. For example, while screening for vision and hearing, the school nurse may discuss with the children, either individually or in groups, the purpose and meaning of the screening and the importance of health care in terms of sight and hearing. As another example, the school nurse may go into the classroom and instruct the students about particular health behavior such as dental health (brushing teeth) or nutrition (good eating habits). However, when health instruction is incorporated in the curriculum of the regular classroom teacher or the special health education teacher, it is referred to as *curricular health education*. In this way health education is either integrated into the classroom curriculum or established as a separate curriculum within the total instructional program of the school.

TRENDS IN SCHOOL HEALTH EDUCATION

Early approaches to curriculum development in health education primarily centered on dealing with some type of acute health problem. In the 1950s it was recognized that the abuse of alcohol had become a serious health and social problem. In an attempt to solve this problem, school personnel were called on to provide instruction, pointing out the dangers and health hazards associated with consuming alcohol. The assumption was that if students knew about these dangers and were told about the health hazards, they would avoid alcohol abuse. Some states went so far as to enact laws requiring public schools to provide instruction in the prevention of alcohol abuse. Schools all over the country responded to this apparent health problem and began providing instruction about alcohol abuse.

It has been demonstrated, however, that even when information is effectively taught, it does not necessarily lead to a change in behavior. Many drug education programs were developed that effectively taught the pharmacologic aspects of drug abuse, legal penalities, and the physical risks of taking certain drugs. When these programs were evaluated, it was found that knowledge about drugs and the dangers involved in drug use did not significantly influence drug-taking behavior.[1,25] The failure of drug education programs in the late 1960s and 1970s helped considerably to demonstrate the weaknesses of health education programs that are primarily based on a cognitive approach.[8]

This failure reinforced what many educators had been suggesting for years—that health behavior is related not only to knowledge but also to factors such as expectations and values associated with health behavior. It also became more apparent that health-related problems could not be effectively dealt with on a crisis basis. If health problems are to be prevented through education, a means of dealing with these problems must be developed long before they reach a state of crisis.

Teaching methods that focus on the learners' attitudes and

feelings fall into the realm of *affective education*. Teaching in this area is related more to personal development than to the learning of facts and concepts. Some of the programs developed in drug education actually had very little to do with information about drugs. Instead, these programs focused on helping children to develop a better understanding of self and interrelationships with others and, for older children, to clarify values.[30] These types of programs hypothesized that children who feel good about themselves, who can develop effective relationships with others, and who have a clear understanding of what is important to them are going to be less likely to have problems related to drug abuse.

As an outgrowth of the increased interest in affective education, many school health education programs in the 1970s were expanded or redirected to focus more on attitudes, feelings, and values.[31] Some suggested programs tended to deemphasize the importance of information, whereas other approaches tended to emphasize an integration of cognitive and affective learning.

In the eighties, school-based interventions were based on a social learning approach, which typically included training students to resist social pressures to engage in negative health behaviors (e.g., smoking) and creating a social environment that may encourage positive health behaviors.[5,8,13,22]

An expansion of the application of social learning theory methods to the design of the health education curriculum led to the development of the "social influences approach." This approach recognized the importance of preparing students to deal with the pressures of an environment that may encourage risk-taking behavior. Teaching strategies used in this approach include the increase of knowledge about short-term consequences of the health risk–taking behavior; peer pressure–resistance training; inoculation against mass media messages; establishment of normative expectations for healthful behavior; use of peer leaders as role models; and the making of a personal commitment to avoid risk-taking behavior or engage in healthful behavior. These methods have been successfully applied to smoking prevention[6,23] and to drug abuse prevention,[21] with evaluations indicating a significant impact on reducing risk-taking behavior.

Another approach that has emerged recently in school health education interventions is the use of skill development methods for preventing health-risk behavior. The skills approach assumes that a set of social and behavioral skills is essential for making effective decisions about health behavior. Further, if students are able to develop these skills, know the consequences of health-risk behavior, and have opportunities to practice these skills, they will be more likely to avoid risk-taking behavior and to develop more healthful patterns of behavior. Types of skills usually addressed in these types of programs include decision-making skills, problem-solving skills, communication skills, and stress management or relaxation skills. The skills approach has been shown to be effective when applied to smoking; it also has been applied to other areas of health behavior.[2,26]

In addition to developments in approaches to the health education curriculum, the concept of school-based health promotion has been expanded to include other components of the school that contribute to influencing or enabling healthful behavior.[11] For example, health promotion programs have been developed to coordinate changes in school food services and physical education with health education classroom instruction to improve the diet and physical activity behavior of elementary school children.[18,19,27] Efforts also have been made to involve parents and to focus on the family as a critical component to influence changes in health behavior through school-based programs.[15,24] Linking school-based programs with community programs and agencies also has shown potential for improving the effectiveness of existing programs concerned with influencing health behavior and preventing health problems.[20,21,32]

Most state guidelines for health education in the schools are organized around content areas, such as nutrition, safety, substance abuse, chronic disease, infectious diseases, mental health, growth and development, and family living. The term *comprehensive school health education* has been used to describe a curriculum that provides a sequence of activities at each grade level to address each designated content area. Thus the predominant approach to health education in the schools today is to present health-related information within each content area with increasing complexity at each grade level.

REASONABLE EXPECTATIONS FOR SCHOOL HEALTH EDUCATION

The health professional may expect that, to be effective, health education must influence behavior to reduce the risk of disease or to improve health status. The educator, however, might argue that the role of the school is to increase knowledge and develop critical thinking and not to change student behavior, which may be greatly influenced by factors outside of the classroom. Both perspectives could be considered correct, but each will be determined by how programs are designed and evaluated.

School health education programs can be effective in helping students learn about their health. Evaluations of school health education programs have demonstrated their effectiveness in influencing a variety of outcomes, including knowledge, attitudes, health practices, behavior, and physiologic indicators.* The program's effect on learning and eventually on behavior depends on the quality of the planning and the input of sufficient resources, including teacher training and adequate classroom instructional time.[4,9] Behavioral change, however, is complex, and simplistic approaches that do not effectively use what has been learned in the field are unlikely to succeed.

It is unreasonable to expect school-based educational programs alone to influence behaviors that are not supported by the larger social environment of the child. For example, how can a child change to a low-fat, low-salt diet when the other family members continue their same eating patterns? How can an adolescent be expected to avoid the social use of drugs or alcohol when the larger social environment not only supports but also encourages the use of alcohol and drugs? How can an adolescent be expected to prevent an unwanted pregnancy when the appropriate counseling and health services are made difficult to access and use? What is needed in the planning of school health education programs is a better match

*References 3, 4, 10, 19, 21, 24, 29, 33.

between what can be expected as reasonable outcomes and the type of program necessary to accomplish those outcomes.[12]

An approach primarily based on providing information can be effective in increasing knowledge about health and health-related problems. Program evaluations, however, suggest that knowledge is an important but an insufficient factor in influencing health behavior. Personal development (reflected in positive feelings toward self, skills in relating to others, and the successful use of coping skills in making decisions, resisting peer pressure, and dealing with stress) is considered the important outcome for health education programs.[14] It is reasonable to expect school personnel to plan and carry out health education programs that can both impart knowledge and foster personal development. The next level of program design is to provide students with activities that will enable them to practice skills such as decision-making and resisting social pressure that can be applied directly to health-related behaviors.[16] Whether students actually develop positive health behaviors will still be influenced by many factors outside the school, but it is possible for schools to assist students in developing the ability to engage in positive health behaviors. It is not reasonable to expect that a single unit on health education placed within the total curriculum will alone accomplish the development of skills needed to adopt positive health behaviors. A more comprehensive approach that provides knowledge, skills development, and practice in a developmental sequence through each of the grade levels is necessary. It also is important to relate the health education program to other parts of the school curriculum and programs. Students will need to have numerous opportunities to experience personal development, and the social environment of the school needs to be structured to provide support for the practice of decision-making and other skills.

THE PHYSICIAN'S ROLE IN SCHOOL HEALTH EDUCATION

The goal of health education is to assist individuals in developing skills and confidence that will enable them to make good choices about their health behavior and appropriate use of health care resources. If this goal is to be achieved through a school health program, it will require a cooperative effort by health care and educational personnel. It is unlikely that any one discipline can accomplish such a formidable task. In both curricular and noncurricular health education activities, the physician can contribute to school health education in five distinct ways: (1) by reviewing content and process of health education activities for accuracy and age appropriateness, (2) by conducting health education activities for children and parents through the school program, (3) by assisting with the training personnel involved in health education, (4) by assisting with the collection of data to evaluate the outcomes of health education activities, and (5) by encouraging support for school health education activities within the community. A discussion in which a physician can contribute follows.

Physician Involvement in School Health Education

In developing a health education curriculum, the physician can play a very important role in identifying the health concerns related to specific age-groups. Physicians see adults and children of different ages for various illnesses and health maintenance. They are aware of the health concerns and needs expressed by their patients. These concerns and needs can be identified and interpreted for educational personnel in planning health education activities. With the physician's help, critical skills can be identified for the various age-groups, and once these skills are identified, activities can be developed to assist children in attaining these skills. Physicians involved in child health care have a unique knowledge about health care needs according to a child's developmental level.

Health professionals need to become involved with inservice training programs in health education.[7] Through their training and experience, physicians are specialists in various aspects of health, illness, and child development. They can assist teachers in understanding normal processes of child development and identifying the developmental needs of children. Teachers are required to deal with a broad spectrum of information related to health behavior; therefore it is difficult for them to keep informed of current knowledge in all these areas. Thus the physician can be especially helpful by imparting recent information to teachers about specific areas of health and can suggest resources for additional information. There almost always is a gap between information generated by the health sciences and the information available for use in instructional programs. The physician can help to narrow this gap.

Physicians may be called on to serve as guest lecturers in classrooms. When a teacher is faced with dealing with complicated or sensitive material, the physician often is asked to visit the classroom to talk to students. The easiest way for physicians to handle such a request is simply to come into the classroom and do the best they can under the circumstances. However, there are some obvious drawbacks to this approach. The physician may not be prepared to present the material at a level appropriate for the students. Also, the physician's time will be limited, and therefore only a small number of students can benefit from the physician's talk. A better approach would be for the physician to work with the teacher to identify more specifically the skills and information that students need to learn. Together the physician and teacher can apply the physician's knowledge to a particular teaching situation and then plan an ongoing program that can be presented by the teacher and carried on at times when the physician cannot be present. In this way a larger number of students can benefit from the physician's contribution over a longer period of time.

Teaching, like the practice of medicine, is an art and requires a certain set of skills, especially communication skills. A good physician is not necessarily a good teacher. Involvement in health education activities requires the physician to communicate effectively. Talking with children is different from talking with adults.

Vocabulary often is a major problem. One should avoid terms or concepts that are inappropriate for the developmental level of the child. The appropriate level can be determined primarily by using a questioning approach rather than a "telling" approach. "Why do doctors give shots?" rather than "Doctors give shots because . . . ." The use of questions has three major advantages: (1) the level of conceptualization can be determined; (2) the degree of understanding can be evaluated; and (3) the children can learn from each other.

The amount of time, effort, and resources devoted to the school health education curriculum will depend on the priority a school district places on health education. When it comes to health, it is obvious that physicians carry considerable influence and prestige in a community. The physician's continuous encouragement and support are essential to gain the necessary resources for doing an effective job of health education. This can be accomplished by spending time with school board members and administrators to encourage a high priority for the school health education curriculum.

AN APPROACH TO DEVELOPING HEALTH EDUCATION PROGRAMS

Each community is different, and modifications in the following suggested approach* may be necessary to accommodate unique situations.

Planning Committees

An initial group consisting of the top school administrators and school staff likely to have responsibility for the program needs to be formed to establish the guidelines and process for program planning. This group would give official approval and support for developing the program. A second group or a subgroup of the first committee is then organized to develop the program. The program planning group should have representation from the administrators, teachers, students, parents, and resource people or consultants from the community. Another typical committee structure would include (1) the establishment of an advisory committee that would have a broad base of representation from several areas of the school and community and (2) a group to design the curriculum.

Assessment of Needs and Resources

The planning group will need information to make decisions about the scope and direction of the program. Useful information can be obtained from a review of the literature and programs from other school districts. However, it is essential to have information about the local situation to aim the program toward local needs. Standardized survey questionnaires can be used to measure the current health knowledge, attitudes, and behaviors of the students. This information can be useful in setting program priorities.

Information should also be obtained regarding the resources available for a health education program, including who has had training and experience in health education, effective educational techniques, the development of interpersonal skills, and social learning methodologies. The following should also be determined: (1) what instructional materials are available from the state education agency, the local state health department, or federal agencies and (2) whether there are any experienced consultants available from university departments, such as health education.

*This approach is an adaptation of the one described for developing a drug education program in Parcel GS: The pediatrician's role in drug education, Pediatr Rev 4:144, 1982. Reproduced by permission of *Pediatrics*, copyright 1982.

Goals and Objectives

Goals, the expected outcomes that will result from the program, should be realistic and achievable. It is preferable that the goals be stated in such a way that their level of achievement can be measured; for example: (1) at the end of 5 years there will be a 30% reduction in the number of youths under the age of 19 years arrested for driving under the influence of alcohol or drugs; or (2) at the end of 3 years there will be a 50% reduction in the number of youths who begin smoking in the eighth grade.

Each example contains a "when," "how much," "of what," and "by whom" to make the goal as specific as possible. Clearly stated goals give more direction and focus for the education program.

The next step is to state for each grade level at which the program is to be taught the objectives to be accomplished by the students. These are usually stated in behavioral terms and can be addressed by asking what the student is expected to be able to do as a result of this instruction. For example, the student will be able to (1) demonstrate how to use techniques to resist peer pressure, (2) apply steps in decision-making to resolve a conflict about food selection in a social situation, and (3) use relaxation techniques to cope with feelings of stress.

Activities

Once the objectives are stated and organized into a logical sequence and structure, the next step is to develop activities to assist students in accomplishing the objectives. Activities include experiences that will provide the knowledge, skills, practice, reinforcement, and confidence for performing the behaviors stated in the objectives. Attention should also be given to activities outside the classroom that will support and reinforce classroom learning. Activities for parents, teachers, and other school staff may be valuable in providing the social support and environment for reinforcing the learning of new behaviors.

Teacher Preparation and Implementation. In-service training for teachers is essential for implementing a new curriculum. Such training should include attitudinal support for the curriculum and specific teaching skills. Attention should also be given to involving other school personnel who might not teach the curriculum but whose support and awareness of the curriculum are important. For example, the school principal, nurse, counselor, or social worker should be involved in planning the implementation of the program.

Pilot Program. Almost any new health education program should be viewed as experimental, since we cannot be certain what the best approach is for a particular community. It is helpful to conduct a pilot program in one school or a few schools before implementing a district-wide program. This provides the opportunity to test ideas and techniques and to make changes. Once a pilot program has worked effectively and has been shown to be acceptable, it is usually easier to implement the program in other schools in the district. It is essential that the pilot program be evaluated in such a way that makes it possible to identify components that may require modification.

IMPLEMENTATION OF CHANGE

Changing old programs and implementing new ones is difficult. The process of change in school systems tends to occur slowly, frequently because of the lack of a systematic approach to effect change. This deficiency is especially relevant to the introduction of innovative school health promotion programs, an area in which change often needs to occur within several components of the total school program. To address this issue, Parcel and colleagues have developed a model for making changes in the schools' organizational structures to implement school health promotion programs.[17] The change includes four phases: (1) organizational commitment, (2) alterations in policies and practices, (3) alterations of roles and actions of staff, and (4) implementation of learning activities. The intent of this model is to provide a systematic approach to change that includes school components that support and enable behaviors addressed by health education programs in the classroom.

In the first phase, commitment is obtained from key decision-makers in the school system to proceed with the planning of a new or modified health promotion program. A top-down approach would involve school board members, superintendents, and program directors arriving at a decision to commit to the proposed program. The proposal for the new program may come from an agency outside the district, such as the health department or voluntary health agency, or from inside groups, such as curriculum planning committees or task force groups appointed to address specified problems. Commitment usually is obtained through a series of meetings with key decision-makers. These meetings typically involve written or verbal presentation on the importance, rationale, and need for the proposed program. Physician involvement in this process can help provide information to establish a high priority for proposed health promotion programs.

Commitment also may be obtained from a bottom-up approach, in which the persons who implement the program (teachers and staff members) are actively involved in making decisions about planning new or modified programs. One method for obtaining this type of commitment has been implemented in several states, and because it is based on a program first conducted in Oregon at a seaside retreat, it has become known as the "seaside model."[28] The seaside model involves the participation of teams from school districts coming together in a conference to explore their own personal health promotion needs as well as those of their students. The process involves planning a health promotion program or activity for their district. Out of this type of experience often comes a strong commitment on a personal and professional level for health promotion programs. Another way to approach commitment at the teacher and staff level is to establish a health promotion program for school personnel.

Once commitment is demonstrated, the next step is to establish a policy-planning group composed of the program directors and key administrators to develop and define policies that support the program's high priority in terms of importance and value. The policies then are given to a second planning group to address the changes that will need to be made in current practices to follow through on the intent of the policies and to implement the new program. This planning group usually consists of program directors and representatives of teachers and staff members who will be implementing the program.

The next phase focuses on preparing the teachers and staff members to implement the program. In-service training, technical assistance, and monitoring and feedback are methods that can be used to alter roles and actions of personnel to implement new programs. Finally, with these changes in place, the school program is ready to provide activities that will assist the students to develop positive, healthful behavior. Student activities should include classroom instruction, practice in school, practice at home, and reinforcement and social support from the school environment for practicing the healthful behaviors.

REFERENCES

1. Berberian RM et al: The effectiveness of drug education programs: a critical review, Health Educ Monogr 4:377, 1966.
2. Botvin GJ: Prevention of adolescent substance abuse through the development of personal and social competence. In Glynn T, editor: Preventing adolescent drug abuse: intervention strategies, NIDA Research Monograph Series, No 47, Washington, DC, 1983, US Government Printing Office.
3. Bush PJ et al: Cardiovascular risk prevention in black school children: the "Know Your Body" evaluation project, Health Educ Q 16:215, 1989.
4. Connell DB, Turner RR, and Mason EF: Summary of findings of the school health education evaluation: health promotion effectiveness, implementation, and costs, J School Health 55:316, 1985.
5. Evans RI: Smoking in children: developing a social pscyhological strategy of deterrence, J Prev Med 5:122, 1976.
6. Flay BR: Psychosocial approaches to smoking prevention: a review of findings, Health Psychology 4:449, 1985.
7. Floyd JD, Lang RM, and Lotsoff AM: Drug education: suggested guidelines for conducting an effective course for teachers, J Am Coll Health Assoc 24:15, 1975.
8. Goodstadt MS: Alcohol and drug education: models and outcomes, Health Educ Manager 6:263, 1978.
9. Green LW: Answering the question "Does health education work?" J School Health 49:55, 1979.
10. Killen JD et al: The Stanford adolescent heart health program, Health Educ Q 16:263, 1989.
11. Kolbe L: Increasing the impact of school health promotion programs: emerging research perspectives, Health Educ 17:47, 1986.
12. Krueter M and Christenson GM: School health education: does it cause and effect? Health Educ Q 8:43, 1981.
13. McAlister A et al: Pilot study of smoking, alcohol and drug abuse prevention, Am J Public Health 70:719, 1980.
14. Nader PR and Parcel GS: Competence: the outcome for health education. In Nader PR, editor: Options for school health, Germantown, Md, 1978, Aspen Systems Corp.
15. Nader PR et al: A family approach to cardiovascular risk reduction: results from the San Diego family health project, Health Educ Q 16:229, 1989.
16. Parcel GS: Skills approach to health education: a framework for integrating cognitive and affective learning, J School Health 46:403, 1976.
17. Parcel GS, Simons-Morton BG, and Kolbe LJ: Health promotion: integrating organization change and student learning strategies, Health Educ Q 15:435, 1988.
18. Parcel GS et al: School promotion of healthful diet and exercise behavior: an integration of organizational change and social learning theory interventions, J School Health 57:150, 1987.
19. Parcel GS et al: School promotion of healthful diet and physical activity: impact on learning outcomes and self-reported behavior, Health Educ Q 16:181, 1989.

20. Pentz MA: Community organization and school liaisons: how to get programs started, J School Health 56:382, 1986.
21. Pentz MA et al: A multicommunity trial for primary prevention of adolescent drug abuse, JAMA 261:3259, 1989.
22. Perry CL: Enhancing the transition years: the challenge of adolescent health promotion, J School Health 52:307, 1982.
23. Perry CL, Murray DM, and Klepp KI: Predictors of adolescent smoking and implications for prevention, MMWR 36:415, 1987.
24. Perry CL et al: Parent involvement with children's health promotion: a one-year follow-up of the Minnesota home team, Health Educ Q 16:171, 1989.
25. Schaps E et al: A review of 127 drug abuse prevention program evaluations, J Drug Issues 11:17, 1981.
26. Schinke SP, Gilchrist LD, and Snow WH: Skills intervention to prevent cigarette smoking among adolescents, Am J Public Health 76:665, 1985.
27. Simons-Morton BG, Parcel GS, and O'Hara NM: Implementing organizational changes to promote healthful diet and physical activity at school, Health Educ Q 15:115, 1988.
28. Stevens N: School health promotion: a study of exemplary districts, doctoral dissertation, Eugene, 1986, University of Oregon.
29. Stone EJ, Perry CL, and Luepker RV: Synthesis of cardiovascular behavioral research for youth health promotion, Health Educ Q 16:155, 1989.
30. Swisher JD: Addiction prevention: future directions, Paper presented at the meeting of the Health Education Bureau, Killarney, Ireland, Nov 1979.
31. Vicary JR: Toward an adaptive developmental education. In Boston RL, editor: Curriculum handbook: the disciplines, current movements, and instruction methodology, Newton, Mass, 1977, Allyn & Bacon, Inc.
32. Vincent ML, Clearie AF, and Schlucter MD: Reducing adolescent pregnancy though school and community-based education, JAMA 257:3328, 1987.
33. Walter HJ: Primary prevention of chronic disease among children: the school-based "Know Your Body" intervention trials, Health Educ Q 16:201, 1989.

62

School Absenteeism

Philip R. Nader

A review[1] of the scant literature on the effects of excessive school absence concludes that school absence patterns are a readily available, easy to use indicator of potentially unmet child health needs. School attendance is a complex phenomenon that tends to be rather stable for a given child and is influenced by many factors, including the prevalence of illness, parental and home influences, and also probably school and educational situations.

Absenteeism has been noted to be higher in lower socioeconomic classes and in children whose parents are under stress, have a chronic illness, have been recently hospitalized, have lower educational expectations, and are worried about their child's health. It is lower among children of well-to-do families that live in less crowded conditions and who "like" school.

The relation between absenteeism and actual school performance and achievement has received surprisingly little attention.[3] The most that can be said at present is that except for those in the higher socioeconomic classes, excessive school absence is most likely associated with poorer educational achievement, less participation in school activities, higher high school dropout rates, and higher rejection rates by the military services.

The relation of absenteeism to health also has not been extensively examined. Children usually are absent from school for "medical" reasons, such as illness or symptoms of illness. It has been estimated that about 75% of absences are accounted for in this way. Children in households with parents who smoke have been noted to miss more school because of minor ailments.[2]

Nonmedical reasons include illness of other family members, taking trips with parents, oversleeping, inclement weather, and inappropriate clothing. However, there is some indication that children excessively absent for medical reasons also are excessively absent for nonmedical reasons.

There may be a relation between school absence and the presence of a health problem. In one study,[5] sixth graders who were absent excessively had more psychosomatic symptoms that necessitated a nurse visit than did a group of similar students with a low absentee rate. In a large prospective study[3] of absenteeism among first and third graders, the high-absentee group had more contacts with the school nurse than did the low-absentee group. These studies show some relation between absence and being referred for a health problem by the school health service. In one study of high school students,[4] a high absentee rate did not lead to identification of students with significant health problems. Another study[6] noted no effect on school absenteeism among children registered for "comprehensive health care" at a Boston neighborhood health center. In an unpublished study conducted in Galveston, Texas, it was found that absence might be increased for students of low socioeconomic status who had to go to a clinic for a medical problem during the school day, whereas more affluent students who required care went to their physician or dentist after school and therefore did not lose school time to attend to a health problem.

School absence patterns represent an underdeveloped area of potential identification of students at risk for school dropout, poor coping with or management of chronic illness, masked depression, teenage pregnancy, substance abuse, inappropriate responses to minor illnesses, or severe family dysfunction.

REFERENCES

1. Barcai A: Attendance, achievement and social class: the differential impact upon social achievement in different social classes, Acta Paediapsychiatr 38:153, 1973.
2. Charlton A and Blair V: Absence from school related to children's and parental smoking habits, Br Med J 298:90, 1989.
3. Douglass JWR and Ross JM: The effects of absence in primary school performance, Br J Educ Psychol 35:28, 1965.
4. Rogers KD and Reese G: Health studies: presumably normal high school students, Am J Dis Child 109:28, 1965.
5. Van Arsdell WR, Roghmann KJ, and Nader PR: Visits to an elementary school nurse, School Health 42:142, 1972.
6. Weitzman M et al: School absence: a problem for the pediatrician, Pediatrics 69:739, 1982.

SUGGESTED READINGS

Fowler M, Johnson M, and Atkinson S: School achievement and absence in children with chronic health conditions, The Journal of Pediatrics. 106:683, 1985.

Klerman L: School absence–A health perspective, Ped Clin North Am, 35:1253, 1988.

Weitzman M et al: High risk youth and health: the case of excessive school absence. Pediatrics. 78:313-322, 1986.

63

Attention-Deficit Hyperactivity Disorder

Esther H. Wender and Mary V. Solanto

A cluster of behaviors, including an excessively high motor activity level and problems with concentration, attention, and impulsivity, which emerge early in the child's life and persist over time, characterizes a behavioral syndrome termed *attention-deficit hyperactivity disorder* (ADHD)[3] referred to in some circles as attention-deficit disorder with hyperactivity (ADD-H). This syndrome, although broadly defined and associated with multiple etiologic agents, is believed to be produced by biologic factors that produce the typical clinical features. These typical behaviors are affected by the environment, which results in considerable individual variation.

In the past this syndrome was designated by a variety of terms, each reflecting a different focus on symptoms or etiology. These terms included, but were not limited to, *hyperactivity,* the *hyperkinetic syndrome,* and *minimal brain dysfunction.* With the publication in 1980 of the third edition of the *Diagnostic and Statistical Manual of Mental Disorders* (DSM III),[2] the focus shifted to attention deficits as the unifying feature, and the syndrome was named *attention deficit disorder* (ADD). At that time the syndrome was said to occur either with hyperactivity (ADD-H) or without (ADD–non H). When the nomenclature was revised in 1987, the belief was that evidence was insufficient to support the existence of two different syndromes; the term for this condition again was changed, this time to the current attention-deficit hyperactivity disorder (ADHD). The 1980 diagnostic criteria for ADD[2] were based on separate assessments of the presence of inattentiveness, impulsivity, and hyperactivity. The criteria established for the diagnosis of ADHD are listed in the accompanying box, which lists the 14 symptoms in the order of how frequently they were reported by parents and teachers in a survey conducted before the nomenclature revision rather than grouped according to categories of behavior. The current nomenclature also includes the category of *undifferentiated attention-deficit disorder,* which is intended to include children who meet many, but not all, of the criteria for ADHD. Some have suggested that those children previously described as having attention-deficit disorder without hyperactivity (ADD–non-H) should now be grouped in this category.

There continues to be considerable controversy concerning other common syndromes that overlap frequently with ADHD: specific learning disabilities, oppositional defiant disorder (ODD), and conduct disorder. With respect to learning disabilities, it appears that many children so identified also display the behaviors of ADHD and qualify for that diagnosis. In one study 25% of a group of children initially identified as learning disabled also qualified for the diagnosis of ADD-H.[8] In another study 45% of a group of children identified as having ADD-H also qualified for a diagnosis of specific learning disability.[10] Both studies have significant flaws and can provide only preliminary evidence of the degree of overlap in these disorders. Much of the current controversy concerns the ability to distinguish between these disorders inasmuch as most children with learning disorders also demonstrate impaired attention. According to current thinking the presence of additional behaviors—that is, hyperactivity and impulsivity—establishes the diagnosis of ADHD in children with learning disabilities.

ODD and conduct disorder are two disruptive behavior disorders commonly seen in conjunction with ADHD. ODD is characterized by the negativistic, hostile, and defiant behaviors described in the box on p. 628. Conduct disorder is a more serious disorder in which the basic rights of others are violated. Specific diagnostic criteria are listed in the box on p. 628.

The relationships among ODD, conduct disorder, and ADHD remain controversial. It is clear that many children with ADHD have additional disruptive behavior problems and, when they are younger, meet ODD criteria. Among older children a smaller, but unknown, percentage meet conduct disorder criteria. Some investigators have proposed that certain behaviors, such as emotional lability and impaired response to discipline, are part of the core symptomatology in a subgroup of ADHD children and lead to disruptive behaviors. Others argue that ADHD leads to poor self-esteem and, in some families, to inadequate parenting, which, in turn, results in conduct problems.

Although these controversies are unresolved, it is clear that many children qualify for more than one diagnosis on the basis of present criteria. If learning disability, ODD, and/or conduct disorder are present, these additional diagnoses have implications for treatment and prognosis and should therefore be diagnosed (see section on natural history and prognosis). These relationships between ADHD and other syndromes are illustrated in Table 63-1.

PRESENTING PROBLEM

The key to diagnosis is an accurate and a comprehensive history. The practitioner, however, usually is overwhelmed

*Diagnostic Criteria for Attention-Deficit Hyperactivity Disorder (ADHD)**

A. ADHD is disturbance of at least 6 months' duration, during which at least eight of the following are present:
   1. Often fidgets with hands or feet or squirms in seat (in adolescents, it may be limited to subjective feelings or restlessness)
   2. Has difficulty remaining seated when required to do so
   3. Is easily distracted by extraneous stimuli
   4. Has difficulty awaiting turn in games or group situations
   5. Often blurts out answers to questions before they have been completed
   6. Has difficulty following through on instructions from others (not a result of oppositional behavior or failure of comprehension), e.g., fails to finish chores
   7. Has difficulty sustaining attention in tasks or play
   8. Often shifts from one uncompleted activity to another
   9. Has difficulty playing quietly
   10. Often talks excessively
   11. Often interrupts or intrudes on others, e.g., butts into other children's games
   12. Often does not seem to listen to what is being said to him or her
   13. Often loses things necessary for tasks or activities at school or at home (e.g., toys, pencils, books, assignments)
   14. Often engages in physically dangerous activities without considering possible consequences (not for the purpose of thrill seeking), e.g., runs into street without looking

B. The onset of ADHD occurs before the age of 7 years

C. ADHD does not meet the criteria for a pervasive developmental disorder

Modified from Diagnostic and statistical manual of mental disorders, ed 3 rev, Washington DC, 1987, American Psychiatric Association.

*Consider a criterion met only if the behavior is considerably more frequent than that of most persons of the same mental age.

*Diagnostic Criteria for Oppositional Defiant Disorder**

A. A disturbance of at least 6 months' duration during which at least five of the following are present:
   1. Often loses temper
   2. Often argues with adults
   3. Often actively defies or refuses adult requests or rules, e.g., refuses to do chores at home
   4. Often deliberately does things that annoy other people, e.g., grabs other children's hats
   5. Often blames others for his or her own mistakes
   6. Is often touchy or annoyed by others
   7. Is often angry and resentful
   8. Is often spiteful or vindictive
   9. Often swears or uses obscene language

B. Does not meet the criteria for conduct disorder, and disturbance does not occur exclusively during the course of a psychotic disorder, dysthymia, or a major depressive, hypomanic, or manic episode

Modified from Diagnostic and statistical manual of mental disorders, ed 3 rev, Washington, DC, 1987, American Psychiatric Association.

NOTE: The above items are listed in descending order of their discriminating power on the basis of data from a national field trial of the DSM-III-R criteria for disruptive behavior disorders.

*Consider a criterion met only if the behavior is considerably more frequent than that of most people of the same mental age.

by a barrage of complaints about many behaviors and has difficulty sorting out those that contribute to the diagnosis. Therefore it is important to group specific behaviors into broader categories that then may suggest the presence of ADHD: (1) hyperactivity, (2) inattentiveness, and (3) impulsivity. The behaviors that appear to underlie disruptive behavior problems include (1) emotional lability and (2) resistance to conditioning. Finally, poor peer relationships and poor school performance are common consequences of all these traits.

Hyperactivity

Hyperactive children are excessively active even in inherently active situations, especially when they are younger (3 to 10 years of age). For instance, instead of running, they run headlong. Instead of dropping objects, they throw them. They tend to talk excessively. When pursuing activities that require sitting still, such as school work or watching television, they especially stand out as exceptionally restless and fidgety. There also is a difference in the quality of motor behavior. From early in life, children with this condition shift more than usual from one activity to another, apparently as a result of their difficulty or refractoriness in sustaining attention. Parents often say that their child is easily bored, and they may inaccurately attribute this boredom to high intelligence. Studies of highly intelligent children, however, reveal that they usually are exceptionally attentive and persistent.

Inattentiveness

Parents and teachers describe affected children as having a short attention span and being easily distracted. However, they also may observe the ability of these children to con-

Diagnostic Criteria for Conduct Disorder

A. A disturbance of conduct of at least 6 months' duration during which at least three of the following have been present:
   1. Has stolen without confrontation of a victim on more than one occasion (including forgery)
   2. Has run away from home overnight at least twice while living in parental or parental surrogate home (or once without returning)
   3. Often lies (other than to avoid physical or sexual abuse)
   4. Has deliberately engaged in fire setting
   5. Is often truant from school (for older person, absent from work)
   6. Has broken into someone else's house, building, or car
   7. Has deliberately destroyed others' property (other than by fire setting)
   8. Has been physically cruel to animals
   9. Has forced someone into sexual activity
   10. Has used a weapon in more than one fight
   11. Often initiates physical fights
   12. Has stolen with confrontation of a victim (e.g., mugging, purse snatching, extortion, armed robbery)
   13. Has been physically cruel to people

B. If 18 or older, does not meet criteria for antisocial personality disorder

Modified from Diagnostic and statistical manual of mental disorders, ed 3 rev, Washington, DC, 1987, American Psychiatric Association.

Table 63-1 *Subgroups of Attention-Deficit Hyperactivity Disorder**

SUBGROUPS (CLINICAL PATTERNS)	ADDITIONAL FINDINGS
ADHD with disruptive behavior problems	Symptoms of oppositional defiant disorder Symptoms of conduct disorder Emotional lability Resistance to conditioning
ADHD with specific learning disability	Perceptual and cognitive deficits Impaired attention associated with above perceptual and cognitive deficits Underachievement in specific academic skills

*Core traits include inattentiveness, impulsiveness, and hyperactivity.

centrate and "attend" in some situations, typically when the activity is one that the child especially likes. In addition, concentration often is strikingly improved when the child is given individual attention by the teacher or parent. Variability in attention, depending on the surroundings and the nature of the task, also has been found in laboratory investigations of this trait, which leads to speculation that problems with attention are closely related to motivation. In other words, children with this syndrome are less likely to be motivated by tasks that engage the attention of most children their age. Activities that particularly provoke inattention are household chores and classroom work. Because these tasks are not inherently interesting to most children, an important element of motivation in the average child would seem to be fear of punishment or a desire to please. These feelings appear to be deficient in children with ADHD. (See section on resistance to discipline.)

Impulsivity

The younger child with ADHD frequently is described as touching everything or rushing to explore things without concern for likely danger or displeasure from others. In the laboratory these children have difficulty delaying their response to a task and thus make errors based on a failure to reflect. In the classroom, written work frequently is done quickly and erroneously or messily, just to be finished. As they get older, these children frequently get into trouble because they act quickly without thinking of the consequences. Some studies have shown that these children suffer accidental injury more often than peers without ADHD.

Emotional Lability

Many children with this attention disorders tend to experience both positive and negative emotions more intensely and with less provocation than do other children of the same age. Parents and teachers report frequent and poorly controlled temper outbursts and overexcitement in response to new or pleasurable activities. Their more easily provoked and more intense anger, combined with a relative lack of fear, leads to excessive fighting, aggressiveness, and impulsive responses to stimulation. This troublesome trait may be the earliest precursor of antisocial behavior seen later in many adolescents with ADHD. Excessive excitability is perceived as a positive quality by these children. Stimulant medication often subdues this excitability, a result that older children and adolescents dislike. This reaction may account for the resistance to taking medications seen in many older patients.

Resistance to Conditioning

Conditioning refers to the general process of reinforcing desirable behaviors and extinguishing undesirable ones. More commonly, parents and teachers refer to this process as discipline. Many children with attention deficit disorder are, compared with their age-group, more difficult to discipline. One component of this resistance seems to be the relative lack of fear and the desire to please others described earlier.

Misbehavior frequently is repeated, despite punishment. Household chores are avoided, and discipline often is ineffective. Teachers report that these children fail to complete classroom work despite loss of privileges and other punishments. Special behavior modification techniques, consisting of close monitoring and immediate and consistent responses, are required for these children; the average child responds to less intensive measures.

Poor Peer Relationships

All the characteristics already described lead to poor peer relationships. Typically these children are outgoing and eager to make friends. Their impulsive behavior, however, often results in knocking others down or pushing them aside. Their emotional lability results in overreacting to the normal teasing and taunting of children; consequently, others pick on them because they are easily riled. In play, these children often are described as "wanting to be the boss." At the other extreme, in large groups they often allow themselves to be led around. Often these children display social interests that are normal for younger children, a characteristic that also impairs social relationships.

Poor School Performance

All the aforementioned behavioral characteristics interact to produce poor school performance. The most important factor appears to be the lack of motivation to persist in the tiresome and repetitive tasks required of children in the classroom. Despite the lack of attention and failure to complete work, these children often do learn, as indicated by their performance on achievement tests. As they become older, however, lack of persistence begins to affect achievement adversely. Children with ADHD also characteristically approach academic tasks impulsively. Rather than analyze a problem, they typically respond to the component that first attracts their attention or put down any answer just to finish tasks they find tiresome.

Children with these behavioral characteristics also may have specific learning disabilities. If so, academic achievement will, by definition, be poor (see Chapter 67). Some children with ADHD have specific problems with handwriting, including poor spacing between words, irregular size and placement of letters, and slow and awkward letter formation. This difficulty in writing appears to result from coordination deficits, which affect the ability to reproduce language-related written material, in contrast with the ability to draw pictures or copy geometric shapes, which may be normal. Eye-hand coordination also may be normal.

DIAGNOSIS

History

The most important aspect of diagnosis is obtaining a careful history from teachers who know the child well and from parents who are careful observers and have some experience with other children of the same age. If any of these aspects of the history is missing, it should be viewed cautiously, and supplemental information—for example, from relatives or baby-sitters—should be obtained.

It should be emphasized that the behavioral characteristics of this disorder are situationally dependent, meaning that there is an important interaction between the biologically determined disorder and the child's immediate environment. Therefore the task of the physician is vastly complicated because the sought-after, nonbiased observer is nonexistent. Varying information frequently is obtained from teachers and parents describing the same child. Knowing how to synthesize these accounts is part of the art of behavioral evaluation. The clinician should ask about each of the behavioral characteristics of ADHD and adapt the questions to the behavioral repertoire typical of the child's age. For example, inattentiveness in a child of nursery school age might typically be seen in play or when being read to, whereas in 9-year-olds such symptoms are more likely to be noted during classroom work or homework. Since the publication of DSM III and DSM III-R, specific behaviors are listed as criteria for the disorder. These behaviors trigger appropriate relevant questions that are then asked of the parent or the older child. This technique has been employed in developing structured, diagnostic interviews such as the Diagnostic Interview for Children and Adults (DICA)[7] and the Diagnostic Interview Schedule for Children (DISC),[15] developed at the National Institute of Mental Health. The clinician can use the same approach, taking care to confirm that the child shows more of any specific behavior than do other children of the same age. To establish the chronicity of the condition, it should be determined when each behavior first appeared. This information tells the clinician whether the behaviors are more likely an acute response to a stress, such as the birth of a sibling or a divorce, or represent a temperamental profile present since early childhood.

It would not be necessary to depend on parent or teacher perceptions if these behaviors could be objectively measured. Equipment designed to test attention and impulsivity has recently become available to the practitioner, but because of the variability of inattentiveness and impulsivity, depending on the nature of the task and the testing situation, such office-based measurements should be viewed cautiously. No single objective measure reliably indicates the diagnosis in the individual child, although differences between ADHD children as a group and normal children often are seen. Behaviors such as emotional lability and resistance to conditioning are difficult to quantify because manifestations of these behaviors depend on the complexity of interaction between the child and others. The best information comes from observers who spend enough time with the child to study his or her behavior over long periods and under many circumstances. Teacher observations are particularly helpful because the teacher can compare this child with a classroom of other children of the same age. However, if the parents or teacher appear to have a negative or positive bias toward the child, the information obtained from that source should be viewed cautiously.

Questionnaires

Questionnaires that have been standardized (i.e., have been administered to large populations of normal and deviant chil-

Table 63-2 *Conners' Abbreviated Parent-Teacher Questionnaire**

	RATING			
	0 NOT AT ALL	1 JUST A LITTLE	2 PRETTY MUCH	3 VERY MUCH
Behavior				
1. Restless in the "squirmy" sense				
2. Demands must be met immediately				
3. Temper outbursts and unpredictable behavior				
4. Distractibility or attention span is a problem				
5. Disturbs other children				
6. Pouts and sulks				
7. Mood changes quickly and drastically				
8. Restless, always up and on the go				
9. Excitable, impulsive				
10. Fails to finish things that he starts				

From Goyette CH, Conners CK, and Ulrich RF: Normative data on revised Conners parent and teacher rating scales, J Abnorm Child Psychol 6:221, 1978.
*Score by adding the rating for each question. Maximum possible score = 30. Usual score for diagnosis of hyperactivity syndrome = 15 or above.

dren) provide useful supplements to the history. A number of such questionnaires have appeared in recent years, the best being Achenbach's Child Behavior Checklist (CBCL).[1] This questionnaire, however, focuses on a broad range of behaviors, and a profile typical of ADHD has not been validated. One of the most useful questionnaires in the diagnosis and management of ADHD was developed by Conners and revised and standardized in 1978 by Goyette et al.[6] The revised questionnaire comes in a 48-question parent version and a 28-question teacher version. Ten questions common to both are referred to as the Conners' Abbreviated Parent-Teacher Questionnaire and can be scored to produce what is known as the *hyperkinesis index*. The scoring instructions and cut-off scores of these questions are shown in Table 63-2. It should be noted that these 10 questions include items that identify disruptive behaviors and emotional lability. The clinician who uses questionnaires should remember that results can be affected by observer bias and distorted by responders who know little about normal children. Also, they do not provide important information about how long the symptoms have been present.

Neurodevelopmental and Other Testing

The usual neurologic examination is not helpful in making the diagnosis of ADHD. However, a neurologic examination that focuses on skills acquired with development frequently reveals developmental delays that have implications for the diagnosis and management of this disorder. For example, the child's physical coordination often is poor for his or her age. The finding of poor coordination should lead to altered expectations of that child's performance in competitive sports and games. Such altered expectations may help prevent the loss of self-esteem that often results when children begin to compete in these areas during elementary school. Another characteristic finding is that of motor overflow, meaning that the child is less able to inhibit motor activity unrelated to the specific motor skill being examined. For example, hopping on one foot may be accompanied by an excessive amount of associated movements for that age. This finding suggests neurologic immaturity, which many but not all children with ADHD display. The child with ADHD also is frequently inattentive during this type of neurologic examination, providing the physician with a concrete example of the dysfunction characteristic of this syndrome. However, the developmentally oriented neurologic examination requires skill to administer and experience to interpret.

All children suspected of having ADHD should have their vision and hearing tested, because deficits in these primary senses can markedly affect behavior and academic performance. An individually administered IQ test is necessary to establish realistic expectations for learning performance. For children between the ages of 3 and 5 years, the most appropriate test is the Stanford-Binet revised test or the Wechsler Preschool and Primary Scale of Intelligence, Revised (WPPSI-R); after 6 years of age the Wechsler Intelligence Scale for Children, Revised (WISC-R) test, should be used. A physical examination is necessary to rule out other illnesses or disorders that may affect behavior or learning.

PREVALENCE

Results of prevalence studies of ADHD vary widely, depending on the particular method of assessment, the informant (the parent, teacher, child, physician, or some combination of these), and the distribution of ages in the sample. Results of all studies indicate a many-times greater prevalence of ADHD in boys than in girls. Studies that rely solely on a score above the traditional cut-off score of 15 on the Conners' teacher questionnaire yield the highest prevalence rates. For example, an overall rate of 15% was reported in a study in the United States[11] and in a study in Canada,[14] 20.6% and 7.5% for boys and girls, respectively. By contrast, Szatmari et al [13] recently reported, on the basis of a questionnaire tailored to DSM III-R symptom criteria, an overall prevalence of 9% of boys and 3.3% of girls, ages 4 to 16. A diagnosis of ADHD was assigned if questionnaire responses of parent or teacher of children between 4 and 11 years of age, or of parent or youth between the ages of 12 and 16, indicated the presence of a sufficient number of ADHD symptoms. If *both* types of informants for each age-group were required to confirm the diagnosis, the prevalence was much lower. This discrepancy among observers frequently has been noted and creates controversy in establishing a diagnosis (see diagnosis section in this chapter). Yet a third approach was used by Costello,[4] who, on the basis of a structured diagnostic interview (the DISC) conducted with 300 children, ages 7 to 11, and their parents, reported a prevalence of 3.4% of boys and 1.1% of girls. Diagnostic criteria in this study could be achieved on the basis of *either* the parents' or the child's report. The DSM III-R states, conservatively, that "as many as 3% of children" may have ADHD.[3]

ETIOLOGY

Many retrospective studies have demonstrated an increase in behavior disorders, including hyperactivity, after diseases or insults that affect function of the central nervous system (CNS).[19] However, prospective studies that specifically assess ADHD syndrome(s) are lacking. Although there appears to be an association between CNS insult and a hyperactive behavior disorder, such a relationship probably accounts for only a small proportion of children identified with this problem.

Evidence suggests that genetic factors can play an important role in the cause of these problems. Speculations regarding the biologic mechanism underlying genetic causation center on dysfunctions in monoamine neurotransmitters active in the limbic brain and the reticular activating system. It has been proposed that the site of CNS dysfunction may be the frontal lobe; this is an attractive thesis because it may help explain the great variability in symptoms in any one child from day to day and from situation to situation.[21]

NATURAL HISTORY AND PROGNOSIS

ADHD usually is detected during the elementary school years. Hyperactivity, as described in this chapter, persists but changes in quality as the child enters adolescence. For example, activity level diminishes and the ability to concentrate improves. However, when these traits are compared with those of matched control subjects, they still are present, although less prominently and disruptively.[17] Antisocial and acting-out behaviors are more pronounced at this age. Emotional immaturity becomes more of a concern to adults, probably because it is a more distressing symptom during adolescence. School performance often is worse because close supervision of academic work diminishes, which increases the adolescent's failure to complete work, resulting in an adverse effect on achievement. In addition, a cumulative effect occurs as a result of a prolonged period of failure to complete work and practice skills. Adolescents are particularly vulnerable to low self-esteem and problems in peer relations, and these are exacerbated in individuals whose ADHD symptoms were not recognized and treated earlier in development. These problems may manifest in adolescence as poor social skills, lack of friends, feelings of not being liked, low self-confidence, frequent fighting, and in some cases, delinquent behavior.

Prospective longitudinal studies of persons diagnosed in childhood as having ADHD reveal that approximately 50% continue to have disabling symptoms of the disorder as young adults that continue to merit the diagnosis.[5,18] Approximately 25%, including some individuals in the persistent ADHD group, exhibit antisocial behavior such as lying, stealing, and aggressive outbursts of the type characteristic of adult antisocial personality disorder. More than half the individuals in this second group also are substance abusers.[5] Persons who do not qualify for diagnosis may experience continued concentration difficulties, distractibility, or restlessness; however, in this group these problems do not interfere significantly with daily functioning.

Follow-up research[16] has revealed that the long-term prognosis in ADHD is better for those children with higher IQs and for those from families of higher socioeconomic status. On the other hand, the triad of aggression, emotional instability, and low frustration tolerance in the child and the presence of a psychopathologic condition in the parent (especially antisocial behavior) have been associated with poor long-term outcome. The impact of pharmacologic and psychosocial treatments on the long-term outcome of ADHD is a subject of continuing investigation.

TREATMENT

ADHD is a complex behavioral syndrome stemming from biologic differences but influenced by environmental factors and the child's underlying temperament. Treatment should be multifaceted in recognition of the importance of biologic and environmental factors. The physician should be competent in the management of medication, especially because only the physician is legally empowered and medically trained to prescribe drugs. However, it is a mistake for the physician to rely exclusively on medication for the treatment of this disorder. Some physicians will wish to pursue aspects of psychological management; others will not. At the very least the physician should coordinate care with special educators and mental health professionals.

Medication

CNS stimulant medication has a striking beneficial effect on behavior in 60% to 80% of children with ADHD. In those children with ADHD and ODD or conduct disorder, stimulant medication often improves all aspects of the disorder. Not only does activity become less frenetic and more goal directed but children also begin to concentrate more and complete their work. Their emotions are less labile, their resistance to discipline is reduced, and the parents may report, for instance, that a scolding, which previously would have been ignored, now produces tears.

The effects of stimulant medication on academic performance are less clear. The problem of visual and auditory perception that is characteristic of a learning disability appears to be unaffected. Handwriting, however, often improves. A short-term improvement in mathematics performance frequently is seen, presumably because learning mathematics particularly depends on the ability to concentrate. Follow-up studies to date have not demonstrated beneficial effects of stimulant medication on long-term academic or occupational outcome. It may be that medication must be combined with other treatment modalities, such as remedial tutoring and

Table 63-3 *Guidelines for Use of Stimulant Medication in Children with Attention-Deficit Hyperactivity Disorder*

MEDICATION	STARTING AMOUNT PER DOSE	SUGGESTED INCREMENTS	DOSES* PER DAY	TIME OF ADMINISTRATION
Methylphenidate (Ritalin)	0.3 mg/kg	0.15 mg/kg	2 or 3	8 AM, noon, 4 PM
Ritalin-SR† (sustained release)	20 mg		1	8 AM
Dextroamphetamine (Dexedrine)				
Tablets	0.15 mg/kg	0.08 mg/kg	2 or 3	8 AM, noon, 4 PM
Spansules	7 yr and younger: 5 mg 8 yr and older: 10 mg	5 mg	1	8 AM
Pemoline (Cylert)	7 yr and younger: 37.5 mg 8 yr and older: 75 mg	18.75 mg	1‡	8 AM‡

*Suggested starting dose of methylphenidate and dextroamphetamine (mg/kg) refers to amount per dose. Amount per day is greater, depending on frequency of administration.

†The sustained-release form of methylphenidate is available, but only in a 20-mg size. If the child's total daily dose is close to 20 mg, this form may be used.

‡Some physicians give an additional dose at 4 PM, 18.75 mg in younger children (7 yr and younger), and 37.5 mg in older children (8 yr and older).

Side Effects of Stimulant Medication

1. Often noted at appropriate doses:
   a. Appetite reduction
   b. Difficulty falling asleep
   c. Pallor
2. Indicates overdose or an adverse response:
   a. Social withdrawal
   b. "Dazed" appearance
   c. Tics or stereotypic movements (if new; or if increased in severity)
   d. Increased irritability and depression

social skills training, to reverse both the primary and secondary deficit associated with ADHD.

Treatment Management

Although many attempts have been made, it has proved impossible to predict which patients will respond favorably to stimulant medication. Therefore, once ADHD is diagnosed and contraindications to medication have been ruled out, a trial of stimulant medication should be arranged. Parents, who often are fearful of psychopharmacologic medications, may be reassured by a trial of medication preceding any decision to pursue long-term treatment. The most frequently used medications, suggested starting doses, and frequency of administration are listed in Table 63-3. The effect of short-acting stimulants usually is immediate, but at least 4 days should pass before the dose is adjusted. If no response is seen at the end of 4 days, the dose should be increased gradually, and each new dosage level should be maintained for 4 to 7 days until a favorable response is seen or significant side effects develop. The accompanying box contains a list of side effects that can be expected and managed and those that indicate that the dose is too high and should be decreased. Once an appropriate dose is established, treatment should continue for at least 1 month to determine the effects on behavior both at school and at home. If significant side effects are seen before benefits are noted, the medication trial should be terminated. Some side effects, however, may subside with time. These often can be managed by adjusting the timing of medication or by changing the time of meals to reduce interference with sleeping or eating.

Contraindications to a trial of medication in the treatment of ADHD are few. First, medication should not be prescribed if there are strong indications that the patient or members of the family will abuse these drugs. The physician who is uncertain if such abuse has taken place should keep a record of the number of pills prescribed and their rate of use to detect any overuse. Explanations that pills have been "lost" should be viewed skeptically. Second, the physician should be reluctant to prescribe medication for children younger than 5 years of age. Beneficial effects have been noted in children at this age, but side effects often are more severe. Also, the diagnosis is more difficult to establish at this age because hyperactive-like behaviors are typical of 2- to 5-year-old children and behavior changes rapidly during this period of development. It is reasonable to delay pharmacologic treatment at this age inasmuch as the child interacts primarily with the parents who, with appropriate help, can learn to manage difficult behavior. In extreme cases medication should be considered. Most pediatricians should refer for more specialized consultation. Third, drug treatment should be delayed in adolescent patients who deny the need for medication and indicate their intention not to comply. Such patients need time to accept the use of drugs for their problem and a treatment approach that will persuade them of the potential benefits of medication. Finally, if the child has any symptoms of Tourette syndrome, stimulants should not be used, and a special evaluation, usually by a neurologist or psychiatrist, should be obtained. Children who come from a family with a strong history of Tourette syndrome but have no evidence of the disorder can be treated with caution.

If the child's behavior improves substantially with medication, treatment should continue until trial periods off the drug indicate that it may no longer be helpful. Children will benefit most if medication is administered regularly, including weekends and holidays, because the behaviors favorably affected by stimulants pose problems for the child at home and at play, as well as at school. Skipping just one or two doses usually will result in an obvious return of problem behaviors such as emotional lability, restless inattention, and resistance to discipline. If, however, missed doses fail to result in deterioration, the medication could be discontinued on weekends or holidays; if no significant deterioration is noted with this type of intermittent administration, a trial period without medication is warranted. Such a trial should last at least 2 weeks because some children show deterioration at first but then improve over time, and others show no change at first but then gradually lose the ability to control their behavior. Medication can be discontinued when a trial of 2 to 3 months off the stimulant results in no substantial behavioral deterioration.

Once medication is begun, if beneficial effects are followed by a gradual worsening of behavior (usually over the first few weeks of treatment), the dose should be increased gradually, because frequently an initial drug tolerance occurs.

When stimulant medication proves helpful, this treatment often is continued for several years. Such children should be seen by the health care provider periodically, at least every 3 to 4 months. The aim of these visits is (1) to monitor the continued need for medication, (2) to assess side effects, and (3) to review the child's and family's understanding and management of drug-related issues.

There is no sudden change in the child's response to stimulants when he or she reaches adolescence. If the adolescent continues to have problems, medication still may be helpful. Particular attention, however, needs to be paid to the adolescent patient's perception of the need for medication. If the youngster understands that medication is for his or her benefit rather than for the benefit of others, compliance will be improved.

Psychological Factors

Attention should be given to the psychological aspects of pharmacologic treatment. Physicians usually discuss the proposed treatment with parents but often fail to include the child in age-appropriate discussions. It is most helpful to explain to children that medications will be given to see whether it helps them control some of their behavior. Without such an explanation, children often perceive that medication is given for the benefit of their parents and teachers because it "makes me be good." This perception is reinforced when adults (or siblings) ask whether the child has remembered to take the medication or administer medication immediately after an episode of misbehavior. Parents should be advised to avoid this response and also to coach siblings and teachers to respond appropriately. If misbehavior reminds the adult that a dose has been missed, the medication should not be administered until the episode of misbehavior has passed.

Growth

The effects of stimulant medication on growth has been raised as a potential contraindication to continued therapy. It has been clearly established that some children show weight loss or a decrease in the rate of weight gain, which may be followed after a period of 6 months to a year by a decrement in the rate of increase in height. This effect on growth varies a great deal from child to child but appears to be most pronounced in children who are large to begin with. It also is clear that discontinuing medication results in catch-up growth. It is not known, however, whether these short-term changes result in any change in long-term growth potential. For example, studies of stature in adults who were treated with stimulant medications for ADHD in childhood do not show deviations from population norms. Also, one study suggested that a return to normal growth rates occurs after prolonged treatment with stimulants. It has been assumed that this effect on growth is due to decreased appetite and resultant weight loss. This causal mechanism, however, has not been established, and there is some evidence to suggest a direct effect of these medications on hormones such as somatomedin and prolactin.

In the absence of evidence for any impact on ultimate stature and because such an impact, if there is one, is likely to be small, it seems prudent to monitor growth carefully, adjust timing of medication and meals to minimize weight loss, and if severe short-term effects on growth are seen, discontinue medication during less stressful periods—that is, the summer. It also may be prudent to use a medication other than stimulants—for example, neuroleptics—when ADHD is seen in a child with significant, preexisting growth problems.

Diet

The notion that sugar and artificial food additives can precipitate or exacerbate hyperactivity in children has been popularized by the media and tenaciously supported by parents who report having observed food-related behavior changes in their children. In a book entitled *Why Your Child Is Hyperactive,* published in 1975, Benjamin Feingold originated the idea that artificial coloring, artificial flavoring, antioxidant preservatives, and all salicylates produce hyperactivity and learning disabilities in children. He claimed that eliminating these substances in the diet would dramatically improve the behavior of 60% of affected children. Controlled research has largely failed to substantiate these claims.[20] The hypothesis that sugar intake contributes to hyperactive behavior also has received little support in research.[12] A recent exception is a well-conducted dietary-replacement study[9] in which artificial additives were eliminated *and* the intake of simple sugars was reduced by 50%. On the basis of parental report on the Conners' questionnaire, the behavior of 50% of the 24 children in the study was reliably improved. This study awaits replication and determination of which dietary alteration was responsible for the behavioral results.

In the absence of research validation of the purported negative effects of food additives and sugar on behavior, it is valid to consider other explanations of the popularity of the dietary approach and parental claims of its effectiveness. First, the diet offers a relatively simple explanation of the cause of the child's problems and an easily effected treatment. Second, and more important, it offers an explanation that is external to the child and therefore releases the child from blame for his or her misbehavior and the parents from frustration and guilt over their possible contribution to the problem. As a result there may be a significant reduction in the tension between parent and child and a significant increase in positive attention toward the child, both of which may bring about marked improvement in the child's behavior. This, of course, may be misperceived by the parent as a direct response to the dietary change.

In response to parents' inquiries about dietary treatment, the physician should be truthful about the status of the scientific evidence. Some families will pursue this form of treatment anyway; if so, they may be reassured that the Feingold diet is safe and that reduction in sugar intake may be beneficial from the perspective of reducing risk for dental caries and obesity. Any improvement, even if based on psychological factors, is desirable, as long as the family continues to pursue other recommended treatment and the child does not rebel against the dietary restrictions.

Behavioral Management

The behavior of children with ADHD is difficult to manage. Resistance to discipline, combined with emotional lability, leads to emotionally charged acts of disobedience. The inattention (or lack of motivation) and emotional immaturity result in failure to complete tasks. When the child is pushed to perform, emotional outbursts are frequent. Inattention and impulsive responses to stimulation often result in unintentional, destructive behaviors. Unless adults are able to manage these problems effectively, their frustration leads to negative feelings toward the child, which ultimately contribute to the child's low self-esteem. Therefore all parents of children with ADHD should learn to recognize the source of the child's misbehavior and how to manage it effectively. Behavior modification techniques should be regularly used, and the parents should learn to focus on preventing misbehavior. Finally, emphatic and clear communication between parent and child is especially important.

Parents should be referred to a program that will train them in behavioral management and communication skills. Unfortunately, this type of training is not well reimbursed by health insurance plans. Another problem is that mental health professionals, who often are involved in such programs, might not understand the interaction between biologic and psychological factors—an understanding necessary for effective management of ADHD. For example, it is helpful for parents to understand not only the psychodynamic determinants of the child's behavior ("He got angry when teased by his sister") but also the biologic or temperamental determinants ("He gets angry more easily than other boys his age, and it takes longer for him to control that anger"). Without this perspective, parents come to feel that they are responsible for all their child's misbehavior and they may drop out of behavior management training. Therefore practitioners should identify professionals in the community who are skilled in providing behavior management counseling and who understand the biologic contribution to these syndromes. They also should become skilled in persuading parents of the need for this kind of therapy. Parents may resist referral that focuses on them when they perceive that the problem is with the child. They should be advised that special skills, beyond those possessed by most parents, are needed to manage these children effectively.

Behavior management training is best begun just after the medication trial has been effected, because the therapist, parents, and child then know the effect that stimulants will have on specific behaviors, a factor that helps clarify the relationship between psychological and biologic determinants. This also allows the therapist to concentrate on those behaviors that are unaffected by medication. It also is helpful for the child to become aware of medication effects. A child who becomes aware, for example, of greater control over emotional responses as an effect of medication also may become aware of his or her low frustration tolerance in the absence of medication and the need to learn to cope with it.

Cognitive behavioral therapy is a variant of behavior therapy in which the focus is on the patient's habitual thoughts or "self-talk" as they relate to clinical problems. Attempts have been made by means of this approach to teach children to self-monitor, self-pace, and self-instruct to achieve greater self-control in academic and social situations; however, this type of intervention is not effective in children with ADHD.

Special Education

Many children with ADHD also show signs of learning disability (see beginning of this chapter). The association between ADHD and learning disability is sufficiently frequent that both disorders should be assessed. If a learning disability is present, special education either in the form of a resource room or special class placement for the learning disability should be considered. The child with ADHD and a learning disability may be much more amenable to special education approaches if medication is prescribed and it helps control inattentiveness and impulsivity.

The child with ADHD also needs special help in the school setting. Unfortunately, however, ADHD is not considered a handicapping condition according to federal guidelines (Public Law 94-142). The educational system recognizes "emotional handicap," and some children with ADHD are placed, often inappropriately, into such classes. What is appropriate is a behavior-modification approach to behavioral problems and to cognitive skills. Within this model the psychologist serves as a consultant who helps the teacher develop and implement a behavioral program tailored to the child's needs. Generally such programs include close monitoring and frequent reinforcement for on-task behavior, accurate completion of assigned work, and appropriate participation in class activities.

Psychotherapy

The symptoms characteristic of ADHD frequently are viewed as arising from emotional conflict as a result of experiences that are stressful to the child. This analysis of causality then leads to recommendations for individual psychotherapy. Genetic data and the effects of stimulant medication, however, suggest that biologic factors play a key role. Therefore, a different approach to psychotherapy has developed out of the recognition that, in ADHD, biology and experience interact to produce emotional symptoms. Children with ADHD typically come to feel inadequate, in part because they cannot do things (e.g., schoolwork and athletics) as well as others their age. In part, they come to view the anger and frustration displayed by parents, teachers, and peers as personally threatening to themselves. The preoccupation with themes of violence in the drawings of children with ADHD and their choice of television shows and stories seem to provide ways of compensating for a sense of vulnerability. These psychological issues, which develop as reactions to their perception of the environment, may best be dealt with in psychotherapy. Children with ADHD need to acquire insight not only regarding their own conflicts and sources of stress but also concerning their temperament. Learning to recognize how medication changes inner experience and outward behavior is part of this process.

Other adjunctive therapies may help the child with social skills training, which typically is conducted in a group and may help the child by modeling and reinforcing appropriate interpersonal behaviors. Family therapy can help address the many strains on family functioning imposed by the child with ADHD. Siblings, for example, who may feel that their needs are being overlooked because of the attention given to the "problem" child, often welcome the opportunity to express these feelings in a supportive context. Marital therapy is indicated when the child's behavior has resulted in deterioration of the marital relationship. Finally, individual psychotherapy may help parents with low self-esteem who often view their child's misbehavior as personally directed toward them. This usually is indicated by a persistently negative reaction toward the child, despite appropriate explanation to the parents of the origins of the child's behavior.

REFERENCES

1. Achenbach TM and Edelbrock CS: Manual for the child behavior checklist and revised child behavior profile, Burlington, Vt, 1988, University Associates in Psychiatry.
2. American Psychiatric Association: Diagnostic and statistical manual of mental disorders, ed 3, Washington, DC, 1980, The Association.
3. American Psychiatric Association: Diagnostic and statistical manual of mental disorder, ed 3 rev, Washington, DC, 1987, The Association.
4. Costello EJ: Child psychiatric disorders and their correlates: a primary care pediatric sample, J Am Acad Child Adolesc Psychiatry 28:851, 1989.
5. Gittleman R et al: Hyperactive boys almost grow-up. I. Psychiatric status, Arch Gen Psychiatry 42:937, 1985.
6. Goyette CH, Conners CK, and Ulrich RF: Normative data on revised Conners parent and teacher rating scales, J Abnorm Child Psychol 6:221, 1978.
7. Herjanic B and Reich W: Development of a structured psychiatric interview for children: agreement between child and parent on individual symptoms, J Abnorm Child Psychol 10:307, 1982.
8. Holobrow PL and Berry PS: Hyperactivity and learning difficulties, J Learning Disabilities 19:426, 1986.
9. Kaplan B et al: Dietary replacement in preschool-aged hyperactive boys, Pediatrics 83:7, 1989.
10. Lambert NM and Sandoval J: The prevalence of learning disabilities in a sample of children considered hyperactive, J Abnorm Child Psychol 8:33, 1980.
11. Langsdorff R et al: Ethnicity, social class and perception of hyperactivity, Psychol Schools 16:293, 1979.
12. Milich R, Wolraich ML, and Lindgren S: Sugar and hyperactivity: a critical review of empirical findings, Clin Psychol Rev 6:493, 1986.
13. Szatmari P, Offord DR, and Boyle MH: Ontario child health study: prevalence of attention deficit disorder with hyperactivity, J Child Psychol Psychiatry 30:219, 1989.
14. Trites RL et al: Prevalence of hyperactivity, J Pediatric Psychol 4:179, 1979.
15. Weinstein SR et al: Comparison of DISC with clinicians' DSM-III diagnoses in psychiatric inpatients, J Am Acad Child Adolesc Psychiatry 28:53, 1989.
16. Weiss G and Hechtman L: Hyperactive children grow up, New York, The Guilford Press, 1986.
17. Weiss G et al: Studies on the hyperactive child. VIII. Five-year follow-up, Arch Gen Psychiatry 24:409, 1971.
18. Weiss G et al: Psychiatric status of hyperactive as adults: a controlled prospective 15 years follow-up of 63 hyperactive children, J Am Acad Child Adolesc Psychiatry 24:211, 220, 1985.
19. Wender EH: Minimal brain dysfunction in children, New York, 1971, Wiley Interscience.
20. Wender EH: The food-additive-free-diet in the treatment of behavior disorders: a review, J Dev Behav Pediatr 7:35, 1986.
21. Zametkin AJ and Rappaport JL: Neurobiology of attention deficit disorder with hyperactivity: where have we come in 50 years? J Am Acad Child Adolesc Psychiatry 26:676, 1987.

64

Dealing with Common Classroom Behavioral Problems

Thomas J. Long

Problems that school-age children have invariably manifest themselves in the classroom, if only because that is where children spend so much of their time. These problems thus become classroom behavioral problems. They can include aggressive behavior, attention deficit disorders, daydreaming, hyperactivity, hypochondriasis, lying, self-stimulating behaviors, stealing, temper tantrums, unacceptable language, and withdrawal. A child's classroom behavior will also be affected if he or she is anxious, has adverse eating habits, suffers from encopresis or enuresis, has imaginary playmates, or is a nail-biter or thumb-sucker.

Not all classroom behavioral problems come to the attention of the physician with equal frequency. Some, such as hypochondriasis, are common among adolescents and adults but rare among young children. Others, such as depression, which has been thought to occur in preadolescent children only rarely, now appear to be on the rise. Incidences of suicide attempts associated with depression in children as young as 2½ years old have been reported, and many professionals see the rise in depression and suicide among school-age children as cause for great alarm.

Because of the multiplicity of behavioral problems that can be evidenced by school-age children and the frequent need for a detailed history when such problems exist, primary care providers should routinely solicit information about all their school-age patients from the classroom teacher. Such information could be conveniently sought for all students, perhaps at the end of each school year or at least at the end of each student's first year of each major school change (to elementary, middle, and high school). Such information should certainly be sought for those evidencing classroom behavioral or learning difficulties as soon as the problem is evident.

This book focuses on the identification and collaborative management of four common classroom behavior patterns: unacceptable language; aggressive, resistant behavior; inhibited, withdrawn behavior; and attention deficit-hyperactivity disorder. The first three of these behaviors are discussed in this chapter; the fourth is addressed in Chapter 63.

UNACCEPTABLE LANGUAGE

When most children reach 3 or 4 years of age, they go through a period of using "bathroom" words, usually to insult one another or to be funny. Such behavior should be considered part of normal development. In such instances parents are advised to ignore such antics, which will run their course in time. If parents become anxious at their child's continued use of such language, a second strategy is to mimic the child's behavior to remove its shock value. Suggesting that the parent say back to the child "ca-ca, poo-poo" with a smile can make the phrase less powerful, unless this is the only time the parent responds to the child. Punishing a child for what is common behavior produces adverse results. Parents should never do more than tell the child to stop, if the behavior is not desired.

When children enter school, they learn slang expressions and swear words, often knowing that such words are unacceptable even before they know what these expressions mean. To appear grown up, they will use these so-called dirty words at home and at school. Parents are often shocked, and teachers sometimes take such language personally. Rather than reinforce the behavior by expressing horror or by punishing the child, it is best to help extinguish such behavior by not responding to it. School-age children often want to elicit the shock value of such words and, if reinforced, will continue using them. Threats or punishments will usually only cause the child to use the language elsewhere.

It goes without saying that if parents and teachers do not want such language used, they should not use it themselves. Children learn the language used by adults who are significant to them. These adults can and should tell children, calmly and firmly, that most people do not use such language and that they would prefer that the child not use it either.

If the child is using unacceptable language in an aggressive way, the language should be treated as though it were aggression. However, ordinarily the use of undesirable language is a problem of learning and habit. Children will normally use language that produces the effect they desire or that expresses exactly what they want to express. As they learn the meaning of slang and swear words and how their use affects others, they will use them to produce a desired effect. Thus children should be taught socially acceptable words that help them express what they want.

AGGRESSIVE, RESISTANT BEHAVIOR

Normal aggression stems from a child's need to feel important and control others. Children also use aggression to let it be known that they are persons in their own right. However, the child who is constantly aggressive is motivated by factors other than a natural desire to be recognized and to control.

A child might be mildly aggressive by being negative or disobedient. Stronger aggressive behavior includes lying or stealing. Extreme aggression involves revenge and harm to others. Such extreme aggression is usually physical, such as fighting and being cruel, destroying property, vandalizing, or setting fires; but when these acts are restricted by the parents or others, the child's aggression may be evidenced through words or glances.

Excessive aggression is often caused by the child's reaction to parental overindulgence or to parental overprotection associated with their rejection of the child or by the child's reaction to unfair or severe punishment.

How to handle a child's aggressive behavior is a common question. The most straightforward answer is that such behavior is to be immediately terminated when it endangers the child or others or threatens serious damage to property. However, mishandling the child causes aggressive behavior to continue. Permitting aggressive reactions in children to gain advantages for them simply reinforces the undesirable behavior and can produce unnecessary anxiety. Unchecked aggressive behavior in children, especially when directed against themselves or a loved one, can produce the fear in the children that there is no limit to the extent of their destructive ability.

In assessing the normality or abnormality of aggressive behavior, the following should be considered: (1) the frequency and duration of the occurrence, (2) the circumstances eliciting the behavior, (3) the form of the behavior, (4) the appropriateness of the behavior for the situation, and (5) the object against which the aggression is directed. As with hyperactivity, both the parents and the teacher can help the physician determine how severe the problem is and arrive at an appropriate diagnosis. It is most helpful to have descriptions of the circumstances surrounding the episodes of aggression against which to apply the preceding considerations. Acting-out behavior is almost always an interactive process, and descriptions of actual episodes can help in understanding second-party contributions to such behavior.

Parents and teachers sometimes help establish patterns of undesirable behavior by unwittingly rewarding it. A child who is behaving well may never be noticed but may be quickly scolded when acting out. The child, preferring negative attention to no attention, learns to continue the behavior for which some attention is obtained. A physician coming to understand the interactive elements of a child's acting out might gain a clue regarding how a change might best be managed.

Acting-out behavior is best corrected by implementing a reward system for desired behavior rather than punishing the undesirable behavior. Punishment, itself aggressive, usually causes the child to cease the unwanted behavior in the presence of the punisher rather than to adopt the appropriate behavior.

A system of well-planned rules and regulations is necessary for controlling behavior. A good rule must (1) serve a useful purpose, (2) be understandable, (3) apply to behavior that is under the child's control, (4) be enforceable, and (5) have a stated consequence if violated. Rules must be applied to clear-cut situations, times, and places.

To improve a child's behavior over time, one should have a consistent program that reinforces desired behavior matched with one that controls unacceptable behavior, without reinforcing it, and a clear set of rules. For such a program to operate effectively, help is needed from the adults with whom the child spends the major portion of the day. Teachers are generally well educated in principles of behavior modification and contingency management. They may also help manage the child at school and work with the parents in home management. It may also be useful to invite the teacher to meet with the physician and the child's parents so that he or she might be better able to coordinate any remedial activities more effectively. A coordinated approach will go a long way in assisting children to gain control over their behavior. Physicians should periodically request follow-up information after the treatment or program has been initiated.

INHIBITED, WITHDRAWN BEHAVIOR

Withdrawal reactions range from mild and occasional shyness to continued avoidance of contact with others. Shyness is not in and of itself pathologic. Follow-up studies of shy children have demonstrated that the shy child, although tending toward shyness during adulthood, does not necessarily manifest adult symptoms of maladjustment. When shy children become adults, they tend to select occupations that offer security and shelter and to marry more outgoing partners. However, given an opportunity to develop their own style, they seem to adjust well to adulthood.

Withdrawal reactions can also be expressions of a child's feelings of helplessness and a safe way to avoid situations that might lead to disparagement or that might demand effort. Such reactions are also self-punitive, since they sustain immaturity and provide no resolution of the child's difficulties.

Signs of withdrawal reactions include excessive crying, isolation, fear, no observable distress or anxiety when threatened with loss of love, and interrupted sleep, nightmares, or sleepwalking after what might be considered a well-controlled demeanor during the day.

Withdrawn children might be quiet, obedient, and undemanding and are often considered "good" and thus not the subject of teachers' complaints. These are children about whom the physician should be concerned, regardless of whether he or she receives complaints. Early identification of children with these problems can be aided by regular descriptive reports of child behavior accumulated at some central location.

Babies who do not protest unfavorable circumstances or who seem to accept them might do so because of damage to the central nervous system. A psychotic child or one with severe auditory processing problems might be recognized by symptoms of isolation, inappropriate affect, uncommon reactions to common stimuli, or extreme difficulty in communication.

With school-age children, especially those with a history of good adjustment and perhaps those who appear to "overconform" and tend toward perfectionism, the onset of a serious pathologic disorder might be gradual, with a progressive loss of interest in people and normal pursuits. Excessive preoccupation with certain abstract subjects and a marked drop in school performance might also be noted.

The shy child who is also evidencing some difficulties in

learning, who repeatedly avoids situations that are "upsetting," who demonstrates few interests, and who garners few friends might be helped in school by a program geared to elevating self-confidence. The teacher can assist a mildly withdrawn child by graduating work to ensure repeated success in school, establishing forums in which the child can experience positive peer interactions, and treating the child kindly rather than harshly.

When withdrawal is a major symptom, the child should be referred to a mental health specialist. When referring such a child, the primary care physician should share some specific observations of the child's behavior with the mental health specialist. These observations should be elicited from parents and school personnel, be gleaned over time, cover many settings, and be as detailed as possible. Every effort should be made to determine whether the withdrawn behavior is situation specific or diffuse. Behavior observed exclusively in the office does not yield sufficient information for referral.

Therapeutic treatment for children with severe withdrawal reactions, whether carried out by a psychiatrist, psychologist, or social worker, will generally focus on the family. Therapy with children is usually aimed at facilitating their learning to accept and express their emotions in the presence of an understanding adult while the offending environment is being realigned. Treatment of the severely withdrawn child has often meant hospitalization and long-term therapy.

SUGGESTED READINGS

1. Carey WB. The difficult Child. *Pediatrics in Review* 8:39, 1986.
2. Dworkin PH. School failure. *Pediatrics in Review* 10:301, 1989.
3. Palfrey JS, Rappaport LA. School placement. *Pediatrics in Review* 8:261, 1987.
4. Wright GF, Nader PR. Schools as milieux. In *Developmental-Behavioral Pediatrics,* eds. Levine MD, Carey WB, Crocker AC, Gross RT. Phila: Saunders, 1983.

65

The Chronically Ill and Disabled Child in School

Linda J. Juszczak and Marcie B. Scheider

It is estimated that 10% to 40% of children have a chronic health problem; the wide range in estimates is due to differing definitions of chronic illness.[6] These school-aged children and adolescents with physical handicaps, chronic illnesses, or long-term transient health problems have the same basic educational and developmental needs as their healthy peers. Well-organized and collaborative efforts among school personnel, health professionals, and families will enhance the education and development of chronically ill and disabled children and should be the basis by which their needs are addressed in the school.

There is wide variation in how special education laws are put into practice by school systems. The need for chronically ill and disabled children to participate in educational programs appropriate for their abilities in the "least restrictive" physical setting possible is mandated by the Education For All Children Act of 1975 (Public Law 94-142). This law, which went into effect in 1977, defines as handicapped those children who are mentally retarded, hearing impaired, deaf, speech impaired, visually handicapped, seriously emotionally disturbed, orthopedically impaired, and multihandicapped and those with specific learning disabilities. As a result of this law, an individualized education program (IEP) that outlines the special education and related services the child needs and will receive must be prepared for each child identified as handicapped. Chronically ill and disabled children whose educational performance is negatively affected by their illness are clearly eligible for special education and related services under Public Law 94-142. It is less evident to what extent services should be provided for those children whose health problems may require support services but who are able to function in a regular classroom.

PROBLEMS OF CHRONICALLY ILL AND DISABLED CHILDREN IN SCHOOL

School is important not only for a child's acquisition of academic skills but for its function as a major socialization experience. Further, the school-related problems and concerns that all children have can be exacerbated for a child with a chronic illness or disability. For example, the child's medical condition may necessitate frequent and occasionally long absences, illness and medications may affect cognitive functioning and physical endurance, and physical limitations may restrict participation in school activities. These obstacles, combined with unreasonable expectations of teachers and parents and social isolation from their peers, can contribute to missed opportunities for academic achievement, psychosocial development, and vocational placement.

Medical Issues

The medical problems of children with chronic illness and disabilities are diverse. Frequent questions asked by school personnel regarding the effects of a child's health problem include restrictions on physical activity; delineation of medications and their side effects; need for special diet, preferential seating, counseling, special equipment, or toileting assistance; need for physical, occupational, or speech therapy; guidelines for emergency situations; prognosis; and the child's understanding of his or her disability.[9]

Examples of common health problems that require guidelines for participation activities include asthma, seizure disorders, and heart conditions. Children with asthma may require medication in order to exercise. Provided wheezing is controlled, they should be allowed to participate in all sports. Recommendations for patients with seizure disorders are that children with petit mal, psychomotor, or frequent seizures should refrain from contact sports. Children with well-controlled, generalized seizures may participate in contact sports, although they should be encouraged to participate to a greater extent in noncontact sports. Children with heart murmurs should have medical clearance to participate in sports. In most cases the diagnosis of an innocent murmur can be made by a primary care provider; those with innocent murmurs can participate fully in sports. The cardiac diagnoses that may preclude participation in collision or contact sports include mitral stenosis, aortic stenosis, aortic insufficiency, coarctation of the aorta, cyanotic heart disease, and recent carditis.[1]

For infectious diagnoses such as tuberculosis or hepatitis, clear precautions and rules for school attendance exist. Acquired immunodeficiency syndrome (AIDS) is an infectious disease that is spread only through *intimate* contact. Although children with AIDS cannot spread the disease through casual contact in school, the subject of children with AIDS attending school remains emotional and controversial. The last policy statement from the American Academy of Pediatrics Task Force on Pediatric AIDS on the issue of school attendance for children with AIDS states that these children should be "admitted freely to all [school] activities, to the extent that their own health permits."[8]

Clearly, most health problems do not require severe activity restrictions. Participation in physical education programs should not be denied because of overprotectiveness or imagined liability restrictions but rather encouraged. Schools are protected by insurance against injuries that occur during sports participation and thus are covered if a chronically ill child who is medically cleared to participate in a sport sustains a sports-related injury. The focus in the classroom and in recreation programs should be on what these children can do as opposed to what they cannot do. This emphasis assists in the child's development of a positive self-image, respect from peers, and a sense of independence.

School Achievement

Although many children with chronic illnesses and disabilities are of normal intelligence, they may not achieve as well as their healthy peers in school.[2,7] Several factors, including the economic, physical, emotional, and intellectual status of the child, contribute to this decreased achievement. Children with chronic illnesses and disabilities may have limited physical endurance. If they must take a 2-hour test but tire within 1 hour, they will not score up to their potential. If endurance is taken into consideration and the test is given in two 1-hour blocks, the children would have a better opportunity to score at their best level. These children frequently miss extended periods of school. The absence rate is reportedly highest among teenagers.[4] Reasons for absence may include physical fatigue or acute physical illness that requires physician visits and/or hospitalization. In most states, special education departments require that children be hospitalized for longer than 2 weeks to be eligible for tutoring. Obviously, if they are hospitalized multiple times for fewer than 2-week intervals, they will miss a great deal of schooling. Those hospitalized for a 3-week period will receive only 1 week of tutoring.

A child's anxiety about a disability and its complications may contribute to diminished academic performance in chronically ill children. A large, but not easily measurable, factor is the expectations of parents and teachers. Lack of knowledge regarding an illness or anxiety about a child's potentially unstable medical condition may lead to lower expectations for academic performance, unnecessary restrictions, and tolerance of inappropriate social behavior. The child, in turn, may increasingly use the illness for secondary gain, which further compounds the problem. This cycle may begin at an early age and may contribute to lowered self-esteem and the child's low expectations of his or her own performance.[5,9,10]

Health professionals can contribute significantly to improving attitudes toward the child's abilities. It is hoped that attitudes can be changed by educating parents and school staff members about the child's assets and strengths, as well as his or her limitations. Testing opportunities can be changed to ensure an opportunity for optimal test-taking situations in keeping with the disabled child's individual limitations. Last, school absence potentially can be decreased with better anticipatory guidance, medical care, and compliance with medical regimens.

Job Achievement

Each year 650,000 chronically ill and handicapped persons are graduated from or terminate eligibility for special education programs. Only 31% of students in high school special education classes have prevocational or vocational objectives in their individual programs. Of the 650,000, 21% will have full-time jobs, 40% will be underemployed and exist at the poverty level, 8% will stay in their homes "idle," 26% will be unemployed and on public assistance, and 3% will be institutionalized.[3]

Employment or further educational opportunities available to chronically disabled young adults are varied. The largest number of chronically disabled young adults (100,000) enter workshops. Vocational rehabilitation, a federally funded, state-operated program, helps approximately 60,000. Other programs include vocational education, higher education, public employment, and training programs.[3] Although legislation is in place and training programs are available, disabled young adults need to avail themselves of the opportunities, and more employers need to be open to hiring them. Both tasks are formidable. It is essential that schools encourage the achievement of goals, including thought to future employment, from the earliest stages. Parental support also is essential. Health care workers who are in contact with these youths from birth can encourage them, their families, and schools to attend to future planning from the earliest years.

COLLABORATION OF SCHOOL STAFF AND HEALTH PROFESSIONALS

Collaboration among school personnel, community-based medical providers, and school health personnel is essential in the management of the chronically ill child in the school. It is only through well-coordinated efforts that educators are aware of the child's medical needs and that health providers are aware of the child's learning needs. The way that health services are delivered in the school and the extent to which the active participation of primary care providers is sought in the evaluation and modification of services for the disabled child vary widely among states and school districts.

The Teacher's Role

Teachers are in a unique position as members of any management team to address the issues that confront chronically ill and disabled children in school, inasmuch as they can implement the recommendations of special education evaluators and health professionals. They also can be objective about the child's school performance, including academic and social achievements and difficulties. Meeting the needs of these children poses many obstacles. Teachers may be unaware of the implication of the medical condition for the child's school performance. Lack of adequate information can result in misunderstanding of the child's condition, which can lead to denial of services, misinterpretation of behaviors, or undue restrictive boundaries being placed on the child. On the other hand, with adequate information teachers can foster not only academic achievement but also social confidence. As the best judge of the appropriateness of the child's educational placement, the teacher can facilitate the child's full academic and vocational potential. Health professionals in the school and in the community should actively seek teacher input in the ongoing evaluation and implementation of medical plans of care for these children.

The Physician's Role

Primary care physicians have the potential to play a vital role as advocates for their chronically disabled patients. The physician's role encompasses direct medical care to patients and guidance about medical issues. In a chronically disabled patient whose illness may cause school absence, it behooves the physician to strive to arrange nonacute medical care after school hours. It also is the physician who can guide the patient to anticipate acute crises and thus prevent school absences to the greatest extent possible. As the professional who knows the patient medically and psychosocially, the primary care physician can encourage the cognitive development and socialization of the child. An important function of the primary care physician is to communicate medical information, including a clear explanation of the child's disability, to the school staff so that it can concentrate on teaching the child rather than worrying about his or her medical state.

Primary care physicians are not subspecialists and thus do not have the final word on what patients with particular diagnoses can or cannot do; however, they often are the ones who fill out school physical examination forms. The physician should not assume that the listing of restricted activities will enable the child to participate in more appropriate sports; allowable activities should be specifically listed. Two sources of activity guidelines for children with chronic illness are the American Academy of Pediatrics' sports medicine handbook by the Committee on Sports Medicine, which contains a chapter that addresses recommendations for participation in competitive sports for children with health problems.[1] Also, individual subspecialists can be contacted to help set guidelines for children with particular limitations.

The School Nurse's Role

The school nurse usually coordinates health services in the school. As previously mentioned, how and what health services are provided to children in schools varies widely. In most school districts the nurse is responsible for communicating with physicians and parents about a child's medical needs. In the case of chronically ill and disabled children the nurse's role as liaison among community health providers, educators, and parents forms the core of collaborative efforts to meet these children's medical needs. The school nurse, who usually is responsible for implementing the recommended medical regimens during the school day, is in an excellent position to assess a child's medical status and need for modified treatment plans. The role of the school nurse and models of school health service are discussed in greater detail in Chapter 68.

School-Based Clinics

The number of school-based clinics is growing rapidly to address the comprehensive health needs of children in the school. These clinics often are located in medically underserved areas with the purpose of increasing access to health services for high-risk populations. Although there are many different models for these health centers, most often they have a multidisciplinary staff (a physician, nurse-practitioner, social worker, and health educator) that provides a myriad of ambulatory health services. The controversy that surrounds school-based clinics, especially those in senior high schools that provide health care related to matters of sexuality, often eclipses the primary care, acute care, health education, counseling, and referral services that are offered in far greater numbers. The potential of these clinics to contribute to the care of chronically ill and disabled children can be overlooked, as a result of the assumption by physicians and educators that the health needs of these children are being met.

Staff members of the school-based clinic are in an excellent position to communicate with school personnel and to function as the patient's advocate. They may serve as the primary care provider for children who do not have access to health services, or they may supplement the role of the community-based provider by making health services available in the school for acute problems. Thus acute medical care (e.g., epinepherine for a child with asthma), ongoing care (such as chest physical therapy for patients with cystic fibrosis), and routine care (yearly physical examinations) can be given with minimal school absence and maximal communication with the school staff. Adolescents, in particular, appreciate school-based services, inasmuch as they are designed to be responsive to their needs, as well as respectful of their confidentiality.

REFERENCES

1. Committee on Sports Medicine: Sports medicine: health care for young athletes, Evanston, Ill, 1983, American Academy of Pediatrics.
2. Fowler MG, Johnson MP, and Atkinson SS: School achievement and absence in children with chronic health conditions, J Pediatr 106:683, 1985.
3. Hippolitus P: Employment opportunities and services for youth with chronic illness. In Hobbs N and Perrin JM, editors: Issues in the care of children with chronic illnesses, San Francisco, 1985, Jossey-Bass, Inc, Publishers.
4. Klerman LV: School absence—a health perspective, Pediatr Clin North Am 35:1253, 1988.
5. Mearig JS: Cognitive development of chronically ill children. In Hobbs N and Perrin JM, editors: Issues in the care of children with chronic illness, San Francisco, 1985, Jossey-Bass, Inc, Publishers.
6. Perrin JM, MacLean WE, JR: Children with chronic illness: the prevention of dysfunction, Pediatr Clin North Am 35:1325, 1988.
7. Rutter M, Tizard J, and Whitmore K, editors: Education, health and behavior, London, 1970, Longman Group Ltd.
8. Task Force on Pediatric AIDS: Pediatric guidelines for infection control of human immunodeficiency virus (acquired immunodeficiency virus) in hospitals, medical offices, schools, and other settings, Pediatrics 82:801, 1988.
9. Walker DK: Care of chronically ill children in schools, Pediatr Clin North Am 31:221, 1984.
10. Weitzman M: School and peer relations, Pediatr Clin North Am 31:59, 1984.

66

School Refusal (School Avoidance Syndromes)

Philip R. Nader

The term *school phobia* or *refusal* usually does not mean a fear of school. Rather it applies to various symptoms of anxiety in a school-aged child who is excessively absent from school. It also differs from truancy, in which the child is neither at home nor at school. Many interacting factors can result in school refusal. Historically, in the preadolescent school-aged child a major psychological factor is an interdependency between a parent and the child: "The umbilical cord pulls at both ends" was Eisenberg's analogy.[3]

School avoidance or refusal, which can be part of a presenting problem or symptom complex, is not a single syndrome. In one series,[1] one group consisted of children who feared separation from dependent, overprotective mothers; another group consisted of perfectionistic and depressed children who manipulated and dominated their mothers, who had been deprived in childhood. A third group was composed of severely disturbed children from multiproblem families. All were fearful and depressed, and they had suffered early deprivation and loss.

Many astute physicians and school nurses are alert to tendencies in parents and children toward overprotection and overresponse to minor illness, which may result in excessive school absence. When the parent or the child is made aware of this situation, it usually improves. Such instances represent the mild end of the spectrum of school refusal.

Most published follow-up studies[2] of school refusal are biased because of the severity of problems referred to child study centers or psychiatrists. These studies, however, show that younger children with school refusal who receive care experience more positive results in overall adjustment than do older children and adolescents referred for the same problem.

DEFINITION OF SCHOOL AVOIDANCE SYNDROME

Primary care physicians often are required to recognize and treat school refusal. To qualify as true school refusal there must be an opportunity to attend school. Excessive absence can be defined as greater than two standard deviations beyond the mean number of days absent per year, which generally is fewer than 5 to 7 days. A significant number of days are involved in a 2-week absence. The absences may be in sequence (all together) or may be intermittent (several days per week absent; e.g., 3 of 5 or 4 of 5 days). Absence longer than 3 months is more difficult to treat.

School refusal is not uncommon, and various studies suggest its prevalence to be around 0.4% of all schoolchildren.[4] Higher percentages of students state that they do not like to go to school or are afraid to go.

Truancy can be part of avoiding school but usually is associated with other delinquent or antisocial behavior in that neither school officials nor parents are able to locate the child.

DETECTION OF SCHOOL REFUSAL

Anecdotal evidence exists that the frequency of school refusal or avoidance is decreasing, with the parallel observation that the severity of the situations identified as school refusal is increasing. Although the reasons are unclear, there appear to be more cases of older, seriously disturbed children who have missed more school and fewer cases of younger children with easily treated separation anxiety. Possible explanations include the following: more children are successful in achieving separation from parents at an earlier age by attending preschools and day-care centers, school personnel are more sophisticated in recognizing and managing the less severe cases, and many schools closely monitor absenteeism and are likely to detect cases early.

School refusal may be identified by a direct complaint from the parent or school personnel that the child will not attend school. More frequently, a variety of psychosomatic complaints are seen by the physician. Organic symptoms of an acute or a chronic illness also may exist, causing parental or other adult reactions that lead to excessive or unwarranted school absence. The truism "It has to be thought of before a diagnosis is made" is applicable in school refusal.

CONFIRMATION OF SCHOOL REFUSAL SYMPTOMS

Termed "the great imitator" by Schmidt,[6] school refusal may manifest many signs and symptoms. The following have been described: insomnia or excessive sleeping and fatigue, pallor, recurrent sore throat, sinusitis, hyperventilation, cough, palpitation, chest pain, abdominal pain, headache, vomiting, diarrhea, dysmenorrhea, bone and joint pain, and syncope. In other words the complaints do not suggest the diagnosis.

Affected children may be of either sex, and the problem occurs in all socioeconomic strata. These children may possess varying degrees of intelligence, often are described as good students, and are bright or average in their school abilities.

The aforementioned interdependency between parent and child may be heard in the parent's comment, "*We* didn't feel good today, so *we* didn't go to school." When a child stays at home with his or her parent during the school day, the parent does not seem to realize how allowing or encouraging this behavior promotes dependency. Such a communication pattern between child and parent should raise the question of why this situation exists and should lead to an assessment of family communication styles.

Because almost all cases of school refusal represent family problems, the primary care physician should be aware of three common patterns of communication found in families in which school refusal occurs: (1) both parents are overconcerned and basically unaware of their contribution to the problem—a situation that often is amenable to short-term counseling, (2) the mother, usually, is overprotective, but the father disagrees completely and is vocal about it—the child responds by being exceptionally manipulative (a situation that probably will respond more quickly to counseling than the third pattern), and (3) the mother is extremely overinvolved, even talking for the child, and the father is absent or might as well be.

The family communication patterns should be assessed. How do the parents see the problem? What happens every morning? Is one or the other parent inadvertently giving a message that it is all right to stay home from school? ("You don't feel like going to school, do you?") The child's perception of and likes and dislikes about school and other significant areas of his or her life should be explored with the child.

Information obtained from the school should include data on previous attendance, performance, and peer acceptance and any reasons why the child might fear school (bullies or extortion). Physicians should be aware of placing importance on a parent's suggesting a change of schools or teachers or even giving realistic reasons why the child might fear going to school. These reasons, although perhaps significant, usually are insufficient to cause school refusal.

A complete and thorough physical assessment with appropriate laboratory examinations is indicated, along with a complete description of all negative findings. Results should be given to both parents and child. Such an assessment should not be omitted even if a physician is virtually certain of the absence of undetected serious organic disease. Unnecessary laboratory tests, however, are not only costly but also serve to reinforce the family's doubts about the real nature of the problem.

MANAGEMENT OF SCHOOL REFUSAL

Management will not be successful unless parents, child, school personnel, and others involved are included in the treatment plan. Successful management requires that the physician clearly identify both short- and long-term goals. These goals dictate the treatment. Follow-up care should be designed to assess the efficacy of the treatment and, if necessary, to revise it, or referral should be considered.

Short-term goals for the treatment of school refusal almost always center on plans to interrupt the pattern of behavior that results in school nonattendance. Therefore, returning the child to school is the major short-term goal. Long-term goals include a gradual reduction in the child's anxiety, an improved self-image, resolution of a precipitating family crisis, improved overall functioning by the child, and improved family communication patterns.

Five general procedures apply to all instances of school refusal:[55] (1) the child should return to school as soon as possible; (2) the child must be helped to obtain relief at school as soon as possible; (3) significant attachment figures at home and significant adults at school should be involved in the treatment plan; (4) persistence and consistency should be encouraged; and (5) if school refusal is secondary to broader coping problems, further evaluation/referral or psychiatric consultation should be carried out.

IMPLEMENTING THE TREATMENT PLAN

In approaching the child, the physician must recognize the veracity of the child's complaints ("The stomachache really hurts"). In the child's eyes, however, "everyone" has now decided it eventually will get better, and "everyone" also has decided that no matter how difficult it is, he or she will return to school. This change in tactics confuses the child, who may react by becoming stubborn. If the parents succeed in returning the child to school, the child's anxiety may initially increase but soon will recede because the more regular the attendance, the more the child's participation in school life will increase. It may be necessary to anticipate possible future difficulties during follow-up care (e.g., a necessary change to a larger junior high school). Counseling and allowing the child to express some concerns may smooth or altogether prevent later transition crises.

In approaching the family, the physician should find out how the family will work together to solve the problem of returning the child to school. The physician must avoid taking sides against one or another of the parents and must recognize and keep any angry feelings toward the offending parent in check. If parents are able to easily recognize the problem and their role in its resolution, management usually will result in immediate success and the lack of need for a referral. Often, however, the physician will have to deal repeatedly with parental doubts and fears and be firm about the diagnosis and management. The physician should discuss with the parents how they can interrupt the child's pattern of behavior; sometimes simple advice regarding normal child rearing and limit setting may be all that is required. The most valuable piece of information the physician can impart to school personnel is that the child is free from any unrecognized serious medical problem. Most teachers, counselors, and nurses can be supportive and firm if they have this reassurance. Ongoing communication is essential not only to assess the success of management but also to minimize the unavoidable resocialization trauma that follows a prolonged school absence. School resources for support and further evaluation of any existing academic or social problems may be required to return the child to optimal functioning.

INDICATIONS AND PROCEDURES FOR REFERRAL

In a preadolescent with school refusal, referral may be required, usually because more severe family or marital problems are interfering with a successful resolution of the problem. Referral of an adolescent with school refusal is almost always made because of a more serious psychopathologic condition in the child (depression or schizophrenia).

Parents whose opinions remain so widely divergent that they seem unresolvable, even after initial counseling, will require referral to some type of family counseling service.

Referral resources are determined by geography, finances, and interpersonal trust. The family will require a great deal of support and confidence that their problem can be solved with the appropriate help. Direct communication between the primary care physician and the source of referral (e.g., private psychiatrist, child development or mental health clinic, social worker, psychologist, or family service agency) is mandatory until it is confirmed that the family has been seen and treatment has been initiated. Either the physician or the referral consultant must keep in contact with the family and school at least until the child is attending school regularly.

REFERENCES

1. Atkinson L et al: Subclassification of school phobic disturbances, ERIC document No 290065, 1987.
2. Coolidge JD, Brodi RD, and Feeney B: A ten-year follow-up of 66 school phobia children, Am J Orthopsychiatry 34:675, 1964.
3. Eisenberg L: School phobia: a study in the communication of anxiety, Am J Psychiatry 114:712, 1958.
4. Granell de Aldaz E et al: Estimating the prevalence of school refusal and school related fears, J Nerv Ment Dis 172:722, 1984.
5. Heath CP: School phobia: etiology evaluation and treatment, ERIC document No 261321, 1985.
6. Schmidt B: School phobia—the great imitator: a pediatrician's viewpoint, Pediatrics 48:433, 1971.

67

School Learning Problems and Developmental Differences

Paul H. Dworkin

School learning problems are complex issues that defy traditional methods of pediatric assessment and management. Learning problems are not, in fact, the exclusive responsibility of the pediatric provider but rather are of multidisciplinary concern. Furthermore, pediatricians neither definitively diagnose nor independently treat learning disabilities. Nonetheless, pediatric providers should assume critical roles when their patients manifest learning problems. Such roles include clarifying the reasons for poor school performance and facilitating appropriate intervention. The importance of such pediatric involvement has been increasingly recognized; parents and educators regard such problems as learning disabilities to be within the pediatric provider's area of responsibility and demand pediatric attention to the needs of children who perform poorly in school. Unfortunately, many pediatric providers view themselves as being inadequately prepared to deal with school learning problems.

REASONS FOR LEARNING PROBLEMS

The British pediatrician Martin Bax noted that a student's learning problems may result from a variety of causes—"from his school burning down to the lack of the appropriate textbook."[1] Causes of school failure may be somewhat simplistically classified into "intrinsic" and "extrinsic." Intrinsic causes of learning problems may be regarded as inherent characteristics of the failing child, such as specific learning disabilities, mental retardation, and sensory impairment. Alternatively, extrinsic causes may be viewed as adverse external influences, such as family dysfunction and social stressors within the home or ineffective schooling. Actually, however, learning problems typically are the consequence of a complex interaction of child-, family-, and school-related variables (Fig. 67-1). For example, a subtle learning disability may be particularly devastating for a child reared in poverty and attending a school of inferior quality. Furthermore, learning problems often coexist with "clusters" of adverse influences. A learning-disabled child, for instance, may be at a particular disadvantage when a "slow-to-warm-up" style of temperament precludes active classroom participation or when the child is confronted with the trauma of parental divorce. Thus the pediatric assessment of school learning problems must include the child's capabilities and weaknesses within the context of social and environmental circumstances.

Specific Learning Disabilities

Of the many causes of school learning problems, specific learning disabilities are the most prevalent and perplexing. Although no uniformly accepted definition exists, learning disabilities have been traditionally defined as biologically based developmental disorders characterized by disturbances in the processes involved in understanding or using language. The hallmark of learning disabilities is a discrepancy between a student's potential for academic achievement, as suggested by cognitive abilities, and actual performance, as documented by achievement tests. The prevalence of learning disabilities is estimated to be 3% to 5% of students.

Although no single cause of learning disabilities has been identified, research has emphasized the critical importance of language development in learning. Because many learning-disabled children have experienced delayed or disordered language acquisition, the belief that learning disabilities may be the expression of a more general linguistic disability has been supported. More recently, the importance of weaknesses in higher-order cognitive functions (i.e., thinking and reasoning processes, memory) has been emphasized. Deficits in so-called metacognitive skills, such as being able to access acquired knowledge when needed and knowing how to apply learned skills, may result in learning-disabled children's inability to focus attention on the salient features of tasks or effectively devise problem-solving strategies. Such children have been described as "passive learners" because of their difficulties with strategy selection and problem-solving.

Learning-disabled children typically display deficits in various areas of developmental functioning. When developmentally assessed, learning-disabled children are more likely than their normally learning peers to be confused by sequences and time relationships (temporal-sequential deficits); to have "right-left confusion" (directional disorientation); to fail to appreciate spatial relationships and visual detail (visuoperceptual difficulties); and to have difficulty integrating auditory and visual stimuli, such as the sounds of words and the visual configurations of letters (deficits in intersensory integration). These children also are more likely to be clumsy and awkward (motor abnormalities) and neurologically immature (i.e., to exhibit neuromaturational delay or so-called soft neurologic signs). In addition, behavioral or emotional problems, such as diminished self-esteem, are more common among such students.

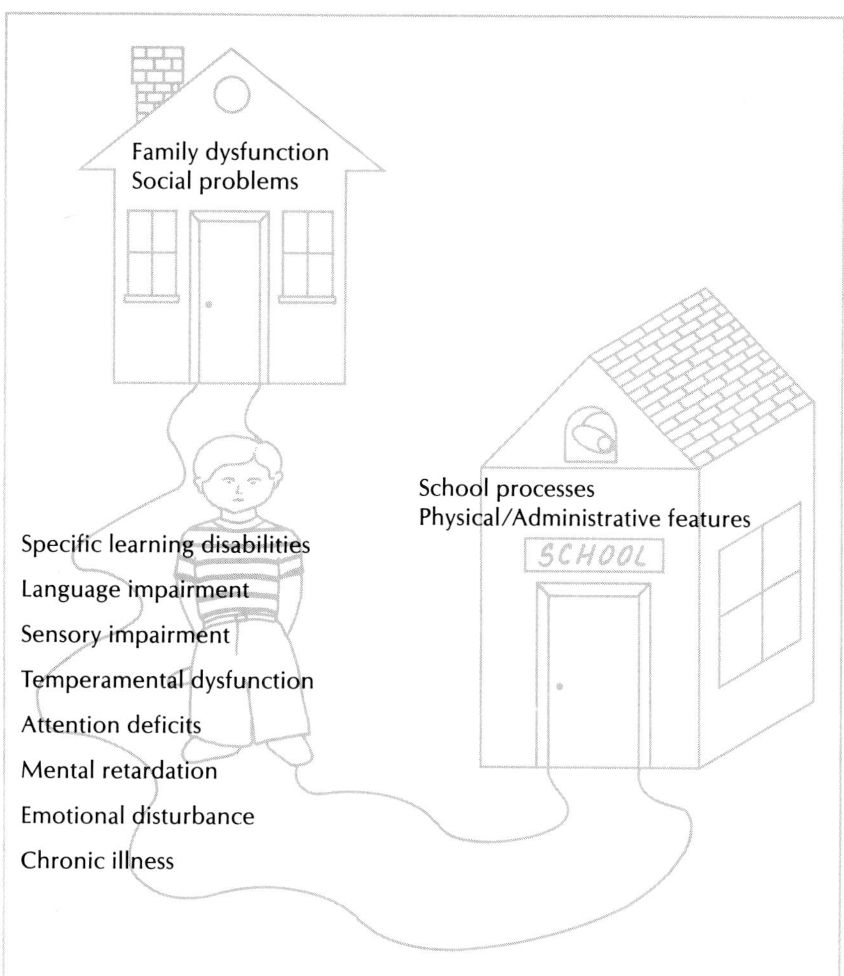

Fig. 67-1 Learning problems are typically the consequence of a complex interaction of child-, family-, and school-related variables.
From Dworkin PH: School failure, Pediatr Rev 10:301, 1989. Used by permission of the American Academy of Pediatrics.

Except for language and cognitive deficits, the extent to which these clinical correlates contribute to, result from, or merely coexist with learning disabilities is uncertain. For example, extensive research fails to substantiate a significant causal relationship between faulty visuoperceptual skills and academic deficits. The presence of such correlates should not form the basis of a learning disability diagnosis. Rather such findings as temporal-sequential deficits and directional disorientation should serve as "red flags" that increase the clinician's suspicion regarding the possibility of learning disabilities and prompt a referral for psychoeducational evaluation to document the potential performance disparity required for diagnosis.

Learning-disabled children most commonly have problems with the language arts—reading, spelling, and written expression—and difficulties with arithmetic and handwriting skills, although isolated problems with arithmetic are less common. A child's pattern of academic performance may change over time. For example, some learning-disabled children may cope satisfactorily during the first 3 years of school, only to experience increasing problems with academic achievement and organization of assignments by third or fourth grade as classroom expectations increase and demands for the rapid retrieval of information and work productivity escalate. Such a pattern of performance, with particular problems in mathematics and written expression, has been termed *developmental output failure*.[4]

Other Reasons for Learning Problems

Whether *attention-deficit disorders* represent a specific syndrome (attention-deficit hyperactivity disorder) or rather result from complex interactions between child-related and environmental factors is highly controversial. Regardless, there clearly does exist a group of children for whom difficulties with inattention, distractibility, lack of persistence, and impulsivity impair school functioning. Such attention deficits often are associated with other causes of learning problems, such as specific learning disabilities.

Mild *mental retardation* usually is not identified until the child is confronted with the cognitive demands of school. The academic performance of such children is characterized by slow learning and acquisition of skills to at most the fifth or sixth grade level. Mental retardation and learning disabilities may coexist, and both contribute to a child's learning problems.

Sensory impairment may contribute to school learning problems. Of the five senses, hearing and vision are the most crucial for academic learning. Of these two, *hearing loss* results in the more profound educational handicap, primarily because of impaired language acquisition and communication skills. The learning problems of hearing-impaired children are characterized by difficulties in reading, as well as in arithmetic reasoning and problem-solving. Deaf students also may experience classroom maladjustment, behavioral problems, and social immaturity. Children with *visual disturbances* usually fare better than their hearing-impaired peers in the classroom. In general, such children tend to perform rather well; thus, their academic achievement has received only limited scrutiny.

Although from 30% to 80% of emotionally disturbed students have problems with academic achievement and classroom behavior, *emotional illness* (such as depression or conduct disorders) is the primary cause of learning problems for only a small percentage of children with school failure. Rather, emotional factors may be far more important in the exacerbation of academic difficulties caused by other problems. For example, the inevitable feelings of diminished self-esteem and frustration that accompany school failure because of learning disabilities may serve to impair classroom functioning even further.

From 25% to 33⅓% of children with *chronic illness* have problems achieving academically. Chronic illness may contribute to school learning problems as a consequence of limited alertness or stamina, chronic pain, medication side effects, absenteeism, altered or inappropriate expectations of teachers or parents, maladjustment, or inappropriate placement in special classes. Low intelligence and learning disabilities may be problems for children with certain neurologic disorders.

A child's behavioral style or *temperament* may contribute to school learning problems. The temperamentally "difficult" child may become easily frustrated and angry when confronted with material not easily mastered. Or the initial reluctance of the "slow-to-warm-up" child to participate and tendency to withdraw may be misinterpreted as anxiety or as a limited capability for learning. Although the "easy" child usually fares well in the classroom, problems may arise when expectations for behavior differ markedly between home and school.

Social and environmental factors also may contribute to school learning problems. These include parental divorce or separation, child abuse or neglect, the illness or death of immediate family members, parental emotional illness, early parenthood, substance abuse, and poverty. Ineffective schooling itself may contribute to learning problems. Some studies have revealed that school processes (e.g., academic emphasis, use of rewards and praise, teachers' actions during lessons) are more important than physical or administrative features.[6] Such factors as school climate and social environment may be particularly important for children from disadvantaged homes who attend schools with limited resources.

PEDIATRIC EVALUATION OF LEARNING PROBLEMS

The goal of pediatric evaluation of school learning problems depends on the specific circumstances of a child's referral. When school-based assessment has already raised the possibility of a child being learning disabled, pediatric evaluation assumes a relatively limited role in excluding medical problems that may contribute to poor school functioning. Alternatively, pediatric evaluation is far more challenging when a child is experiencing unsuspected or unexplained learning problems. The goals of such evaluation include diagnosing "medical" conditions that may contribute to school problems, such as sensory impairment or a seizure disorder, as well as identifying clinical correlates (medical), neurophysiologic, and psychological) of other causes of learning problems, such as specific learning disabilities.

Certain guidelines should be followed in the evaluation of school learning problems, such as consideration of the multiple factors that may contribute to school failure. Communication with school personnel is invaluable in providing information about classroom functioning, past assessments, and school resources. The child must be evaluated within the context of the learning environment; for example, expectations of a 5-year-old entering an academically oriented kin-

Table 67-1 *The Role of History in the Evaluation of School Learning Problems*

ASPECT	FINDINGS SUGGESTIVE OF SPECIFIC LEARNING DISABILITIES
School functioning	
Academic achievement	Discrete delays in select subjects (e.g., language); adequate early performance with difficulties emerging later (e.g., mathematics, writing)
Classroom behavior	Long-standing, pervasive problems with inattention, impulsivity, overactivity; disorganization and poor strategy formation; depression, moodiness
Attendance	Excessive absenteeism; school avoidance
Past psychoeducational testing	Discrepancy between cognitive abilities and academic achievement
Special required school services	Response to "diagnostic teaching"
Perinatal history	"Clusters" of adverse events; maternal alcohol or drug intake
Medical history	Recurrent and/or persistent otitis media; iron deficiency anemia; lead poisoning; seizures; frequent accidents; chronic medication use
Development	Delayed or disordered language acquisition and communication skills; subtle delays in select milestones; "uneven" pattern of skills and interests
Behavioral history	Long-standing, pervasive problems with attention span, impulsivity, overactivity; sadness; acting out; poor self-esteem
Family history	Learning problems, school failure among first-degree relatives
Social history	Child abuse or neglect; other stressors

dergarten class are quite different from those of a child entering a more developmentally and socially oriented program.

History

Important historical information should be sought from parents, teachers, and the child (Table 67-1); questionnaires may greatly facilitate the gathering of necessary information.[3] Certain aspects of *school functioning* should be examined in detail, including the child's academic achievement, classroom behavior, school attendance, past psychoeducational testing, and special school services provided. Findings that suggest the possibility of specific learning disabilities may include (1) discrete delays in select subjects, such as the language arts, or an adequate early performance with the later emergence of difficulties, (2) behavioral problems such as long-standing, pervasive problems with inattention, impulsivity, overactivity, acting out, disorganization, and poor strategy formation or depression, sadness, and moodiness resulting from frustration and diminished self-esteem, (3) school avoidance because of frustration, (4) a discrepancy between cognitive abilities and academic achievement on past psychoeducational testing, and (5) poor responses to special teaching techniques, which suggests special learning requirements.

Further aspects of the traditional medical history also should be examined in detail. The *perinatal history* of learning-disabled children is characterized by a somewhat increased incidence of "clusters" of adverse events, such as anoxic encephalopathy, prematurity, and bronchopulmonary dysplasia, as well as maternal alcohol and drug intake (e.g., substance abuse and anticonvulsants). The *past medical history* may be significant for recurrent or persistent otitis media, iron deficiency anemia, lead poisoning, seizures, frequent accidents as a result of overactivity, or chronic medication use (e.g., phenobarbital, theophylline, or antihistamines). The *developmental history* of learning-disabled children may suggest delayed or disordered language acquisition and communication skills; subtle delays in select milestones such as speaking, sitting, or walking; or an "uneven" pattern of skills and interests, with discrete areas of strength and weakness. The *behavioral history* may reveal long-standing, pervasive problems with attention span, impulsivity, and overactivity; sadness; acting out; or poor self-esteem. The *family history* may corroborate the increased incidence of learning problems and school failure among first-degree relatives of learning-disabled children. The *social history* may reveal such stressors as child abuse or neglect, known to be associated with specific learning disabilities.

Physical Examination

The physical examination has a limited, but important, role in the evaluation of children with learning problems (Table 67-2). The physician's *general observation* of the youngster may suggest sadness, anxiety, a short attention span, impulsivity, or overactivity. Tics may indicate Tourette syndrome, which is known to be associated in some cases with learning disabilities. *Physical features* may be observed that suggest syndromes associated with learning disabilities, such as fragile X syndrome, fetal alcohol syndrome, or Turner syndrome. Alternatively, an increased incidence of so-called minor congenital anomalies (epicanthic folds, hypertelorism, low-set ears, high-arched palate, clinodactyly, and syndactyly of toes) has been observed among some children with specific learning disabilities and attention deficits.

Certain specific aspects of the physical examination deserve special emphasis. Examination of the *skin* should include a search for multiple café au lait spots (neurofibromatosis) and "ash-leaf" spots and adenoma sebaceum (tuberous sclerosis) inasmuch as both conditions are associated with learning problems. Examination of the *tympanic membranes* may suggest signs of recurrent or chronic otitis media. Among older boys, examination of the *genitalia* may reveal delayed sexual maturation, which has been correlated with learning problems. *Growth measurements* may indicate problems such as short stature, microcephaly, and macrocephaly, which also have been associated with learning disabilities. *Sensory screening* should exclude hearing impairment or vision defect.

Examination of Mental Status

Simple projective testing may identify emotional issues as either the cause or, more likely, the consequence of school learning problems. Such techniques as asking the child for three wishes, asking the child to draw a picture of his or her family, or playing the Winnicott Squiggle Game[2] may reveal the child's sadness, diminished self-esteem, or concerns regarding family functioning.

Neurodevelopmental Screening

Surveying the child's functioning in different areas of development may help to identify factors that contribute to learning problems. As previously noted, children with specific learning disabilities are more likely to have deficits in language functioning and cognitive abilities. Furthermore, the

Table 67-2 *The Physical Examination and Evaluation of School Learning Problems*

ASPECT	FINDINGS SUGGESTIVE OF SPECIFIC LEARNING DISABILITIES
General observations	Sadness, anxiety, short attention span, impulsivity, overactivity; tics
Phenotypic features	Stigmata of genetic syndromes (e.g., sex-chromosome abnormalities, fetal alcohol syndrome); minor congenital anomalies
Skin	Multiple café au lait spots; "ash-leaf" spots, adenoma sebaceum
Tympanic membranes	Signs of recurrent or chronic otitis media
Genitalia	Delayed sexual maturation in boys
Growth measurements	Short stature; microcephaly and macrocephaly
Sensory screening	Poor hearing or vision

developmental profile of learning-disabled children is typically characterized by an uneven pattern, with discrete areas of relative strength and weakness.

A few tools have been developed for assessing school-aged children. One is the Pediatric Early Elementary Examination (PEEX),[5] which requires about 45 minutes to administer and surveys the following areas of development: temporal-sequential organization, visuospatial orientation, auditory-language function, memory, fine motor function, and gross motor function. The PEEX also includes a search for minor neurologic indicators of dysfunction (so-called soft neurologic signs) such as dysdiadochokinesia (difficulty with rapid alternating movements), synkinesis (mirror movements), and dystonic posturing of the upper extremities associated with heel walking. An increased incidence of such signs has been observed among boys with attention deficits and, to a lesser extent, specific learning disabilities.

Laboratory Studies

Laboratory tests are of limited value in assessing school learning problems and should be used only in studies of children at specific risk for conditions known to be associated with learning disabilities. Examples include *anemia screening* for children at risk because of nutritional or socioeconomic factors; *lead screening* for those at risk because of their home environment or a history of pica; *thyroid function studies* only if signs or symptoms of thyroid disease are noted; and *chromosome analysis* (including a search for the fragile X site in retarded boys and in retarded girls with a positive family history) in the presence of phenotypic features or multiple congenital anomalies in association with mental retardation. *Drug screening* is recommended for older children and adolescents with a precipitous decline in school performance or in erratic, unpredictable behavior.

Neuroanatomic and neurophysiologic studies should be performed only for specific indications. For example, an electroencephalogram (EEG) should be reserved for children suspected of having a seizure disorder, whereas *computed tomography (CT scan)* or *magnetic resonance imaging (MRI)* is indicated for suspected central nervous system malformations, microcephaly, or macrocephaly.

Further Investigations and Referrals

Referral for *psychoeducational evaluation* is indicated when the pediatric assessment suggests the possibility of learning disabilities as a cause of learning problems. For example, learning disabilities may be suspected if (1) the pediatric history reveals difficulties with discrete subjects such as reading and spelling, (2) developmental testing indicates an "uneven" profile with areas of strength and weakness, and (3) a child demonstrates poor self-esteem and self-image. The goals of psychoeducational evaluation are to examine the child's academic strengths and weaknesses, to determine cognitive ability, to assess perceptual strengths and weaknesses, to examine communicative ability, and to assess social and emotional adaptation. Ideally, such evaluations are performed by the child's school system, although specific circumstances may dictate a private referral. School personnel participating in such evaluations may include psychologists, special educators and learning disability specialists, speech-language pathologists, and social workers. Typically administered tests include those for intelligence, general learning abilities, and academic achievement in reading, mathematics, and writing; perceptual and motor function; and speech and language skills. Diagnostic teaching also may be an effective test mechanism.

Pediatric assessment may indicate the need for referral to a variety of other professionals. For example, concerns about language functioning may result in a direct referral to a speech-language pathologist; emotional disturbance or family dysfunction may suggest the need for referral to a mental health professional (e.g., psychologist, social worker, or psychiatrist). Concerns regarding sensory impairment may suggest a referral to an ophthalmologist, otolaryngologist, or audiologist.

PEDIATRIC INTERVENTION

A variety of actions may follow assessment of the child with school learning problems. Although educational programming is the mainstay of treatment for specific learning disabilities, pediatric participation may involve a variety of traditional and nontraditional roles.

Examples of traditional roles include specific medical intervention for underlying conditions, such as the treatment of a seizure disorder that may contribute to learning problems, as well as the pharmacologic management of attention deficits. Counseling is another traditional role and may include clarifying a child's strengths and weaknesses; alleviating undue concerns, guilt, and anxiety; explaining the legal rights of children and families under state and federal regulations, such as the Education for All Handicapped Children Act Public Law (94-142); offering guidance regarding such alternative treatment strategies as diet, megavitamins, and optometric training; and, depending on the pediatric provider's expertise, giving advice concerning such specific behavioral management strategies as positive reinforcement and "timeout." Arranging for further investigations and referrals is yet another traditional role and may involve coordinating indicated laboratory studies and referring for psychoeducational testing and other evaluations.

A less traditional but nonetheless important pediatric role is serving as ombudsman and helping students and families effectively utilize community services and resources. Specific actions may include facilitating communication with school systems, introducing families to helpful parent and peer support groups, and initiating referrals to mental health and social service agencies. Although pediatricians are unlikely to possess the expertise to directly suggest educational strategies for learning disabilities, participation as a member of a multidisciplinary planning team is both helpful and feasible. Such participation is often reassuring to parents and children, who regard the pediatric provider as an effective child advocate.

REFERENCES

1. Bax M: Looking at learning disorders, Dev Med Child Neurol 24:731, 1982 (editorial).

2. Berger LR: The Winnicott Squiggle Game: a vehicle for communication with the school-aged child, Pediatrics 66:921, 1980.
3. Levine MD: The ANSER system, Cambridge, Mass, 1981, Educators Publishing Service, Inc.
4. Levine MD, Oberklaid F, and Meltzer L: Developmental output failure: a study of low productivity in school-aged children, Pediatrics 67:18, 1981.
5. Levine MD et al: The Pediatric Early Elementary Examination: studies of a neurodevelopmental examination for 7- to 9-year old children, Pediatrics 71:894, 1983.
6. Rutter M et al: Fifteen thousand hours. Secondary schools and their effects on children, Cambridge, Mass, 1979, Harvard University Press.

SUGGESTED READINGS

Dworkin PH: Learning and behavior problems of schoolchildren, Philadelphia, 1985, WB Saunders Co.

Dworkin PH: School failure, Pediatr Rev 10:301, 1989.

Levine MD and Satz P, editors: Middle childhood: development and dysfunction, Baltimore, 1984, University Park Press.

68

Nursing Roles in School Health

Mary Farren and Rosemary K. McKevitt

The school nurse is a key health professional in implementing a viable, effective school health service program. The responsibilities are diverse and require the ability to work collaboratively with children and their families; school administrators, teachers, and other school personnel; and school physicians, other physicians, and community agencies.

VARIETY IN THE SCHOOL NURSE ROLE

The role of the school nurse is multifaceted and complex. Although its origin is the community health nurse role, it varies greatly from one school to another depending on the educational preparation of the individual and the priorities of the school board. In a few schools, licensed vocational (practical) nurses, who have up to 1 year of nursing preparation, provide limited health services; registered nurses may have as little as 2 years of nursing preparation or as much as 4 years. School nurse practitioners, whose expanded role in school health is described later in this chapter, often are prepared in postbaccalaureate or master's degree programs that include specific preparation in school health.

The scope of the school nurse's role is related not only to educational preparation but also to the organizational structure under which the health services are provided. Although some school health services are provided by local health departments or, in a few innovative programs, by a nonprofit corporation,[2] most school nurses are employed by boards of education. The scope of the nurse's role often indicates the school's priority in meeting the health needs of its population and the available resources that the school can commit to that endeavor or that it can secure from other public and private sources. Awareness of some of the variations in the school nurse role can help the physician establish a mutually collaborative relationship with the nurse and become familiar with the existing school health program.

SCHOOL NURSE FUNCTIONS

In most schools with a well-established traditional school health program, high priority is assigned to the three levels of prevention—that is, health promotion and disease prevention, identification and remediation of health problems, and restoration of children with chronic diseases to their optimal level of health. School nurses are responsible for assessing, planning, organizing, implementing, and controlling any health problems they discover in students or that result from the environment. According to the American School Health Association (ASHA), school nurses enhance the capabilities of youth to use their intellectual potential to make worthwhile decisions that affect their present and future health.[1] Priority is assigned to modifying or removing health-related barriers that interfere with student learning. The school nurse ordinarily gathers a health history from parents when the child enters school and verifies the child's immunization status. The school nurse also is responsible for planning a systematic health appraisal of all schoolchildren, although some of the specific activities may be carried out by volunteers or paraprofessional personnel. Screening programs for vision and hearing problems, along with other selected assessment procedures, are routinely conducted at specified grade levels. When health problems are identified, a referral process is initiated that involves counseling the student and family about the nature of the problem, the necessity of further treatment, and the health resources available in the community. After obtaining the family's consent, the school nurse may communicate directly with the family's physician about the problem and, after medical evaluation, discuss any educational implications and follow-up care indicated. The nurse can provide useful information to the physician about a child's response to the treatment, as well as facilitate any temporary or long-term modification of the child's school milieu to meet health needs.

The school nurse works closely with parents and teachers of children with chronic health problems. Because increasing numbers of children with major health problems are "mainstreamed" into regular classrooms, teachers need increased information, advice, and, sometimes, support to promote maximum development and academic achievement for these children. Public Law 94-142, which addresses education of the disabled, has allowed many children to be enrolled in school for the first time, and school nurses have provided physical and rehabilitative nursing care, as well as individual health teaching and counseling to these students and their families, to aid them in coping with chronic health problems.[9]

Emergency care for ill or injured pupils or staff members is viewed as important by the school. First aid policies and procedures ordinarily are developed by the school nursing staff, administration, and medical consultants. Although many school nurses are directly involved in providing some emergency care, teaching basic first aid procedures to all school personnel usually is of high priority. Often the nurse conducts in-service educational training for all staff members regarding emergency care; sometimes only a paraprofessional or a small group of staff members receives specific first aid training from the nurse. Many emergencies can be prevented by analyzing previous accident data, observing health and safety hazards in the school, and ensuring that appropriate protective equipment for students involved in laboratories, workshops, and athletics activities is available.

Such primary, secondary, and tertiary preventive measures usually constitute the common core of the traditional school nurse role, and most nurses view individual and group health education as important responsibilities and, time and energy permitting, become involved in a variety of such educational activities. Virtually every contact with a student is an opportunity for incidental teaching or health counseling. The nurse also may develop special programs in the school for students with similar health needs (e.g., teenagers who need to lose weight). Some nurses are directly involved in the health education curriculum either as primary instructors or as collaborators with a classroom teacher or health educator in specific units of instructions.

EXPANDED SCHOOL NURSE ROLE

In recent years considerable interest has been directed toward the expanded role of the nurse in various primary care settings. Designated by titles such as *nurse practitioner* or *nurse associate,* the expanded role generally involves the acquisition of skills that enable the nurse to provide more comprehensive health care. The notion of the nurse practitioner in the school is a natural extension of the pediatric nurse practitioner role in other ambulatory child health care settings.[5] The nurse practitioner, working with a pediatrician colleague, may assume a primary care role, which involves providing comprehensive well-child care, managing minor illnesses, and making initial assessments of more serious acute and chronic conditions.

Nurse practitioner preparation is obtained within a graduate nursing education program or, alternatively, through a certificate program consisting of a minimum of 4 months of intensive study, including both theory and practice, followed by a preceptorship of 6 to 8 months with experienced nurse practitioners and physicians. In addition to acquiring new assessment techniques, nurses enrolled in practitioner programs expand their understanding of child development and behavioral problems, learn more about common illnesses of children and adolescents, and sharpen their interviewing and counseling techniques.[4] Specific attention is directed toward integrating new and expanded knowledge and skills into the role of the school nurse and into the entire child health care delivery system. Contemporary school nursing demands that the practice focus on principles of epidemiology, case management for aggregates of students, and program management and evaluation.[6] Role reorientation is an important component of the learning, with emphasis placed on an interdependent, collaborative relationship with physicians and a generally more assertive approach in assuming responsibility for children's health care.

The nurse practitioner in an expanded school nurse role has a larger repertoire of assessment skills to use in evaluating a child's health status. Beginning with a health history obtained in interviews with the child and the family, the school nurse practitioner develops a complete data base by using sources of information in the school such as the teacher and by conducting a complete physical examination, including the neurologic component. Diagnostic laboratory tests, as well as developmental and psychological screening procedures to identify behavioral and learning problems, are conducted as indicated. On the basis of the findings, appropriate health teaching and counseling are initiated with the student and family. If referral outside the school is indicated, a report of the nurse practitioner's findings assists in further management of the problem.

The health team concept is particularly important in the implementation of the nurse practitioner role in the school. Unless paraprofessionals are available to assume some of the more routine activities such as minor first aid, clerical tasks, and some screening procedures, nurses may not have enough time to fulfill an expanded role. In the past this applied to school nurses in general; screening and health appraisal procedures often were dictated by tradition, if not mandated by state regulations, and nurses tended to believe that their time was consumed by activities that did not require professional nursing skill.

The school nurse practitioner also collaborates closely with the physician consultant. In fact, the physician-nurse team may provide comprehensive primary health care to a segment of the school population that has no other source of primary care.[11] In demonstration projects in several states, the school has become the base for primary health care for children in the community.[7] More commonly, in communities with a well-established primary child health care system outside the school, the school nurse-physician team serves as the liaison between the school and the primary care physicians.[8]

MODELS OF SCHOOL NURSE SERVICES

Numerous studies[3] have documented the effectiveness of nurse practitioners in improving and maintaining the health of schoolchildren. The school nurse practitioner role has received support from major professional organizations concerned with nursing and school health,[4] and many school districts have demonstrated an interest in an expanded role for the nurse even though these services may be more costly. Reimbursement of some costs to the school district through federal, state, and other third-party payment sources, however, is also more likely when school nurse practitioners provide some primary health care in the school in addition to some of the more traditional school nursing services.

Although the approximate number of nurses who work in schools has remained relatively constant in recent years, the number of students served by one nurse generally has increased, often surpassing the recommended ratio of 1 nurse to 1000 students. A few schools have attempted to meet basic school health needs by employing paraprofessional aids in lieu of nurses or nurse practitioners. Although less costly to the school, these personnel require careful training and supervision by a registered professional nurse to provide safe and effective care. Other schools have used the nursing services provided by local public health departments. In this model of service the nurse's school-related activities may constitute only a part of his or her total community nursing role because the nurse provides care to all age-groups within a geographic district and also may be responsible for health department clinics and other activities. Assigning a high priority to school health activities within the context of community health needs has been a problem because children ordinarily are the healthiest segment of the community's population.

Some schools are trying to achieve an optimal mix of the services provided by the health aide, physician consultant, school nurse, and nurse practitioner to meet the health needs of a diverse school population.[12] This plan allows nurse practitioner services to be concentrated in areas underserved by community primary care resources, frees both nurses and nurse practitioners from activities that can be delegated to health aides, and yet provides backup and consultation for personnel at all levels. In times of rising educational costs and limited resources, however, many schools choose less expensive and thus less comprehensive health services. Studies of cost effectiveness and national trends in the financing of health care may well determine the shape of school nursing services in the future.[10]

THE PHYSICIAN AND THE SCHOOL NURSE

Although communication between the physician and the school may take place in many other contexts, more frequently it is the school nurse who interacts with family physicians. School and health care agencies have different "languages," priorities, and backgrounds. The school nurse can help the physician to bridge the gap; at the same time the nurse may gain valuable consultation and support for health-related activities in the school. The rewards of collaboration in pursuit of common goals outweigh the occasional temporary barriers of frustration and misunderstanding. Mutual respect, open communication, and some understanding of each other's view of the world can enhance cooperation between the physician and the school nurse in improving the health of school-aged children.

REFERENCES

1. American School Health Association: Evaluating *school nursing practice: a guide for administrators. Based on the Standards of School Nursing Practice,* Kent, Ohio, 1987, The Association.
2. Cronin G and Young WM: Posen/Robbins: a model school health care project, Nurse Pract 2:22, 1977.
3. Goodwin LD: The effectiveness of school nurse practitioners: a review of the literature, J Sch Health 51:623, 1981.
4. Guidelines on educational preparation and competencies of the school nurse practitioner: a joint statement of the American Nurses' Association, the American School Health Association, and the Department of School Nurses National Education Association, J Sch Health 48:265, 1978.
5. Igoe JB: Changing patterns in school health and school nursing, Nurs Outlook 28:486, 1980.
6. Igoe JB: What is school nursing? A plea for standardized roles, Matern Child Nurs J 55:142, 1980.
7. Kort M: The delivery of primary health care in American public schools, 1890-1980, J Sch Health 54:453, 1984.
8. Nader PR, editor: Options for school health, Rockville, Md, 1978, Aspen Systems Corp.
9. National Association of State School Nurse Consultants define role of school nurse in "PL 94-142—Education for all Handicapped Children Act of 1975," J Sch Health 52:475, 1982.
10. Oda DS: School nursing: current observations and future projections, J Sch Health 49:437, 1979.
11. Porter PJ: Realistic outcomes of school health service programs, Health Educ Q 8:81, 1981.
12. Sobolewski SD: Cost-effective school nurse practitioner services, J Sch Health 51:585, 1981.

69

Language and Speech Assessment at School Entry

Hiram L. McDade

It is assumed that each child who enters school possesses a fully developed system of spoken language skills, and it is on this system that higher levels of communication are taught. The late talker, the 3-year-old with unintelligible speech, or the child with a limited vocabulary or word-finding difficulties invariably becomes conspicuous again when he or she needs special assistance in the areas of reading, spelling, writing, and mathematics. The failure to provide early remedial services for these children often is the result of a "wait and see" attitude among health professionals. Actually, Johnny, who didn't begin talking until he was 2 years old and whose speech could not be understood until he was 4 years old, never outgrew his problem. It was simply manifested in other channels of language learning. The literature is compelling regarding the relationship between reading and writing failure in the primary grades and a history of earlier communication difficulties. In fact, of the various skills assessed on standardized intelligence tests, those items that are most predictive of later academic performance are language based. For this reason an assessment of a child's readiness for school must give primary consideration to the adequacy of his or her general communicative abilities.

HEARING ASSESSMENT

Inasmuch as normal speech and language development require an intact auditory system, a hearing assessment is an integral part of any developmental screening. It should be noted, however, that children with recurrent otitis media frequently pass pure-tone screenings for two reasons: (1) the resultant hearing loss usually is intermittent and (2) the test signals often are presented at increased levels to compensate for the ambient noise in the examination room. As a result, hearing screenings are inadequate follow-up procedures for children who have been diagnosed as having otitis media. Such children require full audiologic testing. More recently, tympanometry has become a routine component of hearing assessments. When coupled with results from the pure-tone screening, tympanograms help identify a potential conductive component (middle ear problems) that might otherwise be missed.

SPEECH AND LANGUAGE DEVELOPMENT

As in other developmental areas, an important step in assessing a child's oral communication skills involves collecting a thorough history. Because the emergence of certain critical speech and language abilities follows a relatively stable timetable, a child's competency may be compared with these norms, either by history or by direct observation. Inasmuch as the purpose of such assessments is not to make diagnoses but to identify those in need of further testing, children who fail to measure up to normative data should be referred to a speech-language pathologist. By such a referral, two benefits are accrued: (1) those children who are found to be deficient in speech and language abilities are ensured early intervention, and (2) those whose skills remain in question may be followed up and reassessed at appropriate intervals. For children whose skills are in question, the evaluation provides objective baseline data that allow the examiner to measure children's progress over time.

The acquisition of first words (at approximately age 12 months) is the initial evidence of a child's language development. In general, children who remain nonverbal at age 18 months should be referred for further testing. A word of caution should be noted, however, about the achievement of this developmental milestone. Parents, in their eagerness for and anticipation of their child's development of speech, frequently interpret the utterances "mama" and "dada" as meaningful words. Usually these vocalizations are merely a function of the child's advanced babbling stage and, if accepted as words by the examiner, will produce the assignment of a spuriously low age level to the acquisition of first words (e.g., 6 or 8 months). For this reason, more accurate information should be obtained by asking the parents how old their children were when first words other than "mama" or "dada" were spoken.

The emergence of two-word phrases represents a significant milestone in language learning. It is at this stage that the rudimentary rules of grammar are first evidenced. The term *grammar* here refers to (1) those rules that regulate the ordering of individual words into phrases or sentences and (2) the modification of words themselves to indicate higher levels of meaning, such as plural, possession, and verb tense. In English, as in most languages, word order is critical to the meaning of an utterance. For example, the sentences "Mary loves Bob" and "Bob loves Mary" do not carry the same meaning, despite having identical words. A child as young as 18 months displays awareness of grammar in these early two-word phrases, such as "Mommy see" and "See mommy," which are used at different times to express different mean-

Table 69-1 *Ages at Which Children Can Answer Various Types of Questions*

AGE (YR)	TYPE	EXAMPLE
2½	Yes/no	Is this your shoe?
2½	What/do	What are you doing?
2½	What	What is your favorite toy?
2½	Where	Where is your mommy?
3	Whose	Whose doll is that?
3	Who	Who do you play with?
3	Why	Why do we take baths?
3	How many	How many dolls do you have?
3½	How	How do you eat soup?
4	How much	How much can you eat?
4	How far	How far can you walk?
4	What if	What would you do if you got cold?
5	How often	How often do you go to school?
5	When	When do you go to school?

ings. Generally, children should use some two-word phrases by age 24 months, and failure to do so by this age suggests the need for further testing.

By age 3 years most children have a spoken vocabulary of more than 500 words. In addition, their grammatical skills have developed to the point where they routinely speak in three- and four-word sentences. It is at this age that the basic rules of grammar become fine-tuned. Plural, possessive, and past tense forms of words are beginning to be mastered, and the use of pronouns such as *I, me, you,* and *mine* is common. Three-year-olds demonstrate an appropriate understanding of *why* questions (Table 69-1), indicating an appreciation of cause and effect. The speech of 3-year-olds is highly intelligible, and despite their frequent mispronunciations, a stranger has no difficulty understanding the children. In short, 3-year-olds have the capacity to carry on a reasonable conversation with an adult.

The language of 4-year olds approaches adult competency with respect to grammatical skills. Unlike 2- and 3-year-olds, the utterances spoken by 4-year-olds represent complete sentences. Rarely are words omitted from the four- and five-word sentences that these children typically produce. Although 4-year-olds do not have as many different ways as do older children to say the same things, they usually have at least one way to express all thoughts and desires. The vocabulary of 4-year-olds is also quite extensive. By this age most children can recognize and name several colors, count to 10 by rote, understand the prepositions *in, on, under, beside, in front,* and *in back* (but not *behind* until age 5 years), and answer complex questions such as "How much?" "How long?" and "What if . . . ?"

By age 5 years, children have developed most of the language-based concepts that are important for schooling. They can sort and classify objects by category, name all the basic colors, understand the concept of time (which allows them to answer *when* questions), and understand the concept of numbers up to 10 integers. Their skills of articulation are also fully developed by age 5 years. Any residual mispronunciations at this point represent disordered speech and should generate an immediate referral to a speech-language pathologist.

INTELLIGIBILITY OF SPEECH

In the course of normal development, it is common for children to mispronounce certain sounds or to have difficulty producing particular words. The mastery of sounds in the language is a gradual process that takes place over a period of 3 to 4 years. Unfortunately, many children with disordered speech fail to be identified until later years because their deviant patterns of articulation occur during a time when adults expect a certain amount of mispronunciation. There are differences, however, between normal and disordered speech, even as early as 2 to 3 years of age. Our tolerance for errors during this developmental period often prevents us from discerning these differences. The speech-language pathologist is specifically trained to determine if the pattern of misarticulation exhibited by a particular patient is common for normal children or indicates disordered speech and, thus, is not likely to be self-corrected.

One important factor for the health professional to consider is the child's *intelligibility*. Young children, who are acquiring a sound system normally, are easily understood, despite their frequent misarticulation. That is, regardless of the conspicuousness of their speech errors, normal children have little trouble communicating, even with unfamiliar listeners. In contrast, the child who is unintelligible or whose parents report difficulty understanding his or her speech is exhibiting a pattern of misarticulation that is not part of normal development. Such a child is less likely to outgrow the problem and thus requires a thorough evaluation to determine the need for speech therapy.

70

Developmental Approach to Behavioral Problems

T. Berry Brazelton, David M. Snyder, and Michael W. Yogman

Every encounter between pediatrician and child is an opportunity for developmental assessment. The continuous, long-term relationship the pediatrician maintains with the child and the family offers data about physiologic and behavioral functioning under a variety of circumstances. When questions arise concerning the normality of a child's behavior, this data base gives the pediatrician a diagnostic and therapeutic edge, which a consultant can duplicate only with much time and effort.

The spectrum of behaviors about which parents become concerned is broad indeed. Its range encompasses:

1. Nonproblems—the concerns based on simple misinformation, requiring support and corrective information only
2. Normal but frequently "problematic behaviors" to the parents, such as negativism in the second year of life
3. Long-standing, relatively fixed "behavioral problems," such as continued, too-frequent night waking in 2-year-olds
4. Clearly pathologic behavior based on psychopathology or organicity, such as that seen in an autistic child or a child with lead encephalopathy or major psychiatric deviance that is essentially irreversible

This chapter takes a conceptual approach to the assessment of reversible behavioral problems as opposed to the more irreversible ones. The emphasis is on the center of the spectrum: problem behaviors and behavioral problems. These represent both the majority of parental concerns brought to pediatricians' attention and some of the most taxing diagnostic entities in behavioral pediatrics. This section shows how a conceptual approach based on normal development can be applied to these everyday problems in an office practice.

In pediatric practice the diagnosis of a behavioral problem may not be possible in a single encounter. The rush to "make a diagnosis" on the first visit may well be inappropriate. It takes time to assess the dimensions of parental concern as well as the meaning of the behavior to the child. An early diagnosis may miss the appropriate dimensions of each of these. It can lead to extensive diagnostic studies or to referrals that not only may be unnecessary and costly, but may actually make the diagnosis and treatment more elusive by reinforcing parental concerns. This pursuit of a physical diagnosis often will divert the parents from approaching the child's problem. Frequently, the true nature and severity of the behavioral problem emerge only as we observe the parents' responsiveness to counseling or the child's reaction to altered parental approaches. This does not imply an interminable diagnostic phase. Rather, it reflects that, in managing behavioral problems, diagnosis and treatment often proceed in parallel, the diagnostic hypotheses suggesting counseling approaches, the family's response to these generating more precise diagnostic formulations, and so forth.

ETIOLOGY

Behavioral problems arise in the course of growing up as a consequence of the normal stresses of coping with new adjustments.[9] These problems must be viewed as part of the "coping process," the steps through which the child comes to terms with a challenge and successfully masters the difficulties inherent in learning about oneself and about the environment. The coping process may be modified by genetic, biologic, and environmental factors but is always present and needs to be assessed even in those infrequent instances when a severe underlying pathologic condition, such as brain damage, autism, or parental psychosis, is present. The progression from a limited problem behavior to a more global behavioral problem and occasionally even to severe psychopathology depends heavily on how effectively the parent-child unit supports this coping process.

In those few instances when problems are becoming more severe, the parents often show excessive concern about the child's symptom rather than the underlying reason. The symptom may in fact be adaptive and represent a coping response to the stress of growing up or to illness or to somatic defect. Most often the presenting symptom has had its beginning long before, and the parental concerns have reinforced a chain of *behavior→concern→problem behavior→increasing concern→increasing behavioral problem*. To understand the etiology and achieve any change in this ever-lengthening chain, a pediatrician must understand each link in its development.[8]

EVALUATION

The most valuable clinical tool the pediatrician can use to assess developmental behavior in children is observation of the behavior of all participants as they interact with each other.

Clinical judgments about parents and children made at every encounter are based on the physician's observational skills. While formal tests of the child's intellectual and emotional functioning can structure these observations and more clearly articulate clinical judgments, tests can never entirely replace careful observation.

When parents make us, as pediatric observers, feel angry or depressed as they describe a problem, this becomes an important measure of the parent's own depth of reactions to the child and the behavioral problem. Are these feelings representative of their feelings about their conflicts with the child? Why are they generating parallel feelings in us as we observe them? Observations of moments of intense emotion may provide the best clue to the depth of underlying issues. For example, when a mother brightens and becomes animated as she talks about her child's negativism, the pediatrician can be certain that she enjoys it and can identify with it in her toddler and that it will not create a serious problem for either mother or child. Similarly, when a young father begins to hold on grimly to his contention that his 5-year-old son's enuresis is punishable, the depth of tension and frustration created in us becomes our best measure of his inability to react appropriately to this symptom in the boy and indicates that there is a "fixed" problem area between them.

In most instances pediatricians must begin by "listening with a third ear" or observing the behavior and documenting their own reactions to understand clearly what parents mean as they present their children's problem behaviors.[1] As one attempts to gather the necessary information about a disturbing behavior—such as when it was first noted, the circumstances in which it occurs, how the parents react to it, and how the child responds to their reactions—one should be most alert to behavioral signs of deeper concerns. These deeper, often unconsciously controlled, concerns are usually the real reasons the parents seek help. Parents are often reluctant to initiate discussion of their fears regarding brain damage, mental retardation, or psychological disorder in the child, and expressed concerns may really cover up their worries about these issues. These underlying concerns may not be expressed on the first visit. To the degree that they are, they signify that the parents feel the pediatrician is taking them seriously and can be trusted to accept their feelings without censure. Establishing this alliance with the pediatrician is certainly the first step toward solution of the problem they are having with their child.

Evaluation of the Parents

In general, a child's behavior becomes problematic because it does not conform to parental expectations. Evaluation of the parents should start with the assumption that they are concerned about this dichotomy and proceed with specification of the worrisome behavior and how it deviates from their expectations. Insofar as the parents are the focus of attention, we are interested in:

1. How realistic their expectations are
2. How rigid they are in their expectations
3. Whether the child violates these expectations in a narrow or broad area of functioning
4. Whether the violation means abnormality or "badness" in the child or their own failure in parenting

It is also important to determine the origin of their expectations—for example, from their own experiences in growing up, their experiences with their older children, the comments of grandparents, and their cultural expectations.[7]

Parents come to the pediatrician feeling guilty, inadequate, often isolated from their children, and defensive about the difficulties they are having. These feelings, which are invariably an impediment to problem-solving, may well be the tragic result of our cultural biases that blame parents for everything "wrong" with their children. These feelings commonly give rise to questions about the impact of medications taken during pregnancy, genetic factors, and their own child-rearing style as it affects the child's behavior. In some cases these concerns are realistic. In others, the overconcern can be a symptom and measure of the degree of severity of the problem. However, in all cases this concern and guilt interfere with the parents' relationship with their child and need to be brought out and examined in a positive and supportive manner. This entails accepting the parents' concern, validating their right to get help, and above all, feeding back to them a perception of their own basic competence and of their child's strengths, along with an assessment of the child's problem.

Occasionally, signs of markedly unrealistic expectations, such as attributing adult goals to an infant or small child, may come to the surface. Significant parental thought disorders may become apparent. Not infrequently, a parent's own needs and concerns about his or her marriage or about another child may turn out to be the underlying motive for the visit. In any case, the degree to which the parents are conscious of their feelings about their child and his or her problematic behavior, and the ease with which they can express them, can tell us much about the kind of treatment approach that is most likely to work.

If the office assessment of the child reveals that he or she is markedly different from the parents' description, or if their level of concern seems out of proportion to the problem they report, an undiscovered parental concern should be suspected. However, two alternative hypotheses should also be considered: (1) that the behavior observed by the physician is, in fact, not typical of the child; and (2) that the discrepancy represents a real distortion of the child's behavior by the parents.

In the case of significant parental psychological disorder, pediatricians may first sense that their observations do not parallel the expressed complaints. Then they may realize that they cannot reach the parents to help them with their reaction to the child. This, then, may suggest that the primary problem is outside the realm of pediatrics altogether. Even in such situations, the manner in which the pediatrician has talked to the parents about their feelings can have a significant influence on their accepting referral to a source of psychiatric help. If they have learned that a candid expression of their concerns and feelings is met with acceptance and understanding rather than with censure or disinterest, it will be easier for them to make use of psychiatric consultation in this area.

Evaluation of the Child

In evaluating a child's behavior at any one time, pediatricians must take into account the following:

1. How is inborn individual temperament influencing the child's behavior (either overreactivity or underreactivity)?[4]
2. Is the symptom one that is appropriate to the child's age?[5,8]
3. How do the child's reactions to all stress show either adaptive strengths or inadequate coping mechanisms?[9]
4. To what degree has the symptom influenced broad areas of a child's functioning (with the family, peers, in school, etc.)?
5. What is the duration of the symptom as a sign of "fixation"? If the child has not changed over time, one should worry, and if the symptom has increased in severity, the situation becomes even more ominous.[10]

In practice, one evaluates a problem on all five levels simultaneously, but separate discussion may clarify the importance of each level.

Temperament as a Background for a Symptom. An understanding of infant temperament is helpful in assessing the child's contribution to common problems such as crying, feeding, sleeping disorders, temper tantrums, and poor weight gain.[2] Children vary in the rhythmicity of repetitive biologic functions. These include sleep-wake cycles, appetite, and elimination. Parental interviews enable a pediatrician to assess a child's temperamental profile in vital areas of function (activity, intensity, mood, adaptability, rhythmicity, threshold, distractibility, persistence, and approach-withdrawal), as suggested by the longitudinal studies of Thomas, Chess, and Birch.[10] Knowledge of patterns of individual differences such as that of the "temperamentally difficult" (high intensity, low adaptability, low threshhold) child helps a pediatrician to understand the child's intrinsic contributions to a sleep problem, and this understanding can help the parent in turn to manage this "difficult yet still normal" child.

Age Appropriateness of Behavior. A given behavior has different meanings in children of each age. While this is obvious in the case of motor milestones, it is equally true for behavioral problems. Temper tantrums, nightmares, phobias, stuttering, and other types of behavior are regularly seen at certain ages and usually pass without consequence. For example, temper tantrums in an 18-month-old are an appropriate indicator of the child's growing sense of independence.[3] A tantrum of similar intensity at 4 years of age deserves exploration for an answer to why the child's striving for autonomy does not take a more mature form. By being aware of the individual temperamental and maturational differences, a pediatrician not only can better evaluate problems when they arise, but can also use this information preventively to understand the child as an individual and, by sharing this information with the parents, establish an alliance to optimize the child's development.[5]

The Child's Pattern for Coping with Stress. Since the pressures of growing up are a part of everyday life, children's behavioral problems must always be evaluated in the context of how they handle these stresses, as well as others that confront them. A pediatrician can note whether the behavioral symptoms in question provide a way for the child to cope better with the pressures of his or her environment. For example, thumb-sucking and holding onto a bottle or blanket or beloved toy through the stressful second and third years of life seem to be healthy solutions to stress. Unless the parents' concern about such a "lovey" makes it nonadaptive, one should see such behavior as a source of strength for the child and reinforce the parents to see it as such. Assessing a child with a stress model allows one to generalize and view the child's underlying resources available to cope with any challenging situation.

A psychological instrument such as the Denver Developmental Assessment[6] "Screening" can be easily administered in the pediatrician's office, and it may be viewed as just such a stress. Such an assessment can become a way to evaluate the child's "level" of development as well as reaction to the stress of being tested. Then this becomes a way to attend to the child's responses to the stress of testing and how the child is likely to cope with other stresses of life. In other words, we are given an opportunity to see how a child approaches any given problem or item rather than merely whether the test is passed or failed. When a 14-month-old boy turns to his mother to seek help when he is asked to stack blocks, this not only tells us about the child's response to the stress of the test, but also tells us something about the strength of his attachment to his mother and something about his level of autonomy.[9]

The idea of identifying a child's mechanisms for coping is part of the broader principle of being able to list the child's individual strengths, as well as problems in a "problem list." When asked to stack blocks, a 2-year-old may take great delight in knocking them over rather than stacking them. Negativism is a healthy sign of the toddler's growing independence and should not be overlooked.[3]

Influence on Other Areas of Function. In determining the significance of any problem to a child, it is crucial to determine how isolated and discrete the problem is. A 4-year-old's bed-wetting at night may represent a discrete delay in maturation, whereas the same symptom in a 6-year-old may interfere with peer relations (e.g., an inability to spend the night at a friend's house). As children grow and attempt to identify with their peers, such a symptom becomes a real source of anxiety about their own adequacy. This anxiety can begin to interfere with all areas of function. They may begin to show signs of deficit in school performance and in their self-esteem in general. In a small child and in the area of feeding, the problem may range from a discrete attempt to control choices, such as refusing vegetables—a transient, self-limited problem—to a more global feeding disturbance, such as a refusal to eat any solid food. When the problem is no longer confined to feeding and involves other areas of adjustment such as sleep and toilet problems, this suggests an even more global impairment in the parent-child relationship. The degree to which a problem is clinically significant is commonly reflected by the number of functional areas in the child's life that are affected.

Determining the degree to which any symptom affects the child's overall level of function not only has diagnostic implications but also is helpful in managing the problem. A therapeutic plan should account for and support the child's achievement and successful areas while attempting to improve any weaknesses.[7]

Chronicity of a Symptom. Since development implies change over time, any symptom that becomes chronic is worrisome. Crying, for instance, reaches a developmental peak between 3 and 6 weeks of age and tapers off by the age of

3 months.[3] When a 6-month-old shows a persistent problem of "colicky" crying, that child requires evaluation and intervention. Thus, the degree of fixation in a behavior becomes a measure of the degree of the problem.

Finally, behavioral symptoms that become inflexible should arouse even more concern. If appropriate 2-year-old negativism is replaced by intense temper tantrums with persistent head-banging whenever children do not get their way, this constrained, inflexible behavior pattern is a sign of such children's need for therapeutic attention to their relationship with their parents.

Delaying a diagnostic decision while collecting observations at several visits allows a pediatrician to assess the inflexibility of any symptom by observing the parents' and child's responses to various therapeutic suggestions. While an assessment of the parents' concerns, as well as the five areas of child behavior described, aids the pediatrician, no evaluation is complete without the same kind of observation of the parent-child interaction.

Evaluation of Interaction

A pediatrician should evaluate not only parent and child separately, but also the interaction of parent and child over time. The essence of parent-child interaction may be seen in the mutual request for attention and responses by parents with their children. Pediatricians should record observations of these interactions. They can distinguish the mother who sensitively shapes and shows her child how to achieve a task from one who either angrily shoves the child to a task or is completely unavailable to the child. Similarly, pediatricians can distinguish between the child who explores the surrounding environment, using a parent as a secure base, and the child whose interactions with a parent is either minimal or provocative. Value judgments should never substitute for repeated careful observations that attempt to understand the interaction of parent and child on its own terms and in its own culture.

MANAGEMENT

The therapeutic first step may be for the physician to try a simple suggestion. If the parent cannot establish a working relationship with the pediatrician and misuses the suggestion so that the behavioral problem becomes worse or reinforced, this becomes a measure of the depth of the parent's inability to accept help and of the need for more intensive therapy for any solution of the problem. Pediatricians tend to blame themselves when a helping relationship cannot be established instead of recognizing the diagnostic implications of the parents' inability to let down their defenses and to join in a therapeutic effort to help the child.

Pediatric management of childhood behavioral problems usually requires seeing parent and child together. By using the child's behavior as a way of communicating with parents and pointing out the child's behavior and their response to it, the pediatrician can help parents to see their child as an individual with strengths as well as weaknesses. For instance, when parents understand and accept their toddler's negativism as a striving for independence, they can pursue the goal of allowing the child the opportunity to work out negative struggles and to define his or her own capacities and limits. In this way, the pediatrician forms an alliance with parents that supports them in their concern, but gives them a goal that enables them to work together at finding adaptive parental responses to help the child.

A pediatrician who no longer feels able to understand or help a family should consider referral to a psychiatrist or social worker who is trained to work with more difficult parents. Because of the nature of the problem and the nature of their relationships with families, pediatricians should approach such referrals even more sympathetically than they might a referral to another physician. The parents' need for defenses against acknowledging that they have a family problem must be respected. The pediatrician may have to see a family several times to gain a clear idea of what kind of referral they will accept and to outline the questions that should be answered. The pediatrician must remain the primary health worker for the family and must continue to support them after therapy is instituted. The pediatrician not only should remain involved in the assessment, but also must clearly understand the consultant's assessment of the problem, since the pediatrician will most often be left to carry out the consultant's treatment and management recommendations after the diagnostic or therapeutic interval has terminated.

Pediatric management of behavioral problems and active fostering of normal development can be among the most challenging and rewarding aspects of pediatric practice. They need not be especially time consuming, but they do require a knowledge of normal development as a dynamic process, as well as concerned attention in understanding parent's reports and in observing both children's and parent's behavior.

REFERENCES

1. Balint M: The doctor, his patient and the illness, New York, 1972, International Universities Press.
2. Brazelton TB: Crying in infancy, Pediatrics 29:579, 1962.
3. Brazelton TB: Toddlers and parents, New York, 1974, Delacorte Press.
4. Carey WB: A simplified method for measuring infant temperament, J Pediatr 77:188, 1970.
5. Erikson E: Childhood and society, New York, 1950, WW Norton, Inc.
6. Frankenburg WK et al: Revised Denver Developmental Screening Test, J Pediatr 79:988. 1971.
7. Lewis M: Clinical aspects of child development, Philadelphia, 1971, Lea & Febiger.
8. Murphy L: The widening world of childhood, New York, 1962, Basic Books, Inc.
9. Murphy L and Moriarty A: Vulnerability, coping, and growth, New Haven, Conn, 1976, Yale University Press.
10. Thomas A, Chess S. and Birch H: Temperament and behavior disorders in children, New York, 1968, New York University Press.

71

Interviewing Children

David I. Bromberg

In assessing children's problems in which psychosocial and emotional factors are particularly important, a clear understanding of such youngsters and their relationship to their world is essential. This relationship can be viewed as consisting of three interrelated parts: the child's relationship to his or her family, community (mainly school), and peers. The primary method of attaining this understanding is through diagnostic interviewing. A great deal of information is available from parents (see Chapter 6, "The Pediatric History") and from the school (see Chapter 59, "Overview of School Health"). However, a wealth of information and insight that is qualitatively unique is available through a careful interview with the youngster.

The structure of the interview can be divided into three parts: (1) the establishment of rapport, (2) the body of the interview, or data collection, and (3) summation of the session, or closure. While the major goal of the interview is collecting data about the child, there are clearly other important functions. The physician has the opportunity to establish himself or herself as a "helping" person in the relationship with the child by demonstrating an understanding of the youngster's feelings and problems and a willingness to offer constructive help rather than judgmental advice.

STRUCTURE OF THE INTERVIEW

Establishing Rapport

Attempting to teach someone how to establish rapport is somewhat akin to teaching someone how to ride a bike: you have to do it to learn it. Nevertheless, several concepts are useful. Rapport is continually built throughout the interview and the ongoing relationship and is not limited to introductory remarks. Exhibiting a sincere interest in and empathy for what the youngster has to say is essential. Verbalizing the feelings represented by a child's story or using nonverbal behavior can be very helpful in this regard. For example, 11- and 12-year-old youngsters are routinely seen for physical examinations on entry to middle or junior high school. Sitting undressed and draped on an examining table, many of these youngsters appear angry or overly shy. By saying, "I guess it's pretty embarrassing to have to undress and have a physical examination," the physician can aid substantially in establishing rapport with that youngster.

"Reflecting" feelings is generally a useful way for the health care provider to display caring and a desire to communicate. This can involve responding to an "unspoken" message, such as saying, "It sounds like you're pretty angry about that," or summarizing the point of a story, such as saying, "So you've really missed your dad since he moved away but don't want to say so to your mom." The same message can be communicated by "checking back" with the child, prefaced by saying, for example, "Just to be sure we're understanding each other . . . ."

When doing a behavioral assessment, it is important to remember that the consultation is rarely initiated by 8- or 10-year-olds. Such children are often brought to the office with little or no explanation. Exploring their fears and expectations as well as what activities they may be missing by being there can aid in "breaking the ice." For younger children this may involve clarifying that they will not be receiving any blood tests or immunizations. For older children, recognizing how difficult it is to talk about oneself (or to be talked about) is worthwhile. The physician should discuss the format of the evaluation and the demands that will be placed on the youngster. Explicitly stating, "Mary, first I will be talking with you and your family about your school difficulty, and afterwards I will be meeting just with you so we can get to know one another better; then next week I will give you a physicial examination," clearly establishes the format of the sessions.

"Third-person techniques" can facilitate conversation with a child. Rather than attributing feelings or characteristics to the patient, the interviewer can talk about these feelings in other youngsters. The statement "Many 9-year-olds who wet the bed are embarrassed and afraid of sleeping over at a friend's house" allows a youngster to claim these same feelings but does not confront him or her directly. It also shows that the physician will not be shocked or dismayed by this information.

As in all of pediatrics, the interviewer must maintain a developmental perspective in relating to the patient. Complimenting a 3-year-old on climbing the steps to the examining table by himself would be quite appropriate, whereas the same comment to an 8-year-old would be condescending. Erikson, in *Childhood and Society*,[2] describes the "Eight Ages of Man"—critical periods of development. Each of these "ages" is presented as a task in development of the ego. These eight ages are summarized as the accomplishment of the following characteristics: (1) basic trust versus basic mistrust, (2) autonomy versus shame and doubt, (3) initiative versus guilt, (4) industry versus inferiority, (5) identity versus role confusion, (6) intimacy versus isolation, (7) generativity versus stagnation, and (8) ego integrity versus despair. Erikson's tasks of development provide a useful framework for both evaluating and relating to children. Commenting on issues of autonomy in the 3- to 4-year-old, issues of initiative in the

5- to 6-year-old, and issues of industry in the 7- to 9-year-old will often successfully engage the child. It is also important to proceed from very concrete, "here-and-now" discussions with the preschooler and early school-age child to more abstract explanations as the child gets older.

Data Collection

By the conclusion of the interview, the examiner ideally should have accumulated data from three main areas: (1) the child's perceptions about the presenting problem, (2) information about the child's relationship to family, school, and peers, and (3) an assessment of youngster's psychological functioning.

Understanding the child's perception of the presenting problem is probably the most difficult assessment to make. Denial of emotional issues is common in school-age children. The 5- to 12-year-old will frequently claim to be neither worried nor upset about the problem that is being evaluated. The physician must listen with his or her "third ear" and be sensitive to nonverbal cues to understand the youngster's relationship to the presenting complaint. Using third-person techniques may be helpful—for example, "Many children have told me that they feel dumb when they have trouble with reading."

When a child is reluctant to discuss problems, another useful approach is to ask him or her for "both sides of the coin," for example, to state what he or she likes and dislikes about school. The same technique can be applied to assess the child's feelings toward individuals or toward himself or herself; for example, "Can you brag about yourself and then run yourself down?" Social skills can also be evaluated in this manner; for example, "What do your friends like about you? What things do you do that make them mad at you?"

Psychological functioning can be assessed by paying careful attention to both the content and the process of the interview. The assessment should include an estimate of intellectual functioning, an evaluation of the child's approach to problem-solving (e.g., impulsivity, frustration), and the child's fears and fantasies, self-concept, and superego function (conscience). A useful framework for this analysis is the mental status examination. Because a complete discussion of this examination is beyond the scope of this textbook, the interested reader is referred to Simmons' *Psychiatric Examination of Children*.[5]

Numerous assessment techniques are available by which to gather the necessary data. These cover the spectrum from the very unstructured "play" evaluation to the very structured questionnaire. Choice of particular tools depends on the age of the patient, the patient's verbal abilities, the examiner's expertise, and the examiner's style. For the pediatrician evaluating school-age children, a semistructured interview is probably the most appropriate. This combines specific questions about the problem of concern, peer relations, and related issues with the use of projective techniques. A discussion of several diagnostic techniques that can be used by the pediatrician is included in the section on pediatric psychodiagnostics.

Open-ended questions, which leave the respondent a great deal of latitude in interpretation, are most helpful. Some examples include, "What is a typical day at school like?" or "How does everyone in your family get along?" The physician should attempt to be nonjudgmental and allow the youngster maximum leeway in presenting his or her thoughts or feelings. Asking, for example, "You have lots of friends, don't you?" displays the examiner's preference for friendships and closes the subject to the child. A more effective question might be, "Do you have many friends or do you prefer doing things by yourself?" This allows the child to choose either option, without the physician prejudicing the choices.

Closure

At the end of the interview, it is important to summarize for the child. A review of the session, highlighting the important points, is useful. An attempt should be made to offer the youngster honest, positive reinforcement and an optimistic outlook wherever possible. Plans for future meetings should also be discussed. A typical ending statement might be, "Bobby, I know that you really worked very hard today, having to tell me all those things about yourself. It was especially hard to tell me how sad you were when your grandmother died. But now I think that we will be able to make it easier for you to get back to school. I look forward to seeing you and your family next week."

THE PARENTS' ROLE

The relationship of physician, patient, and parents is a complicated one. Children are brought to the physician to have a behavioral problem "fixed." As we have noted previously, the consultation is rarely initiated by the youngster. The pediatrician must define his or her relationship to the child and parents, paying careful attention to the issue of confidentiality and to the patient's therapeutic needs. The initial decision is what format the interview should take and in what order he or she will see the child and parents. Then the physician must decide how to share information among the parties.

Mature preadolescents and teenagers are often seen alone and first in the diagnostic process. The physician thereby demonstrates the primacy of the doctor-teenager relationship. Although the establishment of a similar relationship with a latency-aged or a preschool-aged patient may be equally important, these youngsters may be frightened by an initial separation from parents. I frequently see the child and parents together for the first diagnostic interview. This allows the youngster a chance to become more comfortable with the examiner in a less threatening setting. Parents are occasionally uncomfortable about discussing behavioral or emotional concerns with their children present. Children, however, are usually well aware of these concerns and find an honest discussion much less frightening than their fantasies about the process should they not be included. After an initial joint interview, both parents and child should be seen separately.

The issue of confidentiality is a difficult one to balance. On the one hand, the youngster has the right to tell the examiner specific things that should be held in confidence. On the other hand is the parents' need for information to play an effective role in the therapeutic process. It may be helpful to discuss treatment recommendations with the youngster before the final sum-up session with the family. The parents play a critical role in both the diagnostic process and in executing the therapeutic program. The physician should carefully plan the consultation process so as to maximize an effective relationship with both patients and parents.

PEDIATRIC PSYCHODIAGNOSTICS

Many techniques and types of questions are available to help engage youngsters in an interview as well as to uncover "defended" emotional material. These projective techniques allow the youngster to respond to loosely structured stimuli, giving answers that reflect his or her personality. Examples include, "If a genie were to come and give you three wishes, what would you wish for?"; "If you were stranded on a desert island and could have only one person with you, who would it be?"; "Tell me about your happiest, saddest, and maddest times." The responses to these questions must be evaluated in the context of what is known about the child. Other semistructured projective techniques are described below.

Sentence Completion

Tell children that you are going to play a sentence game with them. You will tell them the first part of a sentence, and they have to finish the sentence with the first thought that comes to mind. You then present the child with short sentence fragments such as, "Boys are . . . ," "Girls are . . . ," "Mothers should . . . ," "I feel bad when I . . . ." The answers may indicate areas of conflict or may introduce other topics of interest to the child.

Drawings

Many children find it easier to express themselves through drawings than through verbal communication. Several formats can be used. You might ask a youngster to draw the best drawing of a person that he or she can. Standards are available in using the "Draw-a-Person" test to make an "IQ" assessment.[4] Kinetic family drawings are obtained by asking the youngster to draw a picture of his or her family doing something.[1] Family relationships and activity can be discussed using this stimulus. Figure placement, size relationships, and use of symbols may all be useful in interpretation. Allowing a child simply to draw a picture and tell you a story about it can also be very helpful.

Storytelling

Stories can be useful for talking about emotions or conflicts. A storytelling format (fables) was developed by Despert and expanded by Fine.[3] Using this technique, the child is told that you both are going to play a storytelling game in which he or she must finish stories that you begin. The child is then given a series of 20 fables that touch on many characteristic areas of conflict. An example is the oedipal fable:

> A boy and his mother go for a nice walk in the park all by themselves. They have a lot of fun together. When he comes home, the boy finds that his daddy is angry. Why is he angry?

The youngster's answer may then be used as a point of departure for other questions about anger; for example, "What do you think the boy's father did when he got angry?" followed by, "What does *your* father do when he gets angry?"

SUMMARY

Engaging children in a helping relationship is the core of pediatric practice. Forming close, empathic relationships with patients clearly begins with the diagnostic interview. It is important, therefore, to be alert to both the process and content of this interview and to select diagnostic tools that will foster development of the desired relationship between physician and child.

REFERENCES

1. Burns RC and Kaufman SH: Actions, styles and symbols in kinetic family drawings, New York, 1972, Brunner/Mazel, Inc.
2. Erikson EH: Childhood and society, ed 2, New York, 1963, WW Norton, Inc.
3. Fine R: Use of Despert fables (revised form) in diagnostic work with children, J Projective Techniques 12:106, 1948.
4. Goodenough FL: Measurement of intelligence by drawings, New York, 1926, World.
5. Simmons JE: Psychiatric examination of children, ed 4, Philadelphia, 1987, Lea & Febiger.

72

Concepts of Psychosomatic Illness

Stanford B. Friedman

The notion that psychological and emotional factors influence a variety of disease states can be traced to antiquity. Only recently, however, has there been systematic observation and scientific study of such relationships. In the 1940s Alexander[1] proposed, from his clinical observations of patients, that specific psychological conflicts could be identified in individuals suffering from seven disease entities: peptic ulcer, ulcerative colitis, regional enteritis, hyperthyroidism, rheumatoid arthritis, essential hypertension, and bronchial asthma. At about the same time, Dunbar[2] proposed specific personality types, rather than the nature of the existing conflict, as being of etiologic importance. Common to both theoretic formulations was a belief that *specific* psychological phenomena caused or predisposed to *specific* diseases, and thus evolved the "theory of specificity." This approach to the conceptualization of "psychosomatic medicine" has led to the common belief that some diseases are significantly influenced by psychological factors and others are "purely" physical. This "either-or" concept represents a simplistic attempt to relate disease, as it exists in a particular individual, to a single cause.

In contrast, Engel emphasized a "multifactorial" concept of etiology and, more recently, has developed the "biopsychosocial model" of disease.[3,4] This model acknowledges that most diseases are the result of the complex interaction of multiple factors—biologic, psychosocial, and cultural—converging at a particular point in the life of an individual.

INFLUENCE OF PSYCHOSOCIAL FACTORS

The degree to which any one etiologic factor contributes to the development of disease depends on a number of considerations. First, some diseases appear to be influenced more by psychosocial factors than are others. The clinical source of ulcerative colitis, for example, may be directly related to the psychological status of the patient. On the other hand, there is little or no evidence that brain tumors in children are affected by such factors. However, the lack of such a relationship *may* be a result of insufficient study of this possibility. Second, just as the virulence and dose of a microorganism affects the development and severity of an infectious disease, so may the nature and intensity of a psychosocial stimulus influence its impact on a disease. Third, individual differences attributable to genetic factors or previous life experiences will modify the impact of etiologic factors on the health status of the individual. Fourth, there are temporal and developmental factors that may alter the role of psychosocial stimuli in disease. Thus, an individual's vulnerability to a particular disease may change with progression from infancy to late adulthood, with biologic and psychological factors interacting to account for such change.

The above discussion of the influence that psychosocial factors may have on the disease process is consistent with clinical observations and, as reviewed by Plaut and Friedman,[5] is supported by experimental findings in infectious diseases that traditionally are not considered "psychosomatic" in nature. There is therefore no *limited* number of diseases that can be identified as psychosomatic, but rather a spectrum of illnesses with varying degrees of susceptibility to psychosocial stimuli. Diseases such as asthma and peptic ulcer, for example, have traditionally been viewed as influenced by psychological factors, but in managing these diseases the clinician should not necessarily assume an etilogic importance of psychological factors in every case. Extreme biologic vulnerability in a given patient may result in disease without the influence of environmental factors or the presence of psychological distress or conflict beyond that normally experienced in everyday life. On the other hand, the presence or absence of psychosocial factors may, in a given individual, determine whether predisposition toward a disease will develop into a clinical problem. Further, psychosocial factors may influence the course of the disease and the response to drugs or other forms of therapy.

ROLE OF THE PEDIATRICIAN

In the evaluation of disease, the pediatrician should always consider psychosocial factors of *possible* etiologic importance. In many instances, however, the benign and infrequent nature of the illness, such as occasional upper respiratory infection, does not warrant an extensive psychosocial assessment of the patient and family. In other instances, the pediatrician would be amiss not to evaluate thoroughly the psychological status of the patient; examples include severe headaches, frequent infections, hypertension, chronic gastrointestinal symptoms, and the onset of many serious childhood diseases.

In the medical evaluation, the physician should be aware of those diseases which frequently appear to be influenced by psychosocial factors (e.g., asthma, ulcerative colitis). In addition, he or she should explore interactions between disease and environmental factors that are characteristic of some diseases, such as exacerbation of asthmatic symptoms secondary to persistent family dysfunction and conflict.

The psychological environment of the child or adolescent should be addressed. This evaluation may be divided into the three major spheres of a child's life—namely, relationship to *peers,* functioning with the *family,* and successes and failures at *school,* work, or both. Basically, the psychological world of the child should be defined, including parental expectations and environmental pressures, as well as sources of psychological and social support. Within the context of the child's social and community environments, is the child experiencing excessive pressure to conform? Are expectations unreasonable? Are these expectations related more to parental needs than to those of the child? The answers to questions such as these should be accompanied by evaluation of the child's past and current coping abilities, psychological strengths, and the existence or lack of social support systems.

The child's psychosocial and cognitive development should be assessed, with a focus on identifying genetic or experiential factors that might predispose him or her to certain diseases that, in general, might make psychological adaptations more difficult. In terms of temperament, was this child's early behavior that of the "difficult child?" Is there a history of hyperactivity or learning problems in the family? Has the patient been abused or rejected by his or her parents? These are merely examples of biologic and psychological factors that may interact with current life experiences to predispose to disease states.

In the overall psychosocial evaluation of a child or adolescent, the developmental status is critical in interpreting the child's "psychological world" ("Theories of Freud, Erikson, and Piaget"). Are the child's behaviors age appropriate? Of at least equal importance, are the expectations of parents (and grandparents) age appropriate for the child? The pediatrician should have an ongoing clinical impression of the "match" between the patient's chronologic age and developmental status.

In conclusion, the concept of a defined number of "psychosomatic diseases" is overly limited. Rather, there exists a spectrum of susceptibility to psychosocial factors that is related to the disease entity, the biologic and psychological makeup of the patient, the psychological and social environment, and the developmental status of the child or adolescent. The *clinical importance* of these considerations must be individualized by the provider of primary health care, and the clinical management, including the advisability of mental health consultation, must be planned accordingly.

REFERENCES

1. Alexander F: Psychosomatic medicine, New York, 1950, WW Norton, Inc.
2. Dunbar HF: Psychosomatic diagnosis, New York, 1943, Hoeber (Harper & Row).
3. Engel GL: Selection of clinical material in psychosomatic medicine, Psychosom Med 16:368, 1954.
4. Engel GL: The need for a new medical model: a challenge for biomedicine, Science 196:129, 1977.
5. Plaut SM and Friedman SB: Psychological factors in infectious disease. In Ader R, editor: Psychoneuroimmunology, New York, 1981, Academic Press, Inc.

73

Prediction of Adult Behavior from Childhood

David S. Pellegrini

It is widely assumed that adult psychopathology has its roots in childhood adjustment difficulties. By extension, it is generally assumed as well that the earlier we intervene in such difficulties the better, since psychopathology is likely to crystallize over time, making subsequent remediation more difficult. Epidemiologic studies suggest that a large proportion of children show some behavioral or emotional deviance at some stage of their development. However, according to Rutter and colleagues,[6] such problems prove to be transitory in the majority of cases. Moreover, a number of well-intentioned early-intervention programs have yielded adverse or mixed results.

Clearly, therapeutic efforts are not without risk. Unnecessary treatment might best be avoided if children would otherwise grow out of their difficulties through the natural process of development. It would be enormously advantageous, therefore, if we could identify those children who are prone to suffer chronic and serious maladjustment across their life span.

Unfortunately, although childhood behavior and early life circumstances show some tendency to predict adult behavior, the correlations are generally too modest to allow useful prediction with regard to individuals.[4]

For example, in a large-scale study published in 1973, West and Farrington[7] obtained a false positive identification rate greater than 50% in predicting deliquency on the basis of early family and child characteristics. Nevertheless, available findings do offer some important and useful clues to guide the primary care physician in referring appropriate children for treatment.

Various symptoms of neurotic or emotional disorder are very common in childhood. These include nail-biting, thumbsucking, bed-wetting, eating and sleeping difficulties, and fears of animals, situations, and places. Such symptoms appear to be of little long-term significance when they are mild in intensity and when they occur in isolation, rather than as part of a general pattern of multiple symptomatlogy. Isolated symptoms of this kind might best be thought of as exaggerations of normal developmental trends rather than as signs of childhood disorder or as precursers of adult disorder. On the other hand, the timing of such symptoms is interesting. Manifestations of emotional distress appear to be less benign when they are age inappropriate than when they occur at ages when the conditions are more common. For example, school refusal or phobia in an 11-year-old typically has a poorer long-term prognosis than the same clinical condition in a child just starting school.

General emotional disorder, in contrast to isolated symptomatology, does appear to have some long-term risk. Rutter and his colleagues[6] observed that children who manifested emotional disorder at age 10 were twice as likely as the general population to show such disorder at age 14. However, even those children who show severe and persistent disorders of this kind appear to have a relatively good adult prognosis, with or without treatment. Moreover, when emotional disorders do persist into adulthood, they tend to remain true to type, rather than evolving into more troubling conditions such as adult sociopathy or psychosis. Finally, it appears that emotionally troubled children respond better to treatment than any other maladjusted group. There is evidence to suggest that appropriate and timely intervention can shorten the course of this kind of disorder.

Childhood depression is one such condition for which the empirical picture is considerably less clear. Unlike most other symptoms of emotional maladjustment, depressive indicators such as sad mood, apathy, and self-deprecation become increasingly prevalent with age, especially among girls. Recent research results[5] suggest that isolated symptoms of depression are much more common among prepubertal children than was once thought. Such symptoms have been increasingly recognized as common corollaries or consequences of physical illness and injury in childhood.

Less consensus is evident regarding the prevalence of depression as a syndrome in childhood, although it is probably much less common before puberty than afterward. Most mood disturbances appear to be so short lived before puberty that some have argued against clinical intervention in all but the most severe cases. However, adequate long-term data are particularly sparse in this area. Although depressive illness arising in adolescence has been shown to have a relatively poor long-term prognosis, possible links between untreated depressive symptomatology in childhood and chronic mood problems or other difficulties in adulthood have not been adequately explored.

In contrast to most indicators of neurosis or emotional disorder, certain indicators of social and behavioral maladjustment in childhood have demonstrated considerable predictive power with regard to adult psychopathology. However, few such predictors exhibit clear continuity with or a direct developmental path to specific and unique outcomes. Rather, they tend to predict a range of adverse outcomes. Moreover, predictive stability of this kind does not emerge until the early school years.

One such indicator pertains to the quality of peer relations. Recent research results suggest that peers play a number of important roles in child development. For example, as agents of socialization, peers help to shape sexual and aggressive behavior. They are also a major source of emotional support, while providing instruction in a variety of social, cognitive, and motor skills. It should not be surprising, then, that poor peer relations in early childhood have been linked with later emotional difficulties, deliquency, substance abuse, suicide, and psychosis. In one classic study, Cowen and co-workers[1] attempted to uncover the early signs of persistent psychiatric disturbance. Of 537 schoolchildren, 33% (180) were identified as being at risk on the basis of ineffective school performance and behavior. By the time of follow-up 11 years later, 19% of this group, compared with only 5% of non-designated children, had received some form of psychiatric care, as indexed by appearance on a cumulative county register. Negative peer evaluations in third grade exceeded a variety of other adjustment indicators (including teacher and school nurse judgments) in predicting later mental health difficulties.

Active rejection by peers seems to be more critical in the prediction and the development of later psychopathology than is social isolation resulting from shyness and social withdrawal. Indeed, shyness alone appears not to be as closely linked to adult disorders, such as schizophrenia, as was once thought. In a long-term epidemiologic study undertaken in the Woodlawn area of Chicago, Kellman and associates[2] found that shyness in first grade was actually correlated with reduced rates of delinquency and substance abuse in adolescent boys and with reduced intake of hard liquor in adolescent girls. However, shyness was related to higher levels of anxiety in adolescent boys.

Early antisocial behavior and aggressiveness appear to be the sturdiest predictors of adult maladjustment. For example, in an exceptionally thorough and well-planned study, Robins[3] followed up some 500 individuals who had attended child psychiatry clinics 30 years earlier. Whereas most neurotic children went on to lead psychiatrically normal lives, children who engaged in early and repeated delinquent or aggressive acts grew up to be, with disturbing regularity, adult sociopaths. Looking backward, Robins noted that 95% of the adult sociopaths had been referred initially for antisocial and aggressive behavior.

In the Woodlawn study,[2] aggressiveness in first-grade boys was clearly linked to heavy drug, alcohol, and cigarette use in adolescence, as well as to delinquency. Although such associations were not apparent for girls, aggressiveness in conjuction with social isolation was associated with the poorest outcome for both sexes. Aggressive behavior has emerged as a primary prognostic component of hyperactivity as well.

Troublesome behavior patterns appear most likely to persist into adulthood when other social, psychological and cognitive handicaps are also present. According to Rutter and associates,[6] parental antisocial behavior or alcoholism, chronic marital discord, and poor academic achievement tend to potentiate emerging behavioral difficulties. Pervasive behavioral problems also tend to be more persistent than situation-specific ones. For example, those few youngsters who demonstrate hyperactivity, poor impulse control, and attentional problems in multiple settings (e.g., school, home, and the community at large) are more likely to show a variety of difficulties later in life (e.g., antisocial behavior, poor academic achievement, and depression) than are youngsters who are hyperactive in only one such setting (the majority of such cases). Similarly, children who engage in a variety of delinquent acts in multiple settings are at greater risk for adult criminality than are those who engage in isolated delinquent acts (see Chapter 103).

Clearly, much more work needs to be done to determine the early precursors, turning points, and contextual influences (family, peer, and community) on psychopathology. In the interim we are left only with general guidelines regarding the appropriate timing of clinical intervention. Available findings to date highlight the particular importance of early treatment for pervasive conduct and relational problems, especially because intervention efforts with antisocial adolescents and adults have so far proved to be singularly unsuccessful.

Early intervention also seems warranted whenever symptoms appear likely to interfere with the acquisition of social and academic skills, which could, in turn, lead to social rejection and school or work failure. Beyond that, intervention may be justified on the grounds of relieving or shortening the immediate distress caused by the presenting symptoms themselves, even when they may bear little or no functional relationship to later difficulties.

REFERENCES

1. Cowen EL et al: Long-term follow-up of early detected vulnerable children, J Consult Clin Psychol 41:438, 1973.
2. Kellam SG et al: Paths leading to teenage psychiatric symptoms and substance use: developmental epidemiological studies in Woodlawn. In Guze SB, Earls FJ, and Barrett JE, editors: Childhood psychopathology and development, New York, 1983, Raven Press.
3. Robins L: Sturdy childhood predictors of adult antisocial behavior: replications from longitudinal studies, Psychol Med 8:611, 1978.
4. Rutter M: Pathways from childhood to adult life, J Child Psychol Psychiatry 30:23, 1989.
5. Rutter M, Izard CE, and Read PB, editors: Depression in young people: developmental and clinical perspectives, New York, 1986, The Guilford Press.
6. Rutter M et al: Isle of Wight studies, 1964-1974, Psychol Med 6:313, 1976.
7. West DJ and Farrington DG: Who becomes delinquent? London, 1973, Heinemann Educational Books, Inc.

74

Options for Psychosocial Intervention With Children and Adolescents

Sheridan Phillips

The pediatrician often is unsure about what therapeutic options exist for children and adolescents with psychosocial problems, as well as about what will actually transpire in the course of treatment. This clearly hampers the effort to refer the patient appropriately and to prepare the child and parents for what to expect. This chapter acquaints the pediatrician with the most common forms of therapeutic interventions currently available and provides a brief review of their efficacy. In the interest of brevity, discussion is focused on treatment rather than on assessment. Also, only "psychological" treatment is described (i.e., chemotherapy is not discussed), although it must be noted that a combination of psychotherapy and chemotherapy is indicated in some instances of severe psychosocial disorders.[11]

Much of the confusion regarding psychotherapy is caused by two confounding variables: the therapist's theoretical orientation and the modality in which it is used. For example, one can take a behavioral approach with a child or with a family. Alternatively, family therapy can be conducted from a "systems" point of view. Thus five major schools of thought, or theoretical orientations, will be described, as well as the modalities in which they are most commonly applied (sometimes in adapted form), as shown in Table 74-1. Each school of thought listed at the left in the table is presented as a separate and distinct orientation. It is important, however, to emphasize that these are artificial divisions. There is much more melding and blending in the actual practice of child therapy, and combinations of approaches are both sensible and common. The modalities in which these theoretical orientations are typically applied are indicated under the appropriate column in the table.

Discussion of each therapeutic orientation includes the basic premises and goals of treatment, its typical course (e.g., length), examples of techniques or procedures used, its most appropriate recipients, and a brief review of the efficacy of that approach. Evaluating the efficacy of treatment, however, is so important yet complex that a general discussion of psychotherapy research precedes the presentation of specific therapeutic orientations.

In an attempt to provide an overview, this review undoubtedly oversimplifies both theories and issues and omits much of the detail and nuance each orientation deserves. It is hoped that there is a clear distinction between data-based statements and personal (or theoretical) bias. Specific discussion of when and how to refer children is not included, since this is provided throughout this section of the textbook for each specific clinical problem, particularly "Consultation and Referral for Behavioral and Developmental Problems."

THERAPEUTIC EFFICACY: GENERAL CONSIDERATIONS

Physicians, consumers, and society at large have an abiding concern to document the usefulness of therapy. The "bottom line" questions are, "Does it work?" and "Is it cost effective?" As with many things in life, these questions are easy to ask but extraordinarily difficult to answer. Conceptual, methodologic, pragmatic, and ethical considerations all appear to conspire against a clear-cut assessment of therapeutic efforts. Before discussing the apparent efficacy of specific orientations and modalities, this section reviews the general types of research strategies used to evaluate therapies and the complexity and problems inherent in such research.

One form of psychotherapy research is focused on the *process* of treatment and examines aspects of therapy as it is unfolding (i.e., what transpires within a session). This large body of literature has yielded very useful information about treatment (e.g., see "Client-Centered Therapy", discussed below).[3] However, for the sake of brevity, this section reviews the other major type of research, *outcome* research, which investigates change that occurs from the beginning to the end of therapy and following the conclusion of treatment. Ideally, such investigations document the nature and extent of change and demonstrate that such outcomes result directly from specific aspects of the intervention.

One approach is a *within-subject* design, whereby the experimental control is internal (i.e., no control groups are used). In this approach each subject or patient serves as his or her own control. Such an evaluation typically begins with a "baseline" period, during which the patient's behavior is recorded before any attempt at intervention. Recording continues during an intervention phase, when specific therapeutic procedures are in effect. One may then cease intervention and return to the baseline condition and subsequently reinstitute treatment. Repeated alternation accompanied by substantial changes in the observed behavior is an indication that

Table 74-1 *Overview of Therapeutic Orientations and Therapeutic Modalities*

	THERAPEUTIC MODALITY					
THERAPEUTIC ORIENTATION	INDIVIDUAL (CHILD ALONE)	PARENTS ALONE	PARENTS AND CHILD	FAMILY	GROUP (CHILDREN AND /OR PARENTS)	RESIDENTIAL
Psychodynamic	X	Adapted		Adapted	Adapted	Adapted
Behavioral	X	X	X	X	X	X
Phenomenologic						
Client-centered	X				X	
Gestalt	X				X	
Systems		X		X		
Eclectic	X	X	X	X	X	X

the treatment is responsible for the behavior change. A variant of this design is to introduce one component of the treatment at a time (e.g., each might be targeted at a different type of behavior) to determine whether a behavior changes when—and only when—the relevant intervention is introduced. The durability of change is assessed at various follow-up points.

The advantages of this design are the degree of experimental control and specificity it offers and its applicability with only a small number of patients or even with a single case (a "single-subject" design). Although internally valid, however, it is difficult to generalize from only one case; replications and extensions are thus required to increase confidence in the efficacy of treatment. Another difficulty is the "irreversibility" of some interventions, either for pragmatic or ethical reasons. It also has been argued that a therapeutic effect should be permanent and not so easily reversible.

In *between-subject* research, the nature of change is compared for a therapy group (or groups) versus a control group (or groups), typically before and after treatment and at various follow-up points (e.g., 6 months and 1 year after treatment). If done well, such research is costly and complex. For example, studies generally include several treatment groups. One group might receive a complete treatment "package" consisting of two components, a second group might receive one component only, and a third group the second component only, with appropriate "fillers" to equate time spent in treatment (note how a three-component package would generate several treatment groups). Alternatively, or in addition, another group might receive a different type of treatment (e.g., behavior therapy versus client-centered therapy). With this approach the difficulty is in controlling for therapist characteristics: using a "switch-hitter" would most likely result in differential levels of skill confounded with therapeutic orientation: using different individuals would confound personal characteristics and therapeutic orientation.

Devising appropriate control groups is no easier. One option is to use a "no treatment," or "waiting list," control group. This is accomplished by collecting a large group of comparable patients who have requested treatment and then randomly assigning them to therapy conditions: (1) immediate treatment or (2) treatment following a waiting period, with a delay at least as long as therapy for the treatment group (and longer if maintenance is to be assessed). It is common to find improvement over time for at least some patients in the waiting-list group. This is thought to occur because the individuals who have requested treatment have come to recognize that they have a problem and have made a commitment to change; deprived of access to professional therapists, they often turn to therapists in their environment (e.g., friends, pastor, self-help groups) or simply apply for treatment elsewhere. With children, one must also consider the effect of maturation during the waiting period.

Another important control is the "placebo," or "attention-control," group, where the therapist is given the challenging task of conducting sessions with patients but not actually doing anything specific. This controls for the patient's expectation that he or she is being helped and for the "nonspecific" aspects of interacting with a sensitive and caring individual. Not surprisingly, placebo groups typically display at least some improvement; in fact, it has been argued that this is the most reliable effect in psychotherapy research. In other words, it appears that the school of thought may account for less of the variance in patient outcome than do the "person variables," or personal qualities of the therapist. To demonstrate its efficacy, then, a therapeutic intervention would ideally demonstrate that it produced significantly greater change than could be accounted for by the nonspecific aspects of treatment.

A host of other difficulties beset research endeavors, such as the selection of appropriate dependent measures (behavior to be recorded) and the reliability and validity of the methods by which behaviors are assessed. Assuming that these challenges can be met and that a large enough pool of comparable patients and comparable therapists is available, the researcher is still confronted by major ethical concerns. Withholding treatment for an extended time and offering placebo intervention or a treatment plan hypothesized to be less than optimal all pose clear ethical obstacles. It is understandable, therefore, to find that some investigators have chosen to conduct *analog* research, which attempts to simulate clinical conditions in the laboratory. Participants are typically undergraduates who volunteer for course credit or monetary incentives or who have minor problems (e.g., mild fear of snakes or dogs, or mild test-taking or speech-giving anxiety). The difficulty with this approach is the trade-off between internal and external validity; although greater experimental control is gained, the ability to generalize to real clinical situations is lessened.

Given the numerous and varied obstacles to be confronted, it is admirable to find investigators who remain undaunted and struggle valiantly to conduct the best possible evaluations of their therapeutic efforts. Accepting this challenge has continued to improve the level of sophistication evidenced in psychotherapy research.[5] Even the questions asked have become more sophisticated and have moved well beyond the question of "Does it work?" Paul has summarized the ultimate outcome question as, "What treatment, by whom, is most effective for this individual, with this problem, under this set of circumstances, and how does it come about?"[3] Clearly, this question cannot be answered by a single study but will represent the cumulative knowledge of multiple efforts to address the efficacy of therapy.

PSYCHODYNAMIC THERAPY

Basic Assumptions

This school of thought covers a wide variety of approaches, from traditional analysis to neofreudian variants such as sociocultural, object relations, and ego psychology. The fundamental assumptions, however, were derived from Freud by his daughter, Anna Freud, by Melanie Klein, and by subsequent analytic theorists who specialized in work with children.[6] The concept of *unconscious conflict* is central: the child's disturbed or abnormal behavior is hypothesized to result from intrapsychic conflict in the same manner that an infection causes the overt manifestation of a fever. Therefore treatment is focused on identifying and resolving the underlying conflict among instinctual urges (id), conscious thoughtful regulation or reality orientation (ego), and self-evaluative thoughts, or "conscience" (superego). If this is accomplished, it is assumed that the overt behavioral disturbance will cease and the child will be free to develop appropriately.

Therapeutic Activities

The therapist first attempts to establish a relationship with the child that will enable the child to feel free to express any thoughts and feelings, such as anger and sadness. In fact, this freedom of expression is seen by many theorists to be therapeutic in itself. With this relationship developed, the therapist comments on the child's expressed feelings, generally interpreting the meaning of symbols revealed in the child's fantasies, dreams, or, most often, free play. Most of the therapeutic work is conducted in a playroom, using materials such as clay and sand, fingerpaints, games, and human figures and a doll house. The "depth" of interpretation provided varies among different theorists. For example, a doll thrown across the room might be seen by Anna Freud as anger toward the situation, whereas others might interpret it as hatred for the mother.

Although interpretation is an important therapeutic device, it is used parsimoniously, especially at the outset of treatment. Most therapists draw on additional devices, such as developing the transference reaction (or reaction to the therapist), "working through" past interpersonal conflicts, and gratifying dependency needs. There are so many different adaptations of psychodynamic treatment, and so much variation among therapists, that it is difficult to provide a unitary picture of therapeutic activities. Many therapists vary the intensity of treatment and their approach, depending on the developmental stage of the child, the nature of the psychopathology, and the family situation.

Certain obvious adjustments have been made to apply psychodynamic treatment to children. Since children find it more difficult than adults to express their inner lives verbally, play is used more often than free association. Also, children do not generally seek therapy themselves; it is thus the therapist's responsibility to develop the child's insight so that he or she understands that a problem exists. Even with these modifications, however, analytic intervention is generally not attempted with children younger than 4 years of age. Adolescents have also usually not been considered to be appropriate candidates for such treatment, since they are too old for play therapy and too young for the traditional analytic couch. However, less traditional forms of psychodynamic therapy have been increasingly used with adolescents.

As shown in Table 74-1, the *traditional* form of psychodynamic treatment has been conducted alone with the child. Whereas Anna Freud believed that it was the therapist's responsibility to educate parents about their child's problems, many psychodynamic therapists deliberately have little contact with the parents and other family members. Such therapists generally consider it inappropriate to work with both the child and any other family member; thus it is quite possible to find a family with three or more therapists: one for the child, another for a second child, and a third for the parents' marital problems. One rationale for this approach is the avoidance of "competition" for the therapist; another consideration is the "transference" problems that are posed.

The disadvantage of separate therapists is the lack of coordination among their efforts, such that they may at times be working at cross-purposes. The absence of contact between the therapist and the child's parents also often results in the parents' ignorance of the child's problems, of the goals and progress of therapy, and of what parents might do to assist with the child's progress. Meeting only with the child may leave parents with the impression that they are expending significant money and effort, often over a period of several years, to enable the child to play with toys such as those he or she has at home. This obviously does disservice to the therapist's efforts. Such problems have prompted adaptations of psychodynamic treatment so that some therapists see the entire family together or meet with the parents separately.

The psychodynamic approach has also been adapted by some for use with groups of children and adolescents (usually from five to eight children). Group therapy has two major assets: it makes more efficient use of professional time and provides therapy in a different setting, where children interact with and learn from each other as well as the therapist. Groups of younger children typically play games or engage in activities such as arts and crafts, with the therapist guiding the group indirectly (i.e., by example). Psychodrama and more "talking" techniques are generally employed with older children and adolescents. The main goals of treatment continue to be achieving insight into and resolving unconscious conflict. Such groups may be homogeneous (e.g., victims of sexual abuse) or more heterogeneous (e.g., including both aggressive and withdrawn children). It is also possible to structure residential treatment with many psychodynamic features, combining individual and group treatment in an accepting, tolerant atmosphere that highlights the use of expressive materials such as paints and clay.

The course of traditional child psychoanalysis is lengthy, typically requiring four or five sessions per week for anywhere from 3 to 5 years. The obvious expense of such treatment and the limited number of children who can receive it have led to the development of less extensive psychotherapy that incorporates many aspects of analysis. Such intervention might involve two sessions a week for 2 to 3 years. The more limited goals of this shorter-term treatment have been described as (1) increasing capacity for reality testing, (2) strengthening object relations, and (3) loosening fixations.

The appropriate adult candidate for psychodynamic treatment has been semijokingly referred to as a "YAVIS"—young, attractive, verbal, intelligent, and salaried. The same point is applicable to children, since the typical patient is only mildly to moderately disturbed and has many assets. Aspects of the analytic approach, however, have been included in other interventions with more universal applicability (e.g., see "Eclectic Therapy," p. 678).

Efficacy

Although a considerable amount of study has been devoted to child psychoanalysis and new adaptations of psychodynamic therapy, the majority of these investigations represent either uncontrolled case studies or investigations of the therapeutic process. Thus there are some data available (1) regarding *process* questions such as who is an appropriate candidate for psychodynamic therapy, both as a patient and as a therapist, and (2) on the effect of therapists' interpretations. However, even these studies have yielded equivocal findings.[1,5,6] As with all forms of therapy, less research has been conducted with children than with adults. For both children and adults, psychodynamic therapists have paid the least amount of attention to *outcome* research, or controlled investigation of actual change or improvement produced by treatment.

Following Eysenck's devastating 1952 critique of the outcome of psychodynamic psychotherapy with adults,[3] Levitt conducted similar analyses of traditional psychotherapy with children (one paper reviewed 17 studies and a second described another 22 studies).[9] This work, published in 1957 and 1963, failed to find any sound support for the contention that traditional psychotherapy facilitates children's recovery from mental illness. These startling reports prompted attempts to broaden approaches to the treatment of children and to develop other alternatives, notably that of behavior therapy.

In the more than 25 years since the Levitt reports, there have been relatively few investigations of analytically oriented therapy with children that have included control groups and/or direct comparisons with other therapeutic approaches. Data that do exist indicate that, at best, the psychoanalytic approach has not been shown to be superior to other less expensive and less time-consuming methods. In fact, analytic therapy may even be inferior to other modalities if judged by the percentage of patients improved among all patients who *began* treatment. Studies of group psychotherapy also have not yielded convincing evidence of beneficial effects, particularly when contrasted with behavioral group methods.[1,5,6,9]

This is not to say that psychoanalysis does no good; the available research merely indicates that clear evidence of efficacy is still lacking. It may in fact be that psychoanalysis has limited applicability to children because of their level of cognitive development. It has been well established that young children have difficulty understanding adult interpretations of social interactions and in taking the other person's point of view and that they often do not understand how others perceive them. Before about 8 years of age, most children have only a primitive understanding of intentions, motives, and feelings. Given these well-documented cognitive limitations, children may have difficulty truly understanding complex psychodynamic explanations of their thoughts and feelings. Alternatively, psychoanalysis may truly be useful with children but merely not as cost effective as other forms of treatment. The remaining possibility is that psychodynamic psychotherapy is in fact the optimum approach but that this has simply not been adequately documented.

Part of the difficulty in conducting scientific research with psychoanalysis lies in the very nature of the concepts used. For example, how can one gain access to an unconscious that by definition is inaccessible? However, the crux of the problem is determining acceptable criteria for measuring outcome: symptom relief is viewed as being too superficial an index of the change brought about in the child. Furthermore, many analysts maintain that each situation or case is unique and therefore that no situation can be replicated and no two patients adequately matched. They also argue that it is impossible to differentiate changes caused by maturation from those resulting from therapy. Finally, most analytically oriented therapists agree with Freud in insisting that psychoanalysis can only be judged by experienced analysts. It should be noted, however, that Freud himself was not optimistic about a scientific study of psychoanalysis.

One must observe that these obstacles have not hindered therapists of other orientations from at least attempting to evaluate the effectiveness of their interventions in a controlled manner. Ultimately, then, the lack of scientific study of psychoanalysis probably reflects the value of its practitioners, who typically are uninterested in research. At this time, evidence regarding the efficacy of psychodynamic psychotherapy seems largely restricted to clinical case material. Although certainly not trivial, such information fails to meet many of the criteria for scientific evidence.

BEHAVIORAL THERAPY

The behavioral approach to treatment has grown with amazing rapidity in the past two decades. For example, the first report of the token-economy theraputic modality was published in 1968; its use was widespread by the mid 1970s. Behavioral therapists who were trained 10 years ago are surprised to find themselves no longer a rebellious, vocal minority but now part of the establishment. Surveys indicate that approximately 50% of all clinical psychologists in the United States and over

60% of clinical child psychologists identify their orientation as behavioral or cognitive-behavioral and that behavioral therapy associations now exist in more than 30 countries.

Basic Assumptions

Behavioral therapy is not, as is often thought, a collection of techniques. Rather it is an *approach* to conceptualizing and changing human behavior, an approach characterized by empirical methodology.[4,7] The key assumption of behavioral therapists is that they must "anchor" their understanding by reference to observable behavior. An abstract concept, such as anxiety, is thus understood by asking questions such as how the patient experiences anxiety, when it is worse and when it is better, what the "trigger" events are, how the patient responds to these anxious situations, and what the consequences are for him or her and for others. Each patient represents a "miniexperiment" in which the therapist examines the presenting problem and its development in the context of the patient's history. The therapist then searches for those variables that control the problem behavior. The resulting *functional analysis* represents an hypothesis that guides the therapist. This hypothesis is tested by the therapist and the patient as intervention proceeds. The therapist also typically relies heavily on data collection to assess the progress of treatment and the adequacy of his or her working hypothesis; the therapist thus often asks the patient to monitor and record specific behavior and will track its frequency over time.

A very early focus for behavioral analysis was a search for the stimuli that prompted the behavior and for the patient's response (hence S-R, or stimulus-response). This fairly rapidly evolved to SORC, which incorporates "organismic" factors such as the patient's perception of the stimulus and the consequences that the response engendered (e.g., the reaction of others). For at least the past 15 years, behavioral therapists have emphasized the importance of the patient's *cognition* as well as his or her overt behavior (hence *cognitive-behavior therapy*). The therapist thus attends to factors such as the patient's expectations for himself or herself and others, how the patient labels an event, and what kinds of statements the patient makes to himself or herself. For example, Kendall has developed and evaluated interventions that focus on altering the ways in which impulsive children think about and work through problems.[8] Increased understanding of such attitudinal and perceptual processes and deliberate attempts to modify them have brought behavioral therapy much closer to other therapeutic approaches, such as ego psychology. In fact, the past few years have seen several laudable attempts to bring about a rapprochement between behavioral and psychodynamic formulations.[5]

In designing therapeutic interventions, the behavioral therapist draws on the principles and models of experimental psychology. Many of these come from learning theory: classic and operant conditioning, observational-social learning (i.e., modeling), and the development of self-control. Other paradigms also are useful, such as research in social psychology regarding the process of attitude change. Probably the broadest theory employed is social learning theory, which presumes a continuity between normal and abnormal behavior, implying that maladaptive behaviors are acquired through the same processes as normal behaviors. Accordingly, specific efforts to learn and use more adaptive behavior are expected to bring about changes in the way patients view themselves and how others see and react to them. Thus intervention is a cyclical process involving change in behavior, attitudes, and cognitions. Bandura's more recent "self-efficacy" theory[2] attempts to synthesize a variety of therapeutic interventions as procedures that gradually convince the individual of his or her ability to cope with difficult and frightening situations.

Therapeutic Activities

It is difficult to state succinctly what a behavioral therapist does with a patient, since the hallmark of the behavioral approach is to tailor intervention to the particular needs of a given patient. Therapy therefore is very different for different problems. Although various treatment "packages" have been developed for specific problems, these are standardized largely for research and demonstration and are subsequently adapted for the individual patient. The key, as noted before, is the functional analysis or behavioral formulation of the problem. Treatment is then logically derived from assessment. For example, one important distinction is that of a behavioral *deficit* versus an *inhibition*. In the case of a deficit of the appropriate skills, the therapist would focus on skill acquisition (e.g., social skill training "Peer Relationship Problems"). Alternatively, a patient might possess the appropriate skills but be inhibited in using them in certain situations because of excessive anxiety or fear of the consequences; therapy would then focus on reducing these inhibitions.

Regardless of the specific problem, there are some commonalities in approach. The focus is largely (although not exclusively) on the present. There is a commitment to experimental evaluation; the behavioral therapist is likely to set concrete goals to be achieved within a relatively short time, with progress then being evaluated by both the therapist and the patient. Therapy is active and involves joint planning and homework assignments for the patient (and sometimes for the therapist). It is assumed that insight is almost always insufficient for satisfactory behavioral change and that it needs to be accompanied by gradual learning and implementation of new behavior in a concrete and deliberate manner. Finally, therapy obviously takes place in an interpersonal context, and practitioner characteristics are an important aspect of therapeutic change. Goldfried and Davison have pointed out that a tough-minded approach to conceptualizing human problems in no way precludes a warm, genuine, and empathic interaction with patients.[7] In fact, patients of behavioral therapists who were asked to describe their therapist identified the same personal qualities that have been found to be therapeutic in other orientations, such as client-centered therapy (discussed below).

Behavioral therapy was initially applied with psychotic, retarded, and autistic populations and with patients who had severe phobias—in other words, people with intractable problems that no one else wanted to treat. This approach to therapy has subsequently been applied to an enormous array of problems and situations and is not restricted by the age of the patient or the type of problem. In some cases it may be applied in conjunction with chemotherapy (e.g., for treatment of hyperactivity), although the goal typically is to withdraw medication gradually whenever feasible. The same basic principles can be applied with a child with conduct disorders and with a group of hospitalized patients who are not functioning optimally.

In fact, a behavioral approach has been applied to many nontherapy situations (e.g., examining the voting behavior of Congress and energy conservation behaviors of the public) and thus is used in businesses and other consultative settings. For example, one could analyze a pediatric clinic to determine whether the existing contingencies in fact promote desired behavior of its users, such as compliance with appointment-keeping. Other general education efforts include self-help books (e.g., regarding toilet training). This broader application of behavioral principles is generally referred to as behavior modification, with behavioral *therapy* referring specifically to clinical problems.

It is important to note that behavioral therapy appears deceptively simple to the neophyte therapist. In fact, the therapist is merely guided by general principles and must rely on considerable improvisation and inventiveness in the clinical situation. Many inexperienced practitioners (and teachers) have failed because of insufficient expertise both with clinical practice and with the theoretical principles on which therapy is based. Thus it is not uncommon to be told before instituting a successful behavioral program, "Oh, we tried behavior modification and that didn't work."

When using behavioral therapy with individual children, therapists typically employ a combination of sessions with the child and parents and, if indicated, the school or other extrafamilial agency. With infants and toddlers, the therapist typically works almost exclusively through the parents, although the child may be present for sessions when the therapist "models" a type of interaction with the child or provides feedback to parents as they attempt to interact with the child in a different manner. With older children and adolescents, the extent to which the parents and other family members are involved depends on the analysis of the problem and the focus of treatment. Seeing all family members together for all sessions is indicated in some situations, whereas in others the therapist may choose to focus on the teenagers and his or her parents. In cases of multiple problems the therapist may alternate family sessions (e.g., to work on communication and problem-solving) with individual sessions (e.g., to address problems with peers). Sessions typically are scheduled once or twice a week, and the length of treatment can be as short as four sessions or can continue for over a year.

Behavioral therapy can also be employed with groups of children or adolescents or with groups of children and their parents. This form of treatment, when appropriate, makes efficient use of professional time and also has the advantage of providing an opportunity to interact therapeutically with peers (e.g., engage in role-playing). Group therapy typically, although not necessarily, is employed with a relatively homogeneous group, such as shy and withdrawn boys, to enable treatment to focus on specific problems. A group approach also has been employed with parents; some parent-training groups are specifically therapeutic, and others are more educational and designed for a "normal" population. In any form, groups are generally limited in time and rarely continue for longer than 6 months. It is not uncommon for two therapists to lead the group, since they offer two models of behavior and also can model interaction with each other (e.g., a male and female therapist with a parent group). In addition, group interactions are so complex that having two therapists is helpful in tracking events in the group and ensuring that all patients receive therapeutic attention.

Behavioral interventions also have had widespread use in the classroom. These range from management tips developed for use in the normal classroom to special classroom programs for children who are hyperactive or have conduct disorders.[6,9] Residential programs also have been developed for a variety of populations. Two examples are Project Re-ED and Achievement Place, the first for emotionally disturbed children and the second for delinquent children and adolescents.[6] Children are placed in an intensive treatment environment that includes sessions with parents and then are gradually returned to the home. (Achievement Place, a community-based program, even enables children to continue attending their own school during treatment.) Currently it is difficult to find residential programs for emotionally disturbed and retarded children that do not make at least some use of behavioral principles. In fact, behavioral therapy's greatest contribution may be the introduction of successful toilet training and management of retarded children, which has released an enormous amount of staff time and enables the reorientation of such programs from being almost completely custodial to emphasizing self-care and education.

Efficacy

With the possible exception of client-centered therapy for adults, no other therapeutic approach has been subjected to as much systematic evaluation as has behavioral therapy. Investigations of behavioral therapy thus dominate most scientific journals reporting professional treatment outcomes, and over 70% of investigations of treatment efficacy funded by the National Institute of Mental Health are conducted by behavioral therapists. Although less research has been conducted with children than with adults, there still have been literally hundreds of outcome studies published in the past 20 years. The majority of these have employed either a single-subject design, with internal controls, or a comparison design, with various control groups, such as a waiting-list or placebo group; fewer studies have directly compared behavioral and other therapeutic approaches. It should also be noted that less scientific evaluation has been conducted in residential programs than in outpatient and classroom settings.

There is now substantial evidence for both the efficacy and the superiority of behavioral therapy for (1) children who are retarded, autistic, aggressive, enuretic (especially those with primary enuresis), introverted and withdrawn, hyperactive, academic underachievers, anxious about tests, or engaging in self-injurious behavior, and (2) classroom management.[6,9] Additional evidence indicates that behavioral therapy is as effective or more so than other modalities for the treatment of specific fears and phobias of children, depression, delinquency, and family problems.[6,9] It should be noted that this is based on reviews of treatment that sometimes combine behavioral therapy with other forms of intervention (e.g., chemotherapy).

Early concern regarding "system substitution" has proved to be unfounded; given appropriate problem analysis and intervention, the substitution of a new symptom for the one that was treated has not been evident. Behavioral therapy has had a more modest degree of success to date with problems such as obesity, addiction, and lack of assertion.[1,4-6,9] A behavioral approach also appears promising, although sufficient documentation is not yet available, for the treatment of headaches and other somatic disorders such as asthma, seizures, and persistent vomiting, as well as for helping children to cope with medical and dental procedures and for promoting compliance with medical regimens.[6,9]

Although its accomplishments to date have been gratifying, much remains to be learned about behavioral therapy. One prominent criticism is that behavioral therapists do not completely understand why successful procedures are successful. For example, relaxation training and desensitization, although clearly efficacious, have been variously explained as counterconditioning (using a classic conditioning model), as operant conditioning, and as a process of cognitive change. Another persistent problem for behavioral therapists has been the generalization of therapeutic effects across different situations and the maintenance of change after the conclusion of treatment. This has led to greater emphasis on problem assessment and suggests, for example, that desensitization may be most appropriate for specific anxiety, whereas a focus on cognitive factors may be best for cross-situational anxieties. Also, behavioral therapists now attempt to design programs that build in long-term maintenance and incorporate expected relapses into the treatment strategy; for example, with patients who have enuresis and those with addictions. It has become clear that generalization must be specifically programmed in the therapeutic plan.

PHENOMENOLOGIC THERAPIES

Phenomenologic (or humanistic) therapy is insight oriented, as is psychodynamic therapy, and assumes that disordered behavior can best be altered by increased awareness of one's own motivations and needs. The distinction of humanistic therapy, however, is its emphasis on free will, attributing considerable freedom of choice to the patient. Phenomenologic therapies focus on promoting the patient's "growth as a person," the primary vehicle for doing so being the patient-therapist relationship.

Client-Centered Therapy

Basic Assumptions. The major phenomenologic model is Carl Rogers' *client-centered* therapy,* which assumes that patients can best be understood by the way in which they subjectively construe events (a phenomenologic perspective) rather than by an objective view of the events themselves.[3] The focus of therapy therefore is to attend to the *client's* perceptions and feelings and to let the client take the lead in the therapeutic process. Rogers postulates an innate tendency to actualize, or to realize one's potential, which is as much a human drive as the reduction of biologic tensions (e.g., hunger).

Because people are assumed to be innately striving for good, total and nonjudgmental acceptance by the therapist is the key to providing an atmosphere in which the client's natural growth may proceed unhindered. Rogers assumes that maximal development will take place when the client does not need to struggle for and be concerned about approval by others. This approach is thus believed to be the appropriate remedy when people have been thwarted in their growth by the evaluations and judgments imposed on them by others, creating "conditions of worth" that force individuals to distort or become unaware of their own real feelings.

Therapeutic Activities. The key therapeutic relationship is based on three vital attitudes of the therapist: (1) *unconditional positive regard* (sometimes also referred to as "warmth"), (2) *empathy,* and (3) *congruence* (sometimes referred to as "genuineness"). To display *unconditional positive regard,* the therapist must convey the message that he or she cares about the client as a person, accepts the client, and trusts the client's ability to change. The therapist is willing to listen and avoid interpretation and value judgments. To display *empathy,* the therapist actively attempts to perceive the client's feelings and to communicate this understanding by "reflecting," or paraphrasing, what he or she believes to be the client's views. It should be emphasized that this is more than merely repeating what the client has said; it represents the distillation and "playback" of the client's feelings. Finally, in displaying *congruence,* the therapist establishes a real, human relationship by abandoning any facade and expressing himself or herself genuinely. In so doing, the therapist leaves the responsibility for the client's life with the client and indicates confidence in the client's ability to handle the therapist's feelings.

This individual, verbal form of client-centered therapy, although developed for adults, is also appropriate for many adolescents. Its course typically consists of one or two sessions weekly, for a period ranging from a few months to several years. Client-centered therapy is generally used for individuals with a mild or moderate disturbance; Rogers himself has warned that it is probably not appropriate for those with severe pathologic conditions. The Rogerian approach has also been applied with groups, most notably with encounter groups. The goals of individual and group treatment are similar: increasing awareness, self-acceptance, interpersonal comfort, and self-reliance.

Client-centered therapy has been adapted by Virginia Axline and others for young children through the use of play therapy, using much the same setting and material as do psychodynamic therapists.[3,6] The key difference is that the Rogerian therapist does not use play to make symbolic interpretations. Analogous to treatment with adults, the therapist encourages the child to lead the session and displays unconditional positive regard by his or her words and actions.

Gestalt Therapy

Basic Assumptions. As with client-centered therapy, Fritz Perls' *gestalt therapy* promotes growth by increasing self-awareness and encouraging patients to assume respon-

*Rogerians refer to "clients" rather than "patients," since they maintain that these individuals are healthy and responsible, not "sick."

sibility for their actions and feelings.[3] Identifying theoretical differences between the two models is difficult, because the language used to describe gestalt therapy is often esoteric and unclear and because it seems to be only loosely related, at best, to principles of gestalt psychology (a laboratory-based study of human perception). Gestalt therapy is most easily discriminated from client-centered therapy by the methods used in treatment, which involve an active, directive therapist, and often, dramatic techniques.

Therapeutic Activities. A major focus of gestalt therapists is to emphasize the present; this therapy takes place in the "here and now." The therapist thus insists that the patient talk in the present tense and discuss current feelings. Use of language is also important in assisting the patient to take direct responsibility for his or her feelings. For example, a patient who says, "It's really aggravating to hear that," might be asked to restate this as, "I am angry with you for saying that to me." Another technique is to ask the patient to project himself or herself into another person or object. For example, if a patient says that it feels like there is a wall between her and her parents, she may be asked to "become" that wall and talk about how it feels.

Possibly the most useful procedure employed by gestalt therapists is to externalize conflicts and feelings. For example, a patient may confront an empty chair, imagine that his father is there, and tell his father those things he has wanted to say but has been unable to say to him. Or, if the patient is stuck in her decision-making (e.g., whether to go to a local college and live at home or to go away to college), she may be asked to alternate sitting in two chairs. When she is in one, she takes the side of staying at home and tells why she wants to stay at home and how she feels about it; sitting in the other chair, she fully experiences and relates to the therapist the part of herself that wants to go away to college. This enables the patient to sort out the emotional aspects of the conflict, and it is fascinating to observe how the balance gradually shifts as one side predominates and the decision begins to resolve.

Gestalt therapy has not been systematically adapted for children and is thus typically employed only with adolescents. As with client-centered treatment, it is generally only appropriate for mildly or moderately disturbed patients. Gestalt therapy is employed both with individuals and with groups. Individual therapy generally consists of one or two sessions weekly for anywhere from a few months to several years. Groups are often begun with an intensive weekend experience and then typically meet for 1 evening a week for 6 months to a year, although some groups continue almost indefinitely.

Efficacy. Largely at Rogers' own insistence, there have been numerous attempts to study and evaluate client-centered therapy.[3,5] In fact, it has been suggested that Rogers can be credited with stimulating the whole field of psychotherapy research. Much of this has been a study of the *process* of therapy, and Rogerians have been responsive to the findings. For example, Rogers no longer calls his therapy "nondirective" (the original label); a careful analysis of his own therapy transcripts has shown that the therapist does "shape," or subtly guide, the client's verbal statements. *Outcome* studies with adults have also shown changes in client's self-perceptions following treatment, in contrast to a normal control group (not in therapy) and a waiting-list control group. This research has been criticized, however, because it is based on clients' self-reports, with no external judgment of how clients actually behave following treatment. Also, it is not clear how much change is attributable to this form of therapy per se and how much to the nonspecific aspects of this and other forms of treatment.

As with all therapeutic modalities, less study of client-centered therapy has been directed to the treatment of children. Investigators have reported positive changes following child therapy, but some of these evaluations suffer from flaws, such as the selective assignment of children to treated and nontreated groups and the use of ratings by observers who were not "blind" to the therapeutic status of the children. The results of these evaluations currently are thus suggestive rather than conclusive.

Much less evaluation of gestalt therapy has been conducted. As with psychodynamic therapists, many gestalt therapists are uninterested in or relatively inimical toward the collection of data. Those who have attempted to study therapeutic outcome have been hampered by the gap between Perls' concepts and his techniques. Gestalt therapy (and to some extent client-centered therapy) has been criticized for being incomplete: by deemphasizing clinical assessment and the patient's history, the therapist may miss diagnostic signs or background facts that could be important in planning treatment. The danger of inadequate screening of group members, for example, can be seen in an estimated 8% "casualty" rate from phenomenologic group experiences (e.g., sensitivity training, encounter groups).[3,4] Although these casualties are not all as dramatic as a psychotic breakdown, there is some evidence to suggest that these participants have been harmed in some way by the experience. This intervention may thus be beneficial for many but not all participants.

SYSTEMS THERAPY

Basic Assumptions

Systems therapy represents an approach to family therapy that views the family as a unit—a dynamic system—rather than a collection of individuals. The relationships among the family members are hypothesized to have developed in the specific manner in which they did so that the family could achieve *homeostasis.* This relatively stable state is periodically disrupted by external events (e.g., geographic relocation) or change within the family (e.g., birth of the first child or new siblings). This triggers changes in the family members' relationships and the subsequent reemergence of a homeostatic state, which may be different from the previous one, in much the same way that a mobile is affected by a gust of wind. Homeostasis may sometimes be achieved in ways that are not beneficial for all members, such as a "problem child" distracting attention from an unhappy marriage.[12]

Systems therapists therefore view the child with behavior problems as merely the *"identified patient"* and believe that treatment is most appropriately focused on the entire family. This form of intervention, conjoint family therapy, treats the family as a group and includes all members who live together except for infants and toddlers. Treatment may focus initially on the "problem child," but the therapist often attempts to move fairly quickly to "reframe," or redefine, the problem as a disturbance in family process, faulty communication, or both. The therapist thus encourages all family members to see their own contribution to the problem and the positive changes that each can make.

The systems approach examines the roles played by family members and the function of the child's problem in maintaining the homeostasis of the family.[12] One goal of treatment is to identify covert family rules that consistently produce the same maladaptive interactions. For example, a stepfather believes his marriage could be threatened by his stepdaughter, who dislikes him; he is thus overly critical of her and promotes conflict between her and her mother to diminish her influence on her mother. Another goal of treatment is to promote appropriate communication, such as providing direct messages, using noncoercive communication, avoiding the use of a "double bind," and minimizing "scapegoating" of the identified patient. Parenthetically, note the similarity of the above to the functional analysis and skill training conducted by behavioral therapists.

Therapeutic Activities

Therapeutic goals are achieved by analyzing and commenting on the verbal and nonverbal messages exchanged by family members. As the family becomes more aware of these maladaptive "rules" and messages, it is assumed that they are better able to change them. The therapist may also ask family members to relabel a behavior more positively (e.g., use the term "independent" rather than "selfish"). Another tactic might be to direct family members to exaggerate their customary style (be the ultimately critical father or ultimately martyred mother) to foster awareness and change.

Minuchin's structural family therapy is an adaptation that emphasizes family "sets" as the target for change.[3,12] These sets refer to the hierarchy, or structure, of family relations and the alliances between members. For example, an *enmeshed* family is one in which the members are overinvolved with one another. Here, the therapist would attempt to strengthen the alliance between the parents and clearly designate their status as parents (e.g., he or she might even say, "You are a child—be quiet; this is a matter for your parents to settle."). The therapist would then encourage members to interact more with others of their own age and would promote more activities outside the family. With a *disengaged* family, there might be an uninvolved father, kept distant by a strong "coalition" between mother and son. The therapist would again attempt to reorder these alliances and reestablish the father in the family structure.

Systems therapy has been used with a variety of problems, both with children and adolescents (although typically not with very young children). Some therapists insist that all family members always attend, whereas others may work with the parents alone for a part of the treatment (e.g., for marital problems). The course of therapy typically consists of one session a week (although this may be longer than the usual 50-minute session), with the active participation of the family between sessions by the use of assigned homework. (Again, note the similarity to behavioral therapy.) Treatment may continue for several months or several years.

Efficacy

Evaluation of "pure" systems therapy to date is inconclusive because of the paucity of appropriately controlled outcome studies. A combined behavioral-systems approach has demonstrated beneficial effects for both the identified patient and other family members (e.g., siblings).[6,10] A combined approach also has been shown to be as effective or more so than individual therapy and client-centered family therapy.[1,6,9]

In general, available data indicate that *conjoint* family therapy, regardless of theoretic orientation, appears superior to other methods, such as providing individual treatment for each family member, particularly when the presenting problems relate to family crises and conflicts about values, lifestyles, or goals. Treatment outcomes have been found to be superior when fathers agree to participate in treatment. Interestingly, this has been shown to be the case when parents are separated as well as when they are together.[6]

ECLECTIC THERAPY

Basic Assumptions

Eclectic therapy is not so much a "school of thought" as the *absence* of an identified school. It has been included in this chapter because surveys of psychologists have indicated that eclecticism is frequently identified as a therapeutic orientation (psychodynamic, behavioral, and eclectic being the most common). As discussed previously, experienced therapists often employ procedures and techniques from a variety of therapies. Furthermore, they may also incorporate *concepts* from orientations other than that of their original training. With increasing borrowing and blending, a therapist may come to believe that his or her orientation no longer can accurately be classified as that of an identified school or theory; such therapists will label themselves "eclectic."

It is important to distinguish between *technical eclecticism* and *theoretical eclecticism*. The former refers to a therapist (1) who is consistently guided by a theoretical framework as he or she conceptualizes and understands a patient, the patient's problems, and his or her attempts to change, but (2) who employs techniques borrowed from other modalities when appropriate for a particular patient. For example, it is not uncommon for a behavioral therapist to be guided by the principles of social learning theory and yet employ gestalt exercises to help an overly intellectual patient identify the emotional factors involved in his or her problem-solving or decision-making. Similarly, a behavioral therapist may use play materials when working with children. These techniques, however, are carefully selected to fulfill a specific purpose, which is part of an overall therapeutic strategy; in other words, the therapist uses them as a *behavioral* therapist. In contrast, *theoretical* eclecticism eschews the guidance of any theoretical system. It is my bias that any theory is better than no theory, since successful therapy requires some purposive stance on the part of the therapist. Meyer has semijokingly said that a theoretical framework is therapeutic for the therapist, since the therapist thinks at least he or she understands what is going on.[7]

Eclecticism may also be an appropriate label for interventions that have been developed for very specific situations or populations, even though they may be loosely associated with some theoretical system. Probably the clearest example of this is Synanon, an intensive, residential program developed to treat drug addiction. Although much of this program is readily translated into social learning (or behavioral) terms, it also makes extensive use of client-centered techniques and encounter group sessions. Other examples abound in community psychology, such as crisis intervention, suicide hotlines, and prevention efforts. Although some programs are explicitly behavioral, many community programs are atheoretical.

Efficacy

Given the plethora of programs and treatments that are essentially eclectic and the general absence of sound evaluative study, no pretense will be made here of discussing the efficacy of eclectic modalities.

SUMMARY

The goal of this chapter has been to increase the pediatrician's understanding of variants of psychotherapy that are available for children and to increase the practitioner's ability to effect an appropriate referral and prepare the patient and family for treatment. In becoming more familiar with the different therapeutic orientations described, it is hoped that the reader will appreciate the extent to which these are not completely separate and distinct. With increasing clinical experience, therapists become more similar to one another, and many combine elements from different schools of thought. Therapeutic orientation is only one of several factors important in the selection of a therapist; quality of training, personal characteristics, general reputation, responsiveness, and ability to work with the pediatrician are clearly vital considerations ("Consultation and Referral for Behavioral and Developmental Problems").

Finally, it is hoped that the reader will appreciate the difficulty and complexity of psychotherapy research and thus be tolerant of the therapist's inability to make categoric and unqualified claims regarding the efficacy of his or her intervention. In fact, it is wise to beware of a lack of humility, both for the individual therapist and for a therapeutic orientation. Even those instances of "demonstrated efficacy" reviewed earlier represent a tentative conclusion based on a number of studies, each of which is imperfect and rarely, if ever, reports unqualified, long-term success with all patients.

REFERENCES

1. Achenbach TM: Developmental psychopathology, ed 2, New York, 1982, John Wiley & Sons, Inc.
2. Bandura A: Reflections on self-efficacy. In Franks CM and Wilson GT, editors: Annual review of behavior therapy: theory and practice, vol 7, New York, 1979, Brunner/Mazel, Inc.
3. Bernstein DA and Nietzel MT: Introduction to clinical psychology, New York, 1980, McGraw-Hill Book Co.
4. Davison GC and Neal JM: Abnormal psychology: an experimental clinical approach, ed 4, New York, 1986, John Wiley & Sons, Inc.
5. Garfield S and Bergin AE, editors: Handbook of psychotherapy and behavioral change, ed 3, New York, 1986, John Wiley & Sons, Inc.
6. Gelfand DM, Jenson WR, and Drew CJ: Understanding child behavior disorders, ed 2, New York, 1988, Holt, Rinehart & Winston, Inc.
7. Goldfried MR and Davison GC: Clinical behavior therapy, New York, 1976, Holt, Rinehart & Winston, Inc.
8. Kendall PC and Braswell L: Cognitive-behavioral therapy for impulsive children, New York, 1985, The Guilford Press.
9. Quay HC and Werry JS, editors: Psychopathological disorders of childhood, ed 3, New York, 1986, John Wiley & Sons, Inc.
10. Robin A and Foster SL: Negotiating parent-adolescent conflict: a behavioral-family systems approach, New York, 1989, The Guilford Press.
11. Wiener J, editor: Psychopharmacology in childhood and adolescence, New York, 1977, Basic Books, Inc.
12. Zuk G: Family therapy: a triadic-based approach, New York, 1981, Behavioral Books.

75

Consultation and Referral for Behavioral and Developmental Problems

Sheridan Phillips, Richard M. Sarles, and Stanford B. Friedman

Certain types of behavior represent such a clear indication of psychosocial problems that a single occurrence should signal the pediatrician to consider referral. Infantile autism, for example, is usually apparent before 30 months of age. These children generally display a lack of responsiveness to other human beings, self-isolation, grossly deficient language development, and peculiar attachments to animals or inanimate objects. Autistic children do vary in symptomatology, and few are totally unresponsive to environmental stimuli, including people; their responses, however, are characteristically irregular (variable) or inappropriate. Similarly, schizophrenic children display such bizarre behavior or preoccupations and such grossly impaired emotional relationships that they are readily identifiable. In fact, a major shortcoming of even relatively successful therapy is the inability to make the psychotic child socially inconspicuous.

Generally, it is also easy to identify certain acting-out behaviors as clear signals for referral. These include suicidal behaviors, vandalism, fire-setting, and cruelty to animals. Family intervention often will be indicated, especially for problems such as child abuse and secondary enuresis. Also, a skilled therapist can help both patient and family to deal with the aftermath of rape.

Unfortunately, the majority of problems cannot be so readily identified by the occurrence of a single behavior. Probably the most difficult determination to make is whether certain behaviors, such as mood swings in adolescence, merely represent the normal developmental process or are manifestations of a more serious problem. One indication, however, is to note any *sudden change in behavior*, such as a significant drop in grades, withdrawal from peers, or withdrawal from family. Such change may be related to a change in environment (e.g., moving to a new school or neighborhood). In such an instance, it is important to reassess the child's status about 2 months after the change is observed. If the situation has not improved substantially at that time, the child probably needs special assistance in adapting to the new environment.

Generally, the difference between "normal" and "problematic" behavior is not the actual behavior (or behaviors) but rather the quantity (number of occurrences), distribution (different manifestations), severity (interference with social or cognitive functioning), and duration (at least 4 weeks).[1] For example, many young boys will occasionally dress up as girls or prefer girls to boys as playmates or say, for example, "I wish boys could have babies." This should be distinguished from genuine cross-sex behavior, which is characterized by a variety of manifestations, by the frequency and duration of such behavior, and by the degree of emotional attachment to the behaviors.

Similarly, all four factors (quantity, distribution, severity, and duration) are relevant in discriminating between the normally energetic child and one who is hyperactive. In other instances, the problem behavior may be more circumscribed but still of concern because of its frequency, severity, or duration, such as with drug abuse, sexual promiscuity, stealing, and poor academic performance. Children often pose conduct problems at home but not at school or at school but not at home.[1] The severity of the behavior, however, may signal a need for intervention despite its being restricted to a single setting. Analogously, fear of animals is prevalent among young children but decreases with age, whereas childhood animal *phobias* persist into adulthood.

The problems most likely to be missed are the "quiet" problems that do not make life difficult for parents or teachers. Examples of these are poor peer relationships, emotional and social withdrawal, apathy, dysphoria, and poor self-esteem. Pediatricians also may not recognize "quiet" parenting problems. Some parents will consistently express concern about their children's behavior or how they manage them. The specific behavior in question may be different at each visit, but the pediatrician may be continually providing brief assurance, which often is ineffective. At such times the pediatrician should consider why these parents are not aware that their children's behavior is well within the norm. Are they isolated from other parents with children of the same age? Do they need education and anticipatory guidance? The parents' questions may indicate that they are excessively protective or concerned or that they have unrealistic expectations of their child. If so, this will continue to be a problem for the child and indicates that intervention is warranted.

Admittedly, it is sometimes difficult to discriminate between problems that do and do not warrant referral. This is especially true for the pediatrician, who must consider not only the current severity of the problem but also the potential benefit of early intervention, which may prevent severe problems or significantly improve the quality of life for a child or family. Some reasons for pediatricians' hesitancy to refer children with behavioral problems and some considerations related to determining whether to refer are discussed in the following section.

SOURCES OF RELUCTANCE TO EMPLOY BEHAVIORAL SPECIALISTS

Physicians are often reluctant to use behavioral consultation or referral for a variety of reasons. One source of hesitation is that the primary care provider may feel pressured to comply with the current medical trend to treat the "total" patient. Any individual physician, however, may not have the time, expertise, or interest to do so. In such cases only the insecure professional will fear consultation from a colleague. Generally, parents will acknowledge a physician's honesty in delineating his or her own area of expertise and concomitant limitations and will appreciate the concern and interest evidenced by the physician's suggesting appropriate consultation or referral.

Conversion reactions illustrate the advisability of simultaneously exploring organic and psychosocial factors.[4] Especially when a patient is admitted to the hospital for evaluation, behavioral consultation should be requested at the outset of hospitalization. Many behavioral specialists have been frustrated by the request to evaluate such a patient on the last day of the hospital stay, when no significant physical findings were obtained. Involvement by a behavioralist at the outset enables a more reasonable and thorough assessment. For example, it provides the opportunity to observe the child's behavior during the hospital stay, thus generating information difficult to obtain in any other way. Also, parents do not see the behavioral assessment as a "last resort."

The tendency to request a behavioral consultation only after a variety of other subspecialty consultations have been conducted poses problems not only for the child and family but also for the consultation service per se. Many insurance and medical assistance plans limit the number of reimbursable consultations per hospital stay which may be reimbursed. Delaying the request for behavioral evaluation thus is one of the reasons consultation/liaison services typically experience difficulty in remaining solvent and viable.

Pediatricians also may avoid referring a child with a behavioral problem because they are reluctant to label a child or adolescent as having such a problem and fear that both parents and child will see the referral as an indication that the patient is "crazy" or seriously disturbed. Thus many physicians tend to be excessively conservative, only recommending referral when there is a blatant and obviously severe problem or when all else has failed. This implicit acceptance of the social stereotype of therapy is unfortunate, since early intervention can be extremely advantageous. For example, it is much easier for a child to catch up, whether with academic or social skills, when the performance gap is small. Similarly, intervening with a 16-year-old who is truly out of control is clearly a different matter from treating the same youngster at age 12.

At other times, it is not clear that the problem will become progressively more serious. Many parents and adolescents survive several stormy years of teenage rebellion and ineffective parental efforts to exert control. However, family disruption and stress can be reduced by a brief series of sessions with a specialist who is skilled in teaching communication and problem-solving skills.[3] It is likely that many parents and teenagers would consider this a worthwhile investment of time and money. The same argument can be made for many other difficulties that are "problem behaviors" rather than "behavior problems."[4] (See Chapter 70, "A Developmental Approach to Behavioral Problems.")

Many behavioral problems reflect a child's lack of skills rather than deep-seated pathologic conditions. It is probably the latter, historical view of behavioral problems that underlies current negative social prejudice regarding psychosocial treatment. Thus many individuals avoid using behavioral services, and yet they will readily turn to experts in virtually every other area of life—lawyers, accountants, physicians, teachers, plumbers—as a natural and clever use of specialists. A pediatrician who is familiar with the nature and purpose of different treatment modalities can encourage families to use behavioral resources effectively.

Pediatricians also may hesitate to recommend referral if they are concerned about the efficacy of behavioral intervention—that is, how much good it will do. A related concern, which is also appropriate, is the effort involved for physicians, parents, and children in going to a different place and person for consultation, then possibly having to adapt to yet another professional. Cost may present another difficulty. In general, it must be considered whether a referral involves more effort and expense than it is worth.

Although no intervention approach or professional can be totally effective, a skilled therapist is generally at least helpful, often very successful, and unlikely to be harmful. Many behavioral specialists now routinely generate a "treatment contract" with their patients, by which both parties agree to an initial series of sessions (usually between four and six), after which they jointly assess whether progress has been made. If the parents or patient believe that the initial experience has been productive, they may continue with the intervention plan; if not, there should be a change in either the plan or the therapist.

This practice ensures that patients will not continue in a long and expensive course of treatment that is deemed unnecessary or unproductive by the therapist or the parent. However, the length and intensity of appropriate intervention vary tremendously with the particular patient and problem. Even a highly effective and responsible therapist will have a range of cases, some requiring four sessions or less and others 100 sessions or more. The key is how to select and use a behavioral specialist to provide optimum care while maintaining contact with the primary care provider.

GENERAL CONSIDERATIONS

The physician can sometimes select a consultant to reduce the chances of a "patient shunt," where the child must first relate to a consultant and then adjust to another professional for intervention. When the primary care provider suspects that treatment is indicated, it is advisable to recommend a consultant who is able to provide both assessment and intervention. In some cases this will not be feasible, nor would it represent the optimum use of specialized skills. Knowledge of behavioral resources that are available, however, can enable the physician to make an appropriate recommendation.

Another consideration is how best to structure interaction with behavioral specialists. One possibility is to include behavioral specialists within general pediatric practices. Increasingly, pediatricians have invited mental health professionals to base their practices in adjacent offices. Even better, such professionals have become members of group practices. This approach has obvious advantages for providing many behavioral services naturally and efficiently. Although any given individual cannot possess the entire range of skills required, he or she can enhance the effective use of other resources in the community.

Preparing Parents

Preparing parents for behavioral consultation begins during the first discussion of the differential diagnosis, when both physical and emotional factors are included as potential causes of the symptoms.[4] Even when the primary care physician has correctly introduced the possibility of emotional issues early in the diagnostic work-up, parents may resist exploring emotional factors. Such resistance is more likely when the symptoms are organic or when there is no overt behavioral disruption.

In some instances parents may not be aware that they foster their child's aberrant behavior; instead, they often blame the school or their child's peers. In other instances, parents may deny any problems with their child, in part to avoid revealing their own interpersonal or marital difficulties or a problem such as alcoholism. Nevertheless, the physician should present an honest appraisal of the situation (with appropriate recommendations for behavioral consultation) without trying to please or appease the parents by avoiding discussing his or her true assessment of the clinical situation.

If parents are reluctant to consider a behavioral consultation, it may help to address their concern for their child's health and welfare. In explaining the need for such consultation, the pediatrician should suggest that this is an additional service for the complete and comprehensive care of their child. It should be emphasized that behavioral consultation does not imply the child is crazy; rather, it suggests that emotional factors may, totally or in part, account for their child's difficulty.

When the complaint is somatic, a useful example most parents can understand is the feeling of "butterflies in the stomach" before an examination, when speaking in public, during a marriage ceremony, or at other times of stress. A tension headache is another common symptom that can be used to demonstrate that a person can experience physical distress or pain without actual structural or physical disease being present.

If the parents agree to the consultation, the pediatrician should inform them of the consultant's name and reasons for this selection, the consultant's credentials, and how closely the consultant works with the primary care physician. It is the pediatrician's responsibility to make the initial contact with the consultant and to discuss the reasons for consultation.

Parents also should be informed that the consultant will probably want to see both parents together to collect important data concerning the child's development and a detailed family history. The number of visits generally required for a consultation and its approximate cost should also be discussed with the parents. Following the consultation, the primary care physician should meet with the parents to discuss the consultant's findings and recommendations. It is often useful to include the consultant and the child in this meeting as well.

If the parents are reluctant to follow a recommendation for intervention, the primary care physician should be careful not to support the parents' hesitation. Such a stance engenders lack of faith in the consultant the physician has recommended. In addition, such a position suggests expertise by the primary care physician in a field in which he or she has just recommended consultation. If, however, both parents and the pediatrician drastically disagree with the findings and recommendations of the consultant, a second opinion is indicated.

Preparing the Child

The young child should be told that his or her parents and the physician are concerned about aspects of the child's behavior, such as an inability to get along with friends, anger, nightmares, or an inability to cope with a physical illness. In the case of a psychosomatic symptom, the child needs to be informed that pain or illness is often caused by emotional feelings or worries. The child should be informed that he or she will be seeing a professional known to the pediatrician who is an expert in helping with these kinds of problems; it should be emphasized that the consultant helps by playing with children and talking with them about their thoughts and feelings.

With an older child or adolescent, the pediatrician begins to prepare the patient for consultation even while obtaining a physical and psychosocial history. As the physician increasingly concentrates on social and emotional aspects, the teenager may become indignant and confront the physician about the personal nature of the questions. The physician should not retreat or become defensive, but should emphasize the need for such probing personal questions in order to understand the symptoms or illness troubling the patient. As with parents, relating everyday examples can help the older child or adolescent to understand the connection between emotions and physical well-being.

Teenagers, since they are struggling with the developmental tasks of adolescence, may be concerned about confidentiality. Also, given the normal mood swings during this period, it is common for teenagers to wonder about their own mental health. Suggesting behavioral consultation can trigger protest that may reflect their own worst fear: that they really are different or even crazy. In most cases, the pediatrician can reassure teenage patients that they indeed are not; however, the physician must convey concern if significant psychopathology is suspected. Not to do so is frightening to the patient or parent, who may recognize that reassurance is premature and inappropriate. If severe emotional problems are present, the pediatrician should explain that the teenager's behavior does signal a departure from normal and indicates some excessive stress, which may be interfering with optimum well-being. Also, it is extremely useful to identify some specific potential benefit of intervention that is likely to be meaningful to the patient (e.g., better relationships with peers) as well as the alleviation of a problem (e.g., reducing conflict with parents or feelings of anxiety).

"Nonargumentative" firmness on the part of the physician concerning the need for referral is essential. While acknowledging the adolescent's anger or dismay, the physician needs to assert professional responsibility to render the best medical opinion, even if it is not to the patient's liking. It is seemingly paradoxical that a sturdy posture in this regard is often reassuring, for it conveys the idea that someone is listening and hearing the patient's troubles and is concerned about his or her behavior.

In most instances the child or adolescent should be informed of the approximate number of visits usually required and the type of interaction to expect. If the patient inquires about the cost of the consultation and evidences concern, the physician can assure the patient that this decision can be made only by the parents. In most cases the physician can emphasize that the patient's parents are concerned enough, and care enough, to be willing to spend whatever it may cost to receive proper help.

In cases of overt psychosis wherein "reality testing" is seriously impaired, psychological preparation of the patient can be ineffective. However, the physician cannot assume that the patient is totally oblivious to the surroundings. In fact, the pediatrician provides a stabilizing, reliable, and predictable influence for the patient. The physician can introduce the consultant as an expert in helping patients whose thoughts are confused or jumbled. It may even be helpful for the primary care physician to offer to be present during the first consultative session as a source of security for the patient.

Selecting a Consultant

Choosing the appropriate professional or agency is probably the most important service provided by the primary care physician to a patient with a psychosocial or learning problem. Although the common practice of suggesting a list of specialists protects the physician from any accusation of favoritism, it is actually not helpful to parents. A specific referral is preferable, which also relieves the family of wondering if they made the best choice.

A common question is whether it is best to use a pediatrician interested and expert in behavioral disorders, a child psychiatrist, a clinical psychologist, or a social worker. Although a thorough discussion of this issue is beyond the scope of this chapter, a brief review of relevant training and credentials may be helpful.

Those pediatricians well-versed in managing behavioral disorders might well have had training in behavioral pediatrics following their pediatric residency. Generally, their specialized training consists of 1 to 3 years of fellowship in behavioral pediatrics and/or child development, including academic and clinical experiences. Such fellowships vary greatly in their emphasis, some focusing almost exclusively on infants and young children, others covering a broad range of ages and problems. The behavioral pediatrician's area of expertise, theoretical orientation, and interests obviously will reflect the specific training received.

Most physicians formally engaged in psychotherapy have been trained in psychiatry. Following a year of internship (usually a rotating, internal medical pediatrics or neurology internship), 2 years of psychiatry residency training are required for board eligibility in psychiatry and neurology. Two additional years of child psychiatry training are needed for board eligibility in child psychiatry. Certification in child psychiatry is typically allowed only after one has been certified in general psychiatry (a small number of experimental programs have recently been initiated that combine pediatric and child psychiatry training).

Psychologists vary greatly in their educational background and may have a master's or a doctoral degree. Those who are qualified to provide clinical service, both diagnostic assessment and therapy, have received a degree in clinical psychology (as opposed to developmental, experimental, physiologic, or social psychology) or have completed a formal, accredited respecialization program. Such training includes, in addition to a dissertation, 3 or 4 years of graduate courses, with accompanying practicum experience, and a year of internship. Graduate programs in clinical psychology and clinical internships are reviewed and accredited by the American Psychological Association (APA).[5] Also, the referring physician may wish to determine whether the consultant is listed in the National Register of Health Service Providers.[2] Finally, most states have licensing procedures for psychologists, and the physician should hesitate to use an individual who is unlicensed in those states. It should be noted, however, that such licensure is generic; that is, it does not distinguish areas of training in psychology (e.g., clinical, developmental, experimental, industrial).

Social workers may have a bachelor's degree (B.S.W.), a master's degree (M.S.W.), or a doctoral degree (D.S.W. or Ph.D.). Social workers are accredited on the national level by the Academy of Certified Social Workers (ACSW), a component of the National Association of Social Workers (NASW), the primary professional association. The ACSW accreditation requirements include (1) a master's degree from a school of social work accredited by the Council of Social Work Education, (2) 2 years of supervised, postmaster's social work practice, and (3) successful completion of a written examination. Many states now have licensing procedures for social workers, with requirements similar to those of the ACSW. The ACSW and most state licenses are generic, however, and do not distinguish among practitioners in clinical social work, administration, and community organization. The NASW maintains a national register of clinical social workers who have demonstrated clinical training and experience. As with all the disciplines discussed above, even clinical social workers vary substantially with regard to orientation and areas of expertise.

Accreditation and organizational affiliations indicate only minimum standards of professional competence. No single mental health profession has sole claim on competence; all fields include individuals who are inadequate and those who are superb. This unevenness of skill simply highlights the importance of the physician's systematic evaluation of resources.

Knowing what behavioral resources are available in a given community and arranging ongoing contact with appropriate individuals require deliberate effort. Pediatricians should meet with an experienced and respected mental health professional to discuss appropriate referral resources within the community. Acquiring appropriate sophistication regarding available referral sources is undoubtedly time consuming, but it will ensure more meaningful referrals and ultimately, save time.

The role of the primary care physician does not cease once the referral has been made. The physician should contact the family to see that an appointment actually has been made. With the appropriate permission, the physician should provide a summary of pertinent information to the professional or agency and in turn *expect periodic reports*. It is helpful for the primary care physician to make a clear statement at the time of referral regarding expectations for feedback: how much detail and how often. Ongoing communication enables the pediatrician to maintain an integral role in providing total care to patients. Over time this will also allow evaluation of the quality of service available from a given professional or agency.

REFERENCES

1. Evans IM and Nelson RO: Assessment of child behavior problems. In Ciminero AR, Calhoun KS, and Adams HE, editors: Handbook of behavioral assessment, ed 2, New York, 1986, John Wiley & Sons, Inc.
2. National Register of Health Service Providers in Psychology, published biannually by the Council for the National Register of Health Service Providers in Psychology, Washington, DC.
3. Robin A and Foster SL: Negotiating parent-adolescent conflict: a behavioral-family systems approach, New York, 1989, The Guilford Press.
4. Sarles RM and Friedman SB: The process of consultation and referral. In Gellert E, editor: Psychosocial aspects of pediatric care, New York, 1978, Grune & Stratton, Inc.
5. Standards for providers of psychological services, Washington, DC, 1977, The American Psychological Association.

76

Colic

Howard R. Foye Jr.

DESCRIPTION

Infantile colic, as classically described, is characterized by episodes of intense fussing or crying, beginning by 2 to 3 weeks of age and resolving by 3 months. Each episode may be brief or last for hours. The episodes are typically worse in the evening, but there is often no predictable pattern, and they may persist well beyond 3 months.

INCIDENCE

The incidence of colic ranged from 13% to 49% in three prospective studies of middle-class infants.[3,11,14] Wessel and colleagues found an incidence of 49% when they defined a colicky infant as "one who, otherwise healthy and well fed, had paroxysms of irritability, fussing or crying lasting for a total of more than three hours a day and occurring on more than three days in any one week."[14] Using a less precise definition that focused on parental distress and infant inconsolability, Paradise found an incidence of 23%.[11] The Paradise criteria are probably closest to the criteria commonly used for a clinical diagnosis of colic.

ETIOLOGY

Several different etiologic proposals for colic have enjoyed cycles of popularity in this century. They may be grouped in the following categories:

1. Food allergy or intolerance
2. Immaturity of the gastrointestinal tract
3. Hypersensitivity of the central nervous system
4. Transfer of tension from caregiver to infant
5. Normal variant

Food Intolerance

The idea that colic is caused by a specific allergic reaction to the protein content of milk, or to lactose intolerance, has been proposed for decades. The common practice of switching formulas in the management of colic is based on this notion. Recent investigations[5,8,9,12] have again thrust this controversy into the spotlight. It appears that food intolerance can cause colic, but when multiple-crossover, blinded, clinical trials are performed, it is not a common cause.[5]

Immaturity of the Gastrointestinal Tract

The term "colic" derived from observations of increased flatus and "doubling up" with apparent abdominal cramps in infants with colic. These symptoms, however, may be a result of air swallowing with crying rather than the initial cause. The common use of antispasmodics for treatment of colic is based on this etiologic assumption. The argument has been made, however, that if ineffective peristalsis resulting from immaturity is the problem, then antispasmodics may exacerbate rather than ameliorate the condition. Furthermore, double-blind studies have had mixed results regarding the effectiveness of antispasmodics.[10,13] Antiflatulents have also been used with the assumption that cramps are caused by air trapping, but evidence is lacking for their effectiveness.[4] The idea that colic is a maturational phenomenon is suggested by the natural history of the syndrome (i.e., typical age of onset and resolution by several months of age).

Hypersensitivity of the Central Nervous System

This etiologic proposal is based on the idea that infants with a low threshold for overstimulation may respond to environmental stimulation with excessive irritability and crying. In support of this hypothesis, Carey found that 11 of 13 infants with colic in the first 3 months of age had a low sensory threshold on a temperament questionnaire administered to their parents when the infants were 4 to 6 months of age.[2] Consistent with the maturational pattern of colic, it has been suggested that colic symptoms resolve as the maturing central nervous system becomes less sensitive to external stimulation.

Transfer of Tension from Caregiver to Infant

Although it is plausible to propose a chain of causation from anxiety and tension in parents to ineffective or inappropriate caregiving, and then to irritability in the infant, it is also plausible to propose a chain of causation in the opposite direction. Regardless of the initial cause, a vicious circle may develop that increases crying and decreases the likelihood of effective caregiving. Two prospective studies[2,11] have provided some evidence that maternal anxiety during the prenatal or neonatal periods is related to the subsequent development of colic, but in both studies the majority of "anxious" mothers did not have colicky babies and most colicky infants did not have "anxious" mothers.

Normal Variant

Another common proposal is that colic is not a distinct clinical entity but merely one end of a continuum of normal crying and fussing behaviors in early infancy. Few discussions of colic include a description of normal crying behavior, yet this is a logical prerequisite for judging abnormal behavior.

Figs. 76-1 and 76-2 present data collected prospectively from diaries kept by parents of 100 healthy, middle-class newborns.[6] The diaries were kept for one 24-hour period per week for the first 3 months. Fig. 76-1 presents percentile data for minutes of crying per day during the first 3 months of life. The data for crying approximate a normal distribution each week. A similar distribution was found by Brazelton[1] in the most frequently cited study of normal crying in early infancy. He reported larger amounts of crying because his data combined crying and fussing. Brazelton also found a similar peak age for average amounts of crying and fussing—2¾ hours per day at 6 weeks of age. As is clear from these data, many infants meet the commonly cited criterion to diagnose colic—at least 3 hours of crying per day. For the infants reported in Fig. 76-1, 35% had at least one diary with more than 3 hours of crying.

Fig. 76-2 presents data on the timing of crying during the day over the first 3 months. About 10% of the crying occurred between midnight and 6:00 AM, 20% between 6:00 AM and noon, 30% between noon and 6:00 PM, and 40% between 6:00 PM and midnight. This pattern was consistent over the 13 weeks of the study, although the total amounts of crying varied, as shown in Fig. 76-1. This pattern is remarkably similar to the pattern reported by Wessel for colicky infants.

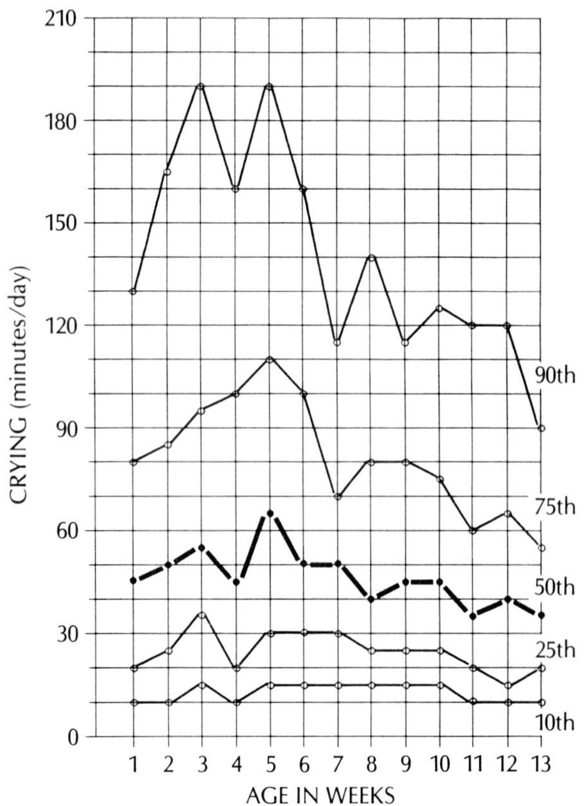

Fig. 76-1 Percentile lines for minutes of crying per day in the first 13 weeks of life. (N = 100)

The similarities between crying patterns reported for colicky infants and for our normative sample (i.e., age of peak crying and timing of crying during the day) support the argument that colic is merely the upper end of the normal continuum.

Regarding etiology, it is clear that no single, simple, cause-and-effect explanation has emerged for the clinical syndrome of colic. Although selected cases may appear to have a clear etiology, it is wise to remember that the natural history of colic is to resolve spontaneously. Resolution is often attributed to clinical maneuvers that happen to precede spontaneous resolution.

As with other behavioral problems, it is likely that multiple factors contribute to the development of colic. Infant factors (e.g., sensory threshold, gastrointestinal function, illness), parental factors (e.g., anxiety, fatigue, responsivity and sensitivity to infant's needs), and environmental factors (e.g., family stresses and social support) probably interact to make "colic" more or less likely. An exclusive focus on possible pathologic explanations in the infant (e.g., food intolerance) will usually miss the mark. Counseling is likely to be more effective when the contributions of a wider range of etiologic possibilities are considered.

DIFFERENTIAL DIAGNOSIS

Of course, all episodes of prolonged, intense crying in the first 3 months of age cannot be attributed to colic. Crying is a nonspecific sign of distress. Feeding problems and many pathologic conditions (e.g., infection, intestinal obstruction, or injury) may accompany increased irritability.

An initial thorough physical examination is important, not only to find the occasional case with a pathologic explanation but also to provide credible reassurance when no pathologic explanation is found.

The history is crucial. It is particularly important to get careful descriptions of the patterns of crying (timing and duration), feeding (timing, quantity, and content), and elimination (vomiting and bowel movement frequency and quality). It is often necessary to have the parents keep a careful diary of these behaviors to clarify the patterns. Additional information of importance includes the caregiving schedule, family stresses and supports, descriptions of the infant's responses to external stimulation, the parents' responses to the infant's crying, and techniques of formula preparation and breast-feeding as appropriate.

MANAGEMENT

Management begins with sympathetic *listening* to the parents' frustration and concerns. Once the clinician is convinced that there is no pathologic explanation for the crying, then *reassurance* is important in shifting the parents' focus away from a search for a pathologic explanation. To be reassured, however, the parents will need to feel that the clinician has given

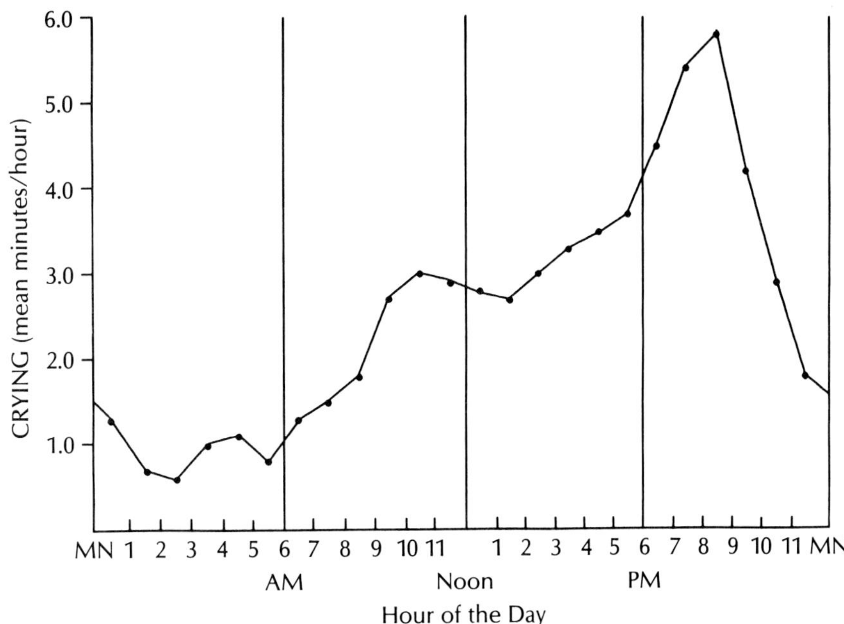

Fig. 76-2 Mean minutes of crying for each hour of the day over the first 13 weeks of life. (N = 80, subjects with ≥ 10 completed diaries)

their concerns specific and thoughtful consideration, not hasty dismissal. *Education* about normal crying patterns, the natural history of colic, and normal temperamental differences in infants can help in providing reassurance. It also may relieve the *guilt* that many parents feel when they have an infant who is difficult to console.

Because there are many factors that may contribute to colic, many different intervention strategies may be helpful. Although success attributed to interventions may result from the placebo effect or the natural course of spontaneous resolution of colic, the pressure to do something makes it very tempting to suggest anything that might help. In this regard it is well to remember the clinical maxim, first do no harm.

Caution is particularly relevant when *pharmacologic interventions* are considered. There are insufficient data to support the use of antispasmodics or antiflatulents in colic. Sedatives may be indicated in extreme cases for a limited time to break the cycle of crying and loss of sleep in all family members that can escalate to a crisis. Diphenhydramine (1 mg/kg) or chloral hydrate (25 mg/kg) 1 hour before the worst period of crying (or before the parents' bedtime) for 1 week may relieve the tension and fatigue. The clinician must be clear with the family that this is a temporary measure intended to diffuse the situation and buy time. It is not a cure. The colic is likely to return when the sedative is discontinued, but the parents will be rested and better able to respond calmly.

Formula changes are perhaps the most common intervention for colic symptoms. Although the evidence shows that food intolerance or allergy is an infrequent cause of colic, the ease of the intervention and the adequacy of many alternative formulas make this seem to be a safe attempt at help. Problems, however, include the expense of special formulas and the frequent erroneous assumption by parents that their child is allergic to cow milk or other items.

Many potentially helpful interventions involve specific *soothing techniques*. These include gentle motion (e.g., automatic rockers, stroller or car rides), continuous monotonous noise or music (e.g., mechanical alarm clock, radio), a pacifier, and a warm water bottle next to the abdomen. One randomized, controlled trial[7] found significantly less crying in a group of infants who were assigned to receive at least 3 hours of carrying each day (either in a caregiver's arms or carrying sack). This preventive strategy is more appealing than techniques that merely respond to crying.

Suggestions about the *quality of interactions* may also be helpful. Parental fatigue or anxiety about the colic may result in inconsistently responsive, abrupt, or tense interactions with the infant. Parents often overstimulate the infant in a frantic attempt to find an effective soothing technique. Suggestions for calm, gentle handling (perhaps gentle rocking in a quiet, dimly lit room) in response to crying and during feedings may help. Feeding in a semiupright position with burping every few minutes to minimize air swallowing may also help.

Suggestions for *parental support and respite* can be very helpful. One of the most effective intervention strategies is a night or weekend away from the infant when the parents are exhausted. An understanding relative or friend can be invaluable as a source of substitute care and emotional support.

REFERENCES

1. Brazelton TB: Crying in infancy, Pediatrics 29:579, 1962.
2. Carey WB: Clinical applications of infant temperament measurements, J Pediatr 81:823, 1972.
3. Carey WB: Maternal anxiety and infantile colic, Clin Pediatr (Phila) 7:590, 1968.
4. Danielsson B and Hwang CP: Treatment of infantile colic with surface active substance (simethicone), Acta Paediatr Scand 74:446, 1985.
5. Forsyth BW: Colic and the effect of changing formulas: a double-blind, multiple-crossover study, J Pediatr 115:521, 1989.

6. Foye HR, Keller B, and Berko JK: Prospective study of crying in early infancy, *Ambulatory Pediatric Association, program and abstracts*, San Francisco, April 30, 1984.
7. Hunziker UA and Barr RG: Increased carrying reduces infant crying: a randomized controlled trial, Pediatrics 77:641, 1986.
8. Hyams J et al: Colonic hydrogen production in infants with colic, J Pediatr 115:592, 1989.
9. Lothe L and Lindberg T: Cow's milk whey protein elicits symptoms of infantile colic in colicky formula-fed infants: a double blind crossover study, Pediatrics 83:262, 1989.
10. O'Donovan JC and Bradstock AS: The failure of conventional drug therapy in the management of infantile colic, Am J Dis Child 133:999, 1979.
11. Paradise JL: Maternal and other factors in the etiology of infantile colic, JAMA 197:123, 1966.
12. Sampson HA: Infantile colic and food allergy: fact or fiction? J Pediatr 115:583, 1989.
13. Weissbluth M, Christoffel KK, and Davis AT: Treatment of infantile colic with dicyclomine hydrochloride, J Pediatr 104:951, 1984.
14. Wessel MA et al: Paroxysmal fussing in infancy, sometimes called "colic," Pediatrics 14:421, 1954.

77

Conduct Disorders

Karen C. Wells and Rex L. Forehand

Conduct disorders of childhood represent the most frequently occurring child psychopathologic conditions. Chief presenting problems of young children with a conduct disorder include aggressiveness toward others (hitting, kicking, fighting), physical destructiveness, oppositional noncompliance to adult figures, temper tantrums, and high rates of annoying behaviors. Older children and adolescents may continue to display these behaviors or may add to their repertoires covert aggressive or antisocial acts, including truancy, stealing, or fire-setting.

Children often display one of these behaviors during the course of normal development. If the behavior is displayed infrequently and in only one situation and is transient, the child is said to have a minor behavioral disturbance. In some children, however, these behaviors cluster together as a primary problematic behavioral dimension or syndrome. In such cases the behaviors usually occur frequently, occur in more than one situation (e.g., home and school), and persist or worsen over time. Such cases are labeled an oppositional defiant disorder or, when the behaviors are more serious and involve community rule violations, a conduct disorder, in the current psychiatric nomenclature. Although some authors view oppositional defiant disorder and conduct disorder as two separate syndromes, others view the former as a developmental precursor of the latter. Despite the controversy as to their syndrome status, empirical studies using sophisticated statistical techniques confirm that aggressive behavior disorders are robust and prevalent conditions of childhood and adolescence.[9]

Noncompliant and aggressive behavior also can occur secondary to other psychological disturbances and thus poses a problem for clinicians and researchers. For example, a high percentage of children who have attention deficit hyperactivity disorder also display secondary conduct problems, and aggressive behavior often occurs in children with psychotic, organic, or emotional disturbances. Our comments in this chapter primarily concern children who display a conduct disorder as their primary behavioral disturbance rather than as an associated symptom of some other pathologic condition.

ASSOCIATED CLINICAL FEATURES

Studies comparing children with conduct disorders and their families with normal children and their families have identified a number of associated features. Those with conduct disorders have a higher rate of *learning problems*, particularly reading disabilities, than do normal children. Children with conduct disorders also display *social skills deficits* and poor peer relationships. Finally, there is accumulating evidence showing an association between aggressive behavior and *depression*, especially in boys; this association has been found in both clinical and empirical studies.[14]

The families of children with conduct disorders also display associated clinical features. Mothers of children with conduct disorders have been found to have less coping ability and tolerance for stress and a higher incidence of anxiety and depression than have mothers of normal children. Maternal depression is a significant factor in the overall clinical picture, because depression adversely affects mothers' perceptions of their children and reduces the probability of a positive treatment outcome. Finally, in addition to maternal psychological adjustment, parental marital maladjustment has been related to conduct disorders in children.[6]

EPIDEMIOLOGY

In a large-scale epidemiologic survey of the population of the Isle of Wight, a small island off the coast of England, 4% of all 10- and 11-year-old children displayed conduct disorders.[12] Clinic population surveys in England and the United States have repeatedly demonstrated that children with conduct disorders represent by far the largest proportion of referred children, with estimates ranging from 47% to 67%.[14] Boys are much more likely to display conduct disorders than are girls, by a factor of at least 3:1. Low income, poor housing, and large families are strongly associated with delinquency, but many authors consider delinquency to be a separate behavioral syndrome in children; it is currently unclear if social and economic factors are related to noncompliant and aggressive behavior in nondelinquent children.[14]

ETIOLOGY

Although most of the theorizing regarding the etiology of conduct disorders in children has emphasized environmental determinants, it is likely that in many children there also may be consitutional or organic predisposing factors.[14] For example, children with impulsivity associated with cerebral dysfunction may have a diminished capacity to inhibit aggressive motor responses, control anger, or delay gratification as compared with normal children. If such a child finds himself or herself in a socially disorganized environment, or one in which the parents fail to reward appropriate behavior and administer firm, consistent consequences for negative behavior, then a conduct disorder is the likely outcome.

On the other hand, with or without constitutional predisposing factors, it is clear that certain environmental processes occurring within the family are strongly related to the development and maintenance of conduct disorders in children. Patterson[10] has emphasized the coercive or controlling nature of problem behaviors displayed by such children and has developed a "coercion hypothesis" to account for their development and maintenance. According to this hypothesis, coercive behaviors (crying, tantrums, etc.) are adaptive in the newborn in that they influence the mother to display behaviors necessary for the infant's survival (e.g., feeding). However, whereas most children learn more appropriate social behaviors for controlling the environment over the course of development, some children continue to employ coercive control strategies.

This can happen in the context of mutually reinforcing reciprocal influence processes occurring in parent-child interactions. In these interactions parents and children reinforce each other for engaging in higher and higher rates of coercive behavior and fail to reinforce each other for more appropriate social behaviors. In addition, parents of children with conduct disorders display poor family management practices, such as (1) not *monitoring* their children's whereabouts and their children's performance of basic expectations, and (2) not *disciplining* the children for violating age-appropriate rules. Patterson[10] has speculated that poor parenting skills occur because of poor grandparental models, parental psychopathology, poor coping skills, and disruptive stresses such as marital crises, poverty, and illnesses.

TREATMENT

The key to successful management of the child with a conduct disorder lies in early identification and intervention. Although oppositional behaviors may be a normal developmental phenomenon in the toddler (hence the label "terrible two's"), persistence of these behaviors much beyond 3 ½ years of age should warn the pediatrician that intervention may be warranted. Treatment is much more likely to be successful for the younger child, in whom coercive behavior patterns have not become overlearned and habitual. Contrary to the once-popular adage that children will "outgrow" their behavioral problems, follow-up studies[11] indicate that a conduct disorder in the 5- to 6-year-old is a pernicious diagnosis, with a poor long-term outcome for untreated children. About 75% of children with conduct disorders continue these disorders in adolescence; a conduct disorder at 6 years of age is a strong predictor of a conduct disorder at age 13 or 14 years. Furthermore, both prospective and retrospective studies[14] have shown that an "antisocial personality" or "sociopathy" in adults is strongly associated with conduct disorders in childhood. It is incumbent on health care providers, therefore, to take conduct disorders in children seriously; advising parents of a 5- or 6-year-old that "he is just a strong-willed boy—he will outgrow it" is neither true (in most cases) nor appropriate.

With this admonishment in mind, it is important for pediatricians to screen for conduct disorders in their patients. There are three primary methods of screening available to the pediatrician: informal observation, interview, and rating scales. Oppositional and aggressive behaviors can often be observed informally in the waiting room, with the strongest indicator being a child repeatedly failing to comply with his or her parent's instructions, requests, and commands. Parents often can be observed to whine and wheedle, cajole, nag, or threaten their children, with the children complying infrequently and then only if it pleases them to do so.

When interviewed, parents will complain that the child is "stubborn," "never listens," "won't mind," "throws fits when she doesn't get her way," "constantly demands attention," "breaks or destroys things," and so forth. If the parent further admits to frequently failing in efforts to manage the child or to get him or her to mind, the pediatrician should strongly suspect that a conduct disorder may be present, and a rating scale should be given to the parent or parents and teacher (if the child is of school age). The Conners Parent and Teacher Rating Scales[4] are suited for this purpose, since each scale includes a primary factor called "conduct disorder," and since a child can be evaluated in terms of his or her position on this factor relative to children in the normal population. In addition, the Teacher Questionnaire asks for a report of school achievement to identify those children who may have learning problems. Finally, because of the relationship of parental depression and marital maladjustment to conduct disorders in children, an adult depression scale (e.g., Beck Depression Inventory)[3] and a marital adjustment scale (e.g., Locke-Wallace Marriage Inventory)[8] can be given to the parent to complete.

Once the presence of a conduct disorder is suspected, the pediatrician's task is to discuss the potential diagnosis with the parents and alert them that the problem may be serious and should not be ignored. A small subset of parents will be able to profit from advice by the pediatrician to reward appropriate behavior in the home (e.g., compliance, cooperative behavior with siblings) and to treat negative behavior firmly and immediately.

Most parents, however, will need to be referred to a clinician skilled in specialized treatment procedures for children with conduct disorders and their families. There are three treatment approaches that have demonstrated efficacy in psychological management of conduct disorders.

Parent Management Training

Parent management training is the most extensively developed and evaluated approach to treatment of child and adolescent conduct disorders.[9] This approach focuses on work with the parents in which they are taught a systematic set of skills for developing age-appropriate rules and expectations for their children, reinforcing compliance with these rules and expectations and decreasing aggressive behavior with effective, nonviolent punishment procedures. Specifically, parents learn attending and rewarding skills for reinforcing prosocial behavior, how to give appropriate directions to their children, and how to use time-out and privilege-removal strategies for noncompliant and aggressive behavior. They practice all of these skills in therapy sessions with the therapist and during prescribed homework sessions at home.[5]

For more "advanced" or serious forms of conduct disorder, parents also learn additional strategies for treating covert behaviors or behaviors that place the adolescent at risk for delinquent or predelinquent acts (e.g., curfew violations, congregating with delinquent friends). For example, when stealing is an issue, parents learn to apply consequences for the *suspicion* of stealing. The actual behavior does not have to be observed. For "at-risk" behaviors, parents learn the importance of tracking and monitoring their children's whereabouts and companions and increasing their supervision of the child. Families may be involved as a unit in developing behavioral contracts.[9]

As mentioned earlier, parent management training has been extensively evaluated and found to be a generally effective approach for treating conduct disorders.[5,9] However, in some cases parents may be unwilling or unable to cooperate in therapy. In these cases another approach to treatment, cognitive therapy, may be indicated.

Cognitive Therapy

Cognitive therapy is a treatment that focuses on individual work with the child. It is based on the general notion that change in behavior can be brought about by change in the child's cognitive processes related to aggressive acts. Some cognitive processes that have been identified as relevant to aggressive behavior include a predisposition to attribute hostile intent to others in social situations; a lack of empathy with others; inability to evaluate the short-term and long-term consequences of behavior; inability to take the perspective of others; and limitations in general problem-solving skills.[13]

In cognitive therapy, children are taught problem-solving skills directly such as generating alternative interpretations and solutions to a problem, thinking consequentially, and taking the perspective of others. Children first observe a competent model perform a task or manage an interpersonal situation while the model talks aloud through adaptive cognitive processes. They perform the same task under guidance while making comparable verbalizations out loud, then perform it alone while whispering or subvocalizing. Once they learn the cognitive skills, the bulk of therapy focuses on situations from the child's own life in which new cognitive skills can be applied, especially in interpersonal situations that might lead to aggression. Reinforcement is used to motivate children to carry out the problem-solving.

Despite some early negative results with cognitive therapy, the approach has recently been shown to lead to significant reductions in aggressive behavior in children when applied systematically and intensively.[7] Cognitive therapy, administered by a therapist skilled in this approach, appears to be a viable alternative to parent management training when parents are not available for treatment.

Functional Family Therapy

Functional family therapy is a therapeutic approach that combines behavioral and systems models of family therapy into a framework that derives the meaning of behavior from an examination of the relational process in which it is embedded. Functional family therapy also looks at the outcomes that behavior evokes from others. The approach assumes that presenting problems are legitimate in their function or outcome, even though the behavior itself may be maladaptive. For example, a child's tantrums may produce a legitimate short-term outcome (contact or closeness with the mother), but in a way that is maladaptive to harmonious family life. In functional family therapy the therapist first tries to determine the interpersonal functions of particular sequences of problem behavior. Then the therapist selects and implements treatment strategies that *maintain* the interpersonal outcome achieved, but less disruptively.[1]

The behavioral-systems family therapy model, from which functional family therapy evolved, has received empirical support for its use with delinquent adolescents who have conduct disorders and their families. The approach has been more effective on measures of behavioral outcome and on recidivism than have other forms of family therapy (e.g., client-centered family counseling, psychodynamic family therapy), not only for adolescents identified as having a conduct disorder but for their siblings as well.[2] Such studies lend strong empirical support to functional family therapy with adolescents who have conduct disorders, a population that is notoriously difficult to treat.

As noted earlier, if parents are unable to reverse family processes contributing to maintenance of aggressive behavior in their children with brief counseling from the pediatrician, then referral should be made to a mental health practitioner skilled in one of the treatment approaches previously described. Consultation or referral should probably occur immediately for children displaying persistent behavior indicating a conduct disorder; for children who, in addition to a high conduct disorder factor score, also obtain high scores on other factors (e.g., hyperactivity or anxiety); and for children whose parents display significant problems of their own. Finally, pediatricians should be acutely aware that children with conduct disorders often have learning problems or learning disabilities. If there is any indication that learning problems are present, the child should be referred for a psychoeducational evaluation. Prolonged school failure exacerbates behavioral problems and leads to low self-esteem. For this reason, children with conduct disorders who are underachieving or have learning disabilities should be referred to remedial programs as early as possible.

REFERENCES

1. Alexander JF and Parsons B: Functional family therapy, Monterey, Calif, 1982, Brooks/Cole Publishing Co.
2. Alexander JF et al: Systems-behavioral intervention with families of delinquents: therapist characteristics, family behavior and outcome, J Consult Clin Psychol 44:656, 1976.
3. Beck AT: Depression inventory, Philadelphia, 1978, Center for Cognitive Therapy.
4. Conners CK: A teacher rating scale for use in drug studies with children, Am J Psychiatry 126:884, 1969.
5. Forehand R and McMahon RJ: Helping the noncompliant child: a clinician's guide to parent training, New York, 1981, The Guilford Press.
6. Griest DL and Wells KC: Behavioral family therapy with conduct disorders in children, Behavior Therapy 14:37, 1983.
7. Kazdin AE et al: Problem solving skills training and relationship therapy in the treatment of antisocial child behavior, J Consult Clin Psychol, 55:76, 1987.
8. Locke HJ and Wallace KM: Short marital-adjustment and prediction tests: their reliability and validity, Marriage and Family Living, 21:251, 1959.

9. McMahon RJ and Wells KC: Conduct disorders. In Mash EJ and Barkley RA, editors: Treatment of childhood disorders, New York, 1989, The Guilford Press.
10. Patterson GR: Performance models for antisocial boys, Am Psychol 41:432, 1986.
11. Robins LN: Follow-up studies: Problems amenable to investigation. In Quay HC and Werry JS, editors: Psychopathological disorders of childhood, ed 2, New York, 1979, John Wiley & Sons, Inc.
12. Rutter M et al: Research report: Isle of Wight studies, 1964-1974, Psychol Med 6:313, 1976.
13. Spivack G, Platt JJ, and Shure MB: The problem solving approach to adjustment, San Francisco, 1976, Jossey-Bass, Inc, Publishers.
14. Wells KC and Forehand R: Conduct and oppositional disorders. In Bornstein PH and Kazdin AE, editors: Handbook of clinical behavior therapy with children, Homewood, Ill, 1985, The Dorsey Press.

78

Cross-Sex Behavior

George A. Rekers

Cross-sex behavior may represent either a normal episodic exploration of sex role behaviors ("tomboyishness" in girls or "sissyish" behavior in boys) or a persistent and compulsively stereotyped pattern indicative of a "gender identity disorder of childhood."[1,5] Although many harmful arbitrary sex role stereotypes for males and females are increasingly being challenged in our culture,[11] and there are changing values regarding fathers sharing child-bearing and household duties, there remains a cultural consensus on certain sex role distinctions that children normally master in early development (e.g., females but not males are normally permitted to appear in public with lipstick, wearing a dress).

In 1980, "gender identity disorder of childhood" first became an official diagnosis in the *Diagnostic and Statistical Manual of Mental Disorders, Third Edition*, (DSM-III) for prepubertal children with persistent and intense distress about their gender role or anatomic sex. In 1987, the new diagnosis of "gender identity disorder of adolescence or adulthood, nontranssexual type" was added in the revised manual (DSM-III-R) for postpubertal individuals who have a persisting discomfort with their assigned sex, who repeatedly cross-dress (but not for the purpose of sexual excitement, as in transvestite fetishism), and who have no persistent desire to change their primary and secondary sex characteristics to those of the other sex.[1] In addition, a new diagnosis of "gender identity disorder not otherwise specified" was added in 1987 for gender disorders without the full diagnostic criteria for transsexualism or the other two gender identity disorders.[1]

Cross-sex behavior in boys[5,9,12] includes dressing in feminine clothing, using cosmetics, avoiding male playmates and rough-and-tumble play, being rather rigidly and exclusively preoccupied with girls' activities,[3,9] taking a predominantly female role in play, talking predominantly about female topics, projecting the voice into a high femalelike voice inflection, and displaying effeminate gait and body movements ("swishing hips") or feminine-appearing gestures such as "limp wrist" (flexing the wrist toward the palmar surface of the forearm), "arm flutters" (rapid up and down movements of the forearm or upper arm or both, while the wrist remains relaxed), or "palming" (touching the palm or palms to the back, front, or sides of the head above the ear level).[10] In some cases of gender identity disorder, the boy persistently repudiates his male anatomy by repeatedly saying (1) that he will become a woman, (2) that it would be better not to have male sex organs, (3) that his penis or testes will disappear or are disgusting. Boys outnumber girls more than five to one in numbers of diagnosed cases of gender identity disorder.[6]

For girls, cross-sex behavior[8] may include chronic rejection of feminine clothing, cosmetics, and jewelry, regular avoidance of female playmates, a stated desire to be "one of the boys," frequent projection of the voice into a low malelike voice inflection, predominant talk about male activities, and habitual attempts to stand, sit, or walk in a hypermasculine manner (e.g., sitting with legs crossed with the ankle of one leg resting on the other knee). In cases of gender identity disorder in girls, a persistent repudiation of female anatomy is evidenced by statements (1) that she will develop into a man, (2) that she is biologically unable to develop breasts or become pregnant, (3) that she will develop a penis, and (4) that she has no vagina.

The gender identity disorder is a rare condition with onset occurring before puberty and cross-sex behavior patterns often beginning before 4 years of age. In later grade school years, overt cross-sex behavior may lessen in public, even though a gender identity disorder is present. Both retrospective and prospective data[2,3,12,14,15] indicate an unusually high incidence of depression and suicide attempts in the adult years for these boys who are untreated, and these reports also indicate that 46% to 64% of boys with untreated gender identity disorders develop *homosexual or bisexual orientation* during their adolescence. A small minority of girls with a gender identity disorder retain a masculine identification, with some also developing a homosexual orientation. These reports further indicate that 5% to 12% of untreated male cases develop adulthood *transsexualism* accompanied by severe depression and suicide attempts, whereas approximately 1% to 5% develop heterosexual *transvestism*. The remaining 6% to 23% have a heterosexual orientation in adulthood.

The formation of gender identity is related to the child's appropriate identification with his or her sexual anatomy and its reproductive function.[3,4,12] Normal child-rearing experiences contribute to identification with the parent figure and peers of the same sex and to development of complementary role behaviors toward members of the other sex.[5] Some reports suggest that excessive and extremely prolonged physical and emotional closeness between mother and infant, coupled with physical or psychological *absence of the father* during early childhood years, may contribute to gender identity disorders in boys.[5,6,12] Similarly, some young girls with unavailable mothers may be at risk for a compensatory identification with the father, contributing to a male gender identity.[8] However, children reared in a single-parent home are not necessarily at risk for a gender identity disorder, especially when the child is afforded the opportunity to develop positive and enduring attachments with adults of both sexes to compensate for the missing parent. It is extremely rare for gender identity disorders to be associated with any detectable abnormalities in genetic constitution, gonads, external sex organ anatomy, internal accessory genital structures, sex endocrinology, or maternal health during pregnancy.[5,7,12]

DIAGNOSTIC CONSIDERATIONS AND ISSUES

Clinicians have found it useful to assess a child with cross-sex behavior across the seven major psychosexual dimensions as outlined in Table 78-1, because a complete diagnosis must consider all these levels of assessment.[5]

The evaluation of cross-sex behavior should involve notation of frequency and setting, as well as the social labeling attached to the behavior pattern.[5,6] The developmental context of the behavior and the child's overall emotional and psychosocial functioning should also be considered. An inquiry should be made regarding the cultural context of the sterotypic behavior, the presence or absence of a compulsive cross-sex behavior pattern, and the significance of the behavior to the child or adolescent.[11] The cluster of behaviors should be considered because it is the ratio of masculine to feminine behavior rather than the exact number of cross-sex behaviors that is diagnostically significant.[9] Parents can be asked:

1. How do you categorize masculine and feminine behaviors?
2. Does your child identify with and model after the parent and peers of the same sex?
3. In what ways does your child relate to boys and girls differently?
4. To what degree does your child identify with his or her sexual anatomy and understand its future reproductive function?
5. What is the history and frequency of the following behaviors in your child: cross-dressing, masculine and feminine gestures, play with cosmetics, avoidance of play with peers of the same sex, play with girls' toys and activities, play with boys' toys and activities, feminine and masculine voice inflection, desire to be called by a name of the other sex, deviant sexual behaviors, masturbation with cross-dressing articles?
6. Does your child insist on being or pretend to be a member of the other sex?
7. Has your child ever asked for a *sex change*, and if so, how often?

The parents can be asked to record the frequency of several key masculine and feminine behaviors daily for 1 or 2 weeks.[4] Parental inquiries with the schoolteacher on how the child relates to other boys and girls may be recommended.[5,9]

In interviewing the child, the pediatrician can simply ask the boy or girl to draw a person and talk about the drawing. In some cases, this is a quick diagnostic screening test that may provide clues to the child's gender identity.[13] After establishing rapport with the child, interview questions[5] can help clarify progress in gender identity development. For example:

1. What are the first names of your friends and playmates at home and school? (Note and compare the number of female and male friends.)
2. Are you more like your mom or your dad? How?
3. If you could have three wishes, what would you wish for?
4. What are your favorite subjects and activities at school?
5. How often do you feel like a boy? How often do you feel like a girl?
6. When you have free time, what are your favorite things to do?
7. Most kids are called names at some time or other; what names do the other kids call you?

Although children under 8 years of age are often open to disclosing truthful answers to such interview questions, older children and adolescents are more aware of the social significance of their gender role behavior and may have gone "underground" with their true interests at home, and they may conceal their cross-gender preferences from the physician as well. In such cases a more comprehensive evaluation with psychological testing by a clinical psychologist is recommended.[3,5]

If appropriate, parallel questions should be asked from the parent interview described previously. Even when the criteria for a gender identity disorder are not all present, a persisting "gender role behavior disturbance" (which can be diagnosed as an example of "gender identity disorder not otherwise specified" as defined earlier) can be detected in a child as young as 4 years of age.[1,5] In cases of chronic cross-sex

Table 78-1 *Dimensions for Psychosexual Assessment*

LEVEL OF ASSESSMENT	DIMENSION	MAJOR CATEGORIES
Sexual status	Physical sex	Male, female or intersexed; Tanner's stages for prepubertal, pubertal or postpubertal development
	Social assignment	Male, female or intersexed; child, adolescent or adult (boy, girl, man)
Intrapersonal behavior	Gender identity	Normal, undifferentiated, cross-gender or conflicted
	Sexual role identity	Heterosexual, bisexual, homosexual, transsexual, transvestite, "queen," "fag," "drag queen," "gay" etc.
	Sexual arousal orientation	Human object choice (male, female, both); animal object choice; magnitude and frequency; fantasies
Interpersonal behavior	Gender role behavior	Masculine, feminine, undifferentiated, androgynous
	Sexual behavior	Human partner (male, female, both); animal partner; inanimate object; intrusive versus receptive roles; group versus individual partner, etc.

From Rekers GA: Psychosexual assessment of gender identity disorders. In Prinz RJ, editor: Advances in behavioral assessment of children and families, vol 4, Greenwich Conn, 1988. JAI Press Inc.

behavior, evaluation should include medical and pregnancy history, physical examination (including external genitalia), chromosome analysis, and sex chromatin studies, even though these diagnostic procedures result in negative findings in the vast majority of cases.[7]

For adolescents, the pediatrician will find it necessary to assess sexual arousal patterns and frequency of specific sexual behaviors by interviewing the adolescent or by asking the patient to make written recordings of the occurrence of sexual urges and sexual behaviors over a 2- to 4-week period.[5]

SUGGESTIONS FOR MANAGEMENT

If psychodiagnostic questions are raised regarding a potential gender identity disorder, refer the child *immediately* for psychological evaluation.[5,11] Early detection and early intervention is the preferred clinical strategy for optimum gender identity adjustment. In cases of cross-sex behavior without conclusive evidence of gender identity disorder, recommend the following management strategies, where appropriate:

1. Encourage the same-sex parent to invest time in positive play and interaction with the child, avoiding criticism of the child.
2. Where a same-sex parent is unavailable, recommend finding a substitute same-sex adult who can be a positive role model.
3. Recommend ignoring cross-sex behavior where possible.
4. Advise parents to reward or praise appropriate "sex-typed" play and mannerisms.
5. Provide appropriate *sex education* where needed.
6. Inquire at regular office visits about the child's sex-typed behavior, and if only limited improvement is apparent after several months, refer the child to a clinical child psychologist or child psychiatrist for behavior therapy.[4,6,8]

Specific *child behavior therapy* techniques have been demonstrated to be effective in the successful treatment of gender identity disorders and other cross-sex behavior problems in childhood.[4] Positive reinforcement for normal sex-typed play, normal speech pattern, and sex-appropriate behavioral mannerisms has been found to be effective in the clinic, home, and school.[5] Positive reinforcement for appropriate sex role behavior has been demonstrated to be effective in the successful treatment of deviant cross-sex behaviors in boys and girls, particularly when the parents are closely trained and supervised by a child psychologist or psychiatrist to carry out behavior-shaping programs in the child's natural living environment.[4]

REFERENCES

1. American Psychiatric Association: Diagnostic and statistical manual of mental disorders, ed 3, revised, Washington, DC, 1987, The Association.
2. Davenport CW: A follow-up study of 10 feminine boys, Arch Sex Behav 15:511, 1986.
3. Green R: The "sissy boy syndrome" and the development of homosexuality, New Haven, Conn, 1987, Yale University Press.
4. Rekers GA: Gender identity problems. In Bornstein PH and Kazdin AE, editors: Handbook of clinical behavior therapy with children, Homewood, Ill, 1985, The Dorsey Press.
5. Rekers GA: Psychosexual assessment of gender identity disorders. In Prinz RJ, editor: Advances in behavioral assessment of children and families, vol 4, Greenwich, Conn, 1988, JAI Press, Inc.
6. Rekers GA et al: Child gender disturbances: a clinical rationale for intervention, Psychother Theory Res Practice 14:2, 1977.
7. Rekers GA et al: Genetic and physical studies of male children with psychological gender disturbances, Psychol Med 9:373, 1979.
8. Rekers GA and Mead S: Female sex-role deviance: early identification and developmental intervention, J Clin Child Psychol 9:199, 1980.
9. Rekers GA and Morey SM: Relationship of maternal report of feminine behaviors and extraversion to clinician's rating of gender disturbance, Percept Mot Skills 69:387, 1989.
10. Rekers GA and Morey SM: Sex-typed body movements as a function of severity of gender disturbance in boys, J Psychol Human Sexuality 2:2, 1989.
11. Rekers GA et al: Sex-role stereotype and professional intervention for childhood gender disturbances, Prof Psychol 9:127, 1978.
12. Zucker KJ: Cross-gender-identified children. In Steiner BW, editor: Gender dysphoria: development, research, management, New York, 1985, Plenum Press.
13. Zucker KJ et al: Human figure drawings of gender-problem children: a comparison to sibling, psychiatric, and normal controls, J Abnorm Child Psychol 11:287, 1983.
14. Zuger B: Early effeminate behavior in boys: outcome and significance for homosexuality, J Nerv Ment Dis 172:90, 1984.
15. Zuger B: Is early effeminate behavior in boys early homosexuality? Compr Psychiatry 29:509, 1988.

79

Depression

Alan E. Kazdin

Depression can refer to different levels of dysfunction or to specific clinical problems. As a symptom, depression refers to sadness or dysphoric mood. Depression can also denote a syndrome or group of symptoms that occur together and may include affective, cognitive, motivational, motoric, and vegetative signs. In adults, depression is often referred to as a disorder, because a great deal is known about the syndrome, including a characteristic natural history, biologic and familial correlates, and a predictable response to treatment. The distinction of depression as a symptom, syndrome, and disorder has been widely recognized in adult psychiatry but only recently has been considered in child psychiatry.

Within psychiatry, views of childhood depression as a syndrome or disorder have varied within the last several years.[2,5,6] For many years the dominant psychodynamic position considered depression in children not to be possible. This position viewed depression as a phenomenon of the superego involving either an inward directedness of aggression or a discrepancy between the real and ideal self. Full depression is not possible because the superego is not completely developed until adolescence. A second view was that depression in children can exist but the manifestations differ from the clinical signs seen in adults. According to this view, depression in children was considered to be "masked" or expressed in "depressive equivalents," that is, other symptoms that are not usually characteristic of depression. Diverse symptoms and syndromes, including tantrums, hyperactivity, phobias, school refusal or failure, and others, were considered to reflect masked depression. A third view was that symptoms of depression are part of normal development and are transitory. The full syndrome may occur at various points in normal development, but its relatively high prevalence at particular points in development makes it normal in children rather than a clinical syndrome.

These views have given way to the current position in the field—that depression is a disorder similar in children, adolescents, and adults. Specific symptoms may vary as a function of developmental level, but the core features that define a mood disorder are similar across the age spectrum. This position has been adopted by most experts in the field. Depression has been successfully diagnosed in children by use of standard diagnostic criteria such as those specified by the *Diagnostic and Statistical Manual of Mental Disorders* (DSM-III-R).[1]

With the availability of assessment devices and improved diagnostic criteria over the years, investigations of prevalence have emerged.[3] Studies of normal children have suggested prevalence rates of depressive disorder from approximately 2% to 5%. Among clinical populations the rates have typically ranged from 10% to 20%. Depression appears to be more prevalent in adolescents than in children. Also, sex differences in prevalence rates tend to emerge in adolescence, during which the rates for girls are much higher than for boys.

DIAGNOSIS AND ASSESSMENT

According to DSM-III-R the criteria to diagnose a major affective disorder in children or adults are the same. These include (1) depressed mood, (2) loss of interest or pleasure in activities, (3) significant change in weight or appetite, (4) sleep difficulties, (5) psychomotor agitation or retardation, (6) fatigue or loss of energy, (7) feelings of worthlessness or excessive guilt, (8) diminished ability to think or concentrate, and (9) recurrent thoughts of death. For the diagnosis to be made, at least five of these symptoms must be present during the same 2-week period; at least one of the symptoms must include either a depressed mood or loss of interest. These symptoms may be evident and hence serve as the diagnostic basis of major depression. Other diagnoses may include depressive symptoms.[1] Dysthymia is a mood disorder in which depressive symptoms may be evident in less severe forms. Separation-anxiety disorder, in which the child shows fear of separation from someone to whom he or she is emotionally attached, may be associated with many symptoms of depression as well. Adjustment disorder with depressed mood may emerge in response to a particular psychosocial stressor, such as divorce of the parents or leaving behind friends when the family moves to another community. Bereavement, too, may include a number of depressive symptoms that must be distinguished from the disorder.

Major depression may also be overlooked, because the symptoms are associated with a variety of nonspecific signs such as generalized anxiety, apathy, school problems, and sleep disturbance—signs that may not initially direct the clinician to suspect depression. Depressed affect or the full syndrome may occur with other syndromes such as a conduct disorder, in which the diagnostic symptoms are overt and more clearly delineated. If the clinician focuses on the behavioral problems, which are often more obvious, the depression may be missed.

Because depression can be easily overlooked, the patient needs to be carefully assessed. Until recently, standardized procedures for soliciting information to make the diagnosis have been unavailable. Several semistructured interviews have appeared that evaluate the large spectrum of symptoms in children and permit diagnosis using DSM-III-R or Research

Diagnostic Criteria.[1] Several other measures of depression have emerged, including self-reports, parent, teacher, and clinician ratings, and peer evaluations.[3] These usually are more easily administered than diagnostic interviews and focus specifically on depression.

ETIOLOGY AND TREATMENT

Etiologic models of adult depression have implicated the role of genetics, biochemical abnormalities, cognitions, life stressors, a paucity of reinforcing life experiences, learned helplessness, and other factors. No single position, however, can fully account for the range of affective disorders. In addition, little research has examined the different models in childhood depression. Yet preliminary research has already suggested close parallels between adult and childhood depression in various biologic markers and in responses to specific pharmacologic treatments.[3-5] Evidence from twin and adoption studies suggests that an affective disorder in children is transmitted genetically, although the mode of transmission is not clear. Psychosocial stressors such as early separation from a parent, parental marital discord, and parental psychiatric illness place the child at risk for depression. Yet these factors have not been isolated as risk factors specific to childhood depression rather than to psychopathology in general. Current evidence suggests that childhood depression bears close resemblance to adult depression. Additional diagnostic issues need to be addressed to help delineate subtypes and their possibly different etiologies.

Several treatments have been effective for adult depression, including pharmacotherapy, cognitive therapy, and select forms of psychotherapy and behavior therapy, alone or in combination with medication. Few controlled investigations, however, have evaluated treatments for childhood depression. The success of tricyclic antidepressants (e.g., imipramine, amitriptyline), monoamine oxidase (MAO) inhibitors (e.g., phenelzine), and lithium for adults has led to their use in children.[4] A few controlled trials have indicated that tricyclics are effective with prepubertal depressed children, particularly if plasma levels are monitored to achieve therapeutic levels. However, the placebo response in control groups that do not receive medication is sometimes high, and the evidence for the effectiveness of tricyclics in relieving depression is sparse and mixed for both children and adolescents. Although medication holds promise of controlling the symptoms, the possibility for side effects (e.g., cardiovascular toxicity) must be closely monitored.

Psychosocial interventions for childhood depression have been reported with only a small number of children. Behavior modification techniques involving modeling, role-playing, rehearsal, and positive reinforcement, used alone or in combination, have increased social behavior and reduced displays of depressive affect. As yet, large-scale investigations of behavioral or cognitive therapy or psychotherapy for clinically depressed children have not been reported. It is likely that effective treatment will require a multifaceted approach. Symptoms of depression might be ameliorated with medication; yet, social deficits that depressed children display apparently remain after successful medication treatment. Hence, both medication and psychosocial interventions may be warranted.

SUMMARY

Considerable progress has been made in identifying childhood depression; advances have been largely a result of the application of specific diagnostic criteria to children. Also, many investigators have adopted the model that childhood depression closely resembles adult depression. This view not only has the advantage of parsimony, but also fosters investigation of known characteristics such as a natural history, clinical course, biochemical correlates, and response to specific treatments, as established with adults.

The diagnostic commonality of childhood and adult depression does not mean that the disorders are identical. Researchers have noted some differences in severity and patterns of symptoms, albeit diagnostic criteria can be applied across the developmental spectrum.

From a clinical standpoint, the important breakthrough is that a major affective disorder can be identified in children through careful interview of the parent and child. The obstacles in identifying depression pertain to the presence of other symptoms or syndromes that may distract the clinician from exploring whether an affective disorder exists. The symptoms of an affective disorder need to be examined explicitly through interview or other assessment procedures.

REFERENCES

1. American Psychiatric Association: Diagnostic and statistical manual of mental disorders, ed 3, revised, Washington, DC, 1987, The Association.
2. Cantwell DP and Carlson GA, editors: Affective disorders in childhood and adolescence: an update, New York, 1983, Spectrum.
3. Kazdin AE: Childhood depression. In Mash EJ and Terdal LG, editors: Behavioral assessment of childhood disorders, ed 2, New York, 1988, The Guilford Press.
4. Puig-Antich J and Weston B: The diagnosis and treatment of major depressive disorder in childhood, Annu Rev Med 34:231, 1983.
5. Rutter M, Izard CE, and Read PB, editors: Depression in young people: developmental and clinical perspectives, New York, 1986, The Guilford Press.
6. Trad PV: Infant and childhood depression: developmental factors, New York, 1987, John Wiley & Sons, Inc.

80

Encopresis

Melvin D. Levine

The condition of encopresis refers to a chronic disorder in which schoolchildren have bowel movements in unacceptable sites (usually their underwear) after the age of 4 years.[5,8] Varying degrees of this problem are common in all cultures, although *precise* prevalence figures are unavailable.[2] For a typical child with encopresis, life's waking hours often are tense, laced with anxiety, guilt, and a fear of being discovered and accused. Such a youngster is preoccupied with his or her incontinence, plagued by the realization that in any place, at any time, he or she is apt to lose control, "mess," and have the shameful secret be revealed.

ORIGINS

Wide-ranging pathophysiologic pathways are known to culminate in encopresis. It therefore is inappropriate to assume a priori that all cases are "psychogenic" or "organic." In fact, it is likely that most children with encopresis have several reasons for their incontinence. In reviewing the histories of such youngsters, one most commonly uncovers clusters of *potentiating factors*.[5] These can be grouped according to their time of occurrence: early infancy, the toilet-training period, and the school years. Potentiators most likely to be accumulated during each of these periods are summarized in Table 80-1. It can be seen that some youngsters manifest risk factors early in infancy. Aggressive or coercive and manipulation (by parents or physicians) or severe gastroenteritis are examples of early life influences that may create an "anal stamp," "setting up" a youngster for later functional bowel difficulties.[1] At the time of training, other types of vulnerability are likely to come forth. Psychosocial stresses at home, irrational fears surrounding the toilet, or ill-conceived toilet-training techniques are common toddler-preschool antecedents of encopresis. In school years, children who have attention deficits (therefore tending to be impersistent at toilet use as well as at other daily performances) may develop encopresis for the first time. School bathrooms, with their lack of privacy and highly charged atmospheres, may be another source of bowel stress. Continuing aggravation of encopresis during the school years may stem from mismanagement, inconsistent approaches to the problem on the part of parents, and the child's denial or unwillingness to acknowledge and deal with the unbearable shame of encopresis. It is interesting that children who experience early predisposing factors seem more vulnerable to the accumulation of later ones. Thus, youngsters with bowel problems in infancy may be more difficult to toilet train, may have more concerns about school bathrooms, and may be less willing or equipped to deal with their problem during the school years.

Some youngsters develop encopresis as a direct or oblique response to psychosocial stresses at home or school. In most cases, however, these too are children who have predisposing factors that cause their stress responses to be bowel registered.

Schoolchildren with encopresis retain their stools, at least intermittently. In many cases the colon is diffusely replete with hard feces. In other instances, retained stools may be relatively soft or "pasty." In a number of cases, only *rectal constipation* is encountered; that is, the youngster may have a vast accumulation of stool localized in the rectal area. In virtually all cases, some degree of functional megacolon or megarectum is present. This tends to weaken bowel musculature, to alter pressure/volume relationships during defecation, and to compromise sensory feedback or awareness of the need to have a bowel movement.[4] Some children may not appear to be constipated at the time they are evaluated, but all victims of encopresis are at least intermittently retentive.

COMPLICATING FACTORS

In evaluating and managing children with encopresis, it is important that the clinician have a lucid understanding of the youngster's predicament. The following observations should help to sensitize health care professionals:

1. Children with encopresis often insist (correctly) that they do not feel the *need* to have a bowel movement—that is, they receive no signal; their incontinence is therefore unanticipated. Their parents may admonish, "At least if you'd come in when you need to go to the bathroom, you wouldn't have this problem. You're just too lazy to come inside while you're playing." This all too common assertion by parents clearly and cruelly overlooks the child's diminished or absent perceptual awareness of the need to defecate.
2. Children with encopresis have difficulty smelling their own "products." Thus parents might state, "If only you would change your clothes after an accident, it wouldn't be so bad." This attitude tends to overlook that children with encopresis often are not particularly aware that they have had an accident, likely because they get used to the odor.
3. Children with encopresis (and their parents) usually have never heard of any other children who have this problem.[6] This is a unique, isolating facet of the clinical

Table 80-1 *Potentiating Factors in the Genesis of Encopresis*

PERIOD	COMMON FACTORS
Infancy and toddler	Simple infant constipation; parental overconcern; congenital anorectal anomalies; acquired anorectal problems (e.g., fissures); coercive physical treatments of constipation
Training (ages 2-5 yr)	Extreme family stress at time of training; overaggressive training; extreme permissive training; continuing painful defecation; idiosyncratic toilet fears
Early school age	Fear of school bathrooms; prolonged or severe gastroenteritis; attention deficit with task impersistence (i.e., incomplete defecation); food intolerance or excess; frenetic lifestyle; psychosocial stresses

Modified from Levine MD: Encopresis: its potentiation, evaluation, and alleviation, Pediatr Clin North Am 29(2):318, 1982.

picture. Most other childhood dysfunctions are publicized and their existence acknowledged widely. Children who wet the bed know of other youngsters with enuresis. Those with attention deficits or learning problems are aware of others who are similarly dysfunctional. In encopresis, however, each child is somehow convinced that he or she is the sole citizen who messes at his or her age.

4. Children with encopresis live in fear of exposure, especially before their peers. Their accidents usually occur late in the afternoon (between 3:00 PM and 7:00 PM). This makes them highly vulnerable on the school bus, while out playing with friends, or at the home of an acquaintance. Nocturnal encopresis is rare. "Accidents" in school, although not unusual, are less common than those in the late afternoon. That children tend to mess in the afternoon sometimes is taken as evidence of a form of "revenge" against parents. Thus parents may be told unfairly that, "You notice he never messes in school. Therefore he only likes to stink when his mother is around." The inferring clinician may have overlooked that the child also has late afternoon accidents on Saturday, Sunday, and vacations. One can torment one's parents just as easily on holidays as in the morning.
5. Children with encopresis often have been victims of erratic management.[6] Parents may be susceptible to conflicting counsel from neighbors, teachers, relatives, physicians, and others. They may feel that they have tried everything, but nothing therapeutic may have been implemented for very long or with much consistency.
6. Children who have encopresis appropriate a wide range of coping strategies intended to help them save face and somehow contain their intense emotions surrounding the problem. Some may act as though indifferent, seeming not to care. Others may retreat strategically, preferring to be alone, avoiding intimate contact as much as possible. Some more furtive copers may hide their underwear or sequester odoriferous garments beneath the family herb garden! All represent efforts to avoid intolerable shame.
7. Often, children with encopresis will develop *secondary* affective responses. A child may become chronically anxious and depressed as a *result* of his or her loss of this primitive form of control. Steeply declining self-esteem is common. At times it can be difficult to decide which came first: Is the child having encopresis because of his or her anxiety, or is anxiety a by-product of incontinence? Since both states require careful management, resolution of this quandary may not be important.
8. Encopresis is likely to become a family problem. For one thing, it can cause considerable resentment on the part of siblings, who may not want to bring other children home because of odors in the house. Or they may not want their clothes cleansed in the same washing machine as the patient's clothes. The family may be reluctant to take the child on a car trip or to a restaurant. Parents may disagree and argue about the appropriate management of the problem. The child may feel guilty about all of the tension and turmoil he or she is generating. In some cases, a child paradoxically may come to enjoy the intensity of feelings his or her problem engenders at home. This can provide a secondary gain that subsequently may thwart effective treatment.
9. When encopresis exists amid marital strife at home, the bowel disorder can become ammunition for either parent. For instance, one parent may stand accused of having caused or perpetuated the problem. In some cases, a mother or father in distress seems to *need* the child to have such difficulty—a possible way of dramatizing shameful inadequacy of a spouse. The child may be caught in the crossfire, the encopresis unconsciously potentiated by the accusing parent.

EVALUATION

Any child with fecal incontinence should have a complete review of his or her developmental, behavioral, and health history. Organic conditions such as hypothyroidism, a spinal defect, abnormalities of calcium metabolism, and aganglionic megacolon usually are fairly easy to rule out without extensive laboratory tests. A systematic review of the origins of the child's problem can shed light on pathophysiologic factors. The time of onset, the accumulation of various "bowel risk factors" (see above), previous methods of management, and the child's own cluster of associated behaviors and coping mechanisms all are relevant. Much of this information can be gathered with the use of standardized questionnaires that summarize the youngster's earlier history, for example, the questionnaire developed by Levine and Barr.[7]

A complete physical examination can help to rule out specific organic disorders. In addition, the physical assessment can enable a clinician to make determinations regarding the frequency or extent of a child's current incontinence. Telltale stains in the perianal area as well as signs of chronic skin irritation may suggest that the child is indeed having frequent accidents. Sometimes intertriginous skin lesions suggest the need for management of the irritation itself. Occasionally, boys with long-standing encopresis (especially those who also have enuresis) may develop meatal stenosis from chronic irritation in and around the urethral meatus. The clinician should also look for signs of hemorrhoids or anal tags. Some pediatricians perform rectal examinations to establish that there is a significant amount of stool in the ampulla. Psychologically, rectal examinations may engender reluctance or apprehension regarding return visits; yet one needs to be done as part of the initial evaluation of all children with encopresis.

Often, although not always, a clinician can palpate stool throughout the abdomen. Some patients have an extensive functional megacolon with considerable stool retention, but this is not always detectable on abdominal palpation. For this reason, it is helpful to obtain a postvoiding supine roentgenogram of the abdomen to document the extent of retained feces. The roentgen rays can then be used as a baseline from which to judge the success of an initial catharsis. Barium enemas are seldom a part of the evaluation; anal manometry may be helpful.

Girls with encopresis tend to have recurrent urinary tract infections as a result of ascending contamination from the perineum. Thus girls with long-standing fecal incontinence should have a urinalysis and culture performed. An intravenous pyelogram may also be indicated in such cases to rule out chronic pyelonephritis.

It is important to evaluate the mental health of children with encopresis. Standardized behavioral inventories can help with this. In particular, it is revealing to delineate the extent to which the child has developed a clinical depression as a result of encopresis, the degree to which maladaptive coping strategies have been applied, and the extent to which the child's feelings about the problem are likely to facilitate or impede a treatment program. In addition, family influences regarding the problem need to be evaluated.

TREATMENT

The management of children with encopresis demands perseverance, consistency, and support. A strong advice-giving, nonaccusatory approach is most likely to succeed. There exist a number of detailed reviews of management in the literature.[3,6,8] The following is a summary of steps that can be used in one model of treatment.

Demystification

The first step in managing a child with encopresis is to educate the child and the parents about the problem. Various diagrams can be used to explain the development of a megacolon and subsequent incontinence. The child should have a clear understanding of what is wrong inside of his or her abdomen. It might be helpful to review roentgenograms with the patient. One can then set up some concrete treatment goals to help rebuild muscles in the child's large intestine. As part of the demystification, the child and parents should understand that many other youngsters have the problem, that it really is no one's fault, and that with some persistent long-term effort, normal bowel function can be restored.

Initial Catharsis

To restore bowel function effectively, the clinician must begin with an empty large intestine. This requires an initial "cleanout." In most cases this can be done over a 10-day to 2-week period. A series of 3-day cycles is instituted. On the first day, the child is given two hypophosphate enemas,* one right after another. On the second day, a bisacodyl suppository is used, and on the third day a bisacodyl pill is taken. Such 3-day cycles are repeated four or five times, and a roentgenogram of the abdomen is taken following this catharsis. In milder cases, an oral laxative may be used for the cleanout instead of the enemas and suppositories. Once it is established that the child has been well evacuated, a maintenance program can be implemented.

In more severe cases, hospitalization may be necessary. A child may require inpatient treatment consisting of twice daily high saline enemas and oral laxative therapies. During an inpatient admission, a child can also undergo a thorough psychological evaluation if indicated. Generally such hospitalizations require 5 to 7 days.

Maintenance Treatment

Maintenance involves training as well as facilitating defecation.[5] The child is asked to sit on the toilet twice a day at the same times each day for at least 10 minutes each time. The best times usually are after meals. In addition, the youngster is placed on light mineral oil (approximately 2 tablespoons twice a day). For the first 4 to 6 weeks, an oral laxative is also given, usually senna or danthron. If the child is doing well after the first 6 weeks, the laxative can be tapered off and the mineral oil continued. In general, a minimum of 6 months is required for moderate cases.

Follow-Up and Monitoring

Depending on the severity of the case, the youngster should be checked by the pediatrician regularly.

On follow-up visits a child should have a physical examination during which his or her abdomen is palpated carefully. The anogenital area should be inspected for evidence of chronic skin irritation that might suggest frequent "accidents." A repeat rectal examination is not required. It should be stressed that often children are not very reliable reporters of how they are doing. The clinician needs to seek physical evidence of improvement or regression. In most cases a return visit at least every 6 weeks for the first 6 months is needed. The physician should spend time alone with the youngster, discussing various setbacks and triumphs. He or she should help the youngster talk about the bowel problem, promising

*All doses are calculated for an average 7-year-old child. The clinician should adjust these, especially for younger or smaller patients. Davidson and co-workers suggest even higher doses.[3]

confidentiality and pursuing a nonaccusatory approach. In a sense, the pediatrician is acting as a "coach," helping the child to build up the muscles and autonomy for good bowel function.

Other Services

Some children who are particularly depressed or whose family situations are perpetuating the problem may require more intensive counseling by a psychologist, psychiatrist, or social worker. This in no way replaces ongoing pediatric management and follow-up.

Affected children seldom, if ever, need any surgical intervention. It should be remembered that many youngsters with encopresis require a long course of treatment. Relatively treatment-resistant cases may require several years of laxative and stool softener therapy. Such cases can really test the physician-patient relationship. Ultimately, professional endurance may be the key to success.

In general, a child who has been cured of encopresis is an eternally grateful patient. In successfully managing this devastating disorder, the physician has lifted from a youngster one of the heaviest burdens that can be borne during the years of growing up. Through sensitive support, the toll on self-esteem can be minimized even before the encopresis is alleviated.

REFERENCES

1. Anthony EJ: An experimental approach to the psychopathology of childhood: encopresis, Br J Med Psychol 30:146, 1957.
2. Bellman M: Studies on encopresis, Acta Paediatr Scand 170(suppl):1, 1966.
3. Davidson M, Kugler MM, and Bauer CH: Diagnosis and management of children with severe and protracted constipation and obstipation, J Pediatr 62:261, 1963.
4. Fitzgerald JF: Difficulties with defecation and elimination in children, Clin Gastroenterol 6:283, 1977.
5. Levine MD: Encopresis: its potentiation, evaluation, and alleviation, Pediatr Clin North Am 29(2):318, 1982.
6. Levine MD and Bakow H: Children with encopresis: a study of treatment outcome, Pediatrics 58:945, 1976.
7. Levine MD and Barr RG: Encopresis evaluation system, Unpublished manuscript, Boston, Mass, 1980, The Children's Hospital Medical Center.
8. Silber DL: Encopresis: discussion of etiology and management, Clin Pediatr 8:225, 1969.

81

Enuresis

Michael W. Cohen

For the primary care provider, the evaluation and management of an enuretic child is a frequent and demanding task. One must consider the various etiologies for enuresis in developing a reasonable, efficient, and successful approach to a "wetting" child and to the child's family.

Enuresis is defined as the involuntary discharge of urine, although it is often used to mean wetting during nighttime sleep *(nocturnal enuresis)*. Daytime wetting is termed *diurnal enuresis*. The diagnosis of enuresis should be reserved for those wetting beyond the age of 5 years in girls and 6 years in boys, the sex-related age differences reflecting developmental variations.

Nocturnal enuresis exists in approximately 15% of all 5-year-olds, 7% of 8-year-olds, and 3% of 12-year-olds. Lower socioeconomic groups, families with lower educational levels, and institutionalized populations have a higher reported prevalence of enuresis. Males predominate at all ages within all enuretic populations, with the differential being greater in older children. Somewhat fewer than 10% of all enuretics also wet in the daytime. Diurnal enuresis infrequently occurs without nocturnal enuresis.[1]

Primary enuresis exists when a child has never achieved consistent dryness. A child with secondary enuresis is generally considered to have had a period of dryness of at least 3 to 6 months and is commonly referred to as a "relapser" or an "onset enuretic." Among enuretic children, secondary enuresis generally increases with age, with over 50% of all enuretics being of the onset type by 12 years of age. Approximately 25% of children will have some relapse in bed-wetting after a period of initial dryness. This form of secondary enuresis is often self-limiting and may occur only at times of illness or emotional stress.

The strong familial aspect of enuresis is well established. If both parents have a history of enuresis, there is approximately a 75% chance that one or more of their children will be enuretic. If one parent had enuresis, there is a 40% to 45% chance that a child in that family will be enuretic. If neither parent was enuretic, the risk decreases to 15%.[2,5]

ETIOLOGY

Enuresis must be considered multifactorial in etiology. Developmental "delays," organic disorders, and psychological factors have all been emphasized as causes of enuresis. Although definitive proof is lacking, many believe that a delay in adequate neuromuscular bladder control is the major etiologic factor in enuretic children. This view is supported by (1) the primary nature of most enuresis, (2) the common familial pattern, (3) the common history of frequent voiding and urgency to void as a manifestation of a small functional bladder capacity, and (4) the high incidence of spontaneous remission (or developmental maturation). Proponents of this theory argue that the persistence of enuresis after neuromuscular maturation is based on the psychological effects of the child's interaction with significant individuals in his or her environment.

Sleep investigations in enuretic children have evolved with the technologic advances that allow study of sleep patterns. Initial studies concluded that enuresis occurred in lighter stages of sleep. Subsequent studies described nocturnal enuresis as a "disorder of arousal," with the voiding episodes beginning in the deepest stages of sleep, from which the patients lightened their sleep but were unable to wake completely. More recent studies conclude that nocturnal enuresis is independent of sleep stage and not specifically related to the depth of sleep. Enuretic episodes randomly occur throughout the night; wetting occurs in each stage of sleep in proportion to the amount of time spent in that stage.[3,4]

Organic explanations have focused primarily on the genitourinary and nervous systems. Obstructive lesions of the distal outflow tract, such as posterior urethral valves, have received particular attention both as a cause of urinary tract infections and as an independent cause of enuresis. A current urinary tract infection or the history of previous infections may be causal factors in enuresis. However, in a primary setting, only about 3% to 4% of enuretic youngsters demonstrate significant urologic pathology.[2]

Nervous system dysfunction may be associated with enuresis, either through lumbosacral disorders that affect bladder innervation or as a reflection of global mental retardation. Although true myelodysplastic disorders may affect bladder function, the radiologic finding of spina bifida occulta has not been shown to be causally related to enuresis.

Recent studies of preadolescent and older teenagers have focused on the contribution of polyuria and diuresis in their nocturnal enuresis. These patients were urodynamically normal. They had a sleep diuresis that exceeded their daytime bladder capacity by up to several hundred percent. In contrast to the normal nighttime increase in antidiuretic hormone (arginine vasopressin), these patients maintained constant serum levels at night. Enuresis for this group of patients appears to be related to polyuria secondary to a lack of circadian rhythm in antidiuretic hormone secretion. This information is consistent with parental reports of multiple nighttime wetting episodes and an apparent excessive urinary output in their children.[4] Diabetes mellitus, sickle cell anemia and sickle cell trait, food allergies, and ingestion of foods or medications with diuretic actions have all been implicated as infrequent causes of enuresis.

Psychological functioning may relate to enuresis at two levels. The enuresis may be only one aspect of a child's general difficulty in behavioral adaptation, or it may be an isolated symptom in a child whose behavioral functioning is otherwise adequate.

The incidence of behavioral problems in enuretic children has been estimated by behavioral inventories, interviews, and observation in children who have been evaluated for their enuresis. These surveys indicate a slight increase in behavioral problems among this population. However, it has also been shown that families who bring their enuretic child for an evaluation perceive more behavioral problems in their child than those who do not seek an assessment. Therefore the true incidence of behavioral problems in enuretic children is difficult to determine. It is reasonable to conclude that most enuretic children are not maladjusted nor are they psychopathologic.[2]

As an isolated phenomenon, enuresis most often is probably the result of poor or deficient learning of a habit pattern during toilet-training. Resistance to initial training efforts, despite the nature of the techniques used, appears to be an important factor.

The evaluation should be considered as the initial phase of therapy. The positive therapeutic value of a complete evaluation that satisfies the concerns and expectations of the enuretic child and the child's family is well documented. Potential parental guilt associated with management failures can be alleviated by a brief explanation of the multifactorial origin of the condition and the common difficulties in management.

HISTORY

The severity of the enuresis should be estimated and expressed as the number of wet nights per week or month (for example, 4/7, 16/30). Quantification of the enuresis allows for a relatively accurate demonstration of a trend and the effect of intervention. A delineation of the type of enuresis (primary versus secondary, nocturnal versus diurnal) should be established. The effect of environmental factors on the severity of the symptoms should also be explored. Parental management techniques should be discussed, beginning with a history of initial toilet-training efforts. The age and response of the child, the attitudes and approach of the parents, and the results of such efforts are important information. The child's perception of family and peer responses to the difficulty should be elicited. An impression about whether the enuresis is limiting age-appropriate activity should also be obtained.

The medical history will reveal any perinatal difficulties that may have led to neurologic trauma; the weight and gestation of the patient can alter developmental expectations. The review of systems should focus on the genitourinary and nervous systems. Delays in perceptual-motor or communication skills might coexist with a delay in bladder control. In addition to frequency and urgency of urination and symptoms of urinary tract infection, dribbling after and between micturition and also dysuria have been found to be more common in enuretic children. Approximately 1 in 10 enuretics will also be encopretic. This association is firmly established and may reflect an underlying deficiency in toilet-training or organic pathology.

PHYSICAL EXAMINATION

A full examination is essential. Renal disease may be reflected in poor growth or elevated blood pressure. Examination of the genitalia should be complete and sensitive to the feelings of a developing youngster or teenager. A search for major and minor anomalies should be followed by an observation of micturition. Anomalies, including undescended testes, underdeveloped scrotum, epispadias, phimosis and abnormalities in the urethral meatus in males, and location and characteristics of the urethral meatus in females should be observed, because they may be associated with internal anomalies. Abnormalities or difficulties in voiding, such as changes in the quality (e.g., size and velocity) of the urinary stream, an inability to initiate or stop micturition voluntarily, and the presence of dysuria or dribbling, should be noted.

A neurologic examination may reveal lower spinovertebral dysfunction that reflects bladder innervation abnormalities. Gait, muscular strength and tone, deep tendon reflexes, sensory responses, and rectal sphincter tone should therefore be examined.

LABORATORY TESTS

A urinalysis provides valuable information about a wide range of organic disorders that may be associated with enuresis, including diabetes insipidus, psychogenic water drinking, diabetes mellitus, urinary tract infection, and various forms of renal pathology. Beyond the urinalysis and urine culture, the indication for further evaluation remains quite controversial.

One author has divided noctural enuresis into uncomplicated and complicated, with the second category requiring additional diagnostic studies. Factors that dictate these studies include persistent secondary onset of bed-wetting, severe voiding dysfunction, associated encopresis, urinary tract infection, and an abnormal neurologic examination. Further studies may include a renal or bladder sonogram, intravenous pyelogram (IVP), a voiding cystourethrogram (VCUG), or urodynamic measurements.[7] If these procedures are indicated, the child must be adequately prepared in a manner that will minimize the psychological trauma. The nature of this preparation will depend on the age, sex, and developmental maturity of the child. A measurement of functional bladder capacity should be obtained if bladder training is the proposed form of treatment. Unless there is a strong suspicion of an undiagnosed seizure disorder, the presence of enuresis does not warrant an electroencephalogram.

At the conclusion of this type of evaluation, the majority of enuretics with significant organic dysfunction or psychopathologic dysfunction will have been discovered. When their needs exceed the expertise of the primary care physician, these patients should be referred to the appropriate specialist. The remaining group, which constitutes the vast majority of enuretics, will present a picture consistent with a basic developmental delay in bladder control with associated psychological factors. This population is best managed by the clinician who is most familiar with the child and the child's family and environment.

MANAGEMENT

An air of optimism is realistic and may have immeasurable therapeutic value. Although a positive clinical response to the process of evaluation and intervention has often been labeled a placebo effect, the benefit of a carefully planned approach has been documented and should be considered a therapeutic response, not the result of a placebo. Optimism is supported by reports of an annual spontaneous cure rate of approximately 15% after age 5.[8] Optimism can also be cultivated by uncovering a history of parental enuresis.

The active participation of the child will enhance the efficacy of any specific mode of therapy and should be solicited. The child's involvement should begin with an explanation of the probable cause of his or her enuresis at the child's level of understanding. A clarification of the involuntary nature of the symptoms will remove any sense of guilt and allow the child to develop an optimistic perspective. Such involvement will also decrease the chances of struggle between child and parents and will promote the child's responsibility for effecting alleviation of the symptoms.[5]

Reassurance may be the therapy for younger children or for children developing transient secondary enuresis in response to environmental stress. For parents who feel compelled to do something while waiting for a remission, various simple measures have been recommended, such as limiting the child's fluid intake, having the child empty his or her bladder at bedtime, or taking the child to the bathroom during the night. If these are suggested, it should be realized that although they may decrease the symptoms somewhat, they have not been shown to hasten a remission. These tactics may also initiate or aggravate a struggle between parent and child.

Supportive counseling may be required as the sole mode of therapy or as an adjunct to other specific regimens. The goals of counseling could include (1) parental understanding of the multifactorial nature of enuresis, (2) parental acceptance of the child and the symptoms in a manner that allows them to provide maximum emotional support, (3) acceptance by the child of the symptom and an appreciation of "individual differences" that many children demonstrate in other areas of functioning, and (4) appreciation by the patient that he or she can have some control over the enuresis. The requirement for counseling depends on the age of the child, the child's general developmental and behavioral pattern, the family's experience with enuresis, the coexistence of emotional problems, intrafamily communication patterns, and the response to the initial management.

If the enuresis is deterring the child's social, emotional, or cognitive development, therapy beyond reassurance and supportive counseling is indicated. Since no one therapy has been consistently superior, the clinician's experience, enthusiasm, and comfort should dictate the choice. Drug therapy, conditioning devices, bladder training, and self-hypnosis have been shown to be effective by various clinicians. However, both parents and child should be alerted to the potential for relapse and thus the need for a "second dose" of treatment.[1]

Several pharmacologic agents have been used to treat enuresis. Sedatives, stimulants, and sympathomimetic agents are not beneficial. Oxybutynin, an anticholinergic agent often prescribed for enuresis, is not significantly better than a placebo in reducing the frequency of bed-wetting.

Tricyclic antidepressants, particularly imipramine, have been used extensively to treat enuresis, with a short-term success rate of up to 40% and a high relapse rate. Three proposed mechanisms of action are (1) a direct relaxation effect on the bladder detrusor muscle, (2) an alteration in the arousal state of the nervous system during sleep, or (3) an antidepressant effect. Since there is no evidence that enuretic children are depressed, and since enuretic improvement can be immediate, whereas antidepressant benefits take more than 7 to 10 days, it is unlikely that antidepression is the mechanism. The arousal proposal is less tenable, since the relationship between depth of sleep and enuresis has been questioned.[7]

Imipramine is generally given ½ to 1 hour before bedtime, with no proven advantage to multiple daily doses. The initial imipramine dose is 25 mg for children under 12 and 50 mg for older children. The maximum recommended dose is 75 mg. The child should be asked to maintain a diary of success. At the first follow-up visit, the drug dosage can be altered and positive feedback can be supplied to the youngster. Once a successful therapeutic response is achieved, the child should be maintained on the medication for approximately 3 months. At the end of this period, a gradual discontinuation of the drug will decrease the likelihood of a relapse. Tapering to once every other night and then every third night should be accomplished over a period of 4 to 6 weeks. The maximum psychological benefit of dryness on "nondrug" nights can be supplied by emphasizing and praising the child's newly developed bladder control, which will, it is hoped, be sustained without medication. The most common adverse drug side effect is nervousness.

Imipramine is well known for its thin margin of safety and toxicity. The triad of coma, convulsions, and cardiac disturbances can occur at relatively low-dosage accidental ingestions in young children and may be fatal. School-age youngsters are vulnerable to overdosage because of magical thinking that leads them to believe that more medication might be more permanently beneficial. A number of deaths have been reported under these circumstances. Great caution must be used in prescribing this agent, and the parents and child must be well aware of the potential dangers involved in, and their control over, its administration.[5] Drug therapy with this agent should be reserved for the older enuretic who has not responded successfully to other modalities of therapy.

The diuresis theory of causality has led to clinical trials with desmopressin (antidiuretic hormone). This agent serves as a substitute for endogenous nocturnal vasopressin, leading to a reduction in overnight urine volume. The dosage is 20 to 40 μg given at bedtime. Most studies have used intranasal administration, although the oral route appears to be just as effective. Desmopressin has been used for 20 years in the treatment of central diabetes insipidus with few adverse effects. Water intoxication and hyponatremia can occur but are not of concern in healthy children given only a bedtime dose. Headaches, nausea, mild abdominal cramps, and vulvar pain have been reported but disappear when the dose is reduced. The drug does not suppress endogenous production of vasopressin nor does it induce destructive antibodies. Desmopressin is effective in 10% to 65% of cases, depending on the particular study. When compared with conditioning devices, desmopressin had a more immediate benefit, but conditioning provided significantly more long-term results with less chance of relapse.[4]

The specific indications for the use of desmopressin have not been defined. It may be most useful in older patients (over 10 to 11 years of age) who have not benefited from prior therapies. It also may help in conjunction with conditioning devices to achieve a rapid improvement while the conditioned response is developing, allowing eventual withdrawal of the medication. Intermittent use when enuretic children are sleeping over with peers may avoid embarrassment while a spontaneous resolution of the enuresis is awaited.

Enuresis conditioning instruments involve a moisture-activated sensor, which is connected to an alarm that provides auditory stimulation to wake the child or parent on initiating of wetting.[5] Older devices involve a mattress pad; the new ones have portable mechanisms that attach to the child's underpants; the auditory sources are contained in a wristwatch or small pin-on battery-powered alarm. Because the temporal relationship between the wetting episode and the alarm is critical for effective conditioning, a refined instrument with adequate sensitivity is required. Several controlled studies have yielded cure rates between 60% and 85%. Permanent responders require an average of 60 days of therapy. A 20% to 40% relapse rate is reported in all studies, but dryness is often obtained more quickly and permanently with a second course of treatment. One author feels that the technique of "overlearning" by increasing fluid intake before bedtime to stress the bladder additionally and increase the waking episode decreases the relapse rate. An intermittent reinforcement program, with the alarm sounding during 70% of the wetting episodes, may also lead to a lower relapse rate. The safety and portable nature of the new devices and the reported successful results of such conditioning therapy make this an attractive therapeutic technique.[1]

Self-hypnosis or self-conditioning has been effective in primary nocturnal enuresis.[6] The enuretic episode is viewed as a habit disorder that allows the wetting episode without the child awakening. The child is taught the technique of self-induced relaxation, to be practiced before sleep. During this "trance," the child (for example, a boy) tells himself that he *will* wake up when he experiences the need to void, thus allowing a dry bed and very happy feelings on waking in the morning. This happiness can be associated with a visual image of some warm, tranquil, and enjoyable experience in the youngster's memory to enhance the desirability of the dry bed feeling. Significant improvement and cure rates (80%) have been reported after only a few training visits. This technique requires special therapy skills, but appears to be a very potent, safe modality with much promise for the future.

Bladder-training therapy is based on the observation that many children with enuresis have a decreased functional bladder capacity. The goal of this training is to transform a functionally infantile bladder into one with adult volume and coordination capabilities. The procedure involves the active participation of the child in holding the urine as long as possible once a day for several months. Increasing urine volumes and number of dry nights are recorded on a calendar, which serves as a reinforcement for the child. The clinician must be cautious that the discomfort caused by urine retention does not discourage the participation of the youngster and create a struggle with the parents.

TREATMENT FAILURES AND RELAPSES

The experienced clinician will attest to relapses and treatment failures being relatively frequent with all modes of therapy. A particular therapy should not be considered a failure until it has been tried for at least 4 to 6 weeks. A failure of one type of therapy might dictate the addition of another mode. If combination therapy fails, the practitioner may have to tell the child and the family that the neuromuscular bladder control mechanisms are still too immature and that the symptoms must be tolerated for several more months, when the treatment can be reinstituted. Reassurance of physical and mental normality *must* accompany this message. However, if any new information concerning organic dysfunction or a psychopathologic problem becomes apparent, further evaluation might be indicated. For example, a treatment failure could result from noncompliance, which reflects either an underlying family interactional pattern that precludes the necessary empathy and understanding or emotional needs of family members that require persistence of the symptom. This aspect should be appropriately investigated by the primary care clinician or a mental health associate. Psychiatric consultation may be handled by explaining to patients that the nervous system–bladder control mechanism is developing but is not yet fully mature and that a few more months of specific therapy will be required. The previously successful mode of therapy is then reinstituted. This approach allows for maintenance of an optimistic posture and, if necessary, the use of several courses of therapy.

REFERENCES

1. Foxman B, Valdez RB, and Brook RH: Childhood enuresis: prevalence, perceived impact and prescribed treatment, Pediatrics 77:482, 1986.
2. McLorie GA and Husmann DA: Incontinence and enuresis, Pediatr Clin North Am 34:1159, 1987.
3. Mikkelson EJ and Rapoport JL: Enuresis: psychopathology, sleep stage and drug response, Urol Clin North Am 7:361, 1980.
4. Norgaard JP, Rittig S, and Djurhuus JC: Nocturnal enuresis: an approach to treatment based on pathogenesis, J Peditar 114 (suppl):705, 1989.
5. Novello AC and Novello JR: Enuresis, Pediatr Clin North Am 34:719, 1987.
6. Olness K and Gardner GG: Hypnosis and hypnotherapy with children, Philadelphia, 1988, Grune & Stratton, Inc.
7. Rushton HG: Nocturnal enuresis: epidemiology, evaluation and currently available treatment options, J Ped Suppl 114:691, 1989.
8. Schmitt BD: Nocturnal enuresis: an update on treatment, Pediatr Clin North Am 29:21, 1982.

82

Failure to Thrive

Lewis A. Barness

Failure to thrive is a convenient label applied to those children who are behind their age peers in physical growth or development. The term is most frequently used in reference to infants under 2 years of age. It is equally applicable, however, to older children or to those at any age with deficient mental development. The present discussion is adapted largely to infants who are below the 3rd percentile for height, weight, or both.

Children most often fail to thrive because of psychosocial difficulties, although they may also suffer from malnutrition and specific physical defects. Those who have a psychosocial etiology require investigation similar to that for children with more obvious forms of parenting problems or child neglect. Children with specific physical abnormalities will, of course, require management of those abnormalities.

NORMAL GROWTH FACTORS

The ultimate growth of a normal child is most closely determined by inheritance, but other factors can alter this pattern.

One external factor affecting growth is malnutrition. Nutritional deprivation in utero may result in permanent growth retardation; effects of nutritional deprivation later in life may cause permanent mental and physical retardation or may be reversible, depending on age and duration of deprivation and the type of rehabilitation utilized. Nutritional deprivation that causes retardation may be caused by lack of calories, lack of protein, or lack of any one of the specific nutrients such as a vitamin or a mineral.

Malnutrition occurs in children whose families do not feed them for psychological or economic reasons, or because of ignorance of how, how often, or what to feed.[1,2,8] However, malnutrition also occurs in those with organic defects that produce excess waste and abnormal metabolism[3] or inanition that decreases ability to eat.

Hormones are necessary for normal growth and include pituitary growth hormone, which induces skeletal muscle and hepatic and renal protein synthesis.[9] Insulin affects carbohydrate metabolism and stimulates amino acid transport, protein synthesis, and cell division. Thyroid hormone influences the rate of cell division and cell size. Androgens and estrogens increase the rate of cartilage cell division, but accelerate maturation and calcification of the epiphyses even more rapidly, so that immediate growth is rapid but the growing period is shortened when these hormones are in excess. Glucocorticoids inhibit cell division. All other known hormones affect growth in some way.

All acute or chronic diseases can slow growth, because of increased catabolism of tissue, increased caloric demands, increased waste, or defective metabolism.

EVALUATION

It is essential that children who fail to thrive be evaluated systematically to conserve time and resources and provide remedial measures as quickly as possible. A history and physical and laboratory examinations are obtained similar to those obtained for other children, although care should be directed to certain areas. In cases with strong psychosocial features, nonroutine laboratory tests may not be indicated.

HISTORY

Birth Weight and Gestational Age

Birth weight in relationship to gestational age may indicate intrauterine growth retardation, causes of which include intrauterine infection, placental insufficiency, chromosomal anomalies, and some of the dwarfing syndromes. Many of these children are born with a smaller-than-normal complement of cells and can never grow normally.

The shorter small-for-gestational-age (SGA) babies born at term are more likely to catch up than the longer babies. They are voracious eaters and usually catch up in the first 6 to 9 months.

Sequential Growth Record

It is important to know if a child has always been of low height or weight for age or if growth slowed at some specified time. If the latter, this points to a disease or phenomenon occurring near the time of the change in growth rate.

Family History

The heights of parents and grandparents and heights and weights of siblings may indicate genetic growth aberration or some factor common to several family members.

Feeding

A careful 1-day feeding history is often revealing. Caloric intake is estimated. Well-motivated parents may restrict intake of fats and calories to prevent obesity or atherosclerosis, but when such a regimen is applied rigidly or at early age, it results in growth failure.[7] A history of massive intake with no growth usually indicates that the informant is fabricating or ignorant of intake, although excessive losses cannot be excluded. A history of pica should be noted.

Stools

Excessive stool losses may be the cause of lack of gain and growth.

System Review

Disease in any system can cause lack of weight and height gain.

Social History

The importance of an adequate social history cannot be overestimated. Family interest and time spent with the child, degree of caring for the child, and realistic concern can be estimated. Economic status and availability of resources should also be determined.[1,6]

PHYSICAL EXAMINATION

A careful physical examination further leads to detection of disease in body systems, any one of which can lead to failure to thrive. Determining the sitting height as a fraction of the total height helps to distinguish specific types of growth failure. Blood pressure measurement should not be forgotten as a screening test for acute or chronic renal disease.

Accurate height and weight measurements are essential. Some parents complain that their children are not growing properly. If the history and physical examination are within normal limits and the child falls within the lower percentiles of the growth charts for height and weight, explanation of normal growth patterns may reassure the parents and child. Some parents who themselves are short may expect excessive growth of their normal children. An explanation of genetic factors and normal growth rates leads to realistic expectations of growth without excessive investigation.

In the young child, head circumference can give valuable clues to diagnosis. In caloric deprivation, weight is lost first, then linear growth slows, and finally, head circumference does not increase. The head circumference below normal for age indicates either severe malnutrition or primary failure of development of the skull or brain.

LABORATORY EXAMINATION

Because many children who fail to thrive have inadequate nutritional or emotional support, early admission to a hospital may prevent rapid deterioration of the child. Laboratory studies should be minimized at this phase so that the child will not be fearful of the hospital environment. These studies include peripheral blood examination, which may suggest iron-deficiency anemia, a hemoglobinopathy, or a hematologic disorder. A tuberculin test can detect an otherwise unexpected infection.

Urinalysis includes pH, which when high in the presence of acidosis suggests renal tubular acidosis. Low specific gravity may indicate diabetes insipidus. Presence of acetone or glucose may indicate dehydration, poisoning (e.g., lead), or diabetes mellitus. Cellular elements are present in renal inflammatory disease, poisoning, or febrile states. Reducing substances other than glucose should be determined, since inborn metabolic errors such as galactosemia can be detected by the presence of a reducing substance in the absence of glucose. Ferric chloride is positive in a host of poisonings and is also a screening test for aminoaciduria.

If the child's problem is failure to gain weight, careful note should be made of the height, weight, and head circumference. The child should then be fed; if he or she gains rapidly, the diagnosis of inadequate feeding is suggested, and careful instruction and discussion with the family are required with frequent supportive follow-up visits. If the child fails to gain within 3 days, further laboratory studies may reveal a specific cause.

The stool should be examined and its appearance noted; examination should include staining for fat, ova, and parasites. Excessive numbers or bulk of stools point to a major enteropathy, though parenteral infections may also be responsible for chronic diarrhea. Dipping a urine dip stick in the stool water reveals the pH and the presence of glucose and protein. Demonstration of alpha-1-antitrypsin in the stool provides a quantitative estimate of stool protein levels. Excessive fat may indicate a malabsorption syndrome, excess protein, or a protein-losing enteropathy, and a stool pH below 5.5 may be the first indication of a disaccharidase deficiency. Some parasites (e.g., *Giardia*) may cause malabsorption syndromes.

A sweat test is performed to determine the likelihood of pancreatic insufficiency; in short girls, a buccal smear or chromosomal analysis is performed to determine genetic sex and the presence of gonadal insufficiency.

Other blood tests, including blood chemistries, should be performed (Table 82-1). These tests may result in a specific diagnosis or indicate involvement of a specific organ or system, after which more definitive tests for that organ or system can be performed.

Skull, chest, and long-bone roentgenograms should be obtained and should include views to determine bone age. Skull films may indicate asymmetry from previous injuries or specific abnormalities; abnormal calcifications suggest intracranial bleeding or intrauterine infections. Chest abnormalities may indicate chronic diseases, such as tuberculosis, cystic fibrosis, or antitrypsin deficiency. Long-bone roentgenograms help diagnose acute or chronic infection or metabolic and hereditary bone diseases. Bone age should be compared with height and chronologic age (Table 82-2).

Other studies that may be suggested include immunoelectrophoresis and special immunologic studies in children with frequent infections; chromosome studies in those with peculiar appearance or a conglomeration of abnormalities; 17-ketosteroids and other biochemical studies for adrenal or gonadal diseases; radiologic and endoscopic gastrointestinal studies for those with enteropathies; radiologic kidney studies for those with renal or adrenal diseases or with abdominal masses; electrocardiograms in those with heart abnormalities; and electroencephalograms in those with seizure disorders. Human growth hormone should not be given to short children

Table 82-1 *Suggested Blood Studies and Diagnoses Indicated by Abnormal Results*

BLOOD STUDY	DIAGNOSES
Hemoglobin, smear	Iron-deficiency and other anemias; hematologic disorders; some hemoglobinopathies
Sodium, potassium, chlorine, blood urea nitrogen	Renal diseases; adrenal disorders; dehydration
Calcium, phosphate, phosphatase	Rickets; thyroid and parathyroid insufficiency or excess
SGOT, prothrombin	Liver diseases; hepatitis; cirrhosis
Albumin	Chronic malnutrition; protein-losing enteropathy
Fasting blood glucose	Diabetes mellitus; adrenal disorders; glycogen storage disease; hypoglycemia syndromes; pituitary insufficiency or excess
Uric acid	Hyperuricemia
T_4, T_3 resin uptake	Thyroid insufficiency or excess
Growth hormone	Pituitary disease
Alpha-1-antitrypsin	Alpha-1-antitrypsin deficiency
Erythrocyte sedimentation rate	Collagen disorders; infections

Table 82-2 *Comparison of Chronologic Age (CA), Height Age (HA), and Bone Age (BA)*

RELATIONSHIP OF CA, HA, AND BA	SUGGESTED DIAGNOSES
HA < BA; BA = CA	Genetic short stature; chondrodystrophies; trisomy 21; gonadal dysgenesis (XO); trisomy 13; Cockayne syndrome; leprechaunism; Seckel syndrome; intrauterine infection; maternal drugs; storage diseases
HA = BA; BA < CA	Normal variant; constitutional delay; familial trait; mild malnutrition; metabolic or other chronic illness
BA < HA; BA < CA	If marked, hypothyroidism; if moderate, hypopituitarism or malnutrition

who are not growth hormone–deficient, even though it can initially increase their height.

Another complaint of failure to thrive occurs in children who approach the age of puberty without the development of secondary sex characteristics. At this time, several other considerations may lead to a definitive diagnosis. The most common cause of delayed adolescence is constitutional delay, including that arising from malnutrition, and requires reassurance of the patient and family. In these, characteristics of prepubertal development are normal and proceed as listed in the left-hand box, p. 707. Male genital development should begin by 14 years of age and should be complete by age 19 years. Female sex development should begin by 10 years of age, and menarche should occur within 5 years. If the developmental order is abnormal or if delay is beyond these limits, then further investigation is required (see also Chapter 164, "Sexual Developmental Alterations").

MANAGEMENT

If a specific cause of failure to thrive is determined, it should be treated as an entity. In most children, this is related to inadequate food intake. Depending on the type of clinic population served, in some series as few as 50% and in others as many as 90% of children who were seen because of not thriving were finally found to be growing poorly or not at all because of inadequate intake (see right-hand box, p. 707). In most series, the cause of inadequate intake[4,5] was almost equally divided among economic, educational, or psychological inadequacy.

Realimentation in a marasmic child may be accompanied by no weight gain for as long as 6 weeks, presumably because of shifting of water between intracellular and extracellular spaces. During the phase of rapid weight gain, the liver may enlarge from fat accumulation, and signs of increased intracranial pressure may occur. These are usually temporary and require no treatment. If, however, refeeding is begun after even a short period of inadequate intake, diarrhea may occur. The child may have developed lactase deficiency during the period of low intake of lactose and must be given lactose in small quantities or not at all. He or she may have developed gastrointestinal motility abnormalities, so that slow increases in feeding are necessary.

After diagnosis and the beginning of treatment, frequent visits serve to determine not only the adequacy of treatment but also the adequacy and completeness of the diagnosis. Regardless of the age at the beginning of treatment, some catching up of growth will occur. The more severe, the earlier, and the longer the insult, the less likely is the child to attain his or her genetic potential. Nonetheless, treatment efforts should be persistent.

If treatment is not maintained after it is begun, the previous inadequate growth and development pattern will likely recur.

PROGNOSIS

In managing the child with nonorganic failure to thrive, the parents should be involved early in both investigation and treatment. A nonthreatening, nonrecriminatory attitude is fostered as the interaction between the child and parents is ob-

Order of Adolescent Development

MALE
Enlargement of testes
Pubic hair
Axillary hair
Facial hair

FEMALE
Growth acceleration
Breast development
Pubic hair
Menarche
Axillary hair

served. A few suggestions or instructions may suffice, but follow-up by a social worker in the home to give continual support is usually helpful. Mental stimulation of the child is necessary.

For those with severe failure to thrive, the prognosis for future growth and development may be poor for as many as 50% of those diagnosed before 5 years of age. The correspondence of statistical outcome of those with failure to thrive and other forms of abuse is striking.

Causes of Failure to Thrive*

IMPROPER FEEDING—50%-90%
Economic—10%-40%[2,4,5,10]
Education—10%-40%[2,4,5,10]
Psychological—30%-40%[2,4,5,10]
Intolerance—<5%[4,5,10]

OTHER CAUSES—10%-50%
Hypothyroidism
Cystic fibrosis
Subdural hematoma
Glycogen storage disease
Celiac disease
Methylmalonic acidemia
Maple syrup urine disease
Mental retardation, unspecified
Urinary tract disease
Diencephalic syndrome
Brain tumors
Chronic liver disease
Congenital heart disease
Ulcerative colitis

*Compendium from various sources. Some obvious causes are missing because the complaint is not failure to thrive, but rather is related to the diagnosis.

REFERENCES

1. Baertt JM, Adrianzen B, and Graham GG: Growth of previously well-nourished infants in poor homes, Am J Dis Child 130:33, 1976.
2. Barness LA: Failure to thrive, Dallas Med J 58:325, 1972.
3. Barness LA and Morrow G: Clinical clues to diagnosis of metabolic disorders, Clin Pediatr 9:605, 1970.
4. Berwick DM: Non-organic failure to thrive, Pediatr Rev 1:265, 1980.
5. Hannaway PJ: Failure to thrive: a study of 100 infants and children, Clin Pediatr 9:96, 1970.
6. Klaus MH, Leger T, and Trause MA: Maternal attachment and mothering disorders, ed 2, Skillman, NJ, 1982, Johnson & Johnson.
7. Lifshitz F and Moses N: Growth failure: a complication of dietary treatment of hypercholesterolemia, Am J Dis Child 143:537, 1989.
8. Mitchell WG, Gorrell RW, and Greenberg RA: Failure-to-thrive: a study in a primary care setting—epidemiology and follow-up, Pediatrics 65:971, 1980.
9. Root AW, Bongiovanni AM, and Eberlein WA: Diagnosis and management of growth retardation with special reference to the problem of hypopituitarism, J Pediatr 78:737, 1971.
10. Sills RH: Failure to thrive: the role of clinical and laboratory evaluation, Am J Dis Child 132:967, 1978.

SUGGESTED READING

Smith DW and Simons ER: Rational diagnostic evaluation of the child with mental deficiency, Am J Dis Child 129:1285, 1975.

83

Fire-Setting

William F. Gayton

The extent of the problem of fire-setting in children is unclear. Available estimates[5] obtained from child psychiatric populations suggest a prevalence of 2% to 3%. The number referred to physicians is also reported to be small. Recent reports[4] suggest that these figures may be underestimates. When parents at a child guidance clinic were asked to fill out a symptom checklist on the child being referred for help, 15% checked the item "sets fires." When 300 adults from the general population were asked, "If you had a child who repeatedly set fires, what would you do?" only 54% responded in a way that would have led to appropriate professional referral. Moreover, only 15% indicated they would seek help from a physician.

These findings suggest that fire-setting in children may be more prevalent than is believed and that parents are confused regarding what is an appropriate referral source. Physicians would seem to be in an ideal position to help with both of these matters. Relating to parents in such a way as to convey an interest in their children's social and emotional development as well as their physical well-being would provide parents with an opportunity to discuss behavioral problems such as fire-setting. Early detection of childhood fire-setting is especially important in view of the potential and life-threatening danger to the rest of the family and community. A willingness on the part of the physician to screen routinely for such problems would facilitate early recognition. Physicians also have an excellent opportunity to help with the confusion concerning an appropriate referral source. It appears that a significant percentage of parents and physicians are unsure how to respond to a child who sets fires. Physicians willing to concern themselves with behavioral problems of their patients are in an excellent position to prevent the inappropriate parental responses that do occur, such as burning children to teach them a lesson or calling the police to give their children a good scare.

ETIOLOGY

Early psychoanalytic theoretic speculations emphasized the relationship between fire-setting and sexual problems. Fire-setting was thought to result from parental prohibitions against masturbation and was viewed as a substitute activity for masturbatory behavior. Direct study[2] of childhood fire-setters has suggested a more diverse picture. In particular, the aggressive elements of fire-setting have received emphasis. Fire-setting is viewed as a means by which children retaliate against those aspects of the environment that have rejected them. Subsequent writers[3,5] have also emphasized the multidetermined aspects of the behavior. While noting that in some instances fire-setting may be a manifestation of sexual problems, they also point out its frequent association with impulse control problems and in some cases with severe emotional disturbance, including psychotic conditions. Failure to find a typical personality profile of childhood fire-setters is consistent with this view.

Severe family dysfunctioning is regularly mentioned in studies of childhood fire-setters.[2,3,5] A high incidence of parental psychopathology is noted, including alcoholism and psychosis. Varying degrees of child abuse and an absent father are also present. In this context, fire-setting is most likely an aggressive response to situational frustration, and the physician will need to approach the problem in terms of the total family. An exclusive focus on what is wrong with the child will not lead to an effective resolution of the problem.

A high incidence of academic difficulties is also reported.[2] Available estimates suggest that underachievement is present in roughly 75% of the cases. These difficulties may result from a personality disturbance associated with the fire-setting behavior. On the other hand, the possibility that fire-setting is a way of handling the frustration stemming from school failure should also be considered. The physician also needs to be alert to the presence of an undetected learning disability.

There have been several attempts to include fire-setting in children as part of a symptom triad (along with enuresis and cruelty to animals) predictive of later violent behavior. The evidence for such a relationship is based on either clinical case studies or retrospective data gathered from adjudicated adult individuals being evaluated for the court.[2] Such studies have considerable methodologic deficiencies, and further evidence is clearly needed before fire-setting in children can be used as a predictor of adult violent behavior. In this context, it should be noted that no long-term follow-up studies of childhood fire-setters are available, and it is unclear whether fire-setting is a self-limiting symptom or whether it carries more serious prognostic implications.

The dynamics of fire-setting in children would therefore appear to be multifaceted. Physicians will need to approach the problem without preconceived notions about the meaning of the behavior. Each child will require an individual approach based on the idea that fire-setting may mean different things to different children.

MANAGEMENT

Approaches to management depend on the physician's assessment of the seriousness of the problem. Key factors include the age of the child and the frequency of the behavior in the past. Although young children (4 to 6 years) may set fires for purposes of experimentation, fire-setting in the older child usually reflects a more serious psychiatric disturbance. The frequency of previous episodes is directly related to seriousness, and a history of repetitive fire-setting is an especially poor prognostic sign. Although fires set by younger children are usually spotted early and extinguished quickly, serious consequences may occur. One investigator[1] found that in 33 children who had been associated with the death of another person, death was caused by fires in six cases, and in 8 of the remaining 27 children, compulsive fire-setting was present.

In cases in which the behavior seems to be related to novelty and curiosity, the following steps are recommended. Discuss with the parents the necessity for "reality" controls. For example, encourage them not to leave the child at home unsupervised or provide the child with easy access to matches. They should communicate clearly to their child that playing with fire is inappropriate, and a full discussion of the dangers of such behavior should be included. Discuss with the parents the necessity for rewarding children when they engage in behavior that is incompatible with fire-setting, such as returning matches they have found without lighting them.

Active attempts should be made to discourage the parents from trying to help children get over their fascination with fire by allowing them to light fires in their presence. Frequently the parents will assign the child the job of lighting the dinner candles or their cigarettes in hopes this will reduce the child's interest in fire. The problem with this approach is that children are not able to discriminate between permissible and nonpermissible opportunities to light matches. Parents should also be warned about the dangers of overreacting, in terms of either excessive alarm or punitiveness. These reactions may paradoxically increase the frequency of the behavior by suggesting to the child that this is an especially effective way of retaliating against the parents.

For more serious cases of childhood fire-setting, the parent will first have to be introduced to the idea that the fire-setting is part of a broader pattern of disturbance. Discussing with the parent other aspects of the child's behavior and illustrating how such behavior fits a broader symptom picture will be necessary. The parents need to recognize that serious cases of childhood fire-setting are often an attempt to communicate distress. The possibility that the incidents are a response to environmental frustration, including family dysfunctioning, needs to be discussed. This ought to be done in a nonaccusatory manner with an emphasis on doing something to help the child. At this point, referral to a mental health professional is appropriate. Because of the potential danger associated with childhood fire-setting, direct contact between the physician and the consultant is recommended. The physician will need to emphasize the seriousness of the problem and the need for quick attention. After referral has been made, the physician should make a routine call to the family to ensure that the referral has been followed through.

In extreme cases, the possibility of hospitalization will have to be discussed with the parents. This will be necessary in cases in which children appear to be out of control and in which the parents are unable to manage the situation. Such a drastic measure as hospitalization is necessary to help children reestablish controls over their behavior. It may help to emphasize to parents that clinical experience suggests that the fire-setting behavior typically terminates soon after hospitalization.

REFERENCES

1. Bender L: Children and adolescents who have killed, Am J Psychiatry 116:510, 1959.
2. Heath AH, Gayton WF, and Hardesty VA: Childhood firesetting: a review of the literature, Can Psychiatr Assoc J 21:229, 1976.
3. Macht LB and Mack JE: The firesetter syndrome, Psychiatry 31:277, 1968.
4. Miller LC: Louisville behavior checklist for males 6-12 years of age, Psychol Rep 21:885, 1967.
5. Vandersall JA and Wiener JM: Children who set fires, Arch Gen Psychiatry 22:63, 1970.

SUGGESTED READINGS

Fineman KR: Firesetting in childhood and adolescence, Psychiatr Clin North Am 3:483, 1980.

Kaufman I, Henis LW, and Reiser DE: A re-evaluation of the psychodynamics of fire setting, Am J Orthopsychiatry 22:63, 1961.

Kolko DJ: Juvenile firesetting: a review and methodological critique, Clin Psychol Rev 5:345, 1985.

Yarnell H: Firesetting in children, Am J Orthopsychiatry 10:262, 1940.

84

Lying and Stealing

Gregory E. Prazar

Acts of lying and stealing by children often evoke strong emotional reactions from parents. Truthfulness and respect for property are two highly valued mores espoused by our society, even though adults frequently violate their own moral codes. Lying and stealing can represent a psychopathologic spectrum from a common transient developmental phenomenon to an ominous indication of severe psychiatric disturbance. Frequently both parents and professionals overreact to symptoms of lying and stealing before analyzing all the relevant information.

Prevalence figures for lying and stealing indicate that these behaviors occur more frequently in boys than in girls and achieve highest rates between 5 and 8 years of age. In one study by MacFarlane,[3] 49% of mothers of 5-year-old boys and 42% of mothers of 5-year-old girls reported lying by their children; stealing among 5-year-old boys was reported for 10% and for 4% of 5-year-old girls. By age 8, 41% of the boys and 19% of the girls exhibited some lying, whereas only 9% of the boys and 5% of the girls exhibited stealing behavior.

Given the prevalence of these behaviors, it is the responsibility of the primary care physician to inquire about symptoms of lying and stealing during regular routine visits and to help families understand and respond to these symptoms if they do occur. To identify and manage these problems adequately, it is necessary to obtain as complete a history as possible from parents and child, encompassing aspects of the home environment (patterns of child rearing, child's interaction with siblings and parents), peer relationships, and school performance.

LYING

When lying by children is presented as a problem to the physician, either directly by the parents or indirectly from questions asked by the physician during a regular visit, it is important that several aspects of the child's functioning be considered before definitive action is taken. Features of the child's life to be considered include the individual's maturational level; the influence of family, peers, and school; and, above all, the situation in which lying occurs.

The child's chronologic age and developmental level greatly influence the extent to which lying should be evaluated. Children under 3 years of age are beginning to establish independence from their parents. For these children, the differentiation between what Stone and Church[5] refer to as "private self and public self" is tenuous. Children at this age have no concept of deception and therefore do not intentionally lie. Their experimentation with concepts of language often is interpreted by adults as lying. The toddler, attempting to understand presence and absence of individuals, may tell the father that "Mommy is not here," when she may indeed be in the next room.[4] Emotionally painful situations are avoided by all children, especially by toddlers under 3 years of age. The child, whose moral code is immature, thinks nothing of denying a misdeed, because admission might bring painful consequences.

The mental life of the preschool child (3 to 7 years) is one filled with fantasy. According to Stone and Church,[5] 20% to 50% of this age group create imaginary companions, pets, or situations. The imaginary companion is usually a helpful, empathic playmate, although he or she may function as a disciplinarian for the child. By serving as a surrogate friend, the imaginary companion helps the child adapt to new social situations. By serving as a disciplinarian, the imaginary companion helps the child to develop a sense of right and wrong. The imaginary companion usually has a very short life span, generally dying of "old age" by the time the child is 5 to 7 years old. For the preschooler, fantasy and reality are frequently not well delineated, evidenced by the existence of imaginary companions and also by the child's love for fairy tales. A 4- to 5-year-old unabashedly tells tall tales, although he or she will, when encouraged, admit to creating a make-believe situation. By the age of 6 or 7 years, children are aware of the morality of lying and stealing. Although they are quick to accuse peers of cheating and lying, they often continue to cheat, seemingly guiltlessly, while playing.

Between the ages of 6 and 12 years, the child understands the concept of lying and its moral implications. However, lying may continue in an attempt to test adult-imposed moral codes. Children may admit to lying but have many rationalizations for their behavior. Rules are more important at this age than is winning, so cheating is less important and therefore more infrequent. "Half-beliefs" become a part of the child's life; children become believers of superstitions, from the dangers of walking under a ladder to stepping on sidewalk cracks. Half-beliefs may extend into adulthood, and they are heavily invested with emotion. Their level of acceptance by the individual is inversely proportional to the individual's level of intellectual development.

Aside from developmental issues, external influences (family, school, and peers) affect the incidence of lying in children. Parents may unconsciously encourage their children to lie if expectations for the children exceed their ability to fulfill them and if truthfulness is not valued by the parents (i.e., if parents frequently lie). Parents who overestimate their child's academic capabilities frequently find that their child lies about grades received. Parents who tell "white lies" to protect the feelings of others, or for personal gain, fail to realize that young children cannot discern the moral issues involved in lying. Parents demanding to know why their son hit his younger sister or why the child broke the cookie jar are not aware that the child often cannot explain these behaviors to himself, much less to them. When interrogated, the confused child, in desperation, lies. According to Ginott,[2] "awkward lies" are told to avoid "embarrassing confessions"—confessions that the child knows from experience parents do not want to hear. For example, after hitting his younger sister, the son knows that his parents do not want to hear that he hit her because he does not like her. The parents want to believe that their children love each other, and they find it difficult to accept verbalizations to the contrary.

The child who is inconsistently disciplined, receives little positive reinforcement from parents, and lives in an inflexible, demanding environment is often the child who lies. Physicians can help parents deal with childhood lying in several ways. First, by apprising parents of what behavior is normal during maturational stages, the physician helps the parents more easily understand why their 5-year-old makes up stories or why their 7-year-old cheats at games. Second, by helping parents become aware of their importance as role models for their child, the physician effectively guides the parents in telling their child the importance of truthfulness. Third, when specific problems arise, the physician, by using gentle and nonpunitive counseling, encourages parents to be as tactful and nonthreatening with the child as possible. For example, Spock believes that the child who spends much time with imaginary companions may need more age-appropriate friends or may be indirectly asking for more parental involvement in play activities.[4]

Children who cheat at games past age 7 (when rules become more important and therefore cheating becomes a form of breaking the rules) need guidance from parents. If the parent is playing with a child who is cheating, the behavior should be calmly identified. The parent should tell the child that everyone likes to win and that losing is difficult to accept. Cheating among children, when identified, should best be settled among the players, without parental "judicial" intervention. Academic cheating is a more serious problem, frequently signaling that unrealistic expectations for performance have been placed on the child. Parents should be counseled to explore with school personnel possible academic problems.

It is vital that parents are made cognizant of their importance as role models for their child and of the child's need for reasonable and clear expectations. Similarly, physicians must understand that they are role models for the parents whom they counsel. The physician who assumes a flexible, constructive, nonthreatening approach to problems raised by parents and who has been honest with the family in the past is more likely to experience success in counseling.

Lying becomes a symptom of more severe psychopathology under several circumstances. If other behaviors concomitantly exist (such as fire-setting, cruelty to animals, sleep disturbances, hyperactivity, phobias), there is a much greater likelihood of significant emotional disturbance. Similarly, if lying or fantasizing becomes a predominant behavior for children, more serious behavior disturbances must be suspected, such as chronically poor self-esteem, endogenous depression, and sociopathic behavior. Children with few friends and limited interest in group activities often suffer from low self-esteem and depression. Children who lie for material gain and, apparently, guiltlessly may be displaying early signs of sociopathic behavior. If these symptoms are present and if attempts at counseling fail to dissipate lying, referral to a psychiatrically oriented professional should be considered.

STEALING

Stealing often represents a much more worrisome symptom to parents than does lying because the former more often involves situations outside the home, represents a much more severe societal taboo, and affects other people more directly. Indeed, especially during school years, stealing can be an ominous sign of psychiatric disturbance. However, it may represent conformity to peer pressure and consequently a transient phenomenon. Children under 3 years of age take things because they want them and have an immature sense of "mine" and "not mine," a concept related to their beginning struggle for independence from parents. Slowly they develop a conception of their own bodies (or property) and those of their parents. By age 3, children have a firmer sense of what belongs to *them*. They become possessive of their things and jealous of those of others, although they have only a tenuous grasp of others' property rights.

Between 3 and 7 years of age, as they begin to develop peer relationships, children become more respectful of property rights. However, they frequently give away their possessions and have not developed a concept of one thing being more valuable than many things. Therefore, 25 hoarded pennies may be treasured much more than one piece of paper currency. The school-age child, though not yet completely mature, has a much more sophisticated sense of property rights. Consequently an 8-year-old may pick up loose change from the table while unsupervised. However, after about age 9, respect for property should be well integrated into the child. Children who steal at this age or beyond are motivated by one or more factors. They may steal in a group, especially during adolescence, to conform to peer pressure. They may suffer from poor self-esteem because they feel unloved by parents or because they have difficulty making friends. Therefore, they may steal to buy friendship, to achieve peer acceptance, or to display to themselves and their parents that they are worthwhile because they can succeed in at least one activity. Stealing as a mechanism to improve self-esteem is especially common with adolescents, who are concomitantly attempting to separate from parents and to establish satisfactory same-sex and heterosexual relationships. If adolescents feel they have failed in both tasks, they frequently steal.

Families exert an important influence with respect to childhood stealing. If parents stole as children, they are more likely to assume a permissive role to intrafamilial stealing. Their reactions to extrafamilial stealing, however, may be extremely punitive, since their child's stealing will unfavorably reflect on them as parents. This value discrepancy between intrafamilial and extrafamilial acts is easily recognized by the child, whose resentment frequently precipitates intensified stealing. Parents giving little attention, affection, or approval to their child will potentiate poor self-esteem, which may result in stealing as the child attempts to attract attention and approval. Punishment may be ineffective, since the child may rationalize that, as Fraiberg[1] states, "Any ensuing punishment will cancel the crime."

Management of stealing, as in management of lying, requires an empathic but firm approach by both physician and parents. Parents should be advised to deal with the specific incident forthrightly. The child over 3 years of age should be confronted with the evidence but should not suffer interrogative techniques (e.g., the parent should say, "I believe you took $5 from my wallet," rather than, "Why did you take $5 from my wallet?"). Immediate restitution of the stolen item is extremely important. If the article has been taken from a friend, the child should return it. If the article has been stolen from a store, the parent should accompany the child to the store and explain to the manager tactfully that the child took an item without paying for it and now wants to return it. The parents should voice their disapproval of stealing to the child, but should also reinforce their belief in the child's basic integrity. A child who has stolen usually has poor self-esteem; punitive measures serve to damage self-concept further and imbue in the child the parent's mistrust.

Several specific questions should come to mind when the child steals, because the answers may aid in management. Is the child receiving a reasonable allowance? If not, the child may feel the need to resort to stealing to obtain spending money. Are there unrealistic academic pressures on the child? As previously stated, children who feel they cannot fulfill academic expectations of parents frequently steal to display at least transiently their success in one activity. Is the child having difficulty making friends? Stealing often occurs in situations in which the child feels that peer group acceptance can be achieved by offering peers stolen material goods. In cases of group stealing, are alternative community facilities available to occupy extracurricular hours? Although structured community activities may not obliterate all acts of group stealing, they may help to discourage such acts by offering alternative activities to occupy adolescents' time.

Stealing assumes more ominous connotations in several situations. As in lying, if other behavioral disturbances coexist, a more psychiatrically sophisticated approach may be necessary. A child who steals without guilt, who compulsively steals (kleptomania), or who seemingly steals in a setting in which apprehension is inevitable may have serious emotional problems. Frequently these are children who received little or inconsistent love and security as infants. Without psychiatric intervention, they will progress to delinquent and ultimately criminal life-styles (see Chapter 103, "Juvenile Delinquency"). Unfortunately, psychic damage to these children is often severe by the time psychiatric referral is finally made.

REFERRAL CRITERIA

Effective referral to mental health specialists for problems of lying and stealing requires several things of referring physicians. The family should be informed of the possible need for referral when the physician first suspects a potential for significant psychopathology. As in managing less severe cases, it is vital that the referring physician be empathic and nonpunitive in the explanation given to parents. The physician should make sure that the parents do not think that their child is "crazy" because he or she is being referred. The parents should also know that the referral does not sever the physician's relationship with the family. Continued communication by the referring physician, both with the family and with the specialist, often solidifies recommendations made to parents by the therapist and encourages compliance with recommendations. It is beneficial if the physician can personally introduce the family to the therapist. In general, a team approach between the referring doctor and specialist increases the treatment plan's efficacy.

SUMMARY

Lying and stealing in childhood usually cause both parents and physicians concern and also create much worry for the involved child. The seriousness of these behaviors depends on many factors: the age of the child; circumstances that precipitate the behavior; psychosocial adjustment of the child in school, with peers, and at home; and the reaction of parents. The physician's approach to the problem greatly influences whether the behavior disappears or intensifies. In dealing with problems of lying and stealing, it is important for the physician to obtain a complete history, to explain carefully to the parents and the patient the significance of the behavior, and to ensure regular follow-up for the problem. If referral to psychologically trained professionals becomes necessary, the physician is obligated to prepare the family for the referral, to maintain communication with the consultant, and to offer the family emotional support before and after the consultation occurs. In most cases lying and stealing represent transient developmental behavioral problems that resolve if an empathic approach is used by parents and physician. However, the symptoms are not to be ignored in hopes that the child will "grow out of it" or because "all children lie and steal."

REFERENCES

1. Fraiberg S: The magic years, New York, 1968, Charles Scribner's Sons.
2. Ginott HG: Between parent and child, New York, 1965, Macmillan Publishing Co, Inc.
3. MacFarlane JW, Allen L, and Honzik MP: A developmental study of the behavior problems of normal children between twenty-one months and fourteen years, Berkeley and Los Angeles, 1954, University of California Press.
4. Spock B: Baby and child care, New York, 1985, Pocket Books.
5. Stone LJ and Church JC: Childhood and adolescence: a psychology of the growing person, ed 5, New York, 1984, Random House, Inc.

85

Mental Retardation

Thomas J. Kenny and Karen Byrne

The prevalence of mental retardation is such that all primary care physicians will be confronted by it. Retardation is defined as significantly subaverage general intellectual functioning that exists concurrently with deficits in adaptive behavior and manifests during the early, mid, and late developmental periods.[7] It is noteworthy that both subaverage general intellectual functioning and deficits in adaptive behavior must coexist in order to fulfill diagnostic criteria.

Subaverage intelligence has been defined as a score that is at least 2 standard deviations below the mean on a standardized intelligence test. This statistically based definition indicates that 2.5% of a given population will be classified as mentally retarded; in the United States, this definition encompasses about 5 million individuals. Actually, however, the number of individuals who are identified as mentally retarded at any given time is far lower.[3,15]

Adaptive behavior means the effectiveness or degree with which individuals meet the standard of personal independence and social responsibility expected of their age or cultural group. Thus, it is possible that a given individual could be considered mentally retarded in one setting (or one age group) but not at another age or in another environment—one that is, perhaps, less competitive or more relaxed, permissive, and accepting.[20] Such a circumstance is much more likely to occur with "educable" (or mildly) retarded persons, who account for 75% of the total population of those who are or may be retarded.

The American Association on Mental Retardation (AAMR) has defined four official levels of mental retardation (see Table 85-1). Mild retardation (encompassing those who are educable) is the most prevalent and is significantly more so among persons of lower socioeconomic status. In this group, the incidence of overt neurologic problems and multiple handicaps is not markedly elevated. In fact, no specific etiology is identified for 75% to 80% of those at this level. In contrast, the more pronounced types of retardation, although less common, are found equally across all socioeconomic groups. Generally, these more markedly handicapped individuals are more likely to be identified early, are more likely to have an identifiable etiology and diagnosis, and are more likely to be associated with other overt neurologic handicaps (e.g., seizures, cerebral palsy).[2,12-14]

In contrast to this categoric definition, the federal government has adopted a functional definition of developmental disability in PL-100-146, the Developmental Disabilities Bill of Rights and Assistance Act amendments of 1987. In short, the law defines seven areas of life function—thinking, economic self-sufficiency, communication, locomotion, capacity for independent living, self-care, and motivation; deficiencies in three or more of these functions caused by physical or verbal impairment that occurred before 22 years of age constitute a developmental disability. Studies have demonstrated that this definition tends to include only some of those persons who would fit the AAMR categoric definition. Since such definitions often dictate eligibility criteria for services, the disparity may create problems for some children in states in which the federal definition has been adopted.[3]

A number of causal factors have been linked with mental retardation. In most cases, particularly in the mildly retarded range, specific etiologic mechanisms are unknown. Risk of mental retardation is associated with a number of contributing social and physiologic factors that have been linked to developmental outcome. Within recent years children known to have one or more of these risk factors have been monitored in an effort toward early identification of delays. Various early intervention programs have been designed to stimulate these children and to offset or modify the effects of deleterious social and physiologic factors. These programs have demonstrated varying degrees of success and have not always had the broad and long-lasting effects that theorists predicted. In general, however, they appear to affect developmental outcome positively.[13,14]

Generally, it is not possible to confirm a diagnosis of mental retardation during the newborn period; Down syndrome (with an incidence of 1 in 800 births) and primary microcephaly are two exceptions. In most other clinical circumstances the diagnosis of retardation is first suspected because the child does not reach developmental milestones when expected rather than because of any specific positive findings. Since developmental differences in early childhood can be difficult to assess, the physician's responsibility in this regard can be burdensome.

Individuals with mild mental retardation are frequently not identified as such during the preschool years. The first real concern about their developmental status may be raised when they encounter academic problems.[10] After leaving school, many of these individuals are assimilated into society. They may obtain jobs, raise families, and be self-sufficient, at least to some degree. Mildly retarded individuals may demonstrate their handicaps most prominently in the academic area and may function quite well in nonacademic activities. Some observers have even charged that mildly retarded children are "manufactured by the school system."

Speech and language problems are characteristic of persons with mental retardation. In general, the greater the degree of retardation, the higher the incidence and the more

Table 85-1 *Official Levels of Mental Retardation and Some Developmental Characteristics**

LEVEL AND TITLE	IQ RANGE	ESTIMATED PERCENTAGE OF TOTAL RETARDED	ADAPTIVE AND DEVELOPMENTAL CHARACTERISTICS		
			PRESCHOOL AGE 0-5 (MATURATION AND DEVELOPMENT)	SCHOOL AGE 6-20 (TRAINING AND EDUCATION)	ADULT ≥ 21 (SOCIAL AND VOCATIONAL ADEQUACY)
1. Profound	<20	5 (Profound and Severe)	Gross retardation; minimum capacity for functioning in sensorimotor areas; may need nursing care	Some motor development present; may respond to minimum or limited training in self-help	Some motor and speech development; may achieve very limited self-care; may need nursing care
2. Severe	20-35		Poor motor development; speech is minimal; able to profit from training in self-help; little or no expressive skills	Can talk or learn to communicate; can be trained in elemental health habits; profits from systematic habit training	May contribute partially to self-maintenance under complete supervision; can develop self-protection skills to a minimum useful level in controlled environment
3. Moderate	36-51	20	Can talk or learn to communicate; poor social awareness; fair motor development; profits from training in self-help; can be managed with moderate supervision	Can profit from training in social and occupational skills; unlikely to progress beyond second-grade level in academic subjects; may learn to travel alone in familiar places	May achieve self-maintenance in unskilled or semiskilled work under sheltered conditions; needs supervision and guidance when under mild social or economic stress
4. Mild	52-68	75	Can develop social and communication skills; minimal retardation in sensorimotor areas; often not distinguished from normal until later age	Can learn academic skills up to approximately sixth-grade level by late teens; can be guided toward social conformity; "educable"	Can usually achieve social and vocational skills adequate to minimum self-support but may need guidance and assistance when under unusual social or economic stress

*Definition of mental retardation: "Significantly subaverage general intellectual functioning existing concurrently with deficits in adaptive behavior and manifest during the developmental period."

marked the degree of speech problems. It is estimated that about 50% of mildly retarded persons and over 95% of severely retarded persons have speech problems. About 50% of profoundly retarded persons are nonverbal.

PHYSICIAN'S ROLE

The primary care physician has a four-part role in the care of the person with mental retardation: (1) identification and diagnosis; (2) provision of comprehensive health care; (3) counseling; and (4) continuity of care, case management, and advocacy.

The most effective way to identify children at risk for mental retardation is to assess developmental status at each health care visit. This assessment should include a history of motor, language, and social development. A screening tool that measures cognitive and behavioral development can also be useful. One standard tool for such screening is the Denver Developmental Screening Test presented in Chapter 18. Repeated studies have demonstrated that this instrument is highly effective and easily administered. Another option is to use the combined vision/developmental screening procedure developed by Sturner,[19] which is both brief and valid.

After identification, the physician's role in health care remains important. Although there is no specific medical treatment for most types of mental retardation, children who are mentally retarded are at increased risk for many medical problems. For example, the child with Down syndrome is at risk for congenital heart disease, thyroid dysfunction, visual problems, obesity, and leukemia. As a group, mentally retarded persons have a higher incidence of delayed speech development, decreased visual acuity, and seizures. It is vital, therefore, that the physician provide comprehensive health care to the affected youngster or see that it is provided.

The third role of the physician involves counseling parents of the child with mental retardation. First, there is a need for simple, clear, effective communication with the parents about their child and issues of mental retardation (see Chapter 89, "Physical Disability"). One of those issues that will surface eventually is that of sexual development and related behavior, often a difficult area for parents to face. Specific issues, such as the management of menstruation, or the general problems of adolescence itself can be difficult to deal with in retarded persons. Similarly, retarded persons will encounter sexual drives; their more limited social heterosexual contacts, however, provide fewer reasonable outlets for these feelings.

The parent or professional with concerns in these areas should contact local agencies, including the local Association for Retarded Persons, where there is likely to be a spectrum of help available. Possibilities include educational programs and appropriate literature. Two very useful books for parents or professionals are Kempton's *A Teacher's Guide to Sex Education for Persons with Learning Disabilities*[11] and Monat's *Sexuality and the Mentally Retarded*.[16]

The fourth role for the physician is that of case manager or advocate. The physician should thus be ready to refer the child for appropriate evaluations (including psychological evaluation) to establish basic data about the child's developmental status, especially in the areas of cognition and social skills. The results of this evaluation should help the physician and parents plan for the child's needs; thus, the child should be evaluated as early as possible. A reasonably accurate assessment can usually be conducted at about 2 years of age, and a comprehensive evaluation should certainly be performed before the child starts school.

The primary care physician's role in care coordination has dramatically increased with the increasing number of mentally retarded children who no longer live in institutions and remain with their families until adulthood. Health care for children with mental retardation often doesn't exceed the level of care necessary for children without disabilities. But mentally retarded children require coordination of allied health, educational, and family support services, which the physician may be in a unique position to provide.[8]

Other evaluations that may be necessary include those for speech and language development, and audiometric evaluation may also be called for. In addition, ophthalmologic and neurologic consultations are frequently indicated.

BEHAVIORAL PROBLEMS

As a group, mentally retarded persons have a greater incidence of behavioral problems than do those in the general population. Foale[6] found the incidence of psychoneurosis in retarded persons to be double that of the general population. Pervasive emotional problems such as psychosis and autism are also more frequent among retarded children.[9,18]

The more severely retarded person often has poor communication abilities and frequently has increased motor activity (i.e., is hyperactive). Mentally retarded persons also tend to have short attention spans and problems focusing their attention. Their behavior tends to be impulsive, repetitive, or stereotypic, and they are at increased risk of engaging in self-stimulatory or self-injurious behaviors.

Mildly retarded children have many of the characteristics of children with an attention deficit disorder. They are usually overactive, have a poor attention span, and are impulsive; they also tend to be aggressive and to "act out their frustrations." Management of these problems is similar to that with nonretarded children. Medications such as methylphenidate hydrochloride (Ritalin) or dextroamphetamine sulfate (Dexedrine) can be useful if used judiciously and carefully monitored, and behavior management techniques have been demonstrated to be effective. There are a number of books that can be used by parents to develop behavior management programs, including *Parents Are Teachers* by Wesley Becker[1] and Gerald Patterson's book, *Families: Application of Social Learning to Family Life*.[17]

Cromwell[4] sees the behavior of retarded persons as a consequence of the frustration related to the many failures they experience. He proposes that this causes the retarded person to (1) perform in a new situation below the level of his or her constitutional ability; (2) be less likely to be moved by failure; and (3) be less likely to try harder after a mild failure—that is, to give up more easily. Cromwell thus describes the retarded child as a "failure-avoider" as opposed to a "success-striver."

MANAGEMENT

Current trends in the management of mentally retarded persons will require increased services from the primary care physician. Improved medical care has extended the life span of the mentally retarded person, which has resulted in a greater need for ongoing health maintenance by the physician as well as for expanded efforts in case management, especially in the psychosocial area.

The current emphasis on "deinstitutionalization" and normalization of living experiences requires a comprehensive and sustained social support system. Increased attention must be devoted to vocational preparation and the development of occupational opportunities. The deinstitutionalization effort necessitates helping the family and the mentally retarded person prepare for alternate living arrangements. More mentally retarded persons are moving into the community in group homes and apartments, which requires a support system that meets their physical, social, and occupational needs.[5] Available data[2,6,12] on the effectiveness of such programs are conflicting but suggest that much remains to be done to facilitate the optimum adjustment of mentally retarded persons and to match settings to individual needs. The physician can help the family and the child prepare for entry into this system of independent living and working.

REFERENCES

1. Becker WC: Parents are teachers: a child management program, Champaign, Ill, 1971, Research Press.
2. Birenbaum A and Re M: Resettling mentally retarded adults in the community—almost 4 years later, Am J Ment Defic 31:323, 1979.
3. Boggs E and Henney RL: A numerical and functional description of the developmental disabilities population (printed booklet), Philadelphia, 1979, EMC Institute.
4. Cromwell RL: Personality evaluation. In Baumeister A, editor: Mental retardation: appraisal, education, and rehabilitation, Chicago, 1967, Aldine.
5. Eyman RK and Arndt S: Life-span development of institutionalized and community based mentally retarded residents, Am J Ment Defic 86:342, 1982.
6. Foale M: The special difficulty of high grade mental defective adolescents, Am J Ment Defic 60:867, 1956.
7. Grossman HJ: Classification in mental retardation, Washington, DC, 1983, The American Association on Mental Deficiency.
8. Guralnick MJ and Bennett FC: The effectiveness of early intervention for at-risk and handicapped children, Orlando, Fla, 1987, Academic Press, Inc.
9. Jacobson J: Problem behavior and psychiatric impairment within a developmentally disabled population. I. Behavior frequency, Appl Res Ment Retard 3:121, 1982.
10. Kappelman M, Kenny T, and Clemmens R: Mild mental retardation: clinical characteristics in early and late identification, Md Med J 23:83, 1974.
11. Kempton W: A teacher's guide to sex education for persons with learning disabilities, North Scituate, Mass, 1975, Duxburg Press.
12. Landesman-Dwyer S: Living in the community, Am J Ment Defic 86:223, 1981.
13. Lazar I and Darlington RB: Lasting effects of early education, Monogr Soc Res Child Dev 47:1, 1982.
14. McKey RH et al: Impact of Head Start on children, families, and communities, Pub No (OHDS) 85-31193, Washington, DC, 1985, Department of Health and Human Services.
15. Mercer J: The myth of 3% prevalence. In Tarjan G, Eyman RK, and Meyers CE, editors: Sociobehavioral studies in mental retardation, Monograph No 1, Washington, DC, 1973, The American Association on Mental Deficiency.
16. Monat RK: Sexuality and the mentally retarded, San Diego, Calif, 1982, College-Hill Press.
17. Patterson GR: Families: application of social learning to family life, Champaign, Ill, 1975, Research Press.
18. Reiss S: Psychopathology and mental retardation: survey of a developmental disabilities mental health program, Ment Retard 20:128, 1982.
19. Sturner RA et al: Simultaneous screening for child health and development: a study of visual/developmental screening of preschool children, Pediatrics 65:614, 1980.
20. Tredgold RF: Mental retardation, ed 12, Baltimore, 1977, Williams & Wilkins Co.

SUGGESTED READINGS

Clarke ADB and Clarke AM: Research on mental handicap, 1957-1987: a selected review, J Ment Def Res 31:317, 1987.

Hill BK, Lakin KC, and Bruininks RH: Trends in residential services for mentally retarded people, 1977-1982, Journal of the Association for Persons with Severe Handicaps 9:243, 1984.

86

Nightmares and Other Sleep Disturbances

Thomas F. Anders

Problems associated with sleep affect almost all children during the course of development. Such problems span the gamut from an occasional awakening following a frightening nightmare to severe and intractable insomnia. Within the spectrum are included such disturbances as fear of the dark, difficulty in falling asleep, night waking, sleepwalking, sleeptalking, and night terrors. Some persist into adulthood. Although we spend approximately one third of our lives asleep, it is surprising how scant are the hard data on sleep disorders in childhood. Only since the 1950s, with the introduction of polygraphic recording techniques, have we been able to investigate physiologic and behavioral activities during sleep. Actual incidence figures and diagnostic criteria for sleep disorders and sleep disturbances are only now being delineated.

As a general introduction to sleep state physiology and sleep cycles, a brief review is warranted. The initial observations of "active," rapid eye movement (REM) sleep states and "quiet," nonrapid eye movement (NREM) sleep states were made in 1924 by two Czech scientists, Denisova and Figurin. Unfortunately, their publication in Russian and the lack of supportive polygraphic evidence precluded widespread recognition of their findings. Since the introduction of polygraphic techniques for studying sleep, it is well established that sleep is not a unitary state of physiologic restitution but rather two cycling states of differing physiologic function and activity.

A description of the adult sleep cycle provides an introduction to an understanding of developing sleep patterns in the infant and young child. Four states of electroencephalographic (EEG) activity during adult sleep have been described by Dement and Kleitman[3]: stage I is typified by low-voltage, fast activity; stage II, by the presence of sleep spindles* and K complexes† against a low-voltage background; and stages III and IV, by varying degrees of slow, high-voltage, delta-wave activity.‡

*Sleep spindles are defined as EEG activity of 12 to 14 Hz, of at least 0.5 second's duration, occurring in runs of greater than 6.

†K complexes are defined as EEG wave forms having a well-delineated negative sharp wave, which is immediately followed by a positive component. The total duration of the complex should exceed 0.5 second. The K complex is generally maximal over vertex regions.

‡Delta-wave activity is defined as waves of 2 cycles per second or slower, which have amplitudes greater than 75 μV from peak to peak.

REM sleep is defined by the occurrence of a stage I EEG pattern in association with binocularly synchronous rapid eye movements, the suppression of muscle tone as recorded from the chin electromyogram (EMG), and accelerated, irregular respiratory and heart rates. NREM sleep lacks REMs and is accompanied by the presence of tonic muscle activity recorded from the chin EMG, a stage II, III, or IV EEG pattern, and slowed, regular cardiac and respiratory rates. Alternating REM and NREM sleep states represent two distinct patterns of neurophysiologic organizations: the REM state is highly activated; the NREM state is basal and highly regulated. They follow each other in a periodic fashion, and together they make up the sleep cycle.

Whereas active REM sleep periods of infants are qualitatively similar to REM periods of adults, three important quantitative differences have been described: whereas adults spend 20% of a night's sleep in active REM sleep, sleeping full-term neonates, recorded for a 4-hour interfeeding sleep period or for an entire 24-hour period, spend 50% of their total sleep in this state. The proportionate amount of time spent in active REM sleep diminishes as the infant becomes older and as central nervous system (CNS) maturation progresses. Second, infants frequently enter sleep through an initial active REM period, in contrast to adults, who enter their first REM period 90 minutes after the onset of sleep. And third, active REM periods emerge more frequently in infants than REM periods in adults, so that the infant's sleep cycle is shorter than the adult's. Active REM periods recur every 50 to 60 minutes during infancy in contrast to every 90 to 100 minutes as reported in adults. The staging of quiet NREM sleep by EEG criteria into four distinct NREM sleep stages becomes possible only after the second 6 months of life.[1] The differences between sleep patterns in infants and adults are outlined in Table 86-1.

PATHOLOGIC SLEEP PATTERNS

A sleep disorders clinic, using modern techniques of polysomnography to record multiple physiologic parameters during a night of sleep, is rapidly becoming an important entity in the diagnostic assessment of sleep disturbances.

For ease of description, clinical sleep disturbances may be divided into five major categories: those in which sleep is

Table 86-1 *Comparison Between Infant and Adult Sleep Patterns*

PARAMETER	INFANT	ADULT
Ratio of REM to NREM	50 : 50	20 : 80
Periodicity of sleep states	50- to 60-min REM-NREM cycle	90- to 100-min REM-NREM cycle
Sleep onset state	REM sleep onset	NREM sleep onset
Temporal organization of sleep states	REM-NREM cycles equally throughout sleep period	NREM stages III and IV predominant in first third of night; REM state predominant in last third of night
Maturation of EEG patterns	Low-voltage, fast EEG pattern High-voltage, slow EEG pattern 1 NREM EEG stage	K complexes Delta-waves 4 NREM EEG stages
Concordance of sleep measures (organization of sleep states)	Poor	Good

shortened (the insomnias); those in which sleep is disturbed by episodic events (the parasomnias: sleepwalking, night terrors); those in which sleep is affected secondarily by illness; those in which the rhythmic organization of sleep is disrupted (phase disturbances); and finally, those in which sleep during the 24 hours is lengthened (the hypersomnias).

In this presentation, the focus is on parasomnias—the sleep disorders characterized by episodic events that interrupt sleep. The insomnias and the hypersomnias, including narcolepsy and the sleep apnea syndrome, are extensively reviewed elsewhere.[5]

An idealized version of a night's sleep is portrayed in Fig. 86-1, which serves as a useful guide for locating the parasomnias and sleep disturbances that are described below.

NREM Parasomnias

The NREM parasomnias include pavor nocturnus (night terrors), somnambulism (sleepwalking), somniloquy (sleeptalking), and possibly, stage IV sleep-related enuresis. The REM parasomnias include nightmares and REM behavior disorder. In the years before "sleep laboratory diagnosis," many children suffering from these disorders were referred to a child psychiatrist. Current evidence suggests, however, that these disorders reflect CNS immaturity or abnormality. The NREM parasomnias have certain features in common: several of the disorders may occur in the same person; there is often a positive family history of the disorders; they are paroxysmal in nature and are characterized by nonresponsiveness to the environment, automatic appearance to actions, and retrograde amnesia for the episode the following morning; and finally, they usually appear at a particular point in the sleep cycle, as indicated in Fig. 86-1.

Most younger children "outgrow" the symptoms of NREM parasomnias as neurophysiologic maturation proceeds. In adolescents and adults, however, when these disturbances persist, secondary psychological conflicts frequently complicate the clinical picture. Although specific medications are available for disabling symptomatology, reassuring support to the family and child, blended with an optimistic and patient attitude, generally suffices. Medications should be prescribed only when the symptoms are so severe that they affect waking behavior, particularly school performance, peer interaction, and family relationships. Parasomnias can most often be diagnosed from a careful history. In rare cases temporal lobe seizures may mimic these disorders, but adequate study in a sleep laboratory readily differentiates epileptic disorders from a sleep disorder. Children with unusual presentations of symptomatology (daytime attacks or attacks between 1:00 AM and 6:00 AM when stage IV NREM sleep is absent) should be referred to a sleep disorders center.

Pavor Nocturnus. Pavor nocturnus, or night terrors, is found with greatest frequency in children 3 to 8 years of age. In some infants, however, symptoms may begin during the second half of the first year of life. And a small number of children will continue to have severe night terror attacks into adulthood.

Night terrors must be differentiated from the more common nightmare or anxiety dream. Nightmares are associated with vivid visual imagery. They occur during REM sleep, and the child is fully aroused following the episode. Recall for the content of the nightmare is excellent. In pavor nocturnus, approximately 90 to 100 minutes after going to sleep, the child suddenly sits upright in bed and screams. Tachypnea, tachycardia, and other signs of autonomic activation are apparent. The child is usually inconsolable for 5 to 30 minutes, then finally relaxes and returns to sleep. If the child arouses, dream recall is fragmentary. Retrograde amnesia for the attack is present the following morning. Attacks frequently occur after stressful or especially fatiguing daytime activities. The diagnosis can be made most often from the history alone. An attack occurring during the latter third of the night with vivid recall is unlikely to be pavor nocturnus (see Fig. 86-1) but rather a nightmare or a spontaneous awakening. Most night terror episodes in young children occur so infrequently that medication is not indicated. For severe cases, however, the drug of choice is diazepam (Valium).

Somnambulism and Somniloquy. Somnambulism and somniloquy present more commonly during the school-age years. According to Kales and colleagues,[6] 15% of all children between the ages of 5 and 12 have walked in their sleep at least once. Persistent sleepwalking occurs in 1% to 6% of the population, afflicting more males than females, and is often associated with nocturnal enuresis. A typical somnambulistic episode consists of the following behavioral sequence: a body movement during stage IV NREM sleep is followed by the subject abruptly sitting upright in bed. Although the eyes are open, they appear glassy and "unseeing." Movements are clumsy, and efforts to communicate with the sleepwalker

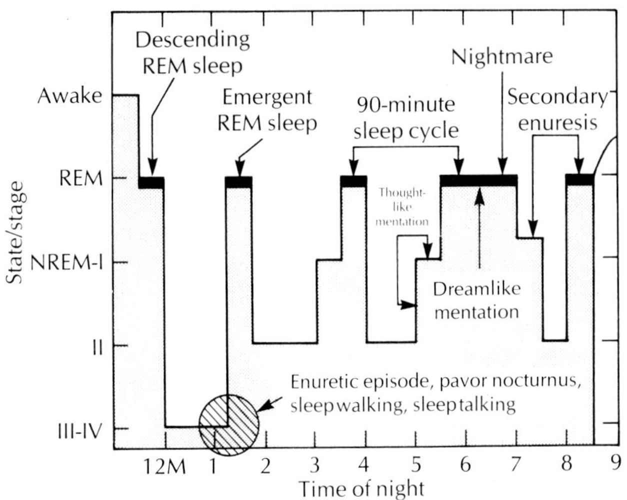

Fig. 86-1 An idealized all-night sleep state histogram. The various disorders and disturbances of sleep are depicted at their usual point of occurrence.

usually elicit mumbled and slurred speech with monosyllabic answers. The total duration of the episode may range from 10 to 30 seconds when sitting in bed to 5 to 30 minutes or more when actually walking. The event is not remembered on awakening in the morning. Severe sleepwalkers may have one to four episodes weekly. The episode occurs most often at the transition point from stage IV NREM sleep to the first REM period. If individuals with a predilection for somnambulism or somniloquy are aroused during stage IV NREM sleep, a walking or talking episode may be precipitated. In contrast, no such response is obtained from unaffected controls.

Several myths about sleepwalking and sleeptalking need to be laid to rest. Sleepwalkers are not acting out dreams and are not in control of purposeful actions. Rather, sleepwalkers are in danger. They frequently hurt themselves and must be protected from self-injury by a secure environment. Likewise, somniloquists do not reveal their deepest secrets while sleep talking. Their utterances are most often incomprehensible or monosyllabic. Meaningful speech and purposeful walking during sleep suggest psychological dissociative disorders rather than physiologic NREM parasomnia symptomatology. Again, as in night terrors, temporal lobe epilepsy must be ruled out. This is so particularly in adults.

As CNS maturation progresses, somnambulistic episodes usually diminish and disappear spontaneously. For severe, intractable cases, diazepam has been used successfully.

Mixed Parasomnias

Sleep-Related Enuresis. Enuresis should not be considered a syndrome, but rather a symptom of a disorder. By careful history, one should determine whether the enuretic symptom has been present from birth (primary) or has occurred after a period of successful training (secondary), whether it is confined to nighttime or occurs during the daytime as well, and whether organic factors are present. In addition, an attempt should be made to localize the episode to a time of night and point in the sleep cycle. Sleep-related enuresis is usually primary and occurs only at night, often during the first third of the sleep period at the transition point from stage IV NREM sleep to REM sleep. Enuretic episodes may occur at any point during the night, however.

Sleep-related enuresis is probably the most common parasomnia of childhood. Broughton[2] has defined an enuretic episode as one that generally occurs 1 to 3 hours after sleep onset as the child shifts from stage IV NREM sleep to the first REM period. The sleep state change is often associated with a body movement and increased muscle tone, followed by tachycardia, tachypnea, erection (in males), and decreased skin resistance. Micturition occurs 30 seconds to 4 minutes after the start of the episode in a moment of relative quiet. Immediately following micturition, children are difficult to awaken and, when aroused, indicate that they have not dreamed. They also do not remember the event. Broughton has demonstrated that enuretics with this disorder have higher resting intravesical pressures, especially during stage IV NREM sleep, have more frequent and spontaneous bladder contractions during stage IV NREM sleep, and have secondary contractions in response to naturally and artificially occurring increases in pressure in contrast to nonenuretic controls, whose bladder functions and capacities are normal.[2] On the other hand, Mikkelsen and Rapoport[8] report that enuresis is not limited to stage IV NREM sleep.

For children with severe sleep-related enuresis, imipramine (Tofranil) has proved to be effective. It is unclear whether it is efficacious primarily because of its anticholinergic properties affecting bladder tone or because of its stimulant effect on the sleep stage pattern. A flexible dosage and slow withdrawal schedule are recommended. Conditioning methods are also effective and recommended as a first choice. (See Chapter 81, "Enuresis," for a more complete discussion of this subject.)

REM Parasomnias

REM Sleep Behavior Disorder. REM sleep behavior disorder (RSBD) is a rare parasomnia characterized by vigorous and sometimes violent self-directed or other-directed motor attacks that interrupt REM sleep. Typically, peripheral muscle tone is inhibited during REM sleep, thus causing sleep "paralysis." In RSBD, however, the tonic inhibition is episodically interrupted leading to motor outbursts. CNS anomalies or lesions are associated with this disorder in both children and adults.[7]

Psychological and Developmental Disturbances of Sleep

The disorders described in this section are characterized by normal polysomnography. Nevertheless, they may be a source of psychological suffering for the child and conflict within the family. Virtually all parents anticipate sleep disturbances in their children. These sleep disturbances are much more common than those described previously. They often reflect normal phases of development and have been loosely labeled as "insomnias" and "nightmares." The majority are transient, and although a source of irritation and concern, are inconsequential. Sometimes, when overwhelming or persistent, they may indicate a more serious psychopathologic condition. Medication, by and large, is not indicated, although the short-term use of chloral hydrate has been advocated to promote peace and quiet in the family and prevent the sleep disturbance from becoming ingrained by "positive" reinforcement. Understanding the source of a child's anxiety, the parental concerns, and the current family situation is most often sufficient to enable the pediatrician to provide supportive guidance until the disturbance subsides.

These sleep disturbances may occur anytime from the imminent approach of bedtime to awakening. Ferber[4] has reviewed these disturbances extensively. They can be classified according to their most common age of appearance. This system of classification affords optimum understanding of the disturbance within the context of the child's developmental stage.

First Year of Life. During the first year of life, sleeping through the night ("settling") and night awakenings are the primary concerns of the family. In England, a comprehensive investigation of sleep patterns of infants during the first year of life reported that 70% of babies slept through the night, or settled, by 3 months of age. Another 13% had settled by 6 months of age, and 10% never slept through the night without interruption. Once settling occurred, night waking recurred in 50% of the infants during the second half of the first year of life.[5] Environmental factors, such as changed sleeping arrangements, separations, minor trauma, and new family members, were reported to be associated with night waking after settling had occurred, although these factors did not seem to affect the age of initial settling.

Second Year of Life. The problems of separation and object permanence confront the immature ego of the 2-year-old child. Lacking the capacity to differentiate between absence and total disappearance of an object, the child attempts to hold on to important ties to avoid the fear of loss. A prevalent disturbance of this age, therefore, is reluctance to go to sleep. Substitute objects, such as teddy bears or blankets, often tide the child over difficult separations. By the end of the second year, with the acquisitions of language and the development of a sense of object permanence, these difficulties often disappear.

Since children of this age are also easily overexcited and frightened by daytime experiences, nightmares also make their appearance in this age group. Nightmares, also called "bad dreams" and "anxiety dreams," occur during REM sleep. Most often, the dream reports represent reenactments of daytime experiences, although the characters are frequently animals or monsters. Since the child at this age has difficulty distinguishing between dreams and reality, fear of going to sleep may be a prominent feature of children with nightmares.

Third to Fifth Years of Life. It is rare to find a child in the age group of 3 to 5 years who is not experiencing some difficulty over sleep, whether it be a tardiness in falling asleep, nightmares, projective fears of ghosts and wild animals, fear of the dark, inability to sleep alone, or ritualistic presleep behaviors. These disturbances are usually associated with daytime frightening or otherwise conflictual experiences. They are most often transient and responsive to minimal environmental manipulation. If refractive, on the other hand, sleep disturbances may represent one symptom of a more profound psychological conflict. In such cases, they usually reflect the child's inability to enter into the widening world of social relationships. Family counseling or individual psychotherapy may be indicated.

USE OF THE SLEEP LABORATORY IN DIFFERENTIAL DIAGNOSIS

More and more, polysomnography in sleep disorder clinics has been useful in diagnosing sleep-related pathologic conditions. The following case report is exemplary:

> Richard, a 7-year-old boy, was referred because of night wakening occurring several times a night, four to five times a week. These attacks started approximately 1 hour after falling asleep and were associated with disorientation, confusion, and screaming. The boy did not remember the event in the morning. Frequently, second and third attacks occurred later in the night. Sometimes these attacks were associated with sleepwalking episodes. Complete physical and neurologic examinations, including two waking EEGs, were unremarkable. A variety of medications, including phenytoin (Dilantin), diazepam, flurazepam (Dalmane), imipramine, and barbiturates, were successful for short periods of time, but then symptomatology worsened once again.
>
> The sleep disorders clinic workup revealed a complex disturbance. Continuous all-night polysomnography and time-lapse video monitoring were carried out. Approximately 65 minutes after the onset of sleep, during the midst of stage IV NREM sleep, Richard sat up glassy-eyed and began screaming. He appeared in obvious distress and was inconsolable. After about 5 minutes, he lay back in his bed and returned to sleep. At 3:30 AM, some 6½ hours after he fell asleep, Richard again aroused and began to cry out. This arousal was from stage I NREM sleep. The arousal was followed by movement and was characterized by a waking EEG pattern. For the next 10 minutes, Richard remained awake with his eyes closed, sobbing and crying out. Finally he returned to sleep, covered by a sheet and curled up in a fetal position. Approximately 1 hour later, another attack resembling the latter occurred. The character of the first attack was markedly different from the two later attacks. In the first attack, Richard seemed disoriented and confused, whereas in the later ones, he awakened and appeared depressed and anxious. Thus, it was apparent from our video monitoring and our polysomnographic recording that we were dealing with two distinct types of sleep disturbances—night terror attacks and night waking episodes. While the various medications had been effective in suppressing the night terror attacks, secondary sleep disturbances repeatedly broke through.

We recommended that, since Richard's anxiety was excessive and inhibiting, family counseling and psychotherapy be instituted. We felt that the secondary sleep disturbance was more important than the night terror attacks and suggested, therefore, that medications be withheld. Six months after evaluation, the family situation had improved and the nighttime disturbances had significantly diminished without medication.

REFERENCES

1. Anders T, Carskadon M, and Dement W: Sleep and sleepiness in children and adolescents, Pediatr Clin North Am 27:29, 1980.
2. Broughton R: Sleep disorders: disorders of arousal? Science 159:1070, 1968.
3. Dement W and Kleitman N: Cyclic variations in EEG during sleep and their relation to eye movements, body motility and dreaming, Electroenceph Clin Neurophysiol 9:673, 1957.
4. Ferber R: Solve your child's sleep problems, New York, 1985, Simon & Schuster, Inc.
5. Guilleminault C: Narcolepsy and its differential diagnosis. In Guilleminault C, editor: Sleep and its disorders in children, New York, 1987, Raven Press.
6. Kales J, Soldatos C, and Kales A: Childhood sleep disorders. In Gellis S and Kagan B, editors: Current pediatric therapy, ed 9, Philadelphia, 1980, WB Saunders Co.
7. Mahowald MW and Rosen GM: Parasomnias in children, Pediatrician 17:21-31, 1990.
8. Mikkelsen E and Rapoport J: Enuresis: psychopathology, sleep stage and drug response, Urol Clin North Am 7:361, 1980.
9. Moore T and Ucko LE: Night waking in early infancy. I, Arch Dis Child 32:333, 1957.

87

Peer Relationship Problems

Sharon L. Foster, David D. DeLawyer, and Heidi Inderbitzen-Pisaruk

Peer relations and positive social interaction are crucial to the normal development of children. A child's relations with peers serve important functions in his or her life, including promoting the development of social skills through interaction and feedback, providing emotional support and security, and sharing information relevant to common situations and events during childhood and adolescence. The importance of peer relations is highlighted by the finding that by the sixth grade, children spend twice as much time with their peers as with their parents.

EPIDEMIOLOGY

A lack of friends is the major identifying characteristic of children with peer relationship problems. This can be manifested in three ways: social withdrawal, social neglect, and peer rejection. Socially withdrawn children interact infrequently. Socially neglected children are those who are ignored by peers and are neither liked nor disliked. Socially rejected children are openly and actively rejected by peers.

Reports of the incidence of peer relationship problems suggest that as many as 6% to 11% of children have no friends in their classrooms, and an additional 12% to 22% have only one classroom friend.[8,9] There is some evidence that rejection is relatively stable, with one investigation[2] finding that about 67% of rejected children assessed in elementary school still had peer problems 5 years later. Neglected children's status was less stable, with only 25% still manifesting peer relationship difficulties over the same interval. Reports[9] indicate that between 40% and 60% of children with few or no friends are socially withdrawn or neglected, whereas the remainder are rejected by peers. Males and females appear to be equally represented in terms of peer relationship problems.

In addition, some evidence indicates that children with poor peer relations (particularly peer rejection) are more likely to encounter adjustment problems later in life, including hyperactivity, conduct disorders, school maladjustment, juvenile delinquency, and dropping out of school in childhood and adolescence, as well as mental health problems, bad conduct discharges from military service, and suicide in adulthood. On the other hand, positive peer relations have been associated with academic achievement and better interpersonal adjustment in later life.[12,16] Unfortunately, causal relationships between early peer problems and later difficulties have not been established. Furthermore, whether withdrawn and neglected children experience serious concurrent or future difficulties is not well-documented and continues to provoke controversy. Nonetheless, the substantial number of associations noted above strongly suggests that intervening early with children who have poor peer relationships may alleviate current dysfunction and prevent dysfunction later in life.

ETIOLOGIC FACTORS

Understanding the etiology of peer relationship problems is complicated by findings that children may lack friends for a variety of reasons. Characteristics of the child, including physical attractiveness, race, sex, and academic competence, may affect his or her social status with peers. The major hypothesis with respect to why children have difficulties in peer relationships, however, is that children with problems possess inadequate repertoires of social skills, which results in ineffective social interaction, causing them to be ignored or actively rejected by their peers.[12] This negative experience may further encourage maladaptive responses such as increased social withdrawal or retaliatory verbal or physical aggression. These behaviors could in turn create a vicious circle by making children even less accepted by their peers.

Various theories of the development of socially skillful behavior have some empirical support but none has unequivocal acceptance. Behavioral theories of etiology speculate that inadequate opportunities or reinforcement for appropriate social behavior results in deficient or inappropriate social behaviors.[4] Others[5] hypothesize that poor social skills result from inadequate development of information-processing skills believed to be prerequisites for effective social intervention. These include perceiving and interpreting social situations correctly; evaluating possible ways of responding; selecting and performing an appropriate response; and monitoring the impact of that response. Related hypotheses emphasize the role of social role-taking (the ability to view situations from others' perspectives) and empathy (actually experiencing another's feelings) in adaptive peer relationships.

Other research[11,14] with preschool and first-grade children highlights the relationship between family experience and children's social competence. Children who are poorly accepted, when compared with peers who are better accepted, interact with their mothers in more negative and demanding ways. Their mothers are less positive and more negative, focus less on feelings, and participate less in play during these interactions.[12,15] Fathers of unpopular children issue more commands and engage less in their child's play.[11] Additionally, mothers of poorly accepted children supervise their children more intrusively than mothers of better accepted children.[10] Finally, deviant maternal values and expectations (e.g., positive endorsement of aggression as a solution to interpersonal problems) are associated both with how children think about social problems and with peers' and teachers' views of children's social competence in the classroom.[13] Together, these findings suggest that early social experiences may play an important role in children's development of social competence. The actual mechanisms by which these early experiences become transformed into extrafamilial social behavior, however, are not yet clearly understood.

CHARACTERISTICS AND DIAGNOSIS

Observations of socially withdrawn and neglected children reveal similar behavioral characteristics. Rejected children display a different constellation of behavior, particularly during preschool and early elementary school years (see the article by Foster and colleagues[6] for a review). Children who spend little time interacting with peers at school also do not initiate interactions with peers and fail to respond to others' initiations. They tend to be less verbal than their classmates. Furthermore, they spend more time in solitary activities and play submissive or deferent roles when they do interact with more sociable partners.[17] Some of these children may experience more anxiety, low self-esteem, and depression than peers,[18] although for what percentage these reactions are outside the normal range is not yet clear.

In contrast, peer rejection in preschool and the primary grades has been associated with more actively negative behavior—higher rates of "off-task" behavior as well as solitary activity, greater dependence on adults, negative statements, interference with ongoing activities, aggression, and failure to conform to classroom rules. Poorly accepted children have difficulty joining ongoing play activities and are more likely than their peers to disengage from the group, to make weak demands, to engage in incoherent behavior (i.e., inaudible, ambiguous, or nonsensical), or to hover near the peer group. They interrupt the flow of social exchange by being disagreeable and demanding.[15] Once engaged in group play, rejected boys engage in more physical and verbal aggression and exclude others more than do better-accepted peers.[3,4] Children also treat rejected classmates differently than they treat their better-accepted peers. Peers initiate relatively few interactions with rejected children and may view their positive behavior less favorably than they do similar behavior by better-accepted peers. In general, researchers document that behavioral differences between rejected and better-accepted peers are more readily apparent during preschool and early elementary than during later primary school years, perhaps because important social behavior is less readily observed as children grow older.

In addition, poorly accepted children differ from their better-accepted peers in how they think about and try to solve social dilemmas. When questioned about handling interpersonal problems, rejected children's responses indicate that their knowledge of appropriate behavior may be deficient. Rejected children may be able to verbalize only one or two appropriate strategies to cope with a problem, and they voice unusual or inappropriate responses when pressed for other options. Furthermore, aggressive boys, as compared with average boys, are less accurate at detecting prosocial intentions but more accurate at detecting hostile intentions, generate a higher proportion of aggressive responses to hypothetical situations, and are less likely to choose appropriate responses when evaluating the possible ways of reacting to problem situations.

Although most studies treat rejected children as a homogenous group, recent findings[7] suggest that there are at least two distinct subtypes of rejected children, aggressive-rejected and nonaggressive-rejected, with different behavioral profiles. Peers view aggressive-rejected children as more aggressive and disruptive than accepted children; teachers report that these children lack self-control and academic motivation and appear anxious. Peers view nonaggressive-rejected children as more withdrawn than others, but teachers do not see them as particularly deviant otherwise.

Detection of peer relationship problems by the physician is complicated by several factors. Most children's problems are first noted by teachers and peers and occur in the school. Parents may be unaware that the child has difficulties because they are uninformed, they ignore the teacher's feedback, or the child behaves differently at home. Although some rejected children recognize their difficulties and will admit to loneliness and low self-esteem, others view themselves no differently than their well-accepted peers[1] and may deny that they have difficulties. Indications that peer relationship problems may be present include reports from the child's teacher, complaints by the child that he or she has few or no friends, evidence that the child is frequently used as a scapegoat by others, or reports of excessive shyness around other children, particularly at school. In addition, interpersonal difficulties have been associated with physical disabilities, learning disabilities, obesity, conduct disorders, hyperactivity, and delinquency; thus, assessment of the child's functioning with peers would seem warranted when any of these correlated problems is present.

MANAGEMENT AND INTERVENTION

The physician's direct intervention with a child having peer relationship problems is of questionable use unless the physician plans to meet regularly once a week with the child, teachers, or parents. However, the physician who only occasionally sees the child can still play an important role in educating both parents and teachers about the importance of developing good peer relationship skills. Furthermore, he or she may be able to advise them of initial strategies to try in attempting to ameliorate the problem. In addition, the physician may be able to identify the cases in which the child's rejection may be a result of poor physical appearance and instruct the parents and child in more appropriate dress or personal hygiene.

For the young child with more minor or circumscribed peer relationship difficulties, advising the parents or teacher to provide the child with toys that require cooperation and sharing (e.g., seesaw, board games, flash cards) can lead to increased positive social interaction. Cooperative parents and teachers can also be advised in these cases to engineer opportunities for the child to interact positively with peers and then attend to and positively reinforce desirable social behaviors, such as cooperative play, while ignoring negative or nonsocial behaviors.

With children whose difficulties are pervasive or whose parents and teachers are uncooperative, more extensive intervention is advisable. Intervention methods with documented-effectiveness vary with the age of the child. With preschoolers and young primary grade–age withdrawn children, modeling can be effective in increasing positive peer interactions. Modeling procedures typically include observation of other children (usually filmed) engaged in positive interaction, followed by opportunities for the child to engage in similar activities with peers. Modeling has been shown to be generally effective, although less so for children from families of lower socioeconomic status. Alternatively, reinforcement programs can be instituted in which the teacher or parent rewards positive social participation with praise, with attention, or with tokens that can be exchanged later for privileges or other rewards. A variant of this procedure appropriate for withdrawn children involves verbally praising peers for interacting with the withdrawn child, which presumably leads others to get to know the withdrawn child better and to begin to include him or her in their activities. This approach, however, is contraindicated for the child whose responses to peers are often negative, as the child's annoying behavior is likely to lead to increased exclusion in other situations.

With older children, intervention frequently consists of one-to-one or group training in specific social skills. Training may focus on teaching specific social interaction skills, such as helping others, conversing, and taking turns. "Coaching" procedures are frequently used to instruct the child in the skill to be mastered. Coaching includes providing a rationale for the target skill, having the child rehearse the skill in a mock situation with an adult or child partner, providing feedback on the child's performance, and sometimes reenacting the scene. In general, social skills training programs are most effective for children who lack positive behaviors and are less effective for children who drive others away with frequent negative behavior.

Coaching usually results in the child learning the trained skills, but generalizing the new skills to ongoing social interactions is a problem for some children and requires additional intervention. Peer-mediated interventions are sometimes used in an attempt to generalize trained skills. Typically, same-sex accepted peers are recruited as "co-therapists" and trained to initiate interactions, to respond to refusals, to maintain interactions, and to respond to the target child's negative behavior in order to engage the target child in the activities of the larger peer group. This procedure needs to be conducted and monitored carefully, however, to avoid even more stigmatization of the rejected child in the peer group.

Changing the child's school is another intervention sometimes considered by parents or teachers. However, research[3] shows that rejected boys quickly reestablish their rejected status when placed in a group of children all unknown to one another. These findings suggest that simply changing a child's school, without a concomitant change in a child's social behavior, will merely perpetuate a child's negative peer relations. Changing the child's school may be indicated, however, if his or her previous negative reputation is making it difficult for the child to be accepted by peers even though he or she is performing new socially appropriate behaviors.

Similar to social skills training are interventions that address more general interpersonal problem-solving skills. In this approach, the child is taught (usually by means of coaching) to handle interpersonal dilemmas by defining the problem, generating several alternatives that might resolve the situation, and selecting the solution most likely to produce desirable results. Although these programs are successful at improving children's social knowledge, their effects on actual social behavior (particularly negative behavior) is less clear.

The health care worker who elects to work directly with the child is best advised to assess the effects of the intervention after approximately six sessions. If progress is not apparent, referral to a child psychiatrist, psychologist, social worker, or school counselor experienced with peer relationship problems would be warranted. In addition, preschools and elementary schools (particularly in urban and academic communities) occasionally include curricula related to social development, and such classrooms are referral possibilities if available in the local area.

REFERENCES

1. Boivin M and Begin G: Peer status and self-perception among early elementary school children: the case of the rejected children, Child Dev 60:591, 1989.
2. Coie JD and Dodge KA: Continuities and changes in children's social status: a five-year longitudinal study, Merrill-Palmer Q 29:261, 1983.
3. Coie JD and Kupersmidt JB: A behavioral analysis of emerging social status in boys' groups, Child Dev 54:1400, 1983.
4. Dodge KA: Behavioral antecedents of peer social status, Child Dev 54:1386, 1983.
5. Dodge KA et al: Social competence in children, Monogr Soc Res Child Dev 51:1, 1986.
6. Foster SL, DeLawyer DD, and Guevremont DC: Selecting targets for social skills training with children and adolescents. In Gadow KD, editor: Advances in learning and behavioral disabilities, Greenwich, Conn, 1985, JAI Press, Inc.
7. French DC: Heterogeneity of peer-rejected boys: aggressive and nonaggressive subtypes, Child Dev 59:976, 1988.
8. Gronlund NE: Sociometry in the classroom, New York, 1959, Harper & Row, Publishers, Inc.
9. Hymel S and Asher SR: Assessment and training of isolated children's social skills, ERIC document reproduction service no ED 136:930, 1977.
10. Ladd GW and Golter BS: Parents' management of preschooler's peer relations: is it related to children's social competence? Dev Psych 24:109, 1988.
11. MacDonald K and Parke RD: Bridging the gap: parent-child play interaction and peer interactive competence, Child Dev 55:1265, 1984.
12. Parker JG and Asher SR: Peer relations and later personal adjustment: are low-accepted children at risk? Psychol Bull 102:357, 1987.
13. Pettit GS, Dodge KA, and Brown MM: Early family experience, social problem solving patterns, and children's social competence, Child Dev 59:107, 1988.
14. Putallaz M: Maternal behavior and children's sociometric status, Child Dev 58:324, 1988.
15. Putallaz M and Wasserman A: Children's naturalistic entry behavior and sociometric status: a developmental perspective, Dev Psych 25:297, 1989.
16. Roff M, Sells SB, and Golden MM: Social adjustment and personality development in children, Minneapolis, 1972, University of Minnesota Press.
17. Rubin KH: Social and social-cognitive developmental characteristics of young isolate, normal, and sociable children. In Rubin KH and Ross HS, editors: Peer relationships and social skills in childhood, New York, 1982, Springer-Verlag New York, Inc.
18. Rubin KH and Mills RSL: The many faces of social isolation in childhood, J Consult Clin Psychol 56:916, 1988.

88

Phobias

James G. Kavanaugh, Jr. and Åke Mattsson

Phobia is fear, to an extreme degree, of objects or events in the natural environment that in reality are not dangerous to the individual and that would not be of concern to most people. Although adults do show phobic reactions, phobias are predominantly an event of early childhood. Indeed, their common occurrence during this period has continued to challenge theoreticians of child development and psychopathology, as therapeutic successes are reported from varying treatment methods based on quite different theoretic ideas about etiology. Incidence and prevalence figures are not available; diagnostic criteria differ, as does the readiness of those affected to seek professional help. An extensive literature dates its origins to Sigmund Freud's 1909 case report, "Little Hans," which describes an animal phobia in a 5-year-old boy.[1]

Practical as well as theoretic issues are involved in the effort to differentiate phobic responses from the universal fears of early childhood. Every neonate displays fearfulness; initially, such a response is elicited by nonspecific sensory disturbances of high intensity and sudden onset—for example, loud noises, extreme levels of illumination, and rapid movements with seeming loss of support. Such responses are related to the new challenges experienced by the infant just beginning his or her adaptation to an environment that, in contrast to the more evenly regulated intrauterine life, is experienced as changeable and unpredictable even without extreme variations.

As infants mature, they gain in ability to discriminate sensory impressions and to direct their locomotion. Early in the first year, they begin to recognize and integrate sensations that give increasing predictability and meaning to the unending stimulation to which they are subjected. Relating in a general way to the stages of intellectual (cognitive) development is a generally predictable sequence of fears, but not phobias. By 8 or 9 months of age, children have formed an early mental representation of their principal care giver, a person so necessary to them that even temporary substitution of someone different is responded to as a threat; this strong negative emotional reaction to unfamiliar persons is predictable enough to have acquired the designation of "stranger anxiety." The 2- to 3-year-old moves in a physically wider world, filled with an increasing array of objects, both animate and inanimate. The common animal fears of this period are in part related to the ubiquity of pets, with their noisy and unpredictable behavior. For many children, concern about the dark, with its strange-appearing shapes and often unidentifiable noises, heightens their other fears and even becomes a specific fear in itself. Children 7 to 9 years of age have sufficient intellectual powers, combined with a degree of worldly awareness, to comprehend death as a permanent condition that also can happen to them. This new awareness can be experienced as transient strong fears of death and dying. Any of the mentioned fears of childhood may become intensified if the child is aware that they also are major concerns of some close family member.

In contrast to these rather predictable fears, childhood phobias are associated with two major distinguishing characteristics: first, the seeming incongruity of the object or situation evoking a response and, second, the normality of the child's behavior when the phobic situation is avoided. Unlike the child exhibiting a tic or showing multiple problems in daily living, the phobic child who is spared confrontation with the "chosen" stimulus is not markedly different from an unaffected peer. Indeed, many observers comment on the phobic child's brightness, pleasantness, and sociability. Such comments indicate the many areas of normal personality functioning that are available for use in therapeutic approaches to the problem.

The primary physician need not be overly concerned with differing theories of personality predisposition and causation in identifying cases of phobia; the clinical picture underlying varying theoretic formulations is similar, and the history elicited is usually straightforward and pathognomonic. (School phobia alone presents sufficient variation to warrant separate consideration; see Chapter 66.)

In the usual case, the parents will describe a situation in which a child without previous behavioral problems suddenly shows an intense fear, for example, of a particular animal, of the toilet, of becoming ill, or of being dirty. At times, there may have been a recent identifiable event associated with these fears. The family has often tried reassurance and encouragement. The child's concerns may have widened with the result that more animals are being feared, or previous activities away from home are being avoided, or the sleep pattern has become disrupted. The child's continued adequate performance in areas not affected by the phobia seems puzzling to the family. At best the child can offer only sketchy explanations of these fears and often none at all.

In trying to understand this behavioral constellation more completely, the pediatrician may find the differing theories less than helpful. However, since therapeutic approaches will be shaped by the therapist's theory of what has "gone wrong" with the child's functioning, a brief mention of two major schools of thought is necessary. The traditional psychodynamic explanation postulates that the child develops internal mental conflict, most often related to sexual and aggressive themes. A solution to this painful conflicted state is reached by the unconscious displacement of negative feelings onto a specific external object or event. This then becomes the repository of the conflicting impulses and affects with which the child was previously struggling. The child is now able to reduce his or her anxiety by avoiding its designated "source." Psychotherapeutic efforts based on this model work to uncover the linkages of the child's initial conflicted state to the avoided object and, through insight and discussion, to help the child master the underlying threatening emotion.

The other major school of thought is often referred to by the general term *behaviorism*. Its continuing relation to learning theory underlies the concept of a phobia as an example of a maladaptive response that can be corrected by various forms of *behavior therapy*. An originally fearful situation is assumed to have been reinforced by repeated *avoidance*, thereby increasing its impact (as possibly corrective positive experiences are phobically avoided). Folk belief supports the value of immediately remounting the horse that throws you. The phenomenon of *generalization* is used to explain the progression of fears to include additional objects with qualities similar to the original stimulus. Behavior therapy often uses techniques of direct suggestion and, in addition, creates special situations for relearning.

"Flooding" or "implosion," techniques that confront the patient with the phobic situation until tolerance is developed, are rarely used with children. Instead, counterconditioning procedures have been found to be efficacious. One form of counterconditioning, systematic desensitization, has often been modified for children by using positive images or stimuli instead of deep muscle relaxation. Other behavioral approaches that have been employed successfully are observational learning (modeling), participant modeling, reinforced practice, and cognitive behavior therapy (which includes coping self-statements).

A comparison of children receiving short-term treatment (three sessions per week for 8 weeks)—either traditional psychotherapy or systematic desensitization—versus those on a waiting list revealed a marked reduction in the target phobia for all three groups. Measures of behavior did not reveal significant differences between the groups, but parents reported the phobias to be significantly less severe for children in either of the two treatment groups. Subdividing the entire group of patients by age also revealed a significant effect of therapy for the younger group (6 to 10 years of age), whereas the older treatment groups (11 to 15 years of age) did not show significantly more improvement than the older control group. A 2-year follow-up study by Hampe and colleagues[2] found that 80% of the children were problem free or significantly improved, and only 7% continued to be severely phobic (it should be noted, however, that many "control" children had received some treatment before the follow-up evaluation). The investigators concluded that the short-term therapies employed were effective for about 60% of phobic children, that different procedures are required for different age groups, and that the major justification for therapy is that treatment greatly hastens recovery.

Once a phobia is identified, a consultation with a child psychiatrist or child psychologist may be helpful in assessing the severity of the symptom and providing a prognosis. Many phobias of childhood are minor disrupters of day-to-day living and respond well to brief interventions. Consultation may also be helpful to clarify the extent of parental involvement in the onset and perpetuation of the symptomatology. (See Chapter 66 for further details regarding school phobia.)

Brief use of sedatives or tranquilizing drugs is often indicated in situations in which there is major disruption of the child's functioning, especially those with target symptoms that involve bedtime behaviors or sleep. Diphenhydramine (Benadryl) is quite effective as a sleep medication for children up to the age of puberty; those as young as 1 or 2 years will readily accept the flavored syrup. It is also an effective mild tranquilizer for anxious and hyperactive children up to age 10 or 11. Chloral hydrate is an equally safe and effective hypnotic. Diazepam (Valium) can be used with anxious preadolescent and adolescent patients. Research studies and clinical case reports continue to define the place of medications in the treatment of these patients.[3,4]

Drugs are most effective as part of the overall management of acute situations, when their use is directed toward specific symptoms and for limited time periods. Specific details of dosage, side effects, and potentiations, as well as any special precautions with young patients, should be reviewed in the current package insert or the *Physicians' Desk Reference*.

In summary, phobias in childhood are common and are not difficult to diagnose when an adequate history is obtained. The majority of phobic children are spared other behavior symptoms, and their many personality strengths make them good candidates for therapeutic interventions, which should be initiated as early as the condition is identified.

REFERENCES

1. Freud S: Analysis of a phobia in a five-year-old boy. In Complete psychological works, vol 10, London, 1955, Hogarth.
2. Hampe E et al: Phobic children one and two years post treatment, J Abnorm Psychol 82:446, 1973.
3. Noys R, Chaudry DR, and Domingo DV: Pharmacologic treatment of phobic disorders, J Clin Psychiatry 47(9):445, 1986.
4. Rifkin A and others: Psychotropic medication in adolescents: a review, J Clin Psychiatry 47(8):400, 1986.

SUGGESTED READINGS

Adams P: Anxiety disorders. In Kaplan HI and Sadock BJ, editors: Comprehensive textbook of psychiatry/V, vol 2, Baltimore, 1982, Williams & Wilkins Co.

Marks IM: Fears and phobias, New York, 1975, Academic Press, Inc.

Nemiah JC: Phobic disorder/phobic neurosis. In Kaplan HI, Freedman AM, and Sadock BJ, editors: Comprehensive textbook of psychiatry/III, vol 2, Baltimore, 1980, Williams & Wilkins Co.

Ross AO: Child behavior therapy: principles, procedures, and empirical basis, New York, 1981, John Wiley & Sons, Inc.

89

Physical Disability and Chronic Illness

Gregory S. Liptak and Beverly A. Myers

DEFINITION AND DEMOGRAPHICS

Children with chronic illness and physical disability (frequently termed children with special health care needs) include those with physical conditions that affect daily functioning for more than 3 months in a year, cause hospitalization of more than 1 month (total) in a year, or are likely to do either of these. Chronic disabling conditions include (but are not limited to) asthma, cerebral palsy, cystic fibrosis, congenital heart disease, diabetes mellitus, hemophilia, meningomyelocele, inflammatory bowel disease, renal failure, epilepsy, cancer, juvenile arthritis, and red cell disorders (such as sickle cell disease).

Although each condition taken individually is uncommon, taken together they affect approximately 10% of all children and constitute an important part of pediatric practice. Over the past 20 years, disease-specific survival rates have improved dramatically; however, many of these survivors have severe limitations of activity and function.

COMMON CHARACTERISTICS

Although these children differ from each other in various ways, they and their families share common characteristics, which are shown in the accompanying box. A widely held generalization is that 85% of the issues with which children and families must deal are common to all chronic disabilities, whereas 15% of the issues are specific to the child's diagnosis.

The negative impact of a chronic condition, which can be manifest as behavioral problems and psychopathology, such as depression, poor socialization, and family disruption, is worsened at all periods of development by low socioeconomic status.

DEVELOPMENTAL CONSIDERATIONS

In addition to understanding the medical condition and commonalities cited above, the health care provider caring for a child with a chronic disability must also understand the interactions between the condition and the developing child and family.

Infancy

Conditions that affect the physical appearance of an infant, such as cleft lip and palate or hydrocephalus, can affect the bonding and attachment between child and caretakers. In addition, once the diagnosis of an abnormality such as a chronic disability is made, the parents will begin to grieve for the lost "normal" child. This bereavement includes shock, denial, anger, sadness/depression, guilt, and anxiety. Parents may go through these stages of mourning at any time in the child's development, especially during transitions, for ex-

Common Features of Chronic Disability in Childhood

Child
- Chronic, often unpredictable course
- No cure
- Pain and discomfort
- Restricted growth and development
- Frequent hospitalizations and outpatient visits
- Painful, embarrassing treatments
- Inability to participate in peer activities
- Daily burden of care

Family
- Loss of "ideal" child
- Daily burden of care
- Expense (financial, time)
- Lost opportunities
- Neglected siblings
- Confusing systems of health and other care
- Social isolation

Community
- Poor understanding of chronic illness
- Inconsistent policies and funding
- Inadequate facilities (including barriers to access)
- Poor communication and coordination within the health care system and with other agencies

ample, when the child begins kindergarten or the family moves. One parent may be primarily experiencing one set of feelings such as guilt while another experiences feelings such as anger. This makes communication between them difficult and decreases their ability to support each other. This grief also interferes with the ability to form a bond or become attached to the chronically ill child. Parents may express their feelings of anger toward the pediatrician or seek multiple opinions because of their denial.

The behavior of pediatricians during this period can have a major impact on the family's acceptance of their disabled child. The words that are used, or simply holding the infant, or encouraging the parent to do so, can improve acceptance. Discussion of parental feelings and counseling about financial assistance and community support can be invaluable to the family's coping.

Whenever a pediatrician informs a family of the presence of a chronic disability in their child, care must be taken to ensure that the family understands and that their needs are met. This requires the ability to listen nonjudgmentally, even to negative opinions and feelings, without providing false reassurances or premature suggestions (before the family feels they understand or have received empathy from the physician). Patience and repetition of information are often required, as is sensitivity to verbal and nonverbal communication.

Preschool

The normal development of preschool children includes the achievement of a sense of autonomy and initiative. One way that children show autonomy is by, literally, walking away. If a child is physically disabled and cannot walk or is bedridden because of illness, he or she cannot express autonomy by walking away and must express it in some other way. This may manifest as negative verbal behavior or disobedience. Allowing the child to show autonomy in acceptable ways, for example, by having the child choose clothing or diet or the arm into which the intravenous line will go can decrease the occurrence of unacceptable behaviors.

The demands of the chronic illness placed on the family, as well as feelings of sympathy for the child (e.g., "She has suffered enough.") may make consistent limit-setting difficult for parents and can lead to behavior problems in the child. One parent (often the mother) may become overinvolved with the child, thus blurring normal family relationships. The father may become isolated from health care decisions, a process that is hastened by the typical Monday through Friday, 9:00 AM to 5:00 PM office hours of most pediatricians. Encouraging parents to achieve a balance in their roles as parents, spouses, and workers by helping them find support in the community (e.g., for spending time as a couple away from the children) can help families cope.

Referring a young child to an early intervention program may provide support for the family and educational and therapeutic treatments that will assist the child's development. It may also encourage the family to increase their contact with their child. Public Law 99-457 is increasing the availability of preschool programs for children at risk for developmental delay. Unfortunately, day care and nursery programs for disabled children who are not at risk for developmental delay, such as those with asthma, are woefully insufficient to meet the demand.

Young children are especially vulnerable to the effects of separation that occur when they are hospitalized. The pediatrician should encourage rooming-in for parents during hospitalizations, as well as frequent visits from all family members. This includes helping the family obtain transportation, child care, or other nonmedical services.

The pediatrician requires an awareness of the child's temperament, as well as his or her abilities and motivations. Children who are intense, persistent, irregular in rhythm, and negative in mood can be especially difficult for families, even without the added stress of a chronic illness. Providing insight to families about the nature of their child's temperament can decrease their guilt and can provide them with more effective ways of coping with their child's behavior.

School Age

Problems with autonomy and initiative from the previous period may become manifest during school age. The dependent, disabled child may have serious difficulty separating from his or her parents to attend school. Separation anxiety can affect the parents, who impose unreasonable restrictions on their child's activities or who may have unreasonable expectations of their child's abilities.

The chronic condition may directly impair the child's cognitive or motor abilities, or the child may miss more school than other children. Both can hinder his or her ability to achieve a sense of industry at school. A wide array of educational and health-related services are mandated by Public Law 94-142, the Education for All Handicapped Children Act, which requires children to receive an appropriate education in their least restrictive environment (see Chapter 65, "The Chronically Ill and Disabled Child in School"). This law authorizes the provision of services such as physical therapy, occupational therapy, speech therapy, and nursing services, including clean intermittent catheterization. The relative value of taking children away from their classrooms to perform these services compared with the benefits of keeping them in the classroom has not yet been documented.

According to social learning theorists, a child's conviction that he or she can successfully execute a behavior required to produce a certain outcome (self-efficacy) determines how much effect will be expended in that activity. Because chronically disabled children may look or act different from others, they are frequently rejected by peers despite their best efforts at socialization. Their repeated lack of success in this regard will lead to decreased efforts in the development of social relations and may produce deviant social and personality development as they grow older. Children with deficiencies in physical and self-help skills have been shown to have fewer coping skills and more difficulty establishing satisfactory social relations than their peers.

If the child's teacher or the school nurse is not knowledgeable about the child's condition, the child's care at school may be impaired. The pediatrician should enlighten school personnel regarding the child's condition, with regular updates, and must be available for intervention during a crisis.

Providing a written assessment of the child's needs and a plan that the school can follow during an emergency can greatly decrease the discomfort of school personnel, improve communication, and enhance care. Parents should also be encouraged to collaborate with school personnel.

During this period the pediatrician can also increase the responsibility given to the child for the management of the condition, for example, ensuring that medications and treatments are received as scheduled or keeping a diary of illness-related events.

Adolescence

Chronic disabilities can profoundly affect the social and emotional development of the adolescent. Issues of major concern during this period are shown in the box below. The presence of a chronic condition significantly increases the risk for behavior problems and psychiatric disorders such as depression. Behavioral problems and emotional distress are not directly correlated with the physiologic severity of the condition, however. Children who are marginally affected—for example, those with low-level spina bifida or minimal arthritis—may have greater difficulty adjusting during adolescence than those more severely affected. Minimally affected children cannot identify with the world of "normals," since they cannot accomplish many normal activities (such as running or achieving continence) nor do they identify with the world of the severely impaired individual, such as a child in a wheelchair.

The adverse effects of chronic conditions are modified by the gender of the child as well as by socioeconomic status. For example, delayed sexual maturation is more likely to lead to depression and social isolation in boys than in girls.

Adolescents develop a sense of identity by emulating role models. Disabled children have few role models. The normative values for concepts such as "beauty," which assail adolescents through printed media and television, are often widely discrepant with their self-images. The lack of role models, isolation from peers, poor self-image, and a pervasive culture that stresses physical appearance make the development of a positive identity difficult at best.

The pediatrician should address the issues outlined in the box below and address the feelings of the adolescent related to his or her self-concept and condition. Most authorities recommend that the adolescent be evaluated by the pediatrician without the parents present in order to build a trusting relationship that inspires independence.

Issues of Special Relevance for Adolescents

- Physical appearance (actual and perceived)
- Social isolation
- Sexual development
  - Physical maturation, including onset of puberty
  - Heterosexual relationship ideations
  - Sexual behavior and contraception
- Vocational planning
- Genetic counseling

SYSTEMS OF CARE

The goal for the management of the child with chronic disabilities should be to *achieve maximum functioning*. For example, the goal of a specific orthopedic intervention should be to help a child walk, not to make the feet straight. Ironically, the specialization that has improved the health and longevity of children with chronic conditions has resulted in fragmentation of care within the health care system. Also, communication between medical personnel and other agencies, such as the educational and legal systems, is often inadequate. Access to services is still difficult for many families, especially those without health insurance, and preventive services may be unavailable. This has resulted in duplication of some services and gaps in others.

Case Management

Achieving optimum functioning requires an organized, coordinated approach to care that is embodied in the concept of case management. Comprehensive case management includes (1) *needs assessment*—identifying and assessing the needs of the child and family; (2) *comprehensive care planning*—planning and arranging for medical and nonmedical services; (3) *facilitating and coordinating services* (including the training of community providers); (4) *follow-up*—monitoring services and patient progress; and (5) *empowerment*—counseling, educating, training, and supporting the child and family. Successful implementation requires knowledge about the child, the family, and the community in which they function.

Possible case managers for children with chronic conditions have been suggested, including the primary care physician, the specialty program, the community health nurse, and governmental programs. However, any professional who cares for a child who has special health care needs must ensure that *someone* is providing this service. Without it these children will receive less than optimum care, and families will face an even greater burden.

The pediatrician who attends the child with a chronic condition in the community can foster the child's development and functioning. Achieving this goal requires knowledge of the needs of the child's family and of the resources available in the community. This does not necessitate the provision of all services by that single provider. It does, however, require time, which is frequently not reimbursed, thoughtful coordination of effort, support of other professionals, and advocacy.

SUMMARY

The physician who cares for the child or adolescent with a physical disability or chronic illness is in a particularly advantageous position to foster the child's psychological development. He or she can do this both at the time of the informing interview with the parents and throughout infancy, childhood, and adolescence. Even when the physician is not in a position to carry out this process directly, his or her support of others, such as social workers, psychiatrists, and psychologists, in their interactions with the parents and the child will help the parents to recognize the importance of psychosocial issues in the child's development. In this way it may be possible to reduce the high prevalence of behavioral and emotional problems that reflect maladaptation to a physical disability or chronic illness.

SUGGESTED READINGS

Apley J and Ounsted C: One child, London, 1982, Spastics International.

Bandura A: The social foundations of thought and action: a social theory, Englewood Cliffs, NJ, 1986, Prentice Hall.

Cadman D et al: Chronic illness, disability and mental and social well-being: findings of the Ontario Child Health Study, Pediatrics 75:805, 1987.

Hobbs N, Perrin JM, and Ireys HT: Chronically ill children and their families, San Francisco, 1985, Jossey-Bass, Inc, Publishers.

Klaus MG and Kennell JH: Parent-infant bonding, St Louis, 1982, The CV Mosby Co.

Myers BA: The informing interview, Am J Dis Child 137:572, 1983.

Pless IB: Clinical assessment: physical and psychosocial functioning, Pediatr Clin North Am 31:33, 1984.

Stein R, Jessop DJ, and Riessman CK: Health care received by children with chronic illnesses, Am J Dis Child 137:225, 1983.

90

Psychosis

Irving B. Weiner

Psychosis refers to a serious degree of psychological disturbance in which a person's grasp of reality is so impaired as to prevent him or her from meeting the demands of everyday living. A psychotic disorder causes people to perceive themselves and their experiences inaccurately. As a result of being out of touch with reality, psychotic individuals often misjudge the consequences of their actions and behave in strange, unpredictable, and sometimes destructive ways. Other people frequently cannot comprehend why psychotics act as they do and consider their behavior "crazy."

In young people, disorders of psychotic proportion appear mainly in three patterns distinguishable by their typical age of onset: early-onset childhood psychosis, known as *infantile autism,* which almost always begins before 3 years of age and interferes with psychological development from infancy on; late-onset childhood psychosis, now commonly called *schizophrenia in childhood,* which usually begins between 7 and 12 years of age and is continuous with adolescent and adult forms of schizophrenic disorders; and *schizophrenia in adolescence,* which begins after puberty and, like schizophrenia in childhood, constitutes a breakdown or regression in psychological functioning following some years of more or less normal development.[6,7,9]

INFANTILE AUTISM

The primary characteristic of infantile autism is a lack of relatedness to people. Autistic children are indifferent and unresponsive to social overtures. As infants they do not clamor for attention, they do not enjoy being picked up, and they do not cuddle or cling when someone holds them. They rarely look or smile directly at other people, and they seem happiest when left alone.

For these reasons, parents of autistic children usually find little pleasure in nurturing them: "It was like taking care of an object; he never seemed to know or care whether I was around, and I never got any feeling of warmth from him." Nevertheless, because autistic infants tend to be physically healthy and to show normal physical development, their serious deficits in social attachment often go unnoticed initially or are attributed to their being placid or reserved.

During the preschool years, however, the detachment and unresponsiveness of these children become noticeably persistent, and they also begin to display a number of other unmistakable abnormalities. Most prominent in this regard are (1) a need to preserve sameness, which makes them intolerant of any change in their environment, such as moving their playpen or taking a piece of furniture out of their bedroom; (2) marked language abnormalities consisting either of failure to develop any communicative speech or of developing speech that is difficult to understand because of peculiar word usage, unusual grammatical constructions, and lack of relatedness to ongoing conversations; (3) repetitive, ritualistic behaviors, such as sitting for hours staring off into space or passing a toy back and forth from one hand to the other; and (4) indices of a developmental disorder such as strange body movements or posturing, neuropsychological abnormalities, and "soft" signs of neurologic impairment.

Infantile autism is a rare condition that is found in four to five live births per 10,000 and occurs three to four times more frequently in boys than in girls. Despite its rarity, autism is noteworthy for its devastating interference with psychological development virtually from birth and for its serious long-term consequences. Some autistic children improve spontaneously, especially if they are among the few who develop near-average intellectual and communication skills. Others respond favorably to specialized treatment programs that combine behavioral, educational, and pharmacologic approaches. The general prognosis for the condition is poor, however. No more than 25% of autistic children make any substantial social or educational progress, and of these, most achieve only fair academic and interpersonal functioning. The remaining 75% do poorly throughout their lives; 50% of these require residential placement by the end of adolescence.[3-5,8] (See Chapter 167 for further discussion of autism as a "strange behavior.")

SCHIZOPHRENIA IN CHILDHOOD

Although schizophrenia can begin as early as the preschool years, many children who are first identified as psychotic between ages 3 and 7 most likely are autistic youngsters with previously overlooked developmental problems dating from infancy.

Children who become schizophrenic develop the same features of impaired personality functioning that characterize adult schizophrenia: disorganized and illogical thinking, distorted perception of reality, inappropriate ways of relating to people, and poor control over feelings and impulses. As a result, these late-onset psychotic children manifest many of the symptoms seen in infantile autism, including compulsive routines and self-preoccupied behavior; incoherent or incomprehensible speech patterns; excessive, diminished, or unpredictable responses to sensory stimulation; body rigidity and strange posturing; poor social skills; and periods of unaccountably severe anxiety or violent temper tantrums.

Schizophrenic children are also likely to develop delusions or hallucinations that detach them even further from reality and from an appropriate relationship to people. Common in this regard are unrealistic fears about other children being "out to get me," bizarre fantasies about possessing special powers, and the conviction of being a machine or some kind of animal rather than a person. Schizophrenic youngsters are more likely than autistic children to have a history of poor physical health and development, but they are less likely to be intellectually or linguistically handicapped.

The distinction between schizophrenia in childhood and infantile autism is based not only on symptom patterns and age of onset but also on differences in etiology and course. Autism appears to be a biogenetic disorder resulting from prenatal, perinatal, or early postnatal damage to areas of the brain crucial to the development of language comprehension and social relationships. Psychosocial factors play no demonstrable role in whether or when autism appears, and the parents of autistic children do not differ in any psychologically significant way from parents of other handicapped children. Schizophrenia is currently best understood as a disorder of interactive origin in which biogenetic dispositions and psychosocial stressors combine to precipitate personality breakdown. Patterns of family interaction, especially the quality of parent-child communications, bear considerably on the severity and duration of these schizophrenic breakdowns.

Once begun, the symptoms of autism run a continuous, unrelenting course, whereas schizophrenia is an episodic disorder in which severe symptomatology alternates with periods of reasonably adequate functioning. Autistic children who do not improve tend eventually to develop primary features of mental retardation, epilepsy, or aphasia; by contrast, approximately 90% of schizophrenic children subsequently present evidence of adult schizophrenia.[1,2,6]

SCHIZOPHRENIA IN ADOLESCENCE

Late-onset childhood psychosis occurs somewhat more frequently than infantile autism, but schizophrenia remains a rare condition until adolescence. Following puberty the incidence of the disorder increases sharply. The population prevalence of schizophrenia is approximately 1%, and most schizophrenic persons experience their first psychotic breakdown in late adolescence or early adulthood (15 to 25 years of age). Schizophrenia is diagnosed in 25% to 30% of 12- to 18-year-olds admitted to public mental hospitals and in about 15% of those admitted to psychiatric units of general hospitals.

In addition to these instances of overt schizophrenia, many adolescents who are destined to become schizophrenically disturbed as adults show prodromal signs of the disorder during their teenage years. This means that pediatricians who care for adolescents will see an appreciable number of young people in whom various kinds of apparently minor behavioral problems in fact constitute the early stages of a schizophrenic disorder.

The adolescent personality patterns from which schizophrenia emerges usually involve either *schizoid* or *stormy* behavior. Schizoid adolescents tend to withdraw into themselves, avoiding activities that would bring them into contact with people and sharing few interests in common with others. They express little or no emotion, and they may appear apathetic and unenthused about life, as if depressed. Stormy adolescents, in contrast, exercise little control over their emotions or actions. They consequently tend to be in constant conflict with their parents, peers, and teachers over such behavior as fighting, stealing, running away, disobedience, truancy, and school failure. Neither schizoid nor stormy personality patterns are by themselves diagnostic of schizophrenia, and both can occur in the context of numerous other behavior disorders. However, either pattern appearing in adolescence, especially if it represents a marked change from a youngster's childhood behavior, should alert the clinician to the possibility of incipient schizophrenia.[9,10]

Generally, the older people are when they develop a psychotic disorder, the better their prospects for improvement and recovery. Hence late-onset psychosis, although often a persistent and disabling disorder, offers better prospects for improvement and marginal social adaptation than does infantile autism. Conversely, with schizophrenic disorder, the earlier in life a breakdown in response to stress occurs, the greater is the constitutional disposition or vulnerability to psychosis. Thus the prognosis in schizophrenia in adolescence is usually less guarded than in cases of schizophrenia in childhood. Among adolescents hospitalized for schizophrenia, about 25% recover, 25% improve substantially but suffer lingering symptoms or occasional relapses, and the remaining 50% make little or no progress and are likely to require continuing residential care.

REFERENCES

1. Cantor S: Childhood schizophrenia, New York, 1988, The Guilford Press.
2. Chambers WJ: Late onset psychoses of childhood and adolescence. In Kestenbaum CJ and Williams DT, editors: Handbook of clinical assessment of children and adolescents, New York, 1988, New York University Press.
3. Cohen DJ and Donnellan AM, editors: Handbook of autism and pervasive developmental disorders, New York, 1987, John Wiley & Sons, Inc.
4. DeMyer MK, Hingten JN, and Jackson RK: Infantile autism reviewed: a decade of research, Schizophr Bull 7:388, 1981.
5. Green WH: Pervasive developmental disorders. In Kestenbaum CJ and Williams DT, editors: Handbook of clinical assessment of children and adolescents, New York, 1987, John Wiley & Sons, Inc.
6. Prior M and Werry JS: Autism, schizophrenia, and allied disorders. In Quay HC and Werry JS, editors: Psychopathological disorders of childhood, ed 3, New York, 1986, John Wiley & Sons, Inc.
7. Rutter M and Schopler E: Autism and pervasive developmental disorders: concepts and diagnostic issues, J Autism Dev Disord 17:159, 1987.
8. Schreibman L: Autism, Newbury Park, Calif, 1988, Sage Publications.
9. Weiner IB: Child and adolescent psychopathology, New York, 1982, John Wiley & Sons, Inc.
10. Weiner IB: Identifying schizophrenia in adolescents, J Adolesc Health Care 8:336, 1987.

91

Self-Stimulating Behaviors

Richard M. Sarles and Alice B. Heisler

Self-stimulating behaviors, such as head-banging, head-rolling, rocking, thumb-sucking, masturbation, and habits of hair-pulling and nail-biting, are issues of concern for both parents and primary care practitioners. It has been suggested that there are commonalities among such behaviors, sometimes classified as "stereotypies," and that they represent an interaction of the stage of neuromotor development and environmental influences (e.g., arousal state, restrictive car seats, and cribs). Many of these behaviors typically appear before 12 months of age, reach a peak soon thereafter, and subsequently decline rapidly. In general, most of these behaviors are self-limited to the preschool period and are usually viewed as normal, common, expected behaviors. As such, these habits do not generally signify psychological maladjustment; thus, they often require little intervention other than reassuring the parents and recommending adequate stimulation of their child.[4]

HEAD-BANGING AND ROCKING BEHAVIOR

Head-banging consists of rhythmic movements of the head against a solid object, such as the crib mattress or occasionally the headboard itself, and is often associated with rocking the head and the entire body. It is most commonly observed at bedtime or at times of fatigue or stress and may vary in duration from several minutes to hours. It has been noted that head-banging often continues even when the child is asleep. The age of onset shows wide variability, but the behavior is most commonly witnessed during the preschool years. The reported incidence of head-banging or rocking behavior varies between 3% and 20%, with a male/female ratio of approximately 3:1. There is occasionally a positive family history of such behavior, but only 20% of siblings of rockers exhibit similar or other rhythmic pattern disturbances.[6]

Various theories have been developed in an attempt to understand these self-limited but often disturbing behaviors. Rocking is thought to be a soothing, pleasurable experience every infant encounters in utero and many from the neonatal period onward. The pleasure from movement is repeated throughout life, from early childhood rocking in mother's arms to childhood jump rope games, to the playground swing, and to dancing in adulthood, for example. Individual constitutional patterns in childhood account for a wide variability in the amount of stimulation any particular child may require. However, in certain children, such as those who are deaf, blind, emotionally disturbed, or severely mentally retarded, marked rhythmic movements are commonly found. In these cases, the movements may represent a compensatory reaction to make up for the lack of, or the inability to integrate, stimuli. In addition, the normal child who is inactive because of physical illness generally shows a need for motor release often manifested in bed rocking or other rhythmic body movements, which generally disappear once normal mobility is restored to the child.

Physical and neurologic examinations show these children to be predominantly within normal limits, and electroencephalographic studies are not indicated, because they have been generally nonrevealing. It appears that these behaviors are linked to maturational patterns and closely correlate with teething and other transitions of growth and development, perhaps as a mechanism of increasing or reducing arousal. Even though psychosocial growth and development are apparently not disturbed in these children and studies indicate no connection between rocking behavior and parental divorce or separation, the question of inadequate stimulation for the child should be raised, or the presence of family turmoil and stress should be investigated.

Treatment is generally directed toward assuring the parents that head-banging cannot cause brain injury and that the child will show no adverse neurologic residual in later life; in fact, "head-bangers" usually "grow up" to be coordinated and completely normal children. Padding the crib and securing the bed to prevent rolling may be helpful during the limited rocking behavior. Sedation in the form of diphenhydramine may prove effective, but psychotropic medication is generally unnecessary and thus discouraged. Consultation with a child psychiatrist or psychologist is indicated if the head-banging or rocking behavior persists beyond 3 years of age. In the child who shows a lack of social interaction or a preoccupation with himself or herself or with self-stimulatory behavior, such as overt, compulsive masturbation, consultation is also indicated.[3]

THUMB-SUCKING AND NAIL-BITING

Thumb-sucking is an almost universal occurrence in infancy. Infants may place virtually every object in the mouth until parents restrict certain objects for reasons of safety.

The pleasurable sensations associated with the double tactile experience of sucking and being sucked and the feelings of security and comfort that this evokes tend to reinforce this type of behavior. Many families substitute rubber pacifiers as a more socially acceptable means of oral pleasure, and children themselves often spontaneously suck a security blanket, a doll, or a stuffed animal. Thumb-sucking usually occurs during times of stress or boredom and at bedtime. Social and family pressures generally limit thumb-sucking to the preschool years. However, the habit may persist into adolescence. An incidence as high as 59% has been reported, and it is estimated that approximately 30% to 40% of American children engage in finger-sucking during the preschool years, and 10% to 20% continue past 6 years of age.

Nail-biting is an extension or permutation of the habit of thumb-sucking. Some consider this behavior a form of more overt aggression directed toward one's self, whereas others would simply define nail-biting as a variation of thumb-sucking, since this behavior is also typically seen during times of stress. It is estimated that 40% of all children over 6 years of age bite their nails at some time or other, and 20% of college students continue to bite their nails. Thus nail-biting, in contrast to thumb-sucking, often continues throughout childhood and into adulthood. There appears to be a family history in most cases, but this habit is so common that such an apparent association may be of no significance. There does not appear to be any correlation with the number of children in the family, the birth order, the type of feeding or type of feeding schedule, or the age or race of the parents. However, there is a significant association with the time of weaning, in that the later the weaning takes place, the less likely the chance of thumb-sucking.[1]

Thumb-sucking, nail-biting, and cuticle-biting or picking generate an increase in the probability of dental malocclusion and an increase in the incidence of digital cutaneous infections. The probability of malocclusion in thumb-suckers appears directly related to the age of discontinuing the habit. Thus, those children who cease the habit only after 6 years of age generally manifest malocclusion to some degree when seen at 12 years of age.

An underlying cause of tension should always be investigated, but often, simple behavior therapy (based on positive reinforcement) is sufficient to alleviate this habit. The parents should be advised to avoid punishment, threats, or demonstrations of anger. Encouragement in the place of restrictions is helpful in engaging the child in his or her own program to decrease or eliminate this behavior. Bitter-tasting commercial preparations applied to the fingers may be used as a reminder for the child but are generally inadequate unless supplemented by consistent positive reinforcement. This choice of reinforcement reward should be the child's and might represent a "Chinese menu" of extra television privileges, dessert, or other special treats. Weekly visits to the physician for the first month of treatment are important to reinforce the change in behavior further. Hypnosis is another treatment that is often quite successful and poses no dangers; psychotropic medications, on the other hand, are of little value. If these habits are linked to other signs of emotional distress, referral to a specialist in behavioral disorders is warranted.

MASTURBATION

Masturbatory activity in children is common and often leads to great parental concern. Such activity may vary from direct manual genital stimulation to movements of the thighs against each other. Rhythmic swaying or thrusting motions of the child while straddling a hobby horse, pillow, stuffed animal, or other objects are also common methods of masturbation. Infants and children are capable of a physiologic orgasmic response similar to that experienced by the adult, except for the absence of ejaculation in the male child. This was demonstrated by the common practice in Europe about the turn of the century of masturbating an irritable child to induce relaxation and sleep. Occasionally, this orgasmic response has been incorrectly thought to represent a convulsive disorder in the preschool child.

Masturbatory activity is generally initiated as a response to the learned pleasure associated with touching of the genitalia first experienced in infancy during normal body exploration. Masturbation will continue as a lifelong pleasurable experience unless suppressed by parents or other adults. It is important for the practitioner to counsel parents concerning masturbatory practices and emphasize that masturbation is a normal, nondamaging healthy practice that helps the child derive pleasure from his or her own body. Myths must be dispelled concerning the belief that masturbation may cause mental retardation, physical deformity, blindness, poor physical and mental health, facial pimples, hair on the palms of the hand, homosexuality, and sexual perversions. Parents should be aware of the normality and almost universal occurrence of masturbation in children and should be encouraged not to punish or shame their child. If parents observe masturbatory activity in their child, they may want to suggest to the child the inappropriateness of manipulating their genitalia in public places or in front of others and inform the child that certain practices such as "toileting" and masturbation are best carried out in private.

Because local genital irritation, candidal infection, or pinworms in rare cases may cause one to masturbate, a thorough physical examination is helpful to exclude such possibilities. Compulsive, overt masturbation in children and adolescents may lead to social isolation and may signify a deeper emotional problem. Consultation with a specialist in behavioral disorders of children and adolescents is indicated if the practitioner suspects that the masturbatory activity is excessive, compulsive, or overt or may indicate the presence of a more complicated, troublesome emotional problem.

The practitioner should be aware that even with the current trend within our society toward sexual openness and enlightenment, myths and feelings concerning masturbation are often deep seated and persistent. Thus, counseling and advice given by the practitioner may be met with covert or overt resistance by parents or school authorities. The practitioner should be well prepared to educate those responsible for the growth and development of children.

HAIR-PULLING AND TWISTING

Hair-pulling and twisting is an extremely uncommon form of self-stimulating behavior and is often indicative of severe psychological stress on the child. The obvious cosmetic damage often results in ridicule by peers and shame for the child. The possibility of a hair ball, or trichobezoar, forming in the stomach if the child ingests the hair is a serious problem that often results in hospitalization for surgical removal of the accumulated matted hair.

This behavior, more frequent in females than males, has been reported in preschoolers, school-age children, adolescents, and adults. A relationship has been suggested between moderate to severe depression and hair-pulling.

Treatment is usually indicated, which varies from initial behavior modification techniques such as a positive reinforcement–reward system, to wearing a cap. Local irritation from a primary dermatologic condition rarely is the cause of this disorder, but the possibility should be investigated. Referral to a mental health professional is often warranted to investigate possible underlying causes of tension, anxiety, or depression. Hypnosis or psychotherapy may be required in many of these cases.

SPECIAL PROBLEMS IN DISTURBED CHILDREN

A broad spectrum of self-stimulating behaviors may be seen in the severely retarded or emotionally disturbed child. The behaviors, including body-twirling or spinning and hand- or arm-flapping, are often seen in cases of infantile autism or childhood schizophrenia. Excessive rocking behavior is common in the severely retarded and emotionally disturbed child. In addition, severe self-mutilating behaviors such as compulsive self-biting, severe head-banging, and skin-gouging may occasionally be seen in these disorders,[2] but are more characteristic of certain metabolic-genetic disorders such as the Lesch-Nyhan syndrome and the de Lange syndrome.

It is felt that these behaviors are part of a symptom complex in a severe disorder, quite in contrast to the generally isolated behavior previously discussed in normal children. The etiology is generally linked to the basic disorder and may also reflect the lack of, or disordered integration of, sensory stimuli.

All of these cases require treatment for the basic disorder and generally demand special treatment beyond the scope and expertise of the primary care physician. Institutionalization is often required, and methods of treatment include (1) the application of aversive behavior modification techniques, (2) the use of arm and neck restraints, head helmets, and major tranquilizers, and (3) the institution of psychotherapeutic programs.[5]

REFERENCES

1. Fletcher B: Etiology of fingersucking: review of literature, J Dent Children 42:293, 1975.
2. Green A: Self-mutilation in schizophrenic children, Arch Gen Psychiatry 17:234, 1967.
3. Kravitz H et al: A study of head-banging in infants and children, Dis Nerv Sys 21:203, 1960.
4. Lourie R: The role of rhythmic patterns in childhood, Am J Psychiatry 105:653, 1949.
5. Singh NN: Current trends in the treatment of self-injurious behavior, Adv Pediatr 28:377, 1981.
6. Werry JS, Carlielle J, and Fitzpatrick J: Rhythmic motor activities (stereotypies) in children under five: etiology and prevalence, J Am Acad Child Psychiatry 22:329, 1983.

92

Stuttering

Doris R. Pastore

The major characteristic of stuttering is a disturbance in the flow of speech. Experts argue not only the definition of stuttering but also its causation, assessment, and management. Throughout history there has been essentially one main controversy: whether stuttering is a physiological or psychological event. Recent studies have raised the issue of whether the essential component is genetic. Between 5% and 10% of all children stutter at some time, and early identification and prompt treatment are important in cases where stuttering persists or becomes progressive.

It is difficult to distinguish early stuttering from *normal disfluency,* which refers to the repetitions, hesitations, and editing of one's thoughts, typical of speech production. During the preschool years, patterns of fluency, rate, and emphasis of syllables are highly variable. There is a sharp increase in disfluencies from 25 to 37 months of age, followed by a decline in the subsequent months.[9] This is generally described as *developmental disfluency* and is commonly a temporary stage in the process of learning speech. It is known that the first words of babies are arrhythmic and that with time, the ability to produce emphasized or stressed syllables develops. The child then will use the right number of syllables and have an understanding of rhythm before speech processes completely develop. For example, a word such as "ferigerator" may be used for "refrigerator." Stuttering occurs most frequently on emphasized syllables, yet little is known about the way in which the distinction between stressed and unstressed syllables develops.[9]

Characteristics evaluated in assessing speech include the frequency of disfluency, the type of repetition, and the nature of its production. Normally speaking 2- to 3-year-olds have about 6.2 disfluencies per 100 syllables, with easily produced single-unit part-word repetitions, revisions (amendments), and interjections (ums, uhs) as the most common.[12] Children who stutter exhibit 21.5 disfluencies per 100 syllables, with significant part-word repetition and rapid and abrupt phonation.[12] It also was observed that stutterers repeated part-word items more than twice per instance, whereas non-stutterers rarely repeated an item more than once. A stutterer is more likely to say "Ca-Ca-Ca-Ca-Can I go?" rather than "Ca-Can I go?" If stuttering persists, children learn to avoid situations in which they struggle with words, and their disfluencies are characterized by increased facial tension and frustration.[5] About 25% of those who become chronic stutterers are delayed in the development of language and articulation.

INCIDENCE AND PREVALENCE

Except in rare instances, stuttering generally begins in childhood. The male to female ratio of stuttering is high, approximately 3 to 4:1.[4] Retrospective studies report an incidence or a chance of stuttering at some point in one's life to be about 5%; the prevalence rate in the United States among all age groups is estimated at 1%.[2] The marked difference between incidence and prevalence means that a majority of children recover spontaneously, without formal treatment.[11] It is reported that 50% to 75% of children who stutter recover spontaneously, most within the year of onset.

There have been no adequate explanations as to why more males than females stutter. Many theories have been proposed, including differences in the rate of speech and language development, as well as conjectured differences of parental responses to stuttering in their male children versus their female children. Others quote differential cultural treatment as an explanation of the sex ratio described.

ETIOLOGY

Early concepts of stuttering are based on work by Johnson, who believed that stuttering developed in response to the way in which others, particularly parents, reacted to a child's hesitations and repetitions.[7] Studies of the 1950s focused on auditory processes in stutterers and attempted to understand the effects of delayed auditory feedback on speech production. It was found that when some stutterers are subjected to delayed auditory feedback, their speech becomes more fluent; however, no auditory system defects have been identified. Studies of the 1960s and early 1970s analyzed stuttering as a learned behavior, meaning that the momentary reduction of anxiety and tension that follows the stuttering was thought to reinforce unadaptive stuttering.

Investigators currently believe that the stutterer inherits a tendency, making him or her particularly vulnerable to the stresses of language development. Although stuttering has long been recognized as a familial disorder, it is unlikely that its genetic component will be characterized by simple transmission. The risk of stuttering among first-degree relatives is more than three times the risk of the population as a whole.[3] The risk for a child with a parent who stutters is 17%, among siblings is 15%, and for monozygotic twins as high as 77%.[8] There also appear to be important prenatal or postnatal factors; genetically identical twins can be discordant for stuttering.

To date, these factors have not been identified.

There is a higher incidence of other speech and language problems in children who stutter as well as a higher incidence of left handedness, mixed cerebral dominance, increased learning disabilities, and atypical patterns on dichotic listening tests.[10] Stutterers have been found to show a three times greater risk of an articulation disorder than do nonstutterers. It may be that a reduced capacity for sensory-motor integration makes one vulnerable to stuttering. Researchers have described minor timing abnormalities even in the fluent productions of stutters.

ASSESSMENT AND INTERVENTION

Developmental disfluency is characteristically observed in a child who has been speaking normally for months who then begins to speak with repetitions, usually repeating the first syllable of a word effortlessly without facial tension or apparent awareness. With most children this period lasts about 3 months, although it may range from a few weeks up to 6 months. The parent can expect periods of inconsistencies and fluent periods mixed with disfluent periods, with a particular increase in disfluency during excitement and stress. Speech-language pathologists commonly advise parents to "ignore it," meaning that the parent should react no differently whether the child is fluent or disfluent; the parent should not advise the child to "slow down" or "think before you speak."

Speech requiring formal evaluation includes persistent or progressive stuttering or stuttering that has additional warning signs. Often the first sign noted in the child having more than the normal difficulty with speech is the increasing repetition of parts of words in unstressed circumstances. A second warning sign is seen in the child who consistently prolongs the first sound of a word or repeats the vowel used to make the "uh" sound in ways that change or distort the flow of speech "uh-uh-uh-over" instead of "o-o-o-over." A third sign a parent may notice is the presence of mouth tremors. The mouth may be held in one position with no sound being expressed. At other times a rise in pitch may be heard as an attempt is made to express a word with signs of increased tension in the lips, jaw, larynx, and chest. A fleeting moment of fear may develop as the child reacts to disturbances in speech.[1] As the disorder progresses, fear of speaking and anticipatory tension become generalized to many interactive situations and the stutterer creates a compensatory convoluted speaking style.[5]

Other language and articulation disorders need to be differentiated from stuttering and require different treatment. *Cluttering* is characterized by speech so rapid that syllables and words are omitted, resulting in unintelligible speech. In contradistinction to stuttering, cluttering may be improved by conscious slowing of speech. *Palilalia* is characterized by whole word, phrase, or sentence repetition associated with neurologic diseases such as pseudobulbar palsy. Also, patients who have had a cerebrovascular insult with dysphasia may experience stuttering-like behaviors.

Parents can promote the fluency of a child who stutters by speaking more simply and slowly to their child than they speak to others. They should listen for content rather than disfluencies, trying not to interrupt their child and maintaining good eye contact. It is important to reduce the tension of a fast-paced household, teaching the family to take turns talking. Children in whom stuttering has developed are at risk for a negative self-image and tend to suffer socially and academically. Parents should not correct or criticize their child's speech, but rather acknowledge their child's strengths.

Indications for immediate referral to a speech-language pathologist include the child who (1) is disfluent more than 6 months, (2) is attempting to avoid speaking, (3) exhibits signs of facial tension or extra movement of the head or body, (4) has anxious parents demonstrating physical or verbal correction as the child speaks, or (5) is of school age.[6]

Current methods of treatment for stuttering depend on the severity of the disorder. Included is indirect treatment in which the parents enhance their family's interactions in ways that promote fluency. Direct treatment is usually with a speech-language pathologist and involves individual stuttering modification therapy and fluency-shaping therapy. The interactive exercises of stuttering modification therapy include a slow and relaxed style of speaking, forming a model for the child to mimic, and learning to handle words that are difficult. Fluency-shaping therapy would begin with short fluent responses, which are gradually increased in length and complexity. Outcome is influenced by such factors as severity and chronicity of the problem, the presence of other disabilities, and the degree of family involvement. Relapse after treatment is decreased by "booster" sessions with the speech-language pathologist.

Although the exact nature of stuttering remains a mystery, the prognosis is generally good. With careful observation, the physician is able to reassure parents and confidently refer them for further assessment and treatment when indicated.

REFERENCES

1. Ainsworth S and Fraser J: If your child stutters, ed 3, Pub No 11, Memphis, Tenn, 1988, Speech Foundation of America.
2. Andrews G, Craig A, and Feyer A: Stuttering: a review of research findings and theories circa 1982, J Speech Hear Disord 48:226, 1983.
3. Andrews G, Neilson M, and Curlee R: Stuttering, JAMA 260:1445, 1988.
4. Debney SJ and Parry-Fiedler BR: The child who stutters: theory and therapy in the 1980's, Aust Paediatr J 24:273, 1988.
5. Guitar BE: Stuttering, Feelings and Their Medical Significance 31:1, 1989.
6. Guitar BE: Stuttering and stammering, Pediatr Rev 7:163, 1985.
7. Johnson W: Stuttering in children and adults, Minneapolis 1955, University of Minnesota Press.
8. Molecular genetics: the key to the puzzle of stuttering? ASHA 30:36, 1988.
9. Starkweather CW: The development of fluency in normal children, Pub No 20, Memphis, Tenn, 1982, Speech Foundation of America.
10. Strub RL, Black AW, and Naeser MA: Anomalous dominance in sibling stutterers: evidence from CT scan asymmetries, dichotic listening, neuropsychological testing and handedness, Brain Lang 30:338, 1987.
11. Van Riper C: The nature of stuttering, Englewood Cliffs, NJ, 1982, Prentice Hall.
12. Yairi E and Lewis B: Disfluencies at the onset of stuttering, J Speech Hear Res 27:158, 1984.

93

Temper Tantrums and Breath-Holding Spells

Gregory E. Prazar

TEMPER TANTRUMS

Temper tantrums represent a behavior that children almost inevitably exhibit during the second through fourth years of life. Therefore, this is generally a "problem behavior" rather than a "behavioral problem." Displays of temper can run the gamut from a verbalized "no" to dramatic breath-holding spells, during which the child may lose consciousness. Helping parents cope with temper tantrums involves anticipatory guidance, sharing information about developmental psychology, and offering strategies to deal with tantrums.

Temper tantrums usually become part of the child's emotional repertoire during the second and third years of life. Early signs of the negativism that is part of tantrums can be appreciated as early as 12 months of age. Some children continue to display occasional tantrums until age 5 or 6. Tantrums then reappear in a slightly less intense form during adolescence, when independence once more becomes an issue for the developing child.

Several aspects of the toddler's development appear to make tantrums almost inevitable. First, because the 1-year-old can walk and climb, the child begins to achieve physical mastery over the environment. This increased physical independence and an insatiable curiosity frequently place the child in dangerous situations that require parental intervention. Imposition of adult safety limits thwarts and frustrates the child, often precipitating tantrums.

Second, the child's increased exploration of the environment immediately creates a conflict because he or she must adapt to rules of an adult world. The child enters a hostile environment of adult social values, where people are expected to use the bathroom appropriately, verbalize their dissatisfactions rather than "act" them out physically, sit quietly while eating, and sometimes subjugate their own wants to those of others. This is too much for the egocentric toddler to bear, and frustration is inevitable.

Third, between the ages of 1 and 4 years the toddler begins to develop an increased awareness of how he or she is separate and different from his or her mother. The child experiences a conflict between desires for autonomy and desires to remain close to the mother. Frustration in dealing with these intense feelings frequently results in tantrums.

Tensions, therefore, are created in "establishing ego boundaries as separate from those of parents," as Brazelton[1] states, and in coping with physical limitations placed on exploring an adult world. Adults frequently deal with their own tensions and frustrations by verbalizing their feelings; the toddler, however, lacks a sophisticated ability to verbalize. A toddler's frustration with the adult world may be displayed in doing the exact opposite of what the adult requests, by saying "no, no" yet following through with the adult request (what Fraiberg[2] refers to as the "cheerful no"), by dawdling, or by displaying physical behavior outright (e.g., kicking, screaming, lying on the floor, hitting, throwing, biting).

Most parents would probably agree that intellectual appreciation of the etiology of tantrums does not necessarily aid in coping with a screaming and inconsolable child. There are understandable reasons for parental frustration. Well-meaning relatives and friends (who have likely forgotten their experience as young parents) may propagate myths about tantrums. These myths intensify parental anxiety and confusion. Myths of causation suggest that children who display tantrums are overindulged, underdisciplined, or parented by inadequate adults. Myths of management suggest that tantrums should be quelled by spanking, dousing with cold water, or convincing the child with threats not to have a tantrum.

Anticipatory Guidance for Tantrums

It is the responsibility of the primary care physician to provide anticipatory guidance about temper tantrums. Such guidance may forestall events that precipitate tantrums and prevent future parental confusion in dealing with negative behaviors. The physician has many opportunities during the child's first 2 years to provide behavioral counseling.

At the 6-month infant visit, the importance of time away from the infant should be emphasized. Parents who occasionally leave their infants and toddlers with responsible babysitters provide their children with the security that adults can leave and *will* come back and provide themselves with important mental health holidays from the rigors of parenting.

At the 9- or 12-month infant visit, environmental engineering should be discussed. The importance of home safety (e.g., safety plugs in outlets, safety latches on drawers), the removal of valuables or breakables from the child's reach, and the availability of a safe place for the child to play (playpen or enclosed area) are examples of such engineering. Therefore this visit not only may reduce chances for childhood accidents, but also may forestall potential adult-toddler power struggles over environmental dangers.

The 15- or 18-month visit provides the physician another opportunity to offer the parent alternatives to negative interactions with the toddler. Afternoon naps (to allow for renewal of toddler and maternal energy), the importance of praising cooperative toddler efforts, and the concept of limited decision-making for the toddler ("Do you want to wear the green or blue shirt today?" versus "Which shirt do you want to wear today?") represent anticipatory issues that may help parents minimize hostile encounters with their toddler.

The approach here should be one that encourages parents to describe how they believe tantrums should be handled rather than one that displays the physician's personal biases about child rearing. Several excellent books describing turbulent toddlerhood can be suggested to parents, including Brazelton's *Toddlers and Parents,*[1] Ilg and Ames's *Child Behavior,*[3] and Schmitt's *Your Child's Health.*[5] Furthermore, *general* guidelines concerning tantrums can be given. Tantrums are best ignored unless, as Fraiberg[2] states, "they encroach on rights of others or potentially endanger." If safety is the issue, either environmental engineering should take place or the child should be restricted to his or her room for 2 to 3 minutes (a kitchen timer is helpful to remind both parent and toddler of the time). If the child hits, bites, or throws in anger, room restriction for 2 to 3 minutes should once again be suggested.

Some parents are reluctant to use bedroom restriction because they worry either that the child will associate the bedroom with unpleasant experiences or that the child will not feel adequately remorseful if placed in a room full of toys. Parents should be reassured that room restriction does not cause bedroom fears. Similarly, goals of discipline are to teach rules and to help the child understand what behaviors are acceptable. Discipline does not need to be severe to be effective.

More specific guidelines for managing tantrums may be necessary in individual situations. Parents should be encouraged by the physician to ventilate their feelings (to the physician) about tantrums and need reassurance that they are doing the best job they can for the toddler.

Management of Problem Tantrums

Although tantrums represent a stage of the normal, developing toddler personality, several factors may suggest that further professional intervention is advisable. Toddlers who display persistent negativism or tantrums may suffer from too restrictive parenting, may receive too little positive reinforcement and affection, or may have parents who place unreasonable behavioral expectations on them.

Children who regularly display tantrums past 5 or 6 years of age may be displaying signs of depression or poor self-esteem, or they may be children who live in a family in which emotional problems exist. When temper tantrums regularly occur at school, academic problems should be suspected, as peer pressure usually inhibits displays of tantrums. Children exhibiting persistent tantrums with other associated behaviors (e.g., inability to concentrate, stereotypic behaviors, unrealistic fears, inability to display affection) are children who may have underlying emotional problems. Similarly, parents who verbalize persistent frustration with tantrums or an inability to cope with age-appropriate tantrums may need more comprehensive counseling than the primary practitioner can provide.

Many parenting groups are now available to help parents cope with negative behaviors. Programs such as Systematic Training for Effective Parenting (STEP) and Parent Effectiveness Training (PET) provide valuable community referral sources for families. If such services are not available, or if it is obvious that more sophisticated professional counseling is warranted, the family should be referred to a psychiatrically trained counselor.

Referral should be discussed as soon as the physician anticipates its necessity and should stress the involvement of *both* parents. The physician should maintain contact with the family concerning their problem after the referral has been made. Such ongoing contact may solidify the family's commitment to obtain and comply with the counseling.

BREATH-HOLDING SPELLS

Breath-holding spells represent a childhood behavior that causes particular anxiety for parents. Spells occur between ages 6 months and 5 years, with most occurring between 12 and 18 months of age. Menkes[4] states that approximately 5% of all children display breath-holding spells. The pathophysiology of such spells, however, is unclear.

Spells are precipitated by anger, frustration, fear, or minor injury (often a very minor head injury) and are categorized as *cyanotic spells* or *pallid spells*. In both types, spells are unlikely to occur more often than once a day and are apparently not associated with an increased predisposition to epilepsy (although brief seizurelike activity can occur as a terminating event in either form of spell).

Cyanotic breath-holding spells are more often precipitated by anger or frustration than by fear or injury. The toddler emits a short, loud cry, takes a deep breath, and holds it. Cyanosis occurs after approximately 30 seconds. Either the attack terminates at this point or the toddler becomes rigid or limp and loses consciousness (loss of consciousness occurs in approximately 50% of all children who have breath-holding spells). In rare situations, mild clonic movements of the extremities follow.

Pallid breath-holding spells are similar to cyanotic spells in most respects, but more often are precipitated by fear or minor injury. The initial cry is brief or silent. The spell then proceeds as with a cyanotic spell. Toddlers who suffer from pallid spells often are from families with a history of syncope and, in fact, themselves have an increased chance of syncopal attacks as adults.

Since both forms of breath-holding spells can potentially terminate with seizurelike movements, differentiation between spells and epilepsy is important. Patients with epilepsy, when they have seizures, display cyanosis *during* or *after* the seizures, not before seizure onset. Furthermore, electroencephalograms performed on patients who suffer from breath-holding spells are normal during non-breath-holding periods; patients with epilepsy often have abnormal electroencephalograms during seizure-free periods.

Management of Breath-Holding

There is no effective medical therapy for breath-holding spells, although some toddlers who experience seizurelike activity with spells are placed on anticonvulsant therapy. However, the decision to use medication remains a controversial issue among pediatric neurologists.

Coping with breath-holding spells can be extremely difficult for parents. Spells that terminate with loss of consciousness or with seizurelike movements are obviously frightening. Convincing parents that no harm will come to their child is important. Nevertheless, parents of a breath-holder frequently will not enforce limits for fear of precipitating the child's anger and then an attack. Such parents need repeated reassurance and encouragement to continue age-appropriate limits on their child's behavior. To do otherwise will create an overindulged child who may subsequently fear loss of parental love *because* limits have been rescinded.

When to refer a breath-holding patient to a neurologist or a psychiatrically trained professional may not be an easy decision for the physician. If parents request further consultation, their wish certainly should be respected, even if the physician is confident that further evaluation is unnecessary. If parents indicate agreement with the physician that spells are of no consequence, yet continue to withhold appropriate limit-setting, referral to a mental health professional should take place. The physician who is unsure of the diagnosis of breath-holding (especially in situations where loss of consciousness or seizurelike activity occurs) should always refer the family to a pediatric neurologist. Referral must not end the physician-parent communication concerning the spells, however, because an ongoing dialogue may ensure compliance with the referral source.

SUMMARY

Temper tantrums and breath-holding spells usually represent benign forms of childhood behavior, evolving from the child's preverbal attempts to express feelings of frustration and anger. Unfortunately, parents frequently find it difficult to appreciate the benign course of such behaviors when they must daily face a screaming, inconsolable toddler who may even lose consciousness and then display seizurelike movements. Parents can best deal with negative behaviors when they are adequately prepared by the physician *before* such behaviors occur and when they are offered empathic guidance and positive reinforcement during regular office visits.

REFERENCES

1. Brazelton TB: Toddlers and parents, New York, 1979, Dell Publishing Co.
2. Fraiberg S: The magic years, New York, 1959, Charles Scribner's Sons.
3. Ilg FL and Ames LB: Child behavior, New York, 1955, Harper & Row, Publishers, Inc.
4. Menkes JH: Textbook of child neurology, ed 2, Philadelphia, 1980, Lea & Febiger.
5. Schmitt B: Your child's health, New York, 1987, Bantam Books, Inc.

94

Tics

John S. Werry

DEFINITION AND CLASSIFICATION

Tics are recurring, nonrhythmic, sudden, rapid, stereotyped, involuntary movements or vocalizations.[1] The muscles affected are mostly those of the head, neck, and respiratory tract. Tics are usually easily distinguishable from chorea (with which they are most often confused) by their centripetal location, fixed form, and site. They are distinguished from most other neurologically based spontaneous movements by their rapidity, fixity, or location. An additional useful diagnostic feature is that tone of the muscles involved in tics is normal.

Tics are exacerbated by emotion, they disappear in sleep, and they can be controlled to a degree but not completely. These characteristics are not as helpful in differential diagnosis as might be supposed, since they are also present in many neurologically based spontaneous movement disorders. Tics are distinguished from self-stimulating behaviors by their later onset, their more restricted localization and complexity, their involuntary nature, and the apparent lack of pleasure associated with the movement (see Chapter 91, "Self-Stimulating Behaviors").

There are three types of tic disorder: transient (duration longer than 2 weeks but less than 1 year); chronic (longer than 1 year); and Tourette syndrome (multiple tics, including vocal tics).[1] It is not known whether these three disorders are simply more or less severe instances of the same disorder, but there is no doubt that Tourette syndrome disorder is much more disabling.[1,8]

FREQUENCY

Tics can begin as early as age 1 year, but the peak prevalence is around 9 to 12 years of age (2 years earlier for those with Tourette syndrome), after which their frequency declines rapidly.[1,8] At peak prevalence, they may affect from 5% to 24% of children, depending on the criteria used for diagnosis. Boys are more affected than girls, especially in severe cases, where the ratio is at least three to one.

ETIOLOGY

The cause of tics is unknown in most cases, although in a small number they reflect or portend a neurologic disorder.[3,8] Such tics are likely to be much more persistent and to be accompanied by signs of the causative disorder.

Some of the factors that have been shown to be associated with tics and thus may give clues to the cause are the following.[1,8]

1. *Developmental stage*. That tics are common in middle childhood and disappear soon after points very strongly to maturational factors in the neuromuscular apparatus that are mirrored in the general high frequency of all spontaneous movements (such as choreiform movements) at this age.
2. *Sex*. The preponderance of boys affected also supports the motor developmental view, since boys are motorically more active than girls at all ages but especially in middle childhood.[8]
3. *Prenatal and perinatal insults*. There is some association between the same group of factors that has been identified in some cases of hyperactivity; as in that condition, however, this association is at best weak and can explain only a small number of tics, since this finding appears only in large-scale epidemiologic studies.[8]
4. *Psychological factors*. Anxiety is clearly associated with many cases of tics, in that it makes existing tics worse and probably precipitates them in some cases; furthermore, children with anxiety disorders or overanxious personalities are overrepresented in clinical cases.[8] However, little is known about the psychological status of the vast majority of children with tics, since most are never seen in clinics and therefore are not studied. There is also a strong relationship between tics and hyperactivity, especially in Tourette syndrome.[1,3,5,6]
5. *Neurobiologic causes*. The low probability that tics are symptomatic of a frank brain disorder has already been noted. Tourette syndrome, however, has long been suspected of having a neurologic basis, despite the failure thus far to demonstrate such a cause. Heredity may be important in Tourette syndrome and tics,[1] but this requires confirmation.[9] The neurobiologic substrate of any abnormality or predisposition remains elusive, although for physiologic and pharmacologic reasons (see below), dopamine and other monoamines have attracted the most interest so far.[3]
6. *Drugs*. Amphetamine induces stereotypic behaviors in rats and can occasionally produce them in children, although they are usually of the dyskinetic type. It was suspected that stimulants given for hyperactivity might precipitate tics or Tourette syndrome in vulnerable children, but this is now thought to be caused by the common association of the two disorders. However, it is prudent not to give stimulants to hyperactive children if there is any history of tics or Tourette syndrome.[5]

Also, stimulants aggravate tics and should therefore not be given if tics are present. If tics emerge subsequently, the stimulants should be stopped and other medications substituted.[5]

In summary, it seems reasonable to posit that, in most cases, tics appear spontaneously as exaggerations of spontaneous movements normal at that stage of development, but that in others they are catalyzed by increased motor activity or excitability interacting with neuromuscular development status, as in hyperactivity or anxiety. In a few cases, notably Tourette syndrome, tics are probably the result of an as yet unestablished abnormality of the neuromotor system. As with any other motor behavior, however, tics may be influenced by learning or conditioning, which may serve to prolong or shorten their course.

Tics should never be assumed to signal a psychiatric disorder unless they are associated with other signs or symptoms of such a disorder that affect other areas of function beyond the motor system. Also, though tics can be controlled to some degree for variable periods (such as in the pediatrician's office), this should not be interpreted as voluntary and thus "psychogenic," since such control requires considerable concentration and emotional energy from the child, which can be executed only for limited periods. As soon as the child forgets, is distracted, or lets up concentration in the least, the tics will reappear.

TREATMENT

As in so much of medicine, the best treatment for most tics is masterly inactivity coupled with authoritative information to child and parents about the condition.[8] Clearly, any unreasonable and avoidable stress on the child should be reduced as a general measure; however, tics should not be a sign to treat the child as though she or he were necessarily overstressed or anxious. First, that presumes a cause that may not be present; and second, if it is, some stress is not only an inexorable part of life but is also one of the ways children learn how to cope. Hyperactivity or attention deficit disorder may also be present and require attention.

Once a tic has been present, unchanged in form or site for more than a year, treatment may be considered—but only if the tic is conspicuous, disabling, or distressing to the child. Treatments that have been shown to be effective are the following:

1. *Behavioral methods*.[2,8] These are the only methods that are of a truly curative nature. They are not always completely successful, although some improvement can be expected even in Tourette syndrome.[2] There is a variety of such techniques (e.g., massed practice, habit reversal, and avoidance learning); all, however, are specialized and best carried out by a psychologist who is used to working with children, since the procedures are difficult and children are passively resistant.
2. *Anxiety-reducing procedures*.[7] These include relaxation training, biofeedback, psychotherapy, and, where possible, general adjustment of the child's life-style. Unlike behavioral methods, however, none of these is of proven value in tics; neither should these procedures be considered specific; rather, they are ancillary and holistic in objective.
3. *Pharmacotherapy*.[3,7,8] Because of the risks involved and the lack of any truly curative value, drugs should be used only when tics are seriously disabling. In practice, this is likely to be in Tourette syndrome or in multiple severe tics. Medication should not be given simply for cosmetic reasons, except for very brief periods in times of social imperative.

Whatever their cause, tics are executed via the basal ganglia and appear to reflect an overactivity, actual or relative, of dopaminergic systems, which inhibit cholinergic systems responsible for the modulation of movement. The caricature of this modulation can be seen in parkinsonian states, in which movement is so restricted that it often becomes impossible. The effect of dopamine is the opposite—that is, it produces unregulated or spontaneous movements. Evidence to support the hyperdopaminergic view is largely inferential, since tics are aggravated by amphetamines, which are dopamine-releasing agents, and almost all tics can be suppressed or greatly reduced with dopamine blockers, notably antipsychotics (neuroleptics), such as haloperidol. There is some recent evidence that noradrenergic mechanisms may also be involved. For example, Tourette syndrome may also respond in some cases to clonidine,[3] although the action of this drug, like that of so many neurotropic agents, is less than pure from a neurotransmitter point of view.

Although neuroleptics are often effective, their action is symptomatic, not curative. The doses that need to be given are often rather high; thus side effects, such as extrapyramidal symptoms, atropinic syndromes, and an unpleasant kind of sedation, are common. In some cases, relief may be obtained with low doses; however, there is still reason for caution because of the risk of developing the irreversible neurologic syndrome of tardive dyskinesia[4] (orolinguobuccal spontaneous movements that sometimes extend to regions or whole sides of the body as hemiballismus). This disorder is thought to result from postsynaptic receptor hypersensitivity resulting from prolonged blockade. There have been a number of successful lawsuits against physicians for this complication, and it is necessary that the risks involved be discussed fully and that informed consent be obtained. It is strongly urged that a second opinion, by a specialist, be obtained before pharmacotherapy is undertaken.

Although it may seem logical to use anxiolytic drugs in the management of tic disorders, their use, too, should occur only in unusual instances. All anxiolytics and sedatives (excluding antipsychotics and antihistamines, which are not true sedatives) produce a general reversible depression in neuronal excitability that affects the highest functions of the brain, such as attention, thinking, judgment, and fine motor coordination.[7] In addition, anxiolytics and sedatives are euphoriants, like alcohol, and can lead to dependence. They can induce seizures on withdrawal and, like anticonvulsants such as phenobarbital and phenytoin, can make children more irritable, explosive, and aggressive. Most important, they can impair learning.[7] The muscle relaxant properties of the benzodiazepines are clinically insignificant in doses that do not also impair brain function, so they cannot be defended on the basis of that property, either.[7]

In summary, then, tics should be treated pharmacotherapeutically only as a last resort. Such treatment should be carefully considered and discussed, closely monitored, and undertaken only with knowledge and consideration of the risks and disadvantages involved.

Referral to Mental Health Specialists

Criteria for referring children with tics to a mental health specialist are as follows: (1) tics associated with other clear evidence of psychiatric disorder, such as overanxiety or hyperactivity; (2) chronic or recurrent tics that seem to have a clear relationship to stress and when there is reason to believe that mental health procedures may be helpful; or (3) chronic, disabling, or discomforting tics for which differential diagnosis or treatment is indicated.

In general, the preferred specialist is a modern, properly trained child and adolescent psychiatrist—that is, one who has a broad biopsychosocial perspective, including a good grasp of neuropsychiatry and pharmacotherapy but a "light" prescribing hand and a capacity to work closely with behavioral psychologists.

PROGNOSIS

Most tics last only a few weeks and disappear spontaneously, though they may flit from one muscle group to another or change their form at irregular intervals.[8] Even chronic tics are likely to disappear in adolescence, although it goes without saying that the longer a tic has been present and unchanged in form or site, the less likely it will be to disappear. It is also obvious that since the prevalence drops sharply after age 13 years, appearance or persistence of a tic after that age is more likely to be chronic.

Tourette syndrome, however, is generally a lifelong condition, but it generally improves somewhat and even sometimes disappears in late adolescence or adulthood.[1,3]

Behavioral methods of treatment can influence the course of tics, but there is no evidence that any other treatment affects prognosis, as opposed to suppressing symptoms.

REFERENCES

1. American Psychiatric Association: Diagnostic and statistical manual (DSM-III-R), ed 3 (revised), Washington, DC, 1987, The Association.
2. Azrin NH and Peterson AL: Behavior therapy for Tourette's syndrome and tic disorders. In Cohen DJ, Leckman JF, and Bruun RD, editors: Tourette's syndrome: clinical understanding and treatment, New York, 1988, John Wiley & Sons, Inc.
3. Cohen DJ and Leckman JF: Tourette's syndrome: advances in treatment and research, J Am Acad Child Psychiatry 23:123, 1984.
4. Gualtieri CT et al: Tardive dyskinesia and other movement disorders in children treated with psychotropic drugs, J Am Acad Child Psychiatry 19:491, 1980.
5. Riddle MA et al: Desipramine treatment of boys with attention-deficit hyperactivity disorder and tics: preliminary clinical experience, J Am Acad Child Adolesc Psychiatry 27:811, 1988.
6. Sverd J et al: Behavior disorder and attention deficits in boys with Tourette's syndrome, J Am Acad Child Adolesc Psychiatry 27:413, 1988.
7. Werry JS: An overview of pediatric psychopharmacology, J Am Acad Child Psychiatry 21:3, 1982.
8. Werry JS: Physical illness, symptoms and allied disorders. In Quay HC and Werry JS, editors: Psychopathological disorders of childhood, ed 3, New York, 1986, John Wiley & Sons, Inc.
9. Zausmer DM and Dewey ME: Tics and heredity: a study of the relatives of child tiqueurs, Br J Psychiatry 150:628, 1987.

SUGGESTED READING

Cohen DJ, Leckman JF, and Bruun RD, editors: Tourette's syndrome: clinical understanding and treatment, New York, 1988, John Wiley & Sons, Inc.

95

Adolescence

W. Sam Yancy

Adolescence is generally defined as the period of psychological growth and development during the transition from childhood to adulthood. Physical growth and development, or pubescence, also occurs during this time. Many changes occur that can be confusing for both teenagers and the adults who care for them. *Rebellious* and *tumultuous* are terms often associated with this age group. *Joyous* and *carefree* are more positive adjectives also used to describe adolescents. With such diverse feelings about teenagers, it is no wonder that the health care of adolescents in the United States has so long been neglected.

Recent efforts on behalf of adolescents have occurred not because of increasing problems of this age group and certainly not because of increasing demands by teenagers themselves, but rather because of the recognition of adolescents' unmet needs. It was formerly believed that this was a carefree, healthy age, one that required no special interest by health care professionals. In spite of morbidity and mortality statistics that are often reported in such a way as to make it difficult to identify the needs of adolescents, impressive data are available to justify an increase in adolescent medicine training programs and to encourage more health care delivery services for this age group.

The prevalence of sexually transmitted diseases, pregnancies, substance abuse, suicides, delinquency, chronic illness, mental illness, and school problems cannot be ignored.[1,3,4] Equally if not more important is the need for practitioners who have knowledge of normal adolescent development and of the behaviors in adolescents of concern to patients and their parents during this time. Diagnosis and treatment of the physical and psychosocial problems of adolescents, as well as early identification of and appropriate intervention for these, should be incorporated into the practices of all primary care physicians.

Although attention was focused on the health care needs of adolescents in England as early as the late 1800s, it was not until the 1930s that significant reports about this age group began to appear in U.S. medical literature. And it was not until 1951 that the first separate hospital inpatient adolescent unit was established, at Boston Children's Hospital.

Progress in this area is outlined in the accompanying box. Pediatricians have taken the lead in health care delivery to adolescents, as evidenced (1) by the report of the Task Force on Pediatric Education[2] calling for increased training in adolescent medicine, (2) by the requirement of the Pediatric Residency Review Committee of the Accreditation Council for Graduate Medical Education that all pediatric residency programs include training in adolescent medicine, and (3) by the fact that 95% of all divisions of adolescent medicine and all of the adolescent medicine fellowship training programs are based in departments of pediatrics. Teenagers, however,

Progress in Adolescent Medicine

1938	Publication of Greulich WW et al: A handbook of methods for the study of adolescent children, Monogr Soc Res Child Dev, vol 3, no 2, serial no 13, Washington, DC, 1938.
1941	Publication of American Academy of Pediatrics: Symposium on adolescence, J Pediatr 19:289, 1941.
1951	First Adolescent Unit, Boston Children's Hospital.
1965	Four adolescent medicine fellowship programs listed in *Journal of Pediatrics.*
1968	Society for Adolescent Medicine founded.
1968	First federal funding for adolescent medicine training programs, Division of Maternal and Child Health, Department of Health, Education, and Welfare.
1975	First International Symposium on Adolescent Medicine, Helsinki.
1977	Adolescent medicine designated as a specialty by American Medical Association (AMA).
1978	National Conference on Adolescent Behavior and Health, Institute of Medicine of the National Academy of Sciences.
1979	Section on Adolescent Health established by American Academy of Pediatrics.
1980	First volume published of the *Journal of Adolescent Health Care.*
1987	International Association for Adolescent Health founded.
1988	First Annual AMA National Congress on Adolescent Health.
1989	Forty-one adolescent medicine fellowship programs listed in *Journal of Adolescent Health Care.*

are cared for by professionals in many disciplines (i.e., internists, obstetrician-gynecologists, psychiatrists, psychologists, family physicians, social workers, nurses, and educators). Indeed, the most effective health care programs for youth depend on the collaboration of several disciplines to provide comprehensive care for these patients.

REFERENCES

1. Blum R: Contemporary threats to adolescent health in the United States, JAMA 257:3390, 1987.
2. Cohen MI: Importance, implementation, and impact of the adolescent medicine components of the report of the Task Force on Pediatric Education, J Adol Health Care 1:1, 1980.
3. Cohen MI: Adolescent health: concerns for the eighties, Pediatr Rev 4:4, 1982.
4. Hein K: Issues in adolescent health: an overview, Washington, DC, 1988, Carnegie Council on Adolescent Development.

SUGGESTED READINGS

Gallagher JR: The origins, development and goals of adolescent medicine, J Adol Health Care 3:57, 1982.

Neinstein LS: Adolescent health care: a practical guide, Baltimore, 1984, Urban & Schwarzenberg.

Thornburg HD: Development in adolescence, ed 2, Monterey, Calif, 1982, Brooks/Cole.

96

Challenges of Health Care Delivery to Adolescents

Sandra R. Leichtman and Stanford B. Friedman

Adolescence refers to that period of physical and psychosocial growth that marks the transition from childhood to adulthood. The beginning of adolescence is characterized by the onset of puberty and the psychological reaction to these developmental changes; the end of adolescence is marked by preparedness for and opportunity to assume an adult role in society. Throughout the adolescent period, the interaction of physical and psychosocial factors creates unique problems and challenges for adolescents, their parents, and their physicians.

With the onset of pubescence, adolescents experience many changes in physical and sexual growth and maturation that may be confusing to them. Among the concerns of adolescents are whether they are "normal" and maturing at a rate similar to that of other adolescents. In their attempts to adjust psychologically to these body changes, adolescents should know that they can turn to their physicians for professional help regarding normal or abnormal issues of growth and development. Many relatively minor problems, such as acne, may be of great concern to body-conscious adolescents. It is important that physicians anticipate adolescents' concerns and encourage them to ask questions that they may be reluctant to pose, lest they appear naive or for fear of the physician's response.

Adolescents often react to the difficult developmental process by purposely opposing requests of adults, deriding parental standards, and imprudently flouting their adult privileges. Adolescents frequently will transfer feelings related to parental authority onto the physician, producing challenging and often frustrating doctor-patient relationships. Concern with being controlled, for example, can lead adolescents to refuse medical recommendations or to counter suggestions with arguments that may appear illogical or unreasonable to the physician. On the other hand, adolescents may actively seek the counsel of physicians because they are viewed as possessing wisdom by virtue of being adult authorities outside of the direct parent-child relationship. In either case, the physician needs to be able to encourage and respect the adolescent's wish to act as an independent individual, while at the same time recognizing that most adolescents still require guidance and control by adults.

Another potential difficulty in providing medical services to adolescents involves the physician's attitudes toward adolescent behavior, especially in the area of sexuality. Included among the common sexual concerns of adolescents are fears of homosexuality and fantasized consequences of masturbation. Any adolescent involved in or contemplating intimate heterosexual relationships should be able to turn to the physician for advice regarding issues such as birth control, pregnancy, and sexually transmitted diseases. It is critical that the physician's own personal beliefs regarding adolescent sexuality not interfere with the ability to provide medical counseling and treatment in a manner that will be most helpful to the adolescent and consistent with the adolescent's value system. The adolescent does not seek out the physician for a sermon.

Finally, the transitional nature of the adolescent period creates complications with respect to adolescent problems and to the question of who should treat the adolescent. The lack of synchronization of the physical and psychosocial changes that characterize the adolescent age group results in the adolescent being neither child nor adult, but unevenly sharing attributes of both. For example, although the adolescent may resemble the adult with respect to biologic aspects of sexual maturity, psychological immaturity can impede prudent judgment, resulting in problems such as sexually transmitted disease and pregnancy. Thus the physician wishing to manage adolescent problems needs to be relatively comfortable with the dual and changing nature of the adolescent.

ADOLESCENT HEALTH CARE

In 1972 a policy statement issued by the American Academy of Pediatrics[1] defined the practice of pediatrics as extending from conception through adolescence, terminating around 21 years of age. Despite this inclusion of the adolescent within the province of pediatrics, surveys of pediatricians have indicated that adolescent health care is one of the most underemphasized areas in residency training and is in fact viewed as an area of deficiency. The apparent failure to accord adolescent health care a sufficient role within pediatric training appears to reflect uncertainty about whether to embrace adolescence as an appropriate subset of pediatric practice.

The management and treatment of adolescents often require not only the knowledge, skills, and attitudes from the discipline of pediatrics, but also expertise regarding the unique characteristics of adolescence. It is during this stage of development, for example, that three of the four leading causes of death (accidents, homicide, and suicide) relate directly to life style rather than to disease or congenital infirmities. Similarly, behavioral factors influence major causes of adolescent morbidity, as evidenced in motor vehicle accidents, sexually transmitted diseases, and substance abuse. In addition, behaviors such as smoking that often begin during adolescence can have negative consequences for adult mortality and morbidity.

Thus the physician's greatest influence on preventing mortality and morbidity may be in his or her ability to recognize clues to potentially self-destructive activity and to provide appropriate counseling or referral to a mental health professional.

The specialty of adolescent medicine has developed in response to the special health care needs of adolescents and the unique characteristics of adolescent health care. The establishment of adolescent medicine as a specialty provides the advantages of promoting and expanding knowledge regarding specific adolescent disorders and promotes training in the interaction of physical development, disease, and the psychological issues of adolescence. However, considering adolescent medicine as a specialty may discourage conceptualization of adolescent health care as a basic and integral aspect of general pediatrics, possibly resulting in decreased commitment by the generalist to serve this population. For the adolescent, treatment by a specialist has the empiric advantage of more specialized health care—that is, care by one who specializes in adolescence. However, a potential disadvantage is that the adolescent has to form a new relationship with the adolescent specialist and then, as an adult, must form still another relationship with an internist or a family physician.

Whether specialist or generalist, the physician's major consideration of whether to treat adolescents must be his or her interest and comfort in dealing with the complicated interactions of physical development, disease, and the psychosocial status of those in this age group. Since adolescents have unique characteristics, advanced training in adolescent medicine through fellowships, postgraduate workshops, or continuing medical education programs is recommended for physicians wishing to provide optimum medical care to this age group.

LOCATIONS FOR ADOLESCENT MEDICAL SERVICES

Outpatient Facilities

If the pediatrician wishes to continue treating a patient through adolescence, alterations in the office or clinic may be needed to respect the adolescent's need not to be treated as a child. The adolescent is likely to feel infantile if made to wait in an office replete with crying infants, murals of Walt Disney characters, and children's books, toys, and furniture. To provide more hospitable surroundings for the adolescent, part of the waiting room might be arranged around a reading area containing material appropriate for teens. Suggestions include magazines on sports, pop music, and fashion and booklets on teenage health issues. In addition, some pediatricians might consider arranging for specific office hours and days devoted solely to their teenage patients.

Many hospitals maintain adolescent clinics with facilities structured and operated in a manner well articulated with the psychosocial needs of the adolescent. Certain adult outpatient clinic personnel, particularly those in obstetrics and gynecology, are becoming increasingly aware of the special needs of the adolescent and have set aside specific hours during which only adolescent patients are seen.

Alternatives to traditional outpatient care are provided through free clinics, which were initially established to serve runaway and disaffected youth, and through school-based programs often located in areas of high unmet needs for health care. A relatively recent development in school-based programs is the availability of on-site comprehensive services that go beyond usual health care delivery practices to include provision of mental health, substance abuse, and family and vocational counseling. In some schools, family planning, day care, and hotlines also are available.

Inpatient Facilities

Hospital confinement can be particularly distressing for both the adolescent and the hospital staff. Constraints imposed by medical treatment and hospital regulations seriously interfere with the adolescent's quest for independence, involving freedom to engage in physical activity ad lib. Also, the need for hospitalization may be interpreted by the adolescent as proof that he or she is not normal. The reactions of the adolescent to being hospitalized, including anger, rebellion, and depression, often create serious problems for the physicians and ward personnel.

Generally, hospitals set relatively firm policies with respect to age of admission for those assigned to pediatric and adult inpatient units. These arbitrary and often inflexible demarcations can impede optimum patient care for adolescents. It is as inappropriate to hospitalize a pregnant 15-year-old on a pediatric ward as to admit a physically and psychologically immature 13-year-old to an adult ward.

Some hospitals have adolescent inpatient wards or have designated sections of the pediatric wards for adolescents. These units provide the benefits of a staff interested in adolescents and trained to support and to counsel them as well as to manage their medical and surgical problems. Often ward facilities are available for games (e.g., pool, table tennis), music, and discussion groups. Adolescent inpatient units require a high staff-to-patient ratio to care adequately for the complexities and difficult behavioral problems so typical of those in such facilities.

Although the adolescent unit is uniquely prepared to treat the total patient, difficulties arise with respect to the medical aspects of patient care. Characteristically, multiple medical and surgical subspecialties (e.g., orthopedic surgery, neurosurgery, and ophthalmology) admit adolescents to an adolescent unit. However, a comprehensive patient-care approach is not always appreciated by subspecialty staff, who would prefer to admit adolescent patients in their own specialty-oriented wards. This difference in orientation frequently creates major friction among services and challenges the best efforts of resolution through communication at all levels. Other potential difficulties for specialists when adolescent patients are segregated include duplication of expensive equipment and complications in schedules of rounds. An adolescent ward, therefore, presents an administrative challenge that, if not met, can actually deter optimum hospital care for teenagers.

HOW SERVICES ARE DELIVERED

General Approach

As stated, adolescents generally wish to be approached as independent individuals with many, if not all, of the rights and privileges of adults. From the vantage point of adults, however, adolescents often seem reluctant to assume the associated responsibilities. In truth, adolescents are neither children nor adults and should not be expected to behave as either. They should be encouraged to make their appointments (and cancel them when appropriate) and assume as much of their medical care as judged appropriate by the health team. It is important, however, to consider the psychological and social "age" of the adolescent, as well as the chronologic age. This is especially true of teenagers with chronic illnesses, who may enter adolescence with many handicaps—both physical and psychological. The latter may include a history of poor school performance, parental overprotection, and difficulties with peer relations.

There is no agreement on how best to manage the adolescent patient and his or her parents. Some physicians tend to relate primarily with the adolescent; others work primarily through the parents. In either case, it is most important to define the ground rules to all concerned and always to allow some opportunity to see the adolescent alone and the parents alone. The adolescent's confidentiality should be protected, but it is also desirable to let the parents, who ultimately are responsible for their child's welfare, know whether satisfactory progress is being made. These issues are often easier to resolve in medical and surgical cases than when managing problems related to teenage difficulties such as pregnancy, sexually transmitted disease, and drug abuse.

The rights of adolescents to seek medical advice and help are discussed in detail in Chapter 4. Increasingly, adolescents in most states are being given the right to obtain medical attention without parental consent or knowledge. This legal right, however, does not contradict the general tenet that teenagers, especially the younger ones, are best helped if at some point their parents are involved. The matter of confidentiality is always relative, and a balance must be struck between preserving the teenager's right to medical care and privacy and the parents' obligation in society to be responsible for their children. In the area of confidentiality, physicians should never promise more than they wish to deliver—an adolescent boy threatening suicide should not be told that his parents will remain uninformed!

Management of Referrals

Even the specialist with advanced training in the physical and psychosocial development of the adolescent often will find it necessary to refer a patient for medical or psychological consultation. As with all referrals, the primary care physician can play a key role in helping the parents and the adolescent select the best possible consultant to manage a particular problem. Such consultation should be arranged with the care most physicians use in selecting medical care for their own family members.

The family should be advised as to why the consultation or referral is desirable and should be informed of the options available. In cases of serious disease or trauma, the primary care physician should introduce the family to the specialist who will be assuming the major medical responsibility. In any event, the primary care physician plays an important role in "translating" to both the teenager and the family the admonitions of the specialist.

Referral for emergency psychiatric consultation should be made when an adolescent has an acute psychiatric episode, such as repeated drug intoxication, serious threats of injury to self or others, or depressive symptoms characterized by suicidal ideation or behavior. For reasons of expediency and legality, it is usually essential that the adolescent's parent or guardian be involved in the emergency referral process.

There will be times, other than emergency situations, when the primary care physician believes a referral is needed for psychological, psychiatric, or social reasons. Often adolescents are not ready to seek psychiatric or psychological help, or they view such treatment as a sign that they are crazy. Thus it is important that before making the referral, the physician meet with the adolescent and in many cases the family to determine whether the patient is willing to seek such help and to discuss ways in which mental health consultation or treatment will be beneficial. The adolescent's strengths as well as problem areas should be included in the discussion. To be ensured of appropriate referral resources, it is useful for the physician to establish relations with a few mental health professionals working with adolescents in the community. Adolescents will often be relieved by the knowledge that the physician is acquainted with and has realistic confidence in the person or resource to whom they are being referred.

Time and Cost

As a youngster reaches puberty, the physician wishing to carry the patient through adolescence may find it useful to set up an appointment to discuss the many physical changes that will be occurring and to encourage the adolescent to ask questions regarding physical or psychosocial issues for which he or she wishes education or guidance. Although the physician may have been following the patient for a number of years, this special appointment is in many ways comparable to an initial visit and should be billed accordingly. Before this appointment is made, it is important that the adolescent and the family be informed of the nature of the visit and the anticipated time and cost involved. The physician may want to have pamphlets available on topics that the adolescent might feel uncomfortable approaching directly. Depending on the adolescent's level of maturity, these pamphlets may include information on common adolescent concerns, such as acne, as well as more sensitive topics, including sexually transmitted diseases and problems related to substance abuse.

For the physician who offers counseling to the adolescent, fees should be apportioned according to the amount of time involved. Primary care physicians are often reluctant to charge appropriately for their time, feeling that for the same money the family could have "real" psychiatric help. What is underestimated is the value of the primary care physician's knowledge of the family.

There are situations in which charging according to the time commitment may not be appropriate. For example, when parents refuse to support their troubled adolescent's desire to seek counseling, the physician may wish to establish a special rate, which the adolescent is able to pay. The matter of charging adolescents, in view of changing laws giving adolescents the right to medical care, is an issue that is still far from resolved.

REFERENCE

1. American Academy of Pediatrics: Policy statement, Pediatrics 49:463, 1972.

SUGGESTED READINGS

Felice ME and Friedman SB: Behavioral consideration in the health care of adolescents, Pediatr Clin North Am 29:399, 1982.

Gallagher JR, Heald FP, and Garell DC, editors: Medical care of the adolescent, ed 3, New York, 1976, Appleton-Century-Crofts.

Millstein SG: Adolescent health: challenges for behavioral scientists, Am Psychol 44:837, 1989.

97

Conversion Reactions in Adolescents

Gregory E. Prazar and Stanford B. Friedman

DEFINITION, INCIDENCE, AND ETIOLOGIC FACTORS

The amalgamation of emotions and physical symptoms in patients challenges the primary care physician to formulate priorities in history-taking, diagnosis, and management. Some somatic complaints, such as headaches, nausea, and vomiting, can result directly from emotional upsets. Indeed, anxiety frequently is associated with palpitations, sweating, and tremulousness; depression frequently is manifested by symptoms of fatigue and weakness. Other somatic complaints reflect organic disorders, such as a peptic ulcer, which may be associated with emotional turmoil. Still other physical problems are attributed to conversion symptoms.

Conversion reactions represent a form of communicating the uncomfortable, or, as Engel[2] writes, "a psychic mechanism whereby an idea, fantasy, or wish is expressed in bodily rather than in verbal terms and is experienced by the patient as a physical symptom rather than as a mental symptom." The idea or wish is psychologically threatening to the individual or is unacceptable for him or her to express directly. A conversion symptom serves as a form of decompression, so that unpleasant affects associated with the acknowledgment of the wish are dissipated through use of a somatic symptom. Because the wish is completely unconscious, the patient in no way relates any psychological stigmata to the somatic complaint. As Hollender[5] succinctly states, "The conversion symptom is a code that conceals the message from the sender as well as from the receiver."

To understand why a wish or thought is represented by a bodily symptom, it is necessary to explore patterns of everyday behavior and infant development. Body activity (i.e., gestures) is used to express ideas during verbal interaction. Common conversational phrases frequently allude, in a metaphoric manner, to the intermixing of emotion and body functioning. "I'm fed up" and "He gives me a pain in the neck" are two such examples. Developmentally, infants express feelings and communicate through visible behavior long before spoken language becomes the dominant mode of communication. Furthermore, infants explore and learn about their environment, including the people in it, by using their bodies as investigative tools (e.g., placing new objects in the mouth) and as a means of making contact.

Any bodily process that can be perceived by the individual can serve as the focus for conversion symptoms. Similarly, somatic symptoms of relatives or close friends can also serve as the source for a patient's complaint. It is the patient's *interpretation* of the other person's symptom that provides a model for the somatic complaint. When the symptom is adapted from one observed in the other person, that person frequently evokes strong feelings in the patient. Because the patient feels guilty about his or her feelings or impulses toward that person, he or she may take the other person's symptoms as a form of self-punishment, while at the same time psychologically expressing his or her own forbidden idea or wish.

All body systems may be invoked in a conversion reaction. The sensory system is frequently involved (e.g., paresthesia, anesthesia, or diffuse pain), although typically these symptoms are not distributed in the correct pattern of innervation of the implicated cutaneous nerves. Motor system involvement can be represented by paralysis, tremors, or weakness of an extremity. Hyperventilation and dizziness are other frequent conversion symptoms, as are nausea and vomiting and visual problems.

A common conversion symptom seen in children and young adolescents is abdominal pain. After an extensive investigation of 100 children with abdominal pain, Apley[1] found an organic cause in only eight cases. Another study, by Oster,[10] revealed abdominal pain in 14% of the children studied. The incidence was highest in those 9 years of age and lowest in those 16 to 17 years of age. Controversy exists regarding recurrent abdominal pain and its etiology. However, it is important to remember that many patients who have recurrent abdominal pain may have emotional concerns about which they are unaware. Many of these patients may be suffering from conversion symptoms.

Although studies have been done concerning the incidence of certain individual somatic complaints, specific overall incidences for conversion symptoms in children and adolescents are not known. Available data suggest an incidence of between 5% and 13%.[4] Lack of more definitive data reflects the difficulty in ascertaining whether a somatic complaint indeed represents a conversion symptom. Conversion symptoms may appear to be more common in adolescents than in children because the former more often have somatic complaints of an alarming nature, such as chest pains and fainting spells, whereas children frequently suffer from more indolent complaints, such as sporadic abdominal pains. Conversion symptoms are two to three times more common in females than in males and may appear as early as 7 to 8 years of age.[2] There appears to be no correlation between occurrence of conversion symptoms and socioeconomic status: less sophisticated patients, however, tend to have bizarre and physiologically unexplained symptoms.

Conversion symptoms can appear as a group phenomenon. Such a situation is often referred to as *epidemic hysteria*. Adolescent girls swooning and fainting at rock concerts represent an easily appreciated example. In this situation the unacceptable wish relates to sexualized thoughts involving rock stars. Other examples of epidemic hysteria are less easily explained. Recently described was an incident involving nausea, dizziness, and fainting in a group of teenagers awaiting a change of trains in an unfamiliar train station. Such examples of epidemic hysteria appear to have several common characteristics: (1) audiovisual cues appear to be important in precipitating such reactions, (2) adolescent girls are more frequently involved than are adolescent boys, and (3) the reaction is more likely to occur if initiated by a group member who is identified either as a leader (of a large subgroup) or as an outsider. Entire school populations may be involved in mass conversion reactions.[6,9]

Although conversion symptoms have no organic basis by themselves, their perpetuation may result in biochemical or physiologic body changes. These are referred to as *conversion complications*. They can include changes such as muscle atrophy secondary to long-standing paralysis and respiratory alkalosis secondary to acute hyperventilation. It is important to differentiate conversion complications from psychophysiologically mediated lesions, such as peptic ulcers, in which physiologic processes concomitant with emotions contribute to altered activity of an involuntary body function.

INTERVIEW TECHNIQUES

Since symptoms caused by conversion and somatic processes can be confused easily, the evaluator of any patient with a somatic complaint should always consider the possibility of a conversion symptom. Attention to personal history (family functioning, school performance, and peer relationships), as well as physical functioning, demonstrates to the patient and family that the physician appreciates without prejudice the importance of all elements that may be contributing to ill health. Showing respect for the importance of emotional-physical interaction is thereby suggested, so that this concept will not be foreign if later presented to the family in a diagnostic framework. Such an approach also contributes to the physician's understanding, as Engel[2] states, "of those personal, family, and social circumstances that are most relevant to the understanding of the illness and the care of the patient, whether or not the ultimate diagnosis is conversion."

Nondirective interviewing proves more rewarding than does direct questioning. For example, asking the patient to describe the pain ("Tell me how it feels") almost always provides insight into the emotions the patient associates with the symptom. Suggesting how the symptom feels to the patient ("Is it dull or sharp pain?") limits his or her possible responses. If the patient spontaneously offers information about recent events, the interviewer should obtain further data related to such changes in the patient's life. However, care should be taken to avoid suggesting a cause-and-effect relationship between the patient's feelings and symptoms. Since the patient with conversion symptoms has no conscious knowledge of such an association, the suggestion of such a relationship may cause alienation and prevent the establishment of a trusting relationship.

DIAGNOSTIC CRITERIA FOR CONVERSION SYMPTOMS

The conversion symptom has a specific, but unconscious, symbolic meaning to the patient. In other words, the conversion symptom is often related to an unconscious wish, and the physical impairment serves to prevent acting out of the wish. For example, the adolescent boy with a hand paralysis may have anxieties about masturbating. The physician treating children and adolescents may not always be aware of the symbolic meaning of the symptom. Indeed, the concept that conversion symptoms have a symbolic meaning to the patient was formulated only after a series of these patients had undergone extensive psychotherapy. Although it may be intellectually rewarding for the physician to be cognizant of the presence of the symbolic meaning, ignorance of the specific symbolism does not prevent adequate treatment of the patient. For example:

> Todd, a 12-year-old boy, suddenly developed an inability to walk. Physical examination, including a neurologic evaluation, revealed no abnormalities. Interviews by a psychiatrist and a pediatrician working as a team revealed no apparent symbolic etiologic factor. The pediatrician formulated a system to reward Todd's progress in walking and implemented this approach in a supportive manner. The psychiatrist was similarly supportive with the patient. Over a period of 3 weeks, the patient regained his ability to walk.

Adolescents with conversion symptoms frequently display characteristic patterns of behavior, sometimes designed as traits of the "hysteric personality." Such characteristics include egocentricity, labile emotional states (quick shifts from sadness to elation and from anger to passivity), dramatic, attention-seeking behavior, and sexual provocativeness (displayed in gestures and in dress). Patients with such characteristics also are usually demanding, display an air of pseudomaturity, and are dependent in personal interactions. Their personal relationships, however, are rarely intimate or satisfying. Although many aspects of the hysteric personality are seen in adolescent patients with conversion symptoms, such characteristics also are demonstrable in adolescents free of such symptoms. Therefore hysteric behavior traits in adolescents are not synonymous with conversion symptoms and, in isolation, are not indicative of psychopathology.

The manner in which patients with a conversion symptom describe their problem is frequently distinctive. The account is graphic, frequently bizarre, and often dramatized. A pain may be described as "thousands of burning needles thrust into my leg" or as "a giant spike being driven into my chest." These patients are suggestible, so any symptom description alluded to by the physician may be readily adopted and thereafter reported, which again emphasizes the importance of a nondirective approach in the interview.

As previously described, conversion symptoms are unconsciously adopted in an attempt to reduce unpleasant affects, especially anxiety, depression, and guilt. Therefore, although the patient may describe incapacitating pain, he or she often affects an air of unconcern. Psychiatrists refer to this as *la belle indifference*. The extent to which the conversion symptom diminishes the unpleasant affect and communicates symbolically for the patient the forbidden wish is referred to as the *primary gain*. Patients with conversion reactions often are stubborn in their belief that the symptom is caused by organic problems. This reflects denial of the underlying emotional problem. Conversely, insistence (especially by an adolescent) that a symptom is psychological in origin may indicate denial of a physical problem. Therefore differentiating between conversion symptoms and physical disease in adolescent patients cannot depend purely on the patient's emotional response.

Conversion symptoms not only effect a primary gain for the patient but also help him or her cope with the environment. In this respect, the conversion symptom achieves a *secondary gain* for the patient. For example, the patient with a conversion symptom defending against homosexual thoughts may be excused from attending school, where anxiety may have been intensified (e.g., in the locker room). Limitations imposed by the symptom may contradict the patient's verbalized wishes to participate in activities, but nevertheless remove him or her from potentially threatening social interactions. Interference with daily activities also provides a secondary gain for the patient in that attention and more frequent expressions of love are elicited from concerned parents and friends. This situation may be quite resistant to change, not only because the symptom is continually reinforced, but also because the symptom meets psychological needs of the parents. In effect, the symptom may provide the parents with a reason for nurturing or infantilizing their child. Consequently the patient and his or her entire family may fall into a vicious circle of dependence on the symptom.

Demonstration of a secondary gain does not ensure a diagnosis of conversion. All illness is involved to an extent with some secondary gain. Bedridden patients must accept increased attention to cope with their physical confinement. Therefore a degree of secondary gain is necessary for adequate adaptation to a physical disability. However, in the case of a conversion symptom, secondary gain not only intensifies symptoms but also may be associated with further occurrence of somatic complaints. Since perpetuation of secondary gain depends on concern from others, a conversion symptom is more readily exhibited in the presence of those individuals meaningful to the patient.

Children and adolescents who develop conversion symptoms are often overprotected and become extremely dependent on their parents. Daily familial communication may have been heavily invested in somatic complaints, the child recognizing how often activities may have been cancelled because of father's headaches or mother's cramps. Therefore the patient's symptom may conform to the unspoken interactional rules of the family. The patient's problem is thus indirectly reinforced by family members, who may even assume an air of indifference with respect to his or her symptoms. For example:

> James was a 13-year-old with severe abdominal pain who was referred to a pediatrician by his family practitioner. Physical examination revealed little objective evidence of abdominal pain in the physician's office. However, his return home quickly resulted in intensified pain. Abdominal pain appeared to be well controlled during a subsequent 4-day hospitalization (all organic tests were unremarkable). His return home again produced an immediate exacerbation of the abdominal discomfort. Furthermore, John, James's identical twin, began exhibiting signs of abdominal pain. The boys' mother admitted feeling trapped by the demands of her children and volunteered that in the past she had been treated for chronic abdominal pain. Appearance of abdominal pain in both twins reassured her that the pain was "probably a virus." She chose not to pursue further counseling for the boys.

Precipitation of a conversion symptom may be related to specific stressful events. A change of school, final examinations, new social experiences, and parental conflict are examples of life events that may induce a conversion symptom. A study by Maloney[8] suggests that unresolved grief reactions may represent a source of stress that can precipitate a conversion symptom. Examples of grief reactions listed in the study include loss of a parent through death, divorce, or moving. Because the patient's association between conflict and conversion reaction is unconscious, a history will be helpful only if details concerning daily activities are elicited by the interviewer. Often the stressful event precipitating a conversion symptom becomes apparent only after many visits by the patient. For example:

> Chip, a 13-year-old, was brought by his mother to his pediatrician because of chronic abdominal pain, which appeared to be precipitated by his competing in horse-riding events. His history revealed the death of a grandparent 4 months previously, but his mother alleged that her son's pain preceded the onset of the fatal illness. Other family stresses were denied. The teenager did not appear for follow-up care but returned 6 months later, primarily because his mother wanted to discuss her son's reaction to her upcoming divorce. At this visit, the mother volunteered that marital stress had been ongoing for several years.

Symptom selection is based on the patient's unconscious remembrance of his or her own body function or on his or her understanding of symptoms in others. The patient's conversion symptom may appear quite dissimilar to that displayed by the other (often a parent or a close relative), since it is the patient's *perception* of disease that governs the display of symptoms. Parents and relatives frequently misinform children and adolescents about diseases, fearing that the truth would be too frightening. However, such misinformation may actually potentiate the adolescent's fantasies and result in the development of a symptom quite different from the one actually experienced by the individual serving as the model. For example:

> During a routine physical examination, Jeff, a 14-year-old, mentioned that he experienced "migraine headaches," which appeared to be focused "behind my left eye" and occurred approximately once a month. Jeff's mother attached more importance to the symptoms than did Jeff. Initially, exploration of the family history proved unremarkable. Persistent questioning regarding stress led the mother to mention almost parenthetically that she had recently been diagnosed as having multiple sclerosis. She felt the case to be mild and had therefore not directly told Jeff and her other children about the diagnosis, although she sensed that the children knew. Her initial symptom that precipitated the diagnosis of multiple sclerosis was temporary loss of vision in her left eye.

The choice of a symptom may also be based on a previous physical illness suffered by the patient. Thus patients with a history of seizures may, after many years of adequate anticonvulsant control, have atypical and physiologically unexplainable seizures. Unfortunately, these patients often receive only a physiologic workup for seizures. The physician assumes, despite the atypical history, that the diagnosis rests "where the money is, or was" in the past. For example:

> Craig, a 15-year-old, had recently been treated for otitis media. Associated with pain was some dizziness. After the ear appeared adequately healed, his dizziness persisted. By encouraging Craig to discuss his daily schedule, it became apparent that he was under significant academic pressure, having recently transferred to an extremely competitive private school. In addition, extracurricular pressures were severe, including his fervent commitment to gymnastics and his hope to achieve professional status. On further questioning, Craig related that he had had dizzy spells in past years just before competitions.

Since the somatic complaint expressed by the patient is based on a model symptom, a physical disease often is mimicked. Close scrutiny of symptom history and description often reveals anatomic and physiologic discrepancies. The child or adolescent with a *stocking anesthesia,* an anesthesia confined to a specific area of an extremity without any relationship to cutaneous nerve innervation, demonstrates an example of such symptom inaccuracy. It is based on the patient's concept of his or her body rather than on anatomic principles.

A thorough history may not only elicit symptom inconsistencies in the present illness, but may also reveal a record of inexplicable or recurrent bouts of illness associated with life events. A history of chronic abdominal pain occurring only on school days, a history of somatic complaints associated with stressful social events, or documentation of abdominal surgery with equivocal findings should raise suspicion that the patient's current problem may represent conversion. A list of the diagnostic criteria for conversion symptoms appears in the following box. No one diagnostic criterion can be confirmatory, and each patient with a conversion symptom may not display every criterion listed. However, the diagnosis of a conversion symptom cannot be made solely on the basis of negative physical and laboratory findings. It is not a diagnosis of exclusion.

Criteria for Diagnosis of Conversion Symptoms

- The symptom has symbolic meaning to the patient.
- The patient frequently exhibits characteristic interpersonal behaviors.
- Conversion symptoms are more common in girls than boys.
- There is a characteristic style of reporting symptoms.
- The symptom helps the patient cope with his or her environment ("secondary gain").
- There is often frequent use of health issues and symptoms in family communication.
- Symptoms occur at times of stress.
- The symptom has a model.
- History and physical findings are often inconsistent with anatomic and physiologic concepts.

From Prazar G: Conversion reactions in adolescents, Pediatr Rev 8:279, 1987.

DIFFERENTIAL DIAGNOSIS OF OTHER PSYCHOSOMATIC DISORDERS

Other psychosomatic disorders may at times be confused with conversion symptoms. Patients exhibiting *hypochondriasis,* a frequent entity especially in adolescents, view their symptoms with extreme concern. There is none of the apparent indifference seen in patients with conversion symptoms. Patients with conversion symptoms frequently seem relieved when an organic cause is considered; patients with hypochondriasis become more concerned if an organic diagnosis is suggested, since they suspect and fear a serious or fatal disease. However, neither type of patient is reassured more than transiently by being informed that he or she has no disease.

Malingering is an infrequently seen problem in adolescents, except in institutionalized adolescents or in those who are in restrictive situations (e.g., the armed forces). Malingering may even be regarded as an appropriate means of avoiding threatening or unpleasant circumstances. Attempts to feign illness are often naive, especially in younger patients. Malingerers exhibit, as Engel[2] states, "an intense need to be nurtured or suffer." Many appear to be accident prone, and many submit to painful procedures readily and without objection. Malingering adolescents are aloof and hostile to the physician; thus delays in the discovery of their deception often result. In contrast, patients with conversion symptoms are often appropriately fearful of procedures and may appear charming and garrulous in the presence of a physician. Patients with conversion symptoms and malingerers are similar in that their parents may have unconscious psychological needs to have their children ill and therefore may reinforce their children's symptoms.

Somatic delusions are symptoms of psychosis, and they are not usually confused with conversion symptoms. Other signs of severe mental illness are usually present, such as an inability to relate to peers, visual or auditory hallucinations, and stereotypic behaviors. Furthermore, the symptoms described are sometimes intermittent and are frequently extremely bizarre. For example, a patient with somatic delusions may verbalize the conviction that his or her heart is shriveling up or that there is something wrong with the blood that is running from the head to the leg.

Psychophysiologic symptoms may occur when conversion symptoms have failed to dissipate anxiety. Thus continuing anxiety activates biologic systems (especially the autonomic nervous system), resulting in physiologic changes such as tachycardia, hyperperistalsis, and vasoconstriction. A patient's cognizance of these changes is manifested by palpitations, diarrhea, and sweating. In this situation the symptom itself has no organic symbolic meaning and results from a reaction to actual body changes. Therefore psychophysiologic symptoms can occur when conversion symptoms have failed.

Similarly, conversion symptoms can replace psychophysiologic symptoms.

CARE OF THE PATIENT WITH CONVERSION SYMPTOMS

Adolescents with conversion symptoms are most often initially seen and eventually managed by pediatricians or other primary care physicians. Families see this as appropriate, since the obvious aspect of the problem is physical. They typically will accept a diagnosis of conversion only from a medical professional they consider an expert in physical disease. Nevertheless, when the physician undertakes a case of suspected conversion, his or her interviewing acumen and sensitivity to the patient's feelings are paramount. The initial interaction between the physician and the patient is crucial to the degree of success achieved in dealing with a conversion symptom. In essence, treatment of the patient begins before a definitive diagnosis is made. Some considerations involved in the initial evaluation of patients suspected of having conversion symptoms appear in the box below.

The physician should advise the patient and family that the cause of any disorder involves both physical and emotional factors. As Schmitt[12] states, the family should be told that "Everyone's body has a certain physical way of responding to emotional stress." Similarly, every individual has an emotional response to physical stress. Simple examples should be given (e.g., most people have learned that headaches are often intensified when they are upset). If the physician communicates an appreciation of the role of emotions in physical disease, the family may more readily volunteer information about psychosocial functioning. Furthermore, an eventual diagnosis involving emotional aspects may be more acceptable, since the family has been prepared for the possibility. Focusing only on an organic diagnosis intimates to the parents that psychological involvement is unlikely, unimportant, and improbable. Turning to psychological issues after all physical tests prove unremarkable implies to parents that this tack was chosen as a last resort because the physician was unable to ascertain an organic cause. A concurrent physical-psychological diagnostic approach not only prepares the physican to consider the problem with some psychotherapeutic intent, but may also save the family time and money, since multiple laboratory tests frequently may be avoided.

After the evaluation has been completed, the physician must develop a treatment plan. Before embarking on this venture, the physician must be satisfied with the completeness of the physical evaluation. Common sense should dictate when he or she feels further organic tests will be futile. Physician uncertainty can often be sensed by the patient and family, especially if the family is averse to accepting a psychological diagnosis. Therefore it is prudent to solicit from the family what additional tests they might expect to have performed and what other diagnoses they may have considered. Involvement of the patient and family in this diagnostic process frequently dissipates anxiety and allows eventual psychological counseling.

Although patients with conversion symptoms are suggestible, reassurance that the symptom will go away rarely is effective and also does not contribute to a psychological investigation of the symptom. On the contrary, suggesting that the symptom will persist allows time to work out a therapeutic relationship with the patient and sometimes has a paradoxical effect. Since the probability of the symptom disappearing after two or three visits is unlikely, the physician's suggestion will be viewed retrospectively by the patient as being sound. Trust in the physician will be more secure, and the patient may be more comfortable in communicating information about his or her feelings. Placebo medication is usually ineffective and raises questions of medical ethics. Tranquilizers may transiently reduce attendant anxiety in some cases of conversion symptoms; however, medication as the sole therapeutic method rarely results in lasting improvement. Because medication does not relieve the underlying conflict responsible for the symptom, another symptom may eventually appear. Furthermore, there is risk that medication side effects may become the model for new conversion symptoms or that new symptoms may be confused with side effects.

At the conclusion of the evaluation sessions, the number and type of counseling sessions that the physician anticipates should be discussed. The number of sessions should be flexible so that renegotiation can occur if needed. Follow-up sessions with the teenager can usually be limited to 20 to 30 minutes every 2 to 4 weeks. More frequent visits may be necessary if the symptom interferes with school attendance, peer relationships, or family functioning.

During follow-up sessions, the teenager should be encouraged to talk about his or her daily life (e.g., school, friends, family, dating). If the teenager volunteers information about recurrence of the somatic complaint, the physician should inquire about events that were concurrently transpiring when the symptom occurred and how the teenager *felt* about these events. In this way the physician can help the adolescent become reacquainted with how daily events and feelings are related.

Important Considerations in the Initial Evaluation of Patients With Suspected Conversion Symptoms

From the outset, parents and patient should be told that every person has an emotional response to physical stress.

Parents and patient should be encouraged to suggest diagnostic tests that they may want performed and to suggest possible diagnoses for consideration by the physician.

Parents and patient should understand that the symptom may persist but that the goal is to help maintain normal daily functioning in school and with peers.

Parents and patient should understand that referral to a psychiatrically trained professional may be necessary if progress is not made in coping with the symptom.

From Prazar G: Conversion reactions in adolescents, Pediatr Rev 8:279, 1987.

Since the physician will serve both as therapist for the teenager and as provider of acute medical care, there may be occasions when the teenager has a new physical symptom or complaint. If the physician suspects a physical illness unrelated to the conversion symptom, he or she must perform whatever evaluation is indicated, including a full or partial physical examination. However, an overzealous search for disease should be avoided. Treatment goals need to be realistic. Complete disappearance of conversion symptoms seldom occurs. However, adolescents often acquire increased coping skills so that daily functioning is unimpaired and dependence on secondary gain is minimized.

Follow-up visits with parents should take place every 4 to 6 weeks. Such meetings should serve to elicit persistent or new concerns that parents may have about their teenager's progress and should attempt to assess parents' reaction to their teenager's continuing complaints. The practitioner should emphasize the validity of the teenager's concerns, so that misconceptions about the symptom being "faked" are dispelled. Furthermore, positive reinforcement needs to be offered so that parents believe they are doing what is best for their child. Selected parent follow-up sessions should include the teenager. Such family meetings not only demonstrate to the patient that confidentiality of individual sessions is not being violated but also offer the physician an opportunity to observe parent-adolescent interaction. Such observation may provide an important index to the effectiveness of ongoing therapy.

REFERRAL

Referral to psychiatrically trained professionals is indicated if symptoms continue to interfere with the patient's daily activities or functioning, or when the physician or school personnel feel that there has been no diminution in the teenager's symptoms. School officials can provide valuable information about the effect of the conversion symptom on school functioning and peer interaction. Referral is dictated if the family feels that inadequate progress has been made after an agreed on duration of therapy.

If the patient's symptom creates uncomfortable feelings in the pediatrician, referral is indicated. Situations involving seductive adolescent behavior in association with a conversion symptom may create feelings in the pediatrician that can prevent effective intervention. It is as unrealistic to assume that a pediatrician can adequately treat all psychological problems as it is to assume that he or she can treat all medical ones. Cognizance of one's own limitations is an important professional attribute. A third situation requiring referral involves the patient or family member who is a social acquaintance or a relative of the pediatrician. Dealing with the emotional problems of friends' or relatives' children is inappropriate. Obtaining personal details of family or sexual functioning is often indicated in the evaluation and may jeopardize the social relationship. Conversely, failure or hesitancy to obtain appropriate data may jeopardize subsequent problem resolution.

In all cases, when referral is suggested, parental and patient compliance with the referral is improved if the possibility has been mentioned as a contingency *early* in the evaluation. The pediatrician should always help families understand that seeing a psychiatrically trained professional does *not* connote "craziness." Rather, the pediatrician may suggest that a psychiatrist could help because a doctor trained in psychiatry can help teenagers understand feelings about unusual symptoms better than can most pediatricians. After the referral is made, continued pediatrician contact with the family concerning the conversion symptom helps assure compliance with the therapy. Indications for referring patients with conversion symptoms are listed above.[11]

Indications for Referral of Patients With Conversion Symptoms

The symptom continues to interfere with daily functioning (school attendance, participation in extracurricular activities, involvement with peers).
Parents and patient believe that no progress is being made in dealing with the symptom.
The physician feels uncomfortable with the patient's symptom or behavior (e.g., patients exhibiting seductive behavior).
The patient's family includes social friend or relative of physician.

From Prazar G: Conversion reactions in adolescents, Pediatr Rev 8:279, 1987.

The prognosis for patients with conversion reactions is unknown. In a report of 74 children with psychogenic pain, Friedman[3] found a large number of patients were judged to be improved after several years, whether or not professional intervention took place. In a 7-year follow-up of patients hospitalized with conversion, 23 of 41 patients no longer suffered from their presenting physical symptom, were free of underlying stress, and had experienced no symptom substitution or new associated complaint.[7] Patients with conversion symptoms may indeed have an encouraging future. On the other hand, there is a group of patients whose adolescent conversion symptoms mark the beginning of a lifelong career of conversion illness.

SUMMARY

Conversion reactions represent an emotionally charged issue, not only in a literal sense for the adolescent but also in a figurative sense for the physician, since patients displaying such symptoms frequently elicit a wide range of emotions from their physician. The physician's emotional response results from his or her frustration in dealing with such difficult patients. Every patient with a somatic complaint has feelings about his or her symptoms. An evaluation of any somatic complaint should involve inquiry into aspects of the patient's family, school performance, and peer relationships. A better understanding of the patient's baseline emotional functioning can be achieved in this way. The physician must advise both parents and patient that it is acceptable to have feelings about somatic complaints. Both family and patient may be much more accepting of primary emotional involvement if permission for expressing feelings is given early in the physician-patient relationship. The diagnosis of a conversion reaction should never be one of exclusion and should follow specific diagnostic criteria.

Care of the adolescent patient with a conversion reaction involves establishing a renegotiable number of regular visits, encouraging the patient to discuss daily activities and interrelated feelings, meeting with parents regularly to provide them with emotional support and counseling, and knowing that palliation rather than a cure may be the optimum goal. When the physician feels uncomfortable handling a patient with a conversion reaction, or when ongoing follow-up care appears to have made no progress in reducing the symptom, referral to a psychiatrically trained professional should be made. However, referral should not end the physician's contact with the patient, since ongoing physician interest may improve patient compliance with the referral source and may increase the physician's ability to resume responsibility later for the patient's care. The patient with a conversion symptom will not usually outgrow his or her symptom and will not permanently respond to placebo medication. Such patients severely tax the primary care physician's diagnostic and therapeutic acumen. However, the physician who respects the involvement of emotions with somatic complaints can serve a vital role in helping patients with conversion symptoms cope with their disorders.

REFERENCES

1. Apley J: The child with abdominal pains, ed 2, Oxford, England, 1975, Blackwell Scientific Publications, Ltd.
2. Engel GL: Conversion symptoms. In MacBryde CM and Blacklow RS, editors: Signs and symptoms: applied pathologic physiology and clinical interpretation, ed 6, Philadelphia, 1983, JB Lippincott Co.
3. Friedman R: Some characteristics of children with "psychogenic" pain; observations on prognosis and management, Clin Pediatr 11:331, 1972.
4. Friedman SB: Conversion symptoms in adolescents, Pediatr Clin North Am 20:873, 1973.
5. Hollender MH: Conversion hysteria—a post-Freudian reinterpretation of nineteenth century psychosocial data, Arch Gen Psychiatry 26:31, 1972.
6. Levine RJ: Epidemic faintness and syncope in a school marching band, JAMA 238:2373, 1977.
7. Maisami M and Freeman JM: Conversion reactions in children as body language: a combined child psychiatry/neurology team approach to the management of functional neurologic disorders in children, Pediatrics 80:46, 1987.
8. Maloney MJ: Diagnosing hysterical conversion reactions in children, J Pediatr 97:1016, 1980.
9. Moffett MEK: Epidemic hysteria in a Montreal train station, Pediatrics 70:308, 1982.
10. Oster J: Recurrent abdominal pain, headache, and limb pains in children and adolescents, Pediatrics 50:429, 1972.
11. Prazar G: Conversion reactions in adolescents, Pediatr Rev 8:279, 1987.
12. Schmitt BD: School phobia—the great imitator: a pediatrician's viewpoint, Pediatrics 48:433, 1971.

98

Counseling the Parents of Adolescents

Muki W. Fairchild and W. Sam Yancy

Most adolescents and their families manage to survive the adolescent years without serious or irrevocable damage to their relationship with each other. Some disagreement and tension appear to be not only common but even necessary and desirable. The essential task for both parents and adolescent is that of separation—enough letting go of each other so that independent lives are possible. How gracefully this is accomplished will vary. Fortunately, the separation process has frequent shifts and interludes, giving all participants opportunities along the way to appraise the situation. There is adequate time to call in outside help if needed.

RATIONALE FOR TREATMENT

Pediatricians have always worked with the parents of their patients. With the young child, evaluation and treatment may be effected entirely through the parents. But as the child moves into adolescence, pediatricians have been taught to shift the responsibility for health care gradually onto the adolescent, thus seeing and working with the parents less often. This significant shift corresponds with the developmental needs of the adolescent. However, the developmental needs of the parents must not be forgotten. Parents should have the same kind of support and counseling they received from their child's physician in earlier years.

The physician who helps parents get through the sleepless nights of infancy, the exasperating days of a 2-year-old's negativity, and the anxiety of entrusting their child to the outside world of day care providers and schoolteachers is ideally suited to continue a trusting relationship with parents while fostering their adolescent's growing independence. Because most parents still decide who sees their adolescent for what and how often, any successful treatment plan will require their approval and cooperation.

Many physicians are comfortable hearing about and treating the problems of the young child but not those of the adolescent. Anthony[1] has pointed out that society has developed several disturbing and conflicting stereotypes of the adolescent, which range from the dangerous "victimizer" who harbors untamed aggressive and sexual drives to the passive victim who is easily exploited by adults and society. These stereotypes cause adults to respond to adolescents as though they were the embodiments of these negative images rather than actual people. If society has such a strong response to this age group, it is hardly surprising that pediatricians may also be reluctant to become too involved with their difficulties.

Behaviorally, the pediatrician is in an excellent position to evaluate parental concerns because he or she has access to developmental, interactional, and emotional data on both parents and child that are unavailable to any other professional. The pediatrician who has always been interested in the child's behavior as well as in the child's physical health and who has effectively communicated this interest to the family is in a particularly good position to establish the counseling relationship.

It is important to communicate this attitude in light of studies demonstrating that although some parents are needlessly concerned about emotional problems in their children, there are many more who are legitimately concerned but are hesitant to mention it to a pediatrician.[5] Another professional, no matter how well qualified, would have to spend a considerable amount of time and effort developing the rapport, confidence, and knowledge that the pediatrician has already acquired through years of office visits and phone calls. Many families are reluctant to accept a referral to anyone designated as a therapist, but are able and willing to discuss troublesome problems and issues with their child's physician.

KNOWLEDGE BASE

Not all pediatricians will choose to work intensively with the parents of adolescents. For those who do, acquiring the following specific skills and knowledge is essential.

Interviewing Skills

The ability to conduct a skillful and empathic interview is the physician's most important diagnostic and therapeutic tool. A working alliance between parents and physician must be developed and maintained for parents to feel free to reveal their concerns and for both parties to begin to understand and address those concerns. The physician's ability to engender rapport and trust is the cornerstone of this alliance and is also the foundation of all "talking" therapies and counseling methods, from behavior modification to psychoanalysis. (See Chapter 102, "Interviewing Adolescents.")

Interviewing consists largely of talking and listening, and because most people think they know how to do both, this tool is least often addressed and taught. Yet studies[3,10,12-14] have consistently shown that doctor-patient communication is frequently unsatisfactory and unproductive, if not outright detrimental to the diagnostic and therapeutic process. By observing skilled interviewers, by having their own interviews observed and supervised, and by becoming familiar with the literature on this subject, pediatricians can significantly improve their ability to communicate sensitively.[6] Self-awareness is an integral part of counseling. The pediatrician needs to be aware of his or her own patterns of communication, attitudes, and blind spots as well as areas of conflict.

Normal Developmental Patterns and Tasks

As with any physical or psychological complaint encountered by the pediatrician, the first step always is to assess the nature of the problem. Adolescence is a lengthy process extending over several years with distinct, although overlapping, phases—early, middle, and late adolescence. The developmental needs, tasks, and behavior of the 13-year-old are different from those of the 17-year-old.[8,9,11] Although well described in Chapter 43, the seven most frequently cited tasks of these years are summarized in the following list:

1. To separate and become independent from one's parents
2. To become comfortable with one's own body and sexual identity
3. To build new and lasting relationships
4. To seek economic and social stability—that is, a vocational commitment
5. To develop a personal moral value system
6. To verbalize conceptually
7. To establish a new relationship with one's parents, based on relative equality

Viewing the adolescent years as a period when the earlier developmental issues resurface is also useful. According to Erikson,[7] the tasks of the preschool years are to establish a sense of trust in people in general, come to believe that one is a separate, autonomous being from one's parents, and acquire the ability to initiate ideas and activities. During the school years, the child should acquire a sense of industry. Children master each of these tasks to a certain degree at the time they are first encountered, but unresolved remnants may persist and become problems in subsequent stages of development. In adolescence these issues typically come up again, to the despair of both parents and adolescents alike. Their reemergence is also cause for hope, because it provides a second chance, the opportunity to redo what was not satisfactorily accomplished earlier.

The pediatrician is the person most likely to see vestiges of problems from the second developmental stage of life—separation-individuation. Much of adolescent behavior is reminiscent of the negativistic, rebellious 2-year-old who, in experimenting with independence, runs away from his or her mother and then comes running back, terrified by the freedom he or she has found. This ambivalent struggle toward independence is the hallmark of adolescence. A reworking of the family "romance" is also frequently encountered. Just as 3- to 6-year-old children become romantically attached to the opposite-sex parent and rivalrous with the same-sex parent ("Daddy, when I grow up I'm going to marry you"), so do adolescents feel that only they can truly understand the opposite-sex parent's needs and become openly critical of the same-sex parent.

The parents' complaints and concerns must be carefully evaluated. The pediatrician must decide when along the developmental ladder the particular adolescent and parents are stuck. Is the physician witnessing a painful but not necessarily pathologic moment in the lives of a family, or is the complaint indicative of a more seriously flawed parent-child relationship? Although the underlying dynamics of adolescent problems such as anorexia nervosa, running away, and substance abuse may still revolve around some of the same developmental tasks and issues, such problems must be considered pathologic adaptations.

Parents' Developmental Phase

Just as the crucial task for adolescents is to separate from their parents, the crucial task for the parents is to let go. Letting go involves loss, and loss is always painful. When the relationship has been ambivalent and the problems in parenting great, the separation is more difficult. The ties may never loosen enough for the child to leave, or they may be cut prematurely before the child is really ready to go.

One of life's ironies is that many parents of adolescents find themselves truly "in the middle." Just as their children are blossoming into youthful, vigorous, sexual beings, their own bodies are beginning to sag and wrinkle, their fertility on the wane. The realities of life have tempered and sometimes destroyed the dreams and hopes of their youth. The wish to prevent their children from making mistakes similar to their own is strong and a source of potential conflict. Simultaneously, they may be losing a once important avenue of support in their own parents. As grandparents age, they turn to their middle-age children, who find themselves in the awkward position of caring for two generations at the same time—their parents and their children. Implicit in this role reversal is the parents' need to face their own mortality. When their parents (the grandparents) die, a generational barrier against death is gone. And support from an adolescent is not likely to materialize. As the adolescent's parents turn to their child, the adolescent turns away from them to form ties with other adults in his or her life.

Thus it is not surprising that adolescence reverberates and stirs up much emotion in the parents. Feelings of envy, loss, hostility, and uncertainty may coexist and intermingle with those of pride, love, joy, and satisfaction. Some parents may use their children as pawns to live out their own hopes and wishes, conflicts, and rivalries. This is probably true to some extent of all parents, but the degree and intensity will vary. A teenager's behavior may well be a reflection and an acting out of a parent's own but unacceptable (and therefore unconscious) impulses and desires. Thus the mother who insists that her children respect adults but who then smiles when hearing how her daughter "told off" a teacher is deriving some satisfaction from the girl's behavior. An adolescent will respond to mixed messages from a parent.

INTERVENTION

To intervene, the pediatrician's first task is always assessment—to gain an understanding of the problem and the people involved. Although physicians are trained to act and act quickly, the assessment phase is a time for patience and restraint. The physician must refrain from giving immediate advice—often given just to be "doing" something—and concentrate instead on listening and observing. Sufficient time must be allowed for gathering this information. Assessment is a continuous process, and all questions do not need to be answered right away. People need time to tell their stories. Encouraging them to tell too much too soon is not helpful, because they may become so embarrassed by what they have revealed that they will not return.

When possible, seeing the adolescent and the parents both separately and together is helpful. Not only can this provide vital information about the ways in which the family members interact and perceive the problems, but seeing both will also help the pediatrician maintain a neutral stance and avoid becoming overidentified with either parents or teenager. Questions about confidentiality may arise. This issue is complicated but usually not insurmountable. Physicians vary in their approach to confidentiality. Whatever stance the pediatrician takes should be discussed with both the adolescent and the parents. If an agreement cannot be reached, the pediatrician may have to work exclusively with either the parents or the adolescent and refer the other to another counselor.

The nature of the problem, the family's circumstances, their motivation, and the personalities of the individuals involved are the factors that will help the pediatrician decide how and where to intervene. A psychologically oriented parent with previous personal experience in counseling may be interested in sorting out his or her own feelings and reactions to the teenager's behavior. A less sophisticated parent may just want to stop the behavior and have no interest in understanding its origins. As Arnold[2] and others have pointed out, parental counseling can cover a whole range of possibilities, from simply providing information and education, through giving advice, to using various psychotherapeutic strategies aimed at revealing and investigating the sources of feelings.

It is useful to start with the simplest form of intervention. This usually means that the problem is presumed to be caused largely by a lack of information or understanding. The role of the pediatrician is then to educate the parents about normal adolescent development tactfully and supportively. Thus the mother who is convinced that her daughter hates her because her previously compliant 13-year-old has refused to participate in the weekly Sunday outing can be helped to see that this relatively minor form of rebellion reflects the girl's struggle to "distance" herself from a loved rather than hated adult.

The pediatrician may decide that the parents need to be educated about the changing needs of their adolescent. Teenagers no longer want parents present during the physical examination and demand increasing privacy at home. Parents need help and support in understanding this as developmentally appropriate so that they will not respond as though rejected. Unless coupled with other signs of disturbance, an adolescent's staying in his or her room for long periods, writing poetry, and listening to music do not indicate a depressive illness or permanent withdrawal from the family.

The educational role may also be indicated when an adolescent has undergone a stressful experience. When an active adolescent boy develops stomachaches after seeing a friend killed in an accident, his parents need to be aware of the psychological impact of such an experience. They can be helped to understand their son's somatic response without compounding the trauma by insisting on unnecessary invasive diagnostic procedures for the abdominal pain. Similarily, the pediatrician is in an ideal position to evaluate and to inform the parents whose children's development is complicated by additional stresses such as adoption, divorce, or parental remarriage.

Close monitoring and follow-up care are vital for any type of counseling. Weekly or biweekly visits should be arranged, if possible. Families that live far away may only be able to manage visits once a month. More frequent visits may be necessary for a family in crisis. The pediatrician may also elect to work primarily with the adolescent and see the parents regularly but infrequently. The work is then focused on maintaining the relationship with the parents so the child's treatment can continue. Parents' sessions would involve listening to the parents' perceptions of how the adolescent is progressing at home, rather than changing the parents themselves. Regardless of session frequency, the pediatrician must be alert to possible feelings of competition, from or with the parents.

If it becomes obvious that the parents have sufficient knowledge available to them but are not able to make use of what they know, a more detailed exploration of their ideas and feelings is a logical next step. It is usual for parents to know that their adolescent still needs rules and regulations; however, they may be unable to establish limits because of pressures from the adolescent and because they are uncertain about what is right and wrong in this rapidly changing world. The pediatrician's firm support and permission to establish flexible but definite limits allow parents the freedom to do what they already feel should be done. Adolescents who have no limits set for them will, despite bragging to the contrary, interpret this freedom as a lack of caring. On the other hand, the parents' ability to control their child lessens as the balance of power shifts. Because of the adolescent's need and ability to act independently, the pediatrician may advise parents to be selective in setting rules and consequences. Influencing rather than "controlling" their child becomes an important distinction.

The pediatrician must phrase advice, when given, so that it is acceptable to the parents. To do so, he or she must be able to understand the parents' point of view and how they arrived at it. The pediatrician should take the time to find out what others have recommended (family, friends, neighbors, or other professionals), what has been tried, and how it did or did not work. Often the family will already have tried and abandoned what the pediatrician recommends. Unless this advice can be presented differently and with a new attitude of hope and faith, it too will fail. Slight modifications can make a great difference. For example, struggles over chores may be reduced to a manageable level of discord by allowing the adolescent some choice about when they have to be done.

When information and judiciously given advice are not sufficient, the physician will want to explore the parents' reservations and feelings in greater depth. A parent may initially attribute failure to set limits as insecurity in the face of conflicting societal trends but later come to discover that his or her own fear of losing the child's love is a restraining factor. Acquiring this insight, coupled with the pediatrician's insistence that the child is less likely to respect and love the parent if no limits are set, may sufficiently ameliorate the problem. If the problem persists, the pediatrician should listen for the prominent underlying themes of the parents' story. Unless these are identified and recognized, no change can take place and little information can be integrated. Often the real issue has little to do with what the participants are wrangling about. After listening to a list of reasons a parent produces to prohibit a child from a new undertaking, the physician may be able to put into words the underlying fear. For instance, "You're afraid he'll make a terrible mistake, which will jeopardize his entire future." The parent may then recognize how difficult it is to sit back and allow the child to make his own mistakes and that this fear has created the conflict.

A further step in parental counseling is to allow and encourage discussion of the parents' own childhood experiences to understand how the parents' faulty reasoning developed. Even those pediatricians interested in counseling may feel uncomfortable in exploring a parent's psychodynamics and past experiences and will often want to refer the parent for individual psychotherapy at this point. Nonetheless, the pediatrician should learn how to deal with those parents who insist on talking about their past, regardless of the pediatrician's comfort. It is helpful to keep in mind that the focus should continue to be on the parent's difficulties with the child. Thus, when a father describes a painful struggle he had at the age of 12 with his father, the pediatrician can refocus the discussion by asking him how he thinks this struggle has influenced his current relationship with his son.

However one chooses to work with parents, the pediatrician will do well to work at helping them achieve what Anthony[1] calls a *good enough reaction* to their adolescents. This means that the parents (and the pediatrician) are able to respond to the child as the child *really* is, in the here-and-now, rather than to a societal stereotype or a transference figure from the past. As Dorothy discovered in the Land of Oz, it takes courage, brains, and heart to make the eventful journey from childhood through adolescence to adulthood. Pediatricians and parents are in equal need of these three precious attributes.

REFERENCES

1. Anthony EJ: The reactions of parents to adolescents and to their behavior. In Anthony EJ and Benedek T, editors: Parenthood, Boston, 1970, Little, Brown & Co.
2. Arnold LE: Strategics and tactics of parent guidance. In Arnold LE, editor: Helping parents help their children, New York, 1978, Brunner/Mazel, Inc.
3. Boyle MP: Evolving parenthood: a developmental perspective. In Levine MD et al, editors: Developmental-behavioral pediatrics, Philadelphia, 1983, WB Saunders Co.
4. Cooper S: Treatment of parents. In Arieti S and Caplan G, editors: American handbook of psychiatry, vol 2, New York, 1974, Basic Books.
5. Costello EJ and Pantino T: The new morbidity: who should treat it? J Dev Behav Pediatr 8:288, 1987.
6. Enelow AJ and Swisher SN: Interviewing and patient care, ed 3, New York, 1986, Oxford University Press, Inc.
7. Erikson EH: Childhood and society, ed 2, New York, 1963, WW Norton & Co, Inc.
8. Felice M and Friedman SB: The adolescent as a patient, J Cont Educ Pediatr 20:15, 1978.
9. Felice ME: Adolescence: general considerations. In Levine MD et al, editors: Developmental-behavioral pediatrics, Philadelphia, 1983, WB Saunders Co.
10. Francis V, Korsch B, and Morris M: Gaps in doctor-patient communication: patients' response to medical advice, N Engl J Med 280:535, 1969.
11. Group for the Advancement of Psychiatry: Normal adolescence, New York, 1968, Charles Scribner's Sons.
12. Korsch B, Gozzi E, and Francis V: Gaps in doctor-patient communication. I. Doctor-patient interaction and patient satisfaction, Pediatrics 42:855, 1968.
13. Korsch BM and Negrete VF: Doctor-patient communication. In Henderson G, editor: Physician-patient communication: readings and recommendations, Springfield, Ill, 1981, Charles C Thomas.
14. Shuy RW: The medical interview: problems in communication. In Henderson G, editor: Physician-patient communication: readings and recommendations, Springfield, Ill, 1981, Charles C Thomas.
15. Sperling E: Parent counseling and therapy. In Noshpitz JD, editor: Basic handbook of child psychiatry, vol 3, New York, 1979, Basic Books.

99

Anorexia Nervosa and Bulimia

Martin Fisher

The eating disorders, a group of conditions primarily affecting adolescents and young adults, have increased dramatically in prevalence during the past 3 decades. Marked by the combination of medical and psychological factors in their etiology and outcome, they predominantly include the well-known entities of anorexia nervosa and bulimia. Anorexia nervosa, viewed most simply as the *purposeful loss of weight beyond that which is healthy,* is now said to affect one out of every 200 adolescent girls in the United States and Great Britain. Bulimia, which is marked by *recurrent episodes of binge eating and/or vomiting,* has been estimated to affect from 2% to 20% of high school and college-age females in these same countries, depending on the criteria used. Although there is much debate about the diagnosis and prevalence of these disorders, and many questions remain regarding their etiology and outcome, the growing prevalence of eating disorders has made it increasingly important for the primary care physician to be aware of the principles involved in the evaluation and treatment of both anorexia nervosa and bulimia.

DIAGNOSIS AND PREVALENCE

Although individual cases suggestive of anorexia nervosa and cultural behaviors suggestive of bulimia have been described from antiquity, neither disorder was specifically defined as a medical condition until the 1880s. At that time, Charles Laseque in France described a condition he called anorexia hysterica; William Gull in England referred to the same condition as anorexia nervosa. Although the latter term is a misnomer, since patients with eating disorders do not simply have a loss of appetite as the name implies, this name has remained in place since that time.

Individual cases of "anorexia nervosa" appear in the medical literature from the 1880s through the 1950s. Beginning in the 1960s, possibly because of an increased emphasis on thin physiques that swept through the developed world, greater numbers of cases of anorexia nervosa began to be seen. At first considered only a component of anorexia nervosa, bulimia (also called bulimia nervosa) became recognized as a separate entity in the 1970s. It is now well known that anorexia nervosa and bulimia may appear as separate syndromes, that they may occur concomitantly or sequentially in the same individual, and that both may be associated with several other entities, including laxative abuse or alternating with obesity. The growing diversity of the eating disorders has accompanied ever improving refinements in the diagnostic criteria for these conditions.

The first officially published criteria for the diagnosis of anorexia nervosa were developed by Feighner and colleagues in 1972.[1] The original Feighner criteria stipulated that an individual considered as having anorexia nervosa must (1) be under 25 years of age, (2) have lost at least 25% of initial body weight, (3) not have an alternative medical diagnosis to account for the weight loss, (4) not have an alternative psychiatric diagnosis to account for the weight loss, (5) display evidence of a distorted body image, desire for extreme thinness, and a preoccupation with food and weight, and (6) have at least two of the following signs or symptoms associated with anorexia nervosa: amenorrhea, lanugo, bradycardia, periods of hyperactivity, episodes of binge eating, and vomiting.

Changes in both the nature of the condition and our understanding of it have occurred in the ensuing years. It is now acknowledged that in rare instances patients may develop the illness beyond 25 years of age. A 25% weight loss may be simply the result of an appropriate diet for those who start out overweight, whereas a 15% to 20% weight loss may be extremely unhealthy for those already underweight. Patients with anorexia nervosa may have other psychiatric diagnoses (such as depression), and a few patients may manipulate the treatment of other medical conditions (such as diabetes mellitus or cystic fibrosis) in order to lose weight because of a concomitant diagnosis of anorexia nervosa. Further, the emergence of bulimia as a distinct entity brought the requirement for specific criteria for this disorder as well. The best current criteria are those listed by the American Psychiatric Association in the third edition (revised) of the *Diagnostic and Statistical Manual* (DSM-III-R). The criteria are given in the box on p. 762. As noted, there are separate criteria for anorexia and bulimia nervosa, with specific requirements for each. In the DSM-III-R, it is acknowledged that there may be other patients with eating disorders who do not meet the strict criteria for either anorexia nervosa or bulimia; therefore, an additional category, "Eating Disorders Not Otherwise Specified," also has been established.

Changes in diagnostic criteria are partly responsible for debates about incidence that have taken place during the past several years. Most researchers in the field believe that eating disorders have increased in both incidence and prevalence during the past 30 years, although others believe it is mostly higher awareness and improved diagnosis that account for an apparent rise. Over 90% of patients are female, and most cases of anorexia nervosa begin in the teenage years; bulimia is apt to begin in the late teens and early twenties. It is generally accepted that 0.5% of all adolescent females meet strict criteria for anorexia nervosa, although not all of these

Criteria for the Diagnosis of Eating Disorders*

Anorexia Nervosa	Bulimia Nervosa
Refusal to maintain body weight over a minimal normal weight for age and height—for example, weight loss leading to maintenance of body weight 15% below that expected; or failure to make expected weight gain during period of growth, leading to body weight 15% below the expected	Recurrent episodes of binge eating (rapid consumption of a large amount of food in a discrete period of time)
Intense fear of gaining weight or becoming fat, even though underweight	A feeling of lack of control over eating behavior during the eating binges
Disturbance in the way in which one's body weight, size, or shape is experienced—for example, the person claims to "feel fat" even when emaciated, believes that one area of the body is "too fat" even when obviously underweight	The person regularly engages in either self-induced vomiting, use of laxatives or diuretics, strict dieting or fasting, or vigorous exercise in order to prevent weight gain
In females, absence of at least three consecutive menstrual cycles when otherwise expected to occur (primary or secondary amenorrhea)	A minimum average of two binge eating episodes a week for at least 3 months Persistent overconcern with body shape and weight

*From The American Psychiatric Association: Diagnostic and statistical manual, ed 3 (revised), Washington, DC, 1987, The Association.

are medically diagnosed. With the criteria for bulimia nervosa being somewhat more vague, some researchers have found prevalences of binge eating and vomiting in 20% to 30% of college-age females; others, using a strict criterion, limit the diagnosis to only 2% to 3% of the same populations. Both diagnoses are far less common in Third World nations and among minorities and those of lower socioeconomic status in industrialized societies.

PRESENTATION AND ETIOLOGY

The patient with an eating disorder may seek medical care in a variety of ways. Some come to their pediatrician or family physician because of concern about weight loss, vomiting, or abnormal eating attitudes noticed by family, friends, or school authorities. Others visit a gynecologist because of the menstrual irregularities that characteristically accompany the disorder. Many are seen first by a psychiatrist, psychologist, or social worker; others may be seen for the first time in an emergency room because of dehydration or other medical complications. Some patients may be seen within weeks of the disorder's onset, whereas others avoid medical care for months or even years. It is common for patients to be brought for their initial evaluation against their will, claiming, "There's nothing wrong with me," although older patients may seek help willingly, saying, "I'm sick of having this problem." Large-scale questionnaire surveys have shown that there are many patients with mild to moderate eating disorders, both anorexia nervosa and bulimia, who avoid medical care altogether by hiding or denying their illness.

There is considerable literature exploring the possible etiologic factors accounting for these disorders. Several key questions are addressed: Why has there been an apparent increase in these disorders during the past 3 decades? Why are women affected predominantly? And, what factors cause any particular individual to develop the disorder? Cultural, psychological, and biochemical factors have all been invoked in responding to these questions regarding etiology.

Several cultural changes that have taken place during the past 30 years may have direct bearing on the increased incidence of eating disorders. Foremost among these is the strong emphasis our society places on the desirability of a thin appearance, especially for females. This factor, along with changes in clothing styles that emphasize the female figure, could explain why certain vulnerable individuals may feel it necessary to choose an unhealthy means, whether it be dieting, vomiting, laxative abuse, or a combination thereof, in striving for a dangerously thin weight goal. Societal changes in sexual mores, which have lowered the mean age of initiating sexual intercourse from the late teens to the mid teens and which have thereby placed increased pressure on adolescent and young adult females, are hypothesized to play an additional role in furthering the psychological vulnerability of some individuals. In addition, the issue of career versus family, which places an added pressure of decision-making on young females, may create another level of vulnerability for some individuals at risk for the development of psychological difficulties. These pressures, which were not faced as dramatically by women in previous generations and which do not affect males in the same ways, may point to why the eating disorders are increasing in frequency so dramatically and why they mostly affect females. Of further interest is the fact that issues of sexual identity have been noted in some males who develop these disorders.

The psychological factors responsible for the development of an eating disorder in any given individual patient are multiple and complex. When anorexia nervosa first came to prominence in the 1960s, it was found that most of the girls with this disorder exhibited a set of similar characteristics, some of which were manifest openly, whereas others emerged with intensive therapy. Specifically, these girls were described as having been excellent students, compulsive workers, and compliant daughters before the onset of their illness. These same girls then became hostile, withdrawn, and depressed after the illness began. In therapy, they revealed exceedingly low self-esteem despite their apparent outward successes. Their families, outwardly healthy and often so-called "pillars of society," were found to have significant hidden psychopathology.

Based on these early findings, three major lines of reasoning, often overlapping, were proposed to explain the psychological basis of the eating disorders. The first concentrated on the psychopathology of the individual. This theory postulates that poor self-esteem in the face of outward success provides a major difficulty, which the vulnerable adolescent tries to alleviate by striving for one achievable goal—the thinnest possible body. The second theory focuses on the family. It postulates that patients with anorexia nervosa come from families in which the natural childhood processes of separation and individuation are not allowed to proceed normally. The refusal to eat represents the ultimate rebelliousness in a teenager who has previously done "everything you've asked of me." A third, older, theory was developed around a series of sexual themes. This theory hypothesizes that the weight loss in anorexia nervosa serves to diminish the female figure on a young lady who is afraid of becoming a sexual adult. The basis of this fear may be sexual taboos in the family, in some cases, or sexual overstimulation in the family in other cases. In the extreme psychoanalytic interpretation of this theory, patients with anorexia nervosa may even be refusing food intake for fear of "oral impregnation."

The concepts inherent in each of these theories have been expressed in therapy by many patients with eating disorders. However, with more recent recognition of many cases of anorexia nervosa in which the patient does not fit the traditional "good girl" mold, and as in many cases of bulimia, it is apparent that a multitude of psychological themes may be found. For instance, although many girls who develop anorexia nervosa are very compulsive, shy, and not involved sexually, those with bulimia may be impulsive, outgoing, and even promiscuous. Furthermore, the previous finding that most girls with anorexia nervosa are excellent students from apparently healthy and intact families is no longer as true as in the past. In fact, increasing numbers of girls with anorexia nervosa are noted to have learning disabilities or mental retardation or to be from broken homes and other difficult family situations. Clearly, the psychological vulnerability that may be one of the precipitants of the eating disorders may come from many directions and be expressed in multiple ways.

The possibility that a biologic vulnerability may be present in the initiation and continuance of the eating disorders has received much attention of late. Because cases of anorexia and bulimia have been associated with depression, addiction, or both in family studies, it is surmised that a biochemical predeterminant may be present in each of these disorders. Changes in either dopamine or serotonin metabolism may play a role in bringing on these disorders, while the cholecystokinin and endorphin systems have been implicated in maintaining them. It is very possible that the biochemical factors that may predispose an individual to begin weight loss or vomiting may be different from those that prevent reversal of these behaviors.

Most likely, several factors converge in the development of an eating disorder. The adolescent girl who is culturally primed, biologically at risk, and psychologically vulnerable may begin dieting or vomiting in response to a particular precipitant (often an insult by family or friends, exposure to another individual with an eating disorder, or a stressful life). The positive psychological feedback that initially accompanies an "improved" appearance and the biochemical changes that occur in response to decreased nutrition may then serve to perpetuate the behavior. It is at this stage that family and friends become concerned, and the individual patient seeks medical care.

EVALUATION

Initial evaluation of the patient with an eating disorder includes a determination of the diagnosis and its severity, an evaluation of other possible causes of weight loss and effects of malnutrition, an analysis of the psychological context of the illness, and a decision regarding treatment planning.

As previously noted in the box on p. 762, specific diagnostic criteria currently exist for the eating disorders. Evaluation of these criteria serves both to elucidate the diagnosis and determine the severity of illness. Distortion of body image, a hallmark in the diagnosis of anorexia nervosa, may be evaluated by exploring the patient's views of her initial weight, current weight, and desired weight. Although this information may provide insight into how distorted the view may be, one must realize that not all patients are truthful. Similarly, establishing the patient's nutritional and exercise patterns and her use of vomiting or medications designed to promote weight loss (including diet pills, laxatives, and/or diuretics) provides hints both to the diagnosis and the possibility of medical complications. Care must be taken to avoid being misled by the patient who is not completely forthright; often the physical examination and laboratory tests suggest the true extent of the patient's disorder.

The first steps in the physical examination of the patient with an eating disorder are calculation of "percent below ideal body weight" and determination of vital signs. Percent below ideal body weight (IBW), which may be calculated by comparing the patient's current weight with the average weight expected for height, age, and sex (as determined by standard growth charts), serves both as one of the diagnostic criteria and as a gross estimate of the degree of malnutrition. In general, one may assume that more than 30% below IBW represents severe malnutrition, that 20% to 30% below IBW represents moderate malnutrition, and that the patient not yet 20% below IBW is mildly malnourished. For example, a 16-year-old female who is 5 feet, 4 inches tall would have an expected body weight of 120 pounds, plus or minus 10%; she would be 20% below IBW at 96 pounds and 30% below IBW at 84 pounds. Vital signs provide further evidence of the degree of malnutrition, for chronic malnutrition is accompanied by decreases in blood pressure and pulse, as well as electrocardiogram (ECG) voltage. Other physical changes associated with malnutrition or its concomitant hormonal changes include the findings of scaphoid abdomen, muscle weakness, lanugo similar to that seen in newborns, decreased reflexes, and dry skin. Few physical findings are associated with the vomiting of bulimia, although tell-tale bite marks on the knuckles (used to induce gagging) may be evident in some patients.

Laboratory tests performed in the patient with an eating disorder further elucidate the severity of illness. Note that most patients with anorexia and bulimia nervosa initially will have normal laboratory results, although all organ systems are probably affected by the malnutrition. Those laboratory abnormalities found on routine testing generally are related to the individual's particular nutritional pattern. Thus the patient with chronic malnutrition will usually have leukopenia, occasionally have thrombocytopenia, and in rare cases will have severe anemia (being protected for some time from iron-deficiency anemia by the presence of amenorrhea). The patient who restricts fluid intake may show evidence of dehydration on blood chemistry determinations (including an elevated sodium or blood urea nitrogen), whereas the patient who drinks excessive fluids to satisfy her hunger or the doctor's scale may show evidence of hyponatremia and a dilute urine. Conversely, the patient who vomits or uses laxatives may show evidence of hypokalemia, often very severe in those who use both methods of weight control. Nutrient values, including levels of zinc, calcium, magnesium, copper, vitamin B_{12}, and folate, may all be altered in the malnourished patient; amylase levels and urinary pH may be elevated in some patients with bulimia.

Hormonal testing may show evidence of dysfunction in endocrine systems. The development of hypothyroidism, which is believed to be an adaptive response to the lack of adequate nutrition, is generally evident in low-normal levels of T3, T4, and thyroid-stimulating hormone (TSH). Amenorrhea, a hallmark of the disorder, generally develops at approximately 15% below IBW but may be seen earlier; it is accompanied by low levels of luteinizing hormone (LH) and follicle-stimulating hormone (FSH). Loss of diurnal variation in cortisol production and abnormalities in antidiuretic hormone may be noted as well, although these tests need not be performed in most patients. Evidence of abnormalities on brain computed tomography (CT) or echocardiogram may be found, but use of these tests is generally reserved for evaluation of other possible etiologies for those in whom the diagnosis is in question. In general, the initial laboratory work-up of eating disorders consists of a complete blood count, urinalysis, and ECG, as well as evaluation of serum electrolytes, liver function, thyroid function, and levels of LH and FSH in patients with amenorrhea. This battery of tests is generally sufficient to provide a barometer of current status, a baseline to follow further changes, and screening for other possible causes of weight loss.

DIFFERENTIAL DIAGNOSIS

The differential diagnosis of the eating disorders includes possible medical causes of weight loss or vomiting and other psychiatric causes of poor appetite. The history, physical examination, and baseline laboratory tests should help to rule out infectious, inflammatory, neoplastic, or endocrine disease; further testing may be necessary if the weight loss or vomiting cannot be adequately explained by medical history from patient and family. A CT scan, gastrointestinal (GI) series, or other testing may be considered in rare cases for patients who claim to be eating well or not vomiting on purpose. Case reports abound in such entities as hypothalamic tumors, inflammatory bowel disease, mesenteric artery syndrome, or GI tract tumors being mistakenly diagnosed as eating disorders in patients whose weight loss or vomiting was not adequately understood. In occasional situations a patient may show obvious pleasure in the weight loss or vomiting brought on by another disorder, but this must not be confused with a positive diagnosis of anorexia or bulimia nervosa.

Psychiatric causes of weight loss can include depression and psychosis (especially schizophrenia). The patient who refuses to eat because of a desire to lose weight must be differentiated from the patient who cannot eat because of depression or the patient who will not eat because of delusional fears (e.g., that the food is poisoned). Although patients may have concomitant depression or psychosis with anorexia nervosa or bulimia, separate criteria must be used to establish each entity. A full psychosocial history must be obtained as part of the initial evaluation to establish both the diagnosis and the psychosocial severity of the disorder. The patient's functioning in the family, in school, and with peers must be determined, and possible psychiatric symptoms such as sleep disorders, hallucinations, delusions, or obsessions should be elicited. It is the rare patient with an eating disorder who does not exhibit psychosocial changes with the onset of the illness. These generally include fighting with the family, withdrawing from friends, and performing differently in school. If additional psychiatric symptoms are found, the possibility of an additional diagnosis should be actively pursued.

The results of the initial medical and psychiatric evaluation play a major role in establishing a treatment protocol for the patient. Although most patients with an eating disorder may be treated as outpatients, those with significant medical findings (including severe malnutrition, electrolyte disturbance, or vital sign abnormalities) will require hospitalization. Patients who are adamant about continued weight loss, whose vomiting is extreme, or whose psychiatric condition is out of control also may require hospitalization. These hospitalizations may be short term on a general medical unit or long term on a psychiatric or adolescent medicine unit. Treatment approaches, both inpatient and outpatient, are aimed at restoring more normal physical and psychological functioning.

TREATMENT

Patients with an eating disorder have been considered by most clinicians to be among the most difficult and frustrating patients to treat. Undoubtedly, several factors are responsible for this perception. The combination of medical and psychological care required in treatment makes it difficult for any single professional to be proficient in all aspects of a patient's care. If the patient is hostile to the physician (e.g., often choosing to ignore suggestions and testing how much she can "get away with"), the physician may find himself or herself in an uncomfortable and adversarial relationship with the patient. The difficult families within which many of these patients live often make the establishment of the most rational treatment plans a challenge. For these reasons it is advisable that no single individual be totally responsible for any patient's care beyond the initial evaluation or for the most straightforward of cases. Rather, it is recommended that a team approach be used. The team may consist of a primary care physician, a psychiatrist, a psychologist, a social worker, and/or a nutritionist, with the exact combination determined by local availability and preference. In general, each member of the team manages specific aspects of care, with frequent team meetings and discussions to avoid miscommunication that can sabotage the treatment plan, and with one member of the team serving as spokesman to the patient and, especially, the family.

Several modalities may be employed by the treatment team. These include nutritional rehabilitation, behavior therapy, individual psychotherapy, family and group therapy, and psychopharmacology. It is generally acknowledged that a "multimodality therapy," in which aspects of each of these approaches are employed, holds the best promise for successful treatment. The degree to which each of these approaches is incorporated into the treatment plan varies, both with the preferences of the treatment team and the requirements of the individual patient. Each of these approaches may be used in the inpatient *and* outpatient settings.

Nutritional Rehabilitation

The malnutrition that accompanies anorexia nervosa is directly responsible for most if not all of the physical abnormalities noted in the disorder and also for some of the deterioration in mental state. Accordingly, nutritional rehabilitation is crucial in the treatment of the patient with anorexia nervosa. Restoration of body weight, generally to an end-point of within 10% of ideal body weight, should be one of the main goals of treatment. For many patients with mild to moderate malnutrition (i.e., 15% to 25% below ideal body weight), this may be accomplished on an outpatient basis; it is the rare patient with moderate to severe malnutrition (i.e., more than 25% below ideal body weight) who can accomplish the required weight gain without hospitalization.

Nutritional rehabilitation can generally be achieved through oral feedings; a daily intake of three substantial meals and three to four snacks is usually sufficient to bring about the required weight gain. On inpatient units, meals are generally provided as part of a strict regimen, and snacks generally consist of high-calorie supplements, available as liquids or puddings in various brands and flavors. Care is taken to not overfeed those patients with severe malnutrition, as a too rapid weight gain has been associated with severe metabolic abnormalities in some patients. In the outpatient setting, an appropriate meal pattern may be developed based on prior eating habits of the patient and her family, or a specific dietary plan may be offered by the physician or a nutritionist. The dietary plan should be specific in order to avoid ambiguities that can lead to family fighting; it should contain approximately 2000 to 3000 calories per day, with up to 1000 calories in the form of high-calorie supplements; it should be well-balanced, including foods from each of the three major food groups: carbohydrates, fats, and proteins. Compliance with the dietary regimen may be evaluated by use of diet diaries; however, many patients do not always fill these out accurately and honestly. With the exception of the high-calorie supplements, a similar dietary plan may be offered to the normal-weight patient with bulimia, who generally will require "nutritional adjustment" rather than nutritional rehabilitation.

Behavior Therapy

Merely offering a nutritious diet to the patient with either anorexia nervosa or bulimia is unlikely to result in a drastic change in the patient's status. For this reason behavioral therapy is normally a necessary component of the treatment plan. The goal of behavior therapy in the treatment of eating disorders is to offer a set of external positive and negative reinforcements to replace those internal sensors that usually control appetite and weight gain but that are currently missing. Behavior therapy is not intended to be definitive, but rather to accomplish specific goals in the areas of weight and diet stabilization, thus allowing the psychological modalities of treatment to proceed in a more "medically healthy" patient.

Various behavioral approaches may be used. Strict behavioral plans employed on some psychiatric units include removal of all "privileges," including use of telephone, television, and regular clothing, if a particular weight goal is not achieved each day. A somewhat less strict plan employed by our own adolescent unit includes four phases of treatment, with patients moving from one phase to another based on achievement of progressively higher weight goals. Each phase incorporates additional privileges into the patient's daily activities in the areas of mobility on the unit, exercise, meals, snacks, and passes, in such a way that improved weight and eating patterns lead to additional privileges and responsibilities for the patient. For those patients unable to respond to the positive reinforcements provided by such a "phased" system the use of an all-liquid diet, provided by mouth or, more rarely, nasogastric tube, may be substituted. Use of such methods will ultimately result in achievement of necessary weight goals in almost all patients. However, it must be borne in mind that behavioral therapy alone cannot be considered an adequate treatment approach and that controlled studies have been unable to distinguish between the effects of the various behavioral approaches.

Application of behavioral principles to patients with anorexia nervosa in the outpatient setting, or for patients with bulimia, may be somewhat more difficult to accomplish. Usual approaches to behavioral therapy in outpatient settings, such as the use of monetary or similar rewards, may not be strong enough to overcome the fear of eating in many patients with anorexia nervosa. Thus fear of hospitalization itself may be the sole motivation in some cases. Similarly, classic approaches may not be effective for the patient with bulimia, since the symptom of vomiting cannot be readily measured. More sophisticated cognitive-behavioral approaches have been developed, therefore, so that the patient with bulimia may understand and play an active role in her own behavioral therapy. These approaches make use of diaries and alterations in daily patterns to effect change in the patient with bulimia.

Individual, Family, and Group Therapy

Individual psychotherapy remains a critical part of the treatment for most patients with an eating disorder. Although therapeutic styles differ based on the treatment team and individual therapist, an exploration of underlying psychological features and possible mechanisms for change will be appropriate for most patients with either anorexia nervosa or bulimia. Although several common themes have been noted in many of these patients, including poor self-esteem, family conflicts, difficulties with friends, and fear of sexuality, there is obviously great individual variety in the way these themes are expressed and manifested. For many patients, it is apparent that the eating disorder serves as a defense against other difficult aspects of life; there also may be important secondary gain. It is generally acknowledged that psychological change is a necessary precursor to significant improvement in the disordered thinking and behavior exhibited by most patients with an eating disorder.

Family therapy has become increasingly more popular as a treatment modality, especially for younger patients, as the major role that family conflicts and problems play in symptom continuation has become more apparent. Family sessions, arranged in varying combinations to include parents and siblings, generally focus on the disordered communication patterns that preceded and presumably contributed to the eating disorder. Resolving specific conflicts arising from the presence of the eating disorder itself also becomes an important area for discussion. It has been found that the course of the eating disorder is much more difficult for adolescent patients whose families are unable or unwilling to make necessary changes in their ongoing patterns of communication and parenting.

Many patients with eating disorders participate in group therapy during the course of their treatment. For some patients with mild anorexia nervosa and for college-age patients with bulimia, this may be the only approach to therapy employed. Groups may be organized in many different ways, with some focusing on a psychotherapeutic approach and others concentrating more specifically on behavioral changes. Initial fears that patients with eating disorders will "learn bad habits" from each other in the group have been outweighed by the apparent benefit most patients derive from group therapy. This is especially true for those patients who have experienced social difficulties during their adolescence.

Psychopharmacology

The use of medication in the treatment of eating disorders has had a long history of decidedly mixed results. Multiple medications have been tried, from thyroid hormone and insulin in the 1940s and '50s to phenytoin (Dilantin) and hydroxyzine (Atarax) in the 1960s and '70s, as attempts were made to improve appetite, increase weight gain, and reverse physiologic abnormalities. More recent pharmacologic treatments of the eating disorders have concentrated on psychoactive medications, including antidepressants, lithium, and antipsychotics. Two specific lines of reasoning have guided the use of these medications. In those patients who are diagnosed as having an eating disorder along with or as part of another psychiatric diagnosis, medication for the associated diagnosis is offered with the expectation that the eating disorder will improve as other depressive or psychotic symptomatology is relieved. Alternately, there are those who believe that use of psychoactive drugs, especially the antidepressants (including the tricyclics, the monoamine oxidase [MAO] inhibitors, and other newer medications), decrease the urge to binge and vomit in patients with bulimia. Although earlier studies failed to show definitive benefits from the use of medication in the eating disorders, more recent studies have attempted to delineate subgroups of patients most likely to improve with their use. Antidepressants remain a controversial treatment in the management of the eating disorders; only those very familiar with their use should consider utilizing these medications as part of the treatment regimen.

OUTCOME AND PROGNOSIS

The eating disorders must be looked upon as a chronic illness, similar to other medical or psychiatric chronic illnesses. A wide range of outcomes may be expected. Some patients improve rapidly with treatment, return to functioning normally, and show no evidence of eating disorder behavior on long-term follow-up. Other patients improve more slowly, showing partial or complete resolution of symptoms but with evidence of relapses at times of stress. Yet others continue to do poorly for a long period of time, retaining the symptoms of their anorexia nervosa or bulimia for many years. Although there are many different approaches used to evaluate outcome, it is estimated that approximately 25% of patients do well in the long term, 50% show varying degrees of improvement, and 25% do poorly despite adequate treatment.

Multiple personal, family, and treatment factors have been considered for their significance in predicting the course of an eating disorder. Several factors have been found to be associated with prognosis, yet none of these may be predictive for an individual patient. For instance, a poorer outcome in anorexia nervosa has been associated with such factors as older age, vomiting, and premorbid personality problems, yet any particular patient with this constellation of findings may still do well with treatment. Further, no specific treatment has been shown by controlled studies to be more effective than others, in general or for any particular type of patient. Thus the eating disorders remain a complicated and challenging set of disorders for the patient, the family, and the treatment team.

REFERENCE

1. Feighner JP et al: Diagnostic criteria for use in psychiatric research, Arch Gen Psychiatry 26:57, 1982.

SUGGESTED READINGS

Anyan WR Jr and Schowalter JE: A comprehensive approach to anorexia nervosa, J Am Acad Child Psychiatry 22:122, 1983.

Comerci GD: Eating disorders in adolescents, Pediatr Rev 10:1, 1988.

Fava M et al: Neurochemical abnormalities of anorexia nervosa and bulimia nervosa, Am J Psychiatry 146:963, 1989.

Garfinkel PE, Garner DM, and Goldbloom DS: Eating disorders: implications for the 1980's, Can J Psychiatry 32:624, 1987.

Garner DM, editor: Psychotherapy for anorexia nervosa and bulimia nervosa, Clin Psychol Spring:12, 1986.

Griffiths RA et al: The treatment of bulimia nervosa, Aust NZ J Psychiatry 21:5, 1987.

Harper G: Anorexia nervosa: what kind of disorder? Pediatr Ann 13:812, 1984.

Herzog DB and Copeland PN: Eating disorders, N Engl J Med 313:295, 1985.

Herzog DB, Franko DL, and Brotman AW: Integrating treatments for bulimia nervosa, J Am Acad Psychoanal 17:141, 1989.

Herzog DB, Keller MB, and Lavori PW: Outcome in anorexia nervosa and bulimia nervosa: a review of the literature, J Nerv Ment Dis 176:131, 1988.

Johnson C, Lewis C, and Hagman J: The syndrome of bulimia: review and synthesis, Psychiatr Clin North Am 7:247, 1984.

Johnson C, Stuckey M, and Mitchell J: Psychopharmacological treatment of anorexia nervosa and bulimia: review and synthesis, J Nerv Ment Dis 171:524, 1983.

Kaplan AS and Woodside DB: Biological aspects of anorexia nervosa and bulimia nervosa, J Consult Clin Psychol 55:645, 1987.

Lippe BM: The physiologic aspects of eating disorders, J Am Acad Child Psychiatry 22:108, 1983.

Oster JR: The binge-purge syndrome: a common albeit unappreciated cause of acid-base and fluid-electrolyte disturbances, South Med J 80:58, 1987.

Rubel JA: The function of self-help groups in recovery from anorexia nervosa and bulimia, Psychiatr Clin North Am 7:381, 1984.

Russell GFM et al: An evaluation of family therapy in anorexia nervosa and bulimia nervosa, Arch Gen Psychiatry 44:1047, 1987.

100

Drug, Alcohol, and Tobacco Abuse

Susan M. Coupey and S. Kenneth Schonberg

The use of drugs, or more precisely, the use of substances that alter the state of consciousness, has become a nearly universal rite of passage for American adolescents. Whereas the use of alcohol has always been widespread among youth, the past two decades have witnessed a dramatic rise in the amount and types of other substances abused by teenagers and young adults. Opiates, barbiturates, cocaine, hallucinogens, amphetamines, glue, cleaning fluid, aerosols, marijuana, and alcohol have all become familiar terms to those who provide care for youth. Only very recently, as the decade of the eighties came to a close, have there been indications of a downturn in the use of some of these drugs, notably marijuana and cocaine.

The pattern of substance use by adolescents is continually evolving. New drugs, new fads, and new epidemics have been an invariable feature of the substance abuse situation. The late 1960s and early 1970s were marked by a major concern with the abuse of opiates and barbiturates. Addiction, overdose, and medical sequelae from these drugs led to frequent hospitalizations, serious illnesses, and significant mortality. By the mid-1970s the use of these "hard" drugs had declined markedly. A variety of hallucinogens appeared, gained widespread popularity, and subsequently faded from the spotlight as their use lessened; however, hallucinogens remained readily available. Among these agents have been peyote (which contains mescaline), lysergic acid diethylamide (LSD), and phencyclidine (PCP, angel dust). Currently, major attention has been focused on the use of milder intoxicants—alcohol and marijuana. Although these drugs are less likely to cause serious somatic illness during the teenage years, their widespread use and frequent association with both trauma and behavioral disruption cause the health practitioner concern. In addition, in the latter part of the 1980s, cocaine use and abuse became quite common among both adolescents and adults. The emergence of "crack" (freebase cocaine that can be smoked) as a major public health problem, especially in inner cities, has been accompanied by greater public awareness of the addictive and destructive properties of the drug.

Traditionally, discussion of drug-related illnesses with teenagers has been approached either by outlining the physiologic consequences associated with the abuse of a particular substance or by reviewing the effects of abuse on different organ systems. Such approaches, however, are at variance with the usual way most teenage drug abusers come in for medical care. The substances now most commonly abused are not associated with frequent illness; therefore teenagers using these agents are most often encountered when they seek routine health maintenance or care for an illness unrelated to drugs. Only through routine questioning is such drug use discovered. Even the adolescent suffering from a drug-related illness seldom seeks care on account of a particular drug habit or the impairment of a specific body organ, but rather because a symptom complex mandates medical attention. In this respect, teenage drug abusers are like other patients: determining the etiologic factors and the pathologic conditions of their illnesses requires a comprehensive analysis of all possibilities. If drug abuse, of either one or several agents, is not considered along with other possible etiologic factors to explain the symptoms, the physician may miss an opportunity for meaningful therapeutic intervention. Therefore, in keeping with the more usual method by which such adolescent patients come to medical attention, drug abuse–related illnesses will be discussed as they initially appear to the primary care health professional.

THE MEDICAL HISTORY

Inquiries about the extent of drug involvement should be made to every teenager during a periodic health examination. Such inquiries should be a natural adjunct to the assessment of other psychosocial indicators, including academic progress, sexual behavior, family and peer relationships, and recreational interests. An accurate drug history can be obtained only in an atmosphere of confidentiality and privacy, with parents excluded from the interview. In the proper setting, positive responses should be expected from the majority of teenagers when queried regarding the use of alcohol and cigarettes. The teenager should be questioned about not only the specific type of drug used, but also about the extent of use, the setting in which use occurs, and the degree of social, educational, and vocational disruption attributable to the drug abuse behavior. The information gathered from such questioning is necessary for a proper appraisal of the need for further intervention. Obtaining such information will depend in large part on the physician's ability to respond to answers without alarm or dismay.

Although over 90% of adolescents will have tried alcohol before graduating from high school, with approximately one third of this group reporting weekly use, teenagers will seldom volunteer information on the extent of their alcohol use unless questioned directly. The medical complications of chronic alcoholism, although severe, do not usually appear until after adolescence. The physician's task is to identify those teenagers who are experiencing psychosocial disruption or who are at greatest risk of becoming alcoholic adults. The youngster who is doing poorly in school, is having difficulty with peer relationships, or is engaging in delinquent behavior, and who is drinking concurrently, is not difficult to identify as one in need of special attention.

The teenager who has not experienced academic or social failure but whose drinking goes beyond experimentation or occasional use represents a more difficult problem. Although there are no specific criteria to determine who is at greatest risk of future difficulty, a history of parental alcoholism and widespread alcohol abuse within the teenager's peer group are factors associated with a poor prognosis. Even for this high-risk group, no specific therapy may be indicated beyond the need for periodic reevaluation of the situation. For most teenagers, their history of alcohol use should be noted, quantitated, and used as a reference point by which to evaluate information obtained during subsequent visits.

All teenagers, including the minority who do not drink at all, need to be counseled regarding the relationship between intoxicants and accidents. Accidents are by far the leading cause of death among adolescents. The majority of these fatal accidents are automotive, and intoxicants are involved in many if not most. A teenager who will not at some time drive while intoxicated or be a passenger in the automobile of an intoxicated driver is rare. Preventive health care for adolescents and their families must include a discussion of alternatives to such risk-taking behavior.

Although fewer teenagers use tobacco than alcohol, nearly 30% of high school seniors do smoke at least monthly. The long-range cardiac, pulmonary, and carcinogenic consequences of cigarette smoking have been well publicized, and this information has not escaped the teenage population. Although the physician may have little to add in the way of warning to what has already been proffered by the schools and the press, it is negligent not to inquire about the adolescent's smoking habits and offer counsel on those health issues regarding tobacco, which have immediate relevance to the life of the teenager. The adverse effect of smoking on pulmonary function may make an impact on the adolescent with athletic aspirations. The pregnant teenager concerned with the welfare of her unborn baby may alter her smoking habits when informed of the possible association between tobacco and low birth weight and neonatal mortality. The adolescent girl who is starting to use oral contraceptives may be counseled that although "the pill" does not cause cancer, smoking certainly does, and she may be motivated to give up cigarettes. Adolescents with a respiratory illness, particularly asthma, must be apprised of the immediate effects of smoking on their day-to-day health. All these issues lend themselves to discussion in the give-and-take atmosphere of the personal history interview.

A teenager's marijuana smoking usually will only come to light when the physician obtains a drug-use history. Only rarely will a young person obtain medical care because of an acute intoxication secondary to marijuana smoking or will a family seek medical attention specifically for their teenager's marijuana problem. Although in recent years there has been a reduction in the panic associated with the discovery of an adolescent's use of marijuana, the physician's role remains to place the teenager's use of this intoxicant in proper perspective so that an appropriate assessment of the need for further intervention can be made. The primary consideration in the evaluation of the marijuana-abusing teenager is whether the use of this intoxicant is but a symptom of more serious underlying psychopathologic conditions. In this regard, the marijuana smoker is like the adolescent drinker. Similarly, there is concern regarding the relationship between intoxication with marijuana and automotive accidents.

The physiologic changes produced by marijuana smoking are mostly benign, rarely require medical attention, and are peripheral to the more important behavioral issues of intoxicant use by adolescents. However, because teenagers and their parents frequently raise questions about the medical side effects of marijuana smoking, the physician should have an understanding of the physiologic effects for appropriate counseling.

Although sore throats and bronchitis are frequent sequelae to marijuana smoking, the teenager seldom seeks treatment for those complications. Other respiratory effects include bronchodilation with acute inhalation and bronchoconstriction with more prolonged exposure. Thus adolescents with asthma may experience either relief or exacerbation of symptoms. Allergic reactions to marijuana do occur and may cause asthmatic attacks. A potential long-term pulmonary consequence in the chronic marijuana abuser is carcinoma of the lungs. Bronchial biopsies of marijuana smokers with clinical diagnoses of chronic bronchitis have revealed lesions characteristic of the early stages of cancer. Cardiovascular effects include both tachycardia and a transient low-grade elevation of systolic and diastolic blood pressure. Neither of these cardiac consequences is of clinical significance.

Marijuana has been reported to have a number of effects on the endocrine system in males with histories of prolonged and frequent use. They include depression of testosterone levels in the blood, diminished sperm counts, impaired sexual function, and gynecomastia. The associated clinical problems of impotence and infertility should respond to abstinence from marijuana. The long-term effects of these endocrine imbalances on the developing adolescent, however, are as yet unclear.

Although marijuana causes electroencephalographic changes and alterations in neurotransmitters, neither structural damage to the brain nor an increase in seizure potential has been demonstrated. In contrast, there are a number of acute behavioral changes that, because of their potential to facilitate trauma, are of clinical significance. In addition to elation, the marijuana "high" causes a loss of critical judgment, distortions in time perception, impairment of tracking (the ability to follow a moving object accurately), and poor performance on "divided attention" tasks, such as driving. The infrequent correlation between marijuana intoxication and accidental trauma is probably because the users show no specific signs of drug abuse and the authorities lack a readily available method to detect marijuana metabolites in body fluids. Other behavioral effects include impaired short-term memory, interference with learning, and difficulty with oral communication. Occasionally a physician will encounter a patient with an acute adverse reaction to marijuana manifested as a toxic psychosis with depression or panic. Both the symptoms and the treatment of these reactions are similar to those noted for hallucinogen abuse. Prolonged (and possibly permanent) personality changes have been reported in chronic marijuana users. This *amotivational syndrome* is marked by lethargy and a lack of goal-directed activity.

A history of marijuana smoking, alcohol consumption, or the abuse of any drug by an adolescent indicates the need for further exploration into the possibility of underlying psychopathologic conditions. Frequently, the psychosocial problems that initiate drug-taking behavior are more important than the specific medical complications of abuse.

PHYSICAL EXAMINATION

The teenager who is heavily involved in the abuse of hard drugs is more likely to come to medical attention with a specific illness associated with drug abuse rather than through a routine physical examination. However, even those adolescents who use less dangerous drugs often have some concern about the potential somatic consequences of their behavior, and they may seek the reassurance of a checkup to prove to themselves that all is well. In such circumstances the teenager may deny a history of drug abuse even when questioned directly so as not to prejudice the results of the examination. The physician must be alert to those physical findings which are either pathognomonic of or associated with illicit substance abuse.

The abuser of either marijuana, cocaine, or amphetamines may have an accelerated pulse rate; these substances are also associated with weight loss and closely mimic the presentation of hyperthyroidism. Pinpoint pupils unresponsive to light are characteristic of opiate abuse. Barbiturates usually produce sluggish pupillary responses, but pinpoint pupils have been observed in many teenagers using only barbiturates. Conjunctivitis and irritation or ulceration of the nasal mucosa may be found in the teenager abusing drugs by inhalation. Glue "sniffers," marijuana smokers, and "snorters" of heroin or cocaine are likely to manifest these conditions.

Dermatologic Presentations

The majority of the specific physical signs of drug abuse are found on the skin and are associated with the subcutaneous or intravenous abuse of opiates and, less commonly, barbiturates. Subcutaneous fat necrosis, similar to that experienced by persons with diabetes receiving insulin injections, is common in teenagers who inject heroin under their skin ("skin popping"). Cutaneous scars ("tracks") following the course of superficial veins are found in teenagers with a prolonged history of injecting drugs intravenously ("mainlining"). They are caused by chronic inflammation associated with repeated injections or by the deposition of carbonaceous material from needles that were briefly "flamed" in an attempt at sterilization. The teenager frequently disguises these tracks by covering them with a self-administered tattoo applied with a needle and india ink. Any tattoo placed by an amateur or professional and found in the antecubital fossa should be examined closely for tracks or needle marks. Plastic surgery for the removal of tracks and tattoos should be suggested to the patient because these stigmata often interfere with later employability and thereby compromise rehabilitative efforts.

Both the intravenous and subcutaneous routes of drug administration are characterized by a lack of sterile technique. Skin abscesses and cellulitis are common among teenage addicts. When these conditions come to medical attention, drug abuse should be considered as a possible cause. The presence of needle marks confirms drug abuse as an etiologic factor.

Localized pain is the most frequent symptom of skin abscesses, with *Staphylococcus aureus* being the most common causative organism. Fever and leukocytosis are relatively uncommon, and regional adenopathy may or may not be present. Treatment involves incision and drainage and the administration of an appropriate antibiotic as determined by isolation of the causative organism by culture.

Skin abscesses and superficial skin ulcers are potential sites for the growth of *Clostridium* organisms, and tetanus has been reported in adult heroin addicts. A similar incidence of tetanus in teenagers has not been encountered, probably because of residual protection from childhood immunizations; nevertheless, the administration of a tetanus toxoid booster should be considered.

Superficial thrombophlebitis, particularly of the upper extremities, is common among intravenous opiate-abusing teenagers and is a cause of both localized symptoms and systemic infection. Treatment includes local soaks and systemic antibiotic therapy. Anticoagulation is not a necessary part of the treatment for superficial thrombophlebitis.

Serious Systemic Infections and Opportunistic Infections

In the course of evaluating the teenager with a systemic infection or a fever of unknown origin, the physician should remember that intravenous drug abuse may be an etiologic factor in the development of the infectious process. The direct injection of bacteria or viruses into the bloodstream during intravenous drug administration or septic embolization from a site of superficial thrombophlebitis will give rise to the hematogenous dissemination of infectious agents to the heart, brain, osseous structures, and, less commonly, other organs.

Human immunodeficiency virus (HIV) is the most serious of such infections transmitted by contaminated injection apparatus. Because of the prolonged asymptomatic period associated with this virus, clinical illness is not often expressed during the teenage years. However, an adolescent with a history of injecting any illicit drug, including opiates, cocaine, or amphetamines, should be offered counseling and testing for HIV. Adolescents with unexplained weight loss, night sweats, generalized lymphadenopathy, oral thrush, recurrent bacterial infections, severe prolonged diarrhea, tuberculosis, or *Pneumocystis carinii* pneumonia should have HIV-related illness considered in the differential diagnosis and should have complete drug abuse and sexual histories taken. Teenagers who are HIV positive and asymptomatic should have their immune function assessed initially and at least twice per year thereafter. Antiretroviral treatment and prophylaxis for opportunistic infections can then be instituted according to current guidelines, based on significantly decreased immunocompetence. Because HIV is transmitted sexually as well as by contaminated needles, adolescent girls who are not themselves drug users but whose sexual partners use drugs intravenously require counseling and testing for HIV infection.

Endocarditis in the intravenous drug abuser may affect either the right or left side of the heart. Beyond fever and occasional pulmonary symptoms, right-sided endocarditis is associated with few if any systemic signs and almost always affects a previously undamaged tricuspid valve. *S. aureus* is frequently the causative organism. Left-sided endocarditis may involve either normal or abnormal mitral or aortic valves and is usually associated with systemic evidence of infection. *S. aureus* and streptococcal species are the most frequently encountered organisms, and fungal infections with *Candida* organisms have also been reported. The teenager with endocarditis must be hospitalized and treated with intravenous antibiotics as determined by the isolation of the causative organism.

Central nervous system (CNS) infection may be associated with endocarditis or may be a primary manifestation of drug abuse–related septicemia. Brain abscess is rare during adolescence, so, when present, intravenous drug abuse should be suspected. Multiple microabscesses are found more frequently than a single large abscess; thus focal neurologic signs may be absent. Since the only manifestation of multiple microabscesses of the brain may be fever or a personality change, lumbar puncture, electroencephalography, transaxial computed tomography and magnetic resonance imaging may be required to reach the correct diagnosis. *S. aureus* is most often found to be the causative organism. The same organism has been associated with the inceased frequency of osteomyelitis among intravenous drug abusers. The treatment and prognosis for CNS infection and osteomyelitis are the same for the user and the nonuser of drugs.

The intravenous injection of starch and talc, which are used as fillers for medicinal preparations designed solely for oral use, may lead to pulmonary angiothrombosis and granulomatosis. Although pulmonary hypertension and cor pulmonale can eventually result from this process, it is unusual for these problems to become clinically apparent during adolescence. Nevertheless, the evaluation of teenagers manifesting unexplained compromise to respiratory function should include the consideration of intravenous drug abuse; thus chest roentgenograms, blood cultures, and tuberculin skin testing should be performed.

Venereal Diseases and Other Urologic and Gynecologic Presentations

Because of the life-style often followed by adolescents who are frequent drug users, venereal diseases are common in this population and may be the reason they seek medical care. Syphilis can be acquired both sexually and via contaminated needles; therefore a serologic test for syphilis should always be obtained, keeping in mind that false positive results are common in heroin users. Gonococcal and nongonococcal urethritis, cervicitis, salpingitis, proctitis, and pharyngitis are often diagnosed in adolescents who abuse a variety of illicit substances. The signs, symptoms, and treatment of these conditions are the same as for patients who do not abuse drugs.

HIV infection transmitted sexually has been noted in adolescents who abuse drugs other than by the intravenous route. Both male and female adolescent "crack" abusers are at particular risk for sexually acquired HIV infection because of the practice of trading sex for drugs. The highly addictive nature and short duration of the crack "high" encourage drug binges that often include frequent acts of sexual intercourse with multiple partners. This has resulted in an increased prevalence among crack abusers of many sexually transmitted diseases, including syphilis and HIV-related illness.

Amenorrhea frequently occurs in teenage girls who are opiate addicts. Since amenorrhea is associated with anovulation, these girls experience no increase in pregnancies despite their often increased sexual activity. Ovulation, menses, and fertility usually return to normal within a few months of cessation of opiate use; thus contraceptive counseling and prescription must be part of rehabilitation.

Unfortunately, no such protection from pregnancy occurs in girls who abuse cocaine and crack. Cocaine use during pregnancy is associated with an increased incidence of spontaneous abortion, abruptio placentae, intrauterine growth retardation, premature delivery, and irritability in the infants. Contraceptive management is particularly important for these girls during the period of assessment and treatment for their drug abuse.

Abdominal Pain

There are many physiologic and psychosomatic illnesses that produce abdominal pain in teenagers. Among them are a variety of illicit drug–related conditions. Severe abdominal pain, anorexia, vomiting, and gastrointestinal hemorrhage may accompany a large and acute ingestion of alcohol. Although the chronic medical complications of alcoholism, such as cirrhosis, are not found in teenagers, acute gastritis and acute pancreatitis may accompany the consumption of a large quantity of alcohol. The pain of acute gastritis will usually subside with the administration of antacids alone. However, persistent bleeding will require vigorous therapy with iced saline lavage, histamine H_2 receptor antagonist, and increased, regular antacid therapy. Specific diagnostic studies to determine the origin of the hemorrhage may be indicated. In addition to severe abdominal pain and profuse vomiting, acute pancreatitis is usually accompanied by elevation of serum amylase and lipase levels.

An increased incidence of peptic ulcer disease has been reported in adult narcotic addicts, although no such increase has been noted in the adolescent. If ulcer disease or any other cause of acute abdominal pain does occur, the addict may falsely attribute the discomfort to withdrawal symptoms and quickly administer opiates as a form of self-treatment. Having thus masked the symptoms of possible intraabdominal pathologic findings, the opiate-addicted teenager may not seek medical attention until gastric perforation has occurred. Similarly, the physician faced with a patient experiencing opiate withdrawal must be cautious not to overlook other serious illness by attributing all of the patient's symptoms to the abstinence syndrome.

Constipation is almost universal among opiate abusers and, at the extreme, will cause symptoms of intestinal obstruction. Hemorrhoids, otherwise uncommon during adolescence, may result and cause rectal bleeding. Constipation responds rapidly to interruption of opiate abuse. Although constipation is one of the more benign complaints, it represents the most common complaint of the young methadone-maintained patient. In most instances the drug-abusing teenager with abdominal pain should be hospitalized for evaluation, since close observation and testing are required to reach a definitive diagnosis.

Jaundice

In evaluating the teenager with jaundice, the physician must consider the possibility of drug abuse as an etiologic factor. Acute viral hepatitis is common among intravenous opiate abusers. Although primarily associated with the mainlining of heroin, hepatitis has also been reported in intravenous abusers of other substances, including cocaine, barbiturates, and amphetamines. In addition, the hepatitis virus can be transmitted via saliva and semen, and cases have been attributed to the sharing of marijuana joints. The inhalation of cleaning fluid fumes, an abuse practiced most often by younger adolescents, can cause acute toxic hepatitis.

The symptoms, signs, and serologic abnormalities found in patients who use drugs do not differ from those of nondrug users with acute hepatitis. These include right upper quadrant tenderness, anorexia, nausea, jaundice, and hepatomegaly. Elevations of the serum transaminases and hyperbilirubinemia are expected, whereas hepatitis B surface antigen is present in over 25% of patients. The assessment of a jaundiced teenager with acute hepatitis should include measurement of the prothrombin time, since a prolongation of greater than 19 seconds (with a control of 12 seconds) may indicate impending hepatic encephalopathy. Transaminase elevations are of little value in predicting this untoward development. Other indications of early hepatic encephalopathy are changes in sensorium and behavior. In the drug-using teenager, belligerence and lack of cooperation are often incorrectly attributed to drug withdrawal or an underlying personality disturbance, rather than to hepatic encephalopathy. This error in judgment may lead to inappropriate treatment with sedatives; the administration of sedatives to patients with acute hepatic failure can precipitate coma.

Dehydration or evidence of impending hepatic encephalopathy is an indication for hospitalization in any patient, but particularly for the drug-abusing teenager with hepatitis, since noncompliance and lack of supportive care at home are more likely. Hepatitis B immunization should be offered to adolescent drug abusers who are antibody negative and who are at high risk for infection by either the intravenous or sexual route.

GENERAL LABORATORY TESTING

The teenager who is clinically well will occasionally demonstrate abnormal laboratory tests that raise suspicion of covert drug usage. Although neither anemia nor total peripheral white blood cell count abnormalities are associated with substance abuse, peripheral eosinophilia may be found in up to one third of heroin users. The cause of eosinophilia in heroin users is unknown.

The routine urinalysis yields no findings specific to drug abuse with the rare exception of mild proteinuria associated with serum glutamic-pyruvic transaminase (SGPT) elevations, which may be present in heroin-abusing adolescents. These patients show evidence of focal glomerulonephritis when evaluated with renal biopsy.

A false positive serologic test result for syphilis may be found for approximately 10% of heroin abusers. Although these false positive test results may occur for any teenager with active liver disease, they have been observed for heroin abusers without evidence of hepatic dysfunction.

Assessment of liver function is not commonly performed as a part of the usual laboratory evaluation in teenagers; however, it represents the most fruitful method of screening for unsuspected opiate abuse because the liver is the best source for chemical abnormality findings in the known heroin abuser. Nearly 40% of clinically well adolescents with a history of heroin abuse have serum elevations of glutamic-pyruvic transaminase and glutamic-oxaloacetic transaminase. Other indicators of hepatic function, including serum bilirubin and alkaline phosphatase levels, are usually normal. The transaminase abnormalities may persist for months or years after heroin abuse has been interrupted and are not associated with signs or symptoms of hepatic dysfunction. Liver biopsies performed on adolescents with enzyme abnormalities documented over a period of 4 months or longer have revealed histologic evidence of chronic persistent hepatitis. The long-term prognosis for teenagers with this disease is as yet unclear. No specific therapy is indicated.

Technologic advances have made it possible to detect drugs of abuse in body fluids accurately. However, the appropriate use of this testing ability has become an issue of some controversy, especially with regard to teenagers. Routine urine screening for drugs of abuse such as marijuana or cocaine on all adolescent patients without their knowledge and without clinical indicators of substance abuse is not advocated by most thoughtful authorities. Under such conditions, with an expected low prevalence of actual use, many false positive tests would result, leading to potentially harmful confrontations with adolescents who are not abusing drugs. In addition, only very recent drug use would be detected, and no information about patterns and frequency of use or degrees of impairment would be obtained. However, urine drug testing may be a very helpful adjunct to the treatment and rehabilitation of adolescents who are known to be drug abusers. Indeed, many drug treatment programs use random urine toxicologic testing, with the knowledge and consent of the patient, as an early warning system for relapse and as an additional way of helping the adolescent to abstain from drugs. Blood and urine toxicologic testing for illicit substances can also help in the assessment of an acutely ill adolescent with altered mental status who is unable to give a history because of coma or psychotic behavior.

CHANGES IN SENSORIUM: INTOXICATION, ACUTE PSYCHOSIS, LETHARGY, AND COMA

The teenager with apparent intoxication, disorientation, lethargy, or coma represents a complex diagnostic and therapeutic problem. Even when head trauma, diabetic acidosis, hypoglycemia, encephalitis, and other causes of coma and confusion can be excluded and the diagnosis of intoxication is clear, the specific causative drug must be determined. Information from the patient, the family, or friends may provide a ready answer, but such information may be unavailable or unreliable. Serum and urine toxicologic screening can be extremely helpful in such a situation. An attempt must always be made to determine the reason for the intoxication. Was it accidental or deliberate? If the patient is suicidal, the physician must offer appropriate protection, assessment, and treatment.

Although the overwhelming majority of mild intoxications never come to medical attention, sometimes a youngster will be brought for care for being "high." A wide variety of substances are capable of producing a high, including inhaled fumes from airplane glue or cleaning fluid, marijuana, alcohol, and cocaine. Teenagers who exhibit euphoria or minimal disorientation require only protection against self-injury. At an appropriate time after the sensorium has cleared, inquiries should be made as to the nature, frequency, and pattern of episodes of intoxication to determine the need, if any, for further psychosocial intervention.

Teenagers with severe alcohol intoxication can usually be distinguished by their ethanolic breath and, except in instances of extremely large or mixed ingestions, are not at serious physiologic risk. Treatment need only be supportive with protection provided against the aspiration of vomitus and observation for the development of respiratory depression, hypoglycemia, or the intestinal complications of a large alcohol ingestion, including acute gastritis and pancreatitis. Even when the teenager is not at risk, a brief hospitalization while sobriety is regained may be preferable to immediate discharge to the care of distraught parents.

The adolescent who comes for medical attention as a result of an acute psychosis is most often suffering from a hallucinogen ingestion or "bad trip." A wide variety of compounds are capable of producing hallucinations, including LSD, peyote, PCP, and occasionally marijuana or hashish. Hallucinations may recur weeks or months after the ingestion of a hallucinogen as part of a "flashback" phenomenon. In addition, large doses of amphetamines or cocaine may precipitate a psychotic state marked by paranoia and aggression. A similar psychotic episode may follow abrupt cessation of amphetamine abuse. Along with the hallucinations, which are almost always visual, the teenager who has ingested one of the above-mentioned drugs will often have dilated pupils, hyperreflexia, hyperthermia, and tachycardia. Identification of the specific abused hallucinogen is difficult. Even when the substance is known, the adolescent seldom has accurate knowledge of its exact concentration because the compounds are frequently adulterated and misrepresented by the seller. Detection of the presence of PCP, tetrahydrocannabinol, or cocaine in the patient's blood or urine can help in the prognosis of acute psychosis.

Regardless of the hallucinogen abused, treatment is nonspecific and directed at allaying anxiety and protecting the patient from injury to self or others. The teenager should be placed in a quiet, nonthreatening environment. Verbal contact should be established and maintained, with frequent reassurance that the hallucinogenic experience is temporary and drug related. If at all possible, physical restraints should be avoided because they are certain to increase anxiety and panic in the already frightened adolescent.

Sedatives should be administered only if verbal contact does not successfully control behavior or cannot be maintained because of limitations of time and staff. Any sedation administered will further compromise sensorium and may thereby increase the severity of hallucinations. All the most commonly used sedative medications carry additional risks. The administration of phenothiazines is potentially dangerous because hallucinogens are often adulterated with anticholinergics, and this combination of drugs may precipitate circulatory collapse. However, small doses of benzodiazepine may help to allay anxiety. Haloperidol in a dose of 2 to 5 mg may be administered intramuscularly to control the agitation of an acute drug-related psychosis. This dose may be repeated as soon as 1 hour later if severe symptoms persist or recur, although the frequency with which extrapyramidal reactions have been associated with this drug mandates that its use be kept to a minimum.

PCP is among the most toxic of the hallucinogenic agents. Toxic reactions, which may be indistinguishable from schizophrenia and include elements of paranoia, agitation, or catatonia, may last for days and in rare cases weeks. With high-dose ingestions, convulsions, opisthotonos, coma, and, very rarely, apnea may ensue. Treatment of overdose reactions includes (1) anticonvulsants for seizures, (2) support of respiration, and (3) enhancement of drug excretion by gastric lavage with half normal saline, the administration of furosemide, and the acidification of the urine by administering ammonium chloride or ascorbic acid.

In most instances teenagers with acute drug-related psychosis should be hospitalized. These adolescents may have brief periods of lucidity and then relapse into hallucinations. It is difficult to determine with certainty if the teenager has fully recovered without an opportunity to observe behavior over at least a few hours. In addition, there is always a question as to whether the drug ingestion unmasked a preexistent psychosis or simply precipitated psychotic behavior in an otherwise healthy individual. The answer to that question is best gained through an opportunity to observe and evaluate the adolescent during hospitalization.

The adolescent with an opiate or barbiturate overdose will have respiratory depression and constricted or sluggish pupils and be lethargic or comatose. In patients with respiratory depression precipitated by an unknown agent, the use of naloxone has both diagnostic and therapeutic potential. Although it is of no therapeutic benefit in the teenager with a sedative overdose, it is free of the effects of respiratory depression common to other narcotic antagonists and therefore can be used without fear of accentuating respiratory compromise in the nonopiate intoxication. Naloxone is also useful in treating propoxyphene ingestions. Failure of the teenager to respond to an initial dose of 0.01 mg/kg of naloxone given intravenously indicates that the symptoms are not due to an opiate. Pupillary dilation, an improved level of consciousness, and an increase in the respiratory rate in response to the administration of naloxone strongly suggests that an opiate produced the syndrome. The presence of clinical signs of intravenous drug use supports the diagnosis of narcotic overdose. Pulmonary edema and hypoxemia may occur in the teenager with an opiate overdose who then requires intubation, assisted ventilation, and administration of oxygen under positive pressure. Even the adolescent who responds dramatically to naloxone alone will require hospitalization for continued observation and continuous naloxone infusion. A relapse with respiratory depression may occur if the infusion is discontinued too early. This is a particular hazard in the patient with a methadone overdose, since its duration of action is between 24 and 48 hours.

As previously noted, the teenager with a sedative intoxication will display clinical characteristics similar to those of one with an opiate overdose. The patient with a barbiturate overdose will have pinpoint or slowly reactive pupils unresponsive to naloxone, whereas the adolescent with a glutethimide overdose will exhibit widely dilated pupils. In either case, treatment is supportive. Gastric lavage should be performed with care and, in those instances in which the teenager is comatose or severely depressed, only after the insertion of a cuffed endotracheal tube to prevent aspiration pneumonia. The respiratory rate and arterial blood gases must be monitored and mechanical ventilation instituted at the first sign of ventilatory failure. Intravenous fluids should be administered to ensure a high urine output. Analeptics have no role in the treatment of sedative overdose, and although hemodialysis may be effective, it is seldom necessary, for the supportive measures described are usually adequate.

Hospitalization for observation is almost always indicated for the teenager with a drug intoxication, although emergency room treatment may negate all immediate medical risks. Even in those instances in which self-destruction was not a motivation, an overdose may signal the loss of the adolescent's ability to control his drug-abuse behavior. The teenager should not be released from care until a concerted effort has been made to minimize future risk.

ABSTINENCE SYNDROMES

The opiate- or barbiturate-addicted teenager who is involuntarily hospitalized requires treatment to prevent the discomfort and danger inherent in a withdrawal syndrome. At times drug withdrawal will not be imposed on the adolescent; rather, some life crises will provide the motivation for voluntary detoxification. In either case, adolescents are often ambivalent regarding their abstinence and require careful, meticulous attention to their symptoms lest they become disruptive in the hospital or interrupt the attempts to free them from addiction.

A teenager must abuse narcotics daily for weeks to months before the risk of suffering an opiate withdrawal syndrome develops. Within 12 hours after the last dose of heroin and 36 hours after the last dose of methadone, the addicted adolescent should begin experiencing a progression of symptoms, including yawning, "gooseflesh," lacrimation, restlessness, dilated pupils, muscle cramps, diarrhea, and tachycardia. Insomnia may be severe during the first week of withdrawal and persist to some degree for up to a month after abstinence from drugs.

Most teenagers who report less than daily heroin usage are not physiologically addicted but rather are psychologically habituated. Nevertheless, they will be quite fearful of becoming ill if their opiate supply is interrupted. Most often, these teenagers will require no specific therapy beyond reassurance that relief for discomfort will be offered if symptoms appear. The adolescent who manifests symptoms and signs of opiate abstinence can be treated in a variety of ways. Methadone may be offered in a dosage of approximately 40 mg/day orally and then withdrawn slowly at a rate of 5 mg every 1 or 2 days over the course of 1 to 2 weeks. An alternative therapy is to administer 10 mg of diazepam every 4 to 6 hours. This medication may be given intramuscularly or by mouth. Better results can be anticipated if the intramuscular route is used at least initially, since the adolescent addict has greater faith in the efficacy of needle-administered drugs.

Diazepam will relieve most symptoms, except diarrhea and insomnia. Persistent or severe diarrhea can be treated with diphenoxylate hydrochloride. No satisfactory treatment for the insomnia associated with opiate withdrawal is available, and addiction-prone adolescents must be cautioned against self-medication with barbiturates in their search for sleep. Diazepam will need to be continued for 4 to 7 days after the last dose of opiate, the longer treatment being reserved for methadone addiction and the shorter course for heroin addiction.

Unlike opiate-addicted adolescents, barbiturate addicts are at grave risk of a life-threatening withdrawal syndrome if their sedative dosage is abruptly discontinued. They will develop restlessness, postural hypotension, and seizures in rapid succession, usually within 36 hours of their last dose. Occasionally, a teenager will not come for medical attention until after a seizure has occurred and may then require large doses of anticonvulsants. The teenager who seeks medical attention for voluntary detoxification before seizures have occurred should be offered phenobarbital as a substitute for the abused sedative, using an initial dose comparable to the barbiturate dose to which the patient is addicted. This should be divided into four equal parts, with each given every 6 hours. The daily dosage should then be reduced slowly at a rate of 120 mg/day to zero. Since this method of detoxification relies on the accuracy of the original estimate by the addict of daily abuse, it is extremely difficult to judge accurately the appropriate initial dose of phenobarbital to be given. If too much medication is offered, the teenager is at risk of iatrogenically induced barbiturate overdose and coma. If too little phenobarbital is given, convulsions may ensue. To be confident that an adequate dose has been administered, it is often necessary to induce mild barbiturate toxicity, which is accompanied by nystagmus, ataxia, and dysarthria, but which stops short of respiratory depression and coma. Treatment within this narrow therapeutic range requires careful observation of the adolescent, particularly during the first few days. Since the teenager may become somnolent during the initial stages of treatment because the initial dose of phenobarbital is set too high, a concomitant interruption of oral intake may develop. Therefore intravenous fluids should be administered routinely and the patient's fluid intake and output carefully monitored.

The high incidence of convulsions during barbiturate withdrawal and the need for frequent reevaluation and adjustment of therapy mandate in-hospital treatment of this abstinence syndrome. In many instances the guidance of a neurologist or a physician with expertise in addictive illnesses may be necessary. The management of the opiate abstinence syndrome can be accomplished on either an ambulatory or an inpatient basis. In general, greater success can be anticipated with hospitalization because this physically separates the addicted teenager from a supply of illicit narcotics and provides him or her continual support and reassurance.

Stimulants such as cocaine and amphetamines are not associated with a dramatic or life-threatening withdrawal syndrome. Nevertheless, they are considered physically addictive because of the biochemical changes in the brain, induced by these drugs, that lead to the intense cravings and compulsive drug abuse behavior noted in both animal and human studies. A stimulant-abstinence syndrome has been described that follows a three-phase pattern. There is an initial crash after a drug-taking binge that is characterized by a craving for sleep, often leading to the use of opiates, alcohol, or benzodiazepines. Following 1 to 3 days of hypersomnolence, the stimulant abuser begins to experience an increasing intensity of symptom withdrawal, including anergia, anhedonia, limited interest in the environment, and marked drug cravings. If abstinence is sustained for 6 to 18 weeks, the anhedonia, fatigue, and dysphoric mood usually improve. In the final extinction phase of abstinence, brief episodes of drug cravings recur with gradually diminishing frequency, often provoked by circumstances or objects that cue conditioned memories of drug euphoria. Treatment for adolescent stimulant abusers is best conducted within a highly structured chemical dependency program and often does not require hospitalization, since the withdrawal syndrome does not need intensive medical management. Inpatient treatment may be necessary, however, if outpatient treatment fails, if the adolescent exhibits suicidal or psychotic behavior, or if he or she is addicted to alcohol, sedatives, or opiates in addition to stimulants.

Delirium tremens, the major withdrawal syndrome from alcohol, is rarely if ever seen in adolescents. In contrast, a more benign withdrawal syndrome consisting of tremors, diaphoresis, agitation, disorientation, and (in rare cases) brief seizures may occur in adolescents who have drunk heavily over weeks or months. Teenagers whose drinking history suggests the possibility of a minor withdrawal syndrome should be hospitalized for observation if they become abstinent.

SUMMARY

Whether the adolescent voluntarily comes for treatment for a drug abuse problem, is compelled to seek medical attention because of a drug- or alcohol-related illness, or is discovered to be using drugs or alcohol during a routine evaluation, the physician is in an advantageous position to intercede beyond the confines of treating somatic illness. The illegality and stigma attached to drug abuse often prevent the teenager from seeking help from clergy, educators, and particularly family members. Protected by federal guidelines that ensure the confidentiality of the physician patient relationship in drug abuse treatment, the physician who uses a nonjudgmental, sympathetic approach to these teenagers may be able to establish trust and thereby gather sufficient information to make a knowledgeable judgment as to the need for further intervention. Such information must include not only the history of past and present drug or alcohol abuse, but also the nature of peer and family relationships, the extent of involvement with law enforcement authorities, the degree of educational or vocational disruption, and the adolescent's own interpretation of the need for subsequent therapy.

Often, the extent of substance abuse and related disruption is so minimal that no further action beyond the counsel of the physician is required. Such counsel should address the potential somatic effects of the teenager's current drug practices, the potential for escalation of drug-taking behavior, and the risks of trauma and death from even occasional intoxication. Alternatives to driving while intoxicated should be discussed with the adolescent and his or her family.

At the other extreme are teenagers with severe psychopathologic conditions who are in obvious need of psychiatric care. A variety of other therapeutic modalities, not all of which may be present in a given community, is available for treatment of substance-abusing teenagers. Group or individual counseling may be indicated for the teenager with less than severe drug involvement but with some evidence of psychosocial disruption. Group residences are available for adolescents from unsupportive homes. They usually offer counseling and a place to stay while teenagers continue their education or employment. Therapeutic communities are appropriate for those teenagers who are more deeply involved in drugs. These residences are often operated on a communal basis and staffed by former addicts, with or without professional support. The retention rate for teenagers within these programs is poor and may reflect the adolescents' inability to tolerate the rigors of relative incarceration and abrasive therapy.

Methadone maintenance treatment programs may be appropriate for the older, opiate-addicted teenager. This treatment modality substitutes a synthetic narcotic, methadone, for the abused opiate. A single daily oral dose of methadone can both prevent narcotic craving and block the euphoric effect of subsequently administered heroin. With the need to obtain illegal opiates interrupted, the adolescent is now free to take advantage of support services and make an effort toward restructuring his or her life. Therapy is aimed toward eventually withdrawing methadone treatment and preparing the patient for a drug-free existence. Unfortunately, although many adolescents do well while remaining in treatment, evidence to date indicates a high incidence of subsequent drug abuse and significant morbidity and mortality after discharge from these programs.

Often, limitations of time for adequate psychosocial evaluation or lack of familiarity with available therapeutic resources prevents practitioners from reaching a meaningful long-term disposition for their patients. In these instances, referrals need to be made to other professionals or agencies with expertise and interest in the field of teenage drug and alcohol abuse. In this regard, substance abuse does not differ from certain other behavioral problems for which specific therapeutic interventions are beyond the physician's professional scope.

SUGGESTED READINGS

Anonymous: Crack, Med Lett 28(718):69, 1986.

Cohen S: The "angel dust" states: phencyclidine toxicity, Pediatr Rev 1:17, 1979.

Committee on Adolescence, American Academy of Pediatrics: Alcohol use and abuse: a pediatric concern, Pediatrics 79(3):450, 1987.

Gawin FH and Ellinwood EH Jr: Cocaine and other stimulants, N Engl J Med 318(18):1173, 1988.

Institute of Medicine, Division of Health Sciences Policy: Marijuana and health, Washington, DC, 1982, National Academy Press.

Johnson LD, O'Malley PM, and Bachman JG: Drug use, drinking and smoking: national survey results from high school, college and young adult populations: 1975-1988, Rockville, Md, 1989, National Institute on Drug Abuse.

King NMP and Cross AW: Moral and legal issues in screening for drug use in adolescents, J Pediatr 111(2):249, 1987.

Kipke MD, Futterman D, and Hein K: HIV infection and AIDS during adolescence, Med Clin North Am 74(5):1149, 1990.

Perry CL and Silvis GL: Smoking prevention: behavioral prescriptions for the pediatrician, Pediatrics 79(5):790, 1987.

Ray O: Drugs, society, and human behavior, ed 3, St Louis, 1983, The CV Mosby Co.

Schonberg SK, editor: Substance abuse: a guide for health professionals, (1988), American Academy of Pediatrics/Pacific Institute for Research and Evaluation.

Shedler J and Block J: Adolescent drug use and psychological health, Am Psychol 45(5):612, 1990.

101

Homosexuality:

Challenges of Treating Lesbian and Gay Adolescents

Donna Futterman and Virginia Casper

Sexuality does not begin in adolescence; however, puberty usually marks the beginning of self-conscious sexual expression, both biologically and psychologically. It brings with it numerous developmental tasks, including the formation of an adult sexual identity and decisions about intimate ties with others. For those adolescents who may be homosexual and for the health providers entrusted with their care, these tasks involve special challenges. These challenges are particularly urgent, considering the health problems, including AIDS, facing today's homosexual youth.

DEFINITIONS

Individual sexual orientation, or sexual preference, refers not only to patterns of physical behavior, but also to sexual feelings toward others: homosexual (same sex), heterosexual (opposite sex), and bisexual (both sexes). Kinsey in 1948 defined sexual orientation on a continuum of zero to six recognizing that behavior and identity contribute to sexual orientation.

Sexual orientation is distinct from core gender identity—the sense of being a man or a woman—which is formed in the first few years of life. It is also different from gender role or sex role behaviors—expressions of femininity and masculinity that are culturally defined and that may coincide with or deviate from those changing norms.

The term *homosexual* is a formal and general term for same-sex preferences. The more popular term is *gay*. It refers both to lesbians and gay men.

Approximately 5% to 10% of the adult population is predominantly homosexual. The figure for males is closer to 10%; for females it is closer to 5%.

Homophobia is a term used to describe social prejudice against gays and lesbians, stereotyping, and the stigmatization of homosexuality. "Expressions of externalized and internalized homophobia are more pronounced during adolescence than at any other time in the life cycle."[8]

Homosexuality has been documented in many diverse cultures throughout recorded history. Societal attitudes toward homosexuality have decisively affected the extent to which individuals have hidden or made known their sexual orientation and the form that its expression has taken.

ETIOLOGY

Researchers have yet to reach a consensus on the etiology of homosexuality. The many theories are representative of two general lines of thought: nature (the biological) and nurture (environmental/psychological). Within each of these schools is a broad spectrum of views—from those reiterating the principle that homosexuality is a nonpathologic variant in the continuum of sexual orientation, to those presenting homosexuality as a deviance from the heterosexual norm. In 1973, homosexuality was removed from the list of "mental disorders" by the American Psychiatric Association.

Early studies on the etiology of homosexuality tended to be based on samples drawn from bars, prisons, and mental health clinical populations. They were all retrospective in nature. Evelyn Hooker in 1957 was the first to draw on nonclinic populations, reporting on mentally healthy homosexuals. In studies during the last 20 years, populations have been drawn from more representative sectors, and at least one prospective study has been published.[5]

Evidence for the biological basis of homosexuality is both direct and indirect. Direct evidence includes the concordance of sexual orientation among identical twins; however, researchers have yet to identify the specific locus of any basic biological differences. In nonhuman species, researchers have induced gender-atypical mating behaviors by exposing the fetus to androgens. These findings suggest the possible impact of the fetal endocrinologic environment on those areas of the central nervous system that govern sexual response patterns.[8]

Indirect evidence comes from studies such as those of Bell, Weinberg and Hammersmith,[1] whose research on a large sample of homosexuals failed to demonstrate any consistent pattern of family life or parental influence. They concluded that on the basis of their data, they could rule out neither a biological basis for homosexual identity nor the role of learned experiences.

The evidence to date supports an interactive approach: both nature and nurture apparently play a role in determining sexual orientation.

COMING OUT: A DEVELOPMENTAL PERSPECTIVE

"Coming out," or recognizing one's homosexual identity, is a complex process "through which gay women and men recognize their sexual preference and choose to integrate this knowledge into their personal and social lives."[7] Several models have been proposed to describe the coming out process, and almost all have been based on retrospective descriptions by adults of the feelings or experiences of their youth. Significantly, nearly all models of homosexual identity development take into account the impact of homophobia, which affects both the formation and expression of homosexual identity.

Most studies of the coming out process refer to discrete stages, but acknowledge that the process may not be linear. Most models describe the following four stages:

Stage One: Sensitization

The initial stage of awareness has been described as "precoming out"[2] or "sensitization."[9] Looking back, many adult homosexuals describe having felt different from their childhood peers. As prepubertal children, these feelings of "differentness" were often not sexual, but, rather, concerned atypical sex-role play choices, such as a disinterest in sports for boys or disinclination to "play house" for girls. When these differences exist, they can foster an early sense of social isolation.

For gay youth, puberty is often the first conscious realization that their strongest sexual attractions are for members of their own sex. In a retrospective study, Bell, Weinberg, and Hammersmith[1] reported that by age 19, 75% of the gay men and women in their sample described themselves as sexually different.

Stage Two: Identity Confusion

These feelings can generate "identity confusion."[9] Initial denial gives way to crisis, as same-sex feelings become strong enough to break through defenses. This crisis may in fact mark an important stage in the coming out process, stemming from the following factors:

Cognitive Dissonance. Adolescents may feel surprise or real distress at the discovery of sexual feelings that depart from their own expectations, as well as those of friends, family, and society.

Absence of Role Models. Gay youth have relatively few open gay role models to emulate. This is in marked contrast to the experience of heterosexual youth, who have a wide variety of openly heterosexual role models.

Inability to Identify with a Stereotype. Gay adolescents who have limited access to accurate information may have difficulty identifying with the only images of homosexuals available to them—the negative stereotypes of popular culture.

Lack of Opportunity for Open Exploration of Homosexual Socialization and Sexuality. Keenly aware of homophobia, and fearing ostracism by parents or peers, gay youth may attempt to hide their emerging identity at just the age when they should be learning to socialize.

Attraction to Members of the Opposite Sex. Many lesbians and gay men report these attractions, which can lead to denial of one's homosexual feelings and to attempts to prove their heterosexuality, including conceiving a child.

Stage Three: Experimentation and Identity Assumption

In an effort to resolve conflict and dispel confusion, gays and lesbians typically enter a period of emotional, social, and sexual experimentation. Gonsiorek notes that in this stage, "dissolution of a first relationship may lead to another period of crisis, during which the individual reexperiences negative feelings about being gay or lesbian. Expectations, issues of identity, and internalized homophobia are reexamined."[4]

Stage Four: Integration and Commitment

Typically, the process culminates in self-acceptance and integration of a gay identity into one's life and personality. An individual's ability to "integrate" may hinge on the availability of accurate information, a support network, and positive role models.

PROVIDER ISSUES

As a group, gay adolescents share many of the characteristics of their heterosexual peers; at the same time, however, they do present providers with some unique challenges, including the following:

Establishing Trust

Fearing disclosure of their sexual orientation or activity, gay youth may avoid health care altogether—missing routine health screenings and other benefits of preventive care—or may approach health care with considerable trepidation. Establishing trust is therefore critical, and begins with the provider's commitment to creating an environment of acceptance. Providers may want to make available, in the waiting room and the office, literature by gay authors or literature describing gay organizations and resources.

Taking the Medical History

A comprehensive medical history includes a sexual history. Gay and lesbian adolescents are more likely to disclose their homosexuality to the provider if they feel the encounter will be supportive or, at least nonjudgmental.

In discussions with all patients, questions about sexuality should not presume heterosexuality. Rather, they should acknowledge the possibility that sexual encounters or fantasies might involve members of the same sex. With younger adolescents, one might say: "When people your age start having sexual feelings, they sometimes have those feelings about members of the same sex. So I ask everyone who comes to see me whether they've had any of those feelings."

Some providers are reluctant to ask this question, because they do not want to upset heterosexual patients. However, the repercussions of posing this question to a young heterosexual patient appear to be far less serious than the possible consequences of failing to raise the issue with a homosexual adolescent.

Protecting Confidentiality

The provider may want to help a patient work out a decision about talking to parents. But since disclosure may prompt strong reactions from parents—ranging from love and support, to passing anger, to fundamental rejection, or even violence—it is suggested that the adolescent's own assessment of parental reaction be given considerable weight.

Providing Information and Referrals

Gay and lesbian youth may benefit from support groups, family support from organizations such as Parents and Friends of Lesbians and Gays, advocacy and education groups, and AIDS education. Those who need special health care (including mental health services) and social services may need help identifying providers who offer sensitive, nonjudgmental care.

Discussing Birth Control and Sexually Transmitted Diseases with Lesbians

Providers caring for adolescent lesbians must deal sensitively with the issue of birth control. Many lesbians who do not wish to disclose their sexual orientation have experienced intense pressure from providers to ascertain their method of birth control, causing them to avoid medical encounters altogether.

Here again, providers should not presume heterosexuality. At the same time, they should not assume that young lesbians are having sex exclusively with women. Because many lesbian adolescents have sex with males, the topics of pregnancy and sexually transmitted diseases (STD) need to be addressed.

Although women who have sex exclusively with other women have a lower incidence of STDs, infections, including trichomonas, herpes, and syphilis, can be passed between women by oral-genital and genital-genital contact. Although not yet documented, there is a theoretical risk that transmission of HIV between women could be facilitated by engaging in sexual activity during menstruation.

Screening for Sexual Diseases

Like other sexually active youth, gay and lesbian adolescents should be screened for STDs. Providers might discuss with all sexually active adolescents the appropriate test sites. They might say, for example: "To make sure you're healthy, we look at all the parts of your body where you've had sexual contact. So let's talk about which parts of your body we should be checking out." Oral, genital, and anal sites should be screened in all sexually active gay adolescents. Vaccination against hepatitis B is also recommended for all sexually active gay males.

AIDS and STDS

The most serious medical problem facing gay male adolescents today is AIDS.[3] Male adolescents who have same-sex intercourse are at particular risk for HIV, given the high prevalence of HIV among gay and bisexual adult men. In September 1990, males who had sex with other males continued to be the leading transmission category for AIDS among adolescents between the ages of 13 and 21 years.

As of 1990, 20% of AIDS cases were seen in adults between the ages of 20 and 29. Given the average latency period of 10 years from the time of infection with HIV to development of AIDS, many of those young adults were probably infected as teenagers.

AIDS prevention efforts may be complicated by all adolescents who engage in same-sex intercourse not identifying themselves as gay or bisexual. Surveys have consistently demonstrated that 17% to 35% of young males have had same-sex experiences to orgasm.

Societal and familial prejudice against homosexuality often interferes with gay youth's ability to build an integrated gay identity through "open" socialization. With this option closed, the gay adolescent frequently explores his sexuality secretively and unsafely.

Additionally, adolescents who do not yet identify as gay or are heterosexual or bisexual frequently ignore the safe sex messages targeted to the gay community. They may reason, for example, "Even though I fool around with guys, I'm not gay, so AIDS has nothing to do with me!"

HEALTH CARE NEEDS OF LESBIANS AND GAY YOUTH

Lesbian and gay youth are a heterogeneous population, representing a wide range of medical and psychosocial characteristics. However, they have the following very basic needs in common:

- An understanding of the stress involved in coming to terms with their sexual identity in a homophobic society
- A nonjudgmental environment in which to receive health care
- Clear, accessible AIDS and STD information and preventive care
- Assurance of confidentiality
- Appropriate referrals for support, information, and social services
- Birth control information
- Appropriate screening for STDs

REFERENCES

1. Bell AP, Weinberg MS, and Hammersmith SK: Sexual preference: its development in men and women, Bloomington, Ind, 1981, Indiana University Press.
2. Coleman E: Developmental stages of the coming out process, J Homosexuality 7:31, 1982.
3. Futterman D and Hein K: Medical management of adolescents. In Pizzo P and Wilfert C, editors: Pediatric AIDS: The challenge of HIV infection in infants, children & adolescents, Baltimore, 1990, Williams & Wilkins.
4. Gonsiorek JC: Mental health issues of gay & lesbian adolescents. In Remafedi, G, editor: Special section on adolescent homosexuality, J Adolesc Health Care 9:114, 1988.
5. Green R: The "Sissy Boy Syndrome" and the development of homosexuality, New Haven, 1987, Yale University Press.
6. Hooker, E: The adjustment of the male overt homosexual, J Project Tech 21:18, 1957.
7. Monteflores C and Schultz S: Coming out: Similarities and differences for lesbians and gay men, J Social Issues 34:3, 1978.
8. Remafedi G: Fundamental issues in the care of homosexual youth. In Adolescent health care, Med Clin North Am 74:5, 1990.
9. Troiden RR: The formation of homosexual identities. In Herdt G, editor: Gay and lesbian youth, New York, 1989, Harrington Park Press.

SUGGESTED READINGS

Bozett F: Gay and lesbian parents, New York, 1987, Praeger Publishers.

Gonsiorek JC, editor: Homosexuality and psychotherapy: A practitioners handbook of affirmative models, New York, 1982, Haworth Press.

Herdt G, editor: Gay and lesbian youth, New York, 1989, Haworth Press.

Remafedi G, editor: Special section on adolescent homosexuality, J Adolesc Health Care 9:93-143, 1988.

RESOURCES

Hetrick Martin Institute for The Protection of Lesbian and Gay Youth, 401 West Street, New York, NY 10014, 212-633-8920. Provides educational materials for gay and lesbian youth and social service providers. Support groups for youth. Training for professionals. Referrals.

National Gay and Lesbian Task Force, 1517 U Street NW, Washington, DC 20009, 202-332-6483. Provides advocacy and lobbying for the rights of lesbians and gay men. Referrals for local resources.

Parents and Friends of Lesbians and Gays, P.O. Box 553, New York, New York 10021, 212-463-0629. Provides resources and support to families with gay family members. Referrals to local support groups.

102

Interviewing Adolescents

Esther H. Wender

The skill of interviewing is put to a strong test in the practice of adolescent medicine because the relationship between the adolescent patient and adults in a position of authority is rapidly changing and is often fragile. Yet good interviewing requires establishing a relationship between the interacting parties that facilitates communication. The information that is most relevant and useful to both people will emerge if the relationship promotes communication. Conversely, the most skillfully formulated questions will not yield useful information if the interaction between the conversing parties is tense or hostile.

WHOM TO INTERVIEW

During adolescence, a transition from dependence to independence should be made by the teenager and should be facilitated by the parents. In early adolescence the parents are still largely responsible for their teens' health care, although by late adolescence these patients are often managing their own medical needs completely. These changes occur over a relatively brief period; therefore the physician is faced with assessing the stage of transition toward independence each time the adolescent patient is seen. Decisions about whom to interview should be made in the context of this transition, and several potential problems need to be considered.

The Adolescent's Developmental Level

Nothing is more upsetting to adolescents than feeling that they are being treated like younger children. This is particularly a problem in early adolescence when lack of sexual maturation on the part of teens causes insensitive adults to underestimate the patients' psychological age. Adolescent patients, when they feel free to comment, resent an office or hospital setting designed only for younger children. Even more upsetting, however, is the adult who talks to adolescents as though they were younger children. Therefore, to gain the respect of adolescent patients, the physician should take a genuine interest in them at the very beginning of the interview.

It is usually best to greet the adolescent patient before greeting the parent. It is also helpful to chat with the patient briefly before the interview begins, being careful to gear the conversation to the appropriate level for that patient. To accomplish this, the physician should know enough about normal adolescent development to judge the appropriateness of this preinterview conversation. Normal adolescent development is reviewed in Chapter 47.

The Parents' Role

In the midst of enthusiasm for making the adolescent feel comfortable, the physician should not ignore the importance of the parents' role. In early and middle adolescence, the parents' input is essential for a thorough evaluation, since adolescents still have only limited insight about themselves and have inadequate perspective on the timing and importance of symptoms. During late adolescence it may be appropriate to see the adolescent without the parents' involvement, if that is the teenager's wish. When the parents are involved, the physician should allow them time to discuss their concerns without the presence of their child. Particularly during adolescence, parents may be reluctant to discuss their concerns openly in the presence of their child.

A younger (12- to 16-year-old) adolescent may request to be seen alone, particularly regarding sexual issues. The physician should be aware of the particular state's laws regarding the adolescent's rights to confidential evaluation, and these rights must be respected. However, because of their limited perspective and their need for emotional and financial support, it is wise in most cases to encourage younger adolescents to involve their parents. Although the adolescents' independence should be encouraged and they should always have some time to see the physician alone, the appropriate role of the parents should not be ignored. The physician should remember that in our culture parents are still responsible for their children through adolescence.

Adolescent Sensitivity to "Parents Only" Interviews

Adolescent patients are often both upset and resentful when the parents and physician talk about them in their absence. This is particularly true if the adolescent disagrees with the parents' assessment of the problem or objects to consulting a physician. Therefore the need to obtain information from the parents may be in direct conflict with consideration for the adolescent's feelings. One way to solve this problem is to see the patient and parents together for the initial portion of the interview. During this session, the physician should tell both the adolescent and parents that each will be able to talk to the physician alone and that these conversations will be confidential. This approach, which allows disagreements between parents and patient to be aired openly, usually reduces the natural paranoia that the adolescent feels when in conflict with the parents' assessment of the problem.

Physician Neutrality

If there is a significant disagreement between the adolescent and parents, it is important for the physician to avoid seeming to take sides on these issues. Again, this can best be accomplished by interviewing the adolescent and parents together. In this type of interview, the physician should concentrate on understanding and clarifying the disagreements, thus conveying an appropriately neutral attitude toward the conflict. The following vignette illustrates this technique. The evaluation has been initiated by parents concerned that their 15-year-old son has behavioral problems.

Mr. Jones: We think his choice of friends leaves a lot to be desired.

Jim: What's the matter with my friends?

Mr. Jones: Most of them have no ambition. They don't care about school and spend their time just hanging around.

Jim: It's just that we're not like you. You don't care about anything except work. At least my friends know how to have fun.

Physician: Jim, you think your father devotes too much attention to work?

Jim: Yeah.

Physician: And, Mr. Jones, you wish Jim were more ambitious and also picked friends who were?

Mr. Jones: Yes. I worry that Jim isn't going to succeed.

Jim: (to his father) I'll succeed in my own way.

Physician: What are your ideas about success, Jim?

In this interaction, the physician has facilitated communication between the father and son without stating an opinion that would appear to commit him to either person's point of view.

• • •

A review of these issues before the interview will help the physician make a reasonable decision about whom to interview first. There can be no rigid rules. The choice depends on the age of the patient, the person who initiates the contact, and whether there is conflict between the adolescent and parents regarding the problem.

PHYSICAL SETTING

Adolescent patients are often quite sensitive to the atmosphere of the physician's office or hospital ward that emphasizes the interests of the young child. Therefore the pediatrician should arrange the office waiting room with a section that contains reading material and decor appropriate for adolescent patients. At least one examining room should be equipped and decorated with the adolescent patient in mind. The hospital ward should also have a section furnished and decorated specifically for adolescent patients, and an interviewing room to be used exclusively for teens should be available.

The need for privacy during the interview is never more important than in the practice of adolescent medicine. If the adolescent sees that there will be interruptions or believes the conversation will be overheard, important information may not be revealed. It may be particularly difficult to find privacy on the hospital ward or in the emergency room, but every effort should be made.

The interview room should be arranged with physician, patient, and parents seated at the same level, at a comfortable conversational distance, and without desks between the physician and the person or persons to whom the physician is speaking. The few moments it takes to rearrange furniture to meet these requirements are well spent.

INTERVIEWING TECHNIQUE

The key to good interviewing is building a trusting relationship between the physician, patient, and parents. This goal can be accomplished if the physician makes an effort to understand how the adolescent patient perceives the problem and relationships with important people in his or her life. Most physicians would say that they do attempt to understand their patients. However, often physicians become involved in their own agenda of obtaining answers to specific medical questions and miss important clues about their patients' feelings.

The following vignette illustrates the insensitivity that results when medical issues are pursued vigorously and the physician becomes more interested in the answers than in the relationship. The patient is a 16-year-old girl with diabetes.

Physician: How much insulin do you take?

Susan: Sixteen units of NPH and 4 units of regular each morning.

Physician: Do you test your urine?

Susan: Yeah.

Physician: How often?

Susan: Every morning and in the late afternoon, when my mother doesn't bug me.

Physician: Do you ever spill sugar?

Susan: Sometimes; not too often.

Physician: How much? One plus, two plus?

Susan: Just one plus a couple of times a week. Mom's always asking me that, but I tell her to leave me alone.

Physician: Do you ever have insulin reactions?

Susan: Not for a long time.

Physician: How's school?

One can sense the physician's need to fill in the blanks of the medical history. In the process, this physician has failed to pick up the clues of the daughter-mother conflict. The physician completed the agenda and then turned to a question about this adolescent's life that will probably be perceived by the patient as a "mechanical" question, since the physician did not "hear" previous comments.

Techniques that promote the acquisition of useful information fall into two main categories: listening skills and facilitative responses. Component aspects of these two skills, reviewed briefly in the following discussion, are as follows:

1. Listening skills
   a. Clarification of meaning
   b. Verbal asides
   c. Nonverbal communication
2. Facilitative responses
   a. Repetition and review
   b. Acknowledgment of feelings
   c. Silences

Listening Skills

Unless physicians pay attention to the meaning of words, they will often think they understand when they really do not. Every time patients use words or phrases that are abstract or unclear, physicians should ask for *clarification*. Skilled interviewers continually ask themselves if they understand what has just been said. In the following vignette, the importance of this technique is illustrated. The patient is a 15-year-old boy with school problems.

Physician: Your parents seem concerned about how you are doing in school. What do you think?

Gary: Sometimes I think I'm a wreck.

Physician: A wreck?

Gary: Yeah, you know, all washed up.

Physician: I don't know, Gary; what does that feel like?

Gary: Like I get these funny feelings, and I think I'm falling apart.

Physician: Tell me about one of these funny feelings.

Gary: Well . . . sometimes it's like my fingers are growing really big, or small. It's weird.

Physician: You mean like parts of your body are changing size?

Gary: Yeah.

Physician: Anything else?

Gary: Sometimes I feel like I'm walking just a little off the ground, like I was floating.

If the physician did not pursue the meaning of Gary's words, he or she might have been left with the vague statement that Gary feels he is a "wreck," which many people would assume means he thinks he is a failure. Instead, the physician now has evidence that Gary is experiencing somatic symptoms of anxiety, and they can pursue the source of these feelings.

Verbal asides are parenthetic statements that often reveal the patient's true feelings but that are stated as though they were unimportant. They usually reflect the adolescent's ambivalence about exposing his or her real feelings. The diabetic patient, described earlier, who said that she tested her urine twice a day "when my mother doesn't bug me" is giving a verbal aside. Statements about her mother constitute unsolicited information. Physicians often focus only on the solicited information and therefore fail to hear such asides. All that is usually required to facilitate further communication is to echo the phrase back to the patient in the form of a question.

Nonverbal communication consists of body movements and facial expressions that reveal a person's feelings. A physician who is preoccupied with asking the right questions and accumulating the answers will miss these important clues. The skilled interviewer learns to divide attention between the words that are being said and the body language of the person being interviewed. Since body language is usually outside the patient's awareness, it may be premature to comment on such observations. Part of the art of interviewing is to sense when such comments may be useful.

A good rule to remember is that when body language reveals something the person seems to be trying to hide, it should be left alone. For example, a person's clenched fists may indicate tension, when his or her words suggest calm. However, when a facial expression suggests an inner thought or feeling, it is often useful to comment. The patient may say something funny, for example, followed by a sad facial expression. In this instance, it is usually helpful to say something like, "It looks as if that thought suddenly made you feel sad."

Facilitative Responses

The person who is talking usually feels good when the listener can synthesize what the speaker has just said into a summary that accurately reflects the thoughts. If, for example, the patient has had difficulty finding the right words to describe his or her symptoms and the physician then restates those symptoms briefly and accurately, the patient realizes he or she has been heard. People like to be understood, and this type of *repetition and review* greatly facilitates further communication.

An important component of repetition and review is the *acknowledgment of feelings,* as well as the recognition of facts. Often, patients make a series of statements that are really meant to build a case for the underlying feelings they are experiencing. If the physician can hear and then acknowledge these feelings, the relationship may be significantly enhanced. The following segment of an interview illustrates this interaction. The patient is a 13-year-old girl brought by her parents because of acting-out behavior.

Physician: Your parents are upset over some of the things you have done. What do you think?

Judy: They really bug me. Last week, Mom wouldn't let me go to the roller rink with my friends. She said that we were too young to go by ourselves, but all my friends' parents let them go. Then, a couple of nights ago, I wanted to stay at Sally's house for dinner and Dad made me come home. He said that it's getting too dark at night. Geez, you'd think I was a baby.

Physician: It sounds like you don't feel your parents trust you.

Judy: I know they don't trust me. It makes me feel like doing whatever I want, since they don't trust me anyway.

Another important facilitative response is the carefully timed use of silence. This is particularly important when the patient has difficulty expressing himself or herself. Physicians are usually highly verbal people and respond to such patients by asking more and more questions. When a question has been asked and the response is not immediate, the interviewer should look closely for cues that the patient is processing the question. If the patient appears to be thinking about the answer, the physician should learn to pause to allow a response. Further statements might include facilitative responses such as, "What thoughts are you having?" or "It's hard, sometimes, to find the right words." Such replies tend to encourage the response.

The periods of silence should not be so long that the patient is made to feel uncomfortable. Sometimes in psychiatric interviews, long silences are purposefully used, but this approach would be too threatening for most medical interviews. What is recommended, instead, is allowing time for the person whose verbal responses are slow.

SUMMARY

The techniques just described are only suggestions. Effective interviewing requires practice. However, the skill is well worth learning, since it leads to better medical histories and improved patient compliance. The result is improved skill in the practice of adolescent medicine.

SUGGESTED READINGS

Felice ME and Friedman SB: Behavioral considerations in the health care of adolescents, Pediatr Clin North Am 29:399, 1982.

Ginott HG: Between parent and teenager, New York, 1969, Macmillan Publishing Co., Inc.

Weiner IB: Psychological disturbance in adolescence, New York, 1970, John Wiley & Sons, Inc.

103

Juvenile Delinquency

Irving B. Weiner

Juvenile delinquency is the legal term for youthful behavior that violates the law. This broad legal definition embraces two specific questions pediatricians must address when dealing with delinquent behavior: Does the kind and extent of a patient's illegal activity call for clinical intervention? If so, what is the cause of the delinquent behavior in which he or she has been involved?

The first of these questions is important because delinquent acts, regardless of whether they have been detected by the police, can range widely in severity and frequency. Young people may have committed major felonies such as assault or armed robbery, or they may be guilty only of misdemeanors, such as running away or disturbing the peace, that have few implications for criminal tendencies. Likewise, a particular kind of delinquent act may have occurred only once or may have become a repetitive pattern of illegal behavior.

The point at which delinquent acts come to professional attention is often influenced by the tolerance level for such behavior in a particular child's family, neighborhood, or community. Generally, however, the more serious the delinquent acts and the more frequently they have been occurring, the more likely they are to require clinical evaluation and treatment.

Regarding the etiology of delinquent behavior, it is a mistake to think of juvenile delinquency in a global sense, as if there were universally applicable explanations of its causes and uniformly appropriate ways of dealing with this behavior. To the contrary, delinquent youngsters are a psychologically heterogeneous group. Some are socialized delinquents who are well-integrated members of a delinquent subculture and display few if any psychological problems; others are delinquent as a result of various psychological maladjustments, some of which are characterological in nature and some of which express neurotic tendencies.

Characterological maladjustments usually begin forming early in life and crystallize during adolescence into various forms of personality disorder. Individuals with personality disorders are satisfied with their basic nature and have no wish to be different; they feel comfortable with themselves and attribute any difficulties they encounter to external events over which they have no control and for which they bear no responsibility.

Neurotic maladjustments, on the other hand, usually do not appear until the elementary school years and may emerge at any subsequent time of life with little previous warning. They constitute immature or unrealistic ways of attempting to solve problems or to reduce anxiety and are uncharacteristic of how the affected person usually behaves. Neurotic individuals are usually concerned about how they are feeling (e.g., phobic or depressed) or acting (e.g., being compulsive or having temper tantrums) and wish they could change themselves back to what they were like before these symptoms began.[12]

DIFFERENTIAL DIAGNOSIS OF DELINQUENT BEHAVIOR

The appropriate response to delinquent behavior in a patient follows from the differential diagnosis of the origin of his or her delinquency as stemming from socialized, characterological, or neurotic patterns of behavior.

Socialized Delinquency

In socialized delinquency, illegal activity emerges among members of a subculture who share antisocial standards of conduct. In contrast to psychological forms of delinquency, which are maladaptive for the individual, socialized delinquency is adaptive behavior, in that it earns delinquents praise and acceptance from their immediate social group and thereby provides them a sense of satisfaction and belonging. Socialized delinquency is usually a group or gang activity, and it seldom accounts for delinquent acts that are committed alone or without the approval of neighborhood or peer groups.[5]

Accordingly, the differential diagnosis of socialized delinquency is suggested by four findings in the clinical history: (1) the delinquent acts will have been performed with valued companions rather than alone or with strangers; (2) these delinquents see themselves as accepted and integral members of their peer group and rarely exhibit feelings of personal alienation or social inadequacy; (3) unlike people suffering psychological disorders, socialized delinquents evidence little neurotic symptom formation or basic character flaws; and (4) these delinquents will typically have enjoyed close and supportive family relationships during their early years—again, in contrast to the kinds of family tensions and disruption that contribute to psychological problems—although their delinquency as adolescents may result in part from inadequate parental supervision.

Characterological Delinquency

The illegal behavior of characterological delinquents reflects a basically asocial personality orientation. These young people manifest many features of what is commonly termed *psychopathy*. Because of prominent guiltlessness (defective conscience) and lovelessness (incapacity for loyalty to others), they are highly prone to committing illegal acts against persons and property.

Characterological delinquents tend to be loners who neither trust nor expect to be trusted by others. They break the law primarily as a result of disregard for the feelings and rights of others and an inability or unwillingness to control their own behavior. Such personality impairments derive from parental rejection early in life, which deprives children of an opportunity to learn to share mutual bonds of affection and attachment with other people, and parental neglect in middle childhood, which deprives young people of the discipline and guidance necessary to inculcate self-control and internal standards of moral conduct. Lacking such parenting, future psychopaths grow from childhood into adolescence loving no one and guided by an external morality according to which acceptable behavior is whatever you can get away with.[7]

The differential diagnosis of characterological delinquency is based on the adolescents' personality style, their behavioral history, and the nature of their past and current family relationships. The more patients appear to be basically aggressive, impulsive, and amoral, with little sympathy for others and little capacity to tolerate frustration for their own wishes, the more likely their delinquency will reflect a psychopathic personality disorder. Because the roots of psychopathy extend far back into childhood, characterological delinquents will usually have a long history of problem behaviors such as fighting, lying, stealing, unruliness in school, and cruelty to people and animals.

The diagnosis of characterological delinquency is rarely justified in the absence of this kind of history, and it should also be avoided for children who appear to have enjoyed close and supportive care from reasonably well-adjusted parents. Evidence of early affective deprivation, on the other hand, especially when combined with a family history of irresponsible behavior, considerably increases the probability that delinquent activity is characterological in origin.

Occasionally the long-term consequences of having had a childhood learning disability produce patterns of misconduct during adolescence that bear a superficial resemblance to characterological delinquency. The blows to self-esteem typically suffered by learning disabled children at home, in the classroom, and on the playground can result in their becoming insecure, short-tempered teenagers who need to bolster their self-image and beat down unwanted criticism. Hence, like characterological delinquents, they tend at times to show the kinds of aggressive, self-centered behavior seen in psychopathic individuals.[8] The basic nature of their difficulties, however, can readily be differentiated from psychopathy by a good clinical history. Instead of early affective deprivation or other family problems, these adolescents will have demonstrated evidence of an attention-deficit hyperactivity disorder in early childhood (including hyperactivity, delayed motor and language development, and impaired perceptual-motor coordination); in elementary school they will have been slow to learn (especially reading) despite having adequate intelligence and will have had strained relationships with their teachers and classmates.

Neurotic Delinquency

Neurotic delinquents commit illegal acts neither as commonplace pursuits shared with their peer group nor as a reflection of a long-standing characterological disorder. Rather, their delinquency emerges without previous warning as a way of expressing needs for recognition or help. In the first case, young people who feel ignored or unappreciated by others may carry out daring or dramatic acts of delinquency to bask, even if only briefly, in the notoriety they achieve. In the second case, children and adolescents who cannot find direct ways of communicating a need for help in dealing with some problem may act delinquently as an indirect means of getting this message across. The kind of distress most frequently associated with such delinquency is underlying depression, and the onset of uncharacteristic misconduct can commonly be traced to feelings of loneliness or discouragement that a young person cannot express or get others to hear through more direct channels of communication.[1,2]

A key to identifying this pattern of delinquency is the regularity with which neurotic delinquents manage to be caught in the act or give themselves away. Because the symptomatic use of delinquency to express underlying concerns serves its purpose only if the misdeeds come to light, successful concealment of law-breaking usually contraindicates neurotic delinquency. The differential diagnosis of neurotic delinquency is also facilitated by certain elements of the history and family circumstances. Unlike psychopathic individuals, neurotic delinquents have little or no history of earlier behavioral problems. Their current misconduct deviates sharply from how they have acted before and how others have come to expect them to act.

Moreover, in their relationships with their parents, neurotic delinquents will ordinarily have enjoyed both the close supervision denied socialized delinquents and the warmth and affection denied characterological delinquents. Nevertheless, specific problems in family communication are often the final factor in prompting otherwise law-abiding youngsters to resort to delinquent behavior as a means of getting their parents to recognize and respond to their needs. The more clearly these or other kinds of specific precipitating events (such as a painful rebuff from peers or loss of a parent through death or divorce) can be identified as occurring just before the onset of delinquent behavior, the more likely it is that the illegal activity constitutes neurotic symptom formation.

DIFFERENTIAL TREATMENT PLANNING IN DELINQUENCY

Differential treatment planning for delinquent youth depends on the type of delinquent behavior manifest. In socialized delinquency, antisocial actions are adaptive group behaviors that neither reflect nor lead to diagnosable psychological disturbance; hence there is little to be gained from efforts at psychological intervention in the practitioner's office. Socialized delinquents need supervision and control; they need guidance and models that can encourage them to exchange their antisocial values for more conventional standards of conduct. And they need help to prepare themselves for an adult life in which they can find ways of enjoying and supporting themselves within the law rather than by breaking it. Accordingly, the indicated treatment plan for adolescents displaying subcultural delinquency will usually be referral to community-based activities or agencies that provide group-oriented programs for developing the talents and redirecting the energies of delinquent youth.[3,6]

Characterological delinquency, because of its integral relationship to psychopathic personality formation beginning early in life, constitutes a serious and usually chronic form of psychopathology. Successful intervention in characterological delinquency accordingly requires intensive, long-term psychotherapy, which even under the best circumstances offers much less hope for a favorable outcome than can be expected for most other child and adolescent behavioral problems. Pediatricians are unlikely to undertake the long and arduous treatment of characterological delinquents themselves, unless they have had extensive training in child and adolescent psychiatry or behavioral pediatrics and can commit large amounts of time to such work. Instead, their usual choice will be to refer these patients to mental health practitioners or agencies, many of whom, in turn, feel that only an extended period of residential treatment can have sufficient impact on these young people to alter their chronic personality disorder,[4,10,11] albeit a trial in a day-treatment center is appropriate for some patients before residential treatment is instituted.

Recent advances in theory and practice have begun to improve somewhat this gloomy prognosis for psychopathy. The likelihood of psychopathic adolescents becoming seriously and persistently delinquent appears related to their lacking social skills that could help them find noncriminal ways of satisfying their needs. Attention is accordingly being directed to modifying the behavior of these delinquents not by attempting to change their character style, but by enhancing their coping capacities through a variety of training exercises designed to increase the person's repertoire of interpersonal skills and his or her capacities for judgment and self-control. Adolescents' parents are frequently brought into this type of treatment program, not for traditional family therapy but to receive training themselves in interacting with their child in ways that will encourage and reward prosocial behavior.[9]

Neurotic delinquency, because of its specific symptomatic meaning and relatively recent onset, frequently responds promptly to brief psychotherapy. Psychotherapy in correctly diagnosed instances of neurotic delinquency offers much greater promise of altering antisocial conduct than any of the known ways of intervening in socialized or characterological delinquency, and pediatricians who conduct psychotherapy can readily provide the necessary treatment in the office. Because the deviant behavior of neurotic delinquents is motivated by needs for attention and help, the very act of hearing them out and offering to work with them can in short order result in their stopping delinquent activity.[13]

Beyond this immediate salutory impact, effective psychotherapy with neurotic delinquents consists mainly of (1) gaining the patient's trust and confidence and (2) adopting the stance of an interested and concerned listener who makes observations from time to time on the apparent significance of what is being said, rather than of someone who passes judgment and gives advice. If these patients can also be helped to recognize connections between the onset of their delinquency and the onset of certain psychological problems they could not express in other ways, the likelihood of their resorting to such indirect channels of expression in the future will be substantially diminished.

REFERENCES

1. Bynner JM, O'Malley PM, and Bachman JG: Self-esteem and delinquency revisited, J Youth & Adol 10:407, 1981.
2. Chiles JA, Miller ML, and Cox GB: Depression in an adolescent delinquent population, Arch Gen Psychiatry 37:1179, 1980.
3. Coates RB: Community-based services for juvenile delinquents, J Soc Issues 37:87, 1981.
4. Doren DM: Assessing and treating the psychopath, New York, 1987, John Wiley & Sons.
5. Freidman CF, Mann F, and Freidman AS: A profile of juvenile street gang members, Adolescence 10:563, 1975.
6. Gottschalk R et al: Community-based interventions. In Quay HC, editor: Handbook of juvenile delinquency, New York, 1987, John Wiley & Sons.
7. Hare RD and Schalling D: Psychopathic behavior, New York, 1978, John Wiley & Sons, Inc.
8. Jacob DH: Learning problems, self-esteem, and delinquency. In Mack, JE, and Ablon SL, editors: The development and sustaining of self-esteem in childhood, New York, 1983, International Universities Press.
9. Kazdin AE: Treatment of antisocial behavior in children: current status and future directions, Psychol Bull 102:187, 1987.
10. McCord W: The psychopath and milieu therapy: a longitudinal study, New York, 1982, Academic Press.
11. Sutker PB, Archer RP, and Kilpatrick DG: Sociopathy and antisocial behavior: theory and treatment. In Turner SM, Calhoun, KS and Adams HE, editors: Handbook of clinical behavior therapy, New York, 1981, John Wiley & Sons, Inc.
12. Weiner IB: Child and adolescent psychopathology, New York, 1982, John Wiley & Sons.
13. Weiner IB: Psychological intervention for disturbed adolescents. In McNamara JR and Appel MA, editors: Critical issues, developments, and trends in professional psychology, New York, 1987, Praeger.

104

Mood Disturbances, Mood Disorders, and Suicidal Behavior in Adolescents

Åke Mattsson

Western societies have adopted a tolerant view of today's adolescents going through a period of "storm and stress" (Sturm und Drang), a developmental phase acknowledged by some writers as early as the 18th century. These writers noted a common, constructive turbulence of adolescence and youth.

In describing themselves, teenagers often emphasize their mood swings, which tend to baffle both themselves and their families. These mood disturbances include fluctuating states of elation, boundless energy, compassion, and idealism, alternating with hours or days of sullenness, self-doubt, irritability, and sadness, that is, signs of a dysphoric mood. Teenage moodiness is especially "noisy" and visible during the early adolescent years, from ages 11 to 14 in girls and from ages 12 to 16 in boys.

The appearance of short-lived mood disturbances among healthy adolescents has to be distinguished from persistent disturbances of mood that often are signs of a true mood disorder, either of a depressive type (unipolar disorder) or a manic-depressive type (bipolar disorder). Mood disorders are increasingly diagnosed in adolescents and in children (see Chapter 79). They are characterized by symptoms, signs, diagnostic criteria, and treatment approaches similar to those of adult patients.[1]

The primary care physician is often called on to evaluate the nature and persistence of a mood disturbance in an adolescent. For instance, is a sad, despairing mood in a teenager an appropriate, adaptive response to a serious loss or disappointment? Or, notwithstanding some psychosocial stressors, does the dysphoric mood imply a depressive mood disorder accompanied by suicidal ideation? The evaluation of mood disturbances requires knowledge of the main aspects of normal adolescent development and of the clinical features of the major mood disorders.

DEVELOPMENTAL ASPECTS OF ADOLESCENT MOOD DISTURBANCES

Puberty and adolescence entail marked developmental strides in biological, psychosocial, and cognitive areas (see Chapter 43). The physiologic changes, including rapid growth spurt and maturation of sexual organs and functions, pose a new body image to the adolescent and may cause anxious concerns, at times akin to those of hypochondriasis. In the psychosocial area, teenagers are struggling to attain emotional independence from their families and to establish a sense of identity in a society that seems to prolong their dependence on family and educational systems. The "breaking away" from the key persons of childhood is often associated with feelings of loneliness and sadness, like being a stranger among one's family.

In terms of cognitive development, the majority of adolescents begin to exercise formal, abstract operational thinking. This implies the ability to be introspective—to reflect on one's own thinking and mental constructs (operations). Adolescents tend to overestimate their emotional and intellectual experiences and believe that no one else can understand the uniqueness of *their* "inner life." The eagerness to construct ideals and ideal persons usually proves disappointing due to the abstract, unrealistic qualities they assign to their ideals. Finally, the adolescents' egocentric preoccupation with their many physical and mental changes is often accompanied by their belief and fear that others are as concerned about their new appearance and behavior as they themselves are. All these cognitive strides help to explain (1) the vulnerability of teenagers to open or implied remarks about them and (2) their proneness to react with self-derogatory, depressed moods, which are often combined with defensive, irritable attitudes toward family and peers. Again, these are age-appropriate mood disturbances.

CLINICAL MANIFESTATIONS OF MOOD DISTURBANCES AND MOOD DISORDERS

The following brief presentation of adolescent mood disturbances proceeds from those with mild impairment of functioning to those with severe impairment, such as the depressive (unipolar) and the bipolar (manic-depressive) mood disorders.[5] Disorders related to organic etiologies are not included. The diagnostic criteria are those described in the latest edition of the Diagnostic and Statistical Manual of Mental Disorders.[1]

1. *Normal mood disturbances in adolescence:* The moodiness and transient periods of elation, alternating with depression and dysphoria, have already been described. They rarely interfere with sleeping and eating patterns and with social and academic functioning.

2. *Adjustment disorders with depressed mood:* These are the most common mood disorders among adolescents. Usually they are related to recent psychosocial stressors, such as loss of a close relative or friend, serious family strife or illness, change of home or school, or a natural disaster. Common signs and symptoms are a dysphoric mood with feelings of sadness and helplessness, a drop in academic or vocational performance, loss of interest in usual activities, indecisiveness and poor concentration, withdrawal from family and peers, appetite and sleep disturbances, and brooding over issues of life and death that may include suicidal ideation. The usual duration of these symptoms is from 1 to a few months. Some mood disorders in this group, however, do not subside within 6 months and become chronic. They may then warrant the diagnosis of a true depressive disorder.
3. *Depressive disorders:* These are also called unipolar disorders because there is no history of manic or hypomanic episodes. Currently, two depressive disorders have well-established diagnostic criteria: (a) dysthymia and (b) major depression.
   (a) *Dysthymia* (formerly called depressive neurosis) is commonly diagnosed among adolescents referred for psychiatric evaluation (a general population prevalence of at least 10% to 15%) and is characterized by a year or more of not feeling well (dysphoria), irritability, low self-esteem, social withdrawal, impaired academic functioning, appetite and sleep disturbances, low energy, avoidance of pleasurable activities, (anhedonia), and poor concentration. Adolescent dysthymia may be secondary to preexisting mental problems, such as anxiety, attention deficit, substance dependence, and conduct, and to serious physical illness such as diabetes, epilepsy, asthma, hemophilia, and cancer. The often chronic course of dysthymia carries a risk for superimposed episodes of major depression, self-destructive acts, and alcohol and drug abuse.
   (b) *Major depression* shares most of the diagnostic criteria for dysthymia. However, its signs and symptoms are more acute, dramatic, all-encompassing, and functionally impairing, such as marked dysphoria and anhedonia, suicidal ideation, psychomotor retardation, fatigue, indecisiveness, loss of appetite, sleep disturbance, and inability to attend school or to work. Feelings of worthlessness, hopelessness, and guilt are common. At times these reach delusional, psychotic proportions, which may prompt a suicidal attempt in order "to end it all." Some seriously depressed adolescents engage in acting-out behaviors, such as truancy, running away from home, bouts of alcohol and drug abuse, sexual escapades, and delinquent acts, all akin to the features of a conduct disorder, which may also be present.[5,6] The self-destructive implication of some of these behaviors is at times obvious to the teenagers themselves.
4. *Bipolar mood disorders:* These were formerly named manic-depressive disorders. They are increasingly recognized in adolescents, often beginning with a manic episode. There may be weeks to months of a state of a euphoric, expansive, and irritable mood, associated with many or all of the following symptoms: decreased need for sleep, increased expenditure of physical and intellectual energy in both goal-directed and aimless pursuits, flight of ideas, distractibility, and grossly inflated self-esteem, which may be associated with grandiose delusions. During a manic episode, the person displays poor judgment and little insight. The young patient frequently engages in idiosyncratic, "foolish" activities such as buying sprees, sexual encounters, stealing, public offenses, elopement, and heavy drinking and drug use. The substance abuse may have a self-medicating, calming purpose, at times acknowledged by the patient. Most manic episodes require hospital admission in order to protect the youngster and to initiate proper psychiatric treatment. Even with treatment, recurrence of manic episodes is common. Eventually, the bipolar nature of the disorder becomes clear, that is, a major depressive episode will occur. A "complete" bipolar disorder is then present, with episodes (cycles) of mania and depression that are likely to continue into adulthood. It requires long-term psychiatric management.

   Many patients with a bipolar mood disorder will show "muted" periods of mania, named *hypomanic episodes* because the symptoms are less severe and neither associated with marked impairment in functioning nor with delusional features as seen in full-blown manic episodes. Ideally, an adolescent patient with a bipolar disorder will learn to recognize the elevated, expansive mood disturbances of a hypomanic episode and to prevent its escalation by consulting his or her psychiatrist for a prompt readjustment of the psychotropic medication.
5. *Cyclothymia* is a chronic, cyclic mood disturbance of at least 1 year duration for children and adolescents; it is characterized by repeated, alternating periods of hypomania and depressed, dysphoric mood. These episodes are not severe enough to meet the criteria of a bipolar disorder or a major depressive disorder. They only mildly interfere with social and school functioning. Yet many follow-up studies show that childhood cyclothymia may be a forerunner of bipolar disorders developing in adolescence or young adulthood. Both cyclothymia and bipolar disorders are equally common in males and in females, with a lifetime prevalence of from 0.5% to 3.5%, and show a clear familial pattern. Thus, some adolescents have a constitutional vulnerability to develop cyclic mood disorders under stressful biological and psychosocial conditions such as those occurring during puberty and adolescence.

Suicidal Behavior

The majority of healthy, well-adapted adolescents will give at least fleeting consideration to ending their lives or to being "non-alive" in an existential or "to Hell with the rest of society" sense, as they experience depressive mood swings or mourn the loss of a beloved person. Rarely do they intend or plan to harm themselves.

Genuine suicidal behavior includes actual suicidal acts, a preoccupation with self-destructive thoughts, and some instances of self-inflicted injuries such as wrist-cutting. The depressive and bipolar mood disorders are still viewed as the prevalent preconditions to attempted and completed suicides by adolescents.[3] However, conduct disorders, antisocial acts, substance abuse, and severe anxiety disorders are common, coexisting (comorbid) conditions, and conduct disorders alone may soon become known as major presuicidal disturbances.[2,4,8,9]

Current mortality surveys suggest that juvenile suicide in the United States presents an increasing public health problem, especially among 15- to 24-year-olds. The 1986 death certificate data[7] show that the number of deaths resulting from suicide in age group 10 to 14 years was 250; in age group 15 to 19, 1986; and in age group 20 to 24, 3224. In age groups 15 to 19, boys outnumbered girls by nearly 5 to 1. The country's total suicide rate in 1986 was 12.8 per 100,000 population. For children below age 14, the rate was 1.5 per 100,000, while the suicide rates among 15- to 19-year-olds was 10.2 per 100,000 and among 20- to 24-year-olds was 15.9 per 100,000. The distribution according to sex and ethnicity shows markedly higher suicide rates for boys than for girls at all ages and in all ethnic groups. Total figures for various ethnic groups indicate higher rates for white adolescents than for black, hispanic, and "other" ethnic minorities. (The lumping together of the nation's many native minorities in the annual mortality statistics unwittingly fails to document the alarmingly high suicide rates among some native groups, particularly, Native American youth).

Between 1976 and 1986 adolescent suicide rates rose sharply among white males (from 12 to 18 per 100,000 for 15- to 19-year-olds) while only slightly among white females (from about 3 to 4 per 100,000). Black adolescent males and females showed no sustained rise in suicide rate over the same period. In 1986 the suicide rate for black males age 15 to 19 was 7.1 per 100,000; for black females, it was 2.1 per 100,000.

While boys outnumbered girls in terms of completed adolescent suicides, the ratio is the reverse for unsuccessful suicide attempts: about four girls to one boy. In regard to suicide methods, the use of firearms has taken the lead for both sexes, while hanging is a common means for boys and jumping from heights for girls.[3,9] Self-poisoning, especially by drug ingestion, remains a favored suicide method among girls, which may allow for a greater chance for successful rescue efforts than do violent means of self-destruction. Overdosing with psychotropic medications, such as antidepressants prescribed for the depressed adolescents or their family members is becoming a common suicidal method. Action should be taken to eliminate the availability of potent drugs in the homes of depressed teenagers, as well as eliminating access to firearms.[3,4]

Current studies of adolescent suicidal behavior commonly report evidence of preexisting childhood psychosocial problems, often in the form of mood disorders, conduct disorders and antisocial behavior, alcohol and drug abuse, and learning disorders.[4,5,8,9] In addition, a family history of mood disorder, suicidal behavior, and substance abuse is present in a large number of suicidal adolescents.[3,5,9]

Most suicide attempts appear to be impulsive, unplanned acts, precipitated by stressful events common to all adolescents, but that cause acute, severe anguish with a wish "to be dead" in those youngsters whose preexisting psychiatric conditions have made them uniquely vulnerable.[4,9] An increasingly common contributory factor is the state of intoxication: the bereft, lonely, or ravingly furious, "non-heard" adolescent drinks or drugs himself into a state of grave cognitive impairment and disinhibition that precludes any rational means at seeking relief.[4] Only self-destruction carries a hope for relief.

Planned suicide attempts in adolescence are less common than in adult populations. The major preexisting psychiatric disorders are: (1) long-standing major depression with a pervasive sense of worthlessness and hopelessness and a preoccupation with suicidal ideation often associated with delusions of guilt, self-accusation, and deserved punishment; (2) schizophrenic disorders with florid psychotic features such as paranoid delusions and command hallucinations that seem to force the patient toward self-destruction; and (3) conduct disorders and antisocial acting-out often associated with angry, assaultive, and attention-seeking behaviors where the suicide attempt represents a manipulative, often repeated act.[2,9]

EVALUATION, DIFFERENTIAL DIAGNOSIS, AND MANAGEMENT

The primary care physician evaluating an adolescent with depressive or manic features must assess the depth of the teenager's mood disturbance and the presence of self-destructive intentions. This requires interviewing the patient and the essential family members (usually the parents). The physician should inquire about the teenager's medical and psychosocial history, individual and family functioning, school performance, and peer relationships. In addition, the following areas should be explored: (1) any recent events that might have precipitated the mood disorder, such as loss of a loved one, a family crisis, academic setbacks, and serious illness in the patient or a family member; (2) evidence of long-standing family, school, and peer problems; (3) signs of an organic brain syndrome resulting from central nervous system disease or substance abuse; (4) the common features of depression; (5) the possibility of a psychotic state with cognitive impairment, preoccupation with feelings of guilt and worthlessness, and evidence of delusions or hallucinations; and (6) signs of hyperactivity, marked irritability, running away from home, reckless driving, antisocial acts, and substance abuse. In the case of a suicide attempt, the physician should determine the details, including the lethality of the act, which often reflects the seriousness of the youngster's wish to die. Lethality is determined by the method used, the self-damage sustained, and the circumstances surrounding the attempt.

The physician should openly discuss the possibility of a mood disorder with the adolescent patient and inquire about any thoughts of self-destruction. Most dysphoric teenagers are relieved to find that their physician understands their painful state and its common occurrence among adolescents.

The evaluation of an adolescent with a mood disturbance should include a complete physical examination and indicated laboratory tests. A school report may help in complementing the family's observations of any changes in behavior and academic performance.

At the conclusion of the evaluation, the physician may decide to undertake the psychological counseling of the adolescent and parents provided the following conditions are present: (1) the mood disturbance is an exaggerated, normal type of adolescent mood swing or an acute depressive reaction caused by clearly recognized personal losses or frustrations; (2) the patient, the parents, and the physician all understand the major reasons for the mood disturbance and feel reasonably certain that the adolescent is not contemplating suicide or engaged in high-risk behaviors such as running away or substance abuse; (3) there is no evidence of a major depressive disorder, manic episode, psychotic features, or conduct disorder; and (4) those in the home and school environment are able to provide psychosocial support to the patient, which includes his attending scheduled counseling sessions. The first aim of these sessions, usually held weekly, should be to encourage the teenager's trust in the primary care physician, who then may help the adolescent examine the reasons for his mood disturbance. Whenever feasible, the emphasis should be on its "normality" and adaptive nature and on the patient's available strengths. The patient's hopeful future should be stressed, based on a realistic appraisal.

A psychiatric referral should be made if the primary care physician is unable to undertake psychological counseling or finds evidence of a serious mood disorder that clearly impairs social functioning, school performance, and vegetative functions. It then becomes the task of the psychiatrist to assess the nature and seriousness of the mood disorder and the suicide risk and to decide whether hospitalization is necessary for further evaluation and treatment. Any need for emergency medical care of a suicidal teenager requires admission followed by a prompt psychiatric consultation.

It should be the responsibility of a psychiatrist to evaluate the indications for drug therapy in adolescents with mood disorders. In most cases of major depressive disorders and bipolar disorders, psychotropic medication is an essential adjuvant to other interventions, such as individual and family psychotherapy. The optimal and safe usage of these potent drugs requires considerable experience with adolescent populations. Therefore, the responsibility for initiating and monitoring antidepressant, antianxiety, and mood stabilizing medications should lie with a psychiatrist.

When a psychiatric referral is made, the primary care physician often assists in the evaluation of the adolescent because of his or her knowledge of the patient's psychosocial and medical history. The physician may also help the family gain confidence in the psychiatrist and may provide follow-up care for the adolescent after the psychiatrist has completed the evaluation or the psychotherapeutic and medication interventions.

SUMMARY

The primary care physician can help prevent adolescent suicidal acts by prompt recognition of serious depressive states and suicidal tendencies among teenagers. Equally important is the physician's role as an identifier of the various types of mood disturbances seen in adolescents, from the normal mood swings to the rare psychotic depressions and manic episodes. Most adolescent depressive states are transient, adaptive, and prepare the teenagers for successful mastery of the inevitable losses and disappointments of adult life. The physician-counselor may then assume the role of an empathetic listener and supporter who takes an active role in explaining the reasons for the depressive condition and charting new courses for the patient and family. Together, the physician and adolescent often find that most mood disturbances are normative, self-limited crises with a potential to promote the teenager's psychological and social growth, attainment of self-reliance, and beginnings of adult independence.

REFERENCES

1. American Psychiatric Association: Diagnostic and statistical manual of mental disorders, ed. 3, revised, Washington, DC, 1987, American Psychiatric Association.
2. Apter A et al: Suicidal behavior, depression, and conduct disorder in hospitalized adolescents, J Am Acad Child Adolesc Psychiat 27:696, 1988.
3. Brent DA et al: Risk factors for adolescent suicide: a comparison of adolescent suicide victims with suicidal inpatients, Arch Gen Psychiat 45:581, 1988.
4. Hoberman HM and Garfinkel BD: Completed suicide in children and adolescents, J Am Acad Child Adolesc Psychiat 27:689, 1988.
5. Kashani JH and Sherman DD: Mood disorders in children and adolescents. In Tasman A, Hales RE, and Frances AJ, editors: Review of psychiatry, Washington, DC, 1989, American Psychiatric Press, Inc.
6. Kovacs M et al: Depressive disorders in childhood. III. A longitudinal study of comorbidity risk and risk for conduct disorders, J Affective Disord 15:205, 1988.
7. National Center for Health Statistics: Vital Statistics of the United States, 1986, Vol II, Mortality, Part A. DHHS Pub. No. (PHS) 88-1122. Public Health Service, Washington, DC, 1988, US Government Printing Office.
8. Pfeffer CR et al: Suicidal behavior in adolescent psychiatric inpatients, J Am Child Adolesc Psychiat 27:357, 1988.
9. Shaffer D et al: Preventing teenage suicide: a critical review, J Am Acad Child Adolesc Psychiat 27:675, 1988.

105

Runaway Youth

Gerald R. Adams

DEMOGRAPHIC ESTIMATES

In the largest and most comprehensive study of the runaway problem in the United States, the National Opinion Research Corporation[10] completed a nationwide probability study of nearly 14,000 households with teenagers. This pioneering study reported that 5.7% of the households had at least one runaway incident in 1976. This incidence rate, extrapolated to the general population, reflects between 985,000 and 1,134,200 runaway acts annually. Recently, Cairns[8] has tracked 695 children over 8 years during the 1980s; she reports that 22% of the children in her sample ran away from home. Furthermore, 29% of the females and 41% of the boys contemplated running away. Such evidence suggests that about one of three children considers running away and that about one of five actually does so.

The *National Statistical Survey on Runaway Youth* included a sample of more than 13,000 households and indicates that instances of running away were highest among 15 through 17-year-olds (median age = 16 years).[10] Slightly more than 50% of all runaways were males. Racial and socioeconomic differences were not apparent, but regional differences were observed. The incidence of runaway behavior tended to be higher in the western and north central states than in northeastern or southern states.

DISTINGUISHING RUNAWAYS FROM THROWAWAYS

In the early 1970s, runaways were considered to be a homogeneous group.[1] However, several investigations have since established that runaway adolescents consist of several subtypes. In a study of Colorado youth, Brennan, Huizinga, and Elliott[7] identified two broad categories of runaway youth. One group consisted of youths who were not delinquent or particularly alienated (Class 1). In general, these youths appeared to be psychologically healthy and had nondelinquent or nondeviant friends. The second group, in contrast, were delinquent and manifested considerable alienation in their attitudes and behaviors (Class 2). These youths experienced considerable conflict with and rejection from parents, had delinquent peers, manifested school alienation, reported low self-esteem, and engaged in deviant behaviors. The Class 1 youths were mostly temporary escapists from a conflict-laden home, had unrestrained peer activities without supervision, and tended to be lonely or isolated from their peers. The Class 2 youths were rejected, rebellious, and unrestrained youths who were labeled in negative terms and pushed away from the family.

In 1985, Adams, Gullotta, and Clancy[3] substantiated the multiple types of runaways in a study of runaway youths who were currently "on the streets." In a YMCA facility with a shelter program, runaway youths were interviewed while still away from home. Three classes of runaways were identified. The first group consisted of runaways who were similar to Brennan and associates' Class 1 youths. These youths left home because of (a) family conflict (hostile, confrontive, and unpleasant but endurable); (b) alienation from family, schools, and sometimes peers; and (c) poor social relationships with others. A second group consisted of "throwaways," children who had been encouraged or forced to leave home and were told not to return. A third group of youths were called societal rejects. These youths were rejected by their families, their neighborhood and school peers, their teachers, and even the justice and public social services. They lived independently, usually through criminal behaviors, and were an integral part of street culture. The "throwaways" and societal rejects were similar to the Class 2 runaways reported by Brennan and associates. Very little is documented empirically on Class 2 throwaways and societal rejects. Because of difficulties in identifying Class 2 youths and obtaining their cooperation, our knowledge base about runaways is primarily limited to information obtained from Class 1 youths.

UNDERSTANDING THE NATURE OF RUNAWAY BEHAVIOR

To speak authoritatively to parents and with adolescents about runaway behavior, medical professionals should be informed about the typical behaviors, psychological characteristics, social and familial circumstances, and the documented negative consequences of running away.

Typical Behavioral Patterns

Reviews by Nye,[11,12] Nye and Edelbrock,[13] and Adams and Gullotta[2] provide similar descriptions of the behavioral patterns of runaways. About 50% of the adolescents who run away do not run far and stay near home. Many runaways stay with friends, relatives, or neighborhood families (sometimes with the knowledge of their parents). Most stay away for just a brief time, with overnight absences the most common occurrence. Adams and Gullotta[2] estimate that approximately 40% of runaways return home in 1 day, with 60% returning after 3 days. More than 80% return in 1 month or less. Furthermore, they report that 52% of runaways stay within a 10-mile radius of home. Only 18% travel more than

50 miles from home. Less than 5% of runaways run away more than three times, and most run away without companions. However, females are slightly more likely than males to run away with a partner. There is some evidence that older runaways are likely to travel greater distances and stay away longer. Cairns[8] reports that males are more likely to only run away overnight or up to 1 week, while females are more likely to run away for extended periods or permanently. Furthermore, while some runaway youths may deliberate over a decision to run away, most do not substantially plan their episode, and usually the quick decision to leave is a result of emotional reactions.

Nye and Edelbrock[12] indicate that more than 50% of these youths report their runaway experience neutrally and as relatively noneventful. Some 25% report a positive adventure resulting in a sense of independence and confidence in their ability to survive on their own. Approximately 20% report negative consequences, with 3% reporting at least one violent experience. According to Nye,[11,12] approximately 40% of runaways return willingly and on their own initiative. Approximately 20% are found by parents and brought home, with another 20% returned by the police. The remaining 20% are returned by relatives and friends or other individuals not known personally by the family.

Psychological Characteristics

The American Psychiatric Association at one time classified the "runaway reaction" as a specific mental disorder. To assess the appropriateness of this decision, Adams and Munro[4] reviewed the numerous investigations comparing runaway and nonrunaway youth. They concluded that runaways are more likely than nonrunaway comparisons to have lower self-esteem, show greater signs of depression, perceive having less control over their environment, and show poor signs of judgment. They also concluded that runaways are more impulsive, easily frustrated, and less tolerant or sustaining of close interpersonal relationships. However, as Walker[14] correctly cautions, we are uncertain whether these psychological characteristics are antecedents or consequences of runaway behavior.

Social and Familial Circumstances

Problems in social and family relationships are important factors in running away from home. Many forms of evidence indicate not only problems between parents and runaways but also between the parents.[4] Family life is generally tense and conflict laden. Evidence summarized in the National Statistical Survey on Runaway Youth[10] clearly indicates that parents of runaways make few positive comments about their children, have more drinking problems, and engage in more physical abuse of their children than do parents of nonrunaways. These same parents are uninvolved in their children's community and school activities, and they show marked problems in communicating with their child.

According to Wolk and Brandon,[15] parents of runaways are commonly unable to exercise effective supervision. Parents of runaway male adolescents seem unable to control them, while parents of runaway female adolescents tend to overcontrol and punish their daughters. According to Gottlieb and Chafetz,[9] this inability to supervise effectively tends to produce a long series of confrontations between parents and adolescents. Furthermore, Gottlieb and Chafetz provide evidence indicating that upon returning home, runaways are likely to experience even more heightened communication problems, which are reflected in increased conflict and withdrawal.[9]

NEGATIVE CONSEQUENCES

Runaways leave home for several reasons, contributing factors including psychological characteristics, home environment, school and peer influences, abuse and neglect (particularly for throwaways), and delinquency. While throwaways are considerably more likely to leave for extended periods or even permanently, thus placing themselves at considerable risk, most runaways return home in 1 to 2 weeks and perceive their experience as relatively benign. However, the greater the distance from home and the longer the youth is on the streets, the greater the risk for negative consequences.

Young, Godfrey, Matthews, and Adams[16] have examined the evidence regarding potential negative consequences for runaway youth. Clearly, the risk factors are substantial. Confrontation with the legal system, substance abuse, coercive sexual behavior, contraction of sexually transmitted diseases (including acquired immune deficiency syndrome) and nutritional and general health problems, loss of educational training opportunities, pregnancy, and early parenting are likely. Furthermore, the negative conditions that may have motivated the adolescent to run away are only likely to be exacerbated, because increased tensions are likely in the home when the adolescent returns.

Of particular concern to the medical profession is the heightened likelihood of illicit drug use and contracting a sexually transmitted disease. Not only are runaways more likely to sell drugs to support their own habits, but their potential for addiction is extremely high. Furthermore, the risk for prostitution is also evident. According to Boyer and James,[6] it is estimated that there are 600,000 prostitutes between the ages of 6 and 16. The majority emerge from runaway and abandonment backgrounds. Unplanned pregnancies commonly result from selling sex. Not only does an early pregnancy have negative health consequences for the teenage girl, but it also places the offspring at risk for numerous medical problems. Indeed, Young and associates[16] summarize evidence indicating that children born of young adolescents are at risk of becoming socially maladjusted, commonly manifesting poor peer relationships and a propensity toward temper tantrums and impulsivity during their childhood.

INTERVENTION SERVICES AND RECOMMENDATIONS

Service provisions for runaway and throwaway youths are intricately related to federal and state statutory definitions of emancipation (see Chapter 4, Legal Aspects in Pediatric Medicine). Running away is referred to as "functional emancipation" when departure is undertaken without the benefit of legal maneuvering. In most states, statutory emancipation can occur if the minor is under a judicial order, by marrying, or upon joining the military. When treating a known runaway, most states require either parental permission or contact with a parent after a designated period. Interested professionals must refer to their own individual state laws and requirements, given the wide variance among states.

Adams and Adams[5] have suggested guidelines for intervening and treating. The first phase consists of *crisis intervention* and *stabilized placement**; the second involves *supportive counseling* and *assessment;* and the third includes *long-term therapy, education and training,* and *support services*. The agency (or physician where appropriate) first interacting with the youth should assume responsibility for crisis intervention and the initiation of a stabilized placement. Assessment and supportive counseling should be undertaken by local mental health providers. Long-term therapy, education and training, and supportive services should be provided through family and social welfare assistance.

The purpose of crisis intervention is to diffuse existing and looming physical, social, and mental crisis. The agency initially accepting responsibility for the care of the youth should conduct the crisis intervention required. The desired outcome is to resolve immediate crises sufficiently to make a stable placement possible. The purpose of stabilization is to provide security, calm the youth, and assure assessment of the situation. The assessment should provide the necessary information to enhance supportive counseling and to determine appropriate long-term treatment and placement. Long-term treatment, education and training, and supportive services should be undertaken to deal with the medical, social, and mental health issues of the youth. The desired outcome is diminution of runaway reactions, increased skill and coping abilities, and reunion of the adolescent with the family, and/or the establishment of alternative care.

*While the *National Statistical Survey on Runaway Youth*[10] found that few runaways use hotlines to contact parents, care providers can encourage the youth to make contact. The current national hotline number is 800-231-6946.

REFERENCES

1. Adams GR: Runaway youth projects: comments on care programs for runaways and throwaways, J Adolesc 3:321, 1980.
2. Adams GR and Gullotta T: Adolescent life experiences, Monterey, CA, 1983, Brooks-Cole Publishing.
3. Adams GR, Gullotta T, and Clancy M: Homeless adolescents: a descriptive study of similarities and differences between runaways and throwaways, Adolescence 20(79):715, 1985.
4. Adams GR and Munro G: Portrait of the North American runaway: a critical review, J Youth and Adol 8(3):359, 1979.
5. Adams PR and Adams GR: In Coleman JC, editor: Working with troubled adolescents, London, England, 1987, Academic Press.
6. Boyer D and James J: Easy money: adolescent involvement in prostitution. In Weisberg K, editor: Women and the law, Cambridge, 1981, Schuckman.
7. Brennan T, Huizinga D, and Elliott DS: The social psychology of runaways, Lexington, 1978, DC Heath and Co.
8. Cairns BD: Emancipation, abdication, and running away: a longitudinal perspective. Paper presented at the 1989 biennial meeting of the Society for Research in Child Development, April, Kansas City.
9. Gottlieb D and Chafetz JS: Dynamics of familial generational conflict and reconciliation, Youth & Society 9:213, 1977.
10. National Opinion Research Corporation: National statistical survey on runaway youth, North Harrison Street, Princeton, NJ, 1976.
11. Nye IF: Runaways: a report for parents. (Extension Bulletin No. 0743), Pullman, 1980a, Washington State University.
12. Nye IF: Runaways: some critical issues for professionals and society. (Extension Bulletin No. 0744), Pullman, 1980b, Washington State University.
13. Nye IF and Edelbrock C: Some social characteristics of runaways, J Fam Iss 1:147, 1980.
14. Walker D: Suburban runaway youth in the 1970's. Paper presented at the 1976 biennial meeting of the American Psychological Association, September, Washington DC.
15. Wolk S and Brandon J: Runaway adolescents' perception of parents and self, Adolescence 12:175, 1977.
16. Young RL et al: Runaways: a review of negative consequences, Fam Rels 32:275, 1983.

106

Sexual Behavior in Adolescents

Sharon B. Satterfield

At the turn of the century, an adolescent could expect to experience approximately 2 years between the onset of puberty and marriage. Today's adolescent, because of an earlier onset of puberty, prolonged education, and prolonged financial and emotional dependency on the family, may experience a transition period of up to 15 years, while also being expected to adhere to multiple cultural taboos against sexual expression. In addition, a variety of options are available today, including choices not to marry or to bear children—options that were formerly not part of the traditional rites of passage. These traditional rites have broken down because of what many people consider positive societal changes—equalization of career opportunities for both sexes, changes in dating practices, and increasing choices for careers and life-styles. These additional choices, however, require teenagers to make more decisions for themselves about their values and take more responsibility for their future. This occurs at a time when many are witnessing their parents' struggle with divorce and are exposed to confusing attitudes about dating and sexual practices. They are also exposed to a culture that is increasingly using the appeal of sex in commercials to sell many products, with much of the advertising directed to teenagers. At the same time, a strong opposition to formal sex education exists in many school systems. Therefore the teenager's decision-making process regarding personal sexual behavior must often occur amidst ignorance and confusion.

A profound influence on adolescent sexual behavior occurs in early family life. Although many families deny that sex education occurred, it is obvious that within the first years of life, children are initiated into nonverbal communication among family members about processes of elimination, caressing, nudity, and how people interact affectionately. They also witness which subjects are not addressed and which questions are not asked because of the embarrassment that parents have about certain topics. Adolescents with sexual problems commonly associate the lack of affectionate touching between family members with their later discomfort with sexuality.

As children explore their own bodies, they notice reactions of family members to masturbation, nudity, and "dirty" words. These reactions continually form attitudes that are internalized and contribute to the identity and body image of an adolescent. Having the genitalia viewed as dirty or shameful does not help the adolescent develop a positive body image or promote ease in accepting the changes of puberty. Families refusing to talk about sexuality is a strong negative message to children and teenagers, as is secrecy or embarrassment about parental sexual behavior.

In addition to the early family years, the attitudes and behavior exhibited by peers have a profound influence on adolescent sexual behavior. Sexual myths are common, and most of these are communicated by peers. Ford and Beach[1] categorized American society as sexually repressive compared with most modern and ancient civilizations, since it prohibits communication about sex as well as prohibiting sexual behavior. Since many adults equate providing information about sex with condoning sexual behavior, it is not unusual that sexual myths persist. A common example of such misinformation is the persistent belief of many people that masturbation will cause insanity or retardation. Sexual ignorance correlates with a higher risk of pregnancy and venereal disease, and the most sexually active teenagers are often ill informed in these matters.

There is no doubt that sexual attitudes have changed dramatically in the twentieth century. A person has only to consider the material in novels, films, and television to realize the United States has experienced an increasing tolerance toward explicit sexuality. The effect of changing attitudes on the sexual behavior of adolescents, however, is less clear.

EARLY ADOLESCENCE

Adolescence is preceded by an intense interest in and practice of sex roles. It has been demonstrated that adolescent sexual behavior is determined to a great extent by the developmental progress of the individual. The areas of cognitive, ego, moral, and personality development may vary a lot and may have little connection with chronologic age.

Cognitively, early adolescence is characterized by an ability to grasp and handle complex situations with increasing flexibility and adaptability. The younger adolescent is less likely to weigh the cost of a decision and more likely to make arbitrary decisions. Early adolescence is characterized by curiosity and consciousness about one's body and an acute embarrassment about sexual topics. Young adolescents are likely to be concerned about their dreams and fantasies. Many, at some time, feel guilty about being preoccupied with sex or are concerned that they might be homosexual as a result of close relationships with those of the same sex. It is often important that they be reassured by professionals that their thoughts and feelings are normal.

Variations in pubertal development may severely disrupt normal psychosexual growth. If puberty is precocious, the adolescent may be expected by adults and peers to act older than his or her chronologic age. When puberty is delayed, an arrest of psychosocial development will probably occur.

If the perceived abnormality is physically evident, the adolescent may withdraw from peers in embarrassment. Adolescents' perceptions of their bodies should be explored so that they can realize that their "problem" may be normal, as, for example, when the right scrotum hangs lower than the left or when there is a discrepancy between the size of the breasts. Teenagers who suffer from chronic disability or disease often feel that they will never be attractive to peers.

Much of the education about sex during this period comes from the peer group. Boys often participate in group forms of exposure, as in seeing who has the largest penis. Particularly in males, orgasmic same-sex liaisons are likely to exist; they are not usually associated with later adult homosexuality but may produce concern in the adolescent about being homosexual (see Chapter 101).

Sex education, particularly from health professionals, is crucial during early adolescence and may alleviate much anxiety.

MIDDLE TO LATE ADOLESCENCE

As teenagers reach middle adolescence, they naturally separate gradually from family influence in their search for identity. At this time the peer group exerts increasing influence, often to the dismay of parents. This is also a time when many health professionals feel less able to influence the adolescent.

It must be remembered that peer influence is exerted on a framework molded by many years of attitudes developed at home and in society at large. It is common to see teenagers following their parents' past behavior. For example, if a girl's mother married at 16, the daughter may have a monogamous relationship involving intercourse with a boyfriend at the same age. Dating patterns are particularly dependent on peer norms and usually begin with group parties before pairing off occurs. In some communities, however, adolescents experience a lot of pressure from adults to conform to premature dating patterns so that they fulfill the parents' social expectations.

The adolescent usually follows a fairly predictable series of behaviors: dating, kissing, deep kissing, breast stimulation over clothes, breast stimulation under clothes, genital apposition, and sexual intercourse. Teenagers vary tremendously regarding how far or how fast they progress on this scale.

Adolescents have been a particularly difficult group to study. However, it is obvious that over the past 30 years there have been significant changes in sexual attitudes and an increase in premarital intercourse. In clinical interviews with adolescents, it appears that the double standard is diminished, that love is not as frequently a prerequisite for a sexual relationship, and that some young women and men are ashamed of their virginity. On the other hand, many adolescents profess to hold their parents' belief that premarital sex is wrong.

Adolescents feel free to try a wider variety of life-styles than did those in previous generations. Some older adolescents choose to live together with or without a sexual relationship; communal living offers an alternative to the extended family. Having children without marriage and having marriage without children are additional options. As early as 1973, Sorenson[3] reported that 72% of all adolescents agreed that two people should not have to get married to live together. It remains to be seen whether society will expand its options or return to a nuclear family (see Chapter 45, "Changing American Families").

Adolescents give many reasons for becoming involved in sexual relationships. For some, sex has become a means of communicating, a step toward a relationship rather than the result. They justify this form of behavior on the basis that sex is "natural," whereas verbal communication is more painful and frustrating. For many, sex represents the communicating of a level of trust or caring within a relationship.

Other adolescents feel that sex for physical pleasure alone is acceptable. They see sex for love, sex for reproduction, and sex for pleasure as being different but worthy motivations. Some adolescents view their sexual behavior as part of a constant search for new experiences. This may represent a healthy index of maturity, or it may result from frustration in the compulsive search for excitement that often accompanies depression. Adolescents may use sex as an escape from loneliness or other pressures. Many report that friends influence their behavior considerably.

Possibly the most difficult adolescents to help are those who use sex as a challenge to parents or what they perceive as an unresponsive society. Sexual behavior is often the signal to adults that communication has broken down in other areas. Much of sexual behavior is still determined by the relationship in which the adolescent is involved. Using sex as reward or punishment is common and is often related to communication patterns learned earlier in life, particularly from the parents.

Biologically, sexual behavior is linked to reproduction. Traditionally, American culture, which has had a strong double standard, has supported the notion that women's drives and reproductive functions have to be linked. "Liberated" adolescents, both male and female, now refuse to accept this doctrine without question. The "unisex movement" has produced teenagers of both sexes who not only dress alike but who share tasks once stereotyped by sex. Dating appears to be oriented toward getting to know one another rather than toward demonstrating success in acquiring a date.

MASTURBATION

Although masturbation occurs commonly, especially in adolescent boys, there is widespread fear, ignorance, and guilt associated with the practice. According to Sorenson,[3] girls are less likely to masturbate than boys and probably will not at as young an age. Only about 33% of adolescent girls report having masturbated. This does not necessarily represent a biologic difference between the sexes but rather the fact that female adolescents are more likely to be discouraged in sexual experimentation by societal pressures and that women may tend to be less genitally focused in their sexuality. However, masturbation has been suggested by sex therapists as not only a healthy alternative for the teenager who does not wish to have intercourse but also, particularly for women, as an important component in the development of normal orgasmic response.

DECISION-MAKING

The most neglected area of adolescent sexuality has been the lack of studies regarding the decision-making process about becoming sexually involved, particularly with respect to boys. It is obvious that as an adolescent matures, decisions about participating in sexual behavior are influenced less by conformity, impulsiveness, and the drive to attain unrealistic goals. These are crucial components in ego development. But an adolescent's moral development leads to a less egocentric view of life that is less concerned with punishment over being caught or what he or she can get out of the experience and more concerned with universal moral principles. Interpersonal communication is an obvious component of sexual decision-making, and as an adolescent matures, communication is more likely to occur within an intimate relationship. Decision-making is also influenced by peer pressures, social norms, family and cultural expectations, and particular interpersonal needs of the adolescent.

PREGNANCY

Sexual behavior in adolescence cannot be discussed without alluding to the incidence of teenage pregnancy and venereal disease. Although the overall birth rate has been dropping in the United States, the number of teenage mothers has increased and their average age has decreased. Teenage mothers create enormous social problems because, emotionally, they are rarely prepared to cope with the demands of a child, the pregnancy interrupts their education, and it may result in estrangement from family or friends.

In many cases adolescents deny the possibility that they are fertile. Often they are embarrassed about seeking contraceptive advice because their parents might find out. Others are reluctant to use a contraceptive because it interferes with spontaneity, or the "naturalness" of the act, or because they do not want to admit to themselves or their partner that they really wished or planned to have intercourse. In many cases, however, adolescents refuse contraception because they wish, or have an unconscious desire, to conceive. Many troubled, lonely teenagers believe that having a baby will finally provide them with someone who will love them.

Often if her mother was a teenage mother and many of her peers have babies, a girl will respond to societal pressures to become pregnant. It is common in some instances for an adolescent's mother actually to encourage the pregnancy, overtly or covertly. Some adolescents, both male and female, feel insecure in their sexual identity and need to prove to themselves or others that they are capable of producing a child.

Many studies have attempted to determine differences between those adolescents who become pregnant and those who avoid pregnancy. Most studies have shown no significant differences in the populations, but there appear to be common themes when looking at individual cases. The need to be loved is a driving reason that many adolescents consciously give for getting pregnant. This may occur out of a lack of a basic trust developed within the family and the feeling of vulnerability so that only an infant is safe as a love object. It can occur out of feeling neglected by parents, whether the adolescent is actually neglected or not. Frequently, in cases in which there has been child abuse, the young woman wants to become pregnant because she has never experienced a loving relationship. Following sexual abuse, an inability to discriminate between sex and love on the part of many victims is common. One of the most neglected yet obvious reasons for getting pregnant is cultural. In subcultures in which the male needs to prove his masculinity by impregnating a girl or she needs to prove her femininity by becoming pregnant, this will likely occur in adolescence. Rebellion against parental values has been implicated in a number of adolescent pregnancies. There are also a variety of other unconscious motivations that need to be explored in understanding teenage pregnancies. The most common and preventable cause of pregnancy is the lack of knowledge among teenagers about sexuality and contraceptive methods. It should be noted, however, that efforts to prevent adolescent pregnancies by providing such knowledge without determining the reason why the sexual behavior is occurring may have little impact on changing pregnancy rates.

PROMISCUITY

Promiscuity is a term frequently used lightly by adults when speaking of adolescents. Often it merely indicates that an adolescent is sexually active. However, if defined as indiscriminate or compulsive sexual intercourse with several partners, the term is usually directed toward females because of society's double standard. Promiscuous behavior is almost always a sign of underlying emotional problems in the adolescent or the result of severe family conflict and discord.

The capacity for intimacy is acquired gradually and often with a certain amount of trial and error on the part of the adolescent. Disappointment over a relationship is common and can be a constructive experience for the adolescent if it does not lead to a compulsive form of sexual activity. Serial monogamy—that is, extended, meaningful relationships without the commitment of marriage—is increasingly common in late adolescence.

Venereal disease is obviously a consequence of sexual behavior and often of promiscuity and is reaching epidemic proportions. Little can be done to eradicate the problem unless the motivation for the behavior leading to it is understood.

Promiscuity or overly seductive behavior is one of the most obvious sequelae of sexual abuse. The possibility of sexual abuse should always be explored, but the physician should be aware that seductive behavior in itself may be only provocative and not indicative of previous sexual abuse.

SEXUAL DYSFUNCTION

Adolescents may seek professional advice about sexual questions or problems; however, they usually go to community agencies such as Planned Parenthood, peer counseling services in school, or neighborhood clinics rather than their pediatrician or family physician. They often seek approval for their behavior or advice on relationships. The judgmental adult will turn them away quickly. Reassurance about the normality of a situational disturbance such as erectile failure may prevent severe dysfunction later in adulthood.

The question "What is normal?" will be debated in medical circles for many years. The answer, "Whatever occurs between consenting adults," is a popular response but is not applicable to most adolescents. The behavior of each adolescent must be put in the context of other measurements of maturity. The extent of the behavior, how publicly it occurs, and the degree of impulsivity involved are useful indicators. For instance, a certain amount of voyeurism occurs in all adolescents, but not to the extent of habitually invading the privacy of others. Sadistic behavior that harms another, either psychologically or physically, should be an indication for psychiatric intervention. Exhibitionism is a common phenomenon in groups of adolescents, but not in a public one-to-one relationship, particularly with an unwilling observer.

Kaplan[2] distinguishes between immediate causes of sexual dysfunction, usually arising from the current relationship or environment of the couple, and the remote deeper causes that individuals carry with them from an earlier stage in life. Immediate causes of dysfunction include sexual ignorance, fear of failure, demand for performance by the partner, an excessive need to please the partner, intellectual defenses against erotic feelings, and communication failures. Deeper causes include intrapsychic conflicts or severe cultural constriction. Other causes of adult sexual dysfunction include traumatic events during adolescence, such as fear of discovery, ridicule by a partner, pressure to perform faster, or severe moralistic prohibitions.

Common forms of dysfunction in the male are premature ejaculation and erectile failure. Retarded ejaculation, though once considered rare, is common in its mild form. These dysfunctions may all occur in the adolescent, and except for those traumatically induced, the cause is rarely organic.

Members of both sexes may report concern about a low sex drive. They should be advised that this is an individual phenomenon dependent on multiple factors, particularly the state of the individual relationship. Low sexual drive, tension, orgasmic dysfunction, and vaginismus all may occur in adolescent girls, although there are no data to determine the incidence. Vaginismus, although seemingly less common, may be diagnosed early in adolescence if the physician is alert for the girl who is unable to insert a tampon or whose vaginal muscles spasmodically contract on pelvic examination. It also may occur secondary to a painful case of vaginitis.

Sexual abuse, both rape and incest, are increasingly reported (see Chapter 57, "Sexual Abuse of Children"). In many cities, more than 50% of all reported victims are children and adolescents. The professional must deal with victims of abuse in a gentle, supportive manner, being particularly aware of the reactions of their families. It is common for the victim and his or her family to have delayed emotional reactions months or even years later. Often secondary sexual dysfunction in the victim or his or her partner is subsequently reported.

SUMMARY

Teenagers require a thorough sex history carefully integrated into the routine history and physical examination, particularly when they have vague complaints or questions about the genitourinary system. The interviewer should ask questions designed to elicit attitudes rather than experiences. For example, asking what the adolescent thinks of abortion usually elicits attitudes and also sexual experiences. The interviewer should be nonjudgmental and empathetic and, most of all, ensure confidentiality.

Adolescence is a time of physiologic and emotional lability when the youth must integrate his or her rapidly changing body and attitudes to form a stable identity, including the ability to relate to others. Emerging sexuality is a significant factor in forming this identity and is influenced by society in general, the family, and the adolescent's peer group.

REFERENCES

1. Ford CF and Beach FA: Patterns of sexual behavior, New York, 1951, Harper & Row, Publishers, Inc.
2. Kaplan HS: The new sex therapy, New York, 1974, Brunner/Mazel, Inc.
3. Sorenson RC: Adolescent sexuality in contemporary America, New York, 1973, World Publisher.

SUGGESTED READINGS

Schofield M: The sexual behavior of young people, Gretna, La., 1968, Pelican Publishing Co., Inc.

Zelnik M and Kantner J: The probability of premarital intercourse, Soc Sci Res 1:335, 1972.

107

The Teenage Parent

Elizabeth R. McAnarney and Barbara N. Adams

In 1982, 1,077,124 pregnancies occurred in 15- to 19-year-old adolescents: 513,758 (48%) eventuated in live births, 418,740 (39%) in therapeutic abortions, and 144,626 (13%) in spontaneous abortions. Of all live births to adolescents, nearly 62% were born to unmarried women. Although in 1987 there were fewer births to all adolescent women (472,623), this decrease resulted primarily from the decline in their numbers.[4]

During the last decade, substantial increases have been made in knowledge about the risks of adolescent childbearing. Teenage women who receive early and consistent prenatal care should not experience more obstetric problems than do adult women of similar socioeconomic status, parity, race, and marital status. Even though adolescents bear more infants weighing less than 2500 g than do adults, the current thinking is that this difference is probably a reflection of teenagers' later entry into prenatal care and their poorer health habits compared with adults rather than the adolescent's biologic predisposition to bear small infants. Adolescent mothers and fathers experience educational and vocational dysfunction, marital instability, and often financial dependence on governmental assistance at least during some portion of their lifetime, thus making them a high-risk population for being inadequate parents.

Teenagers' adequacy to effectively care for their offspring has become the subject of investigation during recent years. Even though some professionals think that adolescents are more likely than adults to abuse their children, the data supporting this contention are far from conclusive. Some professionals are more concerned about adolescents' passive neglect of their children, a more benign neglect caused by their lack of child-rearing experience and ability to think ahead, than active, aggressive abuse.

Current investigations of adolescents as parents are focusing on (1) adolescent mother-infant interaction during the neonatal period and subsequently during the first year of the child's life; (2) adolescent fathers—their strengths, needs, and behavior toward their children; (3) the intellectual, social, and emotional development of the children of adolescents; and (4) intervention programs with adolescent mothers and the effects of these programs on their offspring. These investigations will take time to complete, since a methodology must be developed to study the many variables other than age that affect parenting, such as the adolescent's socioeconomic status, marital status, parity, educational level, and child-rearing experience.

PSYCHOSOCIAL REASONS ADOLESCENTS BECOME PREGNANT

Teenagers become pregnant for many reasons, some of which are conscious and some of which are subconscious. The circumstances are unique for each individual.

Pregnancy may be the teenager's way of trying to resolve acute or chronic depression. Acute, reactive depression may result from the loss of a loved one—parent, grandparents, or a caring relative—through death, separation, divorce, or a move. The teenager may conceive in an attempt to replace the individual who has been removed from her life.

Chronic, unresolved depression may precede the pregnancy by some years. A series of problems starting in childhood, such as poor school attendance, running away, suicidal behaviors, or drug overdoses, may be antecedent behaviors to the pregnancy. New data indicate that young women who report problem behaviors are more likely than women who report no problem behaviors to have a child before age 19 years. Pregnancy, like the other behaviors, reflects the girl's chronic inability to resolve her depression. For example:

> Jeannie, a 13-year-old girl, was 6 months pregnant when she was initially seen in the clinic. Her widowed mother worked outside the home to keep Jeannie and her two older siblings together at home. Jeannie had a history of absenteeism and withdrawn behavior at school. When she was 12 years old, she had run away and was returned to her mother by the authorities. In the year before conception, she had gone to the emergency department of the local hospital twice—the first time with acute alcoholism and the second time after a suicide gesture. Evaluation of Jeannie during the last emergency department visit revealed a depressed teenager who stated that she had been sad for as long as she could remember.

Jeannie's history indicates that she had been chronically depressed over several years and that her multiple attempts to gain attention had failed. Her history of school absenteeism, running away, alcohol ingestion, suicide gestures, and finally pregnancy suggested a long history of unresolved depression.

Peer pressure may be another important reason some teenagers become pregnant. Peer pressure for boys may come from friends of the same sex and for girls from friends of the opposite sex. For example:

> Carrie, a 15-year-old girl, became pregnant during the same time as three of her classmates. She was unable to say why she had become pregnant. The four girls had often talked about having babies. Carrie's boyfriend had not wanted her to use birth control pills, and he was pleased when she told him of the pregnancy.

Pregnancy and parenthood may represent positive accomplishments for teenagers who have experienced few. For example:

> Beth, an 18-year-old school dropout, had a history of school problems and also had few friends. When she was told that she was pregnant, she was very happy. During the last trimester of pregnancy, she began to talk about her baby and all she expected it would be able to do. After the baby was born, she brought her proudly to the clinic to show her baby to the other pregnant girls. One year later, she still talked with great pride about the baby and was trying to become pregnant again. Beth saw her child as her first real achievement and was seeking greater achievement through a second pregnancy.

In some families, an adolescent is encouraged to become pregnant either through overt approval of the young woman's sexual activity or through indirect encouragement. Still other teenagers become pregnant as a direct confrontation of parental authority or as a way of showing their growing independence. The need to show their independence may be most particularly intense for middle adolescents (15 to 17 years old), because they are normally in the midst of struggling for their independence and thus may be most threatened if it is challenged. Adolescents' ignorance about their sexuality and their potential for becoming pregnant are also contributing factors to teenage conception. Although some adolescents are misinformed about the details of sexuality, contraception, and pregnancy, ignorance about coitus possibly resulting in pregnancy contributes to only a limited number of teenage pregnancies.

DIAGNOSIS OF PREGNANCY

The diagnosis of teenage pregnancy poses problems for both the adolescent and the practitioner that usually do not occur with adults. Teenagers concerned about being pregnant may hesitate initially to seek help from their primary care physician. The physician may find it difficult to talk with pregnant teenagers about confidentiality, sexuality, and pregnancy if he or she and the adolescent have not discussed these topics before the pregnancy. In pediatric settings where these issues have been raised before the teenager seeks care for pregnancy, few problems arise between physician and adolescent.

Pregnant girls raise their concerns to the physician in several ways. Some (often older adolescents) who have achieved formal operational thinking state they think they may be pregnant. Other teenagers may complain of vague, somatic symptoms, such as headaches, abdominal pain, or joint pains, when their real concern is pregnancy. Still others expect the physician to guess that they are pregnant and do not indicate that pregnancy is even a possibility. This belief in the physician guessing that they are pregnant may represent the magical thinking of some adolescents. If a reproductive history is included in the general history-taking procedure for all teenage women, the physician will be able to move easily into the question of pregnancy in a situation such as the one just described. Questions about the menstrual cycle, including last menstrual period (LMP) and menstrual irregularities, should be incorporated into the reproductive history. Questions about previous pregnancies, contraceptive use, sexually transmitted diseases, particularly acquired immune deficiency syndrome (AIDS), and tampon use should also be included. If pregnancy is a possibility, the teenager can be asked whether she also considers pregnancy a possibility. Most teenagers are relieved to have the question of pregnancy raised. The physician should then decide how much of the pregnancy evaluation he or she will do and when the teenager will be referred for obstetric care.

Confirmation of pregnancy is clearly within the primary care physician's role. In addition to the medical and reproductive history, symptoms of pregnancy should be explored; a physical examination that includes a pelvic evaluation should be performed. Unless the pregnancy is well advanced, a pregnancy test is needed to confirm the diagnosis.

Serum pregnancy testing may be necessary if there is still question after the urine screen. Urine tests for pregnancy are sensitive enough to give accurate results 6 to 8 days after conception. Laboratory screening is endorsed because many teenagers inaccurately report their LMP.

When pregnancy has been diagnosed, the teenager should be referred to a special program for pregnant adolescents if one is available. If not, the teenager can be referred to a private office or clinic for obstetric care. The primary care physician may then choose to continue seeing the teenager for counseling and education throughout her pregnancy. Practitioners with good counseling skills and knowledge of pregnancy options can also be involved in abortion or adoption counseling. Referral to agencies providing these services is also appropriate.

COUNSELING PREGNANT TEENAGERS

Counseling in the practitioner's office might concentrate on the discussion of immediate considerations such as the course of the pregnancy, labor, and childbirth, as well as on future considerations—the effects of the pregnancy on education, vocation, and finances. Every effort should be made to work with the adolescent father-to-be if he and his partner are still in contact.

Some discussion should be directed toward the circumstances under which the teenager became pregnant and how she and her partner feel about the pregnancy. Problems may include the academic future for both, as well as the possibility of finding day care and funds for day care for their child. Finances are a major concern for most teenagers, and referral to the appropriate social service agency is often helpful.

Group counseling provides an effective method of communication with and education for teenagers. If there are two or more pregnant adolescents in one practice and the health professional is knowledgeable about group processes, group counseling can be provided.

An unstructured format for groups is optimal, since it allows adolescents to choose the subjects to be discussed and to exert some control in that setting. Both tasks are consistent with the developmental tasks of adolescence. Significant others, such as husbands, boyfriends, or labor coaches, can also attend, allowing the group leader to help these people reorder their relationships, a task similar to altering relationships when a new baby is added to the family.

Since some teenagers are not developmentally at the level of formal operational thinking, techniques traditionally used in adult groups need modification. For example, rather than presenting didactic information on a particular subject, role-playing provides an experience that teenagers enjoy. Although adolescents need to consider concrete, nonthreatening information at first, they soon become aware of their personal feelings about the meaning of pregnancy and are able to express these as the group process progresses. Although they may be unable to label their emotions abstractly, they can discuss their feelings by describing the thinking or behaviors of others. Written materials, videotapes, and movies at developmentally appropriate stages can be most helpful. Within groups, teenagers can learn to solve problems, resolve conflicts with their parents, clarify their independent, individual identities, and plan for their future.

POSTPARTUM CARE

Adolescents who become pregnant are at a high risk for repeat pregnancy during adolescence. A major goal in the provision of care to teenagers during pregnancy is preparing both partners for responsible planning of their reproductive future. Ideally, responsibility for contraception after the first pregnancy is shared by both partners.

Adolescent contraception imposes many problems that do not diminish once the baby has been born. Those circumstances which were present before and which contributed to the initial conception may still exist, even though some teenagers are motivated to prevent a second pregnancy. Contraceptive failures caused by noncompliance in pill-taking or sporadic or improper use of condoms or foam, as well as barriers to the use of these inherent in the health care system, may continue to be particular problems for teenagers seeking effective contraception.

Even though all contraceptive methods currently available rely on patient compliance for effectiveness, new products, including subdermal implants of the hormone leveonorgestrel, are now available. Contraceptive methods decreasing reliance on adolescents are more effective than the methods that depend on adolescents. For those young people at risk for AIDS, special emphasis should be placed on counseling and education about condom usage. The primary care practitioner may decide to assume the responsibility for contraceptive education and birth control prescription for adolescent parents.

TEENAGERS AS PARENTS

Teenage parents face multiple problems. Although often experienced in baby-sitting, teenagers are not prepared for the reality of round-the-clock child care. Adolescents may expect to have complacent babies who eat and sleep with regularity; they may become disillusioned easily when the child demands far more time and effort than they are prepared to give.

Attitudes of adolescent mothers suggest the use of physical punishment for discipline and minimal understanding of the need for stimulation. Although these attitudes may reflect sociocultural influences rather than the mother's age, professionals should be aware of this issue. Most teenagers are fond of children, want to be good parents, and are eager to learn about child rearing.

Adolescent parents frequently live with their own parents or other family members. Observing the efficiency with which their relatives care for the child may add to their own lack of confidence. The adolescents' reaction may be to give up parenting and relinquish this task to other caretakers in the home. The child, in turn, may become confused and have difficulty forming a bond with his or her own parents and may not even identify them as the actual parents. Simply teaching about child care and role modeling can help the adolescent parent. Home visits are an effective way to observe the teenage parents with the baby and help them in the care of the infant.

Many teenagers expect their baby to fulfill their own needs for love immediately and are disappointed when the infant does not respond as they had expected. Data indicate that younger adolescent mothers are less accepting of, cooperative with, and accessible and sensitive to their children during the first postnatal year than are older adolescent mothers. For example, a teenager may think her crying baby will be immediately comforted when picked up. If the infant does not respond as anticipated, the young mother may feel rejected and unloved by her child. However, with time and patience, teenagers can be taught about the needs of infants and the variety of responses that meet those needs.

Adolescent fathers who want to be actively involved with the rearing of their children should receive the same support as adolescent mothers. New data indicate, however, that most adolescent males are ill-prepared for fatherhood. In one recent study,[2] academic, drug, and conduct problems were significantly more common among adolescent fathers than among males in general. Teenage fathers may choose to relieve the mother of total responsibility for their child by being available to provide care when the mother needs time for her education, job, or other activities. Even if the adolescent father is not personally available, he may want to ask members of his extended family to provide direct help and support for the mother.

Mixed feelings about parenthood are appropriate for teenagers. They want to be good parents and to love their children, but they also want to engage in normal teenage activities. It is important for the practitioner to remember that teenagers need to gain knowledge and expertise to fulfill their role as parents and also need to move through the adolescent period in concert with their peers. Often families will need help in effecting an appropriate balance for the adolescent mother and father between their duties as parents and their peer, school, and social activities.

LONG-TERM FOLLOW-UP

New data[3] indicate that on long-term follow-up in Baltimore, Md., women who became mothers as adolescents may actually finish their educations and become independent of welfare assistance. In a 17-year follow up of a group of inner city poor adolescents, 67% of the group had obtained their high school diplomas and 35% had graduated from college or had taken some postsecondary courses. Only 12% of those who went on welfare assistance during the first 5 years of the study continued to be on assistance nearly 2 decades later.

SUMMARY

Even though fewer adolescents are choosing to continue their pregnancies than was so in the past (primarily because of the availability of contraception and abortion), the ability of teenagers to care for their children effectively is still an area in which intensive investigation is needed. However, some professionals who have worked with adolescent parents are impressed by their strengths and their ability to learn how to be effective parents when they receive adequate instruction.

REFERENCES

1. Elster AB, Ketterlinus R, and Lamb ME: The association between adolescent parenthood and problem behavior in a national sample of adolescent women, Pediatrics 85:1044-1050,1990.
2. Elster AB, Lamb ME, and Tavare J: Association between behavioral and school problems and fatherhood in a national sample of adolescent youths, J Pediatr 111:932, 1987.
3. Furstenberg FF, Brooks-Gunn J, and Morgan SP: Adolescent mothers and their children in later life, Fam Plann Perspect 19:142, 1987.
4. Moore KA et al: Statistical appendix: trends in adolescent sexuality and fertility behavior. In Hofferth SL and Hayes CD, editors: Risking the Future. Washington, D.C.: National Academy Press; 2:418, 1987.

SUGGESTED READINGS

McAnarney ER and Hendee WR: Adolescent pregnancy and its consequences, JAMA 262:74, 1989.

McAnarney ER and Hendee WR: The prevention of adolescent pregnancy, JAMA 262:78, 1989.

Unger DG and Wandersman LP: The relation of family and partner support to the adjustment of adolescent mothers, Child Dev 59:1056, 1988.

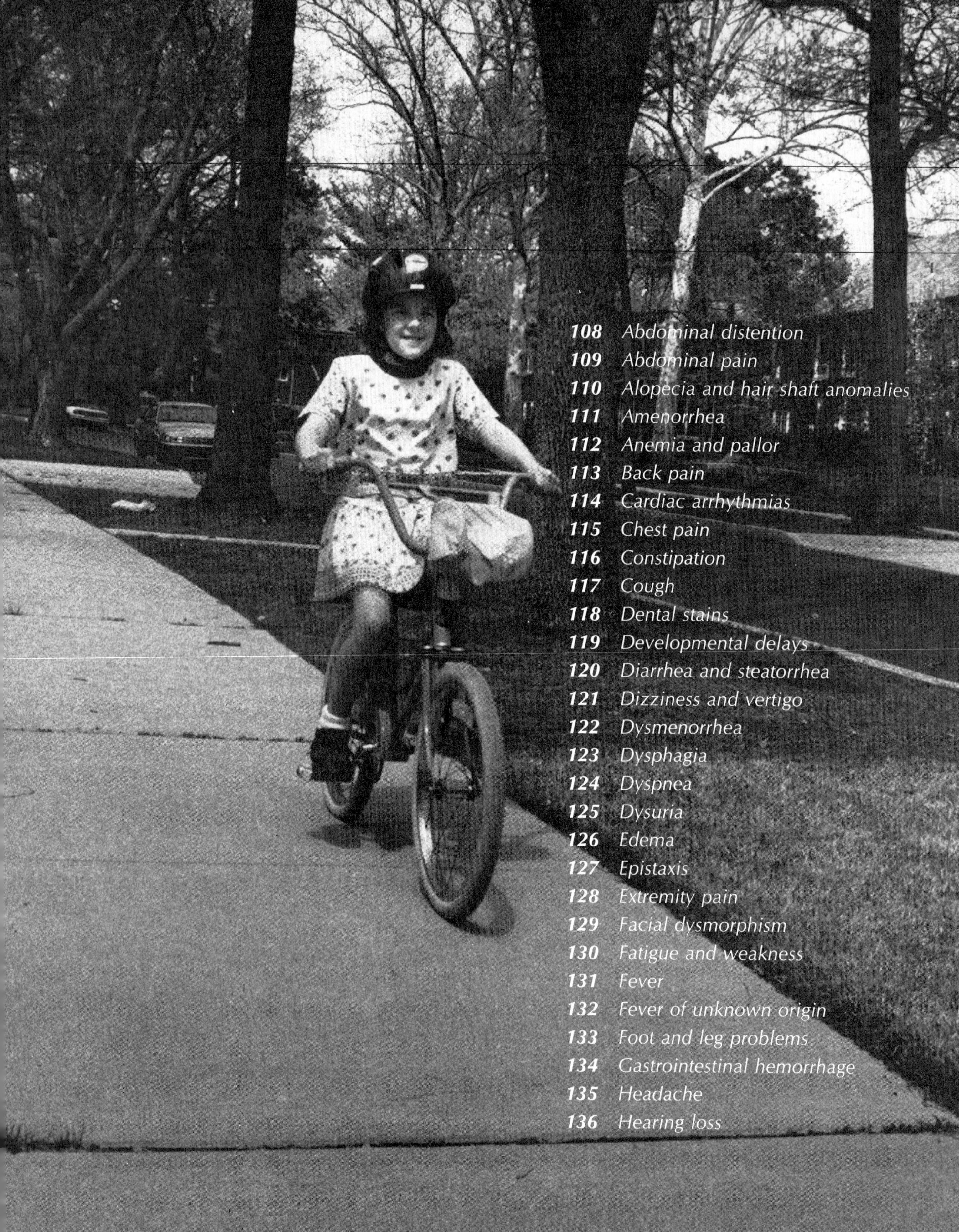

Part Seven

Presenting Signs and Symptoms

108

Abdominal Distention

Henry S. Friedman and Joanne Kurtzberg

DIAGNOSTIC CLUES

Abdominal distention or swelling is a common pediatric complaint; it may be due to a wide variety of disorders, ranging from a simple gastrointestinal problem to a systemic illness with significant consequences (see accompanying box). A complete history addressing the duration and swelling and associated symptoms such as pain, vomiting, diarrhea, and the presence or absence of fever is crucial to an accurate diagnosis and appropriate intervention. The infant or child with the sudden onset of abdominal swelling accompanied by vomiting and pain is likely to have an acute gastrointestinal tract obstruction or peritonitis. Chronic abdominal enlargement or swelling is often associated with less acute but equally serious disorders. Diarrhea may be the clue to an inflammatory process or malabsorption. A dietary history will provide valuable information both for those children who eat poorly and suffer from consequent dietary deficiencies and for those children who seemingly ingest all foods in sight. Abdominal swelling in a female of reproductive age must suggest pregnancy to the physician.

PHYSICAL EXAMINATION

The physical examination of an infant or child with a swollen or protuberant abdomen should follow the same guidelines as the examination of a child with a normal-appearing abdomen. Inspection is important but often cursorily performed. The abdominal contour may help the physician to distinguish the normal "potbelly" of a healthy prepubescent child with a lordotic stance from one with true localized or generalized swelling. A tense, distended abdomen with taut skin and an everted umbilicus often suggests ascites. An epigastric mass with left-to-right peristalsis suggests pyloric stenosis or obstruction, while an enlarged liver or spleen may be seen in the right or upper left quadrant, respectively. The superficial abdominal veins must be noted because with a number of disorders, including peritonitis, these veins are often distended in children.

Auscultation may yield the high-pitched frequent sounds of early peritonitis or intestinal obstruction, whereas auscultation over the liver or spleen may reveal a bruit, which suggests a vascular tumor or lesion.

Percussion may reveal the tympanites of lower intestinal tract obstruction or aerophagia with resultant gastric distention. A distended abdomen without tympany suggests the presence of fluid or a solid mass. Distinction between the two is made by demonstrating a fluid wave or shifting dullness on physical examination.

Palpating a distended abdomen can be difficult. Patients with surgical conditions such as an obstruction or peritonitis may have hard, tense abdomens. The tense abdomen of a crying infant or child should relax on inspiration. Tenderness to palpation may help pinpoint a localized obstruction, infection, or abscess, but also may not correlate with the underlying pathologic condition. Abnormal masses (such as Wilms tumor, neuroblastoma, hydrometrocolpos, polycystic kidneys, or an enlarged uterus) may be readily identified. The liver and spleen can likewise be felt, enabling the practitioner to pinpoint visceromegaly if present. Masses palpable in cases of acute intestinal obstruction include the "olive" of pyloric stenosis (see Chapter 206, "Gastrointestinal Obstruction") and the sausage-shaped tender mass of an intussusception.

DIFFERENTIAL DIAGNOSIS

Obstruction of the gastrointestinal tract generally produces pain, vomiting, absent stooling, and abdominal distention (see Chapter 206). In neonates, one suspects duodenal atresia when vomiting and distention occur shortly after the infant's first feeding. Lower gastrointestinal tract obstructions may present with the same symptoms but a few hours to days later. Meconium ileus, with or without associated peritonitis, produces obstruction and abdominal swelling. The association with cystic fibrosis should be remembered. A premature infant with vomiting, apnea, abdominal distention, and hypothermia should be suspected of having necrotizing enterocolitis, especially if there is a history of asphyxia or other prior insults.

The differential diagnosis of abdominal swelling resulting from an obstructive process in an older child is more limited. A child with crampy, intermittent abdominal pain associated with "currant-jelly" stool and ultimately with abdominal distention has an intussusception. Intestinal malrotation with volvulus, seen with rapid abdominal swelling and vomiting, can occur in an infant or child of any age. Hernias may become incarcerated, producing partial or complete intestinal obstruction with subsequent pain, vomiting, and abdominal swelling.

Gastrointestinal infections such as an intraabdominal abscess, amebiasis, or malaria are rare causes of abdominal swelling. Inflammation of the gastrointestinal tract caused by regional enteritis (Crohn disease) or ulcerative colitis (espe-

Abdominal Distention

GASTROINTESTINAL (GI) TRACT

Obstruction
- Tracheoesophageal fistula
- Duodenal atresia
- GI atresia and duplication
- Annular pancreas
- Gastric perforation
- Meconium ileus
- Hirschsprung disease
- Intussusception
- Incarcerated or strangulated hernia
- Volvulus with malrotation
- Bezoar
- Imperforate anus
- Necrotizing enterocolitis

Infection
- Abscess
- Botulism
- Amebiasis
- Malaria

Inflammation
- Regional enteritis
- Ulcerative colitis

LIVER AND BILIARY TRACT

Hepatomegaly
Liver tumor
Choledochal cyst
Hydrops of the gallbladder

URINARY TRACT

Hydronephrosis
Polycystic kidneys
Wilms tumor
Bladder distention

GENITAL TRACT

Ovarian tumor
Hydrometrocolpos
Pregnancy

SPLEEN

Splenomegaly
Subcapsular hemorrhage

PANCREAS

Cyst
Tumor

PERITONEUM

Peritonitis (bacterial, chemical [bile], or tuberculous)
Ascites
Cysts (peritoneal, mesenteric, or omental)

NEOPLASM

Lymphoma
Neuroblastoma
Rhabdomyosarcoma

NUTRITION OR METABOLISM

Excessive eating
Beriberi
Scurvy
Hypothyroidism
Rickets
Hypokalemia
Carbohydrate intolerance

MUSCLE

Muscle weakness
Prune-belly syndrome

MALABSORPTION

Cystic fibrosis
Gluten enteropathy
Abetalipoproteinemia

MISCELLANEOUS

Poor posture
Aerophagia
Chronic constipation
Pneumoperitoneum
Beckwith-Wiedemann syndrome
Chloramphenicol toxicity
Diabetes mellitus

cially with toxic megacolon) may cause abdominal swelling, but diarrhea, pain, weight loss, and fever are more commonly seen in these disorders.

Chronic and often more insidious abdominal swelling can be caused by hepatic or biliary tree disease. Inborn errors of metabolism, such as mucopolysaccharidoses, Tay-Sachs disease, Gaucher disease, or glycogen storage disease, cause hepatosplenomegaly, often first perceived as abdominal swelling. Biliary disease, such as a choledochal cyst or hydrops of the gallbladder, appears acutely with a right upper quadrant mass and severe pain. However, children with hydrops will appear toxic, whereas those with choledochal cysts are jaundiced.

Genitourinary tract disorders can cause chronic or acute abdominal swelling. Hydronephrosis, polycystic kidneys, pregnancy, and hydrometrocolpos tend to produce chronic swelling; bladder distention, however, can be a more acute phenomenon. Wilms tumor is often diagnosed after a parent notices the child's swollen abdomen. Abdominal pain, painless hematuria, and hypertension are associated findings that may support this diagnosis.

Peritoneal conditions that cause abdominal swelling include peritonitis and ascites. The former, causing severe pain with a boardlike abdomen, is usually of bacterial origin but can be due to the sudden escape of bile into the peritoneal cavity. The latter has its own extensive differential diagnosis, including the Budd-Chiari syndrome, biliary atresia, ascending cholangitis, cytomegalovirus infection, toxoplasmosis, syphilis, chronic active hepatitis, pancreatitis, Wilson disease, galactosemia, and cardiac failure.

Neoplastic disorders causing abdominal swelling include lymphoma, neuroblastoma, and rhabdomyosarcoma. Malabsorptive disorders such as cystic fibrosis and gluten enteropathy may cause steatorrhea or chronic diarrhea, failure to thrive, and abdominal swelling.

Nutritional or metabolic causes of a swollen abdomen include the normal postprandial swelling, beriberi, scurvy, and hypokalemia. Hypothyroidism, which should be diagnosed as early in its course as possible, should be considered in a child with a protuberant abdomen and umbilical hernia. Muscular weakness may be associated with a prominent abdomen, especially in the prune-belly syndrome, in which the abdominal musculature is absent.

Finally, a number of miscellaneous disorders may be associated with a swollen abdomen. These range from benign disorders (e.g., aerophagia or lordotic posture) to more problematic disorders (e.g., chronic constipation) to life threatening disorders, such as the gray-baby syndrome of chloramphenicol toxicity or pneumoperitoneum.

SUMMARY

A multitude of causes ranging from a benign to life-threatening illness can produce abdominal swelling. The history and physical examination remain the keys to an accurate diagnosis. Radiographic procedures and laboratory tests are generally necessary for the diagnostic evaluation. Upright and flat plates of the abdomen may demonstrate air-fluid levels and dilated loops of bowel characteristic of an obstruction; ascites appears as diffuse haziness with absence of psoas lines. Contrast studies and computed tomography may also yield important clues, especially in the diagnosis of tumors and abscesses. Magnetic resonance imaging may similarly provide helpful diagnostic information.

SUGGESTED READINGS

Bates B: A guide to physical examination and history taking, ed 5, Philadelphia, 1991, J.B. Lippincott Co.

Illingworth RS: Common symptoms of disease in children, ed 5, Oxford, 1975, Blackwell Scientific Publications, Ltd.

Tunnessen WW, Jr.: Signs and symptoms in pediatrics, ed 2, Philadelphia, 1988, J.B. Lippincott Co.

109

Abdominal Pain

Ronald G. Barr

Abdominal pain is a common and difficult diagnostic and therapeutic problem. As with many other pediatric complaints, it raises the possibility of potentially life-threatening physical disease on the one hand and significant interpersonal dysfunction on the other. As a result, the problem of abdominal pain includes both diagnosing and treating the pain symptom, as well as understanding and managing the secondary effects of an abdominal pain complaint in a child.

Abdominal pain can take three forms: acute, recurrent, or chronic. To some extent the clinical priorities will be determined by the form in which the complaint first appears. In acute presentations, recognizable organic entities are more common, and the main concern of management is preventing tissue damage. In recurrent presentations, recognizable organic entities are less common, and management must be concerned with the probability that the child will continue living with this symptom without the physician knowing the cause. In truly chronic pain a physical disease usually is recognized and coexists with significant functional disability that is only partially responsive to therapy. Although children seldom are seen initially with chronic abdominal pain, once the complaint is established, the diagnostic and management problem relates to understanding the interaction between the disease process and the pain complaint and to promoting optimal psychosocial functioning.

CLINICAL CLASSIFICATION

For purposes of clinical differentiation, abdominal pain may be considered to include organic, psychogenic, and dysfunctional categories. Organic pain includes those cases in which pain sensations are assumed to originate intraabdominally from a specific disease process of an organ system(s) and in which treatment of the disease results in amelioration of the symptoms. Subcategories include disease referable to the gastrointestinal tract (e.g., inflammatory bowel disease), the genitourinary tract (e.g., pelvic inflammatory disease), and others (e.g., acute intermittent porphyria).

Psychogenic pain includes those cases in which (1) the patient experiences or complains of pain and (2) pain sensations are assumed not to originate in intraabdominal sensory nerve endings. Explicit recognition by the patient of a relationship between the pain events and relevant psychological events contributes substantially to appropriate diagnosis and therapeutic prognosis. Subcategories include pain experiences in response to acute or chronic stress (e.g., loss of a parent), behavioral pain complaints (e.g., complaint modeling, maintenance of pain complaint for secondary gain), pain that occurs as part of a psychiatric syndrome (e.g., depression, conversion reactions), and other behavioral syndromes (e.g., school phobia). The assumption that *associated* stress events are causal is unjustified in the absence of positive evidence for the relationship between the relevant disordered intrapersonal or interpersonal behavior and the pain complaint.

Dysfunctional pain syndromes include those cases in which pain sensations are assumed to originate intraabdominally from normal rather than disordered physiologic processes. The term *dysfunctional* (in contrast to the more common term *functional*) is used to recognize that even in the absence of disease, the pain symptom interferes with normal activity and is a problem for the patient and for those in his or her environment. Dysfunctional pain has two subcategories: *specific* syndromes (e.g., lactose intolerance, Mittelschmerz), in which the mechanism of pain production is identifiable, and *nonspecific* syndromes, in which no apparent mechanism is identified. In this classification, an increase in the frequency or severity of pain episodes in the response to normal variation in daily mood or stress would be distinguished from psychogenic pain and considered a specific dysfunctional pain syndrome.

GENERAL APPROACH TO DIAGNOSIS

In addition to the typical differential list for acute abdominal pain, there are well over 100 entities that may occur as *recurrent* abdominal pain (see box on pp 810-811). Although the approach to diagnosis is relatively simple if one knows the entity causing the symptom, the more typical diagnostic problem occurs when the complaint is presented without clear evidence of its cause. In general, the diagnostic approach will be largely governed by the form and setting of clinical presentation, whereas the management usually will depend on the classification of the complaint.

The apparently simple distinction between acute and recurrent pain is blurred by the following factors: an acute presentation may be only the first episode of a recurrent syndrome, a particular episode of recurrent pain may have an acute presentation, and patients with recurrent syndromes may be equally likely to have an acute intercurrent disease process as one of these manifestations. Despite this caution, a number of general principles are applicable to help structure the general approach to the pain complaint (Fig. 109-1):

1. In acute pain the primary question concerns the necessity for and timing of surgical intervention (a "surgical" abdomen) or specific medical therapy; in recurrent pain, definition of the syndrome, identification of sec-

Clinical Classification of Recurrent Abdominal Pain in Children

ORGANIC (5%)*
Gastrointestinal

Peptic ulcer
Gastritis
Esophagitis
Hiatal hernia
Other hernias
Volvulus, recurrent
Obstruction resulting from bands
Inflammatory bowel disease
  Crohn disease
  Ulcerative colitis
Meckel diverticulum
Neoplasms
Yersinia enterocolitica infection
Intussusception, recurrent
Hirschsprung disease
Infestations (e.g., giardiasis)
Malrotations
Annular pancreas
Polyps, polyposis
Foreign body
Mesenteric adenitis
Malformations—gastric duplication
Hydronephrosis
Lower tract obstruction
  Posterior urethral valves
Pyelonephritis
Renal stones
Ovarian cyst
Testicular or ovarian torsion
Hematocolpos
Endometriosis
Neoplasms
Urinary tract infection
Pelvic inflammatory disease or salpingitis
Ectopic pregnancy
Secondary dysmenorrhea

*Percentages are approximate and may vary significantly with referral practice patterns.

ORGANIC (5%)—cont'd
Hepatobiliary System

Hepatitis
Gallstones, cholecystitis
Pancreatitis (especially familial)

Trauma

Traumatic hemobilia
Pancreatic pseudocyst
Subserosal intestinal hemorrhage
Abdominal wall strain

Metabolic

Lead poisoning
Acute intermittent porphyria
Hereditary angioedema
Familial hyperlipidemia

Miscellaneous

Abdominal epilepsy or migraine
Anorexia nervosa
Sickle cell disease
Familial Mediterranean fever
Riley-Day syndrome
Multiple endocrine adenomatosis
Blood dyscrasias
Lymphomas
Coxsackievirus infection (pleurodynia)
Meconium ileus syndrome
Brain and spinal cord neoplasms
Epilepsy
Hemolytic disease

ondary anxiety sources (e.g., fear of cancer) or dysfunction (e.g., accusations of malingering), and staged evaluation of potential causes are paramount.

2. In acute pain the primary concern is prevention of tissue damage; in recurrent pain, in which tissue damage and resolution of the symptom are less likely, prevention of secondary dysfunction is an appropriate and achievable therapeutic goal.
3. Clinical presentations of disease entities are a function of age. Ulcers tend to be secondary and gastric in infants but primary and duodenal in older children and adolescents.
4. In infants and toddlers, both acute and recurrent pain complaints should be considered organic until proved otherwise. In school-aged children, dysfunctional abdominal pain is predominant. Although dysfunctional abdominal pain remains the most common category in adolescents, both organic pain referable to the genitourinary tract and psychogenic pain are increasingly prevalent.
5. In general, specific diagnostic and therapeutic strategies are relevant for each clinical category. Organic pain is diagnosed in the classic fashion of seeking signs and associated symptoms of disease that might *cause* the pain, and appropriate therapy follows logically from the diagnosis. Dysfunctional pain is identified by directing questions toward constitutional and environmental factors that might *predispose* the patient to pain; therapy is aimed at interrupting the interaction or providing for the consequences (environmental manipulation). Psychogenic pain is elucidated by defining how and why the patient experiences pain; therapy is directed toward modifying the experience (often this is accomplished through counseling).

Clinical Classification of Recurrent Abdominal Pain in Children—cont'd

DYSFUNCTIONAL (85%)

Specific (35%)

Chronic stool retention
Heightened awareness of intestinal motility
Lactose intolerance
Sucrose intolerance
Alcohol sugars intolerance
Intestinal gas syndromes
Menses
Dysmenorrhea, primary
Mittelschmerz
Pregnancy
Reaction to normal stress and anxiety
Overeating
Irritable colon
Chilaiditi syndrome

Nonspecific (50%)

"Spontaneous" resolution
Persistent unresolved

PSYCHOGENIC (10%)

Stress Related

Reaction anxiety
 Acute
 Chronic

Behavioral

Complaint modeling
Maintenance or manipulation for secondary gain
Hypochondriasis

Psychiatric

Depression
Conversion reaction

Other

School phobia
Factitious

*Modified from Barr RG: Recurrent abdominal pain. In Levine MD et al, editors: Developmental-behavioral pediatrics, Philadelphia, 1983, WB Saunders Co.

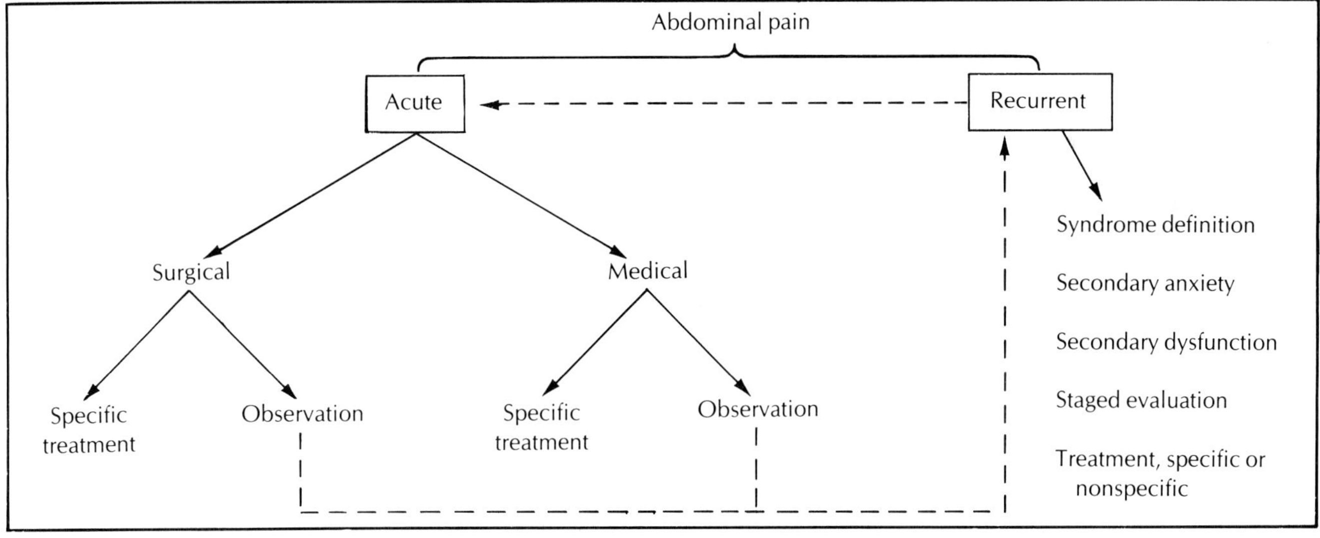

Fig. 109-1 Clinical presentation and clinical priorities in abdominal pain.
From Barr RG: Abdominal pain in the female adolescent, Pediatr Rev 4:283, 1983.

HISTORY

General Considerations

The history should consist of inquiries concerning the nature of the symptom and the source of the concern. Questions about the symptom include a description of the timing, quality, location, radiation, severity, and course of the pain episode(s). In recurrent pain, events surrounding the initial episode and factors associated with subsequent episodes also should be described. Noting the extent to which pain disrupts normal activity, the measures that relieve or exacerbate the pain (e.g., position, food, rest), and the use of previously attempted therapeutic regimens also may be helpful. In acute pain an accurate description of the *course* of the *episode* (start, change of location or severity) is critical, because the timing of surgical intervention may depend on changes within the specific pain episode (e.g., appendicitis). In recurrent pain an accurate description of the timing of *episodes* (e.g., frequent and regular, clusters, infrequent and irregular) is important both to identify precipitating factors and to evaluate subsequent therapeutic trials. Most often it helps to ask the child and the parents for this information separately.

In addition to defining the characteristics of the symptom, explicit questions should be asked to identify the source of concern and the symptom's effect on the child's activity and relationships. This is particularly important for recurrent pain syndromes. Typically the greatest concern is shown by the parent, whereas the child admits to relatively little concern. Often this is due to a fear of a specific disease process about which the parent may be aware, whereas the child is concerned only when the pain is actually present. The presence of the pain symptom may contribute to the child being seen as vulnerable by the parent; on the other hand, the child is aware of, but does not understand, a changed attitude on the parent's part. A more common negative consequence is attributable to the recurrent nature of the symptom. The apparently spontaneous resolution of the symptom when the child is removed from mathematics class, for example, may make him or her liable to accusations of malingering. The natural sympathy of a parent for a child in pain may turn to ambivalence or even anger when its sporadic presence and absence cannot be explained. Because no apparent explanation can be found in a large proportion of dysfunctional pain syndromes, understanding the source and effect of anxiety concerning the symptom is necessary for prevention of secondary dysfunction.

Organic Disease

Certain questions increase the index of suspicion that organic disease underlies the pain.[1] In particular, organic diseases are more likely if pain is well localized, is constant, wakes the child from sleep, or is located in an area other than the periumbilical region. Referred pain should be considered, particularly if the pain is localized in the upper portion of the abdomen. A history of fever, jaundice, change in stool color, persistent vomiting, change in appetite, or weight loss contributes to the suspicion of organic disease. Unfortunately, however, these features are far from specific, and their presence is to some extent age-dependent.[2] Both location of pain and its description are diffuse in infants and toddlers. In school-aged children, pain typically is localized in the periumbilical region. In adolescents, pain is more likely to be localized and nonperiumbilical even in the absence of organic disease. Whether this increasing specificity is due to a different mechanism of pain production or to increasing language facility is not known. Nonorganic pain also may be accompanied by "organic indicators." Both lactose intolerance and stool retention may be associated with nonperiumbilical pain and waking at night, and weight loss may be associated with depression and complaints of pain.

Some conditions, such as urinary tract infections[5] and ulcer disease,[7] deserve particular mention. Urinary tract infections appear differently at different ages. Abdominal pain and fever are more common presenting symptoms in older children, whereas dysuria, urgency, frequency, and vomiting are more common in younger children and infants. Primary ulcer disease usually is seen in older children and commonly manifests as a recurrent pain syndrome. Secondary ulcers are more common in infants and typically occur acutely. Diagnosis of ulcers in adolescents is difficult, partly because the presentation is atypical in more than 50% of patients. The atypicality includes shorter exacerbations and remissions, absence of night and early morning wakening, exacerbation of or no change in pain with eating, and presence of heartburn as an associated rather than primary complaint. In adolescent girls, pelvic inflammatory disease is an increasingly prevalent and important cause of abdominal pain.[11,13] The characteristic presentation (lower abdominal pain and tenderness with accompanying cervical and adnexal tenderness) occurs only in 20% of patients, which makes diagnosis difficult. As these examples illustrate, abdominal pain of organic origin occurs atypically and differently at different ages. As a result, affirmative answers to questions aimed at symptom clusters typical of specific diseases should be confirmed by appropriate tests, but it should be understood that negative answers do not necessarily rule out these causes.

Dysfunctional Pain

Most of the dysfunctional pain syndromes involve recurrent pain. A history directed toward both constitutional (e.g., physiologic maturity) and environmental (e.g., nutrition, medications, social relationships) predispositions is most likely to be rewarding. Increasing evidence indicates that altered gastrointestinal motility may be implicated as a mechanism in pain production.[10,12] Nevertheless, the key to therapy currently appears to lie in identifying the constitutional and environmental factors that set the mechanism in motion.

The most common such condition is chronic stool retention, estimated to occur in 4% to 30% of children with recurrent abdominal pain[1,8] (see Chapter 118). Evidence provided by Dimson[8] of prolonged transit time in 90% of children with positive rectal examination and 40% of the remainder lends credence to this hypothesis. There may be a family history of constipation. Ineffective toilet training or the existence of insufficient or too-exposed facilities may predispose a child to chronic stool retention.

A physiologic decline in small intestinal lactase activity in many population groups predisposes children to lactose intolerance after age 4 to 5 years. Because the symptoms usually do not appear until 2 hours after ingestion of milk, most children do not associate milk ingestion with pain.[3] The person taking the history must inquire about ethnic background, family history of intolerance, timing of the symptoms, and dietary sources of lactose. Typically, pain symptoms do not occur every time milk is ingested, probably because the production of gas and pain symptoms is mediated by many other factors, such as colonic acidity, composition of intestinal flora, and gut motility. Sometimes the identification of pain symptoms with "lactose binges" helps to pinpoint the mechanism.

Dysmenorrhea is one of the most frequent pain complaints referable to the genitourinary tract in adolescent girls, and its association with (or occurrence a few hours before) the onset of menstruation makes recognition easy if menstrual periods are well established.[2] In patients with anovulatory or irregular periods, however, the pain may be absent or sporadic. When dysmenorrhea is suspected, questions also should be directed at identifying secondary dysmenorrhea (i.e., that resulting from pathologic pelvic conditions), which is more likely in the presence of fever, use of intrauterine devices, and failure of response to oral contraceptives or prostaglandin synthetase inhibitors.

The typical syndrome of *nonspecific* dysfunctional pain has been carefully described by Apley,[1] but there is much overlap with the other, specific syndromes already described. The child usually is seen between the ages of 5 and 10 years, although onset of the complaint may be at younger ages. The pain is most commonly periumbilical and severe enough to modify activity. It also is self-limited, and the child usually is completely well between episodes. There is normally a high prevalence of autonomic correlates, such as pallor, nausea, vomiting, headache, perspiration, and prolonged intestinal transit time. In contrast to these fairly constant features, the time of occurrence, severity, duration, and description of the character and the frequency of the pains are inconstant. The concept that this type of pain is associated with a particular personality type or general anxiety is not well substantiated, and the syndrome often occurs in children who are physically and emotionally well. Only one third of mothers are very worried about the recurrent pain episodes, and slightly more than one half of patients see their physician about the complaint.[9] A family history of similar abdominal complaints may or may not be elicited and probably is more relevant if the complaints are occurring in family members concurrently rather than in the past.

Psychogenic Pain

In general, the recognition of primary psychogenic conditions is as difficult as the identification of organic disease entities. In psychogenic pain the pain experience is determined by its affective qualities (e.g., pleasant or unpleasant) and by the special meaning the pain connotes. It may imply anger, separation, or punishment (unpleasant) or the anticipation of increased attention (pleasure and relief). Explicit understanding of how both the patient and those around the patient deal with an episode of pain often is helpful. Because it usually is easier for patients to "discover" emotionally significant feelings than to describe them in response to direct questioning, clear evidence of psychogenic pain may not be elicited at the first interview. Such discoveries may provide the starting point for broader discussions of more central questions. Usually the pain complaint acts as a signal of disordered intrapersonal or interpersonal relationships, which go well beyond the pain symptom itself. In some types of psychogenic pain, the complaint is an integral component of the syndrome complex (e.g., conversion reaction), whereas in others it is peripheral to the syndrome (e.g., secondary gain) and soon becomes unimportant when attention is focused on the patient's (or the parents') more important concerns.

PHYSICAL EXAMINATION

As in other clinical situations, the principles of a good physical examination must be carefully applied in evaluating abdominal pain complaints. Inspection, palpation, percussion, and auscultation should all be performed and the findings carefully described. Studies of traditional signs (such as rebound tenderness and substernal tenderness) have shown them to be less sensitive than usually believed. Although they may not be pathognomonic, the presence of such signs may still be helpful in raising the likelihood of some entities and lessening the likelihood of others. Abdominal examination must include palpation for masses, suggestions of inflammation, and localized tenderness. A rectal examination is important for these reasons, as well as for testing for occult blood. A common error in the rectal examination is missing the presence of significant stool retention, either because of a recent bowel movement or because the stool is plentiful but not hard and impacted. In long-standing stool retention, the rectum tends to be full of stool that is of normal consistency.[4] In adolescent girls, gynecologic evaluation is particularly important and must be performed adequately to be useful.[6] If the practitioner does not have sufficient experience, gynecologic consultation is indicated for this reason alone.

DIFFERENTIAL DIAGNOSIS

Diagnosing the cause of abdominal pain is difficult. Although the diagnostic approach to a disease entity known to be causing a symptom is relatively straightforward, the patient more often has the complaint without specific signposts that indicate the pathogenic mechanism. In the acute presentation the decision as to which tests to use or which therapies to initiate depends almost entirely on presenting symptoms and signs. Usually, the definitive test necessary for making the differential diagnosis (e.g., urine culture, cervical culture of gonococcus) will not be available by the time a clinical decision must be made. In recurrent pain the yield from invasive and expensive tests is lower and more difficult to justify. The problem is compounded by the prevalence of atypical presentations and the similarities in presentation of so many entities.

In the face of these difficulties, the following general principles should facilitate appropriate diagnosis and management:

1. In acute pain presentations, one should first consider entities with potentially severe consequences requiring early definitive treatment (e.g., appendicitis, ectopic pregnancy, gastrointestinal bleeding, ovarian torsion, pelvic inflammatory disease) and move "down" the differential diagnosis list only when there is good evidence that these entities are *not* implicated.
2. In recurrent presentations, one should first consider entities that are most common (e.g., nonspecific recurrent abdominal pain, stool retention) and move "up" the differential diagnosis list to investigate further only when there is good evidence implicating other specific entities.
3. Relatively noninvasive baseline tests should be used to look for occult common disease processes early in the investigation (urinalysis, urine culture, sedimentation rate, complete blood count and smear, and reticulocyte count).
4. More invasive procedures should be used selectively, and the investigation should be "staged" according to relative priorities (Table 109-1).
5. In recurrent pain, further investigation for organic disease seldom will be indicated if the complaint of pain is the *only* symptom.
6. In both acute and recurrent presentations, repeat observation and examinations often are essential once the acute "surgical" abdomen has been ruled out.

Table 109-1 *Laboratory Evaluation of Nonspecific Abdominal Pain*

CONDITIONS TO CONSIDER	TESTS TO BE PERFORMED	LIKELIHOOD OF PRESENTATION	
		ACUTE	RECURRENT
Common causes			
Urinary tract pathologic conditions	Urinalysis, urine culture	++++	++++
Inflammatory process	Sedimentation rate, white blood cell count	++++	++++
Anemia, blood loss	Hemoglobin, hematocrit, reticulocyte count, smear	++++	++++
Liver disease	Liver function tests	++	+
Pancreatitis	Serum amylase	++	+
Lactose intolerance	Lactose breath hydrogen test	+	+++
Stool retention, renal stones, pancreatic calcification, spinal dysrhaphism	Plain supine abdominal roentgenography	++	+++
Intestinal obstruction	Abdominal series	+++	+
Gynecologic condition	Gynecologic consultation	+++	++
Uncommon causes			
Inflammatory bowel disease	Barium enema, upper gastrointestinal series	+	++
Appendicitis	Barium enema	+++	+
Urinary tract pathologic condition	Intravenous pyelogram	+	+++
Pelvic inflammatory disease	Appropriate cultures, ultrasound laparoscopy	+++	+++
Esophagitis, ulcer disease	Esophagoscopy, *C. pylori* culture	+	++
Pregnancy	Human chorionic gonadotropin	++	++
Gallbladder disease	Ultrasound	+	++
Abdominal masses detected on physical examination	Ultrasound	+	+++
Pneumonia	Chest radiography	+	
Strep throat	Streptococcal throat culture	++	
Other intraabdominal pathologic conditions (rare)	Exploratory laparotomy	++	+

TREATMENT

In the presence of identified organic disease, appropriate therapeutic modalities should be instituted. In the absence of organic disease the primary aim of therapy is to deal with the factors predisposing the child to the symptom and to ensure that the existence of the symptom does not become any more incapacitating for the child in terms of his or her relationships with family, peers, and school personnel.

Diagnosis is the first step in therapy and is facilitated by inviting the patient (or parents) to become a coinvestigator with the physician in a search for predisposing conditions. The parents' keeping a calendar or diary of symptoms is helpful. The physician can assume responsibility for the organic disease workup, attempting to relieve the anxiety produced in the parents by the symptom. In addition, the parents should be given specific things to look for (change of pain pattern, associated symptoms such as fever and weight loss) so that an intercurrent organic disease is not overlooked. In general, the aim is to *focus* parental anxiety rather than attempting to dismiss it by "reassurance."

Nonorganic pain should be not be labeled "emotional," inasmuch as this term most often has the effect of implying that the pain is not real, thereby rendering the patient helpless to do anything about it. With the exception of anticonstipation medications, the use of drugs is not indicated. A therapeutic trial of dietary fiber, however, may be helpful for children with nonspecific dysfunctional recurrent pain.[10] Counseling or psychotherapy by the pediatrician or social worker is the treatment of choice and must involve the family as well as the patient. The success of counseling depends on the willingness and interest of the therapist to share the symptom-related experience with the patient. Removal of environmental factors (such as instituting a lactose-free diet) may aid in the therapy.

One cannot be too sanguine about the claim that children with nonorganic pain will "grow out" of their pains. In my experience, the pain will remit in about 20% of cases within three visits. However, available evidence suggests that one third to one half of such children will continue to have abdominal complaints as adults, although they may have a symptom-free period during adolescence.[1] The many similarities between recurrent abdominal pain of childhood and irritable colon syndrome of adulthood imply a common pathogenesis. Nevertheless, reassurance and explanation alone have been associated with more rapid and permanent remission in those who do respond. With increased attention to underlying predispositions, a better prognosis may be obtainable.

REFERENCES

1. Apley J: The child with abdominal pains, ed 2, Oxford, 1975, Blackwell Scientific Publications, Ltd.
2. Barr RG: Abdominal pain in the female adolescent, Pediatr Rev 4:281, 1983.
3. Barr RG, Levine MD, and Watkins JH: Recurrent abdominal pain in childhood due to lactose intolerance: a prospective study, N Engl J Med 300:1449, 1979.
4. Barr RG et al: Chronic and occult stool retention: a clinical tool for its evaluation in school-aged children, Clin Pediatr 18:674, 1979.

5. Carvajal HF: Kidney and bladder infections, Adv Pediatr 25:383, 1978.
6. Cowell CA: The gynecologic examination of infants, children, and young adolescents, Pediatr Clin North Am 28:237, 1981.
7. Deckelbaum RJ et al: Peptic ulcer disease: a clinical study in 73 children, Can Med Assoc J 111:1225, 1974.
8. Dimson SB: Transit time related to clinical findings in children with recurrent abdominal pain, Pediatrics 47:666, 1972.
9. Faull C and Nicol RA: Abdominal pain in six-year-olds: an epidemiological study in a new town, J Child Psychol Psychiatry 27:251, 1986.
10. Feldman W et al: The use of fibre in the management of simple, childhood, idiopathic, recurrent, abdominal pain: results in a prospective, double-blind, randomized, controlled trial, Am J Dis Child 139:1216, 1985.
11. Golden N, Neuhoff S, and Cohen H: Pelvic inflammatory disease in adolescents, J Pediatr 114:138, 1989.
12. Pineiro-Carrero VM et al: Abnormal gastroduodenal motility in children and adolescents with recurrent functional abdominal pain, J Pediatr 113:820, 1988.
13. Shafer MB, Irwin CE, and Sweet RL: Acute salpingitis in the adolescent female, J Pediatr 100:339, 1982.

110

Alopecia and Hair Shaft Anomalies

Henry M. Seidel

Perhaps one of the major lessons of the 1960s was that hair matters. It certainly does not serve an essential functional purpose inasmuch as one can live without it. Nevertheless, the symbolism over the ages, from Samson to John Lennon, and the emotional investment everyone has in his or her hair makes any of its abnormalities a matter of concern. This is particularly so with alopecia: the loss of hair is a disturbing event.

There is a sequence of events in the life of a single hair—from active growth, a busy period known as the *anagen* phase, to passivity, a resting period known as the *telogen* phase. As many as 15% of scalp hairs may be in the telogen phase at any one time. These hairs soon will be lost in the constant turnover, the continuous shedding that is hardly apparent to a casual observer. Surprisingly, about 50% of the hair must be shed for loss to be noticeable.

The rate of loss may increase to as much as 60% during a period known as a *telogen effluvium*. During such a period the situation is much like that of animals, which shed seasonally. In the human being this change in the normal anagen/telogen ratio may occur after a high, relatively prolonged fever, a period of time after pregnancy, or after a severe illness. It may appear in both sexes. The diagnosis of telogen effluvium can be confirmed simply by plucking a group of hairs and examining them microscopically. The number of resting hairs should be increased well beyond the usual 10% to 15%.

The constant ebb and flow of growth and shedding and the extreme activity of the hair follicle—mitotic and metabolic—put the follicle at great risk in the presence of antimetabolites and mitotic inhibitors. In addition, the constant shedding, even at the rate of 10% to 15%, sets the stage for many of the emotional problems associated with hair that the pediatrician may encounter in patients. The ready availability and pluckability of hair, facilitated by the telogen phase, serve to some extent the need of children who are emotionally distressed.

Obviously, then, the loss of hair is a matter for careful attention. A precise, pointed history and physical examination are necessary. The pediatrician may need to consult with the dermatologist. Certainly the pediatrician must not fall into the trap of limiting the examination simply to the site of loss. The *whole* body and all hair-bearing parts of the body must be observed, and the hairs themselves must be examined microscopically. There are unusual congenital alopecias, and under the light microscope the normality of the individual hair can be judged and the ratio of anagen to telogen hairs determined during a telogen effluvium. That ratio can be disturbed, and there may be five to six times as many telogen hairs as anagen hairs.

If a child should lose scalp hair rather suddenly, one must be concerned with the possibility of a toxic event. This is most common in children with malignancy who have been treated with antimetabolites and therefore suffer loss because of the damage done by those drugs during the anagen phase. Occasionally, sudden hair loss is caused by accidental poisoning, as with rat poison that contains thallium or coumarin. Children must be protected from toxins, and parents must be educated in this regard. Fortunately, in most instances, new hairs will replace, over a period of several weeks, those lost—unless the exposure to the toxic element is repeated or chronic.

The prognosis for the return of hair depends in large part on elimination of the toxic stimulus (when the practitioner is aware of what it might be) or on the hair loss not being accompanied by scarring. Loss with scarring (e.g., from iatrogenic scalp injury during delivery or from a burn) is permanent. In children, the various alopecias of both known and unknown causes usually occur without scarring. This is true of alopecia areata, alopecia totalis, and alopecia universalis; drug-induced, postfebrile, and postpartum alopecias; and those alopecias associated with the endocrinopathies (hypothyroidism, hyperthyroidism, and hypoparathyroidism) or nutritional deficiency, particularly deficiencies of vitamins A, B, and C and the protein deficiency that causes kwashiorkor. Occasionally there can be some loss of frontal hair in sickle cell anemia or some patchy, "moth-eaten" loss in secondary syphilis. In parathyroid insufficiency the long-term calcium deficiency is associated with ectodermal abnormalities—not only alopecia and dental abnormalities but also cataracts and pitting and ridging of the fingernails. Hair, too, will not grow in the presence of most nevi and hemangiomas.

When there is scarring, as with the kerion associated with severe tinea capitis, keloid formation, or discoid lupus erythematosus, there is little hope for recovery. (Systemic lupus erythematosus may result in some hair loss, particularly frontally, but scarring does not occur).

MICROSCOPIC EXAMINATION

Appropriate diagnosis mandates the microscopic differentiation of hair and its roots in both the anagen and telogen stages. Deformities of the hair shaft are seen, particularly with aminoacidopathy, in a variety of rare syndromes, including Menkes kinky-hair syndrome. One can differentiate monilethrix (usually an inherited, autosomal dominant disorder in which the diameter of the hair shaft varies) from pili torti (a disorder in which the hair is twisted on its long axis). These aberrations should raise the suspicion of some noxious abnormality. The common causes of hair loss, however, usually are innocuous, and the most common ones are distinctly age-related.

PHYSIOLOGIC LOSS OF HAIR

The first hair made by hair follicles in utero feels "silky," covers the entire body of the fetus, and is known as lanugo. It is most often shed in utero, to be replaced by hair that begins to grow on the scalp in the third trimester and continues to grow after birth. It, too, is lost, a normal process that results in a temporary near-baldness. Often parents will be concerned with the thinning or with a more markedly localized area of loss, usually over the occiput, the result of the movement of the head from side to side as the baby lies in the crib. Finally, however, this hair is gradually replaced by the new, which has more of a "feel" to it. It is thicker, usually darker, and more stable, growing longer before loss and shedding not quite so readily.

CAUSES OF ABNORMAL HAIR LOSS

A variety of congenital and hereditary disorders can be heralded by hair loss—either a total loss or, perhaps, a less obvious thinning. A true congenital alopecia may be inherited as an autosomal recessive trait. If the loss is not due to this genetic circumstance, it most often is accompanied by an equally disturbing possibility of another significant hereditary disorder. The hair may be not only thin or possibly lost but also abnormal in a variety of ways. The pediatrician must look for other signs of ectodermal dysplasia and consider radiographic exploration for skeletal defects (e.g., as with cartilage-hair hypoplasia, congenital ectodermal dysplasia, orofaciodigital syndrome), inherited metabolic disorders such as phenylketonuria or homocystinuria, or congenital problems such as hypothyroidism. These and other clinical pictures that result from serious chromosome defects (e.g., de Lange syndrome, Down syndrome) obviously provide a surfeit of signs and symptoms beyond the simple loss of hair. In addition, significant loss, even baldness, may on occasion follow intense and persistent fever, severe surgical insult, or precipitous weight loss, for any reason, with concomitant malnourishment and hypovitaminosis.

Hair Shaft Anomalies

Anomalies of the hair may result in a stubbly growth—a short, bumpy terrain most often of the scalp alone, the effect of broken hair and usually not true alopecia. There may be accompanying ectodermal defects, brittle fingernails, or perhaps cataracts and tooth anomalies. Actually, the fragility of hair and the resultant breakage (trichorrhexis) and stubble can be seen in a variety of conditions, all of which are rather rare. These may be familial or congenital, as in trichorrhexis nodosa, a familial circumstance in which the hair is fragile but in which there are no associated findings, or as with the stubbly hair associated with argininosuccinic aciduria, the stubbly hair being the least of the problems in a disease that, fortunately, is uncommon. Children with argininosuccinic aciduria show evidence of severe mental retardation in the first year of life.

The feel of the hair may be helpful in finding the source of difficulty. In an infant with hypothyroidism, it may be coarse and brittle and without luster; in progeria and in cartilage-hair hypoplasia syndrome, it may be fine, even silky. In all these circumstances, the hair may break off and there may be baldness. Whenever the hair is abnormal, it becomes weakened, fragile, and fractured, and it may be lost or unevenly shortened, resulting often in a stubbly, ragged alopecia. The various abnormalities—congenital, traumatic, or endocrine—can all lead to such fragility and loss. Referral to a dermatologist is appropriate so that, at the very least, a specific diagnosis can be made.

Loose Anagen Syndrome. Loose anagen syndrome, recently described, is characterized by anagen hairs that are quite easily and painlessly pulled from the scalp.[1] Affected children are generally, but not always, blond and female preschoolers between the ages of 2 and 5 years. Their hair appears sparse. The individual hairs are not fragile and, on examination, have misshapen bulbs with absent external root sheaths. Typically the child's hair is said to be slow growing, seldom requiring cutting. The hair over the occiput often is matted and sticky. Fortunately, the condition seems to wane as time passes. The hair grows thicker and longer, and its pigmentation increases. Still, even in adulthood, it may pull out easily and painlessly. Although a hereditary factor may be involved, it is not conclusive. Diagnosis can be made on the basis of history and examination, the painless "pull test" (when the hair is normal, it may hurt to pull), and light microscopic examination of the recovered hairs. Management is limited to reassurance and allowance for the passage of time.

Trichorrhexis Nodosa. Trichorrhexis nodosa is a common abnormality of the hair shaft that becomes obvious under the light microscope. The "nodes" seen resemble the effect one observes when the ends of two brushes are pushed together. This is most often congenital and results in breakage of hair and a short stubble over the scalp. It is also probably a genetic predisposition in black patients who experience hair breakage over large areas of the scalp and whose hair will not grow beyond a relatively short length. There is usually an accompanying history of hair straightening or repeated vigorous brushing and combing. The avoidance of this kind of steady abuse and a more gentle cosmetic approach can result in some gradual improvement. White and Oriental persons can experience the same difficulty, probably without congenital or familial relationship, and the breakage most often will occur at the distal end of hair. White specks may appear after some physical or chemical injury. Here again, the gentle approach and elimination of any noxious element are appropriate.

Monilethrix. Monilethrix (beaded-hair syndrome) is a condition in which scalp hairs have regularly spaced differences in their circumference, suggesting a chain of beads. The cause is unknown, and there is no known treatment; however, the outlook occasionally is promising in that a degree of recovery may occur spontaneously, particularly after puberty or during pregnancy. This is a long time to wait inasmuch as hair breakage becomes obvious during infancy. Occasionally, there are associated problems—cataracts, brittle nails, faulty teeth—suggestive of a more widespread ectodermal defect.

Pili Torti. Pili torti simply means "twisted hair"; indeed, that is the way it looks under the microscope. The color is "off," and the hair is coarse and lusterless. It is as though straight and curly hair were competing for a place in the same strand. If one looks at a straight hair in cross section, it is round—a curly hair is oval. In pili torti, both configurations may be seen in a single strand. This abnormality can be an important clue to Menkes kinky-hair syndrome, an X-linked disease characterized also by progressive cerebral degeneration, arterial degeneration, and the suggestion of scurvy in the bones. There is a low serum copper level because of poor intestinal absorption of copper. This fatal disease has not, to date, yielded to the administration of parenteral copper.

Alopecia Areata

Alopecia areata, most often seen as an acute problem, results in a rather sudden and total loss of hair in sharply circumscribed, round areas, often several centimeters in diameter, usually on the scalp but possibly anywhere on the body where there is hair. There is no evidence of inflammation. Hairs at the periphery of an area are easily plucked and may be particularly colorless and thin. Sometimes the fingernails may look pitted and ridged, as though nature were trying to tell us that the as-yet undiscovered cause goes beyond the hair to another ectodermal expression. There may be just a few patches of loss or a total absence of body hair (alopecia universalis), including eyebrows and eyelashes. The more extensive the loss and the younger the child, the less likely a full recovery. The prognosis is best when the loss is less widespread and there are only one or two patches. Currently the pediatrician has little to offer, because the cause is unknown. There has been some suggestion of relationships with acute emotional trauma or an autoimmune process. Occasionally, autoimmune antibodies may be identified in patients with alopecia areata when there is no other clinical evidence of autoimmune disease; an increased incidence of alopecia areata also occurs in persons with acute autoimmune thyroid disease and with vitiligo.

As is often the case in a poorly understood process, cortisone has been used with some apparent success, applied topically and with an occlusive covering. It is possible in the older, more cooperative child to inject the hair follicles with corticosteroids. These are relatively insoluble, and the process is painful. It should be performed with a very small-gauge needle and topical anesthesia— for example, an ethyl chloride spray. In any event, the primary care pediatrician should seriously question the need for this procedure, carefully assessing the impact of the disease and of the treatment on the patient and should refer the patient to a dermatologist for further consideration of this procedure. The large areas that require infiltration present obvious difficulty, and the addition of oral steroid therapy can only further complicate the treatment.

There also has been some use of irritants (dinitrochlorobenzene, psoralen, ultraviolet light). These agents should be used only in children older than 12 years of age, and only by a knowledgeable dermatologist in a controlled circumstance. This treatment is possibly justified in alopecia universalis, when all hair is lost. The poor prognosis, however, suggests that although a trial is appropriate, it should not be pushed to unreasonable lengths. It is odd that when hair does regrow after alopecia areata, it may be white. This, however, is temporary, and in the long run it will be impossible for casual observers to identify the formerly affected area.

Common Baldness

There is a genetically determined loss of hair that begins most often with a receding hairline and some thinning over the occiput. This occurs most often in men, but it can happen in women. Fortunately, its fullest expression is most common in the mature adult; the pediatrician rarely is confronted with the problem. There is, unfortunately, no effective therapy.

Trichotillomania

Some children have a considerable compulsive need to pull out their hair, even their eyebrows or eyelashes. Although this may not always have important emotional significance, it often provides a major clue to an underlying psychosocial problem. The pediatrician should begin with that assumption and follow this lead gently. The family structure and the interaction with siblings and parents and with friends at home and at school should be explored. Consulting with a psychiatrist also should be considered. One can paint the attacked areas with collodion in an attempt to frustrate the habit; however, without attention to the possibility of a more basic emotional problem, this approach quite obviously is inappropriate.

The hair that is lost is that which is most accessible to the probing hand. Sometimes enough is pulled to simulate alopecia areata, and the patient who eats hair may accumulate it in the stomach and create a trichobezoar (hairball), which ultimately may lead to acute intestinal obstruction or, most often, to the complaint of abdominal pain. At that point it often is possible to palpate a mass and to demonstrate it on a roentgenogram. Then referral to a surgeon is mandatory.

Traumatic Alopecia

Hair is a relatively fragile adornment. It does not respond positively to assault, and it should be handled gently and without physical or chemical importuning. It is probably best left alone, except for simple washing and, to suit the fashion, simple cutting.

For some, vanity can lead to alopecia. Constant teasing and fluffing and straightening with heat or chemicals may seriously damage hair. Some hairstyles, particularly when one uses barrettes or has ponytails, braids, or corn-rowing, will cause traction that is constant and often tense and prolonged. The hair may then fall out, and there may be an accompanying redness and inflammation with some pustular involvement of the follicles. Generally, a simple discontinuation of the stress will help; the hair almost always will return. Remember, however, that regrowth can be slow. The loss of any hair in this way, because of trichotillomania or because of a simple, excessively playful tug, will be slow to repair. Injured hair follicles do not heal quickly and often may take 3 or more months before they are fully back to an anagen phase.

Hypoparathyroidism

Sometimes hypoparathyroidism is preceded by an acute bacterial infection and sometimes by candidiasis. The nature of the association between hypoparathyroidism and candidiasis is poorly understood. Nevertheless, chronic hypocalcemia and dental abnormalities can abound in this condition, along with other ectodermal defects: pitted and ridged fingernails, cataracts, and a stringy, patchy loss of hair.

Most likely, the candidiasis does not cause the hypoparathyroidism but, rather, follows the hormonal dysfunction; an immune mechanism possibly is common to both. The general pediatrician should consult with the endocrinologist to develop a firm diagnostic and management plan.

Tinea Capitis

Whenever a child has patches of alopecia or stubbly hair growth, even in the absence of crusting, scaling, redness, or other inflammatory signs, the practitioner should consider the possibility of tinea capitis, seborrheic dermatitis, or psoriasis. Obviously, if there is crusting, scaling, or redness, the likelihood of alopecia areata is diminished because inflammation is not a symptom of that condition. In any event, the practitioner should perform a mycologic examination, looking particularly for *Microsporum canis* and *M. audouinii*, fungi that can invade the hair shaft and thereby cause breakage and stubbiness. *M. canis* tends to cause much more inflammation than does *M. audouinii*. Also, the clinician should look for evidence of fungal infection by shining the Wood lamp on the affected area in a darkened room. There may well be a greenish fluorescence, although some chemical treatments in the hair may simulate this fluorescence. In any event, the absence of this finding, while not precluding the diagnosis, may suggest a source other than *M. audouinii* or *M. canis*. Occasionally, for example, tinea capitis may be caused by *Trichophyton tonsurans*, in which case these lesions tend to be more elevated than in other forms of tinea and are characterized by black dots.

On occasion, particularly with *M. canis* or after treatment with an irritant, the area may become secondarily infected and seriously inflamed. Kerion may develop, and the resultant scarring interferes with the regrowth of hair. Early diagnosis and treatment therefore are helpful, although the 2- to 4-week course of oral griseofulvin usually presents difficulties with compliance in the young child. The topical antifungal agents, however, do not effect a cure as readily.

Acrodermatitis Enteropathica

Acrodermatitis enteropathica, an autosomal recessive disorder characterized by abnormal zinc absorption, has several important cutaneous manifestations, simulating, at times, psoriasis, epidermolysis bullosa, pyoderma, or candidiasis. With zinc deficiency there is abdominal pain and diarrhea; there also can be an associated "wispy alopecia" and dystrophic development of the fingernails, suggesting widespread ectodermal involvement. Zinc sulfate given orally is the treatment of choice. The child is committed to a lifetime of therapy; therefore the lowest effective dose should be sought.

Discoid and Systemic Lupus Erythematosus

Discoid lupus erythematosus can be disfiguring to the scalp, and with scarring it can cause a permanent loss of hair. Therefore early treatment is necessary. Scarring can be avoided with repeated injections of steroids by a dermatologist. Systemic lupus erythematosus also can cause alopecia, and the scalp itself can be erythematous; however, the loss of hair generally is temporary and without the scarring characteristic of discoid lupus erythematosus.

Alopecia Mucinosa (Follicular Mucinosis)

The name of this condition is a bit misleading in that the lesions, which are harmless, occur much more often on the face and forehead than above the hairline. They are slightly raised, edematous, slightly reddened plaques and are much more common in older adults than in the young. There is no particular racial or sexual predilection. Because there is no effective therapy, it is fortunate that the lesions usually are self-limited.

Notably, however, this condition can be predictive of an underlying present or future lymphoma, and its presence should alert the pediatrician. However, a biopsy of the lesion itself will show only mucin in the epithelium of the hair follicles. The process usually is benign, and when the lesions disappear, any lost hair grows back.

GENERAL MANAGEMENT

Treatment for alopecia depends, of course, on the cause. Practitioners have become all too accustomed to seeing hospitalized children with a malignancy being treated with antimetabolites and wearing baseball caps to hide their full or partial baldness. However, a noticeable loss of hair at any point is disturbing to both patient and parent; therefore the suggestion that the child wear a baseball cap or some other inobtrusive, concealing adornment is appropriate. Even a hairpiece can be designed for a child. These steps serve only for the interim while practitioners attend to the discovery of a potentially helpful treatment or while they wait expectantly in those circumstances in which they do not have specific treatment and in which their role is diagnostic and supportive. The possibility that regrowth will not occur cannot be discarded when loss (1) follows high fever or chronic toxicity, for example, (2) is accompanied by scarring, or (3) occurs in the areas of nevi, aplasia cutis, or persistent hemangiomas.

Therefore the supportive aspect should not be minimized, because hair loss does matter. It is necessary to talk this through with the child who is old enough and also with the parents, exploring the source of emotional reaction and discomfort and, if recovery of hair is questionable, working with the patient to achieve an emotional balance consistent with reality and to adopt suitable coping mechanisms. Most often this is an achievable goal, and the pediatrician should not back away from it. The practitioner, sometimes frustrated by the lack of a practical and readily successful management regimen, should not forget the value of a willing, listening ear—in this as in all things.

REFERENCE

1. Price VH and Gummer CL: Loose anagen syndrome, J Am Acad Dermatol 20:249, 1989.

SUGGESTED READINGS

Datloff J and Esterly NB: A system for sorting out pediatric alopecia, Contemp Pediatr, 3:53-72, 1986.

Porter PS and Lobitz WC Jr: Human hair: a genetic marker, Br J Dermatol 83:225, 1970.

Price VH: Office diagnosis of structural hair anomalies, Cutis 15:231, 1975.

Rasmussen JE, editor: Symposium on pediatric dermatology, Pediatr Clin North Am 30:417, 1983.

Solomon LM, Easterly NB, and Loeffel ED: Adolescent dermatology, Philadelphia, 1978, WB Saunders.

Stroud JD: Hair loss in children, Pediatr Clin North Am 30:641, 1983.

Weinberg S, Leider M, and Shapiro L: Color atlas of pediatric dermatology, New York, 1975, McGraw-Hill, Inc.

111

Amenorrhea

Alain Joffe

Amenorrhea is a symptom, not a disease, and has a variety of causes. In terms of establishing the etiology of this symptom, it is useful to classify amenorrhea as being either primary or secondary. *Primary amenorrhea* is defined as the failure to initiate menstruation, whereas *secondary amenorrhea* refers to cessation of menses in a female who has had previously normal menstrual function.

PRIMARY AMENORRHEA

The mean age of menarche in the United States today is 12½ to 13 years; 95% of girls will have menstruated by age 16.[3,10] Menstruation usually begins approximately 2 years after breast budding, the earliest sign of puberty. However, the interval between the two can be as short as 6 months or as long as 5¾ years.

Given this broad range of individual variation in the onset of puberty, the physician first must note whether breast budding or pubic hair is present. If one or the other is absent by age 14 years, the patient should be evaluated for delayed puberty (see Chapter 164).

If signs of puberty are present, the age at which they appeared must be determined. If fewer than 4 years have elapsed at the time the patient seeks advice and the findings of a general history and physical examination are normal, the patient should be counseled about the variability of development and reassured that hers is normal, particularly if her mother indicates that she first menstruated at a relatively late age.[5] A urine pregnancy test should first be done if there is any possibility that the patient is sexually active. Otherwise, documentation of growth and sexual development should be comforting to the patient until menarche ensues.

When a period of more than 4 years has elapsed since the onset of puberty, the patient has true primary amenorrhea, and a thorough evaluation is warranted.[2] The major causes of primary amenorrhea are listed in the accompanying box. A careful history and physical examination will, in most instances, help to guide the clinician in the workup.

History

The history should address the presence of significant stress in the patient's life, as well as recent significant weight gain or loss (anorexia nervosa). Queries about drug use (e.g., phenothiazines) and sexual activity also should be carefully pursued. Clues to any of the endocrine abnormalities, as well as a history of past central nervous system insults (e.g., meningitis) or symptoms of an intracranial tumor, need to be sought. The age at which the patient's mother first menstruated also is helpful knowledge because such a pattern may be familial.[5]

Physical Examination

A complete physical examination, including a pelvic examination, should be performed. Previous growth data (both height and weight) should be plotted. Obesity or excessive thinness can result in amenorrhea.[9] Abnormalities of visual field, smell, or cranial nerve function, papilledema, or disturbances of reflexes suggest a brain tumor. Hirsutism, a receding hairline, excessive acne, moon facies, striae, an enlarged thyroid, or buffalo hump suggests an endocrine disorder. A webbed neck, short stature,[5] or widely spaced nipples suggest gonadal dysgenesis (e.g., Turner syndrome). Physical signs and symptoms that suggest anorexia nervosa should be sought (see Chapter 99).

A pelvic examination is critical to ensure the presence of normal internal and external female genitalia.[8] An imper-

Causes of Primary Amenorrhea*

1. Familial
2. Psychosocial stress
3. Obesity or severe weight loss (similarly, thin body habitus associated with strenuous exercise programs, as seen in ballet dancers and in patients with anorexia nervosa)
4. Endocrine
   a. Hypopituitarism
   b. Congenital adrenal hyperplasia; adrenal disease
   c. Gonadal dysgenesis (Turner syndrome or Turner mosaic)
   d. Premature ovarian disease
   e. Testicular feminization syndrome
   f. Hypothyroidism
5. Chronic disease
6. Pregnancy
7. Anatomic anomalies
   a. Vaginal agenesis
   b. Uterine agenesis
   c. Imperforate hymen
8. Brain tumor (e.g., prolactinoma)

*For a more detailed list, see reference 12.

forate hymen will prevent menstrual blood from escaping.[1] If the hymenal opening is patent, the examination should proceed to determine the presence of a normal vagina, cervix, and uterus. If the hymenal opening is very small, palpation of the cervix and uterus can be accomplished through a bimanual rectoabdominal examination. The size of the clitoris should be noted because clitoromegaly indicates the presence of excess androgens (e.g., congenital adrenal hyperplasia).

Laboratory Tests

A few simple laboratory tests are helpful if the history and physical examination results are normal. A normal urinalysis would rule out diabetes mellitus and chronic renal disease. The presence of epithelial cells in a cytologic smear obtained from the wall of the vagina and subsequently fixed and examined as with a Pap smear correlates with the presence of circulating estrogens. Greater than 10% superficial cells demonstrates a definite estrogen effect. Similar information can be obtained by examining the cervical mucus. The cervix is swabbed with a cotton-tipped applicator, and a small sample of cervical mucus is then obtained and spread thinly onto a glass slide and air dried. The slide is then examined for ferning, the presence of which indicates a definite estrogen effect. Its absence, however, does not rule out the presence of estrogen inasmuch as circulating progesterones will prevent ferning from occurring. A pregnancy test should be performed if there is any possibility of pregnancy.

If the vaginal or cervical mucus smear shows the presence of estrogen, little else needs to be done. Thyroxine (T_4) and thyroid-stimulating hormone (TSH) levels probably should be obtained, because the presence of hypothyroidism can be subtle. If this test result is normal, the patient can be reassured that menstruation will begin. The physician at this point should make certain that significant stress or psychosocial problems are in fact not present as a cause of the amenorrhea.

If the vaginal or cervical mucus smear is equivocal, or if superficial cells and ferning are present, several options are now open to the clinician, who at this point may wish to refer the patient to a physician skilled in adolescent medicine, a gynecologist, or an endocrinologist. Alternatively, a trial of progesterone may be given (either 100 mg of progesterone in oil, given intramuscularly, or medroxyprogesterone [Provera], 10 mg twice daily given orally for 5 days). Withdrawal bleeding after this therapy indicates that the uterine lining has been stimulated by estrogens. Again, no further workup, aside perhaps from obtaining T_4 and TSH levels, is necessary.

If there is no withdrawal bleeding, referral already as noted is appropriate. Several of the diagnostic tests now indicated (e.g., measurement of serum levels of follicle-stimulating hormone [FSH] and luteinizing hormone [LH]) need to be performed in highly specialized laboratories to ensure the reliability of the results. Treatment with hormonal therapy consisting of estrogen and progesterone will be necessary.

An algorithm for evaluation of primary amenorrhea is shown in Fig. 111-1.

SECONDARY AMENORRHEA

By definition, secondary amenorrhea implies some previous level of normal menstrual function. Thus certain causes of primary amenorrhea, mainly abnormalities of the genitalia, are not in the differential diagnosis. Most of the other causes of primary amenorrhea, however, also can lead to secondary amenorrhea.

In evaluating an adolescent patient who appears to have secondary amenorrhea, it is important to consider her pubertal status. After the onset of menarche, many teenagers will have sporadic menstruation; regular monthly cycles often are not established until 2 to 3 years after menarche.[6] Clearly, the abrupt cessation of menstruation in a teenager who has had regular cycles is of greater concern than is the absence of menses for 3 to 4 months in a teenager with a history of oligomenorrhea (infrequent periods). The point at which the clinician elects to pursue an evaluation depends on the anxiety of the patient and her family, the possibility of pregnancy, and the physician's assessment of the likelihood that a potentially serious disease is responsible for the amenorrhea. A teenager with previously regular menses should be evaluated endocrinologically if amenorrhea has persisted for 6 months.

History

The history and physical examination again serve as the starting point. The hypothalamic-pituitary-ovarian axis of the teenager is more sensitive to either physical or psychological stress than is that of the adult woman. Stress, emotional upset, fever accompanying viral illness, and changes in weight or environment (e.g., going away to college) all can induce amenorrhea. More severe stresses, such as anorexia nervosa, can produce prolonged amenorrhea. The history also should include questions about drug use, particularly the use of oral contraceptives, which frequently cause amenorrhea. Most women who become amenorrheic while taking oral contraceptives will resume menstruation within 6 months of stopping them. Whether the patient is sexually active also needs to be ascertained. If she is, pregnancy should be a primary consideration. Unfortunately, a negative response does not exclude this diagnosis inasmuch as many teenagers are reluctant to admit to something they feel will be met with condemnation from adults. Sudden cessation of menstruation is more likely to indicate pregnancy or stress as a cause, whereas a gradual cessation suggests polycystic ovarian disease or premature ovarian failure. A history of uterine surgery or abortion raises the possibility of uterine synechiae. With more and more women involved in sports, questions about participation in athletics (frequency, duration, intensity) also are appropriate.[7]

Physical Examination

The physical examination may provide clues to the diagnosis. Hirsutism suggests polycystic ovarian disease or late-onset congenital adrenal hyperplasia,[2] whereas receding hairline, deepening of the voice, or clitoromegaly suggests an androgen-secreting tumor. The breasts should be carefully exam-

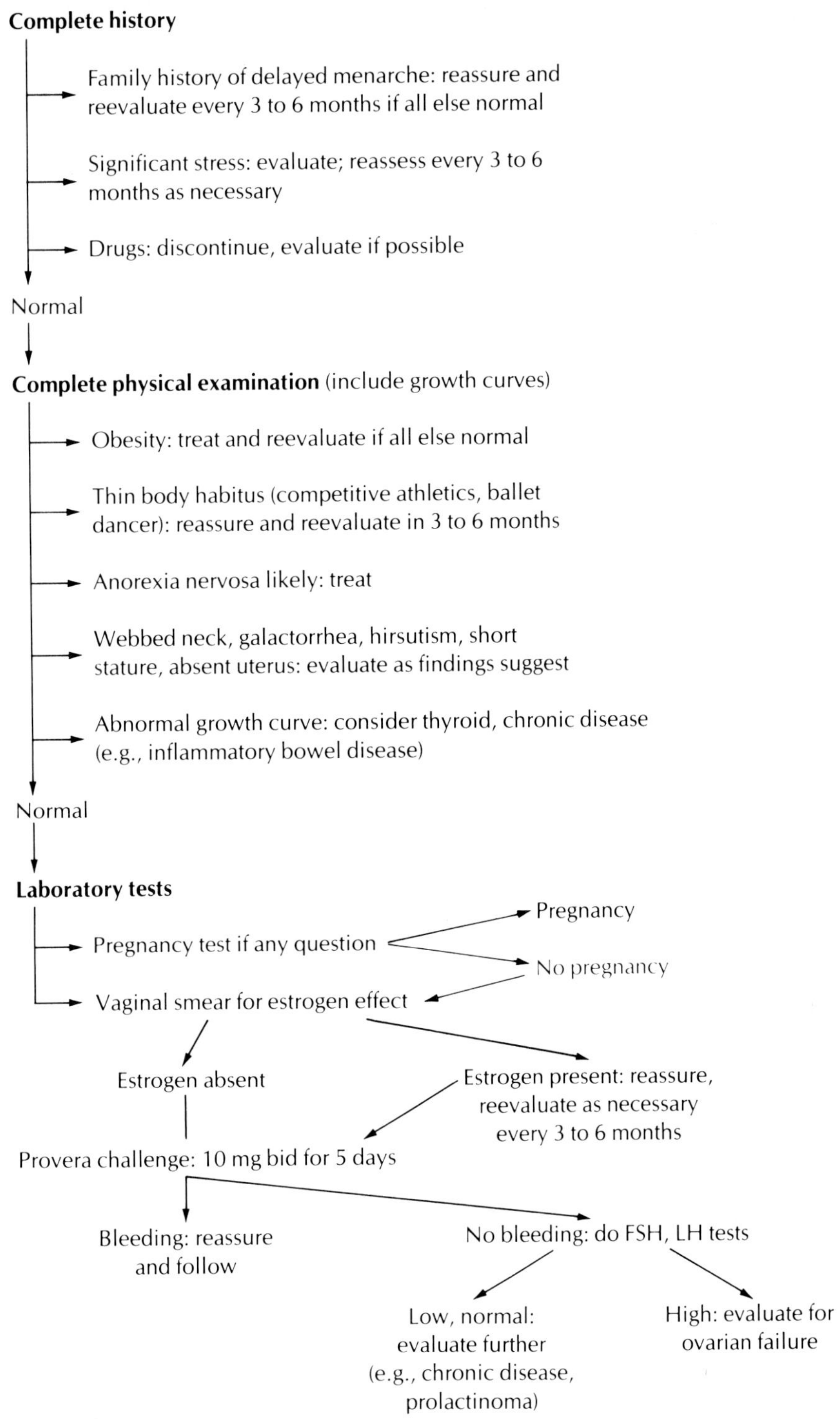
Complete history
Family history of delayed menarche: reassure and reevaluate every 3 to 6 months if all else normal
Significant stress: evaluate; reassess every 3 to 6 months as necessary
Drugs: discontinue, evaluate if possible
Normal
Complete physical examination (include growth curves)
Obesity: treat and reevaluate if all else normal
Thin body habitus (competitive athletics, ballet dancer): reassure and reevaluate in 3 to 6 months
Anorexia nervosa likely: treat
Webbed neck, galactorrhea, hirsutism, short stature, absent uterus: evaluate as findings suggest
Abnormal growth curve: consider thyroid, chronic disease (e.g., inflammatory bowel disease)
Normal
Laboratory tests
Pregnancy test if any question
Pregnancy
No pregnancy
Vaginal smear for estrogen effect
Estrogen absent
Estrogen present: reassure, reevaluate as necessary every 3 to 6 months
Provera challenge: 10 mg bid for 5 days
Bleeding: reassure and follow
No bleeding: do FSH, LH tests
Low, normal: evaluate further (e.g., chronic disease, prolactinoma)
High: evaluate for ovarian failure

Fig. 111-1 Evaluation of patients with primary amenorrhea but with secondary sexual characteristics present.

ined; the ability to express any fluid (galactorrhea) manually strongly suggests a neuroendocrine disorder (e.g., prolactin-secreting tumor). The skin should be examined for the presence of striae and the size of the uterus noted, because enlargement may be an early sign of pregnancy. Enlarged ovaries suggest polycystic ovarian disease. Physical symptoms suggestive of anorexia nervosa should be sought especially if there is a history of weight loss (see Chapter 99).

Laboratory Tests

Again, a normal urinalysis will help to rule out diabetes or chronic renal disease. A negative urine pregnancy test result performed on a first-morning urine specimen makes pregnancy unlikely if the interval since the last menstrual period is at least 6 weeks. If there is any question of an ectopic pregnancy, the more sensitive serum human chorionic gonadotropin test can be performed. Examination of the cervical mucus for ferning can indicate the presence of a normal estrogen effect.

If the results of all these tests are nondiagnostic, the most likely cause of the amenorrhea lies in the hypothalamus and the condition probably is a result of stress. However, serum T_4, TSH, and prolactin levels should be obtained to rule out hypothyroidism and a prolactinoma.

If these test results are normal and the patient is not pregnant, a progesterone challenge should be undertaken. Withdrawal bleeding indicates an intact hypothalamic-pituitary-ovarian axis, and no further workup is needed. The patient's condition should be monitored.

If the amenorrhea continues, withdrawal bleeding should be induced to prevent endometrial hyperplasia.[7] This can be accomplished through use of progesterone alone or with oral contraceptive pills. The latter is particularly useful if the patient is sexually active.

Absence of withdrawal bleeding requires further evaluation. High FSH and LH levels indicate ovarian failure. An LH/FSH ratio greater than 3:1 strongly suggests polycystic ovary syndrome. Evaluation of patients who appear to have an androgen excess is more complex. Useful laboratory tests include obtaining levels of serum testosterone, free testosterone, and dehydroepiandrosterone, as well as measurement of 24-hour urinary excretion of 17-hydroxycorticosteroids and 17-ketosteroids. Individuals differ as to which of these tests are necessary.

The evaluation of secondary amenorrhea can proceed along lines similar to those shown in Fig. 111-1. Particular attention should be paid to pregnancy, hypothalamic causes (weight changes, athletics,[4,11] anorexia nervosa), prior contraceptive use, a prolactinoma (especially if galactorrhea is present), endocrine causes (hypothyroidism, polycystic ovary syndrome, or late-onset congenital adrenal hyperplasia), and chronic disease (inflammatory bowel disease).

REFERENCES

1. DeKoos EB: Primary amenorrhea, Pediatr Ann 5:12, 1975.
2. Emans SJH, Grace E, and Goldstein DP: Oligomenorrhea in adolescent girls, J Pediatr 97:815, 1980.
3. Emans SJH and Goldstein DP: Pediatric and adolescent gynecology, ed 3, Boston, 1990, Little, Brown & Co.
4. Frisch RE et al: Delayed menarche and amenorrhea of college athletes in relation to age of onset and training, JAMA 246:1559, 1981.
5. Hollingsworth DR and Kessler Kreutner AK: Gynecologic problems of adolescent girls, Curr Probl Pediatr 8:9, 1978.
6. Huffman JW: Diagnosis of secondary amenorrhea, Pediatr Ann 5:27, 1975.
7. Mansfield JM and Emans SJ: Anorexia nervosa, athletics and amenorrhea, Pediatr Clin North Am 36:533, 1989.
8. Mashchak CA et al: Clinical and laboratory evaluation of patients with primary amenorrhea, Obstet Gynecol 57:715, 1981.
9. McFarland KF: Amenorrhea, Am Fam Physician 22:95, 1980.
10. Neinstein LS: Adolescent health care: a practical guide, ed 2, Baltimore, 1991, Urban & Schwarzenberg, Inc.
11. Schwartz B et al: Exercise-associated amenorrhea: a distinct entity? Am J Obstet Gynecol 131:662, 1981.
12. Soules MR: Adolescent amenorrhea, Pediatr Clin North Am 34:1083, 1987.

112

Anemia and Pallor

David N. Korones and Harvey J. Cohen

Pallor and anemia are among the most frequently encountered clinical problems in pediatric practice. Pallor is a physical sign; anemia is a laboratory finding. Neither is a diagnosis, and while both may be deviations from the norm, it is incumbent upon the pediatrician to investigate these findings thoroughly and determine their etiology.

PALLOR

Pallor is pale complexion of the skin. Although it may often be a familial trait or a consequence of limited exposure to the sun, pallor is also observed in a variety of pathologic conditions. Vasoconstriction of subcutaneous blood vessels causes the pallor that is associated with shock, exposure to cold, or syncope. Accumulation of fluid in the interstitium causes the pallor sometimes seen in edematous states such as myxedema, hypoproteinemia, and congestive heart failure. When the hemoglobin concentration is low, pallor due to anemia may be apparent.

The assessment of skin color for pallor is often confounded by clinical and environmental factors. Fluorescent lighting, a frequent fixture in physicians' offices, distorts the true hue of the skin. It is particularly difficult to recognize pallor in the dark-skinned patient. The assessment of pallor may also be complicated by coexistant disorders that cause changes in skin color; for example, jaundice and cyanosis may entirely mask pallor.

ANEMIA

Because most pediatricians routinely screen children for anemia in the first or second year of life and in adolescence, they will frequently encounter children with this problem. Like pallor, anemia is not a diagnosis; it is a laboratory value that alerts the health provider to a reduction in red blood cell mass. The physician or nurse practitioner must therefore be familiar with and be prepared to evaluate anemia for a broad range of etiologic possibilities. Armed with a thorough history and physical examination, as well as routine laboratory data that can be obtained in the office, the pediatric health care provider in most instances can determine the cause of anemia.

Definition

Anemia is defined as a decrease in red blood cell mass as determined by a low hemoglobin or hematocrit value. Determining whether a child is anemic is sometimes problematic. Efforts to define a normal hemoglobin level have been hampered by sampling of small or nonrepresentative groups of infants and children, by differences in the normal range of hemoglobin in various ethnic groups, and by failure to exclude patients with mild anemia from the sample populations. In one of the most thorough studies of normal hematological values of childhood,[4] large numbers of children from different ethnic groups, socioeconomic strata, and ages were sampled. Children with findings suggestive of iron deficiency, thalassemia, or hemoglobinopathies were excluded. It was found that normal ranges varied depending on the age, gender, and race (see Table 112-1). Normal hemoglobin levels in Blacks are approximately 0.5 g/dl lower than those in Whites and Orientals.

Normal ranges for hematocrit and hemoglobin values are usually defined as the mean of these values ± two standard deviations. This definition results in the arbitrary classification of 2.5% of children as anemic. Some of these children in fact may not be anemic, while others whose values fall within the normal range may actually be anemic relative to their usual value. For example, a 3-year-old whose hematocrit value has dropped from 40 to 34 still has a value that falls within the normal range, but this decrease in the hematocrit merits further evaluation. A table of normal values serves only as a guideline for the pediatric health care provider. The hematologic values of an individual child should be compared with any previous values obtained on that child and must be evaluated in the full context of the child's age, race, history and physical examination, and general state of health.

HISTORY

Because most children with anemia are asymptomatic, a careful history may reveal clues to the existence of a anemia that would otherwise remain undetected. Demographic factors such as age, gender, and ethnic background define important risk groups for different types of anemias. Toddlers and adolescent females are at highest risk for iron deficiency anemia. Sickle cell disease is observed almost exclusively in Blacks, and thalassemia occurs with increased frequency in Blacks and people of Mediterranean and Southeast Asian descent. A dietary history should be elicited. A poor or unbalanced diet may result in a nutritional deficiency, and young children who demonstrate pica are at risk for lead toxicity. Certain drugs can cause anemia; sulfa drugs can precipitate hemolysis in children deficient in the red blood cell enzyme glucose-6 phosphate dehydrogenase. Acute infections may suppress

Table 112-1 *Values (Normal, Mean, and Lower Limits of Normal) for Hemoglobin, Hematocrit, and MCV Determinations*

AGE (YR)	HEMOGLOBIN (G/DL) MEAN	HEMOGLOBIN (G/DL) LOWER LIMIT	HEMATOCRIT (%) MEAN	HEMATOCRIT (%) LOWER LIMIT	MCV (μ^3) MEAN	MCV (μ^3) LOWER LIMIT
0.5-1.9	12.5	11.0	37	33	77	70
2-4	12.5	11.0	38	34	79	73
5-7	13.0	11.5	39	35	81	75
8-11	13.5	12.0	40	36	83	76
12-14:						
Female	13.5	12.0	41	36	85	78
Male	14.0	12.5	43	37	84	77
15-17:						
Female	14.0	12.0	41	36	87	79
Male	15.0	13.0	46	38	86	78
18-49:						
Female	14.0	12.0	42	37	90	80
Male	16.0	14.0	47	40	90	80

From Nathan DG and Oski F: Hematology of Infancy and Childhood, ed 3, Philadelphia, WB Saunders, 1987.

production or accelerate destruction of red blood cells. The patient should be screened for signs of acute or chronic bleeding in the most common sites for blood loss—the gastrointestinal tract and the female genitourinary tract. Anemia may also be part of an underlying systemic disorder such as juvenile rheumatoid arthritis or Crohn disease. A family history should be taken; family members with jaundice or who have had a cholecystectomy or splenectomy at a young age may have a hereditary hemolytic anemia, such as hereditary spherocytosis, or a hemoglobinopathy.

Signs and Symptoms

Signs and symptoms in children with mild or moderate anemia are limited. Infants and toddlers may present with irritability, longer periods of sleep, changes in behavior, or pallor. Older children may present similarily, or like adults may complain of a decrease in exercise tolerence, weakness or dizziness, fatigue, shortness of breath, or palpitations.

Signs of anemia are often subtle. It is not uncommon for a child to receive a "clean bill of health" at a routine health care visit, only to be called back for reevaluation because of a low hematocrit value on routine screening. Pallor may indicate anemia, but it is not appreciable in mild anemia and may not be detectable until the hemoglobin level is as low as 8g/dl.[9] Careful examination of the conjunctivae, mucous membranes, palmar creases, and nailbeds may reveal pallor when the skin does not. The presence of scleral icterus or jaundice suggests a hemolytic anemia. Frontal bossing and prominent maxillae may represent expansion of bone marrow red blood cell production secondary to a chronic hemolytic anemia such as thalassemia major. Diffuse lymphadenopathy and organomegaly may indicate leukemia or lymphoma. Auscultation of the heart often reveals a pulmonary flow murmur with mild to moderate anemia, and a gallop rhythm may be heard when a profound anemia results in congestive heart failure. Splenomegaly is apparent in patients with certain hemolytic anemias or with infiltrative diseases.

Laboratory Data

In addition to the hemoglobin or hematocrit, three other laboratory tests that can be performed in most offices—the reticulocyte count, the peripheral blood film, and the mean corpuscular volume—provide the clinician with enough information to determine the etiology of most anemias. The reticulocyte count is a measure of red blood cell production and thus provides valuable information regarding the ability of the bone marrow to respond to an anemia. Review of the peripheral blood film allows one to assess the morphology and color of the erythrocytes. The mean corpuscular volume is an index of red cell size and serves as a starting point for the morphologic classification of anemia. Observation of the plasma in a centrifuged sample of blood is a simple test that may provide additional clues: clear plasma suggests iron deficiency, icteric plasma may be secondary to extravascular hemolysis, and pink plasma secondary to intravascular hemolysis. Other laboratory tests may be indicated when particular etiologies of anemia are suspected; these are summarized in Tables 112-2 to 112-4.

CLASSIFICATION OF ANEMIA

Anemias are often classified based on decreased production or increased destruction of red blood cells. Another basis for classification is red cell morphology; the information gained from the peripheral blood film and the mean corpuscular volume enable the clinician to classify an anemia as microcytic, normocytic, or macrocytic. One can then systematically follow an algorithm to evaluate the subtype of anemia (Fig. 112-1) and minimize the number of laboratory tests obtained in arriving at a diagnosis.

Table 112-2 *Laboratory Evaluation of Hypochromic and Microcytic Anemias*

DIAGNOSIS	LABORATORY TEST	EXPECTED RESULT
Iron deficiency	Serum ferritin	Low <25 μg/L
	Serum iron and total iron-binding capacity	Low/high
	% iron saturation	Low <15%
	Bone marrow iron stores	Absent
	Stool for occult blood	Positive (if gastrointestinal bleeding)
	Urine for blood, hemoglobin or hemosiderin	Present (if renal loss)
	Ratio of MCV/RBC	>13
β-Thalassemia trait	Blood film	Basophilic stippling
	Hemoglobin electrophoresis	Increased A_2 or F hemoglobin
	Biosynthetic β/α-globin chain ratio	<1
	Ratio of MCV/RBC	<13
	Family studies	Hb/Hct decreased Blood film Anisocysotis Poikilocytosis Basophilic stippling MCV <70 fL/cell
α-Thalassemia trait	No routine specific test	Normal A_2 hemoglobin
	Family studies	Hb/Hct normal or slightly decreased Blood film Anisocytosis Poikilocytosis MCV <70 fL/cell
	Biosynthetic β/α-globin chain ratio	>1
	Specific genetic probe analysis	Absent genes
Chronic inflammation	Nonspecific tests	
	ESR	Increased
	Acute phase reactants	Increased
	C-reactive protein	
	Fibrinogen	
	Haptoglobin	
	Serum ferritin	Increased
	Serum iron + total iron-binding capacity	Low/low
	% iron saturation	Low
	Bone marrow iron stores	Increased
	Bone marrow sideroblasts	Decreased
Sideroblastic anemia	Serum ferritin	Increased
	Serum iron + total iron-binding capacity	Normal to increased/normal
	% iron saturation	High
	Bone marrow iron stores	Increased
	Bone marrow sideroblasts	Increased sideroblasts plus "ringed" sideroblasts
Lead poisoning	Blood film	Basophilic stippling
	Erythrocyte protoporphyrin	Increased
	Blood lead	Increased

Abbreviations: MCV, mean corpuscular volume; Hb, hemoglobin; Hct, hematocrit. (From Segel GB: Anemia, Pediatr Rev 10:77, 1988).

Microcytic Anemias

There are five causes of microcytic anemia in children: iron deficiency, thalassemia, lead, chronic inflammation, and sideroblastic anemia.

Iron Deficiency. Iron deficiency is by far the most common cause of anemia in children.[5] The clinician must determine whether the deficiency is due to poor dietary intake of iron, blood loss, or other less common causes. Children between the ages of 12 and 24 months are at the highest risk for iron deficiency anemia. Most of these children are no longer taking iron-containing formula, but are drinking cow's milk instead, and their intake of solid foods is erratic. Adolescent girls may also develop an anemia due to poor dietary intake of iron; they may have further loss of iron from blood loss with menses. Iron deficiency anemia is unusual in full-term infants in the first 6 months of life. These infants are born with sufficient iron stores to maintain a normal hematocrit level for 6 months.

When children of any age present with an iron deficiency anemia, it is essential to evaluate them for blood loss. Because the gastrointestinal tract is a common site of occult or chronic blood loss, patients and families should be queried about black or tarry stools, hematochezia, and bloody or coffee-ground emesis. Stool guaiac testing should be done at several different times, because blood loss through the GI tract may be intermittent. Gastric or duodenal ulcers, Meckel diverticula, polyps, hemorrhoids, and aspirin-induced bleeding should be considered. Other possibilties include epistaxis and inflammatory bowel disease. Cow's milk may induce gastrointestinal bleeding.[15] Iron deficiency itself, through damage to iron-dependent enzymes in the intestinal mucosa, may

Table 112-3 *Laboratory Evaluation of Normocytic Anemias**

DIAGNOSIS	LABORATORY TEST	EXPECTED RESULT
Anemias with low reticulocyte percentage		
Diamond-Blackfan anemia	Bone marrow examination	Decreased erythroid precursors
	Fetal hemoglobin and i antigen	± Increased
	Mean corpuscular volume	± Macrocytosis
Transient erythroblastopenia of childhood	Bone marrow examination	Decreased erythroid precursors
Aplastic crises	History	Underlying hemolytic disease
	Bone marrow examination	Decreased erythroid precursors
	Serology and/or viral culture	Parvovirus
Anemias with high reticulocyte percentage		
Extrinsic		
Autoimmune hemolysis	Blood film	Spherocytes
	Antiglobulin (Coombs) test	Positive
	Complement consumption assay	Positive (used if Coombs' test is negative)
	Tests for underlying disease	
Fragmentation hemolytic anemia	Blood film	Fragmented RBC
	Tests for underlying disease	
Intrinsic		
Membrane disorders	Blood film	Characteristic RBC: spherocytes, stomatocytes, elliptocytes
	Incubated osmotic fragility	Increased fragility if spherocytes present
	Autohemolysis	Increased and corrected by glucose
	Membrane protein-structural analysis (investigational)	Abnormal e.g., decreased spectrin in spherocytosis
Hemoglobin disorders	Blood film	Irreversibly sickled cells in severe sickle syndromes: SS, SC, or S-thalassemia Targeting in CC, also in SS, SC, and S-thalassemia
	Hemoglobin electrophoresis	Abnormal hemoglobin(s) present
Enzyme disorders G6PD	Screening tests	Positive
	Enzyme assay	Low activity
Pyruvate kinase and other glycolytic defects	Enzyme assay	Low activity

*From Segel GB: Anemia, Pediatr Rev 10:77, 1988

Table 112-4 *Laboratory Evaluation of Macrocytic Anemias**

DIAGNOSIS	LABORATORY TEST	EXPECTED RESULT
Vitamin B_{12} deficiency	Blood film	Macroovalocytes, Howell-Jolly bodies; nucleated RBC and hypersegmented granulocytes
	Serum vitamin B_{12}	Low <100 pg/mL
	Bone marrow examination	Megaloblastic erythroid and granulocyte precursors
Folic acid deficiency	Blood film	Same as above
	Serum folate	Low <3 ng/mL
	RBC folate	Low <160 ng/mL
	Bone marrow examination	Same as above

*From Segel GB: Anemia, Pediatr Rev 10:77, 1988

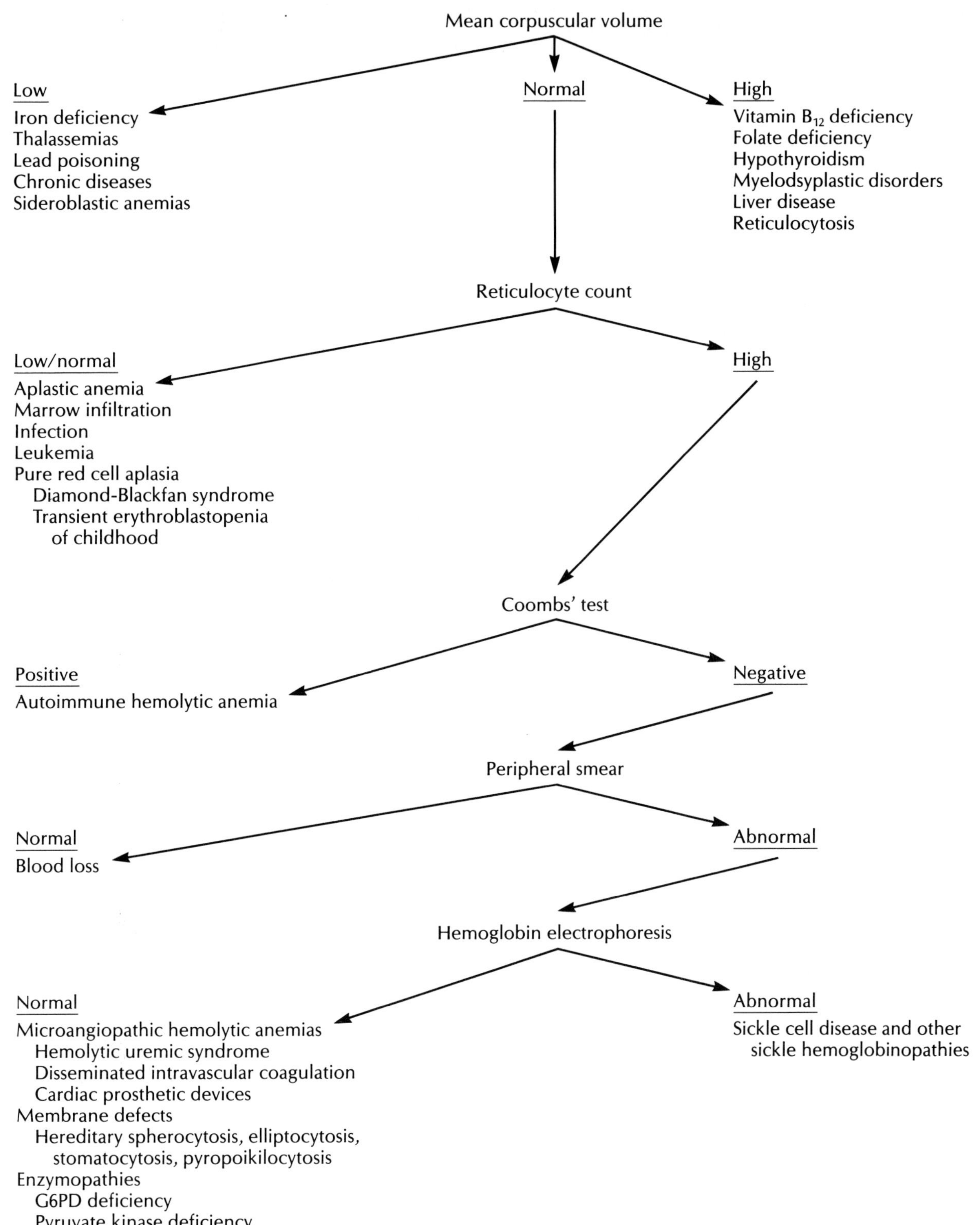

Fig. 112-1 Diagnostic approach to anemia in the child, based on the mean corpuscular volume.

cause occult blood loss.[10] The signs and symptoms of iron-deficiency anemia do not differ significantly from those of any other slowly developing anemia. Irritability, pica, and craving for ice and unusual foods have occasionally been observed with anemia specifically due to iron deficiency.[16]

If the deficiency of iron is enough to cause anemia, changes in other laboratory parameters will be present. The mean corpuscular volume and the absolute reticulocyte count will be low, and the peripheral blood film will show a predominance of hypochromic and microcytic cells. Target cells and elliptocytes may also be observed. These data are usually sufficient to diagnose iron deficiency. When the diagnosis is not certain, confirmatory laboratory tests may include serum ferritin and serum iron levels (both of which are low) and a total iron-binding capacity (elevated). The plasma of patients with iron deficiency anemia is clear rather than the normal, straw-colored appearance, and the anemia is frequently associated with thrombocytosis.

It is reasonable to give a patient a therapeutic trial of supplemental iron (6mg/kg Fe/day) if the patient has laboratory evidence of iron deficiency anemia and his or her age and history suggest poor dietary iron intake. For patients who do not fall into this category, or who are compliant and yet do not respond (or respond only transiently) to supplemental iron, additional evaluations for blood loss are imperative. It must be remembered that iron deficiency anemia is a pathophysiologic state for which an etiology needs to be found.

For individuals with moderate to severe iron deficiency anemia, increases in reticulocyte count should occur within 5 to 7 days after starting therapy. The therapy for iron deficiency requires continuous iron supplementation for approximately 6 months following the correction of the anemia. For a more complete discussion of iron deficiency anemia, see Chapter 20.

Thalassemias

The thalassemias are a heterogeneous group of disorders of hemoglobin production. In alpha thalassemia there is a reduction in the synthesis of the alpha chain; in beta thalassemia there are similar deficits in beta chain production. A decrease in production of one leads to a surplus of the other. This imbalance results in precipitation of the surplus chains and destruction of the red blood cells. As a general rule, the greater the imbalance in production of the two chains, the more severe the clinical syndrome.

Beta Thalassemia. There are two genes (one on each chromosome 11) that direct the synthesis of the beta chain of hemoglobin. An abnormality in one of these genes causes a mild decrease in beta chain production. The associated clinical syndrome is termed beta thalassemia trait (or thalassemia minor) and is commonly observed in patients of Mediterranean descent. These patients are completely asymptomatic and are usually diagnosed incidentally or when undergoing routine screening for anemia. The children are mildly anemic; they have a low mean corpuscular volume (usually 60 to 70 fl), a mild increase in the number of red cells, and a peripheral blood film showing microcytosis, hypochromia, and target cells. Iron deficiency may be confused with this entity because of the similarity of laboratory findings in these two disorders. A useful guideline for distinguishing between them is the Mentzer index,[14] which is based on there generally being greater numbers of red blood cells in beta thalassemia trait than in iron deficiency. Hemoglobin electrophoresis usually shows mild elevation of hemoglobin F or hemoglobin A_2. Genetic counseling is recommended for families of patients with beta thalassemia trait; individuals who inherit this defect from one parent and a similar or second defect from the other parent (e.g., sickle cell trait) may be afflicted with more severe hemoglobinopathies.

Severe beta thalassemia (Cooley anemia, thalassemia major) is the result of defects in both the genes directing synthesis of the beta chain. The marked deficiency in beta chain production that results is reflected in the more severe clinical syndromes. Patients are severely anemic because there is active hemolysis and the compensatory erythropoiesis is inadequate. Erythropoiesis in the maxillary and frontal bones is responsible for the characteristic prominence of the cheeks and for the frontal bossing seen in these patients. Extramedullary hematopoiesis and red blood cell destruction cause marked hepatosplenomegaly. Effective genetic counseling has led to a dramatic decrease in the incidence of this disorder in the United States. Treatment consists of repeated blood transfusions and the administration of deferoxamine to minimize iron overload from the transfusions.

Alpha Thalassemia. There are four identical genes (two on each chromosome 16) that code for the synthesis of the alpha chains. Abnormalities in these genes are most frequently encountered in Blacks and Asians. The silent carrier has a mutation in one of the four genes and is asymptomatic and clinically undectectable. Abnormalities in two genes causes alpha thalassemia trait. Patients with this mutation are also asymptomatic; they have laboratory findings similar to those of patients with beta thalassemia trait. However, they are even less anemic (if at all), and their hemoglobin electrophoresis is normal. The diagnosis of alpha thalassemia trait must therefore be based on a constellation of clinical findings: a patient with the appropriate ethnic background and with a parent having similar laboratory findings—very mild anemia, microcytosis, a normal hemoglobin electrophoresis, and normal iron status. Hemoglobin H disease is the result of abnormalities in three of the four alpha chain genes. Patients are usually asymptomatic but have moderate anemia (hemoglobin 7 to 10 g/dl), microcytosis, hypochromia, and red cell fragments. The hemoglobin electrophoresis shows 5% to 30% hemoglobin H (four beta chains). Abnormalities in all four genes result in no production of alpha chains and are not compatible with life except with extraordinary measures such as intrauterine transfusions.

Other hemoglobinopathies associated with microcytosis and anemia include Hemoglobin E syndromes (common in southeast Asians) and sickle thalassemia (a combination of beta thalassemia trait and sickle trait).

Lead Poisoning. Despite lead having no known physiologic role in humans, virtually everyone has measurable levels because of the widespread use of lead in industrial societies. Lead exerts its hematologic effect at low plasma levels, inactivating heme synthesis by inhibiting the insertion of iron into the protoporphyrin ring. Thus, with lead poisoning, the hematologic picture is similar to that of iron deficiency anemia: there is microcytosis, hypochromia, and a low mean corpuscular volume. In addition, target cells and intense basophilic strippling of red blood cells may be observed. Since iron cannot be inserted into the protoporphyrin ring, this latter compound builds up in the red cell, and levels of free erythrocyte protoporphyrin (FEP) rise.

Children are exposed to lead in the air (from combustion of lead-containing gasoline), in dust, and in old house lead-based paint. Approximately 4% of children ages 6 months to 5 years have lead levels greater than 30 mg/ml,[1] a level that can affect heme synthesis and may even result in lead encephalopathy. Even greater numbers of black and inner city children may be affected. Symptoms of the anemia are nonspecific, but children with associated lead encephalopathy may present with malaise or behavioral changes. Many physicians use the FEP level to screen for lead poisoning because it is a very sensitive indicator of the pathophysiologic effect of the heavy metal. Children with elevated FEPs then have a blood lead level checked. The most important aspect of treatment is the removal of any known sources of lead from the child's environment. Medical treatment consists of chelation therapy with dimercaptopropanol or calcium EDTA, both of which chelate lead and are subsequently excreted with the lead into the urine.

Anemia of Chronic Disease. Patients with a wide variety of chronic illnesses may have a mild microcytic anemia. This anemia can be seen in children with cancer, collagen vascular disease, chronic renal failure, and infection. Although the red cells of these patients are more often normocytic and normochromic, they are sometimes microcytic and hypochromic. The anemia is moderate (hemoglobin 7 to 10 gm/dl) and the reticulocyte count is normal or low. Plasma iron and total iron-binding capacity are low, and ferritin is high. This anemia is believed to be caused by a combination of decreased red blood cell survival, poor marrow response to anemia, and diminished flow of iron from the reticuloendothelial cells to the erythroblasts. The hypochromic microcytic anemia develops when the flow of iron is affected.

Sideroblastic Anemias. These rare forms of anemia are a heterogenous group of disorders caused by retention of iron in the mitochondria of developing erythrocytes. Inherited forms are extremely rare but may be seen in children. Some may respond to pyridoxine. Acquired forms of the disease are encountered more frequently, but almost exclusively in adults.

Normocytic Anemias

Normocytic anemias can be caused by increased destruction or decreased production of red blood cells. The reticulocyte count is a valuable test for distinguishing between these two processes. It is generally high in disorders of increased destruction and low in diseases of impaired red cell production.

Normocytic Anemia with Reticulocytopenia. A normocytic anemia with a low reticulocyte count is uncommon; it may be due to either an isolated problem in the erythroid line or to a disorder that affects all hematopoietic cell lines.

Pure Red Cell Aplasia. Diamond-Blackfan anemia and transient erythroblastopenia of childhood are the most common pure red cell aplasias in children. Diamond-Blackfan anemia is a rare congenital disorder. Children usually present in the first year of life with profound anemia and reticulocytopenia. As many as 25% of affected children have physical abnormalities such as short stature or malformed thumbs.[6] Additional laboratory features may include slight macrocytosis, persistent fetal hemoglobin, and persistence of the fetal "little i" red blood cell surface antigen. The etiology is unknown. Patients usually respond to treatment with prednisone.

Transient erythroblastopenia of childhood is a recently recognized,[13] benign, transient hypoplastic anemia that occurs most frequently in children between the ages of 1 and 4 years. These otherwise healthy children present with marked pallor and are severely anemic with reticulocyte counts of less than 1%. They have normal-appearing erythrocytes that show none of the fetal characteristics of the red cells of Diamond-Blackfan anemia. While the etiology is unknown, several studies suggest there is humoral suppression of erythropoiesis.[11] Recovery is spontaneous; treatment consists only of red cell transfusions when the anemia is profound. Patients sometimes present in the recovery phase with anemia and reticulocytosis. In these instances the diagnosis may be confused with a hemolytic anemia.

Pancytopenias. Because anemia may be but one manifestation of a more global disorder of the bone marrow, a white blood cell count, and differential and platelet counts should always be performed when the hematocrit is low. When these other cell lines are abnormal, serious disorders must be considered in the differential diagnosis. Such disorders include leukemia, primary bone marrow failure syndromes such as aplastic anemia or myelodysplasia, and infiltration of the marrow as is seen with bone marrow metastases or granulomatous diseases. Occasionally a viral illness will cause a transient suppression of all cell lines.

Aplastic Crises. Children with chronic hemolytic anemia (e.g., sickle cell anemia or hereditary spherocytosis) compensate for increased hemolysis with an increase in the rate of red cell production. Occasionally these children have transient suppression of red cell production, while the hemolysis continues at the same rate. The result is a precipitous drop in the hematocrit value, and patients may present with the sudden onset of weakness, fatigue, pallor, and even shock. Laboratory values include a low hematocrit and reticulocytopenia. A patient with a known hemolytic anemia who presents with these findings must be treated immediately. The principal treatment is infusion of red blood cells. The aplasia is transient and in many instances has been associated with acute parvovirus infection.[12]

Other. A normocytic, normochromic anemia is often seen with chronic illness, as noted previously. Acute blood loss may be mistaken for a hypoproductive anemia when the patient is seen shortly after the blood loss, but prior to generating a reticulocyte response.

Normocytic Anemia with Elevated Reticulocyte Count

Normocytic anemias with reticulocytosis are characterized by accelerated destruction of red blood cells and a compensatory increase in erythropoiesis. These hemolytic anemias can be further classified by the nature of the red blood cell destruction: those secondary to destruction of normal red cells by extrinsic forces and those in which intrinsic abnormalities of the erythrocytes result in their premature destruction.

Hemolysis due to Extrinsic Factors. Disseminated intravascular coagulation (DIC), hemolytic uremic syndrome (HUS), certain types of cardiac prosthetic devices, and immune-mediated hemolysis all cause destruction of otherwise normal red blood cells. In DIC and HUS, there is fibrin deposition in the small vessels, and erythrocytes are torn apart as they attempt to flow through the maze of fibrin strands. The peripheral blood film shows red cell fragments (schistocytes). A similar morphologic picture is seen when erythrocytes are destroyed by prosthetic devices such as artificial heart valves or foreign bodies such as arterial or central venous catheters.

Immune-mediated hemolysis is uncommon beyond the neonatal period; when it occurs, it is usually an autoimmune phenomenon. Autoimmune hemolytic anemia may be idiopathic or a feature of an underlying systemic disorder. Idiopathic autoimmune hemolytic anemia is often associated with an antecedent viral infection and occurs in children of all ages. In most instances the red cell destruction will resolve over several months, although children less than 4 or greater than 10 years of age are more likely to develop a chronic hemolytic anemia.[2]

Symptoms of autoimmune hemolytic anemia depend on the rapidity and degree of the drop in the hematocrit level. Patients are usually jaundiced secondary to the hemolysis and often have splenomegaly. Patients with intravascular hemolysis may have pink or red urine due to excretion of free hemoglobin. The hematocrit may range from normal to profoundly low, reflecting the intensity of the hemolysis. The reticulocyte count is usually elevated, but is normal or low in as many as one third to one half of children,[7] presumably because autoantibodies are directed to reticulocytes as well as the mature red blood cells. There is a preponderance of spherocytes on the peripheral blood film. A positive Coomb's test is diagnostic. It is imperative to evaluate the patient with an autoimmune hemolytic anemia for an underlying systemic disorder. Autoimmune hemolysis is seen in association with malignancies, immune deficiencies, collagen vascular disease, certain drugs, and with infections such as *Mycoplasma pneumoniae*, Epstein-Barr virus, and the human immunodeficiency virus.

Treatment of autoimmune hemolytic anemia is directed at correcting the underlying disorder. In cases of idiopathic disease, treatment with prednisone is recommended. Patients should be maintained on a dose of 2 mg/kg/day until the hematocrit value is in the normal range and there is little or no evidence of red cell destruction. Patients who do not respond to steroids may respond to other immunosuppressives or to high doses of intravenous gammaglobulin.[3]

Wilson disease must always be considered in any patient presenting with a nonimmune hemolytic anemia. Hemolysis in Wilson disease is due to elevated levels of serum copper. Early diagnosis leads to early treatment and the prevention of severe liver disease and mental retardation associated with more advanced Wilson disease. Vitamin E deficiency also causes hemolysis. It occurs in premature infants and patients with fat malabsorption (e.g., children with cystic fibrosis).

Hemolysis Due to Intrinsic Abnormalities of Red Blood Cells. There are three types of intrinsic abnormalities of red cells that predispose them to premature destruction: a defective red cell membrane, deficiencies in red cell enzymes, and production of abnormal forms of hemoglobin.

Membrane Defects. Hereditary spherocytosis is the most common of the membrane disorders. The membrane defect is due to a deficiency in spectrin, the main structural protein of the red cell membrane. This deficiency renders the red blood cell more fragile and as a result, more susceptible to hemolysis.

Hereditary spherocytosis is transmitted as an autosomal dominant trait and occurs in at least 1 in 5000 people of Northern European descent. The spectrum of disease is highly variable; classically, patients with hereditary spherocytosis present with anemia, jaundice, and splenomegaly, but in fact, many are identified incidentally on routine screening. Frequently, affected patients report family members with a history of anemia, jaundice, and splenectomy or cholecystectomy at an early age. Laboratory studies reveal anemia, reticulocytosis, and increased numbers of spherocytes on the peripheral blood film. The osmotic fragility of the red blood cells is increased. This test is not diagnostic, however, because spherocytes or red cells in any disorder characterized by unstable membranes show increased osmotic fragility. The hemolytic anemia resolves with splenectomy, because the spleen is the sole site of red cell destruction in this disease. Most patients eventually require a splenectomy in order to avoid such complications of hereditary spherocytosis as aplastic crises, gallstones, or splenic trauma.

Hereditary elliptocytosis and hereditary stomatocytosis and pyropoikilocytosis are less common heterogeneous congenital defects of red cell membranes and are infrequently encountered in children.

Enzyme Deficiencies. Glucose-6-phosphate dehydrogenase (G6PD) deficiency is the most common enzymopathy affecting red blood cells. G6PD generates NADPH by catalyzing the conversion of glucose-6-phosphate to 6-phosphogluconate. The NADPH is utilized by the red blood cell for reduction of potentially toxic oxidizing agents that accumulate with exposure to certain drugs, chemicals, and infections.

Two of the most common types of G6PD deficiencies are a mild variant (Gd^{A-}) that occurs in approximately 10% of American black males and a more severe variant ($G^{Mediterranean}$) observed in people of Mediterranean descent. The disorder is transmitted as an X-linked trait; thus males are more commonly affected than females. Most patients in the United States (those with the Gd^{A-} variant) are asymptomatic, and their deficiency is not apparent unless they are exposed to an oxidant stress such as an infection. Agents most frequently precipitating hemolysis include sulfa drugs and chloramphenicol, antimalarial drugs, aspirin, ascorbic acid, chemicals such as benzene or naphthalene, infection (hepatitis), and diabetic ketoacidosis.

Patients present with jaundice and symptoms of a rapidly falling hematocrit. Because the hemolysis is intravascular they may have hemoglobinuria. Laboratory findings include anemia and reticulocytosis. There may be pitted red blood cells on the blood film, but findings are often nonspecific. Special stains reveal the presence of precipitated hemoglobin aggregates called Heinz bodies. A test for red cell G6PD is often normal or elevated at the time of a hemolytic episode because only the younger, more enzyme replete cells remain. If G6PD deficiency is strongly suspected, the test should be repeated 1 to 2 months after the acute crisis or performed in the mother. Treatment is supportive and consists of eliminating exposure to offending agent and, if necessary, giving the patient a transfusion.

There are many other enzyme deficiencies that predispose the red cell to hemolysis. Perhaps the most frequently occurring (excluding G6PD) is pyruvate kinase deficiency. Patients with this rare enzymopathy suffer from a chronic hemolytic anemia. Routine laboratory studies are nondiagnostic;

specific assays for pyruvate kinase must be ordered if the diagnosis is suspected.

The Hemoglobinopathies. The hemoglobinopathies are a group of hemolytic disorders in which there are abnormalities in the amino acid composition of the alpha or beta chain of the hemoglobin molecule. Sickle cell anemia is the most prevelant disease in this group. The defect in sickle cell anemia is a single amino acid substitution of valine for glutamic acid in position 6 of the beta chain of hemoglobin. This substitution renders hemoglobin susceptible to polymerization when it is exposed to low tensions of oxygen; as a result, the red cell "sickles" irreversibly.

Sickle cell anemia is transmitted as an autosomal recessive trait. Approximately 8% of American Blacks carry this trait. Although 30% to 45% of their hemoglobin is the sickle variant, this is not sufficient to cause their red cells to sickle under normal circumstances. These patients grow and develop normally and have normal hematocrit levels and reticulocyte counts. They may occasionally develop renal papillary necrosis, and when at high altitudes (>10,000 feet) they are at risk for splenic infarction or other manifestations of vaso-occlusive disease. It is important to identify patients with the sickle hemoglobin trait for purposes of genetic counseling.

Homozygous sickle cell anemia occurs in approximately 1 in 650 American Blacks. Although the vast majority of people afflicted with the disease in the United States are Black, it has been occasionally reported in Greeks, Arabs, and Indians.

Children with sickle cell anemia do not usually have symptoms of the disease until they are approximately 6 months of age. From age 6 months to 3 years, however, most affected children have experienced the pain of vaso-occlusive crises; by age 4 years, many already show delayed growth and development. Typically these children have hematocrit values ranging from the low to mid 20s with reticulocyte counts of 5% to 15%. The mean corpuscular volume is normal. The peripheral blood film reveals some irreversibly sickled cells, but there are also target cells, polychromasia, and Howell-Jolly bodies. Hemoglobin electrophoresis is diagnostic: there is usually greater than 90% hemoglobin S and less than 10% hemoblogin F and/or hemoglobin A_2.

Most of the signs and symptoms of sickle cell anemia are a consequence of intravascular sickling and occlusion of blood vessels by the sickled cells. This vaso-occlusion (often referred to as a vaso-occlusive crisis) occurs episodically, usually in association with infection, dehydration, acidosis, or exposure to cold. The most common type of vaso-occlusive crisis is the "painful" crisis that is the result of widespread ischemia and infarction of bone marrow, bone cortex, or other organs. Infants may present with dactylitis; older patients complain of excruciating extremity, back, or chest pain and usually have a paucity of physical findings. Treatment consists of hydration, pain control, and careful monitoring for other complications of vaso-occlusion. Patients may present with focal rather than diffuse bone pain. When this occurs in association with high fevers, it is often difficult to distinguish whether the patient is experiencing a bone infarction or an osteomyelitis.

Patients may also present with chest pain, respiratory distress, high fevers, and an infiltrate on the roentgenogram of the chest. This constellation of signs and symptoms is called the "acute chest syndrome" and may be secondary to pneumonia, pulmonary infarction, or both. Patients with acute chest syndrome are particularly vulnerable to severe, widespread vaso-occlusive crises because the pulmonary involvement can cause hypoxia and exacerbate the sickling. Treatment should include vigorous hydration, supplemental oxygen, antibiotics to treat the presumed pneumonia, and if the patient is hypoxic, exchange transfusion to lower the amount of hemoglobin S and increase the oxygen-carrying capacity of red blood cells. Other complications of vaso-occlusion include stroke, priapism, and splenic infarction.

Younger patients (ages 6 months to 3 years) are susceptible to splenic sequestration, a sudden accumulation of blood in the spleen. The result is rapid enlargement of the spleen and a precipitous drop in the hematocrit level. Treatment consists of blood transfusions and volume expanders. Patients who experience splenic sequestration are at increased risk for subsequent episodes. Splenectomy is advocated by some physicians for patients who have two or more episodes.

As previously noted, patients with sickle cell anemia are also at risk for aplastic crises. Etiology, presentation, laboratory values, and treatment are similiar to aplastic crises with other chronic hemolytic anemias.

Perhaps the most grave threat to patients with sickle cell anemia is their susceptibility to serious bacterial infection. This increased risk of infection is largely due to a hypofunctional spleen; defects in opsonization of bacteria may also play a role.[8] These children are at great risk for overwhelming sepsis, meningitis, and pneumonia secondary to *S. pneumoniae* or *H. influenzae* type b. They may also experience severe *Mycoplasma* pneumonia and are unusually susceptible to osteomyelitis secondary to Salmonella organisms.

So great is the risk of serious bacterial infection in children with sickle cell anemia that in most centers they are started on penicillin prophylaxis at age 3 months. It is also recommended that they receive the pneumococcal, *H. influenzae* type b, and influenza virus vaccines. Patients with sickle cell anemia who develop a fever should be carefully evaluated; if no simple etiology is found, they should be admitted to the hospital and treated empirically with intravenous antibiotics.

Several other hemoglobin defects can occur in combination with the sickle hemoglobin trait and cause a syndrome similar to sickle cell anemia. Patients heterozygous for both hemoglobin S and hemoglobin C may have signs and symptoms of sickle cell anemia, although generally they are less affected than children with homozygous sickle cell disease. Patients who inherit both the sickle and beta thalassemia traits may have signs and symptoms of mild or severe sickle cell disease. Patients with any of these sickle syndromes (as well as those with the more rare types such as hemoglobin SD or SO^{Arab}) should be managed similarly to patients with homozygous sickle cell disease; they should receive penicillin prophylaxis and the appropriate vaccines and should be treated similarly for any clinical manifestations of sickling.

Macrocytic Anemias

Macrocytosis is very unusual in children. It can be seen with deficiencies in folic acid or vitamin B_{12}. Folate deficiency may be secondary to inborn errors of metabolism, poor dietary intake, malabsorption, increased requirements for folate (as

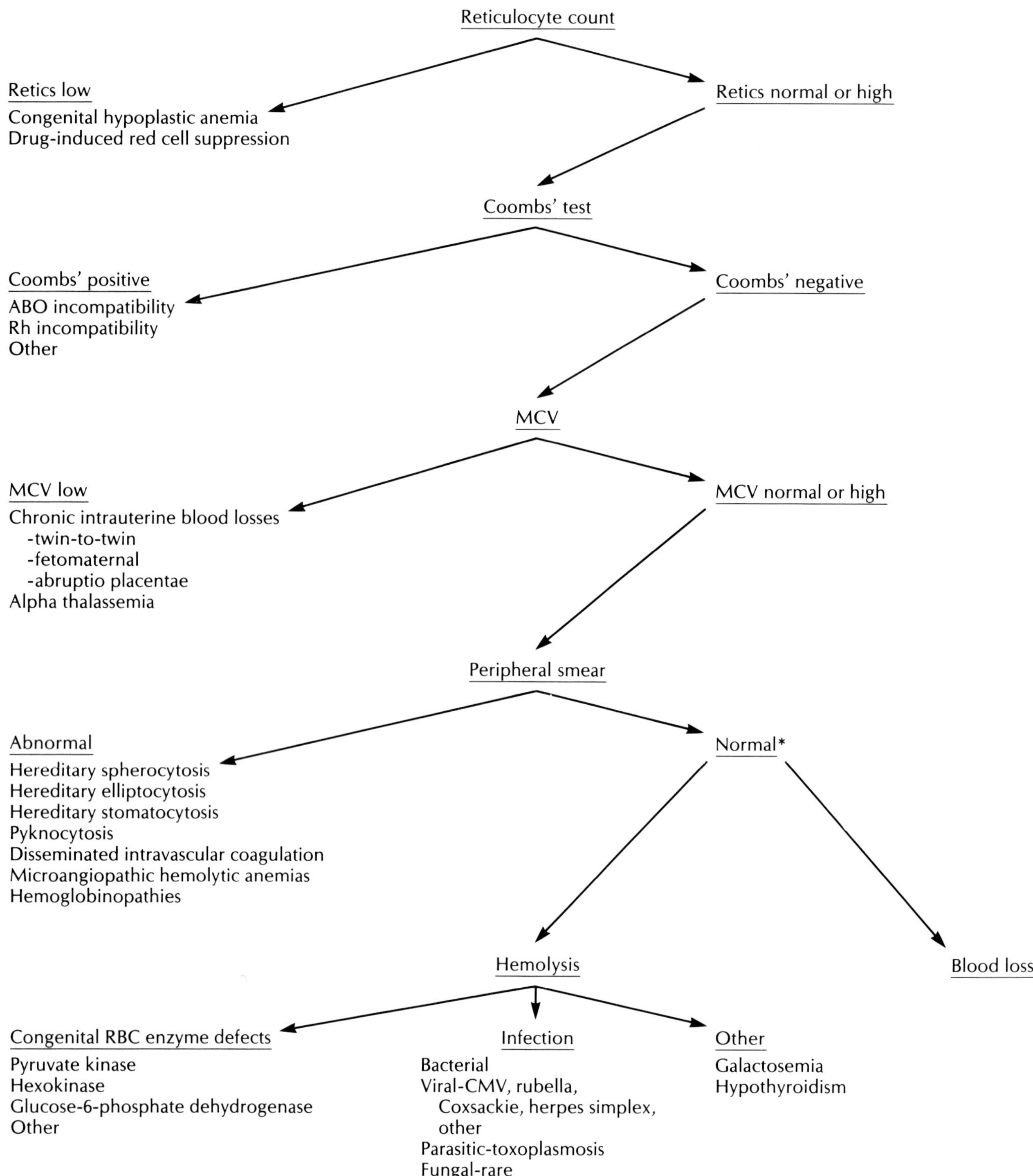

Fig. 112-2 Diagnostic approach to anemia in the newborn based on reticulocyte count. *Indicates a peripheral blood smear with no specifically diagnostic abnormalities.

From Nathan DC and Oski F: Hematology of Infancy and Childhood, ed 3, Philadelphia, 1987, WB Saunders.

in chronic hemolytic anemias), and drugs that inhibit the metabolism of folate (e.g., methotrexate). Vitamin B_{12} deficiency may also be due to inborn errors of metabolism, poor dietary intake, or malabsorption.

The anemia associated with either of these vitamin deficiencies can be severe and the MCV is often 100 to 140 fl. The peripheral blood film shows numerous normochromic macrocytes and hypersegmented neutrophils. The diagnosis can be confirmed with a serum folate or vitamin B_{12} level; as with iron deficiency, once the deficit is documented, the etiology must be determined.

Macrocytosis is also observed in hypothyroidism, myelodysplastic disorders, dyserythropoietic disorders, liver disease, and in patients with a significant reticulocytosis. It is a normal finding in the red blood cells of newborns.

ANEMIA IN THE NEWBORN

The approach to anemia in the newborn must be considered apart from that of anemia in an older infant or child. Many of the etiologies of anemia in the newborn (e.g., isoimmune disease) are unique to this age group. Conversely, some common causes of anemia in older children, such as iron deficiency anemia, are rare in infants. Furthermore, some of the etiologies of anemia common to both newborns and older children may manifest themselves quite differently in the newborn period than at an older age. A useful algorithm for the evaluation of anemia in the newborn is illustrated in Fig. 112-2.

The normal hematologic parameters of a newborn are markedly different from normal values for older children (Table 112-5). The mean hemoglobin of term infants at birth is approximately 19.0 g/dl, but the level falls gradually over 8 to 12 weeks to a nadir of 10 to 11 g/dl. This phenomenon is known as the "physiologic anemia of infancy." The drop is even more pronounced in premature infants in whom hemoglobin levels may fall to 7 to 8 g/dl. This "physiologic anemia" is normal in premature and term infants, and despite the low hemoglobin levels, blood transfusion is not necessary in the asymptomatic, otherwise healthy infant.

There are three broad classifications for the etiology of anemia in the newborn: blood loss, hemolysis, and decreased red blood cell production. Blood loss may occur prenatally or perinatally. Common causes include feto-maternal or twin-to-twin transfusion, placenta previa, placental abruption, and internal hemorrhage due to cephalohematoma, caput succedaneum, or intracranial hemorrhage. Fetomaternal hemorrhage can be confirmed by the Kleihauer-Betke test, which detects the presence of fetal red cells in maternal blood. (The test may result in a false negative if the mother has type O blood and the child does not.) The clinical presentation depends on the rapidity and degree of blood loss. Infants who have experienced chronic blood loss are hemodynamically stable, but pale, and have a microcytic, hypochromic anemia. Infants with acute blood loss are often pale and floppy with tachypnea, tachycardia, and hypotension. The initial hematocrit may be normal, but the infant soon develops a normocytic normochromic anemia with a reticulocytosis.

The most common cause of hemolytic anemia in newborns is isoimmune disease (erythroblastosis fetalis). It is caused by an incompatibility between fetal and maternal Rh, ABO, or minor blood group antigens. In Rh incompatibility, the mother's red blood cells are Rh negative while those of the infant are Rh positive. If the Rh negative mother has been previously sensitized to Rh positive blood (from a previous pregnancy), she may have developed antibodies to the Rh antigen; these antibodies cross the placenta and destroy the Rh positive red cells of the infant. The result is a brisk hemolytic anemia, which occurs in utero and continues after the birth of the child. The hematocrit may fall quickly, and the associated hyperbilirubinemia can cause kernicterus. Rh disease can be prevented by the prenatal administration of Rh immune globulin to Rh negative mothers. Life-threatening Rh incompatibility is rare today, largely because of the routine use of Rh immune globulin. ABO incompatibility (a mother with type O blood and her infant with type A, B, or AB) occurs frequently, but the hemolysis is mild and infrequently causes hyperbilirubinemia or anemia. Hemolysis occasionally occurs when the mother has been sensitized to one of the minor blood groups such as the Kell or Duffy antigen. An alloimmune hemolytic anemia or drug-induced hemolysis may also occur in the newborn secondary to passive transfer of maternal autoantibody or maternal drug.

Hemolytic anemia in the newborn is associated wtih many types of infection. Bacterial sepsis and CMV, toxoplasmosis, herpes, and rubella infections can all cause hemolysis. A microangiopathic hemolytic anemia can occur secondary to disseminated intravascular hemolysis, cavernous hemangiomas (as in Kasabach-Merrit syndrome), and localized thrombi.

Hemoglobinopathies rarely cause symptoms in the neonatal period. Beta chain defects, such as sickle cell syndromes, are not apparent until later in infancy when there are appreciable concentrations of the beta chain of hemoglobin. Similarly, beta thalassemias are not clinically detectable at birth. Newborns with alpha thalassemia major present with erythroblastosis fetalis. Infants with red blood cell membrane defects or enzymopathies are occasionally diagnosed in the newborn period, but more often present at a later age.

Disorders of red cell production are rare in the newborn. Hypoproduction of red cells is most often secondary to drugs or infection. Diamond-Blackfan syndrome is a rare congenital pure red blood cell aplasia, but infants with this disease are not anemic at birth. They are usually not diagnosed until the

Table 112-5 *Normal Hematologic Values During First 2 Weeks of Life in Term Infant**

	CORD BLOOD	DAY 1	DAY 3	DAY 7	DAY 14
Hb (g/dl)	16.8	18.4	17.8	17.0	16.8
Hematocrit (%)	53.0	58.0	55.0	54.0	52.0
Red cells ($mm^3 \times 10^6$)	5.25	5.8	5.6	5.2	5.1
MCV (fL)	107.0	108.0	99.0	98.0	96.0
MCH (pg/cell)	34.0	35.0	33.0	32.5	31.5
MCHC (g/dl rbc's)	31.7	32.5	33.0	33.0	33.0
Reticulocytes (%)	3-7	3-7	1-3	0-1	0-1
Nucleated RBC/ (mm^3)	500	200	0-5	0	0
Platelets (1000/mm^3)	290	192	213	248	252

*Key: MCV = mean corpuscular volume; MCH = mean corpuscular hemoglobin; MCHC = mean corpuscular hemoglobin concentration. (From Nathan DG and Oski F: Hematology of Infancy and Childhood, ed. 3, Philadelphia, 1987, WB Saunders).

anemia is clinically apparent, sometime between the ages of 3 and 12 months; they may be diagnosed earlier if they have one of the characteristic physical anomalies. Congenital leukemia and osteopetrosis are other very rare causes of red cell aplasia and are associated with abnormalities in other cell lines.

REFERENCES

1. Annest JS et al: Blood lead levels for persons 6 months-74 years of age: U.S., 1976-80. Hyattsville, Md, 1982, [U.S. Dept. of Health and Human Services].
2. Buchanan GR et al: The acute and transient nature of idiopathic immune hemolytic anemia in childhood, J Pediatr 88:780, 1976.
3. Bussel JB, Cunningham-Rundles C, and Abraham C: Intravenous treatment of autoimmune hemolytic anemia with very high-dose gammaglobulin, Vox Sang 51:264, 1986.
4. Dallman PR and Siimes MA: Percentile curves for hemoglobin and red cell volume in infancy and childhood, J Pediatr 94:26, 1979.
5. Dallman PR, Yip R, and Johnson C: Prevalence and causes of anemia in the United States, Amer J Clin Nutr 39:437, 1984.
6. Glader BE: Diagnosis and management of red cell aplasia in children, Hemat/Onc Clin NA 1:431, 1987.
7. Habibi B et al: Autoimmune hemolytic anemia in children, A review of 80 cases, Am J Med 56:61, 1974.
8. Johnston RB, Newman SL, and Struth AG: Increased susceptibility to infection in sickle cell disease: defects of opsonization and of splenic function, Birth Defects: Original Articles Series 11:322, 1975.
9. Kay R, Oski FA, and Barness LA: Core Textbook of Pediatrics, ed 3. Philadelphia, 1988, JB Lippincott Co.
10. Kimber C and Weintraub LR: Malabsorption of iron secondary to iron deficiency, New Engl J Med 279:453, 1968.
11. Koening HM et al: Immune suppression of erythropoiesis in TEC, Blood 54:742, 1979.
12. Lefrere JJ et al: Six cases of hereditary spherocytosis revealed by human parvovirus infection, Br J Haematol 62:653, 1986.
13. Lovric VA: Anemia and temporary erythroblastopenia in children, Aust Ann Med 1:34, 1970.
14. Mentzer WC: Differentiation of iron deficiency from thalassemia trait, Lancet 1:449, 1973.
15. Wilson JF et al: Studies on iron metabolism. V. Further observations on cow's milk-induced gastrointestinal bleeding in infants with iron-deficiency anemia, J Pediatr 84:335, 1974.
16. Ziai M: Pallor and anemia *Pediatrics,* ed 4. Boston, 1990, Little, Brown & Co.

SUGGESTED READINGS

Pearson HA: Sickle cell diseases: Diagnosis and management in infancy and childhood, Pediatr Rev 9:121, 1987.
Segel GB: Anemia, Pediatr Rev 10:77, 1988.

113

Back Pain

George R. Kim

Back pain in children is relatively uncommon. Although little information is available regarding its actual incidence in the pediatric population,[4] it generally is observed to be low, increasing in frequency with age.[6]

Etiologic factors are physiologic and developmental. The smaller size, higher flexibility, and greater relative ligamentous strength of the child's spine allow a greater dispersion of traumatic forces and thus a higher tolerance to injury compared with the adult.[1] In addition, the degenerative changes that contribute to adult back pain are, for the most part, absent in the child. As the child grows into adolescence, the spinal anatomy and life-style approximate that of the adult, with a presumptive rise in the factors leading to back pain. During the adolescent growth spurt, many problems, such as scoliosis, become apparent, adding to the frequency of back pain in the older child.

Developmentally, as children age, their ability to relate verbally increases; thus the incidence of complaints such as back pain also increases. In addition, with age the psychological development necessary to present pain for secondary gain and hysteria develops.

Although relatively rare, pediatric back pain is clinically significant. Studies examining etiologic factors of the complaint in children are summarized in Table 113-1.[4,6] In each study an organic cause of the problem was found in a high percentage of children with back pain, unlike back pain findings in adults. It also is notable that in each study the definitive diagnosis was delayed for a period of up to 6 or 7 months after initial presentation.

The causes of back pain are found in the musculoskeletal, respiratory, gastrointestinal, renal, hematopoietic, endocrine, circulatory, reproductive, and nervous systems. Presentation can be acute or subacute, with the potential for great morbidity if not recognized. Thus the condition presents a diagnostic and therapeutic challenge to the clinician, whose persistence in finding a cause should be steered by two guidelines: first, pediatric back pain is rare; second, when it does occur, serious disease needs to be ruled out (Figure 113-1).

DEFINITIONS

The term *back* is a broad one, describing approximately 50% of the body, including structures in the neck, thorax, abdomen, pelvis, and hips. It includes the cervical, thoracic, lumbar, and sacrococcygeal spine and its vertebrae, disks, joints, paraspinous musculature, ligaments, and tendons. All are joined together in an intricate, dynamically growing system. Because the spine also carries the sensory and motor nerve roots to the entire body, "back pain" can be diverse in presentation as well as cause.

The mechanisms of back pain, like pain in general, involve derangements of nerves in relation to their surrounding anatomy. Pain can be caused by *direct nerve injury* (as in trauma), *local irritation* (as in infection or inflammation), *compression* (as in vertebral fracture), *stretching* (as in tethered cord), and *muscle spasm* (as may occur in scoliosis).

These mechanisms may occur *spinally*: *intraspinally* (as in a cord tumor), at the *spinal root* (in which case the pain is characterized as *radicular*), and in the *paraspinous* musculature and adjacent structures. When the source of the back pain is not in the spinal or paraspinal region, the pain is *referred*. In addition, pain may have no organic cause, and it can be *psychogenic* in origin.

Back pain may be grouped according to the pathologic condition responsible for the pain. The causative factor may be *mechanical* (due to macroscopic changes in the structures

Table 113-1 *Etiologic Factors in Back Pain in Children*

	FINDINGS				
AUTHOR (DATE) NO. OF PATIENTS	POSITIVE DIAGNOSES (%)	MECHANICAL (%)	DEVELOPMENTAL (%)	INFECTIOUS/NEOPLASTIC (%)	NO DIAGNOSIS (%)
Hensinger (1980)[3] 100 patients with back pain >2 mo	85	33	33	18	15
King/Tufel (1984)[4] 54 patients <19 yr	63	28	13	22	37
Turner et al (1989)[6] 61 patients <15 yr	53	21	15	16	47
Sponsellar and Tolo (1990)[5] Estimate	75				

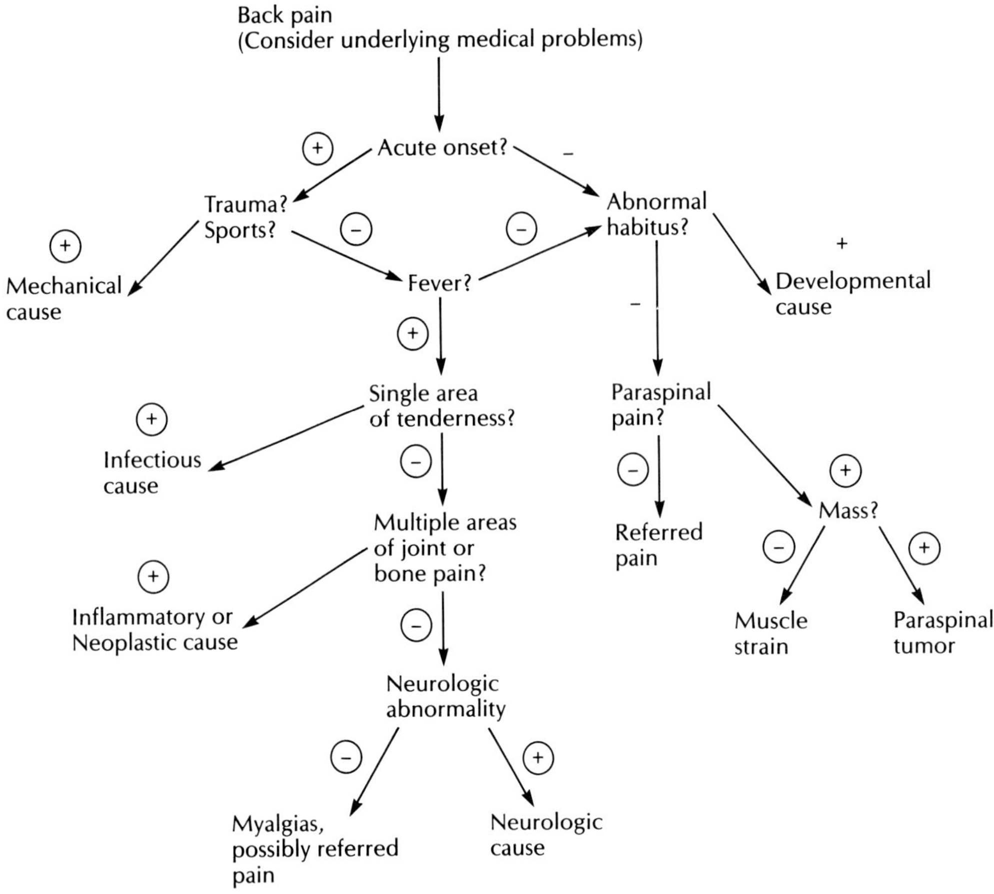

Fig. 113-1 A suggested approach to back pain.

surrounding the nerves), *developmental* (due to defects in growth or formation of those elements), *inflammatory* or *infectious* (both due to microscopic changes in anatomy, causing irritation to the nerves), *neurologic* (due to nerve tissue pathology alone), or *neoplastic* (due to abnormal, noncongenital tissue growth). These categories are by no means absolute, and many disease states will cause back pain by means of several mechanisms (see accompanying box).

CHARACTERISTICS

Circumstances Surrounding Presentation

The most common acute presentation of back pain follows trauma. The complaint may follow, immediately or by several hours, injuries sustained by patients in motor vehicle accidents, falls, sports activities, or fights. The severity and mechanism of the injury may vary, and a neurologic change such as loss of consciousness or posttraumatic seizure may accompany it. Loss of consciousness may occur with intoxication, which in turn may accompany spinal injury.

Occult trauma may cause acute back pain in a child, but so can other causes. Infectious and inflammatory causes may have rapid onset, with the potential for organic destruction if left untreated. Catastrophic processes such as a ruptured ectopic pregnancy or aortic aneurysm, which may occur initially with back pain but no trauma, can lead to hemorrhage, shock, or death, if not recognized.

Nonacute back pain most commonly occurs in athletes as part of an "overuse" syndrome. In this case trauma is again the cause of the pain, but it is repeated mild trauma, the source of which usually can be found in work, sports, or other activities that require repetitive motions. Extreme obesity, poor posture, failure to warm up before activity, improper lifting techniques, or prolonged immobilization can contribute to the problem of lower back pain in the athlete.

A history of repeated mild trauma does not exclude other pathologic conditions. Nonacute, or chronic back pain, in a child may be due to underlying disease that has gone unnoticed or that has been attributed to "overuse."

The preverbal child represents a diagnostic problem. In both acute and nonacute cases the patient may give no verbal clues. A history either is absent or is provided by a caretaker who simply may have noticed a change in some behavior of the child. Fever, irritability, decreased motion of an extremity, change of gait, or a "clutching" of the back may be noted in acute cases. Slow progression of limp, stiffness, progressive weakness, or other neurologic changes may manifest more subtly. The diagnosis rests on a high degree of suspicion and a thorough and sometimes repeated physical examination.

Associated Symptoms and Signs

The symptoms and signs associated with back pain in children are varied but may help in sorting out the diagnosis (Table 113-2).

Causes of Back Pain in Children

I. Mechanical
  A. Spinal
    1. Trauma: fracture, dislocation, contusion
    2. Disk problems: hernation, compression, fracture
    3. Osteoporosis due to
      a. Rickets
      b. Chronic disease: cystic fibrosis, renal failure
      c. Steroids: endogenous, medical, abusive
      d. Parathyroid disease
      e. Metabolic abnormality: osteogenesis imperfecta
      f. Vascular disease: sickle cell anemia
      g. Idiopathic osteoporosis
  B. Paraspinal
    1. "Overuse" syndromes, including strains/sprains
    2. Postural problems, including chronic immobilization
    3. Injuries to the paraspinal skeleton
    4. Contractures due to burns
  C. Referred
    1. Pregnancy: intrauterine or ectopic
    2. Nephrolithiasis
    3. Urinary retention due to any cause
    4. Constipation (severe)
    5. Adhesions due to old surgery/injury/burn
    6. Dissection of aortic aneurysm
    7. Slipped capital femoral epiphysis
    8. Legg-Calvé-Perthes disease
    9. Unequal leg lengths
    10. Splenic injury or infarction
    11. Sciatica or other distal nerve compression
    12. Chest syndrome in sickle cell anemia
    13. Gastroesophageal reflux/esophagitis/hiatal hernia/Sandifer syndrome
    14. Peptic ulcer disease

II. Developmental
  A. Spinal
    1. Congenital anomalies
      a. Spina bifida
      b. Atlantoaxial instability
      c. Klippel-Feil anomaly
      d. Scoliosis/kyphosis
      e. Diastematomyelia
      f. Developmental lumbar stenosis
      g. Sacral agenesis
    2. Kyphosis/lordosis
    3. Scheuermann disease
  B. Paraspinal
    1. Muscle spasm due to scoliosis
    2. Torticollis
    3. Congenital scapula deformity

III. Inflammatory
  A. Spinal
    1. Juvenile rheumatoid arthritis
    2. Ankylosing spondylitis
  B. Paraspinal
    1. Rhabdomyolosis
    2. Sacroiliitis
    3. Myalgia due to generalized viral infection
    4. Juvenile dermatomyositis
  C. Referred
    1. Pancreatitis
    2. Vasoocclusive crisis in sickle cell anemia
    3. Crohn disease
    4. Ulcerative colitis

IV. Infectious
  A. Spinal
    1. Vertebral osteomyelitis
    2. Diskitis
    3. Tuberculous spondylitis
  B. Paraspinal
    1. Retropharyngeal abscess/cervical adenitis
    2. Paraspinal abscess/cellulitis
    3. Psoas abscess
  C. Referred
    1. Pneumonia/asthma
    2. Retrocolic appendicitis
    3. Perirectal abscess
    4. Pilonidal abscess
    5. Salpingitis/tuboovarian abscess/perihepatitis
    6. Pyelonephritis

V. Neoplastic
  A. Spinal
    1. Benign tumors
      a. Osteoid osteoma
      b. Osteoblastoma
      c. Dermoid tumor
      d. Aneurysmal bone cyst
    2. Malignant
      a. Ewing sarcoma/osteosarcoma
      b. Invasive metastatic neoplasia (Wilms tumor/neuroblastoma)
      c. Neurofibromatosis (variable)
  B. Paraspinal
    1. Neck tumors
    2. Neurofibromatosis
    3. Presacral teratoma
  C. Referred
    1. Leukemia
    2. Abdominal tumors
    3. Testicular tumors (older adolescent male)

VI. Neurogenic
  A. Intraspinal/intracranial lesion
    1. Neoplasia
    2. Meningocele
    3. Abscess
    4. Hematoma
  B. Postmanipulation (lumbar puncture) pain
  C. Dystonia/dysautonomia
  D. Guillain-Barré syndrome
  E. Acute transverse myopathy
  F. Muscular dystrophy/atrophy
  G. Muscle imbalance
    1. Spastic diplegia or cerebral palsy
    2. Poliomyelitis
  H. Phenothiazine toxicity

VII. Psychogenic/psychosocial
  A. Child abuse (physical findings inconsistent with history)
  B. Malingering/drug abuse
  C. Conversion reaction/hysteria
  D. Factitious disease (Münchausen syndrome by proxy)
  E. Vulnerable child syndrome

Table 113-2 *Differential Diagnostic Signs and Symptoms of Back Pain*

SIGN/SYMPTOM	POSSIBLE CAUSE
History	
Onset	
Acute	Trauma, infection
Chronic	Posture, congenital problem overuse, tumor
Quality	
Sharp, intermittent	Trauma, infection, renal colic
Dull, gradual	Progressive scoliosis, intraspinal lesion, tumor
Timing	
Worse in morning, stiffness	Inflammatory/juvenile rheumatoid arthritis
Worse with activity	Overuse, trauma
Worse with rest	Tumor, nerve impingement
Aggravating factors	
Cough	Radiculopathy, rib trauma
Bending	Muscle strain, disk herniation
Straight leg raising	Radiculopathy, hamstring tightness, cerebral palsy
Sitting	Tethered cord, sacrococcygeal fracture
Eating	Gastrointestinal lesion
Associated symptoms	
Fever, chills	Pyelonephritis, influenza
Syncope	Asthma, pneumonia, intracranial process, blood loss
Bone pain	Leukemia
Vaginal discharge, dysuria	Pelvic inflammatory disease, pyelonephritis, nephrolithiasis
Anorexia	Gastrointestinal lesion
Progressive weakness	Cord compression, neurologic problem
Urgency	Urinary obstruction
Influenza symptoms	Myalgias
	Malignancy, collagen-vascular disease
Past medical history	
Sickle cell disease	Vasoocclusive crisis
Cystic fibrosis	Secondary vertebral wedging
Missed menses	Pregnancy (normal or ectopic)
Obesity, adolescent	Slipped capital femoral epiphysis
Down syndrome, achondroplasia, mucopolysaccharidosis	Atlantoaxial stability
Drug use	Diskitis, trauma, malingering
Ethanol	Pancreatitis, trauma

The history of back pain should include its acuity and the relationship of the pain to recent trauma and work or sports activities. The specific location, radiation, severity, and quality of the pain should be noted, as well as any fever, weight loss, anorexia, respiratory distress, fatigue, or neurologic deficits. Aggravating or relieving factors may help with treatment as well as diagnosis. Inquiry should be made into any underlying medical problems that may contribute to the problem, as well as inquiry into the use or abuse of medications.

Physical examination should include an evaluation of the general habitus of the patient in regard to posture, spinal or skeletal asymmetries, gait disturbances, and skin lesions, which may help in diagnosis. A thorough examination should be performed systematically to rule out the possibility of referred pain. Special attention should be given to the orthopedic evaluation with regard to spinal symmetry and range of motion, as well as to areas of tenderness. A thorough examination should include evaluation of the lower extremities, including hip motion and leg lengths. Special attention also should be given to the neurologic examination, noting bowel and bladder function, as well as sensory and motor capacity.

DIFFERENTIAL DIAGNOSIS

Infant/Preverbal Child

The presentation of illness may be nonspecific in the infant or preverbal child; thus back pain may not be considered. Fever and irritability may suggest an infectious process, whereas progressive neurologic loss or other physical findings may suggest a congenital lesion. Problems that can occur in this age-group include the following (see box):

1. *Tethering of the cord* results from a thickened filum terminale, which prevents its normal ascent during growth and creates traction on the cord, with subsequent neurologic

Table 113-2 *Differential Diagnostic Signs and Symptoms of Back Pain—cont'd*

SIGN/SYMPTOM	POSSIBLE CAUSE
Physical examination	
Respiratory distress	Pneumonia, asthma, retropharyngeal abscess
Decreased blood pressure	Intraabdominal catastrophe
Fever	Infection, collagen-vascular disease
Abnormal habitus	Structural or developmental lesion
Neurologic loss	Cord compression
Location of pain	
Cervical	Muscular strain, cervical trauma, torticollis/neck mass/retropharyngeal abscess, cervical malformation, atlantoaxial instability
Thoracic	Shoulder pathology/injury, rib fracture/dislocation, scoliosis (muscle spasm)
	Vertebral degeneration due to sickle cell disease, cystic fibrosis, Scheuermann disease, paraspinous muscle strain, pneumonia, asthma
Lumbar	Pneumonia
	Peptic ulcer disease/reflux
	Pregnancy
	Pancreatitis
	Pyelonephritis/nephrolithiasis
	Splenic infarction
	Psoas abscess
	Tuberculous spondylitis
	Osteomyelitis/diskitis
	Retrocolic appendicitis
	Spondylolysis/spondylolisthesis
	Scoliosis (muscle strain)
	Tumor
	Aortic aneurysm
	Juvenile rheumatoid arthritis
	Ankylosing spondylitis
	Ulcerative colitis/Crohn disease
	Constipation
Sacral/hip	Pregnancy/pelvic inflammatory disease
	Urinary obstruction
	Testicular tumor
	Slipped capital femoral epiphysis
	Legg-Calvé-Perthes disease
	Sciatica
	Pilonidal cyst/abscess
	Perirectal abscess
	Sacrococcygeal fracture
	Presacral teratoma
	Spina bifida
	Tethered cord
	Sacroiliac joint inflammation

loss. The diagnosis is suggested clinically and confirmed by computed tomography (CT), magnetic resonance imaging (MRI), or myelogram. The treatment is release of the tether.

2. *Spina bifida* is a congenital failure of the vertebrae to close posteriorly. Neural tissue can be involved, and the presentation and treatment are variable. *Diastematomyelia* is characterized by a lumbosacral hair tuft and is confirmed by CT of the spine. The lesion involves a bony spike that extends posteriorly and splits the cord in two longitudinally. If not treated, it may lead to progressive neurologic loss. The treatment is surgical removal of the spike.

3. *Klippel-Feil syndrome* is a congenital fusion of the cervical vertebrae. It appears as a triad: short neck, limited neck motion, and low hairline. The diagnosis is made by cervical spine roentgenograms. The condition usually is not surgically correctable, given the close proximity to the cord. Treatment is aimed at maintaining cervical flexibility through stretching exercises. *Sprengel deformity* is a related problem in which the scapula fails to descend to its normal anatomic position. The diagnosis, usually made on physical examination, may be confused with Klippel-Feil. Treatment is surgical correction.

4. Intrinsic bone problems, such as *osteogenesis imperfecta*, are rare but may predispose a child to easy fracturing of the vertebrae, leading to back pain. The diagnosis is made clinically, and the treatment is to avoid trauma to these patients.

5. *Sandifer syndrome* is due to gastroesophageal reflux and is characterized by the signs of reflux, torticollis, and opisthotonus. The diagnosis, which is made clinically, should be distinguished from seizures. The treatment is directed toward the underlying cause.

6. *Vitamin deficiencies* that cause bone and connective tissue abnormalities can lead to back pain. *Rickets* may result from a number of medical causes, including vitamin D deficiency. It is characterized by osteopenia and rachitic changes

Differential Diagnosis of Back Pain by Age-Groups

INFANT/PREVERBAL CHILD

May manifest only as irritability, physical deformity, or neurologic loss
Infection
Congenital malformation
Trauma (consider child abuse)
Vitamin deficiency (C, D)
Nephrolithiasis (premature infants receiving loop diuretics)
Presacral teratoma
Cord malformation (tethered cord)

VERBAL CHILD/PREADOLESCENT

Infection
Trauma (consider abuse/neglect)
Phenothiazine intoxication
Tumors
Hip pathology (toxic synovitis/avascular necrosis of the femoral head)
Collagen-vascular disease
Progressive congenital malformation (e.g., tethered cord)

ADOLESCENT

Trauma (acute and chronic)
"Overuse" syndrome
Postural problems
Pregnancy
Salpingitis
Muscle spasm due to scoliosis/failure to stretch
Tumors
Spondylolisthesis/spondylolysis
Scheuermann disease
Ankylosing spondylitis/Reiter syndrome
Slipped capital femoral epiphysis/sciatica
Diskitis
Drug abuse/malingering

in the skeleton, which may be seen on radiographic examination. *Scurvy* (vitamin C deficiency) is characterized by irritability, general tenderness, and "frog" positioned legs. The diagnosis is made clinically; it is treated by reversing the deficiency.

7. *Child abuse* should be considered in any infant with a severe injury or one that is unexplained by history.

Verbal/Preadolescent Child

Progression of an undetected congenital lesion may occur in the verbal or preadolescent child. Trauma and infection play a larger role in the differential diagnosis, as do neoplastic agents. Other considerations follow (see box):

1. *Pathologic condition of the hip*, including *Legg-Calvé-Perthes disease* (avascular necrosis of the femoral head), occurs more often in boys than in girls and is diagnosed by pelvic roentgenogram or bone scan. The treatment usually is rest or casting and is aimed at maintaining the normal anatomy of the femoral head and acetabulum. *Toxic synovitis*, a transient cause of hip pain, is relieved by rest. This condition is to be differentiated from *septic arthritis of the hip*, which is a medical emergency necessitating antibiotics and possible drainage of the infected joint.

2. *Phenothiazine toxicity* can occur acutely with akathisia and oculogyric crisis. The diagnosis and treatment usually are effected with a trial dose of diphenhydramine to reverse the toxic effects.

3. *Infections*, such as *vertebral osteomyelitis*, or *diskitis*, can occur in this age-group. The etiologic agent usually is *Staphylococcus aureus*, but other bacteria may be involved. The diagnosis usually is made by roentgenogram or bone scan, and treatment is directed toward the cause. *Bacterial* or *viral meningitis* may occur with neck stiffness, fever, and toxicity. The diagnosis and treatment are based on findings of cerebral spinal fluid examination. *Tuberculous spondylitis*, which is rare, can occur with progressive spine pain and muscle rigidity. The diagnosis and treatment are based on staining and culture of *Mycobacterium tuberculosis* from aspirated or biopsy specimens obtained from the affected vertebra. *Poliomyelitis*, which involves the anterior horn cells of the spinal cord, may cause neck pain and spinal stiffness, followed by flaccid paralysis and late atrophy of one or more muscle groups.

4. *Leukemia* may occur in this age-group, with bone pain as the initial symptom. Although vertebral degeneration is rare, it may accompany the neoplasm. Diagnosis is made by bone marrow examination, and treatment consists of multiple modalities. Other tumors include *neurofibromatosis*, *osteoid osteoma*, *osteoblastoma*, *aneurysmal bone cyst*, *Ewing sarcoma*, and *osteosarcoma*.

5. *Juvenile rheumatoid arthritis* may manifest in this age-group with sacroiliac tenderness and systemic signs such as weight loss and fever. The diagnosis is made clinically with radiographs that show progressive bony destruction. The erythrocyte sedimentation rate may be elevated, and many of the clinical tests that show positive findings in adults may reveal negative results in children despite active disease. *Crohn disease*, *ulcerative colitis*, *juvenile dermatomyositis*, *polymyositis*, and *myositis ossificans* also may occur, with back pain as part of the disease manifestation.

6. *Torticollis*, or wryneck, is a unilateral shortening of the sternocleidomastoid muscle caused by strain, birth trauma, muscle or nerve defects, neck infection, or central nervous system tumor. The diagnosis is made by physical examination, and the treatment is aimed at the underlying cause. In benign cases the treatment consists of stretching the affected muscle.

Adolescent

Many cases of back pain in adolescents can be attributed to trauma, overuse, or postural problems. Pain may be referred from other organ systems such as the renal and reproductive systems (e.g., pyelonephritis and pelvic inflammatory disease). Other conditions include the following (see box):

1. *Diskitis*, infection of the intervertebral disk space by *Staphylococcus aureus* (usually by hematogenous spread) can manifest with fever, limp, and splinting of the back. The

diagnosis is made by noting a narrowing of the disk space on roentgenogram or bone scan. The treatment is immobilization and appropriate antibiotics.

2. *Ankylosing spondylitis* can manifest (in males, predominantly) with stiffness, back pain, and arthritis when the sacroiliac joint is affected. There is a family association with human leukocyte antigen (HLA)–B27. The diagnosis is made clinically, and the treatment is aimed at prevention of joint destruction by immobilization and surgical intervention.

3. *Slipped capital femoral epiphyses* usually are found in obese males and may occur with limp and buttock pain that radiates to the knees. The diagnosis is made radiologically, and treatment usually consists of surgical correction.

4. *Scoliosis* (abnormal lateral curvature of the spine) and *kyphosis* (anterior curvature) usually are painless, abnormal curvatures in the spine. In severe cases, however, pain may be associated with muscle spasm because of stretching on the convex side and compression on the concave side of the spinal curve. The treatment is prevention of further progression, with bracing or casting; surgical correction may be required.

5. *Scheuermann disease*, or roundback deformity, is associated with severe thoracic kyphosis and anterior vertebral wedging as a result of osteochondrosis, which can be seen on lateral spinal roentgenograms. This condition may be mistaken for poor posture, but in Scheuermann disease there is midthoracic back pain that is accentuated with cough. The treatment is similar to that for scoliosis.

6. *Spondylolysis* is a defect in the pars interarticularis, usually between the fourth and fifth lumbar vertebrae, probably because of genetic predisposition and/or trauma. This is seen in persons who engage in sports such as gymnastics in which there is great potential for a hyperextension injury to the lumbosacral spine. *Spondylolisthesis* is an actual slipping of the fifth lumbar vertebra in relation to the first sacral vertebra. This produces radicular pain with tightening of the hamstrings, which may be noted on straight leg raising. The diagnosis is confirmed by roentgenogram or bone scan, and the treatment is variable, depending on the severity of the lesion.

7. *Bone tumors* may occur at any age, but more frequently they are noted at the time of adolescent growth spurt. The diagnosis is made by roentgenogram, CT scan, bone scan, or MRI. Surgery is the usual treatment. In benign tumors, such as osteoid osteoma, resection may be curative. In malignant tumors, such as Ewing or osteosarcoma, a multifaceted treatment approach may be required.

PSYCHOSOCIAL CONSIDERATIONS

Back pain as a result of *conversion reaction* has been reported in the literature.[4] This pain may be accompanied by "la belle indifférence" on the patient's part. A conversion reaction, however, must remain a diagnosis of exclusion, and the possibility of organic disease must not be discarded. A time lag of months can occur after presentation before the correct diagnosis is reached.[2] Repeated diagnostic tests, such as radiographs, CT scans, or bone scans may be warranted.

If conversion reaction is considered or suspected, psychiatric consultation should be obtained to elucidate the intrapsychic dynamics leading to the complaint. *Depression* may be a primary reason for back pain (a cry for help), or it may be secondary to chronic pain, aggravated by other issues. Intrafamilial dynamics also should be investigated.

In the child with an "organic" diagnosis, back pain may become a family focus if the patient is treated as a "*vulnerable" child* or if the pain becomes a controversial issue between the parents. Another diagnosis that may involve family members is *factitious illness* (Münchausen syndrome by proxy), in which the patient's illness is feigned by caretakers.

Back pain for secondary gain, *malingering*, is unusual in children, but it may be more frequent in adolescents. In this diagnosis a "reason" for the back pain may be apparent. Possible sources of "gain" are recreational drug acquisition, time off from work or school, or simply attention.

Drug and/or alcohol abuse should be considered, but not necessarily implicated, in any adolescent involved in a motor vehicle accident, particularly as the driver. Diskitis and vertebral osteomyelitis are believed to occur more frequently in intravenous drug abusers.

Issues of safety should be addressed in a younger child with traumatic injury. Car seats and protection from falls and other forms of injury need to be stressed before, not after, the injury occurs.

Finally, during the course of ongoing back pain that does or does not have a specific diagnosis, issues of pain management need to be considered. Relaxation, feedback techniques, and hypnosis have been used in treating some patients.

MANAGEMENT

The management of back pain begins with making an accurate diagnosis to determine the appropriate treatment. The acuity and severity of presentation also play a role, inasmuch as they determine the need for rapidity in making a diagnosis and instituting treatment.

Acute Management

In traumatic back or neck injuries, the spine, particularly the cervical spine, must be stabilized. If the trauma is severe, if there is an associated loss of consciousness, or if there is a possibility of an underlying spinal instability, as in Down syndrome, complete immobilization of the neck on a backboard by trained medical personnel is essential until a complete spinal examination is completed. Patients with mild trauma, nuchal tenderness, and no neurologic deficits may be stabilized with a Philadelphia collar until after evaluation is effected.

In cases in which there is traumatic neurologic loss, neurosurgical consultation should be sought to aid in evaluation and treatment of possible central nervous system damage. Certain radiologic procedures such as myelograms to rule out intraspinal tumors are best performed by trained personnel and under the direction of a neurosurgeon.

Radiographic and Laboratory Investigations

In acute traumatic cases, depending on the severity, radiographs of the spine may be warranted. This usually is the case in neck trauma accompanied by nuchal pain and/or neurologic deficits. When back pain does not involve the neck, is mild, and is not accompanied by neurologic loss, radiographs may be deferred. The spinal radiographs usually consist of anteroposterior and lateral views of the area of the spine in question. If oblique views are required, they should be obtained by radiologic technologists trained in the procedure. Chest, abdominal, pelvic, and bone roentgenograms may help in locating sources of referred back pain.

Other studies may elucidate spinal structure and function. By use of *computed tomography* areas of the spine that do not appear on standard roentgenograms, such as the spinal canal and nerve roots, can be visualized. *Bone scintigraphy* shows areas of inflammation such as those in diskitis and osteomyelitis. *Myelography* utilizes a radioopaque dye, such as metrizamide, to visualize masses within the spinal cord. *Magnetic resonance imaging* can obtain detailed views of the spinal canal and its contents.

Laboratory examinations, including urinalysis, complete blood count, and erythrocyte sedimentation rate, may be helpful in arriving at a diagnosis. The leukocyte count and the sedimentation rate may be elevated in inflammatory or infectious processes. Other laboratory tests that may be performed but that probably are less useful include HLA-B27 typing, usually present in juvenile rheumatoid arthritis (JRA) and ankylosing spondylitis, and tests for collagen-vascular disease, such as rheumatoid factor and antinuclear antibodies. In many cases these test results may be negative in the face of active disease in children. A pregnancy test should be performed on any female adolescent with back pain.

Conservative Therapy

Mild traumatic back pain without neurologic loss, including "overuse" syndromes, should be treated conservatively. If the pain does not improve within a reasonable period, further evaluation is warranted. A good rapport between patients and caretakers is needed to maintain follow-up. Conservative treatment consists of uninterrupted bed rest, analgesia, local heat applications, and possibly massage for muscle spasms. In the case of mild trauma, ice applications to the affected area may be helpful during the first 24 hours. Uninterrupted bed rest on a firm surface, with the hips and knees flexed, should be maintained for 1 to 2 weeks. Flexion reduces pressure on the lumbar spine. Occasionally a brace to minimize spinal movement is helpful for short periods.

Medications that can be used include antiinflammatory agents such as ibuprofen and tolmetin. Muscle relaxants such as diazepam and other benzodiazepines and opiate analgesics may alleviate anxiety, muscle spasm, and pain. These should be used in doses sufficient to control symptoms for a short time. Chemical dependency should concern the physician only if malingering for medication is suspected.

Back pain resistant to symptomatic therapy should be reevaluated periodically. The correct diagnosis in many cases may be delayed for months, even with reasonable medical scrutiny. Thus an open mind for a missed diagnosis should be maintained. Referral to an orthopedist is warranted in the case of nondiagnostic back pain that has not improved with compliant conservative therapy after several weeks.

Patient education is important to prevent the factors leading to back pain. The athlete needs instruction on proper warm-up or stretching exercises before physical exertion. Flexion exercises are important to avoid strain in the lumbar spine and to maintain its flexibility. Instruction in proper lifting techniques is helpful in preventing episodes of lower back strain in adolescents. Those patients with underlying spinal problems and their parents should be informed about the particular disease process, along with the precautions to take to avoid situations that can lead to back pain. If a brace is prescribed, instructions regarding its fitting and care should be given by experienced personnel.

REFERENCES

1. Benson D: The spine and neck. In Gershwin ME and Robbins DL: Musculoskeletal diseases of children, New York, 1986, Grune & Stratton, Inc.
2. Ehrlich M et al: Pediatric orthopedic pain of unknown origin, J Pediatr Orthop 6:460, 1986.
3. Bradford DS and Hensinger RM: The pediatric spine, New York, 1985, Thieme, Inc.
4. King H: Evaluating the child with back pain, Pediatr Clin North Am 33:1489, 1986.
5. Sponsellar P and Tolo V: Bone, joint and muscle problems. In Oski F et al, editors: Principles and practice of pediatrics, Philadelphia, 1990, JB Lippincott Co.
6. Turner P et al: Back pain in childhood, Spine 14:812, 1989.

SUGGESTED READINGS

Bunnell W: Back pain in children, Orthop Clin North Am 13:587, 1982.

Fitz C: Diagnostic imaging in children with spinal disorders, Pediatr Clin North Am 32:1537, 1985.

Hoffman H: Childhood and adolescent lumbar pain: differential diagnosis and management, Clin Neurosurg 27:533, 1980.

Stanitski C: Management of sports injuries in children and adolescents, Orthop Clin North Am 19:689, 1988.

Sullivan J: Recurrent pain in the pediatric athlete, Pediatr Clin North Am 31:1110, 1984.

114

Cardiac Arrhythmias

Edward B. Clark

Abnormalities of cardiac rhythm or conduction are a common pediatric cardiac problem. Arrhythmias in children are caused by disturbances in impulse formation or conduction, or both.

DEFINITIONS

Tachycardia is a persistent increase in heart rate greater than required to meet the activity state of the child. Tachycardias occur more frequently in newborns because of the immaturity of the cardiac conduction and autonomic nervous systems. Bradycardia is an abnormally slow heart rate most often caused by congenital heart block. Acquired heart block is exceedingly rare in childhood, usually occurring as a complication of viral myocarditis or of heart surgery.

DIAGNOSTIC METHODS

Children are often unaware of their abnormal cardiac rhythm. However, the physician can recognize them by using the following methods:

1. Examination. Arrhythmias are detected at the time of a physical examination by a heart beat that is irregular, too slow, or too fast.
2. Electrocardiogram. Electrocardiograms (ECGs) taken when the child is at rest and after exercise often document an arrhythmia. However, an individual with intermittent episodes may have a normal ECG between attacks.
3. Monitoring. A 24-hour ECG tape recording (Holter monitor apparatus) can document infrequent arrhythmias. An event monitor can transmit intermittent episodes by telephone to an ECG recorder.

ASSOCIATED SIGNS AND SYMPTOMS

Many children with cardiac arrhythmias are asymptomatic, or the physician notes only occasional skipped beats. In other children, syncope, dizziness, or lightheadedness can occur with the sudden decrease in cerebral blood flow that accompanies the onset of either paroxysmal tachycardia or sudden bradycardia. Congestive heart failure may be precipitated in infants who have sustained tachycardia of 250 to 300 beats per minute. Older children may complain of chest discomfort or of the heart racing when they have paroxysms of tachycardia; however, they rarely develop congestive heart failure.

CIRCUMSTANCES SURROUNDING PRESENTATION

Most episodes of paroxysmal tachycardia occur in the absence of heart disease or detectable electrolyte imbalance. They are found more commonly in males than in females, especially during the first few months of life, and are increasingly being detected in utero by fetal ultrasonic monitoring. Children with heart disease are more prone to arrhythmias than are their normal counterparts. Arrhythmias may also be a late postoperative complication following heart surgery.

ANATOMY AND FUNCTION OF THE CARDIAC CONDUCTION SYSTEM

The cardiac impulse is generated by the sinus node and conveyed by sequential components of the conduction system to depolarize the myocardium. The cardiac conduction system includes the sinus node innervated by the parasympathetic and sympathetic nerve fibers located at the junction of the superior vena cava and the right atrium. Fibers from the three atrial internodal pathways converge at the atrioventricular (AV) node, which is located at the mouth of the coronary sinus just above the insertion of the tricuspid valve. From the AV node, fibers form the His bundle, which branches into left and right ventricular bundles. The two fascicles of the left bundle, the broad posterior fascicle and the slender anterior fascicle, fan out over the endocardial surface of the left ventricle. The right bundle branch extends directly from the His bundle to the right side of the ventricular septum. The Purkinje network of the left and right ventricles is innervated by the left and right bundle branches and is the terminal portion of the conduction system that connects with the myocardial fibers.

TYPES OF DISORDERS

Supraventricular Arrhythmias

Supraventricular rhythm with normal conduction is characterized on the ECG by a narrow QRS complex. The origin of the impulse is indicated by the P wave and by the PR interval. The supraventricular pacemaker is normally the sinus node. An ectopic atrial focus generates an abnormal P-wave axis. With some supraventricular arrhythmias, the QRS complex is abnormal because of aberrant conduction below the His bundle.

Sinus Node

Normal sinus arrhythmia is the most common cause of an irregular heartbeat in a child (Fig. 114-1). The rate periodically slows and accelerates as respiration modulates vagal tone. Sometimes a sinus arrhythmia is so exaggerated that an ECG is needed to clarify the normal P-QRS relationship as the rate changes. *Sinus tachycardia* (Fig. 114-2) during exercise is normal, but during rest and in the absence of fever or cardiac failure it suggests the possibility of hyperthyroidism, ingestion of an atropine-like agent, or myocarditis. The smaller the baby, the higher the normal heart rate at rest. The usual range for a newborn is 110 to 150 beats per minute; for a toddler, 85 to 125; for a preschool child, 75 to 115; and for a child over 6 years of age, 60 to 100.

Sinus bradycardia is normal for a trained athlete but sufficiently unusual in children that possibilities such as hypothyroidism or increased intracranial pressure should be considered. Drugs such as propranolol produce sinus bradycardia by depressing the sinus pacemaker.

A *sinus pause* is an abrupt cessation of sinus node activity characterized on the ECG by the absence of the P wave and QRS complex. *Sinus node dysfunction* (Fig. 114-3) is a disorder in which the sinus node is an unstable pacemaker. During long sinus pauses, a lower atrial focus escapes at a slower rate or with bursts of tachycardia. The patient may have symptoms either with the period of asystole or tachycardia. Treatment may include an artificial pacemaker to prevent extreme bradycardia and antiarrhythmic therapy to control the tachycardia.

Atrium and Junctional Region (AV Node, His Bundle)

The atrium and junctional region possess latent pacemaker properties. They can be a focus of isolated beats or ectopic rhythm.

Ectopic Contractions

Ectopic contractions arise in atrial muscle (Fig. 114-4, *A*) or junctional tissue (Fig. 114-4, *B*). With atrial ectopic beats, the P-wave axis is abnormal. Junctional ectopic beats show no P wave or a P wave with a short PR interval. The ectopic beats occur as escape beats when the sinus node slows, or they may occur prematurely. Although a premature atrial beat may trigger a reentry tachycardia, treatment is usually not necessary.

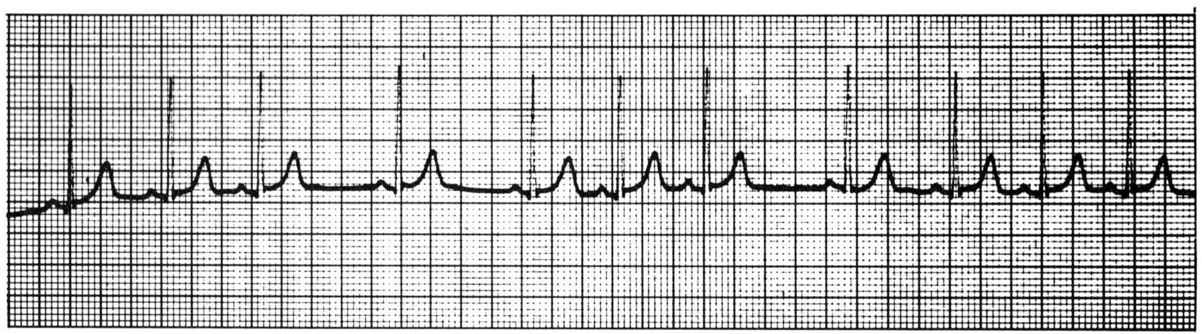

Fig. 114-1 Sinus arrhythmia. Note the regular variation in the RR interval, which varies with respiration.

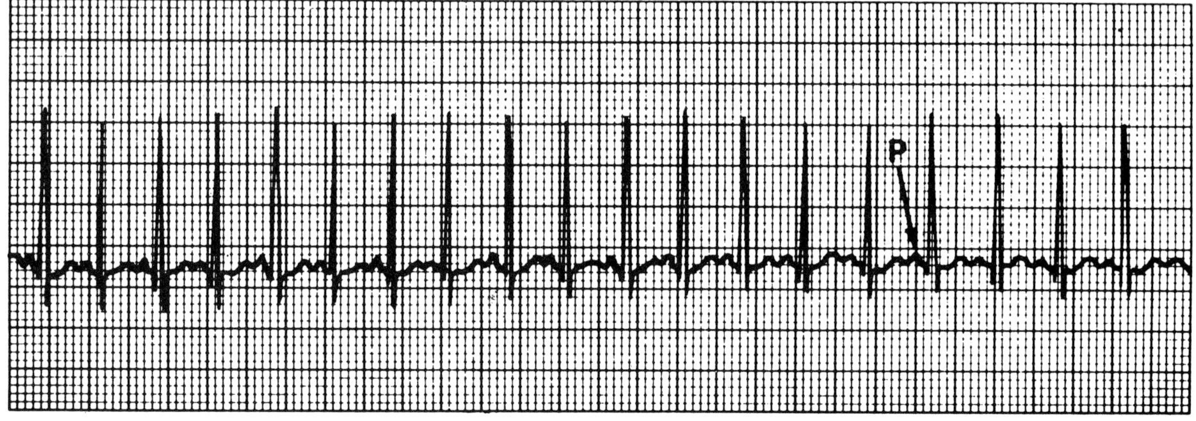

Fig. 114-2 Sinus tachycardia. Each QRS is preceded by a P wave and has a normal PR interval.
From Clark EB: In Cohen SA, editor: Pediatric emergency management, New Jersey, 1982, Prentice Hall.

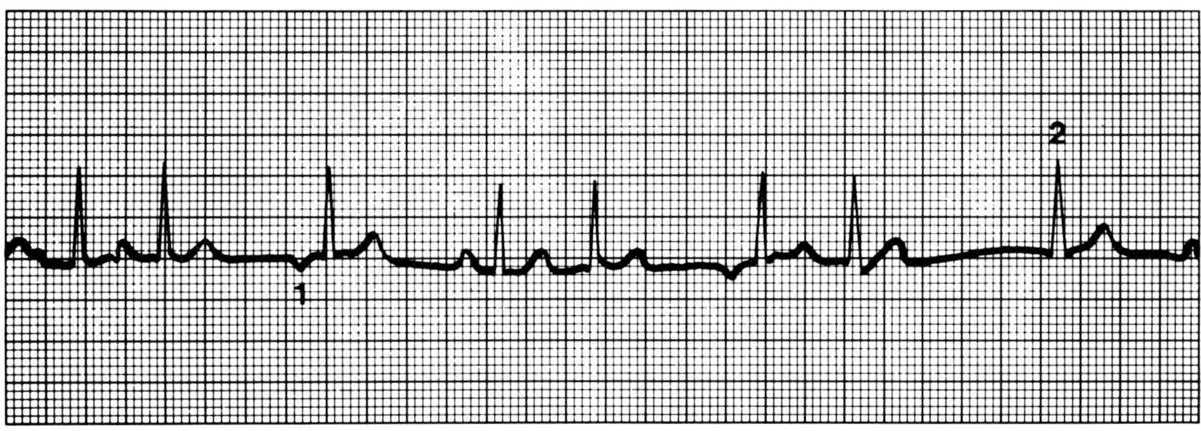

Fig. 114-3 Sinus node dysfunction is characterized by *(1)* ectopic atrial beats and *(2)* junctional escape beats.
From Clark EB: In Cohen SA, editor: Pediatric emergency management, New Jersey, 1982, Prentice Hall.

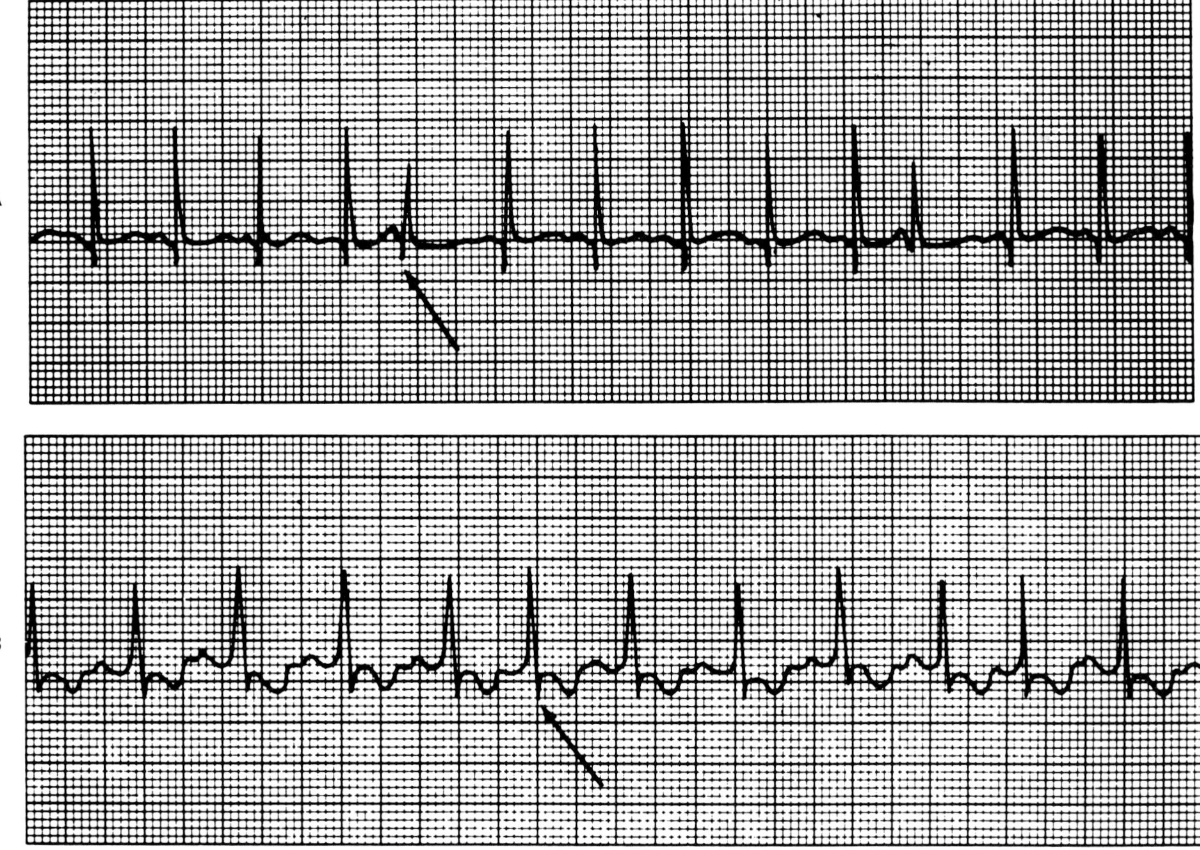

Fig. 114-4 A, Premature atrial contraction has an abnormal P wave *(arrow)* preceding the QRS. **B,** Premature junctional contraction *(arrow)* has no preceding P wave.
From Clark EB: In Cohen SA, editor: Pediatric emergency management, New Jersey, 1982, Prentice Hall.

Supraventricular Tachyarrhythmias

Supraventricular tachycardia (SVT) is the most common tachyrhythmia in children (Fig. 114-5). The heart rate is usually regular and too fast to count (220 to 280 beats per minute), and all leads of the ECG show a narrow QRS and regular RR interval.

Treatment depends on the duration of the tachycardia and the child's symptoms. SVT can often be terminated by an increase in vagal tone from a Valsalva maneuver or by applying an ice-cold washcloth to the face. For tachycardias unresponsive to vagal maneuvers, the child can be treated with adenosine to interrupt transiently the conduction through the AV node. Infants in shock or congestive heart failure should have immediate direct current (DC) cardioversion.

Some infants and children with supraventricular tachycardia have *Wolff-Parkinson-White (WPW) syndrome* (Fig. 114-6). After conversion to sinus rhythm, their ECG shows a short PR interval and a prolonged QRS complex, with a delta wave initiating the QRS. An anomalous connection between the atrium and ventricle serves as a bypass tract for the reentry tachycardia. Children may be treated with digoxin or propranolol to reduce their episodes. Patients with recurrent attacks unresponsive to medical management may require surgical interruption of the bypass tract.

Atrial flutter (Fig. 114-7) is a combination of very rapid atrial activity (280 to 300 beats per minute) and variable AV block. The degree of block may vary but often ranges from 2:1 to 4:1 in the ratio of atrial to ventricular impulses. The ECG shows large sawtoothed flutter waves that undulate along the baseline. *Atrial fibrillation* (Fig. 114-8) is disordered, rapid atrial activity with a slower ventricular rate because of varying AV block. It is the least common of the supraventricular tachyarrhythmias in pediatric practice. No P wave is visible in an ECG, but the baseline may show small, irregular, rapid fibrillary waves and an irregular RR interval. These rhythms can be treated by slowing conduction at the AV node with digoxin and quinidine or by cardioversion.

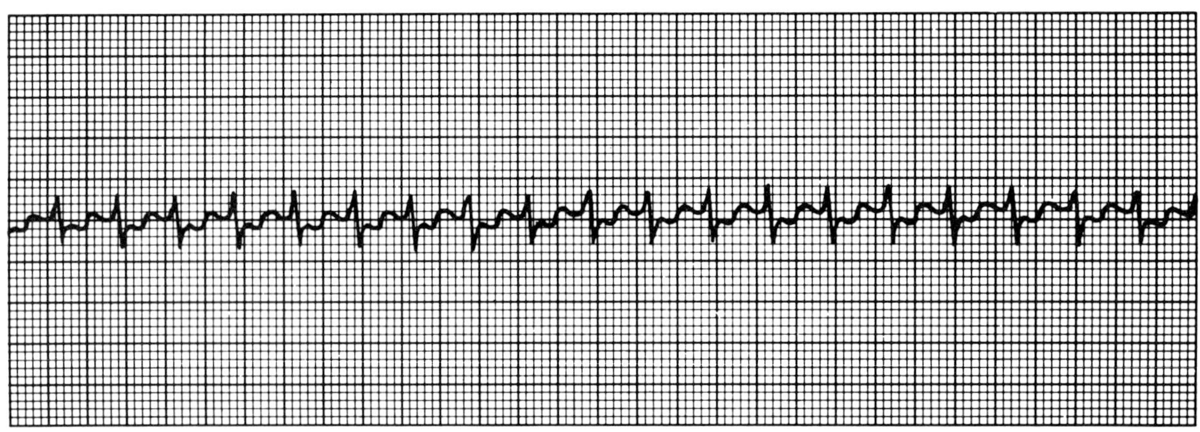

Fig. 114-5 Supraventricular tachycardia is characterized by a narrow QRS complex and no identifiable P wave.
From Clark EB: In Cohen SA, editor: Pediatric emergency management, New Jersey, 1982, Prentice Hall.

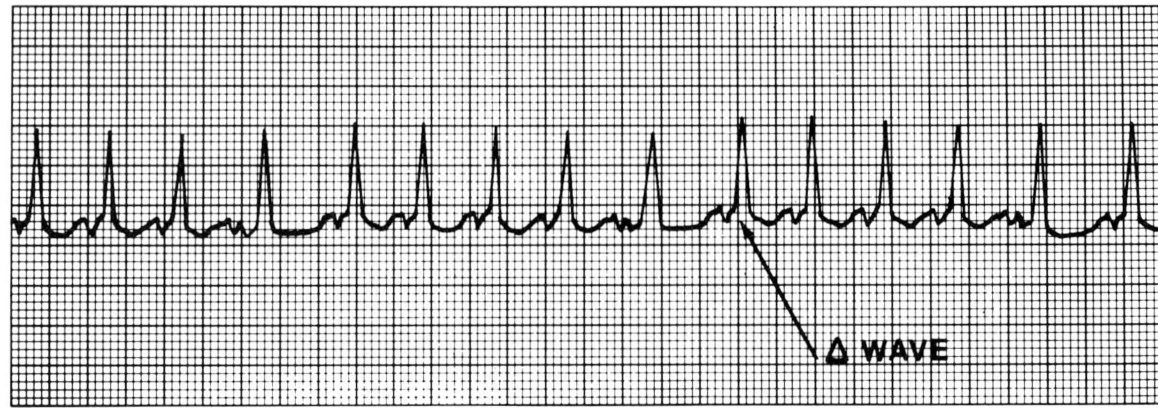

Fig. 114-6 Preexcitation syndrome has a short PR interval and a delta wave *(arrow)*, reflecting early activation of the ventricular myocardium.
From Clark EB: In Cohen SA, editor: Pediatric emergency management, New Jersey, 1982, Prentice Hall.

Ventricular Arrhythmias

Ventricular arrhythmias are almost as common as arrhythmias of supraventricular origin. Most ventricular premature beats are benign when cardiac function is normal.

Ventricular Ectopic Beats

Premature ventricular contractions (PVCs) are usually unifocal (Fig. 114-9); if multifocal, the prognosis is less favorable. Typically the QRS complex is wide and the ST segments and T waves of the repolarization phase are abnormal. Premature ventricular contractions are usually benign if they are (1) unifocal arising from the high right ventricle, (2) suppressed with exercise, and (3) have a fixed coupled RR interval. Premature ventricular contractions may be serious if they are (1) multifocal in origin, (2) increase with exercise, (3) occur in patients with a history of heart surgery, (4) have a variable PR coupling, (5) have an R wave that falls on the T wave, and (6) occur in pairs or triplets. Benign PVCs require no treatment. Multifocal PVCs require investigation and treatment with phenytoin or propranolol.

Ventricular Tachycardia

Ventricular tachycardia is defined as four or more ectopic beats occurring in sequence. Ventricular tachycardia may come and go in bursts (repetitive tachycardia) or may be sustained, usually at a rate of about 150 to 180 beats per minute. A child may notice palpitations, faint, or become hypotensive. Ventricular tachycardia is life threatening because of the possible progression to ventricular flutter or fibrillation. ECG diagnosis of ventricular tachycardia is based on wide, bizarre QRS complexes and the absence of P waves preceding each QRS complex.

Ventricular tachycardia is one complication of long QT

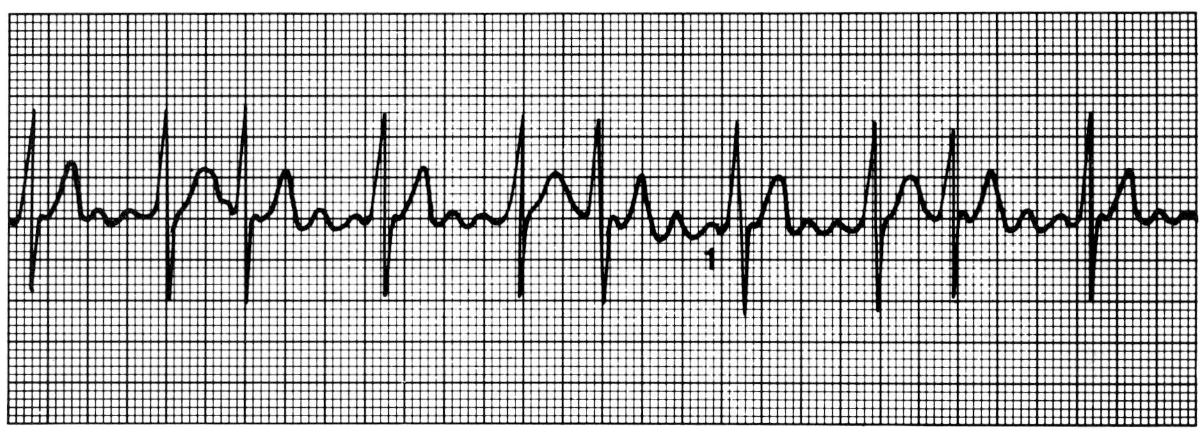

Fig. 114-7 Atrial flutter has coarse, sawtoothed flutter waves (1).
From Clark EB: In Cohen SA, editor: Pediatric emergency management, New Jersey, 1982, Prentice Hall.

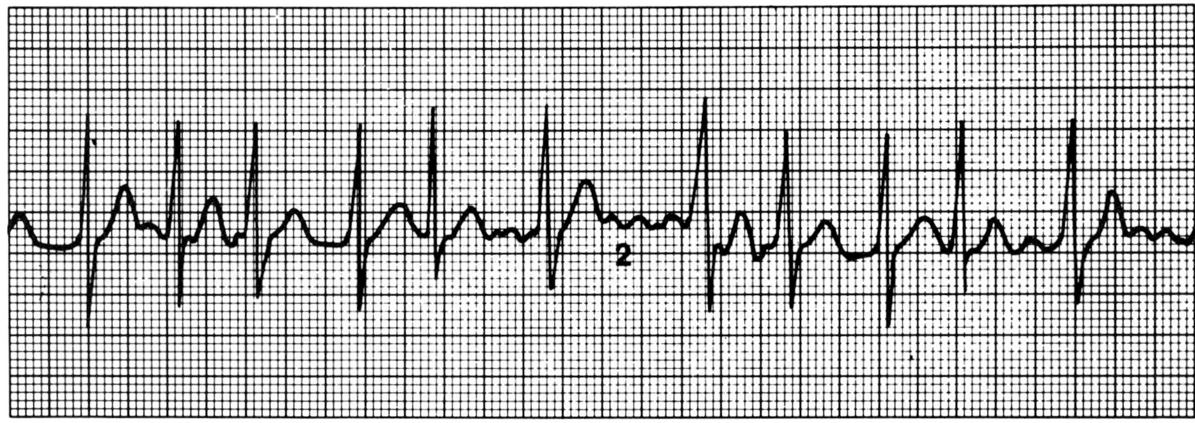

Fig. 114-8 Atrial fibrillation has fine fibrillation waves (2).
From Clark EB: In Cohen SA, editor: Pediatric emergency management, New Jersey, 1982, Prentice Hall.

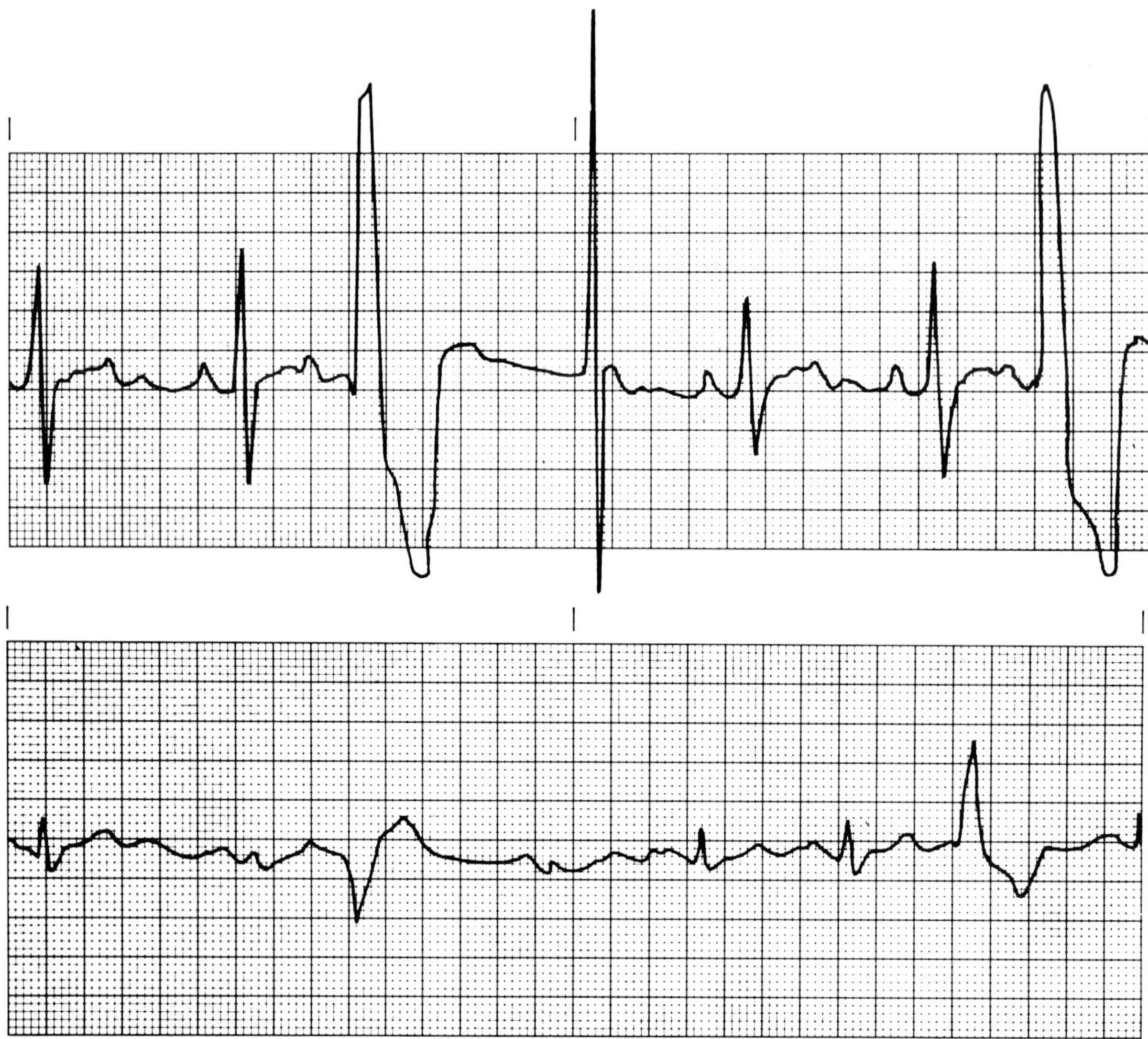

Fig. 114-9 Premature ventricular contractions. Benign unifocal PVC *(top)* and multifocal PVC *(bottom)*.
From Clark EB: In Cohen SA, editor: Pediatric emergency management, New Jersey, 1982, Prentice Hall.

syndrome (Fig. 114-10). Patients with delayed repolarization of the ventricle have a corrected QT interval and may have episodes of ventricular tachycardia that manifest as syncope and atypical seizures. Long QT syndrome may be isolated or familial and sometimes may be associated with sensorineural hearing loss. A child with unexplained syncope or an atypical seizure should have an ECG analyzed for abnormalities of the QT interval. Treatment includes using a beta-blocking agent and sometimes a pacemaker.

Ventricular Fibrillation

Ventricular fibrillation is a chaotic, disorganized, ineffective ventricular rhythm. A patient with ventricular fibrillation must be immediately defibrillated with a direct current precordial shock, because this rhythm is rapidly fatal without therapy.

DISTURBANCES OF CONDUCTION

AV Block

First-degree AV block (Fig. 114-11, *A*) occurs when the impulse is abnormally delayed in junctional tissue so that the PR interval is prolonged, but each impulse is conducted to the ventricles. AV conduction is prolonged if the PR interval exceeds 0.116 second in an infant, 0.18 second in a child, and 0.20 second in an adolescent or adult.

Second-degree AV block (Fig. 114-11, *B*) occurs when some of the impulses fail to conduct to the ventricles. This rhythm can occur with rheumatic carditis, digoxin toxicity, electrolyte disturbance, and in complex heart defects. Mobitz type I block exhibits Wenckebach periodicity—that is, the PR interval gradually lengthens until a beat drops out. Mobitz type II block is an abrupt block, usually of every second beat

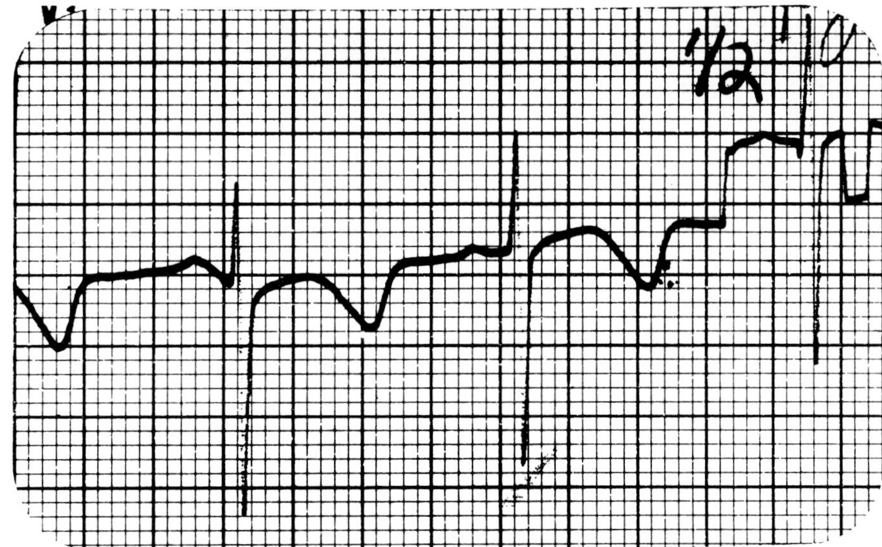

Fig. 114-10 Long QT syndrome has a prolonged recovery of ventricular myocardium.
From Clark EB: In Cohen SA, editor: Pediatric emergency management, New Jersey, 1982, Prentice Hall.

(2:1 block), resulting from a disturbance in the conduction system distal to the AV node (in or below the His bundle).

Third-degree AV block (Fig. 114-4, *C*) is complete heart block. The atrial rate is faster than the ventricular rate. When the QRS complex is narrow, the block is usually proximal to the AV node and His bundle. When the QRS complex is wide, the block may be proximal to the His bundle (in a case of bundle-branch block) or the interruption may be distal to the His bundle. Congenital complete heart block is often noted in children of mothers with lupus erythematosus. In some cases the maternal diagnosis is not made until decades after an affected child's birth. Complete heart block can be a complication of the intracardiac repair of congenital heart defects. Symptomatic patients are treated with a permanent transvenous pacemaker.

MANAGEMENT

Table 114-1 summarizes the drugs, dosages, and toxic effects of the most commonly used antiarrhythmic drugs. Electrophysiologic studies may be needed to guide therapy if an arrhythmia does not respond to the usual drugs. Management of complex cardiac arrhythmias should be referred to a pediatric cardiologist.

Digoxin. Digoxin is used to treat supraventricular tachycardia, atrial flutter, or atrial fibrillation. There is a narrow margin of safety with digoxin. Extreme care must be taken in calculating drug doses and administration frequency.

Quinidine. Quinidine reduces conduction by inhibiting diastolic repolarization; it decreases conduction velocity by lowering the resting membrane potential and decreasing the maximum rate of depolarization. It also prolongs the refractory period by altering the duration of the action potential.

Procainamide. This quinidine-like agent increases the refractory period and conduction time in the atrium, the ventricle, and the junctional region.

Lidocaine. Intravenous lidocaine can be used in the initial treatment of ventricular tachycardia. It converts the rhythm to normal and maintains it that way until the cause can be corrected or until maintenance therapy with another drug in the group of myocardial depressants is instituted.

Propranolol. Propranolol, a beta-adrenergic blocking agent, reduces the heart rate and the contractile force of the heart; thus, it is contraindicated in patients with cardiac failure. Propranolol is effective against ventricular and supraventricular tachyarrhythmias, but its special usefulness is in situations in which there is (1) a central nervous system component to the arrhythmia, (2) a digitalis-toxicity rhythm, or (3) recurrent tachycardia associated with Wolff-Parkinson-White syndrome.

Phenytoin. Phenytoin (Dilantin) is used to treat ventricular arrhythmias and may counteract the depressant effect of procainamide. It depresses ventricular automaticity and enhances AV conduction.

Adenosine. Adenosine produces a transient complete block at the AV node, interrupting reentry tachycardia. Adenosine is the drug of choice for the conversion of supraventricular tachycardia in children.

Increased Vagal Tone

For children with repetitive or sustained supraventricular tachycardia, increasing vagal tone may terminate the attack. Vagal tone can be increased by Valsalva maneuver or ice water dive reflex. Older children and adolescents with infrequent attacks can be taught to manage their attacks themselves. Pressing on the eyeball as a means to increase vagal tone should never be done, because it can produce retinal detachment.

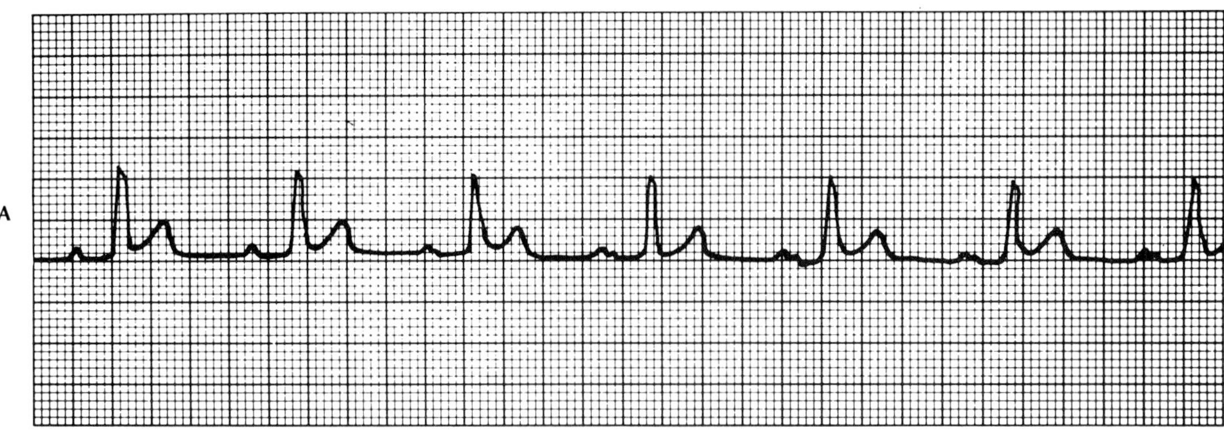

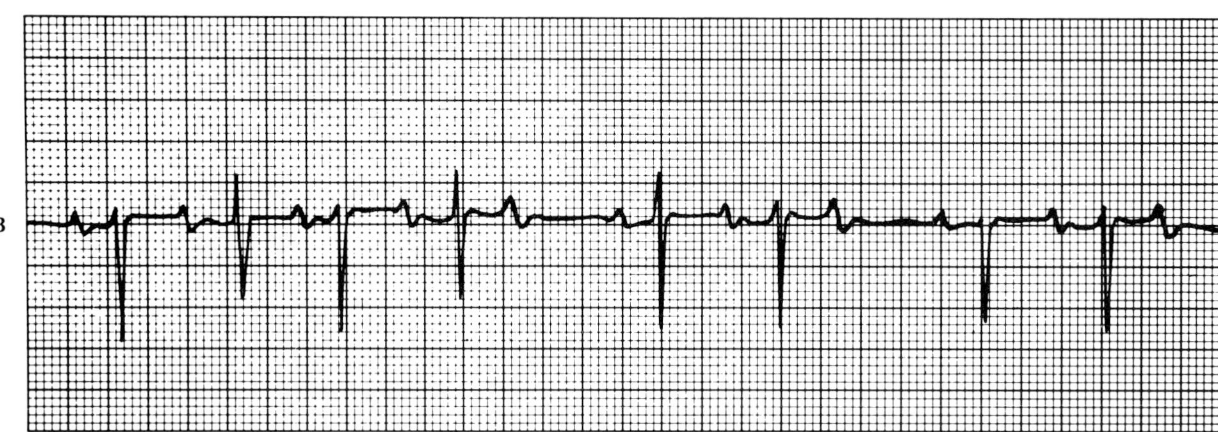

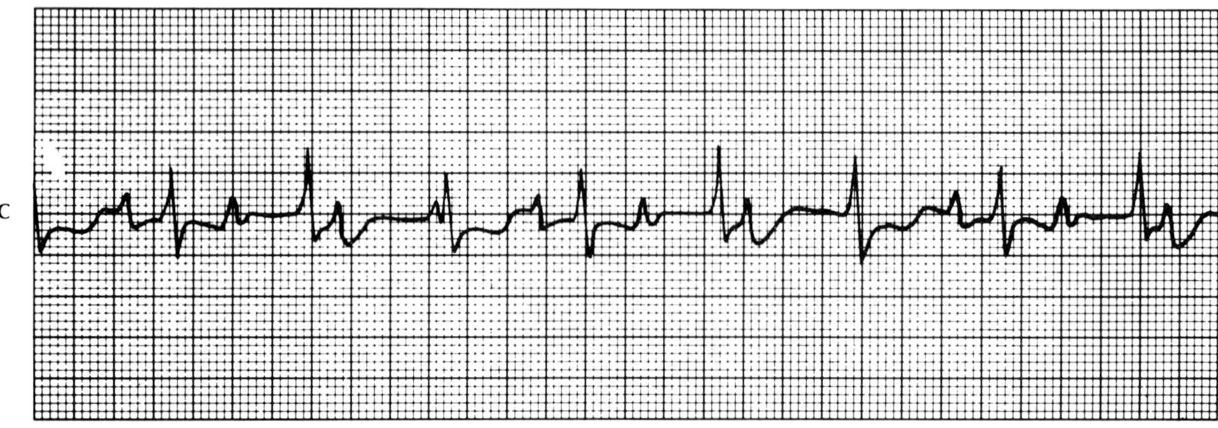

Fig. 114-11 AV heart block. **A,** First degree. **B,** Second degree. **C,** Third degree. See text for details.
From Clark EB: In Cohen SA, editor: Pediatric emergency management, New Jersey, 1982, Prentice Hall.

Table 114-1 *Common Antiarrhythmic Agents*

DRUGS	INITIAL THERAPY	MAINTENANCE THERAPY	TOXIC EFFECTS
Digoxin	Digitalization 20-40 μg/kg divided in four equal doses	PO, 1/4 digitalizing dose/day	Heart block, ectopy
Quinidine	PO, 2 mg/kg every test dose	PO, 4-10 mg/kg every 6 hr	Rash, fever, gastrointestinal (GI) symptoms, purpura, hemolytic anemia, hypotension
Procainamide	IV, 2 mg/kg of 1:10 dilution over 5 minutes	PO, 5-15 mg/kg every 6 hr	Lupuslike syndrome, hypotension, urticaria, GI symptoms
Lidocaine	IV, 1 mg/kg of 1:1000 dilution over 3-5 minutes; up to 5 mg/kg	IV, 0.03 mg/kg/minute of dilute solution of 5 mg/ml; decrease rate as arrhythmia continues to be controlled	Convulsions, drowsiness, euphoria, muscle twitching
Phenytoin	IV, 10-15 mg/kg over 5 minutes	PO, 2 mg/kg tid	Hypotension, ataxia
Propranolol	IV, 0.01-0.15 mg/kg over 3-5 minutes	PO, 0.05-1 mg/kg/day divided, every 6 hr	Bradycardia, hypotension, cardiac failure, asthma
Isoproterenol	IV, 0.1-1.0 μg/kg/minute	Infusion adjusted to maintain stable rhythm and rate	Ventricular ectopic beats, tachycardia
Atropine	IV, 0.01-0.03 mg/kg (0.15 mg minimum; 0.5 mg maximum flushing)		Mydriasis, dry mouth
Adenosine	IV, 0.05-0.25 mg/kg/dose IV push	None	Blocks AV node conduction to convert SVT

Direct Current (DC) Cardioversion

A direct current precordial shock terminates chaotic atrial and ventricular arrhythmias. Elective cardioversion should be accomplished by a team familiar with the cardioverter and with equipment that is checked regularly for proper performance. Patients should be anesthetized while the shock is delivered. Once the tachyrhythmia has been converted, antiarrhythmic medication is often needed to prevent recurrence.

Catheter Pacing

A cardiac pacemaker can be used for the control of cardiac arrhythmias. A transvenous pacing catheter is positioned in the atrial or ventricular chamber, or both, to stimulate the heart sequentially. Indications for permanent cardiac pacing include complete heart block, ventricular tachycardia, and sinus node dysfunction.

Surgery

Surgical ablation of accessory bypass tracts or ectopic foci is effective for managing patients unresponsive to the usual methods of control described above.

SUMMARY

The practitioner plays an important role in identifying children with arrhythmias and directing them to the pediatric cardiologist for evaluation and treatment. The pediatrician also supports the family and provides reassurance to those with benign arrhythmias.

SUGGESTED READING

Adams FH, Emmanouilides GC, and Riemenschneider TA: Heart disease in infants, children, and adolescents, ed 4, Baltimore, 1989, Williams & Wilkins.

115

Chest Pain

Beryl J. Rosenstein

Although not as common or bothersome as abdominal pain or headache, chest pain is frequently encountered in pediatric patients, particularly among preadolescents and adolescents.[1,7,10,11] The major causes are benign; chest pain in children rarely is associated with serious organic disease. However, parents and often the patient are concerned that chest pain indicates heart trouble; if only for this reason, a careful evaluation is indicated. It is important to strike a balance between a cursory evaluation that is less than reassuring to the family and an overly elaborate workup that tends to reinforce the idea of underlying organic disease. In the evaluation of the patient with chest pain, a careful history and physical examination provide the most information. Laboratory procedures, other than a chest roentgenogram, a complete blood count, and an electrocardiogram, usually are not indicated and rarely are helpful.[10,11]

The history should include an accurate description of the pain, including the duration, character, intensity, location, radiation, relation to meals, and precipitating and modifying factors. Pain of pleural origin usually is sharp, stabbing, and superficial. It is accentuated by deep breaths, cough, or movement of the upper portion of the body and tends to disappear when the breath is held in expiration. Parietal pleural pain usually is localized over the involved area, whereas diaphragmatic pleural pain may be referred to the base of the neck or to the abdomen. Pain of pericardial origin may be of three distinct types: pleuritic pain, which is aggravated by a deep breath or cough; steady crushing substernal pain similar to that of a myocardial infarction; or pain along the left heart border and left shoulder that is synchronous with the heart beat. Information should be elicited regarding other somatic complaints, drug use (including cocaine and oral contraceptives), sleep disturbances, school problems, syncope, shortness of breath, history of choking, decreased exercise tolerance, and interferences with usual activities. A history of recent trauma or a temporal relationship to sports activities or exercise sometimes is helpful. A description of psychosocial and environmental factors and family illnesses also is pertinent.

The physical examination should focus on the heart, lungs, and musculoskeletal structures of the chest wall. Findings that are helpful in determining the cause of chest pain include abnormal breath sounds, heart murmurs, tender breast masses, chest splinting, bruising, pericardial and pleural friction rubs, subcutaneous crepitus, swelling of chest wall articulations, and the rash of herpes zoster.

Although it is unusual for serious disease to manifest as chest pain in children and teenagers, chest pain may be associated with pneumothorax, pneumomediastinum, gastritis, esophagitis, peptic ulcer disease, thoracic outlet syndrome, esophageal foreign bodies, Fitz-Hugh-Curtis syndrome, asthma, pneumonia, pulmonary embolus, tumors, hemoglobinopathies, and cardiac abnormalities. In these cases the underlying disease often is readily diagnosed. In about 50% of the patients who seek medical care for chest pain an underlying cause will be found (see accompanying box).

Causes of Chest Pain in Children and Adolescents

CARDIAC DISEASE

Anomalous coronary artery, coronary arteritis
Cardiomyopathy, myocarditis, pericarditis
Left ventricular outflow obstruction
Mitral valve prolapse
Tachyarrhythmias

CHEST WALL SYNDROME

Costochondritis, Tietze syndrome
Hypersensitive xiphoid
Muscle strain, trauma
Slipping rib syndrome
Tender breast masses

GASTROINTESTINAL CONDITIONS

Esophageal burns, foreign bodies
Esophageal dysmotility
Esophagitis, gastritis, peptic ulcer disease

MISCELLANEOUS

Cigarette smoking, cocaine
Fitz-Hugh-Curtis syndrome
Hemoglobinopathy with vasoocclusive crisis
Tumors

PRECORDIAL CATCH SYNDROME

PSYCHOGENIC FACTORS

PULMONARY CONDITIONS

Asthma, cough
Pleuritis, pleurodynia, pneumonia
Pneumomediastinum
Pneumothorax
Pulmonary embolism

The most common identifiable causes of chest pain are related to chest wall abnormalities, including traumatic injuries, muscle strain, a hypersensitive xiphoid bone, and costochondritis.[4,6] *Costochondritis* is most common in female adolescents.[4] There is sharp pain that originates in the anterior chest, may radiate, and may persist for several months; no relationship to position, respiration, or activity exists. Most important, the pain can be reproduced by firm palpation over the involved rib cartilage. Treatment includes reassurance, avoidance of strenuous activity, analgesics, and local heat. In patients with severe pain, local injection of lidocaine or administration of corticosteroids, or both, may help. *Slipping rib syndrome* is an unusual cause of chest pain, probably related to trauma to the costal cartilages of the eighth, ninth, and tenth ribs.[8] The patient feels a slipping movement of the ribs, sometimes accompanied by a clicking or popping sound. The pain can be reproduced by grasping the affected rib margin and pulling it anteriorly.

Chest pain in pediatric patients is infrequently caused by clinically significant *cardiac disease*.[10,11] Adolescents, however, often equate chest pain with a heart attack or heart disease, and chest pain has become a major reason for pediatric cardiology referrals.[3] Organic cardiac disease that produces chest pain can be categorized in three major groups: (1) structural abnormalities such as left-ventricular outflow obstruction, anomalous coronary artery, coronary arteritis (Kawasaki disease), and mitral valve prolapse; (2) acquired myopericardial inflammatory disease; and (3) rhythm disturbances such as supraventricular tachycardia. Pain that occurs fairly consistently with exercise but not at other times should raise concern of heart disease, but it also may be a manifestation of exercise-induced asthma. Except in the case of paroxysmal arrhythmias the history and physical examination usually will exclude most cardiac causes of chest pain. In a patient with suspected *mitral valve prolapse* (Barlow syndrome), it is important to examine the patient in the supine and the upright position to elicit the characteristic midsystolic click and late systolic murmur (honk). The chest pain associated with mitral valve prolapse usually is sharp or "sticking" in quality, midprecordial in location, and unrelated to exercise. The pain usually is mild and requires no treatment. If, however, treatment is necessary, propranolol may be helpful. Echocardiographic examination, Holter monitoring, and exercise stress testing may be necessary in the evaluation of a patient with a suspected cardiac lesion, but in general these procedures add little additional diagnostic information.

In patients with unexplained chest pain it is important to consider a *gastrointestinal* cause, including esophagitis, gastritis, peptic ulcer disease, and abnormalities of esophageal motility.[2] The pain often is described as an uncomfortable burning sensation below the sternum. The symptoms of gastrointestinal-related chest pain often are nonspecific, however, and the underlying cause may be uncovered only by esophageal manometry, esophageal pH probe monitoring, and fiberoptic endoscopy.[2] Before embarking on an extensive gastrointestinal evaluation, a therapeutic trial of an antacid or a histamine-2 (H_2) blocker usually is indicated.

Pleurodynia, caused chiefly by group B coxsackievirus, usually occurs with sudden onset of severe, stabbing paroxysmal pleuritic pain over the lower rib cage and substernal areas. The pain is aggravated by deep breathing, movement, and coughing. It usually is preceded or accompanied by fever, headache, malaise, anorexia, myalgias, and an unproductive cough. With the exception of a pleural friction rub, which is present in 25% of patients, examination of the chest reveals no significant findings. The clinical course of the disease takes from 1 to 14 days, and treatment is directed at the symptoms.

Tietze syndrome, a form of costochondritis, usually occurs in teenagers; it is characterized by chest pain, which often is intense, and a firm, tender, fusiform swelling of one or more of the upper costal cartilages or sternoclavicular joints for which no specific cause can be found.[5] A biopsy specimen of the involved area reveals normal cartilage. The course is prolonged, and recurrences are common. It is important to reassure the patient as to the benign, self-limited nature of the disorder.

Adolescents may experience recurrent brief episodes of sudden, sharp, but not distressing pain localized near the cardiac apex. The pain usually occurs along the left sternal border or beneath the left breast, does not radiate, may have a pleuritic component, and typically occurs at rest or during mild exercise. It may be relieved by shallow breathing, a single deep inspiration, or a change in posture. This symptom complex has been referred to as the *precordial catch syndrome* or *Texidor's twinge*.[12] Treatment consists of reassurance as to the benign nature of the episodes. In adolescents, chest pain may be related to cigarette smoking. Severe chest pain of sudden onset may occur in association with the use of cocaine.[13] A urine toxicology screen will help clarify the diagnosis.

Even after a complete history, physical examination, and pertinent laboratory procedures, a specific cause will not be found in 30% to 50% of cases of chest pain in children.[1,7,10] A cardiorespiratory cause for chest pain is more common in younger children, whereas a psychogenic origin is more likely in adolescents,[10,11] especially girls. The presence of pain that awakens a child, pain of acute onset, fever, and abnormal findings on physical examination suggest underlying organic disease. Constant pain usually is more significant than brief intermittent episodes of pain. The presence of chronic pain of more than 6 months' duration and a family history of chest pain or heart disease suggest nonorganic disease.[10] In general, the longer the complaint of chest pain has been present, the less likely one is to find a specific underlying disorder. Laboratory tests are not generally helpful in establishing a specific diagnosis.[10] They usually reveal previously known or clinically suspected problems or confirm abnormalities uncovered by history and physical examination.[10] Chest roentgenograms and electrocardiograms should not be obtained unless indicated by the history and physical examination. In cases in which a specific cause is not identified, management consists of reassurance and observation. The prognosis for these patients is excellent.[9] Most will become symptom free. It is unusual for organic disease to appear after an initial assessment reveals negative findings, and the appearance of new functional symptoms is uncommon.

In some so-called idiopathic cases, however, there is undoubtedly a *psychogenic* basis for the complaint of chest pain.[1] In these patients a specific stressful situation causally related to the onset of the complaint usually is identified.

There is often a history of other recurrent somatic complaints, school problems, or significant sleep disturbances, along with a history of chest pain or serious illness in other family members. The pain may be associated with hyperventilation that, by itself, may lead to chest pain. The diagnosis of psychogenic chest pain should not be arrived at on the basis of exclusion but rather should be based on a history of a precipitating event along with evidence of significant underlying psychopathologic factors. Therapy consists of appropriate counseling for the patient and other involved family members.

REFERENCES

1. Asnes RS, Santulli R, and Bemporad JR: Psychogenic chest pain in children, Clin Pediatr 20:788, 1981.
2. Berezin S et al: Chest pain of gastrointestinal origin, Arch Dis Child 63:1457, 1988.
3. Brenner JI and Berman MA: Chest pain in childhood and adolescence, J Adolesc Health Care 3:271, 1983.
4. Brown RT: The adolescent with costochondritis, Compr Ther 14:27, 1988.
5. Calabro JJ and Marchesano JM: Tietze's syndrome: report of a case with juvenile onset, J Pediatr 68:985, 1966.
6. Calabro JJ et al: Classification of anterior chest wall syndromes, JAMA 243:1420, 1980.
7. Driscoll DJ, Glicklich LB, and Gallen WJ: Chest pain in children: a prospective study, Pediatrics 57:648, 1976.
8. Porter GE: Slipping rib syndrome: an infrequently recognized entity in children. A report of three cases and review of the literature, Pediatrics 76:810, 1985.
9. Rowland TW and Richards MM: The natural history of idiopathic chest pain in children, Clin Pediatr 25:612, 1986.
10. Selbst SM: Evaluation of chest pain in children, Pediatr Rev 8:56, 1986.
11. Selbst SM et al: Pediatric chest pain: a prospective study, Pediatrics 82:319, 1988.
12. Sparrow MJ and Bird EL: "Precordial catch": a benign syndrome of chest pain in young persons, NZ Med J 88:325, 1978.
13. Woodward GA and Selbst SM: Chest pain secondary to cocaine use, Pediatr Emerg Care 3:153, 1987.

116

Constipation

T. Emmett Francoeur

The term *constipation* refers primarily to a diminished frequency of defecation. In this chapter, *stool retention* is used as a synonym inasmuch as it implies both low frequency of bowel movements and incomplete evacuation. The tendency to retain feces may develop very early in life, may lead to persistent distress through childhood and into adult life, and may predispose the person to a variety of psychological and medical sequelae. The phrase *dysfunctional stool retention* is used to refer to the "problem" of constipation, which includes both the symptom itself and the negative secondary psychosocial consequences. Early identification and successful treatment of this problem may reduce morbidity during later years.

PREDISPOSING FACTORS

A small proportion of children with chronic stool retention have an underlying anomaly or disease. In encountering this symptom, pediatricians most often and primarily are concerned with ruling out aganglionic megacolon (Hirschsprung disease). With increasing age the likelihood that stool retention is the result of aganglionic megacolon becomes increasingly small. Table 116-1 summarizes the clinical differences between aganglionic megacolon and chronic dysfunctional stool retention.

Other congenital abnormalities, however, can predispose a patient to stool retention. Anal strictures and stenoses (very uncommon) may appear early in life and lead to considerable pain and retention of feces. Stool retention or fecal incontinence, or both, may develop in patients who have undergone surgery for imperforate anus. This complication may result from congenital anatomic abnormalities or may be introduced by surgery.

Anal fissures (very common) or hemorrhoids cause pain during defecation and lead a child to retain stool, which in turn makes defecation painful and encourages stool retention. Pain during defecation also can be caused by diaper rashes, dermatitis, and other irritations around the anogenital area. Some young children with diarrhea have strong negative feelings associated with defecation, which may then proceed toward chronic fecal retention, with dehydration often a contributing factor.

In some cases systemic disorders may predispose a child to stool retention. These include celiac disease, hypothyroidism, hypocalcemia, multiple endocrine neoplasia, and lead intoxication. In addition, motility can be reduced by certain medications (especially those containing codeine or phenothiazines). Children with neuromuscular disease (e.g., cerebral palsy, spinal dysraphism, muscular dystrophy) com-

Table 116-1 *Comparison of Aganglionic Megacolon and Chronic Dysfunctional Stool Retention*

CHARACTERISTIC	AGANGLIONIC MEGACOLON	STOOL RETENTION
Prevalence	1 in 25,000 births	1.5% of 7-yr-old boys
Sex ratio	90% males	86% males
Retention as newborn	Almost always	Rare
Problems with bowel training	Rare	Common
Late onset of symptoms (after 2 yr)	Rare	Common
Toilet avoidance	Rare	Common
Incontinence	Rare	Common
Stool size	Often thin "ribbons"	Often large caliber
Frequency of defecation	Greatly diminished	Variable
Abdominal pain	Rare, except in obstruction	Common, especially in cases of recent onset
General appearance	Often chronically ill	Usually healthy
Failure to thrive	Common	Rare
Obstruction	Common	Rare
Abdominal distention	Common	Variable
Stool in ampulla	Often diminished	Often increased
Plain roentgenograms	Narrow rectum	Often dilated, distended rectum
Rectal manometry (internal sphincter)	Contraction or no response	Relaxation
Barium enema	Localized constriction with proximal dilation may be seen	Often diffuse megacolon

monly have refractory chronic stool retention, mostly because of immobility and poor control of the abdominal musculature or the anal sphincter.

Emotional problems may potentiate stool retention. Psychogenic constipation may be seen in a child who is chronically anxious, depressed, or agitated. Such a youngster may be unable to persevere at or attend to the need for defecation. In some cases, more deeply set negative feelings may be associated with the need for stool retention. Failure to defecate may constitute a quiet protest or expression of anger or maladaptive behavior in a toddler of parents who are ambivalent about codes of discipline.

Genetic and constitutional factors, as well as developmental processes, underlie most cases of stool retention. In some families there is a tendency toward ineffective defecation, and concordance for stool retention is four times more frequent in monozygotic twins than in dizygotic twins.[1] Stool retention in children younger than 10 years of age also has been found to be strongly associated with the dermatoglyphic pattern of simple arches.[5] The British have used the term *primary colonic inertia* to describe young infants who, from the earliest days in life, have difficulty with complete evacuation of the rectum. Defecation seems to become a burdensome undertaking for them, and voluntary stool retention is superimposed on an underlying predisposition to poor defecation.

Specific events or situations that occur during development may interfere with normal defecation. Chronic retention may result from overzealous efforts to facilitate an infant's defecation. A newborn with hard stools may be "assaulted" with gloved fingers and suppositories, thus establishing early conflicts over issues of withholding and elimination. Training for stool incontinence may trigger withholding. Parents who train children too early or use methods that are overly coercive may promote reluctance to defecate, although this has not yet been confirmed in large-scale epidemiologic studies. Family stresses such as the birth of a new baby or the loss of a family member, when they occur during training, may engender retentive behavior.

For reasons that often are unclear, some youngsters develop a phobia toward toilets. Some may fantasize about being flushed down the drain. Others may overreact to the odor and be unable to face the reality that they have produced such unattractive waste.

School bathrooms may predispose older children to stool retention. Becoming trained to defecate on a toilet is a major developmental achievement; learning to use a second toilet may represent an even greater challenge. More commonly, absence of doors, toilet paper, and sanitary conditions or the presence of potential pranks and fights results in children postponing defecation until safely at home.

Among children with developmental handicaps of low severity, such as hyperactivity and learning disabilities, there appears to be a high occurrence of dysfunctional bowel disorders. Some children with hyperactivity and a diminished attention span may be as impersistent and as inconsistent about defecation as they are about completing academic assignments.

Usually, more than one factor leads to stool retention. Often it is the final result of an interplay of genetic, psychological, cognitive, and physiologic factors. The box on the left on p. 859 summarizes some of the recognized predispositions to chronic stool retention.

DIAGNOSIS

Chronic retention of stool can be an elusive diagnosis. Both parent and child may be unaware of the existence of constipation and may report a daily bowel movement. In many cases of stool incontinence the parents are unaware of the existence of long-standing stool retention or incomplete defecation, especially in school-aged children. As a result, parents may incorrectly interpret soiling episodes as being related to concurrent stressful events, making diagnosis more difficult. Clues helpful in detecting associated occult stool retention are listed in the box on the right on p. 859. Stool retention can be suspected in infants and toddlers when a parent complains that the child has infrequent defecation or appears in distress while having a bowel movement. With legs hyperextended, fists clenched, and a reddish, nearly plethoric facial expression, the infant may be struggling to inhibit a bowel movement rather than to have one.

The problem of physical diagnosis is further complicated when a child with marked retention has normal findings on physical examination. Palpation of the abdomen and a rectal examination often reveal no abnormal findings because children may retain enormous amounts of pasty soft stool that fail to present rocklike formations to the palpating hand or the inserted finger. Similarly, an easily palpable sigmoid colon or cecum does not necessarily signify stool retention inasmuch as it is normal for stool transit to be slower through the distal colon and for stool to be stored in the cecum.

In questionable cases, demonstration of delayed transit time of orally administered carmine dye through the small and large bowels may be used as a further criterion for underlying stool retention.[4] A supine roentgenogram of the abdomen may reveal retained stool that is granular or rocklike in appearance. There may be a distended rectal ampulla or diffuse megacolon, especially when associated symptoms are present[2] (see following section). For the small percentage of children who have clinical features more typical of aganglionic megacolon (see Table 116-1), the initial diagnostic procedure is rectal manometry. On the basis of the sphincter response results, a small number of these children will require a rectal biopsy (to prove the diagnosis) and a barium enema (to measure the length of colonic involvement) before surgical intervention.[6] Rectal manometry also is indicated in patients with myelodysplasia, patients who have had rectal surgery, and children with severe retention who are unresponsive to an adequate medical therapeutic trial.

ASSOCIATED SYMPTOMS

A wide range of associated symptoms in the school-aged child may accompany chronic stool retention. The presence of such symptoms should elicit a high index of suspicion for dysfunctional problems with defecation. Many children with recurrent abdominal pain have associated chronic stool retention. Often this bowel problem is the source of pain. The stool retention in these children may be occult in that their

Classification of Predispositions to Chronic Stool Retention

ALTERED ANATOMY OR PHYSIOLOGY

Congenital
- Aganglionic megacolon
- Anal stenosis or atresia

Acquired
- Postoperative lesion
- Fissure
- Celiac disease

Metabolic
- Hypothyroidism
- Hypocalcemia
- Multiple endocrine neoplasia
- Drug effects (especially codeinelike medications and phenothiazines)

Neurogenic (myelodysplasia)

DYSFUNCTIONS

Developmental
- Associated with cognitive handicap
- Attentional disorders or hyperactivity

Situational
- Associated with difficult training
- School bathroom induced
- Negative defecation-related experience (e.g., gastroenteritis)

Psychogenic—associated with significant psychopathology

Constitutional
- Primary colonic inertia
- Genetic predisposition

tendency to be retentive is not easily elicited during a routine history and physical examination. Some children with enuresis also are found to have significant stool retention, which may cause or aggravate a child's urinary incontinence; the enuresis subsides when a normal stool pattern is restored. This is more likely to be the case in children with secondary enuresis and daytime wetting. In addition, persistence of recurrent urinary tract infections has been clearly related to underlying stool retention. Perhaps the most common and troublesome symptom associated with chronic stool retention is fecal incontinence, also known as encopresis (see Chapter 80).

TREATMENT

The problem of constipation provides an excellent example of the potential role for prevention within pediatric practice, because often it can be prevented by anticipatory guidance from the physician in working out with the parents an appropriate schedule for bowel "training." It is not uncommon for boys to remain untrained until after 3 years of age.

If uncomplicated dysfunctional stool retention develops, its management depends largely on its severity, the child's age, and the degree of parental anxiety. The clinician needs to achieve a happy medium between overindulgence in reassurance and an excessively aggressive approach; either extreme may aggravate the disorder.

Possible Clues to Stool Retention

1. A period longer than 3 or 4 days without a bowel movement
2. A history of blood-streaked stool (fissure)
3. Straining with small, hard stools (pellets)
4. Occasional presence of very large stools (filling the toilet or requiring mechanical breakup)
5. A child's feet suspended in air when having a movement
6. A child who stays on the toilet for less than 1 minute at a time
7. Enuresis (especially daytime and late onset)
8. History of soiling underwear
9. History of use of laxatives and enemas
10. Onset of recurrent abdominal pain

Stool retention early in infancy should be treated gently. When underlying organic conditions have been ruled out, the physician should proceed to relatively straightforward dietary manipulations. Increasing the osmotic load in the baby's formula with the addition of liquid sugar preparations can be effective. A titrated quantity of prune juice (determined by observation of stool consistency) each day is practical and effective for infants and toddlers. Along with ad libitum water and fruit juices, toddlers can be offered raisins, raw vegetables, and oatmeal cookies at snacktime. The toddler, school-aged child, and adolescent should receive only whole-wheat bread, have adequate daily portions of high-fiber vegetables (broccoli, brussels sprouts, cabbage, corn, and so on), have fruit snacks, and avoid cakes, candies, chips, and soft drinks. Regular exercise is recommended.

In infancy dioctyl sodium sulfosuccinate may be employed in special cases. It is best to avoid the rectal administration of medications. Dilation with a finger, the use of suppositories, and the administration of enemas should be reserved for only the most resistant cases, because these interventions may generate negative feelings about defecation and promote further stool retention. In infants older than 3 months of age, a small amount of a laxative may be administered orally (such as ¼ teaspoon of senna syrup [Senokot] daily, increased to ½ teaspoon per day in toddlers) until soft, easily passed stools occur daily.

Any perianal dermatologic problems or fissures need treatment. In some cases warm baths twice daily with the addition of an emollient solution (e.g., Alpha Keri Lotion or Vaseline Intensive Care Lotion) may alleviate perianal soreness. Steroid creams in infancy tend to make the mucosa even more friable and should be avoided. Simple anal fissures in infants often are alleviated by the anal dilation that occurs when a rectal examination is performed. Rarely, chronic fissures need excision. Parents may need a great deal of support, and clinicians may need to exercise restraint in the management of this problem.

Children in whom stool retention develops during bowel

"training" may improve if there is a scaling down of the process. In such cases training may need to be delayed. Laxative therapy can be initiated during this time.

In older children with chronic stool retention, treatment may be implemented in several stages.[3] First, the degree of retention should be estimated. If there is a considerable amount of retained feces, an initial cleanout is desirable. This is accomplished by (1) administering an adult Fleet hypophosphate enema the morning and evening of the first day of treatment, (2) administering a bisacodyl (Dulcolax) suppository the morning and evening of the second day of treatment, and (3) administering a bisacodyl tablet orally on the third day of treatment. This whole process may need to be repeated two to four times. In milder cases a child might benefit from 1 to 2 weeks of oral laxative therapy (using danthron, senna, or bisacodyl tablets once or twice daily).

After the child is relieved of retained feces, daily doses of light mineral oil may be administered in appropriate dosage (1 to 6 tablespoons per day), with increments in dosage depending on the "daily soft stool." School-aged children, whose pants can become stained by mineral oil, may prefer senna syrup. Such treatment should continue for at least 3 months. In many cases stool softeners will be required for a year or longer.

While the child is receiving treatment, appropriate patterns of toilet use should be encouraged. The child should be encouraged to sit on the toilet twice a day, at the same times each day, for at least 5 minutes each time. A kitchen timer in the bathroom may be helpful, and books or magazines can be offered. The child is welcome to use the bathroom at other times of the day, but such supplementary excursions do not replace the two regular sittings. It is critical to emphasize to the child and parents that these activities do not represent punishment or criticism.

If the child reverts and becomes retentive while taking mineral oil, a short course of laxatives by mouth may be repeated. As a general therapeutic and preventive measure, a high roughage diet is recommended for the entire family.

PROGNOSIS

Although many youngsters with dysfunctional bowel disorders tend to improve with time, there is increasing evidence that these dysfunctions may lead to lifelong disabilities. What begins as simple "colonic inertia" in infancy may progress to chronic stool retention and to fecal incontinence in the school years. These symptoms may resolve and later reappear as the irritable or spastic colon, a major cause of morbidity in adults. The early recognition and comprehensive, continuing management of childhood disorders of defecation must be a seriously regarded component of preventive pediatric care.

REFERENCES

1. Bakwin H and Davidson M: Constipation in twins, Am J Dis Child 121:179, 1971.
2. Barr RG et al: Chronic and occult stool retention: a clinic tool for its evaluation in school-aged children, Gastroenterology 18:674, 1979.
3. Davidson M, Kugler MM, and Bauer CH: Diagnosis and management in children with severe and protracted constipation and obstipation, J Pediatr 62:261, 1963.
4. Dimson SB: Carmine as an index of transit time in children with simple constipation, Arch Dis Child 45:232, 1970.
5. Gottlieb SH and Schuster MM: Dermatoglyphic (fingerprint) evidence for a congenital syndrome of early onset constipation and abdominal pain, Gastroenterology 91:428, 1986.
6. Rosenberg AJ and Vela AR: A new simplified technique for pediatric anorectal manometry, Pediatrics 71:240, 1983.

117

Cough

William A. Durbin, Jr.

Cough is one of the most common symptoms that pediatric practitioners are asked to evaluate and manage. Fortunately, as a symptom, cough generally is innocuous; furthermore, the underlying disease process that produces cough rarely is serious and usually is self-limited. Despite its generally benign nature, however, a cough may be disruptive to the child and often annoying and anxiety provoking for parents.

PATHOPHYSIOLOGY

From a pathophysiologic point of view, cough is a forceful expiration. This "convulsion of the lungs," as Samuel Johnson put it, serves, as do airway cilia and macrophages, to remove secretions and foreign material from the respiratory tract. The cough reflex can be triggered either voluntarily or by stimulation of cough receptors located throughout the respiratory tract—in the nose, the sinuses, the pharynx, the larynx, the trachea, the large bronchi, and the terminal bronchioles. Afferent impulses from the airway cough receptors travel via cranial nerve pathways to the brainstem "cough center"; from there, efferent stimuli activate coordinate closure of the glottis and contraction of diaphragmatic, chest wall, abdominal wall, and pelvic floor musculature.

The cough sequence is composed of three phases. In the *inspiratory* phase there is an initial deep inspiration, followed by closure of the glottis. During the second, *compressive* phase there is a large increase in intrathoracic pressure brought about by contraction of all the expiratory muscles. At the end of this phase the glottis opens suddenly, leading to a sudden, explosive release of intrathoracic air. It is during this *expiratory* phase that material from the respiratory tract is eliminated. In children such secretions often are not expectorated but instead may be swallowed.

CLASSIFICATION

A number of classification schemes of cough have been developed. These focus on aspects such as the duration and descriptive qualities of the cough, the age of the child, and the various types of anatomic lesions and stimuli that can induce cough. The most basic classification is by duration, with cough being characterized as acute or chronic (3 weeks or longer). In evaluating acute coughs, the physician considers infection and foreign body inhalation; in chronic cough, structural, allergic, irritative, and psychiatric causes become more important, as do some chronic infections such as tuberculosis.

A second classification scheme is based on the characteristics of the cough. Thus a staccato coughing paroxysm in infant suggests pertussis or chlamydial infection; a barking or brassy cough and voice changes are associated with laryngotracheal disease; a "hawking" or throat-clearing sound often is heard with postnasal drip; a ringing or grunting cough may be heard with asthma; and a "honking" or "foghorn" cough may suggest a psychogenic origin. In addition, a productive cough usually is associated with lower airway or parenchymal infection, whereas a dry cough may be due to irritation anywhere in the respiratory tract. Children who expectorate purulent sputum may have bacterial pneumonia, a lung abscess, bronchiectasis, or cystic fibrosis. Nighttime coughs suggest the possibility of postnasal drip related to sinus infection or allergy, whereas coughs that cease at night may be psychogenic in origin; productive morning coughs suggest bronchiectasis; coughs associated with feeding suggest aspiration; coughs induced by cold air or exercise may indicate reactive airway disease; and seasonal coughs suggest both reactive airway disease and allergic rhinitis with postnasal drip. Hemoptysis raises concern about diseases such as tuberculosis, cystic fibrosis, bronchiectasis, and pulmonary hemosiderosis; it also occurs occasionally with foreign body aspirations or severe nasopharyngitis. Frequently, blood arising from the gastrointestinal tract is mistakenly thought to be pulmonary in origin.

A third approach to classifying cough is based on age. Infections are a prime concern in all age-groups. In small infants one also considers physiologic or structural alterations—for example, gastroesophageal reflux, tracheobronchomalacia, tracheoesophageal fistula, vascular ring, and other airway anomalies. In toddlers, foreign body aspiration, irritation of airways (e.g., passive smoking), and asthma are all important causes of cough. For school-aged children, asthma, sinusitis, and allergic rhinitis with postnasal drip assume greater importance, whereas in adolescents, smoking and psychogenic cough should be considered.

A fourth classification is strictly anatomic, in which the practitioner considers lesions at all levels of the respiratory tract that can stimulate cough. This includes diseases of the larynx, pharynx, nose, and sinuses (infections, irritations, allergies, foreign bodies, structural anomalies); the trachea and bronchi (infections, irritations, foreign bodies, structural anomalies, asthma, cystic fibrosis); the lung parenchyma (pneumonia, lung abscess, congenital malformations, pulmonary edema); the pleura (effusion, empyema); and the mediastinum (great vessel malformations, adenopathy, tumors). In addition, nonrespiratory tract causes (external auditory canal irritation, diaphragmatic and subdiaphragmatic lesions, and cough tic) should be considered.

Perhaps the most satisfactory classification is one in which the types of stimuli that can produce cough are considered. *Mechanical* stimuli include intraluminal secretions and foreign bodies (including gastric contents, i.e., gastroesophageal reflux or other causes of aspiration). In addition, extraluminal lesions that compress the airway must be considered—both extramural (e.g., vascular rings and other anomalies) and intramural (e.g., the contraction of bronchial smooth muscle, manifested by asthma). *Inflammatory* stimuli include all the infectious conditions of the respiratory tract in which there is edema or exudate involving either the airway or the alveoli. *Chemical* stimuli include irritative gases, such as cigarette or wood stove smoke or allergens, which cause cough on inhalation. *Thermal* stimuli—that is, hot or cold air—also can produce cough, as can *psychogenic* stimuli.

These classification schemes provide the physician a general framework to guide the evaluation of a coughing child. Implicit in the evaluation is the knowledge that most coughs of short duration are related to acute respiratory tract infections, whereas the most common causes of chronic cough are asthma (classical or cough variant), postnasal drip (resulting from recurrent upper respiratory tract infections, sinusitis, allergic and vasomotor rhinitis), and airway irritants (e.g., smoke, dust, chemicals, and aspirated food or gastric contents).

HISTORY

The history should include a description of the cough, including its duration, frequency, quality, timing, and sputum productivity. A history of episodes of cough, respiratory infections, and allergies should be sought. The family history may be helpful in identifying children with diseases such as asthma, cystic fibrosis, and tuberculosis. The environmental history will help identify those children whose symptoms are related to passive smoking or other chemical inhalation, to a respiratory virus that has infected a household, or to an exotic pathogen acquired while traveling. An awareness of family setting and home dynamics may aid in recognizing children at risk for foreign body aspiration or development of a cough tic. It also is important to elicit a history of associated clinical findings. Fever usually suggests an acute infectious process; rhinorrhea may indicate an upper respiratory tract infection, sinusitis, or allergy. Wheezing suggests asthma or a foreign body as the cause of cough; a history of atopic dermatitis or allergic rhinitis provides evidence for the former. Shortness of breath is associated with asthma, upper airway obstruction, pleural effusions, pneumothorax, pneumonias, and congestive heart failure.

PHYSICAL EXAMINATION

In performing the physical examination, the physician is looking for signs of an acute process (fever, tender adenopathy, pharyngitis, or a rash), as well as for signs of a chronic or recurrent process (growth failure or clubbing seen in children with severe asthma, cystic fibrosis, immunodeficiency, or congenital heart disease). The physician also is interested in defining the level of involvement of the respiratory tract; crackles, wheezes, rhonchi, altered breath sounds, and changes in resonance signify lower respiratory tract involvement; stridor and dysphagia indicate laryngeal involvement; and changes in the mouth, nose, ears, and sinuses signify upper airway disease. Observation of color, hydration state, respiratory rate, chest movement, retractions, flaring of the chest, and handling of oral secretions indicate the severity of the process. It always is useful to get the child to cough! Last, inspection for stigmata of allergic disease (e.g., eczema, pale boggy nasal mucosa, clear rhinorrhea, shiners, allergic nasal crease) and for posterior pharyngeal wall cobblestoning (hypertrophic lymphoid follicles seen in chronic postnasal drainage) is important.

LABORATORY TESTS

Most children with coughs do not require any laboratory testing. For those children in whom the cough is chronic or associated with respiratory distress, some investigations may be undertaken. A complete blood count may provide evidence of acute infection, atopy (eosinophilia), or polycythemia. Examination of the sputum, including its macroscopic appearance, cellular composition (polymorphonuclear leukocytes, eosinophils), and bacterial content (Gram stain, culture), should be performed in children who are capable of expectoration. A similar examination of the nasal discharge also may help distinguish allergic rhinitis from purulent rhinitis or sinusitis. Roentgenograms of the chest (including fluoroscopy in children whom may have inhaled a foreign body), neck, or sinuses may yield useful information, as might a barium swallow test in an infant thought to be aspirating mucus, food, liquid, or regurgitated gastric contents. Pulmonary function testing may be carried out in children with suspected restrictive or obstructive airway disease; reversible reactive airway disease (asthma) is indicated either by improvement in an obstructive pattern after bronchodilator administration or by the development of an obstructive airway pattern after exercise or inhalation of such agents as cold air, methacholine, histamine, or specific allergens. Such testing may identify children with cough-variant asthma, whose reactive airway disease is clinically manifested by coughing rather than by wheezing. The performance of pH probe monitoring, sweat testing, tuberculin skin testing, and immunoglobin and alpha-1-antitrypsin measurements may be indicated in children with chronic or recurrent cough and demonstrable pulmonary disease. Bronchoscopy is useful in searching for a foreign body, investigating persistent collapse, confirming anatomic malformations, or obtaining tissue in children with undiagnosed infiltrates or suspected dysmotile cilia syndrome.

MANAGEMENT

The physician, having completed the assessment of the coughing child, is faced with the problem of management. Several caveats are in order. First, the physician often needs to defuse parental anxiety about a cough, particularly when it is part of an acute respiratory infection. An explanation of the normalcy of a cough as part of the disease process, of the protective role that it may play, and of the usually self-limited nature of coughs in children may be necessary. The physician must acknowledge that the cough may be annoying and disruptive but also can reassure the child and parent that coughs in children in and of themselves rarely are harmful.

Second, treating the underlying disorder, thereby reducing the stimulation to cough, is more important than providing nonspecific cough medication. Thus the child with the productive cough of postnasal drip may benefit from antihistamines or decongestants; the child with the barking cough of croup should receive humidification; and the child with allergen- or irritant-induced cough may need environmental alteration or bronchodilators.

Third, the physician who prescribes cough medicines should carefully explain their therapeutic purpose—for example, expectorants to loosen (not diminish) the cough or antitussives to partially suppress (not eliminate) the cough. Such discussion helps avoid unrealistic expectations. Cough medicines generally are contraindicated in the first few months of life because of potential toxicity. Antitussives should be avoided in patients with productive coughs.

There are three categories of cough medicines: expectorants, mucolytics, and antitussives. *Expectorants* are drugs that increase sputum volume and thus promote removal of secretions from the airways. Water is the most commonly used expectorant, given both systemically and by inhalation, methods that probably work because of their demulcent effect in the upper airway; whether administration of water actually affects lower airway secretions is unclear. Another expectorant, guaifenesin (glyceryl guaiacolate), is commonly used in cough preparations; however, although it may reduce sputum thickness, studies have not shown it to reduce coughing. Ammonium chloride and potassium iodide rarely are prescribed for children, in part because of untoward side effects associated with effective dosages.

Mucolytic agents are drugs, such as acetylcysteine, that liquify tenacious secretions. They usually are administered by inhalation for children with bronchiectasis (e.g., cystic fibrosis). Poor taste, the potential for inducing airway reactivity, and uncertain clinical benefit limit their use.

Antitussives are drugs that suppress coughing; they are the most effective cough modifiers. Peripherally acting antitussives work by coating or by anesthetizing irritated oropharyngeal receptors. This group includes the demulcents (e.g., throat lozenges, cough drops, lollipops, honey), as well as topical anesthetics administered by swallowing or spraying. These local measures generally are safe and well tolerated and may be useful in a cough related to upper respiratory tract infections or other pharyngeal irritation; their duration of efficacy is limited, however, because they are quickly washed away. Centrally acting antitussives include both narcotic and nonnarcotic agents that suppress the cough reflex at the brainstem level. Narcotic agents are of proved efficacy in suppressing coughing; codeine and hydrocodeine are the most widely used and have, particularly in children, minimum potential for abuse and associated adverse effects. Among the nonnarcotic drugs, dextromethorphan is the most commonly prescribed; unfortunately, despite uncontrolled studies supporting its efficacy, appropriate objective clinical trials have not been performed. Antihistamines such as diphenhydramine sometimes are classified as centrally acting antitussives, perhaps on the basis of their sedative effect; however, much of their efficacy stems from their drying effect on tracheobronchial secretions.

Most available cough preparations, both prescription and over-the-counter, contain several agents, including antitussives, expectorants, sympathomimetic decongestants, and antihistamines. Such combinations generally are untested and often irrational. Physicians may prefer to seek specific pharmacologic effects by employing preparations that contain agents from just one or two of these groups.

SUGGESTED READINGS

Cough and wheeze in asthma: are they interdependent? Lancet 1:447, 1988.

Curley FJ et al: Cough and the common cold, Am Rev Respir Dis 138:305, 1988.

Holinger LD: Chronic cough in infants and children, Laryngoscope 96:316, 1986.

Irwin RS and Curley FJ: The diagnosis of chronic cough, Hosp Pract 23:82, 1988.

Katz RM, Siegel SC, and Rachelefsky GS: Chronic cough in athletes, Clin Rev Allergy 6:431, 1988.

Leith DE: The development of cough, Am Rev Respir Dis 131S:S39, 1985.

Morgan WJ and Taussig LM: The child with persistent cough, Pediatr Rev 8:249, 1987.

Parks DW et al: Chronic cough in childhood: approach to diagnosis and treatment, J Pediatr 115:856, 1989.

Pruit AW: Rational use of cold and cough preparations, Pediatr Ann 14:289, 1985.

Reisiman JJ, Canny GJ, and Levison H: The approach to chronic cough in childhood, Ann Allergy 61:163, 1988.

Wilmott RW: Persuing the cause of persistent cough, Contemp Pediatr 4:26, 1987.

118

Dental Stains

Lindsey K. Grossman

Parental concerns about changes in tooth color, often the cause of much anxiety, are frequently first brought to the pediatrician. It is important to remember that normal tooth color varies greatly from one tooth to another, from one individual to another, and between the usual blue-white of the primary dentition and the yellowish ivory of the permanent teeth.

EXTRINSIC STAIN

Teeth are often discolored as a result of staining from external deposits on their surface layer. These extrinsic stains usually are removable with careful daily brushing and professional oral prophylaxis (scaling). Chromogenic bacteria in plaque can result in green, orange, or black stains along the gingival margin of the teeth. Although in most cases this is associated with poor oral hygiene, black stains may be associated with good hygiene and a low incidence of caries. Excessive use of certain foods or beverages and smoking can stain the teeth, but the discoloration usually will disappear with oral prophylaxis and avoidance of the staining substance. Children who are receiving certain liquid medications, especially iron preparations, may exhibit teeth with a dark stain. This also resolves with professional sealing after the medication is discontinued but may be completely avoided if the medication is administered through a straw from the onset.

INTRINSIC STAIN

When a staining substance is incorporated into the deep structures of the tooth (i.e., the enamel or dentin, or both), it cannot be removed by scaling and is referred to as an intrinsic stain. Certain problems of the neonatal period, such as erythroblastosis fetalis, biliary atresia, neonatal hepatitis, or other conditions resulting in high serum concentrations of bilirubin pigments, can cause yellow-green or blue-green staining of primary teeth, resulting from pigment deposition in the structures of these teeth. As many as 50% of children with cyanotic congenital heart disease may have dull, pale, bluish-white teeth whose color resembles skim milk. This is believed to be caused, at least in part, by the hypoxemia associated with these conditions.

Intrinsic stains may be associated with certain rare childhood conditions. The erythrodontia, or porphyria, caused by deposition of red-brown porphyrin pigments into the tooth structure, is readily apparent in ultraviolet light if not in daylight. The inherited disorders amelogenesis imperfecta and dentinogenesis imperfecta are associated with hypoplastic enamel and a yellow, opalescent blue-gray, or brown-violet tooth color. Major dental work is required to restore normal appearance in those who have any of these disorders.

Common pedodontic problems often result in a change in tooth color. Tooth trauma and associated bleeding into dentin can cause a pink color that fades first to gray, as pulp degeneration occurs, and eventually to yellow. In certain cases the dentin resorption will result in a permanent pink hue. Active caries in teeth may appear chalky white or yellow but gradually converts to shiny black as the caries converts to the arrested state. An unusual secondary complication of certain childhood infections is Turner tooth. This is a brown or yellow-brown discoloration of a single tooth and is associated with hypoplasia of the enamel in a tooth undergoing odontogenesis at the time of the illness.

Persons who reside in areas where the water contains fluoride have been noted to have increased resistance to caries. However, as the fluoride content rises over 1.5 ppm (parts per million), many individuals in the area will begin to demonstrate hypoplastic enamel, with the characteristic dull, opaque white mottled patches in the permanent teeth. If the fluoride content consumed is extremely high (>5 ppm), the teeth will show a blotchy brown or black-brown color that is highly disfiguring and requires extensive restoration of the dental surfaces.

A similarly involved treatment course often is required for the severe intrinsic staining problems caused by tetracycline. This is a dose-dependent and duration-linked problem caused by the incorporation of tetracycline itself into the mineral complex at the dentinoenamel junction during odontogenesis. If the tetracycline was ingested by the mother before birth or by the child in the first months after birth, the primary teeth will be affected. Permanent teeth will be stained if drug ingestion occurs between 3 months and 7 to 8 years of age. The result may be yellow, gray, or brown tooth discoloration in a linear pattern that, without restoration, may be quite disfiguring. For this reason tetracycline should be avoided in pregnant or lactating women and in young children.

MANAGEMENT

After allaying parental anxieties, the pediatrician should consider referring any child with extrinsic or intrinsic stains. Simple dental office procedures and preventive education can resolve all extrinsic staining problems, and esthetic improvement is possible with the vast majority of intrinsic discoloration problems. Table 118-1 should be helpful in identifying the cause of any staining problem.

Table 118-1 *Common Colorations of Primary and Permanent Teeth*

COLOR	DISTRIBUTION AND PATTERN	CAUSES	TREATMENT
Green	Several teeth; gingival third of crowns; extrinsic stain	Chromogenic bacteria in plaque, associated with poor oral hygiene	Oral prophylaxis; preventive education
Orange	Several teeth; gingival third of crowns; less common than green stain; extrinsic stain	Chromogenic bacteria in plaque, associated with poor oral hygiene	Oral pophylaxis; preventive education
Black	Several teeth; gingival third of crowns; less common than green and orange stains; extrinsic stain	Chromogenic bacteria in plaque, associated with poor oral hygiene	Oral prophylaxis; preventive education
	Several teeth; extrinsic stain	Oral medications, especially iron	Oral prophylaxis after discontinuing medication
	One or several teeth; occlusal or interproximal surfaces; hard, shiny	Arrested caries	Dental evaluation, observation, or restoration
Brown-black	Several teeth; occlusal pits and fissures or smooth surfaces	Accumulation of tin or staining of demineralized enamel after strontium fluoride (SrF_2) topical treatment	None or esthetic restoration
Pink	Single tooth; entire crown	Posttraumatic change	
		Within 1-2 days—bleeding into dentin; changes to gray in 1-3 wk	None or observation
		After several months—internal resorption of dentin	Minor resorption—endodontics; severe resorption—extraction
Gray	Several teeth; linear pattern or entire crown, depending on stage of tooth development	Tetracycline incorporation in tooth and subsequent oxidation by sunlight; exhibits other colors	Esthetic improvement—endodontic therapy and bleaching and/or esthetic restoration
	All primary and permanent teeth; entire crown	Dentinogenesis imperfecta (autosomal dominant)	Esthetic improvement and protection from wear—prosthetic coverage
	Single tooth; entire crown	Posttraumatic change	
		Within 1-3 wk—hemosiderin pigment in dentin	Observation
		After several months—pulpal necrosis	Endodontic treatment or extraction
Yellow	Several teeth; entire crown	Natural color of permanent compared with primary teeth	None necessary
	Several teeth; linear pattern or entire crown	Tetracyclines; systemic infections	Esthetic restoration
	All primary and permanent teeth; entire crown	Amelogenesis imperfecta (various inheritance patterns)	Esthetic restoration and protection from occlusal wear
	Single tooth; entire crown	Posttraumatic change—pulpal obliteration by dentin	Observation or esthetic restoration
	Several teeth; gingival third of crown; extrinsic stain	Food debris and chromogenic bacteria in plaque, associated with poor oral hygiene	Oral prophylaxis; preventive education
	Several teeth; extrinsic stain; part of or entire crown	Tea, coffee, cola, tobacco	Oral prophylaxis; avoid excessive use of substance

Modified from Abrams RG and Josell SD: Common oral and dental emergencies and problems, Pediatr Clin North Am 29:705, 1982.

Continued.

Table 118-1 *Common Colorations of Primary and Permanent Teeth—cont'd*

COLOR	DISTRIBUTION AND PATTERN	CAUSES	TREATMENT
Yellow-brown	Several teeth	Premature birth; enamel disturbance—hypoplasia and hypocalcification	None
	One or several teeth; one or more surfaces with cavitations	Advanced active caries	Restoration
Brown	Several teeth; entire crown	Amelogenesis imperfecta; dentinogenesis imperfecta; premature birth; jaundice	As suggested above under gray and yellow colorations
	Individual teeth; localized area	Turner hypoplasia secondary to infection	None or esthetic restoration
		Hypocalcified or hypoplastic area—traumatized primary tooth affecting permanent crown	None or esthetic restoration
	Several teeth; linear or generalized distribution; associated hypoplasia	Fluorosis; systemic infections, especially with high fever; nutritional deficiencies	None or esthetic restoration
	Several teeth; generalized or linear	Tetracycline	Esthetic restoration
	Several teeth; one or more surfaces; loss of tooth structure	Advanced active caries	Restoration
Red-brown	Several teeth; primary and permanent; generalized	Porphyria	None or esthetic restoration
Blue	Several teeth; extrinsic stain; part of or entire crown	Berries	Oral prophylaxis; avoid excessive use of substance
Blue-green or yellow-green	All primary teeth; entire crown	Bilirubin pigments incorporated into dentin—erythroblastosis fetalis, biliary atresia, neonatal hepatitis	None; generally fades; permanent teeth not affected if condition does not continue
White or cream	Several teeth; linear or entire crown	Fluorosis; systemic infections	None; generally fades; permanent teeth not affected if condition does not continue
	All primary and permanent teeth; entire crown	Amelogenesis imperfecta	None; generally fades; permanent teeth not affected if condition does not continue
	Individual teeth; localized area	Turner hypoplasia	None; generally fades; permanent teeth not affected if condition does not continue
	One or several teeth; occlusal or gingival third of smooth surface	Early active caries—demineralization of enamel	Preventive therapy
	Several teeth; any surface; extrinsic stain	Plaque and food debris (materia alba)—removed easily with gauze	Oral hygiene instruction

SUGGESTED READINGS

Abrams RG and Josell SD: Common oral and dental emergencies and problems, Pediatr Clin North Am 29:681, 1982.

Dayan D et al: Tooth discoloration—extrinsic and intrinsic factors, Quintessence Int 14:195, 1983.

Faunce F: Management of discolored teeth, Dent Clin North Am 27:657, 1983.

Pindborg JJ: Pathology of dental hard tissues, Philadelphia, 1973, WB Saunders Co.

Sweeney EA: Pediatric dentistry, Curr Probl Pediatr 11:1, 1980.

Vogel RI: Intrinsic and extrinsic discoloration of the dentition, J Oral Med 30:99, 1975.

119

Developmental Delays

Rune J. Simeonsson and Michael C. Sharp

A review of current pediatric literature indicates a growing interest in children with developmental delays. This increased interest reflects a decline of infectious diseases, a declining birth rate, and a growth of alternative services and pediatric specialization. More sophisticated screening and assessment procedures and a commitment to early intervention also have contributed to increased involvement with children identified as developmentally delayed (see Chapters 18, Eleven; 75; and 85; and Appendix D).

DEFINITION

Although attention to these children has grown, efforts to define developmental delay and its scope as a problem have not been systematic. In this chapter, developmental delay is defined as a condition in which functional aspects of the child's development are significantly delayed relative to the expected level of development. A reasonable criterion of developmental delay is a discrepancy from the expected rate of 25% or more. Although a child identified as developmentally delayed also may show physical signs and symptoms, it is those symptoms pertaining to developmental functions that are associated with the diagnosis. The major developmental domains and representative signs and symptoms are summarized in the accompanying box. For example, a 20-month-old child whose mental, motor, or other domain of development is that of a 15-month-old or younger would be identified as developmentally delayed. The use of such a discrepancy as a basis for defining developmental delay is more readily achieved in some domains than in others. In domains for which age norms are available (e.g., motor, mental), the label can be objectively supported through motor and mental scales. In other domains (e.g., affective, social), greater reliance is placed on subjective criteria supported by clinical judgment. In either case, however, developmental delay implies a state of discrepant functional development with implications for differential diagnosis and intervention.

In clinical contexts, developmental delay usually is a concept restricted to the preschool child, because neither the presenting problem nor assessment procedures may be as precise as they are with older children, for whom more specific labels such as *learning disabled* or *speech impaired* are applicable. In the absence of disorders associated with specific findings, the term *developmental delay* is used in a generic sense to define preschool children who need intervention. If associated signs indicate a specific disorder, the term *developmental delay* is replaced with an appropriate diagnosis such as cerebral palsy or mental retardation. This approach is consistent with the way in which Tjossem[8] has conceptualized risk status in regard to early intervention. He proposed three categories of vulnerable infants: (1) those with established risk from diagnosed disorders, (2) those at environmental risk from experimental deprivation, and (3) those at biologic risk from potential sequelae of biologic insults. These categories are not mutually exclusive, and each may reflect environmental, as well as organismic, factors in the expression of developmental delay.

SCOPE OF THE PROBLEM

The lack of a widely accepted definition makes it difficult to describe the problem. Drawing on Tjossem's categories and the definition just proposed,[8] reasonable estimates would place the prevalence of developmental delay in preschool children between 5% and 15%. These estimates are consistent

Developmental Delay or Atypical Features: Representative Signs and Symptoms by Domains

MOTOR DOMAIN

Hypertonicity or hypotonicity, poor coordination
Delayed creeping and walking
Persistent primitive reflexes

MENTAL DOMAIN

Delayed or atypical play
Delayed or atypical use of objects
Delayed development of symbolic skills

COMMUNICATION AND LANGUAGE DOMAIN

Articulation and production errors
Immature speech
Absent or delayed speech

SOCIAL AND EMOTIONAL DOMAIN

Lethargy, anxiety
Sleep difficulties, depression
Social withdrawal, selective attention deficits

BEHAVIORAL DOMAIN

Rhythmic habit patterns
Stereotypic behavior
Elevated threshold level
Altered activity level

with empiric and conceptual contributions from the literature. On the basis of neurodevelopmental screening, Drillien and colleagues[1] found that 9% of a preschool population exhibited significant developmental problems. Although epidemiologic studies are clearly needed in this area, the classification label *developmental delay* is essential to obtain valid statistics. It seems reasonable to estimate, however, that 5% to 10% of children in a typical pediatric practice are developmentally delayed.

In typical usage the terms *sign* and *symptom* are used diagnostically in regard to features or characteristics based either on objective or subjective criteria, respectively. With reference to developmental delay, consideration of signs and symptoms is complicated by several qualifications: (1) their significance is relative to development (timing); (2) their significance often is a function of temporal qualities (frequency, duration); and (3) they may be either common to all developmental delays or associated with specific disorders.

Given these qualifications and the lack of a well-established definition, a conceptual framework may be of some value in approaching the developmentally delayed child. Signs and symptoms reflective of delays in functional development lead to an initial diagnosis of developmental delay. This diagnosis is either maintained or replaced after analysis of the history, associated signs and symptoms, and etiologic factors. Management of the developmentally delayed child without a specific disorder involves monitoring of progress and providing supportive interventions for the child and family. Management of children with specific disorders (e.g., cerebral palsy, autism) involves similar activities plus specific medical treatments (e.g., surgery, medication) as indicated.

SIGNS AND SYMPTOMS

An exhaustive discussion of all signs and symptoms associated with developmental delays is beyond the scope of this presentation. There are, however, several issues of particular importance for the pediatrician to consider. One is the diagnostic significance of rhythmic habit patterns such as body rocking and head rolling. Kravitz and Boehm[5] found that the onset, pattern, and decline of rhythmic habit movements can serve to document a developmental delay. A second issue pertains to young children whose motor performance is delayed. Taft and Barabas[7] have advocated systematic evaluation approach to determine if the condition is progressive or nonprogressive and if the site of the lesion is central or peripheral. A third issue is a recognition of the elements of a developmental approach to symptoms. As described by Green,[2] such an approach for a specific phase of development, such as infancy, includes considering signs and symptoms, predisposing factors drawn from the history, and perinatal contingencies. A final issue pertains to signs and symptoms in emotional development, a difficult but important domain to consider. The problem of depression is one that is being recognized increasingly as an entity even in infancy and early childhood, and Herzog and Rathbun[3] have described a diagnostic system that specifies criteria for symptoms by developmental stages. A comprehensive view of symptoms of behavioral abnormalities in children younger than 36 months of age has been presented by Minde.[6]

In approaching a child with a developmental delay, an extensive review of the developmental history may yield a variety of diagnostic clues. Early normality with subsequent slowing of developmental progress may indicate a metabolic defect. Such slowing of mental growth may appear late. The age that slowing becomes evident will vary depending on the nature of the metabolic defect or the diagnosis if a degenerative disease is involved. Another clue to the presence of metabolic disease is the combination of developmental delay and unexplained seizures.

Minor physical anomalies also may predict later behavioral problems. Kaplan and colleagues,[4] for example, have found an increase in physical signs and symptoms in preschool hyperactive children.

Identification of an inadequate environment, poorly educated parents, and other indexes of low sociodemographic status may help to identify children at risk for mild delays associated with lack of stimulation.

A parent's at-risk occupation or a history of pica in the child may suggest lead or another toxin as a cause. Postnatal central nervous system mechanical injury, infection, or damage secondary to hyperosmolar states associated with dehydration also may reveal a cause. Similarly, a review of the neonatal history may suggest a cause of developmental delay if there is a history of asphyxia, hypoglycemia, hyperbilirubinemia, or possible intracranial hemorrhage.

The prenatal history should be reviewed for evidence of maternal infection (the TORCH infections—toxoplasmosis, rubella, cytomegalovirus, and herpes simplex), irradiation, severe malnutrition, or possible toxin exposure—for example, alcohol, anticoagulants (warfarin), or anticonvulsants.

A family history that goes back at least three generations is important and should include a search for miscarriages and consanguinity of parents as diagnostic clues.

Associated Signs

Numerous conditions are associated with developmental delay, many of which may be immediately apparent after a brief examination (e.g., Down syndrome). Many others offer only subtle clues.[4] The eyes are often revealing in a thorough physical examination (e.g., the cherry-red spot of the macula of Tay-Sachs disease). Still others lack any specific signs and symptoms that lead to a diagnosis of their existence (e.g., many inborn errors of metabolism).

In spite of a large number of diagnosable conditions, the pediatrician often finds that, even after elaborate investigation, no specific diagnosis can be reached. Still more rarely will a diagnosis lead to definitive therapy. Proceeding in spite of this rather gloomy perspective is justified on a number of grounds: (1) alleviation of parental concern and provision of supportive services, (2) potential implications for siblings and future generations, and (3) rare instances in which therapy is virtually curative—for example, the child with methylmalonicacidemia that responds to vitamin B_{12} supplementation or a child with biotinidase deficiency.

Some illustrative examples (congenital malformations, motor impairment, and errors of metabolism) of the diagnostic significance of associated signs in developmental delay are provided here. The pediatrician should have additional references to which to turn when faced with a cluster of findings associated with developmental delay.

Congenital Malformations. The child with unusual facies must have the features that make up the atypical appearance precisely defined; philtrum size, eye slant, nasal bridge appearance, positioning of the ears, and the texture of the hair. Discovery of a single, minor congenital malformation necessitates searching for others in a text that describes recognized patterns of human malformations. Specific findings that may suggest the existence of a syndrome or disease include ophthalmoplegia, corneal clouding, cataracts, ectopia lentis, microcephaly or megacephaly, craniosynostosis, abnormal dermatoglyphics, abnormal external genitalia (including male hypogonadism and macrogonadism), abnormal stature, and abnormal spinal curvatures. The frequent association between abnormalities of the ectoderm and the nervous system (phakodermatoses) should lead to a careful examination of the skin, including the use of a Wood light. Tuberous sclerosis, incontinentia pigmenti, and many other neurocutaneous syndromes can thus be diagnosed by referring to the appropriate text.

Motor Impairment. Most children with cerebral palsy eventually develop such marked neuromuscular findings that the diagnosis is evident. The challenge for primary care physicians is early identification. Normal variations exist in the resting muscle tone of infants, and identifying extremes that predict future abnormality is difficult.[5] Movement patterns themselves are an important clue to a diagnosis, and the clinician should be alert for the presence of ataxia, rigidity, athetosis, or abnormalities of posture. Some infants who exhibit severe hypotonia develop normally. Classically, however, a form of athetoid cerebral palsy develops in these children. Occasionally, hypotonia will be the presenting feature of a child with a degenerative neuromuscular disorder such as Werdnig-Hoffmann or Tay-Sachs disease.

The hypertonicity of the spastic forms of cerebral palsy may not become apparent until after the first year of life. This is particularly true of the hemiplegic forms. In such instances the persistence of primitive reflexes combined with developmental delay may be the only clue to the diagnosis. Prominent Moro and asymmetric tonic neck reflexes in a 3- to 5-month-old child are significant signs. With the child's head in a midline position, the physician should be alert to asymmetries of movement. Indication of dominance of one side of the body or of one hand in the child younger than 15 months of age implies hemiplegia of the opposite side, even without increased muscle tone.

Inborn Errors of Metabolism. Perhaps the greatest diagnostic challenge is identifying, from among all children with developmental delays, those who have inborn errors of metabolism. Physical signs and symptoms of the lysosomal storage diseases can be quite distinctive. The approach described earlier for recognized patterns of human malformations might lead the physician to the diagnosis of Hurler syndrome, for instance. Coarse facial features, thick and wiry hair, generalized hirsutism, hepatomegaly, corneal clouding, and a gibbus deformity of the spine combined with short stature would indicate the need for a skeletal survey. Skeletal abnormalities are quite characteristic of the lysosomal storage diseases. Laboratory studies can then be pursued to establish the precise enzymatic defect.

Diagnosing defects in amino acid and organic acid metabolism is considerably more difficult. The neurologic examination provides the most helpful clue, other than the clinical course, to the need for laboratory investigation. Presence of the extrapyramidal syndrome (rigidity, tremor, bradykinesia, and dystonia), intermittent ataxia, chronic progressive ataxia, combined upper and lower motor signs, and the spinocerebellar syndrome, if combined with a clinical course consistent with metabolic disease, suggests the need for a laboratory investigation. Vomiting, if prominent, or the presence of a peculiar odor from the child or the child's urine may be other clues.

MANAGEMENT

The pediatrician's role in the management of children with developmental delays differs somewhat from the role taken in the management of most other disorders. Cure with a return to normality usually is not achievable. Most of the professionals to be consulted for aid in assessment and treatment are nonmedical. This nontraditional approach requires elaboration.

Pediatricians who must inform parents of the presence of a chronic and disabling condition should carefully consider the initial approach. This news should be shared in a quiet, private consultation with both parents present whenever possible. Sufficient time should be allocated to allow a complete and unhurried sharing of both feelings and information.

It is best to clarify the parents' perceptions of the situation at the very beginning. More often than not, the pediatrician will discover that the news confirms long-standing parental suspicions. The parents are likely to be relieved that someone finally is taking them seriously. Support by the physician will do much to form a therapeutic alliance.

Information given to the parents should be as complete and honest as the pediatrician is capable of providing. Withholding information only builds mistrust. The pediatrician must be particularly careful to avoid technical medical terminology. Most professionals believe that if the terms *mental retardation* or *cerebral palsy* apply, they should be used with the parents. Attempting to avoid such emotionally laden terms is, in the long run, a disservice. If the parents react with anger or denial, the physician should avoid arguments or attempts to convince. The parents' perspective on their child's status can evolve in the context of an understanding relationship with a pediatrician. This process may require a number of visits. Providing advocacy for the child and family is essential to the therapeutic process.

REFERENCES

1. Drillien CM, Pickering RM, and Drummond MB: Predictive value of screening for different areas of development, Dev Med Child Neurol 30:294, 1988.
2. Green M: A developmental approach to symptoms based on age groups, Pediatr Clin North Am 22:571, 1975.
3. Herzog DB and Rathbun JM: Childhood depression: developmental considerations, Am J Dis Child 136:115, 1982.
4. Kaplan BJ et al: Physical signs and symptoms in preschool-age hyperactive and normal children, J Dev Behav Pediatr 8:305, 1987.
5. Kravitz H and Boehm JJ: Rhythmic habit patterns in infancy: their sequence, age of onset, and frequency, Child Dev 42:399, 1971.

6. Minde K: Behavioral abnormalities commonly seen in infancy, Can J Psychiatry 33:741, 1988.
7. Taft LT and Barabas G: Infants with delayed motor development, Pediatr Clin North Am 29:137, 1982.
8. Tjossem TD: Early intervention: issues and approaches. In Tjossem TD, editor: Intervention strategies for high risk infants and young children, Baltimore, 1976, University Park Press.

SUGGESTED READINGS

Farmer TW, editor: Pediatric neurology, ed 3, New York, 1983, Harper & Row, Publishers, Inc.

Smith DW: Recognizable patterns of human malformation, ed 2, Philadelphia, 1976, WB Saunders Co.

120

Diarrhea and Steatorrhea

Martin H. Ulshen

Diarrhea, much like vomiting, is a common symptom in the young child, especially during infancy. Therefore it seems surprising that it has been difficult to establish rigid criteria regarding what truly constitutes diarrhea. Loosely defined, diarrhea is characterized by an increase in frequency and water content of stools. The normal daily stool volume varies with the size of the child. Adults and older children have a normal daily stool weight in the range of 100 to 200 g (consisting of 60% to 85% water). Infants weighing less than 10 kg can have approximately 5 g/kg/day of stool. An intermediate range of 50 to 75 g/day is an appropriate approximation for the preschool child. In infancy the frequency and quality of "normal" stools depend very much on diet. During the first weeks of life, the breast-fed infant commonly has up to eight loose stools per day, which at times may contain mucus. These stools frequently follow feedings (as a result of the "gastrocolic reflex") and do not constitute diarrhea. Infants receiving cow milk formula usually have firmer and somewhat less frequent stools. Commonly, the stool of the nursing infant becomes firm when solids or cow milk is introduced into the diet.

Steatorrhea signifies an excess of fat in the stool and is a symptom of malabsorption. Stools that contain an increased quantity of fat can be greasy, bulky, and foul smelling; however, with mild steatorrhea this finding may be insignificant. Fat excretion can be measured with a 72-hour collection of stool. A record of the diet is kept during this period, and fat intake is calculated. The percentage of fat ingested that is absorbed equals (Fat intake − Fat output)/Fat intake × 100, and this is called the *coefficient of absorption*. Absorption of fat by young infants varies with the type of fat that is fed and with the maturity of the infant. A normal premature infant may absorb as little as 65% to 75% of dietary fat, but this improves to 90% in the full-term infant. Furthermore, the neonate absorbs vegetable fat much more efficiently than butterfat. Children and adults typically absorb at least 95% of the fat in a normal diet.

PATHOPHYSIOLOGY

Advances in the understanding of the pathophysiology of diarrhea allow a more rational approach to diagnosis and treatment. Normally large volumes of fluid are processed by the gastrointestinal tract, as illustrated for adults in Fig. 120-1. It is not difficult to see how an infant can rapidly become fluid depleted from diarrhea when large gastrointestinal fluid shifts take place each day. Under normal circumstances about 90% of fluid absorption takes place in the small bowel. However, the colon has a reserve capacity for fluid absorption that must be overcome before diarrhea will result. In adults as much as 2 L of ileal fluid can be reabsorbed by the colon daily without diarrhea occurring.

The movement of water across the gastrointestinal tract mucosa is passive, following osmotic gradients created by electrolytes and other osmotically active solutes (such as glucose and amino acids). Nutrients are absorbed by active transport or passive diffusion; some first require digestion to simpler compounds. There is a bidirectional flux of electrolytes across the mucosa. The net results of absorption and secretion of these osmotically active solutes result in net water retention or loss in the stool. In this sense diarrhea can be thought of as the result of either malabsorption or net secretion of osmotically active substances.

Many nutrients (including glucose and certain amino acids) appear to be absorbed by active, carrier-mediated transport, which is coupled with sodium transport. The osmotic gradient created promotes the absorption of water. Movement of water in turn also carries small solutes, such as sodium and chloride.

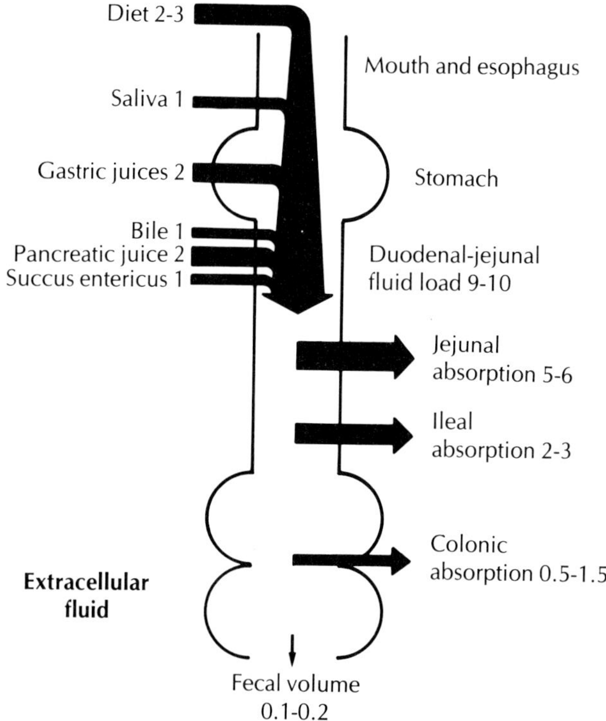

Fig. 120-1 Ingestion, secretion, and absorption of water in the gastrointestinal tract of an adult. Numbers refer to liters of water.

This process is known as *solvent drag* and appears to be an important route for sodium absorption during normal digestion. As noted below, these mechanisms of sodium movement associated with carrier-mediated nonelectrolyte transport are important to preserve normal fluid and electrolyte balance during some episodes of diarrhea.

Active absorption of chloride in exchange for bicarbonate (HCO_3^-) takes place in the ileum. Potassium appears to move passively along electrochemical gradients in the small intestine, but there is both active absorption and secretion of potassium in the colon. The permeability of the intestinal mucosa to passive fluid and electrolyte movement is high in the duodenum and proximal jejunum and decreases distally to the ileum and colon, which are poorly permeable. This feature allows the proximal intestinal contents to equilibrate rapidly with the isotonic extracellular fluid and allows for rapid absorption of water and small solutes by diffusion. Conversely, the ileum and colon are poorly permeable and are able to absorb water and sodium against high electrochemical gradients.

The pathophysiologic mechanisms for diarrhea fall into three basic categories, popularized by Phillips[29]: (1) osmotic diarrhea, (2) diarrhea resulting from secretion or altered absorption of electrolytes, and (3) diarrhea resulting from abnormal intestinal motility. Each mechanism has unique clinical characteristics and requires a different therapeutic approach. Therefore, for the physician considering an individual patient with diarrhea, this framework provides a rational approach for both diagnosis and treatment. Frequently more than one mechanism of diarrhea will be involved in an episode of diarrhea, but this will be apparent.

Osmotic Diarrhea

The ingestion of a poorly absorbable, osmotically active substance and its presence in the bowel lumen create an osmotic gradient that encourages movement of water into the lumen and subsequently into the stool. Electrolyte losses increase because electrolytes will follow water into the lumen through solvent drag and will tend not to be reabsorbed because of unfavorable electrochemical gradients.

There are two main groups of poorly absorbed solutes, the ingestion of which results in osmotic diarrhea. The first group includes normal dietary components that may be either transiently or permanently malabsorbed. For example, disaccharides usually are hydrolyzed to monosaccharides before they are absorbed. If a mucosal disaccharidase (such as lactase) is deficient, the disaccharide (in this case lactose) will be malabsorbed and will represent an osmotic load that will produce diarrhea. In a similar fashion, monosaccharides may at times be poorly absorbed. Medium-chain triglycerides (MCTs) also are osmotically active and may occasionally lead to diarrhea when ingested in high concentration. Such a situation may be found when infants with compromised mucosal function are given an elemental formula containing MCTs. Malabsorption of long-chain triglycerides (LCTs) does not lead to osmotic diarrhea because LCTs are large hydrophobic molecules and therefore have little osmotic activity. Malabsorption of LCTs, however, may lead to diarrhea by mechanisms described below. In addition, any osmotically active solute may produce diarrhea in normal persons if given in quantities great enough to surpass the intestinal capacity for absorption. Thus some infants with normal bowel function will not tolerate the high osmolality of an elemental formula, especially if it is undiluted. Likewise, patients with decreased mucosal surface area may have decreased functional capacity and resultant osmotic diarrhea. This problem is seen in infants after small bowel resection and necrotizing enterocolitis. Protein malabsorption does not appear to be associated with diarrhea except in the rare instance of congenital trypsinogen or enterokinase deficiency. For example, the Hartnup syndrome is a syndrome with malabsorption of primary amino acids that, nevertheless, is *not* associated with diarrhea.

The second group of poorly absorbed solutes includes substances that are transported in limited amounts, even by normal individuals. This group includes magnesium, phosphates, and sulfates. Because these ions invariably lead to diarrhea when given in large enough quantities, they are used as cathartics. The introduction of lactulose in the treatment of hepatic encephalopathy takes advantage of its being a nondigestible disaccharide that leads to acidification of colonic contents by bacterial fermentation of nonabsorbed sugar. Its side effect is diarrhea.

The key characteristic of an osmotic diarrhea is its association with the oral ingestion of the offending solute. When a patient with an osmotic diarrhea is given nothing by mouth, the diarrhea will stop dramatically within 24 hours or less. If the agent is reintroduced (as in a lactose tolerance test), the diarrhea will reappear. The diarrhea is of a moderate volume compared with that in secretory diarrhea. The sodium and potassium ion concentrations and osmolality in the stool fluid are very useful in establishing a diagnosis. As ileal and colonic sodium absorption continues to function against a concentration gradient, stool sodium concentration will be lower than in the plasma. The electrolyte concentration in the stool is roughly twice the combined sodium and potassium concentration. When this value is much less than the measured osmolality of the stool, there must be osmotically active nonelectrolytes in the stool, and an osmotic diarrhea is present. In some instances one may be able to find the osmotic component in the stool (such as a reducing substance in lactose malabsorption).

Diarrhea Secondary to Secretion or Altered Electrolyte Absorption

Net movement of an electrolyte across the intestinal mucosa (i.e., into or out of the bowel lumen) is the sum of the simultaneous bidirectional electrolyte flux across the mucosal surface epithelium. Thus, under normal circumstances, opposing secretory and absorptive processes (both active and passive) take place, and the resulting balance is reflected in normal luminal electrolyte and water content. Secretory diarrhea occurs when there is pathologic stimulation of a physiologic electrolyte secretory process. Under such circumstances there is a net increase in luminal electrolytes and therefore a secondary increase in water. In addition, an associated decrease in absorptive processes may occur. The electrolytes that have been implicated are sodium, chloride, and perhaps bicarbonate. Diarrhea also may result from a decrease in active electrolyte absorption in the absence of any change in secretory function. It should be mentioned at the outset that clinically it is very difficult to distinguish increased electrolyte secretion from decreased absorption; the results are similar. The prototype for the mechanism of secretory diarrhea has been cholera. Cholera enterotoxin has been shown to lead to increased intestinal secretion of chloride and possibly bicarbonate, as well as to inhibition of the absorption of sodium. Cholera enterotoxin appears to stimulate surface epithelial adenylate cyclase, leading to an increase in cellular levels of cyclic 3′5′-adenosine monophosphate (AMP). An important observation has been the normal histologic appearance of the intestinal mucosa during cholera infection or in vitro exposure to cholera enterotoxin. Specifically, there is no evidence of cell necrosis, inflammation, or local bacterial invasion. Similarly, other cell absorptive functions remain normal. The normal absorption of glucose provides a route for secondary sodium absorption. In fact oral glucose- and electrolyte-containing soutions have gained wide use in the management of cholera.

It is now realized that a growing number of infectious agents may be associated with secretory diarrhea. Toxigenic *Escherichia coli* produces an enterotoxin antigenically distinct from cholera enterotoxin, which also activates adenylate cyclase. Infantile diarrhea resulting from this toxin is well known. Other bacteria that have been associated with stimulation of intestinal secretion are strains of *Shigella dysenteriae, Salmonella typhimurium, Klebsiella pneumoniae, Clostridium perfringens, Staphylococcus aureus,* and *Pseudomonas aeruginosa*. Experimental work with viral enteritis suggests that there is a significant secretory component to this diarrhea.[15] Secretion is the result of viral damage to villous epithelial cells in the small intestine and repopulation of the villi with immature crypt cells, rather than toxin production.

There are several noninfectious causes of secretory diarrhea. Malabsorbed bile acids and long-chain fats both have been shown to stimulate a colonic secretory diarrhea. Certain prostaglandins have been shown to activate adenylate cyclase and produce intestinal secretion in experimental models. Because prostaglandins are released during inflammation, it has been hypothesized that diarrhea associated with certain inflammatory states may be caused by these hormones. This is a particularly appealing hypothesis to explain the small bowel secretion that may take place with chronic inflammatory bowel disease. Prostaglandins also have been suggested as possible mediators for the activation of adenylate cyclase by *Salmonella* organisms in the absence of an enterotoxin. Secretory diarrheas may occur in association with increased levels of certain gastrointestinal hormones, most notably vasoactive intestinal polypeptide (VIP).

An isolated decrease of electrolyte absorption is seen much less frequently. The best known example, although extremely rare, is congenital chloride-losing diarrhea.[14] This abnormality results from the apparent lack of normal, active chloride absorption by the distal small intestine. Great quantities of chloride are lost in the stool and lead to diarrhea from birth onward.

The stool in secretory diarrheas tends to be watery and large in volume. As opposed to osmotic diarrhea, secretory diarrhea persists despite discontinuing oral intake. The stool water osmolality will be approximately equal to the electrolyte concentration (i.e., twice the sum of the sodium and potassium concentrations) because there will not be a significant osmotic nonelectrolyte component.

Motility Diarrhea

The intestine has a cyclic, orderly pattern of motility. Increased, decreased, or disordered movement can lead to diarrhea. Rapid intestinal transit often occurs in association with osmotic and secretory diarrheas. Increased intraluminal volume has been implicated in stimulating increased peristaltic action. Increased motility may cause diarrhea by allowing less time for the contact of intraluminal contents with absorptive surfaces. When bowel function is compromised (as with the short bowel syndrome), the time of contact with the limited functioning surface may be a critical factor. In irritable bowel syndrome, disordered motility also may play a role.[10]

Slowed transit and severely disordered motility lead to intraluminal stasis. In normal bowel, steady, progressive movement of chyme is one of the protective mechanisms that prevents the development of bacterial overgrowth, whereas stasis encourages overgrowth. Certain bacteria deconjugate bile acids when present in the upper small bowel and secondarily produce fat malabsorption. In addition, bacterial proteases may damage the small bowel surface. Stasis may result from an anatomic obstruction (e.g., blind loop or stricture), as well as from functional motor disorders. Motility disorder frequently is an associated factor in chronic inflammatory bowel disease. Stools associated with motility disorder, except those secondary to fatty acid malabsorption, tend to be small in volume. The response to feeding is variable, and the gastrocolic reflex may be heightened. In chronic inflammatory bowel disease, many patients find that meals stimulate intestinal activity, resulting in postprandial abdominal cramps and bowel movements.

ACUTE DIARRHEA

Acute diarrhea is common in children, is transient and usually self-limited, and most often is caused by infection. The role of the physician is to rule out causes that require specific treatment, to advise the parents in supportive management, and to provide follow-up for possible complications. The box on p. 874 lists some of the more frequent causes of acute diarrhea. Day-care centers are likely sites for the spread of enteric pathogens; pathogens that have been associated with epidemics include *Giardia lamblia* and rotavirus; *Shigella, Campylobacter,* and *Cryptosporidium* organisms; and *Clostridium difficile*.[1,3,4] Asymptomatic fecal shedding of *Giardia* organisms is common in this setting.

The neonate with acute diarrhea must be considered different from the older infant and child both because of lower tolerance to the associated fluid shifts and because of the greater likelihood of associated infection or congenital anomaly. In addition, signs that suggest necrotizing enterocolitis must be looked for, including gastric retention (frequently bilious), distention, and occult or bright red blood in the stool. Although this disease usually occurs in premature infants, it

Causes of Acute Diarrhea

USUALLY WITHOUT BLOOD IN STOOL

Viral enteritis—reovirus (rotavirus[3,35] and orbivirus), Norwalk agent, and enteric adenovirus[43]
Enterotoxin—*E. coli,*[18] *Klebsiella* organisms, cholera, *C. perfringens,* and *Staphylococcus* organisms
Parasitic—*Giardia*[6] *and Cryptosporidium*[1,42] organisms
Extraintestinal infection—otitis media and urinary tract infection
Antibiotic-induced—especially ampicillin—and *Clostridium difficile* toxin (without pseudomembranous colitis)

COMMONLY ASSOCIATED WITH BLOOD IN STOOL

Bacterial—*Shigella, Salmonella,* and *Campylobacter* organisms, *Yersinia enterocolitica,* invasive *E. coli,*[18] gonococcus (venereal spread), and enteroadherent *E. coli*[40]
Amebic dysentery
Hemolytic-uremic syndrome
Henoch-Schönlein purpura
Pseudomembranous enterocolitis (*C. difficile* toxin)[7,34]
Ulcerative or granulomatous colitis (acute presentation)
Necrotizing enterocolitis (neonates)

also has been reported in ill full-term infants. The presence of pneumatosis intestinalis, gas in the portal vein, or free intraperitoneal gas seen on abdominal roentgenograms supports this diagnosis. Epidemics of diarrhea associated with enteropathogenic *E. coli,* salmonellae, and other organisms, including klebsiellae, have been reported in nurseries. If the onset of diarrhea is associated with early feedings, one must consider congenital digestive defects, especially sugar intolerance. *Hirschsprung disease* may manifest with acute diarrhea and enterocolitis in the neonatal period and should especially be suspected in the infant who has not passed meconium in the first 24 hours. Bloody diarrhea that results from cow milk or soy protein intolerance may develop in infants still in the nursery. Resolution and exacerbation on removal and reintroduction of formula, as well as an atopic family history, are clues to this diagnosis.

In the older infant and child the usual episode of acute diarrhea is transient and benign. On the initial visit the physician must evaluate the course in terms of both possible causes and the status of hydration. The diarrhea usually is the result of viral enteritis, typically occurring with low-grade fever, vomiting, and frequent watery stools. Generally, the stools are without blood or white blood cells. Enterotoxin-producing organisms (such as toxigenic *E. coli*) are associated with watery stools and are without evidence of mucosal invasion (no high fever or blood in the stool). *Giardia lamblia* produces watery diarrhea associated with intestinal gas and crampy abdominal pain. Diarrhea may be present in association with extraintestinal infections, most notably otitis media and pyelonephritis. This has been called *parenteral diarrhea,* and its mechanism is obscure. At least in some cases of otitis media there may be an associated viral enteritis. Certain antibiotics, especially ampicillin, have been associated with transient diarrhea. Less common but of greater danger is the association of pseudomembranous colitis with a number of antibiotics, most commonly clindamycin.[7] In childhood, a pseudomembranous colitis may occur acutely or with a more chronic illness of 1 or 2 months' duration.[34] *C. difficile* toxin, which is considered the cause of most cases of pseudomembranous colitis, also may be associated with chronic diarrhea in childhood in the absence of colitis.[36]

The presence of blood in the stool, especially with symptoms of colonic involvement (tenesmus, urgency, and crampy lower abdominal pain), should make one think of infection with *Shigella* and *Salmonella* organisms. These symptoms of dysentery are typically more striking with *Shigella* species; however, both may be associated with a significant secretory component. When the *Shigella* is an enterotoxin-producing organism, watery diarrhea actually may precede the onset of dysentery. Patients with *Shigella* organisms tend to appear severely ill and may have meningismus or a seizure. The stools tend to be foul smelling. *Yersinia* and *Campylobacter* enterocolitis also may be associated with blood in the stool, but *Yersinia* appears to be less commonly incriminated as an etiologic agent in the United States. *E. coli* can produce diarrhea by a number of pathogenic mechanisms; the enteroadherent, enteroinvasive, and enterohemorrhagic forms can all be associated with blood in the stool.[18] Amebiasis is unusual in the United States, but *Entamoeba histolytica* can produce a picture of acute colitis. Causes of bloody diarrhea that are not obviously infectious include hemolytic-uremic syndrome, intussusception, and chronic inflammatory bowel disease. The last may present with an initial episode of acute dysentery, although when the history is reviewed, there may have been previous episodes, and arthralgia or growth failure may have preceded the diarrhea. The history of recent similar diarrheal illness in family members or friends suggests an infectious diarrhea.

At the initial evaluation (see box on p. 875) the physician should establish the quantity of the diarrhea, the child's ability to maintain oral intake, and the presence of associated vomiting. On physical examination an estimate of the state of hydration should be made. The presence of tears and saliva usually is evidence of adequate hydration. A simple guideline to hydration is that the absence of tears and the presence of a dry mouth suggest 5% dehydration, whereas the addition of sunken eyes, sunken fontanelle, and poor skin turgor suggests 10% dehydration. In the presence of hypernatremia the state of dehydration may be found to be greater than suggested on physical examination inasmuch as extracellular fluid volume tends to be preserved at the expense of intracellular volume. A recorded weight is essential; it can be compared with previous weights and also will be available to reevaluate hydration during the illness. Information about the frequency and quantity of urine is useful, especially if there is a history of good urine output. Parents may underestimate urinary frequency, however, especially when urine becomes mixed with liquid stool.

Evaluation of Acute Diarrhea

1. History
   a. Length of illness
   b. Stools—frequency, looseness (watery versus mushy), and presence of gross blood
   c. Oral intake—diet, quantity of fluids and solids taken, and presence of vomiting
   d. Associated symptoms—fever, rash, and arthralgia
   e. Urine output
   f. Contacts with diarrhea or other infectious illness (including day-care exposure)
2. Physical examination
   a. Hydration status—moist mucosa, presence of saliva and tears, skin turgor, and weight
   b. Alertness
   c. Infant—vigor of suck
3. Laboratory
   a. Stool culture (as indicated), smear for white blood cells, and evaluation for occult blood
   b. Stool ova and parasites and reducing substances (as indicated)
   c. Complete blood count (as indicated)
   d. If hydration status is in question—blood urea nitrogen (BUN) and serum electrolyte levels
   e. Urinalysis
   f. If child is lethargic or has had a seizure, culture for sepsis: measure the BUN and serum electrolyte levels and examine and culture the cerebrospinal fluid (as indicated)

A stool culture should be obtained if blood or leukocytes are noted in the stool or if the child is severely ill. Examination of the stool for leukocytes is helpful in establishing the presence of colitis. A small sample of stool is placed on a microscope slide and mixed with a drop of methylene blue. Multiple fields are then scanned. In the presence of both infectious and noninfectious colitis, white blood cells (WBCs) usually are found in high numbers, in fact, frequently in sheets. Polymorphonuclear leukocytes may account for 60% to 80% of the cells. The presence of only occasional cells is considered a negative finding. The absence of WBCs in grossly bloody diarrheal stool occurs with enterohemorrhagic *E. coli* infection but also should direct attention to entities such as intussusception and Meckel diverticulum when these diagnoses seem clinically appropriate. Amebic colitis also may not be associated with WBCs in the stool, although the trophozoites and numerous red blood cells may be visible on a saline wet mount preparation of the stool. Invasive bacterial diarrhea is frequently associated with a peripheral blood leukocytosis.

The cornerstone of treatment in acute gastroenteritis is good fluid and electrolyte management (see box on p. 876). When the patient has less than 5% dehydration and is able to retain fluids adequately by mouth, outpatient treatment without specialized rehydration solutions is indicated. In the breast-fed infant, gastroenteritis is uncommon; however, it usually is possible to continue nursing, even if diarrhea occurs. It should be kept in mind that human milk is low in sodium content (6 to 7 mEq/L); therefore, when diarrhea is persistent or severe, a clear liquid regimen with a higher sodium concentration should be substituted to avoid hyponatremia. A transient secondary lactose intolerance also may have developed, an indication to discontinue breast milk temporarily.

The goal of treatment for an infant receiving cow milk formula has been to provide a lactose-free oral fluid with low renal solute load (i.e., high free water) and adequate but not excessive electrolyte content. This requires the temporary discontinuation of milk and solids and the initiation of oral clear liquids. Grandmothers, as well as clinicians, have traditionally recommended a diverse group of fluids with wide-ranging electrolyte and carbohydrate concentrations. It is clear that the electrolyte content in diarrheal stool varies widely, with the highest concentrations occurring in secretory diarrheas (e.g., cholera). Fecal sodium levels may range from 40 to 100 mEq/L and occasionally may be as high as 150 mEq/L.

At least 40% to 50% of epidemic diarrhea may be of viral origin (in fact in winter this proportion probably is higher). Viral enteritis has been shown to result in a transient, patchy, mucosal lesion of the small intestine, which may be associated with temporary lactose and fat malabsorption. Decreased mucosal lactase levels may be seen. In experimental viral diarrhea in piglets (transmissible gastroenteritis), intestinal glucose-stimulated absorption of sodium (and therefore water) is impaired because of villus damage.[20] Abnormal glucose absorption also has been observed in infants with rotavirus enteritis. Nevertheless, secretions can be converted to net absorption in most children by providing oral glucose-electrolyte solution, because of the patchy nature of the lesion in viral gastroenteritis.

Oral rehydration solutions have been used safely and successfully to treat acute diarrhea with dehydration.[30,33,37] Infants with diarrhea usually will drink large volumes of liquids ad libitum, appropriate for the stool output. Most episodes of diarrhea in previously healthy, well-nourished children are mild, and the selection of clear fluid is not critical. These liquids can be offered ad libitum, although frequent, smaller amounts may be better tolerated when diarrhea is associated with vomiting. If the episode is more severe, a solution as described in the box on p. 876 should be used. Commercial rehydration solutions are available (e.g., Rehydralyte, Lytren, and Resol). The contents of these solutions have evolved in conjunction with advances in the understanding of optimal absorption during oral rehydration. Therefore the clinician should consult current manufacturer specifications before choosing a product. The timing of advancement from oral fluids to formula is controversial, although recent studies suggest that rapid progression, supplemented with oral rehydration solution, is well tolerated and usually leads to quicker recovery. Vomiting usually is not a contraindication for oral rehydration. This treatment appears to be associated with shorter hospitalization and lower medical costs. Furthermore, infants with hypernatremic dehydration appear to have fewer problems with seizures during oral, as compared with intravenous, rehydration.[30,33] Oral rehydration therapy,

Management of Acute Diarrhea

A. Less than 5% dehydration without significant vomiting
   1. Nursing infant may continue breast-feeding—supplement with clear fluids as necessary; discontinue solids.
   2. Formula-fed infant
      a. Discontinue formula and solids.
      b. Begin clear liquids (e.g., carbonated beverages, Kool-Aid, Jell-O water, Gatorade, Pedialyte, Lytren, Resol). If intake is good without vomiting, offer fluids every 3 to 4 hours; otherwise, offer small quantities more frequently.
      c. As diarrhea resolves, reinstitute formula half strength at first.
      d. If child tolerates half-strength formula for 12 to 24 hours, then go to full strength.
      e. Solids may be introduced as diarrhea resolves (rice, cereal, bananas, crackers, and mashed potatoes without butter).
      f. If reinstitution of formula is not tolerated, continue clear liquids and then try half-strength lactose-free formula (soy formula).
      g. After improvement in diarrhea, increase solids as tolerated.
      h. Reintroduce lactose in patients on lactose-free diet several days to weeks after resolution, depending on severity of original diarrhea; if not tolerated, continue lactose-free diet for several months.
   3. Avoid diphenoxylate (Lomotil), loperamide (Imodium), paregoric, and anticholinergics.

B. Greater than 5% dehydration: either oral or intravenous rehydration
   1. Oral rehydration therapy
      a. Offer rehydration solution *hourly ad libitum:* 50 to 75 mEq/L sodium, 20 to 30 mEq/L potassium, 30 mEq/L bicarbonate or citrate, remainder of anion as chloride, and 20 g/L glucose.
      b. As the diarrhea slows (usually within 24 to 48 hours), begin one-half strength formula (can be lactose free) and advance to regular diet within 24 hours. For ongoing diarrheal losses, supplement with oral rehydration solution.
      c. Infants with signs of shock should be given intravenous Ringer lactate (20 ml/kg body weight per hour) until the blood pressure is normal, followed by oral rehydration solution.
      d. Initial vomiting is not a contraindication to the use of oral rehydration; however, persistent vomiting to the extent of interference with rehydration should lead to the use of intravenous fluids.
   2. Intravenous fluids (see Chapter 25)
      a. Replacement of deficit is based on estimated percentage of dehydration or known weight loss and serum sodium.
      b. There may be ongoing loss through stool and vomitus.
      c. Maintenance should be appropriate for size.
   3. Give half of fluids in first 8 hours, then remainder over next 16 hours (except with hypernatremia, when fluids should be given uniformly with gradual correction over 48 hours; hypotonic fluid should not be used for hypernatremia).
   4. If severe dehydration or shock is present, give isotonic fluid or a colloid (10 to 20 ml/kg body weight, over 1 to 2 hours).
   5. Delay giving intravenous potassium until urine output is established.
   6. As diarrhea resolves, begin treatment as in those patients with less than 5% dehydration, except avoid lactose.

however, requires the nearly constant presence of a caretaker although this individual does not require previous medical experience. Currently, the use of amino acids or starches in oral rehydration solution is being evaluated in an effort to improve sodium and water absorption and to reduce stool output.

There is little indication for medications in the treatment of acute gastroenteritis in infants and children. As already noted, the key mechanisms involved are intestinal secretion and transient malabsorption. Therefore, although medications frequently are used, there is no apparent rationale regarding the pathophysiology of the disorder for medications that slow gut motility—diphenoxylate, loperamide, paregoric, and anticholinergics. In fact, pooling of fluid in the intestinal lumen after treatment may give a false impression that the diarrhea has improved. Diphenoxylate also has been implicated in accidental overdosage and respiratory arrest. This drug is not approved in the United States for children younger than 2 years of age. In the study of Portnoy and colleagues,[31] children with acute gastroenteritis (3 to 11 years of age) were given diphenoxylate; no difference in the amount of change in stool weight or water content could be found during the 2 days after onset of treatment when these children were compared with others who had received a placebo.[31] Although Kaopectate does not carry the hazards of these drugs, it has not been shown to be efficacious in slowing fluid output and also may lead to a false impression that the diarrhea has resolved. There is a concern that slowing intestinal transit with drugs may allow greater mucosal contact with pathogens and thereby allow for local mucosal invasion. Antibiotics are useful in specific situations: *Shigella* dysentery, *Yersinia* or *Campylobacter* gastroenteritis, pseudomembranous colitis, *Salmonella* infections in infants younger than 6 months old, and *Salmonella* infections in older patients with enteric fever, typhoid fever, or complications of bacteremia. For the individual patient, the presence of an *E. coli* serotype previously labeled enteropathogenic correlates poorly with the presence of diarrhea and alone is not an indication for antibiotic treatment.[18]

Most episodes of gastroenteritis are self-limited and of short duration. Symptoms of rotavirus enteritis typically last 4 to 10 days. As the diarrhea resolves, the child may restart solids (especially rice, cereal, bananas, apples, and dry toast) and then the previous formula. It usually is best to begin with half-strength formula. If this is tolerated for 1 to 2 days, full-strength formula then may be resumed. If diarrhea recurs on the introduction of lactose-containing formula, the child may have acquired a transient lactose intolerance. In this situation half-strength soy formula may be offered (the sugar in this formula can be either sucrose or a glucose polymer). In the rare situation in which sucrose is not tolerated, a sucrose-free formula should be used. As noted in the section on disaccharide intolerance, sugar malabsorption can be identified by the determination of reducing substance in the stool (keeping in mind that sucrose must be hydrolyzed first with hydrochloric acid). A secondary lactose intolerance usually lasts only a week or less but at times can persist for months.

If the degree of dehydration is greater than 5%, either oral or intravenous rehydration solution should be instituted in the manner presented in the box on p. 876. For severe dehydration or shock, rapid intravenous administration of 10 to 20 ml/kg of fluid is required initially. Hyponatremia and hypernatremia must be corrected slowly to prevent complications of the central nervous system (CNS). Recent studies suggest that oral solutions may be tolerated with fewer CNS complications than are intravenous solutions in infants with hypernatremia.[30,33] Potassium should not be added to intravenous fluids until adequate urine output is established. Urine specific gravity may be misleading inasmuch as kidney concentration may be poor in the face of the whole body potassium depletion. Complete discussion of intravenous treatment is presented in Chapter 25, "Fluid Therapy."

CHRONIC DIARRHEA

Chronic diarrhea can develop in children of all ages; however, it is most frequent and often most challenging to diagnose in infants. Both healthy and ill infants seem to develop diarrhea in response to a variety of stresses. The younger the infant, the more likely he or she is to enter the cycle of diarrhea and secondary malnutrition that leads to further diarrhea, malnutrition, and susceptibility to infection. Many of the causes of chronic diarrhea may appear at any time during childhood. Certain diseases, however, occur much more commonly in infancy, whereas others are more likely to begin in later childhood. This section discusses illnesses of infancy and older childhood separately. This division is somewhat artificial, but it is helpful as a guide in evaluating the patient with chronic diarrhea. All the causes discussed are listed in the accompanying box.

Causes of Chronic Diarrhea

MORE COMMON CAUSES

Chronic nonspecific diarrhea (irritable colon of childhood)[24]
Disaccharide intolerance[39]
Chronic constipation with overflow diarrhea
Cystic fibrosis
Gluten-sensitive enteropathy (celiac disease)[25]
Inflammatory bowel disease—Crohn disease and ulcerative colitis
Hirschsprung disease
Immunodeficiency states
Chronic enteric infection—*Salmonella* organisms, *Yersinia enterocolitica, Campylobacter* and *Giardia* organisms, *C. difficile* toxin,[34,36] enteroadherent *E. coli,*[40] rotavirus (in immunodeficient patients), and cytomegalovirus
Monosaccharide intolerance
Eosinophilic (allergic) gastroenteritis
Cow milk protein intolerance[5]
Short bowel syndrome
Urinary tract infection
Factitious causes

LESS COMMON CAUSES

Hormonal—adrenal insufficiency and hyperthyroidism
Vasoactive intestinal polypeptide–secreting tumor
Neural crest tumor and carcinoid
Intestinal lymphangiectasia[41]
Acrodermatitis enteropathica[26]
Intestinal stricture or blind loop
Pancreatic insufficiency with neurotropenia[13]
Trypsinogen or enterokinase deficiency
Congenital chloride-losing diarrhea[14]
Abetalipoproteinemia
Microvillus inclusion disease[9]
Intestinal pseudoobstruction

Infants

The physician confronted with an infant with a history of chronic diarrhea must decide first whether the stool pattern is in fact abnormal. A nursing mother who has not been forewarned may become concerned about the appearance and frequency of her child's transitional stools. The infant's weight gain and healthy appearance, combined with an explanation about stools of breast-fed infants, should dispel these concerns. In the latter half of the first year and in the second year, the most common cause for persistent diarrhea is irritable colon of infancy (also called chronic nonspecific diarrhea or toddler's diarrhea). Affected infants have intermittent loose stools with no apparent rhyme or reason. Often the stools occur early in the day and not overnight. These infants appear healthy and are thriving according to weight and length growth curves. This condition represents a stool pattern rather than a pathologic state and requires minimal or no laboratory evaluation. Symptoms may begin initially after an apparent acute enteritis (postenteritis irritable bowel).

Treatment may include (1) restricting the frequency of feedings, whether liquids or solids, in an effort to decrease stimulation of the gastrocolic reflex (in the older infant, three meals and a bedtime snack with nothing by mouth in between), (2) restricting the volumes of fluids ingested, which often are excessive, (3) avoiding excessive intake of juices,[16] and (4) reassuring the parents of the benign nature of this entity. A high-fat diet may be helpful in some children.[8] Cholestyramine (2 g by mouth one to three times daily) also is effective at times; however, the duration of use should be restricted because of the potential for interference with fat-soluble vitamin absorption. Bile acid malabsorption has been described as an infrequent sequel of gastroenteritis that can produce persistent diarrhea. This condition also will respond to cholestyramine therapy.

Protracted Diarrhea of Infancy. This syndrome of chronic diarrhea occurring during infancy is poorly understood[24]; it is somewhat arbitrarily defined as occurring in infants younger than 3 months of age and persisting for more than 2 weeks. Historically, this syndrome, called *intractable diarrhea of infancy,* has been associated with a high mortality secondary to irreversible diarrhea and related malnutrition. However, the outcome has been markedly improved with the advent of total parenteral nutrition and oral elemental diets. Protracted diarrhea of infancy is probably the final pathway for multiple causes, including gastrointestinal infection and perhaps food intolerances. Generally, malnutrition develops and in concert with the persistent diarrhea leads to alteration of gastrointestinal flora sometimes associated with bacterial overgrowth of the small intestine. Both altered mucosal function of the small intestine and pancreatic function have been associated with malnutrition and intractable diarrhea. Bile salt deconjugation as a result of bacterial overgrowth may occur. Commonly the initiating cause is not found, and it is likely that it may no longer be present when the diarrhea has become chronic. The small bowel biopsy specimen may show patchy villous shortening with a decreased villus/crypt ratio and marked inflammation, as well as a damaged surface epithelium. However, the results of the small bowel biopsy also may be normal. Likewise, a rectal biopsy specimen may show evidence of inflammation, including crypt abscesses, or may be normal. The presence or absence of these biopsy findings may not correlate with the severity of the clinical syndrome.[12] Affected infants are severely malnourished with low serum protein, albumin, and hemoglobin levels. Frequently they have had repeated treatment with oral clear liquids and peripheral intravenous fluids, all of which provide inadequate caloric intake.

In evaluating a young infant with protracted diarrhea, the physician must rule out those causes that require urgent treatment while correcting hydration and nutrition. Acute rehydration is similar to the intravenous treatment of acute diarrhea, although it is more difficult to estimate the level of dehydration accurately in the presence of malnutrition. Stool output should be quantitated. If the urine is collected in a urine bag, diapers can be weighed before and after stools to give an accurate measure. Urine specific gravity and volume may be deceiving because of poor concentration by the kidneys in the presence of malnutrition and total body hypokalemia. The infant should be weighed at least daily. It is important to rule out infection as a cause early in the evaluation. Several stool cultures, as well as blood and urine cultures, should be taken initially. The diagnosis of Hirschsprung disease with enterocolitis should be considered early, inasmuch as infants with this disorder are prone to perforation of the colon unless a decompression colostomy is performed. In such babies it is usually possible to elicit a history of the absence of stools in the first 24 hours of life and early obstipation.

In Hirschsprung disease a flat plate roentgenogram of the abdomen may show a dilated colon, although toxic megacolon also may be seen in infectious colitis or in chronic inflammatory bowel disease in infancy. Air-fluid levels throughout the bowel are common in infants with gastroenteritis, and this sign is not helpful in defining a cause. A barium enema under low pressure in the unprepared patient may show the narrow distal segment of rectum; however, this finding may not be present in neonates. Often Hirschsprung disease is more obvious on a delayed roentgenogram (24 to 48 hours).

If the child with chronic diarrhea has recently been fed, stool pH and reducing substance should be determined to evaluate sugar malabsorption. The stool pH is not a good measure of the effect of diarrhea on total body acid-base balance. If stool concentration of sodium and potassium minus chloride is greater than the plasma bicarbonate, the infant is losing bicarbonate. Stool pH also should be determined. White blood cells in the stool suggest colonic inflammation, whereas occult blood in the stool suggests loss of blood across the mucosa in the small or large intestine.

It is important to begin nutritional rehabilitation at once. Currently the best choices in treatment are either enteral alimentation with an elemental or modular formula[22] or total parenteral nutrition (TPN) (peripheral or central) (see Chapter 25, "Fluid Therapy"). Often enteral nutrition is best tolerated by the continuous drip method. Recent studies suggest that recovery may be more rapid when enteral alimentation is used.[28] Nevertheless, unsuccessful attempts at enteral feeding necessitate initiation of TPN therapy in some infants. Initial treatment with TPN and a gradually increasing, continuous enteral drip is a good approach to patients who do not tolerate elemental diet alone. Elemental formulas are composed of predigested components in fixed proportions, whereas modular formulas allow one to vary the components. A small bowel biopsy for diagnosis may help in planning therapy. Severe mucosal damage would make one less inclined to persist with unsuccessful enteral alimentation. Measuring stool output and weight gain may be used to assess the infant's response. If disaccharidase levels are abnormal, the specific disaccharides should be avoided. During the treatment, a further workup, including an upper gastrointestinal series with small bowel roentgenogram, barium edema, proctoscopy, the measurement of sweat electrolytes, and other specific tests to rule out the entities noted below, should be carried out as indicated.

Malabsorption Syndromes. Infants and children with malabsorption syndromes typically have diarrhea, steatorrhea, or growth failure, or a combination of these. Cystic fibrosis is the most common chronic disease that causes malabsorption in the United States. Steatorrhea results from pancreatic insufficiency and secondary maldigestion. Infants with cystic fibrosis who nurse or are fed soy formula (but not cow milk formula) may be seen in the first months of life with protein malabsorption. Although cystic fibrosis is thought of primarily as a respiratory disease, some infants and children will have malabsorption and little history of respiratory symptoms. These patients typically have voracious appetites. The diagnosis may be suspected by the absence of trypsin in the stool and must be confirmed by sweat electrolyte studies. Other diseases much less common than cystic fibrosis may occur with prominent steatorrhea in early infancy, including congenital pancreatic insufficiency with cyclic neutropenia (the *Shwachman-Diamond syndrome*),[13] *intestinal lymphangiectasia,*[41] and *abetalipoproteinemia*. Measurement of serum trypsinogen appears to be a useful screening test for pancreatic insufficiency.[11] Transient steatorrhea may follow an acute enteritis.[19]

In infancy the age at which celiac disease manifests (gluten-sensitive enteropathy) varies with the age of dietary introduction of gluten-containing products (wheat, rye, oats, and barley).[25] Usually the onset is 1 to several months later. Typically infants with celiac disease are irritable and have loose stools, poor appetite, and poor weight gain. They also may have recurrent vomiting. The presentation, however, is quite variable. Steatorrhea does not need to be present, and results of absorptive studies such as the D-xylose tolerance test may be normal. A diagnosis of celiac disease should be made by small bowel biopsy; dietary trials and antigliadin antibody studies may be misleading.[38] A later challenge with gluten and a repeat biopsy will confirm the diagnosis. *Giardia* infection can produce small bowel malabsorption that mimics celiac disease.[6]

Carbohydrate (monosaccharide or disaccharide) intolerance may be primary or more commonly secondary to other gastrointestinal disorders.[39] The congenital form of lactase deficiency is much less common than is congenital sucrase-isomaltase deficiency. The latter disorder typically manifests after introduction of sucrose into the diet in solids. With a carbohydrate intolerance the extent of symptoms varies directly with the quantity of the offending sugar in the diet. Likewise, the age at presentation will vary with the age at which the sugar is introduced into the diet. The diagnosis may be established by conducting standard sugar tolerance tests, measuring hydrogen excretion in the breath, and assaying the enzymes present in tissue obtained by a small bowel biopsy. Examination of the stool for reducing sugar is a good screening test. Sorbitol,[15] an artificial sweetener, as well as fructose,[32] may produce diarrhea when ingested in large amounts.

The congenital deficiency of trypsinogen, the zymogen precursor of the pancreatic protease trypsin, has been reported as a very rare cause of congenital diarrhea. The absence of trypsin in the stool may suggest the diagnosis (in the absence of cystic fibrosis and congenital pancreatic insufficiency), but evaluation of the pancreatic proteases in the duodenal aspirate is necessary to confirm this impression. Congenital deficiency of enterokinase, the intestinal enzyme that activates trypsinogen to trypsin, appears in a similar fashion to that of congenital trypsinogen deficiency and is diagnosed by testing the duodenal aspirate for enterokinase activity.

Infection. It has been mentioned that acute bacterial or viral enteritis may be an important initiator of protracted diarrhea in infancy. If the initial infection is no longer present at the time of evaluation for chronic diarrhea, this association will be difficult to prove. Infections at distant sites, especially urinary tract infections, also have been incriminated as a cause of chronic diarrhea in infancy. A urinalysis and urine culture should be routinely obtained in the evaluation of children with chronic diarrhea. *Salmonella* enteritis commonly is associated with a chronic asymptomatic carrier state, especially in infancy. *Salmonella* infection, however, also may be associated with persistent diarrhea in infants. *Y. enterocolitica* enteritis has been associated with a chronic relapsing diarrhea. *Yersinia* organisms do not appear to be common pathogens in the United States; however, one must be sure that the microbiology laboratory specifically looks for this organism or it will be missed. *Campylobacter* enteritis also can have a protracted course.

Parasites. The principal parasite associated with diarrhea in the United States is *G. lamblia*.[6] It may be associated with watery diarrhea and crampy abdominal pain and may manifest in epidemic form. This protozoon may be difficult to detect in stools, and the best yield of organisms comes from a duodenal fluid aspirate or a small bowel biopsy. Amebic dysentery may be indistinguishable from the colitis of inflammatory bowel disease and must be ruled out along with bacterial colitis before a diagnosis of inflammatory bowel disease can be made.

Hirschsprung Disease. This congenital abnormality involving the submucosal and myenteric plexuses of the colon (rarely small intestine as well) accounts for about 25% of intestinal obstructions in newborns. Such neonates almost invariably fail to pass meconium and have persistent obstipation and recurrent abdominal distention. These features may be overlooked, however, and the infants may subsequently have chronic diarrhea. The diarrhea is secondary to enterocolitis, which can be a surgical emergency that demands rapid diagnosis and treatment. A barium enema in the neonate may reveal false negative findings; anorectal manometric examination may be helpful, but an adequate rectal biopsy specimen showing absence of ganglion cells will confirm the diagnosis. Properly performed, suction biopsy of the rectum is highly reliable.[2]

Food Intolerance. Dietary protein intolerance, especially cow milk intolerance, is a well-known entity in pediatric practice.[5] The frequently inappropriate use of this diagnosis to justify formula changes has made its actual incidence difficult to determine. More objective criteria for the diagnosis are being sought. The syndrome must be considered when an infant with chronic diarrhea has any of the following manifestations: occult or gross blood in the stool (colitis), protein-losing enteropathy, peripheral eosinophilia, or other extraintestinal manifestations of allergy such as eczema, hives, or asthma. Continued manifestations when the infant is fed a cow milk–free, soy formula diet do not rule out the diagnosis, inasmuch as 20% of patients intolerant to cow milk protein also will be intolerant to soy protein. Bloody diarrhea develops in some infants while nursing, which then resolves when they are given a protein hydrolysate formula.[23] Some but not all of these infants respond to the reinstitution of nursing with the removal of dairy products from the mother's diet.

Short Bowel Syndrome. This syndrome of chronic malabsorption and diarrhea follows extensive resection of the small intestine. Short bowel syndrome begins most commonly in the newborn period in association with necrotizing enterocolitis or a congenital anomaly of the small intestine (e.g., malrotation with secondary midgut volvulus, intestinal atresia, or gastroschisis). Occasionally, recovery requires the use of TPN for the first several years of life. The factors that appear to contribute to this entity include a decrease in intestinal absorptive surface, altered intestinal motility, intraluminal bacterial overgrowth (with secondary deconjugation of bile salts and hydroxylation of fatty acids), malabsorption of bile salts secondary to terminal ileal resection, disaccharidase deficiency, and an increase in gastric acid secretion.

Intestinal Lymphangiectasia. This syndrome of dilated intestinal lymphatic vessels is associated protein-losing enteropathy, steatorrhea, lymphocytopenia, and chronic diarrhea.[41] As a result of the bowel protein loss, affected children may have hypogammaglobulinemia and hypoalbuminemia, usually with peripheral edema. Primary intestinal lymphangiectasia appears to be a developmental anomaly of unknown origin and frequently is associated with lymphatic abnormalities of the extremities. Secondary lymphangiectasia may result from chronic volvulus secondary to malrotation, with malfixation of the bowel, constrictive pericarditis, tumor, malformation, or any other factor that leads to obstruction of intestinal lymphatic flow. The diagnosis is suggested by a history of chronic diarrhea and poor growth and the presence of peripheral edema, hypoalbuminemia, hypogammaglobulinemia, and lymphocytopenia. The latter two abnormalities may lead to a decreased immune defense and an increased risk for infections. A radiologic small bowel follow-through study may show generalized thickening of the intestinal folds. The diagnosis is confirmed by the presence of characteristically dilated lymphatics on a small bowel biopsy specimen. The treatment includes the dietary use of medium-chain triglycerides and avoidance of long-chain fat. Protection from and early treatment of infection also are important.

Acrodermatitis Enteropathica. This rare familial disease of poorly understood etiology frequently appears when breast-fed infants are weaned.[26] Typically the infant has chronic diarrhea, intermittent vomiting, and an intractable erythematous, raw, crusty rash, which is most prominent in the perianal and perioral regions. The rash also may be seen on the extremities and responds poorly to local therapy. Alopecia is characteristically present, and conjunctivitis and dystrophic changes of the nails may occur. Infants with acrodermatitis enteropathica are usually irritable and unhappy. Results of the small bowel biopsy have been described as normal, although this has been questioned. The response to therapy is dramatic, with a relapse occurring when treatment is discontinued. The earliest treatment was a breast-milk diet; subsequently iodoquinol was used. Intravenous infusion of polyunsaturated fats has been associated with temporary improvement. However, the disorder is associated with a zinc deficiency (perhaps secondary to malabsorption) and responds dramatically to zinc salts given orally. This appears to be the treatment of choice.[27]

FACTITIOUS DIARRHEA

Factitious diarrhea is more common than pediatricians prefer to recognize. It is reasonable to screen a stool specimen for laxative abuse when an infant is seen with persistent diarrhea that does not seem to fit any known pattern. Inappropriate administration of laxative to an infant is a symptom of the caretaker's psychosocial dysfunction; often problems in other areas become apparent during the social history. Parents who administer laxatives surreptitiously frequently are medically knowledgeable persons (e.g., nurse or laboratory technician background) and often seem to prefer staying in the hospital with their child rather than being at home. They tend to be very helpful to the nursing staff, often to the degree of excessive involvement in the nursing care, and commonly are described by the nurses as caring and concerned parents. The pediatrician may note that the parent seems to encourage invasive diagnostic studies and treatment even beyond the medical plan, rather than showing an appropriate degree of hesitancy.

Hormone-Related Diarrhea. There are several entities that may be included in this group. Adrenal insufficiency secondary to either adrenogenital syndrome or adrenal hemorrhage may be associated with significant diarrhea, as may congenital thyrotoxicosis. Vasoactive intestinal polypeptide (VIP)–secreting tumors of the pancreas have been reported as a rare cause of diarrhea in adults and an even less common cause in children.

Ganglioneuroma, as well as the more malignant ganglioneuroblastoma, has been associated with chronic secretory diarrhea. The tumors usually are abdominal but also have been reported in the mediastinum. Although these are catecholamine-secreting tumors, there is some thought that prostaglandins or VIP may be the mediator of the diarrhea. A workup of the infant with persistent diarrhea of unknown cause but that is clearly secretory in nature should include urinary catecholamine studies, abdominal and chest roentgenograms, and an intravenous pyelogram. Even when the findings of these studies are negative, one must strongly consider a CT scan or arteriographic examination and surgical exploration if a severe secretory diarrhea persists. Plasma prostaglandin and VIP levels may be useful. When a tumor is found and is completely excised, the diarrhea usually resolves abruptly.

Immune Disorders. Immunodeficiency should be considered in any child with chronic diarrhea. In early infancy the two disorders associated with diarrhea are severe combined immunodeficiency and the Wiskott-Aldrich syndrome. The most common association seen in later childhood is late-onset, variable hypogammaglobulinemia. Pure T cell abnormalities (DiGeorge syndrome and other T cell deficiencies) also are associated with diarrhea. There is an increased incidence of celiac disease among persons with selected IgA deficiency; therefore measurement of immunoglobulin levels should be a routine part of the workup of any patient with chronic diarrhea. If the diagnosis remains unclear, a T cell evaluation also should be carried out. Chronic *Giardia* or rotavirus infection can be seen with immunodeficiencies. Diarrhea in association with granulomas of the intestinal tract has been noted in chronic granulomatous disease of childhood. These children can have perianal fistulas; the disorder may be mistaken initially for Crohn disease. Diarrheal illness can be a prominent feature of the acquired immunodeficiency syndrome as well.

IDIOPATHIC INTESTINAL PSEUDOOBSTRUCTION

Idiopathic intestinal pseudoobstruction constitutes a group of rare disorders characterized by widespread gastrointestinal dysmotility.[17] When this syndrome occurs in early infancy, vomiting and diarrhea often are major components. Diarrhea may alternate with constipation. In older children the presentation frequently is more insidious—a long history of constipation may precede the onset of diarrhea. Persons with this syndrome usually have intermittent or constant abdominal distention. The syndrome is characterized by the roentgenographic findings of bowel dilation with disordered motility; urinary bladder dysfunction often is present as well. These disorders can be sporadic or transmitted in an autosomal dominant fashion. They can result from a visceral myopathy or neuropathy, or a combination of both.

MICROVILLUS INCLUSION DISEASE

Microvillus inclusion disease (familial enteropathy) is a recently identified disorder that occurs at birth and causes severe intractable secretory diarrhea with malabsorption.[9] These infants have small bowel villous atrophy and crypt hypoplasia. The villous surface epithelial cells lack a normal brush border, and on electron microscopic examination the microvilli are absent or severely abnormal. These defective cells contain intracytoplasmic inclusions, which in turn contain the components of the brush border suggesting that the cells are either unable to assemble normal brush borders or rapidly dismantle them. There are reports of a number of families with more than one child having this disorder. Microvillus inclusion disease, although a rare disorder, may prove to be an important cause of intractable diarrhea of infancy.

Congenital Chloride-Losing Diarrhea. This very rare, familial, persistent diarrhea results from congenital absence of the normal ileal mechanism for active absorption of chloride in exchange for bicarbonate.[14] These infants have a chronic metabolic alkalosis instead of the metabolic acidosis usually seen in chronic diarrhea. Stool chloride concentration is high, usually exceeding the sum of concentrations of Na^+ and K^+. In children with this disorder, stool Cl^- may be in the range of 100 to 150 mEq/L, although in infants it may be 30 to 100 mEq/L (normally adult stool Cl^- is less than 20 mEq/L). There is no satisfactory treatment, although support with oral fluids and potassium chloride is recommended.

Infant of a Drug-Addicted Mother. The syndrome of neonatal drug withdrawal has become a more common problem, especially in urban areas. Diarrhea may be a prominent manifestation, and this diagnosis should be entertained in newborns with persistent diarrhea, especially when other symptoms of neonatal drug withdrawal are present (see Chapter 33).

Older Children

A pediatrician will see fewer older children with chronic diarrhea than infants, but older children are more likely to have chronic diarrhea associated with significant underlying disease. As in infancy, the association of poor growth, weight loss, or other systemic manifestations suggests a serious organic cause. There is a common tendency in older children to deny symptoms, and the true impact of the disorder may not be apparent except in retrospect after initiation of appropriate treatment. Subtle changes in personality, sense of well-being, and appetite and other systemic clues should be sought. Children may hesitate to talk about their stooling pattern, and the degree of deviation from the norm may only become apparent after improvement occurs.

The etiologic focus differs somewhat after infancy. Many of the causes seen in infancy, even congenital anomalies, may first manifest in childhood and must therefore still be considered. Factors that determine the age at diagnosis include (1) the objective variation in presentation of signs and symptoms, (2) the parental expectations of normality, and (3) the index of suspicion of the physician consulted. Certain diseases, however, including inflammatory bowel disease and chronic constipation with encopresis, are much more likely to be seen in childhood than in infancy. Celiac disease clearly may occur throughout life. Cystic fibrosis may be associated with only mild manifestations in infancy and may be overlooked until frequent, bulky, foul-smelling stools become intolerable at home.

Irritable Bowel. Irritable bowel similar to that occurring in adults may be seen in older children and adolescents.[10] Stools may alternate from diarrhea to constipation. In addition, the patient may have recurrent, crampy, abdominal pain. It is important to rule out late-onset lactose intolerance, which may mimic irritable bowel.

Inflammatory Bowel Disease (IBD). The manifestations and presentation of both Crohn disease and ulcerative colitis are so variable that this group of diseases must be thought of and ruled out whenever one sees an older child with chronic diarrhea.[21] Systemic evidence of inflammation (fever, weight loss, and leukocytosis), abdominal pain, blood in the stool (gross or occult), perianal disease, anemia, or extraintestinal manifestations (arthralgia, arthritis, and erythema nodosum) are helpful in making a diagnosis. Growth failure can occur with or precede other symptoms. An elevated sedimentation rate also is a clue; however, normal sedimentation rates may occur in as many as 50% of patients with IBD. Thrombocytosis has been associated with IBD and may be present in the absence of an elevated sedimentation rate. Suggestive signs and symptoms require a workup, including a complete blood count, platelet count, erythrocyte sedimentation rate, serum protein levels, roentgenographic contrast studies of the upper or lower bowel, with good views of the terminal ileum and proctoscopic or colonoscopic examination with rectal biopsy. The absorptive function of the gastrointestinal tract should be quantitated as appropriate.

Chronic Constipation. Occasionally chronic constipation with overflow incontinence will manifest as diarrhea. A thorough history and physical examination, including a rectal examination, should make the diagnosis apparent. If one goes back in the history, it is usual to find that the problem began with constipation. A large amount of stool usually is palpable in the abdomen, as well as a hard mass of stool in the rectal ampulla. This presentation is treated in the usual fashion of chronic constipation (as noted in Chapter 116).

REFERENCES

1. Alpert G et al: Outbreak of cryptosporidiosis in a day-care center, Pediatrics 77:152, 1986.
2. Andrassy RJ, Isaacs H, and Weitzman JJ: Rectal suction biopsy for the diagnosis of Hirschsprung disease, Ann Surg 193:419, 1981.
3. Bartlett AV, Reves RR, and Pickering LK: Rotavirus in infant-toddler day care centers: epidemiology relevant to disease control strategies, J Pediatr 113:435, 1988.
4. Bartlett AV et al: Diarrheal illness among infants and toddlers in day care centers. I. Epidemiology and pathogens, J Pediatr 107:495, 1985.
5. Bock SA: Prospective appraisal of complaints of adverse reactions to foods in children during the first 3 years of life, Pediatrics 79:683, 1987.
6. Burke JA: Giardiasis in childhood, Am J Dis Child 129:1304, 1975.
7. Buts JP et al: Pseudomembranous enterocolitis in childhood, Gastroenterology 73:823, 1977.
8. Cohen SA et al: Chronic nonspecific diarrhea; dietary relationships, Pediatrics 64:402, 1979.
9. Cutz E et al: Microvillus inclusion disease: an inherited defect of brush-border assembly and differentiation, N Engl J Med 320:646, 1989.
10. Drossman DA, Powell DW, and Sessions JT: The irritable bowel syndrome, Gastroenterology 73:811, 1977.
11. Durie PR et al: Plasma immunoreactive pancreatic cationic trypsinogen in cystic fibrosis: a sensitive indicator of exocrine pancreatic dysfunction, Pediatr Res 15:1351, 1981.
12. Goldgar CM and Vanderhoof JA: Lack of correlation of small bowel biopsy and clinical course of patients with intractable diarrhea of infancy, Gastroenterology 90:527, 1986.
13. Hill RE et al: Steatorrhea and pancreatic insufficiency in Shwachman syndrome, Gastroenterology 83:22, 1982.
14. Holmberg C et al: Congenital chloride diarrhea, Arch Dis Child 52:255, 1977.
15. Hyams JS: Sorbitol malabsorption: an unappreciated cause of functional gastrointestinal complaints, Gastroenterology 84:30, 1983.
16. Hyams JS et al: Carbohydrate malabsorption following fruit juice ingestion in young children, Pediatrics 82:64, 1988.
17. Hyman PE et al: Antroduodenal motility in children with chronic intestinal pseudo-obstruction, J Pediatr 112:899, 1988.
18. Infectious Diseases Committee, Canadian Paediatric Society: *Escherichia coli* gastroenteritis: making sense of the new acronyms, Can Med Assoc J 136:241, 1987.
19. Jonas A et al: Disturbed fat absorption following infectious gastroenteritis in children, J Pediatr 95:366, 1979.
20. Kerzner B et al: Transmissible gastroenteritis: sodium transport and the intestinal epithelium during the course of viral enteritis, Gastroenterology 72:457, 1977.
21. Kirschner BS: Inflammatory bowel disease in children, Pediatr Clin North Am 35:189, 1988.
22. Klish WJ et al: Modular formula: an approach to management of infants with specific or complex food iintolerances, J Pediatr 88:948, 1976.
23. Lake AM, Whitington PF, and Hamilton SR: Dietary protein-induced colitis in breast-fed infants, J Pediatr 101:906, 1982.
24. Larcher VF et al: Protracted diarrhea in infancy, Arch Dis Child 52:597, 1977.
25. Lebenthal E and Branski D: Childhood celiac disease—a reappraisal, J Pediatr 98:681, 1981.
26. Moynahan EJ: Acrodermatitis enteropathica: a lethal inherited human zinc-deficiency disorder, Lancet 2:399, 1974.
27. Neldner KH and Hambridge KM: Zinc therapy of acrodermatitis enteropathica, N Engl J Med 292:879, 1975.
28. Orenstein SR: Enteral versus parenteral therapy for intractable diarrhea of infancy: prospective, randomized trial, J Pediatr 109:277, 1986.
29. Phillips SF: Diarrhea: a current view of the pathophysiology, Gastroenterology 63:495, 1972.
30. Pizarro D et al: Oral rehydration in hypernatremic and hyponatremic diarrheal dehydration, Am J Dis Child 137:730, 1983.
31. Portnoy BL et al: Antidiarrheal agents in the treatment of acute diarrhea in children, JAMA 236:844, 1976.
32. Ravich WJ, Bayless TM, and Thomas M: Fructose: incomplete intestinal absorption in humans, Gastroenterology 84:26, 1983.
33. Santosham M et al: Oral rehydration therapy of infantile diarrhea: a controlled study of well-nourished children hospitalized in the United States and Panama, N Engl J Med 306:1070, 1982.
34. Schwarz RP and Ulshen MH: Pseudomembranous colitis presenting as mild, chronic diarrhea in childhood, J Pediatr Gastroenterol Nutr 2:570, 1983.
35. Steinhoff MC: Rotavirus: the first five years, J Pediatr 96:611, 1980.
36. Sutphen JL et al: Chronic diarrhea associated with *Clostridium difficile* in children, Am J Dis Child 137:275, 1983.
37. Tamer AM et al: Oral rehydration of infants in a large urban U.S. medical center, J Pediatr 107:14, 1985.
38. Tucker NT et al: Antigliadin antibodies detected by enzyme-linked immunosorbent assay as a marker of childhood celiac disease, J Pediatr 113:286, 1988.
39. Ulshen MH: Carbohydrate absorption and malabsorption. In Walker WA and Watkins JB, editors: Nutrition in pediatrics—basic sciences and clinical applications, Boston, 1985, Little, Brown & Co.
40. Ulshen MH and Rollo RL: Pathogenesis of *Escherichia coli* gastroenteritis in man—another mechanism, N Engl J Med 302:99, 1980.
41. Vardy PA, Lebenthal E, and Shwachman H: Intestinal lymphangiectasia: a reappraisal, Pediatrics 55:842, 1975.
42. Wolfen JS et al: Cryptosporidiosis in immuno-competent patients, N Engl J Med 312:1278, 1985.
43. Yolken RH et al: Gastroenteritis associated with enteric type adenovirus in hospitalized infants, J Pediatr 101:21, 1982.

SUGGESTED READINGS

Bishop WP and Ulshen MH: Bacterial gastroenteritis, Pediatr Clin North Am 35:69, 1988.

Ghishan FK: The transport of electrolytes in the gut and the use of oral rehydration solutions, Pediatr Clin North Am 35:35, 1988.

121

Dizziness and Vertigo

Diane L. McDonald

Dizziness as described by adults is a disturbance in one's sense of relationship to the surrounding environment, characterized by feelings of unsteadiness, of random movement within the head, of total loss of concentration and awareness of ongoing activity, and of lightheadedness or confusion.

Dizziness can be difficult for children to describe; it is a vague term that can represent a variety of symptoms. Lightheadedness often is associated with high fever or the ingestion of medications (e.g., antihistamines or decongestants), or it may occur as a presyncopal event. Visual distortion, disequilibrium, and vertigo also can accompany dizziness. Differentiating among the various symptoms will help establish the diagnosis.

The ability to maintain balance depends on the interconnections of the visual, sensory, proprioceptive, and vestibular systems. Dysfunction in any of these can produce a sense of imbalance or "dizziness." For example, a visual disturbance such as diplopia may not be recognized as such by a child. Instead, the child may appear to have difficulty walking or to be confused. Cerebellar dysfunction, associated with ataxia, also can be perceived as dizziness by both the child and the parents. Dizziness experienced as vertigo makes one seem to be in motion when one is not. In the nonverbal child this may appear to be clumsiness and, in some cases, may result in expressions of fear or in vomiting. A thorough history of the present illness, of past and family illnesses, and of possible drug use should be obtained. A complete physical examination with special attention to the neurologic, cardiac, and otologic systems will assist in establishing the diagnosis.

DIFFERENTIAL DIAGNOSIS

Children who complain of *lightheadedness* may be experiencing decreased cerebral perfusion, hypoxia, or hypoglycemia. This may be a presyncopal event. Also, upper respiratory tract infections or "the flu" may make the child feel somewhat lightheaded.

Impaired vision or *diplopia* may be interpreted as dizziness. Refractive errors or tumors involving the optic chiasm (e.g., optic gliomas or craniopharyngiomas) will alter vision. Double vision can occur as a result of trauma or a sixth nerve palsy. When problems of this magnitude are suspected, referral to an ophthalmologist or neurologist most often is required.

The symptom and sign of *unsteadiness* or *disequilibrium* can indicate the initial presentation of a pathologic condition of the cerebellum, for example, a posterior fossa tumor, such as an astrocytoma or a medulloblastoma. Acute cerebellar ataxia can follow a viral illness, for example, varicella or mycoplasma infection. Ataxia also may be caused by drug intoxication, trauma, or an inherited disease, such as Friedreich ataxia.

Vertigo is the sensation of spinning or whirling within one's environment or of the environment doing the spinning or whirling. It may be due to dysfunction in the vestibular system or of the eighth cranial nerve. The evaluation of vertigo therefore should include a thorough examination of the central nervous system and of the ear. Consultation with a neurologic or otologic specialist usually is required. Vertigo may manifest as acute, recurrent, or persistent.

Acute vertigo can be caused by middle or inner ear infections. A middle ear effusion may transmit pressure to the inner ear, leading to a sense of imbalance or vertigo. Chronic otitis media can result in labyrinthitis or mastoiditis and, with severe protracted infections, is associated with cholesteatoma formation. In this event the labyrinth may be seriously damaged, even destroyed. A viral labyrinthitis, vestibular neuronitis, frequently is associated with an upper respiratory tract infection or otitis media. The symptoms of vertigo in this situation last 2 to 3 weeks and usually resolve spontaneously.

Trauma and toxic ingestions also must be included in the differential diagnosis of acute vertigo. Salicylate or alcohol ingestion can cause the sudden onset of vertigo. Ototoxic drugs (e.g., streptomycin and gentamicin) slowly damage the inner ear, and vertigo (and deafness) may result.

Recurrent vertigo is characterized by episodes that usually last less than 30 minutes and can be associated with *basilar artery migraine* or *temporal lobe epilepsy*. A *brain-stem glioma* or an *acoustic neuroma* can affect the eighth cranial nerve, causing recurrent vertigo. Trauma that results in a fracture through the temporal bone, hemorrhage into the middle ear, or a perilymph fistula often leads to recurrent vertigo. Although *benign paroxysmal vertigo* is an entity of unknown cause, it may be associated with migraines. It affects children between the ages of 1 and 3 years. Attacks occur in clusters with symptoms of crying and vomiting and signs of pallor and nystagmus. Although these attacks may occur over a period of months or even years, this disease is self-limited (see Chapter 154, "Nonconvulsive Periodic Disorders" for further discussion of benign paroxysmal vertigo). *Meniere disease* is caused by increased endolymphatic pressure in the inner ear and may result in recurrent vertigo. Dizziness may be the presenting symptom of the demyelinating disease, multiple sclerosis. Congenital syphilis, too, can cause a labyrinthitis.

Chronic persistent vertigo is characterized by episodes of vertigo, each lasting as long as 1 week. Structural lesions—for example, brain-stem glioma or acoustic neuroma, or a variety of demyelinating diseases—must be considered. A computed tomography (CT) scan, magnetic resonance imaging (MRI), or an electronystagmogram may help establish the diagnosis. Psychogenic causes such as hysteria or malingering should be considered if the findings are inconsistent with an organic cause.

MANAGEMENT

The approach to the patient who is experiencing dizziness depends on the diagnosis. Dizziness that occurs as a presyncopal event is discussed in the section on syncope. To determine if refractive error or a visual disturbance is the cause, a vision test and funduscopic examination are needed. The differentiation of cerebellar and vestibular pathology can be difficult. Ataxia and a positive Romberg test reaction are commonly seen with both. However, difficulty in performing rapid alternating movements and an intention tremor suggest a cerebellar abnormality and should prompt a CT scan or an MRI study. A neurology consultation is indicated.

Dizziness associated with the sensation of motion—vertigo—frequently has a benign origin. Special attention should be given to the otologic and neurologic examination. The otologic evaluation should include tympanometry or pneumatic bulb otoscopy examination and also a hearing test. If a middle ear effusion is noted, antibiotic therapy may be needed. If the symptoms persist, referral to an otolaryngologist for a possible myringotomy and tube placement is advised. Other pathologic conditions of the middle ear, such as a cholesteatoma, warrant similar referral for possible surgical exploration and excision.

The neurologic examination should assist in differentiating vestibular disease from other central nervous system causes. If there is evidence of neurologic dysfunction, a CT scan and neurology consultation are advised. Recurrent or persistent episodes of vertigo or vertigo *preceding* trauma also require a referral. An electrocardiogram should be obtained if vertigo is associated with a loss of consciousness or with seizure activity.

The Nylen-Bárány test is used to provoke nystagmus. It may help to distinguish a peripheral from a central vestibular lesion. This test is performed with the child seated on an examination table. The head is dropped over the edge of the table to a position 45 degrees below the horizontal and then turned 45 degrees to one side. The entire test is repeated, turning the child's head 45 degrees in the other direction. Inner ear lesions will result in a 20-second delayed onset of nystagmus, and the rapid phase of nystagmus always will be in the same direction regardless of the direction of gaze. With central lesions the onset of nystagmus is immediate and the direction of the nystagmus changes with gaze. Electronystagmographic examination is a more specific but less frequently used procedure to locate the vestibular lesion.

Finally, if the otologic and neurologic examinations are unrevealing and the episode is of acute onset, the most common cause is vestibular neuronitis. These children may be treated symptomatically and if necessary reevaluated frequently. Meclizine (Antivert) in a dosage of 25 mg every 4 to 6 hours for children older than 12 years of age may provide symptomatic relief.

SUGGESTED READINGS

Busis SN: Dizziness in children, Pediatr Ann 17:648, 1988.

Dunn DW: Dizziness: when is it vertigo? Contemp Pediatr 4:67, 1987.

Farmer TW: Pediatric neurology, Philadelphia, 1983, Harper & Row, Publishers, Inc.

122

Dysmenorrhea

Alain Joffe

Dysmenorrhea, generally meaning painful menstruation, is a syndrome associated with varying degrees of crampy lower abdominal pain and other symptoms such as nausea, vomiting, low back pain, diarrhea, fatigue, and headache. These symptoms may last from 1 to 3 days.[8] The prevalence of this syndrome is not clearly established, but the majority of surveys indicate that at least 40% to 60% of adolescent girls suffer some degree of discomfort during menstruation, and many miss school as a result. Most teenagers will have primary dysmenorrhea, that is, a syndrome not associated with pelvic pathologic conditions; however, before this diagnosis can be made, causes of secondary dysmenorrhea should be excluded. The physician also should ensure that the pain described is not actually indicative of premenstrual tension syndrome, characterized by irritability, fluid retention, edema, and a sensation of bloating, which occurs in the week before menstruation.

SECONDARY DYSMENORRHEA

The causes of secondary dysmenorrhea—an intrauterine device (IUD), pelvic inflammatory disease (PID), or endometriosis—can usually be easily excluded by history and physical examination. Organic pathologic conditions should be suspected in a woman whose pain begins after 20 years of age, who has a history of surgery related to the genitourinary or gastrointestinal tract (including IUD placement), or whose pain is dull and constant rather than crampy.[6] PID and endometriosis generally are characterized by pain that begins 2 or 3 days before menstruation and often is relieved by the onset of menses. Endometriosis often is associated with dyspareunia, tenesmus, and rectal pain.

Endometrial polyps or fibroids are rare in women younger than 20 years old but should be suspected if the bleeding with menstruation is heavy or prolonged or associated with the passage of clots. Whether these entities alone cause dysmenorrhea is unclear. Teenagers with a history of genital tract surgery (including abortions) may have outflow tract obstruction.

A pelvic examination that reveals cervical motion tenderness, adnexal masses, or fixation of the ovaries strongly suggests PID. If the cervical os is stenotic or the cervix or uterus feels atretic or abnormally shaped, outflow obstruction is possible. Small fixed nodules in the rectovaginal septum or cul de sac, fixation or enlargement of the ovaries, or fixation of the uterus indicated by the presence of pain on stretching of the uterosacral ligaments suggests endometriosis.[11]

If any of these causes is detected, consultation with a gynecologist is warranted. Anatomic abnormalities may need surgical correction; endometriosis is difficult to manage (although new drugs for treatment are available), and women with endometriosis are at greater risk for infertility. PID should be treated with standard antibiotic regimens; careful follow-up is critical to ensure cure and because such women are at increased risk for further episodes and infertility. An IUD that causes significant dysmenorrhea will probably necessitate removal.

PRIMARY DYSMENORRHEA[5,14]

Although psychosocial and cultural factors may play some role in the pathogenesis of primary dysmenorrhea,[4,10,11] the preponderance of current research indicates that this symptom complex is caused largely by increased amounts of prostaglandins E_2 and $F_{2\alpha}$ in the endometrium of women with dysmenorrhea in comparison with women without painful menses.[1,13] Such a biologic explanation correlates with clinical observation: women with anovulatory cycles usually do not have dysmenorrhea. The incidence of dysmenorrhea increases with chronologic and gynecologic age (as does the percentage of ovulatory cycles), and the increase in prostaglandin synthesis may be related to changes in serum progesterone levels not seen in anovulatory women. Additional confirmation comes from the dramatic response women experience with the use of either prostaglandin synthetase inhibitors or oral contraceptives (which inhibit ovulation). The increased levels of prostaglandin activity produce myometrial contractions and ischemia, both of which result in pain.

A careful history usually will exclude most pathologic causes of dysmenorrhea. Physicians differ in their opinions regarding what examination is necessary to evaluate the patient with true dysmenorrhea. Some contend that for a teenager with mild to moderate menstrual cramps relieved by nonsteroidal antiinflammatory drugs (NSAIDs), only an external genital examination to rule out hymenal abnormalities is indicated. For any sexually active teenager or for one who is having significant pain unresponsive to NSAIDs, a thorough pelvic examination is necessary. For patients in whom a vaginal examination is not possible (which should be rare if the patient is prepared properly), a rectoabdominal examination usually can exclude pelvic disease.

Although treatment of primary dysmenorrhea is likely to include drug therapy, other considerations are pertinent. The extent to which the pain is interfering with the patient's activity should be explored. Is she missing school, and if so, how often? Does she miss valued activities because the pain and nausea prevent her from participating? The physician also should determine what the mother and daughter's understanding of menstruation is; many teenagers do not fully understand the physiology of menstruation or may have inaccurate beliefs that have been passed on from mother to daughter.[7] In any case such a discussion provides the physician a valuable opportunity to teach the patient and perhaps her family about her body.

Although mild analgesics are all that are necessary for the teenager with mild discomfort,[9] prostaglandin synthetase inhibitors appear to be the treatment of choice for moderate to severe pain.[3,12] The dosage varies from patient to patient. Some need medication only part or all of the first day; others require medication for 3 days or so. Ibuprofen (200 to 600 mg every 6 to 8 hours), available in 200-mg tablets without a prescription or 400-mg tablets by prescription, is highly effective for dysmenorrhea. Alternatively, naproxen sodium (550 mg immediately and then 275 mg every 12 hours) can be used.

Some patients (perhaps as many as 30%) will not respond to these measures. In these women a trial of oral contraceptives used in the same way as for contraception usually will provide relief. Patients should be told that 2 to 3 months may elapse before contraceptives exert their maximal effect.[2]

Other treatment modalities are more controversial. Some authors believe that remedies such as pelvic exercise, general exercise, biofeedback, or relaxation therapy are efficacious; however, other authorities remain skeptical.

Women who fail to respond to any of these measures should be referred to physicians with experience in adolescent medicine or to a gynecologist for evaluation; they probably have secondary rather than primary dysmenorrhea.

REFERENCES

1. Alvin PE and Litt IF: Current status of the etiology and management of dysmenorrhea in adolescence, Pediatrics 70:516, 1982.
2. Coupey SM and Ahlstrom P: Common menstrual disorders, Pediatr Clin North Am 36:551, 1989.
3. Dingfelder JR: Primary dysmenorrhea treatment with prostaglandin inhibitors: a review, Am J Obstet Gynecol 140:874, 1981.
4. Durant RH et al: Factors influencing adolescents' responses for regimens of naproxen for dysmenorrhea, Am J Dis Child 139:489, 1985.
5. Golub LJ, Land WR, and Menduke H: The incidence of dysmenorrhea in high school girls, Postgrad Med J 23:38, 1958.
6. Heinrichs WL and Adamson GD: A practical approach to the patient with dysmenorrhea, J Reprod Med 25:236, 1980.
7. Johnson J: Level of knowledge among adolescent girls regarding effective treatment for dysmenorrhea, J Adolesc Health Care 9:398, 1988.
8. Klein JR and Litt IF: Epidemiology of adolescent dysmenorrhea, Pediatrics 68:661, 1981.
9. Klein JR et al: The effect of aspirin on dysmenorrhea in adolescents, Pediatrics 98:987, 1981.
10. Lawlor CL and Davis AM: Primary dysmenorrhea: relationship to personality and attitudes in adolescent females, J Adolesc Health Care 1:208, 1981.
11. Neinstein LS: Adolescent health care: a practical guide, Baltimore, 1984, Urban & Schwarzenberg, Inc.
12. Owen PR: Prostaglandin synthetase inhibitors in the treatment of primary dysmenorrhea, Am J Obstet Gynecol 148:96, 1984.
13. Rosenwaks Z: New approach to dysmenorrhea, Drug Ther 12:47, 1982.
14. Svanberg L and Ulmsten UP: The incidence of primary dysmenorrhea in teenagers, Arch Gynecol 230:173, 1981.

123

Dysphagia

Steven L. Werlin

Dysphagia is a symptom that something is wrong with the swallowing mechanism.[13] True dysphagia is never psychogenic, and every patient with this complaint requires a thorough evaluation. Globus hystericus, or the feeling of having a lump in the throat, is psychogenic and not true dysphagia. Odynophaghia, pain on swallowing, does not necessarily accompany dysphagia.

Preesophageal dysphagia almost always is accompanied by the signs and symptoms of a more generalized disease such as cerebral palsy, muscular dystrophy, myasthenia gravis, or familial dysautonomia. In these conditions dysphagia is due to primary or secondary involvement of skeletal muscle, which causes difficulty in initiating a swallow.

Esophageal dysphagia is the subjective sensation of a bolus of food failing to be transported down the esophagus. Patients with an esophageal motor disturbance usually have dysphagia for both solids and liquids, whereas mechanical obstruction usually is accompanied by dysphagia for solids alone. In the young child this history may be difficult to elicit; such patients may be slow or "picky" eaters, may prefer liquids, or may refuse feedings altogether.

NORMAL ESOPHAGEAL FUNCTION

Anatomically the esophagus is divided into the upper one third, composed of striated muscle, and the distal two thirds, composed of smooth muscle. Functionally the esophagus is composed of three zones: the upper sphincter, the body, and the lower sphincter. The upper esophageal sphincter (UES), composed of the cricopharyngeal muscle, is contracted at rest. After pharyngeal contraction but before esophageal peristalsis occurs, the UES relaxes, contracting again when swallowing is completed. The cricopharyngeal muscle is contracted at rest by a constant discharge of motor nerves. Each swallow is followed by a monophasic pressure wave that traverses the entire length of the esophagus.[5] Approximately 90% of swallows are followed by this primary peristalsis. Secondary peristalsis is not preceded by a swallow; it is induced by the failure of a bolus to pass into the stomach initially or by reflux of gastric contents into the esophagus. The velocity of a peristaltic wave is 2.5 to 6 cm/sec.

A zone of increased pressure is present at the lower end of the esophagus. The pressure drops promptly with a swallow and remains depressed until the peristaltic wave has ended. During this period of reduced lower esophageal sphincter (LES) pressure, the pressure gradient between the stomach and esophagus remains, preventing reflux of gastric contents. On the basis of studies in adults, it appears that the LES is the major barrier against reflux of acid gastric contents into the esophagus.[5,6] Although it has been shown that gastrointestinal hormones can affect sphincter pressure, the control mechanism for basal LES pressure still is unknown. Anticholinergic drugs and theophylline reduce LES.

METHODS OF STUDY

Radiology

The barium swallow examination is the most diagnostically useful method of evaluating esophageal structure and function. With the use of fluoroscopy and modern videotape recording, the transport function of the esophagus can be well studied; the rate of propagation of the peristaltic wave can be measured, and mechanical and functional obstruction can be differentiated. Unfortunately, the barium swallow does not help to diagnose gastroesophageal reflux very accurately.[11]

Manometry

Intraluminal esophageal manometry has taken an important place in the study of esophageal dysfunction.[5,6,15] Intraluminal, perfused catheters connected via transducers to a recording device allow measurement of upper and lower esophageal sphincter pressures, documentation of sphincter relaxation, and determination of rate and strength of the peristaltic wave. Sedation usually is not required except in young children. The diagnoses of achalasia and diffuse esophageal spasm can be confirmed only by manometric evaluation. At times the use of esophageal manometry also is required to establish the diagnosis of scleroderma. Gastroesophageal reflux cannot be diagnosed by manometry or by measuring the LES pressure.

Esophagoscopy

Flexible fiberoptic esophagoscopic examination can be performed on children on an ambulatory basis. Suspected lesions can be inspected, biopsied, and photographed rapidly and safely.

CAUSES AND MANAGEMENT

The many causes of dysphagia are listed in the box on p. 888.

Structural-Mechanical Disorders of the Esophagus

Even after successful repair of esophageal atresia, swallowing problems usually persist.[16] Peristalsis is nearly always abnormal, and symptomatic gastroesophageal reflux with or without esophagitis is found almost universally. Anastomotic strictures may occur. Congenital strictures and esophageal webs, usually in the proximal esophagus, are uncommon and may be difficult to detect on a roentgenogram. Typically the patient can point to the level of the obstruction. Esophageal foreign bodies frequently are seen in children and can be removed easily.[3] A hiatal hernia (Fig. 123-1) may be associated with gastroesophageal reflux, which is the true cause of the symptoms. Hiatal hernias usually do not produce symptoms. Peptic strictures that result from gastroesophageal reflux with or without symptoms cause dysphagia by obstructing the esophageal lumen (Fig. 123-2). Dysphagia typically is more pronounced with solids than with liquids. The diagnosis of peptic stricture is readily made roentgenographically. The stricture is treated with dilation, but the underlying reflux also must be treated. Esophageal tumors are rare in children. Mediastinal tumors may rarely cause esophageal obstruction. Although vascular rings are not uncommon, mechanical obstruction of the esophagus by this anomaly is extremely rare.[7]

Motor Disorders of the Esophagus

Achalasia, a rare cause of functional obstruction of the distal esophagus, results from failure (1) of the LES to relax and (2) of the peristaltic wave to propagate.[1,14] Its prevalence is about 1:100,000; 10% of cases occur in childhood. It is functionally and pathologically similar to Hirschsprung disease; in both conditions the distal myenteric ganglion cells are absent, causing functional obstruction and proximal dilation. The onset of dysphagia usually is gradual but progressive; weight loss and aspiration will occur if the condition is neglected. Symptoms often are surprisingly mild, and intermittent substernal pain may be present.

A characteristic J-shaped megaesophagus, with a tapered distal beak, is seen on a barium swallow examination (Fig. 123-3). Peristalsis is absent, but sporadic aperistaltic contractions may be seen. Intraluminal manometric examination

Causes of Dysphagia

STRUCTURAL-MECHANICAL DISORDERS
- Atresia
- Foreign bodies
- Hiatal hernia
- Stricture
  - Congenital
  - Inflammatory
  - Caustic
- Tumor
- Vascular ring
- Web

MOTOR DISORDERS
- Primary
  - Achalasia
  - Diffuse spasm
  - Gastroesophageal reflux
  - Scleroderma
- Secondary
  - Dysautonomia
  - Muscular dystrophy
  - Myasthenia gravis

INFLAMMATORY DISORDERS
- Caustic ingestion
- Epidermolysis bullosa
- Esophagitis
  - *Candida albicans*
  - Cytomegalovirus
  - Gastroesophageal reflux
  - Herpes simplex

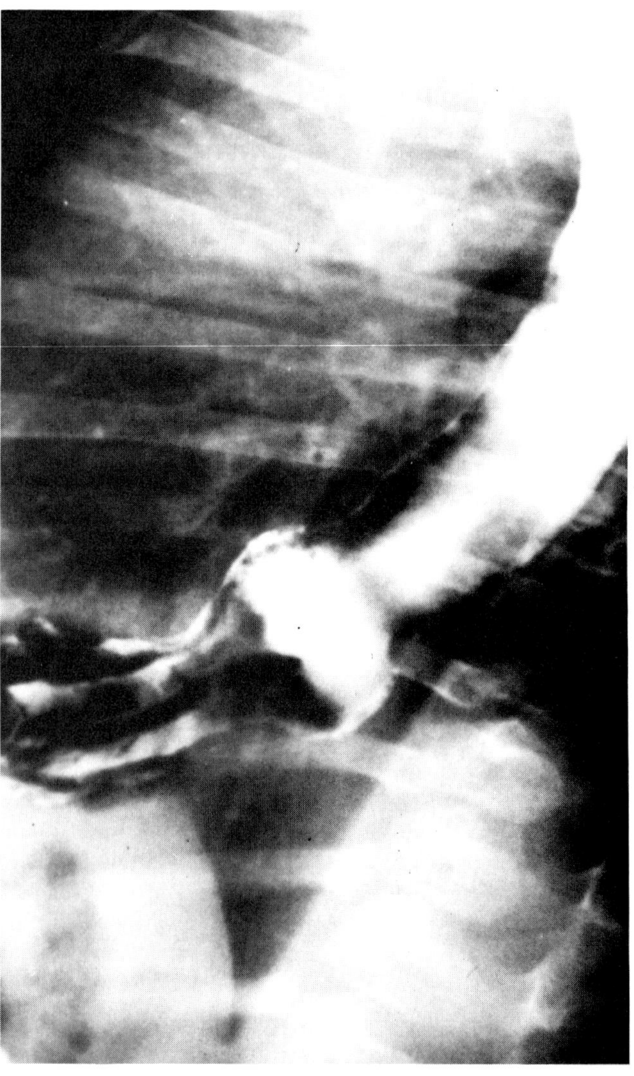

Fig. 123-1 A clearly defined small hiatal hernia.

documents the absence of peristalsis, as well as high resting pressure in the LES and failure of the sphincter to relax after a swallow. The esophagus responds with spastic, high-pressure contractions to an intramuscular injection of methacholine. This test can be quite painful and is not recommended for routine use. In achalasia, cholecystokinin will cause a paradoxical increase of the LES pressure.

Although medical therapy with the calcium channel blocker nifedipine may relieve symptoms, the current treatments of choice are pneumatic dilation and surgical myotomy, which successfully relieve the symptoms in nearly all patients.[1,14] Pneumatic dilation may need to be repeated. The long-term outlook is good, although there may be an increased risk in late adulthood of carcinoma of the esophagus.

Diffuse esophageal spasms in which both dysphagia and pain are present is even less common than achalasia.[13] Symptoms typically wax and wane, often with long symptom-free intervals. Cold beverages frequently exacerbate symptoms. Esophageal spasm is readily demonstrated with manometric study. Barium swallow studies also may demonstrate the spastic contractions. Medical therapy with nitroglycerin is occasionally successful; otherwise, either pneumatic dilation or surgical myotomy is necessary. Neither approach is totally satisfactory.

Dysphagia may be the presenting symptom in a small but significant number of patients with scleroderma. A roentgenographic or manometric examination may show aperistalsis in the distal esophagus. A manometric study can be used to confirm the suspected diagnosis of scleroderma.

Gastroesophageal reflux may be associated with esophagitis, disordered peristalsis, and dysphagia. Dysphagia resolves when the esophagitis is treated.

Generalized muscular and autonomic nervous system diseases such as muscular dystrophy, myasthenia gravis, and familial dysautonomia can cause dysphagia.

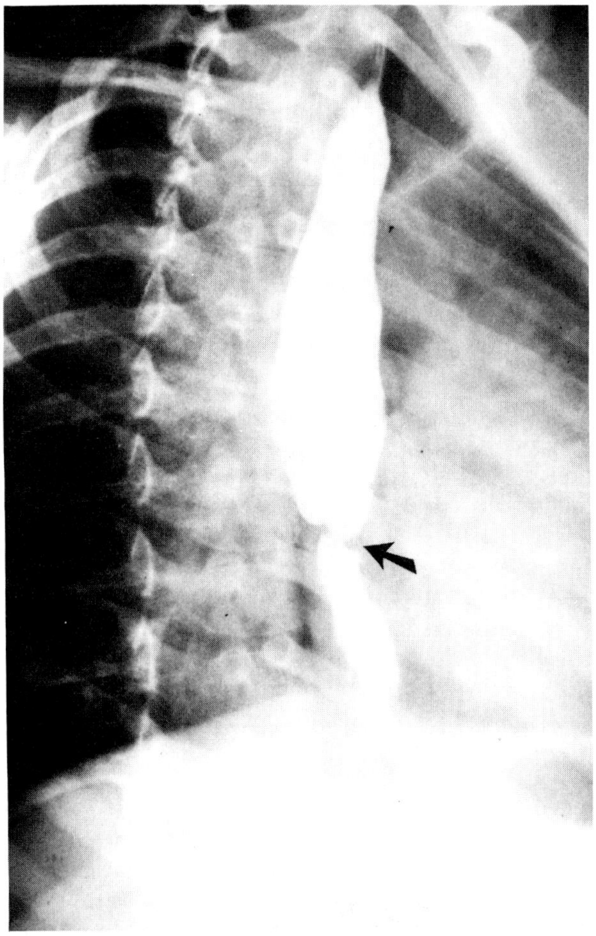

Fig. 123-2 Peptic esophagitis with stricture. There is dilation proximal to the tight stricture *(arrow)*. Note the irregularity of the distal esophageal mucosa.

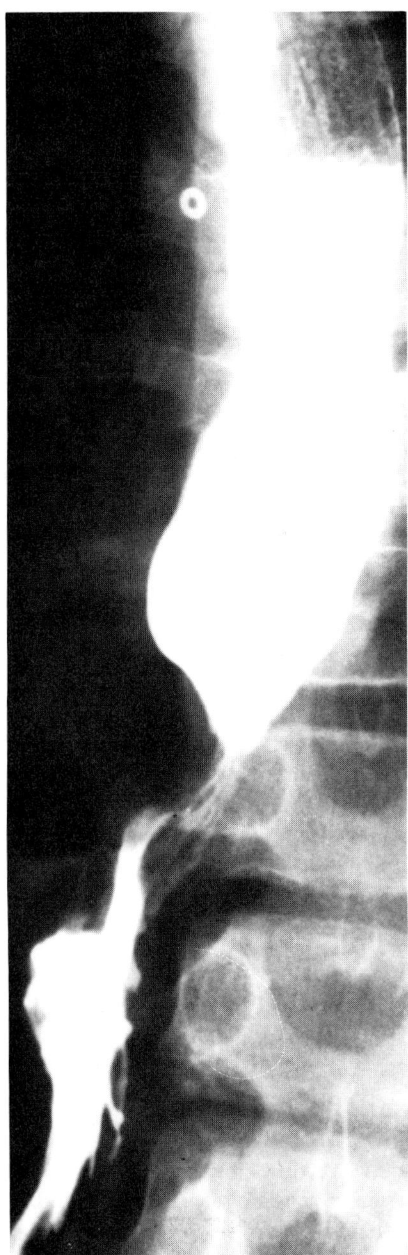

Fig. 123-3 The classic appearance of achalasia of the esophagus. The dilated esophagus ends in a narrow segment.

Inflammatory Disorders

It is now recognized that normal function of the LES is the critical factor in preventing reflux of gastric contents.[6] If the LES responds normally to swallowing and is otherwise intact, reflux esophagitis will not occur.

The presence of a hiatal hernia demonstrated by roentgenographic studies is not an indication for surgical repair.[2] Rather, appropriate diagnostic studies as already described should be instituted. A great deal of confusion has existed about which patients with reflux should have surgery. On the basis of current knowledge it can be stated without hesitation that more than 85% of neurologically intact children referred for evaluation of reflux will respond to medical therapy. Children with neurologic disorders do poorly with medical therapy and usually need surgical intervention.

Gastroesophageal reflux can be demonstrated in many normal infants. This phenomenon was formerly called *chalasia*. Normally reflux and benign regurgitation disappear by the age of 9 to 12 months. Infants who regurgitate chronically should be observed closely and, if symptoms persist, evaluated for esophagitis. Esophageal inflammation and even stricture may occur in the absence of symptoms.

Although the diagnosis of gastroesophageal reflux may be confirmed by a barium swallow study, radiographic studies may not document reflux in as many as 40% of children, even in patients with known esophagitis. This is due to the intermittent nature of symptoms and the brief period of fluoroscopic observation. Esophagitis usually is not seen roentgenographically. Although intraluminal esophageal pH recording and scintigraphic techniques can assist in diagnosing reflux, only esophagoscopic examination and biopsy can definitively document the presence of esophagitis. Diagnostic studies, including a complete blood count, serum iron level, and a stool guaiac test, are useful in documenting bleeding from an inflamed esophagus. A chest roentgenogram may be obtained because chronic reflux has been incriminated as a cause of recurrent aspiration pneumonia, chronic obstructive pulmonary disease, and bronchopulmonary dysplasia.

Although esophagitis is considered uncommon in children, pediatricians are recognizing an increasing number of patients with the classic symptoms of heartburn, foul taste in their mouth, bad breath, and vomiting.[13] Symptoms increase when one is reclining. Infants may only regurgitate, although this finding accompanied by failure to thrive and irritability often indicates that esophagitis is present.

An important factor in the development of esophagitis is the rate that refluxed material is cleared from the esophagus. In patients with esophagitis the normal stripping action of the lower esophagus is impaired, and the distal esophagus remains acidic longer after reflux than in normal patients.

Although a recent study suggests that the prone position may be more effective in infants, traditional medical therapy consists of using a "chalasia chair" to maintain the upright position, as well as thickening the feedings with cereal.[2,12] At times a bottle may be needed and should be filled one third with cereal and two thirds with formula. Bethanechol (1.25 mg, four times daily) and metoclopramide (0.1 mg/kg, four times daily) have been extremely beneficial in the treatment of infants.[8] A new prokinetic agent, cisapride, not yet available in the United States, may be superior to both bethanechol and metoclopramide.[4] Antacids or histamine-2 (H_2) blockers must be administered when esophagitis is documented. Surgery is needed only rarely for medical failure or stricture formation.

Inflammatory lesions of the esophagus are particularly common in association with infection by *Candida albicans*, cytomegalovirus, and herpes simplex virus. Although these agents may appear spontaneously, most pediatric patients who contract them are seen because of immunosuppression such as may occur with cancer chemotherapy and acquired immunodeficiency syndrome (AIDS) and after transplantation. Although the roentgenographic appearance of *C. albicans* and herpes infections may suggest those diagnoses when they are suspected, it otherwise may not be strongly diagnostic, and endoscopic examination and biopsy usually are required to confirm their presence. An infectious agent is not often the cause of esophagitis in uncompromised hosts and therefore not often considered in the differential diagnosis.

The traditional and still most effective medical treatment for esophagitis consists of liquid antacids, avoidance of foods such as coffee, alcohol, and fatty foods that reduce LES pressure, and elevation of the head of the bed at least 8 inches.[13] Anticholinergic drugs, which decrease LES pressure, should be avoided. Bethanechol, metoclopramide, and cisapride have been shown to be clinically effective in decreasing both reflux and symptoms. H_2 blockers may be used to decrease gastric acid secretion. Surgery is indicated only for intractable symptoms and stricture development.

When *C. albicans* infection is documented, the aforementioned therapy should be supplemented by the appropriate dose of nystatin or ketoconazole. Amphotericin B frequently is required. Herpes esophagitis should be treated with acyclovir, and cytomegalovirus esophagitis may be treated with ganciclovir.

Ingestion of caustic agents, especially liquid alkali, causes intense pain and dysphagia.[10] Symptoms commonly resolve after 3 or 4 days, but stricture formation associated with the return of dysphagia may follow after 3 to 8 weeks. Early esophagoscopic examination, preferably 12 to 24 hours after the caustic ingestion, is essential to establish the extent and degree of the burn. If the burn is limited to the mouth, no therapy is necessary. If an esophageal burn is confirmed, many physicians recommend the use of steroids (prednisone, 1 to 2 mg/kg/day or the equivalent for 4 weeks) and antibiotics. The most recent literature suggests that steroids do not decrease stricture formation.[9] Strictures are treated by bougienage. Esophagectomy and colon interposition rarely are necessary.

Although not truly esophagitis, the esophageal lesions that occur in cases of epidermolysis bullosa may be recognized roentgenographically.

REFERENCES

1. Berquist WE et al: Achalasia: diagnosis, management, and clinical course in 16 children, Pediatrics 71:798, 1983.
2. Carre IJ: Management of gastro-oesophageal reflux, Arch Dis Child 60:71, 1985.
3. Christie DL and Ament ME: Removal of foreign bodies from esophagus and stomach with flexible fiberoptic panendoscopes, Pediatrics 57:931, 1976.

4. Cucchiara A et al: Cisapride for gastro-oesophageal reflux and peptic oesophagitis, Arch Dis Child 62:454, 1987.
5. Dodds WJ: Instrumentation and methods for intraluminal esophageal manometry, Arch Intern Med 136:515, 1976.
6. Dodds et al: Pathogenesis of reflux esophagitis, Gastroenterology 81:376, 1981.
7. Eklof O et al: Arterial anomalies causing compression of the trachea and/or oesophagus, Acta Paediatr Scand 60:81, 1971.
8. Euler AR: Use of bethanechol for the treatment of gastroesophageal reflux, J Pediatr 96:321, 1980.
9. Ferguson MK et al: Early evaluation and therapy for caustic esophageal injury, Am J Surg 157:116, 1989.
10. Gaudreault P et al: Predictability of esophageal injury from signs and symptoms: a study of caustic ingestion in 378 children. Pediatrics 71:767, 1983.
11. Leonidas JC: Gastroesophageal reflux in infants: role of the upper gastrointestinal series, AJR 143:1350, 1984.
12. Orenstein SR, Whittington PF, and Orenstein DM: The infant seat as treatment for gastroesophageal reflux, N Engl J Med 29:760, 1983.
13. Pope PE: Heartburn, dysphagia and other esophageal symptoms. In Sleisenger MH and Fordtran JS, editors: Gastrointestinal disease, ed 4, Philadelphia, 1989, WB Saunders Co.
14. Vantrappen G and Hellemans J: Treatment of achalasia and related motor disorders, Gastroenterology 79:144, 1980.
15. Werlin SL et al: Mechanisms of gastroesophageal reflux in children, J Pediatr 97:244, 1980.
16. Werlin SL et al: Esophageal function in esophageal atresia, Dig Dis Sci 26:796, 1981.

124

Dyspnea

Jay H. Mayefsky

Dyspnea is the uncomfortable feeling of not being able to satisfy "air hunger"; patients may complain of not being able to catch their breath or of a suffocating feeling. Dyspnea is a symptom, a subjective complaint by the patient, that describes the sensation caused by an underlying disorder. As with any subjective complaint, the diagnosis of dyspnea and its cause in the infant and young child can be problematic. Therefore, to evaluate fully a child in respiratory distress, the pediatric health care provider must be familiar with the pathophysiology, signs, and common causes of dyspnea. With the aid of the medical history, physical examination, and appropriate laboratory tests, the proper diagnosis can be made and therapy initiated.

PATHOPHYSIOLOGY

Dyspnea is most commonly seen with exercise. In this instance the increased work of breathing necessary to keep up with the body's increased metabolic demands causes the dyspnea.[8] The sensation probably is transmitted from stretch receptors in the chest wall muscles to the central nervous system (CNS). Chemoreceptors, sensing changes in arterial pH, oxygen, and carbon dioxide concentrations, as well as chest wall proprioceptors, lung stretch receptors, and mechanoreceptors in the heart and skeletal muscles, also may play a role.[2,10,19] The transmission is processed in the CNS, and the sensation of dyspnea is experienced. In the example of exercise, the person with dyspnea is aware of an increased ventilatory effort. In addition, a person with obstructive or restrictive lung disease has difficulty breathing. A person with neuromuscular disease feels that he or she is not getting enough air.

To satisfy their oxygen needs, children with dyspnea must either increase their minute ventilation ($\dot{V}_E$) or must work harder than normal to maintain their usual $\dot{V}_E$. Minute ventilation, the product of tidal volume and frequency of respirations per minute ($\dot{V}_E = V_T \times f$), is helpful in diagnosing dyspnea and its causes. In normal breathing, respiratory muscles work only during inspiration and the diaphragm does most of the work. The work of inspiration is the sum of the work necessary to overcome the elastic forces of the lung, the tissue viscosity of the lung and chest wall, and airway resistance.[7] When any of these is increased—for example, elastic force and tissue viscosity in restrictive pulmonary disease or resistance in obstructive airway disease—the work of inspiration must increase to maintain an adequate $\dot{V}_E$. The accessory muscles of inspiration—the sternocleidomastoid, anterior serratus, scalene, and external intercostal muscles—are recruited to accomplish this. The forceful expansion of the thorax by the contractions of these muscles results in an unusually large negative intrathoracic pressure. This negative pressure draws in the soft tissues of the chest wall and creates the classic sign of dyspnea—retractions. Retractions may be seen in the suprasternal, infrasternal, intercostal, subcostal, and supraclavicular areas. An alternative way to maintain an adequate $\dot{V}_E$ is to increase the rate of breathing; hence the second classic sign of dyspnea—tachypnea. Other signs that are seen and heard during inspiration are nasal flaring and grunting.

Little energy is expended during normal expiration. Relaxation of the diaphragm, elastic recoil of the lungs and chest wall, and compression of the lungs by the intraabdominal organs force air from the lungs. In obstructive airway disease the force generated by these processes may not be great enough to effect adequate expiration. In a child with tachypnea the elastic recoil may not be fast enough to allow adequate exhalation between breaths. In either instance the accessory muscles of expiration are used. The abdominal recti contract and force the abdominal contents against the diaphragm to compress the lungs, and the internal intercostal muscles contract to pull the ribs downward and to create a positive intrathoracic pressure to force the air from the lungs. The contractions of these muscles provide the most important expiratory sign of dyspnea.

Although dyspnea is a respiratory symptom, it may be caused by primary disorders in other body systems. Cardiac, hematologic, metabolic, circulatory, and psychogenic causes must be considered in the differential diagnosis of dyspnea. The age of the child also is important, because various disorders occur with different frequency at different ages. The history, including information about associated signs and symptoms, other known illnesses, medication or toxin exposure, and duration of the present illness, is essential. A thorough physical examination always is indicated, with special attention paid to the aforementioned systems. The most useful laboratory tests are the complete blood count and peripheral blood smear, arterial blood gas measurement, and roentgenographic studies of the airways and lungs. The measurement of arterial oxygen saturation by pulse oximetry is invaluable for its ability to provide a quick and noninvasive assessment of oxygenation status. Pulmonary function tests are very helpful as well, but they usually are not available during the evaluation of an acutely ill patient.

ETIOLOGY AND CLINICAL PRESENTATION

Pulmonary Disease

Pulmonary disease that causes dyspnea can be classified as obstructive, restrictive, or vascular.

Obstructive Pulmonary Disease. Obstructive disease is characterized by airway narrowing that can be caused by intraluminal objects (mucus, foreign bodies, or tumor), intramural factors (smooth muscle contraction, edema, or bronchomalacia), or extramural compression (tumor or lymph nodes). The narrowing causes an increase in both airway resistance and turbulent flow in the airways. In the presence of a fixed obstruction, affected areas of the lungs will become atelectatic. With a ball valve type of obstruction (in which air can get into the lungs but not out) there is air-trapping, and affected areas become hyperinflated. In either event an imbalance occurs between pulmonary ventilation and perfusion, and oxygen exchange is adversely affected.[18] All these processes force the patient to work harder to maintain adequate ventilation, and hence dyspnea occurs.

During normal respiration, inspiration and expiration are of equal length. In the presence of a fixed degree of obstruction, both are equally prolonged. If the obstruction is variable and extrathoracic (i.e., above the vocal cords), inspiration is affected more, because the negative intraairway pressure during inspiration tends to collapse the extrathoracic airway. The characteristic sign of such an obstruction is inspiratory stridor.

If the obstruction is variable and affects intrathoracic airways, expiration is prolonged because the positive intrathoracic pressure tends to collapse these airways during expiration. If larger airways are involved, the rhonchi are present. Airflow across an obstruction in smaller airways generates wheezing.

A paradoxical pulse and cyanosis are sensitive but nonspecific signs of severe obstruction. Patients with chronic obstructive disease may be barrel chested and have signs of chronic hypoxia, such as clubbing. Children with a systemic disease, such as cystic fibrosis, also will show the extrapulmonary manifestations of that disease.

The common causes of obstructive airway disease in childhood are shown in the accompanying box. Obstruction in the nose or nasopharynx, especially in infants, should not be overlooked.

Blood gas values may be normal in mild obstructive disease. As the disease progresses, hypoxemia is the first abnormality seen. Hypocapnia initially seen as a reflection of increased $\dot{V}_E$ is replaced by hypercapnia as the maldistribution of ventilation and perfusion increases (increasing dead space), the patient tires, and respiratory failure occurs.

The chest roentgenogram may reveal that the cause of the obstruction is inside or outside of the airway. Often hyperinflation with an increased anteroposterior chest diameter and flattened diaphragm are seen. Atelectasis may appear as a result of a fixed obstruction. Fluoroscopic examination or inspiratory and expiratory roentgenograms may be useful in localizing a ball valve type of obstruction.

Restrictive Pulmonary Disease. The cardinal features of restrictive pulmonary disease are a reduction in lung volume and pulmonary compliance secondary to pathologic changes in the lung parenchyma or the pleura, deformities of the chest wall, or neuromuscular disease. Decreased volume necessitates an increase in respiratory rate to maintain a normal $\dot{V}_E$. The work of breathing must be increased to overcome the reduced compliance. Because it is more energy efficient to breathe rapidly with small tidal volumes than to breathe slowly and attempt to expand the chest against great restrictive forces, children with restrictive diseases characteristically have rapid, shallow respirations.[18] The common pediatric causes of restrictive disease are listed in the box on p. 894.

Observation of the child often reveals skeletal and neuromuscular causes. Pleural and parenchymal diseases are best detected by palpation, percussion, and auscultation of the chest. Tactile fremitus can demonstrate pulmonary consolidation or pleural effusion. Careful percussion reveals effusions, consolidation, and abnormal diaphragmatic excursion. On auscultation, rales characteristic of alveolar disease may be heard, and changes in whispered pectoriloquy and egophony can be detected.

The complete blood count may be helpful in diagnosing an infectious cause. Arterial blood gases have a characteristic pattern of hypoxemia and hypocapnia. The chest roentgenogram is useful in that it can demonstrate decreased lung volume, pleural thickening and effusions, increased intersti-

Causes of Obstructive Pulmonary Disease

NEWBORNS
- Choanal atresia or stenosis
- Dermoid cyst
- Encephalocele
- Hemangioma
- Vocal cord paralysis
- Pierre Robin syndrome

INFANTS
- Foreign body
- Vascular ring
- Tracheal web
- Bronchiolitis
- Asthma
- Cystic fibrosis
- Bronchomalacia
- Pyogenic thyroid[11]
- Accessory thyroid[11]

CHILDREN AND ADOLESCENTS
- Foreign body
- Asthma
- Adenopathy
  - Lymphoma
  - Systemic lupus erythematosus
  - Tuberculosis
  - Sarcoidosis
- Croup
- Epiglottitis
- Retropharyngeal abscess
- Enlarged tonsils or adenoids
- Cystic fibrosis

Cause of Restrictive Pulmonary Disease

NEWBORNS

Hyaline membrane disease
Hypoplastic lungs
Eventration of the diaphragm
Meconium aspiration
Pneumonia (group B streptococci or gram-negative organisms)
Diaphragmatic paralysis
Osteogenesis imperfecta
CNS depression
- Hypoxia
- Congenital
- Maternal drugs

Congenital myasthenia gravis
Aspiration
Pulmonary edema
- Septicemia
- Congenital heart disease

INFANTS

Pneumonia
- Bacterial
- Viral
- Aspiration

Bronchopulmonary dysplasia
Wilson-Mikity syndrome
Hamman-Rich syndrome
Pulmonary edema
Infantile botulism
Congenital lobar emphysema

CHILDREN AND ADOLESCENTS

Skeletal
- Kyphoscoliosis
- Ankylosing spondylitis
- Pectus excavatum
- Crush chest injury

Parenchymal
- Pneumonia
- Hypersensitivity pneumonitis
- Systemic lupus erythematosus
- Scleroderma
- Fibrosis
- Toxin inhalation
- Granulomatous disease
- Drugs (e.g., antineoplastic agents and narcotics)[15]
- Carcinoma
- Fat embolus
- Pneumothorax

Smoke inhalation
Pulmonary infarction
Pulmonary edema
- Congestive heart failure
- Sepsis
- Intracranial disease[4]
- Croup[9]
- Epiglottitis[9]

Neuromuscular
- Cord transection
- Myasthenia gravis
- Muscular dystrophy
- Multiple sclerosis
- Guillain-Barré syndrome
- Pickwickian syndrome
- Toxins

Pleural effusion
- Pneumonia
- Hypoproteinemia
- Renal failure
- Tumor
- Pulmonary infarction

tial markings, parenchymal consolidation, skeletal deformities, and abnormal movement of the diaphragm.

Vascular Pulmonary Disease. Vascular lung disease is characterized by a decrease in the size of the pulmonary vascular bed. In the newborn this most often is due to persistent pulmonary hypertension of the newborn.[5] Microemboli also have been reported in the lungs of infants with severe respiratory distress.[12] In older children the most common cause of vascular pulmonary disease is intimal hyperplasia after persistent left-to-right shunting and resultant pulmonary hypertension. The size of the pulmonary vascular bed also can be reduced by obstruction caused by thromboembolic disease, obliteration (e.g., vasculitis),[6] or destruction, as in emphysema. The reduced blood flow through the lungs results in arterial hypoxemia and hypercapnia, which in turn lead to the symptoms and signs of dyspnea.

In addition to the common signs of dyspnea, the child with vascular lung disease may have signs of pulmonary edema and pleural effusion. Systemic signs of right-sided heart failure secondary to pulmonary hypertension or left-sided failure that was the cause of the pulmonary hypertension may be present. The cardiac findings observed with pulmonary hypertension are an accentuated P_2, paradoxical splitting of S_2, an S_3, a pulmonary ejection click, and a right ventricular heave.

The electrocardiogram is helpful in the diagnosis of right ventricular hypertrophy. The chest roentgenogram may reveal increased right ventricular size, enlargement of the pulmonary artery silhouette, decreased pulmonary blood flow in advanced disease, or increased flow early in the course of disease, with a left-to-right shunt.

Cardiac Disease

Dyspnea occurs with cardiac disease when insufficient blood is being pumped to the lungs as a result of congenital structural anomalies in the heart, pump failure (myocarditis or cardiomyopathy), or, as already described, secondary pulmonary hypertension. Heart disease must be considered in all dyspneic newborns and older children with a history of congenital heart disease. In the neonate, pulmonary disease often can be differentiated from cyanotic heart disease by use of a hyperoxia test. The nature of the cardiac defect can be delineated with the help of a thorough cardiac examination, an electrocardiogram, a chest roentgenogram, and an echocardiogram.

It must be remembered that what would be a trivial respiratory infection in a normal child may cause severe respiratory insufficiency in the child with cardiopulmonary disease. Indeed, the mortality of infants with respiratory syncytial viral pneumonia and congenital heart disease has been shown to exceed significantly the mortality of children with normal hearts.[13]

Hematologic Disease

If the oxygen-carrying capacity of blood is sufficiently reduced, tissue hypoxia will ensue. The resultant drop in arterial pH will signal the CNS and stimulate the onset of dyspnea. Severe anemia, whether chronic or acute, congenital or acquired, is an example of this. The oxygen-carrying capacity also can be lowered when the hemoglobin's ability to bind oxygen is reduced. This is most commonly seen with carbon monoxide poisoning, but it also occurs with cyanide poisoning and methemoglobinemia. In any of these cases the child will not be cyanotic. The blue color of cyanosis is caused by a level of less than 5 g/dl of reduced hemoglobin in the blood.[18] Such a concentration of reduced hemoglobin is not found in anemia uncomplicated by other diseases or in the other conditions cited. Conversely, a polycythemic infant whose blood is hyperviscous may have dyspnea because of poor perfusion. Because such an infant has an increased hemoglobin concentration and removes more oxygen from the hemoglobin because his or her flow is decreased, this child may be cyanotic (having >5 g/dl unsaturated hemoglobin) and not hypoxic.

It should be noted that even though an anemic child may be hypoxic and dyspneic, he or she will probably not be hypoxemic, that is, the arterial oxygen tension (PaO_2) measured by blood gas analysis will be in the normal range.

Metabolic Disease

Disorders that increase the body's rate of metabolism and therefore oxygen consumption can cause dyspnea. Examples are hyperthyroidism and fever. Metabolic disorders that are associated with an increased production of hydrogen ion and carbon dioxide cause a dyspnea-like breathing pattern to help rid the body of the carbon dioxide. The classic example is Kussmaul breathing of those with diabetic ketoacidosis. Aspirin poisoning can have a similar manifestation. In addition, children with various muscle enzyme deficiencies, especially those that affect the mitochondria, may have dyspnea as part of their clinical presentation as a result of their increased acid production and decreased work tolerance.[14,16] In chronic renal failure the kidney's inability to remove acid from the blood adequately is the underlying cause of dyspnea. The history, physical examination, and appropriate laboratory tests should facilitate the proper diagnosis of these diseases.

If oxygen cannot reach the tissues, the body responds with dyspnea, cardiovascular collapse, and shock. This is a medical emergency and should not present a diagnostic problem.

Obesity

Dyspnea, especially with exertion, is a common complaint of the obese child. The obese child is prone to dyspnea because of an increased metabolic requirement for a given amount of work.[20] In addition, the diaphragm of the obese child must move against an increased abdominal pressure and the chest wall is heavier; thus the expenditure of more energy is required to maintain $\dot{V}_E$.

Treatment should include dietary regulation and an exercise program graded to keep pace with the child's level of exercise tolerance.

Psychogenic Cause

Finally, hysteria may cause dyspnea. A thorough history, when available, makes the diagnosis easy. However, inasmuch as fear and anxiety may be present in dyspnea of any cause, hysteria may become a diagnosis of exclusion, although ordinarily it should not be. The physical examination results will be completely normal, and the only laboratory abnormality should be a decreased arterial carbon dioxide tension caused by hyperventilation. Treatment consists of calm reassurance and occasionally mild sedation.

MANAGEMENT

Severe dyspnea is a medical emergency. If not treated promptly, a child with dyspnea may rapidly progress to respiratory failure and death. Initially the adequacy of the airway must be assessed. Foreign bodies must be removed, and anatomic obstructions must be bypassed with endotracheal intubation or rarely tracheotomy. Bronchospasm, when present, should be treated with beta-agonistic drugs.

Subsequently, the efficacy of the child's ventilation must be evaluated. Normally, breathing uses 2% to 3% of the total body energy expenditure. When the work of breathing is increased during dyspnea, this amount may rise to 30% or more.[6] Such a degree of energy expenditure cannot be continued indefinitely, and the child tires. Even after an obstruction is removed, the child will still be unable to effect adequate ventilation. In this instance, or in the case of neuromuscular disease, the child requires mechanical ventilation.

Once ventilation is established, the ability of the cardiovascular system to deliver oxygen to the tissues must be appraised. This includes evaluation of the heart, peripheral circulation, intravascular volume status, and the blood's oxygen-carrying capacity. Therapy with vasopressors, fluids, blood transfusion, or diuretics should be initiated when indicated. Although not all children with dyspnea require supplemental oxygen, until the cause of the dyspnea is known, every child should have oxygen administered.

Once the patient's condition is stabilized, the search for the underlying cause of the dyspnea should progress in an urgent but calm manner. At this point a detailed history can be elicited, a full physical examination can be performed, and a chest roentgenogram and appropriate blood work can be obtained. When the diagnosis is made, specific therapy can be initiated.

When dyspnea is caused by a chronic illness, there may be no satisfactory therapy available for treatment of the underlying disease. Relief of dyspnea alone, however, can significantly improve the child's functional ability and quality of life.[1] Several modalities can be used to treat the symptom of dyspnea in a chronically ill child. Sedatives and narcotics decrease $\dot{V}_E$ and thereby diminish the intensity of the breathless feeling. Several other classes of drugs such as phenothiazines (specifically, promethazine), prostaglandin inhibitors, and beta agonists that may blunt the perception of dyspnea without affecting ventilation currently are being studied.[17] Exercises that increase the strength of the inspiratory muscles and thereby reduce the perceived magnitude of dyspnea also are useful.[1] Finally, inasmuch as dyspnea is a subjective complaint, there is a significant psychological contribution to its perceived severity.[3] Therefore the child's emotional state, behavior, and personality must be monitored because psychosocial intervention may be indicated.

REFERENCES

1. Altose MD: Assessment and management of breathlessness, Chest 88 (suppl 2):77s, 1985.
2. Angelillo VA: Evaluation of dyspnea, Postgrad Med 73:336, 1983.
3. Cherniak NS and Altose MD: Mechanisms of dyspnea, Clin Chest Med 8:207, 1978.
4. Drucker TB, Simmons RL, and Martin AM: Pulmonary edema as a complication of intracranial disease, Am J Dis Child 118:638, 1969.
5. Fox WW and Duara S: Persistent pulmonary hypertension in the neonate: diagnosis and management, J Pediatr 103:505, 1983.
6. Goffman TE, Bloom RL, and Dvorak VC: Acute dyspnea in a young woman taking birth control pills, JAMA 251:1465, 1984.
7. Guyton AC: Textbook of medical physiology, Philadelphia, 1981, WB Saunders Co.
8. Howell JB and Campbell EJM, editors: Breathlessness, Oxford, 1966, Blackwell Scientific Publications, Ltd.
9. Kanter RK and Watchko JF: Pulmonary edema associated with upper airway obstruction, Am J Dis Child 138:356, 1984.
10. Killian KJ and Campbell EJM: Dyspnea and exercise, Annu Rev Physiol 45:465, 1983.
11. Leigh M, Holman G, and Rohn R: Dyspnea as the presenting symptom of thyroid disease, Clin Pediatr 19:773, 1980.
12. Levin DL, Weinberg AG, and Perkin RM: Pulmonary microthrombi in newborn infants with unresponsive persistent pulmonary hypertension, J Pediatr 102:299, 1983.
13. Macdonald NE et al: Respiratory syncytial virus infection in infants with congenital heart disease, N Engl J Med 307:397, 1982.
14. Robinson BH et al: Clinical presentation of mitochondrial respiratory chain defects in NADH-coenzyme Q reductase and cytochrome oxidase: clues to pathogenesis of Leigh disease, J Pediatr 110:216, 1987.
15. Rosenow EC: The spectrum of drug-induced pulmonary disease, Ann Intern Med 77:977, 1972.
16. Scholte HR et al: Defects in oxidative phosphorylation: biochemical investigations in skeletal muscle and expression of the lesion in other cells, J Inherited Metab Dis 10(suppl 1):81, 1987.
17. Stark RD: Dyspnoea: assessment and pharmacological manipulation, Eur J Respir Dis 1:280, 1988.
18. Tisi GM: Pulmonary physiology in clinical medicine, Baltimore, 1980, Williams & Wilkins Co.
19. Wasserman K and Casaburi R: Dyspnea: physiological and pathophysiological mechanisms, Annu Rev Med 39:503, 1988.
20. Wasserman K et al: Principles of exercise testing and interpretation, Philadelphia, 1987, Lea & Febiger.

SUGGESTED READINGS

Burki NK: Dyspnea, Lung 165:269, 1987.

Downes JJ, Fulgencio T, and Raphaely RC: Acute respiratory failure in infants and children, Pediatr Clin North Am 19:423, 1972.

Gandevia SC: Neural mechanisms underlying the sensation of breathlessness: kinesthetic parallels between respiratory and limb muscles, Aust NZ J Med 18:83, 1988.

Mahler DA: Dyspnea: diagnosis and management, Clin Chest Med 8:215, 1987.

Rebuck AS and Slutsky AS: Control of breathing in diseases of the respiratory tract and lungs. In Geiger SR, editor: Handbook of physiology, Bethesda, MD, 1986, American Physiological Society.

Shayevitz MB and Shayevitz BR: Athletic training in chronic obstructive pulmonary disease, Clin Sports Med 5:471, 1986.

125

Dysuria

Fred J. Heldrich

Dysuria is defined as painful or difficult urination. Although this symptom occurs with some frequency in pediatric patients, it is interesting that the term can rarely be found in the index of standard pediatric texts and cannot be found in the *Cumulative Index Medicus*. The reason is that dysuria rarely occurs as an isolated symptom; far more often it manifests with other signs or symptoms of urinary tract pathology and thus is discussed as part of these urinary symptoms. Although occasionally dysuria may be the only complaint, the identification of causes of dysuria is enhanced in many instances by considering the associated symptoms.

Identifying the causes of dysuria requires a thorough history, a careful physical examination, and a planned laboratory evaluation.[1] Failure to follow this routine usually leads to unnecessary expense, an incorrect diagnosis, and improper management.

CLINICAL MANIFESTATIONS

Although older patients may clearly indicate that urination is painful or difficult, infants and young children give other evidence of dysuria. Infants indicate pain on urination in a variety of ways (see accompanying box), with crying being the most typical sign, which should be associated with the act of micturition if the patient experiences dysuria. Just as voiding provokes crying, cessation of voiding provides relief of pain, and crying may stop. Characteristically infants who cry because of the discomfort associated with voiding will flex their thighs. This combination of crying and drawing up of the legs frequently is described as colic. At times the association between crying and voiding is not appreciated, and the infant appears to be hyperirritable without an obvious explanation. The frequency of urination that usually accompanies painful urination in infants results in their diapers seldom being dry.

Young children unable to state accurately that urination is painful or difficult evidence dysuria by other signs (see box). At this age, crying that occurs because of the pain experienced with urination is more readily identified. Because of the discomfort occasioned by voiding, the patient may delay urination as long as possible. This can lead to bladder distention, suprapubic discomfort, and irritability or further crying. Difficulty in either initiating or continuing urination may produce a hesitant or an episodic urine stream, which may be seen or heard when the patient is seated on a potty chair or commode. In an attempt to overcome resistance to urine flow, a patient may assume a squatting position or sit with each act of micturition.

Older children use terms such as "burn," "tingle," or "hurt" to express pain, and "strain," "bear down," or "It's hard to start" to indicate discomfort and difficulty in the act of voiding.

Although dysuria may be the only symptom, other signs and symptoms that frequently occur concomitantly are extremely important and helpful in establishing the cause of dysuria. Regardless of the patient's age, there is considerable similarity in the associated signs and symptoms, and they can be placed in one of two major categories: (1) other specific urinary symptoms, such as hematuria, malodorous urine, or frequency, or (2) nonspecific symptoms, such as fever, abdominal pain, diarrhea, or vomiting. Thus dysuria may be either the primary complaint or simply an associated symptom frequently occurring with other symptoms of greater magnitude.[2]

PHYSICAL FINDINGS

Frequently, positive findings on physical examination are lacking. However, anomalies of the external genitalia may be seen. An obstructive uropathy may be discernible as an abdominal mass (enlarged bladder, ureters, or kidneys). Palpation may elicit pain at the costovertebral angles, above the symphysis pubis, or over the abdomen in general. In male infants a small meatal opening, frequently ulcerated, may be seen. A rectal examination may identify a fecal mass or a tender, swollen prostate. Inspection of the perineum may reveal excoriation of the skin, labia, or meatal opening. Ure-

Indicators of Dysuria

INFANTS

Crying
Colic
Irritability
Flexing of legs
A diaper that is wet more frequently than usual

YOUNG CHILDREN

Crying when voiding
Hesitant stream
Straining
Squatting or sitting to void
Refusing to urinate

thral prolapse is identified by a doughnut-shaped, red, swollen mucosa protruding from the urethral orifice. In addition to erythema, vesicles and a serous, serosanguineous, or purulent discharge may be found in the vagina.

DIFFERENTIAL DIAGNOSIS

Any condition that leads to inflammation or irritation of the urinary tract or obstructs the flow of urine may cause dysuria.[3] Dysuria as the dominant symptom suggests the diagnostic possibilities shown in the accompanying box.

Urinary Tract Infection

Urinary tract infection is the most common cause of dysuria. Pain on urination also may lead to urgency, frequency, hesitancy, and enuresis. The urine may be clear, cloudy, bloody, or foul smelling. Dysuria typically is associated with infection of the lower urinary tract, although it also may occur with upper tract disease. The inability to rule out upper tract disease without resorting to ureteral catheterization, collection of urine by use of the bladder washout technique, renal biopsy, or radionuclide studies impels the physician to evaluate the patient carefully on more basic clinical grounds for evidence of upper tract disease. Here associated symptoms can be helpful. Systemic symptoms such as chills, fever, or abdominal or costovertebral angle pain usually indicate pyelonephritis. Suprapubic discomfort is more consistent with cystitis.

Bacteria are the most common cause of both upper and lower urinary tract infections. Gram-negative organisms predominate, and *Escherichia coli* is found most frequently. A mixed bacterial flora, although unusual, is most apt to exist if infection occurs in a urinary tract with structural abnormalities or if the patient has had persistent reinfections.

In female adolescents with both frequency and dysuria, the persistent recovery of a single organism at colony counts below 10^5/ml of a clean-caught, midstream specimen is consistent with the diagnosis of infection.[4]

Viruses, particularly coxsackieviruses A11 and A12, have been identified as a cause of hemorrhagic cystitis. Dysuria usually is pronounced, and blood clots pass frequently. *Ureaplasma urealyticum, Mycoplasma hominis,* and anerobes are other potential pathogens.[4]

Tuberculosis is an uncommon cause of urinary tract infection today, but when it is the cause, it frequently is accompanied by dysuria and hematuria. Both the upper and lower urinary tracts may be affected.

Fungi, especially *Candida albicans,* are an unusual cause of urinary tract infection, but they may occur, usually as a superimposed infection in a patient taking antibiotic therapy.

Pinworms *(Enterobius vermicularis)* may lead to perineal irritation and discomfort on urination.

Causes of Dysuria

Urinary tract infection
Urethritis
Prostatitis
Balanoposthitis
Meatal lesions
Vulvovaginitis
Stones
Obstruction
Foreign bodies
Tumors
Drugs
Trauma
Sexual abuse
Hematologic disorders
Perineal dermatitis (primary)
Masturbation
Psychogenic factors

Urethritis

Neisseria gonorrhoeae is a major cause of urethritis in sexually active adolescent boys. A profuse, creamy urethral discharge accompanies the dysuria. In prepubertal boys, urethritis frequently is nonspecific; that is, no etiologic agent is recovered.

Chlamydia trachomatis is yet another organism that has been identified as a cause of urethritis and frequently appears as a recurrent infection after the patient has received treatment for gonorrhea. Burning on urination is a common symptom in nongonococcal forms of urethritis.

Prostatitis

Prostatitis is confined almost exclusively to sexually active patients. In addition to dysuria, there often is a sensation of deep, suprapubic discomfort. Urination may be more frequent than usual. A rectal examination reveals a tender prostate, which after massage will yield a urethral discharge. The bacteria involved vary and are determined by culturing the discharge.

Balanoposthitis

Balanoposthitis, infection of the glans penis and prepuce, is an unusual infection that may occur in uncircumcised boys. The diagnosis is readily made by inspection, and the bacterium responsible is isolated by culturing the prepucal discharge.

Meatal Lesions

In the male infant still in diapers, a meatal ulcer may develop as a result of irritation by the wet diaper. An ammoniacal diaper rash also is present in most instances. Bleeding at the site of the meatal ulceration may produce a spot of blood on the diaper covering the area.

A diaper rash also may be associated with dysuria in the female infant. A unique lesion of the female urethra is prolapse, which appears as a circumferential ring of red or bluish mucosa protruding from the urethral orifice.

Vulvovaginitis

Various organisms may cause vulvovaginitis: *N. gonorrhoeae, Haemophilus vaginalis, C. trachomatis, Trichomonas vaginalis,* and herpes progenitalis are the most commonly encountered. A discharge of varying degree is present in all instances. Herpes, an infection that is associated with severe dysuria, is further characterized by the presence of vesicles, or ulcerations after rupture of vesicles, on the vulva and vagina. All these infections are sexually transmitted.

In the prepubertal girl, although any of the aforementioned agents may be identified, the infection usually is nonspecific. Gonococcal infection in the prepubertal girl should be considered as evidence of child abuse until proved otherwise.

Stones

The pain caused by kidney stones usually is "colicky," with associated hematuria. Passage of the stone down the ureter or through the urethra is most apt to produce pain that frequently radiates to the urethral meatus. Bladder stones typically produce pain at the end of micturition. Approximately 80% of kidney and bladder stones are radiopaque and contain calcium. The family history may be positive for nephrolithiasis. Hypercalciuria without stone formation may produce dysuria and hematuria.[5] Diseases that are associated with renal stones include hyperparathyroidism, gout, renal tubular acidosis, hypercalciuria, cystinuria, inflammatory bowel disease, and immobilization hypercalcemia.

Obstruction

Lesions below the bladder (posterior urethral valves, urethral strictures, urethral diverticulum, or meatal stenosis) are almost always found in boys and may produce difficulty in initiating urination. Obstruction in this area also produces dilation of the bladder and both ureters, which can lead to overflow incontinence and suprapubic discomfort.

Obstructive lesions of a ureter (ureteral stricture, ureteroceles, ectopic ureters, ureteropelvic obstruction) lead to unilateral hydronephrosis, which may remain silent or cause dysuria.

Either bilateral or unilateral hydronephrotic changes increase the probability of urinary tract infection, which can then produce dysuria. Hydronephrotic urinary tracts also are easily aggravated by subsequent hematuria and dysuria. Either infection or hematuria may lead to stone formation. Finally, hydronephrotic changes may produce ptosis of urinary tract structures and can be associated with pain that radiates toward the urethra and leads to an urge to urinate. In this instance the pain may be related to changes in body position.

Other Causes of Dysuria

Children may insert foreign bodies in their own urethras or those of their playmates. Evidence of trauma at the urethral orifice and discovery of a foreign body by roentgenogram confirm the diagnosis.

Bladder tumors are rare in children and usually are associated with bleeding. Wilms tumor, the most common renal tumor in children, may produce dysuria with hematuria, but this form of presentation would be highly unusual.

The use of the following drugs has been associated with dysuria: amitriptyline, chlordiazepoxide, imipramine, isoniazid, sulfonamides, cytoxan, heparin, dicumarol, and antihistamines.

Trauma that produces hematuria may result in dysuria. Direct trauma to the perineum or external genitalia may be an obvious cause of dysuria. Irritation of the urethra with a catheter or a cystoscope is a cause of dysuria that is self-limited.

A special form of trauma, sexual abuse, deserves consideration in all instances in which history and physical findings are not compatible with the symptoms or when the accusation is made by the patient or a person bringing the child for treatment.

Dysuria may occur as a result of pain caused by the flow of urine over an irritated perineum. Local lesions may be caused by soaps or bubble bath, local infections such as varicella or candidiasis, and masturbation. Wet diapers may cause perineal irritation when they are not changed frequently.

Cystoscopic examination is to be avoided in the management of most urinary tract infections. It may be useful, however, in identifying a bladder lesion. Often such lesions cause hematuria and dysuria.

Other studies may be indicated to determine renal function and to rule out hematologic disorders and rare forms of renal disease.

MANAGEMENT

The major cause of dysuria is a urinary tract infection, which usually can be managed effectively by the pediatrician. The principles of management are precise diagnosis, adequate evaluation of the genitourinary tract, appropriate antibiotic therapy, and long-term follow-up. Details are discussed in Chapter 264. Sexually transmitted diseases should be treated as discussed in Chapter 254.

Offending irritants such as soaps, powders, or bubble bath should be removed. Tight-fitting diapers that restrict the entrance of air should be avoided. Local medications may be indicated for a candidal infection. If oxyuriasis (pinworm infestation) is present, mebendazole should be effective. (Remember to treat other family members.) Sitz baths in warm water may temporarily relieve acute symptoms of dysuria after catheterization or cystoscopic examination.

When evidence supports the diagnosis of functional dysuria, a positive approach to management begins with minimizing the laboratory workup. For example, imaging studies may not be required initially. Counseling to ensure understanding of the dynamics involved and methods to eliminate factors that are contributing to the symptom are of greatest importance. The patient, when old enough, should be reassured that organic disease does not exist but that the symptom of dysuria is real and steps will be taken to alleviate it. Pediatricians can manage functional dysuria effectively when they are willing and able to spend the time necessary and show appropriate concern for the problem.

Suspicion of sexual abuse requires prompt protection of the child and warrants hospitalization pending adequate evaluation. Appropriate agencies should be notified.

Urologic consultation occasionally is required, notably when the diagnosis of obstructive uropathy, renal calculi, foreign bodies, tumors, or urethral prolapse is suspected or confirmed.

REFERENCES

1. Carlton CE Jr: Initial evaluation: including history, physical examination, and urinalysis. In Harrison JL et al, editors: Campbell's urology, ed 5, Philadelphia, 1986, WB Saunders Co.
2. Kaplan GW and Brock WA: Voiding dysfunction in children, Curr Probl Pediatr 10:41, 1980.
3. Rubin MI and Barratt TM, editors: Pediatric nephrology, Baltimore, 1975, Williams & Wilkins Co.
4. Sobel J and Kaye D: Urinary tract infections. In Gillenwater JY et al, editors: Adult and pediatric urology, ed 1, Chicago, 1987, Year Book Medical Publishers, Inc.
5. Stapleton FB et al: Hypercalciuria in children with urolithiasis, Am J Dis Child 136:675, 1982.

126

Edema

Robert H. McLean

RECOGNITION AND SIGNIFICANCE OF EDEMA

The recognition of edema can be a clinical challenge. Edema, which is swelling caused by excessive fluid accumulation, often is labeled many other things before being recognized as just what it is. Frequently the parents will notice weight gain, chubbiness, the outgrowing of shoes, or irritability in their child, whereas the physician may diagnose allergic problems before a more fundamental cause of the swelling is determined.

Recognizing edema is important because any disturbance of salt and water homeostasis in the body is significant. Water makes up 65% of the adult's body weight and 75% of the newborn's body weight. When edema is detected early, the clinical circumstances usually are dramatic enough to determine its cause. When, however, edema is clinically more subtle, the diagnosis can be delayed, often with serious consequences.

Edema reflects a profound abnormality in body fluid homeostasis because so much metabolic energy is spent regulating the body's water and sodium content. However, the patient's age, sex, and organs involved and the extent and duration of the edema influence its ultimate importance. Edema usually is not idiopathic in children.

PATHOPHYSIOLOGY

The movement of water between the extracellular and intracellular body compartments under normal circumstances is regulated carefully, with the largest quantity of water being located within the intracellular spaces. The appearance of edema results from disturbances in the distribution of fluid between the two extracellular space subcompartments—the intravascular and the interstitial spaces.

At the end of the nineteenth century, Starling[2] proposed the following hypothesis to explain the movement of water between the intravascular and the interstitial spaces: at the capillary and precapillary level, two types of forces cause water to leave the intravascular space (plasma): hydrostatic pressure (blood pressure) and oncotic pressure within the interstitium. (The forces that cause oncotic pressure are discussed below.) Opposing this movement of water out of plasma are two forces: the plasma oncotic pressure and tissue turgor. The forces that create egress of water from plasma slightly outweigh the opposing ingress forces at the arterial end of the capillary bed, but the reverse is true at the venule end of the bed. The result is movement of water, nutrients, and electrolytes through the interstitium at both ends of the network, but no net change occurs in intravascular and interstitial fluid exchanges. Any slight accumulation of water in the interstitial spaces is carried away in the lymphatic system.

In quantitative terms, the most important force opposing movement of water into the interstitium is the oncotic pressure.[3] Plasma contains charged electrolytes (crystalloids such as sodium and chloride) and electrically charged proteins (colloids such as albumin). The osmotic pressure is the function of the total number of such charged particles in any given fluid. A sodium molecule is osmotically as effective as an albumin molecule, even though the latter is much larger. The sum of the positive and negative particles in each body fluid–containing compartment must balance, but the exact composition of these charges varies considerably. For example, because the capillary membrane is semipermeable rather than fully permeable, the protein content of plasma normally is much greater than that of the fluid in the interstitial spaces. Because of the high plasma protein concentration and the characteristics of the capillary membranes, the total number of osmotically active particles present in plasma normally is higher than the number in the interstitium. This slight difference between the osmolarity of the plasma and the osmolarity of the interstitium creates the oncotic pressure. Because this difference is caused primarily (but not exclusively) by the protein content of plasma, determination of the status of protein metabolism is important in evaluating edema. For example, mechanisms that decrease oncotic pressure, such as the excessive loss of protein in the urine or gastrointestinal tract, may lead to edema.

Despite this, the role of body sodium in edema is paramount in most clinical situations. Several forces control sodium balance, including the rates of glomerular filtration and aldosterone production. Simply put, continued intake of the usual amount of sodium will lead to sodium retention if the sodium-controlling factors do not respond appropriately to maintain a proper balance between the intake and output of sodium.

Sodium moves freely throughout the plasma and extracellular water spaces. It constitutes the largest cationic (positively charged) crystalloid and thus exerts the greatest osmotic force for movement of water between these spaces. Therefore it is not surprising that excessive accumulation of sodium in the body will lead to the accumulation of excessive body water.

Primary control of the amount of sodium in the body is

regulated through the process of glomerular filtration and the renin-angiotensin-aldosterone hormonal axis. Normally, most sodium filtered through the glomerulus is resorbed through the renal tubules before it reaches the pyelocaliceal system by a precisely controlled mechanism responding to the amount of sodium consumed each day.

Total body sodium levels become abnormal when the glomerular filtration of sodium becomes so reduced that sodium balance can no longer be controlled via renal tubular resorption or nonresorption. Such is the case in renal failure, in which glomerular filtration becomes too low to excrete sodium to any significant degree. Aldosterone excess, which may occur in intravascular volume–depleted states (such as the nephrotic syndrome), may be a primary cause of edema.

Edema confined to a single extremity or a well-circumscribed area of the body is a special situation. This can occur from obstruction of the vascular or lymphatic system of a limb because of trauma, tumor, embolization, or thrombus formation. Local release of vasoactive substances that cause locally increased vascular permeability may occur in allergic persons and in patients who lack a particular complement system inhibitor.

CAUSES OF EDEMA

Various disorders can lead to edema[1] (see accompanying box). The history, physical examination, and some simple laboratory tests usually point to the most likely cause, although more sophisticated evaluation procedures may be indicated.

Causes of Edema in Children

- Cardiovascular
  - Congestive heart failure
  - Acute thrombi or emboli
  - Vasculitis of many types
- Renal
  - Nephrotic syndrome
  - Glomerulonephritis of many types
  - End-stage renal failure
- Endocrine or metabolic
  - Thyroid disease
  - Starvation
  - Hereditary angioedema
- Iatrogenic
  - Drugs (diuretics and steroids)
  - Water or salt overload
- Hematologic
  - Hemolytic disease of the newborn
- Gastrointestinal
  - Hepatic cirrhosis
  - Protein-losing enteritis
  - Lymphangiectasis
  - Cystic fibrosis
  - Celiac disease
  - Enteritis of many types
- Lymphatic abnormalities
  - Congenital (gonadal dysgenesis)
  - Acquired

It is particularly helpful to classify the cause of edema according to the usual age of onset (Table 126-1). In this regard the pediatrician has an advantage over the internist because this information often is less useful for diagnosis in adults.

The most common cause of chronic renal failure in children is a congenital abnormality. Signs of renal failure, such as edema, usually have their onset during infancy and childhood, unlike congenital heart disease, which so often causes edema and other symptoms at or soon after birth.

Certain forms of gastrointestinal disease result in edema early in life because of protein losses, but some congenital diseases, such as hepatic fibrosis associated with autosomal recessive diffuse cystic disease of the kidneys, will cause signs of fluid retention only as the child grows older.

Vasculitis is a general term that includes anaphylactoid purpura, systemic lupus erythematosus, and a spectrum of inflammatory vascular diseases and syndromes. These diseases are rare in the newborn or infant. Similarly, drug abuse and the overuse of prescribed drugs, such as diuretics (a rare cause of edema), are confined largely to adolescents. Abuse of narcotics or other drugs can produce the nephrotic syndrome and glomerulonephritis. Idiopathic glomerulonephritis and acute poststreptococcal glomerulonephritis are far more common in children and adolescents than in infants.

At all ages the most common cause of edema in hospitalized patients is the excessive parenteral administration of sodium and water. In the confusion of caring for a sick, postoperative, or traumatized child, inappropriate fluid management continues to be a problem.

HISTORY AND PHYSICAL EXAMINATION IN THE EVALUATION OF EDEMA

In trying to establish the cause of edema, several important aspects of the medical history are the rate of accumulation of the fluid, the age and sex of the patient, the location of the swelling, and the association of other medical conditions, including acute intercurrent illness.

The rate of accumulation of edema caused by significant organ damage may be so low as to go unnoticed by the parents or the child. Frequently the associated weight gain is attributed to other causes. A change in shoe size or clothing size often is dismissed as compatible with changes that occur in a growing child.

Knowing the age of the child when the edema first began is extremely helpful. Differentiation of the cause of edema in the newborn often can be clarified by weighing the placenta. Infants with congenital nephrotic syndrome have a large and boggy placenta, which may weigh twice as much as normal. The appearance of edema in the newborn or infant is reason for concern because significant organ damage may be present. Hematologic and infectious disease in utero must be considered in the evaluation of the edematous newborn, whereas diseases of the heart, liver, and gastrointestinal tract are more common in the older infant or child.

Edema caused by the nephrotic syndrome usually becomes noticeable early in the course of the disease (after a few weeks). Careful questioning can establish that subtle signs of fluid accumulation had been present for some time. The pres-

Table 126-1 *Causes of Edema and Age of Onset*

ETIOLOGIC FACTOR	FETAL OR NEONATAL	INFANCY	CHILDHOOD	ADOLESCENCE
Hemolytic anemias	X			
Congenital heart disease	X	X	X	
Congenital kidney disease	X	X	X	X
Gastrointestinal disease	X	X	X	X
Vasculitis			X	X
Drug reactions				X
Infections	X	X		
Acute or chronic glomerulonephritis			X	X
Excessive salt and water administration	X	X	X	X
Hereditary angioedema			X	X

ence of periorbital edema frequently is the first sign noticed by the parents. This is more noticeable in the morning because of nighttime "dependency." For the same reason, presacral edema is the primary edematous site in the nonambulatory child. The "pot-belly" so characteristic of the nephrotic syndrome is a late sign of fluid accumulation (ascites).

Although edema caused by heart disease and chronic renal failure occurs about as frequently in boys as in girls, idiopathic nephrotic syndrome is twice as common in boys. The peak age of onset is between 3 and 4 years. Attacks of hereditary angioedema appear in adolescents and adults, but abdominal pain and swelling also may occur in the preadolescent child with this disease. An acute intercurrent illness often precedes attacks of angioedema and exacerbations of idiopathic nephrotic syndrome.

The family history is positive for edema in more than 50% of the cases of angioedema. A family history positive for nephrosis occurs in less than 4% of cases, but familial forms of glomerulonephritis that lead to kidney failure constitute an identifiable cause of edema.

LABORATORY TESTS IN THE EVALUATION OF EDEMA

The initial steps in the evaluation of edema must include a urinalysis. The presence of protein or abnormal cellular elements will immediately focus attention on a renal cause for edema. Large amounts of protein in a random urine specimen with little or no blood present strongly support the diagnosis of the nephrotic syndrome. The presence of red or white blood cells or casts suggests glomerulonephritis. The further evaluation of renal disease requires testing renal function, including the determination of serum urea nitrogen, creatinine, and total protein and albumin concentrations. If results are abnormal, the (corrected) creatinine clearance and quantitative urine protein should be measured. Consultation with a pediatric nephrologist would be appropriate at this point.

Normal urinalysis and renal function tests associated with a low serum protein concentration should lead one to consider contrast studies of the gastrointestinal tract. Protein-losing enteropathies may be expected to be accompanied by significant symptoms of gastrointestinal aberrations (diarrhea and weight loss).

Performance of a complete blood count and serologic studies for red cell antibodies are emergency procedures in the evaluation of the edematous newborn infant. In the presence of chronic renal disease one can expect to find anemia and an elevated sedimentation rate; in acute infectious processes an elevated white blood cell count or a shift to the left in the differential count should be present.

Edema caused by heart failure can be quickly confirmed with chest roentgenograms or by use of electrocardiography or echocardiography. Unlike the nephrotic syndrome or protein-losing enteropathy, congestive heart failure demands rapid corrective measures.

The particular combination of abdominal cramps with localized edema (such as edema of the hands, feet, or larynx) should prompt the physician to consider measuring the concentration and function of the serum C1 esterase inhibitor (C1INH). Reduced levels of C1INH are present in 80% of cases of hereditary angioedema. However, because 20% of cases of hereditary angioedema have normal or elevated serum concentrations of C1INH but reduced function of the inhibitor, special effort needs to be made to measure C1INH function (some commercial laboratories offer this service).

MANAGEMENT OF EDEMA

When the cause of edema is recognized, treatment begins with the management of the causative disorder. For example, if surgical correction of a cardiac lesion is possible, the appropriate corrective procedure becomes the primary therapeutic maneuver.

Supportive care before beginning specific therapy of a cardiac, renal, or other cause of edema depends on the consequences of the edema collection. Generalized edema with dependency of fluid accumulation in the legs or abdominal or genital areas is not, by itself, reason for treatment. Slow accumulation of edema in nephrosis or cirrhosis generally is well tolerated. Treatment with diuretics or aldosterone inhibitors is only of transient benefit in many of these chronic diseases, although such drugs may be tried if the situation demands such action. For example, if edema involves the lungs, as in heart failure, or if it may lead to a skin breakdown, as may occur in the scrotum in the nephrotic syndrome, then even the temporary relief provided by diuretics is indicated. In situations in which the "effective" vascular volume may be decreased, further shrinkage of that volume may produce acute renal failure. The use of plasma volume expanders with colloid followed by diuretics often is appropriate when plasma volume is low but should obviously be avoided in the presence of heart failure.

Careful assessment of the sodium requirements should be made. Sodium and fluid restriction may be all that is required to correct the edema and is critically important in iatrogenic cases. For chronic edema my practice is to teach patients and parents about the sodium content of foods so that the minimum sodium necessary for palatability of food is ingested. It is good practice to maintain this diet between episodes of edema, inasmuch as patients can adjust well to a low-sodium diet but switching back and forth is difficult.

Acute episodes of edema associated with the nephrotic syndrome occasionally are accompanied by irritability and changes in behavior. The self-image of the child with chronic edema can be seriously affected either because the edema may be interpreted as obesity in the adolescent or the underlying disease may require change in the patient's activity and life-style. Such secondary effects of edema should be recognized by the physician and the parents to minimize the consequences for the child.

Several of the diseases that may cause significant edema require the assistance of a specialist. However, because these patients eventually return home, the availability of the primary care physician is essential for proper continuous care. The specialist should ensure that the patient and family are familiar with the early signs of recurrence or worsening of the process. The importance of accurate record keeping of weights, urine protein excretion, and blood pressure must be explained. Most parents and patients become more comfortable with a chronic disease when they acquire a working knowledge of the disease and can participate in the required care. With such education the primary physician can rely more fully on the parents' observations, which are of immeasurable help in the home management of edema.

REFERENCES

1. Fisher DA: Obscure and unusual edema, Pediatrics 37:506, 1966.
2. Starling EH: On the absorption of fluids from the connective tissue spaces, J Physiol 19:312, 1895-1896.
3. Valtin H: Renal function: mechanisms preserving fluid and solute balance in health, ed 2, Boston, 1983, Little, Brown & Co.

127

Epistaxis

David R. Edlestein and Edward V. Sauris

Epistaxis, which occurs frequently in childhood, can be a frightening experience for a parent or child. Fortunately, most nasal bleeding in childhood is minor. Severe, prolonged or recurrent bleeding, however, can indicate a more critical problem such as a bleeding disorder or nasal tumor. Epistaxis is rare in neonates and infants, increases in incidence in childhood, and again becomes less common during adolescence.[2] It is more common in boys than in girls.[9]

The nose is a highly vascular organ with a large surface area and therefore is predisposed to bleeding. Its function is to move air; to filter pollutants; to humidify, warm, and to serve as a buffer to central structures during trauma; and to function as a resonance box in speech. Its relatively high vascularity serves to increase local blood volume, which helps to warm the temperature of inspired air, to move critical cells like leukocytes or immunoglobulins, and to provide an expansile surface area that aids in filtration and cleaning. The most vascular areas therefore are near the front of the nose in Little's area, where there is a plexus of vessels with branches from the internal and external carotid arteries (Table 127-1). Two other critical areas are the posterolateral portion of nose, which contains large branches of the internal maxillary artery, and a portion high in the lateral nasal vault that contains other branches of the internal carotid artery.

There are many possible causes for nasal bleeding. Fortunately, most are benign. These include mucosal irritation from weather changes and allergies, simple trauma from nose-picking,[4] chronic rhinitis with nose blowing, chronic usage of nasal sprays or drying agents such as decongestants, and viral or bacterial infections. More serious epistaxis may occur after blunt trauma following accidents or nasal surgery. In some cases severe or recurrent bleeds may represent a bleeding diathesis such as von Willebrand disease or a neoplasm such as nasopharyngeal angiofibroma. Differentiating local from systemic causes is very important in order to institute early treatment and to avoid the need for blood transfusion. The correct diagnosis may have implications for the patient's family or community, because some causes of epistaxis may be genetic or result from environmental problems.

CHARACTERISTICS

The type, location, and frequency of nasal bleeding may help the physician understand its cause and danger. In 1988 Katsanis and colleagues[10] devised an *epistaxis scoring system* to help identify children who may need elaborate workups. This system is based on the frequency, duration, amount, and site of bleeding. Those children with high epistaxis scores had a much greater chance of having a clotting abnormality.[10] Standard criteria are important in deciding whether to proceed with an elaborate evaluation for a bleeding disorder. Children for whom there is a high index of suspicion for a bleeding disorder need more diagnostic tests beyond a complete blood count, platelet count, and prothrombin time measurement.

In most instances epistaxis is unilateral and is caused by local irritation or trauma. In contrast, bilateral epistaxis may be due to a bleeding disorder, a posterior bleeding source, or severe craniofacial trauma. Gradual-onset bleeding frequently results from the overuse of medications such as aspirin or ibuprofen in the older child or from slowly growing tumors. In contrast, sudden-onset bleeding usually is due to trauma or nose picking. Intermittent bleeding may be caused by changes in the weather, allergies, or low humidification of inspired air. It also can be associated with menses.

The location of the bleeding may be useful in determining the cause and the treatment. An anterior bleed, which can be viewed with a nasal speculum, can be treated by simple compression. In contrast, a posterior bleed can be visualized only if the anatomy of the nose is normal and adequate premedication and special instruments are used. A high nasal bleed may represent a fracture involving the nasoethmoid

Table 127-1 *Blood Supply of the Nose*

VESSEL	LOCATION
Internal carotid artery	
Ophthalmic artery	
Anterior ethmoid	Anterosuperior septum, anterior lateral wall
Posterior ethmoid	Posterior septum, posterior lateral wall
External carotid artery	
Internal maxillary artery	
Sphenopalatine branch	Posterior septum, posterior lateral wall
Nasopalatine branch	Posterior septum, floor of nose
Descending palatine branch	Posterior lateral wall
Pharyngeal branch	Nasopharyngeal roof
Facial artery	
Superior labial branch	Tip of septum, nasal alar

complex and orbit. Recurrent epistaxis may occur in a patient with a minor bleeding disorder or in one with chronic nasal mucosal irritation.

ASSOCIATED SIGNS AND SYMPTOMS

Although epistaxis is a dramatic symptom, it usually is not the only one related to the nose. Other symptoms can be useful in arriving at a diagnosis. For example, a child with nasal obstruction and epistaxis may have a foreign body or a polyp in the nose. Obstruction also can be caused by a deviated septum, which may predispose the patient to local dryness and cracking of the mucosa. If the nasal obstruction is chronic and related to lower airway symptoms, the child may have perennial allergic rhinitis associated with asthma.

It is important to know if the patient has had facial pain or headaches. Facial pain may be present with sinusitis or an enlarging mucocele of one of the sinuses. It also can be caused by a tumor involving the nose, the sinuses, or the base of the skull, which may bleed intermittently. Headaches associated with epistaxis in infants can be caused by an encephalocele or meningocele.

Children with trauma-induced epistaxis should be tested for visual acuity because injury to the nose or the ethmoid sinuses may disrupt the lamina papyracea and injure the eye, including retroorbital bleeding, orbital fractures, and damage to the eye muscles. A fracture of the cribriform plate also can occur, which can result in meningitis, anosmia (lack of smell), or chronic cerebrospinal fluid leakage through the nose.

Occasionally the only symptom noticed by a parent of a child with chronic mild epistaxis is the presence of unexplained melena. This is due to the child swallowing blood from the posterior nares. Similarly hematemesis can result from epistaxis when the child swallows blood.[8]

All children with epistaxis should have their vital signs taken and monitored closely. Hypotension and syncope-like episodes can occur if the blood loss is significant. Some children who have had chronic nasal bleeding may tolerate a surprisingly low hematocrit. Younger children and infants tolerate blood loss less well than do older children; a blood transfusion may be required in severe cases.

CIRCUMSTANCES

One of the most useful observations the physician can make is whether other persons in the family have bleeding disorders or problems with epistaxis. Although episodes of epistaxis are relatively rare in the general population, they are common in patients with coagulation disorders. Beran and Petruson[3] studied habitual nose bleeders (primarily in adults) and found that 27% had bleeding disorders, such as factor V, VII, or X deficiencies. Kiley and colleagues[11] found a 30% incidence of such disorders in a similar group of children. Families with children who have chronic bleeding may have hereditary hemorrhagic telangiectasia syndrome (Osler-Weber-Rendu disease). This is an autosomal dominant disease associated with increased fragility of small blood vessels. McCaffrey and colleagues[12] reported that 70% of patients with this disease have a family history that is positive for epistaxis.

If a child has epistaxis associated with trauma, it is important to determine the type of injury that occurred. Blunt trauma with a heavy instrument to the nose may point to other facial fractures. A bicycle fall may suggest an "accordion" injury to the nose and a potential septal hematoma, which would require immediate incision and drainage. Recurrent trauma that results in epistaxis may suggest child abuse. It has been estimated that 30% of physically abused children have some form of facial trauma.[1]

DIFFERENTIAL DIAGNOSIS

The easiest way to conceptualize the many causes of epistaxis is to categorize them according to either local or systemic causes (see the box on p. 907). The local causes include trauma, surgery, infection, medications, or tumors. The systemic causes may be divided into bleeding disorders, other major diseases (e.g., leukemia, renal dysfunction, and hypertension), and cancer therapy (radiotherapy or chemotherapy).

Most nasal injuries in children occur at home or during sporting events. Bleeding occurs because of an abrasion of the nasal septum. Intranasal hematomas, abscesses, and lacerations can be overlooked unless the physician looks for them carefully. Failure to recognize an infection or a blood clot lodged in this area may result in pressure necrosis of the nasal septum and eventual external and internal nasal deformities.[15] Major facial fractures also can manifest in this way; thus a complete facial structure examination with roentgenograms should be performed when this diagnosis is considered.

Occasionally epistaxis may occur after surgery. Postoperative bleeding from the tonsils and adenoids can mimic epistaxis. Septal surgery, rhinoplasty, and turbinectomies also can lead to postoperative bleeding among adolescents. Whenever a child undergoes nasotracheal intubation, the nasal mucosa may be torn, which can lead to bleeding.

Chronic nasal irritation as a result of infection, allergies, or drugs can cause epistaxis. Local mucosal cellulitis and failure of the mucociliary lining of the nose to function properly after an infection may cause Little's area to become dry and cracked. Children with chronic rhinorrhea may rub their noses and frequently, thereby, irritate the septum significantly. Chronic irritation also can occur from overuse of topical antiallergic sprays (e.g., cromolyn sulfate and dexamethasone). Schwartz and colleagues[17] have reported that 27% of adolescents who routinely snorted cocaine complained of recurrent epistaxis. Cocaine causes local infection, chronic necrosis of the mucosa and septum, foreign body reactions, and destruction of nasal ciliary function.

Bloody rhinorrhea occurs in children as a result of a variety of nasal masses. Hemangiomas, which are among the most common benign tumors of the nose during childhood, can cause epistaxis. Juvenile angiofibromas should be considered in male adolescents who have unilateral spontaneous epistaxis and a nasopharyngeal mass. Neel and colleagues[14] have reported that 73% of boys with this diagnosis had epistaxis. Angiofibromas can be differentiated from benign choanoantral polyps by computed tomographic scanning with contrast medium. Blind biopsies of the nasopharynx should be avoided because of the risk of life-threatening epistaxis. The most common benign growths of the nose—antral choanal pol-

Causes of Epistaxis in Children

A. Local
1. Trauma: nose picking, surgery (septoplasty, turbinectomy), blunt impact (fist or instrument), foreign body, child abuse, sports, auto accident
2. Infection: viral, bacterial, fungal, parasitic
3. Chronic irritation: allergies, recurrent colds, dry environment, chronic sniffers, smoking, cocaine abuse, ciliary dysfunction, chemicals, caustic ingestion
4. Structural abnormality: deviated septum, vomer spur, septal perforation
5. Drugs: topical sprays (phenylephrine, aerosol steroids), drying agents (decongestants, antihistamines)
6. Neoplasms: polyps, hemangiomas, rhabdomyosarcomas, angiofibromas

B. Systemic
1. Bleeding diseases: von Willebrand, coagulation factor deficiencies, vitamin deficiencies, Osler-Weber-Rendu, idiopathic thrombocytopenia, disseminated intravascular coagulation
2. Infections: rheumatic fever, diphtheria, malaria, measles
3. Neoplasms: leukemia, lymphoma
4. Granulomas: Wegener, midline reticulosis, tuberculosis, sarcoidosis
5. Medications: antiinflammatories (aspirin, ibuprofen), anticoagulants (warfarin), steroids
6. Cancer treatment: chemotherapy (methotrexate), radiotherapy
7. Hormonal influences: menses, birth control pills, pregnancy
8. Cardiovascular disease: hypertension, arteriosclerosis
9. Barometric pressure changes: scuba diving, air flight, elevator rides
10. Miscellaneous: liver disease, renal dysfunction, aplastic anemia, sepsis

yps—and the most common malignant lesions—rhabdomyosarcomas—usually are not associated with epistaxis.[16]

Excessive nasal bleeding may be caused by a variety of acquired or inherited bleeding disorders. Aspirin can cause a relative platelet dysfunction that results in a prolonged bleeding time. Vitamin C and K deficiencies also can predispose a child to epistaxis because of blood vessel changes and coagulopathies, respectively. Thrombocytopenia can occur after the use of sulfasoxazole, chloroquine, carbamazepine, estrogens, and thiazide diuretics. Ingestion of toxic substances and the eating of certain foods such as beans can lead to thrombocytopenia. Viral illnesses may cause idiopathic thrombocytopenic purpura. The most common inherited bleeding disorders that cause epistaxis in children are von Willebrand disease and factor XI deficiency (hemophilia C). Less common disorders include factor VIII deficiency (hemophilia A) and factor IX deficiency (hemophilia B or Christmas disease).[13]

Severe epistaxis is a common feature of Osler-Weber-Rendu disease (hereditary hemorrhagic telangiectasia). Fewer than 9% of a series of patients from the Mayo Clinic with this disease had epistaxis. Usually the disease occurs with bleeding, skin telangiectasias, and a family history of this condition. McCaffrey and colleagues[12] reported that these symptoms can appear in childhood but usually do not begin until after the age of 15 years. Epistaxis is caused by defects in small mucosal vessel walls.

Epistaxis may occur in immunocompromised children. Leukemia and lymphomas that involve the bone marrow can lead to thrombocytopenia and concomitant bleeding. In addition, the chemotherapeutic agents, such as methotrexate and cyclophosphamide, used to treat these malignant diseases can cause thrombocytopenia. Radiotherapy often causes cracking, irritation in the nasal mucosa, and bleeding.

As noted, there are many causes of epistaxis. The age of the patient and the circumstances that surround the onset of bleeding are important clues to the diagnosis. In neonates the most common cause is birth trauma, especially if forceps are used. Frequently the bleeding is caused by deflection of the nasal septum, which can be gently manipulated back into position or left as is if there is no deformity. In childhood, simple nose picking or blunt trauma are the most common causes. In early adolescence, boys have a higher incidence of nasal tumors, such as angiofibromas, than do girls. Pubescent girls may have occasional bleeding during their menses.

MANAGEMENT

The basic approach to treatment of children with epistaxis should incorporate the "two C's"—calmness and compression. The patient should be reassured during the history taking and the assessment of his or her general condition and the amount of blood loss. Most bleeding can be stopped by sitting the child upright and gently squeezing the anterior nose for 5 minutes. Blood pressure and other vital signs should be taken. Blood tests and roentgenograms should be performed only if the bleeding cannot be stopped with simple pressure or anterior or posterior nasal packing. The first few minutes should be used to stem the bleeding while an appropriate assessment of its cause is made.

Once the initial bleeding is slowed, the nose should be more carefully examined with a nasal speculum and headlight. A simple solution of phenylephrine (¼%, ½%) can be sprayed into the nose for local vasoconstriction to control further bleeding and to help clear any clots that may have formed. A 1% epinephrine solution with or without lidocaine can be used for the same purposes if required. Nose blowing should be avoided even though the nose will feel quite congested. Bleeding sites in Little area can be cauterized electrically or with silver nitrate sticks. If either form of cautery is used, the septum should be covered with a petroleum jelly–based antibiotic ointment to provide a moist environment for optimum healing. Care should be taken to clean any excess silver nitrate from the anterior nares, because it will discolor the local skin and may frighten the child and family.

If these simple measures fail to control the bleeding, placement of bilateral anterior nasal packing by use of a ½-inch gauze covered with petroleum jelly should be the next step.

Although this is not a pleasant experience for the child, it is a highly effective way to stop anterior nasal bleeding. Bilateral packing is recommended to provide the greatest compression of the anterior septum. When packing is used, antibiotics should be given to prevent sinusitis. The packing usually is left in place for 3 days. Prepackaged surgical or Avitene-containing gauze can be used as additional hemostatic agents if bleeding persists. These agents may be the treatment of choice for patients in whom standard nasal packing might promote more bleeding by destroying the lining of the nose. This group of children includes those undergoing renal dialysis and those who are severely immunocompromised.

Recurrent anterior nasal bleeding or posterior bleeding can be controlled with placement of either posterior or nasopharyngeal balloons. Posterior packs are made from gauze pads inserted through the mouth into the nasopharynx and secured by ties through the nose. Whenever they are used, an anterior pack also is placed. Unfortunately, these standard packs may cause a drop in oxygenation and patient discomfort.[5] The balloon catheters are easier to position. Small Foley catheters can be used and filled with methylene blue–stained saline. The methylene blue indicates that the Foley balloon has burst accidently. Cook and colleagues[6] reported that the use of balloons decreased the average length of hospital stay from 12.5 to 5.6 days.

Severe bleeding that does not respond to packing should prompt one to consider a different diagnosis and perhaps employ more invasive therapeutic procedures. The use of tests for bleeding disorders, including determination of bleeding time, prothrombin time, partial thromboplastin time, and platelet count, as well as other hematologic studies, should be based on the family history. Roentgenographic studies should be reviewed for mass lesions, bone erosion, and other bony abnormalities. Angiographic examination of the internal and external carotid arteries should be considered.

Embolization with nonresorbable (usually plaster), spherical pellets can be used if a discrete bleeding source or a vascular tumor is discovered. Embolization is a useful procedure in hereditary hemorrhagic telangiectasia, juvenile angiofibromas, hemangiomas, vascular metastatic lesions, arteriovenous malformations, and traumatic arterial tears.[7]

Persistent posterior nasal bleeding from the sphenopalatine artery sometimes requires ligation of the internal maxillary artery.[13] This type of bleeding after trauma, which may be due to a tear of the anterior ethmoid artery, requires surgical ligation for control.

Although the goals of epistaxis management are to stop the bleeding and to determine its cause, the care of the patient often continues after the bleeding stops. Blood replacement or iron supplements may be required, and humidifying medications such as saline nasal sprays and petroleum jelly–based ointments often are needed to promote healing and subsequent adequate nasal mucociliary function. Children who have had severe epistaxis should be reexamined frequently to determine if further therapy is necessary. Recurrence of epistaxis can be prevented only if its many causes are considered and appropriate preventive measures are instituted.

REFERENCES

1. Becker DB, Needleman H, and Kotelchuck M: Child abuse: orofacial trauma and its recognition by dentists, J Am Dent Assoc 97:24, 1978.
2. Behrman RE and Vaughan VC III: Nelson's textbook of pediatrics, ed 12, 1983, WB Saunders Co.
3. Beran M and Petruson B: Changes in the nasal mucosa of habitual nose-bleeders, Acta Otolaryngol (Stockh) 102:308, 1986.
4. Beran M, Stigendal L, and Petruson B: Haemostatic disorders in habitual nose-bleeders, J Laryngol Otol 101:1020, 1987.
5. Cassisi NJ, Biller HF, and Ogura JH: Changes in arterial oxygen tension and pulmonary mechanics with the use of posterior packing in epistaxis: a preliminary report, Laryngoscope 81:1261, 1971.
6. Cook PR, Renner G, and Williams F: A comparison of nasal balloons and posterior gauze packs for posterior epistaxis, Ear Nose Throat J 64:79, 1985.
7. Davis KR: Embolization of epistaxis and juvenile nasopharyngeal angiofibromas, AJR 148:209, 1987.
8. Hutchison SMW and Finlayson NDC: Epistaxis as a cause of hematemesis and melena, J Clin Gastroenterol 9:283, 1987.
9. Juselius H: Epistaxis—a clinical study of 1,724 patients, J Laryngol Otol 88:317, 1974.
10. Katsanis E et al: Prevalence and significance of mild bleeding disorders in children with recurrent epistaxis, J Pediatr 113:73, 1988.
11. Kiley V, Stuart JJ, and Johnson CA: Coagulation studies in children with isolated recurrent epistaxis, J Pediatr 100:579, 1982.
12. McCaffrey TV, Kern EB, and Lake CF: Management of epistaxis in hereditary hemorrhagic telangiectasia, Arch Otolaryngol 103:627, 1977.
13. McDonald TJ and Pearson BW: Follow-up on maxillary artery ligation for epistaxis, Arch Otolaryngol 106:635, 1980.
14. Neel HB III et al: Juvenile angiofibroma: review of 120 cases, Am J Surg 126:547, 1973.
15. Olsen KD, Carpenter RJ, and Kern EB: Nasal septal injury in children, diagnosis and management, Arch Otolaryngol 106:317, 1980.
16. Schramm VL: Inflammatory and neoplastic masses of the nose and paranasal sinus in children, Laryngoscope 89:1887, 1979.
17. Schwartz RH et al: Nasal symptoms associated with cocaine abuse during adolescence, Arch Otolaryngol 115:63, 1989.

SUGGESTED READINGS

Guarisco JL and Graham HD III: Epistaxis in children: causes, diagnosis and treatment, Ear Nose Throat J 68:522, 1989.

McDonald TJ: Nosebleed in children: background and techniques to stop the flow, Postgrad Med 81:217, 1987.

128

Extremity Pain

Michael G. Burke

Extremity pain is a frequently encountered complaint in primary care pediatric practice. Up to 15% of school-aged children report a history of occasional limb pain,[2] and 4.5% have reported interruption of activities of greater than 3 months' duration because of limb pain.[4] Seven percent of office visits to pediatricians are for pain in an extremity.[3] Fortunately, most of these visits are generated by self-limited pain as a result of mild trauma. Occasionally, however, limb pain is the presenting complaint of systemic illness, neoplasm, an infectious process, a nutritional derangement, or a significant orthopedic disease. The challenge for the practitioner is to determine when the pain is significant, without exposing the child either to excessive diagnostic studies or to delay in treatment or referral. Most of this determination is based on the history and physical examination.

HISTORY

The description of the extremity pain by both patient and parents may help in determining its cause. The location of the pain, although usually helpful, may be deceiving inasmuch as pain referred from one part of an extremity to another is common in children. It is important to ask about areas above and below the stated location of the pain. Mode of onset, variability, duration, and frequency of the pain help in determining its cause. Many patients have a clear idea of what makes their pain better or worse, and these strategies may strike a familiar chord for the practitioner. In trauma a report of an audible "pop" or "snap" increases the likelihood of a sprain or fracture. A history of stiffness without trauma should elicit concern about a rheumatic process, whereas a history of trauma, although it provides an explanation, may be deceptive, for example, in the case of a pathologic fracture. As always, if the physical findings of trauma are greater than would be expected from the history, physical abuse must be considered.

The general health history of the child, which can be helpful, usually is more available to the primary pediatrician than to the consultant. Age is important; for example, it might help differentiate toxic synovitis of the hip in a child younger than 10 years of age from a slipped capital femoral epiphysis in an adolescent. As a screen for systemic disease a review of systems (including general health, weight loss, fevers, sweats, rashes, and diarrhea) should be obtained. History of recent medications is important and might reveal a serum sickness–like illness. Even a short course of systemic steroids can predispose a person to aseptic necrosis of the hip or can result in demineralization of bone and the pain associated with osteoporosis. Immunizations, particularly for rubella, may cause joint or extremity pain, and a history of exposure to viral illness might explain myalgia or arthralgia. The prodrome of hepatitis B also can cause significant arthralgia.

The patient's family history may reveal a tendency toward autoimmune disease or recent exposure to infectious diseases. Family history is particularly helpful in identifying hemoglobinopathies. A family history of sickle cell anemia in a 6- to 24-month-old child with painfully swollen hands and feet may lead to the diagnosis of hand-foot syndrome and heretofore undiagnosed sickle cell disease. A sickle cell crisis must always be considered in a child with a painful extremity who is of black or Mediterranean heritage.

Occasionally extremity pain is a symptom of a functional disorder and can serve as an entry to the physician's office for the child or parent with a hidden agenda. The history may be either quite dramatic or highly understated. Pain in a nonanatomic distribution or that disturbs unpleasant but not pleasant activities (waxing on school days and waning on weekends) should raise suspicion of a functional disorder.

Joint pain, especially without a history of trauma, is of more concern than is generalized limb pain. Rheumatologic diseases, including acute rheumatic fever, come to mind. Polyarthritis and arthralgia are major and minor Jones criteria for this diagnosis. Poststreptococcal arthralgia without acute rheumatic fever also has been described. In addition, joint pain can be a manifestation of inflammatory bowel disease; thus, eliciting a careful gastrointestinal history may be helpful.

PHYSICAL EXAMINATION

It is worthwhile to do a brief general physical examination, even if the history points to extremity pain from minor local trauma. Fever, pallor, lymphadenopathy, or organomegaly may be clues to systemic disease, and a rash may indicate a specific exanthematous disease. Dermatomyositis occurs with muscle pain and proximal weakness associated with a vasculitic rash on the extensor surfaces of knuckles, knees, and elbows. Palpable purpura and extremity pain are associated with Schönlein-Henoch purpura.

A complete physical examination can reveal generalized joint laxity, differentiating benign hypermobility syndrome from a focal ligament injury. In benign hypermobility syndrome, joint pain may result from chronic hyperextension of a joint. This is particularly common in gymnasts and dancers. Pain is relieved by exercise aimed at tightening the joints.

Because referred pain is common in children, the physical

examination should include areas proximal and distal to the site of the complaint. Slipped capital femoral epiphysis and Legg-Calvé-Perthes disease—both of which affect the hip—can manifest as knee pain, whereas an abscess of the psoas muscle occurs with hip pain. Further, some abdominal processes and diskitis may manifest as extremity pain.

Examination of a painful extremity should include assessment of peripheral vascular status, muscle strength, and skeletal and joint integrity. Assessment of peripheral vascular status is accomplished by palpating the pulses and determining capillary refill time distal to the pain. Skin color and warmth, pain to palpation, muscle strength, and extent of passive and active range of motion should be ascertained. Point tenderness over a bone raises suspicion of a fracture. Point tenderness in the absence of a clear history of trauma may indicate osteomyelitis. It is helpful to compare the opposite limb in the assessment of swelling, muscle wasting, or joint mobility. Observation of the gait or use of the painful limb when the patient is unaware helps in diagnosing a functional process. In evaluating strength, one should remember that isolated distal weakness is likely to be of neurologic origin, whereas proximal weakness most likely is due to a muscular disease.

LABORATORY AND X-RAY EVALUATION

For most extremity pain, laboratory studies are unnecessary. If, however, the history and physical examination do not lead to a definitive diagnosis, if they raise suspicion of a systemic or an infectious disease, or if the pain persists longer than anticipated, then screening laboratory tests are in order. A basic evaluation should include a complete blood count, a sedimentation rate, and a sickle cell preparation or hemoglobin electrophoresis. Rheumatologic studies should be added if the aforementioned diseases are suspected or if the pain becomes chronic. An elevated sedimentation rate raises suspicions of an infectious, an inflammatory, or occasionally a neoplastic disorder. A complete blood count is useful as a screen for anemia and infectious disease. With leukemia the white blood count is variable, but immature forms may be present in the differential white blood cell count.

Radiologic studies often are unnecessary in evaluating limb pain. The tendency to obtain numerous x-ray views is reinforced, however, because traumatic injury that would ordinarily illicit only a sprain in an adult is more likely to cause a greenstick or buckle fracture in a child. Rivara et al.[5] have proposed criteria for obtaining roentgenograms in extremity pain after trauma. By retrospectively analyzing 189 children with 209 extremity injuries, they concluded that the presence of point tenderness and/or gross deformity in an upper extremity injury identified 81% of children with fractures. Their absence predicted 82% without fractures. For lower extremity injuries, the presence of a gross deformity and/or pain on motion of the leg identified 97% of fractures. Absence of both indicators correctly ruled out a fracture in 97% of cases. The work of Rivara and colleagues speaks for reducing the number of x-ray studies obtained in the evaluation of extremity pain. Posttraumatic pain that fails to resolve as expected, however, should be evaluated radiographically, whether or not those criteria are met.

When there is not a clear history of trauma, roentgenograms help in identifying bony tumors, pathologic fractures, some metabolic defects, and a number of orthopedic conditions. Timing of the roentgenograms will depend on the pediatrician's level of concern, as established by the history and physical examination.

A bone scan is a useful diagnostic tool in evaluating limb pain. One should be obtained when a stress fracture or osteomyelitis is suspected. Bone scans are more sensitive than are plain radiographs for establishing diagnoses.

DIFFERENTIAL DIAGNOSIS

The differential diagnosis of extremity pain is extremely broad (see the box on p. 911). However, most limb pain is benign, requires no intervention, and is self-limited. Characteristic patterns of pain and associated signs and symptoms signal the presence of certain diseases and conditions. A discussion of some of these disorders follows.

Growing Pains

"Growing pains" constitute a time-honored pediatric disorder. They usually are described as intermittent, deep extremity pains that affect the lower more often than the upper extremities. The pain nearly always is bilateral, rarely involves the joints, and is almost universally worse at night, with complete resolution in the morning. Despite their name, growing pains do not occur most frequently during periods of rapid growth. Instead, their onset usually is described at 3 to 5 years or 8 to 12 years of age. Although they usually resolve in 12 to 24 months, they may persist into adolescence.

The etiology of growing pains remains unclear. The previous emphasis on a psychological cause recently has given way to an emphasis on an overuse type of injury. Apparent worsening of the pain during times of increased activity and relief by use of heat and massage seem to support a physical cause. Headache and abdominal pain, however—often associated with emotional illnesses—have also accompanied growing pains.

The diagnosis of growing pains is significant for its lack of associated physical signs. Thus any abnormal finding on physical examination should provoke a search for another cause. Similarly, results of screening laboratory tests and roentgenograms should prove normal. Treatment involves heat, massage, and analgesics.

Sprains

A sprain is a physical disruption of a ligament, a less common occurrence in children than in adults. A child's open epiphyseal plate or plastic bony cortex may give way under tension before a ligament tears. Therefore Salter fractures and buckle fractures should be considered when the history indicates the pressure of a sprain and physical examination reveals tenderness on palpation or pain on stretching the ligament. In addition, joint stability should be assessed. Sprains can be graded according to the degree of associated ligament disruption. A mild, microscopic tear that results in no laxity of the involved joint is a grade I sprain. Grade II sprains involve

Extremity Pain in Childhood: A Differential Diagnosis

CONGENITAL ORIGIN

Caffey disease
Mucopolysaccharidosis
Mucolipidosis
Sickle cell anemia
Hemophilia

ALLERGY/COLLAGEN VASCULAR ORIGIN

Schönlein-Henoch purpura
Serum sickness
Juvenile rheumatoid arthritis
Systemic lupus erythematosus
Dermatomyositis
Mixed connective tissue disease
Polyarteritis nodosa
Familial Mediterranean fever
Rheumatic fever
Inflammatory bowel disease
Scleroderma

NEOPLASTIC ORIGIN

Leukemia
Lymphoma
Neuroblastoma
Histiocytosis X
Tumors of bone
- Osteoid osteoma (benign)
- Osteoblastoma (benign)
- Osteogenic sarcoma
- Ewing sarcoma
- Chondrosarcoma

Tumors of soft tissue
- Rhabdomyosarcoma
- Fibrosarcoma
- Synovial cell sarcoma

Tumors of the spinal cord

NUTRITIONAL ORIGIN

Rickets (vitamins D)
Scurvy (vitamin C)
Hypervitaminosis A
Hypercholesterolemia
Gout
Osteoporosis

TRAUMA/OVERUSE

Myohematoma
Myositis ossificans
Hypermobility syndrome
Compartment syndrome
Shin splint
Fracture
Stress fracture
Sprain
Subluxed radial head
Physical abuse

ORTHOPEDIC ORIGIN

Chondromalacia patellae
Osteochondritis dissecans
Osgood-Schlatter disease
Slipped capital femoral epiphysis
Legg-Calvé-Perthes disease
Köhler disease
Sever disease
Freiberg disease
Pathologic fracture
Osteogenesis imperfecta

INFECTIOUS ORIGIN

Bacterial
- Osteomyelitis
- Diskitis
- Septic arthritis
- Pyogenic myositis
- Arthralgia/myalgia associated with streptococcal infection

Viral
- Myositis
- Myalgia/arthralgia
- Toxic synovitis

Tuberculosis
Lyme disease
Syphilis: periostitis
Trichinosis

PSYCHOSOCIAL ORIGIN

School phobia
Reflex neurovascular dystrophy
Hysteria/conversion reactions
Behavior disorders

IDIOPATHIC ORIGIN

Fibromyalgia
Growing pains
Sarcoidosis

ENDOCRINE ORIGIN

Hypothyroidism
Hyperparathyroidism
Hypercortisolism

Modified from Bowyer SL and Hollister JR: Limb pain in childhood, Pediatr Clin North Am 31:5, 1984.

macroscopic, but incomplete, ligament tears. There is increased laxity of the joint but less than a 5-mm movement differential between the strained and the contralateral joint. Grade III sprains result in greater than 5 mm of increased mobility of the affected joint compared with the contralateral one. Grade I sprains can be treated by the primary practitioner by icing and wrapping the involved joint to minimize swelling. Early range of motion exercises should be encouraged, and a gradual return to activity is allowed. Return of pain indicates too rapid a return to a given level of activity. Grades II and III sprains generally should be referred to an orthopedist for immobilization and consideration of surgical repair of torn ligaments.

Overuse Syndromes

Overuse injuries have become more common as physical fitness has become popular nationally. Localized, gradually increasing, persistent extremity pain that worsens with weight bearing, exercise, and activity but that decreases with rest can indicate a stress fracture. *Stress fractures* are rare in children younger than 12 years of age. They most commonly affect the second metatarsal, the proximal tibia, or the fibula. Although roentgenograms may show normal findings, a bone scan can help establish the diagnosis. Treatment consists mostly of rest and treatment with nonsteroidal antiinflammatory agents. Casting or splinting occasionally is necessary.

Little League elbow is an overuse injury caused by the repetitive motion of pitching a baseball; this motion compresses the radial aspect of the elbow and stretches the ulnar aspect. The result is painful inflammation of the epicondyles. Diminished range of joint motion also may occur. Fragments of bone splintered into the joint may cause the joint to "catch" or "lock." Treatment consists of resting the arm by avoiding the repetitive movement. A change in pitching technique may diminish recurrences. Some Little Leagues limit the number of innings that a youngster may pitch in one game to avoid this problem.

Shin splints also are caused by overuse syndrome. The term originally referred to pain along the posteromedial aspect of the tibia as a result of irritation at the origin of the posterior tibial muscle. *Shin splints* now refer to any of a series of painful overuse syndromes of the lower portion of the leg, including irritation of the posterior or anterior tibial muscle, inflammation of the interosseous membrane located between the tibia and fibula, and both anterior and posterior compartment syndromes. All can cause pain in the lower extremities. The condition, which is exacerbated by running and jumping, occurs most commonly at the beginning of a training season. Although the pain initially occurs after activity, it may occur during or before activity as the syndrome progresses. On examination there may be tenderness over the posteromedial aspect of the tibia, at the site of origin of the posterior tibia, or over the anterior tibia. Treatment involves rest, ice application, and antiinflammatory drugs. For runners, training on a softer surface or with better-quality running shoes may be helpful.

Subluxation of the Radial Head

Nursemaids' elbow is a common injury in toddlers. The injury usually follows sudden, forceful traction of the hand or forearm. The traction briefly pulls the immature radial head from the cuff formed by the annular ligament. Release of the force allows the radius to trap the ligament against the capitellum. The patient who can talk usually indicates that the pain is in the elbow or, occasionally, the wrist. More frequently, the child refuses to use the extremity and holds the arm with the elbow flexed, the forearm close to the chest, and the hand in pronation. The diagnosis usually is made by history alone. Although roentgenograms are not helpful, occasionally they are obtained to rule out a fracture if the history is unclear or if attempts to reduce the subluxation are unsuccessful. The practitioner usually can reduce the subluxation by using one hand to supinate the patient's forearm quickly while simultaneously exerting traction on the forearm and using the thumb of the other hand to create pressure over the patient's radial head. This latter maneuver is accomplished simultaneously with pronation of the patient's forearm; it is completed by placing the elbow through full extension and flexion while maintaining pressure over the radial head. Return of normal use of the extremity usually occurs within 30 minutes. The rapid recovery is dramatic and rewarding to the parents and the physician. Failure of prompt return to normal may occur when the subluxation has been present for some time because of swelling of the ligament. In such instances the affected arm should be placed in a simple sling and positioned across the upper portion of the abdomen for 12 to 24 hours. Referral to an orthopedist rarely is required.

Slipped Capital Femoral Epiphysis

Slipped capital femoral epiphysis is caused by a sudden or gradual dislocation of the head of the femur from its neck and shaft at the level of the upper epiphyseal plate. Characteristic pain is in the affected hip and/or the medial aspect of the ipsilateral knee. The displacement may be sudden, in which case the pain usually is severe and associated with inability to bear weight. Gradual displacement is associated with slowly increasing, dull pain. This condition typically affects sedentary, obese male adolescents. The physical examination may reveal diminished abduction and internal rotation of the hip. The diagnosis is made radiographically. Management involves surgical placement of a pin through the femoral head and the epiphysis to prevent futher slippage. Avascular necrosis of the femoral head is a frequent complication, even with rapid recognition and treatment.

Toxic Synovitis

Toxic synovitis, a self-limited inflammation of the hip joint, commonly occurs in children younger than 2 years of age. The cause is unknown, but inasmuch as it often occurs within 2 weeks after an upper respiratory infection, a viral inflammatory process is suspected. It usually occurs in a toddler who refuses to walk because of apparent pain in the hip. The hip is held in flexion, abduction, and external rotation. Findings may include slight elevation in the white blood cell count and the sedimentation rate—a frustrating occurrence for the practitioner who hopes to rule out septic arthritis, a concern that may lead to consultation with an orthopedist. Treatment consists of bed rest, usually for fewer than 4 days. Avascular necrosis of the femoral head may rarely be a late complication.

Osteochondrosis

Osteochondrosis includes a group of disorders in which degeneration or aseptic necrosis of bone and overlying cartilage occurs at an ossification center and is followed by recalcification. The disorders vary in name and presentation according to their locations.

Legg-Calvé-Perthes disease, or osteochondrosis of the femoral head, results from compromise to the tenuous vascular supply to the area. The condition may be idiopathic, or it can result from a slipped capital femoral epiphysis, trauma, steroid use, sickle cell crisis, or congenital dislocation of the hip. Toxic synovitis also is associated with subsequent Legg-Calvé-Perthes disease, but again this is rare. After compromise of the vascular supply, the bone underlying the articular surface of the head of the femur becomes necrotic. Collapse of the necrotic bone flattens the femoral head and causes a poor fit with the acetabulum even after new bone is formed. The pain associated with Legg-Calvé-Perthes disease, which results from necrosis of the involved bone, frequently is referred to the medial aspect of the ipsilateral knee. A limp may be the presenting complaint. Frequently an early diagnosis eludes the practitioner because roentgenographic findings may be normal or show only swelling of the joint's capsule. A bone scan may demonstrate decreased blood flow to the femoral head compared with the contralateral hip. Later, x-ray studies may show areas of bone resorption, irregular widening of the epiphysis, or dense new bone formation. The goal of therapy is to prevent flattening of the femoral head by allowing it to undergo new bone formation. This is accomplished by keeping the hip abducted so that the head of the femur is held well inside the rounded portion of the acetabulum. Either bracing or an osteotomy may accomplish the goal. Both require referral to an orthopedic surgeon.

Two similar processes affect the knee joint. With *osteochondritis dissecans,* bone and cartilage degenerate at the articular surface of the knee and particularly involve the lateral aspect of the medial condyle of the femur. Knee pain and crepitus, caused by loose bone and cartilage fragments in the joint, can result.

Chondromalacia patellae occurs because of a painful softening or breakdown of the inner surface of the patella. The pain is localized to the knee and increases with activities that require prolonged knee bending and even with prolonged sitting. The pain is described as grinding. It sometimes can be elicited by applying pressure over the patella. Crepitus sometimes can be felt by moving the patella from side to side over the knee joint. Treatment usually is limited to pain relief and reassurance that in time the condition will resolve. Exercise to strengthen the medial quadriceps muscles may promote better alignment of the patella with the knee and thereby diminish the pain. In severe cases, surgical realignment of the patella may be required.

Osteochondrosis of the growth plate of the calcaneus, *Sever disease,* can produce heel pain that worsens with activity. This usually mild process requires only padding of the heel for relief of pain. Avascular necrosis and osteochondrosis of the tarsal navicular *(Köhler disease)* and of the head of the second metatarsal *(Freiberg disease)* can cause foot pain. Treatment usually requires only pain medication and rest.

Osgood-Schlatter disease is a painful degeneration of the tibial tubercle at the site of insertion of the quadriceps ligament. It is characterized by painful swelling of the anterior aspect of the tibial tubercle. Usually it occurs during adolescence. The degree of swelling may be alarming, and the area is tender to palpation. Pain is exacerbated by activity that involves increased use of the quadriceps muscles. The process is self-limited and resolves toward the end of adolescence when the epiphysis at the insertion site closes and the bone becomes stronger than the inserted ligament. Until resolution the condition is treated with rest and analgesics. Rarely, casting or surgical attachment of the quadriceps ligament is required.

Osteomyelitis

Osteomyelitis is a local infection of bone, usually involving one of the long bones, with its greatest incidence in children 3 to 12 years of age. Although infection often occurs by hematogenous seeding, it can be caused by direct entry after local trauma. In both children and adults the most commonly isolated organism is *Staphylococcus aureus*. However, *Haemophilus influenzae* type b, *Salmonella* species, and group A streptococci can all infect the bone. Group B streptococcus is more likely the cause of infection in newborns. Although osteomyelitis caused by *Salmonella* organisms tends to occur more frequently in children with sickle cell anemia than in other children, *S. aureus* is the most common etiologic agent even in this group. In trauma from a puncture wound to the foot, *Pseudomonas aeruginosa* must be considered. In addition, tuberculous osteomyelitis, which has become less common in recent years, still occurs.

Osteomyelitis can manifest as extremity pain alone or extremity pain with signs of a systemic infectious disease (fever, irritability, septic appearance). In the absence of systemic signs it often is difficult to distinguish between osteomyelitis and a traumatic cause of the pain. It may take 2 weeks or longer for roentgenographic evidence of osteomyelitis to develop. A bone scan usually—but not always—is a diagnostic aid. Decreased perfusion because of the pressure generated by the exudative process may result in false-negative findings. In addition, the white blood cell count and sedimentation rate often are elevated. Treatment success can be monitored by following the sedimentation rate serially.

Management involves collection of culture specimens from the blood, the overlying cellulitis, and the bone itself to determine the causative organism, followed by initiation of antibiotic therapy for as long as 6 weeks. Placement of a tuberculin skin test is still recommended, especially in high-risk groups (see Chapter 18, Four).

Neoplasms

A neoplasm rarely is the cause of limb pain; however, the possibility of its presence is a frequent concern in cases of severe limb pain inasmuch as pain is a symptom in benign and malignant bone tumors and systemic malignancies.

Osteoid osteoma is a benign bone tumor that occurs most frequently in adolescents. It usually involves the femur or tibia in a unilateral occurrence. Pain is the presenting complaint, initially dull pain that increases in intensity to become deep and "boring." The pain is more intense at night and at times with weight bearing. X-ray findings of sclerotic bone around a lucent center are diagnostic of this condition; sometimes tomograms are required for confirmation. Surgical excision is curative.

Systemic neoplasms in which extremity pain occurs include leukemia and metastatic neuroblastoma. One third of children with acute lymphatic leukemia have bone pain at the time of diagnosis, and in one fourth, joint or bone pain is a significant presenting complaint.[1] Unrelenting, increasing pain that worsens at night or with rest and that is not relieved by analgesics, heat, or massage may indicate the presence of a metastatic bone tumor. Systemic signs of weight loss, pallor, lymphadenopathy, hepatosplenomegaly, or fever may accompany the pain. In leukemia, examination of the extremity may reveal strikingly little to account for the degree of pain. Radiographic studies of the extremities may show lucent "leukemic lines" in the subepiphyseal area.

Primary malignant tumors of bone may cause severe unilateral pain, with swelling and tenderness at the site. This consideration supports the use of radiographic studies when unilateral limb pain is not adequately explained by a history of trauma and when pain from trauma does not resolve as expected. The peak incidence of both osteogenic sarcoma and the less common Ewing sarcoma occurs in late childhood and during adolescence. The roentgenogram in osteogenic sarcoma may reveal a tumor in the metaphysis with the presence of both radiolucent and radiopaque areas. The characteristic "sunburst" results from extension of calcification into the overlying soft tissue. Although periosteal elevation may be present, it is not diagnostic of the disease.

REFERENCES

1. Leventhal BG. In Behrman RE and Vaughan VC, editors: Nelson textbook of pediatrics, ed 13, Philadelphia, 1987, WB Saunders Co.
2. Naish JM and Apley J: "Growing pains": a critical study of non-arthritic limb pains in children, Arch Dis Child 26:134, 1951.
3. National Center for Health Statistics: Viral and health statistics: patient's reasons for visiting physicians—National Ambulatory Medical Care Survey, U.S., 1977-1978, DHHS Pub No Pt82-1717, Hyattsville, Md, 1981.
4. Oster J and Nielsen A: Growing pains: a clinical investigation of a school population, Acta Paediatr Scand 61:329, 1972.
5. Rivara FP, Parish RA, and Mueller BA: Extremity injuries in children: predictive value of clinical findings, Pediatrics 78:803, 1986.

SUGGESTED READINGS

Landry GL: Why does stretching work for growing pain? Contemp Pediatr, 6(9):9, 1989 (letter).

Szer IS: Are those limb pains "growing" pains? Contemp Pediatr, 6(3):143, 1989.

Tunnessen WW Jr: Signs and symptoms in pediatrics, ed 2, Philadelphia, 1988, JB Lippincott Co.

129

Facial Dysmorphism

Marvin Elliott Miller

The face is the region of the body that reveals our identity to others. Although each person has two eyes, two ears, a nose, a mouth, a chin, and a head, it is the subtle uniqueness of these features in their form and in their relationship to each other that marks each of us as a distinct and identifiable individual. Only monozygotic twins can have apparently identical faces, and even among them facial differences that readily distinguish one from the other often exist.

The face can appear dysmorphic or unusual if any of the facial parts is abnormal in form or function or if a spatial relationship between or among these parts is abnormal.

Physicians and other health care personnel should be sensitive in the use of terminology to describe an individual with a dysmorphic face. The terms "funny looking kid," "FLK," or "funny looking face" add little to the understanding of the situation and may arouse justified parental indignation. In discussing dysmorphic features with parents or describing them in written or verbal communication with colleagues, the physician should be objective in a report that results in an evaluation that is meaningful in establishing a diagnosis and that avoids an insensitive and derogatory approach to the patient.

The dysmorphic face may be quite appropriate in relation to the family's physiognomy, or it may indicate a particular syndrome. Thus it is not surprising to find epicanthal folds and a flat nasal bridge in an Oriental child; if found in a white child, however, the physician should be suspicious of Down syndrome and look for other features that suggest this diagnosis. The child with a large head who has a parent with a large head does not prompt as much concern as the child with a large head whose parents have normal-sized heads. Thus it is critical to evaluate dysmorphic facial features in light of the genetic background of the child.

If the child or baby looks like one of the parents, or if there is a strong resemblance to the baby pictures of one of the parents, then it becomes apparent that the features are familial. It is possible that an autosomal dominant condition, such as Waardenburg syndrome, could explain dysmorphism and parental similarity. If, however, there is no parental or familial resemblance, especially if there are other problems in development or growth or other body symptoms, the physician should consider further evaluation of the individual.

MECHANISMS OF DYSMORPHOGENESIS

There are four general causes of facial dysmorphogenesis: deformation, disruption, primary malformation of the face, and central nervous system malformations that cause secondary facial dysmorphism (anatomic, neuromuscular dysfunction).

Deformations

Deformations are structural abnormalities of newborns, involving the musculoskeletal system, that arise from intrauterine constraint.[1] Any situation that compromises the intrauterine space can cause a deformation; examples of such situations are primigravida pregnancy, nonvertex presentation, multiple births, small mother, large baby, oligohydramnios, and structural uterine abnormality. Deformations are common and occur in 2% of all newborns. Common facial deformations include plagiocephaly (asymmetry of the head); asymmetry of the mandible, nose, ears, or chin; and micrognathia. The natural history of facial deformation is almost always benign, with restoration of the affected tissue to the normal form and function within weeks after birth.

Disruptions

A disruption is the breakdown of previously normal fetal tissue.[2] The most common example is amniotic bands, which are estimated to occur in 1 in 2000 pregnancies. Although they were originally thought primarily to affect limbs, it is now clear that bands can attach to any part of the craniofacial region, causing a vast spectrum of structural defects of varying severity. This diagnosis should be considered in any newborn with bizarre external craniofacial features. Evaluation of the placenta can be helpful in confirming this diagnosis if strands of amnion can be demonstrated or if they are found attached to the affected tissues.

Malformations

Facial. A malformation is a structural defect resulting from an intrinsic abnormality in the cells of the affected tissue.[2] There are a number of potential causes of malformations, including genetic disorders (chromosomes and single genes), drugs, intrauterine infections, metabolic derangements, and hyperthermia. Malformations can involve almost any facial part; examples of these are given in Table 129-1.

Central Nervous System. Malformations of the brain can cause facial dysmorphogenesis in two ways. First, the facial anatomy is, in part, directed by the growth of the forebrain. Any situation that grossly alters the normal development of the brain can alter facial development anatomically. An example of this is holoprosencephaly. When there

Table 129-1 *Examples of Causes of Facial Malformation*

CAUSE	EXAMPLE	FACIAL DYSMORPHISM
Genetic		
Chromosomal	Cri-du-chat syndrome (5p−)	Micrognathia, ocular hypertelorism
Autosomal dominant	Treacher Collins syndrome	Dysplastic ears, maxillary hypoplasia
Autosomal recessive	Hurler syndrome	Corneal clouding, coarse facies
Intrauterine infection	Congenital rubella	Cataracts
Drug induced	Fetal alcohol syndrome	Smooth philtrum, small eyes
Metabolic	Congenital hypothyroidism	Coarse facies; large, protruding tongue

Approach to the Individual with Facial Dysmorphism

1. Describe dysmorphic facial features.
2. Describe any other dysmorphic somatic features.
3. Define growth of the individual in weight, length, and head circumference.
4. Define development of the individual.
5. Review gestational and perinatal history.
6. Review family history.
7. Consider laboratory tests.
8. Determine if the features fit a recognizable syndrome.
9. Communicate findings to the family.

is failure of forebrain septation into the right and left ventricles, secondary midfacial abnormalities may occur. Another example is the upward slanting palpebral fissures in Down syndrome, which is probably secondary to forebrain underdevelopment.

Second, neuromuscular dysfunction of the face resulting from a primary malformation of the brain can cause facial dysmorphism. Whenever there is a primary central nervous system (CNS) malformation, the neuromuscular control of a number of facial functions can be abnormal. These abnormal situations include ptosis, nystagmus, strabismus, and lop ears. Prominent lateral palatal ridges are a sign of intrauterine CNS dysfunction that results from a deficit of tongue thrust into the palate.

APPROACH TO THE INDIVIDUAL WITH FACIAL DYSMORPHISM

The approach to the baby or child with a dysmorphic face is summarized in the accompanying box and is aimed at establishing an etiologic diagnosis.

1. *Describe dysmorphic facial features*. The first task is to describe in objective terms why the face appears unusual. Rather than stating that the distance between the eyes appears increased or the ears appear small, the physician should measure these parameters and compare them with known standards.[2]

2. *Describe other dysmorphic somatic features*. A thorough physical examination should be performed to determine if there are associated somatic abnormalities. Hearing and vision should be evaluated, and fundoscopic examination should be performed. The cranial sutures should be palpated to evaluate for possible craniostenosis, which can cause facial dysmorphism.

3. *Define growth of the individual* in weight, length, and head circumference. Data should be obtained and "plotted" to assess how the individual is growing in these parameters. The growth curves should be interpreted in light of the parental growth curves. Growth excess or, more frequently, growth deficiency can be seen as a part of malformation syndromes in which there is facial dysmorphism; for example, individuals with cerebral gigantism (Sotos syndrome), who have very characteristic facies, are macrocephalic, and are very tall in childhood. Individuals with any of the three common autosomal trisomies (trisomy 13, 18, or 21) all show postnatal growth deficiency.

4. *Define development of the individual*. From the patient's history and the physician's examination and testing, an assessment of development should be made. It is important to know of any developmental delay because it may indicate CNS dysfunction. However, psychosocial deprivation and chronic otitis media, two correctable situations, can cause developmental delay.

5. *Review gestational and perinatal history*. The gestational history should be reviewed for maternal drug exposure, viral illness, fever, and alcohol consumption. Positive findings may suggest an environmental cause of a malformation problem. The history also should include factors that might predispose to deformational problems, such as breech delivery, oligohydramnios, multiple births, or maternal structural uterine anomaly.

6. *Review family history*. The importance of taking a good family history has already been mentioned; this information may suggest a genetic basis for the condition.[3] Some autosomal recessive disorders are found almost exclusively in certain ethnic groups. Ellis–van Creveld syndrome, a rare ectodermal dysplasia, has a high frequency in the Amish population. The offspring of parents who are related to each other, particularly if they are first-degree relatives (i.e., father-daughter, mother-son, brother-sister), are at greater risk for having autosomal recessive disorders. Incestuous matings are probably more common than thought and the couple is at relatively high risk for dysmorphic offspring. An incestuous mating should be considered in any dysmorphic newborn of

a very young mother and no reputed father. A dysmorphic individual born to an older mother may suggest an autosomal trisomy and when born to an older father may suggest an autosomal dominant disorder caused by a fresh mutation.

7. *Consider laboratory tests.* If the dysmorphic features and history suggest a primary CNS problem, then brain imaging should be considered. If multiple systems are involved, chromosomes should be analyzed. Other laboratory tests and imaging studies of other organ systems should be performed when warranted. Magnetic resonance imaging (MRI), computed axial tomography (CT) scanning, and ultrasonography are extremely valuable imaging techniques, which can be selectively used after consultation with a radiologist to evaluate internal structures.

8. *Determine if the features fit a known condition or syndrome after all the information has been gathered.**

9. *Communicate findings to the family.*

**Smith's Recognizable Patterns of Human Malformation*[2] is the most valuable resource to use in this effort. It also is helpful in determining if a particular condition has a genetic basis.

SUMMARY

The physician who is confronted with a patient with dysmorphic facial features must decide whether the patient or family will benefit from a thorough evaluation or referral. The most important task initially is to determine whether the features are consistent with the genetic background of the individual or whether they represent an abnormal phenotype. Through the systematic gathering of information, the physician should attempt to establish an etiologic diagnosis and then convey the implications to the appropriate family members.

REFERENCES

1. Graham JM: Smith's recognizable patterns of human malformation, ed 4, Philadelphia, 1988, WB Saunders Co.
2. Jones KL: Smith's recognizable patterns of human malformation, ed 4, Philadelphia, 1988, WB Saunders Co.
3. McKusick VA: Mendelian inheritance in man, ed 8, Baltimore, 1988, Johns Hopkins University Press.

130

Fatigue and Weakness

Arnold T. Sigler

The signs and symptoms of fatigue and weakness are among the most commonly encountered by practicing pediatricians; yet they are impossible to find indexed or discussed in most current pediatric textbooks. These terms are confused and misused by physicians as well as by patients. Adolescents and children often use other terms to describe their perceptions of somatic weakness or fatigue. Furthermore, pediatric texts have failed to stress that specific complaints, rather than diseases, are what bring most patients to their physicians. Fatigue, in fact, is very different from true body weakness. Therefore it is important to define the terms *weakness* and *fatigue* carefully, even though each definition requires modification to be appropriate for each age-group.

Weakness refers to a decrease in strength of either a part of the body or of the whole body. The definition of true weakness can be fulfilled only by demonstration of abnormal neurologic or muscular functions, by means of history, physical examination, or laboratory techniques. Practically speaking, a history of weakness, on further questioning, will reveal hypotonia in infants and, in older children, trouble running or keeping up in gym class, clumsiness, or lack of agility (see Chapters 121, 145, and 188).

Fatigue may be a normal result of bodily or mental overwork—a feeling of weariness or lassitude, with increasing discomfort and decreasing efficiency for which there may be a biochemical basis. The temporary fatigue of long-distance running, cramming for examinations, or food or sleep deprivation are examples of normal fatigue. In these instances, the amount of fatigue, even when prolonged, will usually be appropriate for the amount of physical or mental exertion.

On the other hand, fatigue may be a pathologic state. The lassitude associated with somatic illness, often with definable physical or laboratory abnormalities, is well known. In contrast, fatigue also may be described as an emotional condition characterized by a state of weariness, boredom, lassitude, and lack of energy and initiative, resulting in the absence of a sense of well-being.

Parents who report that their infant is weak or "floppy" almost always are describing a neuromuscular problem. The term *fatigue*, in fact, is rarely pertinent or appropriate for the very small child.

Older children, too, complain only infrequently of "feeling fatigued." Remarkably, even with chronic organic diseases, fatigue itself often is not verbally expressed by the child. Rather it is the concerned parent who usually observes and reports that the child appears fatigued. Expressions such as "He has no energy," "She lies around all the time," "She seems bored and droopy,""He's sleeping a lot of the time," "She has no pep," "He drags around," and "I can't get her to do a thing" are commonly heard from parents. On questioning, younger children will occasionally express a sense of lassitude and fatigue to a physician. Much of the difficulty in the middle years of childhood (before adolescence), however, is the inability to put into words that which is felt. Fatigue therefore usually is exhibited in terms of a child's physical activity and performance in school, sports, and other organized activities.

Chronic complaints of fatigue are encountered most frequently in adolescents. It is among the adolescent's most common presentation in pediatric practice and one that usually arouses excessive concern from parents. The normal swings in adolescent moods—from excessive exuberance to fatigue— usually are of more concern to parents and teachers than to the patient; thus the parent is most often the complainant. Often the adolescent may vehemently disagree with the parents' view and not share their concern. Adolescents, however, also initiate visits to the pediatrician because they themselves feel fatigue. Parents may be unable or may refuse to recognize the adolescent's symptoms.

FATIGUE ASSOCIATED WITH MEDICAL ILLNESSES

The younger the child, the more likely is the expressed or observed fatigue to have a pathologic cause. The pediatrician often is astounded at the lack of symptoms, such as fatigue, in younger children with profound medical illnesses. Similarly, minor illnesses are more likely to precipitate prolonged fatigue in adolescents compared with younger children. The accompanying box lists those disorders associated with fatigue most likely to be encountered by the pediatrician. Needless to say, any acute illness or trauma may be accompanied by fatigue, but usually only prolonged fatigue is noteworthy.

The most common problem associated with fatigue in children is recurrent or chronic infection. Otitis media, sinusitis, and tonsillitis of a recurrent and often smoldering nature often are overlooked for their systemic effects, among which may be prominent fatigue. Mycoplasmal pneumonia, often low grade and without fever, produces progressive fatigue. In addition, prolonged viral and parasitic illnesses, such as infectious mononucleosis, hepatitis, cytomegalovirus infection, and toxoplasmosis, commonly manifest with fatigue, especially in adolescents.

The terms *chronic infectious mononucleosis* and *chronic fatigue syndrome* have become popular with both physicians and the media. This attention has led to occasional misuse

Disorders Commonly Associated with Prolonged Fatigue

- Severe anemia
- Hypothyroidism
- Chronic upper respiratory tract infections
  - Otitis media and sinusitis
  - Tonsillitis
- Mycoplasmal and other viral pneumonias
- Infectious mononucleosis
- Hepatitis
- Chronic allergies
- Rheumatoid arthritis
- Rheumatic fever
- Diabetes mellitus
- Disseminated malignancy
- Inflammatory bowel disease
- Drug abuse, including alcoholism
- Cyanotic heart disease
- Chronic pulmonary disease
- Chronic renal failure
- Depression
- Severe obesity

of those terms and also, undoubtedly, to mild mass hysteria among young adults and adolescents who now are convinced that they suffer from one of these disorders.

Most adults and many infants and children have been infected with the Epstein-Barr (EB) virus. The clinical manifestations in proved cases are extremely variable: some patients remain symptom free whereas clinical, hematologic, and serologic findings support the diagnosis of infectious mononucleosis in others. The symptoms of infectious mononucleosis usually resolve in several weeks, but an occasional patient may have an atypical or a more prolonged course in which the initial clinical findings either persist or are intermittent over a period of months or, rarely, years. These unusual, but documented, cases of chronic infectious mononucleosis typically include complaints of chronic fatigue.

Another much smaller group of patients has now been described with serious, sometimes lethal, illness associated with EB virus infection. These patients usually do not manifest the classic findings of infectious mononucleosis; very often their conditions are proved to be either acquired or genetically determined immunologic abnormalities. Frequently fatigue manifests as part of allergic rhinitis in children and adolescents. Often mistakenly considered insignificant, upper respiratory tract allergies may cause impressive fatigue, as well as irritability and mild depression.

Of the common endocrine disorders, only hypothyroidism is likely to be associated with fatigue. Certainly the hypothyroid child whose rate of growth has fallen off may manifest increasing fatigue and lassitude—at first subtle—as the only symptoms. Thyrotoxicosis, in contrast, is uncommon in young children, but occasionally it manifests with isolated fatigue in adolescents.

Although any metabolic disorder can cause fatigue, only diabetes mellitus occurs with enough frequency to merit consideration here. Fatigue almost always accompanies the initial or uncontrolled diabetic state.

Collagen-vascular diseases, especially rheumatoid arthritis and other rheumatoid-like disorders, appear frequently in pediatric practice. Many of these disorders are difficult to diagnose precisely and are often eventually self-limited, but many children have significant fatigue, out of proportion to the musculoskeletal complaints. Lyme arthritis, newly described, is one example of this circumstance.

Always unpredictable and often secretive, inflammatory bowel disease may arouse concern initially with unexplained fatigue and a loss of a sense of well-being. Although eventually accompanied by fever, abdominal symptoms, or abnormal stools, this disorder can continue for months with fatigue as the only major symptom.

Congenital cyanotic heart disease and chronic advanced pulmonary disease, as seen with cystic fibrosis, are commonly associated with marked fatigue; in these cases, however, the underlying disease usually is readily evident before the fatigue is severe. In atypical circumstances the pediatrician occasionally may see an older child for the first time with severe fatigue caused by previously undiagnosed hypoxic disorder.

Overall, the condition most often suspected as a cause of fatigue in both children and adults is anemia—and, most often, incorrectly so. Although fatigue often is ascribed to mild to moderate anemia, from whatever source, symptoms usually are not seen in children until hemoglobin levels fall to 6 or 7 g; if red cell levels fall gradually, even lower hemoglobin levels may ensue without clinically evident symptoms. Irritability and attentional problems may be present with mild to moderate iron deficiency anemia, but usually not fatigue. Younger children, especially, seem to tolerate incredibly low hemoglobin levels with no symptoms at all.

Malignancy, particularly leukemia or lymphoma, occasionally develops insidiously, with fatigue as the major symptom. Although always feared, these diseases are infrequently seen in pediatric office practice.

Of more current importance in older children and adolescents is the occurrence of alcoholism and drug abuse—causes of chronic fatigue easily overlooked.

FATIGUE ASSOCIATED WITH EMOTIONAL FACTORS

Most children and adolescents who come to the pediatrician with unexplained chronic fatigue are found to have an emotionally related disorder. Before adolescence the complaint usually centers on parental concern about a child's decreased activity level. The younger child will have been noted to prefer sedentary activities: to "lie around the house a lot," appear tired, lack energy, and shrink from social contacts. These traits may have been long-standing, but a comment from grandparents or a teacher may arouse acute anxiety and for this reason precipitate the first visit to the pediatrician.

At this point the family often is convinced that the child has a serious organic disease. Further evaluation, however, usually reveals that the child is performing at a very satisfactory level, but not up to the excessive expectations of the family. The child may be withdrawing because of failure to compete with an exceptional sibling or because of real or imagined failure in school. In other cases the child may feel a lack of well-being because of parental discord. Similarly, lack of parental involvement with a child may lead to lassitude and boredom. Therefore stress and anxiety in the child of this age usually results in either hyperactivity or withdrawal, and the more common withdrawal reaction may exhibit itself as chronic fatigue.

These observations do not mean that the majority of children do not go through transient periods of lassitude or fatigue, but these instances are brief and usually self-limited.

At the opposite extreme is the child whose chronic fatigue is a sign of true psychiatric depression. Here, as in the adolescent, the more protracted and severe the periods of withdrawal, the more likely that depression and fatigue are pathologically caused.

By far the most frequent and familiar visitor because of protracted fatigue will be the adolescent. The pediatrician can expect to see a generous number who characteristically appear each spring with fatigue, lassitude, lack of energy, and mild depression. This disorder usually appears at times of greatest school-related stress—before examination time. It is "spring fever." Although the patient may have a real fever, usually secondary to infection (e.g., infectious mononucleosis or influenza), the problem usually is emotionally based. All the uncertainties of late adolescence, including identity and sexual crises, may create a "spring fever" during any season of the year, with fatigue often the dominant complaint.

Most of these patients have normal findings on physical examinations and routine laboratory tests; yet some have serologic evidence of EB virus infection. Since 1985 both children and adults have been thought to have a syndrome that included persistent fatigue, headache, myalgias, pharyngitis, lymphadenopathy, depression, inability to concentrate, and defective memory. This "chronic fatigue syndrome" quickly became a popular diagnosis and often was attributed to EB virus infection, although very few patients had documented physical findings or hematologic abnormalities consistent with the diagnosis of infectious mononucleosis. In addition, most had no serologic evidence of active EB virus infection.

Recently, however, a better understanding of the natural course of antibody activity in healthy individuals months and years after an initial illness with infectious mononucleosis indicates that healthy patients who had had infectious mononucleosis years earlier could not be differentiated from fatigued patients with the disease. Instead, analysis of the chronic fatigue syndrome reveals a striking incidence of preexisting depression, phobia, and anxiety. Furthermore, depression commonly accompanies or follows infectious mononucleosis, as well as other acute infectious diseases such as influenza A.

Historically, epidemics of chronic fatigue syndrome or neuromyasthenia have surfaced episodically. Brucellosis and Asian influenza, both prevalent in the 1950s, were implicated as possible causes of a chronic fatigue syndrome. There was also a strong underlying association with emotional disorders during these "epidemics."

Another common circumstance is presented by the adolescent who collapses with marked fatigue after periods of intense and exuberant activity involving schoolwork, extracurricular activity, sports, or social events. These are individuals who also may be short on sleep, with "borderline" eating habits, and an additional variety of hypochondriac symptoms. "Burnout" and fatigue are particularly common in overachieving high school and college students during late adolescence. The emotional reaction actually may be precipitated by a physical illness, particularly an infection.

DIFFERENTIAL DIAGNOSIS AND EVALUATION

Although it may at first appear that the patient with chronic fatigue has an insignificant problem, great care must be taken to rule out underlying medical illness and also to return the child and parents to a state of well-being. The physician must remember that either the child or the parents are worried about the child's fatigued state. Because there may be a lack of agreement among the family members regarding the significance of the symptoms, adequate time and concern must be taken to evaluate the history. The symptoms of chronic fatigue cannot be dismissed casually over the telephone or with a "quick office check."

Inasmuch as most patients who come to the physician with complaints of fatigue have an emotionally based problem, a careful history, with intake from both child and parents (taken separately when appropriate), often will limit the differential diagnosis initially. Discrepancies between the child's and the parents' observations soon will become evident, and the diagnosis of emotionally related fatigue will emerge in most cases on the basis of history alone. Happily, the information derived from a long-standing physician-patient relationship will contribute enormously to increased ease during the evaluation.

Although fatigue may be the only presenting symptom, further questioning almost always uncovers other symptoms of somatic disease. Chronic fatigue alone, in the absence of other physical symptoms, usually is emotionally based. Other supporting complaints will be somnolence, depression, anxiety, boredom, and a decreased activity level. Furthermore, the patient's affect may be inappropriate. Often, emotional stress or some disruption in the patient's life is also part of the history.

A careful physical examination should be performed. A normal examination, patiently performed, may be the only treatment necessary, working miracles to reassure the often fearful child or parent. The child's affect and appearance are usually revealing. The impression that the child "looks well" will invariably prove to be an accurate measure of the child's health. Because in younger children the parent will be describing the child's fatigue, the physician and parent often simultaneously will agree that the child "appears healthy"—again making the presence of organic disease unlikely. The condition of the adolescent, in contrast, may be more difficult to interpret. Although the physical examination may be benign, the adolescent may appear slovenly, uncommunicative, depressed, and unable to express feelings; thus at first the adolescent sometimes will appear to be ill with a physical problem.

In all age-groups a search for sites of chronic latent infection, adenopathy, enlargement or tenderness of the liver and spleen, and abdominal masses should be made. Careful palpation for an enlarged or tender thyroid gland is essential. Mild scleral icterus and petechiae are easy to overlook. Similarly, a patient's pallor (a common finding, especially after long winters indoors) may evade even the most experienced pediatrician. On the other hand, the congested facies of the chronically allergic or infected child, clubbing, and cyanosis will be obvious.

A limited well-selected group of laboratory tests should be performed on most patients with chronic fatigue. These results will reassure the family, the patient, and the pediatrician and usually will serve to erase any lingering doubt about the diagnosis. Furthermore, normal physical examination findings plus a normal laboratory evaluation may provide all the therapy necessary for recovery.

The laboratory evaluation initially should include a complete blood count with red cell indexes, urinalysis, a heterophil screening test, the sedimentation rate, and in some patients, thyroid and liver function tests, a throat culture, and a stool examination for blood. The cold agglutinin test is often a valuable and simple initial screening test for a mycoplasmal infection. Roentgenograms rarely are necessary and should be discouraged.

The critical evaluation of data collected from the history, physical examination, and laboratory tests should enable the pediatrician to ascertain quickly any organic causes of fatigue. Prolonged fever, however low grade, must always be viewed as significant and may suggest infection, inflammatory disease, or malignancy. Pallor suggests the possibility of anemia or hypothyroidism. Cervical adenopathy, even a single enlarged node, in the absence of other findings can be a clue to the diagnosis of infectious mononucleosis. In fact, every pediatrician begins to look for patients with infectious mononucleosis in the autumn and early winter of each year. Remember, however, that infectious mononucleosis is a protean illness, and results of the physical examination sometimes are normal. Children and adolescents with infectious mononucleosis may have no fever or signs of toxicity but may manifest major fatigue.

Furthermore, results of the heterophil antibody test may be negative in many young children and infants and in about 10% of older children and adolescents. The reliability of EB virus antibody testing has now improved to a point at which the diagnosis of acute, active infectious mononucleosis can be confirmed. During the evaluation of chronic fatigue, EB virus antibody titers usually can differentiate long-past infection from recent and active infection, thus eliminating EB virus infection and infectious mononucleosis as causative agents for the fatigue and permitting a search for other likely neuropsychiatric causes. Toxoplasmosis and cytomegalovirus (CMV) infections may closely mimic mononucleosis and manifest with significant fatigue but with only minimal cervical adenopathy and fever. Positive results of a fluorescent antibody test for toxoplasmosis or CMV with negative results of a heterophil antibody test will confirm the diagnosis. Similarly, fatigued children may have hepatitis and may be anicteric (or only slightly icteric), with absent or minimal hepatic tenderness or enlargement. Commonly, other routine but slightly prolonged viral infections, especially during convalescence, will precipitate a prolonged fatigue syndrome accompanied by depression.

A diagnosis of chronic fatigue syndrome should be restricted to patients who meet rigid criteria, including (1) the new onset of persistent or relapsing fatigue in patients with no previous history and (2) the exclusion of other clinical conditions that might produce similar symptoms. In addition, two of the following three physical criteria should be documented on at least two occasions in a 1-month interval: (1) low-grade fever, (2) nonexudative pharyngitis, and (3) palpable or tender postcervical or axillary lymph nodes (less than 2 cm). Furthermore, symptoms must include several of the following: muscle weakness, muscle discomfort, headaches, migratory arthralgia, neuropsychological complaints, and sleep disturbances. After other medical conditions are excluded, some older children and adolescents may meet these criteria for diagnosis. Certainly these patients should not be labeled with a diagnosis of chronic infectious mononucleosis syndrome or chronic EB virus infection, which recently has become a "quick fix" diagnosis for patients with chronic fatigue. At present an etiologic agent for chronic fatigue syndrome has not been found.

Children with a collagen-vascular disease have fatigue and little else at first. Mild articular or periarticular inflammation may be easily missed by the physician. The emphasis must be on a careful examination and the observation of subtle or minimal physical findings inasmuch as children usually do not manifest fulminant findings initially. Children with diseases such as inflammatory bowel disease, arthritis, and arthritis-like illness and some patients with a malignancy—monocytic leukemia, in particular—may have especially prolonged symptoms, including fatigue, without any physical findings whatsoever.

An enlarged, tender thyroid gland and fatigue may indicate thyroiditis with emerging hypothyroidism. However, the thyroid often is palpable and full in healthy adolescents. In any event, chronic fatigue from thyroid disease usually can be quickly ruled out with a T_4 test. Some patients with hypothyroidism also demonstrate mild to moderate anemia, and those with active thyroiditis may have an elevated sedimentation rate.

The diagnosis of pure anemia, to be acceptable as an explanation for fatigue, requires marked reduction of hemoglobin. Red cell indexes and a reticulocyte count will characterize the anemia and probable cause. Anemia with thrombocytopenia, however, suggests leukemia or aplastic anemia. The white cell count may be normal in infectious mononucleosis or hepatitis, but there most likely will be a lymphocytosis with atypical lymphocytes present. The heterophil antibody screening test ("mono test") will be diagnostic in most such circumstances.

The erythrocyte sedimentation rate is the most valuable screening test for inflammatory diseases of all varieties. A normal sedimentation rate almost always rules out collagen-vascular disease, inflammatory bowel disease, chronic smoldering infections, and disseminated malignancies. An elevated sedimentation rate demands further evaluation.

A routine urinalysis almost always reveals diabetes, and most patients with chronic renal failure will have urinary abnormalities as well as significant anemia. In these cases the subsequent measurement of blood glucose in diabetes and of creatinine or blood urea nitrogen in renal disease will provide confirmation.

MANAGEMENT

Inasmuch as significant organic disease will be ruled out in most patients, further management will require a meaningful communication between the pediatrician and the patient and parents. In the instance of the younger child, one must put the variability in performance and behavior of normal children into perspective. Again, emphasis must be placed on appropriate parental expectations. In addition, the child's, as well as the family's, daily schedule should be reviewed. A chaotic life-style, frantic with activity, poorly structured, with inadequate sleep patterns, often will be revealed. Occasionally, true psychiatric depression will be discovered, and a referral to a psychiatrist should then be made.

Older children and adolescents benefit from personal, warm attention. The value of a continuous relationship with one physician becomes self-evident. An understanding, thorough session with the patient's own pediatrician will usually "streamline" the evaluation and eliminate the need for excessive testing. Conversation after the physical examination should attempt to (1) reassure the child or adolescent about his or her basic health, (2) reiterate the common and "normal" occurrence of fatigue, (3) examine the daily routine and stresses on the patient, and (4) suggest modifications of the patient's life-style and approaches to life's situations. It is a time for respectful give-and-take.

It is the pediatrician's responsibility to attempt to establish the probable cause of the fatigue before the patient is referred to a specialist. If emotional fatigue is suspected, the adolescent in particular must be comfortable with the conclusion that organic diseases have been ruled out. The patient then must be made aware of the emotional underlay for the fatigue, and if there is need, the reasons for psychiatric referral must be made clear; otherwise the fatigue, like any psychosomatic symptom, may continue and worsen. The knowledgeable pediatrician therefore will be reassuring but firm in approaching the child or adolescent with both the diagnosis and potential need for further evaluation and referral. Fortunately, such a referral usually is not necessary.

SUGGESTED READINGS

Cassidy J: Textbook of pediatric rheumatology, New York, 1990, Churchill Livingstone.

Hofmann A: Adolescent medicine, ed 2, Menlo Park, Calif, 1989, Addison-Wesley Publishing Co.

Holmes GP, Kaplan JE, and Gantz NM: Chronic fatigue syndrome: a working case definition, Ann Intern Med 108:387, 1988.

Kaplan S: Clinical pediatric and adolescent endocrinology, ed 2, Philadelphia, 1990, WB Saunders Co.

Katz BZ and Andiman WA: Chronic fatigue syndrome, J Pediatr 113:944, 1988.

Klein GL et al: The allergic irritability syndrome, Ann Allergy 55:22, 1985.

MacBryde CM and Blacklow RS: Signs and symptoms, ed 5, Philadelphia, 1970, JB Lippincott Co.

Malmquist CP: Handbook of adolescence, New York, 1978, Jason Aronson, Inc.

Nathan DG and Oski FA: Hematology of infancy and childhood, ed 3, Philadelphia, 1987, WB Saunders Co.

Straus SE: The chronic mononucleosis syndrome, J Infect Dis 157:405, 1988.

Tunnessen WW: Signs and symptoms in pediatrics, ed 2 Philadelphia, 1988, Harper & Row.

131

Fever

Élise W. van der Jagt

For centuries the presence of fever in both human beings and animals has been associated with the presence of illness. Today as many as 30% of all patients seen by pediatricians have fever as their principal complaint, making it one of the most common reasons why children are taken to a physician. If one adds the multitude of telephone calls about fever, which the pediatrician receives night and day, it becomes obvious that the proper evaluation and management of fever is one of the basic and necessary skills of physicians and nurse practitioners.

Even though practitioners have dealt with this common clinical sign for decades, its mechanism, meaning, and management have remained sufficiently unclear and controversial that ongoing research on these matters continues to be conducted by scientists and clinicians. Although advances in neurochemistry and neurophysiology have improved our understanding of the pathophysiology of fever, clinical investigators continue to search for practical knowledge that will directly enhance the care of the febrile patient. Availability of such information would simplify the challenging role of the physician, who must evaluate the patient quickly and effectively, arrive at a diagnosis, institute appropriate therapy, and both educate and support the parents and child during the entire process. The extent to which health care providers accomplish these goals depends on their knowledge of the mechanisms of disease, the various clinical manifestations of disease, and their awareness of the social context in which the disease occurs.

DEFINITION

The word *fever* is derived from the Latin *fovere* (to warm) and commonly means an elevation of body temperature. Although this general definition is acceptable in daily parlance, it should be remembered that fever is more accurately described as a *disorder* of thermoregulation. It must be clearly differentiated from hyperthermia, an elevated body temperature resulting from conditions that overwhelm the normal process of thermoregulation.

The thermoregulatory center resides in the preoptic nuclei of the anterior hypothalamus. These nuclei consist of warm- and cold-sensitive neurons that respond both to the temperature of the blood coursing near them and to stimuli received from peripheral thermal sensors, particularly those in the skin. By regulating peripheral thermoregulatory control mechanisms in response to these stimuli (e.g., sweating, vasoconstriction), the hypothalamic thermostat maintains the core body temperature at about 98.6° F (37° C), the so-called set-point of the hypothalamus.

Excessive body heat generated during strenuous exercise, from excessive coverings, or from high environmental temperatures normally is dissipated by peripheral thermoregulation to maintain the core body temperature at 37° C. If the peripheral thermoregulators are inadequate to accomplish this task, heat will be retained and hyperthermia will occur.

In the case of fever, however, the thermostat itself has been "reset" at a higher set-point, causing the core body temperature to be maintained at a higher level.

The primary substance responsible for elevating the set-point has been known since 1948. It originally was named *endogenous pyrogen* and was believed to originate from leukocytes. It has become evident, however, that endogenous pyrogen is not the only leukocyte product that can induce fever; others, including interferon and tumor necrosis factor (cachectin), also can do this. As additional products of macrophages exhibiting properties almost identical to endogenous pyrogen have been described, they have been grouped and called interleukin-1 (IL-1). Subsequent research with the use of in vitro lymphocyte assays and recombinant IL-1 has shown that IL-1 is a low–molecular weight cytoplasmic protein contained within bone marrow–derived phagocytes (predominantly macrophages and monocytes, although also present in neutrophils and eosinophils), and is released when these phagocytes are active at inflammatory sites. As might be expected, multiple disease processes may precipitate the release of IL-1, including infections, antigen-antibody–mediated reactions, and tumors. After its release, this intriguing substance not only appears to stimulate the production of prostaglandins (primarily prostaglandin E_2), prostacyclins, and thromboxanes (all arachidonic acid metabolites) that directly elevate the set-point of the hypothalamic thermostat (resulting in fever) but also appears to cause T cell proliferation and an increase in B cell–derived antibodies. Thus IL-1 would seem to have a role in immune regulation as well. Although other substances, such as serotonin, norepinephrine, and cyclic adenosine monophosphate (cyclic AMP), also have been implicated in fever production, their precise relationship to IL-1 has yet to be defined.

It is equally important to know the range of normal body temperature. Ever since 1850 when the use of the thermometer was first recommended to measure body temperature, the normal core body temperature has been found to range between 96.8° and 98.6° F (36° and 37° C), although on rare occasions it may be as low as 95.5° F (35.3° C) or as high as 100.4° F (38° C). Young children have higher core body temperatures than do adults, with a temperature slightly greater than 37.8° C occurring frequently in those younger than the age of 2 years. Lowest temperatures occur from 2 to 6 AM and the highest ones from 5 to 7 PM, a diurnal variation that persists even during a febrile illness. Because of the range of normal body temperatures, on occasion it can be useful to know a child's usual body temperature so that an abnormal elevation can be recognized more easily. The degree of body temperature elevation from normal may help in determining the presence and significance of fever, especially if the child customarily has a low body temperature.

MEASUREMENT

Inasmuch as accurate measurement of body temperature is relied on extensively to determine the presence of fever, every physician should ensure that patients and parents are knowledgeable about the techniques for temperature measurement, as well as its rationale. Ideally this discussion should be held at the time of the child's birth, just before hospital discharge.

The traditional locations for measurement of temperature are the rectum, the mouth, and the axilla. Glass thermometers with mercury or alcohol-filled bulbs are commonly used at home, although most physician offices and hospitals now use electronic thermometers with digital readouts and disposable sheaths to reduce the spread of communicable disease. Attempts to facilitate temperature measurement at home by use of a liquid crystal temperature strip applied to the forehead or sensor-containing pacifiers have not been uniformly successful and are not sufficiently reliable. A more recent advance in temperature measurement is the development of a device that is inserted into the outer part of the ear canal and measures infrared radiation from the tympanic membrane,[12] whose blood supply is common with that going to the hypothalamus. Thus core body temperature is measured. This method is not uncomfortable, takes only 1 second, and correlates ($r = 0.98$) with pulmonary artery temperatures. It holds great promise for use in most health care facilities.

Because the rectal temperature generally reflects core body temperature best, this location is preferred unless a specific contraindication to minor rectal trauma exists (e.g., the child with neutropenia). After the procedure is explained to the parent and, as appropriate, to the child, a well-lubricated thermometer should be inserted at least 5 cm into the anal canal. If care is taken that the thermometer stays in the anal canal, peak temperature will be reached in 2 to 3 minutes.

Taking temperatures orally should not be attempted until the child is older than 5 to 6 years of age and is cooperative. After the thermometer has been placed under the tongue for a minimum of 1 minute, a temperature will be obtained that is about 0.5° C less than the rectal temperature. Because hot and cold foods may alter the oral temperature by as much as 1° to 2° C, they should be avoided for an hour before measurement.

Taking axillary temperatures is common in neonates to minimize the risk of rectal trauma. The thermometer must be placed in the axilla for 3 to 5 minutes, and a temperature either equal to or up to 1° C lower than the rectal temperature will be recorded.

ASSOCIATED SIGNS AND SYMPTOMS

Donaldson[4] has noted the behavior of humans and animals to be remarkably similar when fever is present. After IL-1 has elevated the set-point in the hypothalamus, patients will, as much as they are able, attempt to adjust the environment to keep their body at this higher temperature. Young children will seek close contact with a warm person (generally a parent), will wish to be covered by a blanket, will sit near a warm stove or register, and will refuse cold liquids or foods. Although children may be quite comfortable at this elevated body temperature, they will interact less with others, have a decreased ability to concentrate, substitute quieter activities for energetic ones, and become less communicative except to indicate discomfort and distress. This "adaptive withdrawal" often is accompanied by loss of appetite and complaints of headache.

Such a combination of behavioral symptoms is a familiar indicator of illness to most parents and usually results in the "hand on the forehead" maneuver, followed by measurement of the temperature. Unfortunately, parents may not recognize the onset of fever in the younger child because the alterations in behavior are fewer and more subtle. In a small infant, irritability and anorexia may be the sole evidence of fever and disease. If a parent is not familiar with these subtle cues, recognition of serious illness may be significantly delayed.

In addition to the behavioral changes that may accompany fever, the general physical examination may reveal the presence of a pronounced hypermetabolic state. The child may have flushed cheeks, may have an unusual glitter in the eyes, and may be either sleepy and lethargic or exceptionally alert and excited (particularly 5- to 10-year-olds). With rare exception the pulse is elevated by about 10 to 15 beats per degree centigrade of fever, and the respiratory rate is increased. (If the pulse rate is less than expected from the degree of fever, one should think of typhoid fever, tularemia, mycoplasmal infection, or factitious fever.) The skin may feel very hot and dry ("burning up with fever"), although the distal extremities may be cold and pale (vasoconstricted), obscuring a very high core body temperature.

Most children are not particularly uncomfortable, but some may exhibit shivering or sweating, mechanisms by which the body increases or decreases temperature. Sweating may be so excessive that significant dehydration may occur, particularly if the intake of fluids has been poor. Thus a dry mouth and lips may result not only from rapid mouth breathing but also from dehydration. Finally, there may be increased irritability of the central nervous system, reflected in a febrile seizure.

The aforementioned signs and symptoms may be less obvious in a small infant. Shivering does not occur in the first few months of life, and diaphoresis is seen less frequently than in the older child. Because irritability and pallor may be the only suggestions of illness, careful attention should be given to the child if the parent describes these characteristics.

PRESENTATION

How a febrile child comes to the attention of a physician or nurse practitioner will determine the urgency and type of management initiated. Probably the most dramatic and frightening presentation of fever in a child is the sudden occurrence of a seizure. Usually lasting less than 15 minutes and occurring within 24 hours of the onset of fever, a generalized tonic or tonic-clonic seizure may begin without warning. Most parents have not been aware that a fever was present and feel guilty for not having noted it. The pediatrician may be called after the seizure has taken place and often is first alerted when the child has already been transported to the local emergency room. There the child may be postictal with a temperature of 102° to 104° F (39° to 40° C). A careful assessment of the patient is indicated because a seizure may be the first sign of meningitis or encephalitis.

Although some have recommended that every patient with a first febrile seizure automatically have a lumbar puncture, most authorities recommend that diagnostic evaluations be individualized. Reexamination of the child after defervescence and after resolution of the convulsive episode may be more helpful in assessing the need for an examination of the cerebrospinal fluid. However, in children younger than 24 and especially under 18 months of age, it is probably prudent to perform the lumbar puncture, because the telltale signs of meningitis (meningismus, Kernig sign, and Brudzinski sign) may be absent.

More commonly, the patient is first seen when the fever has been present for longer than 24 hours and is associated either with nonspecific symptoms, as mentioned before, or with symptoms referable to a particular organ system. Inasmuch as many of the evaluations of the febrile child take place over the telephone (the first contact with the clinician), the physician must be able to take a pertinent history. Of particular significance are the age of the patient (the younger the child, the more careful the evaluation should be), exposure to illness in the family or community, history of recent immunization, and a history of recurrent infections (e.g., urinary tract infections, streptococcal infections, or otitis media). In addition, the duration and the height of the fever are important considerations. A low-grade fever that has been present for many days usually does not need to be evaluated as urgently as a temperature of 106° F (41° C) that has been present for a few hours. The former is likely to indicate either a chronic or benign illness, whereas the latter has a greater risk of being an acute, perhaps serious, disease.

A visit or phone call for minimal fever and little evidence of disease should prompt a careful assessment of the psychosocial factors that may be contributing to parental concern. Is the main concern about something else—the "hidden agenda"? What knowledge of fever and disease does the caregiver have? Has there been a previous traumatic experience with disease? Could this be a "vulnerable child"? Is this a dysfunctional family in which minor illness either cannot be dealt with or is used as a means to meet other needs? These questions and others may clarify the situation.

DIFFERENTIAL DIAGNOSIS

Innumerable conditions can cause fever; an extensive deliberation about each condition is beyond the scope of this presentation. It is useful, however, to classify these conditions into broad categories: (1) infections, (2) collagen-vascular diseases, (3) neoplasia, (4) metabolic diseases (e.g., hyperthyroidism), (5) chronic inflammatory diseases, (6) hematologic diseases (e.g., sickle cell disease, transfusion reaction), (7) drug fever and immunization reactions, (8) poisoning (e.g., aspirin, atropine), (9) central nervous system abnormalities, and (10) factitious fever. In addition, dehydration, activity, and heat exposure can all cause an elevation in temperature (hyperthermia).

Although any disease in these categories may cause fever at any age, some diseases are more likely to occur at some ages than at others. Collagen-vascular disease and inflammatory bowel disease, for example, are unusual in infants but become progressively more frequent with advancing age. Similarly, febrile immunization reactions are much more common during the first year of life, the time during which immunizations usually are administered.

Infections account for the majority of fevers in all age-groups, primarily affecting the respiratory and gastrointestinal tracts. The majority of these infections are viral (e.g., enterovirus, influenza virus, parainfluenza virus, respiratory syncytial virus, adenovirus, rhinovirus, rotavirus) and generally are self-limited. Knowledge of the seasonality of these viruses will promote correct and efficient diagnoses. In addition, knowledge of the typical physical findings in these infections and their course may help distinguish them from bacterial disease. For example, high fever, irritability, cervical adenopathy, and painful vesicles on the gums and tongue are characteristic of herpes gingivostomatitis. Failure to examine the tongue and gums may result in an unnecessary septic workup in search for a possible bacterial infection. On the other hand, assuming that a high fever in a 2-month-old child is due to roseola (exanthem subitum) would be erroneous because this infection usually does not occur at that age. Failure to evaluate the fever further might result in missing a serious bacterial infection.

Although viral infections can cause significant morbidity and mortality, the more aggressive course and serious outcomes of bacterial infections make early diagnosis especially important, particularly because effective antibiotic treatment usually is available. Bacterial infections may be especially devastating in younger children, who are relatively immunocompromised because of their immature immune system. What remains as a localized infection in the older child may be rapidly disseminated to other soft tissues in the infant and toddler, particularly the blood (bacteremia), the lungs (pneumonia), the meninges (meningitis), the bones (osteomyelitis), and the joints (arthritis). Because these infections may be fatal if not recognized, the physician must be equipped with ways to differentiate bacterial infections from the more benign viral infections.

The younger the child, the more difficult it is to recognize bacterial infection. Complaints cannot be verbalized, and physical signs and symptoms are more subtle and easily missed unless a high index of suspicion is maintained. Of particular concern is the difficulty in diagnosing bacterial disease in children who have no obvious focus of infection. For this reason, there have been many attempts during the last decade to distinguish children in whom fever signals a high versus a low likelihood of a serious bacterial infection.[13] In this regard children between birth and 24 months of age are of special interest because they are particularly difficult to assess. Efforts have focused on three areas: (1) laboratory data,[7] (2) history and physical examination data,[9] and (3) response to antipyretics.[1] As yet no combination of variables in these categories has been found that results in both high sensitivity and high specificity levels. Nevertheless, a considerable amount of information is available that is helpful in both the assessment and the management of the febrile child.

Fever present during the first 4 days of life has been associated with a high incidence of bacterial disease.[14] A temperature above 37° C (98.6° F) occurs in 1% of all newborns; of these children, 10% have a bacterial infection primarily caused by group B streptococcal and gram-negative enteric pathogens.

Although it has been previously believed that febrile infants younger than 3 months of age have a higher incidence of bacteremia, more recent studies suggest that the incidence is similar to that of older infants and children. The presence of bacterial disease ranges between 8% and 15% and that of bacteremia between 3% and 4%. In fact, age, sex, and height of fever have not been reliable predictors of bacteremia or serious bacterial infection. Infants at low risk who are 2 months old and younger have been characterized by the absence of ear, soft tissue, or skeletal infection; a white blood cell count between 5000 and 15,000 cells/mm^3; a band count of <1500 cells/mm^3; and normal urinalysis results (≤10 WBC/HPF on a centrifuged urine specimen).[3] Because the degree of fever is not a reliable predictor of serious disease, a rectal temperature higher than 100.4° F (38° C) in an infant younger than 3 months old should be evaluated promptly. Septicemia has occurred in infants with even such low-grade fevers.[10] Although temperatures higher than 104° F (40° C) in this age-group initially appeared to be associated with serious bacterial disease,[8] subsequent studies have not confirmed this.[2] The potential of serious disease even in the absence of a high fever, therefore, demands a comprehensive evaluation that should include a thorough physical examination, examination of the cerebrospinal fluid, urinalysis, total and differential white blood cell count, and cultures of the blood, urine, and spinal fluid. A urine culture is especially important because urinary tract infections have been noted to be the most common bacterial infection observed in this age-group even in the absence of pyuria.[6] Inasmuch as urinary tract infections have been shown to occur more often in uncircumcised males, notation of this physical characteristic should be made.

In those between the ages of 3 months and 2 years, a fever higher than 100° F (37.8° C) may be associated with bacteremia, even in the absence of localizing signs. *Streptococcus pneumoniae* (pneumococcus) and *Haemophilus influenzae* are the bacteria most commonly implicated in bacteremia and are associated with tissue invasion in 5% of cases of the former and in almost all cases of the latter. To improve the identification of those children who are likely to have bacteremia, a child with a rectal temperature of 39° C or higher should have a white blood cell count and an erythrocyte sedimentation rate determined. If the blood count is greater than 15,000 or the sedimentation rate is greater than 30, a blood culture should be obtained; bacteremia has been diagnosed in 15% of these children. A chest roentgenogram also should be obtained if there is evidence of respiratory distress, including tachypnea.[5]

Children older than 2 years of age are more likely to have signs and symptoms suggestive of a recognizable illness; if they have nonspecific symptoms, an urgent consultation with the physician probably is unnecessary. However, all febrile children with general or localized signs and symptoms, such as swollen joints, meningismus, labored respirations, dysuria, petechiae, and alteration of consciousness, must be seen immediately.

In any child the physical examination may result in major clues to the cause of the fever. Because the majority of infections involve the respiratory tract, this area must be examined carefully. Examination of the tympanic membranes for otitis media, of the pharynx for streptococcal or viral pharyngitis, of the nose for the nasal discharge of sinusitis or a viral upper respiratory tract infection, and of the lungs for evidence of pneumonia or bronchiolitis must be performed in all instances. Conjunctivitis may be a clue to adenovirus infection or conjunctivitis-otitis syndrome; it also is one sign of Kawasaki disease.

The skin is no less important and may demonstrate typical viral exanthems, such as those associated with rubella, roseola, or chickenpox, or it may show the erythema marginatum of rheumatic fever or the rose spots of typhoid fever.

Generalized lymphadenopathy often occurs with viral illnesses, such as infectious mononucleosis, hepatitis, or cytomegalovirus infection, but it also may be a clue to the diagnosis of leukemia or lymphoma. Localized enlargement of lymph nodes should prompt a search for a skin infection or for a tumor. Isolated cervical lymphadenopathy may be associated with tuberculosis infection.

The musculoskeletal system must be examined with care. Localized bone tenderness may suggest osteomyelitis, and a restricted range of motion in a warm joint may suggest arthritis. The latter finding may occur in many different diseases, but a careful examination of the heart is indicated to look for the carditis of rheumatic fever or of infective endocarditis. The spine should be palpated for any evidence of diskitis, and any costovertebral angle tenderness should prompt an examination of the urine for evidence of infection.

A final consideration is factitious fever, an uncommon but nevertheless real entity, even in children. Children as young as 8 years of age have been known to increase artificially the thermometer reading by rubbing the mercury thermometer bulb on the sheets or by exposing it to warm liquids. Clues on physical examination include a pulse that is not correlated with the temperature elevation, inability to document fever when it is measured rectally, and an absence of sweating during defervescence. Investigation of psychosocial disturbances within the family usually is necessary.

MANAGEMENT

During the last decade a large body of evidence has accumulated that appears to support the positive role fever plays as a part of the host defenses. Increased leukocyte mobility, increased leukocyte bactericidal activity, enhanced interferon effect, and decreased available trace metals (notably iron) for pathogenic bacteria are just a few of the ways in which fever improves the body's ability to fight infection. In animals it has been demonstrated that the inability to mount a febrile response in the presence of infection is highly associated with increased mortality.

Provided that an appropriate evaluation has been undertaken and that specific therapy has been instituted for the underlying disease, it is legitimate to question whether it is in the best interest of the patient to eliminate fever through environmental and pharmacologic manipulations. Three factors need to be considered in answering this question: (1) the complication rate associated with fever, (2) the ability of the patient to handle the increased metabolic demands of the fever, and (3) the comfort of the patient.

Complications in children with a temperature below 105.8° F (41° C) are unusual unless the fever is associated with febrile status epilepticus or heatstroke. Of febrile seizures, 1% to 2% last longer than 15 minutes; if they continue beyond 60 minutes, they may be associated with severe brain damage (probably resulting from hypoxia). Heatstroke is uncommon in childhood and usually is associated with a temperature higher than 107.6° F (42° C), coma, and anhidrosis; it has a mortality rate of 80%. In both these instances it is obvious that body temperature should be decreased. Children with a seizure disorder may have an exacerbation of their seizures in the presence of fever and, therefore, may benefit from antipyretic management.

The child who has limited cardiopulmonary reserve, as might occur in congenital heart disease, cardiac infections, cystic fibrosis, or asthma, should be kept as normothermic as possible in spite of some of the benefits of fever in fighting disease. The high metabolic demand induced by fever may otherwise result in irreversible decompensation and death.

Although many children exhibit no discomfort until the temperature is higher than 102° to 104° F (39° to 40° C), discomfort at lower temperatures may be treated with antipyretic therapy. If the child is comfortable, no treatment is necessary up to a temperature of 105.8° F (41° C), except for the administration of additional fluids to prevent dehydration. A complete discussion of antipyretic therapy is provided in Chapter 23.

Finally, it is very important to provide sound education to parents about fever—its definition and meaning, its benefits and disadvantages, when to be concerned about it as an indicator of serious disease, its initial home management, including proper dosing with antipyretics, and when to contact the physician. Such education has been shown to improve home management and to enhance parental confidence in caring for their febrile child.[11]

SUMMARY

Although fever can be a frightening symptom that may be associated with serious illness, its treatment is much less crucial than the evaluation and treatment of the illness causing the fever. It is the responsibility of health care professionals to educate parents about the proper management of their febrile child, emphasizing their role in the observation for symptoms that are more likely to be associated with serious disease. Fever is but one symptom that should be evaluated in the total context of the care of the patient.

REFERENCES

1. Baker RC et al: Severity of disease correlated with fever reduction in febrile infants, Pediatrics 83:1016, 1989.
2. Berkowitz CD et al: Fever in infants less than two months of age: spectrum of disease and predictors of outcome, Pediatr Emerg Care 1:128, 1985.
3. Dagan R et al: Identification of infants unlikely to have serious bacterial infection although hospitalized for suspected sepsis, J Pediatr 107:855, 1985.
4. Donaldson JF: Therapy of acute fever: a comparative approach, Hosp Pract 16:125, 1981.
5. Heulitt MJ et al: Febrile infants less than 3 months old: value of chest radiography, Radiology 167:135, 1988.
6. Krober MS et al: Bacterial and viral pathogens causing fever in infants less than 3 months old, Am J Dis Child 139:889, 1985.
7. McCarthy PL: Controversies in pediatrics: what tests are indicated for the child under two with fever, Pediatr Rev 1:51, 1979.
8. McCarthy PL and Dolan T: The serious implications of high fever in infants during their first three months, Clin Pediatr 15:794, 1976.
9. McCarthy PL et al: Observation scales to identify serious illness in febrile children, Pediatrics 70:802, 1982.
10. Roberts KB and Borzy MS: Fever in the first eight weeks of life, Johns Hopkins Med J 141:9, 1977.
11. Robinson JS et al: The impact of fever health education on clinic utilization, Am J Dis Child 143:698, 1989.
12. Shinozaki T, Deane R, and Perkins FM: Infrared tympanic thermometer: evaluation of a new clinical thermometer, Crit Care Med 16:148, 1988.
13. Teele DW, Marshall R, and Klein JO: Unsuspected bacteremia in young children, Pediatr Clin North Am 26:773, 1979.
14. Voora S et al: Fever in full-term newborns in the first four days of life, Pediatrics 69:40, 1982.

SUGGESTED READINGS

Cone TE: Diagnosis and treatment: children with fevers, Pediatrics 43:290, 1969.

Dagan R et al: Epidemiology and laboratory diagnosis of infection with viral and bacterial pathogens in infants hospitalized for suspected sepsis, J Pediatr 115:351, 1989.

Dinarello CA, Cannon JG, and Wolff SM: New concepts on the pathogenesis of fever, Rev Infect Dis 10:168, 1988.

Jaffe DM et al: Antibiotic administration to treat possible occult bacteremia in febrile children, N Engl J Med 317:1175, 1987.

Kluger MJ: Fever, Pediatrics 66:720, 1980.

Kramer MS, Naimark L, and Leduc DG: Parental fever phobia and its correlates, Pediatrics 75:1110, 1985.

Schmitt BD: Fever phobia, Am J Dis Child 134:176, 1980.

132

Fever of Unknown Origin

Élise W. van der Jagt

One of the more frustrating symptoms for the clinician to evaluate is that of a fever without a discernible cause. Because fever suggests disease, the inability to identify its cause strikes at the physician's *raison d'etre* and may undermine any credibility he or she previously had established with the patient and family. The longer the fever persists, the more concern is raised by the family and the more plentiful the demands made on the physician. A fever that is of only a few days' duration and that is not associated with any localizing signs or symptoms frequently does not even come to a physician's attention unless the child appears quite ill. Fever that continues beyond 5 to 7 days, however, alarms parents sufficiently to prompt a medical consultation. It is these more prolonged fevers and their evaluation that are discussed here.

DEFINITION

The classic definition for a fever of unknown origin (FUO) was proposed by Petersdorf and Beeson[5] in 1961 to be a fever (1) that is higher than 38.3° C on several occasions, (2) that is present for more than 3 weeks, and (3) whose cause is still unexplained after 1 week of evaluation in the hospital. This definition, based on a study of adult patients, has not been completely accepted by most pediatricians, who would prefer not to delay evaluation for 3 weeks. Therefore, an FUO in children has been defined as (1) a fever greater than 38.3° C, (2) lasting for at least 2 weeks, (3) whose cause has not been elicited by simple diagnostic tests, including a good history and physical examination.[2] Some would add that 1 of the 2 weeks of fever should be documented in the hospital.

Careful documentation of fever is necessary before labeling a child with a diagnosis of FUO. A thorough explanation of the range of normal core body temperature for age, with its diurnal variation, may help in excluding patients who are not truly febrile but who instead have a high normal body temperature. The physician should instruct the parents in the technique of taking a rectal temperature and define a day of fever as a 24-hour period in which a temperature greater than 38.3° C occurs at least once. All medications taken and the various activities participated in during this time should be recorded, because these may affect body temperature. However, although in the past much importance has been attached to fever patterns (i.e., remittent, intermittent, sustained), it is not necessary to detail them, since they are rarely diagnostic of a specific disease.[4]

Careful documentation of fever will help to exclude what Kleiman[3] has termed a pseudo-FUO. Children with a pseudo-FUO do not have a true fever when measured accurately and consistently (at times this needs to be done under hospital supervision), but do exhibit a definite constellation of findings that is recognizable and many times diagnostic (see the accompanying box). In addition to the inability to document fever and in the face of a completely normal physical examination, the parents may tell of a previous serious illness and their concerns about its recurrence or lasting effect ("vulnerable child syndrome"). Their child may have missed an excessive amount of school, which does not correlate with the stated degree of illness, but which is associated with fatigue, abdominal pain, and headache in the morning (yet not during the rest of the day). Finally, a sequence of minor illnesses may have occurred, mimicking a single, continuous illness. Only careful questioning and record keeping will clarify this and reassure the parents.

DIFFERENTIAL DIAGNOSIS

The box on p. 929 lists causes of FUO in children. The causes are subdivided into four large categories: infectious diseases, collagen-vascular diseases, malignancies, and miscellaneous. It is clear from this list that the majority of FUOs are even-

Characteristics of the Child with Pseudo-FUO

1. Absence of documented, persistent fever
2. Lack of objective, abnormal physical findings
3. History of significant or near-fatal illness
4. Parental fear of malignant or crippling disease
5. Frequent environmental exposure to illness
6. Absence of persistent weight loss
7. Normal erythrocyte sedimentation rate and platelet count
8. Large number of missed school days because of subjective morning complaints
9. Discordance of fever and pulse rate
10. Medical or paramedical family background
11. Majority have, singly or in sequence, mild self-limited diseases, behavioral problems, parents with misconceptions concerning health and disease, or families under stress

From Kleiman MB: The complaint of persistent fever, Pediatr Clin North Am 29:201, 1982.

Causes of Fever of Unknown Origin in Children

INFECTIOUS DISEASES

Bacterial
- Brucellosis
- Bacterial endocarditis
- Leptospirosis
- Liver abscess
- Mastoiditis (chronic)
- Osteomyelitis
- Pelvic abscess
- Perinephric abscess
- Pyelonephritis
- Salmonellosis
- Sinusitis
- Subdiaphragmatic abscess
- Tuberculosis
- Tularemia

Viral
- Cytomegalovirus
- Hepatitis viruses
- Epstein-Barr virus (Infectious mononucleosis)

Chlamydial
- Lymphogranuloma venereum
- Psittacosis

Rickettsial
- Q fever
- Rocky Mountain spotted fever

Fungal
- Blastomycosis (nonpulmonary)
- Histoplasmosis (disseminated)

INFECTIOUS DISEASES—cont'd

Parasitic
- Malaria
- Toxoplasmosis
- Visceral larva migrans

Unclassified
- Sarcoidosis

COLLAGEN-VASCULAR DISEASES

Juvenile rheumatoid arthritis
Polyarteritis nodosa
Systemic lupus erythematosus

MALIGNANCIES

Hodgkin disease
Leukemia-lymphoma
Neuroblastoma

MISCELLANEOUS

Central diabetes insipidus
Drug fever
Ectodermal dysplasia
Factitious fever
Familial dysautonomia
Granulomatous colitis
Infantile cortical hyperostosis
Nephrogenic diabetes insipidus
Pancreatitis
Periodic fever
Serum sickness
Thyrotoxicosis
Ulcerative colitis

From Feigin RD and Cherry JD: Textbook of pediatric infectious diseases, ed 2, Philadelphia, 1987, WB Saunders Co, p 1057.

tually found to be caused by common pediatric illnesses that are either self-limited or treatable.

An infectious illness is the most common cause for an FUO in children, making up as many as 60% of the reported cases; the second most common cause is collagen-vascular disease, making up about 20% of the cases. Children under 6 years of age are more likely to have an FUO resulting from an infection, whereas collagen-vascular diseases are much more frequently found in children older than 6 years (Table 132-1). Although the majority of infections that manifest themselves as an FUO are an atypical or incomplete presentation of a common infectious disease, unusual infections should be considered. The appearance and increased incidence of human immunodeficiency virus (HIV) infection with its associated acquired immunodeficiency syndrome (AIDS) during the 1980s, should encourage the pediatrician to consider this diagnosis and assess the child carefully for the presence of known risk factors (parental intravenous drug abuse, parental promiscuity, parental sexual contact with individuals who may be HIV positive, an HIV-positive mother, hemophilia requiring transfusion of blood products) and characteristic physical signs and symptoms. Fever alone is not usually the sole manifestation of HIV infection. However, HIV infection should be considered and the appropriate laboratory tests performed if the fever has been present for more than 2 months *and* is associated with one or more of the following: failure to thrive or a weight loss of more than 10% from baseline, hepatomegaly, splenomegaly, generalized lymphadenopathy (lymph nodes measuring at least 0.5 cm present in two or more sites, with bilateral lymph nodes counting as one site), parotitis, and diarrhea that is either persistent or recurrent.[1]

Of the collagen-vascular diseases, juvenile rheumatoid arthritis is the most common. Fever is associated almost 100% of the time with systemic onset juvenile rheumatoid arthritis, frequently preceding the joint manifestations by weeks or months. The typical double quotidian fever (two fever spikes in 24 hours with a normal temperature in between) is a helpful clue to this diagnosis. Other inflammatory diseases that should be considered are lupus erythematosus and regional enteritis. The latter is more common among children over 6 years of age.

Table 132-1 *Diagnosis of Prolonged Fever, Children's Hospital Medical Center, Boston*[6]

AGE	INFECTION "VIRAL"	INFECTION NONVIRAL	COLLAGEN	MALIGNANCY	MISCELLANEOUS	NO DIAGNOSIS	TOTALS
<6 yr	14 (27%)	20 (38%)	4 (8%)	4 (8%)	7 (13%)	3 (6%)	52
>6 yr	7 (15%)	11 (23%)	16 (33%)	2 (4%)	3 (6%)	9 (19%)	48
TOTALS	21	31	20	6	10	12	100

Malignancy, the most anxiety-producing diagnosis, is present in only a small percentage of patients in most studies (1.5% to 6%). This is in contrast to adults with an FUO, of whom 19% are found to have a neoplastic process. Most common in children is leukemia, although solid tumors such as lymphoma, hypernephroma, and hepatoma have all been described. The exact reason for fever in these diseases is unclear, but may be related to endogenous pyrogen produced by the neoplastic cells.

As can be seen from the box on p. 929, there is a whole spectrum of miscellaneous diseases that can cause fevers. In as many as 25% of patients with prolonged fever, however, a true diagnosis is never obtained. These are the genuine FUOs. The majority of these patients appear to do well, and the fever eventually disappears after months or even years.

EVALUATION

Whether the child has a true FUO or a pseudo-FUO cannot be determined without a thorough and precise history and physical examination, with the physician paying close attention to behavioral, social, and environmental factors. Information regarding travel, animal exposure, frequency of exposure to other persons with common febrile illnesses, previous illness, hospitalizations, drug treatments, family history of disease, and the precise course of the presenting symptoms must be obtained methodically and efficiently.

For children over 11 to 12 years of age, a separate interview is indicated to obtain the child's perspective on the illness and to uncover information that may be difficult to express in the presence of parents. School, peer relationships, family functioning, and sexual identity and activity should all be explored.

Once a complete history has been taken, a full physical examination must be performed. Rectal temperature, respiratory rate, heart rate, and blood pressure measurements should not be forgotten. Any discrepancy between heart rate and temperature should suggest factitious fever. A careful examination of the respiratory tract is indicated. Inspection of the pharynx for hyperemia and exudate and the tympanic membranes for chronic otitis media, transillumination of the sinuses for sinusitis, a search for a purulent nasal discharge, and auscultation of the chest for localized wheezing are all important. In the older child, an examination of the teeth to exclude caries and periodontal disease must be included. A new cardiac murmur may be a clue to rheumatic fever or infective endocarditis. Lymphadenopathy, especially if generalized, may suggest a viral infection, such as infectious mononucleosis, cytomegalovirus infection, toxoplasmosis, or HIV infection. Joints must be meticulously examined for swelling, restricted range of motion, and tenderness. Skin rashes may suggest a viral disease or a collagen-vascular disease such as juvenile rheumatoid arthritis. Absence of sweating and a smooth tongue are consistent with familial dysautonomia, a rare genetic disorder of thermoregulation. Finally, a rectal examination with stool guaiac is imperative, because pararectal lymphadenopathy may suggest a pelvic infection and a positive stool guaiac might be consistent with inflammatory bowel disease.

If the history and physical examination disclose no specific findings, simple diagnostic tests are indicated. Routine blood counts and urinalysis have not been shown to be of major benefit, although no one actively advocates their elimination from the workup. A PPD (tuberculin skin test) should be placed to detect tuberculosis, although anergy may occur in active tuberculosis infection. Negative blood, urine, and throat cultures will exclude infections of these areas.

Probably the most useful laboratory tests, however, are the erythrocyte sedimentation rate (ESR) and the albumin/globulin ratio. If the ESR is over 30 or the albumin/globulin ratio is inverted, a high probability of serious disease exists—particularly a collagen-vascular disease or a malignancy—and further evaluation should be pursued vigorously.

How the evaluation should then proceed is variable; it should be individualized. Because infectious causes are the most common, it is reasonable to pursue special serologic tests for such diseases as hepatitis, Epstein-Barr virus infection (infectious mononucleosis), toxoplasmosis, and cytomegalovirus infection. Radioactive gallium scans may be useful in detecting occult abscesses and infections. Total body computed tomography scans may help to delineate tumors. Radiologic studies of the sinuses, the gastrointestinal tract, and the chest may all be appropriate in certain individuals. A bone marrow examination may help in the diagnosis of tuberculosis, leukemia, metastatic cancer, or fungal infections. Finally, if the child is not visibly deteriorating, a period of observation may be necessary until new findings appear that can give more direction.

If the ESR and the albumin/globulin ratio are normal, there is little to be gained from any of the previously mentioned tests. Observation and periodic evaluation are all that are required while remaining alert for the occurrence of new symptoms or signs that might lead the investigation in a specific direction.

SUMMARY

The evaluation of the child with an FUO must be individualized to accommodate the history, the physical examination, and the particular social environment in which the child and family live. An intensive examination of all these factors is the physician's responsibility and is the first stage of management of the patient. Whether hospitalization is part of this approach depends ultimately on the amount of parental anxiety, the necessity to document fever, and the performance of diagnostic tests that cannot be done on an outpatient basis.

REFERENCES

1. Centers for Disease Control: Classification system for human immunodeficiency virus (HIV) infection in children under 13 years of age, MMWR 36(15):225, 1987.
2. Feigin RD and Shearer WT: Fever of unknown origin in children, Curr Probl Pediatr 6:1, 1976.
3. Kleiman MB: The complaint of persistent fever, Pediatr Clin North Am 29:201, 1982.
4. Musher DM et al: Fever patterns—their lack of clinical significance, Arch Intern Med 139:1225, 1979.
5. Petersdorf RG and Beeson PB: Fever of unexplained origin: report on 100 cases, Medicine 40:1, 1961.
6. Pizzo PA, Lovejoy FH, and Smith DH: Prolonged fever in children: review of 100 cases, Pediatrics 55:468, 1975.

SUGGESTED READING

Lohr JA and Hendley JO: Prolonged fever of unknown origin—a record of experiences with 54 childhood patients, Clin Pediatr 16:768, 1977.

133

Foot and Leg Problems

Robert A. Hoekelman

Pediatricians and family practitioners often have to make judgments concerning actual or presumed problems of the feet and legs in infants and children. The frequency of these problems is such that referral to orthopedic consultants is not always appropriate. In most instances the problems presented require no treatment, others can be managed easily without consultations, and only a few require the services of an orthopedist.

The "ped" in pediatrics and orthopedics is derived from the Greek word *paidios*, meaning child, not from the Latin *pedalis* or French *ped*, meaning foot. Therefore, pediatrics is the medicine (Greek *iatrike*) of the child, and orthopedics is the straightening or correction (Greek *orthos*) of deformities of children. Orthopedics has expanded its scope well beyond this initial thrust; nevertheless, the orthopedist and the pediatrician are concerned with many problems involving the feet of children.

SHOES

Anatomy of the Shoe

Because some foot problems in childhood are treated with corrective shoes, understanding the anatomy of the shoe is necessary. The *last* is the wooden or metal form on which a shoe is constructed. Shoes for regular use are built on a straight last; shoes designed to deviate the forefoot outward are built on an out-flare last; and those designed to deviate the forefoot inward built on an in-flare last. Actually, most of the shoes sold for general use in the United States have an adducted forefoot last rather than a truly straight last.

The *sole* is that part of the shoe which covers the ventral surface of the foot. It consists of the *outsole*, usually made of firm leather or rubber that comes in contact with the surface on which the shoe is placed, and the *insole*, made of soft leather or synthetic material that comes in contact with the plantar surface of the foot. The *heel*, also made of leather, rubber, or synthetic material, elevates the rear portion of the shoe. It is usually absent in the shoes of infants and toddlers. It may be low and flat (commonsense), somewhat higher (military), or more elevated and tapered (Cuban or high). The Thomas heel is of medium height with a forward medial extension.

The *shank* of the shoe is that part of the sole between the forwardmost edge of the heel and ball of the foot. A narrow flat piece of steel is sometimes placed between the inner and outer soles to prevent flexion of the shank of the shoe. The *counter* of the shoe is placed above the heel between the outsole and insole and provides a shelf for the rear portion of the foot. It is usually made of firm leather and may be extended forward on the medial aspect of the shoe to provide added support to the instep. The *upper* or top of the shoe may be made of leather or a variety of other materials. The upper of low shoes (Oxfords) rises to a point below the malleoli, and the upper of high shoes extends above the malleoli. The *vamp* is the part of the upper that is attached to the sole.

Functions of Shoes

The physician is often asked by parents when their child should begin wearing shoes and the kind of shoe that should be worn. In answering these questions, the reasons for wearing shoes must be borne in mind. The shoe has two functions, the most important of which is protection of the feet from trauma and temperature change. Protection implies comfort; therefore the shoe must fit properly to avoid discomfort. The second function of the shoe is to provide style. Older children will often sacrifice comfort for style despite parental or medical advice to the contrary.

Support to the foot and ankle is *not* a function of the shoe except when a pathologic condition is present. Low shoes with soft uppers are worn by athletes in all sports that place the feet and ankles under severe strain. Ski boots are worn not to support the foot and ankle but to make them "one with the ski," to ensure response to movements originating in the knee and lower leg. High shoes are usually worn by babies and toddlers not to provide support to the foot and ankle, but to make it more difficult for the child to remove the shoes.

Except for style, there is no reason for a baby to wear shoes at all until he or she begins walking outdoors or is taken out in cold weather. Some babies may gain a certain degree of stability from hard-sole shoes when beginning to stand, but this has not been shown to enhance learning to walk. Properly fitting shoes with firm soles and soft uppers should be recommended initially and subsequently. They need not be expensive. Sneakers are perfectly adequate for summer wear and for winter indoor wear.

Fitting Shoes

There is no great science to determining the proper fitting of shoes. The counter should hug the heel snugly, the length should allow ¾ inch between the tip of the great toe and the front end of the upper, and there should be ¼ inch between the edge of the fifth toe and the lateral edge of the upper when the foot is pushed medially within the shoe. These measurements should be made with the child standing and should apply only to the time the shoes are newly acquired. There is no reason why shoes in good condition cannot be handed down from one child to another.

The frequency with which shoes should be changed depends on the rate of growth of the feet, the quality of the shoes, and the degree of their use. Parents are usually able to tell when shoes become too small (or rather, feet become too large) without professional advice. The toes will be felt to press against the front end of the upper, and there will be increasing difficulty in getting the shoes on or having the child keep them on.

Lightweight cotton, nylon, or wool socks that adjust to the length and width of the foot present no problem in the attainment of maximal foot comfort for children of all ages.

ORTHOPEDIC TERMINOLOGY

Certain terms are used by practitioners to describe positional variations of the lower extremities and are often used in the nomenclature of specific orthopedic conditions.

In general, the joint that is primarily involved in the condition constitutes the first word; the subsequent word or words relate to the positioning of the extremity in relation to the midline of the body. For example, "coxa vara" is a condition of the hip (coxa) that results in a deviation of the leg toward the midline (varus position).

The following orthopedic terms have special reference to abnormalities of the feet (Fig. 133-1):

Talipes—congenital deformities of the foot; if untreated, result in walking on the ankle (talus)
Pes—acquired deformity of the foot
Inversion—foot twisted inward on its long axis
Eversion—foot twisted outward on its long axis
Adduction—deviation toward the midline of the body
Abduction—deviation away from the midline of the body
Varus—heel and forefoot inverted; forefoot adducted
Valgus—heel and forefoot everted; forefoot abducted
Equinus—foot plantar flexed, placing the toes below the level of the heel
Calcaneus—foot dorsiflexed, placing the heel below the level of the toes
Planus—medial longitudinal arch of the foot flattened
Cavus—medial longitudinal arch of the foot elevated

CLINICAL CONDITIONS

A variety of positional deformities of the legs and feet are encountered by the physician who provides primary care for children from birth through adolescence. The distinction between a pathologic and functional cause must be made. The former should be referred to an orthopedist for treatment. When a pathologic deformity of the legs or feet is diagnosed, the physician should look for other congenital anomalies, especially those involving the skeletal system. Most functional deformities of the legs and feet are self-correcting in time without treatment. This must be considered in weighing the results of any treatment prescribed. Unfortunately, studies of those conditions, analyzing treated versus untreated paired control patients, have not been performed; so clinicians are left to their own or others' anecdotal experiences in making therapeutic decisions in individual cases.

Clubfoot

The term *clubfoot* denotes a pathologic deformity that causes the leg and its appended foot to resemble a clubbing instrument. Two varieties occur. The more severe is *talipes equi-*

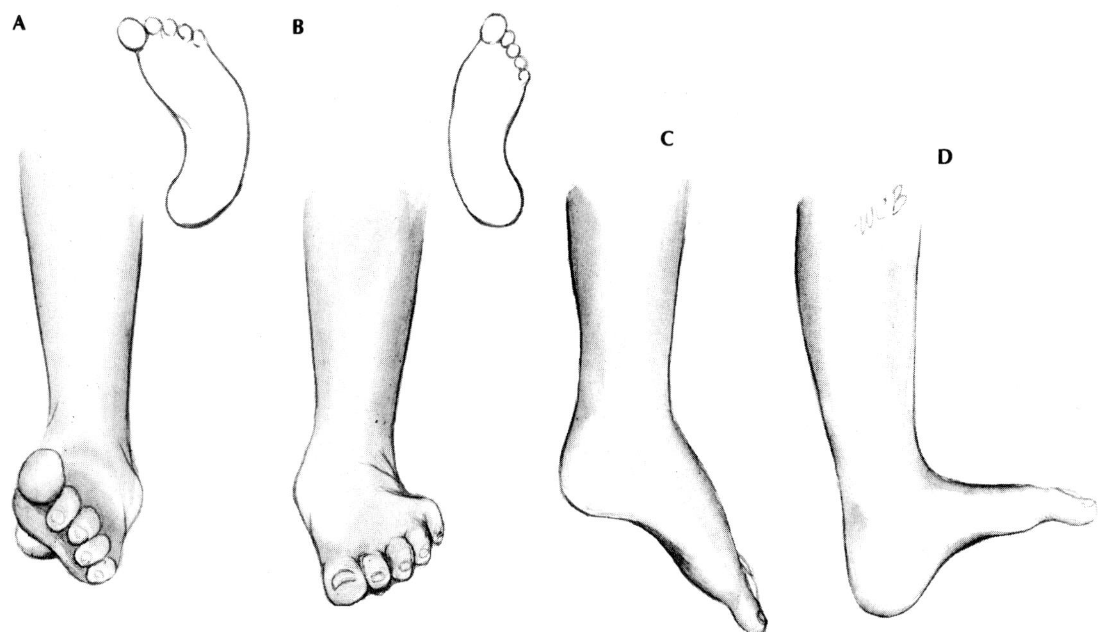

Fig. 133-1 Positional deformities of the foot and ankle. **A,** Varus. **B,** Valgus. **C,** Equinus. **D,** Calcaneus.
From Tachdjian MO: Pediatric orthopedics, 2 vols, Philadelphia, 1977, WB Saunders Co, p 1274.

novarus, in which the heel and forefoot are inverted, the forefoot is adducted, and the entire foot is plantar flexed. Fig. 133-2 shows bilateral clubfoot in a newborn, and Fig. 133-3 shows an untreated right clubfoot. The other, *talipes calcaneovalgus,* is characterized by eversion of the heel and forefoot, abduction of the forefoot, and dorsiflexion of the entire foot (Fig. 133-4). Both forms occur in about 1 of every 200 live births, are bilateral in 50% of the cases, and affect boys almost twice as frequently as girls. When present, associated neurologic, muscular, or other skeletal anomalies should be sought.

Often in the newborn period functional deformities of the feet secondary to in utero positioning will mimic both varieties of clubfoot. These can be readily differentiated in that the functionally deformed foot can easily be brought to a neutral position and overcorrected. This is not possible when pathologic deformities are present, and an orthopedic consultation should be sought immediately. Treatment with casting is usually required for initial correction. In severe cases tenotomies, muscle transplants, and arthrodeses are necessary when the child is older. Functional deformities are self-correcting and require no treatment whatsoever.

Metatarsus Varus

There is much confusion surrounding the incidence and management of metatarsus varus because there are three deformities characterized by adduction of the forefoot: talipes varus (Fig. 133-5) in which the entire foot is inverted and the forefoot is adducted, metatarsus varus (Fig. 133-6) in which the forefoot is inverted and adducted while the hind foot and heel are in the normal position, and metatarsus adductus (Fig. 133-7) in which the only finding is adduction of the metatarsals at the tarsometatarsal joints. The combined incidence of these three forefoot adductive deformities is in the neighborhood of 1 per 100 live births (the most frequent musculoskeletal congenital malformation), with metatarsus adductus being the most common and talipes varus the least common.

Talipes varus and metatarsus varus have been considered lesser degrees of clubfoot and are fixed deformities of the foot that require early treatment. The medial border of the

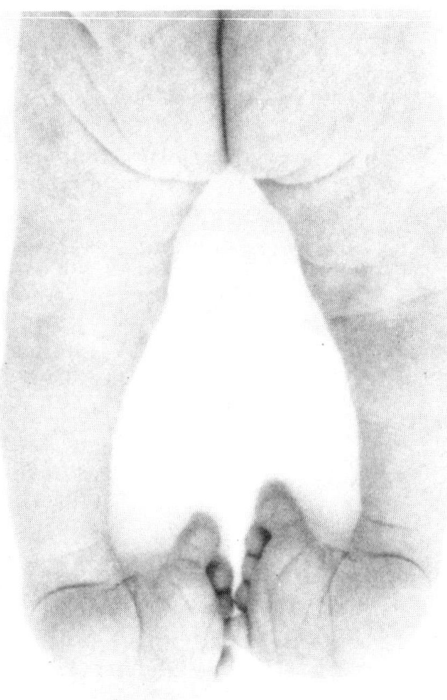

Fig. 133-2 Bilateral talipes equinovarus in a newborn infant.

From Tachdijian MO: Pediatric orthopedics, ed 2, 4 vols, Philadelphia, 1990, WB Saunders Co, p 2449.

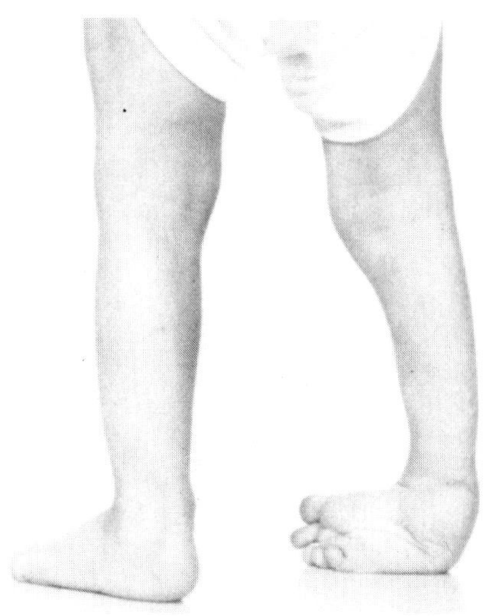

Fig. 133-3 Untreated talipes equinovarus in a 3-year-old child.

From Tachdjian MO: Pediatric orthopedics, ed 2, 4 vols, Philadelphia, 1990, WB Saunders Co, p 2450.

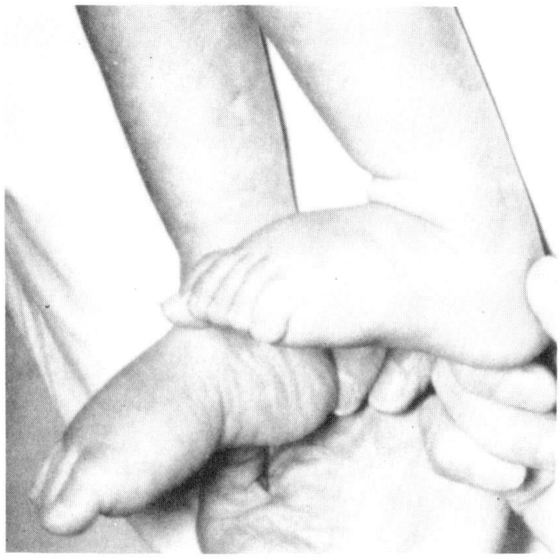

Fig. 133-4 Bilateral talipes calcaneovalgus. The left foot is held dorsiflexed and the right plantar flexed to show the range of ankle movement.

From Sharrard WJW: Paediatric orthopaedics and fractures, ed 2, Oxford, 1979, Blackwell Scientific Publications, Ltd, p 497.

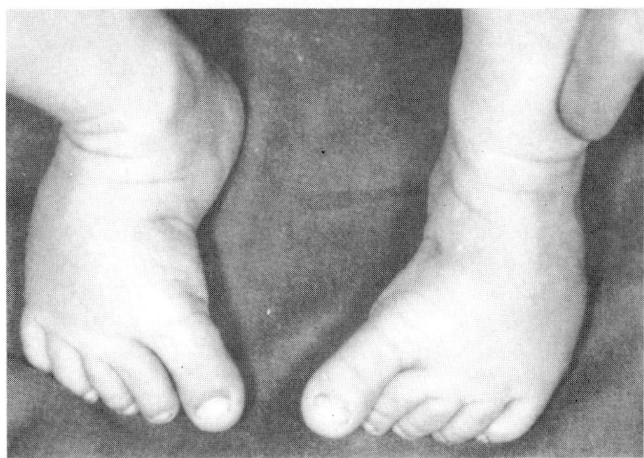

Fig. 133-5 Bilateral talipes varus. The entire foot is twisted inward on its longitudinal axis, and the forefoot is adducted.

From Tachdjian MO: Pediatric orthopedics, ed 2, 4 vols, Philadelphia, 1990, WB Saunders Co, p 2426.

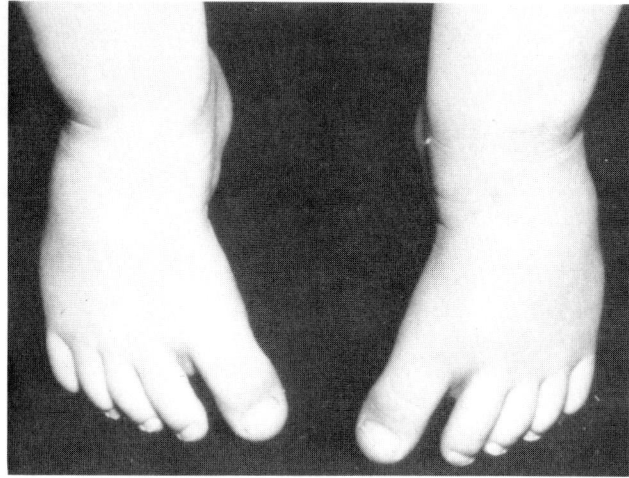

Fig. 133-6 Bilateral metatarsus varus. The forefoot is inverted and adducted, the great toe is widely separated from the second toe, and the lateral border of the foot is convex. The hindfoot is in a neutral position.

From Sharrard WJW: Paediatric orthopaedics and fractures, ed 2, Oxford, 1979, Blackwell Scientific Publications, Ltd, p 543.

foot is concave, with a widening of the space between the first and second toes and a high medial longitudinal arch. The lateral border of the foot is convex, and the base of the fifth metatarsal bone is prominent. Treatment consists of serial casting. Abduction stretching exercises and out-flare–last shoes may be used as an adjunct to cast treatment but should not be relied on as the only therapy.

Metatarsus adductus, a functional deformity, can be distinguished from the two fixed forefoot deformities by observing lateral movement of the infant's forefoot in response to stimulation of the sole. This condition requires no treatment because it corrects spontaneously, usually during the first year. Primary care physicians see metatarsus adductus frequently and observe its resolution without treatment, whereas orthopedists are more likely to see talipes varus and metatarsus through referrals, sometimes unfortunately in late infancy when treatment results are less satisfactory.

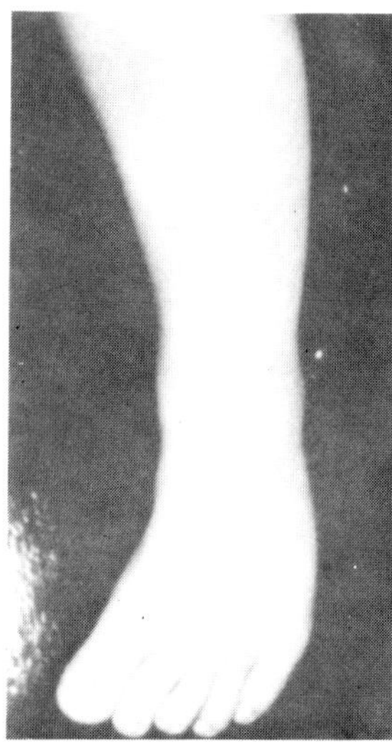

Fig. 133-7 Metatarsus adductus. The forefoot is adducted but not inverted.

From Ferguson AB: Orthopedic surgery in infancy and childhood, ed 4. © 1981, The Williams & Wilkins Co, Baltimore.

Pronation

Almost all children develop some degree of pronation during the early stages of weight-bearing. Pronation is characterized by an outward rolling of the foot with eversion of the heel and abduction of the forefoot. The Achilles tendon is seen to curve inward, and the medial longitudinal arch of the foot, observed without weight-bearing, disappears on standing. These changes occur because a wide-based stance is assumed for balance (accentuated by bulky diapers), causing the weight to be borne on the medial aspect of the feet (Fig. 133-8). Laxity of the ligaments supporting the feet contributes to pronation. Flexible foot, relaxed foot, fatfoot, and flatfoot are also used to describe this condition, leading to considerable confusion in terminology.

Pronation is transient in most children, usually disappears before 2½ years of age, and requires no treatment. In those in whom it persists, treatment is not necessary unless symptoms occur. These include aching of the feet and legs, muscle cramps in the calves at night, easy fatigability, and reluctance to participate in strenuous activity. Symptoms result from the strain caused by the child's continual attempt to shift weight-bearing laterally toward the center of the foot, bringing about some degree of toeing-in. Persistent pronation without symptoms occurs in some children who may have a family history of pronation and often demonstrate hyperextensibility of other joints, including the knees, elbows, wrists, and thumbs.

When symptoms do occur, they may be alleviated by use of corrective shoes with a long medial counter and a Thomas heel. Support to the medial longitudinal arch with a flexible felt, rubber, or leather pad placed beneath the inner sole may

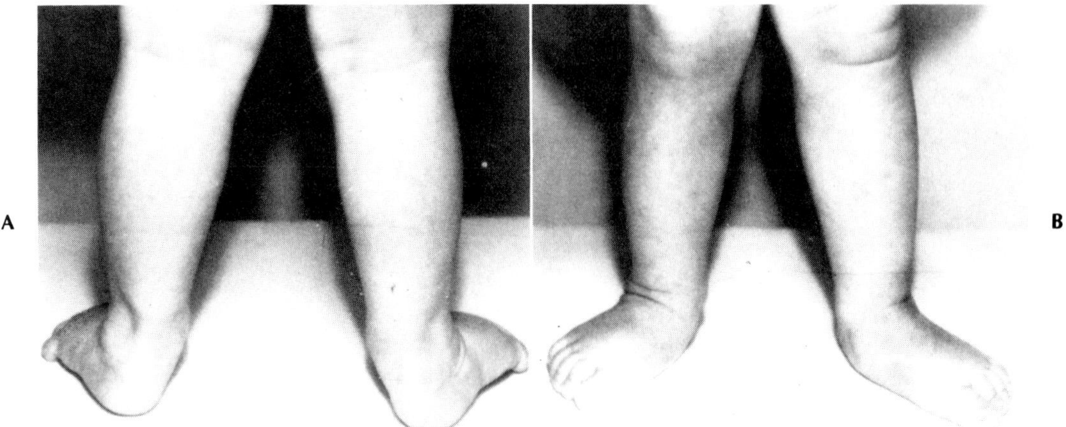

Fig. 133-8 Pronation. **A,** Viewed from behind, there is eversion of the hindfoot. **B,** Viewed from in front, there is eversion and abduction of the forefoot.

From Sharrard WJW: Paediatric orthopaedics and fractures, ed 2, Oxford, 1979, Blackwell Scientific Publications, Ltd, p 506.

help. Wedges ⅛- to 3⁄16-inch thick applied to the medial aspect of the heel and the lateral aspect of the sole of the shoe are sometimes helpful. Steel arch supports placed within the shoe are rarely required, and foot exercises are of no value. Treatment with these simple measures usually brings relief of symptoms but may need to be continued for several years until sufficient maturity of the muscles and ligaments that support the foot occurs.

Planovalgus

There are certain congenital anomalies involving the bones of the foot that will produce flattening of the medial longitudinal arch and eversion of the forefoot. These include vertical talus, accessory tarsonavicular, and fusion of one or more of the tarsal bones (tarsal coalition). The first two conditions usually can be detected in the newborn by the presence of a bony prominence on the medial and plantar aspects of the foot, with limitation of plantar flexion and inversion of the forefoot. Surgical correction should be accomplished early in infancy.

Tarsal conditions usually are not detected until late childhood or adolescence, when they produce pain with walking and inability to invert the foot. The foot is held in a pronated position with eversion of the forefoot. The peroneal tendons stand out prominently when attempts are made to invert the foot. This condition, commonly called spastic flatfoot, is not related etiologically to simple pronation. Treatment in most cases is symptomatic with orthopedic shoes. Surgical correction, usually performed in adulthood, is necessary in only about 10% of cases.

The incidence of pes planovalgus is unknown. Vertical talus and accessory tarsonavicular are very rare. Tarsal coalitions probably occur in 1% of the population and are usually hereditary.

Pes Cavus

Pes cavus is manifested by an equinus deformity of the forefoot in relation to the hindfoot, producing a high medial longitudinal arch (Fig. 133-9). It is referred to as clawfoot when associated with flexion deformities of the toes. The primary pathology is neuromuscular rather than bony, with weakness or paralysis of the intrinsic muscles of the foot and its dorsiflexors, leading to the deformity over time. It is therefore not seen at birth and usually does not manifest itself clinically until late childhood or adulthood, depending on the underlying neuromuscular disease.

Pes cavus is seen in muscular dystrophy, peripheral neuropathies, and disease of the spinal cord, brainstem, and cerebral cortex. Cerebral palsy, meningomyelocele, poliomyelitis, Charcot-Marie-Tooth disease, and Friedreich ataxia are examples of conditions of neurologic origin that produce pes cavus as a late manifestation. Because of the variety of conditions in which pes cavus is seen and its variability as a manifestation of some of these, its incidence in the general population is not known. A family history of pes cavus should be sought because many of the conditions producing this deformity are inherited.

Early treatment includes exercises designed to strengthen the affected muscles and the application of metatarsal pads to the innersoles of the shoes or metatarsal bars to the outersoles. Surgical correction of the fixed deformities, including plantar fasciotomy, tendon transplants, osteotomies, and arthrodeses, may be required later.

Toe-Walking

Walking on the toes or the ball of the foot is a variation of normal gait for many children as they begin to walk. This usually progresses to a toe-heel gait and eventually to the normal heel-toe gait pattern within 3 to 6 months. Reassurance to parents is all that is required.

A congenitally short tendocalcaneus will cause persistent toe-walking even though the child can toe-heel and heel-toe walk. These latter gaits are awkward and are less comfortable for the child until he or she is 6 to 8 years of age, when toe-walking disappears. No treatment is required.

As with pes cavus, certain rare muscular, peripheral, spi-

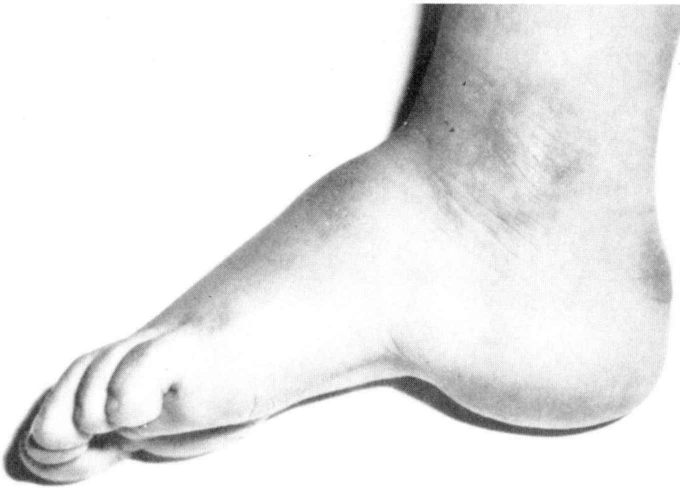

Fig. 133-9 Pes cavus, viewed from the outer side. There is abnormal height of the medial and lateral longitudinal arch.
From Sharrard WJW: Paediatric orthopaedics and fractures, ed 2, Oxford, 1979, Blackwell Scientific Publications, Ltd, p 488.

nal, and central neurologic diseases should be ruled out when toe-walking persists beyond 2 years of age.

Bowed Legs and Knocked Knees

From birth until 18 months of age there is normally a distinct bowing of the lower extremities. This is followed by a transitional period over the next year or so, during which a knocked knee pattern assumes prominence. This persists until later childhood or early adolescence when a balancing and straightening occur spontaneously. Physicians must be aware of this normal developmental pattern to avoid unnecessary treatment of mild to moderate degrees of bowed legs and knocked knees. However, marked degrees of these conditions require investigation to rule out underlying disease that can result in permanent deformity.

Bowing of the legs (genu varum) when extreme or unilateral requires roentgenographic examination to exclude rickets, dyschondroplasia, osteogenesis imperfecta, osteochondritis (Blount disease), or injury to the medial proximal epiphysis of the tibia. Extreme degrees of physiologic bowing of the legs may occur in the young child and resolve over time without treatment (Fig. 133-10).

Knocking of the knees (genu valgum) is often associated with pronation and is more apt to be marked in the child who is overweight. The degrees of knocked knee can be gauged by measuring the distance between the medial malleoli when the child is standing with the knees approximated (Fig. 133-11). Injury to the lateral proximal tibial epiphysis can cause unilateral genu valgum (Fig. 133-12). As with extreme bowing, underlying generalized diseases of the bone can cause marked bilateral genu valgum.

Treatment of severe bowing or knocking of the knees caused by underlying disease is determined by the nature of the condition and may include wedge osteotomy or epiphyseal stapling.

Toeing-In and Toeing-Out

Toeing-in (pigeon toe) and toeing-out (slew foot) are frequently seen at all ages and are caused by a variety of conditions affecting the feet, ankles, legs, knees, and hips. Toeing-in is more common than toeing-out and is more likely to be caused by benign conditions. Protective or compensatory shifting of the body weight to the middle or outside of the foot in pronation and knocked knee, both normal developmental stages, is the most common cause of toeing-in and corrects itself in time.

Developmental bowing of the legs, also self-correcting, may lead to temporary toeing-in. Talipes equinovarus and metatarsus varus are associated with toeing-in, whereas toeing-out is seen with calcaneovalgus and pes planovalgus. Spasticity of the internal rotator muscles of the hip, as seen in cerebral palsy, produces toeing-in; and flaccid paralysis of these muscles results in toeing-out. Anterior and posterior maldirections of the acetabulum produce toeing-in and toeing-out, respectively. The remaining causes of both are related to internal or external torsion of the tibia and femur.

In general, if in cases of toeing-in the child's patellae are noted to be rotated inward while walking, the underlying problem is above the knee; if they face straight forward, the underlying problem is below the knee.

Tibial Torsion. During fetal life the tibia is rotated inward on its longitudinal axis relative to the transverse axes of the knee and ankle joints. At birth, it reaches a neutral position and thereafter gradually rotates outward, reaching 20 degrees of lateral torsion by the time walking is fully established and 23 degrees by adulthood. The degree of internal and external tibial torsion can be determined by observing the relative position of the medial and lateral malleoli while the child is sitting on the edge of a table or chair with the legs dangling, the patellae facing forward, and the feet in their relaxed position (Fig. 133-13). The medial malleolus is placed posterior to the lateral malleolus in internal tibial torsion and anterior to it in external torsion.

Exact measurement of the degree of torsion can be made radiographically or with special instruments but is not required in most cases. The incidence of internal tibial torsion is 12% at birth. This gradually diminishes to near zero at 2 years of age. External tibial torsion develops in most babies shortly after birth and is almost universal by age 2 years. Pathologic

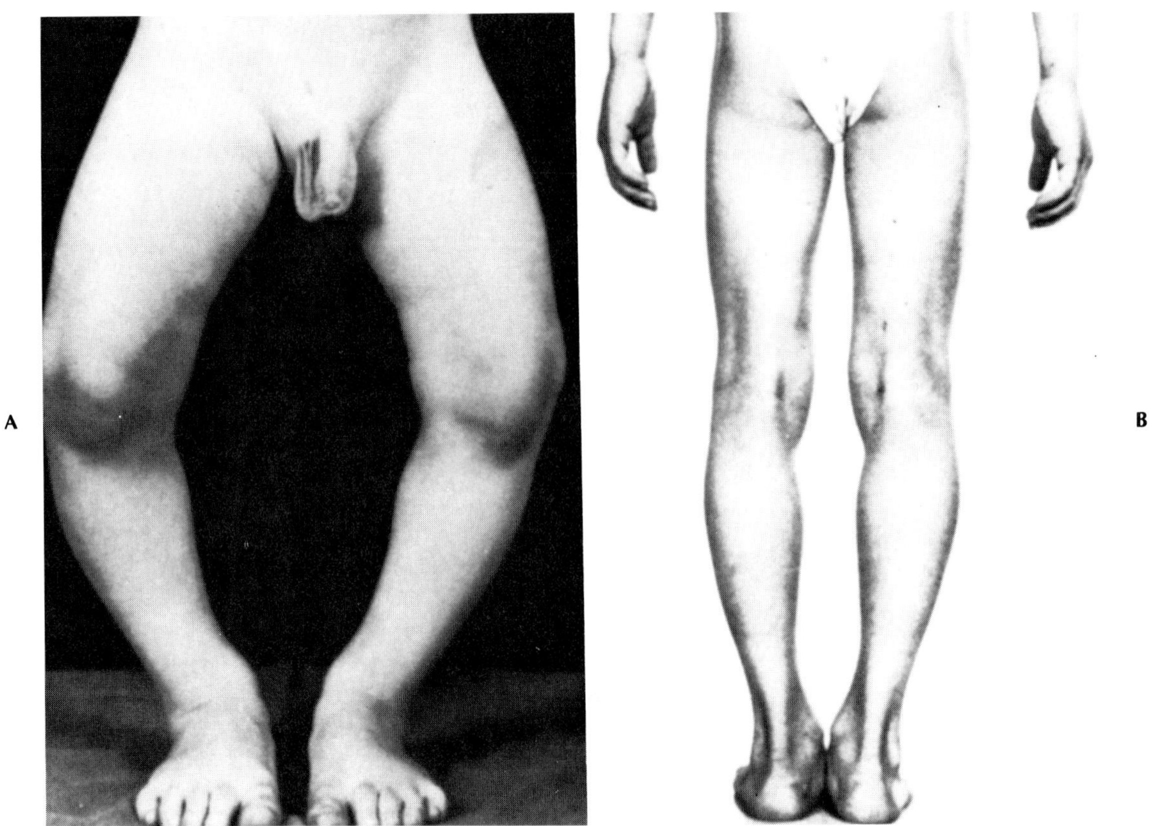

Fig. 133-10 A, Extreme physiologic bowing of the legs at age 18 months. **B,** Spontaneous resolution over time (age 7 years).
From Sharrard WJW: Paediatric orthopaedics and fractures, Oxford, 1971, Blackwell Scientific Publications, Ltd, p 488.

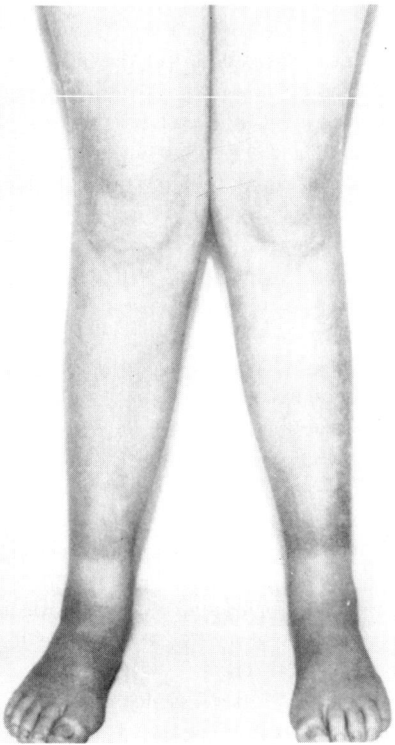

Fig. 133-11 Marked degree of physiologic genu valgum. At age 11 years the distance between the medial malleoli measured 4 inches.
From Sharrard WJW: Paediatric orthopaedics and fractures, ed 2, Oxford, 1979, Blackwell Scientific Publications, Ltd, p 456.

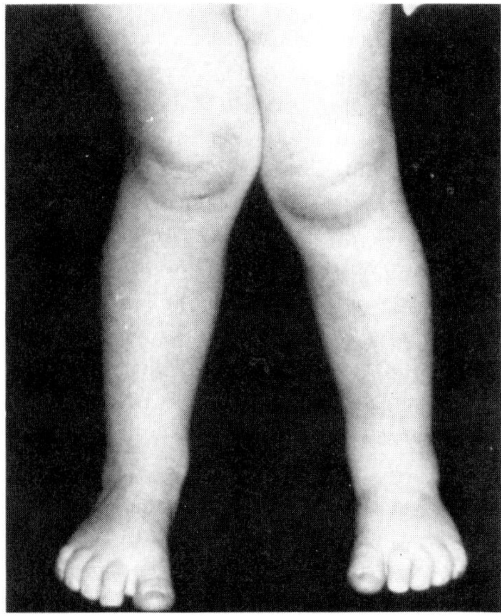

Fig. 133-12 Unilateral genu valgum caused by previous injury to the lateral aspect of the right proximal tibial epiphysis.
From Sharrard WJW: Paediatric orthopaedics and fractures, ed 2, Oxford, 1979, Blackwell Scientific Publications, Ltd, p 454.

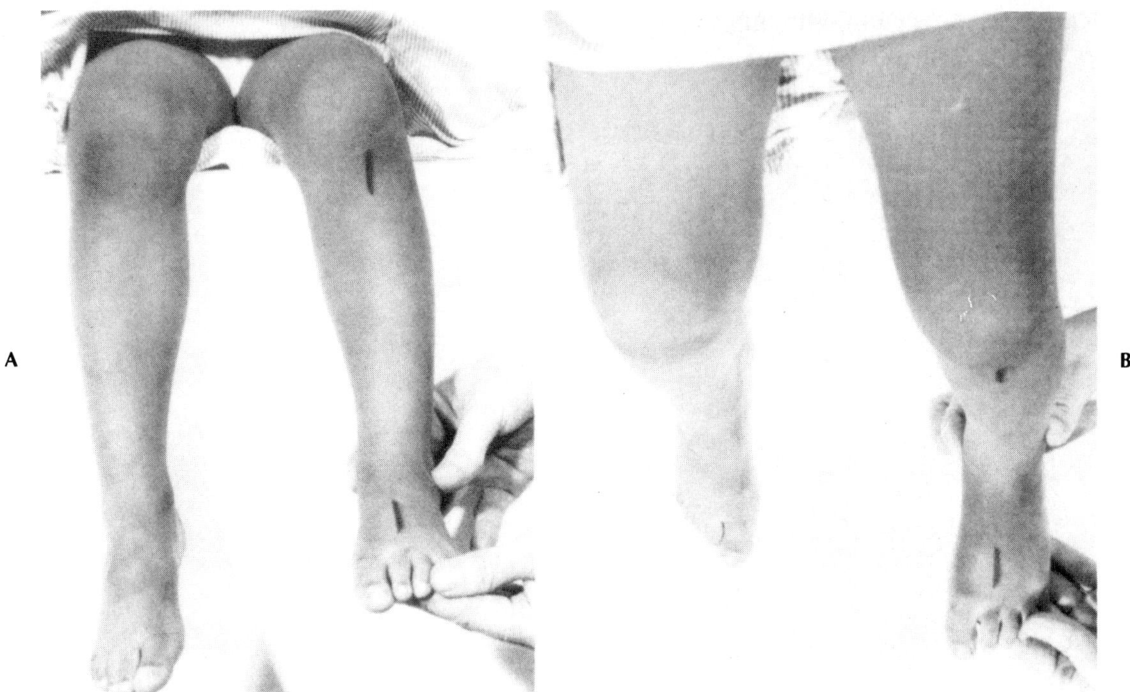

Fig. 133-13 Testing for tibial torsion. **A,** The patient is seated on the examining table with the knees flexed at 90 degrees and the legs hanging over the edge. A mark is drawn along the longitudinal axis of the tibia through the proximal tibial tubercle. Another mark is drawn over the second metatarsal bisecting the foot. The two marks are then aligned. **B,** With the left hand holding the foot in this neutral position, the thumb of the right hand is placed over the lateral malleolus and the forefinger over the medial malleolus. The angle at which an imaginary line joining the malleoli intersects the longitudinal axis will approximate the degree of internal or external tibial torsion.

From Tachdjian MO: Pediatric orthopedics, ed 2, vol 4, Philadelphia, 1990, WB Saunders Co, p 2814.

degrees of internal and external tibial torsion are found only in association with deformities of the feet, ankles, knees, and hips or as a result of improperly applied casts, braces, or Denis Browne splints.

Treatment of primary internal tibial torsion is not required in most cases. Occasionally, if a child trips on his or her feet and falls frequently or if parents are unduly concerned over toeing-in, passive stretching exercises (externally rotating the foot at the ankle), corrective shoes (Thomas heel, longitudinal arch pad, inner-heel and outsole wedges), or application of torque heels may be prescribed. Denis Browne splints should not be used without orthopedic consultation because they may create abnormal stress on the hip joint. Derotation osteotomy of the tibia is rarely required and then almost always when tibial torsion is associated with other orthopedic anomalies of the lower extremity.

Femoral Torsion. The proximal portion of the femur rotates on its longitudinal axis in relation to the transverse plane of the knee when the femoral neck is twisted anteriorly (anteversion) or posteriorly (retroversion) in relation to the femoral condyles. Anteversion produces "kissing knees," toeing-in, and a clumsy gait (Fig. 133-14). With the patella in neutral position, the greater trochanter of the femur lies posterior to the lateral, longitudinal midthigh line. There is decreased external rotation and increased internal rotation of the hip in extension (normally 35 to 45 degrees for both). External rotation of the hip in flexion is normal, however. The findings in retroversion are the opposite of those found in anteversion of the femoral neck.

In utero and postnatal positioning of the legs and hips produces stresses that bring about these rotational deformities of the femoral neck. The true incidence of anteversion and retroversion is not known, but the former is much more common and occurs twice as frequently in girls as in boys. Most femoral torsion deformities correct themselves by 7 years of age. If they do not, orthopedic consultation should be obtained because their persistence may lead to degenerative arthritis of the hip joint. Orthopedic treatment consists of the use of a bivalve lower-trunk and leg cast during sleeping hours or in rare cases a derotation osteotomy of the middle and lower femoral shaft. A simple measure that can be employed by the primary care physician early on for parental concern over toeing-in is to have the child learn to sit in the tailor, modified lotus, or Indian-style sitting position. The use of Denis Browne splints is contraindicated, and corrective shoes are of no value.

Positions Leading to Toeing-In and Toeing-Out. Infants and children often assume certain positions during sleep or while sitting for long periods (watching television) that lead to positional deformities of the femur, tibia, or feet.

Sleeping in the prone, knee-chest position with the legs internally rotated may lead to anteversion of the femoral neck, internal tibial torsion, and varus of the forefoot; having the legs externally rotated may lead to valgus of the feet; and having the legs in a neutral position may lead to equinus of the feet and toe-walking. Sleeping in the prone position with the legs extended and rotated inward may lead to anteversion of the femoral neck, internal tibial torsion, and varus of the

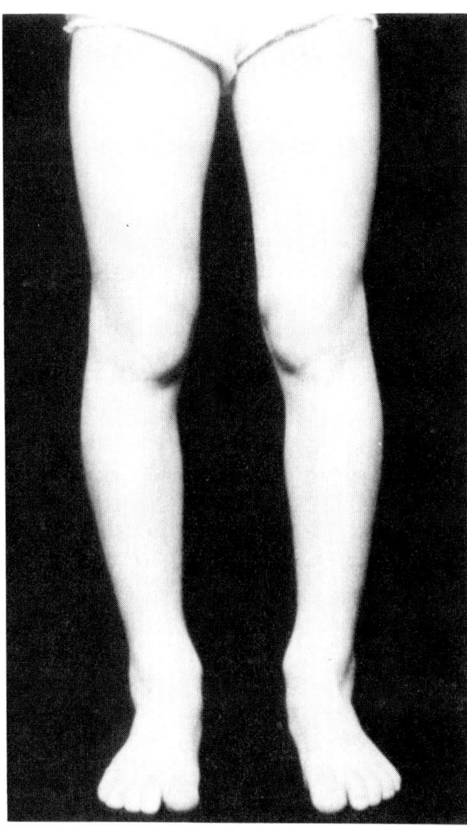

Fig. 133-14 Anteversion of the femoral neck or medial femoral torsion.

From Sharrard WJW: Paediatric orthopaedics and fractures, ed 2, Oxford, 1979, Blackwell Scientific Publications, Ltd, p 416.

forefoot; having them rotated outward may lead to retroversion of the femoral neck and valgus of the feet. Sleeping in the frog-leg position prone or supine may lead to retroversion of the femoral neck and valgus and abduction of the feet.

Sitting in the reversed tailor position (on one's feet) with the feet internally rotated may produce anteversion of the femoral neck, internal tibial torsion, and varus of the forefoot; having the feet externally rotated may produce anteversion of the femoral neck and valgus of the feet.

When these sleeping or sitting positions are noted to occur in conjunction with the positional deformities listed, and when there is concern regarding them, some effort can be made to change the positional sleeping or sitting habit. Success, however, is not often attained.

Although toeing-in or toeing-out may reflect a variety of underlying orthopedic diseases, there is no evidence to suggest that toeing-in or toeing-out of developmental origin will lead to any functional disabilities if left uncorrected.

SUGGESTED READINGS

Bleck EE: The shoeing of children: show or science? Develop Med Child Neurol 15:188, 1971.

Kling TF and Hensinger RN: Angular and torsional deformities of the lower limbs in children, Clin Orthop 176:136, 1983.

Staheli LT et al: Lower-extremity rotational problems in children, J Bone Joint Surg 67:39, 1985.

Tachdjian MO: Pediatric orthopedics, Philadelphia, 1972, WB Saunders Co.

134

Gastrointestinal Hemorrhage

David M. Steinhorn and Wallace F. Berman

Bleeding from the gastrointestinal tract in children requires prompt evaluation and appropriate treatment. The potential severity of this problem is often underestimated, thereby putting some children at even greater risk for life-threatening hemorrhage. A thorough assessment is made possible by taking into consideration basic pediatric principles. The age of the child, the history, and the associated findings, such as vomiting, pain, bruisability, and medication use by the patient or, if nursing, by the mother, will help direct the physician's subsequent workup. Although earlier literature suggested that a cause for gastrointestinal bleeding could not be found in many cases, a diagnosis can now be determined in the majority of cases. This advance in diagnostic ability stems from increasing skill with and widespread use of flexible fiberoptic endoscopy in small children.

AGE AT PRESENTATION

Newborn

Gastrointestinal bleeding in the newborn period usually appears as rectal bleeding or blood suctioned from the infant's stomach during routine immediate postnatal care. There often may be no readily discernible lesion, the cause may remain obscure, and the bleeding may cease spontaneously and permanently. In the first 24 hours it is necessary to evaluate the infant for maternal blood swallowed during delivery. The Apt test, which detects reduced fetal hemoglobin, can easily be performed by mixing 1 part bright red stool or vomitus with 5 to 10 parts water and then centrifuging the mixture; 1 ml of 0.2 N NaOH is added to the supernatant. A pink color developing in 2 to 5 minutes indicates fetal hemoglobin; adult hemoglobin produces a brown color.

Premature and newborn infants with low Apgar scores are at increased risk for developing gastric ulceration and erosions. In young infants one must consider anorectal fissures, enteric infections, and congenital or acquired hemorrhagic disorders occurring from a variety of drugs. Maternal aspirin ingestion within 1 week of delivery, promethazine used during delivery, or maternal use of phenytoin or phenobarbital, all of which lower vitamin K–dependent clotting factors, may be associated with altered platelet function or coagulopathy. The loss of large quantities of blood should suggest an intrinsic structural lesion of the gastrointestinal tract, such as duplication, enteric cyst, erosive mucosal lesions, Meckel diverticulum, intussusception, volvulus, hemangioma, polyp, or enterocolitis. Bleeding associated with a polyp, hemangioma, or Meckel diverticulum is usually not associated with pain. Hemorrhage secondary to intussusception, duplication, enteric cyst, or volvulus tends to occur with abdominal pain, a mass, or distention; however, these findings may be difficult to appreciate in the neonate.

Infants

In infants up to 1 year of age a number of other lesions in addition to most of those already mentioned for the neonate must be considered. Children in this age group are introduced to a wide variety of foods. Food sensitivities, most frequently cow milk and soy protein allergy, can produce a fulminant enterocolitis. This reaction can be seen even in breast-fed infants when the offending agent is consumed by the mother. Children with food sensitivities that produce colitis usually have varying degrees of iron-deficiency anemia from chronic blood loss. Immunodeficiency states are also associated with potentially severe enterocolitis.

As infants become mobile, with improved hand-to-mouth ability, their proximity to small objects on the floor makes foreign body ingestion a significant risk. Other causes of gastrointestinal bleeding tend to be similar to those in older children.

Children and Adolescents

In children and adolescents esophageal varices, peptic ulcer disease, and gastritis must be considered, as well as many of the structural lesions previously described. Cavernous transformation of the extrahepatic portion of the portal vein, leading to portal hypertension, has been associated with umbilical vessel catheterization, omphalitis, or neonatal conditions associated with hypoxia, prolonged jaundice, or sepsis. Intrahepatic causes of cirrhosis, leading to portal hypertension that may first present during childhood or adolescence, include Wilson disease, alpha-l-antitrypsin deficiency, or other forms of chronic liver disease—either metabolic, infectious, or anatomic. These latter diseases may also be associated with coagulopathies and thrombocytopenia secondary to the hypersplenism that usually accompanies them.

In acute variceal bleeding the portal system may be acutely decompressed, emptying an otherwise palpable spleen. If the cause of the portal hypertension is extrahepatic, the bleeding may be remarkably well tolerated in contrast to those patients with cirrhotic liver disease in whom rapid hepatic decompensation may occur. Variceal bleeding may be induced following routine aspirin use, upper respiratory tract illnesses, excessive physical exertion, or the ingestion of rough, bulky foods.

The true incidence of peptic ulcer disease in the general pediatric population is unknown. The reasons for this gap in our knowledge come from the difficulty in separating causes of upper gastrointestinal bleeding—that is, "pill" gastritis, stress ulceration, or acid-peptic disease—as well as from the extremely variable presentation of symptoms that differ according to age group. The classic history of epigastric pain that worsens with an empty stomach and improves with eating is more typical in the adolescent but may be absent in the younger child. Peptic ulcers may present as acute bleeding or as a chronic anemia secondary to ongoing blood losses.

Polypoid lesions of the gastrointestinal tract may present with rectal bleeding. These lesions, which produce painless bleeding as a result of local irritation, usually represent simple, solitary, juvenile polyps of the colon. This bleeding may be seen either as minor streaking on the stools or less frequently as frank, bright red blood. Seventy percent of these polyps are located within 25 cm of the anus and are readily removed using a snare-cautery technique. If bleeding is not a problem, many of these polyps will autoamputate if left alone. Polyps not easily reached by this method can usually be removed using a fiberoptic colonoscope and snare technique after appropriate patient preparation. Adenomatous polyps may present with rectal bleeding as early as infancy. They are managed differently from juvenile polyps.

Many parents will be extremely concerned and anxious over the possibility that their child's rectal bleeding may represent a malignancy. Colonic carcinoma is extremely rare in children, occurring predominantly in older children with long-standing ulcerative colitis or familial polyposis syndromes. The Peutz-Jeghers syndrome consists of diffuse polyps of the gastrointestinal tract that may twist on their stalks and infarct. It is associated with melanotic spots of the oral mucosa and skin.

Hemangiomas and other vascular lesions, such as hereditary hemorrhagic telangiectasia (Rendu-Osler-Weber syndrome), must be considered in the evaluation of painless rectal bleeding. Its most common form is the larger cavernous hemangioma, either polypoid or diffuse, extending several centimeters through the submucosa of the small or large intestine. The large bowel, specifically the rectum, is the area usually involved in the diffuse type. Cutaneous vascular malformations are often present but may require scrupulous searching to detect. Selective arteriography or digital subtraction angiography may aid in demonstrating the abnormal vessels if they are not visible on direct inspection. The clinician must determine whether the patient has indeed bled and whether the discolored vomitus or stools truly represent the presence of blood. This task may be accomplished easily and rapidly by confirming the presence of blood with the Hematest, Hemoccult (guaiac), or Gastroccult test. Some false positive and negative results have occurred with these tests; however, the ability to determine the presence of blood accurately in most cases mandates their use in evaluating suspected gastrointestinal bleeding.

GENERAL APPROACH TO PATIENTS WITH GASTROINTESTINAL BLEEDING

In evaluating a patient with gastrointestinal blood loss, the physician should keep two goals in mind: first, the severity of the blood loss must be quickly assessed (see following section) to institute appropriate resuscitative measures; second, the physician must consider the most likely etiologies to separate the problems requiring immediate surgery from those requiring medical management and evaluation. Thus the workup is based on clinical appearance, age, history, and the physician's familiarity with the patient and on the family's reliability and compliance. A list of lesions commonly associated with gastrointestinal bleeding is provided in the box. These include lesions with upper gastrointestinal (UGI) bleeding and those with rectal bleeding, since blood is a potent cathartic and reduces transit time.

If, on initial assessment, the physician determines that the degree of blood loss is neither enormous nor life threatening, a more leisurely diagnostic approach is suitable. In infants and small children, particular attention should be paid to a history of chronic or familial diseases, allergies, medications the child or nursing mother is receiving, diet, recent behavior pattern, and growth pattern, with particular attention to recent

Causes of Gastrointestinal Hemorrhage

INFANTS UNDER 1 YEAR OF AGE

- Presenting as upper gastrointestinal bleeding
  - Swallowed maternal blood
  - Gastritis, acid-peptic disease
  - Stress ulceration
  - Mallory-Weiss syndrome
  - Vascular malformations
- Presenting as lower gastrointestinal bleeding
  - Anal fissure or trauma
  - Gastroenteritis
    - Enteric infections
    - Enterocolitis
  - Intussusception
  - Coagulation disorders
  - Congenital malformations
    - Malrotation
    - Intestinal duplications, Meckel diverticulum
  - Food allergies

CHILDREN OVER 1 YEAR OF AGE

- Presenting as upper gastrointestinal bleeding
  - Stress ulcers
  - Gastritis, acid-peptic disease
  - Esophageal varices
  - Esophagitis
  - Mallory-Weiss syndrome
  - Swallowed blood from nasopharynx
- Presenting as lower gastrointestinal bleeding
  - Anal fissures
  - Polyps
  - Gastroenteritis, enteric infections
  - Intussusception
  - Inflammatory bowel disease
  - Congenital malformations
    - Malrotation or volvulus
    - Intestinal duplication
    - Meckel diverticulum
  - Henoch-Schönlein purpura

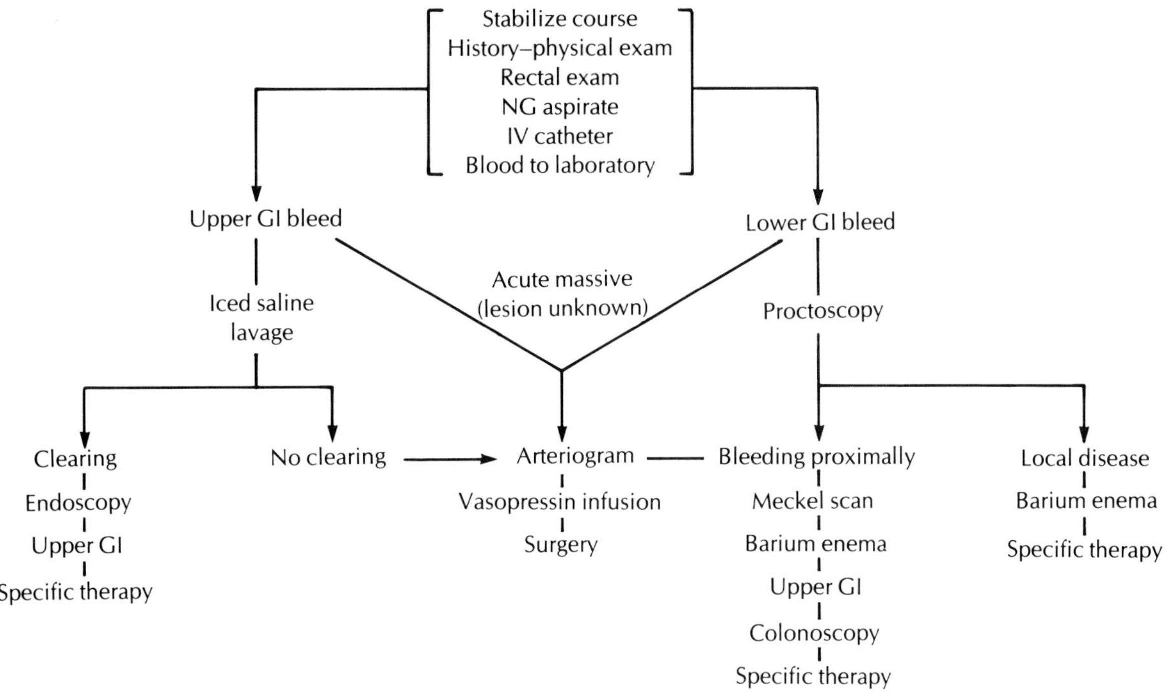

Fig. 134-1 Management of gastrointestinal hemorrhage.

weight loss or failure to thrive. The sequence of diagnostic studies should be designed to determine whether the blood is most likely coming from a site proximal or distal to the ligament of Treitz. From that point, the physician concentrates either on looking for upper gastrointestinal lesions by using endoscopy, a UGI series, or angiography or else examining the lower tract with bacterial cultures, proctoscopy or colonoscopy, barium contrast studies, labeled red cell studies, or a Meckel scan (Fig. 134-1).

For a child having acute massive gastrointestinal bleeding, the approach must be the same as in any other emergency. The physician must approach the patient with an efficient, rational plan in mind that will allow him or her to obtain the pertinent history, perform a brief but adequate examination, stabilize the patient clinically, arrive at a working diagnosis, and institute appropriate therapy or consultations. As soon as possible, cardiovascular status should be evaluated by measuring blood pressure, pulse, and respiratory rate. Skin turgor and the color of the mucous membranes should also be noted.

If signs of shock are present (e.g., orthostasis or frank hypotension, tachycardia, poorly perfused extremities, pale mucous membranes, or altered mental status), a large-bore intravenous catheter should be placed.

If an intravenous line cannot be placed in a patient with evidence of hypotension and hypovolemia or if one of sufficient size cannot be placed to administer 20 ml/kg of crystalloid fluid in less than 30 minutes, then one should consider inserting an intraosseous needle for fluid resuscitation and administering any necessary medications. This technique may be lifesaving and carries an extremely low risk of complications.[1]

Also, 20 ml/kg of lactated Ringer solution, Hetastarch, normal saline, or plasma should be given as rapidly as possible to reexpand the vascular volume. This dose may be repeated once if needed. Additional fluid should be given as needed to make up for equilibration of these solutions with the extravascular space. Red cells should be given as soon as possible, while watching for signs of circulatory overload.

Next, an appropriately sized nasogastric (NG) tube (preferably of the vented sump type) should be placed to help determine the source and estimate the volume of ongoing blood loss. This tube should be left in place and attached to either low-pressure continuous suction, if vented, or to intermittent suction, if nonvented. The only instances when an NG tube may be contraindicated are in patients with documented varices in whom NG placement may aggravate bleeding. Nonetheless, even in these cases an NG tube may be required to quantitate blood loss adequately.

The presence of blood in the stomach, either fresh or acidified (coffee ground appearance), suggests that the bleeding is occurring proximal to the ligament of Treitz. If the pylorus is closed, bleeding may not be apparent from the appearance of the NG tube aspirate. Therefore, duodenal bleeding may present with blood stools rather than with bloody vomitus. Lower gastrointestinal bleeding is characterized on the basis of the appearance of the stools as hematochezia (bright red bloody stools), blood-streaked stools, melena (black, tarry stools), or currant-jelly stools. Hematochezia usually indicates massive upper gastrointestinal or colonic bleeding. Blood streaking is often associated with disease involving the rectum or the perianal region. Melenic- to maroon-colored stools may be seen with small bowel or proximal colonic bleeding. The presence of currant-jelly stools is usually an ominous sign, suggesting impending infarction of bowel with the sloughing of necrotic mucosa; in these cases one may also see signs similar to those associated with an acute surgical abdomen.

With this basic information in hand, the physician can

proceed to a more complete history of the present illness. Pertinent points include the presence of pain, vomiting, diarrhea, or fainting. A history of chronic or predisposing illnesses (i.e., liver disease, bleeding disorders, or familial gastrointestinal disorders) must be sought. The pediatrician should inquire as to all medications and substances taken by the child before or during the episode, particularly emphasizing salicylates, iron, alcohol, or caustic agents, such as household cleaning products. A complete neonatal history, including complications such as hypoxia, umbilical vessel catheterization, prolonged jaundice, and omphalitis, must be obtained. Prior surgery, trauma, and chronic illnesses must be asked about directly.

To expedite the treatment of unstable patients, the physical examination should be performed while taking the history and initiating therapy. Pulse rate, respirations, and postural blood pressure measurements should be recorded. Of particular importance in any patient with bleeding is the presence of petechiae, ecchymoses, or blood in the nares, throat, or urine. The physician must also look for signs of chronic liver disease, such as the presence of telangiectasias, jaundice, hepatosplenomegaly, and a prominent abdominal venous pattern. With lower gastrointestinal bleeding a careful rectal examination should be performed with special attention to (1) the perianal region, observing for skin tags, abscesses, fissures, bleeding points or, much less commonly hemorrhoids; (2) the character of the stool; and (3) the presence of occult blood. It is also necessary to palpate for polyps and pelvic masses during the rectal examination.

Having completed all the above, which in practice usually takes less than an hour, controlling the bleeding and determining the specific diagnosis become the next orders of business. If the nasogastric aspirate contains blood or if the patient has hematemesis, iced saline irrigation may be instituted in an attempt to decrease mucosal blood flow and thereby stop profuse bleeding. Although the efficacy of lavage in decreasing and controlling upper bleeding has not been conclusively demonstrated, it allows easier assessment of the rate of bleeding and helps in removing clotted blood. Iced saline is instilled through an NG tube and is withdrawn after 5 minutes, while signs of blood in the aspirate return are watched for. The procedure is repeated until the aspirate return is clear or if there is no diminution in the blood content of the aspirate return for 30 to 45 minutes.

If the bleeding ceases, gastroduodenoscopy should be performed to demonstrate the bleeding source and to determine the type of lesion present. Upper endoscopy can establish the diagnosis in 75% to 90% of patients. If the bleeding is massive and cannot be controlled with iced saline lavage, it is likely that adequate visualization cannot be achieved with the fiberoptic endoscope. If the bleeding is not immediately life threatening, arteriography can be considered, which may demonstrate bleeding that occurs at rates of 0.5 ml/minute or more.

Of greater sensitivity and reduced invasiveness is the use of a sulfur-colloid isotopic study, which can demonstrate active bleeding at rates as low as 0.1 ml/minute. This method will demonstrate active bleeding using a tracer with a very short half-life. In small infants, a large uptake of the isotope by the liver may mask the right upper quadrant. An additional isotopic method of determining the bleeding site consists of injecting the patient with technetium-pertechnetate–labeled red blood cells. These labeled cells may remain in the circulation for more than a day and allow repeated imaging to locate the site of intermittent bleeding.

If the lesion is one of mucosal erosion or inflammation, antacid therapy with or without the concomitant use of a beta-2-blocker should be instituted. If the bleeding source is found to be variceal bleeding, the cause of these lesions must be considered, with appropriate treatment of the underlying cause. Liver or portal venous disease should be sought. Clotting factors and platelets should be replaced as indicated.

Variceal bleeding requires special mention because of the myriad settings in which varices may be seen. Although the treatment of variceal bleeding continues to evolve, it may be divided into those therapies that can be instituted in most emergency facilities and those requiring a pediatric endoscopist skilled at sclerotherapy. Of the former therapies, balloon tamponade and vasopressin therapy are most common. Although Blakemore tubes are available in pediatric sizes, their use has been associated with an unacceptably high incidence of airway problems and even esophageal rupture. Vasopressin may be used as a mesenteric vasoconstrictor to reduce portal blood flow and thus decrease variceal pressure. Initially, 0.3 U/kg of vasopressin is diluted in 2 ml/kg of 5% dextrose and given over 20 minutes, preferably through a central or intraosseous line. A continuous infusion of vasopressin 0.15-0.35 U/m^2/minute may be continued for 12 hours after bleeding stops; the dose is then gradually tapered. Extreme care must be taken to avoid malignant hypertension in patients receiving vasopressin infusions, and arterial pressure must be monitored continuously.

Endoscopic sclerotherapy has taken its place in recent years as a significant modality for controlling variceal bleeding in children resulting from a wide variety of underlying diseases. The number and magnitude of complications are exceedingly small, with a low incidence of rebleeding when performed for esophageal varices. This technique is somewhat more effective when used for varices associated with extrahepatic portal hypertension rather than those associated with primary liver disease. A major drawback to this technique is the frequent need for general anesthesia and endotracheal intubation when initially performed on small children and the need for a facility skilled at managing critically ill small children. For many patients, however, sclerotherapy offers a relatively less invasive means for controlling variceal bleeding than more risky portal shunting procedures.

The workup for lower gastrointestinal bleeding differs in several aspects from that of upper gastrointestinal bleeding. The abdomen and perianal and rectal region are carefully examined. Stool must be analyzed for the presence of blood, ova and parasites, and enteric pathogens. If diarrhea is present, the stool should be examined microscopically for polymorphonuclear leukocytes and mucus, both of which are evidence of bacterial infection. Proctosigmoidoscopy, which can be performed in even the smallest infants, should follow in an attempt to discover the presence of fissures, polyps, or mucosal disease. It is necessary to look for signs of mucosal friability and edema. The presence of blood coming from above the reach of the proctosigmoidoscope indicates the need to proceed with other diagnostic studies. Depending on the circumstances, these may include (1) an upright and supine view of the abdomen, looking in particular for signs of obstruction or for calcifications; (2) a radionuclide scan, using pentagastrin to enhance uptake in search of a Meckel diverticulum; (3) a sulfur-colloid isotopic scan; (4) arteriography; and (5) an isotope-labeled red blood cell infusion (usually reserved for cases of intermittent bleeding). If the rate of bleeding does not permit the delay necessary to perform these studies, the parenteral administration of vasopressin may be used in an attempt to control the bleeding and to stabilize the patient.

An air contrast barium enema to identify mucosal lesions and an upper GI series with small bowel follow-through should be the last studies performed, since they make the further use of arteriography, isotope scans, and endoscopy impossible for several days thereafter.

In those cases in which vascular compromise of the gut is present or the rate of bleeding is excessive and uncontrollable by more conservative methods, prompt surgical intervention is required. Fortunately, however, most acute episodes of gastrointestinal bleeding can be controlled relatively easily by using conservative measures; in those patients who will require surgical intervention, it can be handled electively at a later time.

REFERENCE

1. Rossetti VA et al: Intraosseous infusions: an alternative route of pediatric intravascular access, Ann Emerg Med 14:885, 1985.

SUGGESTED READINGS

Alavi A and Ring EJ: Localization of gastrointestinal bleeding: superiority of ^{99m}Tc sulfur colloid compared with angiography, Am J Radiol 137:741, 1981.

Caulfield M et al: Upper gastrointestinal tract endoscopy in the pediatric patient, J Pediatr 115:339, 1989.

Donovan TJ, Ward M, and Shepherd RW: Evaluation of endoscopic sclerotherapy of esophageal varices in children, J Pediatr Gastroenterol Nutr 5:696, 1986.

Gryboski JD: The value of upper gastrointestinal endoscopy in children, Digest Dis 26(suppl):17, 1981.

Hyams JS, Leichtner AM, and Schwartz AN: Recent advances in diagnosis and treatment of gastrointestinal hemorrhage in infants and children, J Pediatr 106:1, 1985.

McKusick KA et al: ^{99m}Tc red blood cells for detection of gastrointestinal bleeding: experience with 80 patients, Am J Radiol 137:1113, 1981.

Steffen RM et al: Colonoscopy in the pediatric patient, J Pediatr 115:507, 1989.

Tedesco FJ et al: Upper gastrointestinal endoscopy in the pediatric patient, Gastroenterology 70:492, 1976.

Torsoli A: Gastrointestinal emergencies, Clin Gastroenterol 10:1, 1981.

135

Headache

Henry M. Seidel

Headache—quite literally, a pain in the head—is a common presenting complaint in childhood, increasing in frequency as the child becomes more verbal and, consequently, better able to be explicit about aches and pains. We cannot, of course, accurately appreciate its frequency in the very young. Eventually, virtually every one experiences a headache—probably humanity's most commonly experienced pain—usually, for the first time, at some point during childhood or adolescence. It is a complaint that easily elicits empathy.

It is also a complaint that causes serious concern and frustration. The physician does not want to overlook the relatively infrequent causes that require lifesaving therapeutic interventions. Parents and many older children and adolescents with headaches are often worried about a major disease, particularly a brain tumor. The box on p. 947 includes a partial list of the causes of headache. Because there are several categories of headache (migraine, "abdominal" migraine, tension, and "cluster"), each with imprecise starting and end points, diagnosis and management can be difficult.

Nonetheless, most headaches during childhood are transient, bearable, and associated with the general wear and tear of life—from the nonthreatening viral and upper respiratory tract infection to the results of stress-producing experiences of day-to-day living. The older the child, the more likely the latter is so. However, if an acute episode persists or the intensity of the complaint accelerates, it is necessary to be aware of the possibility of an organic cause for the complaint.

MECHANISM OF HEADACHE

Headache may have either an extracranial or intracranial cause. An extracranial cause is the most common, not surprising in that almost all extracranial structures are pain sensitive. Thus headache is frequently associated with dilation and distention of the extracranial vessels or with spasmodic contracture of the scalp and neck musculature. Infections or other diseases in any of the extracranial structures of the head—eyes, teeth, sinuses, and ears—can cause headache and are usually readily identifiable by the localizing evidence of the particular affliction. However, this is not always the case, and the physician must be aware that extracranial causes of headache may not be made immediately evident by localized signs.

Not all intracranial structures are pain sensitive. Those that are include cranial nerves V, VII, IX, and X; cervical nerves 1 through 3; and the venous sinuses and some of their branches. Most of the rest of the intracranial structures—skull, substance of the brain, and most of the meninges—are not pain sensitive. However, the pressure produced by a mass of any sort, the pulls and displacements of the venous sinuses and their branches, and inflammation from any cause can and do influence those cranial and cervical nerves that are pain sensitive. Much is ascribed to distention, stretching, and compression of these structures, but the exact mechanism by which pain results is not really known, particularly when there are no identifiable anatomic displacements.

CONCOMITANT SIGNS AND SYMPTOMS

Meningismus and fever, for example, may accompany headache and, when present, do increase concern for an acute, treatable condition. Meningitis is an obvious first thought. However, other major conditions may produce a severe headache along with meningismus: retropharyngeal abscess, superior longitudinal sinus thrombosis, and subarachnoid hemorrhage, as well as typhoid fever and pneumonia. And, of course, the common infecting bacteria or viruses may not always be the cause of meningitis or meningoencephalitis. Less likely agents (e.g., cryptococci) must also be considered.

HISTORY AND PHYSICAL EXAMINATION

The history and physical examination are extremely important. They will help immediately to rule out most diagnoses that lead to therapeutic imperatives, thereby obviating the need for laboratory and roentgenographic procedures. Actually, while taking the history, the pediatrician can begin to eliminate (or include) many concerns—for example, by an immediate look to observe the movement of the eyes (for evidence of cranial nerve VI palsy—frequently the first manifestation of intracranial pressure) or an initial question directed to the associated complaint of vomiting (whether it is accompanied by nausea, which is not usually the case with increased intracranial pressure).

Occasionally, the acute presenting circumstance requires great speed to reach even a tentative diagnosis. The patient's physical condition and level of consciousness may direct the diagnostic search. Certainly, the following accompanying complaints and findings will suggest organic causes and, therefore, a less leisurely approach:

Fever
Meningismus
Trauma (even if obscure or distant in time)
Seizures
Severe hypertension
Confusion

- Diminished awareness
- Petechiae and ecchymoses
- Lethargy
- Vomiting, with or without nausea
- Intense irritability
- Great specificity in description of headache
- History of pica

Similarly, the headaches that are characterized by one or more of the following suggest an organic cause:

- Initial, dramatic episode
- Sudden onset
- Intense pain upon awakening from sleep
- A dramatic description (e.g., "jackhammer in the head")
- Occurrence in the morning; subsidence after arising, particularly after vomiting
- Precipitation by cough, sneeze, strain (particularly if headache is of short duration—a few minutes to 30 minutes)

A sharply defined, acute onset is worrisome, and the age

Partial Listing of Causes of Headaches

INTRACRANIAL MASSES (SHARPLY LOCALIZED OR DIFFUSE)

- Intracranial tumor, benign or malignant
- Brain cyst
- Subdural hematoma
- Central nervous system leukemia
- Acute onset of hydrocephalus for any reason caused by obstruction within the ventricular system

VASCULAR CAUSES

- Migraine
  - Classic
  - With ophthalmoplegia or hemiplegia
  - Basilar artery
  - Complicated by tension
  - With ornithine transcarbamoylase deficiency
- Arteriovenous malformation
- Venous sinus engorgement
- Hypertension
- Cranial arteritis
- Intracranial aneurysm
- Subarachnoid hemorrhage
- Vascular occlusion
  - With congenital heart disease
  - With sickle cell disease
- Vascular dilation secondary to fever, hypoxia, hypercapnia, or severe anemia

SPECIFIC FOCAL DISEASE

- Inflammation, new growth, foreign body, or other injury of:
  - Eye
  - Ear
  - Nose
  - Throat
  - Teeth
  - Sinuses
  - Cervical spine

EMOTIONAL CAUSES

- Conversion reactions
- Daily stress, psychogenic causes, familial patterning
- Depression

INFECTIONS

- Meningitis or encephalitis
  - Bacterial
  - Viral
- Sinusitis (less frequent in the younger child with poorly developed sinuses)
- Otitis media
- Mastoiditis
- Retropharyngeal abscess
- Brain abscess
- Cervical adenitis
- Systemic infection

NEURAL CAUSES

- Epileptic equivalent
- Trigeminal neuralgia
- Glossopharyngeal neuralgia
- Excessive auditory, visual, or gustatory sensory stimuli
- Seizures (postictal)

TRAUMATIC CAUSES

- Lumbar puncture (with subsequent decreased intracranial pressure)
- Head injury
  - Concussion
  - Subdural hematoma
  - Subarachnoid hemorrhage
- Other posttraumatic events

NOXIOUS STIMULI

- "Gas leak" syndrome
- Alcohol
- Lead
- Oral contraceptives
- Other drugs (e.g., steroid withdrawal)

OTHER CAUSES

- Allergy
- Hyperaldosteronism
- Hypoglycemia
- Occipital neuralgia with malformation at C1 and C2
- Pseudotumor cerebri (with otitis media, use of vitamin A, tetracyclines, steroids)
- Renal disease
- Unknown origin

of the child is a prime consideration—the younger the child, the greater the risk. Also, the precision of the complaint suggests a more life-compromising diagnosis. Even the young child can point a finger very accurately. A frontal location of the headache suggests frontal or ethmoid sinusitis, cerebral tumors, a migraine, and problems with the eyes; an occipital or suboccipital location suggests a cerebellar tumor, occipital neuralgia, sphenoid sinusitis, or tension. The more severe the complaint, the more likely an organic cause.

Some characteristics of headache particularly suggest increased intracranial pressure. These include headaches that wake the patient from sleep or occur in the morning and that are accompanied by vomiting free of nausea; are related to a change in position from prone to supine and from either of those to the erect position; and are related to physical activity, coughing, sneezing, and straining. Increased intracranial pressure does not provide a warning—a prodrome like that of scotomata (visual "fireworks"), pallor, and abdominal pain that may precede a migraine headache. The headache that wakes the patient from sleep and that does not respond to aspirin, acetaminophen, or other over-the-counter drugs may often have a more serious cause. The simple, transient episode generally responds most readily. Finally, the presence of pica, particularly in the younger child, may suggest lead encephalopathy; the description of "throbbing" may suggest hypertension. A clear history of trauma always requires particular attention.

These considerations underscore the need for eliciting a careful history and sharply dissecting the often intermingled psychosocial and organic variables. Clearly, the family history is important. Children with migraine headaches tend to have parents who have them also. Care should be taken, however; children under stress are apt to mimic their parents' behavior. Beyond that, the description of the headache, its frequency, duration, and location, and the report of prodromata are all very important. There may be clues to stress and tension in the events that precede the headache, such as the experience and thoughts of the patient, the time of day, and the day of the week. Understanding the experiences of the child, both at home and at school; the nature of relations with family, teachers, and friends; reading and television habits; eating patterns; environmental noise; sleep habits; and any recent change in bowel and urination patterns can all help. Even the presence of a gas stove in the home is important, since it may be leaking. The search, then, must be for hints of organic cause and for evidence of emotional stress and tension.

A "concept" of the child emerges from this inquiry. The depiction of behavioral patterns, past coping mechanisms, any recent behavioral change, hints of any change in the flow of normal development, and diminished school performance all aid in characterizing the child. Is the child shy or compulsive, too sensitive to the needs of others, obsessively neat—in all, a possible "worrywart?" These traits may facilitate a migraine or the so-called tension headache. Certainly, it is also important to look for evidence of depression because headache may indeed be the prime complaint of the chronically depressed child.

The physical examination must be precise, including a careful neurologic evaluation and a conscientious attempt at ophthalmoscopy; a visual field check; evaluation of ocular muscle balance and convergence; palpation and auscultation of the skull and mastoid and of the optic globes; palpation and transillumination of the sinuses; a careful check of the teeth, ears, and throat; a blood pressure reading; and a urinalysis. Eye drops may be used to improve the visualization of the fundus, but only after a description of the pupils and their reactions to light and accommodation are carefully recorded. It is, then, rarely necessary to have laboratory and imaging examinations performed.

INTERPRETING INFORMATION

Characterization of the headache is most important. There are two major groups: those with an apparent first acute episode in the absence of a significant prior complaint and those that suggest chronicity and recurrence. This latter group bestows the advantage of hindsight in determining the patterns. However, the acute episode may be the first of many; the boundary can be obscure, at least at the start. A tendency to the diffuse and nondescript may suggest tension or a more "distant" cause—an association, perhaps, with anemia, fever, some infectious process, or hypoglycemia. In any event, it is worth repeating that youth and specificity—the younger the child and the more specific the headache—increase the likelihood of an organic disorder. But make haste cautiously; there usually is time for the careful approach.

The trap to avoid is relying too greatly on a mechanical and unthinking use of the various laboratory tools and diagnostic aids—that is, the workup. Most headaches should be successfully diagnosed and managed without the skull roentgenographic series, computed tomography (CT) scan, magnetic resonance imaging (MRI), lumbar puncture, or arteriogram; most patients are helped by a conscientious history and physical examination, a meticulous explanation, and a ready and willing ear. It is the ability to listen wisely and to respond constructively that will do most for the patient with a rather diffuse, chronic, or recurrent headache—that and, perhaps, a little acetaminophen.

A headache, more than most complaints, tends to force the physician's behavior toward extremes—on the one hand, intervening forthrightly for major problems; on the other, responding gently in a conscientious attempt at understanding the patient's sometimes submerged feelings and needs. The physician must thoughtfully reject mechanistic diagnostic intervention unless the situation clearly calls for it.

DIFFERENTIAL DIAGNOSIS

Given a precise history and physical examination, resorting to the laboratory does become necessary in the presence of a genuine indication of *infection* or *increased intracranial pressure* from whatever source. The choice of studies at the start is relatively simple. The suspicion of infection suggests the need for a complete blood count and, quite often, a lumbar puncture and blood culture. The lumbar puncture should be approached with care and only after assurance that there is no papilledema or other evidence of increased intracranial pressure. A urinalysis is easy to obtain and is certainly indicated in the presence of hypertension. Skull and sinus films can be helpful.

There may be a need to resort to the CT scan, sonography,

MRI, or radioactive isotope brain scans. If so, consultation is indicated with the neurologist and the "imagists"—the radiologists and others who can help determine the best use of varying imaging techniques so that the most helpful information is gained most rapidly and least invasively. Arteriography, still sometimes used in the late 1980s, should be avoided if at all possible, because it does increase morbidity and the risk of hemiplegia.

The electroencephalogram, of itself relatively benign (save for its cost and impressive, intimidating trappings), is of questionable help. Its findings, for example, are often abnormal in patients with a migraine and often normal in those with epilepsy. It is sometimes helpful in localizing an intracranial lesion, but it is not nearly as specific as some of the newer techniques. Some clinicians seem to be bound to the use of electroencephalograms but are not often well served by them. It certainly is not necessary to use them frequently in acute circumstances.

At this point, the individual problem often becomes sufficiently clear so that the appropriate therapeutic pathway is readily evident. Infection can be further defined with appropriate cultures and treated with antibiotics, surgical drainage, or both; expanding lesions and the results of trauma and bleeding are ameliorated with the help of the neurosurgeon. Fortunately, the diagnosis of pseudotumor cerebri can sometimes be made.

However, once the history and physical examination are complete, the pediatrician may still be confronted with a complaint that seems nonspecific and difficult to clarify. There may be some helpful information indicating a behavioral change, for example, even as there may be information eliminating the possibility of organic disease; sometimes the organic and the functional components may be concurrent. If there is a family history of migraine, present about 75% of the time, the physician should turn the evaluation in that direction.

In this circumstance other factors are helpful. Migraine, quite common in childhood, usually begins in children during the early school years—5 or 6 to about 9 years of age. However, it is not uncommon in the younger child. There has often been a history of cyclic vomiting or car sickness. These headaches predominate in males by at least 2 to 1 and are sometimes accompanied, particularly in the classic migraine, by prodromal periods that may include scotomas, abdominal pain, irritability, and paresthesias; prodromes, however, are less common in children than in adults. There is, at times, retroorbital pain, usually on one side.

It is necessary to ask about odd visual phenomena—gaping "holes," dots, lines, and "stars." The older child should be asked to draw the scotoma. The often associated gastrointestinal complaint can be severe, and the occasional transient neurologic finding of aphasia, hemiplegia, or ophthalmoplegia can be very disturbing. This complicates matters and leads to more extensive testing, particularly to the use of the CT scan or MRI and to the investigation of a urea-cycle abnormality (ornithine transcarbamoylase deficiency), believed by some to be a cause of migraine.

A migraine headache may occur on either side of the head and may vary in frequency. There is no consistency. It may often begin during periods of emotional stress, intense use of the eyes (reading, television), menstruation, use of oral contraceptives, or exposure to loud sound (rock music played at high pitch); it may occur when menses have been missed or chocolate and cheeses have been eaten. A period of sleep following the headache often terminates the episode.

Tension headaches usually follow periods of stress, and may last for days or weeks; they are dull (not pulsating) and usually bilateral. There may be some evidence of behavioral change and, particularly, of difficult relations with family, friends, or teachers. These undercurrents and any suspicion of them should have been explored during the history and should prompt the interviewer to go beyond initial denials. An effort must be made to gain a clear understanding of those feelings and attitudes that may provoke anger, hostility, or anxiety. The history may also reveal a disruption of sleep patterns, particularly a difficulty in falling asleep.

Such headaches usually begin at about 8 to 12 or 13 years of age. Females predominate, and they are often overweight. The description of a tension headache is more fuzzy than that of migraine (although it may be compulsively precise), and it is often said to involve the entire head or the occiput. There is no prodromal period akin to that of migraine, and generally there is no conclusion of the episode by a period of sleep. Finally, these headaches do not have associated objective findings, such as an abnormal electroencephalogram.

The depressed child may often have a severe headache that lasts for days or longer. Acute anger and subsequent guilt may underlie the depression. Although there is no particular behavioral pattern that suggests either migraine or tension headache, these children frequently have a demeanor that sharpens the intensity of concerns common to all people; for example, sensitivity to criticism, meeting new people, worry about grades, and precision in doing homework. Such children may seem to be compulsive and to worry very much if they do not meet the personal demands they place on themselves.

Occipital neuralgia, often suggested by tenderness over the cervical spinous processes, usually occurs first during adolescence. A roentgenogram may reveal subluxation or narrowing at the level of the first and second cervical vertebrae. There is no prodrome and no cessation of the pain with sleep.

Finally, vascular headaches, often called "cluster" headaches, begin to occur in older teenagers, predominantly males. When they do occur in females, there is no association with menses. They are usually unilateral and accompanied by ipsilateral tearing of the eye. They are certainly recurrent, tending to occur in clusters, often at night, each one lasting for perhaps an hour and then disappearing. Thus they are briefer and perhaps more frequent than migraines. They are not accompanied by vomiting or nausea.

Headache manifestations, then, are age related. The organic lesion is not confined to any age, yet headache in the very young suggests organicity. Thereafter, there is a sequence of diagnostic possibilities: migraine during the early school years, tension headaches just before the onset of puberty, occipital neuralgia during adolescence, and finally, the vascular headache of the older teenager.

MANAGEMENT

The symptomatic management of headache is made less difficult when there is a specific cause requiring a specific management. The therapeutic task is less certain in the chronic circumstance—the headache is described less precisely, and its true chronicity, severity, and recurrence are often obscured by fuzzy verbiage. The child most often involved is older than 6 or 7 years, and the circumstances almost invariably suggest at least some emotional basis. The desire, then, is to be more specific in getting at the cause, invoking at times the psychologist or psychiatrist, and to use drugs sparingly. In fact, the very process of meticulous evaluation and sympathetic response is often enough to break the cycle of complaint, particularly with the older child and adolescent.

However, although the cautious use of drugs has much to recommend it, it is possible to be too cautious. A limited list of agents is helpful (Table 135-1). Headaches that are not severe, not particularly frequent, and not prolonged are best managed with acetaminophen. Acetaminophen is preferable to aspirin in that there is little risk of developing Reye syndrome, whereas there is such a risk with aspirin. With either drug, the response is not dose related, and an increase in the amount or frequency of the dosage is *not* justified when the headache persists. In addition, a period of rest and sleep (if that is achievable) is synergistic. Again, a migraine headache, particularly, responds to sleep. Thus, although the chronic use of sedatives as an additional management "crutch" should be avoided, short-term daily phenobarbital in low doses may help.

The next steps are guided by the diagnostic conclusion and the age of the child. Some children will persist in experiencing an intense and frequently recurrent headache (one or two times a month) and may, if they have migraine or cluster headaches, require ergot. The primary care pediatrician must then consider consultation with a neurologist or a physician whose specific concern is the treatment of headache. It is uncommon in pediatric practice to use ergot derivatives to treat acute migraine and certainly not in the prepubertal child and in any young person in whom gastrointestinal symptoms predominate. In addition, the cluster headache is often managed more effectively by potentiating the effect of ergot with methysergide. However, the potential toxic effect of methysergide (retroperitoneal fibrosis and fibrotic syndromes) suggests the need for great caution.

Therefore the pediatrician's unfamiliarity with these drugs and occasional inadequate understanding of their toxicity in the young (e.g., ergot will intensify an abdominal complaint) require the direction of a consultant who is more experienced in their use. If the clinical picture includes significant depression, amitriptyline may be prescribed. This, too, requires the advice of a consultant, preferably a psychiatrist.

It may be relatively easy to eliminate certain foods thought to be associated with migraine, such as chocolate, citrus fruits, red wines, and some beans, but it pays first to try to establish some relation between the use of these foods and the occurrence of migrainous episodes. After all, abstinence from some foods can be difficult to enforce in children. Suggested preventive medications for migraine—propranolol and cyproheptadine hydrochloride (Periactin)—should be approached with caution. Propranolol is preferable but *is not* to be used once an attack has begun.

Tension headache is apt not to respond to acetaminophen, particularly if the underlying circumstance goes beyond the usual wear and tear of living and involves a more deep-seated problem, intense anxiety, or depression and if these contributors have been present for some time. In fact, the failure to respond to simple medication strongly suggests a tension headache. The temptation simply to intervene with tranquilizers should be resisted, even though there may be some occasional reason to offer diazepam. However, a frequent need for its use in a particular patient should suggest intense

Table 135-1 *Drug Dosage for Relief of Headache*

DRUG	DOSE	COMMENTS
Acetaminophen	<1 yr: 60 mg q4-6h PO 1-3 yr: 60-120 mg q4-6h PO 3-6 yr: 120-180 mg q4-6h PO 6-12 yr: 240 mg q4-6h PO >12 yr: 325-650 mg q4-6h PO Alternative: 5-10 mg/kg q4-6h Maximum adult dosage: 4 g/day	
Amitriptyline	1-2 mg/kg/day: 1/3 in morning, 2/3 at bedtime	Prescribe only after consultation.
Codeine phosphate	0.5-1 mg/kg PO or SC stat; repeat q4-6h Maximum dosage: 3 mg/kg/day	May be habit forming.
Cyproheptadine	0.25-0.5 mg/kg/day, divided, q6-8h PO Maximum total dose: 0.5 mg/kg/day	Use with caution in asthma because of atropine-like effects; contraindicated in neonates.
Diazepam	0.1-0.8 mg/kg/day, divided, q6-8h PO	
Ergot	<12 yr: no more than 4 mg per episode; preferably 2 mg sublingually	Prescribe only after consultation.
Phenobarbital	2-4 mg/kg/dose PO, IM, or PR; repeat p.r.n. q8h	
Propranolol	<35 kg: 10-20 mg PO t.i.d. >35 kg: 20-40 mg PO t.i.d.	May cause hypotension, nausea and vomiting, and bradycardia; contraindicated in asthma and heart block; caution advised in presence of obstructive pulmonary, renal, or liver disease.

underlying factors that must, if possible, be uncovered. Given this, it is possible, sometimes with the help of a psychologist or psychiatrist, to be more secure in the use of diazepam or, in the instance of the child with chronic depression, amitriptyline. Such a serious and persistent problem, however, requires concomitant psychiatric intervention.

Physicians are occasionally confronted with a patient with a headache episode so severe and persistent that there is a real temptation to resort to narcotics or intramuscular sedative medication. In this event, the physician must be secure in the diagnosis. After all, there may be an unrecognized organic cause that mandates a specific intervention. The primary pediatrician should, therefore, seek consultation at this point. Severity, whether defined by intensity of the episodes, their frequency, or the persistence of an individual episode, often requires the contribution of a consultant. The failure of relatively simple medication also suggests consultation rather than the addition of riskier drugs.

SUGGESTED READINGS

Barlow CF: Headaches and migraine in childhood, Philadelphia, 1984, JB Lippincott Co.

Basbaum AI and Fields HL: Endogenous pain control mechanisms: review and hypothesis, Ann Neurol 4:451, 1979.

Fenichel G: Migraine in children, Neurol Clin 3:77, 1985.

Greene MG, editor: The Harriet Lane handbook, ed 12, St. Louis, 1991, Mosby-Year Book, Inc.

Sullivan JF: Diagnostic imperatives in neurology. In Proger S and Barza M, editors: Diagnostic imperatives, New York, 1981, Thieme-Stratton.

136

Hearing Loss

Michael H. Weiss, Patricia Chute, and Simon C. Parisier

The early identification and remediation of children with hearing loss is highly desirable, so that these individuals may develop normal communication skills.[9] The incidence of congenital hearing loss is approximately 1 per 600 live births. About half of these cases are attributable to a genetic disorder, the great majority of which are autosomal recessive.

Acquired hearing loss in childhood is extremely common.[3] Over 75% of children have at least one episode of otitis media, with concomitant conductive hearing loss. Many of these cases readily resolve with antibiotic treatment over time, but others go on to chronic effusion, which causes hearing loss that requires intervention. Chronic otitis media, cholesteatoma, and otosclerosis are other causes of acquired conductive hearing loss in the pediatric population.

DEFINITION AND CHARACTERISTICS OF HEARING LOSS

Hearing loss is defined and quantified according to the hearing thresholds measured (i.e., the softest tone heard by the test subject at a given frequency) during the performance of pure tone audiometric testing. Zero decibels (0 dB) is the reference standard set by testing a cohort of normal young adults. Normal hearing ranges between 0 and 25 db; mild impairment from 26 to 40 dB; moderate from 41 to 55 dB; moderately severe from 56 to 70 dB; severe from 71 to 90 dB; and profound 91 dB and above.[17] The degree of hearing loss determines the type of treatment required.

ASSOCIATED SIGNS AND SYMPTOMS

The evaluation of hearing loss in an infant or child starts with the history. A family history of congenital hearing loss places all subsequent children at high risk. Prenatal or perinatal infection such as rubella or cytomegalovirus is significant. Birth trauma, anoxia, or both are also important to note. Medications, such as aminoglycosides, may cause ototoxicity. In the older child, behavioral or personality changes may signify hearing loss. A history of frequent ear infections or other nonspecific signs and symptoms (e.g., fever, irritability, or gastrointestinal upset) may accompany otologic pathology. Vestibular problems may well accompany hearing impairment; thus, a history of dizziness or imbalance should be sought. All prior medical problems should be reviewed, as these may shed light on the etiology of the hearing loss.

The physical examination includes careful examination of the entire head and neck to note the presence of any anomalies. Examination of the ear will disclose any abnormalities of the external ear and reveal any middle ear infection or effusion. While examining with the patient, the pediatrician should note his or her responsiveness to auditory and verbal cues.

ASSESSMENT OF AUDITORY AND MIDDLE EAR FUNCTION

Older children are tested with a standard battery of audiometric tests that includes pure tone tests of air and bone conduction. The child signals the tester whenever he or she hears a tone, and a graph of the hearing thresholds at a variety of test frequencies is generated. Speech reception and discrimination testing, as well as tympanometry, are also performed.

Unfortunately one cannot test infants and very young children this straightforwardly, but several tests have been devised to determine hearing thresholds in young subjects. A device called a Crib-o-Gram has been used to attempt to screen infants' hearing; it is still used in some institutions, although evoked response testing has largely supplanted it. The Crib-o-Gram consists of a transducer attached to the infant's crib, which detects movements and records them on a strip recorder. Sound signals are emitted from a test loudspeaker, and the resulting movements of the infant are compared with baseline activity. A common form of behavioral testing uses sound generators and observation of the auropalpebral reflex, the startle reflex, and arousal. However, these behavioral testing techniques provide estimates of hearing acuity only for the better hearing ear.[14] Brainstem-evoked response audiometry (BERA) uses the measurement of electric potentials generated within the brainstem in response to monaural acoustic stimuli. Electrodes are placed on the scalp, and a computer is used to record responses to many auditory clicks. Hearing thresholds for each ear may be generated separately with this method. BERA results should be considered in conjunction with behavioral testing to obtain a total picture of the infant's capabilities.[4]

At 2 years of age, the hearing of 70% of children can be evaluated by play audiometry. With this technique, children are behaviorally conditioned to respond to sounds during play. A skilled tester can elicit responses to threshold-level stimuli, and the percentage of children who can be evaluated by play audiometry rises to 96% by 3 years of age.[16] In addition to pure tone testing, an estimate of speech discrimination can also be obtained by a variety of picture identification tests. Such tests require the child to point to the correct picture in response to an auditory cue. Thus it is possible to obtain an accurate assessment of a young child's hearing ability for pure tones and speech.

Because one of the most common causes of hearing loss in young children is otitis media, an assessment of middle ear function is necessary for this group. Tympanometry is the measurement of the acoustic impedance of the ear as a function of ear canal pressure. It is helpful in identifying abnormalities of the middle ear, particularly problems characterized by high impedance (middle ear effusions).[10,15]

The acoustic reflex has also been employed as a diagnostic measurement. In the demonstration of the acoustic reflex, the impedance meter measures the sudden change in ear canal sound pressure caused by the decrease in compliance of the middle ear system as the stapedius muscle contracts in response to an auditory stimulus. The threshold for the acoustic reflex has been employed to estimate the level of hearing loss in young children.[5] The absence of an acoustic reflex is often noted in conductive hearing loss. An absent or abnormal acoustic reflex is a common finding in the presence of retrocochlear pathology.

DIFFERENTIAL DIAGNOSIS

Following complete testing, hearing loss may be characterized as conductive, mixed, or sensorineural. Conductive losses are those that involve the external or middle ear or both. These losses may be congenital (as in the cases of anomalies of the external or middle ear such as congenital atresia) or acquired. Sensorineural hearing loss implies damage to the cochlea or the acoustic nerve (part of cranial nerve VIII).[13] Such losses may be congenital or acquired. A subset of sensorineural hearing loss is retrocochlear hearing loss, which implies dysfunction of the acoustic nerve or the brainstem, usually secondary to neoplasm. Retrocochlear pathology is rare in children. Mixed hearing loss is a combination of conductive and sensorineural hearing loss.

Central auditory dysfunction is characterized by hearing loss in combination with one or more of the following: deficits in foreground-background discrimination, poor auditory attention, limitations in memory and retrieval, and delays in receptive language development. Finally, there is functional hearing loss. This hearing loss is pretended, exaggerated, or hysterical. It is a diagnosis of exclusion and must be made with caution but has been noted unequivocally in several studies.[7]

With the newer techniques available to test newborns, one can diagnose hearing loss very early in life, but the cost of testing all infants would be prohibitive. The following risk factors are suggested as indications for neonatal testing:

1. Family history of childhood hearing loss
2. Congenital or perinatal infection (e.g., rubella, herpes, or syphilis)
3. Congenital anomalies of the head and neck (e.g., dysmorphic appearance, including syndromal and nonsyndromal abnormalities, overt or submucous cleft palate, morphologic abnormalities of the pinna)
4. Birth weight less than 1500 g
5. Hyperbilirubinemia requiring exchange transfusion
6. Bacterial meningitis
7. Anoxia (including infants with low Apgar scores or hypotonia)[1]

A radiologic workup consisting of a high-resolution noncontrast computed tomography (CT) scan of the temporal bones is often helpful. There are several anomalies of the inner ear, notably Mondini dysplasia, that can be definitively diagnosed in this way. Computed tomography is an important adjunct in the workup of aural atresia, in order to determine if there is a cleft of the middle ear or the ossicles, thus determining suitability for surgical correction.

Individuals with congenital sensorineural hearing loss must be carefully examined for associated anomalies of the head and neck, integument, and internal organs. More than 60 genetic syndromes have been characterized, including Usher, Alport, Pendred, Waardenburg, and many other eponymic syndromes.[6,13] Other cases are caused by prenatal or perinatal insult, such as low birth weight, infection, or anoxia. Appropriate blood serologies are tested and a CT of the temporal bone is ordered.

A substantial number of cases of congenital sensorineural hearing loss will not yield an obvious diagnosis following this workup. Many of these probably occur genetically, although this is difficult to prove.

Acquired sensorineural hearing loss may be caused by ototoxicity, meningitis, labyrinthitis, temporal bone trauma, perilymph fistula, and acoustic trauma.[13]

Conductive hearing loss is usually caused by otitis media or middle ear effusion. Chronic otitis media, cholesteatoma, otosclerosis, and ossicular fixation or discontinuity are less frequent etiologies.

PSYCHOSOCIAL CONSIDERATIONS

Any degree of hearing loss present during a child's early life can impair that child's development of language and communication skills. In the case of a child with a severe or profound hearing loss, this effect can be most pronounced. Early identification of such children therefore is imperative, as it enables the child to be rehabilitated (artificial amplification can often provide some useful hearing), and the special needs of the child with a hearing impairment can be addressed. Most communities and school systems have special agencies or programs for those with a hearing impairment; thus early referral of a child allows for maximal benefit. If a child with a severe impairment remains unidentified for the first 2 or 3 years of life, a severe handicap in all areas of interpersonal communication is the usual result. Such an individual has been understimulated during a crucial phase of language development, and it is extremely difficult to make up for that lost opportunity.

Milder degrees of hearing loss may also induce significant hardship, because children with hearing losses in the 20 to 50 dB range may not fully follow conversations or may miss instructions from teachers. Such children may be thought of as inattentive, antisocial, or unintelligent. Following treatment of such hearing losses, one often sees remarkable improvement in school performance and personality.

MANAGEMENT

Mild and moderate conductive hearing losses caused by middle ear infections are treated with antibiotics. Middle ear effusion is frequently seen after an acute infection, but such effusions often resolve spontaneously. When an effusion lasts several months, or if the tympanic membrane is severely retracted with marked hearing loss, surgical intervention may be indicated. Myringotomy and insertion of drainage tubes is usually performed, along with adenoidectomy if there is concomitant evidence of nasopharyngeal obstruction. (See Chapter 261 for discussion of the indications for adenoidectomy.)

Severe and profound hearing losses require an intensive rehabilitative and educational program.[2] Hearing aid technology has advanced in recent years with miniaturization and improved acoustic characteristics. The child should be fitted with an appropriate device early in life. Frequency modulated (FM) assistive listening devices are excellent adjuncts in the classroom and home. With such a device the individual with a hearing impairment has an FM receiver and earphone, and the speaker has a microphone. The range of the device can extend up to several hundred feet. Speech reading and auditory training help to maximize communication skills. Children who are successful in oral communication have been increasingly successful with "mainstreaming" into a regular classroom. When oral communication is less successful, a manual mode of communication (e.g., sign language) is introduced. For profoundly deaf children who do not benefit from conventional hearing aids, the use of fibrotactile aids may improve communication performance.[13] Cochlear implants have emerged as a new and exciting modality in the treatment of children with a profound hearing impairment.[8,11]

The key to proper treatment of children with hearing impairment is early identification and intervention. Today's technology makes it possible to diagnose hearing loss in infants and children of any age and thus to treat and rehabilitate these individuals at the earliest possible time.

REFERENCES

1. American Speech, Language and Hearing Association, Joint Committee on Infant Hearing: Position statement, ASHA 24:1017, 1982.
2. Erber N: Auditory training, Washington DC, 1982, AG Bell Association for the Deaf.
3. Ginsberg I and White T: Otologic considerations in audiology. In Katz J, editor: Handbook of clinical audiology, Baltimore, 1985, Williams & Wilkins.
4. Hecox K and Galambos R: Brainstem auditory-evoked responses in human infants and adults, Arch Otolaryngol 99:30, 1974.
5. Jerger S et al: Studies in impedance audiometry. II. Children less than 6 years old, Arch Otolaryngol 99:1, 1974.
6. Konigsmark BW and Gorlin TJ: Genetic and metabolic deafness, Philadelphia, 1976, WB Saunders Co.
7. McCanna D and DeLapa G: A clinical study of 27 children exhibiting functional hearing loss, Language Speech Hearing Services in Schools 12:26, 1981.
8. Miyamoto RT et al: Comparison of sensory aids in deaf children, Ann Otol Rhinol Laryngol 99(suppl 142):2, 1989.
9. Northern JL and Downs MP: Hearing loss in children, Baltimore, 1978, Williams & Wilkins.
10. Paradise JL, Smith C, and Bluestone CD: Tympanometric detection of middle ear effusion in infants and young children, Pediatrics 58:198, 1976.
11. Parisier SC, Chute P, and Hellman S: The use of cochlear implants for profound hearing loss, Surgical Rounds 12:15, 1989.
12. Pickett J and MacFarland W: Auditory implants and tactile aids for the profoundly deaf, J Speech Hear Res 28:134, 1985.
13. Schuknecht HF: Pathology of the ear, Cambridge, Mass, 1974, Harvard University Press.
14. Simmons F and Russ F: Automated newborn hearing screening: the Crib-o-Gram, Arch Otolaryngol 100:1, 1974.
15. Terkildsen K and Thomsen K: The influence of pressure variations on the impedance of the human eardrum, J Laryngol Otol 73:409, 1959.
16. Thompson G and Weber B: Responses of infants and young children to behavior observation audiometry, J Speech Hear Disord 39:140, 1974.
17. Yantis P: Pure tone air conduction testing. In Katz J, editor: Handbook of clinical audiology, Baltimore, 1985, William & Wilkins.

137

Heart Murmurs

Edward B. Clark

The normal murmur that most children develop sometime during childhood must be distinguished from a pathologic murmur indicating a structural heart defect. Yet not all patients with heart disease have a murmur; cyanotic patients with pulmonary atresia and healthy-looking children with coarctation of the aorta may have no murmur. Thus the cardiac examination includes what one sees and feels, in addition to what one hears.

INSPECTION

Much can be learned from careful observation. Asymmetry of the chest often reflects long-standing enlargement of the heart. Retraction of the suprasternal notch and grooving of the lower rib cage may be caused by vigorous pulling of the diaphragm in an infant with stiff lungs from pulmonary overcirculation.

PALPATION

Palpation adds to the examination. Thrills felt over the heart or neck vessels reflect high-velocity blood flow. The cardiac thrust or heave correlate with ventricular enlargement. A palpable pulmonary artery signifies pulmonary hypertension.

The peripheral pulses should be palpated simultaneously. A strong brachial pulse and weak femoral pulse suggest the diagnosis of coarctation of the aorta. A water-hammer pulse may be the clue to aortic insufficiency or another cardiac lesion associated with a wide pulse pressure. The plateau pulse of aortic stenosis can be easily recognized. An enlarged liver correlates with vascular engorgement.

AUSCULTATION

The heart sounds relate to the hemodynamic events of the cardiac cycle. The first heart sound is generated by closure of the tricuspid and mitral valves. The second heart sound is produced by closure of the semilunar valves and is particularly important for diagnosis. The first component of the second heart sound (S_2A) is caused by aortic valve closure and the second component by pulmonary valve closure (S_2P). The intensity of S_2A and S_2P and their relationship to each other and to respiration provide information about the pressure at which the valves close and about blood flow across the valves. Other sounds such as systolic click of a bicuspid semilunar valve, an opening snap of the mitral valve, diastolic gallop, friction rub, and bruits over intercostal arteries or an arteriovenous fistula help make an accurate cardiac diagnosis.

TYPES OF HEART MURMURS (Fig. 137-1)

A heart murmur is caused by turbulent blood flow. The timing, intensity, and location of heart murmurs define the anatomic cause of the turbulent flow. A thrill is palpable when the murmur is a grade 4 or more in intensity in the grading system of 1 to 6.

An *ejection murmur* reflects turbulence as blood flows in increased volume through a narrowed orifice or normal semilunar valve. Murmurs arising in the pulmonary outflow tract are best heard in the left second intercostal space. Those arising in the aortic outflow tract radiate to the right second intercostal space.

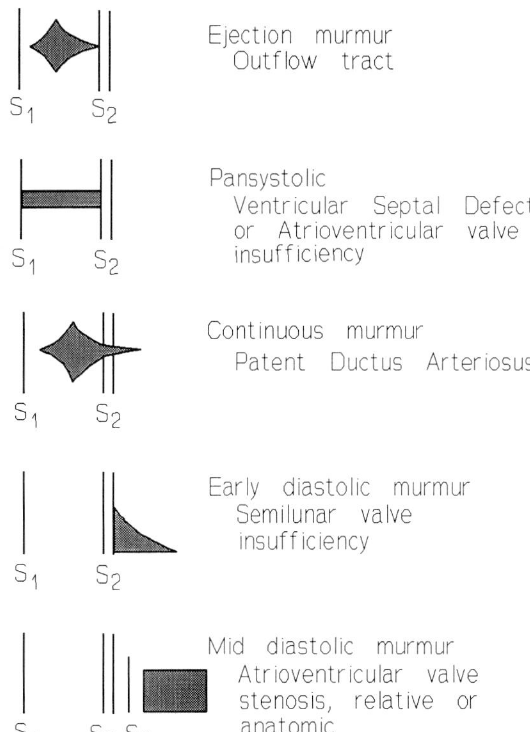

Fig. 137-1 Diagram of the five most common types of cardiac murmurs: ejection murmur, pansystolic murmur, continuous murmur, early murmur, and mid-diastolic murmur. The shaded areas show the timing and intensity of the cardiac murmur in relation to the first (S_1) and second (S_2) heart sounds, and the third heart sound present with a gallop rhythm. (See text for further description.)

A *pansystolic murmur* denotes turbulent blood flow during the isovolemic phase of contraction. Ventricular septal defect (VSD), mitral insufficiency, and tricuspid insufficiency cause such a murmur. The location of maximal intensity distinguishes the murmur of a ventricular septal defect from that of mitral insufficiency. The VSD murmur is heard best along the left lower sternal border and radiates to the right. A mitral insufficiency murmur is heard best at the apex and radiates to the left axilla. The murmur of tricuspid insufficiency is maximal at the fourth left interspace and varies with respiration.

A *continuous systolic and diastolic murmur* arises from turbulent flow across a patent ductus arteriosus or another direct connection between a high- and low-pressure system such as a pulmonary arteriovenous fistula.

An *early diastolic murmur* begins with the second heart sound and is caused by insufficiency of the aortic or pulmonary valve. A high-pitched murmur indicates aortic insufficiency; a low-pitched, soft murmur indicates pulmonary regurgitation.

A *mid-diastolic murmur* heard at the apex is caused by excessive blood flow across the mitral or tricuspid valve. This murmur is heard with large left-to-right shunts such as an atrial septal defect, a ventricular septal defect, or a patent ductus arteriosus.

ASSOCIATED HEART SOUNDS

The *second heart sound* is particularly important in the diagnosis of congenital heart defects. Normally this sound is split, with the aortic component preceding the pulmonary component. The two elements separate on inspiration and fuse on expiration. The louder the pulmonary component and the narrower the splitting, the greater the pulmonary artery pressure. Conversely, delay and diminution of the pulmonary component signify increasingly severe pulmonary stenosis. A wide and fixed split second heart sound occurs with mild pulmonary stenosis and with increased right heart ejection volume, as in the left-to-right shunt of an atrial septal defect.

An *early systolic ejection click* denotes a bicuspid aortic or pulmonary valve. Clicks can also be heard from a dilated aorta or pulmonary artery. A *midsystolic click* and a late systolic murmur at the apex characterizes the mitral valve prolapse.

An intermittent *third heart sound* at the apex is heard in many normal children; a *fourth heart sound,* however, often is pathologic. The S_3 and S_4 gallops reflect blood flow into a stiff ventricle and are often associated with heart failure.

DIFFERENTIAL DIAGNOSIS: INNOCENT MURMUR

Most heart murmurs arise from turbulent blood flow in a normal heart. There are four common kinds of normal murmurs:

1. *A Still murmur:* A short, vibratory, grade 1 or grade 2 ejection murmur heard over the precordium; it is the most common innocent murmur. A Still murmur is noted in at least 50% of normal, healthy children by 3 or 4 years of age.
2. *Venous hum:* A continuous murmur heard above the clavicle when the patient is upright. The murmur disappears when the patient is supine or when the head is turned and the external jugular vein is compressed.
3. *Pulmonary souffle:* A soft, midsystolic murmur heard in the second left interspace (pulmonary area). This murmur is heard in high cardiac output states such as fever, anemia, or hyperthyroidism.
4. Benign *peripheral pulmonary murmur:* An ejection murmur heard in the left second intercostal space that radiates to both axilla. Frequently heard in infants and small children, it represents blood flow turbulence at the branch point of the main and right and left pulmonary arteries.

MANAGEMENT

The only management needed in a child with a normal heart murmur is complete reassurance. A child with an organic murmur merits evaluation by a pediatric cardiologist.

SUGGESTED READING

Park MK: Pediatric cardiology for practitioners, ed 2, Chicago, 1988, Year Book Medical Publishers, Inc.

138

Hematuria

Edward J. Ruley

The diagnostic approach to hematuria in a pediatric patient is quite different from the strategy employed for investigating hematuria in an adult. Having an organized plan of investigation is important if one is to determine the diagnosis most cost effectively so that the child is subjected to the fewest invasive and uncomfortable procedures.

It is helpful to consider the occurrence of hematuria in several clinical scenarios. Some children have a large enough quantity of blood in the urine that the urine is darkened in color, thereby producing macroscopic or gross hematuria. Others may have apparently clear urine, but spots of blood will be found on the underclothing or diapers. Finally, the most common circumstance is the child who has normal-appearing urine that tests positive for blood, a situation termed *microhematuria*. The presence of symptoms, either localized to the urinary tract or more generalized, is variable in each of these circumstances. The most likely etiologies of the hematuria in these clinical scenarios are different; therefore the clinical approach to the diagnosis of each also differs.

GROSS HEMATURIA

Incidence

Gross hematuria is a relatively uncommon urinary symptom, the occurrence of which varies according to the population being cared for as well as certain environmental factors. In a study of more than 128,000 consecutive patients visiting an emergency clinic in a large city in the northeastern United States, the incidence of "red urine" as the chief complaint was 1.4 per 1000 visits. When other causes of a red urine were eliminated, the incidence of true gross hematuria was 1.3 per 1000 visits.[2]

Etiology

Urinary tract infection (either bacterial or viral) is the most common cause of gross hematuria in children, accounting for approximately half the cases. Irritation or ulceration of the perineum or urethral meatus is the next most common cause, constituting about 20% of the cases. Trauma, such as from an automobile accident or a fall, is the third most common etiology. However, when relatively minor trauma results in gross hematuria, the clinician should be alerted to the possibility of an undiagnosed dilated urinary system. Such dilated structures may be fluid-filled cysts associated with various types of congenital cystic kidney diseases or a urine-filled kidney pelvis and ureter caused by obstructive uropathy. These dilated systems are much more susceptible to gross bleeding after minor direct or indirect trauma than is the normal urinary system. Although urinary stones can also produce gross hematuria, they occur less commonly in children than in adults. However, hypercalciuria without lithiasis has been recognized as an important cause of gross hematuria in children. In one study, significant hypercalciuria was found in 43% of the children with gross hematuria.[1] Although coagulopathy has always been included in lists of gross hematuria causes, it is very uncommon. In contrast, gross hematuria is not uncommon in patients with sickle cell trait or sickle cell disease. Glomerulonephritis usually accounts for fewer than 10% of patients with gross hematuria, although the incidence varies considerably depending on whether there is a nephritogenic strain of *Streptococcus* in the community. Even with a complete and thoughtful approach, between 10% and 20% of children will not be found to have discernable etiology.

History

It is important to ascertain the color of the urine observed by the patient or the caretakers. Pink or red urine most often indicates bladder or urethral bleeding; greenish or brown urine is most commonly seen in upper tract or renal parenchymal bleeding. A child, particularly a circumcised male infant, who has generally clear urine but who is noted to have a spot of blood (usually red or pink) on the underclothing or diaper most often has bleeding from the urethra or the meatus. The presence of symptoms, either generalized or localized to the urinary tract, is important in determining the most likely etiology. Generalized symptoms such as fever, abdominal pain, arthralgia, arthritis, and rash imply that the gross hematuria is but part of a more extensive illness. In contrast, urinary frequency, urgency, and dysuria would lead one to consider the lower urinary system and the bladder outlet as the site of the pathology. The past medical history, in particular previous diagnoses, prior episodes of gross hematuria, recent or concurrent illness (especially upper airway infections), as well as the events surrounding the onset of gross hematuria, are obviously important. Certain diagnoses such as sickle cell disease, hypercalciuria, or IgA nephropathy are characterized by recurrent episodes of gross hematuria. The occurrence of antecedent or concurrent upper respiratory tract infections may favor a particular type of glomerulonephritis as the etiology (see Chapter 230, "Nephritis"). Prior voiding habits such as the frequency and style of voiding can be important clues to the etiology. It has been noted that young boys may squeeze or compress the penis in an attempt to thwart an urge to micturate, experienced at a time when they do not want to interrupt their play or activities. Other boys may have the habit of bending their penis over the elastic in their underpants when voiding, causing a sharp bend in the urethra. Both of these practices may lead to urethral irritation from the pressure of the urinary stream and produce gross or microscopic bleeding. In girls, it is important to consider menarche as being misinterpreted as an episode of gross hematuria. Finally, a history of other family members with gross hematuria, urinary stones, sickle cell disease, or coagulopathies can be pertinent.

Physical Findings

A relatively comprehensive general physical examination is appropriate for children with gross hematuria. Specifically, blood pressure measurement, abdominal examination, and direct visualization of the penile meatus or the female introitus, including the urethral meatus, is important.

Laboratory Findings

Obviously the most important laboratory test is the urinalysis. The centrifuged sediment of a freshly voided urine specimen should be examined very carefully under the microscope with attention given to the presence and morphology of any erythrocytes, as well as to the presence of any cellular casts (Fig. 138-1). Should there be only relatively homogenous pigmented casts without significant numbers of erythrocytes, one should suspect hemoglobinuria or myoglobinuria as the cause of the discolored urine. The dip-and-read strips for blood react to both hemoglobin and myoglobin. Some causes of hemoglobinuria and myoglobinuria are given in the box on p. 959. These situations are relatively uncommon in pediatric patients.

When erythrocytes are present, scrutiny of their appearance helps determine their origin.[1] Red blood cells that originate from the urinary structures outside the nephrons look like normal peripheral-circulating erythrocytes on a blood smear. They will be eumorphic; that is, of uniform size and shape. Also, no casts will be seen. In contrast, erythrocytes originating from the kidney parenchyma are dysmorphic; that is, they vary in size and have irregular outlines with blebs of cytoplasm appearing to bud from the cell surface (Fig. 138-2). The reason for the dysmorphic appearance of the erythrocytes remains uncertain. It may be the result of cell damage during extrusion through the glomerular basement membrane, the effect of osmotic forces during the cell's passage down the tubule, or some other as yet undefined factor. In addition to dysmorphic erythrocytes, a variety of casts containing erythrocytes, leukocytes, or tubular cells, as well as casts that appear coarsely and finely granular or hyaline, may be present (see Fig. 138-1). Regardless, dysmorphic erythrocytes and erythrocyte casts are thought to originate only from diseases in the kidney parenchyma. Nowhere in the urinary system from the calyx to the meatus are there conditions that can create dysmorphic erythrocytes or casts. However, there are certain situations in which kidney insult can cause some overlap. One of the most obvious is trauma, in which there can be bleeding from the kidney parenchyma and the urinary system at the same time. In this circumstance, both dysmorphic and eumorphic erythrocytes may be present in the same specimen, as well as erythrocyte casts.

Proteinuria can also be found in urine specimens in which there is gross hematuria. In urine specimens that are isotonic or hypertonic, gross hematuria can result in modest amounts of protein being detectable. In urine specimens that are hypotonic, the degree of proteinuria can be marked. Studies have shown that the protein in this latter circumstance originates from the hemoglobin released from the lysed erythrocytes. Microhematuria does not result in any significant proteinuria.[4] Therefore proteinuria in the presence of microhematuria needs to be investigated as an additional harbinger of significant renal disease.

Because urinary tract infection is so common, a urine

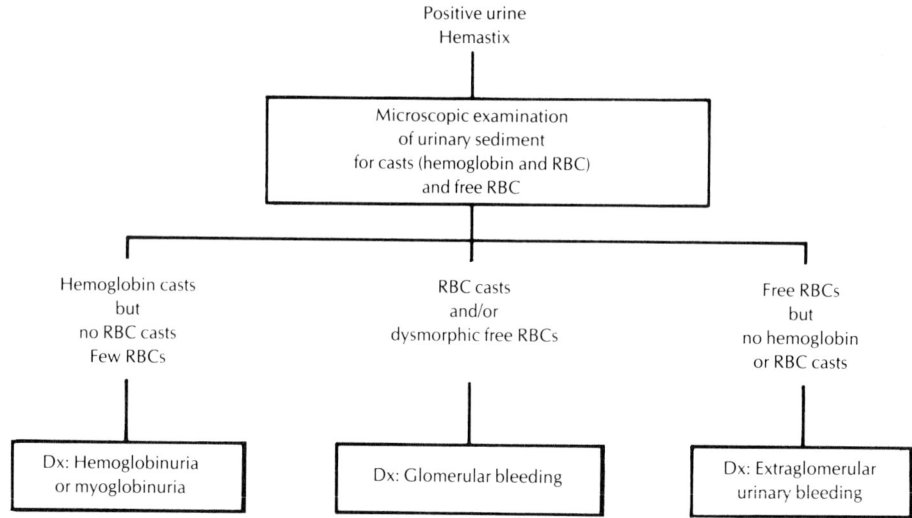

Fig. 138-1 A clinical algorithm for microhematuria in children.

Causes of Hemoglobinuria and Myoglobinuria

HEMOGLOBINURIA

Hemolytic anemia (e.g., glucose 6-phosphate dehydrogenase [G6PD] deficiency, Coombs'-positive hemolytic anemia)
Mismatched blood transfusions
Intravascular coagulation (e.g., disseminated intravascular coagulation [DIC], hemolytic-uremic syndrome)
Infections (e.g., sepsis, malaria)
Freshwater near-drowning
Mechanical erythrocyte damage (e.g., artificial heart valves, cardiopulmonary bypass)

MYOGLOBINURIA

Muscle injury (e.g., crush injuries, electrical burns)
Myositis
Rhabdomyolysis

culture is indicated in all instances of gross hematuria. To investigate hypercalciuria, calcium and creatinine levels should be determined on a random urine specimen. If this ratio is above 0.21 mg/mg, a 24-hour specimen should be obtained to determine the calcium excretion.[3] Imaging of the kidneys and the urinary system by ultrasound is also indicated to investigate kidney size and the character of the kidney parenchyma and to screen for dilated collecting systems. Gross hematuria is one instance in which cystoscopy may be indicated to look for sites of bleeding within the bladder or to determine from which kidney the blood is originating. Obviously, such direct visualization is indicated for selected cases only and must be done when the patient is actively bleeding to be of value. Further investigation and the institution of treatment depend on the working diagnosis as suggested by recent, past, and family histories and the results of the preliminary tests. In contrast to adults, tumors of the urinary system are very uncommon causes of gross hematuria in children.

MICROHEMATURIA

Incidence

Microhematuria occurs much more frequently than gross hematuria in the pediatric population, with a prevalence of 0.05% to 2.0%, depending on the definition of significant hematuria (see Chapter 18, Seven, "Use of Urinalysis and Urine Culture in Screening"). Although the definition of significant microhematuria differs among studies, many investigators have come to consider more than 10 erythrocytes per high-power field in the sediment of a centrifuged aliquot of freshly voided urine a pathologic number of cells.

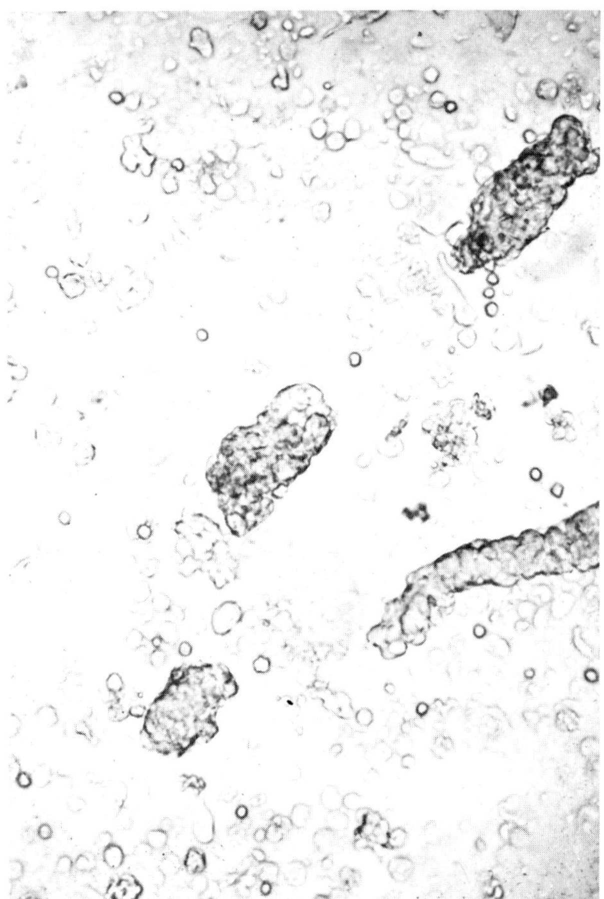

Fig. 138-2 Unstained urine sediment showing a red blood cell cast and dysmorphic red blood cells. (×100.)

Etiology

Many of the causes of gross hematuria may also cause microhematuria, although infection does so less commonly. Microscopic hematuria in the asymptomatic child, usually discovered during a routine well-child examination, is a frequent clinical problem that requires a thoughtful, systematic approach. The same algorithm given for macroscopic hematuria (see Fig. 138-1) can be applied to the child with microhematuria.

History and Physical Findings

The same questions should be asked and a similar physical examination done in the child with microhematuria as that outlined for the child with gross hematuria. Not uncommonly, the history is completely noncontributory and the physical examination unrevealing.

Laboratory Findings

As with gross hematuria, the carefully done urinalysis becomes the critical first test for the child with microhematuria. Pigmenturia should be considered, although significant hemoglobin or myoglobin filtration more often causes macro-

Causes of Extraglomerular Hematuria

Infection (e.g., cystitis, urethritis, balinitis)
Hypercalcuria (e.g., absorptive hypercalcuria, renal tubular hypercalcuria)
Trauma (e.g., vehicular accidents, falls, child abuse)
Urinary lithiasis (e.g., hypercalcuria, cysteinuria)
Malformations (e.g., cystic kidney diseases, posterior urethral valves, ureteropelvic junction obstruction)
Hemoglobinopathy (e.g., sickle cell disease, thalassemia)
Drugs (e.g., antibiotics, cytoxan)
Bleeding diathesis (e.g., Von Willebrand disease, hemophilia)
Instrumentation (e.g., suprapubic aspiration, urinary catheterization, cystoscopy, self-stimulation)
Tumors (e.g., Wilm tumor, rhabdomyosarcoma, bladder papilloma)

scopic urine discoloration. When true hematuria is assured, the morphology of the erythrocytes and the presence of casts assume the same significance as in gross hematuria. Differentiation of the causes of glomerular bleeding often requires hospitalization and more extensive testing (see Chapter 230, "Nephritis"). Should the urine contain only eumorphic erythrocytes and be free of casts, extraglomerular bleeding is most likely. Some of the etiologies are listed in the box below. Random and 24-hour urine specimens should be collected for calcium-creatinine ratios and calcium excretion determination. Specific treatment regimens depend on the etiology of the microhematuria.

REFERENCES

1. Birch DF et al: Urinary erythrocyte morphology in the diagnosis of glomerular hematuria, Clin Nephrol 20(2):78, 1983.
2. Ingelfinger JR, Davis AE, and Grupe WE: Frequency and etiology of gross hematuria in a general pediatric setting, Pediatrics 59(4):557, 1977.
3. Stapleton FB et al: Hypercalcuria in children with hematuria, N Engl J Med 310(21):1345, 1984.
4. Tapp DC and Copley JB: Effect of red blood cell lysis on protein quantitation in hematuric states, Am J Nephrol 8:190, 1988.

SUGGESTED READING

Norman ME: An office approach to hematuria and proteinuria, Pediatr Clin North Am 34(3):545, 1987.

139

Hemoptysis

Beryl J. Rosenstein

Hemoptysis, defined as the expectoration of blood or blood-tinged sputum, is a potentially life-threatening but fortunately unusual occurrence in the pediatric age group. Over a 10-year period at a large pediatric referral center, hemoptysis was diagnosed in only 40 children.[15] In seven of these children, hemoptysis was the sole presenting manifestation; in the remaining patients, hemoptysis was often associated with fever and cough. The amount of bleeding was usually small; only two children experienced a blood loss in excess of 200 ml. Because hemoptysis often is a sign of significant underlying disease and may be life threatening, patients with this condition deserve rapid and complete evaluation. If hemoptysis occurs as something more than blood-tinged sputum or mild bleeding, the evaluation is best carried out in a hospital in collaboration with pediatric pulmonologists and endoscopists.

CHARACTERISTICS AND ORIGIN

The majority of children brought to medical attention because of "spitting up blood" have an identifiable source of bleeding outside the lower respiratory tract, usually epistaxis, gingivitis, pharyngeal ulceration, or trauma to the oropharynx. At times it may be difficult to differentiate hemoptysis from hematemesis.[11] With hematemesis the blood is dark red or brownish in color, may contain food particles, and has an acid pH; bleeding is usually preceded by nausea or accompanied by retching. With hemoptysis the blood is usually bright red and frothy, may be mixed with sputum, and has an alkaline pH; such bleeding may be preceded by a gurgling noise in the large airways and is usually accompanied by coughing. Older patients with bleeding in the lung may describe a vague sensation that enables them to localize the site of the bleeding. It is sometimes difficult to determine the origin of bleeding when there is both coughing and vomiting. In infants, swallowed blood originating in the lungs may be vomited in the absence of coughing. Therefore the possibility of a respiratory tract source of bleeding should be considered in children with unexplained hematemesis, particularly if there are chest radiograph abnormalities. Children under 6 years of age rarely expectorate sputum; in this age group, the presence of hemoptysis may not be apparent unless the amount of bleeding is large. Children who have a hard, forceful cough may produce sputum that has small streaks of blood on the surface but that is not mixed with blood. This finding may be seen in association with respiratory tract infections and is usually of little clinical significance.

The treatment of hemoptysis is the management of the underlying disorder, making a correct etiologic diagnosis mandatory. In adults, hemoptysis is a relatively common occurrence. The leading causes are chronic bronchitis/bronchiectasis, lung cancer, and tuberculosis. However, almost any disease that affects the respiratory tract can result in hemoptysis. The number of disorders associated with hemoptysis is not as large in children as in adults but is still extensive (see the box on p. 962). The most common cause is infection, followed by foreign body aspiration.[15] Many of the underlying conditions occur infrequently and may be difficult to diagnose.

EVALUATION

Evaluation of the patient with hemoptysis should begin with a detailed history and physical examination. The history should be elicited as to underlying illnesses, fever, cough, sputum production, stridor, wheezing, dyspnea, joint pain, weight loss, menstrual history, family illnesses, recent trauma, prior episodes of bleeding, choking episodes, medication use, substance abuse, exposure to toxins, and travel to areas endemic for parasitic infestations and mycobacterial disease. Any history of travel is especially pertinent because of the large-scale immigration from southeast Asia to the United States. Some patients with hemoptysis, however, will be otherwise asymptomatic and given an entirely negative past history.

When confronted with a child with presumed hemoptysis, it must first be determined if the blood originated from the lungs and/or lower airways or from the mouth, upper airway, or gastrointestinal tract. Careful examination of the nasopharynx and oral cavity for bleeding sites is essential. Nasopharyngoscopy and laryngoscopy may be helpful. Pertinent physical findings include saddle-nose deformity, bruits, thrills, unequal chest wall movement and air entry, abnormal breath sounds (especially localized wheezing, heard with bronchial lesions and foreign bodies), pleural rub, heart murmur, hypertension, digital clubbing, lymphadenopathy, hepatosplenomegaly, hemangiomas, telangiectases, neuropathies, deep vein thrombosis, and evidence of trauma to the head, neck, or chest.

Radiographic Evaluation

If the source of bleeding is not apparent on the basis of the history and physical examination, a chest roentgenogram is the next step in the evaluation.[1] The most common abnor-

Causes of Hemoptysis in Children

INFECTION
Bacterial
- Bronchitis
- Lung abscess
- Necrotizing pneumonia
- Tuberculosis
- Bronchiectasis
- Immune deficiency
- Cystic fibrosis
- Immobile cilia syndrome

Fungal
- Actinomycosis
- Aspergillosis
- Coccidioidomycosis
- Histoplasmosis

Parasitic
- Echinococcosis (hydatid disease)
- Paragonimiasis
- Strongyloidiasis

FOREIGN BODIES

CONGENITAL DEFECTS
Cardiovascular
- Congenital heart defects
- Absent pulmonary artery
- Arteriovenous malformation
- Hemangiomatous malformation
- Telangiectasia (Rendu-Osler-Weber syndrome)

Other
- Pulmonary sequestration
- Bronchogenic cyst
- Intrathoracic enteric cyst

VASCULITIS
Periarteritis nodosa

AUTOIMMUNE DISORDERS
Wegener granulomatosis
Pulmonary hemosiderosis
Milk allergy
Goodpasture syndrome
Collagen-vascular disease

TRAUMA
Compression or crush injury
Iatrogenic
- Postsurgical
- Diagnostic lung puncture
- Transbronchial biopsy

Inhalation of toxins

NEOPLASTIC CONDITIONS
Endobronchial metastases
Primary lung tumors
- Benign (hamartoma, neurogenic tumors)
- Malignant (bronchial adenoma, bronchogenic carcinoma, pulmonary blastoma)

Endometriosis

DRUG INDUCED
Propylthiouracil

PULMONARY EMBOLISM

HEMOGLOBINOPATHY WITH PULMONARY INFARCT

FACTITIOUS

malities found on chest roentgenograms are atelectasis and parenchymal and interstitial infiltrates. Other helpful findings include localized air trapping, pulmonary nodules, hilar adenopathy, pleural effusion, pneumothorax, cardiomegaly, and foreign bodies. Ring shadows and parallel lines represent thick-walled bronchi and suggest bronchiectasis. In one third of children with hemoptysis, the initial roentgenogram is normal; however, a pulmonary source for the bleeding eventually is identified in half of those patients with negative chest roentgenograms.[15]

Inspiratory and expiratory roentgenograms help detect any partially obstructing endobronchial foreign body. The lung on the side of the foreign body demonstrates air trapping on expiration relative to the normal side. On a decubitus view, the side that does not deflate normally in the dependent position is the side with air trapping. With complete obstruction secondary to a foreign body, there is obstructive atelectasis or pneumonia. High kilovoltage roentgenograms can help better visualize the upper airway and define mass lesions. Fluoroscopy can be used to (1) confirm questionable parenchymal lesions on plain roentgenogram; (2) localize an identified lesion or mass on a chest roentgenogram to lung parenchyma, pleura, chest wall, mediastinum, or vascular structures; or (3) identify and localize a suspected bronchial foreign body causing air trapping when findings are equivocal or not apparent on chest roentgenogram. An esophagogram may help localize a mass to the middle mediastinum. Based on the results of the roentgenographic evaluation, the diagnostic workup may require a number of laboratory and imaging procedures.

Laboratory Evaluation

A variety of laboratory tests may be helpful. These include a complete blood count and indices; eosinophil count; erythrocyte sedimentation rate; urinalysis; arterial blood gas measurements; skin test for *Mycobacterium, Aspergillus,* and *Echinococcus;* clotting studies; sputum cytology; and cultures for bacteria, fungi, and mycobacteria. Gastric aspirates can be examined for ova, parasites, and hemosiderin-laden macrophages (hemosiderosis) and cultured for mycobacteria. Other helpful procedures include measurement of sweat electrolyte concentration (cystic fibrosis); milk precipitins in serum (milk allergy, hemosiderosis); and antinuclear antibody, lupus erythematosus (LE) cell preparation, and rheumatoid factor (collagen-vascular disease). In patients with hemoptysis and renal involvement (Goodpasture syndrome, collagen-vascular disease, and Wegener disease), renal function studies, measurement of antiglomerular basement membrane antibody, and renal biopsy may be needed for a definitive diagnosis.

Diagnostic Imaging

Computed tomography (CT) may detect radiographically unrecognized parenchymal infiltrates or foreign bodies and is usually the procedure of choice to define further the anatomy of an abnormality found on chest roentgenogram.[1] CT can outline the extent of a mass and properly localize it to the anterior, middle, or posterior mediastinum, lung parenchyma, pleura, chest wall, or spine. The trachea and major proximal bronchi are well defined. Computed tomography is good for the detection of cystic bronchiectasis, broncholithiasis, and endobronchial obstruction secondary to adenoma or blood clot. The use of intravenous contrast identifies vascular structures and can determine if a suspected mass is vascular in nature. The internal characeristics of a mass also can be identified; calcification, hemorrhage, and fat can be differentiated by their relative densities. CT may also be useful in guiding diagnostic procedures.

Magnetic resonance imaging (MRI) gives superior soft tissue contrast resolution and is useful in the evaluation of the mediastinum and hila.[1] Because vessels can be distinguished from other mediastinal structures, this technique can be used to demonstrate arteriovenous malformations and congenital anomalies of the pulmonary arteries.

Conventional angiography is useful for the evaluation of congenital malformations of the lungs and abnormalities of pulmonary vessels—that is, pulmonary sequestration, arteriovenous malformations, pulmonary embolus, and congenital anomalies of the pulmonary vessels. *Digital subtraction angiography* can be used to define the blood supply to a pulmonary sequestration or arteriovenous malformation.

Ventilation-perfusion scanning is helpful in evaluating regional lung perfusion and ventilation. This procedure can detect a decrease in pulmonary blood flow—that is, pulmonary artery agenesis or hypoplasia, and pulmonary embolus. The hallmark of a pulmonary embolus is ventilation without perfusion (V/Q mismatch).

A *technetium radionuclide scan* using radiolabeled red blood cells can be used to identify active bleeding sites (even with bleeding rates as low as 0.1 ml/minute)[4] or ectopic gastric mucosa.

Endoscopy

If the source of hemoptysis is still not apparent after laboratory and radiographic evaluation or if bleeding is recurrent or substantial, endoscopy is indicated.[13] A bleeding site is best localized when bronchoscopy is performed during active bleeding. The availability of the flexible fiberoptic bronchoscope has been a great advance. Compared with the rigid bronchoscope, this instrument has increased maneuverability and is tolerated more readily and for longer periods. The fiberoptic bronchoscope can usually be passed transnasally by use of sedation instead of general anesthesia. It can be used to visualize subsegmental airways that are beyond the reach of the rigid bronchoscope. There is still a role, however, for the rigid bronchoscope; it is better for removing foreign bodies and for maintaining a secure airway while providing adequate suctioning in those patients who have massive bleeding.

Bronchoscopy is particularly useful for the detection of foreign bodies and for the diagnosis of infection and endobronchial lesions. Material can be obtained for cultures, stains, and cytology. Bronchial brushings can be obtained and transbronchial biopsy performed. Old blood can be removed by saline lavage of segmental bronchi; the airway can then be reexamined. The need for bronchography has been virtually eliminated by the availability of computed tomography and high kilovoltage roentgenography. In rare cases it may be indicated as an adjunct to fiberoptic bronchoscopy to define type, site, and extent of bronchiectasis or to identify a congenital abnormality of the bronchus. It may also be used to differentiate an extrinsic from an intrinsic defect in the airway.

DIFFERENTIAL DIAGNOSIS

Among 40 children with hemoptysis who were seen at a pediatric referral center, bleeding was caused by infection in 16 cases and by an aspirated foreign body in six cases.[15] The remaining cases were associated with a variety of other disorders. In some cases, such as those associated with cystic fibrosis, congenital heart disease, or bleeding secondary to surgical procedures, diagnosis of the underlying disorder is usually well established at the time of hemoptysis. In most cases, however, the underlying diagnosis is not immediately apparent. In general, it is rare for children with pulmonary neoplasms or bleeding disorders to have hemoptysis. The diagnoses of bronchial wall neoplasms, mediastinal tumors, and arteriovenous malformations should be considered in young children with massive airway bleeding. Most aspirated foreign bodies occur in children under 4 years of age. Worldwide, echinococcosis and paragonimiasis are probably the most common causes of hemoptysis in childhood. This is not so, however, for hemoptysis occurring in North America.

Foreign Bodies

In children with hemoptysis, it is always important to be aware of the possibility of foreign body aspiration, even in the absence of a suggestive history.[10,12] Although most cases of an aspirated foreign body involve children younger than 4 years of age, teenagers with retained aspirated foreign bodies may have hemoptysis.[10] The major complication of foreign body aspiration is bronchial obstruction, which may result in atelectasis, abscess formation, pneumonia, and bronchiectasis. Hemoptysis is secondary to the extensive neovascularization that may occur in the bronchiectatic portion of the lung.

In many patients the initial choking episode is either not observed or not remembered, and there may be a long latent period between the episode of aspiration and the appearance of symptoms.[12] The likelihood that an aspirated foreign body is the cause of hemoptysis is increased if the episode of hemoptysis is accompanied by pronounced coughing, localized wheezing, and locally diminished or absent breath sounds. On examination, there may be localized rales or wheezes or both, but some patients have a normal examination. Patients commonly have recurrent or incomplete clearing of a focal infiltrate. The chest roentgenogram may be normal (20% of cases) or may show localized air trapping, atelectasis, or signs of unresolved pneumonia. A radiopaque object is seen in approximately 15% of cases. Fluoroscopy may reveal unequal aeration, asymmetric diaphragmatic movement, or mediastinal shift. Inspiratory and expiratory roentgenograms may be useful in demonstrating localized air trapping. Foreign bodies may also be identified by computed tomography. However, normal roentgenographic findings do not eliminate the need for bronchoscopy, at which time the diagnosis is usually confirmed. A flexible fiberoptic bronchoscope may be used for diagnosis, but a rigid bronchoscope is more useful for removal of foreign bodies. Because there may be more than one foreign body, it is important to examine both sides during bronchoscopy.

Hemosiderosis

Idiopathic pulmonary hemosiderosis (IPH) is an unusual and often baffling cause of hemoptysis in children.[2,7] It is a disorder of unknown cause characterized by recurrent episodes of diffuse intraalveolar hemorrhage. Although familial cases have been reported,[2] the inheritance pattern is not clear. Patients usually manifest the disorder during infancy and early childhood with hemoptysis, respiratory distress (cough, dyspnea, wheezing), diffuse parenchymal infiltrates, and iron-deficiency anemia. It is one of the few conditions in which refractory iron-deficiency anemia occurs without an obvious bleeding site.

Hemosiderosis may occur as a primary condition or in association with glomerulonephritis (Goodpasture syndrome), collagen-vascular disease, IgA deficiency and, in rare cases, cow milk protein allergy. The diagnosis of pulmonary hemosiderosis is suggested by the clinical picture along with the finding of iron-laden macrophages in bronchial or gastric washings and confirmed by the demonstration of these macrophages in lung biopsy material. Nuclear scanning of the lungs after injection of radiolabeled red blood cells can be used to confirm that lung infiltrates are secondary to intrapulmonary hemorrhage. Patients with hemosiderosis should have (1) an immunologic evaluation (collagen-vascular disease); (2) renal function studies, including renal biopsy and measurement of antiglomerular basement membrane antibody (Goodpasture syndrome); and (3) measurement of circulating precipitins to constituents of cow milk (milk allergy).

Treatment depends on associated disorders. In patients with cow milk allergy, all dairy products should be eliminated from the diet. Patients with Goodpasture syndrome and collagen-vascular disease are treated with immunosuppressive agents. Patients with persistent pulmonary infiltrates may benefit from an iron-chelating agent such as deferoxamine (Desferal).

Infections

Hemoptysis can occur with a variety of pulmonary infections, including necrotizing pneumonia, tuberculosis, aspergillosis, coccidioidomycosis, actinomycosis, histoplasmosis, and parasitic infestations. Worldwide, echinococcosis and paragonimiasis are probably the most common causes of hemoptysis in children. Bronchiectasis may be seen after lower respiratory tract infections (measles, adenovirus, tuberculosis), after foreign body aspiration, with allergic bronchopulmonary aspergillosis, and with genetic disorders such as cystic fibrosis, immotile cilia syndrome, immunodeficiencies, and alpha-1-antitrypsin deficiency. About 5% of patients with bronchiectasis have significant hemoptysis.[8] This diagnosis should be considered when hemoptysis occurs in conjunction with pulmonary infiltrates, cough, purulent sputum, and localized abnormal breath sounds. Plain roentgenography, computed tomography, and ventilation-perfusion scans may aid in the diagnosis. Bronchoscopy may be helpful in confirming the diagnosis and in obtaining material for stains and culture. In the child with suspected infection, serologic studies, cultures, and skin testing may all aid in arriving at a specific etiology. In some cases needle aspiration of a lesion or open lung biopsy is necessary.

Cystic Fibrosis

In patients with cystic fibrosis and bronchiectasis/chronic suppurative pseudomonas bronchitis, there are dilation, increased tortuosity, and hyperplasia of the bronchial artery circulation.[6] Anastomoses develop between the bronchial and pulmonary circulations in the walls of larger bronchi in chronically infected segments of lung. The right upper lobe is the most common site of bleeding. Secondary to exacerbations of pulmonary infection, there may be erosion of bronchial arteries and episodes of moderate to massive hemoptysis. Although episodes may subside spontaneously, recurrences are common. Bronchoscopy during active bleeding remains the most reliable means of identifying the area of bleeding but may not always be possible. Identification of a hypervascular area of lung by arteriography may also help localize the bleeding site.

Conservative treatment consists of bed rest, sedation, temporary withholding of chest physiotherapy, and intravenous antibiotics. Blood losses should be replaced and vitamin K administered if the prothrombin time is prolonged.

Percutaneous bronchial artery embolization is now accepted as the standard procedure for treating episodes of hemoptysis in patients with cystic fibrosis.[6] Indications for embolotherapy include either massive acute bleeding (300 ml over 24 hours) or chronic bleeding (75 to 100 ml per day) recurring over weeks or months. With this technique immediate cessation of bleeding can be achieved in more than 90% of patients. On long-term follow-up, one can expect recurrent episodes of minor bleeding in 70% of patients and major rebleeding in 20%. In rare cases, as in an unstable patient with cystic fibrosis who has massive hemoptysis, pulmonary resection may be indicated.[9]

Miscellaneous

There are a number of unusual causes of hemoptysis that need to be considered in pediatric patients. Hemoptysis may occur in thyrotoxic adolescents who develop a clinical picture of purpura, nephritis, severe anemia, and hemoptysis (secondary to pulmonary cavitation) during treatment with propylthiouracil.[3]

In rare cases, recurrent episodes of hemoptysis may occur coincident with the onset of menses in patients with bronchopulmonary endometriosis.[5] The chest roentgenogram is usually normal. It is a clinical diagnosis based on the association of unexplained hemoptysis coincident with menses, but the bleeding site can be localized through computed tomography at the time of bleeding.[5]

Factitious bleeding is one of the most baffling of all causes of hemoptysis in children.[14] This represents a form of Munchausen syndrome by proxy in which blood other than the patient's is presented as evidence of hemoptysis. Innovative detective work may be needed in such cases, including video monitoring and blood typing from the patient and caretakers.

MANAGEMENT

Management of the patient with hemoptysis depends almost entirely on the underlying cause and extent of bleeding. Once the underlying cause is found, treatment is directed at the source. In children with massive bleeding (more than 8 ml/kg/24 hours), an aggressive approach is mandatory. Arterial blood gases should be monitored. Once the airway is established, vigorous suctioning may be necessary. Supplemental oxygen, transfusions, and mechanical ventilation may be required. Bronchoscopy is useful, both diagnostically and therapeutically. It can be used to localize the bleeding site, protect and maintain the airway, and prevent asphyxiation. In cases with active bleeding, the open ventilating bronchoscope is preferable. It allows for simultaneous ventilation and inspection of the airway and is better than the flexible bronchoscope for suctioning and clearing the airway. Lavage with iced saline solution or topical application of a vasoconstrictor may be helpful. Control of massive bleeding may require endoscopic tamponade with a balloon catheter, embolization of involved arteries, or thoracotomy with a direct surgical approach to the source of bleeding.

REFERENCES

1. Ablin DS and Newell JD: Diagnostic imaging for evaluation of the pediatric chest, Clin Chest Med 8:641, 1987.
2. Beckerman RG, Taussig LM, and Pinnas JL: Familial idiopathic pulmonary hemosiderosis, Am J Dis Child 133:609, 1979.
3. Cassorla FG et al: Vasculitis, pulmonary cavitation, and anemia during antithyroid drug therapy, Am J Dis Child 137:118, 1983.
4. Coel MN and Druger G: Radionuclide detection of the site of hemoptysis, Chest 81:242, 1982.
5. Elliot DL, Barker AF, and Dison L: Catamenial hemoptysis: new methods of diagnosis and therapy, Chest 87:687, 1985.
6. Fellows KE et al: Bronchial artery embolization in cystic fibrosis: technique and long-term results, J Pediatr 95:959, 1979.
7. Levy J, Kolski GB, and Scanlin TF: Hemoptysis and anemia in a 3-year-old boy, Ann Allergy 55:439, 1985.
8. Lewiston NJ: Bronchiectasis in childhood, Pediatr Clin North Am 31:865, 1984.
9. Marmon L et al: Pulmonary resection for complications of cystic fibrosis, J Pediatr Surg 18:811, 1983.
10. Pattison CW, Leaming AJ, and Townsend ER: Hidden foreign body as a cause of recurrent hemoptysis in a teenage girl, Ann Thorac Surg 45:330, 1988.
11. Putnam JS and Tellis CJ: Hemoptysis, Prim Care 5:67, 1978.
12. Pyman C: Inhaled foreign bodies in childhood, Med J Aust 1:62, 1971.
13. Selecky PA: Evaluation of hemoptysis through the bronchoscope, Chest 73:741, 1978.
14. Shafer N and Shafer R: Factitious diseases, including Munchausen's syndrome, NY State J Med 80:594, 1980.
15. Tom LWC, Weisman RA, and Handler SD: Hemoptysis in children, Annals Otolaryngology 89:419, 1980.

140

Hepatomegaly

Roberta A. Hibbard

As a child grows, so does the liver. Liver mass increases tenfold from birth to adulthood. Normal liver size is described as a function of a child's age but may be influenced by the child's growth status and body habitus. Liver enlargement should prompt an evaluation to distinguish benign, self-limited processes from serious, life-threatening ones. Enlargement may be a manifestation of primary liver disease or of a generalized disease. The complete history and physical examination provide important clues to diagnostic considerations.

Liver size is best estimated by liver span, the height in the right midclavicular line. Liver span is determined by percussion of both upper and lower borders or by percussion superiorly and palpation inferiorly.[1,2,3] Palpation alone is unreliable and can be misleading. The lower border of the liver can be determined by auscultation. The diaphragm of the stethoscope should be placed just above the right costal margin in the midclavicular line. Scratching the skin of the abdomen along the midclavicular line upward from below the umbilicus will first be heard through the stethoscope when the liver's edge is reached and the sound is transmitted through the liver.

The physical relationship of the liver to adjacent structures is also important in assessing liver size. Hyperinflation of the lungs, a pneumothorax, a retroperitoneal mass, or a perihepatic abscess may displace the liver without enlarging it. Narrow costal angles, flared costal margins, pectus excavatum, and accessory lobes may alter the perception of liver size. The liver may not be palpable in a child with wide costal angles but may be normally palpable several centimeters below the right costal margin in a child with normal costal angles. Reidel lobe is a normal tonguelike elongation of the right lobe toward the right lower quadrant. If the upper border of the liver is at or near the fifth intercostal space in the midclavicular line, the palpable margin improves as an index of liver size. Under these conditions a distance from the costal margin of 2 cm in infancy and 1 cm in childhood is acceptable.[1,4] As a general rule, a liver span of less than 7 cm is normal (Table 140-1).

Hepatomegaly may be an unexpected finding in an asymptomatic patient, or it may be one of a constellation of findings in systemic disease. The history and physical examination simplify the evaluation. As noted in the box on p. 967, the age at presentation may provide one clue to etiology. Historical information should include nutritional assessment, exposure to hepatotoxins, and geographic exposure to possible infectious agents. Jaundice commonly accompanies hepatomegaly and is discussed in detail in Chapter 147. Splenomegaly associated with hepatomegaly occurs in all age groups and results most often from increased portal venous pressure, tissue infiltration, and reticuloendothelial cell hyperplasia.

In addition to the size of the liver, the contour, consistency (soft, firm, rock hard), character of the surface (smooth, irregular, nodular), and character of the palpable edge (rounded, sharp) should be noted. The liver edge is often tender and rounded in hepatomegaly because of tissue inflammation or sinusoidal congestion. A carcinomatous liver may be rock hard with or without an irregular border; a cirrhotic liver is firm and nontender. Auscultation may reveal a bruit, which often indicates hepatoma, or a friction rub, which suggests a tumor or perihepatitis. Frequent reevaluation employing percussion, palpation, and auscultation yields information about liver size and patterns of change.

PATHOPHYSIOLOGY

Several pathophysiologic mechanisms may be involved separately or in concert in the evolution of liver enlargement. Sinusoidal congestion associated with increased venous pressure (as in right-sided heart failure and constrictive pericarditis) or postsinusoidal block (as in venoocclusive disease) may cause a rapid and massive expansion of the liver. Kupffer cells—the reticuloendothelial cells lining liver sinusoids—phagocytize antigen-antibody complexes, bacterial endotoxins, and defective red cells. As a filtering system, these cells undergo proliferative and hyperplastic responses to septicemia, hepatitis, hemolysis, and neoplasia.

Inflammatory and cellular infiltrates may enlarge the liver diffusely. Normal erythropoietic tissue may be found within the sinusoids of term infants as a remnant of the major fetal hematopoietic organ. In extramedullary hematopoiesis associated with erythroblastosis fetalis and other forms of neonatal anemia, blood-forming units distend the sinusoids. Leukemic, lymphomatous, and lymphohistiocytic infiltrates may be prominent in the portal and periportal areas. Granulocytes, mononuclear cells, and plasma cells infiltrate the liver as an inflammatory response to hepatocellular destruction or Kupffer cell lysis, each of which can result from viral hepatitis, transplacental infection, drug toxicity, or biliary obstruction.

Storage of glycogen and lipids within hepatic parenchymal cells or Kupffer cells produces a diffuse distortion of the normal hepatic architecture. Inborn errors or acquired defects in the metabolism of glycogen, mucopolysaccharides (as in Hunter and Hurler syndromes), and lipids (as in gangliosidoses) thus produce liver enlargement.

Table 140-1 *Expected Liver Span of Infants, Children, and Adolescents by Percussion*

	MEAN ESTIMATED LIVER SPAN (cm)			MEAN ESTIMATED LIVER SPAN (cm)	
AGE IN YRS	MALES	FEMALES	AGE IN YRS	MALES	FEMALES
6 (mos)	2.4	2.8	8	5.6	5.1
1	2.8	3.1	10	6.1	5.4
2	3.5	3.6	12	6.5	5.6
3	4.0	4.0	14	6.8	5.8
4	4.4	4.3	16	7.1	6.0
5	4.8	4.5	18	7.4	6.1
6	5.1	4.8	20	7.7	6.3

From Hoekelman RA: The physical examination of infants and children. In Bates B, editor: A guide to physical examination and history-taking, ed 5, Philadelphia, 1991, JB Lippincott Co.

Hepatomegaly: Clinical Disease Stages and Age of Presentation

NEWBORN

Intrauterine- and intrapartum-acquired infection
Erythroblastosis fetalis
Biliary tract obstruction
Neonatal hepatitis
Congestive heart failure
Viral hepatitis
Infection, septicemia

INFANT

Cystic fibrosis
Metabolic disorders
- Glycogen storage disease
- Galactosemia
- Gaucher disease
- Alpha-1-antitrypsin deficiency
- Mucopolysaccharidosis
- Wolman disease

Histiocytosis syndromes
Malnutrition
Tumors

INFANT—cont'd

- Intrinsic (hepatoblastoma, multinodular hemangioendothelioma)
- Metastatic (neuroblastoma, Wilms tumor, gonadal tumor)

YOUNG CHILD

Toxic and drug reactions
Parasitic disease (visceral larva migrans)
Leukemia

OLDER CHILD AND ADOLESCENT

Chronic active hepatitis
Liver disease with inflammatory bowel disease
Drug and alcoholic hepatitis
Lymphoma
Wilson disease
Hepatic porphyrias
Congenital hepatic fibrosis, polycystic liver disease
Amyloidosis
Alpha-1-antitrypsin deficiency

Modified from Walker WA and Mathis RK: Hepatomegaly: an approach to differential diagnosis, Pediatr Clin North Am 22:929, 1975.

Fat accumulation in the liver produces symmetric, often striking hepatomegaly; lipid content may increase from 5% by weight to 40%. In the pediatric population fatty infiltration commonly reflects the nutritional disturbances of protein-calorie malnutrition, starvation, or malabsorption (as in celiac disease or cystic fibrosis). In the absence of other pathologic conditions, liver function tests are normal and fat content rapidly normalizes with improved nutrition. A fatty liver and hepatomegaly associated with parenteral hyperalimentation may be independent of cholestasis seen in young infants. An abnormality in carbohydrate metabolism and an increased supply of free fatty acids in both diabetes mellitus and obesity may produce a fatty liver. Drugs and toxins, including tetracyclines, steroids, ethanol, and carbon tetrachloride, cause fat accumulation as a major component of induced liver change. Reye syndrome, inherited metabolic disorders (such as galactosemia, tyrosinosis, and hereditary fructose intolerance), and some lysosomal deficiency diseases (such as Gaucher disease and Niemann-Pick disease) include fatty infiltration as one manifestation of their systemic processes.

Intrinsic liver tumors, benign or malignant, often present with asymmetric enlargement. Liver cell carcinomas in infants and young children are usually hepatoblastomas, which may produce precocious puberty by gonadotropin secretion. Pedunculate and cystic tumors are often benign. Mixed tumors, adrenal rest tumors, hamartomas, teratomas, cavernous hemangiomas, and cysts (such as congenital, ecchinococcal, and traumatic) may have similar asymmetry. The most common metastatic tumors in the liver are neuroblastomas, Wilms tumors, and gonadal tumors.

EVALUATION

The history and physical examination guide the selection of appropriate diagnostic procedures, which in turn provide valuable information about responsible mechanisms and the extent of disease. Alterations in blood counts and sedimentation rate are nonspecific inflammatory responses of many liver diseases. Hepatocellular function is reflected in transaminase levels—serum glutamic-oxaloacetic transaminase (SGOT) and serum glutamic-pyruvic transaminase (SGPT). Elevations in the levels of these enzymes generally parallel the degree of injury and are useful in following the course of disease. Evaluation of bile secretion includes determining serum bilirubin levels, levels of bile acids, a lipid profile, and levels of alkaline phosphatase isoenzymes. As hepatic insufficiency significantly worsens, enzyme levels may actually return to normal or decrease; however, a concomitant prolongation of clotting times, a decrease in the amounts of serum albumin and globulin, and an elevation in the serum ammonia level indicate that liver function is failing.

Other modalities of study include scanning, angiography, biopsy, and tests specific for a single diagnosis. The technetium liver-spleen scan is useful in assessing Kupffer cell function and distribution; it may reveal extensive parenchymal disease, inflammation, or a mass lesion. Ultrasound scanning yields information about homogeneity of tissue and is particularly useful in distinguishing solid and cystic lesions. Magnetic resonance imaging does not yield additional information in most cases. Hepatobiliary scintigraphy can demonstrate biliary patency or abnormal dilation of the bile ducts. These scans help distinguish complete obstruction, as in extrahepatic biliary atresia, from cholestasis associated with neonatal hepatitis. Small intrinsic mass lesions and traumatic liver lesions may best be delineated by hepatic angiography. Needle biopsies and open liver biopsies may be performed when a tissue diagnosis is necessary. The biopsy analysis may include culturing, histochemical studies, electron microscopy, and enzyme or heavy-metal assays. Tests designed to elucidate a specific diagnosis range from hepatitis B antigen and antibody level measurements to sweat tests for cystic fibrosis and urine metabolic screening for inborn errors of metabolism.

MANAGEMENT

Liver enlargement is not an uncommon occurrence in infancy and childhood. Careful evaluation of the patient with an enlarged liver determines the approach necessary to establish a diagnosis. A healthy child with minimal abnormality found in liver function tests and no jaundice or splenomegaly requires only observation; good clinical judgment is reliable and avoids overuse of painful or expensive tests. Emphasis in evaluation is placed on distinguishing conditions that necessitate immediate diagnosis or intervention from self-limited conditions that may resolve with time. Management of the child with hepatomegaly involves the diagnostic evaluation, as considered above, with supportive therapy for the child's clinical status and the appropriate treatment for the underlying condition.

REFERENCES

1. Lawson EE et al: Clinical estimation of liver span in infants and children, Am J Dis Child 132:474, 1978.
2. Reiff M and Osborne LM: Clinical estimation of liver size in newborn infants, Pediatrics 71:46, 1983.
3. Walker WA and Mathis RK: Hepatomegaly: an approach to differential diagnosis, Pediatr Clin North Am 22:929, 1975.
4. Weisman E et al: Clinical estimation of liver size in the normal neonate, Clin Pediatr 21:596, 1982.

SUGGESTED READING

Fitzgerald J: Colestatic disorders of infancy. In Lebenthal E, editor: Pediatric gastroenterology II, Pediatr Clin North Am 35:357, 1988.

141

High Blood Pressure in Infants, Children, and Adolescents

Edward B. Clark

Blood pressure, the dynamic force driving blood flow through the body, varies greatly during each day. Transient increases in blood pressure are essential in meeting the metabolic demands of the body, but a sustained increase in blood pressure can lead to premature vascular changes in the heart, brain, and kidneys. Most physicians suspect that the seeds of adult-onset hypertensive disease are sown during childhood. Therefore, abnormalities in blood pressure are of great interest to all who care for children. Although the highest levels of blood pressure in a child likely correlate with essential hypertension as an adult, data on the long-term outcome in children are only now becoming available.[6] Lauer found that 45% of young adults with high blood pressure had had childhood high blood pressure recorded on at least one measurement; he concluded that although in an individual child there is variable predictability of adult blood pressure, on a population basis early childhood blood pressure elevations are predictive of risk for future high blood pressure.[6] This important, ongoing study and others confirm that regular measurement of blood pressure in childhood is an essential part of good primary pediatric care.

DEFINITION

High blood pressure is a level of systolic or diastolic blood pressure at which there is an unacceptable risk for cardio-

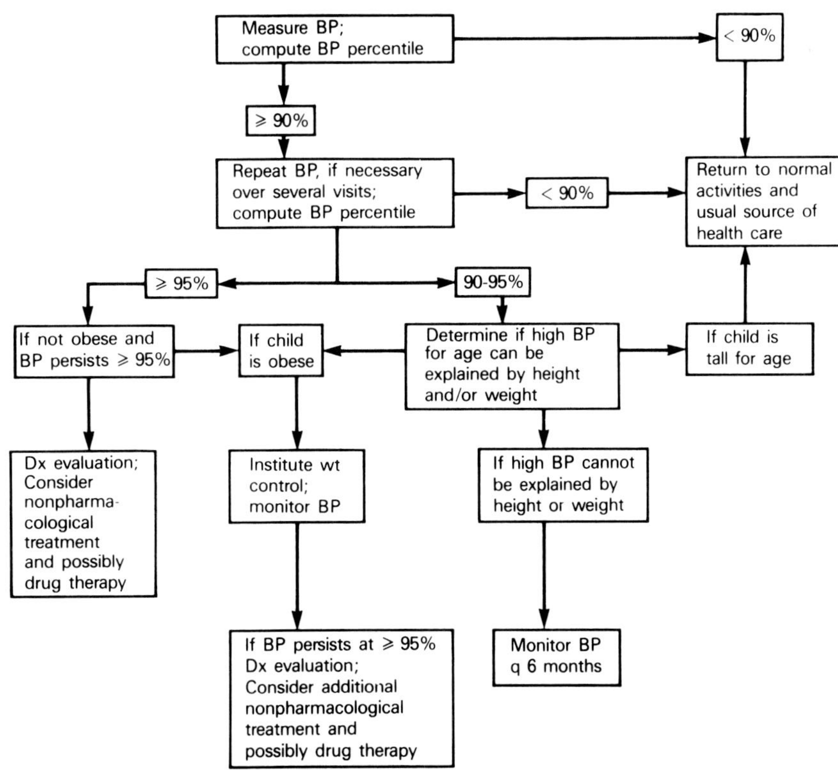

Fig. 141-1 Algorithm for identifying children with high blood pressure.

vascular complications for that individual. Setting that level is difficult, because there are no long-term studies relating blood pressure beginning in childhood to vascular disease arising during adult life. Thus the current definition is statistical and closely correlated with age, gender, physical activity, body size, and sexual maturity.

Primary (essential) hypertension occurs without identifiable pathologic cause and is likely related to genetic factors. Secondary hypertension is caused by chronic vascular, renal, or neuroendocrine causes.

DIAGNOSIS

Most children with high blood pressure do not have symptoms. Therefore recognition requires regular measurements of blood pressure during normal growth and development. The current recommendation is for infants and children to have their blood pressure checked beginning at 3 years of age and annually thereafter. All symptomatic children, including those evaluated in emergency rooms, hospitals, or in critical care units, and high-risk or premature infants should have their blood pressure measured routinely (Fig. 141-1).

Blood pressure must be measured in a quiet, resting infant or child, because the normative data were gathered under these conditions. The blood pressure cuff must cover more than two thirds of the upper arm, the bladder positioned over the brachial artery, and the sensor (Doppler crystal, oscillometer, or stethoscope) placed over the artery.

Systolic blood pressure is the first sound (phase 1 Korotkoff) as the cuff is deflated; diastolic blood pressure is either the muffling (phase IV Korotkoff) or disappearance (phase V Korotkoff) of the sounds. The most frequent "cause" of elevated blood pressure is an improperly taken measurement.

Using the standard blood pressure tables for age, gender, and weight, *normal blood pressure* is a systolic and diastolic pressure less than the 90th percentile; *high normal blood pressure* is the average of three or more systolic and/or diastolic pressure measurements from the 90th percentile to the 95th percentile; and *high blood pressure* is the average of three or more systolic and/or diastolic pressures greater than the 95th percentile. Note that a child who is taller or heavier for age will have a higher blood pressure than a child of average size. (See Figs. 141-2, 141-3, and 141-4 for gender-, age-, and weight-corrected systolic and diastolic blood pressures.)

Severe symptomatic high blood pressure (hypertensive crisis) includes evidence of cardiovascular or cerebrovascular malfunction.

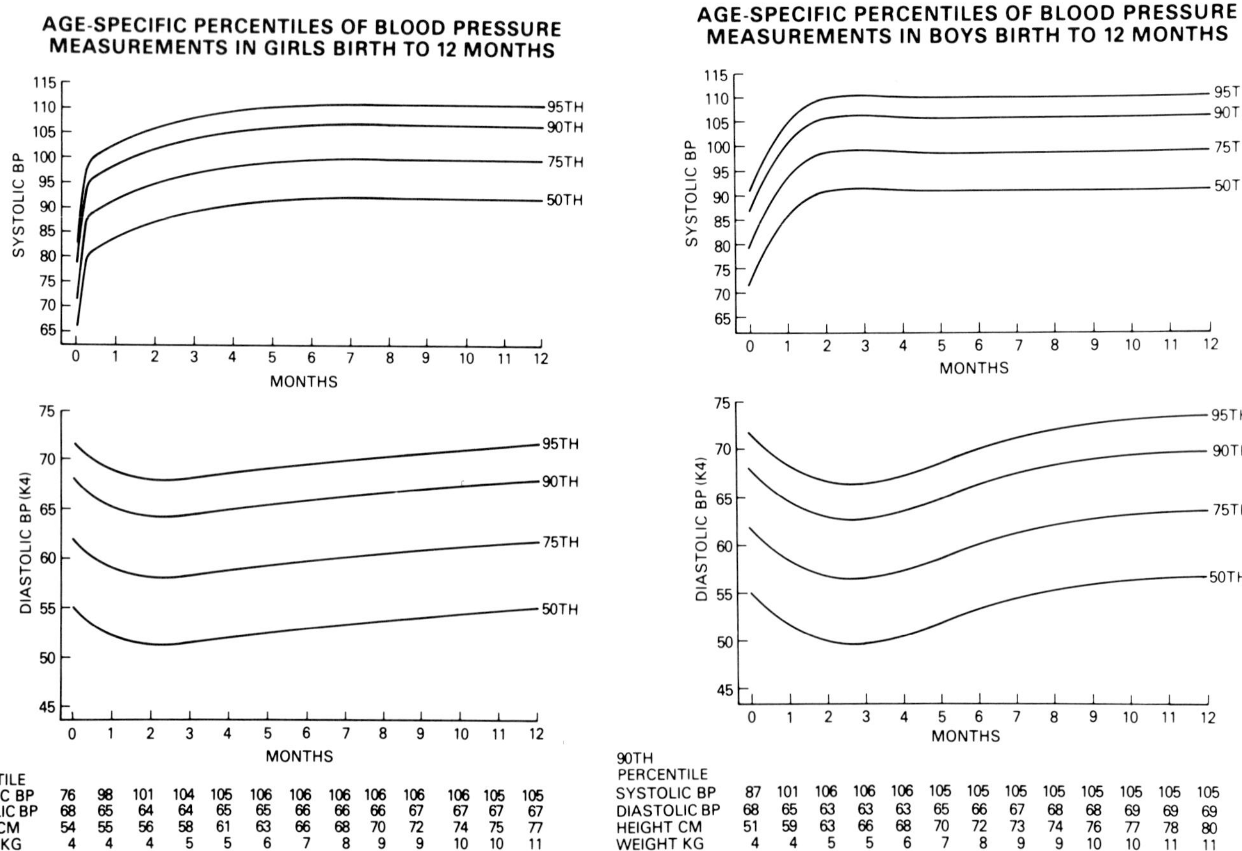

Girls:

90TH PERCENTILE	0	1	2	3	4	5	6	7	8	9	10	11	12
SYSTOLIC BP	76	98	101	104	105	106	106	106	106	106	106	105	105
DIASTOLIC BP	68	65	64	64	65	65	66	66	66	67	67	67	67
HEIGHT CM	54	55	56	58	61	63	66	68	70	72	74	75	77
WEIGHT KG	4	4	4	5	5	6	7	8	9	9	10	10	11

Boys:

90TH PERCENTILE	0	1	2	3	4	5	6	7	8	9	10	11	12
SYSTOLIC BP	87	101	106	106	106	105	105	105	105	105	105	105	105
DIASTOLIC BP	68	65	63	63	63	65	66	67	68	68	69	69	69
HEIGHT CM	51	59	63	66	68	70	72	73	74	76	77	78	80
WEIGHT KG	4	4	5	5	6	7	8	9	9	10	10	11	11

Fig. 141-2 Age-, gender-, height-, and weight-specific percentiles of systolic and diastolic blood pressure for birth to 12 months of age.

DIAGNOSTIC EVALUATION

Patients with normal blood pressure on a single reading require continued annual surveillance. Those with high normal blood pressure on three consecutive measurements separated by at least 3 days should have three extremity blood pressures (right arm, left arm, and a leg) taken to rule out coarctation of the aorta, urinalysis, and a quantitative urine culture to rule out chronic urinary tract infection, counseling for dietary salt and weight reduction where appropriate, and more frequent surveillance.

Children with high blood pressure should be evaluated for a possible treatable cause of secondary hypertension. The evaluation includes the tests listed in Table 141-1. The younger the child and the higher the blood pressure, the more likely is it that renal or renovascular disease or other cause of secondary hypertension is present.

Children with symptomatic severe high blood pressure fitting the criteria for hypertensive crisis should have aggressive treatment to reduce blood pressure to safer levels (see Chapter 280) and a thorough diagnostic evaluation to determine the underlying cause (Table 141-2).

Children with high normal blood pressure and most children with high blood pressure can be evaluated and cared for in the primary physician's office or clinic.[3,7] Children or adolescents with severe hypertension or a perplexing presentation should be referred to a consultant with expertise in the diagnosis and management of pediatric patients. A summary of the approach to such severe and complex cases was published recently.[1]

ASSOCIATED SIGNS AND SYMPTOMS

Symptoms are rare in children with high blood pressure; when present, they are usually associated with either sudden acute or chronic severe elevation in blood pressure. Table 141-3 lists the most common causes of the chronic type. The cardiovascular complications of congestive heart failure and pulmonary edema are often associated with left ventricular hypertrophy (determined on the electrocardiogram) and/or an increase in myocardial mass measured from the echocardiogram. Cerebrovascular complications include persistent headache, blurred vision, coma, convulsions or, in rare cases, stroke. Retinal vascular changes are evidence of chronic severe hypertension.

ETIOLOGY OF HIGH BLOOD PRESSURE

The dynamic control of blood pressure occurs through a complex feedback mechanism regulating cardiac output, vascular

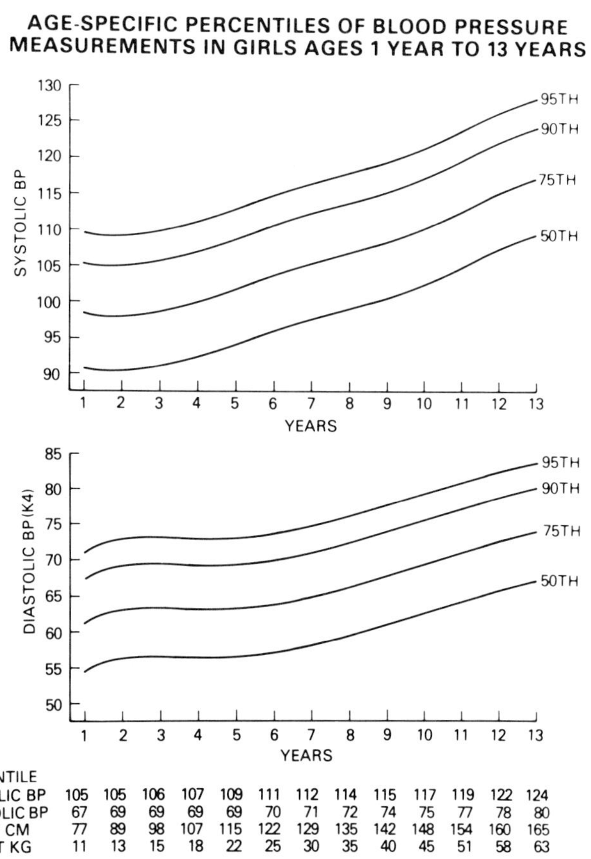

90TH PERCENTILE													
SYSTOLIC BP	105	105	106	107	109	111	112	114	115	117	119	122	124
DIASTOLIC BP	67	69	69	69	69	70	71	72	74	75	77	78	80
HEIGHT CM	77	89	98	107	115	122	129	135	142	148	154	160	165
WEIGHT KG	11	13	15	18	22	25	30	35	40	45	51	58	63

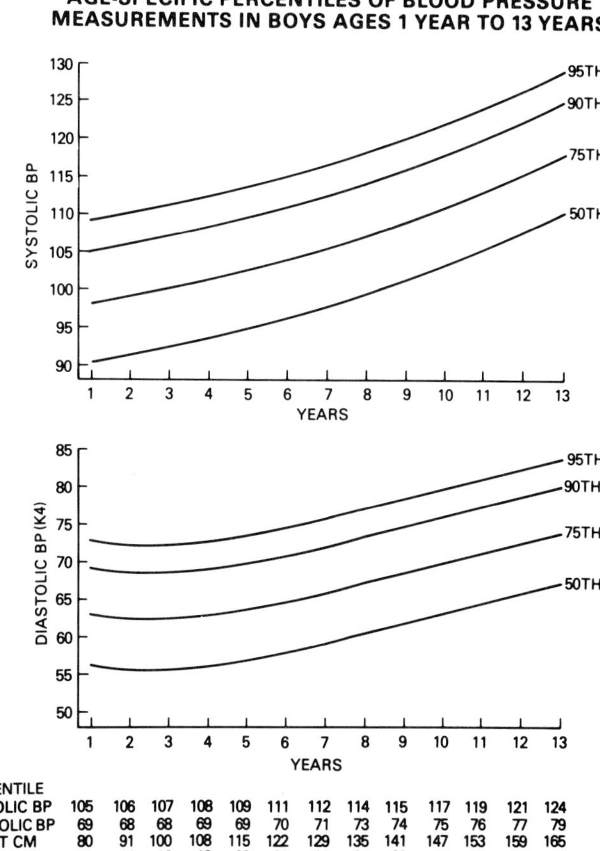

90TH PERCENTILE													
SYSTOLIC BP	105	106	107	108	109	111	112	114	115	117	119	121	124
DIASTOLIC BP	69	68	68	69	69	70	71	73	74	75	76	77	79
HEIGHT CM	80	91	100	108	115	122	129	135	141	147	153	159	165
WEIGHT KG	11	14	16	18	22	25	29	34	39	44	50	55	62

Fig. 141-3 Age-, gender-, height-, and weight-specific percentiles of systolic and diastolic blood pressure for 1 to 13 years of age.

Table 141-1 *A Diagnostic Strategy in the Evaluation of High Blood Pressure*

ITEM	ACTION
Exclude drugs or prior illness	Conduct history, physical examination
Exclude coarctation of the aorta	Measure blood pressure in all extremities
Identify renal causes	Auscultate for abdominal bruits; perform urinalysis; obtain urine culture; measure electrolytes and blood urea nitrogen
Assess for end organ changes	Obtain echocardiogram for evidence of left ventricular hypertrophy; perform ophthalmoscopy
Assess vascular disease risk factors	Obtain family history; perform lipid screen, including high-density lipoproteins and triglycerides
Assess general health	Conduct history and physical examination; obtain complete blood count

Table 141-2 *Commonest Causes by Age Group of Chronic Sustained Hypertension*

AGE GROUP	CAUSE
Newborn	Renal artery thrombosis Renal artery stenosis Congenital renal malformations Coarctation of the aorta Bronchopulmonary dysplasia
Infancy to 6 years	Renal parenchymal disease Coarctation of the aorta Renal artery stenosis
6 to 10 years	Renal artery stenosis Renal parenchymal disease Primary hypertension
Adolescence	Primary hypertension Renal parenchymal disease

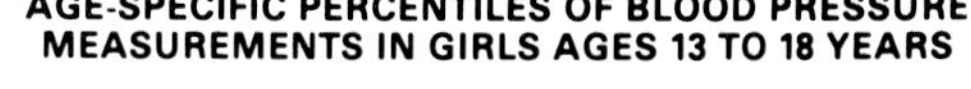
AGE-SPECIFIC PERCENTILES OF BLOOD PRESSURE
MEASUREMENTS IN GIRLS AGES 13 TO 18 YEARS

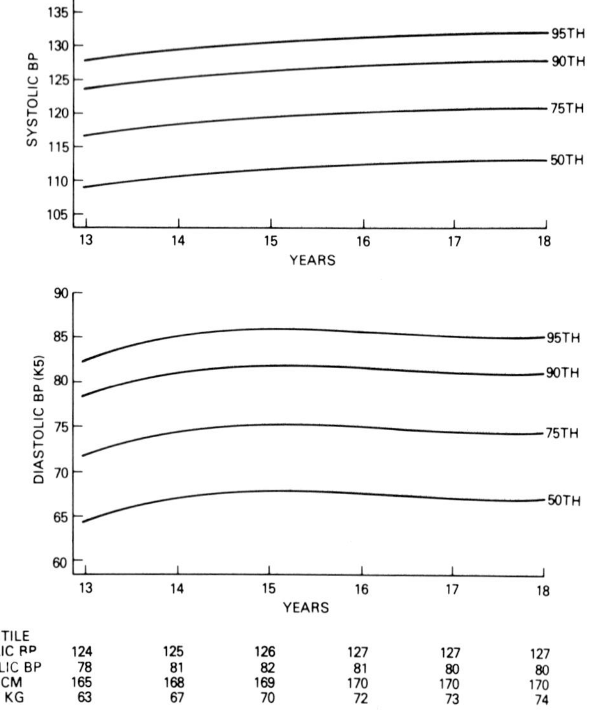

90TH PERCENTILE	13	14	15	16	17	18
SYSTOLIC BP	124	125	126	127	127	127
DIASTOLIC BP	78	81	82	81	80	80
HEIGHT CM	165	168	169	170	170	170
WEIGHT KG	63	67	70	72	73	74

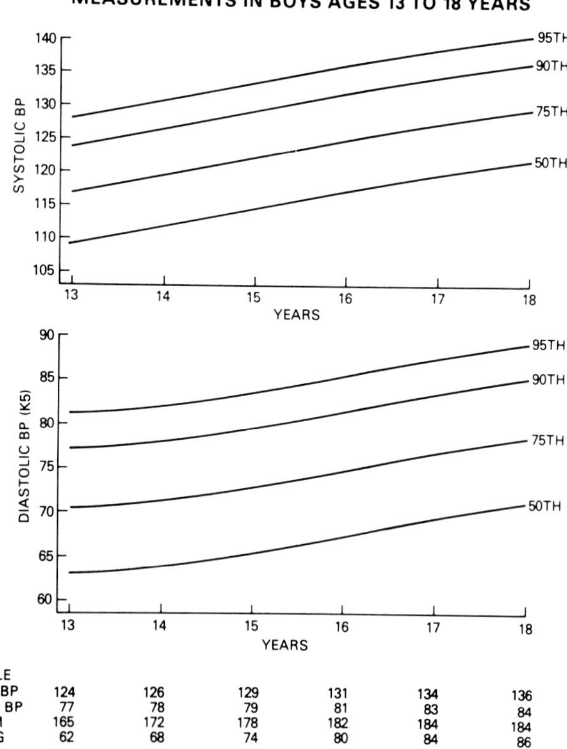

90TH PERCENTILE	13	14	15	16	17	18
SYSTOLIC BP	124	126	129	131	134	136
DIASTOLIC BP	77	78	79	81	83	84
HEIGHT CM	165	172	178	182	184	184
WEIGHT KG	62	68	74	80	84	86

Fig. 141-4 Age-, gender-, height-, and weight-specific percentiles of systolic and diastolic blood pressure for 13 to 18 years of age.

Table 141-3 *Causes of Secondary Hypertension*

CAUSE	MECHANISM
Renal	Renal parenchymal disease
	Glomerulonephritis
	Chronic pyelonephritis
	Polycystic kidney
	Connective tissue disease
	Hydronephrosis
	Renal tumors
Cardiac	Coarctation of the aorta
Adrenal	Cortical
	Mineralocorticoid secreting tumors
	Adrenogenital syndrome
	Medullary
	Pheochromocytoma
Neurogenic	Increased intracranial pressure from a variety of pathologic causes
Drug induced	Oral contraceptives
	Amphetamines
	Sympathomimetic amines
	Cocaine, phencyclidine (PCP), illicit drugs, licorice

resistance, and blood volume.[4] A number of pathophysiologic defects are recognized as causes of *secondary hypertension* (see Table 141-2). In childhood, renal and renovascular disorders are among the most frequent and important causes.

Primary (or *essential*) *hypertension* has as yet no clearly defined pathophysiologic mechanism or mechanisms but likely has a strong genetic component. This concept is supported by studies showing that high blood pressure tends to aggregate in families. Studies in experimental animals, together with human studies of blood pressure in twins, of erythrocyte sodium-lithium transport, and of familial patterns of blood pressure response to stress all demonstrate the importance of genetic factors in control of blood pressure.[2]

Identification of children at risk for primary hypertension is important, because elevated blood pressure is one of the risk factors for stroke, myocardial infarction, congestive heart failure, and renal failure in adults.

PSYCHOSOCIAL CONSIDERATIONS

Although it is important to detect children with high blood pressure, it is equally important to avoid erroneous identification of a child as "hypertensive." The dangers of a false

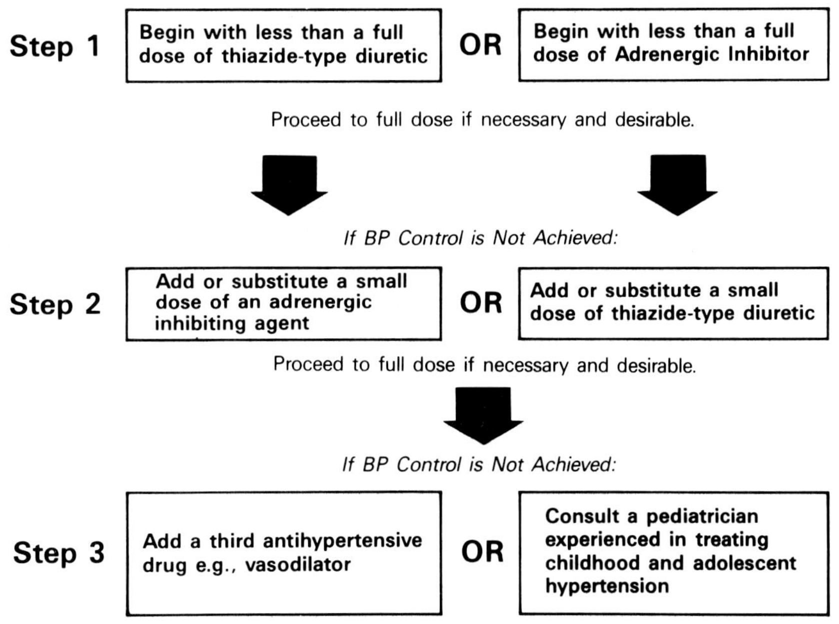

Fig. 141-5 Stepped-care approach to antihypertensive drug therapy (reproduced from Fig. 141-1).

ACKNOWLEDGEMENT: Figs. 141-1 through 141-5 are reproduced with permission from Task Force on Blood Pressure Control in Children: Report of the Second Task Force on Blood Pressure Control in Children in 1987. Pediatrics 79:1-25, 1987. Courtesy of Dr. Michael J. Horan.

Table 141-4 *Antihypertensive Medications**

	DOSE	TIMES/DAY	ROUTE
Diuretics			
Hydrochlorothiazide (Hydrodiuril, Esidrix)	1-2 mg/kg	2	Oral
Chlorthalidone (Hygroton)	0.5-2 mg/kg	1	Oral
Furosemide (Lasix)	0.5-2 mg/kg	2	Oral, intravenous (IV)
Spironolactone (Aldactone)	1-2 mg/kg	2	Oral
Triamterene (Dyrenium)	1-2 mg/kg	2	Oral
Adrenergic inhibitors			
Beta-adrenergic antagonists			
Metoprolol (Lopressor)	1-4 mg/kg	2	Oral
Atenolol (Tenormin)	1-2 mg/kg	1	Oral
Propranolol (Inderal)	1-3 mg/kg	3	Oral
Central adrenergic inhibitors			
Methyldopa (Aldomet)	5-10 mg/kg	2	Oral
Clonidine (Catapres)	0.05-0.40 mg	2	Oral
Guanabenz (Wytensin)	0.03-0.08 mg	2	Oral
Alpha-adrenergic antagonist			
Prazosin hydrochloride (Minipress)	0.5-7 mg	3	Oral
Vasodilators			
Hydralazine (Apresoline)	1-5 mg/kg	2 or 3	Oral, intramuscular, IV (drip)
Minoxidil (Loniten)	0.1-1.0 mg/kg	2	Oral
Diazoxide (Hyperstat)†	3-5 mg/kg/dose		IV (bolus)
Nitroprusside (Nipride)†	1-8 μg/kg/minute		IV (drip)
Angiotensin-converting enzyme inhibitor			
Captopril			
≤6 mo of age	0.05-0.5 mg/kg	3	Oral
≥6 mo of age	0.5-2 mg/kg	3	Oral

*Not to exceed usual adult dosage with all drugs.
†Primary use is in hypertensive emergencies.
Adapted from Task Force on Blood Pressure Control in Children: Report of the Second Task Force on Blood Pressure Control in Children in 1987, Pediatrics 79:1-25, 1987. Courtesy of Dr. Michael J. Horan.

positive diagnosis include labeling within the family and at school, limiting participation in sports, creating an obstacle to obtaining life and health insurance, losing employment opportunities, and risking the potentially harmful side effects of treatment.

Rigorous diagnosis and care of the severely hypertensive child is essential. Careful evaluation and management of the child with normal high blood pressure is judicious.

MANAGEMENT

The treatment of high blood pressure depends on the cause and the degree of elevation. Acute symptomatic severe elevation in blood pressure requires immediate evaluation and treatment. Other forms of secondary hypertension frequently require direct intervention such as surgery for coarctation of the aorta or pharmacologic management for children with chronic renal disease.

The management of high normal or high blood pressure without an identifiable cause is more difficult. The current recommendation is for conservative therapy: weight reduction if obese, exercise, moderate salt restriction (to around 2500 mg of sodium per day), and avoidance of tobacco, particularly cigarette smoking. There is unanimity on the benefits of dynamic exercise; because isometric forms of exercise such as wrestling and weight lifting may lead to elevated blood pressure, these activities are more often questioned. The present consensus is that supervised, graduated isometric exercise is not harmful and may be beneficial.

Weight reduction is particularly important, because tracking data from childhood to adulthood indicates that obesity in a child is most predictive of obesity and hence high blood pressure in an adult. Therefore strategies designed to prevent the acquisition of excess weight during adolescence may be useful in preventing adult hypertension.[5]

There is a small role for drug treatment, because the natural history of blood pressure elevation is obscure, the side effects of lifelong drug treatment are undefined, and the risk of target organ disease is unknown. When pharmacologic therapy is necessary, a stepped care approach traditionally has been used by the pediatrician (Fig. 141-5). Step 1 usually is a thiazide diuretic or adrenergic inhibitor at less than a full dose; step 2 is the addition of a second drug gradually increased to full dose; step 3 is the addition of a third drug, usually in consultation with a physician skilled in treating children and adolescents with more refractory forms of high blood pressure. Table 141-4 provides a list of antihypertensive medications and their doses. Once blood pressure returns to the normal range, discontinuing medication is more often feasible and desirable in the young than in older subjects who already have fixed arterial wall changes.

REFERENCES

1. Balfe JW et al: Hypertension in childhood. In Barness LA, editor: Advances in pediatrics, Chicago, 1989, Year Book Medical Publishers 36:201-246.
2. Burns TL and Lauer RM: Blood pressure in children. In Pierpont MEM and Moller JH, editors: Genetics of cardiovascular disease, Boston, 1986, Martinius Nijhoff.
3. Gifford RW et al: Office evaluation of hypertension: special report—a statement for health professionals by a writing group of the Council for High Blood Pressure Research, American Heart Association, Hypertension 13:283, 1989.
4. Guyton AC: The kidney in blood pressure control and hypertension. In Holliday MA, Barratt TM, and Vernier RL, editors: Pediatric nephrology, ed 2, Baltimore, 1987, Williams & Wilkins.
5. Lauer RM et al: Factors related to tracking of blood pressure in children, Hypertension 6:307, 1984.
6. Lauer RM and Clarke WR: Childhood risk factors for adult high blood pressure: the Muscatine study, Pediatrics 84:633, 1989.
7. National Heart, Lung and Blood Institute Task Force on Blood Pressure Control in Children: Report of the Second Task Force on Blood Pressure Control in Children in 1987, Pediatrics 79:1, 1987.

142

Hirsutism, Hypertrichosis, and Precocious Sexual Hair Development

Cynthia H. Cole

Both hirsutism and hypertrichosis technically imply excessive hair growth. When a patient is seen with an excess of hair, one must decide if it is a normal variant or pathologic. An increase in body hair in areas under sex hormone control increases the likelihood of an endocrine origin. The areas of the body primarily influenced by sex hormone levels are the face, chest, axilla, abdomen, and pubic region. There is little chance of an endocrine cause if the disproportionate hair growth is in or limited to body areas not primarily under sex hormone control. These areas include the extremities, the eyebrows, and the scalp.

DEFINITIONS

Hypertrichosis

Hypertrichosis is excessive growth of nonsexual hair and is associated with normal androgen metabolism. The quantity of total body hair varies considerably among normal individuals and is influenced by the individual's genetic background. Females of Mediterranean origin have more hair than do those of Scandinavian origin, and white people have more than Asians. Therefore the quantity of hair, as opposed to its distribution and type, has little diagnostic significance.

Disproportionate hair growth may also be a feature of various congenital syndromes, including generalized lipodystrophy, fetal hydantoin syndrome, mucopolysaccharidoses, trisomy 18, leprechaunism, and de Lange syndrome, among other disorders of infancy and childhood. In each of these, excessive body hair should be considered in context with other features of the specific syndromes.

Hirsutism and Precocious Sexual Hair Development

Hirsutism is excessive growth of androgen-dependent sexual hair in females, which primarily involves pubic, axillary, facial, chest, and abdominal hair. It is most often associated with increased production of total or free androgen. When an overproduction of androgens cannot be demonstrated, the cause of hirsutism may be related to increased "sensitivity" of the hair follicle to normal levels of androgen. Hirsutism is but one manifestation of virilization and refers to the development of a "male" hair growth pattern in a female.

Pubic hair usually starts after 13 years of age. Development of sexual hair in males before 9 years of age or in females before age 8 years deserves further evaluation. Disorders that result in premature development of sexual hair in prepubertal children include premature adrenarche; precocious puberty; late-onset, virilizing congenital adrenal hyperplasia; Cushing syndrome; and tumors of the adrenal glands, of the ovaries or testicles, or of the central nervous system (CNS). Exogenous administration of androgens may also cause premature or excessive sexual hair development.

Evaluation of a child with premature sexual hair development should include observing for or inquiring about (1) a history of obesity, of an unusual growth spurt, or of electrolyte problems; (2) a family history of infant deaths or of ambiguous genitalia; and (3) the rapidity of onset and progression of symptoms and their duration and severity. It is important to look for the advancement of other secondary sexual characteristics or for signs of virilization. Evidence of virilization in prepubertal males or females includes advanced genital growth (clitoris, penis, testicles), accelerated muscle development, and growth of facial, chest, and abdominal hair in addition to pubic and axillary hair. Hirsutism and virilization in any prepubertal child or in girls of any age are the result of increased androgen stimulation; the source of these signs must be sought.

The sources of excess androgen production include the adrenal glands, the ovaries and testicles, the enhanced peripheral conversion of androgenic precursors to potent androgens, and hypothalamopituitary dysfunction. Hyperandrogenism in some pubescent or postpubescent girls may result from increased androgen production by both the adrenal glands and the ovaries.

DIFFERENTIAL DIAGNOSIS

Premature Adrenarche

Premature adrenarche (PA) is defined as the precocious growth of pubic hair in the absence of other signs of precocious puberty (under 8 years of age in females and under 9 years of age in males). It occurs more commonly in girls than in boys. Axillary hair, oily skin, and acne may also be observed. Height and bone age are usually slightly accelerated. Pubertal development appears to ensue at a normal or slightly early time in children with premature adrenarche.

In many patients with premature adrenarche, the mean androgen concentrations and their metabolites are similar to those in pubertal children. Therefore dehydroepiandrosterone (DHEA), DHEA-sulfate (DHEA-S), testosterone, androstenedione, and urinary 17-ketosteroids are elevated for the age of the child with PA but normal for those at midpuberty. In these patients it has been assumed that PA was caused by a precocious maturation of the adrenal zona reticularis. In other patients with normal androgen concentrations, it is assumed that these individuals have an increased sensitivity to adrenal androgens.

Recently it was demonstrated that some individuals with PA have enzyme defects in steroidogenesis and exaggerated responses to adrenocorticotropic hormone (ACTH) stimulation. Some of the abnormal hormonal responses resembled late-onset 21-hydroxylase deficiency, heterozygosity for classic adrenal hyperplasia, and yet others with evidence of 3-beta-hydroxysteroid dehydrogenase deficiency.[6,8,10]

The differential diagnosis for children with PA should include idiopathic PA, PA with enzyme deficiencies, isosexual precocious puberty presenting with pubic hair, and gonadotropin-producing tumors.

Evaluation of a child with PA should include a complete history and physical examination; an abdominal ultrasound may be needed. Hormonal evaluation of androgens, cortisol, precursor steroids [DHEA, DHEA-S, testosterone, androstenedione, dehydrotestosterone (DHT), 17-OH progesterone (17-OHP), 17-OH pregnenolone (D5-17OHP), desoxycorticosterone (DOC)], luteinizing hormone–releasing hormone (LH-RH)-stimulation, ACTH-stimulation, and dexamethasone suppression tests may also be required.

Periodic follow-up of patients with PA every 3 to 6 months is important to determine growth velocity, bone age, and evidence of precocious development of other secondary sexual characteristics. Repeat hormonal evaluation may be considered if precocious puberty or an androgen-producing tumor is still in the differential diagnosis.

Precocious Puberty

Precocious puberty (PP) should not be confused with hirsutism per se. It includes premature isosexual development of secondary sexual characteristics as well as advanced sexual hair growth. Precocity in sexual development is defined as premature sexual development in boys under 9 years of age and girls under 8 years of age.[4,6]

True precocious puberty results from a disorder of premature maturation of the hypothalamohypophysial complex. Subsequent increased gonadotropin secretion and gonadal maturation ensues. In males, the increased secretion of testosterone produces a hyperandrogenic state. In females, the increased secretion of estradiol produces a hyperestrogenic state. PP occurs less frequently in boys than in girls, with idiopathic precocious puberty more common in girls; CNS lesions are evenly distributed between the sexes.

The clinical course is variable in tempo, although the clinical symptoms are those of normal puberty at an abnormally early age. The evolution of secondary sexual characteristics may be slow or fast. The more rapid evolution is frequently associated with CNS lesions. Linear growth velocity and bone age maturation are accelerated, which leads to premature epiphyseal closure and, ultimately, short stature. Bone age is consistent with the child's pubertal stage.

Hormonal changes may be similar to those observed in normal puberty. Episodic, pulsatile secretion of gonadotropins occurs as in normal puberty but is of lesser amplitude than expected in normal children for the comparable stage of pubertal development. Gonadotropin levels, although usually elevated for the age of the patient, may also overlap with normal levels for the patient's age. Thus, according to the stage of puberty, testosterone, luteinizing hormone (LH) and follicle-stimulating hormone (FSH) are usually greater than normal for age in boys. Likewise, estradiol, LH, and FSH levels are usually elevated for age in girls, although estrogen levels may fluctuate widely.[4]

Idiopathic precocious puberty is a diagnosis of exclusion and may be familial in origin. Sexual precocity may also occur after various CNS injuries (e.g., trauma, meningitis, sarcoidosis, toxoplasmosis, hydrocephalus). Septooptic dysplasia, McCune-Albright syndrome, and neurofibromatosis are other disorders in which precocious puberty is a component. Magnetic resonance imaging has enhanced the diagnosis of CNS tumors (e.g., hamartomas) associated with true precocious puberty.

True precocious puberty must be differentiated from false precocious puberty. False precocious puberty occurs when secondary sexual characteristics develop without maturation of the gonads and when serum gonadotropin levels are normal. False precocious puberty is usually caused by an abnormality of the gonads (e.g., tumors) or of the adrenal cortex. In boys, false precocious puberty may result from congenital virilizing adrenal hyperplasia, a virilizing adrenal tumor, or a virilizing gonadal tumor. False precocious puberty in girls is rarely caused by an estrogen-secreting tumor of the adrenal gland or of the ovaries. It is more commonly a result of exogenous estrogen administration.

Congenital Virilizing Adrenal Hyperplasia

Congenital virilizing adrenal hyperplasia (CVAH) may not be accompanied by hirsutism, virilization, cortisol deficiency, or electrolyte disturbance for varying periods of time (sometimes years), depending on the degree of enzyme deficiency present. The most common adrenal enzyme deficiency associated with CVAH is that of 21-hydroxylase, whereas 11-beta-hydroxylase deficiency occurs in a small percentage (5%) of CVAH cases and may be associated with hypertension.[1] In both types of CVAH, urinary excretion of 17-ketosteroids and pregnanetriol is usually increased.

Depending on the degree of enzyme block, urinary levels of 17-hydroxycorticosteroids (17-OHCS) may be normal or decreased with 21-hydroxylase deficiency, whereas these levels may be increased in 11-beta-hydroxylase deficiency. Urinary metabolites of tetrahydric derivatives of compound S and deoxycorticosterone are usually increased in patients with 11-beta-hydroxylase deficiency.

Twenty-four hour urine specimens are difficult to collect

in some children and, even if properly collected, may yield equivocal results. Plasma hormone determinations of 17-hydroxyprogesterone are reliable and are elevated in both 21-hydroxylase deficiency and 11-beta-hydroxylase deficiency. Normal values for 17-hydroxyprogesterone vary with age.

There are two classic forms of 21-hydroxylase deficiency, salt-wasting and simple virilizing, which tend to appear early in life. The nonclassic variants of congenital adrenal hyperplasia (CAH) can be classified as late-onset symptomatic CAH and cryptic-asymptomatic CAH. Late-onset CAH appears around peripubertal and postpubertal periods with manifestations of hirsutism, menstrual abnormalities, acne, clitoromegaly, and infertility. Although late-onset CAH has been most often associated with 21-hydroxylase deficiency, it has also been described with 3-beta-hydroxysteroid and 11-beta-hydroxylase deficiencies.[9]

Treatment of CVAH consists of hydrocortisone replacement (15 to 30 mg/m^2/day). The dosage may vary, depending on the severity of the enzyme deficiency and the presence of stress factors. Mineralocorticoid replacement (e.g., deoxycorticosterone acetate) is required for patients with the salt-wasting features of CVAH.

Virilizing Adrenal Tumors

A virilizing adrenal tumor (VAT) is uncommon in childhood. When such tumors do occur, they usually appear in early childhood and affect females more often than males. VATs may be associated with other congenital anomalies (e.g., hemihypertrophy), other nonadrenal tumors, and Beckwith-Wiedemann syndrome.[1,5]

The clinical features of VAT include rapid linear growth and advanced bone maturation. In boys, the development of the penis, scrotum, and pubic hair is advanced, but the testicles usually remain small. In girls, pubic hair and clitoral enlargement occur. Some degree of breast development is not uncommon in patients with virilizing adrenal tumors, which also have an associated increased estrogen production. Acne, greasy hair, adult body odor, deepening voice, masculine habitus, and hypertension may be other features of VAT. Rapidly growing carcinomas may develop with abdominal pain, weight loss, fever, or abdominal mass. VATs often are associated with excess glucocorticoid secretion. Therefore features of Cushing syndrome, or glucocorticoid excess, may also be apparent.

Virilizing adrenal tumors produce excessive androgens, primarily DHEA and DHEA-S, although a few may produce testosterone primarily. Serum DHEA levels are usually higher than 20 ng/ml, and serum DHEA-S levels are usually higher than 9000 ng/ml. Depending on the amount of androgen produced by the tumor, 24-hour urinary 17-ketosteroids are significantly increased. Dexamethasone suppression studies usually do not suppress androgen production, but exceptions occur on occasion.[1,5]

In addition, some VATs demonstrate heterogeneous steroid production with deficiencies or enhancement in specific enzyme systems. The hormonal secretion pattern of VAT may change with time, therapy, or both.[5]

Computed tomography (CT) provides more reliable imaging, particularly of small adrenal tumors.

The prognosis is largely related to completeness of surgical removal and the presence or absence of metastases. If the VAT is associated with excess glucocorticoid production, postoperative management may require glucocorticoid support because of the possibility of contralateral adrenal gland suppression. Postoperative follow-up also requires long-term hormonal surveillance for years. Malignant VATs do not respond well to radiation or chemotherapy.

Cushing Syndrome

Cushing syndrome, which results from abnormally high levels of cortisol, usually manifests with a characteristic pattern of truncal and facial obesity, buffalo hump, striae, and hypertension. Virilization caused by excess adrenal androgen production may result in hirsutism, acne, deepened voice, and clitoral or penile enlargement. Linear growth is impaired or arrested.

In infants and young children, adrenocortical tumors (carcinoma, adenoma, and nodular hyperplasia) are most often the cause of Cushing syndrome. Bilateral adrenal hyperplasia, caused by pituitary microadenomas or basophilic adenomas (Cushing disease), is the most common cause of Cushing syndrome in older children. Extrapituitary ACTH-producing tumors are rare in children.[1]

Cushing syndrome must be ruled out in any female with cystic ovaries, obesity, hirsutism, hypertension, and diabetes mellitus. The cystic ovaries in Cushing syndrome may be the result of chronic anovulation with ovarian androgen overproduction and increased peripheral estrogen production.[9]

Laboratory evaluation of Cushing syndrome usually reveals hypercortisolism with loss of the circadian rhythm of cortisol production. Urinary 17-hydroxycorticosteroid and free cortisol levels are elevated. Plasma ACTH levels and the response to dexamethasone suppression will vary, depending on the syndrome's etiology. Lack of cortisol suppression by prolonged (7 to 10 days) dexamethasone administration is presumptive evidence of a tumor. A low or undetectable baseline level of ACTH eliminates Cushing disease as an etiology. CT scanning is helpful in localizing adrenal tumors.[1]

Treatment of Cushing syndrome depends on the cause, but involves either surgery to remove an adrenal or other tumor or bilateral adrenalectomy. Patients with Cushing disease may require pituitary irradiation or transsphenoidal surgery for selective removal of pituitary microadenomas. Adrenocortical carcinoma is highly malignant and frequently has metastasized by the time of presentation.

Androgen-Secreting Testicular Tumors

Androgen-secreting testicular tumors, which are rare in boys under 15 years of age, cause either virilism or false precocious puberty. Levels of blood and urinary androgens are markedly elevated. Leydig cell tumors secrete testosterone, which cannot be suppressed with dexamethasone.

Testicular tumors are usually diagnosed on finding painless, unilateral testicular swelling. Pain is often associated with metastatic disease.[2]

Androgen-Secreting Tumors of the Ovaries

Androgen-secreting tumors of the ovaries, such as Sertoli-Leydig cell tumors, hilus cell tumors, lipid cell tumors, and cystic teratomas are exceedingly rare but need to be considered in girls with hirsutism, virilization, and markedly elevated serum testosterone levels.[3]

The most frequent manifestations are abdominal pain and abdominal mass. Torsion occurs more frequently in young females than in older ones and with benign rather than malignant tumors. The clinical features reflect the predominant hormone secretion pattern: estrogens, androgens, or both. Virilizing tumors are much less frequent than feminizing tumors. In young children with virilizing tumors, the presenting signs and symptoms include precocious development of sexual hair, clitoromegaly, acne, deepened voice, and accelerated growth and bone age. Adolescent girls and young women have abrupt menstrual abnormalities, breast atrophy, hirsutism, clitoromegaly, and male-type muscle development.

Laboratory evaluation of virilizing ovarian tumors reveals marked elevation of plasma testosterone and DHT. CT scans may help identify small tumors.

The differential diagnostic process includes ruling out the two main adrenal disorders causing masculinization in childhood (VAT and CAH) by assessing plasma DHEA, DHEA-S, and 17-OHP. In both VAT and CAH, urinary 17-ketosteroids and ketogenic steroids are elevated. Differentiating between a small virilizing ovarian tumor and a small virilizing adrenal tumor may require selective venous catheterization of ovarian and adrenal veins for hormonal sampling. Adrenal tumors should be strongly suspected in the presence of marked elevation of DHEA-S (over 2000 mcg/dl). Polycystic ovarian disease (PCOD) must also be considered in the differential diagnosis, although patients with PCOD usually do not experience the abrupt onset of virilization and menstrual abnormalities seen with virilizing ovarian tumors.

Optimum surgical and medical management of ovarian tumors depends on the type of tumor.

Polycystic Ovarian Disease

Polycystic ovarian disease is a disorder of androgen excess seen in postpubertal females with manifestations of hirsutism, menstrual disorders (including anovulation), obesity, and cystic ovaries. A number of other endocrine disorders (e.g., CAH, Cushing disease, hypothyroidism, hyperprolactinemia, and ovarian hyperthecosis) may have similar components in their clinical presentations and must be differentiated from PCOD. Hirsutism in PCOD may be mild to severe; virilization is not usual with this disease. Galactorrhea, acanthosis nigricans, and insulin resistance may be seen in PCOD.[7,9] The pathophysiology of polycystic ovarian syndrome is not entirely understood, in part because of the heterogeneity of clinical and biochemical features of the disorder among affected women. The aberrant ovarian steroidogenesis and follicular maturation are related to dysfunctional feedback within the hypothalamopituitary-ovarian-adrenal axis. Hyperandrogenism is one feature of this syndrome. Excessive androgen production from the adrenal gland and the ovary has been documented, as has increased peripheral conversion of androgen precursors to testosterone and dehydrotestosterone, the two most potent androgens. The luteinizing hormone/follicle-stimulating hormone ratio is increased because of increased LH secretion and low or normal FSH secretion. Urinary 17-ketosteroid excretion and total serum testosterone levels are not always abnormal in these patients. Free serum testosterone and 5-alpha-androstane-3-alpha, 17-beta-diol glucuronide (3-alpha-diol G) levels correlate well with hirsutism, but neither of these assays is routinely available to the clinician. Other serum androgens whose levels may be elevated are DHEA, DHEA-S, and androstenedione. An abdominal sonogram is useful in documenting polycystic ovaries.

Treatment of polycystic ovarian syndrome may include suppression of ovarian function with combination estrogen-progestin oral contraceptives to decrease LH secretion and therefore ovarian androgen production. Adrenal suppression has been used in patients in whom the excess androgens appear to originate from the adrenal gland or from a mixed adrenal-ovarian source. Weight reduction should be incorporated in the treatment program of obese women with PCOD. Other agents with antiandrogen effects (e.g., clomiphene citrate, spironolactone, cimetidine, and bromocriptine) have been used in specific circumstances to treat PCOD.[9] The eventual decrease in hirsutism is variable, depending on the duration of hirsutism before treatment and the levels of androgens present during treatment.[7,11]

Ovarian Hyperthecosis

Ovarian hyperthecosis manifests with signs of androgen excess (severe hirsutism, mild clitoromegaly, obesity, temporal balding, and oligomenorrhea). The androgen excess (testosterone, androstenedione) is ovarian in origin. Histologically the ovaries are characterized by theca interna hyperplasia. The ovaries are not usually cystic and may be of normal size. LH and FSH levels can be normal. Diabetes mellitus and hypertension may be associated clinical problems. The diagnosis of hyperthecosis is made by wedge biopsy of the ovary.[9]

Idiopathic Hirsutism

Idiopathic hirsutism (IH) by definition is not associated with other signs of excess androgen secretion (e.g., virilization). Elevated free testosterone (T) and metabolites of T and DHT have been demonstrated in some women with IH. There is other evidence that adrenal function may be abnormal.[9] Ethnic differences do exist with respect to the frequency of IH diagnosis (it is more common among women of Mediterranean background). The diagnosis is made by exclusion of other hyperandrogen disorders. Treatment of IH has included agents with antiandrogenic effects such as diethylstilbestrol (DES), medroxyprogesterone, cimetidine, spironolactone, and cyproterone acetate.[9]

MANAGEMENT

When a prepubertal child prematurely develops sexual hair, or when a postpubertal female has hirsutism, it is imperative to perform a careful clinical and biochemical evaluation to distinguish between pathologically significant and pathologically insignificant causes. This will provide the basis for a rational therapeutic regimen.

Regardless of the pathophysiologic basis and whether the condition is deemed hirsutism or hypertrichosis, there may be some particular advantage to removing the existing excess hair. This can have positive cosmetic and emotional effects. The pediatrician will encounter cases in which the presence of excess hair can be appropriately managed by physical removal. This may be accomplished by bleaching (6% hydrogen peroxide solution), shaving, plucking, or using depilatory agents (sulfides of alkali metals, thioglycolate-containing agents). Electrolysis, if properly performed, is also effective and safe. Since commercial electrolysis is unlicensed in many states, one should choose an electrologist carefully. The use of glucocorticoids and oral contraceptives is beneficial in decreasing the rate of new hair growth but will have no effect on existing hair.

REFERENCES

1. Behrman RE, Vaugh VC, and Nelson WE, editors: Nelson textbook of pediatrics, ed 13, Philadelphia, 1987, WB Saunders Co.
2. Berthelsen JG et al: Testicular tumors in infancy and childhood. In Forest MG, editor: Androgens in childhood pediatric and adolescent endocrinology, vol 19, Basel, Switzerland, 1989, S Karger AG.
3. Forest MG: Ovarian tumors in infancy, childhood, and adolescence. In Forest MG, editor: Androgens in childhood pediatric and adolescent endocrinology, vol 19, Basel, Switzerland, 1989, S Karger AG.
4. Francois R, dePerett E, and Forest MG: Precocious puberty in boys. In Forest MG, editor: Androgens in childhood pediatric and adolescent endocrinology, vol 19, Basel, Switzerland, 1989, S Karger AG.
5. Grant DB: Virilizing adrenal tumors. In Forest MG, editor: Androgens in childhood pediatric and adolescent endocrinology, vol 19, Basel, Switzerland, 1989, S Karger AG.
6. Lobo RA, Goebelsman U, and Horton R: Hirsutism in polycystic ovarian syndrome, Fertil Steril 38:278, 1982.
7. Korth-Schutz S: Precocious adrenarche. In Forest MG, editor: Androgens in childhood pediatric and adolescent endocrinology, vol 19, Basel, Switzerland, 1989, S Karger AG.
8. Pang S et al: Late-onset adrenal steroid 3B-hydroxysteroid dehydrogenase deficiency: a cause of hirsutism in pubertal and post-pubertal women, J Clin Endocrinol Metab 60:428, 1985.
9. St Louis Y, Levy R, and Saenger P: Hyperandrogenism in females: hirsutism and acne. In Forest MG, editor: Androgens in childhood pediatric and adolescent endocrinology, vol 19, Basel, Switzerland, 1989, S Karger AG.
10. Temeck JW et al: Genetic defects of steroidogenesis in premature pubarche, J Clin Endocrinol Metab 64:609, 1987.
11. Yen SSC: The polycystic ovary syndrome, Clin Endocrinol (Oxf) 12:177, 1980.

143

Hoarseness

Susan E. Levitzky

Hoarseness, a symptom of voice dysfunction, is a change in voice quality, often described as harsh, grating, rough, noisy, or raspy. Hoarseness should not be confused with (1) stridor, which is a high-pitched whistling sound, (2) the muffled "hot potato mouth" speech of persons with supraglottic lesions, or (3) the weak "breathy" speech of persons with neuromuscular disorders. The main significance of hoarseness is that some process has affected the structure or function of the vocal cords. This may be an early sign of local disease or a manifestation of a systemic illness.

The following discussion highlights the common causes of hoarseness in newborns, infants, children, and adolescents. For an in-depth discussion, refer to the books and articles listed at the end of this chapter.

According to voice surveys conducted among elementary schoolchildren, the prevalence of chronic hoarseness ranges from 5% to more than 20%.[29] Statistics reflecting the incidence of acute hoarseness are not available because data from outpatient surveys have focused on general diagnostic categories rather than on specific symptoms and diagnoses.

HISTORY

In evaluating a child with hoarseness, it is essential that a thorough history be obtained from the parents. In hoarseness of sudden onset, an inflammatory process should be considered. In acute laryngitis, symptoms of rhinorrhea, cough, and sore throat often precede the hoarseness. Occasionally a history of foreign body aspiration or direct laryngeal trauma may explain acute hoarseness. Gradually progressive or persistent hoarseness implies a more insidious and chronic disease process. Information should be gleaned regarding age of onset, excessive use of the voice, associated allergies, chronic chest congestion with recurrent pneumonias (gastroesophageal reflux), sluggishness and any decrease in the yearly rate of height increase (hypothyroidism), chronic postnasal drip, recent tuberculosis tine test conversion, underlying systemic disease, and change of hoarseness with change in position (mobile lesion). Thus, a thorough review of systems is indicated to uncover any conditions that may be responsible for persistent hoarseness.

PHYSICAL EXAMINATION

A complete physical examination should be performed to detect any unsuspected disease. One should especially observe for any signs of increased respiratory effort (stridor, drooling, nasal flaring, retractions, use of accessory muscles, or tachypnea). If any of these is present, the child should be evaluated promptly by a qualified, experienced physician for potentially life-threatening airway obstruction (see Chapters 168 and 267). If stridor is not present, the physician may proceed with the examination, noting any of the following: neck masses (hemangiomas, lymphangiomas), local adenopathy, tracheal shift, thyromegaly or thyroid nodule, pale boggy nasal mucosa (allergies), chest congestion (gastroesophageal reflux), cardiac murmurs or enlargement, cutaneous hemangiomas, café-au-lait spots, pallor, rash, joint swelling, or splenomegaly.

With clues from the history and physical examination, the physician must decide what further investigation is indicated.

FURTHER INVESTIGATION

Direct laryngoscopy by a skilled endoscopist has become the mainstay in diagnosing laryngeal disease.[4] Categories of hoarseness meriting direct laryngoscopy include (1) congenital hoarseness, (2) possible foreign body in the larynx, (3) progressive, unremitting hoarseness of unknown cause, (4) hoarseness of unknown cause with stridor, and (5) acquired hoarseness persisting for longer than 2 to 3 weeks.[27] Other diagnostic modalities complement but do not replace laryngoscopy. True lateral and anteroposterior roentgenographic views of the soft tissues of the neck, computed tomography (CT) scans, and magnetic resonance imaging (MRI) studies may reveal vocal cord immobility, cysts, foreign bodies, or masses. A chest roentgenogram may demonstrate a mediastinal mass. A recently developed quantitative method for evaluating vocal cord dysfunction is a valuable adjunct in following perturbation (the degree of hoarseness of the voice).[21] This procedure is simple, brief, highly accurate, and cost effective.

CAUSES OF HOARSENESS

Newborns

Increasingly, lifesaving measures are successful in treating premature and newborn infants with respiratory distress, but reports on subsequent laryngeal injuries have also increased. Following intubation, an infant may sustain arytenoid cartilage dislocation, ulceration, or edema of the vocal cords. Unilateral vocal cord palsy may result from birth trauma, with stretching of the neck and the recurrent laryngeal nerve during a breech delivery.

Congenital anomalies causing hoarseness include the following:[9]

1. Laryngeal web, a persistent membrane of tissue usually located at the anterior commissure between the true vocal cords. The thickness and extent of the web are variable and determine the mode of therapy. Webs have been associated with cardiac defects, mainly a ventricular septal defect.
2. Laryngeal cysts and laryngoceles, cysts arising from the laryngeal ventricle and containing either fluid or air. A hoarse cry eventually leads to stridor, especially when air cysts are present. Lateral neck roentgenograms show a supraglottic mass, which may disappear when the child is quiet. The endoscopist must be prepared to deal with complete airway obstruction, because laryngeal edema or hemorrhage into the cyst may occur during endoscopy.
3. Laryngeal fissure or cleft, a rare anomaly characterized by an incomplete closure of the posterior larynx. This vertical slit often extends below the vocal cords with a tracheoesophageal communication; in 20% of cases, a fistula coexists. Feeding-associated respiratory distress usually overshadows the voice disorder.
4. Laryngeal hemangiomas, rare causes of hoarseness in newborns. In 50% of cases, skin hemangiomas are also present. Symptoms worsen with crying or with an intercurrent upper respiratory tract infection. Most of these hemangiomas regress spontaneously, but if airway compromise develops, surgical laser and steroid therapy may avert a tracheostomy.

Infants with Down syndrome have a harsh, flat, low-pitched cry. Infants with de Lange syndrome have a coarse, growling cry. The cry of babies with untreated hypothyroidism has a hoarse, "gravelly" quality resulting from myxedematous infiltration of the vocal cords. Rarer causes of hoarseness with onset in the newborn period include Farber lipogranulomatosis,[7] lipoid proteinosis of Urbach and Wiethe,[22] pachyonychia congenita,[6] and Weaver syndrome.[25] Hypocalcemic tetany may cause laryngospasm with accompanying hoarseness and stridor.

Infants, Children, and Adolescents

Infectious Inflammatory Causes. By far the majority of cases of acute hoarseness in childhood are related to respiratory tract infections, especially those caused by adenoviruses 4 and 7, influenza A, and parainfluenza I. Acute laryngitis and acute laryngotracheobronchitis (infectious croup) result in vocal cord inflammation. Children with postnasal drip associated with the common cold, sinus disease, or adenoiditis are hoarse as a result of bathing of the vocal cords with purulent material. Impaired nasal respiration during a cold leads to mouthbreathing and drying out of the vocal cord mucosa, with resultant hoarseness upon arising in the morning. Children with "spasmodic croup" have recurrent episodes of laryngeal obstruction and awake at night with a harsh voice and inspiratory stridor. Children with epiglottitis are *not* hoarse, and cough is *not* a prominent symptom. As the epiglottis swells, the voice becomes *muffled* and drooling sets in. Laryngeal diphtheria should be considered in the differential diagnosis of progressive hoarseness. With lapses in immunization practices and the recent influx of refugees into the United States, sporadic outbreaks still occur. Laryngeal diphtheria usually develops as a downward extension of the tonsillar-pharyngeal membrane. Sudden death from laryngeal obstruction may also occur. Other causes of hoarseness in this age group are laryngeal candidiasis or tuberculosis,[26,28] especially in the immunocompromised host. Febrile immunocompromised or neutropenic children with hoarseness should have prompt laryngoscopy to rule out fungal involvement.[11,14] Cytomegalovirus (CMV) infection of the laryngeal nerve has resulted in hoarseness in adults with AIDS[24] and should be considered in immunocompromised children with CMV infection who develop vocal cord paralysis. The recent upsurge in maternal and congenital syphilis requires physicians to consider this infection in the evaluation of hoarseness in an infant.[19]

Noninfectious Inflammatory Disease. Gastroesophageal reflux may result in hoarseness secondary to acid or chemical laryngitis.[2] Therapy with thickened feedings, 30-degree prone upright positioning, and antacids usually controls the reflux, and eventually a normal voice returns.

In allergic laryngeal disease, children with documented respiratory allergies and rhinosinusitis develop vocal cord edema and inflammation and the hoarseness that accompanies these changes.[3] Occasionally patients using inhaled steroids for asthma control may develop secondary dysphonia. Discontinuation of this route of treatment or addition of a Volumatic spacer device for administration leads to resolution.[15]

Angioneurotic edema of the larynx occurs either sporadically, triggered by a specific allergen, or as a result of an inherited quantitative or functional deficiency of complement (C1) inhibitor. In the former type, steroids, antihistamines, and epinephrine alleviate the symptoms. In the hereditary type, laryngeal edema is refractory to steroids, and intubation and infusions of fresh-frozen plasma are the usual forms of treatment. Recently, therapeutic trials with infusions of C1 inhibitor concentrate have controlled the life-threatening airway obstruction promptly. Administering short-term prophylaxis with androgen derivatives before performing dental work in these patients will raise C1 esterase inhibitor levels and prevent the feared laryngeal edema.[13]

Inhalation of a caustic or hot gas or ingestion of salicylic acid may lead to vocal cord edema and hoarseness in susceptible individuals.[16] Cricoarytenoid arthritis, sometimes associated with juvenile rheumatoid arthritis, can cause painful hoarseness.

Traumatic Causes. The most common cause of chronic hoarseness in school-age children is the development of vocal cord nodules. The nodules usually occur bilaterally and are whitish protuberances on the free margin of the true vocal cords, located at the junction of their anterior and middle thirds, the area of maximum vibration. Nodule formation is attributed to submucosal hemorrhages caused by screaming or shouting. Organization of the hemorrhages into fibrous nodules or polyps then takes place. Speech therapy may resolve the nodules and alleviate the hoarseness. Surgical removal of the nodules is not usually indicated, but in specific situations, such as several years of hoarseness without improvement, with worsening, or with psychological sequelae, vocal nodule microsurgical removal should be considered.[5]

Acute hoarseness may follow endotracheal intubation, aspiration of a foreign body, or fracture of the larynx. Laryngographic investigation of postoperative hoarseness may be helpful.[17]

Tumors. Juvenile laryngeal papillomatosis is the most common benign laryngeal tumor that occurs during childhood. Such papillomas usually present with hoarseness in children between 2 and 7 years of age, but they may occur in newborns. The tumor consists of wartlike proliferations of stratified squamous epithelium arising in the glottic region, but occasionally it spreads to involve the trachea and the bronchi. Possibly caused by a viral agent, this tumor often undergoes spontaneous involution during puberty. Carbon dioxide laser excision has been very successful in maintaining a patent airway and preserving vocal cord function.[20] Leukocyte interferon administration has shown some promise in inducing remission.[18] Osteochondroma of the cervical spine has resulted in hoarseness caused by edema, erythema, and deviation of the larynx. Surgical excision is curative.[23]

Rhabdomyosarcoma of the larynx is a rare but highly malignant tumor that presents with painful hoarseness. Combined partial laryngectomy, radiotherapy, and chemotherapy have effected very high cure rates.[10]

Miscellaneous Causes. Miscellaneous causes of hoarseness during childhood and adolescence include sarcoidosis, which may cause supraglottic granulomas and compression of the left recurrent laryngeal nerve by enlarged lymph nodes; laryngeal neurofibromatosis, amyloidosis, or lipid proteinosis; and vocal cord paralysis secondary to central nervous system malfunction, such as the Arnold-Chiari malformation. In cardiovocal syndrome, vocal cord paralysis results from impingement on the left recurrent laryngeal nerve by an enlarged pulmonary artery or an enlarged left atrium.[8]

Other causes of hoarseness that occur during adolescence include abusive, vigorous, loud singing and yelling (without vocal cord nodule formation), pubertal voice changes, laryngeal trauma complications of car and motorcycle accidents, smoking, myasthenia gravis, multiple sclerosis, and functional dysphonia (whispering syndrome in girls and falsetto voice in boys).[12]

RESTORING AND PRESERVING NORMAL PHONATION

Speaking in a pleasant-sounding voice is especially important for older children and adolescents, because peers are very cognizant and often intolerant of deviations from the "norm." It is essential that once the cause of a child's or adolescent's hoarseness is determined, every attempt should be made to restore and preserve vocal function. Voice therapy with a speech pathologist is useful for children with functional hoarseness as well as for those with organic hoarseness.

REFERENCES

1. Autier C and Grimfeld A: Endoscopy of the respiratory tract. In Gerbeaux J, Couvreur J, and Tournier G, editors: Pediatric respiratory disease, New York, 1982, John Wiley & Sons, Inc.
2. Bain W et al: Head and neck manifestations of gastroesophageal reflux, Laryngoscope 93:175, 1983.
3. Baker BM, Baker CD, and Le T: Vocal quality articulation and audiological characteristics of children and young adults with diagnosed allergies, Ann Otol Rhinol Laryngol 91:277, 1982.
4. Benjamin B: A new pediatric microlaryngoscope, Ann Otol Rhinol Laryngol 93:468, 1984.
5. Benjamin B and Groxson G: Vocal nodules in children, Ann Otol Rhinol Laryngol 96:530, 1987.
6. Benjamin B, Parsons DS, and Molloy HF: Pachyonychia congenita with laryngeal involvement, Int J Pediatr Otorhinolaryngol 13:205, 1987.
7. Burck U et al: A case of lipogranulomatosis Farber: some clinical and ultrastructural aspects, Eur J Pediatr 143:203, 1985.
8. Condon LM et al: Cardiovocal syndrome in infancy, Pediatrics 75:22, 1985.
9. Cotton RT and Richardson MA: Congenital laryngeal anomalies, Otolaryngol Clin North Am 14:203, 1981.
10. DeGroot TR, Frazer JP, and Wood BP: Combination therapy for laryngeal rhabdomyosarcoma, Am J Otolaryngol 1:456, 1980.
11. Dole M et al: Hoarseness in children with neutropenia, J Pediatr 113:782, 1988.
12. Froese AP and Sims P: Functional dysphonia in adolescence: two case reports, Can J Psychol 32:389, 1987.
13. Gadek JE et al: Replacement therapy in hereditary angioedema, N Engl J Med 302:542, 1980.
14. Hass A et al: Hoarseness in immunocompromised children: association with invasive fungal infection, J Pediatr 111:731, 1987.
15. Henry RL: Inhaled cortiocosteroid agents and dysphonia, Med J Aust 147:365, 1987.
16. Hillerdal G and Lindholm H: Laryngeal edema as the only symptom of hypersensitivity to salicylic acid and other substances, J Laryngol Otol 98:547, 1984.
17. Lesser T and Williams G: Laryngographic investigation of postoperative hoarseness, Clin Otolaryngol 13:37, 1988.
18. McCabe BF and Clark KF: Interferon and laryngeal papillomatosis, Ann Otol Rhinol Laryngol 92:2, 1983.
19. Murphy FK and Patamasucon P: Congenital syphilis. In Holmes KK et al, editors: Sexually transmitted diseases, New York, 1984, McGraw-Hill Book Co.
20. Ossoff RH, Toriumi DM, and Duncavage JA: The use of the laser in head and neck surgery, Adv Otolaryngol and Head and Neck Surg 1:220, 1987.
21. Rontal E et al: Quantitative and objective evaluation of vocal cord function, Ann Otol Rhinol Laryngol 92:421, 1983.
22. Savage MM, Crockett DM, and McCabe BF: Lipoid proteinosis of the larynx: a cause of voice change in the infant and young child, Int J Pediatr Otorhinolaryngol 15:33, 1988.
23. Scher N and Panje WR: Osteochondroma presenting as a neck mass, Laryngoscope 98:550, 1988.
24. Small PM et al: Cytomegalovirus infection of the laryngeal nerve presenting as hoarseness in patients with acquired immunodeficiency syndrome, Am J Med 86:108, 1989.
25. Teebi AS et al: A new autosomal recessive disorder resembling weaver syndrome, Am J Med Genet 33:479, 1989.
26. Varteresian-Karanfil et al: Pulmonary infection and cavity formation caused by *Mycobacterium tuberculosis* in a child with AIDS, N Engl J Med 319:1018, 1988.
27. Vaughan CW: When to refer the hoarse patient, Hosp Pract 24:21, 1989.
28. Vyravanathan S: Hoarseness in tuberculosis, J Laryngol Otol 97:523, 1983.
29. Wilson DK: Voice problems of children, Baltimore, 1979, Williams & Wilkins.

SUGGESTED READINGS

Aronson A: Clinical voice disorders: an interdisciplinary approach, New York, 1980, Thieme-Stratton, Inc.

Grunberg J and Tournier G: Laryngeal disease. In Gerbeaux J, Couvreur J, and Tournier G: editors: Pediatric respiratory disease, New York, 1982, John Wiley & Sons, Inc.

144

Hyperhidrosis

Nancy K. Barnett

Hyperhidrosis, or sweating more than normal, occurs commonly in childhood. The child or the family usually expresses concern because the sweating is either odoriferous or so intense that it interferes with hand or foot functions. Axillary hyperhidrosis usually becomes more of a problem in adolescence because of the odor associated with bacterial degradation of apocrine sweat—the apocrine glands being stimulated at puberty by androgenic hormones. However, palmar and plantar hyperhidrosis secondary to eccrine sweat production may occur at any age.

Palmoplantar hyperhidrosis is thought to be stimulated by anxiety, whereas axillary hyperhidrosis is probably stimulated by both heat and emotion. It is postulated that emotions and the temperature of the blood perfusing the hypothalamus stimulate the secretion of the hormones that regulate the autonomic nervous system's control of perspiration.[1]

Excessive sweating that is not chronic or limited to the palms, soles, and axillae may indicate a systemic disorder, such as infection, lymphoma, thyrotoxicosis, Riley-Day syndrome, hypoglycemia, drug withdrawal, or pheochromocytoma. Diagnostic evaluation for these disorders must be undertaken only in the face of *generalized* increased perspiring.

Systemic anticholinergic agents will control hyperhidrosis, but the side effects of cholinergic blockage preclude their long-term use. For palmar sweating, the application of aluminum salts (Drysol) every other day is probably the most effective treatment. Plantar hyperhidrosis responds also to aluminum salts, and one can use absorbent powders (e.g., Zeasorb) more easily here than on the palms. Whenever possible, the patient should be allowed to go barefoot. For bromhidrosis (malodorous hyperhidrosis) of the soles, cleansing frequently with drying deodorant soaps and applying topical antibiotic creams (erythromycin, tetracycline, or clindamycin) may help.

Axillary hyperhidrosis is troublesome because, in the face of continual sweating, it is difficult to maintain an effective antiperspirant in contact with the axillary skin. One approach consists of applying a saturated solution of aluminum chlorohydroxide in absolute ethanol or isopropyl alcohol to the axillary vault at night under Saran Wrap occlusion. Frequent clothing changes may be necessary, as well as topical antibiotics and deodorant powders, for individuals with axillary hyperhidrosis and bromhidrosis. In extreme cases, when these measures fail and the patient is desperate for relief, local axillary skin excision can be performed with reasonable expectation of success. Because of its attendant complications, ganglion sympathectomy cannot be recommended for most patients with axillary hyperhidrosis.[2,3]

REFERENCES

1. Cage GW, Shwachman H, and Sato K: Hyperhidrosis. In Fitzpatrick TB et al, editors: Dermatology in general medicine, New York, 1979, McGraw-Hill Book Co.
2. Hurwitz S: Clinical pediatric dermatology, Philadelphia, 1981, WB Saunders Co.
3. Shelley WB and Hurley HJ: Studies on topical antiperspirant control of axillary hyperhidrosis, Acta Derm Venereol 55:241, 1975.

145

Hypotonia

Cynthia H. Cole

Infants with hypotonia ("floppy" infants) are born with sufficient frequency to require the pediatrician to have some experience in their initial assessment and eventual management. Often the etiology of hypotonia is apparent based on the history, perinatal events, and physical examination (e.g., hypotonia in an asphyxiated infant). Even in cases in which a careful history and physical examination yield limited information, the etiology of hypotonia may be clarified through diagnostic studies (e.g., muscle biopsies, muscle chemistry analysis, electromyography, nerve conduction studies, or nerve biopsy). The following discussion approaches the topic of hypotonia from the perspective of the clinical presentation (with emphasis on the "anatomic" localization of dysfunction) and laboratory evaluation. In addition, a brief profile of various disorders is provided.

CLINICAL EVALUATION OF HYPOTONIA

Hypotonia is a dysfunction of the motor system and should be suspected in any infant who assumes unusual postures, has decreased resistance to passive movements, and demonstrates relative immobility. Hypotonic infants may have excessive range of joint mobility or joint contractures (e.g., arthrogryposis multiplex congenita). Some hypotonic infants may have additional problems such as difficulty sucking and swallowing; reduced respiratory excursion, which leads to frequent respiratory infections; and delays in attaining motor milestones.

The history and family evaluation are often relevant to specific disorders. The pregnancy history may be significant for polyhydramnios and decreased fetal movement. Perinatal history may reveal intrauterine exposure of the baby to magnesium, obstetric analgesia or anesthesia, or evidence of obstetric trauma. Family history and examination of the parents may be positive for a specific motor disorder (e.g., myasthenia gravis or myotonic dystrophy).

Physical evaluation of the hypotonic infant requires an orderly approach. Consideration of the effects of the major contributors of the motor system is critical for "localization" of the dysfunction. The major levels and components of the motor system, referred to below, include (1) central or "above the lower motor" neuron, (2) the lower motor neuron, (3) the peripheral or cranial nerve level, (4) the myoneural junction, and (5) the muscle itself. Motor dysfunction at any level results in hypotonia.[1,4]

It is also important, from an etiologic perspective, to assess whether *significant* muscle weakness accompanies hypotonia.[1,3,4] Significant weakness is not present if an infant can move spontaneously and withdraw an extremity or raise it against gravity. Hypotonia is often associated with some degree of weakness, such that *complete* absence of weakness is unusual. Therefore one's evaluation distinguishes whether *significant* muscle weakness is or is not associated with hypotonia.

Hypotonia Without Significant Weakness

If significant muscle weakness does *not* accompany hypotonia, then the etiology of the baby's "floppiness" is *central* and involves pathology of the cerebral cortex; the corticospinal-corticobulbar and other spinal tracts; the basal ganglia or the cerebellum; or is caused by a systemic disorder (e.g., connective tissue disorders, endocrinopathies, other metabolic disorders, or malnutrition) that can affect motor function. Other features characteristic of "central" motor disorders include preservation of the deep tendon reflexes and the presence of other signs of central nervous system (CNS) involvement (e.g., altered mental status, seizures). The differential diagnosis of central hypotonia is diverse and includes such entities as hypoxic-ischemic encephalopathy, intracranial hemorrhage or infection, neurodegenerative disorders, developmental anomalies of the central nervous system and spinal cord, and CNS or spinal cord trauma. Systemic disorders, as noted above, should be considered as well. Therefore the diagnostic evaluation will be guided by the clues derived from the patient's presentation. Hypoxic-ischemic encephalopathy, the most common cause of hypotonia in the neonatal period, is usually apparent based on the perinatal history and the neonatal examination.

Hypotonia With Significant Weakness

Hypotonia with weakness is caused by (1) disorders of the lower motor neuron, (2) peripheral neuropathies, (3) disorders of the neuromuscular junction, and (4) disorders of the muscle itself.

Disorders of the lower motor neuron involve the anterior horn cells of the spinal cord and are characterized by hypotonia, muscle weakness, and eventually areflexia. These features are observed in the presence of an alert infant with intact sensory and sphincter function. Fasciculations may be visualized or detected on an electromyogram (EMG). Werdnig-Hoffman disease, glycogen storage disease type II (Pompe disease), and anterior horn cell neurogenic arthrogryposis multiplex congenita are examples of lower motor neuron disorders. Each of these have specific features that may distinguish them from each other. Werdnig-Hoffman disease typically follows a deteriorating course, in contrast to the nonprogressive course of most cases of neurogenic arthrogryposis multiplex congenita. Pompe disease may be distinguished from the other lower motor neuron disorders by the presence of cardiac failure, hepatomegaly, and glycogen in muscle, the tongue, and the anterior horn cells.

Peripheral neuropathies, similar to lower motor neuron disorders, manifest hypotonia, weakness, and hypoactive or absent reflexes. In addition, sensory deficits may be elicited in some peripheral neuropathies. Elevation of cerebrospinal fluid (CSF) protein and reduction of nerve conduction velocities are features of polyneuropathies. The diagnosis of peripheral neuropathy may be established with nerve biopsy. Muscle biopsy shows a denervation pattern, and the EMG reveals fasciculations. Charcot-Marie-Tooth disease is the most common peripheral neuropathy in infants; Guillain-Barré syndrome and infectious and toxic polyneuritis may occur at any age.

Disorders of the neuromuscular junction share common features of hypotonia and weakness. However, they are individually distinguished by differences in onset and evolution, patterns of hypotonia and weakness, characteristic EMG findings, and pathogenesis. Deep tendon reflexes and muscle biopsy results are normal. Examples of myoneural junction disorders include neonatal transient myasthenia gravis and congenital myasthenia gravis syndromes and infantile botulism. Dysfunction of the myoneural junction may also be induced by hypermagnesemia and aminoglycoside antibiotic therapy. Disorders of the neuromuscular junction are important to recognize because supportive and anticholinesterase therapeutic interventions are available. (Clinical profiles of the myasthenia gravis disorders that affect neonates and older infants are given below.)

Disorders of the muscle share nonspecific features of hypotonia, weakness, and depressed deep tendon reflexes. The EMG may reveal a characteristic but nondiagnostic pattern. Muscle enzymes are variably elevated, depending on the particular myopathy. The diagnosis of muscle disorders is often made based on the particular myopathic pattern shown on the muscle biopsy.

Additional Neurologic Evaluation. Assessment of specific neurologic features may help differentiate the etiology of hypotonia. For instance, the pattern and distribution of significant weakness (if present) vary among disorders. Disease of the peripheral nerve is characterized by weakness that often is greater in the distal than in the proximal limbs, whereas the opposite is true for myopathies and variably true for lower motor neuron disorders. The facial muscles may be more prominently involved in disorders of the myoneural junction compared with a late or variable involvement in disorders of the anterior horn cell or in myopathies.

Deep tendon reflexes are normal in "central" and myoneural junction disorders, depressed in peripheral neuropathies and myopathies, and eventually absent in anterior horn cell disease.

Evaluation of the sensory level may differentiate transection of the spinal cord from anterior horn cell disease. Diminished touch and vibratory perception may be found in some peripheral neuropathies.

Cranial nerve function may be abnormal in myasthenia gravis, ocular dystrophies, myotubular myopathy, and Möbius syndrome.

Additional information that influences clinical evaluation of the hypotonic infant includes the age of the patient at the onset of signs and symptoms and the clinical course (nonprogressive or progressive).

DIAGNOSTIC STUDIES

The initial diagnosis of a hypotonic patient may be sufficiently clear from a thorough history and physical examination alone. This occurs more commonly in the group of disorders in which hypotonia is present without weakness. Floppiness resulting from hypotonia associated with weakness usually requires further diagnostic studies.

Muscle Enzyme Levels

Serum levels of creatinine phosphokinase (CPK), serum glutamic-oxaloacetic transaminase (SGOT), serum glutamic-pyruvic transaminase (SGPT), aldolase, and lactic acid dehydrogenase (LDH) help to identify only a few muscle disorders. These levels are moderately increased in Duchenne and Becker muscular dystrophies and less so in the facioscapulohumeral and limb-girdle dystrophies. CPK levels may be slightly increased in spinal muscular atrophy and in many congenital myopathies. CPK levels also are increased during the first few days of life and remain elevated for 4 to 6 weeks. Thus it is not usually helpful to measure muscle enzyme levels in the initial evaluation of infants and young children with hypotonia.

Muscle Biopsy

A muscle biopsy is essential in establishing the diagnosis of a disorder in which weakness is associated with hypotonia. It must be kept in mind that muscle biopsies may be nonspecific or nondiagnostic in newborns and that biopsy results may change with time. It is important that an individual assessing the biopsy specimen of a newborn be expert in the pathologic conditions associated with that age and, specifically, with neonatal muscle biopsies. Various histologic patterns—denervation, myopathy, and inflammation—may shed light on the diagnosis. Proliferation of adipose and connective tissue is common in muscular dystrophy, neurogenic atrophies, and other myopathies. Characteristic morphologic, histochemical, and electron microscopic markers are essential in the diagnosis of congenital myopathies, since these disorders often have similar clinical presentations.

Electrodiagnostic Studies

Electromyography and nerve conduction analysis may help to distinguish between neuromuscular disorders and denervation myopathy. However, both tests have limitations. Electromyograms are often unreliable and difficult to interpret in the newborn period, and the results may change with time. An EMG performed on a muscle at rest in which fasciculations and sharp waves are present may indicate denervation, but these may be seen in the distal muscles of normal infants. An electromyogram may be normal in many congenital myopathies; nevertheless, electromyography is useful in diagnosing myotonia and polymyositis. Nerve conduction studies are also difficult to interpret in small children. Slow conduction velocities may be seen in peripheral neuropathies, and repetitive stimulation is useful in diagnosing myasthenia gravis.

Ultrasound Imaging

Ultrasound imaging has recently been used to differentiate neuromuscular from nonneuromuscular disorders, but its role and limitations require further study.[2]

COMMON DISORDERS OF THE HYPOTONIC INFANT

When all data have been gathered from the available sources, it is often possible to be definitive. The most frequent diagnoses encompass relatively few conditions; it is therefore useful to highlight these more common causes of hypotonia.

Disorders of Hypotonia Without Associated Weakness

Disorders of the Central Nervous System. Disorders of the central nervous system are commonly associated with hypotonia and delayed motor milestones. Mental retardation may be present, along with global developmental delay. In the majority of patients with nonspecific mental retardation, no diagnosis or clinical disorder can be recognized. However, in some (Down syndrome and other genetic syndromes) the clinical features may be sufficient to define a specific disorder. If a child demonstrates loss of acquired developmental milestones, a degenerative CNS disorder resulting from various storage diseases must be considered and investigated. Hypotonia associated with CNS disorders varies in degree and subsequent course. Hypotonic cerebral palsy has features of athetosis and ataxia with or without increased deep tendon reflexes (DTRs) in addition to hypotonia. Various metabolic disorders (aminoacidopathies, organic acidemias, mucopolysaccharidoses, and lipidoses) may manifest with hypotonia, failure to thrive, and other nonspecific symptoms. Acidosis, hypoglycemia, and hyperbilirubinemia may be found with chemical screening tests. The ferric chloride test is a useful metabolic urine screen for some aminoacidopathies. However, specific analysis of blood and urine for amino acids, organic acids, or urinary sulfates (keratan, dermatan, haparan) should be requested if clinical judgment suggests one of these metabolic disorders. Cultured fibroblasts are also used to diagnose the specific enzyme deficiency in mucopolysaccharidoses. Lipidoses (Tay-Sachs disease, metachromatic leukodystrophy, Krabbe leukodystrophy) are disorders of lipid metabolism and are characterized by progressive mental retardation, hypotonia, and possible diminished nerve conduction velocity. Eventually muscle biopsy may reveal degenerative changes. Cerebral trauma, hemorrhage, or anoxic insult will produce varying degrees and durations of hypotonia.

Connective Tissue Disorders. Connective tissue disorders may be associated with lax joints, hypotonia, and delayed motor milestones. Ehlers-Danlos syndrome in addition exhibits hyperelasticity of the skin. Marfan syndrome is characterized by hypotonia, delayed motor milestones, increased joint laxity, tall stature, dislocated lenses, and vascular lesions. Osteogenesis imperfecta varies in presentation depending on the specific form of this disorder's spectrum. Hypotonia, blue sclerae, multiple fractures, and delayed motor milestones are classic features. Congenital laxity of ligaments has no other clinical features in addition to increased joint laxity. Mucopolysaccharidoses may manifest with hypotonia and delayed motor and intellectual milestones. The diagnosis is usually suspected based on characteristic facial and clinical features and is confirmed by appropriate biochemical screening of acid mucopolysaccharides in urine and by cell cultures of lymphocytes and fibroblasts.

Endocrine Disorders. Hypothyroidism, hypopituitarism, and Cushing syndrome may be associated with hypotonia. Clinical features and biochemical analyses of serum electrolytes, glucose, and various hormones usually reveal the specific disorder.

Metabolic Disorders. Many of the previously mentioned disorders have a metabolic basis for the disturbance. Infantile hypercalcemia and renal tubular acidosis may have associated hypotonia and failure to thrive. Serum and urine chemistry analyses are necessary to establish the diagnosis.

Miscellaneous Disorders. It is not practical to discuss here all of the possible causes of hypotonia without associated weakness. However, a few deserve mention. Prader-Willi syndrome manifests in the newborn with extreme floppiness, feeding difficulties, and, in boys, cryptorchism and a small penis. The characteristic facies of this disorder may not be prominent and therefore may be overlooked. Obesity begins around 2 to 3 years of age in association with hyperphagia. Short stature and mental retardation are two additional features. Nutritional disorders (e.g., celiac disease and rickets) may exhibit hypotonia associated with malnourishment and failure to thrive. Some infants defy diagnosis and exhibit hypotonia as an isolated feature with no other demonstrable disorder; in these instances the hypotonia has improved with time.

Disorders With Significant Weakness and Incidental Hypotonia

Spinal Muscular Atrophy Syndromes. Spinal muscular atrophy syndromes are caused by degeneration of the nuclei of the motor cranial nerves and anterior horn cells of the spinal cord. The denervation leads to muscular atrophy. Infantile progressive spinal muscular atrophy (Werdnig-Hoffmann disease) is the most common cause of severely hypotonic, floppy infants. Weakness may have its onset in utero and be apparent at birth or within the first few weeks of life. Other forms of spinal muscular atrophy may not have their onset until after a few months or even after 5 to 10 years of age. Although these disorders usually progress quite rapidly, with many infants dying before 3 years of age, it is difficult to predict the clinical course. These infants characteristically have few spontaneous movements and appear floppy, with poor head, trunk, and extremity control. The alert facial expression is in striking contrast to the general paralysis. Furthermore, the deep tendon reflexes are usually diminished or lost early in the course of the disease. Fasciculations may be seen in the tongue, and muscle enzyme levels are usually normal, except that mild elevation of CPK levels may be present. Biopsy shows a classic denervation pattern: large groups of uniformly atrophic muscle fibers interspersed with single or groups of normal or enlarged fibers. Electromyography reveals a denervation pattern. Supportive treatment is all one can offer. Most of these infants develop complications of contractures and osteoporosis (resulting from immobilization) and are prone to the morbidity of repeated respiratory infections and aspiration pneumonia. Less severe forms of spinal muscular atrophy may manifest with delay in motor milestones, hypotonia, and muscle weakness. In early- or late-onset forms proximal muscles are always affected more than distal muscles. Inheritance is of the autosomal recessive type.

Myasthenia Gravis. Different forms of myasthenia gravis may appear during the neonatal period. These forms are broadly categorized as (1) neonatal transient myasthenia gravis and (2) congenital myasthenia syndromes. Each of these disorders manifests with hypotonia and muscle weakness. Both respond to anticholinesterase therapy and display decremental response to repetitive motor nerve stimulation.

Neonatal transient myasthenia gravis is the most common of these disorders. It is an immune-mediated process that occurs in 10% to 15% of infants born to mothers with myasthenia gravis, presumably as a result of passive transfer of antiacetylcholine receptor antibody across the placenta. Symptoms of feeding difficulties, weak cry, and respiratory problems may rapidly evolve during the first 24 to 72 hours of life. Generalized hypotonia is apparent in approximately 50% of affected infants. Deep tendon reflexes generally are normal. Although facial diplegia is frequently observed, ophthalmoplegia and ptosis are infrequently seen in neonatal transient myasthenia gravis, in contrast to the prominent ocular involvement in congenital myasthenia gravis syndromes. The diagnosis may be confirmed by evidence of the myasthenic phenomena in response to repetitive motor nerve stimulation and by a positive response to anticholinesterase medication (e.g., neostigmine 0.1 mg/kg intramuscularly). The duration of symptoms may be from 2 to 8 weeks. It is recommended that patients with marginal motor deficits receive electrophysiologic therapy to minimize the risk of serious deterioration and morbidity.

Congenital myasthenia gravis syndromes are inherited and demonstrate a variety of defects in the neuromuscular junction. "Congenital myasthenia," the most common of these syndromes, has its onset in the first weeks of life and is characterized by prominent ptosis and evolving ophthalmoplegia. In general, hypotonia and weakness are not pronounced. However, facial diplegia and a weak suck and cry are common. The course is persistent and mild. All features of the disorder, except for ophthalmoplegia, respond to anticholinesterase therapy. Electrophysiologic studies and treatment are as for neonatal transient myasthenia gravis except that therapy is required for life. "Familial infantile myasthenia" syndrome may be dramatically apparent at birth with apnea, feeding problems, facial diplegia, less pronounced ptosis, and no ophthalmoplegia. The course is episodic with natural remissions and relapses. Diagnosis and treatment are as for the other myasthenia gravis syndromes.

Congenital Myotonic Dystrophy. Classic myotonic dystrophy is primarily a disease of early childhood. It is an autosomal dominant inherited disease. The congenital form of myotonic dystrophy manifests with general hypotonia, difficulty in sucking and swallowing, and varying degrees of respiratory difficulties (which may necessitate assisted ventilation), associated skeletal deformities (e.g., scoliosis, talipes equinovarus), and facial diplegia (open, triangular-shaped mouth and open eyes). Mental retardation is another common feature that may subsequently manifest.

The clinical course of congenital myotonic dystrophy is one of gradual improvement in muscle tone over several weeks, such that the infant may be weaned from assisted ventilation and fed from a bottle. Patients subsequently develop the clinical and electromyographic features characteristic of classic myotonic dystrophy.

The explanation for the congenital form of myotonic dystrophy is the presence of an unidentified, maternal intrauterine factor that affects babies who have inherited the dominant gene for myotonic dystrophy. The congenital form is not seen in infants who have not inherited the dominant gene and are born to affected mothers.

Pregnancy history is frequently remarkable for evidence of decreased fetal movement and polyhydramnios, presumably resulting from the inability of the fetus to swallow.

The diagnosis is based on the infant's clinical features and confirmation of myotonic dystrophy in the mother by examination and electromyography.

Congenital Muscular Dystrophy. Congenital muscular dystrophy represents a group of muscle disorders that may or may not have central nervous system involvement along with diffuse hypotonia and weakness. Other features of congenital muscular dystrophy at birth include weakness of face, neck, and limbs (proximal more than distal); the presence of arthrogryposis multiplex congenita; and swallowing and respiratory problems. The progression of the clinical course is variable. Three forms of congenital muscular dystrophy associated with central nervous system involvement differ in the neuropathology associated with each form. The serum CPK is elevated. Electromyography reveals a myopathic pattern. CT scan of the brain is useful in identifying gyral abnormalities and cerebral hypodensity. Muscle biopsy reveals a dystrophic process that may vary in severity in terms of muscle replacement by adipose tissue and connective tissue proliferation. Inheritance is consistent with an autosomal recessive pattern.

Congenital Myopathies. Congenital myopathies include a number of entities that manifest with hypotonia during infancy. Weakness may be proximal or diffuse and can range from mild to severe. Because the diagnosis can be made only by muscle biopsy with detailed histochemical and electron microscopic studies, the names of congenital myopathies have been based on the results of these studies. They include those with (1) *structural abnormalities*—central core disease, nemaline rod myopathy, minicore disease, myotubular myopathy, mitochondrial myopathies, nonspecific congenital myopathies, congenital fiber-type disproportion, and congenital type 1 fiber predominance; and (2) *metabolic abnormalities*—glycogen storage diseases (types II, III, IV, V, VII with variable degrees of muscle, cardiac, and liver involvement, depending on the specific enzyme deficiency); and abnormal lipid metabolism (carnitine deficiency, carnitine palmityl transferase deficiency, and periodic paralysis).

REFERENCES

1. Dubowitz V: The floppy infant. Philadelphia, 1980, JB Lippincott Co.
2. Heckmatt JZ, Leeman S, and Dubowitz V: Ultrasound imaging in the diagnosis of muscle disease, J Pediatr 101:656, 1982.
3. Menkes JH: Diseases of the motor unit. In Avery ME and Taeusch HW, editors: Diseases of the newborn, Philadelphia, 1984, WB Saunders Co.
4. Volpe JJ: Neurology of the newborn, ed 2, Philadelphia, 1987, WB Saunders Co.

SUGGESTED READINGS

Clairezux AE and Lake BD: Muscle disorders in the floppy child. In Rosenberg HS and Bolande RP, editors: Perspectives in pediatric pathology, vol 4, Chicago, 1978, Year Book Medical Publishers, Inc.

Dubowitz V: Muscle disorders in childhood, Philadelphia, 1978, WB Saunders Co.

Hanson PA: Floppy baby (Oppenheim's disease, amyotonia congenita), Pediatr Ann 6:98, 1977.

Low NL: Spinal muscular atrophy syndromes, Pediatr Ann 6:35, 1977.

Paine RS: The future of the "floppy infant": a follow-up of 133 patients, Dev Med Child Neurol 5:115, 1963.

Sarnat HB: Diagnostic value of the muscle biopsy in the neonatal period, Am J Dis Child 132:782, 1978.

Slater GE and Swaiman KF: Muscular dystrophies of childhood, Pediatr Ann 6:50, 1977.

Spiro AJ: Approach to diagnosis in the child with muscle weakness, Pediatr Ann 6:11, 1977.

146

Irritability

Barry S. Marx

Irritability is a common presenting sign in the pediatric age group. Although often associated with other signs or symptoms that strongly suggest a diagnosis, irritability generates the greatest concern when its cause is obscure.

Irritability can be defined as a state characterized by testiness, snappishness, or resentment. By its very nature, the presence of irritability as a complaint may complicate attempts to identify its cause, particularly in the child or adolescent with marked agitation or in the preverbal child. Irritability may be characterized by an increase in protest to maneuvers that affect the involved body part, such as change of position or palpation. The older child or adolescent may describe the source of discomfort or exhibit behavioral or mental status changes to direct further investigation.

The circumstances surrounding the complaint of irritability provide essential clues to diagnosis. This information most commonly is elicited from the parents, but the child may provide important information, especially if interviewed alone. This is particularly valuable in cases of suspected physical, sexual, or psychological abuse, substance abuse, or adjustment disorder. The physical and emotional environment that existed before the complaint, and subsequent changes, should be described. The duration of the complaint, as well as circumstances associated with its exacerbation and amelioration, are key factors. When the complaint has been of significant duration, the effect on the rest of the family should be discussed.

Associated signs or symptoms can help direct the diagnostic workup. Fever may suggest an infectious process such as sepsis, meningitis, urinary tract infection, or otitis media. Failure to thrive, with poor linear growth, poor weight gain, or both may be associated with metabolic disorders (see the accompanying box). Exacerbation of irritability and/or protective withdrawal related to an organ or body part may localize the source of discomfort, as in a fracture, osteomyelitis, dislocation, or testicular torsion. Associated neurologic or mental status changes may suggest central nervous system disease or acute or chronic intoxication. Antecedent or concomitant personality changes, including withdrawal from relationships, deterioration in school performance, risk-taking behavior, and signs of vegetative or agitated depression, suggest psychological dysfunction.

Metabolic Disorders Characterized by Irritability and Failure to Thrive

Acrodermatitis enteropathica
Globoid cell leukodystrophy
Gluten-induced enteropathy
Lipogranulomatosis
Pyruvate carboxylase deficiency
Tryptophan malabsorption
Tyrosinemia
Vitamin B_6 deficiency

A differential diagnosis for irritability would include occult injury, unintentional intoxication, substance abuse (intoxication or withdrawal), infection (especially of the central nervous system), metabolic disorder (including acquired electrolyte imbalance), abuse (physical, sexual, or psychological), and psychological dysfunction. To the extent that some phenomena are age specific (teething, colic, substance abuse), the scope of the differential diagnosis may be narrowed.

Psychosocial considerations are fundamental to the diagnostic investigation and management of irritability. Although the cause of the complaint may or may not be rooted in psychological dysfunction, if the problem is of significant severity or duration, family dynamics are likely to have been affected and need to be assessed.

The management of irritability lies in ascertaining its cause. The range of laboratory studies in pursuit of an etiology is virtually limitless. The history, physical examination, and severity of the complaint dictate the focus and pace of evaluation. Finally, a decision must be made as to whether the child should be placed in a monitored environment, particularly during investigation of possible abuse.

SUGGESTED READINGS

Arena JM: Davison's compleat pediatrician, ed 9, Philadelphia, 1969, Lea & Febiger.

Tunnesson WW Jr: Signs and symptoms in pediatrics, Philadelphia, 1983, JB Lippincott Co.

147

Jaundice

Joel M. Andres

Clinical jaundice, a yellow discoloration of skin and mucous membranes, is the most common presenting manifestation of liver dysfunction in infants and children. This important physical finding is a direct indicator of hyperbilirubinemia, that is, excessive unconjugated and/or conjugated bilirubin in blood and tissues. The spectrum of conditions associated with jaundice extends from physiologic immaturity of bilirubin metabolism in the neonate to life-threatening disruption of liver function in the adolescent using illicit drugs. Jaundice in all age groups stimulates concern and anxiety in the physician, parents, and older child; this always demands an appropriate explanation.

EVALUATION OF THE PATIENT

History

The history is important in determining the patient's age at onset of the illness, defining the chronicity of the hepatic dysfunction, and helping to understand the clinical manifestations, especially jaundice and hepatomegaly. Inquiry may point to prolonged abdominal distention suggestive of longstanding hepatomegaly, splenomegaly, or ascites. Other manifestations of chronic liver disease are easy bleeding or bruising and peripheral edema. The occurrence of jaundice, dark urine, and acholic stools may help date the onset of illness; also, the jaundice usually appears in a cephalad to caudad progression. Pruritus and skin excoriations suggest prolonged cholestasis. Additional areas of inquiry for historical assessment of the liver problem are maternal illness during pregnancy; exposure to sick individuals, blood products, or hepatotoxins; or recent surgery with anesthesia. Since inheritable metabolic disease is a more common cause of liver dysfunction in the infant than in the older child or adult, a careful family history is essential and should include information regarding early childhood deaths, pulmonary problems, and neurologic or liver disease.

Clinical Assessment

The infant liver, a large organ relative to body size during the first 2 years of life, is normally palpable about 2 cm below the right costal margin[37] and should not be felt to the left of the midline. Knowledge of vertical liver span for normal children may provide a guideline for estimating liver size in children less than 2 years of age: a liver span greater than 7 cm should be considered an indication for further evaluation.[39] Changes in structures adjacent to the liver can influence apparent liver size; for example, gas in the hepatic flexure of the colon may obscure hepatic dullness, and hyperinflation of the lungs with subsequent depression of the diaphragm may displace the liver downward so that it is more easily palpable.

The consistency and character of the liver surface may help determine the nature of the underlying liver disorder. The liver edge is normally sharp, but soft and nontender. A large liver secondary to congestive heart failure has a rounded, smooth edge with a firm consistency; the cirrhotic liver is hard and has an irregular surface and edge. Auscultation over the liver area is valuable in detecting increased hepatic arterial blood flow (bruit) caused by primary liver tumors, metastatic disease of the liver, hepatic hemangiomas, or arteriovenous fistulas. A complete abdominal evaluation of the infant with jaundice or suspected hepatomegaly should include palpation of the spleen. In normal infants less than 2 years of age, the spleen can be palpated 1 to 2 cm below the left costal margin; this organ should not be felt in normal children older than 2 years under most circumstances. Splenomegaly suggests portal hypertension, especially in the child with a prominent abdominal venous pattern, peripheral edema, and ascites. Splenic enlargement may be the first manifestation of previously undiagnosed progressive liver disease, since it is not always associated with jaundice. Table 147-1 presents the clinical manifestations of liver dysfunction with associated differential diagnostic considerations for infants and children.

JAUNDICE IN THE NEONATE AND YOUNG INFANT

Because of the unique response of the infant liver to injury (e.g., active fibroblastic proliferation, Kupffer cell hyperplasia, and formation of multinucleated giant cells), in addition to the frequent occurrence of unconjugated hyperbilirubinemia in early life and its relative infrequency after the neonatal period, jaundice in the neonate and young infant (box, p. 993) will be considered separately from jaundice in the older infant and child (box, p. 994).

Unconjugated Hyperbilirubinemia

Unconjugated bilirubin in neonates is hazardous because of the potential for deposition of free bilirubin in neuronal tissues with associated brain damage (kernicterus), especially in the premature infant. Also, more subtle central nervous system abnormalities can occur in infants, although a critical level

Table 147-1 *Manifestations of Liver Dysfunction*

NO JAUNDICE		JAUNDICE		
GENERALIZED HEPATOMEGALY	ASYMMETRIC HEPATOMEGALY	GENERALIZED HEPATOMEGALY	APPARENT HEPATOMEGALY	NO HEPATOMEGALY
"Benign" hepatomegaly	Tumors	Unconjugated hyperbilirubinemia (hemolytic)	Choledochal cyst	Unconjugated hyperbilirubinemia (nonhemolytic)
Congestive hepatomegaly Malnutrition Metabolic liver disease (storage) Infiltrative liver disease (cellular)	Trauma	Bile duct abnormalities Infections Metabolic liver disease (with cell necrosis) Chemical (e.g., drug) injury		
With splenomegaly Metabolic liver disease Infiltrative liver disease		With splenomegaly All conditions except chemical injury	With cholestasis All conditions except hemolytic disease	

From Andres JM, Mathis RK, and Walker WA: Liver disease in infants. I. Developmental hepatology and mechanisms of liver dysfunction, J Pediatr 90:686, 1977.

of serum unconjugated bilirubin, at which there are only physiologic changes rather than brain cell injury, has not been clearly identified. A total bilirubin of 14 mg/dl or greater may be associated with a significant risk of deafness in high-risk preterm infants with a birth weight of 1500 g or less.[9] Others have suggested that moderate hyperbilirubinemia (10 to 20 mg/dl) in full-term infants affects adjoining areas of the brainstem, including both the auditory pathway and cry production pathways.[36]

A persistent unconjugated hyperbilirubinemia suggests excessive production of bilirubin; an inherited or acquired block in bilirubin transport, uptake, or conjugation; or abnormal enterohepatic circulation of bilirubin. Also, more than one mechanism may be operative at any time during the course of an illness. Normally, bilirubin metabolism commences with the breakdown of hemoglobin and subsequent conversion of heme via the enzyme heme oxygenase to biliverdin, which is reduced to bilirubin. This unconjugated molecule becomes bound to albumin and is then transported to the hepatocyte and taken up across the hepatocyte-plasma membrane. Cytoplasmic proteins assist in transportation of bilirubin to the smooth endoplasmic reticulum for conjugation. Only the bilirubin glucuronide conjugates are secreted at the bile canaliculus into bile and subsequently to the small intestine. Because unconjugated bilirubin is not secreted into bile, urobilinogen does not appear in the intestine or subsequently in the urine.

Sepsis is one of the important treatable problems associated with *bilirubin overproduction,* and the hyperbilirubinemia is a consequence of rapid hemolysis. Severe infection eventually causes a more prominent conjugated hyperbilirubinemia because of the bacterial or viral hepatocellular damage. The jaundice associated with hemolytic states such as erythroblastosis occurs during the first 36 hours of life; the risk of kernicterus is high if the infant develops early severe anemia and splenomegaly. Blood group typing and a direct Coombs test will establish the diagnosis of Rh incompatibility. Late hyporegenerative anemia occurs in some of these infants.[14] In a patient with ABO incompatibility, there may be numerous spherocytes noted in the blood smear, in addition to the appropriate blood group typing of infant and mother. The presence of hematoma or polycythemia can lead to hemolysis because of the increased red blood cell mass. Certain drugs administered during pregnancy or to the infant after birth may increase the risk of significant unconjugated hyperbilirubinemia. For example, vitamin K may produce hemolysis by acting as an oxidizing agent. Congenital erythrocyte defects such as spherocytosis cause chronic hyperbilirubinemia in infancy. The diagnosis is suspected when maternal agglutination antibodies are not demonstrated, especially with a family history of splenomegaly or hemolysis.

Most cases of neonatal unconjugated hyperbilirubinemia are secondary to physiologic jaundice, a transient, benign condition. There is no single cause of this common form of jaundice. It results from the interaction of many complex factors and is noted in approximately 15% of normal newborn infants. Bilirubin overproduction is known to occur in these children because of increased catabolism of fetal hemoglobin and shortened red blood cell survival.

Other newborn developmental factors include delayed conjugation of bilirubin secondary to immaturity of the glucuronyl transferase enzyme, poor hepatocellular transport of bilirubin because of decreased cytoplasmic transport proteins, and increased intestinal reabsorption of unconjugated bilirubin. For the full-term infant the serum bilirubin concentration rarely exceeds 10 mg/dl; the onset of jaundice occurs on the second or third day after birth and usually disappears by the fifth to eighth day of life. Bilirubin levels may increase to 12 mg/dl by the fifth to seventh day of life in the premature infant, returning to normal by the fourteenth day. Physiologic

Differential Diagnosis of Jaundice: Neonate and Young Infant

UNCONJUGATED HYPERBILIRUBINEMIA*
(NONCHOLESTATIC JAUNDICE)

Overproduction of Bilirubin

Sepsis
Rh/ABO incompatibility
Hematoma (birth trauma)
Drugs (e.g., vitamin K)
Polycythemia
- Maternal-fetal or twin-to-twin transfusion
- Delayed clamping of umbilical cord

Erythrocyte defects (e.g., congenital spherocytosis)
Hemoglobinopathies
Physiologic jaundice

Impaired Transport of Bilirubin

Hypoxia, acidosis
Drugs (e.g., sulf, aminosalicylic acid [ASA])
Serum free fatty acids
- Breast milk
- Fat emulsions

Hypoalbuminemia of prematurity

Impaired Hepatic Uptake of Bilirubin

Decreased sinusoidal perfusion (e.g., diminished venous flow after birth)
Gilbert syndrome
Physiologic jaundice

Impaired Conjugation of Bilirubin

Breast milk jaundice
Drugs (e.g., chloramphenicol)
Hypoglycemia
Hypothyroidism
High intestinal obstruction
Glucuronyl transferase deficiency (types I and II)
Physiologic jaundice

Enterohepatic Circulation of Bilirubin

Delayed passage of meconium
- Low intestinal obstruction
- Cystic fibrosis

Decreased intestinal motility
Physiologic jaundice
- Negligible intestinal bacterial flora
- Presence of intestinal beta-glucuronidase

*Predominant form of bilirubin.

CONJUGATED HYPERBILIRUBINEMIA*
(CHOLESTATIC JAUNDICE)

Acquired Cholestatic Jaundice

Sepsis
Other infections
- Bacterial
- Congenital (TORCH)
- Viral (e.g., hepatitis A or B)
- Parasitic (e.g., toxoplasmosis)

Chemical liver injury (e.g., drugs)

Idiopathic Cholestatic Jaundice

Hepatocellular cholestatic jaundice
- Neonatal hepatitis

Ductal cholestatic jaundice
- Biliary atresia
- Biliary hypoplasia
- Paucity of intrahepatic bile ducts
- Choledochal cyst

Inherited Cholestatic Jaundice

Familial cholestatic syndromes (e.g., benign recurrent cholestasis)
Metabolic cholestasis
- Galactosemia
- Hereditary fructose intolerance
- Hereditary tyrosinemia
- Cystic fibrosis
- Alpha-1-antitrypsin deficiency
- Glycogne storage disease

Other storage disease
- Niemann-Pick disease
- Gaucher disease

"Noncholestatic" syndromes
- Dubin-Johnson syndrome
- Rotor syndrome

jaundice is of no clinical significance unless additional factors such as prematurity, acidosis, or hemolysis are also present. Odell[23] has outlined four criteria to help distinguish physiologic jaundice from pathologic jaundice; these criteria should prompt careful diagnostic evaluation: (1) jaundice before 36 hours of age, (2) serum total bilirubin concentration above 12 mg/dl, (3) persistent jaundice beyond the eighth day of life, and (4) level of conjugated bilirubin greater than 1.5 mg/dl.

There are numerous other conditions that can cause unconjugated hyperbilirubinemia in the neonate. Drugs such as aspirin and sulfonamides[31] can lead to *impaired transport of bilirubin* because of displacement of the bilirubin molecule from albumin-binding sites. Other albumin-binding sites can also be blocked by free fatty acids, known to be in high concentration in breast milk and the main metabolic product of intravenous lipid (e.g., Intralipid or Liposyn).[2,24] Various cephalosporins[27] and sodium fusidate[6] also increase the risk of bilirubin encephalopathy by altering bilirubin-albumin binding. Although the precise mechanism of action is not known, benzyl alcohol, a bacteriostatic agent used to flush intravascular catheters, has recently been associated with the

Differential Diagnosis of Jaundice: Older Infant

UNCONGUGATED HYPERBILIRUBINEMIA*
(NONCHOLESTATIC JAUNDICE)
Overproduction of Bilirubin
Hemoglobinopathies (e.g., sickle cell disease)
Erythrocyte defects (e.g., congenital spherocytosis

Impaired Uptake of Bilirubin
Gilbert syndrome

Impaired Conjugation of Bilirubin
Glucuronyl transferase deficiency (types I and II)

*When this is the predominant form of bilirubin, consider the following diagnoses.

development of kernicterus in infants.[13] Other changes in care may have contributed to the findings in this latter group of patients (many also had intraventricular hemorrhages), but drug interference with bilirubin-albumin binding was suspected. Bilirubin displacement from albumin is further enhanced in the neonate with hypoxemia and acidosis, especially the premature infant with hypoalbuminemia.

Impaired hepatic uptake of bilirubin occurs in Gilbert syndrome, a common familial condition that is infrequently diagnosed until the second decade of life, and in sick neonates with diminished hepatic sinusoidal blood flow or persistent patency of the ductus venosus. Although alteration of bilirubin-albumin binding is probably the main problem, breast milk jaundice may occur because of pregnanediol in the mother's milk.[11] This hormone is capable of inhibiting glucuronyl transferase activity, which leads to *impaired conjugation of bilirubin*. Clinical jaundice occurs in about 1% of breast-fed infants and usually appears between the sixth and eighth days of life in a normal-appearing, thriving child. The serum concentration of unconjugated bilirubin rarely exceeds 20 mg/dl, recedes following discontinuance of breast-feeding, and usually does not recur if breast-feedings are reinstituted after 2 or 3 days.[15] Even with continued ingestion of breast milk, the serum bilirubin usually decreases over a period of 2 to 3 months. Kernicterus has never been reported with this common form of jaundice; however, a brief discontinuance of breast milk should always be considered because of the small potential for subtle neurologic dysfunction after prolonged exposure to unconjugated bilirubin. This should be done before subjecting the child to a detailed diagnostic evaluation.

The possibility of drug-induced jaundice should again be emphasized; for example, chloramphenicol and novobiocin can decrease bilirubin conjugation by competing for glucuronyl transferase. Hypoglycemia may accentuate jaundice in young infants because glucose is a substrate that participates in the synthesis of the bilirubin-glucuronide conjugate. Prolonged elevation of unconjugated bilirubin is seen in congenital hypothyroidism, presumably on the basis of delay in maturation of the bilirubin-conjugating enzyme.[16] This is a critically important, treatable disease; therefore thyroid function studies are necessary in all children with this type of jaundice. Some infants with intestinal obstruction—for example, neonates with pyloric stenosis or duodenal atresia—develop unconjugated hyperbilirubinemia. The mechanism for jaundice in this circumstance is not known, but there is evidence for diminished glucuronyl transferase activity in these infants, who improve rapidly after the anatomic problem has been surgically corrected.

A rare familial cause of unconjugated hyperbilirubinemia is glucuronyl transferase deficiency.[4] Two forms have been described, depending on the patient's clinical response to phenobarbital. Type I (Crigler-Najjar syndrome) is the rare, severe autosomal recessive disease in which no glucuronyl transferase enzyme can be demonstrated. Nonhemolytic jaundice develops in the first hours of life, and early signs of kernicterus are often present. Transmission of the type II deficiency is autosomal dominant. These infants have decreased glucuronyl transferase enzyme, the action of which is enhanced by phenobarbital; serum bilirubin levels may drop dramatically with the use of this drug. Lower intestinal obstruction syndromes and clinical conditions that lead to decreased intestinal motility promote *increased enterohepatic circulation* of unconjugated bilirubin, especially in the early days of life when the intestinal lumen sequesters bilirubin-rich meconium together with deconjugating glucuronidase enzyme.

Conjugated Hyperbilirubinemia

Immature secretory mechanisms, damage to the hepatocyte canalicular membrane, or an anatomic abnormality of bile ducts contributes to conjugated hyperbilirubinemia. This is always pathologic and usually associated with hepatocellular disease, even though the conjugated molecule is not known to be chemically harmful to body tissues, including the central nervous system. A serum conjugated bilirubin level greater than 1.5 mg/dl should always be considered abnormal and secondary to hepatic injury.

Hepatic excretion of organic anions such as bilirubin is dependent, in part, on movement of bile acid and water across the canalicular membrane. Jaundice is usually closely associated with a reduction in bile flow, or cholestasis; hence the term *cholestatic jaundice*. Various acquired, idiopathic, and inherited conditions that cause neonatal cholestatic jaundice will be briefly enumerated in this section (see the box on p. 993).[18]

Hepatocellular cholestatic jaundice includes neonatal hepatitis and represents the diagnosis for the majority of infants with conjugated hyperbilirubinemia in the early months of life. Symptoms usually occur in the first 2 weeks after birth, and the typical presentation is that of an unwell, jaundiced infant with hepatomegaly. The main differential diagnostic consideration is ductal cholestatic jaundice, especially biliary atresia—that is, determining whether the jaundice is secondary to a surgical or a nonsurgical problem. An evaluation to determine the type of hyperbilirubinemia and to establish an early diagnosis of a treatable disease should always be immediately considered. These studies include total and direct serum bilirubin determinations; hemoglobin count; Coombs test; blood glucose test; serum amino acid determinations (e.g., for tyrosine); serologic tests for toxoplasmosis, syphilis, and HBV (especially anti-HBc); urine test for non-glucose-reducing substances and organic acids (to eliminate galactosemia and hereditary fructose intolerance); and blood cultures. The liver histology may suggest the cause of the infant's problem, but failure to make a specific diagnosis of hepatocellular cholestasis necessitates studies to determine patency of the biliary tree such as hepatobiliary scintigraphy (e.g., DISIDA), duodenal intubation for bile, and percutaneous liver biopsy. Factors related to an unfavorable prognosis are prolonged jaundice and cholestasis, early appearance of portal fibrosis, and coexistence of systemic disease.[8] Approximately 30% of infants with hepatocellular cholestatic jaundice develop progressive liver failure, another 30% survive the early months of illness but have chronic disease (including cirrhosis), and the remainder recover completely. The overall outlook for these patients is now improved because of the success of liver transplantation.

Ductal cholestatic jaundice includes diagnoses such as biliary atresia, biliary hypoplasia, and choledochal cyst. Infants with biliary atresia usually appear well until jaundice persists beyond the first week after birth. Although the theory is controversial, *Reovirus* (type 3) has been implicated as an important etiologic agent for hepatobiliary disease in infants.[21] This virus has been localized in biliary remnants in the inflamed porta hepatis.[22] Jaundice increases with time, and the liver becomes hard and firm as cirrhosis progresses over the first months of life. In the past, the prognosis for infants with biliary atresia correlated best for those who had expert surgical treatment performed by operating teams skilled in biliary microsurgery[7]; however, the long-term outcome for these children is now more strongly related to the skill of the liver transplantation surgeon. In some Japanese surgery units, bile drainage is reported in almost 90% of patients; in North America, the overall success rate of Kasai portoenterostomy is less satisfactory,[26] but this procedure should always be done before consideration of transplantation. Postoperative cholangitis often leads to deteriorating liver function, which continues to be a major problem despite surgical technologic advances; it occurs in over 50% of successful portoenterostomies. Liver transplantation is the only opportunity for survival of many patients with end-stage liver disease.

Biliary hypoplasia is noted in infants with acute infections of the liver, various familial cholestasis syndromes such as arteriohepatic dysplasia,[1] and the more common metabolic cholestasis syndrome, alpha-1-antitrypsin deficiency.[29] The clinical course of infants with biliary hypoplasia is variable, but overall survival is much longer than for children with biliary atresia. Clinical recognition of a jaundiced child with a choledochal cyst depends on cyst size and the presence of biliary obstruction. Use of ultrasonography improves the preoperative diagnosis of this problem, which can be surgically amendable before the occurrence of progressive biliary obstruction and cirrhosis.

Just as rare as the *familial cholestasis* syndromes are the *metabolic hepatocellular* problems (except for cystic fibrosis and alpha-1-antitrypsin deficiency); nevertheless, they are important to diagnose because of the potential for effective treatment. Specifically, infants with galactosemia, fructose intolerance, and tyrosinemia have similar clinical manifestations, usually within days to weeks after birth. Marked jaundice, hepatosplenomegaly, bleeding, and failure to thrive are usually prominent. However, infants with galactosemia may have less apparent findings, after several months developing cataracts, cirrhosis, and psychomotor retardation. Similarly, the tyrosinemic infant may escape the acute phase of illness and be discovered months later to have cirrhosis, rickets, and renal disease; these patients have a high incidence of hepatoma in later childhood.[38] The jaundiced child with cataracts and psychomotor retardation might very well have galactosemia, whereas jaundice associated with a history of vomiting, distaste for sweet foods, and fructosuria would more likely result from fructose intolerance. Each of these metabolic disorders may also cause renal dysfunction manifested by aminoaciduria, glycosuria, and phosphaturia (Fanconi syndrome). Their definitive diagnosis depends on specific tolerance tests and the measurement of enzyme activity in red blood cells (galactosemia), liver, or kidney (fructose intolerance). Analyzing the urine for non-glucose-reducing sugars, organic acids, and amino acids is appropriate for initial screening. The long-term prognosis for all of these metabolic diseases depends on the early introduction of dietary restrictions.

Jaundice is unusual in children with glycogen storage disease[20] except for types III and IV. Hepatocellular dysfunction is more prominent in infants with type IV glycogenosis; jaundice occurs in the first months of life and is usually followed by cirrhosis and death before 2 years of age. Persistent jaundice is unusual in infants with cystic fibrosis, but it may occur when the disease is associated with increased enterohepatic circulation of bilirubin (meconium ileus), drug hypersensitivity, parenteral alimentation, or common duct inflammation secondary to inspissation of biliary secretions. Alpha-1-antitrypsin deficiency,[29] a genetic defect of glycoprotein metabolism, is the most common metabolic disorder associated with liver disease in infants. The usual presentation is that of cholestasis with associated jaundice and hepatomegaly. The diagnosis is suspected if a diminished or absent alpha-1-globulin peak is observed in the serum protein electrophoretic pattern. Diagnosis is then confirmed by a low serum alpha-1-antitrypsin level and protease inhibitor (Pi) typing. No specific treatment is available, but it is essential to identify infants at risk and provide proper genetic counseling to the family. Liver transplantation has been performed in older children with end-stage liver disease caused by antitrypsin deficiency.[12] The prognosis is extremely variable. Despite persistence of mild hepatocellular dysfunction, clinical improvement may occur in infants a few months after birth. Biliary cirrhosis and portal hypertension eventually develop in some older children.

Inherited storage diseases such as Niemann-Pick and Gaucher disease usually cause hepatosplenomegaly in infants, but jaundice is unusual. They are exceedingly rare and should not be considered in the initial evaluation of children with cholestatic jaundice.

Dubin-Johnson syndrome[3] is another type of familial jaundice that probably has an autosomal recessive mode of inheritance. It is considered a benign condition, but the child has a reduced capacity to secrete several organic anions, especially conjugated bilirubin, sulfobromophthalein (BSP), rose bengal, and cholecystographic dye. Interestingly, the excretion of bile acids is normal; therefore the term *noncholestatic jaundice* is applicable and the extrahepatic biliary tree is always patent. Recurrent episodes of jaundice, which can be precipitated by infection, may begin in infancy and can be misdiagnosed as acute hepatitis because of abrupt onset of illness. There is often a family history of jaundice and vague upper abdominal pain in older children. Routine tests of liver function are normal except for increased total bilirubin levels (usually less than 15 mg/dl) with predominance of conjugated bilirubin. Rotor syndrome is similar to (or may be a variant of) Dubin-Johnson syndrome except that pigmentation of hepatocytes has not been demonstrated and secretion of cholecystographic dye is normal. Recognition of these benign "noncholestatic" jaundice syndromes may prevent unnecessary diagnostic evaluations.

JAUNDICE IN THE OLDER INFANT AND CHILD

Unconjugated Hyperbilirubinemia

Unconjugated hyperbilirubinemia in older infants (after maturation of the blood-brain barrier) and children is usually of no pathologic significance. It is uncommon in the older child without underlying hemolytic disease, for example, sickle cell disease or spherocytosis. Gilbert syndrome[25] is a common familial syndrome of autosomal dominant inheritance that may be secondary to an abnormality of bilirubin uptake at the hepatocyte sinusoidal membrane. Mild fluctuating jaundice can be noted during early infancy, but the syndrome is usually not diagnosed until the second decade of life. Fatigue and caloric deprivation accentuate the jaundice. The mechanism is not understood, but it may be related to increased bilirubin production after fasting. Abdominal pain, malaise, and other vague symptoms usually accompany the jaundice. The criteria for diagnosing Gilbert syndrome are a serum unconjugated bilirubin level greater than 1.5 mg/dl but less than 6.0 mg/dl, lack of other demonstrable abnormalities of liver function, absence of overt hemolysis, and no evidence of liver disease on examination except for jaundice. The main differential diagnostic considerations are glucuronyl transferase deficiency (type II) and mild hemolytic syndromes. No treatment is necessary for Gilbert syndrome except for resumption of adequate caloric intake. It is a benign condition but important to recognize so that unnecessary diagnostic investigations are avoided.

Conjugated Hyperbilirubinemia

Acute viral hepatitis is the most common cause of jaundice in older infants and children. Hepatitis A virus (HAV) is usually the etiologic agent, but the majority of these children do not have jaundice. Hepatitis B virus (HBV) produces a similar symptom complex of nausea, vomiting, and anorexia that often precedes the jaundice. In children, liver disease secondary to HBV may be mild, but persistent jaundice and hepatocellular dysfunction with the eventual occurrence of chronic hepatitis can occur. Antigenemia and clinical disease occur frequently in the infant born to a mother with acute hepatitis during the latter part of pregnancy or early in the postpartum period.[28] Another mode of transmission is contact with the HBV-positive mother during infancy, including the ingestion of contaminated breast milk.[5] From a worldwide perspective, the perinatal and postnatal transmission of HBV is an extremely important public health problem. For example, before an extensive, controlled HBV vaccine trial in Senegal, striking evidence of the endemicity of HBV infection was present, with 12% of blood donors being HB_SAg-positive and 80% of 6- and 7-year-old children having at least one serum marker of past or present HBV infection.[19] In those areas where HBV is endemic, the relative risk of hepatocellular carcinoma is much higher in carriers to that of noncarriers.

In the United States and other developed countries, the adolescent user of parenterally administered illicit drugs may develop acute HBV liver disease. The HBV vaccine is now available for patients at risk of developing this serious infection.[33,35]

Sporadic cases of jaundice in childhood may be noted with other infections such as infectious mononucleosis. Jaundice occurs in only a small percentage of children infected with Epstein-Barr virus (EBV) despite hepatic involvement in most patients. This diagnosis should be suspected in the adolescent with acute pharyngitis and splenomegaly with or without hepatomegaly.

Cholecystitis is a rare problem in children; acute disease usually develops in adolescent girls, who often experience jaundice, right upper quadrant pain, vomiting, and fever. Gallbladder ultrasonography will suggest the correct diagnosis and identify the presence of gallstones, which are most commonly seen in children with hemolysis or cystic fibrosis and some children with cirrhosis. Cholangiography may be important to exclude the presence of gallstones in the common bile duct, especially in the patient with hemolytic disease who is acutely ill with fever and abdominal pain. Hemolytic anemia can be the mode of presentation for Wilson disease in children over 5 years of age. Individuals with this important, treatable disease have jaundice during the early hepatic stage of illness when the liver is becoming saturated with copper. A careful evaluation should be made to detect Kayser-Fleischer rings and subtle neurologic dysfunction.

Chronic active hepatitis is probably rare in infants less than 2 years of age. In greater than 25% of these children the illness begins as acute hepatitis with jaundice, and the severity, course, and prognosis are highly variable. An immunologic form of chronic active liver disease ("lupoid" hepatitis) occurs in young girls who develop extrahepatic signs, such as skin rash and arthritis. Exposure to drugs such as isoniazid and methyldopa occasionally leads to liver dysfunction and a histologic abnormality indistinguishable from chronic active hepatitis. The appearance of jaundice can be delayed for months after the institution of isoniazid therapy, and the severity of the liver dysfunction correlates with continued use of the drug.[32]

The anticonvulsant agent valproic acid also causes cholestatic jaundice with diffuse hepatocellular injury.[34] The mechanism for hepatic damage is uncertain; concurrent administration of valproic acid with other anticonvulsants should be carefully monitored. Other common drugs, for example, erythromycin estolate and sulfonamides, are capable of causing jaundice with either a hepatitis-like or cholestatic pattern. Jaundice occurs in children, especially infants, who are receiving total parenteral nutrition (TPN). The precise mechanism is unknown, but the problem may be related to amino acid imbalance and subsequent decreased bile acid synthesis or to inadequate secretin stimulation of bile flow in a child with minimal oral alimentation.

MANAGEMENT

Unconjugated Hyperbilirubinemia

Excellent general reviews in the literature are available concerning the treatment of newborn infants with unconjugated hyperbilirubinemia.[17] An extensive discussion of such treatment can be found in Chapter 40, "Common Neonatal Illnesses." Intravenous infusion of albumin, especially before exchange transfusion, increases the potential binding sites for the unconjugated molecule. A double volume exchange transfusion is infrequently indicated except for hemolytic disease when the serum indirect bilirubin concentration exceeds 20 mg/dl in full-term neonates or 10 mg/dl in ill premature infants, or in any child who experiences a rapid rise (more than 0.5 mg/dl/hour) in serum bilirubin. Phototherapy is more efficacious than exchange transfusion for nonhemolytic jaundice and may help prevent a rapid increase in serum bilirubin. Its effectiveness in terms of prevention of brain injury, however, is unknown, and as noted earlier, it should not be instituted before excluding any underlying pathology. This form of therapy is never considered routine and should be reserved for premature infants or term infants with high serum bilirubin concentrations, as well as the rare patient with type I glucuronyl transferase deficiency who requires continuous therapy. Specific guidelines for commencement of phototherapy include treatment if the bilirubin level exceeds 15 mg/dl at any time of life in the full-term infant,[29] at 12 hours of age in neonates weighing less than 1500 g at birth, and when the serum bilirubin rises to 10 mg/dl in infants weighing 1500 to 2000 g at birth.[27] Phototherapy probably induces increased biliary excretion of photoisomers of bilirubin after the molecule in exposed skin undergoes photochemical reactions.[10,11] There are well-recognized potential side effects, including an increase in insensible water loss, retinal damage, unusual bronzing of skin,[18] higher occurrence of patent ductus arteriosus in premature infants,[34] and even alteration of intracellular deoxyribonucleic acid (DNA).[40]

The effectiveness of agar in treating neonates with jaundice is uncertain, but it may be associated with reduced peak serum bilirubin levels by binding bilirubin in the gut.[16] Recently, a new treatment with tin (Sn)-protoporphyrin has been proposed[15] for infants with unconjugated hyperbilirubinemia. This synthetic metalloporphyrin is a competitive enzyme inhibitor (of heme oxygenase), which blocks the degradation of heme to the bile pigment, biliverdin. The excess heme is not converted to bilirubin, instead, it is excreted in bile. This synthetic compound may prove to be useful, especially if it helps to lessen dependence on phototherapy and exchange transfusion.

Phenobarbital is used for treatment of unconjugated hyperbilirubinemia in older infants with type II glucuronyl transferase deficiency. In this situation, continuous use of phenobarbital is necessary in the early weeks of life when the risk of kernicterus is greatest. Children with Crigler-Najjar syndrome do not respond to phenobarbital. An exchange transfusion is the only effective early therapy to reduce toxic serum bilirubin levels in these patients, but curative treatment has been reported with home phototherapy, followed by orthotopic liver transplantation at an early age.[30]

Conjugated Hyperbilirubinemia

It is not necessary to treat the jaundice of patients with conjugated hyperbilirubinemia because the conjugated molecule is nontoxic. However, the use of choleretic agents such as phenobarbital and cholestyramine may effectively increase bile flow, which in turn lowers the level of total serum bilirubin. Fat-soluble vitamins are also essential in these children with cholestatic liver disease.

REFERENCES

1. Alagille D, Odievre M, and Gautier M: Hepatic ductular hypoplasia associated with characteristic facies, vertebral malformations, retarded physical, mental, sexual development and cardiac murmur, J Pediatr 86:63, 1975.
2. Andrew G, Chan G, and Schiff D: Lipid metabolism in the neonate. II. The effect of Intralipid on bilirubin binding in vitro and in vivo, J Pediatr 88:279, 1976.
3. Arias IM: Inheritable and congenital hyperbilirubinemia: models for the study of drug metabolism, N Engl J Med 285:1416, 1971.
4. Arias IM et al: Chronic nonhemolytic unconjugated hyperbilirubinemia with glucuronyl transferase deficiency: clinical, biochemical, pharmacologic, and genetic evidence for heterogeneity, Am J Med 47:395, 1969.
5. Boxall EH et al: Hepatitis B surface antigen in breast milk, Lancet 2:1007, 1974.
6. Brodersen R: Fusidic acid binding to serum albumin and interaction with binding of bilirubin, Acta Paediatr Scand 78:874, 1985.
7. Danks DM: Biliary atresia: lessons from Japan, Lancet 1:219, 1981.
8. Danks DM et al: Prognosis of babies with neonatal hepatitis, Arch Dis Child 52:368, 1977.
9. deVries LS, Lary S, and Dubowitz LMS: Relationship of serum bilirubin levels to ototoxicity and deafness in high-risk low birth weight infants, Pediatrics 76:351, 1985.
10. Ennever JF, Knox I, and Speck WT: Differences in bilirubin isomer composition in infants treated with green and white light phototherapy, J Pediatr 109:119, 1986.
11. Gartner LM and Arias IM: Studies of prolonged neonatal jaundice in the breast-fed infant, J Pediatr 68:54, 1966.
12. Hood JM et al: Liver transplantation for advanced liver disease with alpha-1-antitrypsin deficiency, N Engl J Med 302:272, 1980.
13. Jardine DS and Rogers K: Relationship of benzyl alcohol to kernicterus, intraventricular hemorrhage, and mortality in preterm infants, Pediatrics 83:153, 1989.
14. Koenig JM et al: Late hyporegenerative anemia in Rh hemolytic disease, J Pediatr 115:315, 1989.
15. Lascari AD: "Early" breast-feeding jaundice: clinical significance, J Pediatr 108:156, 1986.
16. MacGillivray MH, Crawford JD, and Robey JS: Congenital hypothyroidism and prolonged neonatal hyperbilirubinemia, Pediatrics 40:283, 1967.
17. Maisels MJ: Jaundice in the newborn, Pediatr Rev 3:305, 1982.
18. Mathis RK, Andres JM, and Walker WA: Liver disease in infants. II. Hepatic disease states, J Pediatr 90:864, 1977.

19. Maupas P et al: Efficacy of hepatitis B vaccine in prevention of early HB_SAg carrier state in children: controlled trial in an endemic area (Senagal), Lancet 1:289, 1981.
20. McAdams AJ, Hug G, and Bove BE: Glycogen storage disease, types I to X: criteria for morphologic diagnosis, Hum Pathol 5:463, 1974.
21. Morecki R et al: Biliary atresia and *Reovirus* type 3 infection, N Engl J Med 307:481, 1982.
22. Morecki R et al: Detection of *Reovirus* type 3 in the porta hepatis of an infant with extrahepatic biliary atresia: ultrastructural and immunocytochemical study, Hepatology 4:1137, 1984.
23. Odell GB: Neonatal jaundice. In Popper H and Schaffner F, editors: Progress in liver disease, New York, 1976, Grune & Stratton, Inc.
24. Ostrea EM et al: Influence of free fatty acids and glucose infusion on serum bilirubin and bilirubin binding to albumin: clinical implications, J Pediatr 102:426, 1983.
25. Powell LW: Clinical aspects of unconjugated hyperbilirubinemia, Semin Hematol 9:91, 1972.
26. Psacharapoulos HT et al: Extrahepatic biliary atresia: preoperative assessment and surgical results in 47 consecutive cases, Arch Dis Child 55:351, 1980.
27. Robertson A, Fink S, and Karp W: Effect of cephalosporins on bilirubin-albumin binding, J Pediatr 114:291, 1988.
28. Schweitzer IL: Vertical transmission of the hepatitis B surface antigen, Am J Med Sci 270:287, 1975.
29. Sharp HL: The current status of alpha-1-antitrypsin, a protease inhibitor in gastrointestinal disease, Gastroenterology 70:621, 1976.
30. Shevell MI et al: Crigler-Najjar syndrome type I: treatment by home phototherapy followed by orthotopic hepatic transplantation, J Pediatr 110:429, 1987.
31. Silverman WA et al: A difference in mortality rate and incidence of kernicterus among premature infants allotted to two prophylactic antibacterial regimens, Pediatrics 18:614, 1956.
32. Stein MT and Liang D: Clinical hepatotoxicity of isoniazid in children, Pediatrics 64:499, 1979.
33. Stevens CE et al: Yeast-recombinant hepatitis B vaccine: efficacy with hepatitis B immune globulin in prevention of perinatal hepatitis B virus transmission, JAMA 257:2612, 1987.
34. Suchy FJ et al: Acute hepatic failure associated with the use of sodium valproate, N Engl J Med 300:962, 1979.
35. Szmuness W et al: Hepatitis B vaccine: demonstrations of efficacy in a controlled clinical trial in a high-risk population in the United States, N Engl J Med 303:833, 1980.
36. Vohr BR et al: Abnormal brainstem function (brainstem auditory evoked response) correlates with acoustic cry features in term infants with hyperbilirubinemia, J Pediatr 115:303, 1989.
37. Walker WA and Mathis RK: Hepatomegaly: an approach to the differential diagnosis, Pediatr Clin North Am 22:929, 1975.
38. Weinberg AG, Mize CE, and Worthan HG: The occurrence of hepatoma in the chronic form of hereditary tyrosinemia, J Pediatr 88:434, 1976.
39. Younoszai MK and Mueller S: Clinical assessment of liver size in normal children, Clin Pediatr 14:378, 1975.
40. Speck WT, Chen CC, and Rosenkranz HS: In vitro studies of effects of light and riboflavin on DNA and HeLa cells, Pediatr Res 9:150, 1975.

148

Joint Pain

David M. Siegel and John Baum

Those providing primary health care to children are often faced with clinical situations involving musculoskeletal aches and pains; within this group of symptoms is the subset of joint pain. In fact, 1 out of every 6 to 10 pediatric outpatient visits includes a musculoskeletal complaint.[1] As outlined in this chapter, discomfort in a joint can be the result of a wide variety of diagnostic entities that must be sorted out to provide the appropriate evaluation and management. Using a systematic approach to patients with pain and swelling in one or more joints will help the clinician arrive at an accurate diagnosis and course of therapy.

ARTHRALGIA VERSUS ARTHRITIS

As always, a careful and thorough history is indispensable in initially approaching the child with joint pain; the physical examination can then substantiate suspicions raised during the interview. It is essential to distinguish between arthralgia and arthritis. *Joint pain* can, by definition, mean arthralgia—the subjective experience of pain referrable to a locus of bony articulation. In a young child this sensation of pain might be inferred from the patient's refusal to move a given extremity or joint, but the term arthralgia usually refers only to the *discomfort* in the joint. On the other hand, the term *arthritis* (as suggested by the *itis* suffix) should be used only when the joint can be shown to be inflamed, as evidenced by the classic signs of inflammation similar to those found in other parts of the body—redness, warmth, swelling, and pain. In the joint this kind of inflammation is accompanied by loss of motion. Thus all that is arthralgia is not arthritis—an invaluable observation in the differential diagnosis of joint pain.

With these definitions in mind, what would be the characteristics of children with joint pain, and what information must be elicited through the interview and physical examination? Before enumerating specific entities, general characteristics of clinical presentations will be discussed.

The onset of joint pain can be rather sudden or quite indolent (over days or weeks). In cases of sudden onset, an associated history of a fall or direct blow to the joint immediately suggests a traumatic etiology, whereas the presence of fever points toward an infectious process such as septic arthritis or a systemic inflammatory disease such as juvenile arthritis. Often the complaint expressed to the physician is that there is stiffness in a joint with or without obvious swelling. Further clues are found in eliciting the time of day the stiffness occurs and its duration. A child with juvenile arthritis will typically complain of joint stiffness on arising in the morning, which may last from one half to several hours and which may be relieved by gradual exercise. On the other hand, the patient with hypermobility syndrome (a type of traumatic disease) will give a history of pain and stiffness occurring at the end of a vigorous and active day. In addition to fever, other distinguishing signs can include rash, mucous membrane involvement, lymph node inflammation or enlargement, or the presence of some recognizable chronic diseases that can involve the joints, as discussed later.

DIFFERENTIAL DIAGNOSIS AND MANAGEMENT

A useful format for beginning a discussion of the differential diagnosis of joint pain is the division between rheumatic and nonrheumatic diseases. A classic rheumatic disease of childhood involving the joints is juvenile arthritis, sometimes called Still disease.[1,5] This disease typically occurs in the child 1½ to 2 years of age, although onset can also be found through late adolescence. The clinical presentation can be limited to a few (four or less) usually large joints (pauciarticular disease) or might involve a greater number of joints, both large and small (polyarticular disease). There is also a systemic, and at times initially fulminant, form of juvenile arthritis known as systemic-onset disease in which one observes high spiking fevers, a typical salmon-pink, maculopapular, evanescent rash, lymph node and spleen enlargement, anemia, and general malaise. Frequently these more systemic findings precede the onset of any joint involvement, although arthritis must be present for at least 6 to 8 consecutive weeks to establish the diagnosis of the other two subgroups of juvenile arthritis (pauciarticular and polyarticular). The clinician may only glean a history of ill-defined arthralgias and stiffness, whereas on physical examination he or she finds contractures of elbows, knees, and wrists or limitation of cervical motion, all of which provide evidence of former episodes of active inflammation in these joints. Although not a common disease, juvenile arthritis has a prevalence of from 0.1 to 1.0 child per 1000 children worldwide.[1,5]

Diagnosis can be further reinforced using laboratory studies, including the erythrocyte sedimentation rate, the C-reactive protein, and a complete blood count, as well as more specialized studies such as the antinuclear antibody test, rheumatoid factor titer, serum immunoglobulin levels, and others.

Management is focused on subduing inflammation and preserving the normal range of joint motion. Salicylate therapy remains a mainstay, beginning with a daily dosage of 80 mg/kg of body weight in divided doses, whereas other (and more expensive) nonsteroidal antiinflammatory drugs

(NSAID) are increasingly useful in those not adequately responding to their maximum tolerated salicylate dose. Some rheumatologists are now advocating NSAID therapy from the outset.[7] Particularly useful is the enteric-coated form of aspirin, which provides a more gradual rise and fall in blood concentrations while protecting the gastric mucosal lining. Long-acting agents, including gold, hydroxychloroquine, D-penicillamine, and methotrexate have their place in persistent cases, whereas systemic steroid therapy is used only when these other modalities have failed. Surgery is employed mostly in joint reconstruction or prosthetic replacement as a means of dealing with sequelae of synovial inflammation and destruction. (See Chapter 221, "Juvenile Arthritis.")

Another classic rheumatic disease of childhood is acute rheumatic fever (ARF). Although not the scourge that it once was, the incidence of ARF is increasing, and its inclusion in the differential diagnosis of arthritis and arthralgia remains important. The characteristics of the disease are described at length in Chapter 249; suffice it to say that the arthritis usually involves large joints such as the knees and is typically migratory, with the joints being quite tender to palpation. Although signs of inflammation are commonly present, arthralgia alone can be seen in acute rheumatic fever.

Ankylosing spondylitis, which can involve large joints of the lower extremities during childhood and early adolescence, is typified in late adolescence by involvement of the sacroiliac joint (which can be seen on the roentgenogram) and by pain elicited on palpation over the joint. In adulthood there is further axial involvement—the classic "bamboo spine" develops, with its diffuse vertebral fusions and often severe limitation of back motion. The presence of the HLA-B27 transplantation antigen is seen in 90% of patients with ankylosing spondylitis, though the converse is not true. Treatment is usually with one of the nonaspirin nonsteroidal antiinflammatory drugs.

Reiter syndrome is a triad of urethritis, conjunctivitis, and arthritis and can be seen in adolescents and children. In children it often starts with enteritis. It is more common in boys, and making the diagnosis depends on ruling out infectious causes of the inflammation. The arthritis is predominantly of large joints; again, there is a strong association with the HLA-B27 locus in these patients (about 60%). Therapy is through use of antiinflammatory drugs. The majority of children recover within a few months, although some follow a more chronic and relapsing course, occasionally progressing to subsequent ankylosing spondylitis.

Also showing a predisposition for larger joints is an arthritis sometimes seen with psoriasis: the characteristic involvement of the skin is either present, or there is at least a history of psoriatic skin disease.

Systemic lupus erythematosus (SLE) is a cause of chronic joint pain. SLE is a true multisystem disease with potential involvement of almost every organ in the body; the joints, however, may be merely stiff and painful, or they may show frank signs of inflammation. This would, then, be within the differential diagnosis of joint pain in the adolescent girl. Dermatomyositis and polymyositis can also cause inflamed joints in addition to muscle and skin involvement. Other rheumatic diseases that can affect children and cause joint involvement are scleroderma, mixed connective tissue disease, and mucocutaneous lymph node syndrome (Kawasaki disease; see Chapter 222). Each of these entities has its own distinguishing features, as seen on physical examination and in the laboratory findings.

Unlike most of the rheumatic diseases that cause joint pain and tend to be chronic (having waxing and waning courses), many of the nonrheumatic diseases are acute in onset and short in duration (given appropriate therapy). Foremost among this group, and representing something of a medical emergency, is acute bacterial infection of the joint, or septic arthritis (see Chapter 254). The usual presentation is one of a child complaining of a painful joint (rapid onset), often accompanied by fever. The joint itself is red, warm, swollen, and exquisitely tender to palpation or with movement. This clinical situation demands immediate arthrocentesis for diagnosis and therapy. Analysis of the fluid for appearance (opaque), viscosity (usually low), mucin clot (friable), cell count (more than 100,000 WBC/mm^3 with 80% polymorphonuclear cells), glucose (low, much less than serum), and protein (high) helps to establish the diagnosis. Most important, a portion of the fluid must be Gram stained to search for bacterial organisms. Cultures can direct definitive antimicrobial therapy. In the absence of direct (traumatic) inoculation of the joint, the child under approximately 4 years of age is at high risk for *Haemophilus influenzae* infection (seeding from a bacteremia), whereas the older child is more likely to have *Staphylococcus aureus* as the offending organism. Blood cultures may also yield growth of the organism. Systemic bacterial infections can also produce arthritis, notably those caused by *Neisseria gonorrhoeae* and *Neisseria meningitidis,* although the organism is not usually isolated from the joint in these cases. Following joint aspiration and establishment of at least a strong suspicion of a purulent arthritis, hospitalization and appropriate intravenous antibiotic therapy should be initiated. Prompt and aggressive therapy usually brings about recovery without sequelae, although some foci, such as the hip joint, can remain a persistent problem. Because of the tenuous blood supply to the femoral capital epiphysis, purulent arthritis of the hip can lead to chronic problems despite timely intervention.[5]

In addition to bacterial agents, other infectious causes of joint disease occur. Viruses, including rubella, mumps, chickenpox, and adenovirus, as well as Epstein-Barr virus (in infectious mononucleosis), can all affect synovial tissue. Manifestations of the viral syndrome (rash, fever, mucous membrane involvement) usually precede joint involvement. Infectious hepatitis, on the other hand, can produce arthritis before overt hepatic involvement. Rubella immunization is also associated with arthralgias and arthritis in as many as 3% of those children receiving the vaccine—rarely, if ever, with any sequelae.[4] Other infections in which joints can be involved include brucellosis, leptospirosis, tularemia, Rocky Mountain spotted fever, and rat-bite fever. Mycobacteria can cause arthritis, as can various fungal agents, particularly in immunocompromised hosts.

A newly identified offender is *Ixodes dammini,* a tick that harbors the Borrelia burgdorferi. This tick is carried by a number of mammals. The infection and arthritis produce the syndrome of Lyme disease. First described in Lyme, Connecticut, the syndrome is characterized by an initial tick bite that causes a large circular erythematous lesion known as erythema chronicum migrans. Meningoencephalitis, neuritis, and carditis may also occur. The arthritis manifests itself as recurrent attacks of inflammation of the large joints (85% of cases involve the knee), each recurrence usually lasting no more than a week or two. On occasion, symptoms may persist for several months, and chronic persistent arthritis of the knee has been reported in rare instances. A short course of high-dose penicillin therapy seems to be effective in shortening the course of the rash and perhaps in attenuating the arthritis, whereas salicylate therapy can be used for symptomatic relief.[6] (See Chapter 225.)

Congenital syphilis (see Chapter 255) can be seen in the infant as painful bony lesions and refusal to move the involved limb (Parrot pseudoparalysis), along with other associated stigmata. The infant born with this syndrome can in adolescence have bilateral knee effusions known as Clutton joints.

Osteomyelitis is another acute infection of the bone. However, when one of the long bones is involved adjacent to a joint (such as the distal femur and knee), the patient can describe pain in the joint and there may even be a sterile effusion present.[5]

Another infection that can cause joint pain is discitis. In this situation, low-grade fever, back pain, and tenderness over the spinous process contiguous to the involved disk space are present. *S. aureus* has been isolated from the blood and disk space in some instances, but often there is no culture-proven cause. The presentation can involve sensory and motor complications secondary to nerve root impingement, and an epidural abscess must be considered in the differential diagnosis.

Noninfectious origins for arthralgia and arthritis abound. The most common extraintestinal manifestation of inflammatory bowel disease is large joint involvement. This can be pain alone or inflammation as well. The activity of the bowel disease may or may not correlate with joint flare-ups. Sarcoidosis can include arthritis, as can the unrelated diseases of polyarteritis nodosa and Marfan disease. In the group of vasculitic disorders, Henoch-Schönlein purpura is a disease of childhood evidenced by fever, abdominal pain (with or without melena), purpuric lesions of the buttocks and lower extremities, and warm, swollen, painful, and tender joints—usually large joints such as knees and ankles. Hematologic diseases with articular manifestations include hemophilia and sickle cell disease. In the latter, one must consider the hand and foot syndrome type of vasocclusive crisis in the child between 1 and 4 years of age. Although primary gout is exceedingly rare in children, hyperuricemia and subsequent joint disease can be seen in those with leukemia (with chemotherapy producing sudden lysis of cells), hemolytic anemia, glycogen storage disease, and the Lesch-Nyhan syndrome. In the latter, a sex-linked, recessive, genetic, inborn metabolic error results in overproduction of uric acid. Interestingly, polyarthritis and limb pains can be seen in children following traumatic pancreatitis. Infantile cortical hyperostosis, or Caffey disease, occurs in the infant under 6 months of age and includes fever, irritability, increased sedimentation rate, and tender swellings of facial, trunk, and limb bones, with associated arthralgias. Toxic synovitis of the hip can also cause arthralgia.

A fascinating condition seen primarily in children and adolescents that can include arthralgia without arthritis is the hypermobility syndrome. These children have increased joint laxity, and with vigorous activity, especially those activities requiring extremes of joint flexion and extension, they can experience significant arthralgia. Diagnosis is by physical examination and observation of at least three of the following five signs: (1) hyperflexion of the wrist, bringing the thumb in contact with the volar surface of the forearm; (2) hyperextension of the fingers to parallel with the forearm; (3) hyperextension of the elbow to at least −10 degrees; (4) hyperextension of the knee to at least −10 degrees; and (5) hyperflexion of the back such that the palms can be placed flat on the ground with the feet together and without flexing the knees. All laboratory and radiologic studies are normal. Therapy is with nonsteroidal antiinflammatory medication.

In chondromalacia patellae or patellofemoral syndrome the child has knee pain usually related to activity, especially descending stairs. The problem is a roughening of the underside of the patella and subsequent pain as it moves in the patellofemoral groove. Exercises directed toward strengthening the quadriceps femoris muscle can result in marked improvement. Antiinflammatory medication can also be used as an adjunct to the physical therapy.

"Growing" pains are an actual discomfort in the lower limbs and joints (often worse in the middle of the night) experienced by children during a phase of rapid linear growth. A bedtime dose of enteric-coated aspirin can be useful in alleviating this pain until it spontaneously resolves with the slowing of growth.

Physical abuse must be strongly considered whenever signs of trauma are evident, and accidents that represent neglect on the part of parents or guardians need to be recognized and pursued. Any suspicious history or circumstance needs complete investigation.

There are many other orthopedic reasons for arthralgia and arthritis, and these are discussed elsewhere in this text.

MANAGEMENT

Having arrived at a diagnosis and plan of therapy, the practitioner must also offer management for the psychological aspects of joint disease. In those children afflicted with an ongoing joint problem, all the issues of chronic diseases in children must be dealt with. The child may not be able to keep up with peers in physical activity and may also be faced with multiple health care visits. Many clinicians feel that not only does the disease create stress in these patients, but also stress in their environment can exacerbate the disease, as occurs in those with juvenile arthritis. The child faced with hospitalization for an acute problem, such as septic arthritis, is exposed to all the complications of being taken out of his or her family and school environment, as well as those dealing with an institutional setting. Any child with ongoing joint disease, even those with mild disability, should be provided with the expertise and services of a social worker or counselor experienced with this population of patients. Family resources (both emotional and financial) need to be assessed and support provided when needed. Discussion groups composed of these children and their families can be very beneficial, since they offer an opportunity to compare experiences and coping mechanisms. Attention to the physical dimension alone does not provide adequate care in these diseases. A functionally minor disability can cause major problems of body image and feelings of lack of independence, which must be dealt with appropriately.[2,3]

REFERENCES

1. Bass JC: Clinical and diagnostic overview of the child with a musculoskeletal complaint. In Gershwin ME and Robbins DL, editors: Musculoskeletal diseases of children, New York, 1983, Grune & Stratton, Inc.
2. Lowit IM: Social and psychological consequences of chronic illness in children, Dev Med Child Neurol 15:75, 1973.
3. McAnarney ER et al: Psychological problems of children with chronic juvenile arthritis, Pediatrics 53:523, 1974.
4. Phillips P: Viral arthritis in children, Arthritis Rheum 20(suppl 2):584, 1977.
5. Schaller JG: Arthritis and infections of bones and joints in children, Pediatr Clin North Am 24:775, 1977.
6. Steere AC et al: The spirochetal etiology of Lyme disease, N Engl J Med 308:733, 1983.
7. Stiehm ER: Nonsteroidal anti-inflammatory drugs in pediatric patients, Am J Dis Child 142:1281, 1988.

149

Limp

Alain Joffe

A limp in a child is never normal. Its presence suggests that weight bearing on one extremity is either painful or is difficult because of ipsilateral muscle weakness. The causes of limp are legion: they can be as obvious as a foreign body embedded in the foot or shoe or as subtle as appendicitis or discitis.[5]

CAUSES AND CHARACTERISTICS

Table 149-1 lists the causes of limp in children and adolescents.[3] Although the list is formidable, most of the causes can usually be excluded by obtaining a complete history and performing a comprehensive physical examination.

Some of the causes listed in Table 149-1 are likely to be associated with systemic signs and symptoms. Tumors, neoplastic disease, and infections might reasonably be expected to produce constitutional symptoms such as fever, anorexia, weight loss, malaise, and fatigue. Diseases such as infectious myositis, Rocky Mountain spotted fever, dermatomyositis, Gaucher disease, or leukemia, which involve more than one muscle or bone group, will likely produce pain at more than one site, although the pain may be most severe in a lower extremity.

The age of the child is helpful in determining the cause of limp as well. One can anticipate that anatomic causes of limp, such as congenital coxa vara or congenital dislocation of the hip, will become manifest shortly after an infant begins to walk. Occult trauma (toddler's fracture) should always be considered as a cause of limp in the small child, since he or she cannot relate that a significant fall has occurred.[9] Legg-Calvé-Perthes disease occurs most commonly in children 4 to 10 years of age, whereas slipped femoral capital epiphysis and Osgood-Schlatter disease are most common among adolescents.

Whether the limp is associated with pain can help to exclude certain causes.[1] Severe pain is associated with fractures, dislocations, severe trauma, or infections of bones or joints. The various osteochondroses generally produce only moderate pain. A very mild pain in the knee or medial aspect of the thigh above the knee is consistent with slipped femoral capital epiphysis, whereas such pain in the groin or lateral hip is associated with Legg-Calvé-Perthes disease. Pain is likely to be absent if the cause of the limp is solely muscle weakness (as in muscular dystrophy) or a discrepancy in leg length. One should always keep in mind that pain in a child is often referred distally, so that pain in the knee or lower thigh may be caused by a pathologic process in the hip, and pain in the hip may indicate pelvic, vertebral, or spinal cord problems.

HISTORY

Inquiries about the onset of the limp and its antecedents need to be made. A history of trauma may be helpful, but often parents will focus on an insignificant event in an effort to determine the cause of the limp; conversely, a seemingly trivial past trauma may produce a significant injury. If the nature of the injury does not seem to correlate with the clinical illness, child abuse should be suspected. Details of the injury—for example, whether it was a flexion or hyperextension injury—may help to pinpoint what anatomic structures are involved. If the associated symptoms are recurrent, a chronic illness such as juvenile rheumatoid arthritis may be the cause of the limp. Adolescent girls who receive rubella vaccination will often develop a transient but painful arthritis 1 to 2 weeks following vaccination. In a young boy with a swollen painful knee, a family history of bleeding problems suggests a hemarthrosis as the cause of the limp. A history of a flulike illness associated with a large, erythematous skin lesion with central clearing suggests the possibility of Lyme arthritis.[10] (See Chapter 225.)

Athletic individuals are prone to a variety of injuries. Stress fractures caused by overuse, patellofemoral malalignment syndrome (chondromalacia patellae), and Osgood-Schlatter disease are more common among runners than nonrunners.[7,8] A sudden increase in the amount or duration of exercise (e.g., suddenly running 3 miles instead of 1) is frequently associated with injury.[2]

PHYSICAL EXAMINATION

If there is any suggestion of a systemic illness causing the limp, a complete physical examination, including height, weight, and body temperature measurements, should be performed. Obese boys are more likely to develop slipped femoral capital epiphysis. If systemic signs are lacking, most of the physical examination should be directed toward the affected limb. Some useful information may also be gathered by observing the patient walk.

The skin should be carefully inspected for redness, warmth, bruises, or puncture wounds. It is logical to assume that any such findings indicate a process involving the underlying subcutaneous tissue, muscle, or bone. Osteomyelitis of the distal metaphysis of the femur, for example, will produce redness and tenderness in the skin overlying that area of bone.

Each joint should be systematically examined for its range of motion, both active and passive, and for the presence of

Table 149-1 *Causes of Limp*

CAUSES	INFANTS AND TODDLERS	CHILDREN	ADOLESCENTS
Foreign bodies in foot	+*	+	+
Trauma to bone, periosteum, muscle, or ligaments	+	+	+
Infections of bone, joint, or muscle			
Osteomyelitis	++	++	+
Septic arthritis	++	++	+
Myositis	−	+	+
Rocky Mountain spotted fever	−	+	+
Lyme arthritis	+	++	++
Neoplastic diseases			
Leukemia	−	++	+
Tumors of bone (e.g., Ewing sarcoma, osteogenic sarcoma)	−	+	+
Metastatic diseases	−	+	+
Diseases of bone or cartilage			
Osteochondroses (e.g., Legg-Calvé-Perthes disease, Osgood-Schlatter disease)	−	++	+
Slipped femoral capital epiphysis	−	+	++
Neuromuscular disorders			
Spinal cord tumor	−	+	+
Muscle weakness	−	+	+
Muscular dystrophy	−	+	+
Systemic diseases			
Juvenile rheumatoid arthritis	+	++	+
Autoimmune diseases	+	+	+
Rheumatic fever	−	+	+
Scurvy	+	−	−
Hyperparathyroidism	−	+	++
Crohn disease	−	+	+
Gaucher disease	+	−	−
Pancreatitis	−	+	++
Hematologic diseases			
Sickle cell anemia	+	+	+
Hemophilia	+	+	+
Congenital deformities			
Dislocated hip	+	−	−
Leg length discrepancies	++	+	+
Otto pelvis	−	−	+
Miscellaneous causes			
Appendicitis	+	+	+
Inguinal adenopathy	+	+	+
Toxic synovitis	−	+	−
Drug induced			
Steroids	+	+	+
Vitamin A poisoning	+	+	+
Rubella vaccination	−	+	++

Modified from Green M: Pediatric diagnosis, ed 3, Philadelphia, 1980, WB Saunders Co.
*−, Not likely to cause limp in this age group; +, causes limp in this age group; ++, more likely to cause limp in this age group.

redness, swelling, or warmth. If there is any question about whether swelling is present, the examiner can measure the same area on the opposite extremity. Pain with active but not passive motion suggests a muscle or tendon problem. Examination of the knee should also include attention to the patella, since some causes of knee pain and limp are related to problems in the patella or its ligaments.

Unless the site of the pain is evident from a simple examination, it will also be worthwhile to palpate the entire extremity anteriorly and posteriorly. Again, pinpoint tenderness suggests a process involving the structures at that point. If the hip or upper thigh appears to be involved, the lower spine, paraspinal areas, abdomen, and inguinal area should also be examined. A rectal examination may help confirm a diagnosis of appendicitis or some other pelvic pathologic condition.

If examination of the extremity is equivocal or if some kind of congenital anatomic process or neurologic disease is suspected, other physical signs may be present. Discrepancy in leg length can be detected by measuring both legs from the anterior iliac crest to the medial malleolus. Performing the Ortolani maneuver to check for dislocated hips can still be useful in the ambulatory toddler. Asymmetry in deep tendon reflexes or alterations in sensation suggest a spinal cord pathologic condition, and difficulty raising the leg against mild resistance suggests muscle weakness.

MANAGEMENT

If the cause of the limp is obvious from the history and physical examination, treatment should be directed toward it. Causes such as bruises or muscle sprains can generally be managed with mild analgesics, heat, and rest until the injury heals. If slipped femoral capital epiphysis or some of the osteochondroses cause the limp, combined management with an orthopedist may be necessary. Infectious causes such as osteomyelitis or septic arthritis may require drainage in addition to obtaining appropriate cultures and instituting antibiotic therapy.

Often, however, a clear cause may not be obvious. The complete blood count and erythrocyte sedimentation rate (ESR) may be helpful in this context as markers of systemic illness or infection. A normal ESR is generally inconsistent with a systemic disease or an inflammatory process, although some diseases such as osteomyelitis can exist with a normal ESR. An elevated value strongly suggests systemic disease or inflammation.

When the physical findings are ambiguous, consultation with a radiologist can be extremely helpful.[6] Some fractures are difficult to detect with routine anteroposterior and lateral views of the affected part. Specialized (oblique) views are often required, and these views can best be selected if the pediatrician and radiologist jointly review the clinical symptoms. Views of both limbs may occasionally be necessary. The inexperienced examiner can often miss early and subtle signs of a problem such as periosteal elevation or changes in the fat pads surrounding the joints.

In certain situations, such as osteomyelitis or various types of stress fractures, plain roentgenograms will be normal in the early phases of the disease. Recent studies show that bone scans can be helpful in these circumstances, since they become positive before changes occur on plain films.[4] Again, a radiologist can help determine which radionuclide test is most appropriate.

If the initial history does not suggest a systemic illness or infection, if the physical examination is essentially normal, and if radiologic investigation (if it seems necessary) fails to reveal an abnormality, a short period of observation, perhaps 1 to 2 weeks, is appropriate. At that time, the history and physical examination should be repeated if the limp persists. A repeat ESR and radiologic examination will likely establish a diagnosis at that time. If the picture remains confusing, consultation with an orthopedist or perhaps a neurologist is warranted.

REFERENCES

1. Chung SMK: Identifying the cause of acute limp in childhood, Clin Pediatr 13:769, 1974.
2. Garrick JG: Knee problems in adolescents, Pediatr Rev 4:235, 1983.
3. Green M: Pediatric diagnosis, ed 3, Philadelphia, 1980, WB Saunders Co.
4. Hensinger RN: Limp, Pediatr Clin North Am 24:723, 1977.
5. Illingworth CM: 128 limping children with no fracture, sprain, or obvious cause, Clin Pediatr 17:139, 1978.
6. Kaye JJ: Roentgenographic evaluation of children with acute onset of a limp, Pediatr Ann 5:11, 1976.
7. Keller EK: Patellar management syndrome in runners, Nurs Pract p. 27, June 1983.
8. Newell SG and Bramwell ST: Overuse injuries to the knee in runners, Physician Sports Med 12:81, 1984.
9. Singer J and Towbin R: Occult fractures in the production of gait disturbance in childhood, Pediatrics 64:192, 1979.
10. Steere AC, Schoen RT, and Taylor E: The clinical evolution of lyme arthritis, Annals of Internal Medicine 107:725, 1987.

SUGGESTED READINGS

Eichenfield AH et al: Childhood Lyme arthritis: experience in an endemic area, Journ Pediatrics 109:753-758, 1986.

Steere AC, Schoen RT, and Taylor E: The clinical evolution of Lyme arthritis, Ann Intern Med 107:725-731, 1987.

150

Loss of Appetite

Martin H. Ulshen

Loss of appetite (anorexia) is a symptom seen commonly in pediatric practice. Acute illness in childhood is frequently associated with transient loss of appetite. Prolonged loss of appetite associated with poor weight gain or loss of weight usually signifies serious chronic illness, either organic or psychogenic.

The mechanisms regulating hunger and satiety are complex and remain poorly understood.[2,4] Hypothalamic control of the appetite may be influenced by visual and taste sensations, ambient temperature, and changes in blood levels of glucose or other nutrients, as well as by limbic signals from higher central nervous system regions. Satiety appears to be initiated via the vagus nerve by gastric distention, by cholecystokinin release from the intestine following the ingestion of food and from endogenous stores in the central nervous system, and by other possible humoral influences, such as glucagon and endorphins. As no hypothesis appears to explain the mechanism of appetite control fully, it seems most likely that this function is influenced simultaneously by multiple stimuli. Certain physical characteristics of food, such as appearance, aroma, and bulk, undoubtedly contribute to the generation of appetite.

In considering anorexia, the physician must first separate complaints based on unrealistic parental dietary expectations from justified parental concerns over a child's decreased nutritional intake. This is usually not difficult, since children in the former situation thrive and gain weight appropriately. Although significant gastrointestinal disease commonly leads to poor appetite, anorexia may be the result of disease distant from the bowel. In the newborn period, poor oral intake by an infant developmentally capable of feeding may be the only indication of a major disorder, such as sepsis, meningitis, urinary tract infection, congenital viral infection, a gastrointestinal anomaly, central nervous system disease, renal failure, or a metabolic disorder.

During infancy there is a wide spectrum of causes for inadequate caloric intake without an obvious cause. Acute infectious disease is a common cause of transient anorexia in infants. In the absence of an obvious explanation for poor feeding, one should always consider the possibility of an oral disease such as thrush. Emotional deprivation is a common cause of failure to thrive. A careful social history is essential in the evaluation. Early observation of parent-infant interaction in the hospital, including feeding techniques, may be appropriate. Chronic reduction in caloric intake can be established objectively by computing the total calories ingested (most of which will come from formula) and comparing this with the estimated caloric requirements for weight. This becomes more difficult in breast-fed infants, although intake may be established by weighing the infant before and after feedings. If the nursing infant has a decreased intake, one must establish whether maternal milk production is inadequate or the infant is too weak or uninterested to nurse.

In older children and adolescents, an adequate evaluation of nutritional intake requires careful calorie counts. If there is concern about the possibility of malabsorption, the calorie count may be done in conjunction with a 72-hour stool fat collection. It is important at the outset to separate children with poor appetites from children who will not eat for fear of worsening their symptoms. Children with abdominal pain

Causes of Loss of Appetite in Infants and Children

ORGANIC DISEASE

1. Infectious—acute or chronic
2. Neurologic—congenital degenerative disease, hypothalamic lesion, increased intracranial pressure, swallowing disorders (neuromuscular)
3. Gastrointestinal—oral lesions (e.g., thrush or herpes simplex), obstruction (especially with gastric or intestinal distention), inflammatory bowel disease, celiac disease, constipation
4. Cardiac—congestive heart failure (especially associated with cyanotic lesions)
5. Metabolic—renal failure, liver failure, congenital metabolic disease, lead poisoning
6. Nutritional—marasmus, iron deficiency, zinc deficiency
7. Fever—rheumatoid arthritis, rheumatic fever
8. Drugs—morphine, digitalis, antimetabolites, methylphenidate, amphetamines
9. Miscellaneous—rheumatoid arthritis, systemic lupus erythematosus, tumor[1]

PSYCHOLOGICAL FACTORS

1. Anxiety, fear, depression, mania (limbic influence on the hypothalamus)[3]
2. Avoidance of symptoms associated with meals—abdominal pain, diarrhea, bloating, urgency, dumping syndrome
3. Anorexia nervosa (see Chapter 99)
4. Excess weight loss and food aversion in athletes, simulating anorexia nervosa[5,8]

resulting from chronic inflammatory bowel disease or chronic constipation may not eat because this increases their pain. Similarly, children with chronic diarrhea may eat less if doing so seems to lead to improved stools. These patients may not actually have anorexia, and treatment aimed at improving the other symptoms may result in a rapid increase in appetite.

The box on p. 1006 presents a list of causes of loss of appetite applicable to both infants and children. Generally, the best approach to anorexia is treatment of the underlying condition.

Planning diets with the aid of a dietitian can be helpful for maximizing nutritional intake in older children. Nutritional supplements (e.g., high-calorie milk shakes, Carnation Instant Breakfast, Ensure, and Sustacal may be indicated). Other nonspecific treatments include a trial of cyproheptadine, which, although controversial, has been demonstrated in a number of studies to be an appetite stimulant. In some disorders (e.g., congenital heart disease) a nasogastric or nasoduodenal infusion of nutrients may be necessary to promote growth.[7] Parenteral nutrition may be indicated in very specific situations; however, expertise with this modality and close supervision are both required, especially if it is done at home.[6]

REFERENCES

1. Bernstein IL and Sigmundi RA: Tumor anorexia: a learned food aversion? Science 209:416, 1980.
2. Brobeck JR: Nature of satiety signals, Am J Clin Nutr 28:806, 1975.
3. Pugliese MT et al: Fear of obesity: a cause of short stature and delayed puberty, N Engl J Med 309:513, 1983.
4. Robinson PH et al: Gastric control of food intake, J Psychosom Res 32(6):593, 1988.
5. Smith NJ: Excessive weight loss and food aversion in athletes simulating anorexia nervosa, Pediatrics 66:139, 1980.
6. Strobel CT, Byrne WJ, and Fonkalsrud EW: Home parenteral nutrition: results in 34 pediatric patients, Ann Surg 188:394, 1978.
7. Vanderhoff JA et al: Continuous enteral feedings: an important adjunct to the management of complex congenital heart disease, Am J Dis Child 136:825, 1982.
8. Yates A, Leehey K, and Shisslak CM: Running: an analogue of anorexia? N Engl J Med 308:251, 1983.

151

Lymphadenopathy

George B. Segel and Caroline Breese Hall

Lymphadenopathy, or enlargement of lymph nodes, is a common problem in childhood. Lymphadenopathy may be defined as any lymph node enlargement; all lymph nodes that are palpable are technically considered enlarged. However, nodes in the cervical chain and occipital areas drain regions commonly infected in childhood and often are mildly enlarged (diameter less than 1 cm) in children who are otherwise normal.

The clinically relevant problems in assessing lymphadenopathy are (1) whether any lymph node or lymph node aggregate or chain is abnormal and requires further assessment; (2) if abnormal, whether the nodes are benign, primarily inflammatory, or malignant; (3) the appropriate evaluation, diagnosis, and management. The following section will address these problems by considering explicitly: (1) the characteristics of lymph node enlargement; (2) the associated signs and symptoms; and (3) the potential differential diagnosis for the adenopathy.

CHARACTERISTICS OF LYMPH NODE ENLARGEMENT

The Components of the Lymphatic System

The lymphatic system includes not only lymph nodes but also the spleen, thymus, tonsils, Waldeyer ring, and Peyer patches in the intestine as well as the appendix. Potentially palpable lymph node groups and their drainage areas are shown in Table 151-1, which may serve as a guide to palpation of these superficial nodes.

Lymph Node Features

Abnormalities of the palpable lymph nodes are assessed by the node's size, location, mobility, inflammatory reaction, and consistency. Small nodes (less than 1 cm) are found often in the cervical chain and the femoral and inguinal areas. Likewise, nodes less than 0.5 cm may be palpated in the occipital, postauricular (mastoid), and axillary chains (Table 151-1). In the submental or submaxillary regions nodes may become enlarged to over 1 cm from intraoral or facial infections. It is unusual, however, to find lymph nodes of any size in the supraclavicular or epitrochlear areas. Thus the same size lymph node observed in two different regions may have markedly different implications. For example, a 1 cm node in the cervical region is very likely to be benign, whereas a 1 cm supraclavicular node requires a biopsy, since it is unlikely to result from superficial inflammatory disease and may reflect intrathoracic or intraabdominal malignancy.

Fluctuance and signs of inflammation surrounding a group of enlarged lymph nodes are helpful in reaching a diagnosis, particularly if there is an infectious source distal to the node area. These findings strongly suggest an infectious etiology (Table 151-2) usually requiring systemic antibiotic therapy. In the absence of inflammation, the consistency and mobility of the nodes may heighten one's suspicion of underlying malignancy. Nodes that are hard and fixed are more often seen in adults with metastatic carcinoma. The nodes of Hodgkin disease and lymphoma are more matted than hard, although nodes associated with neuroblastoma, rhabdomyosarcoma, and other childhood malignancies may mimic the findings in adults.

DIFFERENTIAL DIAGNOSIS

The major differential diagnostic categories for enlarged lymph nodes include infectious (inflammatory) and neoplastic diseases. A summary of the common and not so common conditions associated with lymphadenopathy is shown in Table 151-2 for newborns, infants, children, and adolescents, because the relative occurrence varies with age. The classification of these conditions is somewhat arbitrary and not all inclusive but does reflect the diagnostic likelihood within a given age group.

Table 151-1 *Palpable Lymph Nodes and Lymphatic Drainage*

NODE AREA	AREA OF DRAINAGE
Occipital	Posterior scalp, neck
Mastoid	Mastoid area
Submental	Apex of tongue and lower lip
Submaxillary	Tongue, buccal cavity, lips, and cheek
Cervical	Cranium, neck, and oropharynx
Axillary	Greater part of arm, shoulder, superficial anterior and lateral thoracic and upper abdominal wall
Supraclavicular	Right: Inferior neck and mediastinum Left: Inferior neck, mediastinum, and upper abdomen
Epitrochlear	Hand, forearm, and elbow
Inguinal	Leg and genitalia
Femoral	Leg
Popliteal	Posterior leg and knee

Table 151-2 *Etiology of Lymphadenopathy*

DIFFERENTIAL DIAGNOSIS	NEWBORN	INFANT	CHILD	ADOLESCENT
Infections				
Bacterial				
Pyogenic		Streptococci/staphylococci, and other gram positive and gram negative organisms		
			Cat-scratch fever →	→
			Typhoid fever →	→
			Tularemia →	→
Spirochetal	Syphilis →	→		Syphilis
				Anaerobes
				Vincent angina
Granulomatous		Mycobacteria →	→	→
		Atypical mycobacteria →	→	→
Viral			Rubella →	→
			Rubeola →	→
			Varicella →	→
		→	→	→ HHV6 syndrome
		Adenovirus →	→	→
		Enterovirus →	→	→
			Epstein-Barr virus (EBV) →	→
			Cytomegalovirus (CMV) →	→
			Herpes simplex virus (HSV) (stomatitis and pharyngitis) →	→
		Human immunodeficiency virus (HIV) →	→	→
Protozoan	Toxoplasmosis →	→	→	→
Fungal		Histoplasmosis →	→	→
		Rarely other fungi →	→	→
Rickettsial			Rocky Mountain spotted fever →	→
Chlamydial				Lymphogranuloma
Parasitic			Toxocara →	→
			Myiasis →	→
Neoplastic				
Endogenous		Leukemia →	→	→
		Lymphoma →	→	→
		Histiocytosis →	→	→
			Hodgkin disease →	→
Exogenous (metastatic)		Neuroblastoma →	→	→
		Wilms tumor →	→	→
			Ewing sarcoma →	→
			Rhabdomyosarcoma →	→
Immunologic		Juvenile rheumatoid arthritis (JRA) →	→	→
			Systemic lupus erythematosus (SLE) →	→
		Serum sickness →	→	→
			Sarcoidosis →	→
Other (Reactive)		Kawasaki disease →	→	
			Hemoglobinopathies →	→
			Hemophilia →	→
			Phenytoin →	→
			Addison disease →	→
			Hyperthyroidism →	→
	Chronic granulomatous disease (CGD) →	→	→	→
	Agammaglobulinemia →	→	→	→

Infections

The infectious problems may be localized or systemic. If localized, the primary site of infection draining to the involved lymph node area should be identified.

The common pyogenic bacteria, atypical mycobacteria, and anaerobic bacteria are most likely to cause localized adenopathy. Generalized adenopathy or regional adenopathy associated with adenopathy elsewhere is more likely caused by infections from viruses, spirochetes, or sometimes toxoplasma. *Mycobacterium tuberculosis* may produce localized or multiple sites of adenitis. Fungal infections, such as histoplasmosis, occasionally may cause generalized lymphadenopathy, but most fungal infections, if associated with adenopathy at all, produce regional enlargement.

Neoplastic Diseases

Primary neoplastic diseases are the other major consideration in both localized and generalized adenopathy. Included in this category are lymphomas, leukemia, histiocytosis, and metastases from solid tumors such as neuroblastoma, Wilms tumor, Ewing sarcoma, and rhabdomyosarcoma.

Immunologic and Inflammatory Diseases

Generalized lymphadenopathy may also be associated with chronic inflammatory conditions, such as collagen-vascular diseases and sarcoidosis or with reactions to certain drugs, such as phenytoin and isoniazid, or serum sickness. Such divergent causes as hyperthyroidism and Addison disease must also be included within the differential diagnosis of generalized adenopathy.

ASSESSMENT

History, Physical Examination, and Chest Roentgenogram

The history and physical examination may reveal a source for a localized infection, such as a dental abscess, mastoiditis, scalp infection, insect bite, or cat scratch. Alternatively, systemic diseases such as infectious mononucleosis, juvenile rheumatoid arthritis, HIV infection, and others may be suggested by other characteristic historical and physical findings. The physical examination should include all the palpable nodes listed in Table 151-1. Furthermore, the assessment of enlarged lymph nodes without an obvious inflammatory explanation requires a chest roentgenogram to evaluate the presence of enlarged mediastinal or hilar nodes. The chest roentgenogram is the most commonly omitted study in the evaluation of patients with lymphadenopathy who are referred to our center. The presence of mediastinal or hilar adenopathy would preclude "trials of antibiotics" with the attendant delay in performing a diagnostic biopsy.

Imaging

The abdominal lymph nodes, including retroperitoneal, periportal, and celiac nodes, as well as the nodes of the splenic hilum, are more difficult to evaluate without more sophisticated imaging techniques. The spleen represents primarily lymphoid tissue and may be enlarged in infectious, immunologic, collagen-vascular, and neoplastic disorders and may be delineated by ultrasound or computed tomography (CT) examination. Abdominal and pelvic lymph nodes may be visualized by ultrasound or may require techniques such as CT and magnetic resonance imaging (MRI). In some special circumstances, lymphangiograms are used to define the iliac and periaortic nodes for the staging of Hodgkin disease.

Complete Blood Count

A number of other studies may be useful in the assessment of lymphadenopathy. The complete blood count may reveal the reactive lymphocytes of infectious mononucleosis or a granulocytosis suggesting systemic bacterial infection. The presence of any cytopenia such as anemia, granulocytopenia, or thrombocytopenia would be a "red flag" that a hematologic malignancy, such as leukemia or lymphoma, or metastatic disease involving the bone marrow, such as neuroblastoma, may underlie the lymphadenopathy. The finding of nucleated erythrocytes and immature granulocytes ("leukoerythroblastic blood picture") on the peripheral blood film is an ominous sign suggesting bone marrow "irritation" and may be seen in metastatic diseases such as neuroblastoma and rhabdomyosarcoma and with immunologic vasculitis.

Infectious Evaluation

The diagnostic workup of potential infectious lymphadenopathy is diverse and depends on the history, age of the patient, location of the nodes, and signs of inflammation accompanying the adenopathy, as previously noted. For acute, inflamed, and localized adenopathy, an infectious etiologic diagnosis is most frequently achieved by obtaining material for culture and histologic or pathologic examination. In children with acute cervical adenitis, needle aspiration of an acutely inflamed, sometimes fluctuant node will demonstrate the infecting organism in two thirds or more of cases. The aspirated material should be cultured aerobically and anaerobically and for fungi and mycobacteria. Histochemical evaluation should include a Gram and acid-fast stain. In certain cases a biopsy may be required. The biopsy may be evaluated by additional special stains, such as the Warthin-Starry silver stain for cat-scratch disease. Intradermal skin tests should be applied when mycobacterial infection is suspected. Although a skin test exists for cat-scratch disease, the antigen is neither standardized nor commercially available at this time. Specific serologic or antigen detection tests may be obtained to evaluate further such infections as syphilis, toxoplasmosis, brucellosis, tularemia, fungi, and some viral infections such as Epstein-Barr virus, HIV, and cytomegalovirus. Viral cultures are also appropriate for the latter and for the common respiratory viruses, such as the adenoviruses and enteroviruses. The erythrocyte sedimentation rate may be useful in assessing underlying inflammation, but it is not unique to infectious diseases, for it may be elevated in immunologic and neoplastic diseases as well.

After initial evaluation by history, physical examination, chest roentgenogram, and preliminary laboratory studies, the clinician may not have an obvious explanation for the node enlargement. If a bacterial source for localized adenopathy (e.g., pharyngitis and cervical nodes) is suggested, a limited course of 7 to 10 days of antibiotic therapy may be tried. However, if the nodes have not regressed significantly, prompt further evaluation is necessary. At this time a chest roentgenogram should be obtained, if it has not already been done, and even in the absence of mediastinal or hilar adenopathy, significantly enlarged, unexplained lymph nodes should be biopsied promptly to permit institution of appropriate therapy.

Biopsy

Biopsy of significant adenopathy should be performed early if there is no evidence suggesting an infection or other etiology, and particularly if there are enlarged mediastinal or hilar nodes present. The biopsy should encompass the central mass of the enlarged nodes to avoid a misdiagnosis of reactive inflammation in adjacent nodes. This is particularly common in Hodgkin disease in which an adjacent smaller lymph node may be more accessible and technically easier to biopsy but may not demonstrate the presence of Reed-Sternberg cells.

It is critical that the biopsy be performed at a medical center specializing in the care of children so that all of the appropriate touch preparations, cultures, special stains, and biochemical studies are obtained. The pathology of Hodgkin disease, lymphoma, and other similar round-cell tumors may be difficult to establish and requires the assessment of a pediatric pathologist with experience in these diseases. The biopsy diagnosis is obviously critical for the subsequent management, which may involve treatment with radiation, chemotherapy, or both.

TREATMENT

Infectious Diseases

Therapy of lymphadenitis depends on determining its etiology or judging the most likely cause. Acute adenitis, particularly in the cervical area, in young children frequently associated with infection from group A beta-hemolytic streptococci or *Staphylococcus aureus*. The latter is particularly likely in adenitis that progresses to fluctuance. In such children with acute adenitis, antibiotic therapy should be directed at these organisms with an antibiotic that covers penicillinase-producing strains of *S. aureus*. For most patients oral therapy with drugs such as dicloxacillin or cloxacillin is adequate. The broader spectrum oral agents such as Augmentin and some of the oral cephalosporins may also be used. The usual course of therapy is 10 to 14 days, but therapy should be continued for at least 5 days after the signs of acute inflammation have subsided. For patients with suppurative adenitis from these organisms, drainage is not only diagnostic (by culturing the exudate obtained), but also therapeutic. A few patients may not respond to oral therapy, even with a drug to which the organism is known to be sensitive. Parenteral antibiotic therapy is then required.

If an anaerobic infection is suspected, therapy depends in part on the location of the adenitis and the type of organism. Most anaerobic infections of the cervical and submental area are associated with mouth flora, most of which are sensitive to penicillin. Occasionally, however, such infections require alternative therapy such as clindamycin.

Both *M. tuberculosis* and atypical mycobacteria may cause adenitis, with the latter being more frequent in children. Differentiating the two may be difficult but is important, because many strains of atypical mycobacteria are resistant to the usual antitubercular chemotherapy, and excisional biopsy may be required. If tubercular infection is suspected, appropriate therapy for *M. tuberculosis* (e.g., isoniazid and rifampin) should be initiated while awaiting identification and sensitivities of the organism. Incision and drainage should not be performed on adenitis suspected to be tubercular.

Cat-scratch adenitis is usually self-limited. Although recently a gram-negative bacillus was identified as the cause of cat-scratch disease, no specific therapy has been identified. For nodes that become markedly enlarged, tender, and fluctuant, aspiration may help relieve symptoms. Incision and drainage, however, should be avoided.

Neoplastic Disease

The treatment of neoplastic diseases today is oriented toward cure in most instances. The effectiveness of treatment for lymphocytic and myelocytic leukemic lymphomas and Wilms and other tumors has markedly improved in the last 2 decades. The specific treatment for childhood cancer often involves combinations of chemotherapy, radiation therapy, and surgery, which depend on the individual diagnosis and are beyond the scope of this presentation (see Chapter 187). However, prompt and accurate diagnosis is essential for the institution of specific treament and the optimum care of these patients.

SUGGESTED READINGS

Filston HC: Common lumps and bumps of the head and neck in infants and children, Pediatr Ann 18:180, 1989.

Freidig EE et al: Clinical-histologic-microbiologic analysis of 419 lymph node biopsy specimens, Rev Infect Dis 8:322, 1986.

Knight PJ, Mulne AF, and Vassy LE: When is lymph node biopsy indicated in children with enlarged peripheral nodes? Pediatrics 69:391, 1982.

Lake AM and Oski FA: Peripheral lymphadenopathy in childhood, Am J Dis Child 132:357, 1978.

152

Malocclusion

Lindsey K. Grossman

The incidence of malocclusion in school-age children and adolescents may, according to some reports, be as high as 90% or more. In evaluating such statistics, however, one must first consider the definition involved, because in the field of orthodontics, any deviation from absolutely ideal tooth alignment is considered to be malocclusion, although probably only 10% to 15% of these at most can be viewed as handicapping.[9] Indeed, the 1963 to 1965 *National Health Survey,* which examined 7400 children 6 to 11 years of age, found 14.2% to have severe or very severe malocclusion.[4] This national survey of malocclusion has not been repeated to date; however, there is no reason to believe that the incidence has changed during the past 2 decades.

Significantly abnormal dental occlusion has been said to predispose individuals to many risks.[2,6,8] Caries, periodontal disease, increased susceptibility to trauma or root resorption, and disturbances of physiologic functioning, including temporomandibular joint disorders, muscular dysfunction, speech defects, and masticatory disturbances, have been linked to malocclusion, although the data supporting such outcomes are either scanty or conflicting.[5] Most patients seek orthodontic treatment because of malocclusion's effect on their appearance. In our society, the individual's own sense of attractiveness can influence behavior and ultimate success in life. However, there is no direct evidence that treatment of dental irregularities positively affects these outcomes.

A major problem hindering objective evaluation of orthodontic treatment is the lack of a universally acceptable classification system. The Treatment Priority Index, which was used in the *National Health Survey,*[4] is a quantitative measure of severity, but because of its complexity has not been widely adopted. The commonly used Angle classification system effectively expresses qualitative but not quantitative differences in dental occlusion; hence it is not helpful in determining the need for referral or in evaluating the treatment outcome.[3] It is therefore difficult to determine objectively which patients require orthodontic correction or to compare the results of various treatments.

The etiology of malocclusion is multifactorial, with both heredity and environment playing a role. Significant evidence exists linking nasal obstruction, especially when caused by enlarged tonsils or adenoids, with the development of a high arched palate and posterior crossbite.[6]

The pacifier and thumb- and finger-sucking habits[7] play a role in malocclusion problems. The majority of children develop such habits during infancy, but by 4 or 5 years of age most have stopped the practice. If sucking continues into the periods of mixed and permanent dentition, the potential for developing malocclusion is greater, although a specific causal relationship may not always hold. Often, abnormal bites revert to normal after the habit is dropped. Anterior open bite, overjet, crossbites, and other malocclusions have been reported in association with oral habits, although other children with such habits may evidence no abnormalities. Thumb-sucking may be preferable to finger-sucking, because fewer physical stresses are exerted on the teeth. A pacifier probably has the least deleterious effects. Most studies show earlier cessation of pacifier use compared with thumb- and finger-sucking.

In the assessment of occlusion, both the maxillary and mandibular arches should be observed with the mouth open to determine if the teeth are crowded or have excess space between them.[9] Crowding almost always increases over time, whereas excess space will either improve or worsen. One should be aware that excess space, especially between the upper lateral incisors and canines and the lower canines and first deciduous molars, is the norm in young children with primary dentition and allows room for the eruption of the larger, permanent teeth.

Occlusion of the posterior teeth is assessed with the teeth set in the biting position. The tongue should not be visible between the upper and lower teeth; the presence of such a space, albeit very small, or the contrasting problem of a deep bite (lower incisors biting on palatal gingiva) nearly always requires treatment. The maxillary teeth should overlap their mandibular partners slightly in the lateral plane and be placed slightly anterior (approximately one-half tooth) to them. The degree of malalignment at this point will determine the need for referral.

Anterior dentition problems, readily apparent when the patient smiles, are the source of many orthodontic referrals. Open bites with space visible between the upper and lower arches, as well as deep bites, are difficult problems to treat whereas over ("buck teeth") or anterior crossbite is often easily corrected. Occasionally one or more of the permanent teeth, often incisors, will erupt before the corresponding primary teeth have been shed, giving the child a double row of teeth and causing much parental concern. Extraction is rarely necessary, since the primary teeth are almost always shed by 8 years of age. Normal tongue movements will usually ensure correct final placement of the permanent teeth.

There are few data linking maloccluded primary dentition with maloccluded permanent teeth. However, the presence of anterior crossbite, wherein the upper lateral incisor erupt behind the lower ones or the upper posterior teeth erupt medial to the lower ones, may interfere with ultimate maxillary growth and tooth position. The absence of normal spacing in primary dentition will almost always lead to severe crowding of the permanent teeth. Children with these conditions should be referred to an orthodontist early.[8,10]

Probably the most important influence that pediatricians have in promoting good dental occlusion is their advice concerning primary dentition. The congenital absence or the loss of one or more of the primary teeth to decay or trauma can seriously affect the spacing required for normal occlusion of the permanent teeth. Thus a dental referral is advisable following failure of eruption or premature loss of any primary tooth.[7]

In general, however, the decision to refer a child or young adolescent for orthodontic treatment may be difficult. There are few objective referral guidelines.[1] Treatment nearly always results in an improved, although not necessarily a flawless, appearance; nevertheless, the pediatrician should assess the patient's and family's expectations as well as their willingness to comply with the discomfort and cost of treatment before arranging for referral.

REFERENCES

1. Currier GF: Fundamentals of orthodontics with criteria for referral, Pediatr Ann 14:117, 1985.
2. Helm S: Etiology and treatment need of malocclusion, J Can Dent Assoc 45:673, 1979.
3. Jago JD: The epidemiology of dental occlusion: a critical appraisal, J Pub Health Dent 34:80, 1974.
4. Kelly JE, Sanchez M, and VanKirk LE: An assessment of the occlusion of teeth of children 6-11 years. National health survey, Series 11, no 130, US Department of Health, Education and Welfare Publications (PHS) 74-1612, 1973.
5. McLain JB and Profitt WR: Oral health status in the United States: prevalence of malocclusion, J Dent Educ 49:386, 1985.
6. Richter HJ: Obstruction of the pediatric upper airway, Ear Nose Throat J 66:209, 1987.
7. Schneider PE and Peterson J: Oral habits: considerations in management, Pediatr Clin North Am 29:523, 1982.
8. Shaw WC, Addy M, and Ray C: Dental and social effects of malocclusion and effectiveness of orthodontic treatment: a review, Commun Dent Oral Epidemiol 8:36, 1980.
9. Smith RJ: Development of occlusion and malocclusion, Pediatr Clin North Am 29:475, 1982.
10. Sweeney EA: Pediatric dentistry, Curr Probl Pediatr 11:1, 1980.

153

Nervousness

Henry M. Seidel and Richard M. Sarles

There are some chief complaints that occasion a sinking feeling when the busy physician first hears them, especially in the midst of a busy afternoon in the office. The nature of the complaint implies that the physician and patients are about to embark on an often murky and abstract search for the root of an evanescent symptom or problem. One such complaint is nervousness, whether it be voiced by an older child or an adolescent or by a parent about the child. Picture, for example, the 11- or 12-year-old who says vaguely, "I don't know. I just feel funny. I feel nervous."

Such moments call for discipline on the part of the physician. They remind us that this may be a circumstance in which an inarticulate patient is literally shouting for help. It is the kind of complaint with which patients may signal that they are among those most in need of help. The physician must look beyond the chief complaint to the "iatrotropic," the "doctor-seeking," stimulus: Why is this patient here with this complaint? What does it mean?

Finding the answer will take time, perhaps a great deal of time. The approach, however, is clear. A good history and physical examination are needed. The circumstance is not life threatening; everything does not have to be done immediately. Indeed, some of the effort may be delayed until a time when the physician is more at ease and less stressed. Certainly the abstraction of the term "nervousness" and the difficulty in defining it more precisely underscore the need and the necessary care.

What accompanies the nervousness—anorexia, restlessness at night, sluggishness, overactivity? A physical problem is implied but quite often is not at the root. Nervousness, for example, is often part of the constellation of complaints in a variety of endocrine disorders (hyperthyroidism, hypoglycemia, Addison disease) and in dermatitis, pinworm infestation, and allergy. Caffeine ingestion (colas and coffee) and a variety of drug abuses can also cause "nervousness." Mitral valve prolapse and paroxysmal auricular tachycardia are cardiac diseases that can create symptoms of nervousness. Clearly, a careful history and thorough physical examination can be productive.

An attention deficit disorder (ADD), with accompanying hyperactivity, and a variety of anxiety disorders (separation anxieties, school phobia, the somatization of depression) are all to be considered. Many more serious problems, such as autism, childhood psychoses, obsessive-compulsive and manic-depressive disorders, and panic attacks, can all be verbalized as nervousness as the parents or patient try to define perceptions and feelings. Such problems, however, are rarely defined as nervousness alone; the history and physical examination can quickly uncover a host of concomitant findings.

It is after the conscientious search has been made and when little if anything more has been discovered that the chief complaint of nervousness becomes more difficult to approach. Time, caring, and sensitive understanding of the patient's needs are required. Unfortunately, little help is available in the literature. Nervousness is not usually defined or described in textbooks and is not listed in the American Psychiatric Association's *Diagnostic and Statistical Manual of Mental Disorders* (DSM-III) or in any standard psychiatric textbook, and a discussion of its implications is not generally included in most medical school curricula.

How, then, is the practitioner to conceptualize, diagnose, and treat nervousness, nervous stomach, or other disorders that occur as a symptom without any readily discernible underlying pathophysiology? First, of course, comes the careful search; then come the devotion of time, the "listening ear," the sensitive exploration, and if necessary, referral to a colleague with expertise in emotional disorders of childhood and adolescence to attempt to unravel the sometimes intricate puzzle.

By this time, the physician may know that the patient has no physical disorder; however, there is evident emotional tension, restlessness, agitation, fearful apprehension, acute uneasiness, undue excitability, or excessive irritability. These manifestations, quite real and requiring care, may need individual attention to the child or work with the family in a group; indeed, the approaches may be as infinite as the variety of complaints. The physician who is unprepared or unwilling to provide this extent of time and effort should refer the patient in order to ease the morbidity inevitably associated with these complaints.

154

Nonconvulsive Periodic Disorders

Sarah M. Roddy

A variety of paroxysmal nonepileptic disorders occur in children. These disorders have a wide range of clinical features that mimic seizures, and it is important to distinguish them from seizures so that the child is not inappropriately treated with anticonvulsants. A careful history is often all that is needed to make the diagnosis, although in a few patients a more extensive evaluation may be needed. Some of the more common paroxysmal nonepileptic disorders are reviewed here.

BREATH-HOLDING SPELLS

Breath-holding spells, or infantile syncope, occur in approximately 5% of children.[11] Most children with breath-holding spells begin having episodes between 6 and 18 months of age, although some may begin in the first few weeks of life. The frequency of episodes ranges from once a year to several times daily. The history of the episode and the surrounding events are the most important part of the evaluation of a child with breath-holding spells. Because there is a high familial incidence of breath-holding spells, the family should be questioned about episodes in other family members.

Two types of breath-holding spells occur. The cyanotic type is more common and is usually precipitated by frustration or anger. The child cries vigorously and then holds the breath in expiration. This apnea is followed by cyanosis with opisthotonic posturing and loss of consciousness. Recovery is usually quick, with return of respiration and consciousness within 1 minute. Pallid breath-holding episodes are usually provoked by sudden fright or minor injuries, especially falling and hitting the occiput. The child gasps or cries briefly and then abruptly becomes quiet, loses consciousness, has pallor, and becomes limp. The child may then develop clonic jerks. Pallid breath-holding spells represent a vasovagal phenomenon. The precipitating event induces a vagal-mediated asystole with a secondary cerebral ischemia. Ocular compression during simultaneous electroencephalographic and electrocardiographic tracing in children with pallid breath-holding spells has shown asystole with flattening of the electroencephalogram without electrical seizure activity.[11,14] The clonic jerks are caused by cerebral hypoxia rather than epileptiform discharges from the brain.

The prognosis for children with either type of breath-holding is excellent; the majority outgrow the episodes by school age. Children with pallid breath-holding spells may later develop syncope.[11] Treatment is directed mainly at reassuring the family of the benign nature of the episodes. It is important to emphasize that the episodes are not seizures and that they do not lead to mental retardation or epilepsy. Because cyanotic episodes are often precipitated by temper tantrums, anger, and frustration, advice about behavior management may be helpful. Anemia has been described as a contributing factor to breath-holding spells, and its treatment may decrease the frequency of episodes.[11] Atropine is effective for pallid breath-holding episodes, but its use is rarely warranted. Anticonvulsants are not effective in the treatment of either type of breath-holding spell and should not be used.

SYNCOPE

Syncope (or fainting) is an acute and transient loss of consciousness resulting from decreased cerebral perfusion. These episodes are relatively common in teenagers. Postural hypotension, which may occur after a sudden change from a sitting or reclining position to a standing position, can precipitate an episode. Emotional upset, fright, or overheating are also common provoking stimuli. Cardiac disorders, including arrhythmias, aortic stenosis, and severe cyanotic heart disease, may cause syncope by decreasing cardiac output. In rare cases, episodes of syncope have been reported with swallowing, coughing, urinating, and defecation.[5,12,16]

Patients have presyncopal symptoms that may include light-headedness, anxiety, sweating, nausea, generalized numbness, and visual changes described as constrictions of vision or darkening of vision. Observers notice marked pallor and clammy skin. These symptoms are followed by loss of consciousness and slumping to the floor. Once the patient is recumbent and cerebral perfusion is restored, consciousness returns within a few seconds. If the patient is held with the head above the body and cerebral perfusion is not restored, clonic movements may occur. As with the pallid breath-holding spells, these movements are secondary to cerebral ischemia rather than epileptiform discharges from the brain. Patients are not disorientated or confused following syncope, although they may be tired.

The history is very important in making the diagnosis of syncope and should include a description of the event by the patient and an observer. Laboratory evaluation is seldom needed, but if there are atypical features such as absence of a precipitating factor or confusion following the episode, an electroencephalogram or a cardiac evaluation, including Holter monitoring, may be necessary. Treatment consists of teaching the patient and family about managing an episode. Because patients have presyncopal symptoms, they should be instructed to sit or lie down as soon as symptoms begin, thereby preventing progression to loss of consciousness. If the patient does lose consciousness, the family should place him or her in a recumbent position with the head lower than the body. Often parents pick up a child who has fainted; they should be cautioned against doing this, because they could prolong the period of unconsciousness. (See Chapter 169, "Syncope," for a more detailed discussion of syncope and its causes.)

BENIGN PAROXYSMAL VERTIGO

Benign paroxysmal vertigo of childhood is a disorder characterized by brief attacks of vertigo. Symptoms usually appear within the first 3 or 4 years of life, although they may begin later. Episodes are characterized by abrupt onset, with the child appearing fearful and unable to maintain normal posture and gait. The child may seek support and clutch the parent or abruptly sit down or fall. In severe cases the child may be limp and incapable of using his or her extremities. Pallor and diaphoresis are usually apparent, with vomiting and nystagmus occurring in some. Typically an episode lasts less than 30 seconds, in rare cases a few minutes. There may be a brief period of postural instability following the episode, but within a few minutes the child is back to normal and playing. There is no alteration of consciousness during the episode or sleepiness following it. The frequency of episodes varies from as many as several weekly to as few as one every 4 months. Audiograms are normal, but caloric testing, which is difficult to obtain in young children, is abnormal with reduction of vestibular sensitivity.[2,10] Radiographic studies of the temporal bone and electroencephalography are also normal. Included in the differential diagnosis of vertigo in childhood are brainstem lesions, posterior fossa tumors, and epilepsy. Usually the history and physical examination differentiate benign paroxysmal vertigo from these more serious disorders. In most cases no treatment is necessary. Anticonvulsants are not effective. Antihistamines such as dimenhydrinate have been used in some patients with frequent episodes, with an apparent reduction in the number of episodes. Because of the variability in the frequency of attacks, it is difficult to assess the effect of therapy accurately. Attacks of vertigo usually cease spontaneously over a period of a few years. Some children with benign paroxysmal vertigo have later developed migraine headaches.[7] (See Chapter 121, "Dizziness and Vertigo," for a more complete discussion of the causes of vertigo.)

SHUDDERING ATTACKS

Shuddering or shivering episodes constitute a benign movement disorder and probably occur in many children at one time or another. The episodes are brief and characterized by paroxysmal rapid tremors primarily involving the head and arms. In some episodes there may be flexion of the head, elbow, trunk, and knees, with adduction of the elbows and knees.[15] There is no alteration in consciousness with the episodes. Their frequency is variable, with some children having more than 100 episodes daily. Emotional factors, including excitement, fear, anger, and frustration, may precipitate episodes. Shuddering episodes may start as early as a few months of age or not until later in childhood. Usually there is a gradual reduction in the frequency of episodes. The pathophysiology of the episodes is unclear, although it has been postulated that the attacks are an expression of an essential tremor.[15] Electroencephalographic monitoring has shown that the episodes are not epileptiform in nature.[8] Because the episodes do not have adverse effects on patients, no treatment is necessary. Anticonvulsants are not effective and should not be used.

BENIGN NEONATAL SLEEP MYOCLONUS

Sudden brief jerks of the extremities are normal in children and adults when falling asleep. In neonates, sleep-related myoclonus has also been observed and called benign neonatal sleep myoclonus. The myoclonic jerks begin in the first month of life, often within the first day of life. The myoclonus is present only during sleep and may be present in both quiet and active sleep states. The jerking movements may start in one extremity and then progress to involve the other extremities, or they may begin bilaterally. They occur every 2 to 3 seconds for several minutes, although they have been reported to last up to 90 minutes.[4] The neonates develop normally and have no neurologic deficit. Electroencephalography is normal with no epileptiform discharges associated with the myoclonus.[13] The major differential diagnosis of neonatal sleep myoclonus is a seizure disorder. A history of episodes only during sleep and a normal electroencephalogram help to differentiate this benign disorder from seizures. The myoclonus usually diminishes gradually during the first 6 months of life. No treatment is necessary.

NIGHT TERRORS

Night terrors are a sleep disorder with some features that mimic partial complex seizures. They occur in up to 6% of children, with a peak incidence in late preschool and early school-age children.[6] There is often a positive family history of night terrors or sleep disorders. The episodes usually occur during the first 2 hours after falling asleep. The child will abruptly sit up in bed and scream or talk unintelligibly. The eyes may be open, and the child has a glazed look. During the episode the child appears to be hallucinating and does not respond to the parents. There is a sympathetic nervous system response with tachycardia and diaphoresis. In some cases the child may sleepwalk. A night terror usually lasts about 10 minutes, with the child relaxing and abruptly falling back to sleep. Upon awakening the child will not remember the episode. Night terrors are caused by a rapid partial arousal from deep, slow-wave sleep. Electroencephalography does not show seizure activity during the episodes. It is important to differentiate night terrors from nightmares, which occur during rapid eye movement (REM) sleep and are associated with easy arousal and recall of the content, or at least the occurrence, of the nightmare. Night terrors usually become less frequent as the child gets older, although episodes may continue into adolescence and adulthood. The nature of the episodes should be explained to the parents. Although parents tend to attempt to awaken and reassure the child, they should be told that the child is not aware of their presence, and attempts to awaken the child are not helpful. Usually no medication is indicated, but if episodes are frequent or severe, diazepam is the drug of choice.[1]

NARCOLEPSY

Narcolepsy is a sleep-wake disorder characterized by excessive and inappropriate periods of sleep during the day. The daytime sleepiness interrupts activities and does not decrease in response to adequate amounts of sleep at night. Naps may last from a few minutes to longer than 1 hour. In addition to the excessive daytime sleep, patients often have cataplexy, sleep paralysis, and hypnagogic hallucinations. Cataplexy is a transient partial or complete loss of tone, often triggered by an emotional reaction such as laughter or fright. There is no loss of consciousness. Sleep paralysis occurs as the patient falls asleep or awakens and is characterized by the inability to move or speak. Hypnagogic hallucinations occur while falling asleep, can be auditory or visual, and may be very frightening to a child.

The prevalence of narcolepsy is between 0.04% and 0.09% in the entire population, but it increases to 50% when there is a positive family history.[9] The age of onset is usually in the second decade, although it has been reported in children as young as 3 years of age. Sleep studies in patients with narcolepsy show that sleep occurs within 15 minutes of sleep onset; in normal subjects, 90 minutes of non-REM sleep precede the first REM period.[17] There is a strong association between narcolepsy and the presence of the HLA-DR2 antigen.[3] HLA typing and sleep studies are important in making the diagnosis of narcolepsy. Included in the differential diagnosis of excessive daytime sleepiness are chronic illness, sleep apnea, hypothyroidism, depression, and seizures.

Narcolepsy is a lifelong condition, but central nervous system stimulants such as methylphenidate help decrease the frequency of naps. Tricyclic medications such as imipramine are used for treating cataplexy and the other associated symptoms.

REFERENCES

1. Anders TF and Weinstein P: Sleep and its disorders in infants and children: a review, Pediatrics 50:312, 1972.
2. Basser LS: Benign paroxysmal vertigo of childhood (a variety of vestibular neuronitis), Brain 87:41, 1964.
3. Billiard M and Seignalet J: Extraordinary association between HLA-DR2 and narcolepsy, Lancet 1:226, 1985.
4. Blennow G: Benign infantile nocturnal myoclonus, Acta Pediatr Scand 74:505, 1985.
5. DiMaria AA Jr, Westmoreland BF, and Sharbrough FW: EEG in cough syncope, Neurology 34:371, 1984.
6. DiMario FJ Jr and Emery S III: The natural history of night terrors, Clin Pediatr 26:505, 1987.
7. Fenichel GM: Migraine as a cause of benign paroxysmal vertigo of childhood, J Pediatr 71:114, 1967.
8. Holmes GL and Russman BS: Shuddering attacks: evaluation using electroencephalographic frequency modulation radiotelemetry and videotape monitoring, Am J Dis Child 140:72, 1985.
9. Kessler S, Guilleminault C, and Dement WC: A family study of 50 REM narcoleptics, Acta Neurol Scand 50:503, 1974.
10. Koenigsberger MR et al: Benign paroxysmal vertigo of childhood, Neurology 20:1108, 1970.
11. Lombroso CT and Lerman P: Breathholding spells (cyanotic and pallid infantile syncope), Pediatrics 39:563, 1967.
12. Proudfit WL and Forteza ME: Micturition syncope, N Engl J Med 260:328, 1959.
13. Resnick TJ et al: Benign neonatal sleep myoclonus: relationship to sleep states, Arch Neurol 43:266, 1986.
14. Stephenson JBP: Reflex anoxic seizures ("white breath-holding"): nonepileptic vagal attacks, Arch Dis Child 53:193, 1978.
15. Vanasse M, Bedard P, and Andermann F: Shuddering attacks in children: an early clinical manifestation of essential tremor, Neurology 26:1027, 1976.
16. Woody RC and Kiel EA: Swallowing syncope in a child, Pediatrics 78:507, 1986.
17. Young D et al: Narcolepsy in a pediatric population, Am J Dis Child 142:210, 1988.

155

Odor (Unusual Urine and Body)

Modena Hoover Wilson

Odor may be relevant in the practice of pediatrics in several ways. Unusual or offensive odor may be the presenting or only complaint. Odor may be a diagnostic clue when other symptoms have prompted a medical visit or may confirm a suspected diagnosis. Unusual odor may be noticed first by the child, the family, others who have contact with the child, or the examiner. Each of these situations suggests a set of possibilities, which may overlap.

UNUSUAL ODOR AS THE CHIEF COMPLAINT

When unusual body odor is the chief complaint, relevant questions include the following: When was the odor first noticed? Of what does it remind the patient or family? Does it seem to come from any particular garments? Does bathing modify it; for how long? What other symptoms have been noted? Does anyone suspect that the child might have an object lodged in a body orifice? Is there drainage from any orifice or skin lesion? Is the child using any medications, either taken by mouth or applied topically? How has the odor affected the child and family?

ODOR AS A CLUE TO DIAGNOSIS

When a particular infection, metabolic defect, or ingestion is suspected for reasons other than odor, the clinician may inquire about or note the presence or absence of an odor that is often associated with the condition in order to clarify the clinical situation.[10,13,18]

An unexpected odor may be detected by the physician during history-taking or physical examination and requires explanation. For example, the lingering odor of feces or urine on a child who should have attained continence may prompt consideration of encopresis or enuresis.

If unusual odor is reported by the patient, especially intermittently, and never detected by others, the possibility of temporal lobe epilepsy should be entertained. On the other hand, if offensive body odor is noted by the clinician and denied by the patient or parent, anosmia affecting one or the other or both should be considered.

ODOR AND THE PHYSICAL EXAMINATION

When an odor needs to be explained, the examiner should observe the character of the odor, the age (and stage of pubertal development) of the patient, the presence or absence of other signs detected during a complete examination with the child unclothed, and localization of the odor to a particular body site.

Of those senses used in conducting the medical examination, the sense of smell is the least used. Satisfactory methods of classifying, quantifying, or even describing odors have been lacking. Gas liquid chromatography techniques now permit more precise identification of odors. Historically and practically, odors have been compared with others for which we have common experience, and their strength is characterized by the distance from which the odor is obvious or by such adjectives as "strong" or "faint." There are individual differences in the ability to detect at least some odors.

CAUSES OF UNUSUAL ODOR

To the careful observer, a myriad of odors are associated with the human body and with personal effects, such as clothing. There are also subtle differences in odor among persons. Therefore the first task may be to decide whether a particular odor is truly peculiar and whether it emanates from the body. It may be a usual body odor brought to attention because of its intensity or because of the complainant's unusual sensitivity or concern.

Usual Body Odor

Usual body odors derive from secretions of the sweat and apocrine glands, vagina, cervix, and respiratory tract and from urine, feces, breath, and flatus.[10] Odor may be modified by the action of normal or abnormal microbial flora. Halitosis refers to offensive breath and bromhidrosis to fetid perspiration.

Body odors often are minimized in our culture by frequent clothing changes, washing, deodorants or antiperspirants, mouthwashes, douches, or scents applied to the skin. If artificial odors are too strong, the clinician may wonder what the patient is trying to hide. On the other hand, when these customs are not practiced, the practitioner may detect odor he or she finds offensive and will need to decide if the patient's failure to comply with these social expectations is either precipitating or precipitated by psychosocial stress.

Body odor changes with puberty and characteristic adult odor may prompt a child or family to seek medical attention. Axillary odor is often the strongest one associated with adolescents and adults.[10] It varies in intensity from individual to individual, with pungency being caused by the action of aerobic diphtheroids on apocrine secretions. Axillary hair appears to retain or spread odor.[9]

Table 155-1 *Abnormalities of Metabolism Associated with Unusual Odor*

DISEASE	DESCRIPTION OF ODOR	CLINICAL FEATURES	METABOLIC DEFECT
Phenylketonuria	Musty, like a mouse, horse, wolf, or barn	Vomiting, progressive mental retardation and microcephaly, eczema, decreasing pigmentation, seizures, spasticity	Phenylalanine hydroxylase
Maple syrup urine disease	Maple syrup, burnt sugar, malt, caramel	Feeding difficulty, irregular respiration beginning in first week, marked acidosis, seizures, coma leading to death in first year or 2 of life Intermittent form without mental retardation but with episodes of ataxia and lethargy that may progress to coma Other variants, including thiamine, are responsive to treatment	Branched-chain decarboxylase
Oasthouse urine disease (methionine malabsorption syndrome)	Yeast, dried celery, malt, hops, beer	Diarrhea, mental retardation, spasticity, attacks of hyperpnea, fever, edema	Kidney and intestinal transport of methionine, branched-chain amino acids, tyrosine, and phenylalanine
Odor of sweaty feet syndrome 1 (isovalericacidemia)	Sweaty feet, cheese	Recurrent bouts of acidosis, vomiting, dehydration, coma, mild to moderate mental retardation, aversion to protein foods	Isovaleryl CoA dehydrogenase
Odor of sweaty feet syndrome 2 (N-butyric and N-hexanoic acidemia; may be same as odor of sweaty feet syndrome 1)	Sweaty feet	Poor feeding, weakness and lethargy developing in first week of life with acidosis, dehydration, seizures, and death in early months of life from bone marrow depression	Green acyldehydrogenase
Odor of cat urine syndrome (beta-methylcrotonylglycinuria)	Cat urine	Neurologic symptoms resembling Werdnig-Hoffmann disease, failure to thrive, ketoacidosis Biotin-response form	Beta-methylcrotonyl–CoA carboxylase
Fish odor syndrome 1	Dead fish	Stigmata of Turner syndrome, neutropenia, recurrent infections, anemia, splenomegaly	Unknown
Fish odor syndrome 2 (trimethylaminuria)	Dead or rotting fish, rancid butter, boiled cabbage	Normal development; has been induced in two premature infants by oral choline	Trimethylamine oxidase
Rancid butter syndrome	Rancid butter, boiled cabbage, decaying fish	Poor feeding, irritability, progressive neurologic deterioration with coma and seizures, death caused by infection in first 3 months	Unknown; hypermethioninemia, hypertyrosinemia, and generalized amino aciduria present; may be a form of acute tyrosinosis

Modified from Mace JW et al: The child with an unusual odor, Clin Pediatr 15:57, 1976; Hayden GF: Olfactory diagnosis in medicine, Postgrad Med 67:110, 1980.

Vaginal Odor

The odor of postpubertal vaginal secretions varies among individuals and with the menstrual cycle. Vulvar secretions, vaginal wall transudates, exfoliated cells, cervical mucus, fluids from the endometrium and uterine tubes, and metabolic products of the vaginal microflora all contribute.[7]

The resulting odor is characterized by many observers as unpleasant, even in the absence of vaginitis. Odor during menses is usually rated as the most offensive.[7] Awareness of these normal odors may cause concern in some individuals.

The "rotten fish" smell of the vaginal discharge associated with bacterial vaginosis is caused by trimethylamine.[1]

Mouth Odor

The odor of the healthy mouth is assumed to be inoffensive in childhood; however, "bad breath" is not uncommon, even in an otherwise well child. Halitosis in the absence of disease is thought to be at least in part caused by volatile sulfur compounds formed when the oral flora metabolize amino acid–containing compounds in saliva or adherent to teeth, tongue, or gums. Halitosis is exacerbated by infrequent eating and drinking, which ordinarily have a flushing action. Halitosis accompanies a variety of childhood respiratory tract and gastrointestinal infections. When it is persistent, halitosis should prompt a search for dental or gingival disease or a nasal foreign body. Infrequently, halitosis may reflect lung disease or gastroesophageal reflux.

Simple oral hygiene can modify mouth odor for about 3 hours. Brushing the teeth, along with the dorsoposterior surface of the tongue, followed by rinsing with water or a mouthwash, supposedly decreases both the concentrations of volatile sulfur compounds and the offensive odor.[17,20]

Foot Odor

Several types of localized dermatitis, including eczema, *Tinea pedis* infection, and pitted keratolysis, have been associated with increased foot odor. Little is known about the causes of excessive foot odor in the absence of apparent skin lesions. One group of investigators found that cultures of particularly smelly feet compared with other feet revealed higher counts of bacteria, especially those that produce lipid- and protein-degrading exoenzymes.[12] Moisture may promote such bacterial growth.

Abnormalities of Metabolism

Certain metabolic defects are associated with unusual odor of the urine,[2] sweat, and other body fluids because odoriferous metabolic precursors or byproducts accumulate. These conditions, although rare among the many possible causes of odor, are those most commonly linked to diagnosis by odor in pediatrics and are presented in Table 155-1.[3,11] They should be suspected when infants have unusual body odor, especially if the infant is doing poorly or is ketotic. Recognition of the odor in a compatible clinical situation may lead to early diagnosis and therapy that may prevent progressive brain damage or death. A specialist in metabolic disease should be contacted and an appropriate diet instituted while blood and urine amino acid analyses are completed.

Foreign Bodies

The retention of a foreign body in an orifice may lead to a fetid or foul smell with or without drainage or to generalized body odor, apparently because odoriferous substances are absorbed and secreted in sweat.[4] Most commonly implicated are nasal foreign bodies.[8,15] Vaginal tampons or diaphragms that have not been removed may promote odor. All orifices must be suspected and inspected.

Inhalations, Poisonings, and Ingestions

When inhalation or ingestion of a toxic substance is suspected, odor may provide a clue to the substance involved. Table 155-2 lists some common associations. When puzzled, the clinician should consult a poison control center.

Penicillin and cephalosporins impart a "medicinal" or musty smell to the urine. Topical benzoyl peroxide has been implicated in at least one case of persistent body odor.[14] Thiourea compounds cause the breath to have a sweet smell, like that of decaying vegetables.[19]

Newborns have smelled spicy after their mothers ingested particular curries before labor.[5]

Table 155-2 *Inhalations, Poisonings, and Ingestions Associated with Recognizable Odors*

ODOR	SITE	SUBSTANCE IMPLICATED
Fruity, like acetone or decomposing apples	Breath	Lacquer, chloroform, salicylates
Fruity, alcohol	Breath	Alcohol, phenol
Fruity, pearlike, acrid	Breath	Chloral hydrate, paraldehyde
Wintergreen	Breath	Methyl salicylate
Severe bad breath	Breath	Amphetamines
Bitter almond	Breath	Cyanide (chokecherry, apricot pits), jetberry bush
Burned rope	Breath	Marijuana
Camphor	Breath	Naphthalene (mothballs)
Coal gas	Breath	Coal gas (associated with odorless but toxic carbon monoxide)
Disinfectant	Breath	Phenol, creosote
Garlic	Breath	Phosphorus, arsenic, tellurium, parathion, malathion
Metallic	Breath	Iodine
	Stool	Arsenic
	Vomitus	Arsenic, phosphorus
Shoe polish	Breath	Nitrobenzene
Stale tobacco	Breath	Nicotine
Hydrocarbon	Breath, vomitus	Hydrocarbons
Violets	Urine, vomitus	Turpentine
Medicinal	Urine	Penicillins
Sulfides or amines	Skin	War gases

Modified from Hayden GF: Olfactory diagnosis in medicine, Postgrad Med 67:110, 1980; McMillan JA, Nieberg PI, and Oski FA: Diseases and poisonings associated with unusual breath odor. In The whole pediatrician catalog, Philadelphia, 1977, WB Saunders Co, p 106; Goldfrank L and Kirstein R: The aromatic vegetarian, Hosp Phys 3:12, 1976, Smith M, Smith LG, and Levinson B: The use of smell in differential diagnosis, Lancet 2(8313):1452, 1982.

Table 155-3 *Odor as a Clue to Infection*

ODOR	INFECTION
Foul, putrid breath or sputum	Lung abscess, empyema (especially anaerobic), bronchiectasis, fetid bronchitis
Severe halitosis	Trench mouth, tonsillitis, gingivitis
Ammoniacal urine	Urinary tract infection with urea-splitting bacteria
Musty or grapelike, especially in a patient with burns or wounds	*Pseudomonas* skin infection
Fetid sweat	Intranasal foreign body
Rancid stool	Shigellosis
Fishy vaginal discharge	Bacterial vaginosis
Foul vaginal discharge	Vaginal foreign body
Pus that smells like feces or overripe cheese	Proteolytic bacteria
Foul cerumen	*Pseudomonas* infection
Putrid smell from skin	Scurvy
Sweetish odor from mouth	Diphtheria
Butcher shop	Yellow fever
Beer odor in peritoneal dialysate	*Candida* infection[21]
Mousy	*Proteus* infection
Rotten apples	*Clostridium* gas gangrene
Stale beer	Scrofula
Fresh-baked brown bread	Typhoid fever
Cerebrospinal fluid smells like alcohol	*Cryptococcus* meningitis
Malodorous newborn	Amnionitis

Modified from Hayden GF: Olfactory diagnosis in medicine, Postgrad Med 67:110, 1980; Smith M, Smith LG, and Levinson B: The use of smell in differential diagnosis, Lancet 2(8313):1452, 1982; Schiffman SS: Taste and smell in disease, N Engl J Med 308:1337, 1983.

Table 155-4 *Some Other Diseases Associated with Specific Odors*

DISEASE	ODOR
Diabetic ketoacidosis, starvation	Ketones are present in breath and smell fruity, like acetone or decomposing apples
Uremia	Fishy smell to urine caused by dimethylamine and trimethylamine Ammoniacal smell to breath caused by ammonia
Acute tubular necrosis	Urine smells like stale water[16]
Hepatic failure	Breath smells like musty fish, raw liver, feces, or newly mown clover; caused by mercaptans and/or dimethyl sulfide
Intestinal obstruction, esophageal diverticulum	Breath smells feculent, foul
Schizophrenia	Sweat smells unpleasant, pungent, heavy; caused by trans-3-methyl-2-hexanoic acid
Skin diseases with protein breakdown	Skin smells foul, unpleasant
Intestinal obstruction, peritonitis	Vomitus smells like feces
Malabsorption	Stool smells foul
Portacaval shunt, portal vein thrombosis	Breath smells sweet

Modified from Hayden GF: Olfactory diagnosis in medicine, Postgrad Med 67:110, 1980; McMillan JA, Nieburg PI and Oski FA: Diseases and poisonings associated with unusual breath odor. In The whole pediatrician catalog, Philadelphia, 1977, WB Saunders Co, p 106; Smith M, Smith LG, and Levinson B: The use of smell in differential diagnosis, Lancet 2(8313):1452, 1982.

Other Diseases

Odor may suggest the presence of an infection or the type of infection (Table 155-3) or may confirm an acquired but noninfectious medical condition (Table 155-4).[6]

SUMMARY

Odor is imprecise. It is not surprising that olfactory cues have been minimized by today's clinicians, who have many other diagnostic aids.[6] Odor, however, should not be neglected, since it may be the chief concern of the patient or the most specific early indication of diagnosis and thereby may guide the choice of diagnostic tools and the prompt institution of therapy.

REFERENCES

1. Brand JM and Galask RP: Trimethylamine: the substance mainly responsible for the fishy odor often associated with bacterial vaginosis, Obstet Gynecol 68:682, 1986.
2. Burke DG et al: Profiles of urinary valatiles from metabolic disorders characterized by unusual odors, Clin Chem 29:1834, 1983.
3. Cone TE: Diagnosis and treatment: some diseases, syndromes, and conditions associated with an unusual odor, Pediatrics 41:993, 1968.
4. Feinstein RJ: Nasal foreign bodies and bromhidrosis (comment), JAMA 242:1031, 1979.
5. Hauser GJ et al: Peculiar odors in newborns and maternal prenatal ingestion of spicy food, Eur J Pediatr 144:403, 1985.
6. Hayden GF: Olfactory diagnosis in medicine, Postgrad Med 67(4):110, 1980.
7. Huggins GR and Preti G: Vaginal odors and secretions, Clin Obstet Gynecol 24:355, 1981.

8. Katz HP et al: Unusual presentation of nasal foreign bodies in children, JAMA 241: 1496, 1979.
9. Leyden JJ et al: The microbiology of the human axilla and its relationships to axillary odor, J Invest Dermatol 77:413, 1981.
10. Liddell K: Smell as a diagnostic marker, Postgrad Med J 52:136, 1976.
11. Mace JW et al: The child with an unusual odor, Clin Pediatr 15:57, 1976.
12. Marshall J, Holland KT, and Gribbon EM: A comparative study of the cutaneous microflora of normal feet with low and high levels of odour, J Appl Bacteriol 65:61, 1988.
13. McMillan JA, Neiburg PI, and Oski FA: Diseases and poisonings associated with unusual breath odor. In The whole pediatrician catalog, Philadelphia, 1977, WB Saunders Co.
14. Molberg P: Body odor from topical benzoyl peroxide (letter), N Engl J Med 304:1366, 1981.
15. Moriarty RA: Nasal foreign body presenting as an unusual odor, Am J Dis Child 132:97, 1978.
16. Najarian JS: The diagnostic importance of the odor of urine (letter), N Engl J Med 303:1128, 1980.
17. Schmidt NF and Tarbet WJ: The effect of oral rinses on organoleptic mouth odor ratings and levels of volatile sulfur compounds, Oral Surg 45:876, 1978.
18. Smith M, Smith LG, and Levinson B: The use of smell in differential diagnosis, Lancet 2(8313):1452, 1982.
19. Stewart WK and Fleming LW: Use your nose (letter), Lancet 1(8321): 426, 1983.
20. Tonzetich J and Ng SK: Reduction of malodor by oral cleansing procedures, J Oral Surg 42:172, 1976.
21. Turney JH: Use your nose (letter), Lancet 1(8321):426, 1983.

156

Petechiae and Purpura

Reggie E. Duerst

Although patency of the body's vascular system is required to ensure continued delivery of nutrients and oxygen to the tissues, immediate steps must be taken to limit any blood loss if the integrity of a blood vessel is disrupted. Primary hemostasis comprises adherence of platelets to the injured endothelium or subendothelium and initiation of thrombus formation. Defects in primary hemostasis are manifested by minute, 1 to 2 mm hemorrhagic spots called *petechiae* following capillary injury. *Purpuric lesions* represent a confluence of petechiae or extravasated blood from a larger vessel; *ecchymoses* result if the extravasated blood extends along a fascial plane.

Many disorders result in the formation of petechiae or purpura or both. Although the underlying etiology may be benign, serious life-threatening illnesses such as meningococcemia, disseminated intravascular coagulopathy (DIC), or purpura fulminans must also be considered. Immediate action should be taken to halt progression of these life-threatening diseases. Also, intracranial hemorrhage must be considered in any child being evaluated for changes in consciousness who also has petechiae or purpuric lesions.

The differential diagnosis of disorders leading to development of petechiae or purpura includes many other serious, potentially life-threatening syndromes or diseases. The pathophysiology of these disorders, although varied, ultimately leads to defective primary hemostasis. These disorders can be manifestations of (1) decreased number of platelets, (2) platelet dysfunction, or (3) defective vessels. An approach for evaluating a patient with petechiae and/or purpura is presented in the box on p. 1024.

The rapidity of onset of purpura and associated signs of systemic illness provide clues that will help in the initial assessment of the gravity of a patient's illness. A well-appearing child with petechiae isolated to a well-circumscribed location may have self-inflicted them by suction (factitious petechiae). A lethargic, febrile patient with rapid onset of diffuse petechiae needs immediate management of sepsis and DIC. As noted above, the distribution of purpuric lesions may also assist in making a diagnosis. Involvement of the buttocks and lower extremities is classic for Henoch-Schönlein purpura; prominence of purpura about hair follicles is characteristic of scurvy.

NORMAL HEMOSTASIS

The pathophysiologic mechanisms underlying formation of petechiae are each associated with different steps in primary hemostasis. Following vascular injury, the subendothelium is exposed, and the blood elements are no longer confined within the vessel. Primary hemostasis, illustrated in Fig. 156-1, is initiated when factor VIII–von Willebrand factor (vWF) is released from endothelial cells and adheres to the exposed collagen matrix. Factor VIII–vWF, in turn, binds to platelets via the platelet surface glycoprotein Ib(gpIb). Next, the platelets that have adhered to the subendothelium release their granule contents. Additional platelets aggregate in response to adenosine diphosphate (ADP) released from the granules. Synthesis and release of thromboxane A_2 (TxA_2) by the platelets results in vasoconstriction and further enhancement of platelet plug formation.

Secondary hemostatic mechanisms include activation of factor X at the platelet membrane surface, prothrombin conversion to thrombin, and thrombin catalyzed polymerization of fibrin. Thrombin also provides positive feedback for primary hemostasis by stimulating platelets to release ADP and synthesize TxA_2. Finally, the clot is stabilized by cross-linking of fibrin strands, a reaction catalyzed by activated factor XIII.

After repair of the damaged endothelium, the clot that has been formed eventually needs to be degraded so that normal blood flow may resume. Plasminogen (which is incorporated into the fibrin clot as it is produced) is converted to the proteolytic enzyme plasmin by the action of plasminogen activators (e.g., tissue plasminogen activator and urokinase). Plasmin cleaves fibrin, forming fibrin degradation products (or fibrin split products) and causing clot dissolution. Thus hemostasis—formation and degradation of a clot—is an ongoing "homeostatic" process designed to maintain vascular integrity and thereby blood flow.

THROMBOCYTOPENIA

Thrombocytopenia is the most frequent cause of bleeding. Regulation of platelet production and maintenance of the normal platelet count (150,000-400,000/μl) is poorly understood. If platelet function is normal, abnormal bleeding will usually not occur unless the platelet count is less than 100,000/μl. Decreases in the platelet count may result from hypoproduction, enhanced destruction, maldistribution, or dilution (e.g., a patient who is hemorrhaging and receiving insufficient platelet replacement). If the decrease in platelet count is caused by excessive platelet destruction despite greatly increased production, symptomatic bleeding will often not develop until the platelet count falls below 20,000/μl. This suggests that the newly produced platelet may have enhanced coagulant function.

Evaluation of Petechiae and Purpura

1. History/Physical Examination
   - Duration/rapidity of onset
   - "Sick versus well"
   - Distribution of lesions
2. Platelet Count
   - A. Low (<150,000)
   - B. Normal (>150,000)
   - *Platelet Dysfunction, Congenital*
     - Glanzmann thrombasthenia
     - Bernard-Soulier syndrome
     - Wiskott-Aldrich syndrome
     - Storage pool defect
   - *Platelet Dysfunction, Acquired*
     - Aspirin or aspirin-like drugs
     - Liver disease
     - Uremia
     - Paraproteinemia—dysgammaglobulinemia, cystic fibrosis
   - *Von Willebrand Disease*
   - *Vascular Defect, Congenital*
     - Ehlers-Danlos syndrome
     - Osler-Weber-Rendu syndrome
   - *Vascular Defect, Acquired*
     - Trauma—lacerations, abuse
     - Factitious
     - Vasculitis
       - Drugs
       - Infection—Bacterial, viral, rickettsial
       - Henoch-Schönlein purpura (HSP)
     - Senile purpura
     - Steroid purpura
     - Scurvy
3. Blood Smear
   - Verify low platelet count
   - Look for *Microangiopathic Changes*
     - Kasabach-Merritt syndrome
     - DIC
     - HUS
     - TTP
     - Liver disease
4. PT, aPTT (±FDP, Fibrinogen)
   - *Abnormal*
     - As above, plus:
     - Histiocytosis X
     - Familial erythrophagocytic lymphohistiocytosis (FEL)
   - *Normal* See Below
5. Bone Marrow Examination
   - *Decreased Megakaryocytes*
   - *Aplasia, congenital*
     - Thrombocytopenia absent radii (TAR)
     - Fanconi anemia
     - Bernard-Soulier syndrome
     - Wiskott-Aldrich syndrome
     - Metabolic disorders
   - *Aplasia, acquired*
     - Idiopathic
     - Nutritional—iron, B-12, folate
     - Drug, chemical, toxin, radiation
     - Rubella, other "TORCH"
   - *Infiltration*
     - Leukemia, lymphoma
     - Neuroblastoma or other metastatic solid tumor
     - Storage diseases
   - *Normal—Increased Megakaryocytes*
   - *Immune destruction*
     - Immune thrombocytopenic purpura (ITP), acute and chronic
     - Isoimmune phenomena
     - Post-transfusion purpura
     - Drug sensitivity
     - HIV-1/AIDS
   - *Other*
     - Histiocytosis X
     - Virally associated hematophagocytic syndrome (VAHS)
     - FEL
     - Intravascular prostheses
     - May-Hegglin anomaly
     - Hypersplenism with sequestration

Hypoproductive Thrombocytopenia

Inadequate production of platelets can be divided between congenital and acquired conditions. Congenital disorders include infants with the syndrome of thrombocytopenia and absent radii (TAR). These infants are readily recognized by their upper extremity deformities. The platelet count is in the 15,000-30,000/μl range, and megakaryocytes are reduced or absent in the bone marrow. There is gradual improvement in platelet production after the first year of life. Congenital amegakaryocytic thrombocytopenia is also present in Fanconi anemia. Patients with Bernard-Soulier syndrome may also be mildly thrombocytopenic secondary to hypoproduction (the functional defect in the platelets in these individuals is more significantly related to bleeding; see below). May-Hegglin anomaly (giant platelets and Döhle bodies in the leukocytes) is rarely associated with thrombocytopenia and bleeding. Wiskott-Aldrich syndrome (WAS) is an X-linked recessive disorder characterized by immunodeficiency, platelet dysfunction, and thrombocytopenia. The combination of thrombocytopenia and platelet dysfunction places the patient at great risk for hemorrhage. Treatment of these disorders is supportive—avoidance of aspirin or aspirinlike drugs and use of protective head gear, the antifibrinolytic agent epsilon-aminocaproic acid (EACA), and if necessary, platelet transfusions.

Marrow aplasia also results in hypoproductive thrombocytopenia. Marrow aplasia following exposure to drugs or other toxic chemicals may be temporary and resolve when the causative agent is withdrawn. Immunosuppressive therapy, bone marrow transplantation, or both may be required for patients with severe aplastic anemia. Extensive infiltration of bone marrow in patients with leukemia, lymphoma, or metastatic solid tumor prevents normal platelet production.

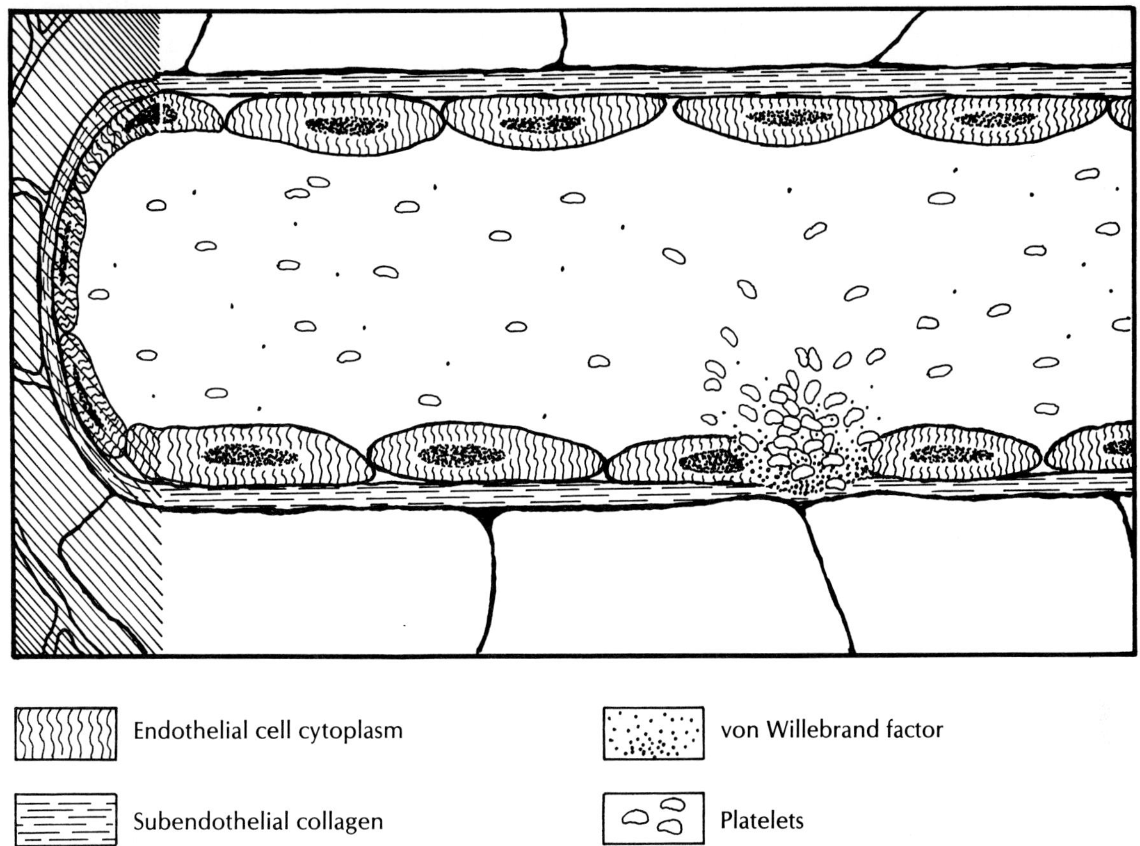

Fig. 156-1 Primary hemostasis comprises platelet adherence to Factor VIII-vWF coated subendothelial collagen followed by platelet aggregation and "platelet plug" formation.

Infectious agents may also produce ineffective thrombocytopoiesis and thrombocytopenia.

Destructive Thrombocytopenia

Acute idiopathic thrombocytopenic purpura (ITP) is the most frequent cause of severe thrombocytopenia and bleeding in childhood. ITP is usually a temporary disorder with 80% to 90% of children completely recovering within 1 year of diagnosis. The incidence of life-threatening hemorrhage or intracranial bleeding is less than 0.1% to 1% and greatest at the onset of the disease. Chronic ITP or other diseases associated with immune dysfunction (i.e., lupus erythematosus, Evan syndrome) develop in 10% to 20% of patients who manifest acute ITP. Thrombocytopenia is a result of increased removal of platelets from the circulation by monocyte-macrophage cells of the reticuloendothelial (RE) cell system. Adherence to the platelet surface of specific antiplatelet autoantiody or immune complexes leads to phagocytosis of the platelets by the RE cells. Bone marrow examination should be performed to exclude an infiltrative process. Treatment with corticosteroids or high doses of intravenous immunoglobulin appears to shorten the initial period of severe thrombocytopenia but has not been shown to affect the long-term prognosis for this generally self-limited disorder.

Isoimmune thrombocytopenia develops in a neonate when maternal antibody is made to a paternal platelet antigen (not expressed on maternal platelets) inherited by the infant. Pl^{A1} is a platelet antigen expressed on 98% of the population's platelets; thus approximately 1% of women are at risk of developing anti-Pl^{A1} antibody during pregnancy. Antibody to the Pl^{A1} antigen has also been implicated in posttransfusion purpura. In this condition, severe thrombocytopenia and mucocutaneous bleeding develop 5 to 8 days after a blood product transfusion. It occurs most commonly in women who have been previously sensitized to Pl^{A1}-positive platelets. Drugs that act as a hapten with platelet surface antigens to form an immunogenic moiety can cause an immune thrombocytopenia. Platelet destruction continues as long as the drug-platelet neoantigen is present. Quinidine, cimetidine, and trimethoprim-sulfamethoxazole have been shown to cause thrombocytopenia by this mechanism.

Destruction of platelets resulting from nonimmunologic platelet injury occurs in children with hemolytic-uremic syndrome (HUS) and adults with thrombotic thrombocytopenic purpura (TTP). These disorders are both associated with microangiopathic hemolytic anemia, endothelial cell injury, and platelet consumption. HUS primarily affects the renal glomerular capillaries, but other organs (including the brain) may be involved. Thrombocytopenia of Kasabach-Merritt syndrome results from platelet consumption in a giant hemangioma. Intravascular prostheses may also cause significant platelet destruction.

Several disorders associated with RE cell proliferation also result in platelet consumption that is not antibody mediated. Patients with histiocytosis X, virally associated hematophagocytic syndrome (VAHS), and familial erythrophagocytic lymphohistiocytosis (FEL) can develop thrombocytopenia as a result of excessive phagocytosis of platelets by abnormal histiocytic cells. If these disease processes are active, splenomegaly is often present, and the spleen is a major site of platelet destruction. Sequestration of platelets in an enlarged spleen (regardless of cause) will also cause a reduction in measured circulating platelet concentration. Bleeding symptoms, however, are infrequent, for the platelet count is not severely reduced.

DEFECTIVE PLATELET FUNCTION

Defects in platelet function can be subdivided by the step in primary hemostasis (platelet adhesion, release, and aggregation) at which the defect is expressed. Adherence of platelets to the exposed subendothelium is mediated by a factor VIII–von Willebrand factor complex. Von Willebrand factor is a glycoprotein of 240,000 molecular weight subunits synthesized primarily by endothelial cells. It is complexed with factor VIII and circulates as multimers of the basic subunit. Larger multimers are more active in promoting coagulation than are monomers or small oligomers. Von Willebrand disease (vWD) is a heterogeneous disorder (at least seven subtypes) involving vWF. Patients may have (1) reduced synthesis of vWF, (2) synthesis of defective vWF, or (3) disordered assembly of the vWF complexes. The inheritance of most forms of vWD follows autosomal dominant transmission. The prevalence of the disease is approximately 3 to 7 per 100,000. The activated partial thromboplastin time and bleeding time are generally prolonged. Factor VIII activity is normal, but ristocetin cofactor activity is reduced. Treatment of active bleeding or prophylaxis before elective surgery involves infusion of desmopressin acetate (1-deamino-8-D-arginine-vasopressin; DDAVP) or cryoprecipitate. DDAVP is effective for most forms of vWD and acts by stimulating endothelial cell release of factor VIII–vWF complexes. Cryoprecipitate provides an exogenous source of factor VIII–vWF and secondarily stimulates further production and release of factor VIII–vWF. However, cryoprecipitate can be associated with transmission of blood-borne viral infections. DDAVP is the current treatment of choice (subtype IIb of vWD is the exception). Bernard-Soulier syndrome is also characterized by a defect in platelet adhesion. Platelet binding to vWF is diminished because of lack of the vWF ligand, gpIb, on the platelet membrane. Platelet transfusion is necessary to correct this disorder, but refractoriness to later transfusions because of development of antibody to platelet gpIb mandates that transfusion be withheld unless absolutely necessary.

Glanzmann thrombasthenia is caused by congenital deficiency or absence of platelet surface antigen glycoprotein IIb/IIIa. This deficiency results in defective binding of platelets to fibrinogen and a decrease in platelet aggregation following activation. Platelet transfusion can be life saving, but its use should be minimized to prevent antibody formation. Deficiency of alpha-granules in the platelets of patients with gray platelet syndrome (named for the platelet appearance on routine blood smears) results in a decrease of coagulation factors available for release following aggregation. Several heterogeneous deficiencies in dense granules are collectively termed *storage pool defects* and result in defective platelet release of ADP and serotonin. This defect is also associated with Wiscott-Aldrich syndrome, Chédiak-Steinbrinck-Higashi syndrome, and Hermansky-Pudlak syndrome. Other diseases associated with defects in platelet granule release include disorders of platelet arachidonic acid metabolism and type 1 glycogen storage disease (glucose 6-phosphatase deficiency). The latter disorder is associated with decreased ADP release during episodes of hypoglycemia.

Acquired platelet dysfunction is characteristic of uremia. Retention of metabolites otherwise cleared by the kidney appears to be causative, and significant bleeding may occur as a result. DDAVP is very useful for prophylaxis against bleeding if a uremic patient requires a surgical procedure. Liver disease and myeloproliferative and lymphoproliferative disorders have also been associated with acquired platelet dysfunction.

VASCULAR DEFECTS

Congenital

A consequence of several congenital vascular disorders is a predisposition to the development of purpuric lesions. The telangiectasia of Osler-Weber-Rendu disease is a consequence of vascular anomalies that include a thin endothelial lining. Thrombocytopenia of Kasabach-Merritt syndrome is a result of consumption within the cavernous arteriovenous malformation. Patients with congenital connective tissue disorders that result in defective collagen or elastin can exhibit "vascular purpura." These disorders include osteogenesis imperfecta, Ehlers-Danlos syndrome, Marfan syndrome, and pseudoexanthoma elasticum.

Acquired

Acquired vascular conditions can be manifested by petechiae or purpura. Vasculitis develops in response to drugs, toxins, or a host of infectious organisms (e.g., meningococcus, yellow fever virus, and rickettsiae). Systemic lupus erythematosus, rheumatoid arthritis, or other collagen-vascular diseases can display purpura resulting from vasculitis. Henoch-Schönlein purpura is a syndrome of widespread acute vasculitis that may cause a rash (vasculitis in the skin) and arthralgia (vasculitis in the joints). Vasculitis in the gastrointestinal tract may cause abdominal pain, bowel wall edema, partial obstruction, and intussusception. Renal complications (proteinuria, hypertension, renal failure) can be observed. Late renal sequelae are confined to patients who have renal involvement during the acute illness.

Vitamin C is required for normal collagen synthesis. Patients with scurvy may develop purpuric lesions as a result of the abnormal collagen in the subendothelium. Prominence of the bleeding at the base of hair follicles is characteristic of scurvy. Senile purpura (purpura of the elderly) is another manifestation of abnormal collagen in the subendothelium. Dysproteinemias and conditions that result in elevated gamma globulinemia (including cystic fibrosis) have been shown to promote formation of petechiae or purpura.

SUGGESTED READINGS

Bell WR and Jackson DP: Bleeding: hemostasis, approach to patient, and vascular defects. In Harvey AM et al, editors: The principles and practice of medicine, 1988, East Norwalk, Conn, Appleton & Lange.

Handin RI: Physiology of coagulation: the platelet. In Nathan DG and Oski FA, editors: Hematology of infancy and childhood, Philadelphia, 1987, WB Saunders Co.

Jackson DP and Bell WR: Disorders of blood platelets. In Harvey AM et al, editors: The principles and practice of medicine, 1988, East Norwalk, Conn, Appleton & Lange.

Marcus AJ: Hemorrhagic disorders: abnormalities of platelet and vascular function. In Wyngaarden JB and Smith LH Jr, editors: Cecil textbook of medicine, Philadelphia, 1988, WB Saunders Co.

Stuart MJ and Kelton JG: The platelet: quantitative and qualitative abnormalities. In Nathan DG and Oski FA, editors: Hematology of infancy and childhood, Philadelphia, 1987, WB Saunders Co.

157

Polyuria

Samuel M. Libber and Leslie P. Plotnick

Polyuria, or excessive urinary volume, is a symptom common to a large number of pediatric disorders. It may be defined as urine production of more than 900 $ml/m^2/day$. It is often associated with frequent urination, nocturia, or enuresis. Sometimes the pediatrician is called on to evaluate this symptom without knowing the exact daily urinary volume; in such situations, a detailed history of fluid intake and urinary habits may help delineate the primary symptom.

A normal homeostatic response to the presence of polyuria is the development of increased thirst; with subsequent liquid intake, then, water balance will remain intact. In the older child, the parent may perceive this symptom to be more prominent than the polyuria. However, in infants who have polyuria and are unable to maintain free access to fluids, negative water balance results, and weight loss, dehydration, and electrolyte disturbances often occur. When chronic or recurrent electrolyte disturbances plague the infant, growth failure and central nervous system (CNS) injury may result.

DIFFERENTIAL DIAGNOSIS

In reaching a diagnosis in the patient with polyuria, the clinician first needs to bear in mind a general overview of the systems that may cause this symptom, as indicated in the accompanying box. A CNS or pituitary lesion may reduce vasopressin secretion; a renal defect may limit the kidney's ability to respond to vasopressin; a compulsion to drink may be the primary cause of polyuria; or excretion of an osmotically active urine may bring about large volume loss.

Central or neurogenic diabetes insipidus is a condition in which the secretion of vasopressin by the posterior lobe of the pituitary gland is limited. Consequently, a dilute urine or large volume is passed, and the crucial function of water conservation in times of volume depletion is lost. In rare cases there may be a familial idiopathic vasopressin deficiency inherited generally as an autosomal dominant trait. More commonly, however, cases are sporadic; in these cases, a search for a specific underlying organic lesion and concomitant anterior pituitary dysfunction is necessary.[2] Injury to the CNS, whether traumatic or surgical, may be associated with a decrease in vasopressin production or release. Likewise, thrombosis or hemorrhage involving the hypothalamus or pituitary gland may result in vasopressin deficiency. Abnormalities in vasopressin secretion may accompany CNS infections. Just as the syndrome of inappropriate antidiuretic hormone (SIADH) may accompany meningitis in the acute states, clinical diabetes insipidus may supervene as a chronic sequela to CNS infections.[8]

Congenital intracranial defects (such as septooptic dysplasia and encephalocele) have also been associated with diabetes insipidus. Brain tumors (craniopharyngioma, glioma, dysgerminoma, metastatic tumor) represent the most frequent etiology for central diabetes insipidus. The recent finding of

Differential Diagnosis of Polyuria in Childhood

- I. Neurogenic vasopressin deficiency
  - A. Idiopathic
    - 1. Familial
    - 2. Sporadic
  - B. Organic
    - 1. Posttrauma
    - 2. Vascular event
    - 3. Following infection
    - 4. CNS tumor
    - 5. Systemic infiltrative diseases (histiocytosis, syphilis, tuberculosis, sarcoidosis)
    - 6. Guillain-Barré syndrome
    - 7. Congenital intracranial defect
    - 8. Autoimmune disorders
- II. Primary polydipsia
- III. Renal vasopressin insensitivity
  - A. Congenital
    - 1. Hereditary nephrogenic diabetes insipidus
    - 2. Other renal tubular defects (cystinosis, distal renal tubular acidosis, Bartter syndrome)
    - 3. Structural defect
  - B. Acquired
    - 1. Postinfectious
    - 2. Postobstructive
    - 3. Drug induced
    - 4. Associated with systemic disease (sickle cell disease, sarcoidosis, amyloidosis)
    - 5. Metabolic (hypercalcemia, hypokalemia)
- IV. Osmotic diuresis
  - A. Diet induced
  - B. Drug induced
  - C. Insulin-dependent diabetes mellitus
  - D. Noninsulin-dependent diabetes mellitus
  - E. Renal glycosuria

vasopressin cell antibodies in some children with diabetes insipidus suggests a possible autoimmune origin.[10,11] Finally, patients with any of a variety of systemic illnesses (histiocytosis, syphilis, tuberculosis, sarcoidosis, Guillain-Barré syndrome) have developed vasopressin deficiency.

An unusual association between diabetes mellitus and diabetes insipidus has been described.[9] A review by Greger et al suggests that in recent years, fewer cases are diagnosed as idiopathic, and a higher proportion has been diagnosed as secondary to CNS infection or intracranial birth defects.[4] The search for an organic lesion must be diligent and persistent; an underlying lesion may not be diagnosed at the initial evaluation.

Primary polydipsia, or compulsive water drinking, is a rare cause of polyuria in childhood.[5] This entity differs from all other diagnoses in that the polyuria is a consequence, not a cause, of polydipsia. It occurs most commonly in older children or adults with emotional disturbances. About 80% of cases are believed to occur in females, and the ailment has a gradual onset as opposed to the more abrupt onset typical of central diabetes insipidus. Although this entity has been thought to be caused by a primary psychiatric disturbance, a recent study of adult psychiatric patients with polydipsia and hyponatremia showed evidence of a defect in water excretion, osmoregulation of water intake, and in vasopressin secretion.[3]

Renal disorders may be associated with polyuria because of an inability of the renal tubule to concentrate urine despite normal circulating levels of vasopressin. This may be a congenital or an acquired abnormality. Hereditary nephrogenic diabetes insipidus is an X-linked, recessive disorder in which polyuria, fever, failure to thrive, and hypernatremic dehydration occur in early infancy. Although a precise defect has not been identified, renal tubular cells lack the ability to respond to vasopressin. Older children and adults may be able to adjust their oral fluid intake to maintain constant serum osmolality, but infants do not have this ability. The condition can be associated with damage to the CNS or even death if the infant develops recurrent hypernatremic dehydration. Thus prompt recognition and treatment are needed so that such sequelae are prevented. Besides the hereditary form of nephrogenic diabetes insipidus, the clinician must also consider other renal tubular defects in which vasopressin resistance has been observed. Patients with cystinosis, distal renal tubular acidosis, and Bartter syndrome may exhibit a clinical picture of polyuria.

In addition to this functional tubular impairment, congenital structural abnormalities that can cause polyuria may also occur. In medullary cystic disease and oligomeganephronia, a condition in which renal tubules are abnormally large and reduced in number, the architecture of the kidney is distorted, with a subsequent abnormality in regulating renal output. In chronic pyelonephritis or in obstructive uropathy, damage to the tubules or disturbance in the medullary osmotic gradient may result in nephrogenic diabetes insipidus. Drugs such as lithium, demeclocycline, and amphotericin have been known to result in functional vasopressin insensitivity. Likewise, hypercalcemia and hypokalemia may each be associated with a nephropathy in which tubular ability to conserve water is lost. Finally, systemic disorders such as sickle cell disease, sarcoidosis, and amyloidosis may cause renal tubular dysfunction and result in polyuria.

The final major group of disorders causing polyuria is that in which renal water loss results from an osmotic diuresis. In rare cases this may be diet induced, as in individuals who are tube fed on a diet high in protein and sodium. Drugs such as mannitol, urea, and glycerol, as well as radiologic contrast agents, may be responsible for this picture. Glycosuria is one of the most frequent findings in children with acquired polyuria; in these patients, insulin-dependent diabetes mellitus is the most likely explanation (see Chapter 197, "Diabetes Mellitus"). Polyuria, polydipsia, polyphagia, and weight loss compose the symptom complex most commonly seen in these patients. Noninsulin-dependent diabetes mellitus is relatively rare in childhood but may occur in the obese child or adolescent. In both situations glycosuria results from diminished carbohydrate utilization, and a loss of water and electrolytes ensues. In renal glycosuria, insulin secretion and activity are entirely normal, but renal tubular cells have a diminished rate of maximal glucose reabsorption. As a result, glycosuria occurs in the absence of hyperglycemia. Glucose, when present in the urine in large amounts, acts as an osmotic diuretic and causes polyuria.

EVALUATION

The initial laboratory procedure of highest yield is a urinalysis performed on a "first morning" voided specimen. A high specific gravity ($\geq$1.020) will generally be found in patients with osmotic diuresis or in normal persons, whereas a specific gravity of $\leq$1.008 is found in patients with nephrogenic or central diabetes insipidus. Patients with damage to renal tubular epithelium—for example, persons with sickle cell disease—are more likely to have isosthenuria with specific gravities in the neighborhood of 1.010. The presence of protein, casts, or formed blood elements in the urine would likewise suggest a renal disorder. In patients with glycosuria, the presence of ketonuria would strongly suggest insulin-dependent diabetes mellitus; if glycosuria without ketonuria is present, one must distinguish further whether the patient has diabetes mellitus or renal glycosuria. A normal serum glucose concentration would point to a diagnosis of renal glycosuria.

Examination of serum electrolytes, glucose, urea nitrogen, creatinine, calcium, and osmolality is also indicated. A hyperosmolar state would suggest vasopressin deficiency or insensitivity, provided the serum glucose concentration is normal. A low serum osmolality would suggest primary polydipsia as the most likely diagnosis. Evidence of renal impairment, hypercalcemia, and hypokalemia will also be uncovered in such an examination.

In polyuric individuals with a low urine specific gravity and without glycosuria, the next step in the evaluation is a water deprivation test, the purpose of which is to determine the capability of the child to conserve water at times when antidiuresis is necessary for homeostasis. After a 24-hour period of adequate hydration, blood is drawn to determine sodium, osmolality, and urea nitrogen levels and to perform a hematocrit; the urine osmolality and specific gravity are measured, the child is weighed, and his or her intake and output are recorded. The child is then restricted from any food or fluid intake for a 6- to 8-hour period. The child is then weighed hourly, at which time urine output and specific gravity are measured and serum sodium is determined. Following the study period, the initial blood tests are repeated, urine osmolality is remeasured, and the final weight is recorded. If at any point the child has lost 5% or more of body weight, the test is terminated, once final blood studies are obtained. Because of the possibility of volume depletion, it is recommended that the study be carried out during the day when supervision is optimal. In normal children and in most children with psychogenic polydipsia, the weight remains constant, the urine specific gravity increases to at least 1.010, the urine volume decreases, and the ratio of urine to plasma osmolality rises to at least 2:1. However, if diuresis continues in the absence of oral intake and if weight loss and a hyperosmolar state develop, one should suspect a diagnosis of diabetes insipidus, either central or nephrogenic.

Performance of the vasopressin test is the next step in the evaluation of a polyuric patient when the water deprivation test shows a specific gravity of less than 1.015 (Table 157-1). The purpose of this test is to determine whether the excessive urine flow responds to exogenous vasopressin. This test is best done immediately following the water deprivation test. Aqueous vasopressin in a dose of 6 U/m^2 is administered subcutaneously, and the patient is allowed free access to water. Subsequently, intake, output, and urine specific gravity are recorded every 30 to 60 minutes. Normal subjects and patients with vasopressin deficiency will evidence a reduced fluid intake and output and a rise in urine specific gravity to at least 1.015. Urine osmolality will likewise increase significantly. Individuals with partial diabetes insipidus will demonstrate a modest rise in urine concentration on water deprivation testing (urinary osmolality less than 400 mosm/kg) but will concentrate their urine after receiving vasopressin. Patients with primary polydipsia will maintain a constant intake but will generally decrease their urine output and increase their urine specific gravity. If no response to vasopressin occurs after 6 hours, the test should be repeated using a dose of 12 U/m^2 subcutaneously. If the patient shows no effect after this double dose, nephrogenic diabetes insipidus is probably the diagnosis.

MANAGEMENT

Patients with evidence of vasopressin deficiency are best referred to an endocrinologist or neurologist to determine the cause of the diabetes insipidus. Skull roentgenograms, visual field examination, full investigation of other pituitary functions, and computed tomography of the head will likely be the next steps in evaluation. Patients should be allowed free access to fluids, and their serum and urine osmolality should be closely monitored. In a severely ill patient, aqueous vasopressin, 0.1 to 0.2 U/kg, may be given subcutaneously every 4 to 6 hours.

Aqueous vasopressin may also be given by constant intravenous infusion. Starting dosages reported vary from 1.3 to 4.6 mU/kg/hour and should be increased or decreased as needed.[1,7] Once the child's condition has stabilized, management consists of desmopressin acetate (DDAVP), a synthetic derivative of vasopressin, instilled intranasally at a dosage of 5 to 20 μg twice daily. The use of thiazide diuretics, chlorpropamide, and clofibrate has met with some success in the management of diabetes insipidus but generally lacks the efficacy of vasopressin derivatives.

In patients with primary polydipsia, once a neurogenic lesion has been ruled out, medical therapy is not indicated. Psychotherapy, however, may be useful in addressing the emotional problem causing the polydipsia.

Patients with structural renal diseases leading to polyuria can be referred to a nephrologist; patients with nephrogenic diabetes insipidus are commonly seen by an endocrinologist or a nephrologist. They should be allowed free access to fluids; parents of infants with this disorder need to offer frequent water feedings to allow their infants to maintain osmotic homeostasis. A low-salt diet has been helpful in reducing urine output; thiazide diuretics cause further reduction in polyuria by reducing the amount of urine delivered to the distal tubule. Recently, indomethacin has been shown to be effective in limiting urine output even further, probably as a result of the enhanced sodium reabsorption caused by inhibition of prostaglandin synthesis.[6]

Osmotic diuresis induced by drugs or diet is generally self-limited. Although renal glycosuria requires no specific therapy, such a diagnosis can be made only when other renal tubular functions are normal. In overweight patients with noninsulin-dependent diabetes mellitus, weight reduction is paramount. This measure alone is usually sufficient to reverse the carbohydrate intolerance. If glycosuria persists, insulin may be prescribed by an endocrinologist. In insulin-dependent diabetes mellitus, patients with polydipsia and polyuria should be hospitalized to stabilize the abnormal carbohydrate metabolism with exogenous insulin, to correct the electrolyte disturbance, and to educate the patient and family about home management (see Chapter 197).

Management of polyuria therefore depends heavily on the underlying diagnosis and must be carefully individualized. Results in most cases are gratifying, but patients frequently are found to have a chronic disease that requires close, long-term surveillance.

Table 157-1 *Interpretation of Vasopressin Test*

	INTAKE	OUTPUT	URINE SPECIFIC GRAVITY
Normal	↓	↓	↑
Psychogenic polydipsia	Unchanged	↓	↑
Central diabetes insipidus	↓	↓	↑
Nephrogenic diabetes insipidus	Unchanged	Unchanged	Unchanged

REFERENCES

1. Chanson P et al: Ultralow doses of vasopressin in the management of diabetes insipidus, Crit Care Med 15:44, 1987.
2. Czernichow P et al: Diabetes insipidus in children. III. Anterior pituitary dysfunction in idopathic types, J Pediatr 106:41, 1985.
3. Goldman M, Luchins D, and Robertson G: Mechanisms of altered water metabolism in psychotic patients with polydipsia and hyponatremia, N Engl J Med 318:397, 1988.
4. Greger N et al: Central diabetes insipidus: 22 years' experience, Am J Dis Child 140:551, 1986.
5. Kohn B et al: Hysterical polydipsia (compulsive water drinking) in children, Am J Dis Child 130:210, 1976.
6. Libber S, Harrison H, and Spector D: Treatment of nephrogenic diabetes insipidus with prostaglandin synthesis inhibitors, J Pediatr 108:305, 1986.
7. McDonald et al: Treatment of the young child with postoperative central diabetes insipidus, Am J Dis Child 143:201, 1989.
8. Moses AM: Diabetes insipidus and ADH regulation, Hosp Pract 12:37, 1977.
9. Raiti S, Plotkin S, and Newns G: Diabetes mellitus and insipidus in two sisters, Br Med J 2:1625, 1963.
10. Scherbaum W et al: Diabetes insipidus in children. IV. A possible autoimmune type with vasopressin cell antibodies, J Pediatr 107:922, 1985.
11. Scherbaum W et al: Autoimmune cranial diabetes insipidus: its association with other endocrine diseases and with histiocytosis X, Clin Endocrinol 25:411, 1986.

158

Proteinuria

Edward J. Ruley

The presence of abnormal amounts of protein in the urine may be asymptomatic or, if severe enough to cause hypoproteinemia, associated with varying degrees of edema. The techniques and pitfalls of detecting proteinuria and determining its prevalence are discussed in Chapter 18, section eight.

The crucial factors in the consideration of proteinuria include (1) its constancy, (2) its quantitation, and (3) its concurrence with other urinary abnormalities. The first two can be determined simultaneously by having the patient collect a 24-hour urine specimen following the instructions shown in the accompanying box.

The constancy of proteinuria in relation to posture and activity can be determined if the amount of protein in each voiding during the 24-hour collection is measured by the patient or parent using dip-and-read strips. Because the collection begins and ends with the first void after waking on consecutive days, two urine determinations after the patient has been supine overnight will be available. More information on the effect of activity on proteinuria can be obtained if the patient is instructed to have periods of both vigorous and quiet activity during the waking hours of the 24-hour collection.

Patient Instructions for Simultaneous Collection of 24-Hour Urine Specimen and Postural Protein Test

This test involves the simultaneous collection of a 24-hour urine specimen (for quantitation of total urinary protein) and the testing of each individual urine specimen for protein. The amount of protein in each urination should be recorded along with the date, time of day, and the activities of the patient since the previous urination. The specific instructions for the patient are as follows:

1. On the day the test begins, urinate immediately after rising (________ AM), test for protein, record the results, and then *discard* the urine.
2. Test each subsequent urination, record the result, and add the entire specimen to the 24-hour collection, which should be kept refrigerated. A good intake of fluid is helpful throughout this test.
3. Sometime during the day, exercise (e.g., bike riding, playing ball), so that there is a urine specimen to test after a period of vigorous activity. Test it, record the results, and add it to the collection as you did with the others.
4. During another time of day (evening is best), remain relatively quiet (e.g., doing homework, watching television) so that there is urine to test after a period of rest. Test it, and add it to the collection.
5. On the next day, rise at the same time, urinate immediately, test for protein, record the results, and add to the 24-hour collection.
6. Bring this paper with the written urine tests results, the unused protein test strips, and the 24-hour specimen to the office. The patient need not come to the office unless an appointment has been scheduled.

Results

Date	Time	Activity	Urine Protein

The total collection should be assayed for volume and the creatinine and protein content. One can determine whether the 24-hour urine was collected properly by calculating the urinary creatinine excretion (mg/kg/day). Children of normal habitus excrete about 18 mg/kg/day of creatinine. If the creatinine excretion is near this amount, one can presume that the 24-hour urine specimen was correctly obtained and that the urinary protein quantitation is a good reflection of the degree of proteinuria. If the creatinine excretion is not near normal, the urine collection should be repeated after the technique of urine collection has been reviewed with the patient and parents. Normally, children excrete less than 150 to 200 mg of protein per square meter, although there may be some variation in quantity between diagnostic laboratories because of different methods of measurement.

The third crucial factor is the concurrence of other urinary abnormalities such as hematuria and cylindruria. The probability that proteinuria represents a more severe pathologic state increases when it occurs with other urinary abnormalities.

An algorithm for the investigation of proteinuria using the 24-hour urine collection in which each individual specimen has been tested is shown in Fig. 158-1. If all specimens are negative and the total 24-hour protein excretion is normal for the size of the child, the previous finding of proteinuria in random urine samples was probably an artifact. Such an occurrence is not unusual in a pediatric practice. The two most common causes of artifactual proteinuria are (1) improper urine collection, in that the cleansing solution or an extraneous source of protein (e.g., vaginal discharge) contaminates the specimen, or (2) collection of a specimen from a person who has had a poor fluid intake. In this latter circumstance, the normal amount of excreted protein that is usually below the range of detection by the dip-and-read strips is concentrated to a detectable level. This occurs commonly in handicapped children (e.g., blind or mentally retarded children) who have limited access to water and apparently adjust to a chronic low intake of fluid. Usually a history of poor fluid ingestion and infrequent voiding can be obtained. In spite of the positive dip-and-read test, the quantitative protein will be normal. High positive dip-and-read tests (3+ and 4+) are not usually caused by poor fluid intake.

One can also find negative urine protein results after the patient has been supine or inactive but positive tests following upright posture or physical activity. A clinical diagnosis of postural, or orthostatic, proteinuria is justified if such a postural effect occurs (1) as an isolated urine abnormality, (2) with a quantitative protein excretion that is less than 5 times the 95th percentile for age, (3) in the absence of symptoms and of a personal or family history of renal disease, and (4) with a normal physical examination and laboratory tests of renal function. Orthostatic proteinuria is usually discovered on routine urinalysis in the asymptomatic adolescent or young adult. The diagnosis of orthostatic proteinuria is a clinical one; therefore renal biopsy and an extensive radiographic investigation are not indicated. When renal biopsies have been performed, they have been normal or have shown only nonspecific changes. Orthostatic proteinuria will resolve in early adulthood in 50% of the patients. Follow-up studies of patients (for as long as 50 years after diagnosis) revealed no tendency for the urinary abnormality to progress to serious renal disease. Regardless, it is advised that the child have a semiannual reexamination and repeat 24-hour urine collection with individual specimen testing. Such a follow-up will then detect any change in the pattern of proteinuria, which may be a harbinger of an underlying serious renal problem.

If all urinary specimens are positive for protein regardless of position or activity, a significant renal pathologic condition is likely. Such pathologic proteinuria is also more frequently associated with hematuria or other abnormalities of the urinary sediment. The nephritic range for total 24-hour proteinuria is usually 5 to 10 times normal and is often associated

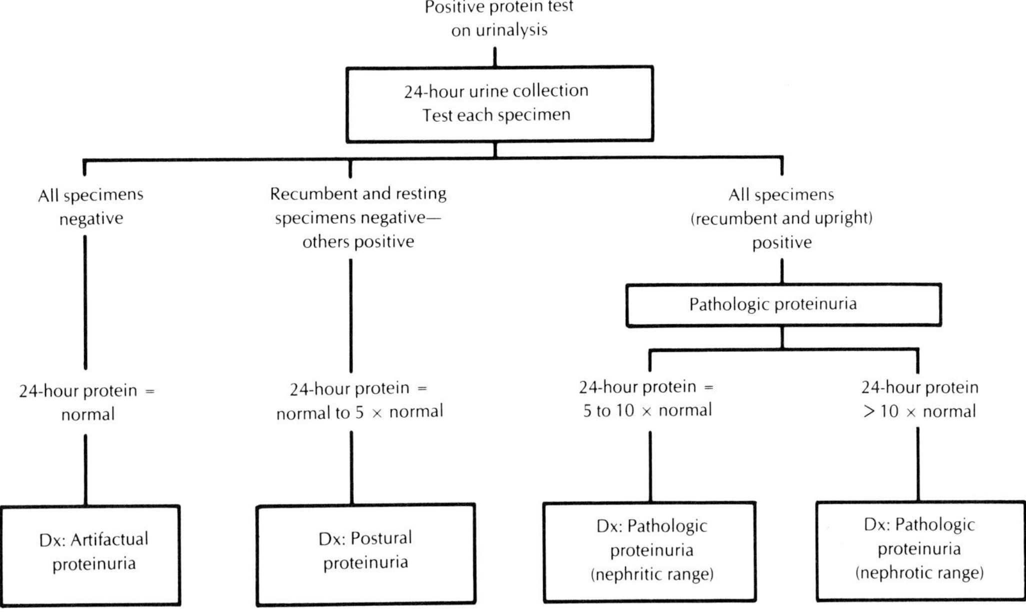

Fig. 158-1 A clinical algorithm for proteinuria in children.

with hypertension, mild edema, and nonspecific generalized symptoms, such as malaise and fatigue. In such patients, a complete renal functional examination and imaging of the kidneys are important. Most of these children should be referred to a pediatric nephrologist for more complete evaluation, which usually includes a renal biopsy (see Chapter 230, "Nephritis").

Pathologic total 24-hour proteinuria greater than 10 times normal can be labeled as being in the nephrotic range. Hypoproteinemia and hypercholesterolemia are often found concomitantly. These patients usually have edema or other obvious signs and symptoms that bring them to medical attention. A complete evaluation is indicated in these circumstances (see Chapter 231, "Nephrotic Syndrome").

SUGGESTED READINGS

Kiel DP and Moskowitz MA: The urinalysis: a critical approach, Med Clin North Am 71:607, 1987.

Norman ME: An office approach to hematuria and proteinuria, Pediatr Clin North Am 34:545, 1987.

Robinson RR: Isolated proteinuria in asymptomatic patients, Kidney Int 18:395, 1980.

Rytand DA and Spreiter S: Prognosis in postural (orthostatic) proteinuria: forty- to fifty-year follow-up of six patients after diagnosis by Thomas Addis, N Engl J Med 305:618, 1981.

Sinniah R, Law CH, and Pwee HS: Glomerular lesions in patients with asymptomatic persistent and orthostatic proteinuria discovered on routine medical examination, Clin Nephrol 7:1, 1977.

Thompson AL, Durrett RR, and Robinson RR: Fixed and reproducible orthostatic proteinuria. VI. Results of a 10-year follow-up evaluation, Ann Intern Med 73:235, 1970.

159

Pruritus

Nancy K. Barnett

Pruritus, or itch, is the subjective perception of a cutaneous disturbance that is relieved by scratching or rubbing. It is not usually brought to the attention of the pediatrician unless it is generalized, chronic, or associated with an eruption. In such instances, however, it must be treated with great respect because severe itching can be physically incapacitating. In addition, scratching or rubbing the itch can produce extensive disfigurement in the form of linear excoriations or lichenified (accentuated skin lines) plaques. The constant scratching can even cause social isolation, for at times the pruritic child is viewed by others as contagious or unclean.

PATHOPHYSIOLOGY

Because it is a subjective sensation, objective evaluation to delineate the pathophysiology of itch has been difficult. However, current thinking implicates a local production of chemomediators that stimulate fine nerve fibers of poorly myelinated C fibers at the dermoepidermal junction.[5] The exact mediators and their release triggers are unknown. Histamine and endopeptidases have elicited itch fairly consistently in experimental settings and may be active in human disease. Experimental triggers that have produced itch are physical pressure, heat, and electric shock.

It is believed that the nerve impulses travel along the anterolateral spinothalamic tract to the thalamus, where they are transferred to the sensory cortex via the internal capsule, where they are interpreted as itch.[3,6] This is the same pathway for pain, and some contend that itch is a mild degree of "pain."

Certain circumstances alter the interpretation of the degree of pruritus. For example, the itch threshold is lowered in and about areas of active dermatitis with psychic stress, with decreased skin hydration or increased skin temperature, and during the night.[1,2]

CLINICAL MANIFESTATIONS

In children, cutaneous rather than systemic disease is by far the most common cause of generalized pruritus. The major differential diagnoses of generalized pruritus with skin lesions in children are infestation (scabies, pediculosis, insect bites, and papular urticaria), atopic dermatitis, miliaria, contact dermatitis, and acute urticaria.[6]

Children may itch with cutaneous diseases such as psoriasis, lichen planus, and bullous disease of childhood. These children should be referred to a dermatologist for evaluation and management, as should a pruritic child who is otherwise healthy and does not have bites, eczema, "heat rash," contact dermatitis, or hives. The child with pruritus, from whatever cause, is at risk for psychological damage, infection secondary to impetiginization, and scarification.

Systemic causes of pruritus in childhood that should be sought in the occasional child with pruritus but no evident skin lesions are hyperthyroidism, leukemia or lymphoma, chronic renal failure, obstructive biliary disease, and xerosis (generalized dry skin).

EVALUATION AND TREATMENT

All of the common cutaneous diseases associated with generalized pruritus can be diagnosed on the basis of a good history and physical examination.

The answers to the following questions may help to diagnose infestation of one sort or another and direct therapy toward topical steroids, long clothes, and repellents: Are there individual pruritic papules with a central punctum? If so, are they on exposed or nonexposed areas? Does anyone else in the family have similar lesions?

A family history of allergy, asthma, or eczema in a child with a chronic eczematous dermatitis over extensor surfaces in infancy and flexural areas in childhood should suggest atopic dermatitis. Hydration and emollients will decrease pruritus and should be the mainstay of therapy, although topical steroids, antibiotics, and cool compresses may be required to bring the scratch-itch cycle under control. A tolerable (nonsoporific) dose of an antihistamine may relieve itch, especially if it is given before bedtime, since the itch threshold is lowered at night. Hydroxyzine seems to be the most effective agent.[4]

Pinpoint crystalline or erythematous papules in areas of occlusion and sweating, that is, miliaria crystallina and miliaria rubra (heat rash), can be controlled by simple measures such as applying dusting powders, avoiding tight clothing, and decreasing exposure to high ambient temperature.

Contact dermatitis is usually readily recognizable because of the linear array of papulovesicular, erythematous lesions and their sharp borders conforming to the shape of the contactant. The use of antihistamines, topical steroids, and compresses is discussed in detail in Chapter 193, "Contact Dermatitis."

Acute urticaria secondary to a drug or other ingestant is indicated by intensely pruritic erythematous and edematous plaques and papules. Careful historical and environmental sleuthing may reveal the cause of contact allergic or contact irritant dermatitis, but the cause of 90% of acute urticaria cases remains a mystery. If there is no question of new drug or food use, and the hives persist despite regular antihistamine use for several days, it is reasonable to obtain a throat culture and a hepatitis screen to rule out occult streptococcal and viral hepatitis infections.

To relieve itching and to prevent scarring (both mental and physical), it is necessary to break the scratch-itch cycle. Scratching only temporarily relieves itching, perhaps by substituting the perception of pain for that of itch. Itching provokes scratching, and when the scratching is stopped, the itching returns. To control itching, the following can be helpful: cut the patient's fingernails short; keep the patient fully clothed, except when applying medications; apply emollients frequently, especially after bathing; apply cool compresses to relieve intense pruritus and to remove crusts and debris; apply topical steroids for short periods (less than 10 days) to control inflammation; increase the dosage of antihistamine until the scratching ceases or marked drowsiness occurs, and then decrease the dosage to a level that controls the scratching; avoid stress, heat, and irritants; and see the patient frequently to provide support and to explain why these methods are being used, if the child is old enough to understand. Topical capsaicin and pramoxine may be indicated in selected cases. Referral to the dermatologist is generally indicated in such a circumstance.

REFERENCES

1. Cormia FE: Experimental histamine pruritus, J Invest Dermatol 19:21, 1952.
2. Edwards AE et al: Pruritic skin disease, psychological stress and the itch sensation, Arch Dermatol 112:339, 1976.
3. Gilchrest BA: Pruritus—pathogenesis, therapy, and significance in systemic disease states, Arch Intern Med 142:101, 1982.
4. Rhoades RB et al: Suppression of histamine-induced pruritus by three antihistamine drugs, J Allergy Clin Immunol 55:180, 1975.
5. Shelly WB and Arthur RP: The neurohistology and neurophysiology of the itch sensation in man, Arch Dermatol 76:296, 1957.
6. Tonnesen MG: Pruritus. In Fitzpatrick TB et al, editors: Dermatology in general medicine, ed 3, New York, 1987, McGraw-Hill Book Co.

160

Rash

Nancy K. Barnett

Rash is an ambiguous term used to describe an acute skin eruption that is usually temporary. It does not define any specific lesion. The term also does not convey information about the evolution or progression of a disorder, data needed to arrive at a logical differential diagnosis.

Tables 160-1 and 160-2 list lesion descriptions and contain historical or characteristic information for particular diagnoses. The tables are not valid for "rashes" that have been altered by therapy. They are not all-inclusive but cover the major acute eruptions that the pediatrician will encounter.

Before reviewing the tables, a few points are worth making. Within all of medicine, a careful history is obviously necessary. However, we are too often prone to look at a rash before exploring its past. We must know when it arose, how it progressed, and whether there were accompanying symptoms or signs—for example, an itch or a fever. A sound history includes the family. It is easy to ask if someone else in the family is scratching or similarly beset now or in the past.

The most important lesson one pediatrician learned early in his career about evaluating a rash involved light: the rash of scarlet fever became evident when he raised the window shade. Make sure the light is adequate when you are performing a physical examination; natural lighting is preferred. Be sure your view of the field is unobstructed. Clothing must be shed. Don't limit your look to a rolled-up sleeve or a lifted shirttail. Feel the rash—is it smooth or rough? Once the site has been inspected and palpated, the rash must be described as accurately as possible. What does it look like (use a magnifier to discern, for example, a burrow or a pinpoint puncture)? Where is it? Are the lesions discrete or confluent, large or small? Use a tape measure to define the lesions accurately by size. Is it oozing or dry; excoriated or relatively untouched in appearance? Describe carefully what is seen and write down the description.

A *macule* is a spot that is set apart from its immediate surroundings by a difference in color. It is a discoloration of the skin that is not elevated above the surface and may be of any color or of many colors. It is small, generally less than 1 cm. Larger areas may be described as *patches*. *Papules* are small (less than 5 mm in diameter), well-circumscribed solid elevations of the skin. A *nodule,* too, is solid and usually elevated or palpable in the subcutaneous area but larger. Its solidity, like the papule, enables it to be detected by touch, although its borders are indistinct. A *vesicle* is a small sac that contains liquid. With respect to the skin, it may be described as a circumscribed elevation of the epidermis containing a serous liquid. As the diameter approaches 1 cm, it is more appropriate to call it a bulla or bleb. A *bulla,* or blister, is, similarly, an elevation above the level of the skin that is filled with fluid, usually serous. It may have either a quite delicate or tough "roof," depending on the level of the skin in which it appears.

Once one has become familiar with Tables 160-1 and 160-2 and their precepts, it becomes evident that many dermatologic diagnoses are not particularly difficult to make. On the other hand, problems of either diagnosis or treatment are sure to arise. Children and adolescents with eczema, acne, and psoriasis, for example, will often benefit from consultation with a dermatologist.

Regardless, for pediatrician and dermatologist alike, *primum non nocere* (i.e., above all, do no harm) should be the rule. Iatrogenic difficulties from the overuse of drugs such as topical corticosteroids and antibiotics must be avoided. There is seldom a need to risk adrenal suppression because of continuous steroid use, and we are already too far along in encouraging bacterial readaptations to the environment. Fortunately, there are some principles of therapy to help guide the pediatrician. First, the least amount necessary of the most effective medication should be given, either by mouth or applied locally. Second, the use of household aids can be convenient and inexpensive; for example, oatmeal can serve as a colloid compress or bath for itching; an emery board will keep the fingernails smooth and short to reduce excoriations from scratching; and tea bags can be used as compresses for odd places (weeping behind the ears). Third, a moistened gauze wrapped twice around atopic areas helps to reduce oozing, to relieve itching, and to potentiate the effect of topical steroids. Fourth, children with generalized itching, as in atopic dermatitis, should be kept fully clothed all the time, using long-sleeved shirts and leotards during the day and pajamas with feet at night. Fifth, emollients, such as Eucerin, Aquaphor, or Dermatology Formula Cream, lubricate and smooth dry skin and diminish itching, whereas powder or cornstarch, dusted on lightly, is useful on moist or oozing surfaces (particularly between the toes and other intertriginous areas) to prevent maceration. And last, precision in instruction is essential; the patient or parent should be asked to repeat the plan for treatment and the steps for its implementation to ensure complete understanding of what is to be done.

Table 160-1 *Descriptions of Lesions*

	NUMBER			PATTERN						DISTRIBUTION									SIZE			SPREAD			OTHER CHARACTERISTICS				
DIAGNOSIS OR DIFFERENTIAL DIAGNOSIS	FEW	MANY	TNTC*	DISCRETE	CONFLUENT	ANNULAR†	LOCALIZED	GENERALIZED	SYMMETRIC	FACE/SCALP	PALMOPLANTAR	TRUNCAL	INTERTRIGINOUS	EXTREMITIES	ACRAL	EXTENSOR	FLEXOR	MUCOSAE	<1 MM	1-5 MM	>5 MM	CENTRIPETAL	CENTRIFUGAL	CAUDAL	SUN EXPOSED	FEVER/ILLNESS	PRURITUS	SCALE	CRUST
Macule																													
Erythematous																													
Dermatomyositis‡					X					X						X									X			X	
Drug reaction‡			X	X	X			X		X	X	X		X				X		X						X			
Erythema infectiosum					X		X			X		X		X						X				X					
Erythema marginatum‡		X				X						X		X							X		X			X			
Erythema multiforme, Stevens-Johnson syndrome	X	X	X	X			X	X	X		X				X	X		X		X	X	X				X			X
Infectious mononucleosis‡					X			X				X		X												X			
Juvenile rheumatoid arthritis‡		X		X	X			X				X		X						X	X					X			
Kawasaki disease‡					X			X		X	X	X		X				X								X			
Rubella			X	X	X			X		X		X		X				X		X						X			
Lyme disease	X	X		X		X	X	X				X									X					X			
Roseola infantum (exanthem subitum)			X	X	X			X				X								X						X			
Rubeola			X	X	X			X		X		X		X				X		X				X		X			
Staphylococcal scalded skin syndrome					X		X	X		X		X	X	X				X								X			
Sunburn, phototoxic reaction	X				X		X	X													X				X				
Toxic epidermal necrolysis					X			X		X		X	X	X				X								X			
Toxic shock syndrome					X			X				X						X								X			
Viral exanthem‡			X	X	X			X		X	X	X		X				X		X						X			
Hypopigmented																													
Pityriasis alba	X	X	X	X	X		X	X		X		X		X						X	X							X	
Tinea versicolor‡	X	X	X	X	X		X	X		X		X		X						X	X			X			X	X	
Vitiligo in evolution	X	X		X	X		X	X	X	X	X	X		X	X	X				X	X								

Table 160-1 *Descriptions of Lesions—cont'd*

DIAGNOSIS OR DIFFERENTIAL DIAGNOSIS	NUMBER			PATTERN						DISTRIBUTION									SIZE			SPREAD			OTHER CHARACTERISTICS				
	FEW	MANY	TNTC*	DISCRETE	CONFLUENT	ANNULAR†	LOCALIZED	GENERALIZED	SYMMETRIC	FACE/SCALP	PALMOPLANTAR	TRUNCAL	INTERTRIGINOUS	EXTREMITIES	ACRAL	EXTENSOR	FLEXOR	MUCOSAE	<1 MM	1-5 MM	>5 MM	CENTRIPETAL	CENTRIFUGAL	CAUDAL	SUN EXPOSED	FEVER/ILLNESS	PRURITUS	SCALE	CRUST
Hyperpigmented																													
Tinea versicolor‡	X	X	X	X	X		X	X		X		X		X						X	X			X			X	X	
Transient neonatal pustular melanosis	X	X	X	X	X			X		X		X	X							X									
Nonblanching (petechiae, purpura)																													
Atypical measles		X	X	X	X			X		X		X		X	X			X	X	X					X	X			
Battered child syndrome‡	X	X		X			X			X		X		X							X								
Leukemia, coagulation defect, ITP	X	X	X	X	X			X		X		X		X				X	X	X									
Rocky Mountain spotted fever‡	X	X	X	X	X			X		X	X	X		X	X		X		X	X		X				X			
Viral exanthem, TORCH infection, drug, hepatitis‡		X	X	X	X			X		X		X		X				X	X	X					X	X			
Papules, nodules																													
Erythematous																													
Atopic dermatitis	X	X	X	X	X		X	X		X		X		X		X	X		X	X	X						X		X
Granuloma annulare	X	X		X		X						X		X	X					X	X								
Insect bites	X	X	X	X			X			X		X	X	X	X					X					X	X			
Miliaria rubra (heat rash)	X	X	X	X			X			X		X	X						X							X	X		
Scarlet fever			X	X	X				X				X	X	X			X		X	X			X			X		
Seborrheic dermatitis	X	X	X	X	X		X	X		X		X	X							X	X							X	
Tinea corporis	X	X		X		X	X			X		X		X					X	X	X			X					
Hypopigmented																													
Lichen nitidus		X	X	X			X					X		X					X	X									
Lichen striatus, linear lichen planus, epidermal nevus		X	X	X	X		X				X			X							X								
Molluscum contagiosum	X	X	X		X		X			X		X		X					X	X	X								

*Too numerous to count.
†Raised border.
‡May be papular in parts.
§May be edematous.

Continued.

Table 160-1 *Descriptions of Lesions—cont'd*

	NUMBER			PATTERN						DISTRIBUTION									SIZE			SPREAD			OTHER CHARACTERISTICS				
DIAGNOSIS OR DIFFERENTIAL DIAGNOSIS	FEW	MANY	TNTC*	DISCRETE	CONFLUENT	ANNULAR†	LOCALIZED	GENERALIZED	SYMMETRIC	FACE/SCALP	PALMOPLANTAR	TRUNCAL	INTERTRIGINOUS	EXTREMITIES	ACRAL	EXTENSOR	FLEXOR	MUCOSAE	<1 MM	1-5 MM	>5 MM	CENTRIPETAL	CENTRIFUGAL	CAUDAL	SUN EXPOSED	FEVER/ILLNESS	PRURITUS	SCALE	CRUST
Violaceous																													
Lichen planus	X	X	X	X	X			X	X			X		X	X			X	X	X	X								
Nonblanching																													
Gonococcemia, SBE	X			X		X					X	X		X						X						X			
Henoch-Schönlein purpura§	X	X	X	X	X			X	X					X		X				X	X	X				X			
Letterer-Siwe disease	X	X	X	X	X		X	X		X	X	X	X	X						X	X					X		X	X
Leukemia cutis/lymphoma	X	X	X	X	X			X				X		X					X	X	X					X			
Mastocytosis (urticaria pigmentosa)§	X	X	X	X	X		X			X		X		X						X	X						X		
Meningococcemia, sepsis	X	X	X	X	X			X		X	X	X		X				X	X	X						X			
Neuroblastoma, TORCH infection, leukemia	X	X		X				X		X		X		X						X	X					X			
Vesicles																													
Contact dermatitis	X	X	X	X	X		X	X		X		X	X	X	X				X	X							X		X
Coxsackievirus hand, foot, and mouth disease	X	X		X		X				X					X			X		X						X			
Dyshidrotic eczema (pompholyx)	X	X	X	X	X		X				X				X				X	X							X		
Flea bites	X	X	X	X			X		X					X	X					X							X		X
Herpes simplex; herpes zoster	X			X	X		X			X		X		X				X	X	X						X	X		X
Miliaria crystallina	X	X	X	X			X	X		X		X	X	X					X						X	X	X		
Tinea pedis	X	X	X	X	X		X				X								X	X							X		X
Varicella		X	X	X			X		X		X		X					X	X	X		X			X	X	X		X

Table 160-1 *Descriptions of Lesions—cont'd*

	NUMBER			PATTERN						DISTRIBUTION									SIZE			SPREAD			OTHER CHARACTERISTICS				
DIAGNOSIS OR DIFFERENTIAL DIAGNOSIS	FEW	MANY	TNTC*	DISCRETE	CONFLUENT	ANNULAR†	LOCALIZED	GENERALIZED	SYMMETRIC	FACE/SCALP	PALMOPLANTAR	TRUNCAL	INTERTRIGINOUS	EXTREMITIES	ACRAL	EXTENSOR	FLEXOR	MUCOSAE	<1 MM	1-5 MM	>5 MM	CENTRIPETAL	CENTRIFUGAL	CAUDAL	SUN EXPOSED	FEVER/ILLNESS	PRURITUS	SCALE	CRUST
Bullae																													
Bullous disease of childhood	X	X	X	X	X	X		X		X		X	X	X	X						X						X		X
Bullous impetigo	X	X		X	X		X			X		X	X	X							X	X				X	X		X
Pustules																													
Acne neonatorum	X	X		X			X		X	X									X	X									
Candidiasis	X	X	X	X	X		X	X		X	X	X	X	X		X		X		X						X		X	
Erythema toxicum neonatorum	X	X	X	X	X		X	X		X	X	X		X						X									
Folliculitis	X	X	X	X			X	X				X		X					X	X									
Transient neonatal pustular melanosis	X	X	X	X	X		X			X		X	X							X									
Plaques																													
Acute urticaria	X	X	X	X	X		X	X		X		X		X				X	X	X	X						X		
Nummular eczema	X	X	X	X			X					X		X		X					X						X	X	X
Psoriasis	X	X	X	X	X		X	X	X	X	X	X		X		X				X	X				X		X	X	

*Too numerous to count.
†Raised border.
‡May be papular in parts.
§May be edematous.

Table 160-2 *Laboratory Studies and Characteristics of Lesions*

DIAGNOSIS OR DIFFERENTIAL DIAGNOSIS	LABORATORY STUDIES	COMMENTS
Macule		
Erythematous		
Sunburn, phototoxic reaction		Look for patterns and sharp edges, e.g., clothing lines after exposure to sun
Rubeola		Koplik spots, preauricular lymph nodes
Drug reaction*	Leukocytosis with eosinophilia	History of drug ingestion
Toxic shock syndrome	Blood, throat, urine, stool, vaginal cultures for *Staphylococcus aureus*	Shock, tampon use
Infectious mononucleosis*	Heterophil antibody; atypical lymphs on smear	Generalized adenopathy, splenomegaly; ampicillin use
Kawasaki disease*	Thrombocytosis 3-5 wk after onset	Conjunctival injection, cervical adenopathy
Staphylococcal scalded skin syndrome	*S. aureus* cultured from focus	Tender erythema, positive Nikolsky sign, bullae
Toxic epidermal necrolysis	*S. aureus* cultures negative	Search for new drug use
Erythema multiforme, Stevens-Johnson syndrome	Skin biopsy may aid diagnosis	Central papule or vesicle, iris lesions; may be bullous
Viral exanthem*	Leukocytosis with lymphocytosis	
Rubella	Fourfold rise in antibody titer	Postauricular lymphadenopathy; monarticular arthritis
Roseola infantum (exanthem subitum)	Leukopenia may be present	Eruption appears with resolution of fever; periorbital edema
Erythema infectiosum	Lymphocytosis, eosinophilia	Reticulated pattern may appear for months with stress
Erythema marginatum*		Acute rheumatic fever with active carditis; fleeting
Juvenile rheumatoid arthritis*	Rheumatoid factor may be positive	Arthritis; lesions may be papular
Dermatomyositis*	Electromyography, creatinine phosphokinase, aldolase	Muscle weakness; periungual telangiectasia; heliotrope eyelid; edema
Lyme disease	Most nonspecific; may look for antibodies to *Borrelia burgdorferi* (see Chapter 225 on Lyme disease)	Erythema chronicum migrans appearing as enlarging rings after tick bite
Hypopigmented		
Tinea versicolor*	Potassium hydroxide (KOH) smear—short, branched hyphae and spores	Chronic; prevalent if immunosuppressed
Pityriasis alba	Wood light—hypopigmented	
Vitiligo in evolution	Wood light—depigmented if vitiliginous; T_4, TSH to rule out thyroid disorder	Observe for scleroderma, melanoma
Hyperpigmented		
Tinea versicolor*	See above	See above
Transient neonatal pustular melanosis	Pustule Gram stain—sterile with polymorphonuclear neutrophils (PMNs)	Pustules; superficial desquamation
Nonblanching (petechiae, purpura)		
Atypical measles		History of killed measles vaccine; pneumonitis; acral petechiae, purpura, vesiculobullous lesions
Viral exanthem, TORCH infection, drug, hepatitis*	Complete blood count (CBC), liver enzymes, viral titers	Drug history

*May be papular in parts.
†May be edematous.

Table 160-2 *Laboratory Studies and Characteristics of Lesions—cont'd*

DIAGNOSIS OR DIFFERENTIAL DIAGNOSIS	LABORATORY STUDIES	COMMENTS
***Macule**—cont'd*		
Nonblanching (petechiae, purpura)—*cont'd*		
Rocky Mountain spotted fever*	Fluorescent antibody screen; OX-19, OX-2; skin biopsy of fluorescent stain	History of tick bite
Leukemia, coagulation defect, ITP	CBC, PT, PTT, platelet count, bone marrow aspirate and biopsy	
Battered child syndrome*		History incongruous with pattern and/or degree of lesions
Papules, nodules		
Erythematous		
Miliaria rubra (heat rash)		Prominent in occluded areas
Seborrheic dermatitis		Intertriginous with yellow greasy scale, cradle cap
Atopic dermatitis	IgE level	Family or personal history of allergies, asthma, eczema; flexural in infancy and extensor in childhood
Scarlet fever	Throat culture, ASP titer	Malar flush, circumoral pallor, Pastia lines, desquamation
Insect bites		Check for central punctae
Tinea corporis	KOH smear—long, thin-branched hyphae	
Granuloma annulare		Lack of scale distinguishes from tinea corporis; no epidermal component
Hypopigmented		
Molluscum contagiosum		Pearly papule with central umbilication containing easily expressed white cheesy core
Lichen nitidus		Check penis for grouped lichenoid papules
Lichen striatus, linear lichen planus, epidermal nevus	Skin biopsy	Linear
Violaceous		
Lichen planus		Purple pruritic polygonal papules
Nonblanching		
Meningococcemia, sepsis	Blood, cerebrospinal fluid (CSF) culture; Gram-stain lesion	Check conjunctivae for hemorrhage
Gonococcemia, SBE	Blood, throat, cervical, rectal cultures	Check for heart murmur, arthritis, tenosynovitis
Henoch-Schönlein purpura†	Stool guaiac, urinalysis, skin biopsy	Abdominal pain, arthritis; crops of lesions
Mastocytosis (urticaria pigmentosa)†	Skin biopsy—mast cells	Wheal and flare on stroking
Letterer-Siwe disease	Skin biopsy—histiocytes	Distinguish from seborrheic dermatitis
Leukemia cutis/lymphoma	Skin biopsy—atypical leukemic infiltrate	Lymphoma, especially Hodgkin disease, may be pruritic
Neuroblastoma, TORCH infection, leukemia	Skin biopsy	"Blueberry muffin" baby

*May be papular in parts.
†May be edematous.

Continued.

Table 160-2 *Laboratory Studies and Characteristics of Lesions—cont'd*

DIAGNOSIS OR DIFFERENTIAL DIAGNOSIS	LABORATORY STUDIES	COMMENTS
Vesicles		
Miliaria crystallina		Superficial
Tinea pedis	KOH scraping of vesicle roof—hyphae	
Herpes simplex; herpes zoster	Tzanck preparation—multinucleated giant cells; viral culture to distinguish simplex from zoster	Grouped vesicles on an erythematous base; simplex labialis, progenitalis, whitlow—zoster usually linear and dermatomal
Contact dermatitis	Patch testing	Sharp borders, linear arrays, bizarre patterns, asymmetric
Varicella		Crops in various stages—macule, papule, vesicle, pustule, and cyst
Coxsackievirus hand, foot, and mouth disease	Throat culture—coxsackievirus A16, 5, and 10	May be recurrent
Flea bites		Treat pet
Bullae		
Bullous disease of childhood	Skin biopsy for hematoxylin and eosin (H&E) stain and immunofluorescence	Refer to dermatologist to rule out bullous pemphigoid and dermatitis herpetiformis
Bullous impetigo	Culture blister fluid for phage group II *S. aureus*	
Pustules		
Erythema toxicum neonatorum	Wright stain of pustule—eosinophils	Pustule in center on erythematous macule
Transient neonatal pustular melanosis	Gram stain of pustule—sterile with PMNs	Hyperpigmented macules; superficial desquamation
Candidiasis	KOH smear of scale or pustule—budding yeast and pseudohyphae	
Folliculitis	Gram stain—staphylococcal or sterile	Follicular, i.e., hair shaft central in pustule
Plaques		
Psoriasis		Well-demarcated erythematous plaque with adherent scale; check family history, arthritis
Acute urticaria	Eosinophil count, throat culture for streptococci, HB_sAG	Erythematous, edematous plaque, drug history, food history (shellfish, berries)
Nummular eczema		Papules and vesicles grouped into plaques

161

Recurrent Infections

John H. Dossett

The notion of frequently recurring infection implies that the child is having infections with such frequency and severity as to be perceived as having more infections than should a generally healthy child. Such a notion is necessarily related to the parents' concept of normal and the acceptable number of infections in children. The prevalence of a truly unusual number of serious infections among children is quite low; however, children whose parents perceive them as having an unusual number of infections are seen often in pediatric practice, so much so that they make up a major part of the practice of consultants in immunology and infectious disease.

It is quite common for generally healthy children to have 6 to 10 separate respiratory virus infections in a year. This is especially true where there is prolonged exposure to large numbers of children in places such as day care centers, nursery schools, and regular schools. A series of new and unrelated respiratory viral infections interspersed among two or three bacterial complications of respiratory virus infections (e.g., otitis media) will make a child appear to be "sick all the time."

Moreover, there are many children with frequent recurrences of rhinitis and cough who appear to be infected but who actually have respiratory allergy and the usual number of respiratory virus infections, making them appear to be "infected all the time."

Other children, commonly labeled as having recurrent infections, are those whose skin is colonized by a virulent strain of *Staphylococcus*, resulting in recurrent episodes of folliculitis or furunculosis.

DEFINITION

Any concise definition of recurrent infection is necessarily arbitrary and very likely to be either too general or too restrictive. Rather than define by some arbitrary criteria whether a child has recurrent infections, it is more appropriate to determine whether the child is generally well and whether there is some specific condition that can be identified and treated.

Recurrent infection has traditionally been viewed as the hallmark of persons with deficiencies in host defense, such as hypogammaglobulinemia, leukocyte-killing defects, or thymic hypoplasia syndromes. However, children with frequent pneumonia secondary to asthma or cystic fibrosis and those with frequent otitis media are much more prevalent than children with immunodeficiency syndromes.

Children who are generally well despite frequent symptoms of infection will usually be thriving, as manifested by normal growth and development. Their infections are usually less severe and are generally limited to the skin and upper respiratory tract. Most often such children have not been hospitalized or were hospitalized only briefly for uncomplicated illnesses.

DIFFERENTIAL DIAGNOSIS

In sorting out the causes of recurrent infection, it is first necessary to establish whether the child's infections are usual and associated with generally good health or whether the infections herald some underlying illness that requires a systematic laboratory evaluation. Careful history-taking is of utmost importance in that it will provide the information with which one decides whether to pursue laboratory evaluation (see box, p. 1046). It will also determine the direction of the laboratory investigation to be undertaken, if one is indicated.

The Generally Well Child

Because the parents of generally well children (category A in box, p. 1046) usually will have already concluded that their child is "sick all the time," it becomes necessary to record the actual dates and duration of each episode. Most often this will demonstrate that there are significant intervals during which the child is well. Moreover, specific episodes of illness can frequently be related temporally to similar illness in other family members. In general, those children whose recurrent infections are limited to the upper respiratory tract, who have intervals of distinct wellness, and who are growing normally do not need a laboratory evaluation of possible immunodeficiency syndromes. Children who have frequent recurrences of otitis media may need chronic prophylaxis throughout the respiratory virus season, namely, November to April (see Chapter 238, "Otitis Media and Otitis Externa"). However, unless they have other manifestations of chronic illness, they do not merit an extensive laboratory evaluation.

The important diagnosis of general wellness should be an early primary diagnosis based on a detailed history, growth records, physical examination, and chest roentgenogram, rather than a delayed diagnosis of exclusion, which one stumbles upon after multiple normal laboratory test results. An astute and sympathetic physician can confidently reassure parents that their child is generally well, even when there have been multiple episodes of respiratory infection or otitis media.

Evaluation of Children with Recurrent Infections

CATEGORY A: GENERALLY WELL CHILD*

1. Normal growth and development
2. Usual illness with common viruses
3. Infections usually of skin and upper respiratory tract, such as furunculosis, otitis media, and rhinitis
4. Infection usually with common pathogens such as respiratory viruses, *Staphylococcus, Haemophilus influenzae,* and *Streptococcus*
5. Usually has periods of complete wellness
6. Chest roentgenogram usually normal
7. Typically has palpable lymph nodes and normal-to-enlarged tonsils

CATEGORY B: CHILD WITH SPECIFIC SIGNS AND SYMPTOMS THAT MAY INDICATE IMMUNODEFICIENCY OR ANOTHER CHRONIC ILLNESS†

1. Failure to thrive
2. Severe disease with common viruses such as chickenpox and measles
3. More than one *serious infection,* such as meningitis, pneumonia, bone and joint infection, or bacteremia
4. May be infected with organisms that are usually of low virulence in the normal host (i.e., *Serratia, Klebsiella, Pseudomonas, Proteus,* etc.)
5. Few periods when child is completely well
6. Chest roentgenogram usually abnormal
7. Physical signs such as the following:
   a. Rales or wheezing
   b. Chronic eczema and alopecia
   c. Small tonsils and nonpalpable lymph nodes
   d. Chronic blepharitis
   e. Opacified sinuses
   f. Clubbing of fingers
   g. Nasal polyps
   h. Chronic mucopurulent nasal or postnasal drainage
8. Chronic diarrhea or stools characteristic of malabsorption
9. Frequent fever

*Children in this category usually need to have their acute complications (otitis media, etc.) treated and their *parents reassured* that they are generally well. Drawing specific attention to each of the items of information that caused one to put them in this category is very comforting to most parents.

†Any one of the items in this category may indicate a need for systematic laboratory evaluation that is specifically designed to *follow the clues.* It is painful, expensive, and reckless to try to rule out every possibility in the differential diagnosis with a "laboratory shotgun" approach.

The Generally Unwell Child

When the detailed history (including family history), physical examination, and chest roentgenogram suggest that the child is not generally well (category B in box, above), the best investigation is that which follows the clues. Clearly, the signs and symptoms listed in category B are not very specific. Most of them may be found in dozens of specific diseases that are associated with recurrent infections. In fact, chronic or recurrent respiratory tract infections are seen in almost every disease that predisposes to recurrent infection. Because of the tremendous overlap in clinical manifestations, one must play the odds as well as follow the clues. Although all the diseases discussed below may seem very similar, asthma and cystic fibrosis are really much more common than are agammaglobulinemia or alpha-1-antitrypsin deficiency.

In the decade of the 1990s, infants and children with human immunodeficiency virus (HIV) infection and acquired immune deficiency syndrome (AIDS) will become increasingly prevalent among those with chronic and recurrent infections. HIV infection should be in the differential diagnosis of every child with manifestations in category B (see box above).

Recurrent Pneumonia or Abnormal Chest Roentgenogram. The box on p. 1047 lists chronic diseases that may be associated with recurrent pneumonia. The most common cause of recurrent lower respiratory infection is respiratory allergy. This diagnosis is easy to make when the child has obvious, frequent asthma attacks; however, many children with bronchospastic disease have never had severe wheezing, and one depends on the family history or a history of mild, exercise-induced wheezing to find a clue. Careful questioning will usually elicit a history of wheezing. Review of all medical records may reveal that another physician has heard wheezing on auscultation or a previous roentgenogram has shown air trapping. The diagnosis is usually supported by an elevated serum IgE level, and the recurrent infections are controlled by the administration of theophylline or other adrenergics.

HIV infection and AIDS are primarily seen at present in children born to women who are drug users, the sexual part-

Chronic Diseases Associated with Recurrent Pneumonia

1. Asthma
   a. Overt wheezing
   b. Subacute bronchospasm with atelectasis
2. Aspiration
   a. Tracheoesophageal fistula
   b. Gastroesophageal reflux
3. Cystic fibrosis
4. Alpha-1-antitrypsin deficiency
5. Immunodeficiency syndromes
   a. HIV infection
   b. Hypogammaglobulinemia
   c. Leukocyte defects
   d. Complement deficiencies
   e. Cellular immunodeficiency
6. Immotile cilia syndrome
7. Bronchopulmonary dysplasia of prematurity
8. Anatomic malformations
9. Bronchiectasis resulting from pneumonia of measles, *Bordetella pertussis,* or *H. influenzae*

ners of drug users, or women who have multiple sexual partners. Even so, HIV testing should be done on any child with only the slightest indication, because many mothers with HIV infection do not know that they are infected. Just as in a previous era when tuberculosis was a major scourge, a sick infant is commonly the first clue that the family harbors HIV. (See Chapter 178.)

Aspiration pneumonia is seen primarily in children who have some form of neurologic impairment. Neurologically, children who aspirate chronically are similar to those alcoholics who vomit and aspirate while drunk, that is, who are temporarily neurologically impaired. Although *gastroesophageal reflux* is quite common, aspiration rarely occurs unless there is accompanying neurologic impairment. Babies who have congenital *tracheoesophageal fistulas* usually start having recurrent pneumonia very early in life and typically cough with feeding.

Cystic fibrosis may be mild or severe and may primarily involve the respiratory tract or the gastrointestinal tract. It is more common than most of the other causes of recurrent pneumonia; consequently, the sweat chloride test should be done early and on minimal provocation.

Alpha-1-antitrypsin deficiency is most often associated with hepatic cirrhosis; however, it is sometimes associated with emphysema and chronic lung disease.

All of the *immunodeficiency syndromes* (hypogammaglobulinemia, leukocyte defects, complement deficiencies, and cellular immunodeficiencies) are likely to result in recurrent pneumonia. In fact, of all the possible sites for infection in the immune-deficient host, the respiratory tract is the most common.

Immotile cilia syndrome is commonly manifest as sinusitis, bronchiectasis, and situs inversus (Kartagener syndrome). Children so affected have a heritable (autosomal recessive) defect of the myofibrils that are responsible for mucociliary motion. The diagnosis is made by nasal biopsy. Motility is assessed by light microscopy and structural abnormalities by electron microscopy.

Bronchopulmonary dysplasia is a form of chronic lung disease often seen in children who have had intensive respiratory support in the neonatal period. The cause is not determined; however, most such children were born prematurely with hyaline membrane disease, requiring oxygen therapy and mechanical ventilation. In the first 2 or so years of life they often manifest severe respiratory distress when infected with common respiratory viruses.

Anatomic malformations, such as congenital anomalies of the bronchial tree and anomalous blood supply to one or more segments of lung (e.g., sequestered lobe), may result in recurrent pneumonia. *Mediastinal tumors* or *enlarged lymph nodes* may compress a bronchus, resulting in atelectasis or recurrent pneumonia. *Foreign bodies* within the bronchial tree usually result in recurrent pneumonia.

Some infectious agents can cause such severe damage to the bronchi that children may recover from an acute infection only to be left with *chronic bronchiectasis*. This is most often seen following infections with measles virus, *B. pertussis*, or *H. influenzae*.

Recurrent Skin Infections. Recurrent furuncles occur quite commonly and are a source of significant discomfort and embarrassment. They are rarely, however, a manifestation of subnormal host defenses. Most often such patients are simply colonized with especially virulent strains of staphylococci that cause recurrent infection of the skin and subcutaneous tissues. Such patients do not need laboratory evaluation; they require only a short course of antistaphylococcal antibiotics and daily baths with a povidone-iodine scrub soap for 2 to 3 weeks.

In rare cases, children with immunodeficiency diseases may have recurrent and chronic skin infections; however, they are associated with other manifestations, such as chronic eczema, alopecia, growth failure, short limbs, and fungal infections of the nails.

Recurrent Otitis Media. Many young children have multiple episodes of otitis media. These are usually children who had their first episode in the first year of life and who may eventually have three to six episodes per year. Most of these children do not have immunodeficiency diseases; rather, abnormal middle-ear mucosa and eustachian tube dysfunction generally cause their frequent recurrences. Although otitis media is a major problem in children with allergies and immunodeficiency, there should be other clues to these diseases before one embarks on a laboratory evaluation. Most children with recurrent otitis media are best served by prescribing sulfisoxazole prophylactically through the respiratory virus season.

Multiple Pyogenic Infections. Children with multiple pyogenic infections, and especially those pyogenic infections caused by bacteria that are usually of low virulence, are more likely to have one of the (rare) immunodeficiency syndromes. The normally functioning host defense system of humoral-mediated immunity requires that there be adequate quantities of normal opsonic antibodies, normal granulocytes, and normal complement components. Deficiencies of opsonic antibodies include the various forms of hypogammaglobulinemia and dysgammaglobulinemia. Granulocyte deficiencies include the various forms of agranulocytosis, intracellular killing defects (chronic granulomatous disease), and the granulocyte migration defects (lazy leukocyte syndrome). Chronic and recurrent infections have been associated with deficien-

Immunodeficiency Syndromes

HUMORAL-MEDIATED IMMUNODEFICIENCY

Antibody Deficiency Syndromes

Transient hypogammaglobulinemia of infancy
X-linked infantile hypogammaglobulinemia
Common variable immunodeficiency or acquired hypogammaglobulinemia
Isolated IgA deficiency
Isolated IgM deficiency
Antibody deficiency with normal immunoglobulins
Miscellaneous dysgammaglobulinemias

Leukocyte Deficiency Syndromes

Decreased number of leukocytes
- Marrow toxicity
- Immune injury to marrow
- Myelothisic suppression of marrow
- Familial hypoplasia

Defective leukocyte function
- Chronic granulomatous disease
- Chédiak-Higashi disease
- Lazy leukocyte syndrome

HUMORAL-MEDIATED IMMUNODEFICIENCY—*cont'd*

Complement Deficiency Syndromes

Isolated C3 deficiency
Isolated C5 deficiency
C2 and C4 deficiencies

CELL-MEDIATED IMMUNODEFICIENCY

Congenital thymic hypoplasia (DiGeorge syndrome)
Chronic mucocutaneous candidiasis

MIXED B AND T CELL IMMUNODEFICIENCY

HIV infection
Severe combined immunodeficiency
Wiskott-Aldrich syndrome
Immunodeficiency with ataxia-telangiectasia
Immunodeficiency with thymoma
Immunodeficiency with short-limbed dwarfism
Cellular immune deficiency with abnormal immunoglobulin synthesis (Nezelof syndrome)

Laboratory Screening Tests for Immunodeficiency Syndromes

1. Antibody deficiency syndromes
   a. Immunoglobulin levels (normal level is age related)
   b. Isohemagglutinin titers
   c. Specific antibody titers (i.e., polio and tetanus)
   d. HIV antibody
2. Leukocyte deficiency syndromes
   a. Granulocyte count (should have 1500 or more granulocytes)
   b. Stained peripheral smear (look at granule size)
   c. Nitroblue tetrazolium (NBT) test
3. Complement deficiency syndromes
   a. Total hemolytic complement
   b. C3 level (radial diffusion kits available)
4. T cell deficiency syndromes
   a. Chest roentgenogram for thymus shadow
   b. Skin test using *Candida* organisms, mumps, SK-SO, and tetanus toxoid
   c. Total lymphocyte count (should have 1500 or more)
   d. HIV antibody

cies of several components of the complement system. Except for deficiencies of IgA and transient hypogammaglobulinemia of infancy, these immunodeficiency syndromes are rare; most of them are listed in the box above.

Children with deficiencies in the system of cell-mediated immunity are likely to have serious infections with viruses and fungi as well as with bacterial disease. The more serious forms are seen at an early age and are likely to be fatal.

It is beyond the scope of this text to detail the unique characteristics of each immunodeficiency syndrome listed in the box above. However, children with the signs and symptoms found in category B of the box on p. 1046 may need to be evaluated for immunodeficiency. Screening tests that are readily available are listed in the box at left. Whether these tests do or do not establish a presumptive diagnosis, the child will be best served by referral to an immunology or infectious disease consultant who has access to specialized tests for pursuing the diagnosis, who has experience with these rare diseases, and who can provide a diagnosis, genetic counseling, and long-term care for a chronic illness.

SUGGESTED READINGS

Insel RA. The child with recurrent infections. In Ziai M, editor: Bedside Pediatrics, Boston, 1983, Little, Brown and Company.

Insel R. Disorders of lymphocyte function. In Hoffman R, Benz EJ Jr, Shattil SJ, Furie B, Cohen HJ, editors: Hematology: Basic Principles and Practice, NY, 1991, Churchill Livingstone.

Johnston RB Jr. Recurrent bacterial infections in children. N Engl J Med 310: 1237, 1984.

Rubin BK. The evaluation of the child with recurrent chest infections. Pediatr Infect Dis J 4:88, 1985.

Stiehm ER, editor. Immunologic Disorders in Infants and Children, 3rd edition. Philadelphia, 1989, WB Saunders.

162

The Red Eye

Carl A. Frankel

The red eye is a descriptive term that encompasses many possible etiologies, only some of which are infectious; all, however, must be addressed. "Pink eye" is a lay term that refers to a subset of the red eye known as conjunctivitis.

The differential diagnosis of the red eye includes (1) conjunctivitis, (2) keratitis, (3) iritis, (4) nasolacrimal duct obstruction, and (5) glaucoma.

CONJUNCTIVITIS

Conjunctivitis means inflammation of the conjunctiva, the etiology of which can be quite diverse. Most types of conjunctivitis do not present an acute risk to the eye; however, chronic, untreated conjunctivitis can endanger vision or even be life-threatening. Conjunctivitis should be evaluated promptly so that appropriate intervention can be instituted. Because of the continuous nature of the bulbar conjunctiva with the tarsal (or palpebral) conjunctiva, as well as the skin of the eyelids, conjunctivitis may also be characterized by injection of the lids. Neonatal conjunctivitis is discussed below in the section on ophthalmia neonatorum.

Allergic Conjunctivitis

Allergic conjunctivitis is a noninfectious form of conjunctivitis characterized by itching, chemosis (conjunctival swelling), conjunctival injection and, frequently tearing. The condition may be unilateral or bilateral and is frequently asymptomatic. Except as noted in the following sections, treatment is tailored to the degree of symptoms and may even be unnecessary. If treatment is indicated, cool compresses and a topical antihistamine for symptomatic relief are usually sufficient.

Contact Allergen Conjunctivitis. Contact allergen conjunctivitis is frequently unilateral, and because of the higher incidence of right-handed individuals, the right eye is more commonly affected. Itching, tearing, and periorbital injection are hallmarks of this condition, but conjunctival injection may be minimal. Treatment consists of good hand washing, attempts to discourage hand-eye contact, and use of topical antihistamines (such as products containing antazoline phosphate, pyrilamine maleate, or pheniramine maleate) for short-term use in more bothersome cases.

Vernal Conjunctivitis. Vernal conjunctivitis is a recurrent inflammation of the conjunctiva that occurs more frequently in boys than girls, is usually bilateral, and is characterized by its springtime occurrence. The age distribution varies from 3 to 20 years but cases typically cluster around 5 to 6 years. A history of atopic disease in the patient or family is frequently obtained. The typical conjunctival injection is bulbar and most noticeable at the limbus. If significant conjunctival edema (chemosis) occurs, the parents and patient are frequently quite alarmed. On examination the upper lids should be everted with the end of a cotton applicator if the patient complains of a foreign body sensation. Conjunctival papillae, often in a "cobblestone" arrangement (Fig. 162-1), suggest significant disease that requires the assistance of an ophthalmologist for successful management.

In mild cases, symptomatic treatment with a mild vasoconstrictor is usually sufficient. Occasionally the use of systemic antihistamines may also be sufficient when used to treat hay fever or other manifestations of atopy. However, when topical treatment is needed, cromolyn sodium (Opticrom 4%) can be invaluable and may obviate the need for chronic topical steroid use. Topical ophthalmic steroid preparations are often initially necessary. However, long-term use of these preparations is associated with herpes simplex keratitis, cataracts, and glaucoma. Therefore steroid-containing ophthalmic preparations should be prescribed with care and probably should be reserved for the ophthalmologist.

Phlyctenular Conjunctivitis. Phlyctenular conjunctivitis and its related keratoconjunctivitis are characterized by a heavily vascularized, whitish yellow, elevated lesion, usually located near the limbus. Left untreated the conjunctival phlyctenule advances into the cornea with its trailing leash of vesicles pointing toward the corneal lesion (Fig. 162-2). In developing nations, tuberculosis is the most common association; however, in industrialized nations an allergic reaction to the *Staphylococcus* exotoxin is the suspected etiology. Treatment with topical steroids is extremely efficacious but should be performed under the care of an ophthalmologist.

Bacterial Conjunctivitis

Most forms of bacterial conjunctivitis are self-limited, but when treatment is indicated, this type of conjunctivitis usually responds rapidly to antibiotic therapy. The appearance is that of a unilateral or bilateral mucopurulent discharge that is typically yellow or green. The discharge may be mild or so copious that the lids may be pasted shut. The conjunctiva is usually mildly to severely injected, and lid edema and erythema may be worrisome. Typical etiologic agents include strains of *Staphylococcus*, *Streptococcus*, *Pneumococcus*, and *Haemophilus influenzae*; strains of *Pseudomonas*, *Klebsiella*, and *Neisseria* are less frequently encountered.

The diagnosis of a bacterial conjunctivitis is generally

made on clinical grounds alone, and treatment is begun. Because most bacterial conjunctivitis responds readily to topical antibiotics, cultures and sensitivity determinations are usually not necessary unless *Pseudomonas* or another particularly virulent organism is suspected. Treatment with ophthalmic solutions is easier than with ophthalmic ointments, and the response is frequently dramatic. Sodium sulfacetamide (10% solution) is useful in most cases although chloramphenicol is occasionally used. Because of the small volume of the conjunctival cul-de-sac, only one drop is needed. Tetracycline, erythromycin, or sodium sulfacetamide ointments can be used, as can polymyxin with bacitracin when ointments are preferred. Gentamycin and tobramycin should be reserved for bacterial conjunctivitis that does not readily respond to

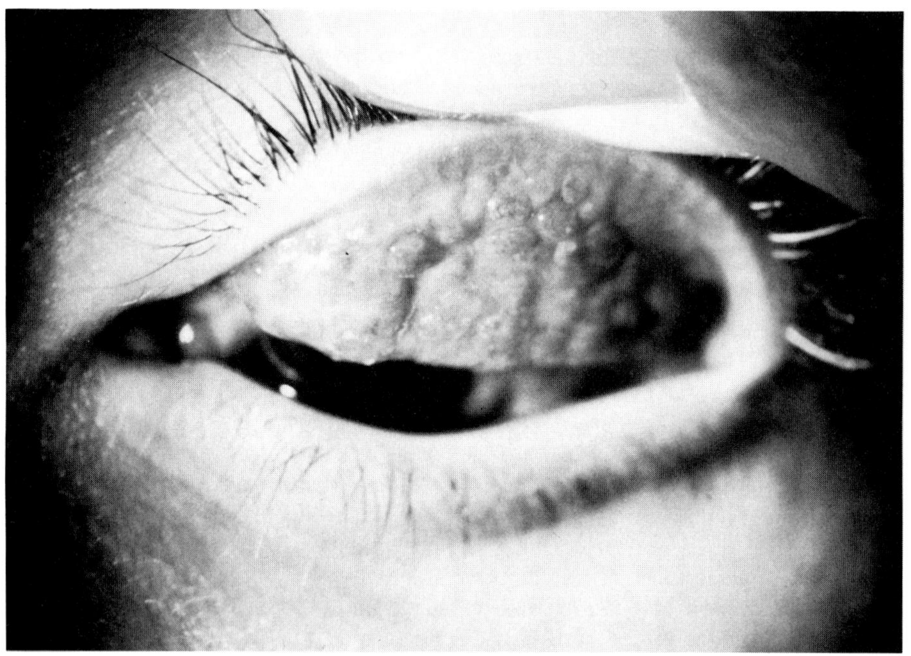

Fig. 162-1 Vernal conjunctivitis with the rather common papillae in a "cobblestone" arrangement.

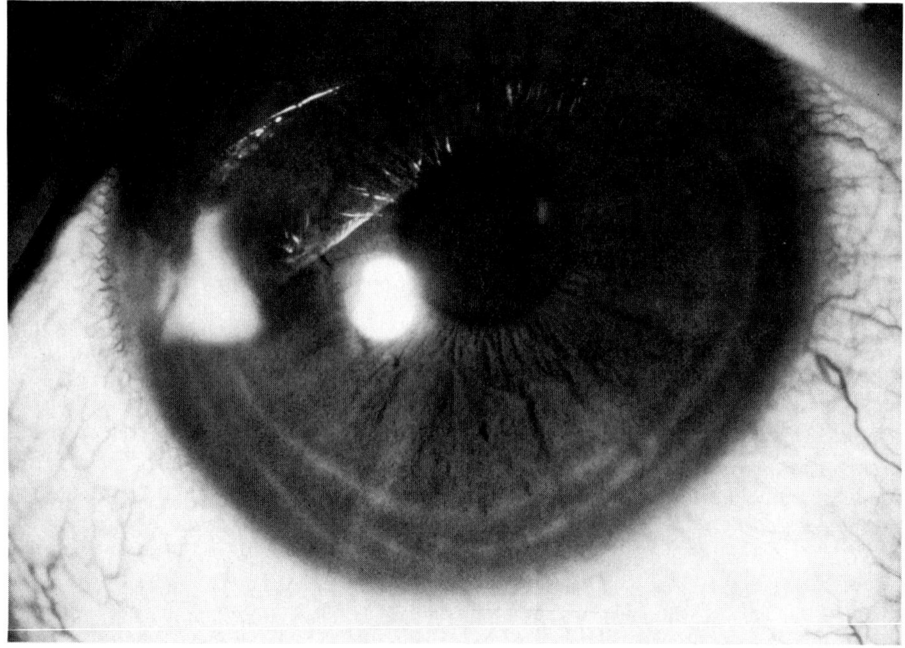

Fig. 162-2 Phlyctenular keratoconjunctivitis with corneal scarring and trailing "leash" of conjunctival vessels.

the less potent alternatives and cases in which culture and sensitivity results justify their use. Treatment should be continued for 24 to 48 hours after the conjunctival injection and purulence have subsided.

Viral Conjunctivitis

Fortunately most cases of viral conjunctivitis are readily suspected because of their association with fairly typical viral upper respiratory infections. As such, this type of conjunctivitis requires no treatment and is self-limited. The typical signs are a watery or mildly mucoid discharge, with mild to moderate conjunctival injection. Lid edema is usually mild, with rare lid erythema. Patients may complain of mild photophobia and discomfort. When a foreign body sensation is reported, a coexisting keratitis must be suspected.

In cases in which a keratitis is suspected, care must be exercised to rule out herpes simplex virus as the etiologic agent because of its potential for severe corneal damage and resultant visual loss. Fortunately fluorescein staining with the use of magnification can prove invaluable when a keratitis is suspected. The keratoconjunctivitis typically associated with an upper respiratory infection or isolated adenovirus infection is characterized by either no corneal staining or diffuse, stippled corneal staining; the keratoconjunctivitis of herpes simplex virus is characterized by an isolated branched lesion known as a dendrite. Dendrites or suspected dendritic keratitis requires referral to an ophthalmologist for definitive treatment.

Chlamydial Conjunctivitis

Chlamydial conjunctivitis is an acute, mucopurulent conjunctivitis often seen in the adolescent population, accompanying sexual promiscuity. Typically the conjunctivitis begins 4 to 12 days after contact with a new sexual partner. If the condition goes untreated, a keratitis, which may lead to corneal scarring, usually begins in the second week. Preauricular lymphadenopathy, reactive ptosis, and photophobia can be associated conditions. The diagnosis is most readily made with direct immunofluorescent antibody testing. Topical therapy alone is ineffective; it must be combined with systemic antibiotics such as tetracycline or erythromycin (1 g daily for 2 weeks). Sexual contacts also must be treated to prevent continued spread to or reinfection from sexual partners.

Fungal Conjunctivitis

Fungal conjunctivitis is exceedingly rare; patients whose conjunctivitis does not respond to standard therapeutic measures should be referred to an ophthalmologist, who can address a possible fungal etiology.

KERATITIS

Inflammation of the cornea (keratitis) indicates significant pathology that needs urgent attention from an ophthalmologist. Because the cornea is relatively avascular, keratitis is usually associated with perilimbal conjunctival injection (ciliary flush), which may simulate conjunctivitis. If the corneal epithelium is damaged, the pain can be quite intense. Otherwise, a mild to moderate foreign body sensation, blepharospasm, and significant epiphora (tearing) are the cardinal symptoms. Under normal conditions the cornea has a bright luster; however, when keratitis is present, the cornea is often hazy (Fig. 162-3) with stromal vessels and a dull corneal light reflex on direct illumination with a penlight. Fluorescein

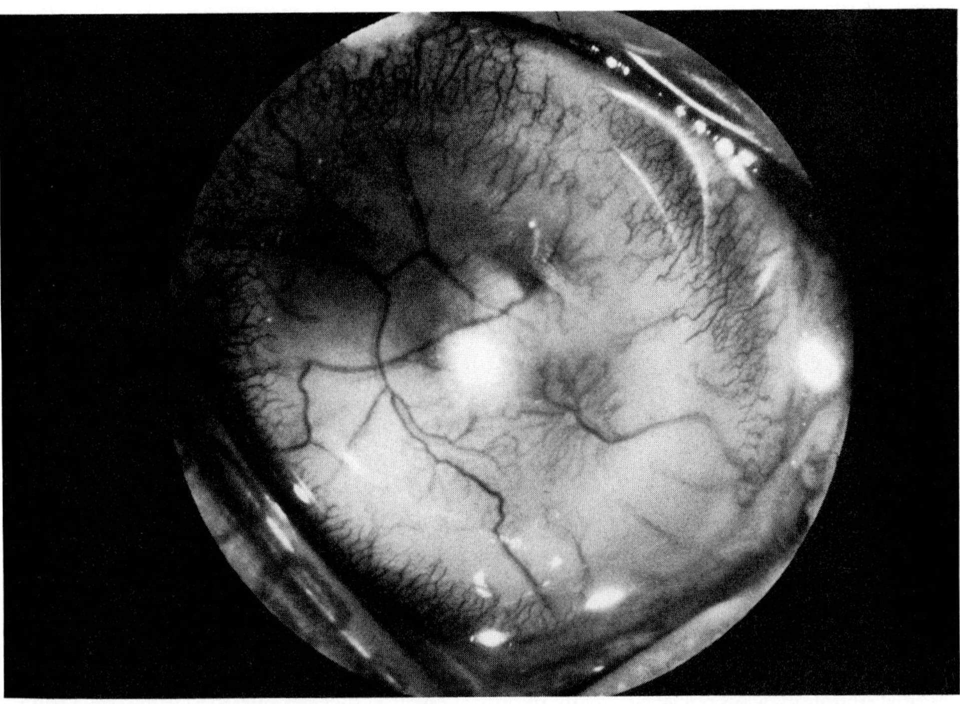

Fig. 162-3 Keratitis of unknown etiology in a newborn infant.

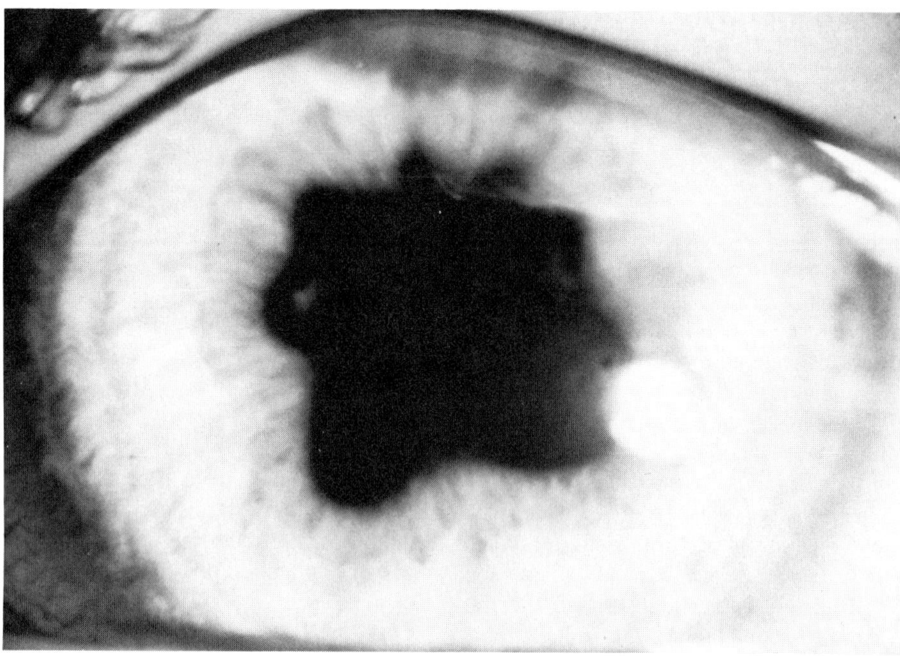

Fig. 162-4 Chronic anterior uveitis treated for 5 months as a chronic "conjunctivitis." Note the irregular pupil due to posterior synechiae.

staining can help distinguish herpes simplex virus keratitis from other forms by the characteristic dendrites.

IRITIS

Iritis is an inflammation of the anterior uvea (iris or ciliary body) and can indicate a severe, vision-threatening condition or even the initial manifestation of systemic disease. As in keratitis, the presenting sign is frequently a ciliary flush or generalized conjunctival injection. Blepharospasm, reactive ptosis, photophobia, epiphora, and pupillary meiosis (secondary to spasm of the constrictor muscle) are common. Iritis may be either unilateral or bilateral, and the more posterior layers of the eye may also be involved. Untreated iritis can result in glaucoma, cataracts, posterior synechiae (adhesions between the iris and the lens), and blindness. Because of the conjunctival injection and epiphora, a diagnosis of conjunctivitis is often first entertained and treatment with a topical antibiotic is instituted; however, the lack of a rapid clinical response soon makes one suspicious. Chronic treatment with an antibiotic may allow the posterior synechiae to become quite advanced (Fig. 162-4); thus any presumed conjunctivitis that does not readily respond should prompt referral to an ophthalmologist to rule out iritis. If iritis is diagnosed, systemic disease should be ruled out. Treatment of iritis is with mydriatic and cycloplegic agents to reduce the ciliary spasm and topical steroid agents (under the care of an ophthalmologist) to reduce inflammation and lessen the risk of posterior synechiae.

NASOLACRIMAL DUCT OBSTRUCTION

Nasolacrimal duct obstruction may be present in as many as 6% to 7% of healthy full-term infants (Fig. 162-5). Fortunately this common condition spontaneously resolves in about 90% of infants by 12 months of age. Occasionally, dacryocystitis (infection in the nasolacrimal sac) (Fig. 162-6) may occur and can progress to preseptal or orbital cellulitis. Treatment of nasolacrimal duct obstruction is varied; ophthalmologic opinion is split between early nasolacrimal duct probing and conservative management with nasolacrimal sac massage and topical antibiotics when purulence is present. Nasolacrimal sac massage is performed with five strokes from just beneath the medial aspect of the brow in a downward direction just nasal to the medial canthus and terminating about ¼ to ½ inch below the level of the medial canthus. The use solely of downward strokes serves to raise the pressure in the nasolacrimal sac in an attempt to overcome the obstruction usually found at the distal nasolacrimal duct. The success rate with conservative treatment is about 90% by 1 year of age, although early nasolacrimal duct probing is often performed to deal with parental unhappiness with the chronic tearing and mucous accumulation in the conjunctival sac.[1]

Referral to an ophthalmologist is indicated by 6 months of age if the condition persists or earlier if the presence of purulence cannot be controlled.

GLAUCOMA

Infantile or congenital glaucoma is usually readily diagnosed by the presence of its hallmark corneal enlargement. However, this rare condition is sometimes mistaken for conjunctivitis or nasolacrimal duct obstruction. The symptomatic constellation of tearing, photophobia, fussiness, and failure to thrive with signs of corneal enlargement (buphthalmos) and cloudiness should prompt urgent referral to an ophthalmologist so that the intraocular pressure can be managed (usually by surgery) to minimize visual loss.

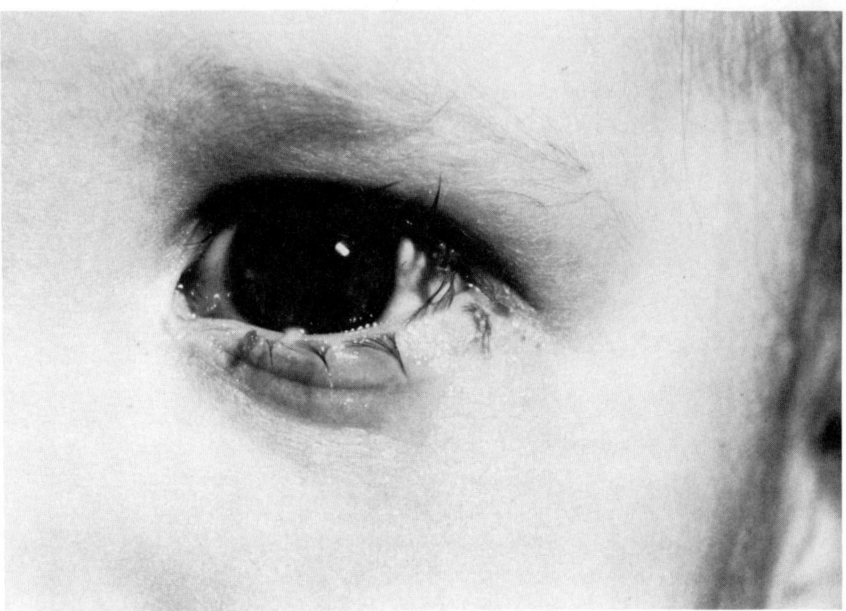

Fig. 162-5 Congenital nasolacrimal duct obstruction. Note the significant discharge, usually accompanied by epiphora. In the absence of conjunctival injection, antibiotic therapy is not indicated and treatment is with nasolacrimal sac massage.

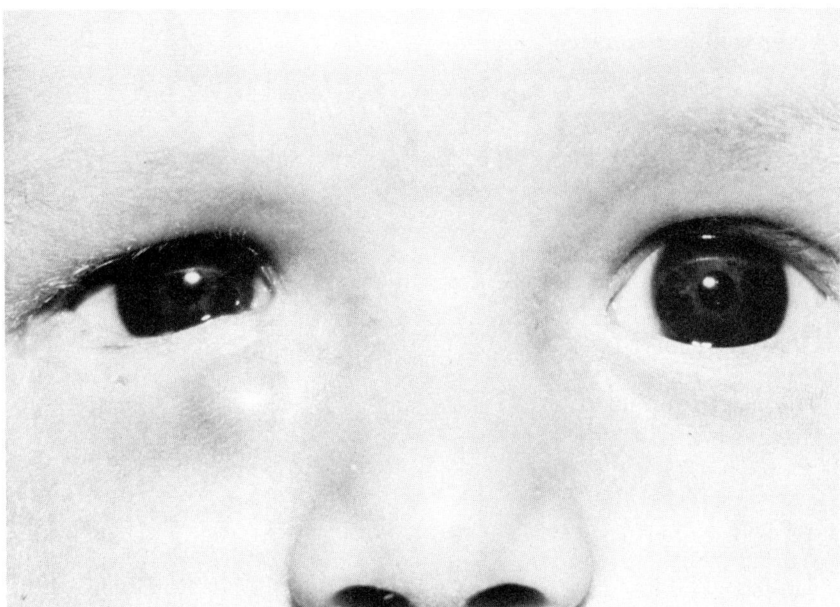

Fig. 162-6 Acute dacryocystitis secondary to nasolacrimal duct obstruction where massage was not performed. Pressure on the tear sac led to mucopurulent reflux from the superior and inferior puncta. Resolution of the dacryocystitis was complete with topical and systemic antibiotics and nasolacrimal sac massage was successful at overcoming the obstruction.

OPHTHALMIA NEONATORUM

Ophthalmia neonatorum is defined as inflammation of the conjunctiva in the first month of life without regard to etiology. The most common cause of ophthalmia neonatorum is a chemical conjunctivitis from the prophylaxis for gonococcal or chlamydial conjunctivitis. This conjunctivitis is usually characterized by conjunctival injection, mild lid edema, and scanty discharge. Fortunately chemical conjunctivitis usually resolves over 24 to 48 hours without sequelae.

The most common infectious cause of ophthalmia neonatorum is inclusion conjunctivitis caused by *Chlamydia trachomatis*. Bacterial ophthalmia neonatorum is usually caused by *Neisseria*, *Staphylococcus*, *Pneumococcus*, or *H. influenzae* organisms. Viral ophthalmia neonatorum caused by *herpes simplex* virus (Fig. 162-7) must also be considered. The bacterial conjunctivitis is characterized by a moderate or profuse purulent discharge with significant conjunctival hyperemia (Fig. 162-8); the lid edema may also be severe. In contrast, inclusion conjunctivitis is usually characterized by

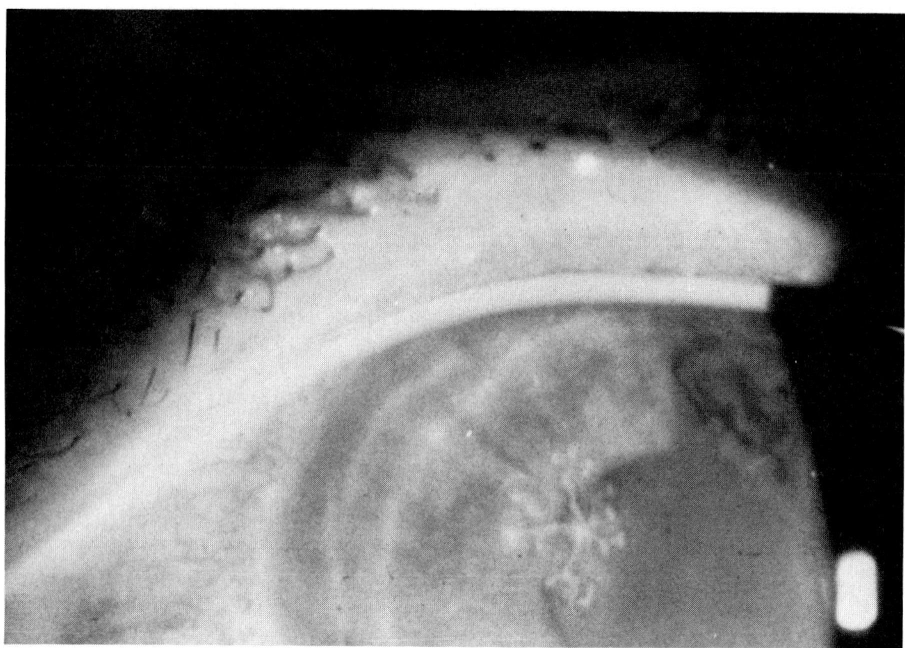

Fig. 162-7 Typical herpes simplex virus dendrites stained with fluorescein and viewed with a cobalt blue light.

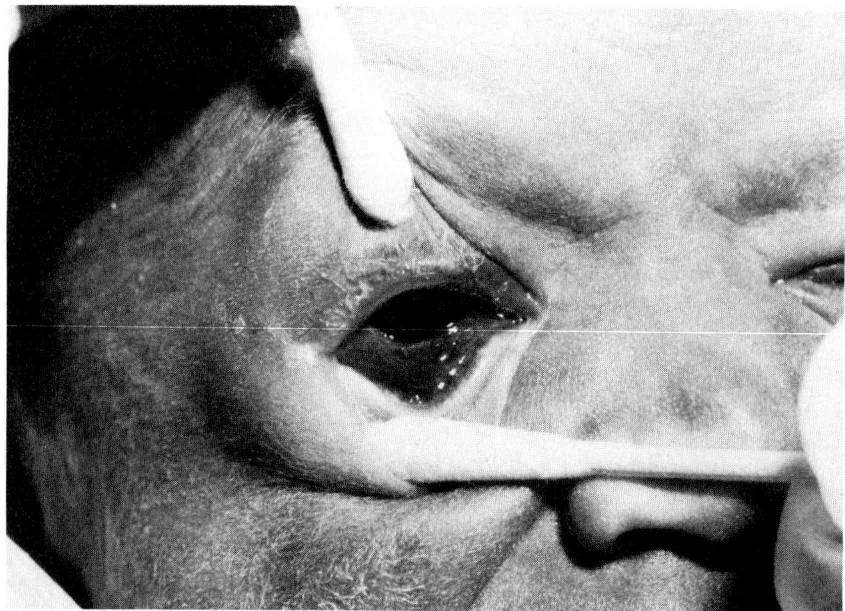

Fig. 162-8 Early bacterial ophthalmia neonatorum that was successfully treated with topical antibiotics.

a mucoid or mucopurulent discharge and mild lid edema with conjunctival injection. Viral ophthalmia neonatorum may be characterized by mild conjunctival injection with a serous discharge, although the cornea may be hazy if there is a simultaneous keratitis.

Diagnosis is determined by direct immunofluorescent antibody testing for *Chlamydia* organisms and by culture (for bacterial and viral ophthalmia neonatorum), with conjunctival scraping and plating markedly superior to the use of a cotton applicator sent to the microbiology laboratory. Treatment is organism specific, with systemic therapy reserved for *herpes virus*, *Chlamydia*, or *Neisseria* infections.

As a guide, gram positive organisms are usually well treated with sodium sulfacetamide 10% solution or ointment, or erythromycin ointment every 4 hours. *Haemophilus* species should also be treated with sodium sulfacetamide, with gentamycin or tobramycin reserved for gram negative organisms. Inclusion conjunctivitis is treated with topical and systemic erythromycin four times a day for at least 4 to 5 weeks. Herpes keratoconjunctivitis is best treated with idoxuridine or trifluridine topically, under the direction of an ophthalmologist, with appropriate systemic antiviral agents. *Neisseria gonorrhoeae* ophthalmia neonatorum is treated with aqueous penicillin G (50,000 U/lsg/day) in two or three divided doses for 7 days. Additionally, some advocate the use of topical aqueous penicillin G (10,000 to 20,000 U/ml), one drop hourly for the first 24 hours and then six times a day. The parents or sexual partners also need to be treated in cases of gonococcal and chlamydial ophthalmia neonatorum.

Previously, etiologic agents were predicted based on the time of onset of the conjunctivitis; however, because of the risk of a misdiagnosis, there is no substitute for appropriate diagnostic evaluation to determine the exact etiology. Additionally, the presence of any corneal findings or any uncertainty should prompt consultation with an ophthalmologist.

REFERENCE

1. Kushner BJ: Congenital nasolacrimal system obstruction, Arch Ophthalmol 100:597, 1982.

SUGGESTED READINGS

Allansmith MR: Vernal conjunctivitis. In Duane TD, editor: Clinical ophthalmology, Philadelphia, 1989, JB Lippincott Co.

Allansmith MR and Ross RN: Phlyctenular keratoconjunctivitis. In Duane TD, editor: Clinical ophthalmology, Philadelphia, 1989, JB Lippincott Co.

Arentsen JJ: Disorders of the conjunctiva in children. In Harley RD, editor: Pediatric ophthalmology, ed 2, Philadelphia, 1983, WB Saunders Co.

Dawson CR: Follicular conjunctivitis. In Duane TD, editor: Clinical ophthalmology, Philadelphia, 1989, JB Lippincott Co.

Flanagan JC, McLachlan DL, and Shannon GM: Diseases of the lacrimal apparatus. In Harley RD, editor: Pediatric ophthalmology, ed 2, Philadelphia, 1983, WB Saunders Co.

Laibson PR and Waring GO: Diseases of the cornea. In Harley RD, editor: Pediatric ophthalmology, ed 2, Philadelphia, 1983, WB Saunders Co.

Rotkis WM and Chandler JW: Neonatal conjunctivitis. In Duane TD, editor: Clinical ophthalmology, Philadelphia, 1989, JB Lippincott Co.

Walton DS: Glaucoma in infants and children. In Harley RD, editor: Pediatric ophthalmology, ed 2, Philadelphia, 1983, WB Saunders Co.

Wilson LA: Bacterial conjunctivitis. In Duane TD, editor: Clinical ophthalmology, Philadelphia, 1989, JB Lippincott Co.

163

Scrotal Swelling

Ross M. Decter

Scrotal swelling, especially if painful, usually prompts urgent pediatric consultation. Evaluation of the pain and concern about the possible effect of an abnormal scrotal process on the development of fertility and masculinity are of paramount concern to the parents. Scrotal swellings can be classified according to the rapidity of their presentation and association with pain (see the list in box). Emergency evaluation is indicated in all acutely painful swellings; chronic swellings tend to be painless.

An understanding of the anatomy of the scrotal contents greatly enhances the examiner's ability to diagnose scrotal pathology accurately (Fig. 163-1); a brief overview of the embryology of the scrotum and testicular descent will serve to review some of the relevant anatomic considerations.[11] The scrotum is derived from the sexually undifferentiated mesenchymal tissue called the labioscrotal folds. In the male fetus, dihydrotestosterone produced locally in these folds by the enzymatic conversion of testosterone prompts normal scrotal development. Early in gestation the scrotum is empty. The testicle is derived from a portion of the intermediate mesoderm known as the genital ridge. The epididymis and vas deferens arise from the mesonephric duct, which served transiently as the excretory tubule of the fetal mesonephric kidney.

Testicular descent occurs during the last 2 months of gestation, but before actual descent, an outpouching of the peritoneal cavity (the processus vaginalis) slowly extends into the scrotum (Fig. 163-2). By mechanisms that are incompletely understood, the testicle descends from its intraabdominal position through the inguinal canal into the scrotum. The processus vaginalis normally obliterates near its abdominal end after testicular descent. The potential space between the two layers of the distal projection of processus vaginalis surrounding the anterior two thirds of the testicle is known as the tunica vaginalis. A patent processus vaginalis, or patent processus, results if normal closure fails. The patent processus provides a communication between the abdominal cavity and the scrotum. Intraabdominal contents or fluids may enter the scrotum by passing through the processus and can cause scrotal swelling.

In the evaluation of any physical sign, an intimate knowledge of the anatomy of the area is a prerequisite to an educated physical examination. However, the examination cannot be limited to the scrotum, since intraabdominal or systemic processes may result in scrotal findings. A careful general examination with special attention to the abdomen (including a rectal examination) will often help define the nature of the scrotal swelling.

An unhurried and considerate approach to the history may set at ease an anxious, uncontrollable child and greatly facilitate the examination. The history of past health problems should be obtained first, with specific attention to genitourinary or abdominal surgery and urinary tract infections or instrumentation. A number of important historical points must be considered when evaluating the current problem: What was the swelling's time of onset? Was it an acute event or has it been intermittent or chronic? Is the swelling painful, and if so, what was the nature of the onset and severity of the pain? Where is the pain localized, and are there any associated problems such as nausea? The temporal relation of the pain, swelling, and erythema can also be helpful in establishing a diagnosis. Other relevant historical points include a specific inquiry about voiding problems, including

Classification of Scrotal Swelling

- Acute Scrotal Swelling
- Painful
  - Testicular torsion (intravaginal)
  - Torsion of testicular appendage
  - Epididymitis
  - Orchitis
  - Hernia*
  - Incarcerated
  - Strangulated
  - Intraabdominal pathology with scrotal findings caused by a patent processus vaginalis
  - Trauma
  - Henoch-Schönlein purpura
  - Idiopathic scrotal edema
  - Insect bites
  - Folliculitis
- Painless
  - Neonatal testicular torsion (extravaginal)
  - Hydrocele*
  - Hernia
  - Tumor*
- Chronic Scrotal Swelling
  - Hernia
  - Hydrocele
  - Tumor
  - Varicocele
  - Spermatocele
  - Sebaceous cyst of scrotal skin

*Variable presentation can be seen with some of these conditions.

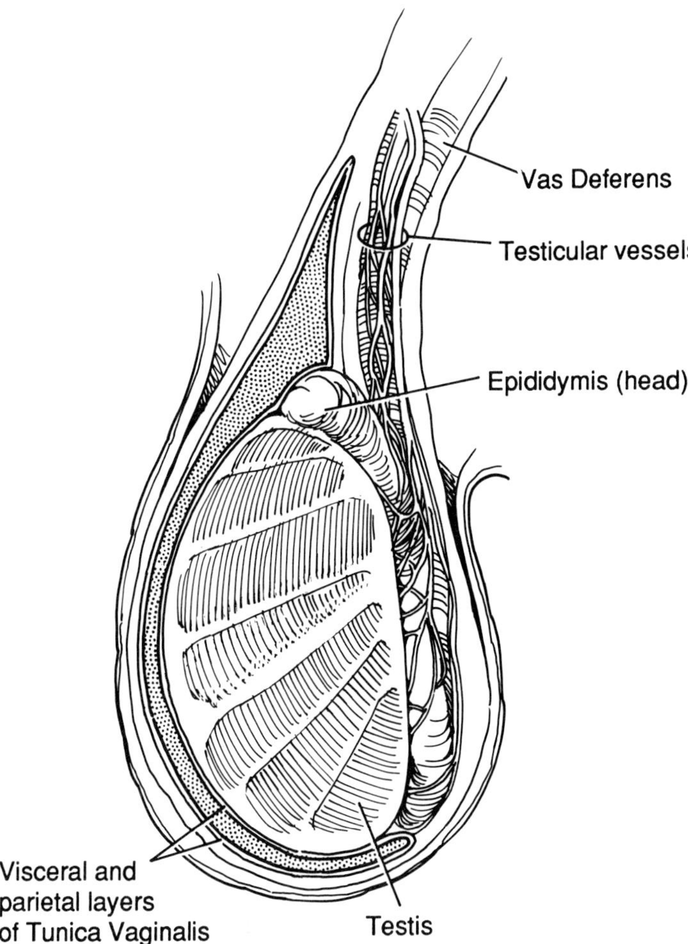

Fig. 163-1 The vas deferens terminates in the epididymis which is closely applied to the posterior aspect of the testicle. The vas deferens and its vessels along with the spermatic vessels comprise the spermatic cord. The tunica vaginalis encircles the anterior 2/3 of the testicle.

urgency, frequency, dysuria, hematuria, or penile discharge.

After establishing a rapport with the patient in the early part of the interview, the pediatrician should continue the questioning while beginning the examination. It can be helpful to start with the abdominal part of the examination, which usually is not painful. Careful inspection of the abdomen and groin may reveal abnormal swellings. The scrotum should be fully visualized, so that the swelling and the nature of the overlying skin can be evaluated. Certain findings characteristic of particular lesions are discussed in the section on each of those problems.

The unaffected testicle and hemiscrotum should be palpated initially—again, in an attempt to set the child at ease and to facilitate the examination. Important information can be obtained by examination of the "normal" side, which can allow one to make inferences about the affected side. While palpating the scrotal contents, it is imperative to evaluate each of the anatomic elements carefully and methodically, much as one listens to each of the heart sounds and the intervals between them to diagnose structural cardiac disease. The examiner must deliberately define the testis, epididymis, and vas deferens sequentially during the examination so that specific abnormalities of each structure can be evaluated. The nature of a mass can often be elucidated by transillumination, which will differentiate cystic or fluid-filled lesions from solid ones. With some conditions, examining the patient in the standing position can be helpful.

In some situations a laboratory evaluation is unnecessary; but in others, it provides essential adjunctive information. The laboratory evaluation often employed in the evaluation of an acutely painful scrotum includes a complete blood count with a differential count, urinalysis with culture, and a Gram stain of a urethral swab. Radiologic tests can be useful in evaluating scrotal pathology. Ultrasound helps to delineate anatomic findings that cannot be clearly defined by palpation, and radionuclide scanning can assess blood flow to the testes and scrotum.[13] Doppler evaluation of blood flow to the testicle has been useful in some cases.[2]

ACUTE PAINFUL SCROTAL SWELLINGS

The overriding concern in the evaluation of any patient with an acutely painful scrotum is to diagnose and treat testicular torsion promptly. The reason for this concern is that delay in diagnosis and treatment of torsion leads to testicular loss.

Testicular Torsion (Intravaginal)

Torsion, or twisting, of the testicle on its spermatic cord can cut off the blood supply to the testicle. The untreated testicle with torsion suffers ischemic necrosis and becomes functionless. The term intravaginal torsion implies that the twisting of the spermatic cord occurs inside the tunica vaginalis; this is the usual type of torsion in nonneonates. Normally the tunica vaginalis invests the anterior two thirds of the vertically oriented testis. In children predisposed to intravaginal torsion, the tunica vaginalis invests the whole testis and epididymis, and these testes tend to have a horizontal lie. The testicle is suspended from the spermatic vessels hanging into the tunica vaginalis; this anatomic variant is called the "bell clapper" deformity (Fig. 163-3). Urgent evaluation and treatment of testicular torsion are mandatory, since even short periods of ischemia damage the testicle, and prompt detorsion may preserve its function.

Intravaginal testicular torsion appears most commonly in the 10- to 14-year-old age group, although it can be seen at any age.[19] The child often awakes from sleep with severe scrotal pain, and a trip to the emergency room ensues. Not infrequently torsion is seen following mild scrotal trauma,[9] and at times a history of prior similar episodes is obtained.[22] Regardless of the history, the child is very uncomfortable and often vomits in association with the pain.

The physical findings vary with the time from onset of symptoms to presentation. The longer the delay to examination, the more swollen the testicle and scrotum become. If the child is seen shortly after the onset of the symptoms, one can often perceive an abnormal transverse testicular position in the unaffected testicle. The affected testicle seems drawn up and fixed in the scrotum. This is because of the twisting and therefore shortening of the spermatic cord. The testicle is very tender to palpation; the discerning examiner may be able to feel the twist in the spermatic cord above the testis.

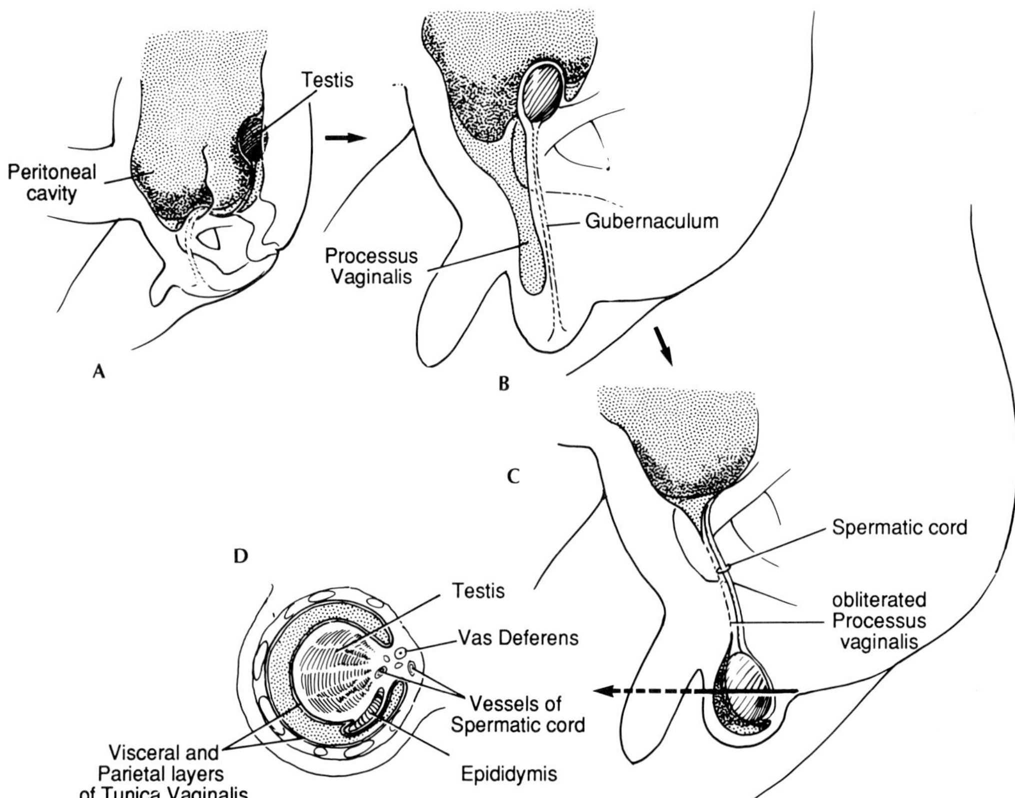

Fig. 163-2 A, In early gestation, a tongue of peritoneum extends through the inguinal canal. By the beginning of the third trimester **B,** this processus vaginalis extends toward the scrotum. **C,** After the testicle descends, the processus vaginalis obliterates having only remnant fibers. **D,** A cross section through the descended testicle demonstrates the relation of the tunica vaginalis to the testicle and epididymis.

In time, scrotal swelling, induration, and erythema become significant. A reactive hydrocele may form, and an accurate assessment of the intrascrotal contents becomes difficult.

Although the diagnosis can at times be straightforward, it is frequently difficult, and rapid laboratory and radiologic evaluation should be performed. The child is usually afebrile with an elevated white blood cell count. Urinalysis is normal. A radionuclide scan of the scrotum usually reveals a "cold spot" which represents the poorly perfused testis.

Once the diagnosis of testicular torsion is reached, prompt surgical intervention is necessary. Scrotal exploration is performed, and the testicle is untwisted. If it appears to be viable after reperfusion, it is sutured in the scrotum in a fashion that precludes further episodes of torsion. Because the contralateral testicle often has the same bell clapper deformity, it is explored and also fixed to the scrotum to prevent subsequent torsion.

Testicular salvage after torsion depends on the time it takes to implement surgical correction and the severity of the torsion. At times the testicle will twist up to three or four complete revolutions, and this immediately cuts off the arterial inflow. Few testicles with this severe degree of torsion are salvaged because of the ischemia that ensues, unless exploration occurs in 4 to 6 hours. However, with less severe degrees of torsion, some testicles have been saved up to 24 hours after the onset of symptoms.[17]

Torsion of Testicular Appendages

There are several vestigial appendages attached to the testis, epididymis, and vas deferens (Fig. 163-4). The appendix testis is the appendage that is present most often, and torsion of the appendix testis is a common cause of acute scrotal pain and swelling.

The peak age of incidence of appendiceal torsion is 10 years.[19] The onset of pain is acute, and although at times the pain is less severe than with the testicle, it is not very dissimilar. Some patients have had prior episodes of intermittent torsion of the appendage.

Physical examination can be diagnostic, especially if the boy is seen early in the process. Careful palpation reveals the testis to be normal and actually nontender. The tenderness is localized to the upper pole, where one can feel a palpable and exquisitely tender mass. Often the torsed appendix, which is gangrenous and therefore black, can be seen through the skin as a "blue dot." This combination of findings is pathognomonic of the torsed testicular appendage. If the boy is seen later in the disease process, the scrotum may have become very swollen and erythematous, so that examination and precise physical diagnosis are more difficult.

The child with torsion of the appendix testis is afebrile, with a normal or elevated white blood cell count and no abnormal findings on urinalysis. If the physical examination is not diagnostic, testicular scanning can be helpful. The scan will show normal to slightly increased perfusion of the testis without a cold spot.

Management of this condition can take two forms. A supportive, conservative approach with analgesics, rest, and reassurance is generally adopted.[14] It is important to let the child and parents know that the discomfort will usually abate within 5 to 10 days. Another option is surgical excision of the appendix,

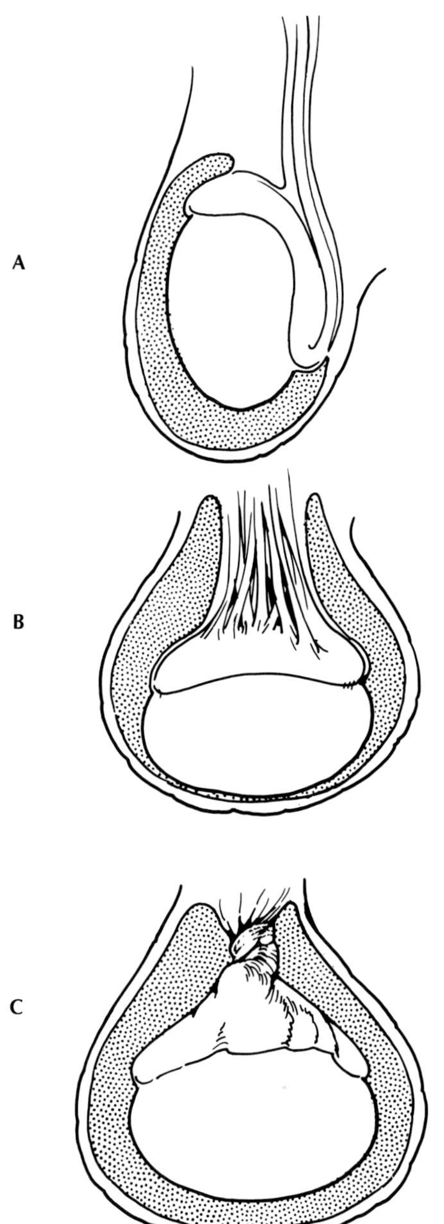

Fig. 163-3 A, The normal anatomical arrangement with a vertically oriented testicle encircled in its anterior portion by the tunica vaginalis. The "bell clapper" deformity is demonstrated in **B**. The testis has a horizontal lie and the tunica vaginalis extends up over the distal spermatic cord. The testis is essentially suspended within the tunica vaginalis by the spermatic cord. **C,** The twist in the spermatic cord demonstrates the typical pathology seen in intravaginal torsion.

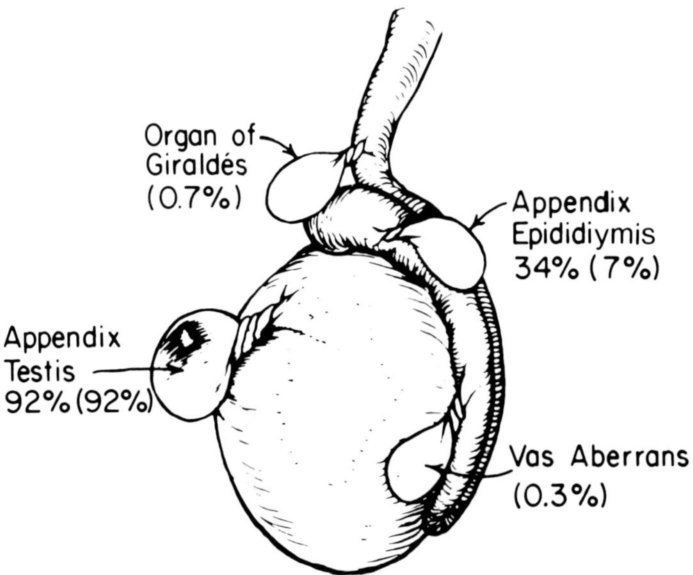

Fig. 163-4 The position of the various testicular appendages is demonstrated. The incidence of torsion of these appendages is shown in brackets. Torsion of the appendix testis is vastly more frequent than torsion of the other appendices.

Used with permission, Sheldon, CA: Surg Clin North Am 65(5):1303, 1985.

which decreases the period of discomfort to 1 to 2 days but exposes the child to the risk of general anesthesia.[10]

Epididymitis/Orchitis

Infection of the epididymis is characterized by scrotal pain and swelling. Although the onset of the pain is less acute than that of torsion, it may progress and become severe. Infections of the epididymis can spread into the testis, causing a concomitant orchitis. At times the testicle is affected primarily. Mumps orchitis is a good example of a primary testicular infection. Mumps orchitis is found almost exclusively in postpubertal boys[1] and can result in postinfectious atrophy.

The boy with epididymitis may have an antecedent history of sexual contact, penile discharge, or itch. In this case the epididymitis is usually caused by *Chlamydia* organisms or gonorrhea.[8] In the younger patient who hasn't had sexual contact, one may at times obtain a history suggesting lower urinary tract infection, although the majority of these patients have a sterile urine culture.[12] It is not known whether viral infections or the chemical irritation of urine passing retrograde up the vas deferens to affect the testicle is important in the causation of these cases of epididymitis.

Physical examination early in the course of epididymitis will reveal tenderness and swelling localized to the epididymis. As the disease progresses, both the scrotal contents and the scrotal wall become swollen; however, this specific finding is difficult to discern. In severe cases the inflammatory process extends not only into the testicle but up the epididymis into the vas deferens and causes an infection of the spermatic cord, or funiculitis.

Boys with epididymitis may be febrile. Laboratory evaluation will show an elevated white blood cell count. Urinalysis will at times show pyuria but is usually normal.[12] Urine cultures are usually sterile in boys who do not have a urethral discharge or obvious anatomic problems such as prior hypospadias repairs or myelomeningocele.

If the examination and laboratory data do not allow for a clear diagnosis, radionuclide scanning can be useful. In boys with epididymitis, the scan will show increased uptake without cold spots. Treatment with antibiotics is generally effective, even with negative urine cultures.

Hernias and Swellings Caused by a Patent Processus Vaginalis

In the male child the term "inguinal hernia" implies the presence of an intraabdominal structure passing from the peritoneal cavity into the processus vaginalis, which is patent for a variable extent toward the scrotum. In most cases the intraabdominal structure passing through the groin toward the scrotum is omentum or intestines. In patients with a hernia, the groin is swollen and the swelling may extend into the scrotum. Hernias are often asymptomatic except for the parent noting an intermittent groin and upper scrotal swelling unassociated with pain. At times, however, an intraabdominal structure gets trapped in the inguinal canal and cannot pass back into the abdominal cavity; these hernias are said to be irreducible or incarcerated. The risk of incarceration is greatest in boys under 1 year of age.[21] The incarceration may cause some groin or abdominal discomfort and, if bowel is involved, stomach upset with vomiting. If a piece of bowel that is incarcerated suffers vascular compromise, it becomes strangulated. In children, incarceration leads to strangulation; therefore incarcerated hernias must be reduced. With strangulation the groin becomes tender in addition to being swollen, and as the process progresses, the area may become red. With tissue reaction and swelling, the incarcerated or strangulated hernia may affect the blood supply of other structures running through the inguinal canal, and at times the testicle can undergo necrosis because of vascular compromise caused by the hernia.

Although most inguinal hernias cause more groin than scrotal swelling, at times the processus vaginalis is open all the way to the testis, allowing intraabdominal contents to herniate into the scrotum. These hernias are characterized by both scrotal and groin swelling (Fig. 163-5).

Hernias are managed by surgical correction. The timing of surgery depends on the type of hernia; surgery may be semielective in the case of an asymptomatic inguinal hernia or emergent in the case of a strangulated hernia.

Intraabdominal Pathology Leading to Acute Scrotal Swelling

The patent processus vaginalis may allow fluids emanating from the peritoneal cavity to cause scrotal swelling. Hydroceles caused by normal peritoneal fluid shifting through the patent processus are discussed below. Intraperitoneal blood can track through the processus and cause scrotal swelling. Bleeding caused by obvious trauma and unsuspected child abuse has been characterized by bluish, nontransilluminating scrotal swelling.[23] Intraperitoneal processes associated with peritonitis and purulent peritoneal fluid can similarly cause scrotal swelling. Cases of primary peritonitis[24] and appendicitis[25] have caused scrotal swelling. As these fluids are infected, the scrotum may become red and tender. Treatment of these cases of scrotal swelling is directed toward the primary pathology and depends on evaluation of the swelling leading to the correct diagnosis.

Less Frequent Causes of Acute Scrotal Pain

Intentional or accidental trauma may be an obvious cause of scrotal pain and swelling. Because the testicle is mobile in the scrotum, significant injuries to the testicle occur relatively infrequently with minor scrotal trauma. If, however, the testicle is damaged by trauma, acute painful swelling will ensue. Even with careful palpation, anatomic definition may be difficult because of the severe swelling and tenderness. Ultrasound is very useful in helping to diagnose testicular rupture. Surgical exploration is necessary in cases of testicular rupture, with debridement of devascularized tissue and reconstruction of the remnant testis if possible. Less significant injuries are treated with bed rest, scrotal elevation, and analgesics.

Henoch-Schönlein purpura (HSP) is a systemic vasculitis of unknown etiology. The multisystem lesions are characterized by nonthrombocytopenic purpura. Scrotal involvement may occur in up to 38% of boys,[3] and scrotal findings have been the initial manifestation of the disease in a few.[5] In the

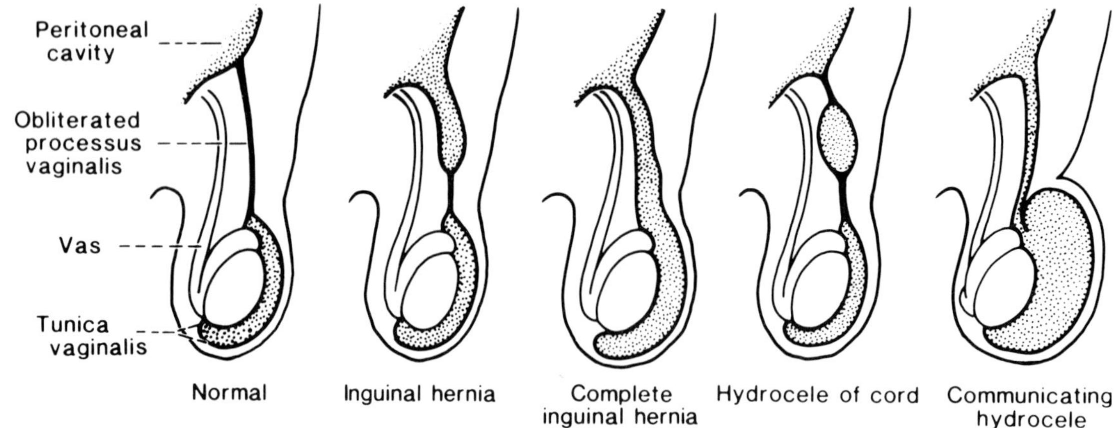

Fig. 163-5 The schematic of the communicating hydrocele demonstrates the patent processus. In the normal situation the processus is obliterated. Varying degrees of closure may lead to either a typical inguinal hernia or if the processus is open all the way into the scrotum a complete hernia. A hydrocele of the cord results if fluid collects between two closed segments of the processus.

Used with permission. Rowe MI. In Welch KJ, Randolph JG, Ravitch MM et al, editors: Pediatric surgery, ed 4, Chicago, 1986, Year Book Medical Publishers, Inc.

latter cases the correct diagnosis was ascertained following scrotal exploration for presumed testicular torsion when other signs of the condition appeared. Although involvement by vasculitis is the most common cause of scrotal swelling and pain in HSP, testicular torsion has been reported,[18] and this possibility must be excluded when the boy is evaluated.

Idiopathic scrotal edema (ISE) is marked by acute scrotal swelling. The skin is characteristically edematous and bright pink. Although the scrotum is uncomfortable, the appearance is more remarkable than the degree of pain. The cause of this condition is not known, although a strong allergic history is observed in some boys.[20] ISE appears at a younger age than does torsion of the testicle or testicular appendages.[19] Skin swelling and erythema are often not limited to one side of the scrotum in ISE and may extend to both sides, the perineum, groin, or penis. The testis is normal in this condition, and the process is self-limited.

An unusual cause of scrotal pain and swelling is thrombosis of the spermatic veins.[6] Only a few cases are reported in children, and the diagnosis is one of exclusion. This condition could result in the diagnosis of ISE.

Primary skin pathology also can cause painful scrotal swelling. In these cases the intrascrotal contents are palpably normal, and the abnormality is limited to the scrotal skin. Severe diaper rash may result in scrotal swelling; this is generally accompanied by extension of the process beyond the scrotum. Insect bites on the scrotum occur, and one can often find the actual site of the bite with the surrounding reaction and secondary infection. In the postpubertal male, a localized infection of hair follicles, or folliculitis, may lead to a swollen scrotum, and a similar complication may result from secondary infection of sebaceous cysts.

Scrotal pain and swelling have been reported to result from scrotal fat necrosis.[16] Children with this condition have been exposed to cold, such as while sledding, and this seems to precipitate the process. The fat necrosis forms palpable tender nodules in the scrotum near a normal testis. The condition resolves with time, but if any question of the diagnosis exists, exploration should be undertaken to avoid missing more significant pathology.

PAINLESS SCROTAL SWELLINGS

The onset of a painless swelling may be difficult to establish. Pain provokes immediate attention, but a painless scrotal process may be occult, especially if the child is out of diapers. Painless swellings are therefore more difficult to classify as either acute or chronic.

Neonatal Testicular Torsion (Extravaginal)

The typical boy with neonatal torsion of the testes has a large swelling of the hemiscrotum at birth. The intrascrotal contents form a firm, smooth mass. There may be fixation to the scrotal skin, and the testicular anatomy cannot be clearly defined. The skin may be minimally red or thickened. The child behaves normally, and no symptoms can be attributed to the mass.[15]

In neonatal torsion there is no anomaly of tunica vaginalis investment of the testis. The torsion, which involves the total spermatic cord, occurs during testicular descent. The twist occurs above the testicle, usually at the external ring, the point at which the cord exits the inguinal canal. Torsion at this point is said to be possible because the loose attachments of the testicular tunics to the scrotum fail to fix the testicle in position.[4]

Although the vast majority of cases of neonatal torsion occur in utero, there are a few instances in which the initial examination showed normal testes and a subsequent examination in the nursery revealed the scrotal swelling. Except in this unusual situation, these testicles have not been found to be viable on exploration, and when followed the testes atrophy, at times becoming impalpable. The risk of contralateral extravaginal torsion with possible resultant anorchia has engendered controversy regarding contralateral testicular fixation. Because of the slightly increased risk of anesthesia in neonates and the rarity of asynchronous bilateral extravaginal torsion, there is no unanimity of opinion regarding optimum management of this problem.

Hydrocele

A hydrocele is a fluid collection between the two layers of the tunica vaginalis. In the pediatric age group this frequent finding[26] is almost invariably caused by fluid from the peritoneal cavity passing via the patent processus vaginalis into the scrotum (Fig. 163-5). This communicating hydrocele is so named because of the connection between the peritoneal cavity and the tunica vaginalis. The usual history of the swelling is that the scrotum looked normal in the morning but became swollen as the day progressed, only to have the swelling disappear by the next morning. Fluid shifts through the patent processus obviously account for the variable findings.

Physical examination reveals a scrotal swelling that may be tense. Often the fluid imparts a bluish color to the affected scrotum. The fluid consistency may be obvious on palpation, but if the hydrocele is tense, brilliant transillumination usually determines its nature. If the testicle is difficult to perceive within the hydrocele, it can be easily imaged with and the diagnosis confirmed by ultrasound.

A patent processus frequently persists after birth, and hydroceles often ensue. The majority of the processus will close spontaneously by 18 months of age. If the hydrocele persists beyond that age or if the swelling seems to be symptomatic, surgical correction is recommended.

Hydroceles may form secondary to primary testicular pathology. These reactive hydroceles occur, for example, in some cases of epididymoorchitis or testicular tumors. An exacting evaluation of the testicle is mandatory to rule out testicular pathology whenever a hydrocele is present.

Tumors

A testicular tumor usually appears as a slowly enlarging scrotal mass. Unless a complication such as bleeding or torsion occurs, the mass tends to be painless. Examination reveals the mass to be firm and free of fixation to the scrotum. The testis is often not discernible by the time of diagnosis, because the tumor usually replaces the testicle. The solid nature of the mass is suspected by a lack of transillumination, although in some cases a reactive hydrocele can be seen. When a question about the examination exists, ultrasound will reliably define the anatomy. After a prompt staging evaluation, which should include serum for tumor markers, the testicle and spermatic cord are excised through a groin incision. Although most testicular tumors in neonates are benign, the same cannot be said in other age groups, and urgent evaluation and treatment are mandatory.

Scrotal swelling may be caused by a mass adjacent to the testicle. If the mass is solid and localized to the spermatic cord, especially if the examination reveals a normal testis, the possibility of paratesticular rhabdomyosarcoma must be excluded. Initial treatment requires a radical inguinal orchiectomy, as in the case of primary testicular tumors.

Varicocele

A varicocele is a dilation of the veins in the spermatic cord. Similar to varicose veins in the legs, these dilations are caused by incompetent valves—in this case, in the internal spermatic venous system. Varicoceles are not seen before puberty. Symptoms caused by a varicocele may include a dull, dragging discomfort in the scrotum; in some patients no discomfort is felt, but the scrotal swelling caused by the veins is noted. The lesion may also be asymptomatic. Observation of the scrotum reveals dilated veins with large varicoceles visible through the scrotal skin. The veins are palpable through the scrotal wall, and they have been likened to a "bag of worms." Characteristically, the varicocele is visible or palpable when the patient is standing; when the patient reclines, the veins collapse and are difficult to perceive. If the varicocele is noted to have an acute onset and if it does not collapse when the patient lies down, then the possibility of a fixed obstruction of the internal spermatic vein where it enters the renal vein must be excluded. In children, such an obstruction could result from a tumor thrombus in the renal vein from Wilms tumor, and this must be excluded. Although varicoceles are commonly associated with infertility, many fertile men have varicoceles. Because fertility potential is not known in the pediatric age group, most surgeons recommend surgical correction of a varicocele only if it is symptomatic or if the testicle on the side of the varicocele is significantly smaller than its mate.

UNUSUAL CAUSES OF PAINLESS SCROTAL SWELLING

A condition in the neonate characterized by scrotal swelling and bruising has been reported as a consequence of a difficult vaginal delivery. In these cases bleeding occurs within the spermatic cord, possibly as a result of forces transmitted to the spermatic veins during the delivery. This leads to bruising and swelling not only of the scrotum but also at the level of the external ring. The testicle reportedly has been unaffected in these instances; however, exploration to establish the diagnosis and drain the hematoma has been recommended.[7]

A spermatocele arises from the ducts draining from the testis into the epididymis. Spermatoceles are cystic structures that may have more than one locule. These lesions are seen in postpubertal males, and the fluid within the spermatocele may contain degenerating spermatozoa. The patient has a painless mass adjacent to or arising from the epididymis. The multiple locules may be evident on examination, and the mass will transilluminate brilliantly. If any question about the nature of the mass exists, ultrasound should be used to define the anatomy. If the mass is asymptomatic and its nature clearly defined, no specific treatment is recommended. At times these lesions can become quite large; if the patient is bothered by this, surgical excision is recommended.

Scrotal skin lesions such as sebaceous cysts are readily diagnosed. In these conditions the lesion is limited to the skin, and the intrascrotal contents are normal.

REFERENCES

1. Beard CM et al: The incidence and outcome of mump orchitis in Rochester, Minnesota, 1935-1974, Mayo Clin Proc 52:3, 1977.
2. Bickerstaff KI, Sethia K, and Murie JA: Doppler ultrasonography in the diagnosis of acute scrotal pain, Br J Surg 75:238, 1988.
3. Byrn JR et al: Unusual manifestations of Henoch-Schönlein syndrome, Am J Dis Child 130:1335, 1976.
4. Campbell MF: Torsion of the spermatic cord in the newborn infant, J Pediatr 33:323, 1948.
5. Clark WR and Kramer SA: Henoch-Schönlein purpura and the acute scrotum, J Pediatr Surg 21(11):991, 1986.
6. Coolsaet B and Weinberg R: Thrombosis of the spermatic vein in children, J Urol 124:290, 1980.
7. Davenport M, Bianchi A, and Gough DCS: Idiopathic scrotal haemorrhage in neonates, Br Med J 298:1492, 1989.
8. Edelsberg JS and Surh YS: The acute scrotum, Emerg Med Clin North Am 6(3):521, 1988.
9. Elsaharty S et al: Traumatic torsion of the testis, J Urol 132:1155, 1984.
10. Flanigan RC, DeKernion JB, and Persky L: Acute scrotal pain and swelling in children: a surgical emergency, Urology 17(1):51, 1981.
11. George FW and Wilson JD: Embryology of the genital tract. In Walsh PC et al, editors: Campbell's urology, Philadelphia, 1986, WB Saunders Co.
12. Gislason T, Noronha RFX, and Gregory JG: Acute epididymitis in boys: a 5-year retrospective study, J Urol 124:533, 1980.
13. Golimbu M et al: Value of scrotal scanning: report of 62 cases, Urology 25(1):89, 1985.
14. Holland JM, Graham JB, and Ignatoff JM: Conservative management of twisted testicular appendages, J Urol 125:213, 1981.
15. Kaplan GW and Silber I: Neonatal torsion—to pex or not? In King LR, editor: Urologic surgery in neonates and young infants, Philadelphia, 1988, WB Saunders Co.
16. Koster LH and Antoon SJ: Fat necrosis in the scrotum, J Urol 123:599, 1980.
17. Krorup T: The testis after torsion, Br J Urol 50:43, 1978.
18. Loh HS and Jalan OM: Testicular torsion of Henoch-Schönlein syndrome, Br Med J 2:96, 1974.
19. Melekos MD, Asbach HW, and Markou SA: Etiology of acute scrotum in 100 boys with regard to age distribution, J Urol 139:1023, 1988.
20. Najmaldin A and Burge DM: Acute idiopathic scrotal oedema: incidence, manifestations and aetiology, Br J Surg 74:634, 1987.
21. Rowe MI and Lloyd DA: Inguinal hernia. In Welch KJ et al, editors: Pediatric surgery, ed 4, Chicago, 1986, Year Book Medical Publishers, Inc.
22. Stillwell TJ and Kramer SA: Intermittent testicular torsion, Pediatrics 77(6):908, 1986.
23. Sujka SK, Jewett TC Jr, and Karp MP: Acute scrotal swelling as the first evidence of intraabdominal trauma in the battered child, J Pediatr Surg 23(4):380, 1988.
24. Udall DA, Drake DJ Jr, and Rosenberg RS: Acute scrotal swelling: a physical sign of primary peritonitis, J Urol 125:750, 1981.
25. Wilkins SA Jr et al: Acute appendicitis presenting as acute left scrotal pain: diagnostic considerations, Urology 25(6):634, 1985.
26. Wilson-Storey D: Scrotal swellings in the under 5's, Arch Dis Child 62:50, 1987.

164

Sexual Developmental Alterations

Robert K. Kritzler and Leslie P. Plotnick

Disorders of pubertal development constitute one of the most frequent referrals to pediatric endocrinology clinics. In many cases no endocrine problem is found. Frequently, a costly referral can be avoided by a careful evaluation, including family history, and a few simple laboratory procedures.

At puberty a series of complex hormonal changes takes place. The hypothalamus secretes pulses of gonadotropin-releasing hormone (GnRH), which stimulates pituitary gonadotropin production of luteinizing hormone (LH) and follicle-stimulating hormone (FSH). Concomitantly, the previously very sensitive gonadal-hypothalamic-pituitary feedback loop becomes less sensitive to the negative effect of gonadal steroids; thus gonadotropin levels increase. This results in the secretion of greater amounts of androgens or estrogens, depending on the sex of the child, leading to the physical changes of puberty. There is also an increase in secretion of adrenal androgens. The mechanism that triggers the maturation of the adrenal cortex at puberty remains poorly understood.

In girls, breast development is usually the first sign of puberty, with the mean age of onset at 10½ years and a standard deviation of 2½ years. This is followed in about 6 months by the appearance of pubic hair. Menarche follows the onset of breast development by about 2 years. A growth spurt accompanies the changes, usually peaking before menarche. The range of normal variation, however, is quite wide.

In boys, testicular enlargement and scrotal thinning are the first signs of puberty, with a mean age of onset at 11½ years and a standard deviation of 2 years; this is followed in about 6 months by pubic hair growth and some penile enlargement. Approximately 2 years after the first changes, axillary hair and then facial hair appear. The male growth spurt peaks 12 to 18 months after that of the female. As with girls, the normal range is wide.

The time of puberty is one of profound change, both physical and psychological. Problems of sexual identity, body image, adolescent independence, and peer acceptance are frequent. When pubertal development is precocious or delayed, many of these problems are compounded.

DELAYED DEVELOPMENT

Few matters are of greater concern to the adolescent than remaining short in stature or sexually underdeveloped. Delayed development demands the immediate attention of the practitioner.

Puberty is considered delayed in girls who have no breast development by 13 years of age or in boys without testicular enlargement at 14 years of age. In girls a delay of more than 5 years from onset of puberty to menarche is also cause for concern. Similarly, maturation arrest in boys warrants evaluation. Delayed puberty is much more common in boys than girls.

Constitutional delay, a slow maturation with appropriate hormonal levels, accounts for more than 90% of all cases of delayed pubertal development. This problem is much more frequently identified in boys, perhaps because of general societal and peer group reaction to short and sexually underdeveloped boys. It is frequently familial. Often, early signs of puberty are found on careful examination, which permits the physician to reassure the child and the parents. Chronic systemic diseases that can lead to delayed puberty may be difficult to differentiate from constitutional delay as a cause for the difficulty; these diseases are given in the box on p. 1064.

The remainder of the differential diagnosis of delayed development relates to failure at either the hypothalamic-pituitary level, shown by low serum gonadotropins (*hypogonadotropic hypogonadism*), or at the gonadal level, shown by elevated gonadotropins (*hypergonadotropic hypogonadism*). Either of these conditions may result from genetic disorders or acquired illnesses (see box on p. 1064). The workup of the patient is directed toward identifying the specific cause.

Treatment should be directed, when possible, toward the cause of the delayed development. If sex steroid secretion is deficient, either primarily or secondary to gonadotropin deficiency, treatment centers on replacing the appropriate sex steroid.

In constitutional delay, waiting is the best course. In males, however, a short course of injectable testosterone may be indicated if the delayed development is affecting the boy's psychological well-being. In girls the use of a padded bra is very helpful. Estrogen therapy is only occasionally necessary. In patients with GnRH or gonadotropin deficiency, fertility may be induced with GnRH or gonadotropin therapy.

In any case, strong psychological support must be provided to the adolescent and sometimes to the family. If the problem is diagnostically difficult or if hormonal therapy is desired, referral should be made to an endocrinologist.

PRECOCIOUS DEVELOPMENT

Precocious puberty is the appearance of secondary sexual characteristics before 8 years of age in girls and before 9 years in boys. It may be isosexual (appropriate for phenotype)

Causes of Delayed Puberty

I. Constitutional delay
II. Deficiency of GnRH secretion by the hypothalamus
  A. Genetic
    1. Isolated deficiency
    2. Kallmann syndrome
    3. Laurence-Moon-Bardet-Biedl syndrome
    4. Prader-Willi syndrome
  B. Acquired
    1. Infection
    2. Neoplasm
    3. Infiltrative disease
    4. Trauma
III. Deficiency of gonadotropic secretion by the pituitary
  A. Genetic
    1. Panhypopituitarism
    2. Isolated deficiency
    3. Fertile eunuch (normal FSH, low LH)
  B. Acquired
    1. Infection
    2. Neoplasm
    3. Trauma
IV. Gonadal disorders
  A. Genetic
    1. Turner syndrome (45, X or structural X abnormalities or mosaicism)
    2. Klinefelter syndrome (47, XXY abnormality)
    3. Noonan syndrome
    4. Syndromes of complete androgen insensitivity (no sexual hair)
    5. Del Castillo syndrome (Sertoli cells only)
    6. Pure gonadal dysgenesis
    7. Myotonic dystrophy
  B. Acquired
    1. Infections
      a. Gonorrhea (male)
      b. Virus (usually mumps)
      c. Tuberculosis (male)
    2. Radiotherapy or chemotherapy
    3. Mechanical causes
      a. Torsion
      b. Surgery
      c. "Vanishing testes"
    4. Autoimmune
V. Adrenal and gonadal steroid enzyme deficiencies
VI. Chronic systemic diseases
  A. Congenital heart disease
  B. Chronic pulmonary disease
  C. Inflammatory bowel disease
  D. Chronic renal failure and renal tubular acidosis
  E. Hypothyroidism
  F. Poorly controlled diabetes mellitus
  G. Sickle cell anemia
  H. Collagen-vascular disease
  I. Anorexia nervosa

or heterosexual (appropriate for opposite sex phenotype). Precocious puberty is much more common in girls than in boys. In girls, idiopathic precocious puberty is the single most common diagnosis, but precocious puberty in boys is more likely (more than 50% of cases) to be secondary to organic causes.

Isosexual Precocious Puberty

Stimulation of the hypothalamic-pituitary axis with gonadotropin secretion and resultant sex steroid secretion is termed precocious puberty. Sex steroid secretion independent of pituitary gonadotropin secretion may be termed peripheral or pseudoprecocious puberty. The left-hand box on p. 1065 lists the causes of these two conditions.

The diagnosis of precocious puberty is based on the physical examination and laboratory evidence of sex steroid secretion. Measurement of serum gonadotropin levels usually allows classification of the condition as either central or pseudoprecocious puberty. In precocious puberty, further workup centers on a search for the cause of the gonadotropin secretion. The diagnosis of idiopathic precocious puberty can be made only after a search for a pathologic cause is negative. In pseudoprecocious puberty, one must search for the source of sex steroid, remembering that exogenous sources (e.g., contraceptive pills in girls) are easily available. In males physical examination of the testes is particularly useful in the differential diagnosis. If both testes are of pubertal size, then it is clear that the patient has gonadotropin-stimulated precocious puberty; if one testis is enlarged, a testicular tumor is probably present; if both testes are small, the androgens are either exogenous or of adrenal origin.

Treatment of the isosexual precocity centers on removal of the underlying cause. The treatment of idiopathic precocious puberty has been approached through pharmacologic suppression of the hypothalamic-pituitary-gonadal axis, initially with medroxyprogesterone acetate (a progestational steroid), danazol (a weak androgen), or cyproterone acetate (an antiandrogen). Although these drugs may successfully suppress menses, they are only variably successful in arresting secondary sexual characteristics, and they have no effect on the rapid osseous maturation that results in early epiphyseal closure and short stature. Greater success has been reported with GnRH analogs. GnRH analogs produce sustained levels of GnRH, which lead to pituitary desensitization and a reduction in gonadotropin secretion. Approval by the Food and Drug Administration is pending. In all cases, psychological support is important. In general, treatment of precocious puberty is a matter for a pediatric endocrinologist.

Variations of Puberty

Two entities not requiring treatment are premature breast development (thelarche) and premature development of sexual hair (adrenarche).

Premature thelarche typically occurs in girls between 6 months and 2 years of age. Breast development is usually moderate, often regresses, and is seen without other signs of precocious puberty. Specifically, estrogen or gonadotropic levels do not increase significantly, and statural and skeletal

Causes of Isosexual Precocious Puberty

I. Central (with pituitary gonadotropin secretion)
  A. Idiopathic
  B. Central nervous system abnormalities
    1. Congenital anomalies (hydrocephalus)
    2. Tumors (hypothalamic, pineal, other)
    3. Hamartoma
    4. Postinflammatory condition
    5. Trauma
    6. Syndromes
      a. Neurofibromatosis
      b. Tuberous sclerosis
  C. Hypothyroidism (severe)
II. Pseudoprecocious puberty
  A. Exogenous sex steroids
  B. Gonadal tumors or cysts
  C. Adrenal hyperplasia or tumor
  D. Ectopic gonadotropin-secreting tumors (chorioepithelioma, hepatoblastoma, teratoma)
  E. Familial Leydig cell hyperplasia
  F. McCune-Albright syndrome

Causes of Heterosexual Precocious Puberty

I. Female
  A. Congenital adrenal hyperplasia
  B. Androgen-secreting tumors
    1. Adrenal
    2. Ovarian
    3. Teratoma
  C. Exogenous androgens
II. Male
  A. Estrogen-producing tumors
    1. Adrenal
    2. Teratoma
    3. Hepatoma
    4. Testicular
  B. Exogenous estrogens
  C. Increased peripheral conversion of androgens to estrogens

maturation accelerates only mildly if at all. Premature thelarche does not progress to complete precocious puberty.

Premature adrenarche usually occurs between 5 and 8 years of age. The development of sexual hair is frequently accompanied by a mild growth spurt (with slight bone age advancement) and signs of increased adrenal androgen (slightly elevated urinary 17-ketosteroids and increased levels of plasma dehydroepiandrosterone and its sulfate); in girls there are no signs of increased estrogen secretion. An abnormal androgen source such as a tumor or adrenal hyperplasia must be excluded.

In both premature thelarche and premature adrenarche, careful follow-up is necessary, because the early stages of complete sexual precocity may appear in a similar way.

Heterosexual Precocious Puberty

Heterosexual precocious puberty is uncommon. The box on the right, top, lists its causes. Exogenous sex steroids (including creams) must be considered. The diagnostic workup must center on the search for a sex steroid–producing tumor. These patients should be referred to a pediatric endocrinologist.

Treatment is aimed at removal of the sex hormone source (exogenous or tumor) or suppression with glucocorticoid replacement therapy (congenital adrenal hyperplasia).

SUMMARY

In most cases of delayed or precocious sexual development, a careful history and physical examination and a few basic laboratory tests will identify those patients likely to have a pathologic etiology requiring referral to a pediatric endocrinologist. In all cases it is extremely important to provide psychological care and support, as well as physical care, particularly in cases in which medical therapy is only partially satisfactory.

SUGGESTED READINGS

Kappy MS, Stuart T, and Perelman A: Efficacy of leuprolide therapy in children with central precocious puberty, Am J Dis Child 142:1061, 1988.

Lee PA and Page JG: Effects of leuprolide in the treatment of central precocious puberty, J Pediatr 114:321, 1989.

Parker KL and Lee PA: Depot leuprolide acetate for treatment of precocious puberty, J Clin Endocrinol Metab 69:689, 1989.

Penny R: Disorders of the testes. In Kaplan SA, editor: Clinical pediatric and adolescent endocrinology, Philadelphia, 1982, WB Saunders Co.

Reindollar RH and McDonough PG: Etiology and evaluation of delayed sexual development. In Cowell CA, editor: Symposium on pediatric and adolescent gynecology, Pediatr Clin North Am 28:2, 1981.

Root AW: Endocrinology of puberty. I. Normal sexual maturation, J Pediatr 83:1, 1973.

Root AW: Endocrinology of puberty. II. Aberrations of sexual maturation, J Pediatr 83:187, 1973.

Rosenfield RL: The ovary and female sexual maturation. In Kaplan SA, editor: Clinical pediatric and adolescent endocrinology, Philadelphia, 1982, WB Saunders Co.

Tanner JM: Growth and endocrinology of the adolescent. In Gardner LI, editor: Endocrine and genetic diseases of childhood and adolescence, Philadelphia, 1975, WB Saunders Co.

Wilson DM and Rosenfeld RG: Treatment of short stature and delayed adolescence, Pediatr Clin North Am 34:865, 1987.

165

Splenomegaly

Allen Eskenazi

The spleen has intrigued physicians for centuries. Pliny the Elder associated it with mirth and laughter, and Galen described it as an organ full of mystery. Over the years the immunologic and hematologic roles of the spleen have been more precisely defined. Understanding the role of the spleen in health and disease will permit the clinician to evaluate rationally the child or adolescent with apparent splenic enlargement.

The spleen is fixed in the left upper quadrant of the abdomen by the splenorenal and phrenosplenic ligaments. Congenital or acquired abnormalities of the support structure can result in *splenic ptosis* and thus allow palpation of a spleen that actually is normal in size. It is estimated that 5% to 10% of normal infants have a palpable spleen tip, whereas a palpable spleen in an adult almost always is a pathologic finding.

A useful framework for evaluating the child with splenomegaly is to consider the four major physiologic functions of the spleen: immunologic, phagocytic, hemodynamic, and hematopoietic. First, the spleen is the major lymphoid organ in the body. It is the primary site of B lymphocyte activity related to antibody production, and it is an important reservoir of T lymphoctyes and natural killer cells, the mediators of cellular immune responses. Second, the spleen serves a major role in the removal of abnormal and senescent blood cells, as well as of circulating particulates. Third, the vasculature of the spleen plays an important role in the regulation of portal blood flow. Finally, the spleen is an important site of hematopoiesis in pathologic conditions in children and adults and of extramedullary hematopoiesis in the fetus.

The accompanying box lists numerous disease states in which splenomegaly is a prominent or associated feature. Splenomegaly caused by recurrent viral infections often is seen in young infants. The degree of splenic enlargement is relatively small and should resolve within a short period of time. A greater degree of splenic enlargement occurs specifically in infectious mononucleosis (Epstein-Barr virus), cytomegalovirus, and human immunodeficiency virus infections. Chronic bacterial infections (such as subacute bacterial endocarditis, syphilis, and tuberculosis) may be associated with splenomegaly. Acute overwhelming bacterial infections with pneumococcus or meningococcus also may result in splenic enlargement. In many areas of the world the spleen may harbor a large burden of protozoan-infected cells.

Inherited and acquired hemolytic anemias generally result in splenomegaly because of either increased phagocytic activity by the reticuloendothelial network (membranopathies, hemoglobinopathies, autoimmune hemolysis) or the devel-

Some Causes of Splenomegaly

INFECTIONS

Viral: Epstein-Barr, cytomegalovirus, human immunodeficiency virus
Bacterial: acute bacterial infections, subacute bacterial endocarditis, congenital syphilis, tuberculosis
Protozoal: malaria, toxoplasmosis
Fungal: candididiasis, histoplasmosis, coccidioidomycosis

HEMATOLOGIC DISORDERS

Hemolytic anemias—congenital and acquired
- Red cell membrane defects: hereditary spherocytosis, hereditary elliptocytosis
- Red cell hemoglobin defects: sickle cell disease and related syndromes, thalassemia
- Red cell enzyme defects: pyruvate kinase deficiency and others
- Autoimmune hemolytic anemia

Extramedullary hematopoiesis
- Thalassemia major, osteopetrosis, myelofibrosis

INFILTRATIVE DISORDERS

Leukemias
Lymphomas
Lipidoses
Mucopolysaccharidosis
Histiocytosis X

CONGESTIVE SPLENOMEGALY

Chronic congestive heart failure
Portal hypertension secondary to hepatic cirrhosis

INFLAMMATORY DISEASES

Systemic lupus erythematosus (SLE)
Rheumatoid arthritis (Still disease)
Serum sickness
Sarcoidosis
Immune thrombocytopenias and neutropenias

PRIMARY SPLENIC DISORDERS

Cysts
Hemangiomas and lymphangiomas
Subcapsular hemorrhage

opment of extramedullary hematopoiesis (thalassemia major). Splenic sequestration of blood is a common, acute event in children with sickle cell anemia, resulting in pallor, irritability, tachypnea, tachycardia, and variable degrees of splenic enlargement. Recognition of splenic sequestration is imperative because hypotension and shock can develop rapidly as a result of accumulation of blood in the spleen.

Infiltrative diseases of the spleen require prompt evaluation. The spleen rarely is the site of metastatic solid tumors but often is infiltrated by leukemias and lymphomas. Nonmalignant infiltration is seen in lipidosis and mucopolysaccharidosis, as well as in histiocytosis X. Autoimmune disorders (e.g., systemic lupus erythematosus and rheumatoid arthritis) and alloimmune disorders (serum sickness) may lead to expansion within the spleen of its lymphoid elements, as well as the phagocytic elements that remove antibody-coated cells and proteins. These conditions often mimic other infiltrative processes and may result in hypersplenism (see below).

EVALUATION

Splenomegaly is diagnosed by physical examination and only rarely requires confirmation by radiographic, ultrasonographic, or radionuclide imaging. These studies, which may be useful in the evaluation of the child with lymphoma, are not indicated in the routine evaluation of splenomegaly. A careful history, including family history, and physical examination permit the clinician to narrow the differential diagnosis to a few of the entities listed in the accompanying box. A complete blood cell count, reticulocyte count, and careful evaluation of the peripheral blood smear are extremely useful studies in the majority of patients with splenomegaly. The results of these simple diagnostic procedures help dictate further diagnostic procedures such as hemoglobin electrophoresis, bone marrow aspiration, or lymph node biopsy.

HYPERSPLENISM

Hypersplenism is not a specific disease entity. The term refers to the condition in which the spleen removes excessive numbers of normal circulating blood cells, resulting in one or more cytopenias. There is active formation of the affected blood element(s) in the bone marrow to compensate for their accelerated destruction in the spleen. Splenectomy will correct the cytopenia(s). It is vital, however, to establish the cause of the hypersplenism inasmuch as other therapeutic modalities may correct the hypersplenism and thus obviate the need for splenectomy.

SUGGESTED READINGS

Crosby WH: The spleen. In Wintrobe MM, editor: Blood, pure and eloquent, New York, 1980, McGraw-Hill, Inc.

Pearson H: The spleen and disturbances of splenic function. In Nathan D and Oski F, editors: Hematology of infancy and childhood, Philadelphia, 1987, WB Saunders Co.

166

Strabismus

Carl A. Frankel

Strabismus is the general term for any misalignment of the eye. The misalignments can be present either under binocular conditions, in which case it is a *manifest strabismus (heterotropia),* or under monocular conditions, in which case it is a *latent strabismus (heterophoria).* Many persons have a small heterophoria, which is of no clinical significance: these latent deviations usually are found on routine ophthalmologic examination. Tropias (manifest deviations) are present under binocular conditions, either intermittently or constantly, and may be alternating or unilateral. Alternating tropias imply equal or near-equal visual acuities, whereas monocular tropias may indicate reduced vision (amblyopia) (see diagram below).

Strabismus occurs in approximately 3% of the population and, while familial tendencies have been well documented, no clear-cut genetic mode of inheritance has been demonstrated. The direction of deviation of one eye with respect to the fixating eye names the deviation. An inward deviation is called an *esotropia;* an outward deviation is called an *exotropia.* A vertical deviation is referred to as a *hypertropia* or *hypotropia* depending on whether the deviating (non-fixating) eye is higher or lower, respectively, than the fixating eye. Torsional deviations are named for *incyclotorsion* or *excyclotorsion* of the twelve o'clock position to the eye, but are usually associated with an abnormality in superior oblique muscle or inferior oblique muscle function with a secondary vertical strabismus; these conditions are usually referred to as *cyclovertical strabismus.*

Congenital or infantile strabismus deviations acquired prior to the maturation of the visual system (between the ages of 7 and 9 years for most children) are not associated with diplopia due to suppression. *Suppression* is the adaptation to strabismus that effectively inhibits the image at the deviating eye from reaching consciousness. In an alternating strabismus, the presence of alternating suppression is evidence for normal monocular visual development (fusion and stereopsis) in both eyes. However, in a youngster with monocular strabismus, monocular visual development in the fixating eye is expected to proceed normally, whereas binocular visual development and monocular visual development in the nonfixating eye can be expected to be impaired. This impairment in monocular visual development leads to amblyopia (poor vision or "lazy eye"), which requires intervention in the form of glasses or patching of the fixating eye to restore normal vision in the nonfixating eye. After the visual acuities have been equalized, surgery may be indicated for the ocular misalignment.

Because one eye is the fixating eye, "bilateral strabismus" is a misnomer. *If both eyes appear deviated when the patient is facing an examiner, visual inattention or visual impairment is suggested,* and further evaluation is indicated to assess the function of the visual system. This assessment can be in the form of the visual evoked potential (VEP) or visual evoked response (VER), electroretinogram (ERG), or forced preferential looking (FPL). The former are electrophysiologic tests that require surface electrodes; the latter requires some demonstrable visual interest for the child.

Acquired strabismus, whether esotropia, exotropia, or a cyclovertical deviation, should prompt concern as to the exact cause, because of the long-term implications for the patient. Poor vision may be the proximate cause, inasmuch as strabismus caused by retinoblastoma (the most common intraocular tumor of children with an incidence of 1:12,000/14,000 live births) is the second most common presenting sign (after leukocoria). Head trauma, either accidental or deliberate, can result in cranial nerve palsies (third, fourth, or sixth) that may result in an acute acquired strabismus. Because of other diagnostic considerations, any patient with

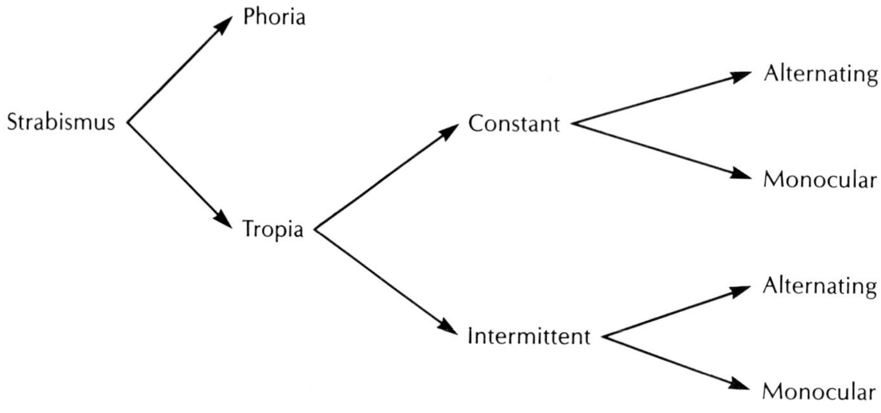

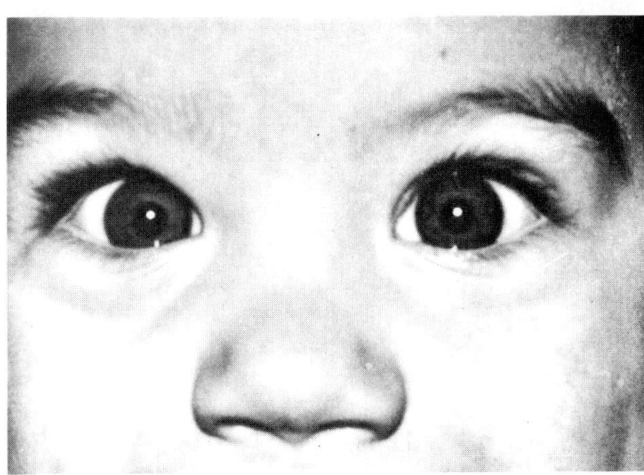

Fig. 166-1 Pseudostrabismus. This child's eyes, in fact, are perfectly aligned, even though the right eye appears "crossed" (esotropic). Epicanthal skin folds produce this illusion, which here is enhanced by the face being turned slightly toward the side. Notice that the corneal light reflections are quite symmetric. If they are displaced at all, it is nasalward, suggesting a divergent (exotropic) deviation.

an acquired strabismus should be referred to an ophthalmologist for evaluation and intervention as needed, including that necessary to restore the integrity of the system of binocular vision.

In a newborn infant, inattention or somnolence is the most common cause of variable ocular alignment. During periods of full wakefulness, the ocular alignment usually is normal. Even in normal infants, however, an intermittent esotropia or exotropia may be noted. This usually represents central nervous system immaturity and typically resolves during the first 2 to 3 months of life. *In any infant in whom strabismus persists beyond 10 to 12 weeks, evaluation by an ophthalmologist is indicated,* earlier if there are other signs of developmental delay or if the strabismus is constant.

DETECTION OF STRABISMUS

Corneal Light Reflection Test

The simplest method to determine the presence of strabismus is the corneal light reflection test (Hirschberg method). In this test a pen-light is directed at the cornea, and the observer notes the position of the corneal reflection with respect to the center of the pupil. If the light reflex is deviated toward the nose, an exotropia may be present; an esotropia should be suspected when the light reflex is deviated toward the lateral side of the visual axis. Although this method is used as a rapid screening test, the high incidence of false-positive findings results in unneeded referrals. On the other hand, the presence of a false-negative result may give a false sense of security (Fig. 166-1).

Alternate Cover Test

A more sensitive test for the presence of a strabismus is the alternate cover test. Although this test targets youngsters with either a heterophoria or a heterotropia, it results in a very low incidence of false-negative findings. To perform this test the examiner uses some bright, pleasant object to attract the youngster's attention and then alternately covers one eye and then the other with the hand, finger, or occluder. *The presence of a shift of one eye while covering or the fellow eye is evidence of a strabismic misalignment* (either a heterophoria or heterotropia) and should prompt referral for further evaluation and intervention as indicated.

PSEUDOESOTROPIA

There is a common misconception among the lay public that children may outgrow "crossed" eyes by the time they are 2 to 3 years of age. Unfortunately, this is not so: what children do tend to outgrow is the "pseudoesotropia" that is caused by the prominent epicanthal folds and broad, flat nasal bridge present in most infants. This condition creates an illusion of esotropia because of the decrease in the amount of nasal conjunctiva visible to the observer (see Fig. 166-1). Because the nasal cornea tends to "dip" under the epicanthal fold on adduction, the parent frequently reports that the eyes are crossed more with right or left gaze and with near viewing (where convergence accentuates the illusion).

ESOTROPIA

The most common type of strabismus is esotropia, which is characterized by a nasal deviation of the nonfixating eye (Fig. 166-2). In patients in whom the visual function is equal, alternate fixation may be present, giving rise to an alternating (*not* bilateral) deviation, whereas a monocular deviation is present in those in whom visual function is better in one eye. The corneal light reflection test will show the light to be centered in the pupil of the fixating eye, with the deviating eye showing the light reflection to be toward the temporal side of the center of the pupil. Because of variation in the location of the visual axis with respect to the center of the pupil, a small deviation may be either accentuated or, of greater concern, minimized. In fact, deviations of up to 7 degrees (15 prism diopters) may be missed. Thus the alternate cover testing is more reliable in the detection of a deviation.

Congenital Esotropia

Congenital esotropia is defined as having its onset within the first 6 months of life. Because the deviation may not be present at birth, a more accurate term is *infantile esotropia*. Infantile esotropia is characterized by a large angle of deviation and, at least initially, by equal visual function and cross fixation. Cross fixation is that condition in which a patient will prefer to look to the left with the already deviating right eye and to the right with the already deviating left eye. Because of cross fixation, a diagnosis of a unilateral or even bilateral sixth cranial nerve palsy may be made. Normal abduction may be demonstrated by occluding one eye and using rotational testing or observing following eye movements of one eye and then repeated for the fellow eye.

In an attempt to normalize the ocular alignment, early surgical intervention is indicated in youngsters with congenital esotropia. Currently, medical opinion recommends sur-

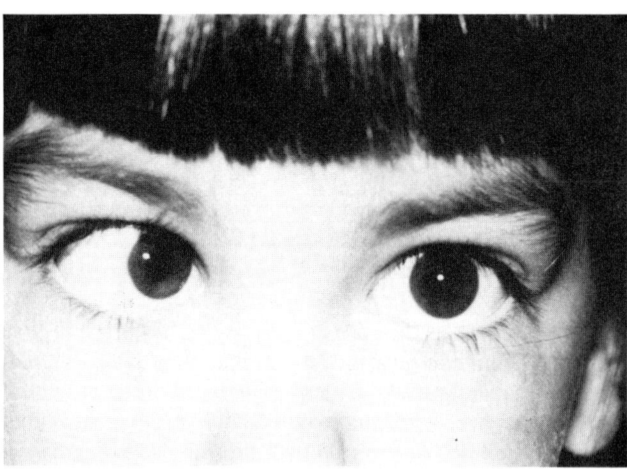

Fig. 166-2 Note the nasal deviation of the right eye with the corneal light reflection temporally displaced on the right eye and centered in the left pupil, indicating an esotropia.

gical intervention between 6 and 18 months (possibly up to 24 months) in an effort to obtain more stable binocular vision than might be possible if the surgery were performed later. Prerequisites for early surgical intervention include stable ocular deviation, treatment of amblyopia (poor vision), and minimal risk for undergoing general anesthesia.

Less common conditions in which an esotropia is present include the congenital abducens nerve palsy (very rare) and Duane syndrome, which typically affects the left eye. Duane syndrome is distinguished from a true sixth nerve palsy by narrowing of the palpebral fissure with retraction of the globe on adduction as a result of contraction of the medial rectus muscle; this is accompanied by an inappropriate simultaneous contraction of the lateral rectus muscle of the same eye.

Acquired Esotropia

Any esotropia first detected beyond 6 months of age is classified as acquired; although it may represent a late-onset form of infantile esotropia, it requires a closer look at possible etiologic considerations. Visual function needs to be assessed inasmuch as *unilateral visual loss in the first several years of life typically results in an acquired esotropia.*

Accommodative Esotropia. This type of acquired esotropia typically has its onset in patients between 2 and 3 years of age. The history is that of an intermittent esotropia which becomes more frequent in its occurrence and is of longer duration. The condition is based on the accommodation reflex. In order for an emetrope (person with no refractive error) to focus at near objects, a synkinetic reflex must occur. *The three components of this synkinetic near reflex include accommodation* (the alteration in the shape of the lens to make it a more powerful refracting element), *accommodative convergence* (nasal movement of the eyes so that the visual axes may be directed to the near object of regard), and *pupillary miosis* (irrelevant to this discussion). In accommodative esotropia, one of two scenarios typically is encountered and depends on the relationship between accommodation (A) and accommodative convergence (AC): the AC/A ratio.

Normal AC/A Ratio. When the deviation (esotropia) of a patient with a normal AC/A ratio is measured and found to be the same for both near and distant targets, a normal linear relationship between accommodation and accommodative convergence is defined. When a refractive error is present, however, the patient often has a moderate degree of farsightedness (hyperopia), characterized by the inability to view distant objects clearly when the lens is in its normal, relaxed state (the usual state for distant viewing). In order to focus, the patient increases the refractive power of the eye by forced accommodation for distant viewing. Accommodative convergence ensues because of the synkinetic near reflex, with a secondary deviation for distance (Fig. 166-3, *A*). Spectacle correction of the refractive error obviates the need for the accommodation reflex during distant viewing (with its secondary accommodative convergence) and promotes normal ocular alignment while spectacles are worn (Fig. 166-3, *B*).

High AC/A Ratio. In those patients with an esotropia only for near vision, an imbalance exists in the linear relationship between accommodation and accommodative convergence. These patients may be treated with bifocal spectacles (with no correction for distance) to relieve the need for accommodation for near vision or with topical ophthalmic preparations (such as isoflurophate or echothiophate iodide) to normalize the high AC/A ratio by decreasing accommodative convergence.

In those patients with an accommodative esotropia for distant vision with a high AC/A ratio, the near deviation exceeds the distance deviation. Patients such as these typically are treated with bifocal lenses or with topical ophthalmic preparations as already described. Fortunately, the AC/A ratio typically begins to normalize by about 8 years of age, and the bifocals or eye drops eventually can be discontinued.

Paralytic. An esotropia secondary to paralytic causes (abducens nerve palsy) is characterized by a deviation that varies with the direction of gaze, depending on whether the patient is fixating with the affected or the unaffected eye. When the patient looks in the direction of the affected side with the unaffected eye, there is an increase in the deviation (horizontal incompetence). For example, in a patient with left-sided abducens nerve palsy, esotropia of the left eye will increase on left gaze and decrease on right gaze in relation to the primary (straight ahead) gaze position.

Additionally, the deviation accompanying fixation by the unaffected eye (primary deviation) is less than that obtained with fixation by the affected eye (secondary deviation), unless the paralytic strabismus is long-standing, in which case the secondary deviation may approximate the primary deviation.

An acquired abducens palsy is a nonlocalizing sign; it may reflect any cause of increased intracranial pressure or may be the benign sixth nerve palsy of childhood.[1,2] An appropriate evaluation to rule out the causes of increased intracranial pressure should be undertaken.

PSEUDOEXOTROPIA

Illusory exotropia occurs much less frequently than illusory esotropia. Because of its strikingly prominent appearance, referral is made much more frequently and at a much earlier age, but the alternate cover test reveals no refixation move-

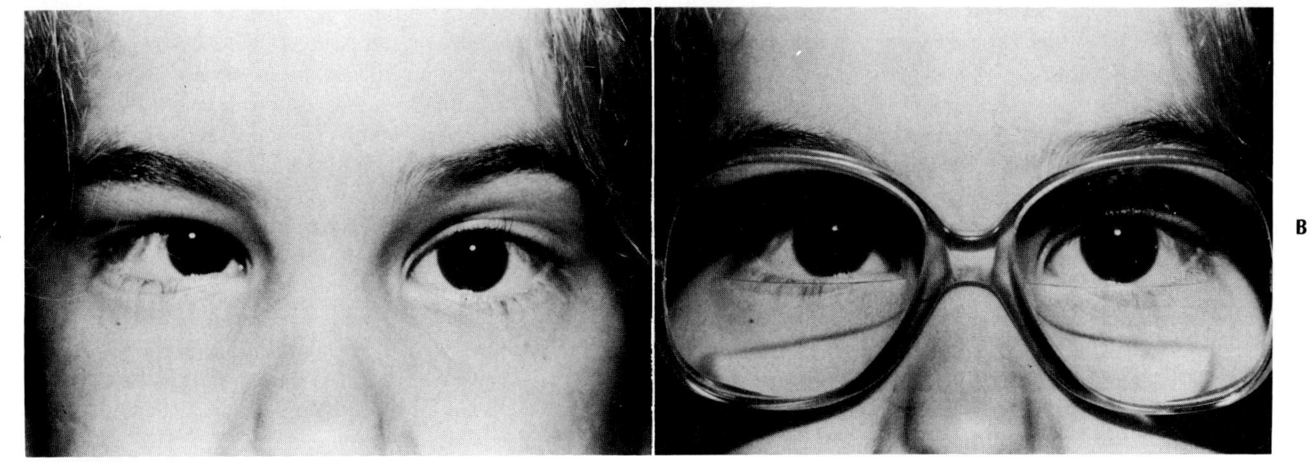

Fig. 166-3 *(A)* Esotropia in a patient with accommodative esotropia. *(B)* Same patient, but now with straight eyes with correction. Note the small increase in pupil size due to the reversal of accommodative miosis with correction.

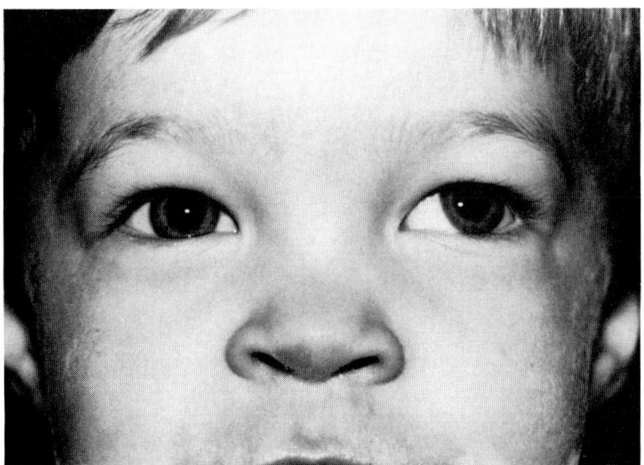

Fig. 166-4 Divergent strabismus of the left eye, defining an exotropia.

ment on uncovering one eye and covering the fixating eye.

EXOTROPIA

Exotropia, or divergent strabismus (Fig. 166-4), occurs less frequently than does esotropia. As with esotropia the deviation may be congenital or acquired and alternating or monocular. Additionally, the exotropia may be constant or intermittent. Careful analysis of all these factors determines the treatment option to be selected by the ophthalmologist.

Congenital Exotropia

This divergent deviation is defined as having its onset in the first 6 months of life and is more appropriately called *infantile exotropia*. Infantile exotropia is much less frequent than is infantile esotropia but is similarly characterized by a large angle of deviation and normal refractive error (mild hyperopia). Pseudoadduction deficit may be present, but full adduction usually is demonstrable on occlusion of one eye and then the other. As with infantile esotropia, early surgery is indicated to improve ocular alignment and binocular vision that is more stable than that obtained with later surgery (after 2 years of age).

Acquired Exotropia

Any exotropia that has its onset after 6 months of age is an acquired exotropia. Visual function must be assessed because the strabismus secondary to visual loss from a retinoblastoma is more likely to be an exotropia than an esotropia.

Intermittent Exotropia. This is the most common type of exotropia seen in children and typically has its initial onset at about 2 to 3 years of age. Late-onset intermittent exotropias typically are diagnosed beyond 3 years of age, although these are perhaps atypical only in the age at which they are first noted.

During periods when the eyes are well-aligned, binocular vision may be developing normally and the presence of binocular vision can aid determination of when, or if, surgical intervention is indicated. If binocular vision is deteriorating or if the frequency and duration of the deviation are increasing, surgical intervention is justified.

Convergence Insufficiency. A subset of intermittent exotropia, convergence insufficiency is characterized by complaints of eyestrain, fatigue, blurred vision, diplopia, headache, tearing or alternate blurring, and diplopia. As a result of the nature of the fusion mechanism, orthoptic exercises for symptomatic convergence insufficiency have a high rate of success as measured by relief of patient symptoms. Orthoptic exercises should not be confused with "vision training," which is of dubious value.

Divergence Excess. This is characterized by a greater degree of exotropia for distant vision, as compared with near vision, and frequently is noted only at extreme distances. Surgical intervention is directed at the distance deviation, and a postoperative overcorrection (esotropia) for near vision usually is obtained.

Consecutive Exotropia. This deviation typically follows surgical correction for an esotropia, in which accommodative esotropia has not been adequately addressed as the cause of the initial strabismus (esotropia); it usually is not seen until early adulthood. Surgical intervention frequently is indicated in an attempt to obtain normal ocular alignment.

Paralytic. Paralytic exodeviations, which usually are seen with acute third cranial nerve palsies, are characterized by pupillary mydriasis, ptosis, an exotropia, and a hypotropia. Head trauma is the most frequent cause, and neuroradiologic imaging (computed tomography and magnetic resonance imaging) usually is indicated. Because of the ptosis, diplopia is not a complaint; thus complete evaluation can be obtained during the wait to see if spontaneous improvement occurs. Special care should be taken in young children, because of the possibility of deprivation amblyopia resulting from the ptotic lid.

VERTICAL AND CYCLOVERTICAL DEVIATIONS

There are four muscles in each eye that contribute to vertical and torsional eye movements: the superior and inferior rectus muscles and the superior and inferior oblique muscles. The two rectus muscles are concerned primarily with vertical eye movement, with secondary actions of incyclotorsion for the superior rectus muscle and excyclotorsion for the inferior rectus muscle. Conversely, the two oblique muscles are concerned primarily with torsional movements: the superior oblique for incyclotorsion and the inferior oblique for excyclotorsion. The secondary actions of the oblique muscles are depression and elevation for the superior and inferior oblique muscles, respectively. As a result of this arrangement the two elevators (superior rectus and inferior oblique) have opposite torsional actions (incyclotorsion and excyclotorsion, respectively), whereas the two depressors (inferior rectus and superior oblique) also have opposite torsional actions (excyclotorsion and incyclotorsion, respectively). Thus *an imbalance in any one of the four muscles of either eye can result in a significant cyclovertical strabismus.*

Superior Oblique Muscle Palsy

The superior oblique muscle is innervated by the trochlear nerve (fourth cranial nerve), and superior oblique muscle palsies are the most commonly undiagnosed forms of strabismus. Although head trauma is a frequent cause of superior oblique muscle palsy, most of these palsies are congenital and bilateral. In a youngster with bilateral superior oblique muscle palsy, fusion is not possible (because of the bilateral excyclotorsion), and the head position typically is normal, giving no clue to the existence of a problem. On right gaze, however, a left hypertropia typically is present because of the relatively unopposed action of the left inferior oblique muscle (Fig. 166-5, *B*). In a similar manner, on left gaze a right hypertropia usually occurs as a result of the action of the right inferior oblique muscle (Fig. 166-5, *B*). In addition, in down gaze a large esotropia is a typical finding, resulting from an absence of the abduction function of both superior oblique muscles.

In unilateral superior oblique muscle palsies, the unopposed excyclotorsion action of the inferior oblique muscle causes the affected eye to rotate outward. In an *attempt to obtain and maintain fusion, a head tilt toward the opposite side from the palsied muscle* results in normal ocular alignment, and fusion may be normal (Fig. 166-6). When the patient's head is straightened, the torsional action of the synergistic incycloductor (superior rectus muscle) results in an upward drift (hypertropia) of the affected eye, which is exaggerated by tilting of the head to the side opposite the naturally occurring head tilt. For example, a patient with a right superior oblique muscle palsy usually will have a left head tilt to overcome the excyclotorsion of the right eye. On forced right head tilt, a large right hypertropia typically becomes obvious. Any patient with torticollis should be evaluated for the presence of ocular torticollis, inasmuch as patients unwittingly may be subjected to such unnecessary treatments as physical therapy and braces for presumed nonocular tor-

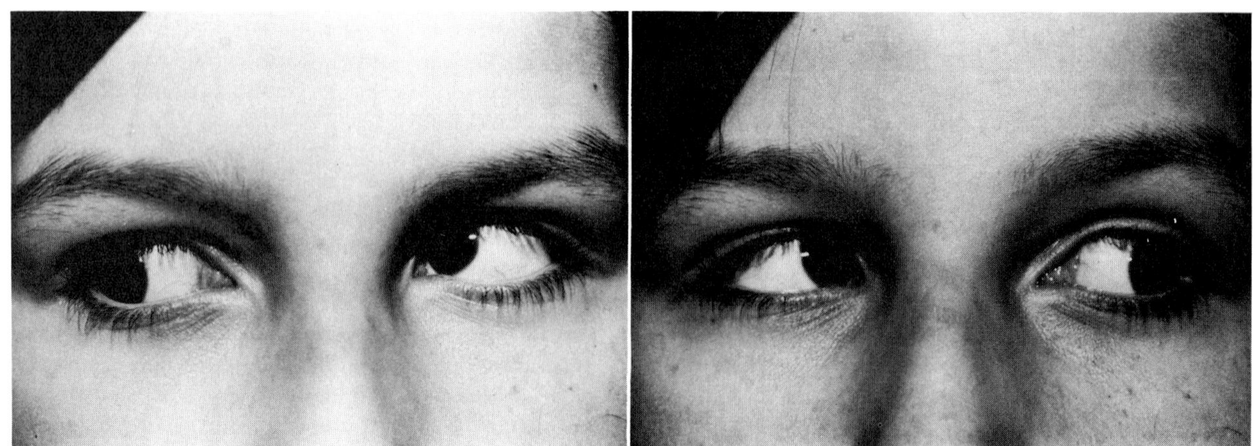

Fig. 166-5 A, Left hypertropia on right gaze characteristic of a left superior oblique muscle palsy. **B,** Right hypertropia on left gaze characteristic of a right superior oblique muscle palsy. This is the same patient shown in **A,** implying bilateral superior oblique muscle palsies.

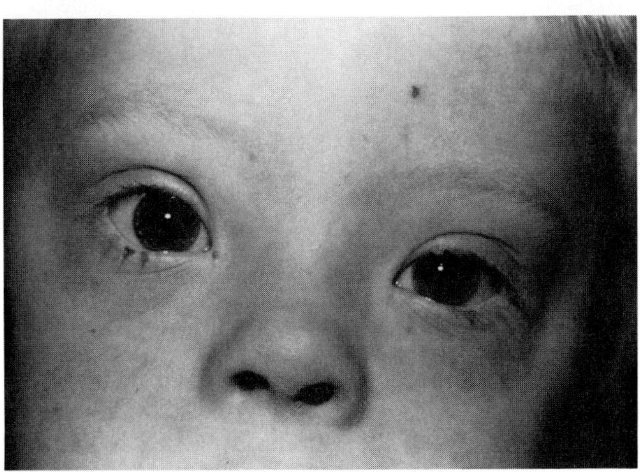

Fig. 166-6 Left head tilt in a patient with a unilateral right superior oblique muscle palsy. Fusion was present, indicating binocular vision.

ticollis. If any doubt exists about a possible superior oblique muscle palsy, the patient should be referred to a pediatric ophthalmologist for further evaluation.

Dissociated Vertical Deviations

Dissociated vertical deviations (DVDs), also termed *alternating hyperphorias* or *double dissociated hyperphorias,* typically are seen in patients with infantile esotropia regardless of whether strabismus surgery has previously been performed. DVDs are characterized by an alternating upward deviation of first one eye and then the other on alternate cover testing.

Occasionally, excycloduction may be noted with a lateral deviation of the eye on its upward movement. The exact cause of DVD is unknown, but both superior rectus and inferior oblique muscle dysfunctions have been implicated. In most patients the deviation is only a clinical curiosity; unless spontaneously present, surgery rarely is indicated. When surgery is indicated, even for unilateral DVDs, bilateral superior rectus muscle recessions usually are performed to prevent the "unmasking" of a bilateral DVD.

Miscellaneous Vertical and Cyclovertical Deviations

Other deviations that may be seen in the pediatrician's office include generalized or isolated congenital fibrosis syndromes, inferior oblique muscle palsies, dysthyroid orbitopathy, double elevator palsies, third nerve palsies, Brown syndrome, double depressor palsies, or inferior rectus muscle restriction or fibrosis secondary to orbital floor fractures. These entities are all unusual, the description of which can be found in any text on pediatric ophthalmology or strabismus.

REFERENCES

1. Knox RL, Clark DB, and Schuster FF: Benign VI nerve palsies in children, Pediatrics 40:560, 1967.
2. Werner DB, Savino PJ, and Schatz NJ: Benign recurrent 6th nerve palsies in children, Arch Ophthalmol 101:607, 1983.

SUGGESTED READINGS

Ernest JT and Costenbader FD: Lateral rectus muscle palsy, Am J Ophthalmol 65:721, 1968.

Greenwald MJ and Parks MM: Amblyopia. In Duane TD, editor: Clinical ophthalmology, Philadelphia, 1989, JB Lippincott Co.

Harley RD: Paralytic strabismus in children, Ophthalmology 87:24, 1980.

Khawam E, Scott AB, and Jampolsky A: Acquired superior oblique palsy, Arch Ophthalmol 88:761, 1967.

Manley DR: Strabismus. In Harley RD, editor: Pediatric ophthalmology, ed 2, Philadelphia, 1983, WB Saunders Co.

Nelson LB et al: Congenital esotropia, Surv Ophthalmol 31:363, 1987.

Parks MM: Ophthalmoplegic syndromes and trauma. In Duane TD, editor: Clinical ophthalmology, Philadelphia, 1989, JB Lippincott Co.

Parks MM and Mitchell PR: Concomitant exodeviations. In Duane TD, editor: Clinical ophthalmology, Philadelphia, 1989, JB Lippincott Co.

Parks MM and Mitchell PR: Cranial nerve palsies. In Duane TD, editor: Clinical ophthalmology, Philadelphia, 1989, JB Lippincott Co.

Parks MM and Mitchell PR: Dissociated vertical deviations. In Duane TD, editor: Clinical ophthalmology, Philadelphia, 1989, JB Lippincott Co.

Parks MM and Wheeler MB: Concomitant Esodeviations. In Duane TD, editor: Clincial ophthalmology, Philadelphia, 1989, JB Lippincott Co.

Rubin SE and Wagner RS: Ocular torticollis, Surv Ophthalmol 30:366, 1986.

Rucker CW: The causes of paralysis of the third, fourth and sixth cranial nerves, Am J Ophthalmol 61:1293, 1966.

167

Strange Behavior

Lois T. Flaherty

Although not a precise term, "strange" usually is the word used to describe behavior that (1) is socially inappropriate, that is, does not conform to that expected in a given situation, and (2) is not understandable in its context. The boy at nursery school, for example, who suddenly, with no apparent provocation, bites or kicks the child standing next to him will be seen as strange. The young adolescent girl who goes to school garishly made up (by standards of her age mates), in a misguided attempt to beautify herself, certainly will be considered "weird" by her peers. The school-aged child who, evidently misinterpreting a friendly "hello" across the backyard fence, shouts back "shut up!" will have a reputation as being odd, to say the least.

Another way of understanding the labeling of behavior as strange is that it reflects a sense of confusion on the part of the observer, which in turn is related to something about the child that does not make sense. The human organism, probably from fetal life onward, is engaged in a constant struggle to impose organization and structure on sensory inputs—in other words, to give meaning to experience. The process by which this occurs involves classification, integration, and storage of information received through sensory channels. Infants and young children are assisted in this process by their parents, with whom they become involved very early in complicated communication processes and who act as modulators of sensory inputs. Defects in children's cerebral integrative functioning, their sensory apparatus, their ability to communicate, or the care they receive can result in impairment of this process by which the child gradually makes sense of his or her world. As a result the child to some degree experiences fragmentation, disorganization, and chaos, which he or she continues to struggle to overcome. From an early age, this child will have difficulty coping with most, if not all, of the major developmental tasks that must be mastered by all children if they are to grow into emotional maturity. The behavior of such a child, reflective of the child's own confusion, appears strange and confusing to others.

These children are considered to have *pervasive developmental disorders.*[1] Although there is some disagreement among experts in the field about this term, it refers to a category of disorders that are characterized by very severe impairment in social interaction, communication, and thinking; it includes disorders that in the past were termed autism, childhood psychosis, atypical development, and borderline states. Once considered to be primarily the result of faulty parenting, these disorders now are recognized to involve serious deficits in neurobiologic functioning, which in turn interferes with many aspects of social, emotional, and cognitive development. No specific locus of abnormality has been found in the brain, and it is possible that similar clinical presentations could result from different kinds of central nervous system abnormalities. Children with pervasive developmental disorders frequently have "soft" neurologic signs, and abnormal findings on computed tomography (CT) scans have been found in some.

Fortunately, the number of such children is small. Although the prevalence of severe emotional disturbance among children in the general population has been estimated at 2% to 5%, the majority of them are not autistic or psychotic. Various epidemiologic studies have consistently placed the prevalence of autism at about 4/10,000[3]; the prevalence of other pervasive developmental disorders is not as easy to pinpoint because diagnosis is less reliable, but it is probably similar. For comparison, the prevalence of schizophrenia, an illness that predominantly affects adults, is about 1% of the population.

AUTISM

Of all "strange" children, those with autism probably are the most strange. The syndrome of early infantile autism was originally described by Kanner[5] in 1943 on the basis of his experience with 11 cases, and this description still stands as a model of careful clinical observation.

The most striking feature of autistic children is the disturbance in their ability to relate to others. They often appear aloof and uninterested in people, preferring inanimate objects. They may avoid eye contact. A concomitant deficit is in communication, both verbal and nonverbal. Some do not acquire speech at all, and those who do tend not to use it to communicate. A variety of speech and language abnormalities have been described, the most common of which are echolalia (rote repetition of what is heard) and pronominal reversal (the use of "you" for "I," for example). Another major deficit is the inability to think flexibly and imaginatively, thought to be related to a basic deficit in conceptualization. This is commonly manifested in a lack of imaginative play. An autistic child may repetitively stack blocks but not *build* anything. Autistic children frequently display poor coordination and motor abnormalities, such as hand flapping, twirling, or head banging, although these are not diagnostic because they occur in other conditions. About 60% have concomitant mental retardation. Autism is three to four times as common in boys as in girls. A variety of metabolic, genetic, and infectious conditions that result in central nervous system damage or dysfunction have been found in association with autism.

These have included maternal rubella, untreated phenylketonuria, tuberous sclerosis, perinatal anoxia, encephalitis, infantile spasms, and fragile X syndrome. It is now recognized that in addition to "classic autism," there is a spectrum of disorders that fall within this diagnostic category, and autistic children vary considerably in their functioning.

Although the cause of classic autism is still unknown, of the "strange" syndromes, it is the most readily recognizable as a discrete entity. Once having observed one of these children, one can never forget him or her, and similarly affected children are easily recognized. Research in the areas of cognitive and biochemical functioning of autistic children has generated some intriguing hypotheses about underlying cerebral dysfunction that may prove fruitful in unlocking the secrets of this condition. Current treatment primarily involves special educational approaches; supportive counseling to families is extremely important.[8] (See Chapter 91 for further discussion of infantile autism as a form of psychosis.)

OTHER PERVASIVE DEVELOPMENTAL DISORDERS

Many of the children who often are described as strange have disorders that are more difficult to diagnose. Unlike the autistic child, who usually shows developmental abnormalities in infancy, their development in the neonatal period and infancy may be described as normal. Somewhere between the second and third year of life they undergo what is apparently a dramatic change, and their developmental progression ceases. They not only fail to acquire new functions but also may lose those previously acquired, such as language or bowel and bladder control. These children may develop some of the features of autistic children, such as engaging in isolated, repetitive play, avoiding eye contact, and being obsessively preoccupied with sameness. They lack self-control and frequently have uncontrolled outbursts of aggressive behavior toward others, as well as severe temper tantrums. Unlike autistic children, these children are extremely attached to their parents—they cling and are overly dependent. They are extremely prone to anxiety and often may not be able to tolerate any separation from their parents, or they may fly into a panic over the appearance of strangers, darkness, or loud noises. Thus, although these children have a better ability than autistic children to form attachments, they have not been able to master the basic developmental tasks of early childhood. Instead of striving for independence like the normal toddler, they fear it. They have been described as resembling toddlers whose parents are perpetually out of the room.[4]

All children regress at times, and most children have fears, temper tantrums, and displays of aggression. What is different about these children is the intensity and prevalence of their disturbed behavior. Their aggression toward another child, for example, involves more than the occasional shove, slap, or bite, and it may be seriously hurtful. Rather than simply having one fear, they have many, and the fears are only part of the whole spectrum of disturbed behavior.

Many of these children are grossly confused about reality and lack a concept of themselves as distinct from others, often confusing their own thoughts with those of others. They may believe, for instance, that they are about to be attacked by another child, when in reality it is their own anger toward the other that is the problem. They tend to be totally preoccupied with trying to protect themselves from what they perceive to be menacing forces all around them, which in reality are their own uncontrolled fantasies and feelings. One child, for example, when asked to draw a person, drew a large stomach, reflecting a preoccupation with eating and being eaten.

Others of this group are in better touch with reality but have only a limited ability to control their own thoughts, feelings, and behavior; they readily become overwhelmed. Typically, children in this group tend to improve with appropriate handling and become dramatically worse with adverse changes in the environment. Placement in a special therapeutic nursery school, for example, may result in a marked improvement in the child's functioning, whereas parental separation may have disastrous effects.

For the severely emotionally disturbed child, a variety of mental health and educational approaches are involved in management. These may range from outpatient psychiatric treatment to inpatient or residential treatment in special facilities. Often special school placement in a class for emotionally handicapped children is required as well. Pediatricians can help families of such children by familiarizing themselves with the resources available in their area and assisting families in finding needed services, as well as supporting and encouraging families to help them persevere in an often discouraging task.

The use of psychotropic medications, including the major tranquilizers, has been of some help in decreasing the extreme anxiety and out-of-control behavior of these youngsters, but they should be prescribed for children only by someone who has extensive experience with their use.

Controversy exists about the diagnosis of childhood schizophrenia and whether it should be considered one of the pervasive developmental disorders.[6] The diagnosis can be problematic, particularly in young children, whose intellectual functioning is not yet sophisticated enough for them to form organized delusions and paranoid thinking, although they show the disorganized thought processes and severe impairment in functioning that are characteristic of the adult forms of this disorder, and they may have hallucinations. Similar to the adult form, the onset in some cases is gradual and insidious and in other cases acute. The older the child the more likely is the disorder to resemble schizophrenia in adults (see Chapter 91).

OTHER CONDITIONS THAT MAY BE ASSOCIATED WITH STRANGE BEHAVIOR

Many other conditions may be associated with strange behavior in children and will occur far more commonly in pediatric practice than those already discussed. These include the following:

1. Organic brain syndromes, including degenerative neurologic disorders, psychomotor disturbances, and petit mal epilepsy
2. Mental retardation
3. Sensory deficits (e.g., deafness and blindness)
4. Speech and language disorders

5. Learning disabilities
6. Child abuse and neglect
7. Underlying chronic illness characterized by failure to thrive (e.g., celiac syndrome and cystic fibrosis)

In addition to the organic conditions previously noted to be associated with autism, various degenerative neurologic disorders can manifest clinically as pervasive developmental disorders. Psychomotor seizures and the staring spells of children with petit mal epilepsy may be mistaken for signs of emotional disorder.

Metabolic disorders often are associated with behavioral disturbances and developmental delays. In a study by Lowe and co-workers,[7] the finding of abnormalities on standard urinary amino acid screening in 3 of 65 children diagnosed as having a pervasive developmental disorder underscores the importance of screening for inborn errors of metabolism. Occasionally, children found to have celiac disease have autistic features; however, what seems to be emotional withdrawal actually is due to severe cachexia.

Mentally retarded children frequently manifest behavioral disturbances. Often what is described as strange is simply behavior that is inappropriate for the child's chronologic age, although it is not necessarily so when one considers mental age—for example, playing with feces by a 6-year-old child with a mental age of 2 years. On the other hand, the prevalence of behavior disorders and emotional disturbances (including psychoses and autism) is greater among this population than among children of normal intelligence. Many of the children who meet all the criteria for autism also are retarded. If one understands both psychoses and mental retardation as developmental disturbances involving delays in cognitive functioning, it is possible to see that they may coexist within the same child.

Congenitally deaf or blind children may show autistic features as a result to their sensory deficits, which hamper communication and reduce stimulation.

Impairment in the child's ability to communicate, associated with hearing or visual impairment or speech and language disorders, inevitably will cause some difficulty in responding to normal social situations. The more severe the child's sensory or language deficit, the more bizarre his or her behavior may seem.

Increasingly it has been recognized that learning-disabled children frequently have difficulty understanding and responding to social cues because of their problems in processing information. Therefore their behavior in social situations may be inappropriate. Although these children are not as impaired as those with pervasive developmental disorders, they often are notably handicapped socially.

Children who have been the victims of neglect or abuse may show autistic or psychotic-like behavior. These children usually improve, often dramatically, on removal from their homes and placement in a good residential treatment facility or foster home. In some cases, several months to a year may be necessary before change is noticed. Their deficits result from failure of their environment to provide the necessary stimulation and nurturance, rather than from any intrinsic deficits in the child. These children can best be understood as reacting to extreme degrees of psychological stress. (See Chapter 47 for a fuller discussion of child abuse and neglect.)

The emotionally disturbed parent may have a distorted view of his or her child and describe the child as strange. In extreme cases this may involve misinterpreting normal child behavior as deviant. A psychotic parent, for example, may see a child as "possessed by the devil." Abusive parents typically ascribe malevolent meanings to their children's actions. For example, an infant's fussiness may be interpreted as "meanness" or a toddler's hyperactivity as being "out to get" the parent. In both cases the parent is attributing something to the child that is, in fact, an anxious preoccupation of the parent's own mind.

EVALUATION OF THE CHILD WITH STRANGE BEHAVIOR

The first task of the pediatrician is to ascertain the accuracy of the description given of the child. Although the parents' description may be exaggerated, one should never dismiss it without attempting to verify it through collateral sources of information. If the child is in a school or day care program or otherwise comes in contact with adults outside the home, this task is simplified. The first step should be to inquire about the setting in which the behavior occurs, the usual reactions of those around the child, and the child's responses to these. As a rule, the more disturbed the child, the more ubiquitous the occurrences of the behavior. One should keep in mind that unless the child is clearly autistic or psychotic, observations made in the clinic or office can be misleading. The child who has violent temper tantrums at home and is described as socially isolated and withdrawn is unlikely to have a tantrum in the pediatrician's office, and his or her poor capacity for social interaction may not be obvious, given a situation that engenders anxiety and reticence in normal children; in some cases, abnormalities in psychological functioning will be apparent only in evaluations by specialists.

The reactions of the child's age mates are a particularly sensitive barometer. Adults may be willing to overlook minor degrees of social ineptness among children, but other children are not. The child who is even a bit strange frequently will be physically avoided by other children in nursery school and later on often will be labeled as weird and treated as a social outcast by school-aged peers, so harsh are the standards of child society.

The evaluation of the child with strange behavior is outlined in Table 167-1. It should address each of the essential components of the process by which children make sense out of their environment. Referral to a special diagnostic clinic within a medical school is one way to facilitate the evaluation, which often necessitates involving several specialists. Another approach that can be used is for the pediatrician to refer the child for psychiatric evaluation and psychological testing and, on the basis of these evaluations, determine whether an additional speech and language evaluation is in order. (See Chapters 13 and 76 for additional discussion of the role of the consultant.)

Evaluation of the *sensory apparatus* includes testing hearing and vision. The *capacity to store, classify, and integrate information* can be assessed through various tests of cognitive functioning. The standard intelligence tests, such as the WISC-R and Stanford-Binet, are helpful, as well as more specialized tests designed to identify difficulties with auditory or visual processing (see Chapter 18). The *ability to com-*

Table 167-1 *Evaluation of the Child with Strange Behavior*

DIAGNOSTIC PROCEDURE	ENTITY IDENTIFIED	PRIMARY SPECIALIST INVOLVED
Developmental history	Developmental delays	Pediatrician
Complete psychosocial history	Problem with child's social and emotional adjustment, family functioning, parent-child relationship	Pediatrician
Physical examination	Growth failure secondary to underlying chronic illness	Pediatrician
Hearing and vision screening	Hearing or visual deficits	Pediatrician
Urinary metabolic screening	Inborn errors of metabolism	Pediatrician
Psychiatric evaluation	Psychiatric disorder	Child psychiatrist
Neurologic evaluation	Degenerative conditions, brain lesions	Pediatric neurologist
Psychologic testing	Abnormalities of cognitive functioning	Child psychologist
Speech and language evaluation	Speech and language disorders	Speech and language specialist

municate is evaluated through a speech and language assessment. The *caregiving environment* is assessed on the basis of information obtained from parents and others as part of the *developmental and social history*, as well as by direct observation of the caregivers and their interactions with the child. Finally, the *psychiatric interview with the child* includes careful observations of the child's behavior, thinking patterns, capacity for relationships, and methods of coping with stress. The synthesis of all available information about the child and family then can be used to arrive at an integrated view of the child's functioning and an assessment of the degree and nature of the psychopathologic condition present. To promote this synthesis it is helpful if the pediatrician can meet with the other specialists who have evaluated the child.

In addition to recognizing that emotional disturbance in parents may lead to misperceptions of normal child behavior, it is equally important to be aware that the disturbed child has a major and often devastating impact on the family's functioning; what may appear to be distortions in the parent-child relationship may in reality be the result of the parents' reaction to the child's emotional disturbance. Autistic and psychotic children, in particular, place an extraordinary burden on families. Typically, families are confused and frustrated in their attempts to manage the child. Focusing only on the parents' apparent psychopathologic condition can blind one to the extent of an emotional disturbance in the child.

During the overall physical examination, the pediatrician should always do a neurologic examination, including an assessment for soft neurologic signs. If a pervasive developmental disorder is suspected, urinary metabolic screening should be undertaken. Because of the likelihood of Rett syndrome, chromosomal studies are indicated in girls who show features of autism. Although abnormal findings on a CT scan and an electroencephalogram (EEG) have been found among children with pervasive developmental disorders, they are not diagnostic and should be obtained only if one is concerned about a degenerative neurologic disorder or space-occupying lesion.

TREATMENT

Treatment approaches obviously need to be determined by the physician's understanding of the type of disorder involved. In the various kinds of developmental disorders, and in those resulting from sensory or cognitive impairments, treatment is aimed at maximizing functioning and teaching skills that will enable the child to be as self-sufficient as possible. These children's needs are complex and require a multipronged treatment approach that includes special education, help in language development, and emotional support for themselves and their parents.[8] Most children with autism or other pervasive developmental disorders are able to be managed at home with appropriate special educational placement and family support. A comprehensive school program that emphasizes structure and behavioral methods is important, and a very high level of individual attention often is necessary. As the child progresses through adolescence, training in skills that will allow for as much independent functioning as possible should be emphasized. Used judiciously, drug treatment can help in some cases to reduce dangerous or extremely bothersome behaviors, such as self-injurious behavior, aggression toward others, or extreme temper tantrums.[2] The most commonly used drugs are the neuroleptic agents, such as haloperidol or thioridazine. These drugs, which have possibly serious side effects such as tardive dyskinesia, may impair the child's ability to learn; they should be used cautiously and prescribed only by a physician experienced in their use.

Psychotherapy can help learning disabled children who suffer social handicaps by giving them a better understanding of their handicaps and helping them develop compensatory strategies.

The importance of emotional support and guidance for parents cannot be overemphasized. The pediatrician is likely to be the professional who has the most long-term relationship with the child and family and is in an excellent position to provide such support. The pediatrician can interpret the findings and recommendations of other specialists to the parents and guide them in the difficult and often frustrating task of obtaining necessary services for their child. In recent years, support and advocacy groups for parents of mentally ill children have developed; such groups also can be extremely helpful.

Awareness of distorted parental perceptions should lead the pediatrician in such a case to intervene immediately to prevent the pathologic influences from irreparably affecting the child.

It is the task of the pediatrician, after listening carefully, to empathize with how difficult things must be for this parent and gently, but directly, suggest that it would be helpful to have someone to talk to in more depth about these problems. If one simply attempts to convince the parent that there is nothing wrong with the child, one almost guarantees that the parent will continue in his or her fixed belief and will seek confirmation of his or her opinions elsewhere.

OUTCOME

Outcome in the pervasive developmental disorders is variable, which should not be surprising given the heterogeneity of these disorders. Outcome has been studied most in autism, which also is the most clearly defined entity of the group. Outcomes have been reported that range from good to very good (5% to 18%), fair (16% to 27%), and poor (60% to 75%). Children with higher intellectual functioning tend to do better; outcome is poor if they fail to develop speech by the age of 6 years. Unfortunately, there are no controlled studies of the impact of various kinds of interventions. In general, children with pervasive developmental disorders will require intensive supportive services throughout childhood and adolescence and into adulthood. Although children who function at a higher level than most and some children with otherwise pervasive developmental disorders may attain economic self-sufficiency, the majority do not.

SUMMARY

Strange behavior may be the manifestation of a variety of different entities, ranging from severe psychiatric disorders to behavioral responses to abuse and neglect. Strange behavior resulting from so many causes underscores the importance of understanding the context in which the behavior occurs, the social environment of the child, and the child's own thoughts and feelings. A careful and comprehensive evaluation is necessary in all cases. Treatment approaches likewise need to be comprehensive and address the complex needs of the child and the family.

REFERENCES

1. American Psychiatric Association: Diagnostic and statistical manual of mental disorders, ed 3, rev, Washington DC, 1987, The Association.
2. Campbell M and Green WH: Pervasive developmental disorders of childhood. In Kaplan HI and Sadock BJ, editors: Comprehensive textbook of psychiatry, vol 2, ed 5, Baltimore, 1989, The William and Wilkins Co.
3. DeMyer MK: The psychoses of childhood. In Noshpitz JD, editor: Basic handbook of child psychiatry, vol 5, New York, 1987, Basic Books.
4. Frijling-Schreuder ECM: Borderline states in children, Psychoanal Study Child 24:307, 1969.
5. Kanner L: Autistic disturbances of affective contact, Nerv Child 2:217, 1943.
6. Kestenbaum CJ, Canino IA, and Pleak RR: Schizophrenic disorders of childhood and adolescence. In Tasman A, Hales RE, and Frances AJ, editors: American Psychiatric Press review of psychiatry, vol 8, Washington, DC, 1989, American Psychiatric Press, Inc.
7. Lowe TL et al: Detection of phenylketonuria in autistic and psychotic children, JAMA 243:126, 1980.
8. Rutter M: The treatment of autistic children, J Child Psychol Psychiatry 26:193, 1985.

168

Stridor

Joanne Kurtzberg and Henry S. Friedman

Stridor, derived from the Latin *stridulus* meaning creaking, whistling, or grating, is a harsh crowing sound associated with obstruction of air flow along the respiratory tract from the pharynx to the main-stem bronchi. It can be acute or chronic, but it always is a pathologic sign or symptom that requires evaluation. On physical examination, stridor generally is audible to the naked ear, but the position of the noise in the respiratory cycle can be best appreciated by applying a stethoscope to the patient's neck. Although stridor is associated with several common pediatric disorders, it also can be an important clue to rarer diagnoses.

DIAGNOSTIC CLUES

Stridor is a distressing symptom to its victims, their parents, and physicians alike. Attention to some of its subtler characteristics can aid in diagnosing its cause. The sounds caused by the stridor, timing of the stridor in relation to the respiratory phase, and the position of the child who is stridorous all potentially provide clues to its etiology.

Stridor characteristically occurs during inspiration but can be heard during expiration as well. The timing of the stridor may help locate the level of obstruction. For example, stridor limited to inspiration usually indicates a supraglottic obstruction, whereas stridor limited to expiration more likely represents a subglottic blockage. Obstruction at the level of the larynx causes stridor that persists through both inspiration and expiration.

The musical pitch of the stridor also may prove helpful in diagnosis. High-pitched stridor is seen with glottic obstruction and low-pitched stridor with supraglottic disease. Stridor plus a barking cough suggests tracheal involvement. The quality of the child's voice or cry also may provide diagnostic clues. A child with hoarseness or a weak or absent voice probably has laryngeal involvement. The child with a normal voice and severe dyspnea is more likely to have tracheal or subglottic disease. One should consider supraglottic pathologic conditions in the infant or child with a muffled cry and involvement of the recurrent laryngeal nerve in the patient with an abnormal cry.

During the physical examination it is important to note the position of the child as he or she breathes. One should suspect extrinsic airway pressure in the child who prefers to keep his or her neck in a hyperextended position.

Finally, the duration of the stridor can provide important information. Relatively few disorders cause acute stridor, but all are potentially life threatening, requiring prompt intervention. Evaluation of a patient with chronic stridor is less urgent but equally important and generally more complicated because of the larger number of potential causes.

CAUSES

Acute Stridor

The most common cause of acute stridor in childhood is viral croup or laryngotracheitis (see box at left on p. 1080). Characterized by a barking cough, as well as by inspiratory stridor, this illness, which usually follows an upper respiratory tract infection, primarily in children between 6 months and 3 years of age, can be frightening. The acute onset, generally low fever, predominant occurrence at night, and absence of other features suggest this illness. Spasmodic or allergic croup, occurring with inspiratory stridor but without a preceding upper respiratory tract infection or fever, may mimic laryngotracheitis. This disorder, which occurs in children older than those with laryngotracheitis, may be recurrent.

These disorders are in marked contrast to epiglottitis, one of the truly life-threatening infections of childhood. It is characterized by the abrupt onset of high fever, stridor, hoarseness or aphonia, drooling, and a toxic appearance in a child, who must sit upright for maximal air exchange. The child who has these symptoms needs direct visualization of his or her airway and immediate intubation if a cherry red, enlarged epiglottis confirms the clinical suspicion. One should avoid unnecessary procedures on and manipulations of the child in whom this diagnosis is suspected until an adequate airway is established (see Chapters 269 and 276).

Other infectious illnesses that can lead to stridor include peritonsillar and retropharyngeal abscesses. Although drooling and dysphagia accompany both, the child with a peritonsillar abscess may have difficulty opening his or her mouth, whereas the child with a retropharyngeal abscess keeps his or her neck hyperextended. Rarely, stridor and even complete airway occlusion can develop in a child with infectious mononucleosis and severe edema of the tonsils and adenoids.

Trauma, such as falls from a bicycle, automobile accidents, or sports-related injuries, may cause laryngeal fractures and consequent stridor. Dyspnea and dysphagia also may occur with one of these injuries. Swelling after intubation may lead to significant acute stridor. Inhalation of a foreign body also can lead to acute stridor and must always be suspected, particularly in young children. Children who ingest corrosives, notably lye, may have swelling of their pharyngeal mucosa, resulting in stridor, and often will have ulceration of the oral mucosa and drooling. One should consider an-

Causes of Acute Stridor

- Croup
  - Laryngotracheitis
  - Spasmodic (allergic)
- Epiglottitis
- Other infections
  - Retropharyngeal abscess
  - Peritonsillar abscess
  - Tuberculosis
  - Diphtheria
  - Laryngitis
  - Infectious mononucleosis
- Trauma
  - Foreign body aspiration
  - Accidents
  - Ingestion of corrosives
  - Trauma after intubation
  - Superior vena cava syndrome
- Metabolic causes
  - Hypocalcemia
  - Rickets
- Angioneurotic edema

gioneurotic edema when faced with a child with stridor, acute facial and tongue swelling, and abdominal pain. This disorder, caused by C1 esterase deficiency, may cause life-threatening airway obstruction.

Chronic Stridor

The causes of chronic stridor in infants and children consist mainly of congenital disorders (see box at right). Stridor may be present from birth or first may be noticed when the baby or child has an intercurrent upper respiratory tract infection. The cause—obstruction of the airway—may be found at the supraglottic, glottic, or subglottic region.

Supraglottic Obstruction. Perhaps the most common of all disorders that cause chronic stridor is laryngomalacia (congenital laryngeal stridor, infantile larynx, or inspiratory laryngeal collapse). Coarse stridor that increases with the intensity of respirations generally is apparent by 4 to 8 weeks of age, but it may be present from birth or the first week of life. It is believed to be caused by collapse of the epiglottis, aryepiglottic folds, and arytenoids over a small and anteriorly placed glottic orifice during inspiration, leaving only a slitlike opening for air exchange. These tissues vibrate as they close, producing the stridor. Expiration, coughing, and crying separate the floppy tissues, and the noise disappears. This stridor is more noticeable in the supine position, with an upper respiratory tract infection, or with any form of increased respiratory effort.

Fortunately, this condition seldom causes significant airway obstruction. It tends to resolve spontaneously, beginning at about 12 months of age and disappearing by 3 or 4 years of age. Conservative management with reassurance of the patient and parents is the best intervention for this condition.

The child with the floppy epiglottis (omega-shaped epiglottis) may have inspiratory stridor that is most severe in the supine position. In this disorder the epiglottis tends to fall back over the larynx to cause a partial obstruction and stridor.

Causes of Chronic Stridor

SUPRAGLOTTIC

- Congenital
  - Congenital laryngeal stridor
  - Floppy epiglottis
  - Cysts
    - Aryepiglottic
    - Dermoid
    - Thyroglossal duct
  - Lingual thyroid
  - Micrognathia
  - Macroglossia
- Other
  - Tonsillar hypertrophy

GLOTTIC AND SUBGLOTTIC

- Congenital
  - Glottic and subglottic stenosis
  - Hemangioma and lymphangioma
  - Vocal cord paralysis
  - Laryngeal web
  - Polyps and papillomas
  - Laryngeal and bronchial cysts
  - Laryngoceles
  - Goiter
  - Vascular ring
  - Cartilage ring abnormalities
  - Esophageal atresia
  - Tracheosophageal fistula
- Neoplastic
  - Thyroid carcinoma
  - Mediastinal tumor
  - Neurofibromatosis
- Traumatic
  - After intubation
  - After tracheostomy
  - Foreign body
- Miscellaneous

Other causes of supraglottic obstruction include aryepiglottic cysts, thyroglossal duct cysts, dermoid cysts, a lingual thyroid, or a supraglottic web. Children or infants with these disorders also have muffled cries and feeding difficulties caused by the presence of a mass. The airways of children with macroglossia, as in Beckwith-Wiedemann syndrome, may be partially obstructed by the tongue. A similar mechanism explains the stridor in children with micrognathia, notably Pierre Robin syndrome, in which the tongue falls back over the supraglottic orifice, producing obstruction. Rarely children with biotinidase deficiency can manifest chronic stridor.

Glottic and Subglottic Obstruction. As in supraglottic obstruction, congenital abnormalities make up the majority of disorders that cause glottic and subglottic obstruction.

Subglottic hemangioma produces a pattern of inspiratory and expiratory stridor with a brassy cough but normal cry. Symptoms are characteristically absent at birth and begin to appear at 1 to 3 months of age. Respiratory symptoms may be severe enough to cause poor feeding and failure to thrive. Similar obstruction may be secondary to subglottic stenosis without the presence of a hemangioma.

Other congenital lesions include laryngeal webs, polyps, papillomas, and cysts. Vascular rings, produced by a double aortic arch, anomalous innominate artery, anomalous left common carotid artery, anomalous left pulmonary artery, or aberrant subclavian artery, may cause airway obstruction and consequent inspiratory or expiratory stridor, as well as emesis and cyanosis.

Vocal cord paralysis that produces stridor includes both unilateral and bilateral palsy. Unilateral palsy, either alone or with other cardiac or neurologic lesions, usually exhibits left-sided involvement secondary to recurrent laryngeal nerve compression. The voice may be normal or hoarse. Stridor and feeding difficulties are the primary findings. Bilateral palsy is occasionally an isolated phenomenon but more often is indicative of hydrocephalus, especially with Arnold-Chiari deformity.

Noncongenital causes of chronic stridor include mediastinal masses, trauma after intubation or tracheostomy, and cricoarytenoid arthritis secondary to juvenile rheumatoid arthritis and vocal cord malfunction as a result of emotional factors.

Evaluation of Chronic Stridor. The diagnostic evaluation of chronic stridor is far more difficult than that of acute stridor. Although the history and physical examination provide useful diagnostic clues, the exact location of the obstruction usually is found via roentgenographic evaluation plus direct airway obstruction through endoscopic examination.

A rational approach includes anteroposterior and lateral roentgenograms of the chest and neck to assess upper airway, epiglottic, retropharyngeal space, laryngeal, and subglottic patency. In addition, fluoroscopy or a barium swallow test may be necessary to observe kinetic changes or to visualize vascular rings. Ultimately, flexible laryngoscopy, with direct visualization of the glottis, and telescopic bronchoscopy may be the tools used to make an accurate diagnosis.

SUGGESTED READINGS

Illingworth RS: Common symptoms of disease in children, ed 5, Oxford, 1975, Blackwell Scientific Publications, Ltd.

Kaye R, Oski FA, and Barness LA: Core textbook of pediatrics, ed 3, Philadelphia, 1988, JB Lippincott Co.

Quinn-Bogard AL and Potsic WP: Stridor in the first year of life: clinical evaluation of the persistent or intermittent noisy breather, Clin Pediatr 16:913, 1977.

Tunnessen WW Jr: Signs and symptoms in pediatrics, ed 2, Philadelphia, 1988, JB Lippincott Co.

169

Syncope

Diane L. McDonald and Archie S. Golden

Syncope is defined as a rapid, transient, complete loss of consciousness and postural tone as a result of cerebral ischemia, hypoxia, or hypoglycemia. In the pediatric population it usually occurs in the older child and adolescent. Within this age-group, syncope (a simple faint) is most frequently caused by a vasovagal reflex. In a recent study by Pratt and Fleisher,[1] 50% of patients examined in the pediatric emergency room for fainting were diagnosed with vasovagal syncope. Other diagnoses included orthostatic hypotension (20%), atypical seizure (7.5%), migraine (5%), and minor head trauma (5%).

Although syncope often is a benign occurrence, an effort must be made to rule out other, more serious causes of a transient loss of consciousness. A thorough history and physical examination must be performed, with added attention to the cardiac and neurologic status. If the cause of the syncopal event is cardiac, the child may be at risk for an arrhythmia or even sudden death. In addition, a child who is lethargic or unconscious is by definition not one with simple syncope and needs to be evaluated for an underlying disorder of the central nervous system. Therefore a child with suspected cardiac disease or one who manifests impairment of consciousness requires immediate attention and intervention.

The history and physical examination are important factors in differentiating among the various causes of syncope. Issues to be noted include the premorbid state of the child, circumstances surrounding the episode, the onset and duration of the loss of consciousness, any associated body movements, and the quality of the recovery period. Any available caretaker or witness should be interviewed for a full description of the event.

The medical history is important in determining the likely cause. A history of congenital heart disease, seizure disorder, or endocrine abnormalities, such as diabetes, may provide significant clues. A history of recurrent syncopal episodes is unusual and may require extensive testing—that is, Holter (cardiac) monitoring, echocardiographic examination, electrophysiologic studies, and/or an electroencephalogram to uncover occult cardiac or neurologic disease. The family history is helpful. Seizure disorders and cardiac disease such as Marfan syndrome, idiopathic hypertrophic subaortic stenosis, or the prolonged QT syndrome, may be inherited. Breath-holding spells, too, have been noted to occur in families.

The history of the present illness should include the circumstances precipitating the event. For example, with vasovagal syncope the child often is standing in a warm, stuffy room and is hungry, tired, or frightened. The prodrome of a seizure may consist of an aura, whereas a cardiac event often is sudden, without warning, or it may be induced by exercise.

The duration of the syncopal episode varies with the diagnosis. A simple faint lasts a few seconds to 1 or 2 minutes, whereas a seizure may be prolonged, often lasting more than 5 minutes. The loss of consciousness during an episode of cardiac arrhythmia may be brief or prolonged, depending on the severity of the disease.

Given an episode, it is necessary to determine if the child was completely unconscious or if there was some degree of responsiveness that suggests hysteria or malingering. A truly unconscious person will not respond if the eyelashes are lightly brushed; a hysterical person will respond, albeit often with just a mild flickering of the lids. Seizure type of movements are important; however, generalized tonic-clonic movements may be seen in all forms of syncope because of cerebral anoxia or hypoglycemia. Also, the duration of the episode should be estimated. In general, the conscious state is regained quickly with vasovagal syncope, whereas the postictal state of a seizure disorder may be characterized by prolonged confusion and fatigue.

DIFFERENTIAL DIAGNOSIS

Syncope can be categorized by its various causes (see accompanying box).

PSYCHOPHYSIOLOGIC SYNCOPE

A fainting episode in which the child has been standing or sitting for a prolonged period of time in an uncomfortable environment suggests *vasovagal syncope*. A noxious event that causes fear, pain, or anxiety also may precipitate the faint. The child may feel dizzy, weak, or nauseated and appear cold and clammy. A rapid drop in blood pressure associated with vagally stimulated bradycardia may lead to the loss of consciousness. It is short-lived and, depending on the degree of cerebral hypoperfusion, may end with tonic-clonic movements. The child usually awakens to full consciousness in a short period of time.

Hyperventilation may occur as a response to anxiety or pain. For instance, the child may hyperventilate in anticipation of venipuncture or in *reaction to fright*. Rapid, short breaths cause hypocapnia and a resultant cerebral vasoconstriction and hypoperfusion. The child experiences a feeling of lightheadedness along with numbness and tingling of the hands and feet. Again, the loss of consciousness is brief and the recovery rapid.

Cyanotic breath-holding spells usually begin around the

Differential Diagnosis of Syncope

- I. Psychophysiologic
  - A. Vasovagal episodes
  - B. Hyperventilation
  - C. Breath-holding spells
  - D. Hysteria
- II. Neurologic factors
  - A. Generalized tonic-clonic seizure
  - B. Atonic seizures
  - C. Complex partial seizures
  - D. Migraine
  - E. Trauma/concussion
  - F. Narcolepsy
- III. Cardiac
  - A. Structural abnormalities
    1. Aortic stenosis
    2. Idiopathic hypertrophy
    3. Subaortic stenosis
    4. Left atrial myxoma
    5. Tetralogy of Fallot
    6. Pulmonic stenosis
    7. Primary pulmonary hypertension
  - B. Arrhythmia
    1. Bradycardia
       - a. Sick sinus syndrome
       - b. Atrioventricular block
    2. Supraventricular tachycardia
       - a. Caffeine/stress
       - b. Wolff-Parkinson-White syndrome
    3. Ventricular tachycardia/fibrillation
       - a. Myocarditis/pericarditis
       - b. Intoxication/medication
       - c. Congenital heart disease
       - d. Postoperative cardiac surgery
       - e. Prolonged QT syndrome
       - f. Ischemic heart disease
- IV. Orthostatic
  - A. Hypovolemia
  - B. Postural hypotension
  - C. Medications
- V. Metabolic
  - A. Anemia
  - B. Hypoglycemia
- VI. Miscellaneous
  - A. Cough
  - B. Swallowing
  - C. Micturition
  - D. Pregnancy

age of 6 months and end by age 6 years. Clinically the child is upset, frightened, or hurt, begins to cry, gasps, and then becomes apneic and cyanotic. Stiffening of the body and a loss of consciousness soon may follow. The pathophysiologic basis is unclear, but it may be that crying during expiration causes increased intrathoracic pressure, which in turn leads to low cardiac output. Hypoxia combined with decreased cerebral blood flow leads to the loss of consciousness. The event is brief, and afterwards the child becomes fully conscious. A pallid type of breath-holding spell *(pallid infantile syncope)* is less common, although it can occur in the same age range as does the cyanotic spell and may begin with the same cry. The mechanism differs. The episode is provoked by pain or crying. The child suddenly becomes pale, limp, and loses consciousness. The pathophysiologic basis is increased vagal tone, which causes an apparent asystole. The event ordinarily lasts only seconds to minutes, and the child awakens to full consciousness (see Chapter 154).

A *conversion reaction* is a means of transforming an unacceptable unconscious desire into a physical complaint. In the older child or adolescent, the conversion reaction may take the form of hysterical fainting. The child often is sitting or recumbent or may exaggerate a fall from a standing position to avoid injury. The child usually responds quickly to a mildly painful stimulus, and the physical examination reveals nothing extraordinary.

NEUROLOGIC SYNCOPE

Generalized tonic-clonic movements can occur with all forms of syncope; therefore the discovery of a specific cause for a seizure may be difficult. Intercurrent fever or a history of seizures, head trauma, or adverse perinatal events may be helpful leads. Frequently there is a family history of epilepsy.

The *generalized tonic-clonic* or *grand mal seizure* is characterized by a rather sudden onset of complete unconsciousness with stiffening of the body and the eyes rolling back. After a tonic phase, clonic movements of the extremities may occur. Although the duration of the seizure may be variable, it usually lasts longer than a simple faint. Incontinence is common, and the postictal recovery period is characterized by prolonged confusion and weakness.

Some *complex partial seizures* can resemble a fainting episode. Partial seizures may begin with an aura, which the child may describe as an uncomfortable feeling or an unusual visual or olfactory sensation. During the seizure the child may be unresponsive and lose postural tone. The complex partial seizure is characterized by semipurposeful yet involuntary action—for example, picking at clothing. In the postictal period the child is tired and slowly returns to full consciousness.

A *basilar artery migraine* may manifest as a syncopal event. It is believed to arise from impaired blood flow to the brain stem during the vasoconstrictive phase of migraine. After the initial spasm the affected artery dilates and a classic or common migraine occurs. A family history of migraine may help in making this diagnosis.

It is not uncommon to lose consciousness for a short time after relatively minor *head trauma* (concussion). Other symptoms such as vomiting, headache, and amnesia also may occur. It may be appropriate to observe the child for a short period, usually overnight, because these symptoms usually resolve quickly without treatment. However, abnormal findings on neurologic examination, clear drainage from the nose or ears, bleeding from the ears, a Battle sign, or a prolonged period of altered consciousness should alert the physician to the possibility of a more serious injury, such as a subdural hematoma, basilar skull fracture, or cerebral contusion.

CARDIAC SYNCOPE

Cardiac syncope is rare in childhood; however, when it occurs, it may be life-threatening. Cardiac disease can cause syncope in a number of ways. Structural heart disease may obstruct blood flow from the left ventricle, with consequent hypoperfusion, or may shunt blood flow from right to left, leading to hypoxia. A person with a diseased or stressed myocardium from hypoxia, myocarditis, toxic drug ingestion, or a congenital heart lesion is at risk for a sudden arrhythmia. Arrhythmias, by decreasing either the cardiac stroke volume or the heart rate, can lead to a reduced cardiac output and cerebral hypoperfusion.

Structural lesions such as *aortic stenosis* and *idiopathic hypertrophic subaortic stenosis* (IHSS) can cause dizziness or fainting after exercise. On auscultation a systolic murmur may be heard at the right sternal border. The murmur of IHSS is accentuated by a Valsalva maneuver, and the electrocardiogram shows signs of left ventricular enlargement. Children with cyanotic congenital heart disease, in particular *tetralogy of Fallot,* may have spells of cyanosis that occasionally lead to unconsciousness. These episodes, "tet spells," are caused by a sudden decrease in pulmonary blood flow and the shunting of deoxygenated blood from right to left through the ventricular septal defect and thence the aorta.

Bradycardia, as seen with *sick sinus syndrome,* is associated with periods of extreme sinus slowing or arrest and may require a pacemaker. Tachycardia, as with *ventricular tachycardia* and *ventricular fibrillation,* is most serious and is usually the result of severe underlying cardiac disease. *Ventricular fibrillation* also may be seen with the *prolonged QT syndrome*. The etiology of this disease is unclear. It may involve an imbalance of sympathetic cardiac innervation. Two inherited diseases characterized by a prolonged QT interval are notable. The *Jervell and Lange-Nielsen syndrome* is autosomal recessive and associated with deafness; the *Romano-Ward syndrome,* on the other hand, occurs with normal hearing and an autosomal dominant pattern of inheritance. Sinus rates of 200 to 300 per minute are possible with *supraventricular tachycardia (SVT),* which can be associated with *Wolff-Parkinson-White syndrome*. In this circumstance an accessory pathway, the bundle of Kent, bypasses the atrioventricular node and speeds conduction from the atria to the ventricles. Stress, coffee, and drugs—for example, amphetamines—also can cause an attack.

ORTHOSTATIC SYNCOPE

Hypovolemia from dehydration or acute blood loss can lead to *orthostatic hypotension* and syncope. Medications (e.g., diuretics, antihypertensives, and antidepressants) also can cause orthostatic blood pressure changes. In addition, *postural hypotension* can occur from rising quickly, prolonged standing, or prolonged bed rest.

METABOLIC SYNCOPE

Syncope caused by *hypoglycemia* most frequently is encountered in the young patient with insulin-dependent diabetes. Better control, with appropriate insulin dosing and an understanding of the warning signs of hypoglycemia, may prevent further episodes. Chronic *anemia* can lead to fatigue, weakness, or a syncopal attack. A thorough search for the source of blood loss is required, and a blood transfusion may be necessary.

MISCELLANEOUS CAUSES OF SYNCOPE

Cough-induced syncope has been described in patients with the paroxysms of pertussis, laryngeal spasm, laryngeal nerve irritation, and asthma. Other rare causes of syncope in childhood are associated with micturition and strenuous swallowing.

Pregnancy always should be considered when an adolescent of childbearing age faints. This is caused by increased estrogen and progesterone levels with consequent decreased peripheral vascular resistance and hypotension.

PSYCHOSOCIAL CONSIDERATIONS

The majority of benign vasovagal fainting episodes occur in places outside the home. It may be that at school or in church the child is forced to sit or stand for long periods of time in an uncomfortable circumstance but at home is more free to move about and alter body position. Thus it may be more significant if the child faints at home or while exercising, suggesting a more serious cause, perhaps cardiac syncope.

Children who manifest an atypical syncopal episode, hysteria, or pseudoseizure should be evaluated for evidence of physical, verbal, or sexual abuse, inasmuch as this may reflect "acting out" behavior. There should be an effort to determine whether the family is subject to unusual stress—for example, marital conflict, divorce, or a recent death.

MANAGEMENT

The approach to the syncopal patient begins with assessment of the neurologic status. A child who arrives unconscious or with depressed consciousness has not had a simple fainting episode and requires immediate care. If the child is alert, a careful physical examination should be performed with special attention to the cardiovascular system. The examiner should listen for murmurs, extra heart sounds, and an unusual rhythm or rate. A simple workup for a first-time fainting episode includes an electrocardiogram and determination of hematocrit, electrolyte, and glucose levels. Vital signs should be taken while the patient is upright and supine (see the box on p. 1085). The electrocardiogram should be evaluated for rhythm disturbances, chamber hypertrophy, abnormal voltage, and a prolonged QT segment. If an abnormality is found on examination or electrocardiogram, monitoring and cardiology consultation are most often mandated. A patient with recurrent syncopal episodes should be evaluated for occult cardiac disease. A referral to a cardiologist for Holter monitoring, an echocardiogram, stress testing, or an electrophysiologic study is indicated. Abnormalities such as a low hematocrit or blood glucose level are rare but, if present, require a vigorous search for the cause. If postprandial hypoglycemia is suspected, a glucose tolerance test may help in making the diagnosis. Children with symptoms of obvious dehydration

Workup for the First Episode of Syncope

History
Physical examination
Vital signs, including orthostatic blood pressure and pulse
Electrocardiogram
Glucose level
Electrolyte levels
Hematocrit measurement
Consider:
  Pregnancy test
  Toxicology screen

Table 169-1 *Relating History to Etiologic Factors*

HISTORY	POSSIBLE CAUSES
Prolonged seizure activity or postictal state	Seizure disorder
Precipitation by crying	Breath-holding spell
Precipitation by cough, swallow, or urination	Cough, swallow, micturition syncope
Precipitation by exercise or a sudden onset of syncope	Cardiac syncope
Head trauma	Concussion
Precipitation by noxious event or environmental stress	Vasovagal syncope
Inconsistent findings or incomplete unconsciousness	Hysteria or malingering

or abnormal orthostatic vital signs require rehydration therapy.

Frequently, the physical examination results are normal and no abnormality is found in the initial laboratory workup. As is so often the case, the history becomes most important in establishing a cause (Table 169-1). A seizure disorder can be particularly difficult to diagnose because seizurelike activity can occur with all forms of syncope, and the electroencephalogram often does not reveal significant findings. Therefore a high index of suspicion and a neurology consultation may be needed.

Most other causes of syncope are benign. Reassurance and common-sense management are required. A child with vasovagal syncope should be placed supine before venipuncture. Children who hyperventilate need to learn its relationship to fainting; attention to the reasons for hyperventilation is required. Breath-holding spells are best treated by educating the parents and by emphasizing the harmless nature of the spells. In severe instances a neurology consultation is warranted, just to make certain that there is no other compelling reason.

The diagnosis of hysteria or malingering may be difficult. Hospitalization for observation and a psychiatric referral may be indicated. Finally, pregnancy always should be considered in the evaluation of an adolescent or postpubertal female with syncope. If in doubt about the validity of the history or if the date of the last menstrual period is unknown, a urine or serum pregnancy test should be performed.

REFERENCES

1. Pratt JL and Fleisher GR: Syncope in children and adolescents, Pediatr Emerg Care B5:80, 1989.

SUGGESTED READINGS

Anderson RH et al: Pediatric cardiology, Edinburgh, 1986, Churchill Livingstone.

Castor W, Skarin R, and Roscelli JD: Orthostatic heart rate and arterial blood pressure changes in normovolemic children, Pediatr Emerg Care 1:123, 1985.

Driscoll DJ and Edwards WD: Sudden unexpected death in children and adolescents, Am Coll Cardiol 5:6 (suppl): 118B, 1985.

Farmer TW: Pediatric neurology, Philadelphia, 1983, Harper & Row Publishers, Inc.

Holmes GL: Breath-holding attacks in children, Postgrad Med 84:191, 1988.

Katz RM: Cough syncope in children with asthma, Pediatrics 77:48, 1970.

Ruckman RN: Cardiac causes of syncopy, Pediatr Rev 9: 101, 1987.

Woody RC and Kiel EA: Swallowing syncope in a child, Pediatrics 78:507, 1986.

170

Torticollis

Beryl J. Rosenstein

Torticollis, or wryneck, refers to abnormal positioning (tilt) of the head and neck. It is a physical finding, not a diagnosis, and an accurate cause must be determined before appropriate treatment can be initiated. It is found in association with many childhood illnesses and, depending on the age of the patient, has a wide spectrum of underlying etiologic factors (see the accompanying box).

DIAGNOSIS

Neonates

When a head tilt is recognized in the early neonatal period, the usual cause is congenital muscular torticollis.[2,6,10] This is characterized by tilting of the head to the involved side and turning of the face to the opposite side, in association with unilateral fibrotic contracture of the sternocleidomastoid *(SCM)* muscle. The head cannot be passively moved into a normal position. Torticollis may be noted at birth and is almost always obvious by 2 to 4 weeks of age. A firm, nontender, discrete fusiform mass ("tumor"), 1 to 3 cm in diameter, may be palpable in the body of the muscle. The mass contains fibrous tissue and does not represent a resolving hematoma. It may increase gradually in size over the first month, but then it regresses; by 4 to 6 months it usually is no longer palpable. By this time only contracture and fibrotic thickening of the involved muscle will be obvious. The cause is not known, but it is postulated to result from trauma to the soft tissues of the neck during delivery, an intrauterine positional deformity, or ischemia secondary to venous occlusion. The family history will be positive for muscular torticollis in 10% of cases.[16] Congenital hip dysplasia, usually occurring on the same side as the torticollis, may be associated in up to 20% of cases.[2,9]

Other causes of congenital torticollis include anomalies of the atlas, odontoid or atlantoaxial articulation; abnormal skin webs or folds (pterygium colli); lesions such as cystic hygroma and branchial cleft cyst in the region of the SCM muscle; vertebral dislocation; and fusion abnormalities associated with cervical hemivertebrae, as seen in Klippel-Feil syndrome or Sprengel deformity.[6,7] When a mass is *not* palpable within the SCM muscle, cervical spine roentgenograms should be obtained. Rarely, the SCM muscle may be absent unilaterally, in which case the head tilt is away from and the chin is rotated toward the side of the absent muscle, compared with the positions associated with muscular torticollis.

Infants

After the newborn period, infants may have abnormal tone and posturing of the head, neck, and upper portion of the trunk in association with gastroesophageal reflux and hiatus hernia *(Sandifer syndrome)*.[1,11] Posturing, which can take the form of torticollis, opisthotonos, or dystonia, has been at-

Causes of Acquired Torticollis

TRAUMA

Injury to cervical musculature (spastic torticollis)
Subluxation (atlantooccipital, atlas-axis [C1-2], or C2-3)
Intervertebral disk calcification

INFECTION

Cervical adenitis
Retropharyngeal abscess
Osteomyelitis of cervical vertebrae
Acute epidemic torticollis

NEUROLOGIC CAUSES

Ventricular shunt malfunction
Dystonic drug reactions (oculogyric crisis)
Tumors (posterior fossa, intraspinal, or extradural)
Syringomyelia
Wilson disease
Dystonia musculorum deformans

OTHER CAUSES

Hiatal hernia with gastroesophageal reflux (Sandifer syndrome)
Benign paroxysmal torticollis of infancy
Vertebral abnormalities
- Atloaxoid instability (nontraumatic dislocation)
- Bone dysplasia
- Eosinophilic granuloma

Strabismus (ocular torticollis)
Nystagmus
Hysteria
Psychogenic
Soft tissue tumors of the neck
Rheumatoid arthritis

tributed to an attempt by the infant to decrease the pain of esophagitis. There may be other manifestations of reflux, including vomiting after feeding, gastrointestinal bleeding, dysphagia, episodes of apnea, recurrent cough, wheezing, pulmonary infiltrates, and failure to thrive. It needs to be emphasized that esophagitis secondary to reflux can occur in the absence of vomiting. Intermittent occurrence and alternating direction of the torticollis, in association with normal SCM muscles and normal cervical spine roentgenographic findings, strongly suggest gastroesophageal reflux as the underlying cause of the torticollis. Esophageal pH probe monitoring and endoscopic examination confirm the diagnosis, and a trial of medical management is then indicated.

Benign paroxysmal torticollis of infancy is a puzzling disorder of unknown etiology characterized by recurring attacks of head tilt and often accompanied by vomiting, pallor, agitation, ataxia, and malaise.[4,5,14] Although usually no specific precipitating factors occur, a familial pattern may exist. The cardinal feature is the periodicity of the attacks; between attacks the infant appears normal. Onset is within the first year of life. Attacks typically last from several hours to several days and usually cease before age 5 years. Apart from the head tilt and ataxia, results of physical and neurologic examinations are normal, as are laboratory tests. Other disorders that need to be considered in the differential diagnosis include recurrent cervical dislocation, posterior fossa tumor, seizure disorder, and gastroesophageal reflux. An electroencephalogram, cervical spine films, esophageal pH probe monitoring, barium swallow, cervical computed tomography scans, and magnetic resonance imaging may help in the diagnostic evaluation. Suggested causes of benign paroxysmal torticollis include episodic vasospasm, migraine, and paroxysmal dysfunction of central vestibular structures. Clinical features of benign paroxysmal vertigo or infantile migraine develop in some patients. Although there is no specific therapy, it is important to recognize this entity and to reassure the family that its course is benign and its prognosis usually good.

Older Children

Acquired torticollis in older children may be secondary to a variety of disorders, as outlined in the accompanying box. Some of these conditions can be adequately managed by the pediatric practitioner; however, patients with cervical spine injuries or with neurologic signs are best evaluated in conjunction with neurology and orthopedic consultants.

Most cases of acquired torticollis seen by the pediatric practitioner are related to ligamentous or muscular injuries of the cervical soft tissues.[6] Their onset is sudden and usually follows strenuous activity, a minor injury, or a sudden change in position. The head is fixed in a tilted position and the affected muscle often has spasms and is tender. Fever and manifestations of systemic illness are absent. Laboratory and roentgenographic studies usually are not indicated.

Sudden onset of difficulty in rotating the head to one side, often after mild trauma or an upper respiratory infection and accompanied by torticollis and muscle spasm, may occur as a result of rotational subluxation of the atlas (C1) on the axis (C2) or C2 on C3. This is seldom accompanied by neurologic signs or symptoms. The diagnosis is confirmed by cervical spine roentgenograms.

Children with bone dysplasia, Morquio syndrome, spondyloepiphyseal dysplasia, and Down syndrome have a high incidence of C1-C2 instability with accompanying torticollis.[7] Asymptomatic subluxation of the atlantoaxial joint secondary to congenital laxity of the transverse atlantal ligaments is estimated to occur in 10% to 20% of persons with Down syndrome.[3] Symptomatic dislocation, which also can occur, is potentially fatal. Children with Down syndrome should have a careful evaluation, including lateral-view roentgenograms of the upper cervical region in full flexion and extension, before being allowed to participate in competitive sports that involve stress to the head and neck.

Spasmodic torticollis can occur as an idiosyncratic dystonic reaction to a variety of drugs, including the phenothiazines, methylphenidate, metoclopramide, and haloperidol. There may be other extrapyramidal manifestations, such as opisthotonos and trismus, sometimes in association with spasmodic conjugate deviations of the eyes (oculogyric crisis).

Torticollis may occur as a result of cervical adenitis in children with an infection of the tonsils and pharynx and with a retropharyngeal abscess. With a retropharyngeal abscess, there also is drooling, sore throat, dysphagia, noisy and difficult mouth breathing, fever, and leukocytosis. The diagnosis can be made by direct finger palpation of a fluctuant mass on the posterior pharyngeal wall or by a roentgenogram of the lateral neck. There also have been reports of epidemic torticollis of acute onset, presumed to be of viral etiology.[12]

Torticollis may occur secondary to *spontaneous calcification of a cervical disk*.[15] Other symptoms include muscle spasm, localized pain, and low-grade fever. Although the cause is unknown, onset may be related to trauma or to an upper respiratory infection. Roentgenograms show fluffy calcification of the nucleus pulposus. Treatment consists of analgesics and a soft cervical collar. Symptoms may last from a few days to several months; the calcification may disappear after 2 to 3 months or may be permanent.

Osteomyelitis of the cervical vertebrae should be suspected in a child who has torticollis accompanied by an unexplained low-grade fever.[17] Leukocytosis may be present, the erythrocyte sedimentation rate may be elevated, and there often is a history of mild trauma. Because of a low index of suspicion, the diagnosis often is delayed until the appearance of neurologic signs. Cervical spine roentgenograms demonstrate bone destruction, but bone scans may help establish an early diagnosis before destruction is detectable.

Torticollis accompanied by motor weakness, muscle atrophy, and fasciculations suggests a spinal cord tumor.[17] There may be neck pain and stiffness, back pain, nerve root pain, impaired gait, and sensory disturbances. Nystagmus may be present with high cervical cord tumors. Cervical spine roentgenograms may show gross bone destruction, erosion of spinal pedicles or vertebral bodies, and widening of the interpedicular spaces. The diagnosis usually is confirmed by a myelogram or by magnetic resonance imaging. Torticollis accompanied by headache, vomiting, nystagmus, or cranial nerve signs suggests a posterior fossa tumor with herniation.

For unexplained reasons, intermittent torticollis may occur because of blockage of a ventriculovenous or ventriculoperitoneal shunt. Revision of the shunt is followed by resolution of the torticollis. Torticollis also may occur as a result of formation of a subcutaneous fibrous cord along the length of a ventriculoperitoneal shunt tract.[13]

MANAGEMENT

In infants with congenital muscular torticollis the prognosis for a good cosmetic and functional outcome depends on the severity of the deformity and the age at which treatment is started.[2,10] All infants, including those with moderate-to-severe deformities and tumors in the SCM muscle, should be prescribed a trial of medical management consisting of passive stretching exercises to the involved muscle and supplemental positioning in which the most interesting aspects of the child's surroundings are placed opposite the side of the contracted muscle.[2,10] This therapy is almost always successful in infants with mild-to-moderate deformities in which treatment is started before 1 year of age. Surgery should be reserved for patients older than 12 months of age who have not responded to a 4- to 6-month trial of medical therapy.[2,10] Surgical management consists of an open tenotomy or resection of the involved muscle and surrounding fibrous bands, followed by neck traction, a soft cervical collar, and passive and active range of motion exercises. After successful medical or surgical therapy, however, potential sequelae include mild residual craniofacial asymmetry (plagiocephaly), intermittent head tilt, decreased range of neck motion, asymmetric motor development, and rarely, scoliosis.[2]

The medical management recommended for gastroesophageal reflux consists of using thickened feedings, drugs such as bethanechol and metoclopramide to enhance gastric emptying, and intensive positional therapy on a reflux board. Patients who do not respond to medical therapy should have the defect corrected surgically (a fundoplication procedure).

Treatment of acquired torticollis as a result of ligamentous and muscular injuries consists of local heat, analgesics, and a soft cervical collar; symptoms usually resolve completely in 7 to 10 days. If rotational subluxation of the atlas occurs, analgesics and light cervical traction followed by the wearing of a cervical collar are usually sufficient. Surgery rarely is required. Patients with anomalies of the occipitocervical junction or of the cervical spine often require surgical stabilization by fusion of the cervical spine.[6-8] Immediate immobilization of the neck, followed by obtaining cervical roentgenograms, should be undertaken in any patient with Down syndrome who manifests neck pain, torticollis, urinary incontinence, or loss of ambulation.[3]

Drug-induced spasmodic torticollis may be treated by discontinuing the offending drug and slowly administering diphenhydramine intravenously at a dose of 1 to 2 mg/kg.

If cervical adenitis and abscess are the causative conditions, treatment consists of surgical drainage and appropriate antibiotics.

REFERENCES

1. Bray PF et al: Childhood gastroesophageal reflux, JAMA 237:1342, 1977.
2. Binder H et al: Congenital muscular torticollis: results of conservative management with long-term follow-up in 85 cases, Arch Phys Med Rehabil 68:222, 1987.
3. Chaudhry V et al: Symptomatic atlantoaxial dislocation in Down's syndrome, Ann Neurol 21:606, 1987.
4. Deonna T and Martin D: Benign paroxysmal torticollis in infancy, Arch Dis Child 56:956, 1981.
5. Hanokoglu A, Somekh E, and Fried D: Benign paroxysmal torticollis in infancy, Clin Pediatr 23:272, 1984.
6. Hensinger RN: Orthopedic problems of the shoulder and neck, Pediatr Clin North Am 33:1495, 1986.
7. Hensinger RN and MacEwen GD: Congenital anomalies of the spine. In Rothman RH and Simeone FA, editors: The spine, ed 2, Philadelphia, 1982, WB Saunders Co.
8. Holmes JC and Hall JE: Fusion for instability and potential instability of the cervical spine in children and adolescents, Orthop Clin North Am 9:923, 1978.
9. Hummer CD Jr and MacEwen GD: The coexistence of torticollis and congenital dysplasia of the hip, J Bone Joint Surg [Am] 54:1255, 1972.
10. Morrison DL and MacEwen GD: Congenital muscular torticollis: observations regarding clinical findings, associated conditions and results of treatment, J Pediatr Orthop 2:500, 1982.
11. Murphy WJ and Gellis SS: Torticollis with hiatus hernia in infancy, Am J Dis Child 131:564, 1977.
12. Neng T et al: Acute infectious torticollis, Neurology 33:1344, 1983.
13. Robb JE and Southgate GW: An unusual case of torticollis, J Pediatr Orthop 6:469, 1986.
14. Snyder HC: Paroxysmal torticollis in infancy, Am J Dis Child 117:458, 1969.
15. Sonnabend DH, Taylor TKF, and Chapman GK: Intervertebral disc calcification syndromes in children, J Bone Joint Surg [B] 64:25, 1982.
16. Thompson F, McManus S, and Colville J: Familial congenital muscular torticollis: case report and review of the literature, Clin Orthop 202:193, 1986.
17. Visudhiphan P et al: Torticollis as the presenting sign in cervical spine infection and tumor, Clin Pediatr 21:71, 1982.

171

Vaginal Bleeding

Alain Joffe

As with other symptoms referable to the female genital tract, physician assessment of vaginal bleeding depends largely on the pubertal status of the patient. In prepubertal girls, vaginal bleeding probably reflects a localized problem in the vagina or uterus; in pubertal females, the differential diagnosis includes disorders affecting the hypothalamic-pituitary-ovarian axis and complications of pregnancy, as well as local causes. In both cases, however, a careful history and physical examination will provide important clues to the diagnosis.

PREPUBERTAL GIRLS

In the neonatal period, a decrease in the circulating maternal estrogens, which diffuse across the placenta, results in a physiologic discharge that can be either blood-tinged or frankly bloody.[5] No treatment, except reassurance, is necessary, and the discharge usually will disappear within 10 days after birth.

A number of factors can result in vaginal bleeding in the prepubertal child:

- Vulvovaginal infections
  - Excoriations secondary to pruritus
- Foreign bodies
- Sexual abuse
- Trauma
- Tumors, including condyloma
- Coagulopathies

A history of exposure to diethylstilbestrol (DES) in utero raises the possibility of a vaginal carcinoma; the patient should be given a careful examination by an experienced gynecologist. If there is any suggestion of sexual abuse, such as bruises, lacerations, or other signs of trauma, careful, nonthreatening questioning of the child or caretaker may reveal whether further referral (to the appropriate social agencies) is necessary. If there is concern about sexual abuse, cultures for *Neisseria gonorrhoeae* and *Chlamydia trachomatis* should be obtained.

Nighttime pruritus may indicate a pinworm infestation. The Scotch tape slide test, to look for pinworm eggs, can help to establish *Enterobius vermicularis* infestation. The review of systems that indicates the presence of petechiae or considerable numbers of bruises on physical examination suggests a bleeding tendency. If so, platelet counts or clotting studies are indicated. A history of foreign bodies elsewhere suggests the presence of a vaginal foreign body as the cause for bleeding. The physician also should make sure that the bleeding *is* vaginal in origin; a prolapsed urethra can mimic vaginal bleeding.

If excoriations, redness, or a rash in the perineal area is noted, vaginitis is a distinct possibility. If a discharge is present and microscopic examination demonstrates the presence of large numbers of white blood cells, vaginitis is certain. If there is concern about sexual abuse, cultures for *N. gonorrhoeae* and *C. trachomatis* should be obtained. Other bacterial cultures may be necessary; for example, a history of diarrhea in the weeks preceding suggests vaginitis caused by *Shigella* organisms.

Vaginal bleeding caused by vulvitis or foreign bodies will respond to removal of the foreign body and proper perineal hygiene. Occasionally, systemic antibiotics may be necessary. Foreign bodies often can be washed out with a flexible red Robinson catheter; sharp objects should be removed carefully, under direct visualization; referral to a gynecologist may be required if the patient is uncooperative.

Bleeding that does not subside within 10 days should be evaluated by a gynecologist. Not all of the foreign body may have been removed, or a tumor, not readily visualized by a primary care provider, may be the actual cause of the bleeding.

PUBERTAL FEMALES

Evaluation

Abnormal vaginal bleeding in pubertal females can indicate a variety of disorders. Evaluation of this symptom depends on the nature of the problem: is she bleeding between normal periods, or have her regular menses become more frequent or heavier? It is also possible that a teenager with prior regular menses will begin to have infrequent but heavy menstrual bleeding. In general, normal periods are 28 days apart (measured from the first day of one period to the first day of the next) with a range of 21 to 35 days and should not last more than 5 days.[4] Thus some teenagers will have only 2 weeks without bleeding between menses. How much bleeding is too much is difficult to quantify objectively. An increase from previous baseline menses is suggestive; Huffman and colleagues[7] recommend that a flow requiring use of more than 6 pads or 10 tampons in a 24-hour period is excessive.

The causes of abnormal bleeding in this age-group are as follows:

- Dysfunctional uterine bleeding
- Complications of pregnancy
- Genital infections, including pelvic inflammatory disease
- Foreign bodies
- Sexual abuse
- Accidental genital injury

Contraceptive-related causes, including intrauterine device
Tumors, including polyps and leiomyomas
Coagulopathies or anticoagulant therapy
Bleeding from coitus

Although anovulatory dysfunctional uterine bleeding is the most likely cause, it is a diagnosis of exclusion; thus the other causes should be eliminated before this conclusion is reached. Menstrual irregularity is frequent during the first year after menarche. In one study of 5000 adolescents, 43% had irregular menses in the first year after menarche and 20% had irregular periods 5 years after menarche.[4,12]

Most of the aforementioned organic causes can be ruled out by history and physical examination. Not all teenagers will admit to sexual activity; a negative response to this question therefore does not rule out complications of pregnancy as a cause of the bleeding. Such is the case for sexual abuse, inasmuch as a discussion of this matter is emotionally difficult for a young woman. A history of in utero exposure to DES should alert the clinician to the possibility of vaginal adenosis or carcinoma, and referral to a gynecologist for a careful examination is warranted in this circumstance. If the teenager describes a discharge that is foul smelling as well as bloody, a foreign body or retained tampon is a likely possibility; however, necrotic tumors can result in similar bleeding patterns. Pruritus or dysuria suggests vaginitis as the cause of the bleeding. Bleeding between periods is common during the first two or three cycles of oral contraceptive use and may require use of an estrogen-dominant pill if the bleeding is in early cycle or a progestin-dominant pill if the bleeding occurs in late cycle. Placement of an intrauterine device (IUD) often increases the amount of menstrual flow. Occasionally women may have a small amount of bleeding or spotting after sexual intercourse, and some women will have spotting at midcycle around the time of ovulation.

Normal findings on physical examination, including pelvic and bimanual rectoabdominal examinations, help to rule out other organic causes. Vulvar or vaginal bruising or lacerations suggest the probability of sexual abuse. Lack of adnexal or cervical motion tenderness generally excludes pelvic inflammatory disease. If the ovaries are of normal size, ovarian tumors or cysts are unlikely sources of the bleeding. A minimally enlarged uterus, consistent with early pregnancy, may not be noted by an inexperienced examiner. Measurement of human chorionic gonadotropin (HCG) level in urine or serum (if ectopic pregnancy is under consideration) will help to include or exclude diagnoses such as a missed or an incomplete abortion or an ectopic pregnancy.[9] Complications of pregnancy (e.g., ectopic pregnancy or incomplete abortion) are more likely if there is a history of amenorrhea, if the prior menstrual period was lighter than normal, if other symptoms of pregnancy are present (breast tenderness or nausea), or if the bleeding is accompanied by crampy lower abdominal pain. A history of "passing tissue" or tissue in the vaginal canal is also suggestive. Although a blood dyscrasia (e.g., thrombocytopenia or von Willebrand disease) can occasionally be present with heavy vaginal bleeding and should be excluded, this condition is often, but not always, accompanied by cutaneous manifestations of easily provoked bleeding.

Pelvic tuberculosis is extremely rare in most practices, but a negative intradermal purified protein derivative (PPD) result is simple to document. A complete blood count with indices and reticulocyte count also should be obtained inasmuch as iron deficiency anemia can cause increased uterine bleeding. Determining whether the anemia, if found, is responsible for or secondary to the heavy bleeding can be difficult, and consultation may be necessary to sort this out. Alternatively, if the bleeding is not heavy and the patient is not severely anemic, a short trial of iron therapy may be instituted and the bleeding followed to see if it persists.

Endometrial polyps or submucous leiomyomas are distinctly unusual in women younger than 20 years of age. They cannot be felt by the examiner on the usual pelvic examination. If the patient has an intractably heavy flow, the presence of one of these entities should be considered. Curettage may be necessary, or an ultrasound examination of the uterus may suggest their presence.[6,7] In either case, referral to a gynecologist for appropriate therapy is necessary.

Normal menstrual function requires that the hypothalamic-pituitary-ovarian axis be intact and functioning properly. When this occurs, the following sequence of events transpires. Follicle-stimulating hormone (FSH) causes maturation of ovarian follicles, which produce estrogen. Rising levels of estrogen stimulate the endometrial lining of the uterus to proliferate. A midcycle surge of luteinizing hormone (LH)/FSH causes the primary follicle to release an ovum, after which LH and FSH levels fall. The remnants of the follicle (termed *corpus luteum*) now produce progesterone, which converts the proliferative endometrium to a secretory phase. At the end of a normal cycle the corpus luteum involutes, and both estrogen and progesterone levels fall. The endometrial lining is now shed, and bleeding occurs.

In adolescents, especially in young adolescents, the hypothalamic-pituitary-ovarian axis is highly sensitive. A number of endogenous and exogenous factors can disturb the axis, and irregular bleeding results. Among young adolescents (but in some older ones as well) the axis has not yet matured, and most cycles are anovulatory.[2] Thus the endometrium proliferates under estrogen stimulation from the maturing follicle, but the midcycle LH surge is absent, ovulation does not occur, and the progesterone-secreting corpus luteum never forms. Toward the end of the cycle, estrogen levels fall and bleeding occurs. Influenced by estrogen only, endometrial shedding is incomplete and irregular, accounting for the excessive bleeding of anovulatory cycles.

Generally, dysfunctional uterine bleeding refers to this anovulatory bleeding pattern, for which no "cause" can be found. A number of other factors, however, can affect the axis and sometimes are included as causes of dysfunctional uterine bleeding:

- Endocrine disorders
  - Hypothyroidism or hyperthyroidism
  - Polycystic ovaries or ovarian tumors
  - Adrenal disorders
- Systemic diseases and infections
  - Diabetes mellitus
  - Iron deficiency anemia
- Obesity or severe weight loss
- Dietary changes (e.g., crash diets)
- Psychosocial stress

Presumably each of these causes affects the hypothalamic-pituitary-ovarian axis at some point, although it is not always possible to determine exactly where. Dysfunctional uterine bleeding usually is painless; therefore the presence of pain suggests a systemic cause for the bleeding.

Any significant stress in the teenager's life can alter the hypothalamic-pituitary-ovarian axis and result in dysfunctional bleeding; thus a general assessment of the patient's overall well-being is valuable. Both obesity and a significant weight loss can affect bleeding patterns, as can adherence to fad or crash diets that are deficient in protein. Hypothyroidism and occasionally hyperthyroidism also can result in excessive bleeding; any symptoms that suggest these conditions should prompt laboratory evaluation. Diabetes as a cause is consistent with a history of weight loss, excessive hunger and thirst, and polyuria. Complaints of excessive facial hair or deepening of the voice indicate polycystic ovarian disease.

The physical examination should include the measurement of height and weight, as well as careful palpation of the thyroid gland. Excessive facial hair would again be consistent with Stein-Leventhal syndrome; striae suggest adrenal disease. Careful palpation of the ovaries may help rule out this syndrome, as well as ovarian tumors.

Relatively few laboratory tests are necessary. Normal urinalysis results would likely exclude diabetes as the cause. An LH/FSH ratio exceeding 2.5 to 3:1 strongly suggests polycystic ovary syndrome. If hormonal treatment of the patient is contemplated, it seems prudent to measure serum thyroxin and thyroid-stimulating hormone levels before instituting such therapy, although the yield is likely to be low.[8] In one series of 59 adolescents evaluated for abnormal bleeding, no cause was found in 74%.[3]

Management

If a specific cause for the bleeding is discovered, treatment should be directed at ameliorating this condition. As the aforementioned series indicates, a specific cause is not found in most instances and the clinician must manage the bleeding without knowing the precise cause. Whether and how to treat is a matter of judgment; some physicians may feel comfortable using hormonal therapy, whereas others may prefer the guidance of a more experienced clinician.

Mild cases of bleeding that do not result in anemia and that do not greatly upset the patient and her parents can be managed expectantly with no immediate, specific therapy. Those with mild anemia (hemoglobin value 11 to 12) should receive iron supplementation. Some will have the problem resolved within three or four cycles.[1]

Hormonal therapy is indicated in those teenagers with moderate bleeding—that is, enough to cause a small decrease in the hemoglobin level or to cause bleeding for 7 to 10 days per cycle. Although there are differences[4] most authorities recommend combined estrogen-progestin therapy. Emans and Goldstein[5] recommend birth control pills, medroxyprogesterone (Provera) or norethindrone (Norlutate), as initial therapy: medroxyprogesterone should be given (10 mg once or twice daily) for 10 days beginning 14 days after the day of onset of the last period. This pattern (beginning the medication 14 days after the onset of menstrual flow) can be continued for 3 to 6 months. Norethindrone (10 mg/day) also can be given using the same schedule. For the sexually active teenager, oral contraceptive pills will abate the bleeding as well as protect against pregnancy.

A significant drop in the hemoglobin level (2 to 3 g) associated with heavy or prolonged bleeding requires alternate therapy. The preferred treatment consists of using an oral contraceptive initially, such as Ortho-Novum (Norinyl), 2 mg daily for 21 days. After the current bleeding stops (2 to 3 days) and withdrawal bleeding occurs (2 to 4 days after the last dose has been taken), cyclic medroxyprogesterone should be prescribed for 3 to 6 months.[5]

Should these methods fail or the hemoglobin level fall below 9 g, gynecologic consultation should be sought, and hospitalization, clotting studies, and a blood transfusion should be considered. Endometrial curettage may be necessary. Even if these measures succeed in controlling the vaginal bleeding, these adolescents require long-term follow-up, because an appreciable number of them will continue to have menstrual abnormalities and will be at increased risk for difficulties in conceiving. Persistent anovulation also may lead to endometrial hyperplasia and carcinoma in later life. In these cases joint management by the pediatrician and a gynecologist is optimal.[1,10,11]

REFERENCES

1. Altchek A: Dysfunctional menstrual disorders in adolescence, Clin Obstet Gynecol 14:975, 1971.
2. Askel S and Jones GS: Etiology and treatment of dysfunctional uterine bleeding, Obstet Gynecol 44:1, 1974.
3. Claessens CE and Lowell CA: Dysfunctional uterine bleeding in the adolescent, Pediatr Clin North Am 28:369, 1981.
4. Coupey SM and Ahlstrom P: Common menstrual disorders, Pediatr Clin North Am 36:551, 1989.
5. Emans SJH and Goldstein DP: Pediatric and adolescent gynecology, ed 3, Boston, 1990, Little, Brown & Co.
6. Gailey TA and McDonough PG: Atypical uterine bleeding, Pediatr Ann 40:66, 1975.
7. Huffman JW, Dewhurst CJ, and Capraro VJ: The gynecology of childhood and adolescence, ed 2, Philadelphia, 1981, WB Saunders Co.
8. Litt I: Menstrual problems during adolescence, Pediatr Rev 7:203, 1983.
9. Little HM: Managing incomplete abortion, Am Fam Physician 9:137, 1974.
10. Southam AL: Disorders of menstruation, Clin Obstet Gynecol 9:779, 1966.
11. Southam AL and Richart RM: The prognosis for adolescents with menstrual abnormalities, Am J Obstet Gynecol 94:637, 1966.
12. Vaughn TC: Dysfunctional uterine bleeding in the adolescent, Semin Reprod Endocrinol 2:359, 1984.

172

Vaginal Discharge

Alain Joffe

Vaginal discharge is a common complaint that confronts the pediatrician. Not all vaginal discharges, however, represent disease; some are physiologically normal, and the physician need only reassure the patient and her parents. The age of the patient and her pubertal status also determine, to a large extent, the cause of the discharge.

NEWBORN PERIOD

In utero the vaginal epithelium of the neonate is stimulated by maternal hormones that diffuse across the placenta into fetal circulation. After delivery these hormone levels fall rapidly, and the parents may note a thick, grayish white or mucoid discharge from the neonate's vagina. Often the discharge is blood tinged or even grossly bloody.[8] No treatment is needed, and the discharge usually resolves by 10 days of age.

PREPUBERTAL GIRLS

The genital area of prepubertal girls is more susceptible to infection than that of older, pubertal girls. The labial folds are smaller, and there is a relatively short distance between the vagina and the rectum in comparison with adolescents and adults. Low levels of circulating estrogen render the vaginal mucosa relatively thin and more susceptible to irritation or infection. The alkaline pH of the vaginal secretions affords a more hospitable environment to bacteria. As such, together with poor perineal hygiene, fecal flora can more easily establish themselves in the genital area.[1,3] (See accompanying box for causes of vaginal discharge in prepubertal girls.)

Evaluation

In evaluating a premenarcheal girl with vaginal discharge, the physician should inquire about the hygiene of the patient. Wiping from the rectum toward the vagina brings intestinal flora to the vaginal introitus. Use of chemicals such as bubble baths or deodorants or of strong detergents to launder underwear can irritate the vulva and vagina. Occlusive nylon or rayon underwear provides a moist environment for potential pathogens, and the material itself can irritate. Although accounting for less than 5% of vaginal discharges, foreign bodies (e.g., toilet paper, coins, and small toys) should be considered and inquiries made regarding the possibility that the girl may have placed some foreign body in her vagina.[5]

The parents should be asked about concomitant illness.

Table 172-1 *Major Causes of Vaginal Infections in Pubertal Girls*

AGENT	DISCHARGE	ODOR; pH	DYSURIA; PRURITUS
Candida albicans	Thick, white, curdlike, "cheesy"	None usually; pH 4.5 (obtained from midvagina with nitrazine paper)	Dysuria frequent; pruritus (4+)
Trichomonas vaginalis	Frothy; yellow-green or gray	Foul-smelling; pH 5.2-5.5	Dysuria frequent; pruritus
Neisseria gonorrhoeae	Purulent, but usually not prominent	None usually; pH <6.0	Occasional dysuria; not usually pruritic
Bacterial vaginosis (formerly *Gardnerella vaginalis*)	Gray or clear, not curd-like*	Fishlike and foul; increased when mixed with potassium hydroxide; pH 5.0-5.5*	No dysuria; slight pruritus
Chlamydia trachomatis	Purulent	None usual; pH > 4.5	Dysuria often; no pruritus

Modified from Amsel R et al: Nonspecific vaginitis: diagnostic criteria and microbial and epidemiologic associations, Am J Med 74:14, 1983; Brunham RC et al: Mucopurulent cervicitis—the ignored counterpart in women of urethritis in men, N Engl J Med 311:1, 1984; and Rein MF and Chapel TA: Trichomoniasis, candidiasis and the minor venereal diseases, Clin Obstet Gynecol 18:73, 1975.
*Must have three of these four criteria to make diagnosis.

Causes of Vaginal Discharge in Prepubertal Girls

Irritative (bubble baths, sand)
Poor perineal hygiene
Foreign body
Associated systemic illness (group A streptococci, chickenpox)
Infections
- *Escherichia coli* with foreign body
- *Shigella* organisms
- *Yersinia* organisms

Infections (consider sexual abuse)
- *Chlamydia trachomatis*
- *Neisseria gonorrhoeae*
- *Trichomonas vaginalis*

Tumor (rare)

Vaginal discharge is associated with streptococcal infection (e.g., scarlet fever) and with *Shigella* infection coincident with or after an episode of diarrhea.[4] Rectal infestations with *Enterobius vermicularis* (pinworms) also can lead to vaginitis if the eggs are deposited around or in the vagina. A history of nocturnal itching accompanying vaginal discharge suggests this diagnosis.

Many organisms, especially *Neisseria gonorrhoeae,* that are sexually transmitted are known to cause vaginal infections in prepubertal girls; thus the possibility of sexual abuse should always be considered in the evaluation. It is unclear whether these organisms can be transmitted in other than a sexual manner—for example, when a girl uses a towel containing infected secretions or sleeps in the same bed with a mother or sister who also has vaginitis. Therefore queries should be made to determine if other family members or sexual partners have venereal infections.

The mother of the child also should be asked whether the daughter was exposed to diethylstilbestrol (DES) in utero. An affirmative response requires thorough evaluation by a gynecologist because of the possibility of vaginal carcinoma.

The physical examination should include the entire genital and rectal area. The condition of the vulva, urethral opening, and vaginal introitus should be noted. Infections in the prepubertal age-group usually involve the vulva and outer vagina as opposed to only the vagina. Bruises, lacerations, or scrapes in the genital area raise high suspicions of some form of sexual abuse. Excoriations around the rectum or vagina suggest itching caused by pinworms. A rash that spares skin folds is consistent with an irritative cause, whereas one that is predominantly within the skin folds suggests candidiasis.

Use of a veterinary otoscope and speculum will allow for examination of the outer portions of the vagina without undue discomfort to the girl.[2] If a foreign body is suspected (because of a thick, yellowish, foul-smelling discharge) but not visualized, irrigating the vagina with use of a red Robinson catheter and tepid saline solution often will flush out bits of toilet paper or small objects.

If sufficient vaginal discharge is present, several drops of the secretion should be placed on three glass slides. If the discharge is scant, a saline-moistened cotton swab can be introduced into the vagina and the material so obtained placed onto the glass slides. To one slide should be added several drops of normal saline solution. The second slide should have several drops of 10% potassium hydroxide added and then gently heated to dissolve epithelial cells. A Gram stain of the material on the third slide also should be made. All slides should be examined as indicated in Table 172-1. A Gram stain that shows gram-negative intracellular diplococci strongly suggests a gonococcal infection, and appropriate cul-

Table 172-1 *Major Causes of Vaginal Infections in Pubertal Girls—Cont'd*

OTHER CLUES	DIAGNOSIS	TREATMENT
Vulva affected; association with use of oral contraceptives and tetracycline	Hyphae on potassium hydroxide examination	Miconazole 100 mg/day or clotrimazole 100 mg/day as a single dose for 7 days; clotrimazole 500 mg as a single dose; or either medication at 200 mg as a single dose for 3 days
Low abdominal pain; "strawberry" cervix; punctate vaginal hemorrhages	Motile trichomonads on wet preparation; avoid drying specimen. PAP smear may indicate trichomonads	Metronidazole 2.0 g as single dose or 250 mg three times daily for 7-10 days; *avoid alcohol*
Partner has discharge or dysuria	Gram-negative intracellular diplococci suggestive; confirm with culture	Aqueous procaine penicillin G, 4.8 million units IM; or ampicillin 3.5 g orally; or amoxicillin 3.0 g orally; each with 1.0 g probenecid; or tetracycline 500 mg four times daily for 4 days. In areas with increasing rates of penicillin resistance, ceftriaxone 250 mg IM should be used
Probably occurs in association with other anaerobic organisms	Clue cells on wet preparation (bacteria-coated epithelial cells)	Metronidazole 500 mg twice daily for 7-10 days; ampicillin 500 mg four times daily, or amoxicillin 500 mg three times daily for 7-10 days
Partner has discharge or dysuria	Purulent material in endocervix, >10 WBCs per field (oil immersion). Endocervix is friable	Doxycycline 100 mg twice daily for 7-10 days; tetracycline 500 mg four times daily for 7-10 days

tures should be obtained. A piece of Scotch tape applied to the rectal area and examined microscopically may reveal the typical eggs of *E. vermicularis* infection.

Management

If the history or physical examination suggests an "irritative" origin, parents should discontinue the offending agent and have the patient wear cotton underpants. Sitz baths will provide temporary relief until natural healing takes place. Removal of a foreign body will result in rapid improvement and cessation of the discharge. Pinworm infestations should be treated in the usual manner (see Chapter 245).[7] Infections caused by poor personal hygiene will respond to the general measures just listed coupled with instructions about proper perineal hygiene. If the discharge is associated with another infection (such as scarlet fever or *Shigella* organisms), it will disappear as the underlying infection is treated.

When the organism causing the vaginal discharge is found to be sexually transmitted, a more comprehensive treatment program is required (see Chapter 255, "Sexually Transmitted Diseases"). Antibiotic treatment adjusted to the girl's weight should be prescribed and a report made to the appropriate agencies that includes a comprehensive evaluation of the social situation of the patient.

PUBERTAL AND POSTPUBERTAL ADOLESCENTS

With the onset of puberty, circulating estrogen and progesterone levels rise, stimulating vaginal mucus production and an increase in the turnover of vaginal epithelial cells. Bartholin and sebaceous glands also are stimulated. Generally the clear mucoid discharge that results will not cause problems. The amount of secretion, however, can increase with sexual excitement, as well as midway through a normal menstrual cycle. It is particularly prominent at the onset of puberty (physiologic leukorrhea). On examination of a wet preparation, only vaginal epithelial cells will be seen. The high protein content of this discharge, absorbed onto underwear, causes yellow staining when the underwear is laundered. Traditionally, occlusive nylon or rayon underpants have been alleged to cause a nonspecific vaginal discharge; recent research, however, suggests that such an association may be spurious.[4]

A wide variety of organisms are normally found in the vagina.[6] These organisms, especially the lactobacilli, help to maintain the normal acidic pH of the vagina that resists infection. Except for *Candida* organisms, virtually all the organisms that cause vaginitis and vaginal discharge in this age-group are sexually transmitted. If the patient denies sexual activity, sexual abuse should be considered. If the patient is sexually active, treatment of her partner should be pursued simultaneously, especially if the infection is due to *Neisseria gonorrhoeae, Chlamydia trachomatis,* or *Trichomonas vaginalis;* otherwise the infection is more likely to recur. The presence of a foreign body (e.g., retained tampon) also should be considered. Because many teenagers fear admitting to sexual activity, a negative response should not rule out consideration of a sexually transmitted organism as the cause of the discharge. As with prepubertal girls, teenagers or their mothers should be queried about the possibility of in utero DES exposure. Those who have been exposed should be referred to a gynecologist.

Table 172-1 lists the major organisms responsible for vaginal infections in pubertal girls. Although the characteristics of each are said to be typical, one should keep in mind that the characteristics of the discharge frequently do not fit the classic presentation. The laboratory methods described are useful; however, they are not very sensitive, and the discharge should be cultured on the appropriate medium if symptoms persist. Cultures for *N. gonorrhoeae* and *C. trachomatis* should be obtained routinely from any sexually active teenager.

Occasionally, herpesvirus infections of the vulvovaginal area and cervix are associated with vaginal discharge. Typically there is pain or a burning sensation in the genital area. The vulva is reddened, and groups of small vesicles are noted on the vulva and occasionally in the vagina. If the vesicles rupture, the examiner sees only small ulcerations. Inguinal adenopathy is present, as are fever and systemic signs such as malaise if this is a first attack (see Chapter 212).

Approximately 50% of women will have recurrent episodes, usually milder than the first. Recently both topical and oral acyclovir have been approved for treatment of genital herpes infections. Women with herpes should have an annual Pap smear.

If the discharge does not appear to fit any of the etiologies described earlier and cultures are negative for *Chlamydia* and gonorrhea organisms, a trial of sitz baths and vinegar douches (15 ml white vinegar in 1 quart of water taken twice daily for 1 week) is warranted.

A teenager with a persistent discharge unresponsive to therapy may not actually be complying with the therapy or may have become reinfected by an untreated partner. If the physician believes that neither is the case, referral to a gynecologist for a more thorough evaluation should be made.

Candidal infections can be especially difficult to treat and may recur. Factors that predispose to candidiasis include oral contraceptive or broad-spectrum antibiotic use and diabetes mellitus.[6] Treatment with one of the medications listed in Table 172-1 for a full 30 days (including during menstruation) may be necessary. Alternatively, 1% gentian violet applied to the vagina and cervix every other day for 2 weeks can be tried. Male sex partners may need treatment.

REFERENCES

1. Caprano VJ and Gallego MB: Vulvovaginitis in children, Pediatr Ann 3:74, 1974.
2. Emans EJH and Goldstein DP: Pediatric and adolescent gynecology, ed 2, Boston, 1982, Little, Brown & Co.
3. Hammerschlag MR et al: Microbiology of the vagina in children: normal and potentially pathogenic organisms, Pediatrics 62:57, 1978.
4. Paradise JE et al: Vulvovaginitis in premenarcheal girls: clinical features and diagnostic evaluation, Pediatrics 70:193, 1982.
5. Paradise JE and Willis ED: Probability of vaginal foreign body in girls with genital complaints, Am J Dis Child 139:472, 1985.
6. Rosenfeld WR and Clark J: Vulvovaginitis and cervicitis, Pediatr Clin North Am 36:489, 1989.
7. Schneider GT and Geary WL: Vaginitis in adolescent girls, Clin Obstet Gynecol 14:1057, 1971.
8. Singleton AF: Vaginal discharge in children and adolescents, Clin Pediatr 19:799, 1980.

173

Visual Disturbance

Earl A. Palmer

Preschool children who painlessly lose vision in only one eye are ordinarily free of symptoms. This results from the very large overlap of the two visual fields, with only a relatively small "temporal crescent" of monocular vision in each eye. This lack of symptoms frequently applies even to older children and adults. This remarkable fact accounts for occasional adolescent or adult patients who suddenly notice poor vision in one eye, despite indications that the visual loss clearly occurred in the past. Typically, pain in the good eye from injury or disease develops and only then, when the better eye is covered or closed in these older patients, do they become aware of poor vision in the symptom-free eye. It is an underemphasized fact that the great majority of serious, treatable eye diseases in children affects vision in the two eyes *unequally,* even if the disease affects both eyes.[5] Thus visual screening examinations are crucial to the detection of treatable eye disease in childhood.

The detection of monocular poor vision generally is far more important among preschool than older children because the primary cause of monocular poor vision in early childhood is amblyopia, a condition that is treatable.[2] Amblyopia affects about 2% to 3% of the population (which is, on average, about one child in every classroom in the United States). This condition is most amenable to treatment during the first 6 to 8 years of life. Thus *visual screening should be performed in every primary practitioner's office*. It should be made clear to the parent, for medicolegal purposes, what a "screening" examination is and that it is possible for some eye diseases to escape detection except by an ophthalmologist. Nevertheless, most treatable eye diseases that cause blindness in childhood can and should be detected by the primary care practitioner. Inasmuch as most intellectually normal children can be satisfactorily tested by age 3½ years, a desirable and achievable public health goal is adequate vision screening for every intellectually normal child to be performed before the fourth birthday.

The key vision screening test is the assessment of visual acuity, which is performed at a testing distance of at least 10, but preferably 20, feet. Distance can be optically simulated by desk-top binocular vision screening devices. For children who know the alphabet or numbers, a Snellen chart is ideal. For younger or less skilled children, a tumbling E chart is used. Single-figure acuity cards are not as discriminating for amblyopia as are charts with figures arranged in lines.[3] To avoid confusion, an assistant or parent may point at each figure for the child. Some younger or handicapped children perform better giving a verbal response, but others prefer the hand signal telling which way the E "points." Teaching the "E game" with a single E card sometimes can be accomplished quickly at a near-fixation distance; the card then is moved farther away, and finally the child's attention is transferred to the testing chart. For some younger children an Allen chart with picture outlines (e.g., cake, car, or duck) sometimes is preferable to the E chart.

Each eye should be covered in turn (Fig. 173-1). By convention the right eye is tested first except when one eye is already known to be the weaker, in which case the weak eye may be tested first to avoid the child's memorizing the eye chart for recall when the good eye is covered.

If visual acuity in a schoolchild is measured as at least 20/20 in each eye, then further screening becomes less important and should concern binocular coordination. In the symptom-free schoolchild who appears free of strabismus (see Chapter 166), the likelihood of detecting treatable eye disease by further screening studies in the primary care office, aside from a routine fundus examination, is quite small.

Reliably comparing the visual acuity of the two eyes is entirely feasible in preverbal or neurologically impaired children—and even in infants—simply by observing the behavior when first one eye and then the other is occluded[3] (usually by the examiner's hand) while the child's attention is attracted to some fixation target, such as the examiner's face. The utter simplicity and extreme value of this "alternate cover test" are remarkable.

Symmetric impairment of visual acuity causes visual inattention and, sometimes, nystagmus. Nystagmus may result from severe visual impairment or may represent a primary ocular motor disturbance. An ophthalmologist usually can distinguish between these two.

A 5-year-old child may normally have 20/30 visual acuity, and a 3-year-old child may test at 20/40. If acuity is symmetric, it is unlikely that these acuities signify serious eye disease. Symmetric reduction of acuity may signify refractive error.

REFRACTIVE ERRORS

Refractive errors are disturbances in the strictly optical properties of the eye and usually can be fully neutralized by the use of "corrective" lenses (glasses or contact lenses). An eye with no problems other than a refractive error usually will be capable of normal vision with the proper lens in place. Although the magnitude of refractive error is related to the thickness of the corrective lens, the clarity of vision without glasses cannot be predicted reliably simply by observing

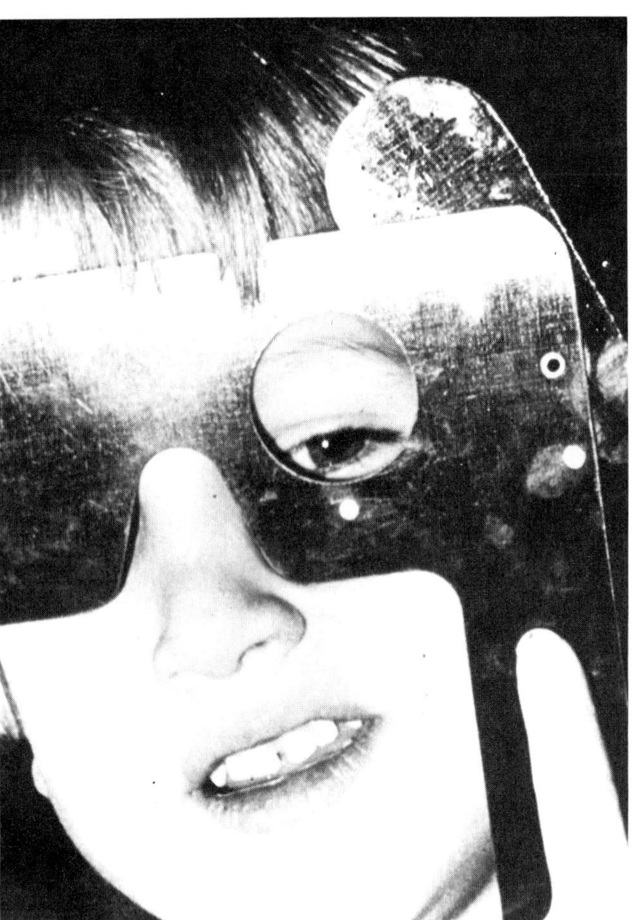

Fig. 173-1 False negative visual acuity test. This schoolboy is severly amblyopic in the left eye but is shown here reading 20/20 figures. He manages to peek with his normal right eye through the occluder gap beside his nose and had passed two previous screening examinations, even though the visual acuity in the left eye is only 20/200. The child is only trying to please the examiner, not deceive. It is the examiner's responsibility to evaluate the validity of acuity test results.

how thick the glasses are. The definition of legal blindness assumes that proper glasses are already in place; therefore it is meaningless to assert, "I am legally blind without my glasses."

It is very important that *near-acuity testing* be performed with the test card at the prescribed distance from the eyes, usually 14 inches. Holding the test card even a few inches closer can give erroneously favorable results. Testing near acuity in patients with reduced distant visual acuity will identify those with myopia (who have normal near-acuity). Other refractive errors can be suspected if acuity improves noticeably when the patient reads the eye chart through an inexpensive standard pinhole device or, more suitable for children, a multiple pinhole device. When near acuity is poor or the pinhole fails to improve the distant acuity, ophthalmologic consultation is indicated.

The four main varieties of refractive error are myopia, hyperopia, astigmatism, and anisometropia.

Myopia

In myopia, objects can be seen clearly if held close enough to the eye (thus the patient is "nearsighted"). At the far point of focus, objects become increasingly blurred as they recede from the patient. When the individual with myopia looks through the proper corrective concave lenses, the far point is extended to optical infinity so that vision becomes clear at distance also. Schoolchildren with myopia typically first complain about an inability to read what is written on the blackboard. It is most unusual for these children to have any difficulty with reading or other close work.

Hyperopia

Hyperopia (hypermetropia) commonly is called *farsightedness*. Normal children have strong focusing ("accommodative") mechanisms that enable them to overcome small amounts of hyperopia and maintain clear vision at all distances. Hyperopia up to 2.00 diopters is considered within the normal range of variation for children and virtually never needs to be corrected as a single defect. Occasionally, however, low degrees of hyperopia need to be corrected as part of the treatment of strabismus. With large degrees of hyperopia, ordinarily more than 3.00 diopters, occasional symptoms of eye fatigue may appear with prolonged close work. The hyperopic individual requires some degree of accommodative ability to see clearly, even at optical infinity, and this effort to focus increases, the closer the viewed object is to the eyes. Adults, who do not have as strong an ability to use their internal eye muscles for accommodative focusing, will have more difficulty with close work, given a similar amount of hyperopia, than will children.

Preschool children with high degrees of hyperopia (5.00 diopters or more) may have an impairment of visual development, and this special form of amblyopia may affect both eyes. If the condition is not detected until the child reaches school age, glasses may not always provide clear vision and visual impairment may be permanent. Fortunately, this last condition is rare. It would be detected in visual acuity screening at age 3 to 4 years.

Astigmatism

This is no more a "stigma" than is any other common refractive error. Astigmatism is present in most normal eyes to a small degree without impairing clear vision. When it is present to a significant degree, however, it can blur vision at all distances in a way that cannot be compensated for by the eye at all. Thus, unlike the eye with modest myopia or hyperopia, the astigmatic eye is incapable of a fully focused image under any circumstance other than with a corrective lens. Children with substantial astigmatism may have impaired school performance and symptoms of eye strain and fatigue. A screening visual assessment will show reduced acuity.

Anisometropia

In anisometropia (unequal refractive errors in the two eyes) the refractive differences may be qualitative (e.g., one eye farsighted and the other nearsighted) or quantitative (one eye with a larger degree of the same type of refractive error as the other). In addition to the problems described for the usual refractive error, patients with anisometropia have difficulty in using the two eyes together. This is most important during the preschool years when binocular vision is being developed. If this condition remains unrecognized, poor visual acuity in one eye that fails to respond to glasses (amblyopia), as well as misalignment of the eyes (strabismus), may develop.

• • •

Refractive errors can be detected at any age, including infancy. If there is any sign of a visual problem in a small child, it must be investigated to ensure that there is no impediment to the development of normal vision.

By the time the child reaches puberty, vision already is fully developed; going without glasses will not cause permanent visual damage. At that age, however, forgoing needed glasses may produce eyestrain, which can result in fatigue and occasional headache.

CAUSES OF UNEQUAL VISUAL ACUITY

Amblyopia, which is the most likely cause of unequal visual acuity, is defined as a reduction of visual acuity (almost always in only one eye) on the basis of disturbance in visual development, for which no explanation can be found on examining the affected eye alone and that responds to treatment during the preschool period.

Amblyopia may result from (1) anisometropia (defined earlier), (2) strabismus (see Chapter 166), and (3) rarer eye problems that impair the formation of an image on the retina of the affected eye, such as a cataract, corneal abnormality, or eyelid tumor.[2-4] These three situations are essentially the only ones that produce amblyopia.

The term *lazy eye,* sometimes defined in textbooks as synonymous with amblyopia, is confusing for many parents who use it to describe the "wandering eye" of strabismus.

Two fundamental points about amblyopia (formerly called amblyopia ex anopsia) need emphasis. First, this is not simply a diagnosis made by exclusion. The ophthalmologist can find evidence to confirm the impression. Second, this condition can arise *only* in the immature visual system. The average age of visual maturity is around 7 years, and visual development may be assumed to be complete by age 12 years; in occasional cases, however, visual maturity can be achieved much earlier, perhaps at age 5. This means that teenagers and adults are virtually "immune" to amblyopia. It also means that the adult with amblyopia is essentially beyond any effective treatment. Exceptions are rare indeed; they may occur when the dominant eye is lost through injury or disease and the amblyopic eye slowly improves over a period of years. The rate of development of the visual system is highest during the first months and years of life, gradually slowing as visual maturity is approached. Thus the younger the patient, the more susceptible he or she will be to the development of amblyopia but also the more likely to respond to treatment.

Examples of other causes of monocular acquired reduced vision are cataract, glaucoma, retinal detachment, retinoblastoma, retinochoroiditis (idiopathic, infectious, parasitic), retinopathy of prematurity, and optic nerve glioma or other intracranial tumor.

Congenital causes of poor vision in one eye may include any in the foregoing list and, in addition, coloboma (choroid and retina or optic nerve), miscellaneous nerve or retinal anomalies, and optic nerve hypoplasia.

Trauma to an eye can cause reduction of vision through a variety of mechanisms—for example, corneal abrasion, hyphema (blood in the anterior chamber between the iris and cornea), cataract, hemorrhage in or under the retina or in the vitreous cavity, optic nerve or retinal contusion, and optic nerve avulsion (as from a stick or finger injury to the apex of the orbit).

Optic neuropathy and neuritis (or retrobulbar neuritis) are rare causes of reduced vision (usually in one eye) in children and may be of postinfectious origin or (very rarely) may accompany a demyelinating disease such as multiple sclerosis.[1]

Possible nonrefractive causes of potentially *symmetric* reduction of visual acuity include, but are not limited to, the following, which are detectable on careful examination: cataract, glaucoma, retinal detachment, and retinoblastoma.

Fortunately rare, an elusive and troublesome potential cause of rather symmetrically reduced visual acuity is a parachiasmal lesion such as pituitary tumor (usually in young adults), craniopharyngioma (usually in school-aged children and adolescents), or glioma, often associated with neurofibromatosis. In early stages the primary manifestation of lesions that affect the optic chiasm is reduced vision, often in the temporal periphery of each eye. Because frequently the two eyes are affected symmetrically, there may be no Marcus Gunn pupil response (see later discussion) even though the optic nerves may be intracranially injured.

Craniopharyngioma and optic nerve glioma are important intracranial tumors of childhood. These tumors may be manifested by unexplained reduction of vision; thus all cases of reduced vision in childhood must be taken seriously even if results of the fundus examination are unrevealing.

The following causes of symmetric reduction of visual acuity are less readily detectable and essentially are untreatable: coloboma, cortical blindness, ocular albinism, bilateral optic nerve hypoplasia, and retinal dystrophies.[1,5]

Conversion reactions (hysteria) and malingering often are difficult to differentiate in children. These conditions occur in children most frequently during the age range of 8 to 10 years. In most cases the episode is of situational origin and does not indicate a serious psychopathologic condition. Treatment by the ophthalmologist involves reassurance of the family and perhaps serial observation, lest an organic problem be associated with the psychosomatic problem. The diagnosis cannot be securely made except by an ophthalmologist.

Migraines typically are preceded by visual disturbances, most often a "scintillating scotoma," in which vision is partially obscured by a shimmering form of light flash that patients compare in appearance to the surface of water. In some cases, however, the scintillating characteristic is lacking and in other cases the headache may never develop. Migraine syndrome may lead to transient visual loss in both eyes. The differential diagnosis usually requires consultation with a neurologist or ophthalmologist.

Pupillary Responses

In any case of suspected asymmetry of visual acuity, pupillary reactions should be tested. Evaluation of the pupillary light responses is extremely useful in children because it is one of the few absolutely reliable and objective signs that can be elicited in virtually all cases; this evaluation also requires minimal cooperation from the patient. An *amaurotic pupil* does not react to a direct light stimulus, but reacts normally when the opposite (seeing) eye is stimulated. *The two pupils remain equal in size at all times*. In cases in which an eye has light perception but is afflicted with optic nerve or retinal disease or damage, the pupil of the affected eye *does* react to direct light stimulus but does not constrict as fully as it does when the opposite eye is stimulated; that is, the direct response is weaker than the consensual response. In such a situation, when the examining light is swung rapidly from the better to the worse eye, both pupils *dilate* because a weaker stimulus reaches the brain through the defective afferent pathways. This paradoxical dilation is the hallmark of the afferent light reflex defect, or Marcus Gunn pupil. It is pathognomonic of a serious optic nerve or retinal lesion and tends to exclude amblyopia, refractive error, cataract, or any other cause of reduced vision in the eye.

Inequality of pupil size indicates a pupillomotor abnormality and may result from a lesion of either the oculomotor nerve, the superior cervical sympathetic chain, or the iris itself.

SUMMARY

Asymmetric reduction of visual acuity is more common than symmetric loss of vision, is more readily detectable in a child, and is far more likely to be amenable to treatment. Thus, even though visual acuity cannot always be measured reliably in a child, visual screening remains highly effective because it readily detects a difference in vision between the two eyes.

REFERENCES

1. Harley RD: Pediatric ophthalmology, ed 2, Philadelphia, 1983, WB Saunders Co.
2. Keech RV: Functional amblyopia. In Fraunfelder FT and Roy FH, editors: Current ocular therapy, ed 2, Philadelphia, 1985, WB Saunders Co.
3. Von Noorden GK: Atlas of strabismus, ed 4, St Louis, 1985, The CV Mosby Co.
4. Von Noorden, GK: Burian–Von Noorden's binocular vision and ocular motility, ed 4, St Louis, 1990, The CV Mosby Co.
5. Weleber RG and Palmer EA: Selected causes of blindness in infants and children, Perspect Ophthalmol 5:13, 1981.

SUGGESTED READINGS

Helveston EM and Ellis FD: Pediatric ophthalmology practice, ed 2, St Louis, 1984, The CV Mosby Co.

Miller NR: Walsh and Hoyt's clinical neuro-ophthalmology, ed 4, Baltimore, 1982, The Williams & Wilkins Co.

Nelson L and Arentson J: Recognizing ocular childhood disorders, Thorofare, NJ, 1985, Charles B Slack, Inc.

174

Vomiting

Martin H. Ulshen

DEFINITION

Vomiting (emesis with effort) is a ubiquitous symptom of acute and chronic illness in childhood. It must be distinguished from regurgitation, which is free reflux of gastric contents into the esophagus and mouth through an important lower esophageal sphincter. Vomiting is a coordinated event usually preceded by nausea in association with increased salivation, gastric atony, and reflux of duodenal contents into the stomach. This phase may not be apparent in infants. Retching immediately precedes the actual vomiting. Increased intragastric pressure from contraction of the abdominal wall musculature, lowering of the diaphragm, and pyloric contraction are associated with elevation and relaxation of the cardia, and vomiting occurs. The total process of vomiting is coordinated in the medullary vomiting center. This center may be influenced directly by visceral afferent stimuli or indirectly via the chemoreceptor trigger zone. The latter region is the site of action of many of the drugs that cause nausea and vomiting, including apomorphine and digitalis, as well as the site of initiation of motion sickness. Higher central nervous system centers also appear able to influence the medullary vomiting center.

CAUSES AND DIFFERENTIAL DIAGNOSIS

The accompanying box lists the most frequent causes of vomiting in infants and children. In infancy, *regurgitation,* or spitting up, is common and most often is a developmental event, called *chalasia,* which has no sequelae and gradually resolves. *Gastroesophageal reflux,* however, can be associated with severe complications (esophagitis with anemia secondary to blood loss, esophageal stricture, aspiration pneumonia, or failure to thrive). *Bilious vomiting* (especially associated with the first vomitus) usually occurs only with serious disease. In patients of any age, it usually suggests gastrointestinal tract obstruction below the ampulla of Vater (in the second portion of the duodenum), although in newborns bilious vomiting also is commonly associated with necrotizing enterocolitis. In older children with persistent vomiting, reflux of bile from the duodenum into the stomach may lead to bilious vomiting without gastrointestinal tract obstruction. Projectile vomiting commonly occurs with *pyloric stenosis.* When this condition persists, however, gastric atony may eliminate the projectile character. A *succussion splash* may be present, as in other causes of gastric outlet obstruction. Vomiting associated with increased intracranial pressure may be projectile and may take place in the absence of nausea or retching.

Persistent vomiting in a newborn or young infant without evidence of infection usually suggests a congenital gastrointestinal anomaly, inborn error of metabolism, or central nervous system abnormality such as hydrocephalus or subdural effusion. If the history and physical examination results do not suggest a cause, it is best to evaluate all three possibilities simultaneously. When the sudden onset of bilious vomiting, especially within the first few days of life, develops in a previously well newborn, one must consider a *malrotation* with secondary *midgut volvulus.* A plain film of the abdomen may show a paucity of gas distal to the upper small intestine; however, the plain film may not be helpful. If a midgut volvulus is suspected, an upper gastrointestinal roentgenographic series done with the controlled introduction of barium through a nasogastric tube after gastric aspiration should be carried out at once. The lack of complete correlation of developmental rotation of the cecum with that of the duodenum makes a barium enema investigation of cecal position an inferior study in evaluating a patient for malrotation. Midgut volvulus is a surgical emergency requiring early diagnosis and surgical intervention. In a sick newborn the diagnosis of *necrotizing enterocolitis* must always be considered in the event of bilious vomiting, especially with blood in the stool. Beyond the first week of life, but within the first 2 months, *pyloric stenosis* is the most common cause of persistent vomiting (but not regurgitation). In the older infant or child, the entire spectrum of causes of vomiting in the accompanying box should be considered. It is interesting that *celiac disease* may occasionally have minimal or no diarrhea but prominent vomiting. When an older child manifests acute vomiting and somnolence, one should always consider Reye syndrome, aspirin toxicity, and meningoencephalitis in the differential diagnosis. Persistent or recurrent vomiting without other symptoms may be the major symptom of an emotional disorder in childhood. Therefore a careful psychosocial history is an important part of the evaluation.

Cyclic Vomiting

Cyclic vomiting is characterized by repeated episodes of vomiting, sometimes occurring in clusters and sometimes associated with abdominal pain.[4] This complex can be a symptom of a number of entities, including abdominal migraine and epilepsy. Uncontrollable vomiting and retching are typical of an attack, but between episodes patients are well. Abdominal

Causes of Vomiting (Arranged by Usual Age of Earliest Occurrence)

INFANCY

Gastrointestinal Tract

Congenital
- Regurgitation—chalasia, gastroesophageal reflux
- Atresia—stenosis (tracheoesophageal fistula, prepyloric diaphragm, ileal atresia)
- Duplication
- Volvulus (errors in rotation and fixation, Meckel diverticulum)
- Congenital bands
- Hirschsprung disease
- Meconium ileus (cystic fibrosis), meconium plug
- Celiac disease

Acquired
- Acute infectious gastroenteritis, food poisoning (staphylococcal, clostridial)
- Pyloric stenosis
- Gastritis, duodenitis
- Intussusception
- Incarcerated hernia—inguinal, internal secondary to old adhesions
- Cow milk protein intolerance, food allergy, eosinophilic gastroenteritis
- Disaccharidase deficiency
- Adynamic ileus—the mediator for many nongastrointestinal causes
- Neonatal necrotizing enterocolitis
- Chronic granulomatous disease with gastric outlet obstruction

Nongastrointestinal Tract

Infectious—otitis, urinary tract infection, pneumonia, upper respiratory tract infection, sepsis, meningitis

Metabolic—aminoaciduria and organic aciduria, galactosemia, fructosemia, adrenogenital syndrome, renal tubular acidosis, diabetic ketoacidosis, Reye syndrome

Central nervous system—trauma, tumor, infection, diencephalic syndrome, rumination, autonomic responses (pain, shock)

Medications—anticholinergics, aspirin, alcohol, idiosyncratic reaction (e.g., codeine)

CHILDHOOD

Gastrointestinal Tract

Peptic ulcer—vomiting is a common presentation in children younger than 6 years old[1]

Trauma—duodenal hematoma, traumatic pancreatitis, perforated bowel

Pancreatitis—mumps, trauma, cystic fibrosis, hyperparathyroidism, hyperlipidemia

Crohn disease

Idiopathic intestinal pseudoobstruction

Superior mesenteric artery syndrome[6]

Nongastrointestinal Tract

Central nervous system—cyclic vomiting, migraine, anorexia nervosa, bulimia

migraine is characterized by the paroxysmal onset of repetitious attacks often relieved with sleep. A strong family history of migraine usually is present. Although headache typical of migraine may occur with episodes, it is not necessarily present. Propranolol is highly effective as prophylactic treatment for abdominal migraine. A careful history of the sequence of events and electroencephalographic evaluation are useful in the consideration of abdominal epilepsy. Anticonvulsants can be tried when this condition is suspected.

EVALUATION

Evaluation of the gastrointestinal tract usually includes an upper gastrointestinal contrast roentgenographic study. *Endoscopy* is feasible in all children, even newborns, if performed by an experienced examiner using a pediatric instrument.[3,8] Esophageal pH monitoring, esophageal biopsies, and gastroesophageal scintiscan all are useful in establishing a diagnosis of gastroesophageal reflux.[7,9] Ultrasound is helpful in diagnosing atypical pyloric stenosis, as is endoscopy.

TREATMENT

The most significant complications of vomiting include aspiration pneumonia, hemorrhage from a tear at the gastroesophageal junction *(Mallory-Weiss syndrome)*, rupture of the esophagus (rare in children), and dehydration and electrolyte imbalance associated with persistent vomiting. Acute intercurrent vomiting without serious underlying disease or significant dehydration should be treated by administering clear liquids by mouth (e.g., in acute gastroenteritis or otitis media). It is usually advisable to start with a period of 4 to 6 hours without oral intake and then begin with frequent small quantities of clear liquids (½ to 1 ounce every hour for infants) with a gradual increase in volume and then an extension of the period between oral fluids. Clear liquids may include Jell-O water (packet of gelatin to 1 quart of water), Kool-Aid, or flat cola or ginger ale. Carbonated beverages may increase vomiting. Fluids of high osmolality, long-chain triglycerides, and anticholinergic drugs all tend to slow gastric emptying and should be avoided. Antiemetic drugs should not be used in infants, although they may at times be useful in older children. The drugs most commonly used are promethazine (Phenergan), prochlorperazine (Compazine), and chlorpromazine (Thorazine). In the controlled studies that have been carried out, trimethobenzamide (Tigan) appears to have been less effective.[2] Rectal suppositories are probably preferable to oral drugs, as nausea is associated with gastric atony and unpredictable absorption. Patients should be monitored for signs of dehydration. *Metoclopramide* can be effective in problems associated with poor gastric emptying.[5] Likewise, for certain patients (e.g., those with severe psychomotor retardation) a nasoduodenal infusion or jejunostomy may circumvent the problem.

Significant vomiting that requires intravenous fluid therapy usually is associated with hypochloremic alkalosis with secondary hypokalemia. Intravenous fluids should repair the deficits (see Chapter 25).

Management of gastroesophageal reflux must be individualized. The extent of treatment depends on the volume of emesis and the presence of any of the complications of reflux (esophagitis with or without esophageal stricture or intractable anemia, failure to thrive, or respiratory manifestations). Medical management includes placing an infant in a prone, head-elevated position for sleep and thickening feedings with cereal (a standard concentration is 1 tablespoonful of cereal for each ounce of formula). Treatment for the older child should include elevating the head of the bed, avoiding snacks or liquids after dinner, and avoiding agents that exacerbate esophagitis (alcohol, caffeine, and smoking). Medications can be used also in an attempt to improve lower esophageal function and gastric emptying (e.g., metoclopramide) and to decrease exposure of the esophageal mucosa to acid (antacids and histamine blockers). A slurry of sucralfate (a cytoprotective agent) four times a day has been used occasionally as well. When a child has severe gastroesophageal reflux, medical management may be unsatisfactory. In this case, antireflux surgery (fundoplication) should be considered. In this group of children the results of surgery generally are good when performed by an experienced surgeon, and the benefits can be long lasting. In children with psychomotor retardation and gastroesophageal reflux, antireflux surgery may not eliminate respiratory symptoms inasmuch as other other factors such as swallowing dysfunction may contribute to these findings. Among all children undergoing a Nissen fundoplication, the risk of a postoperative complication that requires further surgery may be as high as 10% and underscores the need for careful patient selection for this operation.

REFERENCES

1. Deckelbaum RJ et al: Peptic ulcer disease: a clinical study in 73 children, Can Med Assoc J 111:225, 1974.
2. Ginsburg CM and Clahsen J: Evaluation of trimethobenzamine hydrochloride (Tigan) suppositories for treatment of nausea and vomiting in children, J Pediatr 96:767, 1980.
3. Hargrove CB, Ulshen MH, and Shub MD: Upper gastrointestinal endoscopy in infants: diagnostic usefulness and safety, Pediatrics 74:828, 1984.
4. Reinhart JB, Evans SL, and McFadden DL: Cyclic vomiting in children: seen through the psychiatrist's eye, Pediatrics 59:371, 1977.
5. Schulze-Delrien K: Metoclopramide, N Engl J Med 305:28, 1981.
6. Shandling B: The so-called superior mesenteric artery syndrome, Am J Dis Child 130:1371, 1976.
7. Shub MD et al: Esophagitis: a frequent consequence of gastroesophageal reflux in infancy, J Pediatr 107:881, 1985.
8. Ulshen MH: Unique aspects of gastrointestinal procedures for pediatric patients. In Drossman DA, editor: Manual of gastroenterologic procedures, ed 2, New York, 1987, Raven Press.
9. Winter HS et al: Intraepithelial eosinophils: a new diagnostic criterion for reflux esophagitis, Gastroenterology 83:818, 1982.

175

Weight Loss

Carole A. Stashwick

The documentation of weight loss in an infant, child, or adolescent is uncommon and a highly significant event. Weight loss, as the chief complaint or as an incidental finding, should be carefully evaluated and followed. Illingworth[5] ranks the symptom of loss of weight as 1 of 13 that may signal a serious problem in the child.

Parents may have the impression of weight loss on the basis of a decrease in a child's appetite or a change in the fit of clothing. Subjective impressions of weight loss always should be verified objectively before an evaluation is undertaken. True weight loss, however, may be difficult to differentiate from factitious weight loss, even when weights are documented in the medical record. A survey of child health clinics by the Centers for Disease Control revealed that specific errors in weighing children occurred at frequencies ranging from 5% to 20% of all children weighed.[9] Errors were caused by faulty equipment and by poor technique, for example weighing with the clothes on.

NEWBORNS AND YOUNG INFANTS

The normal full-term newborn who is breast-fed is likely to lose about 6% (± 3%) of weight during the first 3 days of life, and at least 7% of infants will lose more than 10% of birth weight.[8] A loss of more than 12% of birth weight in the few days after birth is excessive and is cause for an investigation to ensure that the infant is well, that adequate intake is being provided, and that fluid losses from vomitus, urine, or stool are not excessive.[8] It generally is held that the infant who is breast-fed should have regained the lost weight and thus be at or above birth weight by 2 weeks of age, the time of the first well-baby examination.[7]

The most common reason for the breast-fed infant to have lost more weight than expected or to have failed to regain the lost weight by age 2 weeks is inadequate intake at the breast, not because of "insufficient milk" or milk that is not sufficiently "rich." Rather, inadequate weight gain occurs because of infrequent or short feedings, failure of the let-down reflex, or improper positioning of the infant for an effective suck. The infant will appear well, although perhaps slim, and may or may not act hungry. A number of case reports have documented passivity and infrequent demands to be fed in some infants who are starving at the breast.[4,10]

The breast-feeding mother should be observed during a feeding, if possible, and specific evidence of a let-down or oxytocin reflex should be sought (uterine cramps, milk dripping or spraying from the opposite breast, a pins-and-needles sensation in the breast at the beginning of each nursing, and loud swallowing or occasional choking by the baby at the beginning of the feeding). The mother's motivation to breastfeed and her feelings, positive or negative, about the experience should be discussed; encouragement and support should be given for continuation of the nursing; and specific suggestions should be made for the mother to rest, to nurse frequently (every 2 to 3 hours in the day) to build up the milk supply, and to arrange relaxed, pleasant, and unhurried nursings. Formula or other fluids should not be recommended unless there are serious concerns about the infant's well-being. It is inappropriate for the physician prematurely to recommend discontinuing the nursing.[6,7] A demonstration of an appropriate weight gain in the following few days (120 to 200 g or more each week) is evidence that the infant is well and confirms the diagnosis of initial underfeeding.[6]

The formula-fed infant rarely loses more than 5% of birth weight in the first few days inasmuch as complete nutrition is available beginning a few hours after birth.[7] Because it is unusual for a bottle-fed infant to weigh less than birth weight at the age of 2 weeks, such an infant should be carefully evaluated. An error in feeding caused by maternal inexperience or ignorance is the usual explanation, but a careful search for an organic problem, as well as an evaluation of the family's functioning, support mechanisms, and adjustment to the new infant, is indicated.

Rarely, the newborn will lose weight as a result of (1) inadequate intake for other reasons, such as illness or metabolic abnormality, somnolence from maternal medications or substance abuse, or poor suck resulting from a central nervous system abnormality, or (2) excessive fluid loss, such as vomiting associated with congenital gastrointestinal malformations (duodenal atresia, annular pancreas, volvulus) or polyuria (diabetes insipidus, renal disease).

OLDER INFANTS, PRESCHOOLERS, AND SCHOOLCHILDREN

The infant may lose weight because of excessive vomiting, as in pyloric stenosis or severe gastroesophageal reflux. Tumors of the central nervous system in infancy may manifest with vomiting, anorexia, and cachexia.

The most common reason for weight loss in the somewhat older child is fluid loss as a result of fever, vomiting, and diarrhea. The loss of weight may amount to 5% or more of premorbid body weight and usually is reversed with a few hours of intravenous or oral fluid replacement.

Weight loss also is a frequent concomitant of any severe febrile illness, such as pneumonia, pyelonephritis, septic arthritis, osteomyelitis, or meningitis, as well as less severe illnesses such as stomatitis and pharyngitis. Resolution of the illness often is followed by a period of "catch-up" growth and weight gain. Surgical procedures commonly result in a temporary loss of weight.

Weight loss also may be caused by poor utilization of ingested foodstuffs. Cystic fibrosis, the most common disease in which malabsorption occurs in childhood, may appear in infancy as poor weight gain or actual weight loss. Malabsorption, weight loss, and constipation may occur in the child with Hirschsprung disease. Children with chronic diarrhea or severe immunodeficiency also may have weight loss.

Although emotional reasons often are the basis for an infant's or child's failure to thrive, actual weight loss is much less common than a slowdown or cessation of weight gain and linear growth. Psychosocial dysfunction (poor parent-child interaction, infant or childhood depression, rumination) that results in weight loss in the child requires a prompt and thorough evaluation.[1]

The young child with juvenile diabetes mellitus commonly loses weight (often 10% or more of body weight) despite polyphagia and polydipsia. Hyperthyroidism in childhood, although rare, may occur with weight loss.

A diagnosis of tuberculosis needs to be considered in every child with weight loss, particularly in those with night sweats or cough. Malignancies, such as lymphoma, also may cause loss of weight with few other symptoms initially.

ADOLESCENTS

Planned dieting is the most common cause of weight loss in adolescents, particularly adolescent girls. Commonplace dieting behavior must be carefully distinguished from behavior that indicates an eating disorder, such as anorexia nervosa or bulimia, which may affect as many as 1% of adolescent women in the United States. Anorexia nervosa can be diagnosed when the loss of weight equals or exceeds 25% of the original body weight and when there are distorted attitudes and behaviors about eating or body image.[3] The anorectic adolescent or preadolescent may experience amenorrhea associated with emaciation and overactivity and many demonstrate clinical signs of malnutrition (hypothyroidism, bradycardia, hypothermia, growth of lanugo-like hair on the body and extremities).[11] Nutritional rehabilitation and psychiatric counseling are indicated.

Bulimia is an eating disorder that to some degree overlaps anorexia nervosa. Adolescents with bulimia indulge in binge eating, followed by self-induced vomiting, self-starvation, or the use of cathartics or diuretics to reduce weight. The patient often is depressed and self-deprecating and may seek medical aid when the eating-vomiting pattern becomes compulsive and is out of the patient's control. Psychiatric evaluation and counseling are indicated (see Chapter 99).

Although severe degrees of weight loss during adolescence often can be ascribed to eating disorders, weight loss in adolescence also may result from other psychiatric disturbances, especially affective disorders; central nervous system tumors, particularly those of the hypothalamus, sella turcica, or other midline areas; or gastrointestinal problems, such as undiagnosed inflammatory bowel disease or other syndromes of malabsorption.

Diabetes mellitus may manifest during adolescence with significant weight loss. Tuberculosis should always be considered and ruled out when an adolescent patient reports loss of weight.

INITIAL EVALUATION OF A COMPLAINT OF WEIGHT LOSS

The following should be included in the initial evaluation:

1. A careful *history* and *physical examination,* with special attention to family functioning and the patient's emotional well-being.
2. A *complete blood cell count (CBC)* and *erythrocyte sedimentation rate (ESR).* The CBC screens for oncologic factors and provides an overview of the nutritional state. The ESR may be elevated in rheumatoid diseases, chronic infections, and inflammatory bowel disease; it may be abnormally low in anorexia nervosa.[2]
3. *Serum electrolyte* and *kidney function* tests to diagnose dehydration, to find evidence for pernicious or self-induced vomiting, and to rule out renal disease.
4. *Serum protein levels* to assess liver function, to determine the degree of severity and chronicity of the weight loss, and to rule out protein malabsorption.
5. *Tuberculosis skin test.*
6. *Stool for occult blood* and *tests of malabsorption* to diagnose gastroenteritis, inflammatory bowel disease, and the various causes of malabsorption. The *serum carotene* level may be low in infancy and in malabsorptive conditions, but it often is elevated in anorexia nervosa.[2]
7. *Urinalysis* to rule out diabetes mellitus, diabetes insipidus, dehydration, and renal disease.

REFERENCES

1. Accardo PJ: Failure to thrive in infancy and early childhood, Baltimore, 1982, University Park Press.
2. Anyan WR: Changes in erythrocyte sedimentation rate and fibrinogen during anorexia nervosa, J Pediatr 85:525, 1974.
3. Feighner JP et al: Diagnostic criteria for use in psychiatric research, Arch Gen Psychiatry 26:57, 1972.
4. Gilmore HE and Rowland TW: Critical malnutrition in breast-fed infants, Am J Dis Child 132:885, 1978.
5. Illingworth RS: Common symptoms of disease in children, ed 9, Oxford, 1988, Blackwell Scientific Publications, Ltd.
6. Lawrence RA: Breast-feeding: a guide for the medical profession, ed 3, St. Louis, 1989, The CV Mosby Co.
7. Lawrence RA: Infant nutrition, Pediatr Rev 5:133, 1983.
8. Maisels MJ and Gifford K: Breast-feeding, weight loss and jaundice, J Pediatr 102:117, 1983.
9. Nutrition surveillance, Atlanta, Sept. 1975, p. 10, Centers for Disease Control.
10. Roddey OF, Jr, Martin ES, and Swetenburg RL: Critical weight loss and malnutrition in breast-fed infants, Am J Dis Child 135:597, 1981.
11. Steiner H: Anorexia nervosa, Pediatr Rev 4:123, 1982.

176

Wheezing

Thomas A. Hazinski

The term *wheezing* often is used by parents and children to refer to any noise made during breathing; to avoid ambiguity, however, the term should be used precisely to describe a high-pitched sound heard with a stethoscope during the terminal phases of expiration. Wheezes also may be heard without the use of a stethoscope, usually in patients with chronic asthma, acute foreign body inhalation, or psychogenic asthma.

Wheezing usually implies obstruction of the distal airway, but a wheezelike sound also can be produced by patients with peribronchial edema (e.g., congestive heart failure) and with disorders of the proximal or middle airway. Moreover, the presence or absence of wheezing correlates poorly with the degree of impairment in pulmonary function. As shown in Tables 176-1 and 176-2, the differential diagnosis of wheezing is extensive, so that if one approaches the wheezing patient with only asthma in mind, life-threatening but correctable disorders may be missed.

Airway obstruction usually causes wheezing only during exhalation, because of dynamic changes in airway caliber during spontaneous breathing. During inhalation, normal airways (or even narrowed or poorly supported airways) inside the thorax are expanded by the inspiratory decrease in pleural pressure (as the pressure in the airway becomes positive with respect to pleural pressure). In contrast, narrowed or poorly supported airways will narrow further during exhalation, when intrathoracic pressure begins to exceed the pressure inside the airway lumen. Although small airway closure can thus occur at the end of exhalation, in the normal lung this is counterbalanced by the alveolar walls, which act as springs to hold the small airways open at low lung volumes. In addition, at low flow rates (e.g., as respiratory muscle fatigue in the wheezing child develops), a wheeze may not be generated, despite the presence of severe obstruction. In these patients the appearance of wheezes may actually indicate a beneficial response to therapy as flow rates improve and airways open.

In addition to wheezing, another useful sign of airway obstruction is a prolongation of the expiratory time. During a normal breath the ratio of inspiratory time to expiratory time is approximately 1:1. During airway obstruction, however, expiratory airflow resistance increases, and this ratio approaches 1:2. Indeed, in some wheezing patients with acute tachypnea, the next inhalation actually may occur before complete exhalation has occurred, producing a progressive increase in end-expiratory lung volume, termed *dynamic hyperinflation*.

DIFFERENTIAL DIAGNOSIS OF WHEEZING

Among the anatomic causes of wheezing, large airway "floppiness" is common in infancy and is termed *tracheomalacia*. Most of these infants have had inspiratory *stridor* as a major sign since birth, but wheezing may occur if the lack of airway rigidity is limited to the bronchi. Wheezing develops as the abnormal airway is opened on inspiration but dynamically narrows on expiration, with airflow occurring through the distorted areas. A coarse, low-pitched expiratory sound is generated.

Fixed lesions of the trachea or bronchi may not cause wheezing inasmuch as the degree of obstruction is not influenced by the respiratory cycle. These lesions, however, may cause or be associated with softening of the adjacent airway wall, so that wheezing sometimes occurs. Two examples are a completely circular *tracheal stenosis* or a *vascular ring;* these lesions encircle the airway and are essentially unyielding. Many of these patients have residual tracheomalacia after surgical correction.

In patients with *acute infections* and *asthma,* wheezing is generalized on auscultation, whereas localized wheezing may indicate the presence of a discrete obstruction *(mucus, foreign body,* or *tumor).* Tumors or granulomata may be found in the lumen of the airway, but most lung tumors in children occur outside the lumen and compress the airway to produce obstruction with focal hyperinflation or atelectasis.

Patients with *emphysema* or *interstitial inflammation* may wheeze because damaged alveolar walls cannot act as springs to hold the small airways open. The wheezing of patients with *bronchopulmonary dysplasia* or *cystic fibrosis* may be intermittent and asymmetric because the wheezing is caused by a combination of mucous obstruction, inflammation, loss of airway tone, and bronchial hyperreactivity.

Most of the causes of wheezing in the lower airway are acquired. Infection is the most common cause of acute wheezing, with viral agents being the most frequently implicated. The smaller airways most often are affected by *respiratory syncytial virus* (RSV) or *parainfluenza,* but tracheal involvement, as in viral tracheobronchitis (croup) and *bacterial tracheitis,* may occur. These infections, especially in infants, lead to coarse expiratory wheezes. Bacterial tracheitis can involve the large airway, creating such limited airflow that fine wheezing develops, which leads to its confusion with severe asthma.

Tables 176-1 and 176-2 summarize the causes of wheezing.

Table 176-1 *Causes of Wheezing*

LOCATION	PATHOLOGIC OR ANATOMIC CAUSE	CLINICAL DIAGNOSIS	TYPE OF WHEEZE GENERATED
Trachea	Loss of airway wall rigidity	Laryngotracheomalacia	Generalized, coarse
	Airway inflammation	Tracheobronchitis, bacterial tracheitis	Generalized, coarse to fine
Bronchi	Less airway wall rigidity	Bronchomalacia	Localized, fine
	Foreign body	Aspirated foreign body	Localized, fine
	Inflammation and mucous obstruction	Bronchiectasis	Localized, fine, bubbly
	Extrinsic compression	Mediastinal tumor or nodes	Localized, coarse
	Airway and elastic tissue destruction	Emphysema	Generalized, fine
	Inflammation	Bronchitis	Generalized, fine
Bronchioles	Inflammation and mucous obstruction	Bronchiolitis	Unusual—generalized, fine, but occasionally localized with mucous obstruction
	Airway wall edema, smooth muscle hypertrophy	Asthma	Same as for bronchiolitis
	Peribronchial edema	Congestive heart failure	Diffuse, fine
	Peribronchial hemorrhage	Hemosiderosis	Focal or diffuse, fine

Table 176-2 *Differential Diagnosis of Wheezing as a Function of Age*

AGE-GROUP	ACUTE	CHRONIC OR RECURRENT
Infants	Infection (bronchiolitis), including tuberculosis and opportunistic infection in immunosuppressed patients Congestive heart failure Asthma	Tracheomalacia Cystic fibrosis Tracheoesophageal malformations Vascular ring Tracheal stenosis Congenital lobar emphysema Diaphragmatic hernia Bronchopulmonary dysplasia Gastroesophageal reflux Aspiration pneumonitis Extrinsic compression of airway by tumors (e.g., neuroblastoma) Visceral larva migrans Histiocytosis Hemosiderosis Asthma
Children and adolescents	Infection Foreign body Asthma	Foreign body Asthma Allergic bronchopulmonary aspergillosis Cystic fibrosis Ciliary dysmotility syndromes Tumors, lymph nodes $Alpha_1$-antitrypsin deficiency Sarcoidosis

EVALUATION OF THE WHEEZING CHILD

Physical signs to be recorded are the expiratory time, respiration rate, and the degree to which accessory respiratory muscles are used. Anteroposterior and lateral chest radiographs provide the key laboratory procedure for diagnosis of the wheezing patient, because they allow identification of focal lesions. The clinician should remember that 50% of patients ultimately found to have a *foreign body* have no history of choking or cough. When a foreign body is suspected, additional radiographs should be obtained to demonstrate asymmetric and sustained hyperinflation.

The diagnosis of asthma should not be made in an infant or child during the first episode of wheezing but should be reserved until a pattern of recurrent wheezing responsive to bronchodilator therapy is documented. In infants the differential diagnosis of acute wheezing should include usual or unusual infections, a foreign body, and congenital malformations. Viral and bacterial infections may cause transient bronchial hyperreactivity, and wheezing with respiratory infections can develop in patients with bronchial hyperreactivity. For this reason, patients with respiratory infections often may respond to bronchodilator therapy.

SUGGESTED READINGS

Benjamin B: Tracheomalacia in infants and children, Ann Otol Rhinol Laryngol 93:438, 1984.

Ellis EF: Asthma: current therapeutic approach, Pediatr Clin North Am 34:1041, 1988.

Esclamado RM and Richardson MA: Laryngotracheal foreign bodies in children: a comparison with bronchial foreign bodies, Am J Dis Child 141:259, 1987.

Fireman P: The wheezing infant, Pediatr Rev 7:247, 1986.

Gilbert EF and Opitz JM: Malformations and genetic disorders of the respiratory tract. In Stocker JT, editor: Pediatric pulmonary disease, New York, 1989, Hemisphere Publishing Corp.

Goldenhersh MJ and Rachelefsky GS: Childhood asthma: management, Pediatr Review 10:259, 1989.

Wiseman NE: The diagnosis of foreign body aspiration in childhood, J Pediatr Surg 19:531, 1984.

Wood RE and Gauderer MWL: Flexible fiberoptic bronchoscope in the management of tracheobronchial foreign bodies in children: the value of a combined approach with open tube bronchoscopy, J Pediatr Surg 19:693, 1984.

Part Eight

Specific Clinical Problems

177

Acne

Donald P. Lookingbill

Acne is so prevalent in young adults as to be viewed by some as a physiologic event—a view that may interfere with an appreciation of its impact on the patient and preclude therapeutic intervention. This section addresses acne as a treatable disease that deserves medical attention.[2,10]

ETIOLOGY

Hormones

Acne is a disease of the pilosebaceous unit.[9] Under androgen stimulation, sebaceous glands enlarge and increase their sebum production. Before puberty the responsible androgens are presumed to be of adrenal origin. With puberty the addition of gonadal androgens provides further sebaceous gland stimulation. Inasmuch as most studies to date have not shown patients with acne to have abnormal levels of circulating testosterone, tissue androgen metabolism may be the more important factor in acne pathogenesis.[5] One of the major organs for androgen metabolism is the skin, where the enzyme 5-alpha-reductase metabolizes testosterone to dihydrotestosterone, which has much more potent activity at the tissue level. There is some evidence to suggest that in the skin of acne patients, there is increased 5-alpha-reductase activity. This would be expected to result in increased androgenic stimulation of the sebaceous glands, ultimately causing acne. Increased sebaceous gland activity is necessary for acne to develop, yet it alone is insufficient to cause disease. Additional factors are needed.

Follicular Obstruction

If sebum is allowed to drain freely to the surface, the surface skin becomes oily, but no acne develops. Outlet obstruction of the follicular canal is required for acne to occur. This obstruction is produced by the accumulation of adherent keratinized cells within the canal, forming an impaction that obstructs the flow of sebum (Fig. 177-1). Production of keratinized cells within the lining of the follicular canal is normal, but their accumulation with impaction is not, and it is this follicular obstruction (which also may be influenced by androgens) that is prerequisite to the development of acne.

Bacteria

Proximal to the follicular outlet obstruction, sebum and keratinous debris accumulate. This provides an attractive environment for the growth of anaerobic bacteria, particularly *Propionibacterium acnes*. The role that these bacteria play in the pathogenesis of acne has long been the subject of debate. One early theory held that the lipase enzymes elaborated by these organisms hydrolyze sebaceous lipids, resulting in the release of free fatty acids, which then were presumed to cause irritation. With rupture of the follicle, inflammatory lesions were thought to result. This theory remains controversial. It is possible that bacteria play other roles in the pathogenesis of acne. There is, however, little question of the therapeutic benefit of antibiotics, whatever their mechanism of action.

The pathogenic events involved in acne, then, include (1) androgenic stimulation of sebaceous glands, resulting in increased sebum production, (2) keratinous impaction in the pilosebaceous canal, causing outlet obstruction, (3) accumulation of sebaceous and keratinous debris behind the obstruction, and (4) proliferation of anaerobic bacteria, which possibly alter this milieu in such a way as to contribute to

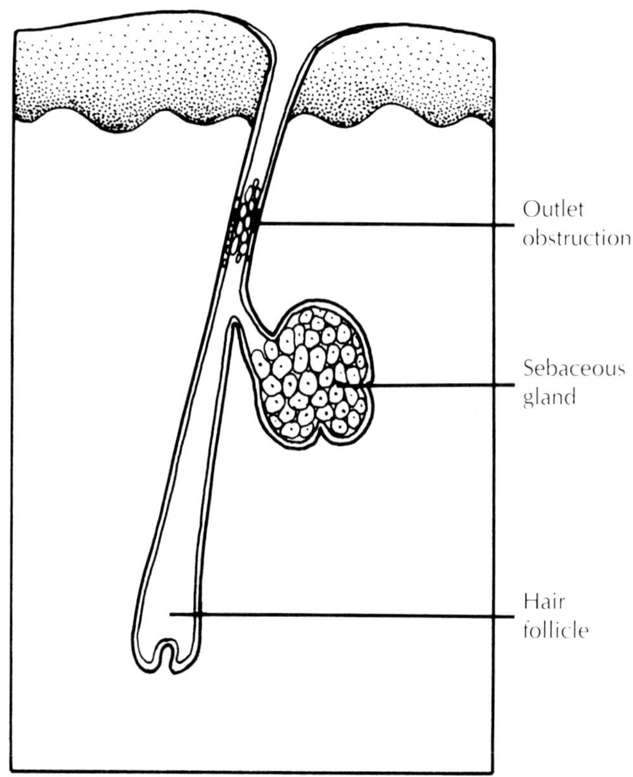

Fig. 177-1 Obstruction of pilosebaceous unit in acne.

the rupture of the dilated pilosebaceous unit with extravasation of its contents into the surrounding dermis, resulting in inflammatory acne lesions.

CLINICAL FINDINGS

The disease process may begin at a surprisingly young age. In one survey of children aged 8 to 10 years, 36% of the boys and 42% of the girls had early lesions of acne. Although the incidence and severity of the disease increase during adolescence, acne is by no means confined to these years. It is not uncommon for acne activity to continue into the third and fourth decades of life, much to the consternation of the afflicted patient.

The pathogenic mechanisms previously described result in the following types of clinical lesions: noninflamed open and closed comedones and inflammatory papules, pustules, nodules, and cysts.

The acne found in prepubertal children usually is noninflammatory and so may easily be overlooked. The open comedo ("blackhead") and closed comedo ("whitehead") represent lesions caused purely by pilosebaceous canal obstructions; there is no accompanying inflammation (Fig. 177-2).

Inflammatory acne in young children is rare and should raise the suspicion of a possible hyperandrogenic condition, such as that associated with congenital adrenal hyperplasia or even a rare androgen-secreting tumor. Examination for virilization (in girls) and precocious puberty (in both sexes) should be undertaken. Screening blood studies should include serum levels of testosterone, dehydroepiandrosterone sulfate (DHEA-S), and 17-hydroxyprogesterone.

With rupture of the obstructed pilosebaceous canal, an inflammatory reaction ensues, resulting in erythematous papules, pustules, nodules, or cysts, depending on the amount of tissue involved, its location, and the magnitude of the inflammatory response. Not surprisingly, acne lesions have a predilection for skin rich in sebaceous glands. Accordingly, the face is the prevailing site, although acne is common also on the chest and back. The lower portion of the trunk, buttocks, and thighs are much less commonly involved, and the distal extremities are always spared.

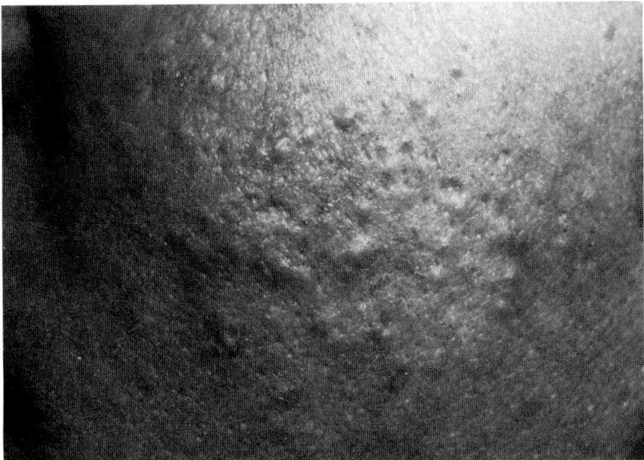

Fig. 177-2 Closed comedones (whiteheads) appear as dome-shaped, flesh-colored papules, which are often overlooked.

DIFFERENTIAL DIAGNOSIS

It is rarely difficult to make the diagnosis of acne. Usually it is made from "across the room," although, as mentioned, the comedonal lesions may require closer inspection (Fig. 177-2). Occasionally acne may be confused with the first three of the entities discussed below. In addition, acne variants may occur and also are included in the following discussion.

Flat Warts

Small flesh-colored warts may be clinically confused with closed comedones. The question usually can be resolved with very close inspection—a flat wart will be seen to have a sharp right-angled edge and a finely roughened surface, whereas the closed comedo will have a dome shape and a smooth surface. Flat warts also vary in size; closed comedones are uniformly small.

Milia

Milia are small epidermal inclusion cysts that are also sometimes confused with comedones and occasionally with inflammatory pustules, especially in infants with neonatal acne.

Adenoma Sebaceum

A misnamed entity (the lesions are actually angiofibromas), adenoma sebaceum represents one of the skin manifestations in tuberous sclerosis. Clinically the lesions appears as pink papules, which occasionally are confused with acne lesions. Correct diagnosis of adenoma sebaceum will be suspected when the papules are (1) clustered primarily in the center of the face, (2) persistent, and (3) resistent to acne therapy.

Acne Rosacea

Acne rosacea is an acneiform eruption distinguished from acne by a background blush of erythema and telangiectasia and by the absence of comedones. Also, rosacea most often occurs in middle-aged adults.

Steroid Acne

Both systemic and topical steroids can induce acne. Acne from systemic steroids usually appears as multiple small, uniform-size papules and pustules, with a predilection for the upper portion of the trunk. The condition slowly involutes spontaneously after withdrawal of the steroid.

Gram-Negative Folliculitis

Gram-negative organisms can rarely produce a pustular folliculitis in patients being treated with systemic antibiotics for their acne. This condition should be suspected in any patient whose disease flares while receiving therapy, especially if the flare is manifested by multiple pustules. Bacterial culture with antibiotic sensitivity studies should be obtained so that the diagnosis can be confirmed and an appropriate change in antibiotic therapy instituted.

PSYCHOSOCIAL CONSIDERATIONS

Acne can be a devastating disease. In an ironic quirk of timing, it occurs at a time of life when personal appearance is of prime concern and self-consciousness is at its peak. Some young people appear to be more affected psychologically by their acne than do others, but no one is comfortable with it. Patients with severe cystic acne may even be socially ostracized. Regardless of the acne's severity, the condition is important to the patient seeking help and deserves serious attention. Patients are not impressed with soothing advice that trivializes their disease and reassures them that they will eventually "outgrow it." Fortunately, an alternative to this advice is possible—excellent and effective medical therapy is now available, the results of which are quite gratifying.

MANAGEMENT

Three methods of treatment have proved efficacious for patients with acne: topical comedolytic agents,[6] topical[13] and systemic[1] antibiotics, and systemic retinoids.[7,8] The most traditional, yet still effective, treatment regimen incorporates comedolytics and antibiotics.

Comedolytics

Topical retinoic acid (Retin-A) and benzoyl peroxide both help disimpact the keratinous plug in the follicular canal. They are most helpful in treating superficial acne lesions—that is, comedones and superficial papules and pustules.[14] Of the two agents, retinoic acid is somewhat more active in its effect on comedones,[15] but the benzoyl peroxide preparations also exert an antibacterial effect. When both agents are used, the patient should be instructed to apply the retinoic acid at bedtime and the benzoyl peroxide each morning.

Both Retin-A and benzoyl peroxide are available in a variety of preparations. The "strength" of a given preparation reflects its irritancy and probably also its efficacy. Benzoyl peroxide gels are marketed in concentrations of 2.5%, 5%, and 10%. For Retin-A, the strength of the preparation depends on both the concentration of the drug and the nature of the vehicle in which it is contained (Table 177-1). Patients are started on the mildest preparations, and the potency of the medication can then be increased at subsequent visits if needed.

Skin irritation, which usually becomes less of a problem with continued use, is the major side effect of the comedolytics. In addition, a true allergic contact dermatitis to benzoyl peroxide develops in about 1% of patients, which necessitates permanent discontinuance of this agent. Topical retinoic acid may make the skin more susceptible to effects of the sun; therefore patients should be instructed to avoid excessive sun exposure and to use sun screens if they need to be exposed to the sun for prolonged periods.

Antibiotics

Antibiotics are indicated in patients with inflammatory acne lesions. Topical agents such as tetracycline, erythromycin, and clindamycin have been commercially formulated. However, for patients already using the two topical comedolytic agents mentioned earlier, the addition of a third topical agent becomes confusing. Accordingly, for most patients, systemic antibiotics are preferred. Tetracycline is the drug of first choice because of its proved efficacy, its relatively low cost, and its record of freedom from side effects, even when given over the long term. Because of dental staining, tetracycline should not be used in patients younger than 9 years of age (albeit acne rarely occurs in children of such age). Food, particularly dairy products, interferes with the absorption of tetracycline; thus this drug needs to be taken on an empty stomach. The most convenient times are on awakening in the morning and on retiring at night. For the occasional patient who does not respond adequately to tetracycline, erythromycin may be used as alternatives. Minocycline also may be substituted, but it is very expensive.

Systemic Retinoids

The systemic retinoid 13-*cis*-retinoic acid (isotretinoin, or Accutane) became commercially available in September 1982 for use in the treatment of severe cystic acne. This drug decreases follicular keratinization, sebum production, and intrafollicular bacterial counts. The net result of these (and possibly other) effects of the drug is a dramatic improvement in acne. The therapeutic effect usually takes several months to begin and often is sustained long after the recommended 30-week course of therapy has been discontinued. Side effects, unfortunately, are common. Almost all patients experience mucocutaneous reactions (cheilitis, conjunctivitis, and dry mucous membranes of the mouth and nose), and extra-

Table 177-1 *Retin-A Preparations*

	MILDEST	MILD	MODERATE	STRONGEST
Cream	0.025%	0.05%	0.1%	
Gel		0.01%	0.025%	
Solution				0.05%

cutaneous complications also occur. For example, systemic retinoids can cause elevation in plasma lipid levels and asymptomatic (to date) vertebral hyperostoses.[3] Most important is the drug's teratogenicity.

Exposure to isotretinoin in pregnancy has been associated with a 25-fold increased risk of major fetal malformation.[4] Thus, it is *mandatory* that female patients exercise strict birth control measures while taking this medication. As mentioned, isotretinoin is recommended only for patients with severe cystic acne, and these constitute a minority of acne patients.

Patient Compliance

Patient compliance is the single most important aspect of a successful acne treatment program. Without patient compliance, even the most effective medications are doomed to failure. To maximize compliance the physician must take time at the initial visit to explain *in detail* the use of each medication, as well as the effects and side effects to be expected. To reinforce these instructions it is extremely helpful to give the patient printed instructions, an example of which is shown in the accompanying box. Medications are used only twice daily. If this activity is centered on an already-established daily habit, such as tooth brushing, it too can become habitual. Given careful and specific instructions, most patients with acne are exceptionally compliant and, given time, will have good results to show for their efforts. In this regard the "it takes time" concept, underlined in the patient instruction sheet, needs to be emphasized to all patients; otherwise they may become prematurely, and inappropriately, discouraged. The acne instruction sheet also can be used to answer several other questions, often unasked, that acne patients or their parents frequently have. The most common of these pertain to diet, cleanliness, cosmetics, and picking at the lesions.[11]

Diet. Although there is some evidence that the usual American diet may have adverse effects on acne,[12] specific foods have not been implicated. For the vast majority of patients it is useful to remember Dr. A.M. Kligman's admonition[9] that "The disease is enough of a curse without gustatory deprivations." For the vast majority of patients a sensible diet is all that is suggested.

Cleanliness. The question of cleanliness is pondered more by parents than by patients; to help maintain peace at home it is useful to dispel the notion that acne is a function of poor hygiene. It is not. In general, acne cleaning agents need not be recommended, because most of these cause irritation, which unnecessarily compounds the irritation from the recommended topical comedolytics.

Cosmetics. Inasmuch as many cosmetics have been implicated as probably contributing to the acne process, it is preferable that they be avoided. If cosmetics are used, they should be water-based and used sparingly.

Acne Instruction Sheet

TOPICAL MEDICATIONS: BENZOYL PEROXIDE AND RETINOIC ACID

A. Action
  1. Both help open up clogged pores.
  2. Benzoyl peroxide also helps kill bacteria in the pores.

B. Method of use (apply to *all* affected areas)
  1. Apply retinoic acid at bedtime.
  2. Do *not* use acne scrub cleaners.
  3. Apply benzoyl peroxide in the morning.

C. Possible problems
  1. May make condition look worse rather than better after several weeks ("bringing acne to surface").
  2. May cause irritation (e.g., redness, dryness, and tenderness). If too much irritation does occur, use every other night until the skin becomes accustomed to it. If irritation is severe, stop medication and schedule a return visit.

TETRACYCLINE

A. Action—helps kill bacteria; particularly useful for deep and inflamed lesions.

B. Method of use—needs to be taken on an *empty* stomach. Therefore take it as soon as you get out of bed in the morning (wait ½ hour before eating breakfast) and at bedtime, at least 1 hour after taking any evening snack.

C. Potential side effects
  1. Uncommon; most patients have no trouble.
  2. May upset your stomach and cause nausea and/or diarrhea.
  3. Occasionally causes a yeast vaginitis, particularly if you are on birth control pills.
  4. Should not be taken if you are pregnant or trying to get pregnant.

GENERAL

A. Diet—for most patients, foods have no effect on acne. If you notice a certain food aggravates the condition, simply avoid that food. Otherwise, no restrictions are necessary.

B. Washing—acne cannot be washed off. Wash your face with regular soap two to three times and bathe or shower daily.

C. Results from medicines—*it takes time,* usually several months, to begin to note their benefit. At return visit in 2 months some improvement should be present, but it is unlikely that the acne will be cleared. The medications and their dose will be altered at that time, depending on the response.

D. Conscientious and *regular* use of medication is essential. They will not do any good if not taken regularly.

E. Cosmetics—they may aggravate your acne. If you must use them, do so sparingly and use only those which are water-based.

F. No picking!

Picking. In many patients with acne, much of the skin damage is self-inflicted. Although the temptation to squeeze a fresh pustule can be overwhelming, the practice must be discouraged. Picking, probing, and squeezing result in more tissue damage and sometimes produce scars. For some acne patients, picking may become so obsessive that excoriations are the only lesions seen.

COMPLICATIONS

The major complications of acne are its psychosocial ramifications. In addition to the cosmetic liability of active lesions, permanent scars further compound and perpetuate the problem in some unfortunate patients—mainly those with inflammatory lesions. Established scars are difficult to treat. Many patients have been disappointed with the results of dermabrasion. Bovine collagen injections have been used in some patients, producing short-term improvement, but repeated injections often are necessary and the long-term results are not yet known. Because scars are more easily prevented than treated, the emphasis in acne is on early and aggressive medical therapy such as that outlined earlier.

PROGNOSIS

With proper therapy the prognosis for acne is good, if not excellent. Patients should understand that most therapies control rather than cure the disease and that improvement does not occur overnight. Improvement, however, will occur, usually within 2 months of starting therapy, and it is at this time that the first revisit is best scheduled. At that visit the acne regimen can be adjusted as necessary. For example, the potency of the comedolytics can be increased (or decreased) and the dosage of the antibiotic altered, depending on the initial response. Continued improvement in the disease is to be expected with continuation of therapy. For many patients the dose of systemic antibiotics can be gradually reduced and eliminated after a number of months, but most patients require prolonged (often over years) maintenance therapy with topical agents and, in some cases, continuation of antibiotic therapy.

Historically, cystic acne has been the most difficult to treat. Isotretinoin now provides a powerful tool to deal with this disastrous disease and further offers the potential for prolonged remissions, sometimes lasting for years after a single course of therapy. As previously discussed, however, this drug is not without serious side effects, and its use is reserved for patients with severe disease that has not responded to standard therapy.

REFERENCES

1. Akers WA et al: Systemic antibiotics for treatment of acne vulgaris, Arch Dermatol 111:1630, 1975.
2. Cunliffe WJ: Acne, Chicago, 1989, Year Book Medical Publishers, Inc.
3. Ellis CN et al: Long-term radiographic follow-up after isotretinoin therapy, J Am Acad Dermatol 18:1252, 1988.
4. Lammer EJ et al: Retinoic acid embryopathy, N Engl J Med 313:837, 1985.
5. Lookingbill DP et al: Tissue production of androgens in women with acne, J Am Acad Dermatol 12:481, 1985.
6. Melski JW and Arndt KA: Topical therapy for acne, N Engl J Med 302:503, 1980.
7. Peck GL et al: Prolonged remissions of cystic and conglobate acne with 13-*cis*-retinoic acid, N Engl J Med 300:329, 1979.
8. Peck GL et al: Isotretinoin versus placebo in the treatment of cystic acne: a randomized double-blind study, J Am Acad Dermatol 6:735, 1982.
9. Plewig G and Kligman AM: Acne morphogenesis and treatment, New York, 1975, Springer-Verlag, New York, Inc.
10. Rasmussen JE: A new look at old acne, Pediatr Clin North Am 25:285, 1978.
11. Rasmussen JE and Smith SB: Patient concepts and misconceptions about acne, Arch Dermatol 119:570, 1983.
12. Rosenberg EW: Acne diet reconsidered, Arch Dermatol 117:193, 1981.
13. Stoughton RB: Topical antibiotics for acne vulgaris: current usage, Arch Dermatol 115:486, 1979.
14. Swinyer LJ, Swinyer TA, and Britt MR: Topical agents alone in acne: a blind assessment study, JAMA 243:1640, 1980.
15. Thomas JR and Doyle AR: The therapeutic uses of topical vitamin A acid, J Am Acad Dermatol 4:505, 1981.

178

Acquired Immunodeficiency Syndrome (AIDS) and Human Immunodeficiency Virus (HIV) Infection

Avril P. Beckford and John H. Dossett

The first case of human immunodeficiency virus (HIV) infection was diagnosed in 1981; the first pediatric case was reported in 1982. The recent pandemic of HIV infection has included many thousands of infants and children. Moreover, the many infected adults who are still in their childbearing years threaten to produce an ever-increasing number of infected children.[6]

DEFINITION AND CLASSIFICATION

HIV infection rather than acquired immunodeficiency syndrome (AIDS) seems to be the best general term to cover the full spectrum of disease, because *AIDS* refers to the most severe end of the spectrum and is defined by strict criteria detailed later in this chapter. The definition for AIDS, developed by the Centers for Disease Control (CDC) (see the box on p. 1116) was established for epidemiologic surveillance only and was not introduced as a clinical tool.[10] This often makes its clinical application difficult. AIDS-related complex (ARC) has been used to describe HIV-infected children who have symptoms but whose clinical manifestations do not satisfy the CDC definition of AIDS.

Although a number of similarities exist between the adult and pediatric clinical manifestations of HIV infection, there are some important differences.

HUMAN IMMUNODEFICIENCY VIRUS (HIV) INFECTION

The definition of *HIV infection* includes the presence of multiple or recurrent bacterial infections and lymphoid interstitial pneumonitis in HIV-seropositive children older than 15 months of age; however, the passive transmission of maternal antibodies limits the interpretation of a positive antibody test result in younger children. The diagnosis in this latter group must be confirmed by a positive viral culture, a positive antigen (such as the P_{24} antigen) or indirect abnormalities, including elevated immunoglobulin levels, lymphopenia, a low T_4 lymphocyte count, or a decreased T_4/T_8 ratio.

Children who fulfill the CDC case definition of HIV infection[7] may be further classified according to the presence or absence of clinical signs and symptoms and subclassified according to the status of their immune function and clinical findings (see box on p. 1117). *Class P-O* includes indeterminate infection in those children who have antibody to HIV, indicating exposure to an infected mother, but in whom the diagnosis of HIV infection has not yet been confirmed. *Class P-1* includes patients who have documented infection with HIV but who have no clinical signs or symptoms. The subclassification of this group relies on immunologic testing, which should include quantitative immunoglobulin determination, complete blood cell count with differential, and T lymphocyte subset quantitation. *Class P-2* includes children with symptoms of more than 2 months' duration, such as the nonspecific findings of *subclass A*, which includes fever, failure to thrive, generalized lymphadenopathy, hepatomegaly, splenomegaly, parotitis, and diarrhea. The lymphoid interstitial pneumonitis noted in *subclass C* is based on either histologic confirmation or a radiologically confirmed chronic pneumonitis present on chest roentgenogram of at least 2 months' duration.

This present (i.e., 1991) definition and classification is based only on current knowledge and diagnostic abilities. Criteria may need to be revised as newer diagnostic techniques are further refined and become generally available.

EPIDEMIOLOGY

HIV infection is now pandemic. Unfortunately, children younger than 13 years of age may represent the fastest growing group of reported AIDS cases.[17] The attack rate in children largely parallels the drug use and sexual habits of adults of reproductive age. This is reflected in the observation that 78% of children with HIV infection acquired the virus perinatally, which may represent transmission during pregnancy, at the time of delivery, or shortly after birth. The majority of these cases can be attributed to intravenous (IV) substance abuse by the mother and/or her sexual partner. Approximately

Summary of September 1987 Revision of Surveillance Case Definition for AIDS

I. Without laboratory evidence of HIV infection (tests not done or inconclusive*), a patient with AIDS:

A. Does not have another cause of immunodeficiency, such as the following:

1. High-dose or long-term systemic corticosteroid therapy or other immunosuppressive-cytotoxic therapy ≤3 months before the onset of the indicator disease
2. Hodgkin disease, non-Hodgkin lymphoma (other than primary brain lymphoma), lymphocytic leukemia, multiple myeloma, other cancer of lymphoreticular-histiocytic tissue, angioimmunoblastic lymphadenopathy ≤3 months after diagnosis of the indicator disease
3. A genetic (congenital) immunodeficiency syndrome or an acquired immunodeficiency syndrome atypical of HIV infection (such as one with hypogammaglobulinemia)

and

B. Has had one of the following AIDS indicator diseases definitively diagnosed:

1. Candidiasis of the esophagus, trachea, bronchi, or lungs
2. Extrapulmonary cryptococcosis
3. Cryptosporidiosis with diarrhea persisting >1 month
4. Cytomegalovirus disease of an organ other than liver, spleen, or lymph nodes in a patient >1 month of age
5. Herpes simplex virus infection causing a mucocutaneous ulcer persisting >1 month, or bronchitis, pneumonitis, or esophagitis in a patient >1 month of age
6. Primary lymphoma of the brain in a patient <60 years of age
7. Kaposi sarcoma in a patient <60 years of age
8. Lymphoid interstitial pneumonia and/or pulmonary lymphoid hyperplasia in a child <13 years of age
9. *Mycobacterium avium* complex or *M. kansasii* disease disseminated to site other than lungs, skin, or cervical or hilar lymph nodes
10. *Pneumocystis carinii* pneumonia
11. Progressive multifocal leukoencephalopathy
12. Toxoplasmosis of the brain in a patient >1 month of age

II. With laboratory evidence of HIV infection, a patient with AIDS:

A. Has had one of the already-listed AIDS indicator diseases definitively diagnosed *or* one of the following AIDS indicator diseases definitively diagnosed:

1. Multiple or recurrent bacterial infections (at least two within 2 years) in a child <13 years of age, including septicemia, pneumonia, meningitis, bone or joint infection, abscess of internal organ or body cavity (except otitis media or superficial skin or mucosal abscesses)
2. Coccidioidomycosis disseminated to a site other than lungs or cervical or hilar lymph nodes
3. HIV encephalopathy
4. Histoplasmosis disseminated to a site other than lungs or cervical or hilar lymph nodes
5. Isosporiasis with diarrhea persisting >1 month
6. Kaposi sarcoma
7. Primary lymphoma of brain
8. Other non-Hodgkin lymphoma of B cell or known immunologic phenotype (small, noncleaved Burkitt or non-Burkitt lymphoma, or immunoblastic sarcoma)
9. Disseminated nontubercular mycobacterial disease involving a site other than lungs, skin, or cervical or hilar lymph nodes
10. Tuberculosis involving at least one site other than lungs
11. Recurrent nontyphoid *Salmonella* bacteremia
12. HIV wasting syndrome

or

B. One of the following AIDS indicator diseases diagnosed presumptively:

1. Esophageal candidiasis
2. Cytomegalovirus retinitis with loss of vision
3. Kaposi sarcoma
4. Lymphoid interstitial pneumonia or pulmonary lymphoid hyperplasia in a child <13 years of age
5. Acid-fast infection (species not identified) disseminated to a site other than lungs, skin, or cervical or hilar lymph nodes
6. *Pneumocystis carinii* pneumonia
7. Toxoplasmosis of the brain in a patient >1 month of age

III. With laboratory evidence against HIV infection (negative test results), a patient with AIDS:

A. Does not have another cause of underlying immunodeficiency (listed in section I, above)

and

B. Has had *Pneumocystis carinii* definitively diagnosed

or

Has had a definitive diagnosis of one of the AIDS indicator diseases listed in section I, above, *plus* a T-helper lymphocyte count <400/mm^3

Modified from Centers for Disease Control: MMWR 36:1S, 1987.

*Includes children with seropositivity who are <15 months of age, who have an HIV-infected mother, and who do not have other evidence for immunodeficiency or for HIV infection.

Summary of the Classification of HIV Infection in Children Younger Than 13 Years of Age

CLASS P-0. Indeterminate infection
CLASS P-1. Asymptomatic infection
Subclass A. Normal immune function
Subclass B. Abnormal immune function
Subclass C. Immune function not tested
CLASS P-2. Symptomatic infection
Subclass A. Nonspecific findings
Subclass B. Progressive neurologic disease
Subclass C. Lymphoid interstitial pneumonitis
Subclass D. Secondary infectious diseases
 Category D-1. Specified secondary infectious diseases listed in the CDC surveillance definition for AIDS
 Category D-2. Recurrent serious bacterial infections
 Category D-3. Other specified secondary infectious diseases
Subclass E. Secondary cancers
 Category E-1. Specified secondary cancers listed in the CDC surveillance definition for AIDS
 Category E-2. Other cancers possibly secondary to HIV infection
Subclass F. Other diseases possibly due to HIV infection

Epidemiology - Pediatric HIV Infection

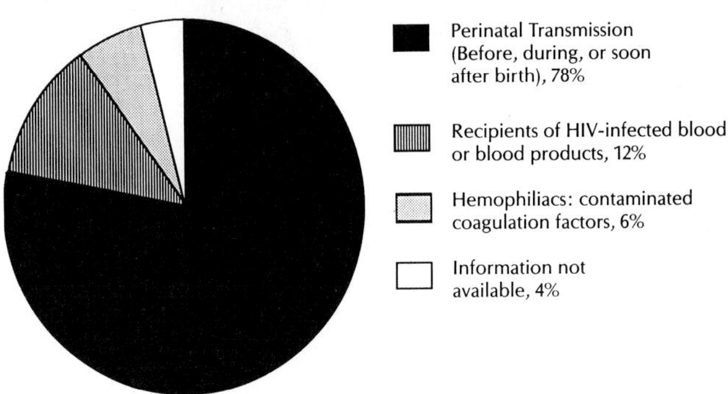

Fig. 178-1 Modes of transmission of HIV infection.

6% represents patients with coagulation disorders such as hemophilia, and 12% represents transmission by the transfusion of blood or blood products before screening for HIV was introduced in 1985. In approximately 4% of cases there may have been one or more risk factors involved; however, the actual method of transmission remains undetermined (Fig. 178-1). Of infants born to infected mothers 30% to 50% will acquire HIV infection.[9]

The epidemiology of HIV infection among adolescents is different from that among infants, in that IV drug use and sexual transmission are the risk factors. The true incidence of HIV infection is difficult to assess. The number of adolescent cases actually reported is small, but the latency time from viral infection to the time of illness is variable (up to 8 or 9 years); thus most infected adolescents may not become ill until they are young adults. This pattern is supported by the observation that the number of cases in the young adult age-group (20 to 29 years) is considerably higher than in adolescents.[16] The lower male/female ratio in the adolescent group compared with adults reflects the higher incidence of heterosexual transmission and IV drug abuse. The epidemiology in the adolescent group emphasizes its enormous infective potential and attitudes about risk-taking behavior.

PATHOPHYSIOLOGY

HIV is a member of the lentivirus family.[21] Presently, two serotypes of HIV (HIV-1 and HIV-2) have been identified; however, the great majority of patient isolates are HIV-1.

HIV predominantly infects cells that possess a CD_4 receptor (most commonly the T_4 lymphocyte). Recent studies, however, have shown that other cell surface moieties may be important for viral entry as well.[20] The virus consists of (1) an outer lipid envelope that has an external surface antigen (gp 120) and an anchoring segment (gp 41), (2) a cylindrical core referred to as P_{24}, and (3) genomic RNA, consisting of polymerase genes, structural genes, and functional genes.

The polymerase enables the transcription of the viral RNA genome into a DNA copy that eventually becomes integrated into the host cell chromosomal DNA. In this form the virus may remain latent for varying periods of time (up to 8 years), during which the patient may be relatively well and minimally infectious. On the other hand, the virus may actively reproduce, leading to cytopathic effects characterized by syncytium formation, degeneration, and lysis. The infected cells may be stimulated to reproduce virus by a variety of factors, such as interaction of the infected cell with other agents (cytomegalovirus [CMV] or herpes simplex virus [HSV]). It is during this period of active replication that clinical symptoms, as well as increased infectivity, may be marked.

Inasmuch as the T_4 cells are particularly susceptible to HIV, this cell group, normally responsible for viral destruction, undergoes dramatic qualitative and quantitative change. This is the basis for the immunologic abnormalities and profound immunodeficiency, with subsequent clinical consequences, seen in HIV infection.[5]

CLINICAL SYNDROME

The most important factor in making the diagnosis of pediatric HIV infection is a *high clinical index of suspicion.* With this in mind, meticulous attention to details in the history and the physical examination will alert suspicion and enable early confirmation. Because most HIV infection in children is perinatally acquired, the disease affects younger children predominantly. In 50% the diagnosis is made within the first year of life and in 82% by 3 years of age.[8] Generally the time between infection and the development of symptoms is shorter in children who acquire the infection perinatally than in those who become infected by blood transfusion.

History

A thorough pediatric history begins with a careful review of the antenatal history. It is clear that the presence of any one of a number of risk factors in women of childbearing age significantly increases the risk of HIV infection. These factors include IV drug use, multiple sexual partners, blood transfusions before 1985, or sexual partners who have known risk factors (known infection with HIV, bisexual practices, history of IV drug use, hemophilia, or blood transfusions before 1985) (see box below).

The important clinical clues that suggest HIV infection in infants and children are prematurity and low infant birth weight,[15] recurrent oral thrush, failure to thrive, recurrent fevers, chronic diarrhea, recurrent infections, opportunistic infections, blood transfusions, and sexual abuse (see box at the bottom of this page).

The adolescent history, as always, needs to address the issues of IV drug abuse and a careful and sensitive approach regarding the details of sexual practices. This information must include not only participation in any sexual activity but also the number of partners, homosexual or bisexual encounters, and the use of contraceptive methods (especially the consistent use of condoms). (See box above). Tattooing also may be a risk factor for HIV infection.

The Antenatal History: HIV Risk Factors in Women of Childbearing Age

Intravenous drug use
Multiple sexual partners
Blood transfusions before 1985
A sexual partner with any of the following characteristics:
- Known infection with HIV
- Bisexual practices
- History of IV drug use
- Hemophilia
- Blood transfusions before 1985

The History: Neonatal and Early Childhood

Prematurity
Low birth weight
Recurrent oral thrush
Failure to thrive
Recurrent fevers
Chronic diarrhea
Recurrent infections
Opportunistic infections
Blood transfusions
Sexual abuse

The History: Adolescents

IV drug abuse
Tattoos
Sexual practices
- Number of partners
- Homosexual preference
- Bisexual preference
- Contraceptive methods

Clinical Signs

After a careful history is obtained, attention should be paid to the details of the examination. The clinical manifestations of HIV infection are numerous and are addressed here systematically.

Nonspecific Findings. These include failure to thrive, recurrent or intermittent fevers, a decreased level of activity, and myalgia. Involvement of the lymphoid system is common, and generalized lymphadenopathy may be the only presenting clinical sign. Although lymphadenopathy generally is a common finding in the pediatric age-group, the presence of more than two lymph nodes that are larger than 1 cm in diameter in two noncontiguous sites and particularly the presence of axillary adenopathy are important indicators of HIV infection.

Pulmonary. Pulmonary disease is responsible for much of the morbidity and mortality in pediatric patients. Lymphoid interstitial pneumonitis (LIP) is common. It manifests clinically with tachypnea and progressive respiratory distress and often progresses to profound hypoxia. Radiographically, peribronchiolar lymphonodular aggregates and interstitial infiltrates are characteristic (Fig. 178-2). Biopsy (which may be required to distinguish this entity from *Pneumocystis carinii* pneumonia [PCP]) classically shows interstitial and peribronchial infiltration by lymphocytes and plasma cells.

Recurrent bacterial pneumonias are common in children with HIV infection. Of the opportunistic pulmonary infections, PCP is the most important pathogen, occurring in more than 50% of children with HIV infection. Clinically it manifests with fever, tachypnea, and sometimes hypoxia. Radiographically it is characterized by a diffuse reticular pattern and pulmonary infiltration. Biopsy sometimes may be necessary to distinguish among LIP, PCP, and other opportunistic infections such as CMV and fungi.

Gastrointestinal. The most common gastrointestinal manifestation is chronic or recurrent diarrhea. This may be secretory diarrhea resulting from primary HIV involvement of the gastrointestinal tract. Alternatively, the diarrhea may be caused by secondary agents such as enteroviruses, sal-

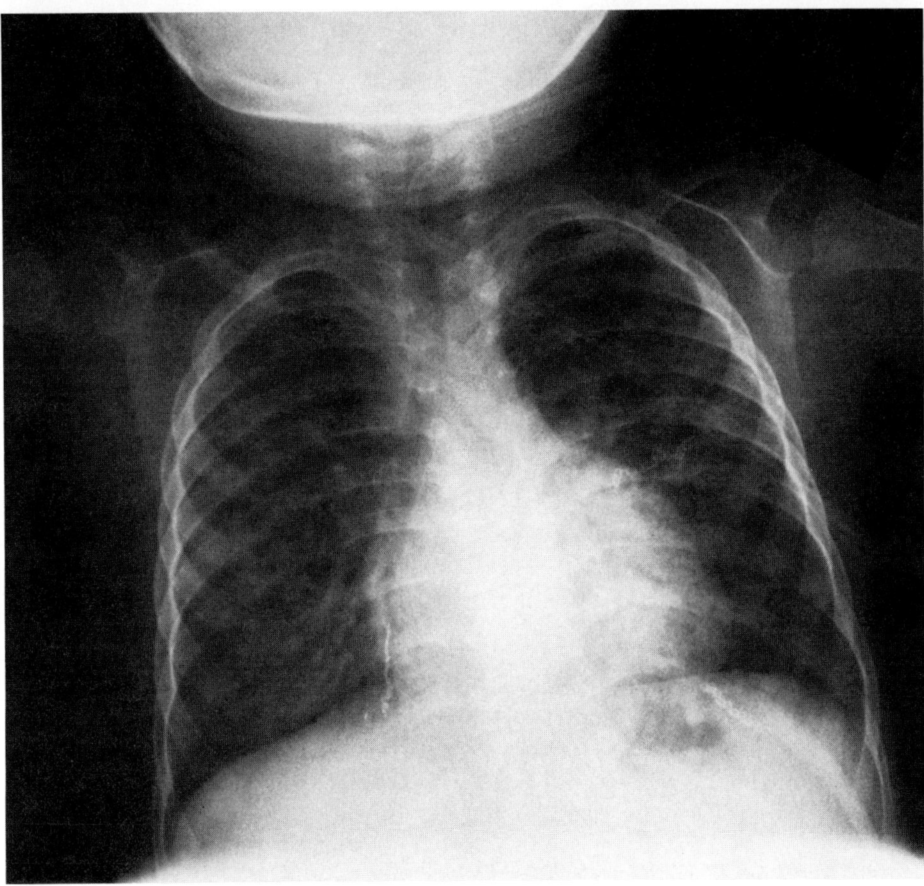

Fig. 178-2 Chest x-ray of a child with lymphocytic interstitial pneumonitis (LIP). The infiltrates are: *(a)* diffuse, *(b)* interstitial, and *(c)* bilateral. The infiltrates have been described as reticulonodular.

monella, or shigella; *Campylobacter, Cryptosporidium,* or *Candida* organisms; CMV or HSV; or *Giardia lamblia, Mycobacterium avium, Isospora belli,* or *Clostridium difficile.* Direct invasion of the bowel by some strains of HIV may induce malabsorption and chronic secretory diarrhea—for example, invasion of the enterochromaffin cells that produce hormones responsible for bowel motility and digestion. Infected macrophages in the stroma may be an indirect source of toxic cytokines that contribute to the secretory diarrhea.[20]

Other gastrointestinal manifestations include parotitis, oral candidiasis, and esophagitis caused by *Candida* organisms, CMV, or HSV.

Hepatitis, manifested by elevated transaminase levels, is commonly seen without serologic evidence of hepatotropic virus infection. Biopsy may show nodular lymphoid aggregates in the portal triads, hepatocellular and bile duct damage, sinusoidal cell hyperplasia, endothelialitis, and changes that suggest chronic active hepatitis. Both HIV and CMV are possible infective causes.[3] Pancreatitis also has been reported in the pediatric age-group.

Neurologic. The prevalence of central nervous system (CNS) manifestations of HIV disease in children has been reported to be as high as 90%. The clinical presentation is varied and includes an encephalopathy characterized by delayed neurologic development or loss of developmental milestones. Seizures may occur but are not typical. Physical examination may reveal extrapyramidal tract signs, paresis, peripheral neuropathy, ataxia, and pseudobulbar palsy.

The encephalopathy seen in HIV infection almost always is due to the presence of HIV in the CNS. Secondary CNS infection, CNS lymphoma, and microvascular accidents occur less frequently in children.

Neuroradiologic studies may show cerebral atrophy, white matter abnormalities, and basal ganglia calcification. Spinal fluid may show pleocytosis and an elevated protein; however, the cerebrospinal fluid frequently is normal. Electroencephalograms may show normal findings or diffuse background slowing.

Pathologic findings include reduced brain weight, consistent with atrophy, as well as microscopic calcifications in the walls of blood vessels. Multinucleated giant cells may be associated with inflammatory cell infiltrates. The inflammatory cells (microglia, mononuclear cells, lymphocytes, and plasma cells) may be found throughout the gray and white matter but are most prominent in the brain stem and the basal ganglia.[14]

Cardiovascular. Cardiomyopathy with congestive heart failure has been seen in a number of children. Arteriopathy characterized by vasculitis that progresses to fibrosis of the intima and media has been reported.[18]

Renal. Children with HIV infection may have renal disease that commonly manifests as proteinuria. The pathology is most consistent with focal glomerulosclerosis or mesangial hyperplasia.[26]

Dermatologic. An eczematoid rash commonly is found early in HIV infection. Infective causes of rashes may include candidiasis, herpetic gingivostomatitis, herpetic whitlow, herpes zoster, molluscum contagiosum, condyloma acuminatum, impetigo, and cellulitis.[25] Kaposi sarcoma is exceedingly rare in children.

Ophthalmologic. Ophthalmologic findings may include a perivasculitis of the retinal vessels where no infectious agent has yet been found. Opportunistic ocular infections include CMV retinitis, *Toxoplasma* retinitis, and fungal infections.

Hematologic. Thrombocytopenia has been reported in 10% to 20% of cases. It usually is an immune thrombocytopenia, although a nonimmune thrombocytopenia has been described.[27] Leukopenia, neutropenia, and anemia (including hemolytic anemia) are common hematologic manifestations.

Infectious. Recurrent bacterial and viral infections are the common initial markers that lead the practitioner to suspect HIV infection. Much like children with congenital hypogammaglobulinemia syndromes, children with HIV infection have frequent infection with common pyogenic bacteria. These may be relatively mild infections, such as pyoderma, recurrent otitis media, sinusitis, and other respiratory infections. More serious bacterial infections, such as pneumonia, bacteremia, meningitis, cellulitis, and empyema, also are common. The bacteria usually responsible for these infections are listed in the box below.

Children with HIV infection are deficient in cell-mediated immunity. This lack is reflected in their having frequent viral, fungal, and protozoan infections. Although PCP (protozoan) is by far the most frequent, other opportunistic infections also are common (see the box at the right). The children are particularly vulnerable to herpes viruses (CMV, Epstein-Barr virus, herpes simplex virus, and varicella-zoster virus). Measles virus infection may result in fatal disease, especially in those children with nutritional deficiency.[4]

Oral thrush is extremely common. Less commonly, *Candida albicans* causes extensive local invasion or severe systemic disease.

LABORATORY DIAGNOSIS

The clinical manifestations of HIV infection are protean and overlap with many other infectious diseases. Moreover, the implications of the diagnosis are of such medical and social significance that *reliable laboratory diagnosis* is essential. Culture of HIV from blood or other tissues is preferable; however, this method lacks sensitivity and is prohibitively expensive. Because HIV culturing is not generally available, the diagnosis depends on less direct methods of virus detection (antigen and antibody).

Methods of Detecting Antibody

Enzyme-Linked Immunosorbent Assay (ELISA). The ELISA is widely used to screen for HIV antibodies. Because it was developed initially for blood donor screening, it is more sensitive (95% to 99%) than specific.[2] Its other advantages include reproducibility, rapid availability, and low cost. Inasmuch as there is a small risk of false-positive results, all positive ELISA reactions must be confirmed by more specific tests such as the Western blot.

Western Blot. This test identifies antibodies to specific antigens (such as the P_{24} antigen) by electrophoretically running the antigen through gel against the patient's sera and identifying specific bands. Standards have been published that enable test results to be identified as positive, negative, or indeterminate. Sera from persons recently infected and with advanced disease may produce an indeterminate pattern.

Crucial principles that bear on the interpretation of the tests for detecting antibodies include:

1. Maternal antibodies cross the placenta and may be detectable in an infant (infected or not) for approximately 15 months. That is, all babies born to seropositive women will have detectable antibodies whether infected or not. Between 30% and 50% of these infants eventually will have confirmed HIV infection.
2. Approximately 75% of seropositive infants who are ultimately found to be uninfected will become antibody-free by 1 year of age.[3] A single negative antibody test result, however, does not confirm that the infant is not infected. Absence of antibody may reflect an inability of the humoral system to respond to antigen or a phase of viral replication that results in binding of the limited amount of circulating antibody. Some infants younger than 6 months of age with very severe disease produce no antibody at all.
3. Children older than 15 months with consistent HIV antibody positivity are presumed to be infected with HIV.

Common bacterial pathogens in HIV

Streptococcus pneumoniae
Haemophilus influenzae
Streptoccocus pyogenes
Salmonella spp.
Staphylococcus aureus
Escherichia coli
Pseudomonas spp.

Opportunistic Infections in Children with HIV

Candidiasis (of the mouth, esophagus, trachea, bronchi, or lungs)
Cryptococcosis
Cryptosporidiosis
Cytomegalovirus infection
Persistent herpes simplex infection
Histoplasmosis
Isosporiasis
Toxoplasmosis
Mycobacteria infections
Herpes viruses (CMV, HSV, Epstein-Barr virus, varicella-zoster virus)

Methods of Detecting Virus

Culture. Because of the large volume of blood needed for culture, it is much more difficult to isolate virus from infected children than from adults. The rate of virus recovery is reported to be less than 50%. In addition, the added disadvantages of time, expense, and intensive labor make this a less practical test for clinical use.

Antigen

1. Antigen capture immunoassay, which relies on viral replication for the detection of HIV antigen (most importantly the P_{24} [core] protein), depends on the quantity of virus present at the time of testing. Therefore P_{24} antigen can be detected most readily early in the course of infection (before or early during antibody production) and very late (when the humoral defense mechanisms may be overwhelmed). The absence of antigen in the blood does not indicate absence of infection. The persistence or recurrence of antigen in the blood of patients with symptomatic disease may be an ominous sign, often heralding clinical deterioration.
2. The indirect fluorescent antibody (IFA) and immunohistochemical techniques are additional tests that may be used to detect viral antigen.

Polymerase Chain Reaction. The polymerase chain reaction is a new technique in which proviral sequences of HIV within host DNA are amplified. This makes small amounts of virus much more readily detectable.[23] This procedure may prove to be an important diagnostic tool in confirming the diagnosis in young infants.

Supplementary Laboratory Investigations

The aforementioned serologic tests plus other studies may confirm the diagnosis (see box at upper right). Immunologic dysfunction is a hallmark. The affinity that HIV has for the lymphocyte explains many of the cellular and humoral abnormalities that are found. Lymphocytes infected with HIV may be killed, resulting in lymphocyte depletion (and reversal of the T_4/T_8 ratio). Those infected cells not killed have altered function, resulting in deregulation of the immune system. These include depressed responsiveness to certain mitogens and absence of cutaneous delayed hypersensitivity responses, such as to *Candida* and mumps antigens. The B lymphocytes also are affected and, despite the frequent occurrence of hypergammaglobulinemia, specific responses to antigenic stimulation are impaired. The hypergammaglobulinemia most frequently includes elevations of IgM and IgG and often will precede an obvious T cell defect. Increased circulating immune complexes also have been reported. The abnormalities of the B lymphocytes help explain the increased autoimmunity.

The immunologic markers may help distinguish seropositive infants who are infected from those who are not. Recent reports indicate that by 3 to 8 months of age, HIV-infected children show significantly higher IgG, IgM, and IgA levels and significantly lower T_4, T_8, and T_4/T_8 ratios than do children who have maternal antibodies but who are not infected. As early as the first month of life, infected infants also may have an elevated β_2 macroglobulin compared with infants who are not infected.

Possible Laboratory Findings in Pediatric Patients with HIV

IMMUNOLOGIC

- B cell abnormalities
  Hypergammaglobulinemia
  Increased circulating immune complexes
- T cell abnormalities
  Quantitative: reversed T^4/T^8 ratio
  Qualitative

HEMATOLOGIC

- Lymphopenia
- Neutropenia
- Anemia
- Thrombocytopenia

HEPATIC

- Elevated transaminase levels

PANCREATIC

- Elevated serum amylase

RENAL

- Proteinuria
- Azotemia

Other laboratory abnormalities might include lymphopenia, neutropenia, thrombocytopenia, and anemia (see box above).

TREATMENT: PRINCIPLES AND PRACTICE

Caring for pediatric and adolescent patients with HIV disease requires a multidisciplinary approach with at least as much emphasis on psychosocial problems and methods of preventing further spread as on the specifics of medical management. Because the majority of children with HIV disease have perinatally acquired infection, appropriate counseling of adolescents and of seropositive mothers becomes critical in attempting to prevent further transmission via this route. Thus physicians need to become comfortable about inquiring into the details of sexual practices, sexual history, and use of contraceptives and drugs.

Social Aspects

Many pediatric patients with HIV infection (more specifically those with transplacentally acquired disease) may be members of families who are unable to care for them. This may result from simultaneous complications of HIV disease in one or both parents, financial or social difficulties, and sometimes the paralyzing effects of drug addiction. Thus an enormous need exists for persons who are willing to provide comprehensive care outside the hospital. This epidemic has brought forward many compassionate heroes who have adopted these children and others who have become foster parents, providing long-term and respite care in their homes.

Parents and alternate caregivers frequently face tremendous lack of support and are commonly alienated from the community (day care, school, religious community, family gatherings). This is due to ignorance and unfounded fear regarding the transmission and communicability of this disease. *One of the most important functions of the pediatrician is to become an advocate for the patient—one who will help the community understand that there is* no *reason why a child infected with HIV should be denied full participation in the school and social environment.*

Physicians commonly are asked to advise schools, churches, and day care centers regarding the risks of HIV transmission in these settings. We are reassured by the observation that HIV has not spread in the families of persons who are infected, except in situations in which the persons are sharing needles with or are sexually active with the index case. Good hand-washing technique and appropriate disposal of debris should apply to *all* hospital and day care settings. Thus no specific precautions are required for persons who are known to have HIV infection.[1,12,13]

Treatment of Infants Born to HIV-Positive Mothers and to Mothers with Risk Factors

As has already been mentioned, all babies born to seropositive mothers will have HIV antibodies. Seropositivity in infants or toddlers may represent passive acquisition of maternal antibody or active HIV infection. An algorithm for determining which of the infants are infected and which have only passively acquired antibodies is shown in Fig. 178-3.

Because HIV can be transferred in breast milk, infants born to seropositive mothers should not be breast fed; it is one of the few situations in which the risk outweighs the benefit. In countries where malnutrition and diarrhea are major causes of infant mortality, breast-feeding may be preferable.

Immunizations

The observation that children with other immunodeficiency syndromes sometimes have serious or fatal complications

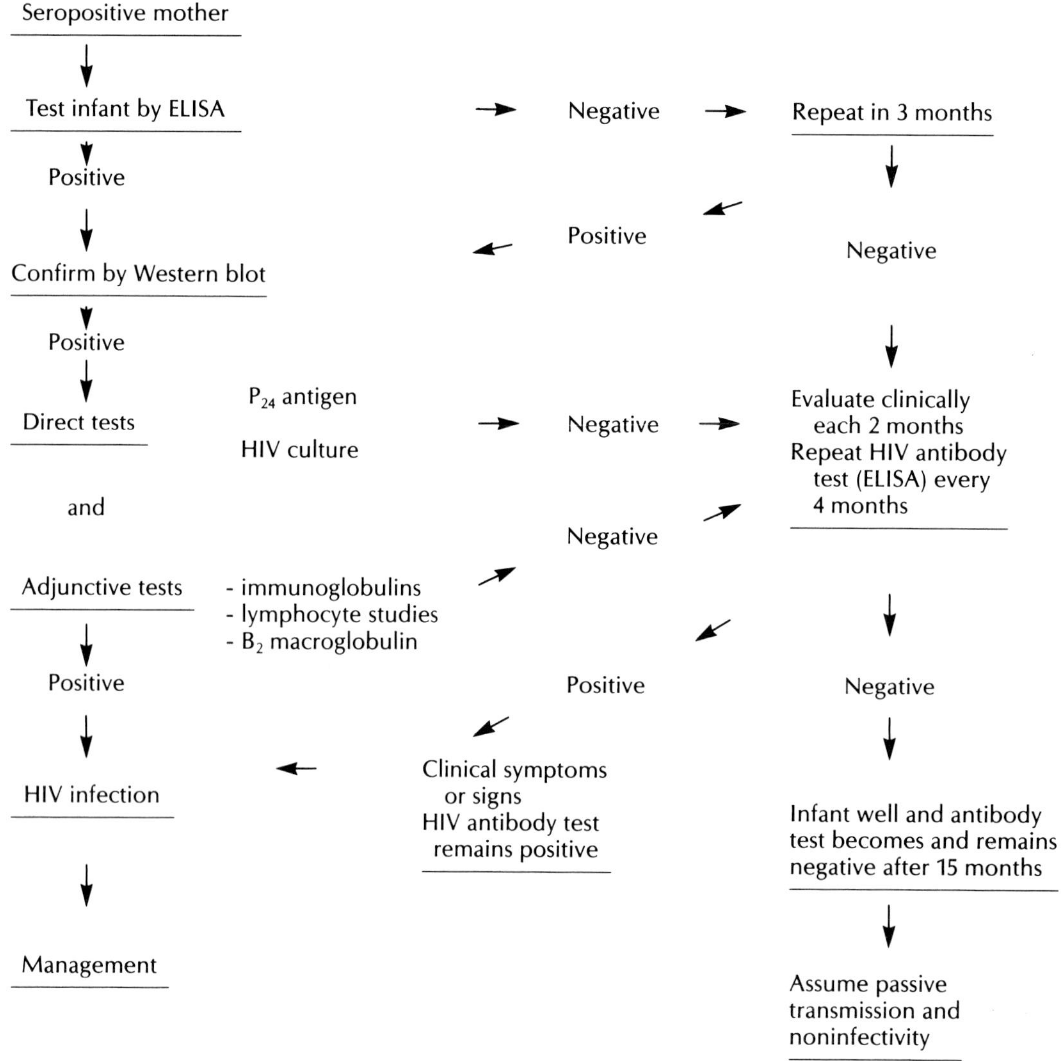

Fig. 178-3 Treatment of infants born to HIV seropositive mothers.
From Dossett JH: AIDS: Perinatal HIV infection. In Nelson NM: Current Therapy in Neonatal-Perinatal Medicine, 2nd ed., Toronto, 1989, BC Decker.

from live virus vaccinations has raised concern regarding the immunization of children with HIV infection.[15] Initially it was recommended that measles-mumps-rubella (MMR) vaccine not be given to children with HIV symptoms. This recommendation has been changed because of reports of serious and fatal measles in HIV-infected children and because there have been no reports of adverse effects in the children who have received this vaccine.[11] In the event of contact with measles, even those children who have received MMR should receive immunoglobulin because their response to the vaccine may have been suboptimal. Inactivated polio vaccine rather than oral attenuated poliovirus vaccine should be given to HIV-infected patients and also to their household contacts. All HIV-infected children should receive diphtheria-pertussis-tetanus (DPT) vaccine, as well as a *Haemophilus influenzae* type b conjugate vaccine, according to the usual schedule. Moreover, we recommend that these children receive pneumococcal vaccine and influenza virus vaccine despite the fact that immunocompromised children may have attenuated responses to some of the vaccines.

Varicella-zoster immunoglobulin should be administered after exposure to chickenpox or herpes zoster infection.

Nutritional Support

In severely ill children with HIV infection, especially those with intractable diarrhea, chronic intravenous alimentation may become essential. Home nursing often can accommodate this procedure without hospitalization.

Treatment of Infectious Complications

Fever is a major manifestation of HIV infection. The cause of fever may be a direct effect of HIV, or it may herald a secondary infection that results from HIV-induced immunodeficiency. Some persons with acute HIV infection have an infectious mononucleosis-like illness, which is characterized by fever, lethargy, and lymphadenopathy. This acute illness typically is mild and usually resolves completely within 1 or 2 weeks. Months to years later there may be recurrences of fever and lymphadenopathy in which no specific infectious agent is found. We believe that such fever is a primary manifestation of HIV.

As has been mentioned, progressive immunodeficiency will eventually develop. Consequently, fever in these children may frequently result from secondary infection with bacteria (often pyogenic), protozoa, fungi, or viruses. Such infections require appropriate antimicrobial therapy. Because of antibody deficiency, these children also may need supplementation with intravenous immunoglobulin (IVIG). Moreover, monthly infusions of IVIG seem to decrease the frequency and severity of recurrent infections. Controlled studies, which will determine the effectiveness of maintenance IVIG, currently are in progress.

Opportunistic infections with PCP, CMV, HSV, *Candida* organisms, and other agents are common. If these infections are to be treated appropriately, the definitive diagnosis must be diligently pursued. This requires aggressive tissue collections and thorough collaboration among the clinician, the pathologist, and the microbiologist. Table 178-1 summarizes some of the important organisms and requirements for their diagnosis and their treatment.[15]

Lymphocytic Interstitial Pneumonitis

LIP is believed to be a primary manifestation of HIV rather than a secondary infection. Exacerbations and remissions are characteristic, making assessment and therapy difficult. Periodic monitoring of oxygen saturation is useful in detecting subtle progression of the disease. Supplemental oxygen therapy may make the children more comfortable, and they adapt well to its long-term administration at home.

Antiretroviral Therapy

Clinical trials to assess efficacy and safety (in children) of antiretroviral drugs are now in progress. The best studied drug is zidovudine (AZT), which prolongs the interval between infection and development of symptoms. It also prolongs the life of persons who are already having symptoms. It does not eradicate HIV and consequently does not cure the disease. Although there are many potential sites for interrupting viral replication, most antiretroviral agents under investigation focus on inhibition of reverse transcriptase.

Zidovudine (3^1-acido-3^1-deoxythymidine) is a nucleoside analogue that becomes incorporated into viral DNA in which it is believed to inhibit reverse transcriptase and possibly result in chain termination. This drug, which can be administered by the oral route, penetrates the central nervous system. Because it inhibits viral replication but has no effect on latent virus, it is likely that therapy will need to be continued indefinitely. Its toxicity is related both to the dose and the duration of therapy. Toxic effects include anemia, neutropenia, thrombocytopenia, headaches, nausea, myalgia, insomnia, and neurologic side effects. Present study doses range from 120 mg/m^2/dose to 220 mg/m^2/dose (orally), but further studies are needed to define better the optimal dose, route of administration, and long-term risk/benefit.

Other agents under investigation include dideoxycytidine (ddc) and dideoxyinosine (ddz).

Vaccines

The development of an effective vaccine is beset by numerous barriers. These include the genetic diversity of HIV, the lack of a good animal model, the appropriate reluctance to experiment with attenuated strains, the lack of evidence that humoral immunity is protective, and the absence of a controllable study population.

Clinical trials of a recombinant HIV envelope vaccine are in progress.

PROGNOSIS

The spectrum of illness caused by HIV infection in children ranges from those who have fully developed HIV-associated immunodeficiency in the first 6 months of life to those who have perinatally acquired infection but still are clinically well at 10 years of age.[19]

For perinatally acquired disease, the mean incubation pe-

Table 178-1 *Pathogens in HIV-infected children*

ORGANISM	SYNDROME	METHOD OF DIAGNOSIS	TREATMENT	COMMENTS
Pneumocystis carinii	Pneumonia	Pneumocysts seen on special stains of respiratory specimen or tissue	TMP-SMX (20 mg/kg TMP component/day IV or PO) or pentamidine isethionate (4 mg/kg/day IV or IM)	Toxic effects of therapy common; treat 21 days, relapses common, prophylaxis may be beneficial
Toxoplasma gondii	Brain abscess	Brain scans; biopsy	Sulfadiazine and pyrimethamine (PO)	Toxic effects of therapy common; use folinic acid; lifelong therapy to prevent relapse
Cryptosporidium sp.	Gastroenteritis	Stool examination (special procedure); biopsy	Best therapy not known; supportive	Chronic infection
Candida sp.	Thrush, esophagitis	Wet mount or Gram stain of lesions (thrush); esophagoscopy and biopsy (esophagus)	Nystatin, clotrimazole, ketoconazole, amphotericin B	Relapses common; consider maintenance
Cryptococcus sp.	Meningitis, fungemia, pneumonia	Cryptococcal antigen tests on blood, CSF; culture of blood, respiratory specimen, CSF; India ink test on CSF	Amphotericin B	Flucytosine can be used if tolerated; chronic suppressive therapy required to prevent relapse
Cytomegalovirus	Chorioretinitis, pneumonitis, hepatitis, colitis, esophagitis, encephalitis, disseminated (including adrenals)	Ophthalmologic examination (retinitis); tissue biopsy; culture (urine, sputum, buffy coat)	Gancyclovir (investigational)	Relapses after therapy; suppressive regimen required; isolation of virus does not alone provide diagnosis
Herpes simplex virus	Stomatitis, perianal infection	Tzanck preparation; culture	Acyclovir (750 $mg/m^2/day$ IV, can treat PO)	Recurrences frequent; chronic suppressive therapy may be needed
Varicella zoster virus	Primary varicella, local or disseminated zoster	Tzanck preparation; culture	Acyclovir (1500 $mg/m^2/day$ IV)	Chronic or relapsing zoster lesions occur; indications for and effectiveness of oral therapy not clear
Mycobacterium avium/intracellulare	Disseminated infection (blood, bone marrow, liver, spleen, gastrointestinal tract, nodes)	Acid-fast blood culture; acid-fast stain or culture of tissue or fluid specimen	Uncertain	Drugs used have included ansamycin, clofazimine, ethambutol, amikacin, rifampin, isoniazid, ethionamide, but efficacy not documented

Modified from Falloon J et al: Human immunodeficiency virus in children, J Pediatr 114:17, 1989.
TMP-SMX, Trimethoprim-sulfamethoxazole; *CSF,* cerebrospinal fluid.

riod is estimated to be 7 to 9 months.[22,24] The range, however, extends to a decade or more. The mean incubation period of transfusion-acquired HIV disease is estimated to be 17 months.[22] These incubation periods may be biased by patients with early symptoms of disease because the patients included were identified by clinical illness rather than by prospective surveillance of seropositivity.[11]

SUMMARY

The pediatric population represents the most rapidly growing group of patients with confirmed HIV infection. Pediatricians need to become familiar with the wide spectrum of clinical manifestation and the subtleties encountered in diagnosing HIV infection. Surely, the principles of clinical care will evolve rapidly over the next two decades; however, the need for social and educational intervention is immediate and compelling.

We abide in the hope that a preventive vaccine or a cure will be found; however, we must continue emphasizing that responsible sexual behavior and avoidance of drug use will prevent the further spread of this incurable disease.

REFERENCES

1. American Academy of Pediatrics, Committee on Infectious Diseases: Health guidelines for the attendance in day-care and foster care settings of children infected with human immunodeficiency virus, Pediatrics 79:466, 1987.
2. Andiman WA: Virologic and serologic aspects of human immunodeficiency virus infection in infants and children, Semin Perinatol 13:16, 1989.
3. Andiman WA et al: Prospective studies of a cohort of 50 infants born to HIV seropositive mothers, Pediatr Res 23:363A, 1988.
4. Beckford AP, Kaschula ROC, and Stephen C: Factors associated with fatal cases of measles: a retrospective autopsy study, S Afr Med J 68:858, 1985.
5. Bowen D, Lane H, and Fauci A: Immunopathogenesis of the acquired immunodeficiency syndrome, Ann Intern Med 5:704, 1985.
6. Centers for Disease Control: Update: AIDS–United States, MMWR 32:688, 1984.
7. Centers for Disease Control: Revision of the case definition of AIDS for rational reporting—United States, MMWR 34:373, 1985.
8. Centers for Disease Control: Immunization of children infected with human T-lymphotropic virus type III/lymphadenopathy-associated virus, MMWR 35:595, 1986.
9. Centers for Disease Control: Public Health Service guidelines for counseling and antibody testing to prevent HIV infection and AIDS, MMWR 36:509, 1987.
10. Centers for Disease Control: Revision of the CDC surveillance case definition for AIDS, MMWR 36(1):1S, 1987.
11. Centers for Disease Control: Supplementary ACIP statement: Immunization of children infected with human immunodeficiency virus, MMWR 37:181, 1988.
12. Centers for Disease Control: Update: Universal precautions for prevention of transmission of human immunodeficiency virus, hepatitis B virus, and other bloodborne pathogens in health-care settings, MMWR 37:June 24, 1988.
13. Centers for Disease Control: Guidelines for prevention of transmission of human immunodeficiency virus and hepatitis B virus to health-care and public safety workers, MMWR 38:June 23, 1989.
14. Curless R: Congenital AIDS: review of neurologic problems, Childs Nerv Syst 5:9, 1989.
15. Falloon J et al: Human immunodeficiency virus infection in children, J Pediatr 114:1, 1989.
16. Hein K: AIDS in adolescence: exploring the challenge, J Adolesc Health Care 10:10S, 1989.
17. Heyward WL and Curran JW: The epidemiology of AIDS in the U.S. Sci Am, p52, Oct 1988.
18. Stewart JM et al: Symptomatic cardiac dysfunction in children with human immunodeficiency virus infection, American Heart Journal, 117:140, 1989.
19. Krasinski K, Borkowsky W, and Holzman RS: Prognosis of human immunodeficiency virus infection in children and adolescents, Pediatr Infect Dis J 8:216, 1989.
20. Levy JA: Human immunodeficiency virus and the pathogenesis of AIDS, JAMA 261:2997, 1989.
21. Levy JA: The human immunodeficiency viruses: detection and pathogenesis. In Levy JA, editor: AIDS: Pathogenesis and treatment, New York, 1989, Marcel Dekker, Inc.
22. Rogers MF et al: Acquired immunodeficiency syndrome in children: report of the Centers for Disease Control national surveillance, 1982 to 1985, Pediatrics 79:1008, 1987.
23. Rogers MF et al: Use of the polymerase chain reaction for early detection of the proviral sequences of human immunodeficiency virus in infants born to seropositive mothers, N Engl J Med 320:1649, 1989.
24. Scott G et al: Analysis of survival in children with human immunodeficiency virus (HIV) infection, Pediatr Res 23:381, 1988.
25. Straka BF et al: Cutaneous manifestations of the acquired immunodeficiency syndrome in children, J Am Acad Dermatol 18:1089, 1988.
26. Strauss J et al: Renal disease in children with the acquired immunodeficiency syndrome, N Engl J Med 321:625, 1989.
27. Weinblatt ME et al: Thrombocytopenia in an infant with AIDS, Am J Dis Child 141:15, 1987.

SUGGESTED READING

Someone at school has AIDS: a guide to developing policies for students and school staff members who are infected with HIV, Alexandria, Va, 1989, National Association of State Boards of Education (pamphlet).

179

Allergic Rhinitis

Kenneth C. Schuberth

Allergic rhinitis is the most common clinical expression of atopic hypersensitivity. It occurs in as much as 10% of the general population and may exist alone or in combination with asthma or eczema. In children it is unusual before age 4 years but increases in frequency thereafter, especially at puberty.[1] The most common form is the typical "seasonal" spring-fall pattern, often referred to as hay fever or pollinosis. Year-round, "perennial" allergic rhinitis triggered by household inhaled allergens is less frequent and more difficult to diagnose.

ETIOLOGY

The tendency to develop allergic rhinitis is clearly inherited. When a child with a genetic predisposition to allergy is exposed to a strong allergic stimulus, antigen-specific IgE molecules are produced and bind to submucosal mast cells located in the respiratory tract epithelium. Once the individual has been sensitized in this way, reexposure to the offending allergen causes an immediate type I hypersensitivity reaction, in which cross-linking of cell surface IgE molecules triggers the release of mast cell mediators such as histamine, prostaglandins, and leukotrienes, along with eosinophil and neutrophil chemotactic factors.[5] Histamine causes immediate local vasodilation, mucosal edema, and increased mucous production. The chemotactic factors summon cells to the area, which accounts for the slower "late-phase reaction," resulting in inflammation and destruction of the mucosal surface, progressing to chronic nasal obstruction.

The severity of symptoms varies tremendously and depends on both the individual's level of sensitivity and the intensity of the antigen exposure.

The allergens most often responsible include the following:

1. Pollens. Wind-borne pollens from trees and grasses in the spring and weeds, especially ragweed, in the fall cause well-defined seasonal symptoms. Most flower pollens are insect borne and rarely cause problems.
2. Molds. In cold climates, outdoor molds produce spores beginning in the early spring and peaking in late fall. In warm climates without frost, molds can grow year-round.
3. Animal danders. Scales from the skin of house pets such as dogs and cats can produce severe intermittent as well as perennial symptoms.
4. Dust mites. The ubiquitous, microscopic insects are the major allergen in house dust. Mites prosper in warm, moist, indoor environments and colonize pillows, mattresses, and carpets. They are the major cause of perennial rhinitis.[2]

CLINICAL FEATURES

The triad of nasal congestion, sneezing, and rhinorrhea is characteristic of allergic rhinitis.[2] Younger children usually have perennial symptoms, whereas pollen sensitivity becomes more common after age 6 years. In the acute, seasonal pollen-related variety, the symptoms may be quite intense and often include itching of the palate and throat, headaches, and itchy, tearing eyes. The patient often can identify the specific allergen responsible. Perennial sufferers may have more non-specific problems such as frequent "colds," recurrent otitis media, nasal speech, mouth-breathing, snoring during sleep, fatigue, malaise, and poor school performance. Epistaxis is common. The rhinorrhea is usually clear unless there is a superimposed infection. Many children will perform the "allergic salute," a maneuver in which they sniff and sweep the palm of their hand upward across the nose in an attempt to open their nasal passages or to relieve nasal itching.

The physical examination usually reveals striking features. The nasal mucosa is pale, bluish, and boggy, with a clear serous discharge. The nasal turbinates are enlarged, sometimes enough to produce almost total airway obstruction. Children with perennial problems often have the typical "allergic facies," consisting of (1) "allergic shiners"—dark discoloration beneath both eyes; (2) "Dennie lines"—extra wrinkles below the lower eyelids; and (3) mouth-breathing. The tonsils and adenoids often are enlarged, and there may be evidence of middle-ear effusion. Nasal polyps are uncommon in childhood allergic rhinitis.

COMPLICATIONS

Early in life, children with allergic rhinitis suffer from an increased incidence of respiratory infections, acute otitis media, and eustachian tube dysfunction, leading to more chronic serous otitis media. Many authors have suggested an association between allergy and chronic serous otitis media, although this is only one of many risk factors. Adenoidal enlargement, nasal speech, and abnormal facial development from chronic mouth-breathing occasionally develop in these patients. Acute and chronic sinusitis are common, probably the result of decreased ciliary clearance and obstruction of sinus ostia. Asthma appears to be a concomitant development in atopic persons and not a complication of untreated allergic rhinitis. There is no good evidence that immunotherapy for allergic rhinitis will prevent the subsequent development of asthma.

LABORATORY FINDINGS

The nasal smear for eosinophils is a simple office procedure that will help confirm the clinical diagnosis.[4] The patient should be instructed to blow his or her nose into a plastic or wax paper wrap, and the secretions are spread onto a glass slide and left to dry overnight. The slide is then prepared with Hansel stain. A cotton swab may be used to obtain secretions if the patient cannot blow. If more than 10% of the cells seen on the smear are eosinophils, an ongoing allergic process is probable. Strongly positive results are most likely during heavy allergenic exposure. Concurrent nasal infection may obscure the results, and eosinophils may be absent during the "off season."

Blood eosinophilia (greater than 5% eosinophils on the differential white blood count or greater than $250/mm^3$ on the proportionate total white blood cell count) occasionally is found. An elevated total serum IgE is suggestive of atopy, but many patients with uncomplicated allergic rhinitis have normal serum IgE levels.

Skin tests and radioallergosorbent tests (RAST) detect the presence of antigen-specific IgE and identify individual allergens in patients who need aggressive managment. Skin tests always should be performed by a physician trained in allergy and interpreted in the light of the clinical history. Screening with RAST has the disadvantages, compared with skin testing, of higher cost and lower sensitivity.

In selected patients, impedance audiometry may help to document eustachian tube dysfunction. Sinusitis, diagnosed on a roentgenogram, is common, especially in older children, and pulmonary function testing occasionally demonstrates reversible obstructive airway disease.

DIFFERENTIAL DIAGNOSIS

There usually is very little difficulty in making the clinical diagnosis of seasonal allergic rhinitis on the basis of family history, clinical presentation, physical examination, and a knowledge of the local pollens. On the other hand, children with nonspecific perennial problems often pose a difficult diagnostic challenge. Two other conditions often confused with allergic rhinitis are recurrent upper respiratory tract infections and vasomotor rhinitis. Children with recurrent viral and/or bacterial infections can be differentiated from those with allergies by their intermittent course, a history of contagion, the presence of fever, purulent nasal discharge, red, inflamed nasal mucosa, and the absence of eosinophils on nasal smear. The family history for allergy is negative, and the serum IgE level is normal.

Vasomotor rhinitis is an ill-defined condition beginning in early childhood, characterized by hyperreactivity of the nasal mucous membranes to a wide variety of irritant stimuli.[2] Perennial nasal obstruction unresponsive to environmental controls and/or medications usually is the most prominent symptom. There is no family history of allergy, the nasal smear and skin test results are negative, the serum IgE levels are normal, and there are no eye signs or other atopic manifestations. Treatment is based on symptoms.

A third variant of perennial rhinitis recently has been described, eosinophilic nonallergic rhinitis—a condition affecting adolescents and adults in which the nasal smear is positive for eosinophils, but serum IgE levels are normal and skin test results are negative.[3]

Other less common conditions that may mimic allergic rhinitis include the presence of a nasal foreign body, choanal atresia, congenital syphilis, enlarged adenoids, rhinitis medicamentosa, cystic fibrosis, and nasopharyngeal tumors.

TREATMENT

Many children manage quite adequately by avoiding allergens and taking medication for symptoms. If symptoms are perennial, are unresponsive to medication, or become worse each year, an allergist should be consulted to confirm the diagnosis, to identify specific allergens, and possibly to prescribe immunotherapy.

Avoidance measures are easier for small children who are confined to the home. Particular attention should be directed to the child's room or other settings in which most time is spent. Dust control measures, removal of animals, and elimination of indoor mold are first steps. Pollen-allergic children can be helped dramatically by closing windows and using a room air conditioner. Forced air heating systems can be improved by adding humidifiers and air filters.

Antihistamines are the mainstay of pharmacologic treatment for allergic rhinitis.[7] They inhibit the histamine effect by blocking its binding to H_1 receptors and are most effective in treating sneezing, rhinorrhea, and nasal itching. They are grouped into several large classes according to structure. The three classes (and examples) used commonly for treating rhinitis are as follows:

Class I: ethanolamines (diphenhydramine [Benadryl])
Class II: ethylenediamines (tripelennamine [Pyribenzamine])
Class III: alkylamines (chlorpheniramine [Chlor-trimeton])

These medications are most effective when given before allergen exposure and often must be used in doses larger than those recommended on the packages. Many are available in long-acting form, which allows twice-daily dosing. Their usefulness sometimes is limited by their sedative side effects or by the development of tachyphylaxis, which can be averted by switching to an antihistamine from another class. Newer, nonsedative antihistamines such as terfenadine (Seldane) and astemizole (Hismanal) provide an alternative for older children who are unable to tolerate the sedative side effects of traditional antihistamines.

Alpha-adrenergic agents such as pseudoephedrine and phenylephrine cause vasoconstriction of the small blood vessels in the nose. They are helpful, either alone or in combination with antihistamines, when nasal congestion is a major symptom. Most of the over-the-counter cold preparations contain a combination of adrenergic and antihistamine compounds. Side effects that limit their usefulness include nervousness and tachycardia. Nasal sprays may provide transient relief, which usually is followed after several days by rebound congestion. Prolonged use of nasal sprays has led to worsening of symptoms, a condition known as rhinitis medicamentosa. Therefore their use should be discouraged. Vasoconstrictor eye drops (naphazoline [Vasocon]) help with ocular irritation.

Corticosteroids usually provide dramatic relief but should be used only in cases unresponsive to less potent medication. The newer fluorinated steroid nasal sprays—for example, beclomethasone (Vancenase) and flunisolide (Nasalide)—reduce mucosal inflammation and shrink nasal polyps with less systemic absorption than do the older dexamethasone preparations.[6,9] They are most useful for short-term treatment of acute seasonal problems. Short courses of oral steroids (e.g., prednisone) should be reserved for severe intransigent cases unresponsive to other therapies.

Patients who do not respond to "avoidance" and medication should be referred for skin testing to identify specific allergens. If the clinical history and skin test results correlate, immunotherapy becomes a logical part of the treatment program.[8] Usually a 3- to 5-year course of regular injections is necessary. Immunotherapy causes the production of IgG antibodies, which block the binding of allergens to IgE-primed mast cells. It is most effective in the treatment of seasonal pollenosis, but it also is beneficial in dust mite and cat dander allergy. As treatment progresses, patients can expect a gradual decrease in symptoms and reduced reliance on medication. Because of the risk of local and generalized reactions to the material injected and because of the inconvenience and expense associated with weekly injections, it is essential that immunotherapy be used selectively.

PROGNOSIS

Allergic rhinitis, like other allergic disorders, is an illness that waxes and wanes over time. Most children tend to improve with time, although very few, probably less than 10%, will lose their sensitivity completely. Remissions of symptoms may result from changes in environment, avoidance programs, and immunotherapy. It is important to counsel patients that allergic symptoms can be controlled but not eliminated entirely and that the success of any treatment program will depend on an understanding of the causes of symptoms and compliance with the regimen prescribed.

REFERENCES

1. Broder I et al: Epidemiology of asthma and allergic rhinitis in a total community: Tecumseh, Michigan. IV. Natural history, J Allergy Clin Immunol 54:100, 1974.
2. Meltzer EO, Schatz M, and Zeiger RS: Allergic and nonallergic rhinitis. In Middleton E Jr et al, editors: Allergy: principles and practice, ed 3, St Louis, 1988, The CV Mosby Co.
3. Mullarkey MF: Eosinophilic nonallergic rhinitis, J Allergy Clin Immunol 82:941, 1988.
4. Mullarkey MF, Hill JS, and Webb DR: Allergic and non-allergic rhinitis: their characterization with attention to the meaning of nasal eosinophilia, J Allergy Clin Immunol 65:122, 1980.
5. Naclerio RM: The pathophysiology of allergic rhinitis, J Allergy Clin Immunol 82:927, 1988.
6. Siegel SC et al: Multicentric study of beclomethasone dipropionate nasal aerosol in adults with seasonal allergic rhinitis, J Allergy Clin Immunol 69:345, 1982.
7. Simons FER: Allergic rhinitis: recent advances, Pediatr Clin North Am 35:1053, 1988.
8. VanMetre TE and Adkinson NF: Immunotherapy for aeroallergen disease. In Middleton E Jr et al, editors: Allergy: principles and practice, ed 3, St Louis, 1988, The CV Mosby Co.
9. Welsh PW et al: Efficacy of beclomethasone nasal solution, flunisolide and cromolyn in relieving symptoms of ragweed allergy, Mayo Clin Proc 62:125, 1987.

180

Animal Bites

Peter G. Szilagyi

It is estimated that annually more than 2 million persons across the United States are bitten by animals.[7] Dog bites account for more than 90% of these injuries, cat bites for most of the remainder, and rodent, rabbit, or, rarely, other wild animal bites for a very small number. Although 50% of these animal bites are trivial, requiring no medical treatment, up to 10% are severe enough to require suturing and about 2% hospitalization.[3] Of the visits to pediatric emergency department, 1% are for animal bites.[1] Children sustain the greatest number of animal bites, probably because of their frequent contact with domestic animals and their lack of experience in dealing with them properly. The peak age for animal bites is 5 to 14 years, and boys are twice as likely to sustain these injuries as are girls.[3,7] Not surprisingly, the vast majority of the animals live in the victim's neighborhood (75%) or own home (15%); in most instances the bites are provoked by humans. With the recent trend toward the purchase of guard dogs by many urban families, including pit bulls, the incidence of dog bites is likely to rise and pediatricians should be familiar with preventive strategies and management of these injuries.[2]

The major morbidity from animal bites results from direct trauma and infection. Although dog bites are more likely to produce lacerations or avulsions, these open wounds can be débrided and cleaned to prevent infection. Puncture wounds, which usually do not require suturing, can result, however, in deep tissue infections.[2,6,10]

Although 75% of all animal bites involve the extremities, facial bites (10% of the total) are relatively common in school-aged children[7] and account for several pediatric fatalities per year.

MICROBIOLOGY

As shown in Table 180-1, the risk of infection varies according to several factors. Hand wounds are most likely to become infected, partly because of the type of wound (frequently puncture), the relatively poor vascular supply, and the vulnerability of the closed spaces of the hand. As noted, puncture wounds, often by cat or human bites, are more likely to become infected than are lacerations. If more than 24 hours has elapsed before medical attention is sought, the risk of infection is substantially increased. Finally, cat and human bites result in a greater risk of infection than do dog bites, partly because these bites more often cause puncture wounds and dog bites frequently cause open lacerations.

The majority of bacteria associated with bite wounds are common organisms that reside in the animal's oral cavity. In addition, bacteria on the victim's skin may contribute to infection. Most infections comprise multiple pathogens[8] and often involve both aerobes and anaerobes. *Pasteurella multocida,* a gram-negative, facultative anaerobe found in the mouths of most dogs and cats, is highly associated with cat bite infections (up to 80%) and, to a lesser extent, with dog bite infections (12% to 50%). Although the exact frequency of other pathogenic bacteria isolated from infected animal bites varies across studies, aerobic gram-negative organisms most frequently are found (e.g., *Pseudomonas, Klebsiella,* and *Enterobacter* spp.). However, gram-positive aerobes (*Staphylococcus aureus, S. epidermidis,* and *Streptococcus* spp.) and anaerobes (e.g., *Bacteroides, Fusobacterium,* and *Peptococcus* spp.) are often noted.[1-3,6-10] Finally, an important group of gram-negative bacteria, classified by the Centers for Disease Control as alpha-numeric organisms, has been frequently isolated from dog bite wounds. Interestingly, human bites rarely are infected by *P. multocida,* but frequently are associated with aerobic gram-positive organisms, gram-negative anaerobes, or *Eikenella corrodens,* a genus that is almost unique to human bites but that occurs rarely in cat bites.

CLINICAL DIAGNOSIS

Important historical points include the length of time since injury, the type of animal (including domestic or wild), the present location and health of the animal, and the prior wound management. The physical examination entails a careful musculoskeletal and neurologic examination to determine damage to underlying structures and a thorough inspection of the wound for signs of infection. Special attention must be given

Table 180-1 *Risk Factors for Infection in Animal Bites*

RISK FACTOR	INFECTION RATES
Location[6] of bite	Hand (18%-36%) > arm or leg (12%-16%) > face (5%-11%)
Type of wound[2,6,10]	Puncture with laceration (17%-26%) > laceration alone (9%-12%)
Time of bite before medical care	If >24 hr, risk of infection is higher
Type of animal	Cat bites (40%-50%) Dog bites (10%-30%) Human bites (13%-40%)[8]

to bites involving the hand because, particularly in deep puncture wounds, superficial signs of infection (redness, swelling, purulent drainage) may be absent. Finally, the clinician should be aware that deep infections of tendons or bones and systemic infections can occur after untreated animal bites.

The time of the infection's onset may be a clue to *P. multocida* infection. Cellulitis from this organism generally develops rapidly, within hours of the animal bite, whereas systemic signs (fever, lymphangitis) usually are absent.[9] A cellulitis that has developed gradually, over days, more likely is due to gram-positive cocci or to other pathogenic bacteria.

A Gram stain of a wound specimen is not useful because findings do not correlate with culture results. Cultures of clinically infected animal bite wounds are reported to have "no growth" in up to one third of cases; conversely, cultures of clinically noninfected bite wounds grow a wide spectrum of oral flora bacteria in up to one third of cases.[11] Moreover, such cultures do not predict the likelihood of subsequent infection; nor do results correlate with culture findings when clinical infection becomes apparent. Cultures of clinically infected wounds, however, may help to ensure that the causative bacteria are sensitive to the antibiotic used.

The clinician should remember that cat-scratch disease is a relatively common complication of cat bites and, less commonly, of bites by other animals. This entity often begins with the development of a red, painless papule at the site of a recent scratch or bite; then, within weeks, a tender, enlarged, regional lymph node appears, usually associated with fever, malaise, and other systemic symptoms. This self-limited illness, caused by a gram-negative bacillus, is diagnosed clinically because the cat-scratch skin test reagent used to substantiate the clinical diagnosis is not licensed and therefore not available for use in most clinical settings. The role of antibiotics in the treatment of this disease is not clear; however, because the disease is self-limited, their use is seldom indicated. Large, tender, fluctuant lymph nodes may require aspiration or incision and drainage.

Animal bites from nondomestic animals require careful attention. Often the animal is not available for examination and observation. The animals most frequently involved are rats, mice, skunks, raccoons, fox, cattle, bats, and a variety of others. One concern of parents and physicians is the possibility of rabies, which is harbored in many areas of the United States in skunks, bats, raccoons, and foxes and in some areas even in domestic animals.[12] In the United States, in all cases of rabies resulting from a dog or a cat bite, the infected animal has been noted to become ill during the standard 10-day confinement and observation period; thus location, confinement, and observation of the animal are important. In cases of wild animal bites, consultation with the local health department is helpful in determining the risk of rabies in a specific animal for a particular geographic region. In general, bats and wild skunks, foxes, raccoons, and other carnivores are considered rabid until proved otherwise by laboratory tests;[12] in the interum, or if the biting animal cannot be found, treatment with human rabies immunoglobulin plus human diploid cell vaccine is recommended.

A variety of rare diseases have been described after wild animal bites, and consultation with the local health department may help establish their diagnosis and manage their treatment. Rat bite fever, a systemic illness caused by *Streptobacillus moniliformis* or *Spirillum minus* after a rat bite, is one such example. The *Red Book* (published by the American Academy of Pediatrics' Committee on Infectious Diseases) contains comprehensive and up-to-date descriptions of unusual diseases transmitted by various domestic and wild animals.

MANAGEMENT

The initial step in treating animal bites is meticulous wound care. This involves gently cleaning with soap and water and vigorously irrigating with saline solution. Saline irrigation of the wound with a syringe and a 19-gauge needle generates increased pressure that facilitates cleansing of the wound and reducing the risk of infection.[5] Devitalized tissue should be débrided. Puncture wounds should be cleansed, but irrigation is ineffective and may result in further damage to underlying structures. Elevation and immobilization are important for significant extremity injuries. The child's immunization status should be assessed and tetanus prophylaxis given if indicated.

Primary closure of lacerations caused by animal (or human) bites is controversial.[5,6] Clearly, infected wounds should not be closed in this way. The general consensus is that most noninfected lacerations can be sutured, after meticulous cleansing and irrigation, for cosmetic purposes or for hemostasis, without increasing the risk of infection. Hand wounds may be an exception[5,10] because of the great likelihood of infection and the risk of serious complications from deep closed-space infections; in these cases, suturing is recommended only for large wounds.

Radiologic studies may be necessary in deep puncture wounds to determine if the periosteum has been penetrated. This includes studies of the calvaria of small children who sustain bites to the head.

The role of prophylactic antibiotics in noninfected animal bite wounds is controversial.[4-6,10] It is prudent to treat, prophylactically (for 5 to 7 days), bites that have a high likelihood of infection, including (1) puncture wounds (particularly from cat bites), (2) human bites, and (3) bites of the hands and face. If infected, bite wounds brought to medical attention after 24 hours should be treated with antibiotics. The choice of antibiotics depends on culture results or, if cultures are not available, on the likely pathogens. Although penicillin is active against *P. multocida* and many oral flora, the addition of a penicillinase-resistant antibiotic provides more effective coverage. Amoxicillin/clavulnic acid (Augmentin) is an excellent choice for empiric treatment of bites from all animals. As mentioned, rabies prophylaxis should be administered, depending on the type of animal and the prevalence of rabies in the community.

ANTICIPATORY GUIDANCE

Although pets provide hours of delight and companionship for children, education about responsible care of a pet is important. Preschool-aged children should not be allowed alone with a pet, and they should be advised never to tease animals, approach strange animals, or play with pets that are eating.[10] Families with children should be advised not to purchase (1) dogs bred for aggressiveness or (2) wild animals. Finally, vaccinations for pets and routine visits to a veterinarian should be encouraged. (See Chapter 21, "Accident Prevention," for a more detailed discussion of animal safety rules for children.)

REFERENCES

1. Aghababian RV and Conte JE Jr: Mammalian bite wounds, Ann Emerg Med 9:79, 1980.
2. Baker MD: Bites and scratches: when pets fight back, Contemp Pediatr 6:76, 1989.
3. Berzon PR: The animal bite epidemic in Baltimore, Maryland: review and update, Am J Public Health 68:593, 1978.
4. Boenning DA, Fleisher GR, and Campos JM: Dog bites in children: epidemiology, microbiology and penicillin prophylactic therapy, Am J Emerg Med 1:17, 1983.
5. Callaham ML: Treatment of common dog bites: infection risk factors, J Am Coll Emerg Med 7:83, 1978.
6. Callaham M: Prophylactic antibiotics in common dog bite wounds: a controlled study, Ann Emerg Med 9:410, 1980.
7. Kizer KW: Epidemiologic and clinical aspects of animal bite injuries, J Am Coll Emerg Phys 8:134, 1979.
8. Lindsey D et al: Natural course of the human bite wound: incidence of infection and complications in 434 bites and 803 lacerations in the same group of patients, J Trauma 27:45, 1987.
9. Lucas GL and Bartlett DH: *Pasteurella multocida* infection in the hand, Plast Reconstr Surg 67:49, 1981.
10. Marcy SM: Management of pediatric infectious diseases in office practice: infections due to dog and cat bites (special series), Pediatr Infect Dis 1:351, 1982.
11. Ordog GJ: The bacteriology of dog bite wounds on initial presentation, Ann Emerg Med 15:1324, 1986.
12. Peter G et al: Report of the Committee on Infectious Diseases [Red Book], Elk Grove, Ill, 1988, American Academy of Pediatrics.

181

Anuria/Oliguria

Edward J. Ruley

Anuria (the failure to excrete any urine) or oliguria (the failure to excrete at least the minimal amount of urine that would be considered normal—defined as <500 ml/1.73 m/BSA (body surface area) in children or <0.5 ml/kg/hr in infants) may represent a physiologic or a pathologic phenomenon. In a water-deprived child the kidney tubules will reabsorb the majority of the glomerular filtrate to maintain the water content of the body. In an extreme case this physiologic response may result in oliguria or anuria. Conversely, there are a large number of acute renal insults or chronic kidney diseases that can reduce glomerular filtration as a result of damage to the kidney parenchyma, thereby producing anuria or oliguria. In clinical practice, oliguria occurs more frequently than anuria.

An organized approach to the child with anuria or oliguria begins with a carefully performed physical examination (Fig. 181-1). The presence of a palpable, enlarged urinary bladder or kidney(s) indicates that urine is being formed but for some reason is not being emptied from the urinary tract. In contrast, if a distended urinary bladder or kidney(s) are not palpable, one must consider the patient's state of hydration in order to assess why urine apparently is not being formed. The systematic approach to these physical findings follows the algorithm in Fig. 181-1.

ACUTE URINARY RETENTION

One of the more common clinical circumstances of anuria in pediatric practice is acute urinary retention. In this situation a distended, often painful urinary bladder can be palpated or percussed just above the symphysis pubis, often extending as high as the umbilicus. Such a circumstance often occurs when the child's regular schedule is interrupted and the child feels that circumstances are not convenient or familiar enough to allow micturition. The child then consciously overrides the urge to micturate, and the urinary bladder becomes progressively more distended. Eventually the child experiences considerable lower abdominal pressure and pain but finds that voluntarily voiding is not possible because overdistention has exceeded the muscular compliance of the bladder, and an organized contraction coordinated with relaxation of the in-

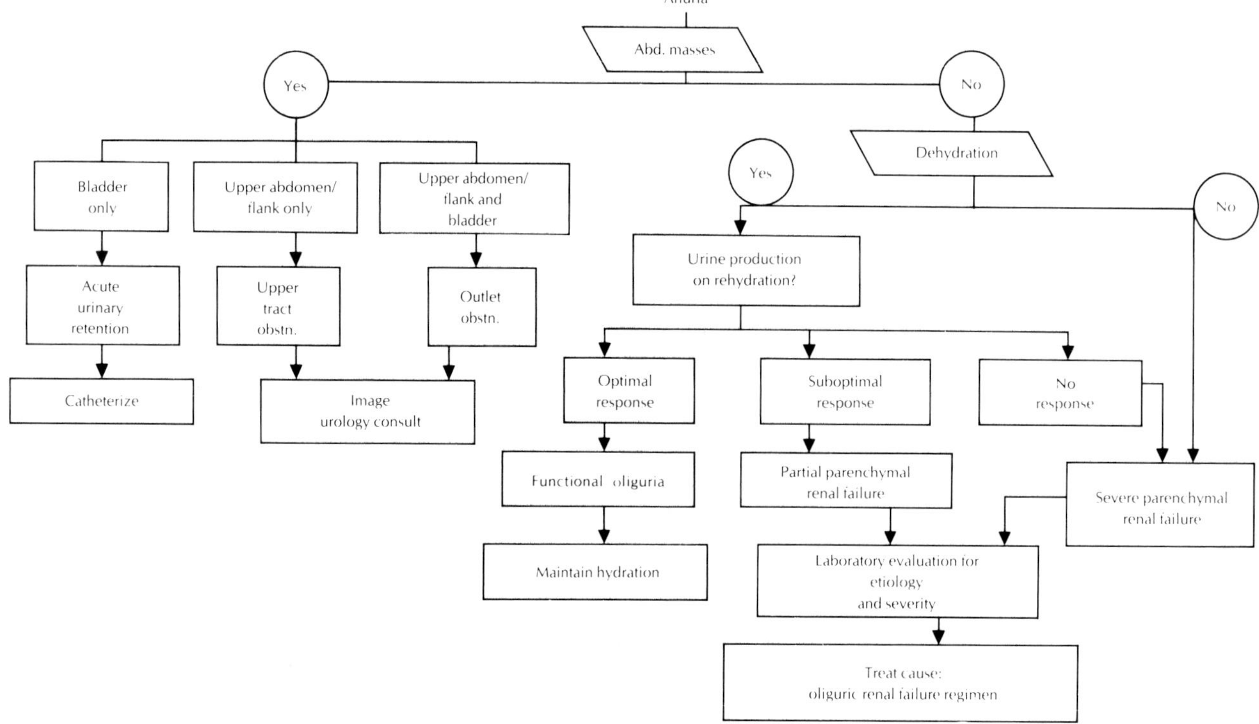

Fig. 181-1 Algorithm of physical examination of child with anuria.

ternal sphincter cannot be achieved. Simple catheterization to empty the bladder usually will relieve the symptoms and restore the compliance of the bladder musculature. It is unlikely that urinary retention will recur, and indwelling bladder catheterization is not indicated. If retention does recur, consideration should be given to a functional or anatomic bladder outlet obstruction, although this is rare.

URINARY OBSTRUCTION

Chronic partial urinary obstruction usually causes polyuria rather than anuria or oliguria. Polyuria in this circumstance occurs because obstruction first affects the medullary functions of the kidney, specifically the ability to reabsorb sodium and water. Chronic partial obstruction can be complicated by an acute complete obstruction that can produce anuria. Occasionally, severe chronic obstruction may so damage the kidney parenchyma that oliguria may develop.

Visualization of the urinary system by the use of ultrasound, computerized tomography, or excretory urography will confirm the diagnosis of obstruction and provide some indication of the site and degree of blockage. Urologic consultation is important in developing a plan for further evaluation and treatment of these children.

DEHYDRATION

In the patient without abdominal masses, the assessment of the state of hydration by clinical examination is the next step (Fig. 181-1). In the presence of significant dehydration, oliguria, or anuria caused by poor perfusion (functional renal failure mediated by a physiologic antidiuretic hormone response) must be differentiated from that caused by established parenchymal renal failure. This is accomplished by assessing the quality of urine remaining in the bladder and then determining the volume and quality of urine produced in response to prompt rehydration. To maximize the value of these studies, the child should be catheterized during rehydration. Catheterization will allow the residual urine to be quantified and renal function to be characterized as to sodium and water resorption capabilities (see Table 287-1). If the residual urine, however small the volume, demonstrates maximal water and sodium reabsorption and there is a prompt increase in urine production during rehydration, it may be presumed that the patient's oliguria or anuria was a physiologic response to dehydration. This should not recur, provided hydration is maintained.

If, however, there is no increased production of urine in the dehydrated patient on rehydration or if oliguria or anuria has occurred in the presence of near-normal hydration, the patient most likely has severe parenchymal renal failure. Most often this will be the result of an extensive parenchymal disease such as acute tubular necrosis or of a sudden renovascular catastrophe such as renal cortical necrosis. Prompt differentiation of functional (prerenal) failure from parenchymal renal failure is extremely important. Significant parenchymal renal failure may result from functional renal failure that goes untreated, as in the dehydrated patient who does not undergo prompt rehydration. The diagnostic evaluation and management of the child with severe renal failure are discussed in Chapter 287.

Finally, a dehydrated patient may have a partial response to rehydration in that the urine output increases but remains suboptimal. Such a patient most likely has partial parenchymal renal failure oliguria (see Chapter 287).

NEWBORNS

Anuria or oliguria in the newborn may represent bilateral renal agenesis or some other major congenital urologic anomaly. Often there is a maternal history of oligohydramnios that reflects a deficient production of fetal urine, a major source of amniotic fluid. Adequate amniotic fluid volume is important in normal fetal development because it promotes lung maturation and acts as a cushion for the fetus. Clues to a major urinary anomaly include a maternal history of small uterine size for gestational age, scanty amniotic fluid passage at delivery, and positional somatic abnormalities discovered on examination of the newborn.

Prenatal fetal sonographic examination may confirm the oligohydramnios and/or demonstrate renal structural abnormalities. Such information is important in parental counseling and in deciding on the optimal delivery date. At birth the blood chemistry test results of the newborn usually are normal because the biochemical status of the neonate is maintained by the mother in utero. Biochemical abnormalities attributable to renal failure usually become evident gradually over the first several weeks of life. Pneumothoraces develop in most of the children with bilateral renal agenesis, and they die of pulmonary immaturity rather than renal failure.

A pediatric nephrologist with experience in renal failure in the newborn should be involved in determining treatment options and in counseling the parents early in the course—prenatally if possible. With the advent of newer dialysis techniques and renal transplantation in small infants, the outlook is not as bleak as before, providing the infant can survive the pulmonary problems that are so common in the first month of life.

182

Appendicitis

R. Scott Strahlman

Although appendicitis is a surgical emergency, the pediatrician has a crucial role in the initial diagnosis and management of this problem and is often the first to suspect appendicitis and to contact the surgical team. The pediatrician's high index of suspicion can be the driving force that leads to an appropriate, timely appendectomy. Prompt diagnosis and preoperative management help to decrease the high morbidity associated with a perforated appendix.

Appendicitis is the most common cause of the acute surgical abdomen in childhood. While the exact incidence is unknown, appendicitis is rare in early childhood and becomes more frequent after age 10. The male to female ratio is 1:1 before puberty and about 2:1 after age 15 years. An increased incidence during the spring and autumn months has also been observed. In addition, appendicitis is more common in children with a family history of appendicitis.[3] Whether this tendency is genetic or diet related is unclear, because the risk of appendicitis may be decreased with a high-fiber diet.[4]

ETIOLOGY AND PATHOPHYSIOLOGY

Appendicitis is always initiated by obstruction of the appendiceal lumen, usually by a fecalith or by lymphoid hyperplasia. Rarely a parasite, tumor, or foreign body may obstruct the lumen. Finally, the inspissated secretions of cystic fibrosis may obstruct the appendiceal lumen (thus, although rarely, cystic fibrosis may present as appendicitis).[13]

As secretions accumulate within the obstructed appendix, the walls become distended. Continued distention causes ischemia and necrosis of the appendix, leading to irritation of the surrounding peritoneum.

Clinically, the initial distention of the appendiceal wall is manifested as a dull, steady periumbilical pain. This pain often shifts to the right lower quadrant after 4 to 6 hours, as local peritoneal inflammation occurs.

Without surgical intervention the appendix eventually ruptures, causing peritonitis. The incidence of rupture increases dramatically 24 to 36 hours after the onset of abdominal pain. A delay in surgery of more than 36 hours has at least a 65% incidence of perforation.[2] Organisms cultured in perforated appendicitis have included both aerobic and anaerobic bacteria.[15] The most common aerobic bacteria are *Escherichia coli*, *Klebsiella*, and *Proteus*. Common anaerobes include *Bacteroides* and *Clostridium* species.

INITIAL ASSESSMENT

History

A thorough history is invaluable in differentiating appendicitis from other disorders. An important component of that history is pain. The onset of symptoms is often heralded by a dull, steady periumbilical pain. The pain is more often suspected of being caused by acute appendicitis if it awakens the patient from sleep. Anorexia is always present. One or two episodes of vomiting may follow, but essentially never precede, the pain. After 4 to 6 hours the pain commonly migrates to the right lower quadrant. Given the many variations in the location of an appendix, however, the location of abdominal pain in appendicitis may vary. There is usually no change in bowel habits. A low-grade fever may be present, but the temperature is rarely above 100.3° F (38.5° C). If the clinical picture suggests but does not convince one of appendicitis, it is best to watch the progression of signs and symptoms carefully over several hours. Because an appendix rarely perforates within 24 hours of the onset of pain, a period of observation can safely differentiate a potentially surgical from a nonsurgical condition.

Physical Examination

A gentle and nonthreatening approach is most effective during the physical examination. One should look for peritoneal signs such as pain with walking or coughing. If the patient is able to jump up on the examining table, he or she does not have appendicitis. Patients may be most comfortable lying supine with the legs flexed. Abdominal tenderness is always present and is often greatest at McBurney's point (two thirds of the distance from the umbilicus to the anterosuperior iliac spine). Rebound tenderness of the abdomen (particularly that which is referred to the right lower quadrant) is often demonstrated, as is hyperesthesia of the skin overlying the painful area. Bowel sounds may be decreased or hyperactive. A rectal examination is essential and may show right-sided tenderness. Examination of the lungs is important to rule out a right lower lobe pneumonia that generates referred pain to the right lower quadrant of the abdomen. A pelvic examination is indicated in any female adolescent with abdominal pain to rule out gynecologic conditions.

Laboratory Tests

The only essential laboratory studies are a blood count and urinalysis. The white blood cell count is in the range of 10,000 to 20,000/mm^3, with a slight increase in the number of neutrophils, particularly younger forms. The erythrocyte sedimentation rate is usually normal. A urinalysis is performed to rule out urinary tract infection or diabetic ketoacidosis as causes of abdominal pain.

If the diagnosis is in doubt, abdominal roentgenograms are occasionally helpful. Radiographic features that suggest appendicitis include a calcified appendicolith or an air-filled appendix, although the absence of abnormalities does not rule out the diagnosis. Ultrasonography or a barium enema may help delineate an appendiceal abscess in cases that are not clear-cut.[9]

The typical progression of signs and symptoms in appendicitis may be summarized as follows: abdominal pain first, followed by nausea, vomiting, and localization of the pain to the right lower quadrant. Low-grade fever, tenderness on rectal examination, and a mild leukocytosis often accompany these symptoms.

DIFFERENTIAL DIAGNOSIS

The differential diagnosis of appendicitis is that of acute abdominal pain and is extensive (see accompanying box). Gastroenteritis can be differentiated from appendicitis on the basis of a benign abdominal examination in the former condition. Vomiting and diarrhea usually occur before the onset of pain, not afterward, as in appendicitis. Constipation can often appear to be appendicitis. However, this pain is usually diffuse, not localized to the right lower quadrant, and there is often a history of constipation. An abdominal flat plate roentgenogram can help in the diagnosis, and a small Fleet enema is often both diagnostic and therapeutic.

With an appropriate initial evaluation, the following nonsurgical conditions can be ruled out in the patient with abdominal pain: urinary tract infection; diabetic ketoacidosis; sickle-cell crisis; right lower lobe pneumonia with referred pain; nephrotic syndrome with primary peritonitis; and inflammatory bowel disease.

Gynecologic disorders can be ruled out on the basis of the history and pelvic examination; pelvic inflammatory disease, ovarian torsion, ectopic pregnancy, dysmenorrhea, and mittelschmerz can all mimic appendicitis.

Unusual conditions such as Henoch-Schönlein purpura and hemolytic-uremic syndrome may be indistinguishable from appendicitis.[8] Even Rocky Mountain spotted fever can mimic appendicitis.[7]

Surgical emergencies that mimic appendicitis (see box at right) can only be ruled out in the operating room.

NEONATAL APPENDICITIS

Appendicitis in the first 2 years of life is rare, comprising less than 2% of all childhood cases.[10] The mortality is high, however, and approaches 100% in cases with perforation.[11] Appendicitis must therefore be considered in any infant suspected of having abdominal pain. The presenting symptoms consist of vomiting and fever, and the baby may appear to be colicky. Physical examination shows abdominal distention with diffuse tenderness. Abdominal roentgenograms can be diagnostically helpful in a neonate by showing an appendicolith, free peritoneal fluid, bowel-wall edema, or free air. With a high index of suspicion, surgery must be performed immediately to prevent perforation and its high mortality.

MANAGEMENT

Once the diagnosis is made, the patient must be prepared for immediate surgery. Nothing is given by mouth, and a nasogastric tube is inserted and placed on low suction. Intravenous hydration is started (e.g., 10 ml/kg/hr of Ringer's lactate), and fever may be controlled with acetaminophen given per rectum. Broad-spectrum antibiotics (e.g., ampicillin, gentamicin, and clindamycin, or a cephalosporin) are administered preoperatively. Antibiotics have been shown to decrease the morbidity even in nonperforated cases.[5] An appendectomy is performed as soon as the patient's condition has been stabilized.

In patients with symptoms for 5 or more days and a palpable mass consistent with an appendiceal abscess, many surgeons prefer an initial nonoperative management.[14] The patient is treated with broad-spectrum antibiotics and, barring interim complications, is brought back in 4 to 6 weeks for an elective appendectomy. This approach lowers the incidence of peritonitis and its associated complications precipitated by surgical manipulation during the acute inflammatory stages of the disease.

Differential Diagnosis of Appendicitis

- Common conditions
  - Gastroenteritis
  - Constipation
- Medical problems
  - Urinary tract infection
  - Diabetic ketoacidosis
  - Sickle-cell crisis
  - Right lower lobe pneumonia
  - Primary peritonitis
  - Inflammatory bowel disease
- Gynecologic problems
  - Pelvic inflammatory disease
  - Ovarian torsion
  - Ruptured ectopic pregnancy
  - Dysmenorrhea
  - Mittelschmerz
- Unusual conditions
  - Henoch-Schönlein purpura
  - Hemolytic-uremic syndrome
  - Rocky Mountain spotted fever
- Surgical emergencies
  - Meckel diverticulitis
  - Intestinal adhesions
  - Intussusception
  - Necrotizing enterocolitis

PROGNOSIS

In uncomplicated appendicitis with prompt surgical repair, the mortality is less than 1% and there is essentially no long-term morbidity. The average hospital stay is about 4 days.[1] Although a ruptured appendix increases the risk of mortality only slightly (with most of that increase occurring in the neonatal age group), the average hospital stay is about 10 days. Complications causing the higher morbidity include peritonitis, postoperative abscesses, and prolonged ileus. A possible long-term complication of a ruptured appendix in women is infertility.[12]

The incidence of perforated appendicitis is about 35%, a disconcertingly high figure.[6] A higher index of suspicion on the part of pediatricians and the general public might lead to earlier diagnosis of the condition and decrease the incidence of appendiceal perforation and its morbid complications.

REFERENCES

1. Berry J and Malt R: Appendicitis near its centenary, Ann Surg 200:567, 1984.
2. Brender JD et al: Childhood appendicitis: factors associated with perforation, Pediatrics 76:2, 1985.
3. Brender JD et al: Is childhood appendicitis familial? Am J Dis Child 139:338, 1985.
4. Brender JD et al: Fiber intake and childhood appendicitis, Am J Public Health 75:399, 1985.
5. Busuttil RW et al: Effect of prophylactic antibiotics in acute nonperforated appendicitis, Ann Surg 194:502, 1981.
6. Cooperman M: Complications of appendectomy, Surg Clin North Am 63:1233, 1983.
7. Davis AE and Bradford WD: Abdominal pain resembling acute appendicitis in Rocky Mountain spotted fever, JAMA 247:2811, 1982.
8. Edmonson MB and Chesney RW: Hemolytic uremic syndrome confused with acute appendicitis, Arch Surg 113:754, 1978.
9. Garcia C et al: Appendicitis in children: accuracy of the barium enema, Am J Dis Child 141:1309, 1987.
10. Grosfeld JL, Weinberger M, and Clatworthy HW: Acute appendicitis in the first two years of life, J Pediatr Surg 8:285, 1973.
11. Kwong MS and Dinner M: Neonatal appendicitis masquerading as necrotizing enterocolitis, J Pediatr 96:917, 1980.
12. Mueller BA et al: Appendectomy and the risk of tubal infertility, N Engl J Med 315(24):1506, 1986.
13. Oestreich AE and Adelstein EH: Appendicitis as the presenting complaint in cystic fibrosis, J Pediatr Surg 17:191, 1982.
14. Powers RJ et al: Alternate approach to the management of acute perforating appendicitis in children, Surg Gynecol Obstet 152:473, 1981.
15. Stone HH: Bacterial flora of appendicitis in children, J Pediatr Surg 11:37, 1976.

SUGGESTED READINGS

Ballantine TV: Appendicitis (review), Surg Clin North Am 61:1117, 1981.
King DR et al: Antibiotic management of complicated appendicitis, J Pediatr Surg 18:945, 1983.
Ravitch MM: Appendicitis (review), Pediatrics 70:414, 1982.
Shaul WL: Clues to the early diagnosis of neonatal appendicitis, J Pediatr 98:473, 1981.
Siler W, editor: Cope's early diagnosis of the acute abdomen, New York, 1983, Oxford University Press, Inc.

183

Asthma

Philip Fireman

Asthma can be best defined as recurrent and reversible obstructive lung disease caused by hyperreactive airways. The obstruction of the hyperreactive airways results from bronchial smooth muscle contraction, increased mucous secretion, and edema with inflammation. Both large and small airways can be involved to a variable degree and are hyperresponsive to a variety of environmental stimuli. Symptoms and signs usually are episodic because of reversible airway obstruction that can improve either spontaneously or as the result of therapy. Although it can occur at any age, asthma usually has its onset within the first 5 years of life and is among the leading causes of both acute and chronic illness in children.[3] It is estimated that 5% to 10% of children have asthma at some time during childhood. In a recent survey conducted at Children's Hospital of Pittsburgh, asthma accounted for 10% of medical emergency room visits and 10% of medical hospitalizations. According to a 1970 U.S. Public Health Service survey, asthma is the most frequent cause of school absenteeism and chronic illness in children younger than 17 years of age.[6] Boys are affected more than girls (3:1 ratio), but the male preponderance does not persist past adolescence. The clinical spectrum of asthma is that of an illness beginning early in life that tends to improve during midchildhood and adolescence but continues on into adulthood in certain patients.[3,8] Of concern is an increase in hospital admissions and mortality during the past decade.[1] Asthma therefore is necessarily of particular interest to pediatricians and to all physicians interested in the care of childhood respiratory illnesses.

ETIOLOGY AND PATHOGENESIS

The pathogenesis is only partially understood, but asthma is a multifactorial respiratory illness involving immunologic, infectious, biochemical, autonomic nervous, and psychological factors to a varying degree in different individuals. Thus respiratory symptoms may develop in the affected individual after exposure to a variety of environmental stimuli, such as specific inhalant antigens, infectious agents, cold air, tobacco smoke, aerosolized chemicals, inert dusts, strong aromas, and the hyperventilation that can be associated with exercise, laughing, or crying. These environmental factors trigger the release or generation of certain mediators of inflammation—such as histamine, leukotrienes, and other agents that can induce smooth muscle contractions, mucous gland secretion, and inflammatory edema to provoke symptoms. Increased levels of plasma histamine recently have been reported during acute asthma in children.[7]

The fundamental abnormality, however, appears to be a genetically influenced hyperreactivity of the airways. Specifically, it has been proposed that the basic abnormality in asthma is that of *a defect in beta-adrenergic responsiveness,* either with or without increased cholinergic activity of the airways.[9] Inhalation challenge with methacholine or histamine to provoke airway obstruction has been proposed as a potential test in persons with asthma, but it is not suitable as a routine test for children. Recent studies have confirmed the impression of many pediatricians that *a history of bronchiolitis or croup is a risk factor for the development of asthma;* approximately 33% to 50% of children who have had more than one episode of bronchiolitis or croup during early life will subsequently demonstrate bronchial hyperreactivity.[2] It is interesting that one third of these patients' first-degree relatives also have airway hyperreactivity, which suggests a genetic predisposition. A relation between allergy and asthma also is proposed whenever specific antigen (allergen) inhalation challenge is documented as provoking signs and symptoms of asthma in the hypersensitive (allergic) host.

CLINICAL MANIFESTATIONS

Asthma in infants and children varies markedly among patients and sometimes even in the same patient. The illness may manifest in several clinical patterns. Patients may have occasional acute episodes of symptoms, which can vary from mild (requiring only minimal medication) to severe and life-threatening attacks of status asthmaticus, which demand hospitalization and treatment in an intensive care unit. Other children may have recurrent episodes every several months, yet appear to be well and symptom-free between episodes. Still others may have chronic or daily symptoms that variably interfere with life-style and have superimposed on this a number of acute episodes that can be severe but may vary in duration from several hours to days. Finally, a small number of patients (probably <1% of all asthmatic persons) have severe daily symptoms that require multiple medications and careful clinical monitoring. Studies indicate that *the most severely affected children have their onset of wheezing during the first year of life* and have a family history of asthma or other allergic disease, especially atopic dermatitis.

Many pediatricians hesitate to diagnose asthma in infancy because of difficulty in documenting the signs and symptoms of reversible obstructive airway disease. Yet, in most children who are subsequently diagnosed as having asthma, suggestive signs appear during the first year or two of life, usually associated with a viral respiratory infection that induces cough and "wheezy," labored respirations. The mechanism of this virus-induced wheezing has been shown to involve virus-specific IgE antibody and increased release of histamine into the secretions of young children infected with respiratory syncytial virus.[10] The infectious agents involved during the preschool years are primarily the respiratory syncytial virus, with fewer episodes being associated with parainfluenza virus; rhinovirus and influenza viruses are more significant in older children and adults.[4] Bacterial infections rarely are associated with acute exacerbations of asthma, except as secondary invaders or as a cause of an associated sinusitis. In many patients *atopic dermatitis (infantile eczema) is either a prior manifestation or an associated condition*. There is no correlation linking the severity of the dermatitis with the severity of the asthma.

An acute episode of asthma may begin with rhinorrhea and fever, then rapidly progress to cough, audible wheeze, and dyspnea. Many pediatricians label these viral respiratory illnesses as "asthmatic bronchitis," "wheezy bronchitis," or "wheezy cold," but such a reluctance or actual failure to recognize the underlying reactive airway disease may delay the institution of appropriate management. Between infections the infant may be relatively free of respiratory symptoms, but cough can persist for longer than the usual 7 to 10 days.

Between the ages of 3 and 5 years, the typical asthmatic child next begins to have episodes without apparent infection. Acute symptoms may commence abruptly and range from paroxysms of cough to severe dyspnea. Symptoms may be seasonal or perennial and can be precipitated by exercise, infection, allergens (e.g., pollens, animal products, and organic dusts), tobacco smoke, fumes, odors, laughter, or other stimuli. In rare instances, food can provoke an asthma attack. Allergic rhinitis, seasonal or perennial, frequently is evident in those children whose asthma has an allergic basis. Between episodes the patient may be free of symptoms or may have latent reactive airway obstruction provoked by forced expiration (elicited by the astute clinician as compression expiratory rhonchi during chest auscultation). *Chronic cough in children or adults may be the only manifestation of airway hyperreactivity*. Sputum production is minimal in children, who usually swallow excess bronchial secretions.

During an acute episode of asthma the patient appears anxious and dyspneic. The pediatrician will recognize the characteristic prolonged expiratory phase of respiration, the raised clavicles, and subcostal retractions. If asthma has been long-standing, there may be a distended or barrel-chested appearance caused by air-trapping. Auscultation of the chest may reveal the characteristic high-pitched musical expiratory rhonchi (wheeze), but both inspiratory and expiratory coarse rhonchi also can be heard. Lack of breath sounds or rhonchi in a dyspneic, asthmatic child should suggest poor air exchange and potential respiratory failure, requiring immediate therapy and close observation in the office, emergency room, or hospital.

LABORATORY FINDINGS

Laboratory studies of pulmonary function in mild cases of asthma during remission may well show no abnormalities. A chest roentgenogram will show hyperinflation during acute attacks, with persistent changes in the more severe and chronic states. *Atelectasis, particularly in the right middle lobe, is a common finding* on chest radiography during acute episodes and should not be misconstrued as pneumonia. Pulmonary function testing may be a valuable adjunct in assessing the degree of pulmonary impairment in children older than 6 years, especially when performed both before and after treatment with an aerosolized sympathomimetic bronchodilator. The long-term management of the chronic asthmatic child may include home monitoring of pulmonary function (e.g., with the mini-Wright peak flow meter). Pulmonary testing after exercise can be helpful in assessing the child with asthma who is involved in athletic pursuits. Monitoring arterial blood gases and pH is essential in the intensive care management of one with severe acute asthma and status asthmaticus.

An allergic evaluation should be undertaken in all children suspected of allergic (immune)-mediated asthma. *Skin testing usually is to be preferred over serologic radioallergosorbent testing (RAST) (IgE antibody) evaluation* because of its greater sensitivity and lower cost. Serum immunoglobulin levels, especially total serum IgE, often are elevated but nonspecifically so. Other allergy tests, including the controversial cytotoxic, sublingual, neutralization, and titration techniques, should be avoided until their sensitivity and specificity are established in controlled studies. Eosinophilia in sputum and blood are frequent findings in the person with asthma, but sputum cultures generally are not helpful.

DIFFERENTIAL DIAGNOSIS

During the first few years of life, other conditions that cause partial airway obstruction and provoke recurrent cough and wheezing must be considered. As already indicated, *bronchiolitis* and asthma often are difficult to differentiate in the infant younger than 1 year of age. *Cystic fibrosis* may cause symptoms that mimic asthma, even in the absence of growth failure. Thus a sweat test is warranted in children with recurrent wheezing. *Congenital anomalies* of the respiratory, cardiovascular, and gastrointestinal tracts may obstruct the airway and produce symptoms that warrant appropriate radiologic studies, especially during the first 2 years of life. *Aspiration* of a foreign body usually produces sudden onset of symptoms, but if the acute event is not appreciated at the time of aspiration, it may result in chronic or recurrent wheezing. Gastroesophageal reflux may be associated with aspiration that causes respiratory symptoms, including wheezing, during infancy and childhood. On occasion an *immunodeficiency* may be associated with repeated respiratory infections accompanied by wheezing. IgG subclass deficiency should be considered in children with recurrent infections and asthma.[5] Yet the child with recurrent episodes of coughing and wheezing will, after appropriate study, most often be shown to have asthma.

TREATMENT

The goals of therapy for asthma are to reverse symptoms and, of course, to prevent their development. To achieve both these goals, appropriate pharmacologic therapy is needed, along with suitable measures of environmental control to reduce or eliminate those specific and nonspecific factors that provoke symptoms. The pharmacotherapy of children with asthma may include four classes of drugs: (1) sympathomimetics, (2) theophyllines, (3) cromolyn, and (4) steroids. The sympathomimetics and theophyllines are prompt and specific bronchodilators, whereas *cromolyn and steroids do not act directly on the airway and provide clinical improvement only over hours or days*. The efficacy of all these drugs can be additive, and they may be used simultaneously. Unfortunately, multiple drug treatment regimens are potentially confusing, not only to the patient but also to the pediatrician.

To simplify the use of appropriate pharmacotherapy, Table 183-1 is presented as a flowchart (Table 183-1) of drug treatment based on the clinical patterns of asthma described above. Efficient reversal of symptoms requires a prompt-acting bronchodilator; thus sympathomimetics are the drugs of choice for the acute, occasional asthma attack. Theophylline does not appear to be as effective during acute asthma. Several of these agents, along with their formulation and appropriate dosages, are listed in Table 183-2. Severe acute symptoms may necessitate the administration of subcutaneous epinephrine or a sympathomimetic aerosol, the latter often seeming to be a faster and safer route of treatment. The *home use of metered-dose inhalers demands proper instruction and bears a potential for overuse and abuse by some children, particularly adolescents*. A sympathomimetic aerosol generated by an air compressor can be used for the child younger than 6 years of age who cannot use the metered-dose inhalers properly; and spacers and holding chambers recently have been devised, which may prove useful in facilitating metered-dose inhaler therapy. Mild acute symptoms may be controlled with oral sympathomimetic agents. If symptoms cannot be managed with one of the sympathomimetics, then an oral, short-acting theophylline should be added to the regimen for more prompt onset of action. If symptoms are severe or unresponsive, then hospitalization is indicated. As an alternative to hospitalization in a known asthmatic child, the administration of a short course of oral steroids may be warranted. Prednisone in a dosage of 2 mg/kg/24 hr (up to a maximum daily dose of 60 mg) can be given in several divided doses for 3 to 5 days; it can then be stopped or tapered as clinically indicated over several days.

The child with episodic (recurrent) asthma may benefit from regular maintenance therapy with a normal form of sustained-release theophylline (Table 183-2), as may also the child who has chronic daily wheezing (Table 183-1). It must be remembered, however, that *there is substantial intersubject variation in theophylline metabolism*. The preschool and primary school–aged child, for instance, metabolizes theophylline faster than does the adolescent or infant. Other factors that can alter theophylline metabolism include liver disease, viral infection, nicotine (from cigarette smoking), and other drugs. Ingestion of sustained-release theophylline with meals can alter its pharmacokinetics and should be avoided. It usually is best to begin with a modest dose (12 to 16 mg/kg/24 hr) and then cautiously increase it at weekly intervals if wheezing persists. Chronically ill children who are to be treated with daily maintenance theophylline probably should have their serum theophylline concentration measured a week after initiation of therapy and thereafter at approximately 6- to 12-month intervals. Still, it may be sufficient to monitor serum theophylline levels only in those children who do not respond to the usual recommended dose or who have adverse symptoms while receiving the usual dosage. Although the therapeutic range for serum theophylline is 10 to 20 μg/ml, it is probably best not to exceed 16 μg/ml in most children. There are several reliable sustained-release theophylline products on the market (Table 183-2). The bead-filled capsules may be particularly useful for the young child unable to swallow a capsule or tablet but who can swallow the beads mixed into or sprinkled on food.

Cromolyn can be an effective drug for the prevention of asthma in the patient who has recurrent or daily wheezing (Table 183-1). It should be used as a prophylactic agent, however, and not as an acute brochodilator for ongoing established episodes of asthma. Cromolyn is available as a metered dose, which is used four times a day or as a powdered

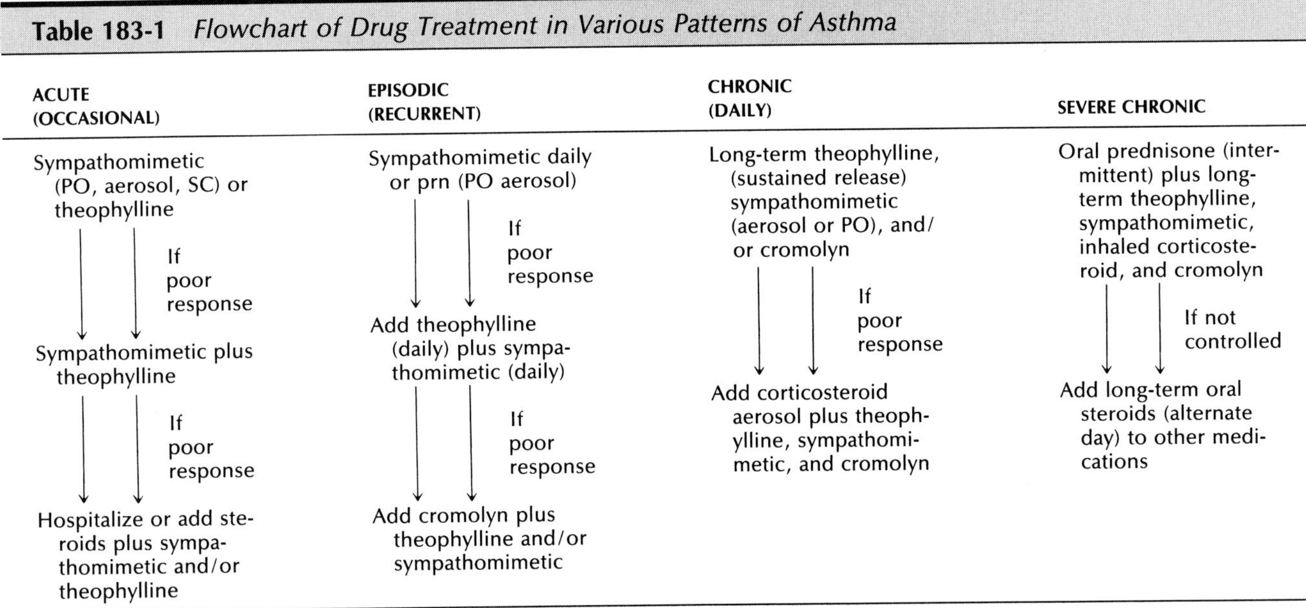

Table 183-1 Flowchart of Drug Treatment in Various Patterns of Asthma
ACUTE (OCCASIONAL)
Sympathomimetic (PO, aerosol, SC) or theophylline
If poor response
Sympathomimetic plus theophylline
If poor response
Hospitalize or add steroids plus sympathomimetic and/or theophylline
EPISODIC (RECURRENT)
Sympathomimetic daily or prn (PO aerosol)
If poor response
Add theophylline (daily) plus sympathomimetic (daily)
If poor response
Add cromolyn plus theophylline and/or sympathomimetic
CHRONIC (DAILY)
Long-term theophylline, (sustained release) sympathomimetic (aerosol or PO), and/ or cromolyn
If poor response
Add corticosteroid aerosol plus theophylline, sympathomimetic, and cromolyn
SEVERE CHRONIC
Oral prednisone (intermittent) plus long-term theophylline, sympathomimetic, inhaled corticosteroid, and cromolyn
If not controlled
Add long-term oral steroids (alternate day) to other medications

Table 183-2 *Selected Bronchodilators Useful in Children with Asthma*

DRUGS	FORMULATION AND ROUTE	DOSE	DURATION (HOURS)
Theophyllines*†‡			
Elixicon	Suspension	300 mg/15 ml	6
Quibron	Syrup (guaifenesin)	150 mg/15 ml	6
Elixophyllin	Elixir (20% ETOH)	80 mg/15 ml	6
Slo-Phyllin	Syrup	80 mg/15 ml	6
	Tablet	100, 200 mg	6
	Gyrocaps	60, 125, 250 mg	8
Theophyl	Chewable tablet	100 mg (scored)	6
Theo-Cur Sprinkle	Capsules	50, 75, 125, 200 mg	8-12
Theo-Dur	Tablets	100, 200, 300 mg	8-12
Slo-Bid	Capsules	50, 100, 200, 300 mg	8-12
Sympathomimetics‡			
Epinephrine	1:1000 SC	0.01 ml/kg up to 0.3 ml	1/2-1
Epinephrine (Sus-Phrine)	1:200 suspension SC	0.005 ml/kg up to 0.25 ml	6-8
Isoetharine (Bronkosol)	Aerosol solution, 1%	0.5 ml/2.5 ml saline	4-6
	Metered aerosol	340 μg/puff	4-6
Metaproterenol (Alupent, Metaprel)	Aerosol solution, 5%	0.25 ml/2.5 ml saline	4-6
	Metered aerosol	650 μg/puff	4-6
	Syrup, 10 mg/5 ml	0.5 μg/kg tid	6-8
	Tablet, 10, 20 mg		6-8
Terbutaline (Brethine, Bricanyl, Brethaire)	SC	0.25 ml/dose	4-6
	Tablet, 2.5, 5 mg	0.075 mg/kg tid	6-8
	Metered aerosol		4-6
Albuterol (Proventil, Ventolin)	Metered aerosol	90 μg/puff	4-6
	Tablet, 2, 4 mg	0.1 mg/kg tid	6-8
	aerosol solution, 0.5	0.5 ml/2.5 ml saline	4-6

* Brand names.
† Usual theophylline dose, 16 mg/kg/24 hr, must be individualized.
‡ Brand names given in parentheses.

Estimation of Severity of Acute Exacerbations of Asthma In Children

SIGN/SYMPTOM	MILD	MODERATE	SEVERE
Respiratory rate	Normal to <1 standard deviation from the norm (S.D.) for age	Normal to <2 S.D. for age	Normal to >2 S.D. for age
Alertness	Normal	Normal	May be decreased
Dyspnea*	Absent or mild; speaks in complete sentences	Moderate; speaks in phrases or partial sentences	Severe; speaks only in single words or short phrases
Pulsus paradoxus	<10 mm Hg	10-20 mm Hg	20-40 mm Hg
Accessory muscle use	No intercostal to mild retractions.	Moderate intercostal retraction with tracheosternal retractions; use of sternocleidomastoid muscles	severe intercostal retractions, tracheosternal retractions with nasal flaring
Color	Good	Pale	Possibly cyanotic
Auscultation	End expiratory wheeze only	Wheeze during entire expiration and inspiration	Breath sounds becoming inaudible
Oxygen saturation	>95%	90-95%	<90%
PCO_2	<35	<40	<40
PEFR	70-90% predicted or personal best	50-70% predicted or personal best	<50% predicted or personal best

Note: Within each category, the presence of several parmeters, but not necessarily all, indicate the general classification of the exacerbation.
*Parents' or physicians' impression of degree of child's breathlessness.

drug (20 mg) inhaled via a device (Spinhaler) that ruptures the capsule. For children younger than 6 years of age, a liquid form of cromolyn is available for inhalation via a nebulizer with compressed air. It may be necessary to stop powdered cromolyn temporarily during an acute exacerbation of asthma. If cromolyn therapy proves beneficial, certain children may be maintained on as few as two or three inhalations per day, and it may even be possible then to reduce or stop administration of theophylline and the sympathomimetics.

Intermittent corticosteroid therapy with prednisone may be necessary in certain children with chronic or severe asthma who have failed to respond to the other drugs (Table 183-1). The judicious use of prednisone in dosages of 1 to 2 mg/kg/24 hr for several days, followed by rapid "tapering" of the dose over 1 week, may prevent frequent hospitalization of the child with severe chronic asthma. An alternative to oral corticosteroids is the prophylactic use of a topical metered-dose steroid (beclomethasone, triamcinolone, or flunisolide) aerosolized by inhaler. At the usual pediatric dose (two inhalations three or four times daily), there are minimal side effects, other than a rare instance of oral candidiasis. Metered-dose triamcinolone or beclomethasone also can be delivered via a spacer or holding chamber to children younger than 6 years of age. At this time, however, a corticosteroid solution is not yet available for aerosol use via an air compressor.

Severely affected children may require alternate-day steroids, which should be tapered to the least dose (given as a single morning dose) that controls symptoms. *Long-term daily oral corticosteroid use should be avoided in children at all costs because of severe impairment of growth and development caused by daily corticosteroids.*

Other aspects of therapy should not be overlooked in planning a comprehensive treatment program. Passive inhalation of cigarette smoke or other respiratory irritants can provoke hyperreactivity in the airways of the asthmatic person. Thus appropriate environmental control measures should be pursued to avoid exposure to known irritants. Appropriate play and exercise are necessary for all children. Should exercise provoke asthma, then prophylactic inhalation of an aerosolized bronchodilator may permit active play and can be especially useful for children engaged in competitive sports.

In certain children, allergic asthma is seasonal. Should identified, offending allergens not easily be avoided, then a trial of hyposensitization by injection with the specific allergen may be considered. The stresses, both emotional and financial, on the family of a child with chronic asthma create an environment conducive to psychological problems. Attention to these potential behavioral problems should lessen the anxiety associated with asthma and improve compliance with the total program of therapy.

PROGNOSIS

In general, the prognosis for the child with asthma is good. Yet *long-term studies of asthmatic patients do show abnormal airway hyperreactivity even in those who have been symptom-free for years.* Many children with intermittent asthma tend to improve during adolescence, with symptoms developing only during viral respiratory infections or strenuous exercise. Of those who experience persistent daily wheezing during childhood, however, fewer than 20% will become asthma free during adolescence. Thus persistent daily bronchospasm may indicate an unfavorable prognosis, and appropriate therapy should be aggressively pursued so that the child with asthma can have a normal life-style, including regular school attendance, uninterrupted rest at night, appropriate recreation, and enjoyment of sports.

REFERENCES

1. Gergen PV, Mulladly DI, and Evans R: National survey of prevalence of asthma among children in U.S. 1976-1980, Pediatrics 81:11, 1988.
2. Gurwitz D, Mindorff C, and Levinson H: Increased incidence of bronchial reactivity in children with a history of bronchiolitis, J Pediatr 98:551, 1981.
3. Martin AJ et al: Natural history of asthma from childhood to adult, Br Med J 280:1397, 1980.
4. McIntosh K et al: The association of viral respiratory infections with wheezing in young asthmatic patients, J Pediatr 82:578, 1973.
5. Page R et al: Asthma and selective IgG subclass deficiency: improvement of asthma following IgG replacement therapy, J Pediatr 112:127, 1988.
6. Schiffer CG and Hunt EP: Illness among children. Data from the National Health Survey, U.S. Public Health Service Pub No 2074, Washington, DC, 1970, US Government Printing Office.
7. Skoner DP et al: Plasma elevations of histamine and a prostaglandin metabolite in asthma, Am Rev Respir Dis 137:1004, 1988.
8. Smith JM: The changing prevalence of asthma in school children, Clin Allergy 1:51, 1971.
9. Szentiavanyi A: The beta adrenergic theory of atopic abnormality in bronchial asthma, J Allergy 42:203, 1968.
10. Welliver RC et al: The development of respiratory syncytial virus specific IgE and release of histamine in nasopharyngeal secretion after infection, N Engl J Med 305:841, 1981.

184

Bacterial Skin Infections

Donald P. Lookingbill

Bacterial infections of the skin are common.[11] Most frequently they are caused by gram-positive bacteria, specifically *Staphylococcus aureus* and group A streptococci.[2,17,19] The clinical diseases that result depend on the location of the infection within the skin. For example, staphylococcal impetigo involves only the most superficial layer of the epidermis, whereas cellulitis represents an infection deep in the dermis, even involving subcutaneous fat. This chapter covers the following bacterial infections: staphylococcal impetigo, streptococcal pyoderma, folliculitis, furuncles and abscesses, and cellulitis.

STAPHYLOCOCCAL IMPETIGO

Etiology

Which bacteria most commonly cause impetigo—*S. aureus* or group A β-hemolytic streptococci? The answer to this question has changed over time. Initially, impetigo was thought to be primarily caused by *S. aureus*, but the studies of children living on the Red Lake Indian Reservation provided evidence that "impetigo" was caused primarily by group A streptococci.[5,8] The work of Dillon supported this thesis.[6] The exception was staphylococcal bullous impetigo, uncommonly encountered in these surveys. Bullous impetigo remains the one form of this disease in which there is uniform agreement regarding bacterial etiology. The roles respectively played by *S. aureus* and group A streptococci in other types of superficial pyoderma are still somewhat clouded, and the medical literature and texts are replete with conflicting opinions and confusing terminology. More recent studies, however, have shown that the majority of cases of impetigo are caused by *S. aureus*.

Perhaps some of the confusion can be resolved by appreciating that *S. aureus* can and does cause superficial skin infection *unaccompanied* by visible bullae. Although the lesions may start with small vesicles, these often are not evident by the time the physician sees the patient. Crusts, usually honey colored, are seen instead. When these crusts are removed, a moist, glistening base is present, representing a very superficial erosion of the epidermis. The culture usually reveals *S. aureus*. This type of impetigo is by far the most common seen in most practices.

The differences between staphylococcal and streptococcal impetigo are summarized in Table 184-1. For the purpose of this chapter the staphylococcus-induced lesion is described as staphylococcal impetigo; although staphylococcal impetigo may be bullous, most frequently it is not. The streptococcus-induced lesion, which will be designated streptococcal pyoderma, is a more inflammatory process and will be discussed later. The relative incidence of the two types of infection varies from one geographic area to another, depending in part on the socioeconomic status of the physician's clientele and the climate.

History

With staphylococcal impetigo there usually is no history of preceding trauma to the skin. Mild to moderate itching may be associated with the lesions. Other family members also may be affected.

Table 184-1 *Features of Staphylococcal Impetigo Versus Streptococcal Pyoderma*

	STAPHYLOCOCCAL IMPETIGO		
FEATURE	HONEY CRUSTED	BULLOUS	STREPTOCOCCAL PYODERMA
Most common location	Face	Trunk	Extremities (usually lower)
Nature of early lesion	Vesicle	Bulla	Pustule
Appearance of crust	Honey colored	Thin, brown, varnishlike	Thick, usually brown
Depth of lesion	Superficial	Superficial	Deep
Appearance when crust is removed	Shallow, glistening erosion	Shallow, glistening erosion	Ulcer
Surrounding erythema	None to minimal	None to minimal	Moderate to marked
History of preceding trauma	No	No	Yes
Other nomenclature	Impetigo	Bullous impetigo	Impetigo, nonbullous impetigo, ecthyma

Physical Findings

The most common location for staphylococcal impetigo is the face, where single or multiple lesions may be present. Lesions scattered elsewhere on the body may occur as well. As mentioned earlier, the usual findings are yellow- or honey-colored crusts, which when removed reveal a pink, superficially eroded, glistening base (Fig. 184-1). It is from this base that the culture should be obtained. With bullous impetigo, intact bullae, if present, will contain deceptively clear fluid. These blisters break easily, leaving behind a superficially denuded skin surface covered with a thin brown "varnishlike" crust, marginated by a thin rim of loose, ragged epidermis that represents the remnants of the blister roof (Fig. 184-2). With staphylococcal impetigo there is minimal surrounding erythema, and regional lymphadenopathy rarely is present.

Laboratory Studies

A Gram stain of either the clear blister fluid or the serum underlying the crusts will show gram-positive cocci. Cultures will grow *S. aureus*, usually resistant to pencillin.

Differential Diagnosis

Herpes simplex infection is the condition most frequently confused with impetigo. Clinical clues that suggest herpes rather than impetigo are as follows:

1. *Intact* vesicles are more likely to be appreciated by both patient and physician in recurrent herpes simplex than in impetigo. In herpes simplex, as the vesicles age, they become cloudy and ultimately result in crusts that also may be honey colored. It is in this crusted phase where the diagnostic confusion most frequently occurs.
2. Herpes simplex tends to be a recurrent condition, with the recurrences usually occurring in the same location. This is not the case with impetigo.
3. In impetigo the Gram stain will show numerous gram-positive cocci. In herpes simplex a scraping from the base of a crust, or preferably a vesicle, will reveal multinucleated giant cells on a Wright stain.

Psychosocial Considerations

Given the potential infectious nature of both staphylococcal and streptococcal skin infections, school nurses are appropriately concerned with this disease, and a child may be asked to leave school until it is treated. Once treatment is initiated, it is probably safe for the child to return to school, even though it will take at least several days for the lesions to heal.

Management

Both topical and systemic antibiotics have been advocated for treating this disease.[7] Traditional topical preparations that contain bacitracin or neomycin, either alone or in combination, have been used, especially for small lesions of staphylococcal origin. The infected area should be washed carefully and the crusts gently removed, if possible, three times daily before the antibiotic cream or ointment is applied. For more extensive lesions—and in the opinion of some physicians for all impetiginous lesions—systemic antibiotics have been employed. Currently most *S. aureus* strains, including those encountered in outpatients, are penicillinase producing[9]; thus penicillin is not appropriate for treating this disease. Oral erythromycin or a penicillinase-resistant penicillin, such as dicloxacillin, is an appropriate drug used for 7 to 10 days.

Of these two agents, dicloxacillin may be preferred because staphylococcal resistance to erythromycin has been increasing.[16] Finally, the use of mupirocin ointment, an expensive new topical antibiotic preparation, recently has been reported to equal or exceed the efficacy of oral erythromycin in the treatment of bacterial impetigo.[1,4]

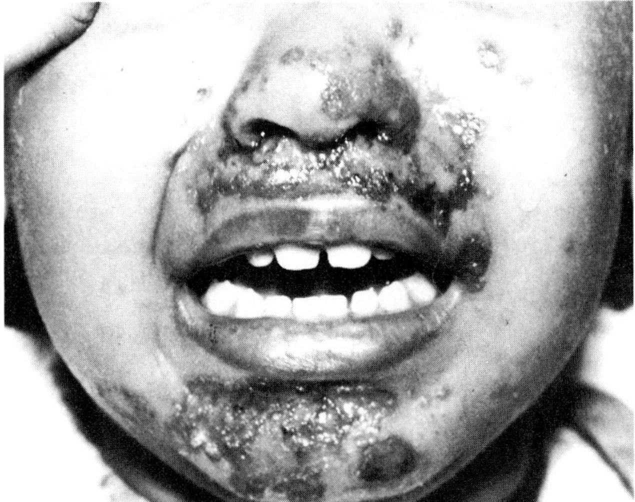

Fig. 184-1 Classic impetigo. Superficial oozing and crusted ulcers. Note involvement of nares—the nose is the likely source of the infective organism.

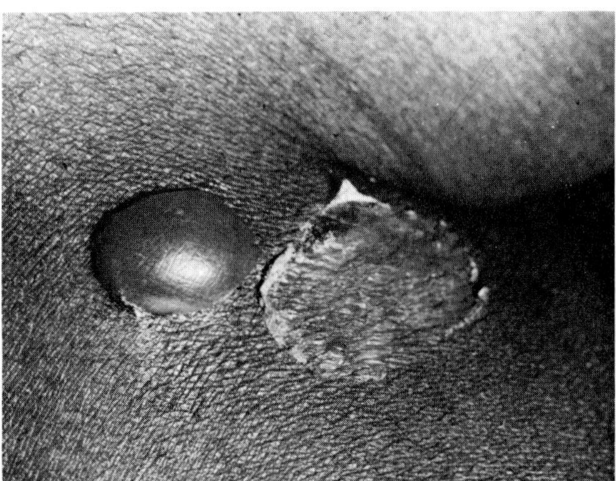

Fig. 148-2 Bullous impetigo. The root of the bulla is thin and delicate; the contents consist of some leukocytes that have settled at the inferior pole and some slightly turbid supernatent fluid. The larger adjacent bulla has already ruptured and its contents discharged. The delicate roof has collapsed onto the base. Lesions of this type may be caused by exfoliatin-producing organisms.

Complications and Prognosis

With appropriate antibiotic therapy, prompt healing is to be expected, with marked improvement occurring in most patients within several days.[13] Bacteriologic cures occur within 7 to 10 days in nearly all cases. If a rapid response to therapy does not occur, it is possible that the infection is caused by an antibiotic-resistant strain. In such instances the result of the initial culture, if obtained, serves as a guide in selecting an alternative antibiotic.

Inasmuch as acute glomerulonephritis is not a sequel of staphylococcal infection, the importance of discriminating between staphylococcal impetigo and streptococcal pyoderma assumes even greater importance. In this regard the features of streptococcal pyoderma should be compared with those of staphylococcal impetigo (Table 184-1).

STREPTOCOCCAL PYODERMA

Etiology

In contrast to the superficial nature of staphylococcal impetigo, which involves mainly the top layers of the epidermis, streptococcal pyoderma frequently extends through the epidermal layer into the underlying dermis. The process may start with small erythematous pustules, at which stage it could be clinically confused with staphylococcal impetigo. Ecthyma is a term used for the more fully developed streptococcal lesion.

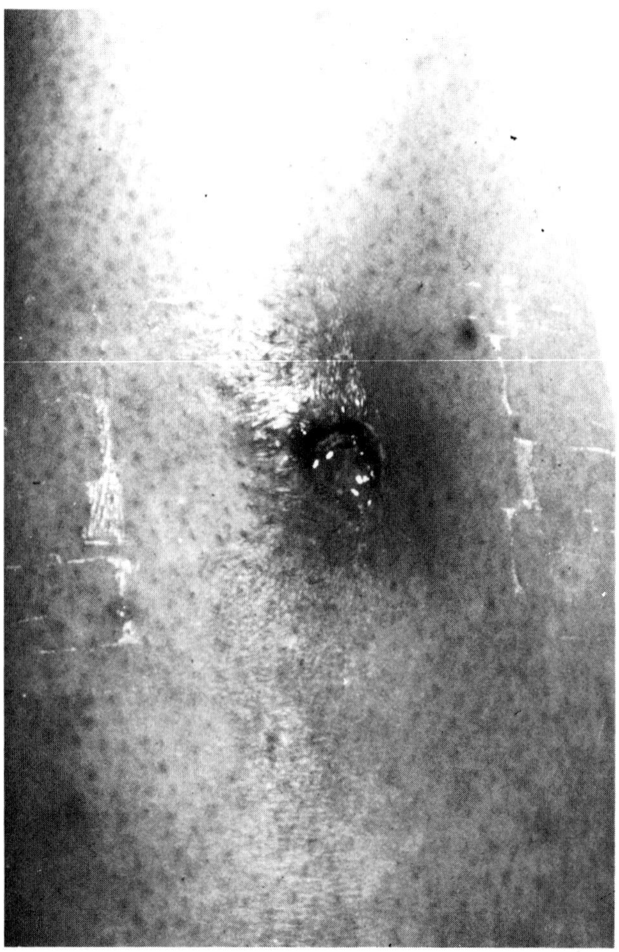

Fig. 184-3 Streptococcal pyoderma (ecthyma). After crust removal, the depth of this ulcerative lesion can be appreciated. The surrounding erythema and lower leg location are also typical for this streptococcal induced lesion.

Streptococcal skin disease occurs more commonly in warm, humid environments. It has been shown that increased humidity favors the survival of group A streptococci on normal skin. It is presumed that trauma to the skin then results in inoculation, which is followed by infection.

History

Streptococcal pyoderma often occurs in epidemics among children of lower socioeconomic status who live in crowded conditions in warm, humid environments. In contrast to staphylococcal impetigo, the streptococcal skin lesions most commonly occur on the lower extremities, where they usually are preceded by trauma such as a scratch or insect bite. This results in bacterial inoculation and subsequent infection. Multiple family members also may be affected.

Physical Findings

The early lesion is a pustule (hence the term *pyo*derma) with surrounding erythema, but the more advanced lesion of ecthyma is more commonly seen. At first glance, this appears as a thick, usually brown crust, surrounded by erythema. When the crust is removed, an actual ulcer is revealed (Fig. 184-3). This is in contrast to the superficial erosion underlying the crust of the staphylococcal lesion. Also in contrast to staphylococcal impetigo, regional adenopathy is often present with streptococcal pyoderma.

Laboratory Studies

A culture taken from the base of the denuded ulcer will grow group A beta-hemolytic streptococci. *S. aureus* is occasionally concomitantly recovered, in which case it is thought to be a secondary invader. Because some strains of group A streptococci are nephritogenic, a screen for renal complications may be done by obtaining a urinalysis 2 to 3 weeks after the onset of infection.

Differential Diagnosis

Ecthyma gangrenosa is an uncommon, but serious, manifestation of *Pseudomonas* septicemia. Clinical features that help to differentiate this lesion from streptococcal ecthyma are (1) the location—usually in inguinal or axillary folds; (2) the appearance of the lesion—a deeper ulcer covered with a tightly adherent, black (gangrenous) crust; and (3) the host—a seriously ill and usually immunocompromised patient, manifesting other signs of sepsis.

Management

Treatment is with antibiotics, although the most appropriate route of administration still is a matter of debate. There is some evidence that topical antibiotic treatment of scratches and insect bites results in a decreased incidence of subsequent pyoderma[4]; thus topical antibiotics may be advocated prophylactically for traumatic skin lesions.[14] Although topical mupirocin has been shown to be effective in impetigo caused by group A streptococci, systemic antibiotics still are recommended for streptococcal infections, particularly if the infection is extensive. Injectable benzathine penicillin G is effective, but a 7- to 10-day course of oral penicillin or erythromycin frequently is used in the compliant patient. Penicillin treatment failures occasionally occur, presumably as a result of the persistence of coexisting penicillinase-producing *S. aureus* organisms.

Complications

Complications are uncommon, although both local and systemic problems can result from streptococcal pyoderma. Cellulitis may develop from the infection extending into larger and deeper areas of skin and subcutaneous tissue. Some strains of group A streptococci produce the toxin responsible for scarlet fever; in fact, streptococcal pyoderma was the most common cause for scarlet fever in one series. But the potential immunologic sequelae from streptococcal infections is the complication of most concern.

Acute rheumatic fever does *not* follow streptococcal infection of the skin, but glomerulonephritis may. It is caused by only a few nephritogenic serotypes of pyoderma-inducing streptococci, and the incidence of infections from these types appears to have been on the decline in recent years. The usual period from onset of infection to development of the glomerulonephritis is 18 to 21 days. Even though treatment of streptococcal pyoderma has not been proved to prevent this nephritic complication, treatment, nonetheless, is recommended. Systemic antibiotic therapy will clear the skin infection and will help to reduce the spread of streptococcal infection to the patient's playmates and family members.

Prognosis

The aforementioned complications are uncommon, and for the majority of patients the lesions heal uneventfully. Streptococcal lesions, because they are deeper, often take longer than staphylococcal lesions to heal; however, bacteriologic cures are usually accomplished within a week. If a prompt response is not achieved, a secondary infection from a penicillinase-producing staphylococcal strain should be considered, particularly if penicillin was used for treatment. Erythromycin-resistant strains of group A streptococci also may be encountered.

FOLLICULITIS

Etiology

Bacterial folliculitis is a moderately common disorder that affects primarily older children and young adults. It is an infection of hair follicles, caused almost exclusively by *S. aureus*. Rarely, infection is caused by gram-negative organisms; this occurs occasionally in antibiotic-treated acne patients.[12] Also, with the recent popularity of hot tubs and whirlpools, some of which become contaminated, *Pseudomonas aeruginosa* has been identified as the cause of an uncommon and unusual type of folliculitis ("hot-tub dermatitis"), causing pruritic papules and pustules on the trunk and proximal extremities. In the usual case, however, *S. aureus* is the responsible pathogen, and it is this type of infection that is discussed.

History

Staphylococcal folliculitis most commonly appears as a chronic and smoldering eruption unaccompanied by symptoms, although an occasional patient will note mild discomfort or pruritus.

Physical Findings

The lesions in staphylococcal folliculitis usually are located on the buttocks and upper portion of the thighs, over which individual small papules and pustules are scattered. The key to the diagnosis is that, on close inspection, hairs can be seen growing out of the very center of many of the lesions.

Laboratory Studies

In the typical case, a culture usually is not necessary. If, however, the presentation is atypical and laboratory confirmation is desired, the contents of a fresh pustule should be cultured.

Differential Diagnosis

Clinically, folliculitis caused by gram-negative organisms differs from staphylococcal folliculitis in its distribution—with lesions occurring primarily on the face and shoulder. "Hot-tub" pseudomonad folliculitis usually occurs on the lower trunk.

Keratosis pilaris is another common follicular disorder that manifests as tiny, rough, scaling papules on the backs of the upper portion of the arms, the buttocks, and the thighs. Although the distribution may be similar to that of staphylococcal folliculitis, the appearance of the lesions is not. In keratosis pilaris, lesions are smaller, more numerous, and scaling, but not pustular.

Management

The usual mild case of staphylococcal folliculitis can be managed with an antiseptic cleanser such as chlorhexidine used daily or every other day for at least several weeks. For more extensive involvement a 7- to 10-day course of systemic antibiotics (e.g., erythromycin or dicloxacillin) is suggested, in addition to the topical regimen.

Complications and Prognosis

Rarely the follicular infection will extend more deeply, resulting in a furuncle. Most patients respond to the treatment outlined above. If not, a bacterial culture should be obtained to rule out infection by gram-negative organisms. Some patients are plagued with recurrences, for which a more prolonged course of antiseptic therapy is recommended.

FURUNCLES AND ABSCESSES

Etiology

Furuncles and abscesses are forms of skin infection (pus-filled nodules or boils) that usually follow folliculitis. *S. aureus* almost always is the responsible organism. Bacteria may also be inoculated into the skin and underlying soft tissue with traumatic injury, including surgery. Gram-negative and anaerobic organisms can be causative.[3,15] In children, anaerobic organisms commonly are isolated from abscesses located in the perirectal area, hand, fingers, and nail beds.

History

A history of trauma may be elicited but frequently is not, especially with furuncles. Immunodeficiency states and diabetes may predispose certain patients to bacterial skin infections, but the typical patient with a furuncle or abscess has no underlying medical disease.

Physical Findings

Furuncles and abscesses are fluctuant masses, filled with pus. They often begin as hard, tender, red nodules, becoming more fluctuant and more painful with time. Abscesses tend to be larger and deeper than furuncles, but sometimes the two lesions may be difficult to differentiate clinically.

Laboratory Studies

A Gram stain of the pustular material may provide a clue to the bacterial etiology, but for precise identification, cultures are required. If anaerobic cultures are desired, material ideally is collected by aspirating the pus, sealing the syringe, and promptly delivering it to the laboratory. If there is insufficient material to aspirate, swab culturettes are available for anaerobic as well as aerobic cultures. Blood culture results rarely are positive and are not indicated unless the patient shows signs of sepsis.

Management

Incision and drainage remain the mainstay of therapy. This results in complete healing in most cases, even in those not treated with systemic antibiotics.[15] Systemic antibiotics may result in involution of early lesions, thereby halting their progression and averting the need for incision and drainage. Erythromycin or dicloxacillin is the antibiotic of first choice. Culture results from abscesses may help in the ultimate selection of the appropriate antibiotic.

Complications

Recurrent furunculosis sometimes prompts a search for an underlying immunodeficiency—a search that almost always goes unrewarded. Many such patients, however, harbor *S. aureus* in a sequestered mucocutaneous site, the most common of which is the nose. The application of an antibiotic ointment, such as bacitracin, to the external nares twice daily may decrease this bacterial colonization and thereby prevent furuncles from recurring. This should be accompanied by an every-other-day total-body scrub with an antiseptic cleansing agent, such as chlorhexidine.

Rarely, a staphylococcal abscess may be the focus of toxin production, resulting in the staphylococcal scalded skin syndrome (most commonly encountered in infants and neonates) or in toxic shock syndrome.

Prognosis

Untreated lesions often spontaneously rupture and drain. After either surgical or spontaneous drainage, uneventful healing is the rule. Larger lesions may leave scars.

CELLULITIS

Etiology

Cellulitis is a deep, locally diffuse infection of the skin with systemic manifestations and life-threatening potential.[10] It usually involves either the face or an extremity. On an extremity the bacteria presumably have been externally inoculated into the deep dermal tissue, although the portal of entry frequently is not clinically detectable. A hematogenous or lymphangitic source also is possible and may explain the development of cellulitis in some cases in which the underlying skin is unbroken. In children younger than 3 years of age, facial cellulitis frequently is associated with an otitis media, *Haemophilus influenzae* type b usually being the responsible organism. *S. aureus* and group A streptococci are more commonly responsible for cellulitis of the extremities. Rarely, other aerobic and anaerobic bacterial organisms, as well as deep fungal agents such as *Cryptococcus neoformans*, can cause cellulitis. These latter infections occur in immunosuppressed hosts.

History

Most children with cellulitis feel and look ill. Fever is present in the vast majority and may precede the clinical skin signs. Patients may complain of pain in the affected area. Symptoms of an accompanying otitis media may be present in buccal cellulitis.

Physical Findings

Fever at the time of presentation is characteristic. The area of involved skin shows the classic signs of inflammation: redness, swelling, heat, and tenderness. *H. influenzae* facial cellulitis has a violaceous hue, and this type of cellulitis frequently is associated with an otitis media and sometimes meningitis, with or without meningismus.

Laboratory Studies

Leukocytosis is usual. Cultures are required to identify the responsible pathogen and should be obtained from skin, blood, and, with facial cellulitis, cerebrospinal fluid. Middle-ear aspirates also may reveal significant findings in patients with otitis media. Skin aspirates from the leading edge of the lesion sometimes help in isolating pathogens when other cultures are negative.[10,20] This procedure is performed by preparing the skin with an antiseptic, introducing an 18- or 21-gauge needle into the deep dermis, and aspirating. If no material is obtained (which is usually the case), 0.5 to 1 ml of nonbacteriostatic saline is injected and then aspirated. All aspirates should be Gram stained as well as cultured.

Differential Diagnosis

Erysipelas sometimes is considered separately from cellulitis. Classic erysipelas has more sharply demarcated borders than does cellulitis and may be caused more commonly by group A streptococci. The distinction between these two entities, however, often is more semantic than real inasmuch as the diagnosis and therapeutic considerations for the two are the same.

A severe, local, confluent contact dermatitis sometimes may be confused with cellulitis in that both may show marked erythema of the skin. The important differences are that with contact dermatitis, the patient complains of itch rather than pain, the skin usually is not tender, and the patient is not febrile. The presence of vesicles also favors contact dermatitis, although vesicles and bullae sometimes may occur in erysipelas as the condition evolves.

Erythema of the cheeks occurs characteristically in erythema infectiosum, in which a "slapped cheek" appearance is noted. Important diagnostic differences between erythema infectiosum and cellulitis are that in the former, the involvement is bilateral, the site usually is not very tender, and the patients do not appear toxic, although they may be mildly febrile.

Management

Systemic antibiotics are the mainstay of therapy. Mild cases of cellulitis on an extremity may be treated with an oral antibiotic, warm soaks, and outpatient follow-up in several days. Inasmuch as cellulitis of the extremity most frequently is caused by gram-positive organisms, erythromycin, dicloxacillin, or cephalexin is an appropriate drug to use. More seriously ill patients in whom sepsis is suspected, as well as most patients with facial cellulitis, should be hospitalized for parenteral antibiotic therapy. Because facial cellulitis most commonly is caused by *H. influenzae* type b organisms, antibiotics must be selected accordingly. In the case of mild involvement, oral therapy can be chosen with agents such as amoxicillin-clavulanate or trimethroprim-sulfamethoxazole. For more advanced disease, parenteral therapy is indicated, and for this a second- or third-generation cephalosporin, such as cefoxitin or ceftriaxone, is recommended.[18]

Complications

H. influenzae type b facial cellulitis often is accompanied by otitis media and, less commonly, by meningitis. Bacterial sepsis frequently accompanies cellulitis, however, and was present in 86% of one series of pediatric cases. Local abscesses and osteomyelitis are rare sequelae. Although cellulitis once was a serious and life-threatening disease, antibiotics have now reduced the fatality rate to nearly zero in otherwise healthy patients.

Prognosis

With appropriate antibiotic therapy, fever usually resolves within 24 hours. If it does not, a change in antibiotic therapy should be considered, optimally guided by early culture results. The skin reaction resolves more slowly than does the fever, sometimes taking a week or longer to subside completely—the outcome to be expected in most patients.

REFERENCES

1. Barton LL et al: Impetigo contagiosa. III. Comparative efficacy of oral erythromycin and topical mupirocin, Pediatr Dermatol 6:134, 1989.
2. Becker LE and Tschen E: Common bacterial infections of the skin, Prim Care 10:397, 1983.
3. Brook I and Finegold SM: Aerobic and anaerobic bacteriology of cutaneous abscesses in children, Pediatrics 67:891, 1981.
4. Coskey RJ and Coskey LA: Diagnosis and treatment of impetigo, J Am Acad Dermatol 17:62, 1987.
5. Dajani AS, Ferrieri P, and Wannamaker LW: Natural history of impetigo. II. Etiologic agents and bacterial interactions, J Clin Invest 51:2863, 1972.
6. Dillon HC: Impetigo contagiosa: suppurative and non-suppurative complications. I. Clinical, bacteriologic, and epidemiologic characteristics of impetigo, Am J Dis Child 115:530, 1968.
7. Dillon HC: Topical and systemic therapy for pyodermas, Int J Dermatol 19:443, 1980.
8. Ferrieri P et al: Natural history of impetigo. I. Site sequence of acquisition and familial patterns of spread of cutaneous streptococci, J Clin Invest 51:2851, 1972.
9. Finnerty EF and Folan DW: Changing antibiotic sensitivities of bacterial skin diseases, Cutis 23:227, 1979.
10. Fleisher G, Ludwig S, and Campos J: Cellulitis: bacterial etiology, clinical features, and laboratory findings, J Pediatr 97:591, 1980.
11. Hayden GF: Skin diseases encountered in a pediatric clinic, Am J Dis Child 36, 1985.
12. Leyden JJ et al: *Pseudomonas aeruginosa* gram-negative folliculitis, Arch Dermatol 115:1203, 1979.
13. Lookingbill DP: Impetigo, Pediatr Rev 7:177, 1985.
14. Maddox JS and Dillon HC: The natural history of streptococcal skin infection: prevention with typical antibiotics, J Am Acad Dermatol 13:207, 1985.
15. Meislin HW et al: Cutaneous abscesses: anaerobic and aerobic bacteriology and outpatient management, Ann Intern Med 87:145, 1977.
16. Mertz PM et al: Topical mupirocin treatment of impetigo is equal to oral erythromycin therapy, Arch Dermatol 125:1069, 1989.
17. Musher DM and McKenzie SO: Infections due to *staphylococcus aureus,* Medicine 56:383, 1977.
18. Santos JI et al: Cellulitis: treatment with cefoxitin compared with multiple antibiotic therapy, Pediatrics 67:887, 1981.
19. Tunnessen WW: Practical aspects of bacterial skin infections in children, Pediatr Dermatol 2:255, 1985.
20. Uman SJ and Kunin CM: Needle aspiration in the diagnosis of soft tissue infections, Arch Intern Med 135:959, 1975.

185

Brain Tumors

Jerome Y. Yager and Robert C. Vannucci

Primary brain tumors, the most common type of solid tumor in childhood, are second only to leukemia as a cause of death from malignancy in children.[4,24] Advances in the fields of neuroradiology, neurosurgery, and cancer chemotherapy have improved the identification, management, and survival of affected children. Accordingly, pediatricians and primary care physicians have become involved in the long-term management of children with central nervous system (CNS) tumors, thereby increasing their need to keep abreast of current trends in cancer diagnosis and treatment.

EPIDEMIOLOGY

The incidence of primary childhood brain tumors has not changed significantly over the years, remaining at 2.2 to 2.4 per 100,000 population at risk per year.[21,25] This figure equates to between 1200 and 1500 new cases identified each year. There is no significant difference in incidence between boys and girls nor among white, black, and other racial or ethnic groups.[25]

Both the incidence and histopathologic typing of brain tumors in children vary with age. In the first year, supratentorial tumors—those of the cerebral hemispheres and the diencephalon—predominate. Thereafter infratentorial tumors—those involving the brain stem and the cerebellum—are more prevalent. The highest incidence of tumors occurs between 5 and 9 years of age; these are predominantly astrocytic in type, with a smaller proportion comprised of medulloblastomas. A slightly lesser number of tumors occurs between birth and 4 years of age; these unfortunately tend to be both clinically and histologically more malignant than those that occur at an older age. Histopathologic types and their respective locations are shown in the accompanying box. Astrocytomas (both cerebral hemispheric and cerebellar) represent 48%, medulloblastomas 23%, brain-stem glioma 9%, ependymomas 8% (both supratentorial and infratentorial), and craniopharyngomas between 6% and 10% of all CNS tumors of childhood. Oligodendrogliomas, optic nerve gliomas, choroid plexus papillomas, and pineal gland tumors each comprise 2% or less.

Primitive neuroectodermal tumors comprise a group of poorly differentiated cerebral malignancies whose classification has yet to be clarified. Because they are of primitive neuroectodermal origin, several investigators include medulloblastomas among them. The tumors arise in either supratentorial or infratentorial regions of the brain, favor the younger age-group, and are rapidly progressive in their growth.

PATHOGENESIS

The etiology of the majority of primary brain tumors in childhood remains unknown. Recent work in the field of molecular biology, however, has brought us closer to an understanding of tumor pathogenesis in general.

Chromosomal abnormalities, manifested as deletions, translocations, and duplications, have long been known to exist in a variety of tumors, including brain tumors.[2,20,21] Highly malignant tumors appear to show extensive heterogeneity in DNA content. Benign tumors, on the other hand, display a more homogeneous cellular karyotype. Extensive evidence also exists, at least in laboratory animals, for a role of both RNA and DNA viruses in the induction of primary intracranial neoplasms.

The mechanism by which either viruses or chromosomal aberrations lead to tumor induction and propagation likely involves oncogenes, a group of genes involved in a cell's growth and differentiation.[22] Activation of these oncogenes releases the cell from its normal growth constraints and allows malignant transformation to occur. One theory proposes that viral genes integrate into host DNA and allow expression of the cellular oncogene; a second proposes that structural chro-

Primary Brain Tumors of Childhood

SUPRATENTORIAL (cerebral hemisphere)
Astrocytoma
Oligodendroglioma
Ependymoma
Choroid plexus papilloma
Meningioma

MIDLINE (diencephalon)
Craniopharyngioma
Pinealoma
Optic nerve glioma

INFRATENTORIAL (brain stem and cerebellum)
Astrocytoma (cerebellum)
Medulloblastoma (cerebellum)
Glioma (brain stem)
Ependymoma

OTHER
Primitive neuroectodermal tumors

mosomal abnormalities predispose a cell to oncogene enhancement.[20]

Several genetic syndromes are associated with an increased risk of CNS tumors. Two of the most common of these are neurofibromatosis (NF) and tuberous sclerosis (TS). Both syndromes exhibit autosomal dominant modes of inheritance with high rates of spontaneous gene mutation. Peripheral neurofibromatosis (NF-I) and central neurofibromatosis (NF-II) have been linked to loci on chromosomes 17 and 22, respectively.[23] The relative risk of benign or malignant CNS neoplasms in NF-I is four times that in the general population,[24] and optic gliomas occur in as many as 15% of affected individuals.[7] A similar rate (15%) has been quoted for the occurrence of giant cell astrocytomas in patients with TS.[14] The vast majority of these tumors are supratentorial gliomas. Whether an association exists between malignant transformation and the genetic abnormalities of these conditions is as yet unknown. Several investigators have suggested a role for neuronal growth factors as a possible cause of oncogenesis in patients with NF-I.[19]

Other mechanisms that likely play a role in the development of childhood CNS tumors include prior radiation[15] and exposure to environmental toxins.[26] Some tumors, often appearing in the first year of life, are congenital in the sense that they arise from embryonic rests (e.g., craniopharyngioma) or are the result of errors in development (e.g., epidermal and dermoid cysts, hamartomas, and colloid cysts). A strong association exists for primary CNS lymphoma and acquired immunodeficiency syndrome.[16]

CLINICAL MANIFESTATIONS

The diagnosis of brain tumor in a child is based on clinical suspicion, a thorough history, and a detailed neurologic examination. Presenting signs and symptoms may be subtle and depend on the age of the child, location of the tumor, and its biologic aggressiveness.

Although there are no pathognomonic features of brain tumors, several general concepts should be kept in mind. Intracranial mass lesions produce symptoms as a result of indirect effects caused by an increase in intracranial pressure (ICP) or of direct effects arising from the displacement or destruction of surrounding tissue. The duration of symptoms before diagnosis is affected by tumor site and growth characteristics. *Symptoms typically are progressive rather than intermittent.* Malignant, rapidly growing lesions have a more explosive presentation than those that are benign and slow growing.

In addition to tissue displacement within a fixed cranial volume, elevated ICP is caused by obstruction of cerebrospinal fluid (CSF) flow and secondary hydrocephalus or more rarely by increased CSF production. *Symptoms appear insidiously;* a change in personality, deterioration in school performance, headache, nausea, vomiting, and lethargy are the most common presenting complaints. Rarely, acute ventricular obstruction leads rapidly to coma.

The *signs of increased ICP* may be subtle. Young infants and children, whose cranial sutures have not yet fused, are able to tolerate a relatively greater expansion of the intracranial contents than are older children and adults. Compensatory head growth and ultimate macrocephaly are presenting features and may be accompanied by (1) failure to thrive from anorexia, (2) lethargy, or (3) irritability. Funduscopic examination may reveal *papilledema*. If increased ICP is long-standing, *optic atrophy* can occur with associated visual loss and nystagmus. Pressure on the sensitive abducens cranial nerve VI causes lateral gaze impairment, resulting in *diplopia*.

Signs and symptoms of intracranial hypertension are common in children with brain tumors inasmuch as the majority of such mass lesions lie in the midline of the posterior fossa and cause ventricular obstruction. Such neoplasms include cerebellar astrocytomas, medulloblastomas, ependymommas, and pineal gland tumors. Choroid plexus papillomas, although rare, cause increased ICP by excessive production of CSF.

Direct symptom-producing effects of a brain tumor vary according to their site of origin. Supratentorial lesions within a cerebral hemisphere lead to headache, unilateral muscle weakness *(hemiparesis)*, visual disturbance, or unilateral sensory loss. *Headaches* may not be localized, but their presence should arouse suspicion, particularly if they worsen while lying down or coughing, sneezing, or straining. Headaches that awaken a child in the early morning hours also are of concern.

Seizures occur rarely as an initial manifestation of brain tumors in children. When present, they typically are focal in nature and tend to be refractory to anticonvulsant medication before definitive therapy. The electroencephalogram shows persistent focal slowing. The tumors usually are benign in nature and slow growing.[1]

Craniopharyngiomas and hypothalamic germinomas, both midline diencephalic tumors, manifest with headache, *endocrine dysfunction* (growth failure, precocious puberty, diabetes insipidus, hypothyroidism), and *visual disturbance*. The accompanying symptoms of abnormal visual fields and hormonal imbalance strongly suggest the presence of a midline supratentorial mass. Infratentorial tumors are associated with increased ICP, usually secondary to hydrocephalus, and brain-stem or *cerebellar dysfunction*, including truncal and limb ataxia, long-tract signs (spasticity and hyperreflexia), and cranial nerve deficits.

The differential diagnosis of intracranial tumors includes less common space-occupying lesions and other causes of increased ICP, such as (1) arteriovenous malformation, (2) subdural hematoma, effusion, or empyema, (3) abscess, (4) infarction, and (5) hemorrhage. Pseudotumor cerebri, especially in adolescents, is a common cause of increased ICP without clinical evidence of a mass lesion. Classic hemiplegic migraine or Todd paralysis after a focal seizure may mimic the signs of an intracerebral mass lesion. The residual signs for migraine or a prior seizure, however, are transient and usually resolve within 24 hours. Occasionally, venous sinus thrombosis manifests with signs of increased ICP.

DIAGNOSIS

The advent of computed tomography (CT) and magnetic resonance imaging (MRI) has revolutionized the diagnosis and subsequent management of CNS tumors. *Initial evaluation should include both an unenhanced and enhanced CT scan.* A noncontrast CT scan affords the opportunity to determine (1) tumor density in comparison with surrounding tissue, (2) the existence of hydrocephalus, and (3) the presence of calcifications or hemorrhage, which may suggest certain tumor types or their aggressiveness. Contrast enhancement delineates tumor margins from surrounding edema and differentiates neoplasms from suspected vascular malformations. Although CT scanning has shown a greater than 90% sensitivity, relevant limitations exist in the assessment of pediatric tumors. In particular, poor resolution of posterior fossa structures (brain-stem and cerebellum) hinders the evaluation of more than 55% of childhood tumors.[11]

Where available, *MRI is now supplanting CT as the imaging procedure of choice.* Greater resolution, the ability to image in more than one plane, and the lack of artifact produced by the surrounding skull make MRI particularly suitable for assessment of posterior fossa structures. MRI has been reported to provide more information than does the CT scan in up to 50% of patients and has proved its superiority for the early detection of neoplasms and determining the limits of their extension.[17] Disadvantages include the inability of MRI to detect calcification and to distinguish tumor from surrounding edema, although contrast enhancement with gadolinium (a paramagnetic contrast agent) can obviate this limitation.[3] MRI requires a much longer scanning time—thus the need for prolonged sedation or even anesthesia, which is potentially hazardous in children with increased ICP. *MRI and CT scans currently are complementary*—both provide important information regarding tumor location, type, and degree of invasiveness.

Once the diagnosis of an intracranial mass is confirmed, further information is required to delineate histologic typing and extent of spread. Angiography, less often required with the advent of MRI scanning, can help differentiate certain lesions from arteriovenous malformations.

Approximately 50% of medulloblastomas have developed seeding along the subarachnoid pathways by the time of diagnosis.[11] CT myelographic examination most accurately detects CSF dissemination and generally is performed as part of the initial assessment of posterior fossa tumors. *Caution must be exercised in performing lumbar punctures* in patients with brain tumors, particularly of the posterior fossa, because of the risk of brain-stem herniation. For the most part such procedures are accomplished postoperatively after decompression of the intracranial contents.

Determination of CSF cytology, although historically of interest in early tissue diagnosis, is presently of little value in the initial investigation of brain tumors. Although cells frequently are present postoperatively in the CSF, it is uncertain whether they are the result of preoperative seeding or intraoperative shedding. Therefore *cytologic examination of CSF rarely is helpful in tumor staging or histologic diagnosis.* Several *biochemical tumor markers* have been shown to be of assistance in the early diagnosis and progression of CNS tumor recurrences. The polyamines, specifically putrescine, are accurate markers for the recurrence of medulloblastomas, whereas CSF alpha-fetoprotein and beta–human chorionic gonadotropin are good indicators of germ cell tumor activity.[8,11]

MANAGEMENT

In the past 10 years substantial gains have accrued in the management of childhood brain tumors through the availability of microsurgical techniques, refined modes of radiation therapy, and chemotherapeutic agents that cross the blood-brain barrier.

Stabilization of the child's neurologic condition through the use of *osmotic agents* and *corticosteroids* to reduce surrounding brain edema and early *CSF shunting* for hydrocephalus is the first step toward comprehensive treatment planning. Histologic diagnosis has been aided by the advent of *stereotaxic biopsy* for most tumors regardless of location, including certain brain-stem gliomas.[10] *Complete excision* and cure are possible for several localized CNS tumors, including choroid plexus papilloma, craniopharyngioma, and cystic cerebellar astrocytoma. Survival generally is aided by a *"debulking" procedure, followed by radiation or chemotherapy, or both.* Operative mortality has been reduced in most centers to less than 5%. Refinement in the use of *microoperative techniques, laser surgery,* and *interstitial radiation* with stereotaxic implantation has further improved outcome, with diminished morbidity.[13]

Most childhood brain tumors that cannot be totally excised will benefit from a combination of surgical debulking and radiation therapy. Medulloblastomas in particular have a high incidence of CSF and meningeal seeding by the time of diagnosis, and affected children should receive craniospinal radiation. Recent reports have suggested prolonged survival of children with brain-stem gliomas after the use of *hyperfractionated radiation therapy.*[9,13]

Substantial evidence now exists that chemotherapy plays a vital role in the treatment of primary childhood CNS tumors. The Children's Cancer Study Group (CCSG) has reported an improved *5-year survival rate of 42% in patients with high-grade astrocytomas treated with combined radiation/chemotherapy* as compared with survival rates of only 10% in patients treated with radiation alone. Unfortunately, similar results as yet have not been forthcoming for medulloblastomas or brain-stem gliomas.[12]

A regimen of eight chemotherapeutic drugs administered in 1 day has shown encouraging preliminary results in children with newly diagnosed brain tumors, including medulloblastomas and malignant astrocytomas. The rationale for this regimen relates to CNS malignant tumors displaying histologic heterogeneity. This *cellular diversification enables a greater degree of drug resistance* to single-drug therapy, whereas multiple drugs attack a tumor by a variety of mechanisms, thereby increasing the likelihood of sensitivity. Studies are in progress to evaluate the effectiveness of "8 in 1" therapy on highly malignant astrocytomas and medulloblastomas.

PROGNOSIS

Prognosis for brain tumors depends on tumor type, size, and location. Overall, 5-year survival rates approach or exceed 50% for all age-groups and tumor types.[4] Less virulent cerebellar and supratentorial astrocytomas have excellent long-term survival rates of 70% to 100%. Survival of patients with medulloblastoma has been variously reported at 40% to 75%. The poorest prognosis occurs in children with brain-stem gliomas, and the survival rate has remained stable at just under 20%. *For all tumor types, survival generally is poorest in affected children younger than 2 years of age.*

The treatment of brain tumors carries with it significant morbidity. Acute effects of radiation and chemotherapy are well known. Bone marrow suppression brings the risk of infection and bleeding diathesis. Cranial radiation is accompanied by hair loss, which though temporary, can be psychologically distressing, particularly for adolescents.

As improvements in therapy lengthen survival, long-term adverse effects of treatment play a greater role. Delayed effects of radiation include progressive demyelination and radiation necrosis. The latter can be misdiagnosed as tumor recurrence. Recent studies have documented a slow decline in intelligence quotients over years in children receiving radiation and chemotherapy.[5] At higher risk are those treated at a young age.[14]

Growth hormone deficiency and subsequent growth deceleration occur frequently in children who receive cranial radiation. Replacement of multiple hormones is required for patients who have been treated for craniopharyngiomas by surgery with or without radiation therapy.[6,18]

FUTURE PROSPECTS

Prospects for improved treatment modalities of childhood brain tumors continue with advances in our understanding of the molecular biology of tumors, sophistication of diagnostic techniques, and the advent of microsurgical procedures and chemotherapeutic programs. The care of children with brain tumors involves a greater number of physicians as long-term survival and neurologic morbidity continue to improve. Therefore management requires an ongoing, multidisciplinary approach with participation by specialists in oncology, neurosurgery, neurology, primary care, social work, psychology, and rehabilitative services.

REFERENCES

1. Blume WT, Girvin JP, and Kaufman JCE: Childhood brain tumors presenting as chronic uncontrolled focal seizure disorders, Ann Neurol 12:538, 1982.
2. Cusimano MD: An update on the cellular and molecular biology of brain tumors, Can J Neurol Sci 16:22, 1989.
3. Dickman CP et al: Unenhanced and gadolinium-DTPA–enhanced MR imaging in postoperative evaluation in pediatric brain tumors, J Neurosurg 71:49, 1989.
4. Duffner PK et al: Survival of children with brain tumors: SEER program 1973-1980, Neurology 36:597, 1986.
5. Duffner PK, Cohen ME, and Parker MS: Prospective intellectual testing in children with brain tumors, Ann Neurol 23:575, 1988.
6. Duffner PK et al: Long-term effects of cranial irradiation on endocrine function in children with brain tumors: a prospective study, Cancer 56:2189, 1985.
7. Dunn DW: Neurofibromatosis in childhood. In Lockhart JD, editor: Current problems in pediatrics, vol 17, Chicago, 1987, Year Book Medical Publishers, Inc.
8. Edwards MSB, Davis RL, and Laurent JP: Tumor markers and cytologic features of cerebrospinal fluid, Cancer 56:1773, 1985.
9. Edwards MSB and Prados M: Current management of brain stem glioma, Pediatr Neurosci 13:309, 1987.
10. Epstein F and McClearly EL: Intrinsic brain stem tumors of childhood: surgical indications, J Neurosurg 64:11, 1986.
11. Finlay JL and Goins SC: Brain tumors in children. I. Advances in diagnosis, Am J Pediatr Hematol Oncol 9:246, 1987.
12. Finlay JL and Goins SC: Brain tumors in children. III. Advances in chemotherapy, Am J Pediatr Hematol Oncol 9:264, 1987.
13. Finlay JL, Uteg R, and Giese WL: Brain tumors in children. II. Advances in neurosurgery and radiation oncology, Am J Pediatr Hematol Oncol 9:256, 1987.
14. Kingsley DPE, Kendall BE, and Fitz CR: Tuberous sclerosis: a clinicoradiological evaluation of 110 cases with particular reference to atypical presentation, Neuroradiology 28:38, 1986.
15. Leviton A: Principles of epidemiology. In Cohen ME and Duffner PL, editors: Brain tumors in children: principles of diagnosis and treatment, New York, 1984, Raven Press.
16. List AF, Greco A, and Vogler LB: Lymphoproliferative disease in immunocompromised hosts: the role of Epstein-Barr viruses, J Clin Oncol 5:1673, 1987.
17. Packer RJ, Batnitzky S, and Cohen ME: Magnetic resonance imaging in the evaluation of intracranial tumors of childhood, Cancer 56:1767, 1985.
18. Rappaport R and Brauner R: Growth and endocrine disorders secondary to cranial irradiation, Pediatr Res 25:561, 1989.
19. Riopelle RJ and Riccardi VM: Neuronal growth factors from tumors of von Recklinghausen neurofibromatosis, Can J Neurol Sci 14:141, 1987.
20. Schmidek HH: The molecular genetics of nervous system tumors, J Neruosurg 16:1, 1987.
21. Schoenberg BS et al: The epidemiology of primary intracranial neoplasms of childhood—a population study, Mayo Clin Proc 51:51, 1976.
22. Shapiro JR: Biology of gliomas: heterogeneity, oncogenes, growth factors, Semin Oncol 13:4, 1986.
23. Sorensen SA, Mulvihill JJ, and Nielsen A: Long-term follow-up of von Recklinghausen neurofibromatosis survival and malignant neoplasms, N Engl J Med 314:1010, 1986.
24. Tomita T and Mclone DG: Brain tumor during the first twenty-four months of life, Neurosurgery 17:913, 1985.
25. Young JL et al: Cancer incidence, survival and mortality for children younger than age 15 years, Cancer 58:598, 1986.
26. Zeller WJ et al: Experimental chemical production of brain tumors, Ann NY Acad Sci 281:250, 1982.

SUGGESTED READINGS

Cohen ME and Duffner PK: Brain tumors in children: principles of diagnosis and treatment, New York, 1984, Raven Press.

Cohen ME and Duffner PK: Tumors of the brain and spinal cord including leukemic involvement. In Swaiman KF, editor: Pediatric neurology: principles and practices, St Louis, 1989, The CV Mosby Co.

Kadota RP et al: Brain tumors in children, J Pediatr 114:511, 1989.

186

Bronchiolitis

Caroline Breese Hall and William J. Hall

Bronchiolitis is an acute infectious respiratory illness of children that usually occurs in the first 2 years of life. The hallmarks of the clinical picture are wheezing and hyperaeration, commonly associated with tachypnea, respiratory distress, and retractions of the chest.

Although the clinical picture of bronchiolitis has been described since the beginning of this century, bronchiolitis was not recognized as a separate entity until Engle and Newns[6] gave it its sovereignty by designating the distinctive infantile disease as *bronchiolitis*.

ETIOLOGY

Viruses and occasionally *Mycoplasma pneumoniae* are now recognized as the causes of bronchiolitis.* As shown as Fig. 186-1, respiratory syncytial virus is by far the most frequently isolated agent, followed by the parainfluenza viruses, the rhinoviruses, and the adenoviruses. In Henderson and colleagues' study[13] of bronchiolitis occurring in children in a private pediatric practice, respiratory syncytial virus, parainfluenza viruses types 1 and 3, adenoviruses, rhinoviruses, and *M. pneumoniae* accounted for 87% of the isolates from children of all ages. Respiratory syncytial virus accounted for 44% of the isolates from children in first 2 years of life, with parainfluenza type 1, parainfluenza type 3, and adenoviruses each accounting for about 13%. In two group practices in Rochester, New York, respiratory syncytial virus was isolated from 55% and parainfluenza type 3 from 11% of bronchiolitis cases. If only hospitalized cases of bronchiolitis are examined, the contribution of respiratory syncytial virus is much higher.[8,26] In the Newcastle-upon-Tyne studies, respiratory syncytial virus was isolated from 74% of hospitalized bronchiolitis patients.[8]

EPIDEMIOLOGY

The seasonal pattern of bronchiolitis reflects the activities of its viral agents, particularly respiratory syncytial virus.[1,7,10] Since respiratory syncytial virus is causative in the majority of cases, bronchiolitis peaks during the winter to spring months when respiratory syncytial virus is epidemic in the community. As shown in Fig. 186-2 on p. 1153, in Monroe County, New York, the greatest number of cases are reported during the yearly January to February peak of respiratory syncytial virus activity. Lesser peaks are seen during the fall when parainfluenza virus type 1 has been present in the community and during the spring period of parainfluenza virus type 3 activity. Cases of bronchiolitis are commonly designated as epidemic or sporadic bronchiolitis, which essentially means cases that are or are not associated with respiratory syncytial virus.

The incidence of bronchiolitis varies according to the age and definition of the syndrome. Over 80% of bronchiolitis cases occur during the first year of life.* The peak attack rate occurs between 2 and 10 months of age and is relatively uncommon during the first weeks of life. The highest reported incidence is from Denny and colleagues' long-term studies[5] in Chapel Hill, North Carolina, in which 115 cases per 100 children up to 6 months of age were detected per year. Because these children in a day care center were examined at regular intervals, and the diagnosis of bronchiolitis did not have to include tachypnea or air-trapping, the mildest cases were included. In subsequent Chapel Hill studies of ambulatory children, the incidence was 11 cases per 100 children per year for both the first and second 6 months of life.[4,13] In both of these studies the incidence fell rapidly during the second year of life to 32 cases per 100 children per year in the day care center and to 6 cases per 100 children per year in the private practice. In hospitalized cases the incidence is highest during the first 6 months of life and in the study by Foy and coworkers[7] was found to be 6 per 1000 children per year. The attack rate in boys is generally one and one-half times greater than that in girls in both outpatients and hospitalized patients.[1,4,10]

PATHOPHYSIOLOGY

Host, environmental, and immunologic factors have all been said to play a role in the development and severity of bronchiolitis. The risk of bronchiolitis appears to be increased in children who (1) come from homes that are in poorer socioeconomic areas, (2) come from crowded surroundings, (3) have more siblings, and (4) have not been breast fed.[2,25] Children with a genetic predisposition to hyperreactive airways appear more likely to manifest their initial respiratory viral infections as bronchiolitis, especially those of respiratory syncytial virus and the parainfluenza viruses, although the role of atopy and an allergic family background is unclear.[2,14,20] Immunologic mechanisms, however, have been suggested in the pathogenesis of bronchiolitis from respiratory syncytial virus and parainfluenza viruses.[23,24] A hypersensitivity of the cell-mediated response to these viral antigens has

*References 1, 4, 5, 7, 10, 13.

*References 1, 4, 5, 10, 13, 26.

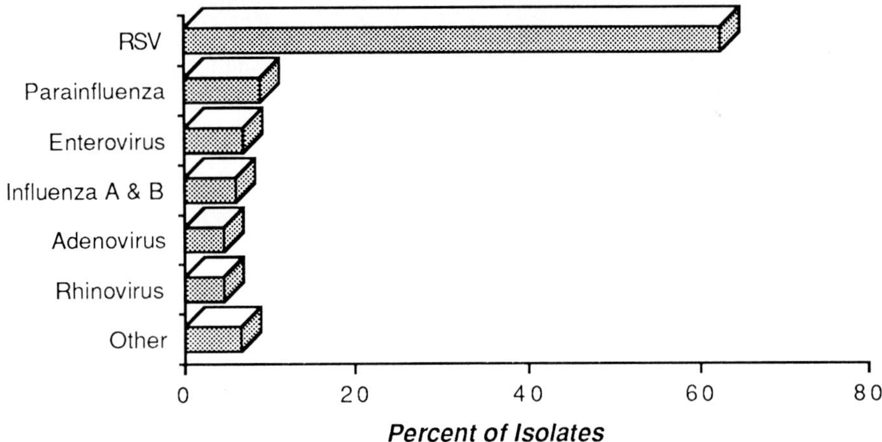

Fig. 186-1 Viral etiology of bronchiolitis from patients in pediatric practices participating in an ongoing community surveillance program in Monroe County, New York, 1983-1988.

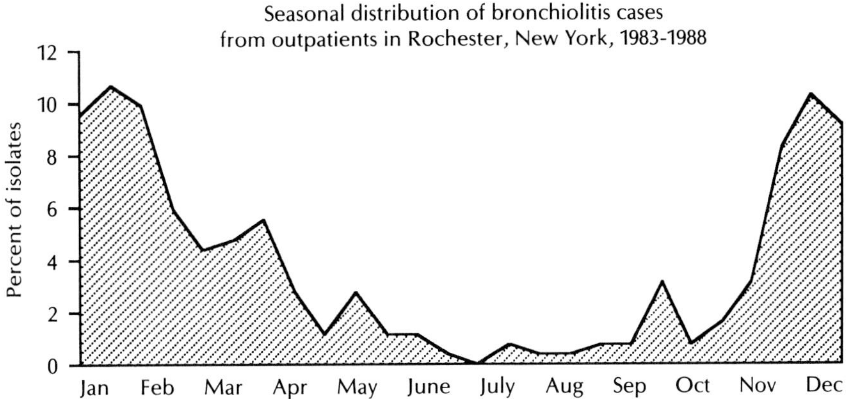

Fig. 186-2 Seasonal occurrence of bronchiolitis cases obtained over a 6-year period from a community surveillance program in Rochester, New York.

been shown in infants with bronchiolitis, which may result in enhanced release of lymphokines, which causes inflammation and hyperreactivity of the airways. Increased production of specific IgE antibody and histamine release in the secretions of infected infants have been associated with the presence, duration, and severity of wheezing.[23,24]

Certainly paramount in the pathogenesis of bronchiolitis is the age of the child and the specific viral agents, particularly respiratory syncytial virus and parainfluenza virus type 3, which infect children early in life and are capable of infecting the lower respiratory tract in a high proportion of young infants. Anatomical and physiologic factors are important in this young age group, such as the small diameter of the peripheral airways, poor collateral ventilation, and the relatively increased number of mucus-secreting glands.[25]

Initially the viral agent usually causes infection of the upper respiratory tract and subsequently spreads to affect the medium and small bronchi and bronchioles. The virus characteristically causes inflammation and necrosis of the respiratory epithelium.[25,26] Histologically, peribronchiolar infiltration and proliferation, mostly of mononuclear cells, are observed. The bronchiolar epithelium subsequently becomes necrotic and sloughs off. In most cases of bronchiolitis, spread of the inflammation beyond the peribronchiolar area is slight, with little involvement of the surrounding alveoli. However, the inflammation of the small bronchi and bronchioles is generalized, but with areas varying in severity. The small diameter of the lumens makes the infant particularly vulnerable to this obstruction caused by the developing edema and exudate. Peripheral to the sites of partial obstruction, air becomes trapped by a process similar to a "ball valve" mechanism. During inspiration the negative intrapleural pressure allows air to flow past the site of partial obstruction. On expiration, however, the positive pressure decreases the lumen's size, causing an increase in the degree of obstruction. The lung, thus, becomes hyperinflated. Expiration, in particular, becomes difficult and prolonged. If the inflammation progresses, complete obstruction will occur. When the trapped air becomes absorbed, multiple areas of focal atelectasis result.

Two important physiologic sequelae occur from these pathologic processes. First, the resistance to airflow markedly increases.[26] This leads to dyspnea and an increased respiratory rate and lower tidal volume. Thus, the amount of each breath reaching the gas-exchanging alveoli diminishes and proportionately more air only ventilates "dead space." This may eventually result in an elevation of the arterial P_{CO_2}. The second sequela resulting from the small-airway obstruction is the marked change in the distribution of ventilation within the lung. The low ratio of ventilation compared with the perfusion of the lung results in arterial hypoxemia. Essentially all infants hospitalized with bronchiolitis have some degree of hypoxemia, which is commonly appreciable and protracted.[11] Despite clinical improvement the hypoxemia may persist for weeks, reflecting the relatively slow resolution of the inflammation and atelectasis.

CLINICAL FEATURES

Bronchiolitis is usually heralded by the signs of a common cold. Rhinorrhea, nasal congestion, a slight fever, and cough may develop over a prodromal period of 1 to 7 days. As bronchiolitis develops, the cough may become more prominent, and an increased respiratory rate, pulse rate, and tachypnea appear. Fever is commonly present during the prodromal period but usually is not high; by the time bronchiolitis has developed, fewer than 50% of the children are febrile.

Physical examination of the infant with bronchiolitis is often striking. Tachypnea is a constant finding, often accompanied by tachycardia; the respiratory rate is usually 45 to 80 breaths/min. The infant may appear lethargic and distressed with circumoral cyanosis. The increased work of breathing is evidenced by flaring of the nasal alae and grunting. Retractions of the chest wall in the subcostal, intercostal, and suprasternal areas and use of the accessory muscles of respiration are notable.

Physical examination of the baby's chest verifies the hyperinflation resulting from the trapping of air peripheral to the small-airway obstruction. The diameter of the chest appears increased, and the percussion note has a hyperresonant ring. The liver and spleen may become easily palpable from the downward placement of the overinflated lungs. Expiration is usually but not always prolonged and may be difficult to detect in a small baby with a rapid respiratory rate. Obstruction to the flow of air also occurs on inspiration, but to a lesser extent. Auscultation usually reveals the diagnostic hallmark of wheezing. The degree of wheezing and the fine moist rales commonly heard on inspiration may vary from hour to hour. A decrease in the auscultatory findings with increasing respiratory distress may indicate progressive obstruction to the flow of air in the small airways and impending respiratory failure. As this stage of respiratory acidosis becomes manifest, the respirations become shallow and ineffective, as if the effort to breathe becomes too great for the infant.

Associated findings that may complicate the infant's course include otitis media (in about 10% to 30% of infants) and dehydration. Babies with bronchiolitis are prone to dehydration because of paroxysms of coughing that trigger vomiting and because of a decreased fluid intake resulting from their respiratory distress and lethargy. In addition, the tachypnea and fever may increase their fluid requirements.

Most infants with bronchiolitis improve appreciably within several days, and the cough and other signs resolve gradually thereafter over a period of 1 to 2 weeks. For some infants the entire course is one of slow, gradual improvement. Most children who worsen and require hospitalization will do so within the first 3 or 4 days.

In most infants the white blood cell count and differential count are within normal limits. However, in the more severely affected and hypoxemic infant the white blood cell count may be elevated and the differential count may demonstrate a shift to the left. In these more distressed infants, determination of the blood gas tensions is helpful.[11] The degree of hypoxemia is extremely difficult to judge clinically, and cyanosis may not be apparent in the face of moderate degrees of hypoxemia. An increasing respiratory rate is the sign best correlated with poor oxygenation.

The chest roentgenogram in most cases of bronchiolitis shows some degree of hyperinflation. An increased anteroposterior diameter of the chest on a lateral film and flat or depressed diaphragm may be present. Increased bronchovascular markings are common, appearing as abnormal streaks or linear densities radiating out from the hila. Scattered small areas of atelectasis and interstitial infiltrates of varying intensity and distribution may also be seen. Differentiation of these areas of atelectasis from those of pneumonic infiltration is often not possible.

DIAGNOSIS

The diagnosis of bronchiolitis is usually made on the characteristic clinical and epidemiologic features; a specific etiologic diagnosis may be made by viral isolation or antigen detection in the nasopharyngeal secretions.[11] Most of the respiratory viruses causing bronchiolitis are identifiable in cell culture within 3 to 7 days. A variety of rapid viral diagnostic techniques, such as immunofluorescence and enzyme-linked immunoassays, are now available to identify some of the viral antigens in the respiratory secretions within hours.[8] Antibody determinations on acute and convalescent sera in the young infant are rarely helpful for several reasons. First, the time required to obtain a convalescent serum excludes its being helpful in the clinical management. Furthermore, young infants will have maternally acquired antibody to most of the viral agents of bronchiolitis, such as respiratory syncytial virus and the parainfluenza viruses, and many infants in the first 3 months of life will not produce an appreciable enough antibody response to be diagnostic, in spite of clinical illness.

DIFFERENTIAL DIAGNOSIS

Asthma is the major consideration in the differential diagnosis of bronchiolitis. Often in a single episode it is not possible to differentiate these two entities; indeed, the two may be combined. A great proportion of wheezing episodes occurring in an atopic child may arise from viral infections. In asthmatic children 1 to 5 years of age, McIntosh and colleagues[16] found 42% of the episodes of wheezing to be associated with a viral infection and respiratory syncytial virus to be the agent most frequently isolated.

Respiratory syncytial virus has an unexplained propensity for producing wheezing in infants. Therefore children who first wheeze during an epidemic of respiratory syncytial viral infections may be less likely to have an atopic predisposition than do children who develop sporadic bronchiolitis at other times of the year. The role of atopy is also apt to be greater in the child older than 18 months and in the one with a family history of allergy and previous episodes of wheezing.

Another diagnostic consideration is gastric esophageal reflux, which in the infant may produce a picture clinically identical to that of bronchiolitis. Aspiration of a foreign body may also result in wheezing and respiratory distress. Wheezing may also occur in congestive heart failure and in cystic fibrosis.

TREATMENT

Management of most infants with bronchiolitis consists mainly of supportive care, including adequate hydration and antipyretics, if necessary. In the hospitalized child the mainstay of care is ensuring of adequate oxygenation, and if the cause of the bronchiolitis is respiratory syncytial virus, therapy with the antiviral drug ribavirin may be used.[12,18] This drug is administered by small-particle aerosol via an oxyhood, tent, or ventilator to the infant for 12 to 20 hours per day, usually for 3 to 5 days. Ribavirin therapy is associated with a more rapid improvement in the clinical symptoms, with the infant's arterial oxygen saturation, and with diminished viral shedding.

In addition, infants in controlled studies treated with ribavirin have been shown to have diminished production in their secretions of specific IgE antibody and leukotrienes associated with inflammation and wheezing.[9,19]

Bronchodilators administered by all routes have been tried but are usually not successful.[26] Therapy with aerosolized bronchodilators has been studied and shown to be of little benefit, as documented by no change in the degree of pulmonary resistance[17]; however, a certain percentage of infants, especially those over 6 months of age, may benefit from bronchodilators.[21,25] For these reasons some experts recommend a trial administration of aerosolized or parenteral bronchodilators in infants who are ill enough to be hospitalized and who can be carefully monitored. The use of steroids in bronchiolitis has been studied and found to be of no benefit.[22,27] On this basis the Committee on Drugs of the American Academy of Pediatrics advises against the use of steroids in those with bronchiolitis. Antibiotics should not be given in bronchiolitis, since bacteria have no role in the etiology. Secondary bacterial infection is rarely observed after bronchiolitis, and unless such is documented, antibiotics should not be used.

COMPLICATIONS AND PROGNOSIS

The prognosis for normal infants with bronchiolitis is good; mortality is less than 1%. In certain children with underlying diseases such as cardiopulmonary disease, bronchiolitis may be accompanied by increased morbidity and mortality.

Pneumonia so commonly coexists with the clinical manifestations of bronchiolitis that the diseases ought to be considered a continuum, particularly in respiratory syncytial viral infection. Bacterial pneumonia is an uncommon complication.

Apnea may complicate the course of approximately 20% of infants hospitalized with respiratory syncytial viral infection.[3] Apnea is most likely to occur in the youngest infants and in premature infants.

Infants with bronchiolitis appear to be at risk for recurrent episodes of wheezing and long-term pulmonary function abnormalities.[20,25,26] However, in one study of ambulatory children with a history of relatively mild bronchiolitis, follow-up examination did not show an increased incidence of abnormal pulmonary function.[15]

REFERENCES

1. Brandt CD et al: Epidemiology of respiratory syncytial virus infection in Washington, D.C. III. Composite analysis of eleven consecutive yearly outbreaks, Am J Epidemiol 98:355, 1973.
2. Carlsen KH et al: Acute bronchiolitis: predisposing factors and characterization of infants at risk, Pediatr Pulmonol 3:153, 1987.
3. Church NR et al: Respiratory syncytial virus related apnea in infants: demographics and outcome, Am J Dis Child 138:247, 1984.
4. Denny FW and Clyde WA: Acute lower respiratory tract infections in nonhospitalized children, J Pediatr 108:635, 1986.
5. Denny FW et al: Infectious agents of importance in airways and parenchymal diseases in infants and children with particular emphasis on bronchiolitis, Pediatr Res 11:234, 1977.
6. Engle S and Newns GH: Proliferative mural bronchiolitis, Arch Dis Child 15:219, 1940.
7. Foy HM et al: Incidence and etiology of pneumonia, croup and bronchiolitis in preschool children belonging to a prepaid medical care group over a four year period, Am J Epidemiol 97:80, 1973.
8. Gardner PS: How etiologic, pathologic, and clinical diagnoses can be made in a correlated fashion, Pediatr Res 11:254, 1977.
9. Garofalo R, Welliver RC, and Ogra PL: Modulation of leukotriene (LT) release with ribavirin during infection with respiratory syncytial virus (RSV), Pediatr Res 25:163A, 1989.
10. Glezen WP and Denny FW: Epidemiology of acute lower respiratory disease in children, N Engl J Med 288:498, 1973.
11. Hall CB, Hall WJ, and Speers DM: Clinical and physiologic manifestations of bronchiolitis and pneumonia, Am J Dis Child 133:798, 1979.
12. Hall CB et al: Aerosolized ribavirin treatment of infants with respiratory syncytial viral infection: a randomized double blind study, N Engl J Med 308:1443, 1983.
13. Henderson FW et al: The etiologic and epidemiologic spectrum of bronchiolitis in pediatric practice, J Pediatr 95:183, 1979.
14. Laing I et al: Atopy predisposing to acute bronchiolitis during an epidemic of respiratory syncytial virus, Br Med J 284:1070, 1982.
15. McConnochie KM et al: Normal pulmonary function measurements and airway reactivity in childhood after mild bronchiolitis, J Pediatr 107:54, 1985.
16. McIntosh K et al: The association of viral and bacterial respiratory infections with exacerbations of wheezing in young asthmatic children, J Pediatr 82:578, 1973.
17. Phelan PD and Williams HE: Sympathomimetic drugs in acute viral bronchiolitis: their effect on pulmonary resistance, Pediatrics 44:493, 1969.
18. Rodriguez WJ et al: Aerosolized ribavirin in the treatment of patients with respiratory syncytial virus disease, Pediatr Infect Dis J 6:159, 1987.

19. Rosner IK et al: Effect of ribavirin therapy on respiratory syncytial virus-specific IgE and IgA responses after infection, J Infect Dis 155:1043, 1987.
20. Sims DG et al: Atopy does not predispose to RSV bronchiolitis or postbronchiolitic wheezing, Br Med J 282:2086, 1981.
21. Soto ME et al: Bronchodilator response during acute viral bronchiolitis in infancy, Pediatr Pulmon 1:85, 1985.
22. Stecenko AA: Treatment of viral bronchiolitis: do steroids make sense? Contemp Pediatr 4:121, 1987.
23. Welliver RC et al: The development of respiratory syncytial virus-specific IgE and the release of histamine in nasopharyngeal secretions after infection, N Engl J Med 305:841, 1981.
24. Welliver RC et al: Parainfluenza virus bronchiolitis: epidemiology and pathogenesis, Am J Dis Child 140:34, 1986.
25. Wohl MEB: Bronchiolitis, Pediatr Ann 15:307, 1986.
26. Wohl MEB and Chernick V: State of the art: bronchiolitis, Am Rev Respir Dis 118:759, 1978.
27. Yaffe SJ et al: Should steroids be used in treating bronchiolitis? Pediatrics 46:640, 1970.

187

Cancers in Childhood

Cindy Schwartz

Advances in the treatment of solid tumors of childhood during the past 20 years have assured the long-term survival of at least two thirds of children with these diagnoses. The pediatrician who initially discovers a solid tumor may not, and need not, know the best treatment regimen available. However, early referral of such a child to the appropriate specialist, a pediatric oncologist, significantly affects the likelihood and the quality of survival. Many common childhood tumors are unique in the pediatric age range. For all solid tumors in children, therapies must be designed to minimize effects on growth and development. Appropriate utilization of the therapeutic modalities—surgery, chemotherapy, and radiation—provides maximum efficacy and minimal toxicity of therapy.

The child, and his or her family, should be encouraged to plan for the future. Educational and developmental needs must be addressed by the pediatric team—generalist and specialist together. Such a team also will best be able to address the needs of the child, the parents, and the siblings if treatment is not successful. Fortunately, most children will be cured and will return to the pediatrician for many years of general pediatric care.

The following solid tumors seen in the pediatric population are described herein: Wilms tumor, neuroblastoma, rhabdomyosarcoma, germ cell tumors and teratomas, retinoblastoma, Ewing sarcoma, osteogenic sarcoma, Hodgkin disease, and non-Hodgkin lymphomas. The role of the pediatrician in the care of these children also is examined.

WILMS TUMOR

Wilms tumor, or nephroblastoma, is a malignant renal tumor of childhood that occurs at an annual rate of 7.6 per 1 million children in the United States. It is the second most common abdominal tumor of childhood.[20] Patients usually are between 2 and 5 years of age, and the incidence of bilateral disease is increased in younger patients. Wilms tumor rarely occurs in teenagers and adults.

The chemosensitivity and radiosensitivity of this tumor, in conjunction with the ability to resect most nonmetastatic tumor, have allowed a multidisciplinary approach to be highly successful. Wilms tumor has become the model for treatment of childhood cancer. The National Wilms Tumor Study (NWTS) has, over the past two decades, evaluated successive therapeutic regimens with the goal of increasing the cure rate and decreasing the toxicity of therapy. The cooperative group approach has made possible the gathering of more data than could have been obtained at single institutions. The findings, such as the superiority of multiagent chemotherapy and the importance of tumor histology, are relevant for many tumors.

Etiology

Wilms tumor has occurred in siblings, cousins, and parent-child pairs, particularly in association with specific congenital anomalies and bilateral disease.[87] Although it has been proposed that 40% of patients with Wilms tumor may have had a genetic predisposition to the disease, a much lower incidence of Wilms tumor in patients with affected relatives has been reported (approximately 1%).[12]

Anomalies are commonly reported in patients with Wilms tumor; most involve the genitourinary tract.[12] Hemihypertrophy is second in frequency, sometimes noted as a component of the Beckwith-Wiedemann syndrome (excessive growth of many body organs). Of children with the sporadic form of congenital aniridia, 33% have Wilms tumor. WAGR syndrome is the association of Wilms tumor–aniridia, genitourinary abnormalities, and mental retardation. Drash syndrome represents the association of Wilms tumor with male pseudohermaphroditism and diffuse glomerular disease.[34] Neurofibromatosis occurs with increased frequency in patients with Wilms tumor.

Clinical Manifestations

Wilms tumor in children usually manifests as a painless mass discovered by a relative, often during bathing.[20] The mass usually is firm, occasionally lobulated, and confined to one side of the abdomen. Rapid abdominal enlargement, anemia, and hypertension (perhaps because of a sudden subcapsular hemorrhage) are occasional presenting features. Hypertension, malaise, abdominal pain, and hematuria each occur in 20% to 30% of patients. Hypertension has been attributed to hyperreninemia.

Table 187-1 presents the differential diagnosis of abdominal and pelvic tumors of childhood that may mimic Wilms tumor.

Evaluation

The evaluation of a patient with presumed Wilms tumor begins with a history and physical examination. Particular attention should be paid to the associated congenital anomalies and the family history. Laboratory studies should include a complete blood cell count, urinalysis, and liver function test-

Table 187-1 *Differential Diagnosis of Abdominal and Pelvic Tumors in Infants and Children*

TUMOR*	AGE	CLINICAL SIGNS	LABORATORY FINDINGS
Wilms	Preschool	Unilateral flank mass, aniridia, hemihypertrophy	Hematuria
Neuroblastoma	Preschool	GI/GU obstruction, raccoon eyes, myoclonusopsoclonus, diarrhea, skin nodules (infants)	Increased VMA; increased HVA; increased ferritin; stippled calcification in mass
Non-Hodgkin lymphoma	>1 yr	Intussusception in >2-year-old	Increased urate
Rhabdomyosarcoma	All	GI/GU obstruction, sarcoma botryoides, vaginal bleeding, paratesticular mass	
Germ cell/teratoma	Preschool, teens	Girls: abdominal pain, vaginal bleeding Boys: testicular mass, new-onset "hydrocele" Sacrococcygeal mass/dimple	Increased HCG; increased AFP
Hepatoblastoma	Birth-3 yr	Large, firm liver	Increased AFP
Hepatoma	School age, teens	Large, firm liver; hepatitis B, cirrhosis	Increased AFP

AFP, Alpha-fetoprotein; *GI,* gastrointestinal; *GU,* genitourinary; *HCG,* human chorionic gonadotropin; *HVA,* homovanillic acid; *VMA,* vanillylmandelic acid.
*Other causes: constipation, splenomegaly, hydronephrosis, kidney cyst, and full bladder.

ing. Bleeding within the tumor may cause anemia.[97] An erythropoietin-secreting Wilms tumor may cause polycythemia. Hypercalcemia occurs in patients with congenital mesoblastic nephroma or a rhabdoid tumor.

A plain radiograph of the abdomen should be obtained. Calcification, if noted in a Wilms tumor, usually is quite coarse, unlike the fine, stippled pattern commonly seen in neuroblastoma. A chest film may reveal pulmonary metastases. An abdominal computed tomography (CT) scan with contrast or intravenous pyelographic examination may reveal an intrarenal mass displacing and distorting the collecting system of the involved kidney. Ultrasonographic examination is particularly helpful in evaluating the renal vein, vena cava, and the right side of the heart for tumor spread. Liver metastases may be diagnosed either by ultrasound or by CT scan. A CT scan of the chest to detect small pulmonary metastases should be performed before surgery inasmuch as postoperative atelectasis can otherwise interfere with the evaluation. Bone scans are indicated in patients with the variant known as clear cell sarcoma, which often spreads to bone.

At the time of surgery the tumor is staged as follows[41]:

1. Stage I: Tumor is limited to the kidney and is completely excised.
2. Stage II: Tumor extends beyond the kidney but is completely resected.
3. Stage III: Residual nonhematogenously spread tumor is confined to the abdomen, such as lymph node involvement, peritoneal contamination before or during surgery, peritoneal implants, residual tumor postoperatively, or incomplete resection caused by local infiltration.
4. Stage IV: Tumor metastasizes hematogenously to areas such as lung, liver, bone, or brain.
5. Stage V: Bilateral renal involvement is found at diagnosis.

Management

In the United States, the initial therapeutic approach is a complete resection by nephrectomy. This requires careful and gentle surgical techniques to prevent tumor spillage. The large transabdominal incision facilitates exploration and excision. The entire ureter is removed, lymph nodes are sampled, and the contralateral kidney and abdominal cavity are examined for evidence of disease. For bilateral disease, nephrectomy of the more involved side, with partial nephrectomy on the opposite side, may be performed. Alternatively, bilateral biopsies are followed by chemotherapy and "second look" excision of residual disease—that is, partial nephrectomies when possible.[65,126]

Actinomycin D and vincristine were both noted to be effective agents in the mid-1960s. The initial NWTS-I study revealed that radiation therapy in combination with a single agent (actinomycin D or vincristine) provided approximately 55% relapse-free survival in patients with localized disease. An 81% relapse-free survival was found when both agents were administered in conjunction with radiation.[21] The two drugs have since been the mainstay of chemotherapy for Wilms tumor. Patients with low-stage disease are now treated with these two agents without the use of radiotherapy.[21,22] For those with high-stage disease, doxorubicin is added to actinomycin D, vincristine, and radiation therapy.[22] The current NWTS-IV is evaluating shorter duration, dose-intensified regimens.

Radiation therapy is initiated within 70 days of surgery to prevent local and regional recurrences in patients with stage II unfavorable histology and with stages III and IV disease, as well as those with the clear cell variant. Lower radiation doses (10 to 20 Gy) and irradiation of the entire width of the vertebrae adjacent to the renal bed have decreased the severity—but not entirely prevented the development—of scoliosis.[119] Peritoneal seeding or tumor rupture necessitates radiation of the entire abdomen. Thoracic radiation is used for pulmonary metastasis.

Prognosis

The prognosis of patients with Wilms tumor is determined by the histopathology of the tumor. In the NWTS-I, 50% of 26 patients with unfavorable histologic findings died, as compared with 6.9% of 376 patients with favorable histologic findings.[6] These findings have been confirmed in succeeding protocols. More intensive regimens are now being studied for those patients with stages II to IV disease and unfavorable histologic findings.

The prognosis also depends on the stage of disease at diagnosis. Most relapses occur within 2 years of diagnosis. Two-year relapse-free survival for stages I and II disease with favorable histologic findings is approximately 91%. For stage III disease, relapse-free survival at 2 years is approximately 76%. The 2-year relapse-free survival rate is 69% for patients with stage IV disease or unfavorable histologic findings (stages II to IV).[23]

Follow-Up

While patients are receiving therapy, they are monitored for disease recurrence at the primary site and in the lungs. Such monitoring continues until approximately 3 years after diagnosis, or until age 5 years (whichever occurs later).

Long-term survival is likely in patients with Wilms tumor. Virtually all have had a nephrectomy and should be discouraged from engaging in contact sports. A kidney guard can be recommended for particularly active children, if only to serve as a reminder of the need for caution.

Scoliosis was a major problem for early survivors treated with moderate-dose radiation (30 to 40 Gy), particularly if the adjacent vertebrae were not included in the field. The scoliosis is less severe in more recently treated patients. Close observation of patients who received irradiation, particularly during the pubertal growth spurt, remains necessary. Prevention of obesity will minimize the asymmetry associated with a decreased quantity of adipose tissue in the radiation field.

Although fertility is preserved in most patients with Wilms tumor, the average size of infants born to female survivors of irradiation is smaller than that of normal women.[73] It is necessary to continue follow-up of these offspring to evaluate the genetic factors involved in the occurrence of Wilms tumor.

NEUROBLASTOMA

Neuroblastoma arises from the fetal neural cells that normally develop into the sympathetic nervous system. It is a tumor that provides insight into the biologic processes of malignancy. Infants may experience spontaneous tumor regression or maturation to benign ganglioneuromas, whereas patients older than 1 year with disseminated disease rarely are cured in spite of aggressive use of active agents.

Neuroblastoma is the most common malignancy of infants, accounting for over half of infantile cancers.[45] Two thirds of patients with neuroblastoma are younger than 5 years of age. Approximately 8.5 white children and 7.4 black children per million in the United States are afflicted with neuroblastoma each year.[128] This accounts for 7% of all children diagnosed with cancer and 15% of childhood cancer mortality.

Etiology

The high incidence of neuroblastoma in early infancy suggests that its development may be related to abnormal maturation of fetal neural crest cells. The finding of microscopic nodules of adrenal neuroblastoma in infants younger than 3 months of age who have died of unrelated causes suggests that spontaneous maturation and/or regression occurs in many children.[7]

Families have been reported in which neuroblastoma occurred in multiple siblings or occasionally in multiple generations.[16,92] It has been proposed that 20% to 25% of neuroblastomas occur in patients with a prezygotic germinal mutation.[67] Neuroblastoma also has been reported to occur with an increased incidence in patients with fetal hydantoin syndrome, von Recklinghausen disease, Beckwith-Wiedemann syndrome, and Hirschsprung disease.

Clinical Manifestations

Neuroblastoma may arise anywhere along the sympathetic nervous system chain, including the adrenal gland (40%), the paraspinal regions of the abdomen (25%), the thorax (15%), the neck (5%), and the pelvis at the organ of Zuckerkandl (5%). The presenting features depend to a large extent on the location of the tumor. A large, firm, irregular abdominal mass that may cross the midline often is the first sign of disease. Disturbances of bowel or bladder function may be due to compression by a pelvic mass. Thoracic masses may cause a persistent cough or respiratory distress and are diagnosed by a chest film. Cervical masses often are initially diagnosed as lymphadenitis, but they do not respond to antibiotic therapy. Horner syndrome or heterochromia iridis should suggest the possibility of neuroblastoma.

Neuroblastomas that arise in the paravertebral ganglia tend to grow into the intervertebral foramina, forming a dumbbell-shaped mass. Paralysis, extremity weakness, or incontinence may result from spinal cord compression by the intraspinal component. This is an oncologic emergency that requires surgical decompression, radiation, or chemotherapy to prevent permanent paraplegia.

Many children with neuroblastoma have metastatic disease at the time of diagnosis. The presenting features are then commonly related to the metastatic tumor rather than to the primary tumor. Infants may have metastatic hepatic involvement. Rapid liver enlargement can cause marked abdominal distention followed by respiratory compromise. Bluish skin nodules, which may release catecholamines if palpated, sometimes are noted in infants with neuroblastoma. An erythematous cutaneous flush occurs, lasting for 2 to 3 minutes, and is followed by blanching because of vasoconstriction.[54]

Older children with metastatic neuroblastoma often have infiltration of the bone marrow, causing pancytopenia. Bone involvement may produce pain, with or without palpable bone masses. Lytic bone lesions are most often found in the skull, orbit, or proximal long bones. A raccoonlike appearance caused by proptosis and eyelid ecchymosis has been described in those with orbital involvement. Intracranial disease usually is due to meningeal metastases.[68] In infants this may manifest as separation of cranial sutures. Intracerebral lesions are extremely rare.

Secretory products of the tumor may be the cause of presenting symptoms. Vasoactive intestinal polypeptide (VIP) has been found in 7% to 9% of children with neural crest tumors, most frequently ganglioneuromas or ganglioneuroblastomas.[107] Intractable diarrhea is caused by this hormone.

An unusual presenting feature of neuroblastoma is the syndrome of opsoclonus-myoclonus.[11] These patients have acute cerebellar ataxia and rapid, dancing-eye movements. Although these patients often have localized disease and usually are cured, residual neurologic dysfunction, including residual ataxia and mental retardation, is common. The etiology of this syndrome is unclear. An autoimmune factor, perhaps an antibody directed against neuroblastoma that cross-reacts with the cerebellar cell antigen, may be causative.

Tables 187-1 to 187-3 present the differential diagnosis of abdominal, pelvic, head, neck, and mediastinal tumors that may mimic neuroblastoma.

Evaluation

Evaluation of a patient with neuroblastoma requires radiologic examination of the area of primary disease, as well as of areas to which neuroblastoma spreads. In addition to the chest film, a CT scan of the abdomen, pelvis, and chest should be performed. For those patients with cervical masses, the CT scan should include this area. Because paravertebral lesions may extend into the intervertebral foramina, any patient with such a lesion should be evaluated by use of myelography or magnetic resonance imaging. A skeletal survey and a bone scan should be performed to detect bony lesions.[64] Radiographs are useful for the detection of small lytic lesions at the end of bones; the bone scan helps find lesions of the skull and tubular bones. A bone marrow aspirate and biopsy specimen should be obtained in all patients because this is a common site of metastatic involvement. The liver should be examined by contrast CT scan or liver-spleen scan in all patients, and biopsy specimens should be obtained in those with abdominal disease.

Neuroblastoma must be diagnosed by histologic examination after biopsy. In patients with localized disease, the biopsy specimen must be obtained from the primary tumor. For those with metastatic disease, neuroblastoma cells can be identified in the primary tumor or in areas of metastases,

Table 187-2 *Differential Diagnosis of Head and Neck Tumors in Infants and Children*

TUMOR*	AGE	CLINICAL SIGNS	LABORATORY FINDINGS
Non-Hodgkin lymphoma	>1 yr	Lymphadenopathy—NR to antibiotics; immunodeficiency; EBV (in Africa)	Increased urate
Hodgkin disease	>10 yr	Lymphadenopathy—NR to antibiotics; weight loss, night sweats, fever, pruritus	Increased ESR
Rhabdomyosarcoma	All	Orbital mass; hoarseness; persistent otitis, sinusitis	
Neuroblastoma	Preschool	Heterochromia iridis, Horner syndrome, myoclonus-opsoclonus, raccoon eyes, skin nodules (infants)	Increased HVA in urine; increased VMA in urine; calcification
Retinoblastoma	Preschool	Cat's eye reflex, strabismus, family history	Calcification

EBV, Epstein-Barr virus; *ESR,* sedimentation rate; *HVA,* homovanillic acid; *NR,* no response; *VMA,* vanillylmandelic acid.
*Other causes: infectious lymphadenopathy, histiocytosis, caffey disease, acquired immunodeficiency syndrome.

Table 187-3 *Differential Diagnosis of Mediastinal Tumors in Infants and Children*

TUMOR*	AGE	CLINICAL SIGNS	LABORATORY FINDINGS
Non-Hodgkin lymphoma	All	Cough, respiratory distress, anterior mediastinal mass, immunodeficiency syndrome	Increased urate; malignant effusion
Hodgkin disease	>10 yr	Middle mediastinum lymphadenopathy—NR to antibiotics; weight loss, night sweats, fever, pruritus	Increased ESR; increased copper
Neuroblastoma	Preschool	Posterior mediastinum; heterochromia iridis, myoclonus-opsoclonus, raccoon eyes, skin nodules (infants)	Increased HVA; increased VMA; calcification
Thymoma	>10 yr	Anterior mediastinum, myasthenia gravis, red cell aplasia, hypogammaglobulinemia	
Germ cell/teratoma	All	Anterior mediastinum (rarely, posterior mediastinum), cough, wheeze, dyspnea	Increased AFP; increased HCG

AFP, Alpha-fetoprotein; *ESR,* sedimentation rate; *HCG,* human chorionic gonadotropin; *HVA,* homovanillic acid; *VMA,* vanillylmandelic acid.
*Other causes: infection, bronchogenic cysts, aneurysms, lipoid tumors, thoracic meningocele.

including the bone, bone marrow, or liver. Neuroblastoma comprises small round cells with scant cytoplasm that must be differentiated from other small cell tumors of childhood, including lymphoma, leukemia, Ewing sarcoma, and retinoblastoma. Neuroblastoma cells often are densely packed and separated by thin fibrils or bundles. Necrosis and calcification may be seen. The small round cells often form clusters surrounded by pink neurofibrillary material called *rosettes*. With increasing maturation, more fibrillary material is present, and ganglionic differentiation may be seen. Cytoplasmic structures consisting of neurofibrils, neurotubules, and neurosecretory granules that contain catecholamines may be noted.[77] Secretion of catecholamines from the granules results in elevated levels of vanillylmandelic acid (VMA) and homovanillic acid (HVA) in 24-hour urine samples or in elevated VMA:creatinine or HVA:creatinine ratios in "spot" urine samples.[48,69] These findings can be used to confirm the diagnosis of neuroblastoma in patients with a small round cell infiltrate in the bone marrow. In addition, elevated urinary catecholamine levels can be used to monitor the response to therapy.

Management

Neuroblastoma is sensitive to both chemotherapy and radiation therapy. For those with localized disease, however, surgical therapy alone may suffice. Complete removal of the tumor offers the best chance of cure. Residual tumor in patients with stages I and II disease may regress spontaneously. Because patients with advanced disease have disease that cannot be completely resected, only a diagnostic biopsy is required initially. Tumor recurrence in such patients often is at the site of the primary tumor. Thus surgical reduction after initial cytoreductive therapy may affect the likelihood of cure.

Chemotherapy is the major modality of therapy in neuroblastoma. Complete and partial responses have been found with the following agents: cyclophosphamide (59%), doxorubicin (41%), cisplatin (46%), epipodophyllotoxin (30%), vincristine (24%), and dacarbazine (DTIC) (14%).[14] Cyclophosphamide and vincristine individually or in combination have been used for the treatment of localized neuroblastoma. A newer, kinetically based regimen uses cyclosphosphamide for 7 days followed by doxorubicin on day 8 or, for those who do not respond, cisplatin followed by epidophyllotoxin. For patients with advanced stage disease, these four agents have been used in combination. An alternative intensive approach uses multiple alkylating agents (nitrogen mustard, doxorubicin, DTIC, cisplatin, vincristine, and cyclophosphamide).[100] Long-term survival for patients with Evans stage III neuroblastoma has improved in recent years, but survival with conventional therapy remains inadequate for patients (older than 1 year of age) with stage IV disease. More intensive regimens that use high-dose cisplatin and other newer agents are being investigated.

Intensive regimens are at the limits of bone marrow tolerance. Total body irradiation and higher doses of chemotherapy may increase the likelihood of long-term survival but require a bone marrow transplantation to restore hematopoiesis. Autologous transplantation using the patient's own bone marrow is preferred to allogeneic transplantation (using another person's bone marrow, e.g., a sibling's), which is limited to human leukocyte antigen (HLA)–matched donors and carries the risk of graft-versus-host disease. A number of long-term survivors of stage IV neuroblastoma have been reported after bone marrow transplantation.[5]

Neuroblastoma is a radiation-sensitive tumor. In early-stage disease, surgery alone or surgery with a small amount of chemotherapy may obviate the need for radiation therapy. Patients with advanced disease may receive radiation therapy to make residual disease surgically resectable or less likely to recur. Emergent situations, such as a large mediastinal mass resulting in respiratory compromise or a dumbbell lesion protruding into the intervertebral foramen that causes cord compression, frequently are treated with radiation. Radiation also is a component of the preparative regimen used before bone marrow transplantation for the treatment of stage IV neuroblastoma. In the terminal stage of neuroblastoma, bone pain or compression of organs such as the trachea, bowel, or urinary tract may require palliative radiation therapy.

Prognosis

Age and stage of disease appear to be the most important predictors of survival. Patients who are younger than 1 year of age do markedly better than those who are older than 2 years of age. Older studies report 2-year survival rates of 80%, 60%, 13%, 7%, and 75% for patients with Evans stages I, II, III, IV, and IVS neuroblastoma, respectively. Patients with IVS neuroblastoma have a small primary lesion in addition to metastatic disease (other than bone involvement). Most are less than 1 year of age. The review of patients treated with more intensive approaches during the decade 1970 to 1980 found survival rates of 100%, 93%, 81%, 23%, and 90% for Evans stage I, II, III, IV, IVS disease.[100] From 2 to 12 years had elapsed since these patients' diagnosis, with a mean follow-up of 46 months for all patients (66 months for surviving patients). Thus intensive multiagent chemotherapy appears to result in improved cure rates.

Follow-Up

Although late recurrences have been reported, most tumors recur while patients are receiving therapy or shortly afterward. Close follow-up with physical examination and radiologic studies should continue for 2 years after completion of therapy. Urinary catecholamine levels may be useful in the surveillance of those who had elevated values at diagnosis. Monitoring for late toxicities (e.g., of cyclophosphamide, doxorubicin, and cisplatin) should be performed.

RETINOBLASTOMA

Retinoblastoma is a congenital malignant tumor of the retina that occurs once in 18,000 live births.[28] Retinoblastoma develops in approximately 200 children in the United States annually, 20% to 30% of whom have bilateral disease. The disorder is diagnosed in 80% before age 4 years, with the median age of diagnosis being 2 years. Patients with bilateral disease appear to have an inherited form of this tumor that manifests at an earlier age. Most patients with unilateral disease have a sporadic form of the tumor.

This tumor is the model for understanding the role of

genetics in the development of malignancy. The pediatrician plays an important role in detecting this disorder initially and in providing support to the family who may carry a genetic predisposition to this malignancy.

ETIOLOGY

Knudson[66] has proposed that two independent mutations must occur in a single retinal cell for retinoblastoma to develop. The initial mutation may occur in a germinal cell (inheritable form) or in the somatic retinal cell itself (sporadic form). Those patients with an abnormality in the germinal cell have one mutation in each retinal cell. A second mutation is relatively likely to occur, causing retinoblastoma (often multiple, bilateral tumors). If the initial mutation arises in a retinal cell, it must be followed by a second mutation in the same cell for the sporadic form of retinoblastoma to arise. The likelihood of two such events is low; hence single, unilateral tumors develop. Because the germinal cell is not involved, the mutation is not inherited.

It is clear that a patient with a family member with retinoblastoma or with bilateral retinoblastoma has a germinal mutation—thus the hereditary form of the disease. The germinal mutation also may have arisen in an affected parent or in one with an undiagnosed retinal lesion. It is recommended that parents have an ophthalmologic examination. If the first child of "normal" parents has unilateral retinoblastoma, their second child has a 1% risk of also being affected. In some families, recombinant DNA techniques may aid in determining which relatives are predisposed to retinoblastoma.[127] All families should be sent for genetic counseling.

Clinical Manifestations

Patients with a family history of retinoblastoma currently are screened by examination under anesthesia every 2 to 3 months during early childhood. These patients therefore are diagnosed before the occurrence of any clinical symptoms. Pediatricians and parents usually detect the abnormality in children with the sporadic form of disease, because young children rarely complain of unilaterally decreased vision. Leukocoria, or cat's eye reflex, describes a whiteness detected in the pupillary area caused by a large retrolental mass. It is the most common presenting sign of retinoblastoma.[108] If a normal red reflex is not present in a young child, it should be investigated. The second most common presenting feature is strabismus. Although this is a common occurrence in childhood because of abnormalities of ocular muscle strength, it rarely arises suddenly in a child with previously normal extraocular movements. Rarely, pain in the eye may occur as a result of glaucoma. New-onset strabismus or an abnormal red reflex requires prompt ophthalmologic evaluation.

The differential diagnosis of retinoblastoma includes Coats disease, retrolental fibroplasia, toxoplasmosis, *Toxocara canis*, persistent hyperplastic primary vitreous, and severe uveitis.[108] In one review,[83] 25% of patients had nonneoplastic disorders at the time of enucleation. Of the patients with retinoblastomas 14% have been found to have had a significant delay from the time of onset of symptoms to diagnosis.[111] Newer methodologies, including ultrasonic examinations and MRI, may help differentiate retinoblastoma from other diseases of the eye. Patients in whom retinoblastoma is a possibility should be referred to an ophthalmologist who has a working relationship with radiation and pediatric oncologists and is experienced in the diagnosis and initial evaluation of these patients.

Evaluation

Examination under anesthesia, after pupillary dilation, is necessary to evaluate the retina in a young child fully. Ultrasonographic examination is useful to evaluate the mass, particularly if the fundal examination is obscured by hemorrhage or retinal detachment.[112] Calcification present in retinoblastoma may be apparent on roentgenogram, ultrasound examination, or CT scanning. The CT scan is useful to demonstrate the extent of intraocular disease and to detect possible extraocular extension. MRI can help evaluate the tumor's involvement with the optic nerve, the subarachnoid, and the brain.

This is not a tumor in which biopsy is a feasible method of diagnosis. Patients with the hereditable form do not need a tissue diagnosis. In most cases of unilateral disease, enucleation is necessary to establish the diagnosis as well as to treat the tumor. During the examination under anesthesia, bone marrow and cerebrospinal fluid specimens are obtained for evidence of dissemination. The extent of local disease (extension beyond the globe or optic nerve infiltration) is assessed at the time of enucleation.

Management

Treatment for retinoblastoma is individualized, based on the extent of disease and the possibility for the preservation of vision.[62] Treatment modalities available include enucleation, cryotherapy, photocoagulation, and radiotherapy. Most patients with unilateral sporatic disease have large lesions and visual compromise. They usually require enucleation, cryotherapy and photocoagulation are used for small lesions, most commonly in those with hereditary bilateral disease. These approaches prevent the need for bilateral enucleation. Radiation therapy is used for those with massive bilateral disease. If vision can be preserved in one eye by photocoagulation or cryotherapy, but not in the other, then a unilateral enucleation may be performed.

Chemotherapy rarely is used for intraocular retinoblastoma. Triethylenemelamine given by intracarotid artery injection in combination with radiotherapy is not clearly superior to radiotherapy alone.[15] The role of adjuvant chemotherapy in those with larger amounts of intraocular disease is not well defined. Combinations of agents such as cyclophosphamide, doxorubicin, vincristine, cisplatin, and epipodophyllotoxins have been used in patients with advanced or recurrent disease with some evidence of success.[95] Bone marrow transplantation for the treatment of recurrent disease has been reported.[36]

Prognosis

Survival of patients with retinoblastoma is excellent; 90% have no recurrence of their tumor.[15] Unfortunately, those with hereditary retinoblastoma have a high incidence of second malignancy. Approximately 50% occur within the radiation field; osteogenic sarcoma or other sarcomas are particularly common. Approximately one third of such patients will have a second malignancy within 15 years. By 30 years, two thirds will have experienced a second malignancy.[3,50]

Follow-Up

Patients who have been treated for retinoblastoma will need close follow-up for evidence of recurrence and for second malignancies. Most recurrences manifest within 3 years of diagnosis. Examinations under anesthesia should be performed every 2 to 3 months during the first year, every 3 to 4 months during the second year, and every 6 months thereafter until age 6 years. Patients with bilateral or familial disease are at great risk of second malignancies and thus should seek medical care promptly for unexplained masses, pain, or other symptoms.

These patients experience a number of long-term complications. After enucleation a prosthesis will be necessary. In young children the orbit will not grow normally after enucleation or radiation. Although bilateral radiation prevents asymmetry, cataract development is likely. Retinal vascular injury also may occur. Growth and pubertal development should be followed after high-dose orbital irradiation, because the pituitary gland or hypothalamus might be affected.

RHABDOMYOSARCOMA

Rhabdomyosarcoma is an aggressive tumor arising from embryonal mesenchyme that has the potential to differentiate into skeletal muscle. It can arise almost anywhere in the body and disseminates early in the course of disease. Before the era of chemotherapy, cure required extirpative surgery of localized disease and then radiotherapy. The rapid progress, with survival rates increasing from less than 20% in the 1960s to 70% currently, has been due to the multidisciplinary cooperative group approach of the Intergroup Rhabdomyosarcoma Study (IRS) teams.[85]

Rhabdomyosarcoma is the most common pediatric soft tissue sarcoma, accounting for 4% to 8% of childhood malignancies and 5% to 15% of childhood solid tumors.[128] It occurs in 4.5 per million white and 1.3 per million black children in the United States; 38% of children are younger than 5 years of age, 47% are 5 to 14 years of age, and 15% are older than 15 years.[85]

Etiology

The cause of this tumor is unknown. It has occurred in association with neurofibromatosis, in families with multiple tumors, and in patients with congenital abnormalities of the central nervous system, the heart, the gastrointestinal tract, and the urinary tract.[105]

Clinical Manifestations

Rhabdomyosarcoma manifests as a painless mass with poorly defined margins.[31] One common site is the orbit, in which swelling, proptosis, discoloration, and limitation of extraocular motion occur. Patients with a tumor of the head and neck may have hoarseness, polyps, obstruction, difficulty swallowing, decreased hearing acuity, persistent otitis, sinusitis, parotitis, or cranial nerve palsies. In parameningeal sites, penetration to the brain may cause headache, vomiting, or diplopia. Retroperitoneal tumor may manifest as a mass or as gastrointestinal discomfort because of partial obstruction. Vaginal bleeding, pelvic or perineal masses, hematuria, urinary frequency, and urinary retention suggest genitourinary tract involvement. A hydrocele, incarcerated hernia, testicular torsion, or testicular mass may be a presentation of paratesticular rhabdomyosarcoma.

Evaluation

The initial evaluation should include a complete blood cell count, liver and renal function tests, and a urinalysis. Roentgenograms, CT scans, and in some instances (e.g., genitourinary tract) ultrasound examination of the involved and adjacent areas should be performed. For those with a parameningeal tumor the spinal fluid should be examined for cellular evidence of meningeal disease. The skull should be examined for erosion into its base. A head CT and dental films may be helpful. A barium enema, voiding cystourethrogram, and cystoscopic and pelvic examinations (sometimes under anesthesia) may be necessary for patients with genitourinary tract involvement. At times an arteriogram or inferior vena cavagram is performed to assess operability of the tumor. If spinal cord symptoms are present, a myelogram or MRI of the spinal cord is necessary. Biopsy of the lesion establishes the diagnosis and should be performed before extensive resection. The bone, bone marrow, and liver must be evaluated for evidence of metastasis. This should be performed before any major surgical resections are attempted. The staging system most commonly used is based on the extent of postoperative disease, including the status of regional nodes and tumor resectiability. This staging system will need revision in the current era of extremely effective chemotherapy inasmuch as extensive surgical approaches often are inadvisable.

Management

Rhabdomyosarcoma is a tumor that requires a multitherapeutic approach, including chemotherapy, surgery, and radiation. Aggressive surgical approaches have become less essential as chemotherapy and radiation therapy have become more efficacious.

The initial surgical procedure should be a diagnostic biopsy. When possible a wide resection of the primary tumor, including surrounding normal tissue, is preferable if excessive morbidity can be avoided.[86] Extensive en bloc lymph node dissection is no longer indicated; however, biopsy for staging purposes is indicated for large regional nodes. At times, second-look surgery is appropriate after chemotherapy or radiotherapy to assess therapeutic responses.

Chemotherapeutic regimens used in the treatment of rhabdomyosarcoma include vincristine, actinomycin D, cyclophosphamide, and doxorubicin.[85] Patients with localized tumors and orbital tumors can be treated with vincristine and actinomycin D alone. Patients with more advanced disease may benefit from doxorubicin, cyclophosphamide, and other agents (cisplatin, DTIC, and etoposide).

Rhabdomyosarcoma is an infiltrative disease, and radiation portals should include the entire extent of tumor volume. Although high doses of radiation (60 to 65 Gy) control local residual disease excellently, substantial late morbidity results.[116] Unfortunately, lower doses of radiation result in an increased recurrence rate. New methodologies utilizing lower total doses of radiation administered twice daily are being examined to determine if disease can be controlled while decreasing late toxicities.[81]

Prognosis

The likelihood of survival for patients with rhabdomyosarcoma is determined by the site and the stage of disease.[71] The prognosis is particularly good for patients with orbital tumors and localized tumors that can be fully resected (90% to 95% long-term survivors). Extremity lesions are particularly difficult to treat, perhaps because many are of the alveolar subtype and tend to metastasize. Treatment of genitourinary primary tumors has improved markedly in recent years with the use of extensive chemotherapy. Pelvic exenteration and other morbid surgeries can now be avoided in most patients. The recent use of cranial radiation and intrathecal chemotherapy in patients with parameningeal lesions has prevented meningeal involvement and has improved survival markedly.[98] Of those patients who do have recurrences, 80% will occur within 2 years of treatment. Local relapse is most common, although distant spread to the lungs, central nervous system, lymph nodes, bone, liver, bone marrow, and soft tissues does occur. Patients with metastatic disease at diagnosis (20%) continue to have a low likelihood of survival.[104] Bone marrow transplantation or the use of new agents may offer hope to these patients.

Follow-Up

Patients with rhabdomyosarcoma should receive close follow-up for evidence of recurrent disease for approximately 3 years from the time of diagnosis. Later recurrences may even occur thereafter. Most of these patients have been treated with high-dose radiotherapy; thus bone films of the area should be obtained periodically. Patients with orbital tumors often have significant cosmetic effects as a result of the radiation therapy. Those with orbital parameningeal lesions have received radiation to the sinuses, hypothalamus, and pituitary gland. Sinusitis is a common complaint. Hormonal levels (e.g., gonadotrophins and growth hormone) may need monitoring. Monitoring for potential late effects of chemotherapeutic agents (e.g., cyclophosphamide and doxorubicin) should be performed (Table 187-4).

GERM CELL TUMORS AND TERATOMAS

Germ cell tumors are growths arising from primordial germ cells. They account for 3% of the tumors in children.[128] The sacrococcygeal teratoma (named from the Greek *teras*, or

Table 187-4 *Long-Term Side Effects of Chemotherapy*

DRUG	POTENTIAL ORGAN DAMAGE	EVALUATION
Anthracyclines, e.g., doxorubicin	Cardiac: myocardial damage, congestive failure, arrhythmias	*Cardiac* History: Exercise in tolerance, palpitations; ECG (QTc interval); echocardiogram (shortening fraction q3-5 yr); Holter monitor; exercise ECG; exercise nuclear angiography
Bleomycin	Lungs: fibrosis, impaired diffusion capacity, exacerbated by increased oxygen (e.g., anesthesia)	*Pulmonary* History: Shortness of breath, dyspnea on exertion, cough. Chest film and pulmonary function tests (with diffusion capacity) q3-5 yr
Cyclophosphamide, ifosfamide	Gonadal damage: infertility, sterility, early menopause	*Gonadal* History: Menses, question of fertility; LH/FSH/testosterone or estradiol during pubertal development, or if there is a problem with fertility/amenorrhea; semen analysis (prn childbearing)
	Bladder: hemorrhagic cystitis	Urinalysis—annually
	Marrow: secondary AML	CBC—annually
Lomustine (CCNU) Carmustine (BCNU)	Gonadal, lungs	Pulmonary, gonadal evaluation (as above)
Cisplatin	Kidney: decreased glomerular filtration rate	Serum creatinine q1-3 yr Creatinine clearance q3-5 yr
	Ears: hearing loss (high frequency)	Audiogram q3-5 yr
Methotrexate	Liver dysfunction CNS: learning impairment (high intravenous dose)	Liver function tests q1-3 yr
6-Mercaptopurine (6-MP), 6-thioguanine, actinomycin D	Liver dysfunction	Liver function tests q1-3 yr

AML, Acute myeloblastic anemia; *CBC*, complete blood cell count; *ECG*, electrocardiogram; *FSH*, follicle-stimulating hormone; *LH*, luteinizing hormone; *prn*, as required.

monster) is benign in 80% of patients. It occurs in 1 per 35,000 live births, more commonly in girls than in boys (2 to 4:1); 60% of childhood germ cell tumors originate in other sites, including the gonads, mediastinum, intracranial region, and retroperitoneum.

Etiology

Germ cells appear in the yolk sac endoderm, migrate around the hind gut to the genital ridge on the posterior abdominal wall of the embryo, and congregate, becoming part of the developing gonad. A slightly aberrant path of migration may account for the occurrence of extragonadal germ cell tumors along the dorsal wall of the embryo in midline sites (sacrococcygeal, retroperitoneal, mediastinal, and pineal regions).[4] Children with sacrococcygeal teratomas have an approximately 15% incidence of associated anamolies (e.g., imperforate anus and rectal stenosis).[51] An association with a family history of twinning resulted in early theories suggesting that teratomas were abortive attempts at the development of twins. Of interest, the common sites of teratomas—the brain, mediastinum, abdomen, and sacrococcygeal region—are all sites of twin attachment. Although most germ cell tumors arise in "normal" individuals, a genetic tendency for abnormal germ cell development may exist in some families. These tumors have been reported to develop in siblings, twins, and subsequent generations. Gonadal dysgenesis has been associated with dysgerminoma or gonadoblastoma.[53]

The type of germ cell tumor that forms is determined by the subsequent development of the germ cell.[117] Those that maintain their total potentiality become embryonal sarcomas. The development of extraembryonic structures results in the formation of choriocarcinomas (placental tumors) or endodermal sinus tumors (yolk sac tumors). Seminomas or dysgerminomas arise when gonadal differentiation occurs. Teratomas form as a result of embryonal differentiation into ectoderm, mesoderm, and endoderm.

Clinical Manifestations

The clinical manifestations of a germ cell tumor depend on the tumor location. Sacrococcygeal tumors occur as a mass between the anus and the coccyx.[124] An abnormality of the overlying skin may be noted. An intrapelvic tumor may be associated with an external tumor or may be the only evidence of disease, noted by the onset of urinary or rectal obstruction. The incidence of intradural tumor extension is 3% to 5%. Maternal polyhydramnios may be associated with infantile sacrococcygeal teratomas.

Ovarian tumors[80] in infants manifest as abdominal masses. Older girls have symptoms of abdominal pain, nausea, vomiting, constipation, or urinary tract obstruction, with palpable masses noted in 50%. Torsion or hemorrhage within the tumor may be responsible for acute abdominal pain; 5% of such children have bilateral tumors. Vaginal germ cell tumors in preschool girls (younger than 3 years old) may cause bloody vaginal discharge.

Testicular tumors[39] most often manifest as a symptom-free scrotal mass, sometimes with a coexisting hydrocele. Torsion of the tumor in an undescended testis may result in acute abdominal pain. Testicular malignancy is 20 to 40 times more common in boys with undescended testes. Because the ipsilateral or contralateral testis may be affected, an intrinsic testicular defect is likely.

Retroperitoneal teratomas that occur in children younger than age 2 years usually are symptom-free abdominal masses. In older children, anorexia, vomiting, or abdominal pain may be noted. Intradural extensions also may occur, and gastric and hepatic tumors have been reported.

The symptoms of patients with germ cell tumors of the anterior mediastinum include coughing, wheezing, dyspnea, and chest pain.[70] Newborns may require immediate intubation for respiratory distress caused by mediastinal, cervical, or oropharyngeal germ cell tumors. Intrapericardial tumors can cause heart failure and cardiac tamponade. Inability of the fetus with an oropharyngeal mass to swallow can cause maternal polyhydramnios. Cranial tumors (80% in the pineal region) cause hydrocephalus and increased intercranial pressure in infants. Teenagers have headaches, lethargy, vomiting, visual disturbance, diabetes insipidus, and seizures.

The differential diagnosis of children with germ cell tumors depends on the location of the primary tumor. For those with sacrococcygeal masses the most frequently alternative diagnosis is meningocele. Abdominal or pelvic masses may be due to neuroblastoma, Wilms tumor, rhabdomyosarcoma, or lymphomas. Nonmalignant disorders such as hydronephrosis, benign ovarian cysts, constipation, and splenomegaly must be considered. Anterior mediastinal tumors include T cell lymphoma or thymoma. The differential diagnosis for an intrascrotal mass includes testicular torsion, epididymitis, and testicular infarction. (See Tables 187-1 and 187-3 for details of the differential diagnosis of germ cell tumors.)

Evaluation

As in any ill child, evaluation includes a careful physical examination. For those patients with a sacrococcygeal mass or abdominal pain, particular attention should be given to the abdominal and rectal examination. A pelvic examination (performed under anesthesia in young girls) will be necessary if an ovarian or a vaginal tumor is suspected.

Careful evaluation by CT or ultrasound examination, or both, is essential in the assessment. A CT scan of benign germ cell tumors often will reveal calcifications. A teratoma frequently shows cystic and solid components on ultrasound examination. A chest CT scan and bone scan should be performed to detect pulmonary and bony metastases.

Malignant germ cell tumors with evidence of extraembryonic differentiation often produce proteins elaborated by the corresponding normal embryonic structure. Serum levels of these markers, alpha-fetoprotein (AFP) and beta–human chorionic gonadotropin (B-HCG), should be assayed before surgery. AFP is found in germ cell tumors with endodermal sinus tumor histology. The evaluation of AFP levels must account for their elevation during fetal development; they do not fall to normal levels until the child is approximately 9 months of age.[120] B-HCG, a glycoprotein normally produced by specialized placental cells, is present in increased quantity in patients with choriocarcinomas and with hydatidiform moles and during pregnancy.

Detection of AFP or B-HCG improves the ability to follow the disease status subsequently. The rate of disappearance after resection reflects the adequacy of the tumor removal. With response to chemotherapy the levels of these proteins fall. A significant rise in these levels suggests disease recurrence.

Management

Germ cell tumors may have components of teratoma, endodermal sinus tumor, embryonal carcinoma, choriocarcinoma, seminoma, or dysgerminoma. Teratomas are classified as mature, immature, or teratoma with malignant components. Mature teratomas (well-differentiated tissues) and immature teratomas (embryonic-appearing neuroglial elements and mature elements) most commonly are found in infants. Malignant evolution may occur years after removal of an apparently benign tumor, particularly in the sacrococcygeal area. For this reason, complete excision of the coccyx often is recommended, and careful follow-up is necessary.

In the past, malignant teratomas, embryonal carcinomas, endodermal sinus tumors, and choriocarcinomas were almost uniformly fatal. Complete surgical resection rarely was attained and was only infrequently curative. Only embryonal carcinoma of the infant testis could be cured by radical orchiectomy. In the 1960s, however, the efficacy of chemotherapy for gestational choriocarcinomas and testicular germ cell tumors was demonstrated.[74] Methotrexate was noted to be effective in gestational choriocarcinoma. Ovarian tumors responded to vincristine, actinomycin D, and cyclophosphamide. In the 1970s, additional agents such as vinblastine and cisplatin were found to have significant single-agent response in testicular germ cell tumors of young men. The combination of these two agents with bleomycin produces a 70% complete remission rate and a 55% long-term disease-free survival for patients with advanced testicular carcinoma.[35]

Prognosis

The regimens already described have been effective in children; 79 children with malignant germ cell tumors, 39% of whom had widely disseminated metastases at diagnosis, were treated with these agents.[1] Of these, 45% remained free of disease 4 years after diagnosis. Newer agents such as ifosfamide, as well as higher doses of cisplatin, are now being incorporated into the treatment regimens. It is hoped that these additions will increase the percentage of cured patients.

The prognosis for a teratoma depends on its degree of maturity. Patients with a mature teratoma do best. Age also is important: sacrococcygeal teratomas usually are benign in children younger than 2 months of age, but thereafter the likelihood of malignant evolution increases rapidly. This may be the reason that intrapelvic teratomas that are not detected early often are found to be malignant. Mediastinal teratomas behave benignly in children and young teenagers; in older patients they are more aggressive. Cervical and intracranial teratomas in infants usually are benign, whereas those in adolescents and adults often are malignant.

Follow-Up

The response of malignant germ cell tumors to chemotherapy is very encouraging. These patients may, however, relapse late in the course of the disease, as many as 10 years from the time of diagnosis. For this reason, close follow-up care is essential, including frequent physical examinations, use of ultrasound, and chest films. Late brain metastases also have been described. Salvage therapy may prolong survival or even provide a cure. Late effects of the chemotherapeutic agent administered (e.g., bleomycin, cisplatin, doxorubicin) should be monitored (see Table 187-4).

EWING SARCOMA

Ewing sarcoma is a malignant nonosseous tumor that usually arises in bone but also may occur in soft tissues. It accounts for 3% of childhood cancers and is the most common bone tumor in children younger than 10 years of age.[128] In the second decade of life it is second only to osteogenic sarcoma in incidence. The peak incidence is between the ages of 11 and 17 years, with a range of 5 months to 60 years of age. Ewing sarcoma is extremely rare in children younger than 5 years of age, as well as in black and Chinese persons.

Etiology

Ewing sarcoma is a primitive small round cell tumor. The cell of origin may be derived from primitive mesenchymal cells.[30] A possible neural origin of Ewing sarcoma is suggested by the finding of a chromosomal abnormality involving a reciprocal translocation of chromosomes 11 and 22 [t(11,22)] in tumor tissue that is identical to that of peripheral neuroepithelioma.[125] There is no evidence of hereditary transmission of Ewing sarcoma. Neither has it been associated with known congenital syndromes nor constitutional karyotypic abnormalities.

Clinical Manifestations

Patients with Ewing sarcoma most commonly consult the clinician for pain.[38] Swelling also may be seen. Symptoms often begin insidiously, several months before diagnosis, and initially are attributed to trauma. At the time of diagnosis a mass is palpable in 60% of patients, resulting from the propensity of this tumor to break through the bony cortex and involve the surrounding tissue.[88] The primary lesion most often is found in the femur (22%), the fibula or tibula (21%), or the pelvis (22%).[25] The ribs and vertebrae are other common sites of origin of this tumor. Demonstrable metastatic lesions are present in 14% to 35% of patients, occurring in the lungs, bones, lymph nodes, and bone marrow.[122] Central nervous system involvement is not common.

The differential diagnosis includes osteogenic sarcoma, osteomyelitis, benign bone tumors, and bone cysts. Other tumors that occasionally involve the bone and have a similar histologic pattern of small round cells include lymphoma, leukemia, neuroblastoma, and rhabdomyosarcoma (Table 187-5).

Evaluation

A roentgenogram should be obtained in a patient with a mass overlying bone or bone pain that is not characteristic of trauma (by lack of history or duration of symptoms). X-ray films of

Table 187-5 *Differential Diagnosis of Malignant Tumors Involving the Extremities*

TUMOR*	AGE	CLINICAL SIGNS	LABORATORY FINDINGS
Ewing sarcoma	≥5 yr	Pain, swelling; GU/skeletal anomaly; weight loss, fever; malaise (metabolic)	"Onion skin" on roentgenogram
Osteogenic sarcoma	Teens	Pain, swelling; familial retinoblastoma; prior radiation to bone; Paget disease	Codman triangle (cortical elevation, new bone formation); "sunburst" ossification of soft tissue; soft tissue mass; elevated alkaline phosphatase level
Lymphoma	All	Pain	
Fibrosarcoma	Infants, teens	Painless mass; prior radiation; plastic implant	
Rhabdomyosarcoma	All	Mass	
Synovial sarcoma	Teens	Mass	Calcification (40%)

*Other causes: trauma, bone cysts, osteomyelitis.

a bone with Ewing sarcoma often show a destructive lesion in the diaphysis. An onion-skin appearance arises from periosteal elevation and subperiosteal new bone formation associated with tumor extension through the cortex. A mottled pattern may be seen as a result of bone destruction, sclerosis, and cystic formation. An associated soft tissue mass occurs in more than 50% of patients with primary tumors of long bones. In addition to a plain roentgenogram of the involved bone, a CT scan and perhaps MRI may help determine the extent of the primary lesion.

Radionuclide bone scanning detects primary and metastatic lesions, but it is not particularly useful in determining the extent of the primary disease. However, it may aid in following the response to therapy. A chest film and a CT scan of the chest are necessary to determine whether pulmonary lesions are present. The possibility of bone marrow involvement should be evaluated by marrow aspiration and biopsy. Cerebrospinal fluid should be examined in patients with parameningeal tumors.

A biopsy of the lesion is necessary to establish the diagnosis. If possible, diagnostic tissue should be obtained from soft tissue rather than cortical bone in order to reduce the potential for pathologic fracture. Ewing sarcoma is characterized by a pattern of monomorphic sheets of small tumors made up of round cells with hyperchromatic nuclei and relatively little cytoplasm.[38] Schiff stains of the cells show positivity, but this finding is not specific for Ewing sarcoma. This sarcoma remains a diagnosis of exclusion, depending on the absence of characteristics specific for other small round cell tumors.

There is no staging system for Ewing sarcoma. Tumors are classified and treated as either localized or metastatic.

Management

Approximately 75% of patients with Ewing sarcoma have apparently localized disease. Localized therapies alone, however, are unlikely to be curative because of the presence of micrometastases. Chemotherapy has made it possible to cure the majority of patients with Ewing sarcoma, and it assists in the treatment of local disease by reducing the need for radical surgery or high-dose, large-volume irradiation.

The choice of radiation or surgery for local control is based on the likelihood of preserving function. Functionally expendable bones should be removed. Aggressive surgical procedures (amputation or radical limb-sparing excisions) are used only when radiotherapy may cause substantial growth impairment or in the presence of severe pathologic fractures. Most often, radiation therapy is used. Local control is attained in 90% of patients with distal extremity lesions, 75% with proximal extremity lesions, and 65% with central lesions.[118] Radiation therapy also may be helpful after subtotal resection of the primary tumor or for treatment of pulmonary or osseous metastases.

Ewing sarcoma is extremely chemosensitive. Active agents, including vincristine, doxorubicin, cyclophosphamide, and actinomycin D, have been used in the most efficacious regimens. Etoposide and ifosfamide, in combination, have elicited good therapeutic responses in many patients with relapsed disease. The integration of these agents into the standard therapeutic regimens currently is being investigated. Dose intensity of the more active agents (cyclophosphamide and doxorubicin) has played a major role in improving disease-free survival.[101] However, the outcome is extremely poor for patients with bone metastases or bone marrow involvement. Bone marrow transplantation currently is being investigated in patients with marrow and bone metastasies. Pulmonary metastases often can be effectively treated with intensive chemotherapy regimens and radiation therapy.

Prognosis

Before the use of multiagent chemotherapy, 85% of children with Ewing sarcoma died within 2 years of diagnosis.[40] Five-year, disease-free survival is now 55% to 70%, influenced by the extent and location of disease.[62,94] Approximately 80% of patients with small, distal extremity Ewing sarcoma tumors survive, compared with only 30% of those with large, central extremity lesions, perhaps because of the difficulties in delivering adequate amounts of radiation therapy. Factors associated with poor prognosis include extensive soft tissue masses, large primary tumors, and high serum levels of lactate dehydrogenase.[37,42,88]

Follow-Up

Patients with Ewing sarcoma require close follow-up for evidence of recurrent disease for approximately 3 years from the time of diagnosis, although later recurrences may occur. Particular attention should be paid to the irradiated field of long-term survivors, because second malignancies may arise (Table 187-6). Bone films should be obtained periodically. Patients with lower extremity lesions whose growth is incomplete should be monitored for evidence of leg length discrepancies, which may need treatment by arresting the growth in the opposite limb. Monitoring for potential late effects of specific chemotherapeutic agents administered (e.g., cyclophosphamide and doxorubicin) is important (see Table 187-4).

OSTEOGENIC SARCOMA

Osteogenic sarcoma is the most common bone tumor encountered in the first three decades of life; there are approximately 2000 to 3000 newly diagnosed patients per year in the United States.[24, 58] Seven teenagers per million are diagnosed annually with osteogenic sarcoma, with a male to female ratio of approximately 1.5:1. The peak incidence occurs at age 14.5 for boys and 13.5 for girls, corresponding to the age of their growth spurts. Taller children appear to be at increased risk.[44]

Etiology

The hallmark of this disease is the production of osteoid or mature bone by proliferating malignant spindle cell sarcoma. The high incidence of this tumor in adolescents who are undergoing rapid skeletal growth, as well as individuals with Paget disease of the bone, suggests that increased bone growth may play a role in the induction of the malignancy.[55] Although patients often report a history of trauma before the diagnosis, it is most likely that injuries allow the recognition of an already proliferating tumor.

Patients at increased risk of osteogenic sarcoma include

Table 187-6 *Long-Term Side Effects of Radiation*

IRRADIATED AREA*	RISKS	MONITORING
Cranium and nasopharynx	Cataracts	Physical examination
	Growth: impaired	Growth charts (bone age, growth hormone)
	Central nervous system: learning impairment	Monitoring of school function; neuropsychological evaluation
	Dentition: abnormal formation	Dental evaluation
	Thyroid: overt or compensated hypothyroidism	Free T_4/TSH levels
	High dose (>2500 Gy)	
	Hypothalamic dysfunction (decreased growth hormone; decreased gonadotropin, hyperprolactinemia)	Growth; pubertal, menstrual, and fertility history (growth hormone, LH, testosterone, estrogen, prolactin levels)
	Hearing (especially with cisplatin)	Audiogram
Neck and mandible	Hypoplasia of bone/soft tissues	Examination of area
	Dentition: abnormal formation, abnormal salivary function	Dental evaluation
	Thyroid: hypothyroidism	Free T_4, TSH
Thorax	Hypoplasia (includes impaired chest wall growth)	Examination of area
	Thyroid: hypothyroidism	Free T_4, TSH levels
	Lungs: fibrosis, decreased capacity	History, pulmonary function tests, chest film q3-5 yr
	Cardiac: pericardial and valvular thickening; possibility of early myocardial infarction	History, ECG, echocardiogram q3-5 yr
	Breasts: impaired growth, possibility of increased malignancy	Breast self-examination, early mammograms
Abdomen/pelvis	Hypoplasia (including scoliosis)	Examination of area, x-ray film of spine during puberty
	Liver (if in field)	Liver function tests
	Kidneys (if in field)	Serum creatinine, urinalysis—protein, (24-hour collection for creatinine, protein)
	Gonads (if in field)	Pubertal, menstrual, and fertility history, LH, FSH, estradiol or testosterone levels during puberty and if fertility is doubtful, semen analysis
	Gastrointestinal tract	Nutritional history
Extremities	Hypoplasia	Examination of area

ECG, Electrocardiogram; *FSH,* follicle-stimulating hormone; *LH,* luteinizing hormone; T_4, thyroxine; *TSH,* thryoid-stimulating hormone.
*All: Consider roentgenograms of bones every 5 to 10 years after ≥35 Gy radiation (risk of secondary malignancy). Examine skin for abnormal pigmented nevi (risk of second malignancy).

those who have received irradiation to the bone, usually for the treatment of malignancy.[109] It is unclear whether x-rays are causative or whether these patients who have already had one tumor are at a higher than normal risk for a spontaneous, second primary malignancy. For example, patients with hereditary retinoblastoma and a constitutive deletion in chromosome 13 have an increased incidence of osteogenic sarcoma; however, only half the sarcomas occur within the radiation field.[2] Thus the abnormality in chromosome 13 itself may predispose to osteogenic sarcoma. Osteogenic sarcoma has been described in sisters with a constitutional translocation between chromosomes 13 and 14.[47]

Clinical Manifestations

The presenting symptom of virtually all patients is pain. Palpable masses, swelling, and limited motion are common signs. Weight loss and other systemic symptoms such as anorexia rarely are seen; if these symptoms are present, overt metastatic disease is likely. A few patients have fractures. Cough, chest pain, or dyspnea may be seen in those with extensive pulmonary metastases at the time of diagnosis, although most patients with such metastases are symptom-free. The metaphyses of bones are common sites of osteogenic sarcoma origin. The lower extremities most frequently are involved, with 60% of tumors occurring around the knee (40% in the distal femur and 20% in the proximal tibia).[122] Three quarters of osteogenic sarcomas occur in the bone of the upper and lower extremities. The sacrum, jaw, and phalanges are less commonly involved. Patients with Paget disease of the bone or those who have had radiation therapy in the area of the orbit may have osteogenic sarcoma of the skull bones.

The presenting symptom, bone pain, is ubiquitous. It is most commonly due to trauma. Prolonged symptoms, or a history inconsistent with trauma, suggest the need for further evaluation. Bone abnormalities that may be confused with osteogenic sarcoma include benign cysts, Ewing sarcoma, lymphoma, or tumor metastases. (See Table 187-5 for the differential diagnosis of osteogenic sarcoma involving the extremities.)

Evaluation

Roentgenograms of the involved bone show bony destruction with periosteal new bone formation. A "sunburst" appearance is characteristic, a result of the eruption of tumor through the cortex with subsequent formation of new bone. Soft tissue swelling often is noted. Adequate biopsy and histologic examination are necessary to establish the diagnosis of osteogenic sarcoma.

Osteoid found within a sarcomatous tumor is the characteristic histologic pattern. Osteogenic sarcoma in the child or adolescent usually is a high-grade tumor characterized by osteoblasts that demonstrate pleomorphism and bizarre mitoses. Necrosis, fibrosis, and calcification may be noted. This classic form usually arises from the medullary cavity. A less aggressive form of osteogenic sarcoma arises in the paraosteal area of the bone and tends to spread along the shaft of the bone without invading the cortex. Periosteal, intracortical, and extraskeletal osteogenic sarcomas also have been described.

It is necessary to obtain baseline lactic dehydrogenase and alkaline phosphatase levels because elevated levels are predictive of a poorer prognosis. The values also may be helpful during follow-up. The extent of the primary lesion is further defined by the use of CT or MRI scanning. Arteriographic examination may be necessary in patients considered for limb salvage procedures, in which the vascular and neurologic integrity of the limb must be ensured. Metastatic disease in the lung should be sought by the use of CT scanning. Bone scans can be helpful both for outlining the primary tumor and for detecting multiple primary lesions and metastasis.

Management

The traditional therapy of osteogenic sarcoma has been amputation of the affected limb. The natural history of disease in such patients is notable for the rapid appearance of pulmonary metastases 6 to 12 months after diagnosis.[24] Five years from the diagnosis, only 10% to 20% of patients are alive. High-dose radiotherapy is even less effective than amputation.[114] In the early 1970s, favorable responses to high-dose methotrexate with leucovorin and to doxorubicin were noted.[19,59] Patients treated with these agents had markedly improved survival rates (40% to 50%) compared with historical control subjects (treated with amputation alone).[19,57] Unfortunately, a report of 50% survival after surgery alone suggested that the improved outcome was a result of improved surgical techniques rather than the chemotherapy.[115] Adjuvant chemotherapy therefore was not recommended by many physicians until the 1980s when a controlled randomized study confirmed that adjuvant chemotherapy improves disease-free survival of patients with osteogenic sarcoma.[75] Adjuvant chemotherapy regimens now being recommended use high doses of methotrexate, doxorubicin, and cisplatin, sometimes in combination with other agents.

The availability of effective chemotherapy has made limb-sparing or subamputative therapies possible for many patients with osteogenic sarcoma.[82] The portion of bone involved with tumor is removed and replaced by an artificial prosthesis or a bone graft. This procedure can be performed only if the vascular and neurologic integrity of the limb is not compromised. Preoperative chemotherapy may effectively reduce the size of the mass so as to make such surgery possible. In many protocols the efficacy of the initially used chemotherapy is evaluated on the basis of the biologic response to therapy.[102] The subsequent chemotherapeutic regimen may be modified. For those with lower extremity tumors, limb-salvage procedures are limited to patients who have achieved most of their growth potential. For patients with lesions of the humerus, any preservation of hand function will significantly improve the patient's life-style.

For patients in whom pulmonary metastases develop, surgical resection of these nodules may result in long-term survival.[84,89] A similar approach has been used in patients with metastatic pulmonary disease at the time of diagnosis, but the frequency of long-term survival of such patients is not well documented.

Prognosis

Two randomized studies have confirmed the role of adjuvant chemotherapy in improving the long-term disease-free survival of patients with nonmetastatic osteogenic sarcoma. Approximately 65% to 75% overall disease-free survival can be achieved.[75,102] The initial biologic response to chemotherapy appears to have prognostic significance, although it is unclear whether subsequent tailoring of therapy achieves a better result than aggressive early chemotherapy for all patients. The advantage of preoperative chemotherapy compared with immediate surgical excision also is unclear. Preoperative chemotherapy, however, allows for the possibility of limb-salvage procedures by decreasing tumor size, as well as by allowing time for a prosthesis to be made.

Prognostic factors in this disorder are related to the site of the tumor (patients with distal tumors do better than those with proximal or central-axis tumors) and the patient's age (prognosis improves with increased age).

Follow-Up

Adjuvant chemotherapy has resulted in an increased number of long-term survivors of osteogenic sarcoma. Virtually all these patients will have undergone either amputation or limb-salvage procedures. It is hoped that at some time, less-disabling therapies will be feasible. Most of these patients, however, maintain a relatively normal life-style, including participation in a variety of sports. Their long-term, follow-up care to detect recurrent disease includes (1) chest films and alkaline phosphatase determinations performed semiannually for 5 years and annually until 10 years from the time of diagnosis, (2) orthopedic evaluations to consider necessary adjustments in prostheses, and (3) monitoring for the late effects of chemotherapeutic agents used (e.g., doxorubicin, cisplatin, bleomycin, and cyclophosphamide).

NON-HODGKIN LYMPHOMAS

Non-Hodgkin lymphoma (NHL) of childhood comprises a heterogeneous group of malignancies arising from lymphocytes and lymphoid precursors. The migratory nature of these cells is reflected by the variable sites at which the tumors occur and to which they spread. Recognition of the systemic nature of disease, even in those patients with only locally detectable disease, has resulted in a marked improvement in survival rates in recent years. Childhood NHL is markedly different from adult NHL both in the immunohistopathologic types that occur and in the better survival rates noted in children.

Lymphomas account for 10% of childhood cancer[128]; 60% are NHLs. The incidence of NHL is low in children younger than 5 years of age and then increases steadily throughout life. It occurs more commonly in males than in females (2 to 3:1). The frequency of NHL itself and of its various subtypes varies markedly in different geographic regions.[78] NHLs of childhood have a high growth rate, approaching 100% in some cases, and short doubling-in-size times (as few as 12 hours). They have a high frequency of dissemination, particularly to the bone marrow and central nervous system. Although the distinction between lymphoma and leukemia is defined by <25% versus >25% marrow blasts, respectively, the distinguishing biologic parameters are not clear. Lymphoid malignancies involving immature thymocytes more frequently occur as leukemia, whereas more mature thymocytes are associated with lymphomatous presentations.[8]

Etiology

Childhood NHL arises from lymphoid precursors in the marrow and thymus. Burkitt and non-Burkitt small, noncleftedcell lymphomas and most large-cell lymphomas are B cell phenotypes, usually manifesting surface immunoglobulin and B cell specific antigens. Lymphoblastic lymphomas almost invariably express the enzyme terminal deoxynucleotidyl (TdT), as well as T cell markers.[8] Specific chromosomal aberrations have been described in Burkitt lymphoma.[9,129]

Different breakpoints of chromosomal translocations may be seen in the Burkitt lymphoma of equatorial Africa, which usually harbors Epstein-Barr virus (EBV), compared with the North American variety, which does so only rarely.[93] The presence of EBV virus in lymphoma specimens suggests that viral infection may play a role in the development of NHL. Immunodeficiency states also are associated with the development of lymphomas, usually of the B cell immunoblastic or large-cell variety.[43] A defect of T cell regulation that permits the expansion of EBV-affected clones of B cells has been hypothesized to result in lymphomas, particularly in immunologically abnormal hosts. Lymphomas occur with increased frequency in children receiving immunosuppressive therapy for renal, cardiac, or bone marrow allografts.

A number of specific, nonrandom chromosomal abnormalities have been reported in lymphoblastic lymphoma and large-cell lymphomas. The variation in subtypes described suggests that these tumors may be more heterogeneous than Burkitt lymphoma.

Clinical Manifestations

Localized lymphadenopathy is a common presentation of NHL. Common areas of involvement are supradiaphragmatic, particularly the cervical, axillary, and mediastinal areas, or Waldeyer ring.[90] The histologic pattern of supradiaphragmatic disease often is lymphoblastic. Dissemination to the bone marrow, the central nervous system, or the gonads is common. Patients with mediastinal masses frequently have a history of cough and occasionally acute respiratory distress. Unless careful attention is paid to the state of the airway, obstruction can occur during evaluation, even in patients with minimal symptoms, particularly with the administration of sedation. The obstruction may involve the lower airway, beyond the reach of an endotracheal tube, resulting in an inability to ventilate the lungs effectively.

An abdominal mass that may involve the iliocecal region, mesentery, ovaries, or retroperitoneum is seen in 30% to 40% of patients.[90] Such tumors are often of B cell origin. Extranodal sites of involvement include the tonsils, lungs, bone, testicles, and soft tissue.

Patients with localized disease often feel well. Those with disseminated disease experience weight loss and malaise, as well as symptoms referable to the primary site of the disease.

The differential diagnosis of cervical adenopathy includes a variety of infectious and inflammatory processes. Malignant processes that cause enlarged cervical nodes include Hodgkin disease, neuroblastoma, leukemia, nasopharyngeal carcinoma, rhabdomyosarcoma, and thyroid carcinoma. Anterior mediastinal masses may be due to T cell leukemia or thymoma. Abdominal masses may be due to constipation, splenomegaly, Wilms tumor, rhabdomyosarcoma, or neuroblastoma. Lymphoma is a rare type of bone tumor. (Tables 187-1 to 187-3 provide differential diagnostic aids in evaluating patients with NHL.)

Evaluation

The diagnosis of NHL should be established by surgical biopsy. Removal of the most suspicious node is recommended. Frozen sections and needle biopsies are to be discouraged in order to ensure proper diagnosis. Although the primary diagnosis is based on histologic findings, immunophenotyping and enzyme studies (TdT) can be helpful. If possible, cytogenetics studies should be performed. A sufficient number of malignant cells may be present in patients with bone marrow involvement or pleural effusions to establish the diagnosis. In this instance a lymph node biopsy may not be necessary. Biopsy may be contraindicated for patients with large mediastinal masses with imminent airway obstruction unless endotracheal intubation will ensure airway patency. If the distal end of the endotracheal tube lies proximal to the mass, localized radiation to the mediastinum may be necessary before the diagnostic specimen is obtained. Alternate sites for obtaining diagnostic specimens must then be considered.

All patients should receive a complete blood cell count and platelet and reticulocyte counts. Serum electrolyte, uric acid, calcium, and phosphorus levels and renal and liver function tests should be obtained. A low serum alkaline phosphatase level predicts a good outcome. A lumbar puncture should be obtained with cytocentrifugation of cerebral spinal fluid to determine if there is meningeal involvement. Imaging studies should include a chest film and a CT scan of the chest and abdomen in all patients. Bone scans and gallium scans can be helpful in selected patients.

A variety of staging systems are used for lymphomas.[78] The most common, the Ann Arbor system used for Hodgkin disease, is not of prognostic significance in pediatric NHL because of noncontinuous patterns of spread. The National Cancer Institute staging system is used primarily for Burkitt lymphoma. The St. Jude system, applicable to most forms of NHL, is devised to reflect the prognostic significance of involvement in various areas of the body.

Management

The majority of patients with NHL have disseminated disease at the time of diagnosis. Even those with clinically localized disease are rarely curable with localized surgical or irradiation therapy alone. The choice of chemotherapeutic regimens is based on the clinical stage and the immunohistologic tumor subtype.

Lymph node biopsy usually is required for diagnosis and characterization of NHL. Removal of the tumor is indicated only for those patients with Burkitt lymphoma whose tumor can be removed en masse (90%) with minimal morbidity.[79] In general, major surgical procedures should be avoided because subsequent healing time may delay initiation of chemotherapy, the most essential component of treatment.

The high incidence of micrometastatic disease at the time of diagnosis necessitates that all children with NHL receive chemotherapy. Many agents are active in lymphomas. Optimal treatment regimens differ for patients with lymphoblastic lymphoma compared with those with nonlymphoblastic lymphoma. For the former, the LSA2L2 regimen, which utilizes pairs of agents in rapid succession, has been the most effective. For patients with nonlymphoblastic lymphoma the most effective regimens include cyclophosphamide, vincristine, prednisone, methotrexate, and doxorubicin used in combination.[61]

Local measures of control rarely are essential in the treatment of childhood NHL. Lymphomas are radiosensitive, but the use of radiation therapy does not improve disease-free survival in patients with advanced disease. Unnecessary morbidity may be added. Radiotherapy is helpful in the treatment of emergent situations such as airway compromise or spinal cord compression and for treating overt meningeal involvement. Radiation therapy also plays a role in the treatment of patients who do not achieve a complete remission after standard chemotherapy. After relapse, radiotherapy is used as part of consolidation therapy before bone marrow transplantation. For terminally ill patients, radiation provides effective palliation for localized pain.

Prognosis

The prognosis is excellent for most children with NHL. Although histologic findings are not of great prognostic significance for outcome, they provide the basis for choice of therapeutic regimen. Clinical staging is of particular relevance because it is determined by a combination of the tumor burden, disease extent, and primary location. New intensive chemotherapy or bone marrow transplantation regimens should improve the likelihood of survival in patients with a poor prognosis.

Follow-Up

Patients with NHL who are disease free 2 years from the time of diagnosis usually are cured. During this initial period they should be monitored on the basis of complete blood cell counts, chest films, and evaluation of the primary site of disease. The follow-up of long-term survivors of childhood lymphomas should reflect the types of therapy (e.g., cyclophosphamide, doxorubicin, methotrexate) administered (see Table 187-4).

HODGKIN DISEASE

Hodgkin disease is a malignancy of the lymphoreticular system characterized by multinucleated giant cells, known as Reed-Sternberg cells, interspersed in an infiltration of normal-appearing cellular elements (lymphocytes, macrophages, histiocytes, plasma cells, and eosinophils).[99] The Reed-Sternberg cells appear to be the mitotically active malignant cell of Hodgkin disease. Controversy exists as to the normal counterpart from which these cells derive.

In the more developed nations there are two age peaks for the incidence of Hodgkin disease, one in young adults (15 to 30 years of age) and one in late adulthood.[52,110] In developing nations the early peak occurs in preadolescence. Hodgkin disease is extremely rare before the age of 5 years. A male predominance is present throughout the preadolescent age range; thereafter the incidence is approximately equal in males and females. Hodgkin disease in older teenagers and young adults is most common in white persons.

Etiology

The role of environment or genetics in the acquisition of Hodgkin disease is suggested by national and racial differences in the epidemiologic features of the disease. First-degree relatives of patients with Hodgkin disease have an increased risk of acquiring the disease.[52] This may be due to similar exposures (viral, environmental) or to genetic susceptibility.

High serum titers to EBV in some patients with Hodgkin disease may reflect a causative role for the virus.[91] Alternatively, patients may have an inappropriate immune response to this virus. The incidence of Hodgkin disease is known to be increased in patients with certain underlying immunodeficiency diseases (e.g., ataxia-telangiectasia and acquired immunodeficiency syndrome).[46,56]

Clinical Manifestations[72]

The most common presenting feature of Hodgkin disease is painless enlargement of the lower cervical lymph nodes. Approximately 50% of the patients with this presentation have mediastinal disease as well. The classic pattern of spread is from the cervical lymph nodes to the mediastinum and then into the spleen and abdominal lymph nodes. Spread via the thoracic duct may result in disease of the right side of the neck and of the abdomen, without mediastinal involvement. Axillary or inguinal adenopathy or extranodal primary sites (e.g., bone) is seen occasionally. Pleural involvement occurs in approximately 10% of patients. Renal, skin, or nervous system involvement is less common. Constitutional symptoms related to Hodgkin disease occur in approximately one third of patients at the time of diagnosis. The symptoms that predict a poor prognosis ("B" disease) are fever (oral temperature >38° C), weight loss (>10% of body weight within 6 months), and drenching night sweats. Absence of these symptoms provides a better prognosis ("A" disease).

Hematologic abnormalities may be present in Hodgkin disease (usually in advanced stages), even in the absence of bone marrow involvement. Hemolytic disease or the anemia of chronic disease associated with impaired mobilization of iron storage may occur. Neutrophilia in the absence of infection occurs in approximately 50% of the patients. Thrombocytopenia caused by immunologically mediated platelet destruction also is seen.

Lymphadenopathy occurs in children for a variety of reasons. Infection with bacteria, viruses, tuberculosis, atypical mycobacteria, and toxoplasmosis may cause lymphadenopathy. Malignancies that can be considered in the differential diagnosis include non-Hodgkin lymphoma, nasopharyngeal carcinoma, soft tissue sarcoma, or in a younger child, neuroblastoma. Histiocytosis and other inflammatory processes also have similar presentations. A chest film, a complete blood cell count, and a sedimentation rate should be obtained in any patient with lymphadenopathy that is atypical for infection. Persistent lymphadenopathy, even after a transient "response" to antibiotic therapy, requires biopsy. (Tables 187-2 and 187-3 provide differential diagnostic aids in evaluating patients with Hodgkin disease.)

Evaluation

Evaluation of the child with Hodgkin disease should begin with a careful history and physical examination. Particular attention should be paid to "B" disease symptoms. Lymphatic areas to be evaluated include Waldeyer ring and the cervical, supraclavicular, axillary, and inguinal lymph nodes. The size of the nodes found should be recorded carefully. It should be noted whether the lymph nodes are tender. In addition, a careful abdominal examination should be performed, particularly to evaluate liver and splenic size. Retroperitoneal lymph nodes are not palpable. The blood cell counts may show anemia (caused by hemolysis or chronic disease), neutropenia, or thrombocytopenia. Elevation of the sedimentation rate and the serum copper level, occurs and may be useful for following response to therapy. Serum hepatic alkaline phosphatase isoenzyme levels also may be elevated.

Radiographic evaluation of a patient with potential Hodgkin disease includes a chest film and CT scans of the chest and abdomen. Bipedal lymphangiography can be used to detect pelvic and paraaortic lymph nodes in institutions in which radiologists commonly perform such tests. Gallium scanning also detects Hodgkin disease and can be useful in detecting disease in obscure sites. Although bone involvement is rare, a bone scan should be considered in patients with advanced disease, particularly those with bone pain or an elevated serum alkaline phosphatase level.

Laparotomy with splenectomy is the only precise way to define the subdiaphragmatic extent of Hodgkin disease.[49] Biopsy specimens of even normal-appearing lymph nodes should be obtained in each of the following areas: splenic hilar, celiac portal hepatic, mesenteric, paraaortic, and iliac regions. In addition, any suspicious lesions should be removed. Evaluation of other organs includes a careful examination of the spleen, with sectioning at intervals of 1 to 3 mm to detect small nodules. Wedge biopsies of the liver are necessary because needle biopsies are unlikely to detect focal lesions. A bone marrow biopsy must be obtained either before or coincidentally with laparotomy. Although bone marrow involvement is not common, the detection of Hodgkin disease in the marrow would be consistent with stage IV disease, obviating the need for a staging laparotomy.

The importance of defining subdiaphragmatic involvement is most clear when radiation therapy will be the primary therapeutic modality. A staging laparotomy with splenectomy allows limited fields to be irradiated, thus preventing the morbidity associated with total nodal irradiation. When chemotherapy is used, the benefits of staging laparotomy with splenectomy can be debated. However, less-intense chemotherapy often is used in those with documented, low-stage disease. Radiation fields and doses may be decreased in this circumstance.

Unfortunately, overwhelming bacteremia with polysaccharide-encapsulated organisms occurs in 10% of patients after splenectomy, with a mortality rate of 50% in these patients.[103] The risk is greatest for young children who have not been previously exposed to these pathogens. All patients who have undergone splenectomy will require presurgical vaccination against pneumococci, *Haemophilus influenzae* type b, and *Neisseria meningitidis*. Prophylactic antibiotics also are recommended throughout their lives.

The extent of disease spread usually is classified by the Ann Arbor staging system[13] by means of either the clinical stage (CS) or the pathologic stage (PS). PS implies that the most extensive degree of involvement has been pathologically confirmed. The stages are as follows:

Stage I—involvement of one lymphatic region only

Stage II—involvement of two or more lymphatic regions on the same side of the diaphragm

Stage III—involvement on both sides of the diaphragm, including nodal regions and/or the spleen

Stage IV—involvement of extranodal organs such as lungs, liver, bone marrow, kidneys, bone, or skin, in addition to lymph nodes

Direct extranodal extension to adjacent tissue is denoted by the subscript E. Stage III disease is subdivided by the degree of abdominal involvement. Stage III_1 involves nodes of the upper portion of the abdomen alone (celiac portal nodes and/or spleen). Stage III_2 involves paraaortic nodes as well; stage III_3 additionally involves iliac nodes.

Four subtypes of Hodgkin disease are described by review of pathologic specimens.[76] The nodular sclerosing type (NS) is most common in childhood. Collagenous bands divide the lymphoid tissues into nodules, and a "lacunar variant" of the Reed-Sternberg cell is seen. Lymphocyte-predominant Hodgkin disease is characterized by destruction of the lymph node architecture with the cellular proliferation of benign-appearing lymphocytes. Reed-Sternberg cells rarely are found in the absence of fibrosis. In mixed-cellularity Hodgkin disease, lymph node architecture is not preserved. Approximately 10 Reed-Sternberg cells are seen per high power field, often with interstitial fibrosis; necrosis is not pronounced. Lymphocyte-depleted Hodgkin disease is characterized by the presence of fibrosis, necrosis, and abnormal cells (but only a rare lymphocyte).

Management

Hodgkin disease responds to radiation or to chemotherapy. Protocols utilizing radiation therapy alone, chemotherapy alone, or both forms of therapy have all been successful, at least in some groups of patients. Choosing an appropriate therapeutic plan necessitates assessing the risk of disease recurrence and the potential for long-term effects in a particular patient.

Contiguous spread of Hodgkin disease via lymphoid organs allows for success with radiation therapy alone.[63] Full-dose radiation therapy (35 to 45 Gy) is used most frequently in the treatment of patients with stages I, II, and III_1 disease. The involved fields, and one field beyond the area of proved disease, are treated. Those patients with large mediastinal masses (more than one third the thoracic diameter) also require chemotherapy for optimal results. Skeletal and soft tissue growth, particularly in the neck and clavicular areas, are severely compromised when these doses of radiation are used. Cardiac and pulmonary complications occur as well. Children who have not achieved most of their growth at the time of diagnosis will have significant skeletal deformity if full-dose irradiation is used to the neck and mediastinum. Low-dose radiation (20 to 25 Gy) to involved fields, in conjunction with chemotherapy, is being used for most younger children.[33]

Hodgkin disease responds to a number of single chemotherapeutic agents, but rarely are durable, complete remissions achieved in this manner. Combination chemotherapy, with active agents that have differing mechanisms of action and nonoverlapping toxicities, is used. The original combination that proved to be successful in the treatment of Hodgkin disease was MOPP (mechlorethamine, Oncovin [vincristine], procarbazine, and prednisone).[29] Cyclophosphamide or a nitrosuria may be substituted for mechlorethamine, or vinblastine for vincristine. Full doses of drugs should be used in as short a period of time as possible. In 1974, 10 years after the initial discovery of MOPP, another combination regimen ABVD (Adriamycin [doxorubicin], bleomycin, vinblastine, and dacarbazine) was devised for the treatment of patients with relapsed disease.[10] The efficacy of this combination has resulted in combined ABVD/MOPP regimens. Chemotherapeutic regimens have been successfully used alone or in combination with radiation for all stages of disease.

Combined therapies (chemotherapy and radiation together) are used (1) to improve cure rates in patients with poor prognoses and (2) to reduce the dose of radiotherapy administered to children with low-stage disease so that skeletal development will proceed more normally. Chemotherapy has side effects as well, including infertility after MOPP chemotherapy, cardiotoxic effects of the doxorubicin of ABVD, and pulmonary toxicity caused by bleomycin.[26,106] Secondary leukemias have been described, particularly after the combination of MOPP and radiation.[17] Second-generation treatment protocols are being devised to decrease the number of courses, to eliminate particularly toxic components of therapy (i.e., bleomycin), and to substitute less toxic agents. In choosing an appropriate regimen for a given patient, the following must be considered: (1) the age of the patient (likely effects on the developing organism), (2) the extent of disease present (how much therapy is necessary), and (3) symptoms that might predict a poor prognosis. Because so many regimens currently appear equivalent in terms of outcome, an experimental protocol should be used (if one is available) to help delineate the best treatment for patients in the future, while ensuring appropriate treatment for those under study.

Prognosis[72]

Radiation therapy alone may cure up to 70% of patients with stage I or IIA Hodgkin disease. The success of this approach varies significantly among institutions. When three to six courses of MOPP are added to radiotherapy, the 5-year disease-free survival rate increases to approximately 90% at all institutions.

Patients with stage IIB or IIIA disease are treated in a variety of fashions, including chemotherapy alone, extended field irradiation, or a combination of the two. Many oncologists use full-dose radiation for fully grown patients. Relapse will occur in approximately 50% of these patients after such treatment. The subsequent use of chemotherapy will enable half of those who relapse after radiation therapy to be cured of the disease.[113,123] Combined modality therapy often is used for younger patients or for those in whom there is an indicator of a poor prognosis (e.g., large mediastinal mass).

Patients with stage IIIB or IV disease are treated with multiagent chemotherapy with or without radiation to areas of bulk disease. Results of recent studies suggest that approximately 50% to 75% of patients will remain disease free 5 years later. In some patients who experience relapse, improvement can be effected with autologous bone marrow transplantation.

Follow-Up

Patients with Hodgkin disease should be monitored for evidence of recurrent disease for as long as 10 to 15 years after the original diagnosis. Useful tests for prolonged follow-up include complete blood cell count, sedimentation rate, and chest film.

After high-dose radiotherapy to the neck and mediastinum, soft tissue and bone growth abnormalities include shortening of clavicles and underdevelopment of the soft tissues of the neck. Sitting height decreases after radiation to the axial skeleton in proportion to the growth potential remaining at the time of radiation.[96] In prepubertal girls, breast development may be impaired. The incidence of breast cancer may be increased after irradiation.[60] Serial mammography examinations beginning at an early age (approximately 25 years) may be appropriate.

Overt hypothyroidism (low thyroxine) occurs in approximately 5% to 10% of patients who have undergone irradiation, whereas compensated hypothyroidism (elevated thyroid-stimulating hormone) occurs in 50% to 90% of such patients.[18] Thyroid function should be assessed for at least 15 years. Thyroid replacement therapy is recommended when the thyroid-stimulating hormone level is elevated.

Patients who receive mediastinal irradiation may have pulmonary fibrosis with variable abnormalities detected by pulmonary function testing.[32] Late cardiac abnormalities include pericardial thickening and, occasionally, valvular dysfunction. Early myocardial infarctions have been reported. These toxicities may be exacerbated by the use of bleomycin and anthracyclines.

Fertility in women is affected by the use of radiation and chemotherapy. Pelvic irradiation of a woman causes infertility unless oophoropexy (moving ovaries to the midline) is performed. After oophoropexy, all teenage girls treated with radiation alone and 88% of those treated with combined modality therapy maintained normal menses.[32] Older women (older than 30 years of age) experience ovarian failure more frequently than do younger women after treatment with MOPP. All should be advised that early menopause may occur. A menstrual history should be elicited at each visit.

Testes are more severely affected by cytotoxic therapies than are ovaries. Fortunately, the radiation fields used in Hodgkin disease spare the gonads in male patients. Six courses of MOPP chemotherapy, however, result in universal male sterility. Approximately 50% of patients treated with three courses of MOPP are sterile.[27] ABVD causes less impairment of spermatogenesis. Men interested in fathering a child may benefit from the monitoring of gonadotropin levels and from semen analysis. Recovery has been documented in previously sterile men.

Acute nonlymphocytic leukemia occurs at the rate of approximately 1% per year for the first 10 years after treatment with MOPP and radiotherapy.[17] Thereafter the risk appears to decrease. The incidence is lower with single modality therapy or after ABVD and radiation. Solid tumors, particularly NHL, may occur after Hodgkin disease.

Patients with Hodgkin disease remain at risk for overwhelming infections secondary to splenectomy.[103] Patients with a high fever should be hospitalized and treated empirically with antibiotics for the potential of sepsis with polysaccharide-encapsulated organisms.

GENERAL ONCOLOGIC CARE

Referral to a Pediatric Oncologist

Children with malignancies fortunately represent a very small proportion of patients in a general pediatrics practice. The treatment of such patients is specialized and changes rapidly each year. Proper care of such patients begins with referral to a pediatric oncologist, even if the initial procedure is surgical. For many tumors, appropriate baseline studies must be obtained before surgical procedures. For example, AFP and B-HCG levels fall rapidly after removal of the germ cell tumor, as do catecholamine levels after removal of a neuroblastoma. Delayed assays for such markers may result in the inability to recognize an important indicator of recurrent disease in a given patient. The chest CT scan should be performed before surgical procedures because perioperative atelectasis may impair the ability to detect metastatic disease in the pulmonary parenchyma.

The tumors of childhood behave differently from those of adults, even when histologically identical. In addition, children tolerate radiation and chemotherapy differently than do adults. Therefore all children should receive the care of a pediatric oncologist. Services available for children and their families at pediatric referral hospitals often ease the pain of being diagnosed with a life-threatening disease. Pediatric social workers, child life workers, and nurses experienced in dealing with children and adolescents who have cancer are available. For patients living at a distance from a center, it often is possible to initiate therapy at a referral center and administer most of the treatments and evaluations closer to the patient's home. At times a local oncologist can assist in administering chemotherapy to children living at a distance from a center, but such oncologists should not be relied on to choose a therapeutic regimen or to evaluate major problems that may arise.

A number of oncologic emergencies exist that general pediatricians must recognize. Cord compression may result from neuroblastoma, Ewing sarcoma, lymphoma, or any other tumor that invades the spinal canal. Such patients will experience incontinence, loss of reflexes in the lower extremities, or decreased ability to use the lower extremities. Rectal spincter tone may be decreased. Rapid institution of therapy may reverse such findings, markedly changing the long-term functioning of the patient. Thus recognition of such findings should prompt immediate referral to a pediatric oncologist who, in conjunction with a neurosurgeon and/or radiation therapist, will be able to deliver emergent therapy.

Patients with infiltration of the bone marrow, particularly those with leukemias (as addressed in another chapter), metastatic Ewing sarcoma, metastatic neuroblastoma, or lymphoma, may have pancytopenia and thus be at risk of infection from neutropenia, bleeding caused by thrombocytopenia, and congestive failure as a result of anemia. Rapid lysis of cells (tumor lysis syndrome) because of the high cell turnover rate of the tumor itself (as is seen in Burkitt lymphoma) or to cytotoxic therapy is characterized by elevated uric acid (risk of urate nephropathy), hyperkalemia, hypocalcemia, and hyperphosphatemia. Medical management includes allopurinol, urinary alkalinization, and binders of potassium and phosphate. Dialysis may be necessary. If delayed arrival to the medical center is anticipated, allopurinol should be started by a referring physician when a tumor with a large cell burden (e.g., leukemia, Burkitt lymphoma, and marrow involvement with either neuroblastoma, Ewing sarcoma, or rhabdomyosarcoma) is suspected.

Role of the Pediatrician During Therapy

The most prominent toxicity that results from chemotherapy is myelosuppression. Infections in neutropenic patients can rapidly result in septic shock, particularly if gram-negative organisms are involved. Primary physicians who follow up these children can help by recognizing the risk of fever and referring the patient immediately to the pediatric oncologist. If the center is at a distance, the pediatrician becomes the frontline caretaker, obtaining proper culture specimens and initiating antibiotics (usually an aminoglycoside and semisynthetic penicillin). In such circumstances the primary pediatrician should discuss aspects of care with the pediatric oncologist to ensure that all appropriate measures are performed. Many patients receiving intensive chemotherapy have indwelling central venous catheters that increase the risk for septicemia with gram-positive organisms. These patients, even in the absence of neutropenia, should have blood cultures performed and the administration of antibiotics considered if fever develops. Any person who is febrile and who has undergone a splenectomy should be given antibiotics empirically to treat polysaccharide-encapsulated organisms.

In the absence of splenectomy and a central line, pediatric treatment of patients whose blood cell counts are normal usually is similar to that of the typical child. The primary pediatrician can be of great assistance in seeing such children for common pediatric complaints, including skin rashes, earaches, and respiratory and gastrointestinal infections inasmuch as these children appear to handle such infections without undue difficulty. Varicella, however, is a major threat to all immunocompromised patients (because dissemination of disease is likely even in the absence of neutropenia). Before the availability of acyclovir, significant morbidity and mortality occurred in such patients. Immunocompromised children who are exposed by a sibling or a close playmate should receive varicella-zoster immunoglobulin within 4 days of the exposure. Should chickenpox occur, the patient should be admitted for treatment for 5 to 7 days with acyclovir. Chemotherapy usually is withheld during treatment of varicella.

Children who are receiving treatment for a malignancy should continue to see their primary pediatrician for well-child visits. This is in anticipation of their ultimate successful treatment and cure. Immunizations are delayed until 1 year after therapy is terminated, because live vaccines may cause disease and inactivated vaccines rarely result in a normal immune response. The pediatrician should remain involved in developmental issues that are ongoing and, at times, exacerbated by the treatment of a malignancy. With the current success rates in treating children with cancer, pediatricians should anticipate the return of these children to their practice for most of their care. Maintenance of a relationship with the patient and family is essential.

Care of Long-Term Survivors

Patients treated for childhood malignancy have, for the most part, received a number of extremely toxic agents, the long-term implications of which are incompletely known. Studies of a therapy's late toxicities are just beginning. Children should continue to return at least annually to the treating institution or to a similar institution elsewhere to be monitored for potential side effects and to be informed of problems occurring in similarly treated patients. Toxicities of radiation to particular areas (see Table 187-6) and of currently used chemotherapeutic agents (see Table 187-4) are listed, and recommended follow-up studies are described. The pediatrician should ensure that his or her patients are being screened appropriately.

Multidisciplinary clinics, which evaluate all survivors for potential late effects, are being formed in a number of hospitals. Subclinical evidence of cardiac damage after anthracycline administration and of pulmonary toxicity (decreased diffusing capacity) after bleomycin administration is found in some survivors, but it is not clear whether the damage will be progressive. The long-term effects on renal function and hearing are not yet known. Fertility has been impaired in some patients who received alkylating therapies, but the incidence of dysfunction is lower than in similarly treated adults. Radiation to the gonads also causes infertility. Affected women need hormone replacement for feminization and to prevent the osteoporosis associated with estrogen depletion. Testosterone levels in treated males usually remain in the normal range, but they should be monitored.

Endocrine dysfunction after radiation may involve the thyroid, hypothalamus, and pituitary. Studies of the mechanism of impairment may help us to treat other affected patients more effectively. Thyroid radiation often causes compensated (increased TSH, normal T_4) or overt (increased TSH, decreased T_4) hypothyroidism and should be treated with thyroid hormone.

Secondary malignancies are reported in long-term survivors. Mutagenic agents such as mechlorethamine and cyclophosphamide, and possibly etoposide and radiation therapy, play a role. A genetic predisposition to malignancy exists for those with certain disorders (e.g., bilateral retinoblastoma).

The psychosocial effects of childhood cancer also differ from patient to patient. Some were so young when they received treatment that they do not remember the ordeal, whereas others had to forsake normal childhood experiences because of their illness. Some have no physical deficits, and others have permanent deformities (amputations, scoliosis, hair loss, scars). Although memories and physical handicaps may linger, survivors usually are cured of their cancer. They are emotionally intact people who are able to live and work normally within the mainstream of society. Unfortunately, certain workplaces and insurance companies continue to discriminate on the basis of a past history of cancer. Because each tumor and treatment regimen is different, businesses and agencies must be educated to accept those who are cured and are likely to have a normal future.

Pediatricians must be advocates for these successfully treated persons. Past medical conditions that will not interfere with future health should not be a barrier to success. However, we must remain aware of potential late effects of therapy. Screening for toxicities will allow for interventions that can maintain health.

REFERENCES

1. Ablin AR et al: Malignant germ cell tumors in childhood: an outcome analysis, Proc Am Soc Clin Oncol 5:213, 1986.
2. Abramson DH, Ellsworth R, and Zimmerman L: Nonocular cancer in retinoblastoma survivors, Trans Am Acad Ophthalmol Otolaryngol 81:454, 1976.
3. Abramson DH et al: Retinoblastoma: survival, age at detection and comparison 1914-1958, 1958-1983, J Pediatr Ophthalmol Strabismus 22:246, 1985.
4. Ashley DJB and Path FRC: Origin of teratomas, Cancer 32:390, 1973.
5. August CS et al: Treatment of advanced neuroblastoma with supralethal chemotherapy, radiation, and allogeneic or autologous marrow reconstitution, J Clin Oncol 2:609, 1984.
6. Beckwith JB and Palmer NF: Histopathology and prognosis of Wilms' tumor, Cancer 41:1937, 1978.
7. Beckwith JB and Perrin EV: In situ neuroblastoma: a contribution to the natural history of neural crest tumors, Am J Pathol 43:1089, 1963.
8. Bernard A et al: Cell surface characterization of malignant T cells from lymphoblastic lymphoma using monoclonal antibodies: evidence for a phenotypic difference between malignant T cells from patients with acute lymphoblastic leukemia and lymphoblastic lymphoma, Blood 57:1105, 1981.
9. Bernheim A, Berger R, and Lenoir G: Cytogenetic studies on African Burkitt's lymphoma cell lines: t(8 14), t(2 8) and t(8 22) translocation, Cancer Genet Cytogenet 3:307, 1981.
10. Bonadonna G et al: Combination chemotherapy of Hodgkin's disease with adriamycin, bleomycin, vinblastine, and imidazole carboxamide versus MOPP, Cancer 36:252, 1975.
11. Bray PF et al: The coincidence of neuroblastoma and acute cerebellar encephalopathy, J Pediatr 76:983, 1969.
12. Breslow NE and Beckwith JB: Epidemiological features of Wilms' tumor: results of the national Wilms' tumor study, J Natl Cancer Inst 68:429, 1982.
13. Carbone PP et al: Report of the committee on Hodgkin's disease staging classification, Cancer Res 31:1860, 1971.
14. Carli M et al: Therapeutic efficacy of single drugs for childhood neuroblastoma: a review. In Raybaud C et al, editors: Pediatric oncology Amsterdam, 1982, Excerpta Medica.
15. Cassady JR et al: Radiation therapy in retinoblastoma, Radiology 93:405, 1969.
16. Chatten J and Voorhees ML: Familial neuroblastoma, N Engl J Med 277:1230, 1967.
17. Coleman CN: Secondary malignancy after treatment of Hodgkin's disease: an evolving picture, J Clin Oncol 4:821, 1986.
18. Constine LS et al: Thyroid dysfunction after radiotherapy in children with Hodgkin's disease, Cancer 53:878, 1984.
19. Cortes EP et al: Amputation and adriamycin in primary osteosarcoma, N Engl J Med 291:998, 1974.
20. D'Angio GJ: Wilms' tumor and neuroblastoma in children, Pediatr Rev 6:16, 1984.
21. D'Angio GJ et al: The treatment of Wilms' tumor: results of national Wilms' tumor study, Cancer 38:633, 1976.
22. D'Angio GJ et al: The treatment of Wilms' tumor: results of the second national Wilms' tumor study, Cancer 47:2302, 1981.
23. D'Angio GJ et al: Results of the third national Wilms' tumor study (NWTS-3): a preliminary report, Am Assoc Cancer Res 25:183, 1984.
24. Dahlin CD and Coventry MB: Osteosarcoma: a study of 600 cases, J Bone Joint Surg [Am] 49:101, 1967.
25. Dahlin DC, Coventry MB, and Scanlon PW: Ewing's sarcoma: a critical analysis of 165 cases, J Bone Joint Surg [Am] 43:185, 1961.
26. Damewood MD and Grochow LB: Prospects for fertility after chemotherapy or radiation for neoplastic disease, Fertil Steril 45:443, 1986.
27. deCunha MF et al: Recovery of spermatogenesis after treatment for Hodgkin's disease: limiting dose of MOPP chemotherapy, J Clin Oncol 2:571, 1984.
28. Devesa SS: The incidence of retinoblastoma, Am J Ophthalmol 80:263, 1975.
29. DeVita VT Jr, Serpick A, and Carbone PP: Combination chemotherapy in the treatment of advanced Hodgkin's disease, Ann Intern Med 73:881, 1970.
30. Dickman P, Liotta L, and Triche T: Ewing's sarcoma: characterization in established cultures and evidence of its histogenesis, Lab Invest 47:375, 1982.
31. Donaldson SS: Rhabdomyosarcoma. In Carter S, Glatstein E, and Livingston RB, editors: Principles of cancer treatment, New York, 1982, McGraw-Hill, Inc.
32. Donaldson SS and Kaplan HS: Complications of treatment of Hodgkin's disease in children, Cancer Treat Rep 66:977, 1982.
33. Donaldson SS and Link MP: Combined modality treatment with low-dose radiation and MOPP chemotherapy for children with Hodgkin's disease, J Clin Oncol 5:742, 1987.
34. Drash A et al: A syndrome of pseudohermaphrodism, Wilms' tumor, hypertension, and degenerative renal disease, J Pediatr 76:585, 1970.
35. Einhorn LG and Donahue JP: Combination chemotherapy in disseminated testicular cancer, Semin Oncol 6:87, 1979.
36. Ekert H et al: Experience with high dose multiagent chemotherapy and autologous bone marrow rescue in the treatment of twenty-two children with advanced tumors, Aust Paediatr J 20:195, 1984.
37. Evans R et al: Local recurrence, rate and sites of metastases, and time to relapse as a function of treatment regimen, size of primary and surgical history in 62 patients presenting with non-metastatic Ewing's sarcoma of the pelvic bones, Int J Radiat Oncol Biol Phys 11:129, 1885.
38. Ewing J: Diffuse endothelioma of bone, Proc NY Pathol Soc 21:17, 1921.
39. Exelby PR: Testicular cancer in children, Cancer 45:1803, 1980.
40. Falk S and Albert M: The clinical and roentgen aspects of Ewing's sarcoma, Am J Med Sci 54:44, 1965.
41. Farewell VT et al: Retrospective validation of a new staging system for Wilms' tumor, Cancer Clin Trials 4:167, 1981.
42. Farley F et al: Lactose dehydrogenase as a tumor marker for recurrent disease in Ewing's sarcoma, Cancer 59:1245, 1987.
43. Filipovitch A et al: Lymphomas in persons with naturally occurring immunodeficiency disorders. In Magrath I, O'Connor G, and Ramot B, editors: Pathogenesis of leukemias and lymphomas: environmental influences, New York, 1984, Raven Press.
44. Frauman JF: Stature and malignant tumors of bone in childhood and adolescence, Cancer 20:967, 1967.

45. Gale G et al: Cancer in neonates: the experience at the Children's Hospital of Philadelphia, Pediatrics 70:409, 1982.
46. Gatti RA and Good RA: Occurrence of malignancy in immunodeficiency disease: a literature review, Cancer 28:89, 1971.
47. Gilman PA et al: Familial osteosarcoma associated with 13;14 chromosomal rearrangement, Cancer Genet Cytogenet 17:123, 1985.
48. Gitlow SE et al: Diagnosis of neuroblastoma by qualitative and quantitative determination of catecholamine metabolites in urine, Cancer 25:1377, 1970.
49. Glatstein E et al: The value of laparotomy and splenectomy in the staging of Hodgkin's disease, Cancer 24:709, 1969.
50. Grabowski EF and Abramson DH: Intraocular and extraocular retinoblastoma, Hematol Oncol Clin North Am 1:721, 1987.
51. Grosfeld JL et al: Benign and malignant teratomas in children: analysis of 85 patients, Surgery 80:297, 1976.
52. Grufferman SL and Delzell E: Epidemiology of Hodgkin's disease, Epidemiol Rev 6:76, 1984.
53. Hart WR and Burkons DM: Germ cell neoplasms arising in gonadoblastomas, Cancer 43:669, 1979.
54. Hawthorne HC et al: Blanching subcutaneous nodules in neonatal neuroblastoma, J Pediatr 77:297, 1970.
55. Hems G: An etiology of bone cancer, and some other cancers, in the young, Br J Cancer 24:208, 1970.
56. Ioachim HL, Cooper MC, and Hellman GC: Lymphomas in men at high risk for acquired immune deficiency syndrome (AIDS): a study of 21 cases, Cancer 56:2831, 1985.
57. Jaffe N: Recent advance in the chemotherapy of metastatic osteogenic sarcoma, Cancer 30:1627, 1972.
58. Jaffe N: Malignant bone tumors, Pediatr Ann 4:10, 1975.
59. Jaffe N et al: Adjuvant methotrexate and citrovorum-factor treatment of osteogenic sarcoma, N Engl J Med 291:994, 1974.
60. Janjan NA et al: Mammary carcinoma developing after radiotherapy and chemotherapy for Hodgkin's disease, Cancer 61:252, 1988.
61. Jenkin R et al: The treatment of localized non-Hodgkin's lymphoma in children: a report from the Children's Cancer Study Group, J Clin Oncol 2:88, 1984.
62. Jurgens H et al: Multidisciplinary treatment of primary Ewing's sarcoma of bone. A 6-year experience of a European Cooperative Trial Cancer 61:23, 1988.
63. Kaplan HS: Hodgkin's disease, ed 2, Cambridge, 1980, Harvard University Press.
64. Kauffman RA et al: False negative bone scans in neuroblastoma metastatic to the ends of long bones, Am J Roentgenol 130:131, 1978.
65. Kay R and Tank E: The current management of bilateral Wilms' tumor, J Urol 135:983, 1986.
66. Knudson AG: Mutation and cancer: statistical study of retinoblastoma, Proc Natl Acad Sci USA 68:820, 1971.
67. Knudson AG and Strong LC: Mutation and cancer: neuroblastoma and pheochromocytoma, Am J Hum Genet 24:514, 1972.
68. Koizumi JH and Dal Canto MC: Retroperitoneal neuroblastoma metastatic to brain: report of a case and review of the literature, Child's Brain 7:267, 1980.
69. LaBrosse EH: Biochemical diagnosis of neuroblastoma: use of a urine spot test, Proc Am Assoc Cancer Res 9:39, 1968.
70. Lack EE, Weinstein HJ and Welch KJ: Mediastinal germ cell tumors in childhood: a clinical and pathologic study of 21 cases, J Thorac Cardiovasc Surg 89:826, 1985.
71. Lawrence W et al: Prognostic significance of staging factors of the UICC staging system in childhood RMS: a report from the Intergroup Rhabdomyosarcoma Study (IRS-II), J Clin Oncol 5:46, 1987.
72. Leventhal BG and Donaldson SS: Hodgkin's disease. In Pizzo PA and Poplack DG, editors: Principles and practice of pediatric oncology, Philadelphia, 1989, JB Lippincott Co.
73. Li FP et al: Adverse pregnancy outcome after radiotherapy for childhood Wilms' tumor, Proc ASCO 5:202, 1986.
74. Li MC, Hertz R and Spencer DB: Effect of methotrexate on choriocarcinoma and chorioadenoma, Proc Soc Exp Biol Med 96:361, 1956.
75. Link MP et al: The effect of adjuvant chemotherapy on release-free survival in patients with osteosarcoma of the extremity, N Engl J Med 314:1600, 1986.
76. Lukes RJ and Butler JJ: The pathology and nomenclature of Hodgkin's disease, Cancer Res 26:1063, 1966.
77. Mackay B et al: Diagnosis of neuroblastoma by electron microscopy of bone marrow aspirates, Pediatrics 56:1045, 1975.
78. Magrath IT: Malignant non-Hodgkin's lymphomas. In Pizzo PA and Poplack DG, editors: Principles and practice of pediatric oncology, Philadelphia, 1988, JB Lippincott Co.
79. Magrath IT et al: Surgical reduction of tumor bulk in management of abdominal Burkitt's lymphoma, Br Med J 2:308, 1974.
80. Mahour GH, Woolley GH, and Landing BH: Ovarian tumors in children: a 33 year experience, Am J Surg 63:367, 1976.
81. Mandell L et al: Preliminary results of alternating combination chemotherapy (CT) and hyperfractionated radiotherapy (HART) in advanced rhabdomyosarcoma (RMS), Int J Radiat Oncol Biol Phys 15:197, 1988.
82. Marcove RC and Rosen G: En bloc resections for osteogenic sarcoma, Cancer 45:3040, 1980.
83. Margo CE and Zimmerman LE: Retinoblastoma: the accuracy of clinical diagnosis in children treated by enucleation, J Pediatr Ophthalmol Strabismus 20:227, 1983.
84. Martini N et al: Multiple pulmonary resections in the treatment of osteogenic sarcoma, Ann Thorac Surg 12:271, 1971.
85. Maurer H, Beltangody M, and Gehan E: The Intergroup Rhabdomyosarcoma Study–1: a final report, Cancer 611:209, 1988.
86. Maurer H et al: Rhabdomyosarcoma in childhood and adolescence, Curr Probl Cancer 2:3, 1977.
87. Meadows AT, Lichtenfield JL, and Koop CE: Wilms' tumor in three children of a woman with congenital hemihypertrophy, N Engl J Med 291:23, 1974.
88. Mendenhall C et al: The prognostic significance of soft tissue extension in Ewing's sarcoma, Cancer 51:913, 1983.
89. Meyer WH et al: Thoracotomy for pulmonary metastatic osteosarcoma, Cancer 59:374, 1987.
90. Murphy SB: Classification, staging, and end results of treatment of childhood non-Hodgkin's lymphomas: dissimilarities from lymphomas in adults, Semin Oncol 1:332, 1980.
91. Nonoyama M et al: Epstein-Barr virus DNA in Hodgkin's disease, American Burkitt's lymphoma and other human tumors, Cancer Res 34:1228, 1974.
92. Pegelow GH et al: Familial neuroblastoma, J Pediatr 87:763, 1975.
93. Pellici PG et al: Chromosomal breakpoints and structural alterations of the c-myc locus differ in endemic sporadic forms of Burkitt lymphoma, Proc Natl Acad Sci USA 83:2984, 1986.
94. Perez CA et al: Radiation therapy in the multimodal management of Ewing's sarcoma of bone: report of the Intergroup Ewing's Study, Natl Cancer Inst Monogr 56:262, 1981.
95. Pratt CB, Crom DB, and Howarth C: The use of chemotherapy for extraocular retinoblastoma, Med Pediatr Oncol 13:330, 1985.
96. Probert JC, Parker BR, and Kaplan HS: Growth retardation in children after megavoltage irradiation of the spine, Cancer 32:634, 1973.
97. Ramsey NKC et al: Acute hemmorhage into Wilms' tumor, J Pediatr 91:763, 1977.
98. Raney R et al: Improved prognosis with intensive treatment of children with cranial soft tissue sarcomas arising in nonorbital parameningeal sites: a report from the Intergroup Rhabdomyosarcoma Study, Cancer 59:147, 1987.
99. Reed DM: On the pathological changes in Hodgkin's disease, with especial reference to its relation to tuberculosis, Johns Hopkins Hosp Rep 10:133, 1902.
100. Rosen EM et al: Neuroblastoma: The Joint Center for Radiation Therapy/Dana-Farber Cancer Institute/Children's Hospital experience, J Clin Oncol 2:719, 1984.
101. Rosen G et al: Ewing's sarcoma: ten year experience with adjuvant chemotherapy, Cancer 47:2204, 1981.
102. Rosen G et al: Preoperative chemotherapy for osteogenic sarcoma, Cancer 49:1221, 1982.
103. Rosenstock JG, D'Angio GJ, and Kiesewetter WB: The incidence of complications following staging laparotomy for Hodgkin's disease in children, Am J Roentgenol 120:531, 1974.

104. Ruymann F et al: Bone marrow metastases at diagnosis in children and adolescents with RMS, a report from the Intergroup Rhabdomyosarcoma Study, Cancer 53:368, 1984.
105. Ruymann F et al: Congenital anomalies associated with RMS: an autopsy study of 115 cases. A report from the Intergroup Rhabdomyosarcoma Study Committee. Med Pediatr Oncol 16:33-39, 1988.
106. Santoro A et al: Long-term results of combined chemotherapy-radiotherapy approach in Hodgkin's disease: superiority of ABVD plus radiotherapy versus MOPP plus radiotherapy, J Clin Oncol 5:27, 1987.
107. Scheibel E et al: Vasoactive intestinal polypeptide (VIP) in children with neural crest tumors, Acta Paediatr Scand 71:721, 1982.
108. Shields JA: Diagnosis and management of intraocular tumors, St Louis, 1983, The CV Mosby Co.
109. Sim F et al: Postradiation sarcoma of bone, J Bone Joint Surg [Am] 54:1479, 1972.
110. Spitz MR et al: Ethnic patterns of Hodgkin's disease incidence among children and adolescents in the United States, 1973-1982, J Natl Cancer Inst 76:235, 1986.
111. Stafford WR, Yanoff M, and Parnell B: Retinoblastoma initially misdiagnosed as primary ocular inflammations, Arch Ophthalmol 82:771, 1969.
112. Sterns JK, Coleman DJ, and Ellsworth RM: The ultrasonographic characteristics of retinoblastoma, Am J Ophthalmol 78:606, 1974.
113. Sullivan MP et al: Intergroup Hodgkin's disease in children study of stages I and II: a preliminary report, Cancer Treat Rep 66:937, 1982.
114. Sweetnam R, Knowelden, and Jedden H: Bone sarcoma: treatment by irradiation, amputation, or a combination of the two, Br Med J 2:363, 1971.
115. Taylor WF et al: Trends and variability in survival from osteosarcoma, Mayo Clin Proc 53:695, 1978.
116. Tefft M et al: Acute and late effects on normal tissues following chemo- and radiotherapy for childhood RMS and Ewing's sarcoma, Cancer 37:1201, 1986.
117. Teilum G: Special tumors of ovary and testis and related neoplasms. In Levine AS, editor: Cancer in the young, New York, 1982, Masson Publishing USA, Inc.
118. Tepper J et al: Local control of Ewing's sarcoma of bone with radiotherapy and combination chemotherapy, Cancer 46:1969, 1983.
119. Thomas PRM et al: Late effects of treatment for Wilms' tumor, Int J Radiat Oncol Biol Phys 9:651, 1983.
120. Tsuchida Y et al: Evaluation of alpha-fetoprotein in early infancy, Pediatr Surg 13:155, 1978.
121. Uribe-Botero G et al: Primary osteosarcoma of bone: a clinicopathologic investigation of 243 cases with necropsy studies in 54, Am J Clin Pathol 67:427, 1977.
122. Vietti TJ et al: Multimodal therapy in metastatic Ewing's sarcoma: an intergroup study, Natl Cancer Inst Monogr 56:279, 1981.
123. Vinciguerra V et al: Alternating cycles of combination chemotherapy for patients with recurrent Hodgkin's disease following radiotherapy: a prospectively randomized study by the Cancer and Leukemia Group B, J Clin Oncol 4:838, 1986.
124. Whalen T et al: Sacrococcygeal teratomas in infants and children, Am J Surg 150:373, 1985.
125. Whang-Peng J et al: Chromosome translocation in peripheral neuroepithelioma, N Engl J Med 311:584, 1984.
126. White JJ et al: Conservatively aggressive management with bilateral Wilms' tumors, J Pediatr Surg 11:859, 1976.
127. Wiggs J et al: Prediction of the risk of hereditary retinoblastoma using DNA polymorphisms within the retinoblastoma gene, N Engl J Med 318:151, 1988.
128. Young JL et al: Cancer incidence, survival and mortality for children younger than age 15 years, Cancer 58:598, 1986.
129. Zech L et al: Characteristic chromosomal abnormalities in biopsies and lymphoid-cell lines from patients with Burkitt and non-Burkitt lymphomas, Int J Cancer 17:47, 1976.

188

Cerebral Palsy

Geoffrey Miller and Steven Couch

The cerebral palsies are neither distinct neuropathologic nor etiologic entities, but are a rather clinically heterogeneous collection of syndromes, classified according to the type and distribution of motor abnormality. They are defined as a group of *disorders of movement and posture due to a nonprogressive lesion of the developing brain.*[1] Although they usually coexist with other manifestations of static brain dysfunction, their diagnosis is important, because it implies specific treatment programs and prognosis, as well as triggering a search for associated disabilities.[17] Despite being uncommon in the general population, the palsies make a major contribution to the ranks of handicapped children. Their prevalence in school children in Western industrialized countries is about 2 per 1000.[28]

ETIOLOGY AND PREDICTION

Ever since the description by Little in 1862[18] of the influence of prematurity and abnormal birth on the development of childhood handicaps, many clinicians and nonmedical personnel have all too easily attributed the cause of cerebral palsy to these unhappy events. This is despite the statement by Freud as long ago as 1897[11] that it is impossible to identify the timing or nature of the event that actually caused the brain damage and that there may be many different factors operating in the prenatal, perinatal, and postnatal periods.

A definite cause for most cases of cerebral palsy is unknown, and even when it can be identified, it is usually of prenatal origin.[24] Intrapartum events play only a limited role,[10] and may have been influenced by preexisting abnormality.[2,21] About 10% are thought to be a caused postneonatally[31] (after 28 days). The most common of these causes are infections (such as meningitis and encephalitis), asphyxia, and accidental injury. Thus, at present, most cases of cerebral palsy are difficult to predict or prevent. There is no evidence that fetal heart rate patterns, pH alterations, or base deficits are markers of later cerebral palsy.[13] Despite sophisticated fetal monitoring, an increased cesarean section rate and falling perinatal mortality there has been little change in the frequency of cerebral palsy.[30]

There are, however, a few conditions known that do contribute to about 10% to 15% of the cases. Severe prolonged peripartum asphyxia is associated with later death or cerebral palsy,[10] and the risks increase with decreasing gestational age. About 10% come from preterm infants, with the risk increasing 20-fold in those less than 1500 grams.[6] Many of these have periventricular leukomalacia, sometimes in conjunction with hemorrhagic infarction. Intraventricular hemorrhage, in the absence of periventricular leukomalacia, is not a good indicator unless followed by persisting posthemorrhagic hydrocephalus. Intrapartum asphyxia, sufficient to contribute to later neurologic deficit,[10] can be predicted by Apgar scores that remain low (less than 3) at 15 to 20 minutes, marked neonatal encephalopathy (which includes stupor, flaccidity, poor suck, and Moro response) in association with signs of damage in other organs as well as the brain, and persisting neurologic signs at 7 days.[8] Poorly controlled early onset neonatal seizures are often present.[7] It should be remembered that a low Apgar score is produced by many factors that, as well as asphyxia, include prematurity, severe neuromuscular disease, cerebral dysgenesis, maternal drugs, and severe illness due to organ failure. In addition, a neonatal encephalopathy may be a result of conditions such as cerebral dysgenesis and seizures or a severe metabolic disorder. Other causes of cerebral palsy include mechanical injury, prenatal ischemic insult,[12,16] prenatal toxins such as mercury, and congenital infection.[27] Bilirubin encephalopathy, leading to choreoathetosis and sensorineural deafness, is now a rare cause in the United States but remains a greater risk for the sick acidotic preterm infant. Breech presentation, but not necessarily breech delivery, increases the risk of later cerebral palsy[24] and is probably due to a prior abnormality in the fetus.[3]

CLASSIFICATION AND DIAGNOSIS

Cerebral palsies are classified according to the type and distribution of motor abnormality (see the box on p. 1180). Spasticity is characterized by passive resistance to joint movement which, (1) when pressure is steadily increased, the involved muscle yields slowly and steadily, (2) when a muscle is stretched beyond its normal length, it gives way quickly (clasp knife); (3) on quick passive movement of the muscle, a sudden resistance (catch) is created. It is associated with characteristic contractures and the classical neurologic signs of upper motor neuron damage such as hyperreflexia and extensor plantar responses. In conjunction with these positive signs are softer, less discriminating ones, such as a pattern of weakness and poor fine motor function. Diplegia is defined as a greater involvement of the lower than upper limbs, quadriplegia as an equal or greater involvement of the upper limbs, and hemiplegia as involvement of one side of the body only. In all the spastic syndromes, some mild dyskinetic signs may be present. Dyskinetic syndromes are characterized by the involuntary movements of athetosis, chorea, and dystonia. Ataxic syndromes involve incoordination of movement and impaired balance.

Cerebral Palsy Syndromes

- Spastic
  - Diplegia
    - Good hand function
    - Poor hand function
    - Asymmetric
  - Hemiplegia
  - Quadriplegia
- Dyskinetic
  - Mainly dystonic
  - Mainly athetoid
- Ataxic
  - Ataxic diplegia
  - Simple ataxia
  - Disequilibrium

Syndromes

In most cases of spastic diplegia the cause is uncertain, but the risk increases with increasing prematurity. Some of these preterm infants with relatively mild periventricular leukomalacia have good hand function and fewer associated disabilities. Full-term infants tend to be more severe; in these infants preexisting brain damage may be a contributory factor.[29] There is also a group with asymmetric function who usually have an increase in associated disabilities. Some of these may be secondary to periventricular leukomalacia plus unilateral hemorrhagic infarction.

The majority of spastic hemiplegia cases are prenatally determined and may be related to circulatory disturbances or maldevelopment.[33] In general, the handicap is usually only moderate or mild. Postnatal causes include trauma, stroke, and infection. In this latter group, the upper limb is often more involved than the lower, and associated disabilities such as intellectual impairment and seizures are greater. About 50% of the children have some cortical sensory impairment. Undergrowth of the affected side is found, and its degree correlating with the severity of motor and sensory deficit. In general, language development is related to cognitive ability.

Babies with spastic quadriplegias are usually term infants who are often small. Extremely low-birth-weight infants are contributing to this group in increasing numbers.[14] This is the most severe of the syndromes and implies a severely multiply handicapped infant. There is marked spastic paresis of all four limbs, and dystonia may also be present, particularly early on. Associated abnormalities include severe mental retardation, little or no speech, pseudobulbar palsy with feeding and respiratory difficulties, microcephaly, hip dislocation, and contractures and scoliosis. Visual impairment may be present, and the majority have seizures.[5]

In the dyskinetic syndromes, obviously detrimental perinatal events may have occurred, with the neuropathologic correlate of "marbling" of the basal ganglia and thalamus.[36] These syndromes are divided into two types[15]: hyperkinetic with varying combinations of athetosis and chorea, and dystonic. The abnormal movements are often induced by emotion, change in posture, or intended movement. Retention of primitive reflexes and facial grimacing with oropharyngeal difficulties are present. There are variable degrees of dysarthria and motor and intellectual disability. These are usually much greater in the dystonic type, who also often have pyramidal signs. Anarthria (difficulty in speaking) is present in about 50% of those with dystonia.

Those with ataxic syndromes are usually term infants with an early prenatal etiology. They are clinically and etiologically heterogeneous.[20] Some of these syndromes are the result of simple genetic inheritance.[19] Although the term ataxia implies an incoordination of cerebellar or sensory origin, in cerebral palsy it is much more likely that it reflects a widespread disorder of motor function control. In practice, the diagnosis is made by exclusion, because all those with cerebral palsy have some incoordination and posture disturbance. The clinician needs to be confident that these are not primarily due to weakness, spasticity, dystonia, or choreoathetosis. Many cases present as hypotonic docile infants with delayed motor skills and language. The ataxia improves in most over time, and in general, but not always, the more severe the motor impairment, the more likely are associated disabilities. Speech acquisition is related to intellectual ability and may be characteristically slow, jerky, and explosive.

Early and Differential Diagnosis

Although the lesion in cerebral palsy is nonprogressive, the clinical signs are not unchanging. Abnormal patterns emerge as the damaged nervous system matures. Evidence of specific spasticity may not be noted until 6 to 9 months, and the dyskinetic patterns are generally not obvious until about 18 months. Ataxia, as opposed to the incoordination and motor delay of mental retardation, may not be apparent until even later. The majority of children are diagnosed after the neonatal period. Aids to early diagnosis are listed in the box on p. 1181. Neurobehavioral signs that should raise suspicion are excessive docility or irritability. Early motor signs include poor head control with normal or increased tone in the limbs, generalized hypotonia with relatively well-preserved muscle power, and persistent or asymmetric "fisting." Gross and fine motor development is not only delayed but also is usually qualitatively abnormal. Failure to suppress early primitive reflexes is a useful sign; such obligatory reflexes are always abnormal.[4] For example, after age 2 to 3 months, when the infant is held in vertical suspension and the feet are placed on a firm surface, plantar flexion occurs. This should return to neutral within a few seconds and is abnormal if it has not done so by 30 seconds. If spasticity is marked, "scissoring" of the lower limbs may be seen.

The diagnosis of cerebral palsy implies that no active disease is present and that the disorder is in the brain. The differential diagnosis includes neurodegenerative disorders, inborn errors of metabolism, developmental or traumatic lesions of the spinal cord, severe neuromuscular disease, movement disorders, spinocerebellar degenerations, neoplasms, progressive hydrocephalus, and subdural hematoma. Repeated examination is necessary to detect any changes that might be consistent with a progressive disorder. However, deterioration can be a result of an increase in contracture

Early Diagnosis

Increased suspicion from neonatal history
Abnormal behavior
Psychomotor delay
Retention or asymmetry of primitive reflexes
Deviant oral motor patterns
Oculomotor abnormalities
Delayed postural reactions

formation, anticonvulsant medication toxicity, and undiagnosed or intractable epilepsy. Hypotonia in association with poor muscle power, and depressed tendon reflexes suggests a neuromuscular disease; rapidly evolving signs, particularly hypertonia becoming hypotonia, imply a neurodegenerative disorder. Extrapyramidal signs in early infancy or marked worsening during periods of starvation or illness also make the diagnosis suspect.

Some infants have motor signs during infancy that later disappear.[25] Although they are no longer designated as having cerebral palsy, they are at risk for expressing other developmental disabilities.

ASSOCIATED DISORDERS

Any type of cerebral dysfunction may occur, including abnormalities of intellect, vision, hearing, and language. Epilepsy is frequently associated, as are defects in gastrointestinal function and growth; a socioemotional disorder is often a particular problem. Nearly 75% of the total cerebral-palsied population have below average mental abilities. About 60% have mental retardation, which is mild in about one third and moderate or worse in one third. In the remainder, who function in the normal range, many have neurobehavioral and educational difficulties.[23] Assessment may be difficult, and mental development is often uneven. Roughly 40% develop seizures, which most often have their onset in the first 2 years of life but may begin later. They are more frequent in the severely intellectually handicapped, in those with gross abnormalities of brain structure, and those with postnatal hemiplegia. Oculomotor anomalies are frequent and include strabismus, refractive error, nystagmus, visual failure, and abnormalities of the pulling and reaching movements. All types of language abnormality may be encountered from aphasia to deviant language. The disorders may be complex. For example, abnormal speech may also be related to hearing, intelligence, experience, language development, the integration of motor mechanisms of the oropharynx, and coordination of breathing patterns. In general, total growth is stunted. Many fail to thrive, especially those with dyskinesia or spastic quadriplegia. This is related to feeding difficulties and recurrent vomiting, with aspiration secondary to pseudobulbar palsy and gastroesophageal reflux. Central factors, however, play an important role. Dental disease (malocclusion and caries) is common. As in other chronic cerebral disorders, some show hirsutism and acne (unrelated to phenytoin) and precocious puberty.

INVESTIGATION

In general, laboratory investigation rarely contributes to the diagnosis, although degenerative and metabolic disorders may need to be excluded. There are no EEG patterns diagnostic for cerebral palsy, but the investigation is an important part of the diagnosis and management of associated epilepsy; brain imaging may be particularly useful. The development of cerebral palsy in a preterm infant is associated with periventricular leukomalacia and sometimes with intraparenchymal hemorrhagic infarction that progresses to cystic leukomalacia; this is readily seen with ultrasound. In the full-term infant following severe asphyxia, a generalized decrease in gray white matter attenuation, as seen on computed tomography (CT), correlates with an adverse neurologic outcome.[9] It reaches a maximum 72 hours after insult and may disappear in 5 to 6 days. Ultrasound may be useful in demonstrating ischemic or hemorrhagic damage to the deep gray matter. In this region, ischemic change may not be apparent on CT, but hemorrhage will.[35] Scanning may also demonstrate cerebral dysgenesis, hydrocephalus, porencephaly, tumor, prenatal ischemic injury, and leukodystrophy. In general, the more severe the cerebral palsy, the more abnormal the scan, although the converse does not necessarily apply. The information gained with brain imaging, while usually not helpful in directing therapy, can be useful to the physician in explaining (or demonstrating) the specific cause of a child's cerebral palsy to the parents, who with this information can set realistic goals for their child and themselves in management and in their expectations of outcome. The presence of dysmorphic features may trigger a search for a chromosomal abnormality. However, an increase in minor congenital anomalies is frequently found in cerebral palsy in the absence of any genetic cause for them.

MANAGEMENT

There is no single professional who can effectively fulfill the multiple medical, social, psychological, educational, and therapeutic needs of a child with cerebral palsy.[34] Comprehensive management requires a multidisciplinary team whose members will instruct and support parents to enable them to achieve maximal potential for self-help and care for their child, and to understand their child's ability and potential for development. According to Public Law 99-457, children at risk for handicapping conditions are eligible for interventional services. These are available at rehabilitation centers where there are facilities for expert assessment, adaptive equipment, training for mobility and living skills, and communication. There is no evidence that physical therapy leads to any radical change in the basic disorder.[26] However, and especially in the very young child, physical therapy sessions enable parents to learn how to position and handle their child, providing more opportunity for play and learning, as well as facilitating feeding and the parent/child relationship.

No muscle relaxant medication is uniformly useful. Diazepam, baclofen, and dantrolene are the most commonly used, but all have potential disadvantages. Various casting and splinting techniques that may maintain muscle length and inhibit increased tone may be helpful. In many cases ortho-

Priorities for Management

Communication
Socioemotional development
Education
Maximal independence in activities of daily living
As normal an appearance as possible
Mobility

pedic procedures such as tenotomies and tendon transfers are necessary. Gastrostomies and fundoplication may improve weight gain and general health, but do not usually improve longitudinal growth when the cause is central. Selective dorsal rhizotomy can decrease spasticity and increase range of motion, and some patients may make functional improvements in sitting and gait, but primitive motor patterns are unaffected. Bearing in mind that most cerebral-palsied children become cerebral-palsied adults, the priorities for management are listed in the box above. An abundance of nonstandard therapies exist but none appears to be an improvement over standard treatment.

Early social and psychological services are vital because chronic grief and the morass of myth, despair, denial, anger, and guilt exact a high price on parents and secondarily on professionals. Parents may become socially limited, stressing the marital relationship and the nurturing of any other children. Whoever breaks the news to parents that their child is handicapped has an unenviable task. Much of what is said may be denied, and information may not be assimilated.[32] Parents frequently express dissatisfaction and at times resentment toward the physician. They react with chronic sorrow, as well as denial, guilt, frustration, anger, and embarrassment. They cannot readily complete their mourning, because they are constantly confronted by the object of their sorrow. Irrational guilt may be countered by an oversolicitous, overprotective attitude. Information should be given honestly and sensitively and delivered skillfully and tactfully. Investigations should be described and a second opinion offered. Early review is vital so that an opportunity to ask questions and ventilate feelings exists. Much of what was originally said may have been forgotten or misunderstood, and the physician must be prepared to repeat information with patience and compassion. It is wise not to be too dogmatic or offer uncertain long-range prognostication. It is important to try to alleviate any guilt that may be felt from fantasies of causation. It is well to remember that parents need to find some cause for the damage, since the unknown, and the feeling of being a victim of fate, is more distressing than being given tangible cause no matter how tangential it might be.

Early active help needs to be offered, as well as specific realistic recommendations on the management of present-day problems. Parental stress is increased by having a child whose handicap is ambiguous and subject to varying professional interpretation; this leads to a delay in obtaining a specific diagnosis and securing appropriate intervention. Stress is also increased by professionals who have limited experience with a handicapped child and limited knowledge of community resources. Initial poor handling of parents may lead to overprotection, denial, and "shopping around," which can be considered valid and appropriate from the parents' perspective. Counseling is a continuous process and its availability is important. Each family will face new stresses and problems at different stages in the development of their handicapped child. These can easily lead to fresh disappointment and the rekindling of grief.

In all, the management of the incurable palsied child will tax the humane resources of the most experienced primary care physician.

PROGNOSIS

Early prognostication may be difficult, except at the extremes of involvement. Social and environmental factors play an important role and accentuate the importance of early support and guidance. In general, prognosis is related to clinical type, pace of motor development, evolution of infantile reflexes, intellectual deficit, sensory impairment, and emotional-social maladjustment.[22] Those who walk under age 2 years are more likely to have normal or borderline IQs; in general, the more severe the motor deficit, the more likely is a significant intellectual impairment, but not always. Those who sit by age 2 years usually become walkers, as do many of those who sit by 4 years. However, most of those who sit between 3 and 4 years walk only with aids or braces, or have restricted functional ambulation. The retention of obligatory primitive reflexes at 18 months makes independent ambulation unlikely. Virtually all children with hemiplegia will learn to walk, as will many with athetosis or ataxia.

Over 90% of infants with cerebral palsy now survive into adulthood. Individual achievement is related to many factors such as intelligence, physical function, ability to communicate, and personality attributes. The availability of training, jobs, sheltered employment, and counseling also contribute to the adjustment of adults with cerebral palsy. The presence of a supportive family and the availability of specialist medical care are further important factors. Long-term planning and preparation is required, particularly when all indications point toward dependency.

Modern technology has created a variety of mechanical devices, computers, and small electric motors, which may replace some motor activities. The use of these, particularly for communication, requires some cognitive ability, thus increasing this developmental dimension's importance in the outcome of cerebral palsy.

REFERENCES

1. Bax M: Terminology and classification of cerebral palsy, Dev Med Child Neurol 6:295, 1964.
2. Brann AW: Factors during neonatal life that influence brain disorder. In Freeman JM, editor: Prenatal and perinatal factors associated with brain disorders, NIH publication No. 85-1149, Washington, D.C., 1985, U.S. Government Printing Office.
3. Braun FHT, Jones KL, and Smith DW: Breech presentation as an indicator of fetal abnormality, J Pediatr 86:419, 1975.
4. Capute AJ et al: Primitive reflex profile: A quantitation of primitive reflexes in infancy, Dev Med Child Neurol 26:375, 1984.
5. Edebol-Tysk K: Epidemiology of spastic tetraplegic cerebral palsy in Sweden. I. Impairment and disabilities, Neuropediatrics 20:41, 1989.

6. Ellenberg JH and Nelson KB: Birthweight and gestational age in children with cerebral palsy or seizure disorders, Am J Dis Child 133:1044, 1979.
7. Ellenberg JH and Nelson KB: Cluster of perinatal events identifying infants at high risk for death or disability, J Pediatr 113:546, 1988.
8. Emond A, Golding J, and Peckham C: Cerebral palsy in two national cohort studies, Arch Dis Child 64:843, 1989.
9. Fitzhardinge PM et al: The prognostic value of computed tomography as an adjunct to assessment of the full term neonate with post asphyxial encephalopathy, J Pediatr 99:777, 1981.
10. Freeman JM and Nelson KB: Intrapartum asphyxia and cerebral palsy, Pediatrics 82:240, 1988.
11. Freud S: Infantile cerebral paralysis (1897). Translated by Russin LA, Coral Gables, Florida, 1968, University of Miami Press.
12. Gilles F: Neuropathologic indicators of abnormal development. In Freeman JM, editor: Prenatal and perinatal factors associated with brain disorders, NIH Publication No. 85-1149, Washington, D.C., 1985, U.S. Government Printing Office.
13. Grant A: The relationship between obstetrically preventable asphyxia, abnormal neonatal neurologic signs and subsequent motor impairment in babies born at or after term. In Kubli F, editor: Perinatal events and brain damage in surviving children, Berlin, 1988, Springer-Verlag.
14. Hagbery B et al: The changing panorama of cerebral palsy in Sweden, Acta Paediatr Scand 78:283, 1989.
15. Kyllerman M et al: Dyskinetic cerebral palsy. I. Clinical categories, associated neurological abnormalities and incidences, Acta Paediatr Scand 71:543, 1982.
16. Larroche JC: Fetal encephalopathies of circulatory origin, Biol Neonate 50:61, 1986.
17. Levine MS: Cerebral palsy in children over 1 year: Standard criteria. Arch Phys Med Rehabil 61:385, 1980.
18. Little WJ: On the influence of abnormal parturition, difficult labour, premature birth, and asphyxia neonatorum on the mental and physical conditions of the child, especially in relation to deformities, Transactions of the Obstetrical Society of London 3:293, 1862.
19. Miller G: Ataxic cerebral palsy and genetic predisposition, Arch Dis Child 63:1260, 1988.
20. Miller G: Ataxic cerebral palsy—clinico-radiologic correlations, Neuropediatrics 20:84, 1989.
21. Miller G: Minor congenital anomalies and ataxic cerebral palsy, Arch Dis Child 64:557, 1989.
22. Molnar GE and Gordon SU: Cerebral palsy: Predictive value of selective clinical signs for early prognostication of motor function, Arch Phys Med Rehabil 57:153, 1976.
23. Molnar GE and Taft LT: Pediatric rehabilitation. Part 1: Cerebral palsy and spinal cord injuries, Curr Probl Pediatr 7:6, 1977.
24. Nelson KB and Ellenberg JH: Antecedents of cerebral palsy: multivariate analysis of risk, N Engl J Med 315:81, 1986.
25. Nelson KB and Ellenberg JH: Children who "outgrow" cerebral palsy, Pediatrics 69:529, 1982.
26. Palmer FB et al: The effects of physical therapy on cerebral palsy. A controlled trial in infants with spastic diplegia, N Engl J Med 318:803, 1988.
27. Paneth N: Etiologic factors in cerebral palsy, Pediatr Ann 15:191, 1986.
28. Paneth N and Kiely J: The frequency of cerebral palsy: A review of population studies in industrialized nations since 1950. In Stanley FJ and Alberman E, editors: The epidemiology of the cerebral palsies, Philadelphia 1984, JB Lippincott Co.
29. Powell TG et al: Cerebral palsy in low birthweight infants. II. Spastic diplegia: Associations with fetal immaturity, Dev Med Child Neurol 30:19, 1988.
30. Stanley FJ: The changing face of cerebral palsy, Dev Med Child Neurol 29:263, 1987.
31. Stanley FJ and Blair E: Postnatal risk factors in the cerebral palsies. In Stanley FJ and Alberman E, editors: The epidemiology of the cerebral palsies, Philadelphia, 1984, JB Lippincott Co.
32. Taylor DC: Counselling the parents of handicapped children, Brit Med J 284:1027, 1982.
33. Uvebrant P: Hemiplegic cerebral palsy aetiology and outcome, Acta Paediatr Scand Suppl 345:78, 1988.
34. Vining PG et al: Cerebral palsy. A pediatric developmentalist's overview, Am J Dis Child 130:643, 1976.
35. Voit T et al: Damage of thalamus and basal ganglia in asphyxiated full term neonates, Neuropediatrics 18:176, 1987.
36. Volpe JJ: Neurology of the newborn, Philadelphia, 1981, WB Saunders.

189

Chickenpox

Evan G. Pattishall III

Chickenpox (varicella) is a common childhood viral disease characterized by a pruritic vesicular rash that appears in crops. It is highly contagious and has been regarded as a relatively benign disease inasmuch as symptoms usually are mild and complications rare in healthy children. However, because of the increasing population of patients who are immunosuppressed or under therapy for malignancies, the educational impact of the disease through days lost from school, the financial impact of days lost from the work force by parents, and the developing possibility of prevention through immunization, the disease is now of greater concern.[41]

The *chicken* part of chickenpox is believed to derive from its likeness to the chickpea *Cicer areitinum,* or from the French for chickpea, *pois chiche*.[16,24] The word *varicella* is derived from a similar-appearing but more severe disease, variola (smallpox). Traditionally, chickenpox has been used to refer to the disease, and varicella, or varicella-zoster virus, to refer to the virus.

ETIOLOGY

Chickenpox is caused by the varicella-zoster virus, a DNA virus and member of the herpesvirus family, along with the herpes simplex virus, cytomegalovirus, and Epstein-Barr virus. It has been established that the same virus causes both chickenpox and herpes zoster, the latter being a reactivation (after a latent phase) of the initial varicella infection.[16] Varicella-zoster virus can be isolated from the vesicles of both chickenpox and herpes zoster. It also has been isolated from blood and tissue during an infection but has proved more difficult to isolate from respiratory secretions. The virus is highly labile, losing its infectivity quickly in the external environment. Inactivation also can be accomplished by heat and trypsin. There is only one serotype of varicella-zoster virus, but different virus strains have been identified by means of restriction endonuclease patterns of DNA.[26]

TRANSMISSION

Chickenpox is highly contagious (only slightly less so than measles and smallpox) and is one of the most contagious viral infections to cause disease in humans. Infection is thought to be spread by respiratory secretions as airborne particles from patients who can transmit infection before onset of the rash.[15] Virus has not been isolated from these secretions, however. Contact with the vesicular fluid of chickenpox or herpes zoster also will result in the transmission of chickenpox infection. Indirect contact (fomite transmission) probably is rare because of the lability of the varicella-zoster virus.

Varicella-zoster virus can cross the placenta during the first and early second trimester of pregnancy to produce a congenital varicella syndrome.[1,11,17,32] Maternal infection during the late third trimester of pregnancy may similarly result in transplacentally acquired varicella in the newborn.[29,37] Transplacentally acquired antibody to herpes zoster virus is partially protective to the newborn, but chickenpox has occurred in young infants born to immune mothers.

EPIDEMIOLOGY

Humans are the only known reservoir, or natural host, of the varicella-zoster virus. Transmission is by droplet or by direct contact in the majority of cases. The communicability period is considered to last from 1 or 2 days before the onset of the rash until 5 days after the onset of the rash or until all vesicles have crusted. Most vesicles have lost virus particles after 5 days. The incubation period is between 10 and 21 days, with an average of 14 to 15 days. With household exposure, clinical disease will develop in approximately 90% of susceptible contacts after one incubation period.[20,36]

Chickenpox, mainly a disease of childhood, has its maximum incidence at 6 years of age; 80% to 90% of children have been infected by 9 to 10 years of age.[16,28,35] Recently in England and Wales the incidence has changed, with the infection most commonly found in the neonate to 4-year-old age-group.[23] Approximately 3 million cases occur each year in the United States. The disease occurs throughout the year, but most cases occur during the winter and spring months. There are epidemic occurrences every 2 to 3 years. It is worldwide in distribution, but children in tropical climates have a lower rate of infection, so that a greater number of susceptible persons remain uninfected among older age-groups in the tropics than is the case in temperate climates.

Subclinical infections with serologic conversion rarely occur. Second clinical infections have been reported but are also rare.[15]

Death rates from chickenpox are estimated to be 2 per 100,000 for children, 50 per 100,000 for adults, 7000 per 100,000 for immunocompromised patients, and 31,000 per 100,000 for neonates.[20]

PATHOGENESIS

Varicella infection is transmitted by droplet or airborne spread with entrance into the susceptible individual through the respiratory tract. The virus migrates to the regional lymph nodes, where primary replication occurs. Approximately 4 to 6 days later a primary viremia spreads the virus to internal organs, where secondary replication occurs. This is followed by a secondary viremia, which spreads the organism to the skin and is followed by clinical chickenpox. Viremia has been documented in blood-borne monocytes after exposure but before onset of the rash or symptoms.[46] The appearance of the rash in crops probably is the result of an intermittent secondary viremia.[18]

The rash at first is macular and then progresses to a papular lesion that contains a minute vacuole. Edema fluid accumulates in the vacuole, causing a vesicle to appear on a reddened base to produce the classic "dewdrop on a rose petal" lesion. Multinucleated giant cells can be identified in the base and on the edges of the vesicle along with eosinophilic type A intranuclear inclusions. As the rash resolves, the vesicle becomes cloudy and fills with fibrinous fluid and leukocytes. A crust develops that may remain attached for 1 to 2 weeks.

When a vesicle occurs on mucous membranes, its roof sloughs to leave a shallow ulcer.

There is evidence that interferon, produced by the polymorphonuclear cells in the lesion, may contribute to resolution of the disease.[44]

CLINICAL MANIFESTATIONS

Normal Children

Chickenpox usually begins with either no prodrome or only a slight malaise and low-grade fever. This is followed in a few hours to days by a macular rash, usually on the scalp, neck, or upper portion of the trunk. The macules progress to a papular, vesicular, pruritic rash usually within 12 to 24 hours. Vesicles appear in crops, with a new crop occurring every 1 to 2 days over the next 2 to 5 days, resulting in two to four crops during the illness. The vesicles turn to pustules and then crust. The case usually runs its course in 5 to 10 days. At the height of the disease, lesions in all phases from early vesicles to crusts can be seen. Fever varies from none to 102° F (38.9° C) at the onset of the disease and may continue until vesicles cease appearing. The rash spreads centrifugally and involves all areas of the skin in severe cases. Vesicles are pruritic, and excoriations frequently are seen. Lesions occur more frequently in areas of irritation, dermatitis, or skinfolds. Occasionally the skin rash will appear as a macular rash in the diaper area or on the trunk and remain for a day or two before becoming vesicular, making early diagnosis more difficult. Vesicles may occur on the mucous membranes of the mouth, conjunctiva, esophagus, trachea, rectum, or vagina. Generally, little scarring occurs, unless the lesions become superinfected or are continually traumatized. Areas where pox have occurred may, however, remain hypopigmented or hyperpigmented months after the rash has resolved. Occasionally lesions are bullous, as a variant of the disease itself, but these more often are caused by a staphylococcal superinfection.

White blood cell counts and other laboratory test results usually are normal.

Older Children and Adults

Chickenpox in older children and adults usually is more severe than in younger age-groups, with a prodrome that may include irritability, listlessness, headaches, chills, anorexia, and myalgias. Fever usually is present and is higher and more prolonged than in the young child. The rash, too, tends to be more severe. There is a 9 to 25 times greater risk of complications; for example, varicella pneumonia has been observed to occur in 15% to 50% of such older patients.[27]

Immunocompromised Children

Immunocompromised children usually have the most severe symptoms and are at greatest risk of death from chickenpox infection, with the exception of the neonate. "Progressive varicella" can be seen in children who are naturally immunocompromised or are being treated by immunosuppression for malignancies.[44] It manifests by a more severe prodrome followed by dissemination of the varicella-zoster virus. This occurs in 30% of cases in which spread to the lungs, liver, pancreas, or central nervous system can be identified. Even if progressive varicella does not develop, these patients still have higher fevers and more prolonged vesicular eruption than the nonimmunocompromised child. Vesicles may be larger and hemorrhagic. All complications of chickenpox are increased in this population, with varicella pneumonia being the most common cause of death. Children receiving steroid therapy for disease other than cancer also are at risk for more severe involvement and complications.

Congenital and Neonatal Varicella

Infants born to mothers who contract chickenpox during the first trimester of pregnancy have a 2% to 17% risk of having congenital varicella. This syndrome includes one or more of the following defects: low birth weight, cicatricial skin lesions, a hypotrophic limb, eye abnormalities, brain damage, and mental retardation.[1,11,19,32]

When mothers have clinical chickenpox immediately before delivery, there is a 24% infection rate among their infants. If the onset of maternal rash is earlier than 5 days preceding delivery or if the onset of rash in the infant is at less than 4 days of age, there seems to be little risk of death. This reprieve probably is attributable at least in part to maternally transferred immunity. If, on the other hand, the maternal rash emerges within 4 days of delivery or if the newborn rash begins at 5 to 10 days of age, there is an associated 21% to 31% mortality.[29,32,37]

The risk for infants who are nursing when the mother contracts chickenpox is uncertain.

COMPLICATIONS

Secondary Bacterial Infection

Secondary bacterial infection is the most common complication of chickenpox. Infection usually is by group A streptococci or *Staphylococcus aureus* and can lead to all the complications associated with these organisms, including scarlet fever, nephritis, cellulitis, abscess, gangrene, pneumonia, conjunctivitis, sepsis, and erysipelas. Bullous lesions caused by *S. aureus* may begin on the second or third day of the rash and manifest as bullous impetigo.[6,16]

Reye Syndrome

The association of Reye syndrome and chickenpox has been publicized and is a frequent cause of parental concern. Approximately 16% to 28% of cases of Reye syndrome are preceded by varicella infection. It is less common, however, for Reye syndrome to follow varicella than to occur after influenza A or B infection. The age distributions of chickenpox-associated Reye syndrome and chickenpox itself are similar, being most common in 5- to 9-year-olds, followed by 10- to 14-year-olds and then 1- to 4-year-olds. Because of the suggested association between Reye syndrome and aspirin, it is recommended that aspirin be avoided in the treatment of chickenpox.

Neurologic Complications

Nervous system complications include cerebral encephalitis—the most common—followed by cerebellar encephalitis, aseptic meningitis, myelitis, and peripheral neuropathy.[22] In a more recent study cerebellar complications were more common than were cerebral infections, occurring in 1/4000 cases of chickenpox.[19] The onset of symptoms has been reported 4 days preceding until 3 weeks after the appearance of the rash. Symptoms are those that would normally be associated with encephalitis, meningitis, myelitis, or peripheral neuropathy. A toxic encephalopathy caused by diphenhydramine toxicity has been reported, which may mimic neurologic complications.[10]

Pneumonia

Varicella pneumonia occurs most often among adults and immunocompromised children.[27] It is one of the more common causes of death. In children it occurs in 1 per 10,000 cases of chickenpox, but in adults it may be present in 30% to 50% of cases of varicella. Manifestations range from a lack of clinical symptoms with abnormal findings on the chest roentgenogram to symptoms that include rales, tachypnea, hemoptysis, chest pain, cyanosis, and respiratory failure.

Hematologic Complications

Febrile purpura, malignant chickenpox with purpura, postinfectious purpura, purpura fulminans, and Henoch-Schönlein purpura have all been described as occurring with varicella infections.[7] Onset occurs from 3 to 5 days to 2 to 3 weeks after the chickenpox rash appears.

Hepatitis

Hepatitis has been reported during chickenpox infections and is marked by the onset of abdominal pain, vomiting, and continued fever on the second to fourth day after the rash appears.[9] Liver function test results become abnormal but return to normal with resolution of the abdominal symptoms. No progression to Reye syndrome occurs, and the blood ammonia level is normal. One study of 39 children with uncomplicated chickenpox found 47% to have a mildly increased level of AST (SGOT) and 29% to have markedly increased AST levels.[33] Whether this condition actually is hepatitis or early Reye syndrome is still not clear.

Zoster

Zoster is the reactivation of the varicella-zoster virus that has remained dormant after clinical chickenpox.[16] It is believed that the virus resides in the dorsal nerve ganglia and is reactivated by periods of decreased host immunity or other unknown stimulus. During reactivation the rash covers the dermatome that corresponds to the infected nerve root. Disseminated zoster, however, can also occur. Zoster has been described in all age-groups, including infancy after prenatal exposure to varicella virus resulting from maternal chickenpox. Children with varicella infections at younger ages, especially when the infection occurs before the child is 1 year of age, have an increased incidence of zoster later in life.[3]

Other Complications

Appendicitis, myocarditis, arthritis, nephritis, orchitis, splenic hemorrhage and rupture, conjunctivitis, necrotizing fasciitis, pancreatitis, pericarditis, optic neuritis, and parotitis have been reported, but rarely.[6,16]

DIAGNOSIS

Usually the diagnosis of chickenpox is made on a clinical basis. There may be a history of exposure. White blood cell counts usually are normal. A Tzanck smear (scraping of the base of a vesicle and staining with Giemsa or Wright stain) will be positive for multinucleated giant cells in varicella-zoster virus infections.[39,40] Herpes simplex types 1 and 2 also produce a positive Tzanck smear.[31] Electron microscopy and viral cultures can be used to demonstrate virus in the vesicular fluid. Viral antigen has been identified in vesicular fluid by countercurrent immunoelectrophoresis. Viral titers during acute and convalescent stages can document a recent infection, if acute titers are obtained early in the illness (preferably day 1 or 2) and titers during convalescence are noted 2 to 6 weeks later.

DIFFERENTIAL DIAGNOSIS

Smallpox (variola) has historically been the most important disease to be differentiated from chickenpox. This can easily be done with a Tzanck smear or other aforementioned laboratory tests, but it has not been necessary since the disappearance of smallpox.

Vaccinia (cowpox) will produce a vesicular rash resulting from exposure to infected livestock or, in former years, from direct contact with a smallpox vaccination.

Disseminated *herpes simplex* can resemble the chickenpox rash, but the history and progression of the disease usually differentiate these two entities. Such a situation is more confusing in newborns because disseminated herpes is rare in normal children. A Tzanck smear will be positive in both diseases.[31,39,40]

Rickettsial pox can resemble chickenpox, but its vesicles are deeper and occur at the same stage of development, and there is a more severe prodrome.

Viral exanthems, especially *coxsackievirus* and *echovirus*, can produce vesicular exanthems that do not usually crust and that follow a distinctly different course. The Tzanck smear is negative in these infections.

Lesions of *Stevens-Johnson syndrome* can resemble chickenpox, but the two diseases follow different clinical courses and the rashes develop differently. A Tzanck smear will again be negative.

Contact dermatitis may produce a rash similar to that of chickenpox (including pruritus) but has a different distribution and evolution.

Insect bites and scabies occasionally cause confusion if they are vesicular. *Bullous impetigo* (especially staphylococcal skin infection) may produce bullae that resemble chickenpox.

TREATMENT

Treatment of symptoms with acetaminophen for control of fever and relief of prodromal symptoms, along with measures to control pruritus, usually are sufficient. However, treatment of children with acetaminophen has been associated with a prolongation of the illness.[8] Pruritus can be controlled with antihistamine (diphenhydramine), calamine lotion, or Cetaphil lotion (containing cetyl alcohol, stearyl alcohol, sodium lauryl sulfate, propylene glycol, butyl, methyl, and propyl parabens, and purified water) with 0.25% menthol lotion. Diphenhydramine, both applied topically in lotions and administered orally, has been associated with encephalopathy in patients with chickenpox.[10,38,42]

Despite the popular belief that bathing is contraindicated, patients should be encouraged to take daily baths to help prevent bacterial superinfection. Adding baking soda to a warm (not hot) bath helps relieve pruritus. Children's nails should be cut and kept clean, and scratching should be discouraged. Occasionally gloves or socks on the hands are required to prevent opening of lesions by scratching.

If superinfection is present, it usually is a result of group A streptococci or *S. aureus*. This may be treated topically with bacitracin ointment or systemically with an appropriate antibiotic. *Aspirin should be avoided* in the treatment of chickenpox, as recommended by the Centers for Disease Control, until its suspected association with Reye syndrome is further defined. Physicians caring for patients on chronic aspirin therapy for juvenile rheumatoid arthritis or other diseases will need to consider the risks versus the benefits of this therapy on an individual basis if chickenpox develops in these patients.

Treatment with adenine arabinoside, acyclovir, transfer factor, and interferon has been attempted in immunosuppressed patients or patients with progressive chickenpox.[4,44] Acyclovir and adenine arabinoside have been effective in varicella therapy. The choice of therapy, however, must be individualized by a consideration of the patient's age, weight, and other concurrent conditions or diseases.[2,14,43]

Occasionally pruritus is so severe that sedation of a patient comes under consideration. If done, this procedure should be regarded with extreme caution because of possible "masking" of central nervous system complications or Reye syndrome.

Hospitalization should be avoided whenever possible because hospital epidemics can occur even when the strictest isolation procedures are followed. These generally have spread by infection of staff members who were thought to be immune or by airborne spread of the virus through ventilation systems. When otherwise unavoidable, hospitalization requires strict isolation. *Hospitalization on an adult ward* with no immunosuppressed patients may lessen the chances of spread in hospitals where effective strict isolation is not available.[12]

PREVENTION

Isolation of the patient to prevent subsequent exposure is the easiest means of prevention. This is not always effective, however, inasmuch as the disease is contagious 1 to 2 days before the appearance of the rash.

Passive prevention may be attempted by giving varicella-zoster immunoglobulin (VZIG) when indicated, within 72 to 96 hours of a known or suspected exposure.[17,20,25,45] With VZIG, disease usually will be prevented in normal children and modified to lessen the severity in adults and immunocompromised patients. Guidelines for the administration of VZIG are outlined in the Feb. 24, 1984, issue of *Morbidity and Mortality Weekly Report*.[20]

The use of interferon and transfer factor in prevention is presently experimental.[44] A live virus vaccine has been developed and successfully tested both in immunosuppressed and in normal children. It has not yet been licensed in the United States, and guidelines for its use are presently being developed. Controversy persists over use of this vaccine.[5,13,21,30,34]

REFERENCES

1. Alkalay A, Pomerance JJ, and Rimoin DL: Fetal varicella syndrome, J Pediatr 111:320, 1987.
2. Arvin AM: Oral therapy with acyclovir in infants and children, Pediatr Infect Dis J 6:56, 1987.
3. Baba K et al: Increased incidence of herpes zoster in normal children infected with varicella zoster virus during infancy: community-based follow-up study, J Pediatr 108:372, 1986.
4. Bean B and Balfour HH: Varicella-zoster infection: advances in prevention and treatment, Minn Med 66:623, 1983.
5. Brunell PA: Varicella vaccine—where are we? Pediatrics 78(4 pt 2):721, 1986.
6. Bullowa J and Wishile SM: Complications of varicella, Am J Dis Child 49:923, 1935.
7. Charkes ND: Purpuric chickenpox: report of a case, review of the literature and classification by clinical features, Ann Intern Med 54:745, 1961.
8. Doran T et al: Acetaminophen: more harm than good for chickenpox? J Pediatr 114:1045, 1989.
9. Ey J, Smith S, and Fulginiti V: Varicella hepatitis without neurologic symptoms or findings, Pediatrics 67:285, 1981.
10. Filloux F: Toxic encephalopathy caused by topically applied diphenhydramine, J Pediatr 108:1018, 1986.
11. Fuccillo D: Congenital varicella, Teratology 15:329, 1977.
12. Gardner P, Breton S, and Charles D: Hospital isolation and precaution guidelines, Pediatrics 53:663, 1974.

13. Gershon AA: Live attenuated varicella vaccine, Annu Rev Med 38:41, 1987.
14. Gershon AA: Live attenuated varicella vaccine, J Pediatr 10:154, 1987.
15. Gershon AA et al: Clinical reinfection with varicella-zoster virus, J Infect Dis 149:137, 1984.
16. Gordon JE: Chickenpox: an epidemiological review, Am J Med Sci 244:362, 1962.
17. Greenspoon J: Fetal varicella syndrome, J Pediatr 223:505, 1988 (letter).
18. Grose C: Variation on a theme by Fenner: the pathogenesis of chickenpox, Pediatrics 68:735, 1981.
19. Guess HA et al: Population-based studies of varicella complications, Pediatrics 78(4 pt 2):723, 1986.
20. Immunization Practices Advisory Committee: Varicella-zoster immunoglobulin for the prevention of chickenpox, MMWR 33:84, 1984.
21. Johnson CE et al: Live attenuated varicella vaccine in healthy 12- to 24-month-old children, Pediatrics 81:512, 1988.
22. Johnson R and Milbourn P: Central nervous system manifestations of chickenpox, Can Med Assoc J 102:831, 1970.
23. Joseph CA and Noah ND: Epidemiology of chickenpox in England and Wales, 1967-85, Br Med J (Clin Res) 296:673, 1988.
24. Lerman SC: Why is chickenpox called chickenpox? Clin Pediatr 20:111, 1981.
25. Lipton SV and Brunell PA: Management of varicella exposure in a neonatal intensive care unit, JAMA 26:1782, 1989.
26. Martin JH: Restriction endonuclease analysis of varicella-zoster vaccine virus and wild-type DNAs, J Med Virol 9:69, 1982.
27. Mermelstein R and Freiveich A: Varicella pneumonia, Ann Intern Med 55:456, 1961.
28. Muench R et al: Seroepidemiology of varicella, J Infect Dis 153:153, 1986.
29. Myers J: Congenital varicella in term infants: risks reconsidered, J Infect Dis 129:215, 1974.
30. Ndumbe PM, Cradock-Watson J, and Levinsky RJ: Natural and artificial immunity to varicella zoster virus, J Med Virol 25:171, 1988.
31. Oranje AP et al: Diagnostic value of Tzanck smear in herpetic and non-herpetic vesicular and bullous skin disorders in pediatric practice, Acta Derm Venereol (Stockh) 66:127, 1986.
32. Paryani SG and Arvin AM: Intrauterine infection with varicella-zoster virus after maternal varicella, N Engl J Med 314:1542, 1986.
33. Pitel PA et al: Subclinical hepatic changes in varicella infection, Pediatrics 65:631, 1980.
34. Plotkin SA: Varicella vaccine: a point of decision, Pediatrics 78:705, 1986.
35. Preblud S and D'Angelo L: Chickenpox in the United States 1972-1977, J Infect Dis 140:257, 1979.
36. Ross AH: Modification of chickenpox in family contacts by administration of gamma globulin, N Engl J Med 267:369, 1962.
37. Rubin L et al:. Disseminated varicella in a neonate: implications for immunoprophylaxis of neonates postnatally exposed to varicella, Pediatr Infect Dis 5:100, 1986.
38. Schunk JE and Svendsen D: Diphenhydramine toxicity from combined oral and topical use, Am J Dis Child 142:1020, 1988 (letter).
39. Solomon AR: The Tzanck smear: viable and valuable in the diagnosis of herpes simplex, zoster and varicella, Int J Dermatol 25:169, 1986.
40. Solomon AR, Rasmussen JE, and Weiss JS: A comparison of the Tzanck smear and viral isolation in varicella and herpes zoster, Arch Dermatol 122:282, 1986.
41. Sullivan-Bolyai JZ et al: Impact of chickenpox on households of healthy children, Pediatr Infect Dis J 6:33, 1987.
42. Tomlinson G, Helfaer M, and Wiedermann BL: Diphenhydramine toxicity mimicking varicella encephalitis, Pediatr Infect Dis J 6:220, 1987.
43. Vilde JL: Comparative trial of acyclovir and vidarabine in disseminated varicella-zoster virus infections in immunocompromised patients, J Med Virol 20:127, 1986.
44. Weller T: Varicella and herpes zoster, N Engl J Med 309:1362, 1984.
45. Wurzel CL, Rubin LG, and Krilov LR: Varicella zoster immunoglobulin after postnatal exposure to varicella: survey of experts, Pediatr Infect Dis J 6:466, 1987.
46. Yoshizo A et al: Viremia is present in incubation period in non-immunocompromised children with varicella, J Pediatr 106:69, 1985.

SUGGESTED READING

Straus SE et al: NIH conference. Varicella-zoster virus infections: biology, natural history, treatment and prevention (published erratum appears in Ann Intern Med 109:438, 1988).

190

Cleft Lip and Cleft Palate

Archie S. Golden and Neil H. Sims

The complex problems associated with cleft lip and cleft palate require that the primary care pediatrician coordinate management, family support, and a variety of medical needs over the years. The goal is a good psychosocial outcome, as well as a satisfactory anatomic result. Cleft lip or cleft palate, or both, occurs in approximately 1 in 750 births. Cleft lip with or without cleft palate is most frequent in native Americans and least so in black persons. Cleft palate alone has similar frequency in all groups. Isolated cleft lip is more common in girls, cleft lip *and* cleft palate more so in boys.

ETIOLOGY AND PATHOGENESIS

The pathogenesis of this malformation is related to hereditary and environmental factors and their interactions. Clefts of the face have been described as a component of more than 250 syndromes. Cleft palate, in particular, occurs more frequently as a constituent of certain syndromes. Because many of these syndromes exhibit single-gene inheritance, their recognition is important so that genetic counseling can be provided. Although a specific environmental cause rarely is identified, several substances are known to increase the risk of this birth defect. Among these are alcohol, some tranquilizers, and a few anticonvulsant medications. Amniotic bands and maternal phenylketonuria also may play a role. Because these deformities may have ramifications far beyond the oral cavity, affected children often present a continuing, complex diagnostic and treatment challenge to a wide range of professionals.

CLINICAL EVALUATION

History

A full family and gestational history is necessary, with particular attention to the maternal use of alcohol, medications, and drugs. A family tree is helpful in identifying those family members with clefts, other congenital anomalies and syndromes, mental retardation, odd speech and dental problems, and parental consanguinity. A physical examination of parents and other relatives can confirm the clues provided in the history.

Physical Examination

All infants must have an examination of their gums, the hard and soft palates, the uvula, and the throat, including palpation in all areas.

The degree of clefting will vary. A cleft lip may manifest as a small notch in the vermilion border or a complete separation extending into the nose. Clefts may be unilateral or bilateral. Isolated cleft palate occurs in the midline and can vary from minimal involvement of the uvula to extension through the soft and hard palates. Associated lip and palatal clefts can involve the soft and/or hard palate on one or both sides, thereby exposing one side of the nasal cavity, or both.

A complete examination is necessary to uncover the existence of possible associated anomalies in the variety of described syndromes. Prognosis varies, of course, with the particular constellation of findings.

COMPLICATIONS

The impact of giving birth to a baby with a facial defect can be emotionally traumatic for parents. The emotions experienced are varied and may include shock, anger and confusion, guilt, anxiety, and sadness. Because most parents are unprepared for the birth of a child with a cleft and are not familiar with the defect, the manner in which the physician first presents the infant and the defect to the parents is of utmost importance. The knowledge, reassurance, and counseling that the primary physician can provide at such a critical time may do much to alleviate the uncertainties and anxieties of the parents. Parents should be encouraged to express their feelings openly and should be reassured that these feelings are normal. The physician should listen attentively and help the parents to understand the importance of their role in the baby's habilitation. Also, the physician should emphasize his or her intent to provide support to the family after the infant is discharged from the hospital. The parents also should be advised that the treatment may take several years and include many types of management. Of paramount importance to the parents is the degree of risk that the cleft will recur in subsequent children. Predictions can be made for individual families with the use of tables that provide risk data for almost every pedigree. Consultation with a geneticist, however, should be sought when available.

Feeding

The most immediate need in the newborn period and during early infancy is the assurance of adequate nutrition. The infant born with cleft lip alone usually has little or no difficulty feeding; however, those who have a cleft palate with or without a cleft lip may have some difficulty. One of the major causes of difficulty in feeding is the inability to generate effective oral suction. Although it has been a common practice to advise a mother against breast-feeding a child with cleft lip or palate, it is possible for some mothers to do so. When breast-feeding the infant is not possible or not desired, a variety of feeding techniques have been found to be effective. The position of the infant while feeding is important. Holding the infant in an upright or semiupright position generally works best and keeps food from coming out the nose. Also, the probability of formula entering the eustachian tubes and causing ear problems is lessened. Because these babies often swallow an excessive amount of air, the feeding period may be prolonged and a great deal of energy used in obtaining a marginal amount of nourishment. The use of a soft nipple with an enlarged crisscross cut often works well. Alternatively, a Brecht feeder or medicine dropper can be tried. Milk should be directed to the inside of the cheek, rather than into the throat. If choking on liquids is a problem, rice cereal may be used as a thickener.

The most important factor in feeding an infant with cleft lip or palate is patience. Smaller but more frequent feedings may help to avoid tiring the infant and frustrating the parents. Parents should be encouraged to be creative, determining what works best for their particular infant. Gavage feedings rarely are needed. It is important that another person (or persons) knows how to feed the infant to enable the mother or other primary caretaker to obtain some rest.

Speech and Language

A hypernasal tone to the voice is the most common speech defect with clefts, particularly of the palate. Functioning of the palatal and pharyngeal muscles is impaired. The development of expressive language and speech may be retarded in children with a cleft palate, and their articulation is less advanced than that of children without such a defect. An associated hearing defect also may play an important role in delayed or abnormal speech development. Because problems may persist even after successful anatomic closure, early referral to a speech therapist should be considered.

Dental and Orthodontic Problems

Irregularities in the upper anterior dental arch associated with cleft lip may result in supernumerary incisors, rotation and malformation of the lateral incisors, or malocclusions. When there is a cleft of both lip and palate, the dental deformities may be greater, involving the canine teeth and the molars. Children with these problems tend to have more cavities, thus requiring meticulous oral hygiene and constant dental care. Orthodontic treatment may be necessary.

Middle-Ear Disease and Hearing Loss

Recurrent otitis media and hearing loss are almost universal complications of cleft palate. A key factor in the cause of secretory otitis in patients with cleft palate is eustachian tube dysfunction. Although middle-ear disease is almost universal in these patients, the hearing loss that often accompanies recurrent disease usually can be avoided under close supervision that results in early recognition and treatment of middle-ear infection. Educating the parents in the recognition of the signs and symptoms of middle-ear disease is important and can be a tremendous aid to the physician.

The likelihood of otitis media decreases after palate repair, but there may continue to be an increased incidence, as compared with unaffected children. Antibiotic prophylaxis should be readily prescribed for these infants and children; referral to an otolaryngologist for possible surgical therapy, tympanotomy tubes, and adenoidectomy is common. Clearly, careful audiologic follow-up is necessary.

Upper Airway Problems

Occasional apneic episodes have been described in children with cleft palate, especially in those with the Pierre Robin malformation.

Psychological Problems

Without question the presence of such a visible defect adds to the burden of child rearing and increases the stress experienced by the child and the parents. However, psychological disorders common to these children have not been found. It is most important that the primary physician, as well as others involved in the medical management, remain sensitive to the emotional needs of these children throughout the total habilitative process.

Explorations should concern the stability of the family, available support, existing emotional problems and those arising from the condition, the possibility of the child being unwanted, and ethnic and cultural beliefs that might affect parental attitudes toward the baby.

Economic status is important because clefts require long-term medical care and rehabilitation, with considerable expense.

In particular, because of our mobile society, pediatricians may "inherit" children with clefts at varying states of repair and rehabilitation. The practical matters of anatomic revisions must be addressed and, depending on age, the psychosocial needs of older children and adolescents and their peer and family relationships.

SURGICAL CORRECTION

A cleft lip usually is repaired in early infancy. Traditionally, most surgeons prefer to wait until the child reaches a body weight of 10 to 12 pounds. However, in an otherwise healthy infant with no complications of general anesthesia expected, the cleft lip may be repaired at birth or at 3 months of age, depending on the preference of the surgeon.

Speech development is of primary consideration in palate repair. The purpose of the operation is to produce anatomic closure of the palate and to minimize maxillary growth retardation with associated dental alveolar deformities. Eighteen months generally is accepted as the latest age for surgical repair of a cleft palate, because frequent speech usually develops soon thereafter. Six months of age is preferable. If the operation is delayed until 3 years of age or older, speech problems are more likely. Revisions of the primary procedure may be necessary by 5 or 6 years of age.

LONG-TERM CARE: THE CLEFT LIP AND PALATE TEAM

Although the pediatrician must assume the responsibility for the child's overall health management and for parental counseling and guidance, referral to an interdisciplinary cleft lip and cleft palate team is essential. There are at least 215 such groups in the United States today, varying in size from some 20 members in major academic centers to 3 in community-based programs—a plastic surgeon, a dentist or pedodontist, and a speech pathologist are the core of the team.

In addition, university-based teams often include an otolaryngologist, a geneticist, a psychologist, a public health nurse, a social worker, a vocational and rehabilitation counselor, an orthodontist, and a prosthodontist. A well-functioning team is cost effective in that it allows a comprehensive group of specialists to evaluate and manage a patient with a minimum of visits closely coordinated over time, thus limiting time lost from school by the patients and work by the parents.

Clearly, the specialization of team members mandates the pediatrician's coordinating effort. This need may continue for decades. The anatomic problems associated with clefts may emerge any time in a patient's life, and the rehabilitative process may be prolonged.

SUGGESTED READINGS

Pashley NRT and Krause CJ: Cleft lip, cleft palate and other fusion disorders. In Symposium on Congenital Disorders: Otolaryngologic Clinics of North America, Philadelphia, 1981, WB Saunders Co.

Rood SR and Stool SE: Current concepts of the etiology, diagnosis and management of cleft palate related otopathologic disease. In Caldarelli DD, editor: Craniofacial anomalies, Otolaryngol Clin North Am 14:865, 1981.

Suslak L and Desposito F: Infants with cleft lip/cleft palate, Pediatr Rev 9:331, 1988.

Tier WC, editor: Symposium on cleft lip and cleft palate, Clin Plast Surg 12:533, 1985.

191

The Common Cold

Mark D. Widome

EPIDEMIOLOGY

Colds are self-limited viral infections of the upper respiratory tract that are anatomically limited to the nasal mucosa and the nasopharynx. Their distribution is worldwide, occurring in all climates and all populations. Among the pediatric population in temperate climates they are extremely common and highly communicable. According to the National Ambulatory Medical Care Survey of 1985, acute upper respiratory tract infection ranked second only to otitis media in frequency of diagnosis by office-based pediatricians, accounting for nearly 3 million office visits annually. Upper respiratory tract illness is the most common cause of school absenteeism.

Children average three to nine colds per year, with a peak incidence in the preschool years. Colds are more common among preschoolers who have school-aged siblings and among large families.

Infection usually is introduced into families by children rather than by adults, and the spread of infection to siblings is twice as frequent as that from child to parent. Therefore parents can expect to have about half the number of colds as do their children. Infants and young children enrolled in day care programs have more colds than do children of similar ages cared for at home; however, colds are no more frequent in large day care settings than in small ones.[4] Fig. 191-1 is useful in illustrating to parents how children in day care appear to get most of their colds "out of the way" at earlier ages.[1]

For reasons not entirely clear, colds are more common in the winter months; contrary to popular belief, however, exposure to a cold environment has no effect on host resistance to the common cold viruses[2]; crowding is clearly a factor. As might be expected, incidence sharply increases in the fall, several weeks after the beginning of school. Additional peaks (in the northern hemisphere) occur at the end of January and again in April. The number of colds varies considerably from child to child. Crowding and pollution may contribute to a child's increased susceptibility. Increased respiratory infections have been associated with passive smoking and other indoor air pollution.

Viruses are shed primarily in nasal secretions. Spread to contacts usually occurs by way of contaminated hands rather than by a direct airborne route.[3] Viruses on skin, fabric, and hard surfaces contaminate the fingers of playmates, who then self-inoculate their respiratory tract by touching their eyes and nose.

ETIOLOGY

Clinically indistinguishable illnesses are caused by a variety of viruses (Table 191-1). In total, more than 100 serologically distinct viruses cause colds; rhinoviruses account for about a third. Parainfluenza and respiratory syncytial virus, frequently responsible for croup and bronchiolitis among infants, causes illness limited to the upper respiratory tract on reinfection of older children and adults. Coronavirus probably also plays a significant role in winter colds.

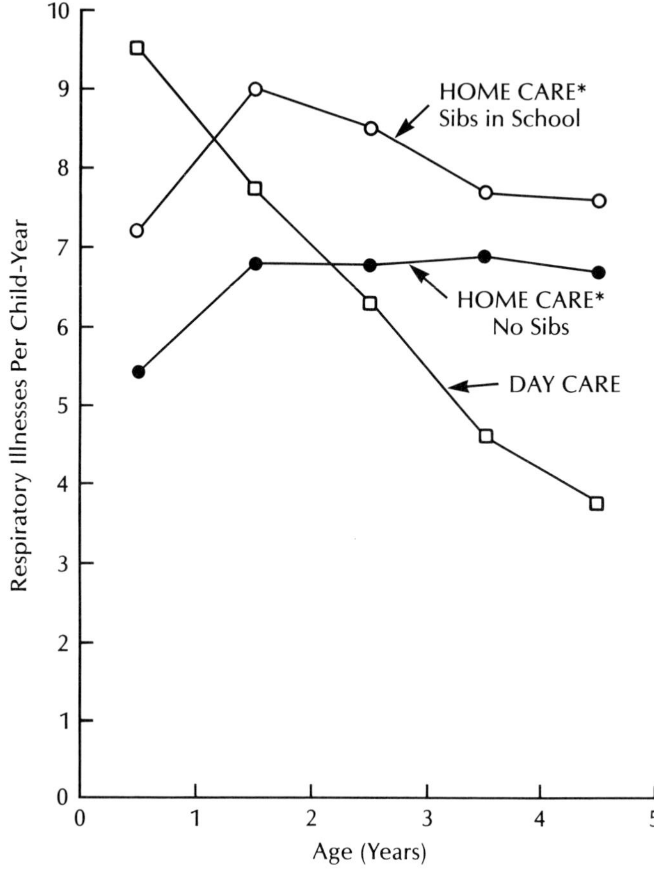

Fig. 191-1 Comparative incidences of respiratory illness in different child care settings.

From Denny FW: Acute respiratory infections in children: Etiology and epidemiology, Pediatr Rev 9(5):135, 1987.

Table 191-1 *Infectious Agents Associated with the Common Cold*

CATEGORY	AGENTS
Common viruses that usually cause the common cold	Rhinoviruses Parainfluenza viruses Respiratory syncytial virus Coronaviruses
Common infectious agents that occasionally cause illness with common cold symptoms	Adenoviruses Enteroviruses Influenza viruses Reoviruses *Mycoplasma pneumoniae*
Unusual causes of common cold-like illness	*Coccidioides immitis* *Histoplasma capsulatum* *Bordetella pertussis* *Chlamydia psittaci* *Coxiella burnetii*

From Cherry JD: The common cold. In Feigin RD and Cherry JD, editors: Textbook of pediatric infectious diseases, ed 2, Philadelphia, 1987, WB Saunders Co, p 156.

Adenoviruses more commonly cause a febrile viral syndrome associated with pharyngitis. The enteroviruses often cause a cold syndrome with additional features that include pharyngitis, aseptic meningitis, exanthemata, diarrhea, and myalgias such as pleurodynia.

CLINICAL ILLNESS

After an incubation period of 2 to 4 days, during which the virus replicates in the nasopharynx, the illness is heralded by nasal stuffiness and a thin nasal discharge. The nasal mucosa appears swollen and erythematous. Postnasal drip and mouth-breathing contribute to throat irritation. Sneezing is prominent by the second or third day. In older children there is little or no fever, whereas infants have a more varied presentation that may include irritability, fever to 102.2° F (39° C), interference with feedings, and mild gastrointestinal disturbance.

Viruses are shed from the nose for about a week. During this period the nasal discharge becomes more purulent as a result of the presence of white blood cells and shed epithelial cells. The duration of illness is usually about 1 week, but lingering cough and nasal discharge may not subside until the end of the second week, when the columnar epithelium has regenerated.

In the typical cold, infection is localized to epithelial surfaces without viremia; therefore constitutional symptoms such as fever, headache, and malaise, although they occur frequently, tend not to be the most prominent aspects of the illness. Likewise, the blood cell count is only mildly affected, with an early slight leukopenia followed by leukocytosis.

DIFFERENTIAL DIAGNOSIS

Diagnosis of the common cold rests on its mode of presentation and epidemiologic consideration rather than on identification of an etiologic agent. The diagnosis can be made with greatest certainty in fall, winter, or early spring in the midst of a community outbreak of acute illness limited to the upper respiratory tract.

If the course of the illness is subacute or chronic, one must consider sinusitis (particularly with prominent fever and cough in the school-aged child or older) and, of course, allergy. Allergy can be differentiated from chronic or recurrent colds by considering allergic history (e.g., eczema), family history, seasonal nature of the illness, and nasal eosinophilia. Upper respiratory syndromes plus evidence of pharyngitis, enanthem, or rash suggest other viral illness. Young infants can have a persistent purulent nasal discharge caused by streptococcal organisms. Streptococcal illness in older children is characterized by pharyngitis in the *absence* of cold symptoms. A unilateral nasal discharge, particularly if it is thick, foul smelling, and blood-tinged, is likely due to be a foreign body.

Early pertussis, measles, and diphtheria can mimic a cold, but each of these illnesses quickly becomes more serious. Auscultatory findings in the chest or tachypnea, with or without auscultatory findings, suggest lower respiratory tract disease of infectious or allergic etiology.

In the adolescent patient, use of cocaine must be considered in the differential diagnosis of persistent congestion and watery rhinorrhea. Chronic abuse of over-the-counter nasal sprays can produce a similar manifestation.

MANAGEMENT

Treatment is symptomatic because the illness is self-limited. Most infants require no treatment at all. Mucosal irritation may be lessened by use of a cool-mist water vaporizer. Saline nose drops or spray will thin secretions so that they may be more easily cleared. Sleeping with the head elevated is also helpful.

Discomfort from fever or throat irritation is best treated with acetaminophen. Aspirin should be avoided because of its association with Reye syndrome. Fluids should be offered as desired, and throat lozenges can be prescribed for older children.

Decongestant nasal sprays should be used cautiously because they tend to cause "rebound" congestion. Phenylephrine (0.125%), if used, should be discontinued after 3 to 4 days, after which it is more likely to cause mucosal irritation and increased congestion. Although many claim symptomatic relief from oral antihistamines and decongestants, there are no controlled studies to support their use.[5] Such medicines should be discouraged in the first 6 months of life because of resultant irritability.

Antibiotics have no effect on the clinical course of a cold, and many studies document their lack of value in preventing complications.

Although vitamin C has been widely used to prevent and treat colds, the various studies show either very small or no differences at all between experimental and control groups in terms of severity symptoms and duration of illness. Because vitamin C in large doses is potentially toxic, its use to change the course of this self-limited illness cannot be recommended.

COMPLICATIONS

Complication by secondary bacterial illness generally is preceded by a fever spike. Otitis media secondary to eustachian tube congestion is common, and is most likely to occur in the youngest patients. Sinusitis as a result of obstruction of ostia in the paranasal sinuses occasionally is seen. Extension of infection, viral or bacterial, to the lower respiratory tract should be considered with fever, tachypnea, or change in character of the cough.

REFERENCES

1. Denny FW: Acute respiratory infections in children: etiology and epidemiology, Pediatr Rev 9(5):135, 1987.
2. Douglas RG Jr, Lindgren KM, and Couch RB: Exposure to cold environment and rhinovirus common cold: failure to demonstrate effect, N Engl J Med 279:742, 1968.
3. Hendley J, Wenzel R, and Gwaltney J: Transmission of rhinovirus colds by self-inoculation, N Engl J Med 288:1361, 1973.
4. Strangert K: Respiratory illness in preschool children with different forms of day care, Pediatrics 57:191, 1976.
5. West S et al: A review of antihistamines and the common cold, Pediatrics 56:100, 1975.

192

Congenital Heart Disease

Edward B. Clark

Most children will have a heart murmur noted on examination sometime during infancy or early childhood. The challenge to the pediatrician is to identify the children who require cardiac care. This chapter is a review of the most common congenital cardiac defects.

EPIDEMIOLOGY

In the United States, eight of every 1000 infants born have a congenital cardiovascular malformation. For some, the defect is of little clinical significance; for others, surgical palliation and repair permits longer life. Some defects are incompatible with life and are fatal in utero or shortly after birth.

ETIOLOGY AND PATHOGENESIS

The etiology of most congenital heart defects is as yet undefined. Many defects are likely the result of single or multiple gene abnormalities, others arise as the consequence of genetic and environmental interaction, and some are chance occurrences in the complex process of cardiovascular development. Of the 2600 infants studied in the Baltimore-Washington Infant Study of Congenital Cardiovascular Malformations, 12% of the cases were associated with chromosomal abnormalities, 8% with multiple congenital malformations, and 80% with isolated cardiac defects.

Abnormalities in cardiovascular development are responsible for a broad spectrum of heart diseases, yet we know relatively little about the process that brings about the shape and function of the heart. The heart begins as a muscle-wrapped tube and becomes a complex four-chambered pump through growth and morphogenesis. Most congenital cardiovascular malformations have their origins during primary morphogenesis in the first 8 weeks after conception. A few defects may arise during later secondary morphogenesis of the heart.

Risk factors for congenital cardiovascular malformations include maternal illnesses such as diabetes mellitus and systemic lupus erythematosus. The known cardiac teratogens include rubella, thalidomide, retinoic acid, and alcohol.

CLINICAL PRESENTATION

Children with a congenital heart defect are recognized because of a heart murmur, cyanosis, congestive heart failure, and/or an arrhythmia. The differential diagnosis of congenital heart defects requires the integration of the history, symptoms, and findings on physical examination, chest roentgenogram, electrocardiography, and two-dimensional Doppler echocardiography. Serious congenital heart disease appears most frequently in infancy, and early prenatal diagnosis can be made by fetal echocardiography. Less severe cardiac abnormalities are identified during childhood. Mild defects may be identified in adulthood or go unrecognized.

LABORATORY STUDIES

Chest Roentgenogram

The chest roentgenogram shows the size of the heart and the amount of pulmonary blood flow. With normal pulmonary blood flow, heart size occupies 50% of the cardiothoracic dimension, and the pulmonary vessels decrease in size from the hilar area through two thirds of the chest. The heart and pulmonary vessels are large and vascular markings are visible in the peripheral one third of the lung fields, with increased pulmonary blood flow. Abnormal size, shape, or location of specific chambers and vessels can be determined from the chest roentgenogram.

Electrocardiogram

The electrocardiogram (ECG) shows cardiac rhythm and myocardial mass. A normal newborn's electrocardiogram has right ventricular dominance that gradually shifts to left ventricular dominance as the child grows and the left ventricular forces increase.

Echocardiography

Echocardiography and Doppler measurement of blood velocity give precise information. It should be used, as should most laboratory data, as an adjunct to careful clinical evaluation of the patient and not as a prediagnostic screening tool.

SPECIFIC DEFECTS

Right-to-Left Shunts

Right-to-left shunts are characterized by cyanosis secondary to decreased pulmonary blood flow. In many defects with right-to-left shunt, pulmonary blood flow depends on a patent ductus arteriosus. As the ductus closes in the first hours to days after birth, the infant becomes progressively cyanotic. If these early signs are ignored, the progressive cyanosis leads to hypoxemia, metabolic acidosis, and death; therefore aggressive initial evaluation and stabilization is essential.

Tetralogy of Fallot (Fig. 192-1, *A*)
Tetralogy of Fallot is characterized by pulmonary outflow tract obstruction, ventricular septal defect, overriding aorta, and right ventricular hypertrophy. Infants with tetralogy of Fallot manifest symptoms in the first days to months of life and may initially have the auscultatory findings of a simple ventricular septal defect. However, as the infundibular obstruction increases, the cardiac murmur changes to reflect pulmonary stenosis. Symptoms are initially cyanotic spells that progress to persistent cyanosis. The ECG shows right axis deviation and right ventricular hypertrophy. The chest roentgenogram shows a normal-size heart with normal to slightly decreased pulmonary blood flow. The echocardiogram defines an intracristal ventricular septal defect, an overriding aorta, and infundibular and pulmonary valve stenosis. For infants with hypercyanotic spells, the knee-chest position increases systemic resistance and decreases the right-to-left shunt. Some infants respond to propranolol, which decreases infundibular obstruction. Surgical management is either a primary repair of the intracardiac defects or, in cases with complex pulmonary artery anatomy, a systemic-to-pulmonary shunt.

Pulmonary Valve Atresia and Critical Stenosis (Fig. 192-1, *B*)
Neonates with pulmonary valve atresia manifest cyanosis in the first hours or days of life as the ductus arteriosus closes and pulmonary blood flow decreases. Physical findings often include a soft murmur of the patent ductus arteriosus. The ECG shows variable right ventricular forces, and the chest roentgenogram shows a normal-size heart and decreased pulmonary blood flow. The diagnosis is established by echocardiography, which defines atresia or critical stenosis of the pulmonary valve. The ventricular anatomy can be that of a single ventricle, two ventricles with a large ventricular septal defect, or a hypoplastic right ventricular cavity with an intact ventricular septum. An infant is initially stabilized with prostaglandin E_1 to maintain ductal patency. Surgical treatment includes a systemic-to-pulmonary artery shunt to increase pulmonary blood flow. Many children eventually undergo surgical repair to reconstruct the pulmonary outflow tract.

Tricuspid Atresia (Fig. 192-1, *C*)
Infants with tricuspid atresia manifest cyanosis and a heart murmur in the neonatal period. The chest roentgenogram shows a normal-size heart with an enlarged right atrium and decreased pulmonary blood flow. The ECG shows left-axis deviation, predominant P wave, and absent right ventricular forces. Echocardiography defines atresia of the tricuspid valve and often a slitlike right ventricle and ventricular septal defect. Initial management includes prostaglandins to maintain ductal patency, followed by a surgical shunt. Many children with tricuspid atresia undergo a Fontan procedure to separate systemic and pulmonary circuits by direct connection of the right atrium to the pulmonary artery.

Ebstein Malformation of the Tricuspid Valve

In Ebstein malformation, the septal and anterior tricuspid valve leaflets are displaced into the right ventricle, often obstructing the pulmonary outflow tract. The clinical presentation varies. In the severe form, an infant may have severe cyanosis because the valve leaflet obstructs the right ventricular outflow tract. In the mild form, a child may have only trivial tricuspid insufficiency. Diagnostic studies include an electrocardiogram that shows left-axis deviation, prominent P wave, and preexcitation (Wolff-Parkinson-White syndrome). (See Chapter 114,[11] "Cardiac arrythmias.") Children with Ebstein malformation are predisposed to supraventricular tachycardia. In severe cases, the chest roentgenogram shows massive cardiomegaly and decreased pulmonary blood flow. Echocardiography defines the displacement of the tricuspid valve leaflets and right-to-left shunt at the atrial level.

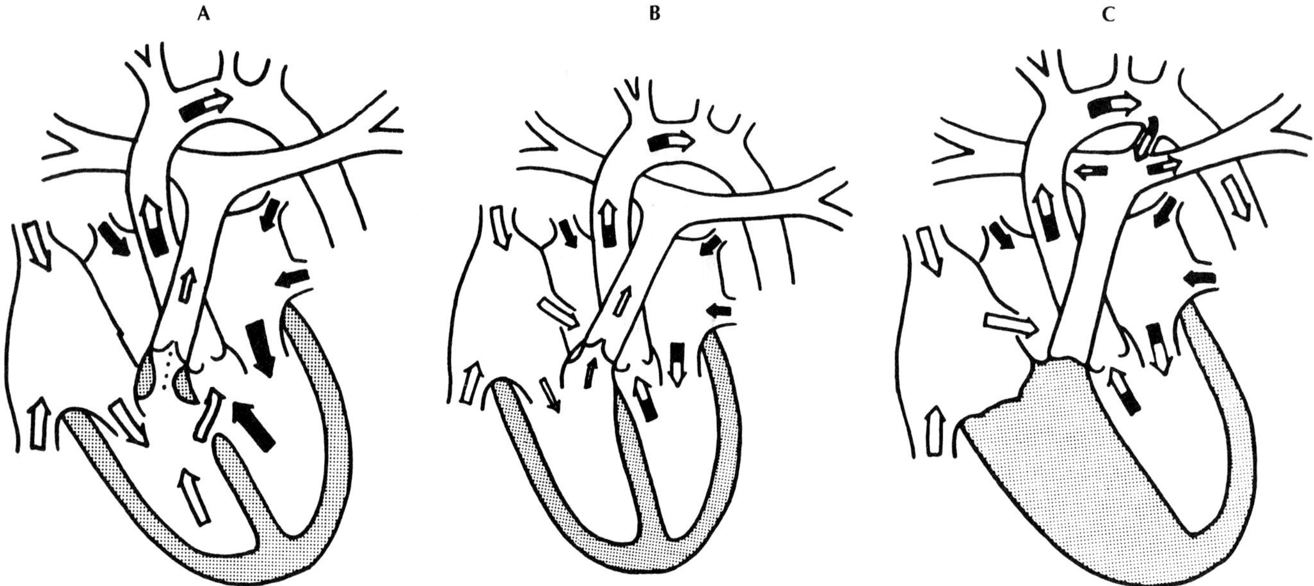

Fig. 192-1 Right-to-left shunts. **A,** Tetralogy of Fallot. **B,** Pulmonary atresia. **C,** Tricuspid atresia. Closed arrows indicate saturated blood; open arrows indicate desaturated blood. (See text for details.)
From Clark EB: Heart disease. In CL Paxson, Jr., editor: Van Leeuwan's newborn medicine, ed 2, St Louis, 1979, The CV Mosby Co.

Infants may require prolonged respiratory support until pulmonary vascular resistance decreases. Some children require chronic antiarrhythmic therapy because of their supraventricular tachycardia. Older patients may require surgical closure of an atrial septal defect and plication of the tricuspid valve.

Admixture Lesions

Admixture lesions are characterized by increased pulmonary blood flow but have mixing of systemic and pulmonary venous return at the cardiac or great artery level. Cyanosis varies depending on the relative amount of pulmonary blood flow.

Transposition of the Great Arteries (Fig. 192-2, *A*) In transposition of the great arteries, the aorta arises from the right ventricle and the pulmonary artery from the left ventricle. Infants with this defect have profound cyanosis in the first few hours or days of life. The clinical examination reveals a soft systolic ejection murmur and profound cyanosis. The chest roentgenogram and ECG are usually normal. Echocardiography defines the origin of the great arteries. Management includes the use of prostaglandins to maintain ductal patency and palliation by atrial septostomy to allow for mixture of saturated and desaturated blood at the atrial level. Surgical repair is either an arterial switch during the first week of life or an atrial baffle (Mustard procedure) before 6 months of age.

Truncus Arteriosus Communis (Fig. 192-2, *B*) In truncus arteriosus communis the septation of the embryonic outflow tract into the aorta and pulmonary artery is incomplete. Infants with truncus arteriosus communis have mild cyanosis and congestive heart failure in the first days or weeks of life. Physical examination characteristics include a hyperactive precordium, bounding pulses, an ejection click from the truncal valve, and a systolic ejection murmur. The ECG shows a normal axis with right or biventricular hypertrophy, and the chest roentgenogram shows cardiomegaly with increased pulmonary blood flow. The right and left pulmonary arteries arise from a higher position than normal. Echocardiography demonstrates a ventricular septal defect, with the truncal root and pulmonary arteries arising distal to the truncal valve. Aortic arch anomalies occur in most cases. Cardiac catheterization and angiography may be needed to define the defect completely. Initial management includes control of congestive heart failure. Definitive management is surgical repair with placement of a conduit from the right ventricle to the pulmonary artery and closure of the ventricular septal defect so that the truncus arises from the left ventricle.

Total Anomalous Pulmonary Venous Return

Children with total anomalous pulmonary venous return usually manifest mild cyanosis and congestive heart failure in the neonatal period. The characteristics include a hyperdynamic precordium, a soft systolic ejection murmur, and a widely fixed, split, second heart sound. This defect can be difficult to diagnose by noninvasive studies alone. Neither chest roentgenogram nor the ECG provides specific information. Echocardiography can be problematic because of the difficulty in identifying individual pulmonary veins. Cardiac catheterization is often required to diagnose total anomalous pulmonary venous return and to define the site of the common pulmonary vein connection. Initial management includes congestive heart failure treatment and ventilatory support. Surgery involves the anastomosis of the common pulmonary vein to the left atrium.

Hypoplastic Left Heart Syndrome: Aortic Atresia with Mitral Atresia or Stenosis

Neonates with hypoplastic left heart syndrome, aortic atresia, and mitral atresia have abrupt onset of shock and cyanosis within a few hours or days of life. Clinical findings include pallor, a hyperdynamic precordium, weak or absent pulses, and congestive heart failure. The echocardiogram shows a diminutive left ventricle, an ascending aorta less than 6 mm in diameter, and retrograde blood flow to the coronary arter-

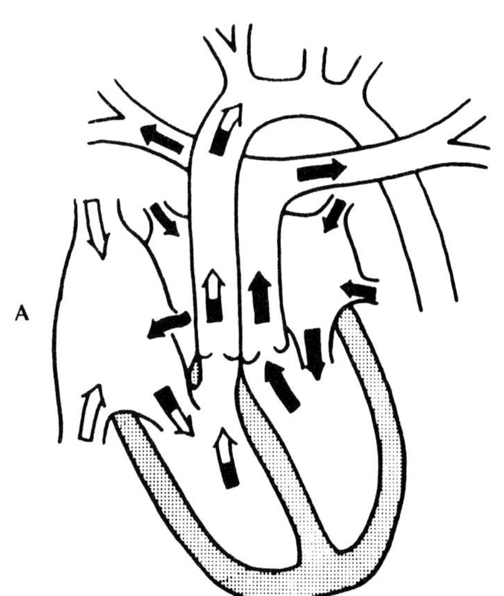

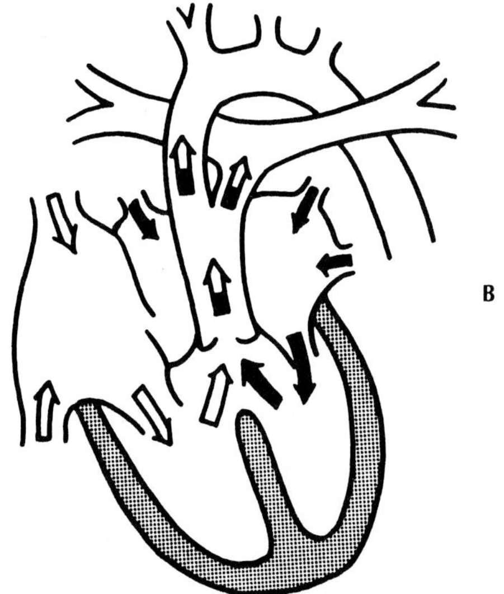

Fig. 192-2 Admixture lesions. **A,** Transposition of the great arteries. **B,** Truncus arteriosus communis. Closed arrows indicate saturated blood; open arrows indicate desaturated blood. (See text for details.)

From Clark EB: Heart disease. In CL Paxson, Jr., editor: Van Leeuwan's newborn medicine, ed 2, St Louis, 1979, The CV Mosby Co.

ies. The infant depends on the patent ductus arteriosus for systemic blood flow. Aortic atresia with mitral atresia is usually a lethal lesion, because death follows closure of the ductus arteriosus. Heart transplantation or surgical palliation (Norwood procedure) is being performed experimentally in some institutions.

Left-to-Right Shunts

Left-to-right shunt defects have increased pulmonary blood flow through a defect at the atrial, ventricular, or great artery level.

Atrial Septal Defect (Fig. 192-3, *A*)
Most children with atrial septal defects have a cardiac murmur. Clinical characteristics include a hyperdynamic precordium, a fixed, split, second heart sound, and a pulmonary ejection murmur. The electrocardiogram shows right-axis deviation and volume-overload right ventricular hypertrophy. The chest roentgenogram shows mild cardiomegaly and increased pulmonary blood flow. The echocardiogram shows a defect in the midportion of the secundum atrial septum and a dilated right ventricle with paradoxic septal motion. The child with an atrial septal defect should have the defect closed before he or she enters school. Closure techniques include direct surgical repair or closure with an umbrella-like device that is positioned on the end of a cardiac catheter.

Ventricular Septal Defect (Fig. 192-3, *B*)
The clinical presentation of a ventricular septal defect varies. The murmur of small defects may be heard in the first few days of life, but large defects may be silent and lead to congestive heart failure at 6 to 8 weeks of age. The physical examination reveals a harsh, pansystolic murmur heard along the left lower sternal border that radiates to the right. Muscular ventricular septal defects may generate a short pansystolic murmur. Noninvasive study results also vary. Although the ECG may be normal with small defects, children with large septal defects show evidence of biventricular hypertrophy. Similarly, the chest roentgenogram shows an enlarged heart only if the left-to-right shunt is large. Echocardiography often shows the location and size of the defect and is important in assessing the prognosis. Small defects are likely to close spontaneously, and even moderate-size perimembranous defects have a greater than 50% chance of spontaneous closure. Large symptomatic ventricular septal defects are closed surgically to reduce the risk of pulmonary vascular obstructive disease.

Patent Ductus Arteriosus (Fig. 192-3, *C*)
Infants with patent ductus arteriosus have a variable presentation. Premature infants have congestive heart failure; term infants may develop heart failure at 2 to 3 weeks of age when pulmonary vascular resistance drops; and older children may be asymptomatic. The physical findings also vary with age. Premature infants often have no murmur but do have bounding pulses and a hyperdynamic precordium. Full-term infants and older children usually have a continuous murmur heard best in the left second intercostal space. The electrocardiogram shows left ventricular hypertrophy, and the chest roentgenogram shows normal to increased pulmonary vascularity and an increase in left atrial and left ventricular size. Echocardiography defines retrograde turbulent blood flow in the main pulmonary artery. Management is surgical closure of the patent ductus. Large defects are closed to prevent pulmonary vascular obstructive disease; small defects are ligated to reduce the risk of bacterial endocarditis.

Atrioventricular Canal Defects

Atrioventricular canal defects make up a spectrum of abnormalities, including complete atrioventricular canal, ostium primum atrial septal defect with mitral valve cleft, and inflow-type ventricular septal defect. These defects are frequently found in children with Down syndrome. Clinical findings include a hyperdynamic precordium and the murmurs of increased pulmonary flow and AV valve insufficiency. The elec-

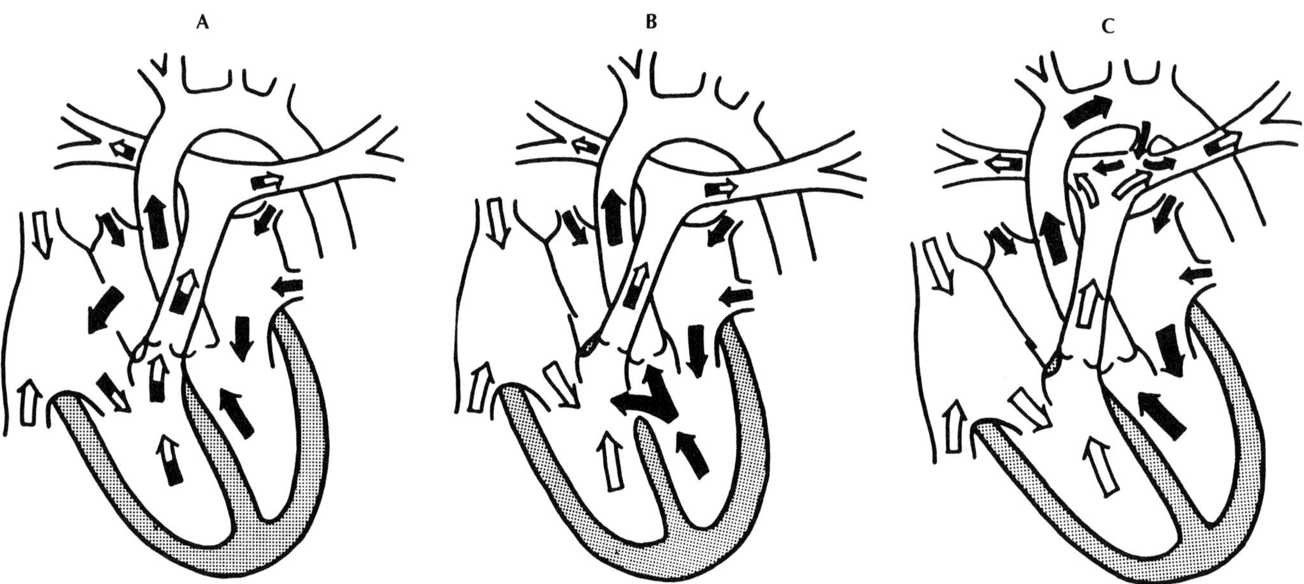

Fig. 192-3 Left-to-right shunt. **A,** Atrial septal defect. **B,** Ventricular septal defect. **C,** Patent ductus arteriosus. Closed arrows indicate saturated blood; open arrows indicate desaturated blood. (See text for details.)
From Clark EB: Heart disease. In CL Paxson, Jr., editor: Van Leeuwan's newborn medicine, ed 2, St Louis, 1979, The CV Mosby Co.

trocardiogram shows a characteristic counterclockwise superior axis in the frontal plane and ventricular hypertrophy. The chest roentgenogram shows cardiomegaly and increased pulmonary blood flow. Echocardiography defines defects in the atrial and ventricular septa and the abnormal position of the atrioventricular valves. Initial management is directed toward control of congestive heart failure. Most children require surgical repair to protect the pulmonary vascular bed from high blood pressure–flow damage. Children with Down syndrome are at particular risk for irreversible pulmonary vascular obstructive disease as early as 6 months of age and thus require early surgical repair.

Obstructive Cardiac Defects

Obstructive cardiac defects are characterized by outflow tract obstruction.

Pulmonary Stenosis (Fig. 192-4)

The pulmonary outflow tract can be obstructed at the infundibulum, the pulmonary valve, the supravalvular area, and the peripheral levels. Pulmonary valve stenosis is the most frequent obstruction. Presentation of pulmonary valve stenosis depends on the severity of the outflow tract obstruction. Mild pulmonary valve stenosis is often found as an incidental condition of little or no clinical significance. Critical valve stenosis can manifest in infancy with profound heart failure and right-to-left atrial level shunt. Clinical examination reveals a systolic ejection click followed by a systolic ejection murmur heard best in the left second intercostal space. The electrocardiogram is normal in mild pulmonary valve stenosis and shows increasing right ventricular forces that parallel the increase in the right ventricular myocardial mass. The chest roentgenogram shows a prominent main pulmonary artery reflecting poststenotic dilation. Echocardiography defines the site of obstruction, and Doppler determination of blood velocity estimates the pressure gradient from the right ventricle to the pulmonary artery. The child with mild pulmonary valve stenosis requires no treatment. Moderate to severe pulmonary valve stenosis can be reduced by transvenous balloon valvuloplasty. Critical valve stenosis or a dysplastic pulmonary valve may require surgical repair.

Aortic Stenosis (Fig. 192-5)

The aortic outflow tract can be obstructed at the left ventricular outflow tract, the subvalve area, and the supravalve region, but the most frequent cause is valve stenosis. The presentation of aortic valve stenosis varies from a benign click and murmur heard on auscultation to profound heart failure associated with critical obstruction of the aortic outflow tract. On physical examination there is a systolic ejection click followed by a systolic ejection murmur heard maximally in the right second intercostal space. The electrocardiogram shows left-axis deviation and left ventricular hypertrophy; the chest roentgenogram may show mild dilation of the ascending aorta. Echocardiography defines the stenotic aortic valve and an increase in ventricular wall mass. The Doppler measure of blood velocity estimates the pressure gradient across the stenotic valve. Long-term management is more complex for aortic valve stenosis. A nonobstructive bicuspid aortic valve can progress to severe stenosis. Thus all children must be followed into adulthood to monitor progression of the disease. Relief of the pressure gradient is achieved by balloon valvuloplasty in some patients, but surgical valvulotomy or valve replacement is often necessary.

Coarctation of the Aorta (Fig. 192-6)

Children with coarctation of the aorta have variable presentations. Neonates can have cardiovascular collapse, whereas older children may have absent femoral pulses as the only sign of disease. The cardiac examination typically reveals a

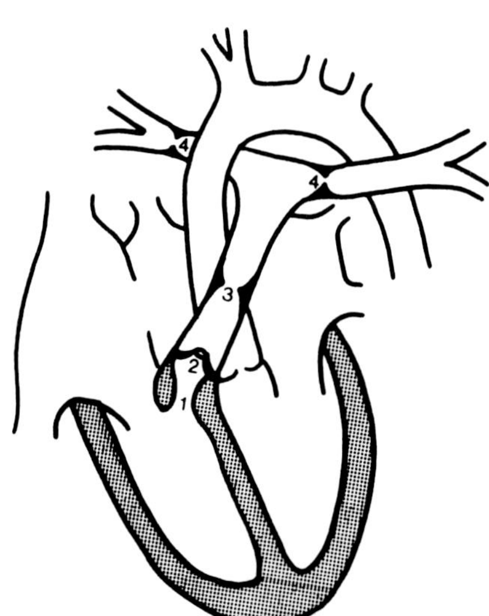

Fig. 192-4 Sites of obstruction to blood flow in right ventricular outflow tract. *1,* Infundibulum; *2,* pulmonary valve; *3,* supravalvular; *4,* peripheral. (See text for details.)

From Clark EB: Heart disease. In CL Paxson, Jr., editor: Van Leeuwan's newborn medicine, ed 2, St Louis, 1979, The CV Mosby Co.

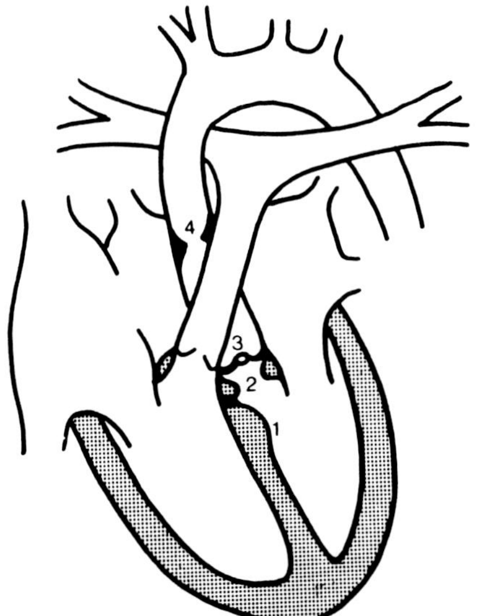

Fig. 192-5 Sites of obstruction to blood flow in left ventricular outflow tract. *1,* Ventricular septum; *2,* subaortic valve membrane; *3,* aortic valve; *4,* supravalvular. (See text for details.)

From Clark EB: Heart disease. In CL Paxson, Jr., editor: Van Leeuwan's newborn medicine, ed 2, St Louis, 1979, The CV Mosby Co.

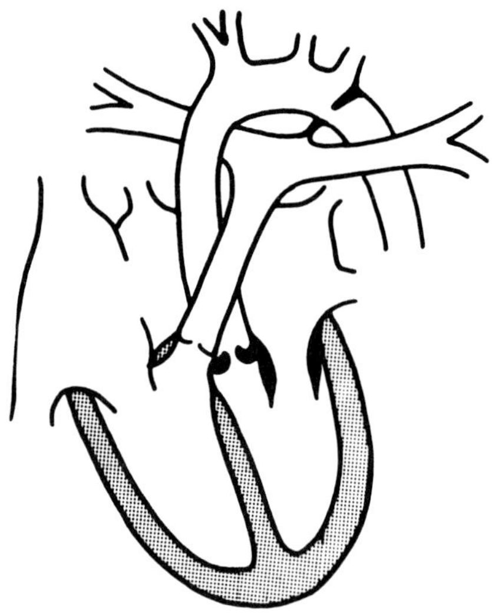

Fig. 192-6 Coarctation of the aorta and associated abnormalities of the mitral and aortic valves. (See text for details.)

From Clark EB: Heart disease. In CL Paxson, Jr., editor: Van Leeuwan's newborn medicine, ed 2, St Louis, 1979, The CV Mosby Co.

systolic ejection murmur that arises from a bicuspid aortic valve and murmurs from the enlarged collateral blood vessels that bypass the site of coarctation. The femoral pulses are decreased or absent, and blood pressure in the legs is less than in the arms. The electrocardiogram shows right ventricular hypertrophy, reflecting the increased work of the right ventricle during fetal life. The chest roentgenogram is usually normal, but older children may have an aortic indentation at the coarctation site and rib erosion caused by collateral intercostal blood vessels. Echocardiography defines aortic valve abnormalities and aortic arch dimensions, and Doppler velocity estimates the pressure gradient across the coarctation site. Neonates with critical coarctation and heart failure can be managed by prostaglandin infusion to reopen the ductus arteriosus, thereby reducing the obstruction. The timing for surgical repair depends on the severity of symptoms and the level of the systemic blood pressure. Elective repair should be accomplished before 5 years of age to reduce the long-term complications of systemic hypertension.

MYOCARDIAL DISEASE

Cardiomyopathy is a primary congenital abnormality of the ventricular muscle that occurs sporadically or as a familial pattern. Cardiomyopathies are classified as either hypertrophic or dilated; each requires thorough evaluation.

Hypertrophic cardiomyopathy usually manifests in children who are asymptomatic and identified either because of a family history of the disease or the discovery of a cardiac murmur. In some adolescents, hypertrophic cardiomyopathy may only be recognized after sudden death. Physical examination is often unremarkable. However, with severe forms of cardiomyopathy, there is outflow tract obstruction that produces a long systolic ejection murmur. The electrocardiogram often shows bizarre ventricular voltages and an abnormal axis. The chest roentgenogram is usually normal. Echocardiography defines a marked ventricular myocardial thickening and obstruction of the left ventricular outflow tract during late systole. There is no definitive treatment. Some patients are treated with beta blocker or calcium channel blocking agents in an attempt to reduce the obstruction. The prognosis varies. Sudden death can occur and is likely related to primary arrhythmias.

Children with cardiomyopathy can manifest in severe congestive heart failure with a dilated and poorly contractile ventricle. The etiology is often undefined, although viral illness sequela or an undefined metabolic abnormality is often suspected. Physical examination findings include congestive heart failure with a prominent gallop rhythm and hepatosplenomegaly. The ECG is often normal or shows diffuse low-voltage and nonspecific T wave changes. The chest roentgenogram shows cardiomegaly. Echocardiography defines a dilated, poorly contractile ventricle. Management is directed toward pharmacologic support of the failing myocardium with inotropic agents, diuretics, and afterload reduction (see Appendix A, "Pediatric Basic and Advanced Life Support"). The prognosis is uncertain, and some patients are eventually considered for heart transplantation.

SUMMARY

The primary care physician is responsible for recognizing the wide spectrum of congenital heart defects. Along with the pediatric heart team, the primary care physician focuses on supporting the child and family and being an advocate for the child in the community.

SUGGESTED READINGS

Adams FH, Emmanouilides GC, and Riemenschneider TA, editors: Moss' heart disease in infants, children, and adolescents, Baltimore, 1989, Williams & Wilkins.

Moller JH and Neal WA: Fetal, neonatal and infant cardiac disease, Norwalk, Conn, 1990, Appleton & Lang.

Pierpont ME and Moller JH: Genetics of cardiovascular disease, Boston, 1987, Nijhoff.

193

Contact Dermatitis

Nancy K. Barnett

When considering the diagnosis of contact dermatitis, the medical provider should distinguish between *contact irritant dermatitis* and *contact allergic dermatitis*. Contact irritant dermatitis is a nonallergic reaction of the skin to direct contact by an irritant. Contact allergic dermatitis is a delayed hypersensitivity phenomenon that requires immunologic sensitization to a contact allergen to become manifest.[3]

Contact irritant dermatitis in childhood is most common in infancy when the skin is thinner. Contact allergic dermatitis is eight times more common in allergic adults than in children, possibly because a mature immune system as well as prolonged exposure to contact allergens is required for it to occur. Contact allergic dermatitis is rare in infancy, less rare in childhood, and approaches adult incidence figures by age 8 years.[2]

The diagnosis of contact dermatitis should be entertained when an eruption (1) is limited to exposed contact surfaces, (2) shows sharp delimitation (i.e., at contactant borders and in linear arrays), or (3) reveals bizarre asymmetric distributions. A good history should provide clues to the offending allergen; if not, a well-kept diary may be helpful.

CONTACT IRRITANT DERMATITIS

There are a variety of common childhood irritants, including soaps, perfumed baby lotions and oils, feces, saliva, food, and detergents. The eruptions vary in severity according to the duration of contact, the strength of the irritant, and the age of the patient. Confluent papular erythema confined to the pattern of contact is the usual manifestation. This will respond readily to the regular (four times a day) application of a topical steroid cream of medium strength over 5 to 7 days. Low-potency steroids should be used on the face whenever possible. In the case of a particularly noxious or potent irritant, an acute dermatitis with erythematous vesiculation, weeping, and crusting may occur. Applying compresses (tepid water, saline, or Burow solution) to the weeping areas for 5 minutes (four times daily) before applying the steroid will help dry the involved areas and remove serous debris. If secondary impetiginization has occurred, then appropriate antibiotic therapy based on Gram stain and culture results should be instituted.

Diaper Dermatitis

Diaper dermatitis is the most frequent contact irritant dermatitis in infancy (see Chapter 198, "Diaper Rash"). The usual irritant is urine or feces that has been in contact with the skin too long as a result of infrequent diaper changes or plastic pants occlusion. Occasionally, detergents used to wash cloth diapers or synthetic components of paper diapers or wipes are direct skin irritants. The dermatitis is usually a confluent papular erythema confined to the areas of contact, with sparing of the inguinal folds. However, contact irritants in oils or lotions applied to the diaper area will usually involve the skin folds. If the irritation is severe, the skin may macerate and erode, leading to oozing and crusting.

In diaper dermatitis the most important aspect of treatment is to dry the involved area (with aeration and powder) while preventing further contact with the irritant. Also helpful at times is the use of a low-potency antiinflammatory steroid cream three times a day, alternating its application with that of an anticandidal cream such as nystatin or clotrimazole two times a day. If the dermatitis persists for more than 3 days (the area usually becomes colonized with *Candida albicans*), the patient probably has a candidal superinfection, which can be recognized as a beefy red dermatitis with frequent satellite papules and pustules; a potassium hydroxide (KOH) preparation of skin scrapings may be positive for pseudohyphae or budding yeast.[4]

Other Irritants

In older children soaps and detergents are frequent irritants. The dermatitis is often limited to those areas of tight contact with clothing (e.g., wrists, axillae, waistbands), where detergent often accumulates. Soaps may be general irritants and cause the most severe eruptions on the face and hands. Bubble bath solution is often a cause of perivaginal dermatitis and vaginitis in young females. Woolens and formaldehyde resins (flame retardants) in clothing can also cause severe irritant dermatitis. In soap or detergent dermatitis, use of the suspected inciting agent should be discontinued. All new clothes should be washed and rinsed twice before initial wearing.

CONTACT ALLERGIC DERMATITIS

In contact allergic dermatitis, it is postulated that the contact allergen penetrates the epidermis as a hapten, which binds to a carrier protein and thus travels via the lymph system to the lymph node where antigen processing occurs in macrophages. T lymphocytes with specific antigen recognition properties presumably proliferate and return in the bloodstream to the skin, where they are available for rapid (6 to 18 hours) antigen recognition and reaction on subsequent contact rechallenges. The time required for sensitization varies with the strength of the allergen—it takes weeks or months in the case of weak allergens and less than a week for strong ones.

The T lymphocytes, on recognition of and reaction to the contact allergen, are assumed to release inflammatory mediators, which cause an acute erythematous papulovesicular eruption confined to the areas of allergen contact. The treatment is the same as that outlined above for acute contact irritant dermatitis. For intense pruritus, liberal use of antihistamines, cool compresses, cool baths, and soothing lotions (e.g., calamine) may be indicated. If the area of involvement is extensive or generalized, a course of oral prednisone may be warranted in otherwise healthy children, beginning with 1 mg/kg/day (maximum 30 to 40 mg) and tapering the dose over 2 to 3 weeks to avoid a rebound resurgence of the dermatitis when the drug is discontinued.

Rhus Dermatitis

The most frequent contact allergic dermatitis seen in children is rhus dermatitis, caused by poison ivy, oak, and sumac. The contact allergen is pentadecylcatechol, an ingredient of the oleoresin, urushiol. The characteristic pruritic, vesicular, red eruption conforming to the typical contact distribution (i.e., on exposed surfaces and in linear patterns where leaves and branches touch the skin) is not always present. The oleoresin can persist on animal fur, clothing, or furniture for months as long as it is not destroyed by heat and can continue to be a contactant, sometimes at unusual sites. Additionally, the burning of rhus leaves can create an airborne contact dermatitis that may be confluent and extensive over exposed sites. Ragweed pollen dermatitis, another airborne contact dermatitis, may be confused with rhus dermatitis in the fall months.

To manage this type of dermatitis effectively, the patient and the family must be educated about the appearance of the *Rhus* plants and how the oleoresin is spread. Specifically, they should be told to wash all garments (including shoes, packs, and purses) and themselves after possible exposure to the oleoresin so as to decrease potential ongoing contact. The transfer of vesicle fluid during scratching does *not* cause the dermatitis to spread.

Other Common Allergens

Nickel sensitivity, a frequent cause of contact dermatitis, is usually seen following ear piercing when nickel studs are placed in the newly formed earring holes. Adolescents and children may also suffer dermatitis from allergens such as parabens, lanolin, and paraphenylenediamine contained in nail polish, hair dyes, perfumes, deodorants, sunscreens, and other cosmetics. Neomycin and ethylenediamine, present in certain topical preparations, also may cause contact allergic dermatitis.

SHOE CONTACT DERMATITIS

Shoe contact dermatitis may be either of the irritant or allergic type. The diagnosis is usually suggested by the presence of a bilateral, symmetric dermatitis involving the dorsum of the toes and feet, with relative sparing of the web spaces. The dermatitis may range in appearance from a chronic eczema with mild confluent erythema and postinflammatory hyperpigmentation of lichenified plaques to an acute papulovesicular eruption with oozing and crusting. Various shoe compounds are irritants or sensitizers; the most common is rubber, but also implicated are dyes and adhesives.

Patients with shoe contact dermatitis should wear loose-fitting, open shoes and go barefoot whenever possible. Plantar hyperhidrosis (see Chapter 144, "Hyperhidrosis") frequently accompanies shoe contact dermatitis and should be managed with frequent changes of socks and the application of absorbent powder and aluminum chloride (Drysol). Acute dermatitis will respond to topical steroids, antipruritic agents, and compresses (see above), but the inciting irritant or sensitizer must be avoided to prevent recurrences.

To determine if the patient is allergic to a shoe component, he or she should be referred to a center where patch testing is routinely performed. Patch testing can be done with a standard shoe patch test tray or parts of the suspected offending shoes. If a shoe allergy is identified, nonallergenic footwear should be recommended.

PATCH TESTING

Patch testing, the process by which dilute quantities of suspected allergens are applied to the skin, should be performed by trained personnel. It can be used to identify many contact allergens, but its results are only significant if there has been exposure to the allergen in question or to a similar compound and if exposure to the identified allergen causes a dermatitis. Care must be taken not to perform the testing when active dermatitis is present. Patch test results are of questionable value in young children. Reliable plant allergens for patch testing are not routinely available.[1]

REFERENCES

1. Adams RM: Patch testing—a recapitulation, J Am Acad Dermatol 5:629, 1981.
2. Fisher AA: Contact dermatitis in childhood. In Contact dermatitis, ed 3, New York, 1986, Lea & Febiger.
3. Hurwitz S: Clinical pediatric dermatology, Philadelphia, 1981, WB Saunders Co.
4. Weston WL: Practical pediatric dermatology, ed 2, Boston, 1985, Little Brown & Co.

194

Contagious Exanthematous Diseases

John H. Dossett

The literal translation of *exanthem* is *to bloom or break out.* Thus those parents speak quite accurately who say that "my child 'broke out' in a rash." Exanthem refers to an eruption or rash that usually is associated with fever and generally implies that the eruption is infectious in origin. These eruptions are extremely common in children and present the clinician with a major challenge in differential diagnosis, inasmuch as many illnesses manifest by rashes that can look very similar. Consequently, the clinical manifestations other than the rash itself often must be explored to distinguish one disease from another. These would include the incubation period, prodromal signs, the age of the patient, immunization history, contact history, distribution and progression of the rash, evidence of other organ involvement, and pathognomonic signs, such as enanthem, peeling, or Koplik spots.

Confusion is further compounded by the knowledge that these rashes may be caused by viruses, bacteria, rickettsia, mycoplasma, and fungi. Moreover, certain allergic and immune complex diseases such as childhood arthritis can mimic the infectious exanthems.

It is not sufficient to conclude that the child with moderate fever and rash has a "viral exanthem" and forget about it. For example, if rubella or erythema infectiosum (human parvovirus) is included in the differential diagnoses, one needs to investigate recent and potential exposures of the sick child to pregnant women, in that fetal infection with these viruses may be devastating. Diseases that might respond to specific therapy require special consideration. These include the exanthem of *Mycoplasma pneumoniae* infection, which will respond to erythromycin, or the exanthem of *Rickettsia rickettsii* (Rocky Mountain spotted fever), which most desperately needs early treatment with tetracycline or chloramphenicol. The rash of streptococcal or staphylococcal scarlet fever (scarlatina) needs specific identification so that it can be appropriately treated, and scarlatina must be differentiated from Kawasaki disease so that the latter receives careful monitoring and specific treatment. Some of the differentiating characteristics of these eruptions are found in Table 194-1 and in Tables 160-1 and 160-2 (see also Chapter 189 for a discussion of chickenpox).

ENTEROVIRAL EXANTHEMS

Inasmuch as rubeola (measles) and rubella have largely been controlled by the administration of effective vaccines, enteroviral infections are now the most common cause of exanthems in children. Many serotypes of echoviruses and coxsackieviruses are associated with rashes; often these are generalized maculopapular rashes with discrete lesions much like those of rubella. They may appear very much like roseola, with an initial 2 to 3 days of fever followed by the eruption. Generally, though, the prodromal fever is much lower than that of roseola.

Although maculopapular rashes predominate, vesicular lesions have been observed in coxsackievirus A5, A9, and A16 infections. Hand-foot-mouth disease is commonly seen with coxsackievirus A16 infection and is manifested by vesicles on the palms and soles and ulcers in the mouth.

Enteroviral exanthems typically occur in the late summer and early fall and are associated with epidemics of aseptic meningitis. These infections are presented in more detail in Chapter 227.

EXANTHEM SUBITUM (ROSEOLA)

On the basis of its clinical course and epidemiology, roseola has long been presumed to be an infectious illness. In 1988 a newly discovered virus called human herpesvirus–6 (HHV-6) was shown to be the infectious agent.[2] Moreover, this virus has been isolated from infants with roseola without a rash—a condition experienced pediatricians have long suspected.[1] Roseola is characterized by 3 or 4 days of high fever (104° to 105° F [40° to 40.6 C]), followed by abrupt resolution ("lysis") of the fever and the eruption of a pink maculopapular rash that begins on the neck and then spreads to the trunk and extremities, usually sparing the face. The lesions are discrete and last only for 1 or 2 days.

The child usually has no other manifestation of illness and does not appear as ill ("toxic") as the severity of the fever might imply.

Roseola occurs year-round and is strikingly limited to children between the ages of 6 months and 3 years.

Complications are limited to febrile seizures, which may be precipitated by the rapid rise in body temperature. Most children who have seizures associated with roseola show normal findings on spinal tap and have an excellent prognosis.

There is no specific treatment for roseola, but affected children can be made more comfortable by controlling their fever. (See Chapter 251 for a more complete discussion of this disease.)

Table 194-1 *Differentiating Common Childhood Exanthems*

DISEASE	CHARACTER OF RASH	PRODROME	PATHOGNOMONIC SIGNS	HELPFUL SIGNS
Enterovirus infection	Maculopapular, generalized to most of body, discrete	May have 3-4 days of mild fever before rash, or rash may appear with constitutional signs	Herpangina, hand-foot-mouth syndrome	Aseptic meningitis, pharyngitis, petechiae with some coxsackievirus strains; occurs in summer and early fall
Exanthem subitum (roseola)	Maculopapular and discrete; begins on the trunk and spreads to face and limbs	3-4 days of high fever and irritability with no other signs	None	Dramatic drop in fever simultaneous with onset of rash
Erythema infectiosum (fifth disease)	Red and flushed cheeks with circumoral pallor; maculopapular rash on extremities (lacelike)	None	Slapped-cheek appearance in an otherwise healthy child	Possible recurrence of eruption with irritation of skin by heat, cold, or pressure
Rubella (German measles)	Pink, maculopapular, discrete; begins on face and spreads to trunk and extremities	Commonly none; adolescents may have 1-3 days of low-grade fever and malaise	None	Tender postauricular and suboccipital lymph nodes; possibly arthralgia in adolescents
Mumps	Maculopapular, discrete, concentrated on trunk; may have urticaria	1-2 days of fever, headache, and malaise	None	Diffuse swelling of parotid glands, with pain and tenderness; aseptic meningitis; orchitis or pancreatitis; erythema of the Stensen duct
Infectious mononucleosis	Macular or maculopapular and discrete; when associated with ampicillin administration, it is confluent (morbilliform) and more intense	2-4 days of fever, pharyngitis, malaise	None	Exudative pharyngitis, lymphadenopathy, splenomegaly, atypical lymphocytes on peripheral smear
Mycoplasma pneumonia	Maculopapular on trunk and extremities in 10% of cases; common spectrum of urticaria, erythema multiforme, and vesicular/bullous lesions	3-5 days of progressive fever, headache, malaise, and cough	None	Pneumonia, cold agglutinins
Rubeola (measles)	Red to brown macular rash that spreads from face and neck to trunk and extremities; confluent (morbilliform), particularly on face; fades after 6-7 days with temporary staining of skin	3-4 days of high fever, conjunctivitis, cough, and coryza	Koplik spots	Always an associated conjunctivitis and cough
Atypical measles	Rash may be maculopapular, purpuric, petechial, or vesicular; prominent at wrists and ankles	2-3 days of fever, headache, and cough	None	History of killed measles vaccine, myalgia, pneumonia

ERYTHEMA INFECTIOSUM (FIFTH DISEASE)

As the name implies, erythema infectiosum is a contagious disease, as manifested by its epidemic occurrence. The infectious agent was identified in 1984 as human parvovirus (HPV). Susceptible persons are infected by droplets via the respiratory tract; in epidemics the attack rate is high.

The diagnosis depends exclusively on the clinical presentation, which is one of rash *without* fever or other systemic signs. The rash first erupts as a bright red erythema of the cheeks and forehead with circumoral pallor. This "slapped cheek" appearance is the result of many large maculopapular lesions that coalesce to form a confluent red rash. These confluent lesions are hot to the touch and commonly palpable, but they are nontender.

After a single day a maculopapular rash next appears on

Table 194-1 *Differentiating Common Childhood Exanthems—cont'd*

DISEASE	CHARACTER OF RASH	PRODROME	PATHOGNOMONIC SIGNS	HELPFUL SIGNS
Scarlet fever	Erythematous papular eruption sometimes associated with generalized erythema; concentrated on trunk and proximal extremities; feels like fine sandpaper	Occurs within 1-4 days of onset of focal infection	None	Focal infections such as pharyngitis, vaginitis, cellulitis, erythema of palms and soles; strawberry tongue; desquamation in recovery phase
Kawasaki disease	Rash ranges from maculopapular to scarlatina form to urticaria; marked erythema of palms and soles	1-3 days of fever and irritability	None	Conjunctivitis, tender lymphadenopathy, strawberry tongue, meatitis, diarrhea, meningitis, prolonged fever, late desquamation, arthritis in recovery phase

the proximal extremities. This then gradually spreads to the trunk and distal extremities, leaving a lacelike appearance as it clears. This stage lasts 2 to 4 days. In a third stage, the rash may transiently reappear when the skin is traumatized by pressure, sunlight, or extremes of hot and cold.

RUBELLA

Our grandmothers knew rubella as "German measles" or "3-day measles." These names served to distinguish the disease from rubeola ("hard measles" or "10-day measles"). The virus was first cultivated in 1962; its clinical spectrum was thoroughly documented in the 1965 epidemic.

The typical clinical illness is mild and brief. In most children the rash is itself the first sign of infection. It is typically a pink, maculopapular eruption beginning on the face and spreading downward to the trunk and extremities. The lesions remain discrete and pink, the appearance of which contrasts with the raised, confluent, and deep red lesions of rubeola. The facial rash clears as the extremity rash erupts, and all are cleared by the third to the fifth day.

Fever is very mild, ranging between 99° and 101° F (37.2° and 38.3° C). Lymphadenopathy frequently is impressive, the nodes most commonly involved being those in the posterior auricular and suboccipital chains. They usually are tender at the onset of rash, but the tenderness resolves rapidly over 2 to 3 days. Although lymphadenopathy is an important sign of rubella infection, it is not pathognomonic, in that other viral infections also may commonly cause enlargement of these same nodes. Some children with rubella have tiny reddish spots on the soft palate. These lesions, however, are themselves not distinguishable from those of scarlet fever or rubeola. The incubation period is 2 to 3 weeks with a peak at 16 to 18 days.

Of all the childhood exanthems it is most important to pursue objective confirmation of suspected rubella, in that the risk of spread to susceptible pregnant women has potential for such devastating consequences.

The rubella virus usually can be grown from the pharynx within 5 days of the onset of the rash. Serologic diagnosis is made by demonstrating an antibody titer rise between acute and convalescent sera. Hemagglutination-inhibition (HI) antibody titers are readily available, and a fourfold rise after 2 weeks indicates recent infection.

Complications of rubella are rare in children, but among adolescents and young adults, a transient arthritis develops in approximately 15%. The arthritis rarely becomes chronic.

The major serious complications of rubella virus result from fetal infection. If a pregnant woman is infected in the first trimester of gestation, there is a very high probability that the fetus will become infected, with involvement of virtually every organ in the body.

INFECTIOUS MONONUCLEOSIS

The exanthem of Epstein-Barr virus (EBV) mononucleosis occurs in approximately 15% of children with infectious mononucleosis who are not treated with ampicillin. The rash is pink to red and macular or maculopapular. The lesions are discrete and have no specific distinguishing characteristic, so that the diagnosis most often is made on the basis of other signs of infectious mononucleosis and confirmed by the peripheral blood smear and serologic tests.

The *administration of ampicillin* to persons with infectious mononucleosis results in approximately 50% of them developing a much more intense rash. This ampicillin-associated rash is deep red and confluent, giving it a morbilliform appearance. This iatrogenic exanthem resolves spontaneously within a week, but its significance extends beyond its mere presence. First, such patients commonly are identified as "allergic to penicillin." Second, administration of ampicillin to a person with infectious mononucleosis indicates that an incorrect diagnosis of antibiotic-treatable disease was made. This happens most often when rash and exudative pharyngitis are observed, a careful examination for generalized lymphadenopathy and splenomegaly is neglected, and a diagnosis of streptococcal or staphylococcal disease is concluded. The full spectrum of EBV infection is discussed in Chapter 218.

MEASLES (RUBEOLA)

Measles is clearly the most serious of the childhood exanthems because of the morbidity of the acute infection and its potential for producing permanent sequelae. The virus is highly contagious, and typical clinical disease begins after an incubation period of 10 to 11 days. The prodromal illness is manifested by increasing fever, cough, conjunctivitis, and coryza. By the fourth day the fever is commonly high (104° F [40° C]) and the rash erupts—typically a deep red macular rash that begins on the face and neck and spreads down the trunk and extremities. The lesions on the face and upper portion of the trunk soon become confluent to produce the characteristic morbilliform rash. By the sixth day the fever subsides and the rash begins to fade; as it fades, it leaves a faint brown stain in the skin and a fine desquamation ensues.

The *enanthem* of measles is pathognomonic. *Koplik spots* begin approximately 2 days before the rash erupts and increase in number until the first or second day of the exanthem. They are tiny bluish white spots on an erythematous base and cluster adjacent to the molars on the buccal mucosa.

The combination of Koplik spots, fever, cough, conjunctivitis, and morbilliform rash is sufficient to make a firm clinical diagnosis of measles. Although the children usually are very ill, they recover rapidly after the eighth or ninth day and most often are back to normal in a few days.

Measles virus induces inflammation throughout the respiratory tract, so that respiratory complications are common; these include otitis media, pneumonia, and croup. The otitis media is treated as any acute otitis media. The pneumonia may be either a primary measles pneumonia or a superimposed bacterial pneumonia. All children with measles need daily examination of the chest and observation for tachypnea. Development of clinical pneumonia is indication for a chest roentgenogram, white blood cell count, blood culture, sputum examination, and treatment with antibiotics because of the probability of bacterial infection.

Acute encephalitis is the major complication of measles infection. It occurs in approximately 1 per 1000 cases and commonly results in death or permanent neurologic sequelae. It manifests by headache, vomiting, drowsiness, personality changes, seizures, and coma. In most cases the cerebrospinal fluid reveals pleocytosis and elevated protein levels. Some of these children have only a mild disease and recover in a few days, but others may have a fulminant course.

Prevention of measles is discussed in Chapter 17.

Atypical Measles

In recent years some children who had been immunized with inactivated measles vaccine have had an atypical presentation of wild measles virus infection. Typically such children have had 2 to 3 days of fever and headache, followed by a rash erupting on the wrists and ankles. The rashes have varied from maculopapular to purpuric to petechial or vesicular. There has been marked myalgia, with swelling of the hands and feet. Pneumonia is common.

The constitutional symptoms and the distribution of the rash may easily be confused with Rocky Mountain spotted fever. Elicitation of a history of having received killed measles vaccine is obviously critical to the diagnosis.

MYCOPLASMA PNEUMONIA

Although cutaneous signs are not major manifestations of mycoplasmal infections, they occur with sufficient frequency to justify attention. A maculopapular eruption may appear on the trunk and extremities of 10% to 15% of persons infected with *Mycoplasma pneumoniae*. It is even more common for these infections to be associated with allergic-type eruptions that display a spectrum of cutaneous lesions ranging from urticaria and erythema multiforme to vesicles or bullae. Such patients frequently have had a prodromal illness of fever, headache, malaise, and cough. The pneumonia may escape physical diagnosis, only to crop up on the chest roentgenogram as an "incidental," accidental finding. Such a combination of symptoms is indication for treatment with erythromycin, whether or not one has access to laboratory confirmation.

MUMPS

An exanthem will develop in fewer than 10% of persons infected with mumps virus, but when a rash does occur, the lesions are maculopapular, pale pink, discrete, and concentrated on the trunk. The virus more typically involves the salivary glands, the testicles (after puberty), the pancreas, and the meninges. After an incubation period of 16 to 18 days, clinical mumps develops in approximately 60% of infected persons. The remaining 40% have inapparent infections, without salivary gland swelling.

The typical illness begins with 1 or 2 days of anorexia, headache, and mild to moderate fever. This is followed by complaints of discomfort when chewing and pain around the ear. There usually is a diffuse but noticeable enlargement and tenderness of the parotid gland, which can be distinguished from lymph node enlargement in that it extends anterior to the ear and below the ramus of the mandible posteriorly to the mastoid bone, usually obliterating the angle of the jaw. Lymph nodes are more discrete and generally submandibular in location. Accompanying the parotitis one commonly sees erythema around the opening of the Stensen duct. The fever usually lasts 2 to 5 days. Rarely, only one parotid gland is involved, or the submandibular salivary glands rather than the parotids will be swollen.

Meningoencephalitis is estimated to occur in 10% of all cases of mumps and is characterized by headache, nausea, vomiting, and mild nuchal rigidity. It may occur before, during, or after the parotitis phase of the disease. It follows a course similar to the aseptic meningitis that is caused by other viruses, and it usually has no sequelae. Some cerebrospinal fluid pleocytosis is present in most cases of mumps without clinical evidence of meningeal irritation.

Orchitis is uncommon in children, but unilateral involvement of the testes and epididymis is observed in approximately 25% of males who are infected with mumps virus *after* puberty. Patients with orchitis usually are quite ill; however, the incidence of sterility in males who experience mumps orchitis is no greater than in those who do not.

The pancreas and other exocrine glands rarely are involved.

Late neurologic complications include nerve deafness and a very rare postinfectious encephalitis.

SCARLET FEVER

The rash of scarlet fever (scarlatina) is caused by a circulating erythrotoxin that is produced by certain strains of streptococci and staphylococci. This rash is characterized by a fine papular eruption on an erythematous base. Often there is a generalized erythema of the skin, including even those areas that are not yet involved with the papular rash. The eruption of scarlet fever is concentrated on the trunk and proximal extremities. It feels rough to the touch like fine sandpaper. The rash commonly is associated with prominent erythema of the lips, soles, and palms. Transverse red streaks (Pastia lines) sometimes are present, usually in the antecubital spaces. Desquamation of involved skin typically occurs in the recovery phase. On the tongue one can observe prominent papillae on a very red base, giving a "strawberry tongue" appearance.

If streptococci are the source of the erythrogenic toxin, then the pharynx is the usual site of focal infection. Other focal infections, however, such as vaginitis or cellulitis, also may be found. When staphylococci are the source of erythrogenic toxin, the infective focus usually is some site other than the pharynx; infected surgical or traumatic wounds have been common sites. The toxic shock syndrome (associated with staphylococcal vaginitis from tampon use) has been a heavily publicized recent cause of scarlet fever rash.

The treatment of scarlet fever is directed toward eradication of the focal infection. Streptococcal infections are treated with penicillin or erythromycin, whereas staphylococcal infections are treated with erythromycin or dicloxacillin. If systemic illness is severe, the patient should be hospitalized to receive parenteral antibiotics and general supportive care.

The eruption that needs most carefully to be differentiated from scarlet fever is *Kawasaki disease*. Its cutaneous manifestations overlap remarkably with those of scarlet fever, but it usually can be distinguished by the additional signs of conjunctivitis, cracking of the lips, very tender lymphadenopathy, meatitis, and diarrhea. These children are profoundly irritable, and their fever persists for more than a week in most cases. Just as in scarlet fever, however, they have erythema of the palms and soles with striking desquamation during the second and third weeks of the disease. Kawasaki disease is presented in more detail in Chapter 222.

REFERENCES

1. Suga S et al: Human herpesvirus–6 infection (exanthem subitum) without rash, Pediatrics 83:1003, 1989.
2. Yamaniski K et al: Identification of human herpesvirus–6 as a causal agent for exanthem subitum, Lancet 1:1065, 1988.

SUGGESTED READING

Feigin RD and Cherry JD: Viral infections. In Feigin RD and Cherry JD, editors: Textbook of pediatric infectious diseases, ed 2, vol 2, Philadelphia, 1987, WB Saunders Co.

195

Cystic Fibrosis

Robert H. Schwartz

Cystic fibrosis (CF) is the most common lethal genetic disease among white children, adolescents, and young adults; it is a generalized disease with numerous secondary complicating features that affect practically every organ system of the body. Its transmission follows an autosomal recessive mode of inheritance, and it occurs once in every 1600 to 2500 live births. Although the incidence in nonwhites is low, it does occur in blacks (1 in 17,000), Orientals, and American Indians; its occurrence in any race is possible. It is estimated that 5% of the white population are carriers (heterozygotes). The genetic pool is diminished by CF male sterility, decreased CF female fertility, and the generally lethal nature of CF before the reproductive years. Genetic laws suggest but do not mandate a heterozygote advantage, which might maintain the high gene frequency. None has yet been detected.[28]

Great strides have been made in understanding the etiology, pathophysiology, and genetics of cystic fibrosis since its original description by Anderson in 1938.[1] Once invariably fatal in the first years of life, a potential cure is now on the horizon for those who live today with an estimated median life expectancy of approximately 20 to 25 years.

ETIOLOGY

The most common CF mutation was identified in 1989.[17,35,37] After extensive DNA linkage analyses in families and in extended kindred, evidence was found for the existence of a single CF locus on human chromosome 7 (region q31). DNA haplotype analyses suggested a small number of mutations in CF at this locus. Approximately 70% of CF chromosomes in affected white North American persons were found to contain a mutation corresponding to a deletion of three base pairs and resulting in the loss of a phenylalanine (F) residue at amino acid position 508 (ΔF508) of the predicted product of the CF gene. This product, the cystic fibrosis transmembrane conductance regulator (CFTR), either serves as an ion channel or regulates ion channel activities. Perturbation of its normal structure presumably results in abnormal transport of chloride ions across sweat duct epithelial cells and across mucosal surface epithelial cells. In the sweat gland there is abnormal reabsorption of chloride and sodium, accounting for the elevation of these ions in sweat, providing the genetic pathophysiologic basis for the diagnostic sweat test. At the respiratory, pancreatic, and hepatic organ levels, there is a block in chloride channel transport to the luminal surface of epithelial cells, resulting in a decrease in water transport to the mucus sol layer. A dehydrated thickened mucus impairs mucociliary clearance and contributes to obstruction of bronchioles, bronchi, pancreatic ducts, and bile canaliculi. In the respiratory tract, mucous viscosity is increased even more by large amounts of DNA from the neutrophilic response to infection and to a lesser extent by exopolysaccharides from infecting mucoid strains of *Pseudomonas aeruginosa*.

Current experimental therapeutic strategies, based on an understanding of the etiology and pathogenesis of CF, consist of (1) gene therapy, including gene transplantation and gene product replacement, (2) pharmacologic correction of the CFTR, and (3) dissolution of the DNA by-product of inflammation.

By the end of 1990 more than 30 different mutations at the CF gene locus had been described, accounting for the different frequencies of the major F508-deletion among different racial and ethnic groups. The F508-deletion is found on 68% to 74% of CF chromosomes in affected North American persons, including French-Canadians, and in affected Scots in Europe.[22] Among the French-Canadians in Saguenay–Lac St. Jean, Quebec province, the frequency is 56%. In southern Europe there is more CF mutation heterogeneity.[12] The F508-deletion is found in 49% of CF chromosomes among Spaniards and in 43% of CF chromosomes of Italians. In the Hutterite brethren of North America there are only three CF mutations; only 35% of CF chromosomes carry the F508-deletion.[19] These differences have important implications for population screening to identify CF carriers. Less common mutations also may account for phenotypic variations such as milder disease in CF patients with pancreatic sufficiency, less severe CF in black persons, and other very mild forms of the disease.[18] Carrier screening of populations other than at-risk families will need to be undertaken with great caution. Most of the CF mutations first will require identification, and their relationship to CF severity will need to be understood. In addition, psychosocial and financial risks and benefits will have to be defined by pilot studies.[7,14]

PATHOPHYSIOLOGY

The pathophysiologic hallmarks of CF are (1) pancreatic enzyme deficiency, (2) progressive chronic obstructive, infectious (usually with *Staphylococcus* and eventually with *Pseudomonas* organisms), and destructive pulmonary disease, and (3) elevated sodium and chloride concentrations in sweat. The pancreatic disease and the pulmonary disease have been attributed to abnormally thick mucous secretions that completely or partially obstruct tubes such as the pancreatic ducts and the conductive airways. Elevated sweat electrolyte concentrations are now thought to be the result of abnormal reabsorption of chloride by sweat duct epithelial cells.[11,32] Other secretory electrolyte abnormalities such as elevated calcium concentrations in both salivary gland and tracheobronchial secretions also have been described, pointing to a possible pathophysiologic link between thick mucous secretions and abnormal electrolyte levels. This link, however, has not been established. Indeed, each may be the independent result of a more basic defect at the secretory and transport membrane surfaces of cells.

An aberration in the immune system, unrelated to the primary genetic defect, has been proposed to account for the inability of CF patients to clear the chronic pulmonary *Pseudomonas* infections that cause most of the morbidity and mortality in this disease.[3] Within the milieu of the *Pseudomonas*-infected and inflammed lung, neutrophil elastase is released into tissue and secretions. It cleaves anti-*Pseudomonas* IgG, rendering it opsonically ineffective. It cleaves antigen-bound IgG, interfering with the activation of phagocytic cells by immune complexes, and it degrades C3b receptors on polymorphonuclear neutrophils and other phagocytes, impairing their ability to kill opsonized *Pseudomonas aeruginosa*. Thus there is a rationale for the use of glucocorticosteroids to modulate the neutrophil inflammatory response and to decrease the local production of elastase. There also is a rationale for the use of intravenous gammaglobulin or *Pseudomonas* immunoglobulin to replace damaged autogenous antibodies.[52] Clinical trials with intravenous and aerosolized alpha-1-antitrypsin (an antielastase) also are in progress.

CLINICAL PRESENTATION

The potential external manifestations of internal disease in CF are numerous.[53] The child who tastes salty when kissed or who has white powdery salt crystals across the bridge of the nose, forehead, and hairline manifests the CF eccrine sweat abnormality. He or she may appear fair skinned and pale because of decreased subcutaneous fat, decreased carotenoid pigmentation of the skin, and subcutaneous blood vessels close to the surface of the skin. Besides chronic cough and sputum production, clubbing of the fingers and cyanosis become apparent and progress with increasing pulmonary disease. Short stature, protuberant abdomen, thin extremities, barrel chest, pectus carinatum, pulmonary osteoarthropathy, and kyphosis are other secondary external manifestations of internal chronic pulmonary infection and intestinal maldigestion. Palmar erythema and spider angiomas may accompany severe multinodular biliary cirrhosis. Purpura, ecchymoses, and bleeding may develop in young children with vitamin K deficiency caused by malabsorption. A deficiency of vitamin K–dependent coagulation factor II (prothrombin) activity also may result from liver disease. Vascular purpura (described as cutaneous necrotizing venulitis and erythema nodosum) may occur, presumably as a result of immune complex phenomena.[46] Transient episodic polyarticular or monoarticular arthritis, usually involving the large joints, also has been described in association with a nodular rash. Goiters have been observed in those CF patients receiving chronic expectorant therapy with iodides. Large goiters occur in those CF patients in whom the rare complication of secondary systemic amyloidosis develops.[36] Pitting edema is observed when right-sided heart failure occurs or in young untreated CF children with hypoproteinemia, edema, and anemia resulting from nutritional protein deficiency. Angular stomatitis may be seen secondary to vitamin B (riboflavin) deficiency. Other features and complications of CF are listed in the accompanying box. It is important to note, however, that the infant, child, and adult with CF may appear entirely normal and may exhibit none of these symptoms or complications.

Although CF affects predominantly pancreatic and pulmonary function, it often has been confused with upper and lower respiratory tract allergy or gastrointestinal allergy.* Chronic rhinitis is eventually a feature in practically all patients. Nasal polyposis occurs in 15% of all those with CF and is observed in even greater frequency in older patients.[16,30,31,39] Chronic ethmoidal and maxillary sinusitis is a constant feature. Chronic cough (occurring eventually in all patients), wheezing and hyperirritability of the airways (occurring in 25% of the patients),[20,25] atelectasis, and allergic bronchopulmonary aspergillosis are associated with CF but also are seen in respiratory allergic disorders.†

The first respiratory symptom of CF is cough, and the first sign of pulmonary involvement is chest hyperexpansion or increased radiolucency of the lung fields on chest roentgenogram. These are due to the earliest lesion of CF, which occurs as bronchiolar obstruction with mucus, predisposing the lung to infection, inflammation, and hyperplasia of goblet cells, progressing with time to the larger airways and destruction of airway walls. Mucociliary clearance becomes impaired. Progressive involvement begins with bronchiolitis and is followed by bronchitis, bronchiectasis, peribronchial pneumonia, peribronchial fibrosis, and large cystic bronchial dilation that eventually involves all subsegmental bronchi. Alveolar destruction ensues, with infection of atelectatic areas or with episodes of patchy pneumonia and hemorrhagic pneumonia. There is progressive loss of pulmonary function, with possible complications from massive hemoptysis, recurrent pneumothorax, hypoxemia, pulmonary hypertension, and cor pulmonale, all of which are poor prognostic signs. The presence of mucoid strains of *Pseudomonas aeruginosa* seems to separate the more severe cases from the milder ones. Although they occur in elderly adult non-CF patients with bronchiectasis, the presence of these pathogens in the lower respiratory tracts of children is almost unique to CF.[44,45,47]

Pancreatic function may be completely ablated, partially active, or normal. Some compromise of exocrine function usually exists. Compared with their counterparts with severe maldigestion (steatorrhea and azotorrhea), patients with near-normal pancreatic function (normal fat absorption without oral pancreatic enzyme replacement) have milder symptoms, lower mean chloride concentration values in sweat, and less lung involvement with better pulmonary function, emphasizing the relation between good nutrition and resistance to infection.[13] From this observation, some investigators infer CF phenotypic differences with a genetic basis. Early destruction of the exocrine pancreas and its progressive deterioration can now be followed by measurement of serum immunoreactive trypsinogen (high levels early and very low levels later). Now

*References 6, 30, 33, 44, 47-50, 54.

†References 15, 23, 24, 29, 34, 38, 40-43.

Features and Complications of Cystic Fibrosis

INTEGUMENT AND EXTERNAL AREAS
1. Pallor
2. Failure to thrive
3. Purpura
4. Telangiectasia
5. Erythema nodosum
6. Digital clubbing
7. Protuberant abdomen
8. Emphysematous chest
9. Short stature
10. Delayed puberty
11. Cyanosis
12. Angular stomatitis
13. Salt crystals on face
14. Paronychia
15. Edema

HEAD
1. Sinusitis
2. Nasal polyposis
3. Optic neuritis
4. Nyctalopia
5. Enlarged submaxillary glands

THORAX AND PULMONARY SYSTEM
1. Bronchiolitis
2. Bronchitis
3. Bronchiectasis
4. Pneumonia
5. *Staphylococcus* organisms in sputum
6. *Pseudomonas* organisms in sputum
7. Allergic bronchopulmonary aspergillosis
8. Pulmonary cysts and abscesses
9. Atelectasis
10. Pneumomediastinum and/or pneumothorax
11. Massive hemoptysis
12. Botryomycosis
13. Empyema
14. Pulmonary insufficiency
15. Pulmonary failure

THORAX AND CARDIAC SYSTEM
1. Pulmonary hypertension
2. Right ventricular hypertrophy
3. Cor pulmonale
4. Right ventricular failure
5. Myocardial fibrosis

ABDOMEN
1. Pancreatic enzyme deficiency
2. Steatorrhea
3. Azotorrhea
4. Pancreatitis
5. Meconium ileus
6. Intestinal atresia
7. Fecal impaction
8. Intussusception
9. Duodenitis and ulceration
10. Mucocele of appendix
11. Cirrhosis of liver
12. Hepatomegaly
13. Splenomegaly
14. Portal hypertension
15. Esophageal varices
16. Ascites
17. Pneumatosis intestinalis
18. Pneumatosis coli
19. Rectal prolapse
20. Inguinal hernia
21. Diabetes

GENITOURINARY SYSTEM
1. Absence of vas deferens
2. Male sterility
3. Thick cervical mucus
4. Cervical polyps
5. Female decreased fertility

72-hour stool fat measurements are used to estimate pancreatic function and to adjust oral pancreatic enzyme replacement, whereas secretin and pancreozymin tests are used less frequently. The pancreatic destructive process eventually affects the endocrine function of islet tissue, and glucose intolerance caused by insulinopenia ensues (30% to 75% of cases). Overt clinical diabetes (hyperglycemia, glycosuria, polyuria, polydipsia, and weight loss) occurs in approximately 1% of cases. The mean age of onset is between 13 and 16 years. The frequency and severity of glucose intolerance correlate with the patient's age but not with the severity of disease, which is most likely correlated with severity of pulmonary involvement. Ketonuria and ketoacidosis, as occur in juvenile diabetes mellitus, are not seen in CF. The concomitant occurrence of excessive urinary glucagon levels in CF may account for this difference.

LABORATORY STUDIES

An early diagnosis of CF requires a high index of suspicion because it is a disease with a wide range of manifestations involving many organ systems, with a variable pattern of onset and a broad spectrum of severity. Once there is a suspicion, only a properly performed sweat test (pilocarpine iontophoresis and quantitative analysis of sweat sodium and chloride in a qualified laboratory) can confirm or rule out the diagnosis of CF in patients with physical features and a history that suggests the disease.[9] Sweat sodium and chloride concentrations greater than 60 mEq/L are required for diagnosis. The indications for sweat testing are listed in the box on p. 1211. False-positive sweat tests occur with adrenal insufficiency diabetes insipidus, glycogen storage disease, and in the hypohidrotic form of ectodermal dysplasia. Other methods

Indications for Sweat Testing

PULMONARY

Chronic cough
Recurrent or chronic pneumonia
Staphylococcal pneumonia
Recurrent bronchiolitis
Atelectasis
Hemoptysis
Mucoid *Pseudomonas* infection

GASTROINTESTINAL

Meconium ileus, steatorrhea, malabsorption
Rectal prolapse
Childhood cirrhosis (portal hypertension or bleeding esophageal varices)
Hypoprothrombinemia beyond newborn period

OTHER

Family history of cystic fibrosis
Failure to thrive
Salty sweat, salty taste when kissed, salt frosting of skin
Nasal polyps
Heat prostration, hyponatremia, and hypochloremia, especially in infants
Pansinusitis
Aspermatism

of prenatal and postnatal diagnosis (including measurement of amniotic fluid protease activity, meconium albumin content, and serum immunoreactive trypsinogen) and more rapid sweat test analyses are still in an investigative stage and cannot yet be relied on.[4]

DIFFERENTIAL DIAGNOSIS

As stated earlier, CF has been confused with upper and lower respiratory tract allergy and gastrointestinal allergy. When CF is mistakenly confused with gastrointestinal milk allergy, the substitution of soybean milk products may contribute to the development of a syndrome of severe failure to thrive, edema, anemia, and panhypoproteinemia.[47] (Soybean proteins are poorly utilized by the untreated child with CF.) CF also can be confused with other chronic pulmonary conditions of infancy, childhood, and adolescence. These are listed in the box on p. 1212.

MANAGEMENT

The natural history of CF has changed in the past 50 years. A disease formerly lethal in the first years of life is now one in which the median age of survival has surpassed 18 years. This improvement has been made possible by (1) medical and public awareness, with earlier diagnosis facilitated by the sweat test, (2) the use of oral pancreatic enzyme replacement, (3) the judicious use of antibiotics, (4) pulmonary physiotherapy, and (5) the establishment of a network of 120 CF care and teaching centers in the United States. Despite progress the ultimate prognosis remains grim. Proper management of these patients requires a broad understanding of the pathology of CF; a knowledge of its secondary physical, psychological, social, and financial manifestations; and a multidisciplinary approach. The most capable physician should no longer be the sole provider of the multiple services needed.

The task of keeping up with the CF literature is a job in itself. One can expect one article per month to appear in the pediatric journals. Because approximately 25% of patients are now in the adult age range, recent advances in knowledge, and therefore in management, also are published in the journals of other specialties.[10] The Cystic Fibrosis Foundation* serves as a clearinghouse for medical information. The medical director and staff members are equipped to triage all inquiries and to direct the health care professional to his or her nearest CF specialist.

The CF specialist, in turn, is trained to make or confirm the diagnosis and to coordinate ongoing care of the chronically ill patient in the context of his or her family and community. The health professional should be prepared and open minded; communication with the specialist and coordination of the patient's nutritional, pulmonary, and psychological care are vital. The open, inquisitive minds of the primary physician and the CF specialist and their attitudes toward the patient and family from the time of diagnosis often determine their future adjustments and attitudes to the vicissitudes of CF. An informed case manager—whether the primary physician, CF specialist, nurse practitioner, family counselor, or other health professional—is a necessity. These persons have the difficult task of providing information, advice, and access to modes of management. They must be able to function effectively despite the following uncertainties: (1) the cause of CF remains unknown; (2) scientific evidence to indicate the best components of the medical treatment program (diet, antibiotics, physiotherapy) is still controversial; and (3) prognosis for the individual patient is difficult to determine.

Patients living near a CF center will rely more heavily on the center for CF management while turning to the primary care provider for all other care. The extent of responsibility of each should be spelled out at the beginning of the relationship and made clear to the patient and family so that lines of communication remain open. Services that CF centers provide include the following:

1. Sweat testing and confirmation of the diagnosis
2. Evaluation and an outline of therapeutic and prophylactic programs
3. Education of the entire family, as well as the patient
4. Instruction in pulmonary physiotherapy and inhalation therapy
5. Instruction in nutrition and diet
6. Genetic counseling
7. Vocational counseling
8. Financial counseling
9. Patient and parent discussion groups
10. Other consultative services, including allergy, otolaryngology, psychiatry, and surgery
11. Personal involvement in research projects by patients and relatives

*6000 Executive Blvd., Suite 309, Rockville, MD 20852.

Chronic Pulmonary Diseases in Children and Adolescents

ALLERGIC
Bronchial asthma
Allergic bronchopulmonary aspergillosis
Hypersensitivity pneumonitis
Hypersensitivity reactions to drugs and chemicals

INFECTIOUS
Chlamydia infections, including psittacosis and ornithosis
Chronic tuberculosis and atypical *Mycobacteria* infection
Histoplasmosis
Other mycoses
Visceral larva migrans
Cytomegalic inclusion disease
Pneumocystis carinii

POSTINFECTIOUS
Bronchiectasis
Bronchiolitis obliterans
Unilateral hyperlucent lung syndrome
Interstitial fibrosis

CONGENITAL AND HEREDITARY
Cystic fibrosis
Alpha-1-antitrypsin deficiency
Immotile cilia syndrome and Kartagener syndrome
Immunodeficiency disorders
Ectodermal dysplasia
Familial dysautonomia
Congenital lobar emphysema
Anomalies of the lung (cysts and sequestration)

ASSOCIATED WITH UNDERLYING SYSTEMIC DISEASE
Sarcoidosis
Collagen diseases
Malignancy
Reticuloendothelioses
  Liporeticuloses
    Gaucher disease
    Niemann-Pick disease
  Histiocytosis X
    Letterer-Siwe disease
    Hand-Schüller-Christian disease
    Eosinophilic granuloma
Wegener granulomatosis

COMPLICATING MANAGEMENT OF PREEXISTING DISEASE
Bronchopulmonary dysplasia
Musculoskeletal disorders
Central nervous system disorders
Radiation pneumonitis

IDIOPATHIC
Pulmonary hemosiderosis
Fibrosing alveolitis (usual interstitial pneumonia [UIP])
Desquamative interstitial pneumonia (DIP)
Lymphoid interstitial pneumonia (LIP)
Giant cell interstitial pneumonia (GIP)
Bronchiolitis obliterans with interstitial pneumonia (BIP)
Pulmonary alveolar microlithiasis

Depending on the particular case, patients will be seen at the CF center as often as every 2 to 4 weeks, but at least once a year. When the situation dictates frequent visits, clinical evaluation is aimed at detecting acute or subacute conditions. In milder cases, seen at 6-month to yearly intervals, routine evaluation consists of (1) measurements of height, weight, and chest width and depth, (2) a full physical examination with emphasis on sinuses, nasal passages, lung fields, heart, liver, spleen, abdomen, and distal phalanges, (3) chest roentgenograms, (4) pulmonary function studies, including response to bronchodilators and arterial blood gas analysis, (5) a complete blood cell count, (6) sputum bacterial and fungal cultures, including antibiotic sensitivities, (7) a urinalysis, including urine glucose levels, and (8) serum chemistries—that is, total protein, albumin, blood urea nitrogen, creatinine, AST (SGOT), ALT (SGPT), alkaline phosphatase, bilirubin, 2-hour postprandial blood glucose level, and prothrombin time. These tests are aimed at assessing the patient's state of health and at detecting complications of CF. Serum immunoglobulin levels (IgG, IgA, IgM, and IgE) sometimes are determined to assess the patient's immune status.* A markedly elevated total serum IgE level indicates the possibility that allergic bronchopulmonary aspergillosis is complicating the CF.[40]

Hospitalization is indicated in three common situations: (1) acute pulmonary deterioration and distress, (2) acute abdominal crisis and distress, and (3) elective nasal, thoracic, or abdominal surgery. Hospitalizations for crises are frequent experiences for those with CF. However, they should be anticipated and avoided if at all possible. Hospitalizations for initial evaluation and education, for reevaluation, and for "tune-ups" may be indicated from time to time, especially when (1) families live far from medical care, (2) outpatient management does not stem the tide of gradual deterioration over a period of 1 to 2 weeks, and (3) family efforts at support and care begin to fail in the face of stress. Timing of the hospitalization, especially when the patient and family sense that "things are not going well," frequently precedes or coincides with major family and social events, such as holidays, birthdays, weddings, trips, vacations, and starting school and college. Things "not going well" may be reflected in one of several messages: (1) "Get me back in shape so I can participate in these events"; (2) "I believe I am too sick to participate in these events"; or (3) "I *am* too sick to participate in these events."

The most common indications for hospitalization are in-

*References 2, 8, 21, 26, 27, 51.

creased respiratory symptoms and decreased pulmonary function. Treatment is aimed at controlling pulmonary inflammation and infection caused by *Staphylococcus aureus* or *Pseudomonas aeruginosa*. The former sometimes can be handled with outpatient oral antibiotic therapy. The latter, however, requires intravenous antibiotics such as the aminoglycosides (tobramycin, gentamicin, amikacin) and the newer penicillins (carbenicillin, ticarcillin, azlocillin, mezlocillin, piperacillin). Treatment may need to last from 1 to 4 weeks or even longer. Because pseudomonal organisms have been almost impossible to eradicate from the respiratory tracts of those patients in whom colonization has occurred, the end point for antipseudomonal therapy is judged by the following clinical criteria: (1) disappearance of fever, (2) decrease in cough and sputum production, (3) normalization of respiratory rate and exercise tolerance, (4) improvement in pulmonary function, (5) improvement in hemoglobin oxygen saturation, (6) clearing of abnormal auscultatory sounds on lung examination, (7) improvement in the chest roentgenogram, (8) normalization of the white blood cell count, (9) increased appetite, and (10) weight gain.

PSYCHOSOCIAL AND GENETIC CONSIDERATIONS

Psychosocial and genetic counseling should be initiated and performed by the health professional with the most thorough understanding of a particular patient and family. A primary physician may need to be assisted by those with special expertise, such as the CF nurse coordinator or CF genetics counselor, who usually is available at the regional CF center. The counseling process begins at the time of diagnosis, when parents learn that CF is an inherited disease and that each is a carrier of a single autosomal recessive CF gene. This knowledge frequently creates feelings of guilt and a need to place blame on oneself, on one's spouse, or on events that occurred before or during pregnancy. Grandparents may attribute CF to the in-law bloodline or may associate the occurrence of CF with other medical conditions that seem to run in the family. To preserve family harmony and cohesiveness, it is imperative to deal with these issues.

It is tempting for the physician to present patients and their families with all the medical information at once and to hide behind the genetic numbers and risk games (Table 195-1). Although the information is necessary, much of it will not be retained because parents are in a period of shock, adjusting to the diagnosis, to the double-edged prognosis (always fatal, but with an unknown life expectancy and rate of deterioration), and to the frequently burdensome therapeutic plan. Conferences should be scheduled at times separate from medical visits, but questions raised at any medical visit should be dealt with at that time. At information and counseling sessions, all primary caretakers (especially mother and father) should be present. They should be guided gently so that all pertinent questions are asked and answered.

The patient with CF and the family develop various mechanisms of coping with the disease. The first reaction of the care provider to overdependence, overprotection, breakdown of family relationships, depression, denial, and noncompliance on the part of the patient and family may be that of rejection and authoritarianism. The care provider must realize that certain behavior patterns, which at first may be considered abnormal, may be valuable for the survival of the affected families. As these patients age, the psychological and social problems that directly affect them and their families change and increase. These problems depend on the severity of disease, its complications, and its rate of progression. The health professional must anticipate these potential psychosocial dangers so that they will be minimized in number and intensity. He or she must also define how much the premorbid psychosocial substrate is contributing to the current problems. Most CF care providers feel that the severe stresses of the disease require that hope not be abandoned and that negative information be presented within the context of that hope. At times, the chronically ill CF patient will engage in avoidance behavior to be able to participate in life. Medical management should work within this framework, the goal being to increase the quality of life as well as its length. The patient advocate must be prepared to guide the family and the patient to function at full potential at each new and progressively degenerative level of physical disability.

Parents frequently are confused and unsure about having more children. Once a couple has a child with CF, the risk of each subsequent pregnancy resulting in CF is 1:4. For some couples this is acceptable. For most, depending on personal, ethnic, and religious convictions, the risk is too high; these parents will ask about prenatal detection (at present unavailable), contraception, abortion, artificial insemination, and adoption. They often will base their decisions about future pregnancies on their experience with the first CF child. Initially they may not appreciate the full potential impact of CF on their own lives. Examples of the best and worst

Table 195-1 *Risks of Producing a Child with Cystic Fibrosis*

ONE PARENT	OTHER PARENT	RISK OF CF IN EACH PREGNANCY (RATIO)
With no CF history	With no CF history	1:1600
With no CF history	With first cousin having CF	1:320
With no CF history	With aunt or uncle having CF	1:240
With no CF history	With sib having CF	1:120
With no CF history	With CF child by previous marriage	1:80
With no CF history	With parent having CF	1:80
With no CF history	With CF	1:40
With sib having CF	With sib having CF	1:9
With CF child	With CF child	1:4

prognoses should be presented to the couple, allowing them to place themselves within this spectrum and to make their own choices. They can be offered the choice of prenatal diagnosis for future pregnancies and the testing of their unaffected children for carrier status. DNA testing to diagnose CF and to determine carrier status is presently limited to those with a family history of CF (with or without a living CF-affected relative for comparison) and to the spouses of CF carriers or "affecteds."[14]

Although sweat testing cannot identify the heterozygote, all siblings of CF patients should be tested because they, too, may have CF. If they do, their disease may have been overlooked because the diagnosis had not been considered previously or because they are at the mild end of the CF spectrum. Each healthy sibling's chance of being a carrier is 2:3 (66%), and the chance of the same parents producing a carrier with each subsequent pregnancy is 2:4 (50%).[28] Healthy siblings carry two burdens: uncertainty about whether they are carriers and a psychosocial burden that may result in maladjustment. Frequently they share silently in the fear, guilt, anger, helplessness, and hopelessness. Efforts should be made to increase their understanding of CF and to improve their self-esteem by including them in a realistic family support system.

As the teenage and adult years approach for CF patients, genetic and vocational counseling becomes an integral part of their medical guidance.[5] The horizons depend greatly on the physical condition of the individual patient. Limitations are imposed by the pulmonary status and the rate of deterioration. When CF is severe, puberty is delayed; even when it is mild, most but not all men are sterile because of ablation of the vas deferens (ductus deferens) system. Men of reproductive age contemplating fatherhood should have sperm analyses; the difference between sterility and penile virility (which is not impaired by CF) should be made clear to them. Many women with CF have had children of their own, although female fertility is impaired because of thick cervical mucus. Their chances of having a child with CF are 1:40 when the carrier status of the father is unknown (assuming a 1:20 carrier rate for the general white population). All non-CF children of a CF mother will be carriers.

Of more importance than the odds and the genetics are the questions of whether the woman with CF can survive a pregnancy, and then if she does, whether her health will be such that she will be able to rear her progeny. Partial assessments can be made by the team of health professionals. Final decisions must be left in the hands of the persons directly involved.

PROGNOSIS

Hippocrates said, "Life is short and the Art long: the occasion fleeting; experiment dangerous; and judgment difficult." For years, this had been true for CF and for those who had provided care for children and adults with this disease. Now, they have entered a new era of scientific and medical optimism. A CF cure is on the horizon. Identification and isolation of all the CF mutations will lead to a complete understanding of CF's pathophysiology, to the development of genetically tailored cellular and animal models of CF, and to the design and use of specific genetic and drug therapies. Life will be longer, the occasion will be permanent, the experiment safe, and the judgment rational.

REFERENCES

1. Anderson DH: Cystic fibrosis of the pancreas and its relation to celiac disease: a clinical and pathological study, Am J Dis Child 56:344, 1938.
2. Berdischewsky M et al: Circulating immune complexes in cystic fibrosis, Pediatr Res 12:830, 1980.
3. Berger M et al: Complement receptor expression at an inflammatory site, the *Pseudomonas*-infected lung in cystic fibrosis, J Clin Invest 84:1302, 1989.
4. Brock DJH: Amniotic fluid alkaline phosphatase isoenzymes in early prenatal diagnosis of cystic fibrosis, Lancet 2:941, 1983.
5. Bywater EM: Adolescents with cystic fibrosis: psychosocial adjustment, Arch Dis Child 56:538, 1981.
6. Carswell F, Oliver J, and Silverman M: Allergy in cystic fibrosis, Clin Exp Immunol 35:141, 1979.
7. Caskey CT et al: The American Society of Human Genetics statement on cystic fibrosis screening, Am J Hum Genet 46:393, 1990.
8. Church JA et al: Circulating immune complexes in patients with cystic fibrosis, Chest 80:405, 1981.
9. Denning CR et al: Cooperative study comparing three methods of performing sweat tests to diagnose cystic fibrosis, Pediatrics 66:752, 1980.
10. di Sant'Agnese PA and Davis PB: Cystic fibrosis in adults: 75 cases and a review of 232 cases in the literature, Am J Med 66:121, 1979.
11. di Sant'Agnese PA et al: Abnormal electrolyte composition of sweat in cystic fibrosis of the pancreas: clinical significance and relationship to the disease, Pediatrics 12:549, 1953.
12. Estivill X et al: ΔF508 gene deletion in cystic fibrosis in southern Europe, Lancet 2:1404, 1989.
13. Gaskin K et al: Improved respiratory prognosis in patients with cystic fibrosis with normal fat absorption, J Pediatr 100:857, 1982.
14. Gilbert F: Is population screening for cystic fibrosis appropriate now? Am J Hum Genet 46:394, 1990.
15. Gorvoy JD: Allergic bronchopulmonary aspergillosis in a patient with cystic fibrosis and prolonged use of marihuana, Cystic Fibrosis Club Abstr 25:79, 1984.
16. Jaffe BF et al: Nasal polypectomy and sinus surgery for cystic fibrosis—a 10 year review, Otolaryngol Clin North Am 10:81, 1977.
17. Kerem B et al: Identification of the cystic fibrosis gene: genetic analysis, Science 245:1073, 1989.
18. Kerem E et al: The relation between genotype and phenotype in cystic fibrosis—analysis of the most common mutation (ΔF508), N Engl J Med 323:1517, 1990.
19. Klinger K et al: Cystic fibrosis mutations in the Hutterite brethren, Am J Hum Genet 46:983, 1990.
20. Larsen GL et al: A comparative study of atropine sulfate and isoproterenol hydrochloride in cystic fibrosis, Am Rev Respir Dis 117:298, 1978.
21. Matthews WJ et al: Hypogammaglobulinemia in patients with cystic fibrosis, N Engl J Med 302:245, 1980.
22. McIntosh I, Lorenzo M-L, and Brock DJH: Frequency of ΔF508 mutation on cystic fibrosis chromosome in the UK, Lancet 2:1405, 1989.
23. Mearns M, Longbottom J, and Batten JC: Precipitating antibodies to *Aspergillus fumigatus* in cystic fibrosis, Lancet 1:538, 1967.
24. Mearns M, Young W, and Batten J: Transient pulmonary infiltrations in cystic fibrosis due to allergic aspergillosis, Thorax 20:385, 1965.
25. Mellis CM and Levison H: Bronchial reactivity in cystic fibrosis, Pediatrics 61:446, 1978.
26. Moss RB: Immunology of cystic fibrosis: immunity, immunodeficiency and hypersensitivity. In Lloyd-Still JD, editor: Textbook of cystic fibrosis, Boston, 1983, John Wright/PSG, Inc.
27. Moss RB and Lewiston NJ: Immune complexes and humoral responses to *Pseudomonas aeruginosa* in cystic fibrosis, Am Rev Respir Dis 121:23, 1980.
28. Nadler HL and Ben-Yoseph Y: Genetics. In Taussig LM, editor: Cystic fibrosis, New York, 1984, Thieme-Stratton, Inc.

29. Nelson LA, Callerame ML, and Schwartz RH: Aspergillosis and atopy in cystic fibrosis, Am Rev Respir Dis 120:863, 1979.
30. Noritake D, Hen J, and Dolan TF: Effects of aspirin on pulmonary function in patients with cystic fibrosis. Cystic Fibrosis Club Abstr 22:144, 1981.
31. Oppenheimer EH and Rosenstein BJ: Differential pathology of nasal polyps in cystic fibrosis and atopy, Lab Invest 40:445, 1979.
32. Quinton PM and Bijman J: Higher bioelectric potentials due to decreased chloride absorption in the sweat glands of patients with cystic fibrosis, N Engl J Med 308:1185, 1983.
33. Rachelefsky GS et al: Coexistent respiratory allergy and cystic fibrosis, Am J Dis Child 128:355, 1974.
34. Ricketti AJ, Greenberger PA, and Patterson R: Serum IgE as an important aid in management of allergic bronchopulmonary aspergillosis, J Allergy Clin Immunol 74:68, 1984.
35. Riordan JR et al: Identification of the cystic fibrosis gene: cloning and characterization of complementary DNA, Science 245:1066, 1989.
36. Ristow SC et al: Systemic amyloidosis in cystic fibrosis, Am J Dis Child 131:886, 1977.
37. Rommens JM et al: Identification of the cystic fibrosis gene: chromosome walking and jumping, Science 245:1059, 1989.
38. Rosenberg M et al: Clinical and immunologic criteria for the diagnosis of allergic bronchopulmonary aspergillosis, Ann Intern Med 86:405, 1977.
39. Schramm VL and Effron MZ: Nasal polyps in children, Laryngoscope 90:1488, 1980.
40. Schwartz RH and Hollick GE: Allergic bronchopulmonary aspergillosis with low serum immunoglobulin E, J Allergy Clin Immunol 68:290, 1981.
41. Schwartz RH et al: Serum precipitins to *Aspergillus fumigatus* in cystic fibrosis, Am J Dis Child 120:432, 1970.
42. Shapira E and Wilson GB, editors: Immunological aspects of cystic fibrosis, CRC Series in Immunology and Lymphoid Cell Biology, Boca Raton, Fla, 1984, CRC Press, Inc.
43. Shen J et al: Specific *Pseudomonas* immunoglobulin E antibodies in sera of patients with cystic fibrosis, Infect Immun 32:967, 1981.
44. Silverman M et al: Cystic fibrosis, atopy, and airways lability, Arch Dis Child 53:873, 1978.
45. Sorensen RU: Immune responses to pseudomonas and other bacteria in cystic fibrosis patients. In Shapira E and Wilson GB, editors: Immunological aspects of cystic fibrosis, CRC Series in Immunology and Lymphoid Cell Biology, Boca Raton, Fla, 1984, CRC Press, Inc.
46. Soter NA, Mihm MC, and Colten HR: Cutaneous necrotizing venulitis in patients with cystic fibrosis, J Pediatr 95:197, 1979.
47. Talamo RC and Schwartz RH: Immunologic and allergic manifestations. In Taussig LM, editor: Cystic fibrosis, New York, 1984, Thieme-Stratton, Inc.
48. Tobin MJ et al: Atopy and bronchial reactivity in older patients with cystic fibrosis, Thorax 35:807, 1980.
49. Warner JO, Norman AP, and Soothill JF: Cystic fibrosis heterozygosity in the pathogenesis of allergy, Lancet 1:990, 1976.
50. Warner JO et al: Association of cystic fibrosis with allergy, Arch Dis Child 51:507, 1976.
51. Wheeler WB et al: Progression of cystic fibrosis lung disease as a function of serum immunoglobulin G levels: a 5-year longitudinal study, J Pediatr 104:695, 1984.
52. Winnie GB, Cowan RG, and Wade NA: Intravenous immune globulin treatment of pulmonary exacerbations in cystic fibrosis, J Pediatr 114:309, 1989.
53. Wood RE, Boat TF, and Doershuk CF: State of the art: cystic fibrosis, Am Rev Respir Dis 113:833, 1976.
54. Zambie MF et al: Relationship between response to exercise and allergy in patients with cystic fibrosis, Ann Allergy 42:290, 1979.

196

Cystic and Solid Masses of the Face and Neck

Peter Szilagyi

The differential diagnosis of a neck mass is broad; it ranges from common inflammatory lymph nodes and cysts to rare neoplasms. Therefore an orderly approach to the workup and management of a neck mass is needed. The most practical approach involves differentiating the anatomic location of the mass into lateral neck masses versus midline neck masses and determining the exact anatomic position of the mass.[9] It is helpful to further localize a lateral neck mass into either the anterior cervical triangle (anterior to the sternocleidomastoid muscle) or into the posterior cervical triangle.

ETIOLOGY

Masses in the neck can be classified into two broad categories: cystic lesions and solid masses.[2] Cystic lesions are either congenital cysts or vascular malformations; however, traumatic hematomas and abscesses may appear to be cystic. Solid neck masses usually are inflammatory lymph nodes or, rarely, neoplastic lesions. In general, a careful history and physical examination will lead the clinician to the correct diagnosis. Carefully chosen laboratory tests or radiologic studies may then confirm the diagnosis.

In the evaluation of neck masses it is important to be familiar with key anatomic structures of the neck. Because most neck masses encountered by pediatricians are lymph nodes and not cysts, it is crucial to understand the location of the different groups of lymph nodes within the anterior and posterior anatomic triangles of the neck. Fig. 196-1 shows the location of the major groups of lymph nodes (in *solid circles*), the sternocleidomastoid muscle, and the typical locations of the most frequently encountered congenital cysts *(open circles)*.

HISTORY

It is important to determine whether the neck mass was observed at birth, whether it has increased or decreased in size, whether it has changed color, and whether there has been any drainage or opening in the lesion. Knowing the age of onset may help because lymph nodes rarely appear at birth, whereas many congenital cysts are noted in the newborn period. Some congenital cysts, however, may not be noted until childhood or beyond and are detected only when they become infected.

The history of pain or tenderness is important. Congenital cysts are nontender unless they become infected. Inflamed lymph nodes are quite tender and painful. Pain during eating suggests parotid gland involvement.

PHYSICAL EXAMINATION

The first step in the physical examination is to determine whether abnormalities exist in other parts of the body, such as the presence of other cysts, lymphadenopathy, hepatosplenomegaly, skin lesions, or signs of infection. The exact anatomic location of the neck mass must be determined, and the clinician should note whether the mass is in the typical location of a lymph node (Fig. 196-1). The consistency, color, and firmness of the mass should be noted, as well as the presence of tenderness. The size of the mass also should be measured.

Midline masses usually are related to a thyroid abnormality. Those that move with swallowing or with tongue protrusion suggest a thyroglossal duct cyst inasmuch as these lesions may be tethered to the foramen cecum by the thyroglossal duct remnant. A mass along the anterior edge of the sternocleidomastoid muscle that moves with swallowing or that has a sinus opening to the surface of the overlying skin is likely to be a branchial cleft cyst. Both cysts and benign lymph nodes are freely mobile, whereas malignant lesions are more likely to be fixed to underlying structures.

Rapidly growing, painless neck masses are worrisome because they might be neoplastic. Additional signs associated with a neoplastic process include fixation of the mass to subcutaneous tissue, firm consistency, or size of greater than 3 cm, and presence of constitutional symptoms. Neck masses in the posterior cervical triangle are more likely to be malignant than are masses anterior to the sternocleidomastoid muscle.

TYPES OF CONGENITAL CYSTS

Thyroglossal duct cysts account for more than 70% of congenital cysts of the neck, branchial cleft cysts for more than 20%, and vascular malformations and other lesions for 4% to 5%.[4]

Thyroglossal duct cysts result from failure of the embryologic thyroglossal duct to degenerate during the fifth week of gestation, leaving a fistula, sinus tract, or cyst at the midline of the neck just below the hyoid bone.[3] Thyroglossal duct cysts are not often detected at birth but are usually first noted

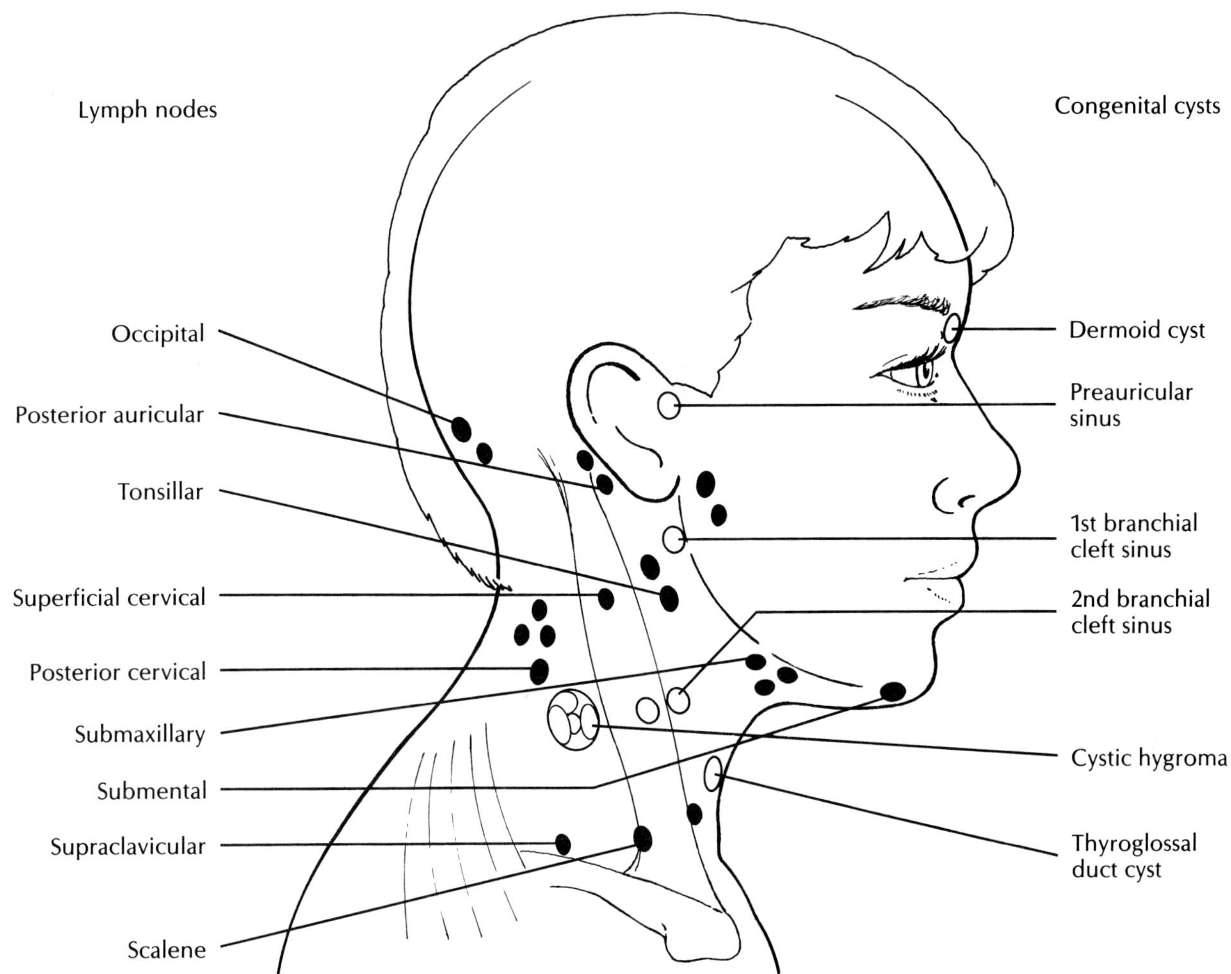

Fig. 196-1 Common locations for cystic and solid masses of the face and neck.

after the age of 2 years; they may first manifest as an inflamed, tender mass. When not infected, they are smooth, firm, mobile, and nontender and move upward with tongue protrusion or with swallowing. The differential diagnosis includes sebaceous cysts, epidermal cysts, submandibular lymph nodes, and lipomas. Unless normal thyroid tissue is palpable, it is important to confirm the presence of the thyroid gland by ultrasonography or technetium scan, because what may appear to be a thyroglossal duct cyst actually may be an ectopic thyroid gland, and its removal would leave the child dependent on thyroid hormone supplementation throughout life.[8] Because the likelihood of infection is high, thyroglossal duct cysts should be surgically removed.

Branchial cleft cysts are congenital remnants of the lateral four branchial pouches and clefts, which, interestingly, correspond to embryologic gill slits in fish.[1] The vast majority of branchial cleft cysts arise from the second cleft or pharyngeal pouch. They appear as a small dimple or opening anterior to the middle portion of the sternocleidomastoid muscle. The cyst is nontender, firm, and mobile and is located just under the skin. A small sinus, which occasionally drains fluid to the surface of the overlying skin, may be present, and a long fistulous tract may extend from it to the tonsil bed.[3,5] Branchial cleft cysts without sinuses often are unnoticed until later childhood when they become infected. Infected cysts can be easily confused with lymphadenitis. Other lesions included in the differential diagnosis are sternocleidomastoid muscle masses associated with torticollis, small cystic hygromas, epidermoid cysts, neurofibromas, lipomas, and an ectopic thyroid gland. Treatment involves surgical removal of the cyst and fistula.

Cystic hygromas are congenital, avascular masses derived from congenital obstruction of lymphatic vessels. They are generally multilocular, fluid-filled, soft, compressible, painless masses located in the posterior triangle just behind the sternocleidomastoid muscle and in the supraclavicular fossa. They usually can be transilluminated. These masses may grow rapidly because of accumulation of lymph and can reach an enormous size, resulting in compression of important structures and in airway obstruction.[4] Although the diagnosis usually is obvious on physical examination, smaller cystic hygromas may resemble hemangiomas or other cysts. Ultrasonographic examination will reveal fluid and multiple cystic components, confirming the diagnosis. Because spontaneous regression is rare and the risk of compression of vital upper airway structures is high, surgical removal is indicated. Often multiple procedures are necessary to remove large lesions in their entirety. Cystic hygromas occur infrequently in the axilla, on the trunk, or on the extremities and in older children within the subcutaneous tissues may be mistaken for a lipoma or a hemangioma.[1]

Cavernous hemangiomas are vascular lesions within the subcutaneous tissues that may appear in any part of the body and that may be difficult to differentiate from congenital cysts. They often are noted in the newborn period and enlarge (sometimes very rapidly) during the first year of life. Cavernous hemangiomas are less firm, more diffuse, and more easily compressible than are cystic masses (except for cystic hygromas). Unlike cystic hygromas, cavernous hemangiomas do not transilluminate, and their size may increase with crying or straining. Often the skin overlying these vascular lesions is bluish in color. Cavernous hemangiomas frequently begin to increase in size during the first few months of life but usually regress spontaneously by school age.[9] Thus surgery is indicated only for masses that compress vital structures or that cause severe cosmetic disfigurement.

Epidermoid cysts are relatively common masses that may arise from an embryologic or fusional defect. They usually are located at midline on the face, most often at the level of the eyebrows. These small cysts feel doughy and smooth and contain sebaceous material and sometimes even hair, cartilage, or bone. One third are present at birth; the remaining two thirds appear by school age.[5] Because these cysts may become infected and may form deep tracts, surgical excision is indicated.

Preauricular cysts and sinuses are the most common anomalies arising from an embryologic fusion failure of precursor tissues that develop into the external ear. The sinuses are pinhole-sized pits usually located anterior to the helix (Fig. 196-1), and they may contain a short sinus tract.[3] Preauricular cysts often are bilateral. These sinuses and cysts are inherited in an autosomal dominant manner with incomplete penetrance and are found more commonly in black than in white persons. They are a far more common cause of preauricular lesions than are first branchial cleft cysts, which are located in the same area.[5] Because they may become infected, elective surgical removal is a preferred treatment. Hearing deficits may be associated with these lesions, but their prevalence is unknown.

Although other congenital masses occur rarely in the head and neck, the aforementioned lesions account for the vast majority of congenital masses. The major challenge in the differential diagnosis involves (1) differentiating congenital masses from lymph nodes and (2) determining the type of congenital lesion. Lymph nodes are found in characteristic locations (Fig. 196-1), are often multiple, are frequently noted in association with an acute infection, have a firm and more solid texture than do most congenital cysts, and usually are not noted at birth. Several excellent articles[6,7,9] discuss the workup and management of cervical lymphadenopathy and lymphadenitis.

MANAGEMENT

As already discussed, all congenital cysts and masses should be followed up closely by the pediatrician. Acute infections must be treated with systemic antibiotics. Patients with thyroglossal duct cysts, branchial cleft cysts, cystic hygromas, and epidermal cysts should be referred to a surgeon who is experienced at excision of these congenital lesions. Elective surgery before a bout of infection is preferable because excision of an entire sinus tract, fistula, or embryologic connection is more difficult after an infection. Many pediatricians and surgeons prefer to delay surgery until the child is beyond infancy and will better tolerate the procedure. For patients with thyroglossal duct cysts, a pediatrician or surgeon should confirm the presence of normal thyroid tissue by ultrasonographic examination or a technetium scan. Hemangiomas can be observed without referral unless they begin to impinge on vital structures.

REFERENCES

1. Feins NR and Raffensperger JG: Cystic hygromas, lymphangioma and lymphedema. In Raffensperger JG, editor: Swenson's Pediatric Surgery, Norwalk, Conn, 1990, Appleton & Lange.
2. Friedberg J: Clinical diagnosis of neck lumps: a practical guide, Pediatr Ann 17:620, 1988.
3. Friedberg J: Pharyngeal cleft sinuses and cysts, and other benign neck lesions, Pediatr Clin North Am 36:1451, 1989.
4. Gray SW and Skandalakis JE: Embryology for surgeons, Philadelphia, 1972, WB Saunders Co.
5. Hogan D, Wilkinson RD, and Williams A: Congenital anomalies of the head and neck, Int J Dermatol 19:479, 1980.
6. Knight PJ and Reiner CB: Superficial lumps in children: what, when and why? Pediatrics 72:147, 1983.
7. May M: Neck masses in children: diagnosis and treatment, Ear Nose Throat J 57:12, 1978.
8. Raffensperger JG: Congenital cysts and sinuses of the neck. In Raffensperger JG, editor: Swenson's pediatric surgery, ed 5, Norwalk, Conn, 1990, Appleton & Lange.
9. Zitelli BJ: Evaluating the child with a neck mass, Contemp Pediatr, 7:90, 1990.

197

Diabetes Mellitus

Robert E. Greenberg

DEFINITIONS AND FREQUENCY

Diabetes mellitus refers to a number of related disorders, all characterized by impaired glucose tolerance associated with a deficiency in either insulin secretion or its metabolic effect. Although disordered glucose homeostasis is the most striking and well-recognized characteristic of diabetes, many other metabolic abnormalities occur, affecting amino acid, protein, and lipid metabolism. The current classification, depicted in Table 197-1, emphasizes the distinction between insulin-dependent and non-insulin-dependent forms of diabetes, as well as the heterogeneity of factors that may underlie hyperglycemia.

The prevalence of type I insulin-dependent diabetes varies strikingly among various populations, with the highest rate in Northern Europeans (1 in 300 to 500 18-year-olds) and much lower rates in black and Asiatic children. The incidence, again in Northern Europeans, approximates 10 per 100,000, with the peak incidence between 11 and 14 years of age. There is some suggestion that type I diabetes mellitus is less common in those groups in which the prevalence of type II diabetes appears to be markedly increasing (American Indians, Polynesians, and blacks).

HETEROGENEITY

Recognition of the heterogeneity within diabetes was a critical step in understanding the separate nature of insulin-dependent and non-insulin-dependent diabetes. This demonstration of heterogeneity has been based on family, twin, hormonal, immunologic, and genetic (human leukocyte antigen [HLA] association) studies. Family studies have indicated that type I and type II diabetes segregate in a completely unrelated fashion. Studies of twins have clearly focused the difference between the two clinical syndromes: only 50% or fewer of monozygotic twins demonstrate concordance for type I diabetes, whereas 100% of twins show concordance for type II diabetes. Hormonal studies have demonstrated deficient insulin secretion in type I diabetes, whereas resistance to the action of insulin appears to predominate in type II diabetes. An altered immune response is associated with insulin-dependent diabetes, in that most type I diabetic patients have islet cell antibodies demonstrable in their sera at the time of clinical diagnosis. Finally, HLA association studies have continued to reveal the striking association between specific alleles in the major histocompatibility locus with type I but not type II diabetes. More than 90% of white patients bear the serologically defined tissue specifications HLA-DR1, HLA-DR3, or HLA-DR4. If the fifty-seventh amino acid on the DQB chain is aspartic acid, occurrence of diabetes is low; a noncharged amino acid at the same site raises the risk.[3] It is now possible to separate completely the two major forms of diabetes. Despite this, they may exhibit some common aspects of their natural history, especially because the vascular and neuropathic complications are a consequence, in part, of similar disturbances in metabolic regulation.[5]

Table 197-1 *Classification of Diabetes Mellitus*

CURRENT TERMINOLOGY	OLDER TERMINOLOGY
Insulin-dependent diabetes mellitus (type I)	Juvenile, growth onset, insulin-sensitive, labile, or ketosis-prone diabetes
Non-insulin-dependent diabetes mellitus (type II)	Maturity onset, insulin-resistant, or ketosis-resistant diabetes
Impaired glucose tolerance	Chemical, latent or borderline, or asymptomatic diabetes
Potential abnormality of glucose tolerance	Prediabetes
Gestational diabetes	Gestational diabetes

ETIOLOGIC MECHANISMS IN TYPE I DIABETES MELLITUS

Genetic and Environmental Interplay

The striking fact that fewer than 50% of identical twins show concordance for type I diabetes strongly suggests that an interplay between genetic and other biologic mechanisms must occur to produce disease.[4,7] Available data indicate that type I diabetes results from autoimmune (self-directed) mechanisms. Evidence for this includes (1) the presence of insulitis (islet inflammation) in the pancreas of newly diagnosed patients, (2) antibodies to cytoplasmic islet cell antigen (ganglioside), to a 64-kilodalton beta–cell membrane protein, and to insulin in the sera of persons with newly diagnosed diabetes, and (3) a strong indication that cell-mediated immune mechanisms underlie the development of type I diabetes. Of importance is the observation that autoantibodies may be demonstrated both in humans and in experimental animal models, long before impaired, detectable carbohydrate tolerance occurs. Further, a marked increase in the incidence of autoantibodies is seen in genetically predisposed, but healthy, first-degree relatives of persons with diabetes. Finally, an increased incidence of other autoimmune phenomena has been shown to occur in either diabetic children or their families. The initiating event(s) for such autoimmune islet cell destruction remain uncertain, but current evidence no longer supports a role for viral infection as a cause.

HISTORY

The classic presentation is that of a child who demonstrates the clinical consequences of reduced glucose utilization (polyphagia, weight loss) and hyperglycemia (polyuria, polydipsia). It is still common for the physician to be confronted with a child in whom the early clinical signs were unappreciated, leading to the classic clinical picture of diabetic ketoacidosis (vomiting, Kussmaul respirations, altered state of consciousness). Diabetic ketoacidosis is discussed in detail in Chapter 271. The coexistence of abdominal pain in the child with diabetic ketoacidosis is extremely common and remains the leading cause of confusion in making the initial diagnosis. Although preexisting infections may be present (as in any child), no convincing evidence exists that newly diagnosed type I diabetic patients are more susceptible to significant infections. Although the majority of affected children have type I diabetes, the occurrence of non-insulin-dependent diabetes (maturity onset diabetes in the young [MODY]) is appreciable. In this circumstance the clinical signs of diabetes usually are more subtle, and ketoacidosis rarely occurs.

Decreased glucose utilization (leading to hyperglycemia) may be found in any severely ill young child, especially in those with reduced blood volume and peripheral perfusion. Hyperglycemia in these circumstances is neither diagnostic nor predictive of insulin-dependent diabetes.

PHYSICAL EXAMINATION

The findings on physical examination are determined by the duration and severity of insulin deficiency. If decreased glucose utilization has been present for weeks or months, then poor weight gain will be an almost universal finding. If glucose utilization has been severely impaired, then dehydration, respiratory compensation for metabolic acidosis, and altered consciousness will be the primary findings.

LABORATORY FINDINGS

Laboratory confirmation of carbohydrate intolerance requires the demonstration of hyperglycemia either in the fasting or in the postabsorptive state. Because of the significant individual variation in the renal threshold for glucose reabsorption, glucosuria alone is not diagnostic. Depending on the severity and duration of insulin deficiency, the laboratory findings of diabetic ketoacidosis—reduced plasma bicarbonate, reduced blood pH, increased anion gap, and hyperlipemia (increased cholesterol or triglycerides)—may be present. Hyperkalemia often accompanies significant metabolic acidosis, whereas hypokalemia in untreated diabetic ketoacidosis may well signify a massive depletion of total body potassium. Hyponatremia may be artifactual, because of the altered water distribution produced either by hyperglycemia or by the water displacement in plasma produced by severe hyperlipemia.

Rapid bedside diagnosis and management of diabetes are facilitated by serial dilution of plasma for the determination of blood glucose (Dextrostix or Chemstrips bG) and ketone bodies (Acetest).

DIFFERENTIAL DIAGNOSIS

Glucose intolerance can result from a number of different conditions: (1) decreased insulin secretion (type I diabetes), (2) defects in the binding of insulin to receptors (altered affinity or numbers of receptors, antireceptor blocking antibodies), (3) defects in the glucose transport system, such as a reduced affinity and number or mobility of glucose transporters, (4) increased secretion of counterregulatory hormones (catecholamines, corticosteroids, growth hormones), and (5) postreceptor defects in insulin action (genetic or nongenetic). A useful path through such confusion is to determine whether the glucose intolerance coexists with a reduced or an increased level of insulin secretion (plasma insulin or C peptide, determined by radioimmunoassay), as measured during a standard oral glucose tolerance test. If insulin levels are increased, then the differential diagnosis of insulin-resistant states may be more confidently undertaken.

MANAGEMENT

Natural History

When the diagnosis of diabetes mellitus is first made, insulin requirements may be high (>1 unit of insulin per kilogram per day). It should be noted, however, that the young child may be exquisitely sensitive to exogenous insulin, especially when the diabetes is diagnosed before the onset of ketoacidosis. Soon after initial stabilization, a respite may occur, wherein requirements for exogenous insulin may fall or even vanish when endogenous insulin secretion resumes (as documented by increased plasma C-peptide levels). This "honeymoon" period may last for weeks or even months, after which insulin requirements are determined primarily by body weight, hormonal changes during puberty, and psychological factors.

The clinical course of the child with diabetes is primarily determined by levels of understanding and the acceptance of the disease, psychological adjustment, family interactions, and stability of life-style. These factors are more significant determinants of metabolic control and frequency of hospitalization and illness than are the strictly biologic factors affecting the action of insulin.

The progression of the natural history of type I diabetes depends on the attack rate and severity of occurrence of the vascular and neuropathic complications. The significance of these long-term complications is made dramatically evident by noting that renal failure caused by diabetes is the most prevalent diagnosis among adults beginning hemodialysis or undergoing transplantation, and that blindness is 25 times more common in individuals with type I diabetes than in the nondiabetic population.

Importance of Metabolic Control

The entire design and implementation of strategies to manage insulin-dependent diabetes effectively are determined by the relation between its metabolic control and the histopathologic events noted during its course. Studies during the last decade have provided strong evidence to support the view that microangiopathy and neuropathy have their origin in the metabolic defects associated with insulin deficiency. This evidence is briefly summarized in the accompanying box. On the basis of this evidence the current approach to management is best characterized as the attempt to achieve as complete metabolic control of diabetes as possible. This newer underlying principle is a marked departure from previous pediatric practice, wherein adequate control was simply defined as normal physical growth and development in the absence of hypoglycemia or ketoacidosis. The practical questions now focus on the best methods to effect such a demanding level of metabolic control.

Monitoring

Short-Term Glycemia. Glucosuria will occur only when the concentration of glucose in blood exceeds the renal threshold for glucose reabsorption (the tubular maximum [Tm] for glucose). Inasmuch as the Tm for glucose normally approximates 180 mg/dl (with wide variations), glucosuria usually cannot occur without significant preceding hyperglycemia, nor does the absence of glucosuria ensure the absence of moderate hyperglycemia or distinguish normoglycemia from hypoglycemia. In brief, if metabolic balance is to be brought under more rigorous control, the glucose concentration of blood, rather than of urine, must be precisely measured. Hence monitoring of the blood glucose level has become the modern cornerstone of diabetes management. Assuming use of proper technique, the self-monitoring of blood glucose has many potential consequences for the patient: (1) it may stimulate interest and motivation in self-control of the disease, (2) it documents the precise nature of metabolic problems, (3) it reinforces learning behavior by demonstrating that metabolic control is possible, (4) it reinforces the acceptance of responsibility, and (5) it teaches through personal experience. Lack of compliance, however, can make home blood glucose monitoring an exercise in self-deception for the physician, as has long been recognized to be the case in home monitoring of the urinary glucose level.

Daily monitoring can easily become an unthinking routine. More effective monitoring may be achieved with the following approach:

1. Determination of the blood glucose level before each meal and before bedtime during 3 days of every week
2. Determination of the blood glucose level whenever symptoms suggest hypoglycemia or hyperglycemia
3. Determination of urine ketone levels whenever the blood glucose level is markedly elevated

This approach provides some incentive for regularity and places responsibility for documentation and interpretation of metabolic control with the patient or parent.[1]

Long-Term Glycemia. When foods are heated or stored in the presence of reducing sugars for long periods of time, a brown color results, which is produced by a direct reaction between the free amino groups of proteins and the reducing sugars (the Schiff reaction of nonenzymatic glycosylation). The demonstration that some minor hemoglobin electrophoretic variants were glycosylated raised the possibility that such variants might be a consequence of nonenzymatic glycosylation, just as in the browning of foods. The detection of elevated levels of the principal glycosylated hemoglobin variant, Hb A_{Ic}, among diabetic patients supported this proposal. The rate and extent of the nonenzymatic glycosylation of any protein in vivo depend, in part, on the concentration of protein and sugar, on the turnover rate of the protein, and on accessibility of sugar to the protein. Thus, if a protein has a rapid turnover rate, it cannot become significantly glycosylated, regardless of the concentration of blood glucose. Similarly, if the concentration of blood glucose is significantly elevated only for a small fraction of time, then the extent of protein glycosylation will be minimal, even if the specific protein has a very slow rate of turnover. The measurement of glycosylated hemoglobin now provides a sort of integrated assessment of the mean blood glucose concentration over the preceding 1 to 2 months. Measurement of fructosamine is a reflection of glycated serum proteins (one half the half-life of hemoglobin).

More than simply providing a handy index of long-term glycemia, nonenzymatic glycosylation may have far greater implications in diabetes—many proteins may exhibit significant changes in their functional properties after glycosylation and thus be responsible for some of the tissue-specific consequences of the diabetic state.[6]

Evidence that Microangiopathy Is a Consequence of Aberrant Metabolic Control

GENETIC ISSUES

Microangiopathy does not occur in monozygotic twins in the absence of clinical diabetes.

Secondary diabetes (i.e., hemochromatosis and pancreatic resection) is accompanied by microangiopathy.

ANIMAL STUDIES

Experimental diabetes is associated with vascular lesions in proportion to the severity of metabolic disturbance.

Vascular lesions can be prevented or reversed by intensive insulin treatment or pancreatic transplantation.

The injured kidney of a diabetic animal may improve when transplanted into a nondiabetic recipient.

HUMAN STUDIES

Histologic changes are not present at the onset of clinical symptoms in type I diabetes.

A normal kidney develops microangiopathic lesions when transplanted into a diabetic person.

Pathologic changes are related to the duration and severity of metabolic derangement.

Effective metabolic control of diabetes limits the rate of progression of microangiopathy.

Monitoring Complications. Within 5 years of onset of type I diabetes, a complete ophthalmologic examination and urinalysis should become regular components of ongoing management.

Patient and Family Education

Critical to the successful management of insulin-dependent diabetes is the extent to which the patient and family are informed. The physician who can transmit the concept that "freedom from diabetes" can be achieved only by mastery of both practical and theoretic aspects of the disease has a much greater chance of supervising optimal diabetic control. Several principles underlie the education of the diabetic family:

1. A natural period of shock and grieving accompanies a new diagnosis of diabetes, during which the family is not easily capable of assimilating extensive information.
2. Education about diabetes must be organized into discrete, separate modules (digestible bites) of information (see box below).
3. Opportunity for self-study, using instructional aids, must be provided.
4. Educational outcome criteria need to be developed and incorporated into the patient's ongoing record.
5. Education must be directed initially toward the more practical procedures of monitoring and insulin administration.
6. Education must be continued as an ongoing, continuous part of patient-physician interaction and management.[9]

Topics for Patient and Family Education

1. Nature of diabetes
   a. Blood glucose regulation
   b. Role of insulin
   c. Significance of hyperglycemia and ketonuria
2. Monitoring
   a. Short term
      (1) Home blood glucose determination
      (2) Urine testing
   b. Long term: glycosylated protein levels
3. Insulin therapy
   a. Types of insulin
   b. Methods of injection
4. Dietary management
   a. Importance of regularity
   b. Exchange lists
5. Effect of environment
   a. Emotional factors
   b. Exercise
6. Special problems and emergencies
   a. Ketoacidosis
   b. Insulin reactions
   c. Illness
7. Informing family, friends, and school personnel about diabetes
8. Resources for diabetics
   a. Peer or family groups
   b. Organizations
   c. Camps

Diet. Of overriding importance to helping children and their families in the management of diabetes is the concept of regularity of diet. When an individual has lost the capacity to modulate the amount of insulin secreted from moment to moment in response to varying stimuli (glucose or amino acids), it obviously becomes essential to keep constant from day to day the magnitude of the substrate load to be metabolized. Fortunately, the average child in a stable family has a uniform pattern of nutrient intake, but when that nutrient intake becomes the prime focus of parental attentions, mealtime can become a center for family anxiety. Soon, regularity in intake is replaced by marked irregularity and variation.

In addition to regularity in the timing and quantity of food intake, several other principles are important:

1. The diet should be nutritionally adequate, just as for the nondiabetic person.
2. The diet prescribed should be within the bounds of cultural patterns and individual preferences and also should be based whenever possible on the usual family pattern of eating.
3. Caloric and protein intake should be sufficient for optimal growth without obesity.
4. Caloric intake in the morning should be proportionally less than at other meals. The "dawn phenomenon" refers to that period between approximately 5 and 9 AM when insulin requirements increase, in the absence of antecedent hypoglycemia, for both diabetic and nondiabetic individuals.[2]
5. Exchange diets, based on individual dietary assessment, may be used as an educational tool for establishing and maintaining a pattern of regularity in nutrient intake. However, there is wide individual variation in the blood glucose response to various food that contain isocaloric amounts of total carbohydrate; thus the basic premise that underlies the older "exchange lists" may not actually be valid.
6. Readily available pure carbohydrate (e.g., candy) makes interpretation of blood glucose patterns difficult and thereby reduces effectiveness of a self-monitoring program.

Insulin Administration

All mammalian insulin is of a similar structure and contains 51 amino acids in two polypeptide chains (A and B). Pork insulin is closer in structure to human insulin than is beef. Allergic reactions to insulin, usually lipodystrophy or IgE-mediated local or systemic reactions, may be stimulated either by the beef or the pork insulin itself or by additives, preservatives, and contaminants. Use of recombinant DNA technology has enabled the synthesis of human insulin, which theoretically should not be immunogenic. Beyond an avoidance of allergic manifestations or antibody-mediated insulin resistance, however, human insulin offers only theoretic advantages over beef or pork insulin.

The proper use of insulin in the management of diabetes currently is restricted by the following considerations.

1. The normal pattern of insulin secretion is one of rapid changes (pulses, almost) in response to substrate stimuli, with a subsequent rapid decline in insulin levels. No current system of insulin administration, including

the newer extracorporeal and implanted pumps, can mimic the rapidly changing secretory patterns found in the normal individual.

2. Fifty percent of endogenous insulin, secreted into the portal vein, is extracted by the liver in a single passage, but when insulin is given parenterally (except by intraperitoneal administration), the liver is bypassed. Thus the hepatic extraction rate for exogenously administered insulin can, theoretically, be only half the physiologic secretory rate without producing peripheral hyperinsulinemia; at physiologic peripheral blood insulin levels, the portal vein concentration remains only half of that seen in the nondiabetic person.

Practical aspects of insulin administration include the following.

1. Insulin absorption from sites of injection is highly variable from day to day, from site to site, and from one individual to another. Furthermore, insulin absorption is more rapid from a site of injection in which vasodilation by exercise has occurred.
2. After administration of either intermediate- or long-acting forms of insulin, a relation between the dose administered and the blood insulin level observed can be demonstrated *only* by measuring the total area under the curve of blood insulin concentrations obtained over a period of 24 to 36 hours; that is, no single time after injection can be selected to measure "peak" levels. Thus intermediate- and long-acting insulins cannot be effectively used where changing levels in circulating insulin are needed to handle sudden changes in substrate load (e.g., after meals).
3. Accordingly, it is generally advisable to give insulin under the following guidelines: (a) in the "established" diabetic (i.e., beyond the honeymoon period) less than 1 U/kg/day of insulin should be given, (b) the usual division of insulin should approximate two thirds of the total before breakfast and one third before the evening meal, and (c) most of the morning insulin should be given as short-acting insulin, whereas increasing amounts of intermediate-acting insulin are given before the evening meal. In some instances additional short-acting insulin may have to be given before the noon meal, if optimal metabolic control is to be achieved.[8]

Physical Activity

Regular physical activity is an important part of diabetic management, not only as an effective means to facilitate glucose utilization but also as an integral component of a life-style designed to minimize the risk of large vessel disease.

Because the physical activity of children often is sporadic and unpredictable, it is wiser to ask the child to take extra calories than to attempt to alter insulin administration in anticipation of exercise, which can improve glucose utilization sufficiently to produce relative insulin overdose.

Psychological Considerations

Diabetes, like any chronic illness, presents new problems that well may affect the diabetic child and his or her family. Many of the normal developmental tasks may be made more difficult and less spontaneous for both child and parents. The family's ability to lead a normal life may be compromised by ignorance of the principles of good control or by unnecessary rigidities that impose excessive restrictions on life-style. In the adolescent period the disease and its quality control may be used by the adolescent as a weapon against his or her parents, whereas the parents, in turn, may use the disease as a mechanism to restrain the normal adolescent's establishment of appropriate independence from them.

The intimate relation that exists between emotional state and the metabolic control of diabetes is well recognized. Numerous studies have demonstrated that emotional disturbances lead to compromised rates of glucose utilization, presumably through increased secretion of counterregulatory hormones. Conversely, emotional well-being of a diabetic patient can be affected by primary disturbances in metabolic control.

Uninformed responses to the child's disease by extended family, friends, and school personnel can all magnify his or her emotional distress. Careful attention therefore must be paid to informing and educating such well-meaning contacts, so that the child's living opportunities are not restricted unnecessarily.

With careful attention to family dynamics, effort should be focused on improving the family's interactions, facilitating the communication of individual and group needs, and allowing both the child and family the opportunity to express the fears, concerns, and frustrations generated by the predictable problems every diabetic family faces.

As the diabetic child grows older, the effect of microangiopathic and neuropathic complications on the emotional state becomes pronounced. Yet many patients remain able to maintain the balance necessary between the demands and excitement of their normal lives and the insistent constraints imposed by their disease.

Future Developments

Insulin Delivery Systems. "Open loop" devices for chronic subcutaneous insulin infusions can provide normal metabolic control in certain patients, but they require, if anything, a higher order of individual responsibility and compliance, and such devices are associated with complications (infection, erratic absorption, localized problems, and ketoacidosis). Therefore the "brittle" and often unmotivated diabetic child usually is not a good candidate for use of these open loop devices.

"Closed loop" infusion devices will require the preceding development of a reliable and implantable glucose sensor before practical use of such a system can occur.

Beta-Cell Transplantation. Islet cell transplantation has not yet been met with prolonged success in maintaining graft acceptance. Attempts to alter the antigenicity of donor cells before transplantation have so far been only partially successful. Modification of the donor tissue is the necessary approach, rather than attempts to inhibit rejection of the graft by the recipient.

Immunosuppressive Therapy. In experimental animal models, islet cell antibodies may appear before the onset of glucose intolerance, and immunosuppressive therapy may forestall or actually prevent the advent of clinical diabetes. A similar approach is being pursued in newly diagnosed type

I human diabetes—an approach that assumes that adequate endogenous insulin secretion may be maintained, once further autoimmune-mediated cytotoxicity is terminated.

Prevention. Development of methods for detecting the autoimmune process that leads to islet cell destruction before the onset of clinical diabetes (such as the 64-K autoantibody) could set the stage for specific preventive immunotherapies: for example, selection and eradication of subsets of T cells that recognize beta-cell antigens.

Biochemical Bases of Diabetic Complications. If the biochemical mechanisms that underlie diabetic complications were completely understood, then specific therapies might be formulated that could forestall or prevent pathophysiologic sequelae. For instance, nonenzymatic glycosylation of proteins leads to increased protein cross-linking, a process that can be chemically impeded. Further, in chronic hyperglycemia, increased shunting of glucose through the sorbitol or polyol pathway occurs (leading to increased tissue concentrations of sorbitol and fructose), and this process can be impeded by inhibitors of the enzyme aldose reductase. Moreover, impaired synthesis of heparin proteoglycan may cause increased permeability of the vascular endothelium to macromolecules, a mechanism that also may be subject to chemical modification. These putative mechanisms exemplify exciting possibilities concerning chemical prevention of the pathologic consequences of diabetes.

COMPLICATIONS

Insulin Resistance

The most common form of insulin resistance is that produced by excessive insulin administration (e.g., the Somogyi phenomenon). When poor metabolic control of the disease is attended by insulin dosages exceeding 1 U/kg/day, then concern should be raised about excessive insulin administration; a stepwise reduction in insulin dose eventually will lead to improved control. Insulin resistance also may accompany use of the same site for repetitive injection. Sequestration of insulin at injection sites is an additional problem that appears more commonly during puberty. Antibody-mediated insulin resistance (commonly diagnosed but rarely present) may respond to human insulin. Futher dissection of rare instances of insulin resistance requires sophisticated study of insulin-binding and postreceptor phenomena. The so-called brittle type I diabetic child, in reality, most often is the child for whom family disruption and emotional factors lead to irregularity in diet, activity, and insulin administration, along with the metabolic consequences of emotional distress. Physiologic insulin resistance can occur during puberty, when insulin requirements may increase to 2 U/kg/day.

Hypoglycemia

Coma or convulsions as a result of hypoglycemia are common complications of diabetes management, which affect up to one third of diabetic children. Hypoglycemia occurs in the presence of unanticipated exercise, diminished food intake, or excessive insulin administration. The loss of glucagon secretion as a counterregulatory factor during the natural history of type I diabetes may be significant.

Organ-Specific Complications

The major goals in diabetic management are the facilitation of normal physical and emotional growth and the development and postponement or actual prevention of the microangiopathic and neuropathic complications of the disease. Signs of microangiopathy are readily observed in many children within 5 to 10 years after the clinical onset of diabetes, although the actual clinical consequences are but rarely seen in childhood. Individuals caring for insulin-dependent diabetic children therefore must constantly recall the consequences of the disease in later life and the resulting overriding importance of establishing and maintaining optimal metabolic control.

REFERENCES

1. Blohme B: Home blood glucose monitoring—the key to good control, Acta Med Scand [Suppl] 671:29, 1983.
2. Bolli GB and Gerich JE: The "dawn phenomenon"—a common occurrence in both non-insulin-dependent and insulin-dependent diabetes mellitus, N Engl J Med 310:746, 1984.
3. Daneman D et al: Severe hypoglycemia in children with insulin-dependent diabetes mellitus: frequency and predisposing factors, J Pediatr 115:681, 1989.
4. Maclaren NK: How, when, and why to predict IDDM, Diabetes 37:1591, 1988.
5. Östman J: Can adequate control of diabetes prevent the development of vascular complications? Acta Med Scand [Suppl] 671:5, 1983.
6. Peterson CM, editor: Symposium on non-enzymatic glycosylation and browning reactions, Diabetes 31(suppl 3):11, 1982.
7. Rotter JI and Rimoin DL: Genetics. In Brownlee M, editor: Diabetes mellitus, vol I, New York, 1981, Garland STPM Press.
8. Tchobroutsky G: Metabolic control and diabetic complications. In Brownlee M, editor: Diabetes mellitus, vol V, New York, 1981, Garland STPM Press.
9. Travis LB: An instructional aid on juvenile diabetes mellitus, ed 6, Austin, Tex, 1980, American Diabetes Association.

SUGGESTED READINGS

Gottesman I, Mandarino L, and Gerich J: Use of glucose uptake and glucose clearance for the evaluation of insulin action in vivo, Diabetes 33:184, 1984.

Olson OC: Diagnosis and management of diabetes mellitus: a clinical manual for medical students, residents, and primary care physicians, Philadelphia, 1981, Lea & Febiger.

Reaven GM: Insulin-dependent diabetes mellitus: metabolic characteristics, Metabolism 29:445, 1980.

Schade DS et al: Intensive insulin therapy, Princeton, NJ, 1983, Excerpta Medica, Inc.

Scherbaum WA: Diabetes insipidus in children. IV. A possible autoimmune type with vasopressin cell antibodies, J Pediatr 107:922, 1985.

198

Diaper Rash

Gregory S. Liptak

Diaper rash is the most common skin disorder of infants and toddlers. In a survey of pediatricians in private practice, 4% of all children seen from birth to 3 years of age were diagnosed as having diaper rash.[11] Similarly, a survey of suburban infants[13] who were not being treated at a health facility revealed that 25% had some diaper dermatitis; 4% of the sample had a rash that was classified as severe. The greatest frequency occurs in infants between 9 and 12 months of age.[1,13] Diaper rash is not a single disorder but represents the reaction of the skin in a local area to a host of factors, both local and systemic, and on occasion may result from serious illness. Despite its high frequency, few scientific studies have been performed on either the causes or treatment of this problem, and old wives' tales regarding both persist.[8]

ETIOLOGY

Four factors have been associated with the occurrence of diaper rash. These include (1) skin wetness, (2) elevated pH level, (3) fecal enzymes, and (4) microorganisms.[2,9,17] Wet skin has been shown experimentally to have greater friction, less cohesiveness, and higher permeability. In one study,[10] infants whose diapers had been changed eight or more times during the day (and presumably were dryer) had less rash than those whose diapers were changed less often. Diapers made with water-absorbent gel material (usually cross-linked sodium polyacrylates) have been shown to decrease the occurrence of diaper rash.[3,12,15]

The normal pH concentration of the skin is between 4.5 and 5.5. Elevated pH levels increase irritation and have been associated with more severe diaper rash. Although ammonia, which once was believed to be the primary irritant causing diaper rash,[14] may play a role in increasing the pH level, it is no longer considered to be the major factor.

Normal stool contains enzymes such as proteases and lipases that inflame skin and increase permeability to substances such as bile salts, which further worsen the inflammation. Infants with more frequent bowel movements have a higher prevalence of diaper dermatitis. Infants who are breast-fed have lower levels of enzymes in their stools and a lower occurrence of diaper rash.

The most important microorganism found on the skin of infants with diaper rash is *Candida albicans*.[4] This yeast, which produces a protease that penetrates the skin, can (1) cause a primary infection, (2) be a secondary invader in systemic conditions such as seborrheic dermatitis, and (3) be found in many infants with nonspecific diaper rash. Even a small number of *Candida* organisms can cause significant infection. The use of oral or parenteral antibiotics can increase the number of *Candida* organisms on the skin (as well as the frequency of stools) and contribute to the occurrence of diaper rash.[7] *Staphylococcus aureus* also has been isolated as a secondary invader of systemic illness such as atopic dermatitis; however, it does not appear to be a common primary pathogen in other forms of diaper rash.[14]

PATHOLOGY

A few histopathologic studies of diaper rash have been described; however, most of these have dealt with unusual or chronic cases. The more common diaper rashes are believed to manifest nonspecific inflammatory changes.

HISTORY

Historical factors that may help determine the cause for diaper rash include duration of the rash; associated symptoms (e.g., diarrhea); type of diaper used; frequency of changing; method of laundering (if cloth diapers are used); use of watertight coverings such as plastic (rubber) pants; past illness (especially dermatologic, allergic, infectious); use of medications (e.g., antibiotics), including the therapy for the rash; exposure to contagious disease (e.g., scabies, varicella); and a family history of illness (e.g., psoriasis, allergy).

PHYSICAL EXAMINATION

Although diaper rashes can be classified by presentation (appearance and location), this approach should be viewed with caution because one agent (e.g., *C. albicans*) can lead to different presentations and a single presentation may be caused by many agents (acting either alone or with other agents).

There are three common distribution patterns for diaper rash. *Chafing* (irritative or ammoniacal) dermatitis (Fig. 198-1) is an erythematous desquamative rash involving the convex surfaces that touch the diaper and spare the inguinal folds. There is mild erythema with or without papules. The skin has a shiny, glazed appearance. This rash is associated with the irritants mentioned previously. Prolonged contact with water (uncontaminated urine) probably facilitates the production of all diaper rashes, especially those in this category. Meatitis (urethritis) may be seen in boys with this type of diaper rash. Diaper rashes that have persisted for more than 72 hours usually are found to have significant *Candida* involvement.

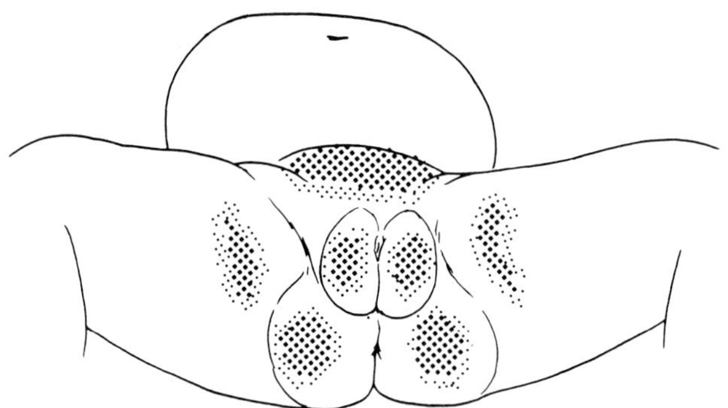

Fig. 198-1 Irritative pattern of diaper dermatitis.

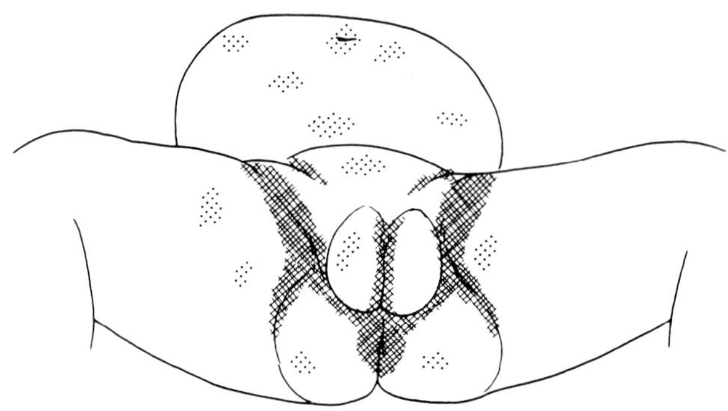

Fig. 198-2 Intertriginous pattern of diaper dermatitis.

Atopic dermatitis may have the same distribution as chafing as can zinc deficiency, Kawasaki disease and Wiskott-Aldrich syndrome. The eczematoid appearance with lichenification (thickening), pruritus, and occurrence of the atopic dermatitis elsewhere on the child should help substantiate this diagnosis. Diaper rash caused by atopic dermatitis is uncommon in children younger than 6 months of age.

The second pattern of diaper dermatitis involves skinfolds and spares convex surfaces (Fig. 198-2). Rashes involving the perianal area only are common in the neonatal period and may be the result of irritation from diarrhea (and are especially common in children with diarrhea secondary to disaccharidase deficiency). They also may be caused by infection with *C. albicans*.

Moist, macerated symmetric eruptions in the skinfolds and creases (Fig. 198-2) may be the result of seborrhea or *intertrigo*, an ill-defined entity. Both commonly are infected secondarily by *C. albicans*, especially when satellite lesions are present. The classic primary candidal (monilial) diaper rash has this pattern with bright red confluent lesions, often with raised borders, and occasionally with pustular-vesicular satellite lesions on the trunk and legs. Other areas, such as the folds of the neck, the postauricular area, and the oral mucosa (thrush), may be involved. Dermatitis caused by *Candida* organisms usually is painful and tender. Letterer-Siwe disease (histiocytosis) may have the same skin rash distribution as seborrhea or *Candida* infections but is more papular and more likely to be ulcerated. It also fails to respond to conventional therapy; the child may have constitutional symptoms such as malaise, and abnormal physical findings such as hepatosplenomegaly may be present. *Seborrheic dermatitis*, which also has been termed psoriaform napkin dermatitis, is characterized by beefy red confluent erythema with scaling involving the entire diaper area; however, the intertriginous areas are more prominently involved. The rash looks worse than it appears to feel to the child. Some of these infants have a family history of psoriasis; true psoriasis will develop in approximately 3% as they get older.

The third major distribution pattern of diaper dermatitis is shown in Fig. 198-3. Erythema in this distribution has been termed *tide mark dermatitis* and is believed to be related to frequent cycles of wetting and drying. Irritation from diapers that are too tight (constrictive) and that may have an elastic band also can lead to a similar rash.

Diaper rashes that do not fit any of these patterns, for example, from herpes simplex virus infection, also occur. In one study the less a rash looked like Fig. 198-1, the more likely it was to be associated with *Candida* organisms.[4] Diaper dermatitis from any cause can become secondarily infected with *Staphylococcus* or *Streptococcus* organisms, leading to impetigo or bullous impetigo.

DIFFERENTIAL DIAGNOSIS

Systemic conditions such as seborrhea, atopic dermatitis, primary herpes simplex infection, psoriasis, varicella, miliaria, and scabies may begin or occur with great intensity in the diaper area. Such predilection for the diaper area probably represents the Koebner (isomorphic) response in which the skin lesions of a systemic illness concentrate on areas previously injured by other factors, for example, friction.[8]

In addition to the aforementioned conditions, histiocytosis (Letterer-Siwe disease), acrodermatitis enteropathica, congenital syphilis, granuloma gluteale infantum, and Wiskott-Aldrich syndrome may lead to rashes that are prominent in the diaper area. Kawasaki syndrome may manifest as a red, desquamating perineal eruption, often during the first week after onset of the syndrome[5] (see Chapter 222). Serious illness always must be considered in the child with an atypical or a severe rash, as well as in the child who fails to respond to customary therapy. For instance, the child with severe "seborrhea" may have histiocytosis; fulminant atopic dermatitis may be the result of Wiskott-Aldrich syndrome; and severe, persistent, and recurrent infections with *Candida* organisms may (albeit rarely) result from immunodeficiency, including infection with human immunodeficiency virus (HIV) or diabetes mellitus. The physician should suspect child (including sexual) abuse or neglect in the child who has lesions in the diaper area (especially burns) that are inconsistent with the history provided.

LABORATORY FINDINGS

Laboratory tests generally are not indicated for most diaper rashs. Those that may be helpful in identifying the cause of a diaper rash include a potassium hydroxide preparation and a fungal culture of skin scrapings for *Candida* organisms, a bacterial culture for *Staphylococcus* organisms, a mineral oil

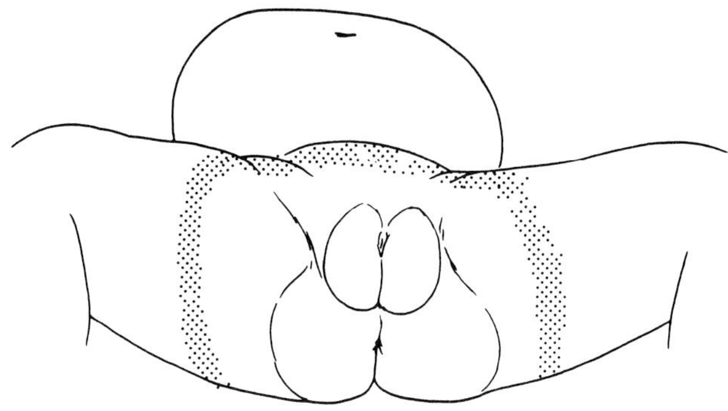

Fig. 198-3 Constrictive pattern of diaper dermatitis.

slide preparation for scabies, a serum zinc level (to rule out acrodermatitis enteropathica), serologic tests for syphilis, and roentgenograms of the skull and long bones for evidence of child abuse. Laboratory studies for atopic dermatitis, Wiskott-Aldrich syndrome, and histiocytosis are discussed elsewhere in this text. Rarely, a skin biopsy in cases in which the diaper rash is atypical or unresponsive to therapy may be useful.

MANAGEMENT

Because most diaper rashes, whatever the cause, are worsened by prolonged contact with wet or soiled diapers, the initial step in their management should be to keep the skin free of such diapers as much as possible. However, total abstinence from diapers is impractical; thus most clinicians recommend that during therapy the diapers be changed frequently (at least eight times a day, using diapers with absorbent gel material) and kept off as much as possible and that plastic pants that retain water not be used.

Most systemic conditions such as scabies, atopic dermatitis, and varicella can be managed for the diaper area as they are for other parts of the skin. Seborrheic dermatitis, however, is an exception. Because it is so often secondarily infected with *Candida* organisms, measures to treat the yeast must be undertaken as well. For this and other diaper rashes in which *Candida* organisms are present, topical nystatin, miconazole, clotrimazole, haloprogin, or ketoconazole should be applied. Miconazole has the advantage of requiring only twice-daily applications, is less irritating than nystatin, and probably is more effective. It also is more expensive. Gentian violet also is effective but is extremely messy. The simultaneous use of 1% hydrocortisone usually hastens healing. Steroids more potent than 1% hydrocortisone should never be used in the diaper area because diapers form an occlusive dressing. Their chronic use may lead to granuloma gluteale infantum (a rash characterized by purple granulomatous nodules), skin atrophy, telangiectasis, striae, irritation, and, systemically, Cushing syndrome. The effectiveness of oral nystatin in the therapy of candidal diaper rash is uncertain. In a controlled study Dixon and coworkers[4] found that oral nystatin did not significantly decrease the recurrence of candidal diaper rash.

For irritative diaper rashes, changing diapers frequently and washing the skin between diaper changes with plain water and allowing it to dry usually are the only interventions needed. The use of diapers with absorbent gel materials has been shown to decrease wetness in the diaper area and may hasten the disappearance of a diaper dermatitis.[12] Scrubbing the rash or diaper area should be discouraged; a soft cloth with water should provide sufficient cleansing in most cases. A barrier ointment that contains zinc oxide or vitamins A and D may help protect the skin from further irritation. Rinsing cloth diapers in methylbenzethonium chloride (Diaperene), a bacteriostatic agent, or in a vinegar solution (1 ounce in a gallon of water) has been shown to reduce recurrences.[6] Agents to acidify the urine (cranberry juice, vitamin C), cornstarch, and ointments with vitamins A and D are widely used; however, there is no experimental evidence that they are effective. Eliminating fabric softeners and changing detergents may be effective in some cases, but this approach also is scientifically undocumented. In cases with significant inflammation, 1% hydrocortisone may promote healing. The meatitis that occurs in this form of rash may be treated with topical antibiotics to prevent stricture by use of an ophthalmic solution applied by partially inserting the tip of the dispensing bottle into the urethra every 4 to 6 hours.[16]

Many more children have been harmed by well-intended diaper rash therapies than have ever been harmed by the rash itself. Boric acid, mercury compounds, and pentachlorophenol used in the treatment and prevention of irritative diaper rash have led to illness and death in infants.[7] Talcum powder never should be used because inhalation of a large quantity can produce serious, even fatal, pulmonary damage. The dangers of topical steroids have already been mentioned. Therefore prudent use of therapeutic agents is necessary to avoid harm. The use of commercial diaper wipes, which contain an emollient and cleansing agent, has been increasing. Their role with regard to diaper dermatitis is uncertain.

PREVENTION

If there were no diapers, there would be no diaper rashes. Because the complete elimination of diapers is unacceptable, alternatives to keep the skin dry such as changing as soon as the diaper becomes wet or soiled and avoiding plastic pants have been recommended.

The importance of the type of diaper in the prevention of diaper rash is controversial. In an uncontrolled study, Wiener[16] found that children who wore cloth diapers had the fewest occurrences of diaper rash when compared with those who wore conventional cloth diapers with plastic pants or those who wore commercial plastic-lined diapers. In an earlier uncontrolled study, however, Grant and co-workers[5] found that infants whose cloth diapers were laundered by a commercial firm were least likely to get rashes and those who wore cloth diapers that were laundered at home were most likely to get rashes; those who wore conventional disposable diapers were between these two groups. In a controlled, blinded study, Stein[16] found that a rash was less likely to develop in infants who wore disposable diapers than in those who wore cloth diapers. None of these studies examined the frequency of diaper changes, which may account for the discrepancies in results. Most recent studies have shown that diapers with absorbent gel are associated with the lowest incidence of diaper rash.[3,10,12,15]

Although plastic diapers with absorbent gel material have been shown to decrease the occurrence of diaper rash, consideration should be given to the effect of plastic diapers on the environment. It is estimated that commercial nonbiodegradable diapers comprise 2% to 3% of landfills. The cost of their disposal, which is borne by all citizens, should be considered when recommending their use.

Breast-feeding and frequent diaper changes have been associated with a lower occurrence of diaper rash. Both should be recommended. Because antibiotics may increase the risk for diaper dermatitis, their use should be carefully monitored. The physician should be certain that other recommendations do not harm the child.

REFERENCES

1. Benjamin L: Clinical correlates with diaper dermatitis, Pediatrician 14(S1):21, 1987.
2. Berg RW, Buckingham KW, and Stewart RL: Etiologic factors in diaper dermatitis: the role of urine, Pediatr Dermatol 3:102, 1986.
3. Campbell RL et al: Effects of diaper types on diaper dermatitis associated with diarrhea and antibiotic use of children in day-care centers, Pediatr Dermatol 5:83, 1988.
4. Dixon PN, Warin RP, and English MP: Alimentary *Candida albicans* and napkin rashes, Br J Dermatol 86:458, 1972.
5. Friter BS and Lucky AW: The perineal eruption of Kawasaki syndrome, Arch Dermatol 124:1805, 1988.
6. Grant WW, Street L, and Fearnow RG: Diaper rashes in infancy: studies on the effects of various methods of laundering, Clin Pediatr 12:714, 1973.
7. Honig PJ et al: Amoxicillin and diaper dermatitis, J Am Acad Dermatol 19:275, 1988.
8. Jacobs AH: Eruptions in the diaper area, Pediatr Clin North Am 25:209, 1978.
9. Jenson HB and Shapiro ED: Primary herpes simplex virus infection of a diaper rash, Pediatr Infect Dis J 6:1136, 1987.
10. Jordan WE et al: Diaper dermatitis: frequency and severity among a general infant population, Pediatr Dermatol 3:198, 1986.
11. Hurwitz S: Clinical pediatric dermatology, Philadelphia, 1981, WB Saunders Co.
12. Lane AT, Rehder PA, and Helm K: Evaluations of diapers containing absorbing gelling material with conventional diapers in newborn infants, Am J Dis Child 144:315, 1990.
13. Leyden JJ and Klingman AM: The role of microorganisms in diaper dermatitis, Arch Dermatol 114:56, 1978.
14. Leyden JJ et al: Urinary ammonia and ammonia-producing microorganisms in infants with and without diaper dermatitis, Arch Dermatol 113:1678, 1977.
15. Seymour JL et al: Clinical effects of diaper types on the skin of normal infants and infants with ectopic dermatitis, J Am Acad Dermatol 17:988, 1987.
16. Stein H: Incidence of diaper rash when using cloth and disposable diapers, J Pediatr 101:721, 1982.
17. Weston WL, Lane AT, and Weston JA: Diaper dermatitis: current concepts, Pediatrics 66:532, 1980.
18. Wiener FW: The relationship of diapers to diaper rashes in the one-month-old infant, J Pediatr 95:422, 1979.

199

Down Syndrome

Eileen PG Vining

Down syndrome (DS) is the most common cause of mental retardation associated with chromosomal aberration, accounting for approximately 20% of persons in institutions for the retarded. Although probably described as early as the seventh century, it was John Langdon Down who, in 1866, recognized the multiple characteristics of the syndrome. He also knew it was common, occurring in more than 10% of the retarded patients he saw. His theory that these children represented a form of retrogression to the Mongoloid race was clearly influenced by darwinian theory and was meant to reflect a belief in the unity of the human species. The more pejorative connotation of mongolian idiocy developed later. Down's description of the physical stigmata of the syndrome was quite accurate, but he went further, recognizing other medical complications (e.g., cardiac anomalies and increased susceptibility to infection) and the capabilities of the children as well.

ETIOLOGY

Down recognized the prenatal origin of the abnormality, but the extra acrocentric chromosome number 21 (trisomy 21) was not defined until 1959 by Lejeune and associates.

There are three different types of DS, based on their cytogenetics: pure trisomy 21, translocation of chromosome number 21, and mosaicism for trisomy 21. Approximately 95% of cases are caused by trisomy 21 in which chromosomes do not separate properly (nondisjunction). The least frequent cause of DS is mosaicism, which occurs in approximately 4% of affected children. This is probably the result of an error in one of the initial cell divisions. There have been no instances in which the clear-cut clinical syndrome has been present without chromosomal corroboration.

EPIDEMIOLOGY

The incidence of DS is in the order of 0.8/1000 live births. Before more extensive use of amniocentesis and therapeutic abortions, more than 3000 children with DS were born each year in the United States. The major factor increasing the likelihood of having a child with DS is advancing maternal age; 20% to 25% of affected children are born to women older than 40 years of age. Thus 1 in 100 children born to these women will have DS and 1 in 250 children born to women older than 35 years of age will have DS. Controversy still exists, however, with respect to the effect of advancing paternal age. Discussion currently is focused on the impact of environmental preconditioning (multiple environmental events increasing susceptibility) and intergenerational effects as important etiologic factors.[9]

The maternal age effect may be explained by a variety of hypotheses: (1) meiotic nondisjunction is constant at all ages, but the older uterus is less selective in rejecting trisomic conceptuses; (2) delays between intercourse and ovulation in older couples result in fertilization of an "aged ovum," which is more likely to experience meiotic nondisjunction; (3) aging itself is responsible for increasing the frequency of errors in the meitotic division of the ovum (as occurs in all cells), thereby increasing the rate of nondisjunction; and (4) cumulative exposure to environmental agents damage the spindle mechanism, eventually producing meiotic errors and nondisjunction.

DIAGNOSIS

Although there has been some evidence that low maternal serum alpha-fetoprotein may serve as a screening test for DS, it is not the direct biochemical test needed, because it lacks both high sensitivity and high specificity. Amniocentesis remains the most sensitive test, although chorionic villus sampling approaches it with 97.8% versus 99.4% accuracy.[15,16] Some children are easily diagnosed when newborns. Those with the recognizable features of a flat facial profile (90%), abundant nuchal skinfolds (80%), short and dysplastic ears (60%), hypotonia (80%), shortened palpebral fissures (80%), an enlarged and protruding tongue, Brushfield spots in the iris, epicanthal folds, and a wide space between the first and second toes provide little in the way of diagnostic dilemmas.[8] However, the syndrome is correctly identified in only about 75% of referrals to genetic clinics or consultants. Clinical criteria have allowed 90% accuracy, but they depend on individual subjective interpretations. A diagnostic index for DS was established by Rex and Preus,[14] with which 95% of patients who are suspected of having DS could be appropriately classified. A definitive diagnosis can be made from peripheral blood analysis; bone marrow cell culture and chromosomal analyses can yield results in 2 to 5 hours.

COUNSELING

The practitioner is faced with two counseling situations when a child is born with DS. The family must be told about the diagnosis, and a referral for genetic counseling usually is indicated.

Sensitive and immediate counseling with both parents

present is advisable.[13] Families quickly perceive the stigmata and are justifiably hostile when their questions about their child are met with evasiveness. Numerous surveys[3] indicate that early discussion of the problem in a controlled, sympathetic, and knowledgeable environment is preferable. The person who brings this news to a family must do so in a way that (1) can help them explore the impact that such a special child will have on the family, (2) will allow the family to understand the medical and intellectual problems of children with DS, and (3) will provide the initial impetus for nurturing, which is so vital to all handicapped children. There is no justification for the physician to make "protective" judgments that would discourage bonding and encourage early institutionalization. Families usually can be sufficiently supported to enable them to care for their child at home.

After the diagnosis is made, it has become common practice to refer families for genetic counseling. Important, practical information should be imparted thereby to a family and the referring physician. In particular, a chromosomal analysis will indicate the specific aberration and the risk for recurrence. In the majority of cases (nondisjunction trisomy 21), the risk of having another child with DS is 1% to 2%. When translocation is the basis for the problem, however, it is necessary to determine whether either parent is a carrier of the chromosome defect. In this instance the risk of recurrence and of having children who are carriers of the defect varies considerably and must be determined on an individual basis. The advent of amniocentesis also has influenced counseling. Prenatal screening for DS has been shown to be cost effective for women 34 years of age or older when therapeutic abortion follows detection. However, the efficacy and impact of genetic counseling must be carefully assessed, inasmuch as it appears to influence subsequent reproductive plans in only about 50% of cases; perhaps only 50% of those families counseled retain concepts and facts over time. The primary practitioner must realize that sending a family for this kind of counseling may not have adequate impact and that subsequent discussions with the family regarding their reproductive plans might prove very effective.

ASSOCIATED MEDICAL PROBLEMS

Although intellectual limitation is an almost universal finding in patients with DS, there is clear evidence that other medical problems are closely linked to the syndrome and seriously affect the patient's life-style and life span. The practitioner must be familiar with these problems to be able to provide comprehensive care for DS patients.

Congenital Anomalies

Congenital heart malformations were found in 40% of patients with DS. Approximately one third have several cardiac lesions.[12] Endocardial cushion defect was found to be the most common (43%), ventricular septal defect (VSD) was noted in 32%, secundum atrial septal defect (ASD) in 10%, tetralogy of Fallot in 6%, and isolated patent ductus arteriosus in 4%. Of these patients 10% died for reasons unrelated to surgical intervention, with 75% of that number succumbing to pulmonary disease or congestive heart failure before 2 years of age. Twenty-five percent of patients underwent surgery. Mortality was 40% in infants younger than 6 months of age, with overall surgical mortality at about 25%. Pulmonary vascular disease developed in about one third of patients with endocardial cushion defect or VSD, with the average age of onset at 4 and 14 years of age, respectively. Routine cardiac evaluation at a young age is therefore advisable for all children with DS.

The other major congenital anomaly seen in DS patients (2% to 3%) is duodenal obstruction caused by atresia. Many also have an annular pancreas.

Immunologic Problems

Children with DS, especially those with congenital heart disease, have a high incidence of infection. This probably is due both to pulmonary abnormalities and to disturbances in defense mechanisms. Some disturbance in neutrophil function appears to exist, and dysgammaglobulinemia (increased IgG, IgA, and IgD, decreased IgM), as seen in the older person with DS, may result from a persistent antigen-stimulating antibody production. A premature aging of the thymus-dependent system also has been noted. Approximately 30% of patients with DS who live in institutions have Australia antigen positivity, and many experience chronic anicteric hepatitis. Serum hepatitis B virus DNA also is seen with increased frequency. There has been little experience with the new hepatitis vaccine in this population, but it may be possible to decrease this incidence of seropositivity and infection. Immunologic abnormalities also may be responsible for the high incidence of leukemia (1%) in children with DS. It is not clear if children with DS who undergo bone marrow transplantation are at increased risk for failure of the procedure; it does appear to be offered less frequently as a therapeutic alternative in this population.[4]

Pulmonary Problems

Compared with children who have similar cardiac problems, children with DS appear to have more pulmonary hypertension, which may be due to abnormal capillary morphology. Small facial and oropharyngeal structures, along with muscular hypotonia, also may produce some upper airway obstruction, which in some infants has led to cor pulmonale and heart failure. This may be helped in severe situations by the temporary use of a tracheostomy.[11]

Endocrine and Growth Disturbances

Thyroid dysfunction, predominantly hypothyroidism, occurs in approximately 20% of patients with DS; thyroid antibodies can be detected in about one third of patients. Growth patterns for children with DS are abnormal: by 36 months of age, most children with DS fall below the third percentile. Growth between 4 and 6 years of age appears to be within the normal range. Growth grids standardized for children with DS should be used to monitor anthropometric change properly.[5] Females with DS may be fertile, and numerous pregnancies have been reported. Males with DS appear to be infertile and have low serum testosterone levels.

Ophthalmologic Complications

Cataracts are observed in more than 50% of DS patients, although they are congenital in only 3% to 11% and may predispose for retinal detachment and poor visual outcome. Keratoconus occurs in 1% to 8% of cases. Myopia is quite common (30% to 35%), as is strabismus (12% to 23%). Approximately 5% are blind.

Hearing and Speech Problems

The external ear is abnormally shaped in more than 50% of children with DS. Often the external canal is very narrow and precludes adequate examination. Possibly as many as two thirds of patients are found to have middle-ear effusion in at least one ear. Mild to moderate hearing loss (15 to 50 dB) has been demonstrated in 40% to 80% of patients. Language development in children with DS often is not commensurate with that of other cognitive skills. Various theories suggest that this deficit is the result of inadequate vocabulary building, inadequate demand on the child to use language to relate to the world, and the disfluency that may result from anatomic abnormalities of the mouth and face. Unfortunately, partial glossectomy does not appear to improve speech intelligibility.

Neurologic and Skeletal Problems

The etiology of muscular hypotonia seen in DS patients has not been established. Investigators have tried to link it to low blood levels of serotonin and have treated infants with 5-hydroxytryptophan without conclusively positive results. Presenile dementia associated with the pathologic changes of Alzheimer disease may develop in older patients with DS; this occurs 6 to 10 times more frequently in this group than in the population as a whole, with 55% of DS persons between the ages of 50 and 59 years experiencing dementia.[10] Atlantoaxial instability is seen in 9% to 31% of children with DS, becoming symptomatic in approximately 1.5%. The American Academy of Pediatrics recommends that children with DS be screened between 5 and 6 years of age. If the distance between the odontoid process of the axis and the anterior arch of the atlas exceeds 4.5 mm or if the odontoid is abnormal, activities that involve hyperextension, radical flexion, or direct pressure should be restricted. Generally a significant history of neurologic signs from cord compression is present more than 1 month before major difficulties ensue. It should be noted that no problems were ever actually reported in children with DS who participated in the Special Olympics before these rules went into effect.[6]

Psychological and Behavioral Complications

Unfortunately, children with DS often are stereotyped as being placid, cuddly, adorable mimics. In reality they have the same chance of developing emotional disturbances as do normal children (approximately 15%). Others have found that 38% of children with DS have a significant behavioral disorder, versus 49% in other forms of mental retardation; children with DS also appear easier to manage. Careful evaluation of the temperaments of normal infants and of those with DS of comparable mental age finds the latter to be equally active, adaptable, distractible, and persistent.[2] Parents must be counseled to consider the developmental stage of their child and to expect the wide range in behavior that is appropriate for their mental age. Parents also must be encouraged to provide appropriate guidelines and discipline for their child's behavior.

INTELLECTUAL DEVELOPMENT

Most children with DS function in the moderately retarded range, with 40% achieving intelligence quotient (IQ) levels in excess of 50. Again, there is no stereotype, and the clinician must realize that the IQs of these children are symmetrically distributed around a mean of 41.7 for males and 49.9 for females. Some studies have indicated that intellectual development peaks at an early age in those with DS and decreases with advancing age. This may be related to the increased incidence of presenile dementia, but it probably reflects the reduction in stimulation that comes with leaving special educational facilities. Families must be told that motor development may lag to a considerable extent behind mental development. This is very important in the early years, when families focus on such feats as crawling and walking. These children must receive stimulation appropriate to their intellectual capacity, regardless of their motor deficits.

TREATMENT AND HABILITATION

Although many drug therapies (some to improve motor abilities and some for cognitive enhancement) have been suggested for the management of children with DS, none has been demonstrated clearly to be of benefit. Clinical therapeutic trials with use of thyroid, vitamins (especially B_6), 5-hydroxytryptophan, glutamic acid, and sicca cell therapy (injection of embryonic cells into muscle) have failed.[17]

Surgical approaches have been increasingly used to improve both function and appearance. These include partial glossectomy; lateral canthoplexy; nose, cheek, or chin augmentation; otoplasty; and cheiloplasty. There is some evidence that these children are subsequently viewed as both more attractive and more intelligent, raising the question of whether appearance may be a barrier to success.[18]

The child with DS must be aided in maximizing his or her potential through more standard means of habilitation. It has become increasingly clear that children raised in a nurturing home with adequate community services and support do better than those who are immediately institutionalized. This has been documented with respect to nutrition, growth, and age at reaching developmental milestones. There are exceptions, as with children who are seriously ill or with the family that has exhausted its resources in dealing with the problems encountered in raising a handicapped child with limited potential.

Considerable controversy exists with respect to vigorous early infant stimulation and developmental training for retarded children, including those with DS. Proponents of this type of intervention argue that the immediate gains, which generally disappear over time, can be perpetuated if these concentrated efforts are sustained throughout infancy and childhood.[1]

OUTCOME

Advances in the treatment of infectious diseases and cardiac defects have improved the prognosis for patients with DS. Nonetheless, an overall death rate five to seven times that of the general population has been observed. However, 20% survive beyond 30 years of age, 8% beyond age 40 years, and 2.6% beyond age 50 years; life span also may be increased in those who have not been institutionalized.[7]

Families worry about how their child with DS will adapt in the real world. The Education for All Handicapped Children Act of 1975 (Public Law 94-142) ensures appropriate public education for the child; group homes for the handicapped have been established in the community as an alternative to living with their own family; and many persons with DS achieve reasonable levels of social function and independence.

REFERENCES

1. Aronson M and Fallstrom K: Immediate and long-term effects of developmental training in children with Down's syndrome, Dev Med Child Neurol 19:489, 1977.
2. Baron J: Temperament profile of children with Down's syndrome, Dev Med Child Neurol 14:640, 1972.
3. Carr J: Mongolism: telling the parents, Dev Med Child Neurol 12:213, 1970.
4. Churchill LR: Bone marrow transplantation, physician bias, and Down syndrome: ethical reflections, J Pediatr 114:87, 1989 (editorial).
5. Cronk CE: Growth of children with Down's syndrome: birth to age 3 years, Pediatrics 61:564, 1978.
6. Davidson RG: Atlantoaxial instability in individuals with Down syndrome: a fresh look at the evidence, Pediatrics 81:857, 1988.
7. Demissie A, Ayres RC, and Briggs R: Old age in Down's syndrome, J Royal Soc Med 81:740, 1988.
8. Hall B: Mongolism in newborn infants: an examination of the criteria for recognition and some speculations on the pathogenic activity of the chromosomal abnormality, Clin Pediatr 5:4, 1966.
9. Janerich DT and Bracken MB: Epidemiology of trisomy 21: a review and theoretical analysis, J Chron Dis 39:1079, 1986.
10. Lai F and Williams RS: A prospective study of Alzheimer disease in Down syndrome, Arch Neurol 46:849, 1989.
11. Levine OR and Simpser M: Alveolar hypoventilation and cor pulmonale associated with chronic airway obstruction in infants with Down syndrome, Clin Pediatr 21:25, 1982.
12. Park SC et al: Down syndrome with congenital heart malformation, Am J Dis Child 131:29, 1977.
13. Pueschel S and Murphy A: Counseling parents of infants with Down's syndrome, Postgrad Med 58:90, 1975.
14. Rex AP and Preus M: A diagnostic index for Down syndrome, J Pediatr 100:903, 1982.
15. Rhoads GG et al: The safety and efficacy of chorionic villus sampling for early prenatal diagnosis of cytogenetic abnormalities, N Engl J Med 320:609, 1989.
16. Schier KJ: Screening for Down's syndrome, Can Med Assoc J 137:989, 1987.
17. Share JB: A review of drug treatment for Down's syndrome persons, Am J Ment Defic 80:388, 1976.
18. Strauss RP et al: Social perceptions of the effects of Down syndrome facial surgery: a school-based study and ratings by normal adolescents, Plast Reconstr Surg 81:841, 1988.

SUGGESTED READINGS

Ferencz C et al: Congenital cardiovascular malformations associated with chromosome abnormalities: an epidemiologic study, J Pediatr 114:79, 1989.

Gath A and Gumley D: Behavior problems in retarded children with special reference to Down's syndrome, Br J Psychol 149:156, 1986.

Schapiro MB et al: Dementia in Down's syndrome: cerebral glucose utilization, neuropsychological assessment, and neuropathology, Neurology 38:938, 1988.

Traboulsi EI et al: Infantile glaucoma in Down's syndrome (trisomy 21), Am J Ophthalmol 105:389, 1988.

van Ditzhuijsen TJ et al: Hepatitis B virus infection in an institution for the mentally retarded, Am J Epidemiol 128:629, 1988.

VanDyke DC et al: Cell therapy in children with Down syndrome: a retrospective study, Pediatrics 85:79, 1990.

200

Drug Eruptions

Donald P. Lookingbill

The clinical expression of drug eruptions is highly variable. Knowing that systemically administered drugs can cause almost any kind of rash leads to the following general principle in dermatologic diagnosis: "For any rash, think of drugs." The types of skin reactions caused by drugs include morbilliform eruptions, urticaria, erythema multiforme, erythema nodosum, vasculitis, photosensitivity reactions, acneform eruptions, alopecia, blistering disorders, fixed drug eruptions, lichenoid reactions, and drug-induced lupus erythematosus.[2,8] Tables in Fitzpatrick and co-workers' general dermatology text[8] conveniently list the drugs most commonly responsible for each of these different types of eruptions. This chapter deals only with the three most commonly found in children. In order of decreasing frequency, they are morbilliform eruptions, urticaria, and erythema multiforme.

Table 200-1 *Allergic Skin Reactions to Drugs*

DRUG	REACTION RATE (REACTIONS PER 100 RECIPIENTS)
Amoxicillin	5.1
Trimethoprim-sulfamethoxazole	3.4
Ampicillin	3.3
Blood	2.2
Cephalosporins	2.1
Semisynthetic penicillins	2.1
Erythromycin	2.0
Penicillin G	1.9
Allopurinol	0.8
Barbiturates	0.4
Diazepam	0.04

From Bigby M et al: Drug-induced cutaneous reactions: a report from the Boston Collaborative Drug Surveillance Program on 15,438 consecutive inpatients, 1975 to 1982, JAMA 256:3358, 1986.

MORBILLIFORM ERUPTIONS

Etiology

A morbilliform eruption, which also is termed *exanthematous* or *maculopapular,* is the most common cutaneous expression of a drug reaction. Although a variety of drugs can cause this reaction, the more common drugs that cause morbilliform or urticarial eruptions are listed in Table 200-1.

History

The onset of a drug-induced morbilliform eruption usually is not immediate; rather it begins within several days of the initiation of the drug. Onset sometimes is delayed up to a week, but seldom longer. Because there are no laboratory tests to identify a responsible drug, heavy reliance is placed on the history. Patients receiving multiple drugs obviously present a problem. When trying to select a single drug from a list of many, the two variables to consider are (1) the temporal relationship between the drug and the rash and (2) the likelihood that a given drug can cause a drug eruption. For the latter, incidence data such as those in Table 200-1 are used.[1]

Itching usually is present but is not helpful as a diagnostic marker. Fever rarely is found.

Physical Findings

The eruption is generalized and comprised of brightly erythematous macules and papules that tend to be confluent in large areas. It usually starts proximally and proceeds distally, with the legs being the last to be involved and also the last to clear. Drug fever has been well described, but most drug eruptions are unaccompanied by an elevation in body temperature.

Laboratory Studies

Laboratory tests usually are not helpful. A peripheral blood eosinophilia sometimes is present and may heighten the suspicion for a drug reaction, but there are no laboratory tests to incriminate a specific drug.

Differential Diagnosis

For a generalized erythematous, "maculopapular" eruption, the major differential diagnosis is (1) a drug reaction, (2) a viral exanthem, or (3) a toxic erythema.

As the name *morbilliform* (measleslike) suggests, a viral exanthem and a drug eruption can be clinically indistinguishable. Often a drug eruption will be much more erythematous and more confluent, but not always. Other clinical information will help, including a drug history and the presence or absence of other viral signs and symptoms. Eosinophilia favors a drug etiology. Acute and convalescent serologic tests can be obtained for some viral infections so as to provide a retrospective diagnosis. In most cases, however, a presumptive diagnosis is made on the basis of the combined clinical data.

Examples of toxic erythema are scarlet fever, staphylococcal-induced scarlatiniform eruptions, and the mucocutaneous lymph node syndrome (Kawasaki disease). Features that help to distinguish these toxic erythemas from drug eruptions include a sandpaper-like roughened texture of the rash, mucous membrane involvement (scarlet fever and Kawasaki disease), the presence of fever, a focus of infection, and the presence of lymphadenopathy. Postinflammatory desquamation from the skin of the hands and feet often follows the rash of toxic erythema, but this is not specific. Drug eruptions and even viral exanthems also can involve the hands and feet, and if the inflammation has been sufficiently intense, desquamation will follow.

Management

When an offending agent is identified, it should be discontinued. If a patient is taking multiple drugs and it is not possible to be certain of the culprit, it is advisable to reduce the number of administered drugs to an absolute minimum and, whenever possible, to change any remaining possible offenders to alternative agents.

Therapy otherwise is directed toward the symptoms, with antihistamines being most commonly used for the pruritus. Topical agents usually are confined to moisturizing lotions, which are most helpful during the later, desquamative phase of the reaction. Topical steroids are of little value, and systemic steroids rarely are required.

Complications

Complications are primarily cutaneous. When large areas of skin are inflamed, increased body heat and water loss occur. In a patient already seriously ill, this could be a problem; for most patients, however, it is not.

There are mainly two consequences of guessing wrong and continuing an offending agent in the face of a drug eruption: cutaneous and renal. The cutaneous risk is that of progressive worsening of the rash, possibly resulting in a toxic epidermal necrolysis condition—a serious problem. Fortunately, this rarely occurs. In fact, sometimes a drug eruption clears even when the offending agent is continued. Of course, it is not desirable to do this if there is an alternative. The renal risk is that of allergic interstitial nephritis, an uncommon development usually associated with penicillins and celphalosporins but only rarely with other drugs.

Course

Drug eruptions clear with *time* after discontinuance of the responsible agent. It is important to realize that the time required for total clearing usually is 1 to 2 weeks and that the eruption actually may worsen for several days after the offending drug has been stopped.

If a responsible drug has been identified, the patient should be advised about the allergy and the medical record should be clearly labeled to that effect.

URTICARIA (HIVES)[4,5,7]

Etiology

Drug-induced hives can be immunologically mediated by either (1) immediate IgE reactions, usually within hours, or (2) delayed immune complexes that result in serum sickness–like reactions after 7 to 10 days. The immediate reactions are more common.

History

A precise cause usually is not found among patients with hives. When it is, it is determined from the history. The drug history is the most important but the most difficult to obtain, at least in outpatients. Because many patients and their parents tend to consider over-the-counter medications as unimportant, it often is helpful to ask about specific medications to help jog their memories. Aspirin is particularly important inasmuch as salicylates cause hives in some patients and aggravate them in as many as one third of all patients with urticaria, regardless of its cause. Whenever a drug is suspected, the physician must be aggressive and persistent in eliciting a medication history. Otherwise, some drugs invariably will be overlooked.

A history of associated symptoms also may be important. Itching nearly always is present. A history of obstructed airway or other anaphylactic symptoms suggests a more serious problem. Fever and arthralgias often accompany hives in serum sickness reactions, in which the two most common causes are drugs and viral hepatitis.

Physical Findings

Hives are skin lesions that are more easily recognized than described. They appear as edematous plaques, often with pale centers and red borders. They frequently assume geographic shapes and sometimes are confluent. The lesions may be scattered but usually are generalized. By definition an individual hive is transient, lasting less than 24 hours, although new hives may continuously develop. In serum sickness reactions, lymphadenopathy, in addition to fever and arthralgias, may be present.

Laboratory Studies

Drug-induced hives may be accompanied by an eosinophilia. To evaluate for hepatitis it is appropriate to obtain liver function tests in patients with hives and fever. In patients without fever, however, laboratory tests rarely are helpful in eliciting a cause, and they are of no help in implicating a specific drug.

Differential Diagnosis

The differential diagnosis of urticaria may be approached in two ways: (1) from the causes of hives per se and (2) from consideration of the cause of lesions sometimes mistaken as hives. As already mentioned, the cause of hives most often will not be determined. When a cause is found, it usually is drug related. Other causes include infections, physical modalities (e.g., cold, pressure, or sunlight), emotions, and, albeit rarely, foods. Tartrazine, a yellow food dye that cross-reacts with salicylates, has been implicated in some patients with chronic urticaria.

Lesions sometimes mistaken for hives include those seen in erythema multiforme and juvenile rheumatoid arthritis. The lesions in erythema multiforme are discussed later. The individual lesions in juvenile rheumatoid arthritis behave like hives in being transient but differ in their size (only 2 to 3 mm), color (typically salmon), and timing (usually appearing with fever spikes).

Management

Any suspected medication, including aspirin, should be discontinued. Symptomatic therapy usually is achieved with antihistamines given on a regular rather than on an as needed schedule. Hydroxyzine is the preferred agent, administered in doses of 10 to 25 mg four times daily.

Complications

Acute urticaria can rarely be accompanied by anaphylactic reactions that require more immediate therapy; usually, however, hives are more a nuisance than a morbid threat.

Course

Drug-induced hives usually clear within several days of discontinuing the responsible medication. As with any drug reaction, if a specific agent has been identified, the patient must be alerted to avoid that drug in the future. Because most hives are IgE mediated, rechallenge with the responsible drug is more likely to result in an anaphylactic response than is rechallenge in a patient with a previous morbilliform eruption.

ERYTHEMA MULTIFORME[3,6]

Etiology

Erythema multiforme has been ascribed to innumerable causes, which are poorly substantiated except for two: (1) drugs and (2) infection, primarily from *Mycoplasma pneumoniae* and recurrent herpes simplex. Circulating immune complexes have been detected in patients with erythema multiforme, a finding consistent with the concept that this distinctive cutaneous disorder represents an immunologic reaction.

History

Sulfonamides, penicillins, barbiturates, and hydantoin have been the drugs most commonly implicated in erythema multiforme; however, a history for all drugs should be elicited. Recurrent herpes simplex infection is the most common cause of recurrent erythema multiforme. The herpetic lesion usually precedes the erythema multiforme by a few days to a week or more. For the more extended intervals, the herpetic lesions may have healed by the time the patient comes for treatment, so that the history will be important. In about 50% of all cases, a cause will not be identifiable. In some patients, a febrile prodrome precedes the cutaneous eruption by 1 to 14 days.

Physical Findings

As the name suggests, this eruption is characterized by a variety of lesions, including erythematous plaques, blisters, and target or iris lesions. Hives sometimes are confused with target lesions. The difference is that a hive has only two zones of color—a central pale area surrounded by an erythematous halo. To meet the criteria for a target lesion, *three* zones must be present: a central dark area or blister, surrounded by a pale zone, surrounded by a peripheral rim of erythema. True target lesions are diagnostic for erythema multiforme. They are more frequently seen on the palms and soles but may occur anywhere. Typically, erythema multiforme is a strikingly symmetric eruption that favors the extremities. The disorder ranges in severity from mild to severe. In the severe form of the disease (Stevens-Johnson syndrome) the skin lesions are more extensive, and severe mucous membrane involvement usually is present, as well.

Laboratory Studies

A chest roentgenogram is appropriate to screen for pulmonary involvement, including that caused by *Mycoplasma* infection, which can be further confirmed by acute and convalescent cold agglutinin titers. For herpes simplex disease, if the responsible vesicular lesion is still present, its fluid can be examined for multinucleated giant cells (a Tzanck preparation) or cultured for herpesvirus. Laboratory evaluation usually is not helpful in drug-induced cases of erythema multiforme.

A complete blood cell count and urinalysis are recommended because erythema multiforme is accompanied occasionally by a leukocytosis and, although it is rare, by renal involvement.

In those cases in which the diagnosis is in doubt, a skin biopsy can be helpful. The blisters in erythema multiforme are subepidermal in location.

Differential Diagnosis

The skin reactions most commonly considered in the differential diagnosis are urticaria, viral exanthems, vasculitis, staphylococcal scalded skin syndrome (SSSS), and other blistering eruptions. The difference in appearance of a target lesion and a hive has already been discussed. In addition, individual hives last less than 24 hours, whereas the lesions in erythema multiforme persist much longer. Viral exanthems usually are monomorphous and tend to be less red, more confluent, and more centrally distributed than in erythema multiforme. Purpura is the distinguishing feature of vasculitis lesions. The skin in SSSS is diffusely red and strips off easily (Nikolsky sign). In the rare instance when erythema multiforme involves the whole skin surface (toxic epidermal necrolysis), a skin biopsy will help to distinguish it from SSSS. In erythema multiforme the split in the skin is subepidermal, whereas in SSSS the split is intraepidermal. Other blistering disorders that might be confused with erythema multiforme are rare in children. An example is bullous pemphigoid, a chronic autoimmune subepidermal blistering disorder characterized histologically by the presence of IgG at the dermoepidermal interface.

Management

There is no convincing evidence that medical therapy favorably alters the course of this disease. Treatment of a precipitating infection seems appropriate, and erythromycin is recommended for *M. pneumoniae* infections even though there is no proof that this alters the course of the skin reaction.

The use of systemic steroids is more controversial. They have been frequently employed in Stevens-Johnson syndrome, but without documented benefit. In fact, Rasmussen's retrospective study[6] found that children with Stevens-Johnson syndrome treated with systemic steroids required more extended hospitalization and experienced more frequent complications (e.g., infection and gastrointestinal bleeding) than did untreated patients. Nevertheless, prednisone given systemically in doses ranging from 40 to 80 mg/m^2 still is frequently employed in patients with severe erythema multiforme. Clearly, a prospective study is needed to determine its benefit.

Although the value of these specific therapies may be unproved, supportive measures are important. These are aimed mainly at (1) restoring and maintaining hydration, (2) preventing secondary infection, and (3) providing pain relief. Patients with severe oral involvement may be unable to drink, so that intravenous fluids are required. When skin involvement is extensive, increased transcutaneous fluid loss occurs and replacement volumes must be adjusted accordingly. Local therapy with antiseptics and dressings may help to prevent secondary infection, and patients with severe involvement may require therapies similar to those for burn patients. Systemic analgesics are used for pain. Topical anesthetics may be used intraorally to provide temporary relief for patients with painful mouth lesions. Viscous lidocaine is one such agent, but dyclonine liquid is easier to use and longer lasting in its anesthetic effects.

Complications

The major complication, occasionally resulting in death, is worsening of the mucocutaneous involvement. The entire skin surface can become involved with the blistering process, a condition for which the term *toxic epidermal necrolysis* often is applied. Mucous membrane involvement can restrict oral intake, resulting in dehydration. Conjunctivitis can leave residual ophthalmic complications of which keratitis sicca is the most common, occurring in about 15% of patients with Stevens-Johnson syndrome. Internal organs are affected less frequently, with pulmonary involvement being reported occasionally and renal involvement rarely.

Course

Patients with mild forms of erythema multiforme usually recover uneventfully within 2 to 3 weeks. The course of the disease is longer (4 to 6 weeks) in patients with severe involvement, and death does occur occasionally in patients with the Stevens-Johnson syndrome, reported rates ranging from 0% to 15%. Erythema multiforme recurs in 10% to 20% of patients and is particularly common in those in whom the disease is precipitated by recurrent herpes simplex infection.

REFERENCES

1. Bigby M et al: Drug-induced cutaneous reactions: a report from the Boston Collaborative Drug Surveillance Program on 15,438 consecutive inpatients, 1975 to 1982, JAMA 256:3358, 1986.
2. Dunagin WG and Millikan LE: Drug eruptions, Med Clin North Am 64:983, 1982.
3. Huff JC, Weston WL, and Tonnesen MG: Erythema multiforme: a critical review of characteristics, diagnostic criteria and causes, J Am Acad Dermatol 8:767, 1983.
4. Joerizzo JL, editor: Symposium on urticaria and the reactive inflammatory vascular dermatoses, Dermatol Clin 3:1, 1985.
5. Monroe EW: Urticaria: an updated review, Int J Dermatol 20:32, 1981.
6. Rasmussen JE: Erythema multiforme in children: response to treatment with systemic corticosteroids, Br J Dermatol 95:181, 1976.
7. Wintroub BU and Stern RS: Cutaneous drug eruptions: pathogenesis and clinical classification, J Am Acad Dermatol 13:167, 1985.
8. Wintroub BU, Stern RS, and Arndt KA: Cutaneous reactions to drugs. In Fitzpatrick TB et al, editors: Dermatology in general medicine, ed 3, New York, 1987, McGraw-Hill Book Co.

SUGGESTED READING

Patterson R and Anderson J: Allergic reactions to drugs and biologic agents, JAMA 248:2637, 1982.

201

Eczema

Howard R. Foye, Jr.

Eczema is a confusing dermatologic term that sometimes is used as a synonym for atopic dermatitis. It is also used as a less specific descriptive label for rashes with a wide variety of etiologies but with similar morphologic characteristics. For management it is helpful to distinguish between acute and chronic eczema. In its acute phase, eczema is characterized by pruritus, erythema, vesicles, exudation, and crusts; in its chronic phase it is characterized by pruritus, dryness (xerosis), scaling, and thickening of the skin (lichenification).

Frequently, terms more specific than *acute* and *chronic* are used to describe eczematous rashes with certain patterns. *Nummular eczema* is a term that is used when chronic eczematous lesions are coin shaped. *Lichen simplex chronicus* is a term used to describe the thickened, scaly (lichenified) skin frequently found over bony prominences, ankles, elbows, wrists, and the occipital area, the result of rubbing and scratching in chronic eczema. Both these patterns are common in chronic atopic dermatitis.

The focus of this chapter is on atopic dermatitis, probably the most common cause of eczema in the pediatric population. Other causes of eczematous rashes are discussed under the differential diagnosis. The principles of local therapy discussed later, under management, are based on morphologic features of the rash and therefore differ according to the stage of the eczematous process. These principles are generalizable to the treatment of eczematous rashes regardless of etiology.

CLINICAL PRESENTATION

Atopic dermatitis is characterized by a number of clinical features that distinguish it from other causes of eczematous rashes. Hanifin and Lobits[3] have categorized the clinical features and associations of atopic dermatitis in terms of major and minor diagnostic criteria, as listed in the accompanying box. Many of those criteria only become apparent when the condition is chronic. Atopic dermatitis is certainly a very common problem, estimated to occur in 3% of the pediatric population. Although it may begin at any age, it usually is described in three stages, each with a characteristic appearance and distribution of rash.

Stages

Infantile Stage. The infantile stage begins at 2 to 6 months of age and resolves in about 50% of patients by 2 to 3 years of age. It has the characteristics of acute eczema—pruritus, erythema, vesicles, exudation, and crusts. The common sites of involvement are the cheeks, forehead, scalp, and extensor aspects of the arms and legs (Fig. 201-1). Initially the lesions have poorly defined margins, but with chronicity they may become thickened and scaly and have well-demarcated margins.

Childhood Stage. The childhood stage usually occurs between 4 and 10 years of age, although it may follow directly from the infantile stage or continue through to adolescence without remission. The lesions are less likely to be exudative and crusted than in the infantile stage and are more likely to have the characteristics of chronic eczema. They usually are dry, scaly, pruritic, papular patches, often well circumscribed. The most common sites of involvement are the wrists, ankles, and antecubital and popliteal fossae (Fig. 201-2).

Adolescent or Adult Stage. The adolescent or adult stage may be an extension of the childhood stage, a recurrence following a remission, or a new problem beginning in ado-

Features Indicative of Atopic Dermatitis

MAJOR FEATURES

Pruritus
Chronically relapsing course
Typical morphology and distribution
  Facial and extensor involvement during infancy
  Flexural lichenification after infancy
Personal or family history of atopy
Immediate skin test reactivity
Abnormal vascular responses
  White dermographism
  Delayed blanch to cholinergic agents
Xerosis

MINOR FEATURES

Dennie infraorbital fold
Keratosis pilaris
Hyperlinear palms
Ichthyosis
Anterior subcapsular cataracts
Elevated serum IgE
Tendency toward nonspecific hand and foot dermatitis
Tendency toward repeated cutaneous infections

Reproduced with permission from Hanifin JM: Atopic dermatitis. In Weinberg S and Hoekelman RA, editors: Pediatric dermatology for the primary care practitioner, New York, 1978, McGraw-Hill Book Co.

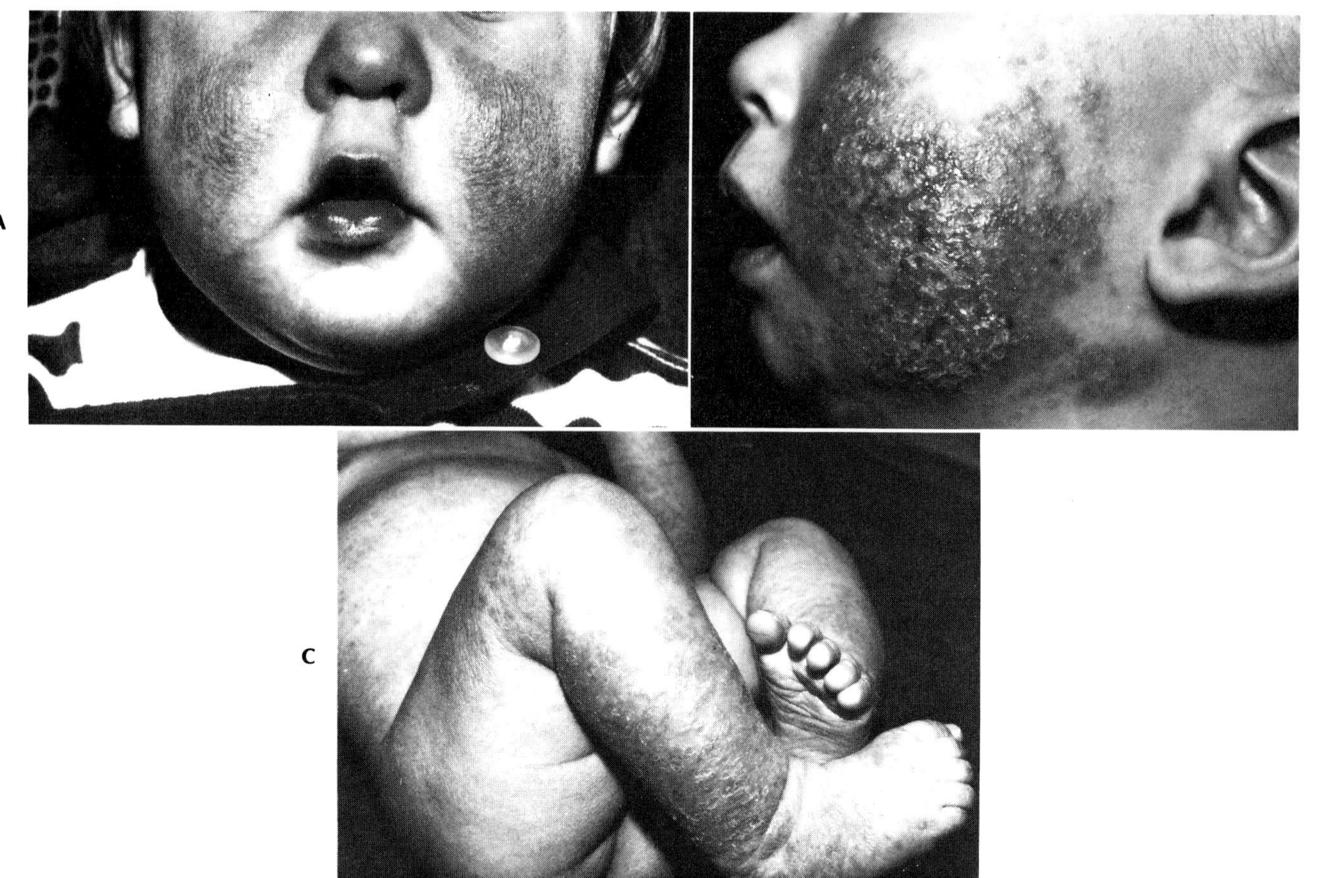

Fig. 201-1 Infantile stage of atopic dermatitis involving the cheeks (**A** and **B**) and legs (**C**).
Courtesy of Alfred T. Lane, M.D., Division of Dermatology, University of Rochester School of Medicine and Dentistry.

lescence and often extending into adulthood. The rash has the characteristics of chronic eczema—pruritus, dryness, scaling, and thickening of the skin, often in large plaques that may have sharp borders. Exudation and crusting may occur, but this usually is a sign of external irritation or secondary infection. The most common sites of involvement are the flexor folds, face, neck, upper portion of the arms, back, and dorsal aspects of the hands, feet, fingers, and toes (Fig. 201-3).

Associated Findings

Skin. In addition to eczematous eruptions, patients with atopic dermatitis have a high incidence of other skin abnormalities. Generally dry skin (xerosis), grouped papules ("goose bumps") over the trunk and nape of neck, accentuated palmar creases, and a lowered threshold to pruritic stimuli are common. Many also have an extra crease in the lower eyelids referred to as a Morgan fold or Dennie pleat. There is an increased tendency to have nonspecific hand dermatitis and repeated cutaneous infections.[4]

White dermographism, instead of the usual red flare, is elicited by stroking the skin with a blunt instrument during the active atopic dermatitis period. Also, patients show a prolonged blanching rather than the usual vasodilatory flare when acetylcholine is injected into the skin.

Other commonly associated cutaneous conditions are pityriasis alba, keratosis pilaris, ichthyosis vulgaris, and dyshidrotic eczema (pompholyx). *Pityriasis alba* is characterized by faintly scaling, hypopigmented patches on the cheeks and upper portions of the back and arms. It is common during the childhood stage of atopic dermatitis and is self-limited, although often lasting 2 to 3 years. *Keratosis pilaris* is a follicular hyperkeratosis manifested by small, scattered papules over the upper posterior arms, anterior thighs, and buttocks. *Ichthyosis vulgaris* is characterized by fine, superficial scales caused by decreased water retention in the stratum corneum. In its milder form it may manifest only as dry and rough skin over the extensor aspects of the arms and legs in the winter. In its more severe form a generalized "fish-scale" rash is seen. *Dyshidrotic eczema* is a term used to describe crops of deep-seated vesicles on the fingertips, thenar and hypothenar eminences, sides of the fingers, and analogous areas of the feet. Irritant contact and fungal infections may look similar.

Atopic History. A family history of atopic disease (atopic dermatitis, allergic rhinitis, or asthma) is present in 60% to 70% of patients, and hay fever or asthma will develop in 30% to 50% of children with atopic dermatitis.[5]

Eyes. Cataracts occur in 5% to 10% of adults with severe atopic dermatitis, but they rarely are seen in childhood. Because it is difficult to differentiate early atopic cataracts from

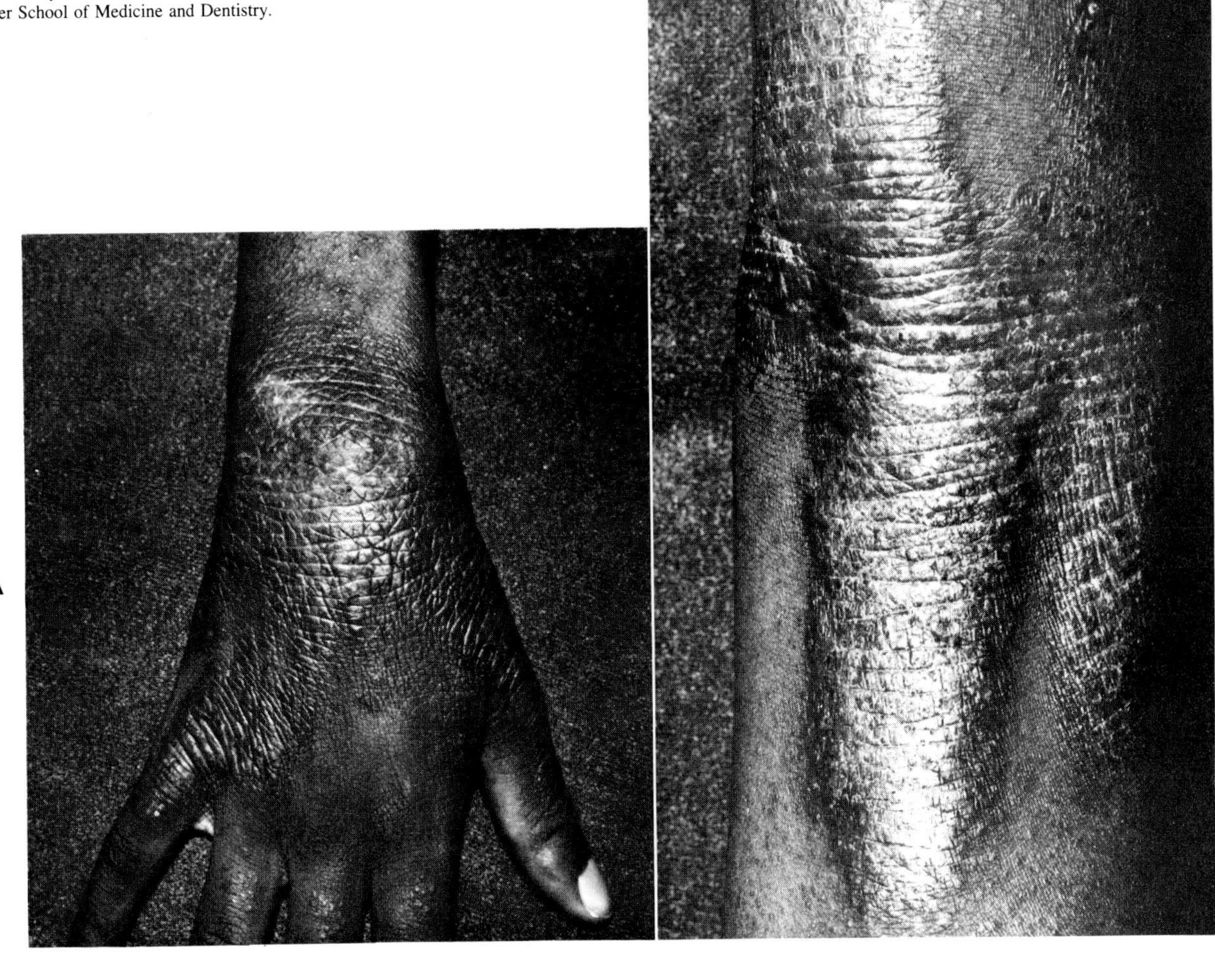

Fig. 201-2 Chronic atopic dermatitis involving the dorsum of the wrist and hand (**A**) and the popliteal region (**B**).

Courtesy of Alfred T. Lane, M.D., Division of Dermatology, University of Rochester School of Medicine and Dentistry.

steroid-induced cataracts, it is possible that some of these are caused by prolonged use of steroids, particularly systemic steroids. An ophthalmologic evaluation is indicated before the prolonged use of systemic steroids. Keratoconus, a conical protrusion of the center of the cornea, has been found in some children. One speculation is that it is a consequence of chronic rubbing of the eyelids.

Immune System. Immunologic abnormalities also are associated with atopic dermatitis. Depressed T cell function and cellular immunity have been demonstrated.[2] Patients have an increased susceptibility to cutaneous infections such as herpes, molluscum contagiosum, warts, and fungi. There also is an increased incidence of serious disseminated viral disease. Contrary to initial expectations, patients with atopic dermatitis were found to have a decreased incidence of sensitivity to poison ivy. This is presumably related to the underlying defect in cellular immunity. Disorders with established defects in cell-mediated immunity such as Wiskott-Aldrich syndrome and ataxia telangiectasia frequently are accompanied by eczematous rashes.

Altered leukocyte function also has been demonstrated in severe atopic dermatitis, which may explain the susceptibility to *Staphylococcus aureus* infection.[3]

Elevated IgE levels are found in patients with atopic dermatitis, but there is little correlation between IgE levels and severity of disease. Also, one report found that when patients with allergic respiratory disease were excluded from the comparison, patients with atopic dermatitis and control subjects had the same IgE levels.[2] Similarly, most patients with atopic dermatitis demonstrate positive skin test reactions to at least one of the common respiratory allergens, but this is not correlated with severity of disease.

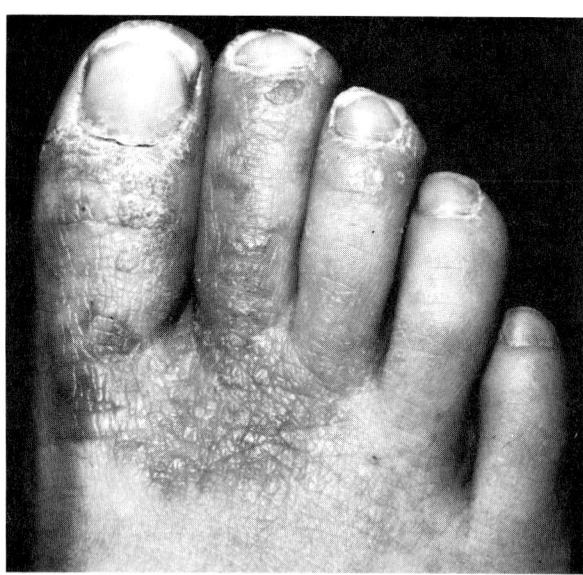

Fig. 201-3 Atopic dermatitis of the foot.

Courtesy of Alfred T. Lane, M.D., Division of Dermatology, University of Rochester School of Medicine and Dentistry.

ETIOLOGY

The etiology of atopic dermatitis remains unclear. Because of its association with asthma, chronic rhinitis, elevated IgE levels, and positive skin tests for common allergens, it is tempting to assume that the mechanism for atopic dermatitis is a specific IgE response to an antigen. The antigen-antibody complex would presumably cause a release of histamine and other pharmacologic mediators from mast cells, producing the itching, rubbing, and scratching that lead to the eczematous rash of atopic dermatitis. Unfortunately, attempts to substantiate this theory have failed. There is no evidence for antibody-antigen complexes, and urticaria, which would be the initial skin lesion in this mechanism, is not observed.

A current theory contends that the underlying defect is a lack of suppressor T cells to suppress the production of IgE. Large amounts of IgE can inhibit rosette formation of normal T lymphocytes and presumably inhibit cell-mediated immunity. Transfer factor, which is known to stimulate T lymphocytes, has been found to improve the eczematous rash in patients with Wiskott-Aldrich syndrome. A similar improvement has been reported in a patient with severe atopic dermatitis.[2] The reason for the deficit in suppressor T cells and the mechanism for the rash, however, are unclear; therefore, before one can place much stock in this theory, the poor correlation between IgE levels and severity of disease must be addressed. The bulk of the findings in this field to date have involved severely affected patients. The applicability of the findings to mild and moderate atopic dermatitis is questionable.

DIFFERENTIAL DIAGNOSIS

Seborrheic Dermatitis

Seborrheic dermatitis may manifest as an erythematous, flaky rash that is difficult to distinguish from atopic dermatitis. Characteristic greasy yellow- or salmon-colored scales make the diagnosis of seborrheic dermatitis more clear, but these are not always present. The typical distribution of seborrheic dermatitis coincides with the areas of highest sebaceous gland concentration—the scalp, face, and postauricular, presternal, and intertriginous areas. The features that distinguish seborrheic dermatitis from atopic dermatitis are the relative lack of pruritus, the lower incidence of a family history of atopic diseases, the characteristic distribution, and more flaking in the acute phase. In infancy the age of onset is helpful information because seborrheic dermatitis usually begins between 2 and 12 weeks of age, whereas atopic dermatitis begins between 2 and 6 months of age.[5]

Contact Dermatitis

Different forms of contact dermatitis cause a variety of eczematous rashes. Mild irritants on repeated contact may cause erythema and scaly, papular eruptions consistent with chronic eczema. Allergic dermatitis or strong irritants such as acids or alkalis may cause an acute eczematous rash with pruritus, vesiculation, erythema, exudations, and crust. The diagnosis of contact dermatitis is made on the basis of a limited area of involvement and a history of contact of that area with an offending agent.

Psoriasis

Psoriasis can be very difficult to distinguish visually and histologically from chronic atopic dermatitis. The classic presentation is that of thick, reddish, well-defined plaques with a silvery scale ("micalike"). The plaques occur most commonly over the extensor surfaces of the arms and legs, other pressure areas, and the scalp. They may merge to form serpiginous patterns, frequently showing greater activity at the periphery and involution centrally. The lesions are minimally pruritic except in advanced stages. Psoriasis also may be seen as a pustular rash of the palms and soles associated with hyperkeratosis and fissuring or with erythema and maceration of intertriginous areas without scaling. Guttate psoriasis occurs with widely disseminated small plaques after a streptococcal infection. Psoriasis may progress to a generalized exfoliative erythroderma. Small, punctate pitting of the nails occurs in 25% to 50% of patients with psoriasis and is very helpful in the differential diagnosis. A different sort of pitting can occur in atopic dermatitis, caused by involvement of the nail bed in the eczematous process, but the pitting is larger and more irregular than the punctate pits characteristic of psoriasis.

Infections

Various superficial infections or infestations can cause an eczematous rash. Dermatophytes may cause infections of the hands and feet that are indistinguishable from dyshidrotic eczema. A culture of fluid from a vesicle may be necessary for differentiation. Intertrigo, particularly with secondary infection from *Candida* organisms, has several of the features of acute atopic dermatitis. Isolated papules, papulovesicles, or pustules at the margin of larger areas of involvement ("satellite lesions") are characteristic of candidiasis. Also, intertriginous involvement is not as common as that of other areas in atopic dermatitis, so the rest of the distribution may help in the differential diagnosis. Impetigo and viral cutaneous infections such as herpes simplex and zoster also have features in common with atopic dermatitis. In general, however, the rapidity of onset, along with other acute features, usually makes the differentiation easy. Scabies frequently is complicated by eczematous changes caused by intense pruritus and scratching. Topical therapy for scabies may contribute to the pruritus. Recognition of burrows, infestation among contacts, and the typical distribution of excoriated papules in the web spaces of the hands and feet, the elbows, sacral area, scrotum, and penis help to distinguish this condition.

One must remember that secondary infection is a common complication of atopic dermatitis. Increased staphylococcal colonization and increased susceptibility to cutaneous bacterial, viral, and fungal infections exist in atopic dermatitis. When increased erythema and exudation occur over chronic eczematous changes, secondary infection must be considered.

Immune Disorders

Eczema is part of the characteristic clinical presentation of several diseases involving immune disorders. Wiskott-Aldrich syndrome is characterized by the triad of severe eczema, thrombocytopenic purpura, and increased susceptibility to infection. There appear to be defects in cellular and humoral immunity. The hyperimmunoglobulin E syndrome is characterized by extremely high IgE levels, recurrent skin infections, defective neutrophil chemotaxis, and a personal or family history of atopic disease. Ataxia telangiectasia is a syndrome that includes progressive cerebellar ataxia, oculocutaneous telangiectasia, recurrent respiratory infections, diminished serum and secretory IgA, diminished immediate and delayed hypersensitivity, hypoplasia, or absence of the thymus, growth failure, and eczema.

Metabolic Diseases

Several metabolic diseases involve eczematous rashes. Acrodermatitis enteropathica is associated with zinc deficiency and is characterized by a vesiculobullous eczematous rash of the distal extremities and perioral region, failure to thrive, diarrhea, alopecia, nail dystrophy, and frequent secondary bacterial or candidal cutaneous infections. Phenylketonuria is caused by a hereditary defect in the enzyme phenylalanine hydroxylase and is characterized when untreated from infancy by mental retardation, seizures, diffuse hypopigmentation, blond hair, eczema, and photosensitivity. Pellagra is caused by a deficiency of niacin and is characterized by the "three D triad" of dermatitis, diarrhea, and dementia. The eczematous rash appears on areas exposed to sunlight, heat, friction, or pressure. Hartnup disease is a hereditary disease in which a defect in the absorption of tryptophan from the gastrointestinal tract seems to be the underlying problem. It involves a pellagra-like light-sensitive eczematous rash.

MANAGEMENT

Acute Phase

The objectives of treatment for the acute phase of atopic dermatitis are to reduce pruritus, to diminish the inflammatory changes in the upper dermis and epidermis, and to remove the accumulated exudates and crusts. The methods of achieving these objectives include wet compresses, topical steroids, and systemic antihistamines.

Wet Compresses. Open, wet, tepid compresses tend to dry weeping lesions, clean crusts, and provide soothing and antipruritic effects. Burow solution (aluminum acetate) frequently is used for its presumed germicidal and astringent properties. It is available without a prescription in the form of Domeboro powder packets and is mixed one packet per pint or, for infants, one per quart. Plain tap water may be equally effective. The wet dressings should be applied for 5 to 10 minutes at a time, four to six times a day for several days to a week during the acute exudative phase. Soft thin cloths (such as thin diapers, handkerchiefs, strips of bed sheeting, or dish towels) are preferable to thick towels, which interfere with evaporation, or gauze, which tends to adhere to the skin. The compresses need to be remoistened during the application to prevent their drying out. Occlusive dressings should not be used in acute eczema, as they may macerate the skin. The purpose of the treatment is the application of moisture and its evaporation. Wet compresses also enhance the penetration of topical steroids by removing crusts.

Topical Steroids. In acute eczema a water-miscible cream is the best vehicle for topical steroids, because of its better miscibility with exudate. An ointment may remain on the surface and possibly increase the maceration by occlusion. The cream should be applied three or four times a day in a thin film after wet compresses and gentle drying.

The choice of steroid potency depends on the location of the rash. It is generally advisable to use 1% hydrocortisone cream or another mild steroid on the face, over extensive acute eczematous areas in small children, and in intertriginous areas. Except on the face, steroids of moderate potency (see the accompanying box, group IV) may be used initially on localized lesions, changing to a mild steroid in a few days.

The side effects of steroids, which are more likely with chronic use of the more potent varieties, include cutaneous atrophy, striae, telangiectasia, and suppression of the pituitary-adrenal axis.[6]

Systemic steroids should not be used in acute atopic dermatitis. Although effective, the risk of side effects is increased. Also, because of the chronic relapsing nature of the condition, patients may become steroid dependent when this relatively easy treatment is used for every exacerbation. A severe, disseminated acute eczematous dermatitis, as may be seen with poison ivy contact, may require systemic steroids.

Antihistamines. Although the rash of atopic dermatitis is not based on histamine-release mechanisms, the sedative and antipruritic effects of antihistamines are helpful in the important task of reducing pruritus. The continued trauma created by scratching and rubbing will exacerbate the acute phase and contribute to chronic changes in the skin. Hydroxyzine is perhaps the first drug of choice because of its excellent antipruritic properties and relatively mild sedative effect. Occasionally the pruritus seems to intensify at night and interfere with sleep. Diphenhydramine may be preferable in these situations because of its greater sedative effect.

Chronic Phase

The objectives of treatment for the chronic phase of atopic dermatitis are to moisten and lubricate the skin; reduce pruritus, hyperkeratosis, and chronic inflammatory changes; and avoid aggravating conditions. The methods for achieving these objectives include the use of lubricating lotions, topical steroids, environmental manipulations, and occasionally, tar preparations or keratolytic agents.

Hydration and Lubrication. In the past, standard treatment of atopic dermatitis has included the paradoxical admonition to avoid bathing for those patients with dry skin. It was believed that bathing, even without soap, would further deplete an already inadequate supply of protective oils in the skin. Current treatment suggestions, however, tend to emphasize rehydration as well as lubrication. Lubrication alone will not soften thick, dry, water-depleted keratin. The addition and retention of water are essential. Rather than being contraindicated, a moderate amount of bathing can be helpful if followed immediately by the application of a lubricating lotion (e.g., Lubriderm, Nivea, or Nutraderm lotions) to produce a water-trapping effect. Minimal use of mild soaps (e.g., Dove, Nutragena, Aveena, Purpose) and the avoidance of very hot water are indicated. Unscented bath oil may be helpful, but not when added at the beginning of the bath when the lipid film may prevent rather than enhance hydration.

Topical Steroids. In chronic atopic dermatitis an ointment base for topical steroids is preferable because its occlusive effect will increase the retention of water in the hydrated stratum corneum. Also, ointment preparations have been found to be more potent than the cream preparations of the same drug in equal concentration (see the box at the right). A thick horny layer will diminish the penetration of steroids and occasionally will necessitate the use of more potent steroids. Potent steroids may be used in small areas for short periods with relatively little risk of side effects. Once the rash is under control, however, it is advisable to taper therapy to a moderately potent steroid and then to a mildly potent steroid as improvement continues. Tapering may avoid a rebound phenomenon when topical steroids are discontinued and will minimize the amount of time more potent steroids will be needed.

Additional measures may be necessary. Tar preparations may help by diminishing the mitotic rate in the epidermis; 2% to 5% crude coal tar, which is black, staining, and malodorous, or liquor carbonis detergens, which is less offensive but also less effective, can be used. Other alternatives are keratolytic preparations that contain 3% to 5% salicylic acid or 10% to 20% urea to reduce the thickness of the horny layer. These agents, however, can be very irritating to the skin of a patient with atopic dermatitis.

Systemic steroids should be reserved for rare, extremely severe cases that cannot be controlled by other means. If this step is anticipated, a previous ophthalmologic evaluation is warranted.

Environmental Manipulations. Environmental manipulations to eliminate unnecessary drying or pruritic stimuli can help to control the itch-scratch cycle that contributes to the chronicity of eczema. Humidified heat in the winter to reduce drying and air conditioning in the summer to reduce the pruritic effect of perspiration can be helpful. The avoidance of soaps, harsh materials such as wool, fuzzy toys, stuffed animals, pets, and activities that induce perspiration may diminish pruritus.

*Topical Steroids in Order of Potency**

I. Cyclocort ointment 0.1%
Diprosone ointment 0.05%
Florone ointment 0.05%
Halog cream 0.1%
Lidex cream 0.05%
Lidex ointment 0.05%
Topicort cream 0.25%
Topsyn gel 0.05%

II. Aristocort cream 0.5%
Diprosone cream 0.05%
Maxiflor cream 0.05%
Valisone ointment 0.1%

III. Aristocort ointment 0.1%
Benisone ointment 0.025%
Cordran ointment 0.05%
Cyclocort cream 0.1%
Kenalog ointment 0.1%
Synalar cream (HP) 0.2%
Synalar ointment 0.025%
Valisone lotion 0.1%

IV. Benisone cream 0.025%
Cordran cream 0.05%
Kenalog cream 0.1%
Kenalog lotion 0.025%
Synalar cream 0.025%
Valisone cream 0.1%
Westcort cream 0.2%

V. Desonide cream 0.05%
Locorten cream 0.03%

VI. Topical agents with hydrocortisone, dexamethasone, flumethalone, prednisolone, and methylprednisolone

From Stoughton RB: A perspective on topical corticosteroid therapy. In Farber EM and Cox AJ, editors: Psoriasis, Proceedings of the Second International Symposium, New York, 1976, Yorke Medical Books. Revised in 1982 by personal communication from the author.

*Group I is the most potent, and potency descends with each group to group VI, which is least potent. There is no significant difference between agents within any given group.

Dietary restrictions are controversial in atopic dermatitis. In a review of the role of diet in atopic dermatitis, Atherton[1] concludes that at least 20% of children with atopic dermatitis will show a beneficial response to elimination of selected items from their diet. Neither skin tests nor IgE radioallergosorbent tests (RAST) are effective in identifying the offending items. Atherton cautions that dietary treatment should be attempted only when simpler treatments have failed. Elimination diets are relatively simple in infancy. Solid foods should be eliminated, and if the infant is receiving cow milk or a cow milk–based formula, a change to a soy-based formula should be tried. If that does not help, a protein hydrolysate formula (e.g., Nutramigen or Pregestimil) should be introduced. After 12 months of age, sequential reintroduction of the excluded foods can be attempted.

After infancy, if other treatment measures have failed, Atherton[1] suggests starting with a simple, empirical elimination diet, excluding foods that contain cow milk, egg, chicken, most artificial food colorings, benzoate preservatives, and other foods that the parents strongly suspect may cause allergic reactions. Nutritional supplements may be necessary, particularly calcium gluconate tablets. If there is no clear benefit in 4 to 6 weeks, the diet should be abandoned. If the dermatitis is improved and nutrition is adequate, the diet should be maintained for about a year before sequential reintroduction of the excluded foods. Consultation with an allergist and a dietitian is advisable for more complex elimination diet trials.

Skin tests and hyposensitization therapy are of little or no value in the management of atopic dermatitis.

Psychosocial Considerations

Children with atopic dermatitis have been characterized as active, restless, irritable, and aggressive. Perhaps some of this behavior is attributable to chronic pruritus and discomfort. Altered interactions with family members and peers also are likely to be significant. Chronic conditions, particularly when a visible abnormality is involved, are known to influence interactions with others, as well as self-concept and self-confidence. In addition, parents can be extremely frustrated and distressed by the chronic, relapsing course of atopic dermatitis. It may be helpful to reassure patient and parents that this condition does not result in scarring, is not contagious, will have remissions, and generally can be well controlled. Also, postinflammatory hypopigmentation is temporary. Openness in receiving their questions may avoid some frightening or counterproductive misconceptions.

Complications

Secondary infection is the most common complication. Patients are more susceptible to bacterial, viral, and fungal cutaneous infections. Eczema herpeticum, or Kaposi varicelliform eruption, is a serious generalized herpesvirus infection that can occur as a complication of atopic dermatitis.

Prognosis

Fifty percent of children with infantile atopic dermatitis will "outgrow" this condition by 2 to 3 years of age; 75% of children with atopic dermatitis will have no recurrences after adolescence.

REFERENCES

1. Atherton DJ: Diet and atopic eczema, Clin Allergy 18:215, 1988.
2. Fellner MJ: Immunology of skin diseases, New York, 1980, Elsevier Science Publishing Co, Inc.
3. Hanifin JM and Lobitz WC: Newer concepts of atopic dermatitis, Arch Dermatol 113:663, 1977.
4. Hurwitz S: Eczematous eruptions in childhood, Pediatr Rev 3:23, 1981.
5. Moss EM: Atopic dermatitis, Pediatr Clin North Am 25:225, 1978.
6. Weston WH: The use and abuse of topical steroids, Contemp Pediatr 57, June 1988.

202

Enterovirus Infections

Jerri Ann Jenista

CLASSIFICATION

Enteroviruses are Picornaviridae, small ribonucleic acid (RNA) viruses. They are classified into three groups: polioviruses, coxsackieviruses, and enteric cytopathogenic human orphan viruses (echoviruses). The paralytic disease of poliovirus was known in ancient Egypt and was clinically described in 1789 in England; three polio serotypes exist. Coxsackieviruses, named for the town in New York State where the first recognized patients lived, are divided into A and B groups, depending on characteristic pathologic changes induced in suckling mice; 23 and 6 serotypes, respectively, are described. Echoviruses were initially thought not to cause disease, but have now been associated with nearly all the enterovirus syndromes; over 30 types are known. In recent years all newly identified enterovirus types have been designated simply as "enterovirus" followed by a number, beginning with 68. The hepatitis A virus, now reclassified as enterovirus 72, is the latest addition to this group.[4]

EPIDEMIOLOGY

In temperate climates, enterovirus infections show a distinct seasonality, occurring from July through October in the Northern hemisphere. In tropical regions, however, infection is noted throughout the year. Although outbreaks of illness associated with a single serotype are often reported, the far more common pattern is endemic infection caused by several enterovirus types. The predominant types may vary yearly and by locality even within the same year. A single serotype may produce variable clinical syndromes in different seasons and communities. Conversely, the same disease may be associated with several serotypes. Pandemic illness is unusual but not unknown. A modern example is the worldwide spread of acute hemorrhagic conjunctivitis caused by coxsackievirus A24 and enterovirus 70, which started in 1969 and affected many millions of people.

Transmission of enteroviruses is nearly always by the fecal-oral route. In the special case of acute hemorrhagic conjunctivitis, spread is often by hand-to-eye contact. The incidence of infection is highest in young children and under poor hygienic conditions. Severe illness may occur at any age but is most often seen in newborns,[12] in agammaglobulinemic patients, and occasionally in bone marrow transplant recipients.

The incubation period for enterovirus infection is ordinarily 3 to 5 days, but it may range from 2 to 20 days. The period of contagion is probably greatest several days preceding and immediately following the onset of symptoms; however, it may be prolonged. Because infection is so commonly asymptomatic and because virus excretion can persist for weeks in the feces following recovery from illness, it is often impossible to identify a patient's contact by history alone. Scrupulous hand washing may decrease the spread of infection but is unlikely to control it completely, given the large pool of asymptomatic "shedders" usually present. Reinfection is frequent and is usually clinically inapparent.[4]

PATHOGENESIS

Infection is initiated by viral replication in the lymphoid tissue of the oropharynx and gut. This phase occurs over 1 to 3 days and is symptom free. There follows a *minor viremia* with spread of virions to the reticuloendothelial system at 3 to 5 days. In a subclinical infection the process is halted at this point by host defenses. A subsequent *major viremia* results in viral dissemination to secondary organs such as the skin, heart, liver, pancreas, adrenal glands, and central nervous system. This phase is most often clinically recognized as a nonspecific febrile illness or the "minor illness" of poliomyelitis. In a very small percentage of cases, viral spread will continue, producing the various forms of paralytic disease most commonly associated wth poliovirus.

Antibody production may be detectable as early as 1 day following exposure to the virus; both serum and secretory forms are induced. Antibody is also found in human milk and may prevent enterovirus infection and successful immunization with oral (live) poliovirus vaccine in the newborn period.[4]

LABORATORY DIAGNOSIS

With the exception of most of the coxsackievirus A group, enteroviruses are easily isolated in cell culture. A presumptive positive culture can be noted as early as 18 hours but more typically requires 2 to 5 days. Specific identification of an individual serotype takes somewhat longer. Suckling mouse inoculation, an expensive and difficult procedure, is currently the only available method of isolating most of the coxsackievirus A group serotypes. Viruses may be isolated from throat swabs, feces, cerebrospinal fluid, serum, skin vesicles, and tissues obtained at autopsy. Specimens from multiple sites will increase the diagnostic yield, since it is not always possible to predict the pathologic stage of infection and thus the most likely source of virus. With the increased availability of virology diagnostic laboratories, efforts to isolate virus may prove cost effective in cases of more severe illness such as aseptic meningitis. Positive identification of an etiologic agent may eliminate the need for further diagnostic tests, reduce the need for antibiotics, shorten the hospital stay, and improve prognostic accuracy.[15]

Because of the prolonged fecal shed of virus following infection, a fecal isolate does not always imply enteroviral etiology of the investigated illness. Indeed, many of the disease associations reported with enteroviruses were probably only coincidental. In cases in which it might be desirable to prove the cause (i.e., in paralytic disease related to a poliovirus vaccine strain), serum-neutralizing antibody titers in acute and convalescent samples may be useful. Unfortunately, because antibody production occurs early, titers may already be high during the acute phase of clinical illness, thus obscuring the diagnosis.

It is not practical to obtain serum for enterovirus antibody titer analysis because of the multiple serotypes and complexity of the procedure. When the clinical or pathologic picture strongly suggests one enterovirus group or a limited number of serotypes (i.e., myocarditis probably related to coxsackievirus B), measurement of neutralizing antibody titers may be feasible.

Several investigators are working on rapid tests to evaluate the presence of enteroviruses in clinical specimens and to detect enterovirus serotype–specific IgM in serum. None of these are commercially available as yet.

CLINICAL SYNDROMES

Large-scale epidemiologic studies of poliovirus infection indicate that probably more than 90% of enterovirus infections are inapparent. When symptoms do occur, a variety of host factors (such as age, genetic background, and antibody status) and viral factors (such as strain virulence and inoculating dose of virions) determine the clinical disease present. Although nearly all the protean syndromes associated with enteroviruses have been noted with serotypes from each group, certain diseases are more frequently associated with specific groups (Table 202-1). For example, a coxsackievirus A is the likely etiologic agent of an outbreak of herpangina.

Any of the enteroviruses may cause a mild nonspecific febrile illness lasting 2 to 5 days. Such seasonal infections probably account for the late summer and early fall peak of office visits noted in community surveillance studies of pediatric febrile illness. A nonexudative pharyngitis with or without lymphadenopathy is frequently observed. In a few cases, this illness may be the first manifestation of more severe disease that will appear following an apparent recovery period of 1 to 3 days. Other respiratory syndromes as listed in Table 202-1 are uncommon and are generally mild.

Herpangina is a disease commonly diagnosed in the young child with mild fever and sore throat or pain on swallowing. An enanthem may be noted early, but it is soon succeeded by small vesicles and then ulcers on the tonsils, pharynx, and soft palate. Occasionally the lesions are firm, tiny white nodules; the illness is then termed *lymphonodular pharyngitis*. Herpangina is differentiated from herpes simplex stomatitis by the milder degree of fever, primarily posterior oropharyngeal involvement, and its epidemic seasonal occurrence.

The hand-foot-mouth syndrome occurs in toddlers and school-age children. The hallmark signs are relatively painless vesicles on a red base, occasionally grouped, appearing on the buccal mucosa and tongue and on the palms and soles. In rare cases the rash may spread to the extremities and

Table 202-1 *Clinical Diseases and Physical Findings Associated with Enteroviruses and the Most Frequently Implicated Etiologic Groups*

	POLIOVIRUS	COXSACKIEVIRUS A	COXSACKIEVIRUS B	ECHOVIRUS	ENTEROVIRUS
Asymptomatic infection	X	X	X	X	X
Nonspecific febrile illness	X	X	X	X	X
Common cold		X			
Pharyngitis	X	X	X	X	X
Herpangina		X			
Parotitis			X		
Croup			X	X	
Bronchitis, bronchiolitis			X	X	
Pneumonia			X	X	
Pleurodynia			X		
Myocarditis, pericarditis			X		
Gastrointestinal symptoms	X	X	X	X	X
Hepatitis			X	X	
Pancreatitis			X		
Diabetes mellitus			X		
Orchitis			X		
Hand-foot-mouth disease		X			X
Exanthem		X	X	X	X
Conjunctivitis		X			X
Aseptic meningitis	X	X	X	X	X
Paralysis, encephalitis	X		X	X	X
Chronic meningoencephalitis				X	
Generalized neonatal disease			X	X	

Reproduced by permission from Amstey MS, editor: Virus infections in pregnancy, New York, 1984, Grune & Stratton, Inc.

buttocks. Patients usually have a low-grade fever and sore throat and recover within a week.

A variety of exanthems may be the sole or major manifestation of enterovirus infection. Epidemics are reported with the classic macular blanching rubella-like rash, the so-called Boston exanthem.[8] It begins on the face and trunk and spreads to the extremities and is distinguished from rubella by the lack of adenopathy. Unusual enterovirus rashes may be maculopapular, vesicular, roseola-like, urticarial, or petechial. When such exanthems occur in conjunction with other enterovirus syndromes such as aseptic meningitis, the illness may be mistaken for more serious disease, such as meningococcal meningitis.

The coxsackieviruses B are often implicated in epidemic pleurodynia, or Bornholm disease. Fever and severe pain in the intercostal and abdominal muscles occur in spasms lasting minutes to hours. The succeeding episodes are milder than the first but may recur days and sometimes even months later. Occasionally symptoms are severe enough to prompt an exploratory laparotomy.

Gastrointestinal symptoms of nausea, vomiting, abdominal pain, constipation, diarrhea, and peritonitis are seen occasionally but almost always with other signs of systemic enterovirus infection such as aseptic meningitis. Hepatitis and pancreatitis are usually part of a generalized enterovirus syndrome. Rare cases of juvenile diabetes mellitus have been related to coxsackievirus B. Orchitis occasionally occurs in postpubertal patients in association with coxsackievirus B enterovirus infection.

Acute hemorrhagic conjunctivitis is an epidemic disease marked by the sudden onset of severe eye pain, photophobia, tearing, dramatic subconjunctival hemorrhage, and swelling. Recovery occurs in a week to 10 days. Illness is most often observed in the middle-aged person. Neurologic residua are not unusual; improvement may take several months. The worldwide pandemic of this disease began in 1969 but only reached the continental United States in 1981.

Of great clinical importance is enterovirus aseptic meningitis. The classic disease presents in the school-age child with headache, nuchal rigidity, fever, and often photophobia, pharyngitis, or a rash. Cerebrospinal fluid analysis shows a moderate pleocytosis with a predominance of lymphocytes, normal glucose levels, and slightly increased protein levels. Occasionally, meningitis (as documented by virus isolation) is present without pleocytosis, especially in the very young infant.[6] Diagnostic dilemmas are not infrequent when such illness occurs in the infant less than a year of age, in sporadic cases, during a course of antibiotic therapy, or with atypical associated findings such as a petechial rash or encephalitis. Spinal fluid obtained early in the course often has a polymorphonuclear cell type predominant; cell counts greater than $1000/mm^3$ are reported. In some patients a second spinal tap following a 6- to 12-hour observation period may clarify the diagnosis.[9,14] In doubtful cases the results of viral cultures may significantly reduce the length of the course of antibiotics and hospitalization.[5]

The course of enterovirus-associated meningitis is usually mild, although complications such as the syndrome of inappropriate secretion of antidiuretic hormone are occasionally seen.[3] Most patients recover within 2 weeks; occasional relapses are seen. Several studies indicate that as many as 10% of survivors of aseptic meningitis occurring before 3 months of age may suffer long-term neurologic sequelae, especially speech and language delay.[13,16] Older children apparently recover completely.[1]

In the United States, paralytic disease still occurs with wild-type poliovirus in unvaccinated populations such as certain religious groups. It is rarely seen associated with vaccine virus strains in young adults or in immunodeficient individuals. Infection with other enterovirus serotypes may also result in paralysis. Nonpolio enterovirus paralysis may be more common in the United States than classic poliovirus-associated disease.[10] Asymmetric weakness and/or paralysis without sensory loss differentiates this illness from Guillain-Barré syndrome. Life-threatening disease usually involves paralysis of the primary and accessory respiratory muscles or bulbar poliomyelitis of the respiratory center. Treatment is entirely supportive; recovery of muscle function may continue for several months.

In the 1980s a new syndrome of progressive weakness and fatigue was recognized in long-term survivors of paralytic poliomyelitis. This "postpolio syndrome" is seen decades following the initial infection. Apparently the previously affected muscles suffer denervation, as overburdened motor neurons eventually "wear out." The long-term outcome of this new syndrome is unknown.[7]

Unusual enterovirus syndromes include encephalitis, often occurring in severely ill neonates, and the chronic meningoencephalitis of hypogammaglobulinemic patients. Myocarditis and pericarditis occur with a high mortality as part of the generalized disease of newborns. Less than 50% of older children and adults with myocarditis die; recovery may be complete, but severe sequelae have been reported.

Enterovirus infection in neonates may occur as any of the syndromes seen in older children.[11] However, premature infants and newborns born without specific passively acquired maternal antibody may suffer a fulminant, rapidly fatal disease. This generalized neonatal infection frequently begins as a syndrome of fever, lethargy, and poor feeding indistinguishable from early bacterial sepsis. Progression is swifter, with multiorgan involvement, including hepatitis, pancreatitis, myocarditis, and encephalitis. Mortality is high in the disseminated forms of infection. The virus in neonates is most often transmitted from mother to infant at or near the time of delivery; however, nursery outbreaks with fatal cases have been reported.

PREVENTION

Attenuated or killed poliovirus vaccines are the only enterovirus preparations currently available. The multiplicity of serotypes and unpredictable epidemiologic behavior of enteroviruses make developing other vaccines impractical.

An enhanced-potency inactivated poliovirus vaccine became available in the United States in 1988. This formulation should be used in immunizing immunocompromised individuals and/or their household contacts. This is of particular importance as infection with the human immunodeficiency virus becomes widespread; there may be households with several severely immunodeficient members. Details of vaccine administration schedules for partially immunized or immunodeficient patients are available from the Centers for Disease Control.[2] In the prevaccine years, 0.2 ml/kg of pooled immune serum globulin given intramuscularly prevented or ameliorated poliovirus infection.[4] In view of the severe disease experienced by neonates, such injections would be justified in nursery epidemics and for infants of mothers suffering probable enterovirus disease within a few days of delivery.

REFERENCES

1. Bergman I et al: Outcome in children with enteroviral meningitis during the first year of life, J Pediatr 110:705, 1987.
2. Centers for Disease Control: Poliomyelitis prevention: enhanced-potency inactivated poliomyelitis vaccine—supplementary statement, MMWR 36:795, 1987.
3. Chemtob S, Reece ER, and Mills EL: Syndrome of inappropriate secretion of antidiuretic hormone in enteroviral meningitis, Am J Dis Child 139:292, 1985.
4. Cherry JD: Non-polio enteroviruses: coxsackieviruses, echoviruses, and enteroviruses. In Feigin RD and Cherry JD, editors: Textbook of pediatric infectious diseases, Philadelphia, 1981, WB Saunders Co.
5. Chonmaitree T, Menegus MA, and Powell KR: The clinical relevance of "CSF viral cultures": a two-year experience with aseptic meningitis in Rochester, New York, JAMA 247:1843, 1982.
6. Dagan R, Jenista JA, and Menegus MA: Association of clinical presentation, laboratory findings, and virus serotypes with the presence of meningitis in hospitalized infants with enterovirus infection, J Pediatr 113:975, 1988.
7. Dalakas MC et al: A long-term follow-up study of patients with post-poliomyelitis neuromuscular symptoms, N Engl J Med 314:959, 1986.
8. Hall CB et al: The return of Boston exanthem, Am J Dis Child 131:323, 1977.
9. Harrison SA and Risser WL: Repeat lumbar puncture in the differential diagnosis of meningitis, Pediatr Infect Dis J 7:143, 1988.
10. Hayward JC et al: Outbreak of poliomyelitis-like paralysis associated with enterovirus 71, Pediatr Infect Dis J 8:611, 1989.
11. Lake AM et al: Enterovirus infections in neonates, J Pediatr 89:787, 1976.
12. Morens DM: Enteroviral disease in early infancy, J Pediatr 92:374, 1978.
13. Sells CJ, Carpenter RL, and Ray CG: Sequelae of central nervous system enterovirus infections, N Engl J Med 293:1, 1975.
14. Singer JI et al: Management of central nervous system infections during an epidemic of enteroviral aseptic meningitis, J Pediatr 96:559, 1980.
15. Wildin S and Chonmaitree T: The importance of the virology laboratory in the diagnosis and management of viral meningitis, Am J Dis Child 141:454, 1987.
16. Wilfert CM et al: Longitudinal assessment of children with enteroviral meningitis during the first three months of life, Pediatrics 67:811, 1981.

203

Foreign Bodies of the Ear, Nose, Airway, and Esophagus

Jay N. Dolitsky and Robert F. Ward

Foreign bodies of the ear, nose, and upper aerodigestive tract represent a common problem among children, particularly those under 5 years of age. The scope of the problem was first underscored by National Safety Council statistics in 1969, which showed that *more children died at home from accidental foreign body ingestion or aspiration than from any other cause.*[1] In 1988 foreign body aspiration and asphyxiation constituted the fourth leading cause of accidents in the home among children under 5 years of age, and it is still a major problem.[2] The severity of the problem depends on several factors, including the site, composition, and duration of residence of the foreign body. The clinical presentation and management of these objects are similarly related to those factors.

Foreign body removal does not usually have to be done emergently, and should be attempted only after the physician has as many factors under control as possible. These factors include appropriate sedation or anesthesia, proper instrumentation and illumination and, most importantly, ability. If these elements are lacking, the problem will very likely be worsened by attempting to remove the foreign body, and the child's well-being may be jeopardized.

FOREIGN BODIES OF THE EAR

Foreign bodies of the external auditory canal are most commonly found in children between 2 and 4 years of age. Curiosity, boredom, and imitation of others are often predisposing factors. Accidental entry of a foreign object through placement in the external auditory canal, either by the child or a companion, can occur during play. Insects can also find their way into the ear canal without any assistance. Das reviewed 233 cases of foreign bodies in the ear and nose and found that the most consistent etiologic factor was chronic irritation or inflammation of these orifices.[4] Thus children with chronic external otitis are more likely to place objects in their ear canals.

Clinical Presentation

Depending on the depth of the foreign object within the external auditory canal, the nature and composition of the object, and its duration in the canal, there may be a wide spectrum of findings. A history of placing an object in the ear canal will usually be absent, because most children are reluctant to admit to this activity for fear of punishment.

Nonreactive substances, such as plastic, that are not completely obstructing the canal and not abutting the tympanic membrane may not cause symptoms. Insects tend to incite local irritation, causing discomfort, erythema, and occasionally drainage. Vegetable matter may also cause local inflammation, which will frequently lead to local pain and itching. Objects touching the tympanic membrane will cause pain, particularly with movement of the drum, as when swallowing. If the entire canal is obstructed, hearing loss will most likely occur.

Recently there have been several reports concerning button-sized alkaline batteries as foreign bodies of the ear canal.[3,10,12] These objects may leak battery acid, causing a severe local tissue reaction with pain, swelling, and discharge. This new type of foreign body should be handled expeditiously to avoid serious injury to the canal or tympanic membrane.

Management

Nonreactive foreign bodies that do not completely occlude the external canal or impinge on the tympanic membrane are nonemergent. These can be removed with a variety of instruments; the most useful will depend on the shape and composition of the object. Often a 6- or 8-mm Frazier tip suction, an alligator forceps, or a right angle hook can be used to retrieve the object. The hook is used by passing it beyond the object, hooking it from behind, and pulling it out gently. Gentle irrigation may also be used on nonvegetable substances; vegetable matter tends to swell when water is applied, thus making its removal more difficult.

When the tympanic membrane cannot be visualized or if there is evidence of inflammation or injury to the external canal, removal of the foreign body should be undertaken immediately. This is particularly important with the presence of an alkaline battery, since tympanic membrane perforations have been reported within only 8 hours of entry.[3] Magnets may be helpful in the removal of metallic objects such as batteries or metal beads.[7]

Insects should be killed before removal, by the instillation of either mineral oil or 4% Xylocaine into the external canal. Extraction with suction or alligator forceps may then proceed.

Following removal of any foreign body, the external canal

and tympanic membrane should be carefully and thoroughly inspected. Aqueous-based acidic ear drops or ophthalmic drops should be used for 5 to 7 days if there appears to be any injury or inflammation to the canal. Water precautions in the affected ear should be encouraged until the ear is completely healed.

In older children who are cooperative, the use of local anesthesia injected with a small-gauge needle into the skin lining the canal may help allow complete foreign body removal and subsequent examination. In younger children or in those who are uncooperative, general anesthesia may be necessary and is certainly preferable to traumatic removal in a child who is unable to cooperate fully.

Complications

Complications can result from the foreign body itself or from traumatic removal. Laceration and inflammation of the external canal is usually not serious and will resolve with instillation of analgesic and antibiotic liquid preparations. Tympanic membrane perforations require careful inspection to ensure that a flap of the membrane has not folded into the middle ear, which may then lead to a permanent perforation or the development of a cholesteatoma. Likewise, when the drum is not intact, there is the potential for contamination of the middle ear space and the development of otitis media.

If it is not possible to remove a foreign object from the ear canal safely or if there is suspicion that the tympanic membrane has been injured by either the foreign body or its removal, the patient should be seen by an otolaryngologist.

FOREIGN BODIES IN THE NOSE

The predicaments that lead to foreign objects in the nasal cavity are quite similar to those of the ear. Boredom, curiosity, and acts of imitation may lead a child to place an object in his or her nose. These objects are typically soft materials such as tissues, erasers, clay, or pieces of a toy. Occasionally a foreign object enters the nose accidentally while the child is attempting to sniff or smell it. Chronic rhinitis was found in Das' study to be the most common underlying factor in children placing objects in their nose.[4]

Clinical Presentation

Children usually will not confess to having placed something in their nose. The most common finding with this problem is unilateral nasal discharge, which is usually foul smelling. In fact, the presence of a unilateral nasal discharge in a young child should be considered evidence of a foreign body until proven otherwise. If possible, the nasal cavities should be examined with a nasal speculum and suction. The key to any evaluation is the use of powerful illumination. Roentgenograms may be helpful if the object is radiopaque or has become calcified. U.S. toy manufacturers are required by law to make toy parts radiopaque, a regulation that proves quite valuable when a physician is looking for foreign objects in the nasal cavity or in any other part of the upper aerodigestive tract. However, toys and toy parts manufactured outside the United States do not have to conform to this regulation.

Management

Nasal foreign bodies should be removed as quickly as possible, particularly in the case of an alkaline battery, which can cause severe local inflammation. Young children tend to detest any nasal instrumentation, and the removal of nasal foreign bodies requires some degree of cooperation. Thus sedation or general anesthesia is usually advised. Topical application of an epinephrine-like decongestant, such as Neo-synephrine, in conjunction with the removal of secretions with a small suction tip will help in visualizing the foreign object.

A foreign body that has been allowed to remain in the nose for a long time may become calcified and thus form what is known as a rhinolith. Removal of rhinoliths is often difficult and bloody.

Various methods of removal have been described that can be attempted in the office. These include using pepper to induce a sneeze while the uninvolved nostril is occluded, or blowing in the child's mouth while the contralateral nostril is held shut. Another method of removal involves use of a Fogarty or small Foley catheter.[6] The catheter is placed beyond the foreign body into the posterior portion of the nasal cavity or nasopharynx and then inflated with 2 to 3 ml of saline solution. The catheter is then drawn gently forward and out of the nose, thus expelling the object. The danger with this technique is that the foreign object may be dislodged by pushing it posteriorly into the nasopharynx, potentially leading to aspiration of the object.

Removal usually can be performed with a Frazier tip suction for soft, friable objects. If the foreign body is rigid, then removal may be accomplished by using a nasal bayonet or Hartman or alligator forceps. After removal, local inflammation manifested by oozing may be controlled with saline nose drops and an antibacterial ointment such as bacitracin or mupirocin (Bactroban).

Complications

Complications of nasal foreign bodies are usually limited to local inflammation and irritation. Occasionally local scar formation may occur, with the development of a scar band or synechia. These can be prevented by placing a splint made of Gelfoam or Silastic over the raw, exposed area. Obstruction of a sinus ostium by a foreign object may lead to the development of sinusitis. This typically manifests pain and tenderness over the affected sinus or clouding and an air/fluid level on sinus roentgenograms. Treatment includes oral antibiotics and nasal decongestant drops.

The differential diagnosis of foreign bodies in the nose includes suppurative rhinitis, adenoiditis, sinusitis, and nasal or nasopharyngeal tumors. Nasal polyps may also manifest a unilateral nasal discharge; in the young child, the diagnosis of cystic fibrosis must be ruled out.

FOREIGN BODIES OF THE AIRWAY

A statistic mentioned earlier bears repeating: Foreign body aspiration and asphyxiation is the fourth leading cause of accidental death in the home of children under 5 years of age.[2] It accounts for approximately 8% of all home accidental deaths of children in this age group. Over 5 years of age the incidence rapidly declines until age 65, when it increases again to an even higher percentage. Overall the incidence of death from foreign body aspiration has declined significantly during the past 2 decades.[2] This is likely the result of increased parental awareness of the risks of leaving small objects within the reach of young children. Consumer education and awareness have been important in the decline of this potential hazard. Also, the development of lifesaving techniques, such as the Heimlich maneuver, that can be performed by people who are not medical personnel accounts for a higher survival rate.

The airway can be divided into three segments with regard to foreign body impaction—the larynx, the trachea, and the bronchial tree. Lima reviewed all airway foreign body admissions to his pediatric hospital from 1980 through 1987.[8] Of the 91 cases, 11 involved a foreign body lodged in the larynx. Of these 11 patients, 5 died and 3 suffered anoxic encephalopathy. It is apparent that although most foreign bodies pass through the larynx, the outcome is grave when one does not.

Etiology

The causes of foreign body impaction in the airway are many. As with foreign bodies of other head and neck orifices, curiosity or boredom may lead a young child to put foreign objects in his or her mouth. Infants in particular are known to explore their world with their oral sense and will attempt to place almost anything they can handle in their mouths. A startle may cause inadvertent ingestion or aspiration. Lack of complete dentition, as well as lack of attention to chewing, allows large food particles to enter the posterior pharynx. Incomplete development of mouth and tongue coordination in young children also may account for a greater incidence of foreign body ingestion or aspiration. Reichert reports that a positive association has been noted between the occurrence of upper respiratory infections and foreign body aspiration.[11] He postulates that the need for continuous mouth breathing when a child suffers a cold interrupts a smooth breathing-swallowing pattern, leading to increased aspirations.

Clinical Presentation

A history of foreign body ingestion or aspiration may or may not be obtained, depending on the age or condition of the patient and whether the suspected incident was witnessed. Classically, when a foreign object is initially aspirated into the respiratory tract, it will produce a choking, gagging, coughing, or wheezing episode. This may be followed by an asymptomatic interval when there is little to suggest the presence of a foreign body. At this time the parent and physician are often lulled into a false sense of security.

Depending on the site of the foreign body within the airway, a patient may manifest a spectrum of findings, from being almost completely asymptomatic to having signs of complete airway obstruction.

Laryngeal foreign bodies are likely to produce the most acute and dramatic presentation. Large objects that completely obstruct the airway may manifest stridor, high-pitched wheezing, cough, dysphonia, or worse—aphonia and cyanosis. Children with smaller, partially obstructing objects that allow adequate air exchange have cough, stridor, hoarseness, pain, or discomfort.

Tracheal foreign bodies are usually associated with cough and some degree of stridor or wheezing and may produce an audible "slap" as the object moves from the carina to the glottis with respiration. Bronchial foreign bodies usually cause wheezing or coughing if they are partially obstructing. Frequently this is misdiagnosed as asthma. With complete obstruction of a bronchus comes an initial asymptomatic period, followed by a postobstructive pneumonitis or bronchiectasis.[9] Sharp objects such as pins or tacks may produce pain or hemoptysis.

If aspiration of a foreign body into the upper airway is suspected, plain roentgenography may help. For objects suspected to be lodged in the laryngeal inlet, upper trachea, or esophageal inlet, anteroposterior and lateral high-kilovolt roentgenograms should be obtained if the patient's condition permits. Bronchial foreign bodies may be suggested by some form of dynamic roentgen ray study—either inspiratory-expiratory roentgenograms or videofluoroscopy. These studies can demonstrate air trapping in the affected lung.

Management

Foreign bodies completely obstructing the laryngeal inlet create a life-threatening emergency and should be expelled immediately by using the Heimlich maneuver (abdominal thrusts). For infants under 1 year of age, four back blows followed by four chest thrusts should be substituted. (See Appendix A, "Pediatric Basic and Advanced Life Support.") If the foreign body cannot be expelled, a large-bore needle or angiocatheter (14 gauge) should be inserted into the cricothyroid space to allow some degree of ventilation until the patient can be taken to the operating room for removal. Alternately, if skilled personnel are present, an emergency tracheotomy may be necessary. Partially obstructing laryngeal foreign bodies should be treated in a way that prevents total airway obstruction; therefore back blows and abdominal thrusts should be avoided.

Tracheal and bronchial foreign bodies should be removed by a physician specifically trained for the task. This usually requires controlled endoscopic removal in the operating room. Usually this is not an emergency; thus adequate preparations can be made.

Complications

Abdominal and chest thrusts may damage intraabdominal contents (e.g., liver, spleen) and ribs respectively. These techniques should therefore be used only in cases of complete airway obstruction that otherwise would cause certain death. Conversion of a partial airway obstruction by a foreign body to a complete obstruction can be best avoided by having skilled personnel retrieve the airway foreign body.

A bronchial foreign body that remains in place for an extended period of time may cause air trapping and irreversible bronchiectatic changes distal to the obstruction.

Prolonged or difficult instrumentation of the airway during

foreign body removal can lead to laryngeal edema or injury, with obstructive symptoms. This may require a period of intubation postoperatively. As an alternative, postoperative edema may at times be avoided by the use of intraoperative and/or postoperative steroids.

FOREIGN BODIES INVOLVING THE ESOPHAGUS

More than half of the foreign bodies in children involve the esophagus, with the highest incidence in children 14 months to 6 years of age.[14] The younger children are inquisitive and tend to explore objects orally. The objects are then intentionally swallowed or are accidentally ingested as the result of a startle. In the United States coins are the most common foreign body to lodge in the esophagus.[13]

The esophagus has four physiologic areas of narrowing—the cricopharyngeal sphincter, the aortic arch, the region of the left main bronchus, and the gastroesophageal sphincter. These correspond to the four most common sites for foreign body obstruction. The cricopharyngeus is the most common, the arch of the aortic region the most dangerous.

Clinical Presentation

The history of foreign body ingestion is often not obtained, and most foreign bodies pass through the normal esophagus undetected. Those that do not pass freely initially stimulate the larynx and cause gagging and coughing. Subsequent symptoms depend on size, composition, and nature of the foreign body. With young children, poor feeding or refusal to eat or drink, as well as increased salivation, are typically present. When the esophagus is completely or almost completely obstructed, choking and vomiting occur. The duration of the foreign body obstruction can affect the clinical presentation: The longer a foreign object is present, the greater the tissue reaction and local inflammation. Thus in the later stages patients can have pain on swallowing, fever, and leukocytosis.

When a foreign body is suspected, PA and lateral roentgenograms, in addition to neck films, will be diagnostic if the object is radiopaque, such as a coin. Contrast studies can be used when an esophageal foreign body that does not show on routine radiographs is strongly suspected.

Management

The presence of an esophageal foreign body does not usually call for emergency measures, but removal should be undertaken as soon as possible after proper evaluation and preparation have.[5] Often children will have eaten recently, and it is generally recommended that an appropriate period of time elapse before they are given general anesthesia. If the foreign body is corrosive, such as an alkaline button battery, removal should proceed as soon as possible to prevent severe inflammation and potential perforation of the esophageal wall.

Endoscopic removal under anesthesia by a trained expert remains the method of choice because of the safety provided. This technique allows for direct visualization of the esophagus, its mucosa, and the foreign body. Removal with a flexible endoscope is also possible without general anesthesia.

Nonendoscopic techniques of esophageal foreign body removal (i.e., with a Foley or Fogarty catheter) have been described.[6] The child is sedated and brought to the fluoroscopy suite. While the child is in a steep Trendelenburg position, the catheter is placed beyond the foreign object and the balloon on the catheter is inflated and withdrawn. This technique can lead to aspiration and airway obstruction and is not generally recommended.

Complications

Esophageal perforation can occur from the endoscopic procedure or from the foreign body itself, especially if it is sharp or caustic. This technique is particularly dangerous with objects that are lodged at the level of the aortic arch. If an esophageal tear is suspected, contrast roentgenography will usually confirm the suspicion.

Foreign bodies that have been in the esophagus for long periods of time can cause a stricture to develop. Again a contrast study should be performed to aid in the diagnosis.

REFERENCES

1. Accident facts, National Safety Council, Chicago, 1969.
2. Accident facts, National Safety Council, Chicago, 1988.
3. Capo JM and Lucente FE: Alkaline battery foreign bodies of the ear and nose, Arch Otolaryngol Head Neck Surg 112:562, 1986.
4. Das SK: Etiological evaluation of foreign bodies in the ear and nose, J Laryngol Otol 98:989, 1984.
5. Giordano A et al: Current management of esophageal foreign bodies, Arch Otol, 107:249, 1981.
6. Henry LN and Chamberlain JW: Removal of foreign bodies from the esophagus and nose with the use of a Foley catheter, Surgery 71:918, 1972.
7. Landry GL and Edmanson MB: Attractive method for battery removal, JAMA 256:3351, 1986 (letter).
8. Lima JA: Laryngeal foreign bodies in children: a persistent life-threatening problem, Laryngoscope 99:415, 1989.
9. Mears AJ and England RM: Dissolving foreign bodies in the trachea and bronchus, Thorax 30:461, 1975.
10. Rachlin LS: Assault with battery, N Engl J Med 311:921, 1984 (letter).
11. Reichert TJ: Foreign bodies of the larynx, trachea, and bronchi. In Bluestone CD and Stool SE, editors: Pediatric otolaryngology, ed 2, Philadelphia, 1990, WB Saunders Co.
12. Skinner DW and Chiu P: The hazards of "button-sized" batteries as foreign bodies in the nose and ear, Laryngol Otol 100:1315, 1986.
13. Turtz MG and Stool SE: Foreign bodies of the pharynx and esophagus. In Bluestone CD and Stool SE, editors: Pediatric otolaryngology, ed 2, Philadelphia, 1990, WB Saunders Co.
14. Witt WJ: The role of rigid endoscopy in foreign body management, Ear Nose Throat J 64:70, 1985.

204

Fractures and Dislocations in Children

R. Scott Strahlman

At first glance the reader may feel that this chapter is unnecessary—that fractures and dislocations are a topic more appropriately discussed by orthopedic surgeons in an orthopedic textbook. The truth, however, is that pediatricians see scores of fractures and dislocations each year. Whether a particular injury is managed conservatively by the pediatrician or referred to an orthopedic specialist is up to the individual primary care provider; regardless, a familiarity with the proper management and triage is essential. This chapter covers the pathophysiology, clinical assessment, and classification of fractures and dislocations, as well as some of the more common conditions encountered in primary care.

ETIOLOGY AND PATHOPHYSIOLOGY

A fracture is defined as a break or crack in a bone. The fracture may occur directly at the site of injury or indirectly when the break occurs at a site different from the applied force. *Stress* fractures result from recurrent trauma to a bone and often occur in athletes (e.g., long-bone fractures in distance runners). *Pathologic* fractures can occur without trauma when a bone is weakened, as with osteogenesis imperfecta or a tumor.

A dislocation is defined as a malposition of bone ends that normally appose one another within a joint. Dislocations are far less common in children than are fractures because a child's ligaments are quite strong; with an injury, it is more likely that a bone will break or a growth plate will separate than that a ligament will tear.

Certain broad generalizations can be made about the pathophysiology of childhood fractures.[1] First, fractures in children heal more rapidly than in adults. For example, a fractured clavicle in a 4-year-old may heal in as little as 3 weeks! Second, the remodeling that occurs in the healing of pediatric fractures often corrects residual bony deformities. Third, children's bones are resilient; they bend instead of break, or they break on one side only (a greenstick fracture). Fourth, a phenomenon called overgrowth occurs in pediatric long-bone fractures. Overgrowth is an accelerated growth rate of bony fragments during healing. Long-bone fractures must therefore be corrected with overriding of the broken ends to prevent length discrepancies with the uninjured side. A final observaton is that one must protect the growth plate in children's fractures. A growth plate injury can result in the loss of growth potential.

INITIAL ASSESSMENT

With any suspected fracture or dislocation, an accurate history is essential. Historical details may give clues about the *mechanism* of injury. One should find out how, where, and when the injury occurred and where any pain is located. Does the parent or child report any loss of function in the affected limb? Is there a previous or recurrent history of trauma?

A complete physical examination, including measurement of the vital signs, should be performed. A neurovascular assessment is important. The examiner should look carefully for any unnatural or deformed position of joints or limbs. Pain with palpation or attempted movement may be a clue. Swelling and discoloration may be seen. One can sometimes elicit crepitus at a fracture site.

Radiography is a mainstay in the diagnosis of fractures and dislocations. Roentgenograms from two angles are indicated to delineate subtle fractures. It is sometimes helpful to include the joint above and below the injury to rule out a dislocation. One may wish to radiograph the unaffected side to provide a comparison view. Stress fractures are often not seen on roentgenograms. If a stress fracture is suspected, a radionuclide bone scan may be indicated.[3]

CLASSIFICATION

Fractures are characterized in various ways to give the orthopedic surgeon information. This information in turn aids in the formulation of a management plan and prognosis for the fracture.

One way that orthopedists classify fractures is according to the clinical appearance. A *closed* fracture has no break in the skin. In an *open*, or *compound*, fracture, a bone fragment is exposed to the air, thereby increasing the risk of infection or injury to adjacent nerves and blood vessels. A *hidden* fracture causes slight pain and swelling but no obvious bone deformity. Roentgenograms are necessary to confirm the diagnosis. An *obvious* fracture or dislocation is an injury easily seen, even with a cursory examination. Immediate medical attention is necessary.

Fractures are also classified according to their radiographic appearance. Breaks in the bone may be described as *transverse*, *oblique*, or *spiral*. A *comminuted* fracture is a bone in three or more fragments. In an *impacted* fracture the bone ends are compressed into each other.

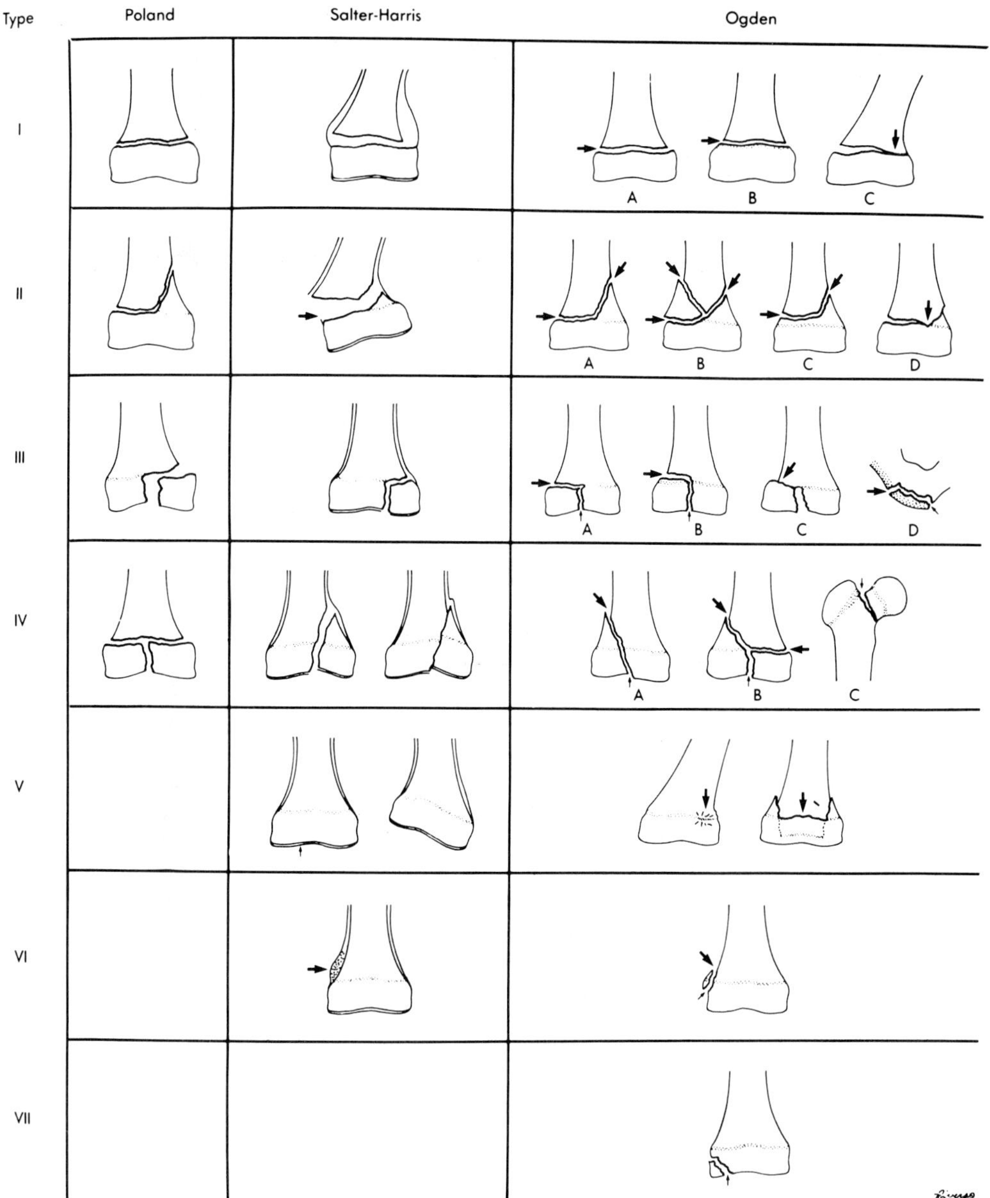

Fig. 204-1 Salter classification of growth plate injuries.

From Canale ST and Beaty JH: Operative pediatric orthopaedics, St Louis, 1990, Mosby–Year Book.

Probably the most important classification of fractures is the Salter-Harris system of describing injury to the growth plate (Fig. 204-1). Growth or epiphyseal plate injuries *only* occur in childhood. They must be treated with care to protect a bone's growth potential. Approximately 15% of all childhood fractures involve the growth plate.[4]

In a Salter I fracture, the epiphysis is separated from the metaphysis without a true break in the bone. Roentgenograms are often normal, and the diagnosis is made on the basis of the clinical picture: tenderness over the area of the growth plate. Usually growth is not disturbed. The treatment is immobilization by cast for approximately 3 weeks.

The most common growth plate fracture is the type II fracture, in which a fragment of metaphyseal bone separates from the epiphysis. Closed reduction of the fracture is usually possible, and with proper casting, growth is not disturbed.

A Salter III fracture involves a *partial* growth plate injury through the epiphysis. An open repair of the fracture in the operating room is indicated to align articular surfaces and preserve joint function.

When a fracture goes *across* the growth plate, injuring both the epiphysis and the metaphysis, it is termed a Salter IV fracture. Perfect realignment of the fracture is necessary to protect growth potential.

In a Salter V fracture, the growth plate is compressed. The prognosis for preserving growth is poor in this case because of a *crush* injury to the growth plate.

MANAGEMENT

Fractures and dislocations should be splinted and immobilized immediately. With most fractures and dislocations, consultation with an orthopedics specialist is then necessary. Most pediatric fractures respond to closed reduction by the orthopedist. If the growth plate is affected, however, open reduction is performed. Close pediatric and orthopedic follow-up are always important. A child in a cast should be comfortable: if pain is persistent, the child needs reevaluation and possibly recasting.

COMMONLY ENCOUNTERED FRACTURES AND DISLOCATIONS

Fractured Clavicle

The "broken collarbone" is the most frequent fracture in children. It can occur at any time during childhood secondary to trauma. This fracture often occurs at birth when there is a difficult vaginal delivery. Physical findings include decreased arm motion on the affected side, crepitus, and swelling at the fracture site. A roentgenogram or ultrasound study may be needed to confirm the diagnosis.[2] If the condition is asymptomatic, there is no treatment; indeed, the diagnosis is often made after the fact when a callus at the fracture site is noted at a well-baby clinic visit. If the fracture causes pain or decreased arm movement, splinting of the clavicle for 2 to 3 weeks is indicated.

In older children the treatment is splinting for 3 to 4 weeks in a figure eight bandage or a shoulder extension harness. Most of the fracture's healing and realignment are spontaneous.

Congenital Hip Dislocation

Congenital hip dislocation is present from birth but is not always detected in the newborn. For this reason children under 1 year of age should be examined for hip dislocation at every routine visit. The disorder may be secondary to abnormal intrauterine positioning; it is more common in breech infants and in infants delivered by cesarean section.

Roentgenograms are of limited value in the diagnosis of congenital hip dislocation. Therefore the physical examination is of utmost importance. To elicit a dislocated hip, one performs the Ortolani test. With the baby on his or her back, the hips and knees are flexed and the knees brought together. The examiner then places a hand on each of the baby's knees, with each middle finger over the greater trochanter and each thumb over the medial thigh. With gentle abduction of the knees, the dislocated femoral head will slip back into the acetabulum; an audible or palpable "clunk" results. The Barlow test is essentially the reverse of the Ortolani test; one feels the femoral head slip out of the acetabulum when the knees are brought back together. An examiner may feel unusual laxity of the hip by pushing up and down on the thigh when the hips are flexed and adducted. The treatment is referral to an orthopedist for a harness or casting.

Nursemaid Elbow

"Nursemaid elbow" is a commonly encountered dislocation in pediatrics. A transient subluxation of the proximal radial head, it is caused by the inadvertent pulling or "yanking" of a child's arm, often by a parent or caretaker. The condition occurs in children between 1 and 4 years of age. The child refuses to move the arm and keeps it flexed and pronated. Roentgenograms are rarely necessary; the history and characteristic posture of the child's arm confirm the diagnosis. The treatment, easily performed by the pediatrician, is rapid, forceful supination of the forearm while pressure is placed over the proximal radial head. Symptoms usually resolve within 30 minutes. The condition is sometimes recurrent, in which case great care must be taken when holding hands with the affected child!

Child Abuse

Unfortunately, fractures and dislocations are all too commonly a presentation of child abuse (see Chapter 46 on child abuse). Child abuse may come to medical attention as an unexplained fracture or an inconsistency between the history and the physical findings in a childhood injury. There may be an unusually long delay between the time of injury and the time that medical attention is sought. On physical examination one may note multiple bruises. If abuse is suspected, a radiographic bone survey should be obtained. Silent fractures, or multiple fractures in varying stages of healing, may be seen.

When child abuse is suspected, the child should be hospitalized to provide protection as well as appropriate orthopedic care. Protective services and social services should be involved. Pediatric care providers are morally and legally responsible for detecting child abuse and reporting all suspected cases.

REFERENCES

1. Chung SMK: Handbook of pediatric orthopedics, New York, 1986, Van Nostrand Reinhold Co, Inc.
2. Katz R et al: Fracture of the clavicle in the newborn: an ultrasound diagnosis, J Ultrasound Med 7:21, 1988.
3. Rosen PR, Micheli LJ, and Treves S: Early scintigraphic diagnosis of bone stress and fractures in athletic adolescents, Pediatrics 70:11, 1982.
4. Salter RB and Harris WR: Injuries involving the epiphyseal plate, J Bone Joint Surg 45a:591, 1963.

SUGGESTED READINGS

Conrad EU and Rang MC: Fractures and sprains, Pediatr Clin North Am 33:1523, 1986.

Mayer TA: Emergency management of pediatric trauma, Philadelphia, 1985, WB Saunders Co.

Sherk HH et al: Congenital dislocation of the hip: a review, Clin Pediatr (Phila) 20:513, 1981.

Tachdjian MO: Pediatric orthopedics, Philadelphia, 1972, WB Saunders Co.

205

Gastrointestinal Allergy

Aubrey J. Katz

Food allergy is a common but often unsubstantiated diagnosis in pediatric practice. Adverse reactions to foods are a feature of many gastrointestinal diseases; however, although food intolerance is caused by allergy in some patients, many other causes should be considered, such as malabsorption (lactose deficiency), toxic effects of contaminants and additives, and psychological factors.

The gastrointestinal tract contains lymphoid tissue capable of mounting an immunologic response to protect against the penetration of antigens across the epithelium. Lymphocytes and plasma cells are present in Peyer patches and the lamina propria of the small and large intestine; IgA-containing plasma cells account for only 2%. The aberrations in immunologic mechanisms that trigger gastrointestinal allergic reactions are unknown.

Allergic disorders of the gastrointestinal tract may be subdivided into two general groups, specific allergens and eosinophilic (allergic) gastroenteritis. Removing specific allergens from the diet results in amelioration of symptoms, which are exacerbated on reintroduction of the allergen. Cow milk protein allergy and soy protein allergy are the best defined. Eosinophilic (allergic) gastroenteritis exists when two or more food sensitivities are present. Usually, several food sensitivities are identified.

COW MILK PROTEIN ALLERGY

The incidence of cow milk allergy is unknown, but estimates vary between 0.5% and 5% of infants under 6 months of age. There is some suggestion that the most antigenic component of cow milk is beta-lactoglobulin. The symptoms and signs of cow milk allergy are listed in the box on p. 1256. Gastrointestinal symptoms predominate in a large number of patients. In other patients, anaphylaxis or pulmonary symptoms occur.[4] Gastrointestinal (GI) manifestations depend on the site of predominant inflammation in the gastrointestinal tract. Esophagitis manifests as recurrent vomiting; gastritis as vomiting, colic, and "GI bleeding"; and enteritis manifest as diarrhea, malabsorption, or protein-losing enteropathy.[2,5]

Enteral gastritis is a common finding in these patients, with increased eosinophils and inflammatory cells in the antrum. Duodenal biopsy reveals patchy changes ranging from normal mucosa to "flat gut" lesions (see Chapter 208, "Gluten-Sensitive Enteropathy"). Esophagitis was recently described, and the biopsies are identical to those for esophagitis associated with gastroesophageal reflux disease. Colitis is common in these patients, who have blood or mucus in the stool. In fact, in those under 6 months of age, allergy is second only to infection as the cause of colitis.

SOY PROTEIN ALLERGY

Soy protein is a very common food additive. Recent studies have revealed that up to 30% of infants allergic to milk protein are also allergic to soy protein.[1] The clinical features of soy protein allergy are similar to those of milk protein allergy in that gastritis, enteritis, and colitis occur.

BREAST MILK COLITIS

The term "breast milk colitis" is a misnomer, but it is now apparent that infants who are breast fed only may develop the same symptoms as patients who are fed formula. It is apparent that allergens cross the breast milk into the baby. The commonest symptom in this group is colitis, with blood or mucus in the stool.[6] These patients are always asymptomatic with no evidence of an acute abdomen, and the findings are confirmed on sigmoidoscopy and rectal biopsy. Rectal biopsy reveals a significant number of eosinophils. Treatment in this instance involves persuading the mother to avoid dairy products completely; 20% of infants respond to this measure. It is extremely rare to have to take these babies off breast milk. Experience has shown that if removing milk from the mother's diet does not alleviate the symptoms, breast-feeding can be resumed, since the colitis is usually mild and self-limited.

EOSINOPHILIC (ALLERGIC) GASTROENTERITIS

Eosinophilic, or allergic, gastroenteritis is a condition characterized by peripheral eosinophilia and infiltration of the gastrointestinal tract with eosinophils.[8] Hypereosinophilic syndromes, which are characterized by infiltration of many organs with eosinophils, are not included in this category. Three types of disease manifestation are described, depending on the site of gastrointestinal involvement: (1) Mucosal disease manifests as protein-losing enteropathy, malabsorption, and gastrointestinal blood loss; (2) submucosal disease usually manifests with pyloric obstruction; (3) serosal disease manifests with eosinophilic ascites. The latter two types are less common in children.

Etiology

The presence of peripheral eosinophilia, systemic allergy, elevated IgE levels, and therapeutic response to steroids indicates an allergic basis for this disease in some patients.

Cow Milk Allergy

Systemic signs
- Anaphylaxis
- Iron-deficiency anemia (secondary to GI blood loss)
- Rhinitis
- Wheezing
- Pulmonary hemosiderosis
- Nasopharyngeal obstruction leading to cor pulmonale
- Peripheral eosinophilia

Gastrointestinal manifestations
- Vomiting
- Diarrhea/malabsorption/protein-losing enteropathy
- Colic
- Gastrointestinal bleeding
- Failure to thrive

Eosinophilic (Allergic) Gastroenteritis

Peripheral eosinophilia (common to all three types of disease)

Mucosal disease
- Protein-losing enteropathy leading to hypoalbuminemia and hypogammaglobulinemia
- Growth failure
- Iron-deficiency anemia secondary to occult gastrointestinal blood loss
- Systemic allergy

Submucosal disease
- May have features of mucosal disease
- Pyloric obstruction

Serosal disease: eosinophilic ascites

Pathology

The small intestine reveals lesions, patchy in distribution, ranging from areas of normal mucosa to a flat villus lesion.[7] Eosinophilic infiltration may be mild or marked. Gastric abnormalities, more commonly found in the antrum, have been described as being consistent in the mucosal form of the disease. The stomach shows evidence of gastritis, with destruction and regeneration of gastric glands and surface epithelium. Eosinophilic infiltration is usually marked. Esophagitis with significant eosinophilic infiltration is a common finding in these patients.[3] Preliminary data indicate that biopsies in these cases are identical to those for patients with reflux esophagitis.

Clinical Features

Peripheral eosinophilia is common to all three types of disease. The mucosal form has many of the features listed in the box at the right, whereas pyloric obstructive disease, especially serosal disease, commonly do not have all these features. Whether these are variants of a similar disease process or distinctly different entities remains to be solved. Pyloric obstructive disease manifests with vomiting, and serosal disease with ascites. Numerous eosinophils are present in the ascitic fluid. Growth failure is a prominent feature of mucosal disease in childhood; diarrhea often is not a feature. These patients usually have evidence of systemic allergy, especially asthma. Thus this syndrome is often missed at initial presentation. Iron-deficiency anemia secondary to gastrointestinal blood loss is another consistent feature, together with protein-losing enteropathy.

Diagnosis

Diagnosis is based on the clinical features and laboratory findings described above. A biopsy of the small intestine reveals both normal mucosa (with or without eosinophilic infiltration) and a flat villus lesion. A gastric antral biopsy appears to be of diagnostic value in the mucosal form of the disease and is usually positive, revealing evidence of gastritis with marked eosinophilic infiltration.

Treatment

Eliminating these allergens, which are found to be highly positive in affected patients, from the diet, may alleviate most of the symptoms. In many cases, corticosteroid therapy may be required intermittently. Pyloric obstructive disease may require surgery.

Prognosis

Extensive follow-up studies are lacking, but evidence appears to indicate that eosinophilic gastroenteritis is a lifelong condition with remissions and exacerbations, often requiring careful dietary manipulation and intermittent steroid therapy. Preliminary data also suggest that younger adolescents go through a phase in which they are much better able to tolerate foods they previously were sensitive to.

REFERENCES

1. Ament ME and Rubin CF: Soy protein—another cause of the flat intestinal lesion, Gastroenterology 62:227, 1972.
2. Gryboski JD: Gastrointestinal milk allergy in infants, Pediatrics 40:354, 1967.
3. Katz AJ, Goldman H, and Grand RJ: Gastric mucosal biopsy in eosinophilic (allergic) gastroenteritis, Gastroenterology 73:705, 1977.
4. Katz AJ et al: Milk-sensitive and eosinophilic gastroenteropathy: similar clinical features with contrasting mechanisms and clinical course, J Allergy Clin Immunol 74:72, 1984.
5. Kuitenen P et al: Malabsorption syndrome with cow's milk intolerance, Arch Dis Child 50:351, 1975.
6. Lake AM, Whittington PF, and Hamilton SR: Dietary protein-induced colitis in breast-fed infants, J Pediatr 101:906, 1982.
7. Leinbach GE and Rubin CE: Eosinophilic gastroenteritis: a simple reaction to food allergens? Gastroenterology 59:874, 1970.
8. Waldmann TA et al: Allergic gastroenteropathy, N Engl J Med 276:761, 1967.

206

Gastrointestinal Obstruction

David L. Dudgeon

Gastrointestinal obstruction (GIO) during infancy, childhood, and adolescence is relatively uncommon but is always a diagnostic challenge. Obstructions occurring distal to the pylorus are surgical emergencies, and the younger the patient, the more ominous the probable cause and the more urgent the required therapy. Therefore the pediatrician must be continually alert for the presence of a GIO to facilitate an early diagnosis and thus prevent a potential tragedy.

HISTORY

The symptoms and signs of a GIO (Table 206-1) vary considerably but involve the following, either singly or in combination: vomiting, pain, abdominal distention (see Chapter 108), a change in bowel habits, fever, abdominal tenderness, and the presence of a palpable abdominal mass.

Vomiting is a ubiquitous symptom seen far more frequently without a GIO in this age group. However, it can frequently be a sign of obstruction, particularly when certain characteristics are noted.

In an infant, a small amount of nonbilious, nonprojectile vomitus is unlikely to be a GIO and commonly denotes a benign, self-limited form of regurgitation or gastrointestinal reflux (chalasia). However, this picture in the newborn can be associated with an esophageal obstruction (atresia).[2] An esophageal block encountered during the attempted passage of a transoral soft catheter into the stomach denotes esophageal atresia. Respiratory distress can be associated with this anomaly, caused by secondary gastric aspiration or the development of acute gastric distention produced by the commonly associated tracheoesophageal fistula distal to the atresia.[2]

Esophageal atresia and the rare entity of pediatric gastric volvulus are uncommon and the only two neonatal instances in which a congenital or early acquired esophageal obstruction is likely to be encountered. Acute gastric volvulus, as opposed to esophageal atresia, is often accompanied by severe pain and can be associated with signs of shock.

The more dramatic, projectile, nonbilious vomiting of early infancy is associated with the semiurgent condition of congenital hypertrophic pyloric stenosis.[14] Bilious vomiting, usually nonprojectile, is a more ominous problem and denotes a GIO below the level of the ampulla of Vater. This concern is caused by the potential associated condition of intestinal nonrotation with a complicating volvulus, which can produce an intestinal block.[7,16] Although a premature infant with an immature pyloric sphincter can have bilious regurgitation without obstruction, related to an underlying septic process, the threat of intestinal vascular compromise caused by an underlying volvulus mandates an immediate diagnostic radiologic contrast study. Other causes of bilious vomiting in the neonate and infant include duodenal, jejunal, and ileal atresias,[8] duodenal stenosis secondary to annular pancreas or Ladd bands (colonic peritoneal bands crossing the duodenum),[20] meconium ileus, colonic atresia, congenital aganglionosis of the colon (Hirschsprung disease),[5] and imperforate anus.[4] The infant or older toddler with bilious vomiting can have a GIO caused by an incarcerated hernia or an intussusception.[13] The etiology of bilious vomiting in an adolescent also includes incarcerated hernias, postoperative adhesions, and meconium ileus equivalent associated with cystic fibrosis,[11] acute inflammation (appendicitis[3] and pelvic inflammatory disease), and chronic inflammation (regional ileitis and ulcerative colitis).

Vomitus with minimal amounts of blood can be seen in infants with congenital hypertrophic pyloric stenosis.[14] Hematemesis, with larger amounts of blood, is rarely associated with a GIO, as in the uncommon occurrence of an acute peptic ulcer obstruction of the newborn or, more frequently, in the older, chronically stressed infant or child.

Abdominal pain, detectable only as irreconcilable crying or irritability in the infant, usually accompanies a GIO. It is likely to be "crampy" or intermittent in character and results in the drawing up of the legs to the abdomen, with crying interspersed with periods of no apparent or obviously decreased levels of distress. This is best exemplified by the toddler who has an intussusception.[13] A complete or chronic partial obstruction of the intestine produces constant abdominal pain, caused by the resultant intestinal distention or peritoneal inflammation or both.

Obstipation in the newborn is a significant finding. Full-term, otherwise healthy infants spontaneously pass normal meconium within the first 24 hours of life. Premature infants, those small for gestational age,[6] and infants of diabetic mothers[12] frequently delay up to 72 hours before having their initial stool. Likewise, a pregnancy complicated by maternal drug abuse (narcotics such as morphine), drug therapy (e.g., magnesium sulfate for toxemia),[15] or neonatal stress (hypoxemia or sepsis) can also produce a delay of the initial bowel movement.

Atresias of the upper gastrointestinal tract do not routinely produce obstipation; however, the meconium passed by these patients is usually sparse, lighter in color, and may be hard and dry. The differential diagnosis of newborn obstipation includes meconium ileus (usually with underlying cystic fibrosis), meconium plug syndrome (30% are associated with

Table 206-1 *Pediatric Gastrointestinal Obstruction: Clinical Findings*

	FINDINGS						
ETIOLOGY	VOMITING	PAIN	STOOL PATTERN	DISTENTION	BOWEL SOUNDS	TENDERNESS	MASSES
Esophageal atresia	Nonbilious (saliva)	No	Normal meconium	No	Absent to normal	No	No
Gastric obstruction	Nonbilious (curdled formula)	Severe with gastric volvulus; none with antral web	Normal meconium	Epigastric	Absent to normal	Severe with volvulus	No
Hypertrophic pyloric stenosis	Nonbilious, projectile	No	Constipation (dehydration)	Epigastric	Hyperactive (epigastric)	No	Yes ("olive")
Duodenal obstruction	Bilious	Minimal	Small meconium stool	Epigastric	Absent to normal	No	No
Volvulus	Bilious	Severe	Hematochezia	Epigastric to generalized	Hyperactive	Yes (severe)	No
Jejunoileal atresia	Bilious	No	Small, hard, light-colored meconium stool	Generalized	Variable	No	No
Intussusception	Bilious	Yes (crampy)	Currant jelly stool	Generalized	Hyperactive	Yes	Yes ("sausage shaped")
Meconium ileus	Bilious	No	Obstipation	Generalized	Variable	No	Yes ("doughy beads")
Meconium plug	Bilious	No	Obstipation	Generalized	Variable	No	No
Congenital aganglionosis	Bilious	No	Obstipation, constipation, and intermittent diarrhea	Generalized	Hyperactive	No	Palpable stool
Obstipation of prematurity	Bilious	No	Obstipation	Generalized	Hyperactive	No	No
Incarcerated inguinal hernia	Bilious	Yes	Diarrhea or constipation	Generalized	Hyperactive	Yes	Inguinal or scrotal
Imperforate anus	Bilious	No	Obstipation	Generalized	Hyperactive	No	No

congenital aganglionosis of the colon),[10] congenital aganglionosis of the colon, imperforate anus, and in rare cases rectal atresia. Strictures secondary to previous episodes of neonatal necrotizing enterocolitis or previous intestinal surgery, as well as extrinsic compression of the gastrointestinal tract caused by congenital cysts, inflammatory masses, and/or malignancies, produce obstipation or constipation in the older infant or child.

In the pediatric patient, particularly in the neonate and infant, diarrhea or alternating diarrhea and constipation can occur as a sign of a partial or an intermittently complete GIO. Congenital colonic aganglionosis or the more critical problem of an intussusception or intermittent volvulus can also produce this picture (usually presenting with hematochezia or melena).

Hematochezia (a grossly bloody stool) in association with GIO symptoms indicates the presence of intestinal vascular compromise. It occurs most commonly in patients with an intussusception or volvulus.[13,16] This currant jelly stool results from the admixture of blood and mucus and is a sign of superficial mucosal slough, but it also can accompany a full-thickness necrosis of the bowel wall. Occasionally darker (mahogany to black), melena-type stools resulting from a more proximal bleeding site are noted, with the same dire potential.

PHYSICAL EXAMINATION

The physical examination of the abdomen includes an evaluation for distention, which is likely to be prominent if the obstruction is distal to the duodenum (see Table 206-1). Gastric obstruction caused by a congenital antral web, hypertrophic pyloric stenosis, or duodenal atresia produces only mild to moderate epigastric distention, whereas lower intestinal atresias or other forms of lower GIO produce generalized distention. The presence or absence of abdominal distention does not aid in the diagnosis of a potential underlying midgut volvulus, because the obstruction can be at the level of the duodenum, with few air- and fluid-distended bowel loops present.

Abdominal auscultation should be performed before any manipulation of the patient. In larger patients, an effort should be made to listen to all the abdominal quadrants. The presence of high-pitched, "tinkling" bowel sounds heard in "rushes" is diagnostic of a complete GIO. However, the bowel sounds are frequently normal in an early obstruction, becoming diminished to absent in a late obstruction or in the case of a GIO produced by an inflammatory process.

If the abdomen is moderately to grossly distended, a mild amount of tenderness or discomfort is to be expected with palpation, because pressure applied to gas- or fluid-filled loops produces pain. However, marked tenderness, especially accompanied by rebound or referred tenderness, clearly indicates an accompanying peritoneal inflammation. This inflammation (or peritonitis) in the face of a GIO means ischemia of the bowel wall with possible necrosis and demands immediate surgical evaluation and treatment.

The presence of multiple, "doughy" compressible, mobile, nontender abdominal masses in a newborn with a GIO is associated with meconium ileus.[9] A tender, palpable, immobile mass is most likely an area of cellulitis or abscess related to visceral perforation—that is, necrotizing enterocolitis or appendicitis in children and adolescents. A nontender, extremely mobile mass producing GIO symptoms is found with congenital intestinal duplication cysts or mesenteric cysts. Malignancies in the intestinal tract are rare and do not commonly produce intestinal obstruction, but lymphomas may do so in older patients. When they cause GIO, intestinal or mesenteric lymphomas in patients over 4 years of age commonly manifest as intussusception.

An incarcerated inguinal hernia is an important cause of GIO in the pediatric age group. Detecting an inguinal hernia in an uncooperative, chubby infant is difficult and requires considerable patience and effort. Sedation using a tranquilizer with or without an added narcotic analgesic may be helpful. These medications must be used very cautiously to avoid excessive sedation, because vomiting and aspiration may occur. If possible, the hernia should be gently reduced and then repaired at a later time when the effects of GIO have subsided. If left unrepaired, repeat incarcerations are likely, with the potential consequences of strangulation and necrosis of the bowel.

Often a rectal examination can clarify the cause of a GIO. In an infant with a suspected incarcerated inguinal hernia, one can often transanally palpate the peritoneal side of the internal inguinal ring and identify an exiting intraperitoneal structure. The rectal examination can be equally important in the diagnosis of any suspected colonic or distal GIO. Previously unsuspected perirectal or presacral pelvic masses, such as hydrometrocolpos or presacral teratoma, can be identified in this manner. Abnormal stool (as in the patient with meconium plug syndrome) or blood found in association with an intussusception or accompanying inflammatory bowel disease may be detected by performing a rectal examination. In rare cases, the palpation of an intraluminal rectal mass, such as in a low-lying intussusception, is possible during a rectal examination.

TREATMENT

Medical Management

The pediatric patient with a GIO requires gastric decompression to avoid continued bowel distention, vomiting, and aspiration. Intravenous fluid therapy to replace the "third space" (i.e., intraluminal and intraperitoneal) fluid loss is required immediately. When replacing the fluid deficit, it must be remembered that luminal GIO losses are high in electrolyte content, requiring administration of higher-than-maintenance concentrations of sodium, chloride, and potassium. Therefore solutions such as lactated Ringer solution will be needed to provide appropriate replacement. A urinalysis, with catheterization if necessary, as well as a complete blood count and blood chemistry studies are mandatory. Because almost all pediatric patients with GIO require emergent or semiemergent surgery, they must be well prepared for anesthesia and the operative procedure. This requires correction of fluid, electrolyte, hematologic, and metabolic imbalances beforehand. Such corrective measures should begin before extensive diagnostic ultrasounds or radiologic studies are begun.

Table 206-2 lists roentgenographic diagnostic studies re-

Table 206-2 *Common Causes of Pediatric Gastrointestinal Obstruction: Roentgenographic Findings*

	FINDINGS				
ETIOLOGY	DILATED AREA	AIR OR FLUID LEVELS	CALCIUM DEPOSITS	NONCALCIUM OPACITIES	FURTHER STUDIES THAT MAY BE INDICATED
Esophageal atresia	Esophagus and stomach	Yes (gastric)	No	No	Esophageal barium instillation*
Gastric obstruction	Stomach	Yes	No	No	Gastric barium instillation*
Hypertrophic pyloric stenosis	Stomach	Yes	No	No	Ultrasound
Duodenal obstruction	Stomach, duodenum ("double bubble")	Yes	No	No	None
Volvulus	Variable	Variable	No	No	Upper gastrointestinal series or barium enema
Jejunoileal atresia	Stomach and small intestine	Yes	Yes (with perforation)	No	Barium enema to rule out nonrotation
Intussusception	Stomach and small intestine	Variable	No	Yes (soft tissue densities)	Barium enema**
Meconium ileus	Stomach and small intestine	No	Yes (meconium peritonitis)	Yes (ground glass appearance)	Water-soluble contrast enema**
Meconium plug	Stomach to colon	Yes	No	No	Barium enema†
Congenital aganglionosis	Stomach to colon	Yes	No	No	Barium enema
Obstipation of prematurity (short left colon syndrome)	Stomach to colon	Yes	No	No	Barium enema†
Incarcerated inguinal hernia	Stomach and small intestine	Yes	No	No	None
Imperforate anus	Stomach to colon	Yes	No	No	Complete evaluation of genitourinary tract

*Should be performed cautiously to avoid aspiration.
**Should be performed cautiously to avoid bowel perforation.
†May be therapeutic and diagnostic.

quired for a patient with a GIO and the expected findings; these studies are dictated by the results of the history and physical examination. However, a plain roentgenogram of the abdomen is obtained in all patients suspected of having a GIO. In a newborn infant, air localized to the stomach and duodenum ("double-bubble sign") is diagnostic of a duodenal obstruction[20] (Fig. 206-1). If there is no distal intestinal intraluminal air, the GIO is usually caused by an atresia; however, if even a small amount of air is located distally, the diagnosis of a malrotation with possible volvulus must be suspected. The use of a barium enema to ascertain cecal position or of an upper gastrointestinal series to determine the relationship between the duodenum and the jejunum and the ligament of Treitz is necessary to rule out a malrotation or nonrotation of the intestine.[16] The presence of even a large number of air-filled loops on the plain roentgenographic study does not eliminate the need for a contrast study, since a volvulus is still possible. The visualization by barium enema of an "unused," small-caliber distal colon (microcolon) located in a normal position makes more likely the diagnosis of intestinal atresia or meconium ileus rather than the presence of an acute volvulus.

Calcifications seen on the abdominal roentgenogram in a neonate with GIO are evidence of an intrauterine intestinal perforation (meconium peritonitis), which is frequently associated with an intestinal atresia. The calcifications may be small, single or multiple, and scattered throughout the entire peritoneal cavity or may be seen to outline the peritoneal cavity (Fig. 206-2). Cystic fibrosis may or may not be associated with such a presentation.

Infants with suspected hypertrophic pyloric stenosis do not usually require an upper gastrointestinal series to confirm the diagnosis. The classic history and the presence of characteristic upper abdominal peristaltic waves and a palpable olive-size mass in the mid to right upper quadrant are diagnostic; roentgenographic confirmation is needless, costly, and potentially hazardous. The hazard results from the routinely ineffective preoperative efforts to lavage the residual barium from a dilated obstructed stomach. This makes the subsequent induction of a general anesthetic hazardous because of possible barium aspiration. The experienced pediatrician or surgeon will be successful in palpating the olive in approximately 80% to 90% of the patients. Diagnostic ultrasound will

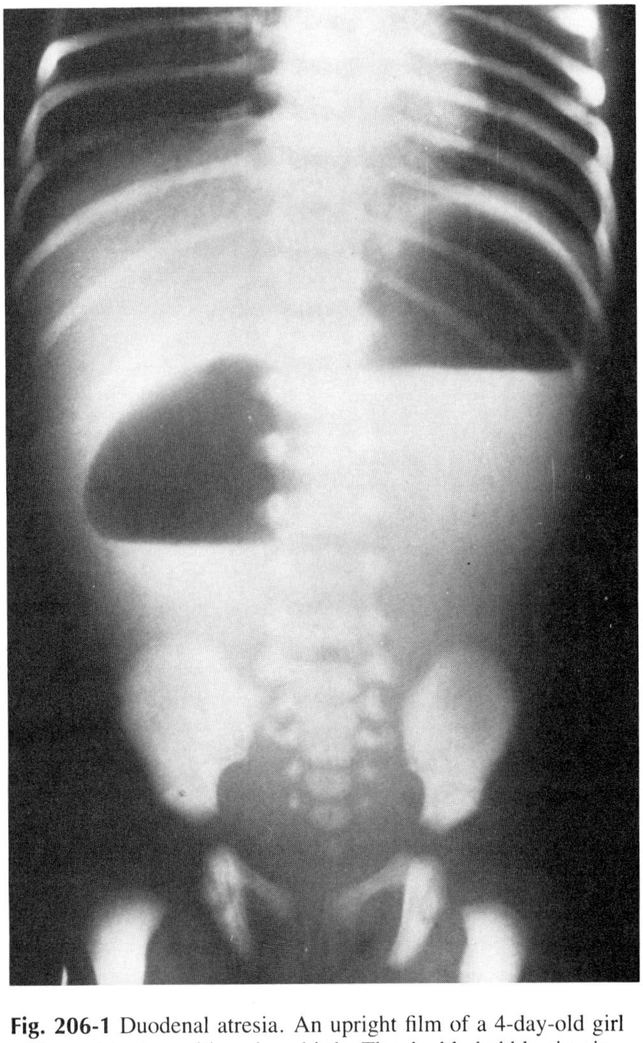

Fig. 206-1 Duodenal atresia. An upright film of a 4-day-old girl with persistent vomiting since birth. The double-bubble sign is classic, showing the large gastric fluid-filled air bubble on the right and the similar duodenal bubble on the left.

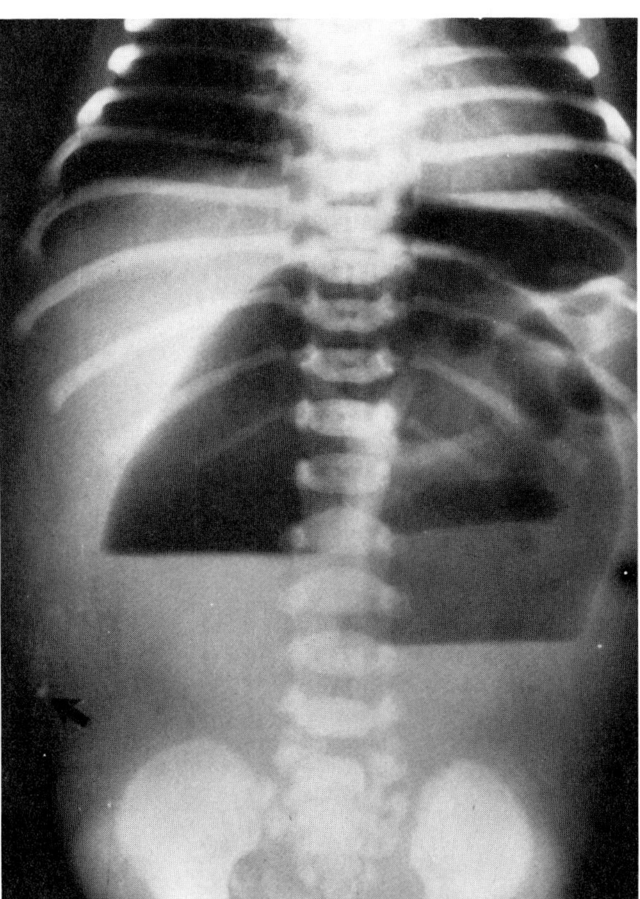

Fig. 206-2 Ileal atresia with meconium peritonitis. An upright film of a 36-hour-old female with persistent vomiting since birth. The numerous dilated loops of small bowel with fluid levels indicate atresia of the ileum; the calcification *(arrow)* is diagnostic of meconium peritonitis caused by prenatal rupture of the small bowel.

achieve a diagnosis in most difficult cases without a palpable mass.[17,19] Contrast studies are rarely required (see Chapter 247, "Pyloric Stenosis").

Frequently an abdominal roentgenogram of a GIO that occurs in association with suspected cystic fibrosis (meconium ileus) will have a peculiar hazy pattern described as a "ground glass" or "soap bubble" appearance (Fig. 206-3). This is caused by the abnormal meconium mixed with air that is inspissated in the bowel lumen. Occasionally this hard, dense, abnormal stool, palpable as multiple abdominal masses, will appear on the roentgenogram as a chain of radiolucencies, or a "string of beads" sign.[9,10] Meconium ileus, like ileal atresia, is associated with a complete GIO; however, air fluid levels are rare in meconium ileus. Meconium ileus and meconium plug syndrome are two neonatal GIO entities that can be diagnosed and frequently treated with the use of a contrast enema. A neonate who has a suspected diagnosis of meconium ileus, without evidence of perforation, and who is well hydrated can be cautiously given a water-soluble contrast enema by an experienced radiologist. This identifies the inspissated meconium, localized to the distal ileum, and may free it from the bowel wall for spontaneous expulsion. This technique is limited in application and duration, with subsequent surgical therapy required in many patients. Uncomplicated meconium plug syndrome, a lower GIO lesion infrequently associated with cystic fibrosis but occasionally associated with congenital aganglionosis, is also diagnosed and successfully treated with a barium enema.[1,10] Unlike meconium ileus, the abnormal meconium in meconium plug syndrome is localized to the distal colon. Contrast enemas in either syndrome are contraindicated when there is intestinal vascular compromise or perforation— that is, peritonitis, free intraperitoneal air, or intraperitoneal calcification.

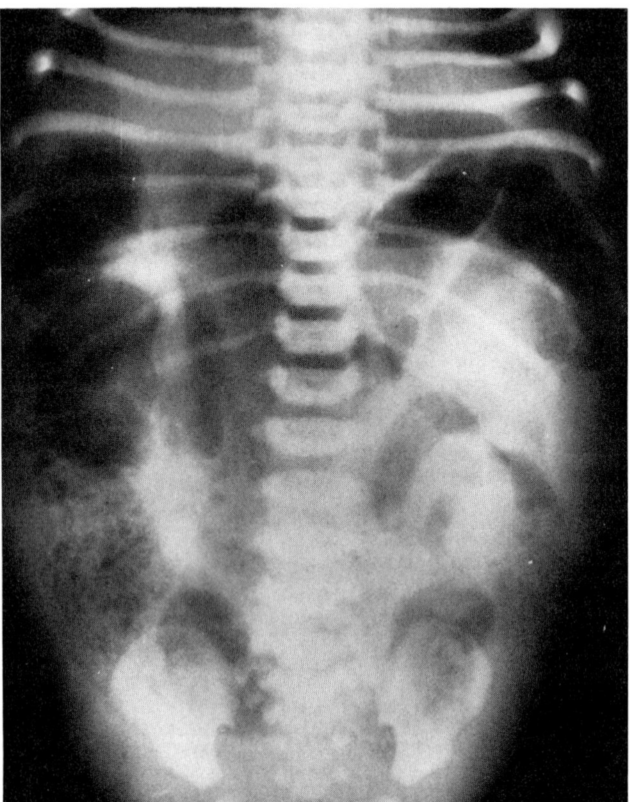

Fig. 206-3 Meconium ileus. An upright film of a 2-day-old male with abdominal distention since birth. The loops of distended bowel of varying size without fluid levels are filled with meconium shadows (radiolucent soap bubbles).

Reproduced with permission from Micro X-ray Recorder, Inc., Chicago, Ill.

Older infants and toddlers with a GIO produced by a suspected intussusception can be diagnosed and sometimes successfully treated with a barium enema.[13] The importance of an experienced radiologist for this maneuver cannot be overemphasized. The study is performed with a limited pressure (3-foot) barium column. The intussusception is slowly reduced by the hydrostatic pressure generated by this barium solution. Because of the potential hazard of a barium perforation, the study should never be performed without a surgical team standing by. The procedure, which can be used in about 75% of the patients, successfully reduces the intussusception in 35% to 50% of cases.[13] The patient is always observed for 12 to 24 hours in the hospital after successful barium reduction.

Surgical Management

The type of surgical procedure performed and the patient's postoperative course and prognosis (Table 206-3) depend on the type of lesion producing the GIO.

ESOPHAGEAL OBSTRUCTION

The presence of esophageal atresia with associated tracheoesophageal fistula (TEF) constitutes an emergency requiring either a primary repair or a staged procedure using an initial gastrostomy for gastric decompression and prevention of aspiration. Subsequent definitive repair, including a division of the fistula and anastomosis of the esophageal ends, is carried out after treatment of any existing underlying pneumonic process. Occasionally the gastrostomy and definitive repair are performed simultaneously or in selected patients; the esophageal repair is performed without a gastrostomy. Complications of the definitive procedure include esophageal leaks, infections, and strictures. There are associated anomalies, particularly of the cardiovascular system, in as many as 50% of cases.[2] Patients with uncomplicated atresia and TEF experience low morbidity and negligible mortality. Associated cardiovascular anomalies and low birth weight lead to a mortality as high as 70%. Late complications of atresia and TEF include congenital hypertrophic pyloric stenosis and chronic gastroesophageal reflux with hyperactive airway symptoms.

GASTRIC OBSTRUCTIONS

Gastric volvulus is usually an acute problem and requires an immediate surgical gastropexy to prevent ischemia and necrosis. If no gastric necrosis is found, recovery is usually uneventful. Gastric necrosis with secondary peritonitis results in high morbidity and mortality rates. A gastric antral web is difficult to diagnose and frequently requires repeated diagnostic studies but is not a critical problem. Surgical therapy

Table 206-3 *Common Causes of Pediatric GIO: Surgery and Prognosis*

ETIOLOGY	SURGICAL PROCEDURE	COMPLICATIONS	PROGNOSIS
Esophageal atresia	Divide tracheoesophageal fistula, perform primary esophageal anastomosis, with or without gastrostomy	Aspiration, leaking anastomosis, stricture	Dependent on associated anomalies; with no cardiac anomaly, ≥95% survival
Gastric volvulus	Gastropexy, gastrostomy, with or without resection	Sepsis, leaking anastomosis	With no necrosis, very good; with necrosis, high mortality
Antral web	Gastrotomy, divide web, modified pyloroplasty	Leaking gastrotomy or pyloroplasty	Good
Hypertrophic pyloric stenosis	Pyloromyotomy	Incomplete procedure, mucosal leak	Good
Volvulus	Detorsion of mesentery, divide Ladd bands, and intestinal resection (if necrosis is present)	Leaking anastomosis, sepsis, short-gut syndrome	With no necrosis, good; with necrosis, guarded
Jejunal atresia	Resection and anastomosis	Strictures, leaking anastomosis, poor gut motility	Isolated anomaly, good; associated with cystic fibrosis, poor
Intussusception	Reduction with or without resection	Ischemic bowel, leaking anastomosis, recurrence	With no necrosis, good; with necrosis, potential short-gut syndrome
Meconium ileus	Intestinal cleansing through enterotomy, possible resection	Sepsis, malnutrition	Immediately after surgery, good; long term, poor
Obstipation of prematurity	Colostomy only for severe cases	Sepsis	Good
Congenital aganglionosis	Colostomy, delayed pull-through procedure	Sepsis, incontinence	Good
Incarcerated inguinal hernia	Reduction, possible intestinal resection	Sepsis	Good to guarded
Imperforate anus	Colostomy, delayed pull-through procedure	Sepsis, incontinence	High defects, guarded; low defects, good

consists of a simple incision of the web and performance of a modified pyloroplasty, resulting in minimal postoperative complications.[18] Hypertrophic pyloric stenosis is a semiurgent surgical problem, with operative therapy following adequate correction of the accompanying dehydration and hypochloremic alkalosis. The procedure is a muscle-splitting pyloromyotomy, leaving the mucosa intact. Acute complications are unusual, with the patient resuming postoperative feedings without sequelae within 8 to 24 hours. Chronic complications such as a stricture related to intraoperative mucosal perforations and adhesions are rare.

DUODENAL OBSTRUCTIONS

Duodenal atresia, stenosis, and annular pancreas constitute semiurgent surgical problems as long as they are not accompanied by an associated volvulus. Surgical therapy consists of a bypass of the obstructed area with a duodenoduodenostomy, a duodenojejunostomy, or a gastrojejunostomy.[20] Moderate feeding problems necessitating a longer hospitalization may be encountered, particularly when a gastrojejunostomy is performed. The prognosis is good; however, in the presence of associated congenital cardiac problems, the mortality rate can be as high as 50%. Growth and development of patients with uncomplicated duodenal obstructions are normal.

JEJUNAL AND ILEAL OBSTRUCTIONS

Jejunal and ileal atresia are also semiurgent conditions, unless they are associated with a volvulus. Surgical treatment involves excision of the atretic bowel and primary anastomosis of the dilated proximal and the narrowed distal segment of bowel.[8] When multiple atretic segments of bowel are present, the overall intestinal length and therefore the absorptive surface may be significantly decreased. Total parenteral nutrition is commonly required after surgery. Overall survival and prognosis is good unless the atresia is complicated by cystic fibrosis or the remaining small intestine is too short for adequate absorption.

Nonrotation with a complicating volvulus is the most critical diagnosis in any pediatric patient with suspected GIO. The twisted bowel mesentery may lead to ischemia and bowel necrosis within 4 to 6 hours after the onset of symptoms. Untreated volvulus has a high initial mortality rate because of associated metabolic imbalances and sepsis, and following successful surgical resection of the involved necrotic bowel, a high long-term morbidity rate can be expected. The entire embryonically derived midgut may have to be resected, leading to decreased intestinal absorption of nutrients and the so-called short-gut syndrome. Thus early diagnosis, rapid correction of fluid and electrolyte imbalances, and surgical reduction of the mesenteric torsion with or without resection of potentially necrotic gut is imperative.[16] Proximal and distal segments of involved intestine that appear ischemic but potentially viable should be retained and abdominal enterostomas created or a second-look operation performed in 24 hours rather than initially performing extensive intestinal resections. Postoperative complications include marked fluid and electrolyte disturbances, local and systemic infections, and malnutrition. Long-term parenteral nutrition, dietary adjustments, and repeated surgical procedures should be expected. Survival with reasonable quality of life can be expected if the remaining viable small bowel is 30 cm or more in length. Survival is improved when the ileocecal valve remains intact. Long-term hospitalization is common.

As previously noted, meconium ileus may respond to water-soluble contrast enemas; however, evidence of an accompanying intestinal perforation or failure of a carefully managed water-soluble contrast enema necessitates surgical therapy.[9] The underlying disease (cystic fibrosis), which is almost certainly present, complicates the postoperative respiratory and nutritional picture. The administration of cleansing solutions via an enterotomy usually frees the intestinal lumen of the inspissated material. Associated atretic or necrotic intestinal segments are excised and primary anastomoses are performed. Enterostomas are created for postoperative lavage of massively impacted meconium or in instances where the viability of the bowel segments is marginal. Operative survival is good; however, the morbidity is high, and the ultimate prognosis is related to the severity of the other manifestations of the accompanying cystic fibrosis.

COLONIC AND RECTAL OBSTRUCTION

An intussusception uncomplicated by a lead point (i.e., a Meckel diverticulum, a polyp, or a malignancy) can be successfully reduced hydrostatically in 50% of appropriately selected patients.[13] Recurrences after hydrostatic reduction range from 5% to 7%. Surgical intervention is required if there is evidence of compromised bowel, such as a free perforation or peritoneal irritation, and in failures of hydrostatic reduction. Most patients with intussusceptions that are reduced intraoperatively do well postoperatively and experience a 2% to 4% recurrence rate. Bowel resection is required when an intraoperatively diagnosed lead point is present or an ischemic complication is found. Early diagnosis and treatment of intussusception result in reduced morbidity and mortality.

Congenital aganglionosis of the colon (Fig. 206-4), or Hirschsprung disease, in infancy can be lethal if complicated by enterocolitis. The disease seldom produces total GIO; when GIO is present, it must be treated as an emergency. The initial diagnosis is made on the basis of clinical suspicion, because it cannot be verified by noninvasive diagnostic procedures (Fig. 206-4). A barium enema is frequently helpful in diagnosing Hirschsprung disease in older children, but either a rectal mucosal or full-thickness rectal wall biopsy specimen is required to confirm the diagnosis in infants. Operative therapy includes creation of a colostomy with the use of a segment of proximal ganglionic colon. This is followed in 6 months to 1 year by excision of the affected segment of aganglionic colon and anastomosis of the normally innervated (ganglionic) bowel to the anus (pull-through procedure).[5] Infant morbidity and mortality rates are high when the disease is accompanied by a complicating enterocolitis; however, patients without such complications do well, with good anal continence, growth, and development following these procedures.

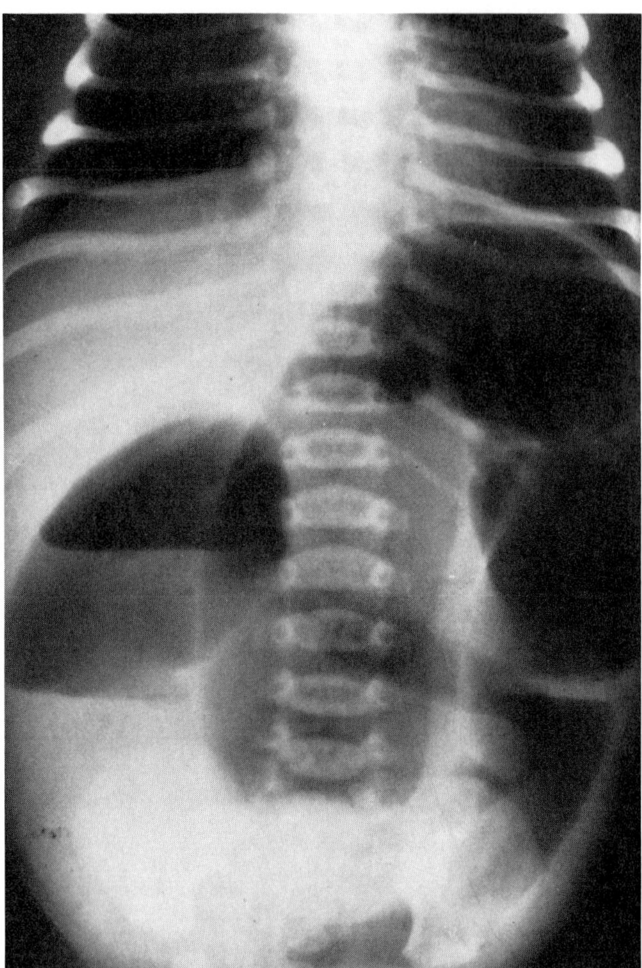

Fig. 206-4 Aganglionic megacolon (Hirschsprung disease). *Left,* An upright film of a 2-day-old male with a distended abdomen and failure to pass anything by rectum shows extreme distention of the colon with several fluid levels. *Right,* A barium enema shows the zone of demarcation between the ganglionic and aganglionic portions of the colon.

Colonic dysfunction of prematurity or short left colon syndrome (SLCS) produces a functional mechanical obstruction that mimics Hirschsprung disease. SLCS can be related to extreme prematurity, maternal diabetes, or prenatal maternal medications for eclampsia $MgSO_4$, $MgSO_2$, hyperthyroidism, or narcotics. SLCS is an R/O diagnosis of exclusion, because its barium contrast appearance resembles long-segment Hirschsprung disease. Surgically, a temporary colostomy is indicated only for failure to respond to careful small-volume saline enema therapy or the presence of signs of peritonitis or intestinal perforation.[12] The prognosis of the uncomplicated patient is excellent.

Rectal atresia and imperforate anus require diagnosis and initial therapy (a colostomy) within 24 hours. Definitive therapy, which includes a pull-through procedure and anoplasty, is performed at approximately 1 year of age.[4] If the lesion is unassociated with other congenital anomalies, survival is good. Such anomalies should be looked for, particularly those of the genitourinary tract (rectovaginal and rectovesicle fistulas, and lower urinary tract obstructions with megacystis, hydroureter, and hydronephrosis). Future stool continence is directly related to the severity of the deformity, which is determined by the degree of normal embryologic descent of the colon through the levator muscle. High lesions, or a colon descent limited to a position above the levator muscle, results in stool continence in approximately 50% to 60% of patients after definitive surgery. Low lesions, in which the colon has descended below the levator muscle, result in a stool continence rate of at least 80% after definitive repair.

REFERENCES

1. Ellis DG and Clatworthy WH Jr: The meconium plug syndrome revisited, J Pediatr Surg 1:54, 1966.
2. Holder TM and Ashcraft KW: Esophageal atresia and tracheoesophageal fistula: collective review, Ann Thorac Surg 9:445, 1970.
3. Janik JS and Firor HV: Pediatric appendicitis: a 20 year study of 1,640 children at Cook County (Illinois) Hospital, Arch Surg 114:717, 1979.
4. Kiesewetter WB et al: Imperforate anus, Arch Surg 111:518, 1976.
5. Kleinhaus S et al: Hirschsprung's disease: a survey of the members of the surgical section of the American Academy of Pediatrics, J Pediatr Surg 14:588, 1979.
6. LeQuesne GW and Reilly BJ: Functional immaturity of the large bowel in the newborn infant, Radiol Clin North Am 13:331, 1975.
7. Lilien LD et al: Green vomiting in the first 72 hours in normal infants, Am J Dis Child 140:662, 1986.
8. Louw JH: Resection and end to end anastomosis in the management of atresia and stenosis of the small bowel, Surgery 62:940, 1967.
9. Mabogunje OA, Wang CI, and Mahour GH: Improved survival of neonates with meconium ileus, Arch Surg 117:37, 1982.
10. Olsen MM et al: The spectrum of meconium disease in infancy, J Pediatr Surg 17:479, 1982.
11. Penketh AR et al: Cystic fibrosis in adolescents and adults, Thorax 42:526, 1987.
12. Philippart AI, Reed JO, and Georgeson KE: Neonatal small left colon syndrome: intramural not intraluminal obstruction, J Pediatr Surg 10:733, 1975.
13. Rosenkrantz JG et al: Intussusception in the 1970s: indications for operation, J Pediatr Surg 12:367, 1977.
14. Scharli A, Sieber WK, and Kiesewetter WB: Hypertrophic pyloric stenosis at the Children's Hospital of Pittsburgh from 1912 to 1967: a critical review of current problems, J Pediatr Surg 40:108, 1969.
15. Sokal MM et al: Neonatal hypermagnesemia and the meconium plug syndrome, N Engl J Med 286:733, 1975.
16. Steward DR, Colodny AL, and Daggett WC: Malrotation of the bowel in infants and children: a 15 year review, Surgery 79:716, 1976.
17. Studen RJ, LeQuesne GW, and Little KE: The improved ultrasound diagnosis of hypertrophic pyloric stenosis, Pediatr Radiol 16:200, 1986.
18. Tunell WP and Smith EI: Antral web in infancy, J Pediatr Surg 15:152, 1980.
19. Weiskittel DA, Leary DL, and Blane CE: Ultrasound diagnosis of evolving pyloric stenosis, Gastrointest Radiol 14:22, 1989.
20. Wesley JR and Majour GH: Congenital intrinsic duodenal obstruction: a twenty-five year review, Surgery 82:716, 1977.

207

Giardiasis

Craig M. Wilson and Donald A. Goldman

ETIOLOGY

A *Giardia*-like organism was described and associated with gastrointestinal symptoms by Dutch microscopist Anton van Leeuwenhoek in 1681,[8] but the true pathogenicity of this flagellate protozoan had been recognized only in the past 30 years. It is now clear the *Giardia lamblia* is one of the most common intestinal parasites in the United States and the world,[1,18] and it has attained a certain notoriety as a result of diarrhea epidemics at fashionable ski resorts, in day care centers, in major metropolitan areas, among campers, and among international tourists. Nonetheless, the prevalence of giardiasis in children is not widely appreciated, and the diagnosis is easily missed by physicians who do not maintain a high index of suspicion.[21]

G. lamblia is an extracellular parasite with no intermediate development outside of the intestinal lumen. This unicellular protozoan exists in two forms: a motile, flagellated trophozoite that causes disease and a dormant cyst that transmits infection. The trophozoite is 12 to 15 μm long and has four pairs of flagella and two prominent nuclei (Fig. 207-1). It lacks many eukaryotic subcellular structures, including mitochondria, Golgi apparatus, or a well-developed endoplasmic reticulum, and has a ribosomal RNA structure suggestive of a very primitive organism.[11,30] A large sucking disk, which the parasite uses to attach to the intestinal mucosa, occupies most of the flat ventral surface. Attachment is regulated by contractile proteins, including actin and myosin, which alter the structure of the disk. It is not clear how the organism evades degradation in the intestinal lumen. The motile trophozoites divide by longitudinal binary fission in the upper small bowel and then encyst as they pass into the colon. Trophozoites are usually only seen in the stool when diarrhea is present. Cysts, the more common form seen in stool specimens, are 9 to 12 μm in length. Recently formed cysts have two nuclei; mature cysts have four.

EPIDEMIOLOGY

Studies in human volunteers have demonstrated the high infectivity of *G. lamblia* cysts. Although one cyst was rarely infectious, infection occurred in virtually all volunteers receiving 100 to 1 million cysts orally and in 36% of those exposed to 10 to 25 cysts.[22]

G. lamblia is one of the most frequently identified pathogens in waterborne diarrheal disease in the United States, where the organism is holoendemic.[3,18] A number of large common-source outbreaks have been traced to contaminated drinking water. Epidemiologic studies have attributed these epidemics to cross-contamination of municipal drinking water supplies with sewage, defective or deficient filtration facilities, and reliance on chlorination as the principal method of water disinfection.[11,27] In mountainous regions, where the prevalence of disease appears to be higher,[4] use of surface water for drinking purposes is the principal problem. It has been suggested that indigenous animal hosts, especially beavers, are responsible for contamination of mountain streams and reservoirs.[10]

As suggested by the occurrence of epidemic giardiasis despite chlorination of municipal water supplies, routine chlorination may not be adequate for killing *G. lamblia*.[26] The level of chlorine necessary for killing cysts depends on many other factors, including pH, contact time, turbidity, and temperature.[16] Thus an adequate water purification system for clearing *G. lamblia* should include filtration, sedimentation, and flocculation systems. Halogen-based, small quantity disinfection methods are also affected by water clarity and temperature.[15]

Because cysts may be shed in abundance in the stool, it is not surprising that *G. lamblia* may be transmitted by the fecal-oral route. This is undoubtedly the main route of spread in families, institutions, day care centers, and among homosexuals. When there is intensive exposure to stool, as in

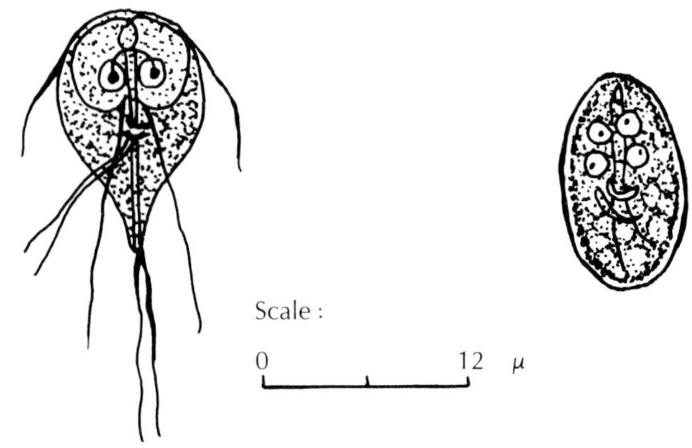

Fig. 207-1 *Giardia organisms.* Trophozoite *(left)* is 12 to 15 μ long and has four pairs of flagella. This form is not usually seen in stools. Cysts *(right)* are 9 to 12 μ in length and may have two to four nuclei.

day care centers caring for infants in diapers, giardiasis may quickly become hyperendemic.[2,25]

Although food-borne giardiasis is a theoretical hazard, only two such outbreaks have been reported—one linked to home-canned salmon, the other to noodle salad.[19,20] In both epidemics the implicated food was probably contaminated during preparation. In one additional report, food handlers appeared to have been intermediaries in the spread of giardiasis from a day care center to an affiliated nursing home.[32]

PATHOGENESIS

Although many mechanisms have been postulated for the diarrhea and malabsorption caused by *G. lamblia,* how this parasite causes disease remains a mystery. It seems likely that the process is multifactorial, with the severity of symptoms dependent on the degree of focal small bowel injury. Infection is associated with injury to the mucosal brush border with disruption of disaccharidase activity and transport mechanisms.[14] There is a basal membrane and intraepithelial inflammatory cell infiltrate,[33] and there is evidence of an increased enterocyte turnover in the murine model.[12] In either case, less efficient villus function would be expected. In the extreme, microvillous atrophy occurs, resulting in the severe malabsorptive diarrhea that is a major complication of giardiasis.[14] Recent studies suggest that parasite-induced prostaglandin E_2 production may play a role in the pathophysiology of this infection.[28] Also, there is now evidence that some *Giardia* strains produce more severe symptoms than others,[17] perhaps on the basis of as yet unidentified virulence factors.

There is little evidence to support several theories of pathogenesis cited frequently in the past. Specifically, physical occlusion or blockade of the mucosa probably does not play a substantial role, because trophozoites preferentially attach to the base of the intestinal villi and inhabit only the proximal small bowel, leaving both the distal villus cells and the entire distal small bowel free of parasites and potentially capable of functioning normally. The existence of a *Giardia* enterotoxin has been postulated but never demonstrated. Although bile salt deconjugation has been associated with giardiasis, in vitro studies have failed to show that *G. lamblia* alone can complete this process. It has been suggested that bacterial overgrowth may be a cofactor in the malabsorption of giardiasis, but bacterial overgrowth has not been found consistently on aspirates of the proximal small bowel cultures.

Host defense mechanisms appear to be relatively inefficient, given the small number of organisms required to initiate infection and the frequency of relapse and reinfection. However, intraluminal secretory antibody response, nonspecific inflammatory responses at the level of the mucosa, and antibody-dependent cell-mediated cytotoxicity (ADCC) appear to be important in limiting the severity of disease.[28] The role of antibody and ADCC in containing giardiasis is supported by the increased incidence and severity of disease in patients with immunoglobulin deficiencies. Underlying IgA deficiency and both X-linked and common variable hypogammaglobulinemia have been associated with more severe or prolonged infection.

G. lamblia should be considered in the workup of diarrhea or malabsorption in patients with human immune deficiency (HIV) infection. The incidence of giardiasis in one adult male homosexual population with HIV infection was an astonishingly high 10% to 15%.[29] On the other hand, the role and extent of *G. lamblia* infections in children with HIV infection have not been clearly established. Of course, diarrhea in patients with acquired immune deficiency syndrome (AIDS) is often multifactorial, and treatment of documented giardiasis may not result in clinical improvement if other pathogens are still present. (See Chapter 178.)

CLINICAL MANIFESTATIONS

Based on experimental studies and point-source outbreak observational data, the incubation period of giardiasis is 7 to 14 days.[22] Most patients infected by *G. lamblia* probably remain asymptomatic, although they do shed cysts in their feces and are probably infectious.[16,22] Children are more likely than adults to have symptomatic disease.

The principal symptoms of giardiasis are gastrointestinal. Diarrhea, abdominal cramps, and nausea are reported most commonly.[26] Vomiting, malodorous stools, flatulence, bloating, anorexia, and even constipation are noted less frequently. Because the colon and rectum are not involved, tenesmus should suggest another diagnosis. Blood is almost never found in the stool, and the presence of mucus is unusual. Gastrointestinal symptoms generally last 7 to 10 days, although a more protracted course is common. Because of the disaccharidase deficiency that accompanies severe infections, some patients complain of milk intolerance, which may last for weeks.

Constitutional symptoms are not prominent in giardiasis, but up to 25% of patients experience fatigue, headache, or low-grade fever.[26] Extraintestinal syndromes, such as urticaria, erythema multiforme, and arthralgia, have occurred very rarely in association with giardiasis.

Some patients, particularly children, develop chronic diarrhea, frank malabsorption, weight loss, malnutrition, and growth retardation. Thus giardiasis must be considered in the differential diagnosis of failure to thrive. Occasionally giardiasis may be misdiagnosed as sprue, food allergy, or psychogenic abdominal pain, and its protean clinical manifestations may mimic a wide variety of gastrointestinal disturbances. Malabsorption leading to an iron-deficiency anemia has also been reported with *G. lamblia.*[7]

Physical examination is generally unremarkable unless secondary malnutrition has developed.

LABORATORY EVALUATION

The diagnosis will frequently escape the physician who performs a casual laboratory evaluation. Unfortunately, one of the hallmarks of parasitic infection, eosinophilia, is generally absent in giardiasis, supporting the observation that *G. lamblia* is rarely invasive beyond the intestinal mucosa.

Careful examination of the stool is of paramount importance in making the diagnosis of giardiasis. Initial microscopic examination should be done on fresh stool suspended in saline or 1% potassium iodide. Trophozoites are more readily detected in fresh, diarrheal specimens. The yield of cyst detection can be increased if the stool is concentrated by either the formyl-ether or zinc sulfate methods. Trichrome-stained, polyvinyl alcohol–fixed specimens are also useful for detecting trophozoites or cysts. At least three stool specimens obtained on separate days should be examined, particularly if diarrhea is not present, as cysts can be passed intermittently. Stool examinations have been sufficient to make the diagnosis in as many as 97% of cases in laboratories in which there is a research interest in giardiasis. However, as many as 50% of cases are missed in less experienced hands, even with repeated stool examinations.

Regardless of the technologist's expertise, a few patients will require additional measures to detect the pathogen. Examination of the duodenal contents will provide the optimum yield in these patients. This can be done either by direct duodenal aspiration or by use of the Entero-Test.[23] In rare patients with chronic symptoms in whom the diagnosis must be excluded, a small bowel biopsy should be performed. Multiple sections of the biopsy specimen stained with Giemsa may have to be examined to find the parasite; *Giardia* organisms are more easily detected in Giemsa-stained mucosal impression smears.

Traditional diagnostic techniques are relatively labor intensive, cumbersome, and slow. Therefore a number of investigators have attempted to develop techniques for detecting *Giardia* antigens directly in stool specimens.[6,13,31] These tests commonly use polyspecific polyclonal antibodies to whole trophozoites or cysts, leading to problems with specificity. Many of these procedures require fresh, untreated specimens, which can pose problems for physicians in the office or investigators in the field. Recently, however, a promising coprodiagnostic kit using antibodies to a specific, abundant, and stable *G. lamblia* antigen (GSA 65) was evaluated.[24] This test appears to be sensitive (96%) and specific (100%) and performed well with specimens treated with many standard laboratory fixatives, with the exception of polyvinyl alcohol. Almost 30% more cases of *Giardia* infection were detected by this method than by standard stool examinations for ova and parasites. Serologic tests are valuable in epidemiologic studies but are of little use diagnostically.

Upper gastrointestinal roentgenograms may reveal mild dilation of the small bowel, edema of the mucosa, segmentation of barium, and either increased or decreased transit times; however, these changes are nonspecific. The sedimentation rate is normal, and as noted above, there is no eosinophilia. There may be biochemical evidence of malabsorption, including disaccharidase deficiency, abnormal absorption of D-xylose and fat, and deficiency of folic acid.

THERAPY[9]

Most authorities agree that giardiasis should be treated when recognized, even if the patient is asymptomatic, since carriers of the parasite are potential transmitters of disease and may have subclinical malabsorption. However, physicians may elect not to treat selected patients, particularly if reexposure to *G. lamblia* seems unavoidable. It is appropriate to approach treatment cautiously, because none of the available drug regimens are universally effective or free of toxicity.

Furazolidone (Furoxone) has the distinct advantages of having a pleasant taste and being available in a pediatric suspension. Side effects, which have been minimal in children, include mild gastrointestinal distress, hypersensitivity reactions, hemolysis in persons with glucose 6-phosphate dehydrogenase deficiency, brown discoloration of the urine, and disulfiram-like reactions (optic neuritis, peripheral neuritis, and/or polyneuritis). Efficacy in children has been as high as 92%, which is comparable if not superior to cure rates seen with alternative agents.[5] The dosage is 8 mg/kg/day (maximum dosage, 400 mg/day) given orally in three divided doses for 10 days. Relapse can occur after the use of any of these regimens. If this occurs, retreatment with the same agent or an alternative drug is often successful.

Metronidazole (Flagyl) has been used widely to treat giardiasis in adults because it is well tolerated (except for the mild metallic aftertaste), has a very low incidence of serious side effects, and has an acceptable cure rate. However, metronidazole is not approved by the Food and Drug Administration for treatment of giardiasis in children. This agent has received considerable adverse publicity, because studies have shown that it is carcinogenic in laboratory animals and mutagenic in bacteria. The relevance of these studies to humans has been questioned, and there are no data suggesting carcinogenicity in humans. The dosage of metronidazole is 250 mg three times a day for 10 days in children weighing more than 27 kg and 15 mg/kg/day in smaller children. The drug is not available as a suspension.

Quinacrine hydrochloride (Atabrine) is an extremely effective agent and is recommended as the drug of choice by some authorities for the treatment of giardiasis in adults. Unfortunately, it has an extremely unpleasant bitter taste and frequently induces nausea and vomiting in young children. Serious side effects, including severe dermatitis and toxic psychosis, have been reported. Other side effects include fever, headache, yellow staining of the sclera (and more rarely of the skin), and blood dyscrasias. Quinacrine is the least expensive agent available for the treatment of giardiasis; it is not available in suspension. The recommended dosage is 8 mg/kg/day (not to exceed 300 mg/day) given orally in three divided doses after meals for 7 days.

PREVENTION

Because giardiasis is so prevalent, total prevention of transmission is virtually impossible. When the disease is known to be present in a household, institution, or day care center, good hand washing is essential to limit spread by the fecal-oral route. Personal hygiene is especially important when infants in diapers are affected. In day care centers with infants in diapers, eradication is difficult unless all *Giardia* excretors, whether symptomatic or not, are treated. Since parasitology examinations of the stool are expensive and diagnosis is often delayed because cysts are not always found in a single specimen, it may be necessary to treat all infants in the center to terminate the outbreak.

As noted above, prevention of waterborne giardiasis is contingent on adequate water purification, including filtration, sedimentation, and flocculation in addition to chlorination. Tourists in endemic areas should avoid drinking tap water. Campers should not rely on chlorination tablets, which are ineffective against *Giardia* cysts. Iodination, boiling for at least 10 minutes (particularly at high altitudes), or filtration (pore size under 3 μm) are satisfactory means for preparing drinking water free of *G. lamblia*.

REFERENCES

1. Beaver PC, Jung RF, and Cupp EW: Clinical parasitology, ed 9, Philadelphia, 1984, Lea & Febiger.
2. Black RE et al: Giardiasis in day care centers: evidence of person-to-person transmission, Pediatrics 60:468, 1977.
3. Centers for Disease Control: Intestinal surveillance: United States 1976, MMWR 27:167, 1978.
4. Centers for Disease Control: Waterborne giardiasis: California, Colorado, Oregon and Pennsylvania, MMWR 29:121, 1980.
5. Craft JC, Murphy T, and Nelson JD: Furazolidone and quinacrine: a comparative study of therapy for giardiasis in children, Am J Dis Child 135:164, 1981.
6. Craft JC and Nelson JD: Diagnosis of giardiasis by counterimmunoelectrophoresis of feces, J Infect Dis 145:499, 1982.
7. DeVizia B et al: Iron malabsorption in giardiasis, J Pediatr 107:75, 1985.
8. Dobell C: The discovery of the intestinal protozoa of man, Proc R Soc Med Section Hist Med 13:1, 1920.
9. Drugs for parasitic infections, Med Lett Drugs Ther 28:9, 1986.
10. Dykes AC et al: Municipal waterborne giardiasis: an epidemiologic investigation—beavers implicated as a possible reservoir, Ann Intern Med 87:426, 1980.
11. Erlandsen SL and Meyer EA, editors: *Giardia* and giardiasis: biology, pathogenesis and epidemiology, New York, 1984, Plenum Publishing Corp.
12. Gillon J, Thamery AL, and Ferguson A: Features of small intestine pathology (epithelial cell kinetics, intraepithelial lymphocytes, disaccharidases) in primary *Giardia muris* infection, Gut 23:498, 1982.
13. Green EL, Miles MA, and Warhurst DC: Immunodiagnostic detection of *Giardia* in feces by a rapid visual enzyme-linked immunosorbent assay, Lancet 2:691, 1985.
14. Hartong WA, Gourley WK, and Arvanitakas C: Giardiasis: clinical spectrum and functional structural abnormalities of the small intestinal mucosa, Gastroenterology 77:61, 1979.
15. Jarrol EL, Bingham AK, and Meyer EA: *Giardia* cyst destruction: effectiveness of six small-quantity water disinfection methods, Am J Trop Med Hyg 29:8, 1980.
16. Jarroll EL, Bingham AK, and Meyer EA: Effect of chlorine on *Giardia lamblia* cyst viability, Appl Environ Microbiol 41:483, 1981.
17. Nash TE et al: Experimental infections with *Giardia lamblia*, J Infect Dis 156:974, 1987.
18. Nelson JD: Etiology and epidemiology of diarrheal disease in the United States, Am J Med 78:76, 1985.
19. Osterholm MT et al: An outbreak of food-borne giardiasis, N Engl J Med 304:24, 1981.
20. Peterson LR, Cartter ML, and Hadler JL: A food-borne outbreak of *Giardia lamblia*, J Infect Dis 157:846, 1988.
21. Pickering LK and Engelkirk PG: *Giardia lamblia*, Pediatr Clin North Am 35:565, 1988.
22. Rendtorff RC: The experimental transmission of human intestinal protozoan parasites. II. *Giardia lamblia* cysts given in capsules, Am J Hyg 59:209, 1954.
23. Rosenthal P and Liebman WM: Comparative study of stool examinations, duodenal aspiration, and pediatric Entero-Test for giardiasis in children, J Pediatr 96:278, 1980.
24. Rosoff JD et al: Stool diagnosis of giardiasis using a commercially available enzyme immunoassay to detect *Giardia*-specific antigen 65 (GSA 65), J Clin Microbiol 27:1997, 1989.
25. Sealy DP and Schuman SH: Endemic giardiasis and day care, Pediatrics 72:154, 1983.
26. Shaw PK et al: A community outbreak of giardiasis with evidence of transmission by a municipal water supply, Ann Intern Med 87:426, 1977.
27. Smith PD: *Giardia lamblia* in Parasitic infections in the compromised host, Walzer PD and Genta RM eds. New York, 1989, Marcel Dekker, Inc.
28. Smith PD: Pathophysiology and immunology of giardiasis, Annu Rev Med 36:295, 1985.
29. Smith PD et al: Intestinal infections in the acquired immunodeficiency syndrome: etiology and response to therapy, Ann Intern Med 108:328, 1988.
30. Sogin ML et al: Phylogenetic meaning of the kingdom concept: an unusual ribosomal RNA from *G. lamblia*, Science 243:75, 1989.
31. Ungar BLP et al: Enzyme-linked immunosorbent assay for the detection of *Giardia lamblia* in fecal specimens, J Infect Dis 149:90, 1984.
32. White KE et al: An outbreak of giardiasis in a nursing home with evidence for multiple modes of transmission, J Infect Dis 160:298, 1989.
33. Wright SG and Tomkins AM: Quantitative histology in giardiasis, J Clin Pathol 31:712, 1978.

208

Gluten-Sensitive Enteropathy (Celiac Sprue)

Aubrey J. Katz

Gluten-sensitive enteropathy (GSE), also called celiac sprue, is a condition characterized by clinical features of malabsorption and pathologic changes in the jejunal mucosa, both of which improve on removal of gluten from the diet and recur on its reintroduction. After cystic fibrosis, celiac sprue is the second most common cause of malabsorption in childhood.

HISTORY

The classic clinical description of celiac disease was given by Samuel Gee in 1888. In 1950 Dicke noted the association between the ingestion of gluten and celiac disease. During World War II, when grain products in Holland were in short supply, the incidence of gluten-sensitive enteropathy was markedly reduced, and children with the disease improved. After the war, when the cereal grain became plentiful, the incidence of gluten-sensitive enteropathy returned rapidly to the prewar level. In 1954 Paulley, studying surgical biopsy material, provided the first accurate description of the intestinal lesion in patients with gluten-sensitive enteropathy. It was not until 1968 that Rubin and co-workers discovered that adult nontropical sprue and celiac disease in childhood were in fact the same disease.

PATHOLOGY

Gluten-sensitive enteropathy affects primarily the mucosa of the small intestine.[5] The submucosa, muscularis, and serosa are not involved. The mucosal lesion of the small intestine in GSE varies in both severity and extent, the lesion in the jejunum being generally more severe than the lesion in the ileum. This variability may explain the differences in the degree of malabsorption seen in some patients. Those with more intestinal area involved presumably have a greater degree of malabsorption. This difference in the distribution of the lesion suggests that the proximal intestine receives a greater exposure of undigested gluten than the distal intestine, since there is no greater sensitivity to gluten in the proximal than in the distal mucosa. In patients with active gluten-sensitive enteropathy, surface epithelial cell damage occurs and the migration rate of cells from crypt to villus region is increased. Thus, compensatory crypt hypertrophy occurs with a marked increase in mitotic activity, and gradual villus flattening develops (Figs. 208-1 and 208-2). The surface epithelial cells demonstrate a loss of the basal nuclei polarity and become more cuboidal. Numerous intraepithelial lymphocytes are now noted, and the lamina propria shows a marked increase in plasma cells and lymphocytes. It should be emphasized at this stage that this flat villus lesion is not pathognomonic of gluten-sensitive enteropathy, since it may be seen in many other diseases.

PATHOGENESIS

Many studies have now established a genetic basis for GSE. The exact mode of inheritance, however, remains unknown.[5] In 1972 Falchuk and co-workers observed the association between histocompatibility antigen HLA-B8 and GSE; 80% of patients had HLA-B8, whereas only 22% of the normal population carried this antigen. A similar incidence of HLA-B8 is observed in patients with dermatitis herpetiformis, a skin disorder characterized by vesicular eruptions and a gluten-sensitive intestinal lesion.

The exact mechanism by which gluten damages the mucosa of the small intestine remains unknown. Two contrasting mechanisms have been proposed: (1) GSE results from the lack of a specific enzyme, perhaps a dipeptidase, which results in accumulation of toxic gluten peptides—evidence for this hypothesis is lacking; and (2) Gluten toxicity is mediated via immunology aberrations associated with the genetically determined cell-surface markers discussed above. Various immunologic abnormalities have been described in GSE: (1) Elevated levels of serum IgA and diminished levels of serum IgM are abnormalities that are reversed by a gluten-free diet; (2) intestinal mucosal immunoglobin synthesis, notably IgA and IgM, is markedly increased in patients with active GSE and returns to normal when remission occurs, and 50% of the elevated IgA is associated with specific antigluten antibody; (3) patients with active GSE respond to treatment with corticosteroids; and (4) in vitro peripheral lymphocyte transformation in response to gluten has been described in GSE patients.[3]

INCIDENCE AND AGE OF ONSET

The precise incidence of gluten-sensitive enteropathy is unknown, because a large number of patients have asymptomatic disease. The disorder is more common in certain European countries than in the United States. This may relate to

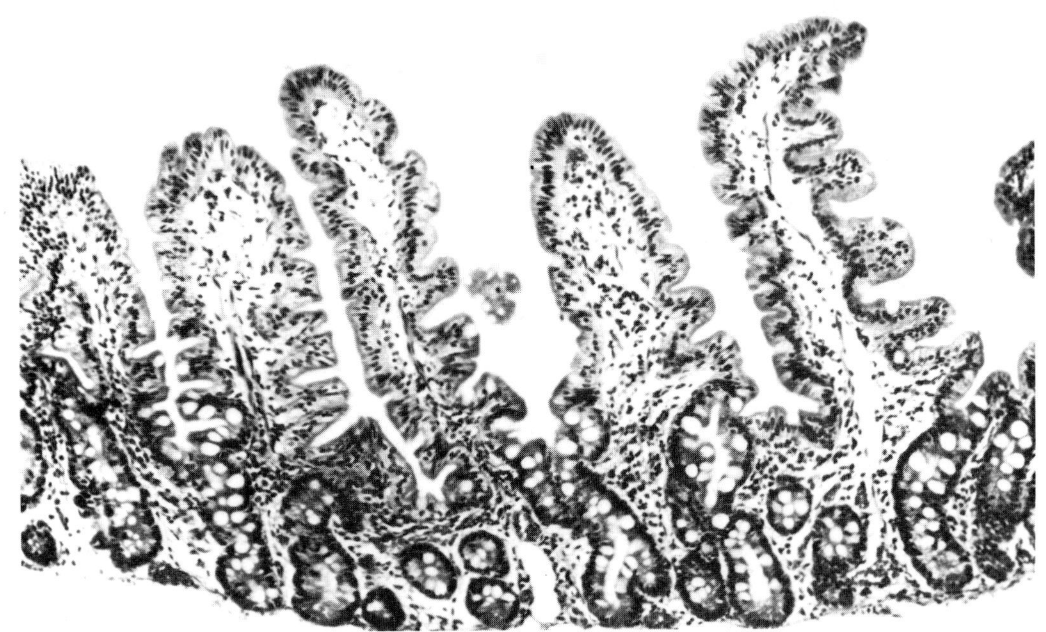

Fig. 208-1 Normal jejunal mucosa. Villi are tall, crypts are relatively short, and the crypt/villus ratio is approximately 1:4. Epithelial cells are columnar, and their nuclei are basally oriented. There are some lymphocytes and plasma cells in the lamina propria. (×160).

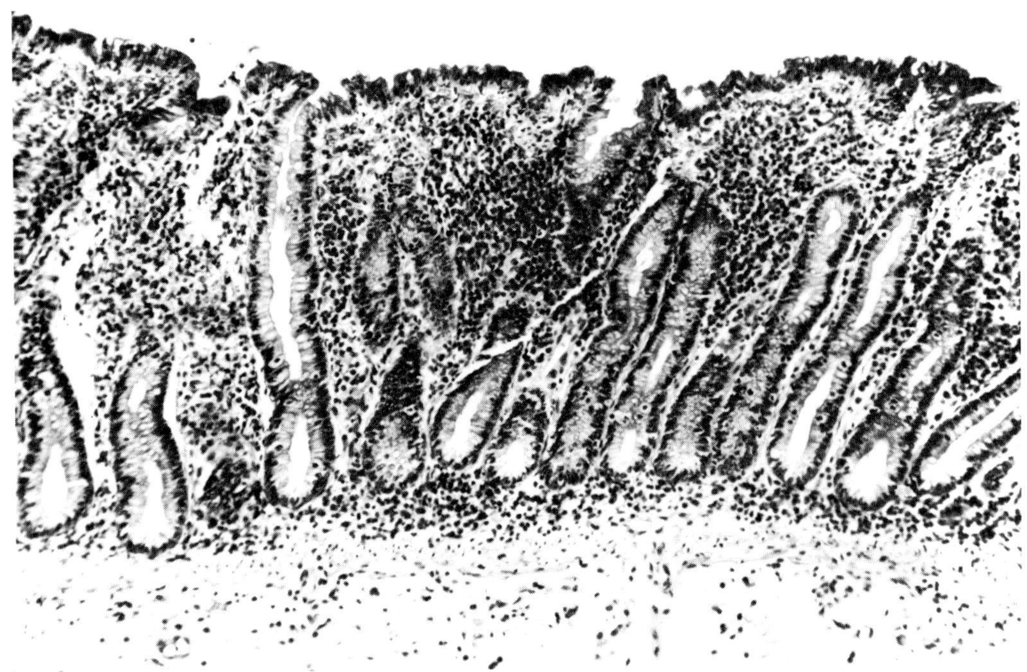

Fig. 208-2 Jejunal mucosa in gluten-sensitive enteropathy (celiac sprue). The mucosa is flat, villi are absent, and crypts are deep. Epithelial cells are cuboidal, and nuclei are not basally oriented. There are increased numbers of mitoses in the crypts. Inflammatory cells, especially plasma cells and lymphocytes, are markedly increased. (×160).

a larger intake of gluten by people in Europe or to the way in which wheat is refined in the United States. The incidence of GSE in the United States is estimated to be 1 case per 3000 people. In certain parts of Ireland, it is as high as 1 in 300. The average age at the time of diagnosis in pediatric patients appears to be between 9 and 18 months, occurring earlier in infants who are fed cereal at an earlier age. The incidence decreases markedly after 2 years of age, and it is uncommon to have a newly diagnosed case of GSE in a teenager. For unknown reasons, clinical but not histologic remission seems to occur during the teenage years. There is a resurgence of clinically manifest disease in adult life, when

GSE may be precipitated by infectious diarrhea, other illnesses, or surgical procedures such as gastrectomy. These patients presumably have had the abnormal histology since infancy.

CLINICAL FEATURES

The patient with an advanced case of GSE typically is an irritable, anorectic child with chronic diarrhea, failure to thrive, pot belly, and muscle-wasting, especially of the buttocks and proximal limbs. These children are usually easy to diagnose; it is extremely important to realize that many patients present atypically (e.g., steatorrhea may be absent). Atypical features of patients with GSE are listed in the box below. These presentations are usually related to selective malabsorption of various nutrients. It is thus not unusual for some patients to have rickets, osteoporosis with bone pain, or pathologic fractures. Also seen are bleeding disorders secondary to vitamin K deficiency, iron-deficiency anemia, and megaloblastic anemia usually secondary to folate deficiency; deficiency of vitamin B_{12} is rare and usually indicates severe disease extending to the terminal ileum. Constipation, rectal prolapse, clubbing of the fingernails, edema, and vomiting have also been described as presenting features. Gluten-sensitive enteropathy should always be considered in patients wtih specific nutritional defects who fail to respond to appropriate replacement therapy.

Atypical Presentations of Gluten-Sensitive Enteropathy

- Growth failure (without gastrointestinal symptoms)
- Anemia
  - Iron deficiency
  - Folate deficiency
  - B_{12} deficiency (rare)
- Rickets, osteoporosis, pathologic features
- Bleeding disorders
- Edema
- Constipation
- Vomiting (under 6 months of age)

DIAGNOSIS

Laboratory Findings

Before a diagnosis of gluten-sensitive enteropathy is made in childhood, a sweat test should be performed to exclude the diagnosis of cystic fibrosis, the most common cause of malabsorption in childhood. A number of reports have described the coexistence of these two disorders. Tests are discussed in detail in Chapter 120, "Diarrhea and Steatorrhea."

Anemia is very common in gluten-sensitive enteropathy and is usually secondary to iron, folate, or vitamin B_{12} malabsorption. Hypoprothrombinemia may be secondary to vitamin K malabsorption. Protein-losing enteropathy may occur in GSE; therefore, serum albumin and globulins should be measured. Electrolyte disturbances, especially hypokalemia, are common; calcium, phosphorus, and alkaline phosphatase levels may be abnormal in patients with rickets. The radiographic findings in gluten-sensitive enteropathy are nonspecific (Fig. 208-3) and include distention of the small intestine and segmentation of barium as a result of hypersecretion of intestinal fluid.

Intestinal Biopsy

Biopsy of the small intestine is the only definitive method for establishing the diagnosis of GSE. Previously, blind biopsies were performed with either the Crosby capsule or the Quinton-Rubin pediatric suction tube; currently, fiberoptic endoscopy is used routinely for the obtaining of biopsies to establish this diagnosis. Various studies have indicated that adequate tissue is obtained with this technique.[1] In addition, endoscopy allows endoscopic visualization of the duodenum. Recent studies have described scalloping of the small intestinal valvulae (valves of Kerckring) as being diagnostic of GSE. This is not classic in very young infants but is found in older children. In young infants, edema of the duodenal mucosa is seen.

Differential Diagnosis of Flat Villus Lesion

In children under 18 months of age, there are many causes of flat villus lesion besides GSE. Many gastrointestinal insults

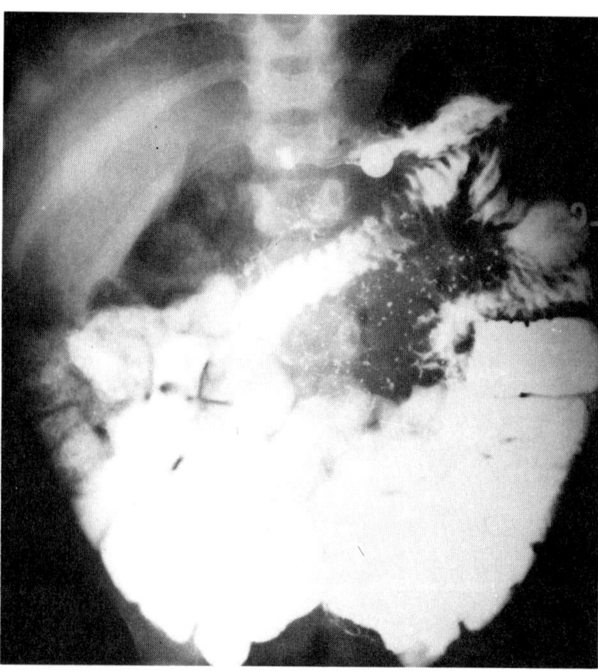

Fig. 208-3 The small bowel follow-through of this child with growth failure shows mild dilation of loops of small bowel, some dilution of barium distally, and mild flocculation. His duodenal biopsy revealed typical celiac sprue, and he responded to a gluten-free diet.

may damage surface epithelial cells, with resultant increased epithelial cell turnover, crypt hypertrophy, abnormal surface epithelial cells, and eventual villus flattening. Other causes of the flat villus lesion are listed in the box below. Thus for a definitive diagnosis of gluten-sensitive enteropathy, the following criteria must be met: (1) demonstration of clinical malabsorption and abnormal intestinal lesion, (2) clinical and histologic response to gluten withdrawal, (3) subsequent gluten challenge which may exacerbate clinical symptoms but always produces abnormal intestinal histology. Since the diagnosis of gluten-sensitive enteropathy means lifelong gluten restriction and, in the untreated patient, perhaps an increased risk for development of gastrointestinal cancer in late adulthood, it is essential that this diagnosis be made with assurance.

Serologic Markers in Celiac Sprue

Some objections have been raised against the necessity for three intestinal biopsies to establish a definitive diagnosis for GSE. Many studies have been performed to attempt to establish serologic markers as a specific diagnostic tool for GSE.[2] These markers included antigliadin, antiendomysium and antireticulin antibodies. Several studies have demonstrated that antiendomysium antibodies have greater sensitivity and specificity in diagnosing GSE compared with the other antibodies; however, this antibody is also positive in patients with dermatitis herpetiformis. More data need to be collected on antiendomysium antibodies as a definitive test for the diagnosis of active GSE. It may well be that in the future initial diagnosis of GSE will be made by a small bowel biopsy and subsequent evaluation and challenge accomplished with antiendomysium antibody.

Common Causes of the Flattened Villus Lesion

Food sensitivity
- GSE
- Cow milk protein allergy
- Soy protein allergy
- Eosinophilic gastroenteritis

Infections
- Viral (rotavirus)
- Bacterial *(Escherichia coli)*
- Parasitic *(Giardia lamblia)*
- Fungi *(Candida albicans)*

Malnutrition (kwashiorkor, not marasmus)
Tropical sprue
Immunodeficiency disorders (most notably B cell abnormalities)
Familial enteropathy
Rarer causes
- Lymphoma
- Crohn disease
- Whipple disease

Common Causes of Flat Villus Lesion

Gluten-sensitive enteropathy
Acute diarrhea
Chronic diarrhea
Tropical sprue
Eosinophilic gastroenteritis
Cow milk protein allergy
Soy protein allergy
Giardiasis
Immunodeficiency disorders
Human immune deficiency virus (HIV)

TREATMENT

The treatment of gluten-sensitive enteropathy is complete withdrawal of gluten from the diet. Various gluten-free diets and recipes are available, and this information should be given to all patients and parents.[4,6] It is important to realize that it may take a number of weeks for symptoms to disappear completely after the withdrawal of gluten. Subjective improvement however, occurs within the first few days. In children, apathy is usually the first symptom to be alleviated, followed by progressive improvement in muscle tone, abdominal distention, and diarrhea. Disaccharidase activities are markedly depressed in untreated cases, and a lactose-free diet is advocated during the initial 4 to 6 weeks of therapy to alleviate the diarrhea. Lactose is gradually reintroduced into the diet providing there is no concurrent infection, severe electrolyte imbalance, dehydration or shock (so-called celiac crisis). Replacement therapy with iron, folic acid, vitamin K, vitamin D, and calcium should be given when appropriate.

REFERENCES

1. Brocci E et al: Endoscopic demonstration of duodenal folds in the diagnosis of celiac disease, N Engl J Med 319:741, 1988.
2. Caffrey C et al: HLA-DP and celiac disease: family and population studies, Gut 31:663, 1990.
3. Calabuig M et al: Serological markers and celiac disease: a new diagnostic approach? J Pediatr Gastroenterol Nutr 10:435, 1990.
4. Hamilton JR, Lynch JJ, and Reilly BJ: Active celiac disease in childhood, Q J Med, 38:135, 1969.
5. Katz AJ and Falchuk ZM: Current concepts in gluten-sensitive enteropathy, Pediatr Clin North Am 22:767, 1975.
6. Sheedy CB and Keifetz N: Cooking for your celiac child, New York, 1969, Dial Press.
7. Strober W et al: The pathogenesis of gluten-sensitive enteropathy, Ann Intern Med 83:242, 1975.
8. Wood MN: Gourmet food on a wheat-free diet, Springfield, 1967, Thomas.

SUGGESTED READINGS

Alper CA et al: Extended major histocompatibility complex haplotypes in patients with gluten-sensitive enteropathy, J Clin Invest 79:251, 1987.

209

Hemolytic-Uremic Syndrome

Edward J. Ruley and J. Ramon Ongkingco

Hemolytic-uremic syndrome (HUS) is characterized by the onset of acute hemolytic anemia in association with thrombocytopenia and acute renal failure (ARF). HUS has been divided into several subgroups based on clinical presentation and suspected etiology.[2] The most common form is called typical childhood HUS (also known as idiopathic, epidemic, or diarrhea-associated HUS). Atypical HUS (also known as sporadic or non-diarrhea-associated HUS) is less frequently seen in pediatric patients and is subcategorized by suspected etiology.

FREQUENCY

Typical childhood HUS occurs worldwide, but its incidence varies among countries. Epidemic outbreaks have been noted in Argentina, Holland, the United States, and South Africa. Typically the illness affects infants and young children of all races and both genders, with most cases occurring in the summer. Even in nonepidemic areas, clustering of cases is common. Although the frequency varies, typical childhood HUS is one of the most common causes of ARF in pediatric patients. Atypical HUS usually affects older children or adults of both genders. Occurrence tends to be sporadic without geographic or seasonal characteristics.

ETIOLOGY

Typical childhood HUS (as well as the other forms of postinfectious HUS) results from toxic damage to the endothelium that initiates platelet activation, fibrin deposition, and microvascular thrombosis. This endothelial damage results most frequently from the effects of verotoxin produced by certain enteric bacteria, particularly *Escherichia coli* subtype 0157:H7. Presently, verotoxin is suspected to be the etiologic agent for more than 75% of the typical childhood HUS cases.[3] This toxin has many characteristics in common with Shiga toxin produced by *Shigella dysenteriae*, an infectious agent known to cause HUS in underdeveloped countries. Other infectious organisms that do not produce verotoxin (e.g., pneumococci, clostridia, and some viruses) have also been associated with HUS. These organisms have in common the production of neuraminidase, an enzyme that can damage platelet, erythrocyte, and endothelial cell membranes.[6,7] Other atypical forms of HUS are presumed to be caused by an imbalance in the local production of prostacyclin resulting from genetic abnormalities caused by endocrine factors (e.g., pregnancy, oral contraceptive use) or from the use of certain medications (e.g., mitomycin, cyclosporin A).[2] Those with genetic imbalances may have recurrent episodes of HUS or multiple cases within a family.[1]

HISTORY

The child with typical childhood HUS usually has a 3- to 10-day history of bloody or watery diarrhea often associated with cramping abdominal pain. Nausea, vomiting, and fever are variably present but not prominent. Extreme pallor and malaise usually occur suddenly in children who appeared to have stabilized or had begun to recover from their gastrointestinal illness. Oliguric ARF usually begins with hemolytic microangiopathy, but symptoms attributable to ARF may take several days to develop. The child may have gastrointestinal bleeding, abdominal distension, or rectal prolapse. Gangrene of the colon and intestinal perforation have occurred.[9] Central nervous system (CNS) abnormalities such as somnolence, convulsions, or hemiparesis may occur; in fact, such symptoms are now recognized to be much more common than was appreciated when the syndrome was first described.[4] In atypical HUS a prodrome is usually absent or consists of an upper respiratory infection. The manifestations at the onset of HUS are similar except that gastrointestinal complaints are less common.

PHYSICAL FINDINGS

Children with HUS usually appear acutely ill with pallor, petechiae, or purpura. They often are irritable or drowsy and may develop hypertension or convulsions. Those with the typical childhood variety may have a distended, tympanitic abdomen with diffuse tenderness and abnormal bowel sounds. The presence of hypertension, congestive heart failure, and pulmonary or peripheral edema results from the ARF and is uncommon in the acute phase; their presence suggests a delay in seeking medical attention or a more prolonged and possibly recurrent form of HUS in which renal failure has been present for a longer time.

LABORATORY FINDINGS

The most striking laboratory findings are the profound Coombs-negative anemia, the presence of fragmented erythrocytes on the blood smear, and the thrombocytopenia. Laboratory evidence of renal failure such as azotemia, hyperkalemia, hyperphosphatemia, and metabolic acidosis are variable in their degree, depending on the magnitude and duration of the ARF. Urinalysis usually reveals severe proteinuria, microscopic or macroscopic hematuria, cylinduria, and pyuria.

DIFFERENTIAL DIAGNOSIS

The features of HUS are not specific, being seen in disseminated intravascular coagulation (DIC), overwhelming sepsis, malignant hypertension, and some instances of vasculitis. The syndrome of thrombotic thrombocytopenic purpura (TTP) may be the adult version of HUS, although some have argued that the presence of fever and neurologic involvement in TTP favors its being a unique entity.[10] HUS can be distinguished from these other disorders by its clinical and laboratory characteristics.

TREATMENT

Management of the oliguric ARF, hypertension, anemia, and CNS abnormalities are the most important issues in all forms of HUS. Prevention of fluid overload, correction of electrolyte imbalances, and control of uremia must be achieved by careful medical management and, if necessary, dialysis. Details of the medical approach to acute renal failure are given in Chapter 287. Early dialysis is very important to prevent the complications of fluid overload (e.g., congestive heart failure, pulmonary edema), to control hypertension, and to create intravascular "room" for intravenous hyperalimentation or packed erythrocyte transfusions. The latter should be given in small quantities as needed to keep the hematocrit around 25%. Platelet transfusions are seldom required and should be restricted to children who have active bleeding or platelet counts below 50,000/mm^3 and who are about to undergo invasive procedures. Convulsions should be treated aggressively, and comatose children may require elective ventilation to protect the airway. The common symptom of irritability cannot be treated but will resolve gradually. Attempts to interrupt the HUS by treatment with corticosteroids and anticoagulants are not effective and present their own hazards. Drugs to minimize platelet aggregation (aspirin and dipyridamole), plasma infusion, plasma exchange, and prostacyclin infusion have been reported to be successful, especially in the atypical forms of HUS. However, there are few controlled studies at present to prove the worth of these interventions.[5] In contrast, plasma infusion has been suggested to be contraindicated in patients with neuroaminidase-associated HUS, because it may worsen the hemolysis. The complexities of acute renal failure management and the rapidly changing concepts in dialysis and treatment for HUS make early consultation with a pediatric nephrologist very important in individualizing patient management.

PROGNOSIS

Over 80% of children with typical childhood HUS will recover without renal or CNS sequela.[5] As many as 10% to 13% may have some persisting renal insufficiency or hypertension.[5,8] Death in the acute phase is directly related to the proficiency in the management of the ARF, hypertension, and the CNS sequela. Children with atypical HUS suffer a much higher frequency of impaired renal function. In those with genetic causes, the recurrent episodes may lead to chronic renal failure, necessitating dialysis or kidney transplantation.

REFERENCES

1. Kaplan BS, Chesney RW, and Drummond KN: Hemolytic uremic syndrome in families, N Engl J Med 292:1090, 1975.
2. Kaplan BS and Proesmans W: The hemolytic uremic syndrome of childhood and its variants, Semin Hematol 24:148, 1987.
3. Karmali MA et al: The association between idiopathic hemolytic uremic syndrome and infection by verotoxin-producing *Escherichia coli*, J Infect Dis 151:775, 1985.
4. Kumudchandra JS, Swick HM, and Haworth N: Neurological involvement in hemolytic-uremic syndrome, Ann Neurol 19:90, 1986.
5. Levin M, Walters DS, and Barratt TM: Hemolytic uremic syndrome, Adv Pediatr Infect Dis 4:51, 1989.
6. Moorthy B and Makker SP: Hemolytic uremic syndrome associated with pneumococcal sepsis, J Pediatr 95:558, 1979.
7. Novak RW, Martin CR, and Orsini EN: Hemolytic-uremic syndrome associated with neuraminidase-producing microorganisms: treatment by exchange transfusion, Helv Paediatr Acta 35:359, 1980.
8. Van Dyck M, Proesmans W, and Depraetere M: Hemolytic uremic syndrome in childhood: renal function ten years later, Clin Nephrol 29:109, 1988.
9. Van Stiegmann G and Lilly JR: Surgical lesions of the colon in the hemolytic uremic syndrome, Surgery 85:357, 1979.
10. Wardle N: What is HUS and what is TTP? Nephron 50:389, 1988.

SUGGESTED READINGS

Fong JSC, Chadarevian J, and Kaplan BS: Hemolytic-uremic syndrome: current concepts and management, Pediatr Clin North Am 29:835, 1982.

Loirat C et al: Hemolytic-uremic syndrome: an analysis of the natural history and prognostic features, Acta Paediatr Scand 73:505, 1984.

Neild G: The hemolytic uraemic syndrome: a review, Q J Med 241:367, 1987.

Remuzzi G: HUS and TTP: variable expression of a single entity, Kidney Int 32:292, 1987.

210

Henoch-Schönlein Purpura

Edward J. Ruley

Henoch-Schönlein purpura (also called HSP, anaphylactoid purpura, or allergic purpura) is a diffuse necrotizing vasculitis whose main manifestations are rash, arthritis, gastrointestinal symptoms, and renal abnormalities.

FREQUENCY

In a recent study of a defined, unselected population in northern Europe over a 13-year period, the incidence was determined to be 13.5 cases of HSP per 100,000 childhood population per year.[3] This illness most often affects children between 3 and 10 years of age with a slight (1.5:1) male predominance. In the Northern Hemisphere most cases appear between November and January.

ETIOLOGY

The etiology of HSP is unknown. Although 75% of the patients have an upper respiratory tract infection preceding the onset of this syndrome, no consistent infectious agent has been identified. The incidence of streptococcal infections is no greater in these children than in those of the same age without this disease. Some have suggested that this syndrome is associated with food allergies, certain medications, bee stings, or prior bacterial infections, but definitive proof of the relationship is lacking. Recent attempts to understand the pathogenesis have focused on abnormalities in IgA production and clearance. At present these studies are inconclusive and at times contradictory.

HISTORY

Approximately 65% to 75% of the patients have a history of an upper respiratory illness 1 to 3 weeks before the onset of the HSP symptoms. The most common initial feature is a petechial rash that gradually becomes purpuric. In the unselected study mentioned previously,[3] 100% of the patients had a rash. Between 60% and 70% of HSP patients will have arthritis, whereas approximately 50% will have some gastrointestinal complaint such as colicky abdominal pain, melena, vomiting, or bloody diarrhea. These abdominal complaints may be severe enough to suggest an acute abdominal emergency. Although many of these complaints do not justify surgical intervention, intussusception is a complication of HSP that may require surgery. Presumably this complication results from bowel wall edema forming a "lead point" that promotes the infolding of the bowel on itself. In about 20% of patients, the gastrointestinal symptoms may precede the rash and arthritis.

A broad spectrum of renal involvement is found in 20% to 70% of patients with HSP. This may range from microhematuria with mild to moderate proteinuria to fully manifested glomerulonephritis or nephrotic syndrome. It has been suggested that if careful urine sediments are repeatedly examined in all HSP patients, nearly 80% will evidence some renal involvement during the course of their illness. In the unselected population mentioned above,[3] only 20% had renal abnormalities. Of these, 45% had coexisting hematuria and proteinuria, 2% had isolated microhematuria, 18% had coexisting nephritis or nephrotic syndrome, and the remaining 15% had nephritis only. The renal manifestations usually coincide with or follow the rash; they rarely precede it. There is a tendency for more severe renal involvement in patients with recurrent purpura or gastrointestinal complaints. Usually the renal abnormality will manifest within 4 weeks of the onset of the nonrenal manifestations, although nephritis has been reported to precede these manifestations in some patients and to occur as late as 2 years afterward in other patients.

Less common are testicular swelling and tenderness, parotiditis, hepatomegaly, and neurologic symptoms.

PHYSICAL FINDINGS

The typical rash begins with symmetrical erythematous macules, which usually start over the malleoli of the ankle but often spread to involve the dorsal aspect of the legs, the buttocks, and the ulnar aspect of the arm. The trunk and face are usually spared. Characteristically the rash evolves rapidly to dusky red maculopapules that coalesce to form ecchymoses within 12 to 24 hours. By 2 weeks the rash becomes purple-brown and then gradually fades. Atypically the rash may not be present initially or may be more urticarial or erythematous in character, which may pose a diagnostic dilemma.

The arthritis, characterized by painful and swollen joints, most commonly involves the knees and ankles and less often the wrists and fingers. These joints are usually not red, warm, or tender. Abdominal findings include distension, direct or rebound tenderness, and abnormal bowel sounds. Physical signs of renal involvement are usually absent early in the illness but may develop later.

LABORATORY FINDINGS

There are no diagnostic laboratory findings for HSP. The platelet counts and bleeding and clotting times are normal. There may be a neutrophilic leukocytosis, and the sedimentation rate is often elevated. Approximately 50% of patients will have a transient elevation in serum IgA. Urinalysis reveals erythrocyturia, proteinuria, leukocyturia, and cylindruria. There is often laboratory evidence of renal insufficiency, and anemia may be prominent. The platelet count is normal. Some individuals have the typical biochemical abnormalities of nephrotic syndrome, including hypoproteinemia, massive proteinuria, and hypercholesterolemia. Usually the complement levels are normal.

DIFFERENTIAL DIAGNOSIS

HSP is a clinical diagnosis based on the rash and the other multisystem findings. Similar rashes associated with renal abnormalities have been reported in poststreptococcal glomerulonephritis and systemic lupus erythematosus. The serum complement levels are usually decreased in these latter two conditions, in contrast to the normal complement in HSP. Other forms of vasculitis such as polyarteritis may be particularly hard to separate from HSP. Although IgG-IgA nephritis is thought to be the monosymptomatic variant of HSP, it is unlikely to be confused with HSP because of the absence of other organ involvement in the former. The biopsy appearances, however, are indistinguishable. Purpura may also be seen in HUS, thrombocytopenia, and sepsis, whereas the arthritis must be differentiated from juvenile rheumatoid arthritis and acute rheumatic fever. Other causes of an "acute abdomen" such as peptic ulcer, volvulus, and so forth must be differentiated from the gastrointestinal complaints of HSP.

TREATMENT

In the past, corticosteroids and immunosuppressive medications have been used in attempts to modify the clinical course. These studies were usually not well controlled; thus at present there is no definitely accepted proved treatment. Supportive and symptomatic therapy is indicated for the renal failure. Although corticosteroids do not apparently affect the renal disease or arthritis, they ameliorate the abdominal pain. Consultation with a pediatric nephrologist is indicated in those children with more severe degrees of renal failure (particularly if it is worsening) and in those in whom a biopsy is contemplated.

PROGNOSIS

The most important determinant of long-term morbidity and mortality of HSP is the degree, type, and persistence of the renal involvement. Even so, the majority of patients recover completely. In a long-term study of unselected patients,[3] all of the children with either isolated microhematuria or hematuria associated with proteinuria had normal urinalyses and renal function on follow-up 8 years later. Of those with either nephritis or combined nephritic and nephrotic manifestations, less than 1% had died of renal complications, and only 2% had continued renal abnormalities. These outcomes are considerably better than the 10% to 15% incidence of chronic renal failure reported elsewhere.[4] This may be explained by the reports of a worse outcome emanating from nephrology referral institutions, in which a selected population of more severely involved patients are being cared for. Clinically the concurrence of nephrotic syndrome and hematuria, especially if associated with hypertension or renal insufficiency, has the greatest likelihood of progressing to chronic renal failure. Careful study has correlated the renal biopsy changes with the clinical manifestations of renal disease and prognosis.[1,2] Generally, a poor prognosis with progression to renal failure has been associated with (1) the onset of HSP nephritis in the child older than 6 years of age, (2) the presence of the nephrotic syndrome, and (3) the presence of crescent formation in the glomeruli. A renal biopsy can help establish the diagnosis and determine prognosis.

The rash of HSP resolves without scarring or pigmentary changes. No permanent deformities result from even the most severe arthritis.

REFERENCES

1. Meadow SR et al: Schönlein-Henoch nephritis, Q J Med 163:241, 1972.
2. Sinniah R, Feng PH, and Chen BTM: Henoch-Schönlein syndrome: a clinical and morphological study of renal biopsies, Clin Nephrol 9:219, 1978.
3. Steward M et al: Long-term renal prognosis of Henoch-Schönlein purpura in an unselected childhood population, Eur J Pediatr 147:113, 1988.
4. Wedgewood RJP and Klaus MH: Anaphylactoid purpura (Schönlein-Henoch syndrome): a long-term follow-up study with special reference to renal involvement, Pediatrics 16:196, 1955.

SUGGESTED READINGS

Austin HA and Balow JE: Henoch-Schönlein nephritis: prognostic features and the challenge of therapy, Am J Kidney Dis 2:512, 1983.

Waldo BF: Is Henoch-Schönlein purpura the systemic form of IgA nephropathy? Am J Kidney Dis 12:373, 1988.

211

Hepatitis

Jay A. Perman and Kathleen B. Schwartz

Approximately 60,000 cases of viral hepatitis are reported annually to the Centers for Disease Control. Not included in these figures are numerous unrecognized anicteric cases, especially in the pediatric population, in whom the anicteric/icteric case ratio is thought to approach 10:1. In addition, an unknown number of subclinical cases must occur, as evidenced by the presence of antibody to hepatitis A in more than 30% of the adult U.S. population and the prevalence of hepatitis B antigen–positive persons identified by bloodbank screening. Two etiologic agents of non-A, non-B hepatitis have been recognized: hepatitis C, which causes most cases of transfusion-associated cases of hepatitis,[7] and hepatitis E, which causes epidemic (enterically transmitted) non-A, non-B hepatitis.[4] Thus acute viral hepatitis continues as a major infectious disease. Although generally a self-limited illness in children, virus A (infectious hepatitis, short incubation period) and particularly virus B (serum hepatitis, long incubation period) and hepatitis C may be associated with significant morbidity and death. In addition, chronic hepatitis, a potential complication of acute viral hepatitis, is being recognized with increasing frequency in children.

ACUTE HEPATITIS

Virus A[8]

Transmission of hepatitis A is predominantly by the fecal-oral route, although saliva and urine are potentially important vehicles, particularly among siblings. Contaminated shellfish, polluted water, and travel to endemic areas have also been identified in the acquisition of type A infection.

Viruslike particles capable of causing hepatitis A infection in primates have been demonstrated by immune electron microscopy in the stools of patients ill with hepatitis A. Antigen can be detected in the stool (as well as in serum and possibly in urine) as early as 2 to 3 weeks before acute illness and as much as 1 week after the onset of illness; recovery in the stool decreases as jaundice becomes evident. Aggregation of the 27 nm diameter viral particles present in stool can be achieved with serum containing anti–hepatitis A. This antibody is recoverable in patients' serum after antigen is no longer found in the stool. Anti–hepatitis A is present at least 10 years after infection and probably confers lifelong immunity to virus A. It is now possible to grow hepatitis A in cell culture, and progress toward a vaccine is under way.

Virus B[5]

Type B is associated with an antigen now designated HB_sAg. Although previously thought to be transmitted only parenterally, hence the designation *serum hepatitis,* it is now accepted that virus B can be transmitted orally. Antigen may be present in saliva and other secretions. Blood-sucking insects have also been incriminated in transmission of the virus, as has ingestion of contaminated shellfish.

Hepatitis B in the Neonate. The neonate delivered of an HB_sAg-positive mother or a mother who has had hepatitis B in pregnancy represents a unique problem. Transmission is more likely if the mother is HB_eAg antigen–positive and appears highly unlikely if maternal antibody to e is present. The risk of infection to the infant appears to be markedly increased (80%) if the mother has had clinical hepatitis in the third trimester of pregnancy. The route of infection may be transplacental by the swallowing of blood at the time of delivery or by close contact postpartum. Evidence for acquisition of antigen after birth is based on conversion from antigen negativity to positivity postpartum. Data linking breast-feeding to the acquisition of antigenicity are equivocal. Infants born to an HB_sAg-positive mother or a mother who has had hepatitis B during pregnancy should be given 0.5 ml of hepatitis B immune globulin (HBIG) intramuscularly immediately after birth, and 0.5 ml of hepatitis B vaccine intramuscularly within the first week of life, and again 1 and 6 months later.

New recommendations may be forthcoming. A preliminary study of neonates born to mothers who were both HB_sAg-positive and HB_eAg-positive demonstrated that administration of recombinant hepatitis B vaccine to infants at birth, 1, and 2 months of age without concomitant immune globulin resulted in a very high protective efficacy rate against the chronic carrier state.[10]

The long-term effects of acquiring antigenicity in infancy are also unknown. It is recognized that infants acquiring antigen tend to become chronic carriers and have features of persistent hepatitis on biopsy. However, infants of carrier mothers have been reported in whom acute fulminant hepatitis occurs in the first 6 months of life.

Hepatitis Delta Virus. Hepatitis delta virus replicates in the liver and is associated with a protein, the hepatitis delta antigen (HDAg), which can be found in both the liver and the serum of individuals with the disease. The virus is unique in that it is defective and requires a coat of Hb_sAg to replicate effectively. The characteristic clinical feature is that it increases the severity of hepatitis B virus infection.

Virus C[5]

Hepatitis C virus (HVC), which was recognized in 1989, is a 30 to 50 nm RNA virus present in serum of infected individuals. Assays for viral antigen are not yet available; however, radioassays and enzyme-linked immunosorbent assays (ELISAs) for anti-HCV have been developed.[7] Preliminary studies have shown the presence of this antibody in 70% to 100% of cases of posttransfusion hepatitis and 50% to 60% of cases of sporadic non-A, non-B hepatitis. In posttransfusion hepatitis, anti-HCV usually becomes positive 6 to 12 weeks after the onset of symptoms.

Virus E[4]

Hepatitis E virus (HEV), a 27 to 34 nm RNA virus, is the cause of "epidemic" or "enterically transmitted" hepatitis, an illness that has been described in outbreaks in India, Pakistan, Nepal, Russia, China, Algeria, central Africa, Peru, and Mexico. Only imported cases have been identified in the United States. The illness usually occurs in areas where the water supply is contaminated by feces, and viruslike particles in stool specimens can be agglutinated by serum from convalescent patients.

Clinical Features

The clinical features of acute viral hepatitis in children are reviewed in Table 211-1. Type A is heralded by an abrupt onset associated with fever, malaise, anorexia, nausea, vomiting, and upper abdominal discomfort. Darkening of the urine and enlargement and tenderness of the liver follow. Shortly thereafter, clinical jaundice becomes apparent. The bilirubin level increases in both direct and indirect fractions but generally does not exceed a total of 15 mg/dl. Aminotransferase elevation generally does not exceed 3 weeks in duration. In general, the clinical and laboratory abnormalities do not persist beyond 4 weeks. The disease is rarely fulminant.

Hepatitis B occurs more often in the adolescent than in the younger age group. It is generally sporadic in occurrence, in contrast to type A, which may occur in epidemics. Occasionally a history of exposure to blood or blood products may be obtained. The onset is usually insidious. Extrahepatic manifestations such as skin rash and arthralgia are common and may be prodromal in nature. In fact, hepatitis B should be kept in mind in the differential diagnosis of serum sickness–like illness. The duration of illness is usually 4 to 6 weeks, generally somewhat longer than in type A. Aminotransferase elevation usually peaks approximately 1 month after the onset of illness. Although more than 90% of children recover without sequelae, fulminant hepatitis is more frequently seen than in type A. Type C hepatitis cannot be rigorously distinguished on clinical grounds from type B hepatitis. However, two characteristic clinical features are (1) fluctuation in the serum concentration of the aminotransferases and (2) progression to chronicity (50% to 70% of patients). Type E hepatitis is clinically similar to hepatitis A. Cholestasis may be more common than with hepatitis A, and elevation of serum aminotransferases is modest. The most unusual clinical feature of the illness is the high mortality rate in pregnant women (approximately 10%). The disease does not progress to chronicity, cirrhosis, or a carrier state.

Table 211-1 *Acute Viral Hepatitis*

CHARACTERISTICS	VIRUS A	VIRUS B	VIRUS C
Age distribution	Children and young adults	All age groups	All age groups
Route of infection	Predominantly fecal-oral	Parenteral-oral	Parenteral-oral
Incubation period (days)	15-40	50-180	20-90
Onset	Acute	Insidious	Insidious
Duration of clinical illness	Weeks	Weeks to months	Weeks to months
Virus present			
Feces	Late incubation, acute	May be present	?
Blood	Late incubation, acute	Late incubation, acute, may persist for months to years	?
Clinical features			
Fever	High, common early	Moderate, less common	Moderate, less common
Nausea and vomiting	Common	Less common	Less common
Anorexia	Severe	Mild to moderate	Mild to moderate
Arthralgia or arthritis	Rare	Common	?
Rash or urticaria	Rare	Common	?
Laboratory findings			
Aminotransferase elevation	1-3 wk	Months	Fluctuates for months
Bilirubin elevation	Weeks	May be months	May be months
HB_sAg	Absent	Present	Absent
Severity	Usually mild	Often severe	Often severe
Progression to chronic hepatitis	Rare	More common	Common
Immunity	Homologous, lifelong (?)	Homologous, lifelong (?)	?
Prevention	Immune serum globulin	Hyperimmune globulin; vaccine	Screen donor blood

Modified from Krugman S and Katz SL: Infectious diseases of children, ed 8, St Louis, 1985, The CV Mosby Co; deBelle RC and Lester R: Current concepts of acute and chronic viral hepatitis, Pediatr Clin North Am 22:948, 1975.

Fulminant hepatitis, which can occur with any of the viruses enumerated above, is heralded by the following laboratory aberrations[11]:

1. Prolonged prothrombin time (>4 s over control) unresponsive to large doses of vitamin K
2. Marked elevation of serum bilirubin (>20 mg/dl)
3. Leukocytosis (>12,500)
4. Hypoglycemia

Fulminant disease may occur in two forms: massive hepatic necrosis or submassive hepatic necrosis. Known as acute yellow atrophy, massive hepatic necrosis is rarely associated with survival; the patient dies within 10 days of onset of illness unless a liver transplant is performed. Submassive hepatic necrosis, often extensive, may lead to death within 3 weeks after the onset of illness or progress to chronic liver disease; a small number of patients recover completely. A characteristic form of "bridging" necrosis—that is, necrosis that extends from one portal area to another—has been described in patients with submassive hepatic necrosis.

Diagnosis

The various types of viral hepatitis can often be discriminated on the basis of their clinical and epidemiologic characteristics, although distinction may be difficult in sporadic cases. Sensitive radioimmunoassay techniques are available for detection of antibody to hepatitis A (anti–hepatitis A). The presence of IgM class anti–hepatitis A coinciding with clinical symptoms confirms the diagnosis of acute hepatitis A. The IgM response is followed rapidly by the development of IgG anti–hepatitis A, which persists for years. The presence of HB_sAg remains the principal means of diagnosing hepatitis B.

The anti-HCV assay does not become positive early enough to be useful in the diagnosis of acute illness. There is a fluorescence test for hepatitis E antigen in hepatocyte cytoplasm; this test has been modified for assay of anti-HEV in the serum of affected patients. However, this assay is not yet commercially available.

If the history, clinical features, and serologic tests leave the diagnosis in doubt, other causes, both viral and nonviral, must be ruled out. Clinical features may help discriminate among other infectious causes—for example, Epstein-Barr virus or leptospirosis. Additional agents associated with inflammation of the liver include cytomegalovirus, toxoplasmosis, herpes simplex, echovirus, coxsackievirus, measles, and adenovirus; in children with acquired immune deficiency syndrome (AIDS), *Mycobacterium avium intracellulare* should be considered. Noninfectious causes include hepatotoxic drugs, as well as metabolic liver disease such as alpha-1-antitrypsin deficiency, Wilson disease, cystic fibrosis, and hepatic involvement in inflammatory bowel disease.

The decision to perform a liver biopsy should depend on the duration of illness and whether the patient conforms to the clinical course of acute viral hepatitis. If the history, clinical features, or laboratory values (persistence in elevation of gamma globulin) suggest chronicity (3 to 6 months), a biopsy should be performed. Similarly, if Wilson disease is suspected, a definitive diagnosis can generally be made by determining the liver copper value. Wilson disease must always be considered in the differential diagnosis of pediatric liver disease, especially since Kayser-Fleischer rings and neurologic findings may be absent and the ceruloplasmin may be normal in juvenile Wilson disease.[13]

Therapy and Prevention

Hospitalization is generally unnecessary for the patient with acute viral hepatitis. However, the infant and young child should be hospitalized and closely observed because of the rapidity with which hepatic failure can ensue in this age group. Regardless of age, if evidence of impending hepatic failure is present, the child must be hospitalized and appropriate measures begun. Although protein restriction coupled with high carbohydrate intake is important in hepatic failure, no benefit of a particular diet has been demonstrated with respect to course and prognosis for the child with an uncomplicated case of viral hepatitis. Similarly, restriction of activity does not appear to affect the course or outcome, although the child with hepatitis will desire increased rest.

Because recovery of virus A in the patient's stool decreases rapidly after the onset of jaundice, return to school at this point, provided the child feels well, does not appear to present an undue risk of infection to others. However, if the child appears noticeably jaundiced, his or her feelings regarding that appearance, as well as the concern of others toward contact, may necessitate staying home from school until the jaundice is reduced.

Although it is likely that household contacts of the patient with hepatitis A are already infected by the time the diagnosis is made, it is reasonable to stress scrupulous hand washing and the use of disposable eating utensils in the patient's home until jaundice clears. Pooled immune serum globulin is of documented benefit in suppressing the clinical symptoms of hepatitis A. Household contacts should receive 0.02 to 0.04 ml/kg body weight intramuscularly as soon as possible after exposure. Children traveling to endemic areas should also be immunized prophylactically.[6] A vaccine against hepatitis A will have to await the cultivation of the virus in cell culture.

Accidentally inoculated persons should receive 0.06 ml/kg of HBIG (maximum of 5 ml) intramuscularly and 1 ml of hepatitis B vaccine intramuscularly, immediately, and again 1 and 6 months later.

Since infants of mothers who are chronic carriers will be continuously exposed to hepatitis B virus throughout childhood, they should receive 0.5 ml of hepatitis B immune globulin (HBIG) and 0.5 ml of hepatitis B vaccine intramuscularly immediately after birth, and 0.5 ml of hepatitis B vaccine again 1 and 6 months later.[12] The most important strategy for control of hepatitis C is screening donor blood for anti-HCV, since preliminary studies have shown that most cases of transfusion-acquired hepatitis C originate from transfusion of donor blood that was anti-HCV positive. No specific therapy exists; agents currently being evaluated for chronic hepatitis C include alpha- and gamma-interferon, ribavirin, and dideoxynucleotides. Prevention of hepatitis E rests on improvement of hygiene in countries where the illness is epidemic.

CHRONIC HEPATITIS

Continuing evidence of hepatic inflammation beyond the period generally expected for resolution of acute viral hepatitis should always suggest chronic hepatitis.[2] However, it is recognized that acute hepatitis may resolve slowly over a period longer than 6 months and, alternatively, that evidence of chronicity may be present earlier than 3 months.

Chronic persistent hepatitis and chronic active hepatitis represent the two forms of chronic hepatitis seen in children. Designated also as chronic active liver disease, chronic active hepatitis has many synonyms: chronic aggressive hepatitis, active chronic hepatitis, lupoid hepatitis, autoimmune hepatitis, subacute hepatitis, plasma cell hepatitis, chronic liver disease in young women, and juvenile cirrhosis. As will be seen, these synonyms reflect many of the features of the disease. Not included in the categories of chronic persistent hepatitis and chronic active hepatitis are other entities associated with chronic hepatic inflammation. These include chronic inflammation secondary to drugs (isonicotinic acid hydrazide or isoniazid [INH], alpha-methyldopa, and oxyphenisatin acetate) and metabolic diseases (alpha-1-antitrypsin deficiency, Wilson disease, and cystic fibrosis).

Type A hepatitis is thought to be infrequently associated with progression to chronic liver disease and cirrhosis. By contrast, type B is more frequently associated with chronicity, at least in the adult population; approximately 10% of patients with acute viral hepatitis type B will develop chronic liver disease, many with the benign clinical pattern associated with chronic persistent hepatitis. It must be emphasized that the hepatitis B carrier state is generally unassociated with overt disease. Further, hepatitis B does not appear to be related etiologically to most cases of chronic active hepatitis. As indicated by the presence of HB_sAg, no more than 25% of adult cases of chronic active hepatitis are related to virus B. This figure appears to be considerably lower in children. Since chronic hepatitis B can evolve to hepatocellular carcinoma, some advocate following serial serum alpha-fetoprotein measurements and liver ultrasound examinations in this setting.

Type C hepatitis progresses to chronicity in 50% to 70% of infected adults; comparable data are not yet available for children.

Chronic active hepatitis has been associated in the pediatric population with immunopathic diseases such as ulcerative colitis, thyroiditis, and systemic lupus erythematosus. Indeed, immunologic mechanisms have been invoked in its pathogenesis. For example, autoantibodies including antinuclear, antimitochondrial, and anti–smooth muscle antibodies have been identified in chronic active hepatitis, although their presence may be an epiphenomenon. Similarly, immune complexes have been associated with the extrahepatic manifestations of both acute and chronic active hepatitis, although no definite role in the perpetuation of liver disease has been identified. Altered cell-mediated immunity to HBAg may also play a role in pathogenesis.

Genetic factors may also be relevant in the establishment of chronicity. A higher incidence of the histocompatibility antigens HL-A1 and HL-A8 occurs in patients with HB_sAg-negative chronic active hepatitis. Characteristics of the etiologic agent may also be important in the establishment of chronicity, as suggested by the association of e antigen with progression to chronic hepatitis.

Chronic Persistent Hepatitis

Although the long-term outcome is unclear, chronic persistent hepatitis is thought to be a benign disorder. The child generally feels well, although enlargement of the liver is occasionally noted. Aminotransferases are usually elevated, and gamma globulin levels may be normal. Mononuclear infiltration of the portal areas is seen on liver biopsy specimens; minimal inflammation and necrosis and little or no fibrosis are seen within the lobules.

Chronic Active Hepatitis

In contrast, significant clinical, chemical, and histologic findings are associated with chronic active hepatitis. Unlike adults, in whom the onset is usually insidious, 50% or more of affected pediatric patients have an acute onset of disease much like that of acute viral hepatitis. Fever, nausea, anorexia, and jaundice are common. An occasional patient may be seriously ill with evidence of portal hypertension or hepatocellular failure. Approximately two thirds of affected children are girls. A summary of clinical findings in 38 patients reported by Dubois and Silverman[3] reveals the following:

Jaundice	87%
Hepatomegaly	79%
Splenomegaly	74%
Ascites	24%
Amenorrhea	18%
Acne	16%
Clubbing	16%
Gynecomastia	5%

Extrahepatic manifestations such as arthralgia, arthritis, and a skin rash are common. Hypergammaglobulinemia is a common laboratory finding, averaging approximately twice the normal level for age. Aminotransferases and the total bilirubin level are elevated to a variable degree. Autoantibodies such as antinuclear antibody are frequently positive. Histologically, portal tracts are infiltrated by lymphocytes and plasma cells. Infiltration by inflammatory cells into the parenchyma often occurs, accompanied by necrosis of cells at the periphery of the hepatic lobule—"piecemeal necrosis" or "destruction of the limiting plate." Fibrosis may be seen to a variable degree, or true cirrhosis may be present. Because chronic active hepatitis may progress, cirrhosis, although not seen initially, may appear later.

Liver biopsy is essential for diagnosis when chronic liver disease is suspected, provided it can be done safely. A needle biopsy is adequate, and the risks are low. An accurate diagnosis is essential because treatment is predicated, at least partially, on the degree of activity seen on biopsy. As emphasized previously, Wilson disease must be ruled out in any child with hepatitis because of the availability of therapy (penicillamine). Demonstration of a normal serum ceruloplasmin level alone is insufficient to rule out this disorder.

Thus a liver biopsy with determination of the hepatic copper level is essential.[9]

Treatment of Chronic Hepatitis

No specific therapy is indicated for chronic persistent hepatitis. Close follow-up of the clinical status and monitoring of liver function and the gamma globulin level are essential for a period of not less than 2 years. If evidence of active inflammation develops, the patient should be reevaluated with a liver biopsy.

By contrast, specific therapy is indicated in patients with chronic active hepatitis.[1] Prednisone alone and in combination with azathioprine is beneficial in prolonging survival of these patients. Although azathioprine alone appears to be no more effective than a placebo in the treatment of chronic active hepatitis, its use in combination with prednisone allows a smaller dosage of the steroid to be used.

Because steroids are associated with growth retardation and other unpleasant side effects, the use of a small steroid dose is critical in the pediatric population. Prednisone is begun in a dosage of 2 mg/kg/day (maximum 60 mg daily). Alternate day dosages appear to be less effective in achieving remission in chronic active hepatitis but may be of value once clinical and biochemical remission has been achieved. Remission is defined as a lack of clinical symptoms, aminotransferase elevation no more than two times normal, decreasing serum gamma globulin levels, and resolution of the aggressive histologic appearance on a liver biopsy specimen.

When evidence of improvement has occurred, the prednisone dosage may be tapered at weekly intervals to a dosage that achieves and maintains clinical and biochemical remission. The patient generally requires between 10 and 20 mg daily. Azathioprine may be added after there is evidence of improvement, especially if unpleasant steroid side effects are noted. Duration of therapy once remission is achieved is controversial. Generally, once remission is achieved, steroids may be tapered over 6 weeks. A role for alternate day steroid therapy in maintaining remission has been suggested.[1]

Clinical remission generally occurs within 3 to 6 months, biochemical remission within 6 to 12 months, and histologic remission within 12 to 24 months. The patient must be watched at 2- to 4-week intervals for approximately 3 months for evidence of early recurrence of disease. If a recurrence does not manifest within that time, the frequency of observation can be decreased.

At least 80% of children appear to achieve initial remission. Although the adult relapse rate is 50% within 6 months, the rate of relapse tends to be less frequent in children. Because of the paucity of affected children, it is difficult to evaluate the long-term outcome of chronic active hepatitis. However, there is good reason to believe that most children will have a prolonged clinical remission and perhaps a cure. Those with severe disease at the time of diagnosis, as indicated by prolonged prothrombin times and morphologic features of extensive necrosis, frequently have already progressed or will progress to cirrhosis. Their prognosis unfortunately remains poor.

Liver Transplantation

Liver transplantation has improved the outlook for children with a wide variety of severe liver diseases, including disease secondary to the viruses discussed in this chapter.

For transplantation in general, 1- to 5-year survival rates in children approach 70% to 80%. Transplantation for liver failure secondary to hepatitis B is complicated by almost 100% recurrence of infection; therefore, transplantation for this indication is controversial. Recurrence of hepatitis C following transplantation is in the neighborhood of 50%. Successful transplantation for fulminant hepatitis has been achieved in a number of centers. The prognosis for transplantation in the setting of viral hepatitis will undoubtedly improve with the development of new, more specific antiviral agents.

REFERENCES

1. Arasu TS et al: Management of chronic aggressive hepatitis in children and adolescents, J Pediatr 95:514, 1979.
2. Czaja AJ: Current problems in the diagnosis and management of chronic active hepatitis, Mayo Clin Proc 56:311, 1981.
3. Dubois RS and Silverman A: Treatment of chronic active hepatitis in children, Postgrad Med J 50:386, 1974.
4. Gust ID and Purcell RH: Report of a workshop: waterborne non-A, non-B hepatitis, J Infect Dis 156:630, 1987.
5. Fulginiti VA, editor: Hepatitis B virus, Infect Dis Newsl 1:25, 1982.
6. Immunization Practices Advisory Committee: Recommendations for protection against viral hepatitis, MMWR 34:313, 1985.
7. Kuo G-L et al: An assay for circulating antibodies to a major etiologic virus of human non-A, non-B hepatitis, Science 244:362, 1989.
8. Lemon SM: Type A viral hepatitis: new developments in an old disease, N Engl J Med 313:1059, 1985.
9. Perman JA et al: Laboratory measures of copper metabolism in the differentiation of chronic active hepatitis and Wilson disease in children, J Pediatr 94:564, 1979.
10. Poovorawan Y et al: Protective efficacy of a recombinant DNA hepatitis B vaccine in neonates of HBe antigen-positive mothers, JAMA 261:3278, 1989.
11. Ritt DJ et al: Acute hepatic necrosis with stupor or coma: an analysis of 31 patients, Medicine 48:151, 1969.
12. Safety of hepatitis B vaccine confirmed, FDA Drug Bull 15:14, 1985.
13. Werlin SL et al: Diagnostic dilemmas of Wilson's disease: diagnosis and treatment, Pediatrics 62:47, 1978.

212

Herpes Infections

Lindsey K. Grossman

Herpesvirus hominis, or herpes simplex virus (HSV), is one of the most common agents infecting humans, and although 85% to 95% of primary infections may be inapparent, the disease in certain circumstances can be fatal. HSV is a deoxyribonucleic acid (DNA) virus with a protein coat. It resembles cytomegalovirus. After an incubation period of 2 to 12 days, the primary infection, if apparent, is usually heralded by constitutional symptoms such as malaise, fever, anorexia, and irritability, as well as by the classic herpetic enanthem or exanthem. This is a painful vesicle, usually several millimeters in diameter, on an erythematous base. Following healing and recovery from the initial infection, the organism is not rid from the host but rather is presumed to remain in a latent phase in the ganglion cells or nerves innervating the region of localized infection. Various stimuli including sunlight, fever, physical or emotional trauma, or menses may induce a recurrent infection. Recurrent infection demonstrates a similar vesicular eruption in the same general anatomic area as the primary eruption but without concomitant constitutional symptoms.

Pathologically, HSV is noted for the presence of multinucleated giant cells and eosinophilic intranuclear inclusions seen in tissue scrapings taken from the base of a vesicle and stained with Giemsa (Tzanck preparation), Pap, or hematoxylin-eosin techniques. Herpes infections can be definitively divided into two immunologic types, which highly correlate with clinical presentations: *herpesvirus type 1* (HSV-1), which is associated with disease above the waist, and *herpesvirus type 2* (HSV-2), associated with disease below the waist and sexually related transmission.[8]

Studies have shown a sharp rise in the prevalence of antibodies to HSV-1 between 1 and 4 years of age and a slower rise of antibody acquisition between 5 and 14 years of age. From adolescence into early adulthood, coincident with the beginning of sexual activity, there is a marked increase in the presence of antibodies to HSV-2. Overall, 80% to 100% of of adults in lower socioeconomic groups, where crowding probably plays an important epidemiologic role, demonstrate antibodies to HSV-1; 60% are positive for HSV-2. Ten percent of those of higher socioeconomic circumstances demonstrate antibodies to HSV-2, and 100% of older prostitutes demonstrate such antibodies.[8]

HERPESVIRUS TYPE 1

Transmission of HSV-1 is presumed to be via person-to-person respiratory spread and probably involves close contact, such as kissing an infected person. Transmission can occur whether or not the contact at the time is symptomatic with an apparent vesicular lesion. The clinical presentation varies with site of entry, and the clinical diagnosis rarely requires laboratory confirmation.

Acute gingivostomatitis is the most common form of HSV-1 seen in children. The peak incidence is between 1 and 4 years of age. It is characterized by an abrupt onset of fever, irritability, poor feeding and, 1 to 2 days later, very tender, red, friable mucous membranes surrounding 2- to 3-mm white ulcerations, and severe halitosis. The vesicular stage is rarely seen, but large, tender anterior cervical and submaxillary lymphadenopathy is common. The duration of the illness varies from 5 to 14 days, and the severity ranges from mild to so severe that oral intake becomes negligible and hospitalization for intravenous hydration is required. The differential diagnosis includes coxsackievirus A herpangina, which results in lesions very similar in appearance to herpes but located in the posterior oral cavity, as contrasted with the anterior clustering of the herpetic lesions.

Herpes labialis (or cold sores) crust and heal without scarring in 7 to 10 days. They may be found on either the upper or lower lip, and recurrence at the same site is extremely common. *Traumatic herpes* is the result of inoculation at the site of local trauma and includes *herpetic whitlow,* an extremely painful syndrome involving herpetic infection of a digit. Although it may resemble a bacterial paronychia, it should not be incised. This condition is common in thumb-suckers who have oral herpes.

Although HSV-1 infections are usually self-limited, certain syndromes are associated with ominous consequences. Ocular herpes can be extremely worrisome and is one of the most common causes of corneal blindness in the United States. The primary infection usually involves *acute keratoconjunctivitis* with intense swelling of the lids, but there is no exudate. Frequently, typical herpetic vesicles are found on the skin surrounding the involved eye. Recurrent disease can be even more severe and may involve superficial or deep epithelial ulceration, stromal damage, or uveitis. Fortunately, treatment is available (see below), but these children should under all circumstances be referred to an ophthalmologist for care. Indeed, the pediatrician should be aware that devastating results can occur with the use of localized steroid preparations in an unsuspected case of ocular herpes. This underlines the necessity of an ophthalmologic consultation before prescribing topical corticosteroids for any use in the eye.

Certain human hosts are at more serious risk for contracting HSV-1 than are others. Individuals with deficiencies in cell-mediated immunity, those undergoing immunosuppressive therapy for cancer or transplantation, and those with extreme malnutrition may be more likely to show serious disseminated disease. The inoculation of herpes into eczematous skin can result in *eczema herpeticum,* which can vary in severity from mild to fatal. Constitutional symptoms are the rule, and the temperatures of 39.4° to 40.6° C may last for a week or more. Wide areas of skin can become denuded, with enormous fluid, protein, and electrolyte losses, which are potentially life threatening. Secondary bacterial infection may complicate the condition. Recurrences, milder than the primary infection, commonly occur on areas of the skin affected with chronic eczema.

HSV-1 is the most common reported cause of viral *encephalitis* in the United States, with an estimated 250 to 500 cases per year. The disease is characterized by a rapidly progressive encephalopathy culminating in death in 1 to 2 weeks in more than 70% of untreated cases. Most often the infection localizes to a single lobe, and a definitive diagnosis can often be made by a biopsy of that area demonstrating the typical morphologic picture of herpes. Treatment is now available (see below) that may improve the prognosis of this disastrous condition.

HERPESVIRUS TYPE 2

As a result of the increase in sexual activity in young adolescents in recent years, pediatricians have been faced with the challenge of diagnosing and treating all types of venereal disease. Genital HSV-2 is of increasing concern to physicians and patients alike because of its symptomatology, lack of cure, and potential for disastrous consequences in the newborn.

Clinically, HSV-2 usually is manifested by typical herpetic vesicles on the penile shaft, prepuce, or glans penis in the male and on the labia minor or majora, mons, or nearby skin, or vagina in the female. Primary infection is accompanied by significant local pain, burning, or paresthesia and constitutional symptoms of fever and malaise, dysuria, and inguinal lymphadenopathy; recurrent bouts are less severe. The 5% to 10% of cases of genital herpes associated with HSV-1 are believed to result from orogenital sex.

Although clinically apparent disease is usually diagnostic in itself, the virus can be shed without the appearance of vesicles; in such cases, the laboratory can be helpful. Since contact with either HSV-1 or HSV-2 will eventually induce the appearance of type-specific antibodies, these tests cannot distinguish the presence of active primary or recurrent disease from latent disease. The previously mentioned cytologic techniques, especially Pap smears, are commonly used to screen and diagnose genital herpes. Although it is highly specific, the Pap smear may result in 30% to 40% false negative values.[8] The only truly adequate test of active disease is tissue culture. If the sample is quickly processed and contains a high titer of virus, a positive result may be obtained in 1 to 2 days but may take up to 7 days in low titer specimens. Tissue cultures may not be universally available.

Genital herpes in infected women is three times more common during pregnancy, and it is then that the most harm can occur.[6] The risk is perhaps 1% of pregnancies in lower socioeconomic groups and less than 0.1% in higher socioeconomic groups.

NEONATAL HERPES

Although most neonatal herpes infections are caused by HSV-2, antibodies to HSV-1 are associated in 25% of cases. Transplacental transmission of HSV can occur and may possibly induce spontaneous abortion or, in rare cases, congenital defects in offspring. More often, however, pediatricians are faced with postnatal herpetic disease contracted by the newborn during the second stage of labor through an infected birth canal. Here the incidence is estimated to vary between 1 clinically affected infant per 3000 deliveries in populations of low socioeconomic status to perhaps an overall risk of 1 case to 20,000 deliveries in the United States, or roughly 160 cases per year.[2,6] The greatest risk occurs when the mother has contracted primary herpes 2 to 4 weeks before delivery, although the disease may be transmitted to the baby in recurrent cases with or without a clinically detectable herpetic lesion. Premature newborns are affected four to five times as often as full-term infants.

The incubation period for neonatal HSV infection may be as long as 4 weeks but averages 6 to 11 days. The clinical presentation is quite variable, although nonspecific signs of poor feeding, lethargy, irritability, and temperature instability, as well as both direct and indirect hyperbilirubinemia, are common.[6,8] Only 50% of all HSV-affected babies demonstrate the typical herpetic vesicular eruption; thus early diagnosis is difficult.

The NIAID Collaboratory Antiviral Study Group[14] classifies cases of neonatal HSV infection into three categories by clinical presentation. Infants with *disseminated disease* involving visceral organs with or without central nervous system (CNS) involvement are most likely to die (more than 80%) without treatment. In disseminated infection, hepatoadrenal necrosis is virtually always found, and microcephaly, hydrocephalus, mental retardation, or seizures occur in many survivors. A second category of disease includes infants with *CNS abnormalities* without involvement of viscera. In this group mortality exceeds 50% and morbidity exceeds 90% without antiviral therapy.[14] A third category includes infants with *skin, eye, or mouth* involvement (SEM) without CNS or visceral involvement. Infants with SEM before antiviral drugs became available were not expected to die, and only 20% to 30% were left neurologically impaired; many who appeared to have SEM, however, went on to develop disseminated or CNS involvement and to suffer disastrous consequences. Classically, more than 50% of all neonatal HSV infections manifested as disseminated disease with only a minority classified as SEM. However, apparently as a result of earlier diagnosis and treatment, 43.4% now manifest as SEM and 22.9% as disseminated disease; the percentage of CNS disease has remained stable (33.7%).[14]

The risk of infection to an infant born vaginally to a mother with active primary genital HSV infection is approximately 40% to 50%, whereas the risk to offspring of women with recurrent genital herpes at delivery is less than 5%. Previously, stringent prenatal screening programs were recommended to attempt to prevent HSV infection in offspring of women with recurrent genital herpes. Such programs proved costly, impractical to administer, and medically ineffective. Current guidelines for managing pregnant women with a positive history of genital herpes suggest (1) vaginal delivery without screening cultures for women with *no* active lesions; (2) culture of all *active* lesions during pregnancy, but vaginal delivery is permissible if no active lesions are apparent during labor; and (3) expeditious cesarean delivery for women with acute lesions near or at term and who are in labor or who have ruptured membranes.[2]

The American Academy of Pediatrics and the American College of Obstetricians and Gynecologists[2] have developed joint guidelines to avoid the less likely possibility of postpartum herpes infection in the baby. These guidelines specify isolation criteria to protect normal babies from their HSV-infected mothers, other infected infants, or infected staff.

TREATMENT

Although there is no universal cure for herpes, the prognosis for many syndromes is improving greatly. One of the earliest successes was with topical idoxuridine (IDU) in the treatment of ocular herpetic infections. Unfortunately, early trials of systemic IDU and cytosine arabinoside (Ara-C) demonstrated little value in the treatment of generalized herpes because of high drug toxicity.

In recent years adenine arabinoside (Ara-A, vidarabine) has been shown to decrease mortality and morbidity markedly without significant drug toxicity in neonatal herpes with CNS involvement.[15,17] This effect is most marked when the diagnosis is made early and treatment begun promptly. Studies of vidarabine in patients with primary and recurrent genital herpes showed effectiveness only in immunodeficient patients.[1,16] Although originally found to be effective in the treatment of HSV encephalitis, more recent data show acyclovir to be superior.[12]

Acyclovir is the newest available weapon against HSV infection. Oral and topical acyclovir (Zovirax) significantly shortens the duration of symptoms and viral shedding in initial or primary genital herpes,[3,4,7] with a lessened effect in cases caused by recurrent disease.[9,11] Clinical trials of chronic suppressive oral acyclovir for patients with primary genital herpes have shown a dramatic decrease in their recurrence rate.[5,11] Oral acyclovir is currently recommended for use in the treatment of initial cases of genital herpes but only for certain patients with recurrent genital herpes who demonstrate very frequent or complicated recurrences. This latter group requires close medical supervision, since the long-term consequences of suppressive acyclovir therapy are unknown. Acyclovir may be particularly useful in treating as well as preventing herpetic infection in immunocompromised patients.[10] Its value in treating neonatal herpes has been demonstrated, although morbidity and mortality are similar to those seen with treatment with vidarabine.[13,18] Earlier diagnosis coupled with the availability of efficacious therapy has contributed to a decrease in mortality and morbidity for this potentially devastating medical problem.[14]

For related discussions of congenital herpes infection, see Chapters 30 and 254.

REFERENCES

1. Adams HG et al: Genital herpetic infection in men and women: clinical course and effect of topical application of adenosine arabinoside, J Infect Dis 133(suppl):A151, 1976.
2. American Academy of Pediatrics and American College of Obstetricians and Gynecologists: Guidelines for prenatal care, ed 2, Elk Grove Village, Ill, 1988, The Academy.
3. Bryson YD et al: Treatment of first episodes of genital herpes simplex virus infection with oral acyclovir, N Engl J Med 308:916, 1983.
4. Corey L et al: A trial of topical acyclovir in genital herpes simplex virus infections, N Engl J Med 306:1313, 1982.
5. Douglas JM et al: A double-blind study of oral acyclovir for suppression of recurrence of genital herpes simplex virus infections, N Engl J Med 310:1551, 1984.
6. Hanshaw JB: *Herpesvirus hominis* infections in the fetus and the newborn, Am J Dis Child 126:546, 1973.
7. Mertz GJ et al: Double-blind placebo-controlled trial of oral acyclovir in first-episode genital herpes simplex virus infection, JAMA 252:1147, 1984.
8. Nahmias AJ and Roizman B: Infection with herpes simplex viruses 1 and 2, N Engl J Med 289:667, 1973.
9. Reichman RC et al: Treatment of recurrent genital herpes simplex infections with oral acyclovir, JAMA 251:2103, 1984.
10. Saral R: Management of mucocutaneous herpes simplex virus infections in immunocompromised patients, Am J Med 85(suppl 2A):57, 1988.
11. Straus SE, Takiff HE, and Seidlin M: Suppression of frequently recurring genital herpes: a placebo-controlled double-blind trial of acyclovir, N Engl J Med 310:1545, 1984.
12. Whitley RJ et al: Vidarabine versus acyclovir therapy in herpes simplex encephalitis, N Engl J Med 314:144, 1986.
13. Whitley RJ et al: Predictors of morbidity and mortality in neonates with herpes simplex virus infections, N Engl J Med 324:450, 1991.
14. Whitley RJ et al: Changing presentation of herpes simplex virus infection in neonates, J Infect Dis 158:109, 1988.
15. Whitley RJ et al: Vidarabine therapy of neonatal herpes simplex virus infection, Pediatrics 66:495, 1980.
16. Whitley RJ et al: Vidarabine therapy for mucocutaneous herpes simplex virus infection in the immunocompromised host, J Infect Dis 149:1, 1984.
17. Whitley RJ et al: Neonatal herpes simplex virus infection: follow-up evaluation of vidarabine therapy, Pediatrics 72:778, 1983.
18. Whitley RJ et al: A controlled trial comparing vidarabine with acyclovir in neonatal herpes simplex virus infection, N Engl J Med 324:444, 1991.

SUGGESTED READINGS

Corey L and Spear PG: Infections with herpes simplex viruses, N Engl J Med 314:686, 749, 1986.

Gold D and Corey L: Treatment of herpes simplex virus infections, Clin Lab Med 7:815, 1987.

Straus SE et al: Herpesvirus infection: biology, treatment, and prevention, Ann Intern Med 103:404, 1985.

Whitley RJ and Hutto C: Neonatal herpes simplex virus infections, Pediatr Rev 7:119, 1985.

213

Hydrocephalus

Robert B. Page

Cerebral ventricular dilation caused by increased intraventricular pressure is called hydrocephalus. Hydrocephalus is not a specific disease entity but rather a response of the brain to many pathologic states that either increase cerebrospinal fluid (CSF) production or impede its resorption. The pediatrician should not be satisfied with the diagnosis of hydrocephalus until its cause has been determined, since appropriate therapy depends on adequate treatment of the cause in addition to effective management of the hydrocephalic state.

ETIOLOGY

The human brain is hollow, and its cerebral ventricles are in communication with the subarachnoid space. CSF is composed of choroid plexus secretions and of brain interstitial fluid that has diffused into the ventricular system.[2] This fluid is pumped through the ventricular system by pulsations of the choroid plexus and brain.[1] It passes from the lateral ventricles through the foramen of Monro to the third ventricle and from there through the Sylvian aqueduct to the fourth ventricle, which it leaves through the foramina of Luschka and Magendie to enter the subarachnoid space. It is carried over the cerebral hemispheres and absorbed into arachnoid villi. The vascular and lymphatic systems make up the first two circulations, and the CSF system may be said to constitute the third circulation.

Theoretically, hydrocephalus may arise from either overproduction of CSF or from obstruction of cerebrospinal pathways, but overproduction of CSF (nonobstructive hydrocephalus) is rare; it occurs with tumors of the choroid plexus, or choroid plexus papillomas. Obstructive hydrocephalus, however, is common and accounts for well over 99% of cases.

Obstructive hydrocephalus may be classified as either communicating or noncommunicating. In communicating hydrocephalus the obstruction of CSF flow is in the subarachnoid space or at the level of the arachnoid villi. Dye placed within the ventricular system will be recovered from CSF sampled by lumbar puncture. Causes of communicating hydrocephalus may be congenital (failure to develop arachnoid villi) or acquired (postinfectious, meningitis; posthemorrhagic, subarachnoid hemorrhage; posttraumatic, subdural hematoma; neoplastic, leukemic subarachnoid spread; idiopathic, cause unknown). In noncommunicating hydrocephalus, the obstruction to CSF flow is within the ventricular system, so that dye placed within the ventricular system cannot be recovered from lumbar CSF. The following are congenital causes of noncommunicating hydrocephalus: (1) aqueductal stenosis; (2) obstruction of the foramina of Luschka and Magendie (e.g., Dandy-Walker syndrome); (3) congenital web within the Sylvian aqueduct; and (4) multiple sites of obstruction (e.g., Arnold-Chiari malformation). Acquired causes include (1) postinfectious, ventriculitis; (2) posthemorrhagic, intraventricular hemorrhage; and (3) neoplastic and associated with tumors of the cerebellum (astrocytoma, medulloblastoma), of the fourth ventricle (ependymoma), of the pineal region (teratoma, pinealoma), and of the hypothalamus (craniopharyngioma).

CLINICAL PRESENTATION AND DIFFERENTIAL DIAGNOSIS

The development of hydrocephalus in neonates may follow intraventricular hemorrhage or gram-negative meningitis. The diagnosis should first be considered on observation of a rapidly expanding head circumference and confirmed by a computed tomography (CT) scan or ultrasound to determine ventricular size. Ventricular dilation following ventricular hemorrhage may be self-limited; hence shunting may not always be required. Neonates born with a meningomyelocele also have a high incidence of hydrocephalus. The hydrocephalus is most often noncommunicating and obstructive, with the obstruction resulting from a malformation in the hindbrain (Arnold-Chiari malformation). This malformation results in obstruction to the flow of fluid out of the fourth ventricle and within the subarachnoid space around the brainstem. It is commonly associated with aqueductal stenosis, resulting in an obstruction to the flow of fluid from the third to the fourth ventricle. The Arnold-Chiari malformation with resultant hydrocephalus is uncommon with a low meningomyelocele lying near the sacrum but is very common with a high defect lying at the thoracolumbar junction or above.

Among infants, hydrocephalus is suspected when the head circumference increases at a rate greater than two standard deviations above the norm. The differential diagnosis of macrocephaly includes congenital glycogen storage diseases, subdural hematoma, and hydrocephalus. In hydrocephalus the head is disproportionately large with respect to the face; there is frontal bossing, the skin is translucent, the veins are prominent, and the eyes may manifest a "setting sun sign" with a visible rim of sclera present above the iris. Skull roentgenograms demonstrate macrocrania with widened cranial sutures. CT scan demonstrates ventricular enlargement, as may ultrasound if the fontanelle is open. Disproportionate enlargement of the lateral and third ventricles with respect to the fourth ventricle allows determination of the site of obstruction, if aqueductal stenosis is present. However, ventriculography or CT scanning following the intraventricular injection of radiopaque dye is necessary to pinpoint the obstructive site. CT scanning with and without intravenous contrast enhancement will determine if the obstruction is secondary to neoplasia.

In infants, communicating and noncommunicating obstructive hydrocephalus occur with equal frequency. In noncommunicating infantile hydrocephalus, the most frequent cause is aqueductal stenosis or the Arnold-Chiari malformation (associated with meningomyelocele). Tumors are infrequent causes of hydrocephalus in this age group but tend to be aggressive when present.

Hydrocephalus in children is recognized by complaints of headache, nausea, and vomiting, all of which are related to increased intracranial pressure. The headache typically occurs early in the morning and is relieved by vomiting. Physical examination may reveal lethargy with irritability, papilledema, and decreased visual acuity. In this age group, tumors commonly obstruct the flow of CSF to produce a noncommunicating hydrocephalus with markedly increased intracranial pressure. Local signs secondary to the tumor may be subtle. Tumors of the cerebellum (astrocytoma, medulloblastoma) may cause unsteadiness of gait; fourth ventricular ependymomas may cause cranial nerve palsies; craniopharyngioma may cause neuroendocrine dysfunction (delayed puberty, short stature). In children acquired aqueductal stenosis may also become manifest with signs and symptoms of increased intracranial pressure. Postmeningitis hydrocephalus may also be seen; thus an appropriate history should be sought.

In adolescents tumors are the most common cause of hydrocephalus. The patient frequently complains of symptoms of increased intracranial pressure (headache, nausea, and vomiting). There may be complaints of decreased visual acuity. Roentgenograms may demonstrate signs of increased intracranial pressure with splitting of the cranial sutures, erosion of the dorsum sellae, and a "beaten silver" appearance to the calvarial bones. Cerebellar astrocytoma, cerebellar sarcoma, craniopharyngioma, and pineal teratoma should be considered in the differential diagnosis. Computed tomography (CT) scanning with and without intravascular infusion of contrast media should be employed to rule out the presence of a neoplasm. Postmeningitis or posttraumatic hydrocephalus should be considered if there is an appropriate history. Aqueductal stenosis may also first become manifest in this age group, but the appearance of hydrocephalus in a teenager must primarily elicit a thorough search for a brain tumor obstructing the flow of CSF.

MANAGEMENT

The management of hydrocephalus is in three phases. The first phase is the search for the cause of hydrocephalus. The second phase is the treatment of that cause, particularly if it is related to neoplasia. The third phase is management of the hydrocephalus itself by placement of a ventriculoperitoneal or ventriculojugular shunt. Progressive ventricular enlargement and increased intracranial pressure in the face of large ventricles are the most commonly employed criteria for shunt placement.

Shunting devices contain three components. First is a ventricular catheter, which is passed into the anterior horn of the lateral ventricle through a right occipital or right frontal burr hole. This is attached to a subcutaneous reservoir, which may be percutaneously tapped to obtain ventricular fluid samples; this in turn is attached to a distal catheter containing a pump and a one-way valve to regulate the pressure or flow in the shunting system. The distal catheter is passed to the right cardiac atrium (ventriculojugular shunt) or to the peritoneal cavity (ventriculoperitoneal shunt).

In infants and young children with shunts, persistent head growth 2 standard deviations above the mean indicates shunt malfunction. Shunt function may be assessed in several ways. The shunt reservoir may be "pumped": *if* it cannot be depressed, then it is blocked distally; if it does not refill, the shunt may be blocked at the ventricular end. However, shunt malfunction may actually be present even if the shunt appears to pump normally, since the examining finger can exert a great deal of pressure on the pump; torr pressures of only 15 can open a sticky shunt, one that does not adequately decompress the ventricles but does "pump" well. Indeed, a shunt may function adequately even when the shunt does not pump well. For instance, a shunt may refill slowly when the ventricles are slitlike in size to give the impression of a malfunctioning shunt. Continued pumping under such conditions may well entrap ependymal cells of the ventricular lining within the ventricular catheter and cause a shunt to malfunction. Shunt function may also be assessed by serial formal tests of mental function. Failure to show developmental gains may indicate malfunction. Serial CT scanning is valuable in the evaluation of shunt function, comparing current ventricular size to earlier sizes. To be helpful, this strategy requires CT scanning shortly after shunt placement or revision so as to establish an adequate baseline. In doubtful cases the reservoir may be tapped and ventricular pressure measured. Injection of a contrast medium into the reservoir and timing of its clearance through the shunt are the final means of assessment.

COMPLICATIONS OF TREATMENT

The major immediate complication of ventricular shunts is intracranial hemorrhage. The hemorrhage may either be in the brain parenchyma along the course of the shunt tract or in the subdural space. Removal of a nonfunctioning ventricular catheter from the cerebral ventricle in order to replace it with another may result in immediate intraventricular hemorrhage if sufficient choroid plexus has grown into the catheter to occlude it.

Delayed complications are numerous in type and frequent in occurrence. The most common complication is malfunction of the shunting system, which requires revision. This occurs in about 50% of cases[4] and is most commonly related to malplacement of the ventricular portion of the shunting system within the ventricular system, which permits subsequent occlusion by the ingrowth of choroid plexus. Malfunction may also result from inappropriate placement of the distal end of the shunting system within the vascular system. This distal end should lie at the level of T6 (within the cardiac right atrium); higher placements (above T5) will result in occlusion. Ventriculoperitoneal shunting procedures are equally as prone to malfunction. The signs of shunt malfunction are, quite simply, those of recurrent hydrocephalus.

Infection is another frequent delayed complication seen in about 20% of ventricular shunting procedures.[5] After ventriculojugular shunting procedures, it is manifested as a low-grade septicemia with malaise, anemia, and modest fever. Signs of shunt malfunction (increased intracranial pressure) may accompany the signs and symptoms of infection. The laboratory workup reveals anemia, leukocytosis, fever, and, frequently, positive blood cultures. CSF tapped from the shunt reservoir may demonstrate organisms on Gram stain or culture. On the other hand, symptoms in infected ventriculoperitoneal shunting systems are frequently related to low-grade ventriculitis with headache, nausea, low-grade fever, and malaise. Anemia is not frequently seen. Blood cultures are usually negative, since the shunt lies outside the ventricular system. Fluid tapped from the shunting system will yield bacterial growth on culture. The most frequent offending organisms are skin contaminants, such as *Staphylococcus epidermidis*.[6] Both infection and hemorrhage can cause an increase in the protein content of ventricular fluid, which in turn can block the shunt and cause it to malfunction.

Less frequent long-term complications of ventriculojugular shunting procedures include "shunt nephritis," pulmonary hypertension secondary to multiple recurrent pulmonary emboli, and dislodgment of the distal portion of the ventricular catheter with migration into the pulmonary vasculature. Infrequent complications related to ventriculoperitoneal shunting systems include perforation of the bowel, cystic fluid collections of CSF in the peritoneum, intraperitoneal abscesses, and renal colic secondary to irritation of the ureters by the shunting system.

PROGNOSIS

The outlook for children with hydrocephalus is directly related to the cause of the hydrocephalus as well as to the management of the hydrocephalic state. In children with obstructive hydrocephalus secondary to the presence of neoplasia, the prognosis is related to the prognosis for the neoplastic state. In children with hydrocephalus secondary to intraventricular hemorrhage in the neonatal period or to neonatal meningitis, the prognosis is as much related to the brain damage sustained during the initial insult as to the subsequent hydrocephalic state.

The prognosis for hydrocephalus itself appears to be related to the efficacy of its management. Children with idiopathic communicating hydrocephalus or aqueductal stenosis with noncommunicating hydrocephalus who are appropriately managed have intelligence quotients within the normal range and an excellent outlook for a productive life. In contrast, there is considerable debate as to the outlook of patients with hydrocephalus complicating an Arnold-Chiari malformation. Some investigators claim that children with meningomyelocele and hydrocephalus have a poor outlook with respect to mental function, regardless of the efficacy of shunt management. Others disagree.[3,7] In any event, the mental function of hydrocephalic children with myelomeningocele will clearly be optimized by maintenance of adequate shunt function through repeated revisions, if necessary.

REHABILITATION

The rehabilitation of patients with hydrocephalus is related to the cause of the hydrocephalus and to the degree of brain damage sustained before treatment of the hydrocephalic state. Rehabilitative measures include special education classes for children whose disabilities are restricted to the mental sphere. In children with associated meningomyelocele, extensive rehabilitation is necessary and must be directed to their paraplegia as well as to their hydrocephalus.

PSYCHOSOCIAL CONSIDERATIONS

In a child with congenital hydrocephalus, psychosocial considerations are related to the mental state of the child. Even if this is normal, there is considerable anxiety on the part of the family and ultimately on the part of the patient about proper maintenance of the shunting system. Persistent support and encouragement are needed. Paraplegic children with myelomeningocele and associated hydrocephalus will need supportive devices, wheelchairs, special transportation devices, and special education classes. The degree of brain damage sustained during intraventricular hemorrhage or neonatal meningitis is the major consideration in the infant with hydrocephalus secondary to such perinatal events, whereas among patients with brain tumors, the tumor itself and its ultimate outlook overwhelm all other considerations.

REFERENCES

1. Bering EA: Choroid plexus and arterial pulsation of cerebrospinal fluid, Arch Neurol Psychiatry 73:165, 1955.
2. Davson H: Physiology of the cerebrospinal fluid, London, 1967, Churchill Livingston.
3. Dennis M et al: The intelligence of hydrocephalic children, Arch Neurol 38:607, 1981.
4. Ignelzi RJ and Kirsch WM: Followup analysis of ventriculo-peritoneal and ventriculo-atrial shunt for hydrocephalus, J Neurosurg 42:679, 1975.
5. Keucher TR and Mealey J: Long-term results after ventriculoatrial and ventriculo-peritoneal shunting for infantile hydrocephalus, J Neurosurg 50:179, 1979.
6. Venes JL: Control of shunt infection: report of 150 consecutive cases, J Neurosurg 45:311, 1976.
7. Young H et al: The relationship of intelligence and cerebral mantle in treated infantile hydrocephalus, Pediatrics 52:38, 1973.

214

Hypospadias, Epispadias, and Cryptorchism

Henry M. Seidel

The male genitalia are much more often a cause of parental preoccupation at the birth of a child than are the female. Untold variables govern this, most of them not readily apparent. The most obvious, of course, is that they are much more accessible. There is usually less concern about the relationship of the penis to the urinary tract than to sexual function. Still, it is as a part of the urinary tract that it serves its immediate purpose at birth; it must wait until puberty to begin to realize its additional potential.

GENITAL ABNORMALITY

An external genital deformity in the newborn boy is usually immediately obvious—for example, hypospadias, epispadias, injury, swelling, and, after careful palpation, undescended testes. It is important to feel both testes. Although frequently of somewhat different size in a newborn, they are generally descended in a full-term infant and frequently still "up" in the premature infant. One cause of parental distress is not often noted at birth but perhaps several weeks later as the baby gains weight. There can be so much of a pubic fat pad that the penis, retracted, may seem to disappear despite its being some 4 cm long. It is important, however, not to belittle the concern. One should assure the parents that the condition will correct itself in time. There is only rarely a real problem, namely, a micropenis, which suggests a dysmorphic abnormality.

Hypospadias

Among the possible penile abnormalities, hypospadias, which occurs in less than 1% of newborn boys, is still the most common. In this event, the urethral meatus opens on the ventral surface of the penis, most often on the glans (first-degree hypospadias), but it may be located at any point along the shaft (second-degree hypospadias) (Fig. 214-1) or as proximal as the perineum (third-degree hypospadias) (Fig. 214-2). The prepuce is incompletely formed, covering only the dorsal surface of the penis. In approximately 5% of cases an associated unilateral or bilateral cryptorchism is present. On rare occasions there may be incomplete scrotal fusion and cryptorchism; this combination should suggest the possibility of an intersex anomaly.

The pediatrician must decide when to refer the patient to the urologist. Obviously the severity of the deformity and the position of the meatus on the undershaft of the penis will greatly influence the surgical decision-making. If the hypospadias is mild, situated at or close to the corona, and if there is relatively little deformity, the need for repair is unlikely if the child's urinary needs and sexual potential are not threatened. This is most often the case. Occasionally there may be a meatal stenosis that can be easily corrected with meatotomy. Chordee, the downward curving of the penis as a result of abnormal ventral fibrous bands, is often present and is one of the factors that may force surgical intervention. A minimal abnormality can be corrected in a single procedure. Although the frequency of an associated anomaly of the upper urinary tract is thought to be low, sonography or excretory urography is often performed. In any event, the urologist should be consulted immediately, because the judgment concerning the necessity for repair is properly shared with the surgeon.

If hypospadias is severe, several reparative operations may be necessary. The decision as to the right time for surgery and the precise approach to use must rest in large part with

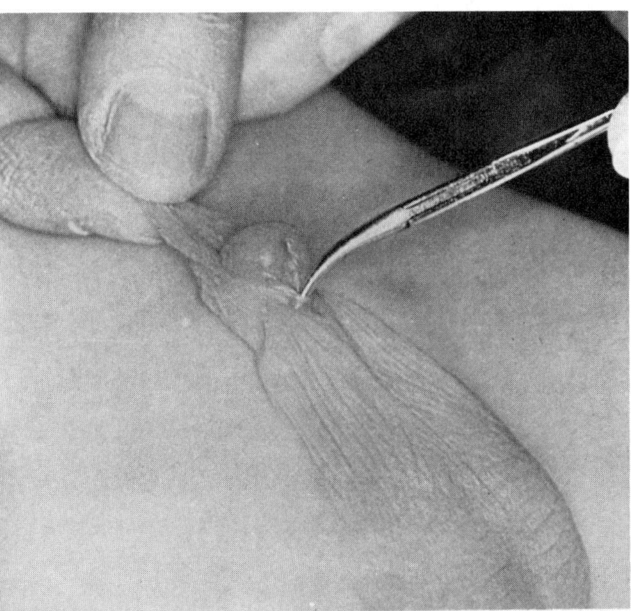

Fig. 214-1 Second-degree hypospadias. The probe is in the urethral orifice located on the ventral surface of the shaft of the penis, below the corona of the glans penis.

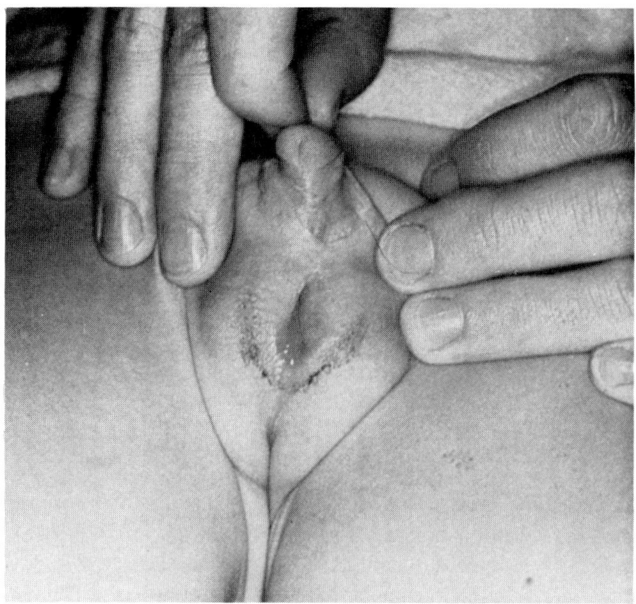

Fig. 214-2 Third-degree hypospadias. The urethral orifice is located at the base of the penile shaft at the anterior border of the scrotum.

Reproduced with permission from Micro X-Ray Recorder, Inc., Chicago, Ill.

the urologist. The pediatrician, however, cannot relinquish responsibility for providing concomitant care; he or she is needed to interpret events and, in a highly charged emotional circumstance, to provide appropriate counseling to parents (and, as the child grows older, to the child). This is especially important when there may be a threat to sexual function and worry about sexual identity. A circumcision should *not* be performed in the presence of hypospadias, however mild. None of the tissue that might be needed for repair should be sacrificed. On occasion, if the hypospadias is severe or if there are associated genital anomalies, a referral for endocrine evaluation is indicated. In the presence of hypospadias alone, aside from an infrequent defect in androgen responsiveness, there is little likelihood of significant hormonal disturbance.

Epispadias

Less frequently, the meatus is formed on the dorsum of the penis at various points along the glans and shaft, on rare occasion so far back as to be beneath the symphysis pubis. More serious deformity may accompany this, including more proximal involvement of the urinary tract (e.g., exstrophy of the bladder), and distortion of the normal architecture of the pubic bones. Epispadias, like hypospadias, may have associated cryptorchism. Early consultation with the urologist is necessary; again, circumcision is to be avoided.

CRYPTORCHISM

Given that the descent of the testes from within the abdomen to the scrotum usually takes place by about week 36 of fetal life, the incidence of cryptorchism (undescended testes) is much higher in the premature infant. Spontaneous descent of the testes after birth, if it is to occur, generally does so well before the end of the first year; if this does not happen by the first birthday, there is need for some concern. This involves the child's potential for childbearing and for sexual function, since with cryptorchism, there is an increasing likelihood of cellular damage with each passing year, damage that is probably not reversible after the age of 4 or 5 years.

On examination, one must be sure that the testis is truly undescended. Occasionally, an overactive cremasteric reflex may make palpation difficult. Moving the infant or the older child into the tailor position (sitting cross-legged) or a kneeling position can help to overcome this. It is important to feel from above downward, "milking" the testis from the inguinal canal into the scrotum. The older patient can help this process by coughing or straining. Cold hands and abrupt palpation can invoke the cremasteric reflex. If one or the other of the testes is not felt, one should search beyond the scrotum and the inguinal canal, feeling the femoral triangle and the inner thigh. Many undescended testes are associated with an inguinal hernia and possibly a hydrocele; these masses can make palpation of the testes even more difficult.

Actually, the testes, if undescended, may have stopped their descent at some point within the inguinal canal or may still be in the abdomen. If a testis has not reached the inguinal canal, there is a greater likelihood that it is abnormal; the lower the testis lies in the inguinal canal, the more likely that it is normal. Sonography or a computed tomography (CT) scan can be helpful in determining location.

A testis that retracts simply because of an overactive cremasteric reflex should obviously not be "repaired." The truly undescended testis needs repair to improve the chance for fertility, provide accessible examination (particularly in the event of malignant change), diminish the possibility of the occurrence of testicular torsion, and prevent the emotional trauma that frequently accompanies the condition.

Given that one or both testes are truly ectopic or "hidden," the management plan raises certain questions: How long should one wait for descent before surgical intervention? Is there a "best" time emotionally? Is there a need to worry about infertility? Can repair help in this regard? If one waits too long, is the child at greater risk for testicular malignancy as an adult?

Certainly no one wants an unnecessary operation. Still, one cannot wait until puberty to see if there will be natural descent. Whenever there is uncertainty about the location of the testis, the potential for natural descent should be explored with a therapeutic trial of human chorionic gonadotropin (HCG), 4000 IU intramuscularly twice a week for 2 or 3 weeks. If the testis is to descend, it generally will at this dosage level and duration. Treating with HCG over a longer period has disadvantages; it can hasten the onset of puberty and cause testicular damage and sterility. Surgery is the desirable alternative if the testis does not descend or goes back up after the HCG trial. For those who do respond to the administration of HCG, the outlook for full sexual maturity is excellent. If the testes lie within the abdomen and are not palpable in the inguinal canal, HCG will not bring them down. However, if a course of HCG (2000 IU/day intramuscularly for 3 days) is given, the functioning of the abdominally placed testes can be determined by detecting a rise in the serum testosterone level on the fourth day.

The optimum age for surgical correction of cryptorchism is still debated. Surgical procedures are generally well tolerated (but also more technically difficult) before school age, and there probably are emotional advantages to correction before the child is plunged into the day-to-day demands of school life and the public nakedness that often accompanies physical education classes. If for some reason surgical correction is delayed until adolescence (e.g., delayed diagnosis), a sperm count should be done to reassure the patient and physician regarding fertility or to prepare them for the realities of infertility. Testicular tumors do occur with greater frequency in undescended testes. Although bringing the testis down does not diminish the potential of malignancy, it obviously increases the likelihood of detection. Periodic examination is important. Finally, if the patient has an associated inguinal hernia with or without a hydrocele, repair of the hernia, along with orchiopexy, should be done immediately. An elective herniorrhaphy is preferable to one done in the face of incarceration and possible strangulation. In any event, surgical repair of cryptorchism should be accomplished by 2 years of age, certainly no later than 3 years, primarily to reduce the risk of infertility.

Surgery may be done on an ambulatory basis when the testis is palpated in the inguinal canal. If it cannot be felt at all, a more extensive procedure with an abdominal incision will probably be necessary. Either way, a demonstrably *abnormal* testis should be removed and replaced with a prosthesis. As with hypospadias or epispadias, the role of the pediatrician in the care of the patient and his family is obvious. The emotional support necessary when such a vital aspect of human function is threatened is enormous. Preparation for surgery requires full discussion about the child's and the parents' fears and concerns; these discussions should continue following surgery, particularly as the child grows older and begins to reflect on the event.

SUGGESTED READINGS

Belman AB and Kass AJ: Hypospadias repair in children under one year of age, J Urol 128:1273, 1982.

Coloday AH: Undescended testes: is surgery necessary? N Engl J Med 314:510, 1986.

Schulze KA and Pfister RR: Evaluating the undescended testis, Am Fam Physician 31:133, 1988.

215

Hypothyroidism

Thomas P. Foley, Jr.

Few diseases affect multiple systems so severely as hypothyroidism and yet are associated with so many nonspecific symptoms and signs. Hypothyroidism can occur at any age and can affect the fetus as early as the first trimester of pregnancy. Its clinical presentation during infancy differs markedly from that of childhood and adolescence; for this reason, we must distinguish between congenital and juvenile hypothyroidism. As a result of screening programs for the detection of congenital hypothyroidism during the preclinical stage of the disease in the first month of life, accurate data on the incidence of congenital hypothyroidism throughout the Western world have been gathered in the past decade.[5] An incidence of approximately 1 congenitally affected infant for every 4000 live births has been reported, whereas the true incidence of juvenile hypothyroidism is not known. Both congenital hypothyroidism and juvenile hypothyroidism occur as familial or sporadic disease with or without enlargement of the thyroid gland (goiter, thyromegaly) and may progress as either a permanent or a transient disorder.

ETIOLOGY

In most instances the causes of hypothyroidism differ during infancy and childhood (see left-hand box on p. 1293).[7] An occasional patient with the mild form of congenital hypothyroidism may not seek treatment until childhood. These children usually have either familial goitrous hypothyroidism (dyshormonogenesis)[4] or thyroid dysgenesis with an ectopic thyroid gland located somewhere between the foramen cecum of the tongue and the anterior mediastinum; in most cases of permanent congenital hypothyroidism, however, the cause of the disease is unknown. Approximately 90% of patients have thyroid dysgenesis, either as an absence of functioning thyroid tissue (athyreosis), as an ectopic thyroid gland, or as a hypoplastic thyroid gland found in the normal anterior cervical location.[5] Recent evidence suggests that antibody-dependent, cell-mediated cytotoxicity (ADCC) was found in 32% of infants and 24% of mothers with permanent sporadic congenital hypothyroidism.[2] There are several inborn errors of thyroid hormone synthesis that are inherited as an autosomal recessive trait and are seen as thyromegaly on physical examination. In rare cases antibodies secreted by a mother with autoimmune thyroid disease may cross the placenta and block the function of the fetal thyroid gland. This form of transient hypothyroidism can persist for several weeks or months and requires thyroxine therapy during infancy. Other types of transient congenital hypothyroidism may occur when drugs prescribed for the mother, such as propylthiouracil, methimazole, or iodides, cross the placenta to block the fetal thyroid gland. Iodine-containing medications therefore should not be applied to the skin or mucous membranes of the neonate for more than a few days, since the iodine is readily absorbed and will block the infant's thyroid gland.

The most common cause of hypothyroidism in children beyond the perinatal period is goitrous or nongoitrous, autoimmune (chronic lymphocytic, Hashimoto) thyroiditis whether goitrous or nongoitrous (see left-hand box on p. 1293).[11] An occasional patient with hypothalamic or pituitary disease may initially be seen with hypothyroidism. These children usually have other clinical features to suggest an abnormality of the hypothalamus or pituitary.

HISTORY AND PHYSICAL EXAMINATION

Since hypothyroidism can affect most organ systems to varying degrees, it is very important that the clinician consider the diagnosis when the patient has many nonspecific or multisystemic complaints. Furthermore, a family history of thyroid and pituitary disease may disclose important diagnostic information. Many of the symptoms and signs of hypothyroidism are different during infancy as compared with childhood.[7,8] These are summarized in the right-hand box on p. 1293. During the first month of life affected infants may have no clinical symptoms or signs of hypothyroidism. Presumably, this occurs because there is some transfer of thyroxine in utero from mother to fetus,[14] because there is incomplete failure of thyroid gland function (as with ectopic thyroid tissue), or because the disease is of short duration, possibly developing during the third trimester of pregnancy.[7] In infants with no functioning thyroid tissue, clinical symptoms and signs may appear as early as the first 2 weeks of life and are certainly present by 6 weeks of age. The difficulty in diagnosing congenital hypothyroidism is evident by comparing the clinical features of three infants (Fig. 215-1). The infant on the upper left was referred at age 8 months with clinical features very suggestive of hypothyroidism, yet her thyroid studies were normal. The infant on the upper right had documented primary hypothyroidism at 4 weeks of age. Her clinical features at this age were minimal and included only mild periorbital edema, an enlarged posterior fontanelle, decreased stooling, and abdominal distention. The 6-month-old infant pictured at bottom center, in contrast, had severe hypothyroidism.

In addition, the clinical symptoms and signs of older children with hypothyroidism may be as nonspecific and insidious in their development as those found in infants with congenital hypothyroidism.[3] If the disease has been present for more

Causes of Hypothyroidism

CONGENITAL HYPOTHYROIDISM

A. Thyroid dysgenesis
   1. Thyroid aplasia
   2. Thyroid hypoplasia
   3. Ectopic thyroid gland
B. Familial abnormalities of thyroid hormone synthesis and metabolism (familial dyshormonogenesis)
C. Maternal disease
   1. Therapeutic doses of ^{131}I
   2. Transplacental autoimmune thyroiditis
   3. Ingestion of goitrogens
D. Endemic goiter and cretinism
E. Hypothalamic-pituitary hypothyroidism
   1. Pituitary agenesis or aplasia
   2. Thyrotropin deficiency: isolated
   3. Hypothalamic hormone deficiency
      a. Isolated thyrotropin deficiency
      b. Multiple tropic hormone deficiencies
      c. Septooptic dysplasia
      d. Anencephaly
   4. Hypothalamic-pituitary lesions

JUVENILE HYPOTHYROIDISM

A. Thyroiditis, autoimmune (Hashimoto)
B. Congenital thyroid dysgenesis
   1. Ectopic thyroid
   2. Hypoplastic
C. Congenital defects in thyroid hormone synthesis or metabolism
D. Iatrogenic thyroid ablation
   1. Surgical
   2. Radioactive iodine (^{131}I)
E. Ingestion of goitrogens
F. Endemic goiter
G. Hypothalamic-pituitary disease

Symptoms and Signs of Hypothyroidism

CONGENITAL HYPOTHYROIDISM

Facial edema
Large posterior fontanelle (>0.5 cm)
Rectal temperature below 35° C
Decreased stooling (less than one stool per day)
Prolonged hyperbilirubinemia (bilirubin above 10 mg/dl after 3 days of age)
Respiratory distress in a term infant
Umbilical hernia
Birth weight above 4000 g
Macroglossia
Bradycardia (pulse below 100 beats/minute)
Feeding problems and lethargy
Cutaneous mottling, vasomotor instability
Hoarse cry
Hirsute forehead

JUVENILE HYPOTHYROIDISM

Growth retardation (below 4 cm/year)
Delayed bone maturation
Delayed dental development and tooth eruption
Onset of puberty: usually delayed; rarely precocious
Myopathy and muscular hypertrophy
Menstrual disorders
Galactorrhea
Increased skin pigmentation
Physical and mental turpor
Pale, gray, cool, mottled, thickened, coarse skin
Constipation
Coarse, dry, brittle hair

than 6 months, growth deceleration should be evident, since normal thyroid hormone secretion is essential for normal linear growth. Hence, most patients with juvenile hypothyroidism have either thyromegaly or a deceleration of growth and are usually short in stature.[3] Deceleration of linear growth should be identified by the physician who routinely measures the height of the patient; its early recognition will prevent the development of long-standing hypothyroidism and short stature. The importance of this easy measurement cannot be overstressed. Frank obesity is, however, an uncommon complaint with hypothyroidism during childhood, since reduction in physical activity, if it occurs, is usually less than the reduction in caloric intake. On the other hand, children with advanced hypothyroidism and myxedema are usually chubby and have periorbital edema.

Inspection and palpation of the anterior cervical area will enable the examiner to identify an enlarged thyroid gland, even in the neonate. The easiest method for examining the thyroid gland of an infant is to place the infant prone with the neck extended and feel for the isthmus of the thyroid, just below the hyoid bone. After identifying the isthmus, one should palpate laterally to delineate the lobes, which are very difficult to define in a normal infant. The examination of the thyroid gland in an older child is easier. Having the patient swallow water will facilitate the identification and delineation of both lobes of the thyroid gland as distinct from other adjacent tissue, since the thyroid rises during swallowing.

LABORATORY DATA

Although the clinical laboratory may offer a wide battery of thyroid function tests, rarely are most of these tests necessary for the diagnosis of hypothyroidism. An elevation of the serum thyroid-stimulating hormone (TSH) value is the single most sensitive test for primary hypothyroidism (thyroid gland failure).[3] The combination of a low serum thyroxine (T_4) value and an elevated TSH is diagnostic of primary hypothyroidism, either permanent or transient, at any age, including term and preterm infants.[11] In patients with hypothalamic or pituitary hypothyroidism, the determination of the T_4 (low) and TSH (usually not elevated) is not adequate for definitive diagnosis, since patients with thyroxine-binding globulin (TBG) deficiency will also have a low T_4 and normal TSH. Hence the free thyroxine (free T_4) and TBG values, as well as specific tests of pituitary function, are usually necessary.[3]

An occasional child or infant with a coexisting and severe illness, such as idiopathic respiratory distress syndrome, may have the so-called euthyroid sick syndrome in which the T_4

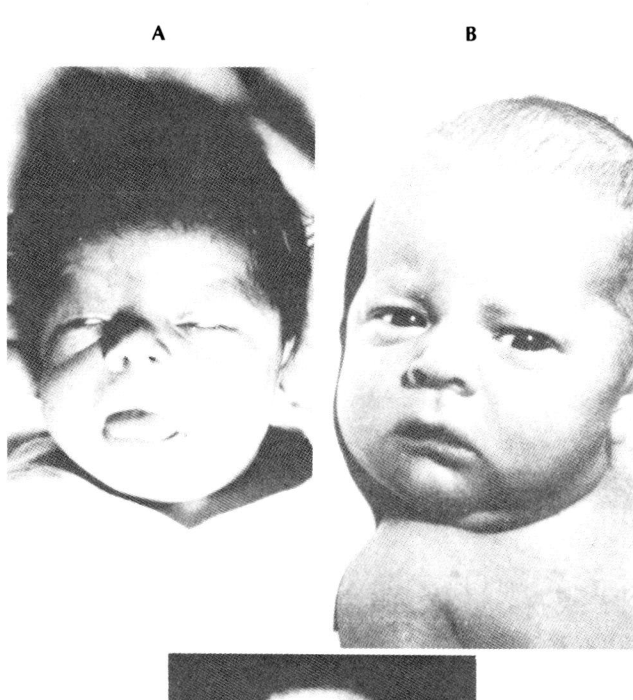

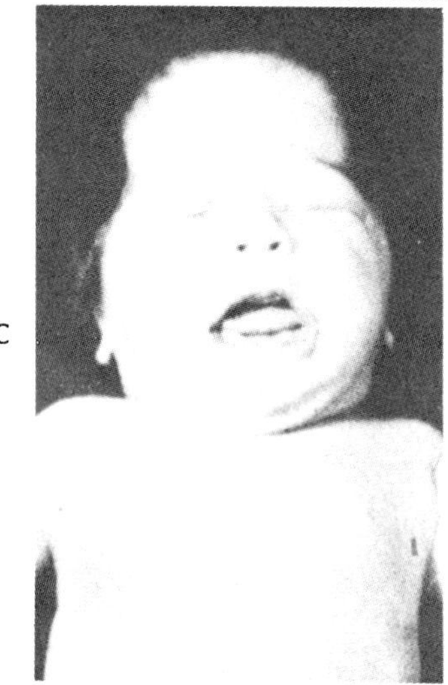

Fig. 215-1 A, Normal infant with clinical signs but no clinical symptoms of congenital hypothyroidism. **B,** Affected infant with athyreosis, age 28 days. **C,** Infant at age 6 months with athyreosis and severe congenital hypothyroidism.

Reprinted from Foley TP, Jr: Sporadic congenital hypothyroidism. In Dussault, JH, and Walker P, editors: Congenital hypothrroidism, New York, 1983, p. 246, courtesy of Marcel Dekker, Inc.

may be low despite normal TBG levels.[4] The serum triiodothyronine (T_3) value is characteristically low and the TSH value normal, while the free T_4 and reverse T_3 levels are either in the upper range of normal or frankly elevated. This problem occurs most frequently in the preterm infant.

Tests other than the serum T_4 and TSH determinations are not often required for children with a suspected diagnosis of hypothyroidism; however, thyroid antibody determinations can be very helpful in determining the cause of juvenile hypothyroidism, since the titers of the serum microsomal or thyroglobulin antibodies are usually elevated in children with autoimmune thyroiditis.[1,6] Transient congenital hypothyroidism may be caused by TSH receptor blocking antibodies (TRAb) acquired from the mother with autoimmune thyroid disease.[10] TRAb levels are diagnostically valuable in these patients. A serum T_3 determination in the infant with congenital hypothyroidism may also be of prognostic value and is often reassuring for parents if the physician can indicate, on the evidence of a normal T_3 value, that therapy was initiated before chemical hypothyroidism developed.[8] The serum T_3 is not indicated, however, in the diagnostic evaluation of juvenile hypothyroidism.

Radioisotopic studies are often inappropriately ordered. It is not usually necessary to perform both a thyroid scan and uptake test. In infants and children, ^{131}I uptake should never be used as a diagnostic test, but a thyroid scan using either ^{131}I or technetium is an important test in infants with abnormal thyroid screening tests for the following reasons:

1. It is the most rapid and definitive diagnostic test on which the initiation of therapy may be decided; the test result can be obtained 2 hours after the dose is administered.
2. The test will distinguish sporadic disease, such as thyroid dysgenesis, from familial disease, a distinction important for genetic counseling.

A thyroid uptake test should not be performed in an infant unless the clinical examination and the thyroid scan demonstrate an enlarged thyroid gland.

An elevated thyroid uptake in an infant with a goiter is very suggestive of an inborn error of thyroid hormone synthesis.[4] Radioisotopic studies are rarely needed in older patients with juvenile hypothyroidism; the thyroid scan is indicated when there is a mass palpated in the thyroid gland, so as to exclude the possibility of thyroid carcinoma.[3] Thyroid uptake studies are indicated when the patient has diffuse thyromegaly and biochemical evidence of hypothyroidism not caused by autoimmune thyroiditis or goitrogen ingestion.[3]

Although not essential, the assessment of skeletal maturation can provide additional data regarding the duration of hypothyroidism. A bone age determination consistent with that of a normal newborn would suggest recently acquired, mild congenital hypothyroidism, whereas notation of the absence of ossification centers at the knee in addition to the presence of only the two ossification centers in the foot indicates that the fetus was affected by hypothyroidism during the third trimester of pregnancy.

THERAPY

The treatment of choice for hypothyroidism in infancy and childhood is the daily administration of oral L-thyroxine (Table 215-1).[7,13] Other thyroid preparations are either more expensive or less reliably monitored for adequacy of dose. The initial dose in an infant is 50 μg (0.05 mg) of L-thyroxine daily for the first 1 to 2 weeks and should be started promptly once the diagnosis of hypothyroidism is confirmed. Infants with hypothalamic or pituitary hypothyroidism should be started on 25 μg/day, since their requirements are less and their hypothyroidism mild. At the end of the first and second week, serum T_4 values should be obtained to determine that the amount of L-thyroxine is adequate but not excessive. Rarely will one find that 50 μg/day is inadequate, but often after 1 or 2 weeks the dose will need to be reduced to 37.5 μg/day and occasionally to 25 μg/day if clinical symptoms of hyperthyroidism develop or the serum T_4 value exceeds 16 μg/dl (the normal range for T_4 in the infant is higher than

Table 215-1 *Dose of L-Thyroxine*

AGE	T_4 DOSE PER DAY (μg)	T_4 DOSE/KG/DAY (μg)
<6 mo	25-50	8-10
6-12 mo	50-75	6-8
1-5 yr	75-100	5-6
6-12 yr	100-150	4-5
>12 yr	100-200	2-3

that in older children and adults), and the serum T_3 value exceeds 250 ng/dl. Therapy should be adjusted to maintain the serum T_4 during infancy above 8 μg/dl, preferably between 10 and 12 μg/dl. Within the first 4 weeks of therapy the serum TSH value should decrease toward normal. But in an occasional infant the TSH value will never return to normal unless the thyroxine dose is excessive and causes clinical thyrotoxicosis; these infants have an abnormality in the feedback set point of TSH secretion. The goal of therapy here should be to maintain normal serum T_4 and T_3 values. Since excessive thyroxine therapy in infancy may cause cranial synostosis and brain dysfunction, frequent monitoring of serum T_4 and TSH levels at 3-month intervals during the first year is essential. Additional determinations may be necessary whenever an adjustment in dose is made. After 2 years of age the need to change the L-thyroxine dose occurs infrequently, so that the annual measurement of serum T_4 and TSH levels should be adequate. If linear growth and weight gain are progressing satisfactorily, no additional studies are necessary.

In contrast to young infants with congenital hypothyroidism, there is not the same degree of urgency in achieving the euthyroid state among older children with hypothyroidism. Although patients with recent onset of mild hypothyroidism may be started on a full replacement dose of L-thyroxine, children with chronic hypothyroidism and clinical symptoms should be started on a low dose (25 μg/day) that is gradually increased every 2 to 4 weeks toward a full replacement dose.[3]

The rapid correction of the hypothyroid state can often be associated with undesirable behavioral side effects. The children act thyrotoxic despite biochemical euthyroidism; they often are restless, have a short attention span, and are emotionally labile. These symptoms, in association with the expected hair loss, may lead to inappropriate discontinuance of therapy by the uninformed parent. In such cases a gradual increase in dose seems to minimize these problems in adjustment from the hypothyroid to the euthyroid state. Adequacy of L-thyroxine therapy can be monitored by serum T_4 and TSH determinations once the patient is receiving a full replacement dose and annually thereafter. Since patients with juvenile hypothyroidism do not have an abnormality in the feedback control of TSH secretion, an elevated TSH with a low T_4 indicates either inadequate therapy or poor compliance; the latter is often characterized by variable serum T_4 and TSH values—for example, the levels are normal on one occasion but discordant (normal or elevated T_4 with elevated TSH) on subsequent determinations despite no change in therapy. In rare cases the medication may not contain the indicated amount of thyroxine. Studies in adults have indicated a reduced absorption of L-thyroxine when administered with meals. Hence it is advisable, particularly in treating infants, that their medication be given an hour before the next feeding.

Since an occasional infant receiving treatment may have had only transient congenital hypothyroidism, therapy should either be reduced or discontinued some time after 2 years of age and serum T_4 and TSH levels determined 2 to 4 weeks later. Temporary cessation or reduction in therapy, however, is not necessary for those patients who previously had had elevated TSH but normal T_4 levels during therapy.

PROGNOSIS

Infants who have been adequately treated for congenital hypothyroidism since the first month of age have an excellent prognosis for normal intellectual function and linear growth.[9] However, delays in diagnosis and in the institution of adequate therapy until after 3 months of age are usually associated with an increased risk of mental retardation.[9] In contrast, no permanent intellectual impairment is found among patients with juvenile hypothyroidism, although adolescents with severe growth retardation may never achieve their full growth potential; often their linear growth response to therapy is not accelerated and the height percentile achieved as an adult is lower than that predicted by their growth before the development of hypothyroidism.[12]

REFERENCES

1. Bachrach LK and Foley TP Jr: Thyroiditis in children, Pediatr Rev 11:184, 1989.
2. Bogner U et al: Cytotoxic antibodies in congenital hypothyroidism, J Clin Endocrinol Metab 68:671, 1989.
3. Dallas JS and Foley TP Jr: Thyromegaly; hypothyroidism. In Lifshitz F, editor: Pediatric endocrinology, New York, 1989, Marcel Dekker, Inc.
4. Delange F, Fisher DA, and Malvaux P, editors: Pediatric thyroidology, Basel, 1985, S Karger AG.
5. Fisher DA et al: Screening for congenital hypothyroidism: results of screening 1 million North American infants, J Pediatr 94:700, 1979.
6. Foley TP Jr: Acute, subacute, and chronic thyroiditis. In Kaplan SA, editor: Clinical pediatric and adolescent endocrinology, Philadelphia, 1982, WB Saunders Co.
7. Foley TP Jr: Sporadic congenital hypothyroidism. In Dussault JH and Walker P, editors: Congenital hypothyroidism, New York, 1983, Marcel Dekker, Inc.
8. Klein AH et al: Neonatal thyroid function in congenital hypothyroidism, J Pediatr 89:545, 1976.
9. Klein AH, Meltzer S, and Kenny FM: Improved prognosis in congenital hypothyroidism treated before age three months, J Pediatr 81:912, 1972.
10. Matsuura N et al: Familial neonatal transient hypothyroidism due to maternal TSH-binding inhibitor immunoglobulins, N Engl J Med 303:738, 1980.
11. Rallison M et al: Occurrence and natural history of thyroiditis in children, J Pediatr 86:675, 1975.
12. Rivkees SA, Bode HH, and Crawford JD: Long-term growth in juvenile acquired hypothyroidism, N Engl J Med 318:599, 1988.
13. Sato T et al: Age related change in pituitary threshold for TSH release during replacement therapy for cretinism, J Clin Endocrinol Metab 44:553, 1977.
14. Vulsma T, Gons MH, and de Vijlder JJM: Maternal-fetal transfer of thyroxine in congenital hypothyroidism due to a total organification defect or thyroid agenesis, N Engl J Med 321:13, 1989 (and editorial, p 44).

216

Iatrogenic Disease

Cheston M. Berlin, Jr.

Iatrogenic (from the Greek word meaning "produced by the physician") illness is the result of the therapy or diagnostic procedures employed with the intent to manage the health needs of a patient. Few comprehensive studies are available to indicate its prevalence, yet a report in 1981 by Steel and associates[3] found that 36% of 815 consecutive admissions to a general medical service had complications during their hospital stay caused by treatment or investigative procedures; 50% of these resulted from drug use.

Pediatric patients are especially vulnerable because of their size, their age, and the use of new therapies with unknown risk for children. This is an especially significant problem in newborn medicine. Raju[2] surveyed a single pediatric journal and reported that 12.7% of articles published between 1965 and 1976 dealt with iatrogenic problems. Principi and coworkers[1] surveyed the use of antibiotics on nine pediatric units (765 patients); *nearly one third of the patients received antibiotics on an "irrational" basis* (no proven infection or positive laboratory test). In 75% of the patients the antibiotic choice was not justified by the given clinical condition. This type of therapy invites iatrogenic disease.

The following is a case report of an iatrogenic illness:

> Keith was referred by his family physician to an allergist at age 8 years for evaluation of continual nasal sniffing, which had been present for years and was attributed to allergies, in part because of a positive family history and because decongestants were ineffective. From age 8 to 10 years he was treated by the allergist with monthly injections of triamcinolone acetate. The parents became concerned at the onset of growth failure during this period. At age 10 he was referred to an endocrinology clinic, where the evaluation revealed his height and weight to be below the 3rd percentile with essentially no absolute gain since 8 years of age. Also noted in the history was enuresis of many years' duration. The clinic note for that visit describes the patient as "hyperactive, with constant small movements of the body and frequent repetitive sounds from the throat." He was evaluated with the following tests, all of which were normal: insulin-arginine stimulation of growth hormone release, serum thyroxine, skull roentgenograms, bone age, and buccal smear. Conclusions of the endocrine consultation were that the growth failure was most likely caused by the administration of steroids; the family was thus advised to stop the steroids. The patient was referred to a urologist for evaluation of his enuresis and to a pediatrician for evaluation of his hyperactivity.
>
> Keith was first seen by the urologist and hospitalized. He underwent an intravenous program with voiding cystourethrogram, cystoscopy with cystometrogram, and cystourethroscopy. All these studies were normal. The patient was given imipramine, 25 mg at bedtime.
>
> The patient was next seen in pediatrics. A diagnosis of Tourette syndrome was made, based on multiple tics and coprolalia. Because of the patient's and family's initial delight in the efficacy of imipramine in controlling the enuresis, drug therapy for controlling Tourette syndrome was discussed but deferred. Six weeks later, with the patient's resumption of frequent enuresis while still receiving imipramine, this drug was stopped and haloperidol, 1 mg twice daily, was started. There was prompt and considerable diminution of his tics and cessation of coprolalia within 2 days. After 1 week on this dosage the patient experienced acute dystonic posturing of the neck and face, which was reversed by intravenous diphenhydramine, 25 mg. The dose of haloperidol was decreased to 0.5 mg twice daily; there were no further side effects.
>
> The patient remained stable for the next 5 years on this dosage. After the initial diagnosis Keith was placed in a special education class; subsequently, his accomplishments and self-esteem both increased. He also became a rifle marksman. The next year he returned to a regular classroom, and 5 years later he graduated from high school with vocational training. His height was at the 20th percentile, and his weight was at the 50th percentile. At 21 years of age he is fully employed. After 5 years of continuous haloperidol therapy at a dose of 0.5 mg twice daily, the patient now takes the medication at the same dosage two or three times per year for 1 to 2 weeks at a time when he is in stressful situations.

Iatrogenic illness in this patient occurred at several levels and for different reasons. First, he was misdiagnosed as being allergic because of frequent sniffing, a common symptom of Tourette syndrome. Second, he received a potent steroid for this symptom, which stopped his growth; this led to a lengthy, expensive, and negative endocrinology evaluation. Third, he was referred to a specialist for evaluation of a common and usually benign developmental condition: enuresis. He received a lengthy, excessive evaluation requiring hospitalization and anesthesia. Fourth, after the correct diagnosis was made, initial drug therapy caused a severe dystonic drug reaction. And finally, failure to diagnose Tourette syndrome early caused serious educational problems.

ETIOLOGY

Every patient contact is capable of producing iatrogenic disease. Infants under the age of 1 year are especially vulnerable to idiosyncratic central nervous system reactions to drugs (e.g., extrapyramidal reaction to prochlorperazine). The risk varies from virtually zero with the insertion of a tongue depressor (the gag reflex can stimulate the vagus to produce asystole) to 100% with the use of intravenous amphotericin

Table 216-1 *Complications that Can Arise from Diagnostic Procedures and Subsequent Therapy*

	COMPLICATIONS
Diagnostic procedure	
Physical examination	
Ears	Laceration of auditory canal; perforation of eardrum
Pharynx	Laceration of soft palate and buccal mucosa
Mouth or rectum (with thermometer)	Broken glass (laceration)
Joints	Dislocation
Abdominal examination	Fractured spleen
Laboratory testing	
Throat culture	Gagging; vomiting; aspiration
Venipunctures	Bruising; arterial spasm
Heel sticks	Lacerated heels; infection, osteomyelitis
Roentgenographic procedures	
Position of patient	Dislocation of joints; infiltration of intravenous lines
Use of radiopaque dyes	Allergic reactions
Sedation	Central nervous system (CNS) depression; drug reaction; cardiac arrhythmias
Radiotherapy	Skin erythema; burns; sterility; alopecia
Therapy	
Drug therapy	Drug reaction; drug interaction; errors in type of drug and frequency and route of administration
Fluids and electrolytes	Overhydration or underhydration; incorrect solution; incorrect route; misplacement of intravenous line
Nutrition (including vitamins)	Deficiency states; inadequate knowledge of formula composition; hypervitaminosis
Equipment	
Infant warmers	Burns
Electric hazards	Shocks
Transillumination (fiberoptics)	Burns
Noise (especially in incubators)	Auditory damage; sleep disturbances
Constant light	CNS dysfunction (?); retinal damage (?); hormonal dysfunction (?)
Temperature control	Hypothermia or hyperthermia
Beds: mesh, rails, objects	Choking; falling out
Surgery	Wrong patient operated on; wrong part of body operated on; complication: infection, contracture, scarring, adhesions, fluid and electrolyte imbalance
Cardiopulmonary resuscitation	Fractured ribs, spleen, or liver
Instructions to patient or family	Overly restricted life at home and school; failure to appreciate impact of illness on family's and patient's life; misunderstanding of oral instructions
Immunizations	Local and systemic reactions

B. The most common but not necessarily the most serious possibilities for iatrogenic disease occur in two broad categories: diagnostic procedures and therapy (Table 216-1).

DATA BASE

Recognition of iatrogenic disorders requires the physician's constant cognizance of the possibility. The history and physical examination are most important; laboratory tests may confirm the clinical impression. Many iatrogenic disorders are obvious: ocular-gyric crisis from prochlorperazine use; sterile thigh abscesses from diphtheria-tetanus-pertussis (DTP) immunization; and a skin burn from touching an overhead warmer. Others are more subtle: rickets in the rapidly growing premature infant from failure to give sufficient vitamins; hypernatremia from using boiled skim milk; and thinning skin from long-term use of steroid cream for diaper rash. A careful review of systems coupled with specific questions concerning recent medications or other therapy (by nonphysicians as well as physicians) will usually uncover problem areas.

DIFFERENTIAL DIAGNOSIS

The diagnosis of the condition is usually straightforward, *once considered,* since awareness and appreciation of iatrogenic causes are frequently difficult. A list of a few iatrogenic diseases with alternative causes may be illustrative (Table 216-2).

MANAGEMENT

The management of iatrogenic disease is no different from that of any other condition, except for investigation of the iatrogenic event. The lesson usually learned is that there has been a breakdown (or even nonestablishment) of patient-physician communication and the mechanisms of health care delivery. Some iatrogenic events are truly unavoidable and, indeed, almost expected: limb atrophy after the application of a plaster cast and postoperative scarring in a person known to form keloids. Other iatrogenic events pinpoint serious deficiencies in medical care technology: failure to recheck the position of a decimal point in a digoxin order and inadequate

Table 216-2 *Differential Diagnosis of Iatrogenic Diseases*

CONDITION (DIAGNOSIS)	CAUSES
Rickets	No vitamin D supplementation Renal disease Rapid growth in a premature infant
Seizure	Seizure disorder Tap water enemas Boiled skim milk Fever
Fever of unknown origin	Urinary tract infection Phenytoin therapy
Hearing loss	Recurrent otitis media Aminoglycoside therapy Incubator noise with concomitant aminoglycoside therapy
Short stature	Heredity Malnutrition Steroid therapy
Loose stools	Enteritis Lactose intolerance Mineral oil and senna products
Increased intracranial pressure	Meningitis Brain tumor Vitamin A intoxication
Hair loss	Emotional Thallium poisoning Vincristine therapy

postmarketing drug surveillance. The following are suggestions for preventing (or at least minimizing) iatrogenic illnesses.

1. *Careful explanation to parents and patient with the institution of any therapy*. Preprinted handouts are helpful in anticipating and recognizing problems—for example, discussion of possible side effects of immunization. Patient information brochures are being developed more and more by practitioners and institutions both for procedures and for drug therapy.
2. *Prompt investigation of any iatrogenic event*. Comments such as "Don't worry, this happens frequently," "We see this occasionally," and "Nobody knows" are hardly reassuring to the family. Corrective measures must be instituted immediately.
3. *Continuing education for all health care personnel*. It is the responsibility of the physician to investigate and report suspected links between therapy and unexpected changes in the patient's condition.
4. *Call for help*. This may mean additional consultative opinions from experts within and without medicine. Electrical engineers can give advice about electric current leaks; social workers and teachers can assist in management of a chronically ill child whose medical regimen does not permit normal school attendance.

Iatrogenic disease may be cause for a medicolegal suit by a family. Such a malpractice risk will be considerably minimized if all of the above management suggestions are followed.

REFERENCES

1. Principi N et al: Control of antibiotic therapy in pediatric patients, Dev Pharmacol Ther 3:145, 1981.
2. Raju TNK: The injured neonate of the seventies, J Pediatr 91:347, 1977.
3. Steel K et al: Iatrogenic illness on a general medical service at a university hospital, N Engl J Med 304:638, 1981.

SUGGESTED READINGS

Koren G, Barzilay Z, and Greenwald M: Tenfold errors in administration of drug doses: a neglected iatrogenic disease in pediatrics, Pediatrics 77:848-849, 1986.

Valdes-Dapena M: Iatrogenic disease in the perinatal period, Pediatr Clin North Am 36:67-93, 1989.

217

Idiopathic Thrombocytopenia

Christopher N. Frantz

GENERAL APPROACH TO THE THROMBOCYTOPENIC PATIENT

In evaluating the patient with thrombocytopenia, the physician must determine if the patient is sufficiently hemostatically impaired to require therapy, and if so, the cause of the thrombocytopenia. Treatment undertaken without knowing the cause of thrombocytopenia is arbitrary and therefore may be unsuccessful. For example, platelet transfusions rarely elevate the platelet count in patients with destructive thrombocytopenias.

The most likely cause of thrombocytopenia may often be deduced before more complex tests need to be undertaken by taking a careful history, performing a physical examination, and knowing the platelet count and the size of the circulating platelets. The history should focus on chronicity of the thrombocytopenia and its effects. The family history is helpful but unlikely to be positive, because thrombocytopenia is much more likely to be acquired than congenital. The hallmark of bleeding as a result of a low platelet count or because of platelet dysfunction is the presence of petechiae. Purpura, ecchymosis, and mucosal bleeding, including epistaxis, gastrointestinal hemorrhage, and menorrhagia, are commonly seen, and bleeding from superficial cuts and abrasions is usually prolonged. In contrast, bleeding caused by plasma coagulation defects usually has a single locus (most often in deep tissues such as joints and muscles) and prolonged bleeding from the oral mucosa.

There are three general types of thrombocytopenia: (1) *destructive,* the most common in children, in which increased platelet destruction occurs; (2) *aregenerative,* in which the production of platelets by the bone marrow is reduced; and (3) *platelet sequestration,* in which the platelets are trapped within the spleen, called hypersplenism. A normal-sized spleen precludes this diagnosis.

Aregenerative thrombocytopenia almost always involves other cell lines, because the underlying disorder involves the entire bone marrow, although there are several rare disorders of isolated decreased platelet production. If one suspects the presence of a destructive thrombocytopenia, one must rule out an aregenerative etiology by determining that the hemoglobin level is normal and that the absolute neutrophil count is greater than 1500.

In destructive thrombocytopenia the platelets usually are large. Patients with destructive thrombocytopenia who are very ill or who have a complex underlying disease may have thrombocytopenia on the basis of disseminated intravascular coagulation, sepsis, or an untoward drug reaction. However, if the patient has none of these, the destructive thrombocytopenia is almost always caused by an immunologic reaction.

IDIOPATHIC THROMBOCYTOPENIC PURPURA (ITP) OF CHILDHOOD

Idiopathic thrombocytopenic purpura (ITP) of childhood is not truly idiopathic; it is caused by the binding of antibody to platelets, which results in their destruction by the reticuloendothelial system. The largest subset of children with ITP has a well-defined clinical syndrome that may be called acute ITP of childhood (AITPC). In other children, the ITP may be related to an underlying disorder that significantly affects the child's long-term prognosis, such as a collagen-vascular disease or hypogammaglobulinemia. Still others may have chronic ITP that has no association with an underlying disorder; chronic ITP is diagnosed when the thrombocytopenia persists for longer than 6 months. Finally, 1% to 4% of children who apparently have classic AITPC suffer recurrent episodes of severe thrombocytopenia for many months or years after an initial return of the platelet count to normal. This disorder is called recurrent ITP of childhood.

The annual incidence of new cases of AITPC is 4 per 100,000 children. There is no sex predilection, and the peak onset occurs between 2 and 5 years of age. Typically, a previously well child suddenly develops easy bruising and petechiae 1 to 3 weeks following a viral illness. Nosebleeds occur in 20% to 30% of those children, but renal, oral, or gastrointestinal bleeding occur in fewer than 10%. Except for the pressure of bleeding, the physical examination is entirely normal. Splenomegaly is not seen in AITPC, although it is commonly seen in patients with chronic ITP or with ITP related to an underlying collagen-vascular disease. A very large spleen suggests hypersplenism rather than ITP. In AITPC, the platelet count is almost always less than 20,000 at the time of diagnosis. Thrombocytopenia is evident on the peripheral blood smear, and the platelets that are present may or may not have bizarre shapes or giant forms or be diffusely increased in size. The red and white blood cells on the smear should be normal; if they are not, other diagnoses should be considered.

The laboratory evaluation of AITPC is quite simple. The complete blood count, including an examination of the blood smear, is usually sufficient in patients who have all the characteristics listed in the box on p. 1300. The typical presentation of AITPC is usually so clear that a bone marrow eval-

Criteria for the Diagnosis of Acute Idiopathic Thrombocytopenia of Childhood

—Platelet count ≤ 20,000
—Normal complete blood count, including the absolute neutrophil count and the examination of red blood cells, white blood cells, and platelet morphology on the blood smear
—Age 1 to 9 years
—Patient is otherwise well
—Acute onset (symptomatic ≤ 2 weeks)
—Preceding viral illness within 1 to 3 weeks
—Spleen is normal size
—No history or family history of other possible autoimmune disorders (e.g., hemolytic anemia, nephritis, thyroiditis, collagen-vascular disease, or frequent infections)

is not ordinarily required. However, bone marrow examination may be necessary to rule out aregenerative thrombocytopenia caused by either aplastic anemia in its earliest stages or acute leukemia. Most pediatric hematologists perform a bone marrow examination for classic onset AITPC to conclusively rule out those aregenerative disorders. A bone marrow examination should always be performed before initiating corticosteroid therapy for presumed AITPC, because steroids can mask the presence of acute lymphoblastic leukemia. Failure to perform a bone marrow examination under these circumstances would delay not only diagnosis but also the identification of leukemic cells that are resistant to the cytotoxic effects of steroids, thus decreasing the likelihood of cure. Indeed, it has been shown that patients with acute lymphatic leukemia who are treated for any reason with steroids immediately before the establishment of the diagnosis have a poor prognosis. Bone marrow aspiration in patients with AITPC should reveal a normocellular marrow with normal erythroid and myeloid maturation. Megakaryocytes are present in normal or increased numbers. It should be remembered that bone marrow examination will not distinguish AITPC from other forms of platelet destruction, including immune-mediated thrombocytopenic disorders other than AITPC. The bleeding time is prolonged and coagulation tests are normal in patients with AITPC. Many hematologists do not perform these tests in the child with classic AITPC. The measurement of platelet-associated immune globulin is elevated in approximately 85% of children with ITP, including the majority with AITPC. Platelet-associated immune globulin levels are also elevated in many other thrombocytopenic disorders, so that the specificity of the test for AITPC is quite low and rarely is diagnostically important.

Additional diagnostic tests for disorders associated with ITP should be performed in all patients who do not completely meet the criteria for the diagnosis of AITPC as outlined in the box on p. 1300. This diagnostic workup is summarized in the box on p. 1301. First, a bone marrow examination should be performed to document adequate production of platelets. Immunoglobulin levels should be measured to rule out hypogammaglobulinemia associated with multiple autoimmune phenomena, especially autoimmune hemolytic anemia, ITP, and autoimmune neutropenia. The remaining tests search for evidence of associated autoimmune phenomena, collagen-vascular disease, or coagulopathies. The reticulocyte count is elevated during compensated hemolysis; the Coombs' test is positive in most cases of autoimmune hemolytic anemia; urinalysis may reveal evidence of nephritis; the antinuclear antibody may identify patients with systemic lupus erythematosus; and the prothrombin and partial thromboplastin and bleeding times may provide clues to the presence of a variety of coagulation disorders. Human immunodeficiency virus antibody tests should be performed because isolated ITP is not an uncommon first manifestation of HIV infection.

PROGNOSIS AND MANAGEMENT

Management of AITPC is based on the natural history of the disease. The vast majority of patients will have a complete remission without therapy and without sequelae (90% as reported in the literature, but considerably more in the experience of most pediatric hematologists, especially when the inclusive characteristics previously listed are documented). Treatment is therefore based on the estimation of short-term bleeding risks in these patients. Less than 1% of patients with AITPC have a poor outcome because of either intracranial or gastrointestinal hemorrhage early in their course. An analysis of patients reported in the literature with intracranial hemorrhage shows that all had a platelet count of less than 20,000 cells/mm^3 at the time of hemorrhage. Most were not receiving corticosteroids. Although many of the reported cases occur during the first month following diagnosis, an equal number occur in later months. It is logical that the risk of serious bleeding is higher in those patients who have more bleeding manifestations. Therefore many pediatric hematologists choose to treat those patients with mucosal or retinal hemorrhages but not those who have only mild petechiae and purpura. Some hematologists treat very young patients whose physical activity cannot be controlled; others treat all patients with AITPC.

Defensive management is most important. Restriction of physical activity and complete avoidance of all contact sports and playground activities are indicated. All medications with any antiplatelet activity should be avoided, including aspirin, antihistamines, phenothiazines, and glyceryl guaiacolate. Intramuscular injections should not be given. Two treatments are effective for immune thrombocytopenia, corticosteroids and high-dose intravenous gamma globulin (IVIG). Advantages of one over the other are not clear at this time. Most patients respond to each, and the use of one does not preclude subsequent trial of the other. Corticosteroids induce the repair of the defects in the vascular endothelium that have been caused by the absence of platelets. Corticosteroids also result in an elevation of the platelet count in patients with ITP. Accordingly, a reduction of the prolonged bleeding time is seen. Although IVIG does not appear to affect vascular stability directly, the increase in platelet count is often more dramatic than that seen with steroids. Prednisone is usually given at 2 mg/kg of body weight/day divided into two or 3 doses a day. It is given for 2 weeks and then tapered during

Diagnostic Workup for ITP

Studies to be performed when a patient with ITP does not fit all the criteria listed in the box on p. 1300 or if apparent AITPC does not resolve within 6 months:
—Bone marrow examination
—Immunoglobulin levels
—Reticulocyte count
—Direct and indirect antiglobulin (Coombs') test
—Urinalysis
—Antinuclear antibody levels
—Prothrombin time and partial thromboplastin time
—Bleeding time
—Human immune deficiency virus antibody

the following week or two, whether or not the patient responds. If the platelet count has risen as a result of the steroids, it may fall during the tapering, but it often does not fall to dangerous levels. Long-term corticosteroid therapy is avoided because of the severe cosmetic effects and growth limitation they cause, especially in the young child. Other well-known adverse effects of steroids include pancreatitis, hyperglycemia, hypertension, fluid and electrolyte disturbances, and psychosis. IVIG is given in two doses of 1 g/kg of body weight each. The infusion should be slow, over a period of approximately 6 hours. The second dose is given 24 hours after the completion of the first infusion. Significant increases in platelet count are usually seen within 24 hours following the second dose of IVIG. The common side effect of intravenous gamma globulin occurs during infusion and is caused by IgG complexes within the preparation. The reaction usually involves headache, nausea, chills, and occasionally fever and hypotension. The risk of an anaphylactic reaction to IgA in an IgA-deficient patient is quite low. The risk of transmission of viral infections by IVIG is also extremely low. Other side effects include the passive transmission of anti-red cell alloantibodies causing hemolytic anemia. Approximately 80% of patients respond to each of these therapies. The cost of IVIG is a few hundred times that of oral corticosteroids, because hospitalization is required for the prolonged infusions and the IVIG itself is quite expensive.

EMERGENCY MANAGEMENT OF BLEEDING

General measures should be directed at the delivery of platelets to the site of hemorrhage. Although the routine use of platelet transfusions in ITP is not indicated, platelet transfusions are useful in an emergency, and a bolus infusion of 6 to 12 U should be administered immediately, as it may exert hemostatic benefit before being cleared by the reticuloendothelial system. Large doses of corticosteroids should be started intravenously (4 mg/kg/day of prednisolone or its equivalent). Intravenous gamma globulin should also be administered at the dose described above. If intravenous gamma globulin fails to raise the platelet count or serious bleeding persists, emergency splenectomy may be indicated, depending on the patient's age (see below). Aminocaproic acid (Amicar), an inhibitor of fibrinolysis, may help prevent serious rebleeding, especially in mucosal areas. Bleeding in the urinary tract is a contraindication to the use of aminocaproic acid. Additional more specific measures depend on the sites of active bleeding.

CHRONIC IDIOPATHIC THROMBOCYTOPENIC PURPURA

Chronic ITP is defined as a platelet count that persists below 100,000 cells/mm^3 for 6 months or more. Approximately 20% of patients with chronic ITP will ultimately recover spontaneously, but it is not possible to predict in which children this will occur. Chronic ITP in children is similar to ITP in adults and is caused by platelet autoantibodies that bind to specific platelet membrane glycoproteins, including IIb/IIIa and Ib. The ratio of females to males with chronic ITP is 3:1. The workup for chronic ITP should include the studies outlined in the box on p. 1301. In addition, a platelet survival test may be very helpful in those patients in whom the diagnosis is uncertain.

Management depends on the overall impact of both platelet count and platelet function on hemostasis in the individual patient. In some patients, the antiplatelet antibody also impairs platelet function. A bleeding time is helpful to estimate hemostatic function at a given platelet count. Whereas splenectomy was once the mainstay of the treatment of chronic ITP, IVIG has now become the initial therapy of choice in most cases, preventing or postponing splenectomy. High-dose intravenous gamma globulin is effective for temporarily raising the platelet count in approximately 80% of children with chronic ITP. The dose is the same as described above for acute ITP. Intravenous gamma globulin results in a permanent remission in only a few children. About 25% of patients eventually become refractory to the effect and require splenectomy. In the remainder of patients, periodic doses of intravenous gamma globulin are effective long-term therapy. These periodic doses are usually given as a single infusion of 0.4 to 1 g/kg of body weight once every several weeks. The interval depends on the patient's platelet count. The infusions can usually be given in the outpatient clinic. Whether to administer intravenous gamma globulin or to perform a splenectomy in the older child with chronic ITP and mild bleeding symptoms is often a difficult decision. The curtailment of activity and inability to engage in contact sports or other peer group activities may affect decisions. It should be remembered that a significant portion of these patients will eventually have a late spontaneous remission.

A very small proportion of children will not respond to intravenous gamma globulin or to splenectomy and will continue to have significant bleeding episodes and low platelet counts. Immunosuppressive therapy may be effective in this situation.

Splenectomy effectively raises the platelet count to levels that prevent bleeding in most children with chronic ITP. There is no definite test by which one can predict this response. Splenectomy itself appears to be safe in patients with chronic ITP, and excessive bleeding during surgery is quite rare. At the time of splenectomy, the surgeon must look carefully for an accessory spleen, because residual splenic tissue may result in the relapse of ITP after surgery. The platelet count usually starts to rise in the immediate postoperative period, and platelet counts over 1 million are not unusual immediately following splenectomy. Since there have been no reported cases of thrombosis at these very high levels, antiplatelet agents are not indicated. Splenectomy should be avoided if at all possible in the younger child, because the risk of postsplenectomy sepsis is the highest in the youngest children. The risk decreases dramatically with age; by 6 years of age, given proper vaccination and postsplenectomy penicillin prophylaxis, the incidence of sepsis appears to be quite low in patients in whom splenectomy has been performed for chronic ITP or trauma. The increased risk of septicemia is limited to encapsulated organisms, pneumococcus, *Haemophilus influenzae* type b, and meningococcus. Rapidly overwhelming sepsis is almost always caused by pneumococcus, so penicillin prophylaxis is important. The efficacy of penicillin prophylaxis has been clearly demonstrated in functionally splenectomized children with sickle cell disease. Many pediatric hematologists recommend lifelong penicillin prophylaxis because (1) penicillin may prevent subsequent exposure and antibody response to pneumococcal polysaccharides to which the patient had not yet been exposed at the time of splenectomy and (2) fatal, overwhelming pneumococcal sepsis does occur, although rarely, in adults who have had a splenectomy. If at all possible, pneumococcal polysaccharide vaccine and *H. influenzae* type b vaccine should be administered at least 2 weeks before splenectomy. The development of fever in children who have had a splenectomy is an indication for parenteral administration of antibiotics (a third-generation cephalosporin to cover all encapsulated organisms) and hospitalization for observation until blood cultures drawn at admission are found to be negative.

OTHER TYPES OF IMMUNE THROMBOCYTOPENIA

Idiosyncratic drug-induced thrombocytopenia is a common cause of unexpected thrombocytopenia in hospitalized patients. Heparin-induced thrombocytopenia is an indication for immediate discontinuation of heparin. Valproic acid (Depakene), a drug commonly used in pediatric patients with chronic seizure disorders, is commonly associated with thrombocytopenia, which probably results from decreased platelet production. Bacterial and viral infections, particularly varicella, may cause thrombocytopenia. Immune thrombocytopenia is acquired in the neonate by the transplacental passage of antiplatelet autoantibodies or alloantibodies. Thrombocytopenia may also occur in a variety of other complex and rare disorders; the reader is referred to pediatric hematology textbooks for information about these disorders.

SUGGESTED READING

Stuart MJ and Kelton JG: The platelet: quantitative and qualitative abnormalities. In Nathan DG and Oski FA, editors: Hematology of infancy and childhood, Philadelphia, 1987, WB Saunders Co.

218

Infectious Mononucleosis and Epstein-Barr Virus Infections

Ciro V. Sumaya

EPIDEMIOLOGY

Infection with Epstein-Barr virus (EBV), a member of the herpesvirus group, is extremely common but not always clinically apparent. In Africa there is a strong association between infection with EBV and development of Burkitt lymphoma and nasopharyngeal carcinoma; this association, however, has been less clearly demonstrated in Western countries despite the demonstration of serologic evidence of past infection by the great majority of children and adolescents. In the United States, interest in EBV infection centers on the typical clinical syndrome, known as infectious mononucleosis, that it produces and on the relationship emerging with an increasing number of tumors noted, for the most part, in immunocompromised patients.

In childhood, EBV infection usually is clinically inappropriate or manifested by a nonspecific, uncomplicated episode of upper respiratory tract infection or pharyngitis.[7] Although EBV antibodies have developed in 70% to 90% of children from low socioeconomic groups by age 5 years, these antibodies occur in only 40% to 50% of those from high socioeconomic groups.[1] Primary infections that do not occur until adolescence and young adulthood are much more likely, for reasons that are unclear, to manifest as infectious mononucleosis. Thus the incidence of infectious mononucleosis is highest among white high school and college students—approximately 1 in 2500 students.

CLINICAL PRESENTATION

After an incubation period of 2 to 6 weeks (normally 20 to 30 days), signs of classic infectious mononucleosis are seen: fever, sore throat, and lymphadenopathy. This constellation of signs can be preceded by vague symptoms of fatigue, malaise, and anorexia.

Because infectious mononucleosis is the result of a systemic viral infection, virtually every organ system may be involved.[5] Fig. 218-1 demonstrates the variety of clinical manifestations compatible with infectious mononucleosis.

The fever usually is not higher than 103° F (39.5° C), but the sore throat, frequently accompanied by exudate and a palatal enanthem, can be excruciating. Lymphadenopathy, perhaps the most striking feature of the illness, can be limited to the cervical nodes but also can be so extensive as to involve virtually all lymph node groups. Posterior cervical adenopathy is most frequently noted. The lymph nodes are not tender nor do they demonstrate signs of adenitis.

Enlargement of the spleen and possibly the liver, together with posterocervical adenopathy, are the physical signs that usually alert the clinician to the diagnosis of infectious mononucleosis. Some patients with this illness, however, do not have any palpable splenic enlargement; massive enlargement of the spleen should suggest an alternative diagnosis. Liver enzyme levels are elevated in virtually all patients, but the frequency of jaundice is low.

The severity of illness is extremely variable, and some individuals may have relatively few signs of infection, whereas others will demonstrate virtually all the findings listed in Fig. 218-1. In general, the clinical manifestations of the illness last approximately 2 to 3 weeks, with peak involvement during the second week. Eyelid edema has been reported by some observers in about 25% of patients.

DIAGNOSIS AND SEROLOGY

The diagnosis of infectious mononucleosis is made by the presence of a triad of typical clinical hematologic and serologic findings. In addition to the clinical profile described in the preceding section, minimal hematologic features should include a relative lymphocytosis of 50% or more and a relative atypical lymphocyte count of 10% or more of all leukocytes. Other general laboratory findings usually include a decline in the number of granulocytes and platelets.

The heterophil Paul-Bunnell antibody, an IgM antibody produced by humans during infection that reacts with horse, sheep, and beef erythrocytes but not with guinea pig kidney cells, is the cornerstone of laboratory diagnosis. This antibody will be present in up to 50% of children younger than 4 years of age.[8] Among school-aged children and young adults, it is detectable 80% to 90% of the time during the second week of clinical illness.[5,8] Occasionally the heterophil response will be brief and minimal or will occur late in the illness and therefore may show negative results at the time of testing. Commercial diagnostic kits, which rely on differential adsorption to detect the heterophil antibody, are readily available and easy to use in a physician's office. They are 96% to 99% sensitive and give a result in 2 minutes.[4] False-positive results have been reported in cases of rubella, hepatitis, serum sick-

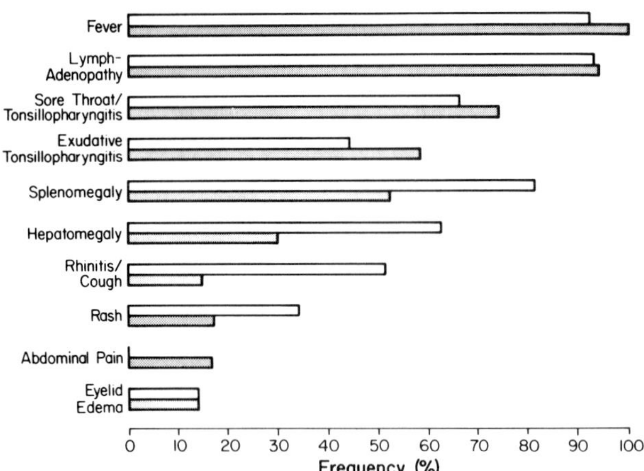

Fig. 218-1 Frequency of clinical findings in two age groups of children with documented EBV infectious mononucleosis: less than 4 years old *(open bars)* and 4 to 16 years old *(dotted bars)*.
From Sumaya CV and Ench Y: Epstein-Barr Virus infectious mononucleosis in children. I. Clinical and general laboratory findings, Pediatrics 75:1005, 1985.

Table 218-1 *Complications Present in 113 Children with EBV Infectious Mononucleosis*

COMPLICATION	NO. OF CHILDREN (%)
Respiratory tract	
Pneumonia	6 (5.3%)
Severe airway obstruction*	4 (3.5%)
Neurologic	
Seizures	4 (3.5%)
Meningitis/encephalitis	2 (1.8%)
Peripheral facial nerve paralysis	1 (0.9%)
Guillain-Barré syndrome	1 (0.9%)
Hematologic	
Thrombocytopenia with hemorrhages	4 (3.5%)
Hemolytic anemia	1 (0.9%)
Infectious	
Bacteremia	1 (0.9%)
Recurrent tonsillopharyngitis	3 (2.7%)
Liver	
Jaundice	2 (1.8%)
Renal	
Glomerulonephritis	1 (0.9%)
Genital	
Orchitis	1 (0.9%)
TOTAL	31†

From Sumaya CV and Ench Y: Epstein-Barr virus infectious mononucleosis in children. I. Clinical and general laboratory findings, Pediatrics 75:1007, 1985.
*Criteria consisted of nasal alar flaring, suprasternal retractions, or stridor.
†Because four children had more than one of these complications, this total is composed of 24 different children or 21.2% of the study group.

ness, drug reactions, and systemic lupus erythematosus and through improper use of the kit or inaccurate interpretation of the agglutination reaction. The magnitude of the heterophil antibody titer does not correlate with clinical severity, and repeat testing, once a positive test result is obtained, provides no additional information beyond that gained from clinical assessment of the patient.

If heterophil test results are negative, confirmation of EBV infection should be sought by other serologic tests. A variety of antibodies directed against various portions of EBV can be detected by numerous hospital, state health, or commercial laboratories. Patients with negative heterophil test results will have antibodies against specific components of the virus if EBV is indeed the cause of the clinical illness. If both test results are negative, other causes for the non-EBV infectious mononucleosis–like illness should be sought.

COMPLICATIONS AND DEATHS

Most persons with infectious mononucleosis will recover uneventfully. Serious complications, however, have resulted from this illness; death occurs in approximately 1 in 3000 cases. The true complication and death rates during this illness are uncertain, because many reports did not include strict diagnostic criteria for infectious mononucleosis.

The relative frequencies of more common complications associated with this illness, as documented in one large study, are listed in Table 218-1.[4] A number of other complications in virtually every body organ also have been reported with this disease.

Of 20 deaths clearly associated with infectious mononucleosis in one series, 9 were of neurologic origin and 3 each were caused by secondary infection or splenic rupture, 2 by hepatic failure, and 1 by probable myocarditis. Because abdominal pain is an infrequent symptom of this illness, its appearance, particularly if severe and in the left upper quadrant, should alert the clinician to the possibility of splenic rupture. Fatal cases of Reye syndrome associated with serologic evidence of EBV infection also have been reported.

MANAGEMENT

Because most patients with infectious mononucleosis recover uneventfully, physicians need do little except establish the diagnosis, explain the nature of the illness, and reassure the family. No specific therapy is indicated. Patients should rest to the extent that they feel necessary. As long as the patient can consume adequate amounts of fluids and calories, hospitalization is unnecessary. To minimize the danger of splenic rupture it seems prudent that ambulatory patients avoid strenuous physical exercise or contact sports until the speen is no longer palpable. Patients with late onset of the heterophil antibody response appear to have a prolonged convalescence.

Corticosteroids are of unproved value in treating this illness.[2] They should not be used routinely merely to make the patient feel better. Most clinicians believe that their use is justified in treating severe hemolytic anemia, significant airway obstruction secondary to tonsillar hypertrophy, and thrombocytopenia. However, controlled studies documenting their efficacy are lacking. Some suggest using them if neurologic involvement is significant, but again, proof of efficacy is not available.

Inasmuch as the pharyngitis of infectious mononucleosis can be indistinguishable from that of true streptococcal pharyngitis, culture specimens of the pharynx should be obtained and those with positive culture findings treated accordingly.

A rash, which can be erythematous, petechial, erythema multiforme–like, urticarial, or scarlatiniform, will develop in approximately 20% of children with this illness. A rash also will develop, however, in 70% to 90% of young adult patients with this illness who are treated with ampicillin. In some cases the ampicillin-related rash will appear after the medication has been discontinued. Although the ampicillin effect has not been well demonstrated in young children with infectious mononucleosis, it is prudent to avoid using this drug under these circumstances.

Infection follows entry of the EBV into the oropharynx, and its recovery from this site can be documented up to 16 months after illness. Transmission from one individual to another occurs most likely through mixing of saliva (thus, its name "kissing disease"). In the absence of such transmission, transfer of infection is unlikely. In a study of families with a childhood index case of infectious mononucleosis, seroconversion occurred in 34.6% of the susceptible siblings over a period of several months after the acute episode.[9] Even though the rate of transmission of the EBV infection was relatively low and slow, however, the development of infectious mononucleosis with the eventual primary EBV infection was quite high (55.6%) in these sibling contacts who showed seroconversion.

Secondary infection in typical college settings is even lower. As such, strict isolation of the patient is unnecessary. Instead, separation of drinking and eating utensils (e.g., avoiding drinking from the same glass) is all that is required.

There are increasing accounts (although still rare) of infectious mononucleosis episodes that are quite severe and fatal or else that result in significant long-lasting problems. Most of these patients had some form of immunologic abnormality—that is, X-linked lymphoproliferative syndrome, renal transplant recipients, and Chédiak-Higashi syndrome, among others. In contrast, the initially suspected etiologic association between EBV, or infectious mononucleosis, and the chronic fatigue syndrome (chronic debilitating illness characterized by extreme fatigue, neuropsychological abnormalities, and a myriad of other problems)[3,6] now appears to be inaccurate. Chronic fatigue syndrome is now thought to be caused by an as yet to be identified retrovirus. The usual EBV serologic findings noted in these chronically fatigued patients is most likely an epiphenomenon related to an immunologic disturbance caused by the retrovirus.

EPSTEIN-BARR VIRUS–NEGATIVE INFECTIOUS MONONUCLEOSIS

Rubella, hepatitis, toxoplasmosis, cytomegalovirus (CMV), and adenovirus infections, systemic lupus erythematosus, and drug reactions can have symptoms similar to those of EBV infection. Negative EBV titers and heterophil antibody responses strongly suggest one of these agents as the cause of the illness under consideration. In hepatitis, in which the heterophil test can give a false-positive result, liver enzyme levels generally are much more elevated than those seen with infectious mononucleosis. Results of serologic tests for hepatitis will be positive, as will rubella titers in rubella infection. CMV can be cultured from urine in those with infection as the cause of their illness. Illnesses that mimic infectious mononucleosis but lack serologic confirmation of EBV infection should be classified as heterophil-negative infectious mononucleosis rather than atypical mononucleosis. Most of these cases are of unknown etiology.

EPSTEIN-BARR VIRUS INFECTION AND MALIGNANCY

Lymphocytes that contain the EBV genome can be subdivided indefinitely. The virus remains dormant in human hosts for indefinite periods of time. These observations, together with the known association of EBV and African Burkitt lymphoma and nasopharyngeal carcinoma, have raised speculation that EBV infection might be oncogenic in the United States as well. Some cases of leukemia occurring shortly after the onset of infectious mononucleosis have been reported. There is no evidence currently available to support this speculation.

Although in the United States the association between EBV and classic Burkitt lymphoma is not strong as in Africa, a number of lymphomas and lymphoproliferative lesions contain EBV markers (including markers of viral replication) in American patients. There also is recent evidence linking EBV with T cell lymphomas and Hodgkin disease. These intriguing findings are the subject of intense investigation.

REFERENCES

1. Andiman WA: The Epstein-Barr virus and EB virus infections in childhood, J Pediatr 95:171, 1979.
2. Collins M et al: Role of steroids in the treatment of infectious mononucleosis in the ambulatory college student, J Am Coll Health Assoc 33:101, 1984.
3. Jones JF et al: Evidence for active Epstein-Barr virus infections in patients with persistent, unexplained illness: elevated anti–early antigen antibodies, Ann Intern Med 102:1, 1985.
4. Karzon DT: Infectious mononucleosis, Adv Pediatr 22:231, 1976.
5. Mandell GL Douglas RG Jr, and Bennett JE: Principles and practice of infectious diseases, vol 2, New York, 1979, John Wiley & Sons, Inc.
6. Straus SE et al: Persisting illness and fatigue in adults with evidence of Epstein-Barr virus infection, Ann Intern Med 102:7, 1985.
7. Sumaya CV and Ench Y: Epstein-Barr virus infectious mononucleosis in children. I. Clinical and general laboratory findings, Pediatrics 75:1003, 1985.
8. Sumaya CV and Ench Y: Epstein-Barr virus infectious mononucleosis in children. II. Heterophil antibody and viral-specific responses, Pediatrics 75:1011, 1985.
9. Sumaya CV and Ench Y: Epstein-Barr virus infections in families: the role of children with infectious mononucleosis, J Infect Dis 154:842, 1986.

219

Insect Bites and Infestations

Nancy K. Barnett

INSECT BITES

Discrete red pruritic papules and nodules should suggest the diagnosis of insect bites. Although mosquito bites are the most common, flies, fleas, gnats, and bedbugs are also potential pests. The lesions may produce discomfort to the unsensitized individual; the sensitized child, however, can develop aggravating, intensely pruritic wheals or even bullae from bites.

On physical examination there are typically a discrete number of scattered erythematous papules and plaques, all in the same stage of development. Some may have central puncta or vesicles; others are capped by a hemorrhagic or serous crust over an excoriation created by scratching. The bites can also be camouflaged by impetiginization or eczematous change. The reactions are usually found on exposed (not covered by clothing) surfaces. In fact, they are often grouped three in a row and referred to as "breakfast, lunch, and dinner bites."

Papular urticaria is a common reaction to insect bites. It consists of recurrent crops of urticarial papules on exposed surfaces and is not caused by bites per se. Papular urticaria occurs seasonally (particularly in warmer months) in certain hypersensitive individuals. Each lesion can last up to 2 weeks, plaguing the child with itch, and can leave an unsightly postinflammatory pigmentary change. We do not know why one family member may be affected and others not; nevertheless, this bit of history may help to rule out scabies or pediculosis (see below).

Insect bites can be controlled by using repellents and by clothing much of the body. Topical antipruritic agents such as calamine and mentholated lotions are sometimes soothing. Topical corticosteroid creams and oral antihistamines can relieve pruritus temporarily. Persons susceptible to mosquito bites should decrease their use of attractants such as bright clothing and aromatic cosmetics.

Flea bites are suggested by vesiculobullous, pruritic erythematous papules and plaques on the distal extremities and in places where clothes bind. These can only be eliminated by treating the source. The pet should be referred to a veterinarian for flea dipping or dusting, and the house should be treated with a veterinary flea "bomb." Bedbugs must be searched for in old bedding, floorboards, and moldings and be appropriately eradicated with insecticides.

INFESTATIONS

Pediculosis

Lice are insects that may infest the scalp as pediculosis capitis, the eyelashes as pediculosis palpebrarum, the body as pediculosis corporis, or the pubic area as pediculosis pubis. They are obligate ectoparasites of humans that create pruritic dermatoses by puncturing the skin and injecting inflammatory saliva. Lice can transmit rare rickettsial and bacterial diseases to humans.

Children with lice infestation sometimes have an itchy scalp, but since lice are spread by close contact and on fomites, the youngsters are more often referred by a concerned school official for evaluation because there is an outbreak of head lice in the classroom. This whitish crawling bug with six legs may be seen in hair, or its eggs (nits) may be found as minute white-gray papules firmly attached to the hair shafts. Family members should be examined especially if they are symptomatic or if combs, towels, and so on are shared. Rarely, pruritic, 1 to 2 mm diameter, erythematous papules will be noted about the nape of the neck and the hairline and occasionally on the body; these usually clear after the head lice are eradicated successfully. These lesions are presumably caused by bites of the head louse.

Nits or the insects themselves may be visible on the eyelashes or pubic hair. The sexually active adolescent usually transmits pubic lice. The affected individual should be screened for other sexually transmitted diseases. Pediculosis palpebrarum is most frequent in the toddler who sleeps with his or her parents, and both parents should be examined for pubic lice.

The body louse is not usually found on the body; rather, it and its nits may be seen in the seams of clothing or in bedding. Pediculosis corporis should be suspected when extreme generalized pruritus is present. The bites consist of erythematous macules and papules. The lesions are often obscured by the results of scratching: excoriation, impetiginization, eczematization, and pigmentation.

The most effective treatment for body lice consists of applying a 1% gamma benzene hexachloride (GBH) lotion or shampoo. The lotion is used for pediculosis corporis or pubis. It should be applied in a light layer over the entire body surface below the neck, left on for 8 to 12 hours, and then washed off. The optimum length of application has not been established, and shorter periods (e.g., 6 hours) may suffice for young children. For head lice GBH shampoo should be worked through wet hair and allowed to remain on for 5 minutes. Then the hair should be shampooed as usual; after rinsing, a fine-toothed comb should be used to remove the nits from the hair shafts. Retreatment may be necessary 1 week after the first application to kill lice that have hatched from viable nits not removed initially.

Nix cream rinse contains permethrin 1% and is probably the most effective agent available for treatment of head lice. A single application is usually sufficient for cure. A vinegar rinse or Step-2 creme rinse (8% formic acid) may be tried to remove stubborn nits.

Pruritus may continue for 1 to 2 weeks after treatments, perhaps because of the continued irritancy of louse antigens or rarely because GBH may cause a primary irritant dermatitis. Patients should be advised that they might continue to itch so that they do not overtreat themselves by repeatedly applying GBH. Antipruritics and topical steroids will help to control severe pruritus.

Pediculosis palpebrarum can be treated by applying petrolatum to the eyelashes twice a day. Treatment is required for about 1 week, and a moustache comb can be used daily to remove lice and nits from the eyelashes.

The controversy over the use of GBH in younger children is largely unfounded and will be addressed below (see "Scabies"). Other effective pediculocides are malathion and pyrethrins. Malathion is available as a 0.5% lotion (Prioderm). It is currently recommended for GBH-resistant lice, which have not been found in the United States. Pyrethrins are found in such over-the-counter preparations as A-200 Pyrinate liquid and Rid.

It is recommended that clothing, bedding, combs, towels, and other items used by lice-infested persons be washed in hot water or boiled to destroy the insects and their eggs.

Scabies

Infestation with *Sarcoptes scabiei hominis* is common. Scabies is a pruritic dermatosis with various manifestations ranging from a few erythematous papules to diffuse scabies-laden crusts (Norwegian scabies). Because of its varied appearance, scabies must be distinguished from insect bites, atopic dermatitis, impetigo, contact dermatitis, urticaria, secondary syphilis, seborrheic dermatitis, pityriasis rosea, and even Letterer-Siwe disease.[1]

Scabies is spread by close personal contact. All family members and sexual partners of index cases should be examined and treated. Frequently, the history will reveal that many people in one household are itching, whereas with papular urticaria, only the patient will be affected. Fomite spread has not been established. However, animal mites can infest humans. Canine scabies is the most common form transferred to humans. It usually lasts but a few weeks because the mite cannot reproduce.

The burrowing of the pregnant female mite into the stratum corneum initiates scabies. She lays ova and defecates in the burrow. Over the next 4 to 6 weeks, pruritus develops gradually as the eggs hatch, increasing the mite population. With reinfestation there is a more rapid onset of pruritus, suggesting a hypersensitivity reaction to mite and excreta antigens.

The burrows created by impregnated female mites are helpful in establishing the diagnosis; however, they are not always obvious and are often disguised by excoriations, eczematous reactions, and impetiginization. They should be looked for in the following locations: digital web spaces, the extensor surface of the elbows, and the flexor aspect of the wrists. Once a burrow is found, mineral oil should be applied to it, and the burrow should be scraped off with a scalpel blade. Ova, mites, or feces can be found by light microscopy in the removed material.

Burrows are not the only scabious lesions. The papules, pustules, vesicles, and hives that can occur in sarcoptic infestation justify the reputation of scabies as being a great masquerader. Therefore, in the face of a gradually worsening pruritus with any of these lesions, the diagnosis of scabies must be considered, particularly if there are close contacts who are also itching. The distribution of lesions can be a clue to the diagnosis. In infants, the face, palms, and soles may be involved with relative sparing of the intertriginous areas, genitalia, buttocks, wrists, and extensor surfaces of joints—areas usually involved in adults.

Treatment. The application of 1% GBH lotion is the treatment of choice for scabies. It should be applied as noted above for lice. Adverse reactions from misuse or agricultural exposure have raised concern about possible neurotoxicity from precutaneous absorption. Nevertheless, when used properly, GBH is a safe and effective scabicide, even in infants.[2] It should *not* be applied following a warm bath because absorption might be enhanced. It should be dispensed in limited quantity, sufficient for but two applications 1 week apart. Parents may be informed about possible neurotoxic complications to deter overtreatment. Animal data[2] suggest that GBH is fetotoxic but not teratogenic. There are no conclusive studies concerning the use of GBH in pregnant women.

Other treatments for scabies do exist. Crotamiton 10% (Eurax) is less efficacious than GBH, however. Precipitated sulfur, 5% or 10% in petrolatum, is a messy and foul-smelling but time-honored therapy. Benzyl benzoate is widely used in developing countries, since it is contained in the inexpensive emulsion recommended by the World Health Organization.[3] However, controlled studies of the toxicity and efficacy of these agents are needed.

Despite the absence of documented fomite spread of scabies, most authorities still recommend that clothing, bed linens, towels, and so on be washed in hot water because epidemiologic studies have demonstrated a higher rate of spread among families in which articles such as these are shared.

Certain postscabietic conditions should be noted. Pruritus can continue for weeks despite adequate treatment; retreatment should be undertaken only when mite manifestation is documented. Certain individuals develop reddish purple, discrete nodules up to 2 cm in diameter on surfaces usually covered by clothing, particularly on the genitalia. These lesions may persist for months. They are, on biopsy, granulomatous histiocytic or lymphocytic infiltrates. This "nodular scabies" is thought to represent a hypersensitivity reaction, since no mites are found. The nodules usually respond to topical applications of steroids or intralesional injections of steroids. Referral to a dermatologist is indicated for treatment of these lesions.

REFERENCES

1. Hurwitz S: Clinical pediatric dermatology, Philadelphia, 1981, WB Saunders Co.
2. Rasmussen JE: The problem of lindane, J Am Acad Dermatol 5:507, 1981.
3. Schacter B: Treatment of scabies and pediculosis with lindane preparations: an evaluation, J Am Acad Dermatol 5:517, 1981.

220

Iron-Deficiency Anemia

James Palis

Iron deficiency is the most common cause of anemia in the world and affects all ages. Iron is needed not only for hemoglobin formation and tissue replacement but also for growth. Iron deficiency, as well as other nutritional deficiencies, is most common in early childhood and during adolescence, when growth rates are maximal. Iron-deficiency anemia is associated with behavioral and cognitive deficits, which may not improve despite adequate iron therapy. This makes the prevention of iron deficiency an important public health issue.

INCIDENCE

Iron deficiency is surprisingly common, even in Western societies where nutrition is generally good and the use of iron-fortified foods widespread. Accurate estimates of iron deficiency are difficult to obtain, because the incidence varies depending on the diagnostic criteria used. Several surveys of infants in various urban areas of the United States reveal a prevalence of between 17% and 44%, the highest being among infants of lower socioeconomic status. Adolescent females are more commonly affected than males, with a prevalence as high as 27%.[7]

IRON-CONTAINING COMPOUNDS IN THE BODY

Iron is the most abundant heavy metal in the body. The multiple iron-containing compounds found within the body can be grouped into two major categories—those serving metabolic functions and those involved with iron storage and transport.

The first category includes heme- and non-heme-containing compounds. Heme is composed of a protoporphyrin ring with noncovalently bound iron in the ferrous form (Fe^{++}). The most abundant heme-containing protein in the body is hemoglobin, which transports oxygen from the lungs to the tissues and accounts for more than 60% of total body iron. Myoglobin, which accounts for 10% of total body iron, is a heme protein that provides oxygen for use during muscle contraction. The other major heme proteins, the cytochromes, are found in the mitochondria and are necessary for the oxidative production of cellular energy. There are also several nonheme iron proteins such as the iron-sulfur complexes and flavoproteins. Many of these proteins are found in the mitochondria and are also involved in oxidative metabolism.

The second category of iron compounds is the iron transport and storage molecules. Transferrin is a β_1-globulin capable of binding two atoms of iron in the ferric form (Fe^{+++}). It transports iron from the serosal surface of intestinal epithelium to the bone marrow for the synthesis of hemoglobin. It also plays a major role in the recycling of iron from senescent red blood cells. In adult males, approximately 95% of the iron needed for red blood cell production is derived from red blood cell breakdown.[1] Ferritin, an iron storage compound found in all cells of the body, is composed of a hollow protein shell encapsulating iron molecules. Hemosiderin, which also serves to store intracellular iron, is thought to be a partially degraded form of ferritin.

ETIOLOGY AND PATHOPHYSIOLOGY

The four most important factors in the development of iron deficiency in children are (1) the iron endowment at birth, (2) the iron needs during rapid body growth, (3) exogenous iron absorption, and (4) blood loss.

During gestation the fetus is able to extract iron efficiently from the mother independently of maternal iron stores.[9] The ratio of iron content to weight in the human fetus remains constant throughout gestation. The healthy full-term infant has sufficient iron stores to last for 6 months, even if little iron is ingested from the diet. The infant's iron endowment can be compromised by blood loss during the pregnancy or the perinatal period. Common causes of blood loss include third trimester bleeding, such as abruptio placentae, placenta previa, fetomaternal hemorrhage, and twin-to-twin transfusions.

Premature infants have a smaller absolute amount of body iron compared with full-term infants because of their lower body weight. Their increased growth requirements after birth coupled with their smaller iron endowment can lead to a rapid depletion of iron stores, resulting in iron-deficiency anemia as early as 3 months of age.[4]

Iron is needed not only for many metabolic functions and tissue replacement but also for growth. Growth rates vary with age and are maximal during infancy and adolescence,[10] the same periods associated with the highest frequency of iron deficiency.

Since there are no mechanisms available for the active excretion of iron from the body, iron balance is maintained by regulation of iron absorption. The amount of iron absorbed depends both on the amount and the bioavailability of dietary iron, as well as on regulation of iron absorption by the intestinal mucosa. Most dietary iron occurs in the nonheme form and is much less bioavailable than that in heme proteins. The iron in hemoglobin and myoglobin is particularly bioavailable; up to 30% is directly absorbed by the gastrointestinal tract.

Breast milk and cow milk contain small amounts of iron (0.5 to 1 mg/1000 ml). However, 50% of the iron in breast milk is absorbed compared with only 10% in cow milk. Full-term infants exclusively breast-fed for the first 6 to 9 months do not become iron deficient.[7] Nonheme iron absorption is inhibited by bran in cereals, polyphenols in many vegetables, and tannins in tea. The addition of solids to an infant's diet can significantly impair iron absorption and puts the infant at risk for developing iron deficiency. The introduced solids therefore should contain abundant amounts of iron (e.g., iron-fortified cereals).

Blood loss causes iron deficiency in children less frequently than in adults. In infancy and childhood iron deficiency caused by blood loss is most commonly associated with the ingestion of unprocessed cow milk and with parasitic infections. Hypersensitivity to whole cow milk causes an exudative enteropathy and frequently leads to gastrointestinal blood loss. Other less common causes of blood loss in children include Meckel diverticulum, intestinal duplication, peptic ulcer disease, hemorrhagic telangiectasia, and the chronic use of medications that prolong the bleeding time (e.g., aspirin).

CLINICAL MANIFESTATIONS

The onset and progression of iron deficiency is usually gradual, and most children will not have major symptoms. Iron deficiency in infants and children is associated with generalized weakness, irritability, easy fatigability, headaches, poor feeding, anorexia, pica, and poor weight gain.[7] The physical examination is usually unremarkable except for marked pallor of the mucous membranes and skin. Other less common physical findings associated with iron-deficiency anemia include mild hepatosplenomegaly, lymphadenopathy, glossitis, stomatitis, and koilonychia (spoon-shaped nails).

Many studies have demonstrated an association between iron-deficiency anemia and lower scores on tests of mental and motor development, impaired learning, and decreased school achievement.[3,6] These findings may be related to the decreased attention span and increased irritability seen in iron-deficient children compared with nonanemic controls. To what degree iron deficiency is responsible for these clinical findings is controversial, since iron repletion may not completely correct the behavioral disturbances or the lower developmental, IQ, and achievement scores.[3] More studies are needed to address and clarify these issues.

STAGES OF IRON DEFICIENCY

Iron deficiency occurs when total body iron content is diminished. Iron is normally absorbed only through the gastrointestinal tract. Sites of iron loss include the skin, the gastrointestinal tract, and the urine. Iron losses also occur during pregnancy and lactation. When absorption exceeds losses, the iron surplus is stored in the reticuloendothelial system, principally the liver, spleen, and bone marrow. As body iron stores increase, the gastrointestinal absorption of iron decreases so that iron balance is maintained.

Iron is removed from the reticuloendothelial storage pool to compensate for negative iron balance. The development of iron deficiency proceeds through a series of overlapping stages. The first stage of iron deficiency is *storage iron depletion*. During this stage, there is no deficit of iron supplied to the erythroid marrow for red cell production. If the negative iron balance continues, then the second stage, *iron-deficient erythropoiesis,* will occur. During this stage, erythroid iron supply is diminished but the hemoglobin concentration remains in the normal range. If the negative iron balance persists, then *iron-deficiency anemia* finally develops. This third stage is characterized by a fall in the hemoglobin concentration and a reduction in red blood cell size and hemoglobin content.

DIAGNOSIS

Specific laboratory findings are associated with each of the three stages of iron deficiency. The hematologic abnormalities and diagnostic tests characteristic of each stage are reviewed in greater depth below and are summarized in Tables 220-1 and 220-2.

Storage Iron Depletion

During this first stage of iron deficiency, the storage pool of iron in the reticuloendothelial system decreases. This can be detected by a fall in serum ferritin levels or by the absence of stainable iron on a bone marrow sample. No red blood cell changes are present at this time, because there is sufficient iron to support normal erythropoiesis.

Serum Ferritin. As seen in Fig. 220-1, serum ferritin levels vary with age during infancy and childhood. In healthy individuals, serum ferritin levels reflect body iron stores; levels below 12 μg/L indicate iron deficiency. Ferritin is an acute phase reactant. Serum ferritin levels are elevated during infections and inflammatory processes as well as in liver disease. Although low serum ferritin is diagnostic of iron deficiency, an elevated ferritin level associated with inflammation or liver disease does not rule out concomitant iron deficiency.

Bone Marrow Iron. The staining of a normal bone marrow aspirate sample with Prussian blue dye reveals the presence of iron in red blood cell precursors (normoblasts) and serves as a reliable index of body iron stores. In iron deficiency there is a decrease in the number of iron granules in normoblasts and an almost complete absence of stainable iron in the marrow aspirate.[2]

Iron-Deficient Erythropoiesis

Iron-deficient erythropoiesis characterizes the second stage of iron deficiency. The serum iron concentration decreases, and serum transferrin levels rise concomitantly. This leads to an increase in the total iron-binding capacity (TIBC), with a decrease in the percent saturation (Iron/TIBC $\times$ 100). Since iron is unavailable for incorporation in the protoporphyrin ring, free erythrocyte protoporphyrin (FEP) in both red blood cells and the plasma increases during this stage of iron deficiency. The plasma loses its usual amber color and becomes

Table 220-1 *Iron Status and Hematologic Abnormalities in the Three Stages of Iron Deficiency*

	STORAGE IRON DEPLETION	IRON-DEFICIENT ERYTHROPOIESIS	IRON-DEFICIENCY ANEMIA
Storage iron	↓	↓↓	↓↓↓
Erythron iron	Normal	↓	↓↓-↓↓↓
Hemoglobin concentration	Normal	Normal	↓-↓↓↓

Modified from Cecalupo AJ and Cohen HJ: Nutritional anemias. In Grand RJ, Sutphen JL, and Dietz WH, editors: Clinical nutrition: theory and practice, Boston, 1987, Butterworth Publishers.
↓, Decreased.

Table 220-2 *Laboratory Abnormalities in the Three Stages of Iron Deficiency*

	STORAGE IRON DEPLETION	IRON-DEFICIENT ERYTHROPOIESIS	IRON-DEFICIENCY ANEMIA
Bone marrow iron	Absent	Absent	Absent
Ferritin	↓	↓↓	↓↓↓
Serum iron	Normal	↓-↓↓	↓↓↓
Total iron-binding capacity	Normal	↑	↑↑-↑↑↑
Percent saturation	Normal	↓	↓↓-↓↓↓
Free erythrocyte protoporphyrin	Normal	↑	↑↑-↑↑↑
Red blood cell indices	Normal	Normal	↓-↓↓↓

Modified from Cecalupo AJ and Cohen HJ: Nutritional anemias. In Grand RJ, Sutphen JL, and Dietz WH, editors: Clinical nutrition: theory and practice, Boston, 1987, Butterworth Publishers.
↑, Increased, ↓, decreased.

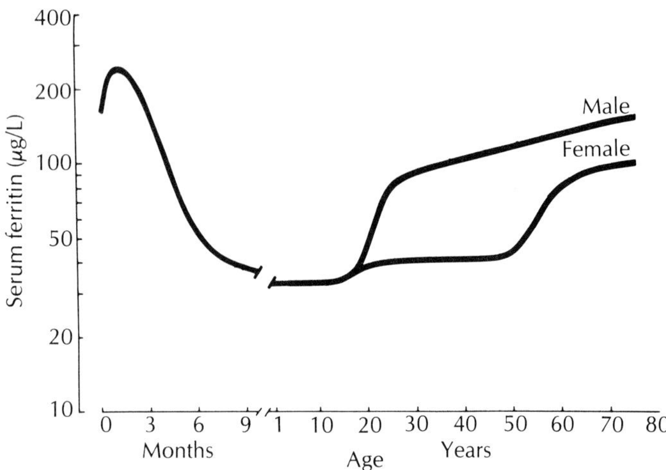

Fig. 220-1 Developmental changes in concentration of serum ferritin.

From Dallman PR, Simes MA, and Stekel A: Iron deficiency in infancy and childhood, Am J Clin Nutrition 33:107, 1980, © Am J Clin Nutr, American Society for Clinical Nutrition.

clear, making inspection of the plasma on a spun hematocrit useful diagnostically.

Iron/TIBC. Serum iron levels normally fluctuate daily, with maximum levels occurring in the morning and minimal levels occurring in the evening. The TIBC varies less than serum iron but is harder to measure accurately.[1] The normal TIBC is 250 to 400 mg/dl, but as serum iron levels decrease, the TIBC increases to 450 mg/dl or more. Iron and TIBC

Table 220-3 *Means and Standard Errors of Measurement of Serum Iron and Iron Saturation Percentage by Age*

AGE (YEARS)	SERUM IRON (μg/dl)	SATURATION (%)
½-2	68 ± 3.6	22 ± 1.1
2-6	72 ± 3.4	25 ± 1.2
6-12	73 ± 3.4	25 ± 1.2
18+	92 ± 3.8	30 ± 1.1

Modified from Koerper MA and Dallman PR: Serum iron concentration (SI) and transferrin saturation (SAT) are lower in normal children than in dults (abstracts), Pediatr Res 11:473, 1977.

measurements are useful in distinguishing iron-deficiency anemia from the anemia of chronic disease. Serum iron levels decrease with both, but the TIBC levels also decrease in chronic disease states.

A useful measure of iron deficiency is the percent saturation—the serum iron divided by the TIBC and multiplied by 100. The normal ranges for serum iron and the percent saturation are shown in Table 220-3. In iron deficiency, the percent saturation is reduced to less than 16%, at which point hemoglobin production becomes limited by the lack of iron. The percent saturation is a more sensitive index of iron status than are serum iron measurements alone. Because of the wide variation in serum iron and iron-binding capacity values, these should be tested in conjunction with at least one other test of iron status (e.g., ferritin, FEP) for reaching a reliable diagnosis of iron deficiency.

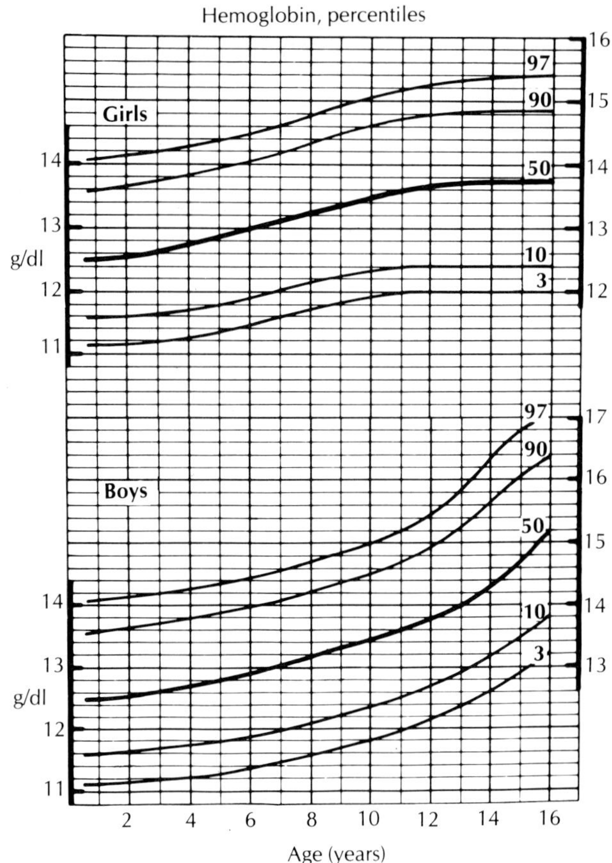

Fig. 220-2 Hemoglobin concentration in infants and children.

Modified from Dallman PR and Simes MA: Percentile curves for hemoglobin and red cell volume in infancy and childhood, J Pediatr 94:28, 1979.

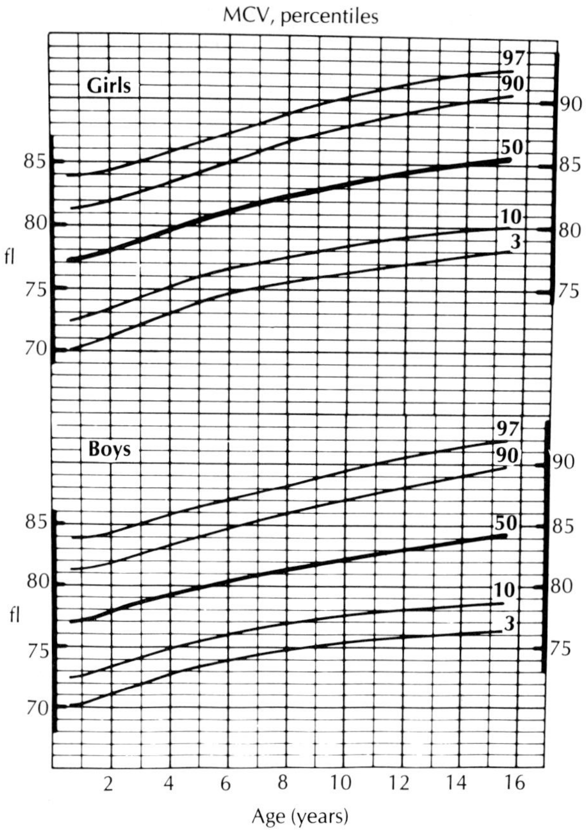

Fig. 220-3 Mean corpuscular volume *(MCV)* in infants and children.

Modified from Dallman PR and Simes MA: Percentile curves for hemoglobin and red cell volume in infancy and childhood, J Pediatr 94:28, 1979.

Free Erythrocyte Protoporphyrin. FEP accumulates in red blood cells when there is insufficient iron to combine with protoporphyrin to form heme. FEP levels are also elevated in lead poisoning, infections, inflammatory diseases, and protoporphyria, but not in thalassemia trait. This makes FEP determinations helpful in distinguishing iron deficiency from α or β thalassemia trait.

IRON-DEFICIENCY ANEMIA

Anemia characterizes the third stage of iron deficiency. Decreased production of red blood cells in the bone marrow leads to a decrease in hemoglobin levels and the hematocrit. The size of the red blood cells, as measured by the mean corpuscular volume (MCV), and their hemoglobin content, as measured by the mean corpuscular hemoglobin (MCH), begin to decrease as the anemia develops. Thus persistent negative iron balance predictably leads to a microcytic, hypochromic anemia.

Hemoglobin. Percentile curves for hemoglobin values of nonindigent children living at sea level are shown in Fig. 220-2. Black children normally have a hemoglobin concentration 0.3 to 1 g/dl lower than that of white children. This difference is not completely explained by differences in socioeconomic status or prevalence of iron deficiency.[1] Anemia, by laboratory definition, is a hemoglobin value below the 95th percentile for age and sex.

Unfortunately, capillary blood hemoglobin determinations vary greatly because of dilution by tissue fluids.[8] Venous blood samples produce more accurate hemoglobin measurements but are more difficult to obtain in infants. These factors limit the usefulness of hemoglobin and hematocrit determinations for the screening of anemia.

RBC Indices. The development of electronic counters has made the use of red blood cell indices widely available for the initial screening of infants and children for iron deficiency. These tests are highly reproducible and less subject to sampling error compared with hemoglobin determinations, since tissue fluid dilution does not affect red blood cell size. Because both the MCV and the MCH normally change during development, it is necessary to consult age-specific reference standards (Fig. 220-3).

Iron deficiency is the most likely diagnosis of anemia characterized by microcytosis and hypochromia. Other causes of anemia with these characteristics include α and β thalassemia trait, hemoglobin E disease, and sometimes the anemia of infection and chronic disease. Most other anemias, however, are characterized by a normal or an elevated MCV.

The Mentzer index, defined as the MCV divided by the RBC count in millions, can help distinguish the anemia of iron deficiency from that of β thalassemia trait.[5] In the former, the Mentzer index is often greater than 13.5; in the latter, it is less than 11.5.

Peripheral Blood Smear. Examination of the blood smear in iron-deficiency anemia reveals hypochromic microcytes, poikilocytes, elliptocytes, and target cells (Fig. 220-4). The presence of basophilic stippling suggests associated lead poisoning. Unfortunately, the red blood cell changes seen on the blood smear are not specific for iron deficiency.

The white blood cell count and morphology in iron-deficiency anemia are usually normal. Both thrombocytosis and thrombocytopenia occur with iron deficiency. The latter is more common in severe iron deficiency and resolves once iron therapy is instituted.

TREATMENT

Therapeutic Trial of Iron

To confirm the diagnosis of iron deficiency, either additional laboratory tests (ferritin, FEP, Fe/TIBC) or a therapeutic trial of iron can be initiated. Since dietary iron deficiency is by far the most common cause of anemia in an otherwise healthy infant, a 1-month therapeutic trial of iron is usually justified. The treatment of choice is the oral administration of ferrous sulfate. Although other iron salts are available, ferrous sulfate is inexpensive and well tolerated. The dose of oral therapy is 3 to 6 mg/kg/day of elemental iron in three divided doses. About twice as much iron is absorbed on an empty stomach as at mealtime. A response to oral iron therapy has been noted within 12 to 24 hours with decreased irritability and increased appetite. The reticulocyte response peaks at 5 to 10 days after the institution of iron therapy. In an otherwise healthy individual, the recovery from anemia is about two thirds complete within 1 month. It is recommended that the hemoglobin measurement be repeated at 1 month to check the therapeutic progress as well as to emphasize compliance.

Once the diagnosis of iron deficiency is confirmed, either by a response to a therapeutic trial or further laboratory tests, oral therapy at 3 to 6 mg/kg/day should be continued for 2 to 3 months after normal hemoglobin levels have been restored. This allows the repletion of body iron stores. Anemia, microcytosis, and elevated FEP levels are completely corrected with 3 months of treatment.

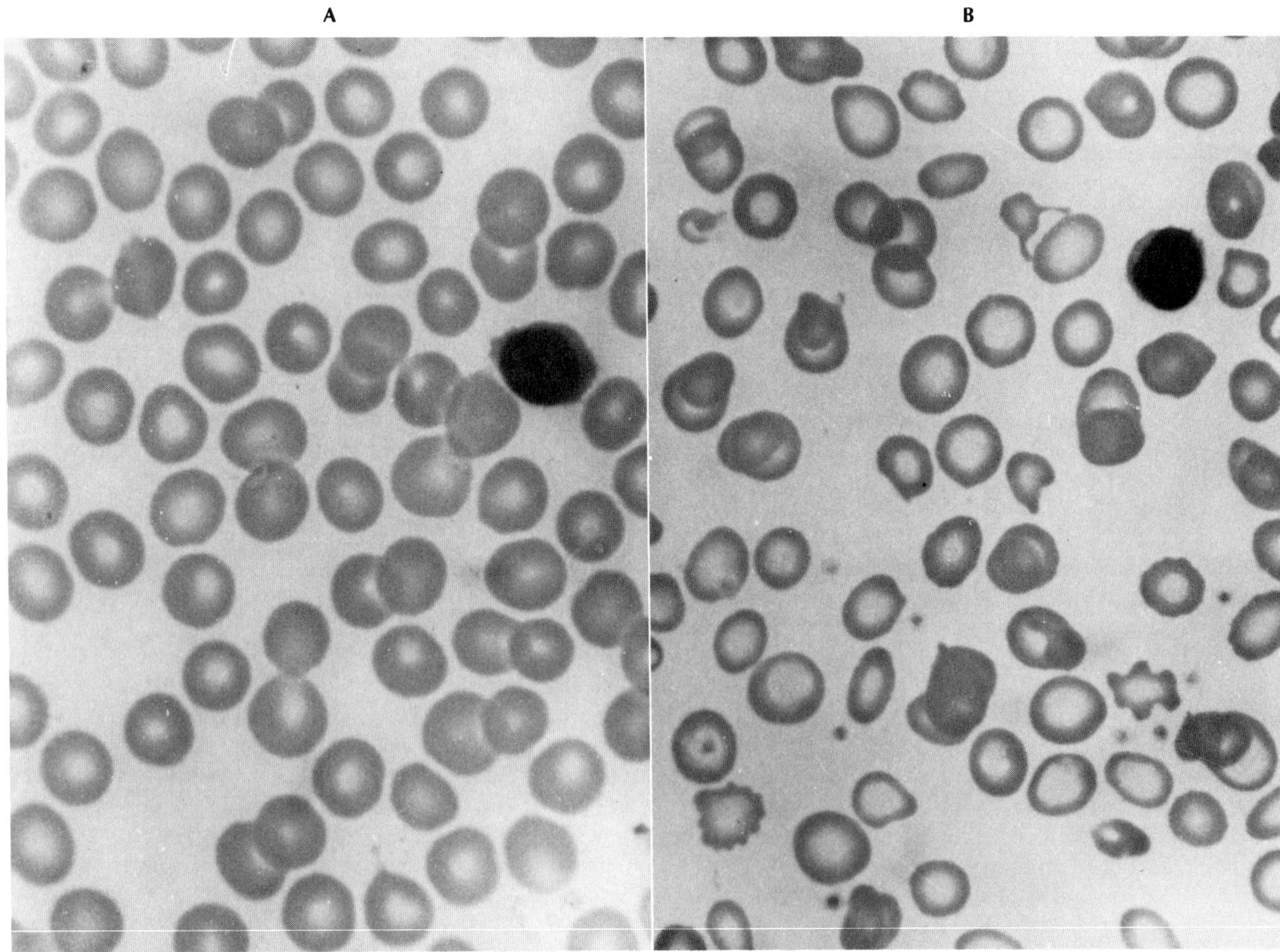

Fig. 220-4 A, A normal peripheral blood smear. The size of normocytic red blood cells is similar to the nucleus of a mature lymphocyte. **B**, The peripheral blood smear from an individual with iron deficiency anemia reveals microcytosis, hypochromia, and poikilocytosis.

Use of intramuscular or intravenous iron is rarely warranted. Intramuscular injections are painful, and skin discoloration is common. Anaphylactic reactions have occurred with both intramuscular and intravenous injection, and deaths have been reported. Parenteral treatment should therefore be used only when oral therapy is not possible—for example, in patients with inflammatory bowel disease.

A blood transfusion is indicated only when severe anemia leads to congestive heart failure and cardiovascular compromise. If a blood transfusion is clinically warranted, then packed red blood cells should be given slowly or a partial exchange transfusion performed. Vital signs should be monitored carefully.

Failure to Respond to Therapy

When a patient fails to respond to oral iron treatment, the following factors should be considered: (1) noncompliance with oral therapy, (2) inadequate iron dose, (3) persistent or unrecognized blood loss, (4) malabsorption of iron—for example, primary gastrointestinal disease, (5) other diagnoses—for example, α or β thalassemia trait and hemoglobin E disease, and (6) poor iron utilization—for example, chronic inflammation, sideroblastic anemia, lead poisoning, and congenital atransferrinemia.

PREVENTION

Although other important nutritional deficiencies of the past, such as pellagra, scurvy, and ricketts, have become rare, iron deficiency remains a current public health problem. Iron-deficiency anemia is associated with behavioral and cognitive deficits, some of which may not improve despite adequate iron therapy. Thus prevention of iron deficiency becomes an important aspect of treatment.

Excessive intake of cow milk during infancy leads to iron deficiency because of the low concentration and poor bioavailability of iron in cow milk. Breast-feeding or the use of milk-based infant formulas supplemented with iron should be encouraged during the first 6 months. The intake of milk thereafter should be limited to less than 1 quart per day. Because the addition of solids to an infant's diet can significantly impair iron absorption, solids should not be started before 4 months of age. The use of iron-fortified cereals should be encouraged once solids are started. Oral iron supplementation is recommended for preterm infants, since they have greater iron needs than full-term infants. In this instance, 2 to 4 mg/kg/day of elemental iron in the form of ferrous sulfate drops should be started at 2 months of age.

REFERENCES

1. Dallman PR: Iron deficiency and related nutritional anemias. In Nathan DG and Oski FA, editors: Hematology of infancy and childhood, ed 3, Philadelphia, 1987, WB Saunders Co.
2. Krause JR: The bone marrow in nutritional deficiencies, Hematol Oncol Clin North Am 2:557, 1988.
3. Lozoff B: Behavioral alterations in iron deficiency, Adv Pediatr 35:331, 1988.
4. Lundstrom U, Siimes MA, and Dallman PR: At what age does iron supplementation become necessary in low birth weight infants? J Pediatr 91:878, 1977.
5. Mentzer WG: Differentiation of iron deficiency from thalassemia trait, Lancet 1:882, 1973.
6. Oski FA: The non-hematologic manifestations of iron deficiency, Am J Dis Child 133:315, 1979.
7. Oski FA and Stockman JA: Anemia due to inadequate iron sources or poor iron utilization, Pediatr Clin North Am 27:237, 1980.
8. Reeves JD: Iron deficiency anemia: cost effective screening and management, Cont Pediatr 1:10, 1984.
9. Rio SE et al: Relationship of maternal and infant iron stores as assessed by determination of plasma ferritin, Pediatrics 55:694, 1975.
10. Tanner JM, Whitehouse RH, and Takaishi M: Standards from birth to maturity for height velocity and weight velocity: British children, Arch Dis Child 41:454, 1966.

221

Juvenile Arthritis

Harry L. Gewanter

Juvenile arthritis (JA or juvenile rheumatoid arthritis) is an uncommon collection of clinical syndromes with the common feature of chronic childhood arthritis. The diagnosis is applied to any child under 16 years of age with persistent arthritis of one or more joints lasting for more than 6 weeks in whom all other diseases have been excluded. JA is further classified into three subtypes (systemic-onset, pauciarticular, and polyarticular), based on the clinical course over the first 6 months of illness.[7]

Many American rheumatologists apply the term *juvenile rheumatoid arthritis* only to those children seropositive for rheumatoid factor. Recent data suggest that many subtypes of pauciarticular and polyarticular JA exist, and it will be a number of years before a universally accepted classification is devised.

Although JA is the most common of the pediatric rheumatic diseases, its true incidence and prevalence are unknown. The peak age of onset is between 2 and 4 years of age, with a smaller peak later in childhood. There is a general female predominance. The best estimate of prevalence is about 0.5 cases per 1000 children; thus approximately 40,000 to 50,000 children in the United States have JA at any given time.[10]

ETIOLOGY

The exact cause of JA is unknown. Recent data on the frequency of certain subtypes of human leukocyte antigens (HLA) in JA (e.g., HLA-DR5 in younger girls with pauciarticular JA, HLA-DR4 in rheumatoid factor–positive polyarticular JA, and HLA-B27 in older boys with pauciarticular JA)[19] have led to the concept of a genetic predisposition for the development of an inflammatory arthritis that may be triggered by any of a number of events, such as trauma, infection,[23] or emotional stress.[15]

Other areas of interesting research include investigations of immunologic abnormalities involving autoantibodies, cytokines, immunoregulation,[4] and the function of and communication between T and B lymphocytes and mononuclear cells. The nature of these interactions and how they result in the development of JA, however, remain to be discovered.

CLINICAL PRESENTATION

Since the diagnosis of JA is based on clinical grounds, the history and physical examination are paramount; no specific diagnostic laboratory tests yet exist. Only by considering all the data on the child's presentation and course is the physician able to diagnose JA.

The presence of arthritis or inflammation within the joint is an absolute criterion for making the diagnosis of JA. Arthritis is defined as being present when there is intraarticular swelling or effusion or when two or more of the following occur: (1) joint pain or tenderness with motion, (2) limitation of joint motion, or (3) increased warmth overlying the joint.[7] Children frequently have arthralgias (pain or tenderness with joint motion), but arthritis is much less common. Other features that may be present in children with JA include fever, rash, lymphadenopathy, hepatosplenomegaly, polyserositis, rheumatoid nodules, vasculitis, and growth retardation. Younger children rarely complain of joint pain but may instead become irritable, stop walking or using an extremity, or regress in their behavior. Other symptoms include decreased appetite, malaise, inactivity, morning stiffness, night joint pains, or failure to thrive.

Any joint of the body may be involved. The pattern and number of involved joints are important in diagnosing the various subtypes of JA.

SYSTEMIC-ONSET JUVENILE ARTHRITIS

Even though the hallmark of systemic-onset JA is its extraarticular manifestations, the presence of arthritis is necessary to confirm the diagnosis. Affecting about 15% of all children with JA, systemic-onset JA is slightly more common in males and usually begins at an early age, although it has even been recognized in adults. The systemic features may persist for months and occur or recur independently of the arthritis.

Daily intermittent fevers are frequent components of systemic-onset JA. Rectal temperature recordings may reach 40° to 40.6° C, most often in the afternoon, and then return to normal or subnormal levels. An evanescent, salmon-colored rash often accompanies the fevers. The lesions are small macules or papules, frequently with central clearing, and often appear in areas of increased heat (e.g., the axilla); they can, however, be induced with mild local trauma (Koebner phenomenon).

Enlargement of the lymph nodes, liver, and spleen is frequent and may be of sufficient size to suggest the presence of a malignancy. Polyserositis in the form of pericarditis or pleuritis is also common. The effusions, however, are rarely symptomatic or clinically significant. Although these children frequently complain of myalgias or arthralgias when they are febrile, they may have few symptoms when the fevers resolve. The arthritis may occur at any time, is more often polyarticular involving both large and small joints, and can be quite severe.

The white blood cell count (WBC) can be quite high, with a shift to the left. Most patients are quite anemic. Thrombocytosis is frequent, as are the acute phase reactants (e.g., erythrocyte sedimentation rate [ESR] and C-reactive protein [CRP]). Rheumatoid factor (RF) and antinuclear antibody (ANA) tests are usually negative. Serum immunoglobulin and complement levels are usually normal but may reflect the degree of inflammation. Evidence of a vasculopathy and an intravascular consumption coagulopathy is sometimes found.[27]

The clinical course is extremely variable. Some children have a single systemic episode that lasts weeks to months and have few, if any, joint problems; others have multiple systemic episodes before developing the arthritis, which can be pauciarticular or polyarticular. About 25% to 34% of these children will develop severe and crippling arthritis.

POLYARTICULAR JUVENILE ARTHRITIS

About 30% to 35% of children with JA have the polyarticular type, which can be subdivided into IgM rheumatoid factor (RF)-positive (about 10% of the total) and IgM-RF–negative (about 25%) forms. So-called hidden rheumatoid factors have been found in all subgroups, but their significance remains obscure.[21] It is extremely rare to find a significantly positive RF in a child under 7 years of age, and it may not be worth ordering this test in younger children. Systemic features are usually mild and include low-grade fevers, easy fatigability, and slowing of growth. The growth problems may be local (e.g., micrognathia) or generalized and can occur regardless of whether the child receives corticosteroids. Discrepancies between height and weight are seen and can be significant. For example, children with polyarticular arthritis may have low weight for height, whereas children with systemic onset tend to be average in weight for height.[3] The arthritis is most often chronic and symmetric and involves five or more joints; any joint of the body, including the temporomandibular joint and the cervical spine, can be affected. Nearly all children have wrist involvement, and small joint involvement of the hands and feet is common. Finally, there is a small chance that these children may develop a chronic uveitis.

Rheumatoid Factor–Positive Polyarticular Juvenile Arthritis

Patients with RF-positive polyarticular JA are most often older than 8 to 10 years of age, are more likely to be girls, and are clinically similar to those patients with adult rheumatoid arthritis. Severe, rapidly progressive, erosive, crippling arthritis, subcutaneous rheumatoid nodules, and rheumatoid vasculitis can develop, just as in adults.

RHEUMATOID FACTOR–NEGATIVE POLYARTICULAR JUVENILE ARTHRITIS

Children with RF-negative polyarticular JA are usually younger and overall have a better prognosis than those who are RF-positive. However, even though children with the RF-negative type typically respond better to therapy and have a lower frequency of severe crippling arthritis than children with the RF-positive form, they may also develop many significant problems. Because their arthritis starts earlier, it can lead to significant deformities and problems as a result of the tendency to develop flexion contractures at the involved joints. Compared with adults, hand involvement more often affects the interphalangeal joints than the metacarpophalangeal joints. Ulnar deviation of the fingers is much less common in children compared with adults, whereas flexion contractures, boutonnière (buttonhole) deformities, and radial deviation of the fingers are more frequently seen. Ulnar deviation and subluxation at the wrist may occur. Arthritis of the apophyseal joints of the cervical spine is common and can lead to rapid and significant limitation of extension and rotation. These children are at the highest risk to develop the local and generalized growth problems mentioned above.

PAUCIARTICULAR JUVENILE ARTHRITIS

Pauciarticular JA involves four or fewer joints, most often the large joints, in an asymmetric distribution. The pattern and course of joint involvement are as important in distinguishing this form of JA from the others as the number of joints involved. With a few exceptions, systemic features are infrequent and mild. Nearly 50% of children with JA fall in this subgroup, and they have the best prognosis.

At least two, more likely four and possibly more, subtypes of pauciarticular JA exist.

Early-Onset Pauciarticular Juvenile Arthritis

Early-onset pauciarticular JA (5% to 10% of all patients with JA) occurs classically in girls under 6 years of age and involves the large joints (knees, ankles, elbows); these girls are at higher risk for developing chronic uveitis.[25] Despite the obvious arthritis, these children generally function quite well and only rarely complain of pain. Little erosive joint damage typically occurs, even though many of these children have ongoing arthritis for many years. Nonetheless, these children are at risk for long-term problems, including leg-length discrepancies and muscle atrophy.[30] Systemic signs and symptoms, except for uveitis, are few. The uveitis is rarely symptomatic until it has progressed to a severe stage and may not occur until years after the onset of the arthritis. It may even occur after the arthritis has resolved. Thus regular ophthalmologic examinations, including slitlamp examinations, should be instituted early, performed every 4 to 6 months, and continued indefinitely. Because the risk of uveitis decreases with time, the interval between examinations can be lengthened after a number of years if no uveitis is present.

Few laboratory abnormalities are noted. Although there may be mild WBC and ESR elevations or a low-grade anemia, these tests may all be normal. Most of these children are ANA positive and many are positive for HLA-DR5 gene markers.[19]

Late-Onset Pauciarticular Juvenile Arthritis

Late-onset pauciarticular JA typically involves boys over 8 years of age. Their arthritis is more frequently in the lower extremities involving the knees and ankles but also occasionally the toes (resulting in a "sausage toe"). Complaints and findings of enthesopathies (i.e., inflammation of the attachment of a tendon, ligament, fascia, or capsule to bone) are extremely common in this group and may antedate the joint problem. There is often a family history of arthritis, and many of these children carry the HLA-B27 antigen. These children also seem to be at increased risk for developing spondyloarthropathies later in life, despite there being no evidence of sacroiliac disease initially. Some patients will progress to fulfill the criteria for ankylosing spondylitis, and some will develop Reiter syndrome. About 10% will develop an acute iritis; in contrast to the chronic uveitis seen in early-onset pauciarticular JA, this is symptomatic, can be treated early, and is usually self-limited. As with the early-onset group, abnormal laboratory tests are found infrequently.

Other Subtypes of Pauciarticular Juvenile Arthritis

At least two other subtypes of pauciarticular JA might exist. The first lies somewhere between the early-onset and the late-onset subtypes. These children seem to have the best prognosis, are ANA negative, and are at a lower risk for eye or other serious, chronic problems. About 10% to 15% of all children with JA make up this last subtype. They have a pauciarticular onset but evolve into a polyarticular course. These children more often start with three or four joints involved and/or have wrist or small finger joint arthritis.

DIFFERENTIAL DIAGNOSIS

Diseases to be considered in the differential diagnosis of JA are given in the accompanying box. The hallmark of JA is its chronicity; frequently, the best diagnostic test is "watchful waiting." Only by meeting the criterion of sustained arthritis for more than 6 weeks and excluding other possible diseases can the physician accurately avoid mislabeling other transient entities as JA.

It is very important to rule out any infectious cause, especially bacterial arthritis. If this is a consideration, arthrocentesis must be performed to establish the diagnosis. *Haemophilus influenzae* type b is the most common organism isolated in children under 2 years of age, *Neisseria gonorrhoeae* is most common in adolescents, whereas various strains of staphylococci may be found at any age. Other infectious agents such as fungi, viruses (including parvovirus, rubella, and hepatitis B), and *Mycoplasma* organisms must also be considered as the cause of arthritis. Lyme disease is a significant cause of childhood arthritis in endemic areas. Osteomyelitis, involving a bone contiguous to a joint, and reactive arthritis from a gastrointestinal (GI) bacterial infection (e.g., *Shigella, Salmonella, Campylobacter,* or *Yersinia* organisms) may also mimic some subgroups of JA. Neoplasms involving the bone, either primary or metastatic (e.g., leukemia, lymphoma, neuroblastoma) can be accompanied

Differential Diagnosis of Juvenile Arthritis

RHEUMATIC DISEASE OF CHILDHOOD
Acute rheumatic fever
Systemic lupus erythematosus
Juvenile ankylosing spondylitis
Polymyositis and dermatomyositis
Vasculitis
Scleroderma
Psoriatic arthritis
Mixed connective tissue disease and overlap syndromes
Kawasaki disease
Behçet syndrome
Familial Mediterranean fever
Reiter syndrome
Reflex sympathetic dystrophy
Fibromyalgia (fibrositis)

INFECTIOUS DISEASES
Bacterial arthritis
Viral or postviral arthritis
Fungal arthritis
Osteomyelitis
Reactive arthritis

NEOPLASTIC DISEASES
Leukemia
Lymphoma
Neuroblastoma
Primary bone tumors

NONINFLAMMATORY DISORDERS
Trauma
Avascular necrosis syndromes
Osteochondroses
Slipped capital femoral epiphysis
Discitis
Patellofemoral dysfunction (chondromalacia patellae)
Toxic synovitis of the hip
Overuse syndromes

GENETIC OR CONGENITAL SYNDROMES

HEMATOLOGIC DISORDERS
Sickle cell disease
Hemophilia

INFLAMMATORY BOWEL DISEASE

MISCELLANEOUS
Growing pains
Psychogenic arthralgias (conversion reactions)
Hypermobility syndrome
Villonodular synovitis
Foreign body arthritis

by musculoskeletal complaints. Arthritis is uncommon and usually transient, but complaints of pain out of proportion to physical findings and complaints of night pain are common and potentially important clues.

The various osteochondroses and avascular necrosis syndromes, musculoskeletal trauma, chondromalacia patellae, Osgood-Schlatter disease, slipped femoral capital epiphysis, discitis, psychogenic arthralgias, and nonspecific musculoskeletal aches and pains can also mimic JA in its early stages.

Hemophilia, sickle cell disease, inflammatory bowel disease, the collagen disorders (e.g., Ehlers-Danlos syndrome, Marfan syndrome), familial Mediterranean fever, and sarcoidosis may also be associated with arthritis.

Juvenile ankylosing spondylitis and Reiter syndrome can be especially difficult to differentiate from JA at their onset, especially in the older child who is HLA-B27 positive. Acute rheumatic fever, although in decline for many years, is now undergoing a resurgence in many areas.[29] Systemic lupus erythematosus has arthritis as one of its major manifestations but can be differentiated from juvenile arthritis by its other systemic features. Although its sex distribution is equal in younger children, there is female preponderance postpubertally. Dermatomyositis is more typically characterized by inflammatory muscle involvement than arthritis. Scleroderma occasionally is associated with arthritis but has classic dermatologic manifestations.

Children with various immunodeficiencies can have arthritis, either from their primary problem or secondary to infections. Serum sickness and the various vasculitides, including Kawasaki disease and Henoch-Schönlein purpura, can produce intermittent arthritis. These illnesses are diagnosed by their individual distinguishing features. Finally, a number of conditions may produce significant arthralgias and myalgias and may mimic an arthropathy. The complaints and disability resulting from the hypermobility syndrome[6] and fibromyalgia (fibrositis)[31] can be sufficient to make one believe that an arthritis is present. A reflex sympathetic dystrophy deserves diagnostic consideration in children with a hot, painful extremity that they refuse to move.[5]

MANAGEMENT

It is always necessary to individualize each patient's management plan in terms of the disease subtype, extent of activity, clinical course to date, and family situation. Although most physicians are accustomed to considering pharmacologic therapy of primary importance, it is only one aspect of the treatment of children with JA. A multidisciplinary team approach is the most effective means to meet the varied needs of a child with arthritis and his or her family.

Currently available drug therapy (see accompanying box), although not curative, can adequately suppress the inflammatory activities in up to 75% of those with JA. Five major categories of drug therapy are available: nonsteroidal antiinflammatory drugs (NSAIDs), slower-acting antirheumatic drugs (SAARDs), corticosteroids, cytotoxic agents, and other therapies (e.g., intravenous immune globulin and plasmapheresis).

Salicylates constitute the classic NSAIDs. Aspirin in divided doses sufficient to achieve a serum salicylate level between 20 and 30 mg/dl may be tried first; no advantage has been found in increasing the level, and toxicity occurs when this is done. For children weighing under 25 kg, this usually requires dosages of between 80 and 100 mg/kg/day; for those weighing more than 25 kg, the dosage is 2.4 to 4.8 g/day. Enteric-coated aspirin is better tolerated by those children who can swallow pills, produces less gastric upset, and delivers adequate serum levels. If a child cannot swallow the tablets or take chewable children's aspirin, both choline salicylate and choline magnesium salicylate are available as liquid preparations. Five to 10 days are needed before steady-

Medications for Juvenile Arthritis

NONSTEROIDAL ANTIINFLAMMATORY DRUGS (NSAIDs) CURRENTLY APPROVED BY THE FDA FOR USE IN CHILDREN

Salicylates
Indomethacin
Tolmetin sodium
Naproxen
Ibuprofen

NONSTEROIDAL ANTIINFLAMMATORY DRUGS (NSAIDs) NOT YET APPROVED BY THE FDA FOR USE IN CHILDREN

Diclofenac Sodium
Fenoprofen
Flurbiprofen
Ketoprofen
Phenylbutazone
Piroprofen
Piroxicam
Proquazone
Meclofenamate sodium
Sulindac

SLOWER-ACTING ANTIRHEUMATIC DRUGS (SAARDs)

Gold

Gold sodium thiomalate
Aurothioglucose
Auranofin

Hydroxychloroquine

D-Penicillamine
Sulfasalazine

CORTICOSTEROIDS

Systemic
Intraarticular

CYTOTOXIC DRUGS

Azathioprine
Chlorambucil
Cyclophosphamide
Methotrexate

OTHER THERAPIES

Pheresis
Intravenous immune globulin
Cyclosporin A

state, therapeutic levels are reached, and it may be a few weeks before the full therapeutic benefit occurs. The physician should always be alert for signs of salicylism, including tinnitus, hyperpnea, GI upset, and central nervous system (CNS) alterations. Serum salicylate levels should be obtained if there is any question of lack of effect or if any persistent adverse effects do not resolve with a decrease in dosage. Given the increased risk of Reye syndrome in children taking salicylates,[16] it is currently recommended that these children receive influenza vaccinations and stop their medications if they are exposed to varicella or develop influenza.

Should a child respond inadequately to salicylates or experience adverse effects, or if the family or physician is uncomfortable using salicylates because of the risk of Reye syndrome, a number of other NSAIDs are available. All these agents are nearly equivalent to aspirin in efficacy, toxicity, and mode of action[17]; unfortunately, they usually are also more expensive. There does seem to be a wide variation of individual response to these agents; therefore, if a child does not improve with one or two of the NSAIDs, it is reasonable to continue trying others for up to 2- or 3-month periods to find an efficacious drug.[18] All seem somewhat superior to aspirin for children with spondyloarthropathies or for older boys with pauciarticular JA. Naproxen and ibuprofen are now available as liquid preparations that can be quite useful in younger children and in those who have difficulties swallowing pills.

If a child continues to do poorly after 6 to 12 months of treatment with NSAIDs or has aggressive disease, the use of additional agents should be considered.[26]

Patients, parents, and physicians should be prepared to allow at least a 6-month trial of one of these drugs.

Three gold preparations are now available for use in the United States: gold sodium thiomalate, aurothioglucose, and auranofin. Gold sodium thiomalate and aurothioglucose are injectable preparations and need to be started on a weekly basis[8]; auranofin is a new oral preparation. Careful monitoring for bone marrow, kidney, or skin toxicity is necessary with preinjection WBC and platelet counts, urinalysis, and physical examination. The presence of adverse effects, such as skin rashes, leukopenia, thrombocytopenia, eosinophilia, hematuria, or proteinuria requires either a dosage adjustment (holding or lowering the dose) or discontinuation of the gold treatment. If the child responds well, the injection interval should be increased as much as possible until it is given on a monthly basis. The dosage for both parenteral preparations is approximately 1 mg/kg/dose to a maximum of 50 mg/dose.

Auranofin is given as a once or twice daily dose of 0.1 to 0.2 mg/kg/day. Since it comes as a 3 mg capsule, it is sometimes difficult to adjust the dose exactly to the child. In addition to the adverse effects noted above with the injectable gold preparations, it may also cause diarrhea. Although it may not be as efficacious as injectable gold preparations, it also does not cause as many serious adverse effects that require discontinuation. After initial biweekly complete blood and platelet counts and urinalyses, laboratory studies may be obtained monthly.

D-Penicillamine has been used quite extensively in Europe,[1] where it is felt to be equally as effective as gold; it has the advantage of being an oral preparation. It is given at a dosage of 5 to 10 mg/kg/day. It should be started at 250 mg or less per day and then gradually increased over a 2- to 6-month period to a maximum dosage of 750 mg or 10 mg/kg/day, whichever is lower. Its adverse effects are similar to those of gold therapy, with the addition of occasional GI upset and frequent dysgeusia. The latter signs often resolve on therapy and are not absolute indications for its discontinuation. Other rare adverse effects include Goodpasture syndrome, lupuslike syndrome, myasthenia gravis, and other autoimmune-induced effects (e.g., hemolytic anemia). Careful monitoring on a schedule similar to that used for gold therapy is necessary.

Antimalarial agents, such as hydroxychloroquine, constitute another therapeutic alternative. Although not as potent as gold or D-penicillamine, these SAARDs have the advantage of producing fewer adverse effects. The dosage for hydroxychloroquine is 5 mg/kg/day given as a single dose. The primary adverse effects that require drug discontinuation are GI upset (e.g., nausea, anorexia, diarrhea), bleaching of the hair, and retinal deposits. Regular ophthalmologic examinations every 6 months are necessary to detect the latter effect early; if found, therapy must be stopped.

Sulfasalazine, a drug first synthesized approximately 50 years ago as a specific antirheumatic agent, has seen a resurgence in recent years.[22] It is given at a dosage of approximately 25 mg/kg/day, usually with food or milk. It should not be used in anyone (1) sensitive to sulfa drugs or salicylates, (2) with impaired renal or hepatic function, or (3) with conditions such as glucose 6-phosphate dehydrogenase deficiency. Adverse effects caused by sulfasalazine include rashes, nausea, vomiting, dyspepsia, and a reversible decrease in sperm count. Bone marrow depression occurs in very rare cases. It seems to be as effective as the antimalarials and auranofin and may be superior in patients who are HLA-B27 positive.

A number of international cooperative trials have been conducted comparing the SAARDs to placebos. D-Penicillamine and hydroxychloroquine have been found variably effective in a number of studies,[9,24] as has auranofin.[11] Many rheumatologists are now reconsidering use of these agents.

Systemic corticosteroid use in JA should follow these maxims: (1) only use when other agents have failed or when the child is seriously ill or has progressive severe chronic anterior uveitis unresponsive to local therapy; (2) use as small a dose as possible; and (3) try to taper and discontinue their use as soon as possible. Corticosteroids are effective antiinflammatory agents but do not alter the course of the disease, are extremely difficult to discontinue in children with JA, and with long-term use are associated with many serious adverse effects, most importantly growth retardation. Alternate-day "dosing" can be tried but is extremely difficult, since many children develop problems on the day they do not receive the steroids. Small (1 to 5 mg) daily doses of prednisone that are tapered by 0.5 to 1 mg/day increments every 2 to 3 weeks can be quite effective. High-dose intravenous "pulse" steroid therapy (e.g., intravenous methylprednisolone 30 mg/kg/dose to a maximum of 1 g given over 2 hours daily for 1 to 3 days) can be useful in dire situations but does not seem to be more effective for chronic therapy.[20]

Intraarticular steroids can be effective in controlling acute problems associated with an active arthritis but are not a substitute for systemic, ongoing therapy. Children with a very painful or swollen joint frequently respond to arthrocentesis and instillation of a long-acting steroid preparation (e.g., triamcinolone hexacetonide).[28] One should be careful not to perform this procedure too frequently (more than three or four times per year) and should be sure there is no concomitant infectious arthritis as the cause of the acute joint problem.

A variety of cytotoxic agents have been used to treat juvenile arthritis. Few good long-term studies have been performed to evaluate these agents, and they should therefore be used cautiously in specific, otherwise unresponsive patients. Chlorambucil has been used extensively in Europe, especially in children with amyloidosis, but the results have been unsatisfactory. Azathioprine, although approved for use in adult rheumatoid arthritis, has not been as extensively studied in children. Methotrexate, however, underwent a double-blind, controlled trial and showed promising results.[12] When given at a dosage of 10 mg/m^2/week as a single dose, it was found over a 6-month period to be significantly superior to either placebo or a lower dose of 5 mg/m^2/week. Slightly higher doses may also be effective without an increase in adverse effects. It is currently approved for use with adults and seems to have a beneficial effect on the arthritis. Careful monitoring for bone marrow, liver, gastrointestinal, hepatic, and pulmonary toxicity is necessary.

A number of other therapies also have been tried for children with juvenile arthritis. Plasmapheresis and lymphopheresis have not been studied extensively, nor do they seem to be very beneficial. Intravenous immune gamma globulin has been used in children with systemic-onset juvenile arthritis, with mixed results.[13] Controlled trials will be necessary before recommendations can be made for this as a treatment.

Pharmacologic therapy, again, is only one aspect of the treatment required by children with JA. Physical therapy and occupational therapy are crucial and important adjuncts to help the child maintain strength and range of motion, to prevent contractures, and to allow the best possible quality of life. All patients should be given a home program of therapy that is reviewed and updated regularly. Heat therapy, such as taking warm baths or using a sleeping bag at night, often help minimize morning stiffness. Swimming is an excellent exercise; thus affected children should be encouraged to swim and to participate in as many other activities as possible. Normal play is the best therapy available.

The orthopedist's contributions for those children with more extensive disease range from the application of splints to operative tendon releases and capsulotomies. Some children may require joint resurfacing or joint replacement surgery as well.[14] Even though most children will not need orthopedic intervention, the orthopedist's perspective is an important part of the management.

JA, in all its forms, is a chronic illness, and none of the current modes of therapy is curative. Further, JA is one of the few childhood illnesses with pain as a primary symptom. Different expectations and attitudes are therefore needed when caring for the patient and family. In addition to a caring and understanding physician, a family counselor, social worker, or similar health professional is of particular value in helping the family to cope with and adjust to this chronic illness. Patients and parents will experience feelings of denial, guilt, and frustration at the time of diagnosis and throughout the course of the disease.[2]

Siblings frequently have a number of difficulties coping with the special and extensive treatment the affected child may receive. Periodic depression and anger are frequent problems, especially in the early stages as the child and the family realize that many changes may be necessary in their life-style and dreams. Despite the frequent episodes of family disruption, families are often able to adapt to their child's chronic illness adequately. All things being equal, most children with JA can do well in school; thus all efforts should be made to keep them enrolled. More recent studies of children's school and family adaptations show that children with juvenile arthritis and their families develop different, albeit generally normal, styles for coping with this chronic illness. Some adjustments may be necessary, including arranging for different transportation and physical education and allowing the child extra time between classes. It may be necessary for the physician or pediatric rheumatology team to act as advocates for these children within the school so they can receive all the necessary services they deserve. Although children with severe disease have a number of obvious problems, it is often the child with mild disease and a "hidden disability" who has more problems coping, adapting, and trying to accomplish the unrealistic goals set by a society that does not recognize the disability. Finally, it should always be remembered that any chronic illness places a financial burden, both directly and indirectly, on the family—a burden that can add a number of further stresses.

COURSE AND PROGNOSIS

JA is rarely a fatal disease, and in general the long-term prognosis is good, regardless of subtype. Approximately 75% of children will undergo a remission at some point, and many children will experience permanent remission. Most children with juvenile arthritis will complete their schooling, be gainfully employed, and raise families, just like their siblings and peers.

Several patterns of disease activity are recognized: (1) persistent active arthritis and destructive arthropathy; (2) active disease, then remission; (3) polycyclic diseases characterized by acute flares of activity followed by temporary remissions; and (4) low-grade continued activity with little if any joint destruction.

Pauciarticular JA has the best prognosis, with 40% to 50% of children undergoing a complete remission, as compared with only 25% to 30% of children with systemic-onset and polyarticular JA. Those children with IgM-RF or ANA positivity, systemic onset, and certain extraarticular manifestations (e.g., subcutaneous nodules, vasculitis) as well as younger children, usually have a poorer long-term articular outcome. Younger children with systemic-onset and polyarticular arthritis have a poorer articular prognosis; children with pauciarticular arthritis without chronic anterior uveitis have the best. Significant risk factors for the development of uveitis include recent onset of disease, female sex, ANA positivity, and younger age. Children with these risk factors should be examined every 4 months for at least 3 to 4 years and then every 6 months for at least another 3 to 4 years. In the absence of these risk factors, children can be examined every 6 months. Because the risk of uveitis decreases substantially 7 to 10 years after the onset of the arthritis, children can be followed yearly at that point if no uveitis has developed. Should chronic anterior uveitis develop, it can become the most significant long-term problem. The increasing awareness of the pediatric rheumatic diseases, which has resulted in earlier diagnosis and treatment, and the rapid advances in understanding the disease and its therapies are encouraging signs that the number of children disabled by these illnesses will decrease in the future.

REFERENCES

1. Ansell BW and Hall MA: Penicillamine in chronic arthritis in childhood, J Rheumatol 8:112, 1981.
2. Athreya BH and McCormick MC: Impact of chronic illness on families, Rheum Dis Clin North Am 13:123, 1987.
3. Bacon MC and White PH: A new approach to the assessment of growth in JRA, Arthritis Rheum 30:S192, 1987.
4. Barron KS et al: Abnormalities of immunoregulation in juvenile rheumatoid arthritis, J Rheumatol 16:940, 1989.
5. Bernstein BH et al: Reflex neurovascular dystrophy in childhood, J Pediatr 93:211, 1978.
6. Biro F, Gewanter HL, and Baum J: The hypermobility syndrome, Pediatrics 72:701, 1983.
7. Brewer EJ Jr et al: Current and proposed revision of JRA criteria, Arthritis Rheum 20:195, 1976.
8. Brewer EJ Jr, Giannini EH, and Barkley E: Gold therapy in the management of juvenile rheumatoid arthritis, Arthritis Rheum 23:404, 1980.
9. Brewer EJ Jr et al: Penicillamine and hydroxychloroquine in the treatment of severe juvenile rheumatoid arthritis: results of the USA-USSR double-blind placebo controlled study, N Engl J Med 314:1269, 1986.
10. Gewanter HL, Roghmann KJ, and Baum J: The prevalence of juvenile arthritis, Arthritis Rheum 26:599, 1983.
11. Giannini EH, Brewer EJ, and Person DA: Auranofin in the treatment of juvenile rheumatoid arthritis, J Pediatr 102:138, 1983.
12. Giannini EH and Brewer EJ Jr. for the Pediatric Rheumatology Collaborative Study Group: Methotrexate (MTX) in the treatment of recalcitrant JRA: results of the double-blind placebo (P) controlled, randomized trial, Arthritis Rheum 32(suppl):582, 1989 (abstract).
13. Greenwald MI et al: Treatment of systemic onset juvenile arthritis with intravenous gamma globulin, Arthritis Rheum 31(suppl):5117, 1988 (abstract).
14. Harris CM and Baum J: Involvement of the hip in juvenile rheumatoid arthritis: a longitudinal study, J Bone Joint Surg 70A:821, 1988.
15. Henoch MJ, Batson JW, and Baum J: Psychosocial factors in juvenile rheumatoid arthritis, Arthritis Rheum 21:229, 1978.
16. Hurwitz ES et al: Public Health Service study of Reye's syndrome and medications, JAMA 257:1905, 1987.
17. Levinson JE et al: Comparison of tolmetin sodium and aspirin in the treatment of juvenile rheumatoid arthritis, J Pediatr 91:799, 1977.
18. Lovell DJ, Giannini EH, and Brewer EJ Jr: Time course of response to nonsteroidal antiinflammatory drugs in juvenile rheumatoid arthritis, Arthritis Rheum 27:1433, 1984.
19. Maksymowych WP, VanKerckhove C, and Glass D: Juvenile rheumatoid arthritis, human leukocyte antigen and other immunoglobulin supergene family polymorphisms, Am J Med 85(suppl 6a):26, 1988.
20. Miller JJ: Prolonged use of huge intravenous steroid pulses in the rheumatic disease of children, Pediatrics 65:989, 1980.
21. Moore TL et al: Hidden 19S IgM rheumatoid factors, Semin Arthritis Rheum 18:72, 1988.
22. Ozgodan H et al: Sulphasalazine in the treatment of juvenile rheumatoid arthritis: a preliminary open trial, J Rheumatol 13:124, 1986.
23. Phillips PE: Evidence implicating infectious agents in rheumatoid arthritis and juvenile rheumatoid arthritis, Clin Exp Rheumatol 6:87, 1988.
24. Prieur AM et al: Evaluation of D-penicillamine in juvenile chronic arthritis: a double-blind, multicenter study, Arthritis Rheum 28:376, 1985.
25. Rosenberg AM: Uveitis associated with juvenile rheumatoid arthritis, Semin Arthritis Rheum 16:158, 1987.
26. Rosenberg AM: Advanced drug therapy for juvenile rheumatoid arthritis, J Pediatr 114:171, 1989.
27. Silverman ED et al: Consumptive coagulopathy associated with systemic juvenile rheumatoid arthritis, J Pediatr 103:872, 1983.
28. Sparling M et al: Radiographic follow-up of joints injected with triamcinolone hexacetamide for the management of childhood arthritis, Arthritis Rheum 33:821, 1990.
29. Stollerman GH: The return of rheumatic fever, Hosp Pract 23:100, 1988.
30. Vostrejs M and Hollister JR: Muscle atrophy and leg length discrepancies in pauciarticular juvenile rheumatoid arthritis, Am J Dis Child 142:343, 1988.
31. Yunus ME and Masi AT: Juvenile primary fibromyalgia syndrome: a clinical study of thirty-three patients and matched normal controls, Arthritis Rheum 28:138, 1985.

SUGGESTED READINGS

Brewer EJ Jr and Cassidy JT, Ed: Rheumatic diseases of childhood, Rheum Dis Clin North Am 13:1, 1987.

Brewer EJ Jr, Giannini EH, and Person DA: Juvenile rheumatoid arthritis, ed 2, Philadelphia, 1982, WB Saunders Co.

Cassidy JT and Petty RE: Textbook of pediatric rheumatology, ed 2, New York, 1990, Churchill Livingstone, Inc.

Jacobs JL: Pediatric rheumatology for the practitioner, New York, 1983, Springer-Verlag New York, Inc.

Lang BA and Shore A: A review of current concepts on the pathogenesis of juvenile rheumatoid arthritis, J Rheum 17(suppl 21):1, 1990.

Miller ML, editor: Pediatric rheumatology, Pediatr Clin North Am 33:1015, 1986.

222

Kawasaki Disease

Michael E. Pichichero

Kawasaki disease, formerly known as mucocutaneous lymph node syndrome, was first described in 1967 by a Japanese pediatrician, Tomisaka Kawasaki.[8] In 1974 the first cases of Kawasaki disease were reported in the United States. Since that time the number of children with this disease has steadily increased nationwide. The Centers for Disease Control estimates of the incidence of this disease for children 8 years old or younger in the continental United States are 2.74 cases per 100,000 in those of Asian or part Asian descent, 1.03 per 100,000 in blacks, and 0.43 per 100,000 in whites. The peak age incidence of Kawasaki disease occurs during the second year of life. More than 80% of all cases occur in children under 5 years of age; the disease is quite uncommon in those beyond 9 years of age. Boys are more commonly affected than girls, with a male/female ratio of nearly 1.5:1. The incidence in siblings is 1.4% and in recurrent cases 3.9%.[1,12,27]

ETIOLOGY

There is no established cause for Kawasaki disease.[2,23] The clinical features suggest a hypersensitivity reaction, exposure to an environmental toxin, or an infectious etiology.[13,19] However, the occurrence of fever and an exanthem as part of an acute although self-limited disease process, seasonality, limited age distribution, and occurrence in communitywide epidemics are most consistent with an infectious cause.[13] In some studies an association between Kawasaki disease and rug shampooing has been observed[21]; no single cleaning product has been identified. A variant strain of *Propionibacterium acnes* has been isolated from both Kawasaki disease patients and mites found in their house dust.[6] It has been postulated that rug shampooing may aerosolize such mites. Case-control studies during Kawasaki disease outbreaks has revealed a tendency for cases more often than not to have an antecedent respiratory, febrile, or gastrointestinal illness within a month of contracting the disease.[13,19] Also, the homes of patients with Kawasaki disease tend to be near stagnant water, which suggests the possibility of water serving as an arthropod vector or an animal reservoir. Initial reports of increased reverse transcriptase activity in supernatants of cocultivated peripheral mononuclear cells from patients with Kawasaki disease, combined with serologic evidence, suggested the possibility that a retrovirus might be involved as an etiology in these patients.[3,20,25] However, subsequent investigations have shed increasing doubt on this hypothesis.

PATHOGENESIS

The pathogenesis of Kawasaki disease is unclear. In some aspects, Kawasaki disease resembles an autoimmune disorder. Immune complexes have been found in some but not all patients; however, the pathogenic role, if any, of these complexes remains to be established. There is a correlation between immune complexes and increased oxygen radical release from activated neutrophils. It has been suggested that thromboarteritis and vascular aneurysm, hallmark findings in Kawasaki disease, could be the result of immune complex deposition leading to neutrophil activation with consequent oxygen radical and liposomal enzyme release.[18]

The effectiveness of high-dose intravenous gamma globulin infusions in reducing coronary vasculitis might result from prevention of immune complex deposition on blood vessel walls or from a reversal of immunoregulatory abnormalities.[11]

CLINICAL MANIFESTATIONS

To make the diagnosis of Kawasaki disease, five of the six major clinical characteristics associated with the condition must be present (see accompanying box), and all other illnesses with similar features must be excluded. Symptoms vary in severity, but greater than 90% of patients fulfill the first five clinical criteria. All the symptoms are not apparent simultaneously, but the timing of their appearance is remarkably constant.

The course of the disease can best be described as triphasic. The acute phase consists of fever, conjunctival hyperemia, oropharyngeal erythema, swelling of the hands and feet, a polymorphous erythematous rash, and cervical lymphadenopathy. Fever, rash, and lymphadenopathy fade after 10 to 12 days of illness, marking the beginning of the subacute phase. The subacute stage is characterized by lip cracking and fissuring, desquamation of skin overlying the tips of the fingers and toes, and the onset of arthralgias (and/or arthritis), thrombocytosis, and cardiac disease. The convalescent stage usually begins about 25 days into the disease process and is characterized by the absence of clinical signs of disease but the persistence of residual inflammation, marked by an elevated erythrocyte sedimentation rate (ESR).

Fever is the most prominent symptom of the acute phase of Kawasaki disease. Temperatures show a high-spiking re-

Diagnostic Criteria for Kawasaki Disease

A. Principal symptoms (At least five of the following six items should be satisfied for diagnosis.)
   1. Fever of unknown cause lasting 5 days or more
   2. Bilateral congestion of ocular conjunctivae
   3. Changes of lips and oral cavity
      a. Dryness, redness, and fissuring of lips
      b. Protuberance of tongue papillae (strawberry tongue)
      c. Diffuse reddening of oral and pharyngeal mucosa
   4. Changes of peripheral extremities
      a. Reddening of palms and soles (initial stage)
      b. Indurative edema (initial stage)
      c. Membranous desquamation from fingertips (convalescent stage)
   5. Polymorphous exanthema of body trunk without vesicles or crusts
   6. Acute nonpurulent swelling of cervical lymph nodes of 1.5 cm or more in diameter

B. Other significant symptoms or findings
   1. Carditis, especially myocarditis or pericarditis
   2. Diarrhea
   3. Arthralgia or arthritis
   4. Proteinuria and increase of leukocytes in urine sediment
   5. Changes in blood tests
      a. Leukocytosis with shift to the left
      b. Slight decrease in erythrocyte and hemoglobin levels
      c. Increased sedimentation rate
      d. Positive C-reactive protein (CRP)
      e. Increased beta-2-globulin
      f. Thrombocytosis
      g. Negative antistreptolysin titer (ASO)
   6. Changes occasionally observed
      a. Aseptic meningitis
      b. Mild jaundice or slight increase of serum transaminase
      c. Swelling of gallbladder

mittent pattern in the range of 38.4° C to greater than 40° C. Fever persists despite the use of empiric antibiotics, corticosteroids, and standard doses of antipyretics. Fever is present on the average for about 12 days, although prolonged courses of up to 5 weeks have been reported. Defervescence occurs over 1 to 3 days. Discrete engorgement of the bulbar conjunctivae blood vessels (without associated discharge, exudate, keratitis, chemosis, or pseudomembrane formation) and an anterior uveitis develop shortly after the onset of fever. The cornea, lens, and retina are not involved. Early oropharyngeal signs include dryness and reddening of the lips and of the buccal and pharyngeal mucosa. The absence of aphthous ulceration or hemorrhagic bullae is noticeable. A "strawberry tongue" is frequently present. Later, as the intensity of the erythema subsides, the lips usually become cracked and fissured.

The most characteristic and unique feature of Kawasaki disease relates to changes that occur in the hands and feet. Early on they become diffusely indurated and swollen, and the overlying skin develops a woody firmness suggestive of acute scleroderma. The palms and soles usually become erythematous or take on a purplish hue. There is fusiform swelling of the fingers, which limits the child's ability to grasp objects. The feet are painful to the touch, and many children will refuse to stand or bear weight. Two to three weeks after the onset of illness and after the early signs involving the extremities have disappeared, an unusual desquamation of the skin beginning at the subungual and periungual regions of the fingertips and toe tips is recognizable in nearly all cases (Fig. 222-1). Progression to complete peeling of the palms and soles may occur, but exfoliation generally does not extend to the remainder of the body surface. During the convalescent phase, deep transverse grooves may appear across the fingernails and toenails, presumably as a result of arrested growth during the illness.

A polymorphous erythematous rash appears 1 to 5 days after the onset of fever; it usually begins on the extremities and spreads centripetally. The three most common patterns of rash are maculopapular (morbilliform), erythema multiforme–like with iris lesions, and scarlatiniform. The rash may be coalescent, producing large, irregular, raised plaques, and it may be pruritic. Vesicles, pustules, and bullae are not seen. The rash is not petechial or purpuric. It usually fades within a week but occasionally either persists longer or is recurrent.

Lymphadenopathy typically involves a single cervical node measuring greater than 1.5 cm in diameter. The node is usually not tender or warm and does not become fluctuant. Generalized lymphadenopathy does not occur. The lymph node diminishes in size with defervescence. This finding is the one least often seen of the major criteria; it occurs in only about 60% of patients in most U.S. series (although it is more common in Japan).

In addition to the six major clinical signs, there are other frequently noted features of Kawasaki disease. Sterile pyuria occurs more often than lymphadenopathy in most American cases. Ten to one hundred white blood cells (WBCs) per high-power field may be observed on a clean-catch voided specimen. No WBCs will be seen on a bladder aspiration specimen, because the sterile pyuria is caused by urethral ulceration or inflammation. Occasionally a patient will demonstrate trace proteinuria or hematuria.

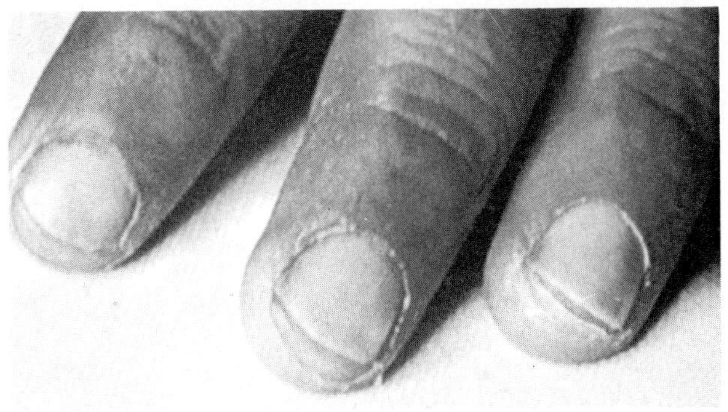

Fig. 222-1 Desquamation of the skin involving the subungual and periungual regions of the fingertips.

From Kawasaki T et al: A new infantile acute febrile mucocutaneous lymph node syndrome (MLNS) prevailing in Japan, Pediatrics 54:273,1974. Copyright American Academy of Pediatrics, 1974.

Irritability, mild meningismus, and lethargy are typically seen in nearly all of these patients, and nearly all probably have aseptic meningitis. When cerebrospinal fluid (CSF) is analyzed, it typically shows 25 to 100 WBCs/mm^3 with normal amounts of glucose and protein.

Diarrhea is seen in about 50% of the patients. Five to 15 stools per day for 2 to 7 days during the acute or subacute phase are not uncommon. Stools do not contain polymorphonuclear cells and are not Hematest positive.

Either arthralgias, arthritis, or both occur in 30% to 40% of the children. Large joints, particularly the knees and ankles, are more often involved. Usually no more than two or three joints will be affected. This symptom occurs 8 to 12 days after the onset of disease. Joint fluid, if analyzed, will reveal findings similar to those of rheumatoid arthritis.

Other findings, such as pneumonia, tympanitis, photophobia, and mild liver dysfunction, are somewhat less commonly observed. Acute hydrops of the gallbladder, jaundice, convulsions, encephalopathy, pancreatitis, orchitis, and pleural effusions are rarely seen but are clearly associated complications of Kawasaki disease.

The most alarming findings of Kawasaki disease are those in the cardiovascular system. Approximately 1% of children with the disease die, usually as a result of coronary artery aneurysms. During the acute phase, tachycardia and gallop rhythms may appear; however, the most serious manifestations of cardiac involvement occur during the subacute phase. These include serious arrhythmias, congestive heart failure, pericardial effusion, mitral insufficiency, and myocardial ischemia or infarction.

LABORATORY FINDINGS

Although there are no pathognomonic laboratory findings in Kawasaki disease, certain laboratory abnormalities are frequently seen and therefore help establish the diagnosis. In the acute phase of the disease, most patients exhibit an elevated white blood cell (WBC) count with an associated left shift; WBC counts of 15,000 to 20,000/mm^3 are not uncommon, and these counts may remain elevated for 1 to 3 weeks. Other laboratory abnormalities in the acute phase usually include an elevated erythrocyte sedimentation rate (ESR) (mean = 55 mm/hr); increased CRP and beta-2-globulin; mild normochromic, normocytic anemia; and slight elevations of the liver enzymes. In addition, as previously stated, many patients will demonstrate sterile pyuria and cerebrospinal fluid (CSF) pleocytosis as well as sinus tachycardia, nonspecific ST segment and T wave changes, and evidence of mild left ventricular hypertrophy on an electrocardiogram. In the second to third week of illness, patients characteristically develop significant thrombocytosis, with platelet counts averaging in excess of 700,000/mm^3. In the subacute phase, myocardial infarction patterns on an electrocardiogram (ECG) can be seen, although infrequently.

Importantly, a number of laboratory studies are negative. Routine cultures of blood, CSF, urine, throat, and lymph node aspirates reveal no growth or normal flora. Serologic studies for bacterial and viral agents are negative, including the ASO titer. Antinuclear antibodies and the rheumatoid factor are absent, as are all other autoantibodies.

DIFFERENTIAL DIAGNOSIS

The clinical picture of Kawasaki disease, after all of the major features have become manifest, is not difficult to differentiate from other mucocutaneous syndromes. In the first days of the illness, a whole spectrum of acute febrile diseases might be considered. Three to five days after the onset, certain clinical features may be singled out as compatible with other diagnoses, for example, strawberry tongue suggestive of streptococcal infection. However, if all the signs and symptoms are carefully considered, the diagnosis is readily apparent.

The clinical features of Kawasaki disease and other mucocutaneous disorders are shown in Table 222-1. Other conditions that share some aspects of Kawasaki disease are ratbite fever, rubella, rubeola, infectious mononucleosis, toxoplasmosis, juvenile rheumatoid arthritis, systemic lupus erythematosus, Behçet syndrome, acrodynia (mercury poisoning), and febrile drug reactions. The similarities between fatal Kawasaki disease and fatal infantile polyarteritis nodosa are striking; pathologically, the two diseases cannot be distinguished. The exact relationship between them, however, remains undetermined. At this time, one is left with the clear differentiating feature that Kawasaki disease is rarely fatal (±1% mortality), whereas infantile polyarteritis nodosa is almost universally so.

MANAGEMENT

The care given to children with Kawasaki disease is primarily supportive. Antibiotics are not beneficial. Corticosteroids are contraindicated, since some evidence suggests that coronary aneurysms occur more frequently in patients receiving these agents. Aspirin, given in high dosages (80 to 120 mg/kg/day), reduces the length and severity of illness during the acute phase of the disease. Aspirin use early in the course of disease also may reduce coronary artery involvement.[5,9,10] Salicylate levels should be checked frequently to avoid toxicity. Defervescence apparently is accompanied by improvement in gastrointestinal (GI) absorption of aspirin; therefore

Table 222-1 *Clinical Features of Kawasaki Disease and Other Mucocutaneous Diseases*

	KAWASAKI DISEASE	STEVENS-JOHNSON SYNDROME	STREPTOCOCCAL SCARLET FEVER	STAPHYLOCOCCAL SCARLET FEVER	TOXIC SHOCK SYNDROME	LEPTOSPIROSIS
Age (yr)	Usually <5	Usually 3-30	Usually 5-10	Usually 2-8	Usually adolescent	Usually >2
Fever	Prolonged	Prolonged	Variable	Variable	Usually <10 days	Variable
Eyes	Hyperemia of ocular conjunctivae; uveitis	Catarrhal conjunctivitis; chemosis; iritis; uveitis; panophthalmitis	No change	Hyperemia of ocular conjunctivae	Hyperemia of ocular conjunctivae	Hyperemia of ocular conjunctivae; uveitis
Lips	Red, dry, fissured	Erosions; crusted, fissured, bleeding	No change	No change	Red	No change
Oral cavity	Diffuse erythema; "strawberry tongue"	Erythema; bullae, ulcers, pseudomembrane formation	Pharyngitis; palatal petechiae; "strawberry tongue"	Pharyngitis	Erythema; pharyngitis	Pharyngitis
Peripheral extremities	Erythema of palms and soles; indurative edema; periungual, palmar, and plantar desquamation	No change	Periungual desquamation	No change	Swelling of hands and feet; dry gangrene	Gangrene of hands and feet (rare)
Exanthem	Erythematous, polymorphous	Erythematous, polymorphous; iris lesions, vesicles, bullae, crusts	Finely papular erythroderma; Pastia lines; circumoral pallor	Finely papular erythroderma; Pastia lines	Erythroderma	Erythematous, maculopapular, petechial, or purpuric
Cervical lymph nodes	Nonpurulent swelling; unilateral (frequent)	Nonpurulent swelling (occasional)	Nonpurulent or purulent swelling (frequent)	Nonpurulent or purulent swelling (occasional)	No change	Nonpurulent swelling (infrequent)
Other	Meatitis; diarrhea; arthralgia and arthritis; aseptic meningitis; rhinorrhea (uncommon); ECG changes	Malaise; cough, rhinorrhea, pneumonitis; vomiting; arthralgia; recurrent episodes	Malaise; vomiting; headache		Headache; confusion; hypotension; icteric hepatitis; diarrhea; coagulopathy; renal injury	Headache; myalgia; abdominal pain; icteric hepatitis; meningitis

dosages should be reduced to 30 mg/kg/day after fever subsides. Aspirin should be continued throughout the subacute phase because of its antiinflammatory and antithrombotic effects. Continued salicylate therapy at 10 mg/kg/day in the convalescent phase until the platelet count and ESR have returned to normal is also recommended.

High-dose intravenous gamma globulin may prevent the coronary artery lesion of Kawasaki disease in some cases. Treatment should commence as soon as the diagnosis is made. A dosage of 400 mg/kg/day for 4 consecutive days has been shown to be effective.[14,17] A single 1 g/kg dose, thereby avoiding the necessity of a 4-day hospital stay, has shown promise in early trials. The composition and manufacturer of the gamma globulin preparation may be important elements for efficacy.

The second critical period in the management of Kawasaki disease occurs during the subacute phase. Once the diagnosis is established, a baseline ECG, chest roentgenogram, and two-dimensional echocardiogram should be obtained to establish ventricular vectors, size, and coronary artery architecture. These studies should be repeated 21 to 28 days from the onset of disease (late subacute stage). If coronary aneurysms are recognized, salicylates (10 mg/kg/day) should be continued until careful follow-up echocardiograms demonstrate aneurysm resolution.

Risk Factors for Coronary Artery Aneurysms in Kawasaki Disease

RISK VERY INCREASED

Fever lasts longer than 14 days
Biphasic fever pattern*†
Biphasic pattern of skin rash
Maximum WBC count ≥30,000
Maximum ESR (mm/hr) ≥101
Time until normalization of ESR or CRP ≥30 days of illness
Biphasic elevation of ESR or CRP†
Increased Q/R ratio in leads II, III, aV_F >0.3
Symptoms of myocardial infarction

RISK INCREASED

Male sex
Age at onset under 1 year
Hemoglobin ≤10 g/dl† and RBC count ≤3.5 million
Maximum WBC count >26,000
Maximum ESR (mm/hr) >50
Cardiomegaly
Arrhythmia
Recurrence of disease

*Separated by afebrile period of 48 hours or longer.
†Causes other than Kawasaki disease must be ruled out.

COMPLICATIONS

The major complication of Kawasaki disease is the development of coronary artery aneurysms.[4,7,24,26] These occur in 15% to 20% of the cases and are usually apparent by echocardiogram during the subacute phase of the illness. Most patients with aneurysms are asymptomatic; in some cases, however, formation of an aneurysm is followed by thrombosis or rupture, resulting in a fatal myocardial infarction.

The coronary artery aneurysms seen in Kawasaki disease develop more frequently in boys than in girls, in children less than 1 year of age, in those with a triphasic fever pattern or prolonged fever (longer than 2 weeks), when a gallop rhythm or other arrhythmia is noted, or when the ESR exceeds 50 mm/hr. See the accompanying box.

A few cases of "incomplete" Kawasaki disease (five of six diagnostic criteria not observed) followed by typical coronary artery involvement have led to the suggestion that an echocardiography examination be undertaken in children with prolonged unexplainable febrile illnesses associated with subsequent peripheral desquamation.[22]

A rare complication of Kawasaki disease is hydrops of the gallbladder. This occurs in approximately 3% of the cases and is seen most frequently in those children who are jaundiced. It becomes evident during the acute phase of the illness and is best diagnosed by ultrasound on recognition of a right upper quadrant abdominal mass. The pathogenesis is unknown. Surgery is not indicated, since the problem spontaneously resolves in convalescence.

PROGNOSIS

Kawasaki disease has a 1% mortality, largely as a result of massive myocardial infarction and cardiogenic shock. Significant morbidity, in the form of coronary artery aneurysms, occurs in 15% to 20% of the cases. One prospective study[15] has shown that 50% of those with aneurysms have complete resolution without apparent sequelae within 1 to 2 years. The remaining children may experience persisting aneurysms, coronary artery stenosis or obstruction, or aortic regeneration.[15,16] Emerging evidence suggests that this latter group of children may be at risk for the subsequent development of significant cardiovascular disease such as coronary arteriosclerosis or persistent aneurysms, placing the patient at risk for sudden death from aneurysm rupture or thrombosis, cardiac arrhythmias, angina, or hypertension.

PSYCHOSOCIAL ASPECTS

Kawasaki disease is typically a self-limited illness without complications, which should be emphasized to the anxious parent. Even if coronary artery aneurysms do develop, these spontaneously resolve in over 50% of the cases. Long-term risks remain largely undefined, and only as we gain prospective experience with the disease will the true incidence of cardiovascular sequelae become evident.

REFERENCES

1. Bell D et al: Kawasaki syndrome in the United States 1976 to 1980, Am J Dis Child 137:211, 1983.
2. Bierman FZ and Gersony WM: Kawasaki disease: clinical perspective, J Pediatr 111:789, 1987.
3. Burns J et al: Polymerase activity in lymphocyte culture supernatants from patients with Kawasaki disease, Nature 323:814, 1986.
4. Daniels SR et al: Correlates of coronary artery aneurysm formation in patients with Kawasaki disease, Am J Dis Child 141:205, 1987.

5. Ichida F et al: Coronary artery involvement in Kawasaki syndrome in Manhattan, New York: risk factors and role of aspirin, Pediatrics 80:828, 1987.
6. Kato H et al: Variant strain of *Propionibacterium acnes*: a clue to the aetiology of Kawasaki disease, Lancet 2:1383, 1983.
7. Kato H et al: Coronary heart disease in children with Kawasaki disease, Jpn Circ J 43:469, 1979.
8. Kawasaki T et al: A new infantile acute febrile mucocutaneous lymph node syndrome (MLNS) prevailing in Japan, Pediatrics 54:271, 1974.
9. Koren G and MacLeod SM: Difficulty in achieving therapeutic serum concentrations of salicylate in Kawasaki disease, J Pediatr 105:991, 1984.
10. Koren G et al: Probable efficacy of high-dose salicylates in reducing coronary involvement in Kawasaki disease, JAMA 254:767, 1985.
11. Leung DYM et al: Reversal of lymphocyte activation in vivo in the Kawasaki syndrome by intravenous gamma globulin, J Clin Invest 79:468, 1987.
12. Morens D, Anderson L, and Hurwitz E: National surveillance of Kawasaki disease, Pediatrics 65:21, 1980.
13. Multiple outbreaks of Kawasaki syndrome: United States, MMWR 34:34, 1985.
14. Nagashima M et al: High-dose gammaglobulin therapy for Kawasaki disease, J Pediatr 110:710, 1987.
15. Nakano H et al: High incidence of aortic regurgitation following Kawasaki disease, J Pediatr 107:59, 1985.
16. Nakano H et al: Clinical characteristics of myocardial infarction following Kawasaki disease: report of 11 cases, J Pediatr 108:198, 1986.
17. Newberger J et al: The treatment of Kawasaki syndrome with intravenous gamma globulin, N Engl J Med 315:341, 1986.
18. Niwa Y and Sohmiya K: Enhanced neutrophilic functions in mucocutaneous lymph node syndrome, with special reference to the possible role of increased oxygen intermediate generation in the pathogenesis of coronary thromboarteritis, J Pediatr 104:56, 1984.
19. Rauch AM: Kawasaki syndrome: review of new epidemiologic and laboratory developments, Pediatr Infect Dis J 6:1016, 1987.
20. Rauch A, Fultz P, and Kalyanaraman V: Kawasaki syndrome: retrovirus serology, Lancet 1:1431, 1987.
21. Rogers M et al: Kawasaki syndrome: is exposure to rug shampoo important? Am J Dis Child 139:777, 1985.
22. Rowley AH et al: Incomplete Kawasaki disease with coronary artery involvement, J Pediatr 110:409, 1987.
23. Rowley AH, Gonzalez-Crussi F, and Shulman ST: Kawasaki syndrome, Rev Infect Dis 10:1, 1988.
24. Shulman ST et al: Risk of coronary abnormalities due to Kawasaki disease in urban area with small Asian population, Am J Dis Child 141:420, 1987.
25. Shulman S and Rowley A: Does Kawasaki disease have a retroviral etiology? Lancet 2:545, 1986.
26. Tatara K and Kusakawa S: Long-term prognosis of giant coronary aneurysm in Kawasaki disease: an angiographic study, J Pediatr 111:705, 1987.
27. Yanagawa H, Kawasaki T, and Shigematsu I: Nationwide survey on Kawasaki disease in Japan, Pediatrics 80:58, 1987.

223

Labial Adhesions

Barbara J. Howard

Adhesions of the labia minora, also called labial fusion, synechia vulvae, or agglutination of the labia, occur commonly in infants and young girls, producing considerable parental concern despite their usual lack of medical significance. What the parents see is a flap of skin formed by the adherence of the labia minora that completely covers all evidence of a vaginal opening. The fear that their daughter may have abnormal sexual anatomy often leads them to ask questions about other problems of the genital area, such as diaper rash, rather than addressing their real concern directly.

The diagnosis of labial adhesions is based entirely on the physical examination. While gently stretching the labia majora apart, a thin flat membrane of variable length is seen in the midline. This extends from the clitoris to the posterior fourchette in 70% of cases, the rest being cases of partial coverage.[2] There is usually a small opening near the clitoris through which the urine passes. The vaginal introitus is obscured, but one could demonstrate the space beneath the flap by inserting a small probe through the anterior opening and directing it posteriorly beneath the membrane. This, however, is not necessary once the thin line of adherence (or agglutination) between the two nonrugated flat labia minora has been identified. Labial adhesions are not present at birth, unlike congenital anomalies of the genitalia such as vaginal agenesis or the ambiguous genitalia associated with the adrenogenital syndrome with which labial adhesions are sometimes confused. Imperforate hymen also differs in that it is apparent within the vaginal introitus and the labia are normal.

The occurrence of the adhesions is ascribed to a combination of inflammation and hypoestrogenization of the labia minora. Commonly, the tissue is irritated (usually so mildly as to go unnoticed) through trauma, infection, or poor hygiene, and the medial edges of the labia adhere to each other as they heal. Urine flow may be partially obstructed, resulting in pooling behind the fusion and further irritation, thereby continuing the cycle of inflammation, adhesion, and obstruction. Labial adhesions are found in infants after 2 months of age and at any time up to menarche irrespective of race. This pattern is presumed to be caused by the relative immunity to inflammation of epithelium exposed to estrogen, such as that of the newborn under the influence of maternal hormones and that of postmenarcheal girls. The only known case found at birth was associated with infection of the infant in utero.[3] Similarly, adhesions are very rare during the reproductive years in females with normal ovarian function,[8] although they have been seen as a result of herpes simplex type II infection.[6] Capraro and Greenberg[3] reported the average age at diagnosis to be 2½ years, with 56% of their patients under 2 years of age and 94% under 6 years. Earlier, Huffman reported the highest incidence to be between ages 2 and 6 years.[3] This shift to an earlier age may be the result of a greater awareness of the condition or perhaps a predisposition to inflammation from the occlusion of the plastic diaper covers often used today.

It has been estimated that 10% to 20% of girls have some period of adhesion before 1 year of age.[12] In one series of 287 girls from birth to 14 years of age admitted to the hospital for other reasons, an incidence of 1.4% was calculated.[4]

An association has been found between labial adhesions and sexual abuse, with two retrospective analyses showing that 3% of children referred for sexual abuse had had adhesions.[2,11] Although this is still infrequent, it represents a threefold to fivefold increase over the baseline prevalence, presumably secondary to trauma or infection. Thus the presence of labial adhesions should alert clinicians at least to examine the child for signs of trauma or infection and to ask about caretaking arrangements and any concerns there may be about inappropriate handling of the child. However, in a study of 500 referrals for suspected sexual abuse, the six girls who had adhesions and were proven to have been abused also had abnormal rectal findings as a clue to the diagnosis.[11]

Examination of the vulvae is recommended during each health maintenance visit to check hygiene, monitor sexual development, and detect problems.[13,14] This is also important for developing a clinical baseline for normal anatomy. With the apparent increase in sexual misuse of children in whom genital complaints may not be reported, skill in this practice becomes especially important.

Parents may be concerned that the normal self-stimulation of the genitalia that starts around 6 months of age and is especially prominent between 18 months and 2½ years of age is damaging to their child. It is helpful to counsel parents routinely about the normality of self-stimulation, particularly when adhesions draw attention to sexual development.[9] An effort must be made to constrain any parental overreaction.

On the other hand, masturbation may be a response to genital irritation from infection or to psychological distress, especially from sexual misuse. These situations should be assessed before providing reassurance about masturbation, particularly if it is insistent or has an acute onset.

Only 20% to 38% of girls with labial adhesions have any symptoms of dysuria, difficulty voiding, or local discomfort.[3] If there is no evidence of obstruction to voiding, repeated urinary tract infection, discomfort, or excessive parental concern, no treatment beyond explanation is needed. Since adhesions completely resolve spontaneously—50% in 6 months,

90% in 12 months, and 100% in 18 months[10]—surgical or mechanical lysis is not only unnecessary in the usual case but is less effective in the long term, is potentially painful, and can be psychologically traumatic and costly. Should treatment be indicated or urgently desired by the parents in spite of counseling, the topical application of estrogen cream (0.1% or 0.01% dienestrol) is effective in about 90% of cases.[3] In addition, recurrence is rare after this treatment, whereas serious readhesion after mechanical lysis has been noted in 20% to 100% of cases.[1] Separation of the labia is achieved in 90% of cases[5] after 2 weeks of twice daily treatment with gentle traction of the labia laterally.[7] This should be followed by nightly application of the estrogen cream for 1 to 2 weeks. Treatment is considered to have failed if separation does not occur within 8 weeks.[1] Occasionally a repeat course of treatment is needed.[7] Several further weeks of application of a bland ointment (e.g., petrolatum) after separation is established is recommended to assure sustained labial separations[3] for as long as a year in the case of recurrences. The older child can be taught to apply the cream herself with supervision. Reversible vulvar pigmentation or erythema and/or breast tenderness has been reported in up to one third of children managed with topical treatment.[2] However, no serious or lasting complications of treatment have been reported. If a urinary tract infection is suspected as either a cause of irritation or a complication of outflow obstruction, urinalysis and culture results will dictate the necessary treatment and follow-up. Although labial adhesions are not known to be associated with congenital anomalies, Capraro and Greenberg[3] found 3 of their 50 affected girls to have urinary tract anomalies (all were symptomatic). Nevertheless, further specific gynecologic or renal evaluation is not needed unless there are indications of persistent urinary tract infections or vulvar irritation or unless there is an unexplained treatment failure.

REFERENCES

1. Ariborg A: Topical oestrogen therapy for labial adhesions in children, Br J Obstet Gynaecol 82:424, 1975.
2. Berkowitz CD, Elvik SL, and Logan MK: Labial fusion in prepubescent girls: a marker for sexual abuse? Am J Obstet Gynecol 156:16, 1987.
3. Capraro VJ and Greenberg H: Adhesions of the labia minora: a study of 50 patients, Obstet Gynecol 39:65, 1972.
4. Christensen EH and Oster J: Adhesions of labia minora (synechia vulvae) in childhood, Acta Paediatr Scand 60:709, 1971.
5. Clair DL and Caldamone AA: Pediatric office procedures, Urol Clin North Am 15(4):15, 1988.
6. DeMarco BJ, Crandall RS, and Hreshchyshyn MM: Labial agglutination secondary to a herpes simplex II infection, Am J Obstet Gynecol 157:296, 1987.
7. Emans SJH and Goldstein DP: Pediatric and adolescent gynecology, ed 2, Boston, 1982, Little, Brown & Co.
8. Goldstein AI and Rajcher WJ: Conglutination of the labia minora in the presence of normal estrogen levels: an exception to the rule, Am J Obstet Gynecol 113:845, 1972.
9. Howard BJ: One approach to anticipatory guidance of sexuality for pediatricians. In Charney E, editor: Pediatric update, New York, 1981, Elsevier-Dutton.
10. Jenkinson SD and MacKinnon AE: Spontaneous separation of fused labia minora in prepubertal girls, Br Med J 289:160, 1984.
11. Muram D: Labial adhesions in sexually abused children, JAMA 259:352, 1988 (letter).
12. Parsons L and Sommers SC: Gynecology, ed 2, Philadelphia, 1978, WB Saunders Co.
13. Singleton AF: The vulvar examination of the premenarchal child, J Natl Med Assoc 78:203, 1986.
14. Williams TS, Callen JP, and Owen LG: Vulvar disorders in the prepubertal female, Pediatr Ann 15:588, 1986.

224

Leukemias

Barbara L. Asselin

Even though many pediatricians are faced only infrequently with a child diagnosed with leukemia, their role in the treatment process is critical. As the primary caregiver, the pediatrician is responsible for ensuring that an accurate diagnosis is rapidly made, that appropriate emergency measures are initiated when necessary, and that referral to a pediatric cancer center is expedited. Once uniformly fatal diseases, the childhood leukemias are now more appropriately considered treatable and potentially curable. However, the aggressive treatment protocols that have played a role in the therapeutic successes to date have resulted in significant acute and long-term toxicities. Pediatric subspecialists are vital members of the health care team that implements these complicated, frequently toxic, multiinstitutional clinical trials. The child's pediatrician will be following his or her patient not only during the stage of acute treatment, but back home during periods of remission and throughout the cure. With the increasing number of long-term survivors of childhood leukemia, the pediatrician, internist, and subspecialists must be knowledgeable about the late sequelae of antileukemic therapy, alert to their recognition, and familiar with appropriate therapeutic interventions.

EPIDEMIOLOGY

Leukemia is the most common form of malignancy seen in children and the second most frequent cause of death in children between 5 and 14 years of age. Almost one third of cancer cases in children will be a leukemia (Fig. 224-1). The incidence of all types of acute leukemia has been reported to be 4.2 per 100,000 white and 2.4 per 100,000 nonwhite children.[82] At these 1985 incidence rates, more than 2000 children under 15 years of age are predicted to be diagnosed with acute leukemia each year in the United States.[82] Despite the remarkable gains that have been made in the treatment of these children, little has been done that has affected this incidence.[32,58]

As shown in Fig. 224-2, acute lymphoblastic leukemia (ALL) predominates, accounting for 80% of all cases of childhood leukemia.[81] Childhood ALL has a peak incidence at approximately 4 years of age.[48] It is more common in boys than in girls.[15,24] The observation that acute leukemia is more common in whites than nonwhites is primarily because of the increased peak incidence of ALL in whites between 3 and 5 years of age.[16,82] In contrast to ALL, acute nonlymphoid leu-

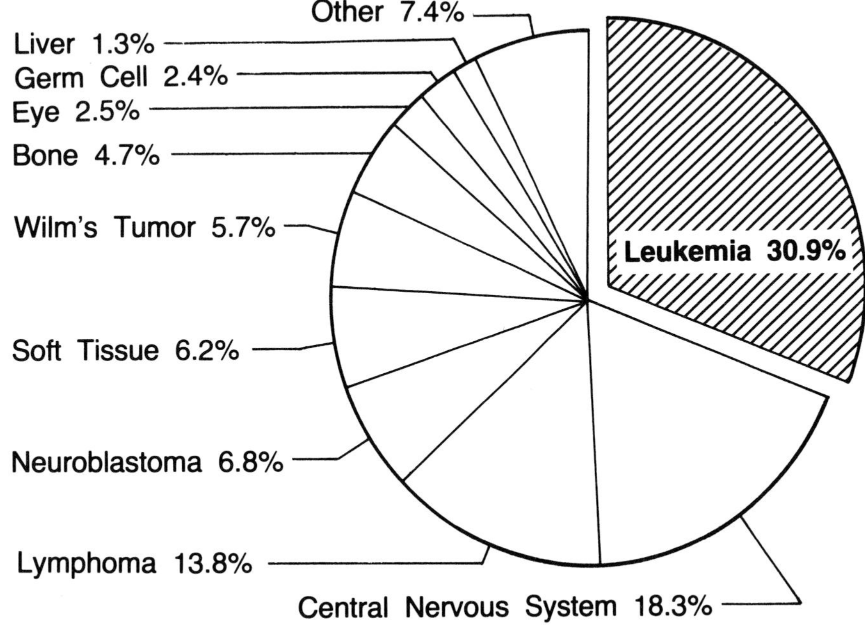

Fig. 224-1 Major forms of cancer in children (U.S. white children).

Modified from Altman AJ and Schwartz AD: Malignant diseases of infancy, childhood and adolescence, ed 2, Philadelphia, 1983, WB Saunders Co.

kemia (ANLL) in the United States shows no marked age peak.

TYPES OF LEUKEMIA

The leukemia syndromes seen in childhood can be classified as acute, chronic, congenital, and preleukemia. Acute leukemias are characterized by a predominance of immature hematopoietic precursors ("blasts") in the bone marrow and a fulminant natural course, resulting in the death of the patient within months unless effective treatment is instituted. In the chronic leukemias, it is the mature bone marrow elements that hyperproliferate, resulting in a condition with insidious onset of symptoms over months. Even without treatment, patients can survive for months to years following diagnosis of these chronic diseases. Congenital leukemia refers to conditions diagnosed in the first 4 weeks of life; they are discussed in more detail at the end of this chapter. The myeloproliferative and myelodysplastic syndromes are characterized by unexplained anemia, neutropenia, and/or thrombocytopenia and distorted maturation of bone marrow hematopoietic elements. These conditions, commonly referred to as "preleukemia" because of their frequent evolution into acute leukemia, are uncommon among children compared with adults.

The leukemias are also classified according to the predominant cell lines involved. This classification broadly divides the acute leukemias into lymphoblastic (ALL) and nonlymphoblastic forms (ANLL). Acute myelogenous leukemia (AML) is the most common subtype of childhood ANLL, followed by myelomonocytic leukemia (AMML), acute promyelocytic leukemia (APML), monocytic leukemia (AMOL), erythrocytic leukemia, and megakaryocytic leukemia. Very few cases are classified as undifferentiated leukemia (AUL) because of recent technologic advances in studies of lineage-specific immunologic surface markers and gene rearrangements. The chronic leukemias can also be divided into lymphocytic and myelogenous forms. Among children, chronic myelogenous leukemia (CML) is seen in 3% to 5% of patients diagnosed with leukemia (see Fig. 224-2). Chronic lymphocytic leukemia is extremely rare.

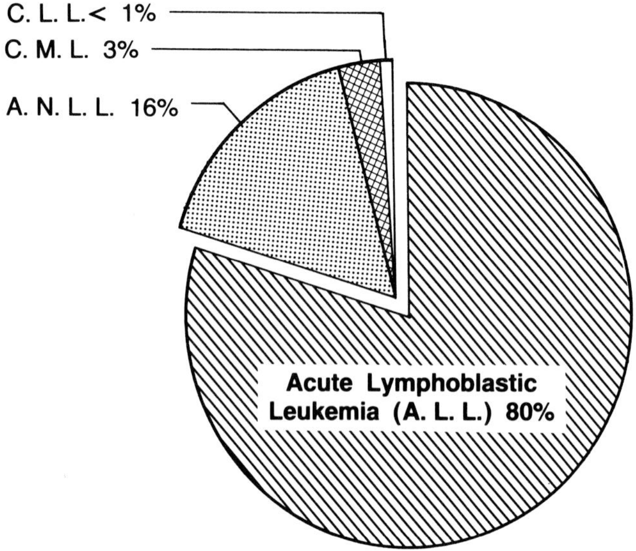

Fig. 224-2 The leukemias of childhood.

From Nathan DG and Oski FA: Hematology of infancy and childhood, ed 3, Philadelphia, 1987, WB Saunders Co.
ANLL, Acute nonlymphoid leukemia; CML, Chronic myelogenous leukemia; CLL, Chronic lymphatic leukemia.

LEUKEMOGENESIS

Normal cell growth is controlled by a complex series of events involving growth factors either produced by the cell itself, produced by other cells, or produced by cells in other tissues. Leukemia is a disorder of growth and proliferation in which one or more of these growth-regulating events go awry within a hematopoietic cell.

Clonal Expansion Theory

It is believed that most cases of leukemia result from a single damaged precursor cell that is capable of continued self-replication but that is unable to undergo further differentiation. The burden of leukemic cells increases, because these cells do not stop dividing. It appears that the disease is a manifestation of the expansion of a single clone of cells. The clonal origin of leukemia is best demonstrated by studies involving the isoenzymes of glucose 6-phosphate dehydrogenase and by cytogenetics.[19,78,84]

Leukemic Clusters

Numerous reports of "leukemic time-space clusters" have attracted intense epidemiologic study. The occurrence of a true leukemic cluster would suggest that a common etiologic factor or horizontal transmission of an infectious agent played a role in the development of leukemia. Careful statistical analysis has failed to demonstrate a truly increased incidence of leukemia in a given area or given time period. Results of intense study suggest that with the exception of Nagasaki and Hiroshima,[4] the reports of epidemics of leukemia can be explained purely by chance.[12,35,56] Inherent to such epidemiologic studies is the difficulty of appropriately defining the population at risk and identifying all the potential confounding events that could influence the outcome.

The exact cause of leukemia remains unknown. A number of contributing factors and possible predisposing conditions have been described, including genetic predisposition, immunodeficiency states, viruses, and environmental exposures. Our current understanding of the complicated nature of normal cellular proliferation and differentiation processes suggests that the etiology of leukemia will be equally complex, resulting from a series of multifactorial events involving "oncogenes," growth factors, and environmental conditions.

Etiology (see the box on p. 1331)

Familial Predisposition and Genetic Factors. The occurrence of familial leukemia,[20,74] the concordance of leukemia in monozygotic twins,[14] and the increased incidence of leukemia seen in patients with certain constitutional chro-

Factors Associated with Increased Risk for Childhood Leukemia[52]

FAMILIAL PREDISPOSITION

Twin of a patient with leukemia
Sibling of a patient with leukemia

GENETIC FACTORS

Down's syndrome
Fanconi anemia
Bloom syndrome
Ataxia telangiectasia
Wiskott-Aldrich syndrome
Neurofibromatosis
Poland syndrome
Klinefelter syndrome
Schwachman syndrome

ENVIRONMENTAL EXPOSURE

Viral infection
Ionizing radiation (atomic bomb and nuclear accidents)
Therapeutic radiation (ankylosing spondylitis, thymic enlargement)
Prenatal diagnostic radiation exposure
Certain drugs (benzene, alkylating agents)

mosomal abnormalities[36,49] are well documented observations suggesting that genetic factors play an important role in leukemogenesis. It is hypothesized that the preexisting chromosomal defect in patients with constitutional chromosomal abnormalities makes them more susceptible than normal to extrinsic environmental leukemogenic factors.[30] The frequent occurrence of one or more chromosomal abnormalities in the leukemia cells of patients is further evidence of the role of genetic events in the development of leukemia.[79,83]

Patients with congenital immune deficiency diseases such as Wiskott-Aldrich syndrome, ataxia telangiectasia, and congenital hypogammaglobulinemia all have an increased risk of lymphoid malignancy.[22,49] In addition, chronic therapy with immunosuppressive drugs has been associated with an increased risk of lymphoid malignancy.[57] The increased risk of malignancy in these individuals is thought to represent a breakdown in normal host "immune surveillance," allowing the proliferation of malignant clones.

Environmental Exposure (see the box above)

Viruses and Leukemias. Certain viruses are known to cause leukemia in animal models,[75] but the relationship of the leukemia that occurs in these species to human leukemia is uncertain. The role of retrovirus in human leukemogenesis has recently been demonstrated by the association of human T-cell leukemia virus (HTLV-1) and adult T-cell leukemia.[5] Epidemiologic studies have failed to show a link between exposure to cats or feline leukemia virus and development of leukemia in humans.[39] Epstein-Barr virus (EBV) infection, which causes infectious mononucleosis in humans, is also clearly associated with the African-type Burkitt's lymphoma.[17] Although a link has not yet been demonstrated, presumably EBV infection may be associated with B-cell leukemia (i.e., Burkitt lymphoma with bone marrow involvement).

The leukemogenic potential in humans of ionizing radiation exposure is well demonstrated by the following observations: (1) in the 1930s, the ninefold increased incidence of leukemia in radiologists compared with physicians who were not radiologists[43]; (2) the tenfold to twentyfold increased risk of leukemia in survivors of the atomic bomb explosions in Hiroshima and Nagasaki in 1945[9]; (3) the high incidence of leukemia in individuals who have received therapeutic radiation to treat ankylosing spondylitis, thymic enlargement, and tinea capitis[7]; and (4) the increased risk of all childhood cancers among children exposed to diagnostic radiation in utero.[34] Controversy persists regarding the role of diagnostic radiation exposure ex utero and development of human leukemia. Diagnostic ultrasound prenatally or postnatally, however, has not been associated with an increased risk for childhood leukemia.

Investigations of adult ANLL have provided considerable information regarding exposures to chemical carcinogens such as solvents and petroleum products that are associated with increased risk.[8,76] In part because of the relatively small number of cases of leukemia in children, a link between chemical exposure and childhood leukemia has not been demonstrated. A study completed by the Children's Cancer Study Group suggests that there may exist an environmental etiologic component in childhood disease similar to adult cases of ANLL.[63]

A number of studies have shown a link between secondary leukemogenesis and chemotherapy, especially alkylating agents, with or without radiation treatment. For example, acute leukemia, usually AML, has been observed in patients with Hodgkin's disease who have received cyclophosphamide or nitrogen mustard as part of therapy, usually with concomitant radiation treatment.[6,55]

Other factors studied for possible association with leukemia include exposure to electromagnetic fields, herbicides, pesticides, and maternal use of alcohol, contraceptives, diethylstilbestrol (DES), or cigarettes. Definitive links between these factors and the risk of childhood leukemia have not been confirmed.[29,52]

CLASSIFICATION

The leukemias of childhood, shown in Fig. 224-2, are actually a very heterogenous group of disorders that can be subclassified in terms of the level of differentiation (acute versus chronic) and the lineage (lymphoid versus myeloid) of the leukemogenic clone. Because the capacity to distinguish these leukemic cells, or "blasts," is therapeutically and prognostically important, various cytologic criteria have been established to differentiate them.[2,3,50,67] Newer approaches involving enzymatic,[21] surface marker,[23] cytogenetic,[42,79,83] and gene rearrangement studies[37,61,75] have also been employed.

Table 224-1 *Clinical and Laboratory Features in Diagnosis of Leukemia*

FEATURE	% OF ALL CHILDREN WITH ALL*	% OF ALL CHILDREN WITH ANLL†
Clinical		
Fever	61	34
Pallor	55	25
Bleeding (i.e., petechiae or purpura)	48	33
Anorexia or weight loss	33	22
Fatigue, malaise	30	19
Bone or joint pain	38	18
Lymphadenopathy	50	14
Hepatosplenomegaly	68	55
Swollen gingivae	—	8
Respiratory symptoms (i.e., sore throat, cough)	—	41
Recurrent infection	—	3
Neurologic	3	10
Laboratory		
Leukocyte count (mm^3)		
under 10,000	53	39
10,000 to 49,000	30	29
over 50,000	17	32
Hemoglobin (g/dl)		
under 7	43	41
7 to 11	45	48
over 11	12	11
Platelet count (mm^3)		
under 20,000	28	15
20,000 to 99,000	47	67
over 100,000	25	18
Coagulopathy	—	17

*Miller DR: Acute lymphoblastic leukemia, Pediatr Clin North Am 27:269, 1980.

†Choi SR and Simone JV: Acute nonlymphocytic leukemia in 171 children, Med Pediatr Oncol 2:119, 1976.

CLINICAL MANIFESTATIONS

Presenting Signs and Symptoms

Leukemia is a process of uncontrolled proliferation of immature hematopoietic cells resulting in suppression of normal hematopoiesis and extramedullary organ infiltration. The common presenting signs and symptoms reflect the degree of bone marrow compromise, the extent and location of leukemic cell infiltration, and the general systemic effects of these processes. In most cases, the presenting complaints have been present a few days, a few weeks, or more rarely, even months. The frequency of presenting complaints among children with ALL compared with ANLL are listed in Table 224-1.

Although fever is the most common feature, in the majority of patients it results from the leukemia itself rather than from infection. Pallor, fatigue, petechiae, pupura, and anorexia are frequently present. Significant weight loss is rare. Bone pain, lymphadenopathy, hepatomegaly, and splenomegaly are more common with ALL than with ANLL. Young children initially may limp or refuse to walk.

Laboratory Findings

Mild anemia and mild thrombocytopenia are common hematologic abnormalities (see Table 224-1). The white blood count (WBC) can be normal, decreased, or increased. Blasts are frequently but not always found in the peripheral blood smear.

Other laboratory studies are frequently abnormal in children newly diagnosed with acute leukemia. In addition to hyperuricemia, serum levels of calcium, potassium, phosphate, and lactic dehydrogenase may be elevated. This constellation of abnormalities is frequently referred to as "tumor lysis syndrome." The severity of these abnormalities is thought to reflect the total leukemic cell burden and the excessive production and rapid turnover of leukemia cells, because they are particularly problematic in patients with high initial white counts and extensive lymphadenopathy and hepatosplenomegaly.

Most patients have some extramedullary disease at the time of diagnosis. An anterior mediastinal mass is present in 5% to 10% of patients newly diagnosed with ALL, making a chest roentgenogram critical in the initial evaluation. Evidence of leukemic infiltration of the periosteum and bone is often present on the roentgenogram (including subperiosteal new bone formation, transverse metaphyseal radiolucent bands, osteolytic lesions, diffuse demineralization, and growth arrest lines), even in patients without complaints of bone pain.

Special Presentations

Central Nervous System (CNS) Disease. The most common site of clinically apparent extramedullary leukemia is the central nervous system; this type is present in up to 10% of patients at diagnosis. Children with CNS leukemia most frequently have increased intracranial pressure (i.e., vomiting, headache, lethargy, and papilledema), occasionally cranial nerve palsies, and in rare cases seizures or meningeal signs. Focal signs related to parenchymal involvement include hemiparesis, hemisensory losses, and seizure activity. Children under 2 years of age and those with T-cell ALL or M4 or M5 subtypes of ANLL have a higher incidence of CNS leukemia. Generally cord compression by epidural leukemic infiltrates is rare; it is more common in AML than in ALL.

Chloromas. Chloromas are solid tumor collections of immature myeloid cells, which can occur in ANLL patients. These tumors frequently involve periosteal and epidural regions of the head and neck but can occur anywhere on the body. Most interestingly, a rare chloroma has been reported to occur months or years before systemic signs of leukemia.

Testicular Leukemia. Although more commonly reported in patients with ALL, leukemic involvement of the testes in males with ANLL has been reported. Testicular leukemia presents with painless enlargement of one or both testes. Although rarely reported as an initial manifestation of ALL (less than 5% of patients) or ANLL, it is not uncommonly (15%) the first identifiable site of leukemia recurrence.

T-Cell Leukemia. T-cell ALL is characterized by several distinctive clinical features. It occurs more often in older males who have a high white blood count and often a mediastinal mass. These patients have a higher incidence of CNS leukemia. In addition they frequently have massive generalized lymphadenopathy and hepatosplenomegaly. This constellation of bulky infiltration of extramedullary sites has historically been referred to as "lymphomatous presentation" of leukemia.

Specific Clinical Features of ANLL Subtypes. Acute promyelocytic leukemia (M3 subtype) is more frequently associated with a spontaneous bleeding disorder than are the other variants of ANLL. Bleeding is the result of disseminated intravascular coagulation (DIC) and secondary fibrinolysis triggered by a substance contained within the cytoplasmic granules of the leukemic cells. Acute monoblastic leukemia (M4 and M5 subtypes) occurs at a younger age and is characterized by extensive extramedullary involvement at diagnosis, CNS involvement, leukemia cutis, lymphadenopathy, gingival hypertrophy, chloromas, DIC, elevated white blood count, and elevated serum muramidase. The M7 morphologic subtype of ANLL, or acute megakaryocytic leukemia, is particularly common in children who have Down's syndrome. The biopsy usually shows hypocellularity with myelofibrosis.

Preleukemia. These children typically will have less than 25% blasts in the bone marrow, circulating blasts, megaloblastosis, chromosomal abnormalities, and quantitative abnormalities of at least two of the three blood cell lines. Such patients may turn out to have juvenile CML, chronic myelomonocytic leukemia, or the monosomy 7 syndrome, which can precede the diagnosis of ANLL.

Diagnosis and Differential Diagnosis

The challenge for the physician in diagnosing pediatric leukemias is not that the symptoms are necessarily subtle, but that subtle differences exist between the symptoms of leukemia and those of more common illnesses or infectious conditions seen in children. The accompanying box lists the most common malignant and nonmalignant conditions that may masquerade as leukemia. Once suspicion is aroused that a patient may have leukemia, the diagnosis must be confirmed by bone marrow aspiration and the type of leukemia determined. Although leukemic cells may be identified in the peripheral blood of many patients at diagnosis, morphologic assessment of these cells may be misleading. Thus examination of the bone marrow is mandatory to establish the definitive diagnosis of leukemia. Bone marrow aspirate usually will provide sufficient material for diagnosis. Occasionally, however, a bone marrow biopsy may be required, particularly in patients with pancytopenia, in which case bone marrow failure must be excluded.

Normal bone marrow contains less than 5% blast cells. By definition, the diagnosis of acute leukemia is confirmed when more than 25% of the nucleated cells in the marrow are blasts; typically, 90% or more of the cells in the bone marrow are blast cells. The presence of 5% to 25% blast cells in the marrow suggests several diagnostic possibilities, including non-Hodgkin lymphoma with leukemic involvement, preleukemia or myelodysplastic syndromes, chronic myelogenous leukemia, or acute monoblastic leukemia, which can manifest with primarily extramedullary disease.

Differential Diagnosis of Childhood Acute Leukemia

NONMALIGNANT CONDITIONS

Juvenile rheumatoid arthritis
Systemic lupus erythematosus
Infectious mononucleosis
Idiopathic thrombocytopenic purpura
Pertussis, parapertussis
Aplastic anemia
Acute benign infectious lymphocytosis
Leukemoid reaction (more common in ANLL)
Bacterial sepsis with or without coagulopathy (more common in ANLL)
Osteomyelitis

MALIGNANCIES

Neuroblastoma
Lymphoma (especially if mediastinal mass, massive adenopathy, and organomegaly are present)
Retinoblastoma
Rhabdomyosarcoma
Ewing sarcoma
Chronic myelogenous leukemia

UNUSUAL PRESENTATIONS

Hypereosinophilic syndrome
Cord compression or cauda equina syndrome
Eosinophilic granuloma
Parenchymal brain lesion

A definitive diagnosis of the specific leukemic cell type is based on review of the morphologic appearance of the blast cells, use of histochemical stains such as myeloperoxidase and nonspecific esterases, enzymatic analysis, immunophenotyping, and cytogenetic analysis. These sophisticated techniques are important in establishing the specific leukemic cell type. It is essential therefore that the bone marrow aspiration or biopsy be performed in a center where cellular-differentiation techniques are routinely performed.

Leukemias must be differentiated from a variety of infectious illnesses. Patients with these infectious conditions may have fevers, rash, generalized lymphadenopathy, splenomegaly, peripheral blood lymphocytosis, and less frequently, thrombocytopenia or immunohemolytic anemia. Usually these diseases can be differentiated in terms of the morphologic appearance of reactive lymphocytes on the peripheral blood smear. Some conditions can be associated with a leukemoid reaction characterized by a reactive leukocytosis (WBC greater than or equal to 50,000 cells/mm^3) with an orderly progression of immature myeloid cells and occasional nucleated red blood cells. Ordinarily, with idiopathic thrombocytopenic purpura, children will not have splenomegaly, anemia, or neutropenia. Juvenile rheumatoid arthritis (JRA) and systemic lupus erythematosus (SLE) may be confused with ALL because of the common complaints of fever, anemia, malaise, and painful, swollen joints. Because there is no reliable, definitive laboratory test for JRA or SLE, a bone marrow aspiration may be necessary to exclude leukemia. The absence of lymphadenopathy and hepatosplenomegaly is an important differentiating feature in diagnosing aplastic anemia. When the bone marrow aspirate is hypocellular, it should be biopsied. Several pediatric malignancies may show bone marrow involvement; these include neuroblastoma, lymphoma, rhabdomyosarcoma, and Ewing's sarcoma. Additional laboratory and clinical evaluation may be necessary (e.g., urinary catecholamine, radiologic imaging) to exclude these malignancies.

TREATMENT

The goal of any antileukemic therapy is to eradicate the invading leukemic cells and their progenitors while preserving the expression of normal blood cell progenitors. Great strides have been made toward this goal as evaluation, primary combination chemotherapy, bone marrow transplantation, treatment alternatives for patients who relapse, and supportive care have become more sophisticated.

Prognostic Factors

Interest in prognostic factors came about in the late 1970s when therapy was successful in a majority of patients. Pediatric oncologists began looking for common features among groups of patients who did well compared with patients whose disease relapsed. Through retrospective analysis of disease-free survival, certain features present at the time of diagnosis were identified that were useful in predicting patients as having a good, fair, or poor prognosis.

A characteristic identified in a group of patients treated one way may not have the same sigificance if a different treatment is used. If therapy is adequate, then the bad prognostic factor will no longer predict a poor outcome. It is significant only to identify patients who need aggressive therapy. The real usefulness of prognostic factors is to allow "tailored therapy," or therapy that is altered for a patient or a group of patients based on clinical features of the disease present in the patient and associated with a higher or lower risk of relapse. Thus "good risk" patients are treated less aggressively in an attempt to minimize toxicity, whereas "poor risk" patients get more aggressive therapy to improve disease control.

In the treatment of ALL, the initial white blood count and age at diagnosis have been the two most reliable indicators of prognosis, both for remission duration and survival.[64] Patients who are very young at diagnosis (under 2 years of age) or older patients (over 10 years of age) have a relatively poor prognosis compared with patients in the intermediate age group.[68] The worst prognosis is for infants under 1 year of age. The presence of the Philadelphia chromosome has been consistently associated with a poor outcome among many study groups. Other clinical features that have been correlated with prognosis include sex, race, degree of organomegaly and lymphadenopathy, presence or absence of a mediastinal mass, cytogenetic features, initial hemoglobin levels, initial platelet count, cell subtype, immunologic subtype, immunoglobulin levels at diagnosis, the presence or absence of CNS leukemia at diagnosis, day-14 bone marrow response, and human leukocyte antigen (HLA) type. Because the prognostic importance is not reproducible among different study groups, the value of these variables remains controversial.

Since it is only recently that more than one third of patients with ANLL survive long term, prognostic factors in ANLL are less clearly defined than in ALL. A variety of clinical features are being examined as potentially important prognostic factors, including cytogenetic features, day-14 bone marrow response, the presence of Auer rods in affected cells, the blast cells' immune phenotype, in vitro growth characteristics, and in vitro response to chemotherapy. The factors accepted by most investigators to be associated with an unfavorable outcome are a white blood count over 100,000, monoblastic leukemia in infants, monosomy 7 karyotype, and presentation with a preleukemia syndrome.

Death from CML usually occurs within months of the acceleration phase. Therefore the major determinant of survival is the duration of the chronic phase. One study found peripheral blood and bone marrow blast counts at presentation to be correlated with survival.[13] The juvenile form of CML is notable for an extremely poor prognosis, with a median survival of less than 9 months from the time of diagnosis.

Acute Management

Initial Evaluation and Referral. The diagnostic evaluation of the child with probable leukemia has become more complex, requiring advanced laboratory techniques to perform appropriate cytogenetic, immunologic, and biochemical assays. The problems and complications in the child receiving leukemia therapy are frequently complex, requiring expert supportive care. A higher death rate has been reported in patients with ALL who were treated outside of a children's cancer center without a standard protocol.[45] For these reasons and because of the intensity of current regimens, children suspected of having one of the leukemias should be referred for diagnostic testing and treatment to pediatric cancer centers using cooperative group protocols.

The goal of initial management, often before the diagnosis has been confirmed, is to assure that the patient doesn't require urgent medical intervention before transfer. The major clinical problems needing to be addressed by the primary care physician and suggested emergency interventions are listed in the box on p. 1335. Many of these problems can be excluded as emergencies by careful history, physical examination, and review of the complete blood count. It is the rare patient who requires specific intervention before transfer to a pediatric oncology center. For most patients, initial management involves consultation with a pediatric oncologist, referral to a pediatric oncology center, and admission to the hospital. Admission to the hospital can be helpful in facilitating evaluation, necessary diagnostic testing, stabilizing metabolic status, starting chemotherapy, beginning patient and parent education, and building the foundation for long-term relationships between family and caretakers. A frequent exception to this is the patient with CML in the chronic phase at diagnosis, who can often be treated as an outpatient if medically stable.

The primary care physician plays a critical role in a smooth transition by preparing the child and family for what may lie ahead. This includes early communication of the facts positively—that is, this may be a "serious illness" and testing

Approach to Acute Management of Leukemia

A. Initial evaluation
History—Fatigue, malaise, anorexia, irritability, fever, bone pain, mouth sores
Physical examination—Pallor, petechiae, purpura, fever, lymphadenopathy, hepatosplenomegaly, respiratory distress, neurologic abnormalities
Laboratory—Complete blood count with differential and platelet count; abnormal results of one or more cell lines

B. Suspicion of leukemia as a possible diagnosis and potential emergency interventions

Observation	Intervention
Temperature over 38° C; neutrophil count under 500; Symptoms of infection	Blood culture; antibodies
Bleeding symptoms	Start intravenous unit for access and delivery of a fluid bolus; transfuse platelets, red cells or plasma
Respiratory distress	Chest roentgenogram; oxygen
WBC over 100,000	Blood urea nitrogen and creatinine, urate, serum potassium, serum calcium, serum phosphate; CXR; start intravenous unit for access and delivery of a fluid bolus

C. Referral to pediatric oncology center
Consult with a pediatric oncologist.
Arrange for transfer of patient to the pediatric oncology center.
Prepare patient and family for what to expect when they get there.

is important to determine the problem so that appropriate treatment can be started, emphasizing the need to enlist the help of other pediatric specialists. Follow-up communication between the referring physician, consulting physician, and family can be critical in establishing and maintaining a strong patient-family-physician relationship.

Supportive Care

Great strides in supportive care, including transfusion therapy, better infection control, and frequent use of indwelling central venous catheters, have contributed immensely to the decreased morbidity and mortality. The specific guidelines followed (i.e., choice of antibiotics, indwelling catheter care, isolation procedures, transfusion indications) may vary among institutions, based partly on the previous experience of the institution or investigators.

Blood Product Support. Myelosuppression with resultant anemia, thrombocytopenia, and neutropenia is frequently observed in these patients secondary to leukemia or chemotherapy-induced bone marrow hypoplasia or both. The radiation of blood products has prevented graft versus host disease in patients with severe bone marrow depression and immune suppression. Administration of cytomegalovirus (CMV)-negative blood products to patients with negative CMV antibody titer has decreased the incidence of transfusion-related CMV infection. More sophisticated techniques to test donor blood for evidence of infection such as hepatitis B, non-A, non-B hepatitis, and human immune deficiency virus (HIV) are effective in decreasing but not eradicating transfusion-transmitted infections.

Unless the anemia is rapid in onset (e.g., because of blood loss or hemolysis), red blood cell transfusion is not necessary until the hematocrit is 25 or less. Frozen deglycerolized or washed red blood cell products are leukocyte-poor and foreign antigen–poor, thus decreasing the risk or sensitization or alloimmunization to minor blood groups.

Platelets generally are transfused when the platelet count falls below 20,000 cells/mm^3, although the use of "prophylactic" platelet transfusion when platelet counts are higher remains controversial. Indications for platelet transfusion in the patient with thrombocytopenia, other than absolute platelet count, include fresh bleeding, fever, infection, or anticipated protracted thrombocytopenia as a result of therapy. The risks of platelet transfusion include alloimmunization and transmission of infection. Patients receiving frequent transfusions may become alloimmunized and refractory, requiring leukocyte-poor, single-donor platelets, or HLA-matched platelets to increase their platelet count.

Granulocyte transfusions are rarely used. Their value is generally limited to treatment of the patient with severe neutropenia with proven gram-negative sepsis or a perirectal abscess unresponsive to appropriate antibiotics. In addition to the risk of infection transmission, white blood cell transfusions are frequently associated with the uncomfortable side effects of fever, rigors, and allergic reactions, caused by sensitization to foreign leukocyte proteins.

Infection. Infectious complications are the most common cause of morbidity and mortality in these patients, second only to relapse of leukemia. Patients with leukemia who are receiving combination chemotherapy should be considered immunocompromised hosts. Neutropenia, which can result from chemotherapy-induced bone marrow hypoplasia, contributes to an increased susceptibility to bacterial and fungal infections.

Any febrile patient (i.e., axillary or oral temperature higher than 38° C—rectal temperatures should not be taken in patients with leukemia) with an absolute neutrophil count [ANC = WBC × (% neutrophils + % bands)] of less than 500 cells/mm^3 must be considered septic. Cultures should be obtained promptly, and the patient should be started immediately on intravenous broad-spectrum antibiotics. Since bowel, respiratory, and skin organisms are commonly identified, antibiotics that cover these gram-negative and gram-positive bacteria are used. Infections in patients with fever and neutropenia are presumably bacterial, although specific etiologic agents are not usually found. Prophylactic oral antibiotics have not proven useful. *Candida* and *Aspergillus* organisms are the major fungal pathogens reported. Prophylactic oral antifungal agents have not proven effective in preventing invasive disease. Amphotericin B is the treatment of choice for such fungal infections. Thus patients with neutropenia who remain febrile after 3 to 7 days of broad-spectrum antibiotics are usually treated empirically with amphotericin B, even before a definitive diagnosis of fungal disease is made.

Viral infections occur frequently in patients with leukemia, but rarely is specific therapy indicated. Before the routine use of varicella-zoster immunoglobulin and acyclovir, chickenpox was frequently complicated by pneumonitis, hepatitis, encephalitis, or even death. Acyclovir in particular has contributed to a notable decrease in morbidity and mortality from varicella-zoster, herpes zoster, and herpes simplex infections.

Pneumocystis carinii is another organism found to cause severe, often fatal interstitial pneumonitis in children receiving multiagent chemotherapy. Trimethoprim-sulfamethoxazole prophylaxis has been clearly demonstrated to reduce the incidence of *P. carinii* infections in the immunocompromised host.

Psychological Aspects. The emotional impact of the diagnosis of cancer is an immediate and lifelong one for both patients and families. No family member is left unaffected. Their lives are changed forever, but it is hoped not irreparably. For most children, leukemia will be chronic, life threatening, and yet treatable. Attention to the child's and family's adaptation to the phases of diagnosis, treatment, returning to "normal," and eventual survival is essential in truly comprehensive oncologic care.

The diagnosis of leukemia is a time of crisis. Feelings of anger, guilt, and loss of control are universal to patients of all ages, their parents, and their siblings. Siblings are often jealous of all the attention given to the patient, which adds to the parents' stress. In the midst of this distress, child and parent are asked to assimilate vast quantities of information regarding diagnosis, prognosis, procedures, treatments, side effects, and hospital or clinical routines. Communication should be gentle, accurate, realistic, hopeful, and above all honest. Several specific techniques can help families in these early adjustments. Frequent repetition of information and encouragement of any and all questions (they should be written down) is important. Whenever possible, the parents should be talked to together to prevent misunderstandings and to avoid making one parent responsible for relaying information and answering questions for the other. Educational materials written in layman's language are helpful supplements to verbal discussions. Information about the child's and the family's previous manner of coping with major events and previous experiences with cancer, serious illness, or death should be obtained from the primary physician and by family interview. Just as for successful medical outcome, a positive psychosocial outcome depends on early assessment, anticipation, prevention, and intervention for complications.

Regardless of the eventual outcome—good or bad—the treatment course is full of ups and downs, discomforts, uncertainties, and both illness- and non-illness-related stress. The patient and family continue to be challenged by the pressures of day-to-day events such as job, school, relocation, marriage, family, financial burdens, and other family illness, injury, or death, which may even precede the diagnosis of leukemia. In addition, illness-related stress factors such as separation of family members, frequent traveling, disruption of normal routine, sleep interruptions, child care arrangements, the high financial cost of care, and the threat of death take an extreme emotional toll on the child and family.

During the course of therapy there are several times that can be extremely stressful and the need for increased support anticipated. Ironically, getting back to "normal" either at the time of hospital discharge, upon return to school, or at the completion of therapy is very anxiety provoking. Every effort should be made to encourage the child to return to normal social, school, and physical activities as soon as possible. Early communication among family, school, and medical personnel is essential to a smooth reentry into normal routines.

Perhaps more devastating than initial diagnosis is the news of disease recurrence or the realization that all treatments have failed and that the child will die. At relapse, families must start the treatment process all over again, although with a smaller chance for successful outcome. They will need, more than ever before, the support of the health care team to enable them to go on. When cure is no longer possible, one must always leave room for hope. Hope can come from changing the focus toward palliative care, with comfort as the goal. Thus the efforts of the health care team—oncologists, psychosocial workers, family physician, and family—must be redirected toward comfort measures. Physical measures would include controlling pain and bleeding without invasive diagnostic or treatment procedures. Frequent reassurances that the child and family will not be left alone are of the utmost importance in providing good, successful palliative care. At this point, perhaps more than ever before, support must be given to staff members who in turn provide the most support for the child and family.

Chemotherapy

Table 224-2 lists the various chemotherapeutic agents used in treating childhood leukemias and the complications associated with their use. The specific indications for their use are described below in the discussions of therapy for each type of childhood leukemia.

Table 224-2 *Use and Complications of Chemotherapeutic Agents in Acute Leukemia*

DRUG	ROUTE	COMMON USE	ACUTE TOXICITY	DELAYED TOXIC EFFECTS
Prednisone	PO	Induction and maintenance of ALL	Hyperglycemia, hypertension, emotional lability, increased appetite, fluid retention, weight gain, striae, cushingoid facies, peptic ulcer, diabetes mellitus	Osteoporosis, growth retardation, aseptic necrosis, cataracts, glaucoma, diabetes mellitus
Vincristine	IV	Induction and maintenance of ALL	Alopecia, constipation, paralytic ileus, peripheral neuropathy, jaw pain, SIADH*, danger with extravasation, in rare cases, myelosuppression	Peripheral neuropathy
6-Mercaptopurine	PO	Maintenance of ALL	Alopecia, nausea, vomiting, diarrhea, myelosuppression, hepatic damage, cholestasis	Hepatic disease, cholestasis
Methotrexate	PO, IM, IV	Maintenance of ALL	Nausea, vomiting, mucositis, rash, myelosuppression, hepatic damage, renal toxicity	Hepatic damage, neurotoxicity
Methotrexate and/or cytosine arabinoside	Intrathecal	CNS prophylaxis of ALL and ANLL	Nausea, vomiting, headache, stiff neck, arachnoiditis, seizures	Cortical atrophy, leukoencephalopathy
L-Asparaginase	IM	Induction and consolidation of ALL	Anaphylaxis, nausea, vomiting, fever, chills, hyperglycemia, diabetes, abdominal pain, pancreatitis (increased amylase), CNS depression, coagulation defects with thrombosis or hemorrhage (i.e., stroke), hypoproteinemia, hepatic damage	Pancreatic or hepatic damage, diabetes mellitus
Doxorubicin	IV	Induction and consolidation of ALL	Myelosuppression, alopecia, nausea, vomiting, mucositis, anorexia, hepatic damage, cardiac arrhythmias, red urine, danger with extravasation	Cardiomyopathy, hepatic damage
Daunorubicin	IV	Induction and maintenance of ALL	Myelosuppression, alopecia, nausea, vomiting, cardiac arrhythmias, hepatic damage, red urine, danger with extravasation	Cardiomyopathy
Cytosine arabinoside	IV	Induction and maintenance of ANLL	Myelosuppression, alopecia, nausea, vomiting, diarrhea, mucositis, conjunctivitis, fever, neurotoxicity	Hepatic damage, neurotoxicity
Etoposide	IV	Induction and maintenance of ANLL	Hypotension, anaphylaxis, myelosuppression, nausea, vomiting, alopecia, mucositis, danger with extravasation	
6-Thioguanine	PO	Induction and maintenance of ANLL	Same as for mercaptopurine but less hepatic toxicity	
Radiation		ALL CNS prophylaxis	Alopecia, nausea, vomiting, skin hypersensitivity, mild myelosuppression	Sleeping syndrome, seizures, leukoencephalopathy, growth retardation

**SIADH*, Syndrome of inappropriate secretion of antidiuretic hormone.

Data compiled from Dorr RT and Fritz WL: Cancer chemotherapy handbook, New York, 1980, Elsevier Science Publishing Co, Inc.

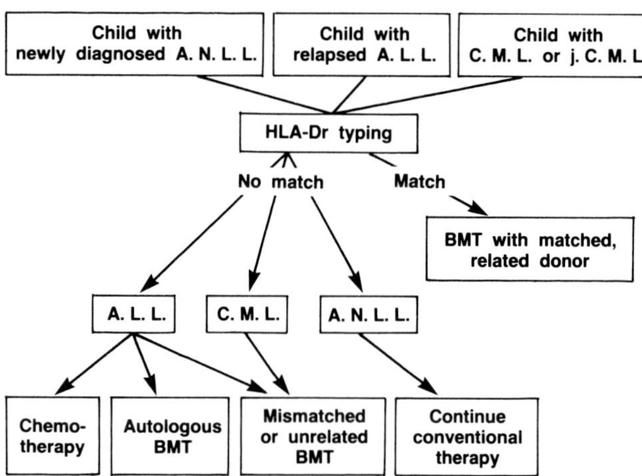

Fig. 224-3 Flow diagram of marrow transplantation for children with leukemia.

From Trigg ME: Bone marrow transplantation and treatment of leukemia in children, Pediatr Clin North Am 35:939, 1988.

Bone Marrow Transplantation

Bone marrow transplantation (BMT) involves the initial administration of intensive cytoreductive therapy—usually total body irradiation and high-dose chemotherapy—designed to eradicate 100% of the leukemia cells. This therapy is so intense that it also is lethal to normal bone marrow cells. Therefore it must be followed by bone marrow rescue with intravenously infused bone marrow from a compatible donor. For allogeneic bone marrow transplant, the donor is an HLA-matched sibling. Unfortunately, only approximately one third of patients who experience a relapse are likely to have an HLA-identical sibling. For these reasons the role of bone marrow transplantation has historically been somewhat limited. With advances of transplantation biology, however, alternatives are being studied, such as autologous donation or transplantation from partially matched related donors (i.e., parents) or from matched unrelated donors. The role of current BMT alternatives for treatment of leukemia in children is shown in Fig. 224-3.

BMT can be associated with significant complications. In addition to the anticipated side effects of the cytoreductive chemotherapy such as nausea, vomiting, mucositis, anorexia, and prolonged bone marrow aplasia, there may be transplant-related problems of graft rejection, graft versus host disease, and hepatic venoocclusive syndrome. As with all the intensive treatment regimens, infections such as bacterial sepsis, invasive fungal disease, cytomegalovirus interstitial pneumonitis, and *P. carinii* pneumonia are a significant cause of morbidity and mortality, particularly during the first 6 months after transplantation.

ACUTE LYMPHOBLASTIC LEUKEMIA

Most ALL treatment regimens divide therapy into three phases: remission induction, CNS prophylaxis and consolidation, and maintenance treatment during remission.

Induction

The aim of the initial treatment of ALL is induction of remission. Complete remission is defined as the absence of clinical signs and symptoms of disease in the presence of a normal blood count and a normocellular bone marrow with 5% or fewer blasts. There is no evidence, however, that clinical disappearance of leukemic cells in the bone marrow indicates their total eradication.

Although the basic two-drug combination of vincristine and prednisone can induce remission in approximately 85% of children with ALL, the addition of L-asparaginase or an anthracycline improves their remission induction rate to approximately 95% and improves remission duration.[25,44,69]

Although 4 weeks generally is required to achieve complete remission, in most cases there is a marked regression of symptoms, organomegaly, and peripheral blasts within the first week of treatment. Hospitalization during this time is common. Pancytopenia is routinely seen as a result of leukemia and chemotherapy-induced bone marrow suppression. These patients are often transfusion dependent for red cells and platelets and often require prophylactic antibiotics for treating fever with neutropenia.

Central Nervous System Prophylaxis

As soon as bone marrow remission has been achieved, CNS prophylaxis is instituted. The optimum and least toxic prophylaxis has not been fully determined. Investigators at St. Jude Children's Research Hospital showed that the administration of cranial spinal irradiation could reduce the incidence of CNS relapse to approximately 10%.[1] Because of the excessive myelosuppression and subsequent growth disturbances associated with spinal irradiation, the use of cranial irradiation plus intrathecal methotrexate was universally adopted as the standard form of CNS preventive therapy in the 1970s. In recent years, however, concern has been raised regarding the apparent adverse effects of this form of CNS preventive therapy on neurologic and intellectual function. Reduction in the dose of cranial irradiation may be as effective, but it is not clear whether a lower dose is associated with a lower incidence of CNS sequelae. Other approaches studied include triple intrathecal chemotherapy with methotrexate, cytosine arabinoside, and hydrocortisone; intermediate-dose systemic methotrexate, either alone or with concomitant intrathecal methotrexate; intrathecal methotrexate alone; or high-dose systemic methotrexate. For patients at standard risk, cranial irradiation does not appear to be necessary; intrathecal methotrexate alone appears to offer adequate CNS preventive therapy.

Maintenance Therapy

The rationale for continuing to treat patients in complete continuous remission is based on historical studies in which therapy was discontinued immediately[26] or 6 months after induction of remission.[41] In both studies, relapse rapidly followed discontinuation of treatment. The backbone of most maintenance regimens includes daily 6-mercaptopurine orally, weekly parenteral methotrexate, postinduction doses of vincristine IV, and oral prednisone at a variety of intervals. These regimens frequently incorporate anthracyclines, asparaginase, and cytosine arabinoside for high-risk patients.

Currently the optimum duration of therapy is unknown. Most centers continue treatment for a period of approximately 2½ to 3 years. For patients who successfully complete a full course of maintenance therapy, the prognosis is generally good. A study from St. Jude Children's Research Hospital demonstrated that approximately 80% of patients who complete therapy following this period remain disease free. Of the 20% who eventually relapse, most do so in the first year of therapy.[27] The risk of relapse after 4 disease-free years is virtually nonexistent.[25]

Relapse Therapy

Most patients who relapse have a grave prognosis. Several factors such as the duration of first remission, whether relapse occurs during or after completion of therapy, and the site of relapse have been identified—factors that have some predictive value in determining the outcome of subsequent therapy. The most common site of relapse in ALL is the bone marrow. Relapse at any site must be presumed to be associated with systemic reseeding of leukemic cells. Therefore patients with clinically localized relapses must be treated both locally and systemically with reinduction therapy and reprophylaxis of the CNS. Most patients who have ALL can readily be induced into a second remission; however, the duration of these remissions is generally less than 1 year, and long-term remissions are infrequent.

Bone Marrow Transplantation

The current role of bone marrow transplantation in the treatment of ALL is for patients who have relapsed and a select few patients during their first remission (i.e., patients who are Philadelphia chromosome positive). For patients who experience a bone marrow relapse and are fortunate enough to have an HLA-identical sibling, bone marrow transplantation should be strongly considered. Patients "transplanted" in remission are better than if the procedure is attempted in relapse; and those transplanted earlier in their disease (i.e., in second remission) do better than those who receive transplantations after multiple previous relapses.[10,11]

ACUTE NONLYMPHOBLASTIC LEUKEMIA

Progress in the treatment of children with ANLL has not kept pace with advances in the treatment of childhood ALL. As a result of new chemotherapeutic strategies, better supportive care, and improved transplantation technology, overall survival has increased for children with ANLL, especially for those with the AML and APML subtypes. In contrast to ALL, current treatment of ANLL is very intensive for all patients.

Induction

Historically, induction therapy has invariably included cytosine arabinoside (Ara-C) and anthracycline, usually daunorubicin.[70] Approximately 70% to 80% of children achieve complete remission with these two drugs. The duration of severe marrow hypoplasia with peripheral pancytopenia during a typical ANLL induction ranges from 21 to 35 days. The leukemic blasts of almost half of the 20% to 30% of patients who fail to achieve remission are refractory to the standard Ara-C and daunorubicin combination. For this group new alternatives for treatment are being studied, including high-dose Ara-C or different drugs (e.g., etoposide, amsacrine, 5-azacytidine).

CNS Prophylaxis

Without some form of CNS prophylaxis, approximately 10% to 30% of children with AML will have an initial relapse in their central nervous system. Apparently effective CNS prophylaxis regimens consist of intrathecal Ara-C or methotrexate and/or cranial radiation. High-dose intravenous Ara-C also probably has some activity against CNS leukemia.

Maintenance Therapy

The principles of treatment in ANLL remission are similar to those of ALL, but the strategy differs. Much more intensive treatment appears necessary. The consequence of such intense chemotherapy programs is severe myelosuppression and its attendant complications. The need for maintenance therapy beyond the induction-intensification phases remains a controversial issue to be addressed by future studies. There are data to support either conclusion. In part, the answer to questions of optimum duration and drug combinations depends on the exact nature and intensity of the therapeutic program used for induction and intensification.

Bone marrow transplantation from an HLA-identical donor is a therapeutic alternative to conventional intensification chemotherapy. Five-year leukemia-free survival is reported to be 50% to 60% of children with AML who are treated by allogeneic transplantation following chemotherapeutic induction of complete remission.[18,72,73] Although leukemia-free survival seems slightly better than that achieved with chemotherapy, the price of bone marrow transplantation in terms of toxicity is high. The best approach is uncertain. Several institutions recommend that children with AML who have donors should first receive a trial of intensive chemotherapy and be transplanted only if they relapse. There are several groups of children such as those with preleukemia syndromes, monosomy 7, and monocytic leukemia (M5 subtype) who have been identified as very high risk for induction failure. For these children, perhaps bone marrow transplantation should be the initial therapeutic approach. It is acceptable practice to perform HLA typing on children and family members when the initial diagnosis of ANLL is made so that options can be established and potentially hazardous transfusions from donors or family members can be excluded. Many centers will harvest bone marrow on all ANLL patients during the first remission and hold it in reserve for use in the event of relapse. As technology improves, bone marrow transplantation from unrelated or partially mismatched family members will become a more reasonable approach for ANLL patients in second remission.

Relapse Therapy

Approximately 50% of children with ANLL who have relapsed or were refractory to initial therapy may be induced into a complete remission with one of a number of investigational treatment regimens such as daunorubicin and cyclocytidine or Ara-C, amasacrine and cyclocytidine, and etoposide and 5-azacytidine.[31,47] The duration of remission has been short for most of these patients. If a second remission is induced, bone marrow transplantation offers the only chance for a cure.

CHRONIC MYELOGENOUS LEUKEMIA

Chronic myelogenous leukemia is rare in children. In childhood, the disorder may appear as two distinct clinical syndromes—adult-type CML, which is virtually indistinguishable from that seen in older patients, and juvenile CML, a disease relatively restricted to very young children and with distinct clinical, laboratory, and cytogenetic features.

Adult-Type CML

The adult form of CML is a clonal myeloproliferative disorder involving all of the blood progenitor lineages and at least some of the lymphoid lineages. It is characterized by expansion of the total body granulocyte pool, myeloid hyperplasia of the bone marrow, extramedullary hematopoiesis, and a specific cytogenetic marker, the Philadelphia chromosome.

The natural history of CML is divided into three phases—chronic, accelerated, and blastic. These phases represent the progressive shift in the nature of the disorder from hyperproliferation, with production of mainly mature blood elements, to production of predominately immature blast cells.

Chronic Phase

The signs and symptoms of CML usually develop insidiously over several months. Patients usually have nonspecific complaints such as fever, night sweats, fatigue, decreased exercise tolerance, weakness, left upper quadrant pain, and early satiation of appetite. Marrow hyperplasia and marrow space expansion may result in bone pain and tenderness. The usual physical findings are pallor, low-grade fever, ecchymoses, sternal tenderness, and hepatosplenomegaly. Neurologic abnormalities, visual difficulties, papilledema, retinal hemorrhages, respiratory distress with tachypnea, or priapism may complicate cases in which there is marked hyperleukocytosis.

Peripheral blood counts typically demonstrate a normochromic, normocytic anemia (mean hematocrit of 25%), marked leukocytosis with "a shift to the left," and thrombocytosis (mean platelet count of 500,000/mm^3). The white blood count at diagnosis ranges from approximately 8000 to 800,000 cells/mm^3. Review of the peripheral blood smear is remarkable for (1) increased numbers of myeloid cells at all stages of differentiation, (2) myeloblasts and promyelocytes accounting for less than 15% of the total white blood cell differential count, (3) basophilia, and (4) eosinophilia.[66] In the bone marrow, granulocytes at all stages of maturation are seen in increased numbers, although their morphologic appearance is normal. The finding of the Philadelphia chromosome in approximately 90% of patients is pathognomonic for CML. The laboratory finding of a decrease in leukocyte alkaline phosphatase (LAP) activity is quite helpful diagnostically. LAP activity is increased in a number of conditions that can be differentiated including infection, leukemoid reaction, during hematologic remission of CML, and a blast crisis of CML. Other common laboratory abnormalities include elevation of serum uric acid and lactate dehydrogenase levels.

Before initiating any specific antileukemic therapy, consideration must be given first to the following special management problems and their treatment: hyperuricemia, hyperkalemia, hyperphosphatemia, priapism, and the neurologic, retinal, or pulmonary complications of leukostasis. The goal of treatment in the chronic phase is to provide symptomatic relief by correcting the leukocytosis and organomegaly. The standard approach to chronic phase CML is with single-agent chemotherapy, usually busulfan or hydroxyurea. Hydroxyurea is the drug of choice in children because of its increased margin of hematologic safety and its decreased systemic toxicity relative to busulfan. Both drugs must be carefully monitored and dosages adjusted according to hematologic response.

Conventional therapy rarely produces a true complete remission. Although the complete blood count may normalize and the organomegaly disappear, the bone marrow continues to show granulocyte hyperplasia and Philadelphia chromosome–positive metaphases. Attempts to ablate the Philadelphia chromosome–positive clone with aggressive multiagent chemotherapy have not been successful. Therapy does not delay acceleration to blast crisis or to prolong survival.

Acceleration Phase

Inevitably, patients develop a more malignant form of their disease. This blast crisis may be heralded by a 3- to 6-month transitional phase referred to as the acceleration phase or metamorphosis. The clinical features observed in this transitional period include basophilia, new-onset thrombocytosis or thrombocytopenia, leukocytosis refractory to previous therapies, anemia, and splenomegaly. Therapy should be instituted to prevent the complications of this accelerated phase of disease—renewed leukostasis, organomegaly, and hyperproliferation. No therapy short of bone marrow transplantation has been shown to prevent the inevitable development of a blastic phase and death in CML.

Blast Crisis

Acute blastic transformation occurs at a median of about 3 years and is responsible for at least 75% of deaths in CML. Leukostasis and very high WBC counts are more common in the blast phase. The blastic phase is quite refractory to chemotherapy regardless of whether the blastic transformation is myeloblastic or lymphoblastic. Median survival after blastic transformation is only 3 to 6 months. Long-term remissions have been reported in patients receiving allogeneic bone marrow transplantation while they are in an accelerated or blastic phase, although the results are generally disappointing.

Bone Marrow Transplantation

Allogeneic bone marrow transplantation is the only curative approach now available for patients with CML. Disease status at the time of transplantation is the most powerful predictor of survival. Most centers, therefore, currently recommend bone marrow transplantation for any child with the adult-type CML in the chronic phase who has an HLA-matched donor, preferably within 1 year of diagnosis. Autologous transplantation has been used as a temporizing approach, the objective being to restore the chronic phase. The bone marrow is reconstituted with Philadelphia chromosome–positive cells. Therefore, although the chronic phase may be reestablished and survival prolonged, this technique is not curative. Advances in bone marrow transplantation technology have allowed successful unrelated donor transplantation and cure for small numbers of patients with CML. For the patient without an HLA-matched sibling, this is the only alternative approach currently available with curative potential.

Juvenile Chronic Myelogenous Leukemia

Juvenile chronic myelogenous leukemia (JCML) is a myeloproliferative disorder seen mainly in infants and characterized by leukocytosis, splenomegaly, and decreased leukocyte alkaline phosphatase activity.[33] Despite these clinical similarities to the adult form of CML, JCML is clearly distinguishable with respect to clinical presentation, hematologic manifestations, cytogenetic analysis, response to therapy, and prognosis (see Table 224-3).

Distinctive clinical features common to JCML at diagnosis include patient under 2 years of age, persistent respiratory infections (with tachypnea, chronic cough, wheezing), prominent lymphadenopathy, skin rash (eczema, xanthomata, and cafe-au-lait spots), bleeding, and failure to thrive. In addition to anemia and leukocytosis, frequent laboratory findings are thrombocytopenia, monocytosis, and nucleated red blood cells in the peripheral blood. Cytogenetic analysis may be abnormal, but the Philadelphia chromosome is never found.

Most patients with JCML die secondary to infection. Chemotherapy is of limited value. Patients with JCML usually do not respond to busulfan or hydroxyurea. Bone marrow transplantation offers the only hope of cure at present and is the treatment of choice for the patient with a histocompatible sibling.

CONGENITAL LEUKEMIA

Congenital leukemia may be apparent at birth or may develop within the first month of life. The majority of patients described with this rare disorder had AML, although ALL has been reported in newborns.[77] The etiology of congenital leukemia is unknown. Leukemia in the neonatal period has been associated with Down syndrome, Turner syndrome, mosaic

Table 224-3 *Differences Between Adult and Juvenile Forms of CML*

AGE AT ONSET	ADULT FORM	JUVENILE FORM
Chromosome studies	Philadelphia chromosome–positive	Philadelphia chromosome–negative
	Usually over 2 years	Usually under 2 years
Physical findings		
Facial rash	Absent	Present
Lymphadenopathy	Occasional	Frequent with tendency to suppuration
Splenomegaly	Marked	Variable
Hemorrhagic manifestations	Absent	Frequent
Hematologic findings		
WBC at onset	Usually over 100,000/mm^3	Usually under 100,000/mm^3
Monocytosis of peripheral blood and bone marrow	Absent	Usually present
Thrombocytopenia	Uncommon at onset	Frequent at onset
Red blood cell abnormalities		
Ineffective erythropoiesis	Absent	Present
I antigen on red blood cell	Normal	Reduced
Fetal hemoglobin levels	Normal	15% to 50%
Normoblasts in peripheral blood	Unusual	Frequent
Other laboratory findings		
Urinary and serum muramidase	Slightly elevated	Markedly elevated
Immunologic abnormalities	None	Strikingly high immunoglobin levels, high incidence of antinuclear antibodies (52%) and anti-IgG antibodies (43%)
Nature of colonies produced in vitro from peripheral blood	Predominantly granulocytic	Predominantly monocytic
Response to busulfan	Uniform good	Poor
Median survival	2.5 to 3 years	Less than 9 months

Modified from Altman AJ and Schwartz AD: Malignant diseases of infancy, childhood and adolescence, Philadelphia, 1983, WB Saunders Co.

monosomy 7, and trisomy 9. No reported cases of congenital leukemia have occurred in infants born to women who had leukemia before or during pregnancy.

The clinical manifestations are similar to those seen with leukemia in older children except that leukemia cutis is more common. These blue-gray skin nodules represent areas of skin infiltration by leukemic cells. Petechiae, purpura, hepatosplenomegaly, and poor feeding are common findings in the newborn with leukemia. The laboratory findings include thrombocytopenia and hyperleukocytosis.

Congenital leukemia must be differentiated from a number of conditions often found in the neonatal period, including congenital syphilis, intrauterine viral infection (cytomegalovirus, rubella, toxoplasmosis), neuroblastoma, congenital thrombocytopenic purpura, leukemoid reaction in response to sepsis, hypoxemia, erythroblastosis fetalis, and the transient myeloproliferative syndrome associated with Down syndrome. Myeloproliferative disorders, which are clinically and hematologically indistinguishable from congenital AML, have been reported in newborns with Down syndrome.[77] These disorders are transient and typically will resolve completely within weeks or months of diagnosis without specific antileukemia treatment. There is no test available that can distinguish infants with this transient disorder from infants with true congenital leukemia. Conservative therapy with close monitoring and supportive care as needed is recommended for 6 to 8 weeks to differentiate between these two disorders.

The treatment of congenital leukemia is identical to treatment for the older child except that cranial irradiation is omitted. The results in general have been disappointing, with many infants dying within a few days to months after diagnosis. A majority of recently reported cases of congenital AML were of the monocytic (M5) subtype. For this group of patients, treatment with etoposide and/or tenoposide has been particularly effective.[54]

LATE EFFECTS: THE AGONY OF SUCCESS

The advent of more successful therapy has been accompanied by a growing concern over the physical and psychological well-being of the survivors of these aggressive protocols. Studies of late effects of the leukemias of childhood and their treatment, but particularly of ANLL and CML, are severely limited because of the small numbers that have been studied. The discussion of late effects pertains to studies of survivors of ALL, because similar data regarding the survivors of ANLL or CML does not exist.

Major areas of concern identified in survivors of ALL include second malignancies, CNS damage, endocrine abnormalities with growth failure and reproductive dysfunction, cardiac toxicity, and psychological morbidity. Preliminary results of clinical research suggest that the likelihood and the type and severity of sequelae are at least in part related to (1) the patient's age at the time of diagnosis and institution of treatment, (2) the specific treatment used, and (3) the treatment intensity. Interpretation of clinical data related to the management of long-term survivors is complicated by uncertainty as to whether a particular problem existed before the diagnosis of cancer, whether the problem is secondary to the treatment or to the life-threatening illness itself, or whether all three scenarios are involved.

Truly successful treatment of childhood cancer must incorporate care of the long-term survivor. This not only involves recognizing what delayed consequences can emerge after cancer therapy but actual follow-up with history, physical examination, and appropriate laboratory testing to monitor the patient's status and provide treatment for any problems that are identified. Unfortunately for both the patient and the physician, there are as yet no firm guidelines as to the best method of monitoring cured patients for delayed physical or psychological sequelae. Recommendations for pertinent follow up must be individualized according to the anticipated problems, based on the patient's disease, therapeutic history, and duration of disease-free, off-therapy survival.

Second Malignancy

The risk of developing a second malignancy following apparently successful therapy of leukemia is estimated to be 3% to 12%.[40,46] Both genetics and treatment have been implicated in this increased risk, which is 20 times greater than the risk observed in the general population. The majority of second tumors seen among survivors of childhood ALL are second leukemias or non-Hodgkin lymphomas. Whether these represent a second carcinogenic event or a different manifestation of the primary malignant process is unknown. Brain tumors account for almost one third of secondary solid tumors, and the prognosis is poor.

In follow-up studies of a child with ALL, especially if cranial irradiation has been employed for prophylactic CNS treatment, the head and neck should be inspected carefully, since most secondary carcinomas (thyroid, basal cell, parotid gland) have occurred in this region.[59] Biopsy is recommended as soon as possible for any suspicious skin lesions, nodules, or firm, enlarged lymph nodes that do not respond completely to a trial of antibiotic therapy. If seizures, severe headaches, or symptoms of increased intracranial pressure occur in the absence of an obvious clinical explanation, computed tomography (CT) or magnetic resonance imaging (MRI) studies should be done before lumbar puncture to ensure that an intracranial mass is not present.

Central Nervous System Damage

Before the use of effective prophylaxis, the central nervous system was the most frequent site of first relapse in children with ALL. Currently, CNS prophylaxis prevents isolated CNS relapse in more than 90% of patients. The functional and structural CNS changes found in long-term survivors of ALL in continuous remission following effective CNS prophylaxis are less frequent and less severe than in patients who relapse with CNS involvement.

The absolute incidence and natural history of long-term neurologic sequelae, including memory and learning problems, in patients treated with intrathecal chemotherapy and cranial radiation therapy is unknown. Both acute and subacute forms of neurotoxicity have been reported in patients treated with the current methods of CNS prophylaxis.[53] These abnormalities include structural changes, as evidenced by ventricular dilation, calcifications, focal areas of parenchymal hypodensity, and cortical atrophy visible on CT scan. Functional changes with intellectual deficits, poor memory skills, low IQ scores, and poor school performance have also been described. Further investigation is required to determine if a correlation exists between these structural and functional CNS changes. Severe permanent neurologic sequelae such as a seizure disorder, residual hearing loss, and hemiplegia are observed almost exclusively in children who are cured after one or more CNS relapses.

In view of the follow-up information currently available, it is clear that ongoing assessment of neurologic function, developmental milestones, school and work performance, behavior, and quality of life must be an integral part of maintaining of health care for the survivor of childhood leukemia.

Endocrine Abnormalities

Endocrine abnormalities involving the hypothalmic-pituitary axis are probably secondary to cranial irradiation, whereas gonadal dysfunction is probably secondary to chemotherapy. Younger age may increase the risk for subsequent growth problems and decrease the risk for gonadal dysfunction.

Abnormally low amounts of growth hormone have been found in children with ALL treated with cranial irradiation. Although growth velocities after therapy is completed are not significantly decreased in these children, their final adult height is reduced.[62] Studies are needed to assess the correlations between various treatments, age at diagnosis, growth hormone secretion, pubertal development, and final height attained. The benefits of growth hormone therapy are unknown, since there are conflicting results from different investigators.[65,80]

Follow-up studies of long-term survivors of ALL treated with cranial irradiation demonstrate approximately a 3% to 5% incidence of hypothyroidism and less than a 1% incidence of secondary thyroid malignancies. Palpation of the thyroid, review of hypothyroidism symptoms, and a low threshold for checking serum triiodothyronine and thyroid-stimulating hormone levels should be incorporated into the routine visit of survivors.

Data on infertility and gonadal function in this group are largely unavailable. Studies in this area are complicated by the young age in the majority of the patients and the lack of an adequate way of measuring eventual reproductive capabilities. The development of secondary sex characteristics does not necessarily mean that germinal cells are present or functional. Oligospermia related to previous chemotherapy frequently improves with time. Patients who received bilateral testicular radiation to treat testicular leukemia are generally sterile. There is virtually no information available about reproductive capabilities of girls. Pubertal progression is more likely to be normal in girls who had leukemia and chemotherapy before the onset of puberty and menarche.

Cardiac Toxicity

The anthracyclines are a vital component of the current antileukemia armamentarium for the majority of patients. The incidence of severe cardiomyopathy has been decreased by limiting the cumulative dose to approximately 350 mg/m^2, frequent monitoring during therapy with electrocardiograms and echocardiograms, and discontinuing the anthracycline if any signs of toxicity (i.e., decreased fractional shorting, arrhythmias) are observed. Unfortunately, in some patients the signs and symptoms of cardiac toxicity do not develop until months after the anthracycline treatment has been discontinued. For many patients, congestive heart failure is reversible or at least controlled with medication.[28,60] More sensitive diagnostic techniques such as stress testing and electrophysiologic studies are likely to increase the frequency of cardiac abnormalities diagnosed. Comprehensive follow-up cardiac evaluation with electrocardiograms, echocardiograms, and stress testing is a crucial part of routine checkups for patients treated with anthracycline with or without chest irradiation.

Psychosocial Changes

Because only a few studies have been designed to focus on the psychosocial status of long-term survivors of ALL, available information on this subject is limited. Those studies of childhood cancer[38,51] survivors have shown a significantly higher incidence among them of behavioral and social adjustment problems than normal, including less participation in physical activities, inadequate social relations, poor school performance, frequent somatic complaints, and behavioral maladjustment. In particular, children treated for ALL had a greater risk for school-related problems, including the number of grades repeated and special education placements. Psychosocial stressors, which continue to be reported long after therapy for ALL has been completed, include anxiety about potential relapse, financial burdens, rejection for employment or insurance coverage, and rejection for military service. No differences in the frequency of major depressive syndromes, suicide attempts, or hospitalizations for psychiatric reasons have been noted between these patients and their siblings and between them and the general population.[71]

REFERENCES

1. Aur RJA et al: Central nervous system therapy and combination chemotherapy of childhood lymphocytic leukemia, Blood 37:272, 1971.
2. Bennett JM et al: French-American-British (FAB) Cooperative Group proposals for the classification of acute leukemias, Br J Haematol 33:451, 1976.
3. Bennett JM et al: Proposed revised criteria for the classification of acute myeloid leukemia, Ann Intern Med 103:620, 1985.
4. Bizzozzero OJ Jr, Johnson KG, and Ciocco A: Radiation-related leukemia in Hiroshima and Nagasaki, 1946-64: distribution, incidence, appearance in time, N Engl J Med 274:1095, 1966.
5. Blattner WA et al: Human T-cell leukemia virus and adult T-cell leukemia, JAMA 250:1074, 1983.
6. Blayney DW et al: Decreasing risk of leukemia with prolonged follow-up after chemotherapy and radiotherapy for Hodgkin's disease, N Engl J Med 316:710, 1987.
7. Boice JD: Cancer following medical irradiation, Cancer 47:1081, 1981.
8. Brandt L, Nilsson PG, and Mitelman F: Occupational exposure to petroleum products in men with ANLL, Br Med J 1:553, 1978.
9. Brill AB et al: Leukemia in man following ionizing radiation exposure: summary of findings in Hiroshima and Nagasaki, Ann Intern Med 56:590, 1962.

10. Brockstein JA et al: Allogeneic BMT after hyperfractionated TBI and cyclophosphamide in children with acute leukemia, N Engl J Med 317:1618, 1987.
11. Butturini A et al: Which treatment for childhood acute lymphoblastic leukemia in second remission? Lancet 1:429, 1987.
12. Caldwell GG and Heath CW Jr: Case clustering in cancer, South Med J 69:1598, 1976.
13. Castro-Malespina H et al: Philadelphia chromosome–positive chronic myelocytic leukemia in children: survival and prognostic factors, Cancer 52:721, 1983.
14. Clarkson BD and Boyse EA: Possible explanation of high concordance for AL in monozygotic twins, Lancet 1:699, 1971.
15. Cooke JV: Incidence of acute leukemia in children, JAMA 119:547, 1942.
16. Court-Brown WM and Doll R: Leukemia in childhood and young adult life: trends in mortality in relation to aetiology, Br Med J 1:981, 1961.
17. De The G et al: Epidemiologic evidence for a casual relationship between Epstein-Barr virus and Burkitt's lymphoma: results of the Ugandar prospective study, Nature 272:756, 1978.
18. Dinsmore R et al: Allogeneic bone marrow transplantation for patients with acute nonlymphocytic leukemia, Blood 63:649, 1984.
19. Dow LW et al: Evidence for clonal development of childhood acute lymphoblastic leukemia, Blood 66:902, 1985.
20. Draper GJ, Heaf MM, and Kennier-Wilson LM: Occurrence of childhood cancers among sibs and estimation of familial risks, J Med Genet 14:81, 1977.
21. Drexler HG et al: Incidence of TdT-positivity in cases of leukemia and lymphoma, Acta Haematol 75:12, 1986.
22. Filipovich ATT et al: Immunodeficiency in humans as a risk factor in development of malignancy, Prev Med 9:252, 1980.
23. Foon KA and Todd RF III: Immunologic classification of leukemia and lymphoma, Blood 68:1, 1986.
24. Fraumeni JF Jr and Wagoner JK: Changing sex differentials in leukemia, Public Health Rep 79:1093, 1974.
25. Frei E and Sallan SE: Acute lymphoblastic leukemia: treatment, Cancer 42:828, 1978.
26. Freireich EJ et al: The effect of 6-mercaptopurine on the duration of steroid-induced remission in acute leukemia: a model for evaluation of other potentially useful therapy, Blood 21:699, 1963.
27. George S et al: A reappraisal of the results of stopping therapy in childhood leukemia, N Engl J Med 300:2269, 1979.
28. Gilladoga AC et al: The cardiotoxicity of Adriamycin and daunomycin in children, Cancer 37:1070, 1976.
29. Greenberg RS and Schuster JL: Epidemiology of cancer in children, Epidemiol Rev 7:22, 1985.
30. Gunz F and Baikie AG: Leukemia, ed 3, New York, 1974, Grune & Stratton, Inc.
31. Hakami N et al: Combined etoposide and 5-azacytidine in children and adolescents with refractory or relapsed acute nonlymphocytic leukemia: a POG study, J Clin Oncol 5:1022, 1987.
32. Hammond DG: The cure of childhood cancers, Cancer 58:407, 1986.
33. Hardisty RM, Speed DE, and Till M: Granulocytic leukemia in childhood, Br J Haematol 10:551, 1964.
34. Harvey EB et al: Prenatal X-ray exposure and childhood cancer in twins, N Engl J Med 312:541, 1985.
35. Heath CW and Hasterlik RJ: Leukemia among children in a suburban community, Am J Med 34:796, 1963.
36. Hecht F and McCaw BK: Chromosome instability syndromes. In Mulvihill JJ, Miller RW, and Fraumeni JF Jr, editors: Genetics of human cancer, New York, 1977, Raven Press.
37. Kirsch IR: Molecular biology of the leukemias, Pediatr Clin North Am 35:693, 1988.
38. Koocher GP and O'Malley J: The Damocles syndrome: psychosocial consequences of surviving childhood cancer, New York, 1981, McGraw-Hill Book Co.
39. Krakower JM and Aaronson SA: Seroepidemiologic assessment of feline leukemia virus infection risk for man, Nature 273:463, 1978.
40. Li FP, Cassady JR, and Jaffe N: Risk of second tumors in survivors of childhood cancer, Cancer 35:1230, 1975.
41. Lonsdale D et al: Interrupted vs. continued maintenance therapy in childhood acute leukemia, Cancer 36:341, 1975.
42. Look AT: The cytogenetics of childhood leukemia: clinical and biologic implications, Pediatr Clin North Am 35:723, 1988.
43. March HC: Leukemia and Radiology 43:275, 1944.
44. Mauer AM: Treatment of acute leukemia in childhood, Clin Lab Haematol 7:245, 1978.
45. Meadows AT et al: Survival in childhood acute lymphoblastic leukemia (ALL): the influence of protocol and place of treatment, Cancer Invest 1:49, 1983.
46. Mike V, Meadows AT, and D'Angio GD: Incidence of second malignant neoplasms in children: results of an international study, Lancet 2:1326, 1982.
47. Miller LP et al: Successful reinduction therapy with amsacrine and cyclotidine in children with acute nonlymphoblastic leukemia, Proc Am Soc Clin Oncol 3:199, 1984.
48. Miller RW: Ethnic differences in cancer occurrence. In Mulvihill JJ, Miller RW, and Fraumeni JF Jr, editors: Genetics of human cancer, New York, 1977, Raven Press.
49. Miller RW: Persons with exceptionally high risk of leukemia, Cancer Res 27:2420, 1967.
50. Mirro J et al: Acute mixed lineage leukemia: clinicopathologic correlations and prognostic significance, Blood 66:1115, 1985.
51. Mulhern RK et al: Social competence and behavioral adjustment of children who are long-term survivors of cancer, Pediatrics 83:18, 1989.
52. Neglia JP and Robinson LL: Epidemiology of the childhood acute leukemias, Pediatr Clin North Am 35:675, 1988.
53. Ochs J and Mulhern RK: Late effects of antileukemic treatment, Pediatr Clin North Am 35:815, 1988.
54. Odom L and Gordon E: Acute monoblastic leukemia in infancy and early childhood: successful treatment with epipodophyllotoxin, Blood 64:875, 1984.
55. Pedersen-Bjergaard J and Larsen SO: Incidence of ANLL, preleukemia, and acute myeloproliferative syndrome up to 10 years after treatment of Hodgkin's disease, N Engl J Med 307:965, 1982.
56. Pendergrass TW: Epidemiology of ALL, Semin Oncol 12:80, 1985.
57. Penn I: Second malignant neoplasms associated with immunosuppression medications, Cancer 37:1024, 1976.
58. Pinkel D: Curing of children with leukemia, Cancer 59:1683, 1987.
59. Pratt CB et al: Carcinomas in children: clinical and demographic characteristics, Cancer 61:1046, 1988.
60. Pratt CB, Ransom JL, and Evans WE: Age-related Adriamycin cardiotoxicity in children, Cancer Treat Rep 62:1381, 1978.
61. Ribeiro RC et al: Clinical and biologic hallmarks of the Philadelphia chromosome in childhood acute lymphoblastic leukemia, Blood 70:948, 1987.
62. Robinson CC et al: Height of children successfully treated for acute lymphoblastic leukemia: a report from the late effects study committee of CCSG, Med Pediatr Oncol 13:14, 1985.
63. Robinson LL et al: Environmental exposures as risk factors for childhood ANLL, Proc Am Assoc Ca Res 28:249, 1987.
64. Robinson L et al: Assessment of the interrelationship of prognostic factors in childhood acute lymphoblastic leukemia, Am J Pediatr Hematol Oncol 2:3, 1980.
65. Romsche et al: Evaluation of human growth hormone treatment in children with cranial irradiation associated short stature, J Pediatr 104:177, 1984.
66. Rowe JM and Lichtman MA: Hyperleukocytosis and leukostasis: common features of childhood chronic myelogenous leukemia, Blood 63:1230, 1984.
67. Sandberg AA: The chromosomes in human leukemia, Semin Hematol 23:201, 1986.
68. Sather HN: Age at diagnosis of childhood acute lymphoblastic leukemia, Med Pediatr Oncol 14:166, 1986.
69. Simone JV: Factors that influence haematological remission duration in acute lymphocytic leukemia, Br J Haematol 32:465, 1976.
70. Steuber CPPC: Therapy in childhood acute nonlymphocytic leukemia (ANLL): evolution of current concepts of chemotherapy, Am J Pediatr Hematol Oncol 3:379, 1981.

71. Teta MJ et al: Psychosocial consequences of childhood and adolescent cancer survival, J Chronic Dis 39:751, 1986.
72. Thomas ED et al: Marrow transplantations for the treatment of chronic myelogenous leukemia, Ann Intern Med 104:155, 1986.
73. Thomas ED et al: Marrow transplantation for patients with acute lymphoblastic leukemia: a long-term followup, Blood 62:1139, 1983.
74. Till MM et al: Leukemia in children and their grandparents, Br J Haematol 29:575, 1975.
75. Todaro GJ and Huebner RJ: The viral oncogene hypothesis: new evidence, Proc Natl Acad Sci USA 69:1009, 1972.
76. Vigliani EC and Forni A: Benzene and leukemia, Environ Res 11:122, 1976.
77. Weinstein HJ: Congenital leukemia and the neonatal myeloproliferative disorders associated with Down's syndrome, Clin Lab Haematol 7:147, 1978.
78. Whang-Peng J et al: Cytogenetic studies in acute lymphocytic leukemia: special emphasis on long-term survival, Med Pediatr Oncol 2:333, 1976.
79. Williams DL et al: Presence of clonal chromosome abnormalities in virtually all cases of acute lymphoblastic leukemia, N Engl J Med 310:640, 1985.
80. Winter RS and Green OC: Irradiation induced growth hormone deficiency: blunted growth response and accelerated skeletal maturation and growth hormone therapy, J Pediatr 106:609, 1985.
81. Young JL Jr and Miller RW: Incidence of malignant tumors in US children, J Pediatr 86:254, 1975.
82. Young JL Jr et al: Cancer incidence, survival and mortality for children under 15 years of age, Cancer 58:598, 1986.
83. Yunis JL and Brunning RD: Prognostic significance of chromosomal abnormalities in acute leukemias and myelodysplastic syndromes, Clin Lab Haematol 15:597, 1986.
84. Zuelzer WW et al: Long-term cytogenetic studies in acute leukemia of children: the nature of relapse, Am J Hematol 1:143, 1976.

SUGGESTED READINGS

Altman AJ and Schwartz AD: Malignant diseases of infancy, childhood and adolescence, ed 2, Philadelphia, 1983, WB Saunders Co.

Green DM: Long-term complications of therapy for cancer in childhood and adolescence, Baltimore, 1989, Johns Hopkins University Press.

Halperin EC et al: Pediatric radiation oncology, New York, 1989, Raven Press.

Nathan DG and Oski FA: Hematology of infancy and childhood, ed 3, Philadelphia, 1987, WB Saunders Co.

Pizzo PA and Poplack DG: Principles and practice of pediatric oncology, Philadelphia, 1989, JB Lippincott Co.

Poplack DG: The leukemias. In Pediatric Clin North Am 35:675, 1988.

225

Lyme Disease

David M. Siegel

EPIDEMIOLOGY, ETIOLOGY, AND PATHOGENESIS

Lyme borreliosis, or Lyme disease, is a spirochetal infection first observed in a group of children living in and around Lyme, Connecticut, on the eastern shore of the Connecticut River. Although initially these patients were mistakenly diagnosed as having juvenile arthritis, the perceptiveness of two mothers and the follow-up epidemiologic work of Steere and others[14] established the infectious etiology and vector of the disease's spread. In their landmark investigation they found a total of 15 patients clustered in the Lyme, Connecticut, region, with an overall prevalence of 4.3 cases per 1000 residents. Since then the disease has been reported on all continents except Antarctica and in 43 of the United States. The major clustering of cases in this country has occurred along the eastern seaboard, in the northern Midwest, and in the Far West. Of cases in the United States 90% have been reported from Massachusetts, Rhode Island, Connecticut, New York, New Jersey, Wisconsin, and Minnesota. Since 1982, 13,825 cases have been reported to the Centers for Disease Control.[5]

Early study revealed a tick vector as consistent with the pattern of spread of the disease.[12,13,15] Specifically the Lyme disease spirochete is transmitted by *Ixodes* sp. ticks, including *I. dammini* in the northeastern and midwestern United States,[13] *I. pacificus* in the western United States,[3] *I. ricinus* in Europe,[10] and *I. persulcatus* in Asia.[10] These ticks go through a 2-year life cycle, with the larval form feeding (on a blood meal) in the late summer and following spring and the nymph in early summer. The preferred host at these times in the life cycle of *I. dammini* is the white-footed mouse, *Peromyscus leucopus*. These mice are able to remain infected with the spirochete without an associated inflammatory response, whereas the spirochete remains in the midgut of the larval tick and later migrates to the salivary glands of the nymph. The adult *I. dammini* prefers the white-tailed deer as a host, although the life cycle of the spirochete does not depend on involvement of the deer.

The discovery of the actual spirochetal etiology of this multisystem disease occurred in Lyme, Connecticut, and came about as a result of two pieces of information. First, the skin rash seen in the majority of these patients was erythema chronicum migrans (ECM)—to be described in more detail later—which previously had been recognized in Europe in the 1950s as an eruption of spirochetal origin. This had been established by visualization of spirochetal structures in the ECM lesions and the subsequent response to penicillin treatment. Second, with this knowledge at hand, and the accumulated epidemiologic evidence implicating *I. dammini* as the vector, Burgdorfer et al.[2] began a careful analysis of the digestive tract of the ticks for spirochetes and were successful in isolating previously unrecognized spirochetes later designated *Borrelia burgdorferi*. These organisms were then consistently isolated from the blood, skin lesions, and cerebrospinal fluid of patients with Lyme disease, confirming the causation. The infection rate of *I. dammini* with *B. burgdorferi* in endemic areas is quite high, with spirochetes being recovered from more than 50% of the ticks on Shelter Island, N.Y.[1]

CLINICAL MANIFESTATIONS

The clinical manifestations of Lyme disease vary with the time that elapses since inoculation by the tick, and the infection has been divided into early and late phases. The former is characterized by two stages. Stage 1 of early infection is seen in 60% to 80% of patients and consists of ECM, sometimes accompanied by fever, minor constitutional symptoms, and regional lymphadenopathy. The ECM rash begins as a red macule or papule (at the site of the tick bite), which expands to form a large annular erythematous patch with a bright red outer border and partial central clearing. In those patients with ECM, its appearance is within days of the tick bite and even untreated will fade within 3 to 4 weeks. Specific antibody to *B. burgdorferi* usually is not present at this time. The spirochete is more easily cultured from the skin during stage 1 of early infection than at any other time in the illness.

Stage 2 of early infection represents dissemination of *B. burgdorferi* and can potentially involve many organ systems (Table 225-1). The most commonly involved areas, however, are the skin, nervous system, and musculoskeletal system. It is in this stage of the disease that patients tend to feel quite ill with significant malaise and fatigue. Smaller annular skin lesions can appear at sites other than the initial ECM eruption. The patient will complain of a transient but severe headache and stiff neck, although the cerebrospinal fluid usually is normal. Arthritis is not present in early disease, but patients experience migratory pain in joints, bursae, tendons, muscles, and bones. It is at this time (3 to 4 weeks after infection) that antibody titers to *B. burgdorferi* will develop.

As stage 2 disease progresses, meningitis can develop, possibly with subtle signs of encephalitis, including somnolence, poor memory, and mood change. Unilateral or bi-

Table 225-1 *Manifestations of Lyme Disease by Stage**

SYSTEM†	EARLY INFECTION: LOCALIZED (STAGE 1)	EARLY INFECTION: DISSEMINATED (STAGE 2)	LATE INFECTION: PERSISTENT (STAGE 3)
Skin	Erythema migrans	Secondary annular lesions, malar rash, diffuse erythema or urticaria, evanescent lesions, lymphocytoma	Acrodermatitis chronica atrophicans, localized scleroderma-like lesions
Musculoskeletal system		Migratory pain in joints, tendons, bursae, muscle, bone; brief arthritis attacks; myositis‡; osteomyelitis‡; panniculitis‡	Prolonged arthritis attacks, chronic arthritis, peripheral enthesopathy, periostitis or joint subluxations below lesions of acrodermatitis
Neurologic system		Meningitis, cranial neuritis, Bell's palsy, motor or sensory radiculoneuritis, subtle encephalitis, mononeuritis multiplex, myelitis‡, chorea‡, cerebellar ataxia‡	Chronic encephalomyelitis, spastic parapareses, ataxic gait, subtle mental disorders, chronic axonal polyradiculopathy, dementia‡
Lymphatic system	Regional lymphadenopathy	Regional or generalized lymphadenopathy, splenomegaly	
Heart		Atrioventricular nodal block, myopericarditis, pancarditis	
Eyes		Conjunctivitis, iritis‡, choroiditis‡, retinal hemorrhage or detachment‡, panophthalmitis‡	Keratitis
Liver		Mild or recurrent hepatitis	
Respiratory system		Nonexudative sore throat, nonproductive cough, adult respiratory distress syndrome‡	
Kidney		Microscopic hematuria or proteinuria	
Genitourinary system		Orchitis‡	
Constitutional symptoms	Minor	Severe malaise and fatigue	Fatigue

From Steere AC: Lyme disease, N Engl J Med 321:586, 1989.
*The classification by stages provides a guideline for the expected timing of the illness's manifestations, but this may vary from case to case.
†Systems are listed from the most to the least commonly affected.
‡The inclusion of this manifestation is based on one or a few cases.

lateral facial palsy (Bell palsy) and/or a peripheral neuritis, which usually is asymmetric and accompanied by motor, sensory, or mixed manifestations, will develop in 15% to 20% of patients in the United States. Cardiac involvement is seen in a smaller group (4% to 8%) and is characterized most commonly by varying degrees of atrioventricular block, but it can include myopericarditis or, rarely, fatal pancarditis. Complete heart block usually is brief, and only temporary cardiac pacing is necessary.[11] It is toward the end of stage 2 (6 months after disease onset) that patients can begin to experience brief attacks of asymmetric, large joint oligoarthritis, most commonly affecting the knee.

During stage 3 of the infection, episodes of arthritis become much more prolonged, with the possibility of chronic arthritis (a year or more of continual inflammation) developing. The arthritis remains confined, however, to one or a few large joints; the knee is the most common site. During stage 3 of infection, patients also can experience neurologic complications, including persistent distal paresthesias or radicular pain. Not well understood, but reported, are cases in which patients who have had classic symptoms of Lyme disease in the past and then later have subtle memory deficits, somnolence, or behavioral changes. These patients present a difficult dilemma, although they certainly should be treated for neurologic Lyme disease if therapy was not given initially.

CONGENITAL INFECTION

The issue of congenital infection with *B. burgdorferi* is only partially understood. Transplacental transmission of the spirochete has been reported in two infants who then died during the first week of life. Spirochetes were seen in tissuesof these infants.[8,16] In a study of 463 infants from endemic and nonendemic areas, however, congenital malformations were not found to be associated with the presence of *B. burgdorferi* antibody in cord blood.[17] Steere[11] has concluded that it is unusual for *B. burgdorferi* to cause an adverse fetal outcome.

SEROLOGIC TESTING

The major diagnostic tool in evaluating a patient for Lyme disease, outside the history of a summer exposure to a tick bite in an endemic area and development of ECM, is the detection of antibody to *B. burgdorferi*. Two serologic tests currently are used: immunofluorescence assay (IFA), which uses fluoroscein-conjugated antihuman immunoglobulins to detect the presence of antibodies in patient sera, and enzyme-linked immunosorbent assay (ELISA). Although IFA is relatively sensitive and specific well into stage 1 disease, it is inadequate in detecting antibody early in the illness. In one study, sera obtained from patients with Lyme disease during the first 3 weeks of their illness showed positivity by IFA in only 38%, whereas patients with neuritis and arthritis had reactive titers 92% to 100% of the time.[7] The ELISA is more sensitive and specific than the IFA in diagnosing early Lyme disease, but the deficiency of both tests is their occasional false-positive results, which are caused by the presence in these patients of other spirochetal infections such as syphilis and relapsing fever, as well as other confounding patient variables as yet to be defined. Another problem with both IFA and ELISA testing is the lack of standardization and quality controls for these tests in most diagnostic laboratories, which results in poor interlaboratory and intralaboratory agreement.[6,9] Early antibiotic therapy also can blunt antibody production. Given these limitations, most laboratories now consider a titer ≥1:256 in a patient with compatible clinical symptoms as sufficient to confirm the diagnosis of Lyme borreliosis.[4] Research into improved serologic testing is focused on antigen detection by use of polymerase chain-reaction techniques.

DIFFERENTIAL DIAGNOSIS

In children who have what appears to be Lyme arthritis, the most likely differential diagnosis to consider (as in the first cases in the Lyme area) is pauciarticular juvenile arthritis. Other considerations include aseptic meningitis, Bell palsy or a peripheral neuropathy not caused by *B. burgdorferi*, multiple sclerosis, septic arthritis, acute rheumatic fever, and fibromyalgia syndrome. Such diagnoses are easily ruled out when a history of a tick bite with ECM is present, but many patients with Lyme disease have no history of these events. Certainly, during the summer in an endemic area, Lyme disease should be considered when consistent symptoms are present.

Table 225-2 *Treatment Regimens for Lyme Disease*

MANIFESTATION	REGIMEN*
Early infection*	
Adults	Tetracycline, 250 mg orally 4× daily, 10-30 days† Doxycycline, 100 mg orally 2× daily, 10-30 days†‡ Amoxicillin, 500 mg orally 4× daily, 10-30 days†‡
Children (≤8 yr)	Amoxicillin or penicillin V, 250 mg orally 3× daily or 20 mg/kilogram of body weight/day in divided doses, 10-30 days In case of penicillin allergy: Erythromycin, 250 mg orally 3× daily or 30 mg/kilogram/day in divided doses, 10-30 days‡
Neurologic abnormalities (early or late)*	
General	Ceftriaxone, 2 g intravenously 1× daily, 14 days§ Penicillin G, 20 million U intravenously, 6 divided doses daily, 14 days§ In case of ceftriaxone or penicillin allergy: Doxycycline, 100 mg orally 2× daily, 30 days‡ Chloramphenicol, 250 mg intravenously 4× daily, 14 days‡
Facial palsy alone	Oral antibiotic regimens may be adequate
Cardiac abnormalities	
First-degree atrioventricular block (PR interval <0.3 sec)	Oral antibiotic regimens, as for early infection
High-degree atrioventricular block	Ceftriaxone, 2 g intravenously 1× daily, 14 days‡ Penicillin, 20 million U intravenously, 6 divided doses daily, 14 days‡
Arthritis (intermittent or chronic)†	Doxycycline, 100 mg orally 2× daily, 30 days Amoxicillin and probenecid, 500 mg each orally 4× daily, 30 days Ceftriaxone, 2 g intravenously 1× daily, 14 days Penicillin, 20 million U intravenously, 6 divided doses daily, 14 days
Acrodermatitis	Oral antibiotic regimens for 1 month are usually adequate

From Steere AC: Lyme disease, N Engl J Med 321:586, 1989.
*Treatment failures have occurred with all these regimens, and retreatment may be necessary.
†The duration of therapy is based on clinical response.
‡The antibiotic has not yet been tested systematically for this indication in Lyme disease.
§The appropriate duration of therapy is not yet clear for patients with late neurologic abnormalities, and it may be longer than 2 weeks.

MANAGEMENT

As a spirochetal infection, Lyme borreliosis can be successfully treated, depending on when in the course of the illness antibiotics are begun. With ECM, oral antibiotic therapy is used; tetracycline, doxycycline, penicillin, amoxicillin, or erythromycin (in the presence of penicillin allergy in a child 8 years old or younger) will shorten the duration of the rash and frequently prevent later complications. Facial palsy or peripheral neuropathy alone also can be treated with antibiotics given orally, but any other neurologic abnormality, such as meningitis or general central nervous system symptoms, should be treated with parenteral ceftriaxone, penicillin G, or chloramphenicol. Although first-degree atrioventricular block usually requires only oral therapy, higher-grade blocks necessitate parenteral therapy with ceftriaxone or penicillin G. Finally, intermittent or chronic arthritis should be treated with either parenteral or long-term oral therapy. Specific dosages and durations are shown in Table 225-2, as recommended by both Steere[11] and others.

The later antibiotic therapy is instituted, the more likely complications and persistent problems will develop. Thus a high level of suspicion, followed by prompt diagnosis and treatment, is rewarded with a high likelihood of a mild and short-term illness with a favorable prognosis. Should chronic arthritis persist, then usual management with antiinflammatory medications and physical therapy will be needed.

REFERENCES

1. Bosler EM et al: Prevalence of the Lyme disease spirochete in populations of white-tailed deer and white footed mice, Yale J Biol Med 57:651, 1984.
2. Burgdorfer W et al: Lyme disease—a tick-borne spirochetosis? Science 216:1317, 1982.
3. Burgdorfer W et al: The Western black-legged tick, *Ixodes pacificus:* a vector of *Borrelia burgdorferi,* Am J Trop Med Hyg 34:925, 1985.
4. Eichenfield AH and Athreya BH: Lyme disease: of ticks and titres, J Pediatr 114:328, 1989.
5. Lyme disease—United States, 1987 and 1988, MMWR 38:668, 1989.
6. Magnarelli LA: Quality of Lyme disease tests, JAMA 262:3464, 1989.
7. Russell H et al: Enzyme-linked immunosorbent assay and indirect immunofluorescence assay for Lyme disease, J Infect Dis 149:789, 1984.
8. Schlesinger PA et al: Maternal-fetal transmission of the Lyme disease spirochete, *Borrelia burgdorferi,* Ann Intern Med 103:67, 1985.
9. Schwartz BS et al: Antibody testing in Lyme disease: a comparison of results in four laboratories, JAMA 262:3431, 1989.
10. Steere AC: Lyme disease, N Engl J Med 308:733, 1983.
11. Steere AC: Lyme disease, N Engl J Med 321:586, 1989.
12. Steere AC, Broderick TF, and Malawista SE: Erythema chronicum migrans and Lyme arthritis: epidemiologic evidence for a tick vector, Am J Epidemiol 108:312, 1978.
13. Steere AC and Malawista SE: Cases of Lyme disease in the United States: locations correlated with distribution of *Ixodes dammini,* Ann Intern Med 91:730, 1979.
14. Steere AC et al: Lyme arthritis: an epidemic of oligoarticular arthritis in children and adults in three Connecticut communities, Arthritis Rheum 20:7, 1977.
15. Wallis RC et al: Erythema chronicum migrans and Lyme arthritis: field study of ticks, Am J Epidemiol 108:322, 1978.
16. Weber K et al: *Borrelia burgdorferi* in a newborn despite oral penicillin for Lyme borreliosis during pregnancy, Pediatr Infect Dis J 7:286, 1988.
17. Williams CL et al: Lyme disease during pregnancy: a cord blood serosurvey, Ann NY Acad Sci 539:504, 1988.

226

Meatal Ulceration

Mark F. Bellinger

Although rarely seen in the uncircumcised child, meatal ulceration may occur if the foreskin is sufficiently loose to allow exposure of a portion of the glans penis. Mackenzie[5] reported a 20% incidence of meatal ulceration at examination 2 to 3 weeks after circumcision but believed that the true incidence was much greater, as indicated by historical data.

ETIOLOGY

It is not surprising that circumcision may expose the thin glanular epithelium to irritation. Irritants include moisture, chemicals (urine, feces, laundry detergents), and trauma from the rubbing of the diaper. A great deal of inflammatory response is evident in the raw, cherry-red surface of the glans after forceful retraction of the prepuce at the time of neonatal circumcision. The foreskin normally fuses to the glanular epithelium during its formation in the fifth month of gestation. Keratinization and desquamation occur naturally and at variable rates, gradually forming a cleft between glans and prepuce. The prepuce is easily retractible in only 4% of newborns, in 20% at 6 months of age, and in 90% at 3 years of age. Once preputial retraction has occurred naturally, the meatus is similarly exposed to mechanical and chemical trauma; however, the epithelium is keratinized and thickened, and ulceration is less common.

HISTORY

Although meatal ulceration may be relatively painless, many infants cry when voiding. Voluntary urinary retention is not unusual when dysuria is severe. Once bladder distention is maximal, overflow dribbling of urine occurs. After a small amount of urine passes, pain usually is diminished and a complete voiding ensues. Meatal crusting during ulcer healing also may cause urinary retention. After repeated ulcerations, scarring can result in meatal stenosis. The urinary stream may become pinpoint in caliber and directed upward, so that the voiding phase is prolonged and the child may have difficulty in aiming his stream.

PHYSICAL FINDINGS

Early ulcers are superficial, clean, and contiguous with the meatus. Spreading of the meatal lips reveals a normal urethral mucosa. Urethral discharge is absent. Meatal ulceration commonly is accompanied by diaper rash, especially when ammoniacal dermatitis is severe, and inguinal adenopathy may be present. Meatal ulcers crust quickly, and the meatus may become occluded, causing bladder distention, evident as a suprapubic midline mass. Crusts rubbed off or removed leave a raw surface, and blood spotting of the diaper may result. Repeated episodes of ulceration and crusting occur until the lesion heals.

DIFFERENTIAL DIAGNOSIS

Penile trauma may result from technical errors during circumcision,[3] and glandular irritation may result from the plastic ring if the Plastibell technique is used. Older children may suffer trauma to the glans; zipper injuries are the most common. Adolescents may sustain glanular injury during intercourse.

Balanitis (inflammation of the glans) or posthitis (inflammation of the foreskin) is seen particularly in the uncircumcised. Edema and inflammation may be severe. Balanitis xerotica obliterans is a chronic inflammatory process of unknown cause that may involve the glans, foreskin, and distal urethra.[6] Although most common in adults, older children may be affected.

It is important to differentiate cutaneous lesions from urethral lesions that may protrude from the meatus. Urethral tumors are rare in children, and most benign polyps occur in the proximal urethra. Condylomata acuminata (venereal warts) are increasingly common and may be seen in sexually active adolescents. These viral lesions may appear on genital skin as small verrucae or may protrude from the meatus if the urethra becomes involved.

Venereal diseases are an increasingly common source of genital lesions in adolescents. Gonorrheal urethritis may occur, with meatal edema and encrustation. Syphilitic chancre is a painless, indurated ulcer with sharply demarcated borders that may occur on the shaft or glans, usually 3 to 6 weeks after exposure. Herpes progenitalis (herpes simplex) may appear as perimeatal vesicles on an erythematous base. Local pain or dysuria may occur, and the vesicles may rupture to form grouped superficial ulcerations.[4] Other meatal ulcerations may result from erythema multiforme, allergic dermatitis, seborrheic dermatitis, drug eruptions, and scabies.

TREATMENT

Prevention of meatal ulceration in the infant requires good hygiene. Care of established lesions must be aimed at removing the irritants: moisture is diminished by more frequent diaper changes; chemical irritation is reduced by frequent changing and proper rinsing of diapers to remove irritating soap residue; mechanical trauma is lessened by pinning diapers as loosely as possible. A change from cloth to disposable diapers, or vice versa, may be beneficial if local irritative factors are substantial. Leaving the infant undiapered for short periods at changing time may help significantly.

Local hygiene of the ulcer is important, and simple cleansing with soap and water usually is sufficient. Petroleum jelly applications may decrease local ulcer pain. Crusts require removal if urinary retention occurs, and associated diaper rash may require topical treatment.

Meatal stenosis subsequent to meatitis may occur.[7] The voided stream must be visualized inasmuch as the appearance of the meatus may be deceiving. A pinpoint stream with pouting of the meatal lips may indicate the need for meatotomy, which usually can be accomplished in the office if local anesthesia is used. After surgery, meatal care is required to prevent restenosis of the raw meatal edges. Balanitis xerotica obliterans may require meatotomy or local excision. Topical corticosteroid therapy has been beneficial in many patients. Condylomata acuminata can be treated by topical therapy (podophyllin) or excision. Urethral lesions may be treated with 5-fluorouracil intraurethral cream. Laser therapy has been used successfully for urethral, as well as for clinical and subclinical, penile condyloma.[2] Other venereal diseases may require antibiotic therapy. Genital herpes, an increasingly rampant disorder, can be treated only symptomatically.[1]

REFERENCES

1. Arvin AM: Oral therapy with acyclovir in infants and children, Pediatr Infect Dis 6:56, 1987.
2. Carpiniello VL et al: Results of carbon dioxide laser therapy and topical 5-fluorouracil treatment for subclinical condyloma found by magnified penile surface scanning, J Urol 140:53, 1988.
3. Gee WF and Ansell JS: Neonatal circumcision: a 10-year overview, with comparison of the Gomco clamp and the Plastibell device, Pediatrics 58:824, 1976.
4. Korting GW: Practical dermatology of the genital region, Philadelphia, 1980, WB Saunders Co.
5. Mackenzie AR: Meatal ulceration following neonatal circumcision, Obstet Gynecol 28:221, 1966.
6. McKay DL, Fuqua F, and Weinberg AG: Balanitis xerotica obliterans in children, J Urol 114:773, 1975.
7. Noe HN and Dale GD: Evaluation of children with meatal stenosis, J Urol 114:455, 1975.

227

Meningitis

Keith R. Powell

The meninges of the central nervous system include three membranes that support, protect, and nourish the brain and spinal cord. The outermost layer, the dura mater, is a tough, poorly extensive connective tissue layer that sheaths the brain and spinal cord and terminates caudally as the coccygeal ligament. The middle and innermost layers, the arachnoid and the pia mater, respectively, are similar in structure and are often referred to singly as the leptomeninges. The arachnoid and pia are partially separated, leaving a subarachnoid space containing cerebrospinal fluid (CSF). The CSF is formed in the choroid plexuses within the ventricles of the brain, which communicate with the subarachnoid space through the foramina of Magendie and Luschka.

Meningitis refers to inflammation of the meninges and is often caused directly or indirectly by an infectious agent.[27] Untreated bacterial meningitis is usually rapidly fatal, and delay in treatment generally increases the chance of death or permanent sequelae. Thus early diagnosis and treatment are essential.

The incidence of bacterial meningitis and the causative organisms are closely related to age. During the first month of life the age-specific incidence is nearly 100 cases per 100,000 live births. The incidence falls to 45 per 100,000 during the second month of life but reaches a second peak at 6 to 8 months with an incidence of nearly 80 per 100,000.

The incidence of aseptic meningitis ranges, in different years, from 1.5 to 4 cases per 100,000 population. The incidence in children is actually much higher because aseptic meningitis is also a disease of the young, with few reported cases occurring in persons over 30 years of age.

The cause of meningitis also changes with age. During the first month of life over two thirds of the cases of neonatal bacterial meningitis are caused by group B streptococci or gram-negative enteric organisms, primarily *Escherichia coli*, with the third most common isolate being *Listeria monocytogenes*. After the first month of life *Listeria* organisms are encountered as the cause of meningitis only in debilitated or elderly persons. The number of cases of different kinds of bacterial meningitis reported by 27 states from 1978 through 1981 and the case fatality rate are shown in Table 227-1.

BACTERIAL MENINGITIS AFTER THE NEONATAL PERIOD

After the age of 1 month, most cases of bacterial meningitis are caused by *Haemophilus influenzae* type b, *Neisseria meningitidis*, or *Streptococcus pneumoniae*. The child between 3 and 12 months of age is at greatest risk for acquiring meningitis; after the neonatal period, 90% of meningitis cases occur in children between 1 month and 5 years of age. Mortality varies with the pathogen, as shown in Table 227-1. These case fatality rates represent cases reported to the Centers for Disease Control and are somewhat higher than actual, since fatal cases are more likely to be reported.

All three of these pathogens can be isolated from the throat or nasopharynx of healthy individuals. Most studies of microorganism carrier states suggest that children at highest risk for disease are also the most likely to be colonized. During an 18-month period, 71% of the toddlers and 48% of the preschool-aged children at a day care center were colonized with *H. influenzae* type b.[24] No invasive *H. influenzae* type b disease occurred. Meningitis usually occurs following bacteremia secondary to infection at another site. The site of primary infection might be apparent, such as otitis media,

Table 227-1 *Total Number of Bacterial Meningitis Cases and Fatality Rates from 27 Participating States: 1978-1981*

ORGANISM	CASES REPORTED (ALL AGES)*	% OF TOTAL	CASE FATALITY RATE (%)*
Haemophilus influenzae	6,756	48.3	6.0
Neisseria meningitidis	2,742	19.6	10.3
Streptococcus pneumoniae	1,865	13.3	26.3
Group B streptococcus	476	3.4	22.5
Listeria monocytogenes	265	1.9	28.5
Escherichia coli	115	0.8	29.6†

*Number of deaths = cases reported × percentage of fatalities.
†Includes *E. coli* and other gram-negative bacilli.
Modified from Schlech WF et al: Bacterial meningitis in the United States, 1978 through 1981: the National Bacterial Meningitis Surveillance Study, JAMA 253:1749, 1985.

sinusitis, pharyngitis, cellulitis, pneumonia, septic arthritis, or osteomyelitis, or the site may be unrecognized.

Meningitis can also occur after head trauma, particularly with fractures of the paranasal sinuses. The pathogens most often associated with meningitis following trauma are *S. pneumoniae* and *H. influenzae*. Posttraumatic meningitis can recur when CSF leakage persists. Meningitis can also occur by direct spread from a congenital dermal sinus that communicates with the central nervous system. Any time meningitis is caused by bacteria that normally reside on the skin or in the gastrointestinal tract, a diligent search of the craniospinal axis should be performed.[25] Meningitis can also follow neurosurgery and is not uncommon after procedures to shunt ventricular fluid. Coagulase-negative staphylococci are the organisms most often associated with shunt infections.

Clinical Manifestations

Children with bacterial meningitis are usually febrile. However, the absence of fever in a child with signs of meningeal irritation does not preclude the diagnosis. Inflammation of the meninges can be manifested by irritability, anorexia, headache, nausea, vomiting, confusion, back pain, nuchal rigidity, and photophobia. The signs on physical examination described by Kernig and Brudzinski can be used to demonstrate meningeal inflammation. The Kernig sign is elicited by extending the leg at the knee while the hip is flexed. This maneuver produces pain in the hamstrings of a person with meningitis. The Brudzinski sign is elicited by flexing the neck of a patient in the supine position and observing involuntary flexing of the hips.

In the young infant, signs of meningeal inflammation can be minimal, and the signs associated with meningitis in the older child can be absent. In infants, irritability (especially in response to actions that are usually comforting), lethargy, poor feeding, and restlessness are often described. The patient may also have signs of increased intracranial pressure such as headache or a bulging fontanelle. However, papilledema is uncommon with bacterial meningitis, and when it is present, other causes should be sought.

Cranial nerve involvement occurs with bacterial meningitis and, although often transient, can be permanent. The auditory nerve is often affected, as manifested by deafness or disturbances of vestibular function. Blindness has been reported but is rare. Children may also have paralysis of extraocular or facial nerves.

The degree of central nervous system derangement observed with bacterial meningitis ranges from irritability to coma. In a prospective series of 124 patients, Feigen[12] found that about 20% of children with bacterial meningitis were comatose or semicomatose at the time of hospitalization. This occurred more often with *S. pneumoniae* or *N. meningitidis* than with *H. influenzae* type b. Seizures occurred before or within 1 to 2 days after admission in about 30% of patients. Focal neurologic signs were present in 14% of the patients and correlated with persistent abnormal neurologic examinations 1 year after discharge. Focal signs at the time of admission also correlated with the presence of retardation later.

Subdural effusions occur in about 50% of children with bacterial meningitis but are seldom clinically significant. Therefore, unless focal neurologic signs or signs of increased intracranial pressure develop, the presence of such effusions need not be sought through the performance of subdural taps or computed tomography (CT) scans. Infection of subdural effusions is extremely rare.

Arthralgia and myalgia often occur in patients with meningitis, particularly those with meningococcemia. Vasculitis can be seen in children with any type of bacterial meningitis, but petechiae and purpura are more commonly associated with meningococcal disease. Children with such rashes should be considered in imminent danger of developing septic shock and should be managed accordingly (see Chapter 283, "Meningococcemia").

Laboratory Findings

When meningitis is suspected in a patient who does not have papilledema, a lumbar puncture should be performed, the opening pressure measured, and the CSF examined immediately. The clinical situation should influence the amount of data required before a therapeutic decision is made. If the CSF from an ill, febrile child is turbid or purulent, antibiotics should be started and the patient managed for bacterial meningitis before further laboratory results are available. In any case, the CSF should be examined as soon as possible. A Gram stain should be performed on a smear of CSF, and the total number of white blood cells should be determined in a counting chamber. A differential cell count should also be performed. The CSF concentrations of total protein and glucose should be determined. A blood glucose determination should preferably be obtained just before the lumbar puncture (since the stress generated by the procedure can cause a temporary elevation of the blood glucose level) to determine the CSF to blood glucose ratio. Characteristic CSF findings are given in Table 227-2.

The CSF should be cultured on chocolate and blood agar plates and in broth. Rapid identification of the etiologic agent is often possible with counterimmunoelectrophoresis (CIE) or agglutination reactions. Soluble capsular antigens can be detected in CSF, serum, and concentrated urine with these methods.

Blood cultures should be obtained on all children suspected of having bacterial meningitis. In one study,[12] blood cultures were positive in 90%, 80%, and 91% of children who had not previously received antibiotics and who had meningitis resulting from *H. influenzae, S. pneumoniae,* and *N. meningitidis*, respectively. Radiographs may be helpful in identifying suspected bone or joint infection. Radionuclide and CT studies have a role in complicated cases of meningitis and may be helpful in making decisions regarding management.

Differential Diagnosis

Signs and symptoms suggesting meningeal inflammation or increased intracranial pressure can also be seen with other infections of the central nervous system. The most common cause of meningeal inflammation is viral meningitis, which is discussed later. Meningitis can also be caused by *Myco-*

Table 227-2 *Characteristic Cerebrospinal Fluid Findings in Patients with Meningitis*

CSF FINDINGS	BACTERIAL	VIRAL	FUNGAL AND TUBERCULOUS
Leukocytes			
Usual	>500	<500	<500
Range	0-200,000	0-2000	
Percent polymorphonuclear neutrophils, usual	>80%	<50%	<50%
Range	20%-100%	0%-100%	
Glucose			
Usual	<40 mg/dl	>40 mg/dl	<40 mg/dl
Range	0-normal	30 mg/dl–normal	
Percent CSF/blood	<30	>50	
Protein			
Usual	>100 mg/dl	<100 mg/dl	>100 mg/dl
Range	Normal–1500 mg/dl	Normal–200 mg/dl	
Stains	Gram stain	—	India ink/acid-fast

bacterium tuberculosis, fungi, or parasites. Meningitis or meningoencephalitis may also be present in patients with Rocky Mountain spotted fever (RMSF), Kawasaki disease, cat-scratch fever, or toxic shock syndrome, and it is often associated with or follows rubeola, rubella, varicella, infectious mononucleosis, roseola, and erythema infectiosum (see the box on p. 1355). A brain abscess, epidural diseases, embolic diseases (like endocarditis or thrombophlebitis), venous sinus thrombosis, space-occupying lesions, reactions to intrathecal medications, ingestion of toxins, spider bites, pemphigus, and Behçet syndrome can mimic bacterial meningitis. CSF abnormalities similar to those seen with viral meningitis occur with RMSF, Kawasaki disease, toxic shock syndrome, and postinfectious syndromes. However, interpretation of the CSF findings in the context of the clinical manifestations usually differentiates bacterial meningitis from other diseases.

Management

When initially examined, children with meningitis may appear only mildly ill with fever and irritability, or they may be profoundly ill with an altered state of consciousness and hypotension. The severity of illness at the time of presentation can predict morbidity and should dictate immediate management. The scoring system devised by Herson and Todd and presented in Table 227-3 has been shown to predict morbidity in children with *H. influenzae* type b meningitis.[17]

Children with a score of 4.5 or higher are significantly more likely to die or to have major sequellae than children with lower scores. This scoring system does not predict deafness.[13,17]

Regardless of the patient's Herson-Todd score, acute bacterial meningitis is always a medical emergency, and all infants and children with an altered state of consciousness should be observed closely and the need for intensive care anticipated.

As soon as bacterial meningitis is diagnosed, intravenous access should be secured and appropriate antibiotics given. Initial laboratory examination should include CSF examination and culture, blood culture, measurement of serum electrolyte concentrations, and measurement of urine specific gravity. If the patient has petechiae or purpura or if the patient is in shock, laboratory tests should also include a partial thromboplastin time (PTT), prothrombin time (PT), platelet count, and measurement of fibrin breakdown products.[8]

Management of the child who is awake and has stable vital signs consists primarily of the administration of antibiotics and fluids and careful monitoring for changes in level of consciousness, development of seizures, changes in vital signs, and development of inappropriate secretion of antidiuretic hormone.

Other therapies should be considered in more critically ill children. If there is evidence of disseminated intravascular coagulation, appropriate blood products, vitamin K, and possibly heparin should be given as indicated by the clinical situation and coagulation test data (see Chapter 283). Pharmacologic doses of steroids probably do have a role in the treatment of septic shock (see Chapter 283). Seizures should be treated with appropriate anticonvulsants, and an open airway that provides good oxygenation should be ensured. Patients who are in profound coma or whose level of consciousness deteriorates while receiving therapy should be evaluated for complications such as a cerebral abscess, obstructive hydrocephalus, or elevated intracranial pressure. A CT scan of the brain is extremely helpful in determining the diagnosis in such cases.

If elevated intracranial pressure is a major concern and treatment has been started or is anticipated, a neurosurgeon should be consulted and an intracranial pressure monitoring device placed. If an intraventricular catheter can be placed, increased intracranial pressure can often be treated by removing CSF. The placement of a pressure transducer affords continuous intracranial monitoring so that mannitol and hyperventilation can be used as necessary to decrease pressure and maintain cerebral perfusion (see Chapter 283). If a cerebral perfusion pressure (mean arterial blood pressure minus intracranial pressure) of 30 to 40 cm of water cannot be maintained, survival is unlikely.[14]

Fluid management and antibiotic therapy are critically important for all patients with bacterial meningitis. Traditionally, fluids were restricted to two-thirds maintenance in patients with bacterial meningitis to minimize brain edema and prevent the syndrome of inappropriate antidiuretic hormone secretion (SIADH). A recent study showed that plasma an-

Etiologic Agents, Factors, and Diseases Associated with Aseptic Meningitis

VIRUSES

Enteroviruses (echoviruses, coxsackie viruses A and B, polioviruses, and enteroviruses)
Arboviruses (In the United States: Eastern equine, Western equine, Venezuelan equine, St. Louis, Powassan, California and Colorado tick fever. In other areas of the world, many other arboviruses are important.)
Mumps
Herpes simplex type 2
Human immunodeficiency (HIV)
Adenoviruses
Varicella-zoster (VZ)
Epstein-Barr (EB)
Lymphocytic choriomeningitis (LCM)
Encephalomyocarditis (EMC)
Cytomegalovirus
Rhinoviruses
Measles
Rubella
Influenza A and B
Parainfluenza
Rotaviruses
Coronaviruses
Variola

POST VACCINE

Measles
Vaccinia
Polio
Rabies

BACTERIA

Mycobacterium tuberculosis
Pyogenic–partially treated
Leptospira spp. (leptospirosis)
Treponema pallidum (syphilis)
Borrelia spp. (relapsing fever)
Borrelia burgdorferi spirochete (Lyme disease)
Nocardia spp. (nocardiosis)

Modified from Cherry JD: Aseptic meningitis and viral meningitis. In Feigen RD and Cherry JD, editors: Textbook of pediatric infectious disease, ed 2, Philadelphia, 1987, WB Saunders Co.

FUNGI

Blastomyces dermatitidis
Coccidioides immitis
Cryptococcus neoformans
Histoplasma capsulatum
Candida spp.
Other: *Alternaria* spp., *Aspergillus* spp., *Cephalosporium* spp., *Cladosporium trichoides, Dreschslera hawaiiensis, Paracoccidioides brasiliensis, Petriellidium boydii, Sporotrichum schenckii, Ustilago* spp., *Zygomycete* spp.

RICKETTSIA

R. rickettsii (Rocky Mountain spotted fever)
R. prowazeki (typhus)

MYCOPLASMA

M. pneumoniae
M. hominis

PARASITES

Angiostrongylus cantonensis (eosinophilic meningitis)
Trichinella spiralis (trichinosis)
Toxoplasma gondii (toxoplasmosis)

PARAMENINGEAL INFECTIONS

MALIGNANCY

Leukemia
CNS tumor

IMMUNE DISEASES

Behçet syndrome
Lupus erythematosus
Sarcoidosis

MISCELLANEOUS

Kawasaki disease
Toxic shock syndrome
Heavy metal poisoning
Intrathecal injections (contrast media, antibiotics, etc.)
Foreign bodies (shunt, reservoir)
Antimicrobial agents

tidiuretic hormone concentrations returned to normal in patients with bacterial meningitis who received replacement plus maintenance fluids for 24 hours while concentrations remained elevated in patients restricted to ⅔ of maintenance requirements.[26] Furthermore, maintenance fluids are necessary to perfuse, oxygenate, and deliver host defenses to the central nervous system, and although SIADH occurs in bacterial meningitis, there is no evidence that fluid restriction *prevents* its occurrence. Therefore it is preferable to give full maintenance fluids and monitor the serum sodium concentration. If the serum sodium level drops below 125 mEq/L, the test should be repeated as soon as possible. If the serum sodium is still below 125 mEq/L, fluids should be restricted to balance urine output and insensible loss until the serum electrolyte concentrations are corrected.

The use of steroids as adjunctive treatment in patients with bacterial meningitis has, until recently, been discouraged on the basis of equivocal results in two clinical trials conducted in the 1960s.[2,10] A recent placebo-controlled double-blind study of children with bacterial meningitis showed that sig-

Table 227-3 *Scoring System for Prediction of Morbidity in Haemophilus influenzae Meningitis*

FACTOR AT ADMISSION	POINTS
Severe coma (apnea, nonreactive pupils, no response to pain)	3
Hypothermia (temperature <36.6° C)	2
Seizures (major motor or generalized)	2
Shock (systolic blood pressure <60 mm Hg)	1
Age <12 mo	1
CSF white blood cell count <1000 × 10/L	1
Hemoglobin <110 g/L	1
CSF glucose	
<1.1 mmol/L	0.5
Symptoms persisting >3 d	0.5

From Gary N, et al: Clinical identification and comparative prognosis of high-risk-patients with *Haemophilus influenzae* meningitis, Am J Dis Child 143:307, 1989.

nificantly fewer children who received an antibiotic plus dexamethasone (0.15 mg/kg/dose given every 6 hours for 4 days) had severe hearing loss compared with children who received antibiotic alone.[20] This difference was observed in children with low Herson-Todd scores (Table 227-3) but not high scores. Another study showed that children with high Herson-Todd scores (≥4.5) who received steroids, with or without osmotic support, had significantly better outcomes than those who did not receive steroids and the outcome of steroid-treated children with high scores was equivalent to that of children with low scores.[13] Thus, there are now studies showing that dexamethasone improves the hearing outcome of children with good prognostic scores and the neurologic outcome of children with poor prognostic scores. Although further studies are needed to confirm these results, the American Academy of Pediatrics Committee on Infectious Diseases currently recommends that dexamethasone, 0.6 mg/kg/day, be given for 4 days starting at the time of the first dose of antimicrobial agents to children 2 months of age or older likely to have bacterial meningitis.[6]

All *N. meningitidis* and most *S. pneumoniae* strains are exquisitely susceptible to penicillin and ampicillin. However, over 20% of *H. influenzae* type b isolates are resistant to ampicillin. All three of these pathogens are susceptible to very low concentrations of the third-generation cephalosporins ceftriaxone and cefotaxime. A survey of the directors of pediatric infectious disease programs, conducted in 1989, showed that nearly 60% treated bacterial meningitis in children over 5 weeks of age with either ceftriaxone (initial dose of 100 mg/kg given intravenously followed by 80 mg/kg/day given intravenously or intramuscularly once daily) or cefotaxime (200 mg/kg/day divided into equal doses and given intravenously every 6 hours). An alternative is to give, intravenously, penicillin (200,000 U/kg/day divided into equal doses and given every 4 to 6 hours) *or* ampicillin (300 mg/kg/day divided into equal doses and given every 6 hours) *plus* chloramphenicol (75 mg/kg/day divided into equal doses and given every 6 hours). Meningitis that is caused by *N. meningitidis* is usually treated for 7 days; meningitis caused by *H. influenzae* type b or *S. pneumoniae* is treated for 10 days. A 7-day course of antibiotic therapy for uncomplicated *H. influenzae* type b and *S. pneumoniae* meningitis has been shown effective.[19,22] If chloramphenicol is used, serum chloramphenicol concentrations should be monitored when possible, and patients treated with oral chloramphenicol should receive the full course of therapy in the hospital. Although most cases of bacterial meningitis are caused by the three organisms mentioned, other bacteria can cause meningitis; in such cases, antibiotic therapy must be individualized.

Most therapeutic failures can be related to delayed diagnosis, inadequate therapy with the correct antibiotic, or resistant organisms. Two potential resistance problems should be mentioned. There have been occasional reports of pneumococci relatively insensitive to penicillin[1] and *H. influenzae* type b resistant to chloramphenicol.[4] Relatively insensitive pneumococci are killed by usual serum concentrations of penicillin but not by concentrations normally reached in the CSF. If pneumococci are isolated from the CSF after a patient has received 24 to 48 hours of intravenous penicillin, the patient should be given chloramphenicol, and the susceptibility of the isolate to other antibiotics should be determined. Although in vitro susceptibility testing suggests that either ceftriaxone or cefotaxime would be effective, there has been little clinical experience in this setting. Chloramphenicol-resistant *H. influenzae* type b strains have rarely been isolated from clinical specimens in the United States. If an isolate is resistant to both ampicillin and chloramphenicol, the use of one of the cephalosporins mentioned previously is indicated. A repeat lumbar puncture on completion of therapy does not reflect the adequacy of therapy or predict the likelihood of recurrence and is not usually indicated. However, a delay in sterilization of the CSF beyond 24 to 36 hours has been associated with adverse outcomes; therefore some experts recommend that a repeat lumbar puncture be performed at that time.[21]

Some contacts of patients with *N. meningitidis* or *H. influenzae* type b meningitis are at increased risk for disease and should therefore receive prophylaxis. Persons at risk for *N. meningitidis* and prophylactic regimens are detailed in Chapter 283. Whether contacts of patients with *H. influenzae* type b disease should receive prophylaxis remains controversial. The American Academy of Pediatrics recommends that rifampin, 20 mg/kg (600 mg maximum), be given once a day for 4 days to all household contacts, including adults, in households with at least one contact younger than 4 years of age. A household contact is anyone who resides with the index patient or a nonresident who has spent 4 or more hours a day with the index patient for 5 of the 7 days before the index patient was hospitalized. Because children younger than 3 years of age are at risk for a second attack of *H. influenzae* type b disease, some authorities recommend prophylaxis for all household contacts, regardless of age, to prevent recolonization on the index patient.[15] The index patient should receive rifampin either during or at the completion of treatment for meningitis.

Complications

Early in the course of the disease, increased intracranial pressure, septic shock, cardiorespiratory arrest, and disseminated intravascular coagulation (DIC) should be anticipated. Subdural effusions occasionally cause seizures or focal neurologic deficits, and in such cases the fluid should be removed by subdural taps. The inappropriate secretion of antidiuretic hormone also can complicate bacterial meningitis; therefore the patient should be carefully monitored for this complication, and if it occurs, fluids should be severely restricted. A brain abscess following bacterial meningitis is extremely rare.

Sequelae

Although the Herson-Todd scoring system can indicate which children are more likely to have a bad outcome, it is not possible to predict long-term sequelae for an individual child at the time of discharge from the hospital. Some children who are apparently normal will subsequently have hearing or learning deficits or develop a seizure disorder. Conversely, some children expected to have a dismal prognosis make remarkable gains. It is therefore important for the practitioner to be optimistic with the family while remaining sensitive to possible sequelae and observing these children closely for the attainment of developmental milestones. Hearing should be formally tested before discharge from the hospital, since most sensorineural hearing loss can be detected at this time.

PREVENTION

In 1985 a purified capsular polysaccharide vaccine against *H. influenzae* type b was licensed for use in the United States. A poor immunogen in children less than 2 years of age, this vaccine was soon replaced by vaccines made by coupling the capsular polysaccharide to a protein carrier. Protein-conjugate vaccines are generally good immunogens in infants, and three are currently available in the United States for administration to children at 15 months of age. One of these vaccines (Lederle-Praxis Biologicals' Hibtiter) was recently approved by the Food and Drug Administration for use in infants at 2, 4, and 6 months of age. Conjugate vaccines in various stages of clinical testing are listed in Table 227-4. If recommendations of the American Academy of Pediatrics Committee on Infectious Diseases to administer Hib vaccine at 2, 4, 6 and 15 months of age[18] are followed, most cases of invasive *H. influenzae* type b disease during the next decade can be prevented by vaccination during infancy. The meningococcal and pneumococcal vaccines currently available are composed of purified capsular polysaccharides, and like the prototype *H. influenzae* type b vaccine, are poor immunogens in infants less than 2 years of age.

Partially Treated Meningitis

Several studies[7,9] have shown that *mean* values for white blood cell counts in CSF, percent of polymorphonuclear cells, and level of glucose and protein concentrations in patients with partially treated bacterial meningitis do not differ from those values in patients not previously treated. However, some patients with partially treated bacterial meningitis will have CSF findings indistinguishable from the classic findings for aseptic meningitis.[7] Unless there is clear evidence of a nonbacterial cause (such as isolation of virus from CSF or blood), antibiotics should be administered to partially treated patients for 7 to 10 days at dosages appropriate for bacterial meningitis.

NEONATAL MENINGITIS

Neonatal meningitis merits separate consideration, because the incidence is high, the etiologic agents are unique, and it is often fatal. The incidence of neonatal meningitis varies with the reporting institute from 0.2 to 1 case per 1000 live births. The age-specific incidence of bacterial meningitis (estimated from 38 states) reported in 1978 was 96 per 100,000 neonates. Case fatality rates range from 15% to 75%, and in a recent report from the Neonatal Meningitis Cooperative Study Group the overall case fatality rate was 30%.[23] In general, mortality is lower for full-term infants than for infants with low birth weight (under 2500 g). Early recognition and treatment are critical, since the case fatality rate falls to about 5% for neonates surviving the first 24 hours of the disease.[23]

The cause of neonatal meningitis has changed in the past decade, and clinicians should be alert to the possibility of future etiologic shifts. During the 1960s, most cases of neonatal meningitis were caused by gram-negative enteric organisms, primarily *E. coli*; gram-positive isolates were likely to be *L. monocytogenes*. During the 1970s, group B streptococci entered the scene; currently this organism and *E. coli* account for 60% to 80% of the cases and *L. monocytogenes* for about 5%. Recent reports have called attention to an increase in the incidence of neonatal sepsis and meningitis caused by non-group D alpha-hemolytic streptococci[3] and coagulase-negative staphylococci.[16]

The clinical signs associated with neonatal meningitis are nonspecific and therefore not very helpful. Neonates often have apneic episodes or feed poorly, and they can be hyper-

Table 227-4 *Haemophilus influenzae type b Capsular Polysaccharide Protein Conjugate Vaccines Under Investigation*

INVESTIGATORS (MANUFACTURER)	CARRIER PROTEIN	SPACER
Schneerson R, Robbins JB, et al (Merieux Institute)	Tetanus toxoid	6 Carbon
Gordon LK (Connaught Laboratories)	Diphtheria toxoid	6 Carbon
Anderson P, et al; Madore DV, et al (Lederle-Praxis Biologicals)	CRM—a nontoxic, mutant diphtheria toxin	None
Marburg S, Jorn D, et al (Merck, Sharpe and Dohme Laboratories)	*N. Meningitidis* 40-kDa OMP (group B)	Complex, containing a thioether

Modified from Weinberg GA, Granoff DM: Polysaccharide-protein conjugate vaccines for prevention of *Haemophilus influenzae* type b disease. *J Pediatr* 113:621, 1988.

thermic or hypothermic, irritable or lethargic, and have respiratory distress or diarrhea; only infrequently do they have nuchal rigidity or a bulging fontanelle. The neonate has a limited repertoire of clinical responses to disease or insult; most sick neonates therefore receive a septic work-up, including a lumbar puncture, and antibiotics are started pending culture results. The cytology and chemistry of the CSF in neonates have a much broader normal range than in other age groups, especially during the first week of life (Table 227-5). When Sarff and co-workers[28] compared CSF values from high-risk infants without meningitis to those with meningitis, no single test results separated the groups. However, only 1 out of 119 infants with bacterial meningitis had normal CSF on examination.

Antibiotic Therapy

The principles of antibiotic therapy for neonatal meningitis are the same as for infants and children, but because the organisms are different, the antibiotic selection must be adjusted. Based on the most common organisms causing neonatal meningitis, the ideal antibiotic would be effective against *E. coli* and other enteric organisms as well as group B streptococci and other gram-positive organisms. Two third-generation cephalosporins, cefotaxime and ceftriaxone, are extremely active against the usual organisms causing neonatal meningitis, with the exception of *L. monocytogenes*. The major difference between these drugs is half-life; cefotaxime has the shortest and ceftriaxone the longest. Data from the Neonatal Meningitis Cooperative Study Group comparing these agents with the combination of ampicillin plus gentamicin or amikacin are not yet available. However, because the drugs are safe, are very active against the common pathogens, and enter the CSF relatively well, one of these agents plus ampicillin should be used to treat documented meningitis. Because some enteric pathogens such as *Pseudomonas aeruginosa* and Enterobacteriaceae readily become resistant to these third-generation cephalosporins, they should not be used empirically for suspected sepsis in neonates. Dosages and characteristics of the antibiotics most often used to treat neonatal meningitis are listed in Table 227-6. Ceftriaxone is highly protein bound and can displace unconjugated bilirubin from albumin. Therefore ceftriaxone should not be used in premature infants at risk for kernicterus or in term infants with hyperbilirubinemia.

The role of intraventricular antibiotics remains controversial; ideally, the newer antibiotics mentioned will bypass this question. Other therapeutic considerations are the same for neonates as for infants and children with bacterial meningitis.

Prognosis

The complications of neonatal meningitis are similar to those seen in older infants and include hydrocephalus, deafness, and blindness. The case fatality rate is 20% to 50%, and long-term follow-up studies[23] have revealed that about 65% of survivors are normal 3 to 7 years after the illness. A brain abscess rarely complicates neonatal meningitis except when the pathogen is *Citrobacter*. For unknown reasons, as many as 80% of neonates with *Citrobacter* meningitis also will have a brain abscess. As with older infants and children, all infants recovering from meningitis should have careful audiology testing and close evaluation for the attainment of developmental milestones.

Table 227-5 *Representative Cerebrospinal Fluid Findings in High-Risk Neonates Without Meningitis*

CSF FINDINGS	FULL-TERM NEONATES—MEAN (RANGE)	PRETERM NEONATES—MEAN (RANGE)
White blood cells per cubic millimeter	8.2 (0-32)	9.0 (0-29)
Polymorphonuclear neutrophils	61.3%	57.2%
Protein (mg/dl)	90 (20-170)	115 (65-150)
Glucose (mg/dl)	52 (34-119)	50 (24-63)
CSF/blood glucose ratio	0.81 (0.44-2.38)	0.74 (0.55-1.05)

Modified from Sarff LD, Platt LH, and McCracken GH Jr: Cerebrospinal fluid evaluation in neonates: comparison of high-risk infants with and without meningitis. J Pediatr 88:473, 1976.

Table 227-6 *Some Characteristics of Antibiotics Useful or Potentially Useful in the Treatment of Neonatal Meningitis*

	DOSE (mg/kg/dose)					
DRUG	AGE 0-7 DAYS	AGE >7 DAYS	GRAM-POSITIVE COVERAGE	GRAM-NEGATIVE COVERAGE	ANAEROBIC COVERAGE	CSF PENETRATION
Ampicillin	50 mg q12h	50 mg q6	Good	Fair	Good	Good
Amikacin	10 mg q12h	10 mg q8	Fair	Good	None	Fair
Gentamicin	2.5 mg q12h	2.5 mg q8h	Fair	Good	None	Fair
Cefotaxime	50 mg q12h	50 mg q8h	Good	Excellent	Good	Good
Ceftriaxone	50 mg q24h	50 mg q24h	Good	Excellent	Good	Excellent

Modified from McCracken GM and Nelson JD: The third-generation cephalosporins and the pediatric practitioner, Pediatr Infect Dis 1:123, 1982.

ASEPTIC MENINGITIS

The syndrome of aseptic meningitis consists of a clinical picture of meningitis with CSF pleocytosis and the absence of bacteria on Gram stain or culture. Although aseptic meningitis is usually a viral disease, it is important that treatable causes of this syndrome be considered in the differential diagnosis. The box on p. 1355 lists a wide variety of infectious and noninfectious agents and diseases that have been associated with aseptic meningitis. Nonpolio enteroviruses cause most cases of aseptic meningitis in the United States, but mumps and polio should be considered in endemic areas. Mycobacteria, rickettsiae, fungi, and parasites can be treated, as can parameningeal infections and intoxications. The CSF findings characteristic of aseptic meningitis are shown in Table 227-2.

Clinical Manifestations

Infants and children with aseptic meningitis are frequently febrile, irritable, and lethargic. The temperature usually is 38.5° to 40° C, rarely higher. Upper respiratory tract symptoms, myalgia, nausea, and vomiting are also commonly present. In general, the child with viral meningitis does not appear as critically ill as the child with bacterial meningitis.

The diagnosis of aseptic meningitis is likely when CSF pleocytosis ranges from 10 to 500 cells, which are predominantly lymphocytes; the CSF protein is mildly elevated—50 to 150 mg/dl; and the CSF glucose level is normal. Early in the course of viral meningitis, polymorphonuclear neutrophils (PMNs) can predominate in the CSF. A transition from a predominance of PMNs to lymphocytes usually occurs rapidly, and a repeat lumbar puncture after 8 to 12 hours may show this transition. Hypoglycorrhachia (low CSF glucose level) can occur with viral meningitis caused by enteroviruses, mumps, herpes simplex, and Eastern equine encephalitis viruses. Hypoglycorrhachia caused by these viruses tends to result in CSF glucose concentrations that equal about 75% of the simultaneous blood glucose concentration, whereas bacterial meningitis usually results in CSF glucose concentrations of less than 30% of the blood glucose. The CSF glucose level can also be low with tuberculous and fungal meningitis.

Many physicians are reluctant to obtain specimens for viral culture because they believe that the isolation of viruses takes too long to affect patient management. A review of patients who had CSF specimens sent for viral culture showed that of 113 patients with a discharge diagnosis of aseptic meningitis, 46 had enteroviral meningitis, 2 had tuberculous meningitis, 2 had herpes simplex meningoencephalitis, 1 had leukemic meningitis, and 1 had toxoplasmosis with central nervous system involvement.[5] It took an average of 3.7 days for CSF cultures to show a typical enterovirus cytopathic effect. The diagnosis of enteroviral meningitis frequently resulted in the discontinuation of antibiotic therapy and early discharge from the hospital. Therefore, when viral meningitis is a possibility, the CSF should be cultured for viruses, as should nasopharyngeal or throat and rectal swab specimens. Although the isolation of a virus from a site other than the CSF could be misleading, if taken in the context of other clinical and laboratory findings, a presumptive diagnosis can often be made when a virus is isolated from one or more of these sites.

The management of viral meningitis is directed to supportive care. Meningoencephalitis caused by herpes simplex or varicella-zoster viruses should be treated with acyclovir.

Outcome

The outcome of aseptic meningitis relates to both the causative agent and the age of the child. Patients with the most common known cause of viral meningitis, enteroviral meningitis, usually recover completely. However, several groups[11,29,30] have reported low intelligence and delayed speech development following enteroviral meningitis in young infants. In light of these findings, the prognosis for an infant younger than 1 year of age is somewhat guarded, and the child's development should be carefully monitored.

REFERENCES

1. Ahronheim GA, Reich B, and Marks MI: Penicillin-insensitive pneumococci, Am J Dis Child 133:187, 1979.
2. Belsey MA, Hoffpauir CW, and Smith MH: Dexamethasone in the treatment of acute bacterial meningitis: the effect of study design on the interpretation of results, Pediatrics 44:503, 1969.
3. Broughton RA, Krafka R, and Baker CJ: Non-group D alphahemolytic streptococci: new neonatal pathogens, J Pediatr 99:450, 1981.
4. Campos J et al: Multiply-resistant *Haemophilus influenzae* type b causing meningitis: comparative clinical and laboratory study, J Pediatr 108:897, 1986.
5. Chonmaitree T, Menegus MA, and Powell KR: The clinical relevance of CSF viral culture: a 2-year experience with aseptic meningitis in Rochester, NY, JAMA 247:1843, 1982.
6. Committee on Infectious Diseases, 1989-1990: Dexamethasone therapy for bacterial meningitis in infants and children, Pediatrics 86:130, 1990.
7. Converse GM et al: Alterations of cerebrospinal fluid findings by partial treatment of bacterial meningitis, J Pediatr 83:220, 1973.
8. Corrigan JJ: Heparin therapy in bacterial sepsis, J Pediatr 91:695, 1977.
9. Davis SD et al: Partial antibiotic therapy in *Haemophilus influenzae* meningitis: its effect on cerebrospinal fluid abnormalities, Am J Dis Child 129:802, 1975.
10. deLemos RA and Haggerty RJ: Corticosteroids as an adjunct to treatment in bacterial meningitis: a controlled clinical trial, Pediatrics 44:30, 1969.
11. Farmer CJ, Carpenter RL, and Ray CG: A follow-up study of 15 cases of neonatal meningoencephalitis due to coxsackievirus B5, J Pediatr 87:568, 1975.
12. Feigen RD: Bacterial meningitis beyond the neonatal period. In Feigen RD and Cherry JD, editors: Textbook of pediatric infectious diseases, Philadelphia, 1987, WB Saunders Co.
13. Gary N, Powers N, and Todd JK: Clinical identification and comparative prognosis of high-risk patients with *Haemophilus influenzae* meningitis, Am J Dis Child 143:307, 1989.
14. Goitein KJ and Tamir I: Cerebral perfusion pressure in central nervous system infections of infancy and childhood, J Pediatr 103:40, 1983.
15. Gray BM: Reinfection with *Haemophilus influenzae* type b. Program and abstracts of the Twenty-fourth Interscience Conference on Antimicrobial Agents and Chemotherapy, Washington, DC, October, 1984.
16. Gruskay J et al: Neonatal *Staphylococcus epidermidis* meningitis with unremarkable CSF examination results, Am J Dis Child 143:580, 1989.
17. Herson VC and Todd JK: Prediction of morbidity in *Haemophilus influenzae* meningitis, Pediatrics 59:35, 1977.
18. Hoekelman RA: A pediatrician's view: Hib vaccination now! Pediatr Ann 19:683, 1990.
19. Jadavji T et al: Sequelae of acute bacterial meningitis in children treated for seven days, Pediatrics 78:21, 1986.

20. Lebel MH et al: Dexamethasone therapy for bacterial meningitis: results of two double-blind, placebo-controlled trials, N Engl J Med 319:964, 1988.
21. Lebel MH and McCracken GH Jr: Delayed cerebrospinal fluid sterilization and adverse outcome of bacterial meningitis in infants and children, Pediatrics 83:161, 1989.
22. Lin TY et al: Seven days of ceftriaxone therapy is as effective as ten days' treatment for bacterial meningitis, JAMA 253:3559, 1985.
23. McCracken GH JR: Perinatal bacterial diseases. In Feigen RD and Cherry JD, editors: Textbook of pediatric infectious diseases, ed 2, Philadelphia, 1987, WB Saunders Co.
24. Murphy TV et al: Pharyngeal colonization with *Haemophilus influenzae* type b in children in a day care center without invasive disease, J Pediatr 106:712, 1985.
25. Powell KR et al: A prospective search for congenital dermal abnormalities of the craniospinal axis, J Pediatr 87:744, 1975.
26. Powell KR et al: Normalization of plasma arginine vasopressin concentrations when children with meningitis are given maintenance plus replacement fluid therapy, J Pediatr 117:515, 1990.
27. Sande MA, Scheld WM, and McCracken GH, editors: Proceedings of a workshop: pathophysiology of bacterial meningitis—implications for new management strategies, Pediatr Infect Dis J 6:1145, 1987.
28. Sarff LD, Platt LH, and McCracken GH Jr: Cerebrospinal fluid evaluation in neonates: comparison of high-risk infants with and without meningitis, J Pediatr 88:473, 1976.
29. Sells CJ, Carpenter RL, and Ray CG: Sequelae of central nervous system enterovirus infections, N Engl J Med 293:1, 1975.
30. Wilfert CM et al: Longitudinal assessment of children with enteroviral meningitis during the first three months of life, Pediatrics 67:811, 1981.
31. Yogev R: Advances in diagnosis and treatment of childhood meningitis, Pediatr Infect Dis J 4:321, 1985.

228

Meningoencephalitis

Margaret K. Ikeda and Richard S. K. Young

Meningoencephalitis is an infection or inflammation of the central nervous system and meninges caused by diverse agents. In the pediatric age-group the most common pathogens are viruses, but other etiologic agents include fungi, parasites, bacteria, and noninfectious agents. Depending on the extent of the infection, the patient may have signs and symptoms of meningitis, encephalitis, or myelitis.

The actual incidence of infectious meningoencephalitis almost certainly exceeds the nearly 12,000 cases reported each year to the Centers for Disease Control as aseptic meningitis and encephalitis.[12] However, the difficulty in identifying the specific agent in each suspected case makes statistical accuracy impossible.

ETIOLOGY OF CHILDHOOD MENINGOENCEPHALITIS

The course of meningoencephalitis may vary from aseptic meningitis with a mild clinical presentation to a fulminant encephalitis with paresis, seizures, increased intracranial pressure, and death.[2] Although the initial signs and symptoms produced by viruses may be similar, differences in seasonal occurrence, clinical course, and outcome allow them to be differentiated.

The family of enteroviruses, including poliovirus, echovirus, and coxsackievirus, is responsible for 85% of cases of aseptic meningitis each year.[4] Enteroviral infection usually is heralded by the development of malaise and gastroenteritis, more often during the summer months (see Chapter 202). Progression to meningoencephalitis is uncommon with most enteroviral infections. When meningoencephalitis does occur, it usually is a mild disease. Poliovirus infections have been virtually eliminated by widespread immunization and now occur primarily in immunodeficient children or among small communities of unimmunized children. Echovirus infections commonly begin with petechial rash; coxsackie infections often start with myalgia and lesions of the palms, soles, and mouth. Although the fetus may be infected transplacentally by an enterovirus, maternal antibodies are protective. An infection of the fetus at term may be severe because delivery of the infant may occur before the development and transfer of maternal antibodies.

Herpes simplex virus infections commonly lead to a severe encephalitis in which 50% to 70% of untreated cases are fatal. As many as 60% of fatal cases are attributed to herpes simplex virus. Although most cases of herpes simplex encephalitis occur in adulthood, there is a bimodal age distribution, with one third of cases occurring in childhood. Neonatal infection results from passage through an infected birth canal. Mothers of infected infants frequently have no symptoms of herpes infection during or before the gestational period, making the diagnosis of a neonatal infection more difficult. Herpes simplex in the neonate may manifest as cutaneous disease, as meningoencephalitis, or as disseminated disease. In all age-groups, herpes simplex infrequently may be the cause of a mild, self-limited meningoencephalitis that resembles the neurologic illness produced by the Epstein-Barr virus. Varicella zoster virus is a herpes virus that causes chickenpox or herpes zoster (shingles).

Arboviral infections caused by Bunyavirus and togavirus are transmitted to human beings by arthropods. Arbovirus meningoencephalitis often occurs in epidemics during the summer and early fall. California virus encephalitis should be suspected in any child in a known endemic region who has signs of fever and cerebrocortical dysfunction. The course usually is mild, with a fatality rate of less than 5%. Western

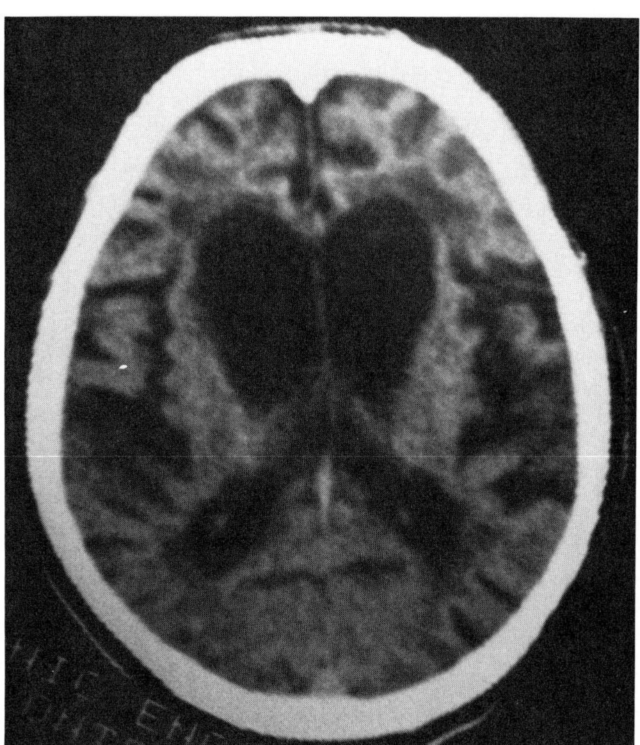

Fig. 228-1 Subacute sclerosing panencephalitis: Marked atrophy of both the cerebral cortex and the deep gray nuclei has occurred in this child with long-standing SSPE.

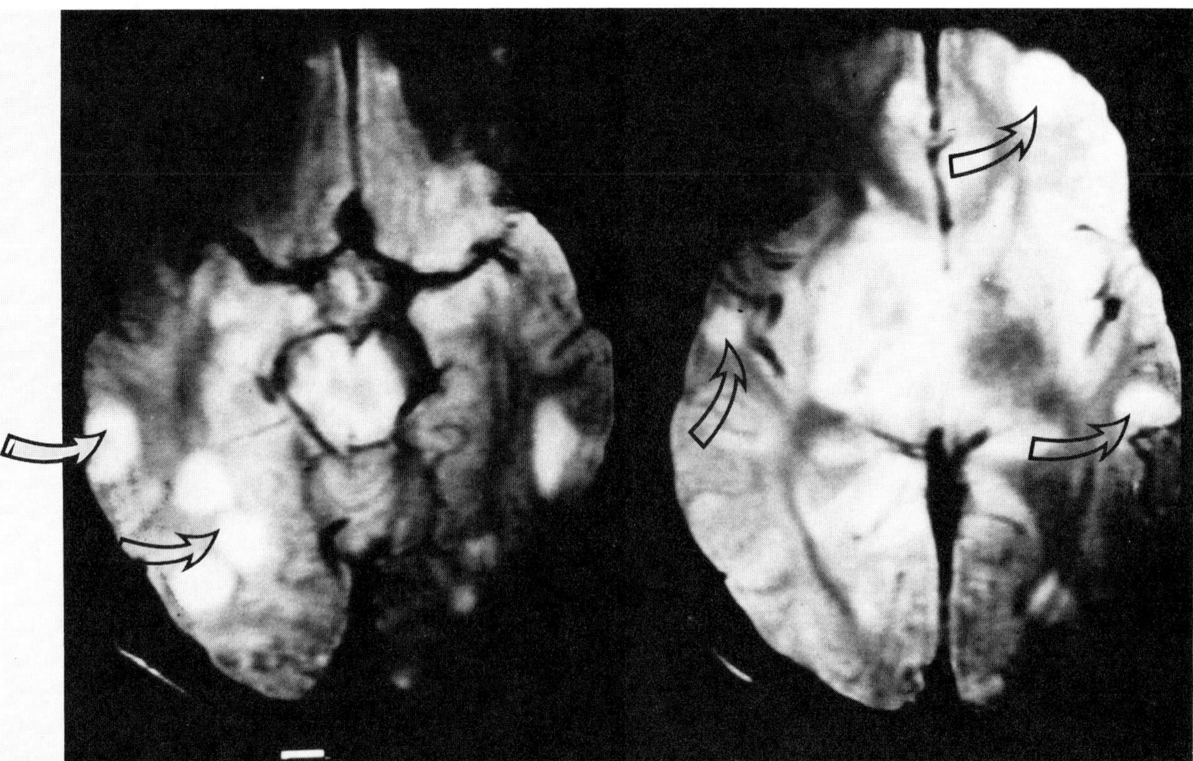

Fig. 228-2 Toxoplasmosis in AIDS: Because they are immunocompromised, patients with AIDS are at risk for opportunistic infections of the central nervous system. This T2-weighted magnetic resonance image shows multiple high intensity lesions caused by *Toxoplasma gondii* scattered throughout the frontal, temporal, and parietal lobes *(arrows)*.

(Courtesy of Dr. G. Sze)

equine encephalitis, an arboviral disease primarily of infancy, causes a more severe syndrome. Eastern equine encephalitis has a predilection for infants and young children and usually is fatal. St. Louis encephalitis occurs most often in epidemic form and produces illness in adults more often than in children.

Other viral diseases are transmitted by vectors. The virus that causes Colorado tick fever is a reovirus transmitted by rodent arthropods and produces a denguelike illness in humans. Viral disease transmitted directly to humans from animals includes lymphocytic choriomeningitis (arenavirus), which is transmitted by infected laboratory or domestic rodents, and rabies, which is transmitted by a bite, scratch, or droplet from an infected wild or a nonimmunized domestic animal. Rabies characteristically has a long incubation period and invariably ends in a fatal meningoencephalitis. Common viral infections such as rubella, adenovirus, influenza, cytomegalovirus, and Epstein-Barr virus (infectious mononucleosis) occasionally can cause meningoencephalitis.

Meningoencephalitis that occurs in the course of childhood exanthems (measles, mumps, rubella, varicella) may result from the host's immunologic response to the virus, as well as from actual infection of the nervous system. Both varicella and measles viruses cause meningoencephalitis in approximately 1 in 1000 cases and within 4 to 7 days after onset of the rash. The severity of the neurologic illness (including irritability, drowsiness, and ataxia) does not appear to be related to the intensity of the systemic illness. Mortality in varicella and measles meningoencephalitis approximates 10%, and up to 50% of survivors may have neurologic re-

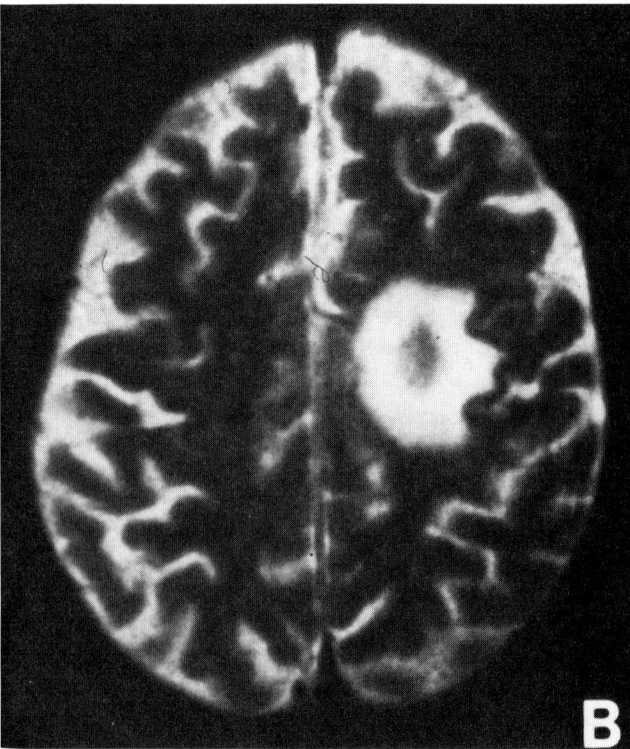

Fig. 228-3 Candida Abscess in AIDS: This T2 magnetic resonance image shows a large left parietal lesion with a mass effect. This lesion is consistent with the diagnosis of toxoplasmosis or lymphoma, but in this patient, proved to be caused by *Candida*.

(Courtesy of Dr. G. Sze)

sidua. A syndrome of dementia and myoclonic seizures can develop in children of school age many years after measles infection or immunization. This disorder results from a persistent measles infection known as subacute sclerosing panencephalitis (SSPE) (Fig. 228-1). Rubella is a less common cause of meningoencephalitis but can result in a more severe illness than measles or varicella. In contrast, mumps meningoencephalitis is a mild illness with a generally good prognosis. Mumps meningoencephalitis may occur without parotitis within a few weeks of exposure to the virus.

Acquired immunodeficiency syndrome (AIDS) is caused by a retrovirus known as human immunodeficiency virus (HIV) and is noteworthy for meningoencephalitides caused both by HIV and by unusual organisms such as *Toxoplasma gondii* (Figs. 228-2 and 228-3) and Epstein-Barr virus. Recovery of more than one organism, whether viral or bacterial, can occur in immunosuppressed patients with AIDS.[10]

Nonviral etiologies of meningoencephalitis include infectious and postinfectious causes and noninfectious conditions associated with cerebrospinal fluid pleocytosis (Table 228-1). These are described more fully by Feigin and Cherry.[5]

SIGNS AND SYMPTOMS

Depending on the extent of the offending virus infection, the patient may have signs and symptoms of meningitis, encephalitis, or myelitis. The patient who has meningitis characteristically will complain of intense headache, stiff neck, and photophobia. Physical findings include meningismus with positive Kernig and Brudzinski signs. The encephalitic patient with lethargy, delirium, or hallucinations may be mistakenly diagnosed as intoxicated or schizophrenic. A central nervous infection should be presumed in every child who has fever and acute mental status change.

Encephalitis may reveal focal neurologic findings. Herpes simplex encephalitis, for instance, is classically heralded by temporal lobe seizures and olfactory hallucinations. Varicella zoster and other viruses may specifically infect the cerebellum, causing acute ataxia. The myelitic form of viral parenchymal disease causes a symmetric limb paralysis, transverse sensory symptoms, and bowel and bladder dysfunction.

Table 228-1 *Etiologies of meningoencephalitis*

INFECTIOUS	POSTINFECTIOUS OR UNKNOWN	NONINFECTIOUS CAUSES OF PLEOCYTOSIS
Viral	Kawasaki syndrome	Intrathecal injections
Enterovirus	Mollaret syndrome	Leukemia
Coxsackie	Reye syndrome	Toxins, e.g., lead
Polio		Trauma
Myxovirus		Lymphoma
Mumps		
Measles		
Inflenza		
Rhabdovirus (rabies)		
Arenavirus (lymphocytic choriomeningitis)		
Bunyavirus (California encephalitis)		
Togavirus		
Eastern equine encephalitis		
Western equine encephalitis		
St. Louis encephalitis		
Rubella		
Reovirus (Colorado tick fever)		
Herpesvirus		
Epstein-Barr virus		
Varicella zoster		
Cytomegalovirus		
Adenovirus		
Human immunodeficiency virus		
Nonviral		
Brain or parameningeal bacterial abscess		
Amebae (*Naegleria and Acanthamoeba* spp.)		
Brucellosis		
Cat-scratch disease		
Fungi (e.g., *Candida and Cryptococcus* spp.)		
Leptospirosis		
Lyme disease (*Borrelia burgdorferi*)		
Lymphogranuloma venereum		
Mycoplasma		
Pertussis		
Rocky Mountain spotted fever		
Syphilis		
Trichinosis		
Tuberculosis		

Table 228-2 *Typical Cerebrospinal Fluid Findings in Meningoencephalitis and Bacterial Meningitis*

CSF FINDINGS	VIRAL MENINGOENCEPHALITIS	BACTERIAL MENINGITIS
Leukocytes	Initial predominance of polymorphonuclear neutrophils, followed by shift to mononuclear cells	Predominantly neutrophils
	Range: 0-2000/mm³	Range: 0-200,000/mm³
Glucose	Greater than 50% of serum concentration	Less than 30% of serum concentration
Protein	Mild to moderate elevation	Marked elevation
	Range: usually <200 mg/dl	Range: usually >150 mg/dl
Gram stain	Negative	Usually reveals bacteria

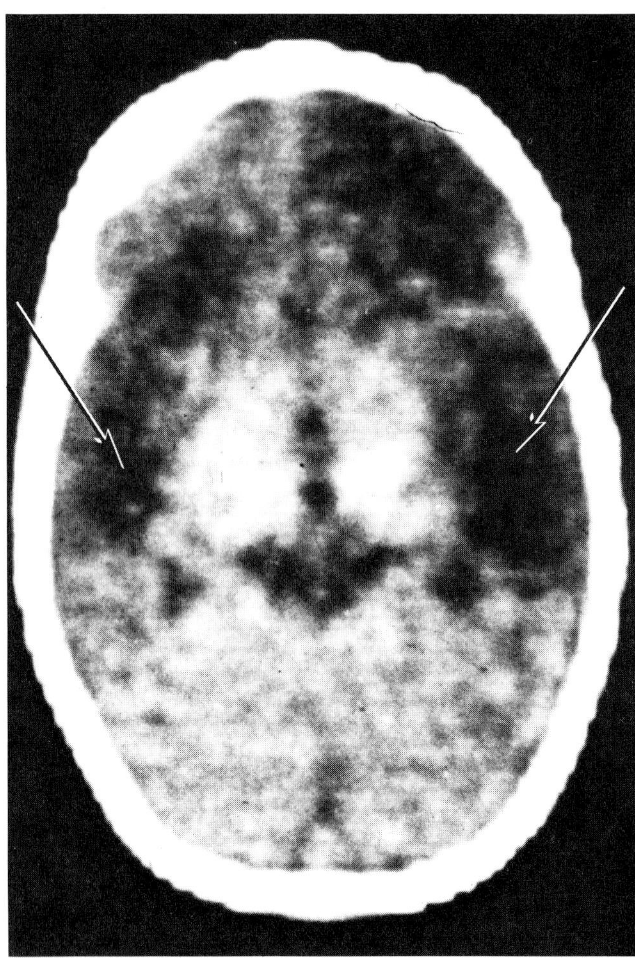

Fig. 228-4 Computed tomographic brain scan of an infant with herpes simplex encephalitis, showing complete necrosis of frontotemporal regions *(arrows)*.

LABORATORY INVESTIGATIONS

Every attempt should be made to identify and to isolate the offending organism to aid in determining the prognosis and to document potential epidemic outbreaks. The cerebrospinal fluid (CSF) examination is crucial. Typical CSF alterations among patients with meningoencephalitis consist of mild pleocytosis, slight increase in protein, and no alteration in glucose concentration (Table 228-2); however, the absence of CSF abnormalities does not rule out encephalitis. The sample of CSF should be refrigerated for later virus isolation and determination of viral antibody titers. Red cells in the CSF may indicate hemorrhagic brain necrosis, commonly seen in herpesvirus infections and eastern equine encephalitis. A predominance of mononuclear cells in the CSF is the exception in acute bacterial meningoencephalitis but may be present with syphilis, Lyme disease,[8] listeriosis, and tuberculosis.

Computed tomography or magnetic resonance imaging of the brain may demonstrate increased intracranial pressure (ventricular compression) or cerebral cortical enhancement. Temporal lobe enhancement or necrosis may be evidence of herpesvirus infection (Fig. 228-4). Electroencephalographic examination is a useful adjunct in the diagnosis of herpes simplex encephalitis.[7]

Specific identification of viruses requires virus isolation by tissue culture. Demonstration of a substantial convalescent antibody rise to a specific virus suggests recent viral infection. Testing the CSF and serum for other organisms may be warranted. A rapid screening test for Epstein-Barr virus (Monospot) is available at most hospitals.

Newborns with cutaneous vesicles who are suspected of having herpes simplex meningoencephalitis need not undergo brain biopsy to establish the diagosis. Rather, attempts should be made to isolate the virus from the throat, eye, or cutaneous lesions. If herpes simplex meningoencephalitis is suspected in older infants or children, a brain biopsy may be indicated for confirmation.[1] In all other nonherpetic meningoencephalitis, blood, urine, stool, and CSF samples should be obtained to facilitate later confirmation of the offending virus. Enteroviruses are isolated relatively easily from throat, stool, and CSF samples. Laboratory diagnosis of mumps meningoencephalitis may be possible within the first week by demonstration of complement-fixing antibodies.

DIFFERENTIAL DIAGNOSIS

Because laboratory tests frequently only suggest rather than confirm the diagnosis of meningoencephalitis, the clinician must carefully consider the differential diagnosis. Subdural empyema (Fig. 228-5) may mimic the course of meningoencephalitis, although the tempo of neurologic dysfunction usually is faster. Focal neurologic signs often are present. Metabolic encephalopathy resulting from Reye syndrome or

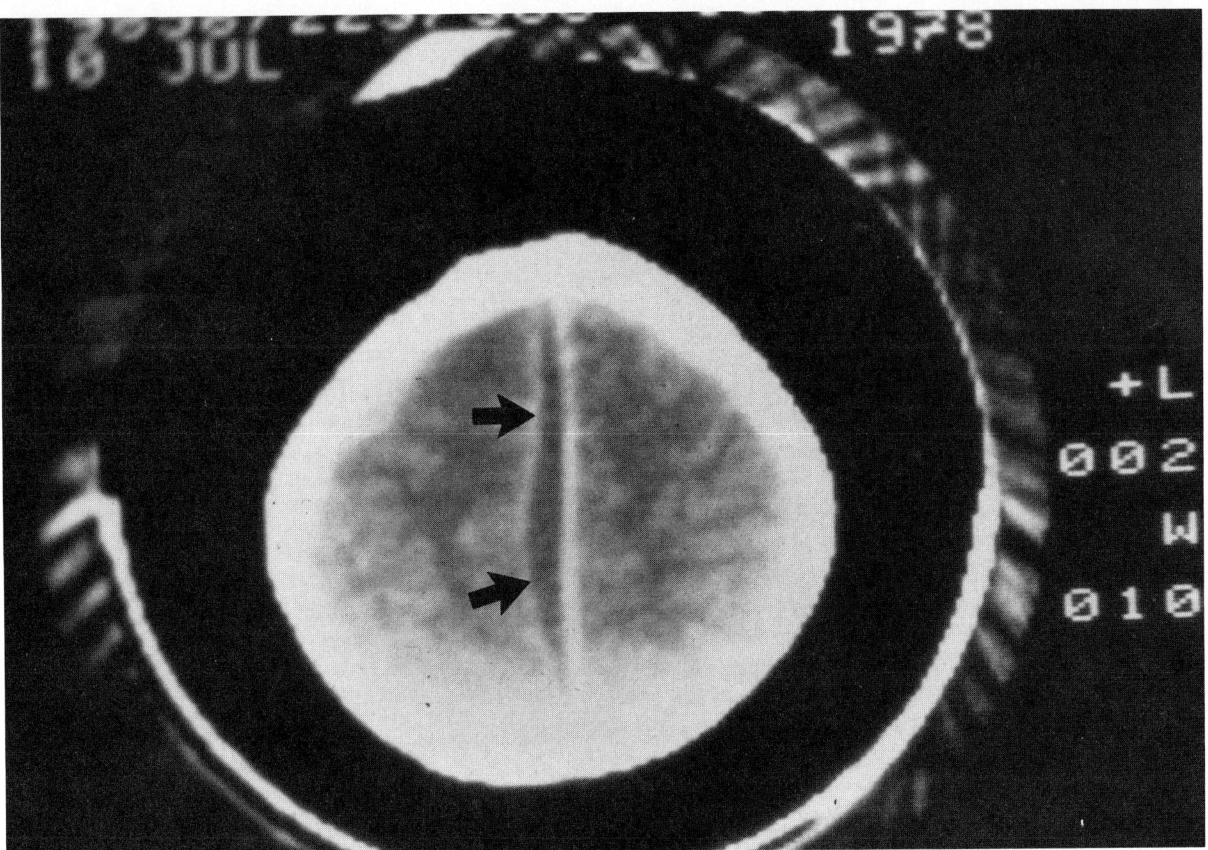

Fig. 228-5 Subdural empyema: This computed tomographic brain scan shows a crescentic empyema *(arrows)* over the cerebral convexity adjacent to the falx cerebri. This child presented with focal seizures of the contralateral foot and leg.

from lead, alcohol, or other toxins can be ruled out by appropriate laboratory investigations. The clinical course of a brain abscess usually is slower, and focal findings may occur; a history of sinus infection, bronchiectasis, or congenital heart disease may be elicited. A myelitic form of viral nervous system infection may be mimicked by demyelinating disease or Guillain-Barré syndrome. Magnetic resonance imaging is superior for ruling out spinal cord tumor, arteriovenous malformation, or infarction.

TREATMENT

Nonspecific treatment of a patient with meningoencephalitis includes reduction of increased intracranial pressure (see Chapter 282), maintenance of fluid and electrolyte balance, respiratory support, and treatment of seizures. Corticosteroids are not of proved benefit in the management of meningoencephalitis and may blunt host defenses.

Specific treatment of acute viral infections of the nervous system exists in herpes simplex infections. Acyclovir has been shown to be superior to vidarabine (ara-A) for parenteral use in herpes infections.[1] Although it is nephrotoxic, acyclovir generally is tolerated by neonates and by children with renal dysfunction or renal transplants. Other antiviral agents (foscarnet, S-HPMPA) are being developed. Ganciclovir, an antiviral agent similar in structure to acyclovir, has been approved for use in cytomegalovirus (CMV) infections.[6] Zidovudine (AZT), an oral preparation, is being administered to symptomatic AIDS patients, although its usefulness is tempered by bone marrow toxicity.[9]

Other drug therapies that may be of potential benefit include intravenous immunoglobulin, which is known to contain viral antibodies for specific viral infections. These nonspecific immunoglobulin preparations have been used as replacement therapy or as adjuncts to treatment of meningoencephalitis in immunodeficient patients. However, immunoglobulin therapy in overwhelming viral sepsis remains controversial. Alpha-interferon has been used as prophylaxis against CMV and varicella zoster in immunocompromised children but not as adjunct therapy in meningoencephalitis.

Prevention is the most cost-effective method of reducing the morbidity and mortality caused by viral meningoencephalitis. Immunization has virtually eliminated poliomyelitis and rubella and has made mumps and measles meningoencephalitis extremely rare. Repeat measles immunizations of older children should further decrease the incidence of measles encephalitis and SSPE. The development of a varicella vaccine holds promise for lowering the morbidity from chickenpox.

PROGNOSIS

The developing nervous system may be more prone to viral infection and more likely to result in serious sequelae. Eastern equine encephalitis, an infectious syndrome more commonly seen in children than in adults, often causes death within 48 hours. Those who survive frequently are severely impaired. Western equine encephalitis is associated with complete recovery in virtually all adults but causes death in 20% of children and a high prevalence of neurologic residua among the survivors. Herpes simplex virus commonly produces a destructive encephalitis in neonates, infants, and children (see Fig. 228-3).

Even the more "benign" meningoencephalitides of infancy, such as those caused by enteroviruses, may produce substantial reductions in head circumference, intelligence, and learning ability. California encephalitis, a relatively mild arbovirus infection, produces emotional learning disorders in 15% of affected children.[3,11] Focal epilepsy may be a sequel of a "mild" encephalitis caused by Epstein-Barr virus.

It is essential that every child with documented or suspected viral nervous system infection be carefully monitored for auditory, visual, and cognitive aftereffects. Carefully performed prospective, sibling-matched controlled studies have shown that these children are at risk for cerebral cortical dysfunction.

REFERENCES

1. Arvin AA et al: Consensus management of the patient with herpes simplex encephalitis, Pediatr Infect Dis 6:2, 1987.
2. Bell WE and McCormick WF: Neurologic infections in children, ed 2, Philadelphia, 1981, WB Saunders Co.
3. Bergman I: Outcome of children with enteroviral meningitis in the first year, J Pediatr 110:705, 1987.
4. Centers for Disease Control: Enteroviral disease in the U.S., 1970-1979, J Infect Dis 146:103, 1982.
5. Feigin RD and Cherry JD: Textbook of pediatric infectious diseases, ed 2, Philadelphia, 1987, WB Saunders Co.
6. Ganciclovir, Med Lett Drugs Ther 31:79, 1989.
7. Mizrahi EM and Tharp BR: A characteristic EEG pattern in neonatal herpes simplex encephalitis, Neurology 32:1215, 1982.
8. Pachner AR, Duray P, and Steere AC: CNS manifestations of Lyme disease, Arch Neurol 46:790, 1989.
9. Pizzo PA: Therapeutic considerations for children with HIV infection, AIDS Update 2(3):1, 1989.
10. Pizzo PA, Eddy J, and Falcon J: AIDS in children, Am J Med 85:195, 1988.
11. Sells SJ, Carpenter RL, and Ray CG: Sequelae of central nervous system enterovirus infections, N Engl J Med 293:1, 1975.
12. Summary of notifiable diseases, U.S., MMWR, 1987.

229

Neonatal Abstinence Syndrome

Loretta P. Finnegan and Karol Kaltenbach

SYMPTOMS IN DEPRESSANT-EXPOSED INFANTS

Infants born to heroin-addicted or methadone-dependent mothers have a high incidence of neonatal abstinence reactions. Less potent opiates have been identified as also precipitating neonatal opiate abstinence syndrome. In addition, a number of nonopiate central nervous system (CNS) depressants have been implicated.

Neonatal opiate or CNS depressant abstinence syndrome is described as a generalized disorder characterized by signs and symptoms of CNS hyperirritability, gastrointestinal dysfunction, respiratory distress, and vague autonomic symptoms, which include yawning, sneezing, mottling, and fever. Infants that are afflicted generally develop tremors, which are initially mild and occur only when the infants are disturbed, but which progress to the point where they occur spontaneously without any stimulation of the infant. A high-pitched cry, increased muscle tone, and irritability develop. The infants tend to have increased deep tendon reflexes and an exaggerated Moro reflex. The rooting reflex is increased, and the infants are frequently seen sucking their fists or thumbs, yet when feedings are administered, they have extreme difficulty and regurgitate frequently because of uncoordinated and ineffectual sucking reflexes. The infants may develop loose stools and therefore are susceptible to dehydration and electrolyte imbalance.

The origin of neonatal abstinence syndrome lies in the abnormal intrauterine environment. A series of steps appears be necessary for its genesis and for the infant's recovery. The growth and survival of the fetus in the intrauterine environment are endangered by the continuing or episodic transfer of drugs of addictive potential from the maternal to the fetal circulation. The fetus undergoes a biochemical adaptation to the presence of the abnormal agent in its tissues. Abrupt removal of the drug at delivery precipitates the onset of symptoms. The newborn infant continues to metabolize and excrete the drug, and withdrawal or abstinence signs occur when critically low tissue levels have been reached. Recovery from abstinence syndrome is gradual and occurs as the infant's metabolism is reprogrammed to adjust to the absence of the dependence-producing agent.[7]

The respiratory systems of the infants are also affected during the withdrawal state, causing excessive nasal secretions, stuffy nose, and rapid respirations, sometimes accompanied by chest retractions, intermittent cyanosis, and apnea. Severe respiratory embarrassment occurs most often when the infant regurgitates, aspirates, and develops aspiration pneumonia.

The effect of heroin withdrawal on respiratory rate and acid-base status has been studied.[14] Infants with acute heroin withdrawal have shown increased respiratory rates associated with hypocapnia and an increase in blood pH during the first week of life. The observed respiratory alkalosis was thought to have a beneficial role in the binding of indirect serum bilirubin to albumin and possibly in the prevention of respiratory distress syndrome, which is rarely observed in infants of addicted mothers. On the other hand, alkalosis can decrease the levels of ionized calcium and lead to tetany.

The high-pitched cry is similar to that of infants with CNS hyperirritability. Blinick has reported on variations in the birth cries of newborn infants from narcotic-addicted and normal mothers.[2] Sound spectrograms of the birth cries of 369 newborns demonstrated a significant increase in abnormal voice changes among 31 babies of addicted mothers.

Sleep patterns are disturbed, and infants have excessive spontaneous generalized sweating. Because newborn infants undergoing narcotic withdrawal have seriously disturbed sleep, Sisson and colleagues studied electroencephalographic (EEG) tracings and electromyographic recordings of eye and mouth movement simultaneously before, during, and after treatment of heroin and methadone withdrawal in 10 infants.[38] Rapid eye movement (REM) and non-REM sleep patterns were correlated with muscular and respiratory activity. These studies concluded that narcotics will obliterate REM sleep in the neonate; withdrawal will prevent normal adequate periods of deep sleep in such infants; proper therapy will cause the return of REM and sleep cycles; and maintenance of therapy can best be regulated by the use of such polygraphic recordings, rather than relying on the observed absence of gross signs and symptoms of withdrawal. Schulman reported the absence of quiet sleep in eight full-term infants whose mothers used heroin until delivery.[36] Heroin-affected infants had evidence of mild withdrawal but did not require medication.

Recent studies by Pinto and co-workers corroborate previous research.[33] Thirteen heroin-exposed babies were studied. Sleep samples were recorded and scored within a few days following birth and repeated 4 to 5 weeks later after recovery from the abstinence syndrome. A significant decrease in quiet sleep and increase of active sleep were found. The same alterations, although less marked, were observed in a follow-up recording performed during the second month of life. Sleep alteration in exposed newborns could be related to CNS distress caused by withdrawal. The authors, however, propose a perturbation of endogenous opiates subsequent to fetal drug exposure as a cause of sleep alterations.

In evaluating the sweating deficit of premature infants, Behrendt and Green noted that 30 of 131 healthy full-size babies and two of 108 healthy low-birth-weight babies demonstrated spontaneous, generalized sweating under standardized conditions.[1] In contrast, eight of 20 low-weight infants of heroin-addicted mothers had spontaneous generalized sweating. In addition, the pharmacologic threshold for sweating was decreased in low-birth-weight infants of addicted mothers as compared to healthy low-birth-weight controls. The authors suggested that this paradox may result from the predominantly central-neurogenic stimulation of sweat glands induced by heroin withdrawal.

At birth, most infants, whether born to heroin- or methadone-dependent mothers, appear physically and behaviorally normal. The time of onset of withdrawal signs ranges from shortly after birth to 2 weeks of age, but for most, signs appear within 72 hours. The type of drug used by the mother; her dosage; the timing of the last dose before delivery; the character of the labor; and the maturity, nutrition, and presence of intrinsic disease in that infant may all play a role in determining the time of onset and in severity, a range of types of clinical courses may be delineated. The withdrawal syndrome may be mild and transient, may be delayed in onset, may have a stepwise increase in severity, may be intermittently present, or may have a biphasic course that includes acute neonatal withdrawal signs followed by improvement and then the onset of a subacute withdrawal reaction.[7]

The occurrence of neonatal seizures associated with opiate abstinence syndrome is also a problem causing concern. Goddard and Wilson reported only one seizure that they could attribute to opiate abstinence syndrome in more than 150 infants born to heroin- or methadone-dependent mothers.[15] On the other hand, other authors have reported a higher incidence of seizures, especially among those infants exposed to methadone in utero.[24,44] Herzlinger and colleagues found that 18 (5.9%) of 302 neonates passively exposed to opiates during pregnancy had seizures that were attributable to withdrawal.[17] Again, the percentage experiencing seizures was higher in the group exposed to methadone alone than in the group exposed to both heroin and methadone. However, there was no apparent relationship between maternal methadone dosage and the frequency or severity of the seizures. In addition, no significant differences were found between neonates with and those without seizures in birth weight, gestational age, occurrence of withdrawal symptoms, day of onset of withdrawal symptoms, or the need for specific pharmacologic treatment. All infants with seizures manifested other withdrawal symptoms before the initial seizure, and the mean age of seizure onset was 10 days. Generalized motor seizures or rhythmic, myoclonic jerks, each of which occurred in seven infants, were the principal seizure manifestations, although in some, the seizure manifestations were complex. Abnormal EEGs tended to occur only during the active seizure phenomenon with normal interictal tracings. The myoclonic jerks observed during neonatal abstinence reactions by many authors may be true seizures.[16,19,29]

More important, the prognosis of abstinence-induced seizures should be considered. Doberczak and co-workers have reported on 14 infants with neonatal abstinence-associated seizures who were assessed neurodevelopmentally during the first year of life.[8] Despite abnormal neurologic examination results in eight of 12 infants at 2 to 4 months of age, nine of 12 infants had normal neurologic examination results at follow-up (two infants were unavailable for follow-up; one infant died of acquired immune deficiency syndrome [AIDS]). Nine neonatal electroencephalograms were abnormal; seven of eight of these abnormal tracings normalized during the first year of life and did not differ from either passively exposed infants without seizures or from published population norms. This short-term favorable prognosis for abstinence-associated seizures differs from that associated with neonatal seizures due to other causes. The authors suggest that this observed improvement in neurologic function may be based on replenishment of neurotransmitters following transient depletion in the neonatal period.

The above symptoms are found secondary to abstinence from the opiate as well as the nonopiate CNS depressants. Although infants born to barbiturate addicts may manifest symptoms similar to those of infants passively exposed to opiates, their symptoms tend to begin at a later age, and undernutrition at birth has not been a usual feature. Since barbiturate withdrawal syndrome may not develop until an infant has been discharged from the nursery, it may not be treated unless suspicion has been aroused by the mother's symptoms or actions. Furthermore, there is a greater risk of seizure activity in infants withdrawing from barbiturates than in those withdrawing from opiates.

Many other aspects of neonatal abstinence have been studied, including brain growth[32]; late presentation of symptoms[24]; delayed excretion with drugs such as methadone[9,34]; abstinence severity with methadone or heroin[11]; sucking behavior[27]; and Brazelton neurobehavioral scale performance.[4,21,25,40,41] These are described in detail elsewhere.[11]

Aside from studies using abstinence scores in evaluating neonatal behavior, the Brazelton Neonatal Assessment Scale has been commonly used.[3] A number of researchers have consistently found that infants born to narcotic-dependent women differ from infants born to non-drug-dependent women in several behaviors.[5,18,25,39,40] Narcotic-exposed infants have been found to be more irritable and less cuddly, to exhibit more tremors, and to have increased tone. Several studies also report that narcotic-exposed infants are less responsive to visual stimulation. However, it has been found that infants undergoing abstinence are less likely to maintain an alert state, so the orientation items of the Brazelton assessment often cannot be completed. Strauss and colleagues report that, when elicited, the orientation behaviors of infants exposed to narcotics were comparable to those of non-drug-exposed infants.[39]

More important, these neonatal behavioral characteristics have implications for mother-infant interaction. A study by Kaltenbach and Finnegan, investigating the effect of neonatal abstinence on the infant's ability to interact with the environment, found that infants born to women maintained on methadone were deficient in their capacity for attention and social responsiveness during the first few days of life.[21] These deficiencies were present regardless of whether neonatal abstinence was severe enough to require treatment. The interactive behavior appeared to be affected until the infant was free of abstinence symptomatology and detoxification was complete. Fitzgerald, Kaltenbach, and Finnegan studied patterns of interaction between drug-dependent women and their infants and non-drug-exposed dyads. Mothers and infants were videotaped at the child's birth and at 4 months of age.[13] Interaction behavior was evaluated by the Greenspan-Lieberman Observational System (GLOS), Newborn GLOS, and the Bayley Scales of Infant Development, including the Infant Behavior Record. The mother's life stress and social support were evaluated by the Social Readjustment Rating Scale and structured interviews, respectively. Drug-dependent mothers and their newborn infants had significantly lower global ratings on dyadic interaction than comparison dyads. Both drug-dependent mothers and their newborns performed poorer on a measure of social engagement. Drug-dependent mothers demonstrated significantly less positive affect and greater detachment, whereas drug-exposed newborns showed fewer behaviors promoting social involvement. At 4 months of age, dyadic interaction quality, social engagement, detachment, and negative affect among drug-exposed infants and their mothers no longer differed from comparisons. However, drug-dependent mothers reported significantly higher levels of stressful events in the past year, which were strongly correlated with their negative affect and detachment scores during interaction. Drug-exposed 4-month-old infants showed significantly greater body tension and poorer coordination on the Infant Behavior Record.

These findings suggest that drug-exposed infants and their mothers experience a difficult early period during which both are less available for, less likely to initiate, and less responsive to social involvement than are comparison dyads. Although better adjusted at 4 months of age, the life stress and infant behavior findings indicate the importance for maternal addiction treatment programs to provide appropriate intervention to facilitate positive mother-infant interaction.

It is clear from numerous studies that despite the maternal choice of drug, neonatal abstinence syndrome may persist in some infants for weeks and in others for months.[7,43] Various investigators have found these infants to have hyperphagia, increased oral drive, sweating, hyperacusis, irregular sleep patterns, poor tolerance to holding or to abrupt changes of position of space, and loose stools.[7] Therefore the clinician not only must assess these infants in the neonatal period, as this chapter describes, but also must realize that long-term follow-up will be essential.

SYMPTOMS IN STIMULANT-EXPOSED NEWBORNS

An epidemic of cocaine use has developed among women. Also, the individual using cocaine frequently uses other psychoactive agents as well. In assessing neonatal abstinence in these cases, the clinician should be aware that abstinence may occur as a result of the narcotics and depressants that the mother may have used concomitantly with cocaine. When cocaine is the primary drug of abuse, most clinicians have not seen symptoms of abstinence significant enough to treat pharmacologically. Infants may react similarly to those exposed to amphetamines and show symptoms of lethargy intermittently with irritability, poor sucking patterns, and sleep disturbances. If narcotics and barbiturates have been used excessively along with cocaine, indications for observation are the same, and the baby should be observed for 4 days. When cocaine is the primary drug, from a purely physical standpoint the infant need not stay in the nursery longer than the general requirement. Unfortunately, family dysfunction, inadequate housing, and lack of infant supplies may often necessitate a longer period of observation.

Studies comparing cocaine as the primary drug of abuse in the perinatal period, but combined with other agents, have been reported. Ryan and co-workers in comparing 36 infants exposed to cocaine and methadone with 43 infants exposed to methadone without cocaine, found that the average frequency of abstinence scores was decreased in 19 of the 21 symptom categories.[35] The exceptions were convulsions and vomiting (Table 229-1).

The data in Table 229-1 suggest that neonatal abstinence symptomatology is not increased by cocaine use. This finding may be related to cocaine's short-lived action and rapid metabolism, or to pharmacologic interactions between cocaine and other drugs used. Despite the cocaine group's lower scoring frequencies for 19 of the 21 symptom categories, statistical significance was not established partly because of the large standard deviations of scores from mean values. However, this study does show that maternal cocaine use concomitantly with methadone does not appear to increase the

Table 229-1 *Average Frequency of Abstinence Scores*

SYMPTOMS	COCAINE/ METHADONE (n = 36)	METHADONE (n = 43)
Cry—high pitched	7.79	15.56
Sleep	17.86	18.12
Hyperactive Moro	9.94	15.07
Disturbed tremor	109.86	144.21
Undisturbed tremor	28.50	41.28
Tone	104.25	137.74
Excoriations	5.42	8.30
Myoclonic jerks	0.53	0.91
Convulsions	0.06	0.02
Sweating	5.61	6.65
Fever	27.53	38.60
Yawning	2.03	3.51
Mottling	24.67	50.49
Nasal stuffiness	35.17	65.16
Sneezing	7.58	15.04
Nasal flaring	0.78	1.05
Respiratory rate	35.97	43.14
Sucking	12.11	14.30
Poor feeding	7.75	10.16
Vomiting	6.72	6.67
Loose stools	13.28	21.18

Finnegan LP and Ehrlich S: Maternal drug abuse during pregnancy: evaluation and pharmacotherapy for neonatal abstinence: In Modern Methods in Pharmacology, vol 6, Testing and evaluation of drugs of abuse, 1990, New York, Wiley Liss, Inc.

severity of neonatal abstinence. Studies by Kosten in adult males and rats have shown similar findings.[28]

Chasnoff and co-workers found increased fetal morbidity when assessing cocaine exposure in comparison to exposure to methadone.[5] Although neonatal gestational age, birth weight, length, and head circumference were not affected by cocaine use compared to methadone use, the Brazelton Neonatal Behavioral Assessment Scale revealed that infants exposed to cocaine had significant depression of organizational response to environmental stimuli (state organization) when compared to methadone-exposed infants.

Doberczak also studied neonatal outcome after cocaine exposure in utero.[8] Thirty-nine infants were examined for neurologic and EEG abnormalities. Of the 39 infants, 34 displayed (CNS) irritability, but only two of the infants required sedation. The EEGs were abnormal in 17 of 38 infants during the first week of life; abnormalities were characterized as showing CNS irritability. The EEG abnormalities could not be predicted on the basis of clinical neurologic dysfunction or perinatal variables. On follow-up, nine of the 17 abnormal EEGs remained abnormal during the second week of life. One infant had an abnormal first EEG at 13 days of age. By 3 to 12 months of age, however, nine of the 10 previously abnormal tracings had normalized and one is pending. The author suggests that these transient clinical and EEG abnormalities may be the result of changes in neurotransmitter availability and function.

The neonatal auditory system has been evaluated by Shih and colleagues subsequent to maternal cocaine abuse.[37] Eighteen neonates born to cocaine-abusing mothers were tested for peripheral and brainstem auditory dysfunction using auditory brainstem responses (ABR). Their data were compared to ABRs from 18 normal neonates. The ABR data were analyzed to determine if ABR parameters were abnormal in neonates born to cocaine-abusing mothers in comparison to normal neonates. ABRs from neonates exposed to maternal cocaine abuse show prolonged interpeak latencies and prolonged absolute latencies. Abnormalities indicate neurologic impairment or dysfunction that warrants further audiologic and neurologic follow-up.

The recent dramatic increase in the use of alkaloidal cocaine (crack) has led to concern about possible deleterious fetal effects associated with its use during pregnancy. Crack, which is not destroyed by heating, can be smoked and delivers a large quantity of cocaine to the vascular bed of the lungs, producing an effect similar to that from intravenous injection. To describe the association of crack use with pregnancy outcome, Cherukuri and colleagues conducted a retrospective matched cohort study of 55 women who admitted to using crack during pregnancy and 55 women who did not use drugs who delivered during the same period.[6] In spite of considerable morbidity in the mothers and a 3.6 times more likely chance of having intrauterine growth retardation, a minority of the infants had abnormal neurobehavioral symptoms and these were mild.

Recognition of a distinct amphetamine-induced abstinence syndrome in adults has been impeded by a common tendency to expect all drug withdrawal reactions to resemble those caused by the CNS depressants. Kalant recognized in 1973 that a syndrome of depression, prolonged sleep, and voracious appetite is characteristic of amphetamine withdrawal.[20] These effects would be expected as rebound phenomena of physical dependence on stimulant and anorexiant drugs.

In contrast, Oro and Dixon compared perinatal cocaine and methamphetamine exposure.[31] Maternal and neonatal growth, behavior, and physiologic organization were evaluated in 104 mother-infant pairs with positive results of urine toxicology screens. An ANOVA comparison of cocaine, methamphetamine, and cocaine plus methamphetamine groups revealed no significant difference perinatal variables. The Finnegan withdrawal scoring schema demonstrates that all three groups of infants had altered neonatal behavioral patterns characterized by abnormal sleep patterns, poor feeding, tremors, and hypertonia. Although the investigators in the previous study found the Neonatal Abstinence Score beneficial in their research, it generally is not an appropriate instrument to assess the subtle symptoms observed in the primarily cocaine-exposed infant nor to identify other risk factors more relevant than clinical symptomatology. Furthermore, negative results in a study in Philadelphia suggest that a different tool is needed to assess the outcome of in utero cocaine exposure.

These results suggest that infants exposed to cocaine but no opiates either are generally symptom free or that the assessment tool is not sensitive enough to evaluate subtle symptoms manifested in them. The response of those exposed to cocaine and methadone reflects that when infants are exposed to methadone and cocaine, they display symptoms that are readily identified by the assessment tool. Furthermore, the assessment tool discriminated between mild, moderate, and severe symptoms, and when using the tool to make the treatment decisions, 40% required pharmacotherapy. In looking at the group exposed to methadone but not cocaine, 100% of the infants exhibited symptoms and once again the assessment tool discriminated between mild, moderate, and severe symptoms, with treatment necessary in 33% of the infants.

Therefore research developing the reliability and validity of the Neonatal Cocaine Exposure Risk Scale is under way. This scale addresses not only neonatal symptomatology, but relevant maternal and infant physical, psychological, and sociological issues. Such a risk scale is important not only to define the prognosis for the infant but also possibly to initiate appropriate discharge planning. Aspects to be scored include maternal prenatal care, concomitant other drug use, maternal drug abuse treatment, maternal physical and psychological symptomatology, homelessness, evidence of positive maternal caretaking abilities, infant morbidity, preterm birth, severe infant lethargy, infant irritability, infant sucking and/or feeding disturbances, excessive and/or high-pitched cry, infant sleep disturbance, and the infant's inability to achieve an alert state and exhibit orienting behavior.

ASSESSMENT OF THE SYMPTOMATOLOGY OF NEONATAL ABSTINENCE

Neonatal Abstinence Score

The Neonatal Abstinence Score is used to monitor the passively depressant-exposed neonate in a comprehensive and objective way; it is essential for assessing the onset, pro-

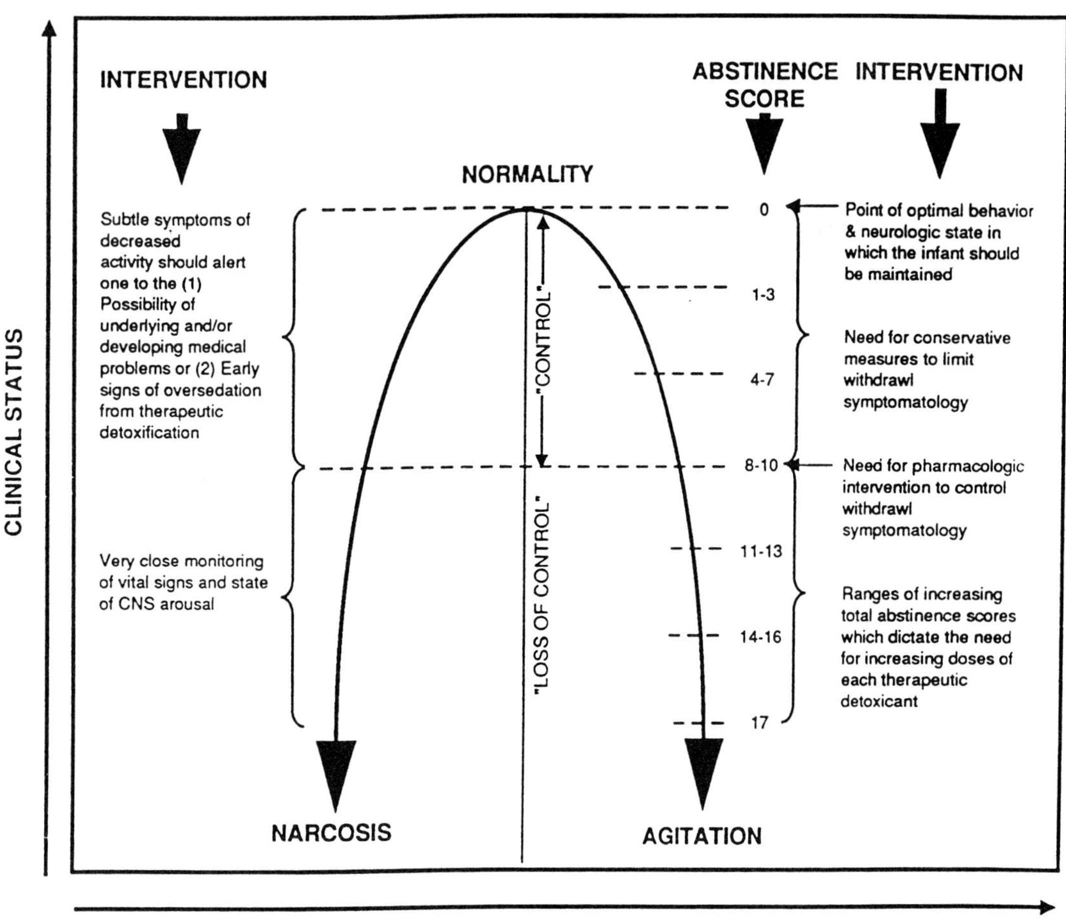

Fig. 229-1 Management of neonatal abstinence syndrome.

(From Finnegan LP: Neonatal abstinence syndrome. In Nelson N, editor: Current therapy in neonatal-perinatal medicine, ed 2, Ontario, 1990, BC Decker, Inc.)

gression, and diminution of symptoms of abstinence. The score is used to monitor the infants' clinical response to the pharmacotherapeutic intervention necessary to control withdrawal symptoms and achieve detoxification (Fig. 229-1).

The abstinence score lists 21 symptoms most commonly seen in the exposed neonate. Signs are recorded as single entities or in several categories if they occur in varying degrees of severity. Each symptom and its associated degree of severity have been assigned a score. Higher scores are assigned to symptoms found in infants with more severe abstinence with consequent increased morbidity and mortality. The total abstinence score is determined by adding the score assigned to each symptom observed throughout the entire scoring interval. The scoring system is dynamic rather than static; that is, all of the signs and symptoms observed during the 4-hour intervals at which infant symptoms are monitored are point-totaled for that interval. Infants are assessed 2 hours after birth and then every 4 hours. If at any point the infant's score is 8 or higher, scoring is done every 2 hours and continued for 24 hours from the last total score of 8 or higher. If the 2-hour scores continue to be 7 or less for 24 hours, then 4-hour scoring intervals may be resumed.

If pharmacotherapy is not needed, the infant is scored for the first 4 days of life at the prescribed 4-hour intervals. (In evaluating several hundred babies exposed to depressants, it was found that 96% of those needing treatment were identified by 4 days of age. The remaining 4% were identified between 5 to 10 days of age by careful follow-up through outreach services). If pharmacologic intervention is required, the infant is scored at 2- or 4-hour intervals, depending on whether the abstinence score is less than or greater than 8, as described above, throughout the duration of the therapy. Once therapy is discontinued, if there is no resurgence in the total score to 8 or higher after 3 days, scoring may be discontinued. If there is a resurgence of symptoms with scores consistently equaling 8 or higher, then scoring should be continued for a minimum of 4 days following discontinuation of therapy to ensure that the infant is not discharged prematurely, with the consequent development of abstinence at home.

The Neonatal Abstinence Scoring Sheet is shown in Fig. 229-2. Symptoms are listed on the left, with their respective scores listed to the right. The time of each evaluation is given at the top, and the total score is shown for each evaluation. A new sheet should be started at the beginning of each day. The complete scoring system allows scoring as frequently as every 2 hours for a full 24-hour period on each sheet.

DATE: **DAILY WEIGHT:**

SYSTEM	SIGNS AND SYMPTOMS	SCORE	AM	PM	COMMENTS
	Excessive High Pitched (other) Cry Continuous High Pitched (other) Cry	2 3			
	Sleeps < 1 hour after feeding Sleeps < 2 hours after feeding Sleeps < 3 hours after feeding	3 2 1			
	Hyperactive Moro reflex Markedly Hyperactive Moro reflex	2 3			
	Mild Tremors Disturbed Moderate-Severe Tremors Disturbed	1 2			
	Mild Tremors Undisturbed Moderate-Severe Tremors Undisturbed	3 4			
	Increased Muscle Tone	2			
	Excoriation (specific areas)	1			
	Myoclonic Jerks	3			
	Generalized Convulsions	5			
	Sweating	1			
	Fever<101 (99-100.8F./37.2-38.2C) Fever>101 (38.4C and higher)	1 2			
	Frequent Yawning (>3-4 times/ interval)	1			
	Mottling	1			
	Nasal Stuffiness	1			
	Sneezing (>3-4 times/interval)	1			
	Nasal Flaring	2			
	Respiratory Rate>60/min Respiratory Rate>60/min with retractions	1 2			
	Excessive Sucking	1			
	Poor Feeding	2			
	Regurgitation Projectile Vomiting	2 3			
	Loose Stools Watery Stools	2 3			
	TOTAL SCORE				
	INITIALS OF SCORER				

Evaluator should place a check next to each sign or symptom observed at various time intervals, then add scores for total score.

Fig. 229-2 Neonatal abstinence score sheet.

(From Finnegan LP: Neonatal abstinence syndrome: assessment and pharmacology. In Rubatelli FF and Granati B, editors: Neonatal therapy: an update, New York, 1986, Excerpta Medica.)

A "Comments" column has been provided so that the nursing and medical staff can record important notes regarding the infant's scoring and treatment and can make reference to relevant progress notes recorded in the infant's chart. Some important points to remember when using the score sheet are:

1. The first abstinence score should be recorded approximately 2 hours after the infant is admitted to the nursery. This score reflects all infant behavior from admission to that first point in time when the scoring interval is completed (this is the first time indicated on the score sheet). The times designating the end of the scoring intervals (whether every 2 or every 4 hours) have been left blank to permit the nursing staff to choose the most appropriate times for the scoring intervals in relation to effective planning and implementation of nursing care.
2. All infants should be scored at 4-hour intervals, except when high scores indicate more frequent scoring.
3. All symptoms exhibited during the entire scoring interval, not just at a single point in time, should be included.

4. The infant should be awakened to elicit reflexes and specified behavior, but if the infant is awakened to be scored, one should not score for diminished sleep after feeding. Sleeping should never be recorded for a scoring interval except under extreme circumstances when the infant has been unable to sleep for an extended period of time—that is, 12 to 18 hours. If the infant is crying, he or she must be quieted before assessing muscle tone, respiratory rate, and the Moro reflex.
5. Respirations are counted for 1 full minute.
6. The infant is scored if prolonged crying is exhibited, even though it may not be high pitched.
7. Temperatures should be taken rectally (mild pyrexia is an early sign indicating heat produced by increased muscle tone and tremors).
8. If the infant is sweating solely because of conservative nursing measures (e.g., swaddling), a point should not be given.

Before pharmacotherapy is initiated, other common neonatal metabolic alterations that can mimic or compound abstinence must be ruled out (e.g., hypocalcemia, hypomagnesemia, hypoglycemia, and hypothermia). Serum glucose and calcium tests may be indicated before therapy is initiated. Toxicologic examination of the urine, for a total of 25 ml collected immediately after birth, is necessary to ensure appropriate choice of pharmacotherapy. Urine collected after 24 to 36 hours of life is likely to be negative for qualitative toxicologic assessment. Maternal urine toxicology may be necessary if the infant's quantity is inadequate or initially discarded.

Pharmacologic intervention is not indicated if consecutive total abstinence scores or the average of any three consecutive scores continues to be 7 or less during the first 4 days of life.

The total scores have been categorized into ranges of scores indicating the severity of abstinence in relation to functional disturbances in various physiologic systems. The total abstinence scores dictate the specific dose of the pharmacotherapeutic agents used to detoxify infants in two management regimens. In the score-dose titration approach, the initial dose of a specific pharmacotherapeutic agent (i.e., paregoric or phenobarbital) and all subsequent doses are determined by and titrated against the total abstinence score. In the phenobarbital loading dose approach, an initial dose of 20 mg/kg is administered in an attempt to achieve an expected therapeutic serum level with a single dose.

The need for pharmacologic intervention is indicated when the total abstinence score is 8 or higher for three consecutive scorings (e.g., 9-8-10) or when the average of any three consecutive scores is 8 or higher (e.g., 9-7-9). Once an infant's score is 8 or higher, the scoring interval automatically becomes 2 hours, so that the infant exhibits symptoms that are out of control for no longer than 4 to 6 hours before therapy is initiated.

If the infant's total score is 12 or higher for two consecutive intervals or the average of any two consecutive scores is 12 or higher, therapy should be initiated at the appropriate detoxicant dosage for that score before more than 4 hours elapses.

In summary, it is important to remember that all infants who meet the scoring criteria for pharmacologic intervention should have the prescribed detoxicant regimen started no later than 4 to 6 hours after loss of control. The severer the abstinence, as reflected by the total score, the greater the need to initiate pharmacotherapy as soon as possible. Finally, the longer the delay in initiation of appropriate pharmacologic intervention, the greater the risk of increased infant morbidity.

GENERAL MEASURES IN THE TREATMENT OF AN INFANT EXPOSED TO DRUGS

While the infant is being assessed with the Neonatal Abstinence Score for potential initiation of pharmacotherapy, general treatment measures should be considered. Overall comfort should be maintained by swaddling, use of a pacifier for excessive sucking, nasal aspiration when necessary, frequent diaper changes (exposure of hyperemic buttock in severe cases for air drying), use of soft sheets or sheepskin to decrease excoriations, positioning to reduce aspiration if vomiting or regurgitation is a prominent symptom. Consideration of weight change patterns is also a key issue and demand or reduced feeding is frequently recommended.

Early weight-change patterns were studied in 101 passively addicted neonates by Weinberger and colleagues.[42] Newborns showing mild abstinence and not requiring pharmacologic treatment lost an average of 4% of birth weight, reached a weight nadir on day 3, and regained birth weight by days 7 to 8. Newborns treated with either paregoric or phenobarbital for more severe signs of abstinence lost an average of 6.3% of birth weight, reached a nadir on days 6 to 7, and regained birth weight only by days 13 to 14. Despite comparable birth weights and energy intakes, treated newborns weighed 95 g less than untreated neonates on day 10 when the untreated neonates were discharged. These investigators suggested that in light of abnormal early weight-change patterns seen with more severe abstinence, both strict control of abstinence and provision of additional individualized nutritional support seem warranted.

Recently, Oro and Dixon have recommended waterbeds as a useful adjunct to supportive care of narcotic-exposed neonates.[31] They described the neonatal course of 30 antenatal narcotic-exposed newborns, half of whom were randomly assigned to nonoscillating waterbeds and half to conventional bassinets. The infants were comparable at birth regarding drug exposure, ethnicity, maternal medical factors, gestational age, growth, and severity of withdrawal at the time of onset. Evaluation of total and subscores of the abstinence syndrome showed a lower total score and a significantly lower CNS subscore on day 5 for infants on waterbeds. The waterbed group demonstrated a significantly earlier onset of consistent weight gain compared with the control group. The authors suggested that nonoscillating waterbeds are an inexpensive and effective component of supportive therapy in the care of narcotic-exposed neonates.

PHARMACOLOGIC AGENTS IN THE TREATMENT OF NEONATAL DEPRESSANT ABSTINENCE

Many pharmacologic agents have been used in the treatment of neonatal abstinence, and some appear to be effective in relieving symptoms. In a review of several studies that included a total of 590 infants, the majority evaluated the effectiveness of paregoric (camphorated tincture of opium), phenobarbital, and diazepam in treating and controlling symptoms of abstinence. The advantages of paregoric use were reported as follows: (1) It can be orally administered, (2) it has no known adverse effects, and (3) there is a wide margin of error because of the low dosage of opiate and a short half-life. Paregoric can also provide a level of sedation that inhibits bowel motility, thereby diminishing the loose stools frequently accompanying abstinence. Among paregoric-treated infants, nutritive sucking has been found to be much closer to normal than among those treated with phenobarbital or diazepam. In opiate-exposed babies, paregoric has been found to control seizure activity better than phenobarbital.[17] However, in comparison with other drugs used, a paregoric regimen has the disadvantage of requiring larger doses and a longer duration of therapy.[13]

Phenobarbital is especially effective in controlling two of the more commonly occurring symptoms of abstinence, irritability and insomnia, through a nonspecific CNS depression. Although phenobarbital may be as effective as paregoric in controlling some of the signs of abstinence, occasionally an infant can become more irritated after treatment.[19] Disadvantages include considerable depression of sucking and less effectiveness than paregoric in alleviating seizures in narcotic abstinence.[27] Loose stools are not prevented, and control in infants may not be fully accomplished, even at doses that produce plasma levels considered to be in the toxic range.[30]

Diazepam has been reported to be safe and effective in a short course of therapy. However, infants treated with this drug have become severely obtunded, and their nutritive sucking is markedly diminished in comparison with infants treated with other drugs.[27] Because of its severe depressant effect on the central nervous system, transient sedation has been noted and, if given intramuscularly, potential effects on neonatal jaundice must be considered.[30] Seizures have been seen more often in infants treated with diazepam than in infants treated with paregoric.[17]

In those instances where one drug emerges as superior, the results are not easily replicated nor can they necessarily be compared with previous findings. In actuality, a more precise approach in evaluating pharmacotherapeutic effectiveness is to consider the specific interaction of the treatment drug with maternal drug use. In our clinical research studies, we have investigated the effectiveness of paregoric, phenobarbital, and diazepam in the treatment of neonatal abstinence while considering the type of maternal drug use, prenatal drug exposure during the last few weeks before delivery, and complications in the detoxification process that might have influenced neonatal abstinence and/or its treatment. In assessing the number of days to control abstinence symptoms, paregoric was most successful when the infant was exposed to opiates only (Table 229-2). When exposed to nonopiates, phenobarbital was most successful. There appeared to be no significant difference between phenobarbital and paregoric when the infants were exposed to both opiates and nonopiates. In assessing the mean total length (days) of treatment of abstinence, paregoric was most successful when the infant was exposed to opiates, and phenobarbital most successful with nonopiate exposure. With exposure to opiates and nonopiates, no significant differences were found between the three treatment drugs.

When assessing the three treatment regimens with regard to success or failure, defined as the need for only one drug to control abstinence, it is clear that paregoric was successful in treating abstinence when infants were exposed to opiates (87% versus 57% with phenobarbital and 12% with diazepam). Phenobarbital and diazepam seem to be effective with regard to nonopiates (98% with phenobarbital and diazepam, and 33% with paregoric), although a smaller number of infants were treated with diazepam. With opiate and nonopiate exposure, paregoric was the most successful (88%) compared to 60% with phenobarbital and 22% with diazepam.

Since sucking behavior is such a prominent symptom in neonatal abstinence, the dependence of sucking behavior on the type of detoxicant treatment has been analyzed. Paregoric-treated infants tended to suck more vigorously than infants treated with sedatives such as phenobarbital and were even superior to those who received no therapy at all. The paregoric group approached control levels on most of the parameters. The averages for the no-treatment group were consistently lower than those for the paregoric babies, despite the fact that

Table 229-2 *Maternal Drug Use and Pharmacotherapy in 176 Infants Undergoing Abstinence*

	MATERNAL DRUG USE		
TREATMENT DRUG	OPIATES (n = 45)	NONOPIATES (n = 25)	OPIATES/NONOPIATES (n = 106)
Mean days to control abstinence			
Phenobarbital (n = 96)	6.7	3.5	8.6
Diazepam (n = 20)	9.5	4.7	11.6
Paregoric (n = 60)	4.9	7.0	9.4
Total infants (n = 176)	6.4	4.8	9.2
Mean days for treatment of abstinence			
Phenobarbital (n = 96)	20	18	32
Diazepam (n = 20)	30	28	33
Paregoric (n = 60)	24	46	34
Total infants (n = 176)	27	29	33

Finnegan LP and Ehrlich SM: Maternal drug abuse during pregnancy: evaluation and pharmacotherapy for neonatal abstinence, In Modern methods in pharmacology, vol 6, Testing and evaluation of drugs of abuse, 1990, New York, Wiley-Liss, Inc.

their withdrawal symptoms were judged to be quite mild and did not indicate the need for drug therapy. Diazepam-treated infants were greatly depressed in feeding behavior. Of the six diazepam subjects, five hardly sucked at all (however, the high sucking scores of the sixth subject brought up the group mean).[26]

Additional data with regard to the safety and usefulness of paregoric and phenobarbital have been presented by Kaltenbach and co-workers.[23] The purpose of this study was to evaluate the developmental outcome of infants born to women maintained on methadone and to determine if developmental status is affected by severity of abstinence and/or type of pharmacotherapy.

In this study, 69 of 85 infants evaluated for abstinence required pharmacotherapy and were assigned to one of three treatment agents: paregoric, phenobarbital, or diazepam. When treatment was not successful with the assigned agent (i.e., abstinence symptomatology was not controlled), one of the other agents was used.

Of those infants treated with paregoric, treatment was successful (i.e., did not require an additional agent) for 91% of the infants, whereas phenobarbital was much less successful and diazepam was never successful.

At 6 months of age the developmental status of the infants was assessed with the Bayley Scale of Mental Development. Based on treatment regimens for neonatal abstinence syndrome four groups were defined: (1) paregoric ($n = 21$); (2) phenobarbital ($n = 17$); (3) more than one agent ($n = 31$); and (4) no treatment ($n = 16$).

The data were analyzed using a one-way analysis of variance. Results revealed no differences in developmental status between groups ($p > 0.10$, $f = 0.25$), and the scores for all groups were well within the normal range. Infants who were treated with paregoric had a mean MDI of 103; those treated with phenobarbital had a mean MDI of 104; infants who required a combination of treatment regimens had a mean MDI of 103; and infants whose symptomatology was so mild that no treatment was required had a mean MDI of 101.

These findings have several important implications. Foremost, they suggest the importance of careful assessment, with a neonatal scoring system and appropriate treatment, in bringing the infants into a general state of good health. Second, they provide specific information regarding the relationship between the severity of neonatal abstinence syndrome and developmental outcome. The fact that no differences were found in developmental scores for infants with mild neonatal abstinence syndrome and those with the severe form of the syndrome indicate that with appropriate pharmacotherapy, severity of neonatal abstinence syndrome does not adversely affect developmental outcome, at least as measured in this study when the infants were 6 months of age. Infant performance on the Bayley assessment showed that these infants do not exhibit any demonstrable developmental sequelae at 6 months of age, since scores were well within the normal range of development.[23]

Although several treatment drugs have been identified in the past as successful in controlling neonatal abstinence, treatment should be limited to one agent that can rapidly control symptoms without harmful side effects.

Clinicians have found that other depressant agents such as morphine, methadone, and laudanum have successfully treated neonatal narcotic abstinence, but limited data exist to recommend these agents at this time.

Additional evaluations of paregoric and phenobarbital and potential recommendations are in progress. (personal communications Elizabeth Brown, M.D., Boston City Hospital 1990). Until the latter are available, the recommendations herein, which have been used over the past decade or so, will be useful to the clinician in the assessment and management of neonatal abstinence. The basic principle in management of the infant undergoing abstinence is that he or she should be able to sleep comfortably and suck with minimal difficulty, and weight gain should progress normally.

The evaluations described above, in addition to our previous investigations and clinical experience in the management of over 1000 infants, have led us to the conclusions regarding treatment principles that should be used for the infant undergoing abstinence: (1) An abstinence scoring system is essential in the assessment of any infant undergoing abstinence; (2) evaluation of the drugs used prenatally will permit more specific drug choices for treating neonatal abstinence; (3) combining a scoring system with specific drug recommendations provides a more objective method of management; (4) paregoric is most effective if the infant has had prenatal exposure to opiates or a combination of opiates and other agents; (5) phenobarbital is most effective if the infant is prenatally exposed to non-opiates only; (6) diazepam is not an appropriate drug for neonatal abstinence, regardless of whether it is a case of prenatal exposure to opiates only, opiates and nonopiates, or nonopiates only.[10,11]

PHARMACOTHERAPEUTIC REGIMENS

Score-Dose Titration Approach with Paregoric

Once the criteria are met to initiate pharmacotherapy (indicated by the total abstinence scores), the total scores dictate the detoxicant dose as prescribed in Table 229-3. Because "steady state" levels of paregoric are not achieved, serum concentrations are not helpful in managing the infant.

Dosage adjustments and timing of dosage changes must be carefully monitored. An increase in a detoxicant dose is necessary at any time after the initiation of therapy when there have been three consecutive total scores of 8 or higher or an average of any three consecutive total scores of 8 or higher.

Table 229-3 *Paregoric Titration Dosage Schedule According to Abstinence Scores*

ABSTINENCE SCORE	DOSE (EVERY 4 HOURS)
8-10	0.8 ml/kg/day
11-13	1.2 ml/kg/day
14-16	1.6 ml/kg/day
17 or above	2.0 ml/kg/day
	continue at 0.4-ml increments until control is achieved

When a change in dose is indicated, the time intervals for administration of the next dose should remain the same as the prescribed dosing schedule. For example, if the total withdrawal score indicates that an increase in dose is needed, the adjusted dose should be given on schedule (i.e., 4 hours after the previous dose) until the total abstinence scores consistently fall below 8.

Substantial changes in the infant's weight indicate a need to recalculate the base dose. This will necessitate weight-related dosage adjustments during any phase of pharmacologic intervention (i.e., dosage increases, maintenance doses, and dosage reductions).

Once abstinence is controlled using the prescribed dosage schedule, the following procedures should be implemented to maintain control for 72 hours and start the detoxification process. The dose administered to achieve control should be maintained for 72 hours before a dosage reduction schedule (i.e., detoxification) is initiated. Detoxification is achieved by decreasing the total daily dose by 10% every 24 hours. When dosage levels reach 0.5 ml/kg/day, paregoric may be discontinued. If an infant's abstinence scores remain low (1 to 3) after a minimum of 72 hours of detoxification (usually a rare event) the detoxification rate may be increased, *with caution,* to 15% to 20% and should never exceed 20%.

Loading Dose Approach with Phenobarbital

If phenobarbital is used, the dose administered to achieve the phenobarbital serum level necessary to control abstinence should be noted. Serum levels of phenobarbital should be determined using micromethod blood samples every 24 hours throughout the treatment phase and until the serum concentration reaches a homeopathic level during administration.

If the infant is metabolizing and excreting phenobarbital at an expected rate, the infant should have a 1:1 ± 2 ratio between milligrams of phenobarbital administered and micrograms per milliliter of phenobarbital in the blood serum. This ratio or an increase in the blood serum provides the data necessary for detoxification from phenobarbital.

The objective in detoxifying an infant with phenobarbital is to allow the phenobarbital serum level to fall approximately 10% every 24 hours.

Important definitions include:

Loading Dose: The administration of a single priming dose of phenobarbital (i.e., 20 mg/kg/day) in a quantity sufficient (i.e., achieving a serum level of 18 to 22 μg/ml) to provide for drug distribution throughout the body compartments as well as a therapeutic level in the brain and cerebrospinal fluid.

Steady State: A state in which the amount of phenobarbital absorbed and distributed per dosing interval is equal to the amount eliminated (excreted and metabolized) per dosing interval, resulting in a constant therapeutic level, as determined by serial measurements of plasma concentration.

Maintenance Dose: Once the effective dose of phenobarbital is determined (i.e., control of abstinence with plasma concentrations between 20 and 70 μg/ml) the maintenance dose is the amount of phenobarbital (usually 2 to 6 mg/day) administered every 24 hours to maintain the effective steady state level.

Dosage Increase: Once the loading dose has been administered, it is often necessary to increase the plasma concentration of phenobarbital to attain control. This may be accomplished by administering phenobarbital (10 mg/kg) as frequently as every 12 hours until control or a plasma concentration of 70 μg/ml has been reached, or signs of clinical toxicity appear.

In some atypical infants, the amounts of phenobarbital prescribed in this protocol are insufficient to either maintain an effective steady-state level or increase the serum levels at the predicted rates. See Fig. 229-3 for the dynamics of the phenobarbital loading-dose regimen.

If an infant meets the criteria for initiation of therapy, a loading dose of 20 mg/kg followed by micromethod blood samples is given to determine phenobarbital serum levels at 12 and 24 hours after administration of the loading dose. A loading dose of 20 mg/kg should be administered *only once* and should result in the desired therapeutic serum phenobarbital level of 20 μg/ml ± 2 μg/ml (i.e., 18 to 22 μg/ml). Occasionally levels ranging from 15 to 25 μg/ml are observed following the loading dose.

If the total withdrawal score is less than 8 (i.e., control is achieved) after the desirable therapeutic serum level (i.e., 18 to 22 μg/ml) is attained, the level is maintained for 72 hours. Dosing following the loading dose is considered maintenance and is initiated 24 hours following the initial dose.

The desirable therapeutic serum level is maintained by a daily dose of 4 to 6 mg/kg/day. Maintenance should be started with 5 mg/kg/day every 24 hours, and this dose is adjusted as necessary (i.e., increased to 6 mg/kg/day or decreased to 4 mg/kg/day) to maintain the desired steady-state phenobarbital level of 18 to 22 μg/ml, determined by 24-hour serial measurements of plasma concentrations.

If the total score continues to be over 8 (poor control) after the loading dose and the desired therapeutic level of 18 to 22 μg/ml is achieved, the serum phenobarbital level should be increased by increments of 10 μg/ml per 12-hour period until control is achieved. This can be accomplished by administering phenobarbital at 10 mg/kg every 12 hours (12 hours after administering the loading dose of phenobarbital) concomitant with verification of expected plasma concentrations of phenobarbital. This stepwise increase of 10 mg/ml should be continued every 12 hours only until (1) control is attained (i.e., the total score is less than 8), *or* (2) the serum level reaches 70 mg/ml, *or* (3) the infant demonstrates signs of phenobarbital toxicity. If the total serum phenobarbital level reaches 70 μg/ml or higher and control still has not been attained, the choice of detoxicant should be reevaluated before attempting to exceed this level.

After 72 hours of steady-state maintenance in a clinically controlled situation (verified by constant serum levels and total scores of less than 8), detoxification can begin by allowing the phenobarbital serum levels to decline at a rate of 10% to 20% per 24 hours, ideally 15% by administering phenobarbital at a dose of 2 mg/kg/day. If serum phenobarbital levels indicate that detoxification is too rapid (greater than 20% in 24 hours), the maintenance dose should be increased to 3 mg/kg/day. If total abstinence scores escalate to 8 or higher, detoxification is stopped. The phenobarbital dose should be increased to achieve the serum level at which

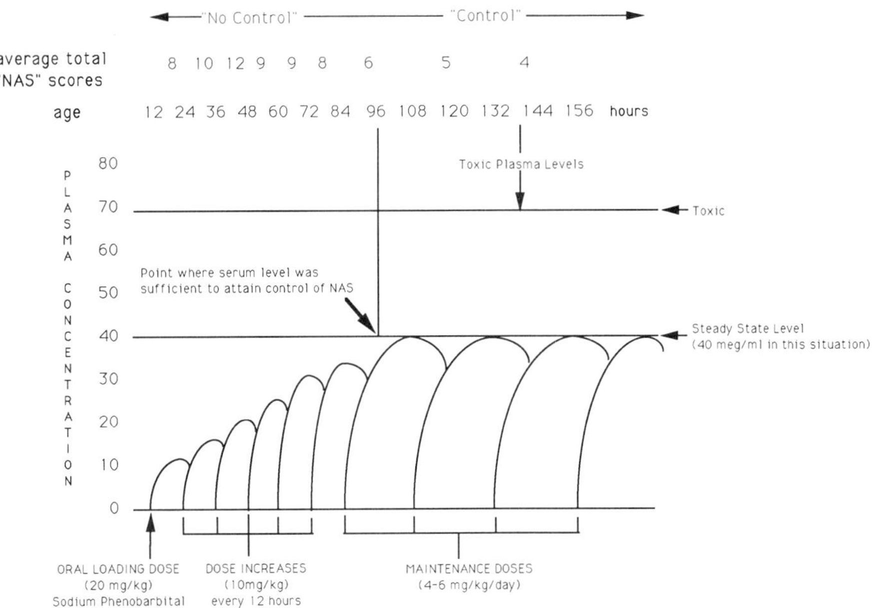

Fig. 229-3 Dynamics of the phenobarbital loading dose regimen (case sample).
(From Finnegan LP: Neonatal abstinence syndrome. In Nelson N, editor: Current therapy in neonatal-perinatal medicine, Ontario, 1985, BC Decker, Inc.)

the infant was previously controlled. This level should be maintained, assuming the infant is controlled again, for 48 hours before detoxification is started again. If detoxification is too slow 10% per 24 hours) the maintenance dose should be decreased to 1 mg/kg/day. Once the serum level falls below 10 μg/ml, and the total score is less than 8, the phenobarbital should be discontinued.

After the phenobarbital is discontinued, the infant is observed for 72 hours for increased withdrawal symptoms. If the total score continues to be less than 8, the infant can be discharged. If the score escalates to 8 or higher after discontinuation of therapy, the infant is observed until control recurs or he or she is reevaluated for further pharmacologic intervention.

Cautions During Pharmacologic Treatment

1. Diminished or absent reflexes—Moro, sucking, swallowing, Galant, Perez, tonic neck, corneal, grasp (palmar or plantar)
2. Truncal (central) or circumoral cyanosis or persistent mottling not associated with ambient temperature decreases
3. Decreased muscle tone with passive resistance to extension of extremities or decreased neck or trunk tone
4. Altered state of arousal (e.g., obtunded or comatose)
5. Diminished response to painful stimuli
6. Failure at visual following
7. Hypothermia
8. Altered respirations—irregular (periodic breathing in full-term infants), shallow (decreased air entry), decreased respiratory rate (less than 20 per minute), apnea
9. Cardiac alterations—irregular rate, distant heart sounds with peripheral pulses, heart rate of 80 to 100 beats per minute, poor peripheral perfusion (pale, gray, mottled), cardiac arrest

Any infant who exhibits a precipitous drop in a total score of 8 points or higher should be monitored for vital signs immediately.

It is important to determine whether any underlying medical problems are developing such as sepsis, meningitis, hypocalcemia, or hypoglycemia. Detection of underlying medical problems may be difficult because poorly controlled abstinence may mimic and/or disguise many common neonatal problems.

An infant may be increasingly depressed by a pharmacotherapeutic agent that is not drug specific for abstinence. This situation may be reflected in the gradual development of symptoms of depression with concomitant poorly controlled abstinence and requires reevaluation for appropriateness of pharmacologic intervention.

The pharmacologic intervention must always be assessed for efficacy in a particular infant. Two common situations indicate that pharmacotherapy must be reassessed: (1) CNS depression, and (2) failure to achieve "control" despite aggressive pharmacotherapeutic intervention and/or near-toxic serum levels of therapeutic agents. In these situations the following measures are indicated:

1. Evaluate the infant for metabolic derangements, sepsis, and CNS disturbances to detect underlying problems compounding the clinical picture. Laboratory evaluations, including serum electrolyte, calcium, and glucose determinations, and blood cultures, should be obtained.
2. Review the maternal drug history, along with both maternal and infant urine toxicology results, to ensure appropriate pharmacotherapy. If the mother has abused barbiturates along with other psychoactive agents not including narcotics, phenobarbital is always the drug of choice. If the maternal drug history and toxicologic findings indicate that only opiates were administered

prenatally, therapeutically administered nonopiates (even at high plasma concentrations) may be ineffective in controlling the symptoms of narcotic abstinence. A change to paregoric may be indicated. If maternal drug history and toxicologic findings indicate that narcotics are the primary drug of maternal abuse, although other addicting agents were also used, paregoric will be most efficacious.

3. If a single pharmacotherapeutic agent is ineffective in controlling abstinence symptoms, a combination of therapeutic agents should be considered.

In conclusion, rapid recognition, careful assessment, and appropriate treatment of neonatal abstinence will augment the satisfactory initial and long-term outcome of drug-exposed infants.

Acknowledgements: The author wishes to acknowledge the contributions of those individuals who assisted in the development of the Neonatal Abstinence Score and those who have been involved in the clinical trials in the evaluation of infants undergoing abstinence using the scoring system. These include Reuben Kron, M.D., Bonnie MacNew, B.S.N., M.S.N., the neonatal nursing staff of the Philadelphia General Hospital and the Thomas Jefferson University Hospital, the neonatology staff and the resident staff of the Philadelphia General Hospital, the Children's Hospital of Philadelphia and the Thomas Jefferson University Hospital.

REFERENCES

1. Behrendt H and Green M: Nature of sweating deficits of prematurely born neonates: observationss on babies with heroin withdrawal syndrome. N Engl J Med 286:1376, 1972.
2. Blinick G: *Soc Biol* 18:534, 1971.
3. Brazelton TB: Fertility of narcotic addicts and effects of addiction on offspring, Neonatal behavioral assessment scale, Philadelphia, 1973, JB Lippincott Co.
4. Chasnoff I, Hutcher, Burns W: Polydrug and methadone addicted newborns: a continuum of impairment? Pediatrics 70:210 1982.
5. Chasnoff IJ et al: Maternal nonnarcotic substance abuse during pregnancy: effects on infant development Neurobehavioral Toxicology and Teratology 6(4):277, 1984.
6. Cherikuri R et al: A cohort study of alkaloidal cocaine ("Crack") in pregnancy, Obstet Gynecol 72(2):147, 1988.
7. Desmond MM and Wilson GS: Neonatal abstinence syndrome: recognition and diagnosis, Addictive Diseases, 2:113, 1975.
8. Doberczak TM et al: One year follow-up of infants with abstinence-associated seizures, Arch Neurol 45(6):649, 1988.
9. Dole VP and Kreek MJ: Methadone plasma level: Maintained by a reservoir of drug in tissue, Proc Natl Acad Sci USA 70:10, 1973.
10. Finnegan LP: Neonatal abstinence. In Nelson N, editor: Current therapy in neonatal-perinatal medicine, Ontario, 1984, BC Decker, Inc.
11. Finnegan LP: Neonatal abstinence syndrome: assessment and pharmacotherapy. In Rubatelli FF and Granati B, editors: Neonatal: therapy an update, Amsterdam-New York-Oxford, 1986, Exerpta Medica.
12. Finnegan LP and Ehrlich S: Maternal drug abuse during pregnancy: evaluation and pharmacotherapy for neonatal abstinence, Modern methods in pharmacology, vol 6, Testing and evaluation of drugs of abuse, 1990, Wiley-Liss, Inc.
13. Fitzgerald LP and MacNew BA: Care of the Addicted Infant, Am J Nurs, 74:685, In Nelson N, editor: 1974.
14. Fitzgerald E, Kaltenbach K, and Finnegan LP: Patterns of Interaction Among Drug Dependent Women and Their Infants. Pediatric Research, Vol. 24 #44, 1990.
15. Glass L and Evans HE: Narcotic withdrawal in the newborn, Am Fam Physician 6:75, 1972.
16. Goddard J and Wilson GS: Management of neonatal drug withdrawal, 1978. J Pediatr 92:861, 1978.
17. Harper RG et al: Effects of methadone treatment programs upon pregnant heroin addicts and their newborn infants, Pediatrics 54:300, 1974.
18. Herzlinger RA, Kandall SR, and Vaughan HG Jr: Neonatal seizures associated with narcotic withdrawal, J Pediatr 91:638, 1977.
19. Jeremy RJ and Hans SL: Behavior of neonates exposed in utero to methadone as assessed on the brazleton scale, Inf Beh and Dev 8:323, 1985.
20. Kahn EJ, Neumann LL, and Polk GA: The course of heroin withdrawal syndrome in newborn infants treated with phenobarbital or chlorpromazine, J Pediatr 75:495, 1969.
21. Kalant OJ: The amphetamines: toxicity and addiction, *ed 2,* Toronto, Canada, 1973, University of Toronto Press.
22. Kaltenbach K and Finnegan LP: The influence of the neonatal abstinence syndrome on mother-infant interaction, In Anthony EJ and Chiland C, editors: The child in his family: perilous development, vol 8, Child raising and identity formation under stress, 1988, Wiley Interscience.
23. Kaltenbach K, and Finnegan LP: "Perinatal and Developmental Outcome of Infants Exposed to Methadone In-Utero", Neurotoxicol Teratol 9:311, 1987.
24. Kaltenbach K and Finnegan LP: Neonatal abstinence: pharmacotherapy and developmental outcome Neurobehavioral Toxicology and Teratology, vol 8, ANKHO International Inc., 1986.
25. Kandall SR and Gartner LM: Late presentation of drug withdrawal symptoms in newborns, 1974. Am J Dis Child 127:58, 1972.
26. Kaplan SL et al: Brazelton neonatal assessment at three and twenty-eight days of age: a study of passively addicted infants, high risk infants and normal infants. Schecter A, Alksne H, Kauffman E, editors: Critical concerns in the field of drug abuse, New York, 1976, Marcel Dekker.
27. Kron RE et al: Assessment of behavioral changes in infants undergoing narcotic withdrawal: comparative data from clinical and objective methods, Addictive Diseases, 2:257, 1975.
28. Kron RE et al: Neonatal narcotic abstinence: Effects of pharmacotherapeutic agents and maternal drug usage on nutritive sucking behavior, Pediatrics 88:637, 1976.
29. Kosten TA: Cocaine attenuates the severity of naloxone-precipitated opioid withdrawal, Life Sci 47:1617, 1990.
30. Lipsitz PJ and Blatman S: Newborn infants of mothers on methadone maintenance, NY State J Med 74:994, 1974.
31. Mitros TF, Hopkins L, and Finnegan LP: Pharmacotherapy for the newborn infant undergoing narcotic abstinence, Clin Res 26:593A, 1978.
32. Oro AS and Dixon SD: Perinatal cocaine and methamphetamine exposure: maternal and neonatal correlates, J Pediatr 111(4):571, 1987.
33. Pasto M et al: Ventricular configurations and cerebral growth in infants born to drug-dependent mothers, Pediatr Radiol 15:77, 1985.
34. Pinto F et al: Sleep in babies born to chronically heroin-addicted mothers: a follow-up study, Drug Alcohol Depend 21(1):43, 1988.
35. Reddy AM, Harper RG, and Stern G: Observations on heroin and methadone withdrawal in the newborn, Pediatrics 48:353, 1971.
36. Ryan L, Ehrlich S, and Finnegan LP: Cocaine abuse in pregnancy: effects on the fetus and newborn, neurotoxicology and teratology Zoltan A. (Ed.), July/August, Volume 9, Issue 4, Pergamon Press: New York, 1987.
37. Schulman CA: Alteration of the sleep cycle in heroin addicted and "suspect" newborns. Neuropaediatrie 1(1): 89-100, June-July, 1969.
38. Shih L, Cone-Wesson B, and Reddix B: Effects of maternal cocaine abuse on the neonatal auditory system, International Journal of Int J Pediatr Otorhinolaryngol 15(3):245, 1988.
39. Sisson TRC et al: Pediatr Res 8:451, 1974.
40. Strauss ME et al: Behavior of narcotic-addicted newborns, Child Dev 46:887, 1975.
41. Strauss ME et al: Behavioral concomitants of prenatal addiction to narcotics, J Pediatr 89:842, 1976.
42. Van Baar: Neonatal behavior after drug dependent pregnancy. Arch Dis Child 64 (2) 235-40, February, 1989.
43. Weinberger SM et al: Early weight-change patterns in neonatal abstinence, Am J Dis Child 140(8):829, 1985.
44. Wilson GS: Somatic growth effects of perinatal addiction, Addictive Diseases 2:333, 1975.
45. Zelson C, Rubio E, and Wasserman E: Neonatal narcotic addiction: 10 year observations, Pediatrics 48:178, 1971.

230

Nephritis

Edward J. Ruley

Nephritis is the general term for noninfectious inflammation of the kidney parenchyma. This inflammation may primarily involve the glomerulus (glomerulonephritis) or the interstitium (interstitial nephritis). Historically, the former has been the subject of more intense interest, so that when the term *nephritis* is used, many practitioners think only of glomerular lesions. Even though glomerulonephritis is more common than interstitial nephritis in the pediatric population, it is important for the clinician to be aware of the latter.

CLASSIFICATION OF THE GLOMERULOPATHIES

In the past, glomerulopathies have been classified according to a variety of schemes, including the clinical course (such as acute, subacute, and chronic glomerulonephritis), the major clinical symptoms (such as Ellis types I and II), or some measurable serum abnormality (such as normocomplementemic and hypocomplementemic nephritides). All these classifications have proved to be of limited use. An ideal classification system based on cause is not possible as a result of the incomplete understanding of the pathogenesis of many types of glomerulonephritis. Furthermore, only a limited number of clinical presentations can be caused by a great variety of different renal insults. Currently, the preferred method of classification is based on glomerular morphologic traits.

To understand morphologic classification, one should have a knowledge of normal renal and glomerular anatomy and understand the descriptive terms *diffuse, focal segmental,* and *global*. These terms are used to describe the distribution of disease in the biopsy specimen and are portrayed in Fig. 230-1. In nephritis, diffuse and focal apply to the distribution of disease among the glomeruli present in the biopsy specimen; *diffuse* means that all the glomeruli are involved, and *focal* means that only some glomeruli are involved. Similarly, in interstitial nephritis the inflammation can be diffuse (i.e., general and uniform) or focal (i.e., patchy and irregular).

Segmental and global apply only to glomerular disease in which they describe the extent of disease involvement in each individual glomerulus; *global* means complete glomerular involvement, and *segmental* means irregular involvement with some loops being normal. Thus glomerular lesions may be described as being diffuse and segmental, indicating partial involvement of all the glomeruli in the biopsy specimen, or focal and global, indicating complete involvement of some of the glomeruli, and so on.

One classification scheme based on glomerular morphology is given in the box on p. 1380. In this scheme the category of minimal glomerular lesions includes those with normal or minimally abnormal glomeruli. The minimal abnormalities usually consist of a mild increase in the amount of mesangium or number of cells (mild hypercellularity). The category of specific glomerular lesions includes those more severe lesions characterized by morphologic changes attributable to a defined cause. The largest category is that of nonspecific lesions in which there are definable pathologic patterns, but the causes may be multiple. Finally, a category of unclassifiable glomerulopathies is included.

The following discussion deals with the common patterns of presentation in an effort to develop a structured way of thinking about the diagnostic possibilities for each clinical problem. It should be recognized that this is only one way of conceptualizing an approach. Furthermore, these clinical patterns are only crude categorizations, and a specific etiology may manifest in a variety of ways. The clinical patterns to be discussed include (1) the acute nephritic syndrome, (2) intermittent gross hematuria and proteinuria syndromes, and (3) chronic glomerulonephritis syndromes. In each disease the classification by glomerular involvement will be in-

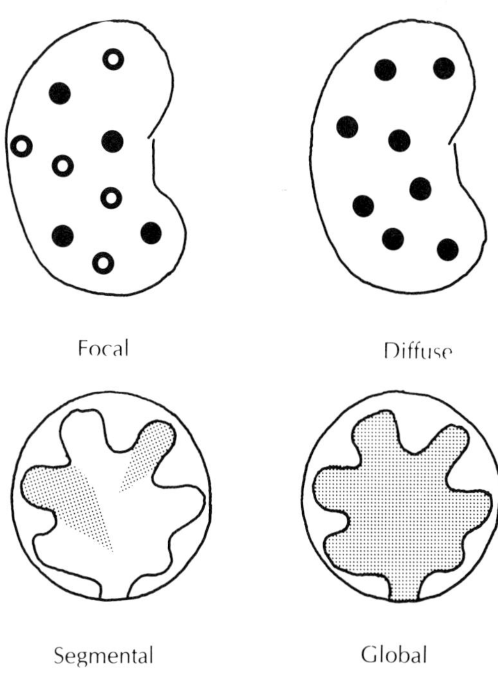

Fig. 230-1 Diagrammatic portrayal of the terms *diffuse, focal, segmental,* and *global,* as used in describing glomerular pathologic conditions.

Morphologic Classification of Glomerulopathies

A. Minimal glomerular lesions (e.g., idiopathic nephrotic syndrome, asymptomatic proteinuria, and asymptomatic hematuria
B. Specific glomerular lesions (e.g., malarial nephropathy, amyloidosis, diabetic glomerulosclerosis, and thrombotic microangiopathy of hemolytic-uremic syndrome)
C. Nonspecific glomerular lesions
   1. Diffuse glomerular lesions
      a. Nonproliferative (e.g., membranous nephropathy)
      b. Proliferative (e.g., mesangial proliferative glomerulonephritis, membranoproliferative glomerulonephritis, and endocapillary and extracapillary glomerulonephritis with and without crescents)
   2. Focal glomerular lesions
      a. Nonproliferative (e.g., focal glomerulosclerosis)
      b. Proliferative (e.g., focal and segmental proliferative glomerulonephritis
D. Unclassified glomerular lesions (e.g., Alport syndrome, focal membranoproliferative glomerulonephritis, and lesions too advanced to classify)

Modified from Habib R: Classification of glomerular nephropathies. In Rubin M and Barratt TM, editors: Pediatric nephrology, Baltimore, 1975, The Williams & Wilkins Co.

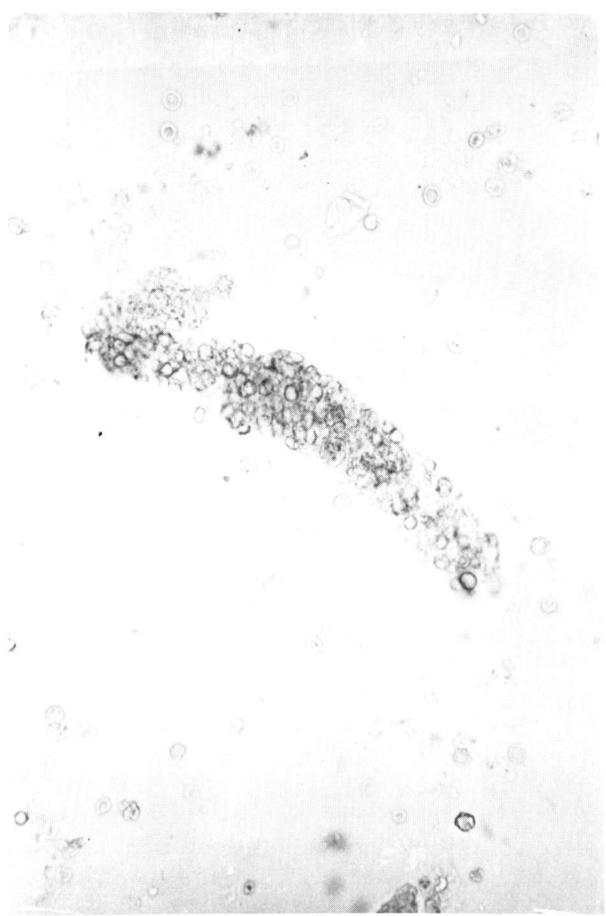

Fig. 230-2 Red blood cell cast—unstained.

dicated. The entities of minimal change disease, membranous glomerulopathy, focal glomerular sclerosis, and the nephropathy of chronic bacteremia are discussed in Chapter 231 on nephrotic syndrome, which is their most common pattern of presentation.

ACUTE NEPHRITIC SYNDROME

The acute nephritic syndrome is characterized by hematuria, hypertension, and edema. The hematuria usually is grossly evident, although in some children it may be microscopic[1] only. Red blood cell casts and dysmorphic red blood cells are always present, although multiple urine samples may have to be examined to demonstrate them (Fig. 230-2). The edema usually is periorbital in location and rarely severe. This syndrome will be discussed as two clinical presentations: acute nephritis syndrome with minimal to mild renal failure and acute nephritic syndrome with rapidly progressive renal failure.

Acute Nephritic Syndrome with Minimal to Mild Renal Failure

Acute nephritic syndrome often is the initial symptom in the renal diseases listed in the box on p. 1381.

Acute Poststreptococcal Glomerulonephritis. Acute poststreptococcal glomerulonephritis is a common form of glomerulonephritis in childhood. The true incidence is unknown inasmuch as only a minority of patients with this illness have symptoms. Although poststreptococcal nephritis may happen at any age, the peak occurrence is at age 7 years, with a slight male predominance. It is uncommon before age 3 years and in adults.

Etiology. Poststreptococcal nephritis occurs as a consequence of the immune response of the host to a nonrenal infection with group A beta-hemolytic streptococci (GABHS). Not all GABHS strains are nephritogenic. Type 12 is the most common nephritogenic strain, whereas types 1, 4, 45, 47, and 55 occur less frequently. The nephritogenicity of types 3, 6, and 25 is less certain. Recent work[7] has suggested that endostreptocin, a cytoplasmic protein found in large quantities in nephritogenic streptococci, may be the antigen to which the patient reacts. Furthermore, recent evidence[7] suggests that immune complex formation occurs in situ in the kidneys rather than as a passive filtration of preformed immune complexes. Infection with a nephritogenic strain does not guarantee an episode of nephritis, because a variety of incompletely understood factors determine the host response. Renal involvement characteristically manifests 1 to 3 weeks after a pharyngeal or skin infection with the nephritogenic streptococci.

Pathology. Grossly, the kidneys are enlarged and pallid. The typical glomerular morphology is that of diffuse, uni-

Diseases That May Have as a Symptom Acute Nephritic Syndrome with Minimal to Moderate Renal Failure in Children

MORE COMMONLY PRESENT

Acute poststreptococcal glomerulonephritis
Henoch-Schönlein purpura with nephritis
Postinfectious (nonstreptococcal) glomerulonephritis
Interstitial glomerulonephritis
Radiation nephritis

LESS COMMONLY PRESENT

Acute episodes in patients with chronic glomerulonephritis
Hemolytic-uremic syndrome (milder cases)
Membranoproliferative glomerulonephritis (some)
Nephritis of systemic lupus erythematosus (some)

form, cellular proliferation, although it is difficult to determine the type of cell involved. The glomerular tufts are larger than normal, and the capillary lumens are reduced. Polymorphonuclear leukocytes may be present. There is an increase in mesangial matrix, but the basement membranes are normal. On immunofluorescent microscopy examination deposits of immunoglobulin and complement can be seen. With the use of electron microscopy, electron-dense structures (presumed to be immune deposits) can be seen on the epithelial side of the basement membrane. With healing, the increased cellularity and immune deposits become limited to the mesangial region and then gradually resolve.

Clinical Presentation. Most patients with acute poststreptococcal nephritis have an acute nephritic syndrome, with macroscopic hematuria in about 50% of the cases. Approximately 60% to 70% of the patients will have hypertension to some degree. Patients with severe hypertension may have symptoms of headache, drowsiness, vomiting, personality and visual changes, and convulsions. Although arteriole spasm is commonly present on funduscopic examination, papilledema and hemorrhages are rare, even with severe hypertension. Edema usually is periorbital and rarely severe. Patients may show cardiovascular disturbances similar to congestive heart failure. Patients usually have oliguria (urine output less than 240 $ml/m^2/day$) and, rarely, anuria. Anorexia and pain in the abdomen or flank are common although palpation of the abdomen usually reveals no significant findings. Costovertebral angle tenderness often is present. Although a history of preceding skin or pharyngeal infection supports the diagnosis, such a history cannot be elicited in many cases. Patients rarely have joint symptoms or urinary outlet symptoms such as frequency, urgency, or dysuria. Rarely, a patient with convulsions or symptoms of cardiovascular dysfunction as the primary complaint actually has unrecognized poststreptococcal nephritis.

Laboratory Findings. The urine usually is tea colored. The specific gravity generally is increased, and hemoglobin levels can be detected by chemical testing. Any proteinuria that is present usually parallels the degree of hematuria and rarely is the level seen in nephrotic syndrome. Microscopic examination usually reveals erythrocyturia, pyuria, and granular or cellular casts. The presence of identifiable erythrocyte casts and dysmorphic erythrocytes may be variable; thus serial urine specimens may need to be examined. A rare patient will have a normal urinalysis despite having all other signs of acute glomerulonephritis.

Determination of the serum complement will show a reduction of C3 in 80% of the patients and C4 in 50%. The erythrocyte sedimentation rate (ESR) usually is elevated. With severe oliguria there may be azotemia and acidosis. The plasma volume usually is expanded, producing a decrease in serum protein, hemoglobin, and hematocrit levels. Hemolysis, a shortened erythrocyte half-life, and decreased erythrocyte production may contribute to these hematologic changes.

Evidence of a preceding streptococcal infection is important to support the diagnosis. The antistreptolysin O (ASO) titer will be elevated in 80% of patients, although rises in titer occur less frequently in patients with skin infection and in those who receive early treatment with antibiotics. If other streptococcal antibodies (antihyaluronidase, antideoxyribonuclease B) are measured, 95% of patients have serologic evidence of preceding streptococcal infection. Cultures are often negative for GABHS by the time nephritis develops and are particularly affected by pretreatment with antibiotics.

Radiographs of the chest in those patients with hypertension usually reveal a large heart with prominent pulmonary vasculature, pulmonary edema, or rarely, hydrothorax.[3] Excretion urographic examination usually reveals bilaterally enlarged kidneys with poor function.

Course. The oliguria and hypertension usually last 4 or 5 days, although in some patients it may be much longer. The onset of diuresis usually heralds the resolution. Gross hematuria resolves within 1 or 2 weeks, although urinary abnormalities may persist for 6 to 12 weeks. Some patients have microscopic hematuria for as long as 2 years and still recover completely. Complement levels should rise gradually to normal by 3 to 6 weeks.

Treatment. Acute poststreptococcal glomerulonephritis most often heals spontaneously and is not affected by corticosteroids or immunosuppressive agents. Even so, the practitioner must be aggressive in treating hypertension, oliguria, and the resulting vascular congestion, pulmonary edema, and encephalopathy that occur in the acute phase of the illness because these can be fatal.

Although mild hypertension may resolve spontaneously, more severe degrees of hypertension should be controlled with antihypertensive agents that have a rapid onset. Although potent diuretics (furosemide and ethacrynic acid) are logical choices, because an expanded vascular volume is theorized to be the determinant of hypertension in the acute nephritic syndrome,[5] diuretics frequently are ineffective when used in conventional doses. Nifedipine (0.15 to 0.6 mg/kg) can be used sublingually; the approximate amount of drug is removed from a nifedipine capsule, mixed with one half to 1 ml water, and placed with a syringe beneath the tongue. Diazoxide (2 to 5 mg/kg) injected rapidly intravenously and oral minoxidil (0.1 to 0.2 mg/kg/dose) may be employed. Slower-acting, less potent antihypertensive drugs are not good choices. Oliguria should be allowed to follow its course of natural resolution and cannot be hastened by administration of fluid boluses. Furthermore, excessive fluid administration is contraindicated because it worsens hypertension. The signs of congestive heart failure usually resolve with control of the hypertension. Occasionally acute renal failure severe enough to require dialysis will develop in some patients.

A 10-day course of antibiotics usually is given to eradicate any remaining GABHS and thus prevent spread of the organism to others. There is no evidence that such treatment affects the course of nephritis in the patient.

Hospitalization for patients with this disease needs to be determined individually. Although many children with mild episodes do well as outpatients, the sudden development of hypertension and oliguria may produce life-threatening symptoms quite rapidly. Bed rest may be indicated as a precaution in the patient with hypertension and may be associated with a decrease in the degree of hematuria, but there is no evidence that it affects the healing of the glomerular lesion. Therefore hematuria alone is not an indication for bed rest. After the acute phase the child may be allowed to gradually resume normal activities. Every child should be followed up regularly until the complement values return to normal. To be certain of the diagnosis a renal biopsy, usually not necessary, may be indicated in the child with atypical clinical or laboratory findings. Every child whose C3 value does not return to normal within 8 weeks should have a kidney biopsy.

Prognosis. Studies have shown that more than 90% of children with acute poststreptococcal glomerulonephritis recover from their illness. For most children the critical period is early in the illness when there is danger of fatal hypertension or fluid overload. Occasionally patients with severe involvement will have some residual damage, although the recovery potential of the kidney in this disease is outstanding.

Henoch-Schönlein Purpura with Nephritis. This illness may have an acute nephritic onset (see Chapter 210).

Postinfectious (Nonstreptococcal) Glomerulonephritis. A variety of viral agents have been suggested to cause an acute nephritic syndrome, including infectious mononucleosis, varicella, echovirus 10, measles, mumps, and coxsackieviruses. Significant renal involvement, however, is unusual in infections with these agents. Children with such involvement are characterized by normal complement levels and the absence of serologic evidence of recent streptococcal infection. In most cases there is a gradual spontaneous resolution of the acute nephritic syndrome and complete recovery of renal function. There is no effective way to differentiate the nonstreptococcal postinfectious glomerulonephritides from the other normocomplementemic nephritides that progress to renal failure except by observation of the clinical course.

Other Renal Diseases That Less Commonly Have as a Symptom Acute Nephritic Syndrome with Minimal to Moderate Renal Failure. Occasionally patients with undiscovered chronic renal failure will suffer a sudden deterioration that may be interpreted as an acute nephritic syndrome (see the box at right). Evaluation of these patients often reveals evidence of preexisting chronic renal failure, such as osteodystrophy or hyperphosphatemia. Hemolytic-uremic syndrome (see Chapter 209) characteristically occurs as an acute nephritic syndrome. Systemic lupus erythematosus may appear to be an acute nephritic syndrome but more often is discovered coincidentally during evaluation of other complaints related to the lupus syndrome. Likewise, membranoproliferative glomerulonephritis or the nephritis of chronic infection may initially manifest acutely with low complement values. However, more often this disease appears to be nephrotic syndrome or chronic glomerulonephritis.

Acute Nephritic Syndrome with Rapidly Progressive Renal Failure

This variant of the acute nephritic syndrome is characterized by symptoms of acute nephritis associated with the relentless progression to renal failure over days or weeks. Although acute interstitial nephritis as a result of pyelonephritis or hypersensitivity may occur in this way, the majority of cases result from glomerular disease, giving rise to the term *rapidly progressive glomerulonephritis* (RPGN). As shown in the accompanying box, RPGN can be classified into three categories on the basis of immunopathologic findings as seen in kidney biopsies.[2]

The most common cause of RPGN in pediatric-age patients is poststreptococcal glomerulonephritis. The diagnosis depends on obtaining the history of a recent sore throat or skin infection and finding reduced serum complement values as-

Classification of Acute Nephritic Syndrome with Rapidly Progressive Renal Failure

IMMUNE COMPLEX

- Postinfectious reaction
  - Streptococcal infection
  - Visceral abscess
  - Other
- Collagen vascular disease
  - Systemic lupus erythematosis
  - Henoch-Schönlein purpura
  - Mixed cryoglobulinemia
- Primary renal disease
  - IgA nephropathy
  - Membranoproliferative glomerulonephritis
  - Unknown cases (i.e., idiopathic)

NO IMMUNE DEPOSIT

- Unknown cause
- Vasculitis
  - Polyarteritis
  - Wegener granulomatosis
  - Hypersensitivity vasculitides

ANTI-GBM ANTIBODY

- With lung hemorrhage (Goodpasture syndrome)
- Without lung hemorrhage
- Complicating membranous nephropathy

Modified from Couser WG: Rapidly progressive glomerulonephritis: classification, pathogenetic mechanisms, and therapy, Am J Kidney Dis 11:449, 1988.

sociated with serologic evidence of a recent streptococcal infection. A large portion of patients with poststreptococcal RPGN will recover spontaneously, provided their courses are well managed during the acute phase.[5]

RPGN may be caused by Henoch-Schönlein purpura, although this occurs considerably less frequently than the poststreptococcal and idiopathic (nonstreptococcal) varieties in children. The multisystem clinical presentation, negative streptococcal serologic findings, normal serum complement values, and renal biopsy findings characterize this cause. Some reports suggest that high-dose intravenous corticosteroid drugs, if given early in the course, promote recovery in these patients. Of the primary renal disease group, IgA nephropathy and membranoproliferative glomerulonephritis (types I and II) will, rarely, occur this way.

RPGN without immune desposits is much less common in pediatric-age patients, and anti-GBM antibody-mediated RPGN is even more rare. Hemolytic uremic syndrome (HUS) and disseminated intravascular coagulopathy (DIC) must be included in the differential diagnosis inasmuch as hematuria and rapidly progressive renal failure are common features of their presentations. Hypertension, however, is less common in these latter two diagnoses. Although the characteristic clinical and laboratory features of these diseases may suggest specific etiologic factors, a renal biopsy usually is indicated to make the diagnosis and to determine the extent of the disease.

INTERMITTENT GROSS HEMATURIA AND PROTEINURIA SYNDROMES

The proteinuria in recurrent gross hematuria syndrome is in excess of that expected from bleeding alone. Between episodes, microscopic hematuria and proteinuria often are present, although in some patients the urine will be completely normal. The more common illnesses that can cause these syndromes are IgA-IgG nephropathy (of Berger), familial (benign) hematuria, hereditary nephritis, and Henoch-Schönlein purpura syndrome.

IgA-IgG Nephropathy

IgA-IgG nephropathy was first described by Berger in 1969 and has been termed *Berger disease*. The cause is unknown.

Pathology. The typical lesion is a focal segmental proliferation of mesangial cells with an increase in mesangial matrix. Immunofluorescent examination reveals mesangial deposits of IgA, IgG, and C3. Morphologically, it is difficult to differentiate this lesion from that of Henoch-Schönlein purpura, which has led to the speculation that the former is a partial clinical expression of the latter.

Clinical Presentation. Characteristically, these children have the sudden onset of asymptomatic gross hematuria and proteinuria occurring without intercurrent illness or concomitant with a nonstreptococcal upper respiratory tract infection.[6] Hypertension usually is not present. The simultaneous onset of the upper respiratory tract infection and the gross hematuria helps differentiate this disease from acute poststreptococcal glomerulonephritis, in which a delay between infection and hematuria is the rule. The absence of rash, abdominal pain, and arthritis helps differentiate IgA-IgG nephropathy from the nephritis of Henoch-Schönlein purpura nephritis. Atypically, patients with IgA nephropathy can have nephrotic syndrome or acute renal failure.

Laboratory Findings. IgA-IgG nephropathy is characterized by a lack of abnormal laboratory findings except for urinalysis. In particular, there is no azotemia, hypocomplementemia, or serologic evidence of recent streptococcal infection. A renal biopsy may be indicated in selected patients to confirm the diagnosis and to be more certain of the prognosis.

Course. The gross hematuria usually resolves spontaneously as the upper respiratory tract infection abates. Many patients will continue to have microscopic hematuria and small amounts of proteinuria, although in some the urinalysis will revert to completely normal findings. With future intercurrent illness the gross hematuria tends to recur.

Treatment. No treatment has yet proved effective for IgA-IgG nephropathy.

Prognosis. Although the prognosis originally was considered excellent, now it is anticipated that about 10% of pediatric patients will progress to renal failure. Progression has been related to the severity of histologic changes on the kidney biopsy.[4]

Familial Hematuria

Familial hematuria is a benign condition inherited as an autosomal dominant trait. Undoubtedly, many of the early reports included patients with IgA-IgG nephropathy because of the similarities of clinical presentation and because renal biopsy specimens were not often obtained. This condition also has been termed *benign recurrent hematuria*.

Etiology. The cause of familial hematuria is not known.

Pathology. Usually light and fluorescent microscopic examinations reveal that renal biopsy specimen findings are normal. Focal or diffuse thinning of the basement membranes often is present on electron microscopy examination.

Clinical Presentation. Most often children with familial hematuria have episodes of asymptomatic gross hematuria and minimal to mild proteinuria.

Laboratory Findings. All laboratory test results usually are normal except for the urinalysis. The presence of hematuria in family members suggests this diagnosis. The absence of notable proteinuria, deafness, ocular defects, and renal failure in older family members with hematuria differentiates this from the hereditary nephritides.

Course. Recurrent microscopic hematuria with intercurrent infections occurs commonly, so that familial hematuria cannot be differentiated clinically from IgA-IgG nephropathy. Microhematuria is usually constantly present, although it can vary in degree. Proteinuria is never severe and can be present only during episodes of macrohematuria.

Treatment. No treatment is indicated for familial hematuria.

Prognosis. The prognosis is excellent.

Hereditary Nephritis

Hereditary nephritis often manifests as recurrent episodes of hematuria. Best known is Alport syndrome, in which a hereditary nephritis is associated with neurogenic deafness and (occasionally) ocular abnormalities. The majority of patients with the classic form of Alport syndrome inherit it as an autosomal dominant trait. Alport features associated with macrothrombocytopenia are known as Epstein syndrome. In addition, some forms of hereditary nephritis are not associated with deafness. Classification of all these hereditary diseases currently is the subject of molecular genetic study, and their interrelationships should become obvious in the future. A variety of pathologic changes have been reported in kidneys obtained from patients with hereditary nephritis. The most common glomerular alterations include cellular proliferation, focal scarring, focal basement membrane thickening, and periglomerular fibrosis. Often the tubules show varying degrees of atrophy with mononuclear cell infiltration. So-called foam cells may be seen but are by no means pathognomonic of hereditary nephritis, as originally thought. On immunofluorescent studies that findings often are negative, although C3 deposition has been noted in a few cases. Attempts have been made to subclassify familial nephritis by its appearance on electron microscopic examination.

The most common clinical presentation in the child and adolescent is one of recurrent macrohematuria, usually occurring with upper respiratory tract infections or exercise and associated with varying degrees of proteinuria. Microhematuria persists between the episodes of macrohematuria, although its severity is also variable. Severe degrees of proteinuria usually do not occur until late in the disease, although in an occasional patient it may precede the hematuria, producing the nephrotic syndrome when the patient is seen initially. In classic Alport syndrome high-frequency nerve deafness is more common in male patients and usually develops after the onset of renal disease. It is recognized in 75% of the patients before age 15 years. The hearing impairment may not be noticed at first because the conversational ranges are spared initially. The impairment usually is bilateral but can be asymmetric. Deafness may skip some generations only to reappear in later ones and can occur in carriers of the disease who do not have the nephropathy. Detection of a hearing impairment in female patients often requires the use of audiometry. The ocular abnormalities are variably present and include cataracts, lenticonus, spherophakia (which can produce myopia), nystagmus, and retinitis pigmentosa. In Epstein syndrome abnormally large platelets associated with defective platelet function have been noted.

Abnormal laboratory findings are variable and nonspecific. Serum complement values usually are normal. A renal biopsy may help to establish the diagnosis in some patients.

The progression of hereditary nephritis to chronic renal failure varies but tends to be the same within a family. The disease generally is more severe in male patients, although occasionally a female patient will progress to end-stage renal failure. Increasing proteinuria is considered to be evidence of progression. The presence of deafness generally indicates more severe renal involvement and thus a worse prognosis for both sexes. Hypertension usually is not prominent. No specific therapy is available. Chronic renal failure is treated in the usual manner, and dialysis and transplantation have been used in some patients. Hearing aids and surgery are of no value for the deafness.

Henoch-Schönlein Purpura with Nephritis

Commonly, patients with Henoch-Schönlein purpura have periodic recurrences of hematuria and proteinuria often associated with recurrent infections. The presence of rash and evidence of involvement of other organ systems besides the kidney help differentiate this syndrome from IgA-IgG nephropathy.

CHRONIC GLOMERULONEPHRITIS SYNDROME

The chronic glomerulonephritis syndrome consists of diminished renal function associated with signs of the detrimental effects of this abnormality on other organ systems. It may be discovered under almost any clinical circumstance but most often is found as the practitioner investigates nonspecific complaints such as anorexia, intermittent vomiting, and malaise that are found to result from undiagnosed chronic renal failure. The more common entities are nephritis of systemic lupus erythematosus, membranoproliferative glomerulonephritis, and "chronic glomerulonephritis." Nonnephritic causes such as renal dysplasia and obstructive uropathies with significant unrecognized parenchymal damage should be considered in the differential diagnosis.

Nephritis of Systemic Lupus Erythematosus

Nephritis of systemic lupus erythematosus (SLE) is a multisystem disease that occurs mostly in female patients (80% to 90%) during their adolescent years. There is an increased familial incidence of the disease.

Etiology. SLE is considered a classic immune complex disease resulting from autoimmunity to endogenous DNA. Both familial predisposition and viral infection have been suggested as important factors.

Pathology. Although the renal disease can be quite variable, several common patterns have been identified. These include a focal segmental proliferative, a diffuse proliferative, and a membranous lesion. On fluorescent antibody examination, deposition of immunoglobulin and complement components usually is seen. Complement deposition often can be demonstrated even in glomeruli that appear normal on light microscopic examination. Electron microscopy examination often reveals evidence of immune complex deposition, cellular proliferation, and basement membrane thickening. The use of renal biopsies has allowed the subcategorization of many of these cases, and attempts are being made to correlate these subcategories with the clinical course.

Clinical Presentation. Although renal involvement in this multisystem disease is both common and important as the eventual cause of morbidity and mortality, symptoms of renal involvement usually are not severe enough at the onset to prompt the patient to seek medical attention. More commonly, the patient has complaints related to skin rash or joint or cardiac involvement. Even if renal disease is not present at the onset, some renal abnormalities develop in most patients as their disease continues. These abnormalities may fit any of the described clinical patterns, including nephrotic syndrome or acute nephritic syndrome.

Laboratory Findings. Serologic evidence of SLE can be obtained by a variety of tests that determine the presence of

DNA antibodies in the serum of the patient. These tests include the LE cell test (positive findings in approximately 60%), the fluorescent antinuclear antibody (FANA) test (positive findings in approximately 94%), and the circulating DNA antibody tests (positive findings in more than 95%). None of these tests is specific for SLE.

Serum complement values usually are decreased with acute renal disease and correlate with the activity of the SLE. Other common serologic abnormalities include positive test results for rheumatoid factor and false-positive test results for syphilis, cryoprecipitable proteins, and Coombs antibodies.

The severity and type of renal involvement (e.g., nephrotic syndrome, chronic renal failure) determine the degree of hypoproteinemia, azotemia, and other manifestations of renal failure. These changes are nonspecific.

Urinalysis usually reveals proteinuria, hematuria, cylindruria, and pyuria. A "telescoped sediment" that consists of every type of element is not pathognomonic of SLE. Changes in urinary sediment are *not* a good indication of disease activity.

Course. The course of SLE is quite variable. Renal manifestations can wax and wane with changes in disease activity, intercurrent illness, and type of therapy.

Treatment. High-dose corticosteroid therapy can reduce the morbidity and mortality from the nephritis of SLE. A renal biopsy should be performed *before* beginning therapy. Treatment usually is associated with variable degrees of steroid-induced side effects that can be as troubling to the patient as the SLE. Other immunosuppressive agents such as intravenous cytoxan currently are being investigated. The danger of overwhelming sepsis in these immunosuppressed patients is constantly present. The effectiveness of therapy can be based on changes in serologic parameters, blood chemistries, and complement levels. Care of the patient with lupus is a highly specialized endeavor requiring knowledge of current treatment modalities, the availability of highly specialized tests, and the willingness to deal with a patient who has a chronic, severe, life-threatening illness, whose treatment often is disfiguring. These patients are best managed by someone trained in dealing with these aspects.

Prognosis. There is a high incidence of renal involvement in childhood SLE, and the survival rate of persons with such involvement is much poorer than for those without it. Although nephrotic syndrome generally is associated with a poor prognosis, renal biopsy provides the best means to anticipate outcome. For this reason it is important to obtain a biopsy specimen early in the course of the illness. Persons with focal glomerulonephritis rarely progress to renal failure. Diffuse proliferative glomerulonephritis, however, is associated with nephrotic syndrome in more than 50% and hypertension in 33% of the cases; it commonly progresses to renal failure. The membranous lesion also is commonly associated wiith nephrotic syndrome and may progress to renal failure, although progression usually is slower than in the diffuse proliferative lesion.

Membranoproliferative Glomerulonephritis

Membranoproliferative glomerulonephritis occurs most commonly in older children and young adults, with a slight seasonal predilection for winter. It accounts for 20% to 25% of chronic glomerulonephritis in the pediatric age-group. It also has been called chronic hypocomplementemic glomerulonephritis and mesangiocapillary nephritis.

Etiology. The cause of membranoproliferative glomerulonephritis is unknown, and there is no evidence that it is the sequela of streptococcal nephritis.

Pathology. Typically the glomeruli are enlarged and lobulated because of increased mesangial cellularity and matrix. There are irregular areas of capillary wall thickening and hyalinization produced by the presence of nonargyrophilic material. On fluorescent examination there usually is extensive capillary loop complement deposition (particularly C3) with lesser amounts of IgG and IgM. Several subtypes have been described.

Clinical Presentation. Many children with membranoproliferative glomerulonephritis initially have nephrotic syndrome or an acute nephritic syndrome, although the disease can be discovered as part of an evaluation of microscopic hematuria. In those patients with nephrotic syndrome, hypertension and hematuria are common. The acute nephritic syndrome onset cannot easily be differentiated from acute poststreptococcal glomerulonephritis, particularly because both may be associated with hypocomplementemia at the onset. Hypertension may be prominent at the onset in some patients but eventually develops in nearly all patients who progress to renal failure.

Laboratory Findings. Abnormal laboratory findings vary with the general clinical presentation syndrome. Renal function often remains normal for a long time. The most typical finding is the persistent reduction in serum C3 with normal C1, C4, and C2 levels. Continual C3 reduction even after clinical recovery has been described and called the *silent phase*. Reduced C3 for longer than 6 to 8 weeks after an acute nephritic syndrome should alert the practitioner to the possibility of membranoproliferative glomerulonephritis. Many patients also will have anemia of a severity out of proportion to the degree of azotemia. If renal failure develops later, the patient will have all the usual nonspecific abnormal laboratory findings associated with insufficient renal function. Occasionally C3 levels will rise at this time, although they may not become completely normal.

Course. The course of membranoproliferative glomerulonephritis is variable, but 50% of the patients will progress to renal failure by the eleventh year after diagnosis.

Treatment. Currently there are no generally accepted treatment regimens, although a variety of drugs are under investigation. Pediatric nephrology consultation is advised for patients suspected of having this diagnosis (e.g., those with persistent hypocomplementemia). It is important to provide long-term follow-up care for patients with this diagnosis because of the documented asymptomatic silent phases and the potential for late renal failure.

"Chronic Glomerulonephritis"

Chronic glomerulonephritis is a general category for less understood, progressive renal lesions that produce renal failure. Often patients with severe renal lesions that have progressed so far that the initial process no longer can be recognized are grouped here. It can be anticipated that in the future specific entiries will be recognized and separated from this heterogeneous group.

REFERENCES

1. Birch DF et al: Urinary erythrocyte morphology in the diagnosis of glomerular hematuria, Clin Nephrol 20:78, 1983.
2. Couser WG: Rapidly progressive glomerulonephritis: classification, pathogenetic mechanisms, and therapy, Am J Kidney Dis 11:449, 1988.
3. Fleisher DS et al: Hemodynamic findings in acute glomerulonephritis, J Pediatr 69:1054, 1966.
4. Gallo GR et al: Prognostic pathologic markers in IgA nephropathy, Am J Kidney Dis 12:362, 1988.
5. Hogg RJ: IgA nephropathy: clinical features and natural history—a pediatric perspective, Am J Kidney Dis 12:358, 1988.
6. Lange K, Seligson G, and Cronin W: Evidence for the in situ origin of poststreptococcal glomerulonephritis: glomerular localization of endostreptosin and the clinical significance of the subsequent antibody response, Clin Nephrol 19:3, 1983.
7. Lange K et al: A hitherto unknown streptococcal antigen and its probable relation to acute poststreptococcal glomerulonephritis, Clin Nephrol 5:207, 1976.

231

Nephrotic Syndrome

Edward J. Ruley

The nephrotic syndrome is characterized by massive proteinuria, hypoproteinemia (particularly hypoalbuminemia), hyperlipidemia, and edema. The incidence of nephrotic syndrome is 1.2 to 2.3 per 100,000 population per year,[7] with the occurrence 15 times more common in children than adults. Two thirds of children with nephrotic syndrome will have the onset between 1 and 5 years of age. In early childhood nephrotic syndrome develops two to three times more frequently in boys than in girls. By the middle teens, the occurrence is equal in both sexes.

ETIOLOGY

The nephrotic syndrome is not an entity but rather a true syndrome in that it can result from diverse causes. Nephrotic syndrome may occur in association with (1) metabolic diseases such as diabetes mellitus and amyloidosis, (2) immune and hypersensitivity diseases such as systemic lupus erythematosus and periarteritis nodosa, (3) nephrotoxin administration such as mercury and trimethadione, (4) allergies resulting from contactants and envenomations, (5) infections such as tuberculosis and malaria, or (6) it can be of undetermined (idiopathic) cause.

In the past the syndrome has been subclassified by a variety of systems in an effort to detect patterns of cause, response to therapy, and prognosis. One of the most definitive classifications was developed by the International Collaborative Study of Kidney Disease in Children based on the findings of renal biopsies.[3,5] In broad terms the pathologic appearance of the kidney in nephrotic syndrome has been divided into two groups: those with moderate to severe morphologic abnormalities and those with mild or no abnormalities. In pediatric patients the former often is part of a defined syndrome (such as systemic lupus erythematosus); therefore the group frequently has been called *secondary nephrotic syndrome*. This group constitutes approximately 10% of childhood cases of nephrotic syndrome. In contrast, biopsy specimens that show no disease or only mild changes often have been equated with the clinical terms *idiopathic nephrotic syndrome of childhood* or *lipoid nephrosis,* which is characterized by a clinical response to corticosteroids. This variety comprises approximately 90% of cases of childhood nephrotic syndrome and is of unknown cause.

PATHOPHYSIOLOGY

The principal pathophysiologic abnormality in nephrotic syndrome is an increased permeability of the glomerulus to protein. Whereas the electrochemical properties of the basement membrane of the glomerular capillary usually functions as a highly efficient barrier for serum proteins during ultrafiltration of the blood, in nephrotic syndrome there is a defect in the barrier so that a massive loss of protein occurs. In the nephrotic syndrome characterized by insignificant morphologic change, this loss is principally albumin. In contrast, in the instances of nephrotic syndrome associated with notable morphologic abnormalities, most of the serum proteins are lost to some degree. The former pattern of protein loss has been termed *selective,* whereas the latter pattern has been termed *nonselective*. Determination of the type of protein loss in the urine has been suggested to be of diagnostic and prognostic value in cases of this syndrome. Recent work also has suggested that tubular reabsorption and catabolism of filtered protein may contribute to the hypoproteinemia.

The liver responds to the low blood protein level by increasing protein synthesis. If the protein loss is mild or moderate, the liver usually can maintain the serum protein at normal or near-normal values. If, however, the loss is greater, the increased synthesis of protein is insufficient and hypoproteinemia ensues. As the hypoproteinemia develops, there is a gradual decrease in the serum oncotic pressure, which allows fluid to exude from the intravascular space into the intracellular space, causing edema. The blood volume often becomes contracted, which stimulates the production of aldosterone by the adrenal gland, which acts to increase renal tubular reabsorption of sodium and water. Although such hemeostatic response ordinarily would serve to correct the abnormal vascular volume, it is ineffective in nephrotic syndrome because the reduced oncotic pressure allows the fluid to continue to leak from the vascular space. It has been suggested that the secondary hyperaldosteronism further contributes to edema formation and the oliguria that commonly is seen in nephrotic syndrome. The pathophysiology of the hyperlipidemia is less clear. Although it has been suggested that hyperlipidemia occurs secondary to the hypoproteinemia, it has been noted to occur before hypoproteinemia in experimentally induced nephrotic syndrome in animals and to persist even after the resolution of proteinuria in human beings.

CLINICAL FORMS OF NEPHROTIC SYNDROME

Idiopathic Nephrotic Syndrome of Childhood

Idiopathic nephrotic syndrome of childhood (minimal change disease, NIL disease) is the most common variety of nephrotic syndrome in pediatric patients.[2] Although it may occur at any age, 90% of cases of idiopathic nephrotic syndrome occur between the ages of 1 and 5 years, with the peak ages between 2 and 3 years. There is a male predominance.

Clinical Presentation. The majority of children have complaints relating to the sudden development of dependent edema (Fig. 231-1). The parents may notice that their child has periorbital edema on rising in the morning, which gradually diminishes with upright activity, only to be followed by ankle and pedal edema later in the day. This ankle edema may manifest as a tight fit of the child's shoes as the day progresses. At first the dependent edema will vary in degree from day to day, but gradually it will become more consistent and severe, so that facial or lower extremity edema may be present regardless of the activity and position of the patient. As edema becomes more generalized, ascites and hydrothorax may develop. If the ascites is gradual, it may be noted as an increase in abdominal protuberance, producing the inability to button pants that previously had fit well. Severe ascites often is associated with labial or scrotal edema (Fig. 231-2). Respiratory difficulty in the form of tachypnea, flaring of the ala nasi, or dyspnea may develop as a result of hydrothorax or the pressure of ascites on the diaphragm.

With the development of edema the child may be anorexic, listless, and pale. The appearance is that of a chronically ill, rather than an acutely ill, child. Diarrhea and vomiting are common at this stage, although it is uncertain whether these symptoms are caused by edema of the bowel as has been proposed. Prolonged hypoalbuminemia may result in muscle wasting, malnutrition, and growth failure. Most patients are normotensive, although mild hypertension may occur.

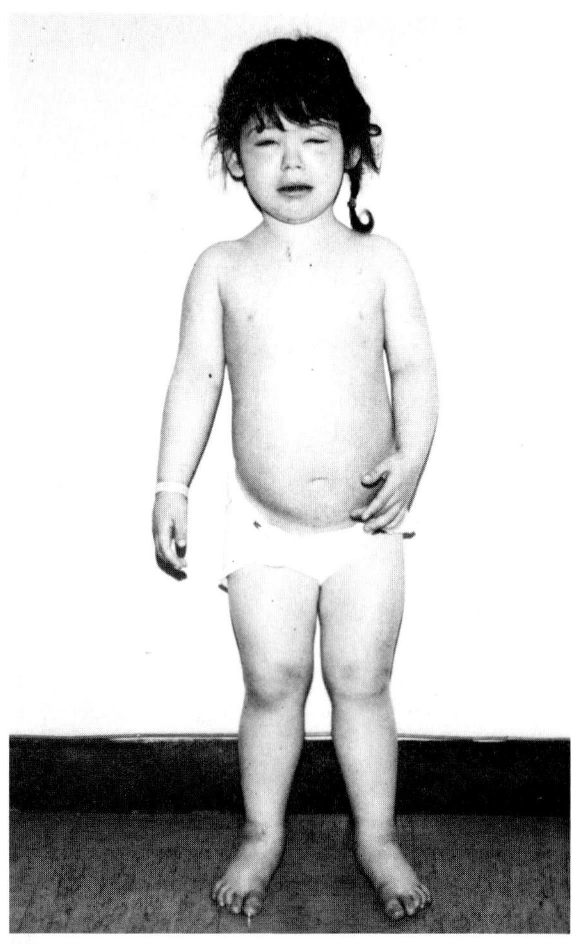

Fig. 231-1 Two-year-old girl with nephrotic syndrome in relapse.

Diagnosis. The urinalysis in idiopathic nephrotic syndrome characteristically contains large amounts of protein and many hyaline and finely granular casts. Microscopic hematuria, which may occur in 33% of patients, is almost never grossly apparent. Cellular casts are seen occasionally. The urine usually is of high specific gravity, and doubly refractile fat bodies may be visualized with polarized light. Quantitative urinary protein determinations often exceed 5 to 10 g/day.

Examination of the serum usually reveals severe hypoproteinemia (serum albumin below 2 g/dl) associated with an increase in triglycerides, high-density lipoproteins, and cholesterol. The hyperlipidemia usually is severe enough to cause the serum to be lactescent on direct examination. This lactescence may interfere with some serum biochemical determinations. The serum calcium level usually is lowered because of the decrease in serum protein. Hyponatremia also may be found. This is usually artifactual inasmuch as sodium is restricted to the aqueous phase of serum, which is relatively diminished in the nephrotic patient as a result of the increase in the nonaqueous phase because of elevated serum lipid levels. Anemia may be present. The serum complement level is usually normal. A diagnosis of idiopathic nephrotic syndrome can be made with 95% certainty on the basis of the clinical impression. Characteristically, these children are between 1 and 10 years of age and have the typical clinical features of the syndrome. They may have either hypertension or hematuria, but not both. Azotemia and hypocomplementemia usually are absent. The presence of selective proteinemia also supports the diagnosis.

Biopsy findings in children with idiopathic nephrotic syndrome reveal grossly normal glomeruli, although some may

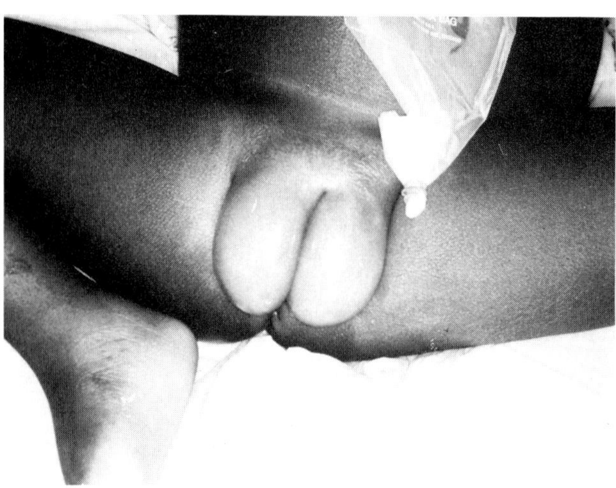

Fig. 231-2 Severe labial edema in 3-year-old girl with nephrotic syndrome.

have slight mesangial hyperplasia (Fig. 231-3). Typically the biopsy specimen, when examined by immunofluorescent techniques, shows no deposits of immunoglobulin or complement proteins and examination by electron microscopy reveals only simplification of the foot processes of the epithelial cells. This latter change generally is considered to be a consequence of proteinuria. If there is strong clinical and laboratory evidence of idiopathic nephrotic syndrome of childhood, renal biopsy usually is unnecessary. However, biopsy is indicated (1) in children who have both hypertension and hematuria, (2) when there is hypocomplementemia or nonselective proteinemia, or (3) when the nephrotic syndrome occurs in an older child or adolescent. Older children and those who fail to respond to a course of corticosteroids are likely to have a renal disease other than idiopathic nephrotic syndrome of childhood.

Occasionally a child will have a complication of an unrecognized nephrotic syndrome such as thromboembolism or signs of infection. The former is related to the propensity to form thrombi in nephrotic syndrome. Furthermore, children with nephrotic syndrome are particularly susceptible to peritonitis. The presence of fever in any patient with nephrotic syndrome requires a careful evaluation for sepsis.

Differential Diagnosis. Nephrotic syndrome of any cause needs to be differentiated in general from the hypoproteinemia and edema found in conditions of decreased protein production, such as starvation, liver disease, and protein-losing enteropathy. The absence of notable proteinuria in these diseases differentiates them from nephrotic syndrome.

Idiopathic nephrotic syndrome usually can be differentiated from the nephrotic syndrome caused by morphologic glomerular disease by the nonselective proteinuria, the tendency for hematuria and hypertension to coexist, and the tendency for onset in older children in the latter condition.[4,5,8] An exception is the child with a focal sclerosing type of glomerular lesion, who initially may have symptoms similar to those of the child with idiopathic nephrotic syndrome. These children usually are detected by their incomplete response to corticosteroid treatment.

Treatment. General aspects of treatment include provision for activity, diet, and diuretic therapy. Children kept at bed rest often will have a mild spontaneous diuresis with a subsequent fall in weight and decrease in edema. However, because a major complication of nephrotic syndrome of any cause is thromboembolism, the wisdom of inactivity and the attendant increased risk of thrombosis must be considered. Traditionally, a diet high in protein has been prescribed, although it usually has a minimal effect on the serum protein level. Salt limitation usually is unnecessary if the patient is not hypertensive. Salt intake by children usually is not excessive, and severe salt restriction may make the diet unpalatable, thereby defeating the attempt to promote a balanced

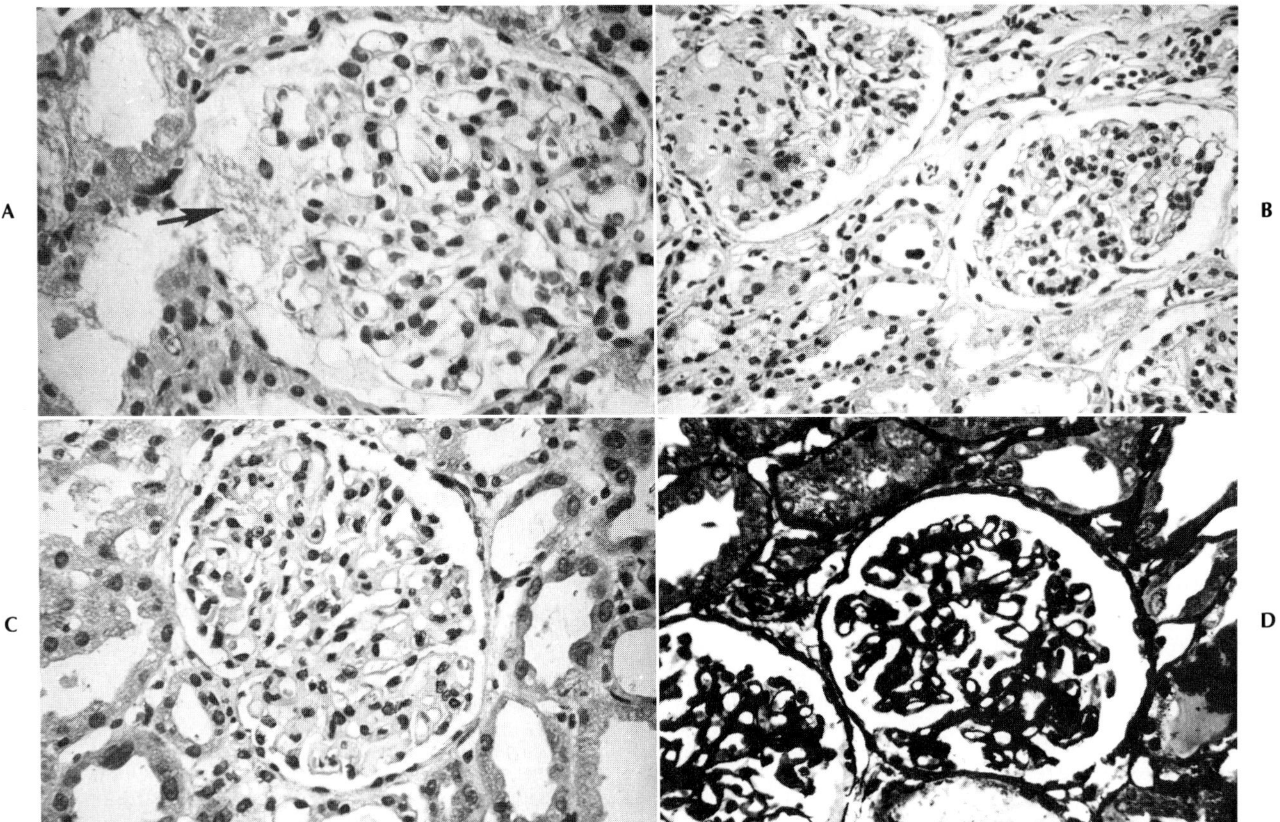

Fig. 231-3 Renal disease in nephrotic syndrome. **A,** Minimal change disease. Arrow indicates proteinaceous material in Bowman space. (Hematoxylin and eosin stain.) **B,** Focal glomerulosclerosis. Note segmental acellular involvement of one glomerulus and virtual sparing of the other. (Hematoxylin and eosin stain.) **C,** Membranous glomerulopathy. Note thickening of basement membranes. (Hematoxylin and eosin stain.) **D,** Membranous glomerulopathy. Thickening of the basement membranes is better seen on silver stain.

intake. Restriction of salt to the amount in a "regular" diet with no added salt at the table and the elimination of foods known to be highly salted (e.g., peanuts and potato chips) are all that is usually necessary. Likewise, limitation of fluids also is unnecessary except in the severely hypertensive patient. Marked limitation of fluids in the patient with hemoconcentration and oliguria may aggravate the hypoperfusion and contribute to the risk of thromboembolism.

Diuretic therapy may be indicated for the patient who has incapacitating edema. However, the response to diuretics usually is less than expected because of the hypoproteinemia in these patients. At best, diuretic therapy can produce only a short-term reduction in the edema. The same is true for intravenous albumin infusion, because the albumin is lost in the urine nearly as rapidly as it is given. A greater effect results from the combined use of albumin (1 g/kg/day intravenously) and diuretics (furosemide, 1 to 2 mg/kg/day orally or intravenously), although the duration of effect is limited. Albumin infusion can be associated with a risk of overexpansion of the vascular space and congestive heart failure. Although such complications are uncommon in nephrotic patients, care always should be exercised in the administration of albumin.

It generally is agreed that a course of corticosteroids can induce a remission in most children with idiopathic nephrotic syndrome. Prednisone is used most often because of its effectiveness and low cost. Usually the child is begun on a daily dose of 2 mg/kg (60 mg/m^2) given either once daily or in two divided doses, with a maximum daily dose of 60 mg. Such treatment should induce a remission in most patients within 6 to 14 days after starting therapy. Remission usually will be heralded by a rather abrupt diuresis associated with a decrease and then absence of urinary protein. Continuing steroids at a high dosage for long periods produces a variety of drug-induced side effects, including increased appetite, weight gain, truncal obesity, moon face, acne, and stria. As with all high-dose continual steroid therapy, serious infections may be masked. At high doses, growth in height is markedly decreased, so that prolonged treatment may result in severe stunting. Thus to reduce these side effects, steroids should be changed to an every-other-day schedule after there is evidence of a response to the daily regimen. Furthermore, the alternate-day steroids should be gradually discontinued because many patients do well for long periods without steroids. There is no general agreement, however, as to the best method or the rapidity with which to make changes in steroid administration.

Patients who respond to corticosteroids are termed *steroid sensitive*. Patients who fail to respond to prednisone after 4 weeks of daily administration are considered to be *steroid resistant*. In other patients a pattern of steroid dependency may develop wherein they remain in remission so long as a particular dose of prednisone is given but relapse as soon as the dose is reduced below the "critical level." Other patients respond to the corticosteroid but have *frequent relapses* (defined as more than three relapses within a year while not receiving steroids).

Patients who are steroid resistant, steroid dependent, or frequent relapsers should be referred to a pediatric nephrologist for consideration for renal biopsy and other forms of drug therapy. At present, effective drug regimens for these children are the subject of investigation. Most of the drugs employed have additional side effects about which the parents need to be informed. It is inappropriate for a pediatric practitioner to institute a course of therapy with one of these unproved drugs in a sporadic case of nephrotic syndrome.

Infections in children with nephrotic syndrome should be treated with appropriate antibiotics. Prophylactic antibiotic therapy is not indicated. Immunization should be delayed until the child has not relapsed for 6 months to 2 years without steroid therapy.

Prognosis. The overall prognosis for steroid-sensitive nephrotic syndrome is good.[6] Because relapses are the rule, however, parents need to be educated about the natural history of the illness. An occasional relapse should not be portrayed as either a severe setback or a condition to be ignored. Most children remain steroid responsive, and the disease can be controlled with additional courses of therapy. Furthermore, it is helpful if the parents are given some means of testing the urine for protein, which involves them directly in the child's care and allows them to feel more in control. Finding no proteinuria will reassure the parents; thus every change in the physical and emotional state of the child will not be viewed as a subtle symptom of a relapse. Furthermore, when relapse does occur, the parents often will be able to discover the proteinuria before the development of clinical edema. Prompt reinstitution of corticosteroids often will produce a remission before clinical symptoms appear and thereby obviate the need for hospital admission. Relapses in most children should be treatable without hospitalization.

It should be stressed that nephrotic syndrome is a chronic disease during which there is a great need for patient and parent education. Side effects of the disease and the therapy—particularly the corticosteroids—need to be taught. Even in the most uncomplicated case, it may be helpful to seek consultation periodically with a pediatric nephrologist. In particular, the use of corticosteroids for this syndrome is constantly changing as various regimens are developed that effectively control the disease with a reduction in side effects. Periodic advice as to the management of these drugs should allow the design of a program that provides the best possible control of the disease with the least treatment side effects, resulting in a child who can lead as normal a life as possible.

Focal Glomerulosclerosis

In the young child, focal glomerulosclerosis can manifest with signs and symptoms identical to those of idiopathic nephrotic syndrome. This illness should be suspected in any nephrotic child who is unresponsive to steroid treatment or who develops steroid resistance, steroid dependence, or frequent relapses after having been steroid sensitive. In addition, azotemia, hematuria, and nonselective proteinuria occur more frequently in these children. On the basis of serial biopsy observations, it has been suggested that focal glomerulosclerosis may be an unfavorable evolution of idiopathic nephrotic syndrome. The diagnosis of focal glomerulosclerosis can be made only by renal biopsy. Typically there are focal acellular hyalinized areas in the glomerular segments, although several patterns of disease have been described based on the degree of involvement (Fig. 231-3). The prognosis of this condition generally is poor, with progressive renal failure developing in most patients. Patients with focal glomerulosclerosis *and* interstitial inflammation tend to have a more rapid rate of deterioration.[1] Definitive drug therapies currently are under investigation. The disease has recurred in some children who have received renal transplants. Because of the complexity in establishing the diagnosis, the probability for development of renal failure and the uncertainty of beneficial effects with drug therapy, these cases are best managed in consultation with a pediatric nephrologist.

Membranous Nephropathy

Membranous (extramembranous) nephropathy usually has a manifestation similar to that of idiopathic nephrotic syndrome, although it more often affects older children. It too is characterized by steroid resistance. Diagnosis can be made only by renal biopsy, in which the specimen reveals diffuse thickening of the glomerular capillary walls without significant proliferation (Fig. 231-3). On electron microscopic examination, subepithelial deposits are found in the capillary loops. As seen by immunofluorescent examination, these deposits usually consist of IgG and C3 and are thought to represent small immune complexes. Although there is no definite therapy of proved benefit, the prognosis in children generally is much better than in adults, with spontaneous remission occurring in about 50% of the children. A complete infectious hepatitis serology study should be performed in these children because many will be found to be carriers of hepatitis-associated antigens. Controlled trials of various agents currently are under investigation. The disease of these children also is best managed in consultation with a pediatric nephrologist.

REFERENCES

1. Ellis D et al: Focal glomerulosclerosis in children: correlation of histology with prognosis, J Pediatr 93:762, 1978.
2. Grupe WE: Primary nephrotic syndrome in childhood, Adv Pediatr 26:163, 1979.
3. Habib R and Kleinknecht C: The primary nephrotic syndrome of childhood: classification and clinicopathologic study of 406 cases. In Sommers SC: Pathology annual, East Norwalk, Conn, 1971, Appleton-Century-Crofts.
4. Habib R, Levy M, and Gubler MC: Clinicopathologic correlations in the nephrotic syndrome, Paediatrician 8:325, 1979.
5. International Study of Kidney Disease in Children: Nephrotic syndrome in children: prediction of histopathology from clinical and laboratory characteristics at time of diagnosis, Kidney Int 31:1368, 1987.
6. Koskimies O et al: Long-term outcome of primary nephrotic syndrome, Arch Dis Child 57:544, 1982.
7. Rothenberg MB and Heymann W: The incidence of the nephrotic syndrome in children, Pediatrics 19:446, 1957.
8. White RHR, Glasgow EF, and Mills RJ: Clinicopathological study of the nephrotic syndrome in childhood, Lancet 1:1353, 1970.

SUGGESTED READINGS

Chesney RW and Novello AC: Forms of nephrotic syndrome more likely to progress to renal impairment, Pediatr Clin North Am 34:609, 1987.

Kher KK, Sweet M, and Makker SP: Nephrotic syndrome in children, Curr Probl Pediatr 18:199, 1988.

Strauss J et al: Less commonly recognized features of childhood nephrotic syndrome, Pediatr Clin North Am 34:591, 1987.

232

Obesity

Modena Hoover Wilson

Obesity has been called an epidemic disease. It does not spare children. Few topics have provoked as much controversy; the prevalence of obesity varies with definition, its causes are complex, its medical outcome is unpredictable, and the results of its treatment often are discouraging.

ETIOLOGY

Obesity results when energy intake exceeds energy needs. The excess is stored as fat. This explanation is at once elegantly simple, inasmuch as it leads immediately to the two therapy choices—decreasing intake and increasing expenditure—and yet superficial. Interest really lies in why a given person's metabolism regulates his or her weight at an apparently inappropriately high level.

Although obesity corresponds to a "maladaptive increase in the size of the adipose organ,"[28] clarification of the origins of this increase continues to challenge researchers. It is overly simplistic to dismiss obesity as a straightforward consequence of undisciplined overeating.[27] Indeed, some obese individuals appear to eat less than their lean peers but remain obese.[4] Neither can the contribution of increased energy intake to the maintenance of obesity be denied. Obese individuals must eat more than those who are not obese to maintain their weight.[14]

As a group, obese children are less active than the nonobese.[4] They are less frequently involved in vigorous activities and move less when they are involved.[31] It is not clear whether this is the cause of obesity for these children or a consequence that perpetuates it. Indeed, because energy expenditure during activity increases with weight, total energy expenditure may be greater for the obese. Activity not only affects weight by using energy; it may help to regulate appetite.

An understanding of hypothalamic processing of cognitive, visceral, and metabolic signals to produce feeding behavior is not yet complete. The mechanisms by which genetic, environmental, and psychological factors are translated into too much food or too little exercise are not known.

Excessive weight at birth, which is related to maternal size and weight gain during pregnancy, may be a predictor, albeit a weak one, of future obesity. Likewise, rapid weight gain during infancy has been repeatedly implicated; however, most fat infants become lean.

If one parent is obese, a child has a 40% chance of becoming obese. If two parents are obese, this possibility rises to 80%.[23] These figures do not rule out environment as a contributor to this strong link, but the following factors support genetic contribution: monozygotic twins show more concordance for fatness than do dizygotic twins, and children reared by adoptive parents are less likely to resemble those parents in terms of fatness than are nonadopted children.[2]

A study[30] of adults who had been raised by adoptive parents found no correlation between weight class of adoptees and the body-mass index of adoptive parents, but a strong relationship to that of biologic parents.

Family expectations, feeding methods, and eating and activity patterns that promote or sustain obesity certainly can be identified in intervention attempts with obese children. There is, for instance, an association between obesity and number of hours spent watching television in childhood.[11]

Finally, obesity may be clearly related in some instances to psychopathology in the individual or in family functioning.

PREVALENCE

Body weight has been increasing in the United States, and so have skinfold thicknesses of children and adolescents.[19] Prevalence rates depend on definition and demographic factors.[17] Perhaps 10% of infants younger than age 1 year are obese. If 120% of normal body weight is the criterion for obesity, 12% of preschool children in New York City are obese.[18] Adolescent obesity prevalence rates are at least 10% to 20%.[24] Whatever the definition, obesity is common, and prevalence increases with age: 30% to 40% of adults in the United States are classified as obese.

COMPLICATIONS

Few obese children suffer serious medical consequences of their obesity in childhood. Orthopedic problems may result from the stress of the weight, and skin irritation may occur in fat folds. Obese children's tolerance for exercise and heat is reduced, and they may be hypertensive.[21]

A few *very* obese children do not keep up with the increased work of breathing and thus develop the obesity-hypoventilation (Pickwickian) syndrome, characterized by high carbon dioxide levels, somnolence, and the risk of cor pulmonale.

Medical abhorrence of childhood obesity is founded primarily on the belief that it leads to adult obesity, which some studies suggest is life shortening.[29] Controversy over this point continues.[20] Certain cardiovascular risk factors such as diabetes, hypertension, and an elevated serum cholesterol level are more prevalent among more than mildly obese adults. Weight reduction may diminish these risks.

The most severe consequences of childhood obesity in a culture that idealizes thinness but provides a life-style that promotes fatness are psychological. A fat child is treated as ugly, weak, and inferior. He or she may be the center of family debate and scorn, ridiculed, excluded by peers, harangued by the family physician and teachers, and discriminated against.[5] Although research results thus far are inconclusive, obese children may develop passive modes of coping and low self-esteem, which is further damaged by unsuccessful attempts to lose weight. Obesity produces isolation, which increases obesity.

ADOLESCENT OBESITY

Adolescent obesity deserves special mention. Unlike younger children, obese adolescents are likely to remain obese as adults.[33] Even lean adolescents may believe they are fat. When an adolescent is truly obese, peer pressures can be devastating. Such a patient may be particularly attracted to crash diets and especially impatient for results. Few are satisfied with the tedious process and continuing self-denial of weight reduction programs. Nevertheless, an approach that combines diet, structured physical activity, and behavioral techniques is indicated. Psychological support is crucial; group therapy may contribute to success.

DIFFERENTIAL DIAGNOSIS

Although obesity is a feature of several endocrinopathies and a number of syndromes (see accompanying box), these are rare causes of obesity.[8] Delayed bone age also is a feature of a number of these syndromes, which need not be pursued if an obese child is of average or above average height and is without other expected signs or stigmata of specific syndromes. Hypogonadism is a particularly suspicious positive finding. Central nervous system damage and certain neuroactive drugs may cause weight gain.

A number of reversible metabolic and hormonal abnormalities such as decreased glucose tolerance, increased insulin resistance, hyperlipidemia, increased corticosteroid levels, and decreased growth hormone response may result from obesity. These are not the causes but rather the results of obesity.

DIAGNOSIS

Although obesity clearly refers to excessive fatness, it is not easy to measure how much fat is present or to decide where in the fatness continuum obesity, the "disease," begins.[32] Some children are clearly obese by appearance alone. However, more discriminating measures must be applied to most children, especially to identify those in the process of becoming obese.

The child's weight can be related to an "ideal" or median weight for children of the same sex, height, and age. Weight-for-height above the 95th percentile or weight greater than 120% of normal (i.e., 50th percentile for height often is considered diagnostic[24].)

Increased weight, however, can represent increased lean body mass rather than fat alone; thus measures based solely on weight and height may be misleading, especially because these change rapidly during adolescence. Body fat can be estimated more closely by measuring the skinfold of the triceps; the 85th or 95th percentile generally is considered the dividing line.[15]

Because normal body weight and the criteria for obesity

Diseases Associated with Obesity

CENTRAL NERVOUS SYSTEM DISEASES

Damage (Fröhlich Syndrome)

Trauma
Tumor
Postinfectious effect
Vascular accident

Drugs

Phenothiazines
Tricyclic antidepressants
Lithium
Cyproheptadine

ENDOCRINE DISORDERS

Hypothyroidism
Cushing syndrome (adrenal hypercorticism)
Exogenous corticosteroids
High insulin level
  Insulinoma
  Diabetes with excessive insulin administration

Modified from Merritt RJ: Obesity, Curr Probl Pediatr 12(11):28, 1982.

CONGENITAL SYNDROMES
Associated with Hypogonadism

Prader-Willi (slow intellectual development, short stature, dysmorphic facies, small hands and feet, skin problems, scoliosis, strabismus)
Laurence-Moon-Biedl (mental retardation, short stature, polydactyly, retinitis pigmentosa)
Alström (deafness, diabetes mellitus, retinitis pigmentosa, short stature)
Vasquez (male, X-linked short stature, mental retardation, gynecomastia)

Chromosomal

Klinefelter syndrome
Turner syndrome
Multiple X syndromes

Others

Pseudohypoparathyroidism
Pseudopseudohypoparathyroidism

are statistical constructs, it would be helpful to know at what level of obesity medical morbidity begins. Unfortunately, that is not known; however, it is known that the threshold for psychosocial consequences appears to be much lower.

TREATMENT

Once obesity is established, long-term remission is difficult to achieve at any age. The longer the duration of the obesity, the more pessimistic the outlook for permanent leanness. The first treatment decision to be made is whether treatment should be undertaken. Indications for considering treatment probably are strongest with *very* obese infants and young children and children who are obese at puberty, in both cases especially if they are from obese families.[16,25]

The treatment of choice is a reduction in caloric intake (a calorie-deficit diet) and an increase in energy expenditure. All techniques of therapy are designed to accomplish one or both.[3,7,10] The weight goal will depend somewhat on the degree of obesity and the patient's age. Because caloric restriction will decelerate linear growth, this is undertaken with extreme caution in young children. For the obese infant or mildly obese older child who is growing rapidly, weight stabilization is appropriate; for the more obese older child, a slow weight loss of 0.5 to 1 kg a week is recommended. Occasionally, middle and late adolescents may try programs for rapid weight loss, which might not necessarily be healthy; therefore, in such instances, an attempt should be made to inculcate good nutritional habits to last a lifetime. Steps in the management of a mildly to moderately obese child might include the following:

1. Establishing that obesity is perceived as a problem by the child or family
2. Agreeing on a reasonable weight goal
3. Determining present eating habits, level of consumption, and commitment to therapy by use of a diet diary
4. Developing a reasonable diet (see below) and a practical activity plan and providing nutritional education
5. Considering the use of behavioral therapy techniques to complement the diet and activity plans
6. Identifying and modifying family functioning styles that jeopardize weight loss or stabilization
7. Seeing the patient frequently for follow-up to monitor and reinforce progress
8. Maintaining a relationship with the patient that enhances the patient's self-esteem whether or not weight is lost

Diet

Few physicians feel competent to design a diet[26]; thus the expertise of a nutritionist, when available, is invaluable. A weight reduction diet for a child must provide the nutrients necessary for growth and development while it maintains a caloric deficit.

Because the caloric value of a kilogram of fat is 9000 calories, a weight loss of approximately 0.5 kg/wk can be predicted from a diet that supplies a weekly deficit of 4500 calories. Because the caloric needs vary for each individual, the recommended daily allowance for age and sex minus the intended loss is only an initial approximation. Results will suggest modifications.

When calories are restricted, protein requirements increase. Children on weight reduction diets should receive about 150% of the recommended daily allowance of protein. This will be roughly 1.5 to 2.5 g/kg of ideal body weight per day, depending on age.[24] When the adequacy of the diet is in question, a multivitamin, trace-element supplement is indicated.

In almost every case, rapid weight loss diets are condemned in pediatrics. They are nutritionally inadequate for children and adolescents and lead to unsound eating habits. Lean body mass is sacrificed, and the lost weight usually is regained rapidly. Extended use of liquid protein diets has been blamed for some adult deaths. Appetite suppressants also are to be avoided for most pediatric patients. However, both moderate fasting and appetite suppressants have been used successfully in very obese patients, usually adolescents, as part of special, often inpatient, pediatric programs for weight reduction. Needless to say, close clinical monitoring is essential.

Behavioral Treatment

Behavioral therapy may be a useful adjunct in accomplishing both weight loss and the changes in eating and activity that permanent weight control usually requires. Applying the principles of social learning to the problem of obesity began with adult patients; few pediatric trials have been reported. Techniques employed include combinations of self-monitoring, stimulus control, slowing of the act of eating, and reinforcing and rewarding behavior changes and weight loss.

Surgery

Surgical treatments for obesity include gastric and intestinal bypass procedures. Both have been applied to selected pediatric patients, most often adolescents with massive obesity. Intestinal bypass, although successful in producing weight loss, is associated with a number of side effects that are especially grave during growth and development. Even gastric bypass surgery probably should not be considered unless the patient is two to three times normal body weight, suffers medical consequences, and has failed to maintain weight loss with vigorous dietary programs. Many would prohibit the use of surgery to treat pediatric and adolescent obesity altogether.

Success of Treatment

Reports vary, but follow-up statistics are moderately to very discouraging. Obesity is complex in origin and remarkably difficult to cure.[28] Although many programs have helped individuals to lose weight, it appears that not more than 20% of patients have maintained the loss at long-term follow-up.

Obesity is a chronic disease. About 20% of obese infants (compared with fewer than 10% of nonobese infants) become obese children. About 70% of obese children become obese adolescents, and most of these become obese adults. Conversely, only 33% of obese adults were obese during infancy and/or childhood.

The role that the number of fat cells plays in this inexorable march is controversial. It has been demonstrated that obese infants have more and larger fat cells than nonobese infants. Abnormal adipose hyperplasia can also be precipitated in those whose obesity begins at older ages. Whether there is a critical period during which overfeeding can make lifelong obesity practically inescapable is not yet clear.[12]

PREVENTION

Obesity is so difficult to modify that it would be much better prevented. Unfortunately, it is not known who should get the intervention and what it should be. Current knowledge supports the notion that infants who have a very high birth weight,[13] gain weight rapidly, have excessive weight in their early months,[6] or have at least one obese parent may be at additional risk, although many of these infants eventually will be lean. Supporting evidence is at best incomplete; however, currently it is suggested that breast-feeding be encouraged and that the introduction of solid foods be delayed to provide more control over intake. Furthermore, an active life-style should be promoted for children of all ages.[9] Although counseling about nutrition is a part of almost every well-baby examination, counseling about appropriate activity probably is rare.

SUMMARY

Established obesity is modified poorly. This is unfortunate because the psychological damage that attends obesity is clear. Evidence that mild obesity is medically harmful, however, is sparse.[22] Perhaps cultural and medical attitudes should be shifted[1] so that lean babies and mildly fat older children are perceived as being more attractive than they are at present. (See also Chapter 16, Three, for further discussion of obesity.)

REFERENCES

1. Barness LA: Obesity, Am J Dis Child 141:486, 1987 (editorial).
2. Biron P, Monegeau JG, and Bertrand D: Familial resemblance of body weight and weight/height in 374 homes with adopted children, J Pediatr 91:555, 1977.
3. Brownell KD, Wadden TA, and Foster GD: A comprehensive treatment plan for obese children and adolescents: principles and practice, Pediatrician 12:89, 1983.
4. Bullen BA, Reed RB, and Mayer J: Physical activity of obese and nonobese adolescent girls appraised by motion picture sampling, Am J Clin Nutr 14:211, 1964.
5. Canning H and Mayer J: Obesity—its possible effect on college acceptance, N Engl J Med 275:1172, 1966.
6. Charney E et al: Childhood antecedents of adult obesity: do chubby infants become obese adults? N Engl J Med 295:6, 1976.
7. Collipp PJ, editor: Childhood obesity, Littleton, Mass, 1980, PSG Publishing Co, Inc.
8. Collipp PJ: Differential diagnosis of childhood obesity. In Collipp PJ, editor: Childhood obesity, Littleton, Mass, 1980, PSG Publishing Co, Inc.
9. Committee on Nutrition: Nutritional aspects of obesity in infancy and childhood, Pediatrics 68:880, 1981.
10. Dietz WH: Childhood obesity: susceptibility, cause and management, J Pediatr 103:676, 1983.
11. Dietz WH and Gortmaker SL: Do we fatten our children at the television set? Obesity and television viewing in children and adolescents, Pediatrics 75:807, 1985.
12. Edelman B and Maller O: Facts and fictions about infantile obesity, Int J Obes 6:69, 1982.
13. Fisch RO, Bilet MK, and Ulstrom R: Obesity and leanness at birth and their relationship to body habitus in later childhood, Pediatrics 56:521, 1975.
14. Forbes GB and Brown MR: Energy need for weight maintenance in human beings: effect of body size and composition, J Am Diet Assoc 89:499, 1989.
15. Frisancho AR: Triceps skinfold and upper arm muscle size norms for assessment of nutritional status, Am J Clin Nutr 27:1052, 1974.
16. Garn SM: Continuities and changes in fatness from infancy through adulthood, Curr Probl Pediatr 15(2):1, 1985.
17. Garn SM and Clark DC: Nutrition, growth, development and maturation: findings from the Ten State Nutrition Survey of 1968–70, Pediatrics 56:306, 1975.
18. Ginsberg-Fellner F et al: Overweight and obesity in preschool children in New York City, Am J Clin Nutr 34:2236, 1981.
19. Gortmaker SL et al: Increasing pediatric obesity in the United States, Am J Dis Child 141:535, 1987.
20. Knapp TR: A methodological critique of the "ideal weight" concept, JAMA 250:506, 1983.
21. Londe S et al: Hypertension in apparently normal children, J Pediatr 78:569, 1971.
22. Mallick MJ: Health hazards of obesity and weight control in children: a review of the literature, Am J Public Health 73:78, 1983.
23. Mayer J: Genetic factors in human obesity, Ann NY Acad Sci 131:412, 1965.
24. Merritt RJ: Obesity, Curr Probl Pediatr 12(11):28, 1982.
25. Mossberg H: 40-year follow-up of overweight children, Lancet 2:491, 1989.
26. Price JH et al: Pediatricians' perceptions and practices regarding childhood obesity, Am J Prev Med 5:95, 1989.
27. Rolland-Cachera MF et al: Adiposity and food intake in young children: the environmental challenge to individual susceptibility, Br Med J 296:1037, 1988.
28. Rosenbaum M and Leibel RL: Pathophysiology of childhood obesity, Adv Pediatr 35:73, 1988.
29. Simic BS: Childhood obesity as a risk factor in adulthood. In Collipp PJ, editor: Childhood obesity, Littleton, Mass, 1980, PSG Publishing Co, Inc.
30. Stunkard AJ et al: An adoption study of human obesity, N Engl J Med 314:193, 1986.
31. Waxman M and Stunkard AJ: Caloric intake and expenditure of boys, J Pediatr 96:187, 1980.
32. Weil WB: Current controversies in childhood obesity, J Pediatr 91:175, 1977.
33. Zack PM et al: A longitudinal study of body fatness in childhood and adolescence, J Pediatr 95:126, 1979.

233

Obstructive Uropathy and Vesicoureteral Reflux

Edward J. Ruley and J. Ramon Ongkingco

OBSTRUCTIVE UROPATHY

Frequency

The exact frequency of urinary tract obstruction is unknown. An autopsy study suggests that it occurs in 2% to 3.8% of children. More important is that it accounts for approximately 20% of renal failure in childhood and that early diagnosis and treatment may delay or prevent the need for dialysis or kidney transplantation, or both, later in the child's life.

Etiology

Although urinary tract obstruction may result from an acquired lesion, congenital anomalies of urinary development are much more common. Obstructive urinary lesions can be divided into those of the lower and upper urinary systems, with the bladder outlet being the dividing point.

Lower Urinary Tract Obstruction. Although lower tract lesions most often are structural in nature, functional lesions occasionally can cause obstruction as well. Anatomic obstruction to the bladder outlet occurs most often in boys because of the length of their urethra and the embryologic complexity of its development.

Posterior urethral valves are the most common obstructive lesions of the lower urinary system. It is believed that abnormal migration of the terminal end of the wolffian ducts results in the persistence of obliquely oriented ridges along the posterior urethral wall or a diaphragm-like structure that acts to obstruct urine flow from the bladder. These valves occur almost exclusively in boys. Urethral obstruction usually results in bladder enlargement and muscular hypertrophy as a result of the work involved in emptying against the obstructive resistance in the urethra. Hypertrophy of the interwoven bladder muscle fibers gives the appearance of a thickened bladder wall, with trabeculation on cystographic examination.

Urethral strictures as a cause of bladder outlet obstruction most often result from urethral trauma such as a straddle injury, a pelvic fracture, instrumentation, or in adolescents, the consequence of urethritis, particularly that caused by a sexually transmitted disease. Congenital strictures are rare.

Bladder outlet obstruction was in the past a very common urologic diagnosis, one most often made in children with vesicoureteral reflux or recurrent urinary infections. Transurethral resection or bladder neck revision often was performed, usually with little benefit. This disorder currently is believed to be unusual and limited almost exclusively to boys.

Meatal stenosis in boys and *distal urethral stenosis* in girls were commonly diagnosed in the past as causes of bladder outlet obstruction. The role of these abnormalities in obstructing urine outflow is still debated. From a practical point of view it is known that the visible size of the meatus does not correlate with its calibrated size. Furthermore, in girls there is an inverse correlation between urethral diameter and urinary infection so that infection is more common in individuals with larger urethral lumens.

Phimosis can cause urethral obstruction, although probably not as frequently as was once thought. It may be a developmental anomaly or an acquired condition.

Anterior urethral valves, urethral diverticula, müllerian *duct cysts,* and *megalourethra* are all rare structural causes of outlet obstruction.

Neurogenic bladder can cause obstructive changes functionally. It may occur as a result of meningomyelocele, an absent sacrum, or hemivertebrae or with spinal cord injury.

Voiding dysnergia, or *nonneurogenic* or *neurogenic bladder,* is another functional cause of urinary obstruction. This condition is a form of incorrectly learned behavior associated with voluntary retention of urine and stool. In this circumstance the child constricts the internal sphincter of the bladder rather than relaxing it when voiding, creating a functional obstruction at the bladder neck. This disorder is considered to be psychogenic in origin.

Upper Urinary Tract Obstruction. *Ureteropelvic junction obstruction* is the most common obstructive lesion of the upper urinary system. The ureteric lumen may be constricted either intrinsically from a congenital narrowing of the lumen or extrinsically from pressure of a crossing blood vessel or a fibrous band or adhesion. It occurs in both genders equally, most often on the left side. It is bilateral in 10% of cases.

Ureterovesical junction obstruction is the second most common supravesical obstructive site. It is more common in boys than in girls and is unilateral 80% of the time, usually on the left. In this condition the distal ureter usually is aperistaltic, producing functional obstruction and a markedly dilated, tortuous ureter. Occasionally, periureteral diverticula can produce ureteric obstruction by external impingement on the ureter.

Ureteral obstruction also can result from congenital ureteral valves, polyps, a retrocaval position of the ureters, or as a consequence of retroperitoneal fibrosis. All of these are rare.

History

The symptoms associated with urinary tract obstruction depend primarily on the degree and the duration of the blockage. In the neonate the severely obstructed urinary system may be dysplastic at birth. In such circumstances there may be a history of oligohydramnios, inasmuch as fetal urine makes up most of the amniotic fluid volume. In a somewhat less severely obstructed system, fetal urine is produced in large quantities because of the damage to the normal medullary sodium and water reabsorptive mechanisms. In this circumstance there may be a history of polyhydramnios.

In the postnatal period the most common symptoms of children with lesser degrees of obstruction are related to the occurrence of infection. Urinary tract infection in infants can be associated with nonspecific symptoms and signs such as failure to thrive, diarrhea, vomiting, feeding problems, or recurrent fever. Each infant with urinary infection should be examined for urinary obstruction. Occasionally an infant or child with obstruction will come to medical attention because of a voiding abnormality such as a poor urinary stream or polyuria. Others will have gross hematuria, often occurring after only minor trauma. Dilated urinary systems are particularly prone to bleeding after even a slight blow to the abdomen or back. Finally, older children may have been symptom-free until later childhood or adolescence when they are found to have azotemia or are referred for the investigation of enuresis or recurrent urinary tract infection.

Physical Findings

An abdominal mass is the most common finding in infants and children with urinary obstruction. In the neonate, half of all abdominal masses are caused by malformations of the urinary system; approximately 65% of these result from obstruction. Upper tract lesions usually result in a unilateral mass, whereas lower tract obstruction often is associated with three masses—the dilated bladder and both hydronephrotic kidneys. In the child with significant but undiagnosed obstruction, recurrent infection usually is associated with poor nutrition, which affects physical growth. Such children may be of normal length at birth but achieve only gradually decreasing percentiles on the growth chart during the first year. Obstructive uropathy should be included in the differential diagnosis of any child with failure to thrive.

Laboratory Findings

Inasmuch as infection occurs commonly in children with an obstructed urinary system, a positive urine culture is one of the most frequently encountered abnormal laboratory findings. In addition, the subtle finding of isosthenuria or hyposthenuria as a result of damage to the renal medullary concentrating mechanism often is present. Such findings are constant when the obstruction is bilateral but may not be present when the abnormality is unilateral. In addition to obtaining a urine culture, the urine specific gravity or osmolality should be measured in any patient with an undiagnosed fever. A low specific gravity or osmolality in such a child, particularly if dehydration is present, is a clue to urinary tract obstruction or urine infection, or both. Patients with severe obstruction may have some degree of azotemia. In the neonate this may not be evident at birth because the maternal kidney functions for the fetus. Azotemia often will become evident during the first week or two. With more severe degrees of renal failure, other abnormalities, such as hypocalcemia, hyperphosphatemia, and anemia, may occur.

Differential Diagnosis

The differential diagnosis of children with urinary tract obstruction relies primarily on various imaging techniques. In pediatric patients these usually include abdominal ultrasound, voiding cystourethrography, and radionuclide renal scans. These studies should allow the clinician to determine the site of the obstruction, the effect on renal function, and the potential for surgical correction. Direct visualization of the lower urinary system by cystoscopic examination also may be necessary. Occasionally intravenous urographic examination is necessary, although its use in pediatrics has declined considerably with the development of newer imaging techniques. Examination by retrograde ureterography is required only under the most special circumstances and should not be part of the routine workup.

Treatment

The initial management of the child with a newly diagnosed obstruction should be directed toward the aggressive treatment of urinary infection and sepsis and the correction of any abnormalities in hydration and blood chemistry values associated with renal failure. Lower tract obstruction may be relieved by catheterization. Early consultation with a urologist skilled in the care of children with obstructed urinary systems is crucial. The surgical correction of the obstructing lesion will depend on the age and the size of the child, as well as the site and cause of the obstruction. Definitive surgical treatment such as dilation of urethral strictures, fulguration of urethral valves, or pyeloplasty of ureteropelvic junction obstructions may be possible. Children with complex anomalies may need several "staged" corrective surgical procedures. In infants, urinary diversion by vesicostomy or nephrostomy may be the more prudent early approach, with deferral of definitive correction until the child is older and larger. Nonsurgical management by self-catheterization or double voiding often are effective in children with neurogenic conditions of the bladder who have little to gain from surgical approaches.

Prognosis

The prognosis of any particular child is related to the degree and duration of the obstructive lesion, as well as to the number of urinary infections that have occurred. Early diagnosis is the most important aspect in minimizing damage. This may be particularly difficult given the nonspecific nature of symptoms of moderate urinary tract obstruction and infection in the infant. The earlier the diagnosis is made, the better the prognosis. Early diagnosis allows prompt treatment of active infection and consideration for surgical correction, thereby preventing future infections through the provision of good urinary drainage and prophylactic antibiotics. In very severe obstruction, because of the severity of the renal damage at the time of diagnosis, even early diagnosis and treatment may not affectively avert the need for dialysis and transplantation in the future. Prenatal diagnosis of obstruction now provides a means for intervention at birth. Intrauterine corrective surgery has not yet been shown to be practical.

VESICOURETERAL REFLUX

Ureteral reflux is not an obstructive lesion but rather the failure of the normal insertion of the ureter into the bladder that acts as a valve to ensure unidirectional urine flow. This anomaly is diagnosed by the finding of contrast material backflow or radioisotope up the ureter from the bladder during a voiding cystourethrogram. A grading system has been developed based on the contrast cystourethrogram that classifies reflux as being minimal (grade I) to severe (grade V). In the former the contrast rises no higher than the distal third of the ureter; in the latter the contrast completely fills the urinary collecting system and demonstrates hydronephrosis and loss of significant renal parenchyma. Reflux may be unilateral or bilateral. Although the lower grades of reflux of sterile urine probably do not produce parenchymal damage, there is evidence that sterile reflux associated with very high intravesicle pressures may damage the renal cortex. In contrast, reflux of almost any degree associated with concomitant infection produces pyelonephritis, the resolution of which may lead to renal scarring. From 30% to 50% of children with vesicoureteral reflux have renal parenchymal scarring at the time of presentation. Extensive scarring can cause chronic renal failure or hypertension, or both. As many as 45% of siblings also will be found to have vesicoureteral reflux, most of whom will be symptom-free. Therefore it is recommended that all siblings younger than 5 years old be screened, because they compose the group most susceptible to renal scarring with infection.

Ureteral reflux can be either primary or secondary. Primary reflux can be caused by (1) congenital anomalies at the ureterovesical junction, (2) ectopic insertion of the ureter either alone or as part of a duplicated ureter, or (3) associated with other anomalies such as the so-called prune belly syndrome. This syndrome includes bilateral hydroureteronephrosis with reflux, deficient abdominal musculature, and undescended testes.

Secondary ureteral reflux can occur as a result of (1) inflammation at the ureterovesical junction, (2) distal anatomic obstruction, for example, in urethral valves, or (3) distal functional obstruction, such as a neurogenic condition of the bladder. Vesicoureteral reflux associated with inflammation—which occurs, for example, in cystitis—usually is low grade and often resolves with the treatment of the infection. This may take weeks to months, during which time the urinary system is susceptible to reinfection. Such patients should receive prophylactic antibiotics after the initial course of treatment and have routine follow-up urine cultures performed periodically thereafter.

Primary reflux of a lesser degree (grades I through III) can be managed medically by low-dose antibiotic prophylaxis. Approximately 60% to 80% of these patients' vesicoureteral reflux will have resolved on follow-up. Surgical correction more often is necessary for grades IV and V and in the rare patient with a lower grade of reflux who has "break-through" infections despite medical management. Radionuclide cystograms, because of their high level of sensitivity and the low dose of radiation they generate, are particularly useful in follow-up on the resolution or correction of reflux.

SUGGESTED READINGS

Arant BS Jr: Reflux nephropathy, The Kidney 21:19, 1989.

Belman AB and Skoog SJ: Nonsurgical approach to the management of vesicoureteral reflux in children, Pediatr Infect Dis J 8:556, 1989.

Bernstein GT et al: Ureteropelvic junction obstruction in the neonate, J Urol 140:1216, 1988.

Glassberg KI: Current issues regarding posterior urethral valves, Urol Clin North Am 12:175, 1985.

Hulbert WC and Duckett JW: Current views on posterior urethral valves, Pediatr Ann 17:31, 1988.

Kaplan GW and Brock WA: Urethral strictures in children, J Urol 129:1200, 1983.

Reinberg Y and Gonzalea R: Upper urinary tract obstruction in children: current controversies in diagnosis, Pediatr Clin North Am 34:1291, 1987.

Steele BT et al: Follow-up evaluation of prenatally recognized vesicoureteric reflux, J Pediatr 115:95, 1989.

Van den Abbeele A et al: Vesicoureteral reflux in asymptomatic siblings of patients with known reflux: radionuclide cystography, Pediatrics 79:147, 1987.

Warshaw BL et al: Prognostic features in infants with obstructive uropathy due to posterior urethral valves, J Urol 133:240, 1985.

234

Ocular Foreign Bodies

Carl A. Frankel

Considering the diversity of foreign bodies to which we are exposed daily, it is truly amazing that the incidence of foreign bodies lodging in the eye is as low as it is. The likely reasons for this low incidence include the rapidity with which the blink reflex occurs and the copious flushing action that occurs almost immediately after contact with the corneal or conjunctival epithelium. Careful examination, preferably with magnification, is necessary for all but the most superficial ocular foreign bodies, with referral to an ophthalmologist of all patients who present a history of invasion of the eye with explosive or high-velocity objects.

Foreign bodies can be classified as (1) surface, in which case they are either nonadherent or only loosely adherent to the corneal or conjunctival epithelium, (2) penetrating, in which case the foreign body partially enters a layer of the eye, or (3) perforating, in which case a layer of the eye or the globe itself is completely traversed. Although the terminology can be confusing, once it is learned, it allows more accurate description of the problem.

SURFACE FOREIGN BODIES

In children the most likely sources of surface foreign bodies are small objects that can be thrown by a child (e.g., dirt, sand, and grass) and small wind-blown particles. Considering the profuse nature of epiphora (tearing) associated with surface foreign bodies, it is truly the exceptional patient who requires medical care for one of these "flying" objects. In fact, even when care is sought after the acute incident, the offending agent often is absent and the cause of the ocular findings usually is unknown.

When a patient consults a clinician with the complaint of a foreign body sensation—or in a nonverbal or preverbal patient with a history of pain, photophobia, epiphora, or rubbing of the eye(s)—the initial examination usually is accomplished more easily if a drop of topical ophthalmic anesthetic is instilled in each eye (unless a perforated or open globe is suspected, in which case no medications should be used). Then an assessment of visual acuity should be attempted. Once this is completed, the lids and lashes should be inspected to see if any foreign bodies can be observed and removed. Uncooperative or frightened children may need sedation to allow an adequate examination.

Attention next should be turned to the corneal and conjunctival surfaces to ascertain if a foreign body can be identified (Fig. 234-1). At this time, magnification, either with a loupe or a slit lamp, is preferred. It may be possible to irrigate or wipe away readily observed foreign bodies with the stretched-out fibers of a cotton applicator. In a cooperative patient sitting quietly by the slit lamp, manual removal of surface foreign bodies usually can be readily accomplished with a fine, toothless forceps. After this procedure the tarsal conjunctival surfaces should be examined. The clinician usually can pull the lower lid down with one finger placed on the middle aspect of the lid just beneath the lash line and another applying gentle traction inferiorly. Again, foreign bodies generally can be irrigated or brushed out and, if adherent, can be removed with an oblique scraping movement with a spud or 20-gauge needle or forceps. Attention then should be turned to the upper lid, which should be everted as follows: the lashes should be gently grasped between the thumb and forefinger; with the noncotton end of a cotton applicator placed at the superior margin of the tarsal plate, the lashes should be pulled out and up to evert the lid onto the cotton applicator (Fig. 234-2, *A*). After the lid is everted, the lashes can be pinned against the superior orbital rim and the cotton applicator removed (Fig. 234-2, *B*). Any foreign bodies that are present usually can be readily seen and removed.

After the foreign body or bodies have been removed, the eye should be checked for a corneal abrasion. This is best accomplished with a minimal amount of sterile fluorescein instilled and the eye examined with a cobalt blue light (although a pen light may suffice if a blue light is not available). If an abrasion is present (it appears as a green line or patch), an antibiotic ointment should be instilled; if the pain was

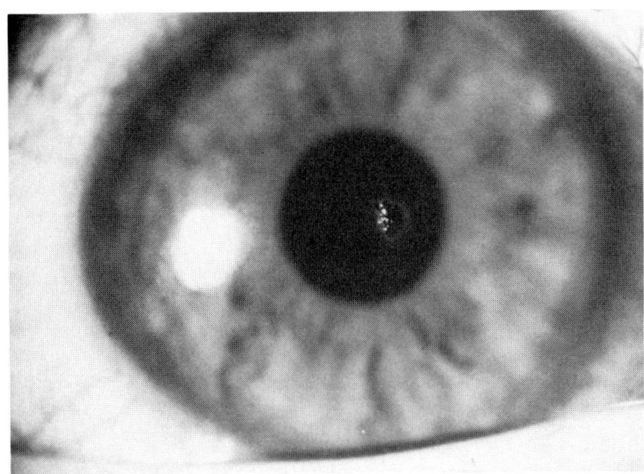

Fig. 234-1 Metallic foreign body on the surface of the cornea. Note the surrounding rust ring, which should be removed to reduce intraocular inflammation from metal breakdown.

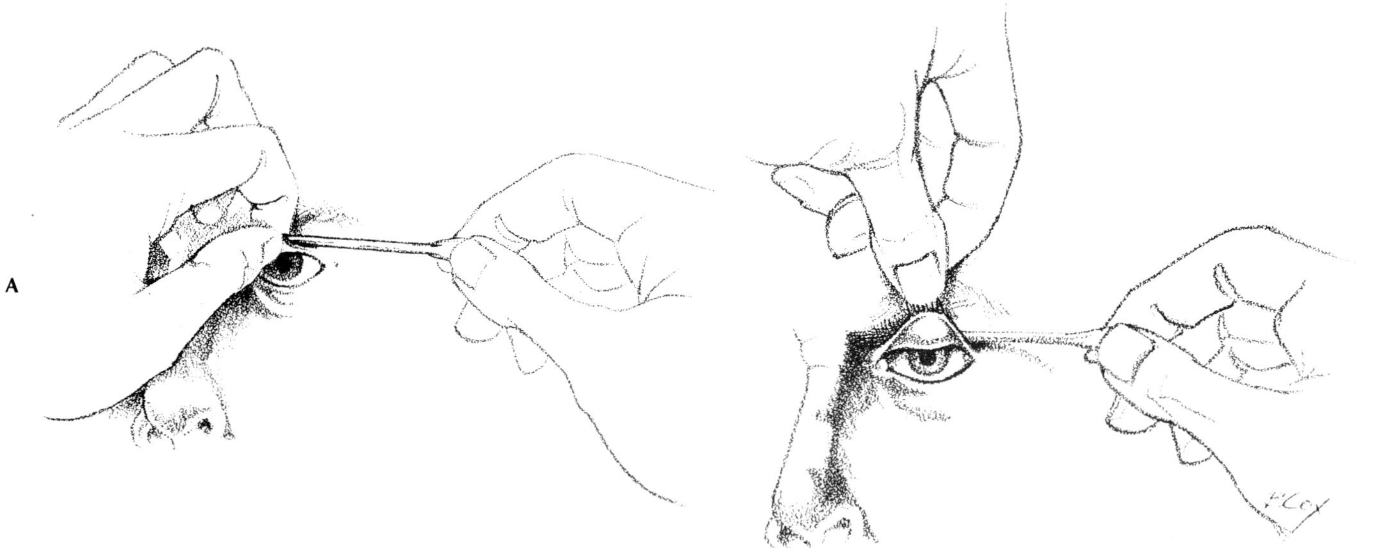

Fig. 234-2 A, Demonstration of an easy method for everting a patient's upper eyelid with the lashes and lid being pulled out and up from the globe. **B,** After the eyelid has been everted, the lashes are pinned against the superior orbital rim prior to removal of the cotton applicator. After the everted lid is examined, the lashes can be pulled inferiorly and released to reposition the lid.

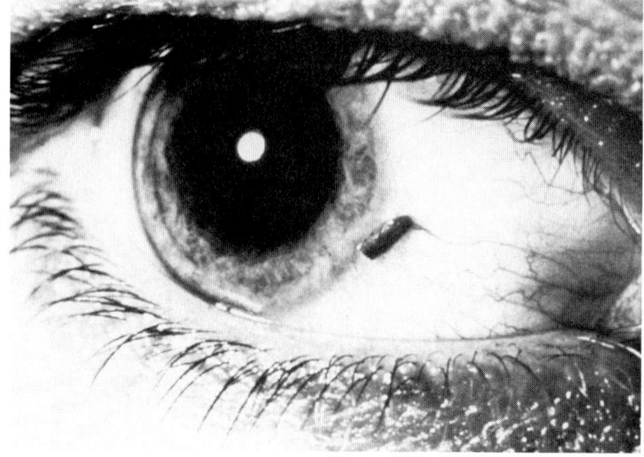

Fig. 234-3 Metallic foreign body that has penetrated the conjunctiva and the underlying sclera. Care must be taken in determining whether this foreign body has actually perforated the sclera and entered the orbit. When in doubt, an ophthalmologist should remove such foreign bodies.

severe before instillation of the anesthetic drops, a sterile eye patch should be taped in place for 6 to 12 hours. Arrangements should then be made for follow-up the next day to ensure that the abrasion has resolved. If it has not, or if significant pain persists, the patient should be referred to an ophthalmologist to be certain that an iritis, which may require more aggressive intervention, has not supervened.

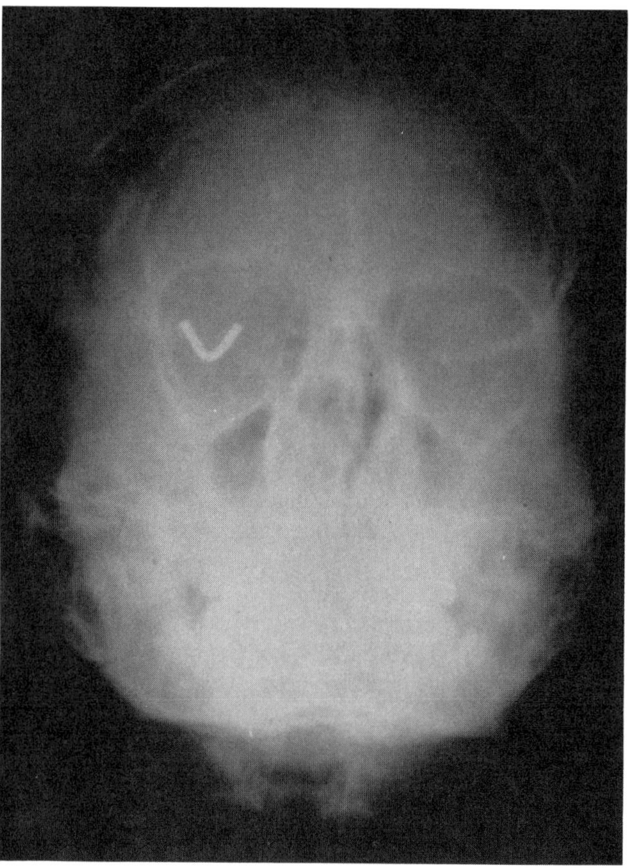

Fig. 234-4 A plain x-ray film of the patient's eye shown in Figure 234-3, showing that the metallic foreign body had penetrated the orbit. Subsequent films taken in varying positions revealed its exact intraorbital position.

PENETRATING FOREIGN BODIES

When a foreign body is imbedded in the conjunctiva, cornea, or scleral tissue (Fig. 234-3), concern must be raised about its removal. Foreign body injuries of low-to-medium velocity usually do not cause significant damage to the eye and typically do not result in derangement of ocular structures or visual loss, unless infection supervenes or corneal scarring occurs in the central visual axis. Whenever a penetrating foreign body is suspected, there should be concern about the possibility of a through-and-through laceration of the cornea or sclera, allowing bacteria to gain access to the intraocular space. In these instances, visual acuity can be surprisingly normal. The examiner therefore must maintain a high index of suspicion and have the patient evaluated by an ophthalmologist.

PERFORATING FOREIGN BODIES

Perforating foreign bodies, the result of high-velocity injuries, usually are devastating to ocular integrity (Fig. 234-4) and frequently result in severe derangement and permanent visual loss, although initial visual acuity and cursory examination findings may be normal. Visual loss can be minimized in some instances by prompt referral to an ophthalmologist skilled at intervention in corneal, anterior segment, and vitreoretinal trauma.

SUMMARY

Fortunately, most ocular foreign bodies are inconsequential, even if painful, when appropriately evaluated and treated. The treatment of most ocular foreign bodies is simple and straightforward and is predicated on identification and removal of all foreign bodies. In any patient in whom the severity of the injury is obvious or if there are questions about the seriousness of the injury, referral to an ophthalmologist is advised.

SUGGESTED READINGS

Augsburger JJ, Goldberg RE, and Magargal LE: Retinal and choroidal vascular abnormalities and fluorescein angiography. In Harley RD, editor: Pediatric ophthalmology, ed 2, Philadelphia, 1983, WB Saunders Co.

Deutsch TA and Feller DB: Paton and Goldberg's management of ocular injuries, ed 2, Philadelphia, 1985, WB Saunders Co.

Simon JW: Trauma to the globe and adnexa: anterior segment trauma. In Harley RD, editor: Pediatric ophthalmology, ed 2, Philadelphia, 1983, WB Saunders Co.

Slusher MM: Trauma to the globe and adnexa: posterior segment trauma. In Harley RD, editor: Pediatric ophthalmology, ed 2, Philadelphia, 1983, WB Saunders Co.

235

Ocular Trauma

Carl A. Frankel

Evaluation of the patient with ocular trauma requires a thorough knowledge of the anatomy of the eye and orbit, as well as an understanding of the types of injuries that may result from specific types of trauma. Although it is unusual, normal or near-normal visual acuity may even be achieved after a rupture of the globe. As a result, a high index of suspicion must be maintained for each patient who is seen for ocular or orbital trauma. In addition, because many children with orbital or ocular injuries are in considerable pain with significant photophobia and fear, the very act of examining or attempting to examine a child's eye can create greater damage than that produced by the original injury. In these cases, sedation should be considered, but because of the time-limited action of sedative agents such as chloral hydrate, an ophthalmologist should be consulted to perform a more thorough evaluation.

ANATOMIC CONSIDERATIONS

The orbit is shaped roughly as a quadrilateral pyramid with walls formed by the frontal bone (superiorly), the zygomatic bone (laterally), the frontal process of the maxilla and frontal bone (medially), and the zygomatic and maxillary bones (inferiorly). The orbital rim tends to absorb the impact of most large-object injuries, which may lead to fractures of the orbital bones with preservation of the integrity of the globe itself. Small-object injuries that have a direct impact on the globe itself tend to cause primary injuries to the globe with secondary injury to the thinner bones of the orbit (i.e., orbital floor and medial wall). Intermediate-sized objects usually have their primary effect on the orbit but also may have a significant effect on the globe. Examples of large objects include soccer balls, softballs, and kickballs, with objects of intermediate size represented by tennis balls, a fist, baseballs, and racquet balls and small objects represented by golf balls, squash balls, small rocks, and the like. Further, the contour of the object can predispose to penetrating or perforating injuries.

EVALUATION

In the evaluation of any child with ocular injury, a careful history should be obtained, realizing that independent or unsupervised play (coupled with guilt and fear) may make the information obtained suspect. As many details as possible should be obtained, specifically highlighting the source of injury, which may suggest the nature of potential injuries. Additional history should include the date of the last tetanus immunization, prior ocular history, medications, allergies, and when the patient last had something to eat or drink (in the event surgical intervention is necessary). After the history has been obtained, with specific regard to symptoms, the examination should then proceed in an orderly manner to ensure that nothing is omitted or overlooked. In a child who is old enough to cooperate, beginning with the nontraumatized eye usually will allay anxiety sufficiently to examine the traumatized eye next. When the traumatized eye is tested, care must be taken not to put any pressure on the globe itself. The examination should begin with testing visual acuity. Although normal visual acuity has been reported in patients with severe injuries, the presence of significantly impaired vision is a sign that the injury is likely to be severe and the services of an ophthalmologist are needed. Appropriate visual acuity charts are invaluable, but even if they are unavailable, a fairly reliable estimate of visual acuity can be obtained by the responses of the traumatized eye compared with those of the other eye. This alternative certainly is preferable to not testing vision at all.

Visual Acuity

Visual function can be measured by use of the following schema, arranged in order of decreasing specificity, in which one eye at a time is tested.

Ability to Identify Objects or Pictures. Depending on the patient's age and ability or willingness to respond, magazine or textbook pictures of common objects such as coins or keys should be presented to the child in an attempt to assess visual acuity. If possible, objects of various sizes should be kept on hand for just such situations.

Recognition of Faces and Facial Features. If a youngster is able to answer specific questions about facial features—such as "Are my eyes open or closed?" or "Do I have a beard?"—valuable information can be obtained. If a child is unable to recognize facial features, the child can be asked to identify the face of someone he or she knows, providing further information about visual function.

Finger Counting. Most children 3 to 4 years of age are able to count fingers; the ability to do so can be correlated with the distance of the presenter's hand from the child. Clearly, the ability to count fingers at 10 feet implies better visual function than the same finger counting at 2 feet. In younger children only one or two fingers should be presented to keep things simple.

Object Motion. The ability to perceive hand motion when illumination is constant indicates the depth of visual impairment. Care should be taken to ensure that the source of illumination is not behind the examiner's hand or else the patient will really be responding to the intermittent shadowing caused by the hand blocking the light source. Again, specifying the distance from the patient is helpful.

Light Perception. The ability to perceive light is a function of the retinal photoreceptors and is less dependent than is a Snellen acuity test on normal clarity of the cornea, anterior chamber, lens, or vitreous. Light perception can be further divided to give some idea of retinal function. The ability to identify two lights separated by a distance is a measure of retinal discrimination and is evidence of better retinal function than not being able to so identify the presence of two lights. Decreasing visual function is evidenced by an inability (1) to identify the direction of light movement, (2) to localize the light, and (3) to be aware of the light's presence.

Although these measures of visual function are less complete and certainly less exact than a Snellen visual acuity test, such assessment of visual function is necessary and need only take about 3 to 4 minutes to perform.

Physical Examination

External Examination. As with the examination of any patient, observation and inspection are important first steps. Key signs to be noted include the presence or absence of edema or ecchymosis of the lids and ocular adnexal structures, proptosis or enophthalmos, the presence of foreign bodies (see Chapter 234), subconjunctival hemorrhage, laceration(s), or the suspected rupture of intraocular contents (including iris, ciliary body, vitreous, and retina). As part of the external examination the site of laceration (such as lid or conjunctiva [not sclera]) and a description of the laceration (including its length and depth), as well as a sketch of its location and course, should be made.

Motility. Motility of the globe should be checked with attention to both ductions (monocular eye movements) and versions (conjugate, binocular eye movements) in all gaze positions, with note made of any abnormalities. The presence of diplopia should be noted, and if possible, the examiner should attempt to obtain a description from the patient of the location of the two images with respect to each other.

Pupils. The presence of round pupils should be noted; if a pupil is not round (Fig. 235-1) (oval, teardrop, or pear shaped, for instance), a drawing of the abnormality should be made. Next, the reactivity of the pupils should be checked, both directly and consensually, looking for an afferent pupillary defect (Marcus Gunn pupil). When this test is performed, the patient should be instructed to fixate on a distant point so that the accommodation reflex (with its secondary pupillary meiosis) does not influence the assessment of pupillary function. The reactivity of the pupils (both direct and consensual) gives important information about both the afferent and efferent limbs of the visual pathway. The absence of an afferent pupillary defect on the *swinging flashlight test* is reassuring confirmation that significant optic nerve and/or retinal damage has not occurred.

A fixed, dilated pupil (no response on direct or consensual testing) indicates damage to the efferent motor limb of the pupillomotor system; it is nonlocalizing in that the site of injury may be anywhere from the Edinger-Westphal nucleus (in the brain stem, rostral to the superior colliculus) to the iris. The afferent limb of the visual system may be normal, however; visual function would likewise be expected to be normal. If the consensual reflex is normal, but the direct reflex is reduced on the swinging flashlight test, presumptive evidence of damage to the optic nerve and/or retina is present, implying a worrisome or grave visual prognosis. An extreme example of this occurs in the amaurotic (blind) pupil in which the pupil is totally unresponsive on direct testing but a normal consensual reflex exists. In the event of posttraumatic iridoplegia, both the direct and consensual reflexes would be diminished because of impairment in the terminal efferent pupillomotor organ (iris).

Anterior Segment. If a slit lamp is available (assuming the examiner is skilled in its use) and if the patient is able, the conjunctiva, cornea, anterior chamber, iris, lens, and red reflex should be examined. Particular attention should be directed to evaluation of (1) the conjunctiva, for subconjunctival (*not* scleral) hemorrhage, conjunctival lacerations, or foreign bodies, (2) the cornea, for the presence of epithelial defects (abrasions), lacerations, or foreign bodies, (3) the anterior chamber, for depth (shallow or deep) or the presence of red blood cells (hyphema), (4) the lens, for the presence of cataract or dislocation (Fig. 235-2), and (5) the retrolenticular red reflex, the absence of which might indicate a vitreous hemorrhage or retinal detachment. If a slit lamp is unavailable, if the examiner is uncomfortable with its use, or if the patient cannot be brought to the slit lamp, then the direct ophthalmoscope can be used to perform an adequate anterior segment examination.

Fundus. A fundus *examination always should be attempted except if a ruptured globe is suspected* and pressure may have to be placed on the eye to open the lids. In those circumstances, increased pressure on the globe (externally applied) would be expected to result in extrusion of intraocular contents, potentially making it impossible to restore the integrity of the visual system. In case of doubt, the examination should be delayed until the arrival of an ophthalmologist.

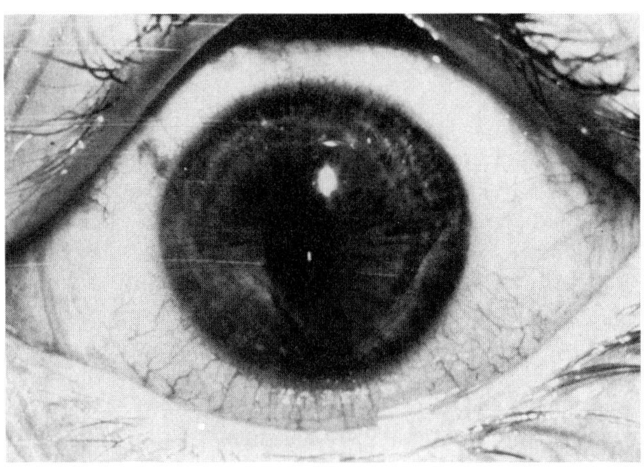

Fig. 235-1 Photograph showing an inverted tear-drop-shaped pupil due to an inferior corneal laceration with the iris drawn to the wound.

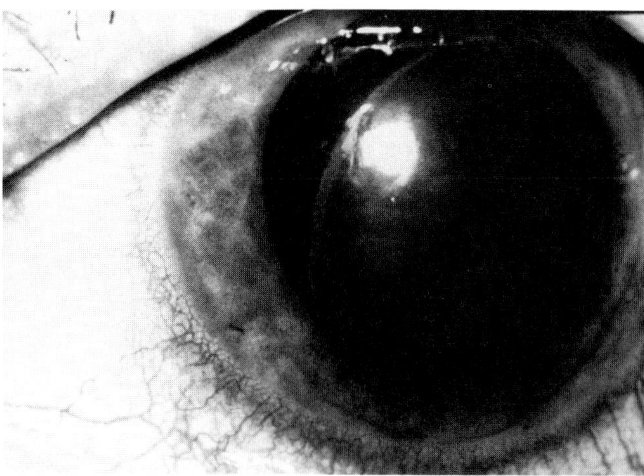

Fig. 235-2 Ocular injury from a fist with inferior lens subluxation and minimal cataractous changes.

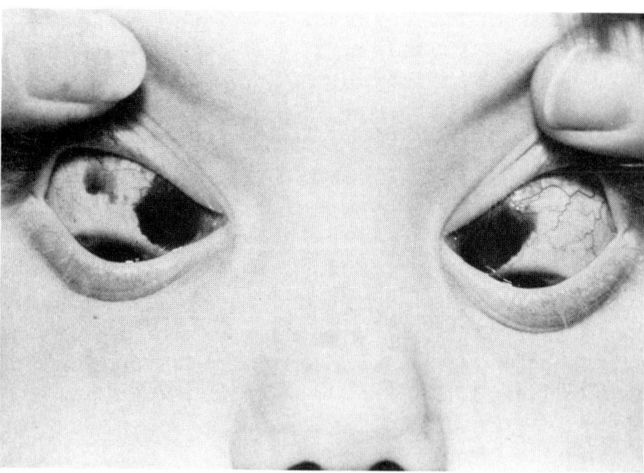

Fig. 235-3 Bilateral subconjunctival hemorrhages after prolonged sneezing.

SPECIFIC INJURIES

It must be kept in mind that just as there is a continuum in the orbital relationships, so too is there a continuum in the extent of orbital and ocular injuries. The result of this is that *when one portion of the orbit or globe is injured, further injury may be present.*

Ecchymosis

Ecchymosis, or bruising, of the periorbital region results in the typical "black" eye. The blunt contusion injury that results in ecchymosis may be either isolated or associated with other orbital and/or ocular injury. An uncomplicated black eye is treated as a contusion anywhere else: cold compresses for the first 24 hours, followed by warm compresses until the swelling subsides, with elevation of the patient's head to help resolve the edema. The patient or parents should be advised that because of gravity, the ecchymosis and edema may appear to spread down the cheek or even to the fellow eye. Although frightening in appearance, this type of spread is not dangerous and resolves spontaneously.

Orbital Hemorrhage

When a contusion injury occurs, ecchymosis of the periorbital region may occur simultaneously with hemorrhage within the orbit itself (orbital hemorrhage). Because the orbit is a bony structure open on only one end, an increase in volume of the orbital contents (as would occur in orbital hemorrhage or orbital edema) increases the intraorbital pressure, which can be relieved only with anterior displacement of the globe, resulting in *proptosis*. If the proptosis is severe, compression of the optic nerve and/or acute glaucoma can permanently impair visual function. If progressive proptosis is noted, emergency lateral canthotomy (and possible orbital decompression) is indicated, inasmuch as time is the worst enemy. Steroids often are used, but their effectiveness has not been demonstrated. In the absence of signs of optic nerve compromise, treatment consists of ice packs for the first 24 hours, followed by warm compresses, with elevation of the head to reduce edema.

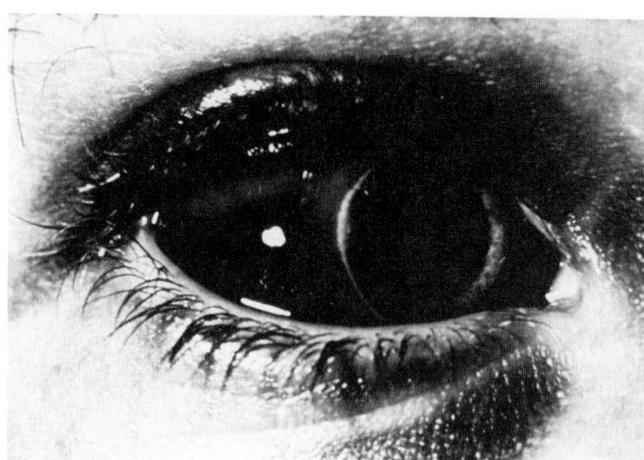

Fig. 235-4 Severe subconjunctival hemorrhage after blunt trauma.

Conjunctival Injury

Conjunctival injury typically manifests with only mild to moderate pain because of the relative paucity of a sensory nerve supply. Most conjunctival injuries take the form of a subconjunctival hemorrhage (Fig. 235-3), which can be quite frightening but actually is harmless, unless associated with more extensive ocular injuries. Because of the potential space between the clear conjunctiva and the underlying white Tenon capsule, a small amount of blood will diffuse over a large area, much as a drop of blood on a microscope slide does when a coverslip is positioned: the effect is very dramatic and causes concern to the uninitiated (Fig. 235-4). No treatment is necessary for isolated subconjunctival hemorrhages, although the patient or parents should be cautioned that a brownish discoloration may result (caused by absorption of hemosiderin).

Small isolated conjunctival lacerations do not require intervention, although a thorough ophthalmic examination must be performed to rule out a laceration of the underlying sclera, choroid, or retina.

Conjunctival *acid or alkali injuries are emergencies* that require copious irrigation as soon as possible. Further details on acid and alkali injuries can be found in the next section on corneal injuries.

Corneal Injuries

The corneal epithelium is a multilayered structure (five cells thick) that rests on a tough basement membrane layer (Bowman membrane). The corneal epithelium is laced with numerous fine sensory nerve endings, resulting in exquisite pain when the epithelium is disrupted. This epithelial disruption is easily observed with the use of a cobalt blue light after the instillation of sterile fluorescein. Fortunately, most corneal abrasions (characterized by injury to all or part of the five-cell layer without encroachment on Bowman membrane) heal extremely rapidly. In the absence of infection, most corneal abrasions (even if quite extensive) tend to heal within 12 to 24 hours, with the most extensive abrasions usually healed by 48 hours after injury.

The initial phase of healing is characterized by migration of the remaining corneal epithelial cells over the defect, with subsequent reestablishment of the normal cell-to-cell and cell-to–basement membrane adhesions over a period of several weeks to months. In extensive corneal abrasions in which no corneal epithelium remains, conjunctival cells migrate over the corneal surface and then undergo transdifferentiation to become, eventually, indistinguishable from normal corneal epithelium.

During the healing phase, a tight patch after instillation of an ophthalmic antibiotic ointment may allow the patient to experience only a mild foreign-body sensation that typically resolves after the epithelial surface of the abraded area has been restored. Typically, the period of time that the eye is patched is 12 to 24 hours; in young children the occlusion may be more distressing than the injury itself. Should the abrasion not be substantially healed by 24 hours after injury, referral to an ophthalmologist should be made to rule out infection or other reasons for nonhealing.

In extremely young children and infants the plasticity of the visual system should be kept in mind so that occlusion amblyopia (poor vision in the eye under the patch because of visual deprivation) does not ensue: the *susceptibility to the development of occlusion amblyopia is inversely proportional to the patient's age*. In addition, as a result of impairment of the fusion mechanism, a latent deviation of an eye (typically an esophoria or exophoria (see Chapter 166) may convert to a manifest deviation (either an esotropia or an exotropia, respectively) because of patching of an injured eye for as short a period as 1 to 2 days. Surgical intervention may be necessary to restore the ocular alignment.

Under no circumstances should any patient be discharged from the office or emergency room while still affected by topical anesthesia. These agents are to be used only in an acute setting for the diagnosis of ocular disorders or in an attempt to relieve patient discomfort for examination or for brief procedures.

Corneal lacerations (either full or partial thickness), no matter how well approximated, require immediate referral to an ophthalmologist. Patients with corneal lacerations should have the eye covered with a shield to reduce the likelihood of prolapse of the intraocular contents. If a shield is unavailable, the bottom of a cup can be taped to the skin (Fig. 235-5) to prevent pressure on the globe.

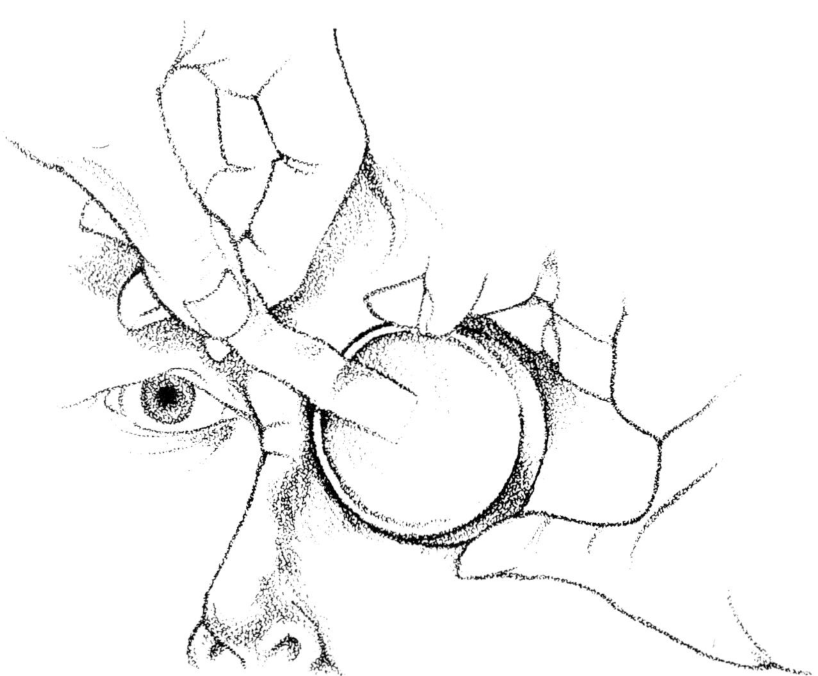

Fig. 235-5 Taping the bottom of a cup to the skin when a shield is not available to protect a suspected open globe from externally applied pressure.

Chemical injuries, with either acid or alkali, are acute emergencies that require copious irrigation, with notification of an ophthalmologist if any corneal or conjunctival damage is indicated. If the patient does not complain of discomfort, the sensory nerves have been severely burned, as in a severe thermal injury. If the patient complains of pain, instillation of a topical anesthetic will reduce the discomfort from the injury and the irrigation itself. If blepharospasm is a problem, a lid speculum should be used to keep the eye open. Overirrigation is not a problem, although the use of pH indicator paper can serve to show when the offending solution has been neutralized.

Hyphema

In blunt trauma to the globe, the shearing forces transmitted to the intraocular structures by the noncompressible fluid contents of the globe may result in avulsion of the blood vessels at the iris root or the face of the ciliary body. When this happens, grossly visible blood enters the anterior chamber of the eye and a hyphema is formed (Fig. 235-6). When a hyphema occurs, the patient requires the care of an ophthalmologist because of potential associated complications. The purpose of this section is to provide guidelines for initial management.

With the presence of a hyphema, some physicians dilate the patient's pupil in an attempt to relax the ciliary body and decrease the likelihood of traction on the injured blood vessels, which occurs with normal pupillary meiosis and mydriasis. In addition, an iritis often develops, and most patients are more comfortable with cycloplegia, because ciliary spasm is prevented. If dilation is to be used, phenylephrine should be avoided because of its action on active contraction of the dilator muscle, possibly increasing traction on the injured vessel(s) and increasing the likelihood of rebleeding. Accordingly, a long-acting mydriatic-cycloplegic agent (such as atropine 0.5% ophthalmic solution) may be used for at least 5 to 6 days. The anticholinergic action of atropine on the constrictor is believed to create passive pupillary dilation, while its action on the ciliary body results in cycloplegia (paralysis of the ciliary body). It should be kept in mind that the use of atropine is by no means widely accepted, and some have reported acute rebleeding associated with its use.

If the hyphema is small and the patient/family are reliable, home management usually is successful; however, for significant hyphemas (greater than one third of the anterior chamber) or if keeping the patient quiet is not possible at home, hospitalization is justified. In uncomplicated hyphemas, management consists of observation for 5 to 6 days, because of the possibility of a rebleed (typically between the third and fifth day as a result of clot resorption). Sedation may be necessary to reduce any agitation, although the hyphema itself tends to have a sedative effect on patients (by an unknown mechanism). Neither unilateral nor bilateral patching is indicated. A hard shield should be taped in place to reduce the likelihood of additional trauma that could precipitate a rebleeding episode. A shield with holes in it should be used so that the patient can use the eye in an attempt to maintain binocular vision.

Because of the violent nature of the saccadic (voluntary) eye movements used for reading and other near activities, near-vision activities should be avoided during the critical 5-day period, in an attempt to reduce the likelihood of an acute rebleeding episode. Distance viewing and television watching are acceptable inasmuch as they allow more stable ocular positioning with fewer saccadic eye movements.

Because of the possibility of rebleeding due to clot resorption, some ophthalmologists use epsilon-aminocaproic acid in an attempt to slow clot resorption, although its use is contraindicated in very large hyphemas (greater than 75% of the anterior chamber). If this antifibrinolytic agent is used, it is continued through at least the sixth postinjury day, if bleeding has not recurred. Although this agent has been shown to reduce the incidence of rebleeding significantly, gastrointestinal side effects (including nausea and vomiting) may prompt some to hold off on its use, except in high-risk situations in which the patient cannot be maintained in a state of quiet. It should be kept in mind that the visual prognosis after acute rebleeding episodes is quite guarded. Most hyphemas are associated with a moderate to severe iritis, so that

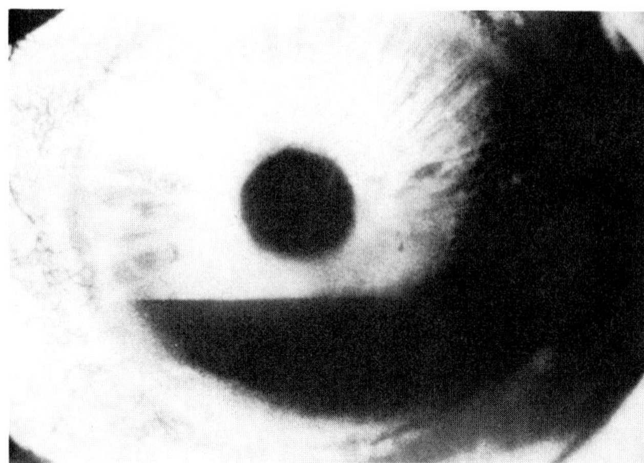

Fig. 235-6 Acute hyphema secondary to blunt ocular injury. Acute glaucoma ensued, which resolved when the hyphema cleared.

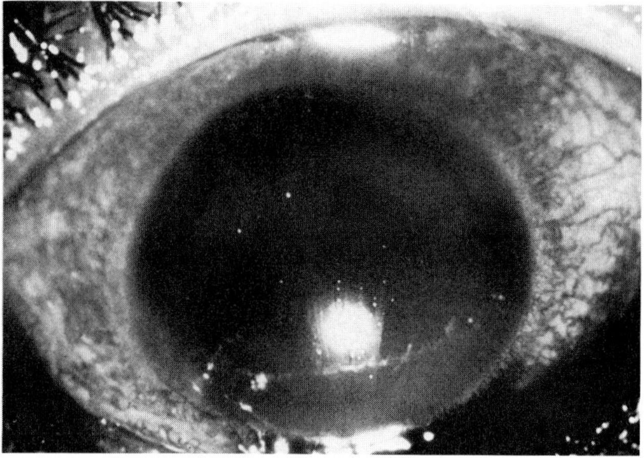

Fig. 235-7 Corneal blood staining following a hyphema in which secondary glaucoma was unable to be controlled.

some ophthalmologists recommend topical or systemic corticosteroids to reduce the inflammatory response and possibly to reduce the incidence of rebleeding.

Secondary glaucoma may result from one of two mechanisms, either of which can result in corneal blood staining (Fig. 235-7), which can severely limit vision and result in deprivation amblyopia in young children (typically younger than 8 years of age). The first mechanism is through damage to the filtration angle that does not resolve with clearing of the hyphema, typically requiring either medical and/or surgical intervention to prevent glaucomatous optic atrophy and visual loss. The second mechanism is due to obstruction of the filtration angle from the red blood cells and usually resolves after the blood is totally absorbed, although emergency medical management may be indicated. Patients with sickle cell anemia or trait are at much higher risk for these complications and need earlier intervention. Any patient with a hyphema needs daily (and sometimes twice daily) intraocular pressure checks to detect the presence of glaucoma in an attempt to reduce the likelihood of permanent visual loss.

Associated injuries with hyphema frequently include lens subluxation and choroidal rupture (Fig. 235-8) or retinal rupture, the latter two of which may result in permanent visual impairment without rupture of the sclera. With severe trauma a ruptured globe also may occur.

Blow-out Fracture

When a broad concussive force is delivered to the orbit in a manner that rapidly increases the intraorbital pressure above a critical amount, one or more of the orbital bones may explode because of the relative incompressibility of the orbital contents. The orbital floor is the most common site for a blow-out fracture, with the medial orbital wall the next most common.

These injuries are seen more commonly in adolescents than in younger children and frequently result from motor vehicle accidents or a blow from a fist; as most people are right-handed, the left orbit is involved more often than the right. The patient frequently complains of diplopia and pain, with clinical signs of proptosis (if orbital hemorrhage occurs) or enophthalmos if the fracture is large, limitation of movement of the affected eye (typically limitation of upgaze because of inferior rectus muscle entrapment in the fracture), lid edema, and ecchymosis.

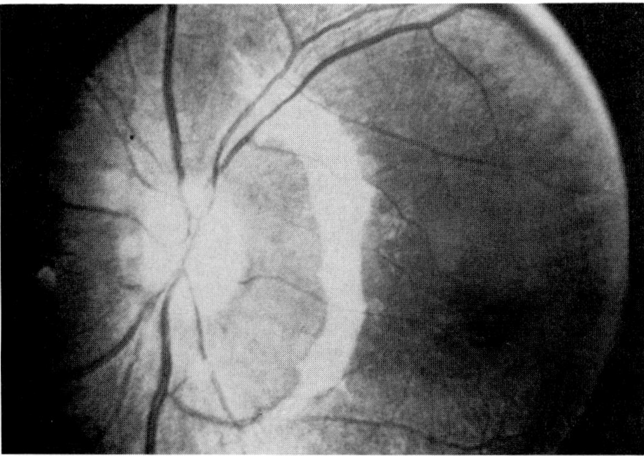

Fig. 235-8 Choroidal rupture following blunt injury to the globe. The overlying retinal vessels are intact but note the crescent-shaped area due to absence of choroid overlying the white sclera. The typical location for choroidal and retinal ruptures is between the macula and optic nerve.

The evaluation of a patient with a suspected blow-out fracture requires the use of orbital computed tomography (CT) scanning to delineate the presence and extent of the fracture most accurately. Appropriate positioning of the patient with 3 to 4 ml slices and adjacent sections is necessary for accurate imaging.

Because of the nature of the orbital injury, the possibility of a coexisting injury to the globe must be considered, and ophthalmologic evaluation should be performed before any other specialist is consulted. The concurrent presence of a ruptured globe and blow-out fracture requires delayed treatment of the fracture until the integrity of the globe is restored.

Treatment of blow-out fractures is not emergent. Indeed, allowing the edema and ecchymosis to resolve may lead to resolution of proptosis and diplopia. Frequently, diplopia is due to a muscle contusion, and the symptoms may resolve over 3 to 4 days. If surgical intervention need be undertaken for entrapment of orbital contents and diplopia, it can safely be performed 5 to 7 days after the injury. Enophthalmos alone is insufficient reason for surgical intervention, inasmuch as the results of surgical intervention for enophthalmos have not been shown to be particularly successful and intractable diplopia may result from orbital and ocular manipulation. Patients with an orbital blow-out fracture should be managed by, or co-managed with, an ophthalmologist (preferably an ophthalmic plastic surgeon). Under no circumstances should an orbital blow-out fracture be repaired by a nonophthalmologic practitioner without prior evaluation by an ophthalmologist.

When surgical intervention is indicated, the goal is to restore the anatomic location of prolapsed orbital contents. On occasion, an artificial floor needs to be created with the use of implanted material.

Ruptured Globe

If a ruptured globe is a possibility (and one must always be suspicious of its occurrence), early involvement of an ophthalmologist is essential. Patients with a ruptured globe may have surprisingly normal vision (extremely unusual), although telltale signs include hemorrhage with chemosis, a shallow anterior chamber, and a low intraocular pressure (0 to 10 mm Hg), although the intraocular pressure should not be measured if a ruptured globe is suspected. Prolapsed intraocular tissue (lens, iris, ciliary body, retina, choroid, or vitreous) may be seen if the rupture occurs at the limbus or if the injury perforates the conjunctiva. In addition, the anterior chamber structures typically are distorted, with a hyphema frequently present. If the site of rupture is beneath an extraocular muscle or posterior to it, few overt signs may be present. The amount of anterior segment derangement may be remarkably small if the globe is penetrated with a sharp object.

A ruptured globe is an acute emergency that requires the

services of an ophthalmologist. In the time before the ophthalmologist's arrival, the patient should be treated as follows:

1. Be kept quiet with sedation as needed
2. Not lie on the injured side
3. Have a shield placed over the orbit to reduce the likelihood of further injury
4. Have nothing to eat or drink in anticipation of the need for general anesthesia
5. Have *no* eye drops or ointments instilled until the globe is repaired
6. Probably receive parenteral antibiotics in an attempt to reduce the likelihood of an endophthalmitis

Lid Lacerations

Lid lacerations and avulsion injuries typically occur without significant injury to the globe; however, suspicion is always warranted. In any situation in which ocular injury is suspected or cannot be ruled out, the ophthalmologist should be contacted before any attempt to repair the laceration is undertaken: a ruptured globe either missed altogether or not detected until after a lacerated lid has been repaired is indefensible.

Simple lid lacerations that do not involve the lid margin, orbicularis muscle, or other structures (such as the medial or lateral canthal tendon, the levator palpebrae superioris muscle, or the lacrimal gland and ducts) can be readily repaired with local anesthesia and the use of a size 6-0 to 7-0 suture, which usually is removed 5 to 7 days after injury. If the lid laceration involves deeper orbital structures or the lid margin (Fig. 235-9), an ophthalmologist should be consulted to assess the integrity of the eye and to repair the lacerations. It is not acceptable for a physician who is not an ophthalmologist to repair the laceration and to notify an ophthalmologist as an afterthought.

Nonaccidental Trauma (Child Abuse)

The ocular manifestations of child abuse are diverse and can encompass any type of ocular trauma; the explanation of the

Ocular Manifestations of Child Abuse

Cataracts
Cigarette burns (lids, cornea, conjunctiva)
Cyanoacrylate tarsorraphy
Esotropia
Intraocular hemorrhages (any type)
Nystagmus
Optic atrophy
Papilledema
Periorbital ecchymosis
Periorbital edema
Retinal detachment
Retrobulbar hemorrhage
Subconjunctival hemorrhage
Subluxated lens

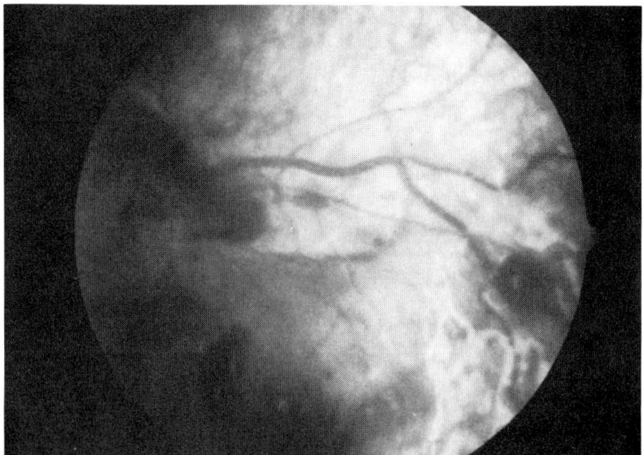

Fig. 235-10 Fundus photograph showing retinal hemorrhages in a victim of the "shaken baby syndrome."

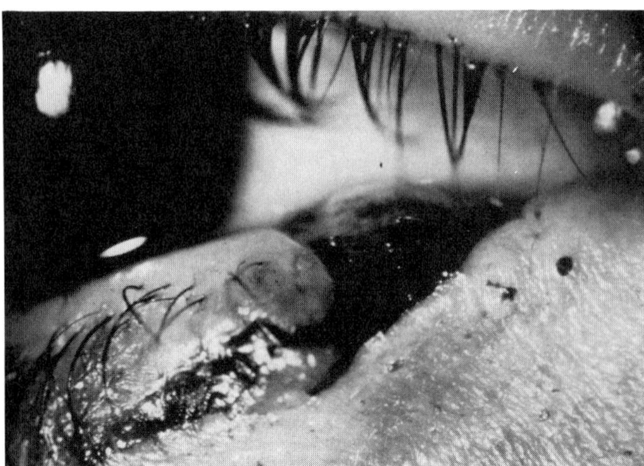

Fig. 235-9 Laceration of the lower lid that was found to involve the inferior canaliculus. Oculoplastic surgical repair was undertaken to restore the function of the inferior tear collection system.

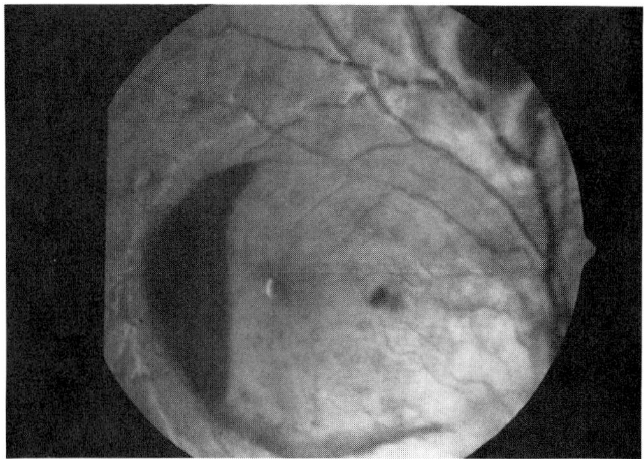

Fig. 235-11 Fundus photograph of the same patient shown in Figure 235-3 with pre-retinal hemorrhage. The patient was lying on his side, hence the orientation of the pooled blood.

injury often is either inappropriate or insufficient. In addition, the ocular manifestations of child abuse may not be readily observable (see the accompanying box). Perhaps the most important (because of its impact on child development) and most often missed (because of its frequent lack of external signs of injury) type of child abuse is the whiplash *shaken baby syndrome,* characterized by intraocular hemorrhages (usually retinal) (Figs. 235-10 and 235-11), subdural or subarachnoid hemorrhages, and minimal or absent signs of external trauma. A patient with these signs needs to have a complete systemic evaluation, preferably by an ophthalmologist familiar with the ocular manifestations of child abuse.

In any case of suspected child abuse, the opthalmologist should be involved to document and treat ocular injuries as appropriate and to assist in any investigation to locate and prosecute the perpetrator(s). It is only through the vigilance of the primary physician and the maintenance of a high index of suspicion that child abuse may be diagnosed.

SUMMARY

Most ocular injuries are relatively minor and easily treatable without sequelae. The circumstances surrounding some trauma, however, increase the likelihood of significant ocular or orbital injury. When such significant injury can be ruled out, involvement of the ophthalmologist may not be necessary. However, in any situation in which the primary examiner cannot readily determine the structural integrity of the globe, an ophthalmologist should be consulted.

SUGGESTED READINGS

Agapitos PJ, Noel LP, and Clarke WN: Traumatic hyphema in children, Ophthalmology 94:1238, 1984.

Caffey J: On the theory and practice of shaking infants: its potential residual effects of permanent brain damage and mental retardation, Am J Dis Child 124:151, 1972.

Deutsch TA and Feller DB: Paton and Goldberg's management of ocular injuries, ed 2, Philadelphia, 1985, WB Saunders Co.

Friendly DS: Ocular aspects of physical child abuse. In Harley RD, editor: Pediatric ophthalmology, ed 2, Philadelphia, 1983, WB Saunders Co.

Kraft SP et al: Traumatic hyphema in children, Ophthalmology 94:1238, 1984.

Nelson LB and Parlats CJ: Systemic and ophthalmic manifestations of child abuse. In Duane TD, editor: Clinical ophthalmology, Philadelphia, 1989, JB Lippincott Co.

Newell FW: Ophthalmology: principles and concepts, ed 6, St Louis, 1986, The CV Mosby Co.

Smith B and Lisman RD: Blow-out fractures of the orbit. In Harley RD, editor: Pediatric ophthalmology, ed 2, Philadelphia, 1983, WB Saunders Co.

236

Osteochondroses

Edward M. Sills

The ossification centers of growing bones may develop irregular mineralization during childhood. Varying degrees of discomfort and dysfunction ensue associated with varying degrees of deformity. In this group of osteochondroses (Table 236-1), the disorders occur in bones preformed in cartilage and ossified from a central nucleus of ossification. Careful study has revealed that the generally assumed causes of interruption of blood supply to the affected areas, damage to cartilage, and inflammation are likely inaccurate. The exact causal agents and mechanisms are not known. Excessive mechanical endogenous stress appears to play an important role in each of the disorders, and the degree of deformity and disability depends on the duration and degree of the stress to which the softened fibrous parts are subjected. The disorders that result from these alterations have been referred to as juvenile osteochondroses. Since damage to cartilage is not an instigating factor in these disorders, the root *chondro* is inaccurate.

The more commonly involved areas of clinical significance include the femoral head, tibial tuberosity, tibial shaft, tarsal navicular, metatarsal heads, carpal semilunar, and lower thoracic vertebral epiphyses.

FEMORAL HEAD

Two distinctly different affections of the hip joint that occur in childhood involve damage to the femoral head. In Legg-Calvé-Perthes disease, the blood supply to the ossification center of the femoral head is interrupted, resulting in aseptic necrosis of the center. The femoral head, neck, and acetabulum become deformed and, in time, extensively reconstructed. The basis of treatment is to encourage the regaining of a spherical femoral head and to prevent irregular contour, flattening, or mushrooming of the head; shortening and broadening of the neck; and flattening of the vertical wall of the acetabulum. If these occur, the patient will develop osteoarthritis at an early age. In the second common disorder, slipped capital femoral epiphysis, the femoral head begins to slip gradually off the femoral neck, disrupting the epiphyseal cartilage plate. In this disorder, treatment is directed at immediately restoring normal anatomic relationships and preventing further slippage.

Legg-Calvé-Perthes Disease

Legg-Calvé-Perthes disease has its onset in the early school-age years and occurs in boys four times more frequently than in girls. In the vast majority of instances the disorder is unilateral. In those rare instances (less than 10%) when both hip joints are involved, the two joints are involved successively rather than simultaneously.

The earliest sign is an intermittent limp, noticed especially after exertion. This limp may be associated with hip and ipsilateral knee pain. The quadriceps muscles and adjacent thigh soft tissues atrophy, and the hip may develop adduction flexion contracture. The child will experience discomfort in

Table 236-1 *Osteochondroses*

SITE	PEAK AGE OF APPEARANCE (YEARS)
Upper extremity	
Humeral head	2-8
Humeral capitulum	4-10
Lower ulna	13-20
Carpal navicular	16-24
Carpal semilunar	16-20
Bilateral entire carpus	10-14
Metacarpal heads	9-15
Basal phalanges	8-14
Lower extremity	
Femoral epiphysis slippage	9-16*
Femoral epiphysis	3-12†
Greater trochanter	6-11
Primary patellar center	8-15
Secondary patellar center	8-10
Shaft of tibia	1.5‡
	6-12§
Tibial tubercle	10-15
Distal tibial epiphysis	4
Calcaneal epiphysis	3-18
Astragalus	2-8
Tarsal navicular	3-7
Second metatarsal	8-17
Fifth metatarsal	8-16
Spine and pelvis	
Vertebral epiphysis	13-20
Vertebral disk	Over 16
Vertebral body	
Eosinophilic granuloma (?)	2-11
Symphysis pubis	12-18
Iliac crest	12-19
Ischial apophysis	13-18
Ischiopubic synchondrosis	12-19

*Girls are younger.
†Maximum is 6-8 yr.
‡Infantile form.
§Adolescent form.

the hip or knee when attempts are made to internally rotate the hip. Associated muscle spasm that anchors the hip to slight external rotation may cause distal thigh or knee tenderness. A roentgenogram taken early in the course of the disease will show widening of the hip joint and, occasionally, metaphyseal demineralization. This "acute phase" generally lasts for a week or two and is followed by the "active phase," which can last for 12 to 40 months, during which time there are no clinical signs or symptoms; however, the process of reparative revascularization causes an increased radiodensity in the femoral head ossification center (seen on roentgenograms), caused by resorption of dead trabecular bone. During this remolding phase, orthopedic care should be directed to maintaining the femoral head abducted and internally rotated in relation to the acetabulum. Use of orthotic devices or surgical approaches can accomplish this goal.

Slipped Capital Femoral Epiphysis

A slipped capital femoral epiphysis causes hip and leg pain in early adolescence, at slightly younger ages in girls than in boys. The sex incidence is nearly equal, with some studies indicating a slight male preponderance. There is a greater prevalence of tall, overweight youngsters among those with this condition than among the general population of young teenagers. About 75% of cases are unilateral, and the left side is more often involved.

Hip pain is the initial complaint, often referred to the thigh or knee in association with a gait that is assumed to protect the hips. In the early "preslipping stage," the pain often commences following a strain or minor injury. There is a sense of tiredness or mild pain in the hip or knee, with mild limping or loss of mobility. The "preslipping stage" is followed by an "acute slip," with sudden acute pain, pronounced limitation of mobility, and difficulty bearing weight on the affected leg. On examination, the hip is externally rotated, with limited internal rotation and flexion. Earliest roentgenographic abnormalities are seen on a lateral view, with dorsal displacement of the capital epiphysis and widening of the zone of radiolucency between the femoral head and neck. If untreated, there will be further posterior and medial slippage. The hip must be placed in Russell traction and surgically pinned. Manipulation of the hip joint in an attempt at closed reduction may aggravate the slipping and should be avoided. The earlier the slippage is treated and the less the amount of unnecessary manipulation, the greater the likelihood that osteoarthritis can be avoided.

TIBIAL TUBEROSITY

Osgood-Schlatter disease results from avulsion of part of the patellar ligament and attached bony and cartilaginous fragments from the tuberosity. Its incidence is higher in boys, but the age of onset is earlier in girls, since ossification of the tibial tuberosity occurs earlier in females. About 25% of cases have bilateral involvement.

The child's complaint is that of local pain and tenderness in the region of the knee, particularly the tuberosity. The pain is most severe at the end of active flexion or extension of the knee. If the condition has been present for several months, the tuberosity is enlarged, and on its anterior aspect one may find a bony prominence. The roentgenographic changes vary, depending on the size of the avulsed fragments, cartilage, and bone and on the duration of the condition. The best view is one with the knee rotated inward, giving a tangential view of the tibial tuberosity. One sees soft tissue swelling, an opaque patellar ligament, and a fragmented tuberosity. Treatment is directed at decreasing the stress on the tubercle until there is bony fusion of the tuberosity with the tibial metaphysis. This occurs at about 15 years of age in girls and 17 years in boys. Depending on the degree of pain, strenuous activities involving deep knee bending and jumping may have to be restricted, or casting to immobilize the knee totally may be required. The former approach is usually sufficient.

TIBIAL SHAFT

Infants usually have some leg bowing until 18 months of age, after which time the legs straighten and then progress to a slight degree of knock-knee. Bowing of the legs that persists or progresses beyond 2 years of age should be evaluated. The differential diagnosis lies between tibia vara (Blount disease) and renal or nutritional rickets. In Blount disease, cartilage has failed to transform to bone at the medial aspect of the epiphysis. The metaphysis beneath the epiphyseal ossification center becomes demineralized, and the medial aspect of the proximal tibia fails to grow as rapidly as the lateral aspect, resulting in a bowleg deformity. In rickets, calcification and growth of the epiphyseal cartilage of the long bones are suppressed, their metaphyses become softened, and they flare at both ends with resultant bowing. Appropriate treatment with vitamin D will produce roentgenographic evidence of healing within a few weeks and eventual straightening of the bones. Most children with Blount disease that persists beyond 6 years of age require an osteotomy for correction of the bowing.

TARSAL NAVICULAR

Köhler disease of the tarsal navicular bone results from an interruption of the blood supply to the developing navicular bone, causing necrosis of its ossification center. The navicular is in a crucial position in the arch of the foot; thus symptoms can be alarming. The condition is self-limited, and the ossification center becomes revascularized and completely reconstructed. The disorder is seen primarily in boys between 3 and 7 years of age, but predominantly in the younger children.

Pain is localized to the inner aspect of the midtarsal part of the foot. The foot is held in a slight varus position, and the child walks on the outer side of the foot or flat-footedly. The skin over the navicular may be warm, red, and swollen, and palpation of the bone elicits tenderness. Lateral roentgenograms of the feet show a very narrowed, waferlike, irregular navicular ossification center, with increased radiopacity and loss of trabecular markings. The process of revascularization and reconstruction takes from 1 to 3 years. Treatment is primarily directed to reassuring the child and family. Various orthotic pads can be used to absorb weight and pressure forces until the healing occurs. Surgical intervention is to be avoided.

METATARSAL HEADS

Freiberg disease is a condition in which a part of the head of a metatarsal bone undergoes aseptic necrosis and becomes sufficiently weakened to be susceptible to functional trauma (running, jumping), which may cause compressional collapse of the metatarsal head. The second metatarsal bone is most often involved; the third metatarsal bone is the next most likely to be so. Females are affected more often than males.

Pain occurs in the region of the affected metatarsal on walking. Plantar pressure elicits tenderness, as does abrupt release of this pressure. Swelling occurs over the dorsum of the involved metatarsophalangeal joint, plantar flexion becomes limited, and the transverse arch of the involved foot becomes flattened. A callus develops on the plantar surface of the foot, overlying the involved metatarsal head. A deformed, broadened metatarsal head is seen on roentgenogram. High heels should not be worn and long walks should be avoided until symptoms subside. Symptomatic use of nonsteroidal antiinflammatory agents is recommended.

CARPAL SEMILUNAR

Aseptic necrosis of the lunate bone (Kienböck disease) weakens the bony structure and usually leads to a compression fracture. The lunate bone of the right hand (the usual working hand) is more frequently involved than that of the left, and males are more frequently affected than females.

There is pain on movement of the wrist, and in longstanding cases the pain may be present at rest. There is often swelling over the dorsum of the wrist and tenderness over the affected bone. The roentgenogram shows a flattened fragmented lunate bone with variations in its radiodensity. The lunate, lying adjacent to the radius, is subjected to great forces and pressures; hence treatment includes wrist immobilization. On occasion, fusion of the lunate with the bones of the wrist that surround it is required for stabilization and relief of pain.

LOWER THORACIC VERTEBRAE

Scheuermann disease is a common cause of kyphosis in teenagers, occurring in about 5% of that population. The lower thoracic vertebrae are most often affected. The pathologic condition involves a swelling of the intervertebral disks that exerts pressure on the cartilage plates covering the vertebral bodies; this causes the plates to thin and interferes with endochondral bone formation. The disk spaces become narrowed (more anteriorly than posteriorly), and pressure is exerted on the anterior portions of the contiguous vertebral bodies, which impedes their longitudinal growth and thus leads to kyphosis.

An aching pain aggravated by physical exertion is present in the affected portion of the vertebral column. The affected area is tender to palpation. Assuming a stooping position will often cause the pain to increase. Within a year or so, the kyphosis is easily apparent as a round back deformity. In many instances, the pain is so minor that the patient's complaint is that of poor posture rather than backache. Roentgenograms reveal narrowing of the anterior disk spaces and defects on the surfaces of adjacent vertebrae. In some children the condition progresses to cause severe deformity and dysfunction; in others the condition stabilizes and the deformity disappears. Treatment is aimed at prevention of further deformity, occasionally with the use of casting or bracing. In those rare instances of rapid progression or of persistent, severe pain, spinal fusion is necessary. The majority of youngsters, however, require only careful observation.

SUGGESTED READINGS

Bowen JR and Abrams JS: Legg-Calvé-Perthes disease, Contemp Orthop 10:27, 1985.

Riseborough E and Herndon JH: Scoliosis and other deformities of the axial skeleton, Boston, 1975, Little, Brown & Co.

Stulberg SD, Cooperman DR, and Wallenstein R: The natural history of Legg-Calvé-Perthes disease, J Bone Joint Surg 63A:1095, 1981.

Tachdjian M: Pediatric orthopedics, ed. 2 Philadelphia, 1991, WB Saunders Co.

237

Osteomyelitis

Edwards P. Schwentker

The vast majority of cases of osteomyelitis are secondary to pyogenic infection. They can result from the direct bacterial contamination of bone, which may occur with an open fracture or during operative procedures or from direct extension from an adjacent soft tissue infection. Most commonly, however, childhood osteomyelitis is hematogenous in origin.

Hematogenous osteomyelitis may occur at any age, but its incidence is higher in children than in adults. Unless promptly diagnosed and aggressively treated, it may lead to severe complications, resulting in lifelong disability. Because the diagnosis of osteomyelitis may at times be difficult, a high index of suspicion is required.

Pyogenic osteomyelitis intitially may manifest as either an acute or a subacute form. In childhood these two entities are sufficiently distinct to require separate discussion. Chronic osteomyelitis will be discussed with acute osteomyelitis, inasmuch as the chronic form of this disease develops from the inadequate treatment of an acute osteomyelitis.

ACUTE OSTEOMYELITIS

Pathogenesis

The pathogenesis and, consequently, the clinical manifestation of acute pyogenic osteomyelitis depend on the anatomy of bone, particularly its pattern of vascular supply. This anatomy is sufficiently different among the infant (birth to 18 months), the older child (18 months to skeletal maturity), and the adult, to cause a different form of acute osteomyelitis in each of these three age-groups.[9] The concern here is with bone infection only as it occurs during infancy and childhood.

Infancy. In anatomic studies, Trueta[9] demonstrated the presence of vessels that penetrate through the growth plate to connect the metaphysis with the epiphysis. These vessels most commonly are seen before the infant is 6 months of age, but they may be present up to 18 months. When present, infectious spread through the metaphyseal side of the growth plate (physis) into the epiphysis is facilitated by these penetrating vessels. Infection is thus able to damage the growth plate and the epiphysis itself; it also is much more likely to penetrate into the adjacent joint. In infancy therefore *acute osteomyelitis commonly results in an associated septic arthritis*.

As in the older age-group, destruction of the bone of the metaphysis and the diaphysis also can occur in infancy, with subsequent formation of sequestrum and involucrum. The richness of blood flow and the natural resilience of the young infant provide an enormous capacity for repair. The development of chronic osteomyelitis is less likely in the infant than in the older child, but irreparable damage to joint surfaces and to growth potential is far more likely.

Childhood. Hematogenous osteomyelitis in childhood (approximately 18 months to skeletal maturity) virtually always arises in the metaphyses of the long bones, gaining entrance to the bone by way of its nutrient vessels. The vasculature on the metaphyseal side of the physis is characterized by vascular loops that extend up into the layer of calcified cartilage of the physis to provide nutritional support for the formation of bone associated with growth. Invading bacteria present within the bloodstream gain their bony foothold on the venous side of these vascular loops. It generally is believed that a relatively sluggish blood flow within these venous sinusoids favors bacterial proliferation. Rang,[6] however, points out that there is a relative lack of reticuloendothelial cells in the metaphyses of actively growing long bones, and he postulates that bone defenses against infection are weakest in this area.

Trauma also may play a role. The presentation of an *acute osteomyelitis frequently is associated with the history of a recent injury* to the affected extremity. Morrissy and Haynes[5] have presented experimental evidence in an immature rabbit model to support injury to the physeal plate as a factor in the development of acute hematogenous osteomyelitis. Whatever the cause or combination of causes, *the metaphysis is the predominant site of origin of hematogenous osteomyelitis* in childhood.

By 18 months of age there are no direct vascular connections between the metaphysis and the epiphysis. The physis consequently forms a barrier to infection, which effectively prevents its spread into the epiphysis.

As bacteria proliferate, local thrombosis occurs, resulting in devascularization of bone. This loss of vascularity further interferes with natural body defenses and prevents the penetration of circulating antibiotics as well. The result is an abscess. Untreated, infection spreads through the haversian system and Volkmann canals, eventually reaching the subperiosteal space. The periosteum then may be elevated by the infection, stripping the periosteal vascular supply from the cortex and causing further bone death.

Rupture through the periosteum at this point may result in a septic arthritis of the adjacent joint if that portion of the metaphysis happens to be intraarticular. This event is most likely in those joints in which capsule attaches circumferentially well down on the metaphysis of the infected bone. Thus a proximal femoral osteomyelitis may result in septic arthritis of the hip. Similarly, sepsis of the elbow can result from infection of the proximal radius.

If treatment is delayed or inadequate, the infection also may track outward to result in a spontaneously draining sinus. Devascularized bone, the *sequestrum,* becomes a fortress for the bacteria, against which antibiotics and natural body defenses can accomplish little more than to prevent further spread of infection. Meanwhile, the elevated hypervascular periosteum lays down a surrounding wall of new living bone known as the *involucrum.* An inadequately treated or untreated acute osteomyelitis thus becomes a chronic osteomyelitis.

In acute childhood osteomyelitis *the growth plate is seldom damaged.* Growth is unlikely to be retarded and may, in fact, be stimulated, possibly secondary to the hypervascularity that attends inflammation.

Clinical Findings

In older infants and children, osteomyelitic infection is *most likely to involve a single bone.* Fever and sepsis may be prominent, but systemic signs and symptoms usually are mild (or even absent), with the major signs being localized to the affected part. This is especially true in the infant. *Localized tenderness* generally is present and often is exquisite. There may be other local signs associated with inflammation, which include *swelling, redness,* and *warmth.* Characteristically, the child is reluctant to or refuses to move the adjacent joint and, when a lower extremity is involved, may refuse to bear weight. In the young infant the loss of active movement in an extremity may mimic neurologic damage, a condition known as *pseudoparalysis.*

The diagnostic workup should include a complete blood cell count and erythrocyte sedimentation rate, blood cultures, and roentgenograms; however, findings here also may be misleading. The white blood cell count often is normal. An elevation in the sedimentation rate usually is present but is nonspecific. The sedimentation rate often is of greatest help in monitoring clinical response.

Early in the clinical course, no bony changes are seen roentgenographically, the earliest detectable signs being those of blurred soft tissue planes secondary to edema spreading into fatty tissues. The earliest roentgenographic changes to occur within bone itself are those of *bone destruction or lysis, which generally is not apparent until at least 10 days after the onset of symptoms.*

The differential diagnosis of acute osteomyelitis includes septic arthritis, acute rheumatic fever, rheumatoid arthritis, cellulitis, leukemia, and bone tumors. In the case of septic arthritis the urgency for prompt treatment is, if anything, more acute (see Chapter 254). Acute osteomyelitis is differentiated from most of these entities by the severity of the localized signs, particularly tenderness, and by the discrete localization of involvement to the metaphyseal area of the involved bone.

Radionuclide scanning is not necessary in most cases of acute osteomyelitis, but if signs and symptoms are inconclusive, it may help in establishing the diagnosis. Scanning is far more sensitive than is radiographic examination in the early stages of the disease and is capable of differentiating most cases of soft tissue cellulitis from infection of the bone itself. Scans are most helpful when signs of localization are poor, when multiple sites of involvement are suspected, or for the localization of sites within the axial skeleton. Technetium pyrophosphate scintigraphy is the most commonly employed scanning modality. Technetium scans provide results within 3 to 4 hours and are most helpful when performed with a three-phase protocol to evaluate blood flow, blood pool, and bone uptake.[2]

The use of gallium scans and scans with radionuclide-labeled leukocytes may be even more sensitive and specific; unfortunately these tests require 24 to 48 hours to complete, rendering them of limited usefulness in a situation in which early diagnosis is critical. Of the two techniques, indium-labeled white cell scanning may be the most useful and should be considered when needle aspiration and three-phase technetium scan both show negative results.[2]

Under no circumstances should treatment be delayed to perform a scan when clinical suspicion is high. Both false-positive and false-negative results with all scanning methods have been reported.[8]

Blood culture results are positive in 40% to 50% of cases of acute osteomyelitis. *Needle aspiration of the subperiosteal space and of the metaphysis* provides a positive identification of the infecting organism in most cases. The predominant offending pathogen (in up to 70% of acses) is *Staphylococcus aureus.* A multitude of other pathogens may be responsible, however, including coliform, pneumococcal, *Salmonella,* and *Pseudomonas* organisms. In infants and younger children, acute osteomyelitis often is due to *Haemophilus influenzae* type b and *Streptococcus pyogenes* (group B).[4]

High-risk, low-birth-weight infants present a special set of problems with respect to acute osteomyelitis. They often have multiple portals for bacterial entry into the systemic circulation, including infection of other organ systems, indwelling catheters, and heelsticks. They frequently are debilitated; as a result, osteomyelitis often develops at several sites, including the facial bones. Extension of infection from the bone into adjacent joints occurs commonly. *S. pyogenes* (group B) is a frequent offender.

The search for multiple sites of involvement in the neonate would seem to be an ideal application of radionuclide scanning. Unfortunately, false-negative results are more common in this age-group.[1] It may be possible to reduce the incidence of false-negative scan results in the neonate with the use of the latest generation of cameras and the application of spot and pinhole views.[2]

Skeletal infections caused by *Candida albicans* may develop in *severely debilitated infants* and children who have required prolonged antibiotic therapy or hyperalimentation by central venous catheter.

Another special group is composed of *patients with sickle hemoglobinopathies;* when osteomyelitis occurs in these patients, it is difficult to differentiate it from bony infarction. *Salmonella* spp. are the most common infecting organisms. Differentiation of osteomyelitis from bone infarction can be accomplished by operative exploration and direct culture of bacteria from the involved bone or by culture of the organism from the blood.

Because the physical signs are more difficult to interpret when osteomyelitis involves the spine or pelvis, diagnosis becomes more complex. Technetium scans are particularly helpful in making the diagnoses in such cases.

Management

Needle aspiration is the most helpful procedure for diagnosing infections of bones and joints. However, it should not be used as a therapeutic measure. All children with suspected osteomyelitis with localized signs should undergo aspiration of the subperiosteum with a large-bore needle and, if results are negative, of the metaphyseal bone. Aspiration of the metaphysis of a long bone can be performed quickly without the use of general anesthesia. Aspiration confirms the diagnosis, determines the necessity for operative decompression, and provides a specimen for pathogen identification by culture, as well as material for immediate Gram stain.

Once blood cultures and aspiration have been performed, antibiotics should be given parenterally. Unless a gram-negative organism has been identified on Gram stain, a penicillinase-resistant penicillin should be used. In the young child with osteomyelitis it may be appropriate to include an agent effective against *H. influenzae* type b. In patients younger than 2 years of age suspected of having an osteomyelitis caused by this organism, examination of cerebrospinal fluid should be considered, because associated meningitis may well be present.

Antibiotics should be continued for at least 3 weeks and must be maintained at adequate concentrations in the blood. It may be possible to achieve adequate bactericidal titers with oral antibiotics. Oral antibiotics, however, should be used only if the patient is responding to treatment, the parents are reliable, the antibiotic does not cause a gastrointestinal disturbance that interferes with absorption, and adequate monitored blood levels can be obtained. *The erythrocyte sedimentation rate is helpful in monitoring the clinical response* and should return to normal values before therapy is discontinued.

Surgical drainage must be undertaken whenever an abscess is detected or suspected. An abscess may be considered as present whenever there has been a loss of vascularity, and hence viability, in any part of the skeletal tissues. If a situation exists in which body defenses or antibiotics are ineffective, operative decompression must be used. The aspiration of frank pus is another absolute indication for surgical drainage. Similarly, lytic changes within the bone or periosteal new bone formation, as seen on *initial* roentgenograms in previously untreated patients, also are indications for operative drainage. On the other hand, in patients already under treatment and responding favorably both clinically and in terms of a falling sedimentation rate, the appearance of radiographic bone changes does not necessarily indicate that an abscess is present, because such changes occur in treated patients as recovery progresses.

A negative aspiration finding is not absolute evidence that operative decompression is not needed. The site of aspiration may have been inaccurate, or pus may be present but too thick to pass through even a large-bore needle. Clinical suspicion alone is an appropriate indication, and failure to respond to nonoperative therapy is an absolute indication. The risks of unnecessary surgery in the child with acute osteomyelitis are far less than those of necessary surgery not performed.

SUBACUTE OSTEOMYELITIS

Subacute osteomyelitis in childhood is a clinical entity entirely distinct from acute osteomyelitis. The clinical course is far more benign, both systemically and with respect to the presence of localized signs and symptoms. The sites of subacute osteomyelitis are *not restricted to metaphyses* but may occur virtually at any site within the bony skeleton. Because of its *mild clinical course,* the diagnosis of subacute osteomyelitis often is delayed. This entity occurs with a variety of roentgenographic manifestations and frequently is confused with a variety of benign and malignant bone neoplasms.

Pathogenesis

Gledhill[3] has hypothesized that subacute osteomyelitis develops as the result of an *altered host-pathogen relation.* As in acute osteomyelitis, bacteria appear to gain entrance to the bone through the circulation. After the infection gains a foothold, it is largely brought under control by body defenses and prevented from spreading within the bone. It may be speculated that this situation occurs when bacterial virulence is decreased, either naturally or secondary to antibiotics administered early in the infection. The acute infection also might be aborted by increased host resistance, such as is to be expected within the diaphysis or epiphysis, as compared with the metaphysis. Subacute osteomyelitis may occur in any of these three areas, whereas acute osteomyelitis arises hematogenously almost exclusively in the more susceptible metaphysis.

Whether such an "attenuated" infection occurs because of decreased virulence of the pathogen, increased natural defenses of the host, or a superimposed factor (such as the administration of suboptimal doses of antibiotics), the establishment of the subacute process is characterized by a pathologic stand-off between pathogen and host, wherein *the infection is effectively contained within a small area of bone.* Although the bacteria cannot expand their foothold rapidly, natural body defenses are unable to eradicate the infection completely.

Clinical Findings

Subacute osteomyelitis is of insidious onset. The pain that results is mild to moderate and often intermittent. There is little to no functional impairment, and the systemic signs and symptoms of fever, malaise, anorexia, and weight loss are minimal to nonexistent. Thus the interval between onset of symptoms and the establishment of the diagnosis often may be measured in months, whereas delay in the diagnosis of acute osteomyelitis generally is no longer than a few days.

By the time medical consultation is sought, enough time generally has elapsed since onset of the infection that roentgenograms reveal positive findings. The radiographic appearance may vary considerably and may closely mimic a variety of benign and malignant neoplasms. Roberts and coworkers[7] have proposed an expansion of a system for radiographic classification originally proposed by Gledhill.[3] They describe three different types of metaphyseal lesions, only one of which clearly suggests a subacute osteomyelitis. A lytic defect within the metaphysis surrounded by a dense sclerotic margin suggests the classic form of subacute osteomyelitis, a so-called Brodie abscess. This variety is described as type IB. Type IA is similar in size and location but lacks the sclerotic rim. It is most frequently confused with an eosinophilic granuloma. Type II subacute osteomyelitis is associated with erosion of the metaphyseal cortex, and its appearance may be confused with that of an osteogenic sarcoma. A type III lesion is seen as a localized defect within the cortex of the diaphysis and resembles an osteoid osteoma. The type IV lesion is characterized by onion-skin periosteal reaction and suggests Ewing sarcoma. The type V lesion occurs within the epiphysis and may suggest a chondroblastoma. Finally, the type VI lesion involves a vertebral body, and the roentgenographic appearance is that of erosion or destruction.

The white blood cell count and sedimentation rate in cases of subacute osteomyelitis are likely to be minimally elevated or normal. *Blood culture results rarely are positive*. Findings on a technetium bone scan may be positive, but if a lesion is already visible on plain roentgenograms, the scan will add little in establishing the diagnosis.

Management

A definitive diagnosis of subacute osteomyelitis can be made only by isolating an organism on culture of the bone or by histopathologic findings consistent with infection. When the lesion involves the long bones of the extremities, curettage generally can be performed easily. Material obtained will establish the diagnosis by culture or histology findings. *S. aureus* is the most commonly isolated pathogen. Operative curettage followed by a course of antibiotic therapy, similar to that used in the treatment of acute osteomyelitis, usually is curative.

When the infection involves a vertebral body, a biopsy specimen may be obtained with a closed-needle technique. If there is a high suspicion of infection, treatment may be undertaken with antibiotics and cast immobilization of the spine without resorting to biopsy or aspiration. Again, prognosis for cure is excellent.

REFERENCES

1. Ash JM and Gilday DL: The futility of bone scanning in neonatal osteomyelitis: concise communication, J Nucl Med 21:417, 1980.
2. Demopulos GA, Bleck EE, and McDougall IR: Role of radionuclide imaging in the diagnosis of acute osteomyelitis, J Pediatr Orthop 8:558, 1988.
3. Gledhill RB: Subacute osteomyelitis in children, Clin Orthop 96:57, 1973.
4. Jackson MA and Nelson JD: Etiology and medical management of acute suppurative bone and joint infections in pediatric patients, J Pediatr Orthop 2:313, 1982.
5. Morrissy RT and Haynes DW: Acute hematogenous osteomyelitis: a model with trauma as an etiology, J Pediatr Orthop 9:447-456, 1989.
6. Rang MC: The growth plate and its disorders, Baltimore, 1969, The Williams & Wilkins Co.
7. Roberts JM et al: Subacute hematogenous osteomyelitis in children: a retrospective study, J Pediatr Orthop 2:249, 1982.
8. Sullivan JA, Vasileff T, and Leonard JC: An evaluation of nuclear scanning in orthopaedic infection, J Pediatr Orthop 1:73, 1981.
9. Trueta J: The three types of acute hematogenous osteomyelitis, J Bone Joine Surg [Br] 41:671, 1959.

238

Otitis Media and Otitis Externa

Rickey L. Williams

OTITIS MEDIA

Ear infections most frequently involve the middle ear (otitis media) or outer ear (otitis externa). Otitis media is one of the most common diagnoses made by the practicing pediatrician. The scope of this problem is enormous, especially when one considers the time used in treating this disorder and the costs involved for office visits, medications, and surgery.

Acute Suppurative Otitis Media

Epidemiology. Approximately 75% of children will develop at least one episode of otitis media before 10 years of age, and many children suffer numerous bouts of the disease. Younger children are more prone to otitis, especially between 6 and 24 months of age. A second smaller peak occurs between 4 and 7 years of age. Boys develop otitis more frequently than do girls, and there are racial differences in the incidence and prevalence of the disease. White children are affected more commonly than blacks, and the craniofacial anatomy of American Indian and Eskimo children is thought to explain in part their high risk for otitis. Children with craniofacial abnormalities such as cleft palate are also at especially high risk for developing acute otitis media, as are those with Down syndrome. Lower socioeconomic status is also associated with a higher risk for otitis media.[11] Allergic rhinitis is also a risk factor for middle ear disease.[4]

The illness occurs most commonly in the winter months in temperate climates, presumably in association with respiratory viral infections.

Some children are plagued with numerous bouts of otitis media. Howie and co-workers[7] have found this "otitis-prone" condition to be associated with a first episode of otitis before 6 months of age, especially if *Streptococcus pneumoniae* is the bacterial pathogen.

Pathogenesis. The middle ear cavity is normally filled with air and is sterile. During swallowing, air enters the middle ear through the eustachian tube. When the eustachian tube malfunctions, normal ventilation of the middle ear cavity does not occur, and negative pressure builds up as the air is absorbed. Effusion of fluid into the middle ear occurs, and bacteria from the nasopharynx may be drawn into the cavity, leading to the suppuration found in acute otitis media.[3]

Eustachian tube malfunction occurs because of obstruction or abnormal mechanical factors. Obstruction can result from inflammation of the tube itself or from hypertrophied nasopharyngeal lymphatic tissue. Mechanical factors that lead to malfunction of the eustachian tube include diminished patency, poor muscular function, and increased tortuosity.[2]

Microbiology. *S. pneumoniae, Haemophilus influenzae,* and *Branhamella catarrhalis* account for most bacterial pathogens isolated from middle ear fluid in older infants and children.[9] Other organisms less frequently found include *Staphylococcus aureus,* group A beta-hemolytic streptococci *(Streptococcus pyogenes),* and various gram-negative organisms.

Combinations of organisms can be recovered from middle ear fluid in acute otitis media, and a patient can have one pathogen in one ear and a different pathogen in the other ear. Cultures of the nasopharynx do not correlate well with those of middle ear fluid.

In infants during the first few months of life, *S. pneumoniae* and *H. influenzae* are the organisms recovered most often, although the proportion of cases caused by gram-negative enteric organisms is higher than in older children, especially if the infant was in an intensive care nursery.

In about one third of the cases in which fluid is obtained for culture, no pathogenic bacteria can be identified, leading to speculation concerning the contribution of anaerobic bacteria or viruses to acute otitis media. That viruses are associated with the development of acute otitis media was demonstrated by Henderson and co-workers[5] in a 14-year longitudinal study of a day care center. Acute otitis media was closely linked in time with viral infections, especially respiratory syncytial virus, adenovirus, and influenza viruses.

Mycoplasma pneumoniae was formerly thought to cause bullous myringitis, but the data are inconclusive.

Clinical History. In the usual case of acute otitis media, a young child who has had an upper respiratory tract infection for a few days develops fever, becomes irritable, and eats poorly. Other signs and symptoms can include vomiting, diarrhea, vestibular disturbances, a bulging fontanelle and, in older children, complaints of ear pain or hearing loss. Pulling at the ears is an unreliable sign, and it should be noted that fever may be absent in over one third of children with bacteriologically proven otitis media.

Diagnosis. Examination of the tympanic membrane by otoscopy is the most common method used by practitioners to make the diagnosis of otitis media. The normal tympanic membrane is translucent, and the short process and handle of the malleus are visible through the tympanic membrane. A cone of reflected light is present. The drum moves laterally and medially with negative and positive pressure respectively during pneumatic otoscopy.

Pneumatic otoscopy is performed by using a speculum of a size that will ensure an airtight seal in the external auditory canal. Gentle negative pressure followed by gentle positive pressure using a tube with an attached mouthpiece or rubber bulb allows the examiner to observe motion of the tympanic membrane.

The diagnosis of acute otitis media is based on changes in the tympanic membrane's contour, color, and mobility. A bulging, yellow or red, immobile ear drum in which the bony landmarks and the light reflex are distorted is usually seen in cases of acute otitis media. Redness of the tympanic membrane alone can be caused by crying and is not a reliable sign of acute otitis media.

Tympanometry is being used more frequently as an aid in the diagnosis of otitis media. As described by Paradise,[10] the tympanometer (electroacoustic impedance bridge) gives one an estimate of tympanic membrane compliance (Fig. 238-1). After an airtight seal is ensured when the probe is placed in the external auditory canal, a tone of constant frequency is emitted into the closed air space. Pressure in the external auditory canal ranging from +200 to −400 mm H_2O is then applied variously by a pump. As the tympanic membrane moves, sound reflected from it is measured with a microphone and displayed on the tympanogram (Fig. 238-2). A normal tympanogram can be found in the early stages of acute otitis media, so otoscopy should also be performed whenever otitis is suspected.

Acoustic reflectometry has recently been described as another possibly helpful adjunct in diagnosing middle ear disease.[17] Tympanocentesis or myringotomy provides definitive proof of the presence of acute otitis media if fluid is obtained and examined by Gram stain and microbiologic culture. These techniques, described in Appendix B, are helpful when dealing with severe illness (especially in infants), otitis that is unresponsive to routine antibiotic treatment, and complications such as mastoiditis and meningitis. Fluid draining into the two external canals after tympanic membrane perforation is frequently contaminated with organisms from the external canal, so culture of this fluid is seldom helpful in assessing the cause of otitis media.

Treatment. Since the microbiologic cause of acute otitis media in children is usually not determined, the condition should under almost all circumstances be considered of bacterial origin and treated with antibiotics (Table 238-1). Amoxicillin or ampicillin is the treatment of choice in children who are not sensitive to penicillin in geographic areas where the prevalence of beta-lactamase–producing strains of *H. influenzae* and *B. catarrhalis* is small.[9] Cefaclor combinations of erythromycin-sulfisoxazole, amoxicillin–potassium clavulanate, or trimethoprim-sulfamethoxazole are also effective in the treatment of acute otitis media. Trimethoprim-sulfamethoxazole should not be used if infection with group A streptococci is suspected or proven.[9] Cephalosporins are being investigated for use in acute otitis media. The advantages of some of these newer agents include once daily therapy, which should improve treatment compliance, and a broad spectrum of antibacterial activity. Cost considerations currently preclude use of these agents as first-line therapy.[9]

Use of antihistamines or decongestants in the treatment of acute otitis media remains controversial; therefore routine use of these drugs is unwarranted.

Myringotomy has not been proved to be effective in treating acute otitis media, although it may help relieve the severe pain associated with a bulging eardrum.

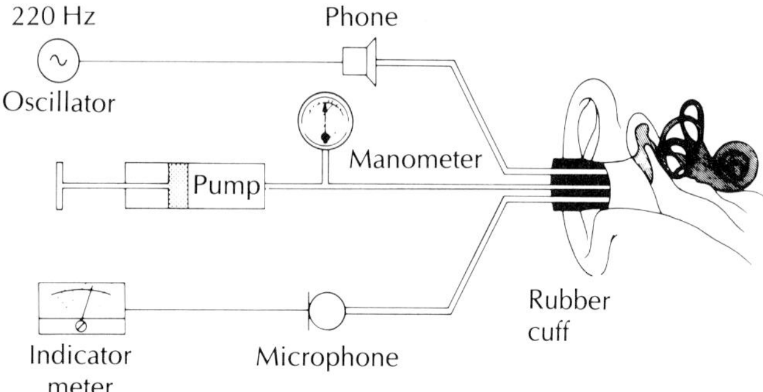

Fig. 238-1 The electroacoustic impedance bridge.

From Paradise JL, Smith CG, and Bluestone CD: Tympanometric detection of middle ear effusion in infants and young children, Pediatrics 58:198, 1976. Copyright American Academy of Pediatrics, 1976.

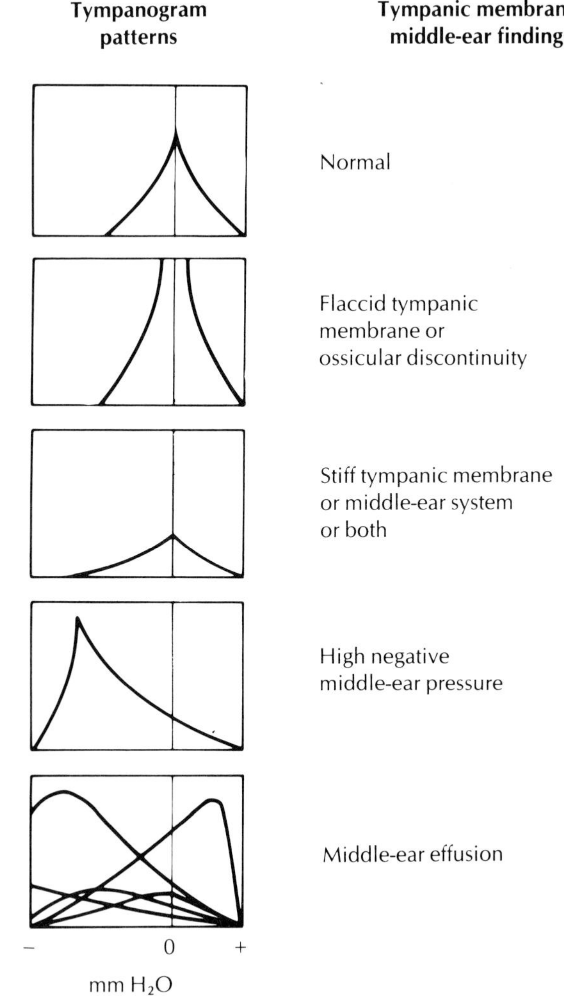

Fig. 238-2 Examples of tympanograms related to tympanic membrane compliance and middle-ear pressure (mm H_2O).

From Bluestone CD: Recent advances in the pathogenesis, diagnosis, and management of otitis media, Pediatr Clin North Am 28:727, 1981.

Table 238-1 *Antibiotic Treatment of Acute Otitis Media*

DRUG	DOSAGE (mg/kg/day)	FREQUENCY OF ADMINISTRATION
Amoxicillin	20-40	tid
Amoxicillin–potassium clavulanate	20-40	tid
Ampicillin	50-100	qid
Trimethoprim-sulfamethoxazole	8 and 40	bid
Erythromycin-sulfisoxazole	50 and 150	qid
Cefaclor	20-40	tid

It is important to tell parents that their child's symptoms will not resolve immediately with initiation of antibiotic therapy and to advise the parents to give an analgesic such as acetaminophen. Because parents frequently discontinue antibiotics when their child's symptoms improve, they must be advised to continue the antibiotics for a full 10-day course.

Persistent Otitis Media. Inadequate resolution of acute otitis media can be attributed to organism(s) involved, the antibiotic regimen, compliance with medication administration, or a number of other factors.[13]

If after 48 hours of antibiotic treatment the child has not improved, Teele and co-workers[19] recommend that tympanocentesis be performed. The antibiotic should be changed, although most recovered organisms will prove to be sensitive to the initially prescribed antibiotic.

Routine follow-up is recommended near the end of the antibiotic course. Persistence of effusion after 10 days of therapy has been demonstrated in about 40% of affected children. If the child is asymptomatic at that time, a repeat examination in 6 weeks is reasonable. Some physicians prefer to treat again with an antibiotic effective against resistant organisms.

Recurrent Otitis Media. Tympanostomy tube placement is performed frequently, although the controversy over the efficacy of this procedure rages. Immediate improvement in hearing occurs with tube placement and continues until the tube is extruded or removed. Less evidence is available to confirm the efficacy of tympanostomy tubes in preventing recurrences of otitis media. Present evidence suggests that tympanostomy tubes should be inserted for recurrent otitis media after failure of medical management with prophylactic antibiotics or in the presence of significant conductive hearing loss.

Prophylactic antibiotics are helpful in decreasing recurrences of acute otitis media in children who suffer numerous infections, especially when used during the winter "otitis season." Perrin and co-workers[14] found that giving sulfisoxazole (75 mg/kg/day) every 12 hours decreased recurrences by 81%.

Prevention. No therapy is yet available to eliminate the occurrence of acute otitis media, although some methods may decrease its frequency. Breast-fed babies suffer fewer episodes of otitis than do bottle-fed babies, especially those bottle fed in a recumbent position. It is postulated that swallowing while lying down allows nasopharyngeal fluid to enter the middle ear, with subsequent infection. Because children exposed to cigarette smoke have more frequent ear infections, parents should be encouraged to avoid having their children around smoke.[6]

Immunization against both the major bacterial pathogens and the viruses associated with acute otitis media is under investigation. Polyvalent pneumococcal polysaccharide vaccines reduce the incidence of pneumococcal otitis media by 50% in children older than 2 years of age, but the vaccine is not effective in infants, who do not develop antibodies to the polysaccharide vaccines.

Nonsuppurative Otitis Media

Nonsuppurative otitis media, also called secretory otitis media and glue ear, is a common sequela to acute suppurative otitis media. The exact incidence and prevalence of this disorder are unknown, although approximately 20% of children with allergies are said to have nonsuppurative otitis media.

This condition, caused by eustachian tube malfunction, usually follows an episode of acute otitis media. Negative pressure in the middle ear leads to effusion of fluid into that cavity. Although the effusion was formerly thought to be sterile, bacterial pathogens can be recovered in approximately one third of cases.

On physical examination, the tympanic membrane appears retracted. An air-fluid level or bubbles of air may be seen behind the tympanic membrane if it is translucent, although it is more often opaque. Mobility of the drum is decreased, and tympanometry frequently reveals high negative pressure in the middle ear cavity.

No satisfactory treatment is available for nonsuppurative otitis media, and spontaneous improvement occurs in nearly all cases, although this may take many months. A course of antibiotics as used for acute suppurative otitis media is reasonable since the same bacterial pathogens are frequently recovered.[8] Antihistamines and decongestants have not proven to be of value in this condition. A combination of prednisone and trimethoprim-sulfamethoxazole may be effective in the treatment of chronic middle ear effusion.[1] Myringotomy with or without tympanostomy tube placement should be considered if no improvement is seen after several months, especially if hearing loss is present.

Complications

Hearing loss is the most common complication of suppurative and nonsuppurative otitis media. Much concern has been expressed that this hearing loss occurs at the time youngsters are developing language skills, and it is postulated that a "critical period" for learning language skills will be missed during the time the child is experiencing hearing loss.[12] Conflicting data exist regarding the impact of recurrent otitis media on speech and language development.[18,21] The long-term effects of middle ear disease on overall cognitive development have not yet been studied.

Suppurative complications of otitis media such as meningitis and mastoiditis are much less common now than before the antibiotic era.

OTITIS EXTERNA

Acute otitis externa, or "swimmer's ear," is an infection in the external auditory canal that can be localized or diffuse. Localized infections occur when a hair follicle in the outer third of the canal becomes infected, usually with *S. aureus*. Diffuse infection of the canal follows swimming, aggressive cleaning of the canal, or trauma. *Pseudomonas aeruginosa* is the leading cause of diffuse otitis externa, although other organisms, including fungi, may be the infecting agent.

Clinical Presentation

Patients are seen clinically with ear pain, ear swelling, and occasionally hearing loss. On physical examination, one finds exquisite tenderness when pressure is placed on the tragus or when the pinna is moved. A furuncle may be seen in localized otitis externa, and moist debris is present on inspection of the ear canal in the diffuse form. The tympanic membrane, if visualized, is usually normal.

Treatment

Treatment of localized infection may require incision and drainage of the furuncle. Diffuse infection is treated by cleaning the debris from the external auditory canal, with suction if possible. A cotton wick may be inserted into the canal to facilitate contact of medication with the skin. Ear drops containing combinations of polymyxin, neomycin, hydrocortisone, and propylene glycol have been found to be effective in combating the infection and decreasing inflammation.[20] Neomycin may cause skin sensitivity in some patients. The patient should lie down with the affected ear upward while the drops are instilled and stay in that position for 5 minutes to allow the drops to penetrate the cotton wick and ear canal. Systemic analgesics are often required to decrease the pain caused by this condition.

Otitis externa may be prevented in persons with frequent recurrences by instilling 2% acetic acid into the external auditory canal twice daily and after each contact with water.[15] Avoiding swimming and thus keeping the external auditory canal dry is also helpful.

Malignant Otitis Externa. Malignant otitis externa is a more severe form of the illness seen in patients who are susceptible to infections, usually patients with diabetes mellitus. *P. aeruginosa* is the offending organism in most cases. Extension of the infection to the middle and inner ear and to the central nervous system may occur and cause severe sequelae. Computed tomography or radionuclide scanning may be necessary to make the diagnosis. Treatment includes antibiotics administered intravenously and, often, surgical intervention.[16]

REFERENCES

1. Berman S, Grose K, and Zerbe GO: Medical management of chronic middle-ear effusion: results of a clinical trial of prednisone combined with sulfamethoxazole and trimethoprim, Am J Dis Child 141:690, 1987.
2. Bluestone CD: Recent advances in the pathogenesis, diagnosis, and management of otitis media, Pediatr Clin North Am 28:727, 1981.
3. Bluestone CD and Doyle WJ: Anatomy and physiology of eustachian tube and middle ear related to otitis media, J Allergy Clin Immunol 81:997, 1988.
4. Fireman P: Otitis media and its relationship to allergy, Pediatr Clin North Am 35:1075, 1988.
5. Henderson FW et al: A longitudinal study of respiratory viruses and bacteria in the etiology of acute otitis media with effusion, N Engl J Med 306:1377, 1982.
6. Hinton AE and Buckley G: Parental smoking and middle ear effusions in children, J Laryngol Otol 102:992, 1988.
7. Howie VM, Ploussard JH, and Sloyer J: The "otitis-prone" condition, Am J Dis Child 129:676, 1975.
8. Mandel EM et al: Efficacy of amoxicillin with and without decongestant-antihistamine for otitis media with effusion in children, N Engl J Med 316:432, 1987.
9. McCracken GH Jr.: Management of acute otitis media with effusion, Pediatr Infect Dis J 7:442, 1988.
10. Paradise JL: Testing for otitis media: diagnosis *ex machina*, N Engl J Med 296:445, 1977.
11. Paradise JL: Otitis media in infants and children, Pediatrics 65:917, 1980.
12. Paradise JL: Otitis media during early life: how hazardous to development? A critical review of the evidence, Pediatrics 68:869, 1981.
13. Paradise JL: Inadequate resolution of acute otitis media following antimicrobial therapy, Pediatr Ann 13:382, 1984.
14. Perrin JM et al: Sulfisoxazole as chemoprophylaxis for recurrent otitis media: a double-blind crossover study in pediatric practice, N Engl J Med 291:664, 1974.
15. Raymond L, Spaur WH, and Thalmann ED: Prevention of diver's ear, Br Med J 1:48, 1978.
16. Rubin J, Yu VL, and Stool SE: Malignant external otitis in children, J Pediatr 113:965, 1988.
17. Schwartz DM and Schwartz RH: Validity of acoustic reflectometry in detecting middle ear effusion, Pediatrics 79:739, 1987.
18. Teele DW et al: Otitis media with effusion during the first three years of life and development of speech and language, Pediatrics 74:282, 1984.
19. Teele DW, Pelton SI, and Klein JO: Bacteriology of acute otitis media unresponsive to initial antimicrobial therapy, J Pediatr 98:537, 1981.
20. Walike JW: Management of acute ear infection, Otolaryngol Clin North Am 12:439, 1979.
21. Wright PF et al: Impact of recurrent otitis media on middle ear function, hearing and language, J Pediatr 113:581, 1988.

239

Parasitic Infestations

Richard Owen Proctor

Parasitism of humans is common. Not all parasites, however, cause disease, and among those which do, light infestations are frequently asymptomatic. Recent estimates of global prevalence make it amply clear that there has been little relief from parasitism in modern times. This is true in spite of a relatively clear understanding of most transmission patterns and the availability of effective therapeutic weapons against most of the offending parasites.

The majority of persons harboring either protozoan or helminthic parasites do so with little or no complaint of illness and with little risk of serious sequelae. Therefore, we must distinguish between infestation and disease. Infestation occurs when a pathogenic parasite enters or resides on the body and either multiplies or develops there. Disease implies some associated host dysfunction that manifests itself by the presence of signs or symptoms. When an infestation becomes disease, some change has taken place in the delicate balance between maintenance of the host and survival of the parasite. This may stem from alterations in host, agent, or environmental factors.

HOST FACTORS

The host may be at greater risk of disease as a result of age, sex, race, occupation, concurrent infection, immunologic disorder, malnutrition, or exposure to irradiation, cortisone, or other immunosuppressant agents. For example, disease caused by pinworms and dwarf tapeworms is far more prevalent among children than adults, and amebic abscess is more common in adults than children. Sex differences are largely a function of occupation and social habit, as illustrated by the increased rates of *Diphyllobothrium latum* (fish tapeworm) infestation in Jewish females because their habit of sampling gefilte fish during its preparation for the table. Certain races appear to have developed a measure of genetic immunity to certain parasites, such as the relatively immune status of some black Africans to malaria. Shepherds are at increased risk of contracting hydatid disease because of handling their dogs, whose feces disseminate the disease agent. Patients suffering from typhoid fever are more likely to develop invasive amebiasis than are persons whose bowel contains *Entamoeba histolytica* as the sole pathogen. Persons with impaired cellular or humoral immunity are at greater risk of developing severe or fatal disease from certain parasites, as seen most recently in cases of acquired immune deficiency syndrome (AIDS).[3,4] Patients taking cortisone while harboring *Strongyloides stercoralis* are at high risk of developing progressive overwhelming infestation with this parasite.

On a global basis, no other variable is as fundamental to preventing the adverse effects of a parasite infestation (i.e., limiting its resident space and invasiveness) as an adequate diet. Protein and iron are frequently deficient in the diets of children in tropical countries where the monoculture of coffee, bananas, sugar cane, and similar products has replaced subsistence farming. It is here that the risk of severe morbidity and mortality from overwhelming parasitism is most evident. In the United States, parasitic disease rates vary chiefly with the level of public understanding of transmission and the degree to which personal hygiene is practiced.

AGENT FACTORS

Our knowledge concerning parasitism allows us to assume that a parasite residing in the gastrointestinal (GI) tract attempts to remain as superficial in the bowel wall as is compatible with feeding. In this way, it avoids triggering additional defense systems of the host. When the host's defenses have been compromised by disease, nutritional deficiencies, or therapies (e.g., irradiation or steroids), the parasite can perhaps move to deeper layers of the bowel wall or enter the lymphatic system and bloodstream for transport to distant sites.

Parasites that normally enter the deeper tissues of the body as part of their life cycle do so by becoming encysted or by living intracellularly for protection against defense mechanisms. This type of arrangement is used by the agents of toxoplasmosis, trichinosis, visceral larva migrans, hydatid disease, and others. Because of the biochemical complexity of human parasites, a spectrum of antigens is available to which the host responds with antibody production, cellular immunity, hypersensitivity, and inflammation. Only to a few parasites (such as *Toxoplasma gondii*) does previous infestation with the same agent provide any lasting immunity like that seen in viral illnesses. Some measure of immunity is probably developed against all parasites and, while seldom eliminating them, serves to limit their activity and site of residence. Nematodes, which pass through the lungs during development in humans, elicit a hypersensitivity to their presence that probably destroys many larvae.

ENVIRONMENTAL FACTORS

The spectrum of transmission modalities used by the protozoan and helminthic parasites of humans is indeed wide but can be largely encompassed by the following categories: direct, soil-dependent, arthropod-borne, and food- or water-dependent types.

Direct

The direct group includes pinworms, dwarf tapeworms, amebas, *Giardia lamblia*, and other parasites that are able to infest humans as soon as they are passed into the environment. Children disseminate such parasites readily among their peers and, to a lesser extent, to adults. Under common circumstances, members of this group can be transmitted in food and water through simple contamination. Superinfestations can occur in members of this group because of direct reinoculation by way of the fingers, from anus to mouth (autoinfestation).

Soil Dependent

Simple. Some parasites, such as *Trichuris trichiura*, *Ascaris lumbricoides*, and the oocyst of *T. gondii*, require a period of development in the soil following passage in the feces. Only then are their ova infestive on ingestion by another host.

Skin Penetration. Some parasites depend on a soil-based incubation period to undergo transformation from ova to rhabdiform larva. After molting, the infestive-stage larva penetrates exposed skin to reach its adult-stage habitat in humans. *S. stercoralis* and the hookworms are typical of this type.

Arthropod Borne

Filariasis, malaria, onchocerciasis, leishmaniasis, Chagas disease, and sleeping sickness are all examples of the arthropod-borne group. Except for Chagas disease, these parasites are delivered by an insect bite. In Chagas disease the feces of the vector are thought to be rubbed into the bite wound, abrasions, or the conjunctiva after the insect bite causes itching.

Food or Water Dependent

Simple. The simple group includes parasites requiring a period of development in an intermediate host (insects, snails, crustaceans, fish, or mammals), which is later ingested in food or water. Examples include *Trichinella spiralis* and the endocyst form of *T. gondii*; beef, pork, and fish tapeworms; and the guinea worm.

Skin Penetration. The *Schistosomae* are typical of the skin penetration mode of transmission because their eggs must reach water that contains snails, their intermediate host. The embryo (miracidium) released by the egg enters a snail, develops into the cercaria form, is liberated from the snail, and must penetrate a human's skin to reach its final site of development.

DIAGNOSIS AND MANAGEMENT

The diagnosis of a parasitic disease depends on maintenance of a strong index of suspicion, especially in the child at high risk. The child whose family is rural dwelling, of lower socioeconomic status, undernourished, and ignorant of transmission possibilities is at high risk. Children with a history of pica, those who are institutionalized because of mental subnormality, and those who visit or reside in an endemic area are at greatest risk.

A systematic and exhaustive attempt to determine the precise parasites, developmental stages present, locations in the body, and number of parasites is warranted for those with significant signs or symptoms and those with compromised body defenses. This information is necessary to manage the patient with maximum safety while effecting the most complete cure of the infestation. Many antiparasite drugs are toxic or near-toxic in the therapeutic dose range. In an asymptomatic or minimally ill patient, the risk of treating some pathogens may be greater than the risk of doing nothing.

It is generally stated that one need not treat light (asymptomatic) infestations of *T. trichiura*, or hookworm, because the worms have a recognized life expectancy and thereby produce a self-limited infestation in the absence of reinfestation. With the newer broad-spectrum antihelminths, which have a wide margin of therapeutic safety, this concept is outmoded. Certainly there are some parasites that should always be eliminated because of their potential for inflicting serious complications. For example, *S. stercoralis* through autoinfestation produces overwhelming disease. Untreated intestinal amebiasis may proceed to liver abscess formation. The eggs released from a pork tapeworm may be moved retrograde in the intestinal tract during vomiting and so reach the upper GI tract, where the shells are digested and the larvae released. These subsequently produce cysts (cysticercosis) in the liver, lungs, brain, and elsewhere that are far more serious than the presence of the tapeworm in the intestine.

Consideration must be given to the effect of the treatment on each stage of the parasite that may be present. A drug that kills an adult worm in the intestine may have no effect on its larvae in the tissue. Even though an available drug will kill a filaria in the eye, the allergic reaction to the dead parasite may blind the patient; left alone, the parasite may be less apt to cause blindness. Although effective against amebiasis in the bowel, some drugs do not eliminate the same organism in the liver. The clinician who lacks experience in treating parasitic infestations would be well advised to seek consultation with an expert in tropical medicine or a qualified medical parasitologist.

The following questions should be answered when the diagnosis of an endoparasite is entertained:

1. What parasites are present?
2. What stages of each parasite are present?
3. What is the site of each stage of each parasite?
4. Is any parasite present that has priority for treatment? (NOTE: *Ascaris* organisms, if present, must be treated first or simultaneously with the treatment of other parasitic infestations.)
5. Is there any stage of a parasite situated at a site where its death could result in an unacceptable tissue reaction?
6. What drugs must be employed to effect death of all stages of all parasites present? (NOTE: Where one drug is highly effective against several parasites present, it is to be preferred.)
7. What temporal sequencing of a drug or drugs will rid the body of the parasite permanently? (NOTE: Retreat-

ment is necessary for elimination of parasites such as pinworms or dwarf tapeworms because their eggs, present at the time of first treatment, are not killed and can reinfest the host. The second dose should be given after the worm reaches the drug-susceptible adult stage but before it deposits additional eggs.)

8. Is the risk from treating the patient greater than the risk of the parasite in the host?

The diagnostician must know the life cycle of a parasite if the history of exposure is to be intelligently sought. Adequate care of the patient and protection for the family and community depend on knowing how the parasite reaches and enters its human host and how soon, how long, and under what conditions the host is capable of transmitting the disease to other humans.

When a parasite is identified in the patient's stool, blood, or biopsy material and a diagnosis of parasitism is entertained, a warning light must flash for the clinician. Does the parasite adequately explain the findings, or could another disease (such as a malignancy) coexist? Close follow-up is essential to determine the disappearance of the parasite and symptoms following therapy. Stool examination, blood eosinophilia determinations, and repeated serologic tests are often helpful in this regard.

For a discussion of giardiasis (*Giardia lamblia* infection), see Chapter 207.

AMEBIASIS (ENTAMOEBA HISTOLYTICA)

Epidemiology

Entamoeba histolytica is a protozoan that inhabits the intestinal tract of at least 5% to 10% of the world's population. Its prevalence is higher in areas of poor hygiene and inadequate water sanitation and where human waste is used to fertilize food crops. Transmission occurs when amoebic cysts, shed in the stools of infected animals, are ingested by another animal host, including humans. Direct inoculation of injured skin or of mucosal surfaces through contact with an infected carrier may also result in infection.

Fewer than 5000 cases of *E. histolytica* are reported annually in the United States, but because of erratic shedding of cysts and the asymptomatic nature of most infections, case reporting and prevalence surveys underestimate the true number of cases. Widespread endemicity is the rule in tropical agrarian societies, but pockets of high prevalence occur in temperate industrial societies as well. Clusters in the latter have been associated with hotels, mental institutes, child care settings, nursing homes, prisons, and male homosexual enclaves. Prevention rests in improved sanitation, public education, and the identification and treatment of hosts who pass cysts in their stools.

E. histolytica cysts are highly resistant to environmental destruction. They survive for months at the temperature of household freezers and may withstand the chlorine concentrations used in city water supplies. However, they are filtered out by modern water purification plants and can be killed by treating drinking water with tetraglycine hydroperiodide (Globaline) or by holding water at a rolling boil for at least 5 minutes.

Pathogenesis and Life Cycle

The slightly ovoid cysts of *E. histolytica* measure 10 to 20 μ and contain one or four nucei (usually four). They may also contain dark-staining, blunt-ended chromatid bodies, which are refractile. The infected person with diarrheic or dysenteric stools usually passes only trophozoites in the stool. These are not infective, because they have poor environmental survival, do not encyst outside the host, and are destroyed by gastric acid and digestive enzymes if ingested.

When an amoebic cyst is ingested, the cyst wall is digested in the small intestine, liberating four metacystic trophozoites, each of which divides into two mature trophoites. These can continue to divide by binary fission. The amoeba exhibits unidirectional movement by the extension of clear pseudopodia. The cytoplasm is granular, with recognizable debris of bacteria and red blood cells in some cases. The amoeba tends to favor the cecal and rectosignoid bowel as a habitat. In the presence of slow-moving, relatively well-formed stools, trophozoites transform into a precyst and then a smaller, true cyst, before being passed in the stool.

Under certain circumstances, not yet clear, the trophozoites may invade the bowel wall, producing varying size, sharply defined ulcers with a granular base and undermined borders. Only with secondary bacterial infection is there much inflammatory response. Trophozoites can be found in the thin exudate, especially near the ulcer border. In severe cases, as seen at times in patients with immunosuppression, the amoeba extend into adjacent tissue; perforate the visceral peritoneum, causing peritonitis; or are hematologically disseminated to the liver, lungs, pericardium, and in rare cases, the brain. The presence of a toxic hepatitis in the absence of demonstrable trophozoites has prompted speculation that products elaborated by the amoeba may induce this phenomenon. It appears either to lead the frank abscess or to resolve with treatment. Trophozoites can be found in the abscess, especially at the periphery, near healthy tissue. *E. histolytica* cysts are not found in the tissues.

Clinical Manifestations

Invasion of the bowel wall is estimated to occur in only 10% to 25% of persons infected clinically with *E. histolytica*. Clinical presentations include an acute abdominal illness with cramps, abdominal pain, distention, diarrhea or dysentery, fever, toxicity, and lower abdominal tenderness.[7] Examination may also reveal hepatomegaly. In older children and adults the onset may be more insidious, with intermittent flatulent, watery diarrhea and constipation plus tenderness in the lower abdominal quadrants. Constitutional symptoms may be few. Tenesmus may be pronounced, especially with ulcerations in the rectosigmoid area.

When trophozoites invade the liver, they may produce a hepatic abscess (85% to 90% occur in the right lobe). This may develop with 2 weeks of symptoms or over a period of months. Symptoms of abscess formation include pain in the right hypochondrium, fever, weight loss, anorexia, cough, and fatigue. Most patients will have a tender, enlarged liver. Bacterial infection occurs with greater frequency as the abscess ages. Amoebic abscesses extend or rupture into the lung and pleural space, the peritoneum and, particularly from the left lobe, into the pericardium. All such events carry a much higher mortality than an uncomplicated amoebic liver abscess, especially if secondary bacterial infection is present. Abscess formation is less common in children than in adults.[1] In rare cases the amoebae are carried to the brain, kidneys, and other distant sites.

The granulomatous response to *E. histolytica* locally in the bowel may result in constrictions of the bowel, simulating Chron's disease, perforation with peritonitis, or the formation of a large granuloma (ameboma) that may be mistaken for cancer.

Diagnosis

The fastest method of diagnosing acute-phase amebic dysentery is in the course of endoscopy to obtain exudate from a colonic ulcer. Material from the periphery of an ulcer is quickly placed in a drop of normal saline on a microscopic slide, with or without stain (e.g., D'Antoni) and observed immediately under high power on a light microscope. Kits are currently available to prepare slides for later transfer to an appropriate laboratory. A negative report for *E. histolytica* should only be considered accurate after at least three stool specimens taken on separate days have been reported to be negative. Extraintestinal infections with *E. histolytica* can occur in the absence of intestinal cyst shedding.

Serologic tests for *E. histolytica* are likely to be positive only when tissue has been invaded by the trophozoites. Therefore tests are usually positive only in the presence of dysentery and with extraintestinal disease. The indirect hemagglutination test is 85% to 95% positive (titer 1:256 or higher) with deep ulcerations or extraintestinal infection. Counterimmunoelectrophoresis and immunofluorescence tests are all acceptable but must by interpreted in light of the history and findings on physical examination.

Liver imaging (including ultrasonography, CT scans, and portal system angiography) has proven useful in defining the location and size of liver abscess formation. It must be remembered that these modalities cannot distinguish between pure amoebic abscess, a pyogenic abscess, or a combination of the two. Chest roentgenograms usually demonstrate an elevated diaphragm, with or without pleural effusion and atelectasis. The costophrenic angle may be obliterated. Upper abdominal films may show hepatic enlargement and, if the abscess is in the left lobe, deformation of the stomach shadow.

Treatment

The treatment of *E. histolytica* infections depends on the location of the organism in the body, the severity of symptoms, and coexisting conditions such as pregnancy, secondary bacterial infection, and drug-related contraindications. Table 239-1 gives current pediatric drugs of choice and their alternatives. Patients who pass cysts in their stools should always be treated unless specific contraindications exist, since they constitute the main reservoir of human infection. If both luminal and tissue disease are present, they must be treated for a cure to be achieved. Percutaneous aspiration of an amebic abscess should only be performed when a diagnosis cannot otherwise be achieved, when the patient has not responded to treatment with appropriate levels of an amebicidal agent for 3 to 5 days, or when a large abscess, especially of the left lobe, threatens to rupture before it can be controlled with systemic amebicide treatment. Surgical drainage should never be performed unless secondary bacterial infection is proven. Amebicidal agents should be given before surgery.

AMOEBIC MENINGOENCEPHALITIS (NAEGLERIA FOWLERI AND ACANTHAMOEBA SPECIES)

General

Three known genera of amoebae produce central nervous system (CNS) disease. *Entamoeba histolytica* is a recognized and rare cause of brain infection that usually occurs in the presence of coexisting amebic liver abscess. *E. histolytica* produces tissue necrosis in the brain, with nonspecific pleocytosis and purulent exudate. Signs of meningeal irritation and hemiplegia

Table 239-1 *Treatment of Amebiasis*

SEVERITY OF DISEASE	DRUG(S)	ADMINISTRATION SCHEDULE	TOTAL DAILY DOSE
Asymptomatic carrier (cyst passer) and Mild intraluminal disease	Iodoquinol	Three times daily for 20 days (PO)	40 mg/kg/day (maximum: 2 g)
	OR		
	Diloxanide furoate	Three times daily for 10 days (PO)	20-30 mg/kg/day (maximum: 1500 g)
	OR		
	Paromomycin	Three times daily for 7 days (PO)	30 mg/kg/day (maximum: 1500 g)
Moderate to severe intestinal disease (dysentery)	Metronidazole	Three times daily for 10 days (PO)	35-50 mg/kg/day
	(followed by one of the three drugs listed for asymptomatic carriers, above)		
Extraintestinal amebiasis or ameboma	Metronidazole	Three times daily for 10 days (PO)	35-50 mg/kg/day
	(followed by one of the three drugs listed for asymptomatic carriers, above)		
	OR		
	Dehydroemetine	Twice daily for 10 days (M)	1-1.5 mg/kg/day (maximum: 90 mg)
	PLUS		
	Chloroquine	Twice daily for 21 days (PO)	10 mg base/kg/day (maximum: 300 mg base)

may occur before lethargy, seizures, coma, and death intervene. Therapy with metronidazole is indicated, but the case fatality rate with cerebral involvement approaches 100%.

Two genera of free-living amoebae that inhabit fresh and brackish water and moist soils have caused CNS infection in humans. These are *Naegleria fowleri* and several species of *Acanthamoeba*, notably *A. castellanii*, *A. polyphaga*, *A. culbertsoni*, and *A. astronyxis*. The infections caused by these pathogens are rare but have a fatality rate approaching 100% when the central nervous system is involved. Each genus produces a typical pathologic picture.

Naegleria fowleri

Naegleria fowleri produces a rapidly fatal disease that mimics acute pyogenic meningitis but fails to respond to antibiotics. Patients give a history of swimming in fresh or brackish water that has a temperature over 30° C. The clinical course is short. There is an incubation period of 3 to 7 days between exposure and the onset of symptoms. Headache, nausea, and vomiting are prominent. Evidence of meningeal inflammation, lethargy, coma, and death follow within a few days. The cerebrospinal fluid (CSF) reveals a moderate number of red blood cells (RBCs) and white blood cells (WBCs) with polymorphonuclear cells predominating. The CSF protein content may be elevated and the glucose moderately reduced. *Naegleria* trophozoites can frequently be found on wet mounts of cerebrospinal fluid or can be grown on salt-free, nutrient-free agar that has been inoculated with *Escherichia coli*. The pathogen enters the brain by way of the olfactory nerves, traversing the cribriform plate. An autopsy will reveal that lesions are especially evident in the olfactory bulbs, posterior fossa, and the frontal and temporal lobes.

Treatment should be instituted as soon as the history and clinical picture suggest the diagnosis. In spite of the nearly uniform fatality rate, treatment with amphotericin B intravenously, intrathecally, and possibly intraventricularly is usually instituted. There is some evidence for a synergistic effect when oral rifampin and intraspinal miconazole are administered along with amphotericin B. However, the prognosis has remained dismal even with combined therapy.

Acanthamoeba Species

Acanthamoeba species produce a subacute to chronic granulomatous disease that generally begins with primary lesions of the skin, pulmonary tract, or eye. When this agent is atomized in the nasal passages of animals, it is inhaled and produces pulmonary lesions that result in hematogenous spread to the central nervous system. No history of swimming or other recognizable exposure has been found for *Acanthamoeba*. It has been noted, however, that victims of *Acanthamoeba* meningoencephalitis are usually immunosuppressed or otherwise debilitated (e.g., alcoholics or patients with malignancy or AIDS, or those taking large doses of corticosteroids).

Symptoms of flulike disease may precede signs of CNS involvement. Headache, fever, nausea, vomiting, hemiparesis, cranial nerve palsies, cerebellar ataxia, and other signs suggestive of multifocal brain abscesses may occur. The course of *Acanthamoeba* infection may last weeks or months, but the outcome has so far been uniformly fatal. The typical victim has multifocal granulomatous lesions in the brain and leptomeninges. Giant cells, monocytes, and plasma cells can be found. Both trophozoites and cysts are found in deep tissues only with *Acanthamoeba* species. The cerebrospinal fluid reveals a pleocytosis with polymorphonuclear and lymphocyte cells. An elevated protein and normal-to-reduced glucose values have been reported. Wet preparations of cerebrospinal fluid should be examined for trophozoites or cysts or both, but their absence does not rule out *Acanthamoeba* infection. Sinusitis; otitis media; granulomatous lesions of the skin, lungs, and genitourinary tract; and corneal ulcers have also been noted.

Treatment with a variety of antimicrobial agents, including amphotericin B, miconazole and rifampin in combination, and numerous other experimental drugs has not produced survivors of CNS disease. Surgical excision of isolated lesions in the eye or brain, when accessible, has been used as an alternative to drug therapy. All cases of CNS infections from *E. histolytica*, *Naegleria*, or *Acanthamoeba* should be treated in a medical setting where neurologic, neurosurgical, and infectious disease expertise can be brought to bear on the case. Life support systems are essential.

TOXOPLASMOSIS (TOXOPLASMA GONDII)

Epidemiology

Toxoplasma gondii, believed to be a member of the subphylum Coccidia, is an obligate intracellular parasite capable of infesting a vast spectrum of animals, including avians and some reptiles. Although members of the cat family alone can play host to the entire life span of this disease agent, humans become host to the asexual (extraintestinal) cycle on ingesting either the oocyst from cat feces or the tissue cyst in inadequately cooked meats. Serologic surveys in the United States indicate an increasing seropositivity with advancing age.[5] Thus, although only 5% of children under 5 years of age have had infestation with *T. gondii*, 65% of adults over 40 years of age have been infested. For humans the most costly and tragic form of the disease is that which is congenitally acquired. An estimated 3000 infants annually are born in the United States with toxoplasmosis. Between 30% and 50% have clinical disease, and up to 450 die of the disease.[2] About 85% of those surviving experience some degree of permanent impairment. Often the infestation, acquired in utero, remains undiscovered until months or years later when mental retardation, loss of visual acuity, or seizures prompt the performance of tests leading to the diagnosis. Worldwide, an estimated one third of the population has been infested, with some communities showing a 75% infestation rate before the twentieth birthday.

Pathogenesis and Life Cycle

The sexual (intestinal) cycle begins when a member of the cat family (Felidae) ingests infestive oocysts from an environment contaminated with cat feces or flesh of an infested animal (such as a mouse) (Fig. 239-1). The intestinal mucosa

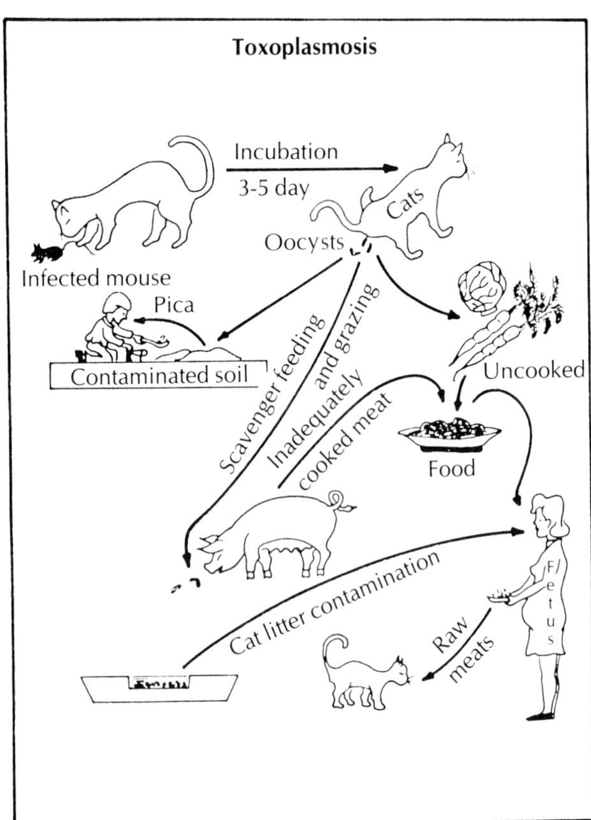

Fig. 239-1 Life cycle of *Toxoplasma gondii.*

is invaded, and within 3 to 5 days the cat begins to pass oocysts in its feces. The oocysts require 1 to 5 days after passage before becoming mature (infestive). The oocyst can then remain viable in the soil for months to years under favorable environmental conditions. These oocysts, passed in cat feces, can contaminate children's playground and sandboxes, gardeners' hands and fingernails, garden vegetables, and the forage for grazing animals who will later serve as food for humans.

On ingestion of oocysts by humans (or other animals), the asexual cycle begins by the release from the oocyst of eight sporozoites, which enter intestinal mucosal cells and develop into trophozoites. Rapid spread of the agent occurs by cell-to-cell movement of the rapidly proliferating form of trophozoite (the tachyzoite). Furthermore, macrophages pick up these organisms and carry them to all parts of the body. At first the macrophages are unable to destroy the parasite, and the macrophages rupture into parenchymal cells when 8 to 16 new organisms are present in their cytoplasm. On release, these new tachyzoites attack other cells, and multiplication continues by endodyogeny (formation of two daughter cells in each trophozoite).

Since humans and other animals do not shed oocysts in their feces, dissemination can occur only by having their flesh consumed by a predatory animal. Thus, in the absence of cannibalism, spread from person to person is assumed not to occur. The exception to this is transplacental spread and transmission during the birth process. Under certain conditions blood transfusion, organ transplantation, sharing of needles by drug users, or accidental inoculation of infested blood in the diagnostic laboratory can occur.[13]

Tissue damage is believed to occur through two mechanisms. The first is the necrosis of cells caused by intracellular multiplication of the organism. Initial multiplication outside of the intestine apparently favors the liver and lung, but a 2-week period of parasitemia probably ensures the involvement of all tissues. As circulating antibodies develop, the tachyzoites disappear from all areas of the body except the brain and eye. Here they continue to produce damage, possibly because of protection from deadly levels of antibody. Tissues not provided with regenerative capability manifest infestation more severely. Meanwhile, within cells the trophozoites transform into a slowly proliferating form (the bradyzoite). These can remain viable indefinitely, perhaps for the life of the animal. As the bradyzoites multiply in a cell, the entire cell is eventually replaced by an encysted collection of organisms. The periodic rupture of these tissue cysts (endocysts) causes the second type of injury observed in toxoplasmosis—that is, necrosis of surrounding cells caused by a hypersensitivity reaction. Damage from either type mentioned above can produce infarction when occurring as a vasculitis of end arteries. Although the macrophages ultimately develop cellular immunity, it is uncertain whether parenchymal cells ever do so.

Clinical Manifestations

Congenital Infestation. The risk of a fetus contracting toxoplasmosis from an infested mother increases with age of gestation (17% in the first trimester to 62% in the third trimester). The risk of serious outcome, however, is greatest following fetal infestation in the first trimester and decreases thereafter. Some infants with in utero infestation remain asymptomatic following birth. Others manifest acute febrile illness with a wide spectrum of organ involvement and findings that include hydrocephaly or microcephaly, intracerebral calcifications, seizures, neurologic deficits, hepatomegaly, jaundice, rash, splenomegaly, and anemia. The cerebrospinal fluid (CSF) may show xanthochromia, increased protein (as high as 2 g/dl in the ventricular fluid), and increased numbers of red blood cells and white blood cells. The latter are predominantly mononuclear. At autopsy, widespread vasculitis, as well as parenchymal cell necrosis, is found, including myocarditis, encephalitis, pneumonitis, and polymyositis. Stillbirths occur, and in those infants born live with the classic picture, mortality in the first few months of life is high. A third type of congenital clinical picture is the infant who appears normal at birth but proves to have had slowly progressive lesions of the brain or eye that are detected much later. As noted earlier, the vast majority of survivors of congenital toxoplasmosis go on to develop sequelae, usually serious, involving the brain or eye. (See Chapter 31 for further discussion on congenital toxoplasmosis.)

Acquired Infestation. Even in the acquired form of toxoplasmosis, the greatest concern centers on the fetus because 25% of women who acquire the disease before menopause do so during the childbearing years (15 to 45 years). When acquired later, especially in adults, the disease tends to be asymptomatic in most. However, 50% of children who have this type of infestation have been found to have residual lymphoid hyperplasia. When clinically evident, however, toxoplasmosis may mimic several other diseases in part. Described are a tick typhus–like syndrome consisting of fever, pneumonitis, and a maculopapular rash that spares the palms and soles. It may be preceded by a prodrome lasting up to 10 days. Death may come within 2 to 4 weeks. Other diseases mimicked are an infectious mononucleosis–type illness with generalized lymphadenopathy and isolated encephalitis or retinochoroiditis. This latter problem accounts for a considerable amount of the residual morbidity in the acquired form of the disease and is to be considered in the differential diagnosis of the "white pupil." Persons with malignancy or who are taking immunosuppressive drugs appear to be at increased risk of having symptomatic disease.

Diagnosis

The clinical triad of hydrocephaly or microcephaly with intracerebral (periventricular) calcifications and retinochoroiditis strongly suggests congenital toxoplasmosis. In fatal cases, impression smears of brain tissue that show tachyzoites confirm the diagnosis. The presence of cysts in biopsy tissue or centrifuged body fluids may only demonstrate prior exposure and does not establish a causal relationship of *T. gondii* with the present illness. Isolation in mice is impractical, time consuming, and dangerous to laboratory personnel.

Serologic tests of sufficient sensitivity and specificity to be of value include the methylene blue dye test, the indirect hemagglutination test, and the indirect fluorescent antibody (IFA) test. All these tests become positive about 10 to 30 days after onset of infestation and remain elevated for 20 to 30 years. A titer of 1:64 indicates past infestation, and titers of 1:256 and higher suggest recent infestations.[5] A very high titer or serial rises in titer are strong evidence of current infestations. The IFA is the test best suited for the diagnosis of congenital toxoplasmosis. The complement-fixation test is sometimes useful in determining the meaning of lower titers of the other tests. It rises in about 2 weeks and disappears in about 2 years. A low positive titer is 1:4; recent infestation is indicated by one of 1:8 or greater. Where the serum titers of mother and newborn are positive at the same level, the presence of IgM antibody specific for *T. gondii* in the baby's serum indicates fetal infestation. The IFA test is generally replacing the dye test because of its lower cost and greater safety, but provision of comparable information. In suspected cases of congenital toxoplasmosis, the CSF should also be examined. Since the dye test and IFA may have reached maximal titers at the time of diagnosis and remain high for long periods, the change in IgM may be followed for determining progress.[9] The double-sandwich test of Naot[8] is useful in avoiding misinterpretation caused by false positives and false negatives.

Treatment

Current therapy for toxoplasmosis is not ideal, nor is its mode of action well understood. It consists of the use of two drugs believed to have a synergistic effect against *T. gondii*. Pyrimethamine (Daraprim) is given in a dosage of 1 mg/kg/day orally divided into two doses at 12-hour intervals. The total daily dose should not exceed 25 mg. If the patient is symptomatic and no drug toxicity is evident, the dosage may remain the same. Otherwise it must be reduced to one-half this dose after 3 days. The patient should be hospitalized because of the near-toxic dosages that must be used. Folinic acid should be added in a single daily dose of 1 mg/kg orally to help prevent bone marrow toxicity by pyrimethamine. Sulfadiazine or one of the other intracellular sulfonamides is given concomitantly in a dosage of 150 mg/kg/day in four divided doses. Both drugs must be given for at least 4 to 6 weeks or until immunity is established. Pyrimethamine is contraindicated during the first trimester of pregnancy. Platelet counts and white blood cell counts should be monitored closely.

Prevention

Suggestions offered for preventing toxoplasmosis include attention to personal hygiene, especially after contact with soil or cats; avoidance during pregnancy of cats and soil that is likely to have been contaminated by cats; and daily emptying of cat litter boxes by a nonpregnant person. Since oocysts require at least 1 day to mature after evacuation from the cat bowel, a major source of potential oocyst infestation is then removed. All meats should be cooked adequately before consumption by humans or pets. House cats should not be allowed outside during the pregnancy of any woman living in the household, and outdoor or stray cats should be kept away from pregnant women.

TAENIASIS (TAPEWORM, CYSTICERCOSIS)

Epidemiology

Taenia solium (pork tapeworm) and *Taenia saginata* (beef tapeworm) are acquired by humans when they consume inadequately cooked meats containing the larval form of one of these cestodes. As a definitive host, humans harbor the adult tapeworm in the small intestine. This produces some abdominal discomfort, increased hunger and food consumption, and weight loss. If a human happens to ingest eggs of the pork tapeworm, as by contamination of food or drink with feces from a person harboring the worm, the eggs release larvae that form cysts in the tissues of the victim. Both parasites have a worldwide distribution, the actual prevalence varying greatly depending on the numbers of animals, meat-eating habits, and amount of human fecal contamination of range land. Neither is common in the United States, although both are common in Mexico. Tapeworm disease caused by *Taenia* organisms can be prevented by adequately cooking all meats (i.e., temperatures of at least 150° F [65.5° C] measured at the center of the meat with a meat thermometer). Persons harboring pork tapeworms are dangerous to all contacts. They should be identified and treated.

Pathogenesis and Life Cycle

The adult worms are segmented and consist of a head (armed with a rostellum and 22 to 32 hooklets in *T. solium*), a neck, and proglottids. These latter may be immature, mature, or gravid and contain both male and female reproductive organs and large numbers of eggs. These proglottids eventually drop off, or strings of them may break off the worm and be carried or migrate out of the anus. *T. saginata* proglottids are more muscular, but either may actually crawl after exiting the body.

The eggs may leave the proglottid before or after it detaches from the rest of the strobila. They are infestive for several weeks in soil or on plants, where they may be ingested by the proper intermediate host (swine or cattle). The larvae released by such ingested eggs penetrate the intestinal mucosa, reach the lymphatic or blood vessels, and are carried to all parts of the body, especially muscles and connective tissues. In 2 months or more, they become infestive worms. These mature to adult tapeworms after the meat is ingested by humans. Both beef and pork tapeworm reach maturity in the human intestine by 12 weeks, reaching lengths of 2 to 7 m and 5 to 15 m, respectively. The eggs of the two species of tapeworms cannot be differentiated.

Clinical Manifestations

A single tapeworm of either pork or beef origin is likely to be silent in an otherwise healthy host. Either can produce abdominal pain or epigastric hunger pains, an increased appetite, weight loss, weakness, and general malaise. Less commonly elicited findings are diarrhea, upper abdominal distention, postprandial vomiting, and rarely, intestinal obstruction. Tapeworms have been known to live up to 25 years. Cysticercus produces few general symptoms, unless very large numbers of larvae develop simultaneously. Localized findings are largely a result of the expanding mass and vary with the location. The most serious threat to life occurs when a cysticercus develops in the brain, eye, heart, or spinal cord. Seizures, neurologic problems, visual disturbances, headache, and evidence of increased intracranial pressure in a potentially exposed child should raise the suspicion of cysticercus.

Diagnosis

Eggs in the stool foretell the presence only of taeniasis. Study of a gravid proglottid for the number of main lateral uterine branches confirms the species. *T. solium* has 7 to 13 such branches per side; *T. saginata* displays 15 to 20 on each side. Cysticercosis is diagnosed by finding calcified "rice grains" on roentgenograms of any part of the body. A negative series of films does not rule out the infestation, however, since calcification usually occurs 5 or more years after the initial invasion of tissues. Excision of a cyst provides the opportunity to examine the evaginated scolex (head) of the larva and to look for the typical rostellum and hooklets of *T. solium*. The indirect hemagglutination test has been valuable in the serologic diagnosis of difficult cases. The indirect fluorescent and counterimmunoelectrophoretic tests are promising. Since cysticercosis may be a result of regurgitation of eggs to the upper gastrointestinal tract where their shells are digested and the invasive larvae released, *T. solium* should always be treated.

Treatment

Taeniasis is currently treated with niclosamide. Niclosamide is given as a one-time dose of chewable 500 mg tablets as follows: adults, 4 tablets; children weighing more than 75 lb (34 kg), 3 tablets; and children weighing 24 to 75 lb (11 to 34 kg), 2 tablets. Niclosamide is not effective against extraintestinal stages (cysticercosis).

HYDATID DISEASE (ECHINOCOCCUS GRANULOSUS)

Echinococcus granulosus is a small tapeworm of canines that infects herbivorous animals, especially range animals that feed on grass contaminated by canine feces. The egg develops into a cystic larval form in these intermediate hosts. Members of the dog family are reinfested by feeding on dead carcasses or when fed inadequately cooked tripe from infested herbivores.

Shepherds and children contract the intermediate-stage parasite (tissue cyst) when eggs are transferred to their mouths after handling diseased dogs or other items contaminated with their feces. The embryo emerges from the ova in the human duodenum, penetrates a small blood vessel, and is filtered out in the liver (60%), the lung (20%), or by the capillaries of other tissues (20%). The bladderlike cyst (larva) expands at about 1 mm/month until body defenses overwhelm it or its size causes symptoms or direct detection of physical examination. It may manifest as an expanding mass (e.g., intracranial), as an inflammatory mass (e.g., pulmonary), or as anaphylactic shock if the cyst leaks. The diagnosis is made by serologic tests and tissue scanning techniques. Treatment is by surgical extirpation. When the location of the cyst precludes surgery or when the cyst recurs after surgery, large doses of mebendazole may be advised. The Centers for Disease Control should be consulted. Prevention lies in control of infestation in dogs through deworming and proper feeding.

Alveolar hydatid disease (*Echinococcus multilocularis*) has a similar life cycle but is found in a wild animal cycle in the Northern hemisphere and produces multilobed cysts with metastatic tendencies.

HYMENOLEPSIS NANA (DWARF TAPEWORM)

Epidemiology

Hymenolepsis nana is a tapeworm of rats and mice. It is, however, well adapted to humans, and transmission occurs directly from child to child or through contamination of food and drink with human feces. The parasite is found worldwide, with a much higher prevalence among children than adults. At special risk are children who are under 3 years of age, on a protein-deficient diet, immunodepressed, or living in a crowded, unhygienic environment infested with rodents. The decreasing prevalence with age reflects a decreased exposure, but serologic studies suggest also that previous exposure evokes a measure of resistance against recurrent infestation. Current world prevalence is estimated to be about 50,000,000 cases.

Pathogenesis and Life Cycle

H. nana is the smallest tapeworm infesting humans. It requires no soil or water cycle, and the eggs become infestive before leaving the human gut. This allows internal autoinfestation as well as transfer from anus to mouth in the same host. After ingestion of a viable egg, its onchosphere (embryo) is released in the stomach or upper small intestine. This stage penetrates an intestinal villus and matures into the cysticercoid stage. This larval stage emerges to attach itself in the small intestine. Maturation to the adult stage is evidenced by the appearance of eggs in the stool several weeks later. The adult worm measures 25 to 40 mm by 0.5 to 0.7 mm. The scolex (head and neck) is provided with four suckers and armed with 20 to 30 hooklets arranged in a single crown. The egg is 30 to 40 μm in length and is characterized by a wide clear space between its outer membrane and its centrally placed embryo. There are four to eight polar filaments in the embryo.

Clinical Manifestations

Although light to moderate infestations are not generally associated with expressed complaints, the heavily infested child often complains of abdominal pain, headache, and loss of appetite. Diarrhea, abdominal distention, and pallor may also be present. Diarrhea seldom occurs in patients with less than 15,000 eggs per gram of feces.

Diagnosis

The diagnosis is made by detecting typical worms or eggs in the patient's feces. A moderate eosinophilia is present in heavy infestations. Serologic tests are not of any real value in the diagnosis of *H. nana*.

Treatment

H. nana has been a difficult parasite to eliminate from the child, but now niclosamide has been shown to be 90% effective. The drug is given for 7 days in the following daily dosage of chewable 500 mg tablets: adults, 4 tablets (2 g); children weighing more than 74.8 lb (34 kg), 3 tablets on the first day, followed by 2 tablets daily for 6 days; and children weighing 24.2 to 74.8 lb (11 to 34 kg), 2 tablets on the first day, followed by 1 tablet daily for 6 days. All tablets should be chewed thoroughly. The drug is active only against the adult worm, and newly emerging adults from the villi of the bowel must be destroyed before they deposit eggs. Stools should be examined 2 weeks and then 3 months after initiation of therapy. Retreatment is instituted if required. A saline purge is indicated following each 5-day treatment with niclosamide.

TRICHURIASIS (WHIP WORM)

Epidemiology

Trichuris trichiura is an intestinal roundworm with a fine hairlike anterior and a thicker posterior body, giving it the appearance of a whip. It is acquired, like *Ascaris lumbricoides*, through ingestion of the egg following its embryonation in soil. Because of their indiscriminate and repeated play in soil, thumb-sucking, nail-biting, and pica, children are more prone to become infested and to accumulate heavier worm burdens. The worldwide prevalence of this parasite has been estimated recently to be 500,000,000 cases. Selected communities in the United States have shown a prevalence as high as 36% of the population. Often, in the moist, warm tropics, the prevalence exceeds 50%. Humans, the only natural host of *T. trichiura*, may pass eggs in their stools for up to 10 years after a single ingestion of eggs.

Pathogenesis and Life Cycle

The ova of *T. trichiura* are barrel shaped with slightly elongated ends containing a mucoid plug and measuring approximately 50 by 22 μm. The outer of the two shells of the egg is generally bile stained. After ingestion and embryonation in the small bowel, migration downward to the large bowel is attended by maturation to the adult stage, which measures 30 to 50 mm in length. The adult threads its anterior body into the mucosa of the cecum, ascending colon, or rectosigmoid areas. This elicits no inflammatory response unless competition for nutrients forces deeper burrowing in the mucosa. This latter triggers infiltration with lymphocytes, plasma cells, and eosinophils down to the muscularis mucosae. This parasite neither causes the degree of blood loss from oozing that hookworms do nor uses blood as a major portion of its diet; however, it can produce significant anemia when 800 or more worms are in residence. One month after ingestion the fertilized female begins laying about 3000 to 7000 eggs per day. When these fertile eggs are passed into a warm, moist, shady soil, they become infestive within 10 days minimally, but usually about 21 days.

Clinical Manifestations

Light infestations generally go unrecognized. With infestations producing 30,000 or more eggs per gram of stool, symptoms are likely to include abdominal pain, headache, pallor, tenesmus, and diarrhea or dysentery. Increased motility and tenesmus, whether caused by physical or chemical irritation, have been blamed for cramping pains, decreased absorption of nutrients, and complications such as volvulus, intussusception, and rectal prolapse. Irritability and other emotional manifestations are reported but are difficult to relate directly to the presence of the parasite. Rectal prolapse, presumably secondary to straining in response to tenesmus, occurs in about 1% of diagnosed symptomatic cases. Intense inflammation in the cecum has occasionally led to a symptom complex mimicking appendicitis. Appendicitis has, in fact, occurred as a result of edema and direct worm obstruction of the appendix. Heavy infestation in the presence of a chronic, debilitating infection and malnutrition carries a grave prognosis. The invasiveness of both amebiasis and typhoid appears to be enhanced by the presence of *Trichuris* organisms in the same patient. In the absence of reinfestation or treatment, the infestation will usually subside after about 3 years, although sometimes the parasite may live more than three times that long.

Diagnosis

The diagnosis must be suspected and the stool examined for the characteristic eggs. The worms may be observed at autopsy, during bowel surgery, or at sigmoidoscopy. When prolapsed rectum occurs, the parasite is frequently visible on the mucosa. The stool should be examined in any case of prolapsed rectum, far advanced abdominal tuberculosis, disseminated histoplasmosis, certain malignancies of the abdomen, and severe malnutrition. A skin test antigen is available (from the Centers for Disease Control) that is positive in 93% of proved *Trichuris* infestations of at least 1 month's duration. This can be valuable in determining the prevalence of *Trichuris* infestation in a community. Probably the most reliable serologic test is the latex flocculation test. Serum from a known case should be used simultaneously for comparison of the degree of flocculation present.

Treatment

In the past it was often recommended that light infestations not be treated. The reason was at least partly because of the potential toxicity of the treatments available. With the effectiveness and safety record of mebendazole, treatment should not be withheld except for specific contraindications. Mebendazole is the drug of choice and is given in a dosage of 100 mg twice daily for 3 days. It is not recommended for children under 2 years old and is contraindicated in pregnancy. In severe infestations, transfusion and general supportive measures should not be neglected. When a prolapse occurs, the rectum must be inspected for foreign bodies, injury (including perforation), and infarction. Where a surgical consultation can be rapidly obtained, this is appropriate. A healthy rectum should be returned to the pelvis using a gloved, lubricated finger while the patient is on the knees with the chest flat on the examining table. When the physician is very concerned or when the distance from medical care is great, it may be prudent to observe the child in the hospital for 24 hours.

ANCYLOSTOMIASIS (HOOKWORM)

Epidemiology

Necator americanus is the cause of almost all hookworm disease found in the United States today. The few diagnosed cases of *Ancylostoma duodenale* infestation are found in travelers and immigrants. The disease in this country is largely confined to an area stretching from the mid-Atlantic coast through the Southeast to the costal plains of Texas. In spite of a general decrease in prevalence, there are still pockets of hookworm transmission in the areas mentioned. On a global basis, hookworm constitutes one of the more serious economic and health problems. Its economic importance can be appreciated by recognizing that it attains a peak prevalence among men in their teens and twenties. The ideal transmission environment for hookworms is sandy loam soil located in a shady, warm area of high humidity.

Pathogenesis and Life Cycle

When a hookworm egg is deposited on the soil, it hatches in about 24 hours, releasing a rhabdiform larva. Within a week, the third-stage (infestive) larva appears. This stage dies in the soil when its stored food supply is exhausted (up to 6 weeks under natural conditions) unless it is successful in attaching to and penetrating human skin. Effective contact by humans can be made by walking barefoot, sitting, or lying on contaminated earth or working in the soil with the hands. *A. duodenale* is apparently also infestive when ingested. During their brief sojourn in the skin, the larvae evoke a reaction characterized by edema, vesicular erythematous or papular rash, and pruritus. Those larvae not killed by the reaction in the skin enter lymphatic or blood vessels and are carried to the lungs. *N. americanus* develops further here, thus evoking a more serious reaction than that of *A. duodenale*. The larvae eventually migrate upward to the epiglottis and are swallowed. They undergo final development to the adult stage in the small bowel, where attachment to the second or third portion of the jejunum takes place. The worm feeds by grasping a small piece of the mucosa, sucking it into its buccal cavity, and digesting it with enzymatic action. Because of slippage of the mucosa out of the buccal cavity during feeding, migration to new feeding sites, and the secretion of anticoagulants by the worm, a considerable loss of blood may occur. This blood loss is estimated at 0.03 ml/worm/day for *N. americanus* and 0.06 to 0.1 ml/worm/day for *A. duodenale*. The latter parasite produces greater bowel damage and blood loss. The female lays eggs that are passed in the feces. The female of *N. americanus* measures 9 to 11 mm, and the female of *A. duodenale* reaches 10 to 13 mm. The eggs, which are ovoid and contain a two- to eight-segment embryo surrounded by an irregular clear zone, are about 40 by 60 μm. It is impossible to determine which type of hookworm is present by observing the ova. The female *N. americanus* worm deposits just under 10,000 eggs per day. *A. duodenale* females deposit 15,000 to 20,000 eggs per day.

Clinical Manifestations

Hookworm infestation must be distinguished from hookworm disease. A single exposure even to moderate numbers of larvae may proceed without notice by the patient, except for the pruritic maculopapular rash ("ground itch") produced by migration of the larvae through the skin. This usually subsides in 1 to 2 weeks. In heavy exposure occurring at one time, there may be sufficient response in the lung to produce asthmatic or pneumonitis-type symptoms and signs.

The symptoms of adult hookworm disease are then largely based on blood loss and gastrointestinal irritation. The worm burden and patient's diet, especially iron and protein, become important determinants of clinical presentation and course.

Findings may include weakness, pallor, tachycardia, tachypnea, palpitations, and abdominal discomfort mimicking a duodenal ulcer or cholecystitis. In far-advanced cases, emaciation, edema of the extremities, a protuberant abdomen, and high output failure of the heart may be observed. The anemia of hookworm disease is generally microcytic and hypochromic unless complicated by other causes. Some circulating antibody formation occurs, probably in response to the migratory larvae. Untreated, about 70% of the hookworms will be dead within 1 year.

Diagnosis

Diagnosis of hookworm infestation rests on identifying hookworm eggs or larvae in the stool specimen. If the stool specimen is left sitting 24 hours or more before examination, only larvae may be present. Should this occur, the larvae must be distinguished from the larvae of *S. stercoralis* and other nematodes. Hookworm eggs can be hatched on special media to identify the species. If more than 20 hookworm eggs are present on a direct 2 mg fecal smear, clinical symptoms can be expected.

Treatment

Because of its effectiveness against several of the more common intestinal worm parasites in American children, mebendazole is the drug of choice in mixed helminthic infestations and solitary hookworm infestation. Treatment consists of one 100 mg tablet morning and evening (200 mg/day) for 3 days. The drug is not recommended for children under 2 years of age and is contraindicated during pregnancy. Nutritional and metabolic disorders should be treated before or during the administration of mebendazole. Pyrantel pamoate in a single dose of 11 mg/kg body weight (maximum of 1 g) may be used as an alternate treatment. Anemia should be treated as for iron-deficiency anemia.

CUTANEOUS LARVA MIGRANS (CREEPING ERUPTION)

Epidemiology

Creeping eruption is caused commonly by *Ancylostoma braziliense* (experimentally by *Ancylostoma caninum* and others), which wanders aimlessly in the skin, producing raised, erythematous, pruritic tracks. It is acquired by children when their exposed skin comes into contact with soil or sand contaminated with animal feces containing nonhuman hookworm eggs. It is most prevalent where warm, moist sandy soil with a high humus content is used by dogs and cats for defecation. Rates of infestation in the United States are highest in the Southeast.

Pathogenesis and Life Cycle

Although ground itch caused by human hookworm and *Strongyloides* larvae is a form of cutaneous larva migrans (CLM), it differs from nonhuman hookworm larvae invasion because the latter cannot effectively penetrate and complete their life cycle. The tunneling migrations of these larvae evoke an intense neutrophilic and eosinophilic infiltrate and produce edema and vascular congestion. The tunnel fills with serum. It is believed that the larva advances with the aid of enzymatic action and that an antienzyme-type antibody formation is triggered in the host.

Clinical Manifestations

The serpentine trails, usually located in the basal layer of epidermis or upper dermis, are intensely pruritic and at times painful, especially on soles and palms. This triggers uncontrolled scratching with subsequent excoriation and sometimes secondary skin infection. When the number of larvae incurred is large, insomnia, emotional irritability, and even weight loss have been noted. The condition often continues for months after a single exposure.

S. stercoralis may produce an area of CLM in the perianal area when infestive larvae are being passed in the stool.

Diagnosis

The causal larva can rarely be precisely classified even when a biopsy specimen shows the parasite. The longevity of symptoms does not invariably distinguish between human and nonhuman parasites. Pulmonary infiltrates appearing a few days to a few weeks after the onset of skin lesions and the sudden appearance of hookworm eggs or *S. stercoralis* larvae in the previously negative stool at 5 to 10 weeks will help distinguish among the causes.

Treatment

Since the larva commonly travels several centimeters per day, the inflammatory response lags behind the parasite. Thiabendazole suspension or tablets are given orally twice daily for 2 days, according to a weight scale in the *Physicians' Desk Reference*.[11] If cure is not evident by 2 days after therapy is completed, treatment should be repeated. As an immediate antipruritic, diphenhydramine may be helpful, especially at bedtime.

ENTEROBIASIS (PINWORM)

See Chapter 245, "Pinworm Infestation."

ASCARIASIS (LARGE ROUNDWORM)

Epidemiology

Ascaris lumbricoides is the largest of roundworms infesting the human. It is contracted by ingestion of the fertile embryonated egg in soil (e.g., pica), food (such as salad greens), or water (e.g., surface wells) contaminated with human feces. The parasite progresses from egg to adult in humans, including migration of the larval stages from intestine to lungs and back before maturity. Although humans are the only host necessary, the egg requires an incubation period in the soil for development of the infestive-stage larvae in the egg. On a global basis, this is thought to be the most common parasitic worm of humans, infesting as much as one third of the world's population. It is probably second only to pinworms in frequency of infestation in the United States. Because of their habits of thumb-sucking, nail-biting, and dirt-eating (pica), children are more likely to harbor sizable numbers of the worm at one time. Regions where modern sewage systems are not in use or where human excreta are used as garden fertilizer have a higher prevalence and larger worm burdens per person.

Pathogenesis and Life Cycle

Once swallowed, a fertile *Ascaris* egg hatches in the small intestine. The larva penetrates the mucosa, enters a portal venule or the lymphatic system, and is carried to the lungs. Since most of the larvae cannot negotiate the capillary bed, they rupture into the alveoli and migrate up the airways to the epiglottis where they are again swallowed. This time in the small bowel, they develop into adults. The larger female commonly reaches 20 to 35 cm in length and 3 to 6 mm in diameter. The male is slightly smaller, and its posterior end curves ventrally. From egg ingestion to appearance of eggs in the stool requires 2 to 2½ months. The female lays approximately 200,000 eggs per day throughout her 6- to 17-month life span. The eggs measure 88 to 95 μm by 44 μ if infertile or 45 to 75 μm by 35 to 50 μ if fertilized. Eggs reaching a favorably moist, warm, shady, clay soil develop after about 3 weeks into infestive larvae, which remain viable inside the ova for many months.

Clinical Manifestations

Most cases of ascariasis are asymptomatic or so mild that medical attention is not sought. The severity of illness is determined in part by the number of infestive eggs ingested, the degree of hypersensitivity that exists, and the general state of health and presence of other parasites in the host. Two types of uncomplicated clinical presentations can occur. The first occurs concomitant with the migration of the larvae. This is characterized by a dry cough, asthmatic wheezing, mild to severe dyspnea (with or without cyanosis), fever, and auscultatory findings compatible with asthma or bronchopneumonia (Löffler syndrome). Urticaria and, in a few very sensitive children, angioneurotic edema may occur. During this phase, the stool may contain no eggs, but peripheral eosinophilia is common, and a chest roentgenogram may reveal patchy central infiltrates or confluent areas of lobar pneumonia or bronchopneumonia. In heavy infestations, bronchial secretions are increased, and larvae can sometimes be identified in the sputum. During passage of larvae through the liver, especially in the host with prior exposure to ascarids, acute hepatitis may occur, and eosinophilic granulomas may result around larvae that die in the hepatic tissue. In rare cases, larvae may pass the pulmonary capillary bed and lodge in other tissues (e.g., the brain), creating a picture compatible with visceral larva migrans. Adult worms may be vomited, be passed in the stool, or appear at other body orifices. A small number of adult *Ascaris* organisms in the small intestine rarely produces clinical disease, although they unquestionably rob the host of some dietary protein and other nutrients. When the adult organisms are present, little more than periodic cramping abdominal pain with some distention, nausea, and vomiting occurs. Headache has also been noted with some regularity in the absence of other detectable causes for it. In rare cases right upper quadrant tenderness, pain, and mild transient jaundice occur secondary to migration of worms in the biliary tract. Complications are more likely to occur in children because of their visceral lumens, resulting is relatively larger worm burdens. Complications arising from the adult *Ascaris* organism include obstruction (from single worms or masses of them) of the intestine, bile duct, pancreatic duct, and appendix. Unless transient, such obstructions can lead to biliary, pancreatic, and appendiceal stasis and to secondary bacterial infection. Bowel obstruction by *Ascaris* organisms is characteristically incomplete and may manifest as a soft mass of variable size. Under certain conditions (e.g., high fever, anesthesia, and selected drug therapy), the worms may migrate indiscriminately through tissue or into the lumens of the bile and pancreatic ducts. This may result in hemorrhage, tissue reaction, and physical damage or perforation of a viscus, with subsequent infection (such as peritonitis or liver abscess) or shock. Adult worm migration through tissue is frequently attended by allergic phenomena. Infestations with 48 or more worms are accompanied by a measurable decrease in fat and protein absorption. During the intestinal phase of ascariasis, eggs can usually be identified in the feces. If no recent migratory activity has taken place, the eosinophilia will probably be absent or nearly so. Abdominal roentgenograms may reveal swirling patterns or air-contrast evidence of the worms. Following a barium meal, the worms may be outlined or identified by the examiner seeing barium in the worms' guts.

Diagnosis

During the migratory phase the diagnosis must be suspected and the blood examined for eosinophils. Finding larvae in the sputum is conclusive evidence of infestation, but their absence does not rule out ascariasis. The presence of *Ascaris* eggs in the stool confirms the presence of the parasite, but the clinician must always be alert to the coexistence of other causes for the illness, especially in areas endemic for ascariasis. An all-male or sterile-female infestation will fail to show eggs when the stool is examined. The presence of a single female worm can usually be detected by examining the stool. Serologic tests, although generally not required, may become useful in cases where male worm infestation may be responsible for biliary tract obstruction and other uncommon expressions of roundworm infestation.

Treatment

Although the evidence for perforation of an otherwise healthy bowel wall by *Ascaris* worms is controversial, the potential of certain drugs to stimulate visceral wandering of these worms should be remembered. When multiple parasites are present, *Ascaris* worms should always be treated first or simultaneously with others. Currently, the drug of choice for treating combinations of *Ascaris* with *Trichuris* or hookworm disease is mebendazole. The dosage for adults and children is 1 tablet (100 mg) every morning and evening for 3 days. A second course is advised if cure is not complete 3 weeks later. Pyrantel pamoate is a reasonable alternative. For pure ascariasis, piperazine citrate in a dose of 75 mg/kg (maximum of 3.5 g) per day for 2 days or pyrantel pamoate in a single dose of 11 mg/kg (maximum of 1 g) is effective in a high percentage of cases.

In children, *Ascaris* worms should generally be treated when discovered, since treatment is quite safe and complications can occur with a single worm. Because of the potential for a negative stool examination in the presence of an infestation, a therapeutic drug trial is occasionally justified when Ascaris infestation is suspected. Where evidence of ductal (nonbowel) obstruction exists, surgery without prior ascaricidal therapy is indicated. Worms dying in bile or pancreatic ducts or in vital tissue can pose life-threatening illness. If only bowel obstruction is present, a course of medical management is generally warranted. Piperazine suspension (given by nasogastric tube) paralyzes the ascarid muscles, often allowing peristaltic action of the bowel to evacuate the worm or worms. The hospitalized patient can be treated with nasogastric suction and intravenous fluids while being administered an effective ascaricidal drug. If this is unsuccessful after 48 hours, surgery is recommended. At laparotomy, small bowel obstructions can usually be "milked" down into the cecum without opening the bowel itself and the patient treated sometime postoperatively for final removal of the parasites. Entering the bowel should be a last resort. Patients going to surgery for any cause who are likely to harbor *Ascaris* worms should be screened preoperatively if possible. Prevention of ascariasis depends on sanitary disposal of human excreta, reasonable personal hygiene, and avoidance of foods potentially contaminated with human feces. Where treatment of a large population is desirable, the most effective season is during a drought, when desiccation of *Ascaris* eggs minimizes transmission and hence reinfestation.

TOXOCARIASIS (VISCERAL LARVA MIGRANS)

Epidemiology

Toxocara canis (the dog ascarid), *Toxocara cati* (the cat ascarid), and in rare cases, other nonhuman nematodes are capable of producing a syndrome in humans similar to that produced during the migratory phase of *A. lumbricoides* but more widely distributed in the body.

In their natural host, these animal ascarids follow a developmental pattern comparable to that of *Ascaris* organisms in humans, eventually maturing in the bowel and depositing eggs in the feces. Puppies and kittens in the early months of life are more heavily infested and thus disseminate more eggs capriciously into the environment than do older dogs. A sizable percentage of domestic pets is infested and routinely contaminates school grounds, yards, and sandboxes used by children for play. Small children, especially those in the 1- to 4-year-old age group, are particularly prone to eating dirt and putting soiled hands or toys into their mouths, thus increasing the risk of ingesting *Toxocara* eggs. The eggs become infestive 2 to 7 days after being deposited outside the animal host. No accurate human prevalence data of these parasites exist. They are believed to be more prevalent, however, than reported (at least 20% of dogs in the United States are believed to be infested).

Pathogenesis and Life Cycle

When ingested by a human, the egg hatches and the larva penetrates the upper gastrointestinal mucosa and either begins wandering erratically through the tissues or reaches the lung or liver via the venous system before doing so. A larva appears to rupture out of the vascular system whenever its size (14 to 20 μm in diameter) is too large to negotiate the vessel in which it is traveling. It cannot complete its maturation cycle and so continues to migrate through the tissues until the host encapsulates it. At first, there may be only a mild inflammatory response or an eosinophilic abscess formation about the parasite and its tunnels in the tissue. Eventually, a granuloma, with eosinophils, lymphocytes, plasma cells, and some giant cells, forms about the larva. The larvae have been identified most frequently in the liver but also in the lung, kidney, brain, heart, skeletal muscle, eye (ocular larva migrans), and other tissues.

A thick fibrous capsule forms around the larva. In this state it may remain viable with no significant change for several years. Under certain unknown circumstances, it appears to be capable of breaking out of the capsule to wander again. In pregnant bitches, this has led to transplacental infection of unborn puppies. In time, many of the encapsulated larvae will die and become hyalinized. The larva does not mature beyond the second (rhabdiform) stage and measures approximately 350 to 450 μm by 18 to 21 μm (*T. canis*) and 350 to 450 μm by 15 to 17 μm (*T. cati*). The eggs found in animal feces are spheroid, are dark brown, and have a rough outer shell surface. They measure 75 to 80 μm (*T. canis*) and 65 to 70 μm (*T. cati*).

Clinical Manifestations

The severity of the illness in visceral larva migrans (VLM) is determined in part by the number of fertile viable eggs ingested, the organ system targeted by the migrating larvae, and the immunologic status of the host. Obviously, multiple larvae could be encysted in the liver with minimal or no symptoms, whereas even a single larva in the brain or eye could be devastating. Infestation is probably underdiagnosed by a wide margin. Toxocariasis can manifest in a spectrum of ways (as discussed below), and a high index of suspicion is essential in making the diagnosis.

Asymptomatic Type. Mild constitutional symptoms may be present but apparently do not prompt a clinic visit. Until a skin test of sufficient sensitivity and specificity is available, the true prevalence of infestation cannot be assessed. The presence of eosinophilia is over 25% in diagnosed cases, and silent hepatomegaly occurs in some cases without systemic symptomatology.

Hepatopulmonary Type. This form involves primarily the liver and lungs but should be distinguished from migration of lung-phase nematodes (e.g., *A. lumbricoides*, hookworm, and *S. stercoralis*). The child may be mildly to severely ill. Typical findings include episodic fever to 40° C with night sweats, hepatomegaly, and pulmonary problems (wheezing, dyspnea, cough, and evidence of patchy pneumonitis or confluent pneumonia). Transient gastrointestinal disturbances that may be recurrent are anorexia, nausea, vomiting, and abdominal pain and distention. A variety of rashes has been described, but urticaria is the most common. Other common findings include marked leukocytosis with fluctuating eosinophilia (usually 20% to 90%), hypergammaglobulinemia, elevated isohemagglutinins, anemia, a positive test for blood in the stool and Charcot-Leyden crystals, and eosinophils in the sputum. Chest roentgenograms demonstrate the pulmonary infiltrates. No form of the parasite is found in the sputum or stool.

Generalized Type (VLM). When larvae migrate directly from the intestine or reach the left ventricle, they may then enter virtually any organ system, with subsequent development of corresponding clinical signs and symptoms. These include myalgias, arthralgias, subcutaneous nodules, loss of weight or failure to gain weight, myocarditis, neurologic dysfunction including grand mal or petit mal seizures, and nephritis.

Ocular Type (OLM). This form is most commonly found in persons over 4 years of age and is not associated with concomitant systemic manifestations or eosinophilia of any degree. In one series of 245 cases the average age was 7½ years old.[14] Sprent[12] listed 36 species of nematodes responsible for VLM in Australia. The most common cause in the United States is probably *T. canis*, since 20% of adult dogs and 98% of puppies in the United States are infected.[6] It presents as insidious or sudden impairment of vision in one eye. The ophthalmoscopic examination reveals a raised, rounded, or umbilicated granuloma frequently near the macula. If the larva protrudes into the vitreous, there may be serious inflammation farther anteriorly, carrying with it a high likelihood for impaired vision. This lesion is usually painless and must be distinguished from retinoblastoma. Ophthalmologic consultation is advised in questionable cases.

Diagnosis

A syndrome comprising prolonged hypereosinophilia, elevated isohemagglutinins and gamma globulins, hepatomegaly, intermittent fever, and episodic pulmonary symptoms should suggest the diagnosis. A history of pica, a pet dog or cat, and poor hygiene are corroborative. The diagnosis is confirmed by finding the causative agent in association with the disease site in biopsy or autopsy specimens. The use of a liver biopsy (preferably open) has been advocated by most experts, although these may be negative in the presence of the disease. A large number of tissue sections must be viewed, and it must be remembered that the larvae, because of their mobility, may be found away from areas of inflammation. Many serologic tests are hindered by cross-reactivity with other conditions, especially ascariasis and *Strongyloides*. The presence of negative serologic tests for *Toxocara* organisms should cause serious doubts about the diagnosis. Use of antigens prepared from the third-stage *Toxocara* or *Ascaris lumbricoides suum* larvae have proved to be superior to former test antigens prepared from the adult worms. The best test now used in the United States is a sensitive enzyme-linked immunosorbent assay (ELISA). This test, which is both sensitive and specific, is believed capable of distinguishing between VLM and ascariasis. A skin test is available but cross-reacts with other members of the family Ascaridae.

Treatment

No therapeutic agent has been uniformly successful in destroying the larvae and controlling symptoms. Great caution must be exercised in treating larvae in tissue because of potential damage from hypersensitivity and migration. Thiabendazole[10] and diethylcarbamazine have both been used with equivocal results. The Centers for Disease Control Parasitic Disease Drug Service* should be consulted for current recommendations.

The use of cortisone-type agents, especially in severe cases, apparently provides some symptom relief. Most cases improve after months to several years. It is probably important to break the continued exposure of the child by periodic worming or removal of pet animals from the home, by preventing pica, and by decontaminating potentially contaminated play areas by turning the soil under.

TRICHINOSIS

Epidemiology

Trichinella spiralis is a nematode that infests humans, pigs, rats, and a wide variety of other animals. Humans contract the disease by ingesting the encysted larvae in inadequately cooked meat (usually pork). Children are rarely infested and infants virtually never. The United States and Europe constitute the major endemic zones of transmission, although trichinosis has been found in the tropics. The prevalence of trichinosis in the United States, as determined by diaphragm histology subsequent to autopsy, has shown a marked decline in the last several decades.[15] Only 3% of those infested are believed to develop clinical disease. The fatality rate of cases in the United States reported to the Centers for Disease Control had fallen to less than 1% by the 1970s. Outbreaks have occurred secondary to ingestion of pork, bear, and walrus meat in North America. Except for cannibalism and instances in which humans become carrion for wild animals, humans are terminal hosts for *T. spiralis*.

Pathogenesis and Life Cycle

Larvae ingested in meat are released by the time the duodenum or upper jejunum is reached. The sexes mate, and the males apparently die shortly thereafter. The females either burrow into the mucosa or remain in the mucoid coating. About the third day after ingestion they begin depositing larvae at regular intervals (about 50 per day) until they die some weeks later. It is estimated that a single female can deposit more than 2000 larvae. These larvae reach muscle (striated and cardiac) via the lymphatic and later the vascular system. They burrow into muscle bundles and develop to a final length of 0.8 to 1 mm. Larvae that fail to reach the muscle, and some that do, die and are absorbed. However, some larvae are thought to remain viable in the muscle for 30 years or more.

Clinical Manifestations

Most infestations are light and produce minor or no symptoms. In heavier infestations, three phases may be recognized. Invasion of the upper gastrointestinal tract by the female worm may occasion anorexia, nausea, vomiting, diarrhea or constipation, and mild fever. These symptoms develop 2 to 12 days after ingesting the contaminated meat. Before the end of the second week, high fever, severe myalgias, edema (especially noticeable in the eyelids), and a striking eosino-

*Atlanta, GA 30333. Weekdays, telephone 404-329-3670; at night, on weekends, or on holidays, telephone 404-329-2888.

philia develop. The presence of inflammation in the brain, heart, kidneys, and lungs may cause serious signs related to those organs. These may occasion death about the fourth to sixth week, but if this phase is survived, convalescence is entered, with amelioration of symptoms over a period of weeks.

Diagnosis

The triad of myalgia, eosinophilia (20% to 90%), and edema of the eyelids in the presence of fever and a history of eating inadequately cooked meat is highly suggestive. If others who shared the food are ill with similar symptoms, the diagnosis is strengthened. Available serologic tests are numerous, but most provide a diagnosis late in the course of acute infection and lack adequate sensitivity or specificity. The bentonite flocculation test may be positive by the end of the first week of symptoms and currently is probably the best test, although the fluorescent antibody test and the counterimmunoelectrophoretic test using an antigen of the mature encysted larva are promising. A skin test that can be recommended for clinical use does not yet exist. A biopsy specimen, which provides the definitive diagnosis, is usually acquired from the deltoid biceps or gastrocnemius muscle. Fresh muscle should be examined after compressing it between two glass slides. Additional specimens can be processed by the usual fixation and staining or digested by using an aqueous solution of pepsin and hydrochloric acid. The larvae, if present, can then be readily identified.

Treatment

Treatment is primarily supportive, since only the very heavily infested cases are fatal. Although corticosteroids are effective in reducing symptoms, their safety may be questionable, since they appear to increase the number of larvae reaching the tissues. Analgesics are frequently necessary to control severe myalgia. Thiabendazole is the drug of choice and, if given early enough, may reduce symptomatology and presumably the extent of the infestation. Its effect on larvae that have reached the muscles is questionable. The dosage is 25 mg/kg given orally twice daily for 2 to 4 days. Prevention requires the cooking of meats to 65.5° C throughout before consumption by humans, enforcement of current laws requiring swill to be thoroughly cooked before it is fed to pigs, and rodent control on pig farms.

MALARIA

Epidemiology

Despite major worldwide efforts at controlling the spread of malaria, it is believed to remain the single greatest infestatious cause of morbidity and mortality in the world. A resurgence since 1965 in many countries can be attributed to a disruption of control programs and the debilitation of exposed populations. These have been brought on by war, famine, growing resistance of the agent and vector to chemicals, laws restricting use of chemicals, and decreased budgetary support for antimalarial campaigns. Even Turkey, the gateway to Europe, had 37,000 reported cases in 1976 compared with 1000 in 1970.

Malaria is prevalent throughout much of the developing world between 40° N and 45° S latitude. It is transmitted from person to person by the bite of female *Anopheles* mosquitos. More than 70 million live births occur annually in countries where malaria is endemic; most of those not living in a major metropolis will become infested within a few years. At least a million of these will die from the disease or its complications.

There is no test suitable for mass measurement of prevalence or incidence rates among the populations of endemic areas. One can, however, obtain a crude estimate of prevalence by extrapolation from the proportion of 2- to 9-year-olds who have splenomegaly. Likewise, a rough estimate of the incidence of transmission can be obtained from the percent of randomly selected infants whose blood smears reveal the parasite.

Four species of plasmodia infect humans (*Plasmodium falciparum*, *Plasmodium vivax*, *Plasmodium malariae*, and *Plasmodium ovale*). *P. falciparum* is the most dangerous; *P. vivax* is the most widely distributed; *P. malariae* is the least common, tending toward the cooler climes; and *P. ovale* is uncommon and largely found in Africa.

Pathogenesis and Life Cycle

When a female *Anopheles* mosquito feeds on a human who has circulating gametocytes (sexual stage malarial parasites), the male microgametes fertilize the female macrogametocyte to begin the sporogony phase. In 1 to 3 weeks the sporozoites (infestive stage) are found in the mosquito saliva and can enter the bloodstream of humans bitten subsequently. Each sporozoite enters a liver parenchymal cell (extraerythrocytic stage) and divides into thousands of tiny merozoites. The merozoites ultimately rupture the liver cell and enter the circulation, where they penetrate erythrocytes (erythrocytic stage) by a complex process that produces abnormalities on the RBC surface. Infested cells lose some of their ability to distort during passage through capillaries and become more vulnerable to osmotic change. They have an increased tendency to stick to vascular endothelium. These RBC changes appear related to the major symptoms and complications of malaria.

Clinical Manifestations

The type of plasmodia in the reservoir population, the seasonality or continuous nature of local transmission, the status of nutrition, the presence of concomitant illnesses, and the child's age are all major factors influencing the nature of the signs and the symptoms seen in childhood malaria. A mother who maintains a high rate of natural immunity through repeated exposure will pass some protection to the fetus. This passive immunity of the newborn disappears in several months to be followed by several years of high vulnerability unless the infant has received some active immunity through exposure while still protected by maternal antibodies.

Malaria in the first several years of life is apt to be manifested by general irritability, periodic fever, vomiting, diarrhea, respiratory symptoms, and poor appetite. The spleen and liver may be enlarged and tender. Drowsiness is common, especially during high fever. Cerebral malaria (usually P. *falciparum*) must be suspected if the patient is lethargic or comatose. Fatalities are most common with *P. falciparum* infestation and may be preceded by renal failure, cerebral ischemia countercurrent infection, or severe prostration with cardiovascular collapse.

Because of its release of massive numbers of merozoites from its one extra erythrocytic phase and its ability to attack all ages of RBCs, *P. falciparum* may rapidly be fatal in the nonimmune host. Inadequately treated *P. vivax* may recur for several years, since it can remain latent in liver cells, with "periodic bursts" into the circulation. Under favorable conditions *P. malariae* can reappear in the blood periodically for up to 40 years following a single infestation.

Diagnosis

Examination of a thick blood smear (Giemsa stained) is the most reliable method of confirming the diagnosis. In *P. falciparum* infestation the "ring" forms (early trophozoites) predominate in peripheral smears, and gametocytes appear later than in other species. Parasitemia rates of over 500,000/mm^3, as may be seen in *P. falciparum* infestation, are a grave sign. In partially treated or immune patients the parasitemia rates may be low, requiring repeated examination of blood smears. A thick blood smear is used to detect the malarial parasite, although identification of species can be done using a thin smear. Although specie-specific serologic tests are available, they only indicate that infestation has occurred at some time.

Treatment

No one drug meets all the requirements for malaria prophylaxis and treatment. The single most important aspect of managing malaria is early recognition and treatment of *P. falciparum* to prevent cerebral malaria, which can result in rapid death. Only *P. vivax* and *P. ovale* have potential for recurrent attacks after the initial circulating disease is treated, since these two species continue to release new crops of merozoites from infected liver cells. Persons traveling or living in areas of the world where *P. falciparum* is developing resistance to chloroquine must use additional drugs for prophylaxis and therapy. When a diagnosis of malaria is entertained, but the specie is unknown, treat for *P. falciparum* immediately and continue the diagnostic workup. Posttreatment recurrence of malaria suggests drug resistance or the presence of *P. vivax* or *P. ovale*. Drugs used in the management of malaria are given in Table 239-2. Consultation with the CDC is advisable when questions of drug resistance or adverse reactions are involved. (404) 488–4046 during daytime and (404) 639–2888 on nights, weekends, and holidays.

THE FETUS AND MATERNAL PARASITISM

When parasites invade a pregnant women, the attending physician must consider the effect of both the infection and its treatment on two patients, the mother and the fetus. The effects on the fetus may be direct (e.g., toxoplasmosis) or indirect through damage to the mother (e.g., hookworm anemia). Parasites may cause abortion (e.g., malaria, toxoplasmosis), or the immunosuppression seen in pregnancy may favor invasiveness of preexisting parasites (e.g., intestinal amebiasis). The placental barrier is remarkably effective in preventing transmission of some parasitic diseases (e.g., malaria) and fairly ineffective in stopping others (e.g., toxoplasmosis). The buildup of parasites capable of autoinoculation is a special threat to the pregnant woman, because her immune system may be somewhat less competent at this time. *S. stercoralis*, *H. nana*, and *Enterobius vermicularis* are all capable of autoinoculation.

One must weigh the risk of treating a parasitic infection against the risk of the parasite to both mother and fetus. Many intestinal helminths pose minimal risk when their numbers are not excessive during pregnancy. It may therefore be possible to postpone treatment until after delivery. Malaria (particularly that caused by *Plasmodium falciparum*), invasive amebiasis, trypanosomiasis (both African and American), and visceral leishmaniasis are more dangerous to the mother during pregnancy. These diseases, plus toxoplasmosis, are quite dangerous to the fetus. All except American trypanosomiasis should be treated expeditiously. Some therapeutic agents are not recommended, because adequate studies of the effect on the mother and/or fetus have not been done, even though for some no complications have been reported (e.g., niclosamide). Other agents are not recommended because they have been found to be mutagenic, teratogenic, or carcinogenic in one or more animals, despite no apparent harm having occurred in humans in whom they have been used (e.g., possibly metronidazole). Accordingly, the wise practitioner employs the agent in question only when a safer agent is not available and only when, after all factors considered, the risk of not treating is greater than the risk of treating.

In malaria, the risk of abortion, stillbirth, and neonatal death and the risk of recrudescences in the second half of pregnancy with maternal hypoglycemia, anemia, and renal impairment justify the use of standard agents (with the possible exception of Fansidar [a combination of sulfadoxine and pyrimethamine]) in nonimmune and semiimmune mothers. Chloroquine is generally considered safe in pregnancy after the first trimester—safe for prophylaxis in areas without chloroquine-resistant strains of *P. falciparum*. Mefloquine may be the safest alternative in areas of chloroquine resistance. Suppression of the disease is recommended in susceptible pregnant women during the second half of pregnancy. With symptomatic disease, blood schizontocidal drug treatment is indicated.

In amebiasis, emetine and its derivatives should not be used. Metronidazole may be required in invasive disease. The dose should be kept low (800 mg three times a day for 5 days). Patients who are passing cysts in their stools may be simply observed without treatment if reasonable monitoring is possible. Invasive disease should always be treated with a tissue amebicidal agent and an intraluminal agent such as iodoquinol, chloroquine, diloxanide furoate, or paromomycin.

Symptomatic giardiasis may not allow delay in treatment. In this case, metronidazole in low-dose regimens, as given for amebiasis, should be used. Palliative treatment should be tried before resorting to metronidazole, if possible.

Treatment of toxoplasmosis in the mother who has acquired the infection for the first time during the current pregnancy is essential. Determination of current infection in the fetus is difficult and depends on finding IgM antibody specific for *T. gondii* under circumstances that preclude contamination with maternal blood and laboratory artifacts and false positives resulting from antinuclear antibodies or rheumatoid fac-

Table 239-2 *Management of Malaria*

SPECIES	PREVENTION OF OVERT DISEASE		TREATMENT OF ACUTE MALARIA	ERADICATION OF EXTRA ERYTHROCYTIC STAGE
P. falciparum	Chloroquine phosphate (as below) plus Pyrimethamine/Sulfadoxine (3 tablets single dose if presumptive diagnosis made) OR Mefloquine 250 mg PO weekly × 4 wks, then every other week until 4 wks after exposure ends	Chloroquine-resistent strains	Quinine 650 mg TID × 3 da PO or parenteral plus Pyrimethamine 25 mg/BID × 3 da plus Sulfadiazine 500 mg/QID × 5 da OR Quinine plus	N/A
P. vivax	Chloroquine phosphate 5 mg/kg base (8.3 mg/kg salt) once weekly UP TO 300 mg base (500 mg salt) once weekly BEGINNING 1 wk before exposure and continuing 6 wks after exposure ends	Chloroquine-sensitive strains	*Orally* Chloroquine phosphate: 10 mg base/kg (max 600 mg base) 6 hr later: 5 mg base/kg (max 300 mg base) 24 hr after initial dose: 5 mg base/kg (max base) OR *Parenteral:* Quinine dihydrochloride: 600 mg in 300 ml normal saline IV over 2-4 hrs: Repeat every 8 hr until oral therapy can be started OR Quinidine gluconate: 10 mg/kg loading dose (max 600 mg) in normal saline slowly over 1 hr followed by continuous infusion of 0.02 mg/kg/min for 3 days OR Chloroquine phosphate: 200 mg base (250 mg salt) IM q 6 hr to max of 1.5 gm if oral therapy not possible	Primaquine phosphate 0.3 mg/kg/da × 14 da UP TO Maximum of 15 mg base (26.3 mg)/day × 14 days OR 45 mg base (79 mg)/wk × 8 wk as a single weekly dose
P. ovale *P. malariae*	Same as for *P. vivax*		Same as for *P. vivax*	N/A

tor. IgG transfers from mother to fetus readily, but should plateau after birth and show a tenfold decline every 3 months thereafter. Multiple repeated negative serologic tests cast doubt on the diagnosis. Isolation of the organism from fetal or infant tissues establishes the diagnosis but is a dangerous test to conduct in the laboratory.

REFERENCES

1. American Academy of Pediatrics: Report of the Committee on Infectious Diseases, ed 22, Elk Grove, Ill., 1991, The Academy.
2. Frankel JK: Toxoplasmosis in and around us, Biosci Rep 23:342, 1973.
3. Hopewell PC: Diagnosis of *Pneumocystis carinii* pneumonia, Infect Dis Clin North Am 2:409, 1988.
4. Israelski DM and Remington JS: Toxoplasmic encephalitis in patients with AIDS, Infect Dis Clin North Am 2:429, 1988.
5. Krugman S and Ward R: Infectious diseases of children and adults, St Louis, 1973, The CV Mosby Co.
6. Levine ND: Nematode parasites of domestic animals and of man, ed 2, Minneapolis, 1980, Burgess Publishing Co.
7. May JM: The ecology of human disease, New York, 1958, MD publications, Inc.
8. Naot Y, Desmonts G, and Remington JS: IgM enzyme-linked immunosorbent assay test for the diagnosis of congenital *Toxoplasma* infection, J Pediatr 92:32, 1981.
9. Naot Y, Guptil DR, and Remington JS: Duration of IgM antibodies to *Toxoplasma gondii* after acute acquired toxoplasmosis, J Infect Dis 145:770, 1982.
10. Nelson JD, McConnel TH, and Moore DV: Thiabendazole therapy of visceral larva migrans: a case report, Am J Trop Med Hyg 15:930, 1966.
11. Physicians' desk reference (PDR), ed 45, Oradell, NJ, 1991, Medical Economics Co, Inc.
12. Sprent JFA: Nematode larva migrans, NZ Vet J 117:39, 1969.
13. Swartzberg JE and Remington JS: Transmission of toxoplasmosis, Am J Dis Child 129:777, 1975.
14. Warren KS: Helminthic diseases endemic in the United States, Am J Trop Med Hyg 23:723, 1974.
15. Zimmerman WJ, Steel JH, and Kagan IG: Trichinosis in the US population, 1966-1970: prevalence and epidemiologic factors, Public Health Rep 88:606, 1973.

SUGGESTED READING

Warren KS and Mahmoud AAF: Tropical and geographical medicine, ed 2, New York, 1990, McGraw-Hill, Inc.

240

Pectus Excavatum and Pectus Carinatum

J. Alex Haller, Jr.

Significant chest wall deformities in children may cause physiologic, structural, and cosmetic problems that often require surgical correction. The most common abnormalities are pectus excavatum (funnel chest) and pectus carinatum (pigeon or chicken breast)(Figs. 240-1 and 240-2).

The cause of these chest deformities is unclear, but the primary defect is due to an overgrowth of the anterior costal cartilages. Such cartilaginous tissue, for some reason, appears to grow excessively and distorts the entire chest wall, either by fixing the sternum posteriorly (pectus excavatum) or by thrusting it anteriorly (pectus carinatum). Overgrowth of the ribs occurs in utero for pectus excavatum; therefore a sunken chest usually is noted at birth or shortly thereafter. Overgrowth in pectus carinatum usually occurs during the pubertal growth spurt; therefore this diagnosis most frequently is made in early adolescence. The cartilage in both conditions appears to be histologically normal.

The surgical repair of both these abnormalities involves

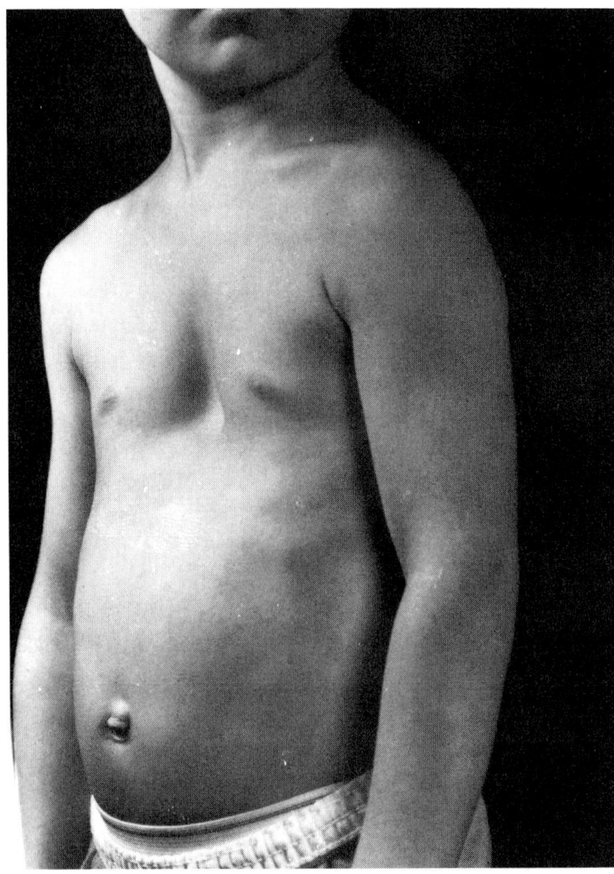

Fig. 240-1 Pectus excavatum.

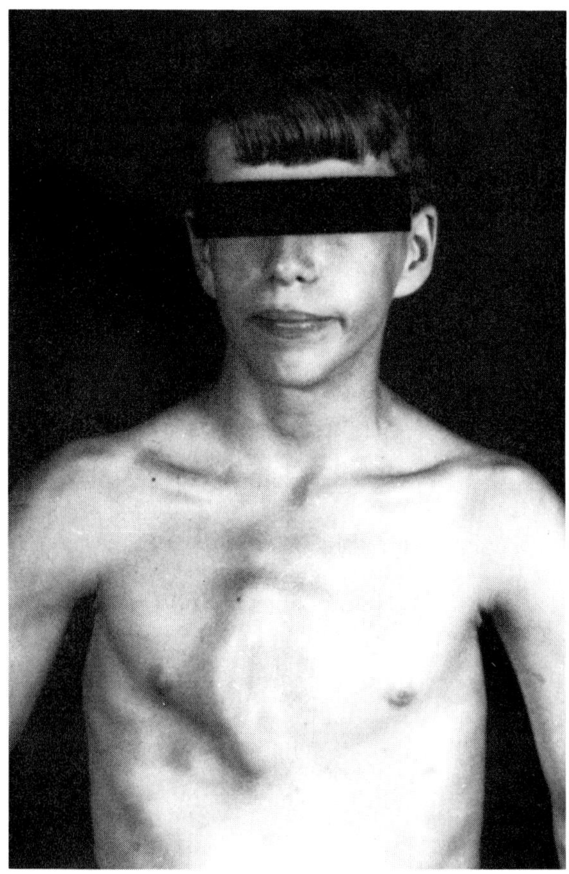

Fig. 240-2 Pectus carinatum.

removal of the overgrown rib cartilage, which allows the sternum to be repositioned.[4] The cartilage then regenerates from the remaining perichondrium. The chest wall is solidly healed and is fully stable after 6 to 8 weeks.

A major difficulty in assessing chest wall deformities in children is deciding which of them require surgical intervention. Unfortunately, there are no absolute criteria. It is important to evaluate each child frequently so as to monitor chest wall growth and development. Sequential evaluations include (1) measurement, with calipers, of the anteroposterior diameter of the chest and (2) determination of any limitation of central thoracic expansion, of abnormalities in posture, and of structural changes in the upper portion of the abdomen.

PECTUS EXCAVATUM

The majority of chest wall deformities seen by primary care physicians are some variation of pectus excavatum. If the deformity is severe, it should be repaired in early childhood for three important reasons: (1) chest wall growth and development will be abnormal if correction is not effected; (2) pulmonary and cardiac function will be adversely affected during adolescence, even though this may not be apparent during childhood; and (3) the cosmetic abnormality will be of increasing concern to the patient. A cosmetic concern is not the primary indication for repairing a pectus excavatum deformity because the structural deformity will always be significant enough in and of itself to require intervention.

Generally, with pectus excavatum a significant structural problem is considered to be present if the depression is greater than 2 cm. Such measurements, however, are not often absolute. By the time a child reaches 5 to 6 years of age, deformities severe enough to cause difficulties usually are obvious. Fortunately, this is early enough to alleviate cosmetic concerns, and the condition can be repaired before any significant psychological problems associated with the deformity occur.

Physiologic derangements in breathing and cardiac function can be documented in teenagers and young adults with severe deformities,[1,2] but such derangements are more difficult to demonstrate in children because of the invasiveness of the evaluative procedures.[3,7] In severe forms of pectus excavatum, the heart is shifted laterally in the left hemithorax, and thoracic compliance is compromised; these changes are reversible, however, if the repair is effected before adolescence. It is important to repair the pectus excavatum deformity before the teenage growth spurt if normal growth and development of the chest wall are to be achieved. Thereafter the deformity can be cosmetically corrected to a certain degree, but the basic abnormal chest wall configuration and posture will not be altered. The surgeon can employ some new plastic surgical procedures to fill the defect with prosthetic material and provide cosmetic correction, but these methods do not correct the physiologic and structural aberrations.

It is important to wait until a child reaches 5 to 6 years of age before performing elective repair of pectus excavatum, so that the child is more mature emotionally and thus can have a better hospital experience and, to some extent, can participate in the decision for surgical repair of the deformity. Even for young children, alterations in the configuration of the body may significantly affect their perceptions of their body image in later years. Postoperative management of 5- to 6-year-olds is far easier than that of 2- to 3-year-olds, and earlier repair has no technical surgical advantage.

The surgical correction has become standardized in most children's centers.[6,8] The operation is essentially bloodless when electric cautery is used, and blood transfusions are not needed. The operation, nevertheless, is major and requires 3 hours of anesthesia followed by considerable discomfort, which requires sedation and analgesia. Children recover within 48 hours and usually are discharged by the fifth or sixth day after surgery.

Surgery yields excellent results in more than 90% of patients.

Complications are extremely uncommon; they include (1) collection of serosanguineous fluid in the substernal and subcutaneous spaces, (2) infection, and (3) bleeding. None of these is life-threatening.

The only postoperative precaution necessary is avoidance of vigorous activities (including contact sports) for 6 to 8 weeks until the cartilages have all regenerated.

PECTUS CARINATUM

Pectus carinatum is much less common than is pectus excavatum, occurring in only 5% to 8% of all children with chest wall deformities. It also appears to result from abnormalities in growth of the involved costal cartilage, which pushes the sternum into an exaggerated anterior position.

Unlike pectus excavatum, which usually is noted in infancy, carinatum deformities occur during rapid pubertal growth. This abnormality is purely cosmetic and does not appear to be associated with any physiologic abnormality. Unlike pectus excavatum deformities, recurrence of pectus carinatum is likely after repair in early childhood because of subsequent chest wall growth in which the regenerated cartilage replicates the initial abnormal growth pattern. It is preferable therefore to wait until the patient is 15 or 16 years old, by which time maximal growth has occurred and the deformity can be corrected with little chance of recurrence. The surgical procedure for the correction of pectus carinatum requires removal of the abnormal costal cartilages and repositioning of the sternum posteriorly by means of a transverse osteotomy, which produces a greenstick fracture of the sternum.[5] Healing occurs within 6 to 8 weeks, after which the patient can participate in contact sports.

REFERENCES

1. Beiser GD et al: Impairment of cardiac function in patients with pectus excavatum, with improvement after operative correction, N Engl J Med 287:267, 1972.
2. Bevegard S: Postural circulatory changes at rest and during exercise in patients with funnel chest, with special reference to factors affecting the stroke volume, Acta Med Scand 171:695, 1962.

3. Cahill JL, Lees GM, and Robertson HT: A summary of preoperative and postoperative cardiorespiratory performance in patients undergoing pectus excavatum and carinatum repair, J Pediatr Surg 19:430, 1984.
4. Haller JA et al: Operative correction of pectus excavatum: an evolving perspective, Ann Surg 184:554, 1976.
5. Haller JA et al: Pectus carinatum: results of surgical therapy, J Pediatr Surg 14:228, 1979.
6. Haller JA et al: Evolving management of pectus excavatum based on a single institutional experience of 664 patients, Ann Surg 209:578, 1989.
7. Peterson RJ, Young WG, and Goodwin JD: Noninvasive assessment of exercise cardiac function before and after pectus excavatum repair, J Thorac Cardiovasc Surg 90:215, 1985.
8. Ravitch MM: Congenital deformities of the chest wall and their operative correction, Philadelphia, 1977, WB Saunders Co.

241

Periorbital and Orbital Edema

Carl A. Frankel

A sagittal section through the eyelids reveals an extension of the periorbita (periosteum of the orbit) known as the *orbital septum*. The orbital septum extends from the orbital rim to the lid margins and provides a natural resistance to the spread of most inflammatory processes to the opposite side of the septum. This anatomic barrier thus creates a natural separation in the discussion of edema into periorbital (preseptal) edema and orbital (postseptal) edema.

PERIORBITAL (PRESEPTAL) EDEMA

As defined by the orbital septum, periorbital edema is limited to the eyelids, although there is, in reality, a continuum between preseptal and postseptal processes. The etiology of periorbital edema is diverse and comprises both systemic and local causes (Table 241-1).

The most common source of nontraumatic periorbital edema is periorbital cellulitis (Fig. 241-1). Occasionally an insect bite or puncture wound may be found to be the origin of this localized infection, but usually no proximate cause is found. Periorbital cellulitis typically occurs with a 12- to 24-hour history of increasing swelling, ptosis, erythema, and edema that is localized to the eyelids. The area is warm to the touch and usually nontender. Early on, the patient may be uncomfortable but rarely shows toxicity. Left untreated, periorbital cellulitis will progress rapidly to orbital cellulitis with possible meningitis, cavernous sinus thrombosis, and death. The most likely organisms associated with periorbital cellulitis are *Staphylococcus, Streptococcus, Haemophilus influenzae* type b, and *Pneumococcus*. Appropriate antibiotics should be chosen.

Periorbital cellulitis is treated by either enteral or parenteral antibiotics, depending on the clinical appearance and age of the child. Surface and blood cultures are not indicated in this disease. Because of the rapidity with which toxicity develops in children younger than 3 years of age, hospitalization of these patients should be considered, with treatment with intravenous antibiotics.

Periorbital cellulitis in a patient in whom toxicity does not appear to have developed can be managed with outpatient care, consisting of antipyretics, enteral antibiotics, and daily follow-up examinations until significant improvement is noted. Antibiotics should be used for a minimum of 10 days. The condition of these patients may worsen 12 to 24 hours after initiation of antibiotics, but in the absence of toxicity, undue alarm (and hospitalization) is unnecessary and rapid improvement should ensue. No clinical sequelae are to be anticipated with appropriately treated preseptal cellulitis.

ORBITAL EDEMA

Orbital edema originates from inflammation, hemorrhage (secondary to trauma), or cellular infiltration, with the most common cause being trauma. All types of orbital edema are characterized by the presence of proptosis and depending on the degree and cause of orbital involvement, diplopia (because of secondary strabismus), exposure keratitis (resulting from

Table 241-1 *Periorbital Edema*

CAUSE	TREATMENT
Trauma	Provide local care, with ice for first 24 hours, then warm compresses. Elevate head to reduce edema. May require ophthalmologic examination if vision and/or ocular motility is disturbed.
Infection	
Preseptal	Administer enteral antibiotics if mild and intravenous antibiotics if patient becomes "toxic" or worsens on enteral therapy. Consider broad-spectrum topical antibiotic therapy (sulfacetamide sodium 10% ophthalmic solution) with mild edema believed to be reactive, as opposed to true preseptal cellulitis.
Conjunctivitis	Culture discharge, and begin topical therapy with erythromycin or polymyxin B/bacitracin, pending results of culture if lid edema is significant.
Dermatitis	
Allergic	Provide symptomatic care, antihistamines.
Poisonous plants	Provide symptomatic care: diphenhydramine, systemic steroids for severe cases.
Sunburn	Provide symptomatic care: systemic steroids for severe cases.
Systemic disease	
Nephrotic syndrome	Manage systemic disease.
Congestive heart failure	Manage systemic disease.
Infectious mononucleosis	Observe.

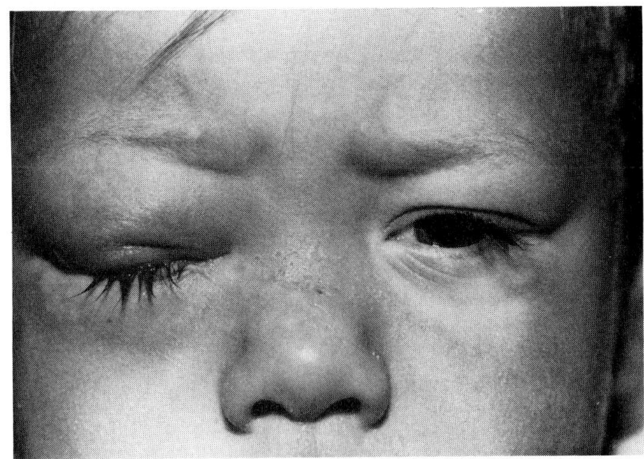

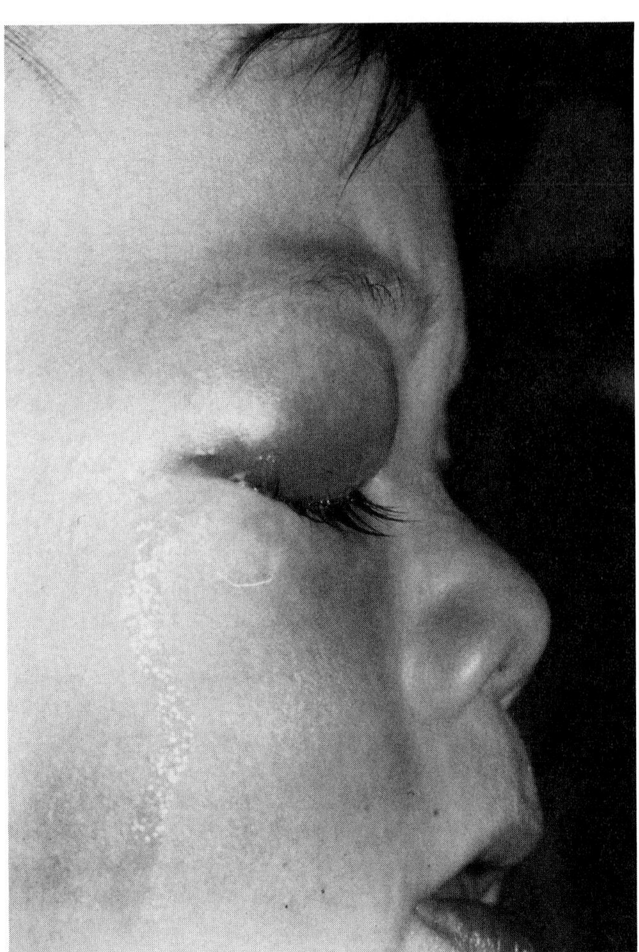

Fig. 241-1 A, Frontal view of a patient with bacterial preseptal cellulitis. When the lid was elevated, no evidence of pain on, or restriction of, motility was noted. The patient's condition readily resolved with systemic antibiotics.
B, Lateral view of the same patient shown in *A*. Note the significant lid edema, however; when the lid was elevated, no evidence of proptosis was noted.

an inability to close the lids over the cornea), pain, or limitation of motion of the globe, optic nerve compression, and visual loss.

Orbital Cellulitis

Orbital inflammation because of infection is the most common form of orbital edema and usually *is due to spread from adjacent paranasal sinusitis*. Children with orbital cellulitis typically have *proptosis, moderate to severe lid edema, and ptosis* (Fig. 241-2, *A*). When the lid is elevated, the eye typically is deviated with respect to the fellow eye (Fig. 241-2, *B*). While the patient's lid is elevated, the patient may report diplopia, pain on attempted eye movement, or an inability to move the globe; visual acuity may be significantly reduced. When visual acuity is reduced, optic nerve compression is present and aggressive management must ensue to prevent visual loss. These patients usually appear acutely ill and almost always have fever, with a leukocytosis with left shift. Blood cultures should be obtained because bacteremia or septicemia may be present.

Patients with orbital cellulitis should be hospitalized and placed on a regimen of broad-spectrum, age-appropriate, intravenous antibiotics. An ophthalmologist should be consulted to follow and manage potential ophthalmologic complications; otorhinolaryngology consultation should be obtained if sinus disease is suspected or documented. Axial computed tomography (CT) scanning should be performed, with contiguous cuts of 3 to 4 ml through the orbits to assess the degree of orbital involvement (contrast enhancement usually is not necessary). If the patient's ocular involvement is not severe (as indicated by normal retinal vasculature and an absent afferent pupillary defect on the swinging flashlight test), the patient should initially be observed, even if CT scanning reveals an orbital subperiosteal abscess. The abscess should be drained only if the patient's condition worsens in spite of appropriate antibiotic therapy. Reliable correlation has not been shown between orbital subperiosteal abscesses as suspected by CT scanning and the actual clinical findings at the time of surgical drainage.[1,2]

The condition of patients with orbital cellulitis may worsen for the first 24 hours; thereafter they usually improve dramatically. Intravenous antibiotics should be continued until the patient is afebrile for 24 hours; oral antibiotics should then be substituted. If the patient remains free of fever for 24 hours on an oral antibiotic regimen, discharge from the hospital is reasonable, with oral antibiotics continued so that the patient receives antibiotics for 3 weeks.

Hyperthyroidism

The second most common cause of proptosis in children is Graves ophthalmopathy (Fig. 241-3) associated with hyperthyroidism, although the ophthalmopathy is likely an autoim-

A 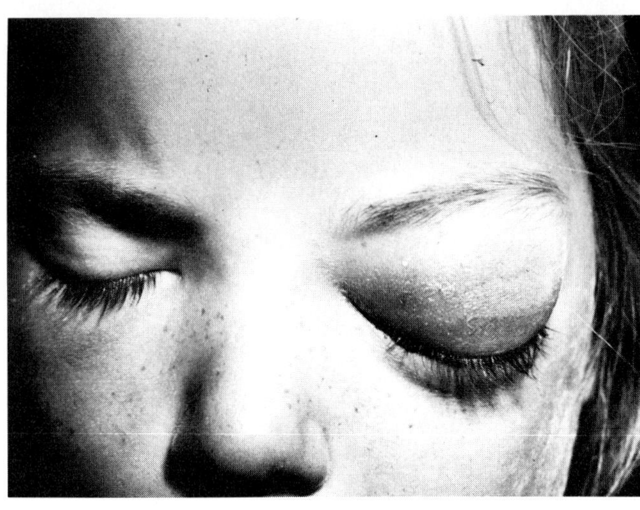

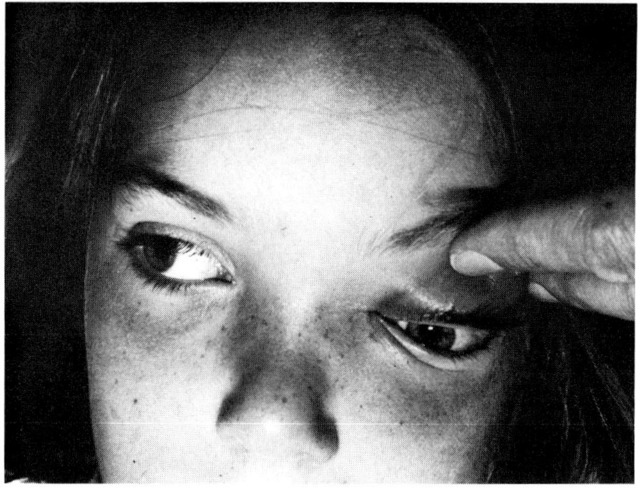 B

Fig. 241-2 A, Photograph of a school girl presenting with severe periorbital inflammatory edema with a suggestion of inferior displacement of the globe. **B,** Photograph of the same patient shown in *A*. On elevation of the eyelid, proptosis and limitation of movement of the eye were noted. These patients also may complain of pain on attempted eye movement and may have decreased vision due to optic nerve compression.

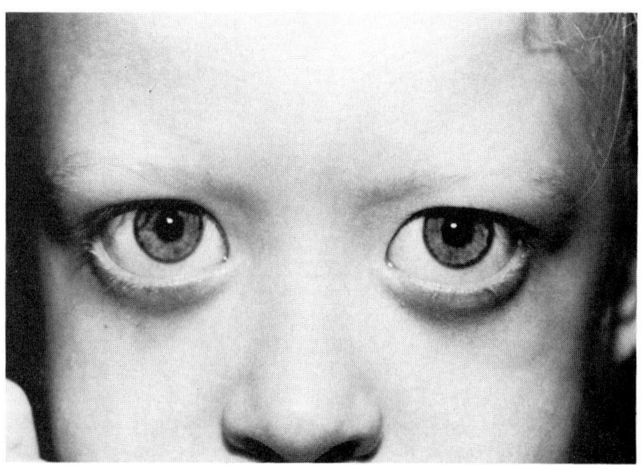

Fig. 241-3 Proptosis and lower lid retraction in a patient with Grave's ophthalmopathy secondary to hyperthyroidism.

mune phenomenon distinct from the thyroid disease. The extraocular muscles are involved with edema, lymphoid infiltration, and necrosis of muscle fibers, with increased orbital volume leading to proptosis. The progression of Graves ophthalmopathy is not as fulminant in children as in adults. Of the children affected, 80% are between 10 and 15 years of age, with girls affected approximately five to six times more frequently than boys. If the proptosis is progressing to produce corneal exposure (because of an inability to close the lids), orbital decompression should be considered.

Orbital Trauma

The third most common cause of orbital edema is secondary to trauma and is discussed in the section on orbital hemorrhage in Chapter 235. In the absence of compromise of the eye, symptomatic treatment usually is all that is needed; resolution tends to be rapid and complete, unless the ocular injury is more extensive than originally recognized. Evaluation by an ophthalmologist is recommended; a suspicion of child abuse must, unfortunately, always be entertained.

Other Causes of Orbital Edema

The presence of proptosis in the absence of orbital trauma or infection encompasses a diverse differential diagnosis of possible causes, almost all of which are highly unusual. When a patient has orbital edema that is either atypical or nonresponsive to the usual treatment of orbital edema, the physician must consider other causes of proptosis (see box below).

Differential Diagnosis of Proptosis in Children

Orbital cellulitis
Hyperthyroidism
Trauma
Craniostenosis
Histiocytosis X (especially Hand-Schüller-Christian disease)
Leukemia
Cavernous hemangioma
Neuroblastoma
Orbital sarcoma
Chloroma
Optic nerve glioma
Hypertelorism
Dermoid/epidermoid tumor
Sturge-Weber syndrome
Idiopathic inflammatory orbital pseudotumor
Glaucoma (with secondary buphthalmos)
Rhabdomyosarcoma

Extremely Rare Causes of Proptosis in Children

Ethmoid mucocele
Chronic granuloma
Rickets
Fibrous dysplasia
Infantile cortical hyperostosis
Melanoma
Lacrimal gland tumor
Teratoma
Lymphosarcoma
Nasopharyngeal carcinoma
Ethmoid sarcoma
Retinoblastoma
Neurofibromatosis
Carotid-cavernous fistula
Hemophilia
Subdural hematoma
Orbital myositis
Meningioma

Extremely rare causes of proptosis are listed in the box above.

The presence of orbital edema should prompt an evaluation of the patient by the ophthalmologist, although ultimately treatment may be rendered by another specialist (e.g., otorhinolaryngologist or neurosurgeon). Only under unusual circumstances should a biopsy specimen of orbital tissue be obtained without an ophthalmologic consultation.

SUMMARY

Periorbital and orbital edema are not two distinct entities; rather they are merely two ends of a continuum. Keeping these thoughts in mind will allow for more appropriate diagnostic and therapeutic intervention and optimal outcome.

REFERENCES

1. Rubin SE et al: Medical management of orbital subperiosteal abscess in children, J Pediatr Ophthalmol Strabismus 26:21, 1989.
2. Tannenbaum M et al: Medical management of orbital abscess, Surv Ophthalmol 30:211, 1985.

SUGGESTED READINGS

Brook I et al: Complications of sinusitis in children, Pediatrics 66:568, 1980.

Chandler JR, Langenbrunner DJ, and Stevens ER: The pathogenesis of orbital complications in acute sinusitis, Laryngoscope 80:1414, 1970.

Eustis HS et al: Staging of orbital cellulitis in children: computerized tomography characteristics and treatment guidelines, J Pediatr Ophthalmol Strabismus 23:246, 1986.

Gold SC, Arigg PG, and Hedges TR III: Computerized tomography in the management of acute orbital cellulitis, Ophthalmic Surg 18:753, 1987.

Goldberg F, Berne AS, and Oski FA: Differentiation of orbital cellulitis from preseptal cellulitis by computed tomography, Pediatrics 62:1000, 1978.

Goodwin WJ Jr, Weinshall M, and Chandler JR: The role of high resolution computerized tomography and standardized ultrasound in the evaluation of orbital cellulitis, Laryngoscope 92:728, 1982.

Haik BG and Ellsworth RM: Pediatric orbital tumors, pediatric ophthalmology and strabismus. In Transactions of the New Orleans Academy of Ophthalmology, New York, 1986, Raven Press.

Hammerschlag SB, Hesselink Jr, and Weber AL: Computerized tomography of the eye and orbit, East Norwalk, Conn, 1983, Appleton-Century-Crofts.

Harr DL, Quencer RM, and Abrams GW: Computed tomography and ultrasound in the evaluation of orbital infection and pseudotumor, Radiology 142:395, 1982.

Hirst LW, Thomas JV, and Green WR: Periocular infections. In Mandell GC, Douglsa RG Jr, and Bennett JE, editors: Principles and practice of infectious diseases, ed 2, New York, 1985, John Wiley & Sons, Inc.

Kaban LB and McGill T: Orbital cellulitis of dental origin: differential diagnosis and the use of computed tomography as a diagnostic aid, J Oral Surg 35:682, 1980.

Krohel GB, Krauss HR, and Winnick J: Orbital abscess: presentation, diagnosis, therapy, and sequelae, Ophthalmology 89:492, 1982.

Macy JI, Mandelbau SH, and Minckler DS: Orbital cellulitis, Ophthalmology 87:1309, 1980.

Moloney JR, Badham NJ, and McRae A: The acute orbit. Preseptal (periorbital) cellulitis, subperiosteal abscess and orbital cellulitis due to sinusitis, J Laryngol Otol Suppl 12:1, 1987.

Morgan PR and Morrison WV: Complications of frontal and ethmoid sinusitis, Laryngoscope 90:661, 1980.

Mottow LS and Jakobiec FA: Idiopathic inflammatory orbital pseudotumor in childhood. I. Clinical characteristics, Arch Ophthalmol 96:1410, 1978.

Rubinstein JR and Handler SD: Orbital and periorbital cellulitis in children, Head Neck Surg 5:15, 1982.

Schramm VL, Myer EN, and Kennerdell JS: Orbital complications of acute sinusitis, evaluation, management, and outcome, Trans Am Acad Ophthalmol Otolaryngol 86:221, 1978.

Teele DW: Management of the child with a red and swollen eye, Pediatr Infect Dis 2:258, 1983.

Watters EC et al: Acute orbital cellulitis, Ophthalmology 94:785, 1976.

Weiss A et al: Bacterial periorbital and orbital cellulitis in childhood, Ophthalmology 90:195, 1983.

242

Pertussis (Whooping Cough)

Fred J. Heldrich

Few illnesses have such a characteristic clinical picture as does pertussis. At the height of the illness, the harsh, persistent cough occurring in paroxysms and ending with an inspiratory whoop and vomiting certainly suggests pertussis as the most probable diagnosis. Although undoubtedly a disease of antiquity, pertussis was first described in 1906 by Bordet and Gengou, who associated it with the *Bordetella pertussis* organism. Although pertussis is one of the communicable diseases of childhood that can be prevented with proper immunization, it nonetheless still occurs, usually in preschool-age children. It has been well documented that a recent decline in levels of pertussis immunization has led to an increased incidence in pertussis in several countries, including the United States,[2,3,10] where the annual incidence rose from 0.82 per 100,000 population in 1982 to 1.74 per 100,000 in 1986.[5]

ETIOLOGY

B. pertussis, a motile gram-negative rod, is the etiologic agent in most cases. A special medium (Bordet-Gengou) and special care in obtaining the specimen of this fastidious organism are required to obtain a positive culture. Either coughing directly onto the culture media or inoculating the medium directly from a nasopharyngeal swab gives the best results. Of the two methods, the nasopharyngeal culture is preferred, especially for younger patients. A more sensitive and rapid diagnostic procedure available is the direct fluorescent antibody (DFA) test, which increases the ability to get laboratory confirmation.[2,3]

PATHOLOGY

The area of involvement is the respiratory epithelium, extending from the upper respiratory tract to the trachea, bronchi, and bronchioles. Histologically, the organisms are lodged in the cilia of the epithelial cells, with underlying epithelial cell changes consisting of edema and necrosis; there is also infiltration of the interstitial tissues by inflammatory cells. A mucopurulent exudate, which may cover the respiratory epithelium, can lead to airflow obstruction. Alveolar exudate is thought to be caused by secondary bacterial invasion. The ability of pertussis to elaborate an endotoxin may be responsible for lymphocytic predominance in the peripheral blood count, local tissue damage, and hypoglycemia.

CLINICAL PICTURE

Typically the child with pertussis will progress through three stages, characterized by varying symptoms and clinical severity: the catarrhal stage, the acute stage, and the stage of convalescence. Each stage lasts approximately 2 weeks. The illness may extend longer than the usual 6 weeks, especially the acute stage. In such instances, other causes of persistent cough should be seriously considered and sought.

The incubation period is from 7 to 14 days, with an average of 10 days. The illness is ushered in with symptoms of a "cold"—sneezing, rhinitis, lacrimation, and cough. The cough soon becomes more pronounced than is customary with the usual cold and becomes a dominant feature by the end of the first week. Fever, if present, is low grade. Systemic, nonspecific symptoms of malaise and anorexia are also seen. Unless exposure to pertussis is known, it shouldn't be seriously considered until the second week of illness or until the cough has become more persistent and annoying. The cough occurs in bursts or paroxysms and has been described as harsh, dry, irritating, and rapid. It accompanies the expiratory phase of respiration and may be especially prominent at night, disturbing the child's (and the parents') sleep. When these bursts of explosive coughing increase in frequency and are followed by an exaggerated inspiratory effort or "whoop," the acute, or paroxysmal, stage has begun.

When coughing is of this magnitude, the patient also shows signs of respiratory distress. The face becomes suffused and red or cyanotic. Neck veins become more prominent, and the child becomes alarmed and anxious. The face appears swollen, the eyes prominent. The tongue may protrude, and perspiration is prominent. The child vomits thick, tenacious material, appearing to be "strangling." Facial petechiae, conjunctival hemorrhage, and epistaxis may occur because of the severe coughing episodes. Paroxysms may last 10 to 15 seconds, and following these episodes the child is frequently exhausted and obtunded. The frequency of these paroxysmal outbursts may range from several per day to several per hour and may be precipitated by eating or drinking. External stimuli such as smoke, examination of the pharynx, or pressure on the trachea also may precipitate the attack.

In younger patients the inspiratory whoops may be absent; however, these patients are at risk for developing respiratory arrest and may require resuscitation.

After approximately 2 weeks of severe distress (by the

fourth week of illness) symptoms begin to abate; the vomiting and whoop clear first. By the sixth week the cough usually has diminished markedly and, barring complications, the patient is well on the way to recovery. After recovery the patient may experience bouts of paroxysmal coughing, with further episodes of respiratory tract infection for the next few months or longer.[7]

Partial immunity provided by inadequate primary immunization or a prolonged interval since immunization, leading to a deficiency in immunologic protection, may produce an atypical or attenuated form of illness characterized primarily by a persistent cough.

The physical examination in patients with uncomplicated pertussis may reveal, in addition to signs of upper respiratory tract infection, a low-grade fever and on auscultation of the lungs, rhonchi.

LABORATORY FINDINGS

Success in culturing *B. pertussis* from the nasopharynx is greatest in the prodromal stage of the illness. A cotton swab wrapped on an aluminum wire allows easy access to the nasopharynx. Positive growth of the organism on a Bordet-Gengou plate should occur in 3 days; it can be identified by the use of specific antiserums to produce agglutination. Serologic diagnosis of pertussis is most readily accomplished by the DFA test or by the enzyme-linked immunosorbent assay (ELISA).[3,8]

The most distinctive, though nonspecific, finding is a marked leukocytosis, with over 50% of the cells being lymphocytes. When associated with a cough, a total white blood count greater than 20,000 strongly suggests pertussis. The total white count may rise as high as 100,000, of which 90% may be lymphocytes.

Acute and convalescent serums may be compared and should demonstrate a rise in pertussis antibody titers; this test, however, is most useful for a retrospective assessment of the illness. Ten to 14 days should elapse between the collection of specimens.

COMPLICATIONS

Death from pertussis, although extremely rare today, is most likely to occur in affected infants. Permanent damage to the lung may lead to bronchiectasis. Bronchopneumonia, usually resulting from secondary invaders, is the most common complication. Although petechiae or purpura, subconjunctival lesions, or epistaxis may occur secondary to the increase in venous pressure associated with the paroxysmal cough, intracranial hemorrhage is a more ominous complication. Inguinal hernias and rectal prolapse have also been reported.

DIFFERENTIAL DIAGNOSIS

Conditions to be considered and ruled out by history, physical examination, and appropriate laboratory studies are chlamydial pneumonia, those conditions caused by other infectious agents, foreign body aspiration, paratracheal lymph node enlargement, and allergic cough. Although not an extensive list, these conditions share a common feature—a persistent, irritating cough.

Chlamydial Pneumonia

Frequently found in infants, chlamydial pneumonia is characterized by a dry, staccato-like cough and a chest roentgenogram that reveals pneumonic infiltrates. Patients are usually afebrile. Eosinophilia may be noted on the peripheral smear. Chlamydiae can be grown on tissue culture from respiratory tract secretions. A serologic study reveals an elevated antibody titer.

Other Infectious Agents

The adenovirus has been associated with a clinical syndrome indistinguishable from pertussis. Organisms that may produce an illness similar to pertussis include *Mycoplasma pneumoniae, Bordetella parapertussis,* and *Bordetella bronchiseptica*. Marked lymphocytosis is usually not found.

Foreign Body Aspiration

Although there is not always a history of aspiration, a definite choking episode usually ushers in this condition. Localized changes may appear on the chest roentgenogram secondary to obstruction, or the foreign body may be radiopaque and easily visualized.

Paratracheal Lymph Nodes

If paratracheal lymph nodes are enlarged, diseases such as tuberculosis, histoplasmosis, infectious mononucleosis, or malignancies of the reticuloendothelial system must be considered.

Allergic Cough

In the allergic individual, a persistent, irritating cough may be the earliest manifestation of bronchospasm. A family history of allergy or a history of allergic manifestations in the patient should strengthen the diagnostic suspicion. Upper respiratory tract symptoms, such as clear nasal discharge, sneezing, conjunctivitis, or "allergic shiners," may also be suggestive. Frequently the serum IgE level will be elevated. A therapeutic trial with a bronchodilator will relieve symptoms and thus confirm the diagnosis.

TREATMENT

Supportive care is the mainstay of therapy for the acute phase of pertussis. The patient should be disturbed as little as possible. The paroxysms of coughing, especially in younger patients, may necessitate the removal of secretions via aspiration. Hypoxia, as manifested by cyanosis, may indicate a need for oxygen. Optimum hydration and adequate nutrition can usually be maintained by frequent but small feedings. In infants, intravenous fluid therapy may be required. Antibiotics have not been found useful in ameliorating the symptoms of the disease, but they have been shown to reduce the period during which *B. pertussis* can be recovered from the respiratory tract. Erythromycin is the antibiotic of choice.

A human immunoglobulin is available (passive immunization) for attempts to ameliorate the severity of the symptoms. However, controlled studies have failed to confirm its effectiveness.

Fortunately, a vaccine is available for active immunization and, when administered at appropriate intervals, affords excellent protection. Routine immunization procedures call for pertussis vaccination—usually combined with diphtheria and tetanus (DPT)—at 2 months, 4 months, and 6 months of age.[9] In the event of a community outbreak, immunization may be started at 2 weeks of age. Graduates of intensive care nurseries who had chronic pulmonary disease are at great risk of significant morbidity or mortality should they develop pertussis. For these infants, pertussis immunization should be initiated when they are 2 months old, even while in the hospital.[6]

The risk of complications secondary to routine use of pertussis vaccine has recently been reevaluated, and the benefits with proper use of the vaccine outweigh the risks; thus its continued use is warranted.[4] Trials are presently under way evaluating the efficacy of acellular pertussis vaccines for future use. These vaccines promise to reduce vaccine side effects and produce effective immunity.[1]

Complications of the disease require specific therapy. Antibiotics should be prescribed for secondary bacterial infections such as pneumonia or otitis media. Bronchial aspiration may be required to relieve segmental atelectasis. Pneumothorax secondary to obstructive emphysema caused by tenacious secretions in the bronchial tree may necessitate the use of closed-tube drainage. Patients may develop seizures because of tetany precipitated by alkalosis, which is caused by severe vomiting. Correction of blood pH abnormalities is indicated. Direct damage to the central nervous system by anoxia or hemorrhage may occur and requires anticonvulsant medication.

Although the prognosis for those few patients who acquire the infection is good, the treatment is not specific. The proper management is prevention, and this can be accomplished by adhering to recommended immunization schedules.

REFERENCES

1. Aoyama T: Efficacy and immunogenicity of acellular pertussis vaccine by manufacturer and patient age, Am J Dis Child 143:655, 1989.
2. Broome CV and Fraser DW: Pertussis in the United States, 1979: a look at vaccine efficacy, J Infect Dis 144:187, 1981.
3. Centers for Disease Control: Pertussis—Maryland, 1982, MMWR 32:297, 1983.
4. Cody CL et al: Nature and rates of adverse reactions associated with DPT and DT immunizations in infants and children, Pediatrics 68:650, 1981.
5. Fulginiti VA: The current state of pertussis and pertussis vaccines, Am J Dis Child 143:532, 1989.
6. Koblen BA et al: Response of preterm infants to diphtheria-tetanus-pertussis vaccine, Pediatr Infect Dis J 7:704, 1988.
7. Krugman S and Katz SL, editors: Pertussis (whooping cough). In Infectious diseases of children, ed 8, St Louis, 1985, The CV Mosby Co.
8. Mertsola J et al: Serologic diagnosis of pertussis: comparison of enzyme linked immunosorbent assay and bacterial agglutination, J Infect Dis 147:252, 1983.
9. Report of the Committee on Infectious Diseases (Red Book), ed 21, Evanston, Ill, 1988, American Academy of Pediatrics.
10. Robinson RJ: The whooping cough immunization controversy, Arch Dis Child 56:577, 1981.

243

Pharyngitis and Tonsillitis

Mark D. Widome

According to the National Ambulatory Medical Care Survey (1985), the diagnosis of acute pharyngitis by the office-based pediatrician is surpassed in frequency only by that of otitis media and undifferentiated upper respiratory tract infection.

Throat infection usually involves the tonsils to a greater or lesser extent. Where tonsillar involvement is prominent, the term tonsillitis applies. Cherry[5] has chosen to divide throat infection into tonsillopharyngitis and nasopharyngitis, pointing out that the latter usually is of viral etiology. Although pharyngitis tends to be an acute infectious illness, it may at times run a subacute or chronic course or may be caused by noninfectious agents, such as an ingested or inhaled irritant.

EPIDEMIOLOGY

Glezen et al[8] analyzed the experience of two private pediatric practices in Chapel Hill, North Carolina, and found that a third of the cases of pharyngitis were diagnosed in 6- to 8-year-old children. This is also the age range in which group A beta-hemolytic streptococcus (GABHS) is most likely to be the etiologic organism (Fig. 243-1). The frequency of cases in which GABHS is cultured depends on the patient's age, the time of year, and the physician's criteria for performing a culture. In primary school–aged children with acute pharyngitis, cultures of throat specimens of 25% to 50% may be expected to be positive for GABHS, whereas a viral cause occurs more frequently among preschoolers.[8] GABHS is distinctly uncommon in those younger than 2 years of age, accounting for only 3% or 4% of all cases of pharyngitis (Fig. 243-1).

Breese and co-workers[3] found GABHS throat infections to predominate in the months from December to May (in upstate New York), with a peak in March. Respiratory viruses responsible for pharyngitis are seen throughout the cold months, although enterovirus is most frequently seen in the summer and fall. The common etiologic agents generally are spread by respiratory particles and contaminated hands. Food-borne outbreaks of streptococcal disease can occur, however, with inadequate refrigeration after contamination by food handlers.

ETIOLOGY AND SYMPTOMS

Bacteria

Streptococcus pyogenes. The bacterium *Streptococcus pyogenes* accounts for perhaps one third of all pharyngitis (Fig. 243-2).[18] It assumes clinical importance primarily because of its nonsuppurative complications (rheumatic fever and acute glomerulonephritis).

Streptococci may be categorized by their ability to cause hemolysis when cultured on sheep's blood agar; colonies of *S. pyogenes* are surrounded by a clear zone of complete hemolysis (beta-hemolysis). Beta-hemolytic streptococci are divided into groups A through D, based on the C-substance carbohydrate in the cell wall. GABHS causes virtually all disease and may be conveniently differentiated from other groups by inhibition of its growth on agar by a bacitracin disk; less than 7.5% of the other groups ("non–group A") show such bacitracin sensitivity.[1,2]

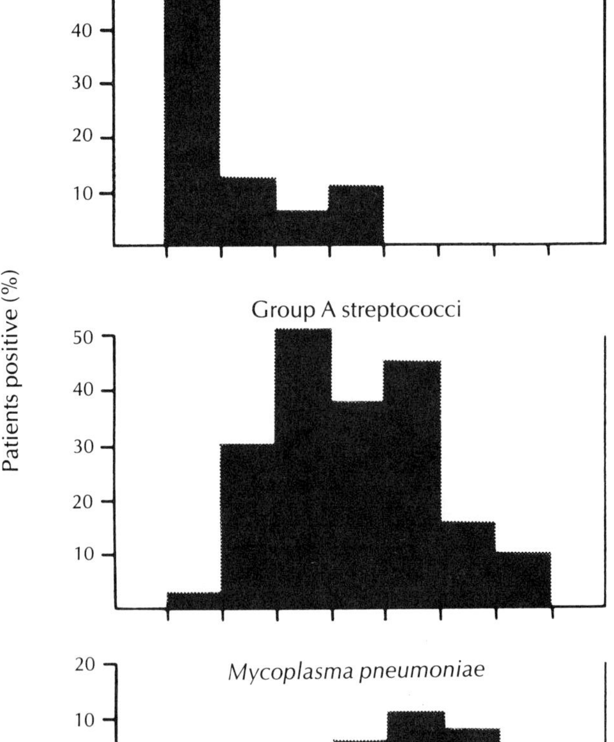

Fig. 243-1 Recovery of microbial agents from persons with pharyngitis, by age.

From Glezen WP et al: Group A streptococci, mycoplasmas, and viruses associated with acute pharyngitis, JAMA 202:457, 1967.

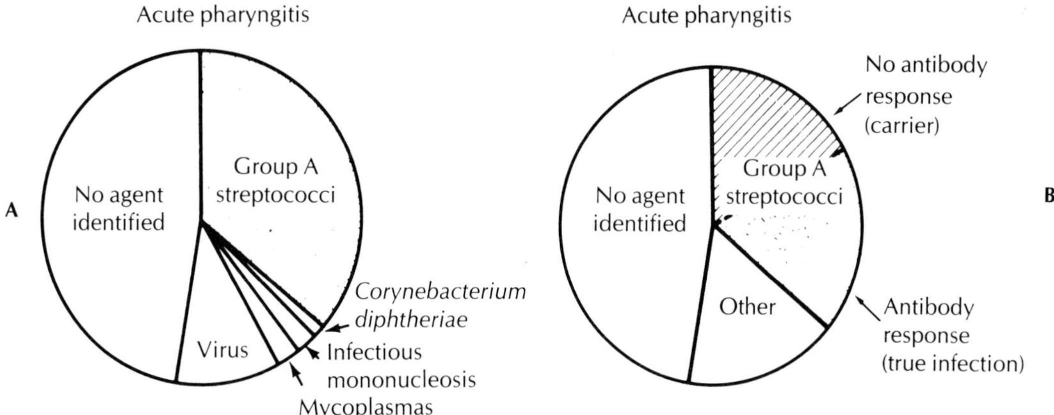

Fig. 243-2 A, Proportion of acute pharyngitis associated with various microbial agents. **B,** Proportion of children with clinical pharyngitis who develop a streptococcal antibody response.

From Wannamaker LW: Perplexity and precision in the diagnosis of streptococcal pharyngitis, Am J Dis Child 124:353, 354. Copyright 1972, American Medical Association.

The GABHS may be divided into approximately 70 distinct M protein types, based on surface antigens. Virulence and likelihood of antibody response depend on the presence and amount of M protein. In recent years an increasing proportion of GABHS has proved to be nontypable and of low virulence.[1]

After a 2- to 5-day incubation period, a GABHS throat infection is characterized by the relatively abrupt onset of pain, dysphagia, and fever, often associated with headache, nausea, and abdominal discomfort, but without nasal symptoms. The pharynx appears red, and exudate often is seen on the tonsils. Cervical lymph nodes are most often tender. The systemic manifestations of streptococcal disease are the result of extracellular toxins released by the organism, such as streptolysin O, hyaluronidase, and deoxyribonuclease B. These are particularly useful in documenting a previous GABHS infection, inasmuch as each of them induces a measurable antibody response. Another extracellular product, erythrogenic toxin, results from the action of a bacteriophage on certain strains of the GABHS and causes the rash and other toxic manifestations of scarlet fever.

Fever, malaise, sore throat, and rash, when present, typically last 4 days. With or without antibiotic treatment, symptoms subside. In the absence of treatment, however, GABHS remains in the throat, and antibody response to the extracellular products (e.g., ASO antibody titer) occurs.

Neisseria gonorrhoeae. Pharyngitis is one of the several extragenital manifestations of gonorrhea and may mimic streptococcal pharyngitis or run a subacute course. The diagnosis should be considered in sexually active adolescents or in younger children who may have been sexually abused. Throat cultures should be planted on Thayer-Martin or a similar medium.

Corynebacterium diphtheriae. Although infrequent, outbreaks of diphtheria are likely to occur among unimmunized, low socioeconomic groups.[19] Crowding and suboptimal hygiene may contribute to the spread of illness. The illness has a gradual onset, consisting of nasal discharge, sore throat, low-grade fever, tachycardia, and nausea with vomiting. Exudate and, eventually, a pseudomembrane appear on the surface of the tonsils and the oropharynx. Depending on the degree of the individual's immunity, the disease may remain mild or may progress to a more serious phase, characterized by marked cervical adenitis, laryngeal involvement, palatal and pharyngeal paralysis, myocarditis and peripheral neuritis, and toxemia. Prompt treatment with antitoxin should begin when the disease is suspected. Penicillin or erythromycin will eliminate this organism as well as GABHS, which often is a coinvader, but is no substitute for antitoxin therapy.

Haemophilus influenzae Type B. Pharyngitis is a poorly recognized manifestation of *Haemophilus influenzae* infection, possibly because of the often rapidly invasive nature of the disease in the preschool-aged group. Walker[17] found that 75% of children with *Haemophilus* bacteremia or meningitis had a diffusely erythematous pharyngitis.

Viruses

A wide range of nonbacterial agents may cause pharyngitis. Moffet et al.[13] were able to isolate viruses in 37% of a group of children with nonstreptococcal pharyngitis. Specific viruses occasionally can be suspected on the basis of clinical presentation, although most often they appear in a nonspecific way. Viral pharyngitis typically is gradual in onset, often with nasal symptoms, low-grade fever, and minimal to moderate toxicity. The more commonly encountered viruses and some distinct clinical presentations follow.

Adenoviruses. Adenovirus is the most common cause of nonstreptococcal pharyngitis. In their review of nonstreptococcal pharyngitis, Moffet et al.[13] recovered adenovirus from 23% of cases. Adenoviruses can cause either a nasopharyngitis or exudative tonsillitis that is indistinguishable from streptococcal pharyngitis and tonsillitis. *Pharyngoconjunctival fever* is a clinically distinct illness caused by adenovirus type 3. A sore throat is accompanied by high fever, by nonpurulent conjunctivitis, which may be unilateral, and by cervical lymphadenopathy.

Enteroviruses. Acute respiratory illness associated with pharyngitis is caused by the coxsackievirus and echovirus, most prevalent during the late summer and early fall. *Herpangina* is a distinct clinical syndrome attributable to several coxsackieviruses, group A.[15] There is a sudden onset of fever, sore throat, dysphagia, and vomiting. Small vesicles that rupture and ulcerate appear on the soft palate, tonsils, and pharynx. The ulcers are pale gray, are several millimeters in diameter, and have a surrounding erythema. The illness may be sporadic or epidemic and lasts 4 to 6 days.

Lymphonodular pharyngitis is a similar coxsackievirus illness in which white-yellow nodules appear on the tonsils and the posterior pharynx. These lesions are not vesicular and do not ulcerate.

Epstein-Barr Virus. Pharyngitis occurs in 85% of patients with *infectious mononucleosis*.[16] An exudative pharyngitis develops in approximately 33% of patients. Older children present the more classic clinical picture of high fever, adenopathy, malaise, headache, anorexia, and chills. Petechiae on the soft palate, which in combination with exudative pharyngitis, mimics streptococcal pharyngitis develop in 50% of these patients (see Chapter 218).

Mycoplasma pneumoniae. *Mycoplasma pneumoniae*, most commonly associated with pneumonia in the adolescent and young adult, frequently causes nonpulmonary symptoms when it occurs in the school-aged child. Although mycoplasmas are uncommon among preschoolers, 5% of pharyngitis in the 6- to 19-year old age-group may be attributable to this agent. Only when nonexudative pharyngitis accompanied by fever, headache, and malaise progresses to cough and pneumonia, particularly in the older child, should mycoplasma be suspected.

Candida albicans. *Candida albicans* should be suspected in cases of exudative pharyngitis in the immunocompromised patient or in the child whose normal throat flora has been disrupted by antibiotic treatment.

Kawasaki Disease. Kawasaki disease, an illness of uncertain cause, occurs primarily in preschool children; its incidence then declines up to 10 years of age. A diffusely erythematous pharynx is associated with other oral findings, including "strawberry tongue" and erythema with fissuring of the lips. In addition to fever unresponsive to antibiotics, the most characteristic feature of the illness is induration of the hands and feet, with palmar erythema and eventual desquamation (see Chapter 222).

DIFFERENTIAL DIAGNOSIS

The determination of the cause of pharyngitis depends on the clinical presentation, epidemiologic considerations, and selective use of the clinical laboratory. Viral throat infections occur year round and are the more likely diagnoses among preschool children and those with nasal symptoms.[3] Streptococcal infection should be considered in the child older than age 2 years who has pharyngitis with or without exudate in the absence of a cold. It is more common in the winter months. Exudate should suggest streptococci, Epstein-Barr virus (infectious mononucleosis), or, occasionally, adenovirus infection. Soft palate petechiae are seen in both infectious mononucleosis and GABHS infection. Vesicles or ulcers on the pillars and posterior fauces should suggest enterovirus. Ulcers anteriorly, with marked adenopathy, suggest herpesvirus.

Influenza and parainfluenza cause erythema without exudate or ulcers. With evidence of lower respiratory tract disease, parainfluenza and mycoplasmas are both likely. Splenomegaly or rash should suggest infectious mononucleosis.

Tracheitis may manifest as a "sore throat," although prominent cough and absence of objective signs of pharyngitis indicate that the soreness is not in the pharynx. Postnasal drip from viral upper respiratory tract infection, allergy, or sinusitis also may cause a sore throat without pharyngitis.

Epiglottitis causes severe sore throat and dysphagia. The rapid onset of symptoms, with evident toxicity and respiratory distress, usually indicates the nature of the illness (see Chapters 168, 269, and 276).

LABORATORY PROCEDURES

Culture

Pharyngitis with or without exudate in the absence of cold symptoms may result from GABHS, adenovirus, Epstein-Barr virus, or other agents. Because of substantial overlap in symptoms (Fig. 243-3), diagnosis of GABHS pharyngitis on clinical grounds alone is unreliable; thus a throat culture or "screen" (see below) should be performed whenever this diagnosis is considered.[8]

Culture specimens obtained with a cotton swab are plated on commercially available 5% sheep's blood agar. The swabbed plate is streaked with a wire loop, which then is stabbed into the agar in several spots to determine subsurface hemolysis. The plate is incubated at 96.8° F (36° C) for 24 hours and observed for characteristic white-gray colonies 1 mm in diameter and surrounded by a broad clear zone of

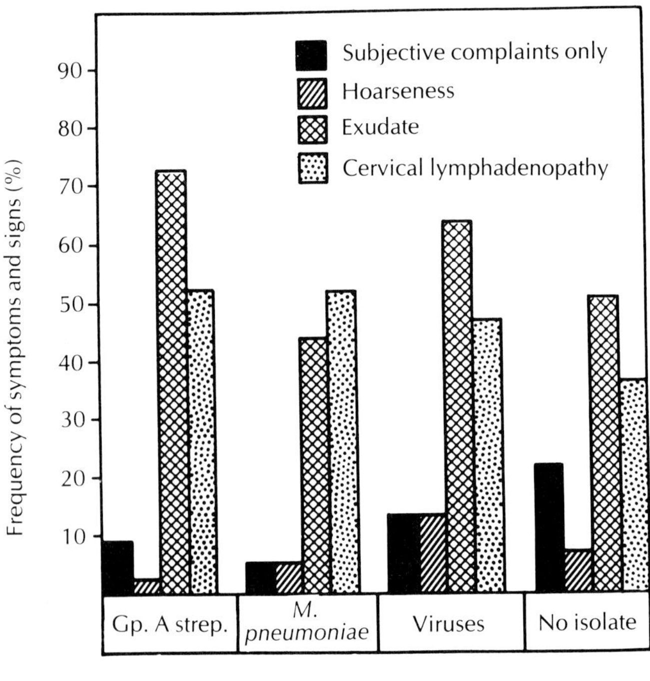

Fig. 243-3 Occurrence of clinical manifestations of pharyngitis in persons yielding microbial agents.

From Glezen WP et al: Group A streptococci, mycoplasmas, and viruses associated with acute pharyngitis, JAMA 202:458, 1967.

hemolysis. Additional diagnostic precision may be achieved by placing a bacitracin disk on the agar. The colonies are presumptively GABHS if their growth is inhibited by this antibiotic. Although the culture findings of most children with GABHS pharyngitis show strong positivity, treatment is instituted by most clinicians when 25% or more of colonies present on the plate are GABHS.

Recovery of GABHS from the throat does not necessarily indicate that it is the cause of infection. As shown in Fig. 241-2, 50% of the "apparent" cases of GABHS pharyngitis are not associated with an antibody rise, suggesting the presence of a different etiologic agent with coincident carriage of GABHS.[18]

Rapid Streptococcal Identification Tests

In the late 1970s, methods were developed to detect the presence of group A streptococci from throat swabs before a culture was obtained.[10] Today a variety of commercial tests are available for office use. Streptococcal antigens are extracted from the throat swab either chemically or enzymatically. Group-specific polysaccharides from the streptococcal cell wall are then detected by agglutination of latex particles or by equivalent techniques. The tests are attractive in that they can permit identification of infection and antibiotic decision-making all in one visit. The rapid tests generally have a better specificity than sensitivity (95% versus 85% to 90%). It appears that they are least sensitive in detecting patients whose throat cultures have the fewest organisms. These patients with false-negative results are sometimes carriers, but a significant percentage have true infection as indicated by a rise in convalescent titers.[7] Therefore most authorities currently recommend that when results of the rapid screen are negative, a culture be obtained from a clinically suspect patient.

Other Serologic Tests

The heterophil antibody test frequently is employed to diagnose suspected infectious mononucleosis. Antibodies are found in greater than 80% of young adults with the clinical diagnosis but far less frequently in children. A positive heterophil antibody test result is uncommon in the preschool child. A number of rapid slide heterophil antibody tests are commercially available.

Documentation of past streptococcal disease is possible by detecting antibodies of the various streptococcal enzymes (e.g., streptolysin O, streptokinase, hyaluronidase). Antibodies to these enzymes are found in almost all cases of untreated streptococcal disease and in 90% of cases of rheumatic fever and acute glomerulonephritis caused by GABHS.

White Blood Count

Blood counts have little diagnostic value in distinguishing among the causes of pharyngitis unless infectious mononucleosis is suspected. Patients with infectious mononucleosis have a relative and absolute lymphocytosis, with 10% to 20% atypical forms having a basophilic, vacuolated, and foamy cytoplasm (Downey cells).

MANAGEMENT

In children, early antibiotic treatment of GABHS pharyngitis has the potential to shorten the duration and severity of symptoms.[12] In addition, it eliminates the streptococci from the pharynx and prevents a rise in the titers of the streptococcal antibodies. The primary rationale for detection and treatment of a GABHS throat infection is to prevent the subsequent development of rheumatic fever. Secondary benefits include prevention of suppurative complications, symptomatic relief, and prevention of the spread of illness to contacts. There is no convincing evidence that treatment affects the incidence or severity of acute glomerulonephritis.

Generally, in the absence of a positive rapid screening test result for streptococci, antibiotic treatment can await the results of the throat culture. Rheumatic fever can be prevented if treatment is started as late as the ninth day of symptoms. The decision to treat with antibiotics before culture results depends on individual circumstances. For example, the physician might be prompted to do so in the light of classic findings and if there is concern that the patient will not return for treatment.

Intramuscular benzathine penicillin G may be given as a single injection in doses of 600,000 units for children weighing less than 60 pounds, 900,000 units for children weighing 60 to 90 pounds, and 1.2 million units for children and adults weighing more than 90 pounds. Preparations that contain additional procaine penicillin are no more effective but are less painful.

Alternatively, oral potassium penicillin V may be given in dosages of 250 mg, 3 or 4 times a day for 10 full days for children weighing more than 10 kg; those less than 10 kg may be given half that dosage. The disadvantage of oral treatment is that even in the middle-class private-practice setting, nearly 50% of children have been shown to be noncompliant with a 10-day course of treatment.[4]

Patients allergic to penicillin may be given erythromycin, 30 to 50 mg/kg/day in divided doses for 10 days.

Routine follow-up cultures after therapy generally are unnecessary. Bacteriologic treatment failures with or without clinical relapse occur in as many as 25% of individuals.[6] Although treatment failures may result from poor compliance with taking oral medication or reinfection from household or other close contacts, many are believed to be evidence of the carrier state. Carriers may be defined as individuals in whom colonization but not infection with GABHS has occurred. Neither an antibody response nor a risk of rheumatic fever development occurs. Likewise, their condition is considered relatively noncontagious. Recently, antimicrobial tolerance and the coexistence in the pharynx of beta-lactamase–producing bacteria have been postulated as explanations for true treatment failures.[6] With clinical relapse a second course of treatment should be given, and specimen cultures of family members may be indicated. With repeated relapse, or persistent failure to eradicate streptococci from the throat, recent evidence[11] indicates that a beta-lactamase–resistant antibiotic might be effective.[11]

Pharyngitis proved to be caused by *N. gonorrhoeae* can be treated with ceftriaxone as a single intramuscular injection (125 mg for children weighing less than 45 kg, 250 mg for adults). Amoxicillin plus probenecid may be used as an alternative therapy. Follow-up of contacts is always indicated, and consideration of sexual abuse is essential.

The course of viral pharyngitis is not affected by antibiotics, and their use has not been shown to be effective in preventing secondary bacterial infection. Acetaminophen may be used to treat discomfort from pain or fever. Aspirin is best not used for symptomatic treatment of respiratory illness in children because of its association with Reye syndrome. Gargles are of no antiseptic value but may ease discomfort.

Tonsillectomy does not reduce the overall incidence of undifferentiated upper respiratory tract infections but may reduce the incidence of GABHS throat infection and certainly prevents tonsillitis.[15] Possible benefits must be weighed against the risks of surgery and anesthesia.

COMPLICATIONS

Rheumatic fever and acute glomerulonephritis are late complications of streptococcal infection and are related to a rise in streptococcal antibodies. The incidence of rheumatic fever has dropped dramatically over recent decades until the mid-1980s, when multiple centers throughout the United States began reporting an as-yet unexplained increase in the disease.[9] Of particular concern is the observation that many of the patients in the current outbreaks have no recent history of symptomatic respiratory infection.

Suppurative complications of streptococcal pharyngitis and tonsillitis can include cervical adenitis, sinusitis, otitis media, and pneumonia. Direct extension of the infection also may occasionally cause retropharyngeal or paratonsillar abscess. Hematogenous spread of the organism can result in bone or joint infection or meningitis.

REFERENCES

1. Breese BB: Beta-hemolytic streptococcus, its bacteriologic culture and character, Am J Dis Child 132:502, 1978.
2. Breese BB and Disney FA: The accuracy of diagnosis of beta-streptococcal infections on clinical grounds, J Pediatr 44:670, 1954.
3. Breese BB, Disney FA, and Talpey W: The nature of a small pediatric group practice, Pediatrics 38:264, 1966.
4. Charney E et al: How well do patients take oral penicillin? A collaborative study in private practice, Pediatrics 40:188, 1967.
5. Cherry JD: Pharyngitis. In Feigin RD and Cherry JD, editors: Textbook of pediatric infectious disease, ed 2, Philadelphia, 1987, WB Saunders Co.
6. Denny FW: Current problems in managing streptococcal pharyngitis, J Pediatr 111:797, 1987.
7. Gerber MA et al: Antigen detection test for streptococcal pharyngitis: evaluation of sensitivity with respect to true infections, J Pediatr 108:654, 1986.
8. Glezen WP et al: Group A streptococci, mycoplasmas and viruses associated with acute pharyngitis, JAMA 202:455, 1967.
9. Kaplan EL: Return of rheumatic fever: consequences, implications, and needs, J Pediatr 111:244, 1987 (editorial).
10. Kaplan EL: The rapid identification of group A beta-hemolytic streptococci in the upper respiratory tract, Pediatr Clin North Am 35:535, 1988.
11. Kaplan EL and Johnson DR: Eradication of group A streptococci from the upper respiratory tract by amoxicillin with clavulanate after oral penicillin V treatment failure, J Pediatr 113:400, 1988.
12. Krober MS, Bass JW, and Michels GN: Streptococcal pharyngitis: placebo-controlled double-blind evaluation of clinical response to penicillin therapy, JAMA 253:1271, 1985.
13. Moffet HL, Siegel AC, and Doyle HK: Non-streptococcal pharyngitis, J Pediatr 73:51, 1968.
14. Paradise JL et al: Efficacy of tonsillectomy for recurrent throat infection in severely affected children: results of parallel randomized and nonrandomized clinical trials, N Engl J Med 310:674, 1984.
15. Parrott RH et al: Clinical and laboratory differentiation between herpangina and infectious (herpetic) gingivostomatitis, Pediatrics 14:122, 1954.
16. Rapp C and Hewetson J: Infectious mononucleosis and the Epstein-Barr virus, Am J Dis Child 132:78, 1978.
17. Walker SH: The respiratory manifestations of systemic *Hemophilus influenzae*, J Pediatr 62:386, 1963.
18. Wannamaker LW: Perplexity and precision in the diagnosis of streptococcal pharyngitis, Am J Dis Child 124:352, 1972.
19. Zalma VM, Older JJ, and Brooks GF: The Austin, Texas diphtheria outbreak: clinical and epidemiologic aspects, JAMA 211:2125, 1970.

244

Phimosis

Dennis M. Super

Phimosis (derived from the Greek word for muzzling) occurs when the tip of the foreskin becomes scarred (Fig. 244-1). This scarred foreskin loses is suppleness and can no longer be retracted over the glans penis. The incidence of phimosis in uncircumcised males ranges from 2% to 10%. The signs and symptoms of a child with a scarred, unretractable foreskin are dysuria, hematuria, poor urinary stream, and foreskin tenderness. If the tip of the foreskin is severely scarred and if the opening of the foreskin is stenotic, the child will develop ballooning of his foreskin during urination. If the stenosis progresses, the child will develop hydronephrosis and renal failure from the atretic opening of the foreskin.

The actual cause of a scarred, unretractable foreskin is unknown. Some of the proposed theories for the etiology of phimosis are trauma from forcible retraction of the foreskin, irritation from soiled diapers, improperly performed circumcision, congenital anomalies, and recurrent infection of the foreskin.

Not all children who have unretractable foreskins have phimosis. Almost 96% of male neonates have foreskins that cannot be retracted over their glans. These infants do not have phimosis because their foreskins are still supple. The difficulty in retracting their foreskin is caused by adhesions between the foreskin and the glans. These adhesions are actually remnants of the tissue plane that normally bridges the area between the foreskin and the glans. By the time these children are 3 years of age, 90% of them will have enough of a disappearance of this tissue plane to permit the retraction of their foreskin.[2] If these adhesions are prematurely lysed, the foreskin may become scarred and phimotic.

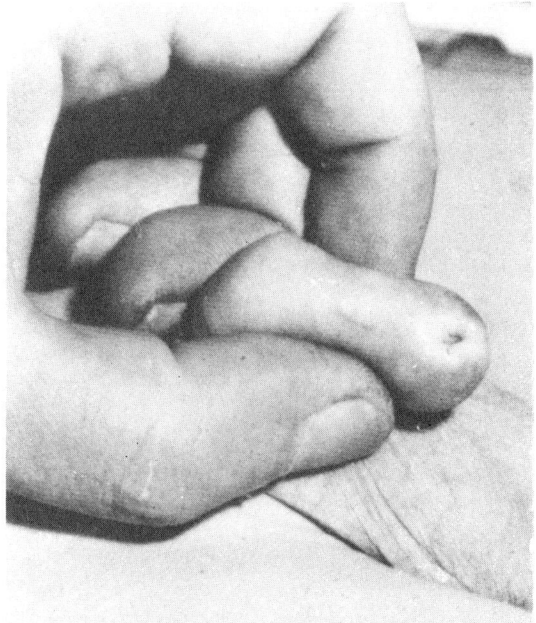

Fig. 244-1 In phimosis the tip of the foreskin is whitish, scarred, and stenotic.

From Rickwood AMK et al: Phimosis in boys, Br J Urol 52:147, 1980.

DIFFERENTIAL DIAGNOSIS

Balanoposthitis

Balanoposthitis is an inflammation of the glans (balano) and the foreskin (posthe). This inflammation begins when a few drops of urine remain trapped between the foreskin and glans. Also trapped in this area is a cheesy substance called smegma, which is composed of desquamated epithelial cells and the secretions of sebaceous glands. In this intertriginous area the trapped moisture and smegma begin to macerate the delicate surfaces of the glans and the foreskin. If proper foreskin hygiene is not maintained, the moist, macerated skin will become infected. The foreskin and the glans may be tender, warm, erythematous, edematous, and suppurative. The child may suffer from dysuria and urinary frequency, and he may be febrile. Some of the organisms that can cause this secondary infection are *Staphylococcus aureus*, groups A and D streptococci, coliforms, *Pseudomonas aeruginosa*, *Candida albicans*, and *Trichomonas vaginalis*.

Children with recurrent balanoposthitis or with phimosis secondary to balanoposthitis may have diabetes mellitus. The glucose in the diabetic child's urine enhances the chance for secondary infections in this intertriginous space. In their retrospective review, Cates and co-workers[1] reported that their adult patients who had recent onset of phimosis secondary to balanoposthitis had a tenfold increase in the prevalence of diabetes mellitus over the general population. Almost 20% of these patients were previously undiagnosed diabetics.

Another type of balanoposthitis that may lead to phimosis is balanitis xerotica obliterans. This type of balanoposthitis is a chronic inflammation of the foreskin and glans. It begins as an erythematous lesion and eventually forms a thickened white plaque that may erode into the urethral meatus. These lesions histologically resemble lichen sclerosus et atrophicus, and there is some evidence linking balanitis xerotica obliterans with squamous cell carcinoma of the penis. Balanitis xerotica obliterans was previously thought to occur only in adults, until Rickwood and co-workers[4] published a prospective review of phimosis in children. In this study they found histologic evidence of balanitis xerotica obliterans in 20 of 21 phimotic foreskins. Except for the phimosis, the preoperative physical examination of the glans and the foreskin was normal in all of their patients except one, who had a lesion that may have involved the meatus.

Paraphimosis

Paraphimosis is a condition in which a snugly fitting foreskin or a foreskin with a partially scarred tip is retracted over the glans and becomes trapped behind it. This incarcerated foreskin begins to obstruct venous return from the tip of the penis, which results in further edema and ischemia. This condition resulted in 0.9% of all childhood admissions per year to the Royal Victoria Infirmary, which serves an area of London in which 88% of the males are uncircumcised.[2] Paraphimosis is a medical emergency because with each passing minute, the amount of edema and the degree of ischemia increase. If the incarcerated foreskin is not released soon, paraphimosis can lead to necrosis of the tip of the penis.

MANAGEMENT AND NEONATAL CIRCUMCISION

The treatment for phimosis is circumcision.

In balanoposthitis, a wet mount preparation, a potassium hydroxide preparation, and a Gram stain of the exudate may help determine which organism is causing the infection. Because of the association of balanoposthitis and diabetes mellitus, children with balanoposthitis should also be tested for diabetes mellitus by either a urinalysis or a glucose tolerance test.

The treatment for balanoposthitis consists of elevation of the penis and warm soaks to the glans. Broad-spectrum systemic antibiotics may be needed if the infection is severe. If the KOH preparation contains hyphae and budding, the treatment would also include topical nystatin for *C. albicans*. The patient should be treated with metronidazole (Flagyl) if the wet mount preparation or urinalysis contains *T. vaginalis*.

Untreated balanoposthitis can cause severe edema, resulting in an ischemic glans. A dorsal slit of the foreskin will reduce this strangulation of the glans. After the edema and the ischemia have resolved, the slitted foreskin can be electively removed by performing a circumcision. Circumcision can also prevent recurrent episodes of balanoposthitis in children who cannot maintain proper penile hygiene.

The treatment of balanitis xerotica obliterans is circumcision, especially if the patient presents with phimosis. The treatment of penile lesions is surgical removal. If removal of the lesion is impractical, the treatment is topical or intralesional corticosteroids.[4]

In paraphimosis the trapped foreskin is released in an anesthetized patient by applying outward traction on the foreskin while pushing on the glans. Another method that is very successful in reducing paraphimosis is the iced-glove technique. In this method, the foreskin is lubricated and anesthetized by applying lidocaine jelly to the foreskin for 2 minutes. The foreskin is retracted, and the glans is placed in the thumbhole of a glove filled with ice water. The glove is pushed down the shaft of the penis until it rests on the symphysis pubis. The glove is held in place for about 5 minutes or until the edema is reduced. Finally, the constricting foreskin is slipped over the glans. If the above two techiques fail, the strangulation of the tip of the penis can be relieved by making a dorsal slit in the foreskin. After the acute episode has resolved, the child should be circumcised to prevent the recurrence of paraphimosis.[3]

REFERENCES

1. Cates JL, Finestone A, and Bogash M: Phimosis and diabetes mellitus, J Urol 110:406, 1973.
2. Gairdner D: The fate of the foreskin: a study of circumcision, Br Med J 2:1433, 1949.
3. Houghton GR: The "iced-glove" method of treatment of paraphimosis, Br J Surg 60:876, 1973.
4. Rickwood AMK et al: Phimosis in boys, Br J Urol 52:147, 1980.

245

Pinworm Infestations

Donald A. Goldmann and Craig M. Wilson

ETIOLOGY

Pinworm *(Enterobius vermicularis)* infestation is exceptionally common. When looked for carefully, the parasite can be found in at least 30% of children worldwide, and infestation rates may approach 100% in boarding schools and institutions. Good sanitation and advanced socioeconomic status are feeble deterrents to pinworms. Adults frequently are infested—in one study, 31% of army recruits were found to be infested—and it is not uncommon to find pinworms in all members of a family. The discovery of *Enterobius* eggs in human corpolites from the Hogup and Danger caves in Utah (10,000 BC) proves that the parasite was no stranger to our ancestors.

E. vermicularis is a white, threadlike worm, 1 cm in diameter, that resides primarily in the cecum and adjacent bowel. The gravid female migrates to the perianal area to deposit her eggs and dies shortly thereafter. Thus the infestation would be self-limited were it not for reinfestation. Unfortunately, the eggs, which are 50 × 30 μg in size, oval, flat on one side, and thin shelled, become infestive in about 6 hours. Autoinfestation readily occurs through ingestion of eggs if the host scratches the perianal area or does not thoroughly wash the hands after defecating. Moreover, *Enterobius* eggs are rather hardy and may survive for weeks in dirt, house dust, clothing, and bed sheets, although most die in less than a day. Eggs are easily swept into the air and may cause infestation if inhaled. Pets may carry eggs in their fur. Occasionally, eggs hatch on the perineum, and larvae migrate back into the intestine, where they mature.

Rarely, pinworms will invade tissue and cause a granulomatous reaction. Inflammation associated with the parasite has been found in cases of appendicitis, but in such patients it is difficult to be certain whether the acute attack was actually caused by *E. vermicularis*. Pinworms occasionally wander beyond the perianal area, and granulomas containing worms have been an incidental finding in the fallopian tubes, peritoneum, and bladder. It must be stressed, however, that serious problems rarely, if ever, can be directly blamed on the pinworm. Perianal pruritus and recurrent urinary tract infections seem to occur frequently in infested patients, but some studies have questioned whether the parasite causes any symptoms at all.

CLINICAL MANIFESTATIONS

The patient may have perianal pruritus with secondary excoriation and dermatitis. Restlessness and fitful sleep are common complaints. A history of masturbation, enuresis, vaginitis, urinary tract infections, nausea and vomiting, diarrhea, and vague abdominal pain may be elicited, but it is seldom clear that the pinworm is the cause of these problems. As mentioned, it is doubtful whether the pinworm is at the root of any cases of acute appendicitis.

LABORATORY EVALUATION

Occasionally, adult pinworms may be noted near the anus, particularly in the morning. Eggs are found in the feces of a minority of patients even if concentration techniques are employed. The best way to make a diagnosis is to use the cellophane tape technique. When the child awakens in the morning, the adhesive side of a 2-inch strip of cellophane tape should be pressed against the perianal skin. The tape should then be placed on a microscope slide with the adhesive side down and scanned for the presence of eggs. A drop of toluene placed on the slide beneath the tape may make the preparation easier to read. A single test should detect at least 50% of infestations, three tests will detect 90%, and five tests will detect virtually 100%.

PREVENTION AND THERAPY

The zealous physicians who try to eliminate pinworm from their patients are doomed to frustration and failure. The ubiquity and infestativity of the parasite and its persistence in the environment make eradication extremely difficult. Moreover, vigorous pursuit of a permanent cure may provoke needless turmoil and anxiety in the family. When the diagnosis is confirmed in a patient with symptoms, the following approach seems reasonable.

The entire family should be treated with one of several drug regimens. A single dose of 100 mg mebendazole is extremely effective and has virtually no side effects. Pyrantel pamoate administered as a single dose of 11 mg/kg (maximum 1 g) also is effective; some physicians give a second dose after 2 weeks. Transient headache and abdominal complaints have been reported. Pyrvinium pamoate, 5 mg/kg (maximum 250 mg) in a single dose, sometimes repeated in 2 weeks, is another alternative. This drug has the disadvantage of staining clothes and stool red, but it is the least expensive therapy available.

It is probably fruitless and unnecessary to boil clothing and bed sheets. Simple measures, however, such as clipping the fingernails (a favorite repository for eggs), frequent hand washing, and daily showering are prudent. Tight-fitting cotton pants and bland ointment applied to the perianal region may limit dispersal of eggs. The most important aspects of therapy, however, are humility on the part of the physician and reassurance of the family.

SUGGESTED READINGS

Drugs for parasitic infections, Med Lett Drugs Ther 25:9, 1986.

Hoekelman RA: Pinworm infestation. In Berkow R, editor: The Merck manual, ed 16, Rahway, NJ, (in press), Merck, Sharp & Dohme.

Warren KS and Mahmoud AAF: Algorithms in the diagnosis and management of exotic disease. V. Enterobiasis, J Infect Dis 132:229, 1975.

246

Acute Pneumonia

Preston W. Campbell and Thomas A. Hazinski

Acute respiratory infections are the most common illnesses in the pediatric age-group. Although pneumonia accounts for only 10% to 15% of all respiratory infections, it causes significant morbidity and mortality among children. This is particularly true during the fall and winter months when parainfluenza, respiratory syncytial virus (RSV), and influenza virus epidemics occur. Pneumonia is distinguished from the more common upper respiratory tract infection by the presence of lower respiratory tract signs (i.e., tachypnea, rales, and cyanosis) and an associated area of infiltration on the chest radiograph. The challenge for the primary care provider is to make the correct diagnosis, to rule out associated serious conditions, and to begin rational treatment.

ETIOLOGY

The causes of pneumonia in children vary with age and season. Knowledge of which agent is most likely in a particular case will guide both the diagnostic workup and initial therapy.

Colonization of the maternal genital tract with group B streptococci and gram-negative organisms (e.g., *Escherichia coli* and *Klebsiella pneumoniae)* occurs most commonly during the neonatal period. Other perinatally acquired infections may cause illness later in infancy. For example, perinatally acquired *Chlamydia trachomatis* may cause a characteristic afebrile pneumonitis in children aged 4 to 11 weeks.[1] Other causes of the afebrile pneumonitis syndrome of infancy include the genital mycoplasmas, in particular *Ureaplasma urealyticum* and *Mycoplasma hominis*. In the infant with congenital or acquired immunodeficiency, cytomegalovirus and *Pneumocystis carinii* may occur.[5]

Between 2 months and 4 to 5 years of age, the most common cause of pneumonia in infants and young children is viruses. RSV is the major cause of pneumonia and bronchiolitis in children, with a peak incidence occurring between 2 and 5 months of age. It occurs in winter and early spring epidemics, with as many as 40% of children becoming infected during their first exposure. Next in importance are the parainfluenza viruses, which cause infection primarily in the fall in slightly older children. Influenza A and B viruses can become the predominant isolate in hospitalized patients during wintertime influenza epidemics. Adenoviruses and rhinoviruses have been less frequently associated with pneumonia. After 5 years of age, viruses become less important as a cause of pneumonia and *Mycoplasma pneumoniae* replaces them as the most common etiologic agent.

Although a potential cause of serious illness, bacterial pneumonia at present actually becomes less common after the neonatal period. *Streptococcus pneumoniae* (pneumococcus), *Haemophilus influenzae* type b, and *Staphylococcus aureus* are the usual offending organisms. Although *S. pneumoniae* has been the most common bacterial agent, recent evidence suggests that *H. influenzae* type b is increasing in importance.[3,4] This, however, should change dramatically with the universal use of *H. influenzae* type b vaccine during infancy.

Several other infectious agents deserve consideration. Although the incidence of all forms of tuberculosis has diminished significantly over the last 50 years, it remains a significant problem in native American Indians, residents of urban ghettos, and recent immigrants from third world countries where tuberculosis is endemic. Further, pulmonary mycoses may mimic tuberculosis and are important considerations in endemic regions. Histoplasmosis is endemic to the central United States, and coccidioidomycosis is endemic to the southwestern United States.

It is important to remember that noninfectious diseases can also mimic pneumonia. Gastroesophageal reflux with aspiration, tracheoesophageal fistula with aspiration, asthma-associated atelectasis, hypersensitivity pneumonitis, and pulmonary hemosiderosis are but a few examples. Finally, a number of conditions can mimic pneumonia radiographically: a prominent thymus, atelectasis, congestive heart failure, and congenital lung malformations. Patients with these noninfectious disorders may seek medical attention during intermittent, nonpulmonary infections; thus their underlying conditions may be misdiagnosed as pneumonia.

CLINICAL MANIFESTATIONS

The signs and symptoms of pneumonia vary greatly and depend on the pathogen, the age of the child, and the child's ability to mount an immunologic response. Although it may not be possible to differentiate clearly between a viral and bacterial pneumonia in an individual case, it is helpful to understand the differences in presentation among the various pathogens.

Viral pneumonia typically begins with upper respiratory tract symptoms of several days' duration, including fever, rhinorrhea, and cough. The onset of respiratory distress usually is gradual. Generalized mucous membrane involvement usually is seen and occurs in the lower respiratory tract as well, accounting for the coarse rhonchi that often are heard along with rales. The presence of wheezing strongly suggests a viral genesis. The classic radiographic appearance of viral pneumonia is that of a patchy bronchopneumonia. In the infant a perihilar pattern associated with hyperexpansion and atelectasis often is seen. The presence of lobar pneumonia should suggest a bacterial process. Peripheral white blood cell counts usually are elevated and not a particularly helpful diagnostic marker, but a signficantly elevated count increases the likelihood of a bacterial cause.

Features that suggest bacterial pneumonia include acute onset, toxic appearance, productive cough, and pleural pain. Lower lobe involvement with diaphragmatic irritation may cause severe referred abdominal pain. Often, rales will not be heard; instead there are diminished breath sounds over the involved segment, with dullness to percussion and tactile fremitus. In fact, in some cases the only discernible findings may be fever and increased respiratory rate. Radiographic features of consolidation, pleural fluid, pneumatoceles, or abscess indicate bacterial causes. Finally, associated extrapulmonary bacterial involvement, such as meningitis or arthritis, strongly suggests bacterial disease.

In *M. pneumoniae* pneumonia, coryza is unusual. Fever and cough develop first and usually are followed by malaise and headache. Cough is the most persistent symptom and can last 3 to 4 weeks. Rales, pharyngitis, and wheezing, in decreasing order of frequency, are the most common physical signs. The roentgenographic changes vary and often correlate poorly with the clinical status, but most common is an interstitial pattern.[2] Other patterns such as lobar or alveolar, or a combination of any of these, are possible.

The characteristics of chlamydial pneumonia are now well described.[6] The children usually are between 3 and 11 weeks of age and have a persistent staccato cough, rales, and wheezing without fever. Laboratory findings include a mild peripheral eosinophilia and elevated IgM and IgG levels. Ureaplasma, cytomegalovirus, and pneumocystis can cause a similar illness now termed *the afebrile pneumonitis syndrome of infancy*.

Recurrent pneumonia often presents a challenging dilemma. Some conditions responsible for recurrent pneumonia are listed in the accompanying box.

Causes of Recurrent Pneumonia

Aspiration
- Gastroesophageal reflux
- Tracheoesophageal fistula
- Altered consciousness (i.e., seizures)
- Foreign body
- Abnormal swallowing reflex

Structural
- Pulmonary sequestration
- Tracheal or bronchial stenosis/web
- Extrinsic compression of the airway
  - Vascular ring
  - Lymph nodes

Immunologic deficiency
- Acquired: AIDS, chemotherapy, malnutrition
- Congenital: humoral, phagocytic

Metabolic
- Cystic fibrosis
- Alpha$_1$-antitrypsin deficiency

Altered mucociliary clearance
- Immotile cilia syndrome

Other
- Asthma
- Hypersensitivity pneumonitis

DIAGNOSIS

Optimal treatment ideally requires precise identification of the offending agent. This may be relatively simple during an RSV epidemic but can prove complex at other times and in patients with underlying chronic disease. The diagnostic workup therefore is tailored to the age of the child, the season, and the nature and severity of the illness.

Although a bacterial cause may be suspected, it may be difficult to make a specific diagnosis because a child younger than 5 years old is unable to produce an adequate sputum sample. Even when sputum is available, the results may be difficult to interpret because of bacterial colonization in some patients with viral infections. In these cases a blood culture may provide a bacteriologic diagnosis. When available, the sputum should be Gram stained and cultured. On the Gram stain a predominant organism associated with polymorphonuclear leukocytes suggests bacteria as the pathogen. Bacterial antigens can be identified in tissue fluids (i.e., urine or pleural fluid) by use of counterimmunoelectrophoresis, latex agglutination, and enzyme-linked immunosorbent assay (ELISA), even after antibiotics have been started. More invasive approaches, such as bronchoscopy, lung puncture, transtracheal aspiration, or open lung biopsy, may be indicated in the child whose condition is deteriorating, is critically ill, or is immunosuppressed. When tuberculosis is suspected, a purified protein derivative (PPD) test should be used; a positive reaction calls for obtaining a culture specimen.

The ability to diagnose nonbacterial pneumonias rapidly has improved remarkably in recent years. Virologic isolation is available in most major medical centers and public health laboratories. Rapid diagnosis of influenza A virus, parainfluenza viruses, respiratory syncytial virus, and *Chlamydia* infections by ELISA assays and fluorescent antibody techniques is now available. Although *M. pneumoniae* can be cultured, the specific diagnosis usually is based on serologic conversion. A four-fold rise in antibody titer to *M. pneumoniae* by complement fixation test is diagnostic. Although false-positive results occur, a cold agglutinin titer of 1:32 or greater strongly suggests mycoplasma. A rapid screening test for cold agglutinins can be performed by placing four drops of blood into a tube with sodium citrate or other anticoagulant. Then it should be placed in ice water for 30 seconds and observed for agglutination by rolling it on its side. When warmed afterward the agglutination should resolve. The diagnosis of fungal pneumonia such as histoplasmosis or coccidioidomycosis is established by isolating the organism from sputum or tissue or by performing serologic tests.

TREATMENT

Despite advances in rapid diagnosis and the rarity of bacterial pneumonia beyond the neonatal period, patients with signs and symptoms of pneumonia are treated with antibiotics. This approach is both practical and reasonable even though it may not alter the course and some experts believe that the use of antibiotics in patients witih viral illness increases the risk of secondary bacterial infection.

Antibiotic therapy in the neonatal period requires coverage of both gram-positive and gram-negative organisms. Ampicillin plus an aminoglycoside provides excellent coverage. An afebrile pneumonia in the patient between the ages of 4 and 11 weeks should be treated with erythromycin. When erythromycin is used concomitantly with theophylline in wheezing infants, theophylline clearance is reduced and theophylline toxicity may occur. These two drugs probably should not be prescribed together.

Amoxicillin is the drug of choice in those older than 3 months and until 5 years of age. An antibiotic with activity against beta-lactamase–producing hemophilus and staphylococcus, such as amoxicillin/clavulanic acid (Augmentin), should be used in the sicker child. In children older than 5 years of age, when hemophilus is less likely and mycoplasma becomes the most likely agent, the drug of choice is erythromycin. If intravenous antibiotics are needed, a second-generation cephalosporin, nafcillin, or chloramphenicol provides excellent coverage in most cases. When an organism is identified, therapy is guided by that organism's sensitivity pattern.

The treatment of viral pneumonia is primarily supportive. As with all pneumonias, close observation, monitoring of heart rate and oxygen saturation, oxygen supplementation, high humidity, bronchodilators, and chest physiotherapy are used as needed. Specific antiviral therapy is available for RSV (i.e., ribavirin) and influenza A (i.e., amantadine) and should be considered for children with chronic lung disease or congenital heart disease.

The decision to hospitalize a patient with pneumonia depends on the severity of the illness, the age of the child, the suspected organism, and the adequacy of the home environment. The majority of older children can be treated at home, but there should be a low threshold for admitting the young infant. Certainly, moderately severe respiratory distress, hypoxia, apnea, poor feeding, posttussive emesis, dehydration, deterioration of clinical status on therapy, or an associated complication such as empyema should prompt hospitalization.

Children with pneumonia should be reevaluated after 2 or 3 weeks. The child who has returned to baseline status needs no further intervention. Repeat chest radiographs are indicated in children who have persistent respiratory difficulties, have had previous pulmonary disease, or have had complicated courses. Persistent radiographic abnormalities may merely reflect the inherently slow resolution of lung inflammation; thus films should be compared with previous films and interpreted in the context of the clinical course. After an acute pneumonia the chest radiograph may remain abnormal for 4 to 6 weeks.

PROGNOSIS

The complications of bacterial pneumonia include empyema and lung abscess. Long-term alteration of pulmonary function is rare even when these complications are seen. Death occurs almost exclusively in patients with underlying conditions. The incidence of long-term complications after viral or mycoplasmal disease is unknown. Significant sequelae have been noted after adenoviral, influenza, and measles pneumonias. These include bronchiectasis, chronic pulmonary fibrosis, and desquamative interstitial pneumonitis. Evidence is accumulating to indicate that recurrent viral pulmonary infections in childhood, in association with environmental irritants (i.e., passive smoking), can lead to chronic lung disease in adults.

REFERENCES

1. Beem M and Saxon E: Respiratory-tract colonization and a distinctive pneumonia syndrome in infants infected with *Chlamydia trachomatis*, N Engl J Med 296:306, 1977.
2. Brolin I and Wernstedt L: Radiographic appearance of mycoplasma pneumonia, Scand J Respir Dis 59:179, 1978.
3. Jacobs NM and Harris VJ: Acute *Haemophilus* pneumonia in childhood, Am J Dis Child 133:603, 1979.
4. Potter AR and Fisher GW: *Haemophilus influenzae*, the predominant cause of bacterial pneumonia in Hawaii, Pediatr Res 11:504, 1977.
5. Stagno S et al: Infant pneumonitis associated with cytomegalovirus, *Chlamydia, Pneumocystis* and *Ureaplasma:* a prospective study, Pediatrics 68:322, 1981.
6. Tipple MA, Beem MO, and Saxon EM: Clinical characteristics of the afebrile pneumonia associated with *Chlamydia trachomatis* infection in infants less than 6 months of age, Pediatrics 63:192, 1979.

SUGGESTED READING

Peter G: The child with pneumonia: diagnostic and therapeutic considerations, Pediatr Infect Dis J 7:453, 1988.

247

Pyloric Stenosis

Arnold H. Colodny

Pyloric stenosis is one of the more common surgical problems of infancy, and its management delights the pediatric surgeon because surgical treatment is decisive. Untreated, the patient's condition will deteriorate. The parents are usually young, inexperienced, and distraught; the operation is simple and curative; and there are few complications if the pathophysiology is understood. The mortality has steadily declined from approximately 50% at the turn of the century to well under 1% today.

CLINICAL FEATURES

About 80% of infants with hypertrophic pyloric stenosis are boys. There may be a positive family history in 15% of the patients. Vomiting is the cardinal sign of trouble in most cases. The age of onset may be variable. Although the average onset is between 3 and 4 weeks, vomiting from pyloric stenosis has been encountered in the newborn period and during the fourth month; this, however, is unusual. In the typical case, an infant will begin to regurgitate a small amount of formula immediately after feeding, although continuing to gain weight at first. Later the vomiting becomes more frequent and more forceful—in a projectile manner—and eventually follows all feedings. The baby will continue to be hungry. The vomitus does not contain bile, but if vomiting has occurred for a considerable period of time, there may be brownish discoloration of the vomitus caused by the presence of blood secondary to gastritis. Weight loss, dehydration, and metabolic alkalosis are the inevitable results of the prolonged vomiting, and in neglected cases the infant may develop an extreme degree of nutritional depletion.

The cause of pyloric stenosis is unclear. Various theories, such as alterations in gastrin levels,[23] changes in breast-feeding practices,[13] changes in infant milk formulas,[34] neurophysiologic alterations,[4] and others, have been suggested. The gastrointestinal tract harbors several populations of peptide containing nerve fibers including the neuropeptides, vasoactive intestinal peptide (VIP), substance P, enkephalin, and gastrin-releasing peptide (GRP). Studies in specimens from patients with pyloric stenosis have shown a reduction of VIP and enkephalin fibers in their smooth muscle, suggesting that impaired neuronal function may be involved in the pathophysiology of pyloric stenosis.[16]

Congenital hypertrophic pyloric stenosis has been reported in association with malrotation, Hirschsprung disease, ovarian cysts, icthyosis,[28] and deletions of the long arm of chromosome eleven.[18] An increased incidence of offspring of women who took significant amounts of benedictine in the first trimester of pregnancy has been reported.[1,6] However, a dissenting view has also been reported.[17]

DIAGNOSIS

A positive diagnosis is best made by feeling the firm, enlarged pylorus. This can be done in approximately 90% of the cases, if the baby's abdominal musculature is relaxed by giving the baby a sugar nipple and elevating the feet. Emptying the distended stomach with a feeding tube may facilitate the physical examination. Palpation should be carried out in the right upper quadrant and adjacent to the midline. One might conceivably mistake a transverse process of a lumbar vertebra, a piece of fecal material, or the lower pole of the right kidney for the pyloric mass, but with experience there should be no mistaking the typical sensation and movement of the enlarged pylorus, which is like feeling a peanut under a blanket.

Examination of an infant suspected of having pyloric stenosis in whom a pyloric tumor is not readily palpable, as is often the case early in the clinical course, is best done during a sugar-water feeding, and infants with pyloric stenosis are usually eager eaters. Gastric contractions may easily be seen moving across the upper abdomen from left to right, much like a golf ball would appear if it were moved slowly beneath the abdominal wall in the same direction (Fig. 247-1). These contractions increase in size and frequency (working against a hypertrophied, closed pylorus) until projectile vomiting occurs. It is at this point that the pyloric mass is most easily felt, with the patient in either the supine or the prone position.

It is interesting that, in a recent study, even when a palpable pyloric mass was present (85%), most patients (80%) still had some unnecessary diagnostic imaging procedure performed. Such imaging is redundant in the vast majority of infants with pyloric stenosis. It should be reserved for those infants with persistent vomiting in whom careful and repeated physical examinations fail to detect a palpable pyloric mass.[8]

Real-time ultrasonography should be the first imaging technique used in vomiting infants who are thought to have pyloric stenosis but do not have a palpable mass. Multiple observers[2,26,32] have confirmed Teele's original observation[30] of its value. The thickness, diameter, and length of the pyloric muscle are measured. If the thickness is greater than 4 mm, the diameter is greater than 15 mm, and the length is greater than 20 mm, a diagnosis of hypertrophic pyloric stenosis is made. In fact, if the length is greater than 20 mm, pyloric stenosis is invariably present.[35] The overall accuracy of ultrasonography in detecting the presence or absence of pyloric

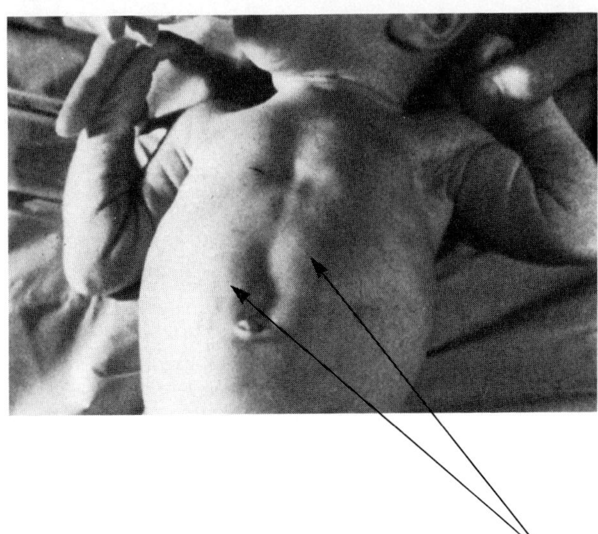

Fig. 247-1 Peristaltic waves seen in upper abdomen, moving from left to right in a baby with pyloric stenosis.

Reproduced with permission from Hoekelman RA. The Physical Examination of Infants and Children. In Bates B, editor. A Guide to Physical Examination and History Taking, ed 5. Philadelphia, 1991, JB Lippincott.

stenosis is 97%.[12,32] Postoperative ultrasonography has shown that these values have returned to normal within 6 months.[7] One study showed return to normal values in 2 to 12 weeks.[19] Since there are some false negatives, a barium swallow and gastrointestinal (GI) series should be obtained (if the ultrasound is negative) to be certain that pyloric stenosis is not present and also to seek other lesions that could account for the vomiting.[5,22]

The GI series is a less satisfactory method of establishing the diagnosis. When the pyloric mass cannot be felt or the diagnosis cannot be demonstrated on ultrasound examination, roentgenograms with contrast material will serve to rule out alternative diagnoses, such as esophageal stenosis, chalasia, hiatal hernia, antral spasm, gastric duplication, or pyloric diaphragm. The three criteria for the roentgenographic diagnosis of pyloric stenosis are (1) delayed gastric emptying, (2) persistent narrowing, and (3) persistent elongation of the pyloric canal. The double-track, or "railroad-track," sign, which consists of two or more parallel linear streaks of barium extending through the elongated pyloric canal, is often seen (Fig. 247-2).

When a diagnosis of pyloric stenosis cannot be established in a baby who has persistent vomiting, a normal ultrasound examination, and a normal GI series, the possibility of sepsis, poor feeding regimen, intracranial disease, renal failure, or adrenal insufficiency should be considered. In these cases, it may be crucial to make a prompt diagnosis. Infants with congenital adrenal hyperplasia who are "salt losers" may be in critical condition and may require immediate therapy. Clues to the correct diagnosis are (1) the baby will be sicker than expected, (2) genitalia may be abnormal (e.g., an enlarged clitoris and labial fusion in females or penile enlargement and scrotal hyperpigmentation and hyperrugation), and (3) the serum sodium level will be low and the serum potassium level high. Otherwise, the infant should be reevaluated in a week or 10 days when the pyloric mass may become palpable or the ultrasound examination or GI series may become diagnostic.[10]

Establishing the diagnosis may be difficult when pyloric stenosis develops in a postoperative period, as it occasionally does in babies who have been operated on for esophageal atresia.[20] This may manifest itself by high residual gastrostomy aspirations or persistent leakage from the gastrostomy site, if the tube has been removed.

COMPLICATIONS

The fluid and electrolyte disturbance in pyloric stenosis is similar to that seen in a patient with an obstructing duodenal ulcer. Loss of acid gastric juice results in a deficit of sodium, potassium, chloride, and water.[11] Since the gastric juice contains more chloride than sodium, a hypochloremic, hypokalemic alkalosis develops. Potassium shifts out of the cell and sodium into the cell; much of the potassium loss is in the urine and a lesser amount in the vomitus.

Although metabolic alkalosis has been regarded as the classic electrolyte derangement, a recent study[31] has shown that a spectrum may be seen, and variations from this expected pattern are not unusual.

The cardinal point to be emphasized in the management of a depleted alkalotic baby with pyloric stenosis is that this is not a surgical emergency. Even though this is a form of intestinal obstruction, gangrene and perforation of the stomach do not occur. *No infant should be operated on for pyloric stenosis until the fluid and electrolyte deficits have been corrected.* If infants come to surgery with uncorrected alkalosis, the profound effect of surgical stress on the urinary excretion of sodium may intensify the hypokalemic alkalosis with disastrous results.

In patients with mild to moderate dehydration, correction can usually be carried out within 24 hours, using intravenous replacement with a solution of one-third saline in 10% glucose; potassium chloride is added at the rate of 40 mEq/L of solution after urine output has been initiated. The volume replaced depends on the degree of dehydration, the history (intake and degree and duration of the vomiting), the physical examination (depression of fontanelle, skin and tissue turgor, filling of veins, state of the mucous membranes, mental status, type of cry, weight loss, recession of eyes, state of pe-

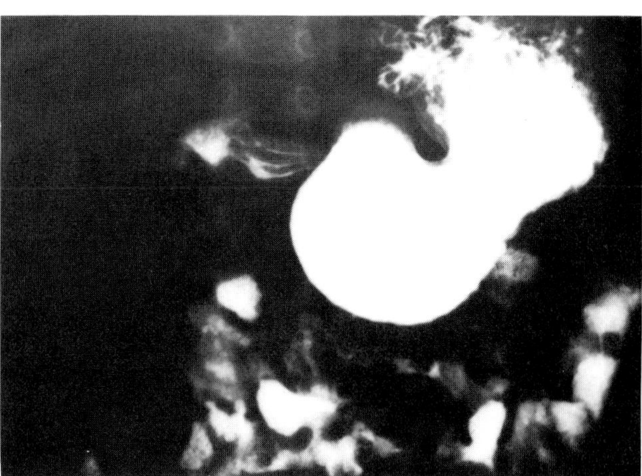

Fig. 247-2 The major features of pyloric stenosis seen on upper gastrointestinal series include elongation of the pyloric canal, "railroad-tracking" sign of the compressed pyloric mucosa, and a mass effect on the gastric antrum and duodenal bulb.

ripheral circulation, type of breathing, and general activity), and the laboratory examination (amount and specific gravity of the urine, electrolyte determinations, and hematocrit).

In the severely depleted, lethargic infant, therapy must be more vigorous. In addition to the electrolyte fluid, plasma may be given rapidly in the amount of 5 ml/kg. If the hematocrit is low following hydration, a small blood transfusion (10 to 15 ml/kg) may be indicated. Even though these severely depleted babies may look remarkably better at the end of 24 to 48 hours and their serum electrolytes may be approaching normal, it is wise to continue the same therapy for another 24 to 36 hours, since their intracellular electrolyte status may not have returned to normal.

Infants with pyloric stenosis who vomit blood or coffee-ground material are assumed to have severe gastritis. Approximately 8% of patients have hematemesis.[27] They also frequently have significant postoperative vomiting. In these infants it is beneficial to omit oral intake preoperatively and for the first 24 hours postoperatively. Infants will then tolerate feedings with much less vomiting.

Jaundice is seen in association with pyloric stenosis, but recedes rapidly on performance of a satisfactory pyloromyotomy. The hyperbilirubinemia results from indirect, unconjugated bilirubin. As many as 2% of patients have jaundice, with bilirubin in the range of 6 to 12 mg/dl, the indirect fraction ranging from 5 to 10 mg/dl. Bilirubin values return to normal within 7 to 20 days after operation.[14] The jaundice is probably related to the nutritional deficits and depression of glucuronyl transferase activity in the liver.

TREATMENT

Preoperative Management

If hematemesis has not occurred and the baby is alert and vigorous, occasional oral feedings of glucose and electrolyte solutions may be given before surgery. Although these babies may not vomit, considerable gastric retention can develop. The stomach must be emptied immediately before the operation; otherwise, relaxation of the cardia may also occur when the stomach is delivered into the incision, if it has not been decompressed preoperatively.

Operation

The operative management of an infant with pyloric stenosis is usually straightforward. Bypass procedures were abandoned at the turn of the century, when the extramucosal muscle-splitting pyloromyotomy was introduced.[21] This may be performed through the standard right upper quadrant gridiron incision or a transverse rectus incision.[25] Significant wound complications now have virtually disappeared. The major intraoperative complication is a duodenal perforation, where there is an abrupt change from the narrowed pyloric lumen to the normal duodenal lumen. Perforation is not catastrophic unless it is unrecognized. Suture closure of the perforation and omental reinforcement and maintenance of nasogastric suction for 24 to 36 hours will prevent further complications.

Reoperation for pyloric stenosis is unusual. Because of the abrupt change between the pyloric mass and the duodenum, most surgeons pay great attention to the distal end of the pylorus. In addition to a noticeable color change from pink to white, there is a distinct ring at the gastroduodenal juncture. This can be felt by drawing a finger up the soft duodenum onto the firm, rubbery pylorus. This ring will feel broken when an adequate pyloromyotomy has been done. This split should be carried well proximally onto normal stomach. In the majority of cases requiring reoperation, the pyloromyotomy has been inadequate at the proximal end.

Postoperative Management

A significant number of babies may vomit postoperatively; thus it requires discretion to select those who require reoperation. Approximately one third of infants will have a day or two of vomiting in the postoperative period. Most of these can be fed, and the vomiting will cease. If vomiting persists, oral feedings should be withheld for 24 to 36 hours and then started again. If the vomiting recurs, the stomach should be put at complete rest for another day or two by nasogastric suction. Feeding with clear liquids may then be started for 1 to 2 days, followed by dilute formula. If this is retained, full-strength formula may be started. A "chalasia chair" may be helpful. Feedings should be small in amount until they are being retained without difficulty.

Methylscopolamine nitrate (Skopyl) has been used with success in the medical treatment of some babies with mild symptoms of pyloric stenosis[9] and has been tried in patients with persistent postoperative vomiting. Metoclopramide (Reglan) may be helpful. If the mother has been breast-feeding, she should be encouraged to continue this in the immediate postoperative period; breast milk seems to be tolerated better than commercial formulas.

If vomiting persists in spite of the above measures, one should obtain roentgenograms. Babies with pyloric stenosis have a 3% to 12% incidence of other congenital anomalies. Most of these are minor, but distal intestinal obstruction in patients with pyloric stenosis does occur. The GI series may be difficult to interpret, since narrowing and elongation of the pyloric canal usually is persistent in the early postoperative period even in babies without postoperative vomiting. A return to normal pyloric opening time is the expected response. Reoperation for pyloric stenosis should not be undertaken hastily; the physician should wait 10 days to 2 weeks to make this decision, unless the infant's condition deteriorates. The increased thickness, length, and diameter of the pyloric muscle take up to 6 weeks to return to normal after a successful operation.[24]

Hypoglycemia. Reactive hypoglycemia has been recorded in depleted infants with a wide variety of medical and surgical conditions. This may cause unexpected respiratory arrest and unexplained death. Increases in insulin secretion by constant infusion of glucose can result in severe hypoglycemia if the infusion is stopped suddenly before oral alimentation is adequate. This is particularly likely to happen when the glycogen stores of the liver have been depleted. Liver biopsies performed in babies with pyloric stenosis and severe postoperative hypoglycemia have revealed depletion of hepatic glycogen stores. Fatalities from postoperative hypoglycemia in babies with pyloric stenosis have been reported.

Apnea. Babies with pyloric stenosis may be hard to anesthetize. After the operation has been completed and anesthesia terminated, apnea may become a problem in the immediate postoperative period in the recovery room. When the painful stimulus of the operative procedure is no longer present, the level of anesthesia deepens. Hypoventilation may then proceed to respiratory arrest. Careful attention to respiratory efforts as the baby enters the recovery room is necessary, and stimulation or assisted breathing may be necessary during this period. Administration of naloxone may be helpful.[3]

Long-Term Follow-up

A study of pyloric function revealed an increased rate of gastric emptying and an increase in duodenogastric reflux in some patients who had a pyloromyotomy for pyloric stenosis 5 to 7 years previously.[29] This might account for the increased incidence of peptic ulcer disease and gastritis in some of these patients. A more recent long-term follow-up study has not shown a significant increase in gastrointestinal difficulties.[33]

CAUSES OF DEATH

The mortality in patients with pyloric stenosis is well under 1% at present.[36] Although this is a satisfactory figure, it would be desirable to prevent these deaths altogether. Modern anesthetic management has contributed to these improved results.[15] The tragedy is that almost all deaths are avoidable. On review of 754 consecutive patients with pyloric stenosis, eight causes of death could be identified: (1) delayed diagnosis, (2) inadequate preoperative preparation (rehydration and restoration of a normal electrolyte balance), (3) pulmonary aspiration, (4) unrecognized perforation, (5) hypoglycemia, (6) persistent obstruction, (7) hemorrhage, and (8) other congenital anomalies.

REFERENCES

1. Aselton P et al: Pyloric stenosis and maternal benedictine exposure, Am J Epidemiol 120:251, 1984.
2. Ball TI, Atkinson GB, and Gay BB: Ultrasound diagnosis of hypertrophic pyloric stenosis, Radiology 147:499, 1983.
3. Beilin B et al: Naloxone reversal of postoperative apnea in a premature infant with pyloric stenosis, Anesthesiology 63:317, 1985.
4. Belding HH and Kernohan JW: A morphologic study of the myenteric plexus and musculature of the pylorus with special reference to the changes in hypertrophic pyloric stenosis, Surg Gynecol Obstet 97:322, 1953.
5. Bell MJ: Antral diaphragm, J Pediatr 90:196, 1977.
6. Benedictine and pyloric stenosis, FDA Drug Bull 13:14, 1983.
7. Bourchier D, Dawson KP, and Kennedy JC: Pyloric stenosis: a postoperative ultrasonic study, Aust Paediatr J 21:189, 1985.
8. Breaux CW et al: Changing patterns in the diagnosis of hypertrophic pyloric stenosis, Pediatrics 81:213, 1988.
9. Corner BD: Hypertrophic pyloric stenosis treated with methyl scopolamine nitrate, Arch Dis Child 30:377, 1955.
10. Geer LL et al: Evolution of pyloric stenosis in the first week of life, Pediatr Radiol 15:205, 1985.
11. Graham JA: Water and electrolyte imbalance in pyloric stenosis, Gut 10:1056, 1969.
12. Keller H, Waldmann D, and Greiner D: Comparison of preoperative sonography with intraoperative findings in congenital hypertrophic pyloric stenosis, J Pediatr Surg 22:950, 1987.
13. Knox EG, Armstrong E, and Haynes R: Changing incidence of pyloric stenosis, Arch Dis Child 58:582, 1983.
14. Lippert MM: Pyloric stenosis presenting as severe prolonged jaundice, S Afr Med J 69:446, 1986.
15. MacDonald NJ et al: Anaesthesia for congenital hypertrophic pyloric stenosis, Br J Anaesth 59:672, 1987.
16. Malmfors G and Sundler F: Peptidergic innervation in infantile hypertrophic pyloric stenosis, J Pediatr Surg 21:303, 1986.
17. Mitchell AA et al: Birth defects in relation to benedictine use in pregnancy, Am J Obstet Gynecol 147:737, 1983.
18. O'Hare AE, Grace E, and Edmunds AT: Deletion of the long arm of chromosome 11, Clin Genet 25:273, 1984.
19. Okorie NM et al: What happens to the pylorus after pyloromyotomy? Arch Dis Child 63:1339, 1988.
20. Qvist N et al: Development of infantile hypertrophic pyloric stenosis in patients treated for oesophageal atresia, Acta Chir Scand 152:237, 1986.
21. Ramstedt C: Zur operation der angeborenen pylorus-stenose, Med Klin 8:1702, 1912.
22. Rober JM and Bleicher MA: Surgical management of duodenal duplication cyst stimulating pyloric stenosis, Mt Sinai J Med 51:702, 1984.
23. Rogers JM: Plasma gastrin in congenital hypertonic pyloric stenosis, Arch Dis Child 50:467, 1975.
24. Sauerbrei EE and Paloschi GG: The ultrasonic features of hypertrophic pyloric stenosis, with emphasis on the postoperative appearance, Radiology 147:503, 1983.
25. Schuster SR and Colodny AH: A useful maneuver to simplify pyloromyotomy for hypertrophic pyloric stenosis, Surgery 55:735, 1964.
26. Shkolnik A: Applications of ultrasound in the neonate, Radiol Clin North Am 23:141, 1985.
27. Spitz L and Batcup G: Hematemesis in infantile hypertrophic pyloric stenosis, Br J Surg 66:827, 1979.
28. Stoll C et al: Hypertrophic pyloric stenosis associated with X-linked ichthyosis in two brothers, Clin Exp Dermatol 8:61, 1983.
29. Tam PK et al: Pyloric function five to seven years after Ramstedt's pyloromyotomy, J Pediatr Surg 20:236, 1985.
30. Teele RL and Smith EH: Ultrasound in the diagnosis of congenital hypertrophic pyloric stenosis, N Engl J Med 296:1149, 1977.
31. Touloukian RJ and Higgins E: The spectrum of serum electrolytes in hypertrophic pyloric stenosis, J Pediatr Surg 18:394, 1983.
32. Tunell WP and Wilson DA: Pyloric stenosis: diagnosis by real time sonography, J Pediatr Surg 19:795, 1984.
33. Vilmann P et al: A long-term gastrointestinal follow-up in patients operated on for congenital hypertrophic pyloric stenosis, Acta Paediatr Scand 75:156, 1986.
34. Webb AR, Lari J, and Dodge JA: Infantile hypertrophic pyloric stenosis: effects of changes in feeding practices, Arch Dis Child 58:586, 1983.
35. Wilson DA and Vanhoutte JJ: The reliable sonographic diagnosis of hypertrophic pyloric stenosis, J Chicago Univ 12:201, 1984.
36. Zeiden B et al: Recent results of treatment of infantile hypertrophic pyloric stenosis, Arch Dis Child 63:1060, 1988.

248

Reye Syndrome

Rebecca E. Ribovich

Reye syndrome, as a distinct clinical and pathologic entity, was first reported from Australia by Reye and co-workers[8] in 1963, when they described a syndrome of encephalopathy and fatty degeneration of the liver. Cases of this syndrome have since been reported from all over the world.

The incidence of Reye syndrome in the United States has been steadily decreasing since 1981 and is reported to be 0.15 cases per 100,000 in populations under 18 years of age.[4] A temporal and geographic association of Reye syndrome with cases of varicella, influenza B, and influenza A has been observed.

Reye syndrome has occurred in infants and children of all age groups, and cases have been reported in adults. The highest incidence is in the 5- to 14-year-old age group. There is no sex predilection. Ninety percent of the cases have occurred in whites and 8% in blacks.

Finally, there have been case reports of recurrent Reye syndrome, familial Reye syndrome, and Reye syndrome following live virus vaccination.

DEFINITION

The case definition for Reye syndrome as established by the Centers for Disease Control[3] in 1980 is as follows:

1. Acute noninflammatory encephalopathy with one of the following:
   a. Microvesicular fatty metamorphosis of the liver confirmed by biopsy or autopsy
   b. A serum glutamic-oxaloacetic transaminase (SGOT), a serum glutamic-pyruvic transaminase (SGPT), or a serum ammonia (NH_3) that is greater than three times normal
2. Cerebrospinal fluid, if obtained, with less than eight leukocytes per cubic millimeter
3. No other more reasonable explanation for the neurologic or hepatic abnormalities

PATHOLOGY

In Reye syndrome, pathologic changes have been described in the liver, brain, kidney, heart, pancreas, and skeletal muscle. The liver has a diffuse yellowish appearance caused by lipid accumulation within the cytoplasm of the hepatocytes. Glycogen stains show the diffuse depletion of glycogen. There is no necrosis or inflammatory infiltrates. The mitochondria of the hepatocytes are swollen, and their outer cellular membranes are deformed.

The brain, on gross examination, is swollen, with flattening of the gyri. Microscopic examination shows cerebral edema. The ultrastructural abnormalities include focal areas of swelling in myelin sheaths and accumulation of edema fluid in glial cells. The brain mitochondria show variable changes, namely matrix distortion and swelling.

Lipid accumulation has also been described in the kidney, the heart, and skeletal muscle. Evidence of mitochondrial injury has also been reported in cardiac and skeletal muscle. Focal necrosis, hemorrhage, and inflammatory changes have been described in the pancreas.

BIOCHEMICAL ABNORMALITIES

Since the original report of Reye syndrome, in which elevated serum transaminases and hypoglycemia were described, numerous other metabolic abnormalities have been documented. The serum ammonia level is elevated in virtually all patients with Reye syndrome, but this is transient, with levels returning to normal in 24 to 48 hours. Levels greater than 350 μg/dl are usually associated with a less favorable prognosis for survival.

There are various explanations for the hyperammonemia. Reductions in the hepatic activities of ornithine transcarbamoylase and carbamyl phosphate synthetase, which are mitochondrial enzymes of the urea cycle, may explain the hyperammonemia. Also, because of the anorexia and vomiting that occur, the patient is in a catabolic state, which results in an increased release of amino acids from muscle; this, too, may lead to the hyperammonemia.

The serum transaminase levels are always elevated, but the bilirubin is normal or only minimally elevated. Hypoglycemia occurs in about 40% of patients and is seen primarily in children under 4 years of age. The hypoglycemia is thought to result from deficient hepatic gluconeogenesis.

Elevated serum lactic acid concentrations are frequently found and may be related to impaired oxidative metabolism of glucose or to accelerated production by extrahepatic tissues such as muscle. Total serum free fatty acids with specific short-chain fatty acids are elevated in patients with Reye syndrome. In some studies, clinical improvement has been associated with the clearance of these short-chain fatty acids. Possible explanations for the fatty acidemia include an increased release from adipose tissue secondary to the anorexia and vomiting or a lipolytic response to a virus.

Coincident with the increased free fatty acid concentrations, dicarboxylic acids appear in urine and serum. This finding suggests that mitochondrial beta oxidation of fatty acids is compromised or overwhelmed by a massive influx of fatty acids. Alternative routes of oxidation are then utilized.

Other reported abnormalities include elevations in serum amino acids, creatinine phosphokinase, uric acid, blood urea nitrogen (BUN), amylase, and serum osmolality. Transient acute renal failure has been described on occasion.

The prothrombin time is prolonged, but the platelet count is usually normal in patients with Reye syndrome. Fibrin split products are usually absent from the circulation, and decreased coagulation factors (except for factor VIII) have been observed. Disseminated intravascular coagulation has been described only rarely.

Respiratory alkalosis is present as a result of primary stimulation of the respiratory centers in the brainstem. A mixed metabolic acidosis is often found in addition to the respiratory alkalosis. The hyperthermia that is present early in the disease may be the result of hypothalamic dysfunction.

ETIOLOGY AND PATHOGENESIS

The cause of Reye syndrome remains unknown, but various theories have been advanced. It may be that the clinical disease recognized as Reye syndrome is the result of a number of different processes producing a common metabolic derangement.

An increased incidence of Reye syndrome has been reported during outbreaks of varicella, influenza B, and influenza A. Both influenza A and B infections have been demonstrated serologically in many Reye syndrome patients. Adenovirus, coxsackieviruses A and B, echovirus, Epstein-Barr virus, parainfluenza virus, reovirus, rubella virus, rubeola virus, type I poliomyelitis virus, and herpes simplex viruses have also been linked to Reye syndrome.

Children with Reye syndrome have either a similar response to many viral infections or a reaction to initial exposure to a certain virus.

Environmental toxins have also been suggested as being important in the etiology of Reye syndrome. Aflatoxins (metabolites of *Aspergillus flavus,* a mold commonly contaminating corn and peanut products) have been found in the tissues and body fluids of some Reye syndrome patients. However, additional work has failed to demonstrate a significant difference in aflatoxin concentrations in children with Reye syndrome compared with controls. Insecticides and related chemicals have also been implicated in the etiology of Reye syndrome. However, there is no evidence showing the accumulation of these chemicals in tissues or serum of patients with Reye syndrome.

Much attention has been given to the role of salicylates in the origin of Reye syndrome. Epidemiologic studies,[6,12,15] including a Public Health Service study,[7] have found a higher rate of salicylate ingestion (by history) in Reye syndrome patients as compared with control children with similar antecedent illnesses. These reports have resulted in the recommendation that the use of salicylates be avoided for children with varicella infections and during influenza outbreaks until the association between salicylate use and Reye syndrome is clarified. Since the publicity about the association between Reye syndrome and aspirin began in late 1980, much of the decline in the reported incidence of Reye syndrome has been attributed by some to the reported decrease in the use of salicylates in treating children with viral illnesses.[1,2] The role of salicylates in the pathogenesis of Reye syndrome remains unresolved.

A final hypothesis for the etiology of Reye syndrome is that of a virus-host–exogenous toxin interaction, the toxin being either a medication or an environmental agent. It is possible that the syndrome develops after an insult to the liver, as may occur with a toxin exposure, followed by a virus-mediated generalized reaction.

The pathogenesis of the encephalopathy in Reye syndrome remains unclear. Some etiologic factors that have been suggested are hyperammonemia, lactic acidemia, short-chain fatty acidemia, and direct brain cell mitochondrial damage paralleling that seen in the liver cells.

It has also been suggested that generalized mitochondrial insult and dysfunction are the bases of the metabolic abnormalities found. As noted, there is strong evidence for insult to hepatic mitochondria in terms of both morphologic and enzymatic abnormalities. The evidence for a similar primary mitochondrial dysfunction in brain cells is less substantial. As yet, the hypothesis of widespread mitochondrial disease is not well supported.

CLINICAL FEATURES

Patients with Reye syndrome have a viral prodromal illness usually consisting of an upper respiratory tract infection, gastroenteritis, or varicella. The child appears to be recovering from such illness, but then develops repetitive vomiting. Within 24 to 48 hours, the child becomes agitated, combative, and disoriented and behaves irrationally. Periods of lethargy may alternate with the combative behavior. Hyperventilation may also be prominent and is probably a result of primary stimulation of the medullary respiratory centers.

Approximately 85% of patients have hepatomegaly, but jaundice is absent. Pancreatitis is found in up to 22% of autopsied cases. The pancreatic involvement can be so severe as to produce hemorrhagic necrosis and death. Seizures can occur at any time during the encephalopathic stages.

The child may begin to recover spontaneously or may deteriorate further into full obtundation. Central nervous system dysfunction progresses from stupor to coma with intact brainstem function, to decorticate or decerebrate posturing, and finally to a flaccid and areflexic state.

Various systems have been devised to stage the severity of the illness in Reye syndrome. The National Institutes of Health Consensus Development Conference on the Diagnosis and Treatment of Reye Syndrome held in 1981 generated the revised staging system, shown in Table 248-1. This was done in an attempt to introduce a uniform staging system for use by all treatment centers.

The clinical presentation of Reye syndrome in infants is somewhat different from that previously outlined, such that early recognition is more difficult. Following the prodromal illness, vomiting may be minimal or absent. Diarrhea, however, is a frequent occurrence. Seizures are also frequently present, can occur early in the course of the illness, and may be the presenting sign. Respiratory disturbances, such as hyperventilation and apnea, are prominent and also may occur early in the course of the illness.

Table 248-1 *Staging of Reye Syndrome*

	I	II	III	IV	V
Level of consciousness	Lethargy; follows verbal commands	Combative/stupor; verbalizes inappropriately	Coma	Coma	Coma
Posture	Normal	Normal	Decorticate	Decerebrate	Flaccid
Response to pain	Purposeful	Purposeful/nonpurposeful	Decorticate	Decerebrate	None
Pupillary reaction	Brisk	Sluggish	Sluggish	Sluggish	None
Oculocephalic reflex (doll's eyes)	Normal	Conjugate deviation	Conjugate deviation	Inconsistent or absent	None

From National Institutes of Health Consensus Development Conference: Diagnosis and treatment of Reye's syndrome, JAMA 246:2442, 1981.

Diagnosis

The diagnosis of Reye syndrome, then, should be considered when a history of an antecedent viral illness is followed by vomiting, progressive lethargy, agitation, and obtundation. Early diagnosis is important because prompt treatment may provide a better chance for complete recovery.

Laboratory Tests. Laboratory tests that should be obtained to help establish the diagnosis include serum ammonia, serum transaminases, bilirubin, prothrombin time, blood glucose, and urine and blood toxicology screens. A lumbar puncture should not be performed routinely if Reye syndrome is suspected, because of the associated cerebral edema and increased intracranial pressure. If meningitis is suspected, a lumbar puncture should be performed using a small-gauge needle, with removal of as little cerebrospinal fluid as possible to minimize the likelihood of cerebral herniation. A cerebrospinal fluid specimen containing less than eight leukocytes per cubic millimeter and normal protein and glucose concentrations, except when there is concomitant hypoglycemia, is consistent with Reye syndrome.

Special Studies and Computed Tomography. A liver biopsy is not essential to diagnose most cases of Reye syndrome, since the clinical and laboratory features are typical. However, a liver biopsy to establish the diagnosis firmly should be considered in patients under 1 year of age, in children with recurrent episodes, in familial cases, in atypical cases without antecedent viral infection or vomiting, and when new and potentially dangerous therapeutic regimens are planned.

Computed tomographic (CT) brain scanning is not needed for diagnosing Reye syndrome. A CT scan performed early in the course of the illness will either be normal or show evidence of diffuse brain edema. Likewise, the electroencephalogram will be nonspecific and will not help in establishing the diagnosis, altering treatment regimens, or determining prognosis.

DIFFERENTIAL DIAGNOSIS

The conditions that should be considered in the differential diagnosis of Reye syndrome are as follows*:

1. Meningitis
2. Varicella, hepatitis, encephalitis
3. Toxins: salicylates, methyl bromide, hypoglycin, isopropyl alcohol, aflatoxin, lead, valproic acid
4. Anoxic encephalopathy
5. Inborn metabolic defects: systemic carnitine deficiency, hyperammonemia syndromes, organic acid disorders

Meningitis may follow an upper respiratory tract infection and can produce vomiting and lethargy. Transaminase elevations may occur in children with varicella without Reye syndrome and in hypoxia resulting from a wide variety of causes. Excessive salicylate ingestion can cause vomiting, seizures, obtundation, hyperventilation, hypoglycemia, and abnormal liver function. A serum salicylate level of 25 mg/dl or more suggests salicylism rather than Reye syndrome. Other toxins, such as methyl bromide, hypoglycin, isopropyl alcohol, aflatoxin, lead, and valproic acid may produce disturbances of consciousness and elevation of serum transaminase levels.

An increasing number of metabolic disorders have been described that may mimic Reye syndrome, especially in infants and younger children.[5,9,10] These disorders are also associated with vomiting and altered consciousness. The inborn errors of ureagenesis that may mimic Reye syndrome include partial ornithine transcarbamoylase deficiency and partial carbamoyl-phosphate synthase deficiency. Defects of fatty acid metabolism, such as systemic carnitine deficiency and various acetyl-CoA dehydrogenase deficiencies, can also resemble Reye syndrome in presentation. Clinical features that suggest an underlying metabolic disorder include an atypical prodrome with rapid onset, age under 2 years, and familial or recurrent episodes of Reye syndrome–like illness.

It has been observed that as the incidence of Reye syndrome declines, an increasing proportion of patients who seem to have its "typical" features may have one of the metabolic disorders that mimic this syndrome.[10] Therefore it has been recommended that investigations to exclude metabolic disorders be seriously considered in all patients suspected of having Reye syndrome.

TREATMENT

Once the diagnosis of Reye syndrome is suspected, the severity of the patient's illness should be staged, using a staging

*From Trauner DA: Reye's syndrome, Curr Probl Pediatr 12:1, 1982.

system such as the one shown in Table 248-1. All patients, regardless of their stage of disease, should be hospitalized for careful observation, since neurologic deterioration can progress rapidly. The primary care physician should arrange for transfer of the patient to a regional pediatric intensive care unit (PICU) as soon as possible, using a transport team prepared to provide support for all vital functions.

Supportive care for patients in stages I and II includes frequent evaluations of neurologic status. A 10% dextrose solution containing balanced electrolytes should be administered intravenously at the rate needed to deliver daily maintenance fluid requirements. The use of a high-glucose concentration is designed to decrease lipolysis. Any abnormalities in the serum electrolytes and fluid balance should be corrected.

Children at later stages of the disease require intensive monitoring and aggressive therapy directed toward correction of metabolic abnormalities and reduction of increased intracranial pressure.

Some authorities recommend that fluids be given at two-thirds maintenance; others recommend full maintenance fluid volumes, with adjustments according to electrolyte levels and urinary output. A nasogastric tube and Foley catheter should be inserted so that accurate intake and output can be calculated. An arterial catheter, which permits continuous blood pressure measurement and arterial blood gas sampling, should be placed. Temperature should be maintained at normal levels with a cooling blanket. Endotracheal intubation should be performed and assisted ventilation instituted in comatose patients. Intravenous phenytoin should be used for seizure control. Barbiturates should be avoided, since they will alter the level of consciousness and the neurologic status.

Mannitol (0.25 g/kg, given intravenously over 30 minutes) should be administered in an attempt to reduce cerebral edema, provided that the serum osmolality level is not over 320 mOsm. The use of mannitol requires careful monitoring of the patient's fluid balance.

Neomycin sulfate enemas have been used by some authorities to reduce serum ammonia levels. Vitamin K (5 mg, given intramuscularly) can be administered in an attempt to correct the clotting abnormalities. If a significant amount of bleeding occurs, the administration of fresh-frozen plasma (10 ml/kg) may be helpful.

Arterial blood gases, serum osmolality, glucose, electrolytes, BUN, and hematocrit should be monitored closely.

Once the patient is admitted to a PICU, more definitive therapeutic measures can be undertaken. A central venous catheter should be placed to monitor blood volume and cardiac function. In addition, it is recommended that patients receive hypertonic glucose solutions of 15% dextrose, and a central line is required for administration of such hypertonic solutions. For seriously ill children, a pulmonary artery catheter may be required to monitor pulmonary artery pressure and cardiac output.

Some centers recommend the use of high-dose glucose and insulin to decrease serum free fatty acid concentrations. Insulin blocks fatty acid release from adipose tissue by inhibiting the enzyme lipoprotein lipase. One unit of insulin per 5 g of glucose is administered intravenously every 4 hours. The insulin dose is adjusted to maintain the serum glucose concentration between 125 and 175 mg/dl. There is no evidence, however, that this therapy improves the clinical course.

Exchange transfusion and peritoneal dialysis have been used to clear the hyperammonemia and to remove "unknown toxins." There is no evidence that the use of these techniques improves outcome either. A double-volume exchange transfusion with fresh blood has also been used to replenish coagulation factor deficiencies.

The most significant adjunct to the management of cerebral edema and increasing intracranial pressure in Reye syndrome has been the development of techniques to monitor intracranial pressure. Most centers recommend that children beyond stage II have an intracranial pressure monitor inserted. Monitoring provides a mechanism to titrate management of the patient and is designed to maintain the intracranial pressure within normal ranges until the illness resolves. The monitoring device can be either an intraventricular cannula or a subarachnoid bolt, and it should be placed after the prothrombin time is brought to normal levels. Intracranial pressure greater than 20 mm Hg should be treated. The cerebral perfusion pressure should be maintained above 50 mm Hg to prevent cerebral ischemia. Cerebral perfusion pressure is equal to the mean arterial pressure minus the intracranial pressure.

The following measures can be undertaken to treat elevated intracranial pressure:

1. Mannitol, 0.25 g/kg/dose, should be administered intravenously. Hyperosmolality is a complication of osmotherapy. Adequate fluid replacement should be carried out to keep the serum osmolality below 310 mOsm and thereby prevent any compromise of renal function.
2. Controlled hyperventilation by a mechanical respirator should be used to maintain a P_{CO_2} of 25 to 30 mm Hg. A P_{CO_2} above this leads to increased pressure from vasodilation, and values below this range can be correlated with inadequate cerebral flood flow.
3. Pancuronium bromide, 0.1 to 0.2 mg/kg/dose, should be administered to immobilize the patient.
4. If an intraventricular catheter is used, small amounts of cerebrospinal fluid can be released through the catheter for immediate control of intracranial pressure elevations.
5. Chest physiotherapy, if performed carefully, will remove mucous plugs and decrease intrathoracic pressure, resulting in better control of intracranial pressure.

Corticosteroids have not been shown to be effective in controlling the intracranial pressure.

If the above measures are unsuccessful, high-dose barbiturate therapy may be indicated, although its use remains controversial.[11,14] Varying success rates have been reported with this therapy. Barbiturates are thought to decrease cerebral metabolic demands and cerebral blood flow and thereby control intracranial pressure. This therapy involves the administration of intravenous pentobarbital to maintain a blood level of 30 to 50 μg/dl and is carried out until the intracranial pressure returns to normal. Since possible complications of this therapy include a drop in arterial blood pressure, a change in cardiac output, or unexplained hypoxia, monitoring devices are necessary to measure these indexes accurately.

Some centers have used hypothermia when the above therapeutic measures have failed to control the elevated intracranial pressure.[13] Surface body cooling to a target body temperature of 32° C is achieved with hypothermia blankets. However, this therapy increases the risk of infection, because the immune system does not function as well during hypothermia.

A final mode of therapy that has been used for patients with increased intracranial pressure refractory to all other measures is decompressive craniectomy. Since there are potential risks of infection and bleeding with this therapy, it should be reserved for the most difficult cases.

PROGNOSIS

Early reports indicated that the mortality from Reye syndrome was 80%. This rate has decreased to less than 30%. Some of this decrease may be the result of increased recognition of the illness, especially of mild cases, in addition to greater use of intensive medical support.

Recent studies have attempted to evaluate neurologic sequelae in survivors of Reye syndrome. It is estimated that 10% of survivors are left severely brain damaged. Several studies suggest that those children with the most severe illness (as evidenced by the degree and duration of increased intracranial pressure) and those who are under 2 years of age when affected are most likely to suffer sequelae. However, the vast majority of children over 2 years of age who develop Reye syndrome and survive appear to recover completely.

Neuropsychological testing has shown that some children who have recovered from Reye syndrome have difficulties with school achievement, visual motor integration, sequencing, tactile problem-solving, and concept formation. These more subtle deficits may persist for many months or years. In general, extensive psychological and educational testing of Reye syndrome survivors appears to be unnecessary.

Overprotectiveness of the child by the family should be avoided, since this can contribute to behavioral or school problems. Family guidance and counseling are essential in this regard.

REFERENCES

1. Arrowsmith JB et al: National patterns of aspirin use and Reye syndrome reporting—United States, 1980 to 1985, Pediatrics 79:858, 1987.
2. Barrett MJ et al: Changing epidemiology of Reye syndrome in the United States, Pediatrics 77:598, 1986.
3. Centers for Disease Control: Follow-up on Reye syndrome—United States, MMWR 29:321, 1980.
4. Centers for Disease Control: Reye syndrome surveillance—United States, 1986, MMWR 36:689, 1987.
5. Greene CL, Blitzer MG, and Shapira E: Inborn errors of metabolism and Reye syndrome: differential diagnosis, J Pediatr 113:156, 1988.
6. Halpin TJ et al: Reye's syndrome and medication use, JAMA 248:687, 1982.
7. Hurwitz ES et al: Public Health Service study of Reye's syndrome and medications: report of the main study, JAMA 257:1905, 1987.
8. Reye RDK, Morgan G, and Baral J: Encephalopathy and fatty degeneration of the viscera: a disease entity in childhood, Lancet 2:749, 1963.
9. Robinson RO: Differential diagnosis of Reye's syndrome, Dev Med Child Neurol 29:110, 1987.
10. Rowe PC, Valle D, and Brusilow SW: Inborn errors of metabolism in children referred with Reye's syndrome, JAMA 260:3167, 1988.
11. Shaywitz BA, Lister G, and Duncan CC: What is the best treatment for Reye's syndrome? Arch Neurol 43:730, 1986.
12. Starko KM et al: Reye's syndrome and salicylate use, Pediatrics 66:859, 1980.
13. Swedlow DB and Schreiner MS: Management of Reye's syndrome, Crit Care Clin 1:285, 1985.
14. Trauner DA: What is the best treatment for Reye's syndrome: Arch Neurol 43:729, 1986.
15. Waldman RJ et al: Aspirin as a risk factor in Reye's syndrome, JAMA 247:3089, 1982.

SUGGESTED READINGS

Boutras AR et al: Reye syndrome: a predictably curable disease, Pediatr Clin North Am 27:539, 1980.

DeLong GR and Glick TH: Encephalopathy of Reye's syndrome: a review of pathogenetic hypotheses, Pediatrics 69:53, 1982.

Heubi JE et al: Reye's syndrome: current concepts, Hepatology 7:155, 1987.

Huttenlocher PR and Trauner DA: Reye's syndrome in infancy, Pediatrics 62:84, 1978.

National Institutes of Health Consensus Development Conference: Diagnosis and treatment of Reye's syndrome, JAMA 246:2441, 1981.

Sullivan-Bolyai JZ and Corey L: Epidemiology of Reye's syndrome, Epidemiol Rev 3:1, 1981.

Trauner DA: Reye's syndrome, Curr Probl Pediatr 12:1, 1982.

249

Rheumatic Fever

Sylvia P. Griffiths

Acute rheumatic fever is a systemic connective tissue disorder that is clinically manifested by polyarthritis, carditis, or chorea. It would be an illness of little consequence except for its potential for causing inflammatory cardiac valvular involvement and the development of rheumatic heart disease. The arthritis clears without sequelae of joint dysfunction or deformity, and the chorea leaves no neuromuscular impediment. Although rheumatic fever is a self-limited disease during an acute attack, it has a strong predilection to recur in succeeding years.

Since it has been established that group A beta-hemolytic streptococci play a part in the etiology of rheumatic fever, it has been shown in pediatric populations, as previously demonstrated in military establishments, that the incidence of the first attack of rheumatic fever can be reduced by adequate penicillin treatment of all cases of streptococcal pharyngitis.[8] In contrast to the high incidence of rheumatic fever observed in epidemics of streptococcal pharyngitis (approximately 2% to 3%), the attack rate following sporadic streptococcal upper respiratory tract infection is only about one tenth of that figure. In those who have already had one or more attacks of rheumatic fever, the recurrence rate rises to about 15% following subsequent streptococcal infection.[9]

Numerous community primary prevention programs have demonstrated the efficacy of identifying streptococcal infection by culturing the throats of susceptible children and treating them early. Further, the widespread application of secondary prevention in the form of antistreptococcal prophylaxis programs for patients after their first attack has significantly reduced the recurrence rate and the possible additive effects of repeated bouts of carditis.

Fortunately, the severity of acute rheumatic fever in a first attack, as well as the incidence of both initial and recurrent attacks, has steadily declined in the past 4 decades in the United States and Europe, particularly in communities with high socioeconomic levels. Still, in other parts of the world, including the Orient, India, and the developing countries, rheumatic fever is not uncommon in childhood and may be a fulminating disease, with acute carditis leading to death during a first attack. With the increase in travel by Hispanic families from the Caribbean Islands and South America, as well as refugee population groups from Southeast Asia, rheumatic fever may also be on the rise in certain cities of the United States to which they migrate. A resurgence of rheumatic fever in certain areas of the United States, both urban and suburban, was reported between 1984 and 1988.[5,10]

DIAGNOSIS

Since there are neither pathognomonic clinical findings nor specific laboratory tests for rheumatic fever, the designation of this diagnosis must be somewhat arbitrary and empiric. Guidelines like those historically noted as Jones criteria, are necessary to minimize both overdiagnosis and underdiagnosis.[1]

The tendency to label as rheumatic fever a low-grade febrile illness with myalgia or arthralgia for which no obvious cause can be found should be strenuously avoided. The distress and anxiety that may lie in the wake of the false diagnosis of rheumatic fever may be even greater than the possible harm of missed recognition in questionable cases. The institution of effective prophylactic regimens requiring prolonged administration of antistreptococcal agents places a grave responsibility on the physician in diagnosing this illness. It is advisable to admit a youngster with arthritis or carditis to the hospital for careful observation and appropriate documentation of a poststreptococcal illness. Because of the specificity of Sydenham chorea with rheumatic fever, hospitalizing a child with this manifestation should not be mandatory if abnormal neuromuscular activity is mild and unlikely to cause self-inflicted injury.

Age

Rheumatic fever is predominantly a disease of school-age children, with most first attacks occurring between 5 and 15 years of age.[6] It is very uncommon under 5 years of age; when it occurs in this age group, it is usually associated with severe carditis and congestive heart failure.

Polyarthritis with rheumatic fever is extremely rare in the preschool-age group, where rheumatoid and other diseases with arthritis become, statistically, much more likely diagnoses. Chorea also is uncommon in early childhood; most of the cases occur in those over 8 years of age.

Host Susceptibility

The tendency for rheumatic fever to occur in more than one member of a family has long been recognized. The observation is noted even when family members are not concurrently living in the same household; thus environmental influences are not solely responsible. Many investigators have sought to define genetic factors, although none has yet been clearly established.

There is no sex predisposition in the incidence of arthritis or carditis in childhood, although chorea has always been noted to be more common in girls. There are, however, sex differences in the type of valvular lesions that may develop with carditis and ultimately with rheumatic heart disease: men have a higher incidence of aortic regurgitation; and, in young adults, mitral stenosis is more common in women.

STREPTOCOCCAL INFECTION AND LATENT PERIOD

Streptococcal pharyngitis presumptively precedes an attack of rheumatic fever, even though some patients fail to report such a history. Scarlet fever occasionally will be followed by signs of polyarthritis or carditis, but suppurative streptococcal disease, such as skin infection, is not a rheumatic fever precursor. Throat cultures, however, are of limited value in the workup of patients suspected of having rheumatic fever, since the streptococcal infection antedates the common manifestations of polyarthritis and carditis by periods varying from 3 to 8 weeks; only 50% or fewer of patients with rheumatic fever continue to harbor streptococci during the course of their illness.[9]

The most reliable evidence of a preceding streptococcal infection is obtained by demonstrating an antibody response to one or more of the streptococcal antigens.[11] The most common of these, the antistreptolysin O (ASO) titer, reaches maximal levels 3 to 5 weeks after infection and gradually declines to preinfection levels 6 to 12 months later. The ASO titer is elevated in about 85% of patients with rheumatic fever. Serologic evidence of an antecedent streptococcal infection rises to 95% if other streptococcal antibody tests (including antihyaluronidase, antideoxyribonuclease B, and antistreptokinase) are performed.[9]

The relationship between time of onset of the common manifestations of rheumatic fever and the antecedent streptococcal infection is illustrated in Fig. 249-1. As noted, polyarthritis and carditis usually occur 3 to 8 weeks after infection. The streptococcal antibody titer (ASO) peaks before the onset of the clinical symptoms and then declines very gradually.

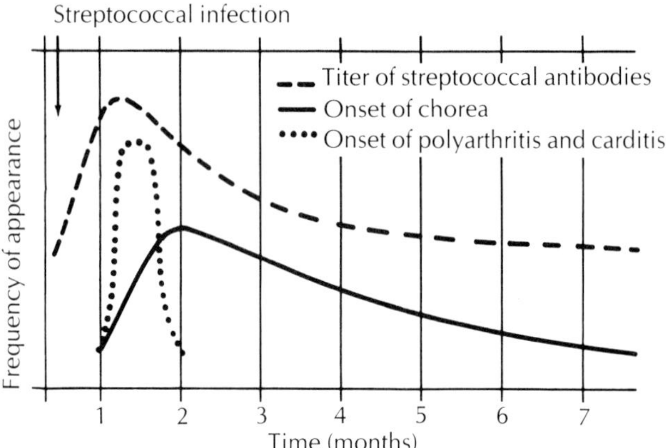

Fig. 249-1 Onset of rheumatic manifestations in relationship to antecedent streptococcal infection and ASO titer.

Modified from Stollerman GH: Rheumatic fever and streptococcal infection, New York, 1975, Grune & Stratton, Inc.

The longer latent period for chorea is indicated by the majority of cases beginning 2 months following streptococcal infection, with episodes still developing up to 6 months afterward.

The sequence of the manifestations themselves is noteworthy: polyarthritis, if it is to occur, usually is present before the onset of carditis. Although carditis may occur without the preceding arthritis, if it is to follow the latter, an obvious apical systolic murmur of mitral valvulitis usually occurs within 2 weeks. It is frequently observed, however, that the diastolic murmur of isolated aortic valvulitis takes longer to present itself and may not be heard for 6 to 8 weeks after the joint signs and symptoms appear.

Chorea not infrequently develops during the convalescent phase of carditis, though more often than not it has an even longer latent period and appears as an independent manifestation of rheumatic fever long after the initial streptococcal infection. Though chorea and carditis may coexist, it is of interest to note that chorea and polyarthritis rarely appear concurrently, presumably because of the differences in their latent periods.

CLINICAL MANIFESTATIONS

Polyarthritis, carditis, or both may be apparent in the context of a febrile illness associated with the nonspecific laboratory sign of inflammation—that of an elevated erythrocyte sedimentation rate, with values in the range of 60 to 120 mm/hr. Occasionally, abdominal pain is the conspicuous symptom after a streptococcal infection for which medical or surgical evaluation is sought and may overshadow or precede signs of joint or cardiac involvement. An uncommonly observed but severe manifestation is so-called rheumatic pneumonia, which almost invariably coexists with, or is hard to differentiate from, congestive heart failure with pulmonary venous congestion.

Electrocardiographic evidence of prolongation of the PR interval strongly supports the diagnosis of acute rheumatic fever but is not in itself an indication of carditis. Delayed atrioventricular (AV) conduction, most commonly first-degree heart block with PR prolongation but occasionally second- or third-degree block, may indicate heightened vagal tone, perhaps more pronounced in the rheumatic state than in other acute illnesses.[2] It is an invaluable early clue to the diagnosis of rheumatic fever, most commonly noted while arthritis is apparent. By the time auscultatory evidence of carditis with murmurs is obvious, the electrocardiogram is usually not remarkable.

When chorea occurs as an isolated manifestation, the patient is usually afebrile, and the sedimentation rate is normal. Because of the long interval following the initiating streptococcal infection, the ASO titer is typically normal or only mildly elevated.

Subcutaneous nodules and erythema marginatum, originally included by Jones[1] as major criteria for establishing the diagnosis of rheumatic fever, are rarely encountered in the United States today. The absence of these previously observed manifestations has been concurrent with the declining severity of acute rheumatic fever. Subcutaneous nodules, characteristically pea size, may be located on the occiput and around the elbows or extensor surfaces of other joints and usually reflect a long-standing, or smoldering, illness following severe carditis. Skin manifestations, notably erythema marginatum, now are also extremely uncommon in association with rheumatic fever, whereas they are not infrequently seen with juvenile rheumatoid arthritis.

Polyarthritis

Polyarthritis, the most common manifestation of rheumatic fever, usually involves large joints of the lower extremities, particularly ankles or knees, though wrists or elbows may also be involved in migratory fashion. An affected joint is characteristically hot, swollen, and exquisitely sensitive to touch, as well as painful on motion. Arthralgias, or pain in the joints without objective signs of inflammation, are highly suggestive of but not specific for rheumatic fever.

Carditis

Involvement of the heart may be expressed as myocarditis, endocarditis (valvulitis), or pericarditis. The characteristic presence of murmurs in rheumatic carditis is caused by endocarditis, secondary to mitral or aortic valvulitis. Implicit in the auscultatory diagnosis of valvulitis is the concurrent existence of myocarditis, which gives rise to tachycardia, heart sounds of poor quality, and in some cases, a gallop rhythm. Pericarditis typically is diagnosed by distant heart sounds, usually because of the presence of some effusion, and a friction rub. Whereas viral inflammation of the heart, such as infection by coxsackievirus B or Kawasaki disease, may be associated with myocarditis and pericarditis, these entities do not cause valvulitis.

Carditis, clinically diagnosable by the presence of valvulitis with obvious murmurs, may arbitrarily be designated in a first attack of acute rheumatic fever as mild, moderate, or severe. Such a categorization is useful in the approach to management and expectations in prognosis for developing rheumatic heart disease. It should be remembered that auscultation of the heart and evaluation of murmurs are influenced by fever and tachycardia; therefore, observations should be carried out, if possible, after the patient has been given acetaminophen to reduce any temperature elevation.

Mild carditis is characteristically defined by the presence of a prominent apical systolic murmur. This usually is of grade 2 to 3 (on a scale of 1 to 6) intensity and occupies all or most of systole. It is consistent with mitral valvulitis; the implication of fixed mitral regurgitation must await a long follow-up period after the acute episode has subsided. Heart size on chest roentgenogram is usually normal.

Moderate carditis designates patients who have (1) both long systolic and prominent middiastolic apical murmurs, reflecting a higher degree of mitral valvulitis; (2) a basilar diastolic murmur of aortic valvulitis; or (3) a combination of mitral and aortic valvulitis. An aortic diastolic murmur, which is high pitched and decrescendo in character, is usually best heard with the diaphragm of the stethoscope in the third left intercostal space; in the early stage of aortic regurgitation, the pulse pressure is not widened. Chest roentgenogram may reflect mild cardiac enlargement because of some dilation associated with more extensive myocarditis and valvulitis.

Severe carditis is defined by the presence of either pericarditis or congestive heart failure in addition to mitral or aortic valvulitis. The quality of the heart sounds will be poor either because of pericardial effusion or low cardiac output and associated gallop rhythm. Murmurs may become more intense as cardiac compensation improves. The chest roentgenogram will show obvious cardiomegaly and possibly will show pulmonary vascular congestion compatible with left-sided heart failure and pulmonary edema. Consultation with a pediatric cardiologist would be most desirable for this small group of patients to confirm the diagnosis and to make recommendations for management with cardiotonic and steroid drug therapy.

Echocardiography is invaluable for the documentation of pericardial effusion. However, the interpretation of valvular regurgitation by Doppler ultrasound should not constitute the basis of a diagnosis of carditis without auscultatory evidence of significant mitral or aortic murmurs.

Chorea

The clinical picture of Sydenham chorea includes that of poor neuromuscular coordination, often first detected by a change or sloppiness in handwriting. A wide variety of jerky, involuntary movements may occur during the period of 6 to 8 weeks that most cases of chorea are active. Neurologic testing may give evidence of specific deficiencies, particularly in trunk and upper extremity control of movements. A protective environment is recommended while the process is active. Occasionally, mild sedation with phenobarbital is indicated; the role of other agents, such as clonazepam (Clonopin) or haloperidol (Haldol), for more severe movement disorders has not been established.

MANAGEMENT

The three major therapeutic approaches include (1) antistreptococcal therapy, (2) antiinflammatory agents, and (3) limitation of activity.

Antistreptococcal Therapy

Intensive antibiotic administration to eradicate group A beta-hemolytic streptococcal infection (even in the absence of a positive throat culture) is the foremost important principle in management, to be immediately followed by a prophylactic program to prevent reinfection. Penicillin is the drug of choice to be prescribed in dosage and duration to maintain therapeutic blood levels for 10 days. Several treatment schedules, which are periodically revised, are outlined by the American Heart Association.[4]

The intramuscular administration of the long-acting repository benzathine penicillin G (Bicillin) is the preferred treatment method, since it ensures continued treatment for a sufficient length of time. A single injection of 1.2 million units for children 5 to 15 years of age is recommended, to be followed in 10 days by monthly prophylactic injections of 1.2 million units. Alternate methods include (1) oral penicillin, 200,000 or 250,000 units (penicillin G or V), given three or four times a day for a full 10 days, followed by the same dose twice daily thereafter, or (2) a combination of oral and intramuscular penicillin.

In patients sensitive to penicillin, erythromycin may be employed for antistreptococcal therapy. The sulfonamide drugs, which are bacteriostatic rather than bactericidal, are not effective for streptococcal eradication, though in rheumatic prophylaxis programs they are helpful in preventing reinfection.

Antiinflammatory Agents

Salicylates are invaluable in the presence of acute, painful arthritis or during the febrile phase of mild or moderate carditis associated with tachycardia. The duration of salicylate therapy in polyarthritis or carditis in childhood is not established and usually ranges from 1 to 8 weeks; the average initial amount prescribed should be approximately 100 mg/kg/day, given in divided doses.[6]

The administration of steroid hormones, most commonly prednisone (1 mg/kg/day), is indicated for severe carditis manifested by pericarditis or congestive heart failure. In this circumstance (particularly in a first attack), it is projected that the myocarditis, which causes the congestive failure, may be fulminant and life threatening and should therefore be vigorously suppressed. In addition, specific therapeutic measures to control congestive failure may need to be employed, namely, diuretics and digitalis. The use of a potent diuretic such as furosemide is critical in the management of pulmonary edema with left ventricular failure. Digitalis (usually in the form of digoxin) should be cautiously administered, remembering that the threshold for toxicity may be lowered because of the presence of inflammatory myocarditis. It may be wise to withhold digitalis for 1 or 2 days until there has been some suppression of myocarditis by steroid therapy. Before steroids are started, the result of the tuberculin test should be determined, and, if positive, a course of isoniazid should be given concomitantly.

Potassium supplementation is advisable to lessen the risk of hypokalemia (from the administration of steroids), predisposing to digitalis intoxication. The duration of steroid therapy may frequently extend upward from 1 to 3 months, with varying schedules of tapering the dosage and possibly adding salicylates.

The ultimate development of rheumatic heart disease, following a first attack of rheumatic fever, may be correlated with the severity of the acute carditis. It has been noted in the 10-year follow-up report on the international study of treatment begun in 1951 that approximately 30% of those with mild carditis and 50% of those with moderate carditis developed rheumatic heart disease (mitral and/or aortic regurgitation).[7] With "severe" carditis, nearly 75% of the patients may be expected to develop residual heart disease. Any claim of superiority of a given regimen of antiinflammatory agents for rheumatic carditis must therefore be evaluated in terms of altering the expected amount of residual rheumatic heart disease.

Limitation of Activity

The importance and duration of bed rest for optimum management of acute rheumatic fever has not been established: guidelines for bed rest and ambulation in patients with acute rheumatic fever have been outlined by Markowitz and Gordis.[6] After resolution of painful arthritis, it is usually satisfactory to start ambulation when the sedimentation rate shows a steady decline, even though not to a normal level. Most children with polyarthritis as their sole major manifestation of rheumatic fever may return to school in 6 weeks.

The period of bed rest recommended for carditis varies according to the estimate of its severity, with the broad range of 2 to 12 weeks for mild and moderate cases. For those with severe carditis, the length of bed rest and restricted activity must be individualized.

EVOLUTION OF RHEUMATIC HEART DISEASE

In the months and years that follow an attack of rheumatic fever, the auscultatory findings frequently change from those heard during the acute episode. For instance, many apical systolic murmurs completely disappear; not infrequently, however, an aortic diastolic murmur may first appear in the follow-up period. "Carditis" having been diagnosed initially does not imply progression to permanent heart damage. When a child is labeled with "history of acute rheumatic fever," the additional appellation of "rheumatic heart disease" must be continually reevaluated.

The majority of children who develop rheumatic heart disease after a single attack of rheumatic fever have mitral regurgitation. The remainder either have mitral and aortic regurgitation or aortic regurgitation alone. The combination of mitral regurgitation and mitral stenosis is uncommon in the United States, and isolated mitral stenosis is rare before early adulthood.

The issue that arises in the follow-up of children with rheumatic heart disease is the amount of physical activity permitted. In general, those who have mitral regurgitation with normal heart size should be allowed to engage in all sports activities, except perhaps for the most strenuous competitive games or track. Those with aortic regurgitation or mitral regurgitation with cardiomegaly should have some program restriction. For the very few children or adolescents with progressive cardiac enlargement, even in the absence of recurrent rheumatic fever, an intensive cardiotonic program with digitalis maintenance should be prescribed. If in spite of medical management symptoms of fatigue or exercise intolerance persist, surgical intervention with valvuloplasty or valve replacement should be considered.

PROPHYLAXIS

The major thrust of prophylaxis in a known rheumatic subject is that of protecting against a recurrence of rheumatic fever through prevention of group A streptococcal infection. However, among the group that develops rheumatic heart disease with valvular involvement, additional prophylaxis must be given at the time of dental and surgical procedures to protect against bacterial endocarditis.[3]

Recurrence of Rheumatic Fever

One of the most striking characteristics of rheumatic fever is its tendency to recur. Before the introduction of preventive measures, the majority of patients with an initial attack of rheumatic fever had one or more recurrences. The recurrence rate is highest during the first 3 years following an initial attack; it diminishes with time since the original episode, as well as with the advancing age of the patient.[6]

Continuous antimicrobial prophylaxis should be carried out in all children with a history of rheumatic fever, including chorea.[7] If by the time of high school graduation or 18 years of age there is no auscultatory evidence of heart disease, then prophylaxis may be discontinued. If, however, there is mitral or aortic valvular disease, prophylaxis should be maintained into adulthood.

The method of choice and the most effective protection in reducing the incidence of streptococcal infection and rheumatic recurrence are afforded by an intramuscular injection of long-acting penicillin (benzathine penicillin G, 1.2 million units)[4] every 28 days. Acceptance of parenteral therapy is noteworthy in the adolescent age group, when adherence to a program of daily oral medication is difficult if not impossible. Some transient discomfort at the injection site (anterior thigh or buttock) may be relieved by a hot bath and aspirin on the evening after injection.

The alternate methods of secondary prophylaxis include the oral administration of penicillin G (200,000 or 250,000 units, twice a day) or sulfisoxazole (Gantrisin, 0.5 g twice a day). For the exceptional patient who may be sensitive to both penicillin and sulfa, daily prophylaxis with another agent (such as erythromycin) is not essential in the absence of rheumatic heart disease. Successful oral prophylaxis is hard to maintain, and if employed, its value and need for compliance should be constantly reinforced by the pediatrician.

Bacterial Endocarditis

Individuals with a history of rheumatic fever without evidence of significant murmurs on follow-up examination are not susceptible to bacterial endocarditis because they do not have damaged heart valves. However, those who do have rheumatic heart disease should have specific antimicrobial coverage before dental manipulation or extraction in addition to their regular rheumatic fever prophylaxis. In the case of dental work or oropharyngeal surgery, including tonsillectomy and adenoidectomy, large doses of penicillin should be administered to protect the patient from *Streptococcus viridans* bacteremia. The latest recommendation of the American Heart Association for patients over 60 pounds in weight is to give 2 g of penicillin V within 1 hour of the procedure and 1 g 6 hours later.[3] For genitourinary manipulation, appropriate antibiotic coverage should be directed against the enterococci and gram-negative organisms.

CONTRACEPTION AND PREGNANCY

The adolescent girl with rheumatic heart disease should be counseled in regard to contraceptive methods. Prescribing oral medication with a low level of estrogen would be satisfactory, as would be instruction on how to use a diaphragm. An intrauterine device, however, should be avoided because of the risk of bacteremia.

If pregnancy occurs and early termination is sought, therapeutic abortion should be carried out in the hospital and prophylaxis against bacterial endocarditis given, using intravenous antibiotics.

Should pregnancy go to term, antibiotics should be employed during delivery to protect against maternal bacteremia. Because of the added cardiovascular burden during pregnancy, obstetric care throughout pregnancy should be provided, as well as prophylaxis against recurrences of rheumatic fever. Psychosocial support is especially needed for the pregnant teenager with rheumatic heart disease, who may face medical complications during pregnancy as well as the added responsibilities of child rearing afterward.

REFERENCES

1. Ad hoc committee to revise the Jones criteria (modified) (of the Council on Rheumatic Fever and Congenital Heart Disease, American Heart Association): Jones criteria (revised) for guidance in the diagnosis of rheumatic fever, Circulation 69:203A, 1984.
2. Clark M and Keith JD: Atrioventricular conduction in acute rheumatic fever, Br Heart J 34:472, 1972.
3. Committee on Rheumatic Fever and Infective Endocarditis (of the Council of Cardiovascular Disease in the Young, American Heart Association): Prevention of bacterial endocarditis, Circulation 70:1123A, 1984.
4. Committee on Rheumatic Fever and Infective Endocarditis (of the Council of Cardiovascular Disease in the Young, American Heart Association): Prevention of rheumatic fever, Circulation 78:1082, 1988.
5. Kaplan EL: Return of rheumatic fever: consequences, implications and needs, J Pediatr 111:244, 1987 (editorial).
6. Markowitz M and Gordis L: Rheumatic fever, ed 2, Philadelphia, 1972, WB Saunders Co.
7. Rheumatic Fever Working Party of the Medical Research Council of Great Britain and Subcommittee of Principal Investigators of the American Council on Rheumatic Fever and Rheumatic Heart Disease: Ten-year report of a cooperative clinical trial of ACTH, cortisone and aspirin, Circulation 32:457, 1965.
8. Siegel AC, Johnson EE, and Stollerman GH: Controlled studies of streptococcal pharyngitis in a pediatric population, N Engl J Med 265:559, 1961.
9. Stollerman GH: Rheumatic fever and streptococcal infection, New York, 1975, Grune & Stratton, Inc.
10. Veasy LG et al: Resurgence of acute rheumatic fever in the intermountain area of the United States, N Engl J Med 316:421, 1987.
11. Wannamaker LW and Ayoub EM: Antibody titers in acute rheumatic fever, Circulation 21:598, 1960.

250

Rocky Mountain Spotted Fever

Fred J. Heldrich

Rocky Mountain spotted fever (RMSF), an acute infectious disease caused by *Rickettsia rickettsii,* is characterized by the symptoms of fever, headache, myalgia, and distinctive exanthem. The major pathologic lesion—a vasculitis—makes RMSF a multisystem disease. Most important, it is a disease that requires a clinical diagnosis and treatment before a confirmatory laboratory diagnosis.

The disease was first reported in patients from the Rocky Mountain region. Today, however, the incidence of the disease is greatest east of the Mississippi River, with the most cases being reported from the Southeastern and South Central states. Although the disease occurs predominantly in the United States, it has been reported from other areas in the Western hemisphere, specifically Canada, Central America, and South America. The reported frequency of the disease has increased slightly over the past several years.

EPIDEMIOLOGY

Ticks serve as a vector for the infectious agent *R. rickettsii.* Transmission to humans occurs when the tick takes a blood meal or when the abraded skin is contaminated by tick feces or a crushed tick, which may occur when ticks are removed. Two specific ticks serve as major carriers: the wood tick, *Dermacentor andersonii,* is the more important vector in the west; in the east, the dog tick, *Dermacentor variabilis,* is the usual vector. Ticks, in turn, acquire the rickettsias by feeding on infected wild mammals. In addition, infection of laboratory workers has been reported independent of exposure to ticks.

The seasonal incidence of RMSF—primarily occurring in spring, summer, and fall—is in accordance with the activity of the tick.[5] Dog ticks infected with *R. rickettsii* have been found in urban areas, which suggests this tick's ubiquitous nature and places patients at risk without travel to endemic areas.[7] In adults, occupational or recreational exposure to ticks increases the risk of infection; however, children are affected with greatest frequency, and boys are affected more often than girls.

Exposure to a tick is not elicited in every case, although a history of removing a tick before the onset of illness is usual. The tick bite is painless and leaves no local lesion or regional lymphadenopathy; thus it is important to question specifically about prior tick removal or activities that increase the risk of exposure (e.g., removal of a tick from a pet dog and camping or picnicking in a high-risk area).

CLINICAL PICTURE

After inoculation with the rickettsias, the incubation period ranges from 3 to 12 days; the usual period is 5 to 7 days. In general, the shortest incubation period is associated with the most serious disease.

In the typical case,[4] there is a short prodromal period of 2 to 3 days with low-grade fever, chills, and muscle aches predominating. Headache is also an early symptom. Younger patients indicate muscle pain and headache by crying. Malaise, anorexia, vomiting, and photophobia are also frequently present. This brief period is followed by accentuation of these symptoms, especially the fever, which remains elevated and reaches as high as 40° to 40.6° C. The lowest temperatures, although still elevated, are recorded in the mornings. Lethargy and mental obtundation become prominent. Even the severity of symptoms seen at this stage is not diagnostic, and only the history of a tick bite indicates that RMSF is the likely diagnosis.

It is the rash that is most distinctive. It usually appears on the fourth day of fever and begins peripherally on the wrists, ankles, hands, and feet. Initially the lesions are macular, discrete, and erythematous and blanch on pressure. This rash rapidly spreads centrally, involving the arms, legs, axillae, buttocks, trunk, neck, and face. The lesions deepen in color, becoming dusky red and papular to palpation; in several days, they are petechial. These petechial lesions may coalesce and form large ecchymotic areas. Before the frank appearance of petechiae, a tourniquet applied when obtaining blood may produce petechial lesions. In severe cases and when treatment is delayed, these ecchymotic areas may ulcerate, and distal regions (e.g., fingers and toes) may become gangrenous. Nonpitting edema, especially notable around the eyes, face, hands, and feet, also occurs frequently.

Tachycardia and an elevated pulse rate are noted early and are proportional to the degree of hyperpyrexia. A sudden increase in pulse rate or fall in blood pressure is ominous and may indicate peripheral circulatory collapse, severe bleeding, or myocardial failure.

Photophobia is associated with conjunctival ecchymosis involving both bulbar and palpebral conjunctivae. Petechial hemorrhages may also be seen.

Abdominal pain and vomiting, with generalized abdominal tenderness, may be found.[2] Hepatomegaly and splenomegaly may be present. Jaundice is usually not seen, except in the most critically ill patients.

Fever, poor fluid intake, and vomiting all contribute to a diminished urinary output. Mild azotemia should respond to rehydration.

In addition to the lethargy and obtunded state of consciousness, the patient may exhibit nuchal rigidity. Disorientation and confusion, as well as seizures, may occur. Vasculitis, hemorrhage, or secondary metabolic changes are responsible for these neurologic manifestations.[1] When these symptoms occur early in the course of RMSF, they may mask its diagnosis.

DIFFERENTIAL DIAGNOSIS

Illnesses to be considered and differentiated from RMSF are listed as follows:

- Measles, rubeola (atypical)
- Meningococcemia
- Henoch-Schönlein purpura
- Idiopathic thrombocytopenic purpura
- Leukemia
- Typhus
- Infectious mononucleosis

Of these, atypical measles and meningococcemia are the most frequently confused; meningococcemia, because of its severe consequences, requires immediate differentiation.

The petechial rash of *meningococcemia* differs from that of RMSF in its distribution, rapid extension, and coalescence of lesions into larger hemorrhagic, purpuric areas. Prostration is either noted on admission or may develop rapidly if untreated. Absence of myalgia and an extremely abrupt onset are helpful differential points. Although the white blood cell count may be elevated, the sickest patients are frequently leukopenic. Meningitis with spinal fluid pleocytosis, low glucose levels, and organisms of the cerebrospinal fluid (identified by Gram stain) may be found also.

Atypical measles has a prodromal period similar in duration to RMSF but differs in that upper respiratory tract symptoms are usually prominent. Atypical measles occurs in patients who have been previously immunized with killed vaccine, and an Arthus response may be noted at the site of prior inoculation. Additionally, joint pain is common in atypical measles, but is not found in RMSF.

Rubeola is characterized by a macular rash (infrequently becoming hemorrhagic), which always begins on the face and neck and is preceded by an exanthem—Koplik spots. The coryza and cough in the prodromal stage of illness are not consistent with RMSF. A history of adequate immunization with rubeola vaccine should help eliminate this possibility.

Henoch-Schönlein purpura may produce a petechial or purpuric rash, frequently concentrated on the lower extremities and buttocks. These cutaneous lesions may be multiform and occur on other parts of the body. Frequently, there is an arthralgia with periarticular swelling and accompanying signs and symptoms of upper respiratory tract inflammation, gastroenteritis, or nephritis.

Other illnesses that produce petechiae must also be mentioned, even though they lack the distinctive distribution of the rash. Idiopathic thrombocytopenic purpura is seen as a petechial rash in an otherwise healthy patient. Leukemic patients with fever and petechiae at initial presentation would be expected to be anemic and have lymphadenopathy or hepatosplenomegaly. Patients with infectious mononucleosis, if they have a petechial eruption, usually have lymphadenopathy, hepatosplenomegaly, and a more gradual onset.

Typhus is a rickettsial infection to be excluded. Murine typhus produces a milder disease, with a rash that is macular and not petechial. Epidemic typhus may produce a petechial rash that typically begins proximally and extends peripherally, but usually does not involve the palms or soles. History of a tick bite is lacking.

LABORATORY EVALUATION

The diagnosis of RMSF is made clinically, and treatment should be started before laboratory diagnosis is sought. Fluorescent antibody studies of petechial lesions may provide the first positive proof of RMSF, but these studies are not readily available to most clinicians. Identification of rickettsias in the blood by immunofluorescent techniques, if available, offers another way to make an early diagnosis.[3]

Complement fixation studies will identify patients with RMSF, but these do not become positive until the second week of illness or later if early antibiotic therapy has begun.

The Weil-Felix reaction, agglutination of *Proteus vulgaris* by the patient's serum, is at best a nonspecific test for RMSF. Again, acute and convalescent serums must be compared, although *Proteus* agglutinins may appear by the end of the first week of illness.

Rickettsias can be isolated from body fluid or tissue specimens when grown in laboratory animals or chick embryos. However, the high rate of disease transmission to laboratory technicians makes such techniques feasible only in laboratories engaged in rickettsia-related research in which all workers are immunized; thus culture identification of rickettsias is not available in most clinical settings.

Leukocyte counts and differential counts are usually within normal limits. Thrombocytopenia is a complication seen in the later stages of the disease. In seriously ill patients, metabolic derangements, such as hyponatremia and hypochloremia, may occur but are nonspecific findings. Only with the complication of intravascular coagulation will such tests as prothrombin time, partial thromboplastin time, fibrinogen, and fibrin split products become abnormal.

In patients with neurologic symptoms, the cerebrospinal fluid pressure, the number of white and red blood cells, and the level of protein in the cerebrospinal fluid may all be elevated.

COURSE

The disease has a mortality of approximately 5% in recognized cases, but patients have recently been identified with serologic evidence of having had RMSF without clinical detection, suggesting that the disease may occur in a mild ol even subclinical form.[6] The importance of abdominal pain mimicking an acute abdominal condition and dominating as an early symptom before the development of or even in the absence of a rash must be emphasized. Rocky Mountain *spotless* fever has also been described.[8]

It is appropriate to consider RMSF a potentially lethal illness, even though younger patients are likely to be less severely affected. Early diagnosis and prompt therapy lessen disease severity. Under such circumstances death would be extremely unusual, and in the majority of patients, early clinical diagnosis and adequate therapy shorten the duration of illness appreciably. Normal temperatures within the first 3 to 4 days may be expected, and rapid recovery from other signs of illness (e.g., headache, myalgia, and lethargy) also occurs. Extension of the rash ceases.[4]

Experience with RMSF before effective therapy indicated that the illness persisted for 2 to 3 weeks and that there was an overall mortality of 20%. Today, a delay in initiating appropriate therapy will lengthen the duration of illness and increase the likelihood of complications. Although mortality of approximately 5% still remains, recovery from the illness is accompanied by permanent immunity.

COMPLICATIONS

The major complication of RMSF is disseminated intravascular coagulation. Patients in whom the diagnosis has been delayed are those at greatest risk. This complication may prove lethal or result in local gangrene, with loss of tissue, appendages, or both.

Myocardial failure may result from myocarditis and arrhythmias. Edema may be generalized as a result of an increase in capillary permeability secondary to the vasculitis, heart failure, or iatrogenic fluid overload.

Neurologic complications, in addition to the lethargy, have already been discussed.

Hematuria and anemia may also occur.

TREATMENT

Specific therapy with either chloramphenicol (100 mg/kg/24 hr; maximum 4 g/24 hr) or tetracycline (20 mg/kg/24 hr; maximum 2 g/24 hr; tetracycline should not be used in children under 8 years of age) should be started on the basis of the clinical diagnosis. The intravenous route is indicated for patients moderately or severely ill or for those who are vomiting. Oral medication should be reserved for the mildly ill.

Hospitalization is desirable initially for all patients, both to ensure an adequate differential diagnosis and to ascertain that therapy is effective. Therapy should be continued until improvement has occurred and the patient is afebrile for 48 hours.

Supportive therapy includes maintenance of hydration and nutrition by appropriate intravenous fluids, oral feedings if tolerated, or both. Management of disseminated intravascular coagulation remains unsatisfactory, but therapeutic maneuvers such as fresh-frozen plasma, transfusion of fresh platelets and packed RBCs, and the administration of vitamin K may be helpful. The use of corticosteroids is believed to be warranted in those patients most severely ill and toxic. Seizures may require the use of anticonvulsant medications.

PREVENTION

The use of vaccine is not indicated except in those individuals at highest risk for exposure. Even then, the availability of effective therapy reduces the need for vaccination.

A search should be made for ticks daily, and for those in tick-infested areas, twice daily. Careful inspection at bath time is an excellent way to discover the presence of ticks. They may be removed by gentle traction with forceps or tweezers, but care must be taken not to crush the tick.

REFERENCES

1. Bell WE and Lascari AD: Rocky Mountain spotted fever: neurologic symptoms in the acute phase, Neurology 20:841, 1970.
2. Davis AE and Bradford WD: Abdominal pain resembling acute appendicitis in Rocky Mountain spotted fever, JAMA 247:2811, 1982.
3. Fleisher G, Lennette ET, and Honig P: Diagnosis of Rocky Mountain spotted fever by immunofluorescent identification of *Rickettsia rickettsii* in skin biopsy tissue, J Pediatr 95:63, 1979.
4. Haynes RE, Sanders DY and Cramblett HG: Rocky Mountain spotted fever in children, J Pediatr 76:685, 1970.
5. Lange JV, Walker DH, and Wester TB: Documented Rocky Mountain spotted fever in wintertime, JAMA 247:2403, 1982.
6. Marx RS et al: Rocky Mountain spotted fever: serological evidence of previous subclinical infection in children, Am J Dis Child 136:16, 1982.
7. Salgo MP et al: A focus of Rocky Mountain fever within New York City, N Engl J Med 318:1345, 1988.
8. Westerman EL: Rocky Mountain spotless fever: a dilemma for the clinician, Arch Intern Med 142:1106, 1982.

251

Roseola

Jerri Ann Jenista

Roseola is a classic childhood exanthem. The illness also is known as roseola infantum, exanthem subitum, 3-day fever, sixth disease, and pseudorubella. Exciting new information has dramatically changed our thinking about this common malady.

ETIOLOGY

The etiologic agent of roseola is now believed to be a newly discovered virus, human herpesvirus 6 (HHV-6).[5] Previously called human B-lymphotrophic virus (HBLV), HHV-6 is classified as a herpesvirus on the basis of its physical and genetic similarity to others of the group: herpes simplex virus–1, herpes simplex virus–2, cytomegalovirus, Epstein-Barr virus, and varicella-zoster virus. HHV-6 can be distinguished from the others by DNA hybridization or by reactions with virus-specific monoclonal antibodies. Sophisticated antigen detection methods demonstrate virus in many healthy persons, including those with HHV-6 antibody. The questions of possible virus latency and reactivation are unanswered.

EPIDEMIOLOGY

Roseola infantum (exanthem subitum, 3-day fever, sixth disease, pseudorubella) is so frequent an illness that fully 30% of children will suffer the clinical disease between the ages of 6 months and 2 years. The diagnosis is unusual, however, at other ages in children; rare cases in adults have been reported. Most cases are sporadic, although family and institutional epidemics occasionally are noted.[2]

The incubation period is probably between 5 and 15 days; however, the mode of transmission and the period of communicability are unknown. The virus has been isolated from saliva, plasma, and many cell lines. Either the rate of subclinical disease is high or the illness is not highly contagious, because most patients have no known exposure.[2]

Serologic surveys show that virtually all term infants have passively acquired maternal antibody at birth. The prevalence of antibody falls, reaching a nadir by 6 months of age. By 1 year of age, nearly 90% of children have detectable antibody. These levels persist unchanged through adolescence and then decline slightly with age. Prevalence surveys of blood donors show antibody detection rates up to 97%.[6]

DIAGNOSIS

Recognition of roseola is based almost entirely on the observation of a classic clinical course. Typically, a fever as high as 102.2° to 105.8° F (39° to 41° C) suddenly develops in a previously well infant. Except for irritability, the child does not seem as sick as the temperature indicates. Physical findings are sparse and include only painless posterior auricular and suboccipital lymphadenopathy with slight eyelid edema, giving a "sleepy-eyed" or "droopy" appearance. Rarely, a pharyngeal exudate, mild coryza, otitis media, or a bulging fontanelle is observed.

After a 2- to 5-day course, the fever dramatically resolves and a rash appears almost simultaneously. With defervescence, the child seems recovered despite the rash. The typical exanthem occurs as macular or maculopapular blanching patches surrounded by a lighter halo. The eruption usually begins on the neck and spreads to the trunk and extremities, sparing the face. It fades within 4 to 48 hours and probably is frequently missed if it is faint or occurs at night.

Clinically inapparent infection certainly occurs. Roseola also may occur in a young infant as an afebrile exanthem or as a nonspecific fever without the characteristic rash.[1,4]

HHV-6 infection in adults rarely causes a roseola-like illness. Three cases of nonroseola HHV-6 infection in adults were reported by Niederman et al. in 1988.[3] The mild disease lasted several weeks and was associated with slight fatigue, headache, sore throat, and cervical lymphadenopathy. The levels of liver enzymes were transiently elevated.

The only helpful laboratory finding is a leukopenia with a nadir count as low as 2000 white blood cells per cubic millimeter on the third day of fever. A relative lymphocytosis or monocytosis is typical. Results of the cerebrospinal fluid examination, urinalysis, and chest roentgenogram are normal. Neither antibody detection methods nor virus isolation techniques are standardized for HHV-6. Because roseola is an inconsequential illness, there rarely is any need to confirm the specific diagnosis.

DIFFERENTIAL DIAGNOSIS

Roseola often is confused with other exanthematous diseases. In rubella the rash and fever are concurrent, and enlarged lymph nodes often are tender. Coryza, respiratory symptoms, and Koplik spots distinguish rubeola. Enterovirus exanthems usually occur in epidemics, involve older as well as younger children, and are more common in the large summer and fall. Erythema infectiosum, of fifth disease, affects the school-aged child and involves most prominently the face. Scarlet fever has a more confluent rash and is associated with marked pharyngitis. Drug eruptions, especially those resulting from sulfa-containing preparations, are not regularly preceded by fever and tend to be more diffuse.

TREATMENT

Management is based entirely on symptoms. Acetaminophen is quite effective in controlling the fever. Reassuring the parents that the rash is a sign of recovery often is comforting to them and may prevent unnecessary office visits.

OUTCOME

Complications are distinctly unusual. Febrile convulsions occasionally are seen, and thrombocytopenic purpura and encephalopathy associated with roseola have been reported.

REFERENCES

1. Asano Y et al: Human herpesvirus type 6 infection (exanthem subitum) without fever, J Pediatr 115:264, 1989.
2. Breese BB Jr: Roseola infantum (exanthem subitum), NY State J Med 41:1854, 1941.
3. Niederman JC et al: Clinical and serological features of human herpesvirus 6 infection in three adults, Lancet 2:817, 1988.
4. Suga A et al: Human herpesvirus 6 infection (exanthem subitum) without rash, Pediatrics 83:1003, 1989.
5. Yamarishi K et al: Identification of human herpesvirus 6 as a causal agent for exanthem subitum, Lancet 1:1065, 1988.
6. Yoshikawa T et al: Distribution of antibodies to a causative agent of exanthem subitum (human herpesvirus 6) in healthy individuals, Pediatrics 84:675, 1989.

252

Seborrheic Dermatitis

Howard R. Foye, Jr.

Seborrheic dermatitis is a term used for a variety of erythematous, scaly rashes ranging from the mildly erythematous, flaky desquamation commonly called dandruff to plaques of yellowish red, greasy scales that may be sharply demarcated. These rashes have a predilection for areas that are dense with sebaceous glands—the scalp, face, ears, chest, and intertriginous areas. This condition is common in early infancy and after the onset of puberty. The term *seborrhea* simply refers to excessive oiliness of the scalp, face, and other areas of the body.

ETIOLOGY

The cause of seborrheic dermatitis is unknown. The most popular theory has been that the sebaceous gland has an abnormal sensitivity to normal levels of circulating sex hormones. The distribution and natural history of seborrheic dermatitis are consistent with this theory. The occurrence in early infancy coincides with the presence of transplacentally derived maternal hormones, and the recurrence in adolescence coincides with the increased production of endogenous hormones. No abnormality in the structure or function of the sebaceous gland has ever been shown, and circulating hormone levels are not abnormal in persons with this condition. Therefore the idea of abnormal end-organ sensitivity has been proposed.

Because there are many similarities between seborrheic dermatitis and atopic dermatitis in the distribution of the rash, skin biopsy findings, and even association with subsequent atopic disease, some consider the two to be clinical variants of the same underlying condition.[2] Another etiologic theory attributes the rash of seborrheic dermatitis to *Pityrosporum ovale,* a fungal organism found on the skin and in the hair follicles of normal adults, which is uncommon in children.[1,3,4]

CLINICAL PRESENTATION

Infancy

Seborrheic dermatitis in infancy usually begins between 2 and 12 weeks of age and resolves spontaneously by 8 to 12 months of age. The most common site of involvement is the scalp, where the rash may take the form of erythematous, flaky, poorly demarcated patches, or thicker, yellowish, greasy scales over an erythematous base. The latter often is referred to as *cradle cap*. The rash frequently extends beyond the scalp to adjacent areas of the face and neck. Flexural and intertriginous areas also are commonly involved and may be secondarily infected with *Candida* organisms.

Puberty and Beyond

Seborrheic dermatitis is not common in late infancy and childhood. The most common period of onset is between puberty and middle age. It usually begins on the scalp as dandruff and may be limited to this type of rash. In more severe cases, yellowish red greasy scales may progress to involve the entire scalp. Other frequent areas of involvement include the forehead, eyebrows, nasolabial folds, pinnae, external auditory canals, and postauricular, presternal, flexural, and intertriginous areas. The lesions may be characterized by irregularly shaped, erythematous, flaky patches, with or without yellowish, greasy scales.

DIFFERENTIAL DIAGNOSIS*

Atopic Dermatitis

The differentiation between atopic dermatitis and seborrheic dermatitis in infants may be difficult. Both appear commonly as erythematous, scaly eruptions on the scalp and face. Some differentiating points in favor of a diagnosis of atopic dermatitis include onset after 2 month of age, marked pruritus, greater vesiculation, and a family history of atopic disease in 70% of those affected. A diagnosis of seborrheic dermatitis is more likely when the rash involves the diaper area or other areas of increased sebaceous gland density in addition to the scalp and face. In adolescence and adulthood the natural history of the condition and the distribution of the rash usually make the differentiation easier. Although involvement of the face, neck, and flexural areas is common in both conditions, atopic dermatitis commonly involves several areas that are unusual in seborrheic dermatitis, such as the hands, feet, upper portion of the arms, and popliteal and antecubital fossae. Also, the chronic lesions of atopic dermatitis generally are thicker, drier, and more pruritic than the lesions of seborrheic dermatitis. The scalp is a less frequent site of involvement for atopic dermatitis, especially after infancy.

Psoriasis

Psoriatic lesions usually are thicker, more sharply demarcated, and less greasy than seborrheic dermatitis lesions. The classic psoriatic lesion consists of a thick, reddish plaque with thin, silvery, "micalike" scales that, when present, make the diagnosis easier. Psoriasis can involve the scalp and inter-

*See also Chapter 160.

triginous area and can be so similar in appearance to seborrheic dermatitis that some dermatologists use the term *sebopsoriasis* when psoriatic lesions occur in areas of high sebaceous gland density. Psoriasis typically involves lesions over the extensor surfaces of the arms and legs and other pressure areas. In addition, 25% to 50% of patients with psoriasis have characteristic punctate pitting of the nails.

Contact Dermatitis

Contact dermatitis, particularly around the eyes and nasolabial folds, can look like seborrheic dermatitis. Vesicles, edema, pruritus, and a history of contact with a potentially offending agent help in the differentiation. Cosmetics and acne preparations are examples of possible causes.

Tinea Corporis

Tinea lesions, particularly in the inguinal area, may be confused with the erythematous, scaly patches of seborrheic dermatitis. In tinea corporis, however, the scale usually is finer, not greasy, and lesions frequently have raised active borders with central clearing. A potassium hydroxide (KOH) preparation and culture for identification of the fungal agent will confirm the diagnosis.

Candida Intertrigo

Candida intertrigo, particularly in infancy in the diaper area, can look like or be a complication of seborrheic dermatitis. Satellite lesions are characteristic of *Candida* intertrigo and will aid in the diagnosis, along with a KOH preparation.

Pityriasis Rosea

Seborrheic dermatitis of the trunk occasionally may look like pityriasis rosea, which is characterized by small, uniform, oval, erythematous, scaly lesions on the trunk. The classic appearance of pityriasis rosea lesions in a Christmas-tree shape several days after the appearance of a herald patch on the trunk will make the differentiation easy.

Lupus Erythematosus

Lupus often involves the face and occasionally the scalp and appears as dry, erythematous, scaly, well-defined lesions. The scales are removed with difficulty, and the scarring and pigmentary changes that are common as the lesions evolve help differentiate them from seborrheic dermatitis.

Histiocytosis X

Histiocytosis X is a rare proliferative disorder of the reticuloendothelial system that may manifest in infancy as a dermatitis with a distribution similar to that of seborrheic dermatitis. A biopsy may be indicated to rule out histiocytosis X if the dermatitis fails to respond to usual therapy or has features unusual in seborrheic dermatitis, such as petechiae, purpura, erosions, or ulcerations.

TREATMENT OF SEBORRHEIC DERMATITIS

For patients with only oily skin and dandruff, frequent washing and the daily use of a commercially available shampoo with a desquamating agent (e.g., Head and Shoulders, Selsun Blue, Sebulex) may be all that is necessary. The patient must be instructed, however, that the shampoo needs to be in contact with the scalp for 5 to 10 minutes to have time to soften and loosen the scales. These same preparations can be used on scalp seborrhea in infants, but shampoos once every 2 or 3 days are recommended.

For more severe seborrheic dermatitis, removal of scales with a desquamating shampoo or oil is still beneficial and may enhance the efficacy of steroid applications. Seborrheic dermatitis usually is responsive to topical steroids; 1% hydrocortisone cream (3 times a day for 1 to 2 weeks) usually is sufficient for treatment. If a steroid application is necessary on the scalp, 1% hydrocortisone lotion is preferable. When the external auditory canal is involved, application of 1% hydrocortisone cream with a cotton-tipped swab is indicated.

New evidence suggests that ketoconazole 2% cream is as effective as hydrocortisone 1% cream in the treatment of seborrheic dermatitis.[2,4] This discovery is consistent with the theory that the fungus *P. ovale* plays an etiologic role.

The most common complication of seborrheic dermatitis is secondary infection with *Candida* organisms. KOH preparations and cultures will indicate whether nystatin (Mycostatin) must be added as a therapeutic measure.

REFERENCES

1. Broberg A and Faergemann J: Infantile seborrhoeic dermatitis and *Pityrosporum ovale*, Br J Dermatol 120:359, 1989.
2. Green C, Farr P, and Shuster S: Treatment of seborrhoeic dermatitis with ketoconazole. II. Response of seborrhoeic dermatitis of the face, scalp and trunk to topical ketoconazole, Br J Dermatol 116:217, 1987.
3. Podmore P et al: Seborrhoeic eczema—a disease entity or a clinical variant of atopic eczema? Br J Dermatol 115:341, 1986.
4. Stratigos J et al: Ketoconazole 2% cream versus hydrocortisone 1% cream in the treatment of seborrheic dermatitis: a double-blind comparative study, J Am Acad Dermatol 19:850, 1988.

SUGGESTED READING

Williams ML: Differential diagnosis of seborrheic dermatitis, Pediatr Rev 7:204, 1986.

253

Seizure Disorders

Sarah M. Roddy and Margaret C. McBride

Seizures are caused by abnormal discharges of neurons and may have a wide variety of clinical manifestations. A seizure should be considered a symptom of systemic or central nervous system dysfunction. Management consists not only of seizure control, but also of diagnosing any potentially treatable underlying condition. Acute conditions associated with seizures include metabolic disturbances, fever, meningitis, encephalitis, and toxic encephalopathy. The terms *seizure disorder* and *epilepsy* are synonymous and are applied to the condition in which there is a tendency for recurrent, unprovoked seizures. Care of patients with epilepsy includes managing the psychosocial impact of epilepsy on the child and family.

CLASSIFICATION OF SEIZURES

Classification of seizures has provided a means to study seizures with similar pathophysiology and to determine which medications are effective for which seizure types. Electroencephalographic (EEG) monitoring has aided in the current classification,[5] which is based on characterization of seizure onset and progression. Seizures are divided into partial or generalized. Generalized seizures result from involvement of both cerebral hemispheres simultaneously from seizure onset. Types of generalized seizures include absence, myoclonic, atonic, tonic, clonic, and tonic-clonic. Partial seizures are caused by seizure discharges that begin in one hemisphere. Partial seizures are further divided into simple partial seizures, in which consciousness is preserved, and complex partial seizures, in which consciousness is impaired. Partial seizures of either type may progress to become secondarily generalized.

Epilepsy syndromes have also been defined in terms of a cluster of signs and symptoms, including age of onset, severity, diurnal or nocturnal occurrence, clinical course, associated neurologic dysfunction, inheritance, and EEG findings.[4] Generalized epilepsy syndromes include juvenile myoclonic epilepsy, Lennox-Gastaut syndrome, infantile spasms, and childhood absence epilepsy. A common partial epilepsy syndrome is benign partial epilepsy of childhood. Neonatal seizures can be generalized or focal and are therefore considered separately, as are febrile seizures. The accompanying box outlines the classification of the various seizure types and epilepsy syndromes.

GENERALIZED SEIZURES

Absence Seizures

Absence seizures are generalized, nonconvulsive seizures characterized by interruption of activity, staring, and unresponsiveness, which usually last between 5 and 15 seconds. The episode starts abruptly, without warning, and ends abruptly with resumption of the child's preictal activity. The child may be unaware that the episode occurred. At times, unresponsiveness is accompanied by eyelid fluttering and upward rotation of the eyes and occasionally by mild clonic movements or automatisms such as lip smacking, grimacing,

Classification of Seizures and Epilepsy Syndromes[4,5]

PRIMARY GENERALIZED

Seizure Types

Absence
Myoclonic
Atonic (also called astatic)
Tonic-clonic

Epilepsy syndromes

Infantile spasms (West syndrome)
Lennox-Gastaut syndrome
Childhood absence epilepsy
Juvenile myoclonic epilepsy

PARTIAL

Seizure Types

Simple partial
Complex partial
Partial seizures with secondary generalization

Epilepsy Syndromes

Benign partial epilepsy of childhood
Epilepsia partialis continua

UNCLASSIFIED

Neonatal seizures
Febrile seizures
Pseudoseizures

or swallowing. Seizures may occur over 100 times per day and may interfere with the child's learning ability. The age of onset is generally between 4 and 8 years of age; rarely does it occur before 3 years or after 15 years. Girls are more commonly affected than boys. The influence of genetic factors in the etiology of absence seizures is suggested by the fact that 15% to 44% of first-degree relatives have a history of absence seizures, paroxysmal EEG abnormalities, or both.[1]

The classic finding on the EEG in patients with absence seizures is bilaterally synchronous 3 Hz spike and wave discharges. Hyperventilation may be used to precipitate the electrical discharge as well as a clinical seizure. Photic stimulation during the EEG will also induce the seizure discharge in some patients. Generalized tonic-clonic seizures may occur in some children, especially those with onset of absence seizures after 8 years of age. The prognosis for remission is good for children in whom absence is the sole seizure type but is less favorable for those with associated tonic-clonic seizures.

Monotherapy with ethosuximide or valproate usually controls absence seizures effectively. Valproate is the drug of choice if there are associated tonic-clonic seizures. Benzodiazepines are also effective in controlling absence seizures, but their adverse effects on behavior make them second-line therapeutic agents. Phenytoin, phenobarbital, and carbamazepine are usually ineffective for treatment of absence seizures and may exacerbate them.

Myoclonic Seizures

Myoclonic jerks are characterized by brief, sudden muscle contractions that may involve only part of the body or may be generalized. They may occur in clusters, especially during the period of falling asleep or shortly after awakening. There may be no alteration in consciousness associated with the jerks.

Atonic Seizures

Atonic, or astatic, seizures have also been termed "drop attacks." They are characterized by a sudden decrease in muscle tone, which may result in head nodding or mild flexion of the legs. More significant decreases in muscle tone may cause the patient to slump to the floor. There is usually no detectable alteration in consciousness with these seizures.

Generalized Tonic-Clonic Seizures

Generalized tonic-clonic seizures are also known as grand mal seizures and consist of motor manifestations and loss of consciousness. The tonic phase is characterized by a sustained contraction of muscles, and as a result the patient falls to the ground, usually in opisthotonus. There is usually extensor posturing with tonic contraction of the diaphragm and intercostal muscles. This halts respirations, which in turn produces cyanosis. The tonic phase lasts less than 1 minute and is followed by the clonic phase, which consists of bilateral and rhythmic jerking. The jerks may be accompanied by expiratory grunts produced by diaphragmatic contractions against a closed glottis. The frequency of the clonic jerks decreases as the seizure progresses, although the intensity may actually increase. The tongue may be bitten, and bowel and bladder incontinence may occur. The clonic activity usually stops after several minutes. The seizure may be followed by vomiting, confusion, and lethargy, with gradual recovery of consciousness over a period of minutes to hours.

Generalized tonic-clonic seizures may be primary generalized or secondarily generalized. Primary generalized seizures are usually idiopathic or genetic in origin and are associated with bilaterally synchronous electrical discharges on EEG. Secondarily generalized seizures begin as partial seizures but may generalize so rapidly that any suggestion of focal origin is lacking. The EEG may demonstrate a focal discharge that may spread to both hemispheres or may show only bilateral synchronous discharges. History that is helpful in determining that a seizure is secondarily generalized is the presence of an aura, head or eye deviation, or focal clonic movement at the onset of the seizure. Neurologic examination may reveal subtle focal signs such as a mild hemiparesis or visual field defect. Complete seizure control is less likely in secondarily generalized epilepsy than in primary generalized epilepsy.[1] Effective antiepileptic medications for the treatment of generalized tonic-clonic seizures include phenobarbital, phenytoin, primidone, and carbamazepine. Valproate is also an effective anticonvulsant for generalized tonic-clonic seizures with or without focal features.

Infantile Spasms (West Syndrome)

Infantile spasms are a unique form of epilepsy, with onset during the first year of life. The seizures are characterized by a sudden contraction of neck, trunk, and extremity muscles. The spasms may be flexor, extensor, or mixed flexor-extensor and last only a few seconds each, but they often occur in clusters of up to 100 individual spasms. A typical episode is characterized by dropping of the head with abduction of the shoulders and flexion of the lower extremities. A cry may occur during or following the spasm. Pallor, flushing, grimacing, laughter, and nystagmus are observed during some episodes. Episodes are common on awakening from sleep, during drowsiness, and with feedings but are rare during sleep. The peak age of infantile spasm onset is between 3 and 7 months of age,[1] with an estimated incidence of 1 per 4000 to 6000 infants.[9] Males are more likely to be affected than females.

Infantile spasms are usually divided into symptomatic and cryptogenic groups based on the presence of a predisposing etiologic factor. Included among symptomatic infantile spasms are infants with abnormal neurologic development before the onset of spasms. Etiologies include structural abnormalities of the brain, hypoxic-ischemic insults, central nervous system infections or hemorrhages, and inborn errors of metabolism. Children with tuberous sclerosis account for up to 25% of patients with infantile spasms.[1] The cryptogenic group includes those patients in whom no etiologic factor can be found. Infants in this group tend to be older at the onset of infantile spasms compared with infants in the symptomatic group.

The EEG pattern associated with infantile spasms is known as hypsarrhythmia and is characterized by high-voltage slow waves with irregularly interspersed multifocal spike and sharp waves. Hypsarrhythmia may precede the onset of clinical manifestations, or it may occur later or not at all. Over time the hypsarrhythmia usually evolves into other focal or generalized abnormalities. In some cases the EEG may normalize.

Infantile spasms are resistant to treatment with most anticonvulsants. The most commonly used treatment is adrenocorticotropic hormone (ACTH). ACTH in a long-acting form is administered as a single daily intramuscular dose of 20 to 40 IU. Adverse effects of ACTH and steroids are significant and include Cushing syndrome, hypertension, susceptibility to infections, hyperglycemia, gastrointestinal bleeding, and electrolyte disturbance. The benzodiazepines are also effective in controlling infantile spasms. Nitrazepam seems to be more effective that clonazepam or diazepam. Valproic acid is also effective therapy of infantile spasms in some infants.

The prognosis for infants with infantile spasm remains grave. Even in recently reported series, the average mortality is approximately 20%, with aspiration pneumonia being the most common cause of death.[9] Mental retardation is associated in approximately 80% of survivors. The spasms usually remit by a few years of age, but 55% to 60% of patients subsequently develop other forms of seizures.[1] The prognosis is more favorable in those infants who have normal neurologic development before the onset of the spasms.

Lennox-Gastaut Syndrome

Lennox-Gastaut syndrome is a severe epileptic encephalopathy characterized by a variety of primary generalized seizures. Tonic seizures cause sudden, sustained contraction of the muscle groups, at times causing the patient to fall. Atypical absence seizures consist of a brief period of staring and immobility. The onset and recovery of atypical absence seizures are less abrupt than those of typical absence seizures. The episodes may be associated with mild tonic motor manifestations, automatisms, or loss of postural tone. Atonic seizures occur and may be preceded by myoclonic jerks. Tonic-clonic seizures and partial seizures may also occur in patients with Lennox-Gastaut syndrome.

The majority of these patients have onset of seizures between 3 and 5 years of age,[20] with boys slightly more often affected than girls. Many patients have neurologic deficits before the onset of Lennox-Gastaut syndrome, including mental retardation and cerebral palsy, which may be related to hypoxic encephalopathy or other insults to the brain. Patients may have a past history of infantile spasms. The EEG typically shows an irregular, high-voltage, slow (2.5 Hz or slower) spike-wave pattern. The discharges are bilaterally synchronous.

The treatment of the seizures associated with Lennox-Gastaut syndrome is disappointing. Valproic acid has been the most successful in treatment of the different seizure types and is felt to be the drug of choice. The benzodiazepines have also been successful in controlling atonic, myoclonic, and atypical absence seizures. Unfortunately, with increasing doses, the frequency of adverse effects also increases. The development of tolerance is also a problem associated with their use. Ethosuximide can help control the atypical absence episodes, and phenytoin can be used for tonic seizures. The ketogenic diet has also been beneficial in seizure control, but because of the nature of the diet, compliance is poor. Generally, the goal of treatment is to achieve reasonable seizure control with as few medications as possible in order to minimize adverse effects. Sometimes the seizures typical of Lennox-Gastaut syndrome occur in otherwise normal preschool-age children, associated with normal background and fast polyspike and wave changes on EEG. These children have a much better prognosis for seizure control and cognitive development.

Juvenile Myoclonic Epilepsy

Juvenile myoclonic epilepsy is a primary generalized epilepsy with an age of onset of 12 to 18 years. It represents 4% of all epilepsy and is characterized by myoclonic jerks that mainly affect the upper extremities and less commonly the lower extremities. The jerks usually occur shortly after awakening, and patients may complain of clumsiness or difficulty holding objects early in the morning. Approximately 80% of patients have generalized tonic-clonic seizures, and 25% have absence seizures in addition to myoclonic seizures.[8] Myoclonic jerks almost always precede the onset of generalized tonic-clonic seizures by months to years. A teenager who has generalized tonic-clonic seizures should be carefully questioned regarding myoclonic jerks. Both the myoclonic jerks and the tonic-clonic seizures may be precipitated by sleep deprivation, stress, alcohol, and hormonal changes. Patients remain neurologically normal. Juvenile myoclonic epilepsy is genetic; a locus on the short arm of chromosome 6 has been identified. Fifty percent of probands report seizures in first- or second-degree relatives, and EEG changes in relatives are even more prevalent.[6] The ictal EEG typically shows generalized, symmetric polyspike and waves at 4 to 6 Hz. Photic stimulation precipitates the electrical discharges in some patients. The recommended treatment for juvenile myoclonic epilepsy is valproate. In over 80% of patients, valproate will control the myoclonic jerks, absence seizures, and generalized tonic-clonic seizures. Other anticonvulsants may control certain seizure components of the syndrome, but valproate controls all of the seizure components. There is a high rate of seizure recurrence in patients who discontinue valproate. Juvenile myoclonic epilepsy is therefore considered a chronic, probably lifelong, condition that requires continuous treatment.

PARTIAL SEIZURES

Simple Partial Seizures

Simple partial seizures are characterized by seizure activity restricted to one side of the body, with preserved consciousness. The symptoms may be motor, sensory, or cognitive, depending on the location of the neuronal discharge. Motor seizures may be restricted to part of the body, such as the face or a limb, or they may spread to involve the entire side. If the seizure discharge spreads to structures involved in consciousness, the seizure will become a complex partial seizure. The seizure activity may also spread to the opposite side of the brain, causing a generalized seizure. A partial seizure may be followed by Todd paralysis, a weakness of the limbs involved in the seizure. Partial sensory seizures most often are manifested by paresthesias lasting less than 1 to 2 minutes. Seizure discharges from one occipital lobe may cause visual symptoms such as scintillating colored spots or scotomata in the visual field contralateral to the discharge. Seizures with more complex visual hallucinations often progress to complex partial seizures with diminished consciousness. Auditory seizures are manifested by hearing noises and less commonly by elaborate but usually nonverbal auditory hallucinations such as music.

Although simple partial seizures are caused by focal epileptiform discharges, a focal structural lesion may not be found in 30% to 50% of patients.[9] Causes associated with these seizures include prenatal and perinatal insults, central nervous system malformations, and metabolic disturbances such as hypocalcemia, hypoglycemia, and inborn errors of metabolism. Carbamazepine, phenytoin, and valproic acid are effective drugs in the treatment of simple focal seizures.

Complex Partial Seizures

Complex partial seizures are seizures that originate in a limited area of one cerebral hemisphere and result in impaired consciousness. A complex partial seizure may begin as a simple partial seizure that progresses to consciousness impairment, or there may be impairment of consciousness from the onset of the seizure. The initial portion of a seizure that occurs before consciousness is lost is referred to as the aura. The aura may consist of any of a wide variety of symptoms, depending on the location of cortical discharges. There may be auditory, olfactory, or visual illusions or hallucinations. Affective symptoms such as fear or other unpleasant feelings can occur. Anger or rage are extremely rare as a seizure manifestation but may occur during postictal confusion if the patient is restrained. Déjà vu, the feeling that an experience has occurred before, and jamais vu, the feeling that previously experienced sensation is unfamiliar and strange, have been described. Young children have difficulty describing déjà vu and may only say that there was a "funny feeling" that occurred in the head or stomach. Staring and automatisms, which are involuntary coordinated motor activity, occur when there is clouding of consciousness. Automatisms include simple phenomena such as chewing, lip smacking, swallowing, and hissing and more complicated activities such as picking at clothes, searching, or ambulating. Automatisms are usually followed by postictal amnesia. The child may become tired and go to sleep.

Complex partial seizures must be distinguished from absence seizures, which are also characterized by staring and unresponsiveness. Episodes of absence seizures have an abrupt onset and termination, compared with complex partial seizures, which have a more gradual onset and termination. Absence seizures last less than 30 seconds and are not associated with postictal confusion. Automatisms can occur if absence episodes are prolonged, but they are often just a continuation of motor activity present before the onset of seizure.

The most frequent EEG finding in complex partial seizures is an anterior temporal lobe spike discharge, although some patients will have spike discharges from other areas.[9] Interictal EEGs are often normal. Repeating the EEG increases the likelihood of demonstrating the abnormal discharge. Nasopharyngeal or sphenoidal electrodes rarely add information that is not obtained by scalp recordings that include special temporal placements.

Causes of complex partial seizures include perinatal insults, head trauma, encephalitis, and possibly status epilepticus, all of which may be associated with scarring of the temporal lobe. Indolent tumors such as hamartomas and low-grade gliomas also can cause complex partial seizures and are found in approximately 20% of persons with intractable partial seizures. Genetic factors play a secondary role in the etiology of complex seizures.[1]

Anticonvulsant drugs used in the treatment of complex partial seizures include carbamazepine, phenytoin, phenobarbital, primidone, and valproate. Carbamazepine is the drug of choice because of its efficacy and relatively mild adverse effects. If seizures are not controlled with carbamazepine, the addition of acetazolamide may result in improved seizure control.[17] Patients with medically intractable partial seizures should be evaluated at a comprehensive epilepsy center to determine their candidacy for surgical intervention, which results in complete seizure control in 40% to 70% of patients.[11]

Benign Partial Epilepsy of Childhood

Benign partial epilepsy of childhood is also known as rolandic epilepsy, sylvian seizures, and centrotemporal epilepsy. This epilepsy syndrome is a common type of partial motor epilepsy in childhood. The onset is usually between 5 and 8 years of age. Males are more often affected than females. Genetic factors play a role in the etiology. The seizures typically occur during sleep, although patients may occasionally have an episode during wakefulness. Episodes are characterized by the child awakening with one side of the face twitching. The oropharyngeal muscles are often also involved, causing the child to make unintelligible gurgling sounds. The ipsilateral upper extremity may be involved, but only rarely is the lower extremity involved. In rare cases a seizure episode will become generalized. Consciousness is often retained during the seizure, although the child may not be able to speak. Most seizure episodes last less than 2 minutes. The frequency of seizures is low, with 25% of patients having a single seizure episode and 50% having less than five episodes.[1] The typical EEG findings are midtemporal or centrotemporal spike discharges that are usually unilateral, often very frequent, and present in light sleep. Neuroradiologic studies show no abnormalities to correlate with the EEG focus. If a child has infrequent episodes, no treatment may be needed. If the episodes are frightening to the child and a decision is made to initiate treatment, carbamazepine is the drug of choice.[9] Other effective drugs include phenytoin and valproate. The seizure episodes remit around 9 to 12 years of age, but no later than 17 years. Remission is long lasting, and no developmental or neurologic impairment is associated with the seizures.

Epilepsia Partialis Continua

Epilepsia partialis continua is a rare type of seizure in which there is continuous twitching limited to one side of the body. The twitching frequently involves only a few muscles and occurs most often in the hand or foot. Consciousness is preserved, but there may be weakness of the extremity involved by the seizure activity. Seizure activity may persist for hours to months. Focal encephalitis and tumor have been associated with this type of seizure. Medical treatment of epilepsia partialis continua is generally unsuccessful, although carbamazepine, phenytoin, and benzodiazepines have been used with varying degrees of success.[9]

UNCLASSIFIED SEIZURES

Neonatal Seizures

Seizures are the most common manifestation of neonatal neurologic disease and occur in approximately 0.5% of all newborns.[16] The manifestations of seizure activity in neonates differ from those in older children. Volpe[24] has delineated five major seizure types in neonates:

1. *Subtle seizures* occur in both full-term and premature infants and are often overlooked. These seizures consist of eye deviation, blinking, sucking, swimming movements of the arms, pedaling movements of the legs, and apnea. EEG recordings do not always show correlation of electrical seizure discharges with the clinical seizure activity. This has raised the possibility that the seizure discharges arise from regions of the brain that cannot be detected by surface electrodes.
2. *Tonic seizures* are characterized by tonic extension of the limbs. Less commonly, flexion of the upper extremities and extension of the lower extremities occurs. There may be accompanying subtle seizure activity such as blinking or apnea. These seizures are more common in premature infants, especially in those with intraventricular hemorrhage.
3. *Multifocal seizures* are characterized by clonic activity in one extremity, which randomly migrates to another area of the body. These seizures occur primarily in full-term infants. The EEG shows multiple areas of sharp activity that discharge independently.
4. *Focal clonic seizures* occur in both full-term and premature infants. The seizure activity is characterized by clonic jerking, which remains localized. Although focal clonic seizures can result from focal central nervous system lesions such as cerebral infarction, they can also occur with metabolic disturbances.
5. *Myoclonic seizures* are flexion jerks of the upper or lower extremities. They may occur singly or in a series of repetitive jerks. Infants with these seizures may later develop infantile spasms. These myoclonic seizures should be differentiated from benign myoclonic jerks that occur during sleep in neonates and are accompanied by a normal EEG.

Jitteriness is a movement in neonates that may be confused with seizure activity. The movement is a tremor that is stimulus sensitive and can be stopped by passively flexing the affected limb. There is no associated eye deviation or other abnormal eye movements. Some investigators advocate identification of neonatal seizures by EEG recording, maintaining that only electrical seizures are "true" seizures and require treatment. However, this remains controversial, since identical clinical seizures in the same infant may at times not be associated with electrical seizures.[25] It is clear, however, that electrical seizures may not have clinical correlates, and hence EEG recording should be done for all infants at risk for seizures in order to identify these silent electrical seizures.

Etiology. There are multiple etiologies of neonatal seizures; however, only a few causes account for most cases. Determining the etiology of neonatal seizures is important, because specific treatment may be indicated. The etiology of the seizures is also an important factor influencing prognosis. Some of the most common causes of seizure are described below:

1. Hypoxia-ischemia is the most common cause of seizure in both premature and full-term infants.[24] These seizures usually begin within the first 24 hours of life and may be very difficult to control. Metabolic disturbances in the infant may also complicate seizure control.
2. Intracranial hemorrhage is another cause of seizures in both premature and full-term infants. Intraventricular hemorrhage is seen mainly in premature infants within the first 3 days of life. Generalized tonic seizures may be associated with severe hemorrhage invading the brain parenchyma. Infants who have a primary subarachnoid hemorrhage may not have any clinical symptoms or may develop seizures on the second day of life. These infants are often term infants who are neurologically normal except for the seizure. Subdural hemorrhage is associated with trauma and may result in focal seizure activity.
3. Metabolic disturbances, especially hypoglycemia and hypocalcemia, are also associated with seizures in neonates. Infants who are small for gestational age and infants of diabetic mothers are at risk for hypoglycemia, and blood glucose should be closely monitored. Low-birth-weight infants and infants of diabetic mothers are at risk for hypocalcemic seizures, which occur when calcium levels drop below 7 mg/dl during the first 2 to 3 days of life. Often, infants who have hypocalcemia also have a history of hypoxia, which contributes to the risk of seizure. Hypocalcemic seizures that occur later are usually related to low calcium–high phosphate intake. Late hypocalcemic seizures are now rare as a result of the development of formula with an appropriate ratio of calcium and phosphorus supplementation. Other metabolic disturbances that are less frequently associated with seizures in neonates include hyponatremia, hypernatremia, local anesthetic intoxication, pyridoxine dependence, and disorders of amino acids, organic acids, and the urea cycle.
4. Infection, including bacterial and viral intracranial infections, is an important cause of neonatal seizures. The most common bacterial etiologies are group B beta-streptococcus and *Escherichia coli*. Onset of seizures with meningitis is usually after the first 3 to 4 days of life. Prenatal nonbacterial infections causing neonatal seizures include toxoplasmosis, rubella, herpes simplex virus, coxsackie B virus, and cytomegalovirus.
5. Malformations of the brain can cause seizures at any time during the newborn period. The malformations most commonly associated with seizures are the ones with cortical dysgenesis such as lissencephaly, pachygyria, and polymicrogyria.[24]

Management of Neonatal Seizures. Treatment of neonatal seizures is urgent, since repeated seizures may result in brain injury.[24] The following outline is an approach to the diagnosis and treatment of seizures:

1. Ensure adequate ventilation and perfusion.
2. Obtain blood for glucose, calcium, magnesium, and electrolyte studies. Check a Dextrostix for an immediate determination of glucose.
3. Correct any associated metabolic abnormality: (a) Hypoglycemia: If glucose is low by Dextrostix (below 40 mg/dl), immediately give 10% dextrose intravenously in a dose of 2 ml/kg. Maintain blood glucose levels above 40 mg/dl by continuous intravenous infusion with monitoring of the levels in both full-term and premature infants. (b) Hypocalcemia: Correct by administering 5% calcium gluconate solution, 4 ml/kg intravenously at a rate of 1 ml/minute to maintain serum calcium levels above 7 mg/dl while monitoring cardiac rate and rhythm. (c) Hypomagnesemia: Correct serum magnesium levels to 1 mg/kg with 50% magnesium sulfate solution, 0.2 ml/kg intramuscularly.
4. For continued seizure activity, anticonvulsants should be administered: (a) Phenobarbital is given in a loading dose of 20 mg/kg intravenously over 10 minutes. Additional doses of 5 mg/kg can be given, up to a total of 40 mg/kg. (b) Phenytoin is given in a loading dose of 20 mg/kg intravenously with cardiac monitoring. (c) Lorazepam can be given in doses of 0.1 mg/kg intravenously for persistent seizures.[7,19] Respiratory status should be monitored.

After seizures are controlled with loading doses of anticonvulsants, infants may be continued on maintenance doses of anticonvulsants. In asphyxiated and premature infants, the half-life of phenobarbital is very prolonged and doses no higher than 1 to 2 mg/kg/day may be appropriate. There is no consensus as to the duration of treatment for neonatal seizures. The seizure etiology and EEG findings can help determine the duration of treatment. Infants with seizures resulting from a metabolic disturbance or infection may not need to be sent home on anticonvulsants; those with a central nervous system malformation may need continued treatment. If clinical seizures are no longer present and the EEG does not contain paroxysmal activity, it is reasonable to taper the anticonvulsants.

Prognosis. The prognosis of neonatal seizures relates mainly to the underlying diseases that caused them. Mental retardation and cerebral palsy are more common sequelae than are seizures. Infants with seizures related to hypoxic-ischemic encephalopathy, hypoglycemia, or bacterial meningitis have a 50% chance of normal development; those with seizures from late-onset hypocalcemia and primary subarachnoid hemorrhage have a greater than 90% chance of normal development.[24] The interictal EEG is helpful in determining the prognosis. A normal background EEG pattern is usually associated with a good neurologic outcome; a markedly abnormal background pattern such as burst-suppression or marked suppression of voltage is associated with a high risk of neurologic sequelae.

Febrile Seizures

Febrile seizures are seizures that occur in young children with fever but with no evidence of intracranial infection or acute neurologic illness. Simple febrile seizures are generalized tonic-clonic convulsions that last less than 15 minutes and do not recur within 24 hours. Complex febrile seizures are less common and are focal or prolonged beyond 15 minutes or recur within 24 hours. Febrile seizures occur in children between 3 months and 5 years of age; the median age of occurrence is 18 to 22 months. Approximately 2% to 5% of children will experience a febrile convulsion; boys are more susceptible than girls. Genetic predisposition plays a role in the etiology of febrile seizures, with 60% of patients having a relative who has had at least one seizure.[9]

A febrile seizure may be the first sign that a child is ill. It is not known whether the seizure activity is triggered by the rapid rise of fever or the actual height of temperature. Febrile seizures can be triggered by any illness that causes fever, most frequently by otitis media and upper respiratory infections. There is a high rate of febrile seizures with shigellosis, salmonellosis, and roseola, possibly related to a direct effect they have on the central nervous system or to a neurotoxin they produce.

One third of children who have a febrile seizure will have another one with another febrile illness. The younger the child at the time of the first episode, the greater the risk of recurrence. Approximately 50% of the recurrences occur within 6 months of the initial seizure; 75% occur within 1 year.

Usually seizure activity has stopped by the time the child is evaluated. However, if the seizure continues, lorazepam or diazepam should be administered (see Chapter 290, "Status Epilepticus"). The temperature should be brought down by using rectal antipyretics, removing blankets and clothing, and sponging. Once seizure activity is controlled, evaluation is directed toward finding the cause of the fever. If the child is under 1 year of age or if the child has not rapidly returned to normal, a lumbar puncture should be strongly considered to evaluate for meningitis.

The EEG is generally not helpful in the evaluation of children with febrile seizures. EEG tracings recorded within 1 week of the seizure often show posterior slowing. Paroxysmal activity is seen in the EEGs of 35% to 45% of patients who are followed-up for several years.[1] These EEG abnormalities do not predict recurrence of febrile seizures or the development of epilepsy.

Treatment of febrile seizures includes family education that addresses the benign nature of the seizures, the use of antipyretics, and first aid for seizures. Administration of phenobarbital at the onset of a febrile illness is not effective in the prevention of seizure activity, because therapeutic blood levels are not achieved. Prophylactic treatment with anticonvulsant agents should be considered if there is abnormal neurologic development, a complex febrile seizure, or the child is under 1 year of age. Phenobarbital administration in doses that achieve blood levels of 15 μg/ml is effective in preventing the recurrence of febrile seizures. Valproate also appears to be effective in prophylaxis; phenytoin and carbamazepine do not prevent recurrences. The adverse effects of anticonvulsant therapy must be weighed against the possible benefits. There is no evidence that prophylactic treatment reduces the risk of subsequent epilepsy.

The risk of subsequent epilepsy in children with febrile seizures is 2.4%. Factors associated with subsequent development of afebrile partial seizures include focal seizures, prolonged seizures, and repeated episodes of seizures with the same febrile illness. Factors associated with development of afebrile, generalized seizures include more than three febrile seizures, a family history of afebrile seizures, and age over 3 years at the time of the first febrile seizure.[2]

Pseudoseizures

Pseudoseizures are uncommon but must be recognized to prevent inappropriate treatment. They differ from true epileptic seizures in several respects. The movements are usually not clonic but may be quivering or random thrashing movements. There is usually no incontinence, injury, or tongue biting with pseudoseizures. Episodes may be dramatic, with screaming and shouting. Episodes may also vary greatly in the same patient. Usually there is no postictal period. Pseudoseizures can occur in early childhood but are more frequent in adolescents, especially females.[1] Pseudoseizures are most likely to occur in children who have true epileptic seizures. A detailed history and observation of an episode is often all that is needed to diagnose pseudoseizures. EEG monitoring can be used in patients in whom the distinction cannot be made clinically. Once the diagnosis is established, treatment is directed toward the psychosocial issues involved.

APPROACH TO AN INITIAL SEIZURE

The first step in treatment of the child with an initial seizure is making the correct diagnosis.

The risk of seizure recurrence is important in deciding whether to initiate antiepileptic therapy. Some types of seizures, such as absence, myoclonic, akinetic, and infantile spasms, have a recurrence rate of virtually 100% and have usually recurred by the time the child is seen by the physician. These types of seizures require treatment. However, children who have a generalized tonic-clonic or partial seizure have a recurrence risk of 50% to 60%.[3,14] Factors that increase the risk of recurrence include a partial complex seizure, an abnormal neurologic examination, and focal epileptiform abnormalities on the EEG. The best prognosis is in those children with a generalized seizure, normal neurologic examination, and a "nonepileptiform" EEG. Many patients who have a single seizure should be observed for recurrence but should not be started on antiepileptic medication. Over 50% of the recurrences occur within 6 months, up to 90% within 1 year. If a second seizure occurs, initiation of antiepileptic medication should be considered, since approximately 80% of children who have a second seizure will have further seizures.[3]

Diagnostic Procedures

Laboratory Tests. Laboratory tests usually performed at the time of the initial seizure include measurement of serum electrolytes, calcium, and magnesium, and blood glucose. In some cases the history or examination may indicate that a more extensive laboratory evaluation is required.

Electroencephalography. The EEG, which measures physiologic function of the brain, changes throughout childhood, reflecting brain maturation. The EEG is important in the evaluation of a child with seizures because it helps to define the seizure type. An epileptiform EEG may support the diagnosis of epilepsy, but a normal tracing does not exclude the diagnosis. Other abnormalities such as slowing and background disorganization are much less specific. Repeat tracings increase the likelihood of detecting epileptiform discharges in patients with seizures. Procedures such as hyperventilation, photic stimulation, and sleep should be used when obtaining EEG recordings. Nasopharyngeal and sphenoidal electrodes may be used to detect mesial temporal discharges, but they rarely add information to that obtainable by special scalp electrode placements. Video EEG monitoring is useful in correlating clinical symptoms with electrical seizure activity and may be useful when clinical manifestations are atypical. Although the EEG provides electrophysiologic evidence to support the diagnosis of epilepsy, EEG abnormalities must be interpreted in view of the clinical symptomatology. Some individuals have epileptiform discharges and other EEG abnormalities without ever having a clinical seizure. Treatment is not indicated for such individuals.

Neuroimaging Studies. Plain skull roentgenograms can detect calcifications that may be seen in some syndromes, but they are rarely helpful in the evaluation of children with epilepsy. Computed tomography (CT) and magnetic resonance imaging (MRI) have replaced skull roentgenograms in the evaluation of seizures. CT and MRI scanning detect structural abnormalities; MRI is more sensitive than CT in the detection of low-grade tumors, changes in myelination, and heterotopic gray matter. Neuroimaging studies are not warranted in every child with epilepsy; however, MRI or CT should be performed in children who have focal neurologic abnormalities on examination or have intractable epilepsy. Positron emission tomography (PET) is useful in evaluating metabolic alterations with seizure activity, but the clinical relevance of PET in individual patients is not clear, and its availability is limited at present.

Lumbar Puncture. The cerebrospinal fluid should be examined in patients in whom meningitis or encephalitis is suspected. In other patients, the lumbar puncture is rarely helpful and is not routinely indicated.

TREATMENT WITH ANTIEPILEPTIC MEDICATION

Once the child has had recurrent seizures and antiepileptic medication is indicated, the physician is faced with the decision of which medication to prescribe. Making the correct diagnosis of seizure type is the critical first step in treatment, since some seizure disorders respond to certain medications. In choosing among potentially effective antiepileptic agents, the drug with the least adverse effects should be selected. The medication is started at a dose that will result in a low therapeutic blood level. The dose should be increased until seizures are controlled or adverse effects become intolerable. If the initial medication is not fully effective, a second medication may be added. Consideration should be given to discontinuing the first medication if seizures are fully controlled with the second medication. It is important to use monotherapy if possible, since polytherapy often does not improve seizure control but may dramatically increase toxicity.

To devise an optimum dosing regimen, it is important to consider the pharmacokinetics of the various antiepileptic medications. The dosing frequency is determined by the half-life, defined as the time in which the serum level falls to 50% of the initial value. The dosing interval should be no longer than the half-life of the medication, which means that most antiepileptic agents may be administered twice a day and some need be administered only once daily.[9] The efficacy of an antiepileptic medication should be evaluated only after five half-lives have elapsed, since this period of time is required for the medication to reach a steady state. In antiepileptic medications that induce hepatic enzymes (e.g., carbamazepine), the half-life decreases over the first weeks of treatment. If breakthrough seizures occur at times of low (trough) serum drug levels or if toxicity occurs at times of peak serum drug levels, the frequency of dosing should be increased.

Patients requiring higher antiepileptic medication levels usually need more frequent dosing to avoid toxicity.

Serum drug levels can guide the adjusting of doses of antiepileptic medications. A baseline level should be obtained when the patient has been on an appropriate dose long enough to have stable levels. Other indications for obtaining levels include verification of compliance, breakthrough seizures, and toxic effects. Levels may also be checked when other medications have been added or deleted from the patient's regimen. The timing of the sample in relation to the last dose is important in the interpretation of the levels, especially in drugs with short half-lives.

SPECIFIC ANTIEPILEPTIC MEDICATIONS

Table 253-1 outlines commonly used antiepileptic medications and their properties.

Table 253-1 *Common Antiepileptic Medications*

DRUG	INDICATIONS	HALF-LIFE (hours)	USUAL DOSE (mg/kg/day)	THERAPEUTIC LEVELS (μg/ml)	ADVERSE EFFECTS
Carbamazepine	Partial, secondarily generalized	3-23 (18-55 initially)	5-25 5-10 (monotherapy)	4-12	Allergic rashes, nausea, diplopia, blurry vision, dizziness, hypersensitivity hepatitis, aplastic anemia
Phenytoin	Partial, secondarily generalized, primary generalized	7-42 (nonlinear kinetics)	5-7	10-20 (occasionally lower)	Rashes, hirsutism, gingival hyperplasia, coarse features, psychomotor slowing neuropathy, folate deficiency, myelosuppression, drug-induced lupus
Valproic acid	Primary generalized, absence, myoclonic, akinetic, febrile, infantile spasms, some partial	6-16	10-30 20-50 (infants and in polytherapy)	50-100 (150 if tolerated)	Nausea, tremor, weight gain, hair loss, thrombocytopenia, hepatic failure, pancreatitis
Phenobarbital	Neonatal, febrile, partial, secondarily generalized, primary generalized, akinetic	36-120	3-5 (<25 kg) 2-3 (25-50 kg) 1-2 (>50 kg)	10-40	Sedation, inattention, hyperactivity, irritability, cognitive impairment, rare hypersensitivity reactions
Ethosuximide	Absence, myoclonic, akinetic	15-68	15-40	40-100	Nausea, abdominal discomfort, hiccups, drowsiness, behavioral problems, dystonias, myelosuppression, drug-induced lupus
Primidone	Partial, secondarily generalized, primary generalized	3-20	5-10 (1-2 initially)	5-12	Sedation, irritability, psychomotor slowing, rare hematologic and hypersensitivity reactions
Clonazepam	Absence, primary generalized, infantile spasms	20-36	0.01-0.2	0.01-0.07	Sedation, hyperactivity, inattention, aggressiveness, tolerance, ataxia, withdrawal seizures
Acetazolamide	Absence, myoclonic, akinetic, partial	10-12	10-20	10-14	Diuresis, paresthesias, sedation, CO_2 retention, rashes

Phenobarbital

Phenobarbital is one of the oldest antiepileptic agents still in use. Because of its long half-life, it has the advantage of requiring dosing only once or twice a day. The recommended dose per kilogram decreases as the weight increases. Failure to decrease the per kilogram dose levels in older children will result in toxic levels. Because phenobarbital is a relatively safe medication in terms of serious toxic effects, monitoring of parameters other than serum levels is usually not necessary. The major disadvantage of phenobarbital is its effect on behavior and cognitive function, including hyperactivity, irritability, and attention deficits. Maintaining serum levels at the minimum level for seizure control may help decrease these adverse effects. Phenobarbital administration will lower the serum levels of carbamazepine and valproate. Administration of valproate will increase phenobarbital levels; therefore phenobarbital doses should be decreased by 25% to 50% to prevent toxicity when prescribed concomitantly with valproate.

Phenytoin

Phenytoin is also among the older antiepileptic medications and has been widely used. Because of its pharmacokinetics, blood levels vary dramatically with small changes in dosage. Therefore changes in dosage should be monitored with serum levels, and only very small dose changes should be made when serum levels are close to or within the therapeutic range. Phenytoin is commonly used for treatment of status epilepticus, since intravenous administration results in rapid penetration into the central nervous system. Although phenytoin is an effective antiepileptic agent in generalized tonic-clonic and partial seizures, its adverse effect limits its use. Cosmetic adverse effects include gingival hypertrophy, hirsutism, and coarsening of the facial features. Also of concern are its effects on mood and cognitive function, which include depressed mood, slowed psychomotor functioning, and in a few, depressed IQ scores.[23] Other adverse effects include folate-deficiency anemia, cerebellar degeneration, and allergic dermatitis. Valproic acid may lower total serum phenytoin, but the free phenytoin level transiently increases and then returns to its original level; thus no adjustment in dosage is necessary. Phenytoin may decrease carbamazepine levels and increase phenobarbital levels.[18]

Carbamazepine

Carbamazepine is one of the new antiepileptic agents and is now widely used because of its relatively few effects on cognitive function. It may also positively affect behavior.[23] The most serious adverse effect associated with carbamazepine has been aplastic anemia. This is extremely rare, occurring at a rate of less than 1 case per 200,000 treatment years.[13] A complete blood count should be obtained before initiating carbamazepine therapy and should be repeated after 2 to 3 weeks. It is not clear whether further blood counts are useful when the initial counts are normal, but they should be obtained more readily when the child is ill and are often repeated biannually or annually. Neutropenia as low as 3000/mm^3 may occur, but this does not predict more serious myelosuppression. The dose of carbamazepine may need to be changed during the course of treatment, because the drug tends to induce its own metabolic breakdown. Phenobarbital, phenytoin, primidone, and clonazepam decrease carbamazepine serum levels.

Valproic Acid

Valproic acid is also one of the new antiepileptic medications and has a broad spectrum of efficacy. It also has the advantage of minimal cognitive adverse effects. Tremor may occur with high serum levels. Other adverse effects include increased appetite, weight gain, transient hair loss, nausea, and vomiting. Fatal hepatotoxicity has also been associated with valproic acid. Most cases occur during the first 3 months of treatment. Those patients at greatest risk for hepatotoxicity are children under 2 years of age who receive valproic acid as part of antiepileptic polytherapy.[10] Successful treatment of valproic acid–associated hepatotoxicity with N-acetylcysteine has recently been reported.[12] Valproic acid should be administered to patients with preexisting hepatic dysfunction extremely cautiously. Liver function should be monitored in patients on valproic acid, especially those in the high-risk group. Valproic acid raises the level of phenobarbital; therefore the dose of phenobarbital must be decreased by 33% to 50% if valproic acid is added. Carbamazepine, phenobarbital, and phenytoin decrease valproic acid serum levels.

Ethosuximide

Ethosuximide has a limited spectrum of efficacy; it is used mainly for treating absence seizures and some forms of myoclonic seizures. Behavioral disturbances also can occur in some children, and pancytopenia has been associated with chronic administration. Therefore periodic blood counts may be necessary.[9] Ethosuximide does not significantly interact with other antiepileptic medications.

Primidone

Primidone is not a commonly used antiepileptic agent, because it has no specific advantage over other agents. Primidone is metabolized to phenobarbital and phenylethylmalonamide and has many of the same characteristics of phenobarbital, including behavioral and cognitive adverse effects. It may be more sedating than phenobarbital. Since one third of primidone is metabolized to phenobarbital, phenobarbital levels should be monitored. Phenobarbital levels may be 1.3 to 2 times higher than primidone levels. Valproate increases primidone serum levels. Phenytoin and carbamazepine increase the phenobarbital to primidone ratio.

Clonazepam

Clonazepam, a benzodiazepine, is not a first-line antiepileptic medication because of its adverse effects. It causes significant behavioral changes, including hyperactivity, decreased attention, aggressiveness, and restlessness. Because withdrawal of the drug may cause irritability, myoclonus, and increased seizures, it should be done slowly. Treatment with clonazepam is usually reserved for absence and myoclonic seizures that are refractory to ethosuximide and valproic acid.

Acetazolamide

Acetazolamide is an inhibitor of the enzyme carbonic anhydrase. It is an effective adjunctive therapy for treatment of several types of seizures, although its antiepileptic properties are not well understood. Acetazolamide can be used in combination with valproic acid for treatment of absence, myoclonic, and akinetic seizures. Adding acetazolamide to carbamazepine may improve control of partial seizures.[17] Acetazolamide metabolism is not significantly affected by other medications.

DISCONTINUATION OF ANTIEPILEPTIC MEDICATIONS

After seizures have been controlled for a period of 2 years, consideration should be given to discontinuing antiepileptic medications. Studies have shown that 75% of children who were seizure free for more that 2 years remained seizure free after antiepileptic medications were discontinued.[21] The EEG can be helpful when considering discontinuing antiepileptic medications. If the EEG shows no epileptiform discharges, the prognosis is excellent. However, if the EEG demonstrates spikes or slowing, there is a higher risk of seizure recurrence.[21] The risk of recurrence is not increased if medication is tapered over a period as short as 6 weeks.[22] Long-term follow-up of children after withdrawal of medication has shown that 50% of the recurrences occur within 6 months and 60% to 80% within 2 years.[15]

REFERENCES

1. Aicardi J: Epilepsy in children, New York, 1986, Raven Press.
2. Annegers JF et al: Factors prognostic of unprovoked seizures after febrile convulsions, N Engl J Med 316:493, 1987.
3. Camfield PR et al: Epilepsy after a first unprovoked seizure in childhood, Neurology 35:1657, 1985.
4. Commission on Classification and Terminology of the International League Against Epilepsy: Proposal for classification of epilepsies and epileptic syndromes, Epilepsia 26:268, 1985.
5. Commission on Classification and Terminology of the International League Against Epilepsy: Proposal for revised clinical and electroencephalographic classification of epileptic seizures, Epilepsia 22:489, 1981.
6. Delgado-Escueta AV et al: Mapping the gene for juvenile myoclonic epilepsy, Epilepsia 30(suppl 4):S8, 1989.
7. Deshmukh A et al: Lorazepam in the treatment of neonatal seizures, Am J Dis Child 140:1042, 1986.
8. Dreifuss FE: Juvenile myoclonic epilepsy: characteristics of a primary generalized epilepsy, Epilepsia 30(suppl 4):S1, 1989.
9. Dreifuss FE: Pediatric epileptology: classification and management of seizures in the child, Boston, 1983, John Wright/PSG, Inc.
10. Dreifuss FE et al: Valproic acid hepatic fatalities: a retrospective review, Neurology 37:379, 1987.
11. Engel J Jr, editor: Surgical treatment of the epilepsies, New York, 1987, Raven Press.
12. Farrell K et al: Successful treatment of valproate hepatotoxicity with N-acetylcysteine, Epilepsia 30:700, 1989.
13. Hart RG and Easton JD: Carbamazepine and hematological monitoring, Ann Neurol 11:309, 1982.
14. Hirtz DG, Ellenberg JH, and Nelson KB: The risk of recurrence of nonfebrile seizures in children, Neurology 34:634, 1984.
15. Holowach J, Thurston DL, and O'Leary J: Prognosis in childhood epilepsy: follow-up study of 148 cases in which therapy had been suspended after prolonged anticonvulsant control, N Engl J Med 286:169, 1972.
16. Mellits ED, Holden KR, and Freeman JM: Neonatal seizures. II. Multivariate analysis of factors associated with outcome, Pediatrics 70:177, 1981.
17. Oles KS et al: Use of acetazolamide as an adjunct to carbamazepine in refractory partial seizures, Epilepsia 30:74, 1989.
18. Penry JK, editor: Epilepsy: diagnosis, management, and quality of life, New York, 1986, Raven Press.
19. Roddy SM, McBride MC, and Torres CF: Treatment of neonatal seizures with lorazepam, Ann Neurol 22:412, 1987.
20. Roger J, Dravet C, and Bureau M: The Lennox-Gastaut syndrome, Cleve Clin J Med 56(suppl 1):S172, 1989.
21. Shinnar S et al: Discontinuing antiepileptic medication in children with epilepsy after two years without seizures, N Engl J Med 313:976, 1985.
22. Tennison MB et al: Rate of taper of antiepileptic drugs and the risk of seizure recurrence, Ann Neurol 26:439, 1989.
23. Trimble MR and Cull CA: Antiepileptic drugs, cognitive function, and behavior in children, Cleve Clin J Med 56(suppl 1):S140, 1989.
24. Volpe JJ: Neurology of the newborn, ed 2, Philadelphia, 1987, WB Saunders Co.
25. Weiner SP, Scher MS, and Painter MJ: Neonatal seizures: electroclinical disassociation, Epilepsia 30:691, 1989.

254

Septic Arthritis

Edwards P. Schwentker

Septic arthritis most commonly involves lower extremity joints and characteristically affects young children and infants. Septic arthritis constitutes a *true clinical emergency,* since its complications may include dissolution of articular cartilage, necrosis of the underlying epiphysis, destruction of the adjacent growth plate, and dislocation of the joint itself. Complications can only be minimized by a high index of clinical suspicion, prompt diagnosis, and aggressive treatment.

PATHOGENESIS

Bacteria may reach a joint by any one of three routes. Direct introduction may occur through percutaneous puncture, with the needle being either purposely introduced into the joint or wandering from adjacent structures such as from blood vessels during an attempted venipuncture. Second, hematogenous bacterial seeding may occur directly to the membrana synovialis. Finally, septic arthritis may develop from a contiguous metaphyseal osteomyelitis that decompresses into the joint capsule. In young infants, bone infection may extend from the metaphysis into the epiphysis via transepiphyseal vessels and then from the epiphysis directly into the joint. For a more complete discussion of osteomyelitis, the reader is referred to Chapter 237.

With few exceptions, the organisms most commonly responsible for septic arthritis are the same as those in acute osteomyelitis; thus the leading offender is *Staphylococcus aureus*. Particularly in very young children, *Haemophilus influenzae* type b and streptococci of various types are seen. Gonococcal arthritis is fairly rare; when it occurs, however, it often involves several joints. Meningococcal arthritis can also occur and may develop without meningitis or meningococcemia.[2]

The consequences of an established septic arthritis can be severe. Enzymes destructive to both cartilage matrix and collagen are released by leukocytes and synovial cells as part of the inflammatory process. With infections caused by *S. aureus* and some of the gram-negative bacteria, the potential for destruction of joint surfaces is increased, because these organisms also produce proteolytic enzymes. By raising intraarticular pressure, intracapsular infection may obstruct blood flow, leading to necrosis of the epiphysis and the underlying growth plate. Finally, an untreated joint infection can result in joint instability through destruction of the ligamentous fibers of the capsule. Dislocation is particularly likely with the hip and shoulder.

Considering the possible consequences and, particularly in the young child, the potential for permanent deformity and disability, the need for accurate diagnosis and expeditious treatment of a septic arthritis cannot be exaggerated.

CLINICAL FINDINGS

The source of a hematogenous septic arthritis may be a preexisting infection elsewhere in the body, but frequently none is recognized. As the septic arthritis develops, there is generally an acute onset of fever, malaise, and marked localized signs and symptoms.[1,3] Swelling, erythema, and tenderness are often prominent but may be hard to detect in a deep joint such as the hip. The most characteristic finding is pain with joint motion. When a lower extremity joint is involved, the patient usually refuses to bear weight.

The joint will be held immobile in a particular position by muscle spasm so that movement of the joint is minimized; this leads to increased intracapsular volume and, overall, decreased intraarticular pressure. For the hip the preferred position is a combination of moderate flexion, abduction, and external rotation; for the knee, gentle flexion; and for the shoulder, adduction against the trunk. It is not at all unusual for a child to appear entirely well and in no distress so long as the affected joint is allowed to remain undisturbed.

The pediatrician should rely most on the physical examination. The only absolutely reliable laboratory tests are a gram stain and culture. White blood cell (WBC) counts may be within normal limits or only mildly elevated. The erythrocyte sedimentation rate is more consistently elevated, but even this test may be unremarkable in the newborn. Blood cultures should be drawn when septic arthritis is suspected, since they are frequently positive for the offending organism.

Early in the course of septic arthritis, radiographs are negative for any bone change but frequently demonstrate soft tissue changes, including swelling and edematous infiltration into fatty tissue planes. Radionuclide scanning is not necessary if there are clear-cut localizing signs. Scans are contraindicated if they delay appropriate treatment in any way. Scanning may help find or rule out other sites of involvement, particularly in very sick or very young children.

Ultrasonography has proven useful in determining the capsular distention that accompanies septic arthritis of the hip.[4] In the hands of an experienced radiologist, this noninvasive test can accurately exclude the presence of a joint effusion or, if one is present, assist the pediatrician in accurate needle placement during diagnostic aspiration.

Joint aspiration with a large-bore needle is the most important diagnostic maneuver. This can generally be performed in most joints without using an anesthetic. An orthopedist should be consulted to aspirate suspected joints, unless the primary care physician is skilled in this procedure. Fluoroscopy or possibly ultrasonography should be used to confirm entrance into the relatively inaccessible hip and shoulder joints. A diagnostic aspiration yields fluid with a white blood cell count exceeding 100,000 with a percentage of polymorphonuclear leukocytes greater than 75%. Lower counts can be found early in the course of a septic arthritis. Effusion with a low WBC count may also be associated with acute osteomyelitis of an adjacent metaphysis, the effusion being sympathetic. In most instances in which septic arthritis is present, the aspiration will yield frank pus. In any case, aspirated fluid should be cultured and gram stained.

In septic arthritis, as in osteomyelitis, the neonate presents a unique challenge.[1] Systemic signs may be absent, and laboratory findings may be within normal limits. Nonetheless, localized signs are almost always prominent, particularly pain with motion of the involved joint. The failure of an infant to move an infected joint is a condition known as *pseudoparalysis* and may be seen in a child who otherwise appears completely normal. The clinician may be misled into seeking a neurologic deficit on the assumption that the lack of motion is caused by true muscle paralysis. The pattern of motor dysfunction, however, is usually atypical for a neurologic deficit, and almost invariably passive movement of the affected extremity will elicit severe pain, a finding not characteristic of true paralysis. To make the diagnosis of septic arthritis, the pediatrician must suspect infection, and any infant's failure to move an extremity spontaneously must be considered a result of septic arthritis until proven otherwise.

MANAGEMENT

Following an expeditious clinical, roentgenographic, and laboratory evaluation, the suspected joint should be aspirated with a large-bore needle. Blood cultures should be obtained. If pus is obtained from the joint, the material should be gram stained and cultured, and parenteral antibiotics should be begun immediately on the basis of the gram-stain findings. If bacteria are not seen, antibiotic therapy should be instituted while culture results are pending. An antistaphylococcal penicillin alone is appropriate therapy for a child over 5 years of age. In younger children, coverage for ampicillin-resistant stains of *H. influenzae* should be added. Once confirmed, a septic joint should be operatively drained, debrided, and thoroughly irrigated with sterile saline as soon as possible.

Aspiration of the joint should be considered a diagnostic and not a therapeutic maneuver. Treatment with antibiotics and repeated percutaneous aspiration is inappropriate. Operative drainage is unquestionably more effective, and the consequence of prolonged joint sepsis may be permanent disability. The findings at the time of arthrotomy often indicate the futility of attempting to eradicate an abscess through a needle, since heavy fibrin deposits are frequently encountered. Such deposits cannot be debrided by needle aspiration.

A negative aspiration of a joint that is otherwise suspected of harboring sepsis must be viewed with skepticism. Fibrin debris or thick pus may prevent aspiration. Exquisite pain with passive joint motion, discretely localized soft tissue swelling and tenderness, and evidence for joint effusion should overrule the negative aspiration and indicate operative exploration. The risks of an unnecessary exploration are minimal compared with the certainty of joint damage that attends a neglected septic arthritis.

Parenteral antibiotics should be continued and adequate blood levels maintained following operative drainage. The choice of antibiotics should be adjusted after the results of cultures are obtained. If methods are available for determining bactericidal activity, it may be possible to substitute oral medications for the parenteral antibiotics. Oral antibiotics, however, should be used only if the patient is responding to treatment, the parents are reliable, the antibiotic does not cause a gastrointestinal disturbance that interferes with absorption, and blood levels can be monitored adequately. Antibiotic therapy should continue for a minimum of 3 weeks, but treatment should not be discontinued until the clinical response indicates that the condition has been corrected and the erythrocyte sedimentation rate has returned to normal.[2]

Immobilization is the final principle of treating septic arthritis.[3] Splinting should be provided for comfort and rest of the affected distal joints of the upper and lower extremities after drainage, but it need be continued only while swelling, tenderness, and pain with motion persist. Neglected infection of a shoulder or hip may lead to subluxation or frank dislocation; thus, these joints should be immobilized long enough for the capsule to restabilize. If diagnosis and treatment are accomplished soon after the onset of the disease, 2 to 3 weeks of immobilization may be adequate. A prolonged infection, particularly of the hip, may require immobilization for 2 to 3 months. The shoulder can be adequately protected with a simple sling and swathe. The hip may be immobilized in a spica cast or, once pain has subsided, protection may be provided by a simple Pavlik harness or any similar device that maintains reduction by centering the hip deeply within the acetabulum. The need for immobilizing a joint should be determined according to the individual's condition, so as to maximize joint stability while avoiding unnecessary stiffness.

REFERENCES

1. Griffin PP and Green WT Sr: Hip joint infections in infants and children, Orthop Clin North Am 9:123, 1978.
2. Jackson MA and Nelson JD: Etiology and medical management of acute suppurative bone and joint infections in pediatric patients, J Pediatr Orthop 2:313, 1982.
3. Paterson DC: Acute suppurative arthritis in infancy and childhood, J Bone Joint Surg 52B:474, 1970.
4. Wingstrand H et al: Sonography in septic arthritis of the hip in the child: report of four cases, J Pediatr Orthop 7:206, 1987.

255

Sexually Transmitted Diseases

Alain Joffe

For a variety of reasons, teenagers are at high risk for acquiring sexually transmitted diseases (STDs) (see box below). Over the past few decades, rates of sexual activity have increased dramatically among adolescents, especially white adolescents; hence, many more teenagers now are exposed to these infectious agents. Furthermore, by virtue of their cognitive developmental level, many adolescents feel invulnerable and minimize their potential for becoming infected. They may ignore symptoms or believe that as long as they are symptom free, they are neither infected nor infectious.

A large body of evidence now indicates that barrier methods of contraception (diaphragm, condom) when used with a spermicide, provide excellent protection against STDs.[15] Yet teenagers, when compared with adults, are poor users of these methods, relying instead on oral contraceptives or nothing at all. Oral contraceptives may protect against some STDs but may actually increase susceptibility to certain agents. Adolescents have difficulty discussing sexual matters with partners or with parents and so are reluctant to reveal that they are infected or have been treated. They may postpone a visit to a physician because they are embarrassed, fear a lecture, are concerned about the physician maintaining confidentiality, or lack the money or social skills to get to a source of health care.

Some physicians fear treating adolescents with a sexually transmitted disease, because they are uncertain about an adolescent's capacity to consent to treatment without parental involvement. Currently all 50 states have laws that specifically permit a physician to treat most minors seeking treatment without parental consent or notification.

Finally, there may be a physiologic basis for adolescent girls being particularly susceptible to infection upon exposure. The transformation zone of the cervix, which is relatively large among pubertal girls, is particularly vulnerable to infection with *Chlamydia trachomatis* and human papillomavirus (Fig. 255-1).

Not surprisingly, therefore, current data indicate that adolescents and young adults have higher infection rates than any other age group in the United States. The most recent data from the Centers for Disease Control (CDC) for syphilis and gonorrhea are shown in Table 255-1. From 1981 to 1988, gonorrhea rates for girls 10 to 14 years of age and for boys 10 to 19 years of age actually *increased*. Infection rates for syphilis have also *increased* among girls ages 10 to 24 since 1981.

Since *Chlamydia trachomatis* infections are not reportable to state or city health departments, accurate data about the extent of the problem are scant. However, several studies have shown that a greater percentage of 15- to 19-year-olds are infected than are those 20 or over.

The list of infectious agents that are potentially sexually

Why Adolescents Are At Risk for STDs

- Increased prevalence of sexual activity at earlier ages
- Sense of invulnerability ("It can't happen to me.")
- Lack of information ("If I don't feel sick, I can't be sick.")
- Infrequent use of barrier methods of contraception
- Poor communication skills with partners and physicians
- Barriers to care (legal obstacles, concerns about confidentiality)
- Poor compliance
- Physiologic changes associated with puberty

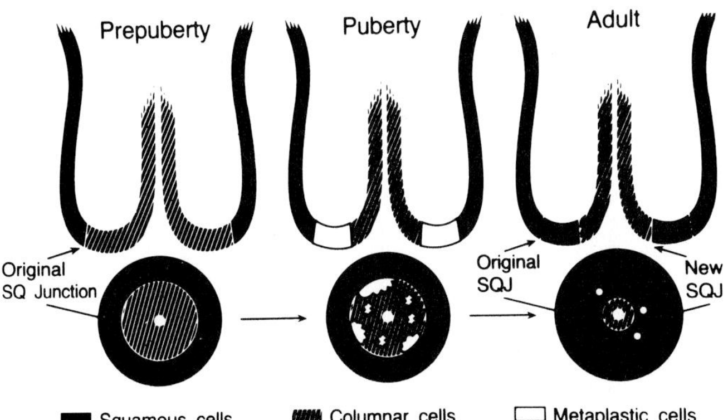

Fig. 255-1 Cervical development: In most prepubertal females, the original squamocolumnar junction is located well onto the ectocervix. During puberty, uncommitted germ cells of the columnar epithelium differentiate into squamous cells during a process called squamous metaplasia. This process begins at the original squamocolumnar junction at various areas and continues caudally. Thus the pubertal cervix is in a transitional state. By adulthood the transformation results in a new squamocolumnar junction, now found near or in the ectocervix.

(From Moscicki B and Shafer MB: Normal reproductive development in the adolescent female, J Adol Health Care 7:505, 1986.)

Table 255-1 *Infection Rates for Syphilis and Gonorrhea (1981 compared to 1988)**

		GONORRHEA		
		RATE		
AGE	SEX	1981	1988	% CHANGE 1981-1988
10-14	M	22.7	35.7	+ 57%
	F	71.6	96.3	+ 34%
15-19	M	965.9	978.4	+ 1.3%
	F	1396.0	1175.0	− 16%
20-24	M	2139.0	1444.6	− 32%
	F	1445.8	1048.5	− 27%

		SYPHILIS		
		RATE		
AGE	SEX	1981	1988	% CHANGE 1981-1988
10-14	M	0.6	0.3	− 50%
	F	1.4	1.8	+ 29%
15-19	M	21.2	16.2	− 24%
	F	18.8	27.7	+ 47%
20-24	M	62.0	58.3	− 6%
	F	23.5	48.4	+ 106%

*Per 100,000 population.
From Blount J: Personal communication, Centers for Disease Control, 1990, Division of Sexually Transmitted Diseases.

Sexually Transmitted Infectious Agents

Neisseria gonorrhoeae
Chlamydia trachomatis
Herpes simplex virus (HSV)
Mycoplasma hominis
Ureaplasma urealyticum
Trichomonas vaginalis
Gardnerella vaginalis (?)
Treponema pallidum
Human immune deficiency virus (HIV)
Human papillomavirus (HPV)
Hepatitis B
Cytomegalovirus (CMV)

Signs, Symptoms, and Clinical Entities Suggesting Sexually Transmitted Disease in Adolescents

MALES
Dysuria, urethritis
Epididymitis (scrotal pain, swelling)

FEMALE
Mucopurulent cervicitis
Vaginitis
Dysuria
Right upper quadrant pain
Pelvic inflammatory disease (low abdominal pain)

BOTH
Genital ulcers
Genital warts
Hepatitis B infection
HIV infection
Proctitis
Septic arthritis

transmitted is increasing. The box above lists the most common of these. Gonorrhea, chlamydia, herpes, human papilloma virus, and syphilis are discussed in detail in this chapter. The reader is referred to Chapter 212 for further discussion of herpes infections and to Chapter 178 for discussion of human immune deficiency virus (HIV) infections. Information about the other agents should be sought through the Index.

An alternative way of conceptualizing the spectrum of problems attributable to STDs is to focus on symptoms or diseases rather than on specific agents. More than one STD can produce various signs, symptoms, or syndromes, and many teenagers will deny sexual activity for the reasons outlined above. Hence when an adolescent has a symptom or sign that may be caused by such agents, the physician must proceed with appropriate diagnostic tests or therapy, even though the history may appear to exclude an STD. Most teenagers, however, will admit to sexual activity when questioned considerately with appropriate guarantees about confidentiality. The box above lists a variety of symptoms and clinical entities that are frequently caused by sexually transmitted agents.

SPECIFIC AGENTS

Chlamydia Trachomatis

The obligate, intracellular, cytomegalovirus microorganisms cause a wide spectrum of disease and are currently the most common sexually transmitted agents in the United States. Of greatest importance is their causative role in urethritis and epididymitis in males and cervicitis and pelvic inflammatory disease in females.[10]

Although data are limited, it appears that 30% to 50% of symptomatic nongonococcal urethritis among adolescent males is caused by chlamydia. Recent data indicate that approximately 10% to 20% of asymptomatic sexually active males will be culture positive for sexually transmitted agents, and almost 75% of them will have chlamydial infection. Males may complain only of mild dysuria, or they may have a scanty, mucoid discharge that is easily ignored. Having the male strip his urethra may produce some discharge if none is apparent. A profuse, purulent discharge should raise the possibility of *Neisseria gonorrhea* causing a coinfection or as the single causative agent. Males may also complain of testicular or scrotal pain or both, suggesting that urethral infection has spread to the epididymis.

Because the organism can infect the urethra as well as the cervix, a female may complain of dysuria as the primary manifestation of infection. Hence *Chlamydia trachomatis* infection should be considered in any adolescent female suspected of having a urinary tract infection. She may also complain of vaginal discharge or, if the infection has spread to the upper genital tract, of low abdominal pain or right upper quadrant pain (Fitz-Hugh and Curtis syndrome). The latter is caused by organisms tracking up the abdominal cavity and causing a perihepatitis. Lower abdominal pain suggests the possibility of pelvic inflammatory disease (see p. 1506).

As with males, females are often asymptomatically infected. On pelvic examination, however, clues to infection are the presence of mucopurulent discharge from the cervical os ("mucopus"—Fig. 255-2), cervical erythema, and friability.[2] A cervical Gram stain will reveal the presence of 10 to 30 or more polymorphonuclear (PMN) white blood cells per oil immersion field in three or more fields. Occassionally, a Papanicolaou (Pap) smear result will reveal the presence of inclusion bodies, suggesting the presence of infection. However, some patients lack signs of infection; given the high prevalence of infection among adolescents and the serious morbidity associated with untreated disease, every sexually active teenager should be screened for chlamydia annually. Such an approach becomes cost effective at a prevalence of 7% (when rapid test kits are used) or 14% (when cultures are used).[20]

Culturing cells for chlamydial infection remains the "gold standard" for detecting infection, although a single swab may be only 50% to 90% sensitive. To culture the organism, endocervical or urethral cells must be obtained; the organism cannot be grown from discharge alone. When a culture is not available or is too costly, direct fluorescent antibody tests or an enzyme immunoassay is acceptable. Compared with a culture test, these tests are 70% to 98% sensitive and 97% specific. For males, use of the "first-part voided" urine technique is extremely valuable for detecting asymptomatic infection (see box on p. 1496).[1] A nonsterile urine cup is marked at the 15 ml line with a wax pencil, and the male is instructed to collect only the first few drops (15 ml) of urine that he

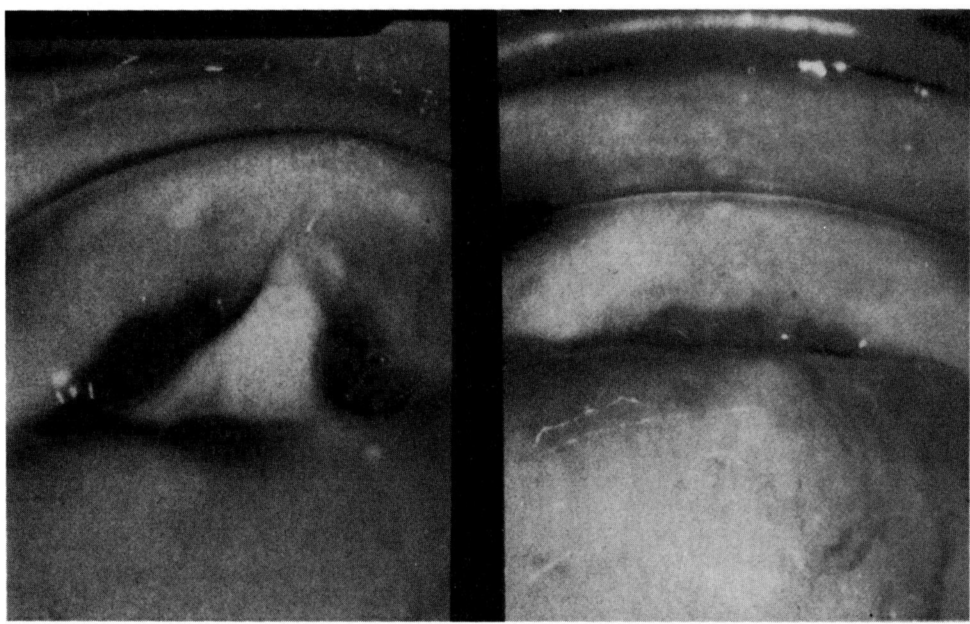

Fig. 255-2 Colpophotograph showing mucopurulent cervicitis before and 2 weeks after treatment with 500 mg of tetracycline four times daily for 7 days. Note disappearance of endocervical exudate after therapy.

(From Brunham RC et al: Mucopurulent cervicitis-the ignored counterpart in women of urethritis in men. N Engl J Med 311:2, 1984.)

Collection of First-Part Voided Urinalysis in Males[1,23]

1. Mark a urine collection cup at the 15 ml line.
2. Instruct the patient to *begin* urinating *into* the cup (no skin preparation is necessary).
3. When the urine reaches the 15-ml line *(no more than 15 ml)*, the patient should finish voiding into the toilet.
4. To look for white cells: centrifuge urine at 500 g for 10 minutes; decant supernatant. Resuspend sediment in remaining 0.5 ml. Ten white blood cells per high-power field is considered positive for urethritis.
5. Alternately, dip *unspun* urine with leukocyte esterase test strips within 10 minutes of collection. A result of 1+ or higher is positive for urethritis.

produces. Once the urine in the cup has reached the line marked, he is to finish urinating into the toilet. The urine is then centrifuged and the supernatant poured off. The residual is examined for white cells: 10 or more leukocytes indicates urethritis and correlates highly with positive cultures. Recently, several investigators have demonstrated that leukocyte esterase dipsticks used on a similarly obtained specimen can suggest chlamydial urethritis if they register 1+ or higher. The dipstick eliminates the need to centrifuge the urine and count cells.

Uncomplicated cervical or urethral chlamydial infection should be treated orally with doxycycline (100 mg bid), tetracycline (500 mg qid), or erythromycin (500 mg qid for 7 to 10 days) (see the box on p. 1497). The bid dosage of doxycycline likely improves patient compliance. As with any sexually transmitted organism, it is imperative to have the patient refrain from intercourse until his or her partner is notified and treated.

Complications of chlamydial infection include epididymitis and pelvic inflammatory disease. Long-term complications include Reiter syndrome and the sequelae of pelvic inflammatory disease. Cervical dysplasia may also be a complication of this infection. Of course an untreated, infected woman can pass the infection to her infant through colonization during birth.

Neisseria Gonorrhoeae

Infection with the gonococcus produces a constellation of symptoms very similar to that produced by chlamydia.[11] Approximately 45% of males with urethral discharge will have gonococcal infection. In general, patients who are symptomatic with gonococcal infection tend to have more pronounced symptoms and usually seek health care within a shorter period of time than those infected with chlamydia. However, many patients will have no symptoms at all. In large-scale studies, approximately 2% of sexually active males have been shown to be infected with gonorrhea; 70% of these were asymptomatic. The proportion of asymptomatic women with infection is unclear; estimates range from 25% to 80%. The gonococcus can cause pharyngitis and proctitis; females may harbor the organism in the rectum even though they do not engage in anal intercourse.

The diagnosis of gonococcal infection rests on culture and on the classic Gram stain with gram-negative intracellular diplococci. Even under ideal conditions, the organism can be difficult to grow, and each physician should be familiar with the yield from the laboratory he or she uses. In the male, a typical Gram stain from a urethral discharge is diagnostic (Fig. 255-3). For females, it is more difficult to sort out gram-negative organisms that are truly intracellular versus those that may be overlying the cells. However, Wald had shown that when at least eight pairs of such diplococci are seen in at least two PMNs, 96% of cultures are positive.[25] The gonococcus can be grown from urethral or cervical discharge, from swabs of the cervix, urethra, pharynx, or rectum, and in many instances from urine sediment.

Uncomplicated gonococcal infection should be treated with a single dose of ceftriaxone (250 mg intramuscularly) and doxycycline (100 mg orally twice daily for 7 days) (see the box on p. 1497). This CDC recommendation is based on the increasing prevalence of beta-lactamase–producing organisms. Because of the high likelihood that coinfection with chlamydia is present, treatment should include an effective regimen for *Chlamydia trachomatis* as well.

Gonorrhea may also produce epididymitis and pelvic inflammatory disease. However, the organism also has the capacity to become blood borne and can lead to what has been called the arthritis-dermatitis syndrome, or disseminated gonococcal infection (DGI).[18] About 1% to 3% of untreated patients will develop DGI. Typically, the patient will develop fever (although not always) and may have anorexia or malaise or both. Skin lesions then appear, generally distributed on the extremities (arms more than legs). These lesions typically are erythematous macules less than 5 mm in diameter; they become pustular and occasionally hemorrhagic or necrotic. They are most often noticed near the small joints of the hands and feet. Such lesions last several days and at this point, blood cultures are positive in 25% of cases. Accompanying the dermatitis is a tenosynovitis that again tends to occur over the extensor and flexor tendons of the hands and feet.

In general, once the tenosynovitis and dermatitis clear, the patient develops polyarthralgias but usually seeks care only at the point that an oligoarthritis develops. The knee is the most commonly infected joint, followed by the elbow, ankle, and small joints of the hands and feet. Hence, among adolescents, DGI should be actively considered in the differential diagnosis of septic arthritis. Aspirates of joint fluid will reveal the typical changes of a septic arthritis, but cultures will usually be negative.

Although the causative organisms are usually exquisitely sensitive to penicillin, patients with true arthritis should be hospitalized for treatment (see box on p. 1497). Those with only skin lesions or who have tenosynovitis may be treated as outpatients if careful follow-up can be assured; otherwise, inpatient treatment is also justified.

Guidelines for Treatment of Sexually Transmitted Diseases

CHLAMYDIAL INFECTIONS

Treatment of Uncomplicated Urethral, Endocervical, or Rectal *C. trachomatis* Infections

Recommended Regimen

Doxycycline 100 mg orally 2 times a day for 7 days

or

Tetracycline 500 mg orally 4 times a day for 7 days.

Alternative Regimen

Erythromycin base 500 mg orally 4 times a day or equivalent salt for 7 days

or

Erythromycin ethylsuccinate 800 mg orally 4 times a day for 7 days.

If erythromycin is not tolerated because of side effects, the following regimen may be effective:

Sulfisoxazole 500 mg orally 4 times a day for 10 days or equivalent.

GONOCOCCAL INFECTIONS

Treatment of Adolescents and Adults

Uncomplicated Urethral, Endocervical, or Rectal Infections

Recommended Regimen

Ceftriaxone 250 mg IM once

plus

Doxycycline 100 mg orally 2 times a day for 7 days.

Some authorities prefer a dose of 125 mg **ceftriaxone** IM because it is less expensive and can be given in a volume of only 0.5 ml, which is more easily administered in the deltoid muscle. However, the 250-mg dose is recommended, because it may delay the emergence of ceftriaxone-resistant strains. At this time, both doses appear highly effective for mucosal gonorrhea at all sites.

Alternative Regimens. For patients who cannot take ceftriaxone, the preferred alternative is **Spectinomycin** 2 g IM, in a single dose ***(followed by* doxycycline).**

Other alternatives, for which experience is less extensive, include **ciprofloxacin*** 500 mg orally once; **norfloxacin*** 800 mg orally once; **cefuroxime axetil** 1 g orally once with **probenecid** 1 g; **cefotaxime** 1 g IM once; and **ceftizoxime** 500 mg IM once. All of these regimens are ***followed by* doxycycline** 100 mg orally, twice daily for 7 days. If infection was acquired from a source proven *not* to have penicillin-resistant gonorrhea, a penicillin such as **amoxicillin** 3 g orally with 1 g **probenecid *followed by* doxycycline** may be used for treatment.

Doxycycline or tetracycline alone is no longer considered adequate therapy for gonococcal infections but is added for treatment of coexisting chlamydial infections. Tetracycline may be substituted for doxycycline; however, compliance may be worse since **tetracycline** must be taken at a dose of 500 mg 4 times a day—between meals, whereas **doxycycline** is taken at a dose of 100 mg 2 times a day without regard to meals. Moreover, at current prices, tetracycline costs only a little less than generic doxycycline.

*Quinolones, such as ciprofloxacin and norfloxacin, are contraindicated during pregnancy and in children 16 years of age or younger.

Pharyngeal Gonococcal Infection

Patients with uncomplicated pharyngeal gonococcal infection should be treated with **ceftriaxone** 250 mg IM once. Patients who cannot be treated with ceftriaxone should be treated with **ciprofloxacin** 500 mg orally as a single dose. Since experience with this regimen is limited, such patients should be evaluated with repeat culture 4-7 days after treatment.

Disseminated Gonococcal Infection (DGI)

Hospitalization is recommended for initial therapy, especially for patients who cannot reliably comply with treatment, have uncertain diagnoses, or have purulent synovial effusions or other complications. Patients should be examined for clinical evidence of endocarditis or meningitis.

Recommended Regimens—DGI Inpatient

Ceftriaxone 1 g, IM or IV, every 24 hours

or

Ceftizoxime 1 g, IV, every 8 hours

or

Cefotaxime 1 g, IV, every 8 hours.

Patients who are allergic to beta-lactam drugs should be treated with **spectinomycin** 2 g IM every 12 hours.

When the infecting organism is proven to be penicillin-sensitive, parenteral treatment may be switched to **ampicillin** 1 g every 6 hours (or equivalent).

Patients treated for DGI should be tested for genital *C. trachomatis* infection. If chlamydial testing is not available, patients should be treated empirically for coexisting chlamydial infection.

Reliable patients with uncomplicated disease may be discharged 24-48 hours after all symptoms resolve and may complete the therapy (for a total of 1 week of antibiotic therapy) with an oral regimen of **cefuroxime axetil** 500 mg 2 times a day *or* **amoxicillin** 500 mg with clavulanic acid 3 times a day *or,* if not pregnant, **ciprofloxacin** 500 mg 2 times a day.

Gonococcal Infections of Infants and Children

Gonococcal Infections of Children. Children who weigh ≥45 kg should be treated with adult regimens. Children who weigh <45 kg who have uncomplicated vulvovaginitis, cervicitis, urethritis, pharyngitis, or proctitis should be treated as follows:

Recommended Regimen

Ceftriaxone 125 mg IM once.

Patients who cannot tolerate ceftriaxone may be treated with:

Spectinomycin 40 mg/kg IM once.

Patients weighing <45 kg with bacteremia or arthritis should be treated with **ceftriaxone** 50 mg/kg (maximum 1 g) once daily for 7 days. For meningitis, the duration of treatment is increased to 10-14 days and the maximum dose is 2 g.

From Centers for Disease Control 1989 Sexually transmitted diseases treatment guidelines, MMWR (suppl) 38:8, 1989.

Continued.

Guidelines for Treatment of Sexually Transmitted Diseases—cont'd

GENITAL WARTS

External Genital/Perianal Warts

Recommended Regimen

Cryotherapy with liquid nitrogen or cryoprobe.

Alternative Regimen. **Podophyllin** 10%-25% in compound tincture of benzoin. Limit the total volume of podophyllin solution applied to <0.5 ml per treatment session. Thoroughly wash off in 1-4 hours. Treat <10 cm^2 per session. Repeat applications at weekly intervals. Mucosal warts are more likely to respond than highly keratinized warts on the penile shaft, buttocks, and pubic areas. ***Contraindicated in pregnancy.***

Trichloroacetic acid (80%-90%). Apply only to warts; powder with talc or sodium bicarbonate (baking soda) to remove unreacted acid. Repeat application at weekly intervals.

Electrodesiccation/electrocautery. Electrodesiccation is contraindicated in patients with cardiac pacemakers, or for lesions proximal to the anal verge. Extensive or refractory disease should be referred to an expert.

Cervical Warts

Recommended Regimen

For women with cervical warts, dysplasia must be excluded before treatment is begun. Management should therefore be carried out in consultation with an expert.

Vaginal Warts

Recommended Regimen

Cryotherapy with liquid nitrogen. (The use of a cryoprobe in the vagina is not recommended because of the risk of vaginal perforation and fistula formation.)

Alternative Regimen. **Trichloroacetic acid** (80%-90%). Apply only to warts; powder with talc or sodium bicarbonate (baking soda) to remove unreacted acid. Repeat application at weekly intervals.

Podophyllin 10%-25% in compound tincture of benzoin. Treatment area must be dry before speculum is removed. Treat <2 cm^2 per session. Repeat application at weekly intervals. ***Contraindicated in pregnancy.*** Extensive or refractory disease should be referred to an expert.

Urethral Meatus Warts

Recommended Regimen

Cryotherapy with liquid nitrogen.

Alternative Regimen. **Podophyllin** 10%-25% in compound tincture of benzoin. Treatment area must be dry before contact with normal mucosa, and podophyllin must be washed off in 1-2 hours. ***Contraindicated in pregnancy.*** Extensive or refractory disease should be referred to an expert.

Anal Warts

Recommended Regimen

Cryotherapy with liquid nitrogen. Extensive or refractory disease should be referred to an expert.

Alternative Regimen

Trichloroacetic acid (80%-90%).

Surgical removal.

Oral Warts

Recommended Regimen

Cryotherapy with liquid nitrogen.

Alternative Regimen

Electrodesiccation/electrocautery.

Surgical removal. Extensive or refractory disease should be referred to an expert.

GENITAL HERPES SIMPLEX VIRUS INFECTIONS

First Clinical Episode of Genital Herpes

Recommended Regimen

Acyclovir 200 mg orally 5 times a day for 7-10 days or until clinical resolution occurs.

Recurrent Episodes

Most episodes of recurrent herpes do not benefit from therapy with acyclovir. In severe recurrent disease, some patients who start therapy at the beginning of the prodrome or within 2 days after onset of lesions may benefit from therapy, although this has not been proven.

Recommended Regimen

Acyclovir 200 mg orally 5 times a day for 5 days

or

Acyclovir 800 mg orally 2 times a day for 5 days.

Daily Suppressive Therapy

Daily treatment reduces frequency of recurrences by at least 75% among patients with frequent (more than six per year) recurrences. Safety and efficacy have been clearly documented among persons receiving daily therapy for up to 3 years. Acyclovir-resistant strains of HSV have been isolated from persons receiving suppressive therapy, but they have not been associated with treatment failure among immunocompetent patients. After 1 year of continuous daily suppressive therapy, acyclovir should be discontinued so that the patient's recurrence rate may be reassessed.

Recommended Regimen

Acyclovir 200 mg orally 2 to 5 times a day*

or

Acyclovir 400 mg orally 2 times a day.*

*Dosage must be individualized for each patient.

Continued.

Guidelines for Treatment of Sexually Transmitted Diseases—cont'd

SYPHILIS

Early Syphilis

Primary and Secondary Syphilis and Early Latent Syphilis of Less than 1 Year's Duration

Recommended Regimen

Benzathine penicillin G, 2.4 million units IM, in one dose.

Alternative Regimen for Penicillin-Allergic Patients (Nonpregnant). **Doxycycline,** 100 mg orally 2 times a day for 2 weeks

or

Tetracycline, 500 mg orally 4 times a day for 2 weeks.

Doxycycline and **tetracycline** are equivalent therapies. There is less clinical experience with **doxycycline,** but compliance is better. In patients who cannot tolerate doxycycline or tetracycline, three options exist:

- If follow-up or compliance cannot be ensured, the patient should have skin testing for penicillin allergy and be desensitized if necessary (see Appendix).
- If compliance and follow-up are ensured, **erythromycin,** 500 mg orally 4 times a day for 2 weeks, can be used.
- Patients who are allergic to penicillin may also be allergic to cephalosporins; therefore, caution must be used in treating a penicillin-allergic patient with a cephalosporin. However, preliminary data suggest that **ceftriaxone,** 250 mg IM once a day for 10 days, is curative—but careful follow-up is mandatory.

Follow-Up. Treatment failures can occur with any regimen. Patients should be reexamined clinically and serologically at 3 months and 6 months. If nontreponemal antibody titers have not declined fourfold by 3 months with primary or secondary syphilis, or by 6 months in early latent syphilis, or if signs or symptoms persist and reinfection has been ruled out, patients should have a cerebrospinal fluid examination and be retreated appropriately.

PELVIC INFLAMMATORY DISEASE

Inpatient treatment

One of the following:

Recommended Regimen A

Cefoxitin 2 g IV every 6 hours, or **cefotetan*** IV 2 g every 12 hours

plus

Doxycycline 100 mg every 12 hours orally or IV.

The above regimen is given for at least 48 hours after the patient clinically improves.

After discharge from hospital, continuation of:

Doxycycline 100 mg orally 2 times a day for a total of 10-14 days.

Recommended Regimen B

Clindamycin IV 900 mg every 8 hours

plus

Gentamicin loading dose IV or IM (2 mg/kg) ***followed by*** a maintenance dose (1.5 mg/kg) every 8 hours.

The above regimen is given for at least 48 hours after the patient improves. After discharge from hospital, continuation of:

Doxycycline 100 mg orally 2 times a day for 10-14 days total.

Continuation of **clindamycin,** 450 mg orally, 4 times daily, for 10 to 14 days, may be considered as an alternative.

Ambulatory Management of PID

Recommended Regimen

Cefoxitin 2 g IM ***plus*** **probenecid,** 1 g orally concurrently ***or*** **ceftiaxone** 250 mg IM, ***or*** equivalent **cephalosporin**

plus

Doxycycline 100 mg orally 2 times a day for 10-14 days

or

Tetracycline 500 mg orally 4 times a day for 10-14 days.

Alternative for Patients Who Do Not Tolerate Doxycycline. **Erythromycin,** 500 mg orally 4 times a day for 10-14 days may be substituted for doxycycline/tetracycline.

This regimen, however, is based on limited clinical data.

Genital Warts (Human Papilloma Virus)

Soon, infections with human papilloma virus (HPV) will likely be the most common sexually transmitted infection in the United States. Such infections have always raised concern, because they cause unsightly warts; however, new data suggest that infection with HPV is closely associated with the development of cervical neoplasia, and among adolescent girls represents the most common cause of abnormal Pap smears.[7,19]

More than 50 different types of HPV have been identified: "benign" genital warts usually are caused by types 6 and 11; types 16, 18, 31, 33, and 35 are most commonly associated with cervical intraepithelial neoplasia (CIN) and malignant changes on Pap smear. These types have the oncogenic potential to transform normal cells into malignant ones. An

Guidelines for Treatment of Sexually Transmitted Diseases—cont'd

NONGONOCOCCAL URETHRITIS (NGU)/NONCHLAMYDIAL URETHRITIS (NCU)

Most urethritis in males is caused by *Neisseria gonorrhoeae* and *Chlamydia trachomatis*. Other organisms that cause 10% to 15% of cases include *Ureaplasma urealyticum, T. vaginalis,* and herpes simplex virus. The cause of other cases is unknown.

Recommended Regimen

Doxycycline 100 mg orally 2 times a day for 7 days

or

Tetracycline 500 mg orally 4 times a day for 7 days.

Alternative Regimen. **Erythromycin** base 500 mg orally 4 times a day or equivalent salt for 7 days

or

Erythromycin ethylsuccinate 800 mg orally 4 times a day for 7 days.

If high-dose erythromycin schedules are not tolerated, the following regimen is recommended: **Erythromycin ethylsuccinate** 400 mg orally 4 times a day for 14 days

or

Erythromycin base 250 mg orally 4 times a day or equivalent salt for 14 days.

Recurrent NGU/NCU Unresponsive to Conventional Therapy. Recurrent NGU/NCU may be caused by lack of compliance with an initial antibiotic regimen, to reinfection resulting from failure to treat sex partners, or to factors currently undefined. If noncompliance or reinfection cannot be ruled out, repeat doxycycline (100 mg orally 2 times a day for 7 days) ***or*** tetracycline (500 mg orally 4 times a day for 7 days).

If compliance with the initial antimicrobial agent is likely, treat with one of the above listed regimens.

If objective signs of urethritis continue after adequate treatment, these patients should be evaluated for evidence of other causes of urethritis and referred to a specialist.

individual can be infected with more than one type. Cervical HPV infection has been associated with more than 90% of cervical dysplasia.

As with other STDs, infection rates among adolescents and young adults are quite high—up to 30%. Detection of infection is not always easy. Although 50% to 60% of women with external warts will have cervical infection, only 3% to 6% of those with cervical disease will have external genital warts. Hence the use of the Pap smear in any sexually active female is of extreme importance in screening for infection, even among those without visible signs of infection.

Males likely constitute a significant reservoir of undetected and untreated HPV infection.[14] In one study only 21 of 156 male partners of HPV-positive women had clinical evidence of warts. However, with use of magnification and acetic acid "soaks" to produce the "acetowhite" changes seen in HPV-infected skin, 77% of males were shown to be infected (Fig. 255-4). All these males were over 20 years of age; virtually no data exist on adolescent males.

Overt warts will develop in roughly two thirds of persons having intercourse with an infected individual. Visible warts will develop in 6 weeks to 8 months, but the range of the incubation period may be even wider. The typical pedunculated wart with a keratotic and irregular surface is usually easy to recognize, but warts may also be flat and more difficult to detect. Use of a hand-held magnifying glass or even a colposcope is extremely helpful. Among males, warts are usually seen on the shaft, prepuce, frenulum, corona, and glans but may also be present on the skin of the scrotum and the anus (Fig. 255-5). The presence of anal warts is often associated with anal receptive intercourse, but warts in this location have been described in males who deny this type of behavior. Occasionally warts will be seen at the urethral opening.

The posterior vaginal introitus, labia minora, and vestibule represent the most common sites of infection among females; again, however, warts can be seen anywhere on the external or internal genitalia. Subclinical disease is most likely to occur on the cervix; the relatively large transformation zone of the maturing adolescent cervix affords a hospitable site of infection for the virus (Fig. 255-6).

Evidence continues to accumulate linking the presence of HPV with the development of dysplastic and malignant changes in the cervix. Hence the role of the routine Pap smear in the care of sexually active teenagers has assumed increased importance. Any patient with evidence of HPV on Pap smear, usually indicated by the presence of koilocytic changes, should be referred for colposcopic examination, as should any woman with visible evidence of cervical infection. This is necessary because it is impossible to tell from the Pap smear or from visualization without magnification whether the infected areas contain cervical intraepithelial neoplastic (CIN) changes, which require vigorous treatment. If such changes cannot be ruled out by colposcopy alone, biopsy may

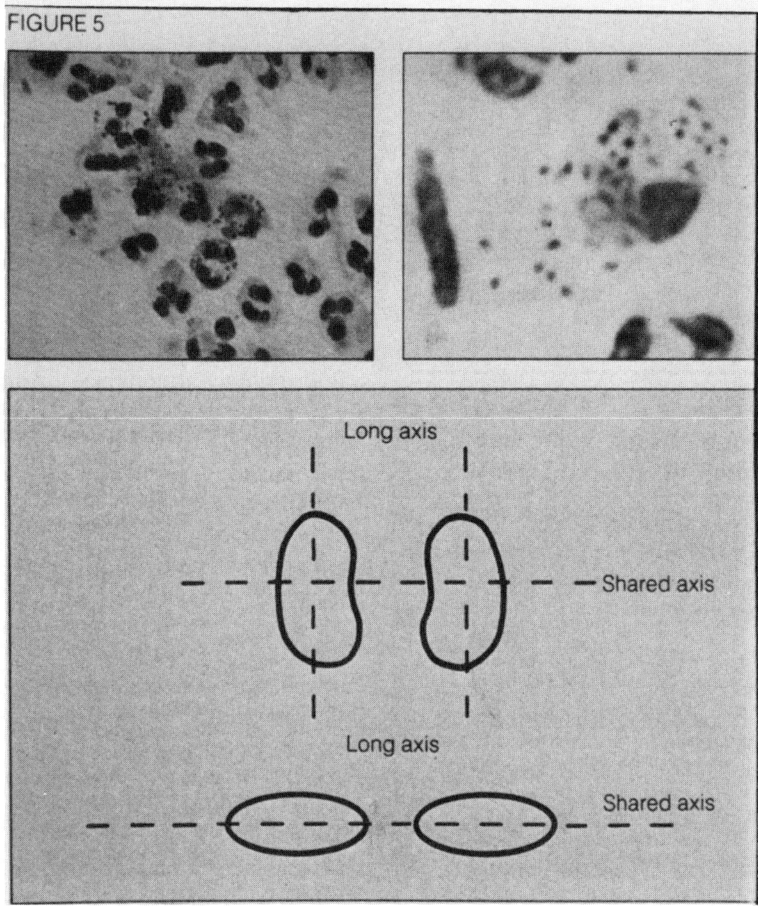

Fig. 255-3 *Neisseria gonorrhoeae* on Gram stains of male urethral smears (1500 × and 4000 × magnification) appear as tiny gram-negative diplococci within polymorphonuclear leukocytes (pink-stained nuclei). *Neisseria* organisms are kidney bean shaped, and their long axes are perpendicular to the shared axis, as shown in the diagram.

(From Gilchrist MJR and Rauch JL: Office microscopy: low-cost screening for STDs, Cont Pediatr 4:54, 1987.)

be necessary. Of untreated cervical infections, 15% to 20% may progress to true CIN changes.

A variety of treatment regimens for genital warts exist (see the box on p. 1498). The Centers for Disease Control recommend the use of liquid nitrogen. A cotton swab or cryoprobe is used to apply the liquid to the wart with firm pressure until the skin whitens. When the skin returns to normal color, the process is repeated two to three times. Applications are made weekly until the warts disappear, usually after four to six treatments. Liquid nitrogen should not be applied to the vaginal mucosa with a cryoprobe. Regardless of which treatment is elected, careful follow-up is needed, both to assure treatment success and because of the potential for disease progression.

The benefit of treating subclinical HPV infection is unclear. However, some authorities do recommend the treatment of subclinical cervical disease and localized sites on the penis or scrotum in an attempt to control sexual transmission.

Herpes Genitalis

Herpes simplex viral infections of the male and female genital tract are particularly distressing to patients because of the high likelihood of recurrence following an initial episode.[4] Both herpes simplex type 1 (HSV-1) and type 2 (HSV-2) can cause genital tract disease, although type 2 infections still tend to predominate. Infection rates have increased in the past 2 decades, especially among those 20 years of age or over. Although genital herpes infections were at one time believed to be associated with the development of cervical cancer, current evidence indicates that HSV more likely acts as a cofactor.

Infections with the virus can be classified as primary or nonprimary. Primary infection refers to the first exposure to HSV-1 or HSV-2 in an individual without any prior exposure to either virus. Nonprimary infection occurs in those with prior antibody to either type 1 or type 2 who become infected with the other strain. This type of infection, most commonly occurring in individuals with existing antibody to type 1 who become infected with type 2, tends to be less symptomatic.

In primary infection, symptoms usually occur within 2 to 20 days after sexual exposure. The patient usually experiences burning or itching at the site of inoculation, followed by erythema and the development of discrete vesicles. Initially the vesicles contain clear fluid, but they rapidly form pustules with an erythematous base. Typically, a patient may have 15

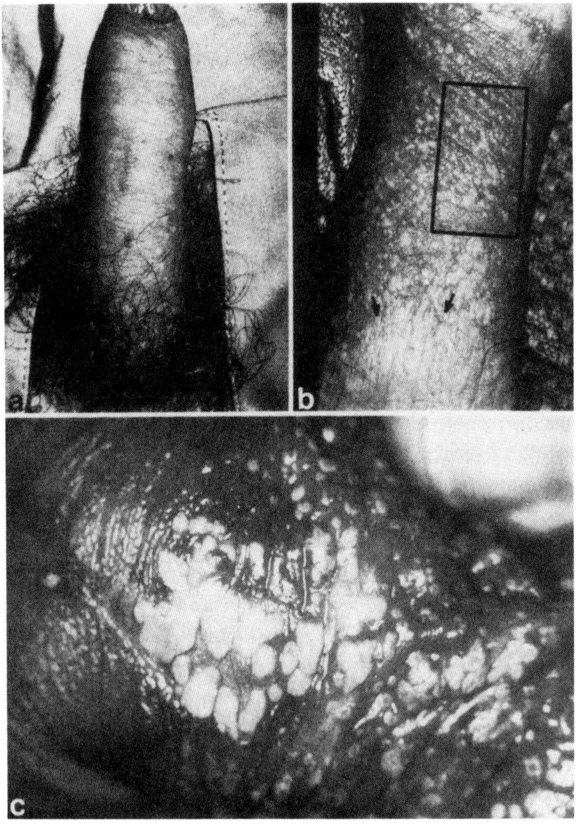

Fig. 255-4 Demonstration of subclinical lesions. **A,** Appearance of penis before acetic acid application. **B,** Penis after 5-minute application of gauze soaked in 5% acetic acid. Note coalescing sheets *(arrows)* and discrete dots of acetowhite staining *(inset)*. **C,** Magnified view of apparent subclinical human papillomavirus infection shown in *B*.

(From Ketelaris PM et al: Human papillomavirus: the untreated male reservoir, J Urology 140:302-303, 1988.)

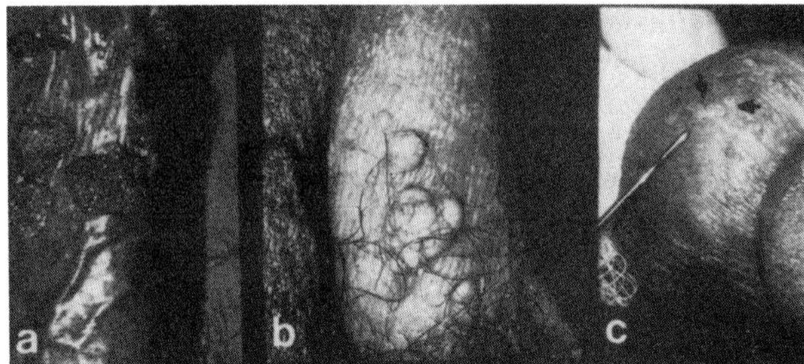

Fig. 255-5 Morphology of macroscopic warts. **A,** Condylomata demonstrated by preputial retraction. **B,** Verrucous wart at penoscrotal junction. **C,** Small, flat warts *(arrows)* on distal third of penis.

(From Ketelaris PM et al: Human papillomavirus: the untreated male reservoir, J Urology 140:302-303, 1988.)

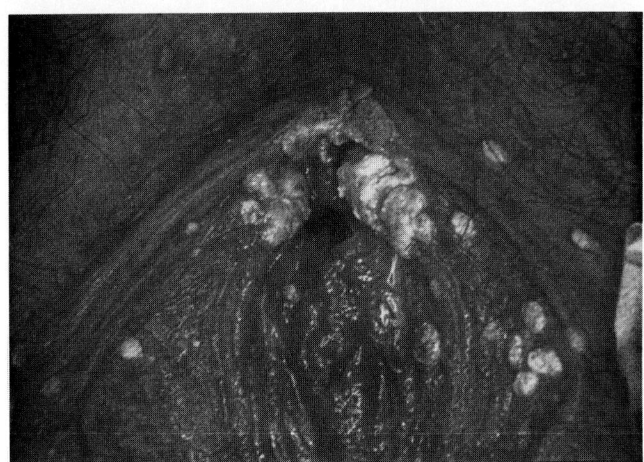

Fig. 255-6 Condyloma accuminatum of the vulva appears as a polypoid mass with a keratotic fissured, and irregular surface.
(From Moscicki B: HPV infections: An old STD revisited, Cont Pediatr 6:24, 1989.)

to 30 vesicles, each full of infectious viral particles. Lesions are located on the vulva, cervix, clitoris, or perineum. In males they may occur on the shaft, glans, or prepuce. Infection can also involve the urethra (leading to dysuria or urinary retention). Vesicles can also be seen on the thighs, buttocks, groin, or anus as a result of autoinoculation or anal receptive intercourse.

Because primary infection represents a first exposure to the particular virus type, systemic symptoms such as fever, malaise, and/or headache are common. About 50% of patients will have tender inguinal lymphadenopathy.

After about 2 to 4 days, the vesicles break open and coalesce to form wet ulcers. This is usually the time at which patients are seen by physicians. New lesions may still be developing at this point, but within 20 days all the lesions have crusted over and the pain and other symptoms have disappeared. Herpetic lesions heal without scarring.

The diagnosis of herpes genitalis is most often made on clinical grounds. Cultures of intact vesicles will generally be positive, as may cultures of the cervix. A Tzanck preparation of a scraping from an ulcer site will demonstrate the presence of multinucleated giant cells.

Following resolution of the infection, the virus remains latent in the sacral ganglia and may reactivate at any time. This reactivation is referred to as recurrent disease. Recurrences may occur in association with stress, local trauma, fever, or menstruation and tend to be shorter in duration, less symptomatic, and lacking in systemic symptoms. Vesicles usually occur near the initial infection site but tend to be fewer in number. Just before the recurrence, the patient may experience burning or itching at the site of infection. Healing takes from 1 to 2 weeks.

Females whose only site of recurrence involves the cervix may be unaware of the recurrence; during this period they are shedding the virus. About one third of males may also have inapparent recurrences but are still infectious. Hence unless sex partners reveal their history of infection, many exposures to the virus occur without an individual being aware that he or she has come into contact with the virus.

The risk of recurrence depends on a number of factors. Males are more likely to have recurrent disease, as are those individuals whose infection was caused by HSV-2. In one study, 12 of 14 patients (about 86%) with HSV-1 infection *did not* have recurrences, compared with only 40% of those with HSV-2. Once a second episode occurs, the patient will likely have recurrences.

Development of the antiviral drug acyclovir (Zovirax) has dramatically altered the nature of herpes therapy.[16,17] Acyclovir tablets, (200 mg) taken five times daily for 10 days significantly reduces the symptoms associated with primary episodes of genital herpes and decreases both the duration of viral shedding and the time to resolution of lesions (see box on p. 1498). However, once acyclovir is stopped, recurrences occur at the same rate as in those not treated for their initial infection. This same daily dose, given for 5 days, also shortens the duration of recurrent episodes, particularly when patients initiate treatment themselves at the first sign of a new episode. Daily use of acyclovir for up to 3 years reduces by at least 75% the risk of recurrence among those with more than six episodes per year (see box on p. 1498).

Syphilis

Syphilis is on the rise, perhaps because of decreased public health efforts directed toward it in this age of acquired immune deficiency syndrome (AIDS), and certainly because more women, addicted to crack cocaine exchange sex for drugs. Hence its diagnosis and management remain important for those caring for sexually active teenagers.

The prevalence of syphilis among those 10 to 19 years of age is 0.13%—0.06% for whites and 0.39% for blacks. In one study, however, 2.5% of incarcerated adolescent girls tested positive for syphilis. Table 255-1 provides data on syphilis infection rates in the United States.

The typical chancre of syphilis develops at the site of intimate sexual contact 10 to 90 days after exposure, with the average occurring within approximately 3 weeks. This lesion, varying from a few millimeters to a few centimeters in size, is clean based, painless, and has sharply demarcated, indurated borders. Unilateral, regional lymphadenopathy is usually present. Because the ulcer is painless, its appearance in the vagina or rectum or perhaps in the mouth is likely to go unnoticed. While the ulcer is present, the exudate overlying it is highly infectious.[1] Untreated, the chancre disappears in 2 to 8 weeks.

Six weeks to 6 months after the chancre appears, the rash of secondary syphilis appears in the untreated patient. The rash and the chancre may coexist. Because the spirochetes spread hematogenously from the site of initial infection, constitutional symptoms such as fever, malaise, sore throat, and generalized lymphadenopathy may be present.

The rash is typically papulosquamous but can be macular or pustular. Annular papules can appear on the face, and the rash can resemble impetigo or eczema. Sometimes, moist, fissured papules or elevated, thickened papules (condyloma lata) are seen; both are highly infectious. Finally, loss of scalp or eyebrow hair can be associated with secondary syphilis.

At the time the chancre is present, a darkfield examination of the nonbloody exudate should be performed by someone expert in darkfield microscopy. If performed on 3 successive days, the likelihood of obtaining a positive result from an infected individual is extremely high. If the results of all three examinations are negative, the diagnosis of primary syphilis should be reconsidered.

If the darkfield examination is unavailable, a serologic test for syphilis should be obtained. A variety of tests for detecting syphilis are available; their relative sensitivities and specificities are outlined in Table 255-2.[6] If the examiner is relatively certain that the chancre is one of primary syphilis, he or she should specifically request the fluorescent treponemal antibody-absorption (FTA-ABS) test, since the sensitivity of the flocculation (VDRL) and rapid plasma reagin (RPR) tests at this point is relatively low. Alternatively, a second specimen can be obtained 2 to 4 weeks later.

Recently, Cox and others reviewed the presentation of syphilis in adolescents: 14% had primary syphilis; 43%, secondary syphilis; 39%, latent syphilis; and 4% were undetermined.[5] A minority of patients had a chancre (14%) or a rash (18%); 47% had no signs or symptoms of the disease. Hence all sexually active adolescents should routinely be screened for syphilis.

The recommended CDC treatment guidelines for primary and secondary syphilis are outlined in the box on pp. 1499. Follow-up with repeat serologic tests should occur at 3, 6, and 12 months after treatment. Typically, VDRL titers should decline by fourfold at 3 months and eightfold at 6 months. The FTA-ABS test will always remain positive. Criteria for reevaluation or retreatment include persistence or recurrence of clinical signs and symptoms, a sustained fourfold or greater rise in titers, or the persistence of a higher than 1:8 titer for more than 1 year after adequate treatment.

Congenital Syphilis

Sadly, *congenital syphilis* is on the rise in the United States. In 1988, 691 cases of this preventable disease were reported to the Centers for Disease Control, the highest number since the 1950s, when penicillin became widely available.[3]

The clinical manifestations of congenital syphilis are protean.[13] Infected infants may be identified early in life via routine serologic screening or on the basis of various symptoms (early congenital syphilis). Alternatively, some may escape detection and appear after 2 years of age with the sequelae of untreated infection (late congenital syphilis).

Most infected liveborn infants (congenital syphilis is a major cause of stillbirths) are asymptomatic.[12] Common signs of infection include hepatomegaly (with or without splenomegaly or jaundice), nephrotic syndrome (limb edema and proteinuria), eye abnormalities (chorioretinitis, glaucoma, uveitis), generalized nontender lymphadenopathy (especially involving the epitrochlear nodes), anemia, and/or thrombocytopenia, persistent rhinitis (which can be clear, blood tinged, or purulent) and intrauterine growth retardation. Involvement of the central nervous system can mimic bacterial meningitis, although the cerebrospinal fluid (CSF) generally shows a monocytosis with an elevated protein and a normal glucose level.

Skin manifestations are also extremely important. Congenital syphilis should always be considered in an infant with a persistent diaper rash or with an exanthem involving the

Table 255-2 *Comparison of Diagnostic Tests for Syphilis*

SENSITIVITY AND SPECIFICITY OF SEROLOGICAL TESTS FOR SYPHILIS* AT DIFFERENT STAGES

	PERCENT SENSITIVITY (SENS.) AND SPECIFICITY (SPEC.)							
	VDRL		RPR		FTA-ABS		MHA-TP	
STAGE OF SYPHILIS	SENS.	SPEC.	SENS.	SPEC.	SENS.	SPEC.	SENS.	SPEC.
Primary	80 (59-87)	98 (80-99)	86 (81-100)	98 (80-99)	98 (93-100)	98 (84-99)	82 (64-90)	99 (98-100)
Secondary	100 (99-100)	98	100 (99-100)	98	100 (99-100)	98	100 (96-100)	99
Latent	96 (73-100)	98	99	98	100 (96-100)	98	100 (96-100)	99
Late	71	98	73	98	96	98	94	99

*Theconsensusfiguresforthesensitivityandspecificityarefortestsdoneinthe CentersforDiseaseControlReferenceLaboratoryonsamplesderivedfromawell-runSTDclinic.Thefiguresinparenthesesdemonstrate the variability in published reports. Responsible factors include *(a)* study of populations with different prevalences of syphilis and other confounding illnesses, *(b)* variable performance by the laboratory, and *(c)* different clinical criteria for the diagnosis of syphilis.

From Dans PE: Syphilis. In Barker LR, Burton JR, and Zieve PD, editors: Principles of ambulatory medicine, ed 2, Baltimore, 1986, Williams & Wilkins.

Surveillance Case Definition for Congenital Syphilis

For reporting purposes, congenital syphilis includes cases of congenitally acquired syphilis in infants and children, as well as syphilitic stillbirths.

A CONFIRMED CASE of congenital syphilis is an infant in whom *Treponema pallidum* is identified by darkfield microscopy, fluorescent antibody, or other specific stains in specimens from lesions, placenta, umbilical cord, or autopsy material.

A PRESUMPTIVE CASE of congenital syphilis is either of the following:

A. Any infant whose mother had untreated or inadequately treated* syphilis at delivery, regardless of findings in the infant;

OR

B. Any infant or child who has a reactive treponemal test for syphilis and any one of the following:
   1. any evidence of congenital syphilis on physical examination†; or
   2. any evidence of congenital syphilis on long-bone radiograph; or
   3. reactive cerebrospinal fluid VDRL‡; or
   4. elevated CSF cell count or protein (without other cause)‡; or
   5. quantitative nontreponemal serologic titers that are fourfold higher than the mother's (both drawn at birth); or
   6. reactive test for FTA-ABS-19S-IgM antibody‡.

A SYPHILITIC STILLBIRTH is defined as a fetal death in which the mother had untreated or inadequately treated syphilis at delivery of a fetus after a 20-week gestation or of a fetus weighing more than 500 g.

*Inadequate treatment consists of any nonpenicillin therapy or penicillin given less than 30 days before delivery.

†Signs in an infant (under 2 years of age) may include hepatosplenomegaly, characteristic skin rash, condyloma lata, snuffles, jaundice (syphilitic hepatitis), pseudoparalysis, or edema (nephrotic syndrome). Stigmata in an older child may include: interstitial keratitis, nerve deafness, anterior bowing of shins, frontal bossing, mulberry molars, Hutchinson's teeth, saddle nose, rhagades, or Clutton joints.

‡It may be difficult to distinguish between congenital and acquired syphilis in a seropositive child after infancy. Signs may not be obvious and stigmata may not yet have developed. Abnormal values for CSF VDRL, cell count, and protein, as well as IgM antibodies, may be found in either congenital or acquired syphilis. Findings on long-bone radiographs may help, since these would indicate congenital syphilis. The decision may ultimately be based on maternal history and clinical judgment; the possibility of sexual abuse also needs to be considered.

From Congenital syphilis—New York City, 1986-1988, MMWR 38:825, 1989.

palms and soles. About 30% to 60% of infected infants have skin lesions, the most common being a large, round, pink macule that turns "coppery" and fades in 1 to 3 months without treatment. The lesions tend to spare the anterior trunk. A fine scale may cover the involved areas. The rash can also be vesiculobullous or, lacking bullae, can manifest as desquamation. Eczematoid, often impetiginized lesions have a predilection for the perineum, for the intertriginous areas, and for the middle third of the face (including the tongue and palate).

Some two thirds of infants also have bony involvement, although in many cases this can only be detected by radiologic means. The epiphyses most commonly involved are those of the radius, femur, humerus, and fibula, with infection generally in multiple, symmetric sites. Bony tenderness can lead to decreased movement of the affected limb and thus a false diagnosis of paralysis secondary to birth trauma (pseudoparalysis of Parrot).

Recently, Dorfman and Glaser[8] reported on seven infants with congenital syphilis diagnosed between 3 and 14 weeks of age, six of whom were RPR negative at birth. In four cases, the mothers had a negative serologic test at delivery; the other three were not tested because of a negative test before delivery. All the infants had hepatomegaly and elevated serum transaminase levels, but other physical findings were inconstant.

The accompanying box lists the CDC criteria for surveillance case definition for congenital syphilis. The diagnosis is more difficult in an asymptomatic infant with a positive treponemal test for syphilis whose mother also has a positive test. In this case, consultation with an infectious disease specialist may be warranted to differentiate active infection from passive transfer of maternal antibody.

Infants classified as confirmed or presumptive cases of congenital syphilis according to the CDC criteria should be treated for 10 to 14 days with either aqueous crystalline penicillin G (100,000 to 150,000 U/kg/day intravenously every 8 to 12 hours) **or** procaine penicillin G (50,000 U/kg/day intramuscularly once daily).[22] If the infant's mother has not been adequately treated, if it cannot be determined whether the treatment was adequate, or if the infant's mother is HIV antibody positive, a similar regimen should be used. If the mother has been adequately treated, the decision to treat the infant depends on assurances regarding careful follow-up and a normal CSF examination. Under optimum circumstances, no treatment is needed at birth, but serial antibody titers should be obtained at 1, 2, 4, 6, and 12 months. Infants who cannot reliably be followed but who have normal CSF should receive a single dose of benzathine penicillin (50,000 U/kg intramuscularly).

SYNDROMES ASSOCIATED WITH SEXUALLY TRANSMITTED DISEASES

Pelvic Inflammatory Disease

Pelvic inflammatory disease (PID) refers to infection involving the upper genital tract (uterus, fallopian tubes, ovaries, and pelvis) occurring as a result of undetected or inadequately treated sexually transmitted infections of the lower genital tract (endocervix). In the short term, PID can lead to such problems as a ruptured tuboovarian abscess. In the long run, infertility, chronic pelvic pain, and increased risk for ectopic pregnancy can also be attributed to this condition, even when the acute episode has been managed appropriately. Among all sexually active females, teenagers under 19 years of age are at greatest risk for development of this disease; because a major risk factor for development of PID is a prior episode, adolescent girls who experience this illness early in their reproductive life cycle are at great risk for having further significant problems.[24]

Even though this condition is common, the diagnosis of pelvic inflammatory disease is imprecise. Signs and symptoms can be nonspecific, and the only sure method for diagnosis—laparoscopy—is not routinely performed for diagnostic purposes in this country. Hence pediatricians must maintain a high index of suspicion when appropriate and must obtain a thorough history and perform a careful physical examination to avoid the pitfalls of diagnosis.

When eliciting the history from a patient with lower abdominal pain, it is worthwhile to keep in mind those factors that place an individual at risk for infection. Hence failure to use barrier methods of contraception, the presence of an intrauterine device (IUD), numerous sex partners, a recent new partner, and/or history of other STDs or PID should raise concern. The presence of a new vaginal discharge (or a change in odor, color, or amount), abnormal menstrual bleeding (increased or prolonged or occurring at the wrong time in the cycle), and/or dyspareunia all suggest PID. Although oral contraceptive pills protect against the development of gonococcal PID, the evidence for protection against *C. trachomatis* PID is uncertain. Oral contraceptive pills actually increase the likelihood of acquisition and persistence of chlamydial infection.

Other symptoms include dysuria, dysmenorrhea (usually more severe than normal), nausea, vomiting, diarrhea, fever, and malaise. Except for dysmenorrhea, these symptoms also can be seen in patients with diseases of the urinary tract (e.g., pyelonephritis) or gastrointestinal tract (e.g., appendicitis).

Depending on the extent of upper genital tract involvement, physical signs may include pain on cervical movement and endometrial and/or adnexal tenderness. Fever is present in *fewer than* 50% of patients with documented PID. If the infection has "tracked" up to involve the capsule of the liver, right upper quadrant tenderness may also be elicited. With extensive infection, signs of peritonitis, particularly rebound tenderness, are present. The palpation of an adnexal mass raises the concern of a coexisting tuboovarian abscess. Mucopus visible in the cervical os strongly suggests the presence of infection, but its absence does not rule out the diagnosis.

Acute-phase reactants lack the necessary sensitivity and specificity to be routinely helpful in establishing the diagnosis of PID. Although 60% to 80% of patients will have an elevated white blood cell count, sedimentation rate, or C-reactive protein, so will many patients with pyelonephritis or appendicitis.

In an attempt to guide clinicians and minimize the potential for diagnostic confusion, several investigators have suggested diagnostic criteria for infections localized to the female pelvic organs.[9] The criteria for making the diagnosis of salpingitis are indicated in the box below. These criteria may also be used for more extensive infections of the pelvic organs, or PID. Nonetheless, several studies have indicated that there is a substantial false positive and false negative rate in the diagnosis of PID. It is particularly important to note that certain surgical emergency conditions can mimic PID in their presentation. Hence it is useful to keep in mind the differential diagnosis, as outlined in the top box on p. 1507. Because many teenagers at risk for PID are similarly at risk for pregnancy and because ectopic pregnancy can mimic PID, serum pregnancy tests should be routinely obtained at the time of evaluation. If a mass is palpated in the adnexa, an ultrasound should be obtained to determine if a tuboovarian abscess is present. Cultures for *C. trachomatis* and *N. gonorrhoeae* should be routinely obtained.

Salpingitis: Clinical Criteria for Diagnosis

Abdominal direct tenderness, with or without rebound tenderness Tenderness with motion of cervix and uterus Adnexal tenderness	All three necessary for diagnosis
	plus
Gram stain of endocervix—positive for gram-negative, intracellular diplococci* Temperature (over 38° C) Leukocytosis (greater than 10,000) Purulent material (white blood cells present) from peritoneal cavity by culdocentesis or laparoscopy Pelvic abscess or inflammatory complex on bimanual exam or by sonography	One or more necessary for diagnosis

*A cervical gram stain that shows 10 to 30 polymorphonuclear white blood cells per oil immersion field is highly suggestive of cervicitis, even in the absence of gram-negative, intracellular diplococci.

From Hager WD et al: Criteria for diagnosis and grading of salpingitis, Obstet Gynecol 61:114, 1983.

Many authorities recommend the hospital admission of any teenager with PID in an attempt to minimize future reproductive sequelae and because teenagers often comply poorly with the lengthy regimens needed for successful treatment. Others argue that if careful follow-up can be assured, outpatient management can be attempted. The other indications for admission are shown in the bottom box on p. 1507.

Treatment is directed toward eradicating the organism responsible for the infection. Unfortunately, there is great difficulty in establishing with certainty the nature of the infection. Cultures obtained from the cervix do not necessarily reflect the nature of the tubal infection. Many organisms felt to play a role in PID are difficult to grow; thus studies that did not use state-of-the-art culture techniques may not have identified all relevant organisms. Those studies that have been carefully performed point to the polymicrobial nature of the infection. Both *N. gonorrhoeae* and *C. trachomatis* have been recovered from approximately 25% to 50% of patients. Nongonococcal, nonchlamydial anaerobes (bacteroides and peptostreptococcus spp.), facultative aerobes *(Gardnerella vag-*

Differential Diagnosis of Acute Lower Abdominal Pain in the Adolescent Female by Organ System

URINARY
Cystitis
Pyelonephritis
Urethritis
Other

GASTROINTESTINAL
Appendicitis
Constipation
Diverticulitis
Gastroenteritis
Inflammatory bowel disease
Irritable bowel syndrome
Other

REPRODUCTIVE
Acute PID
Cervicitis (?)
Dysmenorrhea (primary/secondary)
Ectopic pregnancy
Endometriosis
Endometritis
Mittelschmerz
Ovarian cyst (torsion/rupture)
Pregnancy (intrauterine, ectopic)
Ruptured follicle
Septic abortion
Threatened abortion
Torsion of adnexa
Tuboovarian abscess

From Shafer M and Sweet RL: Pelvic inflammatory disease in adolescent females, Pediatr Clin North Am 36:513, 1989.

Indications for Hospitalization of Patients with Pelvic Inflammatory Disease

Perhaps *all* adolescents with PID
Unable to tolerate oral medications
Uncertainty regarding follow-up
Failure to improve (or worsening of disease) within 48 hours of outpatient treatment
Adnexal mass (tuboovarian abscess)
Fever and/or other signs of peritonitis (rebound tenderness)
Uncertainty regarding diagnosis
IUD in place
Pregnancy

inalis, Escherichia coli, Haemophilus influenzae) and genital tract mycoplasms have also been recovered to varying degrees.

As a result of the uncertainty concerning the nature of the infecting organisms and the lack of controlled treatment and outcome studies, the CDC treatment regimens outlined in the box on p. 1499 reflect empiric therapy based on the assumption that the infection is polymicrobial. The need to use doxycycline or tetracycline as part of therapy underscores the need for obtaining a pregnancy test before treatment. If outpatient therapy is to be attempted, careful follow-up at 48 hours must be assured, and a mechanism for hospitalizing the patient before that time if symptoms worsen must be in place. Otherwise, admission should occur at the time of diagnosis.

Once therapy is initiated, the patient should improve within 48 hours. Failure to see this improvement should raise concerns about the accuracy of the diagnosis or the presence of complications. The pelvic examination should be repeated in order to look for a tuboovarian abscess if one has not already been detected. Approximately 10% to 20% of patients with PID will develop a tuboovarian abscess; 3% to 15% of these abscesses will rupture. If an abscess is detected or if the patient fails to improve, the physician should seek gynecologic consultation (or surgical consultation if appendicitis is suspected).

The patient may be discharged from the hospital 48 hours after she becomes afebrile or after 4 days of intravenous therapy, whichever is longer. Treatment must include a total of 10 days with doxycycline. Follow-up at the end of treatment is important. The patient should be instructed not to have intercourse until her therapy is completed, and her partner must be notified and treated. Because an episode of PID is a major risk factor for development of a second episode, the use of barrier methods of contraception must be stressed to the patient.

Even with optimum diagnosis and treatment, the long-term morbidity from a single episode of PID is significant. After one episode of PID, 11% of women are infertile; a second episode triples that rate to 34%. Westrom and colleagues have reported a sevenfold to tenfold increase in risk for subsequent ectopic pregnancy following PID. Chronic pelvic pain is also an unfortunate sequela.

Nongonococcal, Nonchlamydial Urethritis

Some men with overt or subclinical urethritis will be culture negative for both *N. gonorrhoeae* and *C. trachomatis*.[21,26] *Ureaplasma urealyticum* has been implicated as the cause in approximately one fifth of these cases; the cause of the remaining infections is unclear. *Staphylococcus saprophyticus*, herpes simplex virus, and *T. vaginalis* may occasionally be responsible. It has recently been suggested that some of these males may have prostatitis.

Treatment should be directed toward an agent, if identified. If none exists, the treatment should be doxycycline or tetracycline (see the box on p. 1500). Compliance with the full course of treatment should be stressed, and the sex partner(s) must be treated concomitantly.

Perihepatitis (Fitz-Hugh and Curtis Syndrome)

Perihepatis associated with gonococcal salpingitis was described in 1920. Subsequently, Fitz-Hugh described a patient with "violin string" adhesions between the liver and anterior abdominal wall, and Curtis described localized peritonitis of the liver's anterior surface in a woman with upper abdominal pain and tenderness who was undergoing laparotomy for suspected gallbladder disease. Since then, it has been well documented that *C. trachomatis* infections can cause a similar picture.

Onset of upper abdominal pain usually follows the onset of lower abdominal pain, but it can precede it. The pain is generally right sided and can radiate to the shoulder. Fewer than 50% of patients will have mildly elevated liver enzymes. Treatment for pelvic inflammatory disease will also successfully eliminate the perihepatitis.

Enteric Infections

The syndromes of proctitis, proctocolitis, and enteritis are mostly limited to adolescent males who practice anal receptive intercourse. Symptoms include anorectal pain, tenesmus, constipation, and discharge. Those with proctocolitis or enteritis will have diarrhea.

Patients with proctitis should be examined with anoscopy and evaluated for *C. trachomatis, N. gonorrhoeae,* and *Treponema pallidum*. Treatment should be with standard doses of ceftriaxone and doxycycline.

Those with symptoms suggesting proctocolitis or enteritis should receive more extensive evaluation. Such organisms as *Campylobacter jejuni, Shigella* species, and *Giardia lamblia* can be sexually transmitted.

Vaginitis

As discussed in Chapter 172, "Vaginal Discharge," *T. vaginalis,* an important cause of vaginitis in sexually active adolescents, is a sexually transmitted infectious agent. There is some evidence that bacterial vaginosis, associated with the overgrowth of *Gardnerella vaginalis,* is also sexually transmitted. Male sex partners of women with bacterial vaginosis more often have *G. vaginalis* recovered from the urethra than do controls. However, this same organism can be recovered from approximately 15% of females who have never been sexually active. Treatment of male partners does not appear to influence recurrence risks for females who are treated for bacterial vaginosis.

Vaginitis, in and of itself, can be distressing enough to females. However, current concerns about these two agents center on their possible roles in the pathogenesis of pelvic inflammatory disease. Because trichomonads are motile organisms, it has been postulated that as they ascend into the uterus, they may serve as a vector for other agents to gain access to the upper genital tract. Nongonococcal, nonchlamydial pathogens associated with PID are recovered more often from the endometrium of women with bacterial vaginosis than from those without. Bacterial vaginosis has been causally related to postpartum endometritis.

Hence aggressive treatment of women with either of these two infections is warranted. Male partners of women with trichomoniasis should be treated routinely; whether the same is true for partners of women with bacterial vaginosis is uncertain.

REFERENCES

1. Adger H et al: Screening for *Chlamydia trachomatis* and *Neisseria gonorrhoeae* in adolescent males: value of first-catch urine examination, Lancet 2:944, 1984.
2. Brunham RC et al: Mucopurulent cervicitis—the ignored counterpart in women of urethritis in men, N Engl J Med 311:1, 1984.
3. Congenital syphilis—New York City, 1986–1988, MMWR 38:825, 1989.
4. Corey L and Spear PG: Infections with herpes simplex viruses. I. and II., N Engl J Med 314:686, 749, 1986.
5. Cox J et al: The changing epidemiologic spectrum of syphilis in urban adolescents. Paper presented before the Society for Adolescent Medicine, San Francisco, 1989.
6. Dans PE: Syphilis. In Barker LR, Burton JR, and Zieve PD, editors: Principles of ambulatory medicine, ed 2, Baltimore, 1986, Williams & Wilkins.
7. Davis AJ and Evans SJ: Human papillomavirus infection in the pediatric and adolescent patient, J Pediatr 115:1, 1989.
8. Dorfman DH and Glaser JH: Congenital syphilis presenting in infants after the newborn period, N Engl J Med 323:1299, 1990.
9. Hager WD et al: Criteria for diagnosis and grading of salpingitis, Obstet Gynecol 61:113, 1983.
10. Hammerschlag MR: Chlamydial infections, J Pediatr 114:727, 1989.
11. Hook EW and Holmes KK: Gonococcal infections, Ann Intern Med 102:229, 1985.
12. Ikeda MK and Jenson HB: Evaluation and treatment of congenital syphilis, J Pediatr 117:843, 1990.
13. Ingall D, Dobson SRM, and Musher D: Syphilis. In Remington JS and Klein JO, editors: Infectious diseases of the fetus and newborn infant, ed 3, Philadelphia, 1990, WB Saunders Co.
14. Katelaris PM et al: Human papillomavirus: the untreated male reservoir, J Urol 140:300, 1988.
15. Kelaghan J et al: Barrier-method contraceptives and pelvic inflammatory disease, JAMA 248:184, 1982.
16. Mertz GJ et al: Double-blind placebo controlled trial of oral acyclovir in first-episode genital herpes simplex virus infection, JAMA 252:1147, 1984.
17. Mertz GJ et al: Long-term acyclovir suppression of frequently recurring genital herpes simplex virus infection JAMA, 260:201, 1988.
18. Mills J and Brooks GF: Disseminated gonococcal infection. In Holmes KK et al, editors: Sexually transmitted diseases, New York, 1984, McGraw-Hill Book Co.
19. Mosicki B: HPV infections: an old STD revisited, Contemporary Pediatrics 6:12, 1989.
20. Phillips RS et al: Should tests for *Chlamydia trachomatis* cervical infection be done during routine gynecologic visits? Ann Intern Med 107:188, 1987.
21. Rosenfeld WD and Litman N: Urogenital tract infections in male adolescents, Pediatr Rev 4:257, 1983.
22. 1989 Sexually transmitted diseases treatment guidelines, MMWR 38(S-8):9, 1989.
23. Shafer M et al: Urinary leukocyte esterase screening test for asymptomatic chlamydial and gonococcal infections in males, JAMA 262:2562, 1989.
24. Shafer M and Sweet RL: Pelvic inflammatory disease in adolescent females, Pediatr Clin North Am 36:513, 1989.
25. Wald ER: Gonorrhea, Am J Dis Child 131:1094, 1977.
26. Wong ES et al: Clinical and microbiological features of persistent or recurrent nongonococcal urethritis in men, J Infect Dis 158:1098, 1988.

256

Sinusitis

Rickey L. Williams

Infection of the paranasal sinuses in children occurs frequently, although the exact incidence and prevalence of this disorder are unknown. This is partially the result of the difficulty in making the diagnosis with certainty, especially in younger children.

PATHOPHYSIOLOGY

The paranasal sinuses arise during fetal development as outpouchings beneath the turbinates in the nasopharynx. Only the maxillary and ethmoid sinuses are present at the time of birth, and the sinuses continue to develop and grow until adulthood (Table 256-1). The growth is frequently asymmetric, and some individuals lack one or more sinuses altogether. Various functions have been ascribed to these sinuses, including warming and humidifying inspired air, trapping inspired particles, secreting mucus, and reducing the weight of the skull.[5]

The lining of the mucosa of the sinuses is similar to that of the nasopharynx, with pseudostratified, ciliated, columnar epithelium interspersed with goblet cells and submucosal glands. The cilia beat toward the ostium of the sinus to expel the mucus and particulate matter contained therein into the nasopharynx.[5]

When the ostia become occluded, the sinus is prone to infection. Sinusitis occurs most frequently after a viral upper respiratory tract infection. The inflammation and edema of the mucous membranes lead to obstruction of the ostium, and the normally sterile sinus cavity is invaded by bacteria.

Nasal allergy is another major cause of sinusitis in children. The associated tissue edema, vasodilation, and increased vascular permeability obstruct the ostia of the sinuses, which results in a sinus infection. Other disorders associated with sinusitis in children are listed in the box on p. 1510.

Bacterial pathogens implicated in acute sinusitis are the same as those found in acute otitis media, with *Streptococcus pneumoniae, Branhamella catarrhalis,* and *Haemophilus influenzae* predominating.[7] Anaerobes have been found by Brook[1] to be prevalent in chronic sinusitis, presumably because of the low oxygen content and low pH of fluid retained in the sinus for a long time.

CLINICAL PRESENTATION AND DIAGNOSIS

Children with either severe or prolonged upper respiratory tract infections are most likely to have sinusitis.[6] Cough and nasal discharge are the most common clinical manifestations of acute sinusitis. The cough occurs in the daytime and is frequently worse at night or at any other time when the child is lying supine. The nasal discharge can be clear or purulent. In the infant or young child, fever and irritability following a viral upper respiratory tract infection may be the only manifestations. Malodorous breath, headache, sore throat, a feeling of fullness or pain in the face, and a disturbed sense of smell also suggest the present of sinusitis.

The nasal mucosa is erythematous and swollen on physical examination. Mucopurulent material can sometimes be seen draining into the nasopharynx. Palpation of the bones overlying the sinuses may elicit pain. Microscopic examination of nasal secretions may show polymorphonuclear cells and bacteria.[2]

Transillumination of the maxillary and frontal sinuses is helpful in making the diagnosis of sinusitis in adults; however, the accuracy of transillumination in children is questionable.

Table 256-1 *Sinus Development*

SINUS	FIRST APPEARANCE	SIZE (cc) BIRTH	3 YEARS	10 YEARS	14 YEARS	AGE OF CLINICAL IMPORTANCE
Maxillary	3 wk of fetal life	0.13	2.5	10.4	11.6	Birth
Ethmoid	6 mo of fetal life	0.06	0.16	2.4	4.8	Birth
Sphenoid	3 mo of fetal life	0.02	0.68	1.8	2.1	5 yr
Frontal	1 yr of life	—	0.08	1.0	3.6	10-12 yr

Modified from Schaeffer JP: The embryology, development and anatomy of the nose, paranasal sinuses, nasolacrimal passageways and olfactory organ in man, Philadelphia, 1920, Blakiston.

Disorders Associated with Paranasal Sinusitis

1. Anatomic
   a. Nasal malformations
   b. Nasal trauma
   c. Tumors and polyps
   d. Cleft palate
   e. Foreign bodies
   f. Dental infection
   g. Cyanotic congenital heart disease
2. Physiologic—barotrauma
3. Abnormalities of local defense mechanisms
   a. Allergy
   b. Cystic fibrosis
   c. Immotile-cilia syndrome and Kartagener syndrome
4. Abnormalities of systemic defense mechanisms—immunodeficiency, primary or secondary

From Shurin PA: Etiology and antimicrobial therapy of paranasal sinusitis in children, Ann Otol Rhinol Laryngol 90(suppl 84):72, 1981.

A dark room and bright light are used for this technique. To examine the maxillary sinus, the light is placed in the patient's mouth and the lips are closed. Normal sinuses transmit light to the anterior wall of the antrum, giving a "jack-o'-lantern" effect. The frontal sinuses are examined by placing the light below the floor of each sinus. The two sides should be compared, with the examiner keeping in mind that sinus development is asymmetric in many individuals.[5]

Sinus roentgenograms can be helpful in making the diagnosis of sinusitis. When clinical signs and symptoms suggest acute sinusitis and maxillary sinus roentgenograms are abnormal, bacteria will be present in a sinus aspirate 75% of the time.[8] With acute inflammation, thickening of the mucous membranes and fluid buildup within the sinus lead to complete or partial opacification, which can be seen roentgenographically. Crying *does not* lead to abnormal roentgenograms.[3] Cysts and polyps can also be seen on sinus roentgenograms.

Ultrasound has been examined recently as a method of detecting fluid in the sinuses. Technical difficulties in using this method on children under 3 years of age have been experienced, however, and further improvements in this technology will be necessary before this method can be recommended.[5]

The diagnosis of sinusitis can be made with certainty only by obtaining a positive culture from sinus aspiration. Nasopharyngeal culture results correlate poorly with sinus culture results. Sinus aspiration and lavage are indicated in children who fail to respond to conventional antibiotic therapy, in immunosuppressed patients, and in those with severe or life-threatening illness.

COMPLICATIONS

Complications of sinusitis most commonly occur because of local extension of the disease.

Orbital cellulitis is the most common serious complication of sinusitis. The ethmoid sinus is separated from the orbit by the thin *lamina papyracea*. Erosion of this bone leads to invasion of the orbit by bacterial pathogens. Staging of orbital cellulitis is described in Table 256-2. The eyelids appear intensely red and swollen on physical examination. Fever, malaise, and an increased white blood count are present. Orbital pain, proptosis, and limitation of eye movement (ophthlamoplegia) help distinguish this condition from periorbital cellulitis, although computed tomography (CT) scanning may be needed to differentiate the two. Treatment of orbital cellulitis involves parenteral antibiotics; an ophthalmologist and an otolaryngologist should be consulted to determine whether surgical drainage is indicated.[9]

Intracranial infection, most commonly subdural empyema, is the second most common complication of sinusitis. This can occur by direct extension through necrotic bone or by bacterial spread through the venous system. The frontal sinuses are most often involved, making the peak age of incidence of this complication between 10 and 20 years, although it can develop in younger children. Patients will have a low-grade fever, malaise, and a frontal headache. Vomiting and a decreased level of consciousness appear as the disease progresses.

In a patient suspected of having an intracranial abscess, CT scanning should be performed. A lumbar puncture should be avoided because of the possibility of brainstem herniation. Treatment in the form of high-dose parenteral antibiotics is required. Neurosurgery is indicated to drain the abscess and to debride necrotic bone. Steroids and hypertonic agents such as mannitol or glycerol are used to control intracranial hypertension.

Other less common complications of sinusitis in children include meningitis, osteomyelitis ("Pott's puffy tumor"), and cavernous sinus thrombosis.

TREATMENT

Treatment of sinusitis in children involves antimicrobial therapy, symptomatic relief measures, and drainage if necessary. Antibiotics used in treating sinusitis are the same as those used for acute otitis media (see Table 238-1). Amoxicillin is the drug of choice in those with uncomplicated sinusitis in geographic areas where the prevalence of beta-lactamase–producing strains of *H. influenzae* and *B. catarrhalis* is low.[6] Trimethoprim-sulfamethoxazole should not be used if infection with group A streptococci is suspected or proven. Clinical improvement can be expected within 48 to 72 hours. If the patient's symptoms fail to resolve completely, a second 3-week course of antibiotics is called for.[4] Decongestants, antihistamines, or both are used frequently in an attempt to promote drainage of the sinuses, but no proof of the efficacy of these agents exists. In unusually severe cases, parenteral antibiotics are required and otolaryngologic support is indicated. As with chronic otitis media, surgery is sometimes required in cases of chronic sinusitis.

Table 256-2 *Classification of Orbital Cellulitis*

STAGE	DESCRIPTION
I Inflammatory edema	Inflammatory edema beginning in medial or lateral upper eyelid; usually nontender with only minimal skin changes. No induration, visual impairment, or limitation of extraocular movements.
II Orbital cellulitis	Edema of orbital contents with varying degrees of proptosis, chemosis, limitation of extraocular movement, and visual loss.
III Subperiosteal abscess	Proptosis down and out with signs of orbital cellulitis (usually severe). Abscess beneath the periosteum of the ethmoid, frontal, or maxillary bone (in that order of frequency).
IV Orbital abscess	Abscess within the fat or muscle cone in the posterior orbit. Severe chemosis and proptosis; complete ophthalmoplegia and moderate to severe visual loss present (globe displaced forward or down and out).
V Cavernous sinus thrombosis	Proptosis, globe fixation, severe loss of visual acuity, prostration, signs of meningitis; progresses to proptosis, chemosis, and visual loss in contralateral eye.

From Wald ER et al: Sinusitis and its complications in the pediatric patient, Pediatr Clin North Am 28:787, 1981; modified from Chandler JR, Langenbrunner DJ, and Stevens ER: The pathogenesis of orbital complications in acute sinusitis, Laryngoscope 80:1414, 1970.

REFERENCES

1. Brook I: Bacteriologic features of chronic sinusitis in children, JAMA 246:967, 1981.
2. Furukawa CT, Shapiro GG, and Rachelefsky GS: Children with sinusitis, Pediatrics 71:133, 1983.
3. Rachelefsky GS: Chronic sinusitis: the disease of all ages, Am J Dis Child 143:886, 1989.
4. Rachelefsky GS, Katz RM, and Siegel SC: Chronic sinusitis in the allergic child, Pediatr Clin North Am 35:1091, 1988.
5. Rachelefsky GS, Katz RM, and Siegel SC: Diseases of paranasal sinuses in children, Curr Probl Pediatr 12:1, 1982.
6. Siegel JD: Diagnosis and management of acute sinusitis in children, Pediatr Infect Dis J 6:95, 1987.
7. Wald ER: Management of sinusitis in infants and children, Pediatr Infect Dis J 7:449, 1988.
8. Wald ER et al: Acute maxillary sinusitis in children, N Engl J Med 304:749, 1981.
9. Wald ER et al: Sinusitis and its complications in the pediatric patient, Pediatr Clin North Am 28:777, 1981.

257

Spina Bifida

Gregory S. Liptak

Meningomyelocele (myelomeningocele) is a serious and dramatic congenital malformation, occurring at a rate of 0.4 to 4 cases per 1000 live births.[4,10,23] The incidence is higher in females, in those of lower socioeconomic status, and in families of English, Irish, or Welsh extraction. The incidence of meningomyelocele (and other neural tube defects) has been declining for the past several decades, but whether the rate will reach zero or remain at a fixed baseline is uncertain.[23]

ETIOLOGY

Meningomyelocele belongs to the family of neural tube defects that includes abnormalities of the head (anencephaly, cranial meningocele, encephalocele) and of the spine (spina bifida occulta, meningocele, and meningomyelocele). In spina bifida occulta, which occurs in 5% of the population, the spinal cord and soft tissues are normal, but the vertebral arches are incomplete. In meningocele the spinal cord is normal, but the meninges protrude through abnormal vertebral arches and soft tissue. On rare occasions the meningocele may appear as an anterior mass in the pelvis, abdomen, or thorax. In meningomyelocele, malformed spinal cord and nerve roots protrude through abnormal vertebral arches and soft tissue. Lipomas or dermoid cysts may accompany the meningomyelocele.

The cause of neural tube defects is unknown, although faulty closure of the neural groove by the twenty-eighth day of gestation seems to be the primary mechanism. The most recent etiologic hypothesis is that neural tube defects result from the interaction of many genes (polygenic expression) that can be modified by factors in the fetal (maternal) environment. Given an overall incidence of 1 per 1000, the risk for a second affected child from the same parent is 2 or 3 per 100; for a third, it is 10 per 100. An adult with meningomyelocele has a 2% to 3% chance of having a child with a neural tube defect, the same risk that exists for the sibling of an affected child.

Environmental factors such as potato blight, organic solvents, aminopterin, valproic acid, and ethanol have been implicated in the origin of neural tube defects; however, maternal malnutrition (especially folate deficiency) appears to be the most important variable.[13] Meningomyelocele may be seen with certain syndromes, including trisomy 13, maternal thalidomide and valproate ingestion, and cat cry syndrome. It may also be associated with cryptorchism, imperforate anus, ventricular septal defect, cleft palate, inguinal hernias, tracheoesophageal fistula, renal anomalies, and diaphragmatic hernia.[4] Most cases, however, are isolated occurrences.

PATHOLOGY

As shown in Figs. 257-1 and 257-2, four major malformations account for the findings of meningomyelocele—soft tissue malformation, brain malformation, vertebral body malformation, and spinal cord malformation.

Soft Tissue Malformation

The failure of skin and other soft tissues to close leaves the spinal cord open to infection. The lipomas that occasionally accompany the defect may grow larger, compressing the spinal cord, and may cause progressive neurologic symptoms as the child grows. The surgery to cover the cord may itself result in loss of neurologic function and may lead to scar tissue that tethers the cord and results in further neurologic deterioration as the child grows. Failure of normal morphogenesis of the conus medullaris can also result in tethering or compression of the spinal cord.

Brain Malformation

Malformation of the brain includes the Arnold-Chiari (type II) deformity, in which the pons and medulla are distorted and elongated and the cerebellar vermis is displaced inferiorly into the spinal canal. This abnormality is often associated with progressive hydrocephalus, usually of the communicating type (although with narrowing of the sylvian aqueduct, noncommunicating hydrocephalus may occur). Brainstem malformations may also lead to laryngeal nerve palsy and difficulty in swallowing, as well as hypoventilation, apnea, and sudden death. Brain malformations also result in the 15% incidence of grand mal seizures experienced by adolescent patients with spina bifida.

About 25% of children with meningomyelocele are born with evidence of hydrocephalus, with an additional 25% to 60% developing such signs within the first year of life.[20] The higher (i.e., the more cephalad) the spinal lesion, the greater is the likelihood that hydrocephalus will develop. In addition to the usual manifestations of hydrocephalus and complications of shunt placement, strabismus secondary to abducens nerve palsy or to pressure on the centers that control conjugate gaze occurs in about 50% of children who have hydrocephalus and meningomyelocele.

Sudden shunt malfunction in children shunted for hydrocephalus may produce life-threatening elevations of intracranial pressure requiring emergency intervention. Signs and symptoms of acute shunt malfunction include headache, leth-

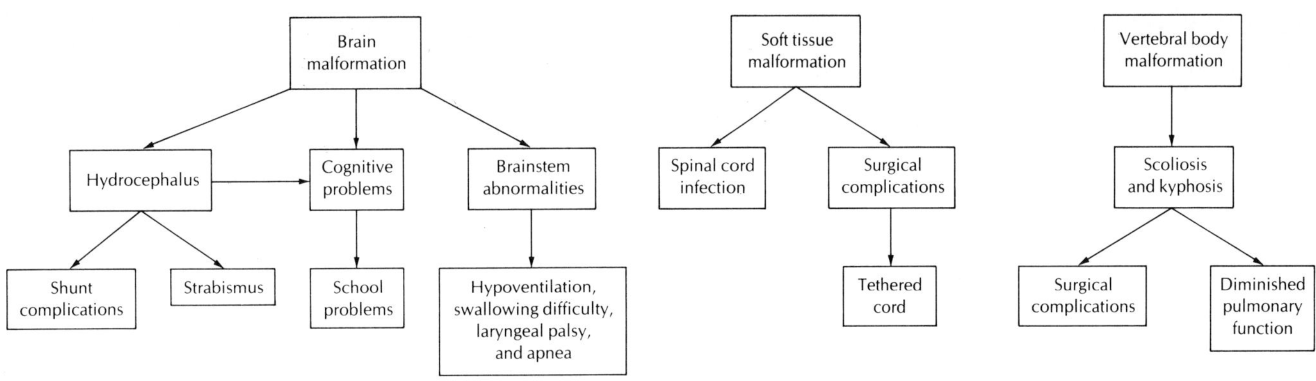

Fig. 257-1 Problems related to meningomyelocele with brain, soft tissue, and vertebral body malformations.

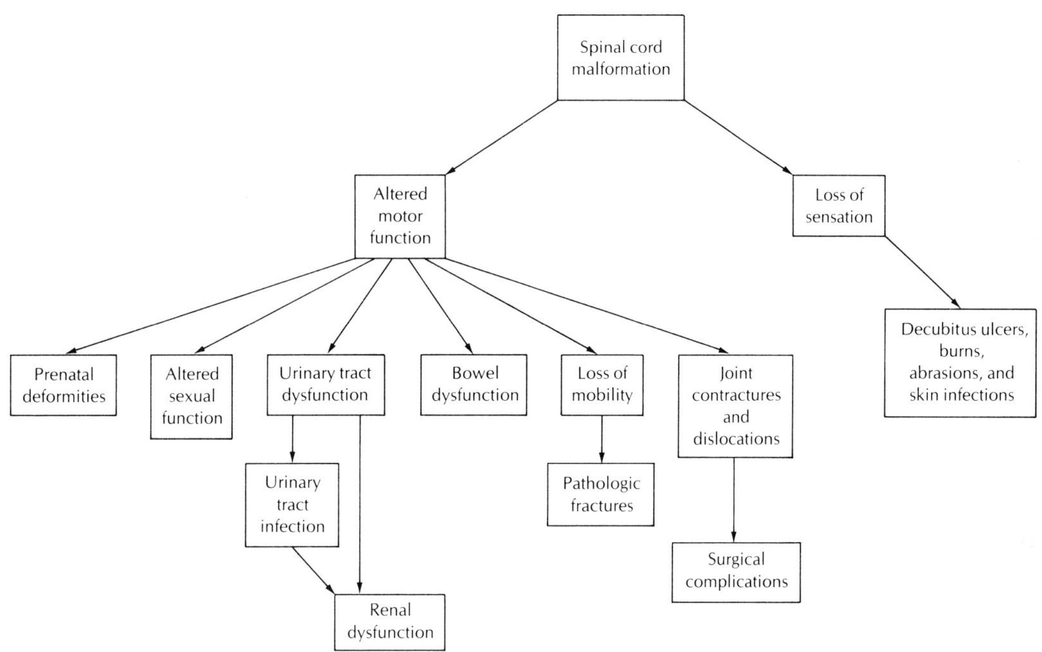

Fig. 257-2 Problems associated with meningomyelocele with spinal cord malformation.

argy, irritability, paralysis of upward gaze, sixth cranial nerve palsy, a bulging fontanelle (in infants), and vomiting. Progression to loss of consciousness, abnormal pupillary reflexes, papilledema, deterioration of vital signs, and death may occur rapidly.[8]

Most children with meningomyelocele have normal overall intelligence quotient (IQ) scores. Yet most of these youngsters have selective cognitive disabilities and score better on verbal than on performance scales. Even those children who have very low performance scores may have surprising verbal fluency, a trait sometimes referred to as the "cocktail party syndrome."[21] Specific cognitive testing often reveals deficiencies of selective visual attention, visual-spatial perception, tactile perception, and auditory concentration. Children with hydrocephalus and higher spinal lesions are more likely to have these deficits. Manifestations seen in school include a short attention span, distractibility, and difficulty with subjects requiring visual-motor integration, such as arithmetic.

Vertebral Malformation

Vertebral malformations caused by abnormal segmentation or formation include absent vertebrae, fused vertebrae, hemivertebrae, and butterfly vertebrae. Occasionally, bony or ligamentous spurs may lead to diastematomyelia. Ten percent of children with thoracic lesions are born with kyphosis; by adolescence this rate increases to 33%. Children with lumbar lesions have a 5% occurrence of kyphosis by adolescence. In addition to cosmetic deformity, severe kyphosis can lead to back pain, pulmonary dysfunction, and recurrent skin ulceration; it also interferes with walking.[15]

The occurrence of scoliosis is related to the level of the lesion, with curves of 30 degrees or more appearing in 81% of adolescents with thoracic lesions and 23% of those with lower lumbar lesions. The consequences of scoliosis are similar to those of kyphosis. Lordosis also occurs, but is much less common.

Spinal Cord Malformation

Spinal cord malformation results in both loss of sensation and loss of motor function. Loss of sensation leaves these children vulnerable to burns and abrasions. Decubitus ulcers also occur, especially in adolescents and adults who spend large amounts of time in wheelchairs. All three skin lesions are susceptible to infection and may lead to osteomyelitis.

Loss of motor function leads to decreased movement in utero, which may lead to deformities seen at birth such as clubfoot (talipes equinovarus) and dislocated hip.

Loss of efferent nerve stimuli to the urinary bladder and sphincter results in neurogenic voiding dysfunction in virtually all children with meningomyelocele. Most children demonstrate passive filling of the bladder, with low-pressure intermittent overflow leaking (incontinence) as a result of mixed upper and lower motor neuron abnormalities. However, some of these children may have "spastic bladders" (i.e., a spastic detrusor muscle) and have bladders with small volumes. Others may have no sphincter tone and may leak urine constantly. Another group may have the even more troublesome combination of hypotonic bladders with spastic sphincters; these infants are at grave risk for hydronephrosis at birth or within the first year of life. In addition to incontinence and hydronephrosis, these children also have frequent urinary tract infections. These problems lead to chronic renal damage, the most common (spina bifida–related) cause of death in these children beyond the first year of life.[1]

Altered sexual function also occurs, especially in males. Approximately 25% of males with meningomyelocele are unable to have erections, and of those who can, most have retrograde ejaculation with decreased fertility. Although females have decreased sensation, most can experience orgasm and have normal fertility.

Children with meningomyelocele often have fecal incontinence as a result of diminished function of the external rectal sphincter and the levator ani muscle. Most children have intact internal rectal sphincter function, and many have intact rectal sensation. Abnormal migration of neural cells in utero can lead to bowel immotility similar to that seen in Hirschsprung disease.[16] Abnormal rectal function, immobility, and the use of a low-fiber diet because of fear of incontinence may lead to constipation or obstipation with overflow soiling.[22]

Loss of motor function in the lower extremities leads to loss of mobility. The degree of mobility is closely related to the level of the lesion; thus children who have intact quadriceps (L2-4) are much more likely to be ambulatory through adolescence than are those who lack such function.[15] As Table 257-1 illustrates, muscle function around the joints is directly related to the level of the lesion. Contractures and dislocations are more likely to develop in children who have an imbalance of forces around a joint than in those who either have full function or no function. For example, children with a lesion at the L4-5 level are more likely to develop foot and ankle contractures than are those with L1-3 or S2-3 lesions. Loss of mobility and innervation also increases the risk for pathologic fractures in the lower extremities.

HISTORY

Because meningomyelocele is inherited in a polygenic fashion, affected newborns may have a family history of neural tube defects or spontaneous abortions (miscarriages). Other historical facts worth noting in the newborn period include length of gestation, type of delivery, complications with and length of labor, maternal nutrition and environmental exposures, current family functioning (including social support and stress), and parental expectations and understanding of the problem. For the older child, information regarding current and past therapies for neurosurgical, orthopedic, urologic, dermatologic, and gastrointestinal problems should be obtained. Educational and social functioning at school, relations with peers and with family members, and the child's sexual function and understanding of sexuality should be ascertained. An assessment of the child's growth, development, mobility, and activities of daily living (personal hygiene, ability to feed oneself, self-help skills) should also be made. The onset of new neurologic symptoms such as weakness, change in bowel and bladder function, tripping, and clumsiness should be sought, since these may indicate deterioration.

PHYSICAL EXAMINATION

The backs of *all* children should be examined for pigmented spots, hairy patches, and sinuses that extend into the spine, since these may be signs of occult spinal dysmorphism.[2]

Table 257-1 *Correlation Between Function and Level of Motor Involvement*

			FOOT	
FUNCTIONAL AREA—LEVEL OF LESION	BOWEL AND BLADDER FUNCTION	TOE INTRINSICS	DORSIFLEXION—INVERSION	PLANTAR FLEXION—EVERSION
S2-3	±*	±	+*	±
S1-2	−*	−	+	±
L5-S1	−	−	+	−
L4-5	−	−	±	−
L3-4	−	−	−	−
L2-3	−	−	−	−
L1-2	−	−	−	−

*±, May be present; +, present; −, absent.

These children are at high risk for meningitis and neurologic deterioration secondary to diastematomyelia and tethering of the spinal cord.

Children with meningomyelocele should have a complete physical examination with special emphasis on the following. The neurologic examination should include motor function (see Table 257-1) and sensory level. A rectal examination and assessment of anal wink can assist in the evaluation of lesions at S2-4. Upper extremity strength, including grip, should be assessed because deterioration may indicate syringomyelia. Palpation of the anterior fontanelle, visualization of the eyegrounds with an ophthalmoscope, assessment of the cranial nerves (especially of extraocular movements), and palpation of the shunt valve and tubing can assist in the evaluation of shunt functioning.[20]

The orthopedic examination should include an assessment of posture (scoliosis, lordosis, kyphosis) as well as joint mobility and stability. Erythema and swelling of a joint or bone in an area that lacks sensation represent a fracture until proven otherwise.[15]

Formal and informal developmental assessments should be part of the routine examination of these children and should include assessment of visual-spatial functioning, verbal, performance, and educational measures, as well as of the more standard areas—fine motor, gross motor, language, and social-adaptive skills.

LABORATORY DATA

Laboratory assessments of the newborn should include measurement of length, weight, and head circumference—the latter, daily. Ultrasound or computed tomography (CT) scan or both of the head, roentgenograms of the spine and hips, ultrasound or intravenous pyelography (IVP) or both of the kidneys, and a urine culture should also be performed. As the child grows, routine urinalysis and urine culture and measurements of head circumference, height, and weight should be done. Some clinicians recommend substituting arm span for height, since growth below the waist is disproportionately slow. A CT scan of the head, especially if the child develops difficulty in school, should be performed routinely. The condition of the spine and joints should be monitored by roentgenograms, renal ultrasound (or IVP), and voiding cystourethrograms should also be done on a routine basis.

Specialized studies that may be indicated include (1) urodynamics to assess detrusor and sphincter function (especially in those children who have reflux or hydronephrosis or do not respond to clean intermittent catheterization,[9] (2) grip strength measurement to monitor for syringomyelia, (3) skin fold thickness measurements, (4) thermography of the skin to look for impending ulcers, (5) magnetic resonance imaging (MRI)[18] or CT scan or myelogram of the spine, and (6) injection of radiopaque dye into the shunt with pressure measurements to determine its function.

PSYCHOSOCIAL CONSIDERATIONS

The birth of a child with meningomyelocele is a potentially devastating event. Most parents are shocked and begin a journey through a series of phases characteristic of people undergoing a loss (in this case a loss of the expected normal child). These stages include shock, denial, sadness, anger, and guilt and ultimately acceptance and equilibrium.[12] In addition to grieving, parents must share in difficult medical decisions. For these reasons parents require tremendous support from medical professionals and others. An evaluation of their current stores of social support and the presence of other stressors is critical in helping them through this time.

Because most children with meningomyelocele have multiple medical problems, they require the expenditure of large amounts of money,[3] time, patience, and understanding.[6] Such demands may "fragment" parents and can lead to isolation of one from the other. This isolation is reinforced by a medical system that sees patients during working hours and that is content to deal exclusively with mothers.[5] The stresses may also affect siblings, who have been shown to have an increased occurrence of behavioral problems.

Parents may begin the stages of mourning and never reach equilibrium, and the clinician will notice manifestations of denial, guilt, or anger. In addition, one spouse may be able to reach equilibrium but be emotionally unavailable to the spouse still struggling with the earlier stages.[12]

The child with meningomyelocele may have difficulty at home with parents unable to provide affection or set consistent limits. They may have difficulty with peers who see them as "cripples" rather than as children with disabilities. They may have difficulty performing academically and may lose interest in school because of frequent negative reinforcement. They

KNEE		HIP			
EXTENSION	FLEXION	FLEXION	ADDUCTION	ABDUCTION	EXTENSION
+	+	+	+	+	+
+	+	+	+	+	±
+	±	+	+	+	−
+	−	+	+	−	−
+	−	+	+	−	−
±	−	±	±	−	−
−	−	−	−	−	−

may have no adult role models. Finally, they may lose self-esteem from frequent visits to clinicians—visits that are often characterized by the identification of new problems without any positive reinforcement of their successes.[1]

MANAGEMENT[14,20]

The two goals in the management of these patients are (1) to prevent dysfuntions (e.g., physiologic and biochemical defects) from becoming disabilities (the functional consequences of the impairment, e.g., "can't walk") and (2) to prevent the disabilities from becoming handicaps (the social disadvantages experienced from the disabilities, e.g., "can't get a job").[11] Achieving these goals requires comprehensive, coordinated care.

In the newborn period the child and family should be evaluated by a pediatrician, nurse, social worker, neurosurgeon, orthopedist, physical therapist, and, when indicated, urologist. Once the child has been examined and given supportive care, central nervous system infection must be prevented. Parenteral antibiotics that provide coverage against gram-negative bacilli and *Staphylococcus aureus* organisms and surgery to close the open defect should be provided as soon as possible. When microsurgical techniques are used, neurologic function should not be further impaired during the closure.

Daily measurement of the head circumference and ultrasound or CT scan of the head should be used as guides for ventriculoperitoneal shunt placement to reduce hydrocephalus. No universally accepted criteria exist to determine the need for or the timing of shunt placement. Furosemide (Lasix) and acetazolamide (Diamox) may be administered to delay the insertion of the shunt.[19]

Deformities such as clubfeet or dislocated hips should be managed with range-of-motion exercises, splinting, and casting. The urologic system should be evaluated by urine culture and IVP or renal ultrasound. Baseline roentgenograms of the skin and hips should be taken.

Genetic counseling and social support should be provided to the family, and assistance with finances should be a priority.

As the child grows, the primary care physician should coordinate the child's care and be his or her advocate.[6] Enhancing environmental stimulation for the maximization of cognitive development should be another goal in the management of these children. In many instances, children may benefit from formal early intervention programs. Opportunities for interactions with people and objects (toys) should be provided. Similarly, the child should be encouraged to develop the best social interaction and self-help skills possible, including developing independence in hygiene and eating.

According to Bronfenbrenner[5]:

> Learning and development are facilitated by the participation of the developing person in progressively more complex patterns of reciprocal activity with someone with whom that person has developed a strong and enduring emotional attachment and when the balance of power gradually shifts in favor of the developing person.

A child with a disability has the same psychosocial needs as healthy children, and the clinician should help the family achieve this shifting of power. Although the child's environment should be conducive to learning and exploration, exclusive concern with direct teaching or special programs may actually inhibit those self-directed activities that should be encouraged.

Orthopedic management may include surgery for joint contractures, scoliosis, or kyphosis. To prevent contractures and dislocations, regular passive range-of-motion exercises, splints, body jackets, and casts may be used.[15]

Various exercises and orthoses (braces) may be used to enhance locomotion. The parapodium, a standing brace that allows the child to be in an upright position with hands unencumbered, has been used for about 15 years. The child in the parapodium can move with several different gaits and can also sit with the knees bent. Crutches or walkers with more standard bracing may be used, and some treatment centers advocate early use of the wheelchair, especially for those children with quadriceps paralysis. Adaptive equipment such as carts and hand-pedaled tricycles can also enhance the function and self-esteem of these children.

Goals of urologic management include prevention of renal damage and attainment of continence.[7] In the past, urinary diversion with ileal loops was performed in most children with meningomyelocele to achieve these goals. Clean intermittent catheterization, introduced in 1972, is safer, is more acceptable, and results in better renal function than does urinary diversion. Most families are able to perform clean intermittent catheterization when the child is 4 to 5 years of age, and many children, even those this young, are able to perform the procedure themselves. Clean intermittent catheterization has also been used in children under 3 years of age, and it can be helpful in the management of vesicoureteral reflux with or without hydronephrosis or in those with frequent urinary tract infections. The addition of drugs that relax the detrusor muscle or increase sphincter tone, such as imipramine hydrochloride, oxybutinin chloride, and pseudoephedrine, can enhance continence. For older children with minimal sphincter tone in whom catheterization does not provide continence, the use of an artificial sphincter or other surgical procedure with or without clean intermittent catheterization, may provide continence.

Obtaining regular urine cultures to detect urinary tract infection and administering prophylactic antibiotics in those children with frequent infections may prevent renal damage. Trimethoprim-sulfamethoxazole, sulfisoxazole, nitrofurantoin, and cefaclor given in less than the therapeutic dosage have been used for prophylaxis.

Bowel continence after 4 years of age with the avoidance of severe constipation is often difficult to achieve. However, high fiber diet, stool softeners, regular toileting, regular stimulants, and biofeedback in those children with rectal sensation may be used singly or in combination to attain these goals. Regular high colonic saline enemas are used by some treatment centers, although their efficacy has not been assessed scientifically.[22]

Impotence in the male may be managed surgically with penile implants. Retrograde ejaculation may also be surgically corrected. Pregnant women with meningomyelocele may need to have their babies delivered by cesarean section because of hip contractures. They may also develop herniation of their intervertebral disks with neurologic sequelae and should have frequent neurologic evaluations throughout pregnancy.

Even though the execution of all these interventions requires tremendous resources and effort, they may still be inadequate in the absence of social changes. To prevent disabilities from becoming handicaps, society's attitudes and practices must be altered. The clinician can be an advocate for these children by helping remove architectural barriers in the community, which will allow disabled people access to places such as banks, public buildings, transportation, and recreation areas. Altering the attitudes of nondisabled people may be more difficult, but the clinician can help to enable the disabled child and adult to serve as role models in the community—for instance, by encouraging the hiring of disabled workers. Performing all the above tasks requires constant effort and can be achieved only with a multidisciplinary team that is willing to collaborate with the family.

PREVENTION

Because the cause of neural tube defects is uncertain, primary prevention is difficult. Yet a reduction in incidence has been demonstrated in infants of mothers who have improved their diets or who have been given either multivitamins or folic acid in the first trimester of pregnancy.[13]

Prenatal diagnosis of open neural tube defects may be made by measuring alpha-fetoprotein levels in maternal serum between 14 and 16 weeks of gestation, coupled with ultrasound confirmation of the diagnosis.[23] Amniocentesis is being advocated for those with elevated alpha-fetoprotein levels. The prenatal detection of a neural tube defect can allow the family to make rational plans, whether or not they elect to continue the pregnancy.[17] If they elect to deliver, the fetus should be monitored for the development of hydrocephalus, which may be treated in utero, and the infant may benefit from cesarean section to avoid trauma to the head and back. Social support should be provided to these families, whatever their decision.

REFERENCES

1. Action Committee on Myelodysplasia, Section on Urology: Current approaches to evaluation and management with meningomyelocele, Pediatrics 63:663, 1979.
2. Albright AL, Gartner JC, and Wiener ES: Lumbar cutaneous hemangiomas as indicators of tethered spinal cords, Pediatrics 83:977, 1989.
3. Anonymous: Economic burden of spina bifida—United States, 1980-1990, MMWR 38:264, 1989.
4. Bamforth SJ and Baird PA: Spina bifida and hydrocephalus: a population study over a 35-year period, Am J Hum Genet 44:225, 1989.
5. Bronfenbrenner U: The ecology of human development, Cambridge, Mass, 1979, Harvard University Press.
6. Colgan MT: The child with spina bifida: role of the pediatrician, Am J Dis Child 135:854, 1982.
7. Ehrlich O and Brem AS: A prospective comparison of urinary tract infection in patients treated with either clean intermittent catheterization or urinary diversion, Pediatrics 70:665, 1982.
8. Frigoletto RD, Birnholz JC, and Greene MF: Antenatal treatment of hydrocephalus by ventriculoamniotic shunting, JAMA 248:2496, 1982.
9. Ghoniem GM et al: Bladder compliance in meningomyelocele children, J Urol 141:1404, 1989.
10. Golden GS: Neural tube defects, Pediatr Rev 1:187, 1979.
11. Hirst M: Patterns of impairment and disability related to social handicap in young people with cerebral palsy and spina bifida, J Biosoc Sci 21:1, 1989.
12. Irvin NA, Kennell JH, and Klaus MH: Caring for the parents of an infant with a congenital malformation. In Klaus MH and Kennell JH, editors: Parent-infant bonding, ed 2, St Louis, 1982, The CV Mosby Co.
13. Lawrence KM: Neural tube defects: a two-pronged approach to primary prevention, Pediatrics 70:648, 1982.
14. Liptak GS et al: The management of children with spinal dysraphism, J Child Neurol 3:3, 1988.
15. Menelaus MB: The orthopaedic management of spina bifida cystica, New York, 1980, Churchill Livingstone, Inc.
16. Merkles RG, Solish SB, and Scherzer AL: Meningomyelocele and Hirschsprung disease: theoretical and clinical significance, Pediatrics 76:299, 1985.
17. Milunsky A: Prenatal detection of neural tube defects. VI. Experience with 20,000 pregnancies, JAMA 244:2731, 1980.
18. Rindahl MA et al: Magnetic resonance imaging of pediatric dysraphism, Magn Reson Imaging 7:217, 1989.
19. Shinnar S et al: Management of hydrocephalus in infancy: use of acetazolamide and furosemide to avoid cerebrospinal fluid shunts, J Pediatr 107:31, 1985.
20. Shurtleff DB: Myelodysplasia: management and treatment, Curr Probl Pediatr X(no 3), 1980.
21. Tew B: The "cocktail party syndrome" in children with hydrocephalus and spina bifida, Br J Disord Commun 14:89, 1979.
22. Wald A: The use of biofeedback in treatment of fecal incontinence in patients with meningomyelocele, Pediatrics 68:45, 1981.
23. Windham GC and Edmonds LD: Current trends in the incidence of neural tube defects, Pediatrics 70:333, 1982.

258

Spinal Deformities

Edward M. Sills

Back pain in children usually is a sign of an underlying disorder. Postural abnormalities may or may not indicate an underlying disorder, and the challenge to the physician is to determine whether the child's posture is caused by an underlying skeletal deformity or is merely a habit that exaggerates increases or decreases in the normal spinal curves. Abnormal curvatures and protrusions merit careful investigation. The thoracic spine normally has some kyphosis, and the lumbar spine normally has slight lordosis. If either condition is excessive, progressive, or painful, concern is appropriate. Scoliosis, a side-to-side curve, always is abnormal. (See the accompanying box for a classification of spinal deformity.)

CONGENITAL MALFORMATIONS

The newborn is relaxed when placed prone in the examiner's palm. The infant's back falls into slight flexion, allowing detection of meningomyelocele, congenital scoliosis, kyphosis, or dorsolumbar hyperflexion. Lumbar spinal deformity may be indicated by a hair tuft, dimple, discoloration, or a palpable spina bifida lamina defect.

Congenital scoliosis is the result of asymmetric growth. It is characterized by a lateral curvature of the spine caused by the asymmetric structural vertebral deformity. The curve is fixed and inflexible. When located near the middle of the spine, the segments of the spine above and below compensate for it by curving in the opposite direction. The result is a balanced spine and a straight back. There is no need for treatment.

When, however, the asymmetric vertebra is at the base of the spine, the compensatory curve that develops above is insufficient, and a curvature progresses as the patient grows. This condition requires surgical correction before adolescence.

When the deformity occurs in the cervical spine, a "wryneck" deformity results, and thoracolumbar compensatory curvature severely distorts posture. Unilateral surgical fusions are required to minimize deformity.

Congenital kyphosis is caused by lack of segmentation of vertebral bodies anteriorly or by lack of formation of a vertebral body. Surgical fusion is required to prevent paraplegia.

Other congenital malformations of the spine include the *Klippel-Feil* syndrome, which is characterized by a short neck, limitation of head motion, and a low posterior hairline. Spina bifida often is present in the cervical spine; it is caused by failure of the two lateral halves of the vertebral arch to fuse. Exercises to maintain the neck's functional range of motion are indicated, but surgery is contraindicated because of the danger of producing injury to the cervical spinal cord.

Spina bifida can be mild and of no clinical significance (occulta), or it can be severe (vera) with meningeal and neural elements protruding posteriorly. When the protrusion includes bony elements, it may transfix the spinal cord. This transfixing spur is called *diastematomyelia*. These severe forms of spina bifida require prompt neurosurgical correction.

Congenital vertebral anomalies also are seen in several syndromes in which other anomalies may be present. These include the following:

1. Larsen syndrome—vertebral, joint, facial, and palate
2. Waardenburg syndrome—spine and ribs
3. Goldenhar syndrome—oculoauriculovertebral dysplasia
4. Morquio syndrome (mucopolysaccharidosis, type IV)—odontoid dysplasia with atlantoaxial subluxation

ACQUIRED ABNORMALITIES

Scoliosis

Scoliosis can be nonstructural (corrects with side bending) or structural (no improvement with position change). Nonstructural scoliosis results from posture habit, splinting because of pain, muscle spasm, or hysteria. Of the structural forms of scoliosis, the congenital (e.g., absent or fused spinal segments), metabolic (e.g., juvenile osteoporosis), or neuromuscular (e.g., poliomyelitis or cerebral palsy) types are less common than idiopathic scoliosis, which accounts for 75% of all cases. Although most cases are idiopathic, there is an increased familial risk for scoliosis. Idiopathic scoliosis can appear clinically at any age, although the majority of cases begin in adolescence and affect mostly girls, who usually exhibit a right thoracic or right thoracolumbar pattern. The infantile form begins before age 3 years, is predominant in boys, and usually resolves without treatment because of vertebral compensations above and below the area of curve. The juvenile form occurs between ages 6 and 10 years, has no sex predilection, and usually consists of a right thoracic curve. Although some of the mild curves will not progress, the juvenile and adolescent curves tend toward rapid progression during growth spurts.

The condition usually is painless and is discovered on routine physical examinations or at school scoliosis screening programs. When the patient bends forward, prominence of one scapula, of one side of the rib cage, or of the lumbar paraspinous muscles can indicate the site and direction of the

Classification of Spinal Deformity

A. Idiopathic
   1. Infantile
   2. Juvenile
   3. Adolescent
B. Neuromuscular
   1. Neuropathic
      a. Upper motor neuron lesion
         (1) Cerebral palsy
         (2) Spinocerebellar degenerations
         (3) Syringomyelia
         (4) Spinal cord tumor
         (5) Spinal cord trauma
      b. Lower motor neuron lesion
         (1) Poliomyelitis
         (2) Other viral myelitis
         (3) Trauma
         (4) Spinal muscular atrophy
         (5) Meningomyelocele (paralytic)
      c. Dysautonomia (Riley-Day)
   2. Myopathic
      a. Arthrogryposis
      b. Muscular dystrophy
      c. Fiber-type disproportion
      d. Congenital hypotonia
      e. Myotonia dystrophica
C. Congenital
   1. Congenital scoliosis
      a. Failure of formation
         (1) Wedge
         (2) Hemivertebra
      b. Failure of segmentation
         (1) Unilateral bar
         (2) Bilateral bar
   2. Congenital kyphosis
      a. Failure of formation
      b. Failure of segmentation
      c. Mixed

C. Congenital—*cont'd*
   3. Congenital lordosis
   4. Associated with neural tissue defect
      a. Meningomyelocele
      b. Meningocele
      c. Spinal dysraphism (diastematomyelia)
D. Neurofibromatosis
E. Mesenchymal
   1. Marfan syndrome
   2. Ehlers-Danlos syndrome
F. Traumatic
   1. Fracture or dislocation
   2. After irradiation
   3. After laminectomy
G. Soft tissue contractures
   1. After thoracoplasty
   2. Burns
H. Osteochondrodystrophies
   1. Achondroplasia
   2. Spondyloepiphyseal dysplasia
   3. Diastrophic dwarfism
   4. Mucopolysaccharidosis
I. Scheuermann disease
J. Infection
K. Tumor
L. Rheumatoid disease
M. Metabolic
   1. Rickets
   2. Juvenile osteoporosis
   3. Osteogenesis imperfecta
N. Lumbosacral anomalies
O. Hysterical
P. Functional
   1. Postural
   2. Secondary to short limb
   3. Secondary to pain

Modified from Scoliosis Research Society.

scoliosis. An erect anteroposterior spinal roentgenogram determines the degree of curvature and the structure of the vertebrae.

Treatment is undertaken because pulmonary restriction, significant back pain, and cosmetic deformity are the sequelae of unrecognized and untreated scoliosis. Exercises are of no benefit in retarding or reversing the progress of scoliosis. A curvature in excess of 40 degrees requires surgical fusion regardless of the patient's age. Curves between 20 and 40 degrees should not require treatment if skeletal maturation is complete, but they should be braced in the growing child. A curve milder than 20 degrees should be observed for possible progression but does not require treatment.

Kyphosis

An acquired dorsal hump can be secondary to a spinal tumor, radiation, infection, or surgery. The most common cause of acquired kyphosis is an osteochondrosis known as Scheuermann disease, which occurs in 5% of the population. The most common site is in the lower thoracic vertebrae, but this condition can occur in any site in the vertebral column. The initial event is a bulging of the intervertebral disks in the direction of contiguous vertebral bodies, which exerts pressure against the cartilage plates covering the bodies, causing thinning of the plates. This interferes with endochondral bone formation on the growth surface of the plates, causing gaps that are the basis for the herniation of the disk into the bodies, isolating the apophyseal ossification center from the vertebral body. The disk space narrows, more so anteriorly, causing increased pressure on the anterior portions of contiguous vertebral bodies and impeding their longitudinal growth anteriorly, resulting in attendant kyphosis.

An aching pain aggravated by physical exertion is present in the affected part of the vertebral column. There is tenderness to palpation of the affected area. Having the patient assume a stooping position often will cause the pain to increase. Once the backache has been present for a year or so, the kyphosis is easily apparent as a round-back deformity. In many instances the pain is so minor that the patient first complains to the physician about pain caused by "poor posture," and then the kyphosis is noted. Roentgenograms reveal a narrowing of the anterior disk space and defects on the surfaces of adjacent vertebrae at sites where the disk tissue has penetrated into the bodies. The prolapsed disk tissue, in time, becomes walled off by osseous tissue, forming a bulbous mass of extruded tissue appearing as an area of lucency in the affected body (Schmorl nodule). In some children the deformity can progress to cause severe deformity and dysfunction; in others, the condition stabilizes and the deformity may disappear. Treatment is aimed at prevention of further deformity, occasionally by use of casting or bracing. In those rare instances of rapid progression or very severe pain, spinal fusion is necessary. The majority of youngsters, however, require careful observation and intervention only if progression of the deformity is noted.

BACK PAIN

Although scoliosis and kyphosis can be painful, they usually are painless postural deformities. There are several painful disorders related to spinal deformity of which the pediatrician should be aware. (See also Chapter 113.)

Spondylolysis and Spondylolisthesis

Spondylolysis, a defect in the continuity of the pars interarticularis of the posterior portion of L4 or L5, may result in forward slippage of the vertebral body, known as spondylolisthesis. The horizontal slippage usually involves the fifth lumbar vertebral body moving anteriorly in relationship to S1. This deformity, however, can occur anywhere in the vertebral column. Spondylolysis often causes back pain before the spondylolisthesis develops. Trauma, causing disruption of the pars interarticularis, is believed to be the cause of spondylolysis in a genetically susceptible host. The propensity for spondylolysis to become spondylolisthesis with forward slippage is exaggerated during growth spurts.

A flattening of the normal lumbar lordosis with posterior tilting of the pelvis is noted in spondylolysis. An oblique roentgenogram reveals the effect of the pars interventricularis on spondylolysis; a standing lateral roentgenogram demonstrates spondylolisthesis. Activities that cause hyperextension of the lumbar spine should be avoided, and exercises to reduce lumbar lordosis relieve the pain of spondylolysis. Once slippage occurs, surgical spinal fusion is necessary.

Infections

Infections involving the spinal structures are exceedingly rare. Acute pyogenic osteomyelitis and tuberculosis cause bone destruction, initially in the anterior portion of the vertebrae, leading to collapse. Vigorous antibiotic therapy and immobilization are indicated.

Disk space inflammation, or *diskitis,* can appear as a fever of unknown origin accompanied by a limp or low back pain. Narrowing of the disk space is the usual roentgenographic finding. In all cases, blood cultures are indicated. The majority of younger patients do not show evidence of bacterial infection and require only immobilization. Children older than age 8 years occasionally are found to have a staphylococcal disease. The indications for using antibiotics include positive blood culture results, recurrences of back pain with systemic signs such as fever, leukocytosis with a "left shift" in the differential white blood cell count, or clinical advancement of disease despite immobilization.

Tumors

Bone tumors occur most commonly in adolescence and usually appear at the end of growth peaks. Of the group of malignant bone tumors, none primarily involves the spine, although chondrosarcomas and the marrow tumors (leukemias, lymphomas, Ewing tumor, and histiocytic lymphoma) often invade the pelvis early and can cause low back pain in adolescence. Roentgenograms display bony lesions with surrounding soft tissue mass. Calcification of periosteum lifted away from bone causes a characteristic sunburst appearance.

Of the nonmalignant tumors, the osteogenic group often involves the spine. Both osteoid osteoma and osteoblastoma are reparative rather than infiltrative. Osteoid osteoma occurs in long bones and in the posterior position of the vertebrae; osteoblastoma occurs in the neural arches of the vertebral column. Pain, usually occurring at night, is the common complaint and is quickly relieved by aspirin. On roentgenogram, the examiner sees a hyperostotic lesion surrounding a nidus of sclerotic bone separated by a radiolucent zone. Surgical excision is curative.

SUGGESTED READINGS

King HA: Evaluating the child with back pain, Pediatr Clin North Am 33:1489, 1986.

Letts M et al: Fractures of the pars interacticularis in adolescent athletes: a clinical-biomedical analysis, J Pediatr Orthop 6:40, 1986.

Papanicolaov N et al: Bone scintigraphy and radiography in young athletes with low back pain, Am J Roentgenology 145:1039, 1985.

Portenoy RK et al: Back pain in the cancer patient: an algorithm for evaluation and management, Neurology 37:134, 1987.

Riseborough E and Herndon JH: Scoliosis and other deformities: deformities of the axial skeleton, Boston, 1975, Little, Brown & Co.

Schmorl G: The human spine in health and disease, New York, 1959, Grune & Stratton, Inc.

Sills EM: What's causing the back pain? Contemp Pediatr 5:85, 1988.

Tachdjian M: Pediatric orthopedics, Philadelphia, 1979, WB Saunders Co.

Williams HJ: Vertebral epiphysitis, Am J Roentgenol 90:1236, 1963.

259

Sports Injuries

David E. Hall

More than 5 million young people participate in high school sports each year. According to one study, more than 2% of all visits to pediatric offices are for recreational injuries.[9] Estimates of the frequency of injuries vary widely.

It has been estimated that 10% to 20% of high school athletes sustain an injury that keeps them out of participation for longer than a week.[15] Wrestling and football have the highest significant injury rates per participant in high school, followed by softball, gymnastics, track and field, and soccer. Tennis and swimming produce the fewest injuries.[7] Other sports fall somewhere in between. Frequency of injury, however, is not always the best measure of a sport's risk. The trampoline, for example, accounts for a disproportionately large number of injuries that cause paralysis.[6]

Most injuries occur during practice, but competitive events have the highest hourly injury rate.[7] The most important determinant of injury is lack of conditioning and recent entry into a sport.[6] The lower extremities are the most commonly injured.[3] Soft tissue injuries, especially sprains and strains, account for the vast majority of injuries and thus may be treated by the primary care physician who has learned basic anatomy and the principles of treatment. Many physicians, unfamiliar with the demands of a particular sport, overtreat and keep the patient out of competition too long. On the other hand, the physician may be pressured by overzealous parents or patients to allow the child to return to activities too soon. Another common mistake is failure to provide appropriate exercises for rehabilitation, because many physicians are ignorant of this aspect of care.

Sports medicine is a discipline in itself. This chapter can only serve as an introduction to some of the more common problems. The reader is referred to a text on sports medicine for information on treatment and exercises for rehabilitation. Sports medicine centers, present in many urban areas, provide consultation and continuing education for interested physicians.

GENERAL PRINCIPLES OF PREVENTION

Pediatricians have become aware that the organization of sports leagues for children—for example, in baseball, football, and soccer—has become so much a part of middle-class American life that, in some ways, it has become the driving force in the experience of many children and adolescents—a force that has thrown out of context the reasons for participating in athletics. A potentially marvelous contribution to a child's physical, emotional, and social well-being is distorted by overemphasis, the drive to excel within overorganized, highly structured leagues, the sometimes rabid participation of parents, and the push to win. Some believe that this overemphasis and distortion require Draconian measures, to the extent of abolishing the leagues. This is not necessary. Pediatricians, however, can contribute to prevention if they work with the families they serve to provide a context for the participation of children, a context that allows for vigorous effort, enthusiastic participation, and a reawakening, perhaps, of the old Grantland Rice advice that it's how one plays the game that matters, not winning. Given this proper context, the child and the family can anticipate a happier time with less emotional battering and less likelihood of physical injury. This requires taking a sensitive history and subsequently developing insights that can lead to better understanding and therefore better management. See Chapter 19, "Physical Fitness in Children," for further discussion of the presentation of sports injuries.

CLASSIFICATION OF INJURIES

Ligaments connect one bone to another. *Sprains* are injuries to ligaments. *Strains,* on the other hand, are "tearing" injuries to a muscle or its tendon. Sprains are usually caused by an outside force and are most common in contact sports, whereas strains are dynamic injuries not caused by an outside force and are most often encountered in "timed" sports such as swimming or running. Strains and sprains may be classified as grades 1 through 3 (Table 259-1). Primary physicians can usually treat grade 1 and most grade 2 injuries.

Most fractures that occur in athletes are not complicated, but many primary care physicians do not feel comfortable treating them and depend on the orthopedist for definitive treatment. Few fractures heal in less than 4 to 6 weeks.

Other types of injuries include *overuse syndromes,* such as Little League elbow, which are associated with excessive or inappropriate use of a body part; *contusions,* which result from a blow to a muscle or bone and result in a painful, swollen area; and *dislocations.* Dislocations may cause significant damage to surrounding ligaments. Joints with range of motion in few planes (e.g., the knee) are more severely damaged when dislocated than are joints with range of motion in several places (e.g., the shoulder). Dislocations usually result from an outside force.

DATA BASE

The wise physician obtains a detailed history of the mechanism of injury. Orthopedists use this information, for ex-

Table 259-1 *Classification of Sprains and Strains*

GRADE	SPRAIN	STRAIN
1	Minimal tearing of ligament; no instability of joint	Minimal tearing of musculotendinous unit
2	Appreciable tearing of ligament (5%-99% of fibers disrupted) with moderate joint instability; testing stability of joint causes pain	Moderate tearing of musculotendinous unit, with partial less of function
3	Complete tear of ligament with absolute joint instability; testing stability of joint causes little pain	Complete tear of musculotendinous unit; painless initially, but dramatic initial sensation of injury

ample, to reduce a fracture or dislocation by reversing the force that led to the injury. Other important information includes the location, character, severity, and radiation of any pain. Was the onset sudden or insidious? What relieves or aggravates the pain? Has the injury occurred before? The sensation or sound of a pop or snap suggests a serious injury. A brief medical history should be obtained to rule out illnesses hat might complicate treatment. On physical examination, the physician should look for any disorders of alignment that may have predisposed the patient to the injury. The location of swelling, tenderness, or discoloration should be noted. Abnormal bulges in muscle groups may signify a ruptured muscle. The physician should also determine the range of motion of the affected joints and look for instability. The integrity of veins and blood vessels should always be evaluated.

During the physical examination, the physician should keep in mind the possibility of anabolic steroid use. An extensive survey of steroid use in the United States found a prevalence of 6.6% among twelfth grade males.[2] Signs of anabolic steroid use include sudden flare ups of acne, evidence of liver disease such as jaundice, rapid gains in muscle mass and weight, and aggressive behavior. Other effects include decreased spermatogenesis and premature closure of the epiphyses. The doses used by bodybuilders are several times those used for replacement in patients with delayed puberty.[11] Steroid use is most common in participants in football, power lifting, shot putting, wrestling, and swimming.

GENERAL PRINCIPLES OF TREATMENT

Much of the disability of soft tissue injuries is increased by soft tissue swelling. Edema, for example, interferes with joint mobility and may keep ligament ends apart, which may cause them to heal with a fibrous scar between the ends, rather than directly together. This makes the ligaments more lax and predisposes to reinjury. Swelling may be minimized by the use of rest, ice, compression, and elevation (RICE), which are the mainstays of initial treatment for virtually all athletic injuries.

Rest is especially important for the first 24 to 72 hours of a significant injury. For lower extremity injuries, crutches should be used to avoid weight bearing.

Randomized studies have demonstrated that athletes return to full activity faster with the use of cryotherapy begun immediately after the injury.[10] The application of ice seems to work by (1) decreasing pain by diminishing nerve impulses and conduction velocity, (2) decreasing muscle spasm by diminishing muscle spindle firing, and (3) decreasing edema by inducing vasoconstriction and decreasing capillary permeability. In addition, cryotherapy decreases the oxygen demand of the cells by slowing down their rate of metabolism. This minimizes tissue death, which causes cell breakdown and further edema. Continuing cryotherapy beyond 30 minutes, however, can cause a reflex vasodilation.[10]

Ice should be applied for 20 minutes at a time every 4 to 6 hours. This is best done by applying a layer of bandage to the skin, preferably wet to conduct cold better, then applying the bag of ice and, finally, wrapping it with an elastic or other bandage. The initial layer of cloth reduces the chance of frostbite. Heat should not be applied early in the injury, nor should the patient be advised to "run it off." Cryotherapy should be used for at least the first 24 to 48 hours, but many trainers and sports medicine physicians recommend that it be continued until the swelling has disappeared completely, which may be much later. An alternate way to apply ice is to freeze water in a paper cup, then rub the cup on the injury in a circular motion. As the ice melts, the top layers of the cup are peeled off, and the ice is rubbed on the skin until it becomes bright pink, which usually takes 7 to 10 minutes.[4]

Compression may be applied with an elastic bandage. Sometimes it is necessary to use gauze pads or disposable diapers to fill in the hollow spaces where edema fluid is most likely to accumulate (see ankle injuries below). The injured extremity should be elevated above the level of the heart whenever possible.

Aspirin should not be used to relieve pain, because it may lead to increased hemorrhage, which in turn may delay healing by causing further inflammation. Acetaminophen or nonsteroidal antiinflammatory medications should be used for pain.

Rehabilitation is the most neglected aspect of injury treatment, yet it is extremely important to ensure a safe return to activities and to prevent reinjury. Resting the injured part leads to muscle weakness and atrophy. If the physician is not well versed in rehabilitation for specific injuries, referral to a physical therapist is advisable. Most rehabilitation involves gradual strengthening exercises for appropriate muscle groups.

SPECIFIC INJURIES

Ankle Sprains

Eighty percent to 90% of ankle sprains are inversion injuries that affect the anterior talofibular ligament and the calcaneofibular ligament on the lateral ankle (Fig. 259-1). Medial injuries usually involve the deltoid ligament. The interosseous

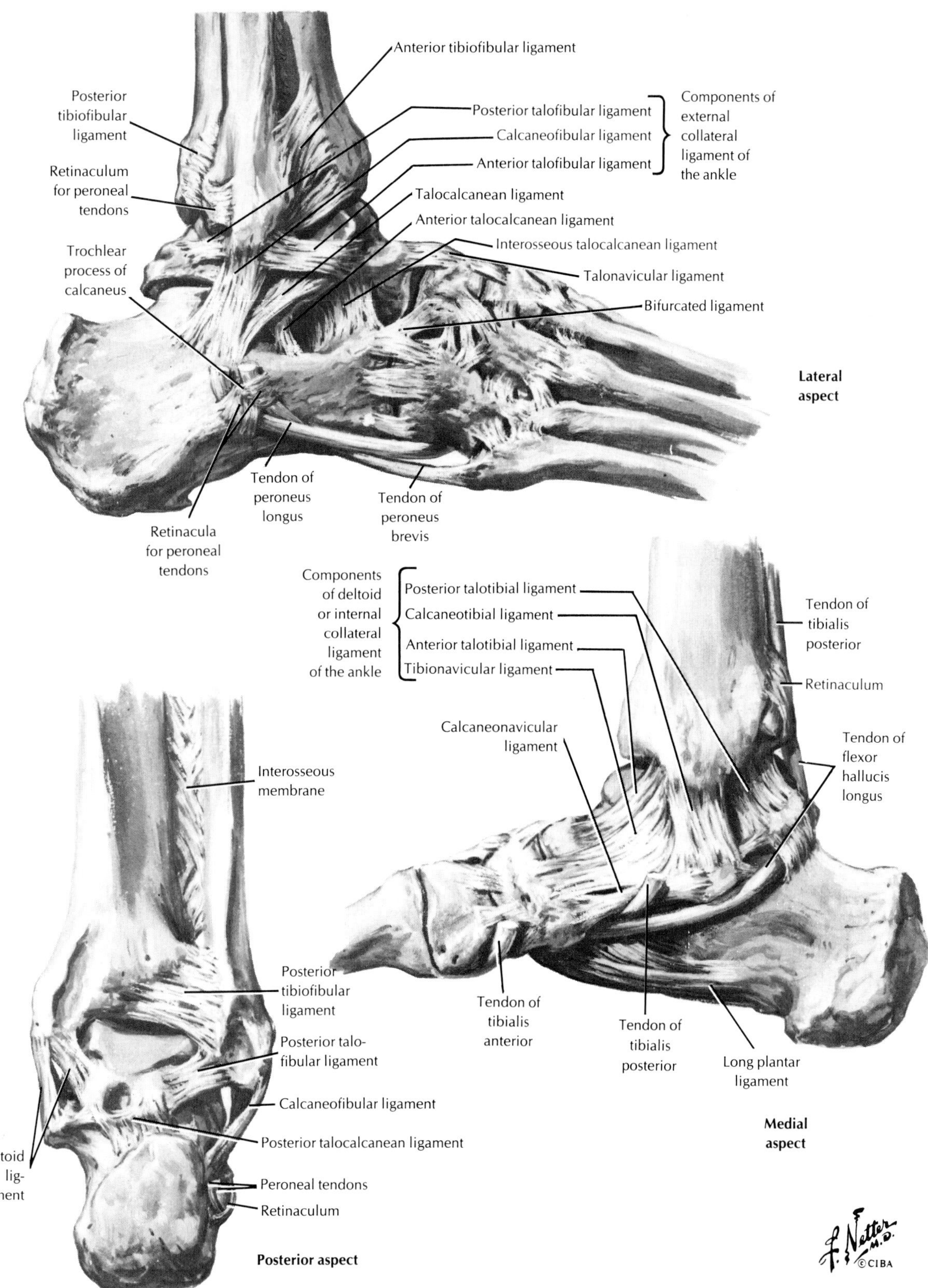

Fig. 259-1 Ligaments of ankle and foot.

ligament, along with the anterior and posterior tibiofibular ligaments, binds the lower ends of the tibia and fibula together. On examination of the normal foot, the prominence of the fibular malleolus, the talus, and the cuboid on the lateral side can be felt. When the foot is maximally inverted, the calcaneofibular ligament may be felt as a firm band. It is usually possible to determine the injured ligaments by palpation, especially if the physician is fortunate enough to examine the ankle before edema has obscured the findings. Avulsion fractures of the malleoli cause local tenderness over the bone. Pain with compression of the tibia and fibula together suggests a fracture. Patients with more serious fractures (e.g., transverse fracture of the tibia or fibula) usually will not even attempt to walk on the ankle. Athletes with "garden variety" ankle sprains and tenderness over the appropriate ligaments without bony tenderness or instability do not always require roentgenograms. If a severe ligamentous injury is suspected, the patient should be referred to an orthopedist. Radiographs with stress views are extremely difficult to interpret and are probably of no value unless the results of the films will alter the management of the ankle sprain. Indeed, regardless of the severity of sprains, it is possible to treat them in similar fashion, thus almost always negating the need for such films. Ice, compression, elevation, and rest with the use of crutches work well to reduce swelling in the beginning. Most physicians do not wrap the ankle properly to reduce swelling. An elastic wrap alone is not sufficient, because it puts maximal pressure over the malleoli and leaves the surrounding soft tissues free to swell. To apply pressure over the ligaments, where most swelling occurs, a disposable diaper should be cut in a U shape to fit around the malleolus (with the bottom of the U facing downward); an elastic bandage should then be applied. If disposable diapers are not available, several pieces of gauze can be used.

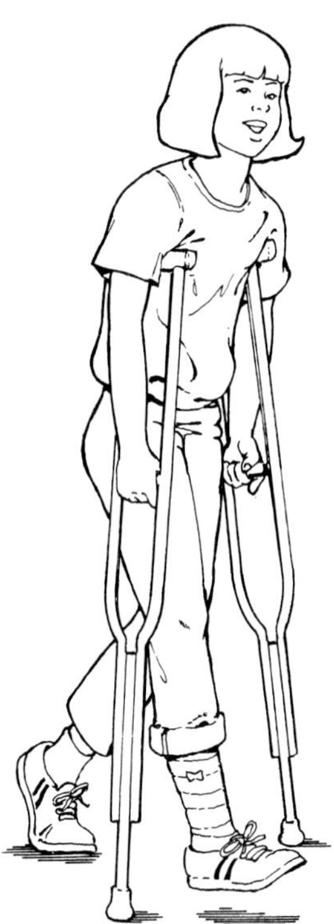

Fig. 259-2 Three-point gait crutch.

Once the swelling and severe pain have decreased, rehabilitative exercises should begin. Before the initial exercises, ice should be applied as described above. When the ankle feels numb after the application of ice, the patient should perform passive dorsiflexion and plantar flexion exercises. The foot should be flexed as far as possible, then held in this position for 10 seconds. After this, the foot maximally should be extended for 10 seconds. This maneuver should be performed 10 times. This exercise is for plantar flexion and dorsiflexion only, not inversion or eversion. After the exercise, the patient should wear an ankle support or brace. The Air Stirrup brace* works well for this purpose.[13] It allows the patient mobility in an anteroposterior plane but restricts inversion and eversion. It also provides compression to reduce swelling. The patient should begin walking with crutches. He or she should be instructed to use a three-point crutch gait (Fig. 259-2). With this method the patient ambulates with both crutch tips and the injured foot touching the ground simultaneously.[14] The idea is that the patient puts some weight on the injured foot and does not carry it off the ground. Once the pain on walking is minimal, the patient should walk with only one crutch, on the uninjured side. Once the patient can walk without a limp, he or she may discard the crutch. At this point more rehabilitative exercises should be added. The patient should stop the exercises if he or she experiences pain. The following are useful exercises[14]:

1. Toe raises: The patient should spread his or her feet about 1 foot apart, toeing in. The patient then rises on the toes as high as possible without pain. This may be repeated with the toes pointing straight ahead, then pointing out.
2. Resistance press: The patient should move the foot in all four planes of motion against resistance, holding each position for 10 seconds. For upward resistance, the patient may put the foot under a piece of furniture and press up; for the other directions, he or she may press against a wall. Alternatively, the patient may use surgical tubing (Fig. 259-3).
3. Running exercises: The patient should not be allowed to run until he or she can balance on the toes of the injured foot for at least 20 seconds and hop on the toes at least 10 times without dropping the heel to the ground. Useful running exercises include zig-zags and figure eights. He or she can start with figure eights 10 yards long, gradually reducing the length of the "eight." Once the patient can do quick right angle cuts in both directions, he or she can return to active sports.

The ankle brace may be worn for weeks to months when exercising or participating in athletics to prevent reinjury.

Knee Injuries

Knee injuries are the most common pediatric sports injuries and may cause serious lifelong disability. The medial and lateral collateral ligaments stabilize the knee on each side; the anterior and posterior cruciate ligaments provide stability in the anterior and posterior planes.

*Air Stirrup ankle brace, Aircast Inc., 92 River Road, Summit, New Jersey 07901. 1-800-526-8785.

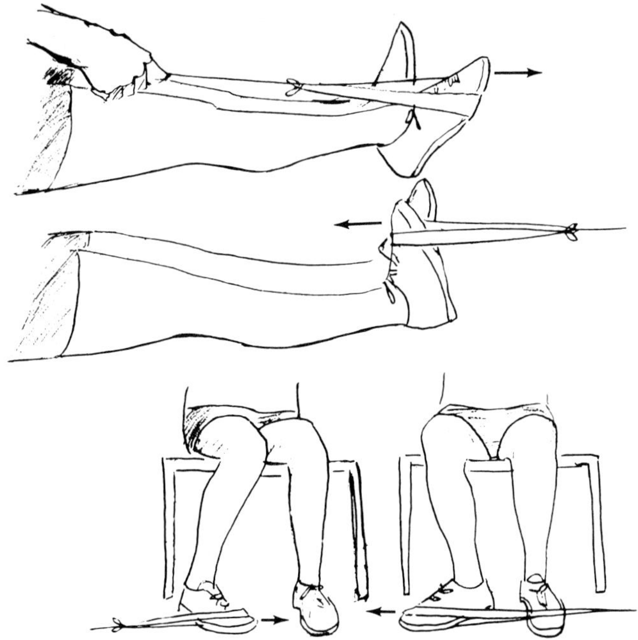

Fig. 259-3 Surgical tubing exercises.
Modified from Garrick JG: The athlete's ankle and other injuries, Emerg Med 14:178, 1982.

A precise diagnosis is often difficult in knee injuries, but a detailed history may help. A pop or snap that occurs during deceleration or cutting often signals an anterior cruciate tear. A rip or tearing sound from a partially bent position often means a patellar dislocation. The tearing sound results from tearing of the patella's supporting structures as it dislocates. A history of locking may be a sign of a loose bony fragment or torn cartilage in the knee. True locking refers to an inability to extend the knee because something "gets in the way" inside the knee. The sensation appears abruptly and may disappear just as quickly. Patients with patellofemoral dysfunction may also complain of locking, but they are actually referring to stiffness in the knee after being in one position for a long time. This feeling may go away after a few seconds or minutes and is probably related to muscle spasm.[5] A sensation of looseness in the knee may denote a torn medial collateral ligament. In this situation, a feeling of instability may be more prominent than pain.

Inquiring about the site of initial pain is helpful, for the pain occurs at the site of the injury. Later the discomfort may be more diffuse and less helpful in establishing the diagnosis. Medial collateral ligament injuries cause pain on the medial aspect of the knee. Meniscus tears are tender along the joint line at the tibial plateau. Anterior cruciate tears cause pain on either side of the patellar tendon at the front of the tibial plateau. Dislocation of the patella causes pain along its medial aspect, because it dislocates laterally and in doing so tears the soft tissue medially.

An immediate hemarthrosis may indicate an intraarticular fracture or dislocation of the patella. A moderate hemarthrosis occurring over the first 24 hours is a sign of an anterior cruciate ligament tear. A small effusion with swelling over the medial aspect of the knee points to an injury of the medial collateral ligament.[5]

The stability of the anterior cruciate ligament should be determined by using the drawer test (Lachman test). The knee should be flexed 30 degrees, and the leg rotated externally to relax the hamstrings and adductor muscles. The proximal tibia should be pulled anteriorly and the physician should look for (1) excessive motion compared with the opposite extremity, and (2) lack of a firm end point to the anterior displacement of the tibia. In all tests of ligament stability, the lack of a firm endpoint is a sign of a significant tear. To test the posterior cruciate ligament, the knee should be flexed 90 degrees, and the physician should look for sagging of the tibia posteriorly or for excessive laxity.

To test the collateral ligaments, the knee should be flexed 30 degrees while a valgus stress is applied to it to test the medial ligaments; then a varus stress is applied to test the lateral ligaments. It is helpful for the examiner to place his or her thumb in the joint space while resting the four remaining fingers on the patient's leg above the knee as this test is performed. If the opening of the medial joint is large (more than 1 cm), then the cruciate ligaments may have also been torn.[4] The most common serious knee injury is a sprain of the medial collateral ligament; the most common *severe* injury is a torn anterior cruciate ligament.

Patients with a dislocation of the patella may show a positive "apprehension test." With the knee flexed 20 to 25 degrees, the patella should be pushed laterally. The patient will be anxious and resist the movement by tensing the quadriceps. This test may be difficult to perform in any patient with an injured, painful knee. Radiographs may be indicated to rule out osteochondritis dissecans or fractures but they are usually normal, since most knee injuries involve soft tissues. When obtaining radiographs, it is helpful to request a tangential view of the patella in addition to the usual anteroposterior and lateral views. The tangential view may reveal fractures of the femoral condyles or the patella.

Patients with grade 1 collateral ligament strains may be treated by the primary care physician as described above under general principles of treatment. Patients with grade 2 or 3 collateral ligament sprains or suspected meniscal or cruciate cartilage injuries are best referred to an orthopedic surgeon.

Overuse Injuries of the Knee

A common condition in the pediatrician's office is the adolescent athlete with recurrent or chronic knee pain. Treating these patients may be more frustrating for the pediatrician than treating the acute injuries, because the source of the pain is less obvious. The roentgenograms are usually normal, and there is nothing to suggest a medical cause for the condition. There may be no obvious history of trauma.

Most of these athletes have overuse syndromes of the knee.[8] A careful history usually reveals some change in the patient's activities—the beginning of a new sport, or a new activity within that sport. Running or playing sports on a hard surface such as concrete may precipitate problems. Some patients may have conditions that interfere with the mechanical function of the leg such as ligamentous laxity and excessive valgus of the knee or foot pronation. Sometimes knee pain follows injuries that do not involve the knee, such as those involving an ankle or hip. The disuse following the injury leads to atrophy of the quadriceps muscles, which causes patellofemoral dysfunction. The most common finding in any of these conditions is loss of tone and muscle mass in the vastus medialis,[5] which is palpable proximal to the knee on the medial side. The vastus medialis ensures proper alignment of the patella in the femoral groove. To examine for this, the patient should sit with the legs extended and tighten the quadriceps, including the vastus medialis. The quadriceps' size and tone are compared with the quadriceps of the other leg.

The most common overuse syndromes of the knee are chondromalacia of the patella, Osgood-Schlatter disease, and patellar tendinitis. At first the pain occurs only after athletic activity. As it worsens, the pain begins during or toward the end of the activity.

Patients with chondromalacia of the patella tend to have vague symptoms. They may complain of diffuse knee pain around and behind the patella but may be unable to point to a specific area. There is usually no swelling. Sometimes the pain is aggravated by walking up and, especially, down stairs or hills. Sometimes sitting with the knees bent for long periods causes pain, as in a car on long trips, in a theater, or in class. Sometimes patients will complain of constant anterior knee pain, which is worse after activity.

Osgood-Schlatter disease is most common in the early years of puberty. The powerful quadriceps muscle causes avulsion or microscopic disorganization of the tibial tubercle in an area of developing bone. The patient complains of knee pain, which is aggravated by extending the knee against resistance or applying pressure over the tibial tubercle. Occasionally the region of the anterior tibial tubercle swells. Radiologic abnormalities do not correlate well with symptoms. Radiographs may be indicated, however, to rule out more serious conditions, such as osteomyelitis, arteriovenous malformation, or osteosarcoma, all of which have been reported to cause symptoms similar to Osgood-Schlatter disease.[1] Hip problems such as Legg-Calvé-Perthes disease or slipped capital femoral epiphysis may also cause chronic knee pain.

Patellar tendinitis causes extremely well-localized pain at the lower pole of the patella. It is caused by a partial rupture and inflammation of the tendon where it attaches to the patella. It typically affects athletes in jumping sports such as basketball and volleyball.

Treatment of these conditions involves using ice after athletic activities, nonsteroidal antiinflammatory medications, and exercises to strengthen the quadriceps muscle. When the pain is severe, rest from the activities that cause pain (and *only* those activities) is helpful. For patients with severe pain from patellar tendinitis or Osgood-Schlatter disease, using a Velcro knee immobilizer will rest the knee. A knee immobilizer, however, has the disadvantage of further weakening the quadriceps from disuse and is recommended for only the most severe cases. An Osgood-Schlatter pad that has a hole in the middle and fits around the tender tibial tuberosity will prevent repeated painful trauma during sports activities. Sometimes a Neoprene sleeve with a pad placed laterally over the patella is helpful in managing chondromalacia of the patella, because it helps keep the patella properly aligned. These devices may be obtained from orthopedic supply companies.*

*Orthopedic Technology Inc., 14670 Wicks Boulevard, San Leandro, CA 94577.

*PRO Orthopedic Devices Inc., P.O. Box 1, King of Prussia, PA 19406.

Patients with excessive pronation of the foot may benefit from cushioned, full-length arch supports, which are available in many sports-oriented shoe stores.

Garrick[5] recommends an isometric quadriceps-strengthening program emphasizing the vastus medialis for patients with these conditions. These exercises may be performed throughout the day, as often as the patient can think about it for a total of 20 to 24 times a day—while waiting for the bus, while in class, or just before meals. To perform these exercises, the athlete should extend the knee and tighten the quadriceps for 5 or 6 seconds, relax it for 2 to 3 seconds, and then repeat the process three times. The patient should palpate the vastus medialis to make sure it tightens during the exercise. It is useful to demonstrate this technique in the office. Alternatively, these patients can be referred to a physical therapist to initiate and monitor a rehabilitative program. Sometimes it is necessary to use an electrical muscle stimulator to strengthen the vastus medialis. Most patients will improve within 2 to 3 months if they comply with the management plan. Patients who fail to improve require referral to an orthopedic surgeon.

Other Injuries

Shin Splint. The term *shin splint* refers to pain along the medial aspect of the distal two thirds of the tibia. This condition usually develops in poorly conditioned runners and is associated with running on hard surfaces, with the use of improper shoes, or with abnormal foot alignment. Its presence may create abnormal forces on the tibialis posterior tendon and the interosseous membrane between the tibia and fibula as the patient tries to shift weight to diminish the pain while running. At first, patients have pain only while running, but eventually pain is present after running as well. Ice, rest, and antiinflammatory medications are effective during the acute stage; better shoes and conditioning should prevent recurrences. Sometimes the use of orthotic devices helps to reduce discomfort. A stress fracture should be considered in the differential diagnosis.

Little League Elbow. Little League elbow is an overuse injury of the elbow that may result in separation, fragmentation, or irregularity of the medial epicondyle apophysis.[1] The condition may be less frequent than before, as a result of Little League rules that limit players to pitching no more than six innings per week. Pain develops first; later there is tenderness over the medial aspect of the elbow. If the pain is severe, the patient may develop contractures and limited range of motion. The mainstay of treatment is prevention but in patients with symptoms, resting the elbow is mandatory.[12] Many patients require flexibility exercises and progressive arm strengthening, arranged in cooperation with an orthopedist and physical therapist.

Stress Fractures. Stress fractures occur most commonly in the fibula and the second metatarsal. The onset of pain may be sudden or gradual, and there is no history of direct trauma. Tenderness is present over the fracture site. Radiographs may not show any abnormality until 6 to 8 weeks after the injury. A bone scan will reveal the fracture much sooner. Treatment consists of significantly reducing activity until the patient is pain free for a period of 7 to 10 days. Then, after reexamination, activities may be resumed gradually. Patients with severe pain may require the application of a cast.

Finger Dislocation. Finger dislocations are frequently reduced immediately after the injury by a trainer or a friend. Because of this, the patient may underestimate the degree of ligamentous damage. Obtaining radiographs is important to rule out avulsion fractures.

Contusions and Hematomas. A contusion to the iliac crest (commony called a "hip pointer") causes disability out of proportion to the severity of the injury because several muscles are attached to the iliac crest at the injury site and cause pain as they contract during any movement of the hip. In addition to ice, compression, and rest, some patients require crutches. If pain is severe, the injection of an anesthetic agent or a steroid compound locally may be required.

A subungual hematoma results from a sudden blow to the fingernail or toenail. To provide instant relief for the exquisite pain that sometimes results from the accumulation of blood beneath the nail, a hole can be burned through the nail with a red hot paper clip. This allows the blood to escape immediately.

REFERENCES

1. Adams JE: Injury to the throwing arm: a study of traumatic changes in the elbow joints of boy baseball players, Calif Med 102:127, 1964.
2. Buckley WE et al: Estimated prevalence of anabolic steroid use among male high school seniors, JAMA 260:3441, 1988.
3. Dehaven KE: Athletic injuries in adolescents, Pediatr Ann 7(10):96, 1978.
4. Dyment PG: Athletic injuries, Pediatr Rev 10:291, 1989.
5. Garrick JG: Knee problems in adolescents, Pediatr Rev 4:235, 1983.
6. Garrick JG and Requa RK: Girls' sports injuries in high school athletics, JAMA 239:2245, 1978.
7. Garrick JG and Requa RK: Injuries in high school sports, Pediatrics 61:465, 1978.
8. Garrick JG and Webb DW: Decisions in sports medicine, Philadelphia, WB Saunders Co (in press).
9. Goldberg B et al: Children's sports injuries: are they avoidable? Physician Sportsmed 7:93, 1979.
10. Hocutt JE et al: Cryotherapy in ankle sprains, Am J Sports Med 10:316, 1982.
11. Moore WV: Anabolic steroid use in adolescence, JAMA 260:3484, 1988.
12. Stanitski CL: Common injuries in preadolescent and adolescent athletes: recommendations for prevention, Sports Med 7:32, 1989.
13. Stover CN: Air Stirrup management of ankle injuries in the athlete, Am J Sports Med 2(31):63, 1983.
14. Stover CN: Functional sprain management of the ankle, Ambulatory Care 6(11):25, 1986.
15. Strong WB and Linder CW: Preparticipation health evaluation for competitive sports, Pediatr Rev 4:113, 1982.

260

Sudden Infant Death Syndrome

Susan F. Woolsey

Defined as "the sudden death of any infant or young child, which is unexpected by history, and in which a thorough postmortem examination fails to demonstrate an adequate cause of death,"[2] sudden infant death syndrome (SIDS) is the leading cause of death in postneonates during the first year of life.

EPIDEMIOLOGY

Infants between 1 month and 1 year of age make up 98% of SIDS cases; 90% of the victims are under 24 weeks of age. The overall incidence is considered to be 2 to 3 per 1000 live births, although the rate for blacks and native Americans is only 4.5 to 8 per 1000. Most infants die during the night, while they are apparently asleep. More cases occur during the winter and early spring. When compared with living, healthy babies, SIDS infants are more likely to have had a recent bout of diarrhea or vomiting or an upper respiratory infection. They are more likely to have had noticeable tachycardia and as a group are less likely to have been breast-fed. Also at increased risk are infants from high-risk pregnancies; that is, those whose mothers smoked, used drugs, or were teenagers, or who had inadequate prenatal care, a short interval between pregnancies, a previous fetal loss, or an illness during pregnancy. Other infants considered at high risk for morbidity and mortality are those who were born prematurely or were small for gestational age. Infants of multiple-birth pregnancies, whether monozygous or dizygous, are at special risk, and males are at greater risk than females. Subsequent siblings of SIDS infants are also at increased risk, although to what extent is uncertain.

It is important to remember that SIDS can and does occur in families that meet none of the high-risk criteria and that many of the known risk factors for SIDS are also associated with recognized causes of most neonatal and infant deaths.

A comprehensive book, with papers by 50 leading experts, that includes risk factors identified by the National Institute of Child Health and Human Development's case control study is available for more in-depth reading.[5]

Prevention

Although SIDS is generally considered unpreventable, the findings of some researchers indicate that under certain circumstances, the incidence of SIDS can be lowered. Based on their study of 85,000 babies, Carpenter and colleagues[3] concluded that with a few extra resources for identified high-risk mothers and babies, unexpected infant mortality can be reduced by 25%. Their interventions include regular home visits and weighing of the baby, simple interventions already considered good community health care for high-risk families. In this country, Myerberg and his group,[7] using the Carpenter model, also demonstrated a significant positive outcome—a 15% decrease in postneonatal deaths after providing intensified primary health care for high-risk infants.

THEORIES OF CAUSE

Most authorities now agree that SIDS is probably the common outcome of several etiologic pathways, but there are some broad categories within which we can consider the various etiologic theories. None of these theories has been consistently confirmed by research. Theories involving *airway obstruction* are the oldest. In the Bible, reference is made to "overlaying" as a cause of infant death. Today those deaths would probably be attributed to SIDS. Some theorists have held that the mechanism of death is a laryngeal reflex or spasm, abnormal displacement of jaw and tongue, an esophageal air bubble that obstructs the airway, or the position in which the baby was sleeping. None of these opinions has been supported by research.

From histories given by some families, it may appear that SIDS is *genetically transmitted*. However, published studies have failed to demonstrate, conclusively, abnormal ventilatory control or cardiac function in parents and siblings of SIDS victims. *Metabolism* has long been under scrutiny as a possible etiologic factor in SIDS. Studies in this area have examined deficiencies of vitamins such as biotin, thiamine, and vitamins E, C, and D and the neurophysiologic roles of these substances. Various hormones have also been studied, including cortisol, insulin, growth hormones, thyroid-stimulating hormones, triiodothyronine, and thyroxine. Glucose levels, glycemic factors, biogenic amines, endorphins, and various minerals, such as chloride, potassium, sodium, copper, calcium, magnesium, selenium, and zinc, have been considered as well. None of these studies provides conclusive evidence of a relationship of any of these factors to SIDS.

Mild *infections* precede death in 40% to 75% of SIDS cases. These include diarrhea, vomiting, and upper respiratory tract infections. A full range of respiratory viruses has been isolated from secretions, but not at levels judged sufficient to have caused death. A small number of SIDS victims has been reported to have actually died from *Clostridium botulinum* infection. The source of spores was thought to be honey, which subsequently led to the recommendation by the American Academy of Pediatrics that infants younger than 1 year of age not be given honey. SIDS has also been associated with intrauterine septicemia, which could explain the signs of chronic hypoxia (e.g., hyperplasia of blood vessels in heart and lung, abnormal retention of immature fat, underdeveloped carotid body, and altered brainstem structure) that are found, depending on the study, in 20% to 60% of SIDS cases. Studies of levels of immunoglobulins, splenic germinal centers, the thymus, and the secretory components in bronchial tissue are inconclusive. Thus, although it appears that in some cases a mild infection triggers acute ventilatory or circulatory failure, the actual mechanism is unknown. Somewhat related is concern on the part of some that the death may have been triggered by diphtheria-tetanus-pertussis (DTP) immunization. This has been refuted in a well-controlled study.[4]

In recent years much research has been based on the hypothesis that SIDS infants are *chronically hypoxic,* possibly as a result of prolonged apneic episodes, before their deaths. This hypothesis has led to the establishment of numerous sleep-study and apnea monitoring programs. Schwartz, Southall, and Valdes-Dapena[9] have compiled numerous papers describing work in this area. Use of home apnea monitors can be lifesaving for infants in whom episodes of apnea have been identified; however, most SIDS victims do not appear to have experienced apneic episodes, and home monitoring programs have not lowered the SIDS death rate. Basic research is looking at immature brainstem development as a contributor or precursor to SIDS death.[6]

It is important for the pediatrician to remember that these research findings and risk factors are characteristic of SIDS infants as a *group* and thus do not permit prediction of risk for SIDS in an *individual* infant. An increasing number of experts have concluded that SIDS occurs in response to multiple etiologic factors that are not the same in all SIDS victims. A special issue on SIDS was published in *Pediatrician* in 1988 that includes 342 references.[6,10]

FAMILY REACTIONS TO SIDS

In cases of SIDS, intervention is necessarily focused on surviving family members. Familiarity with typical grief reactions is vital in providing support to the family in the aftermath of SIDS. Family members are often fearful of the intensity of their reactions and need to be reassured that their feelings are normal and that they are not "going crazy." Reactions vary considerably from individual to individual, and it is important to give "permission" for each person to react in his or her own way. Grief is a necessary human reaction to loss and allows the person to ventilate feelings. This ventilation and subsequent reorganization allow the person to adapt to the loss in a healthy manner. Studies have indicated that maximal family reorganization may not occur for as long as 2 or 3 years, with mothers usually requiring the most time to complete the grief process. Family members are often discouraged from full expression of their feelings by those around them who are either uncomfortable with this expression or underestimate the period of time required for grieving. The physician who can establish rapport with family members that permits crying and open discussion of personal feelings may well be providing the family one of the few available outlets for a positive expression of grief. Open sharing and discussion among family members and their close friends and relatives should also be encouraged to promote mutual understanding of needs and the healthy recovery of all who are affected by the loss.

Immediately after the death, most parents experience a period of shock, disbelief, numbness, or denial. This may be mistaken for an "uncaring" attitude, because emotions may be constricted during this period. Shock eventually gives way to a variety of grief reactions, which may include sadness, crying, a tearless and dazed appearance, mood swings, despondency, listlessness or inability to concentrate or make decisions, and inability to function in "normal" routines.

There may be problems in family interactions, such as difficulty in communicating about the death, confusion, and resentment about different modes of expressing grief, sexual dysfunction, separation (temporary or permanent), disagreement between parents on how to relate to other children in the family (particularly about the death), and disagreement between parents about whether to have another child.

Somatic complaints commonly experienced, particularly by mothers, include arms aching to hold a baby; feelings of emptiness, weakness, and exhaustion; loss of appetite and weight (or *increased* appetite and weight gain); sleep disturbance; exacerbation of preexisting medical conditions; "heartache"; stomach pains; headaches; nausea; sensations of whirling and dizziness; and feelings of body pressure or constriction.

Hostility and anger are common reactions to the loss of a child. Anger may be directed toward the last person attending the baby (family member, baby-sitter, grandparents, or neighbor). Family members may be angry with themselves, God, or "the world," or they may be confused about where to direct their hostility. Anger may be directed toward the physician, the rescue squad, or the individual who last checked the baby medically. Family members may be angry or feel let down by a physician whose personal frustration or feelings of helplessness in response to the case take the form of bluntness or callousness with the family.

Even with an intellectual understanding that SIDS cannot be prevented, guilt is the most pervasive reaction. Family members repeatedly ask themselves, "What could I have done to prevent this?" and "What did I do to cause this?" They may feel guilty about their resentment toward well-meaning but misinformed relatives and friends who try to help. Parents who did not initially want the baby may need to work through this additional source of guilt. Many times, younger siblings who have wished the baby dead or wished it would "go away" believe that their wishes magically came true and that they are responsible for the death. They may therefore experience guilt as well.

The family usually experiences high levels of anxiety and fear. Parents may fear for the health and safety of their other children and become overprotective. Or they may question their ability to care for their other children and even abdicate some parental functions. Fear of being alone is common. Family members may find it especially disturbing to be alone in the same house or apartment in which their baby died. Another common fear in reaction to the loss is, "Now that this has happened, what other catastrophe may occur?" This sense of heightened vulnerability can greatly increase anxiety.

Other children in the family may be afraid because of the explanation given them. If they were told that the baby "went to sleep forever," they may be afraid to go to bed. Or if they were told that God wanted the baby because she was so good and beautiful, they may be fearful when told that they are good or beautiful.

Other normal reactions include a preoccupation with the image of the deceased and a desire to search for the baby. Things touched, seen, smelled, or felt elicit memories of the baby and may cause intense pain. Parents may have strong sensations that the baby is still present or have "visions" of the baby as he or she appeared either before or after death. The baby's cry is often "heard." Parents also may automatically continue previous routines (e.g., preparing formula), only to realize once again that the baby is dead. These experiences can be extremely anxiety provoking to parents who have not been reassured that such sensations are to be expected.

Parents often express an intense desire to move. There may be circumstances in which relocation is beneficial, such as when the environment severely lacks family support to the point of hindering recovery. In general, however, an early relocation should be discouraged because it may be used to avoid coming to terms with the loss. For siblings, relocation itself can be experienced as another severe loss. This should be seriously considered by parents contemplating moving.

Family members often have recurring reactions on monthly or yearly anniversaries of the baby's death or birth and on holidays and other significant days for the family. A subsequent pregnancy usually triggers a period of increased anxiety, which decreases as the new baby's age surpasses that of the SIDS victim.

Differentiating normal grief reactions from pathologic processes can be difficult, particularly in the acute phase. This is due to two factors: (1) grief is an intensely stressful experience that elicits a wide variety of reactions, and (2) many of these reactions, when seen in a person who has *not* experienced a severe and sudden loss, suggest a psychopathologic disorder. The physician must be alert to signals of personality disturbance, particularly in families with previous psychiatric histories, but it is best to avoid transmitting a "pathologic" model of grief to the SIDS family. As a rule of thumb, the duration of severe reactions should be noted, as well as the level of disruption or deviance from customary behavior before the loss. For example, any of the following would indicate the need for mental health referral: inability to return to daily routine several months after the death; total lack of affect; auditory and visual hallucinations or suicidal ideation persisting past the acute stage; parental neglect or extreme overprotection of other children; significant alcohol or drug abuse; violent behavior; and prolonged social withdrawal.

CASE MANAGEMENT FOR THE GRIEVING FAMILY

SIDS presents a number of unique management problems for the pediatrician. First, the death is totally unexpected by the family and all who relate to them. Thus those who would normally be available to provide support under other circumstances will have their own reactions to the loss and may be unable to reach out to the family. In addition, not all physicians are comfortable with death. Second, as a result of increasing national emphasis on detection of child abuse, police, fire, and rescue personnel, emergency room staff, and others may directly or indirectly accuse the parents of neglect or abuse. Third, even though considerable research has been conducted to identify a cause, SIDS continues to be a death that is, in the usual sense, unexplained. Finally, there are no consistent, established criteria for determining the at-risk population, and even when an infant is identified as being at risk, there is no accepted management protocol. If the physician cannot provide the support needed by the family, knowledge of referral resources is vital. Counseling bereaved families is time consuming and frequently involves "after hours" appointments. The physician's own feelings of guilt and helplessness may be elicited in the process. Decisions about fees for this service, therefore, may be difficult. However, the pediatrician has a unique opportunity to give anticipatory guidance, assess the family's progress toward resolution of the loss, and promote open communication. In contrast to clinical situations where progress is very slow or nonexistent, appropriate family counseling will usually result in immediate positive responses from family members, which can be highly rewarding for the physician. The following suggested protocol for case management is based on key transition points in the grief process, when family needs may change.

Initial Contact

During the immediate crisis the pediatrician should do the following.

1. Ensure that parents have had the opportunity to see and hold the infant after pronouncement of death. Although the physician may be tempted to prescribe sedatives or tranquilizers, this is generally not recommended, because it can impede the grief process.
2. Give the family basic information about SIDS and provide answers for any immediate questions. They should be given the names and phone numbers of persons who can help them resolve their concerns (e.g., a talk with the medical examiner may greatly help to allay concerns about the cause of death). Many states have SIDS information and counseling projects, with well-established protocols and literature available on request from the National SIDS Clearinghouse (see Resources, p. 1532).
3. Facilitate contact with other SIDS parents, who may be of great help. The list of resources at the end of this chapter includes groups that can be helpful.
4. Determine the plan for care of surviving siblings. Excellent literature is now available to assist the family in making decisions and explaining death to children.
5. Determine if there are other significant persons who will need support during this time, such as grandparents or a baby-sitter.
6. Identify the support system available to the family. It is crucial for someone to facilitate establishment of such supports (if not readily available) because isolation often compounds family difficulties.
7. Assist the family in making decisions about the funeral.

8. Make an office appointment for 7 to 10 days after the death, at which time the initial shock will have passed and family members can benefit from added discussions of SIDS.

Second Contact (7 to 10 Days After Death)

Because grief reactions interfere with cognitive processes, repetition of information may be required. It may also help to include significant support persons (such as grandparents, siblings of parents, and close friends) in this meeting. Having all key persons present to hear the same information can prevent later confusion and misinformation. Tasks for the second contact can be summarized as follows:

1. Restate basic information about SIDS. A discussion of the autopsy report can be helpful. Reassure the family that they did not contribute to the death. The family will probably share concerns about having another baby, request information about future SIDS risk, and ask about monitoring. It is *not* recommended that families be encouraged to "have another baby right away," because a short interval between pregnancies is a SIDS risk factor. It is also important for the parents to make some progress in resolving their loss before embarking on the anxiety-laden experience of a subsequent pregnancy. With a short interval between pregnancies, there is greater risk for seeking a child to replace the one lost to SIDS.
2. Describe the grief process. Coming to grips with the reality that their infant is dead will enable the family to proceed with their grieving. It is helpful to refer to the baby by name and to use the words *death* and *died* (e.g., "since Johnny died . . .") rather than euphemisms. Open discussion about grief reactions is useful. Usually it is necessary to express thoughts and feeling about losses verbally. However, some parents prefer to work through their grief in a solitary manner by increasing physical exercise or by writing poetry, stories, or books, painting, or otherwise engaging in creative activity. An overview of the variety of normal reactions provides parameters within which parents can view their experiences as normal. Such anticipatory guidance will increase their confidence that they are not "losing their minds," which is a common fear of bereaved parents. The physician should also feel free to express personal feelings about the loss. The family will judge professionals on their human caring rather than on their medical expertise at this time. Many families appreciate their physician's expression of emotion about their loss.
3. Counsel parents about the needs of siblings and other significant persons.
4. Encourage the family to delay making irrevocable decisions until they have resolved their loss, at least to some extent. This usually takes 6 months or longer.

Third Contact (6 Weeks to 2 Months)

By this time, parents will usually make statements indicating that they have passed the shock and denial stage, such as, "I finally realize that the baby is really dead and that I must come to grips with that." This is a time when support is greatly needed by the family and when they are least likely to receive it from friends and relatives, who expect parents to be "back to normal." If they have not been in contact with other SIDS parents, it is a good time to suggest this again. The parents will probably need to review the SIDS diagnosis and the grief process once again and to engage in open discussion of feelings and concerns. Mothers in particular may be ready to do some reading, and several commendable booklets are available. Questions about activities of daily living will help the pediatrician determine the intensity of grief still being experienced. If daily habit patterns are still disrupted, more intensive counseling or referral to a mental health professional may be indicated.

Although this protocol appears to emphasize what the pediatrician *says,* the most important factor is the *listening*. Often long periods of silence or crying occur. Spending time in this way can be quite difficult, particularly on a busy day. Scheduling the visit outside of usual office hours is helpful. This also permits participation by family members whose schedules may preclude day visits.

Fourth Contact (4 to 6 Months)

Usually by 6 months, fathers feel that they are back to their former state of well-being. However, grieving by mothers often persists for 18 months to 2 years. It is essential, therefore, that these differences be discussed. In general, family members should be considering future-oriented issues by the end of 6 months. The mother may go back to school, get a new job, or begin volunteer work, or the couple may begin to consider another pregnancy, in which case more counseling and information about apnea monitoring may be needed.

Fifth Contact (Anniversary of the Birth or Death)

Anniversaries often elicit intense feelings and memories about the baby's life and death. Some recognition from the pediatrician that this is a significant time will provide parents with much needed support. When a child dies, all of his or her future is lost as well. Each year parents are reminded that their baby would have been a year older and wonder what he or she would have been like at this age. It is helpful when someone else also remembers and provides the means for open reminiscence.

RISK IDENTIFICATION, INFANTILE APNEA, AND HOME MONITORING

The practitioner is faced with a serious dilemma when managing infants with apnea or those who may otherwise be considered at risk for SIDS. Experts in the field have reached no consensus as to appropriate evaluation and management and have conflicting opinions, largely because of the inadequate data available as to the efficacy of one protocol over another. An American Academy of Pediatrics Task Force on Prolonged Infantile Apnea has emphasized the following points[1]:

1. Physicians must be responsible for all evaluation and management of infants with prolonged apnea.

2. A thorough initial evaluation to determine possible treatable causes of apnea is mandatory.
3. Asymptomatic infants, including those with previous apnea or those with statistically increased risk of SIDS, may be candidates for home monitoring, but there are no tests that will reliably determine risk status. Physicians should prescribe monitoring if they feel that that method of management is in the best interest of their patient.
4. Monitoring technology is still being developed and refined. Most authorities feel that both cardiac and respiratory functions should be monitored electronically. Some feel monitoring cardiac function alone is equally effective. Ability to produce a permanent record, when needed, is desirable.
5. When home monitoring is elected, parents should be advised that monitors cannot guarantee against SIDS. A plan for periodic reevaluations and termination of monitoring should be developed and explained to parents.
6. Because the etiology and optimal management of prolonged apnea are not clear and because a causal relationship between prolonged apnea and SIDS has not been established, continued research is essential.

The problem was also addressed by the National Institutes of Health (NIH), at a special conference[8] and at an international meeting.[9]

SUMMARY

The pediatrician is challenged on several fronts when providing care for families who are experiencing SIDS or SIDS-related situations. Sensitive help and support supplied during the crisis will be remembered and treasured by the family. It is estimated that at least 100 people are affected by each SIDS loss. Although these cases are difficult and uncomfortable for health care providers, the rewards easily outweigh the effort to ensure that the family receives the best possible care.

RESOURCES

For Assisting Grieving Families

Mutual help groups for parents

Compassionate Friends, P.O. Box 1347, Oak Brook, IL, 60521; 302-323-5010.

National SIDS Foundation (NSIDSF), 10500 Little Patuxent Parkway, Suite 420, Columbia, MD 21044; 301-964-8000, 800-221-SIDS.

SHARE (Source of Help in Airing and Resolving Experiences) St. Elizabeth's Hospital, 211 South Third Street, Belleville, IL 62222; 618-234-2120.

Printed materials for families

Available from NSIDSF (address above):

FACTS about sudden infant death syndrome

The subsequent child

Available from the National SIDS Clearinghouse (address below):

Fact Sheet: Parents and the Grieving Process

Fact Sheet: The Grief of Children

Fact Sheet: Apnea and Other Apparent Life-Threatening Events

Available from SHARE (address above):

Bittersweet . . . Hello, Goodbye: A resource in planning farewell rituals when a baby dies

Thumpy's Story (for surviving siblings)

Available from the Pregnancy and Infant Loss Center, 1415 East Wayzata Boulevard, Wayzata, MN 55391; 612-473-9372.

Grieving Grandparents . . . After Miscarriage, Stillbirth or Infant Loss.

Available from the Centering Corporation, Box 3367, Omaha, NE 68103-0367; 402-553-1200:

A Most Important Picture: A Manual for Taking Pictures of Infants Who Die.

Information for Professionals:

National SIDS Clearinghouse, 8201 Greensboro Drive, Suite 600, McLean, VA 22102; 703-821-8955.

REFERENCES

1. American Academy of Pediatrics Task Force on Prolonged Infantile Apnea: Prolonged apnea, Pediatrics 76:129, 1985.
2. Beckwith JB: The sudden infant death syndrome, Pub No (HSA) 80-5251, 1975, Washington, DC, US Department of Health, Education, and Welfare.
3. Carpenter RG et al: Prevention of unexpected infant death: a review of risk-related intervention in six centers, Ann NY Acad Sci 533:96, 1988.
4. Griffin MR et al: Risk of sudden infant death syndrome after immunization with DTP vaccine, N Engl J Med 319(10):618, 1988.
5. Harper R and Hoffman H: Sudden infant death syndrome, risk factors and basic mechanisms, New York, 1988, PMA Publishing Corp. Available from PMA, 1 Linden Place, Suite 307, Great Neck, NY 11021.
6. Kinney HC and Filiano JJ: Brainstem research in sudden infant death syndrome, Pediatrician 15:240, 1988.
7. Myerberg DZ et al: The West Virginia (WV) birth score: predicting and preventing postneonatal mortality, Pediatr Res 23:293, 1988.
8. NIH Consensus Development Conference on Infantile Apnea and Home Monitoring, 1987. Available from the National SIDS Clearinghouse.
9. Schwartz P, Southall D, and Valdes-Dapena M, editors: The sudden infant death syndrome: cardiac and respiratory mechanisms and interventions, Ann NY Acad Sci 533:1-474, 1988.
10. Valdes-Dapena M: Suddent infant death syndrome: overview of recent research developments from a pediatric pathologist's perspective, Pediatrician 15:222, 1988.

SUGGESTED READINGS

Bergman A: The "discovery" of sudden infant death syndrome: lessons in the practice of political medicine, Seattle, 1988, University of Washington Press.

261

Tonsillectomy and Adenoidectomy

Robert A. Hoekelman

The most frequently performed operation in children in the United States requiring general anesthesia is the removal of the tonsils, the adenoids, or both. In 1987 these procedures were performed on 172,000 children under 15 years of age (29,000 tonsillectomies, 13,000 adenoidectomies, and 130,000 tonsilloadenoidectomies [T&As]).[7] These statistics represent more than half of such procedures performed on persons of all ages during 1987. Most striking is the marked decline in tonsil and adenoid removal in recent years, as demonstrated in Table 261-1. It is clear from these data that in 1987, tonsillectomy was more prevalent among older persons, whereas adenoidectomy and T&A were more prevalent among children. The decline in the frequency of these operations is the result of the controversy regarding the indications for performing them that has raged within the medical community for more than 2 decades.[2] This is so for two reasons. First, the function of tonsils and adenoids, which constitute the major elements of Waldeyer ring within the nasopharynx, is not well understood; second, evaluative studies of the worth of T&A have suffered from a host of methodologic difficulties and have therefore been inconclusive until just recently. Consequently, each practitioner has had to rely on "clinical judgment and individual experience" in determining the rationale to be used in recommending that a given child have a T&A. Naturally, these approaches vary considerably and form the basis for much of the controversial discussion surrounding these surgical procedures.

INDICATIONS AND RISKS

The indications for T&A that have been advanced seriously by practitioners are listed in the accompanying box, beginning with the more generally accepted ones and moving down to those that are more suspect or even capricious. This listing is probably incomplete but does illustrate the range of indications that have been used from both physician and parental viewpoints to rationalize removal of the tonsils and adenoids. There probably would be little argument given to any surgeon who performed a T&A for those absolute indications listed at the top of the box; however, all those listed below (in some relative order of validity) are controversial and subject to some or serious question.

Of particular note is the recent development of a method to measure the severity of obstructive sleep apnea (OSA)[4] quantitatively and to relate that score to abnormalities in right ventricular function, even before clinical signs of cor pulmonale are present.[10] OSA scores higher than 3.5 are highly predictive of the need for T&A (see the box on the right).

Indications Advanced for Tonsillectomy, Adenoidectomy, or Both

ABSOLUTE INDICATIONS

- Alveolar hypoventilation (obstructive sleep apnea) or cor pulmonale, secondary to airway obstruction
- Dysphagia
- Malignancy (radiotherapy alone preferred in most cases)
- Uncontrollable hemorrhage from tonsillar blood vessels

CONTROVERSIAL INDICATIONS

- Peritonsillar abscess
- Chronic cervical lymphadenitis
- Hyponasality, "hot potato" voice, or both
- Chronic or recurrent otitis media
- Chronic or recurrent tonsillitis
- Sensorineural or conductive hearing loss
- Chronic mastoiditis
- Cholesteatoma
- Chronic sinusitis or nasopharyngitis
- Diphtheria or streptococcal carrier state
- Chronic bronchitis or pneumonia
- Mouth-breathing, snoring, or both (without obstructive sleep apnea)
- Rheumatic fever, when compliance with anti-streptococcal prophylaxis cannot be assured
- Parental anxiety
- Frequent colds with loss of time from school
- Adenoidal facies
- Allergic respiratory diseases
- Chronic cough
- Failure to thrive
- Poor appetite
- Focus of infection
- Halitosis
- Scarred or cryptic tonsils
- Routine procedure

The ultimate measure of the worth of T&A must be made by weighing the gains it may bring to the patient against the risks involved. In general, the morbidity and mortality from T&A are poorly documented. The mortality has been estimated in the past to be as high as 1 in every 1000 operations[1] and as low as 1 in 27,000 operations.[2] However, under current

Obstructive Sleep Apnea Score

OSA Score = 1.42D + 1.41A + 0.71S − 3.83
D = Difficulty of breathing during sleep (0 = never, 1 = occasionally, 2 = frequently, and 3 = always)
A = Apnea observed during sleep (0 = No and 1 = yes)
S = Snoring (0 = never, 1 = occasionally, 2 = frequently, and 3 = always)
Scores of >3.5 are highly predictive of the need for T&A
Scores of <−1 rule out OSA
Scores of −1 to 3.4 require polysomography to determine whether OSA requiring T&A exists.

circumstances of modern anesthetic techniques and high technology and professional competence in monitoring and managing postoperative complications of hemorrhage, shock, and airway obstruction, mortality and severe morbidity following T&A surgery should be extremely rare.

The morbidity rate from T&A, however, is unknown, since no nationwide reporting mechanism is available. In the most recently reported series of T&A surgery performed under the best circumstances, 13 (14%) of 95 patients had surgically related complications. Of these, six required one or more extra days of hospitalization. None of the complications was considered serious, and all were easily managed or self-limited.[5] Otitis media has been reported to be a frequent sequela of adenoidectomy,[6] but the incidence of otitis media in children with similar indications for adenoidectomy who did not have surgery was not assessed over the same time interval. The incidence and severity of psychologic complications are unknown, but asocial and aggressive behavior, excessive dependency, night terrors, and enuresis have been attributed to emotional trauma surrounding hospitalization, separation, anesthesia, and discomfort associated with T&A.

On the other hand, the gains that can be attributed to tonsillectomy, adenoidectomy, or both, although attested to by many parents and physicians, were not demonstrated in adequate, prospective, randomized, controlled studies until the late 1970s and the early 1980s in a study conducted at the Children's Hospital of Pittsburgh.[8] In this study, 95 children severely affected with recurrent throat infections were subjected to tonsillectomy or tonsillectomy with adenoidectomy, whereas 92 children with similar histories and "matched" with the "tonsillectomized" children (through both randomized and nonrandomized techniques) were not subjected to surgery. During the subsequent 2 years, the surgical group had a significantly lower incidence of throat infection than did the nonsurgical group. On the other hand, many of the children in the nonsurgical group had fewer throat infections during the 2-year follow-up period than previously, and most of these episodes were mild. During the third year of follow-up, the surgical group had fewer throat infections, but these differences were not statistically significant in most cases.

The criteria for tonsillectomy in the Pittsburgh study[8] were recurrent throat infection (tonsillitis, pharyngitis, or tonsillopharyngitis) characterized by:

1. At least three episodes in each of 3 years, or five episodes in each of 2 years, or seven episodes in 1 year
2. Each episode having been characterized by one or more of the following:
   a. Oral temperature 38.3° C or higher
   b. Enlarged (>2 cm) or tender anterior cervical lymph nodes
   c. Tonsillar or pharyngeal exudate
   d. Positive culture for group A beta-hemolytic streptococci
3. Apparently adequate antibiotic therapy having been administered for proven or suspected streptococcal episodes
4. Each episode having been confirmed by examination and its qualifying features described in a clinical record at the time of occurrence

Those who received concurrent adenoidectomy met *one* of the following criteria:

1. Recurrent suppurative or serous otitis media, if myringotomy and insertion of tympanostomy tubes had been performed at least once previously
2. Persistent nasal obstruction
   a. Manifested by stertorous breathing or mouth-breathing, with or without episodes of obstructive sleep apnea, and by hyponasal speech
   b. Accompanied by both clinical and roentgenographic evidence of adenoid hypertrophy
   c. Apparently not caused by allergy
3. Chronic sinusitis or nasopharyngitis
   a. Accompanied by both clinical and roentgenographic evidence of adenoid hypertrophy
   b. Apparently not caused by allergy
   c. Persisting despite appropriate antimicrobial and other medical therapy

Although the Pittsburgh study provided evidence of the efficacy of tonsillectomy (with or without adenoidectomy) in reducing the number of throat infections using these criteria, the efficacy of T&A performed for less stringent criteria (those used for most T&A surgery in the United States) remains to be proven. A nationwide collaborative study on a larger sample representative of all socioeconomic and geographic childhood populations would also be desirable, but the difficulties in mounting and conducting such a study reliably would be formidable.

Until the results of such studies are available to us, it is likely that the controversy over indications for T&A will continue. There are data indicating that some overall restraint and discrimination in the removal of tonsils and adenoids have been exercised in recent years (see Table 261-1).

The Pittsburgh group has also investigated the efficacy of adenoidectomy for children at high risk for otitis media who had had tympanostomy tube placement and had experienced recurrent suppurative or secretory otitis media after the tubes had been removed.[9] Adenoidectomy proved to be beneficial overall during 2 years of follow-up, although many of the adenoidectomized children continued to have recurrent otitis media. The efficacy of adenoidectomy in reducing episodes

Table 261-1 *Frequency, in Thousands, of Tonsillectomy, Adenoidectomy, and T&A for Inpatients Discharged from Nonfederal, Short-Stay Hospitals: United States, 1971-1987*

YEAR	TONSILLECTOMY	ADENOIDECTOMY	T&A	TOTAL
1971	227	52	740	1019
1975	221	73	464	758
1979	198	83	303	584
1983	170	53	255	478
1987	101	15	143	259

Data from National Center for Health Statistics: National Hospital Discharge Survey (From Paradise JL: Tonsillectomy and adenoidectomy. In Bluestone CD et al, editors: Pediatric otolaryngology, ed 2, Philadelphia, 1990, WB Saunders Co.

of otitis media in children who have not had tympanostomy tube placement beforehand and of T&A in both groups is currently under study by the Pittsburgh investigators.

The probability of a child receiving T&A surgery may be determined more by parental and physician opinion regarding the worth of T&A than on the basis of the child's health status. Since at least 25% of all visits to pediatricians' offices are for upper respiratory tract infections, including tonsillitis and otitis media, it is not surprising that parental and physician attention is frequently focused on decisions concerning the removal of tonsils and adenoids.

The decision to recommend the removal of the tonsils or adenoids should be an individual matter, taking into consideration not only the frequency with which they become infected, but also possible relationships to (1) mechanisms of speech, hearing, and swallowing, (2) airway obstruction, and (3) cardiorespiratory function. Many of these relationships, it must be emphasized, are at best hypothetical. Since the worth of T&A using less stringent criteria than those used in the Pittsburgh study has not been demonstrated conclusively, conservatism in recommending such surgery is indicated. Under certain circumstances, reasonable alternatives such as antibiotic prophylaxis or placement of tympanostomy tubes should be considered.

Although it is not the purpose here to recommend specific indications for T&A, it seems that tonsillectomy or adenoidectomy, or both, should not be performed on any child whose criteria for operation(s) do not approximate those employed in the Pittsburgh studies. In addition, there are certain indications that are considered "urgent," whereas others are considered "reasonable" but in need of verification.

The "urgent" indications are so considered because (as in cor pulmonale) surgical intervention is of established value for a serious or life-threatening condition or because surgery, although of uncertain benefit, *may* help prevent worsening of the impairment. They are as follows:

1. Alveolar hypoventilation with or without cor pulmonale and secondary to severe chronic upper airway obstruction. (See the box on p. 1533.) Depending on the respective size and anatomic relationships of the tonsils and adenoids, this condition may call for either tonsillectomy or adenoidectomy, or both.
2. Tonsillar enlargement sufficient to cause significant difficulty in swallowing. This finding warrants tonsillectomy only.
3. Uncontrollable tonsillar bleeding.
4. Tonsillar malignancy.
5. Nasal obstruction caused by hypertrophied adenoids and resulting in manifest discomfort in breathing and severe distortion of speech. Adenoidectomy alone is the recommended operation.

The "reasonable" indications are any *one* of the following:

1. Recurrent peritonsillar abscess.
2. Chronic (minimum 6 months) tonsillitis, persisting despite appropriate antimicrobial therapy.
3. Muffled, "hot potato" voice if the child is at least 6 years old.
4. Chronic (minimum 6 months) enlargement (larger than 2 cm) or tenderness of anterior cervical lymph nodes, persisting despite appropriate antibiotic therapy.

CONTRAINDICATIONS

Removal of the adenoids is contraindicated in children with hypernasality resulting from velopharyngeal insufficiency. The most frequent cause of this is complete or incomplete cleft palate. Removal of the adenoids in this circumstance may result in a marked increase in hypernasality. Children with a cleft palate, repaired or unrepaired, should not be subjected to adenoidectomy without consultation with specialists in the management of cleft palate. All children scheduled for adenoidectomy should be examined carefully to rule out the presence of a submucous cleft, which involves the palatal muscles but not the overlying mucous membrane. The presence of a bifid uvula, a shortened and widened median raphe of the soft palate, and a palable V-shaped midline notch (rather than a smooth, rounded curve) at the junction of the hard and soft palate is diagnostic of a submucous cleft (see Fig. 7-26 in Chapter 7). When hypernasality resulting from velopharyngeal insufficiency is suspected, irrespective of the physical findings, consultation with a speech pathologist for palatal function studies should be sought.

The presence of local infection is considered a contraindication to T&A because of the patient's increased risk for anesthetic complications, systemic spread of the infection, and hemorrhage during and after the surgery. Ordinarily, surgery should be delayed for at least 3 weeks following an acute local infection, except in cases in which prolonged antibiotic therapy has been ineffective and in which severe obstruction to the upper airway is present. Some physicians believe that tonsillectomy should be performed immediately as one aspect of the treatment of peritonsillar abscess.[3]

The presence of respiratory allergy is considered by some physicians to be a contraindication for T&A, for fear that the surgery may precipitate bronchial asthma. Although such a relationship has not been proven clinically, these physicians advocate at least 6 months of antiallergic treatment for the patient's symptoms before T&A is performed.[1]

PRIMARY CARE PHYSICIAN'S ROLE

The pediatrician's responsibility does not end once a decision has been made in favor of T&A. The risks of the hospitalization, the anesthesia, and the surgery itself, in terms of morbidity and mortality, must be minimized. The pediatrician must assume responsibilities in this regard by choosing a surgeon and anesthesiologist and a hospital that will provide the best expertise[1] and facilities available in the technical performance of the surgery and administration of the anesthesia and by working closely with them in providing the preoperative and postoperative care for the child and the parents. The role of each physician and that of supporting professionals in preparing the child for hospitalization and caring for the patient during hospitalization and in the follow-up period should be discussed and agreed on beforehand, so that a coordinated team approach to care can be effected, misunderstanding among the involved professionals and between them and the parents can be avoided, and the experience for the patient and parents can be as pleasant as possible.

Parents and their child should be well informed of the circumstances of the hospitalization and surgery beforehand through preadmission visits to the hospital and age-appropriate literature (see Chapter 22, "The Ill Child"). A rooming-in arrangement for parents, especially those of younger children, is extremely important in minimizing the potential for psychological trauma. It is particularly important to have one or both parents present just before their child's anesthesia induction and when their child first awakens following surgery.

Assessment of the patient for surgery, anesthesia, and risk for complications should be shared by the team of physicians. Under ordinary circumstances, this requires only a careful history and physical examination and hematologic bleeding and coagulation studies. Minimum studies should include prothrombin time, partial thromboplastin time, a hematocrit or hemoglobin measurement, and a platelet estimate. Radiographic examination of the chest and prophylaxis against bacteremia are not necessary on a routine basis. Children with underlying cardiac anomalies, who are therefore at risk for bacterial endocarditis, should receive antibiotic prophylaxis.

Tonsillectomy and adenoidectomy carry the potential of grave risks for each child subjected to them. The physician must consider these and weigh them against the potential benefits to be gained from the operation in reaching a decision to recommend that tonsillectomy, adenoidectomy, or both be performed. If this is done carefully and conservatively, the benefits of surgery in relation to cost will be maximized.

REFERENCES

1. Avery AD and Harris LJ: Tonsillectomy, adenoidectomy, and tonsillectomy with adenoidectomy: assessing the quality of care using short-term outcome measures. In Quality of medical care assessment using outcome measures: eight disease-specific applications, Santa Monica, Calif, 1976, Rand Corp.
2. Bluestone CD et al: Workshop on tonsillectomy and adenoidectomy, Ann Otol Rhinol Laryngol 84(suppl 19):1, 1975.
3. Brandow EC Jr: Immediate tonsillectomy for peritonsillar abscess, Trans Am Acad Ophthalmol Otolaryngol 77:412, 1973.
4. Browlette R et al: A diagnostic approach to suspected OSA, J Pediatr 105:10, 1984.
5. Giebink GS and Thell TE: Tonsillectomy and adenoidectomy practice patterns in Minnesota: a retrospective multi-hospital audit, Minn Med 63:421, 1980.
6. McKee WJE: A controlled study of the effects of tonsillectomy and adenoidectomy in children, Br J Prev Soc Med 17:49, 1963.
7. National Center for Health Statistics: Personal communication to Jack L Paradise, MD, 1988.
8. Paradise JL et al: Efficacy of tonsillectomy for recurrent throat infection in severely affected children: results of parallel randomized and nonradomized clinical trials, N Engl J Med 310:674, 1984.
9. Paradise JL et al: Efficacy of adenoidectomy for recurrent otitis media: results from parallel random and nonrandom trials, Pediatr Res 21:286A, 1987 (abstract).
10. Tal A et al: Ventricular dysfunction in children with obstructive sleep apnea (OSA), Pediatr Pulmonol 4:139, 1988.

SUGGESTED READING

Paradise JL: Tonsillectomy and adenoidectomy. In Bluestone CD, Stool SE, and Sheetz MD, editors: Pediatric otolaryngology, ed 2, Philadelphia, 1990, WB Saunders Co.

262

Toxic Shock Syndrome

Michael E. Pichichero

Toxic shock syndrome (TSS) was defined as a distinct clinical entity in 1978 by Todd and associates[9] as an acute illness of adolescent children characterized by fever, diffuse nonexudative mucous membrane inflammation, vomiting and profuse diarrhea, generalized myalgia, scarlatiniform erythroderma, hypotension, and shock associated with multiple organ system failure: renal, myocardial, pulmonary, hepatic, hematologic, and central nervous system (CNS). Two years later, a series of epidemiologic studies demonstrated that TSS occurred most often in menstruating females of childbearing age, particularly in those who regularly used tampons.[3,8] Highly absorbent brands of tampons were shown to be especially problematic. With this epidemiologic discovery and the dissemination of this information to physicians and the public, the frequency and pattern of tampon use changed, with a consequent substantial drop in the incidence of TSS. Currently 85% of TSS cases occur in females and 15% in males. Among cases in females, 55% occur during menses. Other risk factors in females include use of barrier contraceptives and the immediate postparturient time frame. Nonsurgical and surgical wounds infected with particular strains of *Staphylococcus aureus* (see below) account for about 10% of female cases and nearly all male cases. The overall incidence of TSS is 0.53 cases per 100,000 population, although wide variations exist in different geographic regions. TSS occurs more often in Caucasians than in non-Caucasions for both menses-associated and non-menses–associated cases.[4]

CLINICAL PRESENTATION

Strict criteria for case definition have been established by the Centers for Disease Control (see box). The time sequence of the clinical manifestations of TSS is outlined in Fig. 262-1.[3] Patients are usually healthy before the onset of symptoms. Occasionally there is a prodrome consisting of low-grade fever, malaise, myalgia, or vomiting in the week preceding the beginning of the acute illness. Then the patient abruptly develops a spiking fever of 39° to 41° C, chills, and severe gastrointestinal symptoms consisting of nausea, vomiting, profuse watery, nonbloody diarrhea, and abdominal cramps. Many patients will also complain of headache, myalgia, and a sore throat. At this stage of the illness a diagnosis of acute viral gastroenteritis may well be incorrectly entertained and the youngster treated symptomatically. However, over the next 24 to 72 hours the patient develops additional clinical signs suggestive of the diagnosis of TSS. A diffuse, blanching, macular erythroderma (sunburnlike) or scarlatiniform rash erupts. The rash may be faint or evanescent and is therefore sometimes missed or attributed to high fever. The rash is not pruritic but occasionally is petechial. Patients demonstrate bilateral conjunctival hyperemia without discharge and may complain of photophobia. Oropharyngeal inflammation, sometimes with an associated strawberry tongue or buccal ulcerations, and vaginal erythema with minimal clear watery discharge also occur.

Within 24 to 72 hours of the onset of illness most patients experience orthostatic dizziness or syncope or both because of orthostatic hypotension. This symptom can become manifest abruptly and may be premonitory of the development of hypovolemic shock. The peak of illness in the clinical syndrome occurs on the second or third day and involves multiple organ systems. CNS dysfunction may appear as headache, confusion, disorientation, hallucinations, and complaints of paresthesias of the hands and feet. Some patients have a stiff, tender neck. If a lumbar puncture is performed, normal values for CSF glucose and protein will be found, although some patients have up to 100 white blood cells per cubic millimeter, 50% of which may be polymorphonuclear cells. Abdominal musculature tenderness, absent or hyperactive bowel sounds, and radiologic evidence of a nonobstructive ileus are common. Azotemia and a diminished creatinine clearance occur as evidence of renal involvement. Oliguria is typical; complete renal shutdown occurs rarely. The musculoskeletal system is nearly always affected. Exquisite muscle tenderness and severe myalgias are common. Arthralgias and joint effusions may be seen. Nonpitting edema over the wrists and ankles and synovitis of the small joints of the hands and feet have been reported to occur in a few patients. Patients may experience shock lung or adult-type respiratory distress syndrome. Hematologic involvement includes a progressive normochromic normocytic anemia, thrombocytopenia, and leukocytosis. Arrhythmias or prolonged shock may lead to eventual myocardial failure.

LABORATORY FINDINGS

No laboratory test is available for confirming the diagnosis of TSS. Initial laboratory findings of TSS often include a leukocytosis, with a striking increase in the percentage of immature neutrophils, a progressive anemia, and thrombocytopenia. These hematologic abnormalities are self-correcting during the convalescent stage. Thrombocytopenia may be accompanied by prolongation of prothrombin time and partial thromboplastin time and the appearance of increased fibrin split products. However, neither serious bleeding during the acute phase of illness nor thrombosis resulting from rebound

Case Definition of Toxic Shock Syndrome

Fever: temperature 38.9° C
Rash: diffuse macular erythroderma; desquamation of palms and soles 1 to 2 weeks after onset of illness
Hypotension: systolic blood pressure 90 mm Hg for adults or below 5th percentile by age for children under 16 years of age; orthostatic drop in diastolic blood pressure 15 mm Hg from lying to sitting, or orthostatic syncope
Multisystem involvement—three or more of the following:
- Gastrointestinal: vomiting or diarrhea at onset of illness
- Muscular: severe myalgia or creatinine phosphokinase level at least twice the upper limit of normal for laboratory
- Mucous membrane: vaginal, oropharyngeal, or conjunctival hyperemia
- Renal: blood urea nitrogen (BUN) or creatinine at least twice the upper limit of normal for laboratory or urinary sediment with pyuria (>5 white cells per high-power field) in the absence of urinary tract infection
- Hepatic: total bilirubin, serum glutamic-oxaloacetic transaminase (SGOT), or serum glutamic-pyruvate transaminase (SGPT) at least twice the upper limit of normal for laboratory
- Hematologic: platelets $<100,000/mm^3$
- CNS: disorientation or alterations in consciousness without focal neurologic signs when fever and hypotension are absent

Negative results on the following tests, if obtained:
- Blood, throat, cerebrospinal fluid (CSF) cultures
- Rise in antibody titer: Rocky Mountain spotted fever, leptospirosis, and rubeola

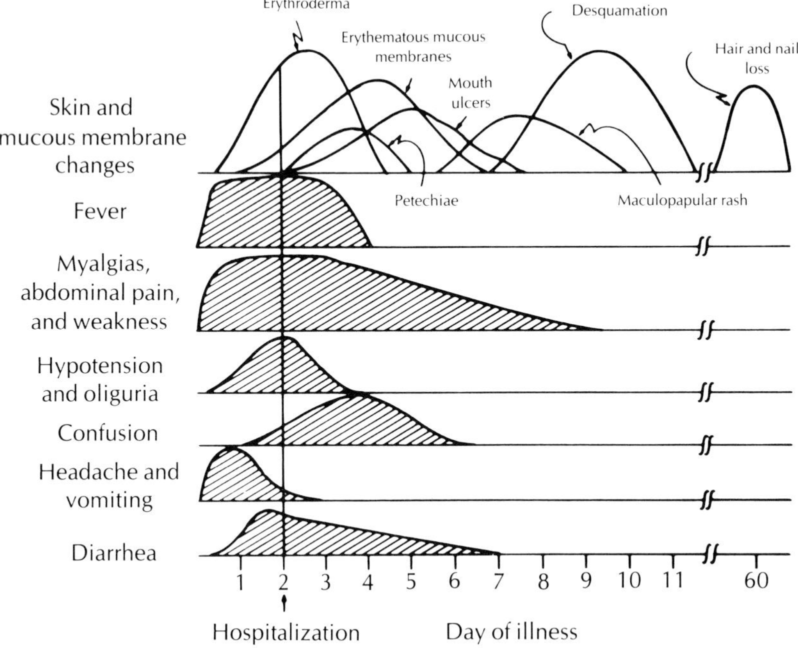

Fig. 262-1 Major systemic, skin, and mucous membrane manifestations of toxic shock syndrome.
From Chesney PJ et al: Clinical manifestations of toxic shock syndrome, JAMA 246:743, 1981.

thrombocytosis during recovery has been a significant clinical problem. A majority of patients have hypoproteinemia and hypoalbuminemia, probably as a consequence of increased capillary permeability because of exotoxin-mediated vascular cell membrane change (see section below on etiology). A number of patients also experience metabolic acidosis from inadequate tissue perfusion, and this may be complicated by hyponatremia and hypokalemia as a result of accompanying persistent vomiting and diarrhea. Serum concentrations of calcium may appear dangerously low; however, tetany is rarely seen. The BUN and creatinine are usually elevated early in the illness. Peak abnormal values occur after 5 to 7 days and then rapidly return to normal. However, some patients have required acute hemodialysis or peritoneal dialysis to correct these and other metabolic imbalances. Despite the abnormal renal function, hypophosphatemia is typically present in the first days of illness. The creatinine phosphokinase level is often quite elevated, and occasionally patients will experience myoglobinemia. These findings normalize with resolution of the myalgias, usually between the fifth and tenth day of disease. Hepatic enzyme and bilirubin levels are typically elevated initially but tend to revert to normal in convalescence. The relative frequency of these abnormal laboratory findings is presented in Table 262-1.

ETIOLOGY

Almost all patients who develop TSS are colonized or infected with *S. aureus*. While only 7% to 10% of normal menstruating females have vaginal or cervical staphylococci, over 90% of girls who develop TSS have been colonized or infected. Similarly, all of the known male cases have had clinical evidence of a staphylococcal soft tissue infection, pneumonia, or osteomyelitis. Furthermore, a specific staphylococcal protein, known as TSS toxin 1 (TSST-1) has been identified as a cause, or a mediator of, the pathophysiologic events associated with TSS.[7] Apparently, colonization with TSST-1–producing *S. aureus* and concomitant antibody formation is common, whereas TSS is not. The unique feature in patients with TSS is that they have sequestered focal sites of *S. aureus* colonization (e.g., the vagina during menstruation with tampon use) or infection (surgical and nonsurgical wounds) where growth conditions are established that promote TSST-1 production.[14] Of note regarding the tampon association, more highly absorbent tampons and tampons with certain fibers seem to create such an environment more effectively. The magnesium-binding capacity of tampon absorptive fibers may be the relevant variant, because low magnesium concentrations in vitro promote TSST-1 production.[5] There is speculation that higher estrogen levels (as produced by oral contraceptives) alter vaginal conditions in such a way that growth of *S. aureus* is inhibited.[1] TSST-1 cannot be the only toxin associated with TSS.[2] Numerous studies have shown that some isolates of *S. aureus* from patients with nonmenstrual TSS do not make TSST-1. Evidence in support of a role for staphylococcal enterotoxins (A through E) as alternative TSS toxins in the appropriate clinical setting (usually nonmenstrual TSS) has accumulated. Some clinical manifestations of TSS may be consequences of secondary mediators—for example, tumor necrosis factor and interleukin-1, released by the host in response to *S. aureus* toxins.[6]

MANAGEMENT

The initial steps in management of TSS are outlined in the accompanying box. Nearly all patients should be hospitalized, although a few with a very mild form of the illness may be cautiously managed as outpatients. The first and major re-

Table 262-1 *Summary of Clinical and Laboratory Data Associated with TSS*

PARAMETER	RELATIVE FREQUENCY OF OCCURRENCE (%)
Clinical	
Fever	100
Temperature >40° C (>104° F)	70
Rash	100
Diffuse erythema	87
Desquamation	90
Myalgia	99
Hypotension (orthostatic hypotension or syncope)	95
Disorientation, irritability, or lethargy	89
Diarrhea	83
Vomiting	82
Sore throat	80
Strawberry tongue	80
Headache	78
Abdominal pain and tenderness	70
Vaginal hyperemia	67
Conjunctivitis	65
Vaginal discharge	42
Stiff neck	36
Arthralgia	15
Joint effusion	12
Adult respiratory distress syndrome	10
Laboratory	
Hematologic	
Increased fibrinolytic split products	100
Immature neutrophils	95
Anemia	82
Leukocytosis	76
Prolonged prothrombin time	70
Decreased fibrinogen	68
Thrombocytopenia	64
Prolonged partial thromboplastin time	60
Metabolic	
Hypoproteinemia	95
Hypoalbuminemia	85
Hypocalcemia	83
Hypokalemia	75
Hypophosphatemia	62
Hyponatremia	47
Hepatic	
Elevated hepatic enzymes	67
Hyperbilirubinemia	63
Renal	
Pyuria	100
Increased creatinine	82
Increased BUN	75
Proteinuria	70
Microscopic hematuria	50
Musculoskeletal	
Increased creatinine phosphokinase	75
Metabolic acidosis	75
Myoglobinuria	66

suscitative goal is to administer large volumes of crystalloid (Ringer lactate) or colloid (fresh-frozen plasma or albumin) solutions to restore normal intravascular volume and correct hypotension, since shock is the initial threat to intact survival. Patients may require enormous volumes of fluid (two to four times normal daily maintenance) to maintain tissue perfusion. Adequate treatment of hypotension may also require vasopressor therapy such as dopamine or dobutamine. Much of the administered fluid is sequestered outside the intravascular space, and many patients become markedly edematous. Therefore it is frequently advisable to have a central venous pressure line or a Swan-Ganz catheter to monitor left ventricular end-diastolic pressure to avoid the development of congestive heart failure caused by overvigorous fluid resuscitation. If significant hypotension exists, it is likely that multiple organ system failure is imminent. The management outlined in the box at the right should be pursued while transport to a tertiary care medical facility is arranged. There, continued management will be largely supportive and dictated by the degree of organ dysfunction.

A multidisciplinary approach may well be required to manage the patient with TSS. The pulmonary specialist may be needed to manage adult-type respiratory distress syndrome or shock lung, since endotracheal intubation and ventilatory assistance with positive end-expiratory pressure and high oxygen flow rates may be required. The hematologist may be of assistance in the treatment of DIC. Peritoneal dialysis or hemodialysis may be necessary to manage renal failure or severe electrolyte and acid-base abnormalities. In this area, services of a nephrologist may be needed. Ventricular ectopy is common, and refractory ventricular arrhythmias have been a frequent cause of death in severely ill patients. The cardiac monitoring and management of this aspect of the patient's care can be facilitated by a cardiologist's input.

Since TSS appears to be an exotoxin-mediated disease, the importance of antibiotics could be questioned. However, 1% to 2% of patients with TSS have an *S. aureus* bacteremia,

Management of Toxic Shock Syndrome

1. Consider other possible diagnoses.
2. Remove potentially infected foreign bodies (e.g., tampons).
3. Obtain cultures of blood, throat, vagina, nares, rectum, and other appropriate sites.
4. Drain and irrigate infected sites.
5. Give an intravenous antistaphylococcal β-lactamase–resistant antimicrobial agent at maximum dosage for weight and age.
6. Consider methylprednisolone for severe cases.
7. Treat aggressively and monitor for the following:

Hypovolemia and inadequate tissue perfusion
Adult respiratory distress syndrome
Myocardial dysfunction
Acute renal failure
Cerebral edema
Hypocalcemia/hypophosphatemia
Metabolic acidosis
Disseminated intravascular coagulation
Fluid and electrolyte abnormalities

Table 262-2 *Differential Diagnosis of Toxic Shock Syndrome*

DISEASE	HYPOTENSION	RASH	LIPS	ORAL CAVITY
Toxic shock syndrome	Yes	Diffuse erythroderma; −Nikolsky sign	Red	Erythematous
Staphylococcal scalded-skin syndrome	No	Erythroderma; bullae; ±Nikolsky sign	—	—
Stevens-Johnson syndrome	No	Erythema multiforme	Bleeding, fissured	Bullous enanthem
Kawasaki disease	No	Polymorphous	Red, fissured	Erythematous, strawberry tongue
Scarlet fever	No	Diffuse erythroderma; circumoral pallor; Pastia lines	—	Strawberry tongue
Measles	No	Morbilliform	—	Koplik spots
Leptospirosis	Sometimes	Erythematous, macular, petechial, purpuric	—	±Pharyngitis
Toxic epidermal necrolysis (drug related)	Sometimes	Painful erythroderma; bullae; +Nikolsky sign	—	—

for which antibiotic therapy would be crucial. Further, it appears that antistaphylococcal antibiotics may reduce the recurrence rate of TSS in girls who have menstrual-related illness. Therefore a 7- to 10-day course of nafcillin (100 to 200 mg/kg/day divided into six equal doses and given intravenously) or other antistaphylococcal antibiotic is probably a prudent part of patient management.

Two somewhat controversial aspects in the management of TSS are the use of corticosteroids and intravenous immunoglobulin (IVIG). Many physicians have elected to use high-dose methylprednisolone (30 mg/kg every 4 hours) during the initial 24 hours of illness. This therapy is based on experimental evidence that steroids may be beneficial in the treatment of shock induced by bacterial toxins. Anecdotal reports of TSS have suggested that steroids have some efficacy in this regard.

High levels of antibody to TSST-1 have been found in IVIG preparations. Animal model studies suggest that administration early in the course of disease can reduce morbidity and mortality of TSS. However, it is also possible that IVIG could diminish the immune response to *S. aureus* toxins, thereby increasing the risk of recurrent episodes. The risk-benefit ratio of this controversial empiric therapy therefore must be carefully considered in each patient.

DIFFERENTIAL DIAGNOSIS

In some aspects TSS might be confused with staphylococcal scalded-skin syndrome, Stevens-Johnson syndrome, Kawasaki disease, streptococcal scarlet fever, measles, leptospirosis, or toxic epidermal necrolysis. The differentiating features among these diagnoses are presented in Table 262-2. The strict case definition presented in the box on p. 1538 is particularly useful for epidemiologic purposes and serves to exclude patients with other diseases. However, recent experience suggests that this strict definition may exclude patients with milder forms of TSS, and this should be kept in mind when confronted with a patient demonstrating some but not all of the clinical findings of TSS.

PROGNOSIS AND CONVALESCENCE

The majority of patients with TSS recover within 7 to 10 days. The case fatality rate is 3.3%. Convalescence is marked by a characteristic desquamation of the palms and soles within 1 to 2 weeks after the onset of illness. Some patients also experience hair and nail loss. Prolonged fatigue and weakness for as long as 3 months may be observed in the recovery phase.

TSS can be recurrent in menstruating girls, and multiple recurrences have been reported to occur. The incidence of recurrent TSS may be as high as 28% if antistaphylococcal antibiotics are not employed. The criteria for recurrent disease are less stringent than those required for defining an initial episode. The use of appropriate antistaphylococcal therapy and discontinuation of tampon use reduces the risk of recurrences. An absent or delayed immune response to TSST-1 frequently is associated with susceptibility to recurrent TSS. Physicians who care for adolescent girls having a febrile illness of uncertain cause that occurs during menstruation, is recurrent, or is associated with an exanthem should seriously consider the diagnosis of TSS.

EYES	HANDS AND FEET	DESQUAMATION	OTHER FINDINGS	DIAGNOSIS
Nonpurulent conjunctivitis	Erythematous, edematous	Hands and feet—can be generalized	Diarrhea; renal, hepatic, CNS, hematologic abnormalities	Clinical; culture of *S. aureus* from nasopharynx, vagina, or wound
± Purulent conjunctivitis	Relatively spared or grossly involved	Gross	—	Clinical; culture of *S. aureus* from nasopharynx or wound; skin biopsy
Purulent conjunctivitis	Involved	Involves only individual lesions	Respiratory and GI tract involvement	Clinical; skin biopsy
Nonpurulent conjunctivitis	Erythematous, edematous	Fingertips	Coronary aneurysms; generalized vasculitis	Clinical; no diagnostic test
—	Relatively spared	Fine, flaky	Rheumatic fever; glomerulonephritis	Clinical; culture of group A streptococci from pharynx; serology
Conjunctivitis	Involved	Fine	Respiratory tract involvement	Clinical; serology
Conjunctivitis	Relatively spared	—	CNS, renal, hepatic involvement	Clinical; serology
± Conjunctivitis	± Involved	Gross	—	Clinical; serology

REFERENCES

1. Best GK et al: Hormonal influence on experimental infections by a toxic shock strain of *Staphylococcus aureus,* Infect Immun 52:331, 1986.
2. Crass BA and Bergdoll MS: Toxin involvement in toxic shock syndrome, J Infect Dis 153:918, 1986.
3. Davis JP et al: Toxic-shock syndrome: epidemiological features, recurrence, risk factors, and prevention, N Engl J Med 303:1429, 1980.
4. Gaventa S et al: Active surveillance for toxic shock syndrome in the United States, 1986, Rev Infect Dis 11:S28, 1989.
5. Kass EH: Effect of magnesium on production of toxic-shock-syndrome toxin-1: a collaborative study, J Infect Dis 158:44, 1988.
6. Kass EH and Parsonnet J: On the pathogenesis of toxic shock syndrome, Rev Infect Dis 9:S482, 1987.
7. Schlievert PM: TSST-1: structure, function, purification, and detection—role of toxic shock syndrome toxin 1 in toxic shock syndrome: overview, Rev Infect Dis 11:S107, 1989.
8. Shands KN et al: Toxic-shock syndrome in menstruating women: association with tampon use and *Staphylococcus aureus* and clinical features in 52 cases, N Engl J Med 303:1436, 1980.
9. Todd J et al: Toxic-shock syndrome associated with phage-group-1 staphylococci, Lancet 2:1116, 1978.
10. Todd JK et al: Influence of focal growth conditions on the pathogenesis of toxic shock syndrome, J Infect Dis 155:673, 1987.

263

Tuberculin Skin Test Positivity

Ciro V. Sumaya

The tuberculin skin test is an extremely important tool for the control of tuberculosis in children. Although bacteriologic confirmation should be attempted, a positive skin test offers a simple and practical means of detecting tuberculosis in children with clinical manifestations or a history compatible with this disease. Moreover, most children with tuberculosis are characteristically asymptomatic and are detected only by means of the skin test. If not found early, a small but meaningful number of these infected children will proceed to develop severe disseminated disease.

As a result of the gradual decline in the incidence of tuberculosis in adults and children, various medical bodies have made modifications in their recommendation for routine tuberculin skin-testing of children. The American Academy of Pediatrics Committee on Infectious Diseases[5] recommends annual tuberculin skin-testing in high-risk children (from high-prevalence settings), such as those living in families with a case of tuberculosis, American Indian children, and children of parents who have recently immigrated from Asia, Africa, the Middle East, Central and South America, or the Caribbean. The committee further states that although annual testing of low-risk groups is not indicated, an alternative approach may be to perform routine skin-testing at three important stages of childhood: (1) 12 to 15 months of age, (2) before school entry, and (3) in adolescence. Awareness of the prevalence of tuberculosis in the community by consultation with local and state health departments is a useful guide in considering the frequency of tuberculin skin-testing.

ETIOLOGY

A tuberculin skin test employing five tuberculin units of purified protein derivative (PPD) injected intradermally (Mantoux technique) and eliciting an induration equal to or greater than 10 mm almost always signals a tuberculous infection (see Chapter 17). False positive reactions are extremely rare with the intradermal test. False negative reactions are also very uncommon but may occur in children with overwhelming tuberculous infections, immunodeficiency, recent viral infection, or following immunization. It has been suggested recently that individuals with a human immune deficiency virus (HIV) infection (see Chapter 178) should have a lower cutoff point, 5 mm, to indicate a positive reaction.

False reactions are more common with multipuncture skin tests that are commonly used as screening devices. Of the multipuncture skin tests available (Tine, Aplitest, Mono-Vacc), the plastic-pronged liquid-tuberculin containing Mono-Vacc preparation may have the least number of false reactions.[2] A positive reaction by a multipuncture skin test should always be confirmed by the intradermal test, unless a severe reaction from the multipuncture test occurs. Skin test positivity should occur within 3 to 12 weeks after being exposed and infected with the tubercle bacillus.

HISTORY

The child with the positive skin test should be questioned for malaise, anorexia, cough, fever, and other problems, although the majority will not have any specific recognizable manifestation.

Since children with tuberculosis are characteristically noncontagious, it is imperative to search for the actively infected adult who transmitted the infection to the child with the positive skin test.[8] Infective adults are usually found within the family setting and may be symptomatic or asymptomatic. A detailed history of prior tuberculosis, other chronic chest infections, prolonged cough, recurrent fever, weight loss, and night sweats should be obtained on all adult family members. Siblings of the infected child should also be included in the history-taking, since they are at increased risk for having been infected by the same adult.

PHYSICAL EXAMINATION

Unless symptomatic, a child with primary tuberculosis detected by a positive skin test usually displays no abnormal physical findings. However, during the general examination, the clinician should look, in particular, for abnormalities in the growth pattern, lymphadenopathy, pulmonary problems, and less frequently, erythema nodosum.

Laboratory Findings

A chest roentgenogram (anteroposterior and lateral views) should be obtained on every child with a positive skin test, although only a minority will yield an abnormal finding. Again, symptomatic patients are more likely to have some pulmonary abnormality. The more frequent roentgenographic abnormalities detected in manifest primary pulmonary tuberculosis are a parenchymal lesion with or without hilar (sometimes paratracheal) lymphadenopathy, or such lymphadenopathy alone.[4] Pleural effusions, calcifications, and miliary lesions are seen less frequently; cavitary formation is rare except in the adolescent. Lymph node involvement is a characteristic roentgenographic finding in childhood tuberculosis, in contrast to adult patients. A pulmonary complex in classic primary tuberculosis, consisting of a combination of clinical-pathologic findings, has been described: primary parenchymal focus, lymphangitis, and regional lymphadenitis, often with pleural effusion.

The erythrocyte sedimentation rate may be elevated in acute primary tuberculosis. This variable and nonspecific finding appears to have no value in predicting the outcome or in monitoring the activity of the disease.

DIFFERENTIAL DIAGNOSIS

Other chronic granulomatous diseases, such as coccidioidomycosis and histoplasmosis, may produce similar pulmonary lesions and symptomatology as primary tuberculosis. Chronic intrathoracic diseases, such as cystic fibrosis, persistent bronchopneumonia, pulmonary changes following measles or pertussis, a lung abscess, aspiration of foreign bodies, parasitic infiltrations, or tumors, also should be considered in the differential diagnosis.

Disseminated forms of tuberculosis may result in clinical pictures that simulate those produced by other persistent bacterial, parasitic, or fungal infections. Appropriate serologic, culture, and histopathologic analyses of body fluids and tissue should aid in determining the etiologic agent.

PSYCHOSOCIAL CONSIDERATIONS

Tuberculosis has for centuries been considered a socially unacceptable illness. This attitude has prevailed mainly because of the contagious nature and prominent symptomatology associated with adult patients. Fortunately, most children with tuberculosis have a less dramatic clinical course, are relatively noncontagious, and can be treated as ambulatory patients. Except in severe illness, children with tuberculosis should be able to continue schoolwork.

The chronicity of the disease process in all ages, however, with its attendant multiple patient visits and extended chemotherapy, can produce significant psychologic problems. Parents of children with tuberculosis and the children themselves should be surrounded by an atmosphere of optimism. They should also be educated about the disease and the importance and effectiveness of appropriate chemotherapy and chemoprophylaxis.

MANAGEMENT

When the clinican sees a child who has a positive tuberculin skin test, it is important to ascertain if this is the only finding of primary tuberculosis or whether there also are clinical, radiologic, and bacteriologic signs of this disease. It is also helpful to ascertain how recent in onset the infection is. A child with a positive skin test but with an absence of symptomatology and a normal chest roentgenogram is classified as a "reactor." This tuberculous infection has been categorized variously as asymptomatic, inactive, latent, quiescent, and nonmanifest. A "convertor" is an individual whose reaction to a tuberculin skin test changed from a negative response to a positive response (minimal increase of 6 mm) within a 2-year period. This child may or may not have other signs of primary tuberculosis.

Children with clinical, radiologic, and bacteriologic signs of tuberculosis, alone or in combination, have a manifest (also called patent or "active") form of primary tuberculosis. Most children with manifest tuberculosis have an abnormal finding on the chest roentgenogram, often accompanied by some symptoms. The diagnosis of pulmonary tuberculosis is then established by demonstration of tubercle bacilli in gastric contents, aspirated bronchopulmonary secretions, or sputum. In contrast to specimens from adults, gastric contents are the most common specimens obtained for laboratory diagnosis of pulmonary tuberculosis in children.[6] Sputum is rarely obtained during coughing episodes, except in older children. The gastric contents and pulmonary specimens are cultured in appropriate media, whereas the pulmonary specimens may in addition be placed on a slide and stained (by fluorescent and nonfluorescent techniques) for the presence of tubercle bacilli. The analysis of stained smears is not appropriate for gastric contents because of the common presence of atypical mycobacteria. The laboratory detection of tuberculous infection in extrapulmonary sites may require analysis by stains, culture, and the histologic appearance of other body fluids or biopsied tissue. The natural course and development of the best-known complications of manifest tuberculosis in children are described in Fig. 263-1.[9]

Children whose only sign of a tuberculosis infection is a positive skin test should receive chemoprophylaxis with isoniazid (INH) alone. Several studies have documented that INH, in a single daily dose ranging from 5 to 20 mg/kg over a 12-month period, can prevent the development of active pulmonary or disseminated disease.[3] The current daily dose for prophylaxis recommended by several health agencies is 10 mg/kg, not to exceed 300 mg/day.

Manifest or active cases of tuberculosis should be treated with a two- or three-drug regimen, depending on the severity and extent of the disease's dissemination. INH, the cornerstone of antituberculous therapy, should always be included in the drug regimen. Single-drug treatment of manifest or active forms of tuberculosis is not used because of the rapid buildup of resistance by the tubercle bacillus.

It is currently recommended that children with evidence of pulmonary (other than miliary) tuberculosis can be adequately treated with a 9-month regimen of INH and rifampin.[1,5] During the first month of treatment, INH is given in a daily dose of 10 to 20 mg/kg, and rifampin is given in a daily dose of 10 to 20 mg/kg. Thereafter, the dosages are 20 to 40 mg/kg twice weekly of INH and 10 to 20 mg/kg twice weekly of rifampin for 8 months. Careful supervision of drug compliance throughout the course is extremely important. When INH and rifampin are combined and higher doses than those stated above are administered, an appreciable incidence of liver toxicity may occur.

Extrapulmonary tuberculous infections or miliary tuberculosis of the lungs usually requires treatment with three drugs—INH, rifampin, and either ethambutol (15 to 25 mg/kg/day), streptomycin (20 to 25 mg/kg/day), ethionamide (15 mg/kg/day), or pyrazinamide (20 to 40 mg/kg/day). (A fourth drug is sometimes used, particularly if there is significant drug resistance to tubercle bacilli in the region.[7] One of the drugs—the parenteral one, if used—is often discontinued after 1 or more months, whereas the remaining two

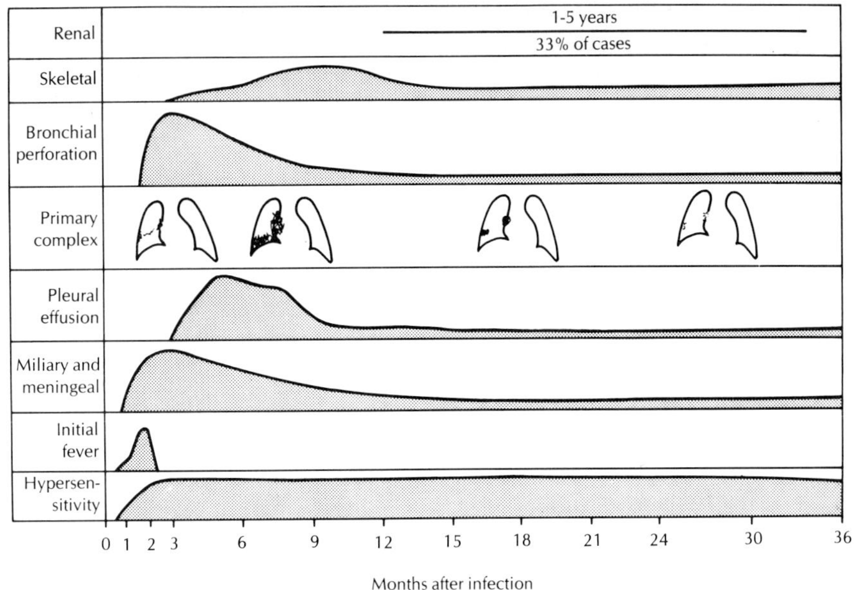

Fig. 263-1 Natural progression of manifest primary tuberculosis, including the more common complications.
After data from Wallgren A: The time-table of tuberculosis, Tubercle 29:245, 1948.

drugs are administered for 1 to 2 years. Although recent data show that the combination of INH and rifampin appears to be adequate drug treatment for most forms of tuberculosis, including extrapulmonary disease, this two-drug combination may not provide adequate coverage for patients living in areas where drug resistance is common. The susceptibility pattern of the tubercle bacillus isolated, it is hoped, from the patient or even the suspected adult source of the child's infection should guide the physician in the proper selection of the chemotherapy used. Shortened versions of the traditional 18-month to 2-year treatment of extrapulmonary or miliary tuberculosis have not been adequately evaluated. Ethambutol has a potential side effect of optic neuritis and therefore is not routinely recommended for children unless visual acuity can be satisfactorily monitored. However, the severity of the tuberculous process or susceptibilities of the tubercle bacillus may make the administration of this drug in younger children necessary.

The evaluation of a child with a positive skin test is not complete without a careful search for an actively infected adult who was the source of the child's infection. In addition to history-taking, this usually entails skin-testing the entire family and other intimate adult contacts, such as grandparents and baby-sitters. Any contact person with a positive skin test should receive a physical examination and a chest roentgenogram. To expedite the search for adults with active tuberculosis, a chest roentgenogram may be obtained on them at the time of skin testing. If an adult source is found, it is important to determine the drug susceptibilities of the tubercle bacilli isolated. These findings may affect the selection of drug therapy to use in the diseased child.

When the actively infected adult is found, all family contacts, whether their skin test result is positive or negative, should receive chemoprophylaxis.[7] Excluded may be those skin test—positive individuals who have previously received purportedly adequate doses of INH for prophylaxis or treatment of tuberculosis. The latter, however, should be investigated for evidence of current active disease. Chemoprophylaxis consists of a single daily dose of INH, 10 mg/kg (maximum 300 mg) for children and 300 mg for adults. Those who remain skin test negative when retested 3 months later may discontinue the drug, assuming the adult with the active infection is receiving adequate treatment. The individuals with positive skin tests who were placed on INH should continue the drug for 9 months (recent change in duration). Even shorter courses of chemoprophylaxis with INH are being evaluated.

There is an ethical need to educate the family about tuberculosis and its potential spread to children from adults with active infections. The family should realize that there are effective drugs available for the prophylaxis and treatment of this disease. Adequate communication between physician, patient, and the patient's family is vitally important to the control of tuberculosis.

PROGNOSIS

Most children with primary tuberculosis go unnoticed, and their infection usually resolves, with or without treatment. However, primary tuberculosis may produce progressive pulmonary lesions that, if untreated, may result in serious disease. Young children, particularly those under 3 years of age, also are at increased risk for widespread dissemination of tubercle bacilli from the primary tuberculous focus. Moreover, reactivation during adult years of untreated childhood infection may lead to further health problems, besides potential transmission of the infection to other susceptible persons.

The development and use of effective antituberculous drugs have produced a significant improvement in prognosis for tuberculosis. Adequate treatment of pulmonary tuberculosis has reduced the rates of chronic pulmonary lesions and complications resulting from hematogenous dissemination of tubercle bacilli to other organs. The rare deaths in children with tuberculosis usually occur in those with meningeal involvement. Even here, a decrease in mortality and neurologic sequelae is seen in those treated earlier in the course of meningitis.[8] The effective use of INH as a chemoprophylactic agent in children has produced a significant reduction in the rate of new infections and in the extension of dissemination of inapparent or even localized lesions. Unfortunately, in populations in which medical care and drug treatment are not readily accessible, the prognosis from tuberculosis is much bleaker.

REHABILITATION

Activity is dependent on the tolerance threshold of the individual child. Bed rest is warranted only for those with significant symptomatology. Nutritional intake should be adequate, but forced feedings should be avoided. Surgical correction of prior pulmonary damage from tuberculosis or orthopedic correction of skeletal deformations is rarely needed because of the uncommon development of these complications with the use of effective chemotherapy. Children with neurologic sequelae following tuberculosis meningitis, however, may require an extensive rehabilitation program.[8]

REFERENCES

1. Abernathy RS et al: Short-course chemotherapy for tuberculosis in children, Pediatrics 72:801, 1983.
2. Donaldson JC and Elliott RC: A study of co-positivity of three multipuncture techniques with intradermal PPD tuberculin, Am Rev Respir Dis 118:843, 1978.
3. Hsu KHK: Thirty years after isoniazid: its impact on tuberculosis in children and adolescents, JAMA 251:1283, 1984.
4. Kendig EL Jr: Tuberculosis: In Kendig EL Jr and Chernick V, editors: Disorders of the respiratory tract in children, Philadelphia, 1983, WB Saunders Co.
5. Report of the Committee on Infectious Diseases (Red Book): Tuberculosis, Evanston, Ill, 1988, American Academy of Pediatrics.
6. Smith MHD: Tuberculosis in children and adolescents, Clin Chest Med 10:381, 1989.
7. Starke JR: Modern approach to the diagnosis and treatment of tuberculosis in children, Pediatr Clin North Am 35:441, 1988.
8. Sumaya CV et al: Tuberculous meningitis in children during the isoniazid era, J Pediatr 87:43, 1975.
9. Wallgren A: The time-table of tuberculosis, Tubercle 29:245, 1948.

SUGGESTED READINGS

Sewell EM, Lincoln EM, and Gutman LT: Tuberculosis. In Krugman S and Katz SL, editors: Infectious diseases of children, St Louis, 1985, The CV Mosby Co.

Smith MHD and Marquis JR: Tuberculosis and other mycobacterial infections. In Feigin RD and Cherry JD, editors: Textbook of pediatric infectious diseases, Philadelphia, 1987, WB Saunders Co.

264

Umbilical Anomalies

Roberta A. Hibbard

The umbilicus serves as a reminder of fetal development. The connection to mother is a complex and central one in the early development of the human infant. Major congenital anomalies of the umbilicus and abdominal wall (e.g., omphalocele and gastroschisis) are discussed elsewhere (see Chapter 41, Critical Neonatal Illness); minor anomalies are discussed here. In addition to anomalies of the umbilicus, tumors and infections (omphalitis) may occur.[3]

EMBRYONIC UMBILICAL REMNANTS

Embryologic variations in the normal development of the umbilical cord explain many of the abnormalities observed. The primitive umbilical cord consists of the umbilical blood vessels, the vitelline duct, and the remnants of the allantois. The vitelline duct is the connection of the yolk sac to the midgut. This duct normally closes at 6 weeks of fetal development but may persist as a Meckel diverticulum, a vitelline cyst (enterocystoma) between the midgut and umbilicus, or an enteric (vitelline) fistula from the midgut to the umbilicus (Fig. 264-1, *A* to *C*). The allantois is continuous with the urinary bladder. As the allantoic lumen disappears, it becomes a fibrous cord (the urachus) connecting the apex of the bladder with the umbilicus. A persistent urachal band has been observed to cause inversion of the umbilicus and abdominal pain with urination.[5] Persistence of the lumen along the length of the urachus results in a urachal fistula, which drains urine. When the lumen only partially closes, a urachal sinus or cyst forms (Fig. 264-1, *D* and *E*). These cysts may become infected and manifest with signs of infection and a lower midline abdominal mass.[1] Enteric and urachal fistulas (Fig. 264-1, *F*) discharge feces and urine, respectively, both resulting in erosive periumbilical dermatitis. Bladder infections may result from a urachal fistula. Neonatal urine ascites from a

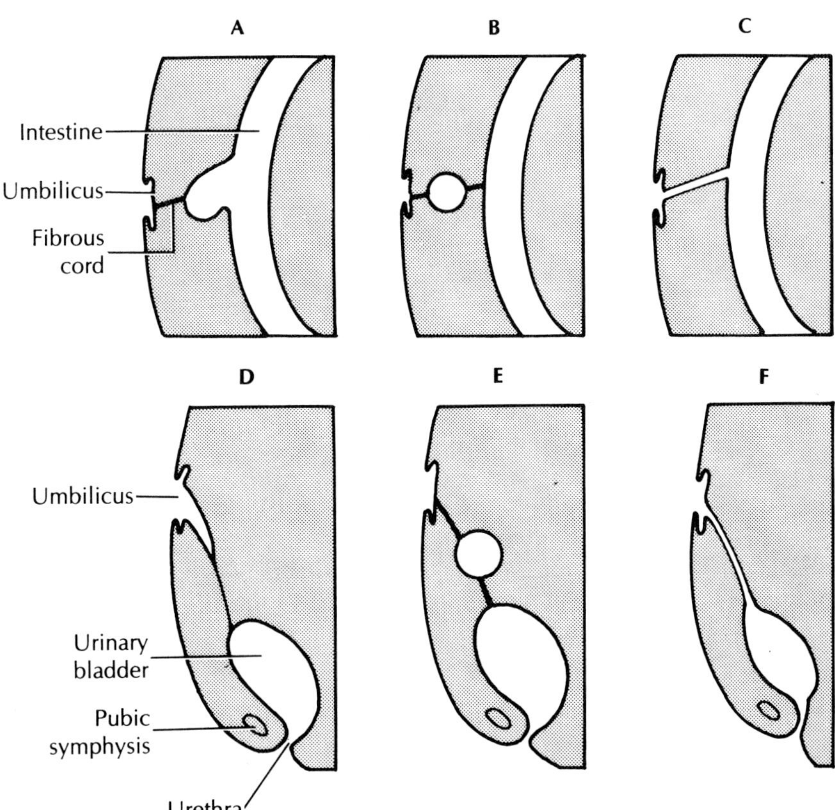

Fig. 264-1 A, Meckel diverticulum. **B,** Enterocystoma. **C,** Enteric (vitelline) fistula. **D,** Urachal sinus. **E,** Urachal cyst. **F,** Urachal fistula.

transected urachus has been reported as a complication of umbilical cutdown procedures. Methylene blue dye instilled at the umbilicus and seen in voided urine demonstrates patency of the urachal fistula. Carmine red dye given orally is discharged at the umbilicus when an enteric fistula is present. These lesions are all treated by surgical excision.

UMBILICAL GRANULOMA

At birth the normal umbilical cord contains only the umbilical vessels surrounded by the protective Wharton jelly. The umbilical stump dries and separates from the abdomen in approximately 2 weeks; it is completely covered by skin in 3 to 4 weeks. Delayed healing with the accumulation of excessive granulation tissue produces an umbilical granuloma, a small, reddened mass sometimes with scant purulent discharge. This lesion may be associated with infection at the base or with a foreign body such as talcum, but it recedes and disappears rapidly after repeated topical applications of silver nitrate. Persistence of a granulomatous-appearing lesion, erosive dermatitis surrounding the umbilicus, or the egression of gas, feces, or urine from it suggests the persistence of an embryonic remnant.[2]

UMBILICAL POLYPS

Polyps at the umbilicus originate from remnants of intestinal mucosa or from sinuses of the vitelline duct or urachus. They often are larger than granulomas, bright red with a mucoid discharge, and unaffected by silver nitrate applications. Histologic examination confirms their origin.

UMBILICAL HERNIA

Umbilical hernias often appear in the first months of life. Lateral connective tissue plates from the umbilical cord fail to close, and a defect in the midline fascia underlying the umbilicus allows peritoneum and viscera (usually small bowel) to protrude through the opening. Contents of the hernia are easily reduced by palpation and frequently pop in and out with changes in intraabdominal pressure.

Umbilical hernias are common, particularly in black children, among whom the prevalence has been reported to be as high as 40% to 60% in the first year of life. Boys and girls are equally affected. Although associated with many syndromes and conditions (e.g., Beckwith-Wiedemann, Down, Hurler, hypothyroidism), an umbilical hernia alone should be considered a normal variation of development.

Most umbilical hernias close spontaneously; many do so within the first year and the majority by the fifth year. A cross-sectional study of black children has suggested that at least 50% of the umbilical hernias present in 4- to 5-year-olds close spontaneously by age 11 years.[4] Incarceration of umbilical hernias is rare and strangulation even more so.

Strapping of the umbilicus was at one time a favored treatment but has been abandoned as ineffective. With incarceration being rare, cosmetic deformity remains the argument for surgical intervention and may be reasonable in selected patients. The low complication rate and evidence to suggest spontaneous closures, at least up to the preteen years, make it reasonable to resist surgery until near puberty in the absence of incarceration or psychological sequelae of the cosmetic deformity.

REFERENCES

1. Boyle G, Rosenberg HK, and O'Neill J: An unusual presentation of an infected urachal cyst, Clin Pediatr 27:130, 1988.
2. Cresson SL and Pilling GP: Lesions about the umbilicus in infants and children, Pediatr Clin North Am 6:1085, 1959.
3. Elhassani SB: The umbilical cord, South Med J 77:730, 1984.
4. Hall DE, Roberts KB, and Charney E: Umbilical hernia: what happens after age 5 years? J Pediatr 98:415, 1981.
5. Knoll LD et al: Periumbilical pain secondary to persistent urachal band, Urology 32:526, 1988.

SUGGESTED READING

Nix TE and Young CJ: Congenital umbilical anomalies, Arch Dermatol 90:160, 1964.

265

Urinary Tract Infections

Edward J. Ruley

INCIDENCE

Urinary tract infection is the most common nephrologic condition seen in pediatric practice, ranking second only to respiratory infections in terms of infection frequency. In the newborn the incidence has been determined to be 1.4 to 5 per 1000 live births. Boys are affected more than five times as frequently as girls. The majority of infections in neonates are sporadic, although outbreaks that suggest epidemics have been reported.

The exact incidence of urinary tract infections in infants and children is unknown. Beyond the neonatal period there is a decline in the incidence of these infections in boys to less than 0.1%, whereas in girls the frequency rises to tenfold that in males. In adolescence another rise in the frequency of urinary tract infection occurs in females coincident with their participation in coitus.

ETIOLOGY

The etiology of urinary tract infections can be considered in terms of those factors that predispose the patient to these infections and the organisms that actually cause the infection.

It has been suggested that the male predominance in the neonatal period is a result of the higher frequency of congenital urinary anomalies in the male. This probably is not the sole reason, however, because many affected male infants have normal urinary tracts. Infection at this age usually is "hematogenous" rather than "ascending" in origin. Inasmuch as the ratio of sepsis in boys compared with girls is similar to the ratio of urinary tract infection, the former may be important in explaining the gender difference. The incidence seems to be inversely related to gestational age, being greatest in low-birth-weight and premature infants. This has led to the speculation that the more immature kidney allows the bacteria to pass the filtration barrier more readily than does the mature kidney.

In the infant and child, most urinary tract infections are "ascending." The high frequency in girls has been attributed to anatomic features of the lower urinary tract, including the short urethra, its proximity to the anus, and its exit within the folds of the vulva. In the adolescent it has been demonstrated that during coitus, bacteria are introduced into the urethra and the urethra often becomes inflamed and swollen, rendering the female adolescent susceptible to ascending infection.

A variety of other factors have been identified that predispose an individual to urinary tract infection. The most common and serious predisposing factors are those that produce incomplete drainage and/or stasis in the urinary system. Poor urodynamics not only contribute to the recurrent nature of urinary tract infection but also promote renal parenchymal damage by allowing infected urine in the lower tract to reach the parenchyma. Even in the absence of parenchymal damage, incomplete urinary drainage is a major factor in the resistance of infections to treatment and infection recurrence. Obstructive urinary lesions can be congenital or acquired. The congenital lesions that predispose to urinary tract infection result from failure of the urinary structures to differentiate normally, with the most common being posterior urethral valves and ureteropelvic junction obstruction. Acquired obstructive lesions include urinary lithiasis, urethral strictures, retroperitoneal fibrosis, voiding dysnergia, and neurogenic bladder. Vesicoureteral reflux is an extremely important factor in urinary tract infections because of its common occurrence and its role in pyelonephritis and renal scarring. (Obstructive urinary lesions and vesicoureteral reflux are discussed in Chapter 233.)

Nonobstructive renal malformations also are associated with an increased incidence of urinary tract infections. These include renal hypoplasia, dysplasia, ectopia, and both autosomal dominant and recessive polycystic kidney disease. The reason for the increased incidence of infection in these conditions is unknown. A variety of metabolic disorders have been associated with an increased frequency of urinary tract infections. Although severe malnutrition is of considerable worldwide importance, other disorders associated with an increased frequency of urinary tract infections include hypokalemia, nephrocalcinosis, vitamin A deficiency, diabetes mellitus, and uremia.

Another factor related to urinary tract infection is urethral instrumentation, particularly bladder catheterization. The need for bladder catheterization in the hospitalized patient is the primary reason that urinary tract infection is the most common nosocomial infection.

A variety of behavioral factors have been implicated in the occurrence of urinary tract infections in the female, including voluntary deferral of micturition and failure to void promptly after coitus. In addition, certain aspects of hygiene such as "wiping forward" after bowel movements, chemical irritation from soaps and detergents, masturbation, the presence of foreign bodies in the introitus, and bowel infestation with *Enterobius* organisms have all been suggested to favor the occurrence and recurrence of urinary tract infections in girls. Finally, it is known that the degree of bacterial virulence is also an important determinant in urinary tract infections.

Bacteria account for the majority of urinary tract infections, with *Escherichia coli* being the infecting organism in 75% to 80% of cases. Less common enteric pathogens are *Enterobacter aerogenes*, *E. cloacae*, and the *Klebsiella* and *Proteus* spp. Of the nonenteric gram-negative pathogens, *Pseudomonas aeruginosa* is the most common. In the sexually active adolescent, gram-positive *Staphylococcus saprophyticus* is the most common pathogen after *E. coli*. Infection with *Neisseria gonorrhoeae* should be suspected in males who have a urethral discharge or purulent balanitis. Furthermore, urinary outlet symptoms may result from gonococcal vulvovaginitis in females. Although the presence of gram-negative intracellular diplococci in a stain of the discharge strongly suggests gonococcal infection, a positive culture result is necessary to confirm the diagnosis. Other causes of the urethritis syndrome (see below) include such sexually transmitted organisms as *Chlamydia trachomatis* and *Ureaplasma urealyticum*.

Viral pathogens are relatively unimportant except for the adenovirus in acute hemorrhagic cystitis. Fungal infections rarely are significant except in immunodeficient, immunosuppressed, or diabetic patients. Fungal overgrowth, however, may complicate antibiotic treatment of the child with a normal immune system whose urodynamics are abnormal or who is catheterized. Although protozoan infections are important in many parts of the world, they are rare in the United States. *Mycobacterium tuberculosis* infections occur rarely as part of secondary tuberculosis and should be considered when sterile pyuria is found. Tuberculosis currently is increasing, presumably as a result of the rise in human immunodeficiency virus (HIV) infection.

CLINICAL FINDINGS

History

Urinary tract infections may occur without symptoms, with symptoms that direct attention to the urinary system, or with symptoms that divert the attention of the clinician to other organ systems. Therefore a high degree of suspicion and continual awareness of potential urinary tract infection must be maintained by all pediatric health practitioners. This concept cannot be overemphasized.

Urinary tract infections in newborns and infants usually are associated with manifestations that are nonspecific or are referable to systems other than the urinary tract. These nonspecific symptoms include malaise, anorexia, difficulty in feeding, unexplained jaundice, failure to thrive, fever of inapparent origin, and malnutrition. To confound diagnosis further, it is common for newborns and infants with urinary tract infection to have gastrointestinal symptoms such as diarrhea or vomiting (sometimes so severe as to mimic hypertrophic pyloric stenosis), as well as neurologic symptoms such as irritability, lethargy, seizures, or hypertonicity. Specific urinary tract symptoms in this age-group, if not absent, are subtle and therefore easily overlooked. They include changes in the caliber and force of the urinary stream, dribbling of urine, or constant wetness of the diapers. Occasionally, parents will report observing an abdominal protuberance and feeling the palpable masses, which later are discovered to be obstructed and distended urinary organs.

In older children, specific urinary tract symptoms are more common and include dysuria, urinary frequency or urgency, burning on urination, foul-smelling urine, pain in the abdomen, back, or loin, or the development of nocturnal enuresis or daytime wetting. Urinary tract infections, however, may not produce symptoms, particularly in children older than 5 years or in those with recurrent urinary tract infections. It has been noted that untreated patients with urinary tract infection may have resolution of fever and urinary symptoms after several weeks, even though persistence of the infection can be demonstrated by culture. Investigators have reported that spontaneous cures in such circumstances are uncommon in spite of the resolution of symptoms.

Physical Findings

Findings in infants with urinary tract infections may be normal except for fever and irritability. In addition to fever and specific urinary complaints, the older child may report direct tenderness to palpation of the abdomen, suprapubic area, or costovertebral area. Those patients with urinary tract obstruction may have palpable abdominal masses, whereas females with sexually transmitted infections often have a concomitant vulvovaginitis.

Laboratory Findings

Although the urinalysis may suggest infection, urine cultures are mandatory for the appropriate diagnosis of urinary tract infections in pediatric patients. In general, the urine for culture should be collected by the simplest and least painful method.

Proper collection of a clean-caught specimen from a female requires that a midstream sample be obtained after the individual has had the vaginal vestibule, vulva, and perineum thoroughly cleansed with a nonirritating antiseptic solution. This cleaned area should be rinsed with sterile water or saline and gently wiped dry with a sterile towel before voiding. Care should be taken not to get the cleaning solution into the urine culture. In males, a midstream urine should be obtained after the glans penis has been cleaned with an antiseptic solution, taking care to retract the foreskin in the uncircumcised individual. Of even greater importance is the handling of the urine after it is obtained. Cultures should be promptly transported on ice to the laboratory, where they should be plated out as soon as possible. Specimens can be kept for 48 hours before plating if kept at 39.2° F (4° C).

Contamination of the urine collection by bacteria from the external genitalia is the most confounding problem in evaluating the results of a positive urine culture result. The technique of colony counting has been suggested to circumvent this problem. A positive diagnosis of bacterial urinary tract infection is based on a colony count of more than 100,000 per milliliter grown from a clean-caught, midstream urine specimen. Colony counts of this magnitude rely on the premise that bacteria thrive in urine at body temperature and multiply significantly in the bladder before voiding takes place. Certain conditions that may produce low colony counts in spite of significant infection are given in the accompanying box. Bacterial counts of 50,000 to 100,000 colonies per milliliter in untreated patients are considered highly suggestive

Factors That Can Cause Low Colony Counts in Spite of Significant Infection

High-volume urine flow
Low urine pH (<5.0) and specific gravity (<1.003)
Recent antimicrobial therapy
Fastidious organisms
Use of inappropriate culture techniques
Bacteriostatic agents in the urine
Complete obstruction of a ureter
Chronic or indolent infection

but not diagnostic of urinary tract infection. Counts of less than 50,000 colonies per milliliter are considered due to contaminants. However, certain organisms such as enterococci and *Staphylococcus saprophyticus* are slow growing and thus may be pathogenic, although the colony counts are less than 100,000 colonies per milliliter.

Consideration of the types of organisms isolated in a colony count is also important. Single ("pure") isolates are more commonly seen in actual infections, particularly of the acute variety, whereas multiple species on culture usually indicate contamination. Multiple isolates, however, are more common in recurrent infections or in cultures taken from sites of urinary diversions.

Suprapubic needle aspiration of the bladder is the preferred method of obtaining urine (1) in the infant or neonate who will not void, (2) when a urine specimen is urgently needed because of the severity of the illness, and (3) to confirm suspected infection in the child with equivocal results on several colony counts. Direct bladder aspiration of urine through puncture of the aseptically prepared suprapubic skin is a safe and reliable technique. (See Appendix B, "Special Procedures," for the techniques used for this procedure.) Any bacteria grown from urine obtained by this method are significant; thus colony counts are not only *not* necessary but may be misleading inasmuch as the bacteria obtained by suprapubic tap may not have had sufficient time to multiply to significant numbers in the bladder. Occasionally no urine will be obtained by suprapubic aspiration because the bladder is empty from recent voiding. A repeat attempt at aspiration after a small oral fluid feeding frequently will render the next attempt more successful. Suprapubic aspiration is contraindicated in patients with bleeding tendencies. Some patients, particularly male neonates, may have transient hematuria after suprapubic aspiration, which usually resolves spontaneously. Although there is minimal risk of entering the bowel if the bladder aspiration is properly performed, in instances in which the bowel has been entered inadvertently, there seems to be little risk for peritonitis. Catheterization of the bladder can be used for the same indications as suprapubic aspiration. In many ways this is more useful than bladder aspirations because more likely it will result in a specimen for culture.

The use of sterile plastic bags that are attached to the washed perineum is unsatisfactory for the collection of urine cultures, because the bags are easily contaminated by skin or fecal bacteria. In addition, the time of voiding usually is unknown, and the urine-filled bag may remain attached to the child in a warm environment for a prolonged period of time. Thus, if the bags are not removed for a colony count soon after voiding, any value of the count is negated.

DIFFERENTIAL DIAGNOSIS

Urinary tract infections may present an identifiable clinical scenario. Discussions of the most common ones follow.

Urethritis

The urethritis syndrome (with or without fever) may be sudden or insidious in onset but usually varies somewhat in intensity from day to day. The complaints primarily are related to urinary outlet irritation. The patients, usually female, void small volumes of urine with symptoms of frequency, urgency, dysuria, and burning. Occasionally patients will have suprapubic or back pain. Although microscopic hematuria is common, gross hematuria is unusual, and casts are never seen. Fever is uncommon.

Such symptoms usually are attributable to irritation of the vulva. Poor hygiene, vulvitis, vaginitis, chemical irritation (from soaps or bubble bath), foreign bodies, masturbation, urethral trauma (bicycle seat hematuria), and *Enterobius* infestations can be the cause. In these circumstances the child has burning on urination because of the urethral or vaginal irritation. This pain causes the child to stop and start the urinary stream, leading to frequent small voidings, hesitancy, and urgency. In the male, such "stop and start" voiding may lead to dilation of the urethra and subsequent microhematuria. Urinalysis may reveal pyuria and bacteriuria as a result of local infection and denudation. Careful examination of the urethral opening is important in making this diagnosis, although urine cultures are still necessary because bacterial infection can cause this syndrome.

Cystitis

In the cystitis syndrome the outlet symptoms are more severe, and back and suprapubic pain as well as fever are more common. Gross hematuria (without casts) is a frequent finding in this syndrome. Bacterial infection, particularly with *E. coli*, is the most common cause of this syndrome in girls. An adenovirus infection is a frequent cause of the syndrome in boys, producing dysuria and urinary frequency with terminal hematuria. The urine culture will reveal the offending organisms in the former instance and will be sterile in the latter.

Pyelonephritis

In the pyelonephritis syndrome the patient usually has generalized symptoms such as a toxic appearance, high fever, chills, vomiting, diarrhea, and abdominal pain in addition to the urinary outlet symptoms. Hypertension more often is seen with infection of the renal parenchyma. Urinalysis usually reveals pyuria and bacteria, and occasionally white blood cell casts will be seen. Granular casts are common in the patient with dehydration and are not specific. There may be isosthenuria, which can persist for 8 to 12 weeks after infection because of medullary dysfunction produced by an ascending infection. Urographic evidence of the loss of renal parenchyma, noted in a patient during an episode of pyelonephritis, indicates *previous* kidney infection or congenital structural maldevelopment, inasmuch as such scars take time to form. Blood cultures should be obtained in all patients suspected of having pyelonephritis, because septicemia is common. A renal biopsy in this syndrome, as in all the urinary infection syndromes, is of limited usefulness because of the patchy nature of a kidney infection and the nonspecificity of the pathologic change.

Radiographic studies are important in the clinical approach to urinary tract infection both from the view of (1) localizing the infection and (2) ruling out urinary anomalies. Currently, the most sensitive way to detect pyelonephritis is to perform a ^{99m}Tc dimercaptosuccinic acid (DMSA) renal scan. The scan will show diminished isotope uptake with preserved renal contour in children with acute parenchymal infection. This imaging test appears to be the "gold standard" for diagnosing pyelonephritis.

Imaging also is the most important tool for investigation of urinary anomalies. It has been recommended that all children whose first urinary tract infection occurs when they are younger than 8 years of age be investigated. The initial test should be a contrast voiding cystourethrogram (VCUG). If this test does not show vesicourethral reflux, the patient should have a sonogram of the bladder and kidneys. If results are normal, no further evaluation is necessary. If the VCUG shows reflux or if the ultrasound findings are abnormal, renal scans with DMSA and ^{99m}Tc diethylenetriaminepentaacetic acid (DTPA) should be performed. The former is the most sensitive means to detect renal scarring; the latter assesses the urinary tract obstruction.

Low-grade vesicoureteral reflux may be a transient abnormality secondary to the effect of the infection on bladder and ureteral muscular function or a more permanent congenital anomaly. Greater degrees of reflux are nearly never transient. As mentioned in Chapter 233, if the child being evaluated has vesicoureteral reflux, any siblings younger than 5 years of age should be studied because of the high familial incidence of this anomaly.

Recurrent Urinary Tract Infections

Recurrent urinary tract infections are seen most commonly in girls. Most often their symptoms are associated with fever, but as aforementioned, they can develop insidiously. Recurrences will develop within the first year in approximately 33% of girls with first urinary tract infections. The risk of recurrence within 2 years of the first infection is 80% in white girls and 60% in black girls. The reason for this racial difference is unclear. Recurrences are infrequent beyond 2 years from the initial infection.

In some children physical or psychomotor developmental delay may be the only manifestation of the recurrent infection. Urinalysis may reveal abnormal medullary function as in the pyelonephritis syndrome, although in more severe or frequent infections there may be abnormalities of glucose and sodium reabsorption, producing glucosuria and natriuresis. Occasionally there will be evidence of glomerular damage, as reflected by a lowered glomerular filtration rate. The degree of functional impairment has been shown to correlate with the histologic severity of the lesion. Similar medullary dysfunction, however, can develop from obstruction without infection. Particular attention should be paid to the possibility of urologic abnormalities in the child with recurrent urinary tract infections. In addition, there is some suggestion that lower urinary tract allergy, *Enterobius* infestation, and poor vaginal hygiene may promote recurrent infections.

TREATMENT

The goals of the treatment program are the eradication of infection, the correction of any anatomic or functional abnormalities, and the prevention of recurrences. Achievement of these goals requires the cooperation of the parents and the patient in diagnostic evaluation and treatment.

Before antibiotic therapy is begun, a properly collected clean-caught urine culture and colony count should be obtained. In cases that are symptomatic of acute infections, treatment may begin before culture data are available. Because most first infections are caused by *E. coli*, trimethoprim-sulfa sulfisoxazole, or ampicillin are good drugs of first choice. If the initial culture is sterile, antibiotics can be discontinued and causes other than a bacterial infection should be considered. A second culture should be taken 48 to 72 hours after beginning therapy and should be sterile if the choice of antibiotics was correct. The antibiotic can be changed if (1) the initial culture shows an organism unresponsive to the initial antibiotic, (2) the 48-hour culture is not sterile, or (3) the patient has not improved clinically. The antibiotic sensitivities of the initial urine culture will be useful in deciding on the best alternative antibiotic. Although various investigators have advised treatment courses from 1 week to 6 weeks in duration, there appears to be little advantage in prolonging initial antibiotic treatment for longer than 2 weeks.

Investigation of the efficacy of shorter courses (or single doses) of therapy in children remains controversial. For bacterial urinary tract syndromes thought to be limited to the lower urinary tract, oral antibiotics usually are sufficient. In patients with suspected renal parenchymal infection (the pyelonephritis syndrome) or in patients with vomiting, the antibiotics should be given parenterally.

In addition to the antibiotics, the patients should be encouraged to have a good oral fluid intake (in the absence of vomiting) and to void frequently. Every preadolescent female with a urinary tract infection should have a cellophane tape test for *Enterobius* infestation and treatment if infestation is present. Advice also should be given on vaginal and vulvar hygiene and the avoidance of irritants (such as perfumed soaps and bubble bath). Besides the initial and 48-hour urine cultures, follow-up cultures should be obtained several days after treatment is completed and monthly thereafter for the next 24 months to detect those patients who have recurrences.

Antibiotic sensitivity of the organism should guide antibiotic choice in persistent or recurrent urinary tract infections, especially those associated with urinary tract obstruction and after instrumentation. Sensitivities of previous infecting organisms may be helpful in selecting an effective antibiotic if one presumes reinfection; the definite choice of an antibiotic again depends on the results of the antibiotic sensitivities of the pretreatment culture. Children with recurrent urinary tract infections should be given chronic prophylactic therapy. Prophylaxis should be continued for at least 6 months with several intratreatment urine cultures. The drugs can be discontinued at the end of 6 months to determine if the problem of recurrence has resolved. Posttreatment cultures are again necessary to ensure the absence of recurrences in the symptom-free patient. The local measures in female patients continue to be important during and after this period of prophylaxis.

PSYCHOSOCIAL CONSIDERATIONS

The patient (if old enough to understand) and the parents should be advised of the overall treatment plan (including the follow-up cultures) at the very beginning. This should be done frankly but in a way that should not create undue anxiety. The necessity to complete the full course of antibiotics and the reasons for the long follow-up with cultures should be stressed. In addition, the patients and parents should know that urine cultures should be performed in the event of fevers for which there is no apparent origin.

REFERRAL

Although usually not needed, a urologist can be helpful in evaluating children with urinary tract infections and should be able to perform a complete urologic evaluation of the child, with a minimum of psychological stress. Many of the urologic abnormalities will require surgical procedures, and one can expect joint follow-up of such patients. Urologic assistance is vital in any child with a urinary diversion and a history of urinary tract infections. In addition, consultation with specialists in pediatric nephrology and infectious disease often are helpful with the patient who has persistent and recurrent infections and in whom urinary tract obstruction has been ruled out or corrected.

SUGGESTED READINGS

Bauchner H et al: Prevalence of bacteriuria in febrile children, Pediatr Infect Dis J 6:239, 1987.

Belman B: Urinary imaging in children, Pediatr Infect Dis J 8:548, 1989.

Hanson L: Prognostic indicators in childhood urinary infections, Kidney Int 21:659, 1982.

Marild S et al: Fever, bacteriuria and concomitant disease in children with urinary tract infection, Pediatr Infect Dis J 8:36, 1989.

266

Verruca*e* (Warts)

Donald P. Lookingbill

ETIOLOGY

Warts are virus-induced tumors of the skin.[2,4,5,7] The wart virus is a human papillomavirus[2,4] (HPV) that infects epidermal cells to cause focal epidermal proliferation, clinically expressed as a verrucous papule.

In recent years deoxyribonucleic acid (DNA) hybridization analysis has been used in identifying different types of human papillomaviruses. To date more than 50 types have been so characterized, and the number increases almost monthly. Specific DNA types have been associated with certain types of warts. For example, HPV type 1 is found in plantar warts, HPV type 2 in common warts, HPV types 6 and 11 in "benign" genital warts, and HPV types 16 and 18 in genital warts with malignant potential (e.g., cervical carcinoma). Thus HPV typing holds promise in helping to identify premalignant warts as well as sources for wart transmission.[8,11]

HISTORY

The wart virus is presumably inoculated into the skin from some external source, but neither the source nor the event of inoculation is usually elicitable. Frogs and toads have been unfairly incriminated as carriers.[9] It is reasonable, however, to ask about and search for warts on other areas of the body—for example, patients with warts on the lips frequently have them on the fingers. Since warts are transmissible, they may also be present in other family members.

In young infants, warts (including those in laryngeal and genital locations) are assumed to have been acquired from the mother's vaginal tract during delivery. *Genital warts in children raise the possibility of sexual abuse*.[3,8,10] If available, HPV typing may help determine if the warts were likely to have come from a genital site, as has been reported with HPV types 6, 11, and 16.[8] But with or without HPV typing, the history and physical examination in children with genital warts should include investigation for possible child abuse.[10] If abuse is suspected, consultation with an appropriate child protection resource should be obtained.

Patients with systemic defects in self-mediated immunity have a heightened susceptibility to warts, which are frequently recalcitrant to therapy.[1] Cellular immune responses in the skin have been shown to be impaired in atopic dermatitis, so that these patients have more difficulty with warts and other viral infections of the skin.

PHYSICAL FINDINGS

Warts vary in their clinical appearance, depending on their type and their location on the skin. The common wart, or verruca vulgaris, is familiar to us all as a superficial light-colored papule with a course, roughened surface. Warts are often studded with black specks, which many patients call "seeds" but which are actually small superficial dermal capillaries. Sometimes warts will be found in linear array, presumably a result of autoinoculation from scratching. (Fig. 266-1).

Not all warts appear as verrucous papules. The following variants may also occur: flat (planar) warts, plantar warts, periungual warts, and genital warts. These are described more fully below.

LABORATORY FINDINGS

The diagnosis is almost always made clinically. If there is doubt, a skin biopsy can provide histologic confirmation.

DIFFERENTIAL DIAGNOSIS

The distinctive clinical appearance of the common wart usually presents no problem in diagnosis. Epidermal nevi, which are epidermal hamartomas, may be confused with warts, but they are usually softer, more pigmented, more persistent, and much less common.

Flat (planar) warts appear as small, flesh-colored papules (Fig. 266-1). When located on the face, they are often confused with the closed comedones (whiteheads) seen in acne. On *very* close inspection, however, flat warts will be seen to have sharp borders and a finely verrucous surface, whereas closed comedones are smooth, dome-shaped lesions.

Plantar warts are so named because they appear on the plantar surface of the foot (Fig. 266-2). They are often confused with calluses and corns, although corns are much less common in children than are warts. Large plantar warts are often composed of confluent smaller ones, forming a mosaic wart, around which satellite lesions often occur. Additionally, plantar warts differ from corns by having a verrucous surface that interrupts the skin markings and is often punctuated with black specks. Sometimes the two entities can only be distinguished by paring down the surface, wherein the wart tissue

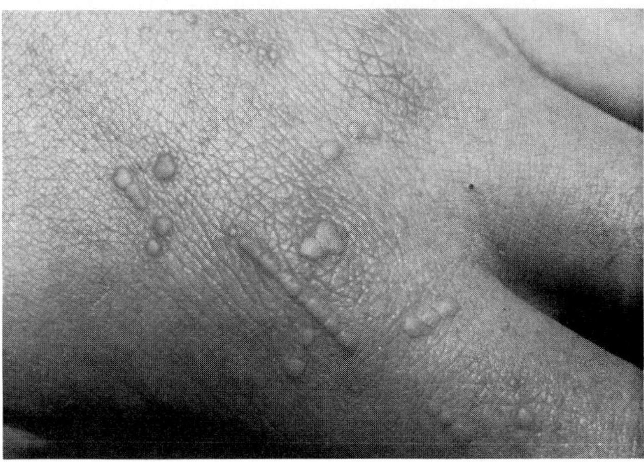

Fig. 266-1 Flat warts. The streaks of warts are due to autoinoculation from scratching. When smaller and located on the face, flat warts may be confused with comedones.

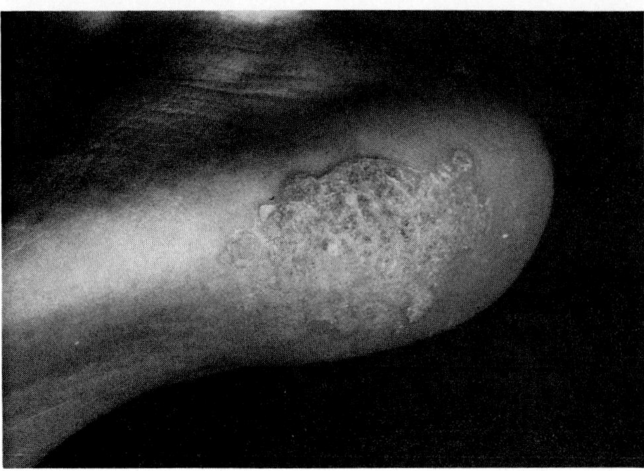

Fig. 266-2 Mosaic plantar wart showing roughened surface punctuated with black specks.

continues to have a roughened texture and a corn is smooth. A corn also becomes smaller in diameter as it is pared; a wart does not.

Periungual warts occurring around the nail fold should not cause diagnostic difficulty. Warts under the free edge of the nail can, however, cause the nail plate to separate from the nail bed and may be confused with fungal infection. On close inspection, the verrucous nature of the wart can usually be appreciated.

Genital warts (condyloma acuminata) are sometimes but not always acquired by sexual contact.[3,5,8,10] They are usually easily identified as verrucous papules (Fig. 266-3), but sometimes they are small and/or flat and therefore more difficult to see. In this situation, the acetowhitening technique can aid in the diagnosis. A compress of 5% acetic acid is applied for several minutes to the suspected area, which then is reexamined, under magnification if desired. With this technique, warty tissue turns white and is thus more easily visualized.

Genital warts may be confused with the less common condyloma lata, a skin lesion found in secondary syphilis. In general, condyloma acuminata are drier and usually more verrucous than condyloma lata, which are flat and moist. If there is doubt, a serologic test for syphilis should settle the issue.

PSYCHOSOCIAL CONSIDERATIONS

Among schoolchildren, warts often serve as a focus for teasing and insensitive remarks. Consequently, when children ask that their warts be treated, they usually do so because of social pressure. Successful therapy provides patients with the opportunity to feel better about themselves and their appearance.

As previously noted, in children with genital warts, the possibility of child abuse needs to be considered and investigated.

MANAGEMENT

Over the years a wide variety of treatments have been recommended, including some particularly interesting approaches, such as that used by Mark Twain's Tom Sawyer. Therapies such as these probably "worked" because most warts eventually undergo spontaneous regression. This fact must be kept in mind when we credit our therapy for a successful result. Nonetheless, when a patient requests wart treatment, we are usually inclined to oblige. But because we still lack a specific antiviral medication for warts, we continue to rely on nonspecific destructive techniques for therapy, of which the following are most commonly used.

Cryotherapy

Tissue is frozen by liquid nitrogen applied either by swab or by a more sophisticated system. The freezing should extend beyond the wart to include a 1 to 2 mm rim of normal skin. For enhanced tissue destruction, the wart may be refrozen after the initial thaw. The patient must be advised that the frozen area will be sore for several days, that a blister may form, and that it will usually take several weeks for the wart to turn dark and "drop off." This is a favorite office therapy for common warts. For small warts, a single treatment is often successful, but large warts frequently need to be refrozen at about 3-week intervals. Scars may result but are uncommon. Hypopigmentation of the skin may also occur. In freezing warts on the fingers, care must be taken not to freeze too deeply, because underlying structures such as digital nerves can be damaged.

Electrodesiccation and Laser Therapy

Electrodesiccation of a wart can be preceded or followed by curettage. One advantage of this technique is that the patient leaves the office without visible evidence of the wart, although

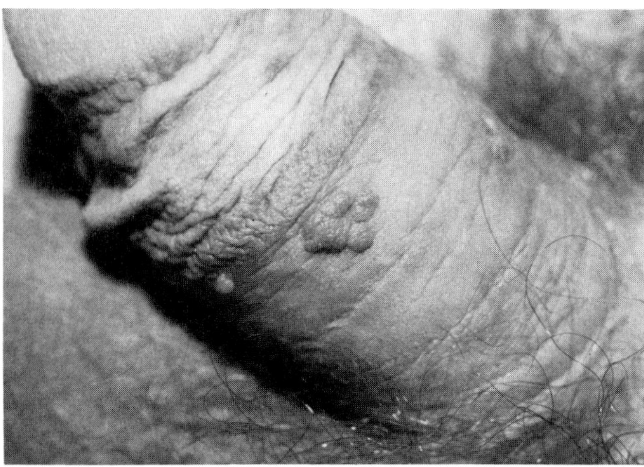

Fig. 266-3 Condyloma acuminata, shown here as verrucous papules on the penis.

the cure rate is probably no higher than with cryotherapy. Disadvantages are that the procedure must be preceded by an injection of a local anesthetic and scarring is more likely to occur. Carbon dioxide laser therapy destroys warts via an expensive, "space-age" method, which for most cases provides only a minimal advantage over electrodesiccation.

Acid Therapy

Acid therapy is slower and involves more patient participation, but it is less immediately painful and is least likely to scar. A variety of acids are available for treating warts. A convenient outpatient medication includes a combination of salicylic acid and lactic acid in a flexible collodion base (Duofilm and Viranol). The collodion dries rapidly to prevent spread of the acid onto surrounding skin. The patient is instructed to apply the medication to the surface of the wart at bedtime and to cover the area with a bandage. At the end of each week, superficial necrotic tissue should be pared. This can usually be done at home either with a sharp blade or emery board. Because of the minimal discomfort involved in this approach, it is useful with multiple warts and those in very young children.

Plantar warts often require a stronger acid, such as a 40% salicylic acid plaster. These can be bought "over the counter," but the patient needs instruction in application. A piece of plaster the size of the wart is cut, and after stripping the backing, the medicated side is applied to the wart and held in place with the tape. The plaster is changed every 24 hours and the macerated wart pared weekly, as described above.

Flat warts are often successfully treated with vitamin A acid (Retin A), which probably acts as a "peeling" agent in this situation. Retin A gel or liquid is applied nightly to the entire affected area. Irritation may occur, necessitating less frequent use.

These home acid therapies usually require a minimum of a month of continuous use to be effective. If no progress has been made after several months, other treatments should be considered.

All these treatments are nonspecific and none is foolproof. Sometimes different modalities are used in sequence. It must be remembered that warts commonly regress spontaneously, although the time required for this is enormously variable. In some patients therapy may only serve to amuse the patient while nature takes its course; in others, perhaps the destructive techniques initiate an inflammatory reaction, exposing the wart viral antigen to the body's immune system, which then finally rejects the wart. This may explain the phenomenon observed by some, wherein by "treating the mother wart, the baby goes away." In any event, whenever we treat warts, we must remember to guard against doing harm by being overzealous. Accordingly, surgical excision should usually be discouraged, and radiotherapy is contraindicated.

COMPLICATIONS

The major complications of warts are those produced by overzealous therapy, resulting in short-term discomfort or long-term scarring. One must balance the risk of a wart, which is usually temporary, against a scar, which is usually lifelong, may be unsightly, and sometimes is tender, particularly if present on a pressure-bearing surface such as the sole of the foot.

PROGNOSIS

As mentioned, most warts eventually involute spontaneously, probably via immunologic rejection.[1] Because the time required for this is greatly variable, it is impossible to predict for an individual patient when this might occur. The goal of therapy, then, is to shorten the time it takes for the wart to disappear. The therapies outlined above result in clearing in the majority of cases, but patients with resistant, persistent warts will continue to be plagued. It is especially for these patients that we need more specific therapy.

REFERENCES

1. Adler A and Safai B: Immunity in wart resolution, J Am Acad Dermatol 1:305, 1979.
2. Androphy EJ: Human papillomavirus: current concepts, Arch Dermatol 125:683, 1989.
3. Bender ME: New concepts of condyloma acuminata in children, Arch Dermatol 122:1121, 1986.
4. Birkett DA: Warts and their management, Practitioner 226:1251, 1982.
5. DeJong AR, Weiss JC, and Brent RL: Condyloma acuminata in children, Am J Dis Child 136:704, 1982.
6. Lutzner MA: The human papilloma virus, Arch Dermatol 119:631, 1983.
7. Rees RB: Warts—a clinician's view, Cutis 28:175, 1981.
8. Rock B et al: Genital tract papillomavirus infection in children, Arch Dermatol 122:1129, 1986.
9. Ross MS: Warts in the medical folklore of Europe, Int J Dermatol 18:505, 1979.
10. Schachner L and Hankin DE: Assessing child abuse in childhood condyloma acuminatum, J Am Acad Dermatol 12:157, 1985.
11. von Krogh G, Syrjanen SM, and Syrjanen KJ: Advantage of human papillomavirus typing in the clinical evaluation of genitoanal warts: experience with the in situ deoxyribonucleic acid hybridization technique applied on paraffin sections, J Am Acad Dermatol 18:495, 1988.

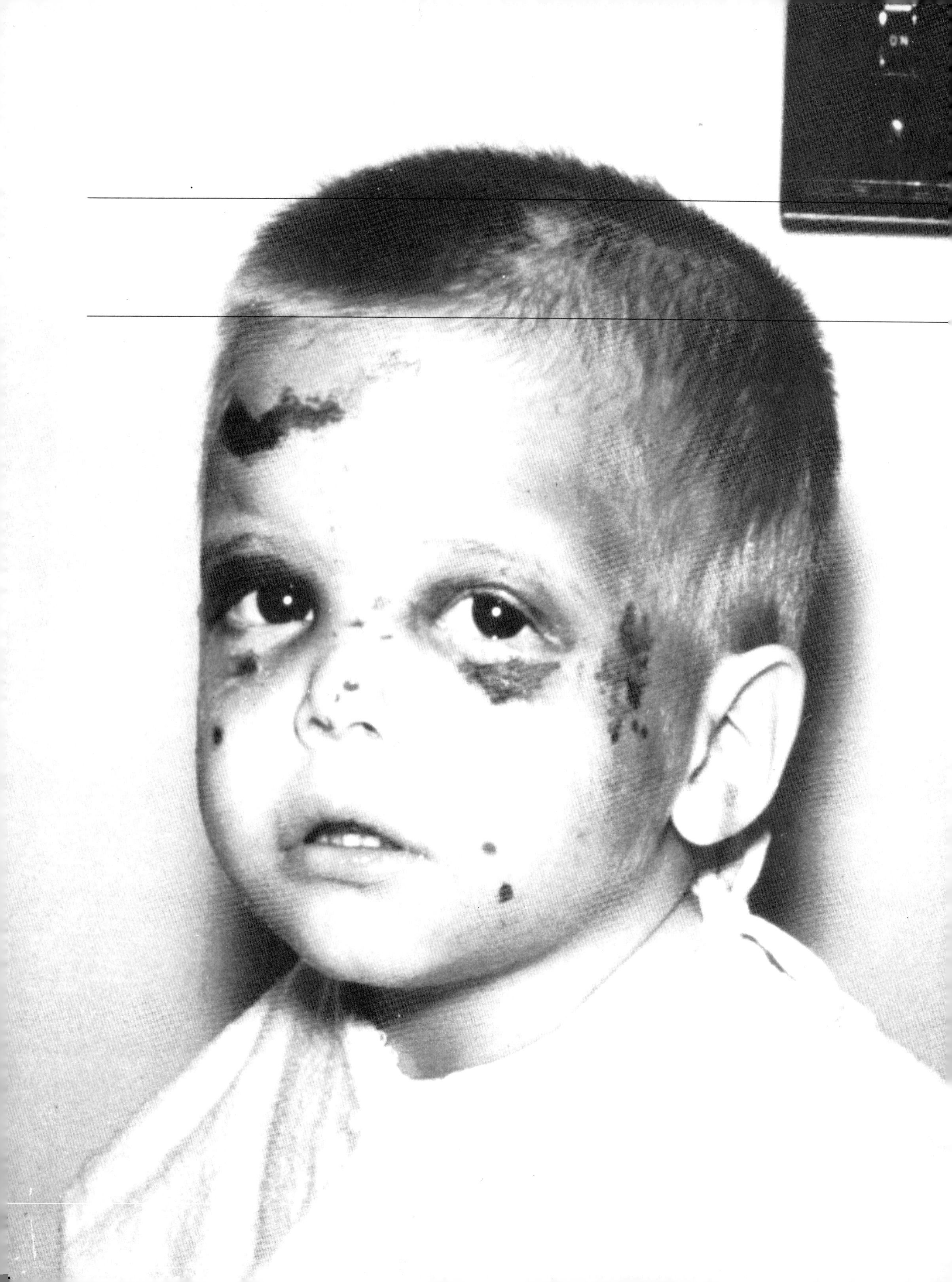
ON

Part Nine

Critical Situations

267

Airway Obstruction

Helen W. Karl

An infant or child with acute upper airway obstruction presents a major challenge to the skills of all those involved in his or her care. The smaller the child, the more the size and shape of the airway predispose him or her to upper airway obstruction. With complete obstruction and death an ever-present possibility, the patient's survival depends on accurate and rapid assessment of the degree of respiratory distress and the approximate level of the obstruction. Appropriate and careful management throughout the hospital course is necessary to ensure a satisfactory outcome.

Stridor, the sound produced by air flow during respiration through a partially obstructed upper airway, was the cause of 1.3% of pediatric medical admissions in one large study.[1] Of 250 children admitted with stridor, 74% were found to have infectious croup, whereas 16% had a congenital anomaly of the airway, 4% had acute epiglottitis, 0.4% had aspirated a foreign body (8 others had foreign body aspiration with symptoms other than stridor), and the remainder suffered from a variety of other problems. Foreign body aspiration is the second leading cause of accidental death at home in children younger than 6 years old[21] and accounted for more than 600 deaths in 1980.[12]

ASSESSMENT OF THE THREAT TO SURVIVAL

Progressive hypoxemia is the cause of brain damage and death in patients with acute upper airway obstruction.[7,8] Because brain damage begins to occur after 3 minutes of complete airway obstruction, the immediate concern of the clinician who first sees the patient must be to provide oxygen and then to assess rapidly the severity of respiratory distress. In acute situations the history and physical examination are the major diagnostic tools. Upsetting the child or delaying treatment to obtain arterial blood gas levels, roentgenograms, and other studies often is hazardous.

HISTORY AND PHYSICAL EXAMINATION

The clinician should perform most of the physical examination at a distance, so as to disturb the child only minimally, thereby preventing the increases in airway obstruction and oxygen consumption produced by crying; the child's condition will not be worsened by use of this approach, and the observations will be more reliable.[4] The parent should be asked to remove the child's shirt to facilitate more rapid assessment of general appearance. Simultaneously, the examiner can obtain a brief history of the onset and symptoms of obstruction, as well as of other major medical problems. The patient then may be approached gently to auscultate the chest and to estimate heart rate and temperature. The following abridged alphabet provides a helpful mnemonic of the salient features in the physical examination:

A. Appearance and accessory muscles
B. Breath sounds
C. Consciousness, color, and cough
D. Drooling
P. Posture
Q. Quality of voice
R. Retractions and flaring
S. Stridor
T. Temperature, tachycardia, and tachypnea

A variety of scoring systems have been developed to help gauge the degree of upper airway obstruction; the use of such a system will help to focus observation and to provide a guide to the effects of therapy (Table 267-1). It is important to note that although stridor usually increases as airway obstruction

Table 267-1 *Scoring System for Upper Airway Obstruction**

	SCORE		
SIGNS	0	1	2
Stridor	None	Inspiratory	Inspiratory and expiratory
Cough	None	Hoarse cry	Bark
Retractions and nasal flaring	None	Flaring and suprasternal retractions	As in 1 plus subcostal and intercostal retractions
Cyanosis	None	In air	In 40% oxygen
Inspiratory breath sounds	Normal	Harsh with wheezing or rhonchi	Delayed

From Downes JL and Goldberg AT: Airway management, mechanical ventilation and cardiopulmonary resuscitation. In Scarpelli EM, Auld PAM, and Goldman HS, editors: Pulmonary disease of the fetus, newborn and child, Philadelphia, 1978, Lea & Febiger.
*A score of 4 or more indicates significant airway obstruction.

Table 267-2 *Clinical Features of Acute Upper Airway Disorders**

CLINICAL FEATURE	SUPRAGLOTTIC DISORDERS	SUBGLOTTIC DISORDERS
Stridor	Quiet and wet	Loud
Voice alteration	Muffled	Hoarse
Dysphagia	+*	−
Postural preference†	+	−
Barking cough	−	+ Especially with croup
Fever	+	+ Usually with croup
Toxicity	+	−
Trismus	+ Usually with peritonsillar abscess	−
Facial edema	−	+ Usually with angioedema

From Davis, HW, et al.: Acute upper airway obstruction: croup and epiglottitis, Pediatr Clin North Am 28:860, 1981.

*+, Present; −, absent.

†In epiglottitis the patient characteristically sits bolt upright, with neck extended and head held forward: with retropharyngeal abscess, the child often adopts an opisthotonic posture; with peritonsillar abscess the patient may tilt his head toward the affected side.

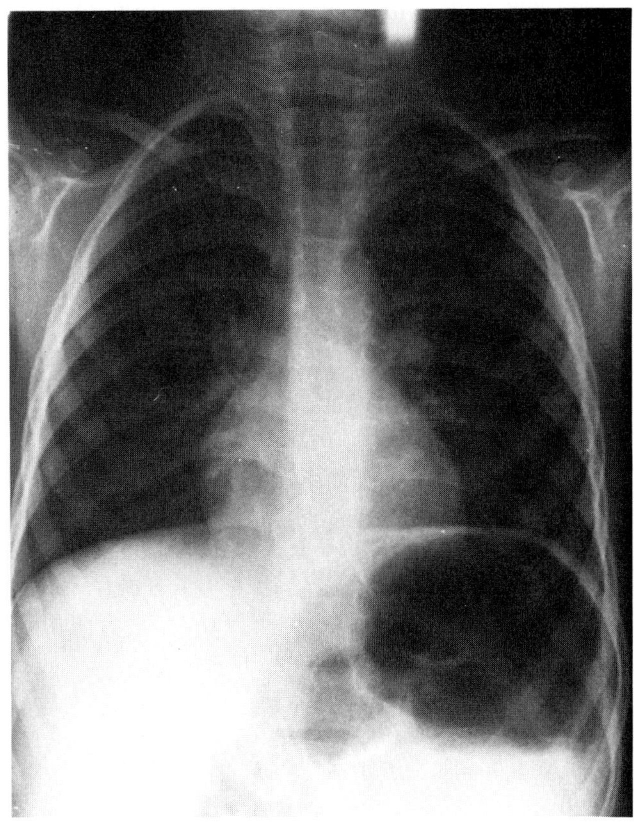

Fig. 267-1 "Steeple sign": subglottic narrowing of the tracheal air shadow seen in patients with croup.

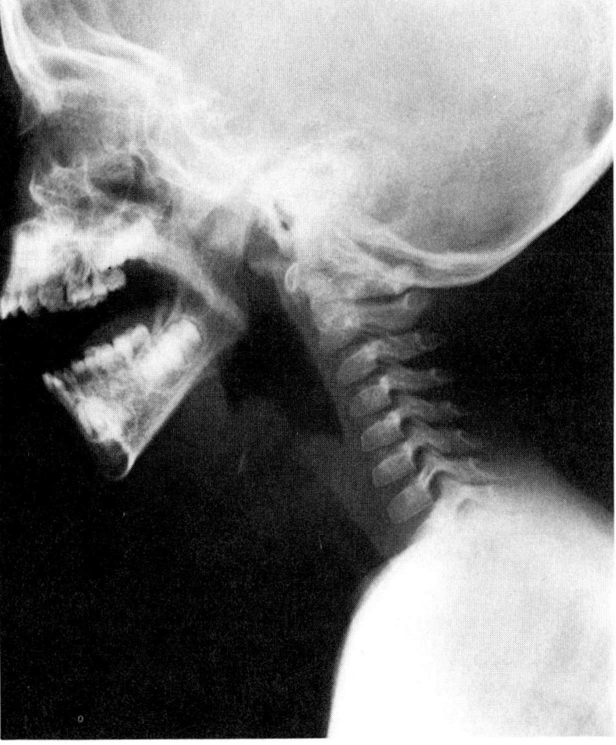

Fig. 267-2 Acute panglottitis ("epiglottitis"). Fullness of the epiglottis and aryepiglottic folds is specific; hypopharyngeal distention is seen in any form of severe airway obstruction.

worsens, in children with extreme respiratory distress and delayed inspiratory breath sounds, stridor and cough actually may be decreased because of the small tidal volumes achieved. A diagnosis of cyanosis, which is a sign of relatively severe hypoxemia ($PaO_2 \sim 40$ mm Hg), is based on the clinical presence of at least 5 g of unsaturated hemoglobin per deciliter of blood. Pulse oximetry now is considered to be the standard of care for patients at risk for hypoxia.[15] Earlier, although less specific, indicators of hypoxemia include restlessness, tachypnea, and tachycardia.[4]

The level at which the airway is obstructed is an additional factor in determining the threat to the patient's survival; the patient's age and history will guide the diagnosis. Although infectious croup is by far the most common cause for stridor, other appropriate possibilities must be kept in mind, because their natural histories may vary widely. Stridor, retractions, tachypnea, and tachycardia are seen in all patients with acute upper airway obstruction, but many other clinical features vary with the cause of obstruction and provide clues to its level. As a guide to management, Davis and colleagues[4] have categorized the major causes of airway obstruction (Table 267-2): those involving supraglottic structures (severe tonsillitis with adenoid enlargement, peritonsillar and retropharyngeal abscesses, epiglottitis) and those affecting areas below the larynx (croup, foreign body aspiration, angioedema).

CLINICAL PRESENTATION, WORKUP, AND DIAGNOSIS

The most common difficulty in diagnosis occurs in the preschool child with a history of progressive respiratory difficulty. The young child who has had an upper respiratory tract infection over the last several days, with the subsequent development of stridor, barking cough, and mild temperature elevation, probably has viral croup. The slightly older child who complains of an acute onset of sore throat, high fever, muffled voice, unwillingness to swallow, and rapidly progressive respiratory distress more likely has acute bacterial epiglottitis. In practice, many children have some combination of these features or, worse, a child with a cold may have aspirated a toy unobserved, and a definitive diagnosis may need to await radiographic evaluation or examination under anesthesia.

Radiologic examinations of the neck may be useful in a moderately ill child of any age with acute upper airway obstruction. On the other hand, even if these roentgenograms are available, diagnosis may not be clear-cut, and the delay in obtaining these studies may be lethal if the child is severely ill.[2,7] An anteroposterior roentgenogram of the chest and neck may show narrowing of the tracheal air shadow in the subglottic area ("steeple" or "hourglass" sign of the patient with croup—Fig. 267-1), whereas, in acute epiglottitis, the inspiratory lateral roentgenogram of the neck is likely to display a fullness of the epiglottis and aryepiglottic folds (Fig. 267-2). A radiopaque foreign body also may be localized. Distention of the hypopharynx will be seen in the lateral neck roentgenogram in a patient with a significant airway obstruction from any cause. A barium swallow and fluoroscopic examination of the neck may be particularly helpful in evaluating congenital stridor.[20]

Blood sampling is of low priority in a child with airway obstruction, inasmuch as the crying elicited by sampling increases both the metabolic rate and the difficulty of breathing through the obstructed airway. A mild lymphocytosis may be expected in croup, whereas an elevation of the polymorphonuclear leukocyte count occurs in patients with epiglottitis. Many children with croup or epiglottitis have hypoxemia out of proportion to or in the absence of hypercapnia.[3] Blood for culture should be obtained before antibiotic therapy for epiglottitis is begun, because the organism, usually *Haemophilus influenzae* type b, more often is isolated from the blood than from the larynx or trachea.[2,7] This is easily performed while the child is anesthetized for endoscopic examination and intubation.

The differential diagnosis[18,20] can be roughly categorized according to the patient's age at the time of presentation (see the accompanying box). The larynx should be examined immediately only when air exchange is inadequate; otherwise, controlled endoscopic examination should be performed in the operating room.[20]

MANAGEMENT

A child with significant airway obstruction from any cause, as well as anyone suspected of having a supraglottic disorder, foreign body aspiration, or airway injury, should be hospitalized immediately, preferably in a pediatric intensive care unit staffed by a health care team experienced in dealing with these problems in children. If these facilities are not readily available, it may be preferable to stabilize the child in the nearest hospital and then transfer him or her to a larger center. Many centers now have multidisciplinary teams for the management of airway problems in children. Contacting a pediatrician or emergency room physician in advance of the child's arrival at the center will help to ensure the presence of an anesthesiologist and endoscopist in the emergency room.

The child with a significant airway obstruction should be transported by ambulance and should continuously receive oxygen. In addition, he or she must be accompanied at all times in the hospital and during transport by a parent and by the available person most skilled in airway management. For example, the primary care physician should accompany the child until responsibility can be transferred directly to the anesthesiologist. Emergency airway equipment always must be immediately available.

Initial Stabilization

Any child with significant airway obstruction—for example, a score of more than 4 on initial inspection (Table 267-1)—should be monitored with a pulse oximeter and receive high inspired oxygen concentrations during evaluation and initial therapy. Allowing the child or parent to hold the oxygen mask will make this unfamiliar equipment less frightening. The child should maintain that position that is most comfortable; most children with an obstructed airway will prefer to sit up. No one with a significant airway obstruction should be allowed to eat or drink, because general anesthesia may be required for intubation or endoscopic examination and because the presence of additional fluid or food in the stomach will increase the risk of aspiration pneumonitis. (Whether the child will drink is not a reliable test for the presence of epiglottitis.)

If croup is a likely cause of the obstruction, racemic epinephrine (2.25%, 0.5 ml in 5 ml of normal saline) or L-epinephrine (0.1%, 5 ml in 5 ml of normal saline) may be nebulized and administered in oxygen via face mask. This should be given only if it does not delay further necessary diagnostic and therapeutic maneuvers and does not unduly upset the child. Nebulized epinephrine usually will produce a dramatic, although often temporary, improvement in the symptoms of patients with croup. Despite this rapid improvement, patients who have received nebulized epinephrine should be hospitalized and observed for "rebound" respiratory distress. Although this drug will be of little value in patients who have acute epiglottitis or in those who have aspirated a foreign body, epinephrine is unlikely to harm them, provided it does not delay further care. The major risks of epinephrine

Differential Diagnosis of Airway Obstruction According to Age

NEWBORN

1. Choanal atresia
   a. Complete obstruction during quiet breathing
   b. Normal cry
2. Craniofacial dysmorphism: Pierre Robin and Treacher Collins syndromes
3. Macroglossia: Beckwith-Wiedemann syndrome, congenital hypothyroidism, glycogen storage diseases, Down syndrome, diffuse muscular hypertrophy, or tumors
4. Congenital laryngeal web
   a. Part of a spectrum that includes laryngeal atresia
   b. Varying degrees of respiratory distress
   c. Usually an abnormal cry
   d. May need forced tracheal intubation in the delivery room to allow survival
5. Vocal cord paralysis
   a. May be bilateral (~30%) or unilateral
   b. Diagnosed in 21% of children with stridor in the first year of life in one study[20]
   c. May be associated with birth trauma
   d. Associated with neurologic diseases and increased intracranial pressure
   e. Abnormal cry and feeding problems
6. Congenital tracheal anomalies
   a. May be malacic or stenotic
   b. Rare
   c. Stenosis usually visible on neck and chest roentgenograms; confirm by endoscopy
   d. Therapy very difficult
7. Birth trauma
   a. Difficult delivery may result in dislocation of laryngeal cartilages
   b. Usually improves spontaneously, but short-term intubation may be required

FIRST FEW DAYS OF LIFE

1. Laryngotracheoesophageal cleft
   a. Present in 1 of 63 infants with stridor in one study[20]
   b. Usual initial symptom is respiratory distress while feeding; aspiration a frequent complication
   c. Abnormal cry
   d. Diagnosis by laryngoscopy and esophagoscopy
2. Vocal cord paralysis: see section on newborns
3. Congenital cysts and laryngoceles
   a. Present in 4 of 63 infants with stridor in one study[20]
   b. May also cause feeding difficulties
   c. Diagnosis by endoscopy
4. Vascular rings and slings
   a. Anomalous segments of embryonic aortic arch causing external compression of trachea, esophagus, or both
   b. Present in 11% of infants with stridor in one study[20]
   c. Stridor, cough, respiratory difficulties with feeding; may have recurrent URI
   d. Diagnosis by contrast esophagography and endoscopy
5. Congenital tracheal anomalies: see section on newborns
6. Reflex laryngospasm
   a. Abnormal vagal reflex postulated
   b. Diagnosis by exclusion of anatomic problems by roentgenography and endoscopy
   c. Anticholinergics and gavage feedings may help symptoms

FIRST FEW MONTHS OF LIFE

1. Laryngomalacia
   a. Immature, "floppy" larynx
   b. Present in 14% of infants with stridor in one study[20]
   c. May be associated with feeding problems, respiratory distress, and frequent respiratory tract infections
   d. Diagnosis by endoscopy
   e. Usually improves with no specific therapy
2. Congenital subglottic stenosis
   a. A symmetric subglottic narrowing that may not cause airway obstruction until a superimposed URI causes some mucosal edema

URI, Upper respiratory infection.

Continued.

inhalation are ventricular arrhythmias, tachycardia (see Chapters 114 and 279), and hypertension; arrhythmias become increasingly likely as hypoxia and hypercapnia worsen.

Most children with tracheobronchial foreign bodies are not in respiratory distress by the time they arrive in the hospital: only 3 of 68 children in one series required emergency endoscopy.[19] A child who has aspirated a foreign body and who can speak or cough requires oxygen therapy, close observation, and referral for urgent removal under controlled conditions. In the very rare instance in which the patient is moribund, back blows, chest thrusts, or Heimlich abdominal thrusts may be performed if foreign body aspiration is deemed likely. If these are not indicated or are unsuccessful, an emergency cricothyrotomy with insertion of an endotracheal tube must be carried out.[5,11-13,21] (See discussion of aspiration accidents in Chapters 21 and 203.)

Motor vehicle accidents, strangulation injuries, and blows to the neck all may cause significant blunt trauma to the

Differential Diagnosis of Airway Obstruction According to Age—cont'd

   b. Suspect in a child younger than 6 months of age with "croup"
   c. Present in 19% of infants with stridor in one study[20]
   d. Diagnosis by endoscopy
   e. May be "outgrown"
   f. May require tracheostomy followed by surgical reconstruction or repeated dilations
3. Subglottic hemangioma
   a. Another cause of "croup" in a child younger than 6 months old
   b. Present in 1 of 63 infants with stridor in one study[20]
   c. May be associated with cutaneous hemangiomas, coagulopathy, thrombocytopenia
   d. Diagnosis: subglottic soft tissue mass seen on lateral neck roentgenogram; confirm by endoscopy
   e. Usually regresses spontaneously after 1 year of age; steroids often improve symptoms until regression occurs
   f. Artificial airway may be required
4. Retropharyngeal abscess
   a. Usually caused by beta-hemolytic streptococcal lymph nodes
   b. Relatively rare; usually occurs in children younger than 3 years
   c. High fever, difficulty swallowing, and respiratory distress after a preceding URI
   d. Diagnosis: by direct visualization in operating room; red bulge seen in posterior nasopharynx
   e. Treatment: drainage; may require tracheostomy
5. Foreign body aspiration: see section on toddlers
6. External or internal trauma: see section on school-aged children and older

TODDLER

1. Viral croup (laryngotracheobronchitis)
   a. Subglottic edema caused by parainfluenza or influenza virus
   b. By far the most common cause of airway obstruction in children
   c. Loud stridor and barking cough
   d. Usually begins at night after preceding URI
   e. Unusual in children younger than 3 months or older than 4 years; presence of a congenital anomaly should be considered in patients younger than 6 months old
   f. Treatment: see text below
2. Membranous laryngotracheobronchitis[6,16,22]
   a. Also called bacterial tracheitis, pseudomembranous croup
   b. Appears to have increased in frequency over the last few years
   c. History similar to that for croup, but progressive toxicity occurs
   d. Most also have evidence of pneumonia
   e. Lateral neck roentgenograms show subglottic narrowing; may see mucosal irregularities that can mimic a foreign body
   f. Endoscopy: normal supraglottic structures; subglottic narrowing; copious purulent secretions or loosely attached membrane; may require repeat endoscopy to remove membranes
   g. *Staphylococcus aureus* usually is cultured from secretions
   h. Treatment: early endotracheal intubation, vigorous humidification and suctioning, appropriate antibiotics; more likely than other infectious processes to require tracheostomy because of thick secretions
3. Foreign body aspiration
   a. Variable presentation depending on level of obstruction[8]; any child with stridor, croupy cough, respiratory distress, hemoptysis, wheezing, or choking should arouse suspicion of foreign body aspiration
   b. History and physical may be negative
   c. Radiologic and fluoroscopic studies are helpful
   d. The object may change position; injudicious attempts to remove it may cause asphyxia
4. Acute spasmodic laryngitis
   a. Diagnosed in 3% of children with stridor in one study[1]

Continued.

airway. Any patient who exhibits respiratory distress, a change in voice, subcutaneous emphysema, or hemoptysis after such an injury must be evaluated for laryngeal or tracheal disruption. A surgeon with experience in pediatric tracheostomy and bronchoscopy must be called immediately. The patient must be treated as though he or she has fractured the cervical spine until this associated injury has been ruled out. Laryngoscopy alone is not adequate for making the diagnosis. Endotracheal intubation through the injured area may not be possible or may cause further trauma. A tracheostomy under controlled conditions in the operating room is the safest way to manage the airway before definitive therapy for these injuries has been instituted.[23]

Definitive Therapy

Definitive therapy of viral croup, epiglottitis, and aspirated foreign body is very different. Most patients with croup (see

***Differential Diagnosis of Airway Obstruction According to Age**—cont'd*

b. Recurrent nocturnal awakening with inspiratory stridor and croupy cough
c. Afebrile
d. May be associated with "nervousness" and allergies
e. Diagnosis: by history; laryngoscopy, if done, shows "watery" edema, no inflammation
f. Supportive therapy

5. External trauma; see section on school-aged children and older
6. Thermal and chemical trauma: see section on school-aged children and older
7. Laryngeal papillomatosis
   a. Present in 2% of children with stridor in one study[18]
   b. Multiple, recurrent rough-surfaced laryngeal tumors thought to be viral in origin
   c. Hoarseness and respiratory distress progressing over weeks
   d. Diagnosis by direct laryngoscopy
   e. Surgical excision required; immunologic therapy may help
   f. Most children outgrow this after puberty
8. Diphtheria: see section on school-aged children and older

CHILD OF SCHOOL AGE AND OLDER

1. Hereditary angioneurotic edema
   a. Sudden onset after eating, bee sting, or environmental exposure
   b. Often a family history
   c. Associated rash
   d. Intubation may be very difficult because of grossly swollen larynx
   e. Early airway support; nebulized or parenteral epinephrine may be helpful, but emergency tracheostomy may be necessary
2. External trauma[23]
   a. Blunt or penetrating neck trauma may dislocate laryngeal cartilages, produce a hematoma or edema that compresses the trachea, or fracture the larynx
   b. Any neck bruises, change in voice, or subcutaneous emphysema following trauma must be investigated immediately
   c. Endotracheal intubation relatively contraindicated
   d. Diagnosis by radiology, bronchoscopy, or surgical exploration
   e. May require artificial airway and/or surgical correction
3. Thermal and chemical trauma
   a. Ingestion of corrosive substances and inhalation of smoke or chemical fumes may produce laryngeal and tracheal edema
   b. Associated pulmonary problems are common
   c. Must be considered after any fire in a closed space
   d. Inhaled nebulized epinephrine and steroids may be helpful
4. Acute epiglottitis or supraglottitis
   a. *H. influenzae* type B infection of epiglottis, aryepiglottic folds, arytenoids, and/or uvula
   b. Diagnosed in 4% of children with stridor in one study[1]
   c. May occur at any age, including adulthood, but is most common between 2 and 7 years
   d. Rapid onset of high fever, dysphagia, and respiratory distress in a previously well child
   e. Drooling in the absence of spontaneous cough is particularly likely[7,17]
   f. Treatment: see text, p. 1564-1566.
5. Peritonsillar abscess
   a. Usually in older children
   b. Sudden increase in temperature and unilateral throat pain after an episode of tonsillitis
   c. Diagnosis and therapy by surgery
6. Diphtheria
   a. Rare infection, but still occurs in unimmunized children
   b. Gradual onset of hoarseness and respiratory distress after several days of URI
   c. Visualization of gray membrane in pharynx; confirm by culture
   d. Diphtheria antitoxin and antibiotics required for treatment
   e. Airway support as needed

Chapter 269) respond to supportive medical treatment ranging from the coolness of damp night air to inhalation of epinephrine every 30 minutes, an oxygen and mist tent, systemic hydration, and observation in an intensive care unit. The use of steroids remains controversial.[2,7] Moreover, 3% to 6% of patients with croup require the airway support of an endotracheal tube or tracheostomy for progressive fatigue despite optimal medical management. A decreasing response to epinephrine or the development of hyperpyrexia and toxicity may be taken as evidence of bacterial superinfection (usually by *Staphylococcus aureus*).[6,16,22] Instrumentation of the airway in viral croup is performed as infrequently as possible, inasmuch as manipulation of this narrow and inflamed area produces a higher incidence of postextubation complications[8]; however, an endotracheal tube or tracheostomy is almost always required if the child has membranous laryngotracheobronchitis.[6,16,22] Helium rather than air has been used as a carrier gas for oxygen (Heliox) to decrease the work of breathing in patients with critical upper airway narrowing after intubation or from viral croup; placement of an artificial airway may thus be avoided.[9] It is important to note, however, that increasing the helium concentration in the mixture requires a decrease in the oxygen concentration; continuous oxygen saturation monitoring is helpful in determining an appropriate combination. Heliox is not a therapy in itself; it is only a way to relieve acute symptoms and "buy time" until definitive therapy is effective.

The optimal treatment in all cases of acute epiglottitis is to secure the child's airway either by nasotracheal intubation or, increasingly infrequently, by tracheostomy.[7,8] Inspection and intubation are carried out in the operating room with the patient under general anesthesia and an endoscopist standing by, fully prepared to perform either rigid bronchoscopy or tracheostomy, should intubation not be possible. The endotracheal tube is left in place for 24 to 48 hours until parenteral antibiotics effective against *H. influenzae* have controlled the infection. Ampicillin (200 mg/kg/day) and, because of the emergence of ampicillin-resistant strains, chloramphenicol (100 mg/kg/day) are both used until the antibiotic sensitivity of the organism is known.[2]

Similarly, foreign body removal should be undertaken only after institution of deep general anesthesia; excellent communication between well-trained anesthesiologists and endoscopists is required for this hazardous procedure.[10] After removal of the object, intubation is initiated in preparation for the child's emergence from anesthesia; extubation may take place when the patient awakens or, if significant trauma to the airway has occurred, after a variable period of time postoperatively. Additional supportive measures include the administration of humidified oxygen, close observation, and perhaps inhaled nebulized epinephrine, steroids, and Heliox.

Further Care

After the diagnosis has been made and appropriate therapy begun, many things still must be done. A child whose life depends on the patency and stability of a nasotracheal tube or newly created tracheostomy requires the constant attention of a nurse experienced in pediatric intensive care. A physician able to replace these devices must be immediately available. The child needs humidified oxygen and systemic hydration to keep secretions moist, as well as frequent suctioning (with use of sterile technique) to prevent obstruction of the tube. A program of chest physical therapy is helpful in preventing secondary pulmonary problems in those patients who are unable to cough effectively.[8] If airway obstruction has been severe, pulmonary edema may be seen after relief and observation, even in children with no underlying heart or lung disease.[14]

To minimize the incidence and severity of complications such as infection and subglottic stenosis, any artificial tracheal airway should be removed as soon as possible. The duration of intubation very much depends on the cause of the obstruction. For example, most patients with epiglottitis require approximately 48 hours of airway support, those with croup require 5 to 6 days, and some with congenital anomalies may have tracheostomies for years at home. Before extubation is attempted in one who has needed short-term support, the patient should be alert, be afebrile for 24 hours, and have air leaking around the tube at a lung inflating pressure lower than that measured at the time of intubation.

After extubation, the patient should not be allowed to eat or drink for at least 6 hours or until once again able to talk and cough well. He or she should continue to be watched closely during the immediate postextubation period, as obstruction may recur or postextubation "croup" develop. Inhaled nebulized epinephrine, Heliox, and, perhaps, steroids are useful in this setting, but reintubation may be required.

The cooperation of well-trained and careful pediatricians, anesthesiologists, endoscopists, and nurses is required for optimal care of the infant or child with acute upper airway obstruction. The risks are great, but so is the satisfaction in seeing a healthy child return home.

Iatrogenic Dangers

1. *Do not make the situation worse.* Everything possible must be done to avoid upsetting the child. Crying caused by overzealous examination, laboratory studies, separation from parents, or the enforcement of a supine position increases the degree of obstruction and the rate of oxygen consumption. In acute epiglottitis, for instance, it is possible to precipitate complete airway obstruction or severe bradycardia by attempting to examine the pharynx[13]; a quick look to see if the patient has epiglottitis[22] can be dangerous. If the child has aspirated a foreign body and has partial airway obstruction, probing the mouth or performing air-flow maneuvers may produce complete obstruction.
2. *Do not underestimate the patient's distress.*
3. *Do not leave the patient unattended by skilled personnel.* Airway obstruction, particularly when it is caused by acute epiglottitis or aspiration of a foreign body, may rapidly become worse; a parent or the radiology technician will not be able to provide adequate care.

REFERENCES

1. Arthurton MW: Stridor in a paediatric department, Proc R Soc Med 63:712, 1970.
2. Barker GA: Current management of croup and epiglottitis, Pediatr Clin North Am 26:565, 1979.
3. Costigan DC and Newth CJL: Respiratory status of children with epiglottitis with and without an artificial airway, Am J Dis Child 137:139, 1983.
4. Davis HW et al: Acute upper airway obstruction: croup and epiglottitis, Pediatr Clin North Am 28:859, 1981.
5. Day RL, Crelin ES, and DuBois AB: Choking: the Heimlich abdominal thrust vs. back blows: an approach to measurement of inertial and aerodynamic forces, Pediatrics 70:113, 1982.
6. Denneny JC and Handler SD: Membranous laryngotracheobronchitis, Pediatrics 70:705, 1982.
7. Diaz JH: Croup and epiglottitis in children: the anesthesiologist as diagnostician, Anesth Analg 64:621, 1985.
8. Downes JJ and Goldberg AI: Airway management, mechanical ventilation and cardiopulmonary resuscitation. In Scarpelli EM, Auld PAM, and Goldman HS, editors: Pulmonary disease of the fetus, newborn and child, Philadelphia, 1978, Lea & Febiger.
9. Duncan PG: Efficacy of helium-oxygen mixtures in the management of severe viral and post-intubation croup, Can Anaesth Soc J 26:206, 1979.
10. Friedberg SA and Bluestone CD: Foreign body accidents involving the air and food passages in children, Otolaryngol Clin North Am 3:395, 1970.

11. Greensher J and Mofenson HC: Emergency treatment of the choking child, Pediatrics 70:110, 1982.
12. Greensher J and Mofenson HC: Aspiration accidents: choking and drowning, Pediatr Ann 12:747, 1983.
13. Heimlich HJ: First aid for choking children: back blows and chest thrusts cause complications and death, Pediatrics 70:120, 1982.
14. Kantner RK and Watchko JF: Pulmonary edema associated with upper airway obstruction, Am J Dis Child 138:356, 1984.
15. Kelleher JF: Pulse oximetry, J Clin Monit 5:37, 1989.
16. Liston SL et al: Bacterial tracheitis, Am J Dis Child 137:764, 1983.
17. Mauro RD, Poole SR, and Lockhart CH: Differentiation of epiglottitis from laryngotracheitis in the child with stridor, Am J Dis Child 142:679, 1988.
18. Maze A and Bloch E: Stridor in pediatric patients, Anesthesiology 50:132, 1979.
19. O'Neill JA, Holcomb GW, and Neblett WW: Management of tracheobronchial and esophageal foreign bodies in childhood, J Pediatr Surg 18:475, 1983.
20. Quinn-Bogard AL and Potsic WP: Stridor in the first year of life, Clin Pediatr 16:913, 1977.
21. Torrey SB: The choking child: a life-threatening emergency, Clin Pediatr 22:751, 1983.
22. Weinberg S, Nakajo M, and Rao M: Airway management in children with bacterial tracheitis, Anesth Analg 63:860, 1984.
23. Yarington CT: Trauma involving the air and food passages, Otolaryngol Clin North Am 12:321, 1979.

268

Coma

Harry C. Dietz

Although coma, an unarousable state of complete unconsciousness, is rarely encountered in pediatric practice, it must be appropriately recognized as the opposite extreme from alert wakefulness along a complex and dynamic continuum. Many labels, such as lethargy, obtundation, and stupor, attempt to define distinct gradations along this spectrum, but for the purposes of most practitioners, these definitions prove burdensome and imprecise and lack immediate significance for diagnosis and management. It is more important to identify promptly *any* state of altered consciousness, especially when associated with a reduced capacity for arousal to a baseline level of functioning. A comatose child would universally be considered a medical emergency; a child with a lesser degree of impairment should invoke no less concern or command no less immediate intervention until the etiologic process has been convincingly determined to be static or self-limited.

INITIAL ASSESSMENT

When confronted with a comatose patient, there is an understandable tendency for the pediatrician to become immediately focused on the complexities of neurologic assessment. Such concerns should never take precedence over meticulous attention to the vital processes of ventilation and tissue perfusion.

Airway and Breathing

Considering the relative frequency with which infants and young children develop respiratory compromise and that hypoxemia and hypercarbia may be primarily involved in the pathogenesis of coma, it is not surprising that many patients with an altered level of consciousness require some form of respiratory assistance. Alternatively, many central nervous system (CNS) insults, either encephalopathic or mechanical, can involve brainstem centers responsible for ventilatory drive or airway protective reflexes. Airway patency and breathing can be initially assessed rapidly and accurately by "looking, listening, and feeling." Inspection should be focused on the color of the skin and mucous membranes for signs of cyanosis and on chest wall movement as a marker of central respiratory drive. The observer should then listen and feel at the nose and mouth for evidence of air movement. Simply counting the respiratory rate by watching chest movement will not suffice, because such effort may not translate into effective air exchange in the event of airway obstruction. Isolated deficiency of tidal volume, as one might see with narcotic intoxication, might also be missed. Finally, auscultation with a stethoscope should be briefly performed to assess ventilatory symmetry.

Even relatively low levels of hypercarbia are intolerable for a comatose patient with the potential for intracranial hypertension. Resulting cerebral vasodilation can have rapidly devastating consequences. Once hypoventilation is suspected, it must be acted upon quickly and decisively. If chest wall motion is present but ventilation is diminished, optimization of airway patency with the jaw thrust maneuver should be attempted. *Any significant flexion of the neck must be avoided until appropriate radiologic studies have ruled out cervical spine fracture or dislocation.* If adequate spontaneous ventilation is not established, clearing the airway of any foreign material should be attempted and assisted ventilation should ensue. Bag and mask ventilation can be established easily in the absence of airway obstruction. Early anticipation of the need for endotracheal intubation will allow for summoning of the most qualified personnel to perform this task. Critical issues include: (1) establishing aspiration precautions in a patient with a potentially full stomach and impaired airway protective reflexes, (2) avoiding neck flexion until the cervical spine has been shown to be stable, (3) preventing prolonged periods of apnea during intubation attempts, and (4) avoiding excessive noxious stimulation or the use of certain agents such as succinylcholine or ketamine that may exacerbate underlying intracranial hypertension.

Circulation

The hemodynamic status of a comatose patient can be assessed quickly by measuring the pulse rate and blood pressure. Tissue perfusion can be estimated by gauging capillary refill and skin temperature. Potential causes for hypotension in a comatose patient include hypovolemia secondary to dehydration or traumatic hemorrhage; decreased systemic vascular resistance, heart rate, or cardiac contractility secondary to infection, intoxication, or interruption of sympathetic discharge with spinal cord injury; and primary cardiac arrhythmia or failure. Maintenance of cerebral perfusion pressure (i.e., mean arterial pressure minus intracranial pressure) greater than 40 to 50 mm Hg is a prime goal of neurologic intensive care; therefore, even a mild reduction in blood pressure cannot be tolerated. Fluid restriction as a prophylactic measure against cerebral edema never takes precedence over hemodynamic stabilization of the patient. The selection of an appropriate fluid (normal saline, Ringer lactate, colloid, or blood) should be tailored to the specific clinical situation, but rapid expansion of intravascular volume is the primary immediate concern. Once the clinician is reasonably confident of adequate intravascular volume, vasoactive drugs may be considered for the ongoing management of refractory hypotension. Continuous electrocardiogram (EKG) monitoring is mandatory to guard against intermittent or recurrent arrhythmia. Any patient with a significant impairment of consciousness should have a secure intravenous line established regardless of the initial hemodynamic status.

Initial vital sign assessment should not be limited to the identification of hypoventilation or hypoperfusion states. Hypothermia might suggest prolonged circulatory arrest or environmental exposure. Hyperthermia might indicate infection, heat prostration, or toxic ingestion. Hypertension with associated bradycardia and irregular respiratory pattern (Cushing triad) suggests intracranial hypertension with brainstem compression. This finding is cause for immediate alarm, but its absence does not preclude a significant and threatening elevation of intracranial pressure.

Emergency Neurologic Assessment

Coma can be the result of either a bilateral insult to the cerebral hemispheres or functional disruption of the brainstem reticular activating system. Mechanical lesions that cause brainstem compromise place a patient at extreme risk for rapidly progressive and irreversible loss of neural integrity in a region that controls vital vegetative functions. Clearly, a portion of the emergency phase of assessment should be focused on the identification of brainstem involvement with ongoing observation for signs of progression. The components of this directed neurologic examination include assessment of cranial nerve function, observation of the quality of homeostatic mechanisms with special attention paid to respiratory pattern, and assignment of a Glasgow coma scale score.

A rapid survey of cranial nerve function includes assessment of pupillary size, symmetry, and reactivity to light; examination for the presence of a gag reflex; and testing of the corneal response to tactile stimulation. Such an examination assesses cranial nerves II, III, V, VII, IX, and X with adequate representation along the brainstem course. Careful analysis of the pupillary examination can yield specific localizing information as outlined below.

Many alterations in respiratory pattern can result from CNS injury of varying location and degree. Certain patterns have specific diagnostic value. Cheyne-Stokes respiration, characterized by crescendo-decrescendo breathing alternating with brief periods of apnea, suggests a deep hemispheric or diencephalic lesion. Injury to the midbrain or upper pons produces sustained hyperpnea, whereas medullary disease produces gasping respirations with prolonged apnea termed agonal or ataxic breathing.

The Glasgow coma scale (Table 268-1) is a relatively simple and universally understood method for describing the momentary status of a comatose patient. It involves observation of the patient's language, motor, and eye opening response to varying levels of stimulation. First, spontaneous activity is recorded. If the patient fails to respond in any category, then verbal stimulation is attempted. Finally, it may be necessary to invoke noxious stimulation in the form of

Table 268-1 *Glasgow Coma Scale*

OBSERVATION	POINTS	INFANT MODIFICATION
Eye opening		
None	1	None
To pain	2	To pain
To voice	3	To voice
Spontaneous	4	Spontaneous
Verbal response		
None	1	None
Nonspecific sounds	2	Moans to pain
Inappropriate words	3	Cries to pain
Confused conversation	4	Irritable spontaneous cry
Oriented conversation	5	Coos and babbles
Motor response		
None	1	None
Extension to pain	2	Abnormal extension
Flexion to pain	3	Abnormal flexion
Withdraws to pain	4	Withdraws to pain
Localizes pain	5	Withdraws to touch
Obeys commands	6	Normal/spontaneous
Maximum score	**15**	

supraorbital, ungual, or sternal pressure. The intent of this scale is to provide quick, accurate transfer of information among the various caretakers following the progress of a given patient. However, although the results of sequential examinations may provide some prognostic information, the Glasgow coma scale should not be used at the initial assessment to determine the futility of aggressive intervention. A sustained score in the 7 to 9 range or below usually signifies severe head injury and should prompt endotracheal intubation. Observation of the motor response to pain is particularly informative. Decorticate posturing, defined as nonlocalizing upper extremity flexion usually accompanied by lower extremity extension, signifies a cortical or subcortical disturbance with relative sparing of the brainstem. Upper and lower extremity extension (decerebrate posturing) suggests upper brainstem dysfunction but is also commonly seen with global metabolic processes. Flaccidity may be seen with diffuse disease or lesions localized to the lower brainstem or upper spinal cord.

One of the immediate goals of neurologic assessment during emergencies is prompt identification of herniation syndromes wherein structural shifts within the fixed compartments of the skull cause tissue damage either by direct parenchymal compression or local ischemia. Contrary to popular practice, this goal is not realized by isolated examination of the pupils; rather, it relies on proper interpretation of all aspects of the rapid neurologic examination previously described. Transtentorial or "central" herniation syndrome is seen when diencephalic structures are displaced downward into the posterior fossa through the rigid gap in the tentorium cerebelli, with subsequent impairment of more caudal structures. Physical signs expected during the initial stage of diencephalic injury include Cheyne-Stokes respiratory pattern, small but reactive pupils, and decorticate rigidity. Midbrain and upper pontine involvement is characterized by sustained hyperpnea, midposition and fixed pupils, and decerebrate posturing. Damage to the lower pons leads to pinpoint pupils, and terminal involvement of medullary centers is manifested by ataxic respirations, dilated and fixed pupils, and flaccidity. Rapid recognition of and response to this rostral to caudal degeneration will minimize tissue morbidity and allow for maximal recovery. Uncal herniation syndrome is seen with unilateral medial displacement of the uncus and hippocampal gyrus caused by an enlarging temporal mass lesion. Early impingement of the oculomotor nerve produces ipsilateral pupillary dilation, loss of light reactivity, diminished ability for eye adduction, and ptosis. A contralateral hemiparesis may be apparent. As with transtentorial herniation, the untreated patient will show progressive destruction of caudal brainstem structures.

By this point the pediatrician has taken a few moments to assure adequate ventilation and tissue perfusion. The patient's risk for rapid neurologic decline has also been assessed. Any significant abnormality has been managed, with priority given to stabilizing the airway, breathing, and circulation. Specific details concerning the appropriate care of neurologic emergencies follows in the "Management" section of this chapter. Simultaneous with these efforts, specific members of the health care team should be instructed to gather pertinent historical data (to be discussed in a later section) and to obtain certain readily available and immediately significant laboratory information, such as Dextrostik, hematocrit, and arterial blood gas results. Assessment for the potential of life-threatening multisystem organ damage is essential. If available historical information cannot absolutely exclude this possibility, a general surgical service should be consulted immediately. Neurosurgical consultation may also be warranted. It is rare that a newly presenting comatose patient will not require computed tomography (CT) imaging of the head. This should be scheduled early in the evaluation, despite the need for initial stabilization of the patient.

ETIOLOGY

An extensive differential diagnosis of coma is presented in the box on p. 1567. Head trauma with resultant parenchymal damage, hemorrhage, and secondary cerebral edema is the leading cause of coma in childhood. The other major causes include cardiorespiratory insufficiency, environmental exposure, infection, intoxication, an intracranial lesion, a metabolic disturbance, and a seizure disorder. As the pediatrician proceeds through the stages of early stabilization, history gathering, physical examination, and laboratory evaluation, this list should be carefully considered, limited, and modified to best accommodate the clinical situation at hand. The patient's age can provide valuable information. During early infancy, children are especially prone to respiratory compromise and invasive infection, including septicemia and meningitis. A child who has been abused may show a paucity of clinical findings at this age, and cerebral damage caused by "shaken baby" syndrome must be considered. A fundoscopic examination for retinal hemorrhage and CT imaging of the head should be performed to support this diagnosis. Although rare in older age groups, inborn errors of metabolism and herpes encephalitis should be high on the differential list for a comatose newborn. It is particularly unfortunate to miss these diagnoses because of their treatable nature and the brief period in which to effect a positive outcome. Toddlers have a high tendency for pica, and accidental self-intoxication should be considered strongly. At this developmental stage, a child's intense curiosity and new-found mobility set the stage for other forms of inapparent injury such as falls and electrocution. During the second half of the first decade, a child is at the greatest risk for developing a primary CNS tumor. During adolescence there is a risk of self-poisoning, either in the form of recreational drug use or suicide attempts. Age is a nonbinding clue, and overlap certainly exists; it helps to establish an initial hypothesis, which must then be tested and either adopted or abandoned.

HISTORY

Even minimal historical information can prove invaluable in narrowing the differential diagnosis. An abrupt onset of coma suggests trauma, cerebrovascular disease, arrhythmia, toxic ingestion, or primary seizure. A slowly progressive decline in mental status culminating in coma is more suggestive of infection, an expanding intracranial mass lesion, or metabolic perturbation. A recurrent pattern of alteration in mental status suggests the possibility of episodic toxic ingestion, a seizure disorder, or an inborn error of metabolism. This finding in a female child should prompt consideration of the heterozygous state of ornithine-transcarbamoylase deficiency. The general historical examination also should elicit information regarding the baseline level of functioning, recent or remote traumatic events, chronic illness, medication or illicit drug use, recent immunizations, change in school performance or social functioning, travel, nutritional status, hydration status, systemic signs of infection, health status of close contacts, and family history of inheritable disease. A comprehensive, systems-oriented history should be obtained on any patient with altered mental status without obvious cause. A list of particularly useful questions is presented in Table 268-2.

PHYSICAL EXAMINATION

Many aspects of the neurologic examination of the comatose patient have been discussed in the section on "Initial Assessment." Review of the vestibuloocular responses, traditionally discussed in this context, was intentionally omitted as part of the emergency evaluation because testing requires significant neck manipulation and some time for preparation. Although assessment of these reflexes can provide detailed anatomic information about brainstem function, findings have little impact on the early phases of patient stabilization. The oculocephalic or "doll's eye" reflex is tested by observing eye movement while rapidly turning the patient's head to the

Differential Diagnosis of Coma

CARDIORESPIRATORY CAUSES

- Cardiopulmonary arrest
- Cardiovascular abnormalities
  - Arrhythmia
  - Hypertension
  - Hypoperfusion states
    - Congestive heart failure
    - Impaired cardiac contractility
    - Left heart obstruction
      - Aortic stenosis
      - Coarctation of the aorta
  - Hypotension
    - Perioperative
- Respiratory abnormalities
    - Hypercapnia
    - Hypoxemia
    - Sudden infant death syndrome (SIDS)

CENTRAL NERVOUS SYSTEM TRAUMA

- Cerebral edema
- Child abuse
- Concussion
- Hemorrhage
  - Epidural
  - Parenchymal
  - Subarachnoid
  - Subdural
- Increased intracranial pressure
- Subdural effusion

EXPOSURE

- Heat prostration
- Hypothermia
- Sunstroke

INFECTION

- Abscess
- Empyema
- Encephalitis
  - Herpes
  - Other viral agents
- Meningitis
  - Bacterial
  - Fungal
  - Tuberculous
- Postinfectious encephalomyelitis
  - Measles
  - Other viral agents
- Sepsis

INTOXICATION

- Analgesics
- Anticonvulsants
- Antihistamines
- Benzodiazepines
- Digoxin
- Ethanol
- Heavy metals
- Hydrocarbons
- Hypnotics
  - Barbiturates
- Insulin
- Lithium
- Organophosphates
- Perioperative causes
  - General anesthetics
  - Muscle relaxants (apparent coma)
  - Sedatives/analgesics
- Phencyclidine
- Phenothiazines
- Salicylate
- Tricyclic antidepressants

INTRACRANIAL LESIONS

- Cerebral tumors/metastases
- Cerebrovascular events
  - Hemorrhage
  - Infarction
    - Embolic phenomenon
    - Thrombosis
  - Thrombophlebitis
  - Vasculitis
  - Venous thrombosis
- Hydrocephalus

METABOLIC CAUSES

- Abnormalities of salts and water
  - Dehydration
  - Hypercalecemia/hypocalcemia
  - Hyperkalemia/hypokalemia
  - Hypermagnesemia/hypomagnesemia
  - Hypernatremia
  - Hyponatremia
    - Water intoxication
- Acid/base abnormalities
  - Metabolic acidosis
  - Metabolic alkalosis
- Endocrine disorders
  - Addison disease
  - Congenital adrenal hyperplasia
  - Cushing disease
  - Diabetic ketoacidosis
  - Thyroid/parathyroid disease
- Hepatic failure
- Hypoglycemia
- Inborn errors of metabolism
  - Acid/base disturbances
  - Hyperammonemia
  - Hypoglycemia
- Malignant hyperthermia
- Porphyria
- Reye syndrome
- Uremia

SEIZURES

- Postictal state
- Status epilepticus

Table 268-2 *Systems-Oriented History Relevant to Coma*

SIGN OR SYMPTOM	SUGGESTED ETIOLOGY
Central nervous system	
Headache	(Mass lesion, infection, hydrocephalus)
Altered vision	(Mass lesion)
Ataxia/clumsiness	(Mass lesion, intoxication)
Seizure	
Respiratory	
Bronchospasm	
Infection	
Upper respiratory infection	(Bacteremia, meningitis)
Otitis media	(CNS invasion)
Pneumonitis	(Respiratory insufficiency)
Chronic lung disease	(Hypercapnia, hypoxemia)
Hyperpnea	(Metabolic disease/acidosis)
Skeletocutaneous	
Rash	(Infection, vasculitis, neurocutaneous syndrome, bleeding diathesis)
Arthralgia/arthritis	(Infection, vasculitis)
Diaphoresis	(Endocrine/metabolic disease, dehydration, infection)
Gastrointestinal	
Gastroenteritis	(Dehydration, toxin {shigellosis})
Pica	(Lead poisoning, other intoxication)
Fad diet, chronic malabsorption	(Vitamin/cofactor deficiency)
Genitourinary	
Polyuria/polydipsia	(Diabetes mellitus, diabetes insipidus, water intoxication)
Precocious sexual development	(Endocrine disorder, CNS tumor)
Cardiovascular	
Palpitation	
Documented arrhythmia	
Congestive heart failure	
Congenital heart disease	
Cardiomyopathy	
Endocarditis risk/prophylaxis	
Early coronary deaths	

side from a midline position. In a comatose patient with intact brainstem function, the eyes will show transient conjugate deviation in the direction opposite to head turning. This finding constitutes a "positive" response. In an alert patient or in the event of brainstem dysfunction at the level of the third nerve nuclei, the direction of gaze will move along with head turning, thus maintaining a forward stare. The normal newborn or alert patient with visual fixation before the maneuver may show a positive oculocephalic reflex. The oculovestibular, or "cold caloric," reflex is performed by slow instillation of a large volume (up to 120 ml) of ice-cold water into the external auditory canal. This test should not be performed on an alert patient, because the sensation of vertigo and nausea may be quite disturbing. The normal response is horizontal nystagmus with the rapid component occurring in the direction opposite the side of stimulation. In a comatose patient with intact brainstem function, the observer would notice conjugate eye deviation toward the side of the stimulus. Brainstem dysfunction abolishes eye movement in response to cold water stimulation. For additional details on the subacute neurologic evaluation of the comatose patient, the reader should refer to any comprehensive textbook of neurology; review of the classic treatise by Plum and Posner is particularly rewarding.[1]

The list of physical findings that might support the many potential etiologies of coma is quite extensive and will not be discussed in detail. A meticulous and comprehensive physical examination is imperative, and every abnormality should be carefully considered in the light of an emerging differential diagnosis. Once again, it is imperative not to become overly focused on the intricacies of neurologic assessment and thereby miss a goiter, butterfly rash, or café-au-lait spot.

LABORATORY AND RADIOLOGIC ASSESSMENT

Unselective investigation of the many possible causes of coma generates an extensive list of laboratory tests. Clearly it is prudent to assimilate all available information into a truncated list of potential etiologies and then to proceed in an orderly and calculated fashion. Certain tests, however, are useful for screening by virtue of their rapid results, physiologic significance, and relatively high yield. Dextrostik, hematocrit, and arterial blood gas determinations should be performed as part of the initial patient assessment. Once vascular access is obtained, the following should be measured: serum electrolytes (including calcium and magnesium), blood urea nitrogen, creatinine, liver enzymes, complete blood cell count with differential, and serum ammonia. When evaluating a comatose infant, the practitioner should be quick to analyze plasma for amino acids and urine for organic acids. All patients should have their urine examined for glucose, blood, ketones, specific gravity, and cellular components. If infection cannot be reliably excluded, then cerebrospinal fluid (CSF) should be examined and cultures taken of blood, urine, and CSF. A focal neurologic examination or low Glasgow coma scale score suggests intracranial hypertension, and CT imaging of the head is warranted before lumbar puncture and secondary decompression of the caudal subarachnoid space. In the absence of focal neurologic findings, the blood and urine of any patient with a depressed sensorium without obvious etiology should be "sent" for a toxicologic screen.

CT imaging of the head is routinely performed on a patient with altered mental status. This procedure may aid in establishing a diagnosis or may be used to define the extent of brain injury and the likelihood for progression. Although a nonenhanced study demonstrates cerebral edema and tissue shift, a contrast study should be considered when it is not informative or when definition of a mass lesion is required.

MANAGEMENT

The mainstay of emergency management of intracranial hypertension with impending herniation is intubation and hyperventilation. This action will effect cerebral vasoconstriction and subsequent reduction in the volume of intracranial contents. The P_{CO_2} should be maintained between 20 and 25 mm Hg. Immediate benefits are seen, but these commonly diminish within the first day of therapy. Other useful therapies include the administration of furosemide, mannitol, or both which promote diuresis and therefore diminish the interstitial fluid component of the intracranial contents and perhaps slow the rate of postinjury parenchymal swelling. Judicious fluid restriction should also be considered in a hemodynamically stable patient. These interventions do not obviate the need for prompt neurosurgical consultation. Inducing a barbiturate coma has limited application and considerable associated risk. This treatment should not be considered by nonexperienced personnel or outside the intensive care setting.

The subacute management goals of treating a comatose patient revolve around maximizing cerebral nutrient delivery and minimizing nutrient demands of the tissues. In this regard, temperature elevation, seizure activity, and noxious stimulation of the patient should be aggressively avoided. CT results and sequential examination will determine the need for invasive intracranial pressure monitoring.

When emergency intervention and acute management do not lead to reversal, chronic care of the comatose patient requires instituting postural drainage, aspiration prophylaxis, skin and eye care, and long-term nutritional management.

OUTCOME

Little precise and useful information can be provided concerning the outcome of coma in pediatric patients. The factors that influence prognosis include the underlying etiology, degree of parenchymal damage, patient's age, duration of coma, simultaneous failure of other organ systems, and the effectiveness of therapy. Fortunately, pediatricians deal with a patient population that has considerable plasticity and resilience. This may allow for the expression of guarded optimism in the early phases of assessment but should not preclude timely discussion with the parents of concerns, setbacks, or an emerging sense of catastrophic and irreversible damage. The family should be helped to prepare for a negative outcome when that event appears to be likely.

REFERENCE

1. Plum F and Posner JB: The diagnosis of stupor and coma, ed 3, Philadelphia, 1982, FA Davis Co.

SUGGESTED READINGS

Fisher CM: The neurological examination of the comatose patient, Acta Neurol Scand 45 (suppl 36):1, 1969.

Kanter RK: Evaluation and stabilization of the critically ill child, Clin Chest Med 8:573, 1987.

Margolis LH and Shaywitz BA: The outcome of prolonged coma in childhood, Pediatrics 65:477, 1980.

Mickell JJ et al: Intracranial pressure monitoring and normalization therapy in children, Pediatrics 59:606, 1977.

Seshia SS, Seshia MMK, and Sachdeva RK: Coma in childhood, Dev Med Child Neurol 19:614, 1977.

Shaywitz BA: Management of acute neurologic syndromes in infants and children, Yale J Biol Med 57:83, 1884.

269

Croup (Acute Laryngotracheobronchitis)

Caroline Breese Hall and William J. Hall

DEFINITION

Viral croup, or acute laryngotracheobronchitis, is an age-specific syndrome caused by a number of different viral agents. It is characterized by subglottic swelling, respiratory distress, and inspiratory stridor. This syndrome, recognized and respected by physicians for centuries, inherited its name, croup, from an old Scottish word *roup*, which meant to cry out in a hoarse voice.

Spasmodic croup is a term sometimes used to denote recurrent episodes of croup that affect some children. Allergy or airway hyperreactivity may play a role in predisposing these children to repetitive bouts of croup.

Recent years have seen important advances in our understanding of the etiology, pathophysiology, and treatment of croup, resulting in better management and outcome for these distressed children. Understanding of the physiologic abnormalities underlying the child's distress is basic to proper management.

ETIOLOGY

As shown in Table 269-1, a variety of agents may be associated with croup. However, the parainfluenza viruses are the most frequently identified agents that cause this disease, and parainfluenza virus type 1 is the major single agent.[6-8] In an 11-year study of croup in a private practice in Chapel Hill, North Carolina, the parainfluenza viruses constituted 75% of all the viral isolates obtained from children with croup; 65% of the parainfluenza viral isolates were parainfluenza virus type 1. Respiratory syncytial virus, influenza viruses A and B, and *Mycoplasma pneumoniae* were the only other agents isolated with appreciable frequency in this study.

Table 269-1 *Agents Causing Croup*

AGENT	EPIDEMIOLOGY
Most frequent	
Parainfluenza type 1	Epidemic, fall
Less frequent	
Influenza A	Epidemic, winter
Influenza B	Epidemic, winter
Respiratory syncytial virus	Epidemic, winter-spring
Mycoplasma pneumoniae	Endemic
Parainfluenza type 2	Occasionally epidemic, fall
Parainfluenza type 3	Spring to summer
Uncommon	
Adenoviruses	Endemic
Rhinoviruses	Endemic, fall, spring-summer
Reoviruses	Endemic
Coronaviruses	Epidemic, winter
Herpesvirus hominis	Endemic

EPIDEMIOLOGY

Croup occurs primarily in children between 3 months and 3 years of age, with the peak incidence being in the second year of life. Studies of both hospitalized and ambulatory patients have shown that boys tend to be affected more commonly than girls.[6-8] The incidence of croup varies not only according to age but also according to geographic location and season. In a prepaid group practice in Seattle, the annual incidence of croup was 7 per 1000 children under 6 years of age.[7] However, between 1 and 2 years of age, this incidence approximately doubled. In the Chapel Hill practice, the attack rate during the second year of life was 4.7 per 100 children per year, and the yearly incidence per 100 children for all ages was 1.82 for boys and 1.27 for girls.

The seasonal flourishes of croup depend on the epidemiologic personality of the viral agents (Table 269-1, Fig. 269-1). Parainfluenza virus type 1, the most frequent cause of croup, has the distinctive pattern of producing epidemics of croup and other associated respiratory illness every other year in the autumn. Overall, the parainfluenza viruses constituted about 75% of the viral isolates obtained from outpatients in private practices in an ongoing surveillance program conducted in Monroe County, New York, from 1983 to 1988 (Fig. 269-2). Smaller peaks of croup are associated with outbreaks of influenza, respiratory syncytial virus, and parainfluenza virus type 3.[6,8] Thus cases of croup seen in the fall are most likely related to parainfluenza type 1 and occasionally to parainfluenza type 2. Winter cases are most frequently associated with influenza and, to a lesser extent, respiratory syncytial virus. In the warmer months of spring and summer, parainfluenza type 3 is the agent isolated most prevalently.

Croup in children 5 years of age or older is most likely to

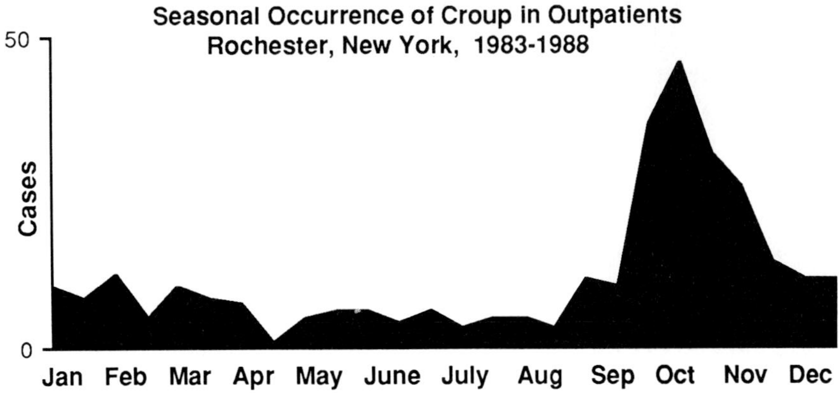

Fig. 269-1 Seasonal occurrence of croup from 1983 to 1988 in patients in pediatric practices participating in an ongoing community surveillance program in Monroe County, New York. Most cases observed in the fall resulted from outbreaks of parainfluenza virus type 1 occurring during odd-numbered years.

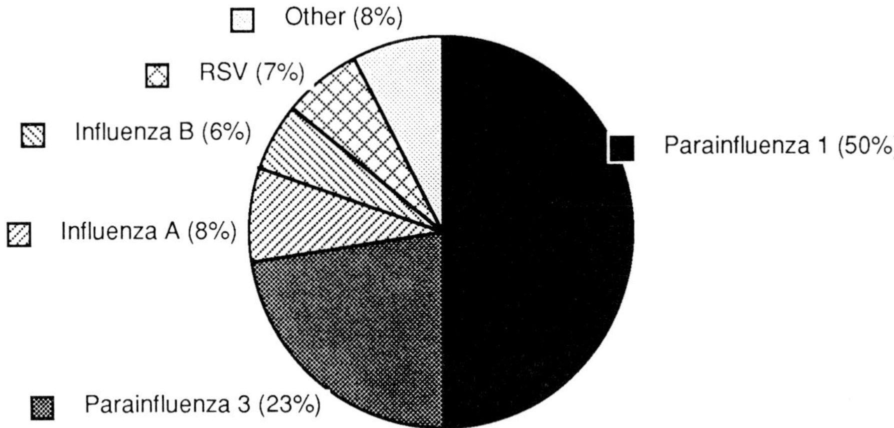

Fig. 269-2 Viral etiology of croup (1983 to 1988) in patients in pediatric practices participating in a community surveillance program in Monroe County, New York.

be associated with the influenza viruses or *Mycoplasma pneumoniae*.[6] Respiratory syncytial virus tends to cause croup in younger children, and the parainfluenza viruses, although predominately causing croup in toddlers, may infect both younger and occasionally school-age children.

PATHOPHYSIOLOGY

Infection with one of these viruses usually occurs through close person-to-person contact and occasionally through contact with infected secretions. The upper respiratory tract serves as the route of inoculation. The respiratory epithelium offers fertile fields for most of these agents, and viral multiplication occurs easily. Subsequently, the infection spreads further down the respiratory tract. Involvement of the subglottic tissue appears particularly pronounced. Nevertheless, the infection may extend from the large airways to the alveoli. Inflammation at the subglottic area is especially apt to cause major obstruction to airflow because this area is both the narrowest and the least distensible part of the larynx, as a result of the anatomy of the cricoid and thyroid cartilage. Inflammation, however, commonly affects the conducting airways at all levels. Necrosis of the epithelium is prominent, and the inflammatory exudate and secretions may add to the obstruction.

The age predilection of viral croup can be explained in part by the anatomy of the airway. In a young child the subglottic trachea is relatively smaller and more pliable than that of older individuals. The narrowing that occurs with inspiratory effort may therefore be exaggerated in croup. In addition, obstruction above the subglottic area, such as may occur with nasal congestion, increases the collapsing force, and an increased respiratory rate associated with crying or anxiety may further compromise the child's ventilation.

Other host factors, as yet poorly defined, such as genetic and immunologic mechanisms are likely to contribute to the development and severity of croup. Atopy or hyperreactivity of the airways has been suggested as playing a role in spasmodic or recurrent croup by the higher incidence of a family history of allergy and positive skin tests for allergens in such children.[10,22] Serum IgA levels have also been noted to be lower in these predisposed patients.[23] Abnormalities in the immune response to parainfluenza viral antigens have also been observed in children who developed croup versus those who had upper respiratory tract illness with parainfluenza virus infection.[20]

CLINICAL FEATURES

Symptoms of an upper respiratory tract infection usually precede the laryngotracheobronchitis. As the infection progresses, the characteristic cough develops. The cough may be spasmodic with a deep "brassy" or "barking" tone. This classic sign has therefore aptly earned the name "seal's bark" and is likened to the notes of a "brass bell" and even to a "crowing cock" or "braying ass." Laryngitis with a raspy-sounding voice may also develop. Fever is commonly present, particularly with influenza A and parainfluenza viral infections.

These signs herald the usually abrupt onset of the inspiratory stridor. The child may awaken at night with a spasmodic cough and respiratory distress. Although the flow of air is impeded during both inspiration and expiration, it is most marked on inspiration. Because the subglottic region is outside the pleural cavity, the negative pressures generated on inspiration tend to narrow the passage further, much like sucking on a plugged straw. The distress of the child is audibly marked by each stridulous note of inspiration and is visibly accentuated by the retractions of the accessory muscles of the chest wall. The suprasternal, supraclavicular, and substernal retractions are particularly characteristic of the inspiratory obstruction. Further distress may be marked by asynchronous movements of the chest wall and abdomen.

The respiratory rate is increased but usually not more than 50 breaths per minute. This is in contrast to bronchiolitis, in which the picture of respiratory distress may be accompanied by respirations of 80 to 90 breaths per minute. Auscultation of the chest reveals a prolonged inspiration, often accompanied by coarse rales. Wheezes and rhonchi may be heard on expiration. With more severe obstruction, the breath sounds may be diminished. Cyanosis may occasionally be noted, particularly about the lips and nail beds.

The variable intensity of the respiratory distress is characteristic of croup. The child may appear severely compromised and an hour later appear improved, only to worsen over the next hour. Often, for unknown reasons, the symptoms appear to abate with the morning light but may worsen again as the day progresses. For most children, the signs of croup may extend over 3 or 4 days, but the upper respiratory tract signs and cough may last longer.

In a few children, the respiratory distress may be unremitting or associated with significant pneumonitis and hypoxemia.[16] As the child tires, his or her respirations may become more rapid but also shallow, indicating the need for ventilatory assistance.

DIFFERENTIAL DIAGNOSIS

Most importantly, viral croup must be differentiated from epiglottitis, which without immediate therapy may be rapidly fatal. The differentiating features are described in Chapter 276, "Epiglottitis." The rapidly progressive and unrelenting course, the drooling, and the toxicity of epiglottitis tend to distinguish it from croup. A lateral neck roentgenogram will show the swollen epiglottis, which appears shaped like a thumb viewed anteriorly.

Bacterial tracheitis is the second emergency entity that needs to be differentiated from viral croup.[5,11,14] Bacterial tracheitis is an uncommon infection that may affect children of any age, resulting in the acute onset of respiratory stridor, high fever, and often copious, purulent secretions. Similar to epiglottitis, the child may appear toxic and the respiratory obstruction rapidly progress, such that tracheal intubation is necessary. The pathogens most frequently involved are *Staphylococcus aureus,* group A beta-hemolytic streptococci, and *Haemophilus influenzae* type b. The diagnosis may be confirmed by direct laryngoscopy, which shows the purulent secretions and inflammation in the subglottic area, and sometimes by a lateral neck roentgenogram, which may reveal an area of subglottic narrowing with a shaggy, purulent membrane.

Other infectious agents that may mimic croup are, fortunately, now rare. Diphtheria may be excluded by a history of adequate immunizations and by the absence of the characteristic gray pharyngeal or laryngeal diphtheritic membrane. Occasionally, an aspirated foreign body may cause stridor. The abrupt onset of the stridor, respiratory distress, and the lack of preceding respiratory symptoms and fever should suggest this diagnosis. Laryngeal edema resulting from an allergic reaction may cause abrupt and severe respiratory distress, occasionally with stridor. The history of the circumstances of the abrupt onset, the lack of previous respiratory signs, and manifestations of an allergic reaction elsewhere should help to differentiate laryngeal edema from other causes of croup.

DIAGNOSIS

The diagnosis of croup is usually made on the basis of the characteristic clinical findings and a compatible history. In cases that are atypical or apt to be confused with other syndromes characterized by stridor, the diagnosis of croup may be confirmed by a lateral inspiratory and expiratory roentgenogram or by a posteroanterior roentgenogram of the neck.[4,17] The air shadow of the larynx will be seen to narrow like an "hourglass" in the subglottic region, as a result of the characteristic inflammation in this area (Fig. 269-3).[17]

The diagnosis of spasmodic croup has been applied by some to children who have recurrent episodes of croup in which allergic diathesis is believed to play a role.[22] However, the illness in almost all instances is still triggered by a viral infection, and clinically spasmodic croup cannot be differentiated from the usual cases of croup.

Laboratory findings are not specific for the diagnosis of acute laryngotracheobronchitis; rather, they are more helpful in the management of these patients than in their diagnosis. The total white blood cell count and differential in children with croup may be normal or shifted slightly to the left in the more distressed child. Children with hypoxemia may have an increased proportion of bands in their peripheral count. Most hospitalized children with acute laryngotracheobronchitis will have an abnormally low PaO_2.[16] The $PaCO_2$ is usually within the normal range but rises in severely distressed children as they tire.

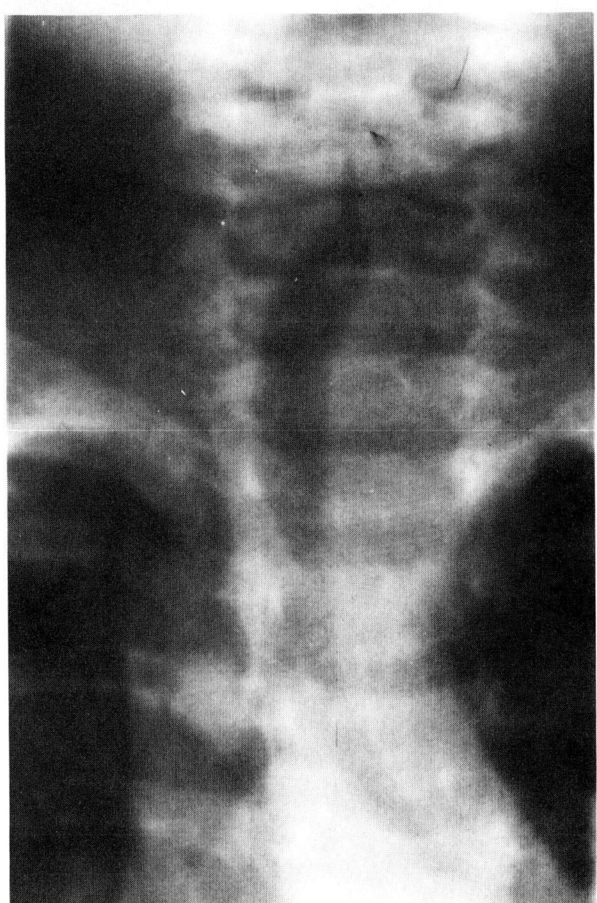

Fig. 269-3 Roentgenogram of the posteroanterior neck of a child with viral croup, showning narrowing in the subglottic area.

MANAGEMENT

Basic to the management of these patients is an understanding of the physiologic changes that occur during acute laryngotracheobronchitis.[1,13] As depicted in Fig. 269-4, the infecting virus causes inflammation in the subglottic area and lower in the respiratory tract, which results in two different types of physiologic abnormalities. Obstruction at the subglottic area forces the child to increase his respiratory effort, producing a rise in his respiratory rate. This increased ventilation compensates for the impeded flow of air and results in a normal arterial Pco_2. A few children will become fatigued from the increased effort of breathing. As their respirations become shallow, the carbon dioxide can no longer be adequately eliminated, and the arterial Pco_2 rises.

The inflammation of the airways and lung parenchyma causes concurrent physiologic abnormalities that often are not adequately appreciated.[16] Infection of the parenchyma results in an abnormally low ratio of ventilation to perfusion. This produces hypoxemia, observed in over 80% of hospitalized cases.[16] In contrast to the abnormalities associated with obstruction at the subglottic area, the child with lower respiratory tract inflammation has little means of compensating. Raising the arterial Po_2 requires therapeutic intervention—the administration of supplemental oxygen. In the severely distressed child, the hypoxemia contributes to the fatigue. The resulting hypercarbia aggravates the hyoxemia, and respiratory failure may ensue.

The first phase of management, therefore, must be to evaluate which children may be managed at home and which require hospitalization. Severity is often difficult to determine in this fluctuating disease. Few clinical signs are indicative of hypoxemia. Cyanosis, when present, is usually indicative of an artierial Po_2 level below 60 mm Hg. However, considerable degrees of hypoxemia may occur without overt cyanosis. The best clinical sign of hypoxemia is an increasing respiratory rate. The severity of the stridor and retractions is better correlated with the degree of subglottic obstruction and the respiratory effort than with hypoxemia. Dehydration and fatigue are also indications for hospitalization.

Those children who are to be managed at home should be made comfortable to avoid unnecessary anxiety and fatigue. Crying and anxiety tend to make the young child take rapid, short breaths, which aggravate the narrowing of the airway and the metabolic need for gas exchange. Fluids should be encouraged, and antipyretics should be given for fever. Despite a cornucopia of cures passed down from generation to generation, few other home therapies have proved to be of benefit. Because of the fluctuating nature of this disease, a number of unverified therapeutic modalities may appear to work. Vaporizers and home-devised mist tents from showers to teakettles are commonly tried. However, the water particles produced by these devices are too large to reach the lower respiratory tract and can only humidify the nares and oropharynx. If the mist is cold, however, it may help to cool the airway, which appears to be beneficial in croup. This might also explain the improvement some children experience when taken out in the cold night air. Cold-dry, cold-mist, and warm-dry air all tend to cool the airway and therefore may be beneficial in croup. This has been supported by animal studies.[21]

In the hospital, the child may be evaluated by the objective criteria of arterial blood gases. The degree of hypoxemia may be determined from arterial or capillary blood or by a noninvasive technique such as oximetry. However, laboratory evaluation should be kept to a minimum to avoid upsetting the child further.

Humidification in the hospital may be achieved by use of an ultrasonic nebulizer fitted to either a mask or an oxygen tent. This device can produce water particles of a size small enough to reach the bronchioles. The value of such therapy, however, has not been proven.

In one small, controlled study, humidification could not be shown to provide any therapeutic benefit for children hospitalized with croup.[3] Aerosolized bronchodilators, especially racemic epinephrine, are frequently used.[2,18] Clinical improvement in the degree of stridor and retractions, probably from local vasoconstriction, occurs in most cases. Such an agent, therefore, should be considered for the distressed child to ward off fatigue. However, it should only be used with the understanding that (1) the amelioration of the clinical signs is transient and the child may worsen within 2 hours, and (2) the arterial Po_2 is not affected.[18] Thus, despite clinical improvement, the degree of hypoxemia remains unchanged. Bronchodilators administered by other routes have not been of benefit and may have unwanted cardiovascular side effects.

The use of corticosteroid therapy is controversial.[2,12,19] A 1980 review of the many studies examining the use of steroids in croup noted that all had some defect in design that would not allow a definitive answer.[19] Steroid therapy probably

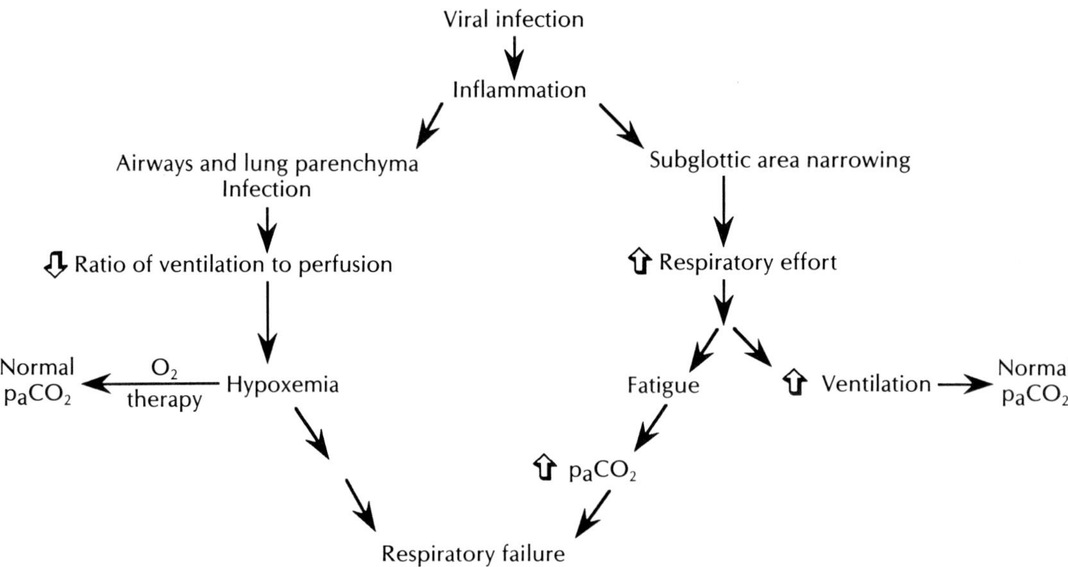

Fig. 269-4 Roentgenogram of the posteroanterior neck of a child with viral croup, showing narrowing in the subglottic area.

should only be considered for the hospitalized child who is severely ill. Antibiotics are usually not indicated in viral croup. Secondary bacterial infection is unusual, and antibiotics should be reserved for such episodes.

Despite these supportive measures, a few children worsen and require assisted ventilation. An elevated arterial PCO_2 (higher than 45 mm Hg) warns that the child needs close monitoring. General guidelines for determining when the child requires a mechanical airway are (1) progressive carbon dioxide retention, (2) hypoxemia unresponsive to supplemental oxygen administration, and (3) copious secretions not mobilized by coughing.

PROGNOSIS

The severity of croup is related in part to the type of infecting virus and in part to unknown host factors. In the great majority of children, croup is a self-limited disease that resolves within a few days. Several studies have suggested, however, that children who have had croup have a high incidence of bronchial reactivity in subsequent years.[9,15,22]

REFERENCES

1. Barker GA: Current management of croup and epiglottitis, Pediatr Clin North Am 26:565, 1979.
2. Bass JW, Bruhn FW, and Merritt WT: Corticosteroids and racemic epinephrine with IPPB in the treatment of croup, J Pediatr 96:173, 1980.
3. Bourchier D, Dawson KP, and Fergusson DM: Humidification in viral croup: a controlled trial, Aust Paediatr J 20:289, 1984.
4. Currarino G and Williams B: Lateral inspiration and expiration radiographs of the neck in children with laryngotracheitis (croup), Radiology 145:365, 1982.
5. Davidson S et al: Bacterial tracheitis—a true entity? J Laryngol Otolaryngol 96:173, 1982.
6. Denny FW et al: Croup: an 11-year study in a pediatric practice, Pediatrics 71:871, 1983.
7. Foy HM et al: Incidence and etiology of pneumonia, croup and bronchiolitis in preschool children belonging to a prepaid medical care group over a four-year period, Am J Epidemiol 97:80, 1973.
8. Glezen WP and Denny FW: Epidemiology of acute lower respiratory disease in children, N Engl J Med 228:498, 1973.
9. Gurwitz D, Corey M, and Levison H: Pulmonary function and bronchial reactivity in children after croup, Am Rev Respir Dis 122:95, 1980.
10. Hide DW and Guyer BM: Recurrent croup, Arch Dis Child 60:585, 1985.
11. Jones R, Santos JI, and Overall JC: Bacterial tracheitis, JAMA 242:721, 1979.
12. Koren G et al: Corticosteroid treatment of laryngotracheitis v spasmodic croup, Am J Dis Child 137:941, 1983.
13. Lenney W and Milner AD: Treatment of viral croup, Arch Dis Child 53:704, 1978.
14. Liston SL et al: Bacterial tracheitis, Am J Dis Child 137:764, 1983.
15. Loughlin G and Taussig LM: Pulmonary function in children with a history of laryngotracheobronchitis, J Pediatr 94:365, 1979.
16. Newth CJL, Levison H, and Bryan AC: Respiratory status of children with croup, J Pediatr 81:1068, 1972.
17. Rapkin RH: The diagnosis of epiglottitis: simplicity and reliability of radiographs of the neck in the differential of the croup syndrome, J Pediatr 80:96, 1972.
18. Taussig LM et al: Treatment of laryngotracheobronchitis (croup): use of intermittent positive-pressure breathing and racemic epinephrine, Am J Dis Child 129:790, 1975.
19. Tunnessen WW and Reinstein AR: The steroid-croup controversy: an analytic review of methodologic problems, J Pediatr 96:751, 1980.
20. Welliver RC, Sun M, and Rinaldo D: Defective regulation of immune responses in croup due to parainfluenza virus, Pediatr Res 19:716, 1985.
21. Wolfsdorf J and Swift DL: An animal model simulating acute infective upper airway obstruction of childhood and its use in the investigation of croup therapy, Pediatr Res 12:1062, 1978.
22. Zach M, Erban A, and Olinsky A: Croup, recurrent croup, allergy, and airways hyperreactivity, Arch Dis Child 56:336, 1981.
23. Zach M and Messner H: Serum IgA in recurrent croup, Am J Dis Child 137:184, 1983.

270

Dehydration

Harry C. Dietz

Dehydration is best defined as a state of negative water balance that occurs when pathologic processes diminish or overwhelm homeostatic mechanisms. Although clinically common, excessive body water loss is not central to this definition. Rather, aberration of a host of basic bodily functions may affect water balance, including ventilation; thermoregulation; thirst, alimentation, and absorption; and renal solute and water clearance. Add to these all factors that influence the basal rate of caloric expenditure, such as environment, activity level, or endocrine metabolism, and it becomes clear that the causes of dehydration are protean. One can take in too little, need too much, or lose too much. It is that simple and that varied.

A further contradiction to the popular "working" definition of dehydration is that negative water balance can occur without depletion of the circulating fluid volume. In fact, certain mechanisms of dehydration preferentially spare the intravascular space at the expense of remaining body water stores. The classic symptoms of dehydration, which manifest intravascular hypovolemia and tissue hypoperfusion, may not be evident, but the potential for morbidity remains high. Effective therapy depends on a firm understanding of all factors that affect the delicate equilibrium of water and solutes among body fluid compartments. A compositional, anatomic, and physiologic discussion of body water homeostasis and implications for therapy of the dehydrated child is presented in Chapter 25. This chapter focuses on the evaluation and management of the critically ill patient with dehydration.

PATHOPHYSIOLOGY

A brief review of the physiology of fluid balance is warranted, with emphasis on the compensatory mechanisms involved in the response to dehydration and significance for therapy.

Compartmental View of Dehydration

Total body water (TBW) constitutes approximately 70% of the lean body mass (LBM) and is distributed between two major compartments, intracellular fluid (ICF) and extracellular fluid (ECF). ICF, which accounts for 65% of TBW, is potassium rich and sodium poor. ECF, which accounts for 35% of TBW, is sodium rich and potassium poor. This compartment can be subdivided into the intravascular fluid (IVF) and the interstitial fluid (ISF), which account for 7% and 28% of TBW, respectively. As a general rule the IVF and ISF are in passive equilibrium, allowing free movement of solutes and water between them. As previously mentioned, however, the ICF and ECF have dramatically different compositions and a relatively impermeable barrier is required to preserve these gradients. The cell membrane, replete with highly selective and energy-dependent transport mechanisms, serves this purpose.

Dehydration traditionally is divided into three subgroups on the basis of the serum sodium (Na) concentration, each with clinical and therapeutic significance. Isotonic or isonatremic dehydration (defined as serum Na, 130 to 150 mEq/L) is the most common form. Fluid losses from the gastrointestinal tract, respiratory tract, and skin generally are hypotonic (contain lower Na concentrations) in relation to serum. These losses, however, commonly are offset in part by avid thirst and a generous intake of sodium-containing fluids; thus isonatremia and normal osmotic gradients among body fluid compartments are preserved. Therefore free water is lost from both the ECF and ICF to a degree proportional to the relative size of each compartment. Therapy must address the fluid and electrolyte needs of all compartments and must account for resistance to the flow of osmoles (and hence free water) from the intravascular to the interstitial space and from there to the intracellular space. Water moves freely when exposed to an osmotic gradient. Charged electrolyte particles move much less easily, which takes time. This is the basis for allowing 24 hours for complete replacement of a fluid deficit in isonatremic dehydration.

Hypertonic or hypernatremic dehydration (defined as serum Na >150 mEq/L) may occur when replacement of hypotonic fluid losses is negligible or when the replacement fluid is hypertonic (contains higher Na concentrations) in relation to serum. This form of dehydration was seen more frequently when boiled milk preparations were commonly used to replace gastrointestinal fluid losses. In hypernatremic dehydration the ECF is hyperosmolar compared with the ICF. An osmotic gradient has been created that favors movement of free water into the intravascular compartment at the expense of cellular stores. Therefore, at any given level of dehydration, the intravascular volume is relatively preserved and clinical symptoms are less pronounced. The compartment needing the most repair (ICF) requires less sodium than does the intravascular space and is "guarded" by membranes that are relatively impermeable to charged particles. More time is necessary for the replacement volume to reach its destination. At least 48 hours should be allowed for reparation of the fluid deficit in hypernatremic dehydration.

Hypotonic or hyponatremic dehydration (defined as serum Na <130 mEq/L) can occur when fluid losses are sodium rich (such as excessive sweating with cystic fibrosis) or when a large volume of hypotonic replacement fluid is provided. The ECF is hypoosmolar compared with the ICF, and an osmotic gradient is created that favors movement of free water out of the intravascular space with relative preservation of cellular stores. Therefore, at any given level of dehydration, the intravascular compartment is more severely diminished and clinical symptoms are more pronounced. The compartment needing the most repair (IVF) requires relatively large amounts of sodium. Fluid can be supplied directly to this compartment with no delay in effective placement of osmotic particles and equilibrium of free water. In severe cases, rapid delivery of isotonic (or hypertonic) fluid is mandatory to preserve vital tissue functions. Repletion of modest deficits in other compartments is of secondary concern and will take time. There is, of course, a finite amount of rapid repletion that the intravascular compartment can accommodate. In general, isotonic fluid should be given at a maximal rate until clinical improvement is seen. The remainder of the deficit should be supplied over a 24-hour period.

Compensatory Mechanisms for Dehydration

The slightest degree of intravascular volume depletion will stimulate a wide array of compensatory processes. An increase in heart rate because of decreased baroreceptor tone will be the first clinically obvious response. This enhancement of sympathetic discharge and decrease in vagal tone also will promote an increase in contractility, stroke volume, and systemic vascular resistance. The most sensitive, powerful, and important homeostatic mechanism is the activation of the renin-angiotensin-aldosterone system. A decrease in renal blood flow stimulates renin release by the juxtoglomerular apparatus. Elevated renin levels prompt angiotensin I formation, with subsequent conversion to angiotensin II in the pulmonary vascular bed. Angiotensin II acts as a potent vasoconstrictor and also stimulates aldosterone release from the adrenal medulla. Aldosterone stimulates distal renal tubular reabsorption of sodium and thereby increases the tonicity of the peritubular capillary fluid, with secondary increase in free water reabsorption. Simultaneous with these changes, the hypothalamus secretes vasopressin, which augments systemic vascular tone and diminishes free water excretion by the kidney. The cumulative effect of all these compensatory mechanisms is to preserve cardiac output, increase systemic vascular resistance, and realize a maximally concentrated urine in the face of severe dehydration.

The body often sacrifices other homeostatic processes in an attempt to repair a dehydrated state and maintain perfusion to vital organs. Preservation of electroneutrality is necessary during aldosterone-stimulated sodium reabsorption. This is initially accomplished by wasting body potassium stores. Subsequently, an anion, either chloride or bicarbonate, will be reabsorbed in union with sodium. Metabolic alkalosis will ensue, and this effect will be intensified if abnormal body fluid losses create a chloride-deficient state. Thus mild and chronic volume contraction might produce hypokalemic, hypochloremic metabolic alkalosis. This identical chemical profile can be seen with pyloric stenosis or chronic administration of a glomerular-loop diuretic. Dehydration accompanied by metabolic acidosis is of particular concern because it suggests that the predictable alkalosis has been overwhelmed. Explanations include excessive bicarbonate loss through the gastrointestinal tract, endogenous production of acid as seen with diabetic ketoacidosis or an inborn error of metabolism, intoxication such as salicylate ingestion, or compromise of tissue perfusion with subsequent lactate production. In extreme circumstances, the increased sympathetic tone created by the baroreceptor response, by angiotensin II, and by vasopressin contributes to the production of lactic acid by shunting blood flow to the brain and coronary circulations at the expense of liver, kidney, gut, and musculocutaneous perfusion.

ASSESSMENT

The initial assessment of a dehydrated child should attempt to determine the cause of the illness, severity and type of dehydration, adequacy of tissue perfusion, and presence of end-organ damage.

History

The most accurate way to determine the degree of dehydration is to compare the premorbid weight with the weight at presentation. Every attempt should be made to obtain this information, including parental questioning, referral to medical records, or communication with other care providers. It is necessary to assess fluid intake since the onset of illness, paying attention to any deviation from usual feeding patterns, frequency of drinking, volume taken, and nature of the fluid provided. Questions also should focus on (1) quantity, frequency, and duration of excessive sensible fluid losses (vomiting and diarrhea), (2) insensible fluid losses (exposure to extreme environments, height and duration of fever), and (3) the possibility of recent blood loss. Inquiring about thirst, urine output, tear production, activity level responsiveness and alterations in consciousness will help to determine the clinical severity of dehydration. The parents may have specific insight as to the cause of illness, including knowledge of chronic disease, medication use, toxic ingestion, infectious exposure, or pertinent family history.

Physical Examination

Although a comprehensive physical examination is necessary to evaluate the many possible causes of dehydration, only features that will affect the initial management of a critically ill child with dehydration are discussed here.

The respiratory pattern of a dehydrated child should be carefully observed. Hyperventilation might be the primary cause of dehydration, or it can be a manifestation of metabolic acidosis (ketones, lactate, excessive bicarbonate loss) or toxic ingestion (e.g., salicylate). Hypoventilation indicates metabolic alkalosis (volume contraction, pyloric stenosis, diuretic abuse) or a moribund state. Examination of the nervous system can be informative; extreme irritability and exaggerated deep tendon reflexes suggest hypernatremia, and seizure activity is most commonly seen with severe hyponatremia.

A list of the physical findings expected at varying degrees of isotonic dehydration (expressed as percentage of body weight lost) is presented in Table 270-1. In hypotonic dehydration all manifestations appear at lesser degrees of deficit;

in hypertonic dehydration, findings are less pronounced for a given amount of fluid deficit. Signs of 10% dehydration or greater herald impending cardiovascular collapse or shock. Immediate and aggressive fluid replacement therapy *parenterally* is mandatory.

Laboratory Evaluation

A list of laboratory tests pertinent to the immediate management of severe dehydration is presented in Table 270-1. Many other studies can be helpful and should be performed when clinically advised.

ETIOLOGY

The causes of dehydration are nearly as varied as the spectrum of human disease. The entries in the box on p. 1582 represent the more common causes and those that may require specific therapy. The reader may refer to this differential diagnosis when the cause of dehydration is not readily apparent or when the condition is refractory to conventional therapy.

MANAGEMENT

Early Stabilization

The cardinal findings in critical dehydration are rapid and diminished pulse, decrease in blood pressure, oliguria or anuria, metabolic acidosis, and altered consciousness. The central theme is impairment of tissue perfusion. Initial therapy must address restoration of the circulating volume and oxygen-carrying capacity. It is necessary to begin this task without the aid of specific laboratory results. These values can be used for fine-tuning later therapy. The recommendations presented in this section should be generalized to all patients with critical hypovolemia regardless of the type or cause of dehydration.

First the clinician should assess ventilatory adequacy. Supplemental oxygen or assisted breathing may be necessary. A member of the health care team should be charged with ongoing monitoring of the patient throughout resuscitation. Use of an electrocardiogram monitor and pulse oximeter also is recommended.

A secure, large-bore intravenous line must be established, which may not be easy in a severely dehydrated child. Temporary infusion through a 24- to 26-gauge needle or catheter might allow for placement of a larger device once venous dilation has occurred. An inordinate amount of time must not be wasted trying to secure venous access. If difficulty is encountered or if cardiovascular collapse seems imminent, an intraosseous infusion should be given and if necessary, a venous cutdown should be performed (see Appendix B). It may be necessary to establish more than one intravascular access route to accommodate the required fluid rate.

Once access is obtained, 20 ml/kg of fluid should be administered as quickly as possible. "Pushing" the fluid by hand generally is recommended. If the physician does not see clinical improvement within minutes after this initial fluid bolus, then an additional 20 ml/kg should be provided. Although precipitation of congestive heart failure is a theoretic concern with rapid-fluid administration, it is much more common that too little fluid is provided during the acute phase of therapy. Adverse overhydration is highly unlikely in a child with a healthy heart and kidneys. If, however, the patient's condition fails to stabilize after the administration of 40 ml/kg, then impaired heart function or excessive ongoing losses (such as internal hemorrhage) should be suspected and investigated. Use of invasive hemodynamic monitoring, such as central venous pressure and Swan-Ganz catheters, might be considered in the intensive care setting. These devices

Table 270-1 *Laboratory Studies in Severe Dehydration*

STUDY	SIGNIFICANCE
Arterial blood gas	Adequacy of oxygenation/ventilation; acid/base status
Complete blood count	Anemia indicative of blood loss; polycythemia indicative of fluid loss; leukocytosis suggestive of bacterial infection
Electrolytes	
Sodium	Type of dehydration
Potassium	Full body stores; acid/base status (shift of potassium ion in response to hydrogen ion concentration)
Chloride	Full body stores: identification of gastrointestinal losses (vomiting), skin losses (cystic fibrosis), renal losses (renal disease, diuretic abuse, mineralocorticoid deficiency)
Total carbon dioxide	Acid/base status
BUN/creatinine	Marker of hemoconcentration; hypovolemia vs. renal failure: BUN:Cr < 10:1 suggests acute renal failure, BUN:Cr > 10:1 suggests prerenal azotemia
Anion gap	Increased with endogenous production of acids (lactate/ketones/organic acidemias) or ingestion (salicylate, others)
Urinalysis	
Specific gravity	Approximation of osmolality (may be falsely elevated with increased glucose/protein)
Glucose	Increased with diabetes mellitus
Ketones	Increased with diabetic ketoacidosis, prolonged starvation
Protein	Increased with primary renal disease
Cellular elements	May indicate renal disease or infection
pH	Marker of acid/base status; may reflect proximal tubular dysfunction (bicarbonate wasting despite acidosis)

BUN, Blood urea nitrogen; *Cr*, creatinine.

Differential Diagnosis of Dehydration

DECREASED FLUID INTAKE

Primary adipsia (CNS abnormality)
Psychogenic adipsia
Secondary causes
- Altered consciousness
- Dysfunctional swallowing: excessive drooling
- Lack of available fluids
- Oral/pharyngeal/esophageal lesions
- Starvation: abuse/neglect; improper mixing of formula; self-imposition

EXCESSIVE GASTROINTESTINAL LOSSES

Diarrhea
- Drugs/toxins: antibiotics, chemotherapy, laxatives (especially inorganic phosphates), radiation
- Endocrine disease: adrenal insufficiency, hyperthyroidism
- Food allergy
- Immunodeficiency
- Inborn errors of metabolism: galactosemia, tyrosinemia, Wolman disease, other
- Infection: bacteria, parasite, virus
- Infectious toxins: cholera, *Escherichia coli,* food poisoning (staphylococci), pseudomembranous colitis
- Inflammatory bowel disease
- Liver disease
- Malabsorption syndromes: glucose/galactose malabsorption; gluten-sensitive enteropathy; hereditary fructose intolerance; lactase deficiency
- Nutritional deficiency
  - Isolated: folic acid, niacin, zinc
  - Protein-calorie malnutrition
- Pancreatic insufficiency
- Postinfectious state: acquired lactase deficiency, starvation (villous atrophy)
- Short-gut syndrome

Vomiting
- Adrenal insufficiency
- Food allergy
- Gastritis
- Gastroenteritis
- Gastroesophageal reflux
- Inborn errors of metabolism: hyperammonemia, metabolic acidosis, primary effect
- Increased intracranial pressure: hemorrhage, hydrocephalus, tumor, vascular event
- Intestinal obstruction: adhesion, bezoar, congenital band, intussusception, volvulus
- Liver disease
- Malabsorption
- Peptic ulcer disease
- Pregnancy
- Pyloric stenosis
- Urinary tract infection/obstruction

EXCESSIVE RESPIRATORY LOSSES

Decreased humidity of inspired gases: environment, general anesthesia, mechanical ventilation, oxygen administration
Hyperventilation (any cause)
Increased temperature of inspired gases: environment, mechanical ventilation

EXCESSIVE SKIN LOSSES

Excessive sweating
- Cardiorespiratory failure
- Chronic infection
- Cystic fibrosis
- Diencephalic syndrome
- Endocrine/metabolic disease: carcinoid syndrome, hyperthyroidism, hyperpituitarism, pheochromocytoma
- Environmental heat exposure
- Exercise
- Familial dysautonomia
- Fever
- Malignancy
- Pain
- Spinal cord injury
- Toxins: drug withdrawal, mercury, organophosphates, salicylate
- Prematurity
- Skin inflammation: atopic dermatitis, burns, desquamating diseases (e.g., staphylococcal scalded skin syndrome), Stevens-Johnson syndrome
- Trauma: chemical, physical
- Weeping infections

EXCESSIVE URINARY LOSSES

Diabetes insipidus: central, nephrogenic
Diabetes mellitus
Drugs: caffeine, diuretics, osmotic agents (intravenous contrast), salicylate, theophylline
Mineralocorticoid deficiency state
- End-organ resistance
- Hypothalamic/pituitary insufficiency
- Primary adrenal insufficiency: adrenal agenesis/hemorrhage/infection/trauma; congenital adrenal hyperplasia; idiopathic causes
- Renin deficiency state

Renal disease
Diuretic phase of acute renal failure
Proximal tubular dysfunction
- Renal tubular acidosis: hereditary/sporadic causes; Fanconi syndrome (drugs, dysproteinemias, genetic disease [many], heavy metal exposure, idiopathic, interstitial nephritis, malignancy, nephrotic syndrome, renal transplantation)
- Renal glycosuria
- Salt-losing renal disease: Bartter syndrome, parenchymal damage
- Urinary tract infection

INTERNAL LOSSES (INTRAVASCULAR DEHYDRATION)

Abdominal third spacing: ascites, postsurgical, trauma
Chest third spacing: adult respiratory distress syndrome, chylothorax, pleural effusion, pulmonary edema
Hyponatremia
Hypoproteinemia: liver failure, nephrotic syndrome, protein-losing enteropathy
Increased systemic venous pressure: pulmonary hypertension, right-sided heart failure, tricuspid regurgitation
Systemic capillary leak: hypoxemia/ischemia, sepsis

measure right and left ventricular preload, respectively. In general, low filling pressures suggest the need for continued volume replacement, whereas high values indicate obstruction to forward flow or intrinsic pump failure.

There is much debate in the literature as to the composition of the ideal fluid for the emergent phase of intravascular volume repletion; a simplified view is that there are many bad choices and only a few good ones. The goal is to keep as much of the fluid in the intravascular compartment as possible; hypotonic preparations must be avoided. Popular alternatives include normal saline, Ringer lactate, colloid solutions (e.g., plasmanate, 5% albumin), or blood products. With few exceptions, use of the standard isotonic crystalloid preparations is preferable because they are effective, readily available, inexpensive, and free of infectious risk. The use of whole blood or packed cells is indicated when the hematocrit level is below 30 or if acute blood loss has occurred. Current opinion, based on infection control (hepatitis C and acquired immunodeficiency syndrome [AIDS]), recommends withholding transfusion therapy until the hematocrit falls below 25 or until the patient shows symptoms of hypovolemia at higher hematocrit levels. Although not experimentally confirmed, normal saline probably should be avoided in the presence of metabolic acidosis, because resulting hyperchloremia might decrease sodium-coupled bicarbonate reabsorption in the renal tubules and therefore would delay correction of acidosis. The buffering capacity of lactated Ringer solution depends on the liver's ability to convert lactate to bicarbonate. This fluid should not be used in the presence of liver failure. A modified solution with bicarbonate substituted for lactate can be used. Potassium should not be added to any intravenous fluid until urine output has been observed. Thereafter it is likely that significant amounts will be needed because of full body potassium depletion. With metabolic acidosis, hypokalemia might not be apparent because of the extracellular shift of potassium in exchange for hydrogen ion. The basal requirement for glucose is 4 to 6 mg/kg/min for most children and 7 to 8 mg/kg/min for premature newborns. Provision of a 5% dextrose solution at maintenance rate or higher will satisfy this need outside the newborn period. Higher concentrations of glucose have a theoretic advantage because their increased osmotic activity will draw fluid into the intravascular space. Any benefit is lost once the renal threshold for glucose has been exceeded. Glucose-containing fluids should be avoided in the initial phase of rapid fluid resuscitation unless hypoglycemia has been documented.

Clinical Estimate of Fluid Deficit in Isotonic Dehydration*

% DEHYDRATION	CLINICAL OBSERVATION
5%	Increased HR (10-15% above baseline) Dry mucous membranes Concentration of the urine Poor tear production Normal sensorium
10%	Increased severity of above signs Decreased skin turgor Oliguria Sunken anterior fontanelle Sunken eyes Lethargy
15%	Markedly increased severity of above Decreased blood pressure Poor tissue perfusion (delayed capillary refill and acidosis) Obtundation/coma

*In hypotonic dehydration (Na < 130 mEq/l) all manifestations will appear at lesser degrees of deficit. In hypertonic dehydration (Na > 150mEq/l) less circulatory disturbance is seen for a given amount of fluid deficit.

Ongoing Care

The management of a patient with hyperosmolar dehydration represents a considerable therapeutic challenge. The most common causes are hypernatremic dehydration and hyperglycemia secondary to diabetes mellitus. As previously discussed, during the evolution of hyperosmolar dehydration the intravascular space has gradually leached free water from the interstitial and intracellular compartments. Rapid infusion of hypotonic fluid or a precipitous fall in the level of serum glucose will create an osmotic gradient receptive to movement of free water into the intracellular space. Although all body tissues will be affected, the most clinically significant impact will be seen on brain parenchyma. Tremendous influx of free water will lead to cellular swelling and damage. A common clinical finding is transient improvement in mental status at the onset of fluid therapy, with subsequent decline. This process can culminate in seizures, coma, or brain death. Although this consideration should not influence the emergent stabilization of a patient in shock, certain safeguards should be followed thereafter. Rapid infusion of hypotonic fluids should be avoided, a minimum of 48 hours should be allowed for replacement of the fluid deficit, serum sodium should not fall more than 0.5 mEq/L/hr, and the rate of glucose fall from baseline in severe hyperglycemia should not exceed 80 to 100 mg/dl/hr. Adherence to these recommendations does not ensure safety, and ongoing patient assessment is required. Therapy must be titrated in response to its clinical effect.

Conversely, rapid correction of severe hyponatremia can cause cerebral desiccation. The use of hypertonic fluid preparations is not indicated unless the patient has status epilepticus. Even at this extreme the use of 3% sodium chloride should be halted after symptomatic treatment, generally to a serum sodium concentration in the mid-120 mEg/L range. Although correction of electrolyte imbalance over a 24-hour period usually is safe, a longer period should be allowed in severe cases or for a chronically ill patient with long-standing hyponatremia.

Once emergent intravascular volume repletion has been accomplished, the physician must address replacement of the "full body" deficit of salt and water, compensation for ongoing losses, and provision of maintenance fluid and electrolyte requirements. The calculations necessary to estimate the patient's needs are based on weight, body surface area, caloric expenditure, and the mechanism, type, and severity of dehydration. (See Chapter 5 for a comprehensive discussion of fluid therapy.) Once a patient has begun to recover, the physician should reconsider prohibition of drinking. In most circumstances the instincts of an alert child, when coupled with healthy kidneys and an appropriate oral fluid, can provide convincing contradiction to the physician's "precise" calculations.

OUTCOME

The most common long-term sequelae of severe dehydration include renal failure, thrombosis of the renal vein or sagittal sinus, hepatic necrosis, brain injury, and intestinal dysfunction. Fortunately, these complications generally are rare and transient. Despite an ominous presentation, the vast majority of patients with severe dehydration enjoy a full recovery when therapy is rapid and appropriate.

SUGGESTED READINGS

Feld LG, Kaskel FJ, and Schoeneman MJ: The approach to fluid and electrolyte therapy in pediatrics, Adv Pediatr 35:497, 1988.

Finberg L: Dehydration in infants and children, N Engl J Med 276:458, 1967.

Finberg L, Fleischman AR, and Kravath RE: Water and electrolytes in pediatrics, Philadelphia, 1982, WB Saunders Co.

Kanter RK: Evaluation and stabilization of the critically ill child, Clin Chest Med 8:573, 1987.

Oh W: Disorders of fluid and electrolytes in newborn infants, Pediatr Clin North Am 23:601, 1976.

271

Diabetic Ketoacidosis

Robert E. Greenberg

Ketoacidosis may often be the initial event leading to the diagnosis of diabetes mellitus. Coexistence of coma is a much less common occurrence. As clinical recognition of the diabetic state has improved, however, diabetic ketoacidosis is now becoming forestalled. Yet intercurrent episodes of ketoacidosis remain a frequent occurrence, especially among those diabetic children whose psychosocial and biologic factors impose barriers to effective diabetic management or impede the metabolic response to insulin. Although the mortality rate is low, even from coma, meticulous management of diabetic ketoacidosis is required to prevent or detect complications.

DEFINITION

Diabetic ketoacidosis occurs when the rate of endogenous glucose production continues unrestrained, despite the presence of markedly curtailed peripheral glucose utilization. The resultant increase in the breakdown of fat leads to the accumulation of nonesterified fatty acids and, in the subsequent hepatic conversion of fatty acids to ketone bodies, to the release of hydrogen ion. The combined effects of osmotic diuresis and increased generation of protons lead to both dehydration and acidosis. If these events are prolonged or severe, then stupor, drowsiness, and coma may occur.

ETIOLOGY

Glucose Metabolism

The concentration of glucose in blood is remarkably constant in the normal child, even during periods of fasting. Fasting involves the physiologic suppression of insulin secretion, with consequent reduction of peripheral glucose utilization and mobilization of substrate (free or nonesterified fatty acids) from triglyceride stores. The reduction in insulin secretion leads to a marked curtailment of glucose utilization by insulin-sensitive tissues. Worse, glucose utilization is further compromised during fasting by the direct inhibiting effects of both free fatty acids and ketone bodies (Fig. 271-1); it may be still further impeded during severe metabolic acidosis, when the binding of insulin to membrane receptors is impaired.

The reduction in glucose utilization that normally occurs during fasting is necessary to conserve body protein as effectively as possible. Were ongoing glucose utilization not curtailed, then increased rates of new glucose formation (gluconeogenesis) would be mandatory to replace missing exogenous carbohydrate. However, gluconeogenesis requires precursor amino acids, so that the duration of a prolonged fast would be markedly restricted were body protein stores not most jealously guarded.

Gluconeogenesis is not finely modulated in diabetic ketoacidosis but, rather, persists at a physiologically uncontrolled rate. This lack of control is the complex result of reduced insulin availability, increased substrate flow from muscle and adipose tissue, and increased counterregulatory hormones (which accelerate glucose production). Thus, at the very time when glucose utilization is compromised, glucose production is paradoxically increased, with resultant hyperglycemia and consequent osmotic diuresis and dehydration.

Alternate Energy Sources

When the availability of glucose as a substrate for intracellular energy metabolism is reduced, then alternate energy sources must be made available. Hence, triglyceride (neutral fat) is broken down into glycerol and fatty acids; the fatty acids release hydrogen ion during their subsequent hepatic conversion to ketone bodies (Fig. 271-2). Ketone bodies thus accumulate in blood as a consequence both of increased production and of reduced peripheral utilization, because turnover rates for ketone bodies are prolonged in diabetic ketoacidosis (Figs. 271-2 and 271-3).

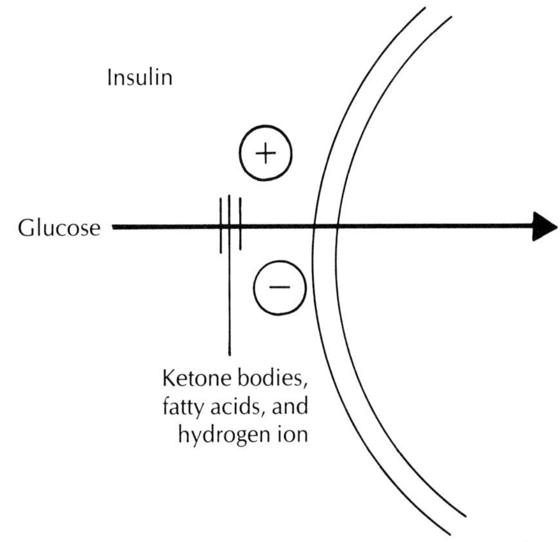

Fig. 271-1 Factors affecting glucose transport across cell membranes. +, Increase; −, decrease.

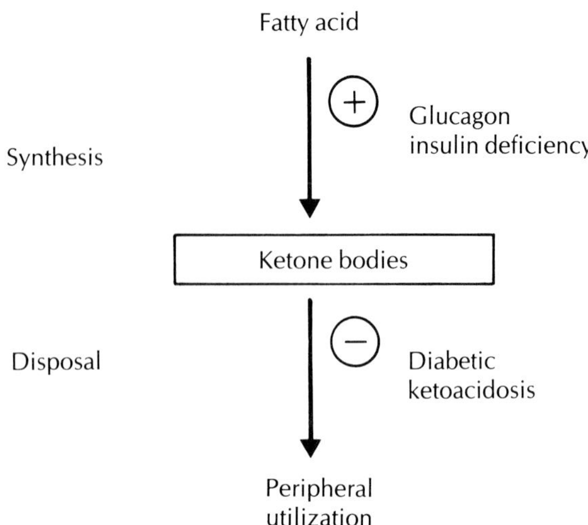

Fig. 271-2 Control of ketone body synthesis and disposal. +, Increase; −, decrease.

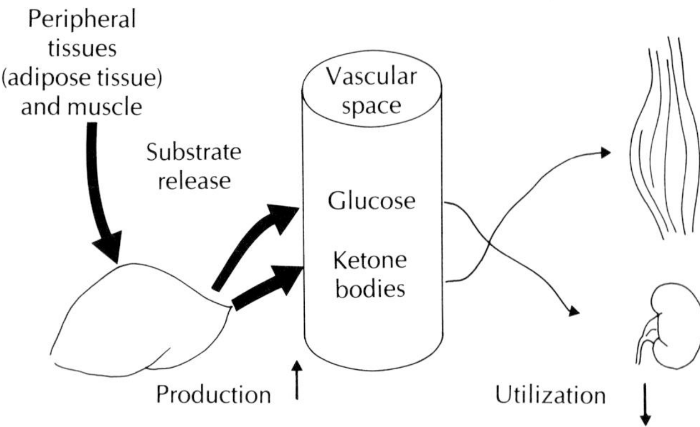

Fig. 271-3 Substrate production and utilization in diabetic ketoacidosis.

Role of Counterregulatory Hormones

There is a resistance to the action of insulin in diabetic ketoacidosis for reasons other than the direct effects of acidosis. One such reason is the increased secretion of counterregulatory hormones, a clear example of which is seen in the control of triglyceride breakdown (Fig. 271-4). Insulin inhibits lipolysis, an aspect of its action that is partially independent of its effects on glucose transport. However, catecholamines, cortisol, growth hormone, glucagon, and thyroid hormones all exert—either directly or indirectly—an opposite effect on fat breakdown so as to enhance lipolytic rates, even in the presence of adequate insulin. Activation of counterregulatory hormone secretion, in response to either biologic or emotional stimuli, leads to accelerated rates of lipolysis, which in persons with diabetes further impairs metabolic regulation. Increased secretion of counterregulatory hormones, in the presence of relative insulin insufficiency, thus compounds the decreased utilization and increased production of glucose and ketone bodies.

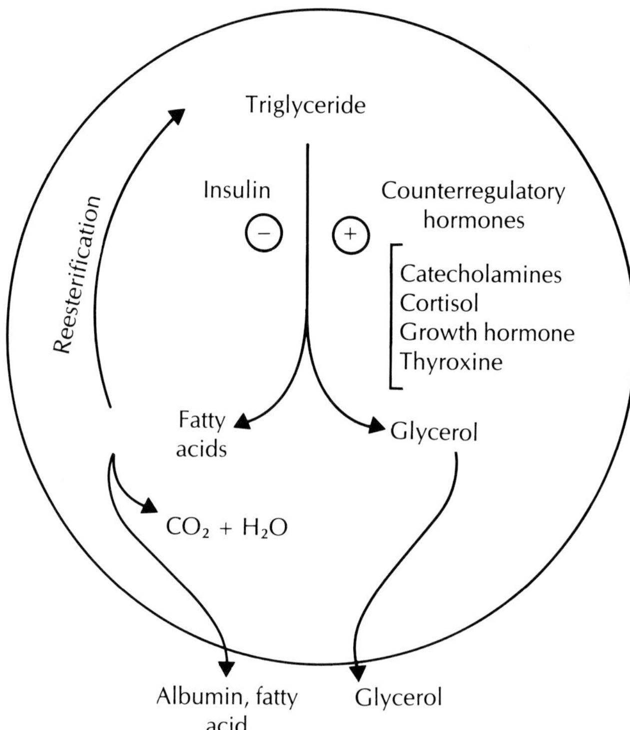

Fig. 271-4 Control of triglyceride breakdown. +, Increase; −, decrease.

INITIAL ASSESSMENT

The severity of acidemia in diabetic ketoacidosis is the summation of increased hydrogen ion generation and reduced hydrogen ion secretion, the latter as a consequence of dehydration. Reversal of this process requires the biologic actions of exogenously supplied insulin and replacement of water and electrolytes. The diagnosis of diabetic ketoacidosis usually is not difficult, except when a previously undiagnosed patient is admitted in coma. The antecedent symptoms of nausea and vomiting, thirst and polyuria, weakness, weight loss, and visual disturbances lead most often to a rapid clinical diagnosis.

In the initial assessment, two urgent issues are (1) the evaluation of effective blood volume and (2) the differential diagnosis of coma. Tachycardia, hypotension, and hypothermia all should suggest reduced blood volume; its rapid expansion with isotonic saline or colloid is essential. The precise cause of stupor, drowsiness, and coma in a diabetic child may be difficult to document (hence, to treat accurately) and might well involve hypoglycemia, ketoacidosis, lactic acidosis, or hyperglycemic-hyperosmolar nonketotic coma. Where there is doubt as to the cause of coma, immediate intravenous administration of glucose (2 to 3 ml/kg of a 50% dextrose solution) may prevent significant neurologic damage; if hypoglycemia is not present, the amount of glucose given under such a policy is insignificant compared with the total pool of available glucose.

When blood volume is markedly depleted or ketoacidosis especially severe, then respiratory compensation for metabolic acidosis may not be clinically apparent; that is, the classic Kussmaul respirations of ketoacidosis may become clinically evident only after blood volume has been at least partially restored.

A confusing problem in assessment often is present because of the notable frequency of abdominal pain as a symptom of diabetic ketoacidosis. In the comatose patient, gastric atony and dilation may lead to vomiting and aspiration; thus immediate placement of an indwelling gastric tube under constant low suction to remove gastric contents is essential.

TREATMENT

Initial Therapeutic Procedures

The suspected diagnosis of diabetic ketoacidosis is rapidly confirmed by use of methods available in any emergency room that demonstrate elevated glucose and ketone body concentrations in both blood and urine. A fairly accurate estimate of serum glucose can be made by diluting serum serially until a reading can be made, using fresh Dextrostix or Chemstrip bG reagent strips; similarly, the severity of ketonemia can be estimated by noting the dilution of serum that still gives a positive test result, with use of crushed or powdered Acetest tablets. Although there are exceptions, it is possible to derive semiquantitative estimates of blood ketone body concentration by multiplying by 0.1 mM the highest dilution still giving a positive test result, to yield a rough estimate of acetoacetate concentration. Because the normal ratio of beta-hydroxybutyrate to acetoacetate is 3:1, multiplying this estimated concentration of acetoacetate by 4 will provide the final estimate for total ketone body concentration. The patient with dehydration, an altered state of consciousness, and Kussmaul respirations, yet with only a minimal rise in estimated serum ketone body concentration, is the one in whom alternate proton donors must be sought, especially lactic acid. A difficult clinical problem may be presented by the dehydrated, acidemic child who has been given parenteral glucose-containing solutions before measurement of blood glucose; in this setting, reduced peripheral perfusion may be associated with impaired glucose utilization to produce "artifactual" (i.e., nondiabetic) hyperglycemia. The correct diagnosis will depend on elicitation of the proper historical evidence to reveal the mechanism producing dehydration.

The severity of blood volume depletion in the child with diabetic ketoacidosis (blood pH <7.2) can be appreciated from the resultant hormonal changes: serum concentrations of arginine vasopressin, plasma renin activity, aldosterone, and norepinephrine are increased threefold to 20-fold, and the concentration of atrial natriuretic peptide is markedly reduced.

After establishing the diagnosis of diabetic ketoacidosis, the physician should quickly center attention on (1) restoring blood volume and (2) initiating a physiologic response to insulin. In the presence of significant hyperosmolality (i.e., hyperglycemia), the rapid administration of hypotonic fluids may cause cerebral edema; accordingly, initial intravenous fluids should be isotonic and rapidly administered (10 to 20 ml/kg/hr), even in the absence of evident blood volume depletion, until the results of laboratory tests can clarify the magnitude of hyperglycemia and the severity of acidemia.

Insulin should be administered as quickly as possible and in doses that achieve physiologic concentrations of insulin in blood. Low-dose *constant insulin infusion* employs 0.1 unit of regular insulin per kilogram as an initial "push" dose, followed by a similar amount administered over an hour by constant infusion.

Two issues are important to note regarding any form of insulin therapy: (1) the physiologic response to insulin must be demonstrated, not assumed and (2) sensitivity to insulin may change during the course of diabetic ketoacidosis, so that a rate of insulin infusion that initially effects stabilization may produce hypoglycemia subsequently. Subcutaneous insulin may be erratically or poorly absorbed by a hypovolemic patient, as compared with intravenous infusion, although insulin administered subcutaneously remains an effective form of therapy.

If clinical evaluation indicates that the blood volume is beginning to be restored and appropriate amounts of insulin are being provided, then the question of patient transfer, if necessary, can be decided. A flow sheet should be started, on which the following should be carefully recorded and monitored: the nature and rate of intravenous fluids administered, insulin dosage, urine output, vital signs, and laboratory data.

Subsequent Therapy

During the 6 to 12 hours after initial stabilization, therapeutic concerns should center on the following series of definable problems.

Prevention of Cerebral Edema. The occurrence of cerebral edema is extremely common as a subclinical finding during therapy for diabetic ketoacidosis; clinically evident cerebral edema represents the primary cause of death. Patients at risk for development of cerebral edema include those whose condition has been in prolonged poor control; those with severe acidemia (blood pH <7.2); those with normal serum sodium concentrations in the presence of hyperglycemia; and those with early signs of increased intracranial pressure. Although blood volume depletion must initially be vigorously addressed, the rate of subsequent infusion of hypotonic fluids should not be excessive and must be carefully monitored.

Management of Acidemia. The definitive approach to the management of ketoacidosis is to reduce the generation of increased hydrogen ion (by insulin administration) and to improve the capacity to excrete an acid load (by blood volume expansion). In the presence of severe acidemia (pH <7.0), the irritability of cardiac muscle increases with resultant increased likelihood of cardiac arrhythmias. Because of negative inotropic effects on the heart, cardiac output may fall. When the pH is markedly reduced, the ability of insulin to bind to its membrane receptors is impaired, reducing still further the physiologic response to insulin.

Correction of severe acidosis with bicarbonate may thus be necessary before insulin can be effective and, certainly, in instances of aberrant cardiac function. However, use of bicarbonate is not without significant hazard; when it is administered in large amounts, serum bicarbonate rises, raising blood pH values and reducing the stimulus for respiratory compensation so that carbon dioxide accumulates. Because carbon dioxide equilibrates across the blood-brain barrier much more rapidly than does bicarbonate, the intracerebral space may become more acidotic, even as extracellular pH values climb. Further, severe hypokalemia may be precipitated by bicarbonate administration, requiring frequent monitoring and potassium supplementation.

Prevention of Hypoglycemia. The occurrence of significant and even dangerous hypoglycemia during management of diabetic ketoacidosis can be a severe complication. It occurs primarily when glucose is not being provided in the intravenous fluids, excessive amounts of insulin are administered, or the patient's changing sensitivity to insulin is not recognized. Early administration of exogenous glucose and use of the low-dose constant insulin infusion technique minimize the risk of hypoglycemia.

Hyperosmolar nonketotic diabetic coma in childhood is a rare condition; when it does occur, however, the mortality is much higher than in diabetic ketoacidosis. Hyperosmolar nonketotic hyperglycemic coma is defined as a marked increase in blood glucose concentration (usually 800 mg/dl), the absence of ketoacidosis, an altered state of consciousness, and significant dehydration. Thus the initial laboratory studies of severe hyperglycemia without significant ketonemia in a child with an altered state of consciousness should alert the physician to the presence of this syndrome. A hyperosmolar state also can develop during treatment and is detected by demonstrating marked hyperglycemia and by noting the excessive rate of diuresis in relation to the observed clinical state of hydration and rate of intravenous fluid administration. Because of the rarity of hyperosmolar coma, relative to the frequency of therapy-induced hypoglycemia, glucose should be incorporated into intravenous fluids just as soon as it is clear that the blood glucose concentration either is not markedly elevated or is falling during insulin infusion.

Replacement of Water and Electrolyte Deficits. The child with severe diabetic ketoacidosis has marked deficits of water and electrolytes. However, in contrast to many other conditions in which dehydration is the presenting problem, ongoing fluid and electrolyte losses in diabetic ketoacidosis may be excessive, as a consequence of osmotic diuresis. Assuming that there is no acute or chronic defect of cardiorespiratory or renal function, it is better to err on the side of excess fluid administration. In most instances the first 24 hours of fluid therapy will require rates of fluid administration in excess of three times the usual maintenance fluid requirements. Careful attention to intake and output records and periodic determination of body weight are necessary.

Osmotic diuresis produces water losses in excess of electrolyte losses. Thus, as soon as blood volume has been expanded and the danger of hyperosmolality assessed, the introduction of hypotonic fluids becomes appropriate. The usual fluid will contain the following approximate contents: Na^+, 30 to 40 mEq/L; K^+, 30 to 40 mEq/L; HCO_3^- 10 to 20 mEq/L; and Cl^-, 50 to 60 mEq/L. Because prolonged use of chloride ion as the only anion is itself acidifying, the administration of bicarbonate in amounts found in extracellular fluid represents physiologic replacement in this case, rather than use of, say, bicarbonate to combat established acidosis.

Prevention of Hypokalemia. Total body potassium losses may well be excessive in diabetic ketoacidosis and may continue during ongoing osmotic diuresis. Further, the reincorporation of available extracellular potassium into the intracellular space may lead to profound hypokalemia. Adequate amounts of potassium used early in the intravenous fluid program and careful monitoring of both serum potassium and electrocardiographic tracings will minimize the hazard of hypokalemia, the danger of which is greatest during the first 12 hours after the initiation of corrective therapy.

Detection of Lactic Acidosis. Lactic acidosis may occur in several situations in diabetes: (1) lactic acid may accumulate, to some degree, as part of ketoacidosis; (2) it may accumulate during therapy as a complication of tissue hypoxia accompanying severe hypophosphatemia; and (3) lactic acidemia may be a presenting problem in the absence of significant ketonemia. This latter occurrence is much more common in adults, especially in elderly persons.

Serum phosphate predictably falls during the management of diabetic ketoacidosis. With significant hypophosphatemia, levels of red blood cell 2,3-diphosphoglycerate also will fall, reducing the ability of hemoglobin to release oxygen. The resultant tissue hypoxia leads to lactic acidosis, which is corrected with phosphate infusions. The presence of lactic acidosis should be suspected whenever the clinical appearance of the child (Kussmaul respirations) or the measurement of blood pH indicates a degree of acidemia unexplained by the measured or estimated concentration of serum ketone bodies.

The Acetest tablet reflects only acetoacetate, however, and does not detect beta-hydroxybutyrate. On initial examination, the patient's degree of ketonemia may be underestimated because the beta-hydroxybutyrate/acetoacetate ratio is increased in diabetic ketoacidosis. Upon correction, on the other hand, the degree of ketonemia may be overestimated, inasmuch as the aforementioned ratio will decrease, so that a greater proportion of the total ketone bodies will be present as measurable (by Acetest) acetoacetate. Thus the occurrence of a significant anion gap and acidemia in the absence of detectable ketone bodies is an important clue to the presence of other causes for persistent metabolic acidosis.

Treatment of Precipitating Conditions. Diabetic ketoacidosis may be precipitated by other events, including infection. Presence of an underlying infection may be difficult to document, because leukocytosis with increased release of nonsegmented leukocytes can occur in diabetic ketoacidosis without infection. Careful observation and repeated physical examination usually will clarify coexistent disease and delineate the significance of concurrent abdominal pain.

IATROGENIC DANGERS

The main predisposing factor in iatrogenic complications is the physician's failure to monitor the child as his or her physiologic state changes under therapy. Attention to the physiology of the primary problems to be ameliorated and careful observation of the child during the first 6 to 12 hours of treatment should minimize the danger of complications. The most important consideration in evaluating the need to transfer a patient is the availability of competent professionals—the expert who is unavailable cannot help.

CONVALESCENT CARE

Subcutaneous insulin can be initiated after oral intake of fluids and nutrition has become adequate. The principal task must then be to focus on exploring reasons for the occurrence of diabetic ketoacidosis. If the onset of ketoacidosis heralded the initial diagnosis of diabetes mellitus, then primary attention must be focused on patient and family education and on helping the family adapt to the new diagnosis of a chronic (and incurable) disease. Where the ketoacidosis represents a recurrent problem in a known diabetic child, primary attention must be focused on determining and resolving the biologic and psychosocial factors that led to aberrant metabolic control.

SUGGESTED READINGS

Barrett EJ et al: Insulin resistance in diabetic ketoacidosis, Diabetes 31:923, 1982.

Baruh S, Sherman L, and Markowitz S: Diabetic ketoacidosis and coma, Med Clin North Am 65:117, 1981.

Cahill GF et al: Hormone-fuel interrelationships during fasting, J Clin Invest 45:1751, 1966.

Hare JW and Rossini AA: Diabetic comas: the overlap concept, Hosp Pract 14:95, 1979.

Harris GD, Fiordalis I, and Finberg L: Safe management of diabetic ketoacidemia, J Pediatr 113:65, 1988.

Keller V and Bergen W: Prevention of hypophosphatemia by phosphate infusion during treatment of diabetic ketoacidosis and hyperosmolar coma, Diabetes 29:87, 1980.

Robinson AM and Williamson DH: Physiological roles of ketone bodies as substrates and signals in mammalian tissues, Physiol Rev 60:143, 1980.

Schade DS and Eaton RP: The temporal relationship between endogenously secreted stress hormones and metabolic decompensation in diabetic man, J Clin Endocrinol Metab 50:131, 1980.

Schade DS et al: Diabetic coma, Albuquerque, 1981, University of New Mexico Press.

Tulassay T et al: Atrial natriuretic peptide and other vasoactive hormones during treatment of severe diabetic ketoacidosis in children, J Pediatr 111:329, 1987.

272

Disseminated Intravascular Coagulation

William E. Hathaway

DEFINITION AND ETIOLOGY

Disseminated intravascular coagulation (DIC) is an acquired pathologic process characterized by activation of the coagulation system, leading to thrombin generation, intravascular fibrin deposition, and platelet consumption. Microthrombi, composed of fibrin and platelets, may produce ischemic tissue damage as well as fragmentation of erythrocytes. The fibrinolytic system is also frequently activated to produce plasmin-mediated destruction of fibrin, fibrinogen, and other clotting factors (factor VIII, factor V). Degradation (split) products of fibrin-fibrinogen (FSP) are formed and function as anticoagulants and inhibitors of platelet function. Clinically these processes may be expressed as diffuse hemorrhage, organ ischemia, or hemolytic anemia. DIC commonly accompanies disorders seen in the critically ill infant and child such as endothelial cell damage (endotoxin, virus), tissue destruction (necrosis, physical injuries), hypoxia (acidosis), ischemic and vascular changes (shock, hemangiomas), and release of tissue procoagulants (malignancies, placental disorders). These conditions or triggers are seen in the specific diseases indicated in the accompanying box.[1,2,8]

RECOGNITION

Physical Findings

Because DIC can occur in any seriously or critically ill infant or child, the process should be suspected whenever the initial assessment indicates one of the diagnoses listed in the box. Physical signs of DIC include (1) a diffuse bleeding tendency (hematuria, melena, purpura, petechiae, persistent oozing from needle punctures or other invasive procedures), (2) circulatory collapse, poor skin perfusion, or early ischemic changes, and (3) thrombotic lesions (major vessel thrombosis, gangrene, purpura fulminans).

Laboratory Findings

The laboratory diagnosis of DIC is relatively straightforward (with the exceptions noted below); laboratory test findings that may be abnormal are listed in Table 272-1. Those tests most useful because they are sensitive, are easy to perform, and reflect the hemostatic capacity of the patient are the partial thromboplastin time (PTT), prothrombin time (PT), platelet count, fibrinogen level, and a test for FSP (the Thrombo-Wellco test for serum FSP), or the protamine precipitation test for plasma monomer–FSP complexes or circulating cross-linked fibrin, D-dimer.[9] If these test results are normal or only slightly abnormal, clinically significant DIC most likely is not present. However, depending on the triggering event for DIC, varying degrees of abnormality may be seen in these screening tests. Patients with an infection may have thrombocytopenia primarily, with only slight prolongation of the PTT and the PT and mildly elevated levels of FSP. Platelets may be consumed during bacterial sepsis without any other evidence for activation of coagulation. Asphyxia (at any

Conditions and Diseases Known to Trigger Disseminated Intravascular Coagulation

ENDOTHELIAL CELL DAMAGE

Bacterial sepsis
Diffuse viral infections
Rickettsial and protozoan infections

TISSUE DESTRUCTION

Trauma (crushing and penetrating injuries, e.g., brain injury)
Thermal burns

HYPOXIA-ACIDOSIS

Asphyxia (perinatal, near-drowning)
Respiratory distress syndrome (neonatal, shock lung)

RELEASE OF TISSUE PROCOAGULANTS

Malignant neoplasms
Leukemia (promyelocytic, monocytic)
Obstetric disorders (abruptio placentae, dead twin fetus)
Venoms (snake, spider)

VASCULAR AND CIRCULATORY DISORDERS

Shock
Vasculitis
Giant hemangioma
Large vessel thrombosis, purpura fulminans

Table 272-1 *Laboratory Tests That May Show Abnormal Findings in Disseminated Intravascular Coagulation*

LABORATORY TEST	MECHANISM FOR ABNORMAL FINDING
Prolonged PTT	Decreased procoagulants, increased fibrin split products
Prolonged PT	Decreased procoagulants, increased fibrin split products
Prolonged TT	Decreased firbinogen, increased fibrin split products, heparin effect
Prolonged reptilase time	Decreased fibrinogen, increased fibrin split products
Decreased platelet count	Platelet consumption
Decreased fibrinogen level	Fibrinogen consumption
Increased FSP; D-dimer	Plasmin degradation of fibrin and fibrinogen
Prolonged BT	Decreased platelets and decreased platelet function
Decreased activity of coagulation factors XXI, prekallikrein, V, VII, VIII, prothrombin (II), AT-III, XIII, plasminogen, protein C	See text for explanation of mechanism

AT, Antithrombin; *BT*, bleeding time; *FSP*, fibrin-fibrinogen split products; *PT*, prothrombin time; *PTT*, partial thromboplastin time; *TT*, thrombin time.

age), on the other hand, may produce significant consumption of fibrinogen and elevated levels of FSP without depression of platelets. In the neonatal period the PTT often is prolonged physiologically and thus is less useful as a screening test for DIC.[4]

In severe DIC virtually all the coagulation factors may be activated as well as inhibited by protease inhibitors (antithrombin [AT]–III, antiplasmins, protein C), resulting in variable and transient alterations of their activity, as indicated in Table 272-1. For this reason, specific factor assays are not often helpful in diagnosis. For example, factor VIII procoagulant activity may be normal, depressed, or even elevated.

Although elevations of FSP, whether measured by the serum test (Thrombo-Wellco test), the "monomer" test (protamine precipitation), D-dimer or the thrombin time, are frequently seen in DIC, normal levels of FSP do not preclude the diagnosis. Further, abnormal test results may be seen in inflammatory conditions or malignancies without other evidence of DIC.

DIFFERENTIAL DIAGNOSIS

The differential diagnosis of a diffuse bleeding tendency in the critically ill patient must include clinical entities other than DIC. Uremic bleeding (because of a platelet function defect), severe hepatic coagulopathy (because of decreased synthesis of clotting factors), and vitamin K deficiency can all mimic DIC or, as well, complicate DIC triggered by other events. Vitamin K deficiency can be easily diagnosed by measurement of noncarboxylated prothrombin (Table 272-2) even after the PT improves. Neither is uremia hard to recognize. The most difficult coagulopathies to manage are those that occur in children with severe liver disease. In fact, fulminant hepatitis and advanced cirrhosis often lead to decreased hepatic production of coagulation factors, as well as to increased consumption of platelets and fibrinogen.[7] The newborn infant with herpes simplex hepatitis is an excellent example of this situation. The usual alterations of coagulation observed in these complex conditions are summarized in Table 272-2.

MANAGEMENT AND COMPLICATIONS

Because the most important aspect of therapy for DIC consists of recognizing and alleviating the underlying disease or triggering event, the management plan must include prompt recognition and efficient correction of shock, hypoxia, acidosis, fulminant infection, and severe anemia. Pertinent examples might include (1) antibiotic therapy, volume replacement, and circulatory support (isoproterenol, dopamine) in bacterial sepsis, (2) relief of hypoxia and correction of acidosis in neonatal asphyxia and respiratory distress syndromes, (3) restoration of blood volume in hemorrhagic shock, and (4) use of antiviral agents in severe viral infections. If the precipitating condition can be quickly corrected (e.g., relief of hypoxia or shock), often no other therapy is needed. Serial determinations of coagulation tests are helpful in deciding when further therapy is indicated.

In most instances, infants and children with significant DIC should be cared for in level III clinical settings (intensive care units). Replacement of depleted coagulation factors and platelets may be necessary, especially if DIC is associated with a bleeding diathesis or potential severe hemorrhage. Initial stabilization of the child suspected of having DIC should include use of fresh frozen plasma (FFP) whenever volume expanders are indicated, so as to replace depleted coagulation factors while replacing blood volume. Fibrinogen and other clotting factors are replaced by FFP; a dose of 10 to 15 ml/kg of FFP will raise the clotting factor level by about 20%. Fibrinogen (and factor VIII) also can be given as cryoprecipitates; 1 cryoprecipitate unit per 3 kg in infants (1 cryoprecipitate unit per 5 kg in older children) will raise the fibrinogen by about 75 to 100 mg/dl. Platelets are replaced with platelet concentrates; in the neonate, 10 ml/kg of platelet concentrate will raise the platelet count by about 75,000 to 100,000 per microliter. In older children, 1 platelet concentrate per 5 to 6 kg is the usual dose. A platelet count of 30,000 to 50,000/μl, a prolongation of the PT by less than 4 seconds, and a fibrinogen level of 100 mg/dl are the minimal acceptable hemostatic target levels for the procoagulants.

The role of the primary care practitioner in the care of seriously ill patients with DIC can be summarized as follows: (1) to recognize the presence of DIC swiftly and to assess its manifestations (bleeding, laboratory evidence for depleted clotting factors, associated thrombotic complications), (2) to institute therapy for the triggering event, (3) to effect stabilization and general support of the patient, (4) to replace depleted hemostatic factors as needed, including administra-

Table 272-2 *Usual Alterations of Coagulation in Conditions That May Be Confused with Disseminated Intravascular Coagulation*

	SCREENING TESTS					OTHER TESTS		
CONDITION	PLATELETS	PTT	PT	FIBRINOGEN	FSP	FACTOR VIII	FACTOR V	FACTORS VII and X
DIC	−	+	+	−	+	− or +	−	0 or −
Uremia	0	0	0 or −	0	0 or +	+	0	0
Hemolytic-uremic syndrome	−	0	0	0	+	+	0	0
Vitamin K deficiency	0	+	+	0	0	0	0	−
Severe liver disease	0 or −	+	+	−	+	+	−	−

+, Increased; −, decreased; 0, normal.

tion of vitamin K (infants, 1 to 2 mg; older children, 5 mg of the K_1 oxide preparation), and (5) to transfer the patient early in the course to an intensive care setting as indicated; for example, the condition of the child with the complex coagulopathy typical of severe liver disease often is difficult to assess and requires the expert hematologic consultation usually available only in a tertiary center.

Occasionally it may be necessary to interrupt the clotting process with heparin, especially in those specific instances in which the triggering event cannot be quickly removed and in which the consumptive coagulopathy and tissue necrosis are ongoing.[3] Examples of these situations include (1) acute promyelocytic or monocytic leukemia, (2) giant hemangiomas, (3) the occasional patient with hemolytic-uremic syndrome and frank DIC, and (4) impending tissue necrosis or gangrene in septic shock, large vessel thrombosis, and purpura fulminans. In these instances, heparin may halt the DIC or at least allow for more effective replacement therapy while the primary disease is being specifically treated. Continuous intravenous administration is the most effective and safe method for giving heparin[5]; a loading dose of 50 U/kg is followed by 10 to 15 U/kg/hr. Unless there is significant tissue necrosis, this dose usually is effective and improvement in coagulation screening tests can be expected in less than 12 to 24 hours.

In purpura fulminans, heparin is absolutely indicated to halt the gangrenous process, often at a higher dose (20 to 25 U/kg/hr). Alternatively, heparin can be given intermittently (75 to 100 U/kg every 4 hours) by intravenous "push." Intermittent therapy may be used when continuous therapy cannot be achieved because of technical difficulties. Monitoring the effect of heparin usually is not necessary in DIC if the desired result in the coagulation process is obtained—specifically, stabilization and improvement in the PT, fibrinogen level, and platelet count. A demonstrable heparin effect on the PTT time or activated whole blood clotting time should be achieved (prolongation of these tests to 1.5 to 2 times normal) by heparin treatment of purpura fulminans. The heparin effect may be enhanced by FFP in severe cases. Note that purpura fulminans in the newborn may be a result of homozygous protein C deficiency[6] and will require replacement therapy with FFP.

Heparinization may rarely be indicated as part of the initial stabilization process. Heparin may possibly prevent tissue necrosis in children with meningococcemia who show severe skin purpura and ischemic changes, as well as in infants with large vessel thrombosis (renal vein, vena cava, aorta).

REFERENCES

1. Bell WR: Disseminated intravascular coagulation, Johns Hopkins Med J 146:289, 1980.
2. Bick RL: Disseminated intravascular coagulation: I, Semin Thromb Hemost 14(4), 1988.
3. Feinstein DI: Diagnosis and management of disseminated intravascular coagulation: the role of heparin therapy, Blood 60:284, 1982.
4. Hathaway WE and Bonnar J: Hemostatic disorders of the pregnant woman and newborn infant, New York, 1987, Elsevier Science Publishing Co.
5. McDonald MM and Hathaway WE: Anticoagulant therapy by continuous heparinization in newborn and older infants. J Pediatr 101:451, 1982.
6. Monlar RA et al: Diagnosis and treatment of homozygous protein C deficiency, J Pediatr 114:528, 1989.
7. Stein SF and Harker LA: Kinetic and functional studies of platelets, fibrinogen, and plasminogen in patients with hepatic cirrhosis, J Lab Clin Med 99:217, 1982.
8. Wilde JT et al: Association between necropsy evidence of DIC and coagulation variables before death in patients in intensive care units, J Clin Pathol 41:138, 1988.
9. Wilde JT et al: Plasma D-dimer levels and their relationship to serum fibrinogen/fibrin degradation products in hypercoagulable states, Br J Haematol 7:65, 1989.

273

Drowning and Near-Drowning

Linda K. Snelling and Richard S.K. Young

Drowning is surpassed only by automobile collisions as the leading cause of accidental death in children and adolescents. Between 1980 and 1985, 8568 drowning deaths were reported among children up to 14 years of age in the United States.[2] The age distribution of drowning is influenced by both race and socioeconomic status. For instance, the incidence of drowning in children 1 to 4 years of age is twice as high for white children as for black children, is highest in western states and Florida, and is strongly correlated with the presence of backyard swimming pools. In other age-groups, as in other causes of accidental deaths, black children are disproportionately affected. Drowning rates for children 10 to 14 years of age are 3.4 times higher for black than for white children and, in this age-group, are especially high in southern states. Drowning in bathtubs accounts for 8% of the total number of deaths caused by drowning.[2] Adolescent and adult drowning incidents frequently are associated with the use of alcohol. The majority of deaths due to drowning are preventable by education of parents as well as children and by barriers preventing access to backyard swimming pools, ponds, and quarries.

Drowning is classically defined as death by suffocation under water. Although the use and definition of the terms *drowning* and *near-drowning* have been somewhat controversial, most authors reserve the term drowning for death occurring within 24 hours of the submersion incident, whether at the scene or in hospital, and define near-drowning as survival for at least 24 hours, whether the patient recovers or subsequently dies. Others have argued that the term near-drowning should be used for all cases of drowning in which the resuscitated victim lives, if only for a short time. We prefer the 24-hour definition because it is not subject to personal interpretation.

PATHOPHYSIOLOGY OF DROWNING

Submersion under water leads to asphyxia. If respiration is prevented, asphyxia leads to myocardial depression and eventually to cardiac arrest. During cardiac arrest the entire body is subject to lack of oxygen and blood flow, a condition known as global ischemia. During ischemia the brain's oxidative metabolism is impaired, leading to interruption of vital cellular processes and accumulation of toxic metabolites. When circulation and perfusion with oxygen are reestablished, the brain begins to restore metabolic processes and corrects its metabolic deficits. In some cases the period of ischemia is so long that the brain is unable to correct metabolic derangements or compensate for cellular injury. Under these circumstances, after the child is resuscitated from the initial insult, it is the reperfusion of the brain that leads to cerebral edema and coma. This postischemic condition in survivors is known as hypoxic-ischemic encephalopathy.

Despite concern about brain injury after near-drowning, the immediate threat to life is hypoxia and pulmonary injury as a result of aspiration of water and material contained therein. Aspirated volumes as small as 2 ml/kg of body weight have been shown to cause hypoxia[11] as well as reflex pulmonary hypertension.[4] Larger volumes may dilute surfactant, leading to alveolar atelectasis, or may cause alveolar inflammation, producing pulmonary edema and exudation. Aspirated foreign material can result in mechanical obstruction of air passages of all sizes, also contributing to atelectasis. These insults lead to severe ventilation-perfusion mismatch, hypoxia, acidosis, and the condition known as *adult respiratory distress syndrome*.

In addition to cerebral and pulmonary injury, multiple other organs may incur damage during the period of ischemia that accompanies drowning.[9] Renal injury may manifest as acute tubular necrosis. Ischemic damage to the myocardium may cause infarction (even in children) or dysfunction (heart failure), or both.

INITIAL STABILIZATION AT THE SCENE OF RESCUE

The most crucial factor in survival after near-drowning is the prompt restoration of respiration and circulation. The following steps should be initiated immediately:

1. Consider all victims of diving-related or unwitnessed submersions to be at risk of head, neck, and other trauma; stabilize the head and neck accordingly.
2. Clear the airway of foreign material and ensure airway patency.
3. Administer oxygen to all spontaneously breathing patients regardless of their level of consciousness.
4. Start mouth-to-mouth resuscitation if the victim is apneic or not breathing adequately to sustain life.
5. Start closed chest cardiac compressions if the pulse is not palpable.

TREATMENT IN THE HOSPITAL

The management of the near-drowning patient in the hospital must be tailored to the child's clinical condition. This discussion begins with a brief review of the initially awake, stable child, followed by a more lengthy description of problems common to the child in shock or coma.

Because evidence of lung injury may not be immediately apparent, it is advisable to monitor the awake and stable child for a period of several hours even if the submersion was brief. Respiratory distress may develop in a child who initially has no symptoms. In instances in which mouth-to-mouth resuscitation was required, the child should be admitted and observed overnight for signs of respiratory or hemodynamic deterioration, regardless of the initial response to resuscitation. In cases of mild respiratory distress, supplemental oxygen may relieve symptoms. If distress progresses, intubation and mechanical ventilation may be required. Pulse oximetry and chest radiographs may be useful in determining pulmonary injury.

In apneic and pulseless children, resuscitation should be continued until successful or until the physician in charge determines it to be futile.

Children who arrive comatose or with cardiorespiratory compromise (shock) have many concurrent needs. Although these crises are discussed by systems, many must be attended to simultaneously.

Vomiting

Vomiting as a result of water swallowed during submersion is very common. Intubation to prevent aspiration should be initiated in a comatose child as soon as possible. Ventilation by mask should be provided until intubation is accomplished. Oxygen should be given at 100% concentration until adequate gas exchange is documented by arterial blood gas analysis. Positive end-expiratory pressure (PEEP) of 10 cm H_2O helps prevent alveolar atelectasis and improves oxygenation in most cases of pulmonary injury. Higher pressures may ultimately be needed.

Circulation and Perfusion

Circulation and perfusion must be restored to normal by all available means. As a guideline, a minimum acceptable systolic blood pressure measurement in an infant up to 1 month of age is 60 mm Hg; for a child 1 month or older the minimum acceptable blood pressure level is $\geq 70 +$ (age in years $\times$ 2).[1] Although blood pressure values are useful as a guide to the adequacy of systemic perfusion, normal pressure alone does not guarantee adequate circulating blood volume or distribution of blood flow. Physical signs such as liver size, capillary refill time, the caliber of distal pulses, and the temperature of the extremities provide a more accurate assessment of the adequacy of perfusion. Pulmonary edema may be due to lung injury alone and does not necessarily reflect fluid overload or an adequate intravascular volume. If perfusion is inadequate by examination, the administration of intravenous fluids, starting with 20 ml/kg, may improve it. If it is not improved by 50 to 60 ml/kg of crystalloid (normal saline or Ringer lactate) or colloid (blood products or commercially available volume expanders), the continuous infusion of an inotropic drug, such as dopamine starting at 5 μg/kg/min, should be considered. If there is no improvement with dopamine at dosages of 15 to 20 μg/kg/min, epinephrine may be administered, starting at 0.1 μg/kg/min and increasing as necessary to obtain adequate perfusion. Central venous pressure monitoring may be useful in guiding fluid therapy, but fluid administration and restoration of normal perfusion cannot be delayed for insertion of central venous catheters. When access to peripheral veins is not immediately possible by direct or cutdown methods, intraosseous infusion should be given (see Appendix B for cutdown and intraosseous infusion methods).

Hypothermia

Hypothermia occurs rapidly after submersion in cold water and may lead to decreased myocardial contractility or bradycardia. Heart block or ventricular fibrillation may occur at temperatures below 28° C. After rescue, wet clothing should be removed and core temperature restored to normal by the administration of warmed intravenous fluids, warming blankets, and lights. In patients suffering from arrhythmias, peritoneal dialysis or bladder and gastric irrigation with warmed fluids will return body temperature to normal more rapidly. In cases of profound hypothermia (temperature less than 28° C with no sustainable cardiac rhythm), rewarming may be accomplished in the operating room by use of cardiopulmonary bypass. Because hyperkalemia and lactic acidosis are common both during and after rewarming, frequent monitoring of serum electrolyte and blood gas values is necessary after hypothermia.

Physical Examination

After resuscitation and initial stabilization, a complete physical examination should be performed to ascertain the presence of injuries previously unrecognized. Victims of unwitnessed or diving-related events may have suffered other traumatic injury. The child should be assumed to have spinal cord injury until proved otherwise. Serious consideration should be given to toxicologic screening in unwitnessed events and in all adolescents.

Baseline Determinations

Baseline determinations of electrolyte, calcium, glucose, and hemoglobin values, as well as markers of renal function (blood urea nitrogen [BUN], creatinine), hepatic function (transaminases), and myocardial injury (creatine phosphokinase [CPK] with isoenzymes), are useful in fluid management and in the continued assessment and management of ischemic injury, even though laboratory evidence of organ injury may not be apparent for several days. Significant electrolyte abnormalities are uncommon after near-drowning[11] and are not likely to require specific treatment. Fluid resuscitation with an inappropriately dilute fluid, such as 5% dextrose in water, may lead to hyponatremia and water intoxication and should be avoided.

Seizure Activity

Seizure activity increases metabolic demands and may lead to extension of brain injury. Seizures after near-drowning usually are due to the effects of cerebral ischemia and should be treated promptly with anticonvulsants. Unless muscle rigidity prevents adequate ventilation, the use of long-acting neuromuscular blockers (e.g., pancuronium) should be avoided because these drugs make the recognition of seizure activity difficult.

Neurologic Injury

The management of neurologic injury and cerebral edema resulting from global ischemia is discussed more fully in Chapter 278. Intracranial pressure (ICP) monitoring, barbiturate coma, and hypothermia have not reduced neurologic sequelae after near-drowning.[3] Although ICP monitoring may be of prognostic value (ICP >20 with cerebral perfusion pressure <50 has been correlated with fatal outcome[12]), outcome also can be estimated on the basis of initial examination.[5,6,8,10,13]

The most important therapy for multiple organ ischemic injury after near-drowning is the prevention of conditions that may lead to extension of the injury,[9] such as hypoxia and hypercapnia. Hyponatremia may contribute to cerebral edema and usually can be prevented by limiting intravenous administration of hypotonic solutions. Hyperthermia increases metabolic demands; treating fever with antipyretics, fans, or cooling blankets is important. In summary the most effective way to care for a child after near-drowning is to maintain homeostasis.

PROGNOSIS OF CHILDHOOD NEAR-DROWNING

Many scoring systems have been shown to be useful in predicting outcome after near-drowning, and all confirm the importance of the child's neurologic condition on first examination. If the child arrives awake or blunted (confused, combative, responsive to voice or pain), chances for good outcome are excellent.[5] In one study all children with a Glasgow Coma Scale score greater than 5 had a normal or near-normal outcome.[6] If a child arrives comatose with fixed and dilated pupils, normal survival is extremely unlikely, although 15% of these children have a normal outcome.[6-8,12] Others state that children who sustain prolonged cardiac arrest (cardiopulmonary resuscitation required on arrival to the emergency department) invariably suffer neurologic sequelae.[14] Other factors that have been correlated with poor outcome after submersion are an age younger than 3 years, initial blood pH <7.0, lack of cardiopulmonary resuscitation (CPR) attempts at the scene, and estimated submersion longer than 5 minutes.[13] Because the majority of these factors reflect cerebral ischemia, it is most likely that the final neurologic outcome of near-drowning patients is related to the severity of brain ischemia occurring at the time of submersion.

A child who drowns in cold water represents a unique exception to outcome predictions and resuscitation. With sufficient acute hypothermia, cerebral oxidative mechanisms may be depressed, offering cerebral protection from hypoxia. Reports of good outcome after rewarming on cardiopulmonary bypass despite prolonged submersion are encouraging.[15] Even after successful resuscitation, these patients frequently have severe, life-threatening pulmonary injury.

CONVALESCENCE AND REHABILITATION

The sequelae of near-drowning are primarily neurologic. Consultation with rehabilitation services personnel should be made as soon as survival is apparent so that, when appropriate, children receive early physical therapy to prevent joint contractures. This may involve splinting the extremities while a child is comatose and intubated. Further intervention will depend on the child's clinical course. Rehabilitation, tailored to the individual child, may be a lengthy process, with neurologic recovery slow and often incomplete.

PREVENTION

Many drowning deaths involving children occur when unsupervised children gain access to pools, excavations, or ponds (see box below). Most of these deaths are preventable by barriers designed to exclude children from these hazards. A fence 4 to 6 feet (1.2 to 1.8 m) high with a self-locking latch is recommended for this purpose. Nothing should be left outside the pool barrier that could be used as a ladder. Because pool and pond barriers are not required in all states, pediatricians must advocate child safety, both by educating the public and by lobbying public officials to pass legislation requiring adequate barriers around both private and public water hazards.

POTENTIAL FOR ORGAN DONATION

Organs have varying tolerances for hypoxic injury. A victim of near-drowning who has satisfied criteria for brain death may have kidneys, heart, liver, corneas, and skin suitable for transplantation. The parents or legal guardians of such a child should be approached to determine their willingness to make such a gift once brain death has been diagnosed.

Swimming and Pool Safety

1. A good test for readiness to learn swimming is the ability of the child to hold his or her breath on command.
2. Young children may panic in times of emergency and for this reason should not be considered "water safe." Do not allow unsupervised or solo swimming under any circumstances.
3. Allow diving only in water of known depth. For swimming pools, 8 feet generally is the minimum recommended depth for use of a diving board. Be aware that this may not be sufficient for diving from docks, rocks, or homemade diving platforms.
4. Keep essential devices such as a life preserver and a rescue pole at poolside. Both children and adults must be taught how to use these devices in the case of emergency.
5. Do not allow tricycles or wagons at poolside.

REFERENCES

1. American Heart Association and American Academy of Pediatrics: Textbook of pediatric advanced life support, Dallas, 1988, The Association and the Academy.
2. Baker SP and Waller AE: Childhood injury: state-by-state mortality facts, Office of Maternal and Child Health, Washington, DC, 1989, US Department of Health and Human Services.
3. Bohn DJ et al: Influence of hypothermia, barbiturate therapy and intracranial pressure monitoring on morbidity and mortality after near-drowning, Crit Care Med 14:529, 1986.
4. Colebatch HJH and Halmagyi DFJ: Reflex pulmonary hypertension of fresh water aspiration, J Appl Physiol 18:179, 1963.
5. Conn AW et al: Cerebral salvage in near-drowning following neurological classification by triage, Can Anaesth Soc J 27:201, 1980.
6. Dean JM and Kaufman ND: Prognostic indicators in pediatric near-drowning: the Glasgow Coma Scale, Crit Care Med 9:536, 1981.
7. Dean JM and McComb JG: Intracranial pressure monitoring in severe pediatric near-drowning, Neurosurgery 9:627, 1981.
8. Frewen TC et al: Cerebral resuscitation therapy in pediatric near-drowning, J Pediatr 106:615, 1985.
9. Hoff BH: Multisystem failure: a review with special reference to drowning, Crit Care Med 7:310, 1979.
10. Modell JH, Graves SA, and Kuck EJ: Near-drowning correlation of level of consciousness and survival, Can Anaesth Soc J 27:211, 1980.
11. Modell JH and Moya F: Effects of volume of aspirated fluid during chlorinated fresh water drowning, Anesthesiology 27:662, 1966.
12. Nussbaum E and Galant SP: Intracranial pressure monitoring as a guide to prognosis in the nearly drowned, severely comatose child, J Pediatr 102:215, 1983.
13. Orlowski JP: Prognostic factors in pediatric cases of drowning and near-drowning, JACEP 8:176, 1979.
14. O'Rourke PP: Outcome of children who are apneic and pulseless in the emergency room, Crit Care Med 14:466, 1986.
15. Saltiel A et al: Resuscitation of cold water immersion victims with cardiopulmonary bypass, J Crit Care 4:54, 1989.

274

Drug Overdose

Cheston M. Berlin, Jr.

Drug overdose, whether from accidental ingestion, a therapeutic misadventure, or a suicide attempt, is a major problem in pediatric practice. In 1987, 1,166,940 case reports of exposure to potentially toxic substances were tabulated by the American Association of Poison Control Centers (AAPCC) National Data Collection System. The participating Poison Control Centers serve a population of 137.5 million; thus the data reported involve approximately 57% of estimated exposures. Children under 6 years of age accounted for 62% of case reports; 47% occurred in children 2 years of age or younger. Thus, well over 1.2 million children are exposed yearly to drugs potentially able to cause toxicity.

DEFINITION

Drug overdose or toxicity occurs when a child accidentally ingests or is given (therapeutically) an amount of a compound that exceeds the recommended dosage or that causes an idiosyncratic reaction within the recommended dosage.

ETIOLOGY

The epidemiology of drug overdose is related to the patient's age, as shown in Table 274-1, which lists the number of deaths from drugs and other compounds according to patient age. The bimodal frequency peaks are at 5 years or below and at 15 to 19 years. The former reflects accidental ingestions; the latter, usually suicidal events. For some compounds, aspirin being the prime example, it is recognized that therapeutic misadventure may play a significant role. As Gaudreault has pointed out,[2] most serious salicylate poisonings occur as a result of the therapeutic administration of aspirin. Young children who are febrile or dehydrated are not able to handle antipyretic doses of salicylate effectively. The incidence of therapeutic salicylate poisoning has dropped markedly in recent years because salicylates are not often used in pediatric patients as a result of the concern regarding the relationship between salicylates and Reye syndrome.

Preventive measures, such as child-resistant bottle tops, are effective in eliminating acute, single-dose accidental exposures. Chapter 285, "Poisoning," provides detailed information on the management of the most common drug ingestions that occur in pediatric practice.

IMMEDIATE ASSESSMENT

An optimum therapeutic response will be achieved if the following steps are taken immediately on encountering the overdosed patient. Detain the person(s) who brought the child to the hospital or office. If initial contact is by telephone, obtain the caller's name and telephone number, and then instruct the caller immediately to proceed with the child to the hospital. Be sure to obtain the precise description of the drug thought to have been ingested: name, dose, pharmacy of origin, and prescription number. Instruct the parents to bring the actual container when they come with the patient. Try to determine the amount of drug ingested. This is frequently impossible, and such information, even if obtained, is occasionally misleading. *Assume maximal exposure unless a precise tablet or liquid count is available.*

Initial Procedures for Stabilization and Life Support

Measure the vital signs—temperature, pulse, respirations, blood pressure, and continuous electrocardiography. Monitor the sensorium frequently; that is, every 15 minutes for 2 hours until the patient's condition is stable. Changes in frequency and duration of monitoring will depend on the drug, dose, and clinical course.

Table 274-1 *Deaths from Toxic Exposure to Substances, by Patient Age (1987)*

SUBSTANCE	AGE (YEARS) <5	5-9	10-14	15-19
Drugs	10	2	2	19
Nondrug solids and liquids	4	0	0	5
Gases and vapors	8	0	5	8
TOTALS	22	2	7	32

Data modified from Litovitz TL et al: 1987 annual report of the American Association of Poison Control Centers National Data Collection System, Am J Emerg Med 6:479, 1988.

Assess the adequacy of the airway. Most drug overdoses will not affect the upper airway (larynx, trachea) but will interfere with air exchange by either depressing the central nervous system or paralyzing neuromuscular transmission. Establish an intravenous line. If danger of respiratory depression or ingestion of drugs that alter cardiovascular status exists, consider placing an arterial line. Cleanse the skin if appropriate. Some compounds, such as insecticides, have significant dermal absorption, especially if the skin is inflamed or abraded. If the patient is alert, induce emesis—except in cases of lye, acid, and hydrocarbon ingestion. Save the vomitus for drug analysis.

DIFFERENTIAL DIAGNOSIS

Considerations of other conditions that can mimic the signs and symptoms of drug overdose will depend on the drug ingested. For patients with alterations in sensorium, head trauma is of prime consideration. Spontaneous intracranial hemorrhages in the pediatric age group are rare; they usually produce focal neurologic signs rather than global depression of consciousness.

Metabolic conditions such as diabetes mellitus, hypoglycemia, and addisonian crises may cause clinical states that resemble drug ingestion. Awareness of these possibilities will help narrow down the diagnostic considerations.

The most thorny area of all is presented by the patient with psychiatric illness, who may develop tremors, hallucinations, or hysterical paralysis. In these patients precise and rapid laboratory analyses are most important in ruling out drug ingestion. If the patient has been receiving psychoactive medications and is having an untoward reaction, management is identical to that discussed in the management section, with special attention directed to the emotional needs of the patient, especially in the recovery phase.

MANAGEMENT

The two factors to consider in deciding location and personnel for management of the patient are (1) expertise of the physician in the management of drug overdose and (2) available hospital support facilities. The latter is of most concern, since even the best-trained physician cannot properly provide care in an institution not equipped with support staff, equipment, and laboratory facilities. The well-trained pediatrician will not always be able to predict the clinical course of a patient who has "overdosed." Will the patient require charcoal perfusion, renal or peritoneal dialysis, or an exchange transfusion? Is the hospital able to offer pediatric intensive care unit monitoring? Can the nursing staff properly monitor intracranial and intraarterial pressure? It is best to decide very early in the clinical course whether specialized facilities will be needed. It is preferable to transfer a stable patient early than a critically ill child requiring mobile life support later on. It is important to maintain frequent and smooth communication with the patient's family. Regardless of cause, these families are in constant need of counseling—especially with regard to any guilt feelings they may be experiencing.

Need for General Homeostatic Support

Thermal monitoring is an important aspect of management in drug overdose. Centrally and peripherally induced hypothermia is a common problem—for example, the hypothermia that occurs with phenothiazine ingestion. Hyperthermia can occur with salicylate and atropine poisoning.

Monitoring fluid balance and electrolyte homeostasis is important. Deficits must be replaced, and the amount of maintenance fluids needed will depend on changes in the vital and physical signs. For example, hyperventilation and increased body temperature require increases beyond normal in the amount of maintenance fluids administered. Continuing losses through vomiting and diarrhea should be replaced as they occur.

Monitoring central venous pressure and arterial pressure to assess vascular volume and tone is important. Evaluate respiratory function and check for an elevation in intracranial pressure to assess the need for treatment of cerebral edema. Consider the need for peritoneal dialysis, hemodialysis, charcoal perfusion, or exchange transfusion to remove the ingested drug.

Nutritional considerations are frequently neglected with patients requiring prolonged intensive care. Feeding via a nasogastric tube or with parenteral alimentation should be considered, especially if coma will exceed 3 days.

Diagnostic Procedures

Assays of blood, urine, and gastric contents for barbiturates, phenytoin, iron, digoxin, salicylate, acetaminophen, narcotics, and propoxyphene must be available. Drug screens should be rapidly available; quantitative analyses should follow as quickly as possible.

A flat plate of the abdomen may be required to identify radiopaque tablets (e.g., iron) or foreign bodies. A computed tomography scan of the head should be performed if intracranial hemorrhage is suspected following amphetamine or cocaine ingestion. A chest roentgenogram is needed if narcotic-induced pulmonary edema or aspiration is suspected.

It is important to remember that trauma may have occurred in any poisoned patient, especially the adolescent. One half of adolescent drownings are associated with alcohol use. Be especially careful of the cervical spine.

Definitive Therapy

Specific antidotes exist for some drugs but unfortunately not for most. Thus definitive therapy consists of intensive supportive care and treatment of signs and symptoms as they develop (e.g., hypotension and hypertension, thermal instability, cardiac arrhythmias).

The following steps should be taken in treating drug overdosage:

1. Stabilize the patient.
2. Identify the drug ingested and determine the amount ingested.
3. Contact the local poison control center for toxicology data and information regarding the signs and symptoms

and clinical course. The "Poisindex" is an excellent comprehensive reference, and the pocket manual by Dreisbach[1] provides essential information in an easy-to-find format.

4. Induce emesis or perform gastric lavage if not contraindicated. Recent work[3] suggests that gastric emptying in the alert patient is not helpful. These authors emphasize the use of activated charcoal and a cathartic.
5. If a specific antidote exists, administer it. It is most helpful to have a table prepared of specific antidotes and their location in the hospital (Table 274-2). The best location is the Emergency Department. All staff members must know the precise location.
6. Give activated charcoal (1 or 2 g/kg) as a slurry with magnesium sulfate (250 mg/kg).[5] Only a very small number of compounds appear not to be adsorbed to the charcoal (acids, alkali, cyanide, DDT, iron salts, N-methyl carbonate, tolbutamide). Repeated doses of charcoal–magnesium sulfate (every 2 to 4 hours) may be very useful in accelerating clearance of many compounds. This technique is referred to as *gastrointestinal dialysis*.[4] Contraindications to repeated use of oral charcoal would be intestinal obstruction, perforation, or poor gastrointestinal motility.
7. Provide supportive care in an intensive or intermediate care unit as appropriate.

Table 274-2 *Common Antidotes*

DRUG	DIAGNOSTIC FINDINGS REQUIRING TREATMENT	ANTIDOTE	DOSAGE
Acetaminophen	History of ingestion and toxic serum level	N-acetylcysteine	140 mg/kg/dose PO, then 70 mg/kg/dose q 4 hr PO × 17
Anticholinergics Antihistamines Atropine Phenothiazines Tricyclic antidepressants	Supraventricular tachycardia (hemodynamic compromise) Unresponsive ventricular dysrhythmia, seizures, pronounced hallucinations or agitation	Physotigmine	Child: 0.5 mg IV slowly (over 3 min) q 10 min prn (maximum: 2 mg) Adult: 1-2 mg IV slowly q 10 min prn (maximum: 4 mg in 30 min)
Cholinergics	Cholinergic crisis: salivation, lacrimation, urination, defecation, convulsions, fasciculations	Atropine sulfate Physostigmine Insecticides	0.05 mg/kg/dose (usual dose 1-5 mg; test dose for child 0.01 mg/kg) q 4-6 hr IV or more frequently prn
Carbon monoxide	Headache, seizure, coma, dysrhythmias	Oxygen, hyperbaric oxygen	100% oxygen (half-life 40 min); consider hyperbaric chamber
Cyanide	Cyanosis, seizures, cardiopulmonary arrest, coma	Amyl nitrite Sodium nitrite (3%) Sodium thiosulfate (25%) Also consider hyperbaric oxygen	Inhale pearl q 60-120 sec 0.27 mL (8.7 mg)/kg (adult): 10 mL [300 mg]) IV slowly (Hb 10 g) 1.35 mL (325 mg)/kg (adult: 12.5 g) IV slowly (Hb 10 g)
Ethylene glycol	Metabolic acidosis, urine Ca^{++} oxalate crystals	Ethanol (100% absolute, 1 mL-790 mg)	1 mL/kg in D5W IV over 15 min, then 0.16 mL (125 mg)/kg/hr IV; maintain ethanol level of 100 mg/dl
Iron	Hypotension, shock, coma, serum iron >350 mg/dl (or greater than iron-binding capacity)	Deferoxamine	Shock or coma: 15 mg/kg/hr IV for 8 hr; if no shock or coma 90 mg/kg/dose IM q 8 hr
Phenothiazines Chlorpromazine Thioridazine	Extrapyramidal dyskinesis, oculogyric crisis	Diphenhydramine (Benadryl)	1-2 mg/kg/dose (maximum: 50 mg/dose) q 6 hr IV, PO
Methanol	Metabolic acidosis, blurred vision; level >20 mg/dl	Ethanol (100% absolute)	1 mL/kg in D5W over 15 min, then 0.16 mL (125 mg)/kg/hr IV
Methemoglobin Nitrate Nitrites Sulfonamide	Cyanosis, methemoglobin level >30%, dyspnea	Methylene blue (1% solution)	1-2 mg (0.1-0.2 mL)/kg/dose IV; repeat in 4 hr if necessary
Narcotics Heroin Codeine Propoxyphene	Respiratory depression, hypotension, coma	Naloxone (Narcan)	0.1 mg/kg up to 0.8 mg initially IV, if no response give 2 mg IV
Organophosphates Malathion Parathion	Cholinergic crisis: salivation, lacrimation, urination, defecation, convulsions, fasciculations	Atropine sulfate	0.05 mg/kg/dose (usual dose 1-5 mg; test dose for child 0.01 mg/kg) q 4-6 hr IV or more frequently prn
		Pralidoxime	After atropine, 20-50 mg/kg/dose (maximum: 2000 mg) IV slowly (<50 mg/min) q 8 hr IV prn × 3

From Barkin RM and Rosen P: Toxicologic emergencies, Pediatr Ann 19:632, 1990.

8. Meet social service needs as indicated (e.g., drug ingestion by a toddler as a symptom of chaotic family structure or by an adolescent as a symptom of depression or as a suicidal gesture or act).
9. Provide counseling concerning the institution of poison control measures in the home.

Complications

Possible complications of drug overdose are many and varied. Therapy itself can have side effects, such as too rigorous treatment of seizures causing apnea and the need for mechanical ventilation. Many poisoned patients require respirator therapy. Such therapy, especially if prolonged, may lead to complications such as pneumothorax, oxygen toxicity, and airway infections. Nosocomial infections are not uncommon—especially hypostatic pneumonia, urinary tract infection (secondary to catheter placement), or septicemia from vascular catheters. Thrombotic and embolic episodes can also result from vascular catheters.

Permanent central nervous system damage sometimes follows periods of hypoxia or hypoglycemia—usually before therapy is instituted. Topical skin, mucous membrane, and deeper tissue injuries often result from acids, lyes, or corrosives. Specific compounds can cause permanent organ damage (e.g., the lungs from hydrocarbons, the kidneys from ethylene glycol, the liver from acetaminophen, and the retina from methanol).

Hazards of treatment for drug overdosage include overtreatment, the wrong treatment, an insufficient period of observation, and failure to appreciate drug ingestion as an indication of child neglect or abuse.

Overtreatment occurs when errors are made in assessing the amount of drug ingested. A nontoxic ingestion may be vigorously but inappropriately treated with potentially toxic antidotes—for example, using sodium nitrate–sodium thiosulfate for the treatment of cyanide ingestion.

The wrong treatment can occur when a mistake is made in identifying the drug ingested—for example, a mislabeled prescription vial.

An insufficient period of observation can worsen the situation. For example, hepatic necrosis may not occur until day 3 after acetaminophen ingestion, and renal disease may not occur until day 7 to 10.

Failing to appreciate drug ingestion as an indication of child neglect or abuse is a further danger. Especially suspect is the child under age 12 months who is admitted with "accidental ingestion" or the child who has a history of repeated drug ingestions.

REFERENCES

1. Dreisbach RH: Poisoning, ed 12, Los Altos, Calif, 1987, Lange Medical Publications.
2. Gaudreault P, Temple AR, and Lovejoy FH Jr: The relative severity of acute versus chronic salicylate poisoning in children: a clinical comparison, Pediatrics 70:566, 1982.
3. Kulig K et al: Management of acutely poisoned patients without gastric emptying, Ann Emerg Med 14:562, 1985.
4. Mofenson HC et al: Gastrointestinal dialysis with activated charcoal and cathartic in the treatment of adolescent intoxications, Clin Pediatr (Phila) 24:678, 1985.

275

Envenomations

Sharon Humiston

An envenomation is the combination of poisonous effects caused by the bite, sting, or effluvia of venomous creatures such as snakes, spiders, scorpions, and insects of the order Hymenoptera (e.g., ants, wasps, and bees). Although not uncommon, venomous bites and stings are usually minor in the United States. In 1985 the 56 members of the American Association of Poison Control Centers received a total of 30,938 bite- or sting-related calls. The patient was 17 years of age or younger in 43% of these cases: the vector was a snake in 5%, a scorpion in 5%, a spider in 30%, and a bee, wasp, or hornet in 41%. There were no symptoms or only minor ones in more than 90% of the cases for which a final outcome was reported.[14] The clinician must be prepared to treat significant envenomations and to avoid overtreating minor ones.

SNAKEBITES

The venomous snakes of North America can be divided into two families, Crotalidae and Elapidae. The Crotalidae family gets its name from the Latin for rattle and includes rattlesnakes, pygmy rattlesnakes (massasaugas), copperheads, and water moccasins (cottonmouth). As a group these snakes are known as pit vipers because of a heat-sensitive pit found behind and below their nostrils. The Elapidae family includes coral snakes as well as the non-indigenous cobras and mambas.

Epidemiology

Type of Snake. In 1985, 39% of the snakebite-related calls to poison centers referred to nonpoisonous snakes; in almost 44% the type of snake was unknown. Indigenous Crotalidae and Elapidae were the vectors in 15% and less than 1%, respectively; nonindigenous snakes were the vectors in less than 3%.[14] Fortunately, although all sea snakes are venomous, none inhabits the coastal waters of North America.[25]

Host Factors. Usually the person bitten is a young adult white male. Approximately 40% of bites occur while handling or playing with a snake; 40% of those bitten have a blood alcohol level over 0.1%.[30] In one study of rattlesnake bites, only 43% occurred before an encounter with a snake was recognized or while the person was attempting to move away from the snake.[9] The incidence of snake venom poisoning by state is illustrated in Fig. 275-1.

Body Area. Most bites are sustained on the upper extremity. A recent review of inpatient and outpatient cases of snakebite in California reported the following site distribution: 70% finger, 15% hand, 2% arm, 12% leg or foot, and 1% torso.[31] Given the high percentage of bites sustained while purposely handling the snake these statistics are less surprising than reports of snakebites to the tongue[10] and the glans penis.[6]

Mortality. Between 1975 and 1980, the number of deaths from snakebite in the United States ranged from 9 to 14 per year.[24] Most snakebite deaths are associated with the absence of medical care, errors in medical management, or the presence of an underlying medical condition. Once bitten by a snake, children are at increased risk of serious sequelae because of the high venom dose per kilogram of body weight.

Prevention

Native Americans used numerous plants, animal tissues, oils, and excrement to prevent snakebites.[24] The box at the left on p. 1603, a summary of more practical suggestions for avoiding snakebites, is based on the epidemiology of these injuries and the nature of snakes.

Snake Venoms

The composition and deadliness of snake venoms vary from species to species. Each venom is a mixture of numerous enzymes (e.g., protease, hyaluronidase, collagenase), polypeptide fractions, and inorganic substances (e.g., sodium, zinc). These substances have two inextricably interwoven chief functions: killing or immobilizing prey and digesting it.

Crotalidae venoms are chiefly but not exclusively digestive, causing necrosis of lymphatics, cells, and small blood vessels. The subsequent excessive permeability of blood vessels can lead to tissue edema, adult respiratory distress syndrome (ARDS), shock, and renal failure. Additionally, pit viper venoms can cause hemolysis, bleeding diathesis, and disseminated intravascular coagulation (DIC). Elapidae venoms, on the other hand, are notoriously neurotoxic, causing paresthesias and paralysis by inhibiting acetylcholine receptors at the neuronal synapse. Some Crotalidae (e.g., the Mojave rattlesnake) also produce a neurotoxic venom.

Pit Vipers

As noted previously, rattlesnakes, copperheads, and water moccasins are members of the pit viper family. Copperheads, which often live in or near cities and suburbs, inflict almost 44% of venomous snakebites in the United States but have

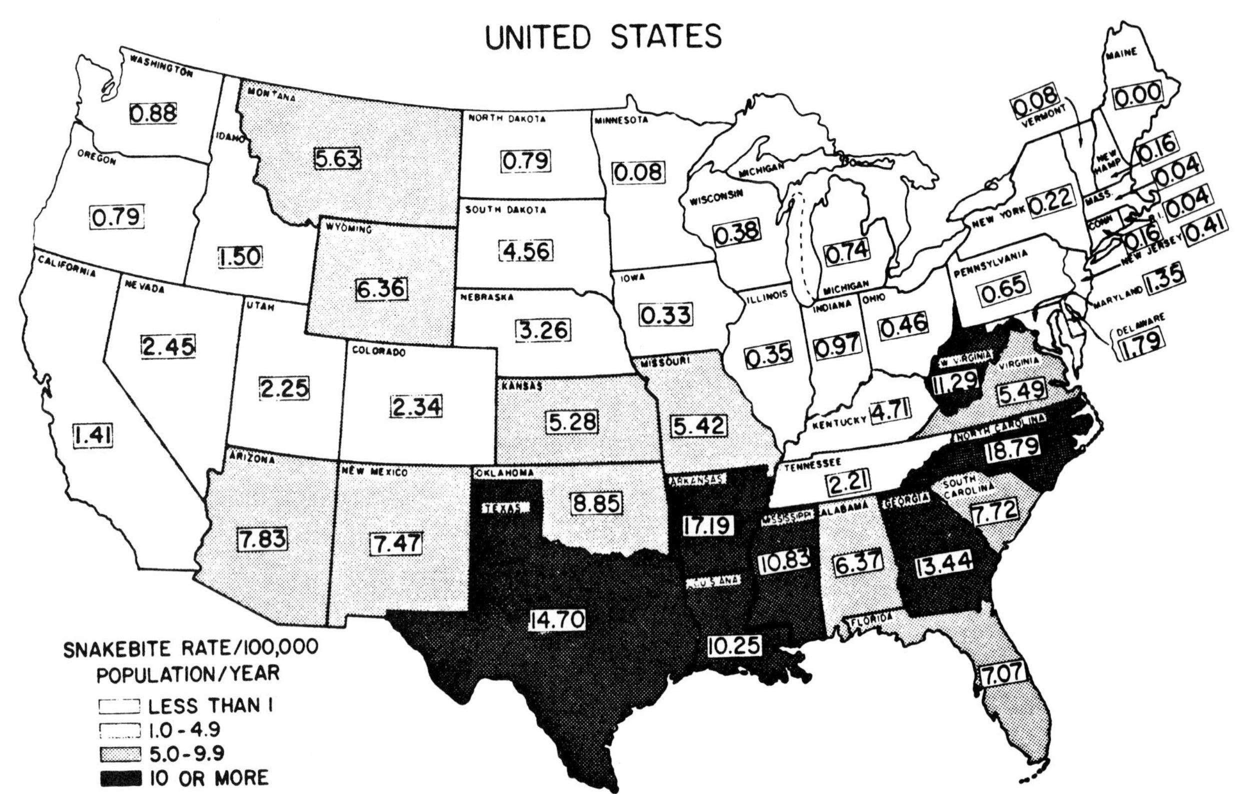

Fig. 275-1 Incidence of snake venom poisoning by state.
From Russell FE: Snake venom poisoning, Philadelphia, 1980, JB Lippincott Co.

a case fatality rate of only 0.01%.[21] Conversely, diamondback rattlesnakes are responsible for only about 10% of venomous snakebites, but 95% of snakebite mortalities.[21] It should be remembered that pit vipers are venomous at birth and as adults can be found in a wide array of sizes that do not necessarily correlate with their deadliness.

Characteristics. Crotalidae are chiefly distinguished from coral snakes by their facial pit. This apparatus is used to locate and estimate the size of prey and predators. The snake thus can estimate a venom dose in accordance with the size of the prey that is to be immobilized and digested.[3]

Pit vipers have retractable, hollow fangs that function much like a hypodermic needle. Usually they penetrate to subcutaneous tissue,[30] but large diamondback rattlesnake fangs can reach a depth of 8 to 19 mm. For an envenomation to take place, the pit viper must be venomous at the time of the strike, penetrate the skin, and inject venom during penetration. Approximately 20% to 25% of pit viper bites are "dry".[13]

Although identification of the type of snake is useful, time should not be lost in getting the victim to medical attention nor should the rescue party expose themselves to risk while trying to find and identify the snake.

Distribution. The list on the right on p. 1603 lists the indigenous locations for North American pit vipers.

First Aid. Commonly accepted guidelines for snakebite first aid are summarized in the box on p. 1604.[3,31] Other forms of first aid are controversial and are discussed here because the physician may see patients less damaged by the snake than by the field treatment of well-meaning, but untrained (and possibly inebriated) attendants.

Cryotherapy. This form of snakebite treatment was used to constrict blood flow and thus diminish systemic venom absorption. Unfortunately, the consequent ischemia is limb-threatening. Cryotherapy is contraindicated.

Incision and Suction. The Sawyer extractor, a syringe-type plunger that develops 1 atmosphere of vacuum, has been shown to be beneficial in removing snake venom in both experimental and clinical settings.[4]

If this device is not available, incision and suction should be instituted only if (1) the procedure does not delay transport to a medical facility and can be started no more than 30 minutes after the envenomation; (2) the nearest medical care is more than 60 minutes away; and (3) the person performing the procedure is knowledgeable about the method and the underlying anatomy and is prepared to continue suction for 30 to 60 minutes. The single incision should be made through the fang marks, no greater than 3 mm deep, 5 to 6 mm long, and parallel to the axis of the limb. A clean suction cup should be used rather than the attendant's mouth for the protection of both parties.[3]

Constricting Bands. Like cryotherapy, use of a tourniquet causes limb-threatening tissue necrosis and is contraindicated. Conversely, wide constricting bands, tight enough to impede lymphatic return but not blood flow, have been found useful according to some studies. It should be remembered that venom spread is not limited to the lymphatic route and that the risk-benefit ratio of this first aid is blurred

Snakebite Prevention

1. It is impossible to differentiate poisonous from nonpoisonous snakes without years of experience. Therefore children should not approach, disturb, play with, capture, or kill *any* snake. These practices are dangerous for the human and annoying to the snake.
2. Children should not put their hands or feet in places they cannot see. Children should not put their hands or feet anywhere without first looking.
3. Snakes can frequently be found under rocks, boulders, fallen trees, fences, and rubbish piles, and in boats that have been left on shore for several hours. They can also be found in tall grass and heavy underbrush and on logs, boulders, trees, walls, or cliffs, sunning themselves. Extra caution should be used in these areas.
4. The striking distance of a snake can be about 17 feet. Children should be taught to keep a good distance from snakes.
5. The striking reflex remains intact for up to an hour after the snake is dead. Therefore even if one is sure that the snake is dead, it must be examined or transported at the opposite end of a long stick.
6. Rattlesnakes are nocturnal feeders and are therefore active after dark. Children should never gather firewood after dark. Camp should be set up on open ground, never near wood, rubbish piles, swampy areas, or the entrance to a cave.
7. Children should not be allowed to walk in an endemic area without boots.
8. Children should not be allowed to walk in an endemic area without another person.
9. Children should not be allowed to swim in waters known to be infested with snakes.
10. If an individual is bitten, everyone should get away from the snake as quickly as possible. The benefit of identifying the snake is small compared with the risk of additional bites.

Indigenous Locations for North American Pit Vipers

Southeast
- Cottonmouths and copperheads
- Eastern diamondback *(C. adamanteus)*
- Timber *(C. horridus)*
- Massasauga pygmy rattlesnakes *(Sistrurus)*

Midwest
- Cottonmouths and copperheads
- Eastern diamondback *(C. adamanteus)*
- Timber *(C. horridus)*
- Prairie *(C.v. viridis)*
- Massasauga pygmy rattlesnakes *(Sistrurus)*

Northeast
- Cottonmouths and copperheads
- Eastern diamondback *(C. adamanteus)*
- Timber *(C. horridus)*
- Massasauga pygmy rattlesnakes *(Sistrurus)*

Northwest
- Great Basin *(C.v. lutosus)*
- Northern Pacific *(C.v. oreganus)*

Southwest
- Western diamondback *(C. atroy)*
- Sidewinder *(C. cerastes)*
- Rock *(C. lepidus)*
- Speckled *(C. mitchelli)*
- Black-tailed *(C. molossus)*
- Twin-spotted *(C. pricei)*
- Red diamond *(C. ruber)*
- Mojave *(C. scutulatus)*
- Tiger *(C. tigris)*
- Prairie *(C.v. viridis)*
- Grand Canyon *(C.v. abyssus)*
- Southern Pacific *(C.v. helleri)*
- Great Basin *(C.v. lutosus)*
- Ridge-nosed *(C. willardi)*

From Banner, W: Bites and stings in the pediatric patient, Curr Probl Pediatr 18(1):1, 1988.

by the likelihood of a "dry" bite, the relatively benign venom of most North American snakes, and the availability of nearby medical care.

If used at all, the constricting band should be used correctly. A blood pressure cuff should be inflated to 15 to 20 mm Hg 15 to 20 cm proximal to the snakebite. Alternately, a wide band may be tied loosely enough to allow two fingers to pass beneath. If swelling occurs, the band should be removed after a more proximal constricting band is placed to prevent sudden release of venom into the system.[3]

History-Taking

Points that should be addressed in the medical history of known envenomations include the size and species of the snake, the circumstances of the bite (e.g., through clothing, alcohol-related), the number and body area of the bite or bites, first aid methods employed, time of bite and transport time, previous snake bite episodes and exposure to horse serum, allergies (e.g., horse serum, antibiotics), and tetanus immunization status.[31]

Physical Examination: Signs and Symptoms

Local. Local signs and symptoms usually include the presence of fang marks as well as pain, edema, ecchymosis, and erythema within 15 to 30 minutes of the bite. Fang marks typically have ragged edges but may be obscured by secondary trauma sustained in the flight from the snake or the first aid attempts. Because of the hematotoxic effects of pit viper venom, blood may ooze from the puncture sites and hemorrhagic bullae develop. Muscle necrosis may also become apparent. The absence of any local signs within 30 minutes makes the likelihood of envenomation low; their presence makes 24 hours of observation important.

First Aid for Snakebites

1. Note the approximate size and characteristics of the snake if this can be done safely—that is, out of the snake's striking range.
2. Minimize movement of the patient.
3. Mark the skin with a pen, denoting the area and time of swelling. Repeat this every 15 minutes.
4. Immobilize the limb by splinting as if for a fracture and keep the limb below the level of the heart.
5. Regardless of early symptoms, transport the victim (at a safe speed) to the nearest medical facility.
6. Do not use ice (tissue damage), aspirin (anticoagulation), alcohol, or sedative drugs (vasodilation).
7. As soon as possible, start basic life support for hypotensive patients, including volume expansion and Trendelenburg positioning.

Systemic. Hemolysis, consumption coagulopathy, and generalized hemorrhage are frequently present in serious envenomations. The physical examination should also be geared toward detecting signs of ARDS, circulatory collapse, and renal failure. Other findings may include weakness, lightheadedness, diaphoresis, visual disturbances, nausea, vomiting, syncope, and metallic taste.[5] Paresthesias (of the scalp, face, or extremities), fasciculations, and the formation of bullae have been shown to increase significantly with the severity of the pit viper bite.[31]

Laboratory Studies

Laboratory studies have been found to be of "minor assistance in assessing the severity of (rattlesnake) envenomation."[31] Creatine kinase levels were the only measure to demonstrate a significant difference in severe bites. Prothrombin times, fibrinogen levels, and platelet counts were often altered, and the urinalysis, when performed, was more likely to show hematuria and proteinuria if the bite was considered serious.

Studies often recommended include a complete blood and differential count, red blood cell morphology to evaluate for spherocytosis, and a bleeding screen (prothrombin time, plasma thromboplastin time, fibrinogen levels, fibrin-split products, and platelet count). For severe envenomations, electrolytes, blood urea nitrogen, blood type and cross-match, serum bilirubin concentration, arterial blood gas, and urinalysis may also be useful. Enzyme-linked immunoassay (ELISA) and radioimmunoassay (RIA) tests for detection of pit viper venom in wound aspirate, serum, and urine are available.[17]

Supportive Therapy

Shock. Because of the increase in membrane permeability, colloid plasma expanders are preferred by many over crystalloid for snakebite victims. Vasopressors may become necessary in the most serious cases.

Fluid and Electrolyte Abnormalities. Extensive third-space losses may cause fluid and electrolyte imbalances. Intravenous fluids and urine output monitoring become essential under these conditions.

Hematologic Complications. Treatment of thrombocytopenia and anemia (caused by hemolysis) may require multiple transfusions. Disseminated intravascular coagulopathy caused by snakebite does not respond to heparin. Antivenin is the drug of choice.

Use of Antivenin

Once venin is bound to the end organ, antivenin has little effect. Therefore as soon as it is determined that the patient has a serious envenomation, antivenin therapy should be considered. Some reserve its use for large rattlesnakes, water moccasins, or unidentified snakes.[27] Antivenin use should proceed simultaneously with the supportive therapy as shown in the box on p. 1605.

Prevention and Treatment of Serum Sickness

Up to 80% of patients develop serum sickness sometime within 4 weeks after being treated with antivenin, but only 3% require hospitalization for this complication. Oral corticosteroids should be prescribed at the first signs (usually urticaria and pruritus) and should be continued until all symptoms have subsided for 24 hours. The steroid should then be tapered over 72 hours. If necessary, diphenhydramine may be added to control pruritus.

Additional Therapeutic Measure

Pain Control. Analgesics should not be overlooked in the management of snakebites. Adequate pain control allows rehabilitation to begin as early as possible in order to prevent contractures.

Infection Control. Although snakes have been found to carry a wide variety of bacteria in their mouths (histotoxic clostridia, *Bacteroides,* many gram-positive and gram-negative aerobes), infection is unlikely in the absence of severe necrosis, and good wound care is thought to be sufficient to prevent secondary infection. Systemic and local changes produced by envenomation and the subsequent vascular damage may be difficult to differentiate from infection. Broad-spectrum antibiotics are generally recommended prophylactically in cases of obvious tissue necrosis.

Tetanus Prophylaxis. *Clostridium tetani* are not part of the mouth flora of snakes. Updating the patient's immunization status is the only necessary intervention.

Surgical Measures. The debridement of hemorrhagic blebs 3 to 5 days after a snakebite is routine if coagulation has returned to normal. Dermotomy is also routine therapy for fingers if digital swelling compresses the neurovascular bundle. Fasciotomy, however, is very controversial. Although usually unnecessary in cases of indigenous snakebite for which sufficient antivenin is given, fasciotomy has a role in cases of dangerously inadequate arterial perfusion caused by elevated intracompartmental pressures.[8,23]

Steps in Using Antivenin

1. *Prepare to manage anaphylaxis.* Because development of an anaphylactic reaction is unpredictable, all patients receiving antivenin should be monitored and have two intravenous catheters, one for the antivenin and one for emergency drugs and fluids. Intravenous epinephrine, diphenhydramine, and plasma expanders, as well as respiratory support, must be readily available.
2. *Test for sensitivity to horse serum.* Skin testing, detailed on the package insert of the antivenin, is not reliable in predicting hypersensitivity.[11] Therefore a negative skin test should not lull one into a sense of false security. However, some physicians have used the antivenin in very serious cases despite a positive skin test. To decrease the risk for allergic reaction in these cases, give the saline-diluted antivenin slowly with diphenhydramine premedication and a simultaneous infusion of epinephrine.[20]
3. *Start the infusion.* In the child over 45 kg, the initial dose should be estimated on the basis of the clinical grading system (see Table 275-1). Children under this weight usually require 50% *more* than this dose. The intravenous antivenin solution infusion should begin at 1 ml/hour and be increased over 30 minutes to a maximum of 150 ml/hour. Practically, "one to two vials per hour is appropriate to avoid the risks associated with higher infusion rates."[3]
4. *Repeat the infusion.* If, after the initial infusion, the local signs progress or the systemic signs persist, the initial antivenin dose (usually five vials in children) should be repeated. Although the incidence of serum sickness is proportional to the person's sensitivity and the volume of antivenin received, morbidity and mortality after serious envenomations are related to giving too little hyperimmune serum or giving it too late. Large doses of antivenin may be associated with metabolic acidosis, because each vial contains 0.25% formalin.[2]

Table 275-1 *Extent of Envenomation and Dosage of Antivenin*

GRADE	SIGNS AND SYMPTOMS	INITIAL TREATMENT
No envenomation	Fang marks present; no local or systemic reactions	No antivenin; local care. Tetanus prophylaxis when indicated. Observation in emergency department for at least 4 hours
Mild envenomation	Fang marks present; local swelling but no systemic reaction. Pain may be present or absent	Three to five vials antivenin
Moderate envenomation	Swelling that progresses beyond the site of the bite with systemic reaction or laboratory changes (e.g., fall in hematocrit and fibrinogen levels or platelets or hematuria)	Six to 10 vials antivenin
Severe envenomation	Marked local and systemic reaction. Bleeding diathesis, DIC, shock, or ARDS with marked laboratory changes	15+ vials antivenin

Coral Snakes

Coral snakes are the members of the Elapidae family that are indigenous to North America. Although their venom can cause a life-threatening paralysis, coral snakes tend to be small, secretive, and mild-mannered unless provoked. Few bites are reported, and mortality is rare.

Characteristics. The Eastern coral snake is often mistaken for the nonvenomous scarlet king snake because of similar colorful bands encircling the body. The mnemonic "Red to yellow, kill a fellow; red to black, venom lack; head of black, step back, Jack!" refers to the color pattern of these snake mimics. The poisonous black-snouted snake has broad red and black bands separated by narrow yellow ones; the nonpoisonous variety's snout is red and its broad red bands are separated by narrow yellow ones bounded on each side by black. Despite these distinctions a large proportion of people bitten by coral snakes thought they were handling a scarlet king snake.[12]

Unlike pit vipers, coral snakes lack facial pits, are diurnal, have fixed fangs and nearly round pupils. Their bites may produce superficial scratches or definite fang marks. Their retroverted teeth gnaw or chew on their prey and make coral snakes difficult to shake off. Because they must stay attached long enough for their venom to be deposited around their teeth, 50% of coral snake bites are dry.

Distribution. Three types of coral snakes are found in the United States: the Eastern coral snake, the Texas coral

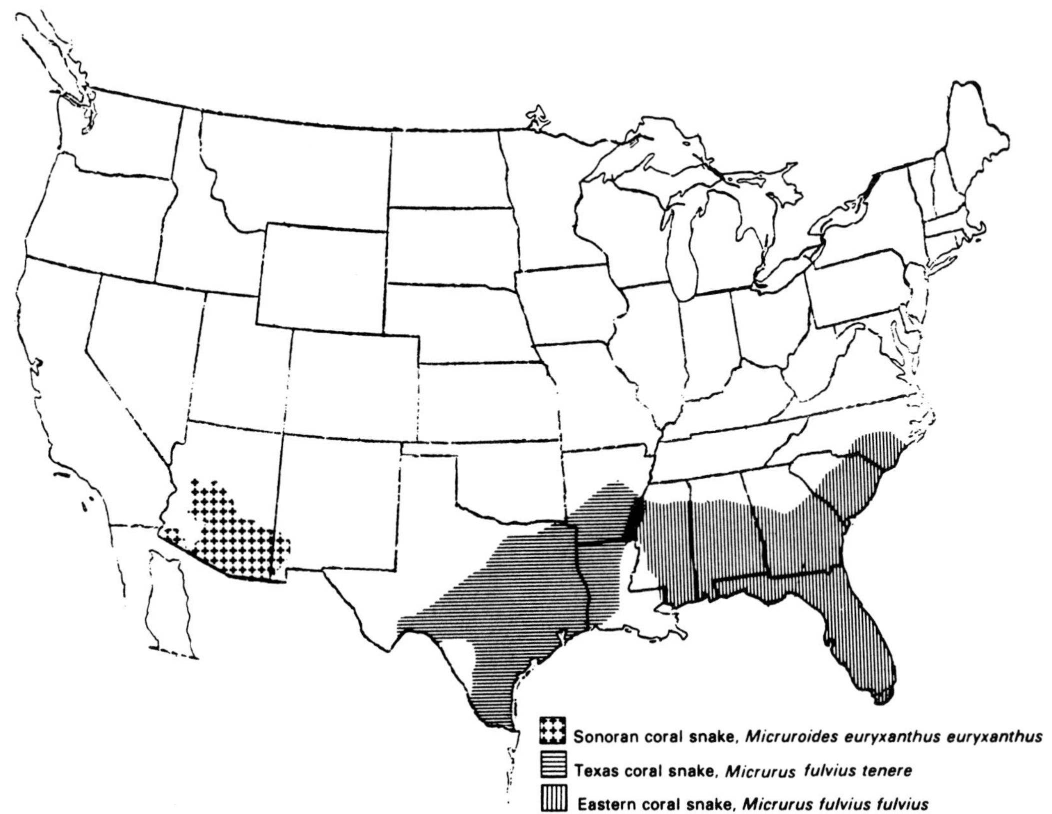

Fig. 275-2 Distribution of coral snakes in the United States, by type.
(From Russell FE: Snake venom poisoning, Philadelphia, 1980, JB Lippincott Co.)

snake, and the Arizona or Sonoran coral snake. Their distribution is shown in Fig. 275-2. The bite of the Sonoran coral snake produces no more than local pain and a small amount of nausea.

First Aid. Cryotherapy, incision and suction (including the Sawyer extractor), and constricting bands have no proven value in coral snakebites. Russell[24] recommends:

> No food or drink should be given. If the victim is more than 1 hour's distance from a medical facility, a tourniquet might be placed immediately proximal to the bite area. It should be released for 1 minute every 10 minutes, and it should be left in place until 3 minutes after intravenous antivenin has been started.

Physical Examination: Signs and Symptoms

Local. Erythema and local pain from a coral snakebite are transient or absent. Although 85% of patients will have evident fang marks, envenomations have been reported that were not associated with apparent fang marks on close examination.[19]

Systemic. Systemic manifestations may be delayed for 12 hours and may appear precipitously. They may include paresthesias, euphoria or apprehension, drowsiness, dizziness, weakness, confusion, nausea, vomiting, diaphoresis, excessive salivation, muscle tenderness or fasciculations, dysphagia, slurred speech, ophthalmoplegias that cause visual disturbances, and bulbar paralysis with ptosis. These may be followed by seizures, respiratory paralysis, and pulmonary hemorrhage. It is often unclear which findings are primary and which are secondary to hypoxia.

Laboratory Studies. Coral snakebites do not mandate laboratory screening.

Supportive Therapy. Elective intubation before impending respiratory paralysis tends to prevent aspiration pneumonia. Elective intubation is recommended if any signs of bulbar paralysis develop.[12]

Use of Antivenin. Russell[24] recommends the use of antivenin effective against Eastern and Texas snake venoms (*Micrurus fulvius;* produced by Wyeth) if a patient has definitely been bitten (five vials) or if any signs or symptoms develop (three vials). These guidelines are based on the judgment that the risks of intravenous hyperimmune horse serum are offset by the potential prevention of respiratory paralysis that may ensue if therapy is not given early in the disease.

As with pit viper antivenin, skin testing yields many false negatives; thus the same precautions must be taken as outlined above. The diluted vials are put into solution with normal saline—250 ml in children or 125 ml in infants. A starting infusion rate of 1 ml/hour is gradually increased until one or two vials are administered per hour.

Additional Therapeutic Measures. Recommendations for infection and tetanus prophylaxis are the same as for pit viper bites. Additional measures may become necessary if aspiration pneumonia develops. Patients should be aware that muscular weakness may persist for 3 to 6 weeks.

Nonindigenous Snakes

The variety of imported snakes is too great to detail in this text. If an exotic species is suspected, the recommended approach includes local wound care, supportive care, and consultation with experts.*

SPIDER BITES

All spiders are venomous. The differences among them are based on the stimulus necessary to provoke and the deadliness of their envenomations. Like snakes, spiders inflict bites noted chiefly for their cytotoxic (necrotizing) or neurotoxic effects.

Epidemiology

The true incidence of spider bites can only be estimated because of the large number of minor bites that go unreported. In 1985 the poison control centers association received 3,906 calls concerning spider bites in children. The spider was unidentified in 88% of the cases, a black widow was involved in 9%, and a brown recluse in 3%.[14] Because of the higher dose of venom per kilogram of body weight, children tend to be overrepresented among the more serious bites.

Prevention

Eradicating brown recluse and black widow spiders is difficult or impossible. Prevention therefore is chiefly focused on being cautious in areas spiders tend to inhabit.

Spider Venoms

Necrotizing venom is produced by many indigenous spiders, including orb weavers, running spiders, jumping spiders, and the commonly implicated brown recluse spider. The latter's venom includes sphingomyelinase, protease, esterase, and hyaluronidase and is potent enough to kill small animals. Its cytotoxic effects are most pronounced in the destruction of endothelial and red blood cells.[32] It causes liquefaction throughout the dermis and subcutaneous tissue.[29] The extent of the associated destruction may be the result of massive local leukocyte infiltration.

In contrast, black widow venom acts on the nerve terminals, producing an excessive motor response. The contraction of uterine muscle, leading to spontaneous abortion, is an example of this venom's effect.

Brown Recluse Spider

Characteristics. As mentioned previously, the brown recluse is the spider most commonly associated with necrotizing bites. It is hardy, living indoors or outside; reclusive, avoiding activity and light; and nonaggressive unless disturbed. Its web is irregular, its looks common. Its body is oval (10 to 15 mm long, 4 mm wide) and light fawn to dark chocolate in color. Its most distinguishing feature is the fiddlehead marking on the cephalothorax.

Distribution. Fifty-four species of *Loxosceles* are widely distributed in North America. The brown recluse, *Loxosceles reclusa,* is chiefly found in the southeastern and midwestern United States, most notably Arkansas and Missouri. *Loxosceles* species in the West tend to deliver less serious bites.

Physical Examination: Signs and Symptoms

Local. The cutaneous manifestations range from local pain and erythema in most cases to full-thickness necrosis. Typically there is an area of induration, erythema, pain, and pruritus with a grey-blue vesiculated center. The vesicle ruptures, becoming a small, dark, necrotic lesion surrounded by a ring of pallor. The remaining necrotic central depression may slowly expand in diameter for weeks, especially in fatty areas with a delicate blood supply.[28]

Systemic. Uncommonly, patients have a flulike illness, including malaise, myalgia, arthralgia, sweats, chills, nausea, vomiting, and a morbilliform to purpuric rash. Acute intravascular hemolysis may lead to hemoglobinuria, renal failure, and death. Convulsions have also been reported.

Differential Diagnosis. Ideally, the spider or some piece thereof could be presented for identification, but this is not often possible. In the absence of a definitive history of spider bite, other diagnostic possibilities must be considered, including emboli, thrombi, focal vasculitis, cutaneous infection, envenomation by other insects or reptiles, fat herniation with infarction, or iatrogenic, abusive, or self-inflicted trauma.

Laboratory Studies. Laboratory studies are useful only in cases of systemic illness that require evaluation for hemolysis.

Therapy. Management is controversial, because the unpredictable natural course of the wounds makes prospective trials difficult. There is no documented efficacy for any specific therapy. Serial observations, cleansing, topical antibiotic prophylaxis, necrotic tissue debridement, cool compresses, immobilization to prevent further trauma, and tetanus prophylaxis are commonly recommended wound care measures. Symptomatic relief with antipruritics, analgesics, and anxiolytics has also been found to be useful. Corticosteroids, dapsone, phentolamine, and early wide excision have been tried and are not promising. Antivenin is not useful, because tissue destruction has usually advanced before the victim is brought to medical attention.

Black Widow Spider

Characteristics. The *Latrodectus* species are found in both temperate and tropical climates. Both sexes have venom, but the male cannot deliver it to humans. Black widows are among the largest spiders in the world, with a leg spread of up to 40 mm. The mature female is black with a red or orange hourglass-shape marking on the ventral surface. The web, usually built in areas with moisture and away from direct sunlight, is distinguishable by its irregular pattern. The venom of the black widow destabilizes cell membranes, releases neurotransmitters, degenerates motor end plates, and causes calcium cellular influx.

History-Taking. The victim should be asked about exposure to areas in which black widows are often found, such as outdoor privies, old clothes, lumber piles, garden tools, and fields. A bite may go unnoticed or may be experienced

*The Arizona Poison and Drug Information Center (602-626-6016); the Oklahoma Poison Control Center (405-271-5454); the Bronx Zoo's herpetology section (212-220-5151).

as a pin prick or burning. Rapid extension of the pain is typical.

Physical Examination: Signs and Symptoms

Local. Two small punctate lesions may be visible. Unlike the bite of a brown recluse, the bite of a black widow usually does not induce an impressive inflammatory response.

Systemic. A retrospective study of patients hospitalized for black widow spider envenomation showed the most frequent systemic signs and symptoms to be abdominal pain (71%), abdominal tenderness or rigidity (71%), and lower extremity weakness (57%).[18] Pain in muscles and bones, bilateral periorbital edema, restlessness, diaphoresis, lacrimation, salivation, increased bronchial secretions, hypertension, tachycardia, and convulsions may develop over the first 48 hours.[22] Respiratory paralysis and heart failure have also been reported. Weakness and pain may persist for weeks.

Laboratory Studies. Laboratory studies show nonspecific changes consistent with increased sympathetic tone (e.g., leukocytosis, elevated blood glucose) and increased muscle activity (e.g., elevated creatine kinase). The blood calcium is normal.

Therapy. The vast majority of black widow spider bites require only cold packs, topical steroid cream, or oral analgesics to relieve the pain. In more severe cases basic life-support measures may be needed. Muscle spasm may be ameliorated by intravenous diazepam. In the extremely rare case of a life-threatening effect, a horse serum–based antivenin is available (Merck, Sharpe, & Dohme).

Tarantula

The tarantula is a relatively harmless desert dweller. Its large fang can deliver a venom that causes local pain and swelling as well as occasional nausea and vomiting. The urticating hairs on its anterior abdomen cause irritation and pruritus if the spider is handled. These hairs should be removed with adhesive tape and the area should be washed. Local cold compresses and mild systemic analgesics are usually sufficient treatment.

Scorpion Stings

The American poison control centers received 600 pediatric calls about scorpion stings involving children in 1985.[14] Scorpion stings may occur in many Southern states, but *Centruroides exilicauda* (also known as *C. sculpturatus*) is the only dangerous species indigenous to the continental United States. This nonaggressive, climbing, photophobic arthropod, commonly called the bark scorpion, is native to Arizona and parts of Texas, New Mexico, California, and Nevada. It is often found clinging to the underside of rocks.

Unlike many tissue-damaging scorpion venoms, the bark scorpion's venom leads to spontaneous depolarization of parasympathetic and sympathetic nerves. The sting of non-*Centruroides* species may produce local pain with minor erythema and heat, but there is usually no inflammatory response at the site of the *Centruroides* sting. Local symptoms of *Centruroides* envenomation—painful tingling and hypesthesia—may manifest as unexplained crying in an infant. In severe cases there may be systemic manifestations, including elevation of all vital signs, generalized muscle fasciculations, and neurologic symptoms (e.g., agitation, disconjugate or roving eye movements, blurred vision, loss of control of pharyngeal muscles and, in rare cases, seizure activity).[3]

Progression of symptoms is not predictable. A review of cases from Arizona's Regional Poison Management Center revealed that progression to serious symptoms always occurred in less than 5 hours if at all. Numbness, tingling, and pain may persist for 2 weeks.[7]

Suggested treatments fall into three categories: supportive (e.g., airway support), symptomatic (e.g., propranolol), and prophylactic (e.g., phenobarbital). Analgesics and application of ice is recommended for the relief of local pain. Corticosteroids, antihistamines, and calcium are ineffective. Sedative/hypnotic drugs and narcotics have been associated with an increase in mortality and morbidity and are contraindicated. Scorpion antivenin, manufactured by the Antivenom Production Laboratory at Arizona State University in Tempe, Arizona, is not licensed or approved by the FDA (personal communication, 1990), but has been used to resolve serious signs and symptoms safely within minutes.[7]

HYMENOPTERA STINGS

Wasps, bees, and ants are venomous insects belonging to the order of Hymenoptera. Although anaphylaxis follows 0.4% to 0.8% of insect stings in children and young adults, few deaths ensue. Large local reactions are common, however, occurring in about 10% of individuals who are stung.

To prevent stings, the following practices should be *avoided* while outdoors; wearing bright colors or floral patterns; wearing scented cosmetics, perfumes, and colognes; leaving food or garbage uncovered; and walking or playing without adequate foot protection. Screens on windows and doors help prevent indoor stings.

When the child is old enough to relate a history, the diagnosis is usually clear. Knowledge of previous exposures and reactions is helpful.

Maguire and Geha[16] divide physical findings into four common categories: local reactions, either small or large, and systemic reactions, either mild or severe. A small local reaction consists of a short-lived, painful, pruritic, urticarial lesion at the site of the sting. Large local reactions are those for which the diameter of the swelling exceeds 5 cm. These tend to persist for up to a week. Mild systemic reactions are chiefly cutaneous and gastrointestinal. Severe systemic reactions also involve the cardiorespiratory system. In rare cases serum sickness, vasculitis, encephalopathy, neuritis, and renal disease are seen.[16]

If a bee's stinger can be seen in the wound, it should be removed by scraping, not squeezing. Local reactions may be treated with ice, calamine, topical corticosteroid creams, oral antihistamines, or oral analgesics. Systemic reactions require subcutaneous epinephrine.* Corticosteroids and antihistamines may also be useful. Supportive measures, especially

*A 0.01 ml/kg dose of 1:1000 aqueous epinephrine solution is injected subcutaneously. The original dose should not exceed 0.3 ml, but it may be repeated in 15 minutes. Alternatively, Sus-phrine (0.005 ml/kg) can be used. It is highly recommended that susceptible individuals carry epinephrine self-administration kits when they are outdoors. After such a kit is used, medical help should be sought because the drug's duration of action is brief.

intravenous fluids, should not be overlooked in severe systemic reactions.

Immunotherapy using insect venoms has been found relatively safe when conducted by experienced physicians; it prevents recurrences of systemic reactions after subsequent insect stings. Although it is unnecessary for most children who are allergic to insect stings, it should be considered for children with a history of severe systemic reactions not limited to the skin.[15,26] Notably, more of the systemic reactions in adults are life threatening; thus all adults with a history of systemic allergic reactions are candidates for immunotherapy.

The extract is injected once or twice each week for several months, then monthly until the skin tests or in vitro tests for specific IgE become negative. Maintenance doses may be necessary thereafter. Immediate access to aqueous epinephrine and a thorough understanding of its administration remain important aspects of care for children undergoing immunotherapy until they reach maintenance doses.[15,26]

REFERENCES

1. Alario A et al: Cutaneous necrosis following a spider bite: a case report and review, Pediatrics 79(4):618, 1987.
2. Bailey WJ: Letter to the editor, J Trauma 25(5):464, 1985.
3. Banner W: Bites and stings in the pediatric patient, Curr Probl Pediatr 18(1):1, 1988.
4. Bronstein AC et al: Negative pressure suction in field treatment of rattlesnake bite, Vet Hum Toxicol 27:297, 1985.
5. Burch JM et al: The treatment of crotalid envenomation without antivenin, J Trauma 28(1):35, 1988.
6. Crane DB and Irwin JS: Rattlesnake bite of glans penis, Urology 26(1):50, 1985.
7. Curry SC et al: Envenomation by the scorpion *Centruroides sculpturatus,* J Toxicol Clin Toxicol 21(4 and 5):417, 1983-1984.
8. Curry SC et al: Noninvasive vascular studies in management of rattlesnake envenomations to extremities, Ann Emerg Med 14(11):1081, 1985.
9. Curry SC et al: The legitimacy of rattlesnake bites in central Arizona, Ann Emerg Med 18(6):658, 1989.
10. Danzl DF and Carter GL: "Kiss and yell," a rattlesnake bite to the tongue, Ann Emerg Med 17(5):549, 1988 (letter).
11. Jurkovich GJ et al: complications of Crotalidae antivenin therapy, J Trauma 28(7):1032, 1988.
12. Kitchens CS and Van Mierop LHS: Envenomation by the Eastern coral snake *(Micrurus fulvius),* JAMA 258(12):1615, 1987.
13. Kunkel DB et al: Reptile envenomations, J Toxicol Clin Toxicol 21(4 and 5):503, 1983-1984.
14. Litovitz TL, Normann SA, and Veltri JC: 1985 Annual Report of the American Association of Poison Control Centers National Data Collection System, Am J Emerg Med 4:427, 1986.
15. Lockey RF: Immunotherapy for allergy to insect stings, N Engl J Med 323:1627, 1990.
16. Maguire JF and Geha RS: Bee, wasp, and hornet stings, Pediatr Rev 8(1):5, 1986.
17. Minton SA: Present tests for detection of snake venom: clinical applications, Ann Emerg Med 16(9):932, 1987.
18. Moss HS and Binder LS: A retrospective review of black widow spider envenomation, Ann Emerg Med 16(2):188, 1987.
19. Norris RL and Dart RC: Apparent coral snake envenomation in a patient without visible fang marks, Am J Emerg Med 7(4):402, 1989.
20. Otten EJ and McKimm D: Venomous snakebite in a patient allergic to horse serum, Ann Emerg Med 12(10):624, 1983.
21. Parrish HM and Carr CA: Bites by copperheads *(Agkistrodon contortrix)* in the United States, JAMA 201(12):107, 1967.
22. Rauber A: Black widow spider bites, J Toxicol Clin Toxicol 21(4 and 5):473, 1983-1984.
23. Roberts RS, Csencsitz TA, Heard CW: Upper extremity compartment syndromes following pit viper envenomation, Clin Orthop 193:184, 1985.
24. Russell FE: Snake venom poisoning, Philadelphia, 1980, JB Lippincott Co.
25. Tu AT: Biotoxicology of sea snake venoms, Ann Emerg Med 16(9):1023, 1987.
26. Valentine MD et al: The value of immunotherapy with venom in children with allergy to insect stings, N Engl J Med, 1990.
27. Wagner CW and Golladay ES: Crotalid envenomation in children: selective conservative management, J Pediatr Surg 24(1):128, 1989.
28. Wasserman GS and Anderson PC: Loxoscelism and necrotic arachnidism, J Toxicol Clin Toxicol 21(4 and 5):451, 1983-1984.
29. Wasserman GS: Wound care of spider and snake envenomations, Ann Emerg Med 17(12):1331, 1988.
30. Wingert WA: Poisoning by animal venoms, Top Emerg Med 2:89, 1980.
31. Wingert WA and Chan L: Rattlesnake bites in southern California and rationale for recommended treatment, West J Med 148(1):37, 1988.
32. Young VL and Pin P: The brown recluse spider bite, Ann Plast Surg 20(5):447, 1988.

SUGGESTED READINGS

Alexander JO: Arthropods and human skin, Suffolk, England, 1984, William Clowes, Ltd.

McLean DC: Insect sting allergy, Prim Care 14(3):513, 1987.

Schuberth KC: How dangerous are insect stings? Contemp Pediatr 6:69, 1989.

Stawiski MA: Insect bites and stings, Emerg Med Clin North Am 3(4):785, 1985.

276

Epiglottitis

Caroline Breese Hall and William J. Hall

Epiglottitis, or supraglottitis, is an acute and potentially fatal respiratory infection that is caused almost exclusively by *Haemophilus influenzae* type b.* Its rapid onset and progression without therapy to a fatal outcome make clinical recognition of this disease essential.

ETIOLOGY

H. influenzae organisms were first discovered by Pfeiffer during the pandemic of influenza in 1890. Believing these to be the cause of influenza, he titled the organism the "influenza bacillus." These gram-negative, aerobic bacilli were later designated *H. influenzae*. In clinical specimens these organisms appear pleomorphic, often coccobacillary. Epiglottitis is caused only by the type b organisms, which are distinguished by their capsular polysaccharide. The organisms may be seen to be encapsulated in clinical specimens by stained smears or by the quellung reaction, which produces capsular swelling with type-specific antiserum. On laboratory growth media and broth, the capsules may easily be demonstrated during the first few hours of growth, but with age the morphology changes.

Epiglottitis may occasionally be caused by other bacteria, such as *Haemophilus parainfluenzae*, beta-hemolytic streptococci, and pneumococci.[2,4,12] Very rarely, even a virus has been implicated.[9] Other agents, however, are unusual, and the clinical features may be atypical. Particularly with pneumococci and streptococci, the epiglottic infection may be secondary to spread from a major nearby focus of infection.

INCIDENCE

H. influenzae epiglottitis is primarily a disease of children 3 to 7 years of age.* In contrast, the peak incidence of viral croup is in the second year of life, and that of other serious disease caused by *H. influenzae* type b, such as meningitis, is 7 to 12 months of age.[22,23] Nevertheless, *H. influenzae* epiglottitis may occur at any age, including infancy, older childhood, and rarely even adulthood.[16]

Epiglottitis has no distinctive seasonal predilection. However, in most areas of the United States, the majority of cases occur from November through March.[17] Clustering of *H. influenzae* meningitis and epiglottitis has occasionally been observed, particularly in settings with close contact among young children.[21]

PATHOGENESIS

Infection with *H. influenzae* type b is very common in young children. Why only a few should develop clinically evident disease, such as epiglottitis, is not completely understood.[22] However, about 3% to 5% of young children at any one time may asymptomatically carry *H. influenzae* type b organisms. Epiglottitis occurs subsequent to infection of the upper respiratory tract. It has been hypothesized that the organisms may become invasive during periods of stress, such as a concurrent viral respiratory tract infection.

The organisms' residence in the upper respiratory tract may be marked by nasopharyngitis. Subsequently, the infection spreads from the pharynx to involve the epiglottis, producing marked inflammation and edema. The inflammation is not limited to the epiglottis, however, but involves the surrounding area, the arytenoids, the arytenoepiglottic folds, the vocal cords, and to some extent the subglottic region. The characteristically rapid and pronounced inflammatory response of these structures causes mechanical obstruction to the flow of air. Inspiratory obstruction is particularly pronounced because of the narrowing force generated by the negative intrathoracic pressure. The edematous epiglottis, like a ball valve, is pulled down into the larynx during inspiration and may cause complete obstruction of the airway. In addition, secretions and exudate are formed by the inflammation, which may include the lower tracheobronchial tree as well. The secretions and edema compound the obstruction to the flow of air. The work of breathing increases, and hypoxemia and carbon dioxide retention may result. Thus, even without total occlusion of the airway by the epiglottis, assisted ventilation is likely to be required.[14,20]

CLINICAL FEATURES

Children with epiglottitis usually have previously been well, although up to one fourth may have had some prior upper respiratory tract symptoms that may or may not be related. The hallmarks of epiglottitis are the abrupt onset of severe sore throat, fever, and toxicity in a formerly active child.[1,2,4,23] With fulminant progression, the other classic symptoms and signs occur: dysphagia, drooling, and respiratory distress.

*References 1,2,5,17,22,23.

Table 276-1 *Characteristic Signs of Epiglottitis Compared with Viral Croup and Bacterial Tracheitis*

	EPIGLOTTITIS	VIRAL CROUP	BACTERIAL TRACHEITIS
Peak age	3-7 yr	3 mo-3 yr	Any age (mostly ≤12 yr)
History	Previously well	Preceding upper respiratory tract infection common; may have had croup previously	Preceding upper respiratory tract infection common; sometimes viral croup; occasionally previous trauma or manipulation of trachea and upper respiratory tract
Onset	Acute (hours)	Less acute (days)	Acute (hours)
Appearance	Toxic; drooling, dysphagia; sitting forward, mouth open	Less toxic; no drooling	Toxic; respiratory distress and stridor; drooling and sitting forward not characteristic
Cough	Unusual	Very characteristic, spasmodic, "seal's bark"	May be absent or may be present from preceding viral upper respiratory tract infection
Temperature	High (usually 39° C)	Lower (usually 39° C or none)	High (usually >39° C)
Pharynx	"Beefy" erythema	Normal or slight erythema	Normal or minimal inflammation
White blood cell count and differential	High; left shift	Normal or slight increase; normal or slight left shift	High; left shift
Roentgenogram of neck	"Thumb" sign on lateral view (edematous epiglottis)	Subglottic narrowing on posteroanterior view	Normal epiglottis; subglottic narrowing with membranous tracheal exudate occasionally visible on lateral view

Stridor usually develops, but toxicity and respiratory distress may be present initially without overt stridor. Retractions of the chest wall become evident, particularly in the supraclavicular and suprasternal areas, and are indicative of high airway obstruction. Cough is usually not a prominent part of the picture, but may develop as the child tries to clear the increasing secretions. As noted in Table 276-1, the preceding spasmodic, brassy cough and laryngitis are more characteristic of viral croup. With progression of the epiglottitis, voice changes do occur, however. These may more correctly be described as dysphonia rather than the "scratchy" or "rasping" hoarseness associated with viral laryngotracheobronchitis.

The general appearance of the child with epiglottitis should suggest the diagnosis. The child with epiglottitis often appears toxic and is in a sitting position, leaning forward with the mouth open, tongue protruding, and drooling. The drooling is a particularly characteristic and helpful clinical sign.

Examination of the child reveals a markedly inflamed, "beefy red" pharynx, bathed by copious secretions. Although the "cherry red" epiglottis often may be seen by examination of the pharynx with a tongue depressor, this generally should not be attempted. Fatal occlusion of the airway may result. Inspiratory stridor and expiratory rhonchi may be heard on auscultation, and with progressive obstruction the breath sounds may become diminished.

Bacteremia with *H. influenzae* type b almost always occurs, and secondary sites of infection may develop.[17] Most frequent of these are pneumonia and cervical lymphadenitis, each occurring in about one fourth of the patients. For reasons, meningitis and septic arthritis are uncommon complications, even in cases occurring in the preantibiotic era.

DIAGNOSIS

Because of the gravity of epiglottitis, the tentative diagnosis must be made on the basis of the history and clinical presentation.[2,20] If epiglottitis is suspected, the child should immediately be sent to the hospital, where the diagnosis may be confirmed and trained personnel and equipment are available for establishing an artificial airway.[8,15] Only with these precautions may visualization of the diagnostic epiglottis be attempted.

If the diagnosis is in question and the child is not severely distressed, roentgenograms of the lateral neck will confirm the diagnosis.[19,20] Nevertheless, at all times the child should be accompanied by personnel equipped to handle an airway occlusion. The roentgenograms of the lateral neck, as shown by Rapkin,[20] are a reliable and noninvasive way of identifying epiglottitis and of differentiating it from viral croup when the posteroanterior views of the neck are compared. As shown in Fig. 276-1, the characteristic swelling of the epiglottis may be seen as an enlarged, rounded shadow that resembles an adult thumb. This has been called the "thumb sign" by Podgore and Bass[19] and may be compared with the "little finger sign" of the normal epiglottis (Fig. 276-2). The normal epiglottis appears narrower, with the configuration of an adult little finger viewed from the side, as seen in the figure. The total white blood cell count is usually elevated (15,000 to 25,000/mm^3) and often contains a pronounced left shift.

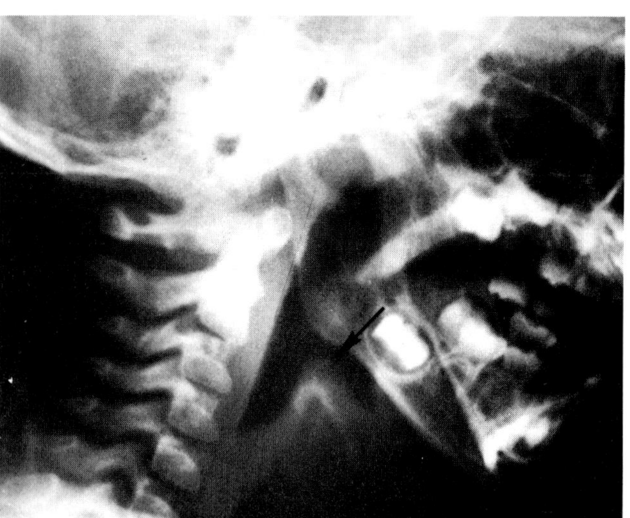

Fig. 276-1 Roentgenogram of lateral neck of a child with epiglottitis. The arrow points to the shadow of the epiglottitis, which is enlarged and resembles the anteroposterior view of a thumb.

From Hall CB and Hall WJ: *Haemophilus influenzae* epiglottitis, Update, 2:665, 1975.

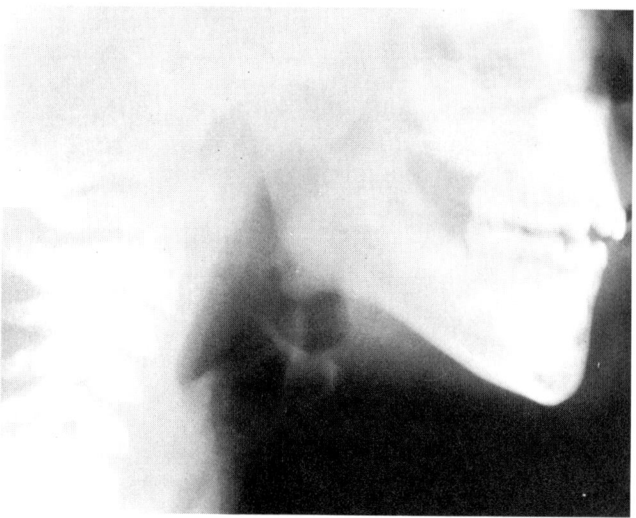

Fig. 276-2 Roentgenogram of lateral neck of a normal child. In contrast to Fig. 276-1, the epiglottis is not enlarged and resembles an adult's fifth finger, viewed laterally.

From Hall CB and Hall WJ: *Haemophilus influenzae* epiglottitis, Update, 2:665, 1975.

More than 80% of children will have band counts of 500/mm^3 or greater. Cultures of the upper respiratory tract and blood will usually demonstrate the pathogen *H. influenzae* type b. One of the rapid diagnostic tests, such as counterimmunoelectrophoresis or latex agglutination, may also reveal the antigen in the blood, secretions, or urine.

MANAGEMENT

Few illnesses in pediatrics require more swift and careful management.[1] As has previously been stressed, suspicion of the diagnosis of epiglottitis is indication enough to rush the child to the hospital. Once the diagnosis is established, an adequate airway must be maintained. In some intensive care settings, with highly trained personnel in continuous attendance, some children with early disease have been managed without an artificial airway. In most centers, however, immediate airway intervention is chosen.[2,3,24] With experienced personnel available, nasotracheal intubation is the procedure of choice. Fewer complications occur with this method, and in most patients extubation is possible within 1 to 3 days.

Intravenous antibiotic therapy also should immediately be started. For years, ampicillin has been the drug of choice. However, the recent insurgence in the United States of *H. influenzae* organisms resistant to ampicillin has necessitated that a drug effective against these resistant organisms be substituted as the initial therapy. Chloramphenicol may be used alone, or in areas where organisms resistant to chloramphenicol have been detected, it may be combined with ampicillin. A more recent alternative is a cephalosporin that is stable against the beta-lactamases, such as several third-generation cephalosporins. If the organism on testing proves sensitive to ampicillin, therapy may be switched to ampicillin or the initial therapy may be continued.

Supportive care in epiglottitis is of the utmost importance. Direct humidification of the airway and mobilization of the secretions should be maintained. As with any mechanical airway, its position and patency should be carefully monitored. A short course of corticosteroids may be used to help reduce the postintubation edema. Antipyretics may be given during the initial period of high fever. Intravenous fluid should be carefully monitored. The acute onset of the disease means that most of these children are not dehydrated and only maintenance fluids are necessary.

PROGNOSIS

The outcome in these children often depends on the primary care physician. The clinical acumen of the physician and high index of suspicion suggesting the diagnosis, even over the telephone, will allow the child to reach the hospital rapidly and will prevent an unexpected calamity. The prognosis of *H. influenzae* epiglottitis is directly related to the speed with which therapy and the precautions against fatal asphyxia are initiated. Once an airway has been established and appropriate antibiotic therapy has been begun, the clinical response is usually rapid. Progression of the infection is usually controlled in less than 24 hours, and the nasotracheal tube may be removed within the next couple of days.

PREVENTION

A vaccine consisting of the purified *H. influenzae* type b capsular polysaccharide was initially licensed in the United States in 1984 for use in children 24 months of age or older.[18] In 1990, conjugated *H. influenzae* type b vaccines capable of eliciting an adequate antibody response in infants as young as 2 months of age were licensed and recommended for universal use.[10] No serious adverse reactions have been reported thus far in clinical trials with these conjugated vaccines, and minor reactions such as fever and local reactions at the infection site are relatively few. Inasmuch as children with epiglottitis are usually older than 12 months of age, these vaccines should virtually eliminate cases of epiglottitis caused by *H. influenzae* type b.

DIFFERENTIAL DIAGNOSIS

The major entities to be distinguished from epiglottitis are viral croup and bacterial tracheitis. The distinguishing features of these diseases are listed in Table 276-1. *Bacterial tracheitis* in particular may mimic epiglottitis in its severity and rapid progression and requires equally prompt treatment.[6,7] This unusual entity may affect children of any age. The onset is similar in its acuteness, fever, and toxicity but is characterized by respiratory stridor, more severe than that usually observed with viral croup, and the production of copious, purulent sputum. The diagnosis is usually made by direct laryngoscopy, which shows the purulent secretions and an exudate localized to the inflamed subglottic area. The epiglottic and supraglottic structures usually show minimal involvement. Roentgenograms of the lateral neck show the subglottic narrowing and occasionally may even demonstrate a fibrinous exudate obstructing the airway.[7] The organisms most commonly causing this syndrome are *Staphylococcus aureus,* group A beta-hemolytic streptococci, and *H. influenzae* type b, which may be recovered usually in almost pure culture from the secretions obtained on laryngoscopy.[6,11]

Diphtheria with pharyngolaryngeal involvement may be confused with epiglottitis. However, the slower onset, other signs of diphtheria, and a pharyngeal grayish membrane may help to differentiate the two. Most helpful in the differentiation is the history of inadequate immunizations. Specific diagnosis of diphtheria may be obtained by Gram-stained smear and culture of the diphtheritic membrane.

Aspiration of a foreign body should be suspected in a child, usually a toddler, with a history of acute onset of choking and respiratory distress. Fever is not present early in the course, and the pharynx does not show the "beefy" erythema characteristic of *H. influenzae* infection. Roentgenograms of the lateral neck will not show the "thumb" sign. Further roentgenographic examination may show the foreign body, if opaque, or endoscopy may be required. In rare cases, thermal injury to the epiglottis has been reported in young children drinking hot beverages, resulting in a clinical picture markedly similar to that of epiglottitis.[13]

REFERENCES

1. Ashcraft CK and Steele RW: Epiglottitis: a pediatric emergency, J Respir Dis 9:48, 1988.
2. Bass JW, Steele RW, and Weide RA: Acute epiglottitis: a surgical emergency, JAMA 229:671, 1974.
3. Battaglia JD and Lockhart CH: Management of acute epiglottitis by nasotracheal intubation, Am J Dis Child 129:334, 1975.
4. Berenberg W and Kevy S: Acute epiglottitis in childhood, N Engl J Med 258:870, 1958.
5. Dajan AS, Asmar BI, and Thirumoorthi MC: Systemic *Haemophilus influenzae* disease: an overview, J Pediatr 94:355, 1979.
6. Davidson S, Yahav BJ, and Rubinstein E: Bacterial tracheitis: a true entity? J Laryngol Otol 96:173, 1982.
7. Denneny JC and Handler SD: Membranous laryngotracheobronchitis, Pediatrics 70:705, 1982.
8. Fulginiti VA: Acute supraglottitis (epiglottitis): to look or not? Am J Dis Child 142:597, 1988.
9. Grattan-Smith T et al: Viral supraglottitis, J Pediatr 110:434, 1987.
10. Hoekelman RA: A pediatrician's view: Hib vaccination now! Pediatr Ann 19:683, 1990.
11. Jones R, Santos JI, and Overall JC Jr: Bacterial tracheitis, JAMA 242:721, 1979.
12. Jones RN, Slepack J, and Bigelow J: Ampicillin-resistant *Hemophilus paraphrophelus* laryngoepiglottitis, J Clin Microbiol 4:405, 1976.
13. Kulick RM et al: Thermal epiglottitis after swallowing hot beverages, Pediatrics 81:441, 1988.
14. Margolis CZ, Ingram DL, and Meyer JH: Routine tracheotomy in *Haemophilus influenzae* type b epiglottitis, J Pediatr 81:1150, 1972.
15. Mauro RD, Poole SR, and Lockhart CH: Differentiation of epiglottitis from laryngotracheitis in the child with stridor, Am J Dis Child 142:679, 1988.
16. Mayo Smith MF et al: Acute epiglottitis in adults, N Engl J Med 314:1133, 1986.
17. Molteni RA: Epiglottitis: incidence of extraepiglottic infection: report on 72 cases and review of the literature, Pediatrics 58:526, 1976.
18. Peltola H et al: Prevention of *Haemophilus influenzae* type b bacteremic infections with the capsular polysaccharide vaccine, N Engl J Med 310:1561, 1984.
19. Podgore JK and Bass JW: The "thumb sign" and "little finger sign" in acute epiglottitis, J Pediatr 88:154, 1976.
20. Rapkin RH: Acute epiglottitis: pitfalls in diagnosis and management, Clin Pediatr 10:312, 1971.
21. Redmond RR and Pichichero ME: *Haemophilis influenzae* type b disease: an epidemiologic study with special reference to day care centers, JAMA 252:2581, 1984.
22. Robbins JB: *Haemophilus influenzae* type b: disease and immunity in humans, Ann Intern Med 78:259, 1973.
23. Todd JK and Bruhn FW: Severe *Haemophilus influenzae* infections, Am J Dis Child 129:607, 1975.
24. Weber ML et al: Acute epiglottitis in children—treatment with nasotracheal intubation: report of 14 consecutive cases, Pediatrics 57:152, 1976.

277

Esophageal Burns

J. Alex Haller, Jr.

Accidental ingestion of powerful corrosive agents is a much more frequent problem in infants and toddlers than in school-aged children and adults. Esophageal burns resulting from ingestion of caustic materials constitute a significant problem, both in immediate management and in subsequent treatment of the serious sequelae of such burns—namely, severe strictures of the esophagus. The ingestion of strong corrosive agents is the most common cause of esophageal stricture in infants and young children. Although progress has been made in the elimination of dangerous caustic materials from the marketplace, much needs to be done to ensure the packaging of such products in child-safe containers.

The goal of therapy is to minimize esophageal injury and to prevent subsequent strictures that may require complicated and dangerous esophageal substitution operations. The most common form of treatment for caustic injury to the esophagus until 15 years ago was the Saltzer technique of immediate and continuing esophageal dilation.[10] For more than a decade the use of systemic steroids and antibiotics and the avoidance of routine dilation has supplanted the Saltzer technique.[1] Pharmacologic treatment controls inflammation and edema and avoids injury that might result from repeated dilations.

MECHANISMS OF CAUSTIC INJURY TO THE ESOPHAGUS

Ingestion of sodium hydroxide is the most common cause of esophageal burns from caustic substances in young children. It is present in toilet bowl, oven, and plumbing cleaners. Recently liquid cleaners have been added to the list of dangerous agents. Weaker alkaline solutions, such as liquid ammonia, can cause esophageal irritation, but they rarely result in significant tissue damage or strictures. Strong acids are more likely to damage the stomach and small intestine than the esophagus.

Strong alkalis are more common in the child's environment than are strong acids. Clinitest tablets and alkaline disk batteries usually lodge in the esophagus and frequently lead to esophageal perforation. Oven and drain cleaners usually contain strong alkalis, as do some toilet bowl cleaners and dishwashing detergents. Bleaches, disinfectants, metal cleansers, and toilet bowl cleansers may be acidic. Household soap, bleaches, and those detergents that are not highly alkaline generally have low toxicity, whereas commercial bleaches may produce caustic burns.[4,11]

Strong alkaline solutions are particularly destructive because they cause *liquefaction necrosis,* which penetrates deep into the wall of the esophagus and may cause perforation into the mediastinum.[5] The inflammatory reaction that accompanies such burns can cause fibrosis, stricture formation, and mediastinitis. Bacteria can invade the injured tissues and lead to mediastinal abscess and sepsis. Acid burns, however, produce *coagulation necrosis,* which prevents penetration into the deeper tissues and protects the esophageal wall from further damage.

Animal models of caustic esophageal burns, particularly those in the cat, have clearly demonstrated the pathologic changes that occur.[6] In the first week after ingestion of sodium hydroxide, the wall of the esophagus is destroyed to varying degrees, primarily from contact necrosis and secondarily from an intense inflammatory process. The inflammatory reaction extends through the muscle layers and may involve the mediastinum. Over the next week, granulation tissue is formed. By the end of the second to third week, the fibroblasts proliferate, causing early esophageal wall contracture. After 3 to 4 weeks the muscle layer is largely replaced by dense, fibrous tissue, and a pseudoepithelium lines the lumen. Contracture then occurs, leading to severe esophageal stricture. The animals show initial dysphagia, caused by muscle spasm at the injury site and by the intense inflammatory edema. Obstruction of the esophagus may lead to aspiration pneumonia and bacteremia. Antibiotics are used to decrease the risk of pulmonary infection and potential bacterial invasion of the blood stream through the injured esophageal wall. Steroids significantly diminish the initial inflammation in experimental animals and thereby decrease scar formation.[5,12]

MANAGEMENT

On the basis of animal experiments and clinical experience, a plan of management should include documentation of the caustic agent ingested, identification of the presence and extent of the esophageal burn by means of early esophagoscopic examination, immediate institution of steroid and antibiotic therapy, serial evaluation of the esophagus to detect early stricture formation, and immediate and continuing dilation if stricture occurs.[2,3]

History and Initial Physical Examination

Caustic ingestion by infants and young children is either accidental or the result of active (rare) or passive child abuse. The caustic agent is immediately regurgitated; for this reason, gastric lavage is not necessary in the initial management. Usually the parent can identify the offending agent. Careful examination of the oral cavity usually reveals areas of edema and superficial burns. Approximately one third of children with oral burns will have esophageal burns as well. If no oral burn is present but the caustic ingestion is positively confirmed, a burn of the esophagus, which can occur with or without oral burns, must be assumed.

Esophagoscopic Examination

All patients with oral burns, as well as those in whom caustic ingestion is strongly suspected, should undergo esophagoscopic examination soon after admission to the hospital.[3,7,9] To obviate the danger of perforation during the procedure, the endoscopist should visualize the oropharynx and upper portion of the esophagus only to the site of the esophageal burn and should not pass the instrument beyond. If there is evidence of an acute esophageal injury, its extent is of no consequence in terms of immediate management, and therapy should be instituted in the hospital. If examination yields negative findings, the patient's care can be managed safely at home.

Steroid Therapy

Steroid therapy should be instituted within 24 hours because a major inflammatory reaction develops within that period. Steroids must be continued throughout the early phases of injury if the complications associated with the inflammatory reaction are to be prevented. Even in young infants a course of steroid therapy should be given for 3 weeks; with significant burns it should be extended to 4 to 6 weeks.

Antibiotic Therapy

Because of the hazards of aspiration pneumonia and mediastinal invasion, especially when steroids are used, prophylactic antibiotic therapy should be instituted. Inasmuch as most of the offending bacteria can be expected to be gram-positive organisms, ampicillin is the most appropriate drug.

Studies of Esophageal Function

Serial barium swallow studies of the esophagus will provide evidence of a developing esophageal stricture. In its present, steroid therapy should be discontinued and esophageal dilation instituted. Barium swallow studies also help in evaluating the extent of esophageal burn during the healing phase of the injury. Any evidence of difficulties with swallowing after the initial treatment period (3 to 6 weeks) indicates the need for repeated barium swallow studies to identify a late-occurring stricture.

Rare and Severe Forms of Caustic Injury in Infants

With the increased use of strong liquid caustic agents (liquid lye), a severe form of caustic esophageal injury has been more frequently reported. These patients have deep second-degree burns or even full-thickness burns (third degree) and inevitable stricture formation. Reyes and Hill[9] introduced a concept of temporary intraluminal stenting in infants with such severe burns, and this technique has been extended to older patients with some good results.[8] Reports indicate that a few teenaged patients ingested liquid lye to commit suicide. Recent experience suggests that the best survival and long-term rehabilitation of these patients is accomplished if the badly burned esophagus is removed immediately, usually by use of transhiatal approach, and a cervical esophagostomy is performed.[3,7] Gastric resection also may be indicated. Ultimately, reconstruction must be individualized, including esophageal replacement after 6 to 8 weeks of recovery. Fortunately, these life-threatening caustic injuries are rare in children.

SUMMARY

The immediate establishment of the diagnosis of esophageal injury is mandatory in all infants and young children in whom caustic ingestion is suspected. Early esophagoscopic examination is necessary to document the presence or absence of an acute caustic esophageal burn. Initiation of steroid therapy and antibiotics to decrease the inflammatory response is the only dependable way to prevent late stricture formation. This form of therapy has significantly decreased the incidence of late esophageal stricture. Signs of early esophageal stenosis require bougie dilitation.

REFERENCES

1. Buttross S and Bronhard BH: Acute management of alkali ingestion in children: a review, Tex Med 77:57, 1981.
2. Cleveland WW et al: The effect of prednisone in the prevention of esophageal stricture following the ingestion of lye, South Med J 15:861, 1958.
3. Estrera A et al: Corrosive burns of the esophagus and stomach: a recommendation for an aggressive surgical approach, Ann Thorac Surg 41:276, 1986.
4. Haller JA: Caustic burns of the esophagus. In Cameron J, editor: Current surgical therapy, ed 3, Toronto, 1989, BC Decker, Inc.
5. Haller JA et al: Pathophysiology and management of acute corrosive burns of the esophagus: results of treatment in 285 children, J Pediatr Surg 6:578, 1971.
6. Haller JA and Bachman K: The comparative effect of current therapy on experimental caustic burns of the esophagus, Pediatrics 34:236, 1964.
7. Meredith JW, Kon ND, and Thompson JN: Management of injuries from liquid lye ingestion, J Trauma 28:1173, 1988.
8. Mills LJ, Estrera AS and Platt MR: Avoidance of esophageal stricture following severe caustic burns by the use of an intraluminal stent, Ann Thorac Surg 28:60, 1979.
9. Reyes HM and Hill JL: Experimental treatment of corrosive esophageal burns, J Pediatr Surg 9:317, 1974.
10. Salzer H: Early treatment of corrosive esophagitis, Klin Wochenschr 33:307, 1920.
11. Temple AR and Veltri JC: Toxicity of soaps, detergents and caustics. In Rumack BH and Temple AR, editors: Management of the poisoned patient, Princeton, NJ, 1977, Science Press.
12. Viscomi GJ, Beekhuis GJ, and Whitten CF: Evaluation of early esophagoscopy and corticosteroid therapy in corrosive injury of esophagus, J Pediatr 39:356, 1961.

278

Head Injuries

David E. Hall

Head injuries are exceedingly common and carry with them a certain mystique, which often leads parents to consult their child's physician. Of hospitalized patients, about 50% admitted with head injury are under 20 years of age.[12] Boys are injured at least twice as often as girls. Interestingly, left-handed children may be more prone to head injury than right-handed children.[9,17]

The causes of severe head injury vary with age. In infants, falls and child abuse predominate; in preschool- and school-age children, auto accidents are more common; and in the adolescent years, sports injuries and assault are more frequently seen. For all ages together, falls are the most common cause of head trauma, but auto accidents are the leading cause of serious injury. In most cases, the child is a pedestrian. As many as 70% of children hit by an automobile were not supervised by an adult at the time of the accident.[28]

Physicians should be familiar with the initial management of the child with severe head injury, but the most common problem faced by the practitioner is distinguishing those patients who require treatment from those who do not. Because these two aspects of care are so different, they are dealt with separately.

INITIAL CARE OF THE SEVERELY INJURED PATIENT

The improved prognosis compared with that in adults,[5] plus the potential for organ donation in those patients with brain death, dictate that the physician providing emergency care make every effort to resuscitate the child with severe head injury.

The level of consciousness is the most important observation in a child with head injury. It should be determined whether the patient obeys commands, cries, speaks understandable words, or opens the eyes spontaneously or in response to pain or to speech. If not, do not perform a complete neurologic examination; rather, evaluate the airway and circulation immediately. The correction of anoxia or poor cerebral perfusion has a far higher priority than detection of an intracranial hematoma.[10,20,27] As Haldane stated in 1919, "Anoxia not only stops the machine but wrecks the machinery.[20] Clear the airway, but avoid extreme flexion or extension of the neck, because a cervical spine injury may also be present. Determine the pulse rate and blood pressure and look for signs of shock. Shock is far more common in head injuries than is the Cushing response of hypertension and bradycardia. Examine the chest for signs of a hemothorax and pneumothorax; then check the abdomen for fullness, rigidity, or other signs of a ruptured viscus. The presence of shock almost always means that a serious injury other than head trauma exists. Infants are rare exceptions to this rule, because they may lose enough blood intracranially for shock to develop; however, even this is less common than shock from other causes.

Only when assured that the airway and circulation are adequate should the examiner proceed to a more detailed neurologic evaluation. The Glasgow coma scale (Table 278-1) is convenient for quantitating mental status and is valuable in assessing prognosis and in following the patient's progress later.[4,19,26] If the scale is not available in the treatment room or committed to memory, the patient's spontaneous actions and response to stimuli should be determined. Terms such as *drowsy, stuporous,* or *comatose,* however, mean different things to different physicians; thus their use is confusing.

Evaluate the pupillary response to light. Unilateral dilation of a pupil signifies compression of the third cranial nerve by a herniating temporal lobe or an optic nerve injury. In the unconscious patient, the physician must make sure that the tympanic membrane is intact and then test the oculovestibular reflex by injecting ice water into the ear canal. If the eyes develop nystagmus with the fast component away from the side of irrigation, the brainstem is intact from the nucleus of the eighth nerve to the nuclei of the third, fourth, and sixth cranial nerves, which control eye movements. The fifth and seventh cranial nerves should be evaluated by testing the corneal reflexes.

Another method to test the oculovestibular reflexes is the doll's eye maneuver. Rotate the head briskly to each side. Normally, when the head moves to the right, the eyes move to the left, and vice versa. Never perform this test until cervical spine trauma has been totally excluded.

Next, look for bruises, hematomas, or other signs of trauma. Ecchymoses behind the ear (Battle sign) or around the orbits (raccoon sign), cerebrospinal fluid (CSF) rhinorrhea, or bleeding from the ear suggests a basilar skull fracture. Papilledema is usually not present in the acutely injured patient, but retinal hemorrhages are common. Skull roentgenograms and cervical spine films are important but of lower priority than stabilizing the patient.

In addition to ensuring an adequate airway and circulation (a large-bore intravenous plastic cannula should be in place), steps to reduce elevated intracranial pressure are important before transfer of the patient to a regional center.[10] Excessive stimulation must be avoided. The patient's head should be elevated with the face looking straight ahead to promote venous drainage from the brain. In the absence of shock, fluids

Table 278-1 *Glascow Coma Scale*

INFANTS		CHILDREN AND ADULTS	
RESPONSE	SCORE	RESPONSE	SCORE
Best motor response		***Best motor response***	
Normal spontaneous movements	6	Obeys commands	6
Withdraws from touch	5	Localizes pain	5
Withdraws from pain	4	Withdraws from pain	4
Abnormal fixation in response to pain	3	Abnormal fixation in response to pain	3
Abnormal extension in response to pain	2	Abnormal extension in response to pain	2
None	1	None	1
Best verbal response		***Best verbal response***	
Coos and babbles	5	Oriented speech	5
Irritable cry	4	Confused speech	4
Cries in response to pain	3	Inappropriate words/vocal sounds	3
Moans in response to pain	2	Incomprehensible sounds/cries	2
None	1	None	1
Eye opening		***Eye opening***	
Spontaneous	4	Spontaneous	4
To speech	3	To speech	3
To pain	2	To pain	2
None	1	None	1

Scores of 10 or less suggest severe head injury.

should be restricted to two-thirds maintenance volumes; 5% dextrose with 0.2% or 0.45% saline solution should be used. Hypotonic solutions such as plain 5% dextrose may increase cerebral edema. A decreased P_{CO_2} level lowers cerebral arterial diameters and thus is very effective in lowering increased intracranial pressure. Initial bag and mask ventilation with 100% oxygen is effective, but if the patient's condition is deteriorating or if he or she is comatose, an endotracheal tube should be placed. If possible, an anesthesiologist should perform the intubation. Usually the anesthesiologist will premedicate with thiopental to induce anesthesia, atropine to control secretions and block vagal responses to tube placement, and pancuronium to induce muscle paralysis. These measures help avoid combative behavior and excessive hypercarbia, which further increase intracranial pressure. The usual goal is to maintain P_{CO_2} at 25 to 30 torr. The benefit of steroids in head injuries is controversial, and evidence of improved outcome with their use is lacking,[14,29] although many medical centers routinely use them. If used, the initial dose is 0.25–1 mg/l of dexamethasone. In a patient with asymmetric neurologic findings or a rapidly deteriorating condition where one suspects herniation, a mannitol infusion (0.25 to 1 g/kg) may be used.

Once the patient is stabilized, computed tomography (CT) is the most useful radiologic procedure in evaluating the patient. If a depressed skull fracture is suspected, ask for bone windows in addition to the usual brain and soft tissue views. Magnetic resonance imaging (MRI) scans require too much time currently to be useful acutely in the severely injured, potentially unstable patient. On the patient's arrival at an intensive care unit, intensivists may add pentobarbital coma to the treatment regimen in an attempt to reduce increased intracranial pressure.

CARE OF THE LESS SEVERELY INJURED PATIENT

Most physicians have little trouble identifying those patients who require intensive care at a regional center. More difficult is making the decision to admit to the hospital the less severely injured child for observation. Information from published studies concerning the indications for such action is scant because most head trauma studies have focused on hospitalized patients only. Evidence to support a decision to hospitalize or not to hospitalize the less severely injured patient is therefore lacking, and each child must be considered individually.[30]

When taking the history, obtain the details of the injury, keeping the possibility of abuse in mind. Children rarelv experience a serious injury when they fall out of bed,[3] so this history when given as the cause of severe injury is suspect.

Loss of consciousness, seizures, and amnesia of the circumstances surrounding the injury are indicators of more severe head trauma. As mentioned, persistent clouding of consciousness is the most reliable sign of a significant injury. Vomiting and headache are common symptoms after head trauma, and their presence is not particularly ominous or suggestive of any particular pathologic finding.[17] The duration of posttraumatic amnesia (inability to remember ongoing events) has repeatedly been found to correlate with the severity of injury.[28] Diplopia may signify sixth nerve compression caused by increased intracranial pressure.

The physician should check the cranial nerves, use of the extremities, the gait, and coordination and reflexes and look for other injuries or signs of serious injuries such as hemotympanum or CSF rhinorrhea. However, it is not true that CSF rhinorrhea may be reliably distinguished from a garden-variety runny nose with the use of glucose oxidase test sticks.

Much has been written about the overuse of skull roentgenograms; physicians consistently overestimate the frequency of fractures.[15,25] With a few exceptions, the finding of a fracture is not helpful. A depressed skull fracture requires surgical intervention, and a fracture of the parietal bone in the region of the middle meningeal artery may increase the likelihood of an epidural bleed. This is less important in small children, because the artery does not lie in a groove on the skull, as in adults. Skull fractures underlying lacerations are important to detect because they may predispose to meningitis. Basilar skull fractures also increase the risk of meningitis but often do not show up on the radiograph. Most of the time, however, the presence of a fracture does not affect treatment or provide prognostic information. Hendrick and co-workers[17] found that only 15% of children with subdural hematomas had skull fractures. Criteria for ordering skull roentgenograms are in the box at right.

The CT scan is excellent for diagnosing intracranial hematoma. The test is indicated when the physician seriously suspects a surgically treatable disorder. Children may require sedation for the examiner to obtain a technically adequate study, and the disadvantage of this must be weighed before ordering the scan. Occasionally, CT scans fail to demonstrate hematomas. This usually occurs between 2 to 6 weeks after injury, when the density of the lesion may equal that of the brain.[13]

Electroencephalograms (EEGs) have little place in the management of acute head trauma. They are neither sensitive nor specific and are usually not available in the emergency room. Rather, a CT scan should be obtained if the examiner is concerned about intracranial bleeding.

Echoencephalography is also of limited diagnostic usefulness in children with head injuries. Lumbar punctures are contraindicated unless meningitis is prominent in the differential diagnosis.

It is prudent to observe the child with posttraumatic amnesia or loss of consciousness until the mental status is back to normal. If this does not occur promptly; the child should be admitted to the hospital. Hospitalization is also indicated for patients in whom there are clear-cut neurologic signs, depressed or compound skull fractures, or a suspicion of child abuse or unreliable parents. Linear fractures do not mandate admission to the hospital if the child is totally asymptomatic, but they do require close observation, since the force required to fracture a child's skull is significant. A reliable observer at home is required.

One complication of skull fractures in children, albeit rare, is the leptomeningeal cyst, or "growing fracture."[22,31] In this condition a portion of leptomeninges or a porencephalic cyst covered by brain tissue squeezes between the edges of a fracture, especially of those involving the suture line. An enlarging defect results in the bone. This may resolve with age, but surgical intervention is sometimes necessary.

Some children experience a brief convulsion within minutes after a head injury. Such seizures do not appear to increase the risk of subsequent epilepsy. Seizures that go on to status epilepticus are more likely to be focal[18] or associated with an intracerebral hematoma.[1] Recurrent early seizures and those associated with intracranial hematomas may be more likely to progress to epilepsy.[21] However, a study of 4465 admissions of children with head injuries found that an early seizure was an isolated event in almost all cases in which it occurred.[16] A population-based study from the Mayo clinic[2] found no association between early posttraumatic seizures (defined as those that occur in the first week after trauma) and later epilepsy, *provided* the severity of head injury was taken into account. There was, of course, an association between the severity of the injury itself and the late development of epilepsy. However, even in children with severe head injuries, the risk of posttraumatic epilepsy was less than 7.5%. In more than 1000 children with mild (defined as unconsciousness or posttraumatic amnesia for less than 30 minutes) or moderate (defined as 30 minutes to 24 hours of unconsciousness or posttraumatic amnesia) head injury, no child who experienced an early seizure had developed posttraumatic epilepsy after 5 years. However, other studies, not population based, have found a higher risk.[18] EEGs cannot predict which patients will develop posttraumatic epilepsy.[18,21] There is no evidence that posttraumatic epilepsy may be prevented by prophylactic treatment with anticonvulsants.[24,32] Thus the use of anticonvulsants in head trauma should be confined to children who have had more than one early seizure or who have evidence of severe brain injury. When anticonvulsants are used, phenytoin is the initial drug of choice because it produces relatively little sedation. Anticonvulsant drugs should be used during the period of acute injury, then tapered as soon as possible, provided late seizures do not develop. When patients are sent home for observation, the parents should be instructed to watch for drowsiness, vomiting, gait disturbance, or severe headache for the next 2 weeks. Most parents are not reliable observers of pupillary size.

Criteria for Skull Roentgenograms in Children with Head Trauma

HISTORY

Age younger than 1 year
Unconsciousness for longer than 5 minutes
Gunshot wound or skull penetration
Previous craniotomy with shunt tube in place

PHYSICAL EXAMINATION

Palpable scalp hematoma
Skull depression palpable or identified by probe in scalp laceration
CSF discharge from ear or nose
Blood in middle ear
Battle or raccoon sign
Persistent clouding of consciousness
Focal neurologic signs

Modified from Leonidas JC, Ting W, and Binkiewicz A: Mild head trauma in children: when is a roentgenogram necessary? Pediatrics 69:143, 1982.

COMPLICATIONS

Even after mild head injuries, children often experience problems such as clinging behavior, irritability, sleep disturbances, hyperactivity, and headaches,[6,11] although how much these symptoms reflect premorbid or concurrent conditions is not certain.[8] Headaches do seem to be more of a problem for mild head injury patients than for "controls" with other types of injuries.[11] Symptoms are transient and generally resolve within 2 to 8 weeks.

Patients with moderate to severe head injuries who recover may experience lingering deficits in memory, speech, and visual perception. Consultation with a psychologist for cognitive testing is often helpful in educational planning.[7,23] Children have remarkable recuperative powers, however, and new methods to control increased intracranial pressure appear to improve prognosis. If treated in a modern, well-staffed pediatric intensive care unit, virtually all patients with a Glasgow coma scale score of 5 or better will recover fully and be able to lead a normal, independent life, and most patients admitted with scores of 3 or 4 will do quite well.[5]

REFERENCES

1. Alessandro R et al: Computed tomographic scans in post-traumatic epilepsy, Arch Neurol 45:42, 1988.
2. Annegers JF et al: Seizures after head trauma: a population study, Neurology 30:683, 1980.
3. Bell RS and Loop JW: The utility and futility of radiographic examination for trauma, N Engl J Med 284:236, 1971.
4. Braakman R et al: Systemic selection of prognostic features in patients with severe head injury, Neurosurgery 6:362, 1980.
5. Bruce DA, Schut L, and Bruno LA: Outcome following severe head injuries in children, J Neurosurg 48:679, 1978.
6. Casey R, Ludwig S, and McCormick MC: Morbidity following minor head trauma in children, Pediatrics 78:497, 1986.
7. Chadwick O: Psychological sequelae of head injury in children, Dev Med Child Neurol 27:69, 1985.
8. Chadwick O and Rutter M: Intellectual performance and reading skills after localized head injury in childhood, J Child Psychol Psychiatry 22:117, 1981.
9. Craft AW, Shaw DA, and Cartlidge NEF: Head injuries in children, Br Med J 4:200, 1972.
10. Davis RJ, Dean M, and Goldberg AL: Head and spinal cord injury. In Rogers MC, editor: Textbook of pediatric intensive care, Baltimore, 1987, Williams & Wilkins.
11. Farmer MY et al: Neurobehavioral sequelae of minor head injuries in children, Pediatr Neurosci 13:304, 1987.
12. Field JH: Epidemiology of head injuries in England and Wales, London, 1976, Her Majesty's Stationery Office.
13. French BN and Dublin AB: The value of computerized tomography in the management of 1000 consecutive head injuries, Surg Neurol 7:171, 1977.
14. Gudeman SK, Miller JD, and Becker DP: Failure of high-dose steroid therapy to influence intracranial pressure in patients with severe head injury, J Neurosurg 51:301, 1979.
15. Helfer RE, Slovis TL, and Black M: Injuries resulting when small children fall out of bed, Pediatrics 60:533, 1977.
16. Hendrick EB and Harris L: Post-traumatic epilepsy in children, J Trauma 8:547, 1968.
17. Hendrick EB, Harwood-Hash DCF, and Hudson AR: Head injuries in children, Clin Neurosurg 11:46, 1964.
18. Jennett B: Epilepsy after non-missile head injuries, ed 2, London, 1975, William Heinermann Medical Books.
19. Jennett B, Teasdale G, and Braakman R: Predicting outcome in individual patients after severe head injury, Lancet 1:1031, 1976.
20. Kalbag RM: Management of head injuries. In Cartilidge NEF and Shaw DA, editors: Head injury, London, 1981, WB Saunders Co.
21. Kollevold T: Immediate and early cerebral seizures after head injuries. IV, J Oslo City Hosp 29:35, 1979.
22. Lende RA and Erickson RC: Growing skull fractures of childhood, J Neurosurg 19:479, 1961.
23. Levine HS, Bento AL, and Grossman RG: Neurobehavioral consequences of closed head injury, New York, 1982, Oxford University Press, Inc.
24. McQueen JK et al: Low risk of late posttraumatic seizures following severe head injury: implications for clinical trials of prophylaxis, J Neurol Neurosurg Psychiatry 46:899, 1983.
25. Phillips LA: A study of the effect of high yield criteria for emergency radiography, Rockville, MD, HEW publication (FDA) no 78-8009, 1978.
26. Raimondi AJ and Hirschauer J: Head injury in the infant and toddler, Childs Brain 11:12, 1984.
27. Raphaely RC et al: Management of severe pediatric head trauma, Pediatr Clin North Am 27:715, 1980.
28. Rutter M et al: A prospective study of children with head injuries, Psychol Med 10:633, 1980.
29. Saul TG et al: Steroids in severe head injury: a prospective randomized clinical trial, J Neurosurg 54:596, 1981.
30. Singer HS and Freeman JM: Head trauma for the pediatrician, Pediatrics 62:819, 1978.
31. Taveras JM and Ransohoff J: Leptomeningeal cysts of the brain following trauma with erosion of the skull: a study of seven cases treated by surgery, J Neurosurg 10:233, 1953.
32. Young B et al: Failure of prophylactically administered phenytoin to prevent late posttraumatic seizures, J Neurosurg 58:236, 1983.

279

Heart Failure

Bradley B. Keller

The infant or child with heart failure presents a diagnostic and therapeutic challenge to the practitioner. The signs and symptoms of heart failure can occur at any age, even before birth. Heart failure usually occurs during the first year of life as a consequence of congenital or acquired heart disease. Heart failure is the result of specific anatomic, physiologic, or metabolic abnormalities, and therapy is directed toward treating the primary cause, as well as toward restoring adequate circulatory function.

DEFINITION

Heart failure is defined as the inability of the heart to meet the circulatory demands of the body. Four factors determine cardiovascular function: heart rate, contractility, preload, and afterload. If cardiac output decreases below metabolic needs, compensatory mechanisms acutely increase heart rate, sympathetic tone, and circulating blood volume to improve nutrient delivery.

Presenting signs and symptoms depend on the time course and severity of heart failure and reflect circulatory compensatory mechanisms (see accompanying box). Decreased cardiac output produces secondary fluid accumulation in the pulmonary and systemic circulations. The infant with heart failure often has a history of diaphoresis, poor feeding, and slow weight gain. Tachypnea and tachycardia are present on examination. Pulmonary vascular congestion results in rales, rhonchi, wheezes, and in premature infants, apnea. Periorbital and peripheral edema reflect systemic venous congestion.

ETIOLOGY

In most patients the primary cause of heart failure can be determined from physical examination and noninvasive studies (see accompanying box). Heart failure as a result of *pulmonary overcirculation,* which causes pulmonary vascular congestion and pulmonary edema, may result in hypoxemia.

Heart failure can occur as the result of *pump dysfunction* of the right or left ventricle. As blood backs up behind the failing ventricle, there is passive congestion of the systemic and pulmonary veins. Cardiac chamber hypoplasia or hypertrophy causes impaired filling and decreases forward output. Primary or secondary tachyarrhythmias reduce ventricular filling time and further decrease stroke volume.

Heart failure may be due to pulmonary or systemic *vascular obstruction.* Chronically elevated pulmonary vascular resistance produces right-sided heart failure in some infants with bronchopulmonary dysplasia. Acute or chronic systemic hypertension can likewise precipitate left-sided heart failure. Pulmonary or aortic valvar stenosis or coarctation of the aorta can cause heart failure.

Heart failure, which can result from intravascular *fluid overload* during renal failure, also can be caused by iatrogenic fluid overload during vigorous intravenous hydration.

Presenting Symptoms and Signs of Heart Failure

- Diaphoresis
- Poor feeding
- Failure to thrive
- Apnea
- Peripheral edema
- Tachypnea
- Tachycardia, gallop rhythm
- Murmur
- Rales, rhonchi, wheezes
- Hepatomegaly

Common Causes of Heart Failure: Differential Diagnosis

PULMONARY OVERCIRCULATION

Ventricular septal defect
Patent ductus arteriosus
Transposition of the great arteries
Truncus arteriosus

DECREASED PUMP FUNCTION

Hypoplastic ventricle
Cardiomyopathy, carditis
Prolonged tachycardia
Sepsis

VASCULAR OBSTRUCTION

Coarctation of the aorta
Aortic valve stenosis
Pulmonary valve stenosis
Pericardial tamponade

FLUID OVERLOAD

Renal failure
Anemia
Overhydration

Table 279-1 *Initial Drug Therapy in Heart Failure*

DRUG	ROUTE	DOSAGE	ONSET OF ACTION
Oxygen	Nasal, endotracheal tube	40%-100%	Immediate
Furosemide	IV, PO	1-2 mg/kg	15-30 min
Digoxin	IV, PO	5-10 μg/kg	5-30 min
Dopamine	IV	5-20 μg/kg/min	Immediate

INITIAL ASSESSMENT AND STABILIZATION

The diagnosis of heart failure begins with a history and physical examination. Assessment may include use of a chest radiograph, an electrocardiogram, pulse oximetry or arterial blood gas sample, and an echocardiogram. Initial therapy maximizes perfusion to vital organs, which limits organ damage from hypoxia and acidosis (Table 279-1). Volume overload is treated with diuretics, and depressed contractility is treated with digoxin or inotropic agents. The treatment of congestive heart failure with respiratory distress includes intubation and ventilation and prompt intravenous or intraosseous drug delivery.

Therapy for heart failure must be individualized. In patients with profound acidosis and circulatory insufficiency, acid-base status must be normalized before inotropic agents can be effective. Prompt arrhythmia management is essential.

DIAGNOSTIC TESTS AND CARDIOLOGY REFERRAL

Medical management includes the immediate care begun by the pediatrician and the diagnostic and therapeutic plan coordinated by the pediatric cardiologist. To initiate definitive therapy the specific cause of heart failure must be identified soon after patient stabilization. Physical examination is supplemented by means of electrocardiography, echocardiography, and in certain cases, cardiac catheterization to yield a definitive diagnosis.

IATROGENIC DANGERS

Careful attention to drug dosage and delivery is critical in the acute management of heart failure. Monitoring patient response to therapy and continued reappraisal of the diagnosis and therapeutic plan are essential. Heart failure is the final common pathway of many conditions, and an encouraging early response to therapy is not necessarily predictive of long-term survival.

SECONDARY NEEDS

Good nutrition with a low-salt, maximum-calorie diet is important. There rarely is a need to restrict total daily fluid volume; to do so usually limits calories. Small, frequent feedings may be necessary in patients with persistent tachypnea and fatigue. The prompt treatment of infections and maintenance of normal body temperature help to limit metabolic requirements.

PLANNING FOR CONVALESCENCE AND REHABILITATION

Home health care, if needed, must be available at discharge. Financial support to help offset uncovered medical expenses can be sought from state and local programs for physically handicapped children. Emotional support for patients and their families is available through social services, family support groups, religious affiliations, and daily interactions with the members of the multidisciplinary care team.

For some children the cause of heart failure is not amenable to medical or surgical management. A long-term medical management plan, which may include cardiac transplantation, should be discussed with the family.

CARDIAC CARE SYSTEM

Care for the infant or child with an acute, life-threatening illness requires the services of a multidisciplinary team. Management of the acute problem is followed by the careful diagnosis of related disorders, and therapy is directed toward prompt discharge home or to a referring hospital. The referring pediatrician remains an integral part of the child's coordinated care and serves as a resource for following the child's recovery and convalescence. Follow-up with pediatric cardiology appointments supplements routine pediatric care and permits individualizing the patient care plan. Home health care may be required to assist in the continued use of diuretics, digoxin, oxygen, and other medications after the acute-management phase of heart failure.

SUGGESTED READINGS

Keith JD: Congestive heart failure. In Keith JD, Rowe RD, and Vlad P, editors: Heart disease in infancy and childhood, ed 3, New York, 1978, Macmillan Publishing Co.

Talner NS: Heart failure. In Adams FH, Emmanouilides GC, and Riemenschneider TA, editors: Moss' heart disease in infants, children, and adolescents, ed 4, Baltimore, 1989, The Williams & Wilkins Co.

280

Hypertensive Emergencies

Edward J. Ruley

Acute hypertensive emergencies are relatively infrequent in the pediatric population as compared with adults, yet acute elevations in blood pressure represent a life-threatening situation that demands prompt evaluation and treatment. The timeliness of intervention depends on the sensitivity of the practitioner to acute hypertensive symptoms and the consideration of this diagnosis in the child who presents with generalized complaints.

ETIOLOGY

Acute hypertension in children and adolescents is almost always secondary to an identifiable cause rather than being a result of an acute exacerbation of primary hypertension, as so often occurs in adults. The probability of secondary hypertension in the pediatric population is directly related to the presence of symptoms of hypertension as well as to the degree and duration of blood pressure elevations.

The accompanying box lists some of the more common secondary causes of acute hypertension in pediatric-age patients. It is not prudent or practical to pursue all these diagnoses in each hypertensive patient. Clinical practice has determined that renal parenchymal diseases, renovascular abnormalities, and coarctation of the aorta make up approximately 93% of the reported secondary causes of hypertension in children. Initial consideration of these three conditions will allow the practitioner to focus the hypertensive workup, thereby limiting invasive and uncomfortable tests and reducing monetary costs. More exotic causes of acute hypertension should be sought only if the initial history and physical examination strongly suggest their presence or after the three more common causes have been ruled out.

HISTORY AND PHYSICAL FINDINGS

The history and physical examination in a pediatric patient being evaluated for acute hypertension often provide clues to the etiology. The clinical presentation of acute hypertension in children usually results from involvement of the neurologic or cardiovascular system or both.

When blood pressure suddenly rises to a high level, the arteriolar autoregulatory mechanisms of the brain fail and hypertensive encephalopathy results. Early symptoms of hypertensive encephalopathy include headache, anxiety, restlessness, dizziness, blurred vision, diplopia, nausea, and vomiting. Later, mental confusion, changing levels of consciousness, cranial nerve palsies, and convulsions can occur. Hypertensive encephalopathy must be considered in every patient having his or her first convulsion. Papilledema and vascular changes in the ocular fundus (Keith-Wagner classification) are much less common in hypertensive children than in adults.

Congestive heart failure can be the predominant manifestation in some patients, particularly neonates and children with underlying heart disease. The diagnosis of acute hypertension is particularly difficult in neonates and infants, in whom the symptoms tend to be vague and nonspecific. In these groups, severe hypertension may manifest as irritability, poor feeding, poor sleeping, restlessness, and vomiting. The diagnosis in these age groups is further complicated by the technical difficulties inherent in accurate blood pressure measurement. A greater awareness by the practitioner is necessary to prevent overlooking this diagnostic possibility.

Clues to the secondary etiology of hypertension can often be discovered in a carefully performed history and physical examination. Acute glomerulonephritis will often be suggested by a history of sore throat or skin infection several weeks before the onset of hypertensive symptoms, as well as by the presence of gross hematuria, which most commonly starts concomitantly with the hypertension. Fever, chills, and urinary outlet symptoms are often seen in pyelonephritis, whereas hemolytic-uremic syndrome may be preceded by a gastrointestinal or upper respiratory tract illness followed by the sudden onset of oligoanuria and microangiopathic anemia.

Renovascular causes are usually much less obvious. Although there may be a history of blunt trauma to the abdomen, such a history is so common in children with hypertension as to be of dubious significance. A more helpful sign is the café-au-lait spots, which suggest neurofibromatosis. The latter condition has a high association of renovascular hypertension. The urinalysis is usually normal in children with renovascular hypertension.

Cardiovascular causes may also be subtle. However, the most common cardiovascular abnormality, coarctation of the aorta, should be suggested by the finding of absent or markedly diminished femoral pulses and the absence of hypertension in the lower extremities.

Endocrine causes of acute hypertension are usually associated with other generalized symptoms in addition to the elevated blood pressure. Pheochromocytoma usually manifests with sweating, palpitations, anxiety, flushing, nausea, vomiting, weight loss, and fatigue. Similarly, such endocrine diseases as hyperthyroidism or Cushing syndrome are usually associated with multiple subjective and objective findings related to the hormonal abnormality.

Causes of Acute Hypertension in Children

RENAL
Acute glomerulonephritis (e.g., poststreptococcal and Henoch-Schönlein purpura)
Hemolytic-uremia syndrome
Chronic glomerulonephritis (all types)
Acute and chronic pyelonephritis
Congenital malformations (e.g., dysplasia, hypoplasia, and cystic disease)
Tumors (e.g., Wilms tumor, leukemic infiltrate)
Trauma
Obstructive uropathy
After genitourinary surgery

CARDIOVASCULAR
Coarctation of the aorta
Renal artery abnormalities (e.g., stenosis and thrombosis)
Takayasu disease

ENDOCRINE
Pheochromocytoma
Neuroblastoma
Adrenogenital disease
Cushing syndrome
Hyperaldosteronism
Hyperthyroidism

IATROGENIC
Intravascular volume overload
Sympathomimetic administration (e.g., epinephrine, ephedrine, and isoproterenol)
Corticosteroid administration

MISCELLANEOUS CAUSES
Immobilization (e.g., fractures, burns, and Guillain-Barré syndrome)
Hypercalcemia (hypervitaminosis D, metastatic disease, sarcoidosis, and some immobilized patients)
Hypernatremia
Stevens-Johnson syndrome
Increased intracranial pressure (any cause)

LABORATORY FINDINGS

The important basic laboratory tests in evaluating the pediatric patient with acute hypertension are a urinalysis (including a carefully performed microscopic examination of the centrifuged urinary sediment), a urine culture, blood urea nitrogen and creatinine, and plasma renin and aldosterone. In patients in whom pheochromocytoma is suspected, a plasma or urine catecholamine quantitation or both should be done. If an acquired glomerulonephritis is suspected, serum complement and streptococcal antibody titers should be obtained. Adolescents with acute hypertension should have urine tests for illicit drug use. It is unnecessary to perform thyroid, adrenal, or other endocrine tests unless the patient has multisystem complaints to suggest such diagnoses.

Imaging studies are very important in sorting out renal causes of acute hypertension. Renal radionuclide scans and ultrasound allow noninvasive assessment of kidney number, size, location, and function. The kidneys of patients with acutely acquired glomerulonephritis may be swollen in size and may have abnormal echogenicity. In renal artery stenosis, the involved kidney often is smaller and has a delay in blood flow and function compared with the uninvolved kidney. Currently there is much interest in performing a radionuclide renal scan in a patient after a brief course of angiotensin II–converting enzyme inhibitor to diagnose more sensitively a critical degree of renal artery stenosis. In this circumstance, the scan done following the converting enzyme inhibitor will often show poorer function on the involved side compared with the function of the same kidney scan done before administering the converting enzyme inhibitor. When these screening tests are abnormal or if the plasma renin value is significantly elevated in the absence of dehydration or any medication that could directly raise renin, a renal angiogram and renal vein renin measurement should be performed.

As mentioned in Chapter 233, imaging studies are important in differentiating the various obstructive conditions of the kidney, most of which can produce hypertension. They also are important in investigating renal tumors.

Physical findings that suggest a coarctation of the aorta should be followed up by echocardiography or cardiac catheterization or both.

TREATMENT

Control of blood pressure is more important than the exact determination of etiology in the child with acute hypertension. Complicated diagnostic tests, which often require transportation to various departments in the hospital, should be delayed until the practitioner believes that the blood pressure is controlled. Blood pressure control is not the same as blood pressure normalization (see below).

The two most important considerations in management of acute hypertension are the chronicity of the blood pressure elevation and the cause. The child who has had his or her blood pressure elevated chronically may have minimal hy-

Table 280-1 *Antihypertensive Drugs for Parenteral or Sublingual Administration in Hypertensive Emergencies in Pediatric Patients*

DRUG	ROUTE	DOSAGE	ONSET	PEAK
Sodium nitroprusside*	IV infusion	0.5 μg/kg/min titrated to a maximum of 10 μg/kg/min	Within 30 sec	—
Diazoxide*	IV bolus injection	1-3 mg/kg repeated q5-15 min until BP controlled (mini-bolus)	1-5 min	1-5 min
Hydralazine	30 min IV infusion or IM	0.15-0.2 mg/kg q6hr	10-20 min	10-90 min
Nifedipine	Sublingual	0.25 mg/kg/dose q4-6hr	10-15 min	60-90 min
Labetalol*	IV infusion	0.5 mg/kg over 2 min. For nonresponse, double dose and repeat every 10 min to a maximum cumulative dose of 5 mg/kg	2-5 min	5-15 min
Phentolamine	IV bolus injection	0.05-0.1 mg/kg	Within 30 sec	2 min

*Manufacturer's warning: safety in children not established.
†*sx*, Symptoms; *Max*, maximum; *BP*, blood pressure; *D/C*, discontinue; D_5W, 5% dextrose in water; *VMA*, vanillylmandelic acid.
‡Vasodilation symptoms include seating, flushing, feelings of warmth, orthostatic hypotension, tachycardia, palpitations, nausea, and vomiting.
§Neurologic symptoms include headache, blurred vision, dizziness, and light-headedness.

pertensive symptoms but may suffer adverse effects if the blood pressure is suddenly reduced. In contrast, the child with a true acute blood pressure elevation would be expected to benefit from rapid blood pressure control. Often it is unclear in an emergency whether the blood pressure elevation is acute or more chronic. In such cases, the reduction of blood pressure by some 30% to 40% is usually well tolerated, regardless of the duration of the elevation. Reduction of blood pressure to absolute normal is probably not advisable until a better understanding of the patient's overall condition can be achieved.

Etiology is important in that some medications may be contraindicated in certain conditions—for example, the use of methyldopa in the child with pheochromocytoma.

Severe acute hypertension should be treated with parenteral therapy so that blood pressure control can be rapid and predictable. Medications that can be titrated to the patient's response are preferred, provided the practitioner has the means to monitor the blood pressure response closely on a continuous basis. Some of the available parenteral medications for blood pressure control are given in Table 280-1. Oral medications should be substituted for parenteral agents as soon as practical. With the determination of cause, the medication that is most specific for the altered pathophysiologic condition that is producing hypertension is preferred. In renovascular hypertension, revision or bypass of the renovascular lesion is preferred to long-term medical therapy or nephrectomy. Consultation with a pediatric nephrologist, cardiologist, or vascular surgeon is important in defining a therapeutic plan to best serve the patient's long-term interests.

PROGNOSIS

The immediate prognosis of the child with acute hypertension depends on the rapidity of recognizing the problem and on blood pressure control. Failure to control blood pressure may result in residual neurologic abnormalities such as seizure disorders, cranial nerve palsies, hemiplegia, or blindness.

DURATION	ADVERSE EFFECTS	RELATIVE CONTRAINDICATIONS	COMMENTS
Length of infusion	Nausea, vomiting; vasodilation sx†‡; neurologic sx§; apprehension, restlessness	Hepatic insufficiency	Solution good for 24 hr; photosensitive (wrap in foil); monitor blood thiocyanate if used >72 hr (D/C for thiocyanate level >10 mg/dl); tachyphylaxis and metabolic acidosis—early cyanide poisoning
Variable; usually <12 hr	Arrhythmias; hyperglycemia; sodium and water retention; vasodilation sx‡; neurologic sx§	Thiazide sensitivity; severe tachycardia; diabetes; coarctation	Ineffective in pheochromocytoma; give diuretics to decrease sodium; hyperproteinemia potentiates effects
3-6 hr	Headache; nausea, vomiting; tachycardia, palpitation	Hypersensitivity to hydralazine ("hyperdynamic syndrome")	Undergoes color change in most infusion fluids, which does not indicate loss of potency
Variable; usually 2-3 hr	Headache; palpitations; flushing	Concomitant use of beta blocking drugs; cimetidine	Dose can be drawn from the 10 mg capsule with a 1 ml syringe and then squirted sublingually
Variable; usually 2-4 hr	Neurologic sx†§; bronchospasm; tingling scalp	Jaundice or hepatic dysfunction; pheochromocytoma; asthma; diabetes	Keep supine for 3 hr after administration; ambulate gradually
15-30 min	Tachycardia; arrhythmias; marked hypotension	None	Specific for pheochromocytoma

The long-term prognosis depends, for the most part, on the underlying cause. Some causes, such as acute poststreptococcal glomerulonephritis, may spontaneously resolve so that the hypertension eventually remits and does not recur. Other causes, such as hypertension associated with chronic glomerulonephritis, may be controlled with continued medication. Regardless, the longevity of the patient and the subsequent development of end-organ damage, such as hypertensive cardiomyopathy, stroke, and so on, are directly related to the adequacy of long-term blood pressure control.

SUGGESTED READINGS

Bertel O and Conel LD: Treatment of hypertensive emergencies with the calcium channel blocker nifedipine, Am J Med 79:S31, 1985.

Cressman MD et al: Intravenous labetalol in the management of severe hypertension and hypertensive emergencies, Am Heart J 107:980, 1984.

Dillon MJ: Investigation and management of hypertension in children, Pediatr Nephrol 1:59, 1987.

Evans J et al: Sublingual nifedipine in acute severe hypertension, Arch Dis Child 63:975, 1988.

Guignard JP, Gouyon JB, and Adelman RD: Arterial hypertension in the newborn infant, Biol Neonate 55:77, 1989.

Sigler R and Brewer E: Effect of sublingual or oral nifedipine in the treatment of hypertension, J Pediatr 112:811, 1988.

Turner ME: What's new in the antihypertensive armamentarium? Pediatr Ann 18:579, 1989.

281

Hypoglycemia

Maurice D. Kogut

Hypoglycemia occurs uncommonly after the first week of life; however, its diagnosis is essential because low blood glucose levels that persist or recur may have catastrophic effects on the brain, particularly in infants. Accordingly, the primary care physician must recognize the clinical symptoms associated with hypoglycemia, document the low blood glucose level, and treat appropriately with glucose. Further, it is necessary to delineate the cause of the hypoglycemia so that effective continuing treatment can be initiated.

DEFINITION

The diagnostic criteria for hypoglycemia, as first established by Cornblath and Schwartz,[8] have now been generally accepted. Hypoglycemia beyond the immediate neonatal period is defined as a serum or plasma glucose concentration less than 45 mg/dl or a whole blood glucose concentration less than 40 mg/dl, measured by a method specific for glucose; values for serum or plasma glucose concentrations are approximately 10% to 15% higher than those for whole blood. If hypoglycemia is suspected, an approximation of the blood glucose level may be obtained quickly by using Dextrostix or Chemstrip bG and later confirmed by an appropriate chemical laboratory test.

CLINICAL MANIFESTATIONS

The clinical findings in hypoglycemia are those caused mainly by cerebral dysfunction and adrenergic discharge. Incoordination of eye movements, strabismus, excessive irritability, motor incoordination, and convulsions may occur after 1 month of age. In the older child, pallor, tachycardia, sweating, limpness, inattention, staring, listlessness, hunger, abdominal pain, ataxia, stupor, coma, and convulsions may be present.

IMMEDIATE MANAGEMENT

In the child with suspected hypoglycemia, it is essential that a diagnostic blood sample for glucose, insulin, growth hormone (GH), cortisol, ketone bodies, lactic acid, and amino acids be obtained at the time of hypoglycemia and before the low blood glucose has been corrected.[1,7] This point is absolutely critical because the cause of hypoglycemia cannot be elucidated by measurement of blood glucose alone and these measurements provide important information rapidly concerning cause. If available blood volume is a limiting factor, judgment must be used in ranking the importance of these tests. At the very least, the blood glucose and insulin levels should be measured. Urinary ketones as well as specific tests for urinary glucose and nonglucose-reducing substances should also be determined. If ketones are present, the urine should be tested further for presence of amino and organic acids.

With the exception of those clinical conditions associated with hyperinsulinism (see box on p. 1627) the administration of glucagon has limited therapeutic value in the treatment of hypoglycemia.[7] For diagnostic purposes, however, the administration of glucagon can be useful; a glycemic response to glucagon strongly suggests hyperinsulinism.[7]

Once these essential diagnostic blood samples are obtained, the child should receive an intravenously administered bolus of 10% to 25% glucose immediately to alleviate acute symptoms. Fluids containing appropriate electrolytes and glucose should then be given intravenously at a rate sufficient to maintain plasma or serum glucose levels above 45 mg/dl. The blood glucose level should be monitored every 2 to 4 hours, and the rate of glucose administered should be adjusted accordingly. Urine is also monitored to detect glycosuria, which can produce osmotic diuresis.

Preparation should be made to hospitalize the child to initiate the diagnostic evaluation. During transport to the hospital, personnel experienced in intravenous techniques and Dextrostix or Chemstrip bG determinations must ensure that adequate amounts of glucose are continuously infused. The previously obtained diagnostic blood sample should be sent with the patient to the hospital. The patient with hypoglycemia should be under the combined care of a pediatric specialist and child's primary physician.

ETIOLOGY

The blood glucose level states the final balance between hepatic glucose production and peripheral glucose utilization. An adequate fasting blood glucose concentration depends on sufficient amounts of endogenous nonglucose precursors (e.g., alanine, lactate, and glycerol), effective hepatic enzyme pathways for gluconeogenesis and glycogenolysis, and normal hormonal activities (insulin, growth harmone, cortisol, glucagon, and epinephrine) for the mobilization of substrates and regulation of these processes.

Many healthy infants and young children, in contrast to adults, cannot maintain normoglycemia during a 24-hour fast.[5,14] The glycogen stores of healthy infants are sufficient only to meet glucose requirements for 8 to 12 hours in the absence of caloric intake,[25] so that after 24 to 36 hours of

Causes of Hypoglycemia in Childhood

HYPERINSULINISM

Nesidioblastosis
Islet cell adenoma
Focal adenomatosis
Microadenomatosis
Beta-cell hyperplasia
Beckwith-Wiedemann syndrome
Normal histologic pancreas (functional beta-cell secretory disorder) (?)
Idiopathic leucine sensitivity

HEREDITARY DEFECTS IN CARBOHYDRATE METABOLISM

Glycogen Storage Diseases

Glucose 6-phosphatase deficiency, types Ia, Ib
Amylo-1,6-glucosidase deficiency, type III
Defects of liver phosphorylase enzyme system

ENZYME DEFICIENCIES OF GLUCONEOGENESIS

Fructose-1,6-diphosphatase (FDPase)
Phosphoenolpyruvate carboxykinase
Pyruvate carboxylase

OTHER ENZYME DEFECTS

Galactose-1-phosphate uridyltransferase (galactosemia)
Fructose-1-phosphate aldolase (hereditary fructose intolerance)
Glycogen synthetase

HEREDITARY DEFECTS IN AMINO ACID AND ORGANIC ACID METABOLISM

Maple syrup urine disease
Propionic acidemia
Methylmalonic aciduria
Tyrosinosis
3-Hydroxy-3-methylglutaric aciduria
Glutaric aciduria, type II

HEREDITARY DEFECTS IN FAT METABOLISM

Systemic carnitine deficiency
Carnitine palmitoyl transferase deficiency

HORMONE DEFICIENCIES

Congenital hypopituitarism or hypothalamic abnormality
Growth hormone
Cortisol
Adrenocorticotropic hormone (ACTH)
ACTH unresponsiveness
Glucagon
Thyroid hormone
Catecholamine

KETOTIC HYPOGLYCEMIA

NONPANCREATIC TUMORS

Mesenchymal tumors
Epithelial tumors
Hepatoma
Adrenocortical carcinoma
Wilms tumor
Neuroblastoma

POISONING OR TOXINS

Salicylate
Alcohol
Propranolol
Oral hypoglycemic agents (e.g., sulfonylureas)
Insulin
Unripe ackees (hypoglycin) (Jamaican vomiting sickness)

LIVER DISEASE

Hepatitis, cirrhosis
Reye syndrome

MALNUTRITION

Kwashiorkor
Starvation
Low phenylalanine diet
Malabsorption
Chronic diarrhea

REACTIVE HYPOGLYCEMIA

Modified from Cornblath MD and Schwartz R: Disorders of carbohydrate metabolism in infancy, ed 2, Philadelphia, 1976, WB Saunders Co. Reproduced with permission from Kogut MD: Hypoglycemia: pathogenesis, diagnosis, and treatment. In Gluck L et al, editors: Current problems in pediatrics, Copyright © 1974 by Year Book Medical Publishers, Inc., Chicago; and Kogut MD: Neonatal hypoglycemia: a new look. In Moss, AJ, editor: Pediatrics update: review for physicians, pp 243-272, Copyright © 1980 by Elsevier Science Publishing Co, Inc.

fasting the young child becomes totally dependent on gluconeogenesis for glucose production.[20]

Because of diminished protein and fat stores, healthy infants and young children during caloric deprivation may not be able to satisfy the glucose requirements of brain and other tissue and still maintain normal blood glucose levels, because of the limited amounts of these substrates for glucose production. Hence, the physician caring for a child requiring surgery or other procedures accompanied by fasting must prevent hypoglycemia by ensuring that extended fasting is avoided, administering parenteral glucose before and after surgery, and monitoring the blood glucose level.

CLINICAL APPROACH

Hypoglycemia in the child is not a disease; rather, it reflects failure of one or more factors that regulate the concentration of glucose in the blood. It may be classified as in the box on p. 1627.

Clinical clues enable the physician to plan a logical approach to the diagnostic evaluation of a patient with hypoglycemia. The age at onset of hypoglycemia is helpful. The inborn errors of carbohydrate, amino acid, organic acid metabolism, and hormonal deficiencies become apparent during the first 2 years of life.[8] Hyperinsulinism has two peak times of onset: during the first year of life and after age 3 years.[8,16] The most likely cause of hypoglycemia with onset after 1 year of age is ketotic hypoglycemia.[8,18] In toddlers, hypoglycemia may result from ingestion of alcohol, aspirin, and other drugs (see box). Hypoglycemia is rare after age 5 years[7].

A *history of other affected family members* or the occurrence of unexplained infant deaths among close relatives suggests the possibility of one of the inherited metabolic disorders. Some disorders associated with hormonal deficiencies and hyperinsulinism may also be familial.[17] The physician should carefully inquire about the frequency of hypoglycemic episodes, the possibility of drug ingestion, and unfortunately, the malicious administration of drugs.[1,7]

The *temporal relation of symptoms to food intake* is very important in assessing hypoglycemia. In idiopathic leucine sensitivity and in hereditary defects of amino acid and organic acid metabolism, hypoglycemic symptoms may occur shortly after the ingestion of protein.[16] Symptoms that occur after the ingestion of lactose suggest galactosemia; those after sucrose ingestion suggest hereditary fructose intolerance (HFI).[16] In contrast, fasting hypoglycemia is characteristic of ketotic hypoglycemia, hormonal deficiencies, hyperinsulinism, glycogen storage diseases (GSD), and fructose-1,6-diphosphatase (FDPase) deficiency (Table 281-1).[16]

Metabolic acidosis, ketonemia, or hepatomegaly in association with hypoglycemia strongly suggests the presence of *an inborn error of metabolism* of carbohydrate, amino acid, or organic acid.[16] Hypotonia and hyperammonemia may also be present in infants with defects in organic acid and amino acid metabolism. The presence of nonglucose-reducing substances in the urine may indicate galactosemia or HFI. Nonketotic hypoglycemia in patients with hepatomegaly, with or without metabolic acidosis, suggests 3-hydroxy-3-methylglutaric aciduria,[24] glutaric aciduria type II,[10] systemic carnitine deficiency,[29] or carnitine palmitoyl transferase deficiency.[3] In contrast, it is usual for hepatomegaly, ketonuria, and metabolic acidosis to be absent in hypoglycemia with hyperinsulinism.[17] Although ketosis may be present in some hypoglycemic patients with hypopituitarism[21] and ACTH unresponsiveness,[15] the findings of ketonuria and hypoglycemia without hepatomegaly in small and underweight males after 1 year of age suggest ketotic hypoglycemia.[8,16,18]

Because children with an inborn error of metabolism may present with a Reye syndrome–like illness, it is important to be alert to the possibility of an underlying metabolic defect, particularly in young children or in a child with recurrence of Reye syndrome–like symptoms.[11]

Table 281-1 *Hypoglycemia in Infancy and Childhood*

	INBORN METABOLIC ERRORS OF CARBOHYDRATE AND AMINO ACIDS	HORMONE DEFICIENCY	HYPERINSULINISM
Family history	+*	Variable	Variable
Hypoglycemia			
Fasting	GSD, fructose-1,6-diphosphatase deficiency	+	+
After lactose	Galactosemia	−	−
After sucrose	Hereditary fructose intolerance	−	−
After protein	Amino acids, organic acids	−	Variable
Hepatomegaly	+	Variable	−
Ketosis	+	Variable	−
Acidosis	+	−	−
Tests	Glucose, glucagon, galactose, fructose tolerance tests; amino acids, gas chromatography	Blood growth hormone, cortisol; stimulation tests	Random blood glucose and immunoreactive insulin; leucine tolerance test
Liver biopsy (enzymes)	Diagnostic for carbohydrate errors (not for galactosemia; use red blood cells)	Not indicated	Not indicated
White blood cells, fibroblasts (enzymes)	Amino acids, organic acids		
Treatment	Specific	Specific	Diazoxide; partial excision of the pancreas

Modified from Cornblath, MD and Schwartz R: Disorders of carbohydrate metabolism in infancy, ed 2, Philadelphia, 1976, WB Saunders Co. Reproduced with permission from Kogut MD: Hypoglycemia: pathogenesis, diagnosis and treatment. In Gluck, L., et al., editors: Current problems in pediatrics, Copyright © 1974 by Year Book Medical Publishers, Inc., Chicago; and Kogut MD: Neonatal hypoglycemia: a new look. In Moss AJ, editor: Pediatrics update: review for physicians, pp. 243-272, Copyright © 1980 by Elsevier Science Publishing Co., Inc.

*+, Present; −, absent; *GSD*, glycogen storage diseases, types I, III, and defects of liver phospharylase enzyme system.

DIFFERENTIAL DIAGNOSIS AND MANAGEMENT OF HYPOGLYCEMIA

Hyperinsulinism

Hyperinsulinism may be caused by any of several abnormalities of the beta-cell (see box, p. 1627) and is the most common cause of persistent or recurrent hypoglycemia in the first year of life.[27]

Infants with *idiopathic leucine-sensitive hypoglycemia* usually do not have symptoms until 1 to 6 months of age.[22] These patients usually respond to medical treatment and do not require surgery.[22]

In *Beckwith-Wiedemann syndrome* (omphalocele, macroglossia, and gigantism), hypoglycemia occurs in 30% to 50% of affected infants, primarily as a result of beta-cell hyperplasia.[2] Some of these infants also have hemihypertrophy. There is an increased incidence of adrenal, liver, and kidney (Wilms) tumors in these patients.

Nesidioblastosis (small nests of beta-cells scattered throughout acinar tissue and neoformation of islet cells budding off from ductile elements) is the most common cause of hyperinsulinism during the first year of life[27] and has been described in siblings.[30] Patients with nesidioblastosis, however, may first manifest symptoms of hypoglycemia during late childhood, adolescence, and adulthood.[13]

Pancreatic *islet cell adenomas* are uncommon in chidren. Although hypoglycemia caused by varying histologic types of insulinoma may have its onset in the newborn period, in 85% of patients symptoms begin after age 4 years.[8]

Laboratory Investigation. Hyperinsulinism in infants and older children is usually characterized by fasting hypoglycemia, even if of only a few hours' duration,[26] and low fasting plasma levels of beta-hydroxybutyrate (β-OHB) and free fatty acids (FFA).[26] Frequent random simultaneous measurements of blood glucose and insulin levels, particularly before feeding and as hypoglycemia occurs, help identify patients with hyperinsulinism (Table 281-1). The diagnosis depends on detecting inappropriate insulin secretion by demonstrating insulin levels disproportionately high relative to blood glucose values, particularly during hypoglycemia.

Abnormalities associated with hyperinsulinism cannot be easily distinguished by available diagnostic tests. Although leucine or tolbutamide may be useful in documenting the presence of hyperinsulinism, their administration is not helpful in delineating its specific cause, since many of these patients may respond to these insulin secretogogues with abnormal insulin release.[16,27]

In any child with intermittent attacks of nonketotic hypoglycemia, it is always extremely important to investigate the possibility of malicious or self-administration of insulin or oral sulphonylurea drugs.[9,19,23] Measurement of C-peptide, insulin, and insulin antibodies in blood may identify the patient with an exogenous source of insulin: in contrast to patients with endogenous hyperinsulinism, C-peptide levels are suppressed, and insulin antibodies may be present in patients to whom insulin has been administered[19,23]; although plasma insulin and C-peptide levels may be misleading in children who have received oral hypoglycemic agents, the drug itself may be detected in the child's blood or urine.[23]

Management. Acute hypoglycemic episodes must be treated promptly and adequately with intravenously administered glucose, and the rate of glucose administration required to maintain normal blood glucose levels among hyperinsulinemic infants can often exceed 12 to 14 mg/kg/min.

Further management of the patient depends on age at onset of disease. Of great diagnostic and therapeutic value in the infant is the response to diazoxide. Diazoxide raises blood glucose levels primarily by suppressing pancreatic insulin secretion.[22] In patients in whom diazoxide results in restoration of normal glucose levels, the drug is continued and the patients are assessed periodically until approximately 5 to 7 years of age.[22] Corticosteroids are of no value. Some patients will remain euglycemic without medication by this age. Because hyperglycemia, ketosis, and hyperosmolar nonketotic coma can occur with diazoxide therapy, the parents should be instructed to monitor urinary glucose and ketones.[16]

If hypoglycemia associated with hyperinsulinism persists or recurs despite diazoxide therapy, the diagnosis of insulinoma or nesidioblastosis must be strongly considered.[17] In these patients, hypoglycemia usually continues or recurs while they are receiving diazoxide.[17] The two disorders cannot be distinguished without surgical inspection. Location of an adenoma has been achieved by selective arteriography of the celiac axis and by ultrasound.[1] However, because islet cell tumors are often so small, it is unlikely that these procedures or computed tomography can detect the presence of tumor preoperatively in most infants and children. Intraoperative ultrasonography, however, may be helpful in identifying adenomas in children.[28] Because the prognosis for subsequent normal mental and neurologic development has been poor among infants with hyperinsulinemia and intractable hypoglycemia, surgical exploration of the pancreas without delay is indicated when there is no response of hyperinsulinism to diazoxide. Finally, the presence of hyperinsulinemic hypoglycemia in an older child without previous evidence of hypoglycemia is very suggestive of an islet cell adenoma; thus, any trial of medical therapy should be limited.

At surgery, the pancreas should be carefully inspected and palpated for the presence of tumor. Removal of a tumor is usually curative. If no tumor is found, 85% to 90% of the pancreas should be removed, but the spleen preserved. Special stains for insulin-containing tissue should be done on the excised pancreas in an attempt to identify nesidioblastosis.

Inborn Errors of Metabolism

Carbohydrate Enzyme Defects. Several enzymatic defects of carbohydrate metabolism result in deficiencies of hepatic glucose formation and release (see box on p. 1627).[16] Glucose 6-phosphatase deficiency is the most common, and the symptoms are more severe than in other glycogen storage disease (GSD) types (see box).[16] Patients with GSD types Ia and Ib have growth retardation, cherubic facies, protuberant abdomen, very large smooth liver, enlarged kidneys, normal intelligence, fasting hypoglycemia of only a few hours' duration, ketosis, lacticacidemia, hyperlipidemia, hyperuricemia, and bleeding diathesis. In type Ib, the patients also have neutropenia and increased frequency of infections. In the infant and young child, poor food intake during an illness may result in severe lactic acidosis and hypoglycemia, and death may result if hypoglycemia and hyperlacticacidemia are not promptly and adequately treated with intravenous glucose and sodium bicarbonate.[16] A dramatic advance in treatment has been the introduction of continuous nocturnal glucose-containing gastric feedings.[12] To maintain normal blood glucose levels during the day, frequent feedings, at least every 3 to 4 hours, are essential. Foods rich in fructose and galactose should be avoided. The daily oral administration of an uncooked cornstarch suspension has been beneficial in older children, but not as effective in infants, in maintaining normoglycemia and attaining adequate metabolic control.[6]

Failure to thrive, jaundice, vomiting, susceptibility to infection, hepatomegaly, edema, ascites, a tendency to bleed, cataracts, proteinuria, aminoaciduria, and galactosuria are characteristic features of the lactose-fed infant with *galactosemia*.[16] Mental retardation, progressive liver failure, and death may occur unless galactose-containing feedings are eliminated. Symptomatic hypoglycemia is not a common finding and is quickly reversed by intravenous glucose. When the diagnosis of galactosemia is suspected, the patient should immediately be given a galactose-free diet. This diet should be carefully maintained while awaiting results of erythrocyte enzyme studies and should be continued if the diagnosis is confirmed.

Clinical manifestations of *hereditary fructose intolerance* (HFI) develop only after fructose ingestion and include vomiting, profound hypoglycemia, and convulsions.[16] Continued ingestion of fructose is associated with failure to thrive, prolonged vomiting, jaundice, hepatosplenomegaly, hemorrhage, abnormal liver function, fructosuria, defects in proximal renal tubular function (including proteinuria, glucosuria, and aminoaciduria), and, in some, hepatic failure and death. The acute episodes of hypoglycemia are promptly reversed by the intravenous administration of glucose. Long-term treatment consists of strict elimination of dietary fructose and of fructose in cough syrups and other drugs.

Patients with *FDPase deficiency* may have episodic hyperventilation, fasting hypoglycemia, lacticacidosis, ketosis, hyperuricemia, and hepatomegaly.[16] Refusal to feed and vomiting, often associated with febrile illness, precipitate the attacks. The disorder is life threatening in the neonate and in young children. In contrast to those with HFI, these patients do not vomit after fructose intake and do not develop an aversion to sweets. Treatment of the acute attack consists of correcting the hypoglycemia and acidosis by intravenous infusion of glucose and sodium bicarbonate. Long-term management should emphasize the avoidance of fasting and the provision of a fructose-free, high carbohydrate diet.

Laboratory Investigation. A suggested outline for the investigation of hypoglycemia caused by inborn errors of carbohydrate metabolism has been included in Tables 281-1 and 281-2. These studies should be done in a pediatric metabolic center, but only when the child's condition is stable and blood glucose level is normal. Judgment must be exercised in choosing the proper diagnostic test to delineate the underlying abnormality. An intravenous galactose test is helpful in the differentiation of some hepatic enzyme defects (Table 281-2) but is dangerous and should not be done to diagnose galactosemia. The presence of specific hepatic enzyme deficiencies may be determined by the use of other tolerance tests (Table 281-2). The *tolerance tests* are done after a variable period of fasting and only with a physician in attendance, who must be prepared to interrupt the test by administering intravenous glucose should symptoms and signs of hypoglycemia occur or should a low blood glucose level be detected. Definitive diagnosis of any of the inherited disorders of carbohydrate metabolism (see box on p. 1627), except galactosemia, depends on assay of specific hepatic enzyme activities (Table 281-2); galactosemia may, on the

Table 281-2 *Differential Diagnosis of Hepatic Enzyme Defects*

BLOOD VALUES	GSD—I	GSD—III	GSD, PHOSPHORYLASE ENZYME SYSTEM	FDPase	HFI
Fasting					
Glucose	↓*	↓ or nl	↓ or nl	↓	nl
Lactic acid	↑	nl	nl	↑	nl
After glucose†					
Glucose	↑	↑	↑	↑	↑
Lactic acid	↓	↑	↑	↓	↔
After glucagon†					
Glucose	↔	↑‡	↑ or ↔	↑ or ↔§	↑‖
Lactic acid	↑	↔	↔	↓ or ↑	↔
After galactose†					
Glucose	↔	↑	↑	↑	↑
Lactic acid	↑	↑	↑	↔	↔
After fructose†					
Glucose	↔	↑	↑	↓	↓
Lactic acid	↑	↑	↑	↑	↑

*↑, Increased, ↓, decreased; ↔, no change; *nl*, normal.
†Tolerance tests done after variable fasting period.
‡Two hours after feeding.
§Variable, dependent on duration of fast.
‖No increase in glucose at time of fructose-induced hypoglycemia.

other hand, be detected by the absence of galactose-1-phosphate uridyltransferase activity in red blood cells, so that liver biopsy is not necessary for its definitive diagnosis.

Amino Acid and Organic Acid Metabolic Defects. Hypoglycemia has been noted in a variety of inborn errors of amino acid and organic acid metabolism (see box, p. 1627).[16] Although symptoms usually begin in the neonatal period, they may occur later. The infants tend to improve when protein feedings are discontinued and 10% glucose is administered intravenously. Occasionally, peritoneal dialysis or exchange transfusion may be lifesaving. Amino acid analysis and gas chromatography of blood and urine are often helpful in detecting these inborn errors (Table 281-1). Diagnosis and treatment of a specific disorder depend on detection of its characteristic metabolites in blood and urine and on assays of specific enzyme activities in skin fibroblasts or white blood cells.

Hormonal Deficiencies

Hormonal deficiencies are not common causes of hypoglycemia (see box, p. 1627), occurring primarily in those with deficiency of GH or cortisol.

Hypopituitarism. Congenital hypopituitarism, caused either by a hypothalamic abnormality or by aplasia of the anterior pituitary gland, is associated with severe, often fatal, hypoglycemia during the first few days of life.[1,8,17] Occasionally, however, hypoglycemia may first appear later in infancy or childhood. A few patients may have midline deformities, including hypotelorism, abnormality of the frontonasal process, and cleft lip or palate. Septooptic dysplasia (optic nerve hypoplasia and absence of the septum pellucidum) is present in some patients and may be accompanied by nystagmus. Some patients with congenital hypopituitarism may have a small penis (microphallus).

The more usual cause of *GH deficiency* is idiopathic hypopituitarism, in which no organic lesions can be delineated. In affected patients there is an increased occurrence of perinatal problems such as breech and forceps deliveries. Symptomatic hypoglycemia occurs in approximately 10% of patients,[4] with onset usually late in infancy or early childhood. Measurement of height and weight is essential for the evaluation of a child with suspected GH deficiency, since these children have significant growth retardation, which may begin within the first 1 to 2 years of life. These children tend to be pudgy, and affected boys may have small genitalia.

Cortisol Deficiency. Deficient cortisol production may be secondary to Addison disease, congenital adrenal hyperplasia, ACTH deficiency, or ACTH unresponsiveness.[1,8,15,17] Patients with ACTH unresponsiveness and Addison disease may have abnormal pigmentation.

Laboratory Investigation and Treatment. Laboratory studies should include determination of GH and cortisol in the blood, particularly when the child has hypoglycemia (Table 281-1). Hypoglycemia is an excellent stimulus for GH and cortisol secretions, so that low values of either hormone in the presence of hypoglycemia indicate the need for additional studies for cortisol or GH deficiency, which should be done only when the child's condition is stable and the blood glucose level normal. A lack of response to a definitive GH stimulation test must be demonstrated to confirm GH deficiency. Tests designed to elicit the normal hypothalamic-pituitary-adrenal responses and measurement of adrenal metabolites in blood and urine should be done to identify the child with either ACTH deficiency, ACTH unresponsiveness, or cortisol deficiency. Correction of hypoglycemia by intravenous administration of glucose makes up the treatment of acute episodes. Specific treatment depends on identifying the underlying hormonal deficiency. Patients should be encouraged to avoid prolonged fasting.

Ketotic Hypoglycemia

Ketotic hypoglycemia is the most common cause of hypoglycemia after 1 year of age.[8,16,18] Symptoms mimicking those noted in ketotic hypoglycemia have occurred in children with GH deficiency, ACTH unresponsiveness, FDPase deficiency, glycogen synthetase deficiency, and Reye syndrome. Before a child is classified as having ketotic hypoglycemia, therefore, careful laboratory investigation to consider these and other disease must be accomplished.

The combination of ketonuria, hypoglycemia, and central nervous system symptoms, which may vary from unresponsiveness, pallor, and vomiting to coma and convulsions, and which often occur in the early morning hours in association with an upper respiratory tract infection or prolonged fast, is quite typical of ketotic hypoglycemia for which there is no known cause.[16] The onset is between 9 months and 5½ years of age, with a peak incidence at 2 years. Hypoglycemic episodes occur at intervals of from a few months to a year or more; they then decrease in frequency, and tend to disappear, usually by 7 to 8 years of age.

Although the pathogenesis of hypoglycemia in ketotic hypoglycemia has not been defined, the evidence suggests that it represents an exaggeration of the starvation state.[8] During hypoglycemia, blood insulin levels are appropriately low; blood alanine levels may also be low; GH, glucagon, cortisol, beta-hydroxybutyrate, and free fatty acid levels in the blood are elevated; urinary ketones are present; and blood glucose levels fail to rise after the administration of glucagon.

It is very important to document hypoglycemic blood glucose levels at the time of symptoms by obtaining a diagnostic blood sample. After the child has had several days to recover from the acute episode and is eating well, the administration of a provocative low calorie, high fat ketogenic diet has been useful in establishing the diagnosis[8,16] if an acute blood sample is unobtainable. The child must be observed carefully for hypoglycemia during the test period.

The acute hypoglycemic attacks are reversed by the intravenous administration of glucose; glucagon usually has no effect. Since the attacks occur infrequently, long-term drug therapy is not indicated. A liberal carbohydrate diet, including a bedtime snack, is recommended. Prolonged overnight fasting, particularly during weekends or holidays and periods of illness, should be avoided. The parents should be encouraged to test their child's urine for ketones each morning and particularly during illness or periods of fasting. Carbohydrate-containing foods, given promptly when acetonuria develops, are usually successful in aborting attacks.

REFERENCES

1. Aynsley-Green A: Hypoglycemia in infants and children, Clin Endocrinol Metab II(1):159, 1982.
2. Beckwith JB: Macroglossia, omphalocele, adrenal cytomegaly, gigantism and hyperplastic visceromegaly. In Bergsma D, editor: Malformation syndromes, Birth Defects 5:188, 1969.
3. Bougneres PF et al: Fasting hypoglycemia resulting from hepatic carnitine palmitoyl transferase deficiency, J Pediatr 98:742, 1981.
4. Brasel JA et al: An evaluation of 75 patients with hypopituitarism beginning in childhood, Am J Med 38:484, 1965.
5. Chaussain JL: Glycemic response to 24 hour fast in normal children and children with ketotic hypoglycemia, J Pediatr 82:438, 1973.
6. Chen YT, Cornblath M, and Sidbury JB: Cornstarch therapy in type I glycogen-storage disease, N Engl J Med 310:171, 1984.
7. Cornblath M: Hypoglycemia in infancy and childhood, Pediatr Ann 10:356, 1981.
8. Cornblath M and Schwartz R: Disorders of carbohydrate metabolism in infancy, ed 2, Philadelphia, 1976, WB Saunders Co.
9. Dershewitz R et al: Transient hepatomegaly and hypoglycemia: a consequence of malicious insulin administration, Am J Dis Child 130:998, 1976.
10. Dusheiko G et al: Recurrent hypoglycemia associated with glutaric aciduria type II in an adult, N Engl J Med 301:1405, 1979.
11. Green CL, Blitzer MG, and Shapira E: Inborn errors of metabolism and Reye syndrome: differential diagnoses, J Pediatr 113:156, 1988.
12. Greene HL et al: Type I glycogen storage disease: five years of management with nocturnal intragastric feeding, J Pediatr 96:590, 1980.
13. Harness JK et al: Nesidioblastosis in adults: a surgical dilemma, Arch Surg 116:575, 1981.
14. Kaye R et al: The response of blood glucose, ketones, and plasma nonesterified fatty acids to fasting and epinephrine injection in infants and children, J Pediatr 54:836, 1961.
15. Kershnar AK, Roe TF, and Kogut MD: Adrenocorticotropic hormone unresponsiveness: report of a girl with excessive growth and review of 16 reported cases, J Pediatr 80:610, 1972.
16. Kogut MD: Hypoglycemia: pathogenesis, diagnosis and treatment. In Gluck L et al, editors: Current problems in pediatrics, vol 4, Chicago, 1974, Year Book Medical Publishers.
17. Kogut MD: Neonatal hypoglycemia: a new look. In Moss AJ, editor: Pediatrics update: review for physicians, New York, 1980, Elsevier Science Publishing Co.
18. Kogut MD, Blaskovics M, and Donnell GN: Idiopathic hypoglycemia: a study of 26 children, J Pediatr 74:853, 1969.
19. Mayefsky JH, Sarnaik AP, and Postellon DC: Factitious hypoglycemia, Pediatrics 69:804, 1982.
20. Pagliara AS et al: Hypoglycemia in infancy and childhood, part 1, J Pediatr 82:365, 1973.
21. Roe TF and Kogut MD: Hypopituitarism and ketotic hypoglycemia, Am J Dis Child 121:296, 1971.
22. Roe TF and Kogut MD: Idiopathic leucine-sensitive hypoglycemia syndrome: insulin and glucagon responses and effects of diazoxide, Pediatr Res 16:1, 1982.
23. Scarlett JA et al: Factitious hypoglycemia: diagnosis by measurement of serum C-peptide immunoreactivity and insulin-binding autobodies, N Engl J Med 297:1029, 1977.
24. Schutgens RBH et al: Lethal hypoglycemia in a child with a deficiency of 3-hydroxy-3-methylglutaryl coenzyme A lyase, J Pediatr 94:89, 1979.
25. Shelly HJ and Neligan GA: Neonatal hypoglycemia, Br Med Bull 22:34, 1966.
26. Stanley CA and Baker L: Hyperinsulinism in infancy: diagnosis by demonstration of abnormal response to fasting hypoglycemia, Pediatrics 57:702, 1976.
27. Stanley CA and Baker L: Hyperinsulinism in infants and children: diagnosis and therapy, Adv Pediatr 23:315, 1976.
28. TeLander RL, Charboneay JW, and Haymond MW: Intraoperative ultrasonography of the pancreas in children, J Pediatr Surg 21:262, 1986.
29. Ware AJ et al: Systemic carnitine deficiency: report of a fatal case with multisystemic manifestations, J Pediatr 93:959, 1978.
30. Woo D, Scopes JW, and Polak JM: Idiopathic hypoglycemia in sibs with morphological evidence of nesidioblastosis of the pancreas, Arch Dis Child 51:528, 1976.

282

Increased Intracranial Pressure

Richard S.K. Young

Increased intracranial pressure is a potentially life-threatening condition that must be rapidly recognized and treated.[9] Raised intracranial pressure frequently occurs with traumatic head injury, hypoxic-ischemic brain injury, and Reye syndrome. Intracranial pressure also may be abnormally elevated during central nervous system infections[5] and diabetic ketoacidosis.[6] The symptoms of intracranial hypertension are protean, and the pediatrician should suspect increased intracranial pressure not only in the child with known brain tumor or head trauma but also in the child with chronic headache, visual complaints, or confusion.

PATHOPHYSIOLOGY

The skull is a rigid container, the principal contents of which include brain tissue (80%), blood (10%), and cerebrospinal fluid (10%). A substantial increase in any one or more of these constituents will cause the intracranial pressure to rise above its normal level (see the accompanying box).

Normal mean intracranial pressure during recumbency is less than 15 mm Hg.[3] Continuous recording of the intracranial pressure shows a pulsatile tracing that results from respiratory and cardiac activity. The relationship between arterial and intracranial pressure is described by the following formula:

Cerebral perfusion pressure =
Mean arterial blood pressure − Intracranial pressure

Under normal circumstances, cerebral blood flow remains constant ("autoregulated") over a wide range of blood pressures.[7,12] Trauma, ischemia, and other brain injuries, however, impair the autoregulatory function, which causes brain blood flow to become "pressure passive," rising and falling in response to the perfusion pressure. If the intracranial pressure approaches the level of the mean arterial blood pressure, cerebral perfusion pressure may become dangerously low, resulting in cerebral ischemia. A vicious cycle ensues in which cerebral ischemia leads to cerebral edema, which further aggravates the intracranial hypertension and ultimately produces brain displacement (herniation). A negative value for cerebral perfusion pressure may indicate brain death.[5]

Causes of Increased Intracranial Pressure

BLOOD

1. Intracranial collections of blood
   a. Epidural hematoma
   b. Subdural hematoma
   c. Subarachnoid hemorrhage
   d. Intraventricular hemorrhage
2. Vascular malformations
   a. Vein of Galen aneurysm
   b. Arteriovenous malformation

BRAIN

1. Cerebral hemispheric tumors
2. Cerebral edema
   a. Cytotoxic (e.g., hypoxic-ischemic, plumbism)
   b. Vasogenic (e.g., brain tumors)
   c. Interstitial (e.g., hydrocephalus)

FLUID

1. Cerebrospinal fluid
   a. Excessive production—choroid plexus papilloma
   b. Communicating hydrocephalus—block at level of arachnoid granulations
   c. Noncommunicating hydrocephalus
      (1) Aqueductal stenosis
      (2) Intraventricular tumors
2. Interstitial fluid—pseudotumor cerebri
3. Extracerebral fluid—subdural effusion

SIGNS AND SYMPTOMS

Elevated intracranial pressure may cause brain herniation through the several dural openings.[10,11] The signs and symptoms of the major herniation syndromes should be recognized by every clinician.

Uncal (transtentorial) herniation is the syndrome most frequently encountered. Swelling of one cerebral hemisphere forces the uncus of the temporal lobe's hippocampus laterally and downward past the medial edge of the tentorium (Fig. 282-1), producing deterioration of consciousness, dilation of the ipsilateral pupil (third nerve compression), and contralateral hemiparesis (compression of the ipsilateral cerebral peduncle).[10] Recent magnetic resonance imaging studies disclose total brain displacement of 6 to 13 mm in stuporous and comatose patients.[11] In extreme instances the contralateral cerebral peduncle and ipsilateral posterior cerebral artery may be compromised to produce an ipsilateral hemiplegia and contralateral hemianopsia, respectively. It is vital that the clinician aggressively treat uncal herniation because once midbrain necrosis has occurred, normal consciousness may be irrevocably impaired.

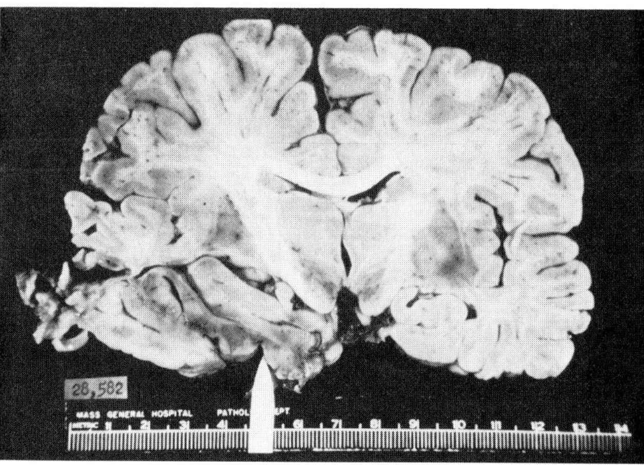

Fig. 282-1 Massive swelling of the right cerebral hemisphere has caused the uncus of the temporal lobe to herniate over the edge of the tentorium (*arrow*).

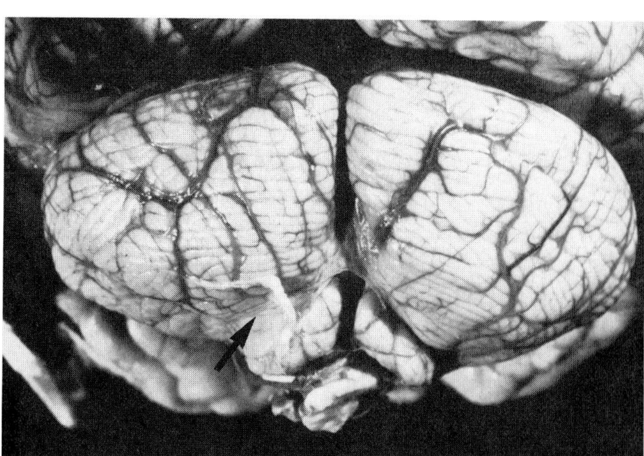

Fig. 282-2 Midline increased intracranial pressure has caused the cerebellar tonsils (*arrow*) to herniate downward with subsequent pressure upon the medullary cardiorespiratory centers.

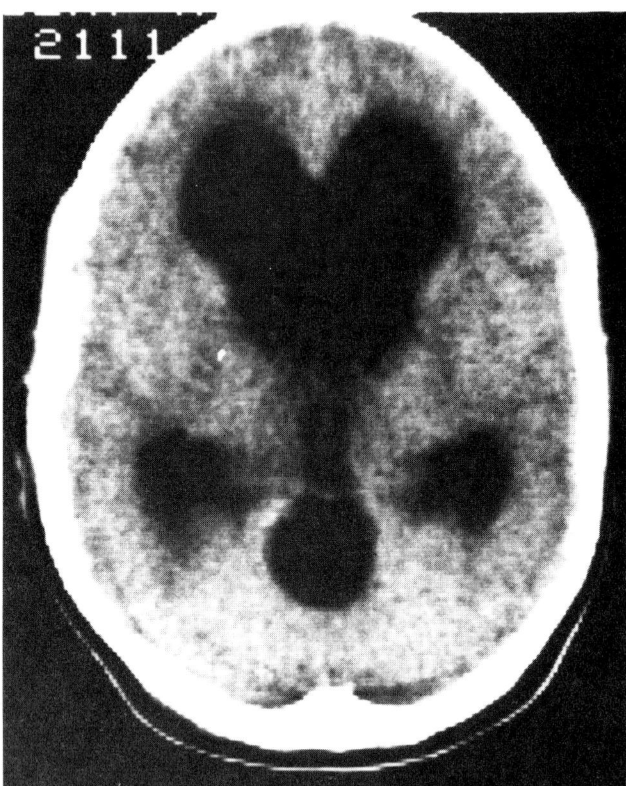

Fig. 282-3 CT brain scan demonstrates (1) marked dilation of the frontal and temporal horns of the lateral ventricles and (2) the third ventricle.

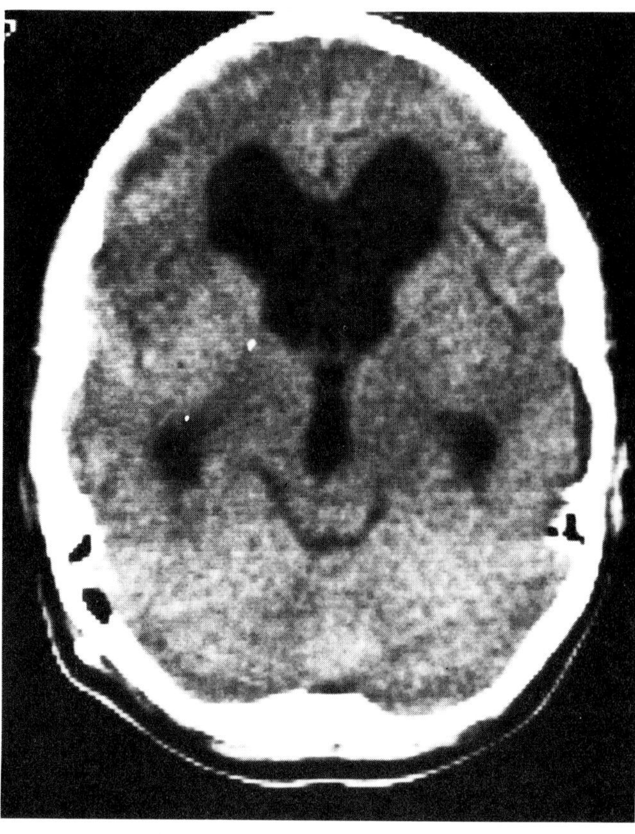

Fig. 282-4 CT brain scan shows partial decompression of the ventricles following placement of a ventriculoperitoneal shunt.

In cerebellar tonsillar herniation, a midline force causes the low brain stem and cerebellar tonsils to herniate through the foramen magnum and crush the respiratory centers in the medulla (Fig. 282-2). The constellation of bradycardia, hypertension, and apnea (Cushing triad) should alert the clinician that there is sufficient pressure on the hindbrain to cause death. The syndrome of upward tentorial herniation is less commonly seen and may be associated with coma, miosis, and oculomotor palsies. This syndrome occasionally occurs in neonates in whom bleeding in the posterior fossa develops, which forces the midbrain and superior pons upward against the tentorium.

In contrast to acute elevations in intracranial pressure, chronic elevations in intracranial pressure allow adjustments in brain compartments to take place. For example, in slowly developing aqueductal stenosis, the cerebral mantle may be compressed (Fig. 282-3) and then reconstituted once pressure has been relieved (Fig. 282-4). Whereas acute elevation of

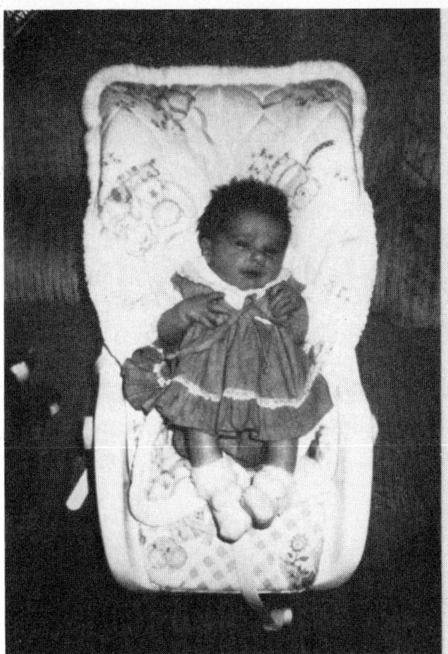
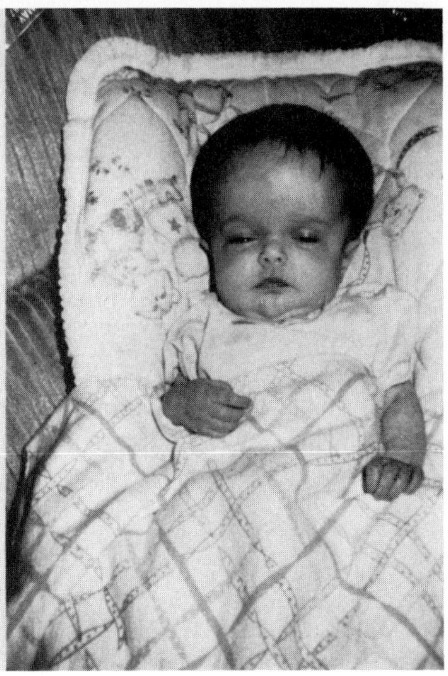

Fig. 282-5 Note the globular appearance of the head ("light bulb" sign), the loss of upgaze, and the distended scalp veins in this infant with slowly developing increased intracranial pressure.

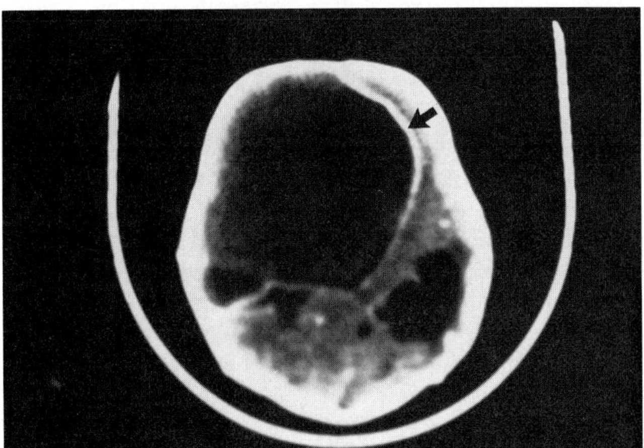

Fig. 282-6 The cause of raised intracranial pressure in the child seen in Figure 282-5 was a large brain abscess. Note enhancement of the rim of the abscess (*arrow*).

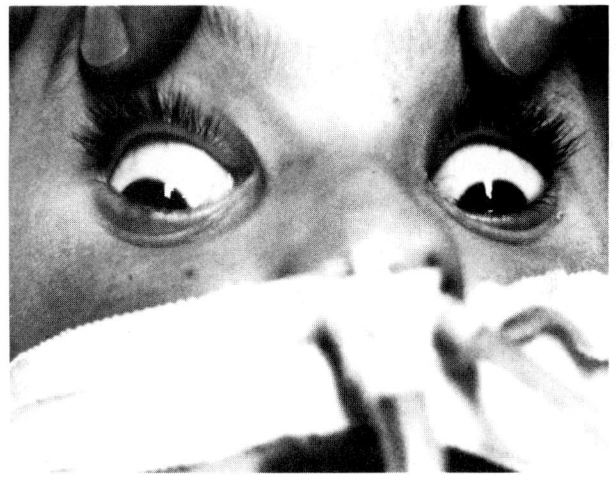

Fig. 282-7 Sunset sign: the eyes are tonically deviated downward.

intracranial pressure frequently occurs with dramatic brainstem signs and coma, the more gradual elevations of intracranial pressure often produce such mild and protean signs and symptoms as headache, visual difficulties, lethargy, dull affect, and episodic blindness.

In the infant, split sutures, increased head size, frontal bossing, and distended scalp veins are clinical clues to intracranial hypertension (Figs. 282-5 and 282-6). Parinaud syndrome results from pressure on the tectum of the midbrain, producing a failure of upgaze and the setting sun sign (Fig. 282-7). Headache as a result of raised intracranial pressure classically occurs in early morning and may be caused by fluid shifts in the brain secondary to assumption of the erect state. Vomiting occurs frequently, as do visual symptoms (blurring, diplopia, decreased acuity). It is essential that the visual fields, acuity, ocular motility, and optic disks be evaluated in every child with headache.

MEASUREMENT OF INTRACRANIAL PRESSURE

Intracranial pressure in the infant can be measured noninvasively by applying a fiberoptic sensing device to the fontanelle (Ladd applanation fontometer).[16] Although not a direct measurement of intracranial pressure, cerebral blood flow velocity may be estimated by the use of pulsed Doppler readings through the open fontanelle.[15] Neither of these methods is entirely satisfactory because the measurements may be affected by variability in applying the sensor.

Once the anterior fontanelle has calcified, measurement of intracranial pressure necessitates craniotomy. A hollow bolt can be placed in the subarachnoid space through a twist-drill hole in the skull, or alternatively, a catheter may be inserted through the brain into the lateral ventricle.[7] The subarachnoid bolt and the intraventricular catheter are subject to periodic malfunction because of occlusion of their lumens by blood or brain. Additional complications of the intraventricular catheter include traumatization of the cerebral tissue if repeated insertions of the catheter are required to localize compressed ventricles, as well as ventriculitis and hemorrhage. However, the intraventricular catheter does have the unique therapeutic advantage of allowing cerebrospinal fluid to drain. Both the subarachnoid bolt and the intraventricular catheter permit continuous pressure recordings, so that these may be correlated with changes in therapy. The computed tomography (CT) brain scan is a useful and noninvasive method for "imaging" the intracranial contents; signs of increased intracranial pressure include effacement, dilation (Fig. 282-3), and shifts of the cerebral ventricles. Although magnetic resonance imaging (MRI) offers superior image quality to that of CT, it has the following disadvantages: it is more difficult to monitor the acutely ill child, it takes longer to perform, and it is necessary to remove all metallic devices from the child's body.

MANAGEMENT

The treatment of increased intracranial pressure must be directed at reversing the primary brain insult that initially produced the increase in pressure.[7,12] In addition, management should be directed toward lowering the pressure by surgical or medical means. Obstruction of the cerebrospinal fluid pathways may respond to diversion of the cerebrospinal fluid by "shunting." Tumors compressing the cerebrospinal fluid pathways may be removed surgically. Collections of blood or pus within the cranial vault may be removed surgically or by aspiration. All too frequently, increased intracranial pressure can be treated only medically. The following general principles should be observed.

1. *Treat hypoxia*. If necessary, intubate and ventilate mechanically. Hypoxia aggravates cerebral swelling and further elevates intracranial pressure.

2. *Do not perform a lumbar puncture* if severely increased intracranial pressure is suspected. Leakage of cerebral fluid from the site of lumbar puncture may contribute to cerebellar tonsillar herniation. If meningitis is suspected as a cause of severely increased intracranial pressure, it may be preferable to obtain ventricular fluid for analysis and culture or treat with antibiotics until the intracranial pressure has subsided.

3. *Apply nursing procedures judiciously*. Pulmonary percussion and drainage and suctioning can cause abrupt increases in intracranial pressure. Nonetheless, pulmonary postural drainage toilet and ventilation must be maintained at optimal levels.

4. *Restrict fluids*. Monitor electrolyte levels, serum osmolality, and urine specific gravity to detect as early as possible the syndrome of inappropriate secretion of antidiuretic hormone (SIADH), which may accompany brain trauma, tumors, or central nervous system infections. A discussion of specific medical therapies for treating children with raised intracranial pressure follows.

Hyperventilation

Carbon dioxide tension has a profound effect on cerebral blood flow. Effective hyperventilation requires that the patient be paralyzed and receive passive ventilation, maintaining carbon dioxide pressure (Pco_2) between 25 and 30 mm Hg. A disadvantage of this form of therapy is that paralysis with neuromuscular blocking agents precludes neurologic evaluation. Extreme hyperventilation should be avoided because it may lead to brain ischemia by markedly decreasing brain-blood flow.

Osmotic Agents

Given as an intravenous bolus, mannitol is effective in temporarily lowering intracranial pressure, even in doses as small as 0.25 mg/kg.[7,8,12,17] The combination of mannitol with a Henle loop diuretic (e.g., furosemide) has been shown to be more effective than mannitol alone in experimental animals.[17] Urea produces a rapid and sustained fall in intracranial pressure but may be followed by a "rebound" of increased intracranial pressure. Successive doses of osmotic agents and diuretics become less effective as blood volume becomes contracted. If the intracranial pressure remains elevated despite an increase in serum osmolality >320 mOsm/L, death usually occurs from the raised intracranial pressure or from renal failure.[7]

Hypothermia

Profound hypothermia protects against cerebral ischemia, because lowering the body temperature reduces cerebral metabolism. However, use of prolonged hypothermia in patients with a variety of cerebral insults has not increased neurologic salvage.[2] Should hypothermia be employed, prevention of shivering with neuromuscular blocking agents is essential. The body temperature should not be lowered below 30° C because of the danger of cardiac arrhythmia.

Acetazolamide

Acetazolamide, a carbonic anhydrase inhibitor, reportedly decreases cerebrospinal fluid production. It also may lead to electrolyte imbalances.

Corticosteroids

Corticosteroids (e.g., dexamethasone, 2 to 4 mg every 6 hours) are of proved benefit in decreasing the cerebral swelling that results from brain tumors. This type of swelling, termed *vasogenic edema*, results from increased capillary permeability. Cytotoxic edema, which may accompany hypoxic injury, results from failure of the adenosinetriphosphate-dependent pump and is not responsive to steroid therapy. The third type of cerebral edema, interstitial edema, is seen in conditions such as obstructive hydrocephalus. Steroids also are ineffective in this type of swelling.[2,14] The disadvantages of high-dose steroid use include the risks of disturbing salt and water homeostasis and inducing hypertension and gastrointestinal bleeding.

Barbiturates

Pharmacologic doses of pentobarbital (sufficient to produce a "suppression-burst pattern" on an electroencephalogram) decrease brain metabolism, brain-blood flow, and intracranial pressure. Because high-dose pentobarbital produces coma, apnea, hypotension, and generalized edema, this therapeutic modality must be employed only in a pediatric intensive care unit equipped to treat these side effects.[18] It is noteworthy that high-dose barbiturate administration has not been of proved benefit in improving the neurologic outcome in humans.[13]

PROGNOSIS

Have aggressive monitoring and treatment of raised intracranial pressure reduced the prevalence of neurologic sequelae? Numerous experimental studies, as well as multicenter clinical studies, have not provided a definitive answer. First, maintenance of a normal intracranial pressure and normal cerebral perfusion pressure does not guarantee good neurologic outcome. For example, in a group of near-drowning victims, 13 of 31 patients who died had intracranial pressure <20 mm Hg.[1] Second, outcome may be predicated more on the cause of the raised intracranial pressure than on the intracranial pressure itself. Mortality correlates with the degree of raised intracranial pressure in central nervous system infections but not in hypoxic-ischemic injury.[5] Finally, raised intracranial pressure because of cytotoxic edema may be intractable to treatment with multiple modalities.[5]

Monitoring and treating raised intracranial pressure have proved beneficial in some disorders. The mortality rate in grade IV Reye syndrome has decreased from 80% to 10% with modern treatment of intracranial pressure.[4] The mortality rate also has been reduced from 52% to 40% in head trauma.[7] Monitoring of intracranial pressure has not proved beneficial in hypoxic-ischemic injury. As a result, some centers no longer routinely monitor it as part of their treatment protocol in near-drowning victims.[2] The current emphasis appears to be centered on optimum support of the cardiovascular system to avoid the potentially devastating effects of secondary hypoxic-ischemic damage.

REFERENCES

1. Allman FD et al: Outcome following cardiopulmonary resuscitation in severe pediatric near-drowning, Am J Dis Child 140:571, 1986.
2. Bohn DJ et al: Influence of hypothermia, barbiturate therapy, and intracranial pressure monitoring on morbidity and mortality after near-drowning, Crit Care Med 14:529, 1986.
3. Bruce DA: The pathophysiology of increased intracranial pressure, Kalamazoo, Mich, 1978, The Upjohn Co.
4. Frewen TC et al: Outcome in severe Reye syndrome with early pentobarbital coma and hypothermia, J Pediatr 100:663, 1982.
5. Goitein KJ and Tamir I: Cerebral perfusion pressure in central nervous system infections of infancy and childhood, J Pediatr 103:40, 1983.
6. Krane EJ et al: Subclinical brain swelling during treatment of diabetic ketoacidosis, N Engl J Med 312:1147, 1985.
7. McGillicuddy JE: Cerebral protection: pathophysiology and treatment of increased intracranial pressure, Chest 87:85, 1985.
8. Mendelow AD et al: Effect of mannitol on cerebral blood flow and cerebral perfusion pressure in human head injury, J Neurosurg 63:43, 1985.
9. Miller JD: Increased intracranial pressure: theoretical considerations. In Pellock JM and Myer EC, editors: Neurologic emergencies in infancy and childhood, Philadelphia, 1984, Harper & Row, Publishers, Inc.
10. Plum F and Posner J: The diagnosis of stupor and coma, ed 3, Philadelphia, 1980, F.A. Davis Co.
11. Ropper AH: A preliminary MRI study of the geometry of brain displacement and level of consciousness with acute intracranial masses, Neurology 39:622, 1989.
12. Safar P: Recent advances in cardiopulmonary-cerebral resuscitation: a review, Ann Emerg Med 13:856, 1984.
13. Shapiro HM: Barbiturates in brain ischemia, Br J Anaesth 57:82, 1985.
14. Shenkin HA and Bouzarth WF: Clinical methods of reducing intracranial pressure, N Engl J Med 282:1465, 1970.
15. Vidyasagar D, Raju T, and Chiang J: Clinical significance of monitoring anterior fontanelle pressure in sick neonates and infants, Pediatrics 62:996, 1978.
16. Volpe JJ: Noninvasive continuous monitoring techniques. In Volpe JJ: Neurology of the newborn, ed 2, Philadelphia, 1987, WB Saunders Co.
17. Wilkinson HA and Rosenfeld S: Furosemide and mannitol in the treatment of acute experimental intracranial hypertension, Neurosurgery 12:405, 1983.
18. Young RSK et al: Pentobarbital in refractory status epilepticus, Pediatr Pharmacol 3:63, 1984.

283

Meningococcemia

Keith R. Powell

Meningococcemia exemplifies fulminant bacterial sepsis. Although occult meningococcemia is occasionally detected, the usual fulminant form of the disease can progress from colonization with *Neisseria meningitidis* to death in less than a day and from a state of good health to death in hours, regardless of whether meningitis is present.

EPIDEMIOLOGY

The pathogen, *N. meningitidis,* is a gram-negative coccus that classically appears in pairs (diplococci) with the adjacent sides flattened. The nasopharynx of 2% to 4% of the population is colonized with this organism at any given time. During epidemics, the overall carriage rate in a population increases, with the highest incidence occurring in household contacts. Humans are the only host for *N. meningitidis,* and its transmission is thought to be from person to person via respiratory secretions. Most persons who become colonized become asymptomatic carriers and develop protective antibodies while still harboring the organism. Colonization with other organisms that induce cross-reacting antibodies also plays a role in the development of natural immunity to *N. meningitidis*. Nonetheless, annual age-specific attack rates of meningococcemia with or without meningitis average 14.4 cases per 100,000 population for infants under 1 year of age, 4.6 for children 1 to 4 years, 1 for children 5 to 9 years, 0.8 for persons 10 to 19 years, and 0.3 for persons over 20 years of age (Fig. 283-1).[1,2]

Although epidemics of meningococcal disease occur where large numbers of susceptible persons live in close quarters (e.g., military barracks, dormitories), the highest attack rate is among young children. Most cases of meningococcemia occur between 3 months and 4 years of age, when passively acquired maternal antibody concentrations reach their nadir and substantial numbers of children have not yet acquired protective antibodies following colonization. The fatality rate in cases of meningococcemia without meningitis reported to the Centers for Disease Control in 1978 was 25%.[1] Other investigations have shown an even higher case fatality rate for meningococcemia without meningitis.[14]

DIAGNOSIS AND DIFFERENTIAL DIAGNOSIS

The early recognition of meningococcemia is probably the most important determinant of survival. Over 50% of children with meningococcemia have fever as their first sign; about two thirds will have a temperature over 40° C.[14] Over 50% of the children will also have rash, vomiting, lethargy, or a combination of these. Less commonly, irritability, delirium, headache, coryza, diarrhea, myalgia, and hypothermia occur.

In a recently reported series of 100 children with meningococcal infections, 71% had a rash.[17] The type and duration

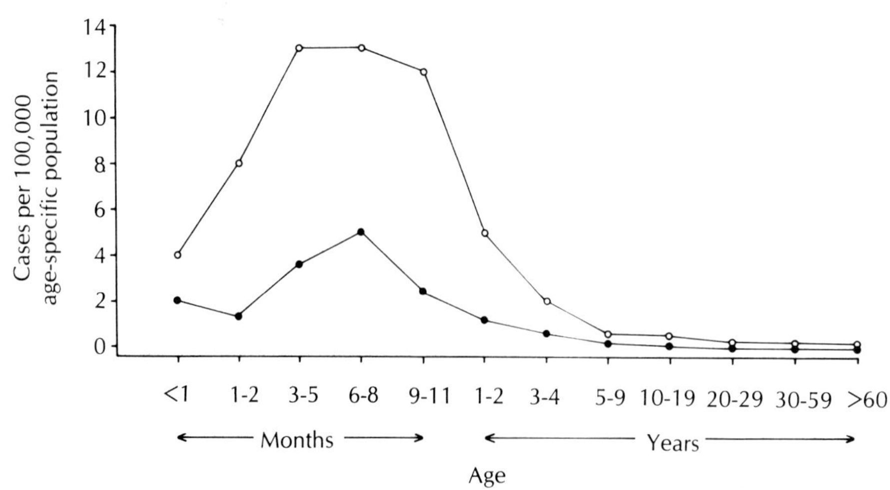

Fig. 283-1 Age-specific incidence of *N. meningitidis* meningitis (○) and meningococcemia without meningitis (●) per 100,000 population in the United States.

Data from Bacterial meningitis and meningococcemia—United States, 1978, Morbid Mortal Week Rep 28:287, 1979.

of the rash may be extremely important clues to the imminent course and the prognosis of the disease.[7,15] A pink maculopapular rash that resembles early varicella, rubella, roseola, secondary syphilis, or disseminated gonorrhea is generalized, appears in crops, is tender, and fades rapidly. Patients with this type of rash are less likely to have a fulminant course.

A generalized petechial rash most prominent on the distal extremities, including the palms and soles, is most commonly associated with meningococcal disease. Initially the lesions are discrete, 1 to 2 mm in diameter, and found in clusters, resembling ecchymoses, where clothing causes pressure on the skin. This rash must be differentiated from that seen with Rocky Mountain spotted fever, bacterial endocarditis, and enterovirus infections (coxsackieviruses A4, A9, and B2 to B4 and echoviruses 4, 7, and 9).[12]

The most ominous rash associated with meningococcemia is ecchymotic or purpuric, with a centrifugal distribution usually present in cases of fulminant meningococcemia. The differential diagnosis includes Rocky Mountain spotted fever, plague, rubeola, chickenpox, septicemia with other bacteria, and Henoch-Schönlein purpura (Table 283-1).

Meningococcemia is the most common cause of purpura. In a series of 151 patients with meningococcal infections, 7 of the 16 patients who had ecchymotic or purpuric lesions died; only 4 of the 135 patients with either maculopapular or petechial lesions or no rash at all did so.[15] In another series of 100 patients, all nine who had purpura fulminans died.[17] The case fatality rate is significantly higher in patients who have petechiae for 12 hours or less. Therefore a febrile child with purpura or petechiae that have been present for less than 12 hours should be managed as a medical emergency.

MANAGEMENT

A child with an acute onset of fever and a purpuric or petechial rash needs intensive care as soon as possible. If the child must be transported to an intensive care unit, blood should be drawn, antibiotics given, and intravenous (IV) access secured beforehand, and the patient should be attended during transport by a physician prepared to treat shock. Initial laboratory tests should include a blood culture, a complete blood count and differential, a partial thromboplastin time (PTT), a prothrombin time (PT), and measurement of fibrin breakdown products and the erythrocyte sedimentation rate (ESR).

As soon as the blood has been drawn, aqueous penicillin G, 50,000 U/kg, and chloramphenicol, 20 mg/kg, or ceftriaxone (100 mg/kg) or cefatoxime (50 mg/kg) should be administered by bolus IV push. If the systolic blood pressure is below 70 mm Hg, crystalloid, colloid, or blood at 20 ml/kg should be infused over about 20 minutes. Although two studies reported in 1987 showed that high-dose corticosteroids did not significantly reduce mortality in adults with septic shock,[4,16] most experts recommend that dexamethasone (3 mg/kg) be given to hypotensive children when meningococcemia is suspected. Dexamethasone can be given again in 4 hours if the blood pressure has not stabilized.

The response to volume expansion should occur during the infusion; response to steroids will take several hours. While the fluids are infusing, catheters should be placed to monitor central venous and arterial blood pressure continuously. The patient also must be ventilated adequately.

If the blood pressure is not maintained after the administration of fluids or if an elevated central venous pressure occurs, a dopamine drip (5 μg/kg/min) should be started and increased gradually until the blood pressure normalizes or the rate of dopamine infusion reaches 15 μg/kg/min. Vasopressor therapy should be aimed primarily at increasing peripheral vascular resistance rather than increasing cardiac output. If the blood pressure does not respond to volume expanders and vasopressors, consideration should be given to administering naloxone hydrochloride (Narcan). A placebo-controlled study has shown that patients requiring

Table 283-1 *Infectious Agents Associated with Illness in Which Petechial and/or Purpuric Exanthems Occur*

INFECTIOUS AGENT	ILLNESS
Varicella-zoster virus	Hemorrhagic chickenpox
Cytomegalovirus	Congenital cytomegalovirus infection
Variola virus	Hemorrhagic smallpox
Coxsackieviruses A4, A9 Coxsackieviruses B2 to B4 Echoviruses 4, 7, 9	Fever, exanthem, and enanthem
Colorado tick fever virus	Colorado tick fever gastroenteritis
Rotavirus	Gastroenteritis
Alphaviruses	Chikungunya fever, O'nyong nyong fever, Ross River fever, Sindbis fever
Rubella virus	Rubella (German measles) Congenital rubella
Respiratory syncytial virus	Bronchiolitis
Measles virus	Hemorrhagic (black measles) Atypical measles
Lassa virus	Lassa fever
Marburg virus	Hemorrhagic fever
Rickettsia typhi	Murine typhus
Rickettsia prowazeki	Epidemic typhus
Rickettsia rickettsii and other tickborne rickettsiae	Rocky Mountain spotted fever
Mycoplasma pneumoniae	Mycoplasmal pneumonia
Streptococcus pneumoniae	Pneumococcal septicemia
Enterococcal and viridans group streptococci	Endocarditis
Neisseria gonorrhoeae	Gonococcemia
Neisseria meningitidis	Meningococcemia
Haemophilus influenzae	*H. influenzae* septicemia
Pseudomonas aeruginosa	Ecthyma gangrenosa
Streptobacillus moniliformis	Rat-bite fever
Yersinia pestis	Septicemic plague (black death)
Treponema pallidum	Congenital syphilis
Borrelia sp.	Relapsing fever
Toxoplasma gondii	Congenital toxoplasmosis
Trichinella spiralis	Trichinosis

Modified from Cherry JD: Cutaneous manifestations of systemic infections. In Feigen RD and Cherry JD, editors: Textbook of pediatric infectious diseases, ed 2, Philadelphia, 1987, WB Saunders Co.

vasopressor therapy for septic shock who received 30 μg/kg naloxone as an intravenous bolus followed by a 30 μg/kg/hr infusion had significantly lower requirements for vasopressors and had late improvements in stroke volume and heart rate. Five of the eight patients treated with naloxone were subsequently discharged from the hospital compared with one of eight in the placebo group.[13] Once the blood pressure has stabilized, a lumbar puncture should be performed.

The febrile child with purpura or with the rapid onset of a petechial rash but who is not hypotensive should be managed expectantly. After obtaining the appropriate laboratory tests, a lumbar puncture should be performed, antibiotics begun, and the arterial blood pressure and central venous pressure monitored closely in an intensive care setting.

Assessment of laboratory and clinical findings can be helpful in making a prognosis. Stiehm and Damrosch[14] reviewed 63 cases of meningococcal disease and found that all patients died who had four or five of the following features: petechial or purpuric rash present for less than 12 hours, shock (systolic blood pressure under 70 mm Hg), absence of cerebrospinal fluid pleocytosis, blood leukocyte count less than 10,000/mm^3, and erythrocyte sedimentation rate of less than 10 mm/hr. Furthermore, six of the seven patients with three of these findings also died, but only 3 of 53 patients with none to two of the findings died. Similarly, Toews and Bass[15] found that patients with a purpuric or ecchymotic rash were statistically different from patients without a rash or with a macular or petechial rash in that they had meningitis and leukocytosis less frequently and more often were hyperpyrexic, were in shock, or had a bleeding diathesis.

More recently, Wong et al found that children who died from meningococcal infections were significantly more likely to have hypothermia, shock, peripheral white blood cell counts of under 5000 cells/mm^3, platelet counts under 100,000/mm^3, purpura fulminans, and seizures.[17] Boucek et al reported that echocardiographic evidence of myocardial dysfunction is associated with fatality in patients with meningococcemia and suggest that early knowledge regarding myocardial function may help direct therapy.[5] It has also been reported that high plasma concentrations of endotoxin predict multiple organ failure and death in systemic meningococcal disease.[6] A simplistic interpretation of the lack of leukocytosis, a low ESR, or lack of pleocytosis in the cerebrospinal fluid is that the pathogen has gained a tremendous head start on the host's immunologic defense mechanisms. The rapidly proliferating organisms release endotoxin, causing vasculitis and disseminated intravascular coagulation (DIC). The aim of the clinician is to eradicate the bacteria and support the patient until the host's defenses can be mustered.

Disseminated Intravascular Coagulation

The reason for obtaining a PTT, PT, fibrinogen level, and platelet count as part of the initial work-up when meningococcemia is suspected is that DIC is a frequent complication. Patients with normal blood coagulation do not require corrective therapy, nor do most patients with abnormal coagulation who are not bleeding.[8] Patients who are normotensive or hypotensive with a restorable blood pressure and bleeding may require vitamin K (5 to 10 mg IV), platelets (1 U/5 kg), and fresh frozen plasma. Patients who are hypotensive and do not respond to therapy should receive platelets for thrombocytopenia, fresh-frozen plasma for prolonged PTT and PT, and cryoprecipitate for hypofibrinogenemia.[8] If the blood pressure normalizes at this time, the consumptive coagulopathy usually stops and coagulation factors return to normal after a variable period of time. If the patient remains hypotensive, the coagulopathy is likely to persist and heparin therapy (50 to 100 U/kg IV every 4 hours) should be started. Heparin therapy may be beneficial in stopping the DIC but does not affect mortality. One of the complications of heparin therapy is bleeding that occurs as the DIC comes under control.

Survival from meningococcemia is usually determined within the first 12 hours after treatment has begun. Meningococci are exquisitely sensitive to penicillin and chloramphenicol as well as to the third-generation cephalosporins ceftriaxone and cefotaxime. Although not widespread, *N. meningitidis* strains with a decreased susceptibility to penicillin have been reported.[10] Antibiotic therapy is generally continued for 5 afebrile days and for a minimum of 7 days.

Continuous arterial blood pressure monitoring should be continued for at least 24 hours after the last dose of steroids and until the patient is normotensive without the use of pressor drugs. The central venous catheter can be removed when fluids and electrolytes are no longer a problem. In patients with meningitis, urine specific gravity and serum sodium concentrations should be closely monitored to detect any inappropriate secretion of antidiuretic hormone.

COMPLICATIONS

In a series of 86 children with meningococcal infections, 27% had complications.[9] It should be noted that 93% of these patients had meningitis; in 8 of the 21 patients with complications, the complications could be related directly to meningitis (7 with hearing loss and 1 each with subdural effusion and empyema).[9] Other early suppurative complications were myocarditis (three patients) and arthritis (two patients). Late-onset vasculitis or arthritis occurred in eight (10%) of these patients. Vasculitis was characterized by pustular skin lesions on the trunk or lower extremities that were negative by Gram stain and culture. Late-onset arthritis was associated with recurrence of fever and symptoms of arthritis. Late-onset vasculitis and arthritis resolved 4 to 14 days after onset. Pericarditis and myocarditis occur fairly frequently in adults, but less often in children.[3] Sterile pericardial effusions develop late in the course of the disease, suggesting a hypersensitivity phenomenon. The course of meningococcal pericarditis is usually benign, although pericardiocentesis is occasionally required. Myocarditis is generally found on autopsy. As more patients who develop extensive areas of avascular necrosis survive, reconstructive surgery and rehabilitation will become an important part of patient management.

PREVENTION

Prophylaxis for persons at high risk for developing meningococcal disease because of exposure to an affected person should be instituted as soon as possible after the diagnosis has been made. These include household or family contacts, contacts in day care centers, and anyone exposed to oral secretions through mouth-to-mouth resuscitation or kissing. Those at low risk (including school contacts, casual contacts, and persons providing routine care for the patient) need not receive prophylaxis. If the sensitivity of the organism is unknown, four doses of rifampin should be given at 12-hour intervals. Adults and adolescents should be given 600 mg/dose; children (1 to 12 years), 10 mg/kg/dose; and infants (less than 1 year), 5 mg/kg/dose. If the organism is sensitive to sulfadiazine, adults should be given 1 g every 12 hours for four doses; children, 500 mg every 12 hours for four doses; and infants, 500 mg/day for two doses.

Capsular polysaccharide vaccines against *N. meningitidis* serogroups A, C, Y, and W135 are commercially available and have been effective in preventing disease in military recruits and during epidemics. A major problem has been that over 50% of meningococcal disease is caused by serogroup B organisms, whose capsular polysaccharide is a poor immunogen. An aluminum hydroxide–adsorbed *N. meningitidis* serotype 2b protein-group B polysaccharide vaccine was recently shown to induce bactericidal antibodies in volunteers and holds promise for future prevention of meningococcal disease.[11]

REFERENCES

1. Bacterial meningitis and meningococcemia: United States, 1978, MMWR 28:277, 1979.
2. Band JD et al: Trends in meningococcal disease in the United States, 1975-1980, J Infect Dis 148:754, 1983.
3. Blaser MJ et al: Primary meningococcal pericarditis: a disease of adults associated with serogroup C *Neisseria meningitidis,* Rev Infect Dis 6:625, 1984.
4. Bone RC et al: A controlled clinical trial of high-dose methylprednisolone in the treatment of severe sepsis and septic shock, N Engl J Med 317:653, 1987.
5. Boucek MM et al: Myocardial dysfunction in children with acute meningococcemia, J Pediatr 105:538, 1984.
6. Brandtzaeg P et al: Plasma endotoxin as a predictor of multiple organ failure and death in systemic meningococcal disease, J Infect Dis 159:195, 1989.
7. Cherry JD: Cutaneous manifestations of systemic infections. In Feigen RD and Cherry JD, editors: Textbook of pediatric infectious diseases, ed 2, Philadelphia, 1987, WB Saunders Co.
8. Corrigan JJ: Heparin therapy in bacterial septicemia, J Pediatr 91:695, 1977.
9. Edwars MS and Baker CJ: Complications and sequelae of meningococcal infections in children, J Pediatr 99:540, 1981.
10. Esso D et al: *Neisseria meningitidis* strains with decreased susceptibility to penicillin, Pediatr Infect Dis J 6:438, 1987.
11. Frasch CE et al: Antibody response of adults to an aluminum hydroxide-adsorbed *Neisseria meningitidis* serotype 2b protein-group B polysaccharide vaccine, J Infect Dis 158:710, 1988.
12. Glode MP and Smith AL: Meningococcal disease. In Feigen RD and Cherry JD, editors: Textbook of pediatric infectious diseases, ed 2, Philadelphia, 1987, WB Saunders Co.
13. Roberts DE et al: Effects of prolonged naloxone infusion in septic shock, Lancet ii:699, September, 1988.
14. Stiehm ER and Damrosch DS: Factors in the prognosis of meningococcal infection, J Pediatr 68:457, 1966.
15. Toews WH and Bass JW: Skin manifestations of meningococcal infection: an immediate indicator of prognosis, AJDC 127:173, 1974.
16. Veterans Adminsitration Systemic Sepsis Cooperative Study Group: Effect of high-dose glucocorticoid therapy on mortality in patients with clinical signs of systemic sepsis, N Engl J Med 317:659, 1987.
17. Wong VK, Hitchcock W, and Mason WH: Meningococcal infections in children: a review of 100 cases, Pediatr Infect Dis J 8:224, 1989.

284

Pneumothorax and Pneumomediastinum

David I. Bromberg

Pneumothorax and pneumomediastinum are defined as the presence of air in the potential pleural or mediastinal spaces, respectively. These conditions are relatively rare in pediatrics, having their greatest incidence in the neonatal period. There are, however, several clinical situations in which pneumothorax is a serious complication and failure to recognize its presence could result in serious morbidity. Pneumothorax may play a prominent role (1) in the neonatal period; (2) as a complication of specific respiratory diseases, especially asthma and cystic fibrosis; (3) as a complication of mechanical ventilation; (4) as a result of trauma; and (5) when it occurs spontaneously.

The classic studies of Macklin and Macklin[1] have helped elucidate the mechanism of pneumothorax and pneumomediastinum. When a pressure gradient exists between the alveolus and interstitial tissue (usually as a result of high inspiratory pressures), alveolar rupture may result, with escape of air into the perivascular interstitium. This accumulation of air travels along the vascular ray (seen clinically as pulmonary interstitial emphysema) to the surface of the lung or to the mediastinum and eventually may result in a pneumothorax or pneumomediastinum. The entities, then, of pulmonary interstitial emphysema, pneumothorax, and pneumomediastinum are all expressions of a single pathologic process.

The clinical presentation varies with the extent of disease. Pain is almost universally present. As the size of the pneumothorax increases, there may be tachypnea, dyspnea, and cyanosis. Physical findings also vary from a normal examination to the presence of hyperresonance to percussion, the absence of breath sounds, and a mediastinal shift to the opposite end.

When air enters the pleural space through a ball valve mechanism, a tension pneumothorax is produced. The pneumothorax increases in size, with each inspiration greatly reducing lung volume. Clinical findings include severe and progressive dyspnea and cyanosis and may include shock. This constitutes an emergency in which thoracentesis can be lifesaving.

Pneumothorax has been demonstrated by radiologic studies to occur in between 1% and 2% of all newborns. Some of these are undoubtedly related to overaggressive resuscitation, but others have been shown to occur spontaneously. Less than half the total number are symptomatic. The incidence of pneumothorax is much greater in neonates with pulmonary disease, especially hyaline membrane disease, meconium aspiration, and pulmonary hypoplasia. An increased incidence of renal anomalies in association with neonatal pneumothorax and pneumomediastinum has been noted.

Pneumothorax in older children, rather than occurring spontaneously, is seen as a complication of an underlying pulmonary disease or as a result of trauma or mechanical ventilation. Although rare, it has been reported in conjunction with asthma, cystic fibrosis, pneumonia (especially staphylococcal), and tuberculosis. Any entity that pathologically includes interstitial emphysema may potentially progress to include pneumothorax or pneumomediastinum as well. In a study of hospitalized asthmatics, over 5% were found to have pneumomediastinum, with the incidence increasing to greater than 15% in patients over 10 years of age. The therapeutic significance of this is clear, contraindicating the use of positive-pressure breathing in these patients. In thoracic trauma cases, a large percentage of patients have pneumothorax, which is usually apparent. These patients may have tension or "sucking" pneumothoraces and require immediate attention.

In late adolescence and young adulthood, in addition to the causes discussed above, spontaneous pneumothorax becomes a significant entity, occurring predominantly in otherwise healthy males with no known underlying respiratory disease. It is believed that these individuals have a pulmonary or pleural site of structural weakness or abnormality, but this is seldom proved. Activity levels appear to have little correlation with the onset of symptoms that may begin while the patient is at rest. Less than 20% will have a recurrence; those who do will frequently have the ipsilateral side involved within a year of the initial attack.

The diagnosis of pneumothorax and pneumomediastinum should be seriously entertained in patients who fall into the clinical categories discussed and who present with sudden onset of sharp chest pain. Confirmation is made by obtaining posteroanterior and lateral chest roentgenograms and demonstrating the presence of free pleural or mediastinal air. Quantification of the pneumothorax also should be attempted. In the neonatal nursey fiberoptic transillumination has proved a valuable adjunctive tool for the rapid bedside diagnosis of pneumomediastinum and pneumothorax.

Iatrogenic causes of pneumothorax must also be considered. Pneumothorax can occur as a complication of tracheostomy, internal jugular puncture, subclavian vein line insertion, and mechanical ventilation. When a patient is given pressurized oxygen, care must be taken to ensure that the system is vented, or a tension pneumothorax could result.

Therapy depends on the size of the lesion, the etiology, and the clinical status of the patient. In neonates, most pneumothoraces are managed with the insertion of a thoracostomy tube attached to a water seal. In symptomatic patients with underlying pulmonary disease, needle aspiration of the pneumothorax is attempted while continuing to direct therapy toward the primary disease. If air reaccumulates in the pleural space, insertion of a thoracostomy tube connected to a water seal is indicated. The therapeutic approach to spontaneous pneumothorax is usually conservative. In the patient who is asymptomatic with a minor pneumothorax, observation alone is sufficient. In the case of larger lesions the physician should perform thoracentesis, removing as much air as possible. In cases of spontaneous pneumothorax without an identifiable cause, the patient and family should be reassured that the initial therapy is curative and that the majority will not recur.

After resolution, no activity reduction is indicated. Pneumomediastinum rarely produces symptoms. When this lesion becomes large enough to produce respiratory or circulatory distress, aspiration under fluoroscopic control is indicated. General supportive care is of the utmost importance in managing both lesions and should include adequate pain control and cough suppression when necessary.

REFERENCE

1. Macklin MI and Macklin CC: Malignant interstitial emphysema of the lungs and mediastinum as an important occult complication in many respiratory diseases and other conditions: an interpretation of the clinical literature in the light of laboratory experiment, Medicine 23:281, 1944.

SUGGESTED READINGS

DeVries WC and Wolfe WG: The management of spontaneous pneumothorax and bullous emphysema, Surg Clin North Am 60:851, 1980.

Melton LJ, Hepper NGG, and Offord KP: Influence of height on the risk of spontaneous pneumothorax, Mayo Clin Proc 56:678, 1981.

Peters JI: When to suspect—and how to treat—a pneumothorax, J Respir Dis 7:17, 1986.

Pollack MM, Fields AI, and Holbrook PR: Pneumothorax and pneumomediastinum during pediatric mechanical ventilation, Crit Care Med 7:536, 1979.

285

Poisoning

Robert J. Nolan

EPIDEMIOLOGY

The ingestion of potentially toxic substances is usually accidental in the child under 6 years of age; in the adolescent and the adult, the ingestion of a potentially toxic substance is generally the result of a willful act, although the resulting toxicity may be either intentional (i.e., attempted murder or suicide) or unintentional (e.g., adverse experience with an illicit drug). The incidence of ingestion episodes, the probability of resulting toxicity, and the agents involved are divergent for those two age groups.

Significant morbidity and mortality occur in both age groups as a result of therapeutic misuse of medications. This may be accidental, as in the multiple dosing of a child by the two parents, each unaware of the actions of the other, or intentional, excessive dosing to achieve an enhanced therapeutic effect (e.g, enhanced antipyresis with aspirin or acetaminophen, enhanced antienuretic effect with imipramine).

The American Association of Poison Control Centers (AAPCC)[4] estimates that more than 2 million human poison exposures occur each year in the United States. More than 60% of the 1,368,748 exposures reported in 1988 were in children under 6 years of age; 75% of these were in children 3 years of age or younger. It can be assumed that many nontoxic or symptomless ingestions are not reported or brought to medical attention. The morbidity in this high incidence age group is small; less than 20% of reported ingestions in children under 6 years of age result in any symptoms. However, more than 75% of adolescent ingestions are symptomatic. Of the 545 fatalities in all ages reported in 1988, only 30 were in children under 6 years of age. Poisoning deaths in adolescents and adults are not unusual and are rarely accidental; poisoning deaths in children are rare and almost always unintended.

Categories of agents most frequently involved in childhood poisonings are medications (41%), caustics and cleaning agents (11%), cosmetics (11%), plants (10%) hydrocarbons (3%), and insecticides or pesticides (3%). A significant incidence of exposure does not imply resultant toxicity; most ingested cosmetics and plants, for example, are harmless. The major categories of agents responsible for fatal poisoning in children under 6 years of age reported by the AAPCC from 1983 through 1988 are medications (50%), carbon monoxide inhalation (14%), insecticides or pesticides (8%), hydrocarbons (7%), and caustics or cleaning agents (6%). Psychotropic agents, ferrous sulfate, and analgesics (salicylates and acetaminophen) in rank order account for over 65% of the fatal *medication* ingestions in children under 6 years of age.

Over the past 20 to 25 years, mortality from accidental poisoning and the agents involved in poisoning episodes have changed significantly. Currently, mortality in the preschool-age child is about 20% of the rate during the mid-1960s. The causes for this decline are not adequately defined but are generally believed to include child-resistant closures (the declining death rate clearly antedated implementation of the Poison Prevention Packaging Act of 1970), increased public awareness of childhood poisoning, improved diagnosis and management of the poisoned child, and a decreased need for certain highly toxic substances (e.g., kerosene, lye) in the home. Aspirin used to be the single substance most frequently ingested by children, but the prevalence of aspirin ingestion has declined both absolutely and as a percentage of total ingestions. Fatalities from salicylates have declined more than tenfold, principally as a result of the legislated use of child-resistant closures and the voluntary restriction (by manufacturers) in packaging quantities for children's aspirin. This trend has accelerated since the early 1980s with declining use of aspirin in children resulting from concerns regarding its association with the onset of Reye syndrome. Childhood ingestions of psychotropic drugs and ferrous sulfate each account for more than twice as many fatalities as does aspirin.

Normal developmental phenomena, such as oral exploration, increasing mobility, and an insatiable curiosity, play a fundamental role in the etiology of accidental poisoning in young children. Young boys poison themselves more frequently than young girls (during adolescence female ingestions predominate). Poisoning reportedly occurs more commonly in children from socioeconomically deprived families. Although recidivism is high (estimates range from 20% to 80%), it has not been possible to identify prospectively the child at risk for an initial ingestion or poisoning episode. Some authorities believe that such poisoning episodes are the result of inappropriate parenting practices, disturbed family dynamics, or both.

Accidental ingestions tend to occur at times of family disorganization, with deviations from normal routines (e.g., household moving, spring cleaning, vacation, or holidays), and during times of family stress (e.g., sickness, death, or divorce). Ingestions occur most frequently in the kitchen, where cleansing products, polishing fluids, and other poisonous household products are commonly stored beneath the sink or on easily accessible lower cabinet shelves. The bathroom is also a common site for an accidental ingestion; agents most commonly involved are medications and cosmetics. In addition to improper storage of toxic products in easily accessible sites, improper storage of solvents and cleaning agents in drinking glasses, cups, or beverage bottles is a contributing epidemiologic factor.

PREVENTION

Prevention of injury from the ingestion of toxic substance is best achieved by preventing the unintended, accidental ingestion. Because the child at risk is effectively identified only after the fact (the recidivist), effective prevention is directed toward the environment of all children and in most instances requires parental compliance. It is therefore not surprising that the only preventive measure of proven efficacy is societal intervention through the legislated requirement of child-resistant closures for toxic household products and drugs.

Appropriate selection of products to be stored in a household with young children, selection of reasonable sites of storage, and prompt, proper disposal of unnecessary toxic materials are facets of the protective parental obligation. The environment may be rendered safer by the use of locked cabinets or boxes for all drugs and for toxic household products. All drugs and household products should be kept in their original containers. Materials no longer required should be discarded in a manner that precludes access by the child, such as flushing them down the toilet.

Advising parents and caretakers of children about these protective measures and alerting parents to the dangers of failing to supervise children during periods of family stress are recommended anticipatory guidance practices. In addition, the physician should limit prescribed drugs to necessary quantities, instruct parents to use the entire prescribed quantities, provide educational materials in the office, and participate in community education programs.

Poisoning in the older child results from failure by parents to meet educational and disciplinary obligations. An understanding of the appropriate use of drugs and medications and an appreciation of the need for adult supervision of drug consumption in childhood are among the more important lessons of childhood.

PRINCIPLES OF MANAGEMENT

General Considerations

The pediatrician should be able to deal effectively with the vast majority of acute ingestions. To facilitate this care, specific textbooks on poisonings should be readily available in the office library. Two excellent books are *Clinical Toxicology of Commercial Products* by Gosselin and associates[3] and *Poisoning* by Arena.[1] The POISINDEX system,[6] a poison information software package, is widely available in emergency treatment facilities.

Prompt removal of the offending agent can obviate the need for future treatment and may ameliorate subsequent developing symptoms. Cleansing from the skin toxins that can produce a local effect or that can be absorbed cutaneously is easily accomplished in the office. Prompt gastric evacuation, using syrup of ipecac to induce emesis, is possible in the office, as is administration of an adsorbent, such as activated charcoal, or of a demulcent, such as evaporated milk or milk of magnesia. Further definitive treatment of seriously poisoned children is more easily accomplished in the hospital or emergency treatment facility.

The physician should be familiar with and have ready access to community resources that may provide information or practical help with acute poisonings. A hospital emergency room or treatment facility should be readily available for the transfer of patients who are in need of care beyond that available in the office. Poison control centers are a good source of information on poisoning for the practicing professional. From 1953 to 1970, local poison control centers were established throughout the United States; improved data retrieval and communication technologies during the 1970s led to regionalization, with a decline in the number of local centers. By 1988 more than 63% of the U.S. population was served by regional poison control centers of the AAPCC. Commercial enterprise has replaced government as the source of toxicologic information for poison control centers. These regional centers offer information 24 hours a day, toll-free telephone access, comprehensive information, and access to a regional treatment facility for patient referral. Protocols for giving advice are used for the initial management of consumer calls.

Pharmacists can sometimes provide helpful information about medications when the name of the medication or the amount dispensed does not appear on the label. Similarly, manufacturers may need to be called to determine the ingredients in a household product. A list of many manufacturers and their addresses can be found in *Clinical Toxicology of Commercial Products*.[3]

Telephone Calls

Most poisoning episodes will be handled over the telephone. Typically, the mother calls and is usually anxious, even frantic. The person answering the telephone needs to be calm and firmly directive. Initially, the practitioner needs to determine the agent, the amount ingested, and the presence or absence of symptoms. From this information, the risk of toxicity can be determined. This may depend on the relative toxicity of the agent involved or on the amount of the agent ingested. Alternatively, the presence of symptoms may suggest that toxicity is a risk, despite neither the agent nor the amount ingested seeming to be toxic.

If there is no toxic risk, the appropriate response is reassurance. If, however, a toxic risk exists, further data must be collected before advice can be given. The resources available to the caller need to be identified—for example, the presence of first-aid drugs in the home (e.g., syrup of ipecac) or the proximity to a pharmacy or to a hospital and whether transportation is readily available. Using this information, the practitioner can recommend appropriate management.

Poisoning and accident prevention should be discussed with the parents within a few days of such a call; experience has shown that addressing prevention at the time of the initial call is less effective than doing so later. A recent accidental ingestion focuses the minds of the parents, providing a valuable opportunity to impart advice on poison prevention.

Approach to the Symptomatic Patient

Diagnosing poisoning in patients who are symptomatic can be difficult when an ingestion has not been observed. Although some poisons produce characteristic signs and symptoms, most do not; they may simulate many acute illnesses seen in pediatrics. The physician should always consider the possibility of poisoning when faced with a puzzling situation in which the diagnosis is not clear. The rapid onset of central nervous system, gastrointestinal, or respiratory symptoms should alert the physician to ask about medications or toxins within the home. Unexplained signs of central nervous system stimulation, such as delirium or convulsions, or of central nervous system depression, such as stupor or coma, should be considered to result from poisoning until proved otherwise. The presence of hyperpnea in a child or a young infant with a febrile illness may be caused by the overzealous use of salicylates by the parents. A characteristic odor of specific poisons on the breath or in the vomitus can sometimes be discerned.

Therapeutic Modalities

The important principles of management with acute poisonings are (1) elimination of the poison from the body, (2) adsorption and inactivation of the poison, (3) administration of specific antidotes, and (4) provision of supportive measures. A calm and reasoned approach is far more effective than overtreatment with stimulants, depressants, or antidotes. Heroic measures are not needed with most poisoning episodes.

Syrup of ipecac is the most efficacious means of inducing vomiting when an ingestion has occurred. Syrup of ipecac is available without prescription in 30 ml containers. Contraindications to its use include neurologic symptoms (depressed level of consciousness, seizures), caustic ingestions, most hydrocarbon ingestions, and antiemetic ingestions. Infants under 6 months of age have a poorly developed gag reflex and should not receive syrup of ipecac. Close medical observation is required when syrup of ipecac is administered to infants 6 to 9 months of age. The dose of syrup of ipecac is 10 ml under 1 year and 15 ml for children; adolescents may receive 30 ml. The dose should be followed by one or two glasses of water and may be repeated if vomiting has not occurred within 20 to 30 minutes. The absence of vomiting after an additional 20 to 30 minutes necessitates gastric lavage.

If there is central nervous system depression, gastric lavage can be done provided the patient has not ingested a strong corrosive agent or a hydrocarbon. As large a plastic catheter as can be passed into the stomach without trauma should be used, and the stomach should be irrigated with small amounts of isotonic or half-isotonic saline until the returns are clear. Tap water should not be used in children because of the danger of producing water intoxication. Before the catheter is withdrawn, it should be either pinched off or the suction maintained to prevent aspiration of material into the lungs.

There has been renewed interest in the use of activated charcoal in the acute management of poisoning in recent years. Activated charcoal is an effective adsorbent for many drugs, including acetaminophen, aspirin, sedative hypnotics, tricyclic antidepressants, stimulants (amphetamines and cocaine) phenothiazines, and others. It is ineffective in iron, alcohol, or cyanide poisonings. It is given as a water slurry (20 to 50 g in children, 50 to 100 g in adolescents). It is effective immediately after ingestion and can be safely given by nonprofessionals. In general, charcoal should be administered as soon as possible, preferably within the first few hours after the ingestion. Activated charcoal should not be used simultaneously with syrup of ipecac, since charcoal adsorbs the ipecac, rendering it ineffective. It should be administered after emesis has been successfully induced.

There are few effective specific antidotes. Oxygen is the specific effective antidote for carbon monoxide poisoning. Naloxone hydrochloride (Narcan) safely and effectively antagonizes the pharmacologic effects of natural and synthetic narcotics. For the treatment of organophosphate poisoning, pralidoxime (2-PAM) is highly effective if used in conjunction with atropine. N-acetylcysteine is effective when administered early in severe acetaminophen poisoning. Of the chelating agents used to treat heavy metal poisonings, deferoxamine mesylate (Desferal) is specific for iron poisoning; dimercaprol (BAL) combines with arsenic, bismuth, lead, and mercury; and calcium EDTA chelates cadmium, copper, iron, and lead. Methylene blue may be lifesaving in drug-induced methemoglobinemia; sodium thiosulfate and inhalation of amyl nitrate combined with intravenous sodium nitrite (both of which may cause methemoglobinemia) may be lifesaving in cyanide poisoning. Although vitamin K effectively counteracts the anticoagulant properties of coumarin and warfarin, its use is rarely needed, since repeated ingestions over a period of days are necessary to produce toxicity.

When poisoning has resulted from an ionizable drug, intracellular and central nervous system drug levels may be reduced and renal excretion increased by therapy directed toward achieving "ion trapping." Ionizable drugs, such as amphetamine, phencyclidine, salicylate, and phenobarbital, cross lipid membranes (the cell wall or blood-brain barrier) only in the nonionized state. Gradients in pH across the membrane "trap" the ionized drug in the milieu, favoring dissociation. A more alkaline pH favors dissociation (and hence, ion trapping) of weakly acidic drugs (e.g., phenobarbital, salicylate); a relatively acidic milieu favors higher concentrations of weakly basic drugs (e.g., amphetamines, phencyclidine). Occasionally in acute salicylism, and almost invariably in chronic salicylism, potassium depletion (with or without hypokalemia) precludes the excretion of an alkaline urine.

Drugs with a small apparent volume of distribution (V_D less than 1 liter per kg) (i.e., most of the drug remains in the blood or extracellular fluid), such as salicylates or amphetamines, can be "cleansed" from the body by hemodialysis, charcoal hemoperfusion, exchange transfusion, or peritoneal dialysis. Drugs with high degrees of tissue binding and a large V_D, such as digoxin and phenothiazines, are poorly removed by those techniques.

Supportive therapy is the mainstay of treatment in most intoxications. This consists of administering intravenous fluids, supporting respiration, and treating shock, congestive heart failure, cerebral edema, and convulsions.

SALICYLATE POISONING

Salicylism is seen in all age groups, including congenital salicylism caused by maternal ingestion of toxic quantities, accidental ingestion in early childhood, and attempted suicide in adolescence and adulthood. Poisoning can also occur following excessive topical application of oil of wintergreen to denuded skin. Over 50% of hospitalized cases of salicylism result from chronic ingestion associated with therapeutic misuse; 25% of patients with salicylism have an associated intercurrent infection. Oil of wintergreen, which contains high concentrations of methyl salicylate, usually produces severe poisoning when it is ingested.

Laboratory Findings

Diagnosis depends on either elicitation of a history of ingestion or recognition of the characteristic clinical findings. A positive urine ferric chloride reaction can confirm salicylate ingestion, but not toxic exposure, since the test is sensitive to ordinary therapeutic doses. The serum salicylate level confirms the diagnosis. Single acute ingestions of greater than 150 mg/kg generally result in clinical symptoms; acute ingestions greater than 500 mg/kg are potentially fatal. The nomogram introduced by Done[2] (Fig. 285-1) correlates the serum salicylate level with the time since ingestion and is essential to assessment of clinical severity following ingestion of a single dose. The serum salicylate level is of no value in assessing clinical severity when the drug has been repeatedly administered or chronically ingested. The clinical picture of salicylism is characterized by vomiting, hyperpnea, and dehydration. Salicylism should be considered in the diagnosis

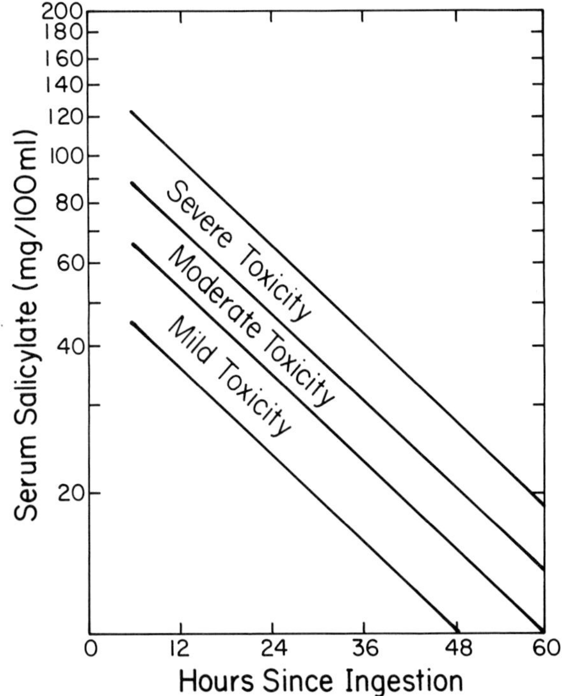

Fig. 285-1 Done nomogram for estimating the severity of poisoning following a single acute salicylate ingestion.

Adapted from Done AK: Salicylate intoxication: significance of measurements of salicylate in blood in cases of acute ingestion, Pediatr 26:800, 1960.

of cryptogenic metabolic acidosis, particularly in the 18-month to 4-year age group.

Clinical Findings

The major toxic effects of salicylate are (1) local gastrointestinal irritation, (2) direct stimulation of the central nervous system respiratory center, (3) increased metabolic rate, (4) interference with carbohydrate metabolism through the inhibition of several Krebs cycle enzymes and the uncoupling of oxidative phosphorylation, and (5) interference with normal blood coagulation mechanisms.

The net disturbance in hydrogen ion concentration in salicylism is the product of two simultaneously occurring challenges to acid-base homeostasis. Central nervous system–mediated inappropriate hyperpnea may lead to respiratory alkalosis. Deranged carbohydrate metabolism and dehydration are potent stimuli for metabolic acidosis. In either event, the carbon dioxide content of the blood is reduced. In children under 4 years of age, metabolic acidosis generally predominates on clinical presentation; in older children and adults, however, the patient frequently has respiratory alkalosis. Profound acidemia in older children and adults heralds a poor prognosis. Hyperthermia, resulting from the increased and disregulated metabolic state, is common.

The clinical findings of hyperglycemia, hyperpnea, polyuria, glucosuria, and ketonuria early in the course of intoxication closely simulate diabetic ketoacidosis. In salicylism, however, it is unusual for the blood glucose to exceed 200 mg/dl. Hypoglycemia may supervene as glycogen stores are depleted. Dehydration causing decreased renal blood flow often results in oliguria later in the course. Hypokalemia is common and total body stores of potassium are often depleted.

Therapy

Therapy has three objectives: (1) prevention of further salicylate absorption, (2) correction of existent solute and fluid deficits, and (3) reduction of tissue salicylate levels. Prevention of further salicylate absorption is achieved by removing salicylate from the gastrointestinal tract through lavage or induced emesis or by binding the medication within the gastrointestinal lumen through the administration of activated charcoal. Gastric emptying should be employed regardless of the time since ingestion.

The initial consideration in fluid therapy is the establishment of an adequate circulating fluid volume. In the presence of shock or impending shock, an isotonic solution should be administered at a rate of 20 ml/kg/hr. This may be safely continued a second hour in the absence of improved tissue perfusion. Lactated Ringer solution may be required for volume expansion in children with moderate to severe metabolic acidosis. Blood pressure, pulse, capillary filling, and in extreme circumstances, central venous pressure are effective monitors of therapeutic efficacy.

The correction of existent solute and water deficits may require total fluid volumes from 115 ml/kg/24 hr to 250 ml/kg/24 hr. A solution containing 40 to 50 mEq/L of sodium should be used. A urine volume of 2000 ml/m^2/day and a specific gravity less than 1.010 (300 mmol/liter) are reasonable goals.

Both hypokalemia and hypoglycemia can present life-threatening situations. A minimum of 25 mEq/L of potassium should be included once adequate renal function has been established; all intravenous fluids should include a minimum of 5 g/dl of glucose; with hypoglycemia or neurologic symptomatology, the use of 10 g/dl of glucose should be considered. Correction of acidemia is essential to the lowering of tissue salicylate levels; moreover, the establishment of an alkaline urine dramatically increases urine salicylate excretion. The use of an osmotic diuretic such as mannitol to ensure a high urine volume engenders the risk of increasing existent fluid deficits and is not recommended. The use of acetazolamide to block urine acidification and to facilitate an alkaline urine engenders the risk of accentuating existent metabolic acidosis, so it is not recommended.

Peritoneal dialysis and hemodialysis are effective therapies for serum salicylate values in excess of 100 mg/dl, coma, renal insufficiency, or failure of response to conservative therapy. Use of these techniques should be limited to physicians experienced with this technical procedure.

ACETAMINOPHEN

Ingestion of acetaminophen is a common cause of death among adults and adolescents with suicidal intent. Although 75% of the acetaminophen ingestions reported by the AAPCC from 1983 through 1988 occurred in children under 6 years of age, less than 5% of the fatalities reported were in that age range. The three fatalities under 6 years of age were a result of therapeutic misuse; one fatal accidental ingestion occurred in a 9-year-old.

More than 90% of an ingested acetaminophen load is inactivated in the liver through conjugation with sulfate or glucuronide. A third hepatic metabolic pathway dependent on cytochrome P-450 detoxifies acetaminophen through conjugation with glutathione. This pathway will produce a variety of hepatotoxic metabolites from acetaminophen if the hepatic glutathione reserves are depleted. Diminished toxicity occurs in children under 6 years of age as a result of relatively increased glutathione stores or lessened metabolic detoxification by the P-450 pathway. Comparable toxic doses are five to 10 times more likely to result in hepatotoxicity in the child over 6 years of age.

Clinical Findings and Therapy

During the first 24 hours after ingestion, the child with toxic plasma levels of acetaminophen may have anorexia, nausea, and vomiting. A latent period follows during which gastrointestinal symptoms resolve concurrent with evolving liver function abnormalities in the untreated individual. The transaminases, bilirubin levels, and prothrombin time peak 2 to 4 days after ingestion; fulminant hepatic failure may intervene. Children who survive the hepatic insult have no clinical or pathologic sequelae.

N-acetylcysteine functions as a specific antidote through its substitution for glutathione in the P-450–dependent pathway. The decision to use N-acetylcysteine is based on the plasma acetaminophen level at least 4 hours after ingestion (Fig. 285-2).[7] Individuals at risk for hepatotoxicity should receive therapy. Maximum benefit is realized if N-acetylcysteine is begun within 16 hours of the ingestion. It is reasonable to begin therapy without a plasma level if a significant ingestion has occurred (greater than 125 to 150 mg/kg in a child under 6 years of age) and if a level will not be available within the first 16 hours after ingestion. A loading of 140 mg/kg of N-acetylcysteine is given orally, followed by 17 doses of 70 mg/kg at 4-hour intervals. Following an ingestion, the gastric contents should be evacuated; catharsis may be considered to remove the drug from the lower gastrointestinal tract. Activated charcoal adsorbs N-acetylcysteine and should not be administered if antidotal therapy is imminently contemplated. However, with mixed drug ingestions, activated charcoal should be administered; if the acetaminophen level proves to be high enough to produce hepatic toxicity, the charcoal can be removed by gastric lavage.

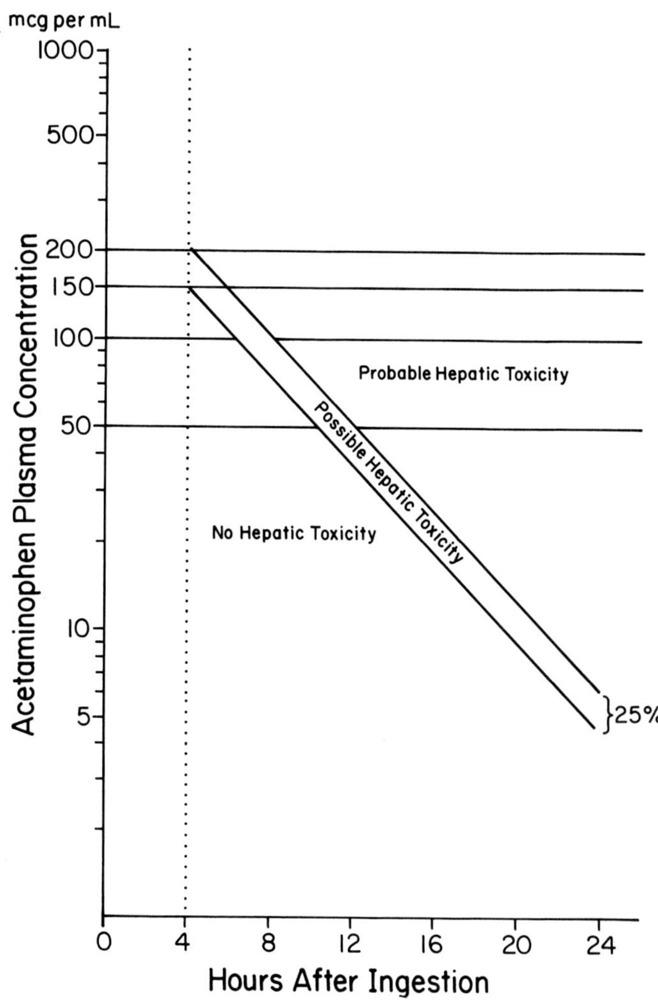

Fig. 285-2 Rumack-Matthew nomogram for estimating the probability of hepatic toxicity following a single acute acetaminophen ingestion. The lower solid diagonal line is placed 25% below the upper solid diagonal line, which divides the "no hepatic toxicity" area. This allows for potential errors in estimating the time following ingestion of the acetaminophen and potential errors in the measurement of acetaminophen plasma levels.

Adapted from Rumack BH and Matthew H: Acetaminophen poisoning and toxicity, Pediatr 55:871, 1975.

ORGANOPHOSPHATES

Pesticides continue to be a source of serious poisoning in children in both rural and urban settings. It is essential that the particular substance be identified or that the particular chemical group into which it falls be identified. Standard references are invaluable in this regard.[3]

Organophosphates account for most reported pesticide exposures and most deaths from such exposures. These insecticides, with few exceptions, are highly toxic to humans. Since organophosphates are readily absorbed from the skin, lungs, and gastrointestinal tract, they need not be ingested to cause symptoms of toxicity. Contaminated clothing can lead to symptoms.

Organophosphate insecticides and their metabolic byproducts inhibit acetylcholinesterase. The result is the accumulation of unhydrolyzed acetylcholine. This causes excessive and continued stimulation and then depression of the parasympathetic nervous system, the somatic motor nerves, and the central nervous system.

Clinical Findings

The clinical manifestations of organophosphate poisoning are protean. Stimulation of the autonomic nervous system leads to increased sweating, salivation, and miosis. Bradycardia may develop. There is an increase in bronchial secretions and bronchial constriction with resultant cough, dyspnea, and cyanosis. Pulmonary edema may occur. Gastrointestinal symptoms include vomiting, abdominal cramps, and intestinal hypermotility. Effects on striated muscle are evidenced by incoordination, tremors, and weakness, then muscle fasciculations followed by paralysis, particularly of the respiratory muscles. Central nervous system manifestations are headache, confusion, anxiety, emotional lability, ataxia, convulsions, coma, and eventual depression of the respiratory and circulatory centers. Hypotension or hypertension may be seen.

Children who are significantly poisoned commonly exhibit pinpoint pupils, excessive respiratory tract secretions, central nervous system excitement or depression, and respiratory arrest. The onset of symptoms may be extremely rapid, and death generally occurs within 24 hours. After sublethal doses, with reversal of inhibition of cholinesterase, the symptoms disappear; the rate of recovery varies with different compounds, from a few hours to several weeks.

Diagnosis

Once thought of, the diagnosis of organophosphate poisoning is not difficult to make. The diagnosis should be made on the basis of (1) history of exposure or a reasonable possibility of exposure, (2) the onset of symptoms within 12 hours of exposure, and (3) a clinical picture consistent with this diagnosis. In addition, these insecticides have a disagreeable garliclike odor, and children who have been poisoned may have a garliclike odor on their clothes or breath. Confirmation of this diagnosis can be made by drawing blood for serum and red cell cholinesterase determinations before therapy is begun. Although serum concentrations (pseudocholinesterase) are measured in most hospitals, many hospitals are not prepared to do the more specific erythrocyte (true cholinesterase) determination. Treatment should be initiated without waiting for laboratory results.

Therapy

Treatment of organophosphate poisoning involves both general measures and specific antidotes. If the skin has been exposed, all clothing should be removed and the skin washed with copious amounts of soap and water. If intoxication has resulted from ingestion, the gastric contents should be emptied. Health care providers should avoid contact with the vomitus or lavage fluid. Activated charcoal absorbs many of the organophosphates. The oronasopharynx should be cleared of secretions and an airway inserted. Endotracheal intubation and mechanical ventilation may be required to treat respiratory depression. Atropine 0.05 to 0.10 mg/kg should be administered every 10 to 30 minutes until complete atropinization (clearing of excessive oral and pulmonary secretions) and the reversal of cholinergic signs has been achieved. Atropinization should be maintained for 24 to 48 hours with intermittent dosing. Atropine blocks the action of acetylcholine without restoring the action of cholinesterase. After atropinization, in moderate to severe intoxication, pralidoxime (Protopam or 2-PAM), a cholinesterase reactivator, 25 to 50 mg/kg (up to 0.5 to 1 g) should be given intravenously in saline solution over 15 to 30 minutes. The dose may be repeated in 1 to 2 hours if muscular weakness does not resolve and every 6 to 8 hours thereafter if symptoms warrant. Pralidoxime does not cross the blood-brain barrier; reversal of central nervous system symptoms is dependent on atropine therapy. Pralidoxime is of minimal benefit if given more than 36 to 48 hours after exposure.

Atropine should be slowly tapered under close observation and reinstituted if symptoms recur. Observation for a minimum of 24 hours is necessary after the cessation of atropine and pralidoxime therapy. The use of aminophyllines, loop diuretics, phenothiazines, and morphine in the management of the signs of organophosphate poisoning are contraindicated. These and other drugs affect acetylcholine metabolism.

PSYCHOACTIVE DRUGS

Sedatives, Hypnotics, Anxiolytics, and Opiates

Clinical Findings. Central nervous system (CNS) depression (e.g., somnolence, stupor, coma) may constitute the presenting signs for patients with toxicity resulting from the ingestion of sedatives, hypnotics, anxiolytics, or opiates. There are frequently no distinguishing clinical features. Occasionally, a constellation of findings may suggest a specific drug class. Hypotension and respiratory depression are frequently seen following ingestion of toxic quantities of barbiturates or a glutethimide; they are occasionally observed with phenothiazine or methaqualone poisoning and are quite unusual with benzodiazepine ingestion. Hypothermia is usually associated with the ingestion of barbiturates or a glutethimide. Pulmonary edema frequently complicates the course of poisoning by glutethimide or methaqualone and occasionally is seen with barbiturate poisoning. Seizures, opisthotonos, and torticollis are frequently observed with phenothiazine poisoning; myoclonus, hypertonia, and increased reflexes are associated with methaqualone intoxication. Focal and rapidly changing neurologic symptoms and signs are characteristic of glutethimide poisoning. Opiate overdose classically shows respiratory and CNS depression and miosis; pulmonary edema, hypertension, and hypothermia also occur. Cyclic variations in the depth of coma with multiple episodes of abrupt onset of apnea are common with poisoning by these drugs; fixed, dilated pupils with anisocoria may also be seen and do not necessarily indicate a grave prognosis.

Central nervous system depression resulting from the opiates or pentazocine is safely and effectively reversed by the narcotic antagonist naloxone hydrochloride (Narcan). Reversal of central nervous system depression by naloxone has also been reported in patients poisoned by diphenoxylate (Lomotil) and propoxyphene (Darvon). Naloxone has no agonist activity. It is administered intravenously, 0.01 mg/kg; this dose can be safely repeated without fear of increasing respiratory depression and can be safely and effectively used empirically in patients with coma of unknown origin.

Therapy. Supportive care is the mainstay of therapy for patients with coma resulting from poisoning that has not responded to naloxone therapy. Immediate attention is directed to stabilization and maintenance of ventilation and perfusion. Patients in coma require intubation. Atelectasis and aspiration pneumonia are frequently complications of coma from poisoning. Gastric lavage late in the course of ingestion-induced coma is hazardous and of questionable efficacy; it should be undertaken only after a protected airway has been carefully secured. Hypotension resulting from barbiturate ingestion is generally caused by decreased peripheral vascular resistance and hypovolemia and usually responds to plasma volume expansion. The frequency of pulmonary edema as a complication of methaqualone or glutethimide poisoning precludes rapid fluid administration in these poisonings in the absence of careful central venous pressure monitoring. In the profoundly ill, comatose, poisoned patient, a central venous pressure monitor is essential. Analeptic drugs are not indicated in the management of poison-induced coma. Forced diuresis, with alkalinization of the urine to achieve ion trapping, is effective in facilitating clearance of phenobarbital but is of no value in treating poisoning from the short-acting barbiturates and is contraindicated in the management of methaqualone poisoning.

Phencyclidine, Amphetamine, and Cocaine

Poisoning by phencyclidine (PCP) is characterized by aggressive, even assaultive, behavior, which may seriously impede evaluation and therapy of the gravely ill patient. Symptoms and signs may include confusion, irritability, hallucinations, tremor, chest pain, palpitations, hypertension, tachycardia, auditory hyperesthesia, sweating, excessive salivation, anxiety, panic, hyperpyrexia, hyperreflexia, and rhabdomyolysis. Coma and convulsions occur with severe poisoning. Psychotic states (which may persist), nystagmus (horizontal or vertical), increased muscle tone (which may be associated with opisthotonos), and fixed staring are prominent features of PCP intoxication.

Amphetamines and cocaine, although structurally different, are powerful CNS stimulants. Abuse of cocaine, particularly the free-base form, "crack," which can be smoked, has reached epidemic proportions. Cocaine deaths reported to the AAPCC more than doubled between 1987 and 1988. Severe morbidity or death may occur from high-dose chronic or "binge" use or may occur after a single exposure. Intoxication results in a sense of enhanced energy, which may progress to violent and bizarre behavior, delirium, seizures, paranoia, agitation, and death. Adverse effects include systemic hypertension, tachycardia and other cardiac arrhythmias, hyperthermia, and respiratory depression. Myocardial infarction, stroke, aortic rupture, and rhabdomyolysis have been reported.

Therapy. Immediate therapy includes careful limitation of sensory stimuli and supportive care. Seizures may be difficult to control. Diazepam is the preferred anticonvulsant. Diazoxide or hydralazine is preferred for the management of hypertension. Additional alpha-adrenergic blocking drugs (phentolamine) may be required. It has been suggested that propranolol has specific antagonist activity for PCP. Chlorpromazine, highly useful in the treatment of amphetamine poisoning, is contraindicated in PCP intoxication. Amphetamine and PCP levels in the central nervous system can be reduced and excretion in the urine increased by acidification to achieve ion trapping. Careful monitoring of serum pH, potassium, and ammonia levels is required. In addition, it is important to interrupt the gastroenteric recirculation of PCP by initiating continuous gastric drainage (independent of the PCP's route of administration).

Tricyclic Antidepressants

The widespread use, accessibility, and toxicity of the tricyclic antidepressants imipramine, amitriptyline, nortriptyline, desipramine, amoxapine, maprotiline, protriptyline, and doxepin make these medications the most common cause of fatal ingestion in individuals under 17. Tricyclics are used for depression in adults and adolescents; several are used to treat enuresis and hyperkinesis in children. In excess of 95% of the fatal ingestions by adolescents reported by the AAPCC between 1983 and 1988 were suicides. Accidental ingestion and therapeutic misuse predominate in the younger population.

Clinical Findings. Patients have anticholinergic effects, such as dry mouth and skin, mydriasis, urinary retention, fever, and delirium; tricyclic poisoning should be suspected when hypotension and cardiac arrhythmias or coma are present. Evidence of central nervous system toxicity may include initial excitement that progresses to coma; myoclonus or choreoathetosis, central respiratory depression, and seizures also occur. The primary cause of death in tricyclic overdose is cardiac malfunction; arrhythmias and myocardial depression are common.

Therapy. Initial treatment of tricyclic ingestion is aimed at removing the gastric contents. The alert patient should have emesis induced; the obtunded patient should receive gastric lavage. The decreased gastric motility secondary to the anticholinergic effects of the ingestion makes gastric decontamination beneficial up to 18 hours after the ingestion. Repeated administration of activated charcoal should follow gastric emptying. All patients should be hospitalized for continuous electrocardiogram monitoring, preferably in an intensive care unit. The pharmacokinetics of tricyclic ingestion are complex. Drug levels should not be used as the sole criterion for therapeutic intervention; initial management should be based on the patient's clinical status. A QRS complex of greater than 100 milliseconds is the most reliable indicator of tricyclic toxicity. This occurs in patients with tricyclic levels greater than 1000 ng/ml. A decreasing QRS interval correlates with decreasing drug levels.

Treatment of intoxication from tricyclics is symptomatic and supportive. Hypotension should be treated initially by intravenous fluid challenges. Norepinephrine is recommended as a pressor agent if volume therapy is insufficient. Because the cardiac arrhythmias are potentiated by acidosis, bicarbonate should be continuously administered to raise the blood pH to 7.45 to 7.5. Phenytoin is the mainstay of antiarrhythmic therapy. Although lidocaine and propranolol may potentiate myocardial depression, they are useful in selected situations. Direct ventricular pacing may be necessary. Procainamide, quinidine, and disopyrimide are contraindicated. Seizures, which may be difficult to control, respond best to intravenous diazepam. Although physostigmine readily reverses the anticholinergic signs of tricyclic overdose, it is generally ineffective in the therapy of arrhythmias and can cause myocardial depression, asystole, and seizures. Its use should be reserved for situations in which other therapies have failed.

HOUSEHOLD CLEANING AGENTS AND CAUSTICS

Household disinfectants and cleaning agents (e.g., ammonia and bleach, laundry detergent, automatic dishwater detergent, and oven, drain, and toilet cleaners) contain variable amounts of acidic or alkaline caustics. The severity of damage to the oropharynx, esophagus, and stomach upon ingestion depends on the volume and concentration of the caustic and its duration of contact with the mucosal surfaces. The concentration of the caustic must be determined through history, examination of the container, or consultation with a regional poison control center if at all possible.

Household bleach (sodium hypochlorite), weak ammonia solutions, and phosphate-based laundry detergents usually don't cause tissue damage but may cause mucosal irritation. Industrial-strength ammonia, bleaches, and detergents brought to the home from the work place constitute a significant hazard. Ecologically sound "low phosphate" detergents containing carbonates and other alkaline agents, such as trisodium phosphate, and dishwater detergents have a high pH and may destroy tissue. Most caustic injuries are caused by ingestion of liquid or particulate alkaline drain or oven cleaners. Recent reductions in the alkali concentration of liquid cleaners to the 8% to 10% range have reduced but not eliminated morbidity.

Clinical Findings

Alkali ingestions generally result in greater tissue destruction than do acid ingestions. The bitter taste and instantaneous burning sensation associated with strong acids limit the volume of the ingestion and prompt immediate expectoration. A greater volume of the relatively tasteless liquid alkaline preparation may be swallowed before the child experiences significant distress. Acid mucosal injury results in a coagulation necrosis, with the formation of a dense eschar that tends to limit tissue penetration. The liquefaction neurosis characteristic of an alkali injury permits deep penetration of the alkali through the mucosa, submucosa, and muscular layers of the upper gastrointestinal tract. Acidic agents generally cause greater damage to the gastric mucosa, particularly the lesser curvature and the prepyloric area; alkaline ingestions result in greater damage to the esophagus. Liquid ingestions often produce circumferential burns; particulate ingestion spotty or streaklike burns. The intense inflammatory response may cause acute or subacute viscus perforation or stricture formation 14 to 28 days after the ingestion.

The patient may be in severe distress, with drooling, inability or refusal to swallow, abdominal pain, and violent retching. Air hunger and stridor may result from burns and subsequent edema of the glottic structures. There may be circumferential or patchy burns or ulcerations of the oral mucosa, with edema of the oral and pharyngeal tissues. Significant ingestions may show minimal symptomatology. Esophageal damage with the potential for stricture formation may occur in the complete absence of oral lesions.

Therapy

Management is supportive and expectant. Induction of emesis is contraindicated. The child should be kept upright to minimize vomiting and reflux. If the child is able to swallow, several ounces of water or milk may be given to dilute the poison. Attempts to neutralize an alkali ingestion with a mild acid such as vinegar are contraindicted because the resulting exothermal reaction will result in further tissue damage.

Endoscopy should be performed on all patients with a history of caustic ingestion. The efficacy of steroids (methylprednisolone 2 mg/kg/day) to reduce the inflammatory response and subsequent potential for stricture formation is based on anecdotal data. H_2-blockers may be used to suppress gastric acid production and secondary gastric or esophageal acid injury. Parenteral fluid therapy and antibiotics are used as clinically indicated. Bougienage may be used to prevent or dilate strictures. Long-term morbidity results from esophageal or pyloric strictures and the attempts to maintain patency through chronic dilation or surgical reconstruction.

HYDROCARBONS

Hydrocarbon ingestion is a leading cause of death from poisoning with household products. Hydrocarbons include petroleum distillates such as gasoline, kerosene, mineral seal oil, lighter fluids, paint thinners, and pine oil derivatives such as turpentine. Deaths from hydrocarbon poisoning are the result of pulmonary involvement.

Pulmonary Complications

The pulmonary complications of hydrocarbon ingestions are the result of aspiration into the tracheobronchial tree. With significant ingestions, symptoms usually begin within 30 minutes and are often associated with choking, gagging, and vomiting. Signs of pulmonary involvement include grunting respirations, a persistent nonproductive cough, intercostal retractions, cyanosis, tachypnea, tachycardia, and fever. Rales, rhonchi, or diminished breath sounds may be heard. Frequently the sensorium is depressed, and the odor of the ingested hydrocarbon can be smelled on the breath. A depressed sensorium signifies hypoxemia. Signs and symptoms of respiratory involvement usually peak in the first 24 hours and then regress over the next 2 to 5 days.

Radiographic Findings

The risk of aspiration depends on the chemical and physical properties of the hydrocarbons ingested. Low surface tension allows a hydrocarbon to spread rapidly over the mucosal surfaces, and low viscosity enables deeper penetration of the fluids into the distal airways. Highly volatile hydrocarbons cause acute chemical pneumonitis. Highly viscous, nonvolatile petroleum distillates such as mineral oil, motor oil, most baby oils, and liquid petrolatum are not often aspirated and do not cause chemical pneumonitis unless large amounts are aspirated.

Chest roentgenographic changes can be seen as early as 30 minutes after ingestion. Initially there are multiple, small, mottled densities in the perihilar area that may extend into the midlung field. The mottled densities may become confluent and give a picture of consolidation. Lower airway obstruction with air trapping is often evident. Pleural effusions may develop. Occasionally, pneumatoceles form. Correlation between the chest roentgenographic findings and the clinical symptoms is poor. Whereas approximately 75% of patients who have ingested hydrocarbons will exhibit roentgenographic evidence of lung involvement, only 25% to 50% of these will have respiratory symptoms.

Therapy

Management of hydrocarbon ingestion is nonspecific, symptomatic, and supportive. Since aspiration is the principal hazard, vomiting should not be induced. Gastric lavage is not recommended. (Hydrocarbons that act as carriers for heavy metals or insecticides, as well as certain halogenated or aromatic hydrocarbons that are toxic systemically such as carbon tetrachloride or benzene, should be evacuated from the stomach.) Patients who are asymptomatic should be observed for up to 6 hours after ingestion. Patients who have respiratory symptoms warrant hospitalization. Oxygen administration, humidification of inspired air, and intravenous fluids should be instituted. The severely symptomatic patient may require mechanical ventilation with positive end-expiratory pressure. Adrenocorticosteroids have not been effective in preventing or ameliorating pulmonary complications and are not recommended. Leukocytosis and hyperpyrexia are common findings in hydrocarbon aspiration without infection. The use of antimicrobial therapy is not routinely warranted. In the very toxic patient with extensive pneumonitis or in the patient compromised by underlying disease or debilitation, the use of antimicrobials during the acute stage of the illness may be justified. Damage to the pulmonary clearance mechanisms and aspiration of oral flora may infrequently cause a secondary bacterial pneumonia.

PLANTS

Because definitive identification of the ingested plant is usually not available, most practitioners find the management of plant ingestions confusing and frustrating. Most plants produce minimal symptoms in the quantities usually ingested. Fatalities are quite rare. In doubtful situations, most physicians prefer to empty the stomach. Activated charcoal adsorbs many plant toxins.

The most commonly reported ingestions involve members of the arum family (dieffenbachia, philodendron, caladium, colocasia). These plants contain needlelike calcium oxalate crystals, which produce intense mucosal irritation. Although treatment at home with a demulcent usually suffices, upper airway obstruction occurs in rare cases and can be life threatening. Corneal damage may result from contact with the crystals. Oleander and lily of the valley contain cardiac glycosides similar to foxglove's digitalis. Digitalis toxicity has occurred following ingestions of these plants, particularly if they are used in the brewing of "herbal" tea.

Jimsonweed (locoweed, angel trumpets) contains belladonna alkaloids that produce anticholinergic symptoms. Therapy with physostigmine may be required but should not be employed for mild symptomatology. Mistletoe berries, Jerusalem cherries, and holly berries represent seasonal hazards and may poison when consumed in quantity; lavage or induced emesis is then indicated. The ingestion of poinsettias usually does not result in symptoms but is occasionally followed by oral or anal irritation or mild gastrointestinal symptoms. Improperly prepared pokeweed (pokeweed salad) produces severe gastrointestinal symptoms and occasionally neurotoxicity. Dangerously poisonous plants occasionally ingested include castor bean, precatory bean (jequirity bean, rosary pea), and lantana berry. Ingestion of water hemlock, a violent plant toxin, may result in the rapid onset of seizures and death.

Most toad stools that grow in the yard are not poisonous. Mushroom poisoning is most common with mycetophiles and their families. Because wild mushrooms are difficult to identify accurately, all such ingestions must be considered potentially toxic. Appropriate supportive management should follow induced emesis, catharsis, and the administration of activated charcoal.

VITAMINS

The accidental ingestion of modest amounts of the routinely used pediatric multiple vitamins with or without fluoride (not containing iron) does not present a toxic risk. Ingestions of fluoride of 8 to 16 mg/kg of body weight has been associated with nausea, vomiting, diarrhea, and abdominal pain. Fluoride ingestions in excess of 32 to 64 mg/kg of body weight result in convulsions, cardiac arrhythmias, and coma and are frequently fatal. The standard toothpaste preparations present minimal risk of acute toxicity. There has been a fatality following failure to comply with a dentist's request of the patient to expectorate 4% stannous fluoride solution, a topical fluoride used to prevent caries.

Toxicity may result from the chronic ingestion of excess quantities of both vitamin A and vitamin D. Excess intake of vitamin D may result in renal damage secondary to nephrocalcinosis, as well as hypercalcemia, bone pain, nausea, and vomiting. Chronic ingestion of excessive vitamin A may result in skin changes, hair loss, cortical thickening of tubular bones, and anorexia.

Acute intoxication with vitamin A results in the abrupt onset of increased intracranial pressure (pseudotumor cerebri). Symptoms include drowsiness, irritability, severe headache, and vomiting. A bulging fontanel may be present in infants. Desquamation, usually beginning around the mouth, may follow over the next few days. Induced emesis or gastric lavage should be considered in patients who have ingested 100,000 units or more of vitamin A.

Toxicity from excessive ingestion of watersoluble vitamins has been reported, usually in association with fad diets or megavitamin "ortho molecular" therapy. Doses of pyridoxine, vitamin B-6, in excess of 2 g per day, cause peripheral nerve degeneration. Excessive dosing of vitamin C may result in chronic diarrhea and kidney stone formation.

IRON

Ingestion of iron-containing medications, particularly the commonly prescribed maternal prenatal 325 mg ferrous sulfate (65 mg elemental iron) tablets, is a major cause of death among accidental ingestions by toddlers. Lack of widespread public appreciation of the toxicity of iron and the close resemblance of prenatal ferrous sulfate to M & M brand candies contribute to the incidence of this common ingestion.

Iron has a direct corrosive effect on the small bowel and gastric mucosa. The lesion is pathologically similar to the coagulation necrosis caused by acid ingestions. Significant ingestions cause severe abdominal pain, diarrhea, vomiting, and gastrointestinal hemorrhage. Shock may ensue as a result of the hemorrhage and attendant coagulopathy; significant hypovolemia can occur secondary to "third spacing" of fluid in the injured bowel in the absence of hemorrhage. Free iron in the circulation causes disregulation of the coagulation cascade. Inhibition of cellular oxidative metabolism and the conversion of ferrous ions to ferric ions in the circulation may intensify the metabolic acidosis. Acute hepatic failure may complicate the course of acute iron poisoning. Scarring and stricture formation, usually at the pylorus, may occur as late as 4 to 6 weeks after the ingestion. The asymptomatic or quiescent period traditionally described as occurring after the gastrointestinal symptoms have subsided and before the onset of shock may represent a failure to recognize early signs of hypovolemia.

Therapy

The minimal toxic dose is 20 to 60 mg of elemental iron per kilogram of body weight. Ingestions in this range or greater should be managed with gastric emptying by induced emesis or gastric lavage. Gastric lavage with disodium phosphate solutions (Fleets enema) is contraindicated; severe phosphate poisoning has resulted. Lavage with a 1% to 5% solution of sodium bicarbonate has been recommended, but this practice is of questionable efficacy. The instillation of 5 to 10 g of deferoxamine following the completion of lavage is controversial. A plain roentgenogram of the abdomen is helpful in detecting residual iron tablets. Large concentrations of iron tablets in the stomach or small bowel may require gastrotomy or whole bowel lavage for removal.

Serum iron concentrations in excess of 500 μg/dl, measured 4 to 6 hours post ingestion, are associated with a significant risk of shock; levels under 300 μg/dl are often tolerated. Ingested doses exceeding 60 mg per kilogram of body weight are usually associated with toxic levels. Symptomatic individuals with levels greater than 300 μg/dl and all individuals with levels greater than 500 μg/dl should receive chelation therapy.

The slow, continuous intravenous infusion of deferoxamine at 15 mg/kg/hr usually causes the color of the urine to change to "vin rose" in the intoxicated individual. Chelation should be continued until the urine color returns to normal. Lack of a urine color change in severely poisoned children (levels greater than 500 μg/dl), particularly in those with early shock or with decreased urine output, can occur. Those children should receive intravenous chelation until the serum iron level is below 300 μg/dl. Supportive care with early intensive management of shock through volume therapy is essential.

LEAD POISONING

Lead poisoning (plumbism) in the young child is a chronic disease. Although leaded gasoline emissions into the atmosphere constitute the preponderant industrial lead burden on society, the ingestion of lead-based paint chips and paint-soaked plaster and putty remain the most significant source of high-dose lead exposure for young children. Dirt contaminated by automobile emissions along congested urban thoroughfares and household dust from crumbling wall fixtures constitute "intermediate dose" sources of lead for the toddler through hand contamination and repetitive mouthing.

Toxicity has resulted from a variety of less common exposures. Water and food contamination can result from lead-soldered plumbing systems or containers. Acidic foods and beverages can be contaminated through storage in improperly lead-glazed ceramic ware. Smelter dust, the contaminated work clothing of lead-acid storage battery factory workers, and the burning of discarded battery casings are a hazard. Slow absorption from ingested lead weights, sinkers, and retained bullets or shotgun pellets may result in poisoning. Certain Mexican-American and Asian Indian folk remedies may contain up to 86% lead by weight. The recurrent intentional inhalation of leaded gasoline for recreation by Native Americans has resulted in encephalopathy.

Physiologic Effects

Blood lead levels reflect the equilibrium among absorption, excretion, and soft tissue and bone pools. A variable percentage of ingested lead, 5% to 10% in adults and up to 50% in younger children, is absorbed. Iron and calcium deficiency and the excessive dietary intake of fat potentiate gastrointestinal lead absorption. Respiratory absorption of lead depends on particle size. Lead is excreted at a relatively limited rate in the urine, bile, and sweat. Ingestion of greater than 5 mg/

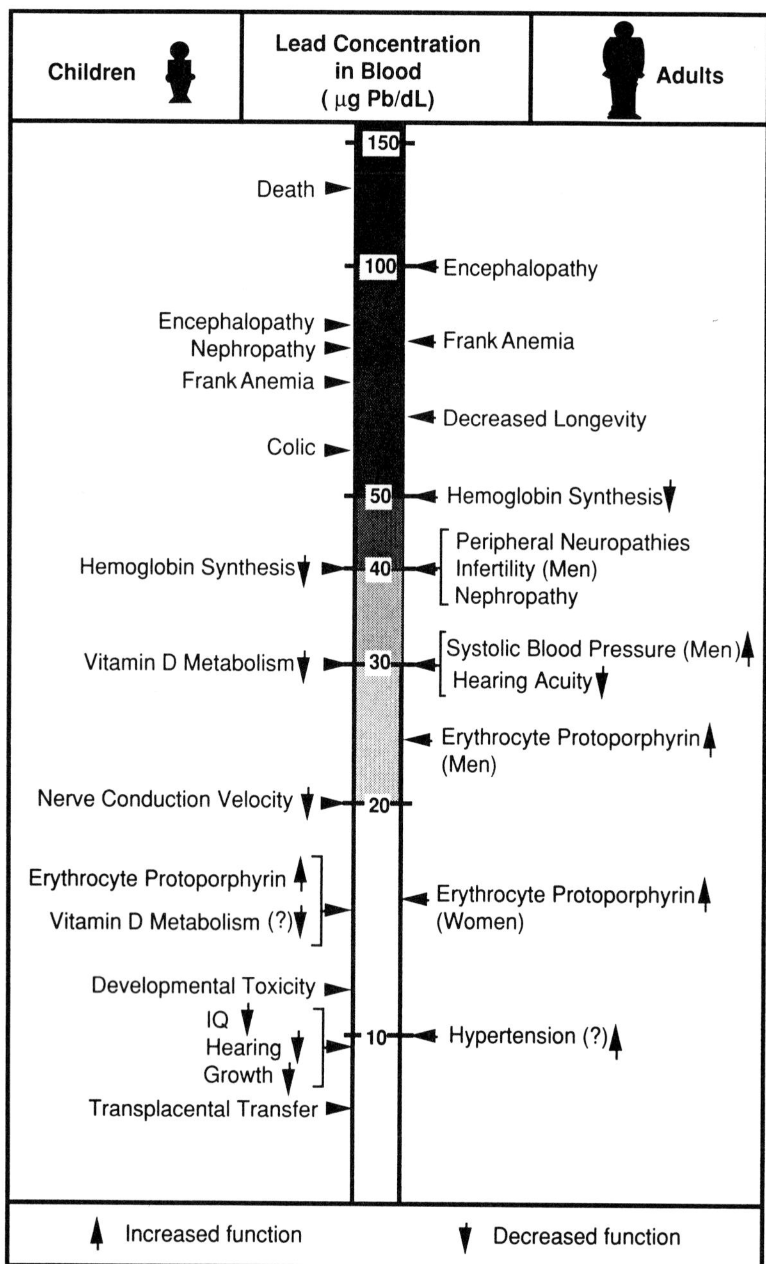

- **Effects in children generally occur at lower blood lead levels than in adults.**
- **The developing nervous system in children can be affected adversely at blood lead levels of less than 10 μg/dL.**

Fig. 285-3 Effects of inorganic lead on children and adults—lowest observable adverse effect levels.
From Agency for Toxic Substances and Disease Registry, U.S. Department of Health and Human Services.

kg of body weight per day will generally result in retention, which will result in increased tissue levels and toxic effects on bone marrow, kidneys, and nervous system and deposition of lead in bone.

Lead in soft tissues has serious but reversible effects on hemoglobin production, renal function, and vitamin D metabolism. Lead interferes with the biosynthesis of heme, leading to decreased activity of delta-aminolevuline acid dehydratase, increased erythrocyte protoporphyrin levels, and increased excretion of coproporphyrin in urine. Globin synthesis is also impaired. The effect on the bone marrow is confounded by the frequent coexistence of iron-deficiency anemia. A reversible Fanconi syndrome (hypophosphatemia with hyperphosphaturia, glycosuria, and generalized aminoaciduria), caused by proximal renal tubular damage, may be seen in acute poisoning.

Lead has irreversible effects on the central nervous system. Severe intoxication causes cerebral edema with resultant acute encephalopathy. Capillary permeability is increased with transudation of protein-containing fluid into the brain. There is necrosis of vessel walls, and petechial hemorrhages may be present. Neurons are irreversibly damaged. Lower-level intoxications result in mild neurologic disabilities. High-level intoxication causes peripheral nervous system injury with a motor neuropathy; lower-level exposure results in an asymptomatic decrease in motor nerve conduction velocity.

Diagnosis and Clinical Findings

The blood lead level reflects the risk of symptomatic lead intoxication and acute encephalopathy. The Centers for Disease Control (CDC) 1985 guidelines list four risk categories based on blood lead levels (PbB): class I ("normal"), PbB under 25 μg/dl; class II (moderate risk), PbB of 25 to 49 μg/dl; class III (high risk), PbB of 50 to 69 μg/dl; and class IV (urgent risk), PbB of 70 μg/dl or higher. Risk of neurologic damage increases, particularly for class III and class IV individuals, the longer the elevated levels are sustained. Erythrocyte protoporphyrin, as an index of the metabolic effect of lead poisoning, is often elevated in association with lead levels greater than 25 μg/dl. The frequent coexistence of iron deficiency in high-risk populations may account for some of the hematologic effects traditionally ascribed to lead intoxication. A minority of iron-sufficient class III and class IV individuals will have anemia or microcytosis.

The symptomatology of chronic lead poisoning is protean, nonspecific, and may wax and wane. Initial symptoms may include anorexia, constipation, and bouts of abdominal pain, nausea, and vomiting. Apathy, lethargy, and irritability may be mistaken for a primary behavioral disturbance. Incoordination, ataxia, and loss of recently acquired developmental milestones may occur. The process may abate or may progress to the gross ataxia, persistent vomiting, lethargy, coma, and intractable convulsions characteristic of acute encephalopathy. Absence of papilledema and vital sign changes does not exclude the possibility of cerebral edema in acute encephalopathy. A child may suffer recurrent symptomatic episodes without developing obvious acute encephalopathy. These nonspecific complaints may seem to be adequately explained by a minor intercurrent illness. A lumbar puncture is generally contraindicated because of the risks associated with increased intracranial pressure. Long-term sequelae of encephalopathy include seizure disorders, nonspecific mental retardation, and hyperkinetic behavior disorders. Widespread public recognition of the dangers of lead intoxication, screening programs, and the reduction of lead content in household paints have led to a dramatic reduction in the incidence of encephalopathy over the past 30 years.

There is a growing appreciation of the effects of low-level lead intoxication. Subtle neuropsychiatric deficits, distractibility, and diminution of IQ scores are statistically associated with lead levels below 25 μg/dl. Intrauterine exposure to maternal PbB levels of 10 to 15 μg/dl may result in quantifiable development delay. The threshold lead level below which adverse biologic effect does not occur has yet to be defined.

For further discussion of the public health problem presented by PbB levels between 10 and 25 μg/dl in our general population, see Chapter 18, Six, "Screening for Lead Poisoning."

Therapy

Chelation therapy is adjunctive to the most imperative intervention in lead poisoning: separation of the child from the source of lead. Acute encephalopathy is a medical emergency. In addition, because the course of encephalopathy is fulminant and its onset unpredictable, any child with an elevated PbB, particularly 50 μg/dl or higher, with symptoms potentially referable to lead should be treated as an emergency. CaEDTA, dimercaptopropanol (BAL), and D-penicillamine are the three chelating agents used to treat plumbism. Piomelli and Chisholm[5] have extensively described the protocols for inpatient chelation therapy of children with lead poisoning. It is essential to consult such a reference before treating children to appreciate the inherent dangers and precautions for such therapy. Their recommendations are summarized in Table 285-1.

The symptomatic or encephalopathic child should be hospitalized without oral intake. After cautious parenteral fluid therapy has established an adequate urine output, chelation may begin. Seizures may be initially controlled with diazepam. If plain roentgenograms of the abdomen demonstrate radiopaque flecks, usually in the region of the colon, signifying recent ingestion of foreign matter containing lead, the bowel should be evacuated. Metaphyseal lead lines present on roentgenogram signifying increased lead storage in bone are not related to the severity of symptoms. Renal and liver function and PbB levels should be monitored daily. Repeated cycles of chelation may be necessary to reduce the PbB levels to acceptable levels.

Initiation of chelation therapy for clinically asymptomatic children with an increased lead burden depends on the lead level. Asymptomatic children with a PbB level under 50 μg/dl should be evaluated with a CaEDTA provocation test. CaEDTA, 500 mg/m^2, is infused intravenously over 1 hour. An 8-hour urine collection should be obtained. A urinary level greater than 0.7 μg lead per milligram of CaEDTA given (CaEDTA provocation test ratio) indicates lead poisoning, and chelation therapy should be performed. This diagnostic test is hazardous in symptomatic cases and should be reserved for asymptomatic children.

Children receiving chelation therapy should not be released from the hospital until lead hazards in their environment are controlled or suitable alternative housing has been arranged. Exposure to aerosolized leaded dust during the deleading of a home containing lead-based paint is particularly hazardous, with the potential for precipitating encephalopathy in the lead-intoxicated child. Children must be excluded from the dwelling until the procedure is complete. Following chelation therapy, children are still at high risk and should have follow-up blood lead or erythrocyte protoporphyrin determinations or both at 1- to 2-week intervals until these levels stabilize or show a decline continually for at least 6 months. Thereafter, they should be followed-up at 1- to 3-month intervals until 6 years of age or longer to prevent repeated poisoning. Neurologic and psychological conditions should be assessed at the time of diagnosis and in the following years. Effective management of each case of lead poisoning should involve the sustained cooperation of health department personnel, the medical social worker, visiting nurse, and pediatrician.

The systematic screening of high-risk toddlers to detect lead deposits in soft tissue before symptoms occur is essential. (See Chapter 18, "Screening for Lead Poisoning.") Therapy does not prevent neurologic sequelae after the onset of encephalopathy.

Table 285-1 *Chelation Therapy of Lead Poisoning*

STATUS	THERAPY	COMMENTS
Encephalopathy	BAL* 75 mg/m² IM every 4 hr for 5 days	Give BAL 4 hr before CaEDTA infusion.
	CaEDTA† 1500 mg/m²/day IV over 6 hr for 5 days	Treat 5 additional days (after 2-day break) if PbB remains high. Additional cycles may be necessary depending on PbB rebound.
PbB of 70 μg/dl or higher or nonencephalopathic symptomatology	BAL 50 mg/m² IM every 4 hr for 3-5 days	Give BAL 4 hr before CaEDTA infusion. BAL may be stopped after 3 days if the PbB falls below 50 μg/dl.
	CaEDTA 1000 mg/m²/day IV over 6 yr for 5 days	Additional cycles may be necessary depending on PbB rebound.
PbB of 50 μg/dl or higher under 70 μg/dl	CaEDTA 1000 mg/m²/day IV over 6 hr for 5 days	Additional cycles may be necessary depending on PbB rebound.
PbB of 25 μg/dl or higher under 50 μg/dl		
CaEDTA provocation test‡ ratio over 0.70	CaEDTA 1000 mg/m²/day IV over 6 hr for 5 days	
CaEDTA provocation test ratio 0.60 to 0.69		
Age under 3 years	CaEDTA 1000 mg/m²/day IV	
Age over 3 years	No treatment	Repeat PbB and CaEDTA provocation periodically.
CaEDTA provocation test ratio under 0.60	No treatment	Repeat PbB and CaEDTA provocation periodically.

*Medicinal iron should not be given concurrently with BAL therapy.
†CaEDTA should never be used as the sole agent with PbB of 70 μg/dl or higher. Adequate diuresis is essential (IV or oral fluid) to minimize renal toxicity.
‡See text.
Adapted from Piomelli S et al: Management of childhood lead poisoning, J Pediatr 105:527, 1984.

REFERENCES

1. Arena JM: Poisoning: toxicology, symptoms, treatment, ed 4, Springfield, 1979, Charles C Thomas.
2. Done AK: Salicylate intoxication: significance of measurements of salicylate in blood in cases of acute ingestion, Pediatrics 26:800, 1960.
3. Gosselin RE et al: Clinical toxicology of commercial products, ed 5, Baltimore, 1984, Williams & Wilkins Co.
4. Litovitz TL, Schmitz BF, and Holm KC: 1988 annual report of the American Association of Poison Control Centers National Data Collection System, Am J Emerg Med 7:495, 1989.
5. Piomelli S et al: Management of childhood lead poisoning, J Pediatr 105:527, 1984.
6. Rumack BH: POISINDEX Information System, ed 62, Denver, 1989, Micromedex, Inc.
7. Rumack BH and Matthew H: Acetaminophen poisoning and toxicity, Pediatrics 55:871, 1975.

SUGGESTED READINGS

Bellinger D et al: Longitudinal analyses of prenatal and postnatal lead exposure and early cognitive development, N Engl J Med 316:1037, 1987.

Braden NJ, Jackson JE, and Walson PD: Tricyclic antidepressant overdose, Pediatr Clin North Am 33:287, 1986.

Clark M, Royal J, and Seeler R: Interaction of iron deficiency and lead and the hematologic findings in children with severe lead poisoning, Pediatrics 81:247, 1988.

Cregler LL and Mark H: Medical complications of cocaine abuse, N Engl J Med 315:1495, 1986.

Gilman AG, Goodman LS, and Gilman A: Goodman and Gilman's the pharmacological basis of therapeutics, ed 8, New York, 1990, Pergamon Press.

Lampe KF and McCann MA: AMA handbook of poisonous and injurious plants, Chicago, 1985, American Medical Association.

Mortenson ML: Management of acute childhood poisonings caused by selected insecticides and herbicides, Pediatr Clin North Am 33:421, 1986.

Needleman HL: The persistent threat of lead: a singular opportunity, Am J Public Health 79:643, 1989.

Peterson RG and Peterson LN: Cleansing the blood: hemodialysis, exchange transfusion, charcoal hemoperfusion, forced diuresis, Pediatr Clin North Am 33:675, 1986.

Report of the Subcommittee on Accidental Poisoning: Co-operative kerosene poisoning study: evaluation of gastric lavage and other factors in the treatment of accidental ingestion of petroleum distillate products, Pediatrics 29:648, 1962.

Rumack BH: Acetaminophen overdose in children, Pediatr Clin North Am 33:691, 1986.

286

Rape

Richard M. Sarles

Rape is a form of violent, physical assault and is not primarily a sexual act. Some professionals argue that any form of sexual abuse of children and adolescents should be considered rape. This is true in the broadest sense, since the one who assaults is usually older, more powerful, and therefore dominant, and the victim is generally younger, powerless, and forced to consent with little opportunity to resist. However, the context in which rape occurs, the dynamics of rape, and the acute and long-term sequelae appear to be distinct from other more common forms of sexual abuse and incest.

The exact incidence of rape during childhood and adolescent years is not known, yet studies indicate that approximately 50% of all rapes occur in females under 19 years of age with the majority occurring in the 14- to 17-year age group; appoximately 10% of rape cases occur in the prepubertal age group. However, it is important to recognize that these estimates are biased in that only one in five to one in ten rapes is actually reported. Contrary to popular belief, most rapes are not interracial, and the attacker is known to the victim in over 50% of all reported cases.

An alleged rape should be considered a medical and psychological emergency. A physical assault nearly always results in physical injury and psychological trauma. The serious connotations of sexual assault, with the invasion of areas of the body held as inviolate by society, creates the need for efficient, empathetic, and sensitive emergency medical and emotional care. Adolescent rape victims, with their particular concerns of body image, self-image, and sexual identity normal for this age, demand the greatest understanding and awareness on the part of the staff in order to preserve their dignity and privacy. Although the victim may be seen in settings ranging from a private practitioner's office to a large urban medical center, and although legal codes may vary in different localities, the physician's and medical team's responsibility is to render treatment for the physical and emotional sequelae of the rape and to collect evidence that can be used in any legal proceedings.

When a female child or adolescent rape victim comes to a medical facility, she and her family should be escorted immediately from the waiting room to a private examining room. Ideally, a female nurse or member of a sexual abuse team should remain with the girl during the entire examination. The nurse should prepare the child or adolescent both physically and psychologically for the physical examination and remain with her until it is completed. If the police accompany the rape victim, they should be asked to wait in a room apart from the victim and other patients, if possible, until the entire examination and collection of all medical and legal data are completed. A written and witnessed consent form must be obtained from the person responsible for the patient to allow the medical team to perform a history and physical examination, take photographs, collect specimens, provide treatment, and release information to law enforcement authorities.

The primary care physician's responsibility in dealing with alleged rape cases is twofold: first, to provide treatment for the acute physical and psychological trauma and outline plans for follow-up care; and second, since rape is not a medical diagnosis but a legal opinion, to gather evidence that can be used in legal proceedings to support the victim's charges or the accused's defense. This evidence should include a careful verbatim history, a complete physical examination, and a collection of laboratory data and specimens.

Special protocols that provide excellent guidelines for the collection of this evidence are used in many large hospitals and rape centers. These forms may be obtained from the American College of Obstetrics and Gynecology or from the National Center for Child Abuse and Neglect.

HISTORY

A history should include a verbatim description of the alleged attack and the current physical and emotional state of the patient. The history should include the exact time and place of the alleged attack, a thorough description of the attacker or attackers, and complete details of the circumstances of the attack, including penile penetration and orgasm of the attacker or attackers. The history should also note whether the victim has changed clothes, bathed or showered, douched, or voided or defecated since the attack. Such practices are not uncommon and can substantially alter the collection and validity of evidence. If the victim is a girl, the history should also include the age of menarche (when appropriate), regularity of menses, date of last menstruation, and parity. Answers to these questions may help the physician when counseling the teenage victim concerning medication to prevent pregnancy.

PHYSICAL EXAMINATION

Ideally, photographs should be taken of the patient fully clothed to document the general physical appearance and to demonstrate soiled and torn clothing. The patient should undress while standing on a white sheet so that falling debris can be collected. All debris and relevant clothing should be collected and placed in separate bags, which must be labeled with the name of the patient, the date, the time and place of collection, and the type and source of material; the bags must then be sealed. Evidence should never be left unattended, and, to maintain a proper chain of custody, all evidence must be personally handed over to law enforcement authorities from whom detailed written receipts must be obtained.

The general physical examination is best carried out by the primary care physician following the cephalocaudal approach of examining the ears, nose, throat, chest, heart, and abdomen to help relieve anxiety and downplay the specific focus on the genital area. Special attention should be given to documentation of all bruises and lacerations anywhere on the body, and sketches or photographs of these lesions are particularly valuable. The examination of the genital area, including the perianal area, should include a detailed description of the presence or absence of bruises, ecchymoses, petechiae, hematomas, or lacerations. When the victim is a girl, the hymen and introitus should be described in terms of their specific appearance and size and not simply as "intact" or "virginal." The presence or absence of menstruation or fluid in the vaginal area should be noted. An examination with a speculum is not necessary for the prepubertal or apparently virginal adolescent. Satisfactory collection of material does not require a speculum or bimanual examination but may be carried out by using soft-tipped cotton applicator sticks and a small medicine dropper.

LABORATORY SPECIMENS

Collection of specimens is very important in cases of alleged rape. Objective scientific evidence is the most revealing and powerful testimony in rape trials. The proper collection and documentation of these specimens are mandatory.

In general, the following materials should be obtained: (1) hair combings from the pubic area, which may contain samples of the assailant's hair (the specimen should be kept separate from cut hair samples of the patient); (2) fingernail scrapings and dried secretions of hair and skin for determining acid phosphatase and AB antigens; (3) Wood lamp illumination for evidence of semen (semen fluoresces under the Wood lamp); (4) a swab of the labia, vagina, and cervix in girls and the anus and mouth in all victims for sperm identification; a swab of vaginal fluid specifically from the posterior fornix should be obtained for (a) an acid phosphatase determination for seminal fluid, AB agglutinogen, and sperm precipitins, (b) a saline wet mount for examination of motile sperm, and (c) a fixed smear to examine for sperm; (5) Gram stains of the genitals, urethra, and anus; (6) *Neisseria gonorrhoeae* cultures from the endocervix, urethra, anus, and throat; (7) a serologic test for syphilis; (8) cultures for *Chlamydia trachomatis* and *Ureaplasma urealyticum* (if available); and (9) a pregnancy test in postmenarcheal girls.

MEDICAL TREATMENT

Treatment of the rape victim includes (1) acute care and repair of any injury; (2) inquiry concerning current tetanus immunization, especially if the skin has been broken or if the rape took place in a contaminated area, such as an alley or old house; and (3) recommendation for prevention of pregnancy, when appropriate, and venereal disease.

Gonorrhea is the most widespread of all the sexually transmitted diseases in children, and the prepubertal female is particularly susceptible to it because of the thin vaginal mucosal wall with its alkaline pH. However, the risk of the rape victim contracting syphilis is very low (0.1%), and the infection of gonorrhea in sexually abused children is only about 4%. Therefore, prophylactic treatment of gonorrhea and syphilis is not recommended by the Centers for Disease Control, although some facilities treat all victims if follow-up cannot be guaranteed. When cultures and Gram stains are positive, the Centers for Disease Control recommends treatment with weight-appropriate dosages of antibiotics, preferably in oral form because antibiotic injections may be perceived as punitive. (See Table 255-5 for treatment regimens.)

Pregnancy occurs in approximately 7% of all rapes, a rate thought to be lower than that which occurs from random single acts of intercourse. The general opinion is that all victims who are adolescent girls, including those in early puberty who are not already pregnant or who are not using oral contraceptives regularly, should be afforded the opportunity to receive therapy to prevent pregnancy.

Pregnancy-preventive drugs are effective in girls who have been raped. Diethylstilbestrol (DES) should not be used as postcoital treatment.[1] Ethinyl estradiol, 25 mg twice a day for 5 days, or Lo/Ovral (0.3 mg/noregestrel and 0.03 mg ethinyl estradiol), four tablets taken immediately and three more tablets taken within 24 hours, may be used.

These drugs may cause nausea or vomiting, which can be counteracted to some degree by the concomitant use of antinausea medication. Another method available to the victim to prevent pregnancy would be determination of the serum human chorionic gonadotropin level several days after the assault and, if possible, performance of a menstrual extraction.

Medical follow-up care should include a repeat culture for *N. gonorrhoeae* and a serologic test for syphilis 6 weeks after the attack.

EMOTIONAL ASPECTS

Victims

Rape is a violent crime that violates the victim's body, emotional well-being, and view of the world. It may change the victim's basic perception about a safe and predictable environment, end his or her trust in others, and also disrupt the sense of self-competency, self-esteem, and self-confidence.

The emotional sequelae of rape are manifested in an array of symptoms, both acute and chronic. *Rape trauma syndrome* best describes the emotional reactions experienced by many rape victims.

The acute phase lasts from a few days to several weeks, during which time the victim may experience a sense of shock and disbelief and notice a decreased ability to make decisions and to concentrate on schoolwork, feeling confused, unsure, and distractible. Sleeplessness and nightmares are common, and generalized fear of strangers and fear of the dark, of being alone, and of leaving home often develop. Withdrawal and isolation from peers and school may result. Somatic

symptoms may include fatigue, loss of appetite, tension headaches, generalized soreness, and abdominal and pelvic pain. Periods of embarrassment, guilt, shame, and humiliation are common, as are periods of irritability, wide mood swings, thoughts of vengeful retaliation, and anger. Fears of being harmed by the accused rapist or his friends are also common, and at times such fears may become generalized to phobic-panic proportions. All these symptoms appear and disappear as a necessary process while the acute trauma is "being worked through" by the victim.

Within a few weeks the "reorganizational" phase usually begins, and most of the acute symptoms diminish and many victims appear to return to their normal behavior and normal lives. However, medical personnel should be aware that many of these victims who insist the rape episode no longer bothers them will continue to have nightmares, insomnia, and a variety of vague psychosomatic complaints, especially those concerned with the genitourinary, gastrointestinal, or gynecologic system. Changes in personal hygiene, such as excessive bathing or douching or, conversely, total disregard of bathing and wearing sloppy clothes to diminish their sexual attractiveness, may indicate unresolved emotional conflicts.

Treatment of the emotional sequelae of rape is usually directed to crisis intervention and supportive counseling where the victim is given the opportunity to discuss feelings of rage, fear, embarrassment, and confusion. Adolescent rape victims often wonder if their behavior was too seductive or if it was seductive at all. They often fear that they may have invited or brought on the rape themselves. The sensitive physician should reassure the victim that he or she did not bring about the rape. In addition, it should be emphasized that seductive behavior is never a license to engage in physical or sexual assault and is never an excuse for rape.

Anticipatory guidance should focus on the types of symptomatology often experienced by rape victims and the normality of such responses following the physical and emotional trauma of rape. The victim should also be alerted to the possibility of chronic unresolved symptomatology and told to return for additional counseling should these symptoms appear. The burden the victim feels in returning to a normal life may be related to the prerape psychological makeup and functioning of the victim and the availability of a psychological support system of family and friends. Psychiatric referral and treatment should be sought in those whose symptoms persist or recur in the form of a posttraumatic stress disorder manifested by recurrent and intrusive recollections or dreams of the rape, hyperalertness or an exaggerated startle response, sleep disturbances, marked numbing of responsiveness, feelings of detachment or estrangement from others, constricted affect, and trouble concentrating.

Parents

The greatest help the rape victim can have is the support and understanding of his or her parents. Therefore the primary care physician must make a special effort to work closely with them. Parents also experience feelings of rage toward the assaulter and often displace this rage onto the community and onto the police for lack of adequate protection. In some instances this rage is even directed toward the victim for transgressing parental rules, such as by staying out late, dressing too provocatively, or associating with the "wrong" crowd. Although parents should advise their children to avoid situations that could place them in jeopardy, it should be emphasized to the parents that dress or behavior that could be considered too seductive even by a female is not license for any male to assault a female physically or sexually and is never an excuse for rape. Parents should also be given the opportunity to discuss their own feelings of guilt over not having provided total protection for their child. They often need to be reassured that the child is not "ruined" or "dirty" and they may require as much support and reassurance as the victim.

Male Partner

When the victim is a girl, many of the same issues and concerns described for her and her parents may be experienced by the victim's boyfriend, fiancé, or husband. Therefore counseling for the partner is also important. The male partner often experiences the same feelings of rage toward the assaulter and tends to blame the victim in ways similar to her parents. In addition, the boy may behave toward the girl in a way that could add to an already stressful situation. It is not uncommon for the male to withdraw from the girl, feeling that she is "dirty" or "damaged"; conversely, he may exhibit hypersexual behavior toward her.

Rape of Males

The rape of prepubertal and adolescent males in noninstitutional settings is apparently increasing in frequency and yet is still quite uncommon. The paucity of information concerning rape of males rests, in part, in the homosexual nature of such attacks, which increases the reluctance of males to report rape and sustains society's failure to establish sufficient facilities for helping male rape victims. The limited information available regarding male rape indicates that male victims experience acute and long-term emotional responses similar to those of female rape victims, including posttraumatic stress disorder.

In institutional settings where rape is often condoned or at least tolerated, this behavior is not viewed as homosexual but rather is often rationalized as a form of normal sexual expression while in confinement. However, it is important to note that such attacks in institutions have the same underlying dynamics as noninstitutional female rape—that is, the fusion of sexual and aggressive feelings to conquer and degrade the victim.

If a male victim of rape is seen by the primary care physician, the same tact and sensitivity shown to the female rape victim and her family must be afforded to the male. The medicolegal aspects remain the same for both sexes, and virtually all the issues discussed concerning the medical and psychological management and treatment of the female may be applied to the male victim with minor variations, but with particular focus on the moral sense of loss of masculinity by being unable to defend himself in a violent attack and by being violated homosexually.

REFERENCE

Physicians' desk reference, ed 45, Oradell, NJ, 1991, Medical Economics Co, Inc.

SUGGESTED READINGS

American Academy of Pediatrics, Committee on Adolescents: Rape and the adolescent, Pediatrics 81:595, 1988.

American College of Obstetricians and Gynecologists: Alleged sexual assault, ACOG Technical Bulletin No 101, Washington, DC, 1987.

Calderwood D: The male rape victim, Medical Aspects of Human Sexuality 21:53, 1987.

Martin GA, Warfield MC, and Brain GP: Physician's management of the psychological aspects of rape, JAMA 249:501, 1983.

Prentky RA and Quinsey VL: Human sexual aggression: current perspectives, Ann NY Acad Sci 528:1, 1988.

Sarles RM: Sexual abuse and rape, Pediatr Rev 4:93, 1982.

Schetky DH and Green AH: Child sexual abuse: a handbook for health care and legal professionals, New York 1988, Brunner/Mazel, Inc.

287

Acute Renal Failure

Edward J. Ruley

Acute renal failure is a syndrome of sudden diminution or cessation of renal function that can result from various causes. The clinical symptoms and signs result from both the inciting disease process and the altered homeostasis produced by cessation of renal function. Acute renal failure may occur at any age but is less common in children and adolescents than in adults. The exact incidence is unknown, since many self-limited episodes may go undetected. This is especially true for the nonoliguric type of acute renal failure (see below).

ETIOLOGY

In general the causes of acute renal failure may be placed into prerenal, renal (parenchymal), and postrenal categories. Prerenal causes are those that diminish renal perfusion without producing renal damage. In the pediatric age group hypovolemia is the most common clinical situation in which this occurs. Usually the hypovolemia is part of a dehydration syndrome associated with abnormal gastrointestinal losses, although it may also be seen in shock that may follow hemorrhage, burns, sepsis, and trauma. Less common causes of prerenal azotemia are congestive heart failure, renal vascular obstruction (that may occur in thrombosis or embolism), and increased renal vascular resistance, as is occasionally seen following anesthesia or surgery. Although the patient develops oliguria and azotemia as part of this prerenal syndrome, adequate renal tubular function usually persists, as evidenced by the high urinary osmolality and urea concentration and the low urinary sodium concentration.

Acute renal failure from intrinsic renal damage may result from lesions that involve either the glomeruli, the tubules, or the interstitium. Glomerular damage may be a consequence of any of the glomerulonephritides or the microangiopathy of the hemolytic-uremic syndrome. Tubular damage can result from prolonged unrecognized inadequate renal perfusion, as seen in hypotensive episodes, severe dehydration, sudden hemorrhage, and sepsis. Tubular toxins (e.g., hemoglobin and myoglobin) and various chemicals (e.g., carbon tetrachloride, diethylene glycol, and heavy metals) may cause acute parenchymal renal failure. Drugs can produce renal failure because of either direct toxic effects or hypersensitivity reactions. Renal cortical necrosis as seen in infection, hemorrhage, or dehydration can produce significant injury to both glomeruli and tubules.

Postrenal causes of acute renal failure are discussed in Chapter 181, "Anuria/Oliguria."

History

The clinician will usually determine the type of insult that caused the renal failure in the patient from recent historical information. It is important to note that the volume of urine production is not part of the definition of acute renal failure in that the patient may be anuric, oliguric (defined as a urine volume under 240 ml/m^2/day), or nonoliguric (defined as a normal or increased urinary output). Some insults, such as hemolytic-uremic syndrome, will tend to cause oligoanuric acute renal failure; others, such as aminoglycoside toxicity, will more often cause nonoliguric renal failure. Determination of the type of insult will provide the clinician with clues to the expected type of renal failure, the probable duration of renal insufficiency, and the overall prognosis. The history

Table 287-1 *Clinical Tests to Differentiate Functional from Parenchymal Oliguric Acute Renal Failure (ARF)*

TEST	FUNCTIONAL ARF	PARENCHYMAL ARF	DISCRIMINATION
Sodium conservation			
Urine sodium concentration (UNa)*	<20 mEq/L	>40 mEq/L	Poor
Fractional excretion of sodium (FENa)	<1	>1	Good
$\left(\text{FENa} = \dfrac{\text{UNa/SNa}}{\text{UCr/SCr}} \times 100\right)$			
Water conservation			
Urine osmolality (Uosm)	>500 mosm/L	>350 mosm/L	Poor
Urine serum osmolality ratio (Uosm/Sosm)	>2	<1.1	Fair
Response to diagnostic challenge with IV mannitol and furosemide (see text)	Urine flow increase	No change	Good

*U, Urine; Na, sodium; Cr, creatinine.

Table 287-2 *Treatment of Hyperkalemia in Pediatric Patients*

AGENT	DOSE	EFFECT	REMARKS
Calcium gluconate (10%)	0.5 ml/kg IV over 2-4 min	Rapid but transient	Monitor ECG for bradycardia during injection; may be repeated but *not likely* to be effective
Sodium bicarbonate (7.5%)	2.5 mEq/kg (approximately 3 ml/kg) IV by slow push	Rapid but transient	Repetition *not* recommended
Glucose (50%)	1 ml/kg IV by slow push	Within 1-2 hr	Attempt to increase blood glucose to 250 mg/dl; may be maintained by infusion of 30% glucose at rate equal to insensible fluid loss
Insulin (regular)	1 U/kg IV	Rapid	Give *only* with hypertonic glucose infusion (30%)
Sodium polystyrene sulfonate (Kayexalate)	1 g/kg PO or PR	Hours to days	Side effects: gastric irritation (nausea and vomiting), diarrhea, *or* fecal impaction; PO more effective than PR; enemas should be retained 4-10 hr for effectiveness—removed by cleansing enema; may cause *hypokalemia;* use cautiously in patients who tolerate sodium loads poorly; also chelates Ca^{++} and Mg^{++}

will also help the clinician differentiate between a true acute renal failure in an otherwise healthy child and an acute deterioration of a child with undiagnosed, smoldering chronic renal failure. A preceding history of fatigue, pallor, sleepiness, poor school performance, and anorexia extending over a period of time would lead the practitioner to suspect the latter.

Physical Findings

Obviously, the child with oligoanuric acute renal failure will have no or markedly diminished urine output. In the child with anuria or oliguria, fluid retention can produce edema, water intoxication, vascular overload with congestive heart failure, pulmonary edema, and hypertension. Fluid overload is often iatrogenic, resulting from attempts to increase urinary output by increasing fluid intake. The retention of fluid is best determined by a gain in weight as seen on serial measurements.

In contrast, acute nonoliguric renal failure may be clinically covert. It is usually suspected only after the laboratory tests reveal azotemia.

Laboratory Findings

The biochemical disturbances that produce the clinical findings in acute renal failure are complex and interrelated. The key in the diagnosis of acute renal failure is the accumulation of nitrogenous waste products as measured by the rise in blood urea nitrogen and creatinine. If hypotonic fluids have been used in excess to hydrate the patient, dilutional hyponatremia, hypoproteinuria, and anemia may result.

Hyperkalemia may result from the inability of the kidney to excrete potassium and is one of the most life-threatening complications of acute renal failure. It can be especially severe where there is cellular damage with release of intracellular potassium as may occur with hemolysis, burns, trauma, or infections. Hyperkalemia produces a state of increased neuromuscular excitability, making the heart liable to arrhythmias. However, there are no reliable physical signs of hyperkalemia. Diagnosis depends on serum measurements of potassium and electrocardiographic evidence of altered cardiac electric activity. Failure to recognize and treat hyperkalemia accounts for many of the deaths of patients early in this disease. Metabolic acidosis develops as a result of failure of the kidney to excrete hydrogen ions and reabsorb bicarbonate. Furthermore, any state associated with increased catabolism such as shock, fever, poor caloric intake, or extensive tissue damage may accentuate the degree of acidosis as a result of increased production of organic and inorganic acid radicals. The acidosis promotes further hyperkalemia resulting from movement of intracellular potassium into the extracellular space as the body attempts to accommodate the higher hydrogen ion concentration. Respiratory compensation for the metabolic acidosis may be evidenced clinically as Kussmaul breathing.

Failure of phosphate excretion can produce phosphate retention. The hypocalcemia that results from the hyperphosphatemia may be manifested clinically as trembling, tetany, or seizures. Other causes of seizures in acute renal failure include hypertensive encephalopathy, uremia, and water intoxication. It is not unusual for a child to present first with the sudden onset of seizures and other central nervous system signs, only to be found to have acute renal failure.

Children with nonoliguric acute renal failure do not have the fluid and electrolyte problems seen with anuric or oliguric renal failure. The former usually have a salt-losing type of urine production that blunts the harmful effects of the renal failure.

DIFFERENTIAL DIAGNOSIS

As mentioned, the sine qua non of acute renal failue is the detection of retained nitrogenous waste products in the blood.

A recommended clinical approach to the child with anuria and oliguria is discussed in Chapter 181 and is portrayed in Fig. 181-1.

In considering prerenal and renal parenchymal failure, it is important to correct the dehydration before beginning an evaluation of the state of renal function. It is inappropriate to begin provocative tests for renal parenchymal failure while the patient remains significantly dehydrated, since the persistent oliguria may merely represent the normal homeostatic response of the kidney to the altered fluid balance.

A variety of tests have been proposed to differentiate prerenal from intrinsic renal failure (Table 287-1). Urine sodium content is usually low in prerenal azotemia, reflecting maximal sodium and water reabsorption by the kidney in an attempt to expand the circulating fluid volume. The normal value for sodium may vary, however, depending on the amount of sodium in the diet.

A more discriminating test is the fractional excretion of sodium (Table 287-1). All tests of sodium conservation are invalid if the child has received large amounts of sodium intravenously, has been given diuretics, or has nonoliguric acute renal failure.

Water conservation is reflected by the urine osmolality or the ratio of urine osmolality to plasma osmolality. Although the latter is more discriminatory, it may be unreliable in children who have received hypotonic intravenous rehydration, in those who have nonoliguric acute renal failure, and in those who are malnourished.

Finally, the renal response to mannitol or furosemide has also been suggested as a means to differentiate prerenal from intrinsic renal disease. Although mannitol (0.5 mg/kg intravenously) and furosemide (1 mg/kg intravenously) were initially evaluated as separate challenges, many clinicians are currently giving them together to decrease the incidence of false negative responses. A good response to these stimuli is the formation of 6 to 10 ml of urine per kilogram over the subsequent 1 to 3 hours. To evaluate the response accurately, the patient should be catheterized. Such a response indicates that the patient needs more mannitol and furosemide. Repetitive doses of mannitol and furosemide in instances of nonresponse may be harmful, with fluid shifts and convulsions being produced by the former and ototoxicity by the latter.

Prompt differentiation of prerenal and intrarenal oliguria is extremely important in view of the effects of further fluid management. If prerenal oliguria is unrecognized, adequate fluids may not be given, leading to the development of intrinsic renal damage as a result of the hypoperfusion. In contrast, if intrinsic renal oliguria is already present but unrecognized, vigorous fluid administration to induce diuresis may make the patient water intoxicated. Determination of acute renal failure and differentiation of its type is one of the most important responsibilities of the physician.

TREATMENT

Management of oliguric parenchymal renal failure, once the diagnosis has been established, requires attention to many details. Hyperkalemia is a particular immediate risk to the patient and must be treated immediately when present. The electrocardiographic changes of hyperkalemia often more accurately reflect the state of potassium balance than does serum potassium measurement. Various means to lower serum potassium are given in Table 287-2. Administration of calcium, sodium bicarbonate, glucose, and insulin is a measure of immediate effectiveness but is of short duration. Potassium-chelating resins are very effective in children.

Strict attention must be given to fluid, electrolyte, and caloric intake in these patients to minimize the development of uremia and related disorders. If acute renal failure persists, the patient may be given intravenous alimentation with essential amino acids that will provide calories, thereby promoting healing and minimizing uremia.

Children with nonoliguric acute renal failure are much easier to manage than are those with anuric and oliguric renal failure, since strict fluid restrictions are not necessary. In addition, the volume of fluid these children require provides the clinician with a means of providing calories, alkalinizing agents, calcium, and other drugs, so that the biochemical abnormalities of the renal failure can be minimized.

Management of the patient with any type of acute renal failure is best done in collaboration with a pediatric nephrologist. With vigorous attention to management details, dialysis may be unnecessary. However, peritoneal dialysis is useful for disturbances resistant to more conservative measures, regardless of the age of the patient. Hemofiltration, hemofiltration-dialysis, and hemodialysis can be used if the patient cannot undergo peritoneal dialysis for some reason. The former two forms of invasive therapy are more suited for use in neonates and smaller infants than is hemodialysis. All of these procedures should be performed in collaboration with a pediatric nephrologist who has experience in these techniques.

COMPLICATIONS

The most common complications of acute renal failure in children, beyond the immediate biochemical and fluid problems already mentioned, are infection and gastrointestinal hemorrhage. Infection is more common in patients who have had trauma or surgery and accounts for up to two thirds of the mortality associated with acute renal failure. The urinary system is the most common site of infection, followed by septicemia and respiratory tract infections. Although urinary catheterization is an important part of the initial evaluation of the oliguric child, prolonged urinary catheterization predisposes the child to infection. Likewise, meticulous care should be given to all intravenous catheters to decrease the incidence of septicemia. Prophylactic antibiotics are not indicated in acute renal failure.

PROGNOSIS

The short-term outcome depends on the ability of the physician to recognize acute renal failure and to construct an individualized treatment plan that will minimize the biochemical abnormalities as well as complications. The long-term prognosis is most dependent on the nature of the underlying condition that produced the renal failure. For example, a patient with acute renal failure following cardiac surgery has a poor prognosis if the cardiac function remains inadequate, whereas a patient with renal failure following hemolytic-uremic syndrome generally has a good prognosis.

SUGGESTED READINGS

Baquero A et al: Dopamine and furosemide in oliguric acute renal failure, Nephron 37:39, 1984.

Dixon BS and Anderson RJ: Nonoliguric acute renal failure, Am J Kidney Dis 6:71, 1985.

Ellis EN and Arnold WC: Use of urinary indices in renal failure in the newborn, Am J Dis Child 136:615, 1982.

Espinel CH and Grefory AW: Differential diagnosis of acute renal failure, Clin Nephrol 13:73, 1980.

Gaudio KM and Siegel NJ: Pathogenesis and treatment of acute renal failure, Pediatr Clin North Am 34:771, 1987.

Schaffer SE and Normal ME: Renal function and renal failure in the newborn, Clin Perinatol 16:199, 1989.

Weiss L et al: Continuous arteriovenous hemofiltration in the treatment of 100 critically ill patients with acute renal failure: report on clinical outcome and nutritional aspects, Clin Nephrol 31:184, 1989.

288

Shock

I. David Todres, Joseph R. Custer, and John H. Fugate

Shock is defined here as a condition in which the perfusion of organs by blood, oxygen, and metabolites is inadequate to meet their metabolic needs. It is important to recognize that hypotension may be only a late-occurring sign. Therefore, a constellation of symptoms and signs, or "shock syndrome," is more appropriate than merely hypotension alone for diagnosing shock. Shock is etiologically classified as follows:

Hypovolemic shock: Hypovolemia caused by loss of blood, plasma, and electrolytes

Cardiogenic shock: Cardiac pump failure caused by hypoxemia, myocarditis, or tamponade

Distributive shock: Loss of peripheral vascular tone as a result of sepsis, anaphylaxis, or drug overdose

This emphasis on a low-flow state (peripheral hypoperfusion) underscores the basic pathophysiology in that type of shock most commonly encountered. Efforts to restore blood flow, by restoration of blood volume, by redistribution of perfusion and oxygen delivery, or by improvement in myocardial contractility will in most situations correct the shock state. However, septic shock usually involves a high-flow state, and factors other than blood flow become critical. Recent work has focused on metabolic change and cell injury, as well as on changes in the body's immune response, in determining the outcome of shock. Humoral and cell-mediated phenomena are especially important factors in septic shock.

SYSTEMIC EFFECTS OF SHOCK

When shock is associated with a low-flow state, as in hypovolemia, oxygen transport to the tissues is reduced and results in cellular hypoxemia and anaerobic glycolysis. The resultant production of lactic acid causes a fall in blood pH and bicarbonate, and poor liver perfusion reduces the body's capacity to metabolize this acid. On the other hand, oxygen transport is not critical in high-flow septic shock, other less well-understood factors being responsible for the serious associated morbidity and mortality; these include tumor necrosis factor, complement activation, endotoxin, prostaglandins, and leukotrienes.

General metabolic changes during shock include increased glucagon production, decreased insulin response to glucose, and marked protein catabolism. Metabolism of the cell is disrupted, and less adenosine triphosphate (ATP) is produced. Cellular changes include the passage of sodium into and potassium out of the cell, as well as intracellular calcium accumulation. Lysozymes are broken down, and the cell is finally destroyed. Some of these cellular changes may be reversed, however, upon restoration of adequate tissue perfusion.

The several organ systems may all be affected by periods of low perfusion during shock. Particularly important is that impairment of lung perfusion leads to a form of respiratory failure known as "shock lung," or adult respiratory distress syndrome (ARDS). This clinical syndrome occurs 24 to 48 hours postshock in the critically ill child and can arise despite the absence of previous lung disease. The child is markedly dyspneic, with significant hypoxemia (reduced PaO_2). A chest roentgenogram reveals "diffuse infiltrates" of both lungs, which resemble pulmonary edema and are often difficult to distinguish from overwhelming pneumonia, massive aspiration, pulmonary hemorrhage, oxygen toxicity, or fluid overload. Roentgenographic changes may be delayed and appear for the first time 12 to 24 hours after the onset of the dyspnea. The interstitial edema that develops appears to be caused by increased permeability of lung capillaries. This complication is life threatening, and mechanical ventilation is required to improve oxygenation and combat respiratory failure. Positive end-expiratory pressure is usually necessary to maintain adequate oxygenation, so that pneumothoraces are a frequent complication of respiratory management and require urgent treatment.

Inadequate perfusion of the heart affects contractility and may lead to a decrease in cardiac output. Underlying cardiac disease will make this more likely. Myocardial depression is commonly encountered in septic shock.

Renal failure is less commonly seen in shock because of modern hemodynamic monitoring techniques and early fluid restoration, but its appearance significantly increases morbidity and mortality. Renal failure is to be suspected when the urine output is less than 0.5 ml/kg/hr; an increase in the blood urea nitrogen and creatinine levels supports this diagnosis. Most often the reduction in urine output is a result of the prerenal factor of hypovolemic hypoperfusion. Hemodynamic monitoring should establish a hypovolemic origin, but in uncertain situations a fluid challenge may be necessary to confirm the presence or absence of hypovolemia. Renal failure will increase the mortality resulting from shock. Its prevention and treatment are thus of paramount importance. Moreover, the level of antibiotics in the blood becomes quite uncertain (usually excessive at the usual dosage); thus antibiotic therapy must be carefully monitored by measuring levels in the blood whenever possible.

The central nervous system is most susceptible to hypoxemia and ischemia because of its high metabolic demands; it is not uncommon for a patient to suffer significant neurologic impairment while other organs are spared. Early central nervous system signs of shock include delirium, irritability, confusion, and coma. Signs of increased intracranial pressure may be delayed after a hypoxemic-ischemic insult as a result of cell death or reperfusion injury.

Liver function may be impaired as a result of inadequate perfusion of that organ. Bilirubin and liver enzymes are elevated, and clotting factors may be diminished. In septic shock, liver perfusion may be adequate, but bacteria or toxins may damage hepatic cells.

Ischemia of the gastrointestinal tract leads to greater absorption of bacteria and toxins; ulceration and necrosis of the bowel may follow.

Adrenal failure is uncommon but may occur in septicemia. Meningococcemia may result in the lethal complication of Waterhouse-Friderichsen syndrome. The common use of steroid therapy in asthma, other allergic states, and immune suppression therapy has produced a population of patients in whom "stress doses" of steroids need to be administered, should such patients be in shock. Such a child exhibits a high cardiac output and low peripheral resistance shock syndrome that is refractory to intravascular volume infusion.

Disseminated intravascular coagulation may occur, especially in septic shock. Early blood-product transfusions to provide clotting factors and red cells for oxygen delivery are necessary to treat this potentially life-threatening complication.

HYPOVOLEMIC SHOCK

Hypovolemic shock is the most common form of shock. Its recognition and treatment should be clearly understood by the primary care physician.

Blood Loss

Traumatic blood loss is the most common cause of shock in children. The bleeding may be obvious or occult, as in intraabdominal rupture of the liver and spleen. Compensatory mechanisms are very active in children, so it is important to appreciate that the injured child with pallor (compensatory vasoconstriction) and confusion has already likely lost 25% of his or her blood volume and that at this stage other compensatory mechanisms, such as tachycardia, may not be evident; later, tachycardia and decreased blood pressure may appear. Infants and toddlers have relatively more body water than does an adult, so that depending on the rate of blood volume loss, the child can better autotransfuse extracellular fluid into the intravascular space.

Because shock is defined by hypoperfusion, not hypotension, it may be present in a child who maintains a normal blood pressure. When the blood pressure has finally fallen below normal in the already vasoconstricted, traumatized child, the situation becomes even more critical, since loss of more than 25% of the child's blood volume has occurred. Although critically ill, such a child may focus his or her attention and complaints on some minimal incidental injury rather than on the more significant underlying major injury.

Significant blood loss may be associated with major surgery. After surgery the attending pediatrician may see evidence of inadequate peripheral perfusion (as demonstrated by poor capillary refill), decreased urine output, or agitation. These conditions suggest that the child may not have had adequate intraoperative blood replacement or may be suffering from continuing blood loss, especially after a tonsillectomy or cardiac or abdominal surgery.

Another common cause of blood loss is gastrointestinal bleeding, which occasionally may be rapid and severe. This may be seen with esophageal varicose ulcerations, Meckel diverticulum, intussusception, or inflammatory bowel disease.

Plasma Loss

Plasma loss is regularly associated with severe burns, and the degree of loss is related to the extent and depth of the burn. Continuing losses can be extremely large until eschar is formed, grafting commenced, or artificial skin placed. Peritonitis produces a significant loss of plasma through the peritoneal surface; this loss, being hidden in a "third space," frequently is underestimated.

Electrolyte Loss

Electrolyte loss and imbalance are most commonly seen in pediatric conditions associated with vomiting and diarrhea. Significant electrolyte loss also occurs in paralytic ileus and intestinal obstruction; large volumes of fluid fill dilated bowel loops, while continuous suctioning removes significant amounts of electrolyte. Excessive diuresis from mannitol or furosemide may also produce significant iatrogenic fluid and electrolyte loss. Hyperosmolar agents, as used especially in radiologic diagnostic and therapeutic procedures, can remove significant quantities of fluid from the body as they are excreted. In the small infant this may produce hypovolemic shock.

In sepsis a generalized capillary "leak" occurs, leading to a loss of both plasma proteins and electrolyte-containing fluids into the interstitial space and resultant significant hypovolemia. Worse, the plasma protein thus leaked into the interstitial space now exerts an oncotic force, which prevents fluid from returning to the intravascular space, while the diminished vascular oncotic pressure further promotes the exit of fluid to the interstitial space. Septic vasodilation and loss of venous tone may produce a relative hypovolemic state that serves to decrease venous return and, hence, cardiac output.

Compensatory Reaction to Hypovolemia

The body's reaction to fluid loss is to maintain adequate perfusion of the vital organs, especially the brain and heart, at the expense of flow to other major organs. Redistribution of cardiac output takes place with diminished flow to the skin from vasoconstriction, which is seen as poor capillary refill. Hypoperfusion of the following other major organs contributes to the clinical picture of shock: kidneys (decreased urine output), gut (ileus and "stress ulcers"), lung (decreased surfactant and ventilation and perfusion abnormalities), and liver (inadequate metabolism of drugs). Frequently, tachycardia occurs in the body's attempt to maintain cardiac output in the face of decreased stroke volume (Cardiac output = Stroke volume × Heart rate). Moreover, cardiac output in the young infant depends on heart rate, since stroke volume is limited by relatively poor myocardial compliance. The infant has twice the oxygen consumption rate of the adult, further compromising the attempt to meet increased metabolic demands.

In addition to the familiar clinical parameters of shock (poor capillary refill; cold, moist extremities; tachycardia; decreased blood pressure; poor urine output; confusion), the blood pH is a valuable indicator of the adequacy of tissue perfusion. Metabolic acidosis reflects inadequate tissue perfusion and the resultant anaerobic metabolism of glucose to form lactic acid, a myocardial depressant; thus this vicious circle further aggravates the already decreased tissue perfusion, and rapid and accurate intervention is necessary to prevent further deterioration.

Management of Hypovolemic Shock

The body's initial but limited response to the loss of significant amounts of fluid is to restore intravascular volume through transcapillary absorption of fluid from the interstitial space (autotransfusion). This process is slow and may take up to 24 hours. Thus rapid restoration of an adequate blood volume is the cardinal principle of management. For this purpose, robust venous access is necessary—that is, a *secure* intravenous line through which isotonic fluids such as blood, fresh-frozen plasma, 5% serum albumin (Albumisol), Ringer lactate solution, or normal saline solution can be rapidly infused. In addition, any continuing bleeding must be stopped. For initial volume resuscitation, the physician should give a bolus of 20 ml/kg of the fluid (Fig. 288-1). Blood is often

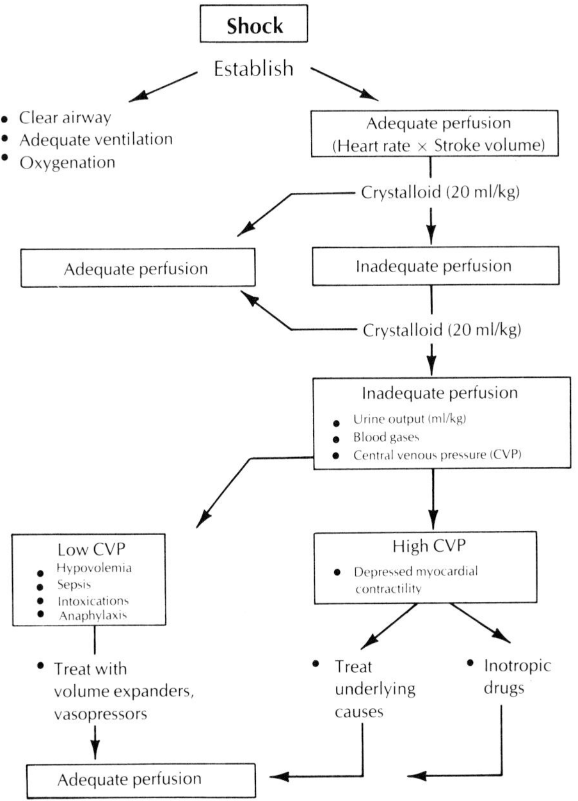

Fig. 288-1 Treatment decision-making plan in the child with shock.

not immediately available when blood loss constitutes an emergency, but Ringer lactate solution rapidly equilibrates with the extracellular fluid and is rapidly excreted in the urine, provided there is good renal function. Hetastarch, an amylopectin, has been used extensively as a 6% solution in adults, but experience with its use in children is limited.

If intravenous access is difficult, especially in the infant or young child, the physician should rapidly obtain access via the intraosseous route. An intraosseous needle may be placed in the bone marrow of the proximal anterior tibia to achieve flow rates into the central circulation that equal peripheral intravenous infusions. Any type of medication or fluid that may be lifesaving can be instilled into the patient via this route.

The adequacy of perfusion is assessed through hemodynamic measurements and clinical indicators of perfusion:

Mental alertness (although head injury may cloud this evaluation)
Capillary refill and warmth of extremities
Heart rate
Blood pressure
Urine output (measured via a Foley catheter)

If the child does not respond to the initial fluid bolus of 20 ml/kg (which should be given as rapidly as possible, usually within 10 minutes), a further bolus of 20 ml/kg of fluid is infused and the above parameters of perfusion are reassessed. Most pediatric patients will respond to two 20 ml/kg boluses of fluid. Patients who do not so respond are generally more ill, require invasive monitoring (at least a central venous pressure catheter), a Foley catheter, and perhaps an arterial catheter; they also will likely require triage to an intensive care unit.

Failure to respond to this therapy also requires a more rigorous pursuit of diagnostic possibilities. Essential is the measurement of the hematocrit (Hct) blood glucose, urea nitrogen and creatinine, serum electrolytes, and blood gases. Of less importance but occasionally useful is the measurement of serum phosphorus, liver function, and coagulation status. The further need for volume requires attention to the composition of the body fluids. Is the Hct less than 35? Is there a metabolic acidosis? Are there extremes of sodium or potassium concentration? Is the patient hypoglycemic? Serious consideration must be given to significant ongoing blood losses (e.g., lacerated liver or spleen), which may require surgical intervention.

Physiologic measurements are made at intervals of 30 minutes or less. These include measurement of urine output, which should be at least 1 ml/kg/hr. Failure of urine output reflects prerenal failure or renal failure. If hemodynamic measurements indicate an adequate intravascular volume, then true renal failure is the more likely condition. In this situation it can be helpful to challenge the kidney by infusing furosemide (Lasix) 1 mg/kg, or mannitol 0.5 g/kg intravenously. Should the response be an increased urine output, then additional crystalloid fluids are required. Mannitol should be used with caution, however, if the central venous pressure (CVP) is elevated. The osmotic effect of the mannitol can lead to a sudden increase in the intravascular volume and the possibility of pulmonary edema. Excessive crystalloid infusions can lead to a marked increase in interstitial fluid volume, resulting in significant peripheral edema.

The interpretation of absolute numeric hemodynamic parameters, such as CVP, may be difficult. For instance, readings may be spuriously elevated in patients receiving positive pressure ventilation or in those with marked abdominal distention. In such situations it is the *trend* in CVP responses to therapy, rather than an absolute number, that is more informative.

In addition to the measures described for replacing lost blood volume in hypovolemic shock, the control of hemorrhage is critical. The use of MAST (military antishock trouser) for children in hypovolemic shock may be beneficial. MASTs generate pressure over the legs and abdomen to redistribute blood to the central circulation (autotransfusion) and thus help restore adequate circulating blood volume to vital organs. In addition, MASTs transmit external pressures to control active bleeding points within the legs and abdomen. The use of MAST devices does not prevent access to the saphenous vein.

Establishing a clear airway and maintaining ventilation and oxygenation are urgent in controlling hemorrhage in the child in shock. Mechanical ventilation and judicious use of positive end-expiratory pressure may be required. Serial monitoring of blood gases is necessary even in the presence of a normal oxygen saturation evidenced by oximetry. Treatment of the patient's abnormal acid-base status is crucial, and the glucose level should be closely monitored.

CARDIOGENIC SHOCK

Causes of primary or secondary cardiac pump failure include myocarditis, overwhelming sepsis (bacterial and viral), hypoxemia, myocardial ischemia from inadequate coronary perfusion associated with hypovolemia, and pericardial tamponade (blood and air). The efficiency of cardiac pump action depends on three factors:

1. Preload (i.e., the filling pressures of the heart)
2. Myocardial contractility
3. Afterload (i.e., the resistance at the arteriolar level of the force [pressure] generated by the myocardial pump)

Management

Monitoring of right-sided or, in some instances, left-sided (i.e., noncardiogenic pulmonary edema) filling pressures (using Swan-Ganz catheters) indicates whether the preload, or filling pressure of the heart, is adequate. This is measured as the central venous pressure (normal is 3 to 6 mm Hg) on the right side of the heart and as the pulmonary "wedge" pressure (normal is 4 to 8 mm Hg) on the left side of the heart. If the CVP rises higher than 12 to 15 mm Hg or the wedge pressure higher than 15 to 18 mm Hg without improved cardiac output, further management will require intensive care. If the filling pressures are abnormally low, expansion of the intravascular volume is indicated. Contractility is enhanced by improving oxygenation of the myocardium and increasing the myocardial contractile force. The Starling curve (Fig. 288-2) reflects the relation between the filling pressures of the heart and its stroke volume; a depressed curve is associated with cardiogenic shock. Clinically, increasing volume support in this situation produces a high CVP without evidence of increased perfusion, such as improved capillary filling, urine output,

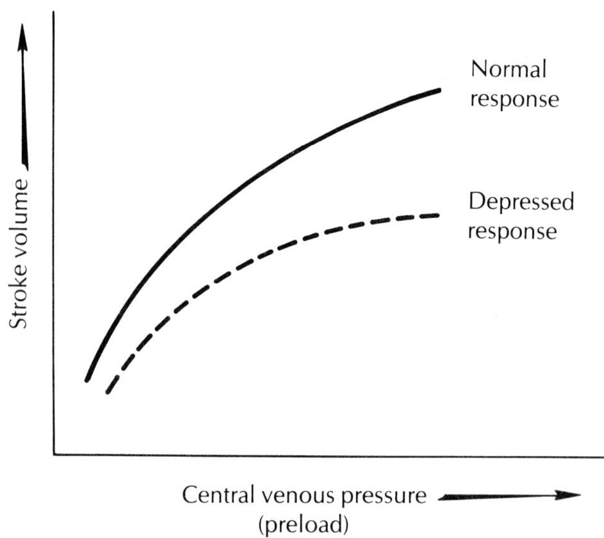

Fig. 288-2 Relationship of stroke volume to preload determining myocardial contractility (Starling curve). A depressed response may be caused by hypoxemia, acidosis, hypocalcemia, sepsis, or drug toxicity.

or improved mental status, and is frequently accompanied by signs of volume overload, especially pulmonary edema.

Therapeutic efforts are aimed at moving the curve from the depressed response pattern to a normal or supernormal response, thus optimizing stroke volume and cardiac output. Various drugs are administered to increase contractility and act on the arteriolar bed to increase vasoconstriction, thus raising blood pressure and perfusion of vital organs—the brain and heart. In special circumstances certain drugs (e.g., sodium nitroprusside) may be given to reduce the afterload by producing vasodilation to lessen the resistance against which the myocardium must work, thus improving its efficiency and increasing cardiac output. The drugs used are classified according to their cardiac and vascular effects (Table 288-1).

It should be emphasized that cardiogenic shock is uncommon in children; the child in shock is much more likely to be suffering from hypovolemic shock.

DISTRIBUTIVE SHOCK

The shock associated with anaphylaxis, sepsis, and drug overdose involves a relative hypovolemia caused by loss of vascular resistance and peripheral vascular tone and consequent dilation of the arteriolar beds. Therapy must be aimed at treating the underlying cause, such as removing the toxin from the body, draining an abscess, or removing necrotic bowel. However, emergency treatment of the impaired circulation is aimed at (1) restoring an adequate intravascular volume to produce an adequate preload and filling pressure for the heart, and (2) counteracting vasodilation by administering vasoconstrictive pressor agents.

Septic Shock

Septic shock may also alter the pulmonary vasculature to produce serious ventilation and perfusion abnormalities. In this circumstance respiratory support by a mechanical ven-

Table 288-1 *Vasoactive Drugs Used in Shock*

DRUG	DOSE	VASCULAR RESPONSE	CARDIAC RESPONSE	COMMENTS
Epinephrine	0.1-0.5 μg/kg/min	Alpha*	Beta-1†	Marked increase in myocardial contractility and rate
Norepinephrine	0.1-0.5 μg/kg/min	Alpha	Beta-1	Marked vasoconstriction; less cardiac effect; less commonly used
Phenylephrine	0.1-0.5 μg/kg/min	Alpha		Marked vasoconstriction and increased systemic vascular resistance; no cardiac effects
Isoproterenol	0.1-0.5 μg/kg/min	Beta-2‡	Beta-1	Positive inotropic and chronotropic effects; peripheral vasodilator; cardiac output directed to skeletal tissue and away from vital organs
Dopamine	2.5-5 μg/kg/min 5-10 μg/kg/min 10 μg/kg/min	Delta§ Alpha	Beta-1	Dilates renal and mesenteric vessels; alpha effect increases with dose of 10 μg/kg/min; infants appear to require relatively higher doses
Dobutamine	1-10 μg/kg/min		Beta-1	Nearly pure inotrope; mild vasodilator

*Alpha effect leads to vasoconstriction.
†Beta-1 effect leads to an increase in cardiac contractility and rate.
‡Beta-2 effect leads to vasodilation.
§Delta effect leads to improved renal perfusion through dopaminergic receptors.

tilator is required to optimize oxygenation and ventilation, and the effects of the ventilator on the circulation must be considered. When high inspiratory and end-expiratory pressures are required, cardiac output may be compromised and additional volume expanders and vasopressor agents may be required.

A special condition of shock that has received a great deal of attention is known as toxic shock syndrome (TSS). It is caused by local infection with toxin-producing strains of bacteria, often *Staphylococcus aureus*. The condition may affect children of any age or sex. However, most reported cases have been associated with the use of tampons by menstruating women. Treatment is aimed at removal of a focal staphylococcal source. The cardiovascular system is supported with fluid volume expanders and vasopressor agents. Therapy with penicillinase-resistant penicillin is indicated. (See Chapter 262, "Toxic Shock Syndrome.")

Another important cause of septic shock in the child is meningococcal disease, which may be fulminating with progressive shock, coma, and evidence of disseminated intravascular coagulation (DIC). (See Chapter 283, "Meningococcemia.") Extensive petechial and purpuric lesions are often seen. Management follows the principles of eliminating the underlying cause (the gram-negative diplococcus, *Neisseria meningitidis*) with appropriate antibiotics (penicillin G) and supporting the circulation by using volume expanders and cardiac and vasoactive drugs—for example, dopamine. (See Table 288-1.) Some children have such a profound capillary leak that even after extensive fluid resuscitation, they still have decreased preload. Blood-product transfusions and even hypertonic saline may be useful in this situation.

Mechanical ventilation may be required to combat the progressive deterioration of gas exchange often seen in septic shock.

Many children in septic shock have a hyperdynamic circulation; that is, the cardiac output is greater than normal and the arteriovenous oxygen difference is narrowed. A hyperdynamic circulation strongly suggests underlying sepsis, in contrast to hypovolemic and cardiogenic shock, in which cardiac output is more typically depressed.

The type of shock following hypoxemic-ischemic insults, a common occurrence in the pediatric age group, is unique. Cardiac output is reduced, oxygen delivery inadequate, and systemic vascular resistance elevated. The poor perfusion and cool, "clamped down" appearance of the child may be interpreted as signs of hypovolemia leading to volume infusion and dopamine administration. High-dose dopamine, a potent alpha-agonist, might increase the high systemic vascular resistance and produce arrhythmias. Volume augmentation might lead to early onset of congestive symptoms such as heart failure and pulmonary edema. (In this situation, administration of dobutamine and/or amrinone through a Swan-Ganz catheter is of diagnostic and therapeutic benefit.)

DRUGS USED IN THE TREATMENT OF SHOCK

Vasoactive drugs are potent agents, so their use must be preceded by a thorough understanding of their benefits and risks (see Table 288-1); close monitoring of the child is mandatory. A vasoactive drug should be infused continuously with a calibrated infusion pump; repeated cardiac and blood pressure monitoring is performed, preferably through an intraarterial line connected to a transducer and displayed on an oscilloscope.

Norepinephrine, epinephrine, and phenylephrine all increase blood pressure by vasoconstriction, which decreases microcirculatory flow and may be disadvantageous to vital tissues, especially the kidneys. These drugs must not be used in hypovolemic shock, where blood and fluid replacement is the cardinal therapeutic principle, but they can be useful in the shock associated with sepsis or cardiac failure. Norepinephrine, when used appropriately, has been a valuable agent. Several studies have demonstrated adequate preservation of renal blood flow when this drug is used alone or in combination with "renal-dose" dopamine, especially in septic shock, where there is significant peripheral vasodilation.

Isoproterenol stimulates beta-receptors in the heart and arterioles, leading to an increase in the rate and force of myocardial contraction and to some arteriolar dilation, with an increase in cardiac output and improvement in tissue perfusion. Isoproterenol may lead to serious tachycardia, so its administration must be carefully titrated. Its rapid onset of action and short half-life make it especially suitable when low blood pressure is caused by bradycardia, or in high peripheral resistance, low heart rate, and low output syndromes, as seen in postoperative cardiac patients.

Dopamine is used frequently to increase cardiac output and augment renal perfusion in the critically ill child. The effects are dose dependent, with renal (dopaminergic) effects seen at the low-dose range (2.5 μg/kg/min). At higher doses (10 μg/kg/min) alpha-adrenergic effects are seen with vasoconstriction and reduced peripheral perfusion. Dopamine causes less tachycardia than does isoproterenol. Dobutamine may be preferred to dopamine because of its enhanced inotropic effect with less chronotropic effect than dopamine; also, it has less effect on systemic vascular resistance.

Digoxin may be indicated in heart failure, but its onset of action is delayed, and the drug cannot be as finely titrated to the individual's needs as can isoproterenol or dopamine. Digoxin's therapeutic index is dangerously narrow. Since renal failure and consequent potassium disturbances are frequently observed in the patient with shock, the use of digoxin in acute situations cannot be recommended.

In experimental settings corticosteroids reduce capillary permeability by stabilizing cell and vascular membranes. They appear to improve survival in the "shocked" animal. In large prospective human trials, steroids in septic shock have increased mortality and the incidence of secondary infection. Therefore steroids are indicated only in patients suspected of having secondary adrenal suppression from prior steroid use.

In selected situations the use of vasodilator drugs (nitroprusside, nitroglycerin) may be beneficial in reducing afterload when increased afterload is detrimental to myocardial performance. This therapy optimizes myocardial contractility and improves cardiac output.

SUMMARY

The pediatrician must be alert to the diagnosis of shock in the child and appreciate that signs and symptoms may be minimal. Attempts should be made to evaluate the cause of shock and remove it (e.g., stop bleeding, drain abscess, remove toxin, treat tension pneumothorax or pericardial tamponade). Aggressive therapy and monitoring are required to prevent serious and potentially lethal effects in major organ systems.

Hypovolemia is the most common cause of shock in children; therefore hemodynamic parameters and vigorous resuscitation with fluids and blood must be monitored in most situations. Drugs are useful in the treatment of shock, but their benefits and risks must be fully appreciated.

SUGGESTED READINGS

Colman RW, Robboy SJ, and Minna JD: Disseminated intravascular coagulation: a reappraisal, Annu Rev Med 30:359, 1979.

Crone RK: Acute circulatory failure in children, Pediatr Clin North Am 27:525, 1980.

Friedman WF and George BL: Treatment of congestive heart failure by altering loading conditions of the heart, J Pediatr 106:697, 1985.

Lucas CE: The renal response to acute injury and sepsis, Surg Clin North Am 56:953, 1976.

Lucas CE: Resuscitation of the injured patient: the three phases of treatment, Surg Clin North Am 57:38, 1977.

Lucking SE, Pollac MM, and Fields AI: Shock following generalized hypoxic-ischemic injury in previously healthy infants and children, J Pediatr 108:359, 1986.

Perkin RM and Anas NG: Cardiovascular evaluation and support in the critically ill child, Pediatr Ann 15:30, 1986.

Perkin RM and Levin DL: Shock in the pediatric patient. I. Therapy, J Pediatr 101:319, 1982.

Perkin RM and Levin DL: Shock in the pediatric patient. II. J Pediatr 101:613, 1982.

Todres ID et al: Swan-Ganz catheterization in the critically ill newborn, Crit Care Med 7:330, 1979.

Zaritsky A and Chernow B: Use of catecholamines in pediatrics, J Pediatr 105:341, 1984.

289

Status Asthmaticus

Nick G. Anas and Paul S. Lubinsky

DIFFERENTIAL DIAGNOSIS AND PATHOPHYSIOLOGY

Asthma, as defined by the American Thoracic Society, is an increased responsiveness of the trachea and bronchi to various stimuli, manifested by widespread narrowing of the airways that changes in severity either spontaneously or as a result of therapy.[1] In the United States asthma represents the most frequent chronic disease of childhood, affecting 5% to 10% of the pediatric population and resulting in more than 400,000 hospital admissions per year. Despite an increasing understanding of the pathophysiology of status asthmaticus and the availability of more effective therapeutic agents, approximately 4000 children died in 1985 as the result of this disorder.[5] The management of status asthmaticus requires intensive therapy in a setting in which trained nurses, respiratory therapists, and physicians are available. A pediatric intensive care unit (PICU) may be required to treat respiratory failure in the child with status asthmaticus; in addition, physicians and hospitals responsible for the care of acutely ill children must establish a stabilization protocol and transport arrangement for the management of the child with life-threatening status asthmaticus.

Status asthmaticus is further defined as an unreversed episode of airway obstruction after three bronchodilator treatments (with either nebulized beta-sympathomimetic agents or subcutaneous epinephrine) that requires further inpatient therapy. Not all children with asthma have wheezing; many report cough, dyspnea, or emesis as their chief symptom. Furthermore, wheezing may be a sign of a variety of clinical problems; the accompanying box presents a differential diagnosis for the onset of acute wheezing in the pediatric patient.

The pathophysiologic features of status asthmaticus include (1) bronchial smooth muscle contraction (bronchospasm), (2) inflammation and edema of the bronchial mucosa, and (3) the production and retention of tenacious secretions. These factors produce increased airway resistance and prolong the expiratory phase of the respiratory cycle, resulting in decreased expiratory airway volume and flow rates and premature closure of small airways. Ventilation-perfusion ($\dot{V}/\dot{Q}$) mismatching occurs, resulting in hypoxemia (reduced arterial oxygen tension or saturation, Pa_{O_2} and Sa_{O_2}, respectively). Hypoxemia so stimulates the central respiratory drive that the child manifests tachypnea and hypocapnic alkalosis (Pa_{CO_2} <35 mm Hg and pH >7.45). Severe airway obstruction in the child with status asthmaticus causes pulmonary hyperinflation and decreased lung compliance, resulting in impaired function of the respiratory muscles and excessive exertion in breathing. Fatigue occurs, minute ventilation is reduced, and hypercapnic acidosis (Pa_{CO_2} >50 mmHg and pH <7.35) develops. Fig. 289-1 summarizes this pathophysiology.

The morbidity and mortality in status asthmaticus are related to a number of anatomic and physiologic features of children: smaller airways, wherein a reduction in radius has a greater effect on airway resistance (Poiseuille law); limited elastic recoil of the lung, resulting in early airway closure and an increased functional residual capacity (FRC); undeveloped collateral channels of ventilation within the alveolar structure, thereby promoting atelectasis; and the propensity for fatigue of the respiratory muscle.[4]

EVALUATION, IMMEDIATE ASSESSMENT, AND GENERAL THERAPEUTIC MEASURES

The initial goals of management include (1) determining the cause, course, and outcome of previous episodes of status asthmaticus in the child, (2) ascertaining the severity of airway obstruction and gas exchange impairment, and (3) anticipating life-threatening hemodynamic and neurologic instability.

One must rapidly review (1) maintenance medications and patient compliance, (2) the therapy and outcome of previous episodes of status asthmaticus, (3) the length of the present illness, and (4) the existence of any evidence of an altered

Differential Diagnosis of Wheezing in the Pediatric Patient

Asthma
Bronchiolitis
Foreign body aspiration
Aspiration pneumonia
Pulmonary edema: cardiogenic and noncardiogenic
Bronchopulmonary dysplasia
Cystic fibrosis
Pulmonary hypertensive crisis
Laryngotracheomalacia
Anomalies of the great vessels
Kussmaul respiratory pattern

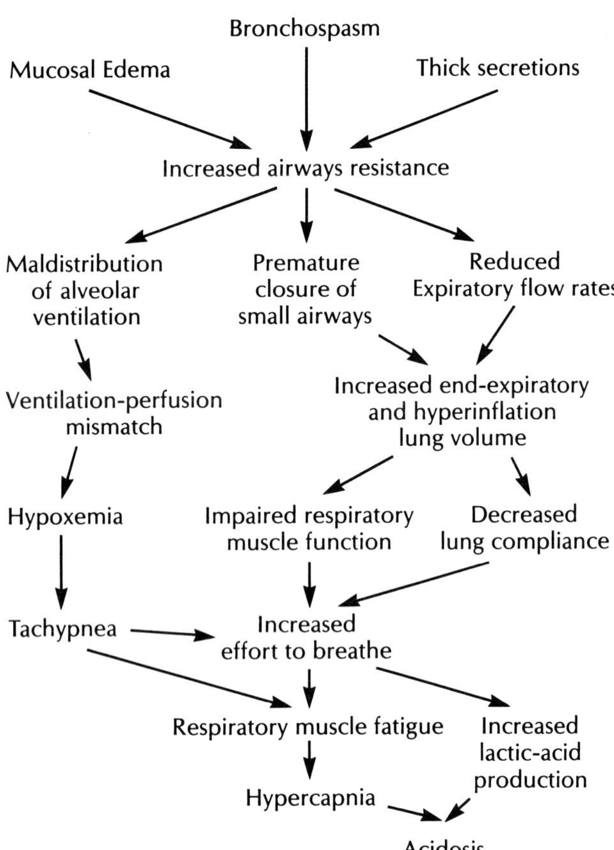

Fig. 289-1 Pathophysiology of status asthmaticus.

level of consciousness. The patient's medical history may contain pertinent information, inasmuch as bronchospasm may also occur in children with cystic fibrosis, bronchopulmonary dysplasia, and hemodynamically significant left-to-right intracardiac shunts (e.g., ventricular septal defects). Underlying chronic cardiorespiratory disease may be a determining factor in the severity of gas exchange impairment.

The severity of status asthmaticus is assessed by the results of initial monitoring, physical examination, and laboratory investigation. Continuous respiratory and electrocardiographic monitoring, as well as pulse oximetry, should be instituted immediately. Supplemental oxygen should be supplied to maintain arterial oxygen saturation greater than 90%.

The child's respiratory effort and pattern are reliable predictors of the severity of airway obstruction and gas exchange impairment. Tachypnea, expiratory grunting, and the use of the accessory muscles of respiration (intercostal, abdominal, and supraclavicular muscles) are evidence of increased work in breathing.[2] Alternating use of the diaphragm and rib cage muscles, paradoxical (upward) movement of the diaphragm on inspiration, or intermittent apnea are signs of respiratory muscle fatigue. Restlessness, agitation, and confusion are nonspecific but important signs of hypoxemia; a depressed level of consciousness (lethargy, obtundation, coma) suggests hypercapnia. Cyanosis is a late sign in the child with status asthmaticus.

Chest auscultation should be performed frequently (i.e., every 15 to 30 minutes). Wheezing signifies obstruction to airflow; prolongation of the expiratory phase of the respiratory cycle (i.e., more than 3 seconds) occurs with physiologically significant obstruction of small airways. Decreased breath sounds or the absence of wheezing in the presence of labored respiratory effort indicates severe disease. Asymmetry of breath sounds suggests atelectasis, tension pneumothorax, or the presence of a foreign body. The physician responsible for making therapeutic decisions should assess the changes in respiratory effort and air movement immediately after the administration of nebulized beta-sympathomimetic agents (discussed later) to gauge the reversibility of the airway obstruction.

Severe airway obstruction in the child with status asthmaticus reduces cardiac output; the development of increased negative pleural pressure during inspiration increases systemic afterload, thereby inhibiting left ventricular output.[3] At the bedside the presence of this phenomenon is ascertained by the measurement of pulsus paradoxus. A reduction in systemic systolic arterial blood pressure of greater than 15 mmHg during inspiration (i.e., when pleural pressure is negative) is abnormal. Pulsus paradoxus greater than 20 mm Hg correlates well with the presence of severe airway obstruction (i.e., forced expiratory volume in 1 second [FEV_1] <60% predicted).[6]

The child's state of hydration should be assessed and assumed to be impaired if the acute attack lasts longer than 8 hours. Initial management includes the administration of intravenous fluids to (1) maintain hydration and (2) replace fluid deficits caused by reduced intake and increased insensible water losses from tachypnea. A total fluid intake of 1800 to 2000 ml/m^2/day (or 120 ml/kg/day) generally is adequate, using a maintenance intravenous solution of D5 0.45% sodium chloride with 30 mEq potassium chloride per liter. The maintenance intravenous rate needs to be adjusted to allow for other infusions and for oral intake. The usefulness of purposeful overhydration to enhance mobilization of secretions has not been substantiated and may result in pulmonary edema.

To assess the adequacy of gas exchange, the physician should obtain arterial blood gas and pH values at the time of initial assessment and management. Alveolar ventilation is inversely and linearly proportional to the arterial carbon dioxide tension ($PaCO_2$); serial measurements of $PaCO_2$ reflect the course of the attack and the effectiveness of therapy. Capillary blood gas measurement, which accurately estimates the $PaCO_2$, is an acceptable alternative to an arterial puncture; it may be less traumatic to the frightened child; and it requires less technical expertise to obtain. An "arterialized" capillary blood gas measurement is obtained by prewarming an extremity to produce vasodilation (usually accomplished by wrapping in a diaper or cloth soaked in warm water) and then puncturing with a lancet the skin of a digit (or the heel in infants) to produce free-flowing drops of blood. The sample is collected in a heparinized capillary tube for analysis. The $PaCO_2$ and pH values of samples thus obtained approximate those of arterial samples, whereas the oxygen tension value (PO_2) does not. Pulse oximetry should be used to assess systemic oxygenation on a continuous and noninvasive basis. To maintain the SaO_2 at a minimum of 92%, supplemental oxygen should be delivered by face mask or nasal cannula to all patients with status asthmaticus. Pulse oximetry is simple to employ and must be available in hospitals responsible for the management of acutely ill children.

A chest roentgenogram should be obtained to assess the degree of hyperinflation and mucous plugging and to check for the presence of pneumonia, pneumothorax, pneumomediastinum, cardiomegaly, pulmonary edema, or an inhaled foreign body. If previous chest roentgenograms are available for comparison, they should be immediately reviewed.

Forced expiratory pulmonary function tests (by use of either a spirometer or a peak flow meter) *should not* be performed. The child with status asthmaticus is too ill to be cooperative; furthermore, the maneuver may worsen the degree of bronchospasm.

A serum theophylline level should be obtained if the child has been receiving a theophylline preparation. During the process of obtaining blood samples, it is reasonable to evaluate the complete blood cell count and serum electrolyte and glucose values.

The accompanying box provides a list of clinical and laboratory predictors of the severity of airway obstruction in the child with status asthmaticus.

SPECIFIC THERAPY

The goal of pharmacologic therapy is to promote bronchodilation by increasing cyclic adenosine monophosphate (cAMP), the active metabolite responsible for bronchial smooth muscle relaxation. This is achieved by stimulating synthesis of cAMP with beta-sympathomimetic agents (e.g., isoproterenol or albuterol) or by blocking its degradation by phosphodiesterase with methylxanthines (e.g., theophylline). The bronchoconstrictor effect of cyclic guanosine monophosphate (cGMP) can be blocked by anticholinergic agents (e.g., atropine). Steroids also increase the sensitivity and number of beta receptors, thereby decreasing the tachyphylaxis that develops to beta-sympathomimetic agents.[6]

Status Asthmaticus: Predictors of Severe Airway Obstruction

- History of previous hospitalizations
- Recurrent episodes in a 24-hour period
- Abnormal vital signs
  - Tachycardia
  - Pulsus paradoxus
  - Tachypnea
- Abnormal respiratory patterns
  - Use of accessory respiratory muscles
  - Respiratory alternans
  - Paradoxical diaphragmatic motion
  - Apnea
- Abnormal air movement
  - Wheezing throughout the expiratory cycle
  - Decreased inspiratory breath sounds
- Abnormal neurologic status
  - Agitation
  - Lethargy
  - Coma
- Abnormal arterial blood gas status
  - Metabolic or respiratory acidosis
  - $PaCO_2$ >50 mm Hg
  - PaO_2 <50 mm Hg

Nebulized Bronchodilators

Aerosol nebulization of beta-sympathomimetic agents, which are safely and effectively administered with minimal patient cooperation, has revolutionized the care of children with status asthmaticus. In addition to promoting bronchodilation, these agents improve mucociliary clearance, thereby enhancing the expectoration of thick sputum. Because of the risk of pneumothorax or pneumomediastinum, these agents should not be administered by positive pressure. Isoproterenol (0.5%) at 0.01 ml/kg, isoetharine (1%) at 0.02 ml/kg, metaproterenol (5%) at 0.01 ml/kg, or albuterol (0.5%) at 0.01 to 0.03 ml/kg may be administered after dilution in 2 ml of 0.9% sodium chloride solution. These are listed in order of increasing beta-2 selectivity (i.e., decreasing cardiac or beta-1 effects) and in order of increasing duration of action; newer and better agents undoubtedly will be marketed in the near future. These medications should be delivered (aerosolized) over a period of 10 to 15 minutes and at intervals of 30 to 180 minutes (as indicated by the patient's clinical course). Atropine (0.01%) at 0.05 ml/kg may also be added to these beta-sympathomimetic treatments every 4 to 6 hours.

Aminophylline

Aminophylline should be administered intravenously to all patients hospitalized with status asthmaticus. If more than two routine oral theophylline doses have been missed or if the patient is not routinely taking a theophylline preparation, then a loading dose of 6 mg/kg needs to be administered over 20 to 30 minutes (a 1 mg/kg bolus will raise the serum level by 2 μg/ml). The serum theophylline level needs to be checked 1 hour after bolus administration to determine that a therapeutic level (10 to 20 μg/ml) has been achieved and again at 12 hours for a steady-state level and thereafter every 12 to 24 hours. Once a therapeutic serum theophylline level is achieved, a maintenance infusion should be started at the rates recommended in Table 289-1. Differences in infusion rates are dictated by the varying volumes of distribution and clearance rates of theophylline as a function of age.[7] The serum theophylline level should be checked any time an inadequate clinical response or toxicity is suspected.

A number of drugs decrease theophylline clearance (i.e., result in an increase in serum levels); most important among these are erythromycin, cimetidine, and oral contraceptives. Liver disease prolongs the half-life of theophylline. Side effects of theophylline include nausea, vomiting, gastritis, agitation, gross tumors, tachycardia, cardiac dysrhythmias, and status epilepticus.

Table 289-1 *Aminophylline Infusion Rate*

AGE	INFUSION RATE* (mg/kg/hr)
Neonate	0.16
1-6 mo	0.50
7-12 mo	0.85
1-9 yr	1.0
>9 yr	0.8

*Add 250 mg aminophylline to 250 ml D_5 so that 1 ml/kg/hr = 1 mg/kg/hr.

Steroids

Intravenous steroids should be administered to all children hospitalized with status asthmaticus. They improve the response to beta-sympathomimetic agents, have antiinflammatory properties, shorten the duration of hospitalization, and do not induce pituitary-adrenal axis suppression if given for fewer than 7 days. Methylprednisolone (Solu-Medrol), 125 mg/m^2/day (or 5 mg/kg/day), or dexamethasone (Decadron), 15 mg/m^2/day (or 0.6 mg/kg/day), in four divided doses is recommended. These medications compared with other steroid preparations exhibit primarily glucocorticoid rather than mineralocorticoid properties. The concurrent administration of antacids or an H_1 receptor antagonist (e.g., ranitidine, 6 mg/kg/day) will minimize the development of stress or steroid-induced gastritis in the patient with status asthmaticus.

TRANSFER OF THE CHILD TO THE PEDIATRIC INTENSIVE CARE UNIT

The development of respiratory failure (i.e., $Paco_2$ >50 mmHg or Pao_2 <50 mm Hg) is an *absolute* indication for the transfer of the child to the PICU for close observation and the institution of life-saving modalities, such as the continuous infusion or nebulization of beta-sympathomimetic agents or mechanical ventilation. Few patients with status asthmaticus will require this degree of intervention, but the following criteria are *relative* indications for PICU admission: (1) the need for placement of an arterial catheter to monitor arterial blood gases and blood pressure, (2) the need for continuous observation and frequent adjustment of therapy as indicated by changes in the patient's clinical course, (3) the failure of the patient to respond rapidly to conventional treatment and anticipation that the patient's course will further deteriorate, or (4) alteration in the patient's normal level of consciousness, as manifested by severe agitation, lethargy, or coma.

The accompanying box provides an outline of the management of the child with status asthmaticus.

Management of the Child with Status Asthmaticus

STEP 1

- History
- Physical examination
- Laboratory evaluation:
  - Arterial blood gas tensions and pH
  - Chest roentgenogram
  - Theophylline level (if appropriate)

STEP 2

- Administer subcutaneous or nebulized beta-sympathomimetic agents
- Decide on the need for hospitalization; if required, initiate the following steps.

STEP 3

- Monitor heart rate and respiratory rate continuously
- Institute pulse oximetry
- Perform physical assessment
- Institute supportive measures: oxygen and intravenous fluids
- Deliver nebulized beta-sympathomimetics as indicated
- Begin intravenous aminophylline
- Begin intravenous steroids

STEP 4

- Reevaluate by physical examination and blood gas analysis
- Check theophylline level
- Assess frequency of need for nebulized medications

STEP 5

- Admit to PICU for:
  - Continuously nebulized or infused beta-sympathomimetics
  - Placement of arterial catheter for frequent ABG analysis
  - Endotracheal intubation and mechanical ventilation
  - Deterioration in mental status

SUMMARY

Status asthmaticus continues to produce significant morbidity and mortality in children. Early intervention, continuous observation, recognition of the clinical signs of severe airway obstruction, use of the many pharmacologic agents now available, and appropriate referral of the high-risk patient to a tertiary pediatric center or ICU are the steps most likely to improve outcome.

REFERENCES

1. American Thoracic Society: Definitions and classification of chronic bronchitis, asthma and pulmonary emphysema, Am Rev Respir Dis 85:762, 1962.
2. McFadden ER, Kiser R, and DeGroot WJ: Acute bronchial asthma: relations between clinical and physiologic manifestations, N Engl J Med 288:221, 1973.
3. Rebuck AS and Pengelly LD: Development of pulsus paradoxicus in the presence of airways obstruction, N Engl J Med 288:66, 1973.
4. Roussos C and Macklem PJ: The respiratory muscles, N Engl J Med 307:786, 1982.
5. Sly M: Mortality from asthma, N Engl Reg Allergy Proc 7:425, 1986.
6. Townley RG and Suliaman F: The mechanism of corticosteroids in treating asthma, Ann Allergy 58:1, 1987.
7. Weinberger M, Hendeles L, and Ahrens R: Clinical pharmacology of drugs used for asthma, Pediatr Clin North Am 28:47, 1981.

SUGGESTED READINGS

Lulla S and Newcomb RW: Emergency management of asthma in children, J Pediatr 97:346, 1980.

Stempel RA and Mellon M: Management of acute severe asthma, Pediatr Clin North Am 31:879, 1984.

Sylbert A and Weiss EB: Status asthmaticus. In Weiss EB, Segal MS, and Stein M, editors: Bronchial asthma, Boston, 1985, Little, Brown & Co.

290

Status Epilepticus

Sarah M. Roddy and Margaret C. McBride

Status epilepticus is defined by the World Health Organization as "a condition characterized by an epileptic seizure that is sufficiently prolonged or repeated at sufficiently brief intervals as to produce an unvarying and enduring epileptic condition."[4] There has been much variability in the interpretation of what constitutes an "unvarying and enduring epileptic condition." The most widely accepted criterion for diagnosis of status epilepticus is any seizure that continues for 30 minutes, or two or more seizures in which the person does not regain consciousness between the episodes.

Status epilepticus can be classified in terms of the type of seizure. Generalized convulsive status epilepticus is the most common and easily recognized form in children. The seizure activity is usually tonic-clonic or clonic and less often is tonic or myoclonic. In partial status epilepticus or epilepsia partialis continua, focal seizure activity is prolonged and restricted to one side of the body without loss of consciousness. Nonconvulsive status epilepticus manifests as a confused, drowsy state in which the patient moves in slow motion. This condition results from continuing or repetitive absence or partial complex seizures.

The incidence of status epilepticus in patients who have epilepsy ranges from 1.3% to 16%.[5] Its relative frequency, based on age, is highest in the younger age groups.[3] Infants and children are also much more likely than adults to have status epilepticus as the manifestation of their first seizure. In one study of children with status epilepticus, 77% had an initial seizure that lasted more than 1 hour.[1] Fever commonly precedes the development of status epilepticus, both in neurologically normal children and in those with a history of neurologic insult before the onset of seizure. Central nervous system infection and electrolyte disturbances are other causes of a status epilepticus that require prompt identification and treatment. A common precipitating factor of status epilepticus in patients with epilepsy is poor compliance with antiepileptic therapy.

Nonconvulsive status epilepticus and epilepsia partialis continua require prompt treatment, but there is less urgency because these seizures do not alter the body's homeostatic mechanisms to the degree that convulsive status epilepticus does. Convulsive status epilepticus is considered a medical emergency, because it is life threatening and is often followed by neurologic sequelae. The longer convulsive status epilepticus continues, the more resistant it is to therapy and the greater the incidence of mortality and morbidity. Experimental studies have shown that continued seizure activity for more than 60 minutes results in permanent cell damage, even in ventilated animals whose metabolic parameters are kept in the normal range. Clinical studies in humans have found that the mean duration of convulsive status is 1½ hours in patients without neurologic sequelae, 10 hours in those with neurologic sequelae, and 13 hours in those who die of convulsive status epilepticus. Mortality rates have gradually dropped over the past century and currently do not exceed 10% to 12%.[2] Death attributable to a seizure is rare, with most deaths resulting from the illness that precipitated the seizure.[5,6]

The objectives of treating convulsive status epilepticus are to maintain vital functions, identify and correct any precipitating factors, and control seizure activity. A plan for management is outlined in the accompanying table. A history should be obtained from an accompanying family member and should include any history of previous seizure, chronic and recent medication usage, intercurrent illness, head trauma, and details of the onset of status epilepticus. On physical examination, any evidence of head trauma, increased intracranial pressure, or infection should be noted. A urine toxicology screen is helpful in determining if the seizures were precipitated by drug ingestion. Computed tomography (CT) scanning may be required to rule out an intracranial lesion if the etiology of status epilepticus remains obscure. If the history or physical examination suggests a central nervous system infection, antibiotics should be administered immediately and a lumbar puncture performed as soon as seizure activity has been controlled. Because neurologic sequelae of status epilepticus can result from complicating factors such as hypoxia, hypotension, and acidosis, attention should immediately be given to the respiratory and cardiovascular status of the child. If the patient is febrile, reducing body temperature is extremely urgent because of the synergism of fever and status epilepticus in producing brain damage. Fortunately, most episodes of status epilepticus are controlled by one or more of the drugs listed in the box on p. 1676.

Once seizure activity is controlled, management should be directed toward preventing recurrence of seizures, including maintaining anticonvulsant therapy. The appropriate duration of therapy following an initial episode of idiopathic status epilepticus is not clear. Recurrence of seizures in this situation may be as low as 25%.[6]

Treatment of Status Epilepticus

A. Assess cardiovascular function by making sure the airway is clear and the patient is breathing. Provide oxygen or respiratory support as necessary.
B. Establish an intravenous line and obtain blood samples for electrolytes, blood urea nitrogen, calcium, a complete blood count, and anticonvulsant medication levels. A blood Dextrostix test should be performed immediately, and if the glucose is under 60 mg%, then 1 to 2 ml/kg of D25W should be administered.
C. One member of the emergency team should obtain a history while another does a brief physical examination.
D. Administer anticonvulsant drugs in the following order until seizure activity is controlled:
   1. Initial therapy
      a. Lorazepam should be the initial anticonvulsant administered intravenously at a dose of 0.1 mg/kg (maximum 4 mg) over 2 minutes; a dose of 0.05 to 0.1 mg/kg may be repeated every 5 minutes if necessary up to a maximum of 0.5 mg/kg, but not over 10 mg in toto.
      b. If lorazepam is not available, diazepam should be administered intravenously at a dose of 0.1 to 0.2 mg/kg (maximum 10 mg) by "pushing" half the dose over 1 minute and the remainder at 1 mg/minute. A dose of 0.1 mg/kg may be repeated in 5 minutes if necessary. Because of diazepam's short duration of anticonvulsant effect, another anticonvulsant such as phenytoin must be administered immediately.
      c. If the patient is known to be receiving phenytoin on a chronic basis, it should be administered as the initial anticonvulsant (see below).
   2. If status epilepticus continues, administer phenytoin 15 to 20 mg/kg intravenously up to a total dose of 1000 mg. A quarter of the dose may be administered during the first 2 minutes and then at a rate of 1 to 2 mg/kg/minute (maximum rate of 50 mg/minute). If the patient is known to be receiving phenytoin chronically, 5 to 8 mg/kg of phenytoin may be administered as the initial anticonvulsant. Monitor the heart rate, and slow the rate of phenytoin infusion if bradycardia occurs. If seizure activity continues despite a full loading dose of phenytoin, correct for presumed acidosis with a modest dose of sodium bicarbonate.
   3. If status epilepticus continues, administer phenobarbital 15 to 20 mg/kg intravenously up to a total dose of 800 mg. Administer phenobarbital over 15 minutes, monitoring respirations and blood pressure, especially if the patient has been given a benzodiazepine.
   4. If status epilepticus persists, administer paraldehyde 0.3 ml/kg mixed with mineral oil (maximum of 5 ml) per rectum.
E. If seizure activity still persists, consult a neurologist to determine the need for other anticonvulsants, general anesthesia, or induction of pentobarbital coma.

REFERENCES

1. Aicardi J and Chevrie JJ: Convulsive status epilepticus in infants and children: a study of 239 cases, Epilepsia 11:187, 1970.
2. Delgado-Escueta AV et al: Current concepts in neurology: management of status epilepticus, N Engl J Med 306:1337, 1982.
3. Dreifuss FE: Pediatric epileptology: classification and management of seizures in the child, Boston, 1983, John Wright/PSG, Inc.
4. Gastaut H, editor: Dictionary of epilepsy. I. Definitions, Geneva, 1973, World Health Organization.
5. Hauser WA: Status epilepticus: frequency, etiology, and neurological sequelae. In Delgado-Esqueta AV et al, editors: Advances in neurology, vol 34, New York, 1983, Raven Press.
6. Maytal J et al: Low morbidity and mortality of status epilepticus in children, Pediatrics 83:323, 1989.

291

Thermal Injuries

L.R. Scherer III

The leading cause of death in children between 1 and 15 years of age is accidental injury. Each year thermal injuries affect an estimated 1 million children in the United States; 10%, or 100,000 require hospitalization.[5] Of these, 3000 die as a result of their injuries, making thermal injuries the third leading cause of accidental death in children, after motor vehicle accidents and drowning. Permanent disability remains a major complication in the long-term rehabilitation of the pediatric patient.

ETIOLOGY

Most childhood thermal injuries occur in the child's home. Approximately 80% to 90% of these injuries are potentially preventable.[5] The pattern of injury is related to the child's age and sex. During the first 2 years of life, 60% of the injuries are caused by scald burns from hot liquids; they involve boys twice as often as girls.[1] This may be because of the seemingly more active and inquisitive nature of males in this age group. Most scald burns occur when a young child accidentally pulls a pan or pot of hot liquid off the stove or table onto the head, chest, and arms. Occasionally a small child may manage to turn on the hot water in the bathtub, or a parent may carelessly or deliberately place a child in a bathtub full of scalding water, causing burns to the arms, buttocks, legs, or feet. Although scald burns more commonly involve only partial-thickness injury, in infants and toddlers the skin is quite thin, and scald burns may result in full-thickness loss.

Because toddlers insist on exploration, the next most common childhood burn results from contact with hot surfaces in the home. These injuries usually involve only the "exploring" surfaces of the extremities.

Flame burn injuries are more common in children over 3 years of age. There is no sex predilection in this age group.[5] Causes include the careless use of matches, space heaters, outdoor fires, and stoves. Governmental restrictions on the manufacture of children's sleepwear have decreased the risk of flame injury in young children, but flammable products are still involved in most flame burn injuries. Because of the intense thermal enrgy in flame burns, full-thickenss injury is more common with major burns, thus increasing the mortality in this age group.

PATHOPHYSIOLOGY

During the assessment of the burn patient, it is necessary to determine the depth and extent of injury in order to develop a treatment plan. Classically, the depth of a burn has been categorized as first, second, or third degree. A first-degree burn is a superficial burn that involves only the epidermis. First-degree burns are erythematous and painful and do not produce blisters. The most common first-degree burn is overexposure to the sun. First-degree burns should not be included in the estimation of the total extent of a burn wound injury. Occasionally, first-degree burns are seen secondary to flash burns from an explosion. A second-degree burn, more commonly regarded as a partial-thickness skin loss, is usually erythematous or appears mottled red. The epidermal and dermal injury is evident with blistering, is moist to the touch, and is extremely painful to touch and exposure. A deep partial-thickness burn appears mottled and waxy because of complete injury to the entire epidermis and dermis, with only skin appendages spared: therefore it may look like a full-thickness injury. A full-thickness injury involves the epidermis, dermis, and subcutaneous tissue. These injuries appear dry or waxlike. There are no blisters, and the skin may be white or black. The texture of the skin is hard, dry, and leathery with no elasticity, and coagulated veins are noticeable. These injuries are painless to touch because of complete injury to all skin appendages.

Injury from partial-thickness and full-thickness burns results in increased capillary permeability and sequestration of large quantities of fluids within the extravascular space. Because of the larger surface area of the infant and child, as well as the thinner skin and subcutaneous tissue, the young subject tends to lose more fluid and body heat than do adults. These greater evaporative water and body heat losses require the use of larger quantities of fluid for resuscitation and external temperature regulation.

Significant morbidity and mortality occur secondary to inhalation thermal injuries. The manifestations of these injuries may not be apparent for the first 24 hours. Major injuries to the respiratory tract result from inhaling products of incomplete combustion and toxic fumes and/or direct thermal injury to the upper or lower respiratory tract.

Inhaling products of incomplete combustion or toxic fumes may lead to chemical tracheobronchitis and pneumonia. Carbon monoxide (CO) exposure in children who sustain burns in an enclosed space should always be assumed. Because of the high affinity of CO for hemoglobin (240 times that of oxygen), CO displaces oxygen from the hemoglobin molecule and shifts the dissociation curve to the left. Carbon monoxide dissociates from hemoglobin very slowly: when breathing 100% oxygen, 50% of the patient's CO will dissociate within 40 minutes; it takes 250 minutes for this to happen when breathing room air. Therefore the patient with suspected smoke inhalation should be treated with 100% oxygen.

Direct thermal injury is caused by inhaling heated gases; it rarely causes injury below the vocal cords except when volatile gases or steam is inhaled. Airway injury produces edema and obstruction, mucosal sloughing, bronchorrhea, and pulmonary edema. Early management of inhalation injuries includes endotracheal intubation and administration of 100% oxygen.

HISTORY

It is extremely important while evaluating a burned pediatric patient to obtain a detailed clinical history. It is important to know when, where, and how the burn occurred and the nature of the burning agent. If it is determined that the injury occurred within an enclosed environment, a smoke inhalation injury should be suspected and aggressive airway management should be initiated. Evaluation should include the child's general health, the preexistence of medical problems, allergies and, most important, immunization status. Recent infection should be noted, especially the possibility of a streptococcal organism. A careful clinical history helps determine the depth of the wound, potential associated trauma, particulate or thermal airway injury, and carbon monoxide poisoning.

The diagnosis of chid abuse can be obtained from detailed information of the injury's history. The physician taking a history that includes the following events should suspect child abuse: (1) an accident that occurs when the child is alone, (2) an injury incurred by a sibling, (3) unclear or inconsistent history, (4) previous history of accidental injury, (5) injury incompatible with description of event, (6) delay in seeking medical attention, and (7) unstable social environment.[2]

CLINICAL FINDINGS

On initial evaluation, all clothing should be removed from the child to stop the burning process and to allow complete assessment of all potential injuries. Airway assessment is particularly important in flame injuries and injuries encountered in an enclosed environment. The child should be assessed for facial burns, singed eyebrows and nasal hairs, carbon deposits in the oropharynx, and carbonaceous sputum, all of which indicate significant airway injury. Early airway management includes endotracheal intubation; delayed intubation may not only be late but more difficult because of upper airway edema. Early and rapid assessment for asociated injuries is necessary when the child has neurologic impairment, a history of trauma, an electrical injury, or evidence of abuse. Unrecognized visceral or long-bone injuries will result in significant morbidity and mortality in the burned child.

At this point a careful, thorough inspection of the burn wounds is necessary. The child should be completely disrobed and all wounds covered with sterile dry linens or towels. Mask, gown, and gloves are worn to inspect the depth and extent of the burn injury. Estimation of the burned surface area in children is determined by using the Lund and Browder chart (Fig. 291-1), because younger children have a relatively larger surface area of the head and small surface area of the lower extremities. Estimation of the surface area is required for the management of fluid therapy and for wound care and prognosis. Pitfalls in estimation occur in chemical and electrical injuries, in which extensive tissue damage may manifest few signs of dermal injury.

OUTPATIENT MANAGEMENT

As stated earlier, approximately 90% of childhood burns can be treated outside of the hospital. Minor burns may be classified as partial thickness burns involving no more than 10% of the body surface or full thickness burns involving no more than 2 percent of the body surface (see the box on p. 1680). Generally, these patients can be treated with oral fluids and burn wound care in the emergency room or the pediatrician's office. The wounds should be cleansed with water or saline and a mild antibacterial solution. Blisters should be left intact as this provides greater comfort and ease of care; however, open blisters should be debrided. Silver sulfadiazine cream is applied to the wound twice daily after cleansing, and dry, sterile, occlusive dressing is applied to the wound. Close observation is required in the initial management of burn wounds, and the child should be seen every 48 hours to evaluate the depth of the burn wound and potential complications. Once intact blisters begin to leak or are no longer tense, the blisters should be debrided. In the overall care of a minor injury, the child should be managed with oral hydration and pain alleviated with acetaminophen or codeine. Most important, the child's tetanus immunization status must be documented and updated if necessary. Facial burns may be treated with open dressings, applying an antibacterial ointment such as bacitracin, neosporin, or polymyxin B to the partial-thickness burn wound areas three times daily. Partial-thickness burn wounds should reepithelize within 14 to 21 days. Follow-up calls for monitoring wound healing and patient compliance with the healing regimen, comfort, and early rehabilitation.

PRIMARY CARE HOSPITAL MANAGEMENT

More extensive burn injuries require hospitalization for wound care and intravenous fluid therapy (see box). Hospital treatment is required in cases of partial-thickness burns involving 10% to 20% of body surface; full-thickness burns involving 2% to 10% of body surface; partial-thickness injury to the face, hands, feet, and perineum; questionable burn wound depth and extent; minor chemical burns; inadequate family support; or suspected abuse. In the emergency room the assessment of a child with a thermal injury involves evaluation of the airway and associated injuries and estimation of the burn wound area and depth of injury. With severe injuries, intravenous fluid resuscitation is required, and one or two peripheral intravenous lines are required for intravenous fluid therapy. In the approach to fluid management, the Parkland formula may be used in burns involving more than 15% of body surface. The formula uses 3 ml of lactated Ringer solution per kilogram per percent burn in addition to the child's regular maintenance fluid during the first 24 hours after the burn injury. Half of the fluid is given over the first

Burn Estimate Age vs Area

Area	Birth 1yr.	1-4 yr.	5-9 yr.	10-14 yr.	15 yr.	2°	3°	Total
Head	19	17	13	11	9			
Neck	2	2	2	2	2			
Ant. Trunk	13	13	13	13	13			
Post. Trunk	13	13	13	13	13			
R. Buttock	2 1/2	2 1/2	2 1/2	2 1/2	2 1/2			
L. Buttock	2 1/2	2 1/2	2 1/2	2 1/2	2 1/2			
Genitalia	1	1	1	1	1			
R.U. Arm	4	4	4	4	4			
L.U. Arm	4	4	4	4	4			
R.L. Arm	3	3	3	3	3			
L.L. Arm	3	3	3	3	3			
R. Hand	2 1/2	2 1/2	2 1/2	2 1/2	2 1/2			
L. Hand	2 1/2	2 1/2	2 1/2	2 1/2	2 1/2			
R. Thigh	5 1/2	6 1/2	8	8 1/2	9			
L. Thigh	5 1/2	6 1/2	8	8 1/2	9			
R. Leg	5	5	5 1/2	6	6 1/2			
L. Leg	5	5	5 1/2	6	6 1/2			
R. Foot	3 1/2	3 1/2	3 1/2	3 1/2	3 1/2			
L. Foot	3 1/2	3 1/2	3 1/2	3 1/2	3 1/2			
					Total			

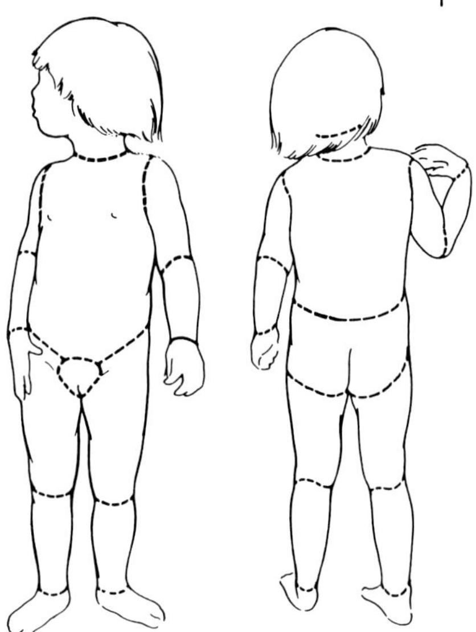

Fig. 291-1 Burn chart for estimating extent of injury. Numbers equal percent of total body surface.

8 hours after injury, and the remaining half is delivered over the following 16 hours. The adequacy of fluid therapy is determined by urinary output, which should be maintained at 1 to 2 ml/kg/hr (measuring output may require the use of a Foley catheter). With extensive burns, a central venous pressure line may be required in the management of fluid therapy. Children with a burn covering 15% or more of the body surface often develop a paralytic ileus, and therefore nasogastric tube decompression is often required. All medications, including antibiotics, analgesics, or sedatives, should be given intravenously since perfusion is unpredictable. Initial management of the wound is similar to the management of minor wounds except for the extent and potential depth of the wound. Therefore early involvement by the surgical team is required for the overall assessment and management of the burned child.

BURN CENTER MANAGEMENT

Thermal injuries of greatest magnitude—that is, partial-thickness burns involving more than 20% of body surface area; full-thickness burns involving more than 10% of body surface area; full-thickness burns of the face, hands, feet, or perineum; a respiratory tract injury; an associated major injury, or major chemical or electrical burns—require the special facilities and personnel of a regional burn center (see box on p. 1680). A burn center offers specialists involved in the long-term physical, psychological, and social needs of these infants and children.[4,7] These centers have produced remarkable improvements in the morbidity and mortality of those with major burns. The injured child needs careful evaluation and adequate resuscitation before transfer to a burn center. Initial evaluation and resuscitation include early airway sta-

Triage Criteria for Thermal Injuries

OUTPATIENT MANAGEMENT

Partial-thickness burn <10% body surface area (BSA)
Full-thickness burn <2% BSA

INPATIENT MANAGEMENT

Primary care hospital
Partial-thickness burn 10%-20% BSA
Full-thickness burn 2%-10% BSA
Partial-thickness burn to face, perineum, hands, or feet
Questionable burn wound depth or extent
Inadequate family support
Suspected abuse

BURN CENTER

Partial-thickness burn >20% BSA
Full-thickness burn >10% BSA
Full-thickness burn to face, perineum, hands, or feet
Respiratory tract injury
Associated major trauma
Significant coexisting illness
Chemical or electrical burns

bilization, adequate intravenous access, fluid resuscitation with lactated Ringer solution, tetanus immunization, and coverage of the burn wounds with sterile, dry linens or towels. To initiate the transfer, it is important that there be telephone communication between the referring physician and the coordinator of the burn center. All pertinent information regarding laboratory evaluation, temperature, pulse, fluids administered, and urinary output should be recorded and a flowchart sent with the patient. Any other information deemed important by either the referring physician or the burn center physician should be sent with the child. At the time of transport, the child must be well prepared with a secure airway, an established and secure intravenous line, burn dressings, adequate pain relief, and a nasogastric tube and Foley catheter in place.

SPECIAL BURN REQUIREMENTS: ELECTRICAL BURNS

Electrical burns result when a source of electrical power makes contact with a person's body.[5] Electrical burns are frequently more serious than they appear externally. A current passing through the body may destroy muscles, nerves, and blood vessels but spare skin and bone because of their high resistance. Rhabdomyolysis results in myoglobin release, which may cause acute renal failure. As with any serious injury, immediate management of the patient includes attention to the airway and breathing, establishment of intravenous access, electrocardiographic monitoring, and placement of an indwelling urethral catheter. If the urine is cola colored, one must assume myoglobin is present in the urine. Fluid should be administered at a rate to ensure urinary output of at least 3 to 5 ml/kg/hr. If the pigment does not clear with increased fluid administration, 500 mg/kg of mannitol should be administered immediately, and 12.5 g of mannitol is added to subsequent liters of fluid to maintain diuresis. Metabolic acidosis should be corrected by maintaining adequate perfusion, and sodium bicarbonate should be used to alkalinize the urine and increase the solubility of myoglobin.

The most common electrical burn in children involves the toddler, when the corner of the mouth is injured by chewing on an electrical cord. Initial management of these injuries involves standard wound care and topical application of an antibiotic ointment. These wounds should be allowed to demarcate and a plastic surgeon should be involved in their early assessment and management.

COMPLICATIONS

A number of complications may occur in the early management of thermal injuries in children[2]; the most catastrophic occurs when an inhalation injury is not recognized. This results in failure to place a secure airway in a child facing severe respiratory distress. If a child suffers thermal injury within an enclosed space, an inhalation injury must be suspected and early endotracheal intubation performed to secure an airway before respiratory compromise develops. The second most common complication arises from underestimating the size and depth of a burn, which is most often seen in scald burns of young children. Early and repeated methodical examination, using a burn chart (Fig. 291-1), helps in estimating the size of the injury. A common unrecognized complication is failure to suspect child abuse. Burns are frequently encountered as part of a spectrum of injuries inflicted on children.

Later complications in the management of children with moderate to severe burns requiring hospitalization include pneumonia,[4] septic thrombophlebitis,[4] burn wound sepsis,[3] peptic ulcer disease,[6] and behavior disorders.[2] The use of appropriate antibiotic therapy, vigorous pulmonary toilet, and intensive ventilatory support are the mainstays of prevention of pulmonary complications in a burn patient.

Potentially lethal infections include suppurative skin lesions or thrombophlebitis when both peripheral and central venous catheters are used. The usual organisms involved are *Staphylococcus aureus, Staphylococcus epidermidis,* or a variety of gram-negative bacterial organisms. Burn-wound sepsis remains a complication with significant morbidity and mortality; thus prevention is essential. Early aggressive debridement and excision of the wound, use of surveillance quantitative culture, and institution of appropriate topical and systemic antibiotic therapy are the cornerstones of prevention and management of burn-wound sepsis. One of the lethal complications in a child with a burn injury is a gastroduodenal ulcer (Curling ulcer). The mortality rate is higher than 60% for children who suffer more than 60% of blood loss over a 24-hour period from peptic ulcer disease secondary to burns. The prevalence, morbidity, and mortality have diminished with the use of antacids, hydrogen-antagonist therapy, and early enteral feeding of burn patients. Because of the severe and chronic nature of burns, psychological changes often occur in children: Characteristically, they regress to earlier stages of development. Behavior changes include hostility and self-destructive behavior. Treatment may require sedation, but usually a great deal of understanding and support for the patient and the family by members of the burn team is required. A cheerful environment, an experienced staff of child-life personnel, and a humane approach to the numerous painful procedures are most beneficial.

PROGNOSIS

The morbidity and mortality of thermal injuries have declined in the past 20 years because of advances in fluid therapy, management of pulmonary complications, control of wound infections by topical antibiotic agents, and advances in surgical wound management, nutrition, and regionalization of care.[3,4,7]

The most remarkable areas of improvement involve burn care. The use of topical antibacterial therapy has changed the LD_{50} from 35% of body surface area (BSA) burn to 65% BSA burn.[4,7] Since the development of early excision and grafting of large body surface area burns, several authors have reported an LD_{50} of greater than 90% BSA burn. Other authors argue that aggressive fluid resuscitation, early excision and grafting, and the overall improved management of the burned child has improved survival.

The early determinants of unnecessary mortality include inadequate volume resuscitation and inappropriate asessment of inhalation injury.[4] Later predictors of mortality include secondary development of renal, cardiovascular, and pulmonary organ failure.

Since the evolution of these new therapies, a child has an excellent prognosis with a burn under 70% BSA, but the morbidity remains high because these children may develop hypertrophic scarring and contractures. Physical and occupational therapy and the use of long-term compressive garments have diminished the morbidity of these wound complications, but further investigation of the prevention of these scars and contractures is required. Again, 90% of children suffering from burns can be treated as outpatients with the expectation of reepithelization of the wound within 5 to 14 days. Further investigation and development of therapies for the 10% who require long-term hospitalization, physical therapy, and rehabilitation of their burn wounds is required to decrease the morbidity of their long-term care, which currently may require 4 to 6 months of hospitalization.

REFERENCES

1. Feldman KW et al: Tap water scald burns in children, Pediatrics 62:1, 1978.
2. Harmel RP, Vane DW, and King DR: Burn care in children: special considerations, Clin Plast Surg 13:95, 1986.
3. Herndon DN et al: A comparison of conservative versus early excision, Ann Surg 209:547, 1989.
4. Herndon DN et al: Determinants of mortality in pediatric patients with greater than 70% full-thickness total body surface area thermal injury treated by early total excision and grafting, J Trauma 27:208, 1987.
5. McLoughlin E and Crawford JD: Burns, Pediatr Clin North Am 32:61, 1985.
6. Prasad JK, Thomson PD, and Feller I: Gastrointestinal hemorrhage in burn patients, Burns 13:194, 1987.
7. Tompkins RG et al: Significant reductions in mortality for children with burn injuries through the use of prompt eschar excision, Ann Surg 208:577, 1988.

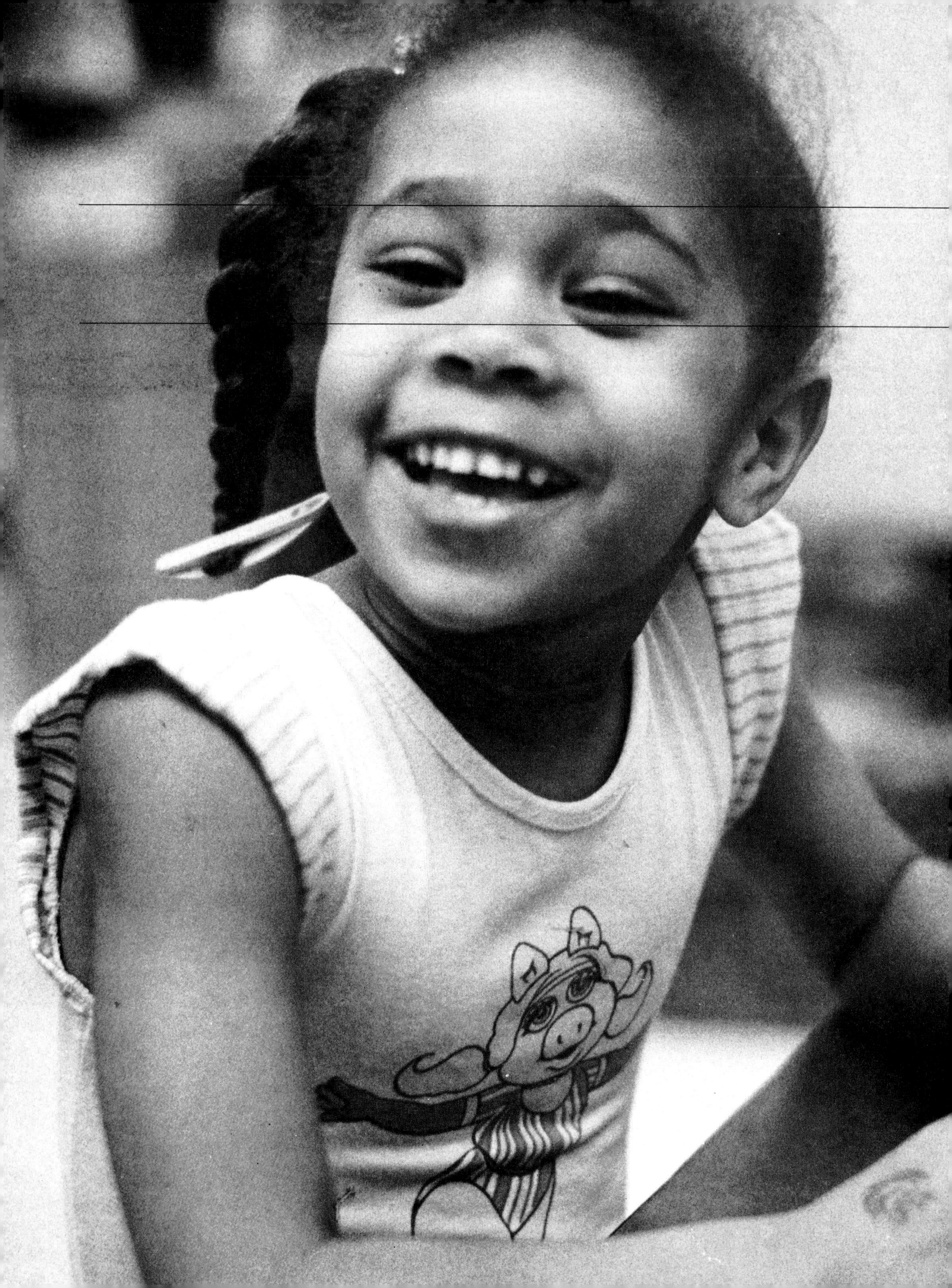

Appendixes

A *Pediatric Basic and Advanced Life Support*

B *Special Procedures*

C *Miscellaneous Values*

D *Common Psychological and Educational Tests*

A

Pediatric Basic and Advanced Life Support

Howard C. Mofenson and Joseph Greensher

An estimated 40,000 infants younger than 1 year of age and 16,000 children between 1 and 14 years of age die annually in the United States from all causes. The majority of deaths in infants younger than 1 year occur before they are 4 months of age.[2] The mortality of infants younger than 15 months who suffer cardiac arrest outside a hospital is almost 100%.[29] Even hospital inpatient cardiac arrests carry a mortality rate of more than 90%, and 50% of the survivors have major neurologic damage.[9]

This appendix reviews and updates the newest guidelines for pediatric basic cardiopulmonary resuscitation and advanced life support. It is not intended as a substitute for participation in the basic and advanced life support courses given by the American Heart Association and the American Academy of Pediatrics. In the discussion that follows, the infant is defined as 1 year of age or younger, the child as 1 to 8 years of age, and the older child as older than 8 years of age.

Cardiopulmonary arrest is the failure of both effective ventilation and circulation. *Respiratory arrest* is the lack of effective ventilation as evidenced by absence of breath sounds or air movement or of thoracoabdominal movement. *Cardiac arrest* is the loss of effective circulation as evidenced by the absence of pulsation in a major artery.

Basic life support is designed to generate perfusion of the vital organs with some oxygenated blood during cardiac arrest. To be successful it must be coupled with advanced life support measures.

In 1985 the National Conference on Cardiopulmonary Resuscitation and Emergency Cardiac Care revised national standards for pediatric basic life support, advanced life support, and neonatal resuscitation. These changes were published in 1986.[15]

DIFFERENCES BETWEEN CARDIOPULMONARY ARREST IN CHILDREN AND IN ADULTS

Adults

The cause of cardiopulmonary arrest (CPA) in adults commonly is an acute cardiac insult, such as myocardial infarction, leading to a disturbance in cardiac rhythm. It usually occurs in patients whose hearts are already damaged. Ventricular fibrillation is common, and unmonitored defibrillation may be attempted to restore normal cardiac rhythm.

Children

The cause of CPA in children usually is severe hypoxia and acidosis or circulatory collapse, or both. Management focuses on prevention of these events with prearrest assessment and anticipatory intervention by means of respiratory ventilation techniques. The establishment of airway patency and adequate ventilation often will make further resuscitative measures unnecessary, if the child is not yet in CPA and is only in respiratory arrest or compromise. Asystole occurs in 90% of pediatric patients with cardiac arrest; unmonitored defibrillation therefore is not recommended.[2]

• • •

Table A-1 summarizes the distinguishing features of CPA in adults and in children.

Children need oxygen more than medications to correct rhythm disturbances; however, they do require medications for some dysrhythmias; for example, epinephrine and bicarbonate for asystole, digoxin for supraventricular tachycardia, and lidocaine for ventricular dysrythmias. The anatomic and physiologic differences of children, compared with adults, present special problems. For example, in pediatric patients major differences exist in the anatomy of the airways, the airway diameter, the methods used for vascular access, and the choice of medication. A special cart with age-labeled equipment and precalculated medication doses should be available.

Cardiopulmonary arrest in children usually is not sudden. It often can be prevented if respiratory failure and shock are

Table A-1 *Differences Between Adults and Children in Cardiopulmonary Arrest*

FEATURE	ADULTS	CHILDREN
Cause	Myocardial infarction	Hypoxia and acidosis
Cardiac status	Damaged heart	Healthy heart
Dysrhythmia	Ventricular fibrillation	Asystole
Defibrillation	Unmonitored	Only monitored
Predominant therapy	Defibrillation	Oxygen

recognized early and therapy initiated promptly.[2,25] Respiratory failure and shock can be recognized within 30 seconds by assessment of the *a*irway, *b*reathing, and *c*irculation (ABC).

RESPIRATORY FAILURE

Respiratory failure occurs when there is inadequate ventilation and oxygenation. Its clinical definition is based on the inability of pulmonary gas exchange to satisfy the body's metabolic demands for oxygen transport and carbon dioxide elimination. Its presence is confirmed by abnormal blood gas (pO_2, pCO_2)and pH levels, not by physical signs, except for apnea. The presence of respiratory failure or impending respiratory failure is determined by the evaluation of airway patency, the quality of breathing, and for signs of hypoxia and hypercardia (cyanosis, central nervous system depression and bradycardia.)

Airway Patency

The airway is clinically determined to be (1) patent, requiring no intervention, (2) maintainable with noninvasive procedures such as positioning, suctioning, or a bag-valve-mask system, or (3) unmaintainable, requiring invasive procedures such as the use of airway adjuncts, endotracheal intubation, cricothyroidotomy, and foreign body removal.

Breathing

The effectiveness of breathing and oxygenation is clinically evaluated by analyzing the respiratory rate, air entry, respiratory effort, skin and muscosal color, and level of consciousness.

The *respiratory rate* is classified as apnea, tachypnea, or bradypnea. The respiratory rate varies and is nonspecific for age. Tachypnea without respiratory distress may result from attempts to compensate for metabolic acidosis ("quiet tachypnea"). Bradypnea is ominous and may be due to fatigue or central nervous system (CNS) depression. Any respiratory rate greater than 60/min or less than 10/min is abnormal at any age.

The adequacy of tidal volume (5 to 7 ml/kg) is best assessed by auscultating for breath sounds and *air entry* at the periphery of the lung fields, over the apices and laterally, and by observing excursions of the chest wall. The minute volume equals the tidal volume times the respiratory rate. Minute volume may be low because of breaths that are too shallow or a respiratory rate that is too slow.

Increased *respiratory effort* indicates respiratory distress and represents compensation for inadequate gas exchange. The minute volume is reflected in the work of breathing. The signs of increased respiratory effort are head bobbing, nasal flaring, grunting, stridor, the use of the accessory muscles, retractions, seesaw movement of the chest and abdomen, and prolonged expiration. These findings mandate measurement of arterial blood gases.

The *skin color* reflects the level of tissue oxygenation. Decreased oxygenation causes an ashen gray or cyanotic color of the skin and mucosa. It is a late sign of hypoxia.

The *level of consciousness* reflects oxygenation and perfusion of the brain. Patients are classified according to their responsiveness as AVPU, or *a*lert, *v*erbal response, *p*ain response, or *u*nconscious. An early sign of decreased cerebral oxygenation and perfusion is failure of an infant older than the age of 2 months to recognize his or her parents.

SHOCK (CIRCULATORY FAILURE)

Shock is a clinical state characterized by failure of the cardiovascular system to perfuse vital organs adequately, resulting in inadequate oxygen delivery. This failure to deliver oxygen and other critical substrates to meet the demands of the tissues and to remove their metabolites results in anaerobic metabolism and the accumulation of acids. Shock may occur with normal, increased, or decreased cardiac output and blood pressure. In *compensated shock* the blood pressure is normal. In *decompensated shock* the blood pressure and cardiac output are low.

Shock is classified as either hypovolemic or cardiogenic. *Hypovolemic shock,* or distributive shock, the most common type in pediatric patients, is caused by a loss of vascular space volume as a result of dehydration or blood loss or a loss of vascular tone, such as occurs in sepsis, anaphylaxis, and acute CNS pathology. *Cardiogenic shock* caused by heart failure or dysrhythmias is relatively rare in pediatric patients, except in postcardiac arrest patients in whom it is the primary cause of shock.

Cardiovascular performance can be evaluated by assessing the peripheral pulses, skin perfusion, the level of consciousness and heart rate, and later the blood pressure and urinary output.

Pulse. Palpation of the peripheral pulse (a reflection of peripheral perfusion) allows estimation of the stroke volume, heart rate, systemic vascular resistance, and blood pressure. The stroke volume is the volume of blood pumped by each heart beat. The cardiac output is the volume of blood pumped by the heart every minute (heart rate times stroke volume). Organ perfusion is determined by the cardiac output and the peripheral vascular resistance.

Skin Perfusion. The skin is a relatively nonessential organ and loses its perfusion first. This is assessed by capillary refill time or the time it takes for normal skin color to return after applying blanching pressure. It should be less than 2 seconds or less than the time it takes to say "capillary refill." In testing for capillary refill the extremity used should be elevated above the level of the heart. Poor perfusion also can be identified by mottled skin color, cool hands and feet, and a line of demarcation that separates the warm from the cool skin of an extremity.

Level of Consciousness. Evidence of decreased brain oxygenation and perfusion is discussed under *respiratory failure,* above.

Heart Rate. Changes in the heart rate reflect changes in cardiac output but unfortunately are nonspecific. Heart rates that are greater than 180 beats per minute in patients younger than 5 years of age, greater than 160 beats per minute in patients between 5 and 10 years of age, and greater than 100 beats per minute in patients older than 10 years of age constitute tachycardia. The presence of tachycardia requires differentiation between its benign and serious causes. When tachycardia fails to compensate for tissue oxygen needs adequately, hypoxia, hypercapnia, acidosis, and bradycardia develop. Bradycardia in a distressed child is an ominous sign of impending cardiac arrest.

Blood Pressure. The blood pressure is a product of cardiac output times the peripheral vascular resistance. Hypotension is a late and ominous finding in patients with shock. The systolic blood pressure should be higher than 60 mm Hg from birth to 1 months of age and greater than 70 mm Hg from 1 month to 1 year. A formula for determining the lower limit for systolic blood pressure in children older than 1 year of age is 70 + (2 times the age in years). This represents a level that is greater than 2 standard deviations below the mean.

Urinary Output. The normal urinary output is 1 to 2 ml/kg/hr. Although this measure is unavailable to help in initial evaluation, it is a valuable indication of kidney perfusion later on. The bladder urine initially obtained should not be used for calculating urinary output.

In respiratory failure the blood is delivered to the body tissues adequately, but the blood delivered is deficient in oxygen content. In shock the blood contains adequate oxygen, but is is delivered poorly. Both conditions can lead to hypoxia, hypercapnia, anaerobic metabolism, acidosis, and cardiopulmonary arrest. Table A-2 summarizes the ABCs of cardiorespiratory assessment.

Table A-2 *Summary of Cardiorespiratory Assessment*

RESPIRATORY ASSESSMENT	CARDIOVASCULAR ASSESSMENT
A. Airway patency B. Breathing 1. Rate 2. Air entry, breath sounds, chest excursions 3. Respiratory effort 4. Color 5. Level of consciousness	C. Circulation 1. Peripheral pulses 2. Skin perfusion 3. Level of consciousness 4. Heart rate 5. Blood pressure 6. Urinary output

Modified from Chameides L, editor: Textbook of pediatric advanced life support, Dallas, 1988, American Heart Association and American Academy of Pediatrics.

PEDIATRIC BASIC LIFE SUPPORTS

In applying pediatric basic life support measures, priorities of management should be based on clinical assessment. Questionable cases, as well as successfully resuscitated cases of cardiopulmonary arrest require frequent reassessment with arterial blood gas determinations and chest films.

The patient's condition should be classified as one of the following:

1. *Stable,* which requires no intervention, but continued reassessment
2. *Questionable,* which requires very frequent reassessment
3. *Definite respiratory failure or shock,* which requires immediate intervention
4. *Cardiopulmonary failure,* which requires basic and advanced life support

General Priorities of Management

1. In upper airway obstruction, the child should be allowed to stay with the parents and to remain in the selected position of comfort, while feedings are withheld, and normal body temperature is maintained, the maximum amount of oxygen tolerated is delivered.

2. Respiratory failure requires securing an airway, establishing adequate ventilation, administering maximum supplemental oxygen, instituting cardiorespiratory monitoring and pulse oximetry, and obtaining frequent arterial blood gas measurements and chest films.

3. Shock requires delivering maximum supplemental oxygen establishing vascular access, expanding blood volume, administering appropriate vasopressors (if necessary), obtaining an electrocardiogram (ECG), and instituting cardiorespiratory monitoring and pulse oximetry.

4. Cardiopulmonary failure requires instituting ventilation and oxygenation, placing the child on cardiorespiratory monitoring and pulse oximetry, gaining vascular access to expand blood volume, and obtaining frequent arterial blood gas values and chest films.

Basic Airway, Breathing, and Circulation (ABCs) of Cardiopulmonary Resuscitation [1,15,25]

If unconscious, the patient should be placed supine, turned as a unit with firm support of head and neck to avoid spinal injury, and placed on a firm, flat surface. The airway should be maintained by using the head-tilt/chin-lift maneuver or, if a neck injury is suspected, by using the jaw-thrust maneuver. If the patient is not breathing, cardiopulmonary resuscitation (CPR) should be performed for 1 minute before help is called. If the patient is conscious and in respiratory distress, the child's position of comfort should be respected and transport in a properly equipped ambulance accomplished without disturbing her or him.

A. Airway

The *head tilt* maneuver consists of placing a hand on the forehead and tilting the head backward into a "sniffing" or neutral position. The *chin lift* maneuver consists of placing the fingers under the chin and lifting it upward. The neck should not be overextended. The *jaw thrust* maneuver is accomplished by placing two or three fingers on each side of the lower jaw at the angle and lifting upward with both elbows resting on the surface on which the victim is lying. If the airway is not maintainable by use of these maneuvers, an oropharyngeal airway or an endotracheal tube should be placed.

B. Breathing

The patency of the airway should continue to be maintained. The examiner should place his or her ear close to the patient's mouth and nose to listen for breath sounds. The chest should be felt for air movement and the chest and abdomen observed for movement.

If the patient is not breathing, mouth-to-mouth resuscitation must be instituted by tilting the head and sealing the mouth and nose of infants and pinching the nose and sealing the mouth of toddlers and older patients. Two slow breaths or puffs (1 to 1.5 seconds' duration) are delivered after each inhalation taken by the examiner, breaking the seal after each puff to allow the patient to exhale. The force and volume of the puff should be sufficient to cause the chest to rise. The use of this volume of air and the slow breaths avoids gastric distention in the patient. If air enters the lungs freely and the chest rises, the airway is proved to be patent. The most common cause of airway obstruction is improper head positioning: It should be readjusted and mouth-to-mouth breathing repeated. If the chest still does not rise, a foreign body lodged in the upper airway should be suspected and the recommendations for its removal (given below) should be followed. As soon as possible, the patient should receive ventilation with a bag (with reservoir) and mask attached to oxygen.

Gastric distention with vomiting and aspiration can be minimized in unconscious patients by applying *cricoid pressure,* using one fingertip in infants and the thumb and index finger in children to occlude the proximal esophagus. The pressure is released once endotracheal intubation is accomplished.

C. Circulation

Inefficient cardiovascular performance is recognized by the absence of the pulse in a large artery or by bradycardia that is unresponsive to ventilation and oxygenation. For patients older than 1 year of age, the practitioner palpates the carotid artery; for those younger than 1 year of age, the brachial artery is palpated. If the pulse is present but respirations are absent, the head tilt and mouth-to-mouth breathing should be maintained.

Chest Compression. Compressions of the chest are performed to effect cardiac compression. Table A-3 summarizes the methods used for chest compression for pediatric patients of varying ages.

The indications for chest compressions are asystole, as evidenced by absent pulses, or bradycardia below 60 beats per minute in a child or below 80 beats per minute in a neonate unresponsive to ventilation and oxygenation.

The patient should be horizontal and supine on a firm surface. In small infants the palm of the rescuer's hand should support the back.

The site of applying compression varies with the patient's age.[8,17,20]

In infants, compressions should be applied one fingerbreadth (fb) below the intersection of the internipple line with the sternum; compression should not be applied over the xiphoid. The middle and ring fingers should be used to compress the chest to a depth of 0.5 to 1 inch (1.3 or 2.5 cm) at a rate greater than 100/min. Pressure is released without lifting fingers off the sternum but allowing it to return to its normal position. The time allotted for each phase (compression and decompression) is equal. In applying compressions for a neonate or a small infant, the hands should encircle the thorax and the thumbs should be placed side by side just below the internipple line over the lower third of the sternum. Chest compressions should then be applied with the thumbs to the same depth and at the same rate as for the older infant.

In children older than 1 year of age, the resuscitator places the heel of one hand two fingersbreadths (fbs) above the sternal notch and uses the pressure generated by his or her arm to compress the sternum 1 to 1.5 inches (2.5 to 3.8 cm) at a rate of 80 to 100 times per minutes, taking care to keep the fingers off the ribs. Again, the compression and decompression phases are equal. The compression rate for children older than 8 years of age also is 80 to 100 times per minute, but the depth of compression is increased to 1.5 to 2 inches (3.8 to 5 cm), with the resuscitator using the pressure generated by his or her whole body, applied through clasped hands just above the sternal notch.

The adequacy of the compressions is determined by palpating the pulse during compression. External cardiac compressions must be accompanied by head tilt and ventilations. At the end of every fifth compression, a pause of 1 to 1.5 seconds should be made to allow for ventilation (5:1 compression to ventilation ratio). The victim should be assessed after 10 cycles of compressions and ventilations (approximately 1 minute) and every few minutes thereafter. With a single rescuer the head tilt maneuver must be performed with each ventilation. The hand performing the head tilt is moved back to its proper position on the chest for compression after each ventilation. As soon as possible ECG monitoring should be instituted and specimens for blood glucose, serum electrolyte, and blood gas analysis obtained.

Relieving Airway Obstruction.[2,6,25] The sequence of managing of an obstructed airway is as follows:

I. Conscious patient
   A. Breathing and coughing → No intervention
   B. Ineffective cough and increasing stridor with a witnessed or suspected foreign body aspiration
      1. Infant → Back blows and chest thrusts
      2. Child → Heimlich subdiaphragmatic abdominal thrusts

II. Unconscious, nonbreathing patient
   A. No spontaneous breathing → Head tilt, chin lift, and assisted ventilation
   B. Assisted ventilation → No chest rise
      1. Reposition head and repeat assisted ventilation
      2. Attempt to relieve obstruction
         a. Infant: 4 back blows and chest thrusts
         b. Child: 6 to 10 Heimlich subdiaphragmatic abdominal thrusts
      3. Perform tongue-jaw lift, and manually remove a foreign body if one is seen

Infant Back Blows and Chest Thrusts. With the infant straddled over the rescuer's forearm, and the head positioned lower than the trunk and the jaw held open by the rescuer's fingers, four back blows are delivered with the heel of the hand between the shoulder blades. If this does not remove the foreign body, the infant should be turned over so that the head, neck, and back are well supported on the rescuer's forearm. Four chest thrusts similar to cardiac compressions are then administered.

The Subdiaphragmatic Maneuver (Heimlich Maneuver)

1. *Standing patient.* From behind, the thumb of one fisted hand is placed in the midline above the navel and well below

Table A-3 *Methods of Chest Compression*

AGE	SITE	APPLICATOR	DEPTH	PRESSURE	RATE/MIN
Infant (<1 yr)	1 FB below internipple line	Middle and ring fingers	0.5-1.0 in (1.3-2.5 cm)	Hand	At least 100
Child (1-8 yr)	2 FB above xiphoid	Heel of the hand	1.0-1.5 in (2.5-3.8 cm)	Arm	80-100
Child (>8 yr)	2 FB above xiphoid	Both hands clasped	1.5-2 in (3.8-5.0 cm)	Body	80-100

FB, Fingerbreadth.

the xiphoid. The fist is grasped by the other hand and a quick upward thrust is administered. Each thrust is separate. Up to 10 thrusts should be completed in an attempt to dislodge and expel the foreign body.

2. *Supine, unconscious patient*. With the child lying supine, the rescuer should kneel at his or her feet. The heel of one hand is placed on the child's abdomen above the navel and well below the xiphoid. The other hand is placed on top of the first and pressed into the abdomen with a quick upward thrust in the *midline*. A series of 10 thrusts are performed—fewer if the foreign body is expelled.

3. *The tongue maneuver*. This maneuver is used if back blows, chest thrusts, and subdiaphragmatic thrusts fail. The child's mouth is opened, and the tongue and lower jaw are grasped between the rescuer's thumb and index finger and are lifted. This maneuver may relieve airway obstruction even with a foreign body still in place. If a foreign body is seen, it should be removed. Blind sweeps of the throat with the examiner's index finger are contraindicated because they may force a foreign body further down the airway.

Table A-4 summarizes the basic life support measures used in infants and children.

PEDIATRIC ADVANCED LIFE SUPPORT

When pediatric basic life support measures such as CPR are ineffective in resuscitating and stabilizing affected infants and children, advanced life support measures must be taken immediately. These measures include airway access and management, oxygen administration, vascular access, fluid and electrolyte administration, and drug therapy. To implement these measures it is necessary to be familiar with the ranges of body surface area, weight, and vital signs for pediatric patients (Table A-5) and the guidelines for the use of resuscitation equipment of various sizes, according to the patient's age and weight (Table A-6). Resuscitation of newborn infants is presented in Chapter 36, One, "Peripartum Considerations."

Airway Access and Management

Assisted ventilation can be given without placing of an endotracheal tube. The purpose of CPR is to get oxygen into the airway. Oxygen delivery systems include an oropharyngeal airway, a nasal cannula, oxygen hoods and tents, and face shields and masks, but these methods, however, do not reliably provide oxygen concentrations over 40%. The most effective noninvasive, assisted ventilation method is the self-inflating bag and mask with a reservoir connected to an oxygen source. Airway patency must be maintained and assessed frequently by observing for adequate symmetric chest movements, adequate breath sounds, and good color.

Oropharyngeal and Nasopharyngeal Airways. The *oropharyngeal airway* can be used in the unconscious patient to support the tongue. It is not used in conscious patients because it may stimulate vomiting. To estimate the proper size, the flange should be placed at the level of the central incisors and the tip of the appropriate-size airway should reach the angle of jaw. The tongue should be depressed with a tongue depressor and the airway should be inserted into the oropharynx in the position of function and rotated into proper position as it approaches the back of oropharynx. Proper head extension must be maintained.

The use of the *nasopharyngeal airway* is better tolerated than is the oropharyngeal airway in conscious patients; however, it may injure enlarged adenoid tissue and produce bleeding in children younger than 10 years of age.

The duration of *suctioning* should not exceed 5 seconds and should be preceded and followed by ventilation with 100% oxygen. The heart rate should be monitored for bradycardia during suctioning.

Endotracheal Airway. The placement of an *endotracheal (ET) tube* should be considered early in the care of the unconscious patient because it prevents aspiration, permits suctioning of the trachea and main bronchi, is a route for administrating of resuscitative medications,[10,11,27] allows for hyperventilation, and permits application of positive end-expiratory pressure when 100% oxygen does not improve oxygenation. Hyperventilation may aid in reducing increased intracranial pressure and can compensate for metabolic acidosis. The positive end-expiratory pressure may increase the functional residual capacity of the lungs and improve ventilation and perfusion. If prolonged ventilation is anticipated or if bag/mask and other airway adjuncts cannot accomplish adequate ventilation, an ET tube should be inserted.

The ET tube should be translucent, uniform diameter (not tapering), and equipped with a standard 15-mm adapter preferably the tube should have an opening on the side wall as well as at the end and distance markers. Cuffed ET tubes should be used only in children older than 8 years of age. An air leak with an uncuffed ET tube should be present when a breath is given at 20 cm H_2O pressure; if it is not, the tube is too large and should be replaced with a smaller one. The internal diameter of the ET tube used should approximate 16

Table A-4 *Summary of Basic Life Support Measures Used in Infants and Children*

	INFANT (>1 YR)	CHILD (>1 YR)
Airway		
Head or neck injury	Head tilt/chin lift/jaw thrust	Head tilt/chin lift/jaw thrust
Foreign body obstruction	Back blows/chest thrusts	Heimlich maneuver
Breathing		
Initial	Two breaths at 1-1.5 sec	Two breaths at 1-1.5 sec
Subsequent	20/min	15/min
Circulation		
Pulse check	Brachial/femoral	Carotid
Compression area	Lower third of sternum	Lower third of sternum
Procedure	Middle and ring fingers	Heel of one hand
Depth	0.5-1 in	1.0-1.5 in
Rate	At least 100/min	80-100/min
Compression	5:1; pause for ventilation	5:1; pause for ventilation

Modified from Chameides L, editor: Textbook of pediatric advanced life support, Dallas, 1988, American Heart Association and American Academy of Pediatrics.

Table A-5 *Ranges of Body Surface Area, Weight, and Vital Signs for Infants, Children, and Adults*

AGE	BODY SURFACE AREA m^2	WEIGHT (kg)	PULSE*/min	SYSTOLIC BLOOD PRESSURE† mmHg	RESPIRATORY RATE‡/min
Newborn	0.19	3.5	90-200	60	30-60
1 mo	0.30	4.0	90-180	65	30-60
6 mo	0.38	7.0	90-180	70	24-30
1-2 yr	0.50-0.55	10-12	70-140	72-74	20-24
3-5 yr	0.54-0.68	15-20	60-120	76-80	16-22
6-9 yr	0.68-0.85	20-28	60-120	82-88	14-20
10-12 yr	1.00-1.07	30-38	60-110	90	12-20
12-14 yr	1.07-1.22	38-48	50-100	90	12-20
15-16 yr	1.30-1.60	53-58	50-100	90	12-18
Adult	1.40-1.70	60-70	50-100	90	12-18

*Pulse range includes sound sleep and crying vigorously.
†Systolic blood pressure less than fifth percentile.

Age	mm Hg
0-1 mo	<60
1 mo-1 yr	<70
>1 yr	Formula: 70 plus 2 × Age in years

Formula for 50th percentile systolic BP at 2 to 10 years is 90 plus 2 × Age in years; the diastolic BP is two thirds of the systolic BP.
‡Respiratory rate >60 or < 10/min is abnormal at any age.

Age	Tachypnea rate	Bradypnea rate
<1 yr	>60	<25
1-5 yr	>40	<15
>5 yr	>30	<10

plus the age in years divided by 4; after 1 year of age the external diameter of the ET tube used should equal the size of the patient's external nasal orifice or the width of the patient's fifth finger.

Straight-blade laryngoscopes are preferred in children. Before laryngoscopy is begun, one should check the equipment and the light source. Attempts at ET intubation should not exceed 30 seconds, and the heart rate and oxygenation should be monitored during the procedure. Bradycardia below 80 beats per minute in a neonate or 60 beats per minute in a child mandates interruption of the procedure and administration of 100% oxygen by face mask and bag. The ET tube should be passed into the trachea to a distance that places the distance marker at the level of the vocal cords.

Once intubation is established, the ET tube should be held securely in position and its position confirmed (1) by observing symmetric movements of the chest, (2) by auscultating the lungs to determine the presence of bilateral breath sounds, (3) by auscultating over the stomach to determine the absence of air-entry sounds, and (4) by looking for condensation in the ET tube during exhalation.

Asymmetric right-sided breath sounds usually indicate intubation of the right main bronchus. When this occurs, the tube should be withdrawn until breath sounds are heard in both lungs; the ET tube should then be withdrawn another 1 to 2 cm to ensure its midtracheal position. *The final position of the ET tube must be confirmed by chest film.*

A properly placed tube but inadequate lung expansion indicates that (1) the tube is too small, (2) there is a large laryngeal air leak (detected by auscultating the neck), (3) the "pop-off" valve on the ventilator bag is not depressed, (4) there is a leak in the bag-valve device, or (5) the operator administered an insufficiently strong puff.

The position of the tube should be verified by noting the distance marker at the lips; it should be secured to the patient's

Table A-6 *Pediatric Resuscitation Equipment Guidelines*[1]

AGE	WEIGHT (kg)	ET TUBE (mm internal diameter*)	LARYNGOSCOPE BLADE (No.)	SUCTION CATHETER (Fr)	DISTANCE FROM MIDTRACHEA TO TEETH (cm)	CHEST TUBE (Fr)	VENOUS CATHETER (gauge)	FOLEY CATHETER and NG TUBE (Fr)
Newborn premature	<1	2.5	0	5 or 6	8	10-14	22-24	5 fdt
Newborn full term	3	3.0	1	6	10	12-18	22-24	6 fdt
6 mo	7	3.5	1	8	12	14-20	22-24	8
1 yr	10	4.0	1	8	12	14-24	20-22	10
18 mo	11	4.0	1	8	14	14-24	20-22	10
3 yr	14	4.5	2	8	16	18-26	20-22	10
5 yr	18	5.0	2-3	10	16	20-32	20-22	10-12
8 yr	25	6.0 cuff	2	10	18	28-34	20-22	12
10 yr	34	6.5 cuff	2	10	18	30-38	18-20	12
12 yr	38	6.5-7 cuff	3	10	20	34-38	18-20	12-14
16 yr	55	7.5-8 cuff	3	12	22	34-38	18-20	12-14
Adult		8-8,5 cuff	3	12	22	34-38	18-20	12-14

Cuff, Cuffed endotracheal tube; *ET*, endotracheal; *Fdt*, feeding tube; *NG*, nasogastric.

*Internal diameter of the ET tube = $\frac{\text{Child's age} + 16}{4}$.

face by the use of benzoin and tape (see Fig. B-21, Appendix B). Its position should be assessed frequently intervals by observing chest wall expansion, listening for bilateral breath sounds, and noting improvement of color and perfusion, obtaining blood gas values, and checking pulse oximeter readings.

Medications can be administered through the ET tube while vascular access is sought. The medications that can be administered by this route are *a*tropine, *N*aloxone, *e*pinephrine, and *l*idocaine (ANEL). The usual intravenous dose (diluted in 1 to 2 ml of normal saline) is administered through a catheter that has been passed beyond the ET tube as deeply as possible into the tracheobronchial tree. The dose of epinephrine, however, should be two to three times the intravenous dose. After the medication has been instilled, several positive pressure puffs should be given.[3,10,11,27]

An *esophageal obturator airway* is not recommended for patients younger than 16 years of age.[2,15]

Cricothyrotomy. In patients younger than 8 years of age, airway obstruction may occur at the cricoid ring, the narrowest portion of the larynx in this age-group. The ring is located below the thyrocricoid membrane; therefore, cricothyrotomy may not be effective in establishing an airway. In general this route is *not recommended* in infants and small children.[13]

Airway emergencies with endotracheal tubes. When emergencies occur, the gas delivery system should be disconnected and the patient should receive manual ventilation with a resuscitation bag and the use of 100% oxygen. Auscultation should be employed to determine the position and patency of the tube. Possible problems that may be encountered include (1) a loss of oxygen supply to the tube, (2) occlusion or kinking of the tube, or (3) displacement of the tube. If obstruction or displacement is the problem, poor breath sounds, no chest movements, and increased resistance to inflation should be observed. Decreased resistance to inflation occurs where the ET tube has been misplaced into the esophagus. If the ET tube is obstructed, it should be irrigated with 1 ml of saline and suctioned for 3 to 4 seconds. After suctioning, the breath sounds, airway resistance, and adequacy of chest movements should be evaluated. If proper position and adequate manual ventilation of the ET tube are ensured, one should assume the problem lies with the gas delivery systems and this should be disconnected and manual ventilation instituted. If it is unclear whether the ET tube has been dislodged, its placement can be determined by direct laryngoscopy; sometimes the tube has to be removed entirely and reinserted.

Oxygen Administration

The rational for administering oxygen is that establishing an adequate airway alone cannot reverse the pathophysiology of hypoxemia. Mouth-to-mouth breathing delivers only 16% fractional inspiratory oxygen (FiO_2) and results in an oxygen tension (PaO_2) of only 80 mm Hg. Normally, when one breathes room air, the PaO_2 is 104 mm Hg. Chest compression generates only 25% to 30% of the normal circulation in adults. Oxygen is indicated in any situation in which hypoxia is suspected. Oxygen should be administered even if the PaO_2

is high, because a low cardiac output may not deliver sufficient oxygen to the tissues. The oxygen concentration should be 100% (preferably humidified and warmed) to achieve an adequate PaO_2 and tissue saturation. Once the airway is established, if the respiration is not adequate, oxygen should be administered through an appropriate-size face mask connected to a self-inflating bag with an attached reservoir that delivers 10 to 15 L of oxygen per minute. When a self-inflating bag is used, the "pop-off" valve should be occluded because the pressures needed to ventilate the lungs may exceed the valve's limit. Administration of oxygen through a nasal cannula, a face mask, or a face shield does not provide reliable oxygen concentrations over 40%.[2,15,25]

Vascular Access

If venous access cannot be established in 90 seconds or after three attempts in children younger than 3 years of age, the intraosseous fluid access route should be used. For patients older than 3 years of age the lesser saphenous vein or a femoral vein should be accessed.[2]

Infusion pumps or minidrip chambers should be used for infusion therapy. Head and neck vessels should be avoided because their use interferes with resuscitative measures. Cannulation of central veins should be supervised by experienced operators.

The intraosseous space is a plexus of noncollapsible veins through which any fluid or medication may be infused.[14,22,24,26] Interosseous infusion is recommended for children younger than 3 years of age if vascular access cannot be established in 90 seconds or after three percutaneous attempts.[2,25] It is an easily learned technique and rapidly accomplished. An 18-gauge short spinal needle with a stylet or a large bore–marrow needle may be used. Intraosseous needles are now available from several commercial distributors. The favorite site is 2 cm below the tibial tuberosity on the medial surface of the tibia. Intraosseous infusions are equivalent to those given intravenously and for medication administration are preferable to the ET route. (Appendix B, "Special Procedures," describes in detail the methods used for intraosseous infusions.)

Resuscitative and Postresuscitative Fluids and Medications

The purposes of the pharmacologic agents used during cardiac arrest and the postresuscitation period are (1) to expand intravascular volume and increase perfusion, (2) to stimulate spontaneous, forceful myocardial contractions, (3) to accelerate the cardiac rate, (4) to correct metabolic acidosis, and (5) to suppress ventricular ectopy. The pharmacologic agents used, their indications and doses, and the precautions that need to be applied in using them are discussed below and presented in Table A-7.

Volume Expansion. The types of fluids available for volume expansion include the following:

1. *Crystalloids*—Ringer lactate or 0.9% saline. Ringer lactate is preferred because if contains less chloride and does not aggravate acidosis. Because only one fourth of crystalloids remain in the vascular space, four times the deficit is required to restore plasma volume.

2. *Colloids and blood products*—albumin, fresh frozen plasma, human plasma protein fraction (Plasmanate), whole blood or packed red blood cells. In general the patient requires one half the amount of the crystalloids to restore plasma volume by use of these products.

3. *Glucose*[2,4,15,23,25] is not administered in the initial resuscitative fluids unless hypoglycemia exists. The endogenous catecholamines in response to stress cause glycogenolysis and increase the blood glucose. Excess glucose may be metabolized to lactate and cause an osmotic diuresis.

Small infants and chronically ill children have limited glycogen stores and hypoxemia-like hypoglycemia may develop. Glucose is a major metabolic substrate for the neonatal myocardium. A rapid blood glucose test should be obtained, and if hypoglycemia exists, glucose should be administered. In children, a D25W solution (dilution of D50W 1:1 with sterile water) should be used and in infants a D10W solution (dilution of D50W 1:4 with sterile water). Sufficient amounts should be given to keep the blood glucose level above 100 mg/dl. Repeated hyperosmolar doses have been associated with intracranial hemorrhage in premature infants.

The principle in fluid resuscitation is to administer a bolus of fluid over a period of 10 to 15 minutes and then reevaluate the state of the patient's hydration. In hypovolemic shock, a 20 ml/kg/dose of crystalloid is administered as soon as vascular access is established. The child with hypovolemic shock often requires 40 to 60 ml/kg of fluid in the first hour of resuscitation, occasionally up to 100 to 200 ml/kg in the first few hours. A three-way stopcock attached to a 20-ml or a 50-ml syringe may be useful in "pushing" fluids with the aid of the syringe. Subsequently, volume expanders such as colloid or blood may be needed; 20 ml/kg/dose of 5% albumin, 1 g/kg/dose of 25% albumin, or 20 ml/kg/dose of fresh frozen plasma may be used. Whole blood (20 ml/kg) is administered if hemorrhage has occurred, and packed red blood cells (10 ml/kg) are given to the patient with chronic blood loss.

Fluid resuscitation should be monitored by frequently reassessing perfusion. Fluid overload is determined by auscultating the chest for signs of pulmonary edema and by noting the size of the heart on chest film. In hypovolemia the heart is of normal or small size; in cardiogenic shock or fluid overload it is usually is enlarged.

Resuscitation Medications.* The resuscitative medications described here are listed in Table A-7, along with their indications for use and the recommended doses. The normal values for arterial blood pH, gases, oxygen saturation, and bicarbonate for newborns, infants, and children are shown in Table A-8.

The vagus nerve, through its neurotransmitter acetylcholine, inhibits conduction at the sinoauricular and atrioventricular nodes. The sympathetic nervous system, through its alpha-adrenergic receptors, enhances perfusion by causing vasoconstriction and increased peripheral vascular resistance. Its beta-1 adrenergic receptors (1) increase heart rate, (2) cardiac conductivity, myocardial contractility, and (3) cardiac contractility, resulting in increased cardiac output. The sympathetic nervous system's beta-2 adrenergic receptors produce vasodilation of skeletal muscle blood vessels and bron-

*References 2, 4, 9, 15, 16, 23, 25, 30.

Table A-7 *Pediatric Resuscitative Medications and Procedures*

MEDICATION	DOSAGE*	COMMENTS	INDICATIONS
Atropine sulfate 1 mg/10 ml (0.1 mg/ml)	0.02 mg/kg IV, IO, ET (0.2 ml/kg) Adolescents: total dose = 1-2 mg	Min 0.1 mg (1 ml) q 5 min up to maximum if needed; max child-dose 1 mg (10 ml) Max adolescent dose = 2 mg (20 ml)	Asystole and bradycardia
Bretylium 500 mg/10 ml *Continue CPR for 2 min before attempting defibrillation*	5 mg/kg (0.1 ml/kg) IV, IO 10 mg/kg (0.2 ml/kg)	Initial dose If VF persists	Ventricular fibrillation and tachycardia
Bicarbonate sodium 1 mEq/ml (8.4%) For Rx acidosis: For Rx hyperkalemia:	1 mEq/kg IV, IO (1 ml/kg) (2 mEq/kg raises pH 0.1 unit) Adolescents: 50 = 100 mEq 0.3 × kg × BE (24-CO²) = mEq 1 mEq/kg	Administer slowly; monitor subsequent doses determined by ABG values (Use only 0.5 mEq/ml solution for infants) Use only if ventilation is established Administer over at least 10 mm	Severe metabolic acidosis (ph<7.20), prolonged (> 10 min) cardiac arrest, and hyperkalemia
Calcium chloride 10% (100 mg/ml) (1.35 mEq/ml)	20 mg/kg IV, IO (0.2 ml/kg) max dose 1 g	Give slowly: <1 ml/min with ECG and BP monitoring; use extreme caution with digitalis. Use only for indications	Hypocalcemia, hyperkalcemia, hypermagnesemia, calcium channel blocker over dose
Defibrillation Cardioversion	2 J/kg 0.5-1 J/kg	Double the dose if first shock fails	Absent pulse, ventricular tachycardia and ventricular fibrillation Ventricular tachycardia with pulses and supraventricular tachycardia
Dextrose 50% 25 g/50 ml *Rx hypoglycemia:* *Rx hyperkalemia:*	0.5-1 g/kg IV, IO 10% <1 yr (4 ml/kg) 25% >1 yr (2 ml/kg) 50% adolescents or adult (1-2 ml/kg IV, IO) 0.5-1 g/kg administered over at least 30 min	Dilute D50W 1:4 = 10% A large dose given too rapidly may cause insulin release Monitor blood glucose	Hypoglycemia and hypokalemia
Epinephrine 1:10,000 (0.1 mg/ml)	0.01 mg/kg/dose IV, IO, ET (0.1 ml/kg/dose) Adolescents: total dose, 0.5-1 mg (5-10 ml)	q5 min if needed; ET dose = 0.2-0.3 ml/kg 0.5 ml, max total dose = 10 ml	Asystole and ventricular fibrillation
Fluid Challenge: Ringer lactate or 0.9% saline Shock: Ringer lactate or 0.9% saline	 20 ml/kg IV, IO in 30-60 min 20 ml/kg IV bolus and reassess		Volume expansion
Dextrose: see above			
Lidocaine 1% 10 mg/ml 2% 20 mg/ml	1 mg/kg IV, IO, ET (0.1 ml/kg 1%) (0.05 ml/kg 2%)	q5-10 min if needed, Max dose = 3-4 mg/kg/hr Toxicity: Seizures, myocardial depression	Ventricular tachycardia and fibrillation

ET, Endotracheal; *IO,* intraosseous; *IV,* intravenous.

ABG, Arterial blood gas; *BE,* base excess; *BP,* blood pressure; *CPR,* cardiopulmonary resuscitation; *CO_2,* carbon dioxide; *ECG,* electrocardiogram; *ET,* endotracheal; *IO,* intraosseous; *IV,* intravenous; *max,* maximum; *min,* minimum; *Rx,* therapy; *VF,* ventricular fibrillation.

*It is useful to have precalculated dose schedules for resuscitative medications.

Some pediatric intensive care units are using "megadoses of epinephrine—10 times the usual concentration by using a 1:1000 dilution (1 mg/ml, but the same volume (0.1 ml/kg) chodilation. They do not play a role in cardiopulmonary resuscitation.

Epinephrine. Epinephrine is an endogenous catecholamine with alpha and beta adrenergic receptor properties. In doses used for CPR, it has alpha, beta-1, and beta-2 effects. Its mechanism of action relates to its alpha effect, which increases systemic vascular resistance, leading to increased coronary artery perfusion pressure and increased oxygen delivery to the myocardium. It is indicated in asystole, unstable bradydysrhythmias, which constitute 90% of rhythm disturbances in pediatric patients, and ventricular fibrillation (VF), which occurs in only 10% of children with rhythm disturbances. Epinephrine renders VF more susceptible to conversion by countershock.

Sodium bicarbonate. Respiratory acidosis is corrected by establishing effective ventilation. By inducing hyperventilation (and thereby reducing the $PaCO_2$), respiratory alkalosis will result and compensate for any metabolic acidosis that may be present because of poor oxygen delivery. The resultant pH will be less acidotic. If acidemia persists in spite of respiratory compensation and the pH is persistently <7.20 to 7.25, sodium bicarbonate should be administered to correct the residual metabolic acidosis. Bicarbonate should not be used in the absence of adequate ventilation. The interpretation of blood pH, gases, oxygen saturation, and bicarbonate determinations is complex and can be simplified in terms of determining the acid-base balance and its origins by applying the following "golden rules:[2]

Rule 1: An acute change in $PaCO_2$ of a 10-torr increase or decrease is associated with an increase or decrease of 0.08 units in the pH.

To assess the respiratory component of acidosis: Determine the amount of the measured partial pressure of carbon dioxide in arterial blood ($PaCO_2$) that falls below or above 40 torr. Calculate the pH, using rule 1. Compare measured pH with the calculated pH; they are reasonably close, all acidotic changes are respiratory in origin.

Rule 2: A pH change of 0.15 units is equivalent to (or the result of) a change in HCO_3 of 10 mEq/L from its 20 mEq/L baseline.

To assess the metabolic component: Determine the calculated pH, using rule 1, and compare with measured pH value. If they are not reasonably close, determine the following: (1) If the measured pH is less than the calculated pH (a negative number), the acidosis is metabolic in origin; subtract the measured pH from the calculated pH to determine base deficit or fixed acid. (2) If the measured pH is greater than calculated (a positive number), metabolic alkalosis is present; subtract the calculated pH from the measured pH to determine the base excess (or negative base excess).

Rule 3: The dose of bicarbonate (mEq) required to correct the metabolic acidosis fully is the base deficit (mEq/L × patient's weight [kg] × 0.3). Usually only one half this amount is administered and then the acid-base status is reassessed, which ordinarily indicates that 1 mEq/kg sodium bicarbonate is needed.

If the arrest is observed and brief, bicarbonate usually is not necessary. Bicarbonate may be required, however, in prolonged arrest (more than 10 minutes) after initial ventilation and perfusion are established and the arterial pH remains below 7.2.

Excessive bicarbonate administration can have adverse effects because it (1) shifts the oxygen dissociation curve to the left and decreases the delivery of oxygen to the tissues, (2) shifts the potassium intracellularly, lowering the serum potassium level (3) decreases the plasma ionized calcium, (4) decreases the fibrillation threshhold, (5) increases the risk of hypernatremia and water overload, (6) increases the risk of hyperosmolality, and (7) may produce paradoxical cerebrospinal fluid (CSF) and intracellular acidosis.

Atropine. Atropine is a parasympatholytic drug by virtue of its competitive antagonism of acetylcholine. It accelerates sinus and atrial pacemaker discharge and atrioventricular conduction. In low dosess (<0.1 mg) a paradoxical CNS vagal nuclei stimulation may produce atrioventricular node slowing. Higher doses are used in asystole to shorten the response time.

Atropine is indicated to treat hemodynamically unstable bradycardia accompanied by poor perfusion or hypotension and asystole. Bradycardia most often results from hypoxia, and initial treatment should be directed at ventilation, oxygenation, and perfusion.

The vagolytic dose is 0.02 mg/kg with a minimum dose of 0.1 mg. The duration of action is 2 to 4 hours; the pupils remain dilated for 6 hours or longer after injection and thus cannot provide a basis for neurologic evaluation of the patient. Repeat doses during asystole can be given every 15 minutes up to 1 mg in a child and 2 mg in an adolescent

Calcium chloride. Calcium has a positive inotropic effect on the heart, but calcium entry into cell cytoplasm is the final common pathway in cell death and may be injurious. *Its use no longer is recommended in cardiac arrest protocols.*

Table A-8 *Normal Values of Arterial pH, Blood Gases, and Oxygen Saturation, and Bicarbonate*

		INFANTS AND CHILDREN			
MEASURE	UNIT	MIXED VENOUS	CAPILLARY	ARTERIAL	NEWBORN
pH	units	7.31-7.41	7.35-7.40	7.40-7.45	7.11-7.30
PCO_2	torr	35-40	40-45	35-40	27-40
PO_2	torr	41-51	45-50	80-100	33-75
O_2Sat	%	60-80	>70	>90	40-90
HCO_3	mEq/L	22-25	22-26	22-26	14-22

Modified from Gordon IB: Reference ranges for laboratory tests. In Behrman RE and Vaughan VC, editors: Nelson's textbook of pediatrics, ed 12, Philadelphia, 1983, WB Saunders Co.

PCO_2, Carbon dioxide pressure; *PO_2;* oxygen pressure; *Sat*, saturation.

The indications for calcium are documented hypocalcemia (total serum calcium levels below 8.1 mg/dl or ionized calcium levels below 2.4 mg/dl), hyperkalemia, hypermagnesemia, and calcium channel blocker overdose. Calcium chloride is used in emergency hypocalcemia because it delivers the ionized calcium directly. Calcium always should be injected slowly concurrently with electrocardiographic and blood pressure monitoring. The injection should be discontinued if bradycardia or hypotension occur.

Lidocaine. Lidocaine in usual doses has no effect on myocardial contractility, blood pressure, or cardiac conduction. Its action suppresses ectopic foci and reduces automaticity, increases the fibrillation threshhold, and inhibits the formation of reentry circuits that lead to ventricular tachycardia and fibrillation. VF occurs in fewer than 10% of pediatric patients with cardiac arrest. If VF is present, a metabolic cause (abnormalities of calcium, potassium, and glucose), hypothermia, and drug intoxication (especially tricyclic antidepressants) should be considered.

The indications for lidocaine administration are (1) ventricular tachycardia, (2) ventricular fibrillation, and (3) frequent (>6/min) or potentially serious premature ventricular contractions (couplets, multifocal), particularly if associated with hemodynamic instability. Lidocaine infusion is recommended after successful conversion of ventricular tachycardia or fibrillation.

To ensure adequate plasma concentrations a bolus of 1 mg/kg should be given when the intravenous infusion is placed. If shock or liver disease is present, beginning doses of 1 ml/kg/hr (20 μg/kg/min) should be used to prevent toxicity from impaired lidocaine clearance. The adolescent dose is a 50- to 100-mg bolus followed by the infusion of 1 to 4 mg/min. The antidysrhythmic effect occurs at a serum concentration of 1 to 5 μg/ml. Concentrations in excess of 6 μg/ml may produce seizures and those in excess of 10 μg/ml, myocardial depression. The practitioner should be prepared to treat bradycardia and hypotension. Lidocaine is contraindicated in severe heart block. Widening of the QRS complex by more than 0.02 seconds or significant ventricular slowing suggests cardiac toxicity. It is important to monitor electrocardiographic activity and plasma lidocaine concentrations because of the erratic pharmacokinetics of lidocaine in patients with CPA.

Bretylium. Bretylium is a quaternary ammonium compound with postganglionic adrenergic properties and antidysrhythmic activity. It has a biphasic effect. Initially, through norepinephrine release, it increases the blood pressure and heart rate; this is followed by adrenergic blockade of norepinephrine and epinephrine, but cardiac output remains unchanged. Bretylium may raise the fibrillation threshhold and prevent reentry. It is a second-line drug to lidocaine and is indicated in refractory ventricular tachycardia or fibrillation. In adults, bretylium improved the susceptibility of the refractory heart to defibrillation, cardioversion, and lidocaine. *It is important to continue CPR for 2 minutes after administrating bretylium* to allow for its circulation before attempting defibrillation. Its adverse effects are nausea, vomiting, hypotension, and transient hypertension; it may worsen dysrhythmias in digitalized patients.

Postresuscitative Medications.* Postresuscitative medications should be administered if the blood pressure or peripheral perfusion remains unstable.

The current teaching is that in a post CPA patient, the following drugs are of importance.

In the presence of hypotension—epinephrine and norepinephrine.

In the presence of normotension and poor cardiac output—dobutamine and epinephrine.

In septic shock with hypotension—epinephrine and norepinephrine.

In septic shock with normotension and poor cardiac output—dopamine and dobutamine.

Dopamine. Dopamine is an endogenous catecholamine that is an immediate precursor of norepinephrine. *At low doses* (2 to 5 μg/kg/min) it binds to dopamine receptors in splanchnic, coronary, renal vascular beds and produces vasodilation with increased contractility without effecting on heart rate and blood pressure. *At higher doses* (6 to 20 μg/kg/min), beta-1 (inotropic and chronotropic) and alpha (vasoconstriction) adrenergic effects are predominant, resulting in an increase in blood pressure as a result of general vasoconstriction and increased cardiac output. At doses *greater than 20 μg/kg/min,* dopamine produces predominantly vasoconstrictive effects without further inotropic effects and should be used with caution. In chronically stressed patients, unpredictible inotropic responses may occur because of variability in the patient's own stores of norepinephrine. The indications for its use are hypotension or poor peripheral perfusion, in the presence of a stable rhythm and with adequate vascular volume.

A reasonable starting dose of dopamine for a patient in shock is 5 to 10 μg/kg/min. It is not recommended that infusion rates above 20 μg/kg/min if a further inotropic effect is needed, epinephrine should be used. Dopamine may produce tachycardia (which increases myocardial oxygen demands), hypertension, dysrhythmias, and extremity ischemia. It should be given in a central vein, if possible. Electrocardiographic activity should be monitored and the skin observed for ischemia; the blood pressure and urinary output also should be closely monitored. Extravasation of dopamine will produce tissue necrosis. Table A-9 summarizes the effects of dopamine infusions at various rates.

Dobutamine. Dobutamine is a synthetic catecholamine prepared by manipulation of isoproterenol. It is a direct-acting catecholamine with selective beta-1 adrenergic action and mild peripheral beta-2 effect (vasodilation) resulting in increased cardiac contractility and heart rate and decreased afterload (systemic resistance); all of this increases the cardiac output. It is less effective in septic shock and in infants younger than 12 months of age. Its major indication is in the treatment of cardiogenic shock. It may produce tachydysrhythmias, nausea and vomiting, hypotension, and hypertension.

Epinephrine infusion. Epinephrine acts directly on adrenergic receptors (not through norepinephrine), and at higher doses (> 0.3 μg/kg/min) alpha-adrenergic effects also occur. It is indicated are in the treatment of hypotension or poor

*References 2, 9, 15, 16, 19, 23, 25, 30.

Table A-9 *Effects of the Infusion Rate of Dopamine on the Cardiovascular System*

RATE OF INFUSION	CARDIAC OUTPUT	INOTROPHY	VASCULAR RESISTANCE	RENAL BLOOD FLOW
2-5 μg/kg/min	0	0	0	+
6-20 μg/kg/min	+ (beta-1)	+ (beta-1)	+/−	+
>20 μg/kg/min	+ (beta-1)	+ (beta-1)	+ (alpha-1)	0

Table A-10 *Effects of the Rate of Epinephrine Infusion on the Cardiovascular System*

DOSE μg/kg/min	CHRONOTROPIC EFFECT	INOTROPIC EFFECT	VASODILATION	VASOCONSTRICTION
0.05-0.3	+	+	+	0
0.3-1.5	+	+	0	+

Table A-11 *Effect of Norepinephrine Infusion on the Cardiovascular System*

DOSE (μg/kg/min)	ADRENERGIC RECEPTORS		
	ALPHA	BETA-1	EFFECT
0.1-0.5	+	+	Vasoconstriction raises diastolic BP and may decrease cardiac output
0.5-1.0	+ + +	+	

perfusion, or both, after stabilization of cardiac rhythm and volume output. An epinephrine infusion is the treatment of choice if the possibility of depleted norepinephrine stores is present, such as in young infants or chronically stressed patients. It should be administered through a well-secured peripheral line or, preferably, a central line. The adverse effects of epinephrine infusion are dysrhythmias, and at doses exceeding 0.5 μg/kg/min profound vasoconstriction that compromises skin and extremity blood flow. Epinephrine vasoconstriction decreases renal blood flow but improves renal function through increased cardiac output and tissue perfusion. Extravasation causes tissue necrosis. Prefilled syringes containing the 1:10,000 epinephrine solution should not be used in preparing the infusion because of the difficulty in dose calculation; 1:1000 (1 mg/ml) solutions contained in prefilled syringes should be used. The effects of epinephrine infusions on the cardiovascular system are summarized in Table A-10.

Norepinephrine infusion. Norepinephrine is an endogenous catecholamine that is derived from dopamine. It has potent alpha-vasoconstriction effects and moderate beta-1 adrenergic receptor effects that stimulate the heart rate and cardiac contractility. Norepinephrine has little action on beta-2 receptors. Because of its pronounced alpha (vasoconstrictive) effects, a reflex bradycardia occurs, offsetting the tachycardia response and resulting in less tachycardia than with epinephrine. The major indication for its use is in the treatment of hypotension after adequate fluid replacement. The initial dose is 0.1 μg/kg/min; it can be increased up to 1 μg/kg/min, with the dose titrated to reach the desired effect. Extravasations should be avoided; if extravasation occurs, the tissue should be infilterated with 5 to 10 mg of phentolamine diluted in 10 ml of saline. Electrocardiographic activity, blood pressure, and urine output should be monitored. The effects of norepinephrine infusion on the cardiovascular system are summarized in Table A-11.

Isoproterenol. Isoproterenol is a nonselective beta-adrenergic agonist. Its beta-1 adrenergic activity increases the heart rate, conduction velocity, and cardiac contractility; its beta-2 adrenergic activity produces peripheral vasodilation in the vascular beds of skeletal muscle. Its use is indicated in hemodynamic unstable bradycardia and in infants younger than 6 months of age whose cardiac output depends on heart rate and whose stroke volume is fixed. Isoproterenol may be used to increase the heart rate if it is less than 80 beats/min in infants with poor perfusion even if the blood pressure is normal. However, epinephrine is preferred in these cases because it does not cause the diastolic blood pressure to fall. Isoproterenol increases myocardial muscle oxygen demand. During the administration of isoproterenol, the heart rate, blood pressure, and electrocardiographic activity should be monitored.

The postresuscitation drugs used for shock and cardiovascular stabilization are listed in Tables A-12 and A-13, along with the indications for their use and the recommended doses.

EMERGENCY PEDIATRIC CARDIAC RHYTHM DISTURBANCES [4]

Emergency pediatric cardiac rhythm disturbances usually result from hypoxemia and acidosis and rarely cause cardiac arrest; thus ventilation and oxygenation are important in their management. The principle of therapy is to initiate treatment only if the rhythm disturbance compromises the cardiac output or can potentially deteriorate into a lethal rhythm. Electrical therapy includes (1) defibrillation, which is an untimed depolarization of the myocardium to allow for a spontaneous organized beat and (2) cardioversion, which is a timed de-

Table A-12 *Medications for Postresuscitation Stabilization*: Types of Shock and the Choice of Vasopressor*

TYPE OF SHOCK	INFANT	CHILD	ADULT
Septic			
First choice	Dopamine	Dopamine	Dopamine
Second choice	Epinephrine	Epinephrine	Norepinephrine
Third choice	Dobutamine	Dobutamine	Dobutamine
Cardiogenic			
First choice	Dobutamine	Dobutamine	Dobutamine
Second choice	Epinephrine	Epinephrine	Dopamine
Third choice	Dopamine	Dopamine	Norepinephrine
Hypovolemic (vasopressors not indicated)			
Hemodynamically unstable bradycardia			
First choice	Epinephrine	Epinephrine	Isoproterenol
Second choice	Isoproterenol	Isoproterenol	

Modified from Seidel JS and Burkett DL, editors: Instructor's manual for pediatric advanced life support, Dallas, 1988, American Heart Association.
*To be administered in patients with stable rhythms and with normal vascular volume status, if blood pressure or perfusion remain unstable.

polarization designed to avoid the vulnerable period in the cardiac cycle.

Table A-14 provides normal ranges for heart rates, PR intervals, and QRS complexes at various ages; these values are important in interpreting electrocardiograms as part of the assessment and management of cardiac rhythm disturbances.

In children younger than 10 years of age, a PR interval >0.18 and a QRS complex duration of >0.10 are abnormal. The P wave is almost always upright in lead II; if it is not, or if it is absent, a normal sinus rhythm is not present. An inverted P wave in lead II most commonly is due to incorrect placement of one of the EKG leads. A wide QRS complex may be of ventricular origin or a result of an aberrantly conducted supraventricular beat. However, *a wide QRS complex should always be considered as ventricular tachycardia because of its serious implications* and the relative rarity of aberrant SVT in the pediatric age-group.[2,18]

A useful *clinical classification* of emergency dysrhythmias in pediatrics is (1) rhythms that are too fast (tachydysrhythmias) or too slow (bradydysrhythmias) associated with hemodynamic instability and decreased cardiac output and (2) rhythms that are disorganized (ventricular fibrillation) or (3) rythms that are absent altogether (asystole). Other dysrhythmias may need evaluation and treatment but usually do not constitute an emergency.[2]

Tachydysrhythmias

Supraventricular tachycardia usually is associated with a heart rate greater than 230 beats per minute in infants; P waves are difficult to find, and the QRS complex is narrow in 98% of cases. If the patient is hemodynamically stable, vagal maneuvers (inverting infant quickly, applying an ice bag to the face, or pressing on the abdomen), IV phenylephrine, or digoxin may be used to convert the rhythm to normal. If these fail, overdrive pacing should be attempted; if that is not successful, synchronized cardioversion should be used with appropriate sedation. If hemodynamic instability and decreased cardiac output are present, synchronized cardioversion (0.5 to 1 joules/kg) should be attempted immediately. If SVT persists, the cardioversion dose should be increased to 2 joules/kg. If it still persists the diagnosis may be incorrect. Verapamil should not be used to treat SVT in infants younger than 1 year of age because cardiovascular collapse has been reported.[2,7,21]

Ventricular tachycardia (VT) usually has wide QRS complexes, absent P waves, and T waves that are the opposite in polarity to the QRS complex. VT may degenerate into ventricular fibrillation.

If the patient is hemodynamically unstable and cardiac output is decreased, synchronized cardioversion (0.5 to 1.0 joules/kg) should be attempted immediately. If a lidocaine bolus can be given without delaying cardiaversion, the success of conversion will be greater. If VT recurs, an infusion of lidocaine given after cardioversion will help to maintain the converted rhythm. If this is unsuccessful, cardioversion at a higher voltage (2 joules/kg) should be used. If success still is not achieved, bretylium should be given initially instead of lidocaine.

Bradydysrhythmias are associated with third-degree heart block. Their management includes ventilation, oxygenation, and volume repletion. If the patient remains hemodynamically unstable with decreased cardiac output, sympathomimetic medications such as an epinephrine infusion, atropine, or isoproterenol should be administered. If the bradydysrhythmia continues, a ventricular pacemaker should be used.

Absent or Disorganized Rhythms

Asystole. It is important in making the diagnosis of asystole to be sure that the clinical picture (no pulse and absent spontaneous respirations) correlates with the electrocardiographic activity that has been monitored. Ventilation, oxygenation, and volume repletion are the standards of treatment. If severe metabolic acidosis is present, an epinephrine bolus followed by vagolytic doses of atropine and sodium bicarbonate may improve myocardial activity.

Ventricular fibrillation is characterized by a disorganized

Table A-13 *Cardiovascular Infusion Therapy**

MEDICATION	DOSAGE RANGE	CALCULATION	INDICATIONS
Dobutamine (Dobutrex) 25 mg/ml 250 mg/10 ml	2.5-5 μg/kg/min mild low BP; 6-10 μg/kg/min moderate low BP; 11-20 μg/kg/min severe low BP	6 mg (0.24 ml) × wt (kg) = mg to add to make 100 ml D5W = 1 ml/hr = 1 μg/kg/min For use in low output CHF, *not* in shock or during CPR; max 30 μg/kg/min	Cardiogenic shock (normovolemic and stable rhythm)
Dopamine (Intropin) 40 mg/ml = 200 mg/5 ml	1-5 μg/kg/min: increases cardiac output and renal perfusion; 6-20 μg/kg/min: increases peripheral vasoconstriction	6 mg (0.15 ml) × wt (kg) = mg to add to make 100 ml D5W = 1 ml/hr = 1 μg/kg/min >20 μg/kg/min peripheral and renal vasoconstriction (alpha-adrenergic action)	Poor perfusion; hypotension (normovolemic and stable rhythm); dilution = 600 μg/ml
Epinephrine (Adrenalin) *Use 1:1000* (1 mg/ml)	0.1-1 μg/kg/min	0.6 mg (0.6 ml) × wt (kg) = mg to add to make 100 ml D5W = 1 ml/hr = 0.1 μg/kg/min; dilution = 6 μg/ml	Hypotension (normovolemic); unstable bradycardia
Isoproterenol Isuprel 1:5000 (0.2 mg/ml-1 mg/5 ml)	0.1-1 μg/kg/min; adolescents: 2-20 μg/min total dose; 1 mg in 250 ml = 4 μg/ml	0.6 mg (3 ml) × wt (kg) = mg to add to make 100 ml D5W = 1 ml/hr = 0.1 μg/kg/min; dilution = 6 μg/ml	Unstable bradycardia due to heart block and resistance to atropine
Lidocaine (Xylocaine) 4% or 40 mg/ml 4 g/100 ml	20-50 μg/kg/hr; adolescents: 4 mg/min, 1 g in 250 ml = 4 mg/ml	120 mg (3 ml 4%) to make 100 ml = 1200 μg/ml; 1 microdrip/kg/min = 20 μg/kg/min 2.5 microdrip/kg/min = 50 μg/kg/min	Ventricular tachycardia; ventricular fibrillation
Norepinephrine (Levophed) 1:1000 (1 mg/ml in 4 ml)	0.1-1 μg/kg/min; start with 0.1 μg and titrate	0.6 mg (0.6 ml) × wt (kg) = mg to add to make 100 ml D5W = 1 ml/hr = 0.1 μg/kg/min, or dissolve 2 ampules 8 ml (8 mg) in 500 ml D5W; start 0.4 ml/kg/hr = 0.1 μg/kg/min; add phentolamine (Regitine) 5 mg to infusion if not in central line	Hypotension (normovolemic and stable rhythm), especially if norepinephrine depletion is suspected.

BP, Blood pressure; *CHF*, congestive heart failure; *CPR*, cardiopulmonary resuscitation; *max*, maximum; *μdrip*, microdrip; *wt*, weight.
*It is useful to have precalculated dose schedules of infusion medications.

Table A-14 *Normal Ranges of Cardiac Function*

AGE (yr)	HEART RATE (beats/min)	PR INTERVAL (sec)	QRS COMPLEX (sec)
<1	90-180	0.07-0.16	0.03-0.08
1-3	70-140	0.08-0.16	0.04-0.08
4-10	60-120	0.09-0.17	0.04-0.07
>10	55-110	0.09-0.20	0.04-0.08

Modified from Garson A: Electrocardiogram in infants and children: a systematic approach, Philadelphia, 1983, Lea and Febiger.

series of depolarizations seen on the ECG with no detectible pulse and decreased cardiac output. The ECG pattern is classified as coarse or fine on the basis of the height of the electrical waves.

Cardiopulmonary resuscitative measures should be continued until defibrillation can be applied, using an initial dose of 2 joules/kg. If this is unsuccessful, the dose should be doubled and repeated twice. If this also is unsuccessful, ventilation and correction of any metabolic disturbance (hypoxia, hypoglycemia, severe metabolic acidosis) should be accomplished, followed by a bolus of epinephrine and another attempt at defibrillation. If this too fails, a bolus of lidocaine and further defibrillation should be attempted. Finally, if that fails, bretylium given initially at a dose of 5 mg/kg and subsequently at doses of 10 mg/kg in place of lidocaine before defibrillation is attempted. The use of lidocaine infusion after cardioversion has been recommended by some.

Electromechanical dissociation is characterized by the presence of organized electrical activity with ineffective myocardial contractions as evidenced by the absence of a pulse. Etiologies include hypoxia, acidosis, volume depletion, tension pneumothorax, and cardiac tamponade. Treatment consists of ventilation, oxygenation, volume repletion, and the administration of an epinephrine bolus.

POSTRESUSCITATIVE CARE OF INFANTS AND CHILDREN [2]

Postresuscitative care involves stabilization, frequent assessment, and care during transport to a tertiary care facility, as well as the care rendered in that facility's intensive care unit. Any infant or child who has suffered respiratory or cardiac arrest should be admitted to a pediatric intensive care unit.

Elements of Postresuscitative Care

1. Cardiovascular function should be assessed by determining tissue perfusion clinically and by monitoring urinary output, blood pressure, and continuous ECG recordings.
2. Ventilation should be evaluated clinically, and by interpretation of arterial blood gas levels and pulse oximeter or transcutaneous Po_2 readings.
3. Serial neurologic examinations should be performed with attention given to the level of consciousness and evidence of increased intracranial pressure and seizures.
4. Humidified warm oxygen at the highest attainable concentration should be administered until arterial blood gas levels are available. Arterial blood gas levels should be measured after a ventilation system has been in use for at least 15 minutes and before the patient's transport. The hematocrit, serum electrolyte and blood glucose levels also should be monitored and determined just before transport.
5. Two well-secured functional venous lines should be placed.
6. A nasogastric tube should be connected to gravity drainage to decompress the stomach, especially if positive pressure ventilation has been used.
7. The cause of the cardiopulmonary arrest should be determined and treated.

Transportation to a Regional Pediatric Intensive Care Unit [5]

Agreements, protocols for specific clinical situations, and protocols for transport to the regional pediatric intensive care unit should be prepared in advance by the directors of the Regional Emergency Medical Services for Children (EMS-C) program.

Information Needed for Interhospital Transport

1. The referring hospital's name, physician's name, and telephone numbers
2. The child's name, age, and weight
3. A history of the present illness and significant elements of the past history, including medications present in the home and medications to which the patient may be allergic
4. The present clinical status, including the level of consciousness, heart rate, presence and adequacy of peripheral pulses, capillary refill time, respiratory rate, air entry status, respiratory effort, skin color, body temperature, and blood pressure
5. Laboratory test data, including all roentgenograms and ECG tracings
6. All medications administered, including dosages and times given
7. The number of intravenous lines and fluids administered, including their infusion rates
8. The ventilator settings if the patient is receiving assisted ventilation
9. The availability of parents or their designates for providing consent for treatment

Brain Death [12]

Brain death, the ultimate criterion for removing life-support mechanisms, is defined as (1) irreversible cessation of circulation and respiratory function or (2) irreversible cessation of all brain functions, including those of the brain stem. Caution should be taken in reaching the conclusion that brain death has occurred in patients who (1) are younger than 5 years of age, (2) have hypothermia, (3) nearly drowned, and (4) have ingested neuromuscular blocking agents or barbiturates, because early in these circumstances electroencephalographic recordings may be unreliable.*

Do Not Resuscitate (DNR) Orders [28]

The purpose of CPR is to prevent of sudden, unexpected death. Its use may not be indicated in circumstances surrounding a terminal, irreversible illness when death is not unexpected or when prolonged cardiac arrest indicates the futility of such efforts, which are a violation of the right to die with dignity. A DNR order should be written on the patient's order sheet, and the physician should explain in a progress note the rationale for the decision and should identify the participants in the decision-making. The use of "partial resuscitation codes" are ethically and legally questionable.[15]

*The determination of brain death is very difficult and must be done precisely. Guidelines for the Determination of Brain Death in Children have been drawn by the Task Force for the Determination of Brain Death in Children (Archives of Neurology 44:587, 1987).

REFERENCES

1. Bardossi K: Newest guidelines on pediatric CPR and first aid, Contemp Pediatr 4:47, 1987.
2. Chameides L, editor: Textbook of pediatric advanced life support, Dallas, 1988, American Heart Association and American Academy of Pediatrics.
3. Chernow R et al: Epinephrine absorption after endotracheal administration, Anesth Analg 63:629, 1984.
4. Committee on Drugs of AAP. Emergency drug doses in children, Pediatrics 81:462, 1988.
5. Committee on Hospital Care, AAP: Guidelines for air and ground transportation of pediatric patients, Pediatrics 78:943, 1986.
6. Day RL: Differing opinions on the emergency treatment of choking, Pediatrics 71:975, 1983.
7. Epstein ML, Kiel EA, and Victoria BE: Cardiac decompensation following verapamil therapy in infants with supraventricular tachycardia, Pediatrics 75:737, 1985.
8. Finholt DA et al: The heart is under the lower third of the sternum, Am J Dis Child 646:649, 1986.
9. Gillis J et al: Results of inpatient pediatric resuscitation, Crit Care Med 14:469, 1986.
10. Greenberg MI: Endotracheal drugs: the state of the art, Ann Emerg Med 13:789, 1984.
11. Greenberg MI and Roberts RJ: Drugs for the heart by way of the lungs, Emerg Med 12:209, 1980.
12. Report of the Medical Consultants of the Diagnosis of Death to the President's Commission for the Study of Ethical Problems in Medicine and Biomedical and Behavorial Research: Guidelines for the determination of death, JAMA 246:2184, 1981.
13. Mace SE: Cricothyrotomy, J Emerg Med 6:309, 1988.
14. Mofenson HC and Caraccio TR: Guidelines for intraosseous infusion, J Emerg Med 6:143, 1988.
15. National Conference on Cardiopulmonary Resuscitation and Emergency Cardiac Care: Standards and guidelines for cardiopulmonary resuscitation (CPR) and emergency cardiac care (ECC), JAMA 255:2954, 1986.
16. Nieman JT and Rosborough JP: Effects of acidemia and sodium bicarbonate therapy in advanced life support, Ann Emerg Med 13:781, 1984.
17. Orlowski J: Optimum position for external cardiac compression in infants and young children, Ann Emerg Med 15:667, 1986.
18. Park MK and Guntheroth WG: How to read pediatric ECGs, Chicago, 1982, Year Book Medical Publishers Inc.
19. Perkin RM et al: Dobutamine: a hemodynamic evaluation in children in shock, J Pediatr 100:977, 1982.
20. Phillips GWL and Zideman DA: Relationship of infant heart to sternum: its significance in cardiopulmonary resuscitation, Lancet 1:1024, 1986.
21. Radford D: Side effects of verapamil in infants, Arch Dis Child 58:465, 1983.
22. Rosetti VA et al: Intraosseous infusion: an alternate route of pediatric intravascular access, Ann Emerg Med 14:885, 1985.
23. Schuman A: Pediatric advanced life support: an update and review, Contemp Pediatr 6:26, 1989.
24. Seigler RS, Tecklenburg FW, and Shealy R: Prehospital intraosseous infusion by emergency medical services personnel: a prospective study, Pediatrics 84:173, 1989.
25. Seidel JS and Burkett DL, editors: Instructor's manual for pediatric advanced life support, Dallas, 1988, American Heart Association.
26. Spivey WH: Intraosseous infusions, J Pediatr 111:639, 1987.
27. Stewart RD and Lacovery DC: Administration of endotracheal medication, Ann Emerg Med 14:136, 1985.
28. Tomlinson T and Brody H: Ethics and communications in do-not-resuscitate orders, N Engl J Med 316:43, 1988.
29. Tsai A and Kallsen G: Epidemiology of pediatric prehospital care, Ann Emerg Med 16:284, 1987.
30. Zaritsky A and Chernow B: Use of catecholamines in pediatrics, J Pediatr 105:341, 1984.

B

Special Procedures

Joseph R. Custer

The information presented here details the methods by which samples of normal and abnormal body fluids are obtained to enhance diagnosis and treatment of pediatric patients, how therapeutic fluids are introduced parenterally, and how endotracheal intubation can be accomplished in children with respiratory difficulties.

PATIENT PREPARATION

General Approach

The first step in the performance of any pediatric procedure is the establishment of an understanding among physician, parents, and child of what is to be done. Failure to do this will compromise the physician-patient-parent relationship. The physician who dismisses parent and patient concerns or fears of an impending procedure will lose their confidence. Procedures that the physician may consider routine and ordinary have great significance to parents and patients. They have a right to know what will be done and why it will be done.

The information to be gained from the simplest procedure must be explained. The parents and the patient should be informed about the indications for each test and procedure. Parents should be given a reason for their child's inconvenience and discomfort. Reassurance that the physician understands the child and the child's perceptions must be conveyed to the parents.

The spectrum of ages and stages of development of pediatric patients dictates that an adaptive approach be taken by the practitioner. Appreciation of both the child's fears and the parents' reservations requires a calm, empathic, reassuring posture. The newborn, toddler, and older child all present different problems. If one forgets the newborn's individuality in the frustration of repeated attempts at venipuncture, normal protective emotions in the parents may be aroused and the physician-parent relationship may suffer.

The toddler, just beginning to develop a new vocabulary and new emotions, may react to painful procedures submissively or obstinately. The toddler's fear of pain, of being handled by strangers, and of separation from the mother must be respected. A calm, authoritative approach will convey to the child that the adults present are in control.

In older children it is important to appreciate their perception of what will happen. Here the expression "blood test" may conjure up all sorts of mysterious images in the child's mind. A more explicit explanation of what is to be done will help to dispel those mysteries. The older child also will respond to contracts of cooperation, such as, "You may cry, but hold your arm still, and we will finish the test quickly," or "You can help by holding very still." One must not violate this contract by denying the child's feelings of pain or discomfort. If the operator sees that the child is terribly upset by a procedure, a few minutes given to reassurance will not be wasted.

Before the performance of any procedure, a decision as to whether the parents should be in attendance during the procedure needs to be made. It will depend on the relative comfort of both the physician and the parents. If their presence causes anxiety for the physician, the success of the procedure may be hampered; on the other hand, children's cooperation may be enhanced by the reassuring presence of their parents. The adolescent may at times feel the presence of parents to be embarrassing.

An "open-door" policy for parents to be present when procedures are performed must never represent a demand for demonstration of parenting behavior. Therefore the wishes of those parents who do not want to be present should be respected. Parents should never be involved in restraining their child or in assisting in the performance of a painful procedure.

Although tradition has kept parents from the bedside and treatment rooms when procedures are performed on their child, this determination should be on an individual basis.

Restraint and Immobilization

It is necessary to immobilize infants and some children to complete quickly and safely most of the procedures described here. Therefore an assistant always is required to help immobilize the child, to observe the child's cardiorespiratory function during the procedure, and to reassure and comfort the child. In general, parents should not be asked to serve as assistants.

For infants and younger children, the "papoose" board can be used effectively for immobilization. Children up to about 5 years of age can be immobilized by mummy wrapping, as demonstrated in Fig. B-1. The assistant stands at the side or foot of the wrapped child, leans lightly on the trunk, stabilizing the patient's thorax with the elbows, and with the hands fixes the patient's head or free arm for the procedure.

Anesthesia

In general, if the procedure involves only a needle puncture, local anesthesia may be dispensed with, inasmuch as it necessitates additional needle punctures.

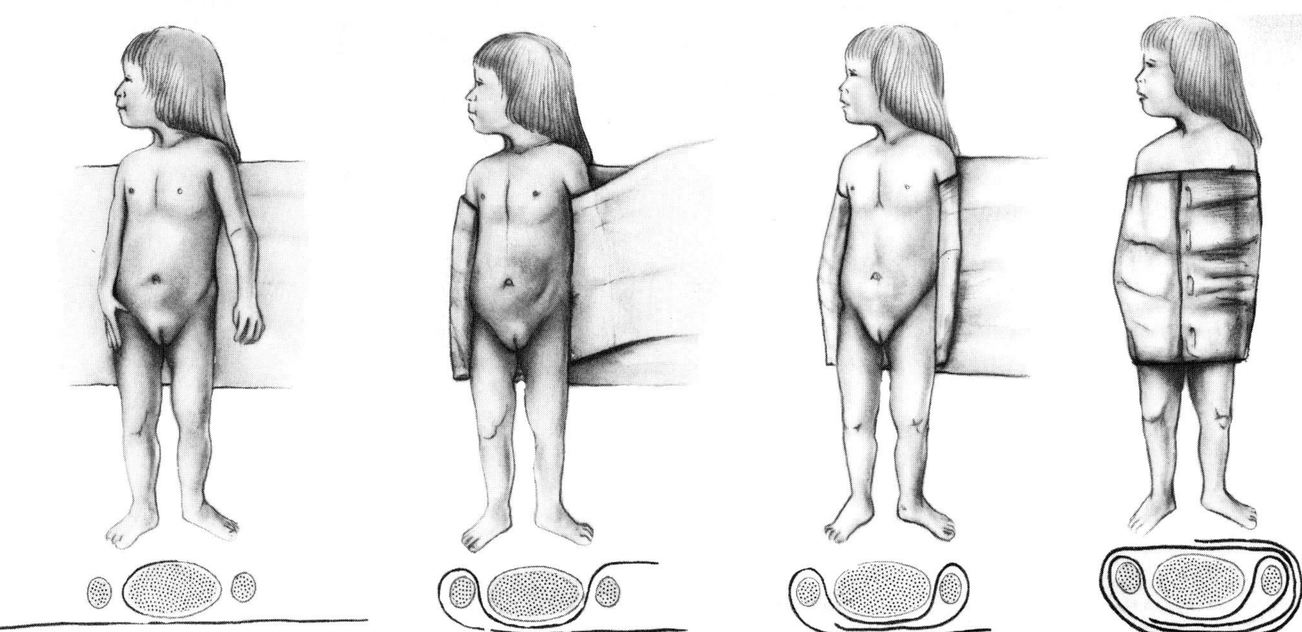

Fig. B-1 Method of mummy-wrapping an infant or child to restrain the upper extremities. The four steps are illustrated with frontal and cross-sectional views. A wider sheet or blanket may be used to restrain the lower extremities.

Local anesthesia usually is produced by infiltration of the skin with lidocaine (1% solution, 10 mg/ml). Lidocaine overdose is uncommon but has the serious consequences of hypotension, seizures, and respiratory arrest. The maximum dose of locally infiltrated lidocaine is 5 to 7 mg/kg.

Deep sedation for invasive procedures may be required. The risks of sedation include respiratory and central nervous system depression, hypotension, and emesis. Therefore patients who are sedated require monitoring of heart rate, respiratory rate and effort, and blood pressure, as well as monitoring of noninvasive pulse oximetry. Judgment is required in the choice of sedative dose. Patients with cardiorespiratory embarrassment will need a reduced dose. The best practice is to titrate the dose to the desired effect while adequately monitoring the patient. A key virtue in sedating a child is patience. One should allow adequate time in a quiet, controlled environment, using a calm voice to gain the confidence of the child. A common error is to start a procedure too soon after giving a sedative. When this happens, the child is inadequately sedated, the physician's impatience is tried by the procedure not going well, and consequently, time is wasted.

Deep sedation can be obtained (in patients who are not in danger of respiratory depression) with a lytic "cocktail," composed of meperidine (Demerol), 2 mg/kg (maximum, 50 mg); promethazine (Phenergan), 1 mg/kg; and chlorpromazine (Thorazine), 1 mg/kg. The drugs are mixed in one syringe and administered by deep intramuscular injection. These doses are appropriate for most procedures that will produce prolonged discomfort or generate high anxiety, but they should be reduced by 50% for precardiac catheterization sedation of children with severe cyanotic congenital heart disease.

When one desires cooperation with relatively pain-free procedures, such as immobilization for an echocardiogram or a computed axial tomographic scan in infants and toddlers, chloral hydrate is the drug of choice. This drug may be given orally or by rectum in doses of 25 to 75 mg/kg. Side effects include movement disorders, respiratory depression, and vomiting.

Diazepam, a commonly used anxiolytic drug in adults, has an application for older children and adolescents, but its use is hazardous in the young infant. It has a narrow therapeutic index—that is, the difference between the effective dose for sedation and that causing apnea is small. The dose is 0.04 to 0.2 mg/kg given intravenously or 0.2 to 0.8 mg/kg by mouth.

Midazolam is a water-soluble imidazobenzodiazepine with rapid onset and short duration of action. The drug produces good anxiolytic effect and retrograde amnesia. Experience with neonates and toddlers is inadequate; however, a dose of 0.05 to 0.2 mg/kg given intravenously is well tolerated in older children and adolescents. Respiratory depression is the drug's most serious side effect.

Morphine, 0.1 to 0.2 mg/kg, is commonly used for sedation in the pediatric population. The drug can be given intravenously, subcutaneously, and intramuscularly. Because the peak effect is delayed for 30 minutes, patience is required for the preprocedure wait. Respiratory depression, hypotension, and bronchospasm secondary to histamine release are commonly encountered complications. Naloxone, 5 to 10 μg/kg given every 5 to 10 minutes, will reverse the hypotension and apnea but must be given repeatedly, inasmuch as its effect is transient.

Fentanyl and ketamine, very useful in specific situations, should be employed under the supervision of an anesthesiologist or a pediatric intensivist.

SAMPLE COLLECTION

Blood

Capillary Puncture. Blood obtained from the capillary bed of a warm finger can be used for blood gas analysis;

blood from the finger, toe, or heel can be used for a wide variety of microdeterminations. After preparation of the skin with alcohol, a firm stab wound is made with a lancet or a No. 11 Bard-Parker blade in the ventrolateral aspect of the terminal phalanx, avoiding the pad and joint. The posterior edge of the heel pad also may be used. Frequent wiping may be needed to prevent clotting and to obtain free flow without squeezing. Local pressure applied with a dry sponge will stop the bleeding after the sample has been obtained.

Venipuncture. Fig. B-2 illustrates the location of superficial veins commonly used to obtain blood samples. For infants the scalp and neck sites provide the easiest access; for older children the veins of the extremities are more accessible, despite the difficulties encountered in restraining movement. The largest superficial veins are those of the cervical and femoral areas, although these should be avoided for routine blood sampling because complications of bloodletting at these sites are more severe than elsewhere. These sites should not be used when bleeding disorders are a factor.

For *venipuncture of the lower arms, lower legs, hands, and feet,* the child is immobilized and the skin is prepared with alcohol. A tourniquet is applied to the extremity (above the point of planned venous puncture) tightly enough to produce venous stasis and distention, yet loosely enough to allow for arterial perfusion. This can be demonstrated if there is capillary refilling after blanching created by direct pressure on the extremity distal to the tourniquet. A 20- or 22-gauge needle or "butterfly" scalp vein infusion needle attached to a syringe may be used. The vein is stabilized by traction on the overlying skin along the axis of the vein. The skin is pierced with the needle bevel up. The needle tip is then advanced subcutaneously, and the vein is entered with a short jab to prevent its rolling away. Negative pressure in the syringe is used to withdraw the amount of blood needed. After the blood is obtained, the tourniquet is released, the needle removed, a dry sponge applied with pressure to the site, and the extremity elevated for a minute or two to prevent bleeding at the puncture site.

For *external jugular venipuncture,* the child is positioned on a table with the head rotated to one side and extended over the edge of the table 45 degrees toward the floor. The assistant, leaning over the mummy-wrapped child, holds the head firmly in this position. Positive intrathoracic pressure created by struggling or crying will distend the jugular vein to make it easily located. After preparation of the skin with alcohol, a butterfly needle is attached to a syringe and used to penetrate the skin in a caudal direction where the vein crosses the sternocleidomastoid muscle. The vein is then entered with a separate thrust, and negative pressure is created within the syringe. If a hematoma appears, the procedure should be discontinued at that site. When the sample is obtained, firm pressure is applied over the venipuncture site for 3 to 5 minutes with the child sitting upright.

Internal jugular venipuncture is a rarely used but accessible site for phlebotomy. This procedure should be reserved as a "last resort" because of the risks of accidental entry into the carotid artery medially and the risk of pneumothorax caused by entering the apex of the lung.

The child is restrained in modest Trendelenburg position, the neck minimally extended at the edge of the table or with the aid of a 2- or 3-inch diameter towel roll at the base of the neck. The child's head is turned 45 degrees away from the proposed side of entry (Fig. B-3).

The internal jugular vein runs lateral to the carotid artery and the trachea. The posterior border of the sternocleidomastoid muscle, as well as its midpoint between the sternal

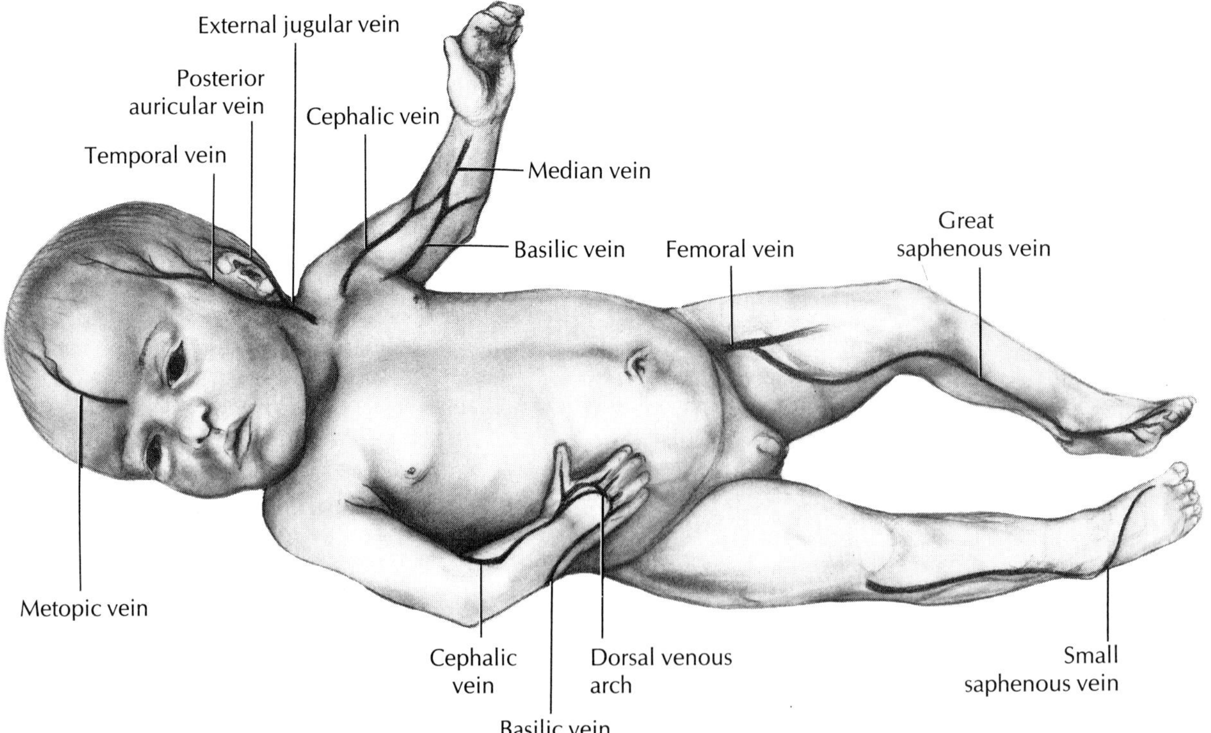

Fig. B-2 Accessible veins for blood sampling and administration of intravenous infusions.

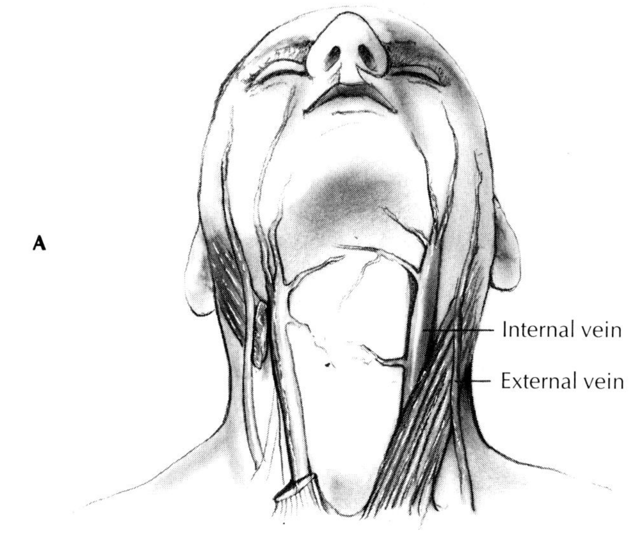

Fig. B-3 Internal jugular venipuncture. **A,** Anatomy of the internal and external jugular veins and their relationship to the sternocleidomastoid muscle. **B,** Positioning of the child, showing the point of the needle overlying the external jugular vein, which must be avoided, and the sternocleidomastoid muscle, beneath which the needle is inserted and thrust toward the suprasternal notch. **C,** Position of the needle and syringe after puncture; negative pressure on the plunger of the syringe should produce rapid filling of the barrel with venous blood.

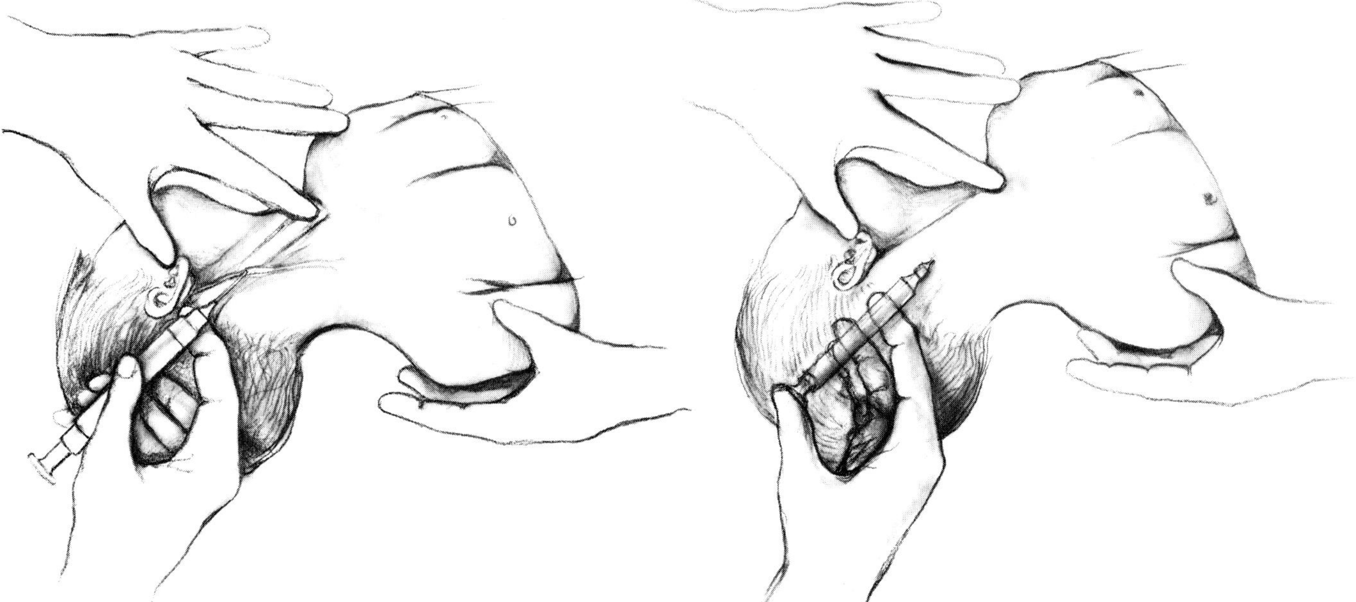

and mastoid insertions, should be identified. A 22-gauge, 1½-inch needle, attached to a 10-ml syringe, is inserted behind and underneath the posterior border of the muscle at the midpoint, aiming for the ipsilateral nipple. Once the skin is pierced, negative syringe pressure should be maintained continuously so that the blood will enter the barrel of the syringe immediately when the vein is entered. Firm pressure should be applied over the site for 3 to 5 minutes after the procedure, with the child sitting upright.

For *puncture of the femoral vein,* the child is placed in the supine position with the leg straight and externally rotated. The assistant holds this position while leaning over the child's trunk from one side. The femoral artery is identified by palpation just distal to the inguinal (Poupart) ligament and medial to the midpoint of the ligament. The femoral vein lies medial and parallel to the artery here (Fig. B-4). The skin is prepared with alcohol, and while the artery is being palpated, the skin is entered 1 to 2 cm distal to the flexion crease of the groin. The needle should be directed medial to the arterial pulsations and cephalad, at a 30-degree angle, while negative pressure is applied to the syringe during insertion and withdrawal. Blood will enter the syringe as soon as the vein is entered. Complications of the procedure, which are caused by faulty needle placement, include septic arthritis of the hip, osteomyelitis of the femur, and femoral arteriospasm (sometimes severe enough to cause gangrene).

Arterial Puncture. Arterial puncture has become a necessary technical skill for physicians who care for critically ill children. Assessment of arterial blood gases is essential in monitoring a variety of cardiopulmonary diseases.

The *right radial artery* is the preferred site for arterial puncture. It is in a consistent anatomic position and is well fixed by surrounding connective tissue. In the newborn the site has the added advantage of providing preductal arterial blood samples. Other available sites are the brachial, femoral, and temporal arteries.

Arterial punctures may be hazardous because arterial laceration, spasm, or insufficiency secondary to hematoma may

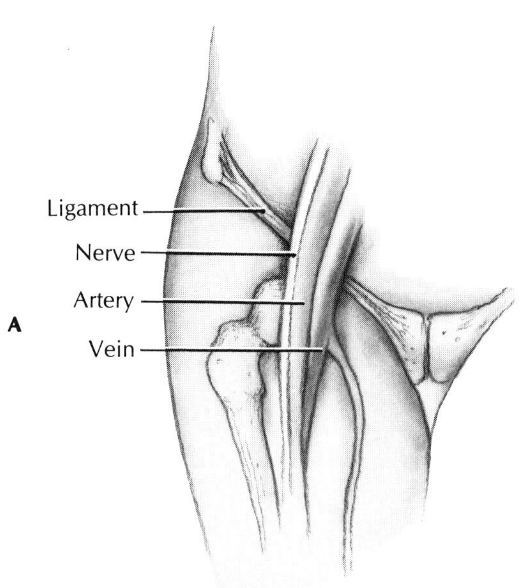

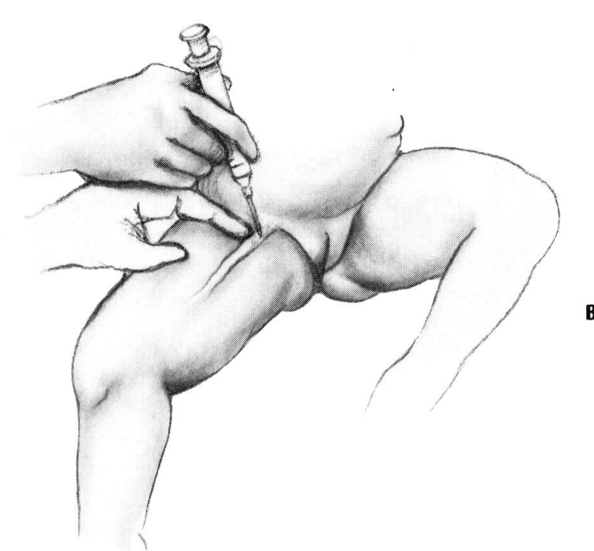

Fig. B-4 Femoral vein or artery puncture. **A,** Anatomic structures. **B,** Positioning of the patient, with needle and syringe poised for piercing the skin, subcutaneous tissue, and femoral vein. The procedure for femoral artery puncture is performed identically except that the needle is aimed more laterally, directly into the pulsating femoral artery.

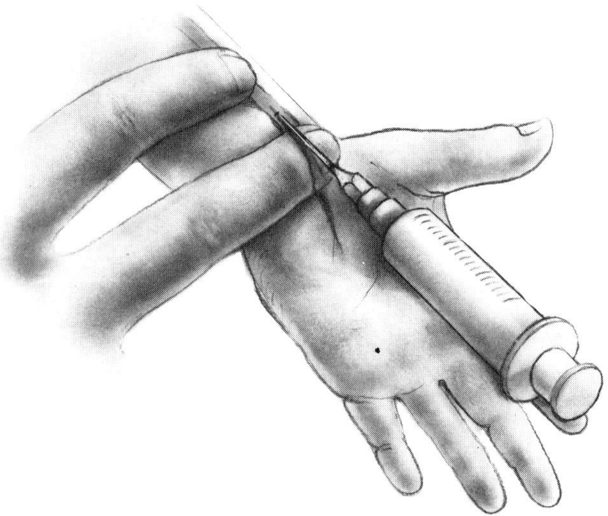

Fig. B-5 Radial artery puncture. The position of the radial artery is determined by palpation, and it is fixed with the index and middle fingers while being punctured with the needle and syringe directed at a 45-degree angle.

occur. The adequacy ot collateral circulation for the radial artery is good, but it may be less so for the femoral and brachial arteries. Septic arthritis of the hip is an infrequent complication of femoral artery puncture. The data from blood gases may be erroneous if venous blood is sampled, if the sample is exposed to air, if the equipment used for analysis is improperly standardized, or if the oxygen concentration to which the patient is exposed during the sampling is not considered.

The wrist is supported in a position of supination and slight dorsiflexion. The artery may be located at the wrist by palpation of the point of maximal pulsation. In newborns it usually is found along the first flexor crease one sixth of the width of the wrist measured from its radial edge (Fig. B-5).

A plastic or glass syringe is rinsed with heparin and emptied. The size of the needle used varies with the patient's age (25 gauge for newborns and infants to 22 gauge for older children and adolescents). Care must be taken to avoid constricting the artery during restraint. The syringe is held as one would hold a pencil or a dart, and the needle is introduced into the artery at approximately a 45-degree angle. A "flash" of blood spurting into the syringe indicates a successful puncture. Gentle aspiration is required when plastic, disposable syringes are used. A butterfly needle may be more easily used with hard-to-restrain patients; in such cases the syringe is rinsed with heparin, and 0.25 to 0.50 ml of heparin is injected into the butterfly tubing to clear it of air. The butterfly needle, without the syringe attached, is then introduced into the artery as described above. A pulsatile flow of blood into the tubing ensures that arterial puncture has been accomplished. The syringe is then connected to the butterfly tubing, and the sample is collected. The sample should be sealed, placed in ice, and sent to the laboratory for analysis. Direct pressure on the puncture site for a minimum of 5 minutes will prevent bleeding and hematoma formation.

The *temporal artery* is an alternative site for arterial sampling. After the scalp is shaved anterior to the ear, the arteries are often visible or, if not, are easily palpated. Gentle traction of the skin with the fingers will fix the artery before puncture. A 23- or 25-gauge butterfly needle is used to enter the skin at a very shallow angle nearly parallel to the plane of the artery (Fig. B-6). The butterfly needle is slowly advanced until a pulsatile flow of blood is obtained, indicating successful arterial puncture.

The *brachial artery* is a less desirable choice for sampling because collateral circulation is not always adequate and because a vein may be mistakenly sampled. The artery is located by palpation. Either a 22- or 25-gauge needle and syringe or, for infants, a 23- or 25-gauge butterfly needle may be used. The needle should be held at a 45-degree angle and the skin punctured at the point of maximal pulsation. Pressure must

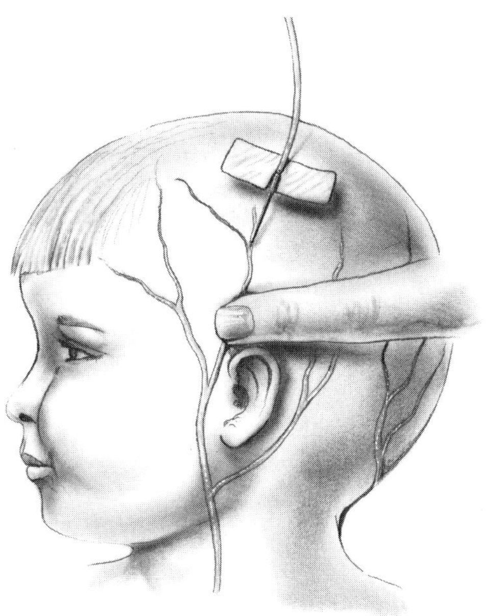

Fig. B-6 Temporal artery puncture. Position of the artery and butterfly needle before arterial puncture.

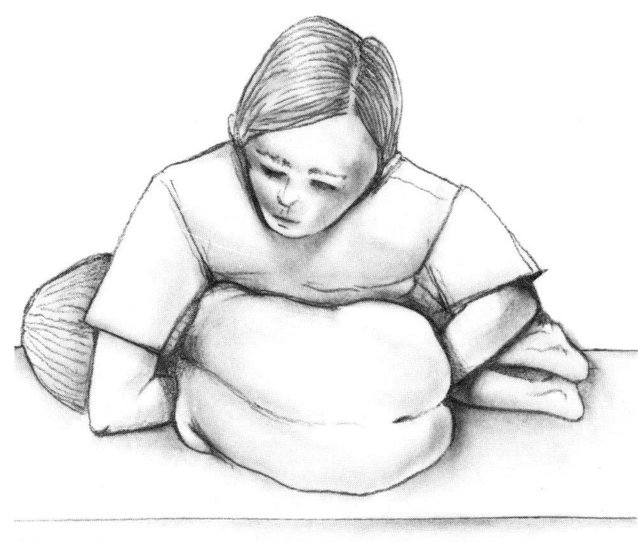

Fig. B-7 Restraint of a child during lumbar puncture. The patient's nuchal and popliteal surfaces are in contact with the antecubital fossas of the assistant.

be applied to the site of puncture for 5 to 10 minutes after the needle is withdrawn.

The *femoral artery* is the least desirable choice for sampling, because the hip joint can be inadvertently entered and contaminated, and collateral circulation is poor should arterial insufficiency result from the procedure. This area is more apt to be contaminated than are other arterial puncture sites; therefore extra attention to skin preparation is required. The puncture site may be found at the point of maximal pulsation, just inferior to the inguinal ligaments (Fig. B-4). The femoral nerve is lateral, and the femoral vein medial, to the artery. The artery should be punctured at approximately a 90-degree angle. Gentle aspiration as the needle penetrates the soft tissue will aid in detecting a successful puncture. Once the sample is obtained, careful pressure on the puncture site for at least 10 minutes is necessary.

Cerebrospinal Fluid

The need to perform a lumbar puncture to rule out meningitis and other central nervous system infections must be weighed against the dangers inherent in performing a lumbar puncture in the presence of a supratentorial space-occupying lesion. Increased intracranial pressure is a relative contraindication to lumbar puncture. Its presence dictates immediate neurosurgical consultation if the collection of cerebrospinal fluid is judged clinically necessary.

The position of the patient during lumbar puncture should be dictated by the mutual comfort of the patient, the assistant, and the operator. Some prefer infants to be held upright; others prefer the lateral recumbent position (Fig. B-7). The use of a local anesthetic is not necessary for infants. Reassurance, explanation of what is to occur, and a tranquil atmosphere may be as important as a local anesthetic for an older child.

The preferred site is the L3-4 interspace. It is located by determining the place at which an imaginary line drawn between the superior edge of right and left posterior iliac crests crosses the spine. The interspace above and below also may be used. The skin is thoroughly prepared with an appropriate antiseptic, the patient is sterilely draped, and sterile gloves are worn.

Care must be taken that the needle will enter the intervertebral space in the sagittal plane. This requires several different perspectives of the proposed line of entry with the needle aimed toward the umbilicus.

Once the skin is penetrated, the needle is advanced slowly in the sagittal plane. Although a distinct "pop," or give, may be felt in the older patient when the dura is pierced, this is not the case in the infant. When the physician suspects that the spinal canal has been entered, the stylet is removed and the needle carefully rotated to maximize the flow of cerebrospinal fluid through the needle. If no flow is obtained, the stylet is reinserted and the needle is advanced further or withdrawn and redirected. Care must be taken to avoid a "bloody tap," or traumatic tap, caused by pushing the needle into the venous plexus along the anterior wall of the spinal canal. A syringe should *never* be used to enhance the aspiration of cerebrospinal fluid, because this will create undue pressure and might produce herniation of the brain stem through the foramen magnum.

A three-way stopcock and manometer are attached to the spinal needle to measure the pressure of cerebrospinal fluid and, in certain instances, to perform manometric tests. These measures are useless with the struggling child. One milliliter of fluid is collected in each of three sterile test tubes to be used for bacteriologic, chemical, and cytologic determinations. In the case of a traumatic tap, the red cells in both the first and the third tubes should be counted. A traumatic tap usually will give fewer red cells in the third tube than in the first. Once the fluid is removed, the needle is withdrawn quickly and the puncture site tamponaded briefly. No dressing is required.

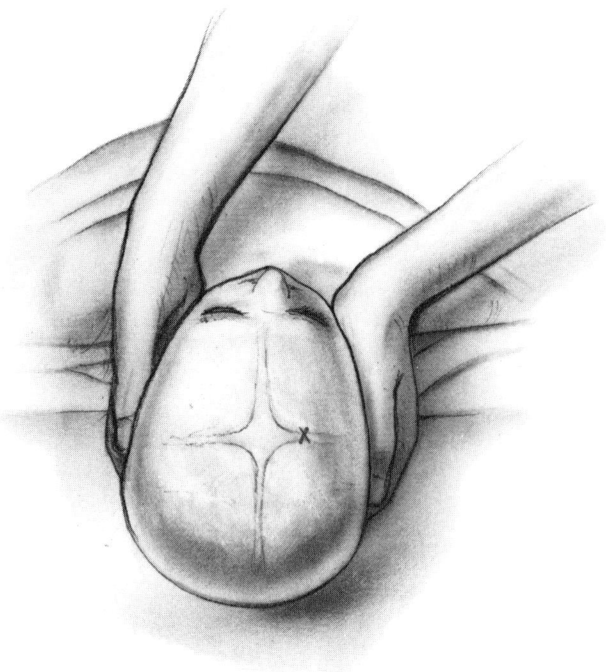

Fig. B-8 Subdural tap. Positioning of the child for a subdural tap. The subdural needle should be inserted in the coronal suture 1 to 2 cm lateral to the edge of the anterior fontanelle.

Subdural Fluid

The purpose of a subdural tap is to determine the existence of a posttraumatic or postinfectious subdural effusion. In the presence of closed sutures and ossified fontanelles, neurosurgical assistance should be sought.

Fig. B-8 illustrates the preferred site of puncture. This is a point in the coronal suture 1 to 2 cm lateral to the anterior fontanelle on an imaginary line drawn posteriorly from the center of the orbit parallel to the sagittal suture.

While the infant is supine, the head should be carefully restrained. The anterior two thirds of the infant's scalp is shaved and cleansed with an appropriate antiseptic. The portion of the unshaved scalp posterior to the planned puncture site should be sterilely draped, and sterile gloves should be used while the procedure is performed.

A short, beveled 19- or 20-gauge lumbar puncture needle or a subdural-tap needle is inserted through the skin perpendicular to the scalp and slowly is advanced 2.5 to 5.0 mm. A hemostat clamped to the shaft of the needle will aid the operator in gauging the depth of insertion and will prevent accidental overpenetration. Perforation of the dura usually is recognized by a sudden decrease in resistance and a sensation of "popping through." A few drops of fluid normally are present and will flow through the needle when the stylet is removed. Negative pressure applied to the needle with the aid of a syringe should be avoided. The procedure usually is performed on both sides of the head. Current practice in the treatment of subdural effusion is to remove no more than 25 ml of fluid from each subdural space per day. Chronic effusions necessitate taps on a daily basis. After the removal of the subdural specimen, the needle is withdrawn and a sterile cotton and collodion dressing is applied.

Urine

Urethral Catheterization. To collect a sterile specimen of urine from a child who cannot produce a midstream, clean-catch specimen, or to monitor the urine output continuously, a catheter is inserted into the bladder through the urethra. The child is placed in the supine frog-leg position and prepared with sterile technique, including drapes, gloves, and skin cleansing with benzalkonium chloride. A small (8 Fr) straight or indwelling catheter should be used for a child; for an infant, a No. 5 feeding tube may be used. The catheter or tube should be coated with sterile lubricating jelly. For a female, the labia majora and minora should be widely separated so that the urethral meatus may be identified, cleansed, and entered with the catheter. For a male, the penis is held at a right angle to the abdomen while the catheter is placed in the urethra and is advanced until urine is obtained. If the catheter is to be indwelling, the retaining balloon should be filled with sterile saline or water. The amount of fluid and the site of filling are shown on the catheter itself. When an indwelling catheter is used, it is necessary to establish a closed, sterile urine-collection system.

Percutaneous Suprapubic Bladder Aspiration. To obtain sterile urine specimens, a percutaneous suprapubic bladder aspiration is especially useful in infants, whose bladders are abdominally placed. Before attempting this procedure, the physician should ensure that the child has not voided for at least 1 hour. An assistant should hold the child in the supine frog-leg position while the operator percusses the bladder above the symphysis pubis and prepares the skin with alcohol. To prevent urination during the procedure, the urethra should be compressed by pressure through the rectum of the female or by direct pressure to the penis of the male. The abdominal wall is entered in the midline 1 to 2 cm above the symphysis pubis with a 22-gauge, 1-inch needle attached to a syringe (Fig. B-9). The needle should be directed slightly cephalad, and negative pressure is maintained in the syringe as it is advanced. Urine entering the barrel of the syringe signals a successful bladder tap.

The procedure may be repeated once if no urine is obtained in the first attempt. If the repeat attempt is unsuccessful, an hour should be allowed to elapse before another attempt is made. When urine is obtained, the needle is withdrawn smoothly, and the entry site is covered with a dry dressing. Complications include transient hematuria and, rarely, perforation of the bowel.

Other Body Cavities

Tympanocentesis. For the bacteriologic diagnosis of otitis media in infants and compromised hosts in whom the identification of gram-negative and other organisms is particularly important, tympanocentesis is required. This maneuver also may be therapeutic because it will reduce middle-ear pressure. The child is mummy-wrapped and restrained by the assistant, who should hold the child's head absolutely immobile. The otic canal is cleansed with cotton swabs and alcohol or benzalkonium chloride. After cleansing and before the puncture, specimens should be taken from the ear canal and cultured to identify contaminating organisms.

The tympanic membrane is visualized through the open-

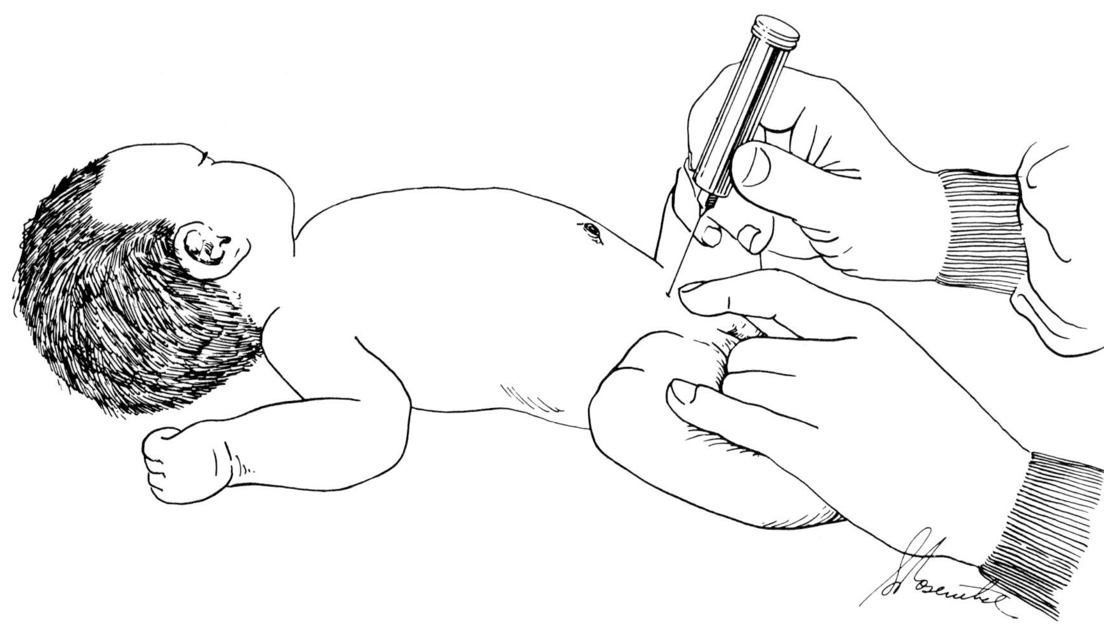

Fig. B-9 Position of an infant before aspiration of urine by suprapubic aspiration. The left index finger of the operator is placed on the symphysis pubis.

ended otoscope. A 3½-inch, 20- or 22-gauge spinal needle with a double bend (Z shape) allows a clear visualization of the tip along its axis (Fig. B-10). The needle is connected directly to a tuberculin syringe. The plunger of the syringe is removed, and one end of the length of tubing is placed over the proximal end of the syringe's barrel. The other end of the tubing is placed in the physician's mouth so that negative pressure can be created within the needle-syringe-tubing apparatus. The needle is used to pierce the posteroinferior quadrant of the tympanic membrane, and negative pressure is applied to withdraw middle-ear fluid. If an adequate amount of fluid has been obtained, a drop should be Gram stained and the remainder cultured appropriately. If there is no visible fluid, the needle should be flushed with 2 to 3 ml of blood culture medium, which may then be Gram stained and cultured. The tympanic membrane should be visualized 2 or 3 days after the procedure to ensure that healing has occurred.

Abdominal Paracentesis and Peritoneal Dialysis Catheter Placement. The physician who encounters a critically ill child in an emergency room or an inpatient unit can easily obtain access to the child's peritoneal cavity. This might be done to sample fluid for possible extravasated blood in a case of trauma; to obtain specimens for a white blood cell count, a differential count, or a Gram stain and culture; to institute peritoneal dialysis for the treatment of renal failure, hyperkalemia, azotemia, or fluid overload; or to remove a dialysable toxin. Peritoneal dialysis also has been used to control body temperature in severe hypothermia or hyperthermia. Relative contraindications include coagulopathy, distended viscera, and local skin infection. Risks are perforation of bowel and bladder, bleeding, and introduction of infection. The removal of large amounts of ascitic fluid can lead to shock. The patient should be sedated and placed in appropriate restraints. The abdomen should be prepared with strict aseptic technique. Three sites are available. The first is in the midline, one third of the distance between the umbilicus and the symphysis pubis. The second and third sites are in the right and left lower quadrants, lateral to the rectus muscle sheath and a few centimeters above the inguinal ligament. The bladder should be emptied. The preferred site is in the midline, 2 to 3 cm below the umbilicus. This should be infiltrated with 1% lidocaine. A catheter placed over a guide wire is recommended because the needle used to gain entry to the peritoneum is "protected" from cutting or perforating by the guide wire.

These catheters are produced by several manufacturers in a variety of lengths and diameters. For paracentesis, lavage, and dialysis in a large multidisciplinary ICU, two sizes of guide wire–placed peritoneal dialysis catheters may be used.* The catheters, available in diameters of 9 Fr and 11 Fr, have multifenestrated tips. The catheter is made with the last few centimeters set at approximately a 30-degree angle, which aids placement. An alternative is a simple plastic intravenous catheter, 4 to 8 cm long, in 20 or 22 gauge sizes.

An incision, 2 to 4 mm, is made with a scalpel to allow easier entry. If a simple intravenous needle and catheter are used, the needle is placed in the incision and, with steady pressure, advanced into the peritoneum. Entry into the peritoneum is easily detected, but the physician must be careful to control the depth of penetration in order to avoid perforating viscera. The plastic cannula now can be advanced and attached to a syringe for aspiration. For lavage, 10 to 20 ml/kg of normal saline, warmed to body temperature, may be instilled before sampling.

The technique for guide wire–aided placement of a dialysis catheter for lavage or dialysis is similar. A needle, supplied with the manufacturer's "kit," is placed through the abdominal wall. Immediately after the peritoneum is entered, a guide

*Cook, Inc, Elletsville, Ind.

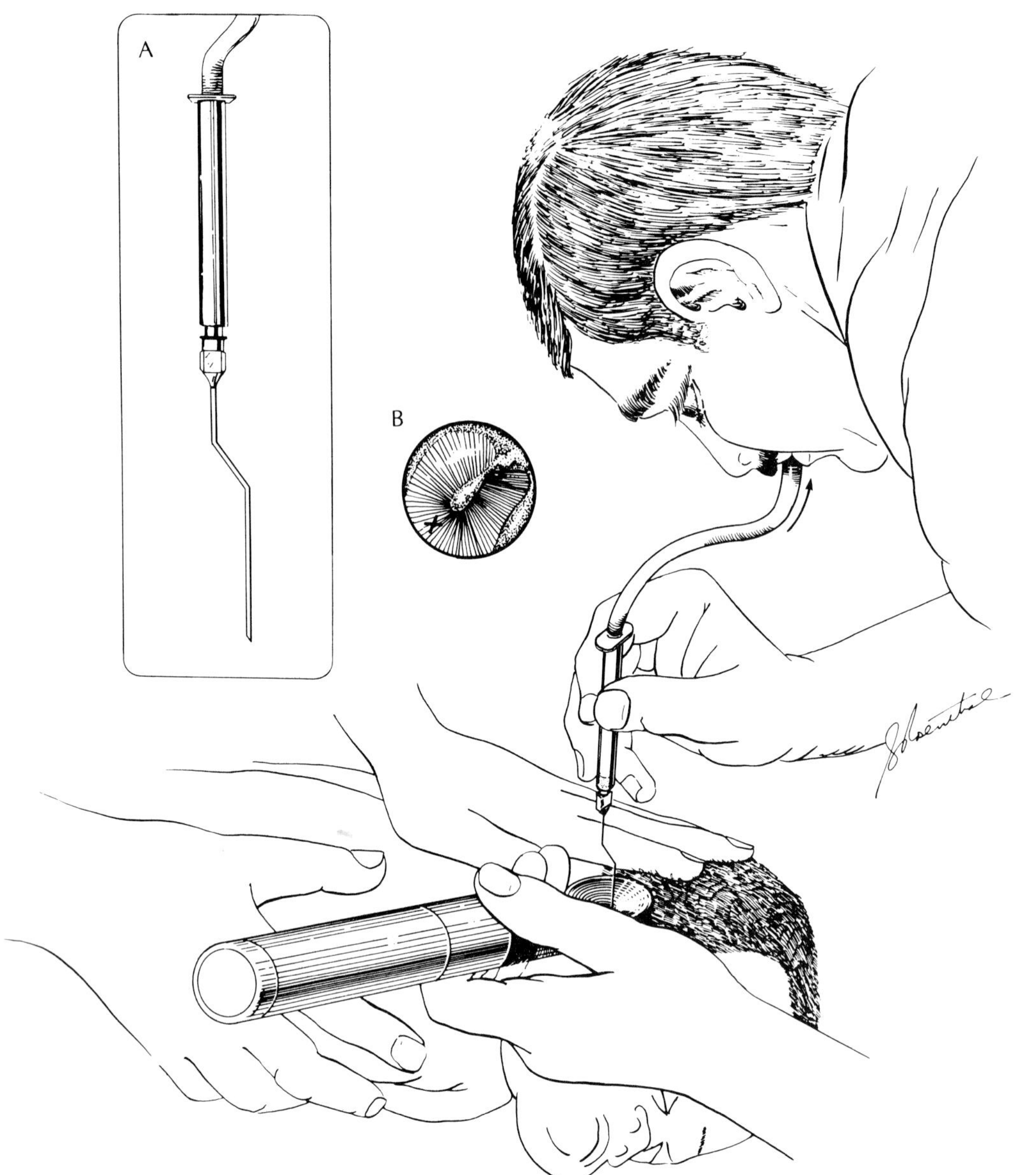

Fig. B-10 Tympanostomy. *A,* A 3-inch, 22-gauge spinal needle that has been shaped to allow direct visualization of the tympanic membrane through the operating otoscope. A tuberculin syringe barrel is attached to the needle, and tubing is attached to the syringe barrel. *B,* The preferred site on the right tympanic membrane for puncture and aspiration of the middle ear. Once the middle ear has been entered, the operator applies negative pressure through the end of the tubing placed in his or her mouth, as illustrated.

wire of appropriate size is placed through the needle and advanced to the left peritoneal "gutter." The dialysis catheter is advanced over the wire and gently steered to the gutter. The wire is then removed, and the catheter can be attached to a syringe or intravenous tubing. A purse-string suture placed around the introduction site helps to prevent leakage. To test the system for patency and to document complete return of instilled fluid, an appropriate instillation volume is 20 ml/kg.

Soft, multihole peritoneal dialysis catheters, which are placed over a large, solid, sharp trocar, are available. The pediatric sizes differ from adult sizes only in that the distance provided for drainage holes at the distal tip is approximately 4 cm for the pediatric size and 8 cm for the adult sizes. Care must be taken in the choice of catheter to ensure that all the side holes will be inside the abdominal cavity. The preferred site is in the midline approximately 2 cm below the umbilicus. Strict aseptic technique should be employed. The site is anesthetized with 1% lidocaine. The catheter-trocar combination is forcibly pushed with a rotary motion perpendicular to the abdominal wall. A small incision made beforehand with a No. 11 scalpel blade through the skin and immediate subcutaneous tissue will help placement. Care must be taken to avoid deep penetration after the peritoneum is entered. The trocar is then directed toward the left peritoneal gutter, the catheter advanced slowly, and the trocar removed. Minimal resistance should be encountered. The catheter is then secured with a purse-string suture and dressed appropriately. A Styrofoam cup can be used to hold the catheter upright over the patient's abdomen. This secures the position of the catheter and improves patient comfort.

Thoracentesis. Thoracentesis is used to remove pleural fluid for diagnosis; the technique also can be used for the emergency relief of tension pneumothorax. The site is determined by roentgenogram and by the findings on physical examination. When fluid is removed from the bases of the lungs, care must be taken that abdominal viscera are not damaged. Anteroposterior, supine, and lateral radiographs should be inspected to determine if the fluid is loculated.

The positioning of the patient depends on whether the anterior or posterior aspect of the chest is to be entered. The patient should be sitting and leaning forward either against the back of a chair, while sitting, or against a bed stand when in bed. An infant or a small toddler may be held in a hugging fashion against an assistant's chest.

The needle is inserted in the anterior, middle, or posterior axillary line in the fourth, fifth, or sixth intercostal space. Other sites may be elected, as dictated by the location of specific loculated collections of fluid.

A wide site is prepared with an appropriate antiseptic, and local anesthetic is infiltrated with a 25-gauge needle over the body of the rib just below the intended puncture site. The needle is inserted in the skin overlying the rib and then moved over the surface of the rib upward to the interspace, while gentle aspiration is alternated with infiltration of the anesthetic solution so that the subcutaneous tissues and the pleura are anesthetized. The intercostal blood vessels and nerves lie along the inferior margin of each rib and therefore can be avoided by means of this approach.

The complications of thoracentesis include pneumothorax, hemothorax, and the introduction of infection. Laceration of the abdominal viscera through the diaphragm can be avoided by careful selection of the puncture site. An 18- to 22-gauge catheter needle combination, such as is used for venous access, a sterile 50-ml syringe, and a three-way stopcock can be used. The stylet, needle, and catheter are advanced along the previously described tract, with suction applied to the syringe. When the pleura is entered, the plastic cannula is threaded over the needle-stylet and advanced. The three-way stopcock is attached to syringe and cannula, and fluid is aspirated and placed in appropriate containers for fungal, viral, and bacteriologic cultures and Gram staining. Pleural fluid also may be examined for its white blood cell and differential counts, its protein, glucose, and LDH levels, and its cytology.

An alternative to tube thoracostomy for long-term drainage of effusions is placement of a pigtail catheter by use of a modified Seldinger technique. An 8.5-Fr, 15-cm polyurethane tube is placed over a 0.035-inch guide wire.* A kit is supplied that contains the pigtail catheter, an 8.0-Fr dilator, a needle, a guide wire, and a "Christmas tree" adapter that Luer locks to the catheter and can be firmly attached to large-bore rubber tubing for continuous suction.

The tube is inserted by advancing the needle over the superior margin of a rib, usually T4 to T6, in the midline or anterior axillary line, into the pleural space. A guide wire is advanced through the needle into the pleural cavity. A small stab wound, 2 to 4 mm in diameter, is made at the site where the guide wire enters the skin. An 8-Fr, hard, polyurethane dilator is advanced over the wire. This enlarges the tract to facilitate the passage of the catheter. With the wire position fixed, the dilator is withdrawn. The pigtail catheter is then threaded over the wire and advanced into the pleural space; then the wire is withdrawn. The pigtail catheter finally is attached to large-bore rubber tubing with the Christmas tree adapter placed on the appropriate suction device. The pressure in the suction device should be set at 15 to 20 cm H_2O. A chest radiograph should be taken to document the catheter's position. The pigtail catheter can be secured to the chest with a small adhesive dressing and/or simply sutured and tied in place. This technique is rapid, simple, complication-free, and easy to teach; it also is especially valuable to transport and emergency room teams for treatment of pneumothorax.

Pericardiocentesis. Pericardiocentesis is a high-risk procedure. Its dangers must be weighed against the urgency of diagnosing a pericardial effusion or an unchecked cardiac tamponade.

Myocardial injury, laceration of a coronary artery, cardiac arrhythmia, and infection are possible complications of pericardiocentesis. The internal mammary arteries are within 2.5 cm of the sternal border, and they also may be damaged.

The alternate points of entry into the chest are illustrated in Fig. B-11. The best site is at the chondroxiphoid angle. The others are in the fourth, fifth, and sixth intercostal spaces, 1 to 2 cm medial to the border of percussable cardiac dullness. Roentgenogram, fluoroscopy, and ultrasound examination also may aid in determining the border of the pericardium.

The patient, who may require sedation, should be supine at approximately a 30-degree angle and carefully restrained. A wide area of the precordium is prepared with an appropriate antiseptic. The chosen site is infiltrated with lidocaine. A 50-ml syringe is then connected to a three-way stopcock and an 18-gauge needle. An electrocardiogram (ECG) V lead, with an alligator clip, is attached to the needle to detect an injury current, should the myocardium or coronary artery be entered.

The needle is directed inward and medially when the intercostal approach is used. When the chondroxiphoid approach is used, the needle is aimed upward and posteriorly.

Gentle negative pressure should be applied to the syringe. The ECG should be monitored constantly and the needle withdrawn if an injury current is detected. The fluid should be aspirated slowly. The needle is then withdrawn, and a simple sterile dressing is applied over the puncture site.

Bone Marrow Aspiration. Bone marrow samples aid in the diagnosis of leukemia, metastatic disease, and several of the "storage" diseases, such as the lipidoses. Culture of the bone marrow occasionally is indicated in cases of suspected sepsis. Bone marrow aspiration has few risks; infection is the greatest. It usually is performed safely in those with thrombocytopenia.

The preferred site is the posterior iliac crest because it is easy to locate, the patient can be easily restrained for its performance, and the site contains active marrow in patients of all ages. Other sites include the tibia, femur, sternum, spinous vertebral process, and anterior iliac crest. The tibia is most useful in children who are younger than 18 months

*Cook, Inc., Elletsville, Ind.

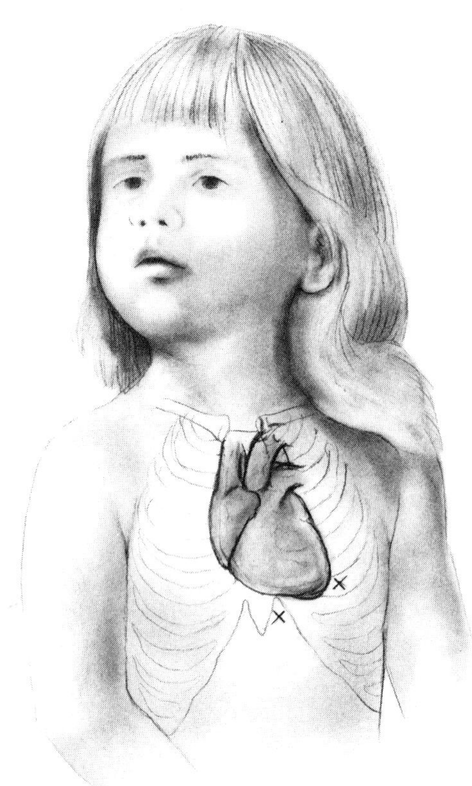

Fig. B-11 Pericardiocentesis. Two sites for aspiration of the pericardial sac. These vary with the extent of the effusion, as determined by examination, contrast study, and/or echocardiography.

of age. The femur also is a useful site in this age-group, but overlying muscle tissue makes the procedure more difficult. The sternum is the least safe site for children. The spinous vertebral process requires exceptional restraint of the patient and is, in general, a technically difficult site to use.

The needle used is a commercially available bone marrow needle and obturator.

The technique for using the posterior iliac crest is described here. The child is restrained in the prone position with a blanket roll or pillow placed under the hips. The use of sedation is effective. The site is scrubbed broadly with antiseptic. The iliac crest is palpable as a bony prominence lateral to the midline above the level of the gluteal cleft.

The site of aspiration is located approximately 1 cm below the lip of the crest. The overlying skin and subcutaneous tissues are infiltrated with local anesthetic down to the periosteum. The aspiration needle with its obturator is then pushed through the skin, angled toward the patient's head, and advanced to the periosteum. A steady, screwdriver-like rotation of the needle with applied pressure forces the needle into the marrow. A decrease in resistance may be felt as the bone's cortex is perforated. The obturator is then removed, and a 20-ml sterile syringe is attached to its hub. Firm and rapidly applied negative pressure will cause a few drops of blood to spurt into the syringe. Negative pressure should be terminated immediately to avoid dilution of the marrow specimen with peripheral blood. No more than 1 ml of bone marrow should be aspirated. The syringe is then carefully removed from the needle, and 6 to 10 meticulously cleaned slides are smeared. The obturator is then reinserted, the needle removed, and a sterile dressing applied over the puncture site.

EMERGENCY THERAPEUTIC PROCEDURES

Emergency Intravenous Access Protocol

Significant delay commonly is encountered in the establishment of intravenous access in the critically ill child. The small size of the pediatric patient, the stress of the situation, and venous collapse make the insertion of a peripheral intravenous device difficult. An algorithmic, protocol approach to the problem of establishing venous access has been suggested.[1] In one series of pediatric resuscitations, more than 10 minutes was required to establish venous access, and in 6% of the subjects no access could be established.[2] In one algorithm suggested for use in cardiopulmonary resuscitation, attempts at peripheral vein insertion would be made for 1½ minutes. If this attempt failed, saphenous vein cutdown or, depending on the available expertise, a femoral vein catheter placement would be attempted. Resuscitation drugs would be administered, when needed, through the endotracheal tube. If after 5 minutes access could not be obtained elsewhere, an interosseous needle would be placed.

Physicians who might encounter critically ill children should consider the development of such venous access protocols and algorithms. These should be tailored to the needs of the institution or site and to those of the practitioner.

INFUSIONS

Percutaneous Intravenous Infusion

Fig. B-2 depicts the location of accessible superficial veins suitable for percutaneous intravenous infusions. The veins of the extremities and scalp are commonly used; the latter have no valves and can be punctured in either direction. Skin preparation should be especially meticulous when scalp veins are used because they communicate by means of emissary veins with the dural sinuses.

The child is positioned and immobilized, and the extremity is immobilized further by being taped firmly to a padded board or sandbag. A tourniquet is applied above the vein to be infused, and the skin is cleansed with alcohol. A butterfly 22- or 25-gauge needle or a 20- or 22-gauge intravenous catheter needle (Longdwel or Medicut) filled with saline and attached to the intravenous tubing and solution bottle is used to enter the vein in the direction of venous flow. When the vein is entered, the tourniquet is removed, and the blood flow is tested by opening the intravenous tubing to allow the solution to be infused to flow or by gently injecting saline through the needle with a syringe.

If the flow is adequate and there is no extravasation of fluid, a piece of tape is placed over the entry site and the wings of the butterfly needle are taped to the skin. A pad may be used under the hub of the needle to maintain the angle that best allows free flow of fluid. A protective cover is taped over the needle, and the adequacy of the retraints is checked (Fig. B-12). If percutaneous needle catheterization is per-

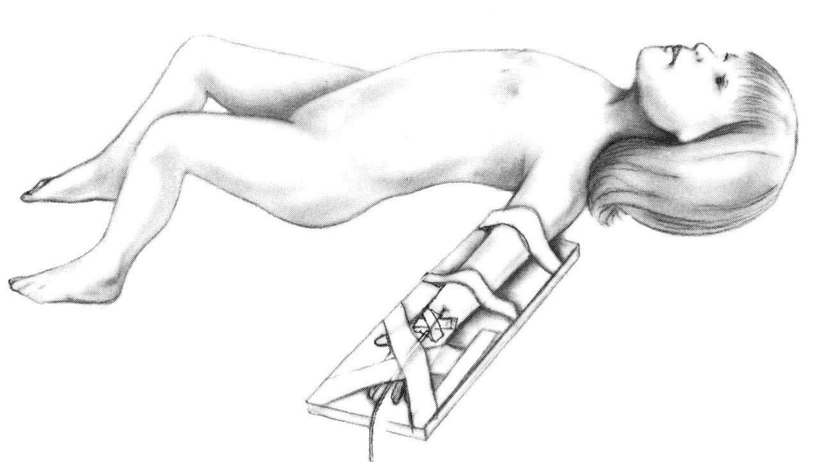

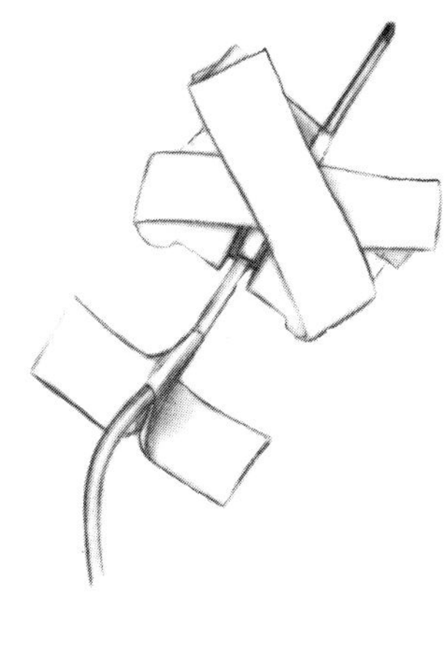

Fig. B-12 Immobilization of the upper extremity for intravenous infusion and method of securing the needle and tubing with tape.

formed, the vein is entered as described above. When blood is seen in the hub of the needle, it is stabilized and the catheter sleeve is advanced up the vein. The catheter is then stabilized, the needle removed, and the blood flow checked before the catheter hub is taped in position and the intravenous tubing attached.

Cutdown Intravenous Infusion

A *cutdown* intravenous infusion may be required in an emergency when rapid fluid and drug administration is needed and a vein cannot be entered percutaneously. The possible sites are, in order of preference, the great saphenous vein at the ankle, the anterior cubital veins, the external jugular vein, the saphenous vein in the femoral triangle, and the femoral vein.

The great saphenous vein is preferred because its position is constant, anterior to the medial malleolus running cephalad, so it may be found even when not visible through the skin. The child is positioned and the limb restrained on a padded board, as for a percutaneous infusion. A tourniquet is applied in the midcalf region, and surgical aseptic technique is observed. Local anesthesia is produced by infiltration of the skin over the site of the incision with 1% lidocaine. A transverse incision, 2 to 3 cm, should be made 1 cm superior and anterior to the medial malleolus, and the skin and superficial fascia should be widely spread. Blunt dissection is used to isolate and identify the vein (Fig. B-13). A curved hemostat is used to scoop the vein off the periosteum and up into the wound. The vein should be freed from connective tissue for 1 to 2 cm along its length by blunt dissection and two No. 000 silk ligatures passed under it. The distal ligature is used to tie off the lower portion of vein and to provide caudal traction on the vein.

An intravenous catheter needle may be used to enter the vein, as described in the section on percutaneous intravenous infusion, or a small nick may be made in the vein and an intravenous cannula threaded cephalad for 2 to 5 cm. The proximal ligature is then firmly tied around the vein and cannula. The wound is closed with fine silk sutures, one of which should be tied around the catheter to anchor it. The wound is dressed with a gauze bandage and cleansed daily. The catheter is removed by pulling it out through the wound and applying local pressure. The wound sutures should be removed 3 to 4 days after they are placed.

An intravenous catheter needle or a plastic indwelling catheter may be converted to *heparin lock* for intermittent administration of medications or drawing of blood samples.

Heparin Lock

Heparin in normal saline solution is used to flush and fill the needle and tubing or the catheter. A concentration of 10 units of heparin per milliliter will avert heparinization of the patient, but it will still prevent clotting within the needle or catheter; an adapter (which has a rubber diaphragm attached for repeated intermittent injections, infusions, or blood drawing, yet protects the needle or catheter orifice from contamination) is attached to the hub of the indwelling needle or catheter. Prolonged use of any indwelling device carries the risk of local and disseminated infection. Care must be taken to sterilize the adapter port with iodophor solution before each use. When the device is used, 1 to 2 ml of blood should be aspirated before sampling to avoid contamination with heparin and the indwelling fluid. Only the volume of the device should be filled with the heparinized saline. The saline should be changed every 12 hours.

Intraosseous Infusions

Intraosseous infusion is a procedure that should be familiar to all who provide care to children. This easily learned technique can be employed in any critically ill child whenever a delay in establishing venous access might compromise the patient. In many situations, venous access is time-consuming. A surgeon, intensivist, or anesthesiologist must be brought in to establish a central venous catheter by guide wire or to perform a cutdown. These actions can cause needless delay in treatment. The ability to place an intraosseous needle allows even a technically inexperienced person to gain immediate access to the intramedullary venous system, which is continuous with the venous circulation (Fig. B-14). Crystalloid and colloid for fluid resuscitation, blood, plasma, cat-

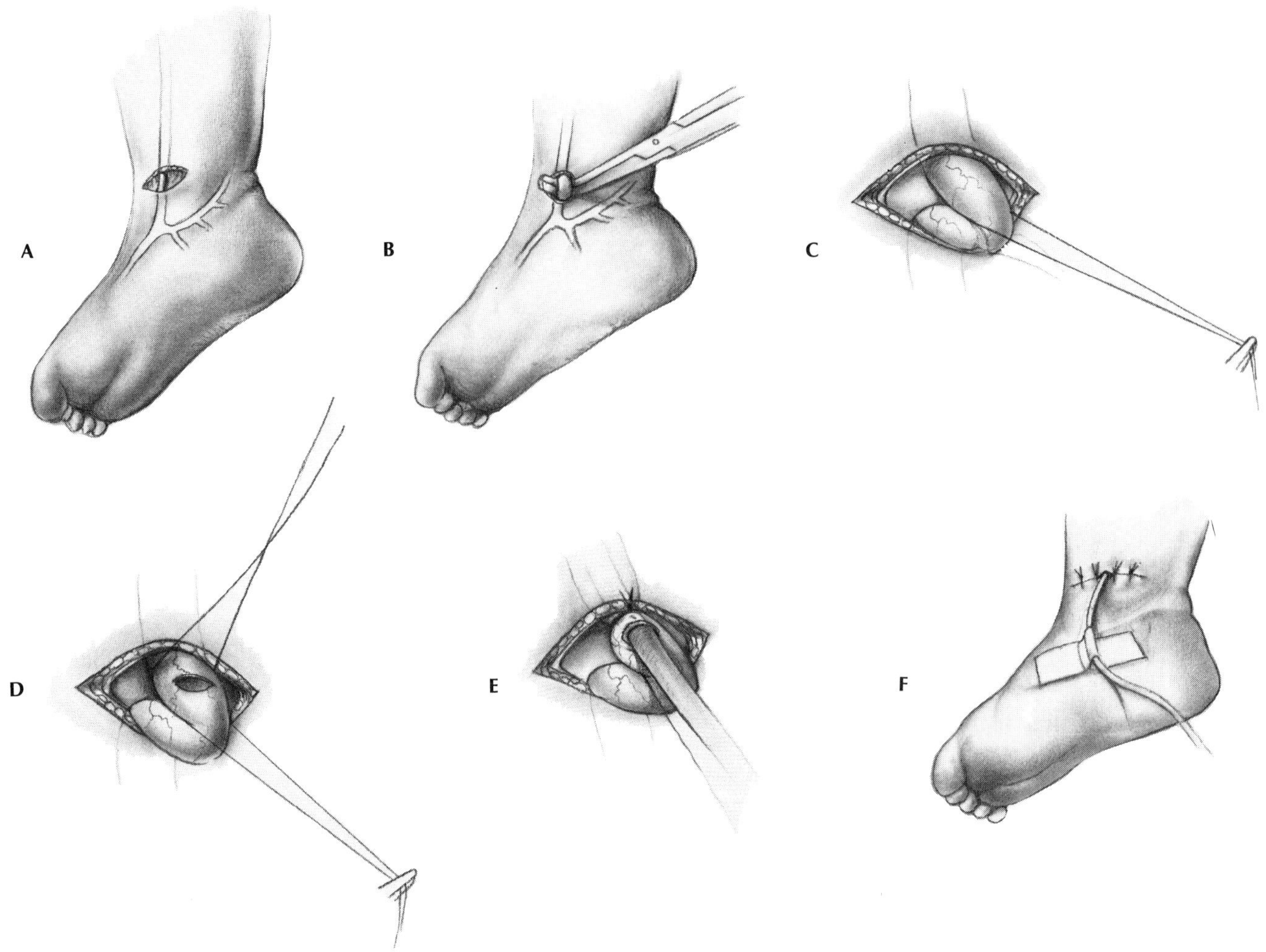

Fig. B-13 Procedure for cutdown of the great saphenous vein. **A,** Site of incision anterior to the medial malleolus. **B,** Elevation of the vein into the wound with a curved clamp. **C,** Application of distal ligature for traction. **D,** Loosely placed proximal ligature and venostomy incision. **E,** Venous catheter tied in place. **F,** Wound sutured and catheter secured.

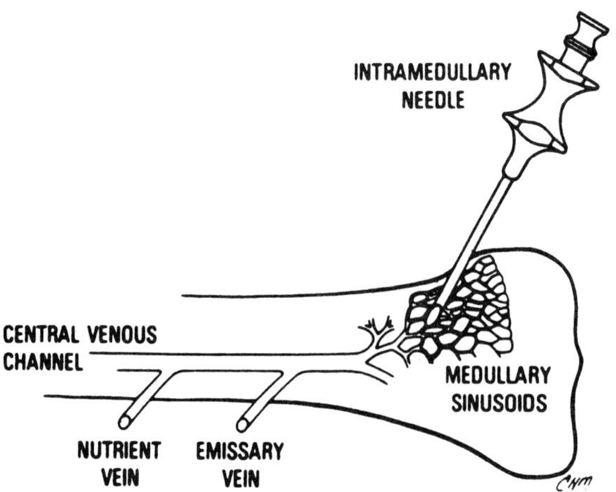

Fig. B-14 The intramedullary venous system demonstrates position of intraosseous needle in the medullary sinusoids. Blood may be aspirated from the sinusoids to confirm position of the needle.
From Spivey WH: Intraosseous Infusions, J Pediatr 5:111, 1987.

echolamines such as epinephrine and dopamine, glucose, calcium, and sodium bicarbonate can all be administered by the intraosseous technique. Although a standard 18- or 20-gauge spinal needle with stylet is ordinarily available, this is somewhat fragile, and although a bone marrow biopsy needle is useful, intraosseous needles, manufactured specifically for this purpose, are now available and are preferred. The proximal and distal tibia are the sites of choice. The iliac crest, sternum, and femur are alternate sites. The anterior medial surface of the proximal tibia or the medial surface of the distal tibia proximal to the medial malleolus are preferred sites (Figs. B-15 and B-16). The epiphysis must be avoided when the proximal tibia is used. The cortex in the midshaft of the tibia is difficult to penetrate, although this is sometimes used in emergencies. In a child older than 6 years of age the thick cortex at the proximal tibia prevents easy use of this site; the distal tibia is recommended in this instance. The site is aseptically prepared. Then the needle is advanced perpendicular to the bone, with firm pressure and rotary motion. Entry to the marrow cavity is detected by decreasing resistance. As-

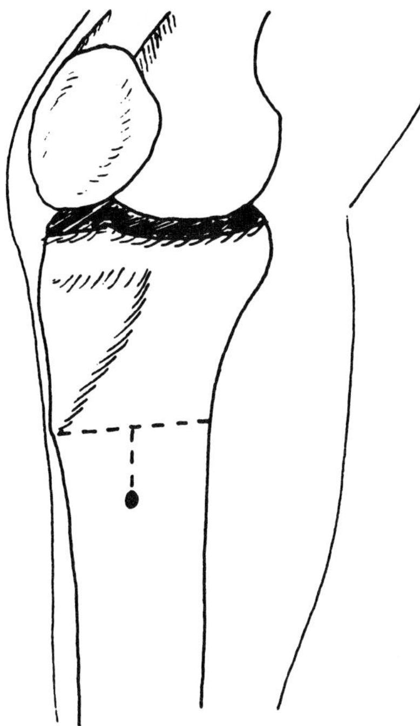

Fig. B-15 Insertion site in the proximal tibia. The tibial tuberosity and medial border of the tibia are palpated. Halfway between these points and 1 or 2 cm distally, the needle is inserted pointing away from the joint space, in a caudal direction.

From Spivey WH: Intraosseous Infusions, J Pediatr 5:111, 1987.

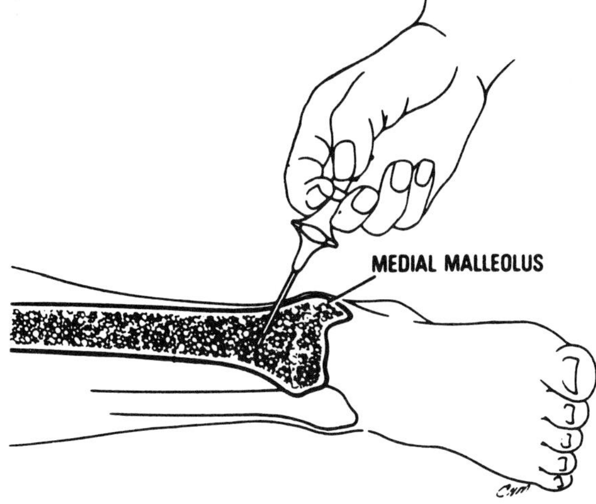

Fig. B-16 The position of an intraosseous needle in the distal tibia. The needle is inserted in the medial surface of the distal tibia at the junction of the malleolus and shaft of the tibia. It is inserted away from the joint space, in a cephalad direction.

From Spivey WH: Intraosseous Infusions, J Pediatr 5:111, 1987.

piration with a syringe should produce blood and marrow. To clear the needle, it should be flushed with 3 to 5 ml of sterile saline in a sterile syringe. The device is now connected to standard intravenous tubing. Although the flow rate will be slower than that observed in a standard device, it should be steady, with no evidence of extravasation at the site. If the needle dislodges or fluid extravasates, the opposite leg should be used. If large volumes are required, two devices should be placed. A second device should not be placed on the same leg after removal of the first device, because leakage will occur. Resuscitative drugs should be "flushed" in after 3 to 5 ml of saline have been injected.

Femoral Venous Cannulation

The femoral vein is a safe, easily accessible vessel for cannulation with a single- or multiple-lumen catheter. The femoral catheter is safe to use for a short time—less than 24 hours—but with reasonable care it can be used for long-term access as well. The consistent anatomy of the area and proximity to the femoral arterial pulse allow the vessel to be easily located, because it lies 1 to 2 cm medial to the artery and 2 to 4 cm below the inguinal ligament. A transcutaneous Doppler device with a hand-held probe and ear phones can help locate the artery when the pulse is difficult to palpate.* When the femoral arterial pulse cannot be located because of obesity or hypotension, as is the case in cardiac arrest, the femoral artery can easily be confused with the vein and inadvertently catheterized. In severe cardiorespiratory embarrassment the color of aspirated blood and blood gas tensions may confuse the operator and prevent discrimination of artery from vein.

Placement is simple and easily learned. The patient should be supine and in four-point restraints. The groin area should be widely prepared with an appropriate antiseptic agent. In young children, placement of a Foley catheter in the bladder will prevent urine from contaminating the site. The femoral artery is palpated 2 to 4 cm below the inguinal ligament, and the vein is 1 to 2 cm medial to the artery. The skin and immediate subcutaneous tissues are infiltrated with 1% lidocaine. Manufacturer-supplied kits that contain an introducer needle, dilator, guide wire, and catheter are available.* The appropriate-size catheter has an outer diameter of 3 to 4 Fr for patients younger than 1 year of age, 5 to 6 Fr to age 7 years, and 7-Fr for children 8 years and older. A syringe that contains 2 to 3 ml of heparinized saline is attached to the introducer needle. The needle is introduced at a 30- to 45-degree angle from horizontal and aimed at the umbilicus. Care should be taken to avoid advancing the needle beyond the inguinal ligament because the peritoneum, bowel, and bladder can be perforated. With continuous gentle aspiration the needle is advanced into the vein. When good blood return is documented, the syringe is removed. The guide wire is then advanced into the vein. There should be minimal resistance to the passage of the wire. If resistance is encountered, the needle and wire must be removed simultaneously to avoid shearing the wire off in the patient's vein. The needle is then withdrawn, leaving the wire in place. An incision, 2 to 4 mm, is made with a scalpel where the guide wire enters the skin. A dilator is now threaded over the wire and passed through skin and subcutaneous tissue into the vessel, then withdrawn, again leaving the wire in place. The catheter is then threaded over the wire. Care must be taken to ensure that at least 1 to 2 cm of the guide wire extends from the proximal end of the catheter before it is threaded into the vein. Otherwise the wire can be "lost" in the vessel. The physician, using caution not to change the position of the wire, slowly advances the catheter over the wire to the desired distance, then removes the wire. For central venous pressure

*Parks Electronics Laboratory, Beaverton, Ore.

*Cook, Inc., Elletsville, Ind.; Arrow International, Inc, Reading, Penn.

measurement the catheter tip should be placed just above the diaphragm. The position should be verified by radiograph. The catheter is then sutured in place.

Complications include bleeding, infection, inadequate venous drainage, thrombus formation, and inadvertent penetration of viscera or vessel wall. These must be weighed against the benefits of obtaining secure, large-bore venous access and needing to determine the central venous pressure.

Subclavian Vein Catheter Placement

The subclavian vein is a readily accessible site that provides a secure central conduit for (1) fluid administration (including hypertonic or irritating solutions that cannot be infused into peripheral veins), (2) maintenance of cardiac output by direct infusions of pressor drugs, and (3) central venous pressure monitoring.

The procedure incurs the risk of pneumothorax or accidental penetration of the subclavian artery, with hematoma formation or thrombosis-induced obstruction of venous return. The operator should first be familiar with the use of the Seldinger technique for percutaneous placement of a catheter over a guide wire placed through an introducer needle.

Catheterization kits* provide a guide wire, catheters, and an introducer needle. The following sizes of catheters are used: 3 Fr in infants, 4 Fr in toddlers, 5 Fr in children 4 to 12 years of age, and 7 Fr for adolescents. The right subclavian vein is preferred over the left because of its more direct entry to the superior vena cava and because there is less risk of pneumothorax (the right lung lies lower in the thorax than the left) and injury to the thoracic duct, which lies in the left hemithorax.

The patient is placed in the Trendelenburg position and is restrained. The child's face is turned 90 degrees away from the intended puncture site. A 3-inch thick towel roll is placed along the long axis of the thoracic spine between the shoulder blades.

The area overlying the puncture site is cleansed widely, and drapes are employed to provide an aseptic field. Masks, gloves, and gowns are used.

The subclavian vein is cannulated by means of the infraclavicular approach. The vein lies approximately parallel to the proximal third of the clavicle and is accessed in a triangle bounded by the medial third of the clavicle, the anterior scalene muscle, and the upper surface of the first rib. The subclavian artery runs posterior to the vein behind the anterior scalene muscle. Through a 1½-inch, 22-gauge needle, the skin overlying the puncture site and intended insertion tract is infiltrated with 1% lidocaine.

The introducer needle is placed just medial to the midclavicular line 2 to 3 cm below the inferior border of the clavicle. The needle is aimed toward the midsternal notch and is advanced to the inferior border of the medial portion of the clavicle. A syringe containing a few milliliters of heparinized saline is attached to the introducer needle, and with negative pressure applied to the barrel of the syringe, the needle is advanced deep to the clavicle on a course nearly parallel to its medial portion. Small cephalad adjustments of the target point (approximately 0.25 cm increments) can be employed if the vein is not immediately entered.

*Available from Cook, Inc., Elletsville, Ind; Arrow International, Inc., Reading, Penn.

When the vein is entered, as evidenced by blood entering the syringe, the hub of the introducer needle is held securely in place by the physician, and the syringe is removed.

Caution must be exercised in a spontaneously breathing patient because air may be introduced into the vein as the patient increases the negative pleural pressure when initiating a breath. Therefore the patient must be instructed to hold his or her breath, or, as with infants and children, the orifice of the needle must be occluded temporarily. The flexible floppy end of the guide wire is now inserted into the introducer needle and advanced through the bore of the needle into the subclavian vein and beyond into the superior vena cava. A minimum of 3 cm of wire length is passed beyond the estimated tip of the needle. A cardiac arrhythmia may signal that the guide wire has been passed too far into the right ventricle, in which case it should be drawn back a bit. The distal end of the wire is now held securely, and the introducer needle is removed.

The catheter is flushed with heparin solution and advanced over the guide wire to the desired position in the superior vena cava; care should be taken not to advance the wire simultaneously. The guide wire is now removed, and the proximal end of the catheter is attached to the desired intravenous fluid–administration system or the central venous pressure–monitoring system.

The position of the catheter should be verified radiographically. The catheter must be placed so that the distal tip is in the middle third of the superior vena cava. This helps to avoid the complications of vessel or atrium perforation.

Umbilical Vein Catheterization

Catheterization of the umbilical vein is useful in newborns for emergency correction of acidosis, hypoglycemia, and hypotension, in the performance of exchange transfusions, and for the measurement of central venous pressure. The complications of umbilical vein catheterization include sepsis and microembolization from catheter-induced thrombosis. An umbilical venous catheter can easily be misplaced into a branch of the portal venous system, and the injection of hyperosmolar solutions containing substances such as glucose and sodium bicarbonate can lead to portal vein thrombosis and hepatic necrosis. Umbilical vein catheters also have been implicated in cases of necrotizing enterocolitis and spontaneous perforation of the large bowel.

A radiopaque catheter must be used in umbilical vein catheterization to allow for verification of its position by roentgenogram. The small premature infant is susceptible to chilling during the catheterization procedure, and the use of a radiant warmer, an Isolette, or a heating blanket is necessary. The equipment found on a cutdown tray, with the addition of fine-toothed pickup forceps, is adequate. The catheter size is selected on the basis of the weight of the baby: a 3.5-Fr catheter should be used for infants weighing less than 1500 g and a 5-Fr catheter for those weighing more. Special attention to aseptic techniques, including surgical scrubbing of the operator's hands, antiseptic preparation of the baby's abdomen and umbilical cord, and maintenance of a sterile field, is essential. The physician should be gloved, masked, and gowned as for any surgical procedure.

The length that the catheter is to be inserted should be

determined by measuring the distance from the infant's shoulder to the umbilicus by the conversion method shown in Fig. B-17. This length ideally will place the catheter at the junction of the inferior vena cava and the right atrium. Care must be taken not to cover the infant's chest in such a manner that apnea or malfunction of the heat probes or monitor leads will go undetected. An assistant now provides gentle traction to the cord stump while the physician transects the cord with a scalpel 1 to 1.5 cm above the skin. Gauze sponges should be available for tamponade to control oozing of blood from the umbilical vein; the amount of oozing usually is insignificant. The cord stump is inspected to locate the thin-walled umbilical vein and the two thick-walled umbilical arteries. The catheter is attached to a three-way stopcock and a syringe containing heparinized saline solution (1 unit of heparin per milliliter of saline), and the catheter is filled. Minimal traction on the superior edge of the cord stump may be helpful in locating the orifice of the umbilical vein; this is gently dilated with pickup forceps or a small probe, and the catheter is introduced the predetermined distance (Fig. B-18). Resistance occasionally is met at the level of the abdominal wall or at the level of the ductus venosus. Very gentle pressure and partial withdrawal and rotation of the catheter usually will overcome this resistance. Force should not be used. The position of the catheter should be verified by roentgenogram except under emergency circumstances.

Care must be taken to avoid iatrogenic blood loss through accidental dislodgment of the catheter. A purse-string suture around the umbilical stump and careful taping of the catheter to the abdominal wall will help to avoid this. Antibiotic ointment and a dressing that will show any significant blood loss from the stump should be applied lightly over the umbilicus after successful catheterization. Current practice discourages keeping umbilical vein catheters in place for long periods of time; however, if neonatal transport requires fixation of the catheter, this can be accomplished with a purse-string suture, a bridge of adhesive tape (Fig. B-18), or umbilical cord tape. Fortunately, these are rarely needed for hemostasis alone. Application of an antibiotic ointment and daily inspection of the umbilical vein and stump for signs of local infection should follow the removal of the catheter.

Umbilical Artery Catheterization

Catheterization of the umbilical artery is accomplished in a manner similar to catheterization of the umbilical vein, and the equipment used is the same. Its purpose is to provide access to the arterial circulation for monitoring blood pressure and blood gases and for infusion of selected solutions. Even in skilled hands the procedure carries risks of embolization, sepsis, extravasation of blood, and distal arterial insufficiency. These complications must be considered in any determination of the risk/benefit ratio before performance of the procedure. Samples from the radial and temporal arteries are of preductal arterial blood and for single-measurement purposes are safer and more precise than is umbilical artery catheterization. Catheter placement at the point of bifurcation of the aorta is desirable to avoid damage to the renal arteries. The shoulder-umbilical length is measured, and the distance to the bifurcation of the aorta is determined by the conversion method shown in Fig. B-17.

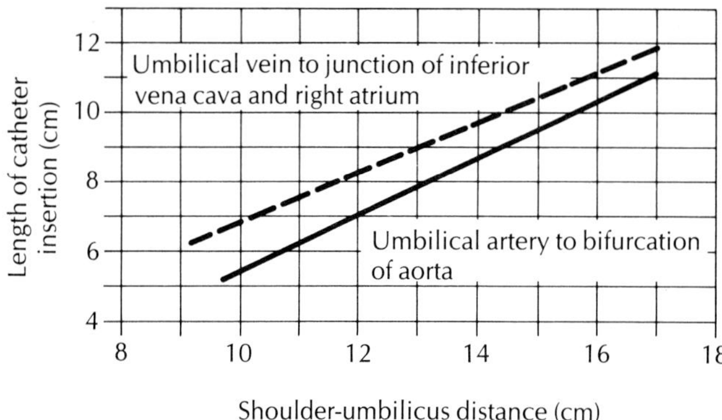

Fig. B-17 Method for determining the optimal length for umbilical catheter insertion.

Attention to aseptic techniques is essential. The heavy-walled artery may be dilated gently. A rim of vessel wall is gently picked up with fine-toothed forceps. The catheter, filled with heparinized saline and attached to a closed three-way stopcock, is then introduced into the artery. Advancement of the catheter may be hindered by vasospasm; this can be overcome by applying slow, gentle pressure. Forceful probing should be avoided. If the catheter cannot be advanced, the other umbilical artery should be used. If resistance is again encountered and gentle pressure fails to advance the catheter, 0.1 to 0.2 ml of 1% or 2% lidocaine, without epinephrine, is instilled into the lumen of the artery. After 2 or 3 minutes the catheter can be more easily advanced.

The position of the catheter at the bifurcation of the aorta should be verified by roentgenogram. The catheter must be carefully fixed to the cord stump with a purse-string suture and to the abdomen with adhesive tape. An antibiotic ointment and a sterile dressing should be applied lightly, so as not to obscure blood loss, and the dressing should be changed daily.

The danger of iatrogenic accidents must be emphasized. Dislodgment of the catheters, stopcock leakage, and inadequate tamponade on removal of the catheter may produce significant blood loss. Failure to record and replace blood removed from the catheter may result in anemia and a deficit of fluid. Catheter removal is indicated when signs of ischemia of the lower extremities are present.

Exchange Transfusion

The indications for exchange transfusion are discussed in Chapter 40. Prepackaged exchange transfusion sets with appropriate four-way stopcocks are commercially available. The operator must take time to become familiar with the function of the stopcock. If two standard stopcocks are used, rather than the four-way, extra care must be taken to prevent accidents.

The equipment needed includes material for an umbilical catheterization, a source of heat (preferably an overhead radiant warmer), surgical drapes, gown, cap, mask, monitors for pulse and respiration, blood matched to infant and mother, resuscitation equipment, and 5 to 10 ml of 10% calcium gluconate solution.

The blood should be warmed with a blood warmer. Contrived hot water baths may cause lysis of red cells and are a potential danger.

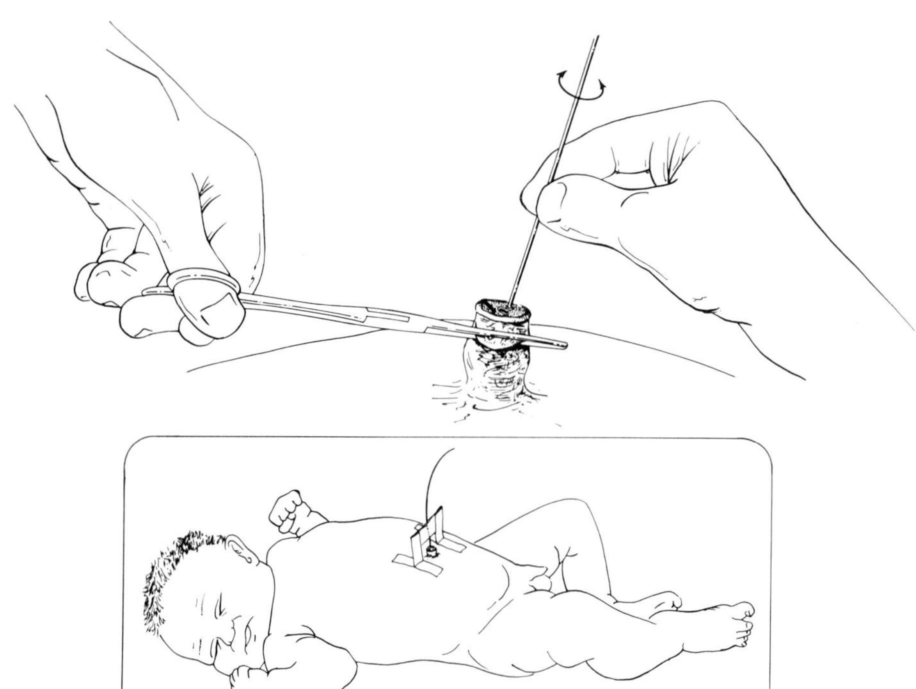

Fig. B-18 Umbilical vessel cannulation. The hemostat is used to grasp the edge of the cord stump, which is then rolled toward the operator to provide visualization and stability. A probe is shown in the operator's right hand. Gentle pressure and a rolling motion are employed to dilate the orifice of the vessel. The lower portion of the figure shows a method of taping that will fix the position of the umbilical catheter, preventing its deeper penetration or dislodgment. A light dressing can be placed over the umbilicus to guard against local infection.

Acid-citrate-dextrose, citrate-phosphate-dextrose, or heparinized preserved blood may be used. The first is adequate and usually available. A two-volume exchange should be performed. The amount of blood required is 170 ml/kg body weight, up to 500 ml. If possible, the blood bank should adjust the hematocrit of the donor blood to 55%. The hydropic infant, however, may require a very slow, careful exchange with packed red blood cells, while central venous pressure is monitored and signs of congestive heart failure are watched for.

The infant should be restrained and the stomach emptied. The umbilicus should be prepared and draped and the venous catheter inserted. Plastic tubing serves to connect the stopcock to the waste bag, the donor blood, and the umbilical vein catheter. The central venous pressure, blood pressure, pulse, and respirations are recorded throughout the procedure.

Blood is initially withdrawn from the baby and sent to the laboratory for a determination of central hematocrit, bilirubin, glucose, total protein, and serum electrolyte (sodium, chloride, carbon dioxide, calcium, potassium, and blood urea nitrogen) values.

Aliquots of 5 to 20 ml may be withdrawn and replaced, depending on the age and cardiovascular stability of the infant. A rate of 3 to 5 ml/kg/min, or 1 to 1½ minutes per aliquot withdrawn and replaced, is desirable.

An assistant is required to record the vital signs, each volume exchanged, and a running exchange total. A person skilled at resuscitation also should be available.

If acid-citrate-dextrose blood is used, 1 ml of 10% calcium gluconate should be given for every 100 ml replaced. Irritability, tachycardia, and prolongation of the QT interval on the ECG are signs of hypocalcemia. If heparinized blood is used, 0.5 mg of protamine is given intramuscularly after the procedure.

Complications of Exchange Transfusions

- Vascular
  - Embolization with air or clots
  - Thrombosis
- Cardiac
  - Arrhythmias
  - Volume overload
  - Arrest
- Electrolyte
  - Hyperkalemia
  - Hypernatremia
  - Hypocalcemia
  - Acidosis
- Hematologic
  - Overheparinization
  - Thrombocytopenia
- Infections
  - Bacteremia
  - Serum hepatitis
- Miscellaneous
  - Mechanical injury to donor cells
  - Hypothermia
  - Hypoglycemia

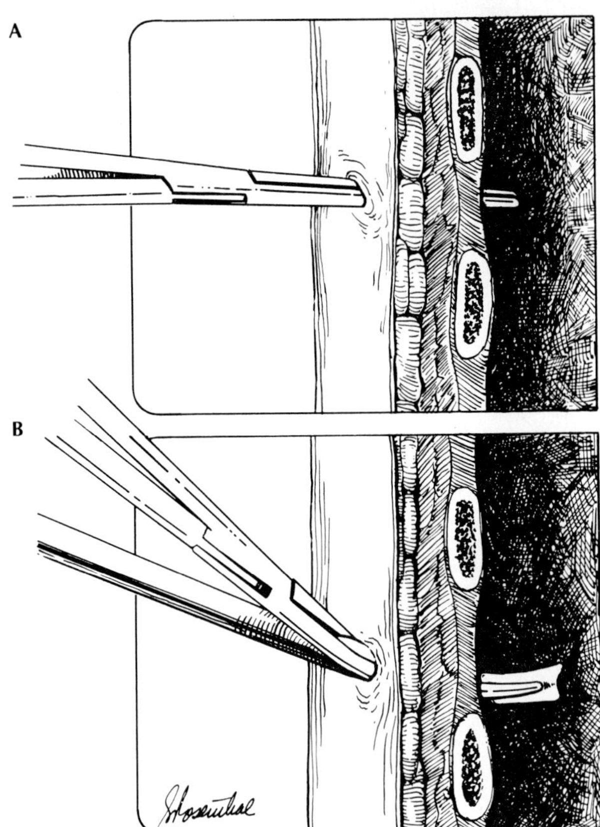

Fig. B-19 Intercostal chest tube placement. **A,** Formation of tract with hemostat. **B,** Insertion of tube with hemostat.

From Wilkins EW Jr: MGH textbook of emergency medicine, ed. 2. © 1983, the Williams & Wilkins Co., Baltimore.

The box on p. 1716 lists the potential complications of exchange transfusions.

The final aliquot of blood removed is sent to the laboratory for typing and cross-matching and for hematocrit and electrolyte determinations. The catheter is then withdrawn, and a sterile dressing is applied to the umbilicus. The infant is monitored intensively over the ensuing 4 hours for cardiovascular stability, pulse, and blood pressure. During this time the infant should receive nothing by mouth and have intravenous hydration. From 4 to 6 hours after the procedure, determinations of hematocrit, bilirubin, and calcium should be repeated.

Tube Thoracostomy

Pneumothorax is a common complication in the delivery of emergency care to infants, children, and adolescents. The placement of a thoracostomy tube (for drainage of air and fluid that has accumulated in the pleural cavity) by blunt dissection of a tract in the intercostal space with a hemostat is more tedious but safer than using a trocar, unless the operator is experienced in the latter technique. A 12-Fr catheter should be used for infants and children up to age 3 years, a 16-Fr catheter for children up to 10 years, and a 20-Fr catheter for older children and adolescents.

The fourth or fifth intercostal space in the anterior axillary line is the appropriate site. The pectoralis muscle, the nipple, and the intercostal arteries (at the inferior aspect of each rib) are to be avoided. The infant or child is placed in the supine position with the arm restrained above the head with appropriate assistance. The site is prepared and draped aseptically. Local anesthetic is infiltrated into the skin overlying the fifth or sixth rib, using a 22-gauge, 1½-inch needle. While the needle is advanced subcutaneously within the fourth or fifth intercostal space, the anesthetic is infiltrated within the soft tissues down to the level of and including the pleura.

A 2-cm skin incision over the intercostal space is made, and with blunt dissection a hemostat is introduced through the previously anesthetized tissues into the pleural cavity, as illustrated in Fig. B-19. The chest tube is then clamped in the curved jaws of the hemostat and advanced through the dissected intercostal space tract to the pleural cavity. The tube ideally should lie anterior to the lung at its apex. The lateral orifices of the catheter must be well within the pleural cavity. The tube is secured with skin sutures, one on either side of the incision, wrapped around the tube and tied tightly enough to crimp the tube slightly. A minimal dressing is applied so that malpositioning may be detected. Bulky dressings are not warranted. The dissected tract heals rapidly.

Common errors in the placement of thoracostomy tubes are their placement subcutaneously as a result of incomplete blunt dissections and dislodgment caused by inadequate securement. Bleeding and infection rarely are encountered. An alternative technique for the immediate placement of a catheter in the chest for drainage is described above in the section on pleurocentesis. This technique employs a guide wire and a pigtail catheter and is useful in emergencies and transport.

Endotracheal Intubation

It is essential for every physician who cares for children to master endotracheal intubation. Several hazards commonly accompany this process; they are listed in the box below.

The key to success in intubation is approaching the procedure in a calm, deliberate way with a much-practiced technique and with equipment that is readily available and properly prepared. The equipment required for intubation is listed in the box on p. 1718. A well-organized emergency tray, which is checked daily, is one of the most important items needed to perform this emergency procedure.

Hazards of Intubation

- Hyperextension or hyperflexion of the neck
- Failure to clear the oropharynx of secretions
- Failure to ventilate the patient manually with mask oxygen before and after unsuccessful attempts
- Prolonged attempts, lasting longer than 30 seconds
- Intubation of the esophagus
- Intubation of the right main stem bronchus
- Faulty or unavailable equipment
- Haste

Preparation of the Patient. Protection of the airway and adequate oxygenation guarantee safe and successful intubations. Intubation always should be accompanied by the administration of atropine, 0.01 to 0.02 mg/kg, with a maximum dose of 1 mg. The use of a muscle relaxant to reduce respiratory effort may be indicated. When employed, it should be accompanied by sedation. Succinylcholine (1 mg/kg given intravenously) is preferred as a muscle relaxant because it is rapidly metabolized. It also can be given intramuscularly (2 mg/kg) but only if the intravenous route cannot be used.

Methohexital (Brevital) may be given as a light anesthetic during intubation (1 to 2 mg/kg intravenously), but it should be used with caution in patients with compromised cardiovascular systems secondary to shock or cyanotic congenital heart disease.

Technique of Intubation. During intubation, care must be taken to avoid damaging the teeth with the laryngoscope blade. A straight laryngoscope blade should be used; Portex or Murphy tubes are recommended because they are uniform in diameter, biologically nonreactive, and less likely to traumatize the vocal cords than are rubber tubes or the narrow-lumen Cole tubes. A slight air leak is to be expected with a tube of appropriate size. The recommended sizes according to patient weight and age are shown in Table B-1.

Fig. B-20 illustrates the relationship of the laryngoscope blade to the epiglottis and the vocal cords. The endotracheal tube ideally should be positioned midway between the vocal cords and the carina. The patient should be placed on a firm surface with head and neck in the so-called flower-sniffing

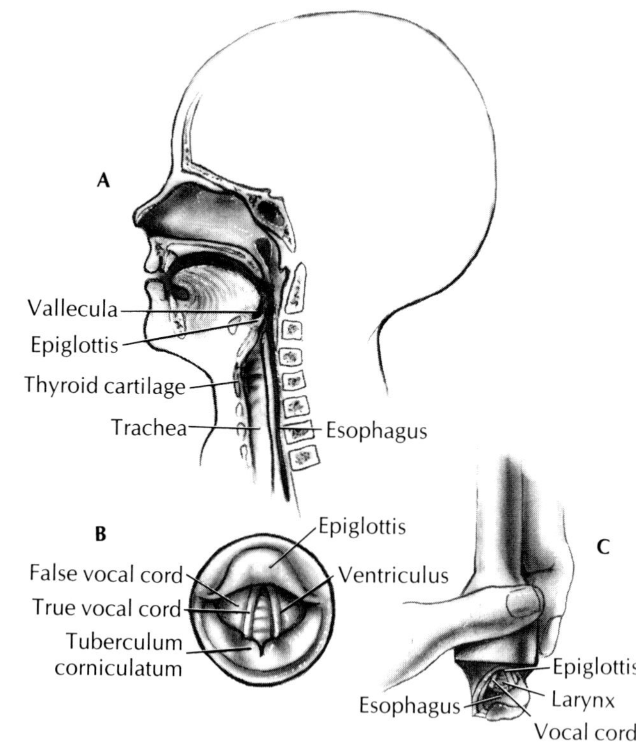

Fig. B-20 Endotracheal intubation. Relationship of the vallecula, the epiglottis, and the base of the tongue; note the cephalad position of the larynx in the infant (**A**); the older child's larynx is positioned more caudally. **B,** The laryngeal structures as viewed from above. **C,** The small size and relative position of the vocal cords, the epiglottis, and the larynx as viewed through the laryngoscope.

Equipment Required for Intubation

- Laryngoscope handle: extra bulbs, batteries
- Blades: Miller, sizes 00, 0, 1, and 2
- Suction catheters: 5, 8, 10, 12, and 14 Fr
- Source of suction
- Endotracheal tubes: one size larger than deemed appropriate by age, one of adequate size, and one size smaller than deemed appropriate by age
- Sterile lubricant
- Oxygen supply
- Ventilator bag with 15-mm universal female adapter (Hope, Ambu, Ohio)
- Mask for ventilator bag: infant, child, and adult sizes
- Tape
- Tincture of benzoin
- Nasogastric tubes

Table B-1 *Recommended Sizes of Endotracheal Tubes**

AGE OF PATIENT	NO. (Fr)	INTERNAL DIAMETER (mm)	LENGTH (cm)	ADAPTER, INTERNAL DIAMETER (mm)
Newborn				
<1 kg	11-12	2.5	10	3
>1 kg	13-14	3.0	11	3
1-6 mo	15-16	3.5	11	4
7-12 mo	17-18	4.0	12	4
13-18 mo	19-20	4.5	13	5
19-36 mo	21-22	5.0	14	5
3-4 yr	23-24	5.5	16	6
5 yr	25	6.0	18	6
6-7 yr	26	6.5	18	7
8-9 yr	27-28	7.0	20	7
10-11 yr	29-30	7.5	22	8
12-14 yr	32-34	8.0	24	8

*Tube should be of material labeled "I.T.-Z79" to satisfy standard tissue-implant tests.

position. The neck is only slightly extended and the jaw pulled only slightly forward. The nose and mouth are gently suctioned, and the patient is given oxygen by bag and mask for no more than 1 minute. The laryngoscope is held in the left hand. The blade is introduced into the mouth to the right of the tongue, so that the tongue will be deflected to the left. The tip of the blade is inserted to the vallecula. As illustrated in Fig. B-20, the handle of the laryngoscope is tilted slightly backward and upward toward the operator. Care must be taken not to use the teeth or alveolar ridge as a fulcrum. The vocal cords should now be in view. The tube can be advanced along the right side of the patient's mouth, inserted between the cords into the trachea, and further advanced to a position below the level of the vocal cords. Immediate auscultation of the lungs for symmetry of air movement is essential. If the right main stem bronchus is accidentally cannulated, the tube can be withdrawn to a safe position above the carina and checked again by auscultation.

Nasotracheal intubation is performed in a similar fashion; however, it is more difficult to perform than orotracheal intubation. It is indicated when long-term intubation is anticipated, inasmuch as the nasoendotracheal tube is more easily stabilized, once placed.

The nasotracheal tube is inserted and guided into the posterior oropharynx. The laryngoscope is then placed as previously described. The distal 1 to 2 cm of nasotracheal tube is then grasped with Magill forceps and poised just above the glottis. An assistant gently advances the external end of the tube 2 to 3 cm while the physician guides and visualizes its passage beyond the vocal cords into the trachea.

Stabilizing the Tube. Stabilizing the tube is primarily a nursing care task and is subject to many variations. Fig B-

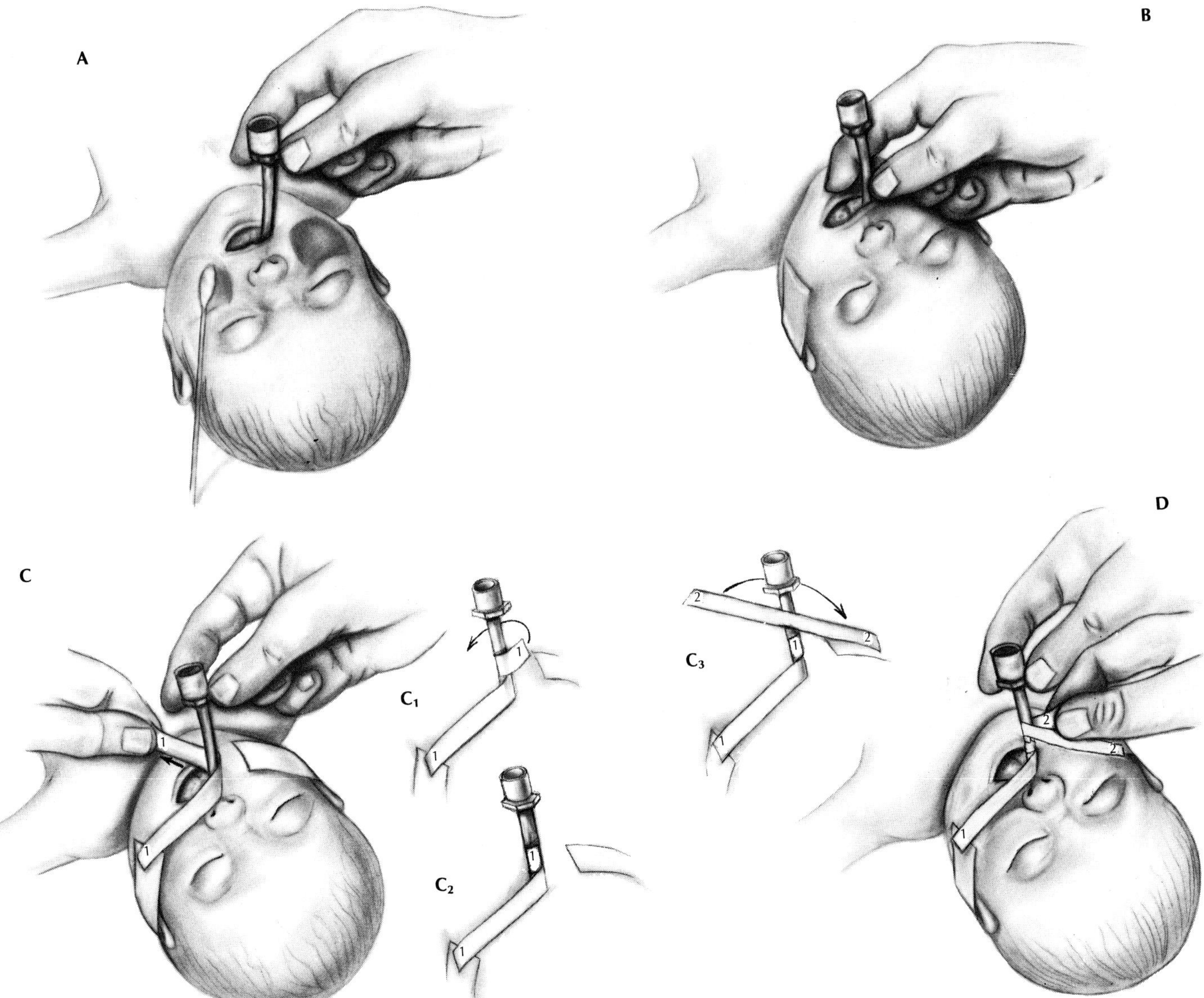

Fig. B-21 Securing the endotracheal tube. **A,** The cheeks and sides of the face are painted with tincture of benzoin (Some neonatal intensive care units currently do not use benzoin because of its absorption and potential toxic effects.) **B,** Wide pieces of elastic tape (Elastikon, Johnson and Johnson, New Brunswick, NJ) are placed over the sides of the face and pinnae. **C** to **C_2,** With the tube pulled to the right side of the mouth, a thin piece of tape (1) secures the tube on the left side of the face. **C_3** and **D,** Another piece of tape (2) then secures the tube on the right side of the face in a similar fashion.

21 illustrates one method. Some common problems encountered include the following:

1. Increased extension or flexion of the neck will cause the tube to move up and down the trachea; therefore care must be taken, in handling the patient, to stabilize the position of the neck. The rule of thumb is that the tip of the endotracheal tube follows the chin up or down.
2. The use of too much tape may prevent adequate nasal and oral suctioning, and inspection for leaks and kinks in the tube may be hampered.
3. Tincture of benzoin may spill into the eyes.

Postintubation Care. The intubated infant or child requires exacting nursing care. The patient will need monitoring of vital signs and frequent physical examinations to ascertain the adequacy of ventilation. The occurrence of pneumothorax, tube obstruction, and dislodgment of the tube must be anticipated in the care of these children.

Suctioning reduces tidal volume and available oxygen. It predisposes the patient to apnea and bradycardia. The physician and nurse should jointly decide how frequently the patient should receive suctioning. Once an hour is a reasonable interval. The need for this type of care is justification enough for referral to an intensive care unit. Suctioning of the tube is primarily a nursing task, but the physician should be aware of certain potential problems. The following is a safe method:

1. The endotracheal tube is disconnected from the ventilator.
2. From 0.25 to 0.5 ml of normal saline is instilled into the tube.
3. The infant then receives ventilation for 60 seconds.
4. The head is turned to one side.
5. A sterile, end-hole catheter is passed a premeasured 1 to 2 cm beyond the tracheal tube's distal orifice.
6. Suction is applied after the catheter has been pulled back 1 cm.
7. Suction is applied as the catheter is withdrawn over a 5-second interval.
8. The endotracheal tube is reconnected to the ventilator.
9. The head is turned to the opposite side, and the procedure is repeated.

REFERENCES

Kanter RK et al: Pediatric emergency intravenous access: evaluation of a protocol, Am J Dis Child 140:132, 1986.

Rosetti V et al: Difficulty and delay in intravenous access in pediatric arrest, Ann Emerg Med 13:406, 1984.

SUGGESTED READINGS

Berg RA: Emergency infusion of catecholamines into bone marrow, Am J Dis Child 138:810, 1984.

Blumer JL, editor: A practical guide to pediatric intensive care, ed 3, St Louis, 1990, Mosby-Year Book.

Butt W et al: Complications resulting from use of arterial catheters: retrograde flow and rapid elevation in blood pressure, Pediatrics 76:250, 1985.

Ducharme F et al: Incidence of infection related to arterial catheterization in children: a prospective study, Crit Care Med 16:272, 1988.

Firestone L, Lebowitz P, and Cook C: Clinical anesthesia procedures of the Massachusetts General Hospital, Boston, 1988, Little, Brown & Co.

Fuhrman BP et al: Pleural drainage using modified pigtail catheters, Crit Care Med 14:575, 1986.

Iserson KV and Criss EA: Pediatric venous cutdowns: utility in emergency situations, Ped Emerg Care 2:231, 1986.

Kanter RK et al: Central venous catheter insertion by femoral vein: safety and effectiveness for the pediatric patient, Pediatrics 77:842, 1986.

Lawless S et al: New pigtail catheter for pleural drainage in pediatric patients, Crit Care Med 17:173, 1989.

Levin DL and Perkin RM: Shock. In Levin DL, Morriss FC, and Moore GC, editors: A practical guide to pediatric intensive care, ed 2, St Louis, 1984, The CV Mosby Co.

Levy L and Pandit SK: Is midazolam a dangerous drug? J Postanesth Nurs 4:40, 1989.

Neish SR, et al: Intraosseous infusion of hypertonic glucose and dopamine, Am J Dis Child 142:878, 1988.

Orlowski JP: My kingdom for an intravenous line, Am J Dis Child 138:803, 1984.

Shapiro JM et al: Midazolam infusion for sedation in the intensive care unit: effect on adrenal function, Anesthesiology 64:394, 1986.

Smith-Wright DL et al: Complications of vascular catheterization in critically ill children, Crit Care Med 12:1015, 1984.

Spivey WH: Intraosseous infusions, J Pediatr 111:639, 1987.

Stenzel JP et al: Percutaneous femoral venous catheterizations: a prospective study of complications, J Pediatr 114:411, 1989.

Swanson RS et al: Emergency intravenous access through the femoral vein, Ann Emerg Med 13:244, 1984.

Tribett D and Brenner M: Peripheral and femoral vein cannulation. In Venus B and Mallory D, editors: Problems in critical care, vol 2, ed 2, Philadelphia, 1988, JB Lippincott Co.

Todres ID et al: Endotracheal tube displacement in the newborn infant, J Pediatr 89:126, 1976.

Venkataraman ST, Orr RA, and Thompson AE: Percutaneous infraclavicular subclavian vein catheterization in critically ill infants and children, J Pediatr 113:480, 1988.

Wetzel RC: Shock. In Rogers MC, editor: Textbook of pediatric intensive care, Baltimore, 1987, Williams & Wilkins.

C

Miscellaneous Values

Kathleen A. Woodin and Gail P. Udkow

BONE AGE

Sontag Method

The Sontag method is used to evaluate the skeletal development of children from 1 to 60 months of age:

1. Take roentgenograms of all epiphyseal centers on the left side of the body: shoulder, elbow, wrist and hand, hip, knee (anteroposterior views before 24 months; lateral views after 24 months), and ankle and foot (anteroposterior views before 48 months; lateral views after 48 months).
2. Count all ossification centers in the left half of the body. A center is counted as soon as it casts any shadow on the roentgenogram.
3. Compare the number of ossification centers with normal values for age in Table C-1.

Gruelich and Pyle Method

The Gruelich and Pyle method is used to evaluate the skeletal development of girls from 5 to 18 years of age and boys from 5 to 19 years:

1. Take roentgenogram of left hand and wrist.
2. Quantitation is based on the order of appearance and maturation of the epiphyseal centers.
3. For normal values, refer to the text of Gruelich and Pyle.[1]

DETERMINATION OF BODY SURFACE AREA

On the basis of the nomogram shown in Fig. C-1, a straight line joining the patient's height and weight will intersect the center column at the calculated surface area.

CONVERSION FORMULAS

Height (Length)

1 millimeter (mm) = 0.04 inch
1 centimeter = 0.4 inch
2.54 centimeters = 1 inch
1 meter (m) = 39.37 inches

Weight

60 milligrams (mg) = 1 grain
28.35 grams (g) = 1 ounce
454 grams = 1 pound
1000 grams (1 kilogram [kg]) = 2.2 pounds

Table C-1 *Mean Total Number of Centers on the Left Side of Body Ossified at Given Age Levels*

AGE (MONTHS)	BOYS		GIRLS	
	MEAN	SD*	MEAN	SD
1	4.11	1.41	4.58	1.76
3	6.63	1.86	7.78	2.16
6	9.61	1.95	11.44	2.53
9	11.88	2.66	15.36	4.92
12	13.96	3.96	22.40	6.93
18	19.27	6.61	34.10	8.44
24	29.21	8.10	43.44	6.65
30	37.59	7.40	48.91	6.50
36	43.42	5.34	52.73	5.48
42	47.06	5.26	56.61	3.98
48	51.24	4.59	57.94	3.91
54	53.94	4.35	59.89	3.36
60	56.24	4.07	61.52	2.69

From Sontag LW, Snell D, and Anderson M: Rate of appearance of ossification centers from birth to age 5 years, Am J Dis Child 58:949, 1939.
* *SD,* Standard deviation.

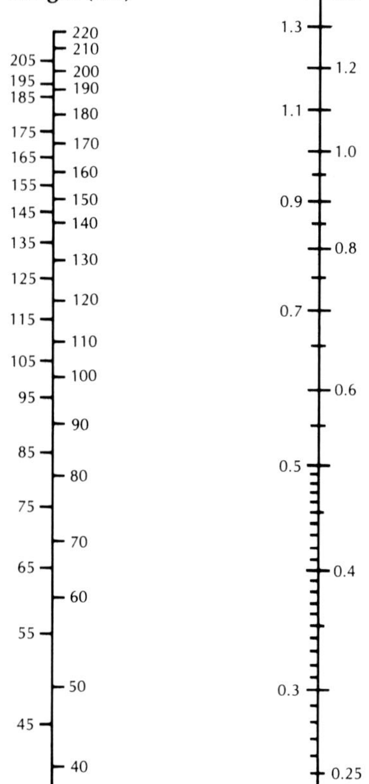

Fig. C-1 Nomogram to determine body surface area.

Redrawn from Cole CH, editor: The Harriet Lane handbook, Chicago, 1984, Year Book Medical Publishers, Inc. Based on data from Gelian EA and George SL: Estimation of human body surface area from height and weight, Cancer Chemother Rep. 54:225, 1970.

Milligram-Milliequivalent Conversions

$$\text{mEq/L} = \text{mg/L} \times \frac{\text{Valence}}{\text{Atomic weight}}$$

$$\text{mg/L} = \text{mEq/L} \times \frac{\text{Atomic weight}}{\text{Valence}}$$

$$\text{Equivalent weight} = \frac{\text{Atomic weight}}{\text{Valence}}$$

Milliosmols

The milliequivalent (mEq) is roughly equivalent to the milliosmol (mosm), the unit of measure of osmolarity or tonicity.

Prefixes for Decimal Factors

Prefix	Symbol	Factor
mega	m	10^6
kilo	k	10^3
hecto	h	10^2
deka	da	10^1
deci	d	10^{-1}
centi	c	10^{-2}
milli	m	10^{-3}
micro	μ	10^{-6}
nano	n	10^{-9}
pico	p	10^{-12}
femto	f	10^{-15}

ACID-BASE RESPONSE IN RESPIRATORY ACIDOSIS AND ALKALOSIS

The nomogram shown in Fig. C-2 provides confidence bands for the normal adjustment in carbon dioxide content and pH made to acute and chronic changes in arterial P_{CO_2}.

1. Determine pH on nomogram from plotted Pa_{CO_2} and carbon dioxide content obtained from blood gas measurement.
2. If pH value is not within confidence bands, then alteration in carbon dioxide content and pH varies from that expected from a pure respiratory condition, and a metabolic abnormality is also present.
3. To estimate the effect of acute and chronic changes in P_{CO_2} on pH, use these formulas:

Acute change in P_{CO_2}:
$(\Delta P_{CO_2})(0.008) = \Delta \text{pH}$

Chronic change in P_{CO_2}:
$(\Delta P_{CO_2})(0.003) = \Delta \text{pH}$

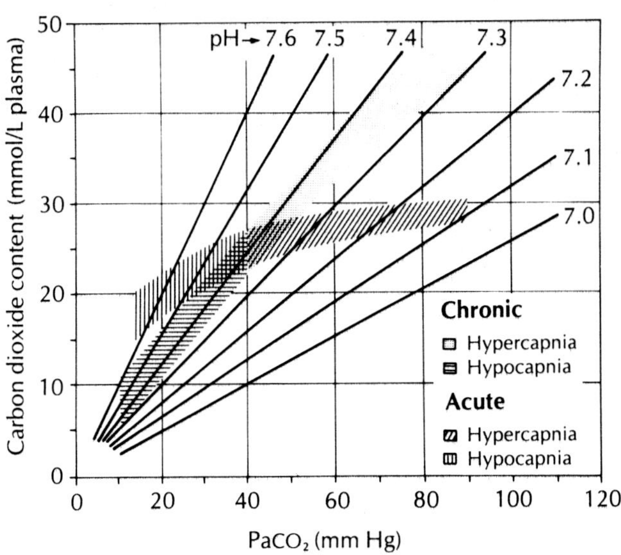

Fig. C-2 Acid-base response in respiratory acidosis and alkalosis.

Modified from Arbus GS: An in vivo acid-base nomogram for clinical use, Can Med Assoc J 109:291, 1973.

Table C-2 *Cerebrospinal Fluid (CSF)*

	MEAN	RANGE	POLYMORPHONUCLEAR CELLS
*Cell count**			
Preterm newborn	9.0	0-29	57%
Term newborn	8.2	0-32	61%
Child >1 mo		0-6	
Glucose			
Preterm newborn	50 mg/dl	24-63 mg/dl	
Term newborn	52 mg/dl	34-119 mg/dl	
Child		40-80 mg/dl	
Pressure, opening			
Newborn	<110 mm H_2O		
Child	<200 mm H_2O		
Protein			
Preterm newborn	115 mg/dl	65-150 mg/dl	
Term newborn	90 mg/dl	20-170 mg/dl	
Child		5-40 mg/dl	
Volume			
Child	60-100 ml		
Adult	100-160 ml		

Modified from Klein JO, Feigin RD, and McCracken GH: Report of the task force on diagnosis and management of meningitis, Pediatrics 78(suppl):959, 1986; Portnoy JM and Olson LC: Normal cerebrospinal fluid values in children: another look, Pediatrics 75:484, 1985; Sarff LD, Platt LH and McCracken GH: Cerebrospinal fluid evaluation in neonates: comparison of high-risk infants with and without meningitis, J Pediatr 88:473, 1976.

*Traumatic lumbar punctures (>1000 red blood cells/mm^3) are uninterpretable because correction formulas may underestimate the true white blood cell count.

Table C-3 *Synovial Fluid Analysis*

	CELLS PER MICROLITER (μl)	POLYMORPHONUCLEAR LEUKOCYTES (PMNL)	GLUCOSE (mg/dl)	MUCIN CLOT	PROTEIN (mg/dl)
Normal	50-200	<5%	>80	Good	1.8
Inflammatory*					
Bacterial	>10,000	>90%	<50	Poor	>4
Nonseptic	<10,000	<90%	50-80	Poor	2-4

Modified from Rudy P and DuPont HL: Infectious arthritis. In Pickering LK and DuPont HL, editors: Infectious diseases of children and adults, Menlo Park, Calif, 1986, Addison-Wesley Publishing Co, Inc, p 238.

*Fluid should be evaluated for the presence of urate crystals that occur in gout and pseudogout.

Table C-4 *Clinical Chemistry*

DETERMINATION	STANDARD UNITS	FACTOR	SI UNITS
Alkaline phosphatase			
Newborn	35-213 U/L	1.00	35-213 U/L
Child	71-142 U/L	1.00	71-142 U/L
Adolescent	106-213 U/L	1.00	106-213 U/L
Adult	32-92 U/L	1.00	32-92 U/L
Aldolase			
Newborn	5.2-32.8 U/L	1.00	5.2-32.8 U/L
Child	2.6-16.4 U/L	1.00	2.6-16.4 U/L
Adult	1.3-8.2 U/L	1.00	1.3-8.2 U/L
Ammonia	15-49 μg/dl	0.7333	11-35 μmol/L
Amylase			
Serum	60-160 U/dl	NA*	NA
Urine	17-200 U/dl	NA	NA
Bicarbonate	18-25 mEq/L	1.00	8-25 mmol/L
Bilirubin (>1 mo)			
Total	<0.2-1.0 mg/dl	17.10	<3.4 μmol/L
Direct	<0.2 mg/dl	17.10	<3.4-17.1 μmol/L
Calcium			
Total	8.8-10.8 mg/dl	0.2495	2.20-2.70 mmol/L
Ionized	4.48-4.92 mg/dl	0.2495	1.12-1.23 mmol/L
Carotene			
Infant	20-70 μg/dl	0.0186	0.37-1.30 μmol/L
Adult	40-130 μg/dl	0.0186	0.74-2.42 μmol/L
Child	60-200 μg/dl	0.0186	1.12-3.72 μmol/L
Chloride	98-106 mEq/L	1.00	98-106 mmol/L
Cholesterol, fasting			
Newborn	53-135 mg/dl	0.0259	1.37-3.50 mmol/L
Infant	70-175 mg/dl	0.0259	1.81-4.53 mmol/L
Child	120-200 mg/dl	0.0259	3.11-5.18 mmol/L
Adolescent	120-210 mg/dl	0.0259	3.11-5.44 mmol/L
Adult	140-250 mg/dl	0.0259	3.63-6.48 mmol/L
Copper			
Infant	20-70 μg/dl	0.1574	3.14-10.99 μmol/L
Child	90-190 μg/dl	0.1574	14.13-29.83 μmol/L
Adolescent	80-160 μg/dl	0.1574	12.56-25.12 μmol/L
Adult	70-155 μg/dl	0.1574	10.99-24.34 μmol/L
Creatinine			
Newborn	0.8-1.4 mg/dl	88.4	70.7-123.8 μmol/L
Infant	0.7-1.7 mg/dl	88.4	61.9-150.3 μmol/L
Adult	0.6-1.5 mg/dl	88.4	53.133 μmol/L
Creatinine phosphokinase			
Female	10-55 U/L	1.00	10-55 U/L
Male	12-80 U/L	1.00	12-80 U/L
Glucose	55-100 mg/dl	0.05551	3.055-5.55 mmol/L
Haptoglobin	40-336 mg/dl	0.01	0.4-3.36 g/L
Iron, serum			
Newborn	100-250 μg/dl	0.1791	17.90-44.75 μmol/L
Infant	40-100 μg/dl	0.1791	7.16-17.90 μmol/L
Child	50-120 μg/dl	0.1791	8.95-21.48 μmol/L
Adult	40-160 μg/dl	0.1791	7.16-28.64 μmol/L

* *NA*, Not available or not applicable.

Continued.

Table C-4 *Clinical Chemistry—cont'd*

DETERMINATION	STANDARD UNITS	FACTOR	SI UNITS
Total iron-binding capacity (TIBC)			
Infant	100-400 μg/dl	0.1791	17.90-71.60 μmol/L
Child	250-400 μg/dl	0.1791	44.75-71.60 μmol/L
Adult	250-400 μg/dl	0.1791	44.75-71.60 μmol/L
Lactate	0.6-1.8 mEq/L	1.00	0.6-1.8 mmol/L
Lactic dehydrogenase			
Newborn	160-450 U/L	NA	NA
Infant	100-250 U/L	NA	NA
Child	60-170 U/L	NA	NA
Adult	45-90 U/L	NA	NA
Lead	<40 μg/dl	0.0483	<1.93 μmol/L
Lipids			
Phospholipids	180-295 mg/dl	0.01	1.8-2.95 g/L
Triglycerides	40-150 mg/dl	0.01	0.4-1.5 g/L
Lipoprotein, HDL	150-330 mg/dl	0.01	1.5-3.3 g/L
Lipoprotein, LDL	28%-53% total		
Magnesium			
Newborn	1.0-1.8 mEq/L	0.5	0.5-0.9 mmol/L
Child	1.5-2.0 mEq/L	0.5	0.8-1.0 mmol/L
Osmolarity	275-295 mosm/kg	1.00	275-295 mmol/kg
pH (arterial)	7.35-7.45	1.00	7.35-7.45
Pco_2	35-45 mm Hg	0.1333	4.7-6.0 kPa
Po_2	83-108 mm Hg	0.1333	11.04-14.36 kPa
Phosphorus, inorganic			
Newborn	5.5-9.5 mg/dl	0.3229	1.78-3.07 mmol/L
Infant	4.5-6.5 mg/dl	0.3229	1.45-2.10 mmol/L
Child	4.5-5.5 mg/dl	0.3229	1.45-1.78 mmol/L
Adult	2.7-4.5 mg/dl	0.3229	0.87-1.45 mmol/L
Potassium	3.5-5.1 mEq/L	1.00	3.5-5.1 mmol/L
Proteins NOTE: Globulin = Total protein − Albumin			
Albumin/total protein			
Newborn	2.4-4.8/4.6-7.0 g/dl	10.0	24-48/46-70 g/L
Infant	3.0-4.5/5.1-7.3 g/dl	10.0	30-45/51-73 g/L
Child	3.8-5.6/6.0-8.0 g/dl	10.0	38-56/60-80 g/L
Adult	3.5-5.5/6.4-8.3 g/dl	10.0	35-55/64-83 g/L
Sodium	136-145 mEq/L	1.00	136-145 mmol/L
Transaminase AST (SGOT)			
Newborn	25-75 U/L	NA	NA
Infant	15-60 U/L	NA	NA
Child	20-50 U/L	NA	NA
Adult	8-40 U/L	NA	NA
Transaminase ALT (SGPT)			
Infant	5-54 U/L	NA	NA
Child	3-37 U/L	NA	NA
Adult	8-45 U/L	NA	NA
Urea nitrogen			
Newborn	4-12 mg/dl	0.3569	1.4-4.3 mmol/L
Child/adult	5-18 mg/dl	0.3569	1.8-6.4 mmol/L
Uric acid	3.0-7.0 mg/dl	0.0595	0.18-0.42 mmol/L
Vitamin A	30-80 μg/dl	0.0349	1.05-2.79 μmol/L
Vitamin E (tocopherol)	0.5-2.0 mg/dl	23.22	11.6-46.4 μmol/L

Table C-5 *Newborn Clinical Chemistry*

DETERMINATION*	CORD SAMPLE	CAPILLARY SAMPLES (RANGE) 1-12 HR	12-24 HR	24-48 HR	48-72 HR
Sodium (mmol/L)	147 (126-166)	143 (124-156)	145 (132-159)	148 (134-160)	149 (139-162)
Potassium (mmol/L)	7.8 (5.6-12)	6.4 (5.3-7.3)	6.3 (5.3-8.9)	6.0 (5.2-7.3)	5.9 (5.0-7.7)
Chloride (mmol/L)	103 (98-110)	100.7 (90-111)	103 (87-114)	102 (92-114)	103 (93-112)
Calcium (mg/dl)	9.3 (8.2-11.1)	8.4 (7.3-9.2)	7.8 (6.9-9.4)	8.0 (6.1-9.9)	7.9 (5.9-9.7)
Phosphorus (mg/dl)	5.6 (3.7-8.1)	6.1 (3.5-8.6)	5.7 (2.9-8.1)	5.9 (3.0-8.7)	5.8 (2.8-7.6)
Blood urea (mg/dl)	29 (21-40)	27 (8-34)	33 (9-63)	32 (13-77)	31 (13-68)
Total protein (g/dl)	6.1 (4.8-7.3)	6.6 (5.6-8.5)	6.6 (5.8-8.2)	6.9 (5.9-8.2)	7.2 (6.0-8.5)
Glucose (mg/dl)	73 (45-96)	63 (40-97)	63 (42-104)	56 (30-91)	59 (40-90)
Lactic acid (mg/dl)	19.5 (11-30)	14.6 (11-24)	14 (10-23)	14.3 (9-22)	13.5 (7-21)
Lactate (mmol/L)†	2.0-3.0	2.0			

Modified from Avery GB: Neonatology, pathophysiology and management in the newborn, ed 3, Philadelphia, 1987, JB Lippincott Co.
*Acharya PT and Payne WW: Blood chemistry of normal full-term infants in the first 48 hours of life, Arch Dis Child 40:430, 1965.
†Daniel SS, Adamsons K Jr, and James LS: Lactate and pyruvate as an index of prenatal oxygen deprivation, Pediatrics 37:942, 1966.

Table C-6 *Hematology*

AGE	HEMOGLOBIN (grams %): mean (−2 SD)	HEMATOCRIT (%) mean (−2 SD)	MEAN CELL VOLUME (fluid) mean (−2 SD)	MEAN CORPUSCULAR HEMOGLOBIN CONCENTRATION (grams/%RBC) mean (−2 SD)	RETICULOCYTES (%)	WBC/mm^3 × 100 mean (−2 SD)	PLATELETS (10^3/mm^3) mean (±2 SD)
26-30 wk gestation*	13.4 (11)	41.5 (34.9)	118.2 (106.7)	37.9 (30.6)		4.4 (2.7)	254 (180-327)
28 wk	14.5	45	120	31	(5-10)	—	275
32 wk	15.0	47	118	32	(3-10)	—	290
Term† (cord)	16.5 (13.5)	51 (42)	108 (98)	33 (30)	(3-7)	18.1 (9-30)‡	290
1-3 days	18.5 (14.5)	56 (45)	108 (95)	33 (29)	(1.8-4.6)	18.9 (9.4-34)	192
2 wk	16.6 (13.4)	53 (41)	105 (88)	31.4 (28.1)		11.4 (5-20)	252
1 mo	13.9 (10.7)	44 (33)	101 (91)	31.8 (28.1)	(0.1-1.7)	10.8 (5-19.5)	
2 mo	11.2 (9.4)	35 (28)	95 (84)	31.8 (28.3)			
6 mo	12.6 (11.1)	36 (31)	76 (68)	35 (32.7)	(0.7-2.3)	11.9 (6-17.5)	
6 mo-2 yr	12 (10.5)	36 (33)	78 (70)	33 (30)		10.6 (6-17)	(150-350)
2-6 yr	12.5 (11.5)	37 (34)	81 (75)	34 (31)	(0.5-1.0)	8.5 (5-15.5)	(150-350)
6-12 yr	13.5 (11.5)	40 (35)	86 (77)	34 (31)	(0.5-1.0)	8.1 (4.5-13.5)	(150-350)
12-18 yr							
Male	14.5 (13)	43 (36)	88 (78)	34 (31)	(0.5-1.0)	7.8 (4.5-13.5)	(150-350)
Female	14 (12)	41 (37)	90 (78)	34 (31)	(0.5-1.0)	7.8 (4.5-13.5)	(150-350)
Adult							
Male	15.5 (13.5)	47 (41)	90 (80)	34 (31)	(0.8-2.5)	7.4 (4.5-11)	(150-350)
Female	14 (12)	41 (36)	90 (80)	34 (31)	(0.8-4.1)	7.4 (4.5-11)	(150-350)

Modified from Greene MG, editor: The Harriet Lane handbook, ed 12, St Louis, 1991.
*Values are from fetal samplings.
†Under 1 mo, capillary Hb exceeds venous: 1 hr—3.6 g difference; 5 days—2.2 g difference; 3 wk—1.1 g difference.
‡Mean (95% confidence limits).

Table C-7 *Conversion of Centimeters to Inches*

cm	in	cm	in	cm	in	cm	in
1	0.39	51	20.08	101	39.76	151	59.45
2	0.79	52	20.47	102	40.16	152	59.84
3	1.18	53	20.87	103	40.55	153	60.24
4	1.57	54	21.26	104	40.94	154	60.63
5	1.97	55	21.65	105	41.34	155	61.02
6	2.36	56	22.05	106	41.73	156	61.42
7	2.76	57	22.44	107	42.13	157	61.81
8	3.15	58	22.83	108	42.52	158	62.20
9	3.54	59	23.23	109	42.91	159	62.60
10	3.94	60	23.62	110	43.31	160	62.99
11	4.33	61	24.02	111	43.70	161	63.39
12	4.72	62	24.41	112	44.09	162	63.78
13	5.12	63	24.80	113	44.49	163	64.17
14	5.51	64	25.20	114	44.88	164	64.57
15	5.91	65	25.59	115	45.28	165	64.96
16	6.30	66	25.98	116	45.67	166	65.35
17	6.69	67	26.38	117	46.06	167	65.75
18	7.09	68	26.78	118	46.46	168	66.14
19	7.48	69	27.17	119	46.85	169	66.54
20	7.87	70	27.56	120	47.24	170	66.93
21	8.27	71	27.95	121	47.64	171	67.32
22	8.66	72	28.35	122	48.03	172	67.72
23	9.06	73	28.74	123	48.43	173	68.11
24	9.45	74	29.13	124	48.82	174	68.50
25	9.84	75	29.53	125	49.21	175	68.90
26	10.24	76	29.92	126	49.61	176	69.29
27	10.63	77	30.31	127	50.00	177	69.68
28	11.02	78	30.71	128	50.39	178	70.08
29	11.42	79	31.10	129	50.79	179	70.47
30	11.81	80	31.50	130	51.18	180	70.87
31	12.20	81	31.89	131	51.57	181	71.26
32	12.60	82	32.28	132	51.97	182	71.65
33	13.00	83	32.68	133	52.36	183	72.05
34	13.39	84	33.07	134	52.76	184	72.44
35	13.78	85	33.46	135	53.15	185	72.83
36	14.17	86	33.86	136	53.54	186	73.23
37	14.57	87	34.25	137	53.94	187	73.62
38	14.96	88	34.65	138	54.33	188	74.02
39	15.35	89	35.04	139	54.72	189	74.41
40	15.75	90	35.43	140	55.12	190	74.80
41	16.14	91	35.83	141	55.51	191	75.20
42	16.54	92	36.22	142	55.91	192	75.59
43	16.93	93	36.61	143	56.30	193	75.98
44	17.32	94	37.01	144	56.69	194	76.38
45	17.72	95	37.40	145	57.09	195	76.77
46	18.11	96	37.80	146	57.48	196	77.17
47	18.50	97	38.19	147	57.87	197	77.56
48	18.90	98	38.58	148	58.27	198	77.95
49	19.29	99	38.98	149	58.66	199	78.35
50	19.69	100	39.37	150	59.06	200	78.74

Table C-8 *Conversion of Pounds to Grams*

OUNCES	1 lb	2 lb	3 lb	4 lb	5 lb	6 lb	7 lb	8 lb
	GRAMS							
0	454	907	1361	1814	2268	2722	3175	3629
1	482	936	1389	1843	2296	2750	3204	3657
2	510	964	1418	1871	2325	2778	3232	3686
3	539	992	1446	1899	2353	2807	3260	3714
4	567	1021	1474	1928	2381	2835	3289	3742
5	595	1049	1503	1956	2410	2863	3317	3771
6	624	1077	1531	1985	2438	2892	3345	3799
7	652	1106	1559	2013	2466	2920	3374	3827
8	680	1134	1588	2041	2495	2948	3402	3856
9	709	1162	1616	2070	2523	2977	3430	3884
10	737	1191	1644	2098	2552	3005	3459	3912
11	765	1219	1673	2126	2580	3033	3487	3941
12	794	1247	1701	2155	2608	3062	3515	3969
13	822	1276	1729	2183	2637	3090	3544	3997
14	851	1304	1758	2211	2665	3119	3572	4026
15	879	1332	1786	2240	2693	3147	3600	4054

Table C-9 *Temperature Equivalents*

CELSIUS*	FAHRENHEIT†	CELSIUS*	FAHRENHEIT†
34.0	93.2	38.6	101.4
34.2	93.6	38.8	101.8
34.4	93.9	39.0	102.2
34.6	94.3	39.2	102.5
34.8	94.6	39.4	102.9
35.0	95.0	39.6	103.2
35.2	95.4	39.8	103.6
35.4	95.7	40.0	104.0
35.6	96.1	40.2	104.3
35.8	96.4	40.4	104.7
36.0	96.8	40.6	105.1
36.2	97.1	40.8	105.4
36.4	97.5	41.0	105.8
36.6	97.8	41.2	106.1
36.8	98.2	41.4	106.5
37.0	98.6	41.6	106.8
37.2	98.9	41.8	107.2
37.4	99.3	42.0	107.6
37.6	99.6	42.2	108.0
37.8	100.0	42.4	108.3
38.0	100.4	42.6	108.7
38.2	100.7	42.8	109.0
38.4	101.1	43.0	109.4

*To convert Celsius to Fahrenheit: (9/5 × Temperature) + 32.
†To convert Fahrenheit to Celsius: 5/9 × (Temperature − 32).

Table C-10 *Laboratory Parameters of Acid-Base Disturbances**

	pH	$Paco_2$	HCO_3^- (mEq/L)	CO_2 CONTENT (mEq/L)
Normal values	7.35-7.45	35-45	24-26	25-28
Disturbances				
Metabolic acidosis	↓	↓	↓	↓
Acute respiratory acidosis	↓	↑	↔	Slight ↑
Compensated respiratory acidosis	↔ or slight ↓	↑	↑	↑
Metabolic alkalosis	↑	Slight ↑	↑	↑
Acute respiratory alkalosis	↑	↓	↔	Slight ↓
Compensated respiratory alkalosis	↔ or slight ↑	↓	↓	↓

*Values obtained by arteriolized capillary blood or direct arterial puncture.

Table C-11 *Ingredients of Infant Formulas*

PRODUCT	PROTEIN[3]	FAT[3]	CARBOHYDRATE	COMMENTS
Alimentum	Hydrolized casein	50% MCT, 10% soy, 40% safflower	Sucrose-modified tapioca starch	For malabsorption syndromes
Cow milk	80% casein, 20% whey	Butterfat	Lactose	
Enfamil	40% casein, 60% whey	45% soy, 55% coconut oils	Lactose	
Enfamil Premature	40% casein, 60% whey	40% MCT oil, soy, and corn oil	Corn syrup solids,* lactose	For premature infants
Evaporated milk based	80% casein, 20% whey	Butterfat	Lactose	Add 17 oz water and 1 tbsp Karo syrup to a 13 oz can evaporated milk; supplement with multivitamins and iron
Human milk	40% casein, 60% whey	Human milk fat	Lactose	
Isomil	Soy protein	60% soy, 40% coconut oils	Corn syrup solids and sucrose	For cow milk protein and/or lactose intolerance
Isomil SF	Soy protein	60% soy, 40% coconut oils	Corn syrup solids	For cow milk protein, lactose and/or sucrose intolerance
Lofenalac	Processed casein hydrolysate to remove phenylalanine	Corn oil	Corn syrup solids and modified tapioca starch	For phenylketonuria—low in phenylalanine
Nursoy	Soy protein	15% soy, 27% coconut and 58% safflower oils	Sucrose and corn syrup solids	For cow milk protein and/or lactose intolerance
Nutramigen	Casein hydrolysate	Corn oil	Sucrose	For sensitivity to intact milk protein or for lactose intolerance

Modified from Greene MG, editor: The Harriet Lane handbook, ed 12, Chicago, 1991, Year Book Medical Publishers, Inc.
MCT, Medium chain triglycerides.
*Corn syrup solids include dextrose, maltose, other glucose polymers.

Continued.

Table C-11 *Ingredients of Infant Formulas—cont'd*

PRODUCT	PROTEIN[3]	FAT[3]	CARBOHYDRATE	COMMENTS
Portagen	Sodium caseinate	88% MCT oil, 12% corn oil	Corn syrup solids, sucrose	For fat malabsorption states, lactose intolerance (liver disease)
Pregestimil	Casein hydrolysate with added L-cystine, L-tyrosine, L-tryptophan	60% corn oil, 40% MCT oil	Corn syrup solids, modified tapioca starch	For many malabsorption syndromes
Prosobee	Soy protein isolate and methionine	45% soy oil, 55% coconut oil	Corn syrup solids	For lactose and cow milk protein intolerance; sucrose intolerance; galactosemia
RCF (Ross Carbohydrate Free)	Soy protein isolate	Coconut and soy oils	None: selected by physician	Contains no carbohydrates
Similac and Similac with Iron	Nonfat cow milk	60% soy and 40% coconut oils	Lactose	
Similac 24 LBW	Nonfat cow milk	MCT, coconut, and soy oils	Lactose, corn syrup solids	Dilute initial feedings; for premature infants with fluid intolerance
Similac PM 60/40	40% casein and 60% whey	60% coconut and 40% corn oils	Lactose	Ca/P = 2:1; for those predisposed to hypocalcemia; low salt content
Similac Special Care	40% casein and 60% whey	MCT, corn, and coconut oils	Lactose, corn syrup solids	For premature infants
SMA and SMA with Iron	Nonfat cow milk, demineralized whey	27% coconut and 58% safflower oils	Lactose	Low salt content
SMA Preemie 24	40% casein and 60% whey	MCT, coconut and soy oils	Lactose and glucose	For premature infants

Table C-12 *Composition of Infant Formulas**

FORMULA	CALORIES PER OUNCE (ml)†	PERCENTAGE OF WEIGHT FOR VOLUME (g/dl)†			Na (mEq/L)
		PROTEIN	FAT	CHO	
Alimentum	20 (0.67)	1.90 (11)	3.80 (48)	6.90 (41)	13
Cow milk	20 (0.67)	3.30 (21)	3.30 (49)	4.70 (30)	21
Enfamil 20‖	20 (0.67)	1.50 (9)	3.80 (50)	6.98 (41)	8
Enfamil Premature	20 (0.67)	2.00 (12)	3.40 (44)	7.40 (44)	11
Evaporated milk with Karo syrup	23 (0.77)	3.04 (18)	3.38 (45)	6.12 (37)	22
Human milk	21 (0.70)	1.00 (6)	4.40 (55)	6.90 (39)	7
Isomil	20 (0.67)	1.80 (11)	3.69 (49)	6.80 (40)	14
Isomil SF	20 (0.67)	2.00 (12)	3.60 (48)	6.80 (40)	14
Lofenalac	20 (0.67)	2.20 (13)	2.60 (35)	8.80 (52)	14
Nursoy	20 (0.67)	2.10 (12)	3.60 (48)	6.90 (40)	9
Nutramigen	20 (0.67)	1.90 (11)	2.64 (35)	9.09 (54)	14
Portagen	20 (0.67)	2.30 (14)	3.17 (41)	7.82 (45)	14
Pregestimil	20 (0.67)	1.90 (11)	3.80 (48)	6.90 (41)	14
Prosobee	20 (0.67)	2.00 (12)	3.60 (48)	6.80 (40)	11
RCF	‖	2.00 (20)	3.60 (80)	0 (0)	14
Similac 20¶	20 (0.67)	1.50 (9)	3.63 (48)	7.23 (43)	10
Similac 24 LBW	24 (0.80)	2.20 (11)	4.49 (42)	8.49 (42)	16
Similac PM 60/40	20 (0.67)	1.58 (9)	3.76 (50)	6.88 (41)	7
Similac Special Care	20 (0.67)	1.83 (11)	3.67 (47)	7.17 (42)	13
Similac whey	20 (0.67)	1.50 (9)	3.63 (48)	7.23 (43)	10
SMA 20	20 (0.67)	1.50 (9)	3.60 (48)	7.20 (43)	6.5
SMA Preemie 24	24 (0.80)	2.00 (10)	4.40 (48)	8.60 (42)	14

Modified from Greene MG, editor: The Harriet Lane handbook, ed 12, Chicago, 1991, Year Book Medical Publisher, Inc.

*Values provided by manufacturers except when indicated otherwise.

†Numbers in parentheses indicate percentage of calories supplied by this substance.

‡Vapor pressure method.

§Freezing point depression.

‖Varies with amount carbohydrate added.

¶Also comes with iron (12 mg/L).

REFERENCES

1. Gruelich WW and Pyle SI: Radiographic atlas of skeletal development of the hand and wrist, San Francisco, 1974, Stanford University Press.
2. Normal laboratory values (case records of the Massachusetts General Hospital), N Engl J Med 314:39, 1986.
3. Queen PM and Wilson SE: Growth and nutrient requirements of infants. In Grand RJ, Sutphen JL, and Dietz WH, editors: Pediatric nutrition: theory and practice, Boston, 1987, Butterworth Publishers.
4. Tietz NW, editor: Clinical guide to laboratory tests, Philadelphia, 1983, WB Saunders Co.
5. Young SD: Normal laboratory values in SI units, N Engl J Med 292:795, 1975.

K (mEq/L)	Ca (mg/L)	P (mg/L)	Ca/P RATIO	Fe (mg/L)	APPROXIMATE SOLUTE LOAD (mosm/L)		
					RENAL	GI‡	GI§
20	71	51	1.39/1	12		370	
39	1190	930	1.30/1	0.5-1.0	220	260	
18	465	317	1.47/1	1.1	100	270	296
19	793	402	2.00/1	1.7	180	220	
35	1165	909	1.28/1	0.9			
13	320	140	2.3/1	0.3	75	273	
24	700	500	1.40/1	12	122	230	238
20	700	500	1.40/1	12	131	140	
18	634	475	1.33/1	13	134	310	
19	630	440	1.40/1	12	122	266	
19	634	423	1.50/1	13	130	430	
22	635	475	1.33/1	13	150	200	236
19	634	423	1.50/1	13	120	310	326
21	634	500	1.26/1	13	130	180	
20	700	500	1.40/1	1.5	131¶	60	
21	510	390	1.30/1	1.5	105	260	307
31	730	560	1.30/1	3.0	161	260	292
15	400	200	2.00/1	1.5	96	240	
24	1200	600	2.00/1	2.5	128	230	
19	400	300	1.33/1	12	101	270	
14	440	330	1.33/1	12.7	126	271	
19	750	400	1.88/1	3	175	300	

D

Common Psychological and Educational Tests

Philip W. Davidson, Jean M. Garrett, and Olle Jane Z. Sahler

Over the past 15 years, there has been a dramatic increase in the number of preschool- and school-aged children seeing allied health professionals for psychological and educational assessment. At the same time the assessment armamentarium of the psychoeducational specialist has expanded to the point that many commonly used materials are unfamiliar to the pediatrician in practice. Frequently, the physician receives reports from psychologists and educational specialists, speech and language pathologists, and pediatric occupational therapists—reports that must be interpreted or explained to the parents. Recognizing that these materials need to be described succinctly to simplify the physician's assignment, a summary is provided in Table D-1.

This table provides a quick reference to a wide range of psychoeducational screening and diagnostic tools commonly used by school health teams, special-child educators, clinical and pediatric psychologists, and other allied health professionals. Included are only individually administered tests, inasmuch as they are less familiar to both parents and physicians than are the group-administered standardized tests used by schools.

The information provided for each procedure is useful in identifying the general nature of each, the usual professional training of the person administering the test, and whether it is "normed." For some procedures, special features or characteristics also are noted.

The list of tests is not all-inclusive. On the other hand, most procedures that are likely to be described in a typical consultant's report are included. Screening procedures are presented because more and more states are requiring preschool and kindergarten readiness screening for all children. These screening tools often trigger more extensive evaluations for those children who do not pass, a decision in which the pediatrician should participate. The diagnostic procedures given include many standard methods, as well as a variety of nonstandard methods designed for children with handicaps that may interfere with routine testing procedures. Finally, some "parent report" procedures also are included, inasmuch as many preschool assessments may depend on such tools.

Clearly, interpreting the results of a screening or complete diagnostic assessment cannot be fully accomplished by referring only to this table. Communicating directly with the evaluator is the only reliable means to clarify results. Such contact often must be initiated by the pediatrician in that personnel from many schools and mental health facilities may not routinely communicate with the primary health care provider.

REFERRAL BY THE PEDIATRICIAN FOR PSYCHOLOGICAL OR EDUCATIONAL TESTING

Under what circumstances should a pediatrician refer a patient for special testing? Often the primary care pediatrician is in the best position to identify a child's developmental or behavioral difficulties, such as developmental delay in the infant or preschool child, learning difficulty or school failure in the school-aged child, or adjustment difficulty in the latency-aged child or adolescent. In these and similar situations the pediatrician quite appropriately might consider initiating a referral for psychological or educational testing, or both.

Several types of resources are available to accept such referrals. One resource is the local school district, which is obliged, under the Education for All Handicapped Children Act (Public Law 94-142), to provide evaluations of children suspected of having educational handicaps. These evaluations usually are performed by school psychologists, who typically specialize in standard educational testing and are less intensively trained in dealing with complex psychoeducational and emotional problems. Unfortunately, the referral may not be acted upon promptly because of the large case loads carried by school psychologists, who usually serve many schools within a district. However, the benefits of this type of referral are that it is free to the patient (because all such evaluations must be provided at public expense) and the results, once available, may be acted on more expeditiously (because the psychologist is a member of the committee on special education, the school district-based decision-making mechanism required by PL 94-142 for addressing the needs of children with educational handicaps).

Another resource is a private practicing psychologist or educational specialist. The reasons for selecting this option might include a need for an independent opinion after a school district evaluation, a limitation on the resources available in the school system for competent studies of children with complex problems, or parental preference.

To determine both cognitive and emotional status by means of psychological evaluations the best resources are licensed psychologists. In most states, psychologists who are eligible for third-party reimbursement must be licensed. In general, licensed psychologists must hold a doctoral degree in psychology and have postdoctoral training. The postdoctoral subspecialization areas of most interest to pediatricians include clinical child psychology, pediatric psychology, counseling psychology, and educational psychology. In some instances, referral to specialists would be appropriate. For example, the child with a closed head injury or other trauma associated with neurologic impairments routinely should be evaluated by a clinical neuropsychologist.

Some psychologists may perform psychoeducational assessments—evaluations of the child's learning styles and determination of the best teaching approaches. Alternative resources for these services include special educators and educational consultants. No licensure is required to practice in this specialty, nor are many of the services provided by educational consultants eligible for third-party reimbursement. Nevertheless, the pediatrician may decide that children with certain complex problems require special education studies to clarify appropriate interventions and consider referral to such consultants as the most appropriate option.

CHARACTERISTICS OF A GOOD PSYCHOEDUCATIONAL OR PSYCHOLOGICAL REPORT

A good evaluation should include a written report to the pediatrician. Because there is no single test that provides a comprehensive assessment, an evaluation of high quality will report the results of a number of measures, including intellectual ability, emotional status, visual-motor and linguistic functioning, and social-adaptive behaviors. Also, a complete report will include suggestions for intervention, including recommendations for placement, curriculum, therapies, and other referrals. Should any of these elements be missing from the report, the pediatrician should request this information from the consultant.

Usually, the psychologist will share the report with the child's parents. In cases in which this practice has not been followed, the pediatrician should ask the psychologist the reasons for withholding the data. It may be that the child refused to allow release of some part of the report to parents, or the psychologist may believe that release of some parts of the report are not in the child's or the family's best interest. Knowing this, the pediatrician is in a better position to preserve requested confidentiality and thus can be discrete in developing an effective management strategy that will be accepted by the child and the family.

Table D-1 *Commonly Used Tests of Educational and Psychological Assessment*

TEST NAME	AGE RANGE	PURPOSE AND DESCRIPTION
Achenbach Child Behavior Checklist	4-16 yr	Screening test for personality and social development in children and adolescents. Social competence and potential behavioral problems are inventoried through a parent questionnaire.
Adaptive Behavior Scale (ABS)	3-69 yr	Diagnostic test of adaptive behavior in children and adolescents that is administered by a trained clinician. Personal independence, social maladaptation, and personal maladaptation are tested. Results of this test can be used for diagnosis, placement, and programming. The instrument has two versions: one for public schoolchildren, the other for mentally retarded children and adults.
Bayley Scales of Infant Development	0-30 mo	One of the most widely used tools to evaluate developmental status in infancy. It is generally administered by a psychologist and measures cognitive, perceptual, and motor behavior. The test yields "normed" developmental indexes that are useful in comparing the child with age peers. It is less useful for predicting later outcome.
Beery-Buktenica Developmental Test of Visual-Motor Integration	2-15 yr	Screening test of visual-motor coordination, involving the copying of geometric designs. Age scores are derived from norms. It usually is administered by a psychologist.
Bender Motor Gestalt Test	4 yr–adult	Widely known and used screening test of visual-motor integration, usually administered by a psychologist. There are two "normed" scoring forms: Koppitz is appropriate for chidren aged 4-12 yr; Hutt is appropriate for adolescents and adults. The test also yields indicators of neurologic and emotional status.
Blind Learning Aptitude Test (BLAT)	6-16 yr	Nonverbal cognitive test for use with blind children that assesses general reasoning and abstraction. The test seems to work best with children ages 6-12 yr. The BLAT should be used in conjunction with a verbal test. It usually is administered by a psychologist or other trained professional.
Brazelton Neonatal Assessment	0-1 mo	Diagnostic test of developmental status in infancy that evaluates early social behaviors. The test results give a profile of infant behavior rather than an overall score. Subscale ratings for different item types (e.g., neurologic development) can be obtained. This test is administered by an examiner who must be certified in its administration and interpretation.
Callier-Azusa Scale–H	Severly and profoundly mentally retarded persons	Developmental scale designed to assess communicative abilities of deaf-blind and severely and profoundly handicapped persons. The scale should be administered by persons who are familiar with the child's behavior.

Continued.

Table D-1 *Commonly Used Tests of Educational and Psychological Assessment—cont'd*

TEST NAME	AGE RANGE	PURPOSE AND DESCRIPTION
Carey & McDevitt Infant Temperament Questionnaire (ITQ)	4-8 mo	Helps to provide a determination of infant temperament. Questions relate to the nine categories of behavior described by Thomas, Chess, and Birch (see Temperament Scales described later in this table). Test time is approximately 30 minutes. This questionnaire, which is completed by parents, can be used to supplement information about parent-child interaction derived from the clinical interview.
Cattell Infant Intelligence Scale	0-48 mo	Diagnostic test of developmental status in infancy that measures cognitive and perceptual adaptive behaviors. This is a well-established tool, but the norms are dated; it has been displaced by the Bayley Scales. It usually is administered by a qualified developmental specialist (e.g., a pediatric psychologist).
Children's Apperception Test (CAT)	2-10 yr	Diagnostic test of personality and social development in children and adolescents that is usually administered by a psychologist and is used to help characterize the child's interpersonal relationships. Two forms of the test exist: one based on picture stories of humans and one on picture stories of animals.
Columbia Mental Maturity Scale	3½-10 yr	Diagnostic test of cognitive ability that usually is administered by a psychologist to evaluate children who have sensory or motor defects or difficulty speaking or writing. A developmental index is derived from norms.
Conners Teacher Rating Scale	School age	Screening test of personality and social development completed by teachers to evaluate possible hyperactivity in students. This tool is widely used in research settings.
Denver Developmental Screening Test (DDST)	0-6 yr	Office screening test of developmental status that evaluates performance in four developmental areas: gross motor, fine motor, language, and personal and social skills. The DDST can be administered by a physician, nurse, or other trained worker. Multiple data points are required, and up to 10% of all results are either abnormal, questionable, or unobtainable. A DDST in shorter form (DDST-R) is available for preliminary screening. (See Chapter 18, Eleven.)
Detroit Test of Learning Aptitude–2	6-18 yr	Diagnostic test of learning potential that was revised in 1988. It is useful as a test of general intellectual ability. Standard scores are used for each of the 11 subtests. It usually is administered by a trained psychologist or special educator.
Draw-a-House-Tree-Person	5 yr–adult	Diagnostic test of personality and cognitive status usually administered by a trained psychologist as a projective device to evaluate self-image and other ego functions.
Draw-a-Man	4-16 yr	Results of this screening test of cognitive ability give a developmental age equivalence. The test also can serve as a projective device to evaluate emotional and personality development. The test can be administered by a psychologist or other trained clinician.
French Pictorial Intelligence Test	3-8 yr	Diagnostic test of cognitive development independent of verbal expression—requires "pointing" responses to visual stimuli. It most frequently is used with speech-, language-, or hearing-impaired children and yields a developmental quotient based on norms. It is administered by a trained psychologist.
Frostig Developmental Test of Visual Perception	Infancy–8 yr	Drawing and copying test of perceptual motor ability that measures five areas of visual perception, including eye-hand coordination, figure-ground perception, form constancy, position in space, and spatial relationships. It usually is administered by a psychologist or specially trained teacher.
Gesell Developmental Schedules	0-36 mo	Physical and mental abilities in the adaptive, gross motor, fine motor, language, and personal-social areas are assessed. Observations of infant performance usually are made by a psychologist. Norms yield an age-equivalent score.
Halstead-Reitan Battery	9-14 yr	Comprehensive neuropsychological battery that is administered by a psychologist and takes approximately 4 to 6 hours to complete. The battery consists of 12 tests, including a variety of sensorimotor and perceptual tests as well as an aphasia test. The battery also includes the Wechsler Adult Intelligence Scale and the Minnesota Multiphasic Personality Inventory (MMPI). Information on the reliability and validity of the test is limited; thus the usefulness of the battery may depend on the sophistication of the examiner.
Hiskey-Nebraska Test of Learning Abilities	3-18 yr	Nonverbal diagnostic test of cognitive ability usually used for deaf and hearing-impaired children. Separate norms for both deaf and hearing children are available. It usually is administered by a trained psychologist.
Illinois Test of Psycholinguistic Abilities (ITPA)	2-10 yr	"Normed" diagnostic test of cognitive ability specifically designed to evaluate verbal abilities and auditory-verbal and visual-motor processing. The test can be administered by a psychologist, speech pathologist, or educator. The norms and the test's usefulness in a psychoeducational battery both have been questioned.

Table D-1 *Commonly Used Tests of Educational and Psychological Assessment—cont'd*

TEST NAME	AGE RANGE	PURPOSE AND DESCRIPTION
Kaufman Assessment Battery for Children (K-ABC)	2½-12½ yr	Diagnostic test that should be administered by a qualified professional. It is intended for use in school and clinical settings to provide a measure of intelligence and achievement. The K-ABC does not include measures of verbal cognitive processes in the composite score.
Key Math Test	Kindergarten–grade 8	"Normed" diagnostic test of arithmetic achievement that can be administered by a teacher or psychologist. Fourteen areas of mathematics content, including operations and applications, are evaluated. The test is weak in the area of computation.
Kinetic Family Drawing	5 yr–adolescence	Diagnostic test of personality and social development that measures, in particular, family interactions. Special features of the test include identification of trends or characteristics commonly seen in various subgroups (e.g., learning disabled, developmentally disabled, or perceptual-motor-handicapped children). This test usually is administered by a psychologist or trained clinician.
Leiter International Performance Scale	2 yr–adult	"Normed" diagnostic test of cognitive development usually administered by a psychologist and particularly appropriate for evaluating speech- and hearing-impaired individuals.
McCarthy Scales of Children's Abilities	2½-8½ yr	Relatively new diagnostic test of cognitive and perceptual ability that yeilds IQ-like indexes of verbal, memory, perceptual, quantitative, and motor function. The General Cognitive Index (GCI), an overall estimate of cognitive function, is derived also. It must be administered by a trained professional. The test is particularly useful for diagnosing learning disabilities.
Merrill-Palmer Intelligence Test	18-71 mo	Diagnostic test of cognitive and adaptive skills usually performed by a psychologist. Because the test contains many timed items, it is highly demanding of the child being examined. It yields a normal cognitive-level score.
Minnesota Child Development Inventory	12 mo–6 yr	Parent questionnaire inventory that assesses general development and fine motor, gross motor, expressive language, comprehension-cognition, self-help, and personal-social skills.
Motor Free Test of Visual Perception (MFTVP)	4-9 yr	Diagnostic test of cognitive ability that measures the same five areas of visual perception evaluated by the Frostig Test, except that the child is not required to give motor responses requiring eye-hand coordination. It is useful in differentiating perceptual-motor problems from purely visual-perceptual difficulties. The test can be administered by a psychologist or teacher.
Peabody Individual Achievement Test–Revised (PIAT-R)	5-18 yr	Achievement test usually administered by an educational specialist or psychologist. It provides wide-range screening in six areas, including general information, reading recognition, reading comprehension, mathematics, spelling, and written expression. The PIAT-R is useful in diagnosing an individual's general level of achievement; however, it does not provide in-depth assessment of specific areas of skill.
Peabody Picture Vocabulary Test–Revised (PPVT-R)	2½ yr–adult	Screening test of receptive vocabulary administered by a speech and language specialist, teacher, or psychologist. It correlates highly with IQ tests but cannot be used in place of a more intensive test of cognitive ability.
Perkins-Binet Tests of Intelligence for the Blind	3-	Test of general intelligence has two forms—one for children with usable vision and one for children with no usable vision. The test yields IQ score based on the same method as that used in the Stanford-Binet intelligence tests.
Personality Inventory for Children (PIC)	3-16 yr	Screening test of personality and social development completed by parents. Areas evaluated include achievement, intellectual screening, somatic concerns, depression, family dysfunction, withdrawal, anxiety, psychosis, hyperactivity, and social skills.
Physician Developmental Quick Screen for Speech Disorders (PDQ)	6 mo–6 yr	Office screening test performed by a physician, nurse, or other trained individual. The test measures various aspects of language, rhythm of speech, articulation, speaking mechanisms, and voice.
Piers-Harris Self-Concept Scale	8-19 yr	Screening test for personality and social development that evaluates six facets of self-concept, including physical, social, family, and school precepts. The face validity of this test appears to be quite good. It usually is administered by a psychologist or teacher.
Preschool Language Scale (PLS)	1½-7 yr	Diagnostic test measuring expressive and receptive language skills. A "normed" age-equivalent score results for each skill. It usually is administered by a teacher, psychologist, or speech and language pathologist.
Prescreening Developmental Questionnaire (PDQ)	0-6 yr	Parent questionnaire used to determine whether DDST screening is necessary. Motor, language, social, and cognitive items are addressed. Either office staff members or parents can complete the items.
Raven Progressive Matrices	5½ yr–adult	Diagnostic test of cognitive ability that relies heavily on visual-spatial abstract reasoning. It is claimed to be culture free. The test usually is administered by a psychologist and is "normed."

Continued.

Table D-1 *Commonly Used Tests of Educational and Psychological Assessment—cont'd*

TEST NAME	AGE RANGE	PURPOSE AND DESCRIPTION
Rorschach Ink Blot Test	2 yr–adult	Projective test of personality and social development specifically designed to evaluate personality structure. It is administered by a trained psychologist. Extensive scoring criteria are required to interpret the results.
School Readiness Survey	4-6 yr	Screening test of learning ability in children that can be administered by a teacher, psychologist, or parent and identifies areas in which a child may be ready for school or deficient with regard to entrance into kindergarten.
Sentence Completion Tests	All ages	Projective tests of personality and social development usually administered by a psychologist. Responses differentiating between adjustment and maladjustment can be identifed. A number of different versions of the technique are in use, some of which have been validated and others in which scoring usually is achieved by clinical interpretation.
Sequenced Inventory of Communication Development	4 mo–4 yr	Test of speech and language ability in children, administered directly by a teacher, psychologist, or speech and language pathologist or completed by the parent. Expressive and receptive language skills are assessed.
Silvaroli Reading Inventory	Preschool–grade 8	Screening test of achievement usually administered by an educational specialist. Word recognition, passage comprehension, and spelling are assessed. Scores for children in kindergarten to grade 6 appear to be somewhat inflated. Reliability of this test appears to be better at the higher grade levels.
Slosson Intelligence Test	0-27 yr	Diagnostic test of cognitive ability usually administered by a teacher or psychologist. It is designed to be a quick assessment, is widely used in schools, and is less well "normed" than the more intensive individual intelligence tests.
Southern California Sensory Integration Test	4-10 yr	Test usually administered by a certified occupational therapist. Eighteen subtests evaluate sensory integration. The findings are not widely accepted by many psychologists or educators, although a sizable literature suggests substantial construct validity.
Stanford Diagnostic Test	2 yr–grade 8	Diagnostic test of achievement usually administered by teachers that particularly addresses achievement in reading and arithmetic.
Stanford-Binet Intelligence Test, fourth edition	2 yr–adult	Well-known diagnostic test of cognitive ability administered by a psychologist. The test yields 15 subtest scores organized into four areas, including verbal reasoning, quantitative reasoning, and short-term memory. The full battery requires more than 2 hours to administer, making it perhaps the longest standardized test of general intelligence. An option to shorten the scales for briefer administration is available, but validity has not yet been established for the shortened version. The test may not be as effective as the WISC-R for diagnosing educational difficulties and for language handicaps. Because of an uneven range of standard scores, any profile analysis should be used with caution.
Sucher-Allred Reading Placement Inventory	Kindergarten–grade 9	Diagnostic test of reading ability containing a word recognition test and an oral reading test. The inventory provides an informal measure of a child's reading ability, not an indepth assessment of reading difficulties. It usually is administered by an educational specialist or a classroom teacher to screen students for placement in reading.
Temperament Scales	Infancy	Nine scales—activity level, rhythmicity, response to new stimuli, adaptability, intensity, threshold of responsiveness, mood, distractibility, and attention span—are used to assess infant temperament. The evaluation usually is performed by a trained clinician.
Test of Language Development–Primary (TOLD)	4-8 to 11 yr	Diagnostic test of language development in children that usually is administered by a speech and language pathologist, but also can be administered by a teacher, psychologist, or other professional. The test measures spoken language, listening, semantics, and syntax. Age scores and language quotients result from norms.
Test of Non-Verbal Intelligence (TONI)	5-86 yr	Language-free measure of intelligence that may be used for hearing-impaired, language-impaired, and motor-impaired persons. It has been suggested that the TONI should be used only as a supplemental test (as part of a battery) and that it should not be used with children younger than 7 years old.
Test of Written Langugue (TOWL-2)	7½-18 yr	Diagnostic test usually administered by an educational specialist. The test helps to determine a student's general writing proficiency and to recognize a student's strengths and weaknesses.
Test of Written Spelling–Revised	5-18 yr	The TWS-2 uses a dictated work format to measure the ability of students to spell words with readily predictable and with less predictable sound-letter patterns. The TWS-2 can provide diagnostic information relative to specific spelling strategies. It is an excellent instrument for assessing written spelling ability. This test can be administered by a teacher, psychologist, or other professional.

Table D-1 *Commonly Used Tests of Educational and Psychological Assessment—cont'd*

TEST NAME	AGE RANGE	PURPOSE AND DESCRIPTION
Thematic Apperception Test (TAT)	School age–adult	Projective test of personality and social development measuring interpersonal relationships and usually administered by a trained psychologist. The test is useful in identifying emotional disorders. Extensive scoring criteria are applied to interpret the results.
Uzgiris-Hunt Ordinal Scales	0-3 yr	Diagnostic test of sensorimotor, perceptual, and cognitive development usually administered by a psychologist. Interpretation of development is based on piagetian theory. It is not "normed" and usually is used in research settings.
Vineland Adaptive Behavior Scale (VABS)	0-19 yr	Test that assesses the social competence of handicapped and nonhandicapped individuals, usually administered by a trained interviewer. There are three versions of the VABS: the survey form, expanded form, and classroom edition. In each version of the scale, adaptive behavior is measured in four domains: communication, daily living skills, socialization, and motor skills. The survey and expanded forms also include a maladaptive behavior domain. The respondent is an attendant, parent, or teacher.
Wechsler Intelligence Scale for Children–Revised (WISC-R)	6-16 yr	The most commonly used school intelligence test. Usually administered by a psychologist, it measures verbal and performance intelligence. Subscales can be used to evaluate learning ability and to diagnose specific learning disabilities. "Normed" IQ scores result.
Wechsler Preschool and Primary Scales of Intelligence–Revised (WPPSI-R)	3-7 yr	Wechsler test designed to be used with preschool children and designed similarly to the WISC-R.
Wide Range Achievement Test–Revised (WRAT-R)	5-64 yr	Screening test of achievement usually administered by an educational specialist. It evaluates word recognition and math and spelling achievement.
Wisconsin Behavior Rating Scale (WBRS)	0-3 yr	The WBRS is an adaptive behavior rating scale designed for persons who function developmentally at or below the 3-year-old level. It assesses basic survival skills, using items that are developmentally arranged and sequenced under several subcategories of adaptive behavior: gross motor, fine motor, expressive communication, play skills, socialization, domestic activites, eating, toileting, dressing, and grooming. It usually is administered by a trained interviewer.
Woodcock Reading Mastery Test	Kindergarten–grade 12	Tests specifically for reading skills usually administered by an educational specialist. The test measures word and letter identification, word attack, and passage and word comprehension. Norms are available.
Woodcock-Johnson Psychoeducational Battery	All ages	Diagnostic test of achievement usually administered by an educational specialist. It measures cognitive ability, achievement, and interest. The test is more reliable at the elementary than at the secondary educational level.

Index

C

H